ORTHOPAEDIC IMAGING

A PRACTICAL APPROACH

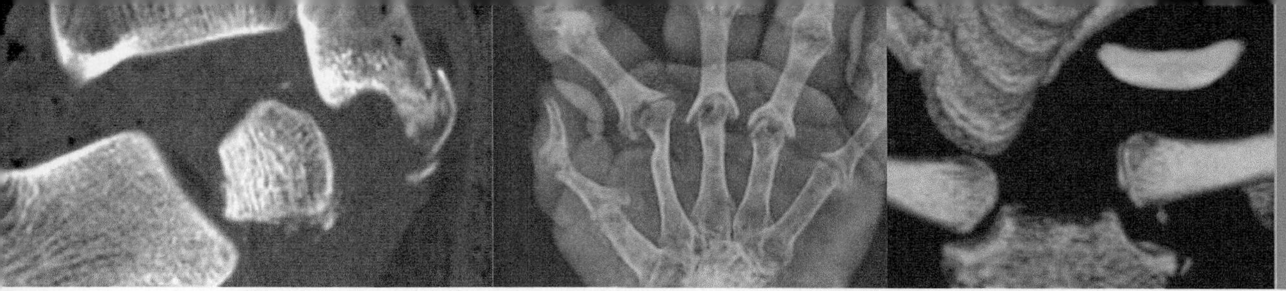

ORTHOPAEDIC IMAGING

A PRACTICAL APPROACH

SEVENTH EDITION

Adam Greenspan, MD, FACR
Professor Emeritus of Radiology and Orthopaedic Surgery
University of California, Davis School of Medicine
Former Director, Section of Musculoskeletal Imaging
Department of Radiology, University of California Davis Medical Center
Former Consultant, Shriners Hospital for Children
Sacramento, California

Javier Beltran, MD, FACR
Professor and Former Chairman of Radiology
Maimonides Medical Center
Brooklyn, New York

Foreword by:

Andrew J. Grainger, BM, BS, FRCP, FRCR
Consultant MSK Radiologist
Cambridge University Hospital
Cambridge, United Kingdom

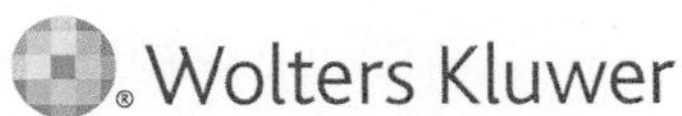

Wolters Kluwer

Philadelphia • Baltimore • New York • London
Buenos Aires • Hong Kong • Sydney • Tokyo

Executive Editor: Sharon R. Zinner
Associate Development Editor: Eric McDermott
Editorial Coordinator: Julie Kostelnik
Marketing Manager: Phyllis Hitner
Production Project Manager: Sadie Buckallew
Design Coordinator: Holly McLaughlin
Illustrator: Luis Beltran
Manufacturing Coordinator: Beth Welsh
Prepress Vendor: Absolute Service, Inc.

7th edition

9 8 7 6 5 4 3 2

Printed in the United States of America

Library of Congress Cataloging-in-Publication Data

Names: Greenspan, Adam, author. | Beltran, Javier (Professor of radiology), author.
Title: Orthopaedic imaging : a practical approach / Adam Greenspan, Javier Beltran ; foreword by Andrew J. Grainger.
Other titles: Orthopedic imaging
Description: Seventh edition. | Philadelphia : Wolters Kluwer, [2021] | Includes bibliographical references and index.
Identifiers: LCCN 2020007727 (print) | LCCN 2020007728 (ebook) | ISBN 9781975136475 (hardcover) | ISBN 9781975136499 (epub)
Subjects: MESH: Bone Diseases--diagnostic imaging | Bone and Bones--injuries | Diagnostic Imaging--methods
Classification: LCC RD734.5.R33 (print) | LCC RD734.5.R33 (ebook) | NLM WE 225 | DDC 616.7/07548--dc23
LC record available at https://lccn.loc.gov/2020007727
LC ebook record available at https://lccn.loc.gov/2020007728

shop.lww.com

MPP1122

To my wife, Barbara;

my children, Michael, Samantha, and Luddy;

and my daughter-in-law, Danielle, with all my love;

and to my grandsons, Avi and Benji,

who are the brightest stars in my life.

A.G.

To my wife, Andrea, and my sons, Xavier and Luis,

for their love and support.

J.B.

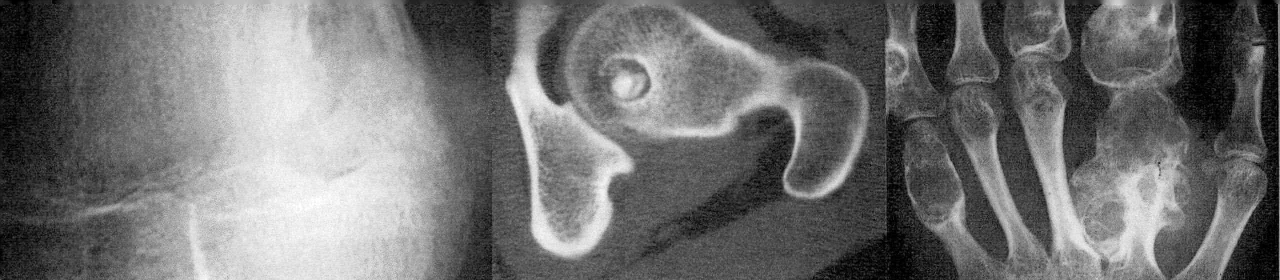

Foreword

It is a great honor to be asked to write this foreword, and as I sit in my office writing, I am conscious of a well-thumbed and now very dog-eared early edition of Dr. Greenspan's book *Orthopaedic Imaging: A Practical Approach* sitting on my bookshelf. This was one of the first books I bought as a radiology trainee and remained a source of reference throughout my training and beyond. Since this early edition of the book, it is amazing to see how the book has developed to become a comprehensive work taking on modern developments in our understanding of the pathology and management of musculoskeletal conditions and their imaging diagnosis. Over this time, the book has also been translated into numerous languages, which is testament to its worldwide appeal and significance.

This latest edition continues the evolution established through past editions, with extensive updating of images, diagrams, and text. In common with the last edition, Dr. Greenspan is joined by Dr. Beltran as a coauthor. Dr. Beltran brings to the book his world-renowned expertise, particularly in magnetic resonance imaging (MRI) imaging. This edition continues to reflect the major role MRI plays in the diagnosis and management of musculoskeletal conditions. It includes discussion of some of the latest advanced MRI sequences and techniques being employed, for instance, in the field of compositional cartilage imaging, alongside up-to-date coverage of other advanced imaging modalities such as ultrasound and positron emission tomography (PET)/computed tomography (CT).

A radiology textbook will always be judged on the quality of the images included by the authors. Past experience shows it is all too apparent when a book fails to keep up with the advances in medical image quality seen by its readers in day to day practice. This is certainly not an accusation that can be made against this book. Once again, Drs. Greenspan and Beltran have meticulously reviewed all the images previously included. They have undertaken extensive replacement of figures and included new examples to ensure that wherever possible the images provided truly reflect the state-of-the-art imaging we expect to see.

The use of illustrations to help explain clinical and pathologic concepts and correlations continues to be one of the strengths of this book. As always, the diagrams and schematics are of the highest possible quality, and it is wonderful that the authors have been able to call on the services of Luis Beltran to continue and maintain the superlative illustrative work brought to the last edition by Salvador Beltran.

One of the joys of Dr. Greenspan's original textbook was its remarkable and comprehensive coverage of the whole field of musculoskeletal radiology through very clear, simple, and succinct text. It accomplished this by emphasizing the conditions that are most important to the clinician and radiologist, showing how imaging is best used to diagnose and provide the most useful information possible for a condition. This has not been lost in the latest edition which remains clear and concise despite embracing the latest developments in the field, including discussion of cutting-edge imaging techniques and roles that are only just starting to find their way from the research arena to clinical practice. These include the expansion of text to reflect the increasing role advanced MRI techniques and that PET and hybrid imaging play in the diagnosis of musculoskeletal conditions. Despite the inclusion of state-of-the-art imaging, the authors have not forgotten that conventional radiographs are fundamental to the majority of musculoskeletal radiologic diagnoses. At a time when many forget the importance of the lowly radiographs and their interpretation often seems to be becoming a dying art, the book emphasizes and explains the techniques and skills that underpin conventional radiographic diagnosis. This inclusion of the newest techniques alongside the established and long-standing allows the authors to admirably fulfill one of their key objectives, showing both the advantages and disadvantages of different imaging modalities in the assessment of musculoskeletal conditions.

Drs. Greenspan and Beltran are both authorities in their field, respected the world over for their knowledge of musculoskeletal medicine and radiology. However, the esteem in which they are held also reflects their ability to communicate the subject to others in a manner, which is easily comprehensible. They provide the facts needed to be not only a knowledgeable musculoskeletal radiologist but also a clinically useful radiologist with the tools to contribute fully in the care and management of patients. This latest edition, of what can now justifiably be considered a classic text, once again overachieves on all its objectives and is to be wholeheartedly commended.

Andrew J. Grainger, BM, BS, FRCP, FRCR
Consultant MSK Radiologist
Cambridge University Hospital
Cambridge, United Kingdom

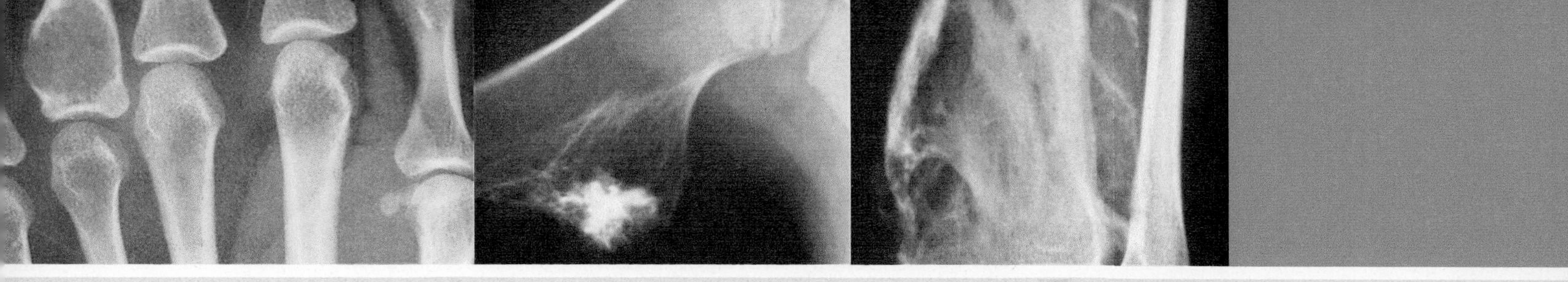

Preface to the First Edition

Orthopedic Radiology: A Practical Approach was written to facilitate the complex process of diagnostic investigation in a broad range of orthopedic disorders. Its underlying concept is threefold: to provide a basic understanding of the currently available imaging modalities used to diagnose many commonly encountered disorders of bones and joints, to help in the choice of the most effective radiologic technique with a view to minimizing the cost of examination as well as the exposure of patients to radiation, and to emphasize the need for providing the orthopedic surgeon with the information required to choose the right therapy. It does not attempt to compete in size and scope with other books on the same subject. Many uncommon entities have been excluded, as have the exact instructions for performing procedures. Likewise, the nature of the volume does not allow inclusion of every detail of a given disorder or full discussion of controversial aspects. These matters are left to the reader's further study of the literature and the many standard and specialized textbooks compiled in the "References and Further Reading" section at the end of the volume.

As its subtitle states, *Orthopedic Radiology* strives to provide its primary audience, medical students and residents in radiology and orthopedics, with a practical approach to its subject. To this end, crucial information within the text of each chapter has been tabulated in a section entitled "Practical Points to Remember" at the end of the chapter. Numerous original schematic diagrams and tables have been developed, detailing, for example, classifications of fractures, the morphologic features of arthritic and neoplastic disorders, and the positioning of patients for the various standard and special radiographic projections, as well as the most effective radiologic techniques for demonstrating abnormalities. Radiographic reproductions, many of which are accompanied by explanatory, labeled line drawings, have been specially prepared to provide high-quality examples of the classic presentations of a wide spectrum of orthopedic disorders. Moreover, most figure captions are written in a case-study format, which, combined with a system of diagnostic notations (explained in Chapter 1) following each legend, is meant to impart an appreciation of the process of radiologic investigations. Although its aim is to teach, *Orthopedic Radiology* should also serve as a convenient reference for physicians interested in bone and joint disorders and those customarily employing radiologic studies in their everyday practice.

Adam Greenspan, MD, FACR

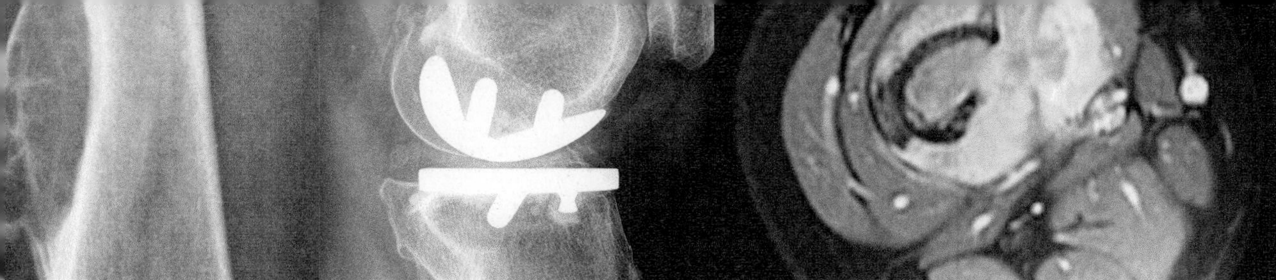

Preface

Continued progress in the field of musculoskeletal imaging has prompted the publication of yet another edition of this book. The constant improvement of existing imaging modalities and increased use of ultrasound (US), positron emission tomography (PET), PET/computed tomography (CT), and magnetic resonance imaging (MRI) in diagnosis and evaluation of a huge variety of orthopaedic conditions motivated us to expand the coverage of these techniques. Again, as in the previous versions of this book, the task of the seventh edition of *Orthopaedic Imaging: A Practical Approach* is not only to familiarize the reader with current applications of a variety of imaging modalities but also to present the constructive and beneficial, as well as negative, aspects of these techniques. The goal, as before, is to help radiologists and referring physicians choose the optimum imaging pathway with the purpose of reducing the cost and time needed to arrive at the correct diagnosis and adequately evaluate a given disorder.

This new edition has many changes, additions, and improvements. Javier Beltran, MD, FACR, Professor and Former Chairman of Radiology at Maimonides Medical Center in Brooklyn, New York, a pioneer of musculoskeletal MRI, remains as a coauthor. Again, his unmatched expertise in musculoskeletal MRI significantly adds to the value of the parts of the text relating to this important technique used in the evaluation of orthopaedic disorders.

The overall design of this book, incorporating full color, has been retained; however, a new interior design has been created, including different color bands for the outside corners of the book, which will enable the reader to easily identify the parts of the book before opening it. The color coding allows the readers to know where they are in the book and easily navigate between sections. The single-volume format, despite an increase in size, once more has been preserved. We substantially decreased the number of references in each chapter, retaining the "old classic" ones and adding only those that are most pertinent and up-to-date. We have deleted technically suboptimal figures and replaced them with better quality images. Specifically, we replaced the majority of magnetic resonance (MR) images with higher quality images obtained on high field strength systems including images obtained using 3 Tesla magnets, and we have added discussion of new pulse sequences in the appropriate sections. We have also included MR arthrographic studies where pertinent. We have deleted some outdated material and have updated the discussion of a variety of conditions. In particular, we have expanded Chapter 3, to include the histology, formation, and growth of the articular cartilage. We added clinical and pathologic information where deemed to be appropriate, including new illustrations, mainly in the chapters devoted to the arthritides, metabolic conditions, and tumors. We have also updated facts related to the molecular genetics and cytogenetics of many musculoskeletal disorders. Almost every chapter contains new sections and new images and schematics. Examples include new material on sports injuries, imaging evaluation of compressive and entrapment neuropathies of the upper and lower extremities, assessment of articular cartilage lesions, detailed MRI anatomy of small joints of the hand, postoperative MRI evaluation of the common surgeries of the shoulder and knee, and many more. We substantially expanded the chapters devoted to the arthritides, adding discussion of the clinical and pathologic evaluation of these conditions and including abnormalities such as SAPHO syndrome, chronic recurrent multifocal osteomyelitis, Wilson disease, and sarcoidosis. We have also integrated the information on advances in the latest medical and orthopaedic therapeutic approaches to many conditions and have significantly augmented the section on prosthetic replacement of the various joints. We have further expanded the text in reference to applications of three-dimensional CT, MRI, US, fluorine 18 (^{18}F)-fluorodeoxyglucose PET (FDG PET), PET/CT, and PET/MRI. We have included information on current imaging of the articular cartilage, discussing the latest techniques such as delayed gadolinium-enhanced MRI of cartilage (d-GEMRIC), T1 in the rotating frame (Th-rho) imaging, and sodium 23 (^{23}Na) MR imaging. We have supplemented the chapter devoted to sclerosing dysplasias of bone with conditions such as endosteal hyperostosis, dysosteosclerosis, Pyle disease, and craniodiaphyseal dysplasia. As in the previous editions, we continue to emphasize the mastery of conventional radiography as the fundamental tool for every radiologist interpreting musculoskeletal images. This technique remains invaluable for the initial evaluation of many traumatic conditions, a variety of arthritides, tumors and tumor-like lesions, and congenital anomalies.

This book has been written primarily for radiologists and orthopaedic surgeons, although it may also be of use for physical therapists, rheumatologists, and other physicians interested in the application of imaging techniques to the musculoskeletal system.

Adam Greenspan, MD, FACR
Javier Beltran, MD, FACR

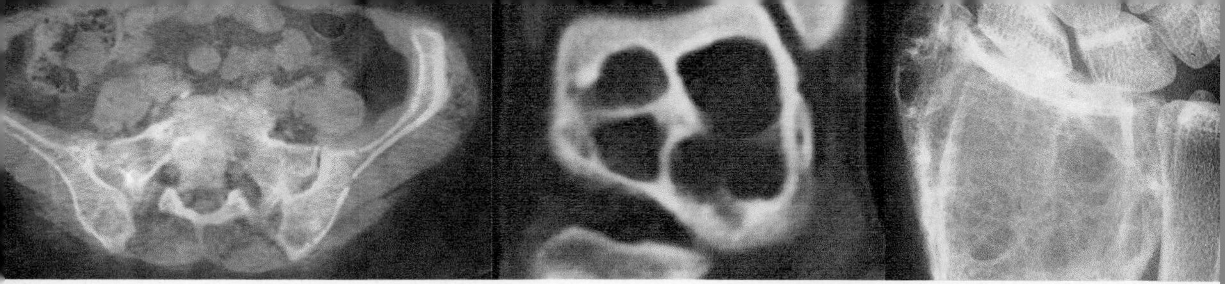

Acknowledgments

We would like to express our thanks to many hardworking on this book individuals from Wolters Kluwer Health who guided us in the preparation of this new edition, but particularly to Sharon R. Zinner, Executive Editor, Medicine and Advance Practice Publishing, for close supervision over this volume. A special note of acknowledgment goes to Eric McDermott, Associate Development Editor; Julie Kostelnik, Editorial Coordinator; and Justin Wright, Senior Production Associate, for attentive review, editing, and restructuring the content of the text. We also would like to thank Holly McLaughlin, Designer Coordinator, for beautiful and artistic design of the cover and interior of this book. Again, we are indebted to Luis Beltran, MD, and Jenny Bencardino, MD, from Hospital for Joint Diseases, New York University, for their help in selecting the best possible images for our book. A very special thanks goes to Luis Beltran, MD, for providing excellent schematics after the unfortunate passing of Dr. Salvador Beltran, contributor to the previous edition. We thank many residents and attendings in the Department of Radiology of Maimonides Medical Center in Brooklyn, New York, for their help in finding good imaging examples of common and less common disease entities from their radiology files. We greatly appreciate the contribution made by Michael J. Klein, MD, Pathologist-in-Chief Emeritus, Professor of Pathology and Laboratory Medicine, Hospital for Special Surgery—Weill Cornell Medical College, and Consultant in Pathology, Memorial Sloan Kettering Cancer Center in New York, who provided us with some excellent examples of photographs of gross pathology specimens and photomicrographs of selected musculoskeletal abnormalities. We also would like to thank Julie A. Ostoich-Prather, Senior Photographer from the Department of Radiology, University of California Davis Medical Center, for help in creating some digital illustrations. We would like to acknowledge Michael Greenspan, Samantha Greenspan, and Danielle Greenspan for their constant help with many technical problems encountered during work on this text. We are grateful to Professor Andrew J. Grainger, BM, BS, FRCP, FRCR, Consultant MSK Radiologist, from Cambridge University Hospital, Cambridge, United Kingdom, for writing the Foreword for this book. Again, we are thankful to all authors who have given permission to reproduce selective illustrations from their books and publications. Finally, we would like to thank Sadie Buckallew, Wolters Kluwer Production Project Manager, and Don Famularcano, Project Manager from Absolute Service, Inc., for their supervision and coordination of the final production stages for our book.

As with the previous editions, this project could not have been successfully and timely completed without the prudent and dutiful efforts of the many individuals acknowledged here.

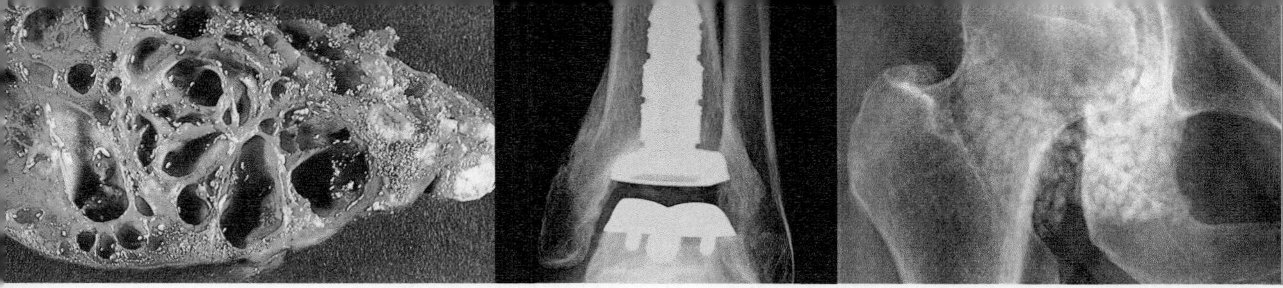

Contents

I

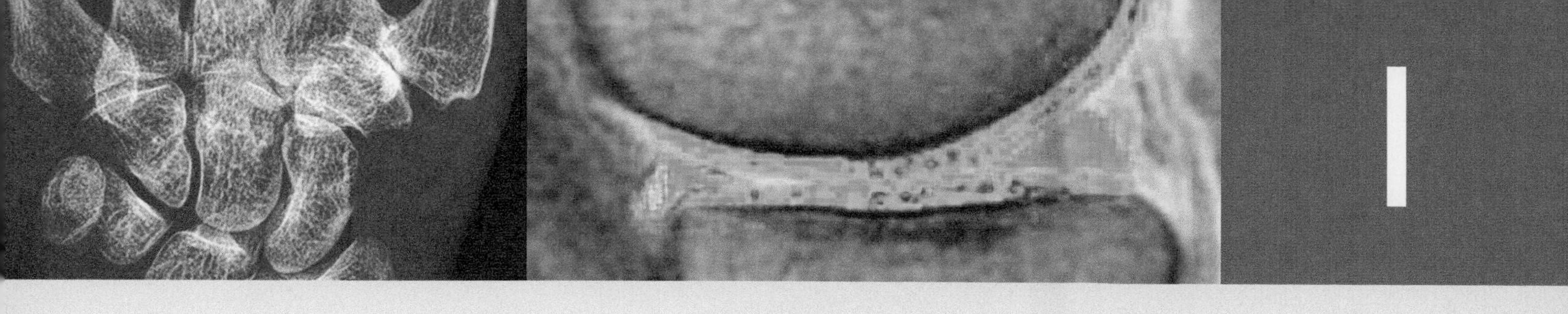

INTRODUCTION TO ORTHOPAEDIC IMAGING

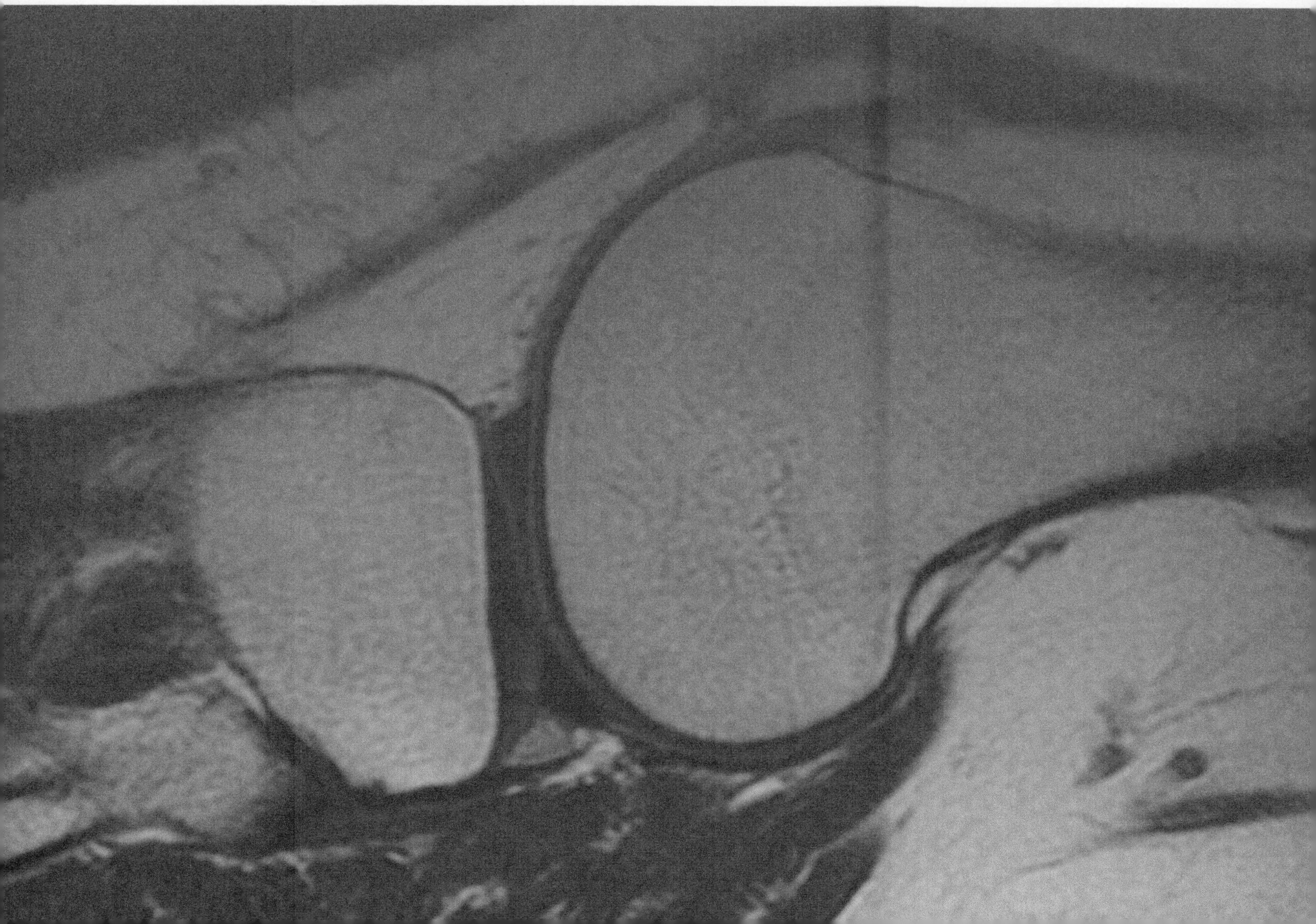

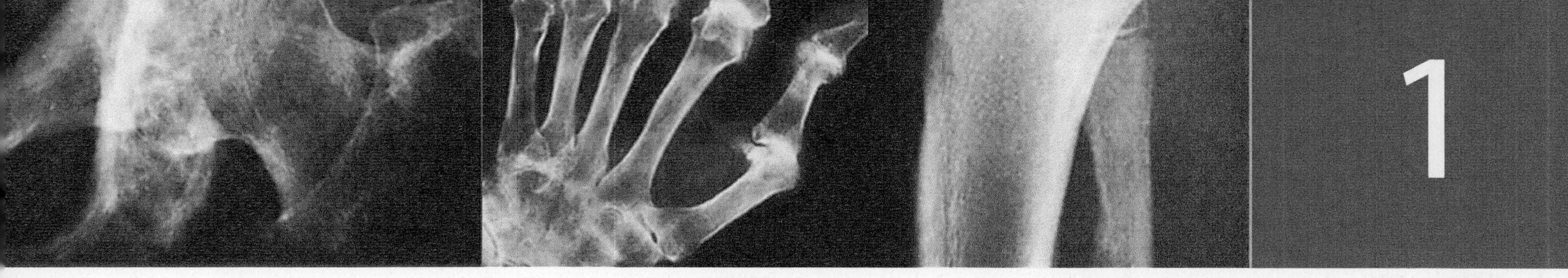

1

The Role of the Orthopaedic Radiologist

Spectacular progress has been made and continues to be made in the field of radiologic imaging. The introduction and constant improvements of new imaging modalities—computed tomography (CT) and its spiral (helical) and three-dimensional (3D) variants, multichannel multidetector row CT (MDCT), dual-energy CT (DECT), cone-beam CT (CBCT), high-resolution flat-panel volume CT (fpVCT), micro CT, 3D CT-angiography, and dynamic four-dimensional CT of the joints; digital (computed) radiography (DR or CR) and its variants, digital subtraction radiography (DSR) and digital subtraction angiography (DSA); 3D ultrasound (US); radionuclide angiography and perfusion scintigraphy; positron emission tomography (PET), PET/CT, and PET/MRI; single-photon emission CT (SPECT); magnetic resonance imaging (MRI) and its 3D variant, delayed gadolinium-enhanced MRI of the cartilage (d-GEMRIC); 3D MRI/CT fusion imaging; magnetic resonance diffusion tensor imaging (MRDTI); diffusion-weighted MRI (DWMRI); magnetic resonance arthrography (MRa); and magnetic resonance angiography (MRA), among others—have expanded the armamentarium of the radiologist, facilitating the sometimes difficult process of diagnosis. These new technologic developments have also brought disadvantages. They have contributed to a dramatic increase in the cost of medical care and have often led clinicians, trying to keep up with new imaging modalities, to order too many frequently unnecessary radiologic examinations.

This situation has served to emphasize the crucial importance of the role of the orthopaedic radiologist and the place of conventional radiography. The radiologist must not only comply with prerequisites for various examinations but also, more importantly, screen them to choose only those procedures that will lead to the correct diagnosis and proper evaluation of a given disorder. To this end, radiologists should bear in mind the following objectives in the performance of their role:

1. To *diagnose an unknown disorder*, preferably by using standard projections along with the special views and techniques obtainable in conventional radiography before using the more sophisticated modalities now available.
2. To perform examinations in the *proper sequence* and to know what should be performed next in the radiologic investigation.
3. To demonstrate the determining *imaging features of a known disorder*, the *distribution* of a lesion in the skeleton, and its *location* in the bone.
4. To monitor the *progress of therapy* and possible complications.
5. To be aware of what *specific information* is important to the orthopaedic surgeon.
6. To recognize the *limits of noninvasive radiologic investigation* and to know when to *proceed with invasive techniques.*
7. To recognize lesions that require biopsy and those that do not (the "don't touch" lesions).
8. To assume a more active role in therapeutic management, such as performing an embolization procedure, delivering chemotherapeutic material by means of selective catheterization, or performing (usually CT-guided) radiofrequency thermal ablation of osseous lesions (such as osteoid osteoma).

The radiologic diagnosis of many bone and joint disorders cannot be made solely on the basis of particular recognizable radiographic patterns. Clinical data, such as the patient's age, gender, symptoms, history, and laboratory findings, are also important to the radiologist in correctly interpreting an imaging study. Occasionally, clinical information is so typical of a certain disorder that it alone may suffice as the basis for diagnosis. Bone pain in a young person that is characteristically most severe at night and is promptly relieved by salicylates, for example, is so highly suggestive of osteoid osteoma that often the radiologist's only task is finding the lesion. However, in many cases, clinical data do not suffice and may even be misleading.

When presented with a patient, the cause of whose symptom is unknown (Fig. 1.1) or suspected based on clinical data (Fig. 1.2), the radiologist should avoid, as a point of departure in the examination, the more technologically advanced imaging modalities in favor of making a diagnosis, whenever possible, based on simple conventional radiographs. This approach is essential not only to maintain cost-effectiveness but also to decrease the amount of radiation to which a patient is exposed. Proceeding first with conventional technique also has a firm basis in the chemistry and physiology of bone. The calcium apatite crystal, one of the mineral constituents of bone, is an intrinsic contrast agent that gives skeletal radiology a great advantage over other radiologic subspecialties and makes information on bone production and destruction readily available through conventional radiography. Simple observation of changes in the shape or density of normal bone, for example, in the vertebrae, can be a deciding factor in arriving at a specific diagnosis (Figs. 1.3 and 1.4).

To aid the radiologist in the analysis of radiographic patterns and signs, some of which may be pathognomonic and others nonspecific, a number of options within the confines of conventional radiography are available. Certain *ways of positioning the patient* when radiographs are obtained allow the radiologist the opportunity to evaluate otherwise hidden anatomic sites and to more suitably demonstrate a particular abnormality. The frog-lateral projection of the hip, for example, is better than the anteroposterior view for imaging the signs of suspected osteonecrosis (ON) of the femoral head by more readily demonstrating the crescent sign, the early radiographic feature of this condition (see Figs. 4.90 and 4.91B). The frog-lateral view is also extremely helpful in the early diagnosis of slipped femoral capital epiphysis (see Fig. 32.39B). Likewise, the application of *special techniques* can help to identify a lesion that is difficult to detect on routine radiographs. Fractures of complex structures such as the elbow, wrist, ankle, and foot are not always demonstrated on the standard projections. Because of the overlap of bones on the lateral view of the elbow, for example, detecting a nondisplaced or minimally displaced fracture of

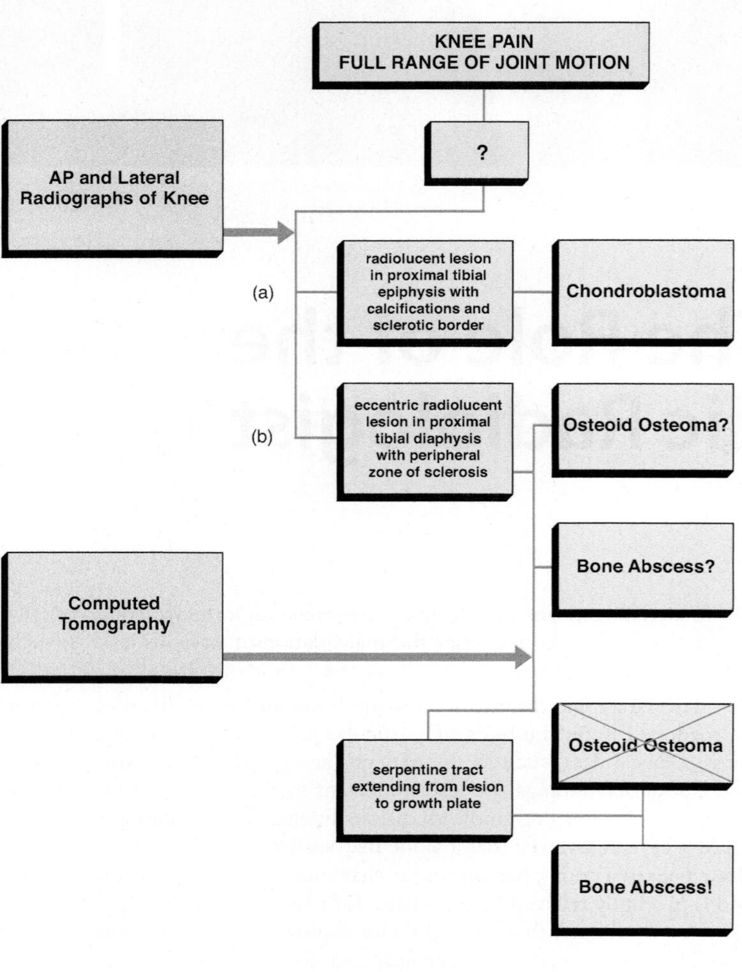

FIGURE 1.1 Cause of symptoms unknown. The patient's history and the results of the clinical examination, supplied to the radiologist by the referring physician, are not sufficient to form a diagnosis *(?)*. Based on conventional radiographic studies, *(a)* the diagnosis is established or *(b)* the studies may suggest the differential possibilities. In the latter case, ancillary imaging techniques, such as scintigraphy, CT, or MRI, among others, are called on to confirm or exclude one of the options.

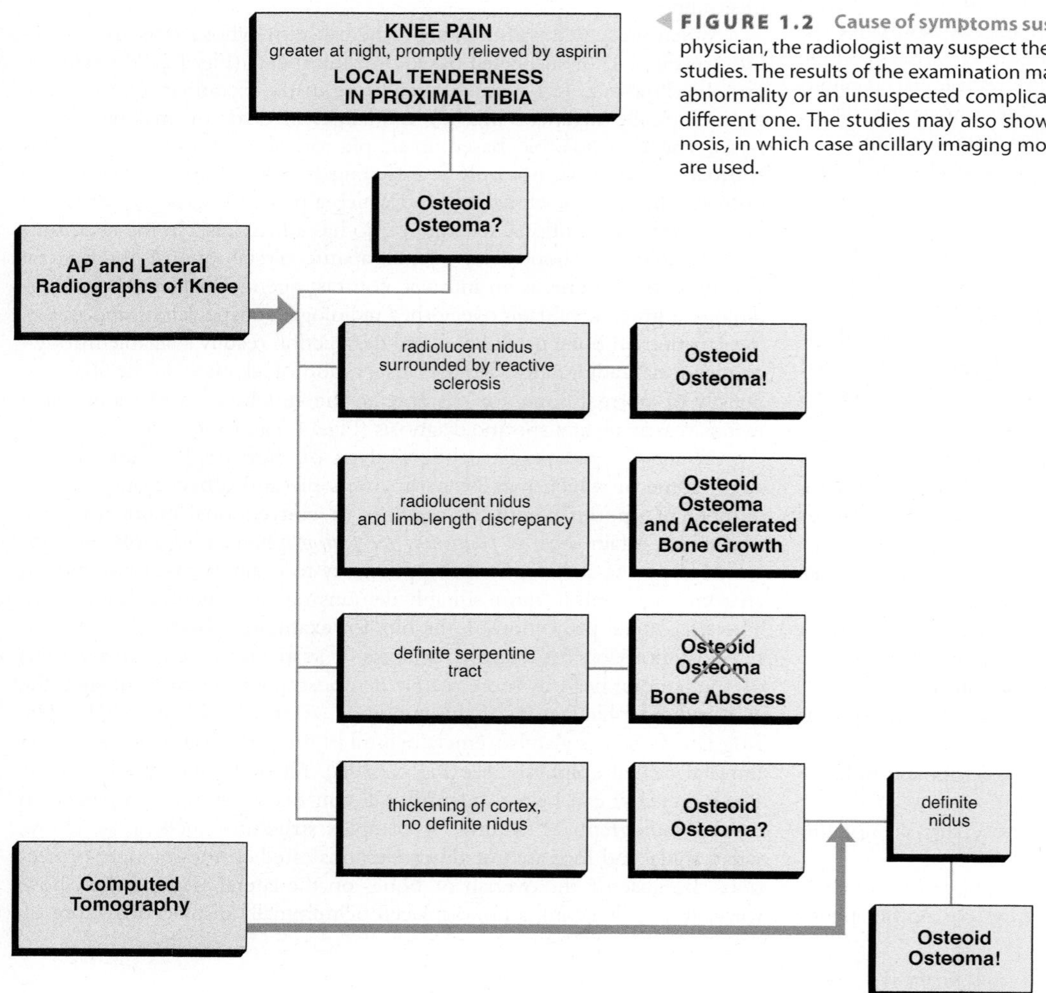

FIGURE 1.2 Cause of symptoms suspected. From the information supplied by the referring physician, the radiologist may suspect the diagnosis and proceed with conventional radiographic studies. The results of the examination may confirm the suspected diagnosis, reveal an additional abnormality or an unsuspected complication, or exclude the suspected diagnosis and confirm a different one. The studies may also show inconclusive evidence of the original suspected diagnosis, in which case ancillary imaging modalities, such as scintigraphy, CT, or MRI, among others, are used.

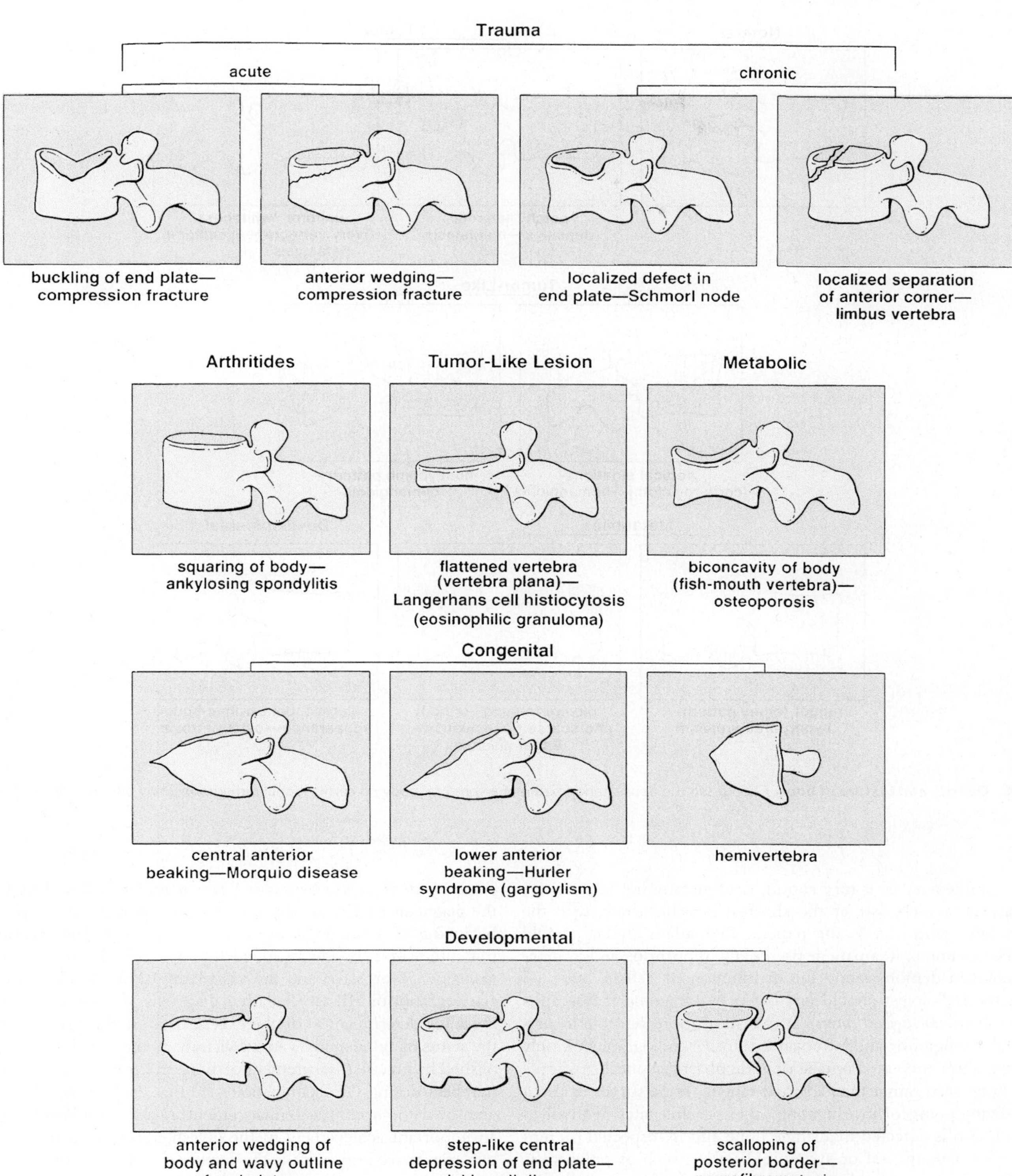

FIGURE 1.3 Shape and contour of bone. Observation of changes in the shape and contour of a vertebral body on conventional radiographs may disclose critical information leading to a correct diagnosis.

the radial head occasionally requires a special 45-degree angle view (called the *radial head–capitellum view*) that projects the radial head free of adjacent structures, making an otherwise obscure lesion evident (see Figs. 6.14, 6.27, and 6.28). Stress radiographic views are similarly useful, particularly in evaluating tears of various ligaments of the knee and ankle joints (see Figs. 9.14, 9.98B, 10.10, and 10.11).

An accurate diagnosis depends on the radiologist's acute observations and careful analysis, in light of clinical information, of the radiographic findings regarding the size, shape, configuration, and density of a lesion; its location within the bone; and its distribution in the skeletal system. Until the conventional approach with its range of options fails to provide the radiographic findings necessary for correct diagnosis and precise evaluation of an abnormality, the radiologist need not turn to more costly procedures.

Knowing the *proper sequence* of procedures in radiologic investigation depends, to a great extent, on the pertinent clinical information provided by the referring physician. The choice of modality or modalities for imaging a lesion or investigating a pathologic process is dictated by the clinical presentation as well as by the equipment availability, physician expertise, cost, and individual patient restrictions. Knowing *where to begin* and *what*

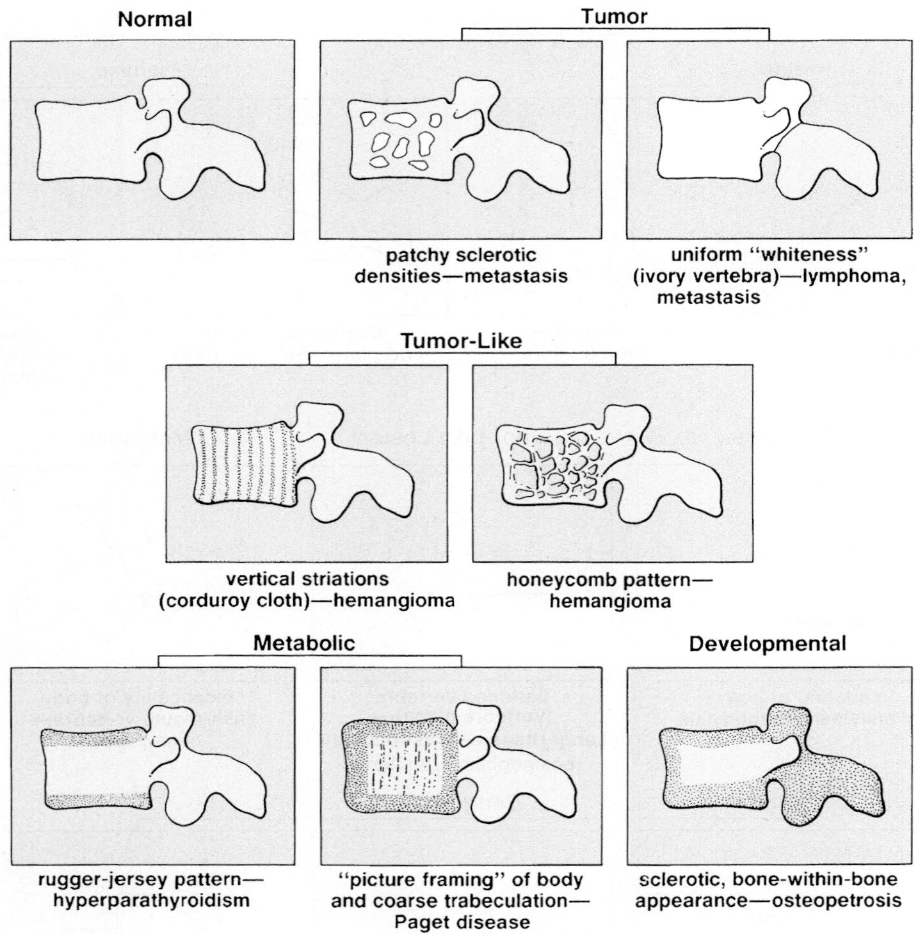

FIGURE 1.4 Density and texture of bone. Changes in the density and texture of a vertebral body on conventional radiographs may offer useful data for arriving at a diagnosis.

to do next, as rudimentary as it may sound, is of paramount importance in reaching a precise diagnosis by the shortest possible route, with the least expense and detriment to the patient. Redundant studies should be avoided. For example, if a patient presents with arthritis and if clinician is interested in demonstrating the distribution of "silent" sites of the disorder, the radiologist should not begin by obtaining radiographs of every joint (a so-called *joint survey*). It is instead more sensible to perform a skeletal scintigraphy and, afterward, to order radiographs of only those areas that show increased uptake of radiopharmaceutical. A simple radionuclide bone scan rather than a broad-ranging bone survey is also a reasonable starting point for investigating other possible sites of involvement when a lesion is detected in a single bone and is suspected of representing part of a multifocal or systemic disorder, such as polyostotic fibrous dysplasia or metastatic disease. Similarly, if a patient is suspected of having osteoid osteoma around the hip joint and standard radiography has not demonstrated the nidus, a radionuclide bone scan should be performed next to determine the site of the lesion. This should be followed up by CT for more precise localization of a nidus in the bone. However, if the routine examination demonstrates the nidus, scintigraphy can be omitted from the sequence of examination. At this point, only CT scan is required to determine the lesion's exact location in the bone and to obtain specific measurements of the nidus (Fig. 1.5; see also Figs. 17.12C and 17.11C). If ON of the femoral head is suspected and the radiographs are normal, MRI should be ordered as the next diagnostic procedure because it is a more sensitive modality than CT, or scintigraphy. The text that follows presents many similar situations in which the proper sequence of imaging modalities may dramatically shorten the diagnostic investigation and at the same time lower the cost.

Reaching a correct diagnosis does not end the process of radiologic investigation because the course of treatment often depends on the *identification of distinguishing features of a particular disorder* (Fig. 1.6). For example, the diagnosis of Ewing sarcoma by conventional radiography is only the beginning of a radiologic workup of the patient. The crucial features of this tumor must be identified, such as intraosseous and soft-tissue extension (by CT or MRI) and the vascularity of the lesion (by conventional arteriography or MRA). Similarly, a diagnosis of osteosarcoma must be followed by determination of the exact extent of the lesion in the bone and the status of bone marrow in the vicinity of the tumor. This can be accomplished by precise measurement of bone marrow density using Hounsfield numbers during CT examination (see Fig. 2.14) or by using MR images with or without contrast enhancement. Diagnosing Paget disease may be an important achievement in the investigation of an unknown disorder, but even more important is the further search for an answer to a crucial question: Is there any sign of malignant transformation? (see Figs. 29.28 and 29.29). *Localization* of a lesion in the skeleton or in a particular bone can frequently be more important than diagnosis itself. The best example of this is, again, the precise localization of the nidus of osteoid osteoma because incomplete resection of this lesion invariably results in recurrence. Determining the *distribution of a lesion* in the skeleton is helpful in planning the treatment of various arthritides and the management of a patient with metastatic disease. Scintigraphy is an invaluable technique in this respect.

Many of the most important questions put to the radiologist by the orthopaedic surgeon concern monitoring the *progress of treatment* and the appearance of possible *complications*. At the stage when the diagnosis is already established, the fate of the lesion, and consequently the patient, must be established. Comparison of earlier radiographic examinations with present findings plays a crucial role at this stage because it may disclose the dynamics of specific conditions (see Fig. 16.6). Likewise, in monitoring the progress of healing fractures, study of the diagnostic sequence of radiographs complemented by CT should decide questionable cases. Ancillary imaging

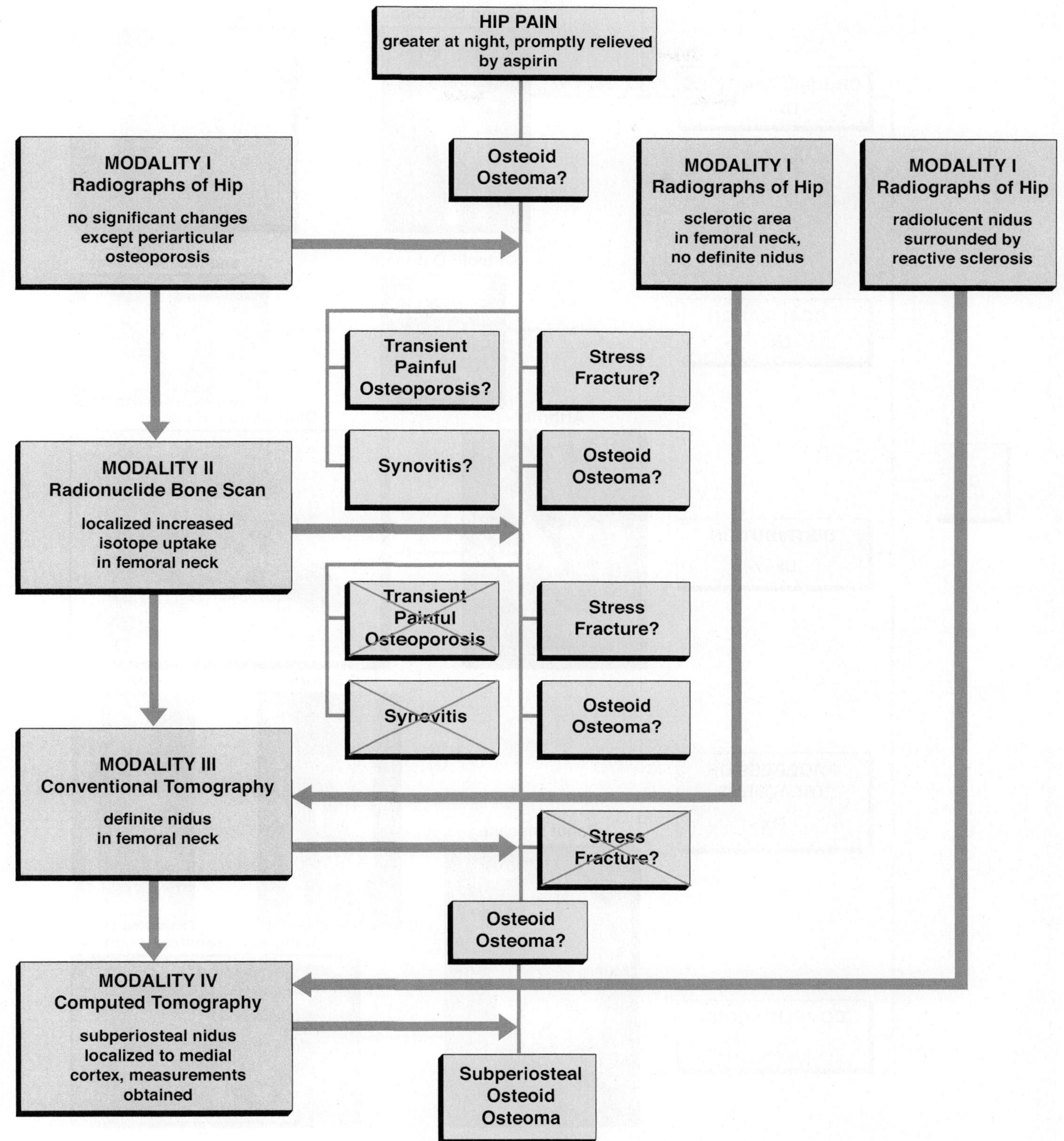

FIGURE 1.5 **Sequence of imaging modalities.** A diagnosis is suspected on the basis of a patient's history and the results of the clinical examination. The radiologist suggests the proper sequence of imaging modalities, eliminating various disorders in the process and narrowing the differential possibilities to arrive at one correct diagnosis. An accurate localization and specific information pertinent to the correct diagnosis are also provided.

techniques such as scintigraphy, CT, PET/CT, and MRI play an essential role in evaluating one of the most serious complications of benign tumors and tumor-like lesions—malignant transformation that may occur in enchondroma, osteochondroma, fibrous dysplasia, or Paget disease.

Providing the orthopaedic surgeon with *specific information* is also an important function of the radiologist at the time when a diagnosis is being established. If, for example, osteochondritis dissecans is diagnosed, the decision on the choice of therapy requires information on the status of the articular cartilage covering the lesion. This information is obtainable by contrast arthrography, alone or combined with CT, or by MRI (see Figs. 6.48 and 6.64). If the cartilage is intact, conservative treatment should be contemplated; if it is damaged, surgical intervention is the more likely course of treatment. Similarly, in contributing to the plan of treatment of anterior dislocation in the shoulder joint, the radiologist should

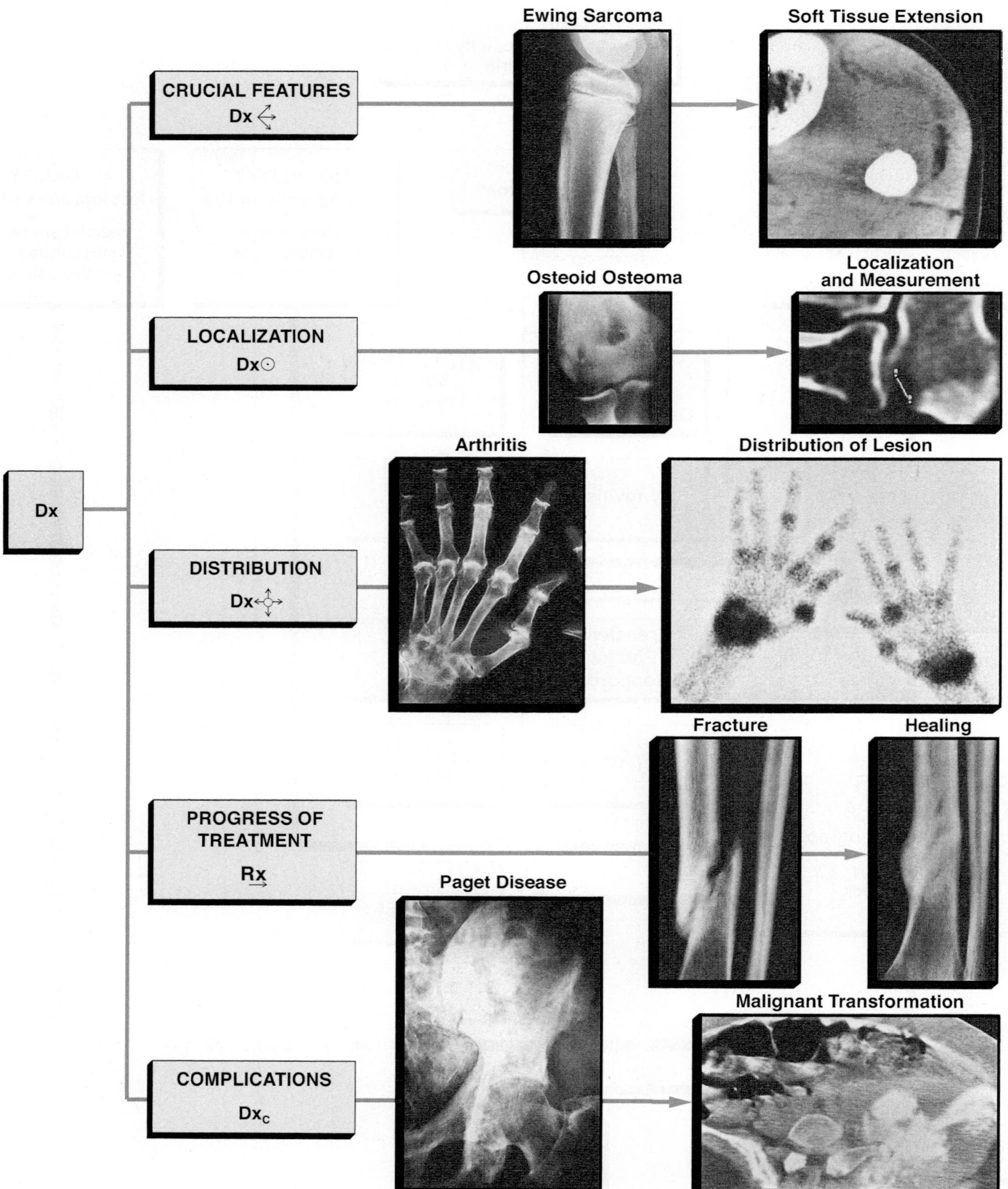

FIGURE 1.6 Distinguishing features of lesion, progress of treatment, and complications. The diagnosis is known *(Dx)*. The clinician is interested in demonstrating (1) the crucial features of the lesion *(Dx)*, that is, its character, extent, stage, and other pertinent data; (2) the location of the lesion in the bone *(Dx⊙)*; (3) the distribution of the lesion in the skeleton *(Dx)*; (4) the progress of treatment *(Rx)*; and (5) the emergence of any complications *(Dx_c)*.

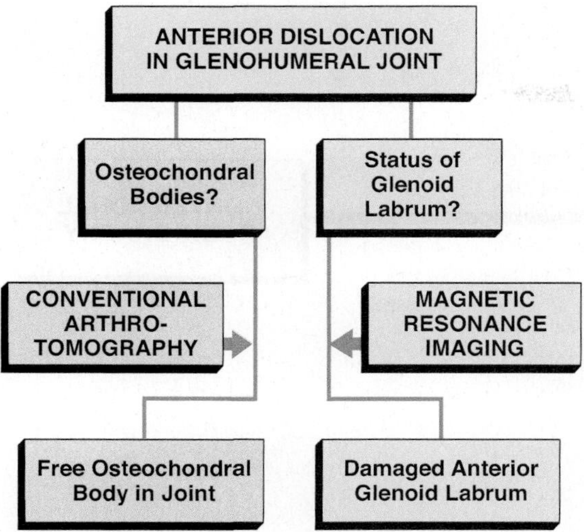

FIGURE 1.7 **Specific information.** The diagnosis is known. The radiologist should be aware of the specific information, for example, regarding the features or extent of a lesion, which is required by the orthopaedic surgeon in planning treatment. The information may also concern the distribution of a lesion and its localization, the progress of treatment, or the emergence of complications. Application of the best radiologic modality for demonstrating the required information is one of the radiologist's primary functions. The modalities may vary depending on the specific information needed.

be aware of the importance to the surgeon of information about the status of the cartilaginous labrum of the glenoid (see Figs. 5.55, 5.56, and 5.64) and the possible presence of osteochondral bodies in the joint. These features must be confirmed or excluded by arthrography combined with tomography (arthrotomography), CT (computed arthrotomography), or MRI (Fig. 1.7).

Recognizing *the limits of noninvasive radiologic investigation* and knowing when to proceed with *invasive techniques* are as important to arriving at a diagnosis and precise evaluation of a condition as any of the points already mentioned. This situation is best illustrated in the case of tumors and tumor-like bone lesions. Many tumor-like lesions have distinctive radiographic presentations that lead to unquestionable diagnoses on conventional studies. In such cases, invasive procedures such as biopsy are not indicated. This is particularly true of a group of definitely benign conditions commonly called *don't touch lesions* (see Fig. 16.60 and Table 16.11). The name *don't touch* speaks for itself. Conditions such as a bone island (enostosis), posttraumatic juxtacortical myositis ossificans, and a periosteal desmoid are unquestionably benign lesions whose determining features can, with certainty, be demonstrated with the appropriate noninvasive techniques without the need for histopathologic confirmation. Obtaining a biopsy of such lesions may in fact lead to mistakes in diagnosis and treatment. The histologic appearance of a periosteal desmoid, for example, may exhibit aggressive features resembling a malignant tumor; in inexperienced hands, this can lead to inappropriate treatment. However, there are times when the radiologist faces the situation in which a battery of conventional and advanced noninvasive techniques has yielded equivocal information. At this point, there is no shame in saying, "I don't know what it is, but I know a biopsy should be performed" (Fig. 1.8). Fluoroscopy-guided or CT-guided percutaneous biopsy can be performed by the radiologist in the radiology suite, eliminating the use of costly operating-room time and personnel. Occasionally, the radiologist may also assume a more active role in therapeutic management by performing an embolization procedure under image intensification or with CT or US guidance, or performing radiofrequency thermal ablation of bone lesion. This more interventional role for the radiologist may shorten the length of a patient's hospitalization and be more cost-effective. Information hidden in the radiologic image, whether it is conventional radiography, scintigraphy, US, CT, MRI, or other modality, can be effectively extracted by knowing the sensitivity of applied technique, spatial resolution, contrast resolution, and distortion among other factors.

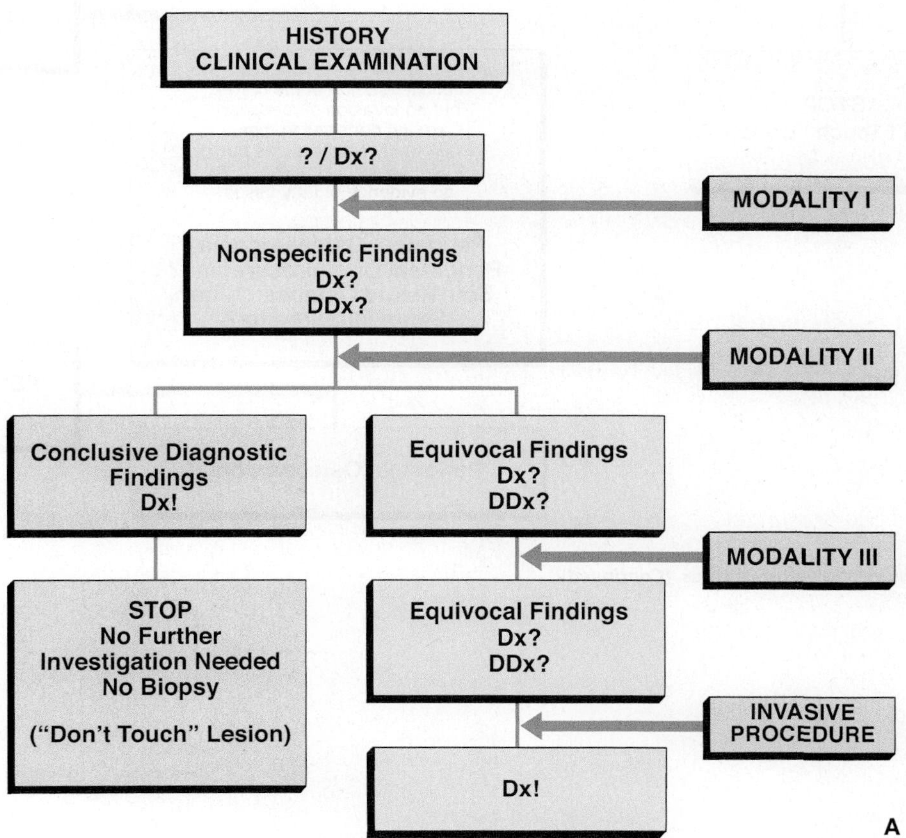

FIGURE 1.8 **Noninvasive versus invasive procedures.** **(A,B)** The diagnosis is unknown *(?)* or suspected *(Dx?)*. Noninvasive radiologic procedures may yield sufficient data to make an unquestionable diagnosis. No further investigation is required, nor is biopsy indicated, particularly if the diagnosis is that of a definitely benign condition commonly called a *don't touch lesion*. However, noninvasive procedures may yield equivocal information at each step in the examination. At this point, proceeding to an invasive procedure such as biopsy is indicated. *(Continued)*

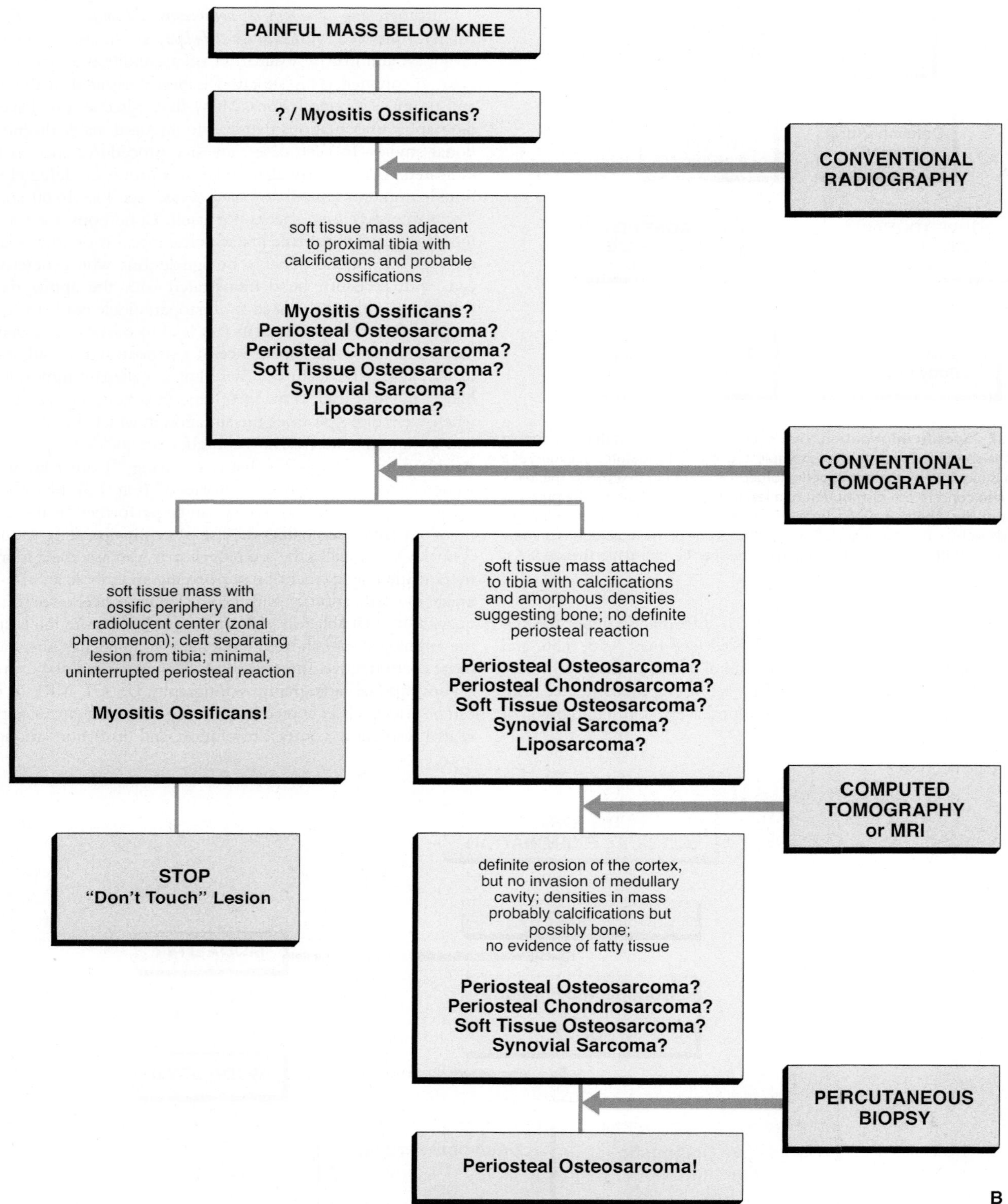

FIGURE 1.8 Noninvasive versus invasive procedures. *(Continued)*

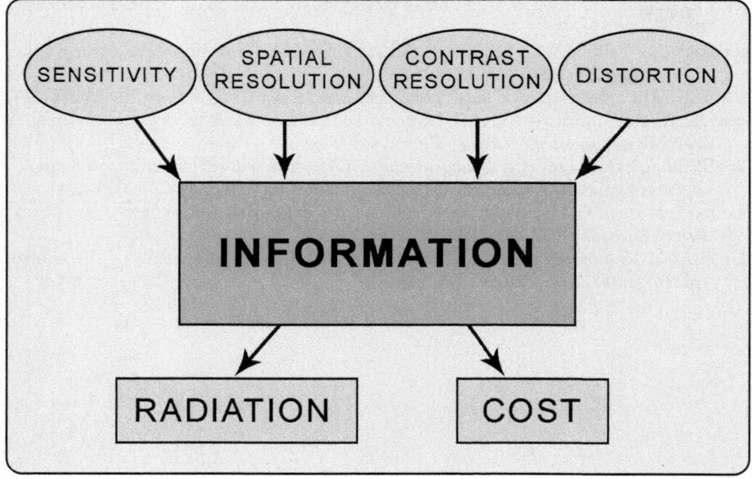

FIGURE 1.9 **Information.** Crucial factors determining the usefulness of information concealed in the radiologic image.

But at the same time, radiologist should never forget the drawbacks of some techniques, such as radiation exposure to the patient or high cost of imaging procedures (Fig. 1.9). Choosing logical diagnostic imaging pathway would not only benefit the patient but would also reduce the cost of radiologic studies and cost of treatment (Fig. 1.10). Therefore, it is mandatory for musculoskeletal radiologist to develop a strategic course of action in pursuing his or her goal to make the correct diagnosis. Radiologist must take into consideration the effectiveness of imaging modalities, their safety, required time to complete the examination, as well as the cost of investigation (Fig. 1.11A). The effectiveness will depend on the use of imaging techniques in proper sequence, and knowledge of which of these techniques is better to demonstrate the lesion, its localization and distribution in the skeleton, and which is the best to monitor the progress of treatment or emergence of possible complications (Fig. 1.11B). In summary, to sufficiently manage the diagnosis and treatment of patients with conditions affecting the musculoskeletal system, the radiologist and the referring physician should be aware of the range of radiologic modalities and their proper uses. This will increase the precision of diagnostic radiologic investigation and reduce the amount of radiation to which a patient is exposed and the cost of hospitalization. The obligation of the radiologist is to:

- Use the conventional radiographic methods, with knowledge of the capabilities and effectiveness of the various techniques, before resorting to more advanced modalities.
- Follow a logical sequence of imaging modalities in diagnostic investigation.

LOGICAL DIAGNOSTIC PATHWAY

- LESSER RADIATION EXPOSURE
- EARLIER DIAGNOSIS
- SHORTER HOSPITALIZATION
- LESSER COST

FIGURE 1.10 **Logical diagnostic pathway.** Benefits of a sensible approach to the diagnostic investigation.

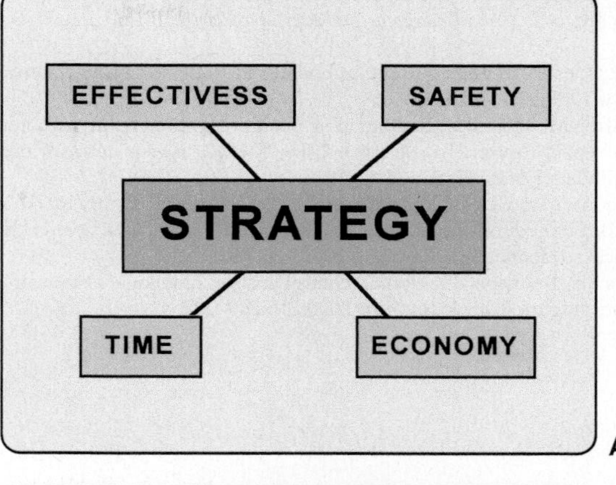

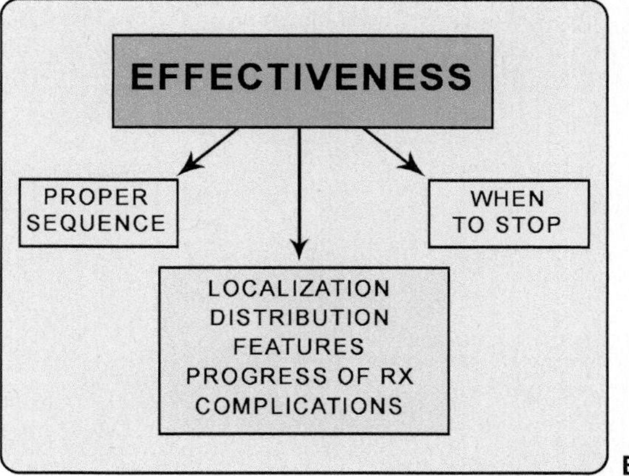

FIGURE 1.11 **Imaging strategy.** Strategic elements **(A,B)** of analytic quest for correct radiologic diagnosis.

- Be as noninvasive as possible at the start but use invasive techniques if they will shorten the diagnostic pathway.
- Improve communication between the radiologist and the orthopaedic surgeon by using the same language and by knowing what the surgeon needs to know about the lesion.
- Provide knowledge to referring physicians about indications, advantages, disadvantages, risks, contraindications, and limitations of the various imaging techniques.

SUGGESTED READINGS

Bolus NE, George R, Washington J, et al. PET/MRI: the blended-modality choice of the future? *J Nucl Med Tech* 2009;37:63–71.

Bone JM. Multidetector CT: opportunities, challenges, and concerns associated with scanners with 64 or more detector rows. *Radiology* 2016;241:334–337.

Cheung AC, Bredella MA, Al Khalaf M, et al. Reproducibility of trabecular structure analysis using flat-panel volume computed tomography. *Skeletal Radiol* 2009;38:1003–1008.

Cohen MD. Determining cost of imaging services. *Radiology* 2001;220:563–565.

Collier BD, Fogelman I, Brown ML. Bone scintigraphy: part 2. Orthopedic bone scanning. *J Nucl Med* 1993;34:2241–2246.

Delfaut EM, Beltran J, Johnson G, et al. Fat suppression in MR imaging: techniques and pitfalls. *Radiographics* 1999;19:373–382.

Gates GF. SPECT bone scanning of the spine. *Semin Nucl Med* 1998;28:78–94.

Gibson DJ. Technology: the key to controlling health care cost in the future. *Am J Roentgenol* 1994;163:1289–1293.

Hamper UM, Trapanotto V, Sheth S, et al. Three-dimensional US: preliminary clinical experience. *Radiology* 1994;191:397–401.

Jackson DW. The cost of diagnostic imaging: on our radar for 2009. *Orthop Today* 2009;29:3.

Johnson RP. The role of the bone imaging in orthopedic practice. *Semin Nucl Med* 1997;27:386–389.

Kaplan PA, Matamoros A Jr, Anderson JC. Sonography of the musculoskeletal system. *Am J Roentgenology* 1990;155:237–245.

Kumar R, Guinto FC, Madewell JE, et al. The vertebral body: radiographic configurations in various congenital and acquired disorders. *Radiographics* 1988;8:455–485.

Levin DC, Spettell CM, Rao VM, et al. Impact of MR imaging on nationwide health care costs and comparison with other imaging procedures. *Am J Roentgenol* 1998;170:557–560.

Margulis AR. Introduction to the algorithmic approach to radiology. In: Eisenberg RL, Amberg JR, eds. *Critical diagnostic pathways in radiology*. Philadelphia: JB Lippincott; 1981.

McDougall IR, Rieser RP. Scintigraphic techniques in musculoskeletal trauma. *Radiol Clin North Am* 1989;27:1003–1011.

Meschan I, Farrer-Meschan RM. Radiographic positioning, projection, pathology and definition of special terms. In: Meschan I, ed. *Roentgen signs in diagnostic imaging*, vol. 4, 2nd ed. Philadelphia: WB Saunders; 1987.

Mezrich R. A contrarian view of X-ray doses: it ain't necessarily so. *Appl Radiol* 2006;35:6–8.

Rogers LF. From the editor's notebook. Imaging literacy: a laudable goal in the education of medical students. *Am J Roentgenol* 2003;180:1201.

Saini S, Seltzer SE, Bramson RT, et al. Technical cost of radiologic examinations: analysis across imaging modalities. *Radiology* 2000;216:269–272.

Siegel E. Primum non-nocere: a call for re-evaluation of radiation doses used in CT. *Appl Radiol* 2006;35:6–8.

Steinbach LS, Palmer WE, Schweitzer ME. Special focus session—MR arthrography. *Radiographics* 2002;22:1223–1246.

Stoller DW. MR arthrography of the glenohumeral joint. *Radiol Clin North Am* 1997;35:97–116.

Swan JS, Grist TM, Sproat IA, et al. Musculoskeletal neoplasms: preoperative evaluation with MR angiography. *Radiology* 1995;194:519–524.

Tam EP, Rong J, Cody DD, et al. Quality initiatives: CT radiation dose reduction: how to implement change without sacrificing diagnostic quality. *Radiographics* 2011;31:1823–2011.

Tratting S, Mosher TJ. High field MR imaging of the musculoskeletal system. *Semin Musculoskelet Radiol* 2008;12:183–183.

Yamanaka Y, Kamogawa J, Katagi R, et al. 3-D MRI/CT fusion imaging of the lumbar spine. *Skeletal Radiol* 2010;39:285–288.

2

Imaging Techniques in Orthopaedics

Choice of Imaging Modality

In this chapter, the principles and limitations of current imaging techniques are described. Understanding the basis of the imaging modalities available to diagnose many commonly encountered disorders of the bones and joints is of utmost importance. It may help determine the most effective radiologic technique, minimizing the cost of examination and the exposure of patients to radiation. To this end, it is important to choose the modality appropriate for specific types of orthopaedic abnormalities and, when using conventional techniques (namely, "plain" radiography), to be familiar with the views and the techniques that best demonstrate the abnormality. It is important to reemphasize that conventional radiography most of the time remains the most effective means of demonstrating bone and joint abnormalities.

The use of radiologic techniques differs in evaluating the presence, type, and extent of various bone, joint, and soft-tissue abnormalities. Therefore, the radiologist and the orthopaedic surgeon must know the indications for use of each technique, the limitations of a particular modality, and the appropriate imaging approaches for abnormalities at specific sites. The question "What modality should I use for this particular problem?" is frequently asked by radiologists and orthopaedic surgeons alike, and although numerous algorithms are available to evaluate various problems at different anatomic sites, the answer cannot always be clearly stated. The choice of techniques for imaging bone and soft-tissue abnormalities is dictated not only by clinical presentation but also by equipment availability, expertise, and cost. Restrictions may also be imposed by the needs of individual patients. For example, allergy to ionic or nonionic iodinated contrast agents may preclude the use of arthrography; the presence of a pacemaker would preclude the use of magnetic resonance imaging (MRI); and physiologic states, such as pregnancy, preclude the use of ionized radiation, favoring, for instance, the use of ultrasound (US). Time and cost consideration should discourage redundant studies.

No matter what ancillary technique is used, conventional radiograph should be available for comparison. Most of the time, the choice of imaging technique is dictated by the type of suspected abnormality. For instance, if osteonecrosis is suspected after obtaining conventional radiographs, the next examination should be MRI, which detects necrotic changes in bone long before radiographs, computed tomography (CT), or scintigraphy becomes positive. In the evaluation of internal derangement of the knee, conventional radiographs should be obtained first and, if the abnormality is not obvious, should again be followed up by MRI because this modality provides exquisite contrast resolution of the bone marrow, articular cartilage, ligaments, menisci, and soft tissues. MRI and magnetic resonance arthrography (MRa) are currently the most effective procedures for the evaluation of rotator cuff abnormalities, particularly when a partial or complete tear is suspected. Although US can also detect a rotator cuff tear, its low sensitivity (68%) and low specificity (75% to 84%) make it a less definitive diagnostic procedure. In evaluating a painful wrist, conventional radiographs should precede the use of more advanced techniques, such as CT-arthrography or MRI. If a tear of triangular fibrocartilage complex, a tear of intercarpal ligaments, or a carpal tunnel syndrome is suspected, MRI is preferred because it provides a high-contrast difference among muscles, tendons, ligaments, and nerves. Similarly, if osteonecrosis of carpal bones is suspected and the conventional radiographs are normal, MRI would be the method of choice to demonstrate this abnormality. In the evaluation of fractures and fracture healing of carpal bones, CT is the procedure of choice, preferred over MRI, because of the high degree of spatial resolution. In diagnosing bone tumors, conventional radiography is still the gold standard for diagnostic purposes. However, to evaluate the intraosseous and soft-tissue extension of tumor, it should be followed by either CT scan or MRI, with the latter modality being more accurate. More recently, positron emission tomography (PET)/CT and PET/MRI have been added to the armamentarium of imaging modalities, especially for detection and staging of variety of osseous and soft-tissue tumors. To evaluate the results of radiotherapy and chemotherapy of malignant tumors, dynamic MRI using gadopentetate dimeglumine (gadolinium diethylenetriamine pentaacetic acid [Gd-DTPA]) as a contrast enhancement is far superior to scintigraphy, CT, or even "plain" MRI.

Imaging Techniques

Conventional Radiography

The most frequently used modality for the evaluation of bone and joint disorders, and particularly traumatic conditions, is conventional radiography. The radiologist should obtain at least two views of the bone involved, at 90-degree angles to each other, with each view including two adjacent joints (see Figs. 4.1 and 4.2). This decreases the risk of missing an associated fracture, subluxation, and/or dislocation at a site remote from the apparent primary injury. In children, it is frequently necessary to obtain a radiograph of the normal unaffected limb for comparison. Usually, the standard radiography comprises the anteroposterior and lateral views; occasionally, oblique and special views are necessary, particularly in evaluating complex structures such as the elbow, wrist, ankle, and pelvis. A weight-bearing view may be of value for a dynamic evaluation of the joint space under the weight of the body (see Fig. 13.36). Special projections, such as those described in the following chapters, may, at times, be required to demonstrate an abnormality of the bone or joint to further advantage.

In the last decade, conventional radiography has evolved into digital radiography in most places (Fig. 2.1), allowing direct acquisition of a digital image that can be transferred to a picture archive and communication system (PACS) workstation permitting change contrast and orientation, choose magnification, and obtain measurements of linear distances and angles, among many others (see discussion in the following text).

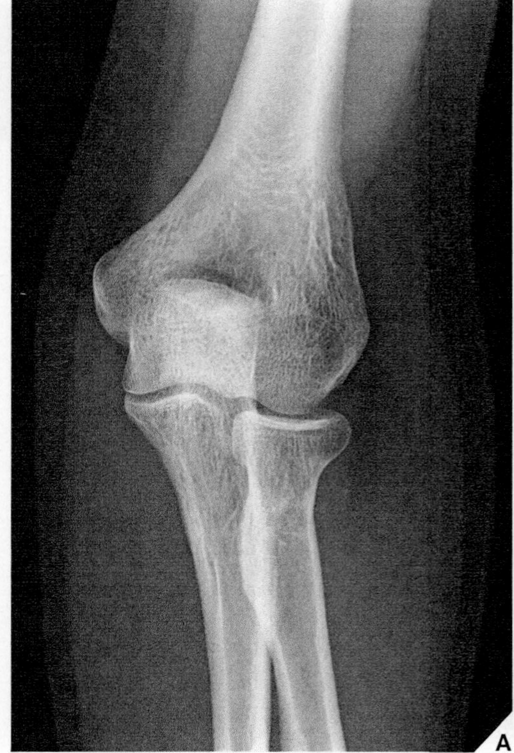

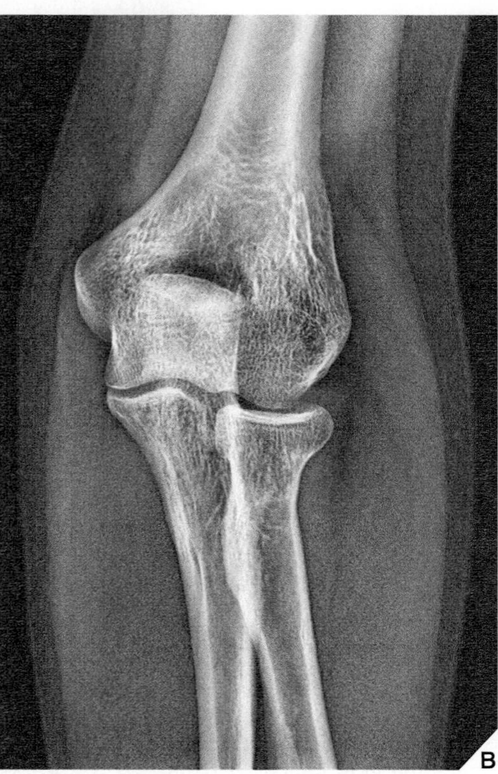

FIGURE 2.1 **Digital radiography.** Digital radiograph of the elbow without **(A)** and with **(B)** edge enhancement. The bone details and the soft tissues are better appreciated than on the standard radiographs.

Magnification Radiography

Magnification radiography was used in the past to enhance bony details not well appreciated on the standard radiographic projections and to maximize the diagnostic information obtainable from a radiographic image. This technique has been replaced using digital PACS viewers, which allow digital magnification without the use of additional radiation exposure. Digital magnification techniques are particularly effective in demonstrating early changes in some arthritides as well as in various metabolic disorders (see Fig. 26.9B). Occasionally, it may be useful in demonstrating subtle fracture lines otherwise not seen on routine projections.

Stress Views

Stress views are important in evaluating ligamentous tears and joint stability. In the hand, abduction–stress film of the thumb may be obtained when a gamekeeper's thumb, resulting from a disruption of the ulnar collateral ligament of the first metacarpophalangeal joint, is suspected (see Fig. 7.127B). In the lower extremity, stress views of the knee and ankle joints are occasionally obtained. The evaluation of knee instability caused by ligament injuries may require the use of this technique in cases of a suspected tear of the medial or lateral collateral ligament and, less frequently, in evaluating an insufficiency of the anterior and posterior cruciate ligaments. The evaluation of ankle ligaments also may require stress radiography. Inversion (adduction) and anterior-draw stress films are the most frequently obtained stress views (see Figs. 4.5, 10.10, and 10.11).

Scanogram

The scanogram is the most widely used method for limb-length measurement. This technique requires a slit-beam diaphragm with a 1/16-in. opening attached to the radiographic tube and a long film cassette. The radiographic tube moves in the long axis of the radiographic table. During an exposure, the tube traverses the whole length of the film, scanning the entire extremity. This technique allows the x-ray beam to intersect the bone ends perpendicularly; therefore, comparative limb lengths can be measured. When a motorized radiographic tube is not available, a modified technique may be used with three separate exposures over the hip joints, knees, and ankles. In this technique, an opaque tape measure is placed longitudinally down the center of the radiographic table. Occasionally, an orthoroentgenogram is obtained. For this technique, the patient is positioned supine with the lower limbs on a 3-ft-long cassette and a long ruler at one side. A single exposure is made, centered at the knees to include the entire length of both limbs and the ruler.

This technique has been replaced by digital scanogram obtained with a CT unit. While the patient lies on the CT table, the tube rotates during advancement of the table, providing a digital image of the extremities. The limb length can then be measured either in the CT console or in a PACS workstation with the advantage of decreased radiation exposure.

Fluoroscopy and Videotaping

Fluoroscopy is a fundamental diagnostic tool for many radiologic procedures, including arthrography, tenography, bursography, arteriography, and percutaneous bone or soft-tissue biopsy. Some of these procedures are no longer in use (tenography, bursography), but fluoroscopy remains a necessary tool for arthrography, MRa, CT-arthrography, biopsy, and drainage. Fluoroscopy combined with videotaping is useful in evaluating the kinematics of joints. Because of the high dose of radiation, however, it is only occasionally used, such as in evaluating the movement of various joints or to detect transient subluxation (i.e., carpal instability). Occasionally, it is used after fractures in follow-up examinations of the healing process to evaluate the solidity of the bony union. Fluoroscopy is still used in conjunction with myelography, where it is important to observe the movement of the contrast column in the subarachnoid space; in arthrography, to check the proper placement of the needle and to monitor the flow of the contrast agent; and intraoperatively, to assess the reduction of a fracture or placement of hardware.

Digital (Computed) Radiography

Digital (computed) radiography (DR or CR) is the name given to the process of digital image acquisition using an x-ray detector comprising a photostimulable phosphor imaging plate and an image reader–writer that processes the latent image information for subsequent brightness scaling and laser printing on film (see Fig. 2.1). The system works on the principle of photostimulated luminescence. When the screen absorbs x-rays, the x-ray energy is converted to light energy by the process of fluorescence, with the intensity of light being proportional to the energy absorbed by the phosphor. The stimulated light is used to create a digital image (a computed radiograph).

A major advantage of CR over conventional film/screen radiography is that once acquired, the digital image data are readily manipulated to produce alternative renderings. Potential advantages of digitization include contrast and brightness optimization by the manipulation of window width and level settings as well as a variety of image processing capabilities, quantitation of image information, and facilitation of examination storage and retrieval. In addition, energy subtraction imaging (also called *dual-energy subtraction*) may be acquired. Two images, acquired either sequentially or simultaneously with different filtration, are used to reconstruct a soft tissue–only image or a bone-only image.

In digital subtraction radiography, a video processor and a digital disk are added to a fluoroscopy imaging complex to provide online viewing of subtraction images. This technique is most widely used in the evaluation of the vascular system, but it may also be used in conjunction with arthrography to evaluate various joints. The use of high-performance video cameras with low-noise characteristics allows single video frames of precontrast and postcontrast images to be used for subtraction. Spatial resolution can be maximized using a combination of geometric magnification, electric magnification, and a small anode–target distance. The subtraction technique removes surrounding anatomic structures and thus isolates the opacified vessel or joint, making it more conspicuous.

Nonvascular DR may be used to evaluate various bone abnormalities and, in conjunction with contrast injection, a procedure called *digital subtraction arthrography* (Fig. 2.2); to evaluate subtle abnormalities of the joints, such as tears of the triangular fibrocartilage or intercarpal ligaments in the wrist; or to evaluate the stability of prosthesis replacement. DR offers the potential advantages of improved image quality, contrast sensitivity, and exposure latitude, and it provides efficient storage, retrieval, and transmission of radiographic image data. Digital images may be displayed on the film or on a video monitor. A significant advantage of image digitization is the ability to produce data with low noise and a wide dynamic range suitable for window-level analysis in a manner comparable to that used in a CT scanner.

Digital subtraction angiography (DSA), the most frequently used variant of DR, can be used in the evaluation of trauma, bone and soft-tissue tumors, and in general evaluation of the vascular system. In trauma to the extremity, DSA is effectively used to evaluate arterial occlusion, pseudoaneurysms, arteriovenous fistulas, and transection of the arteries (Fig. 2.3). Some advantages of DSA over conventional film techniques are that its images can be studied rapidly and multiple repeated projections can be obtained. Bone subtraction is useful in clearly delineating the vascular structures. In the evaluation of bone and soft-tissue tumors, DSA is an effective tool for mapping tumor vascularity.

Tomography

Tomography is a body-section radiography that permits more accurate visualization of lesions too small to be noted on conventional radiographs or demonstrates anatomic detail obscured by overlying structures. It uses continuous motion of the radiographic tube and film cassette in opposite directions throughout the exposure, with the fulcrum of the motion located in the plane of interest. By blurring structures above and below the area being examined, the object to be studied is sharply outlined on a single plane of focus. The focal plane may vary in thickness according to the distance the x-ray tube travels; the longer the distance (or arc) traveled by the tube, the thinner the section in focus. Tomographic units can localize the image more precisely and have aided greatly in the ability to detect lesions as small as approximately 1 mm (see Figs. 7.47C, 7.53B, and 7.54B). Different tomographic techniques were used in the past including linear and hypocycloidal or trispiral machinery. Today, tomography has been completely replaced by multidetector CT with multiplanar reconstructions.

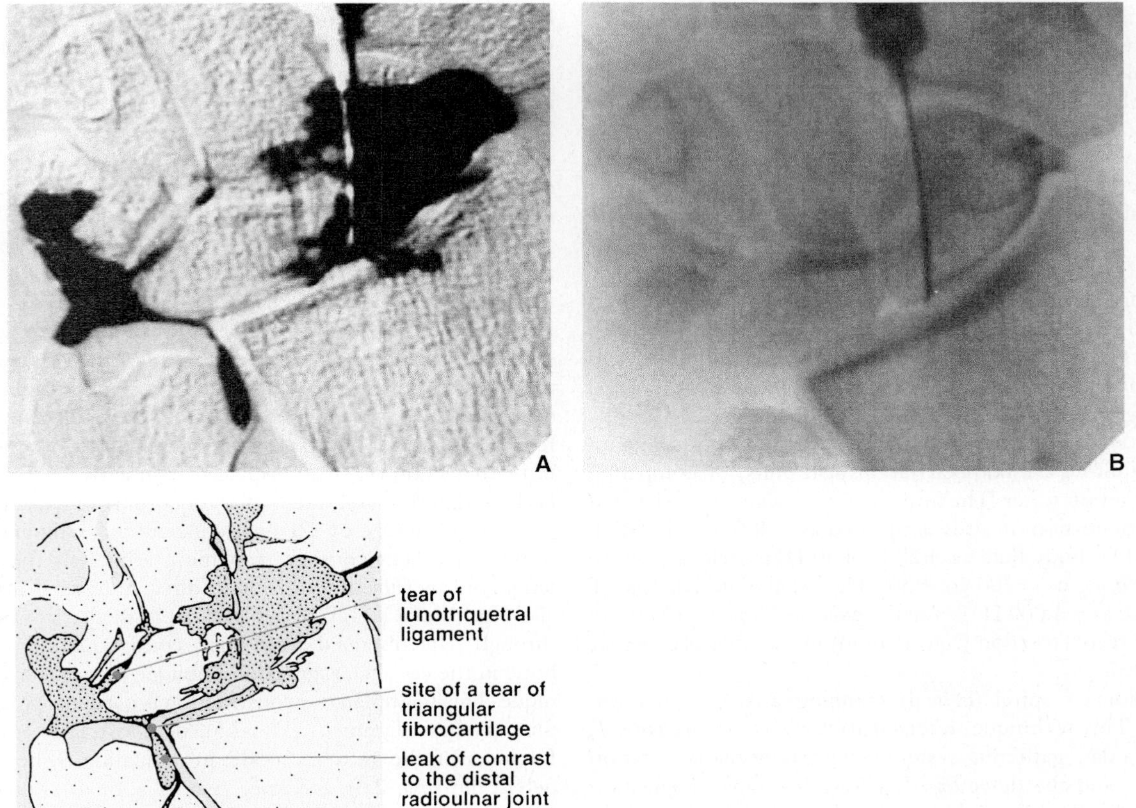

FIGURE 2.2 Digital subtraction arthrography. Digital subtraction arthrogram demonstrates tears of the lunotriquetral ligament and the triangular fibrocartilage complex. **(A)** This image was obtained by subtracting the digitally acquired preinjection image **(B)** from postinjection film. (Courtesy of B. J. Manaster, MD, Salt Lake City, Utah.)

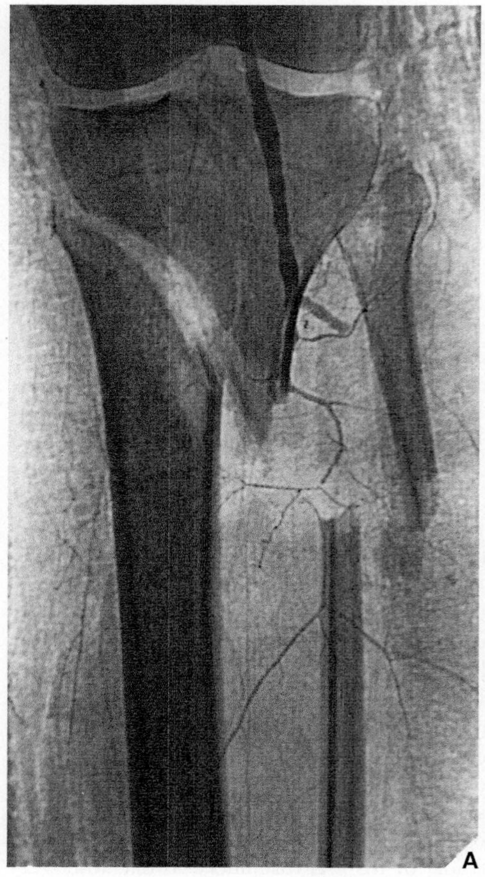

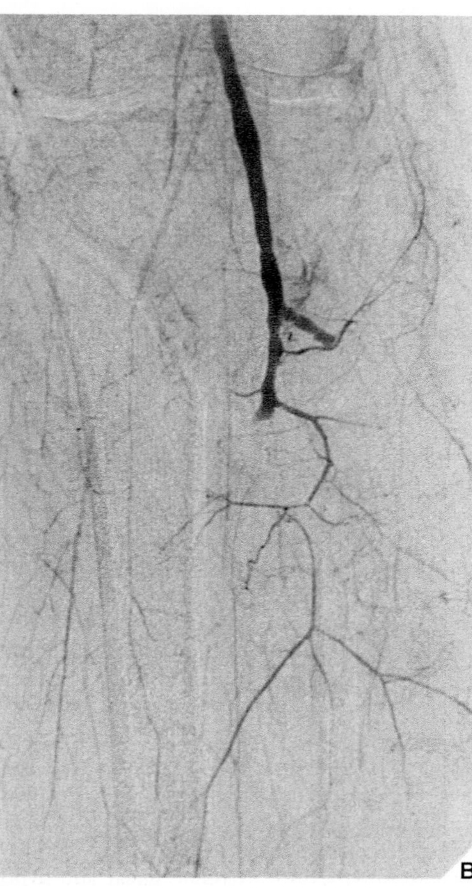

FIGURE 2.3 Digital subtraction angiography. Digital radiograph **(A)** and digital subtraction angiogram **(B)** of a 23-year-old man who sustained fractures of the proximal tibia and fibula show disruption of the distal segment of the popliteal artery.

Computed Tomography

CT is a radiologic modality containing an x-ray source, detectors, and a computer data processing system. The essential components of a CT system include a circular scanning gantry, which houses the x-ray tube and image sensors; a table for the patient; an x-ray generator; and a computerized data processing unit. The patient lies on the table and is placed inside the gantry. The x-ray tube is rotated 360 degrees around the patient while the computer collects the data and formulates an axial image, or "slice." Each cross-sectional slice represents a thickness between 0.1 and 1.5 cm of body tissue.

The newest CT scanners use a rotating fan of x-ray beams, a fixed ring of detectors, and predetector collimator. A highly collimated x-ray beam is transmitted through the area being imaged. The tissues absorb the x-ray beam to various degrees depending on the atomic number and density of the specific tissue. The remaining, unabsorbed (unattenuated) beam passes through the tissues and is detected and processed by the computer. The CT computer software converts the x-ray beam attenuations of the tissue into a CT number (Hounsfield units) by comparing it with the attenuation of water. The attenuation of water is designated as 0 (zero) H, the attenuation of air is designated as −400 to −1,000 H, fat as −60 to −100 H, body fluid as +20 to +30 H, muscle as +40 to +80 H, trabecular bone as +100 to +300 H, and the attenuation of normal cortical bone as +1,000 H. Routinely, axial sections are obtained; however, computer reconstruction (reformation) in multiple planes may be obtained if desired.

The introduction of spiral (helical) scanning was a further improvement of CT. This technique, referred to as *volume-acquisition CT*, has made possible a data gathering system using a continuous rotation of the x-ray source and the detectors. It allows the rapid acquisition of volumes of CT data and renders the ability to reformat the images at any predetermined intervals ranging from 0.5 to 10.0 mm. Unlike standard CT, in which up to a maximum of 12 scans could be obtained per minute, helical CT acquires all data in 24 or 32 seconds, generating up to 92 sections. This technology has markedly reduced scan times and has eliminated interscan delay and hence interscan motion. It also has decreased the motion artifacts, improved the definition of scanned structures, and markedly facilitated the ability to obtain three-dimensional (3D) reconstructions generated from multiple overlapping transaxial images acquired in a single breath hold. Spiral CT allows data to be acquired during the phase of maximum contrast enhancement, thus optimizing the detection of a lesion. The data volume may be viewed either as conventional transaxial images or as multiplanar and 3D reformations.

CT is indispensable in the evaluation of many traumatic conditions and various bone and soft-tissue tumors because of its cross-sectional imaging capability. In trauma, CT is extremely useful to define the presence and extent of a fracture or dislocation; to evaluate various intraarticular abnormalities, such as damage to the articular cartilage or the presence of noncalcified and calcified osteocartilaginous bodies; and to evaluate adjacent soft tissues. CT is of particular importance in the detection of small bony fragments displaced into the joints after trauma, in the detection of small displaced fragments of the fractured vertebral body, and in the assessment of a concomitant injury to the cord or thecal sac. The advantage of CT over conventional radiography is its ability to provide excellent contrast resolution, accurately measure the tissue attenuation coefficient, and obtain direct transaxial images (Fig. 2.4; see also Figs. 11.25C, 11.37B, and 11.66B). A further advantage is its ability—through data obtained from thin, contiguous sections—to image the bone in the coronal, sagittal, and oblique planes using reformation technique. This multiplanar reconstruction is particularly helpful in evaluating the vertebral alignment (Fig. 2.5), demonstrating horizontally oriented fractures of the vertebral body; in evaluating complex fractures of the pelvis, hip (Fig. 2.6), and knee (Fig. 2.7); or in evaluating calcaneus abnormalities, of the sacrum and sacroiliac joints, sternum and sternoclavicular joints, temporomandibular joints, and wrist. Modern CT scanners use collimated fan beams directed only at the tissue layer undergoing investigation. The newest advances in sophisticated software enable 3D

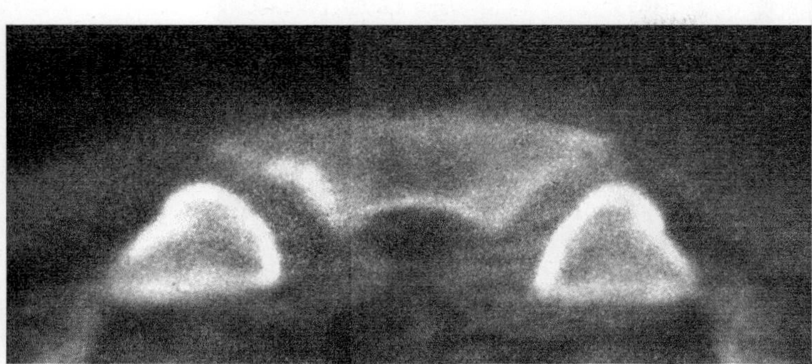

FIGURE 2.4 CT transaxial imaging. In this direct transaxial image, the sternoclavicular joints are well depicted.

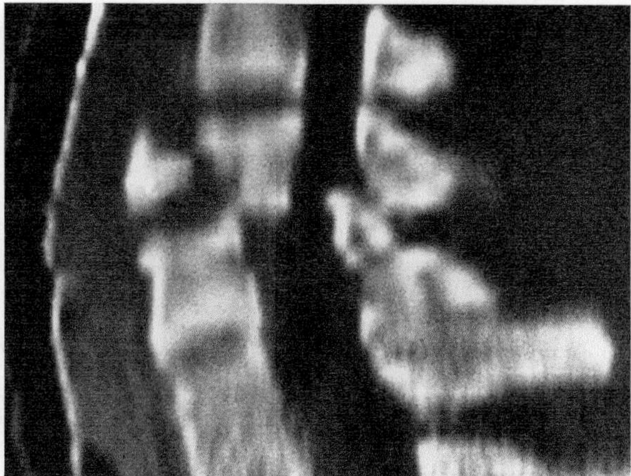

FIGURE 2.5 CT reformatted imaging. Sagittal CT reformatted image demonstrates the flexion teardrop fracture of C5. It also effectively shows the malalignment of the vertebral bodies and narrowing of the spinal canal.

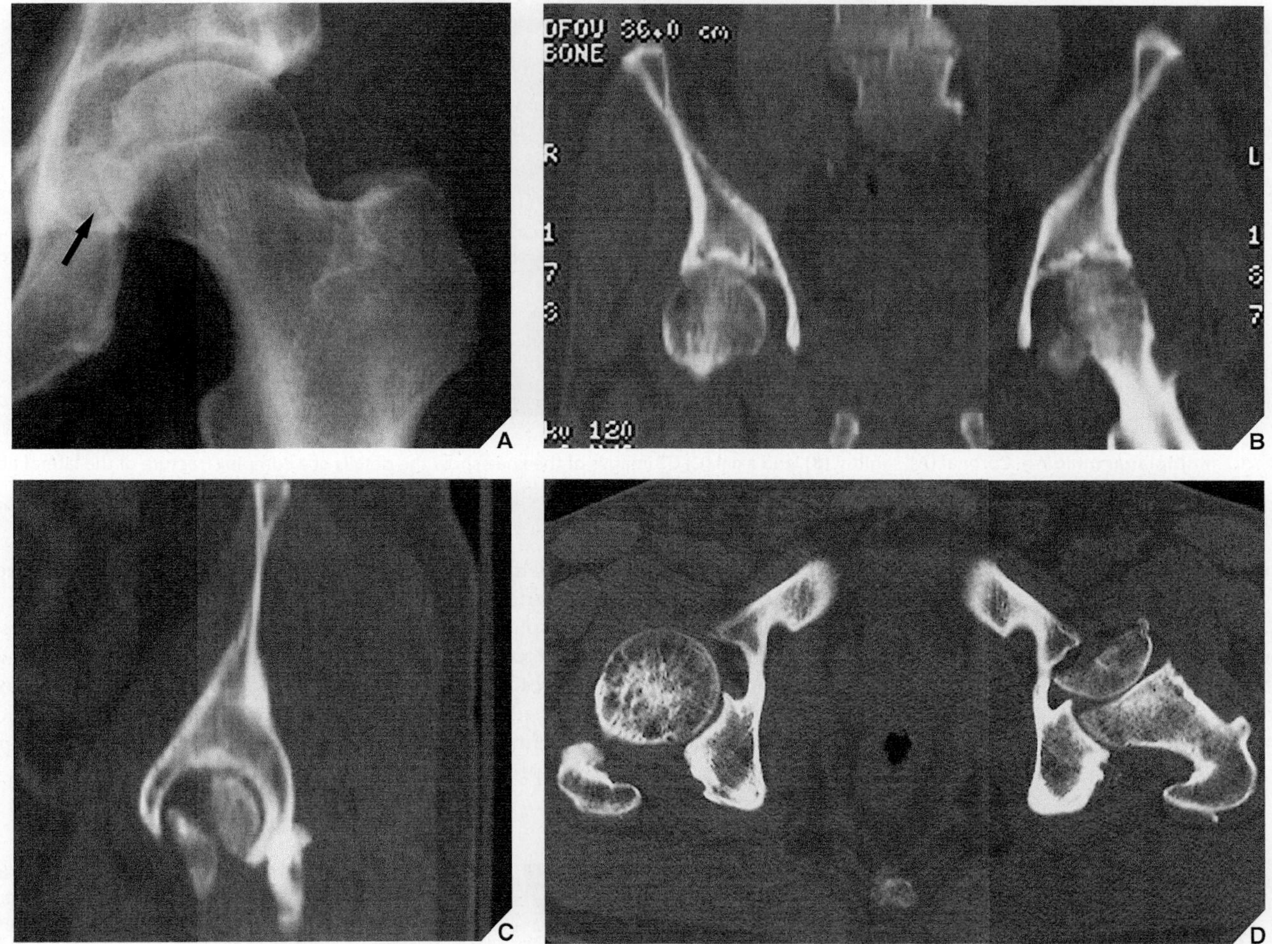

FIGURE 2.6 CT multiplanar imaging. A 62-year-old man sustained a posterior dislocation of the left femoral head. After reduction of dislocation, the anteroposterior radiograph of the left hip **(A)** showed increased medial joint space and distortion of the medial aspect of the femoral head *(arrow)*. To evaluate the hip joint further, CT was performed. Coronal **(B)** and sagittal **(C)** reformatted images showed unsuspected fracture of the femoral head, and axial image **(D)** demonstrated a 180-degree rotation of the fractured fragment.

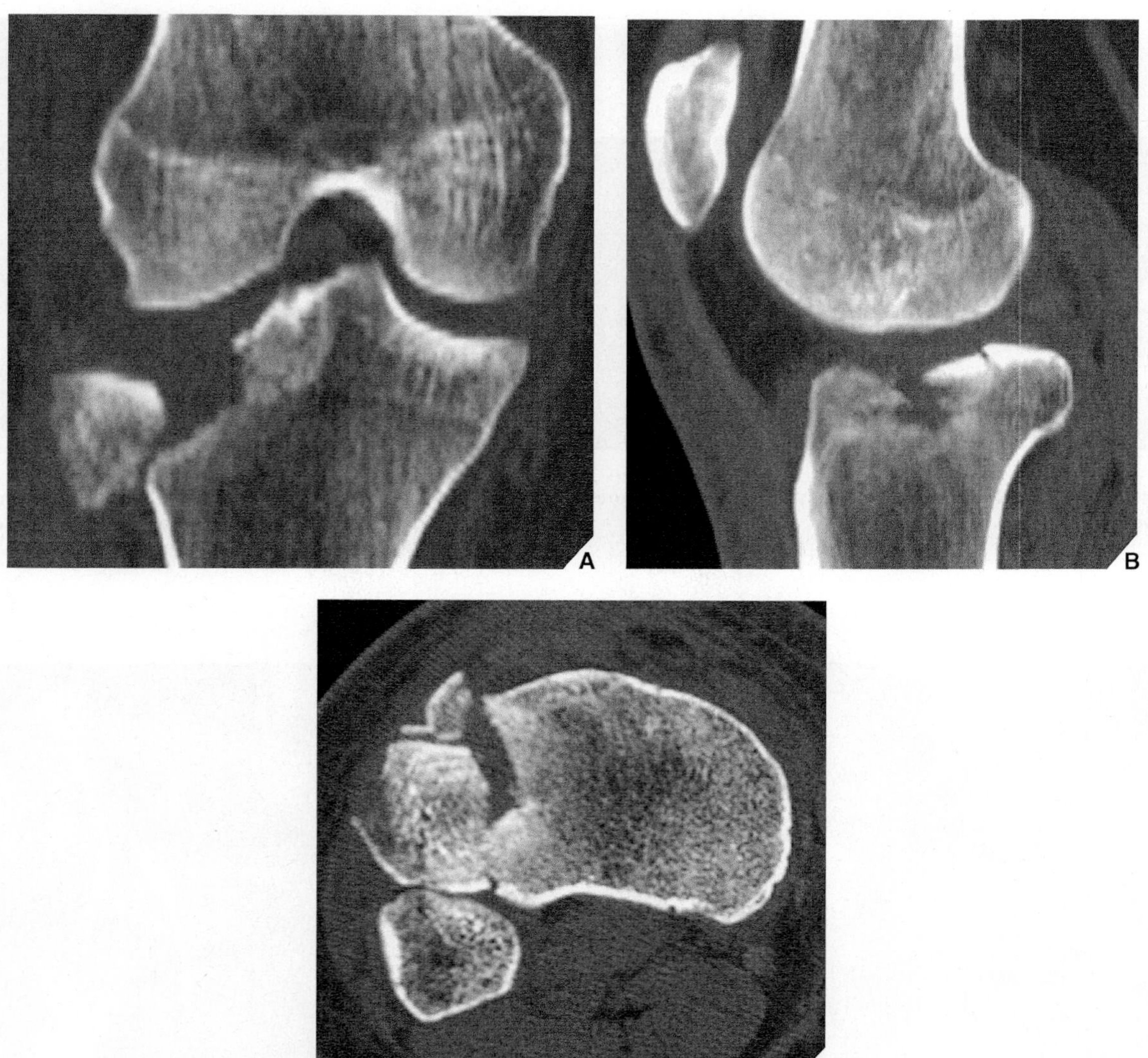

FIGURE 2.7 CT multiplanar imaging. Coronal **(A)**, sagittal **(B)**, and axial **(C)** CT images of the knee show the details of a complex fracture of the lateral tibial plateau.

reconstruction, which is helpful in analyzing regions with complex anatomy such as the face, pelvis, vertebral column, foot, ankle, elbow, and wrist (Figs. 2.8 to 2.11). New computer systems now permit the creation of plastic models of the area of interest based on 3D images. These models facilitate operative planning and allow rehearsal surgery of complex reconstructive procedures.

Most recently, with the advent of multichannel multidetector row CT (MDCT), images can be generated with subsecond gantry rotation times yielding high-resolution volume data sets and at the same time minimizing the radiation dose to the patient. Even more advanced is high-resolution flat-panel volume CT (fpVCT), which uses digital flat-panel detectors and provides volumetric coverage as well as ultra-high spatial resolution in two-dimensional (2D) and 3D projections. Furthermore, it reduces metal and beam-hardening artifacts. In addition to the aforementioned features, fpVCT also allows dynamic imaging of time-varying processes.

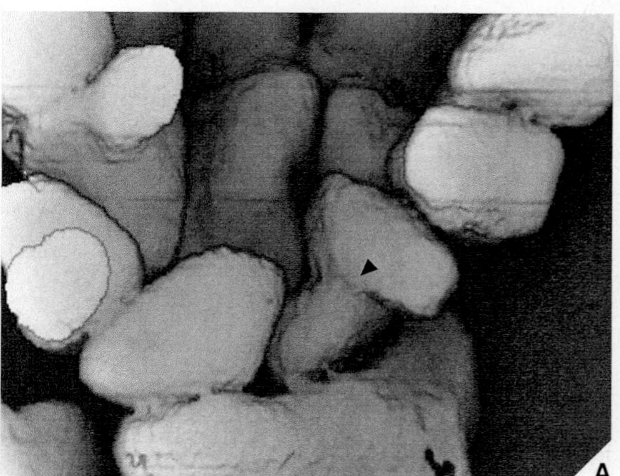

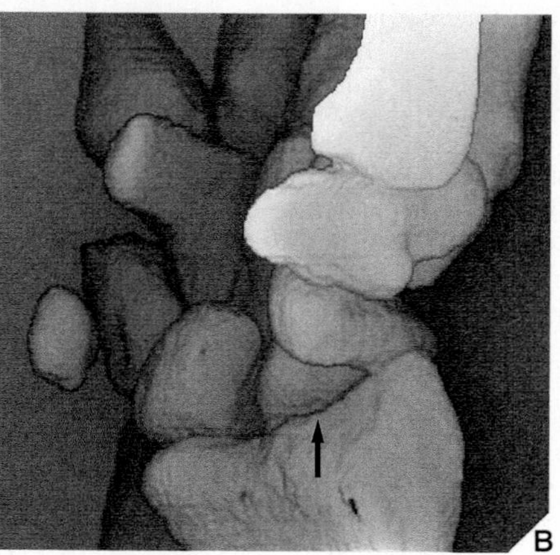

FIGURE 2.8 CT 3D imaging. Anteroposterior **(A)** and oblique **(B)** 3D CT reconstructed images of the wrist demonstrates a fracture through the waist of the scaphoid bone *(arrowhead)*, complicated by osteonecrosis of the proximal fragment *(arrow)*.

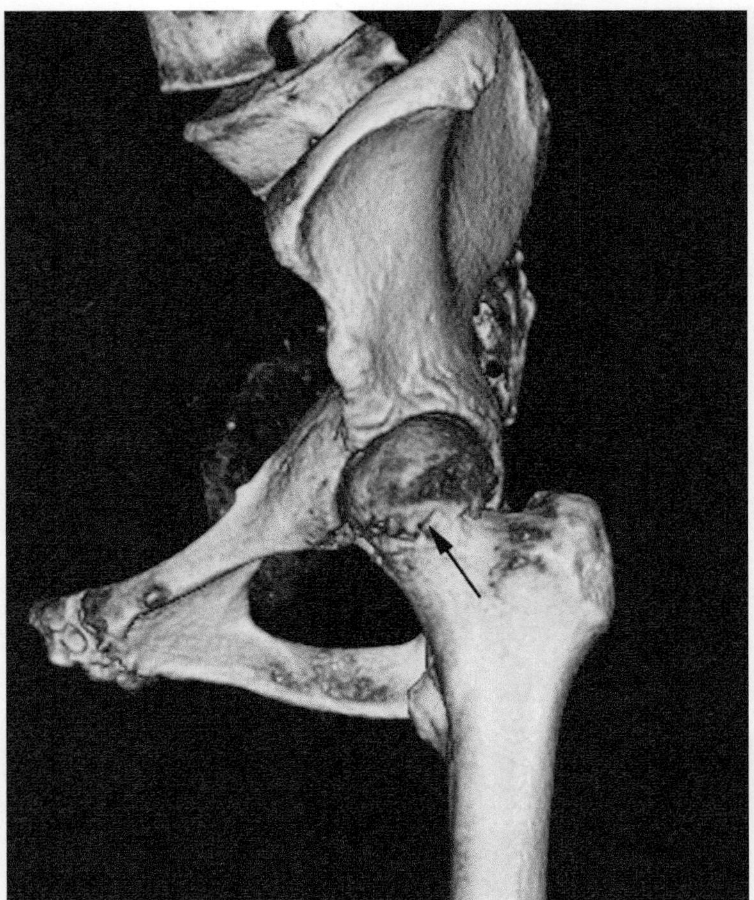

FIGURE 2.9 CT 3D imaging. 3D CT reconstructed image with surface-rendering algorithm demonstrates a subcapital femoral neck fracture with angulation *(arrow)*.

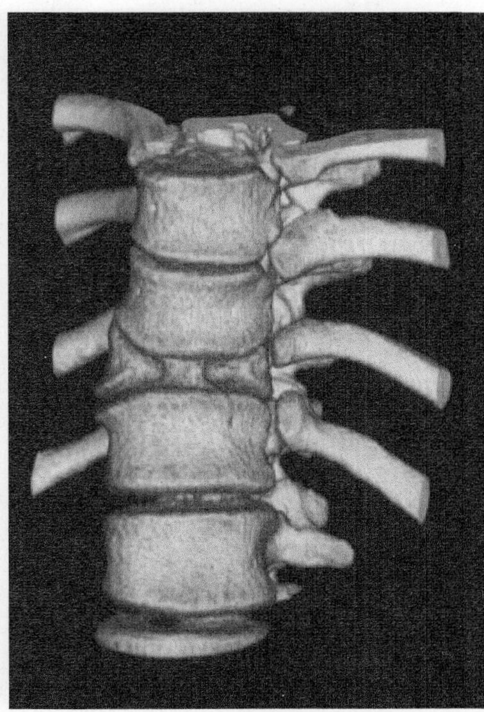

FIGURE 2.11 CT 3D imaging. 3D CT reconstruction of the thoracic spine shows sagittal cleft with an anterior defect of T11, a typical appearance of congenital butterfly vertebra.

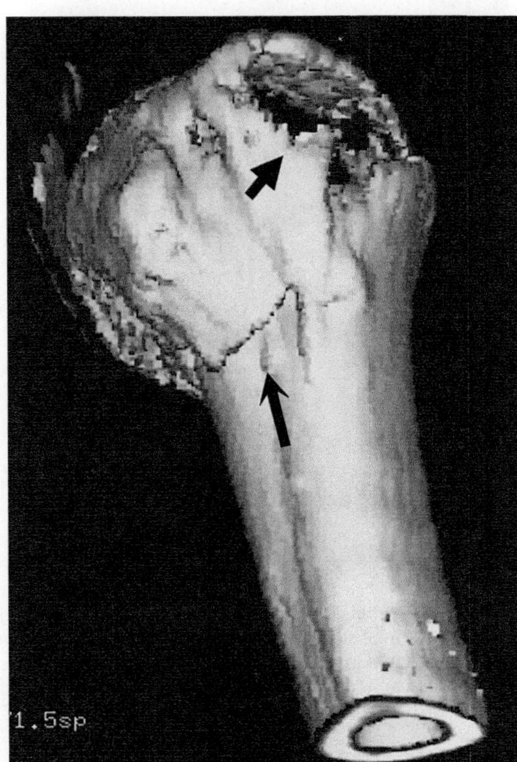

FIGURE 2.10 CT 3D imaging. A fracture of the surgical neck of the humerus *(long arrow)* and a displaced fracture of the greater tubercle *(short arrow)* are well demonstrated.

In the evaluation of traumatic abnormalities, 3D CT-angiography is effectively used to determine the presence or absence of injury to the vessels near the fractured bones (Figs. 2.12 and 2.13).

CT plays a significant role in the evaluation of bone and soft-tissue tumors because of its superior contrast resolution and its ability to measure the tissue attenuation coefficient accurately. Although CT, by itself, is rarely helpful in making a specific diagnosis, it can precisely evaluate the extent of the bone lesion and may demonstrate a break through the cortex and the involvement of surrounding soft tissues. Moreover, CT is very helpful in delineating a tumor in bones having complex anatomic structures, such as the scapula, pelvis, and sacrum, which may be difficult to image fully with conventional radiographic techniques. CT examination is crucial to determine the extent and spread of a tumor in the bone if limb salvage is contemplated so that a safe margin of resection can be planned (Fig. 2.14). It can effectively demonstrate the intraosseous extension of a tumor and its extraosseous involvement of soft tissues such as muscles and neurovascular bundles. It is also useful for monitoring the results of treatment, evaluating for the recurrence of a resected tumor, and demonstrating the effect of nonsurgical treatment such as radiation therapy and chemotherapy.

Occasionally, iodinated contrast agents may be used intravenously to enhance the CT images. A contrast agent directly alters image contrast by increasing the x-ray attenuation, thus displaying increased brightness in the CT images. It can aid in identifying a suspected soft-tissue mass when initial CT results are unremarkable, or it can assess the vascularity of the soft-tissue or bone tumor.

Recently, a lot of attention was directed toward clinical use of dual-energy CT (DECT) for evaluation of tophaceous gout. The DECT system is equipped with two x-ray tubes with different peak kilovoltages (80 and 140 kVp), thus allowing simultaneous acquisition of two sets of images of the desired anatomic region. The material-specific differences in attenuation of various elements enable classification of the chemical composition of scanned tissue, allowing accurate and specific characterization and separation of monosodium urate from calcium-containing mineralizations. DECT data yields color-coded cross-sectional images, clearly depicting the foci of accumulation of urate crystals (Fig. 2.15; see also Figs. 12.10, 12.11, 15.37, 15.38, and 15.39D–G).

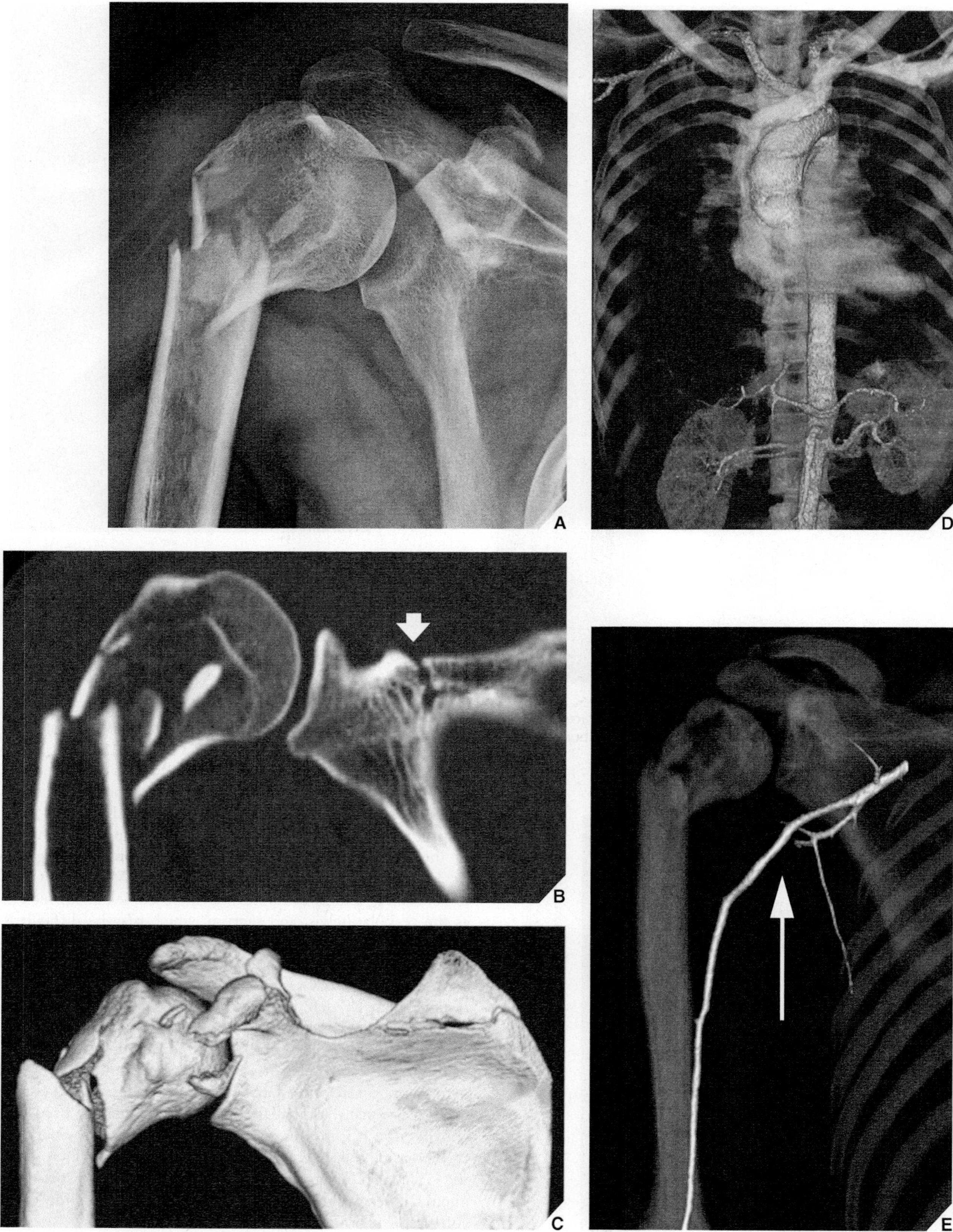

FIGURE 2.12 3D CT-angiography. A 52-year-old man was hit by a car and sustained a chest and right shoulder injury. **(A)** Conventional radiograph of the right shoulder demonstrates a fracture of the proximal humerus. **(B)** Coronal reformatted CT image shows more details of the comminuted displaced fracture of the humerus and, in addition, shows a fracture of the scapular crest *(arrow)*. **(C)** Both these fractures are effectively shown on 3D CT reconstruction image. Because an injury to the vascular structures of the chest and right shoulder was clinically suspected, 3D CT-angiography was performed. **(D)** The great vessels of the chest were intact. **(E)** Anterior view of the right shoulder and arm shows the displacement of intact axillary and proximal brachial arteries *(arrow)* due to a large soft-tissue hematoma.

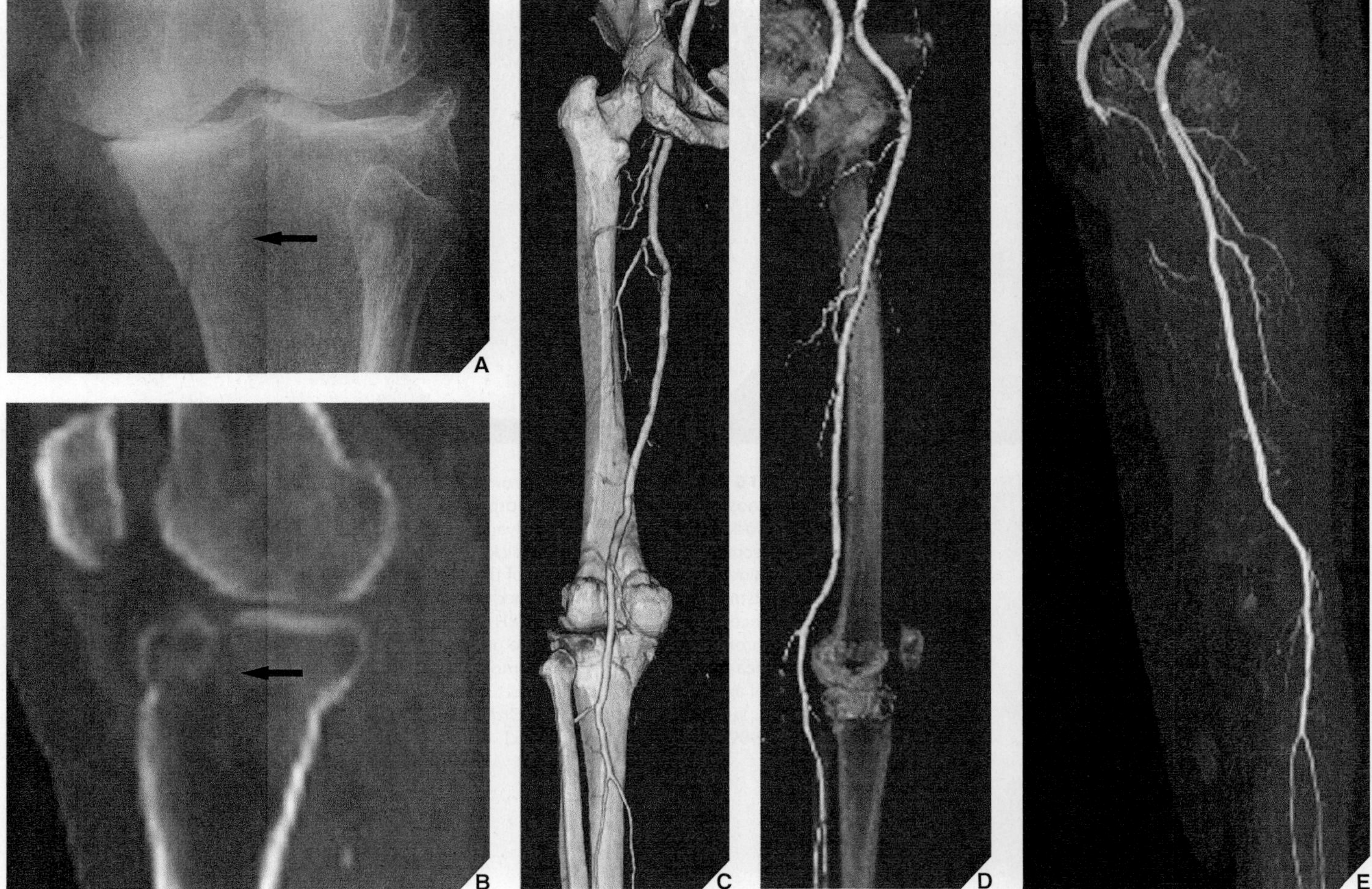

FIGURE 2.13 3D CT-angiography. A 68-year-old man was injured in a car accident. Anteroposterior radiograph **(A)** of the left knee and sagittal reformatted CT image **(B)** show a fracture of the medial tibial plateau *(arrows)*. Note also advanced osteoarthritis of the knee joint. Because an injury to the popliteal vessels was clinically suspected, 3D CT-angiography was performed. Posterior **(C)** and lateral **(D)** views show intact femoral and popliteal arteries, confirmed on the frontal subtracted vascular image **(E)**.

Quantitative CT (QCT) is a method for measuring the lumbar spine mineral content in which the average density values of a region of interest are referenced to that of calibration material scanned at the same time as the patient. Measurements are performed on a CT scanner using a mineral standard for simultaneous calibration and a computed radiograph (scout view) for localization. The evaluation of bone mass measurement provides valuable insight into improving the evaluation and treatment of osteoporosis and other metabolic bone disorders. QCT has been replaced by Dual-Energy X-ray Absorptiometry (DEXA) scanning for the evaluation of bone mineral content, with decreased radiation exposure (see Fig. 26.14).

CT is also a very important modality for successful aspiration or biopsy of bone or soft-tissue lesions because it provides visible guidance for precise placement of the instrument within the lesion (Fig. 2.16).

Some disadvantages of CT include the so-called *average volume effect*, which results from a lack of homogeneity in the composition of the small volume of tissue. In particular, the measurement of Hounsfield units results in average values for the different components of the tissue. This partial volume effect becomes particularly important when normal and pathologic processes interface within a section under investigation. The other disadvantage of CT is poor tissue characterization. Despite the ability of CT to discriminate among some differences in density, a simple analysis of attenuation values does not permit precise histologic characterization. Moreover, any movement of the patient will produce artifacts that degrade the image quality. Similarly, an area that contains metal (e.g., prosthesis or various rods and screws) will produce significant artifacts, although recently, several different acquisition and reconstruction parameters have been developed to significantly reduce artifacts related to the metallic implants. Finally, the radiation dose may occasionally be high, particularly when contiguous and overlapping CT sections are obtained during examination.

Arthrography

Arthrography is the introduction of a contrast agent ("positive" contrast, iodide solution; "negative" contrast, air; or a combination of both) into the joint space. Despite the evolution of newer diagnostic imaging modalities, such as CT and MRI, arthrography has retained its importance in daily radiologic practice. The growing popularity of arthrography has been partially caused by advances in its techniques and interpretation. The fact that it is not a technically difficult procedure and is much simpler to interpret than US, CT, or MRI makes it very desirable for evaluating various articulations. Although virtually, every joint can be injected with contrast, the examination, at the present time, is most frequently performed in the shoulder, wrist, knee, and ankle. It is important to obtain preliminary films prior to any arthrographic procedure because contrast may obscure some joint abnormalities (i.e., osteochondral body) that can be easily detected on conventional radiographs. Arthrography is particularly effective in demonstrating rotator cuff tear (Fig. 2.17; see also Figs. 5.68 and 5.69) and adhesive capsulitis in the shoulder (see Fig. 5.91) and osteochondritis dissecans, osteochondral bodies, and subtle abnormalities of the articular cartilage in the elbow joint. In the wrist, arthrography retains its value

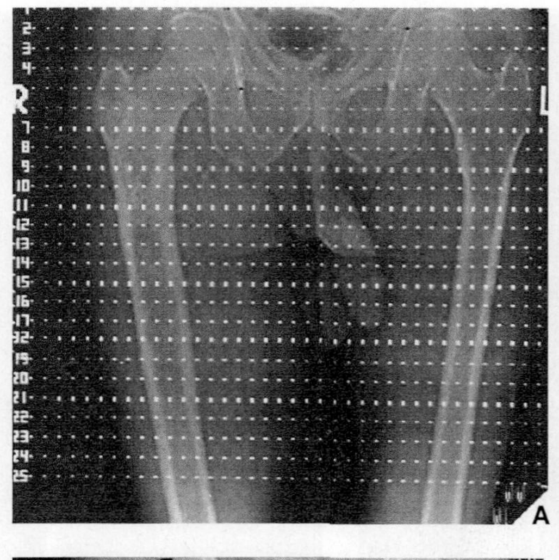

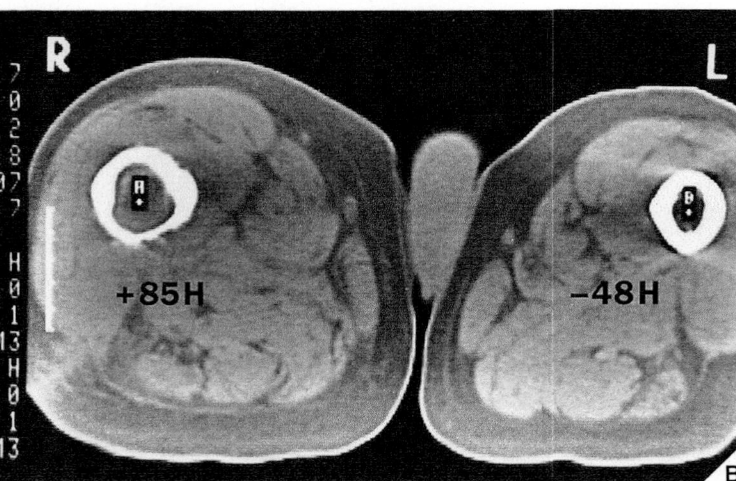

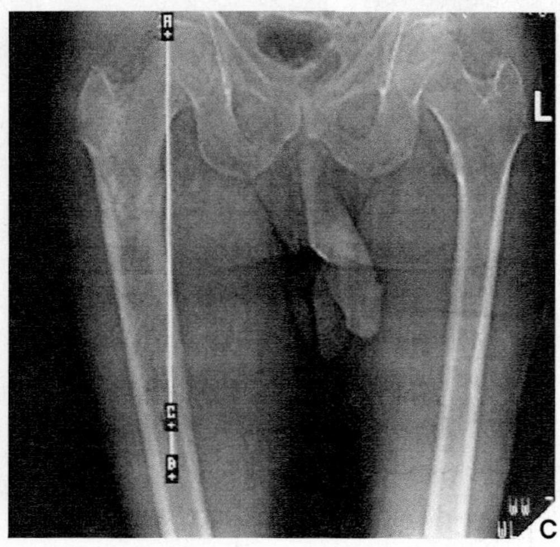

FIGURE 2.14 **CT measurement of Hounsfield values.** CT evaluation of intraosseous extension of chondrosarcoma is an important part of the radiologic workup of a patient if limb salvage is contemplated. **(A)** Several contiguous axial sections, preferably 1 cm in thickness, of affected and nonaffected limbs are obtained. **(B)** Hounsfield values of the bone marrow are measured to determine the distal extent of tumor in the medullary cavity. A value of +85H indicates the presence of tumor; a value of −48H is normal for fatty marrow. **(C)** The linear measurement is obtained from the proximal articular end of the bone *A* to the point located 5 cm distally to the tumor margin *B*. Point *C* corresponds to the most distal axial section that still shows tumor in the marrow. (Reprinted from Greenspan A. Tumors of cartilage origin. *Orthop Clin North Am* 1989;20:347–366. Copyright © 1989 Elsevier. With permission.)

in diagnosing triangular fibrocartilage complex abnormalities (Fig. 2.18; see also Fig. 7.32). The introduction of the three-compartment injection technique and the combination of arthrographic wrist examination with digital subtraction arthrography (see Fig. 2.2) and postarthrographic CT and MRI examinations have made this modality very effective when evaluating a painful wrist.

Although arthrography of the knee has been almost completely replaced by MRI, it still may be used to demonstrate injuries to the soft-tissue structures such as the joint capsule, menisci, and various ligaments (see Fig. 9.69B). It also provides important information on the status of the articular cartilage, particularly when a subtle chondral or osteochondral fracture is suspected or when the presence or absence of osteochondral bodies (i.e., in osteochondritis dissecans) must be confirmed (see Fig. 9.60C).

In the examination of any of the joints, arthrography can be combined with the digitization of image (digital subtraction arthrography) (see Fig. 2.2), with CT (CT-arthrography) (Fig. 2.19), or with MRI (MRa) (Fig. 2.20), thus providing additional information. Recently, the innovative technique of combined cone-beam CT (CBCT) with arthrography was introduced to study the ligament and cartilage injuries. Although the investigations are still in experimental phase, the early results using this modality are very promising.

There are relatively few absolute contraindications to arthrography. Even hypersensitivity to iodine is a relative contraindication because, in this case, a single-contrast study using only air can be performed.

Angiography

The use of a contrast material injected directly into selective branches of the arterial and venous circulation has aided greatly in assessing the involvement of the circulatory system in various conditions and has provided a precise method for defining local pathology. With *arteriography*, a contrast agent is injected into the arteries and films are made, usually in rapid sequence. With *venography*, a contrast material is injected into the veins. Both procedures are frequently used in the evaluation of trauma, particularly if a concomitant injury to the vascular system is suspected (see Figs. 2.3 and 4.15).

In the evaluation of tumors, arteriography is used mainly to map out bone lesions, demonstrate the vascularity of the lesion, and assess the extent of disease. It is also used to demonstrate the vascular supply of a tumor and to locate vessels suitable for preoperative intraarterial chemotherapy. It is very useful in demonstrating the area suitable for open biopsy because the most vascular parts of a tumor contain the most aggressive component of the lesion. Occasionally, arteriography can be used to demonstrate abnormal tumor vessels, corroborating findings with radiography and tomography (see Fig. 16.16B). Arteriography is often extremely helpful in planning for limb-salvage procedures because it demonstrates the regional vascular anatomy and thus permits a plan to be made for the tumor resection. It is also sometimes used to outline the major vessels before the resection of a benign lesion (see Fig. 16.17). It can also be combined with an interventional procedure, such as the embolization of hypervascular tumors, before further treatment (see Fig. 16.18).

Myelography

During this procedure, water-soluble contrast agents are injected into the subarachnoid space, mixing freely with the cerebrospinal fluid to produce a column of opacified fluid with a higher specific gravity than the nonopacified fluid. Tilting the patient will allow the opacified fluid to run up or down the thecal sac under the influence of gravity (see Figs. 11.17 and 11.56). The puncture usually is performed in the lumbar area at the L2-3 or L3-4 levels. For the examination of the cervical segment,

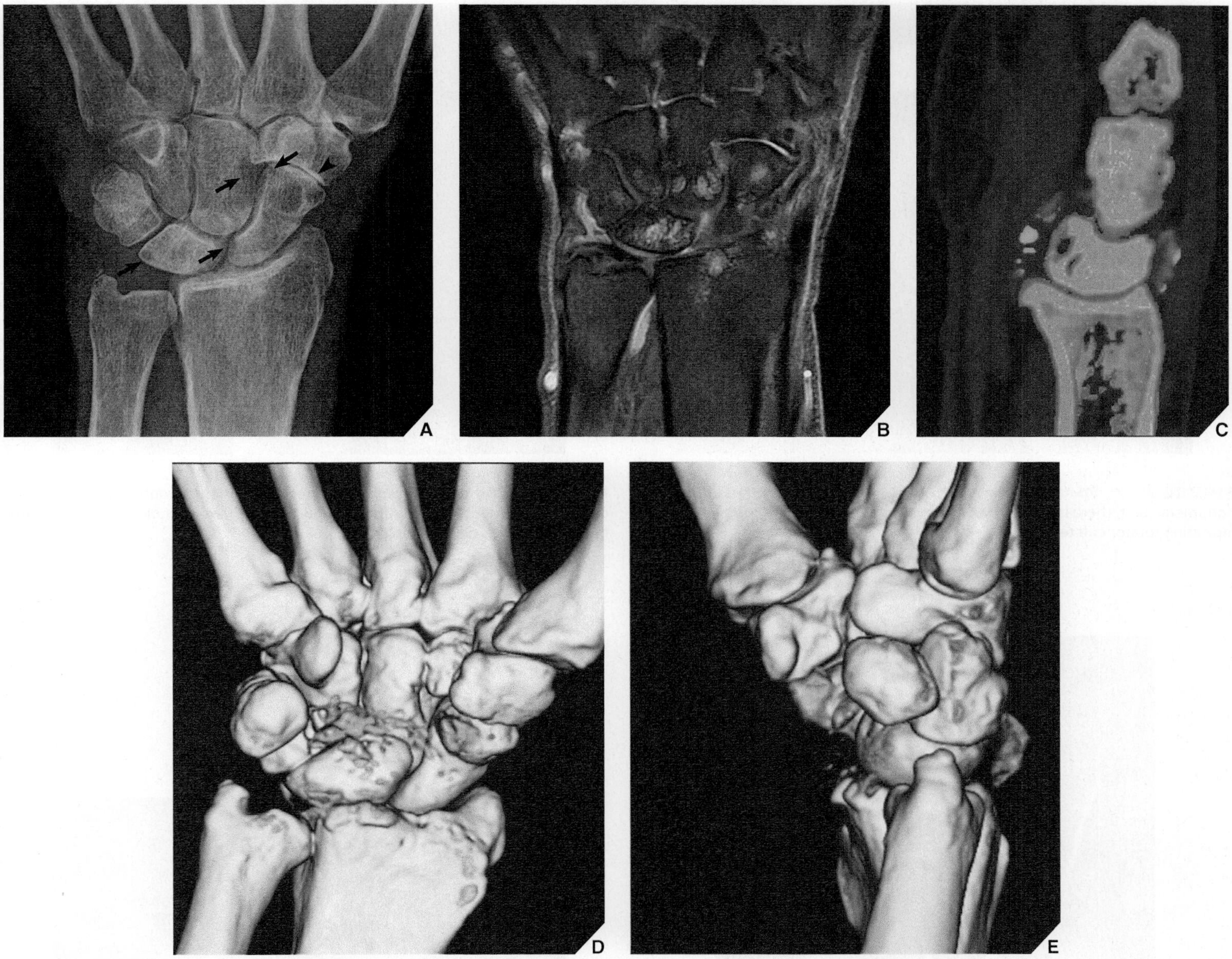

FIGURE 2.15 DECT of the tophaceous gout. **(A)** Dorsovolar radiograph of the wrist of the 72-year-old man shows erosions of the capitate, scaphoid, and lunate *(arrows)*. Osteoarthritis is noted of the scaphoid-trapezium-trapezoid joint *(arrowhead)*. **(B)** Coronal MR image, in addition to erosions of several carpal bones, demonstrates synovitis of the radiocarpal and midcarpal articulations. **(C)** Sagittal DECT color-coded image shows the presence of urate crystals *(green)*, confirming the diagnosis of tophaceous gout. **(D,E)** 3D reconstructed CT images show the exact anatomic relationship between the monosodium urate–containing tophi *(green)* and osseous structures.

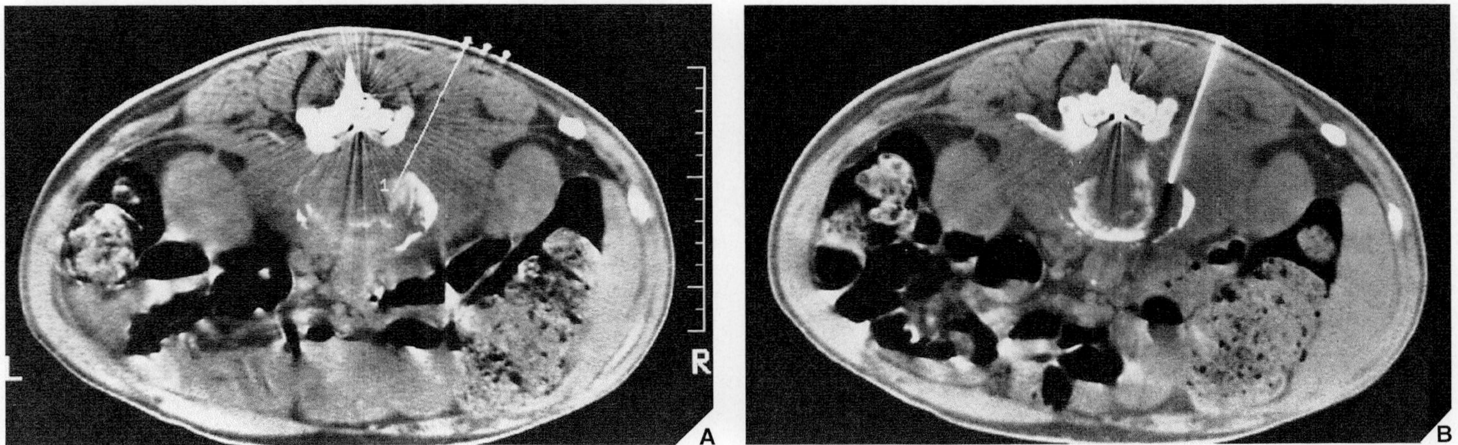

FIGURE 2.16 CT-guided aspiration biopsy. Aspiration biopsy of an infected intervertebral disk is performed under CT guidance. **(A)** Measurement is obtained from the skin surface to the area of interest (intervertebral disk). **(B)** The needle is advanced under CT guidance and placed at the site of the partially destroyed disk.

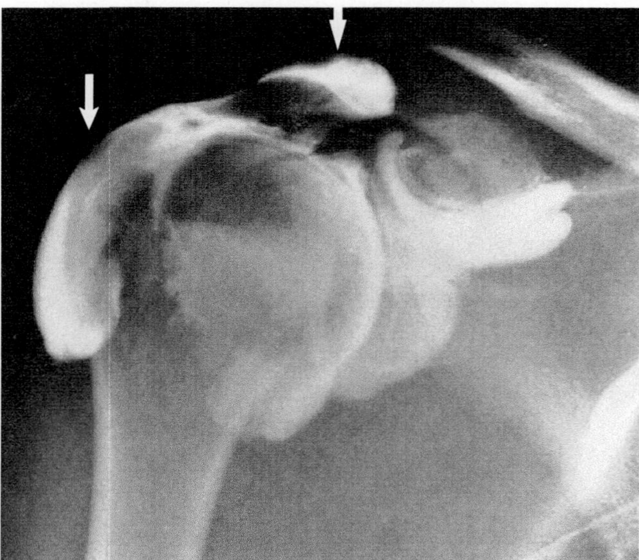

FIGURE 2.17 Shoulder arthrogram. After an injection of contrast into the glenohumeral joint, there is filling of subacromial–subdeltoid bursae complex *(arrows)*, indicating rotator cuff tear.

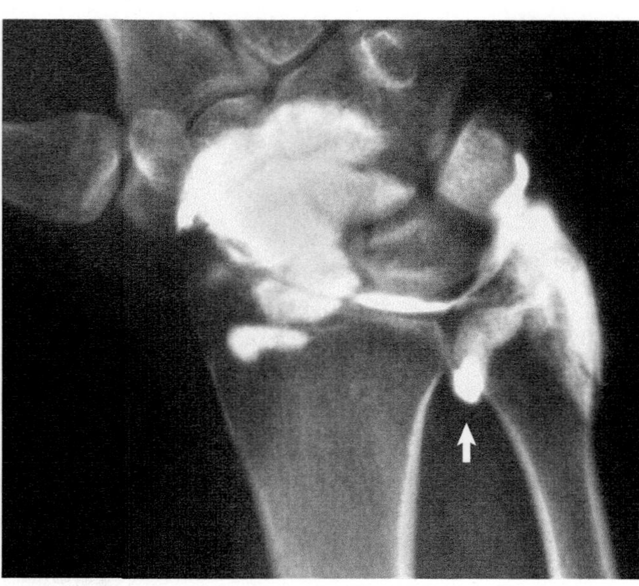

FIGURE 2.18 Wrist arthrogram. After an injection of contrast into the radiocarpal joint, there is filling of distal radioulnar joint *(arrow)*, indicating a tear of the triangular fibrocartilage complex.

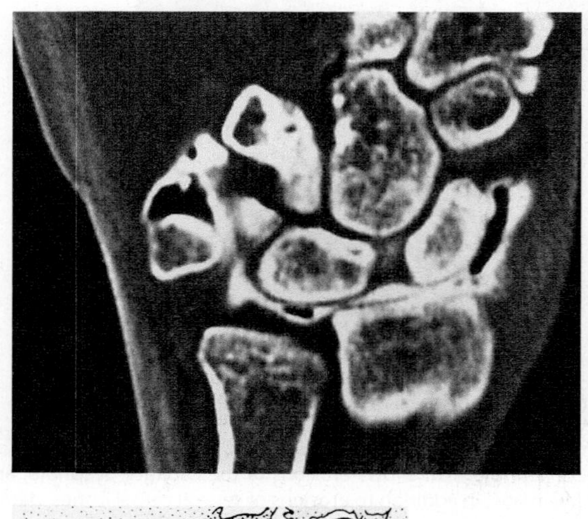

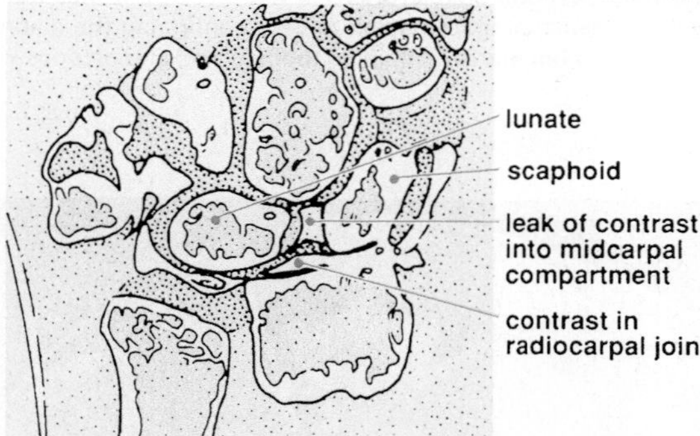

FIGURE 2.19 CT-arthrography. Coronal CT arthrogram of the wrist demonstrates a subtle leak of contrast from the radiocarpal joint through a tear in the scapholunate ligament, a finding not detected on routine arthrographic examination of the wrist.

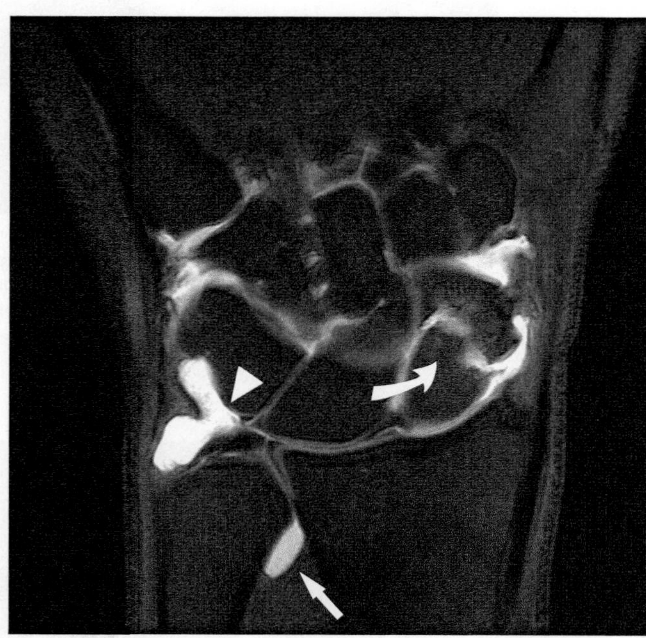

FIGURE 2.20 MR-arthrography. Coronal T1-weighted fat-saturated MR image obtained after an injection of contrast into the radiocarpal joint shows opacification of the distal radioulnar joint *(arrow)*, diagnostic of a tear of the triangular fibrocartilage complex. In addition, noted is a tear of the lunotriquetral ligament *(arrowhead)* and leak of contrast into the ununited fracture of the scaphoid *(curved arrow)*.

a C1-2 puncture is performed (see Fig. 11.17A). Myelographic examination has been almost completely replaced by high-resolution CT and high-quality MRI.

Diskography

Diskography is an injection of a contrast material into the nucleus pulposus. Although this is a controversial procedure that has been abandoned by many investigators, under tightly restricted indications and immaculate technique, a diskogram can yield valuable information. Diskography is a valuable aid to determine the source of a patient's low back pain. It is not purely an imaging technique because the symptoms produced during the test (pain during the injection or pain provocation) are considered to have even greater diagnostic value than the obtained radiographs. It should always be combined with CT examination (so-called *CT-diskogram*) (see Figs. 11.57, 11.102B,C, 11.103, and 11.104). According to the official position statement on diskography by the Executive Committee of the North American Spine Society in 1988, this procedure "is indicated in the evaluation of patients with unremitting spinal pain, with or without extremity pain, of greater than four months' duration, when the pain has been unresponsive to all appropriate methods of conservative therapy." According to the same statement, before a diskogram is performed, the patient should have undergone an investigation with other modalities (such as CT, MRI, and myelography) and the surgical correction of the patient's problem should be anticipated.

Ultrasound

Over the past two decades, US has made an enormous impact in the field of radiology and particularly in skeletal imaging. It has several inherent advantages. It is relatively inexpensive, allows comparisons with the opposite normal side, uses no ionizing radiation, and can be performed at bedside or in the operating room. It is a noninvasive modality, relying on the interaction of propagated sound waves with tissue interfaces in the body. Whenever the directed pulsing of sound waves encounters an interface between tissues of different acoustic impedance, reflection or refraction occurs. The sound waves reflected back to the US transducer are recorded and converted into images.

Various types of US scanning are available. Most modern US equipment displays dynamic information in "real time," similar to information that is provided by fluoroscopy. With real-time sonography, the images may be obtained in any scan plane by simply moving the transducer. Thus, imaging may include transverse or longitudinal images and any obliquity can also be produced. Modern probe technology has extended usefulness of US in orthopaedic radiology (Fig. 2.21). Higher frequency transducers of 7.5 and 10 MHz have excellent spatial resolution and are ideal for imaging the appendicular skeleton.

Applications of US in orthopaedics include an evaluation of the rotator cuff (see Fig. 5.71), injuries to various tendons (e.g., the Achilles tendon), Osgood-Schlatter disease (see Fig. 9.50), and, occasionally, soft-tissue tumors (such as hemangioma and other vascular lesions).

The most effective application, however, is in the evaluation of the infant hip, for which US has become the imaging modality of choice. Contributing factors are the cartilaginous composition of the hip, US's real-time capability for studying motion and stress, absence of ionizing radiation, and relative cost-effectiveness. The newest development in this area is the introduction of 3D US for the evaluation of developmental dysplasia of the hip. 3D sonography provides functional utility in the evaluation of the joint in the added sagittal plane (section image) and craniocaudal projection (revolving spatial image). This technique permits excellent demonstration of the femoral head–acetabulum relationship and femoral head containment (see Figs. 32.19 and 32.20). The important advantage of this technique is not only the acquisition of images in real time but also subsequent reconstruction and viewing at a workstation, allowing further manipulation of the volume image. This permits the extraction of usable measurements and enhancement of the anatomic information obtained from the images.

US has recently been applied to certain areas in rheumatic disorders, particularly to detect intraarticular and periarticular fluid collection, and to the differentiation of popliteal fossa masses (e.g., aneurysm vs. Baker cyst vs. hypertrophied synovium) (Fig. 2.22). US-guided intervention procedures have gained popularity for the treatment of various musculoskeletal conditions including calcific tendinopathy, synovitis, evacuation of fluid collections, and for needle guidance during biopsy of osseous and soft-tissue lesions.

More recent US techniques such as Doppler US or color-flow imaging, which expresses motion from moving red blood cells in color, have found limited applications in orthopaedic radiology. This modality is used mainly to detect arterial narrowing and venous thrombosis (Figs. 2.23 and 2.24). However, there have been a limited number of reports regarding the use of this technology in detecting complications of benign soft-tissue masses, such as a Baker cyst (Fig. 2.25), or in detecting tumor vascularity within malignant soft-tissue tumors.

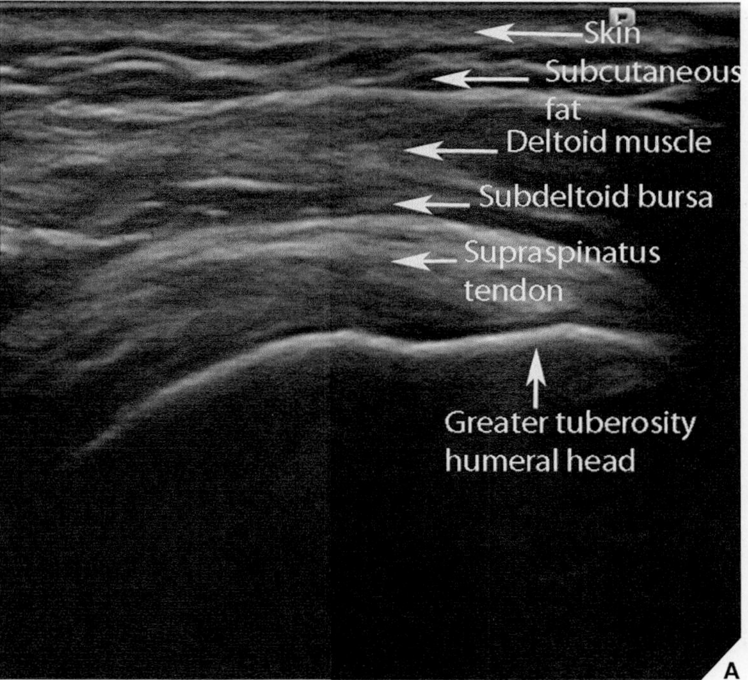

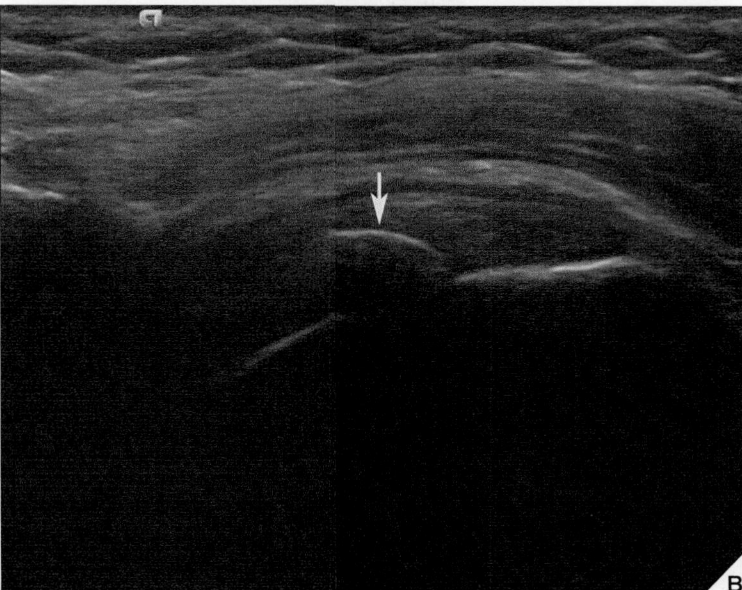

FIGURE 2.21 **US of the shoulder. (A)** Long axis view of the supraspinatus tendon and its attachment in the greater tuberosity of the humerus. **(B)** Long axis view of supraspinatus tendon shows curvilinear echogenic focus with acoustic shadowing secondary to intrasubstance calcification consistent with calcific tendinitis *(arrow)*. (Courtesy of Luis Beltran, MD, Boston and Ron Adler, MD, New York.)

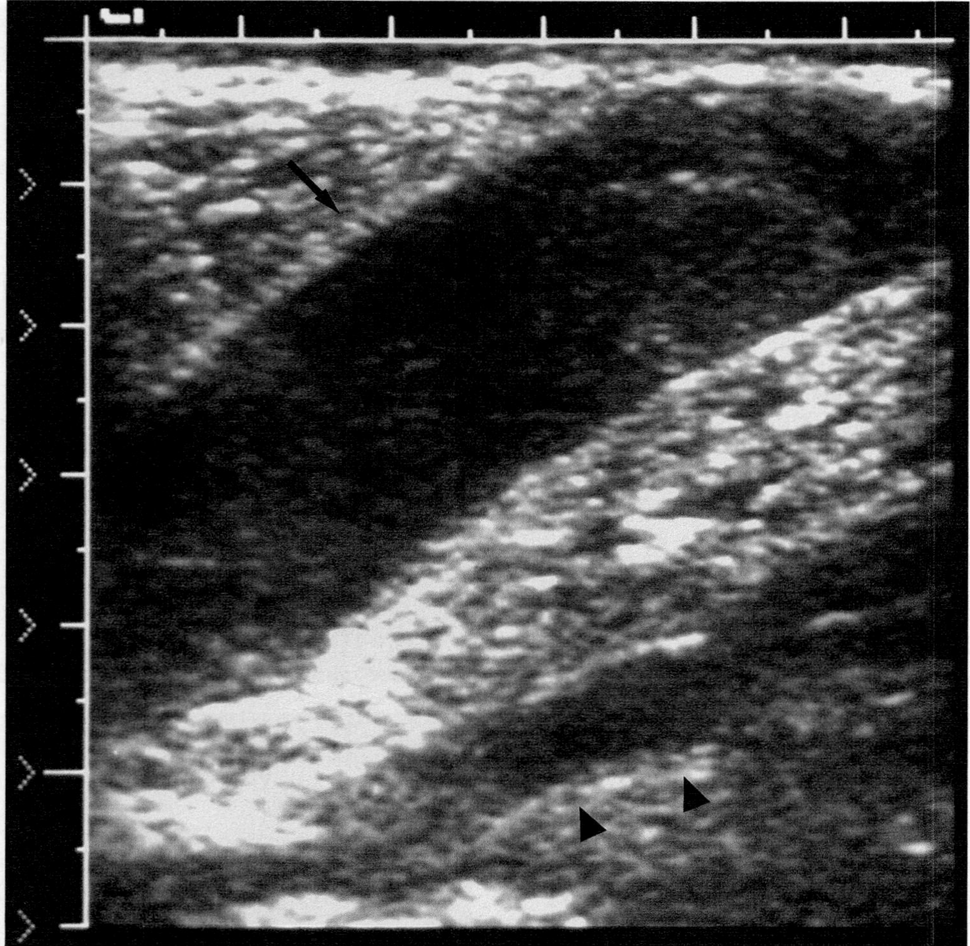

FIGURE 2.22 US of the popliteal fossa. A 45-year-old woman with rheumatoid arthritis presented with pain in the back of the knee radiating to the leg. Clinically, deep vein thrombosis (DVT) was suspected and US was performed. The study was negative for DVT but demonstrated a large fluid-filled Baker cyst *(arrow)*. The *arrowheads* point to the patent popliteal vein.

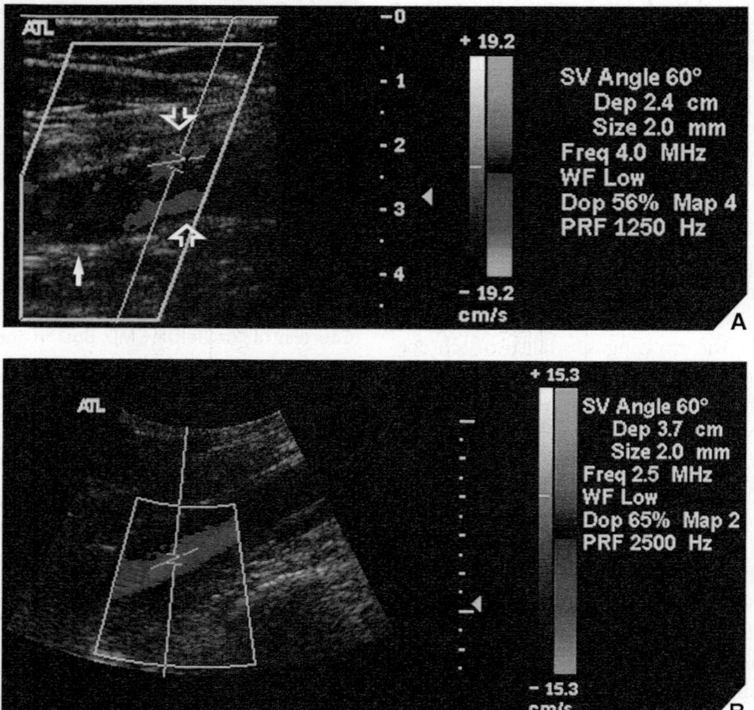

FIGURE 2.23 Color Doppler US of deep vein thrombosis. A 76-year-old man presented with a history of a chronic pain in the left lower extremity. **(A)** Color Doppler image of the popliteal fossa shows hypoechoic area in the popliteal vein *(arrow)* representing an intraluminal thrombus. More proximally noted is diminished blood flow around the blood clot *(open arrows)*. **(B)** A normal color Doppler US of the same region in the right lower extremity is shown for comparison.

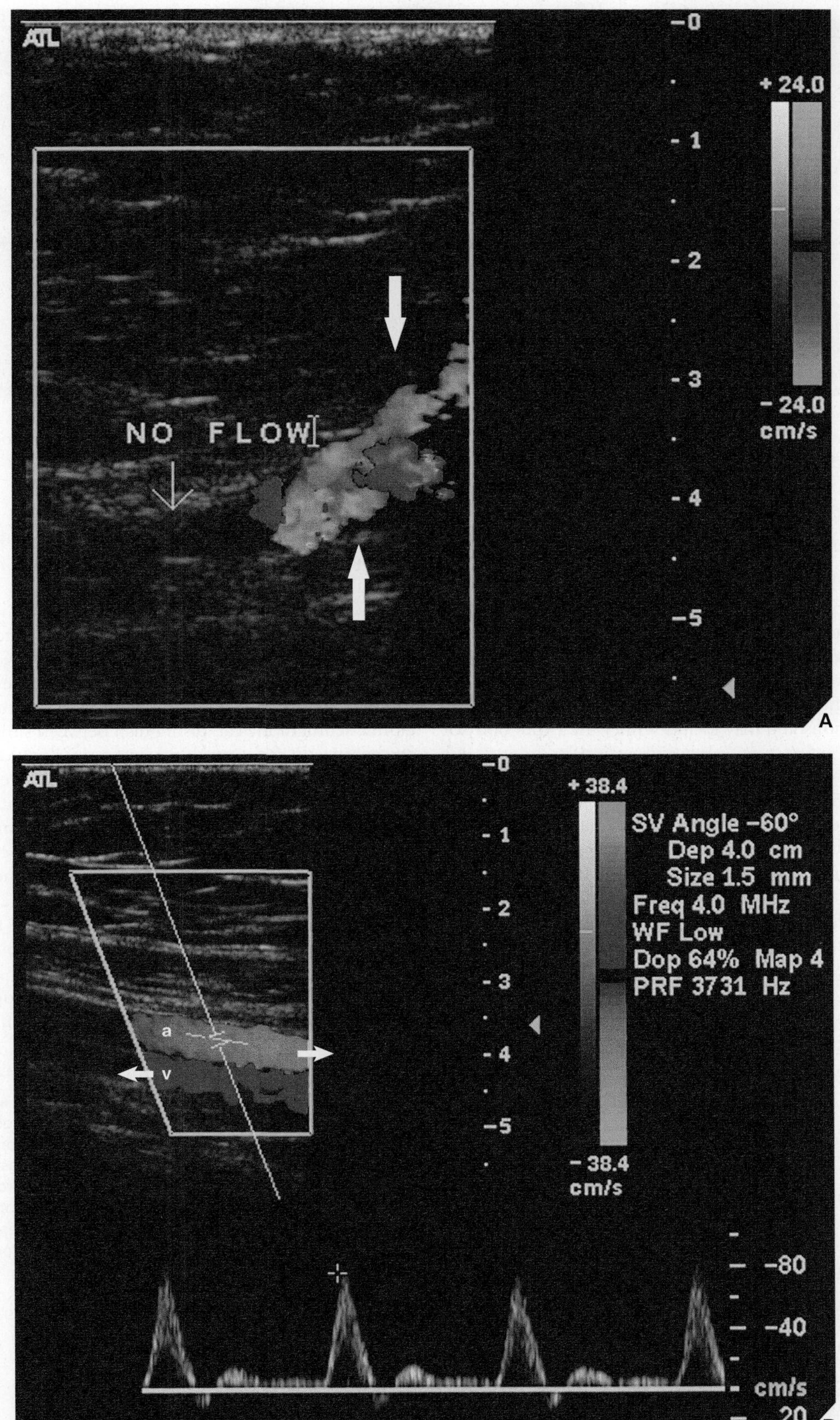

FIGURE 2.24 Color Doppler US of arterial occlusion. A 67-year-old woman presented with a history of claudication worse with exercise. **(A)** Color Doppler image shows complete occlusion of superficial femoral artery. Stream turbulence *(thick white arrows)* is compatible with hemodynamically significant stenosis or occlusion. **(B)** Normal color and pulsed Doppler images are shown for comparison. The *arrows* indicate the direction of blood flow in a vein *(v)* and artery *(a)*.

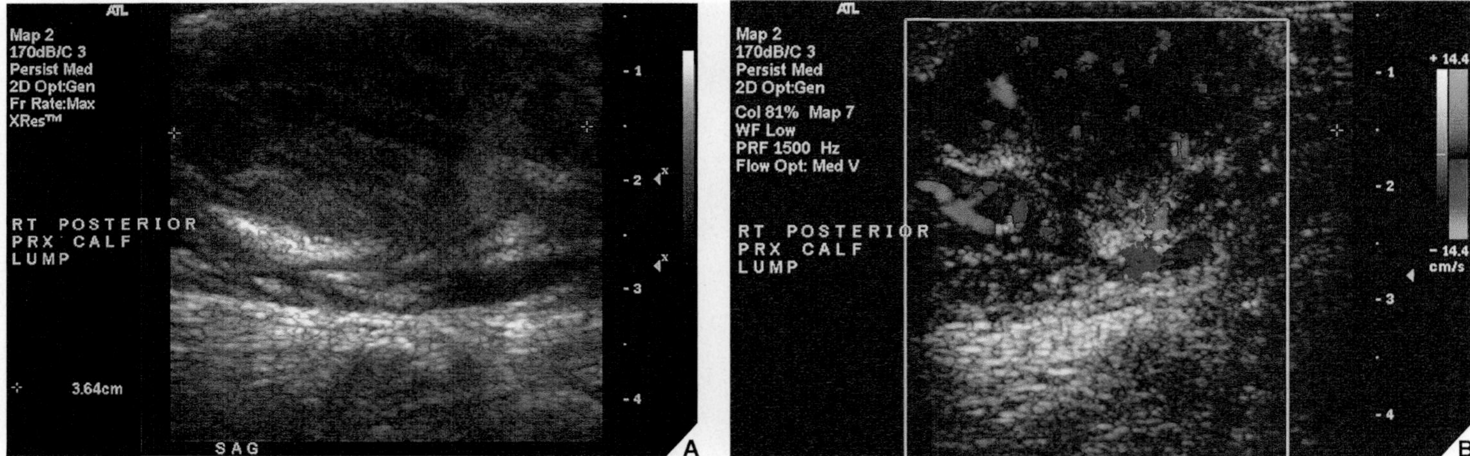

FIGURE 2.25 US of the Baker cyst. A 41-year-old woman presented with painful mass in the popliteal region. Color-flow US shows portion of intact Baker cyst with hyperechoic heterogeneous fluid collection **(A)** and the site of chronic rupture associated with internal debris, secondary inflammatory changes, and hypervascularity **(B)**.

Scintigraphy (Radionuclide Bone Scan)

Scintigraphy is a modality that detects the distribution in the body of a radioactive agent injected into the vascular system. After an intravenous injection of a radiopharmaceutical agent, the patient is placed under a scintillation camera, which detects the distribution of radioactivity in the body by measuring the interaction of gamma rays emitted from the body with sodium iodide crystals in the head of the camera. The photoscans are obtained in multiple projections and may include either the entire body or selected parts.

One major advantage of skeletal scintigraphy over all other imaging techniques is its ability to image the entire skeleton at once (Fig. 2.26). As Johnson remarked, it provides a "metabolic picture" anatomically localizing a lesion by assessing its metabolic activity compared with adjacent normal bone. A bone scan may confirm the presence of the disease, demonstrate the distribution of the lesion, and help evaluate the pathologic process. Indications for skeletal scintigraphy include traumatic conditions, tumors (primary and metastatic), various arthritides, infections, and metabolic bone diseases. The detected abnormality may consist of either decreased uptake of a bone-seeking radiopharmaceutical agent (e.g., in the early stage of osteonecrosis) or increased uptake (such as in the case of fractures, neoplasms, a focus of osteomyelitis, etc.). Some structures under normal conditions may show increased activity (such as sacroiliac joints or normal growth plates).

Scintigraphy is a very sensitive imaging modality; however, it is not very specific, and frequently, it is impossible to distinguish various processes that can cause increased uptake. Occasionally, however, the bone scan may yield very specific information and even suggest diagnosis, for instance, in multiple myeloma or osteoid osteoma. In the search for myeloma, scintigraphy can distinguish between similar-looking bony metastases because in most myeloma cases, no significant increase in the uptake of the radiopharmaceutical agent occurs; however, in skeletal metastasis, invariably, the uptake of the tracer is significantly elevated. In the case of osteoid osteoma, the typical bone scan may demonstrate the so-called *double density sign*—greater increased uptake in the center, related to the nidus of the lesion, and lesser increased uptake at the periphery, related to the reactive sclerosis surrounding the nidus (Fig. 2.27).

Radionuclide bone scan is an indicator of mineral turnover. Because there is usually an enhanced deposition of bone-seeking radiopharmaceuticals in areas of bone undergoing change and repair, a bone scan is useful in localizing tumors and tumor-like lesions in the skeleton. This is particularly helpful in such conditions as Paget disease, fibrous dysplasia,

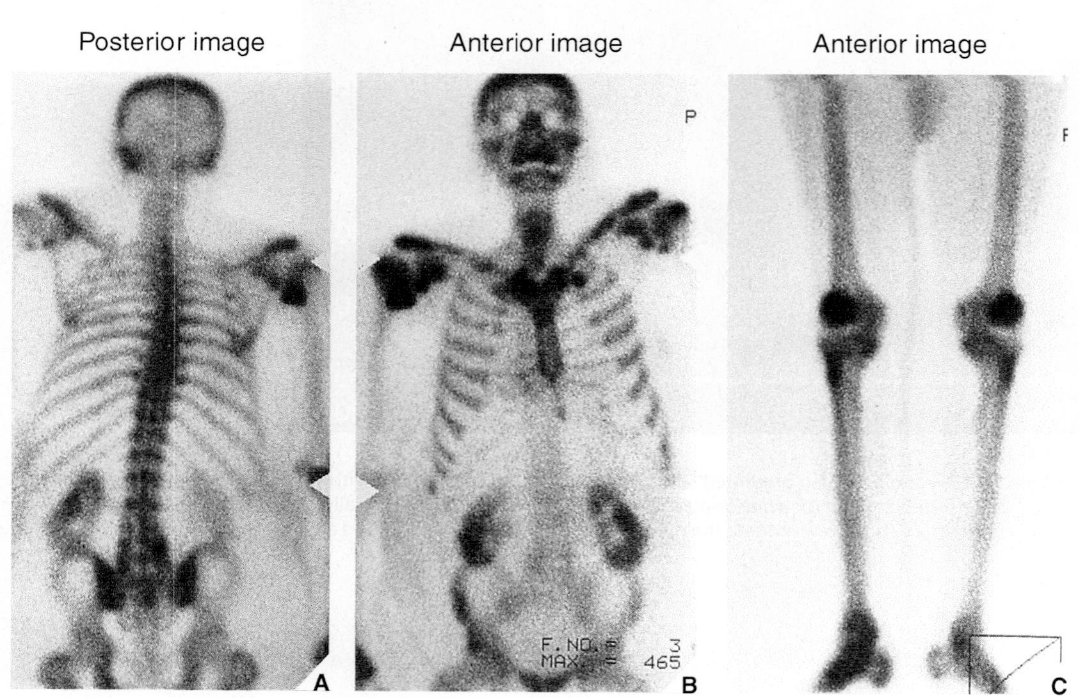

FIGURE 2.26 Radionuclide bone scan. **(A–C)** Scintigraphy obtained in a patient with renal disease and secondary hyperparathyroidism demonstrates several abnormalities: left hydronephrosis secondary to urinary obstruction, resorptive changes of the distal ends of both clavicles, and periarticular soft-tissue calcifications around both shoulders.

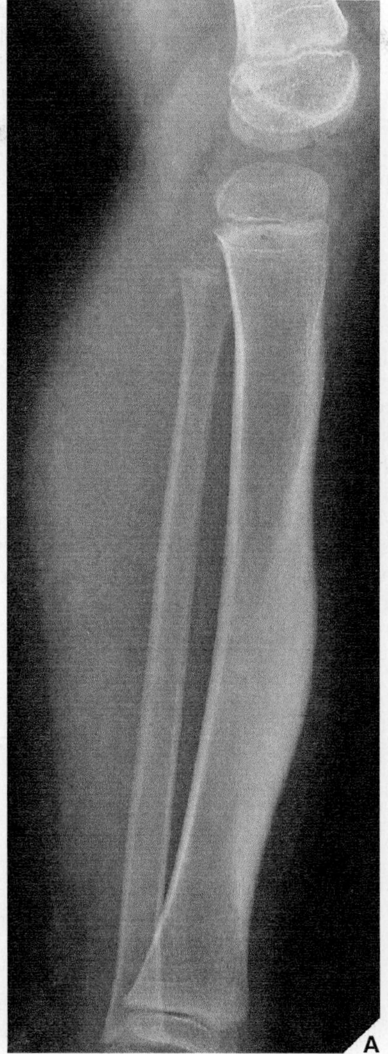

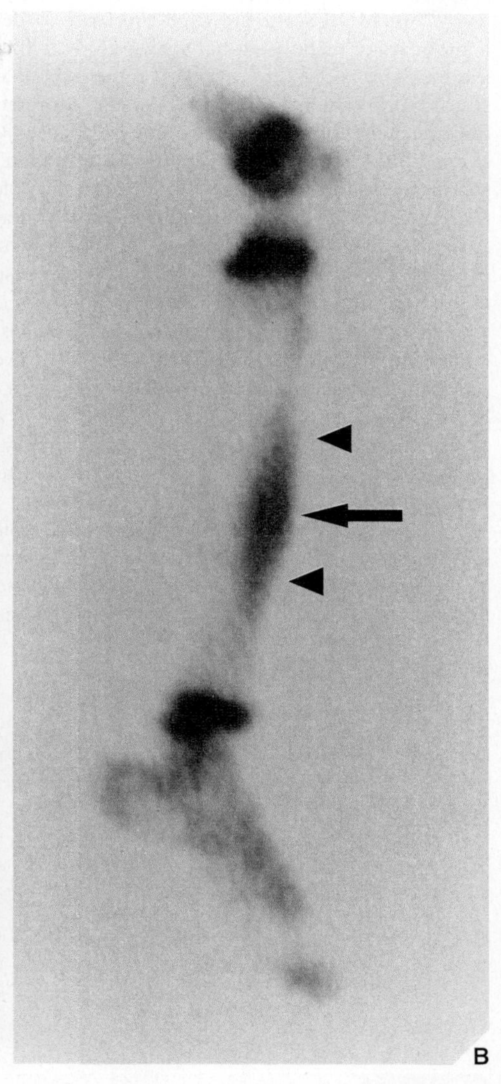

FIGURE 2.27 Osteoid osteoma—effectiveness of scintigraphy. A 4-year-old girl presented with symptoms suggesting a diagnosis of osteoid osteoma; however, a radiograph **(A)** failed to demonstrate the nidus. Radionuclide bone scan that was performed next demonstrates a characteristic "double density" sign **(B)**: More increased uptake of the radiopharmaceutical in the center *(arrow)* is related to the nidus of osteoid osteoma, whereas less increased uptake at the periphery *(arrowheads)* denotes reactive sclerosis.

enchondromatosis, Langerhans cell histiocytosis, and metastatic cancer in which more than one lesion is encountered, and some may represent a "silent" site of disorder. It also plays an important role in localizing small lesions, such as osteoid osteoma, which may not always be seen on radiographs. In most instances, radionuclide bone scan cannot distinguish benign lesions from malignant tumors because increased blood flow with consequently increased isotope deposition and osteoblastic activity will take place in both conditions.

In traumatic conditions, scintigraphy is extremely helpful in the early diagnosis of stress fractures. These fractures may not be seen on conventional radiographs or even on tomographic studies. Scintigraphy is often used to differentiate tibial stress fractures from shin splints. In an acute stress fracture, hyperperfusion and hyperemia are typically present, and delayed images demonstrate band-like or fusiform uptake in the lesion. Conversely, shin splints are characterized by normal angiographic and blood pool phases with delayed images revealing longitudinally oriented linear areas of increased uptake. Radionuclide bone imaging also has value in diagnosing insufficiency fractures of the osteopenic bones in elderly patients when routine radiographic examinations may appear normal.

In metabolic bone disorders, bone scintigraphy is helpful, for instance, in establishing the extent of skeletal involvement in Paget disease (see Fig. 26.10) and assessing response to treatment. Although it is of no value for patients with generalized osteoporosis, it may occasionally be helpful in differentiating osteoporosis from osteomalacia and multiple vertebral fractures resulting from osteoporosis from those occurring in metastatic carcinoma. Radionuclide bone scan has also been reported to be useful in the diagnosis of reflex sympathetic dystrophy syndrome.

Skeletal scintigraphy is frequently used in the evaluation of infections. In particular, technetium-99m (^{99m}Tc) methylene diphosphonate (MDP) and indium-111 (^{111}In) are highly sensitive in detecting early and occult osteomyelitis. In chronic osteomyelitis, imaging with gallium-67 (^{67}Ga) citrate is more accurate in detecting the response or lack of response to treatment than ^{99m}Tc–phosphate bone imaging. For detecting recurrent active infection in patients with chronic osteomyelitis, ^{111}In appears to be the radiopharmaceutical agent of choice. It must be stressed, however, that because the ^{111}In-labeled leukocytes also accumulate in active bone marrow, the sensitivity for the detection of chronic osteomyelitis is reduced. To improve the diagnostic ability of this technique, combined ^{99m}Tc–sulfur colloid bone marrow/^{111}In-labeled leukocyte study has been advocated. The three- or four-phase technique using technetium phosphate tracers can be effectively used to distinguish between soft-tissue infections (cellulitis) and osseous infections (osteomyelitis).

The use of ^{99m}Tc hexamethylpropylene amine oxime (HMPAO)-labeled leukocytes for diagnosing infectious processes has recently been advocated. The kinetics and normal distribution of such leukocytes are similar to those of ^{111}In-labeled white cells. The superior resolution and count density of ^{99m}Tc, however, gives this technique an advantage over the use of ^{111}In-labeled leukocytes.

In neoplastic conditions, the detection of skeletal metastasis is probably the most common indication for skeletal scintigraphy. It also is used frequently to determine the extent of a lesion or the presence of so-called *skipped lesions* or *intraosseous metastases*. It is not, however, the method of choice to determine the extent of the lesion in bone. It is important to stress that scintigraphy alone cannot diagnose the type of tumor; however, it may be useful to detect and localize some primary tumors as well as multifocal lesions (such as multicentric osteosarcoma).

^{99m}Tc MDP scans are used primarily to determine whether a lesion is monostotic or polyostotic. Such a study is therefore essential in staging a bone tumor. It is important to remember that although the degree of abnormal uptake may be related to the aggressiveness of the lesion, this does not correlate well with histologic grade. ^{67}Ga may show uptake in a soft-tissue sarcoma and may help to differentiate a sarcoma from a benign soft-tissue lesion. Although a bone scan may demonstrate the extent of the primary malignant tumor in bone, it is not as accurate as CT or MRI. It may be useful in the detection of a local recurrence of the tumor and occasionally indicates the response or lack of response to treatment (in the case of radiotherapy or chemotherapy).

In the evaluation of arthritides, a bone scan is extremely helpful in demonstrating the distribution of the lesion in the skeleton and has completely replaced the previously used radiographic joint survey (see Fig. 12.12A). Scintigraphy can determine the distribution of arthritic changes not only in large and small joints but also in areas usually not detected by standard radiography, such as the sternomanubrial and temporomandibular joints, among others.

With the development of single-photon emission tomography (SPET) and single-photon emission CT (SPECT), diagnostic precision in evaluating bone and joint abnormalities has increased tremendously. Instrumentation efficacy for SPECT is improving with the introduction of multiple crystal detectors, fan beam, and cone-beam collimators; the detection of a greater fraction of photons; and improved algorithms. In comparison with planar images, SPECT provides increased contrast resolution using a tomographic mode similar to conventional tomography, which eliminates noise from the tissue outside the plane of imaging (Fig. 2.28). It provides not only qualitative information on the uptake of bone-seeking radiopharmaceuticals but also quantitative data. SPECT images are viewed in the transverse, sagittal, and coronal planes as well as the 3D mapping.

The principal benefit of SPECT is the improvement of lesion detection and anatomic localization, hence producing a better diagnostic sensitivity. Bone SPECT has proved particularly useful in the detection of lesions in large and complex anatomic structures, in which it allows the removal of overlying and underlying activity from areas of interest. The widest applications have been found in imaging of the spine, pelvis, knees, and ankles. Using SPECT imaging in the spine, for example, lesions can be localized to different parts of the vertebra (i.e., vertebral body, pedicle, articular process, lamina, pars interarticularis, spinous, and transverse process). In the knee, SPECT imaging has proved to be effective in the detection of meniscal tears.

Over the past decade, SPECT/CT has emerged as a means of correlating functional information from SPECT with anatomic information from CT. Integrated SPECT/CT scanners are gaining popularity as

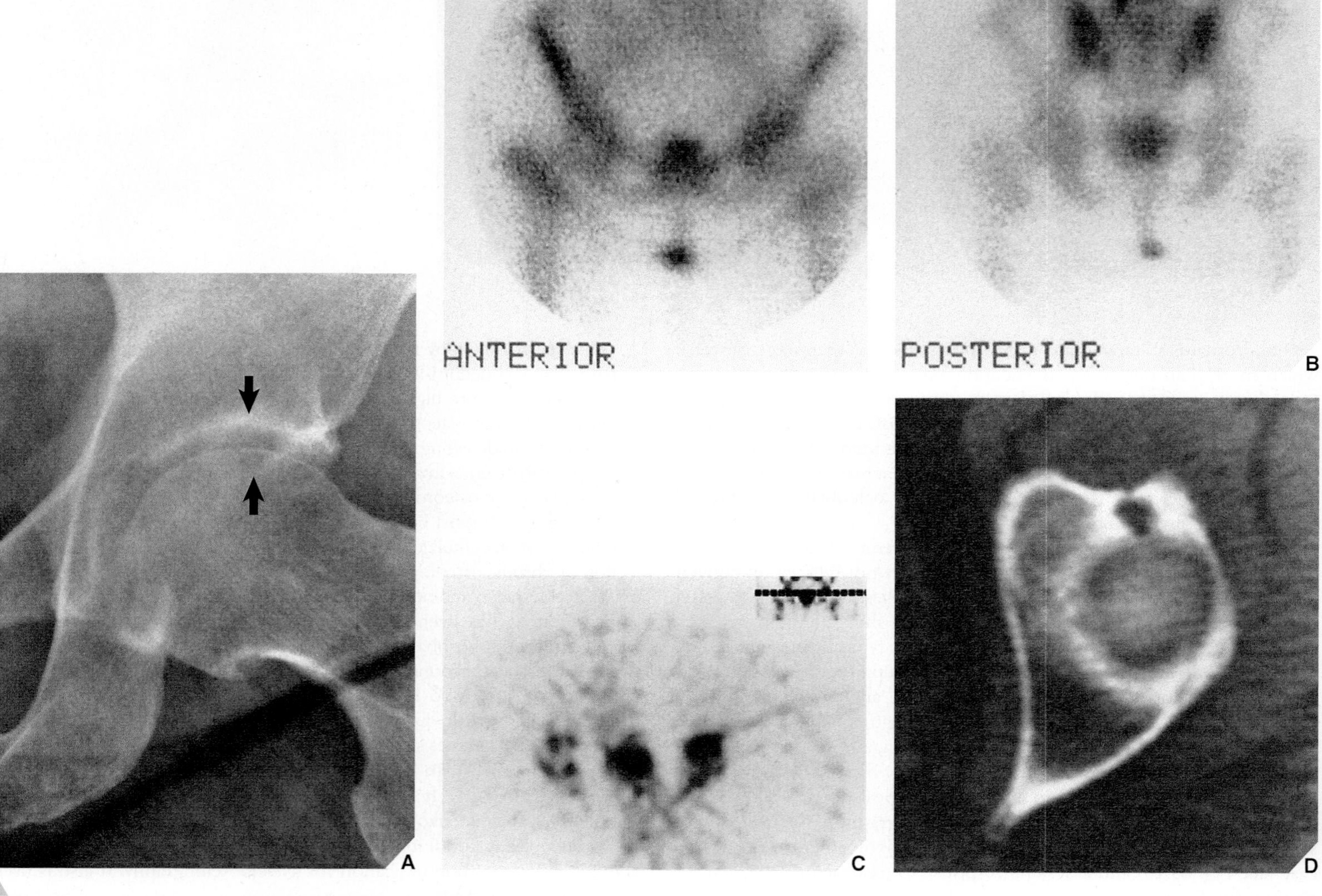

FIGURE 2.28 Effectiveness of SPECT imaging. A 46-year-old woman presented with left hip pain for several month. **(A)** Anteroposterior radiograph of the hip demonstrated only minimal degenerative changes. A small radiolucent focus in the superior portion of the acetabulum *(arrows)* raised some concerns about the diagnosis. **(B)** Conventional radionuclide bone scan in anterior and posterior projection demonstrated a slight increase in the uptake of the tracer localized to the left hip joint. **(C)** On the tomographic cut of the SPECT at the level of the acetabula *(inset)*, there is an area of increased activity localized to the anterosuperior aspect of the left acetabulum and focal areas of activity related to osteophytes of the femoral head. **(D)** CT examination showed a large degenerative cyst (geode) in the acetabulum in the area corresponding to abnormal uptake of the tracer on SPECT section.

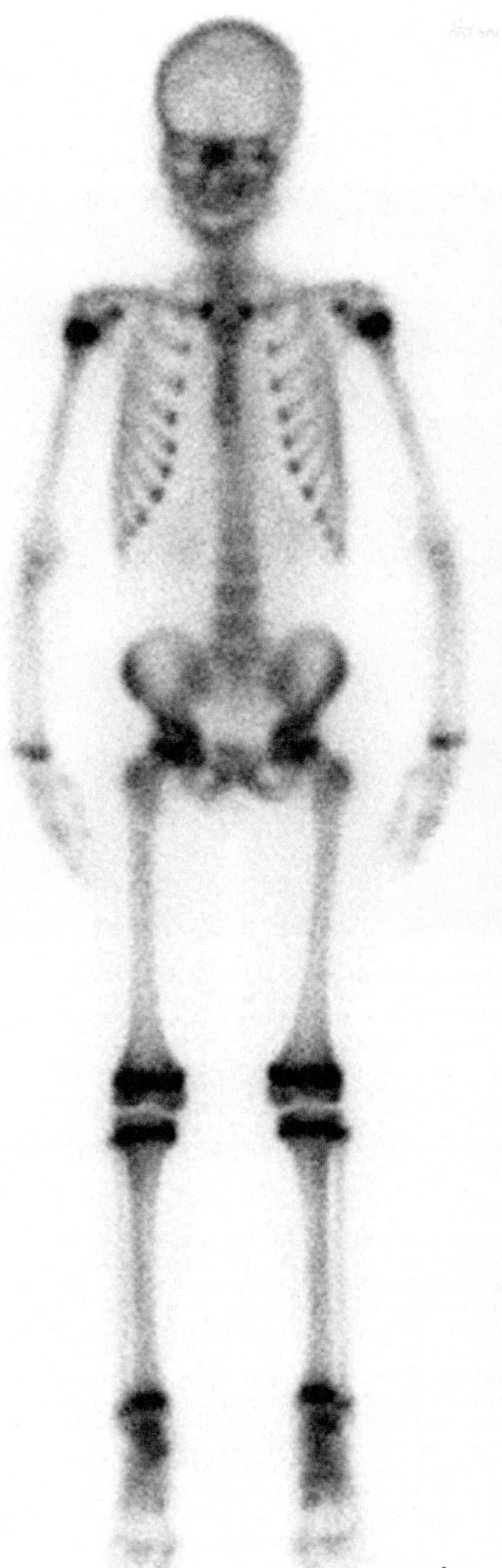

hybrid molecular imaging devices that can acquire SPECT and CT images in single examination (Fig. 2.29). Hybrid SPECT/CT by combining the functional imaging capabilities of SPECT with the precise anatomic characterization provided by CT, enhanced the sensitivity and specificity of scintigraphic techniques and diagnostic accuracy of morphologic abnormalities. By precisely localizing areas of abnormal radiopharmaceutical tracer uptake coupled with ability to generate 3D images, this technique significantly improved sensitivity and specificity of pathologic findings (Figs. 2.30 and 2.31). Recently, high-resolution SPECT and SPECT/CT trials have been attempted to detect osseous alterations in early stages of rheumatoid arthritis (Fig. 2.32) as well as in mechanical (Fig. 2.33) and infectious (Fig. 2.34) loosening of the orthopaedic implants, with promising results.

Several bone-seeking tracers are available for scintigraphic imaging. Those that are most frequently used are as follows.

Diphosphonates

In recent years, there has been remarkable progress in the development of new gamma-emitting diagnostic agents for radionuclide imaging. The radiopharmaceuticals currently in use in bone scanning include the organic

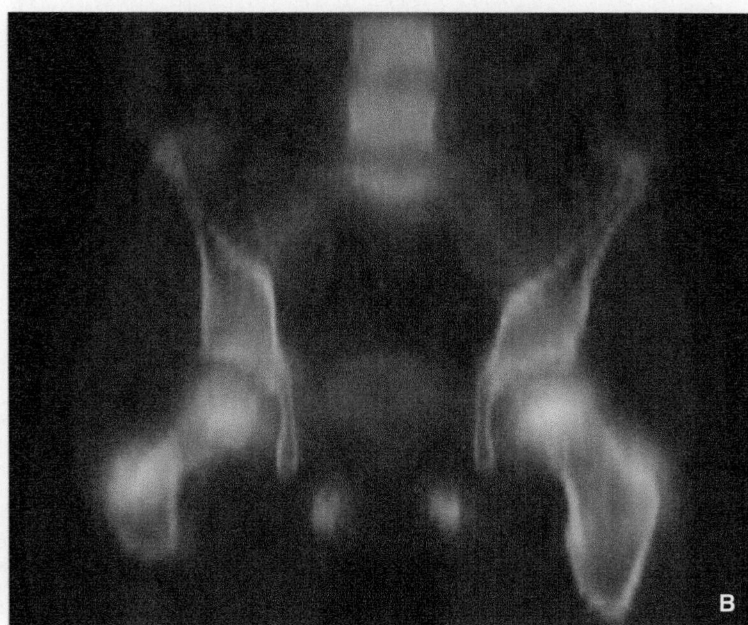

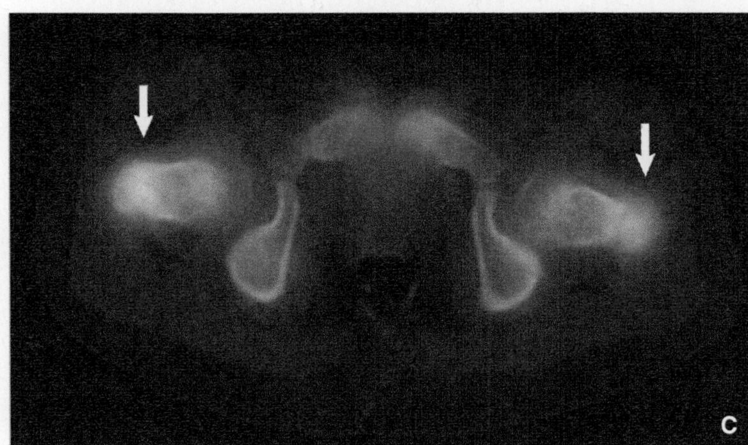

FIGURE 2.29 **Normal SPECT/CT. (A)** A whole-body radionuclide bone scan was performed in this 9-year-old boy who was diagnosed with sickle cell anemia. After intravenous injection of 12.9 mCi of ^{99m}Tc MDP, normal, age-appropriate tracer activity is noted within the visualized bones and soft tissues. Increased uptake of the radiopharmaceutical tracer is present within active growth plates. SPECT/CT of the pelvis in coronal **(B)** and axial **(C)** planes shows no abnormalities. Increased uptake again is seen within the growth plates *(arrows)*.

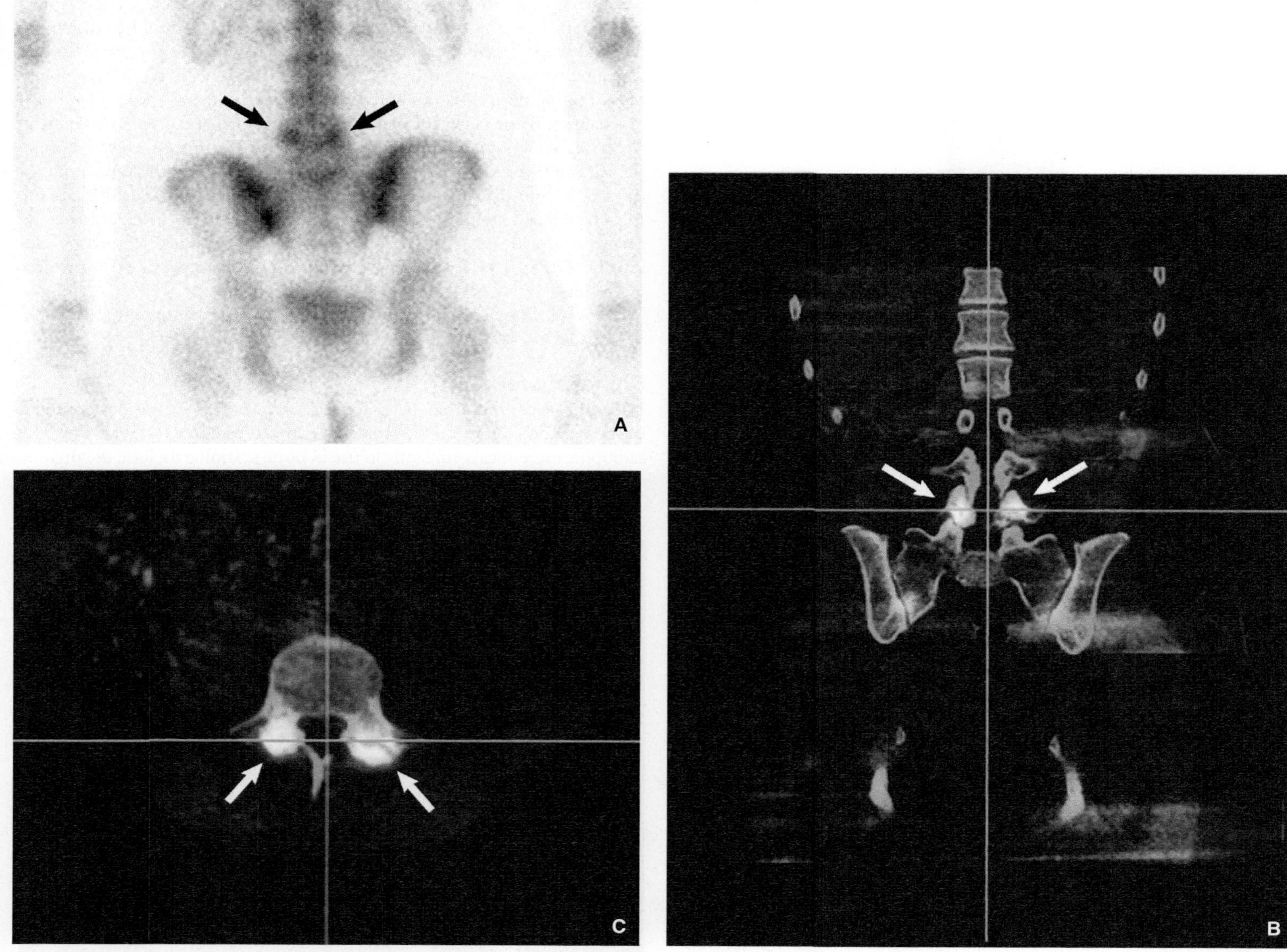

FIGURE 2.30 SPECT/CT of pars interarticularis defect. (A) A radionuclide bone scan of the pelvis and lower lumbar spine of a 14-year-old boy obtained after intravenous injection of 17.2 mCi ^{99m}Tc MDP shows increased activity in the tracer-avid foci at the site of L5 vertebra *(arrows)*. Normal increased uptake is seen within the sacroiliac joints. SPECT/CT in coronal **(B)** and axial **(C)** planes demonstrate increased activity of the radiopharmaceutical tracer localized to bilateral pars interarticularis of L5 *(arrows)*, consistent with pars defect.

diphosphonates, ethylene diphosphonates (HEPDs), MDPs, and methane hydroxydiphosphonates (HNDPs), all labeled with ^{99m}Tc, a pure gamma-emitter with a 6-hour half-life. MDP is more frequently used, particularly in adults, typically in a dose that provides 15 mCi (555 MBq) of ^{99m}Tc. After an intravenous injection of the radiopharmaceutical agent, approximately 50% of the dose localizes in bone. The remainder circulates freely in the body and eventually is excreted by the kidneys. A gamma camera can then be used in a procedure known as *four-phase isotope bone scan*. The first phase, the *radionuclide angiogram*, is the first minute after the injection when the serial images obtained every 2 seconds demonstrate the radioactive tracer in the major blood vessels. In the second phase, the *blood pool scan*, which lasts from 1 to 3 minutes after the injection, the isotope is detected in the vascular system and in the extracellular space in the soft tissues before being taken up by the bone. The third phase, or *static bone scan*, usually occurs 2 to 3 hours after the injection and discloses the radiopharmaceutical agent in the bone. This phase may be divided into two stages. In the first stage, the isotope diffuses passively through the bone capillaries. In the second stage, the radionuclide is concentrated in the bone. The most intense localization occurs in the first and second phases in areas with increased blood flow, and in the third phase, in areas with increased osteogenic activity, increased calcium metabolism, and active bone turnover. The fourth phase is a 24-hour *static image*.

Gallium-67

^{67}Ga citrate is frequently used to diagnose infectious and inflammatory processes in bones and joints. Although the target site of gallium localization is soft tissue, gallium localizes also to some extent in bones because it is incorporated into the calcium hydroxyapatite crystal as a calcium analog, and in the bone marrow, because of its behavior as an iron analog. Gallium accumulates in regions of infection because of an association with bacterial and cellular debris as well as leukocytes. Because white blood cells migrate to the foci of inflammation and infection, some of the gallium is transported intracellularly to these sites. The sensitivity of ^{67}Ga for abscess detection varies from 58% to 100%, and the specificity varies from 75% to 99%. The images are usually obtained 6 and 24 hours after the injection of 5 mCi (185 MBq) of this radiopharmaceutical agent. These images are extremely accurate in following the response to therapy of chronic osteomyelitis and infectious arthritis. In particular, changing activity of ^{67}Ga uptake parallels the patient's clinical course in septic arthritis more closely than the images obtained after the injection of technetium-labeled diphosphonate.

Over the past few years, there has been a considerable change in the role of gallium imaging in infection. Once the mainstay of radionuclide imaging for infection, gallium scanning has now been supplanted by labeled leukocyte imaging. The ^{67}Ga citrate scan, however, enhances and complements the diagnostic value of the ^{99m}Tc MDP scan. In conjunction with the latter, gallium scintigraphy has been used to improve the specificity of technetium imaging. For example, sequential technetium–gallium imaging is superior to technetium MDP scintigraphy alone in distinguishing cellulitis from osteomyelitis and in precise localization of infectious foci.

In neoplastic conditions, gallium scan is used to differentiate a sarcoma from a benign soft-tissue lesion.

Indium

The diagnostic advantage of ^{111}In oxine–labeled white blood cells over other bone-seeking radiopharmaceuticals in detecting inflammatory abnormalities in the skeletal system has recently been advocated. Because ^{111}In

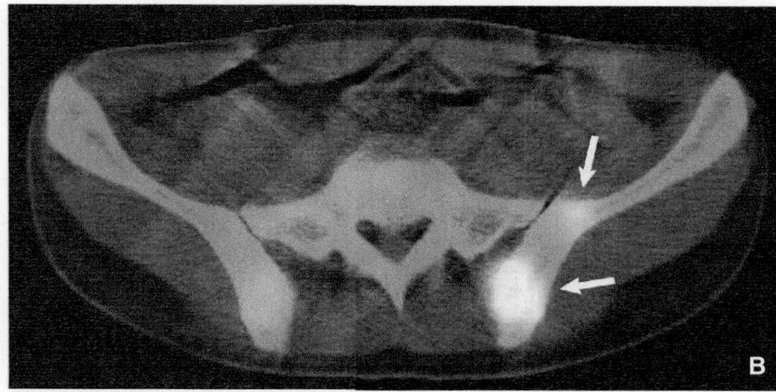

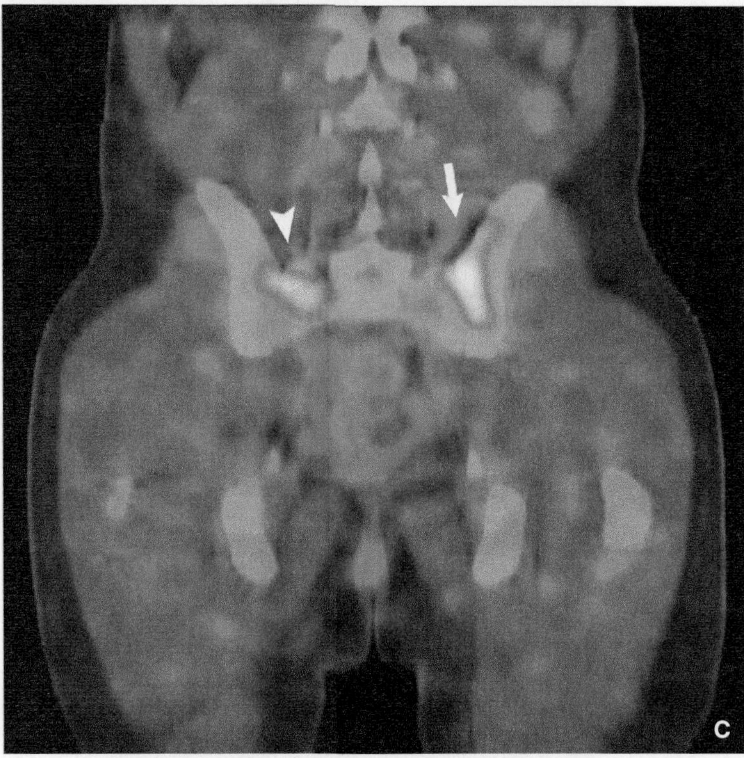

FIGURE 2.31 SPECT/CT of metastatic neuroblastoma. (A) A whole-body radionuclide bone scan of a 17-year-old boy performed after intravenous injection of 24.8 mCi ^{99m}Tc MDP shows increased activity of the radiopharmaceutical tracer in the left iliac bone *(arrow)* and in the right sacrum *(arrowhead)*. Subsequently, SPECT/CT was performed after intravenous injection of 51.43 mCi of iodine-123 MIBG. **(B)** Image in the axial plane shows two foci of increased activity of the tracer within the left iliac bone *(arrows)*. **(C)** Image obtained in the coronal plane shows in addition to the lesions in the left ilium *(arrow)*, a focus of increased activity within the right sacrum *(arrowhead)*, all consistent with metastases from previously clinically diagnosed neuroblastoma.

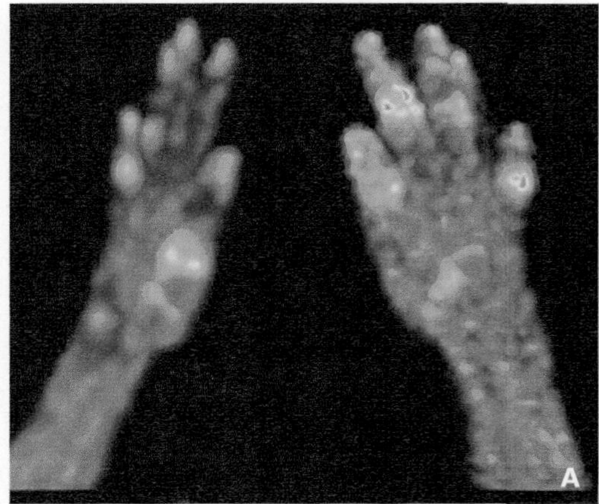

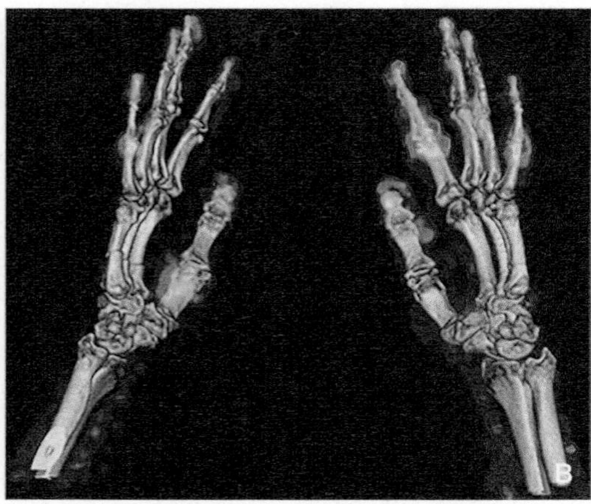

FIGURE 2.32 SPECT/CT of rheumatoid arthritis. ^{99m}Tc-labeled MDP SPECT **(A)** and SPECT/CT 3D reconstructed images **(B)** show inflammatory changes of the several joints of both hands. (Courtesy of PZWL Wydawnictwo Lekarskie, Warsaw, Poland.)

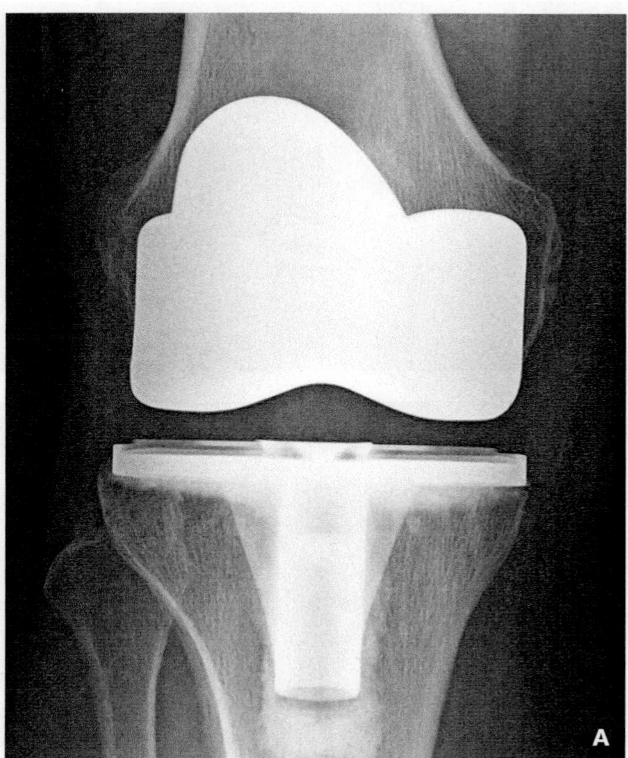

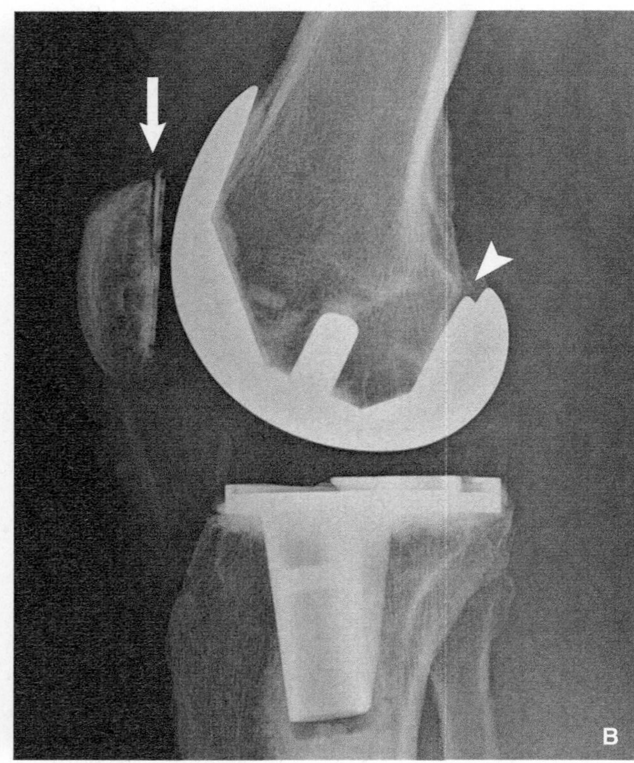

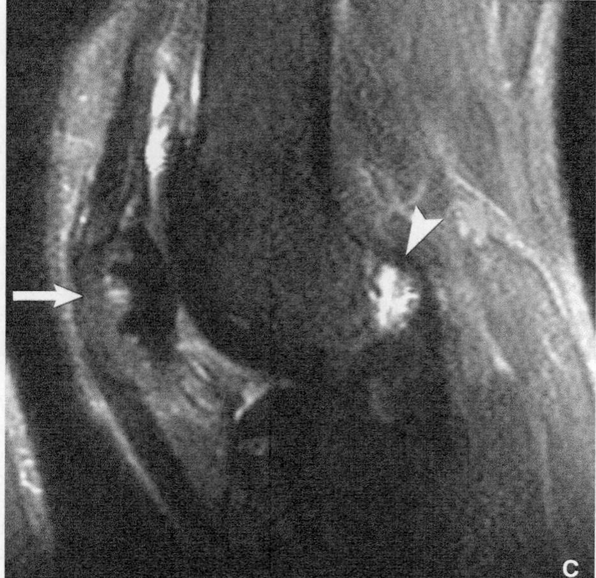

FIGURE 2.33 SPECT/CT of mechanical loosening of prosthesis. A 60-year-old man, who had a three-part cemented nonconstrained total knee arthroplasty performed for osteoarthritis, presented with knee pain for past few weeks. **(A)** Anteroposterior radiograph of the right knee shows no obvious abnormalities of the femoral or tibial components of the prosthesis. **(B)** Lateral radiograph shows a small radiolucent gap at the patellar component *(arrow)* and a similar gap at the posterior bracket of the femoral component *(arrowhead)*, suggesting loosening of the prosthesis. **(C)** Sagittal IR MR image obtained using specialized multiacquisition variable-resonance image combination (MAVRIC) sequence to minimize metallic artifacts around prosthesis shows increased signal at the patellar *(arrow)* and femoral *(arrowhead)* prosthetic components. *(Continued)*

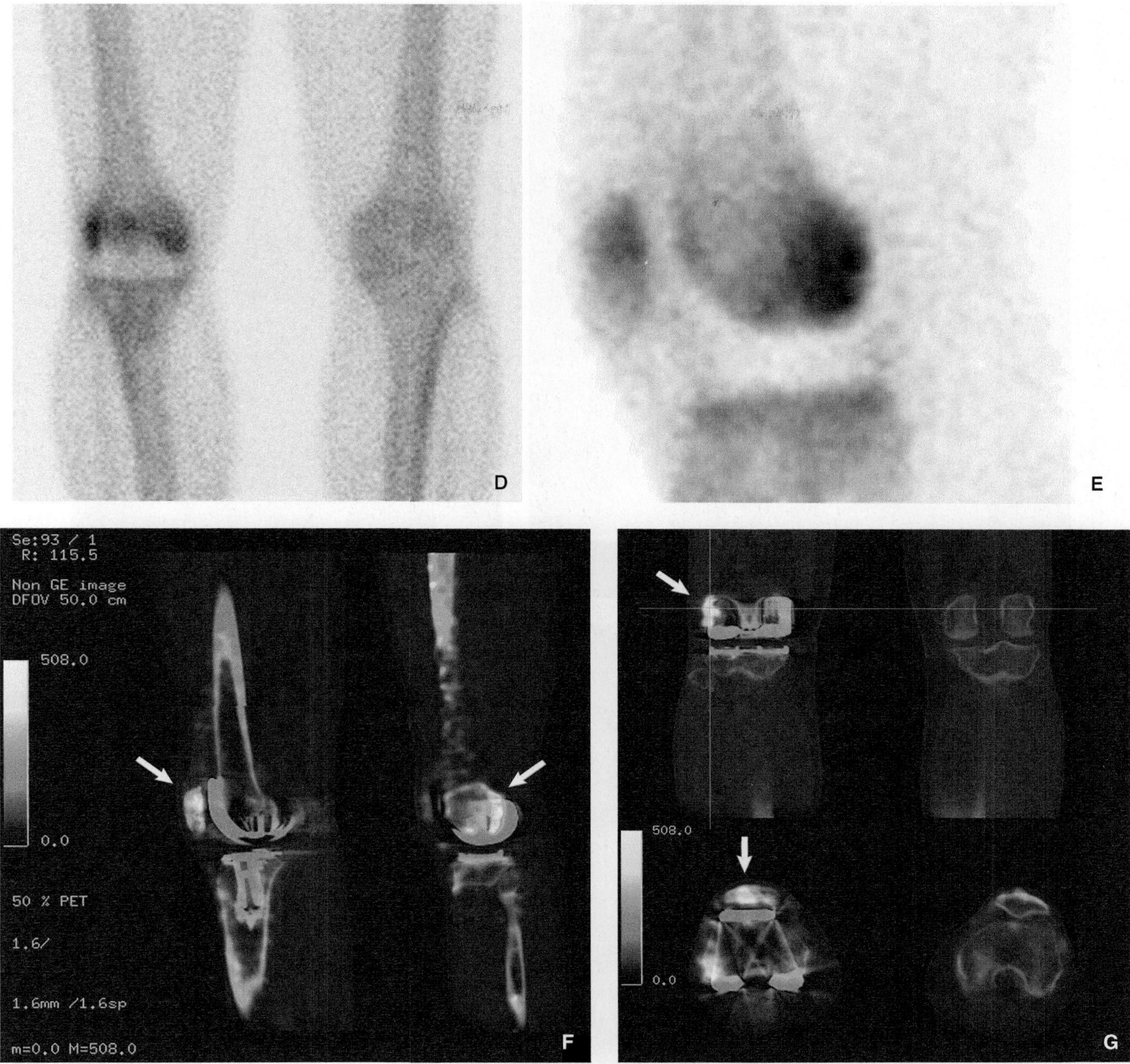

FIGURE 2.33 SPECT/CT of mechanical loosening of prosthesis. ***(Continued)*** Radionuclide bone scan in frontal **(D)** and lateral **(E)** projections, obtained after intravenous administration of ^{99m}Tc-labeled MDP, shows increased uptake of radiopharmaceutical tracer at the site of femoral and patellar components. SPECT/CT images in sagittal **(F)** and coronal and axial **(G)** planes show more accurately the sites of loosening at the superior aspect of the patellar component and at the posterolateral part of the femoral component *(arrows)*. (Courtesy of PZWL Wydawnictwo Lekarskie, Warsaw, Poland.)

leukocytes are not usually incorporated into areas of increased bone turnover, indium imaging presumably reflects inflammatory activity only, and early experience has shown it to be specific in detecting abscesses or acute infectious processes, including osteomyelitis and septic arthritis. The sensitivity varies from 75% to 90%, and the specificity, as recently reported, is approximately 91%. False-negative results are often seen in patients with chronic infections in which there is reduced inflow of circulating leukocytes. False-positive results are seen in patients who have an inflammatory process without infection (such as rheumatoid arthritis mistaken for septic arthritis).

Nanocolloid

Very small particles of ^{99m}Tc-labeled colloid of human serum albumin were tried as a bone marrow imaging agent. Approximately 86% of these particles are 30 nm or smaller, and the remainder are between 30 and 80 nm. This nanocolloid has a sensitivity for the detection of osteomyelitis in the extremities equal to that of indium-labeled leukocytes. The clinical value of this method has not been yet determined.

Immunoglobulins

Recently, radiolabeled human polyclonal immunoglobulin G (IgG) has been used as an agent for imaging infection. This labeled Ig is thought to bind to Fc receptors expressed by cells (macrophages, polymorphonuclear leukocytes, and lymphocytes) involved in the inflammatory response. In a study of 128 patients, polyclonal IgG yielded a sensitivity of 91% and a specificity of 100%. Polyclonal immunoglobulins have a number of advantages, such as availability in kit form and the fact that they do not require in vivo labeling.

Chemotactic Peptides

The same investigators who developed ^{111}In-labeled IgG are also pioneering the use of radiolabeled chemotactic peptides for infection imaging. These are small peptides that are produced by bacteria. They bind to high-affinity receptors on the cell membrane of polymorphonuclear leukocytes and mononuclear phagocytes, stimulating chemotaxis. Rather than using the native peptide, synthetic analogs are created that allow

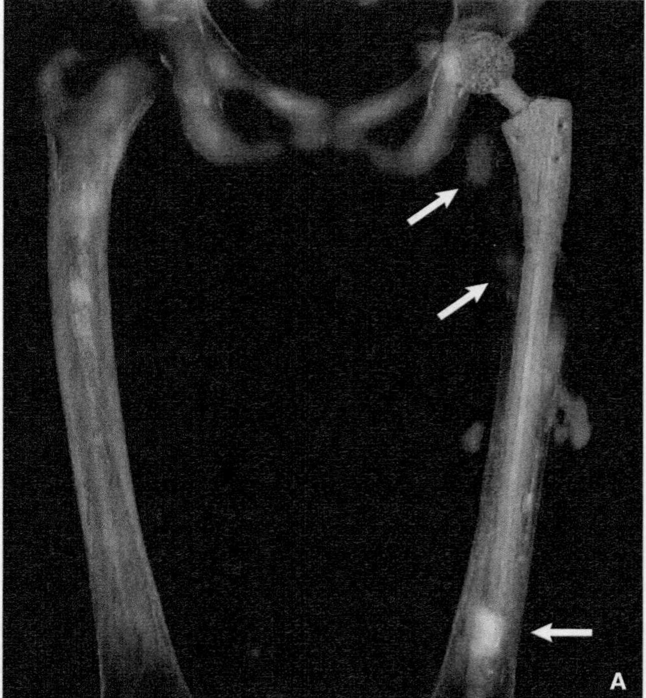

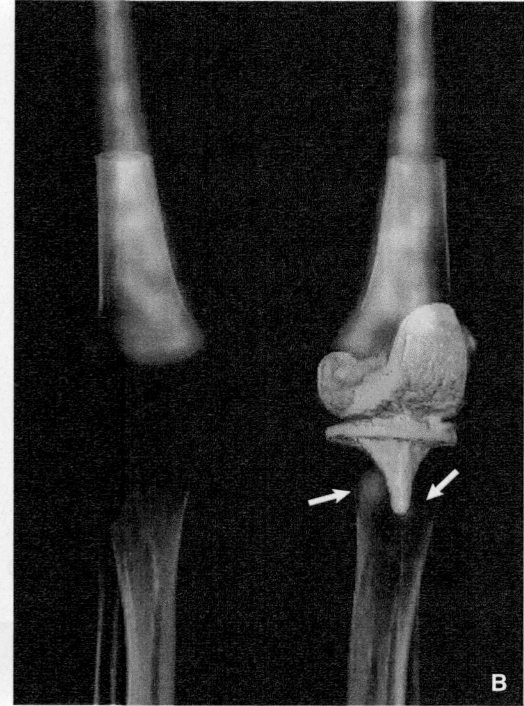

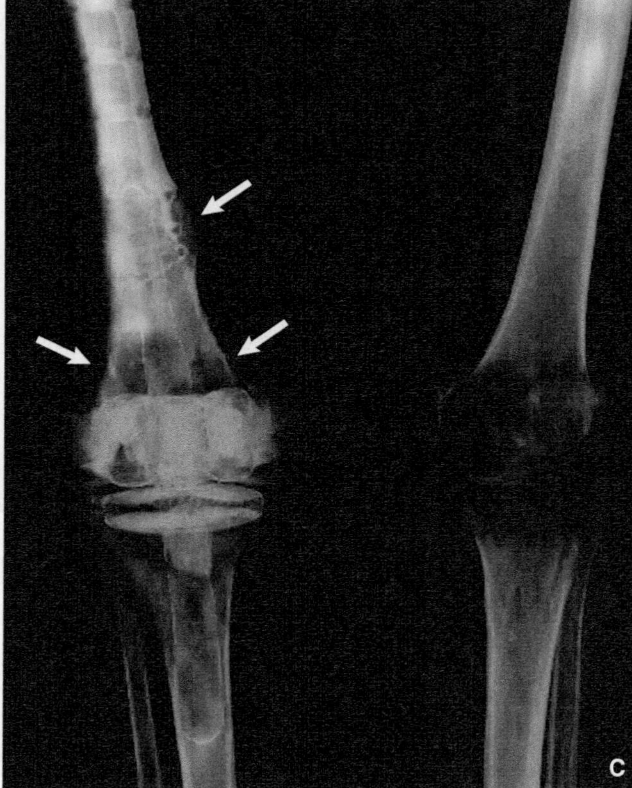

FIGURE 2.34 **SPECT/CT immunoscintigraphy of infected joint arthroplasties.** **(A)** Imaging performed in an 81-year-old woman using antigranulocyte scintigraphy with ^{99m}Tc-labeled monoclonal antibodies shows increased radioactivity at the site of the distal end of the femoral component of the left hip prosthesis as well as within the medial aspect of the proximal part of the stem *(arrows)*. **(B)** Imaging using the same radiotracer, performed in a 75-year-old woman, shows increased activity at the site of the tibial component of the left knee prosthesis *(arrows)*. **(C)** Imaging performed in a 79-year-old woman shows increased activity at the site of the femoral component of the right knee prosthesis *(arrows)*. (Courtesy of PZWL Wydawnictwo Lekarskie, Warsaw, Poland.)

radiolabeling. The small size of ^{111}In-labeled chemotactic peptides allows the component to pass quickly through the vascular walls and enter the site of infection.

Iodine

Iodine-125 (^{125}I) is used in a radionuclide technique known as *single-photon absorptiometry* (SPA) to determine bone mineral density at peripheral bone sites such as finger and radius. This method measures primarily the density of the cortical bone.

Iodine-131 (^{131}I) is used as iodine-123 or iodine-131 metaiodobenzylguanidine (MIBG), also known as *iobenguane*, for detection of neuroendocrine tumors. Occasionally, these tumors metastasize to the bones, and this technique combined with the use of SPECT/CT is very effective in anatomic localization and evaluation of this complication.

Gadolinium

Gadolinium-153 (^{153}Gd) is a radionuclide source used in a technique known as *dual-photon absorptiometry* (DPA), which is also used to calculate bone mineral density. This technique permits the measurement of central sites of bone such as the spine and the hip. ^{153}Gd produces photons at two energy levels, and the images are generated on a whole-body rectilinear scanner. The measurements are obtained for compact and trabecular bones.

PET, PET/CT, and PET/MRI

PET is a diagnostic imaging technique that allows the identification of biochemical and physiologic alterations in the body and assesses the level of metabolic activity and perfusion in various organ systems. The process produces biologic images based on the detection of gamma rays that are emitted by a radioactive substance, such as fluorine-18 (^{18}F)-labeled 2-fluoro-2-deoxyglucose (^{18}FDG). PET differs from other single-photon radionuclide scans in its ability to correct for tissue attenuation signal loss and its relatively uniform spatial resolution. One of the main applications of this technique is in oncology, including the detection of primary and metastatic tumors and recurrences of the tumors after treatment. Only recently has PET scanning been found to be useful in the diagnosis, treatment, and follow-up of musculoskeletal neoplasms (Figs. 2.35 to 2.37). Although some promising results have been reported in using this technique, the detection of bone marrow involvement is still controversial because physiologic bone marrow uptake and diffuse uptake in reactive changes in bone marrow (such as after chemotherapy) can be observed on FDG-PET images. Recently, a significant progress has been made in the application of PET scanning in diagnosing infections associated with metallic implants in patients with traumatic conditions.

PET/CT combines in a single gantry system a PET and a CT, allowing a sequential acquisition of images derived from both systems at the same time and thus combining them into a single superimposed image. The advantage of this fusion image is clear: The functional images obtained with PET that depict the spatial distribution of metabolic and biochemical activities in the tissues are precisely correlated with anatomic images obtained with CT (Fig. 2.38). 2D and 3D image reconstruction may be rendered as a function of a common software and control system.

PET/MRI is a newest hybrid technology with capability of instantaneous fusion of anatomic and functional data that allows an integrated scanning for simultaneous PET and MRI. In order to avoid the interference of magnetic field on PET performance, the traditional PET detectors based on scintillators coupled to photomultiplier tubes were substituted with the avalanche photodiodes and silicon photomultipliers. This technique combines the strength of MRI, including lack of ionizing radiation and high-resolution as well as high-contrast morphologic imaging of soft tissues and osseous structures, with high sensitivity of PET and its ability to obtain functional images depicting metabolic and biochemical activity in the tissues as in PET/CT. Although still an experimental technique at the time of this printing, the limited clinical applications yielded encouraging results, particularly in the field of evaluation of the progress of treatment of some of the inflammatory arthritides (John Hunter, MD, and Stanley Naguwa, MD, UC Davis Medical Center, Sacramento, California, unpublished data and personal communications, 2018; see also text pertinent to Imaging Evaluation of the Arthritides, Chapter 12) and mapping of metastatic disease (Fig. 2.39) (Luis Beltran, MD, Hospital for Joint Diseases—Orthopaedic Institute, New York University, New York, personal communication, 2018).

Magnetic Resonance Imaging

MRI is based on the reemission of an absorbed radiofrequency (rf) signal while the patient is in a strong magnetic field. An external magnetic field is usually generated by a magnet with field strengths of 0.2 to 3.0 Tesla (T). The system includes a magnet, rf coils (transmitter and receiver), gradient coils, and a computer display unit with digital storage facilities. The physical principles of MRI cannot be discussed here in detail because of space limitations; only a brief overview will be given.

The ability of MRI to image body parts depends on the intrinsic spin of atomic nuclei with an odd number of protons and/or neutrons (e.g., hydrogen), thus generating a magnetic moment. Atomic nuclei of tissues placed within the main magnetic field from the usual random alignment of their magnetic poles tend to align along the direction of that field. The application of rf pulses causes the nuclei to absorb energy and induces resonance of particular sets of nuclei, which causes their orientation to the magnetic field. The required frequency of the pulse is determined by the strength of the magnetic field and the particular nucleus undergoing investigation. When the rf field is removed, the energy absorbed during the transition from a high- to low-energy state is subsequently released, and this can be recorded as an electrical signal that provides the data from which digital images are derived. Signal intensity refers to the strength of

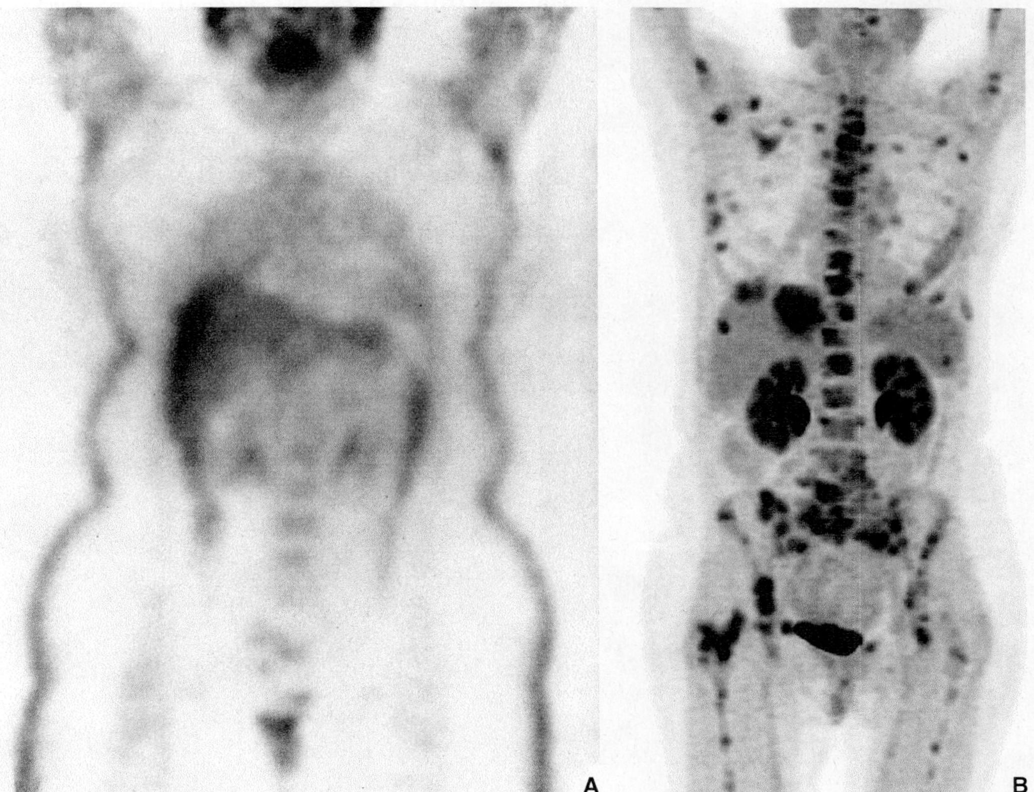

FIGURE 2.35 PET scan. **(A)** A normal whole-body PET scan of 62-year-old woman suspected of having skeletal metastases caused by recently treated breast carcinoma. **(B)** A 65-year-old woman diagnosed with stage IV adenocarcinoma of the lungs developed widespread skeletal and internal organ metastases, as revealed on this PET scan.

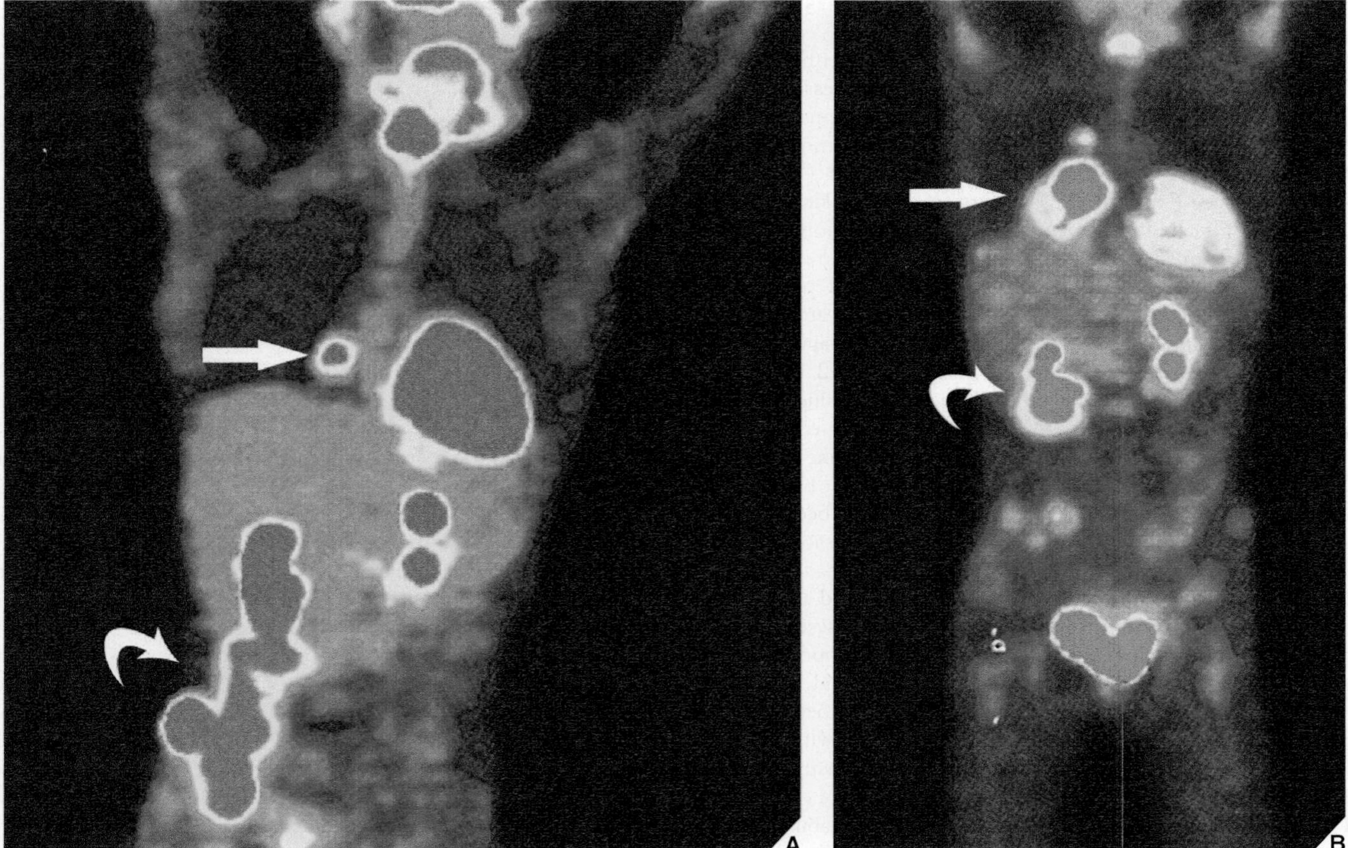

FIGURE 2.36 PET of a malignant tumor. **(A)** A whole-body PET scan of a 9-year-old girl with Ewing sarcoma of the right ilium shows hypermetabolic tumor in the bone *(curved arrow)* and a metastatic lung nodule *(arrow)*. **(B)** After several months of chemotherapy, the primary iliac bone tumor has markedly decreased in size *(curved arrow)*, but metastatic lung lesion has enlarged *(arrow)*. (Courtesy of Frieda Feldman, MD, and Ronald van Heertum, MD, New York.)

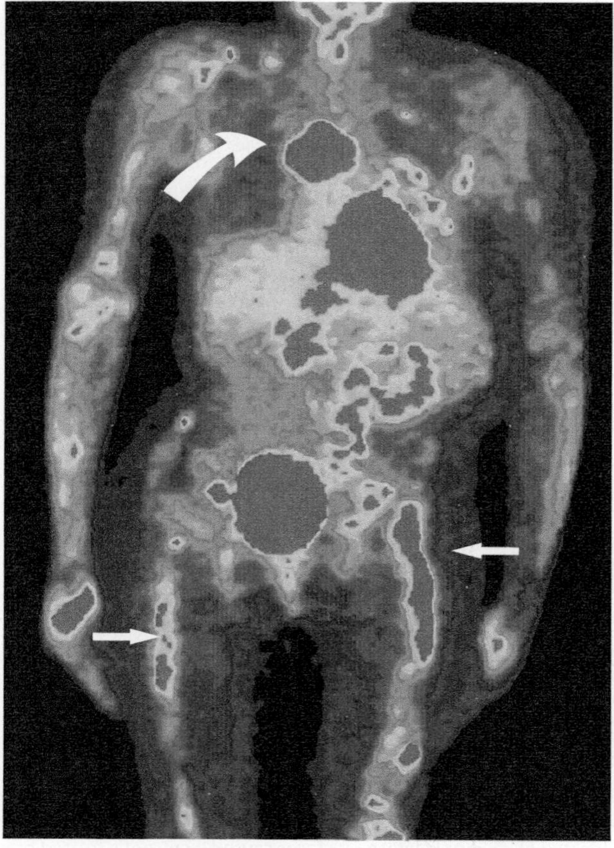

FIGURE 2.37 PET of a benign lesion. A whole-body PET scan of a 37-year-old woman with fibrous dysplasia shows multiple skeletal deformities. The *arrows* point to the lesions in proximal femora, and the *curved arrow* points to a large hypermetabolic focus in the sternum. (Courtesy of Frieda Feldman, MD, and Ronald van Heertum, MD, New York.)

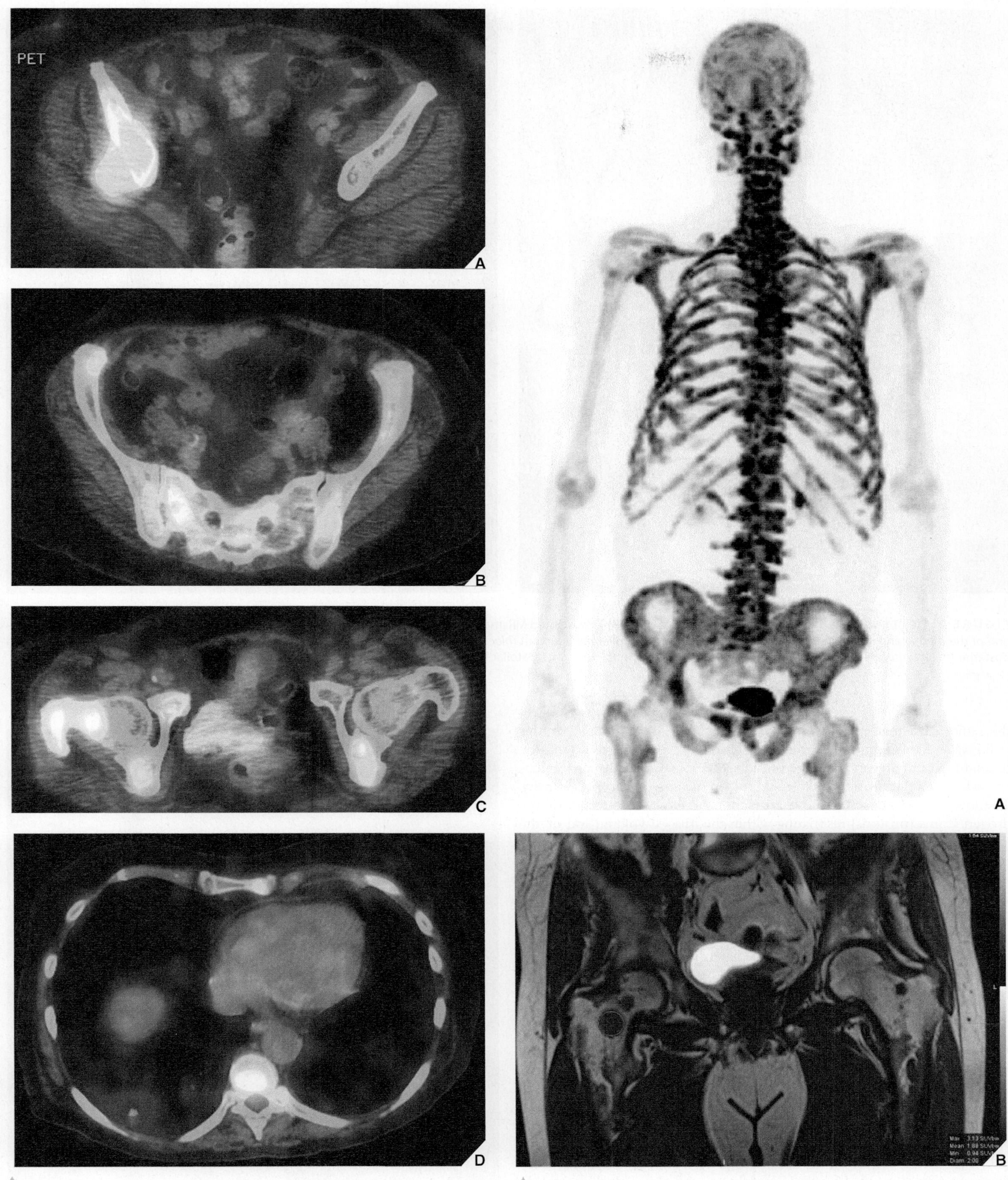

FIGURE 2.38 PET/CT scanning. A 60-year-old woman with breast carcinoma underwent a PET/CT scanning. The axial fused PET/CT images revealed several hypermetabolic foci of skeletal metastases including right ilium **(A)**, sacrum **(B)**, right femur and both acetabula **(C)**, and thoracic vertebrae **(D)**.

FIGURE 2.39 Effectiveness of PET/MRI. **(A)** Sodium fluoride PET demonstrates multiple skeletal metastases in this patient with prostate carcinoma but failed to show a large metastatic lesion in the right femoral neck, clearly shown on the fused PET/MRI **(B)** *(green circle)*. (Courtesy of Luis Beltran, MD, Boston.)

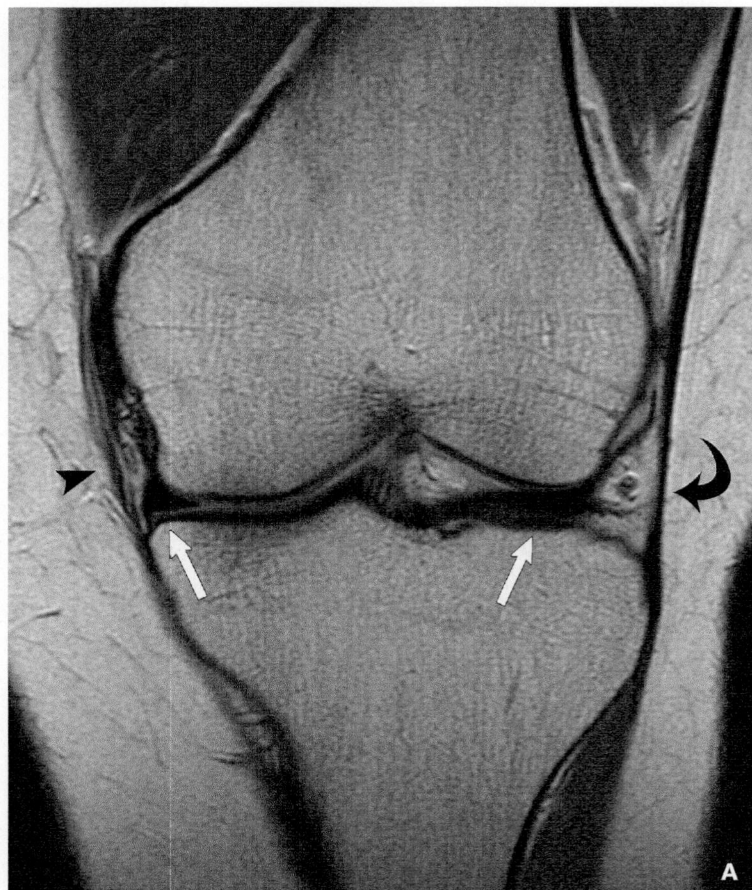

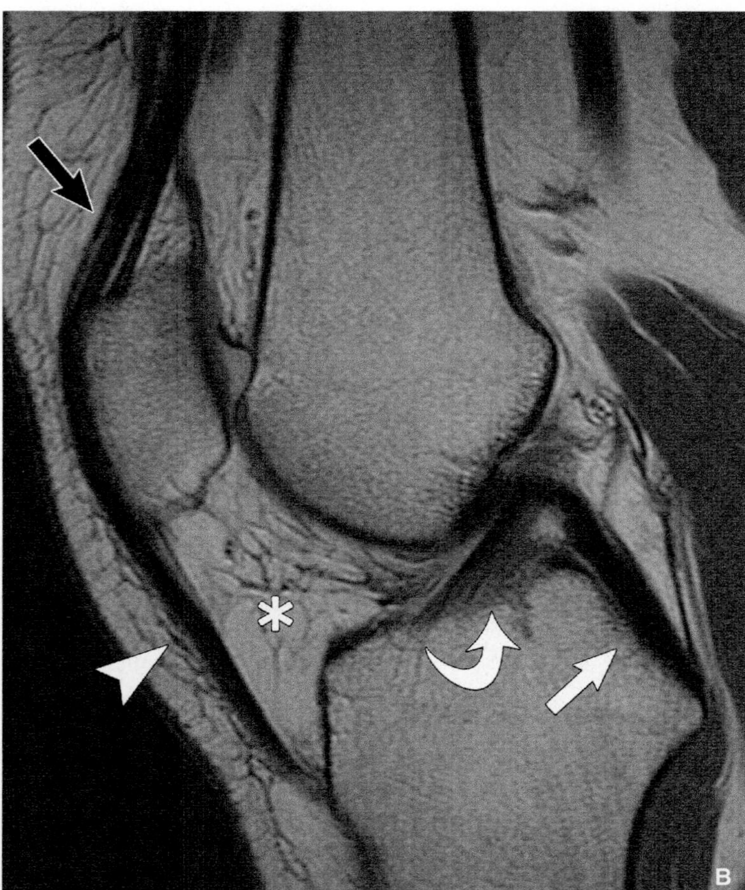

FIGURE 2.40 T1-weighted images. Coronal **(A)** and sagittal **(B)** T1-weighted MR images of the knee are effective in showing the anatomic details. Observe clear definition of the medial and lateral menisci *(thin white arrows)*, medial collateral ligament *(black arrowhead)*, iliotibial band *(black curved arrow)*, anterior *(white curved arrow)* and posterior *(thick white arrow)* cruciate ligaments, quadriceps tendon *(black arrow)*, patellar ligament *(white arrowhead)*, and infrapatellar Hoffa fat pad *(asterisk)*.

the radio wave that a tissue emits after excitation. The strength of this radio wave determines the degree of brightness of the imaged structures. A bright (white) area in an image is said to demonstrate high signal intensity, whereas a dark (black) area is said to demonstrate low signal intensity. The intensity of a given tissue is a function of the concentration of hydrogen atoms (protons) resonating within the imaged volume and of the longitudinal and transverse relaxation times, which, in turn, depend on the biophysical state of the tissue's water molecules.

Two relaxation times are described, termed *T1* and *T2*. The T1 relaxation time (longitudinal) is used to describe the return of protons back to equilibrium after the application and removal of the rf pulse. T2 relaxation time (transverse) is used to describe the associated loss of coherence or phase between individual protons immediately after the application of the rf pulse. A variety of rf pulse sequences can be used to enhance the differences in T1 and T2, thus providing the necessary image contrast. The most commonly used sequences are spin echo (SE), partial saturation recovery (PSR), inversion recovery (IR), chemical selective suppression (CHESS), and fast scan (FS) technique. SE short repetition times (TRs) (800 msec or less) and short echo delay times (TEs) (40 msec or less) pulse sequences (or T1) provides good anatomic detail (Fig. 2.40). Long TR (2,000 msec or more) and long TE (60 msec or more) pulse sequences (or T2), however, provide good contrast, sufficient for the evaluation of pathologic processes (Fig. 2.41). Intermediate TR (1,000 msec or more) and short TE (30 msec or less) sequences are known as *proton or spin density images*. They represent a mixture of T1 and T2 weighting, and although they provide good anatomic details, the tissue contrast is somewhat impaired (Fig. 2.42). IR sequences can be combined with multiplanar imaging to shorten scan time. With a short inversion time (TI), in the range of 100 to 150 msec, the effects of prolonged T1 and T2 relaxation times are cumulative and the signal from fat is suppressed. This technique, called *short time IR* (STIR),

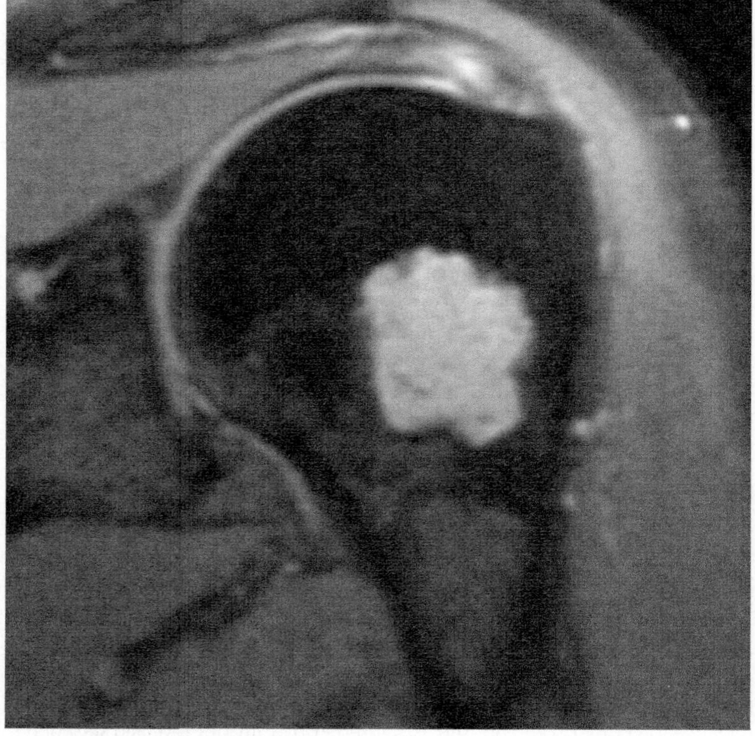

FIGURE 2.41 T2-weighted image. Coronal T2-weighted MR image of the left shoulder demonstrates a high signal intensity lobulated lesion with small low-signal calcifications within it, a characteristic appearance of an enchondroma.

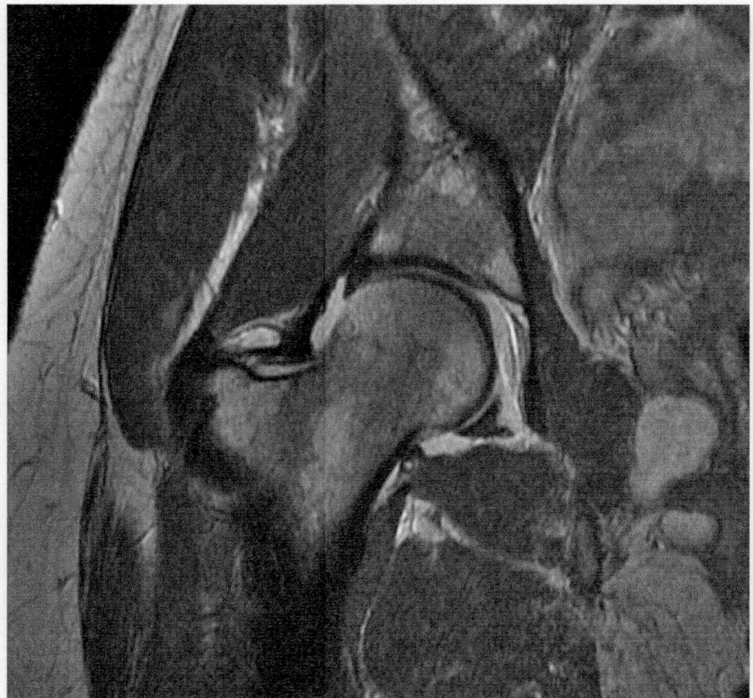

FIGURE 2.42 PD-weighted image. Coronal PD-weighted MR image of the right hip shows normal appearance of the bones, joint, and surrounding muscles.

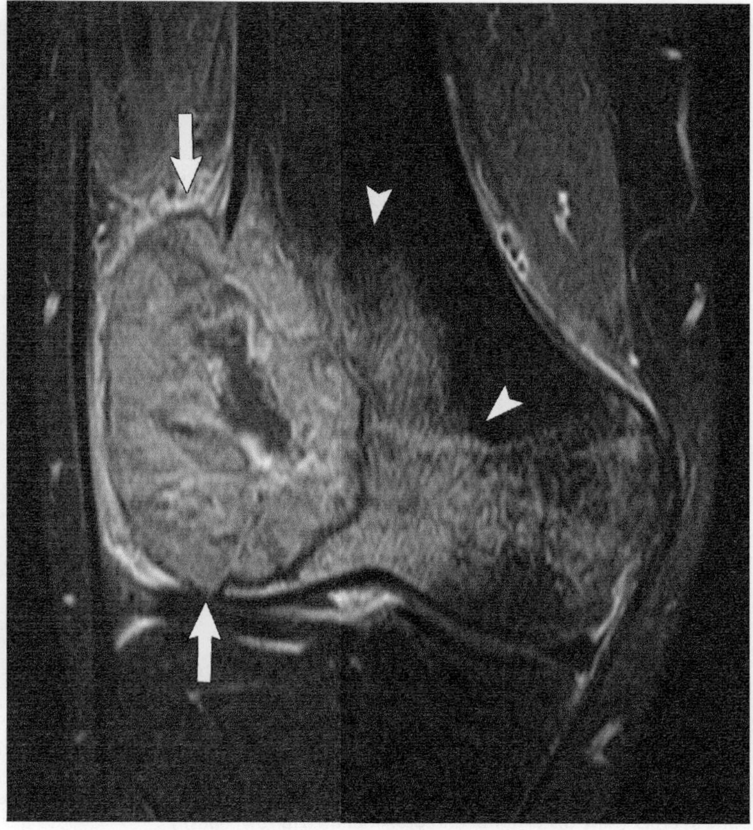

FIGURE 2.43 STIR image. Coronal STIR MR image of the right knee shows a large heterogenous mass occupying the entire lateral femoral condyle *(arrows)* that on an open biopsy proved to be a giant cell tumor. Observe high signal peritumoral edema *(arrowheads)*.

has been useful for evaluating bone tumors (Fig. 2.43). CHESS is a sequence also used for fat signal suppression. In this sequence, the chemical shift artifacts are removed, and the high-intensity fat signal is suppressed; thus, the effective dynamic range of signal intensities is increased, and contrast depiction of anatomic details is improved.

Fat suppression technique is commonly used in MRI to detect adipose tissue or suppress the signal from adipose tissue. There are three methods to achieve this goal: frequency-selective (chemical) fat saturation, inversion–recovery imaging, and opposed-phase imaging (Table 2.1). The selection of one of these methods depends on the purpose of fat suppression, whether it is used to enhance the contrast or to characterize the tissue and the amount of fat in the tissue under investigation. *Fat saturation* methods are usually chosen for the suppression of signal from large amounts of adipose tissue and to provide a good contrast resolution. This technique can be used with any imaging sequence (Fig. 2.44). It is useful to visualize small anatomic details, for example, in postcontrast MRa (see Figs. 2.57 and 2.58). *Inversion–recovery* method (such as STIR sequence) allows homogeneous and global fat suppression; however, the generated images have low signal-to-noise ratio, and this technique is not only specific for fat (see Fig 2.43). *Opposed-phase* method is recommended for the demonstration of lesions that contain only small amounts of fat. The inability of this technique to detect small tumors embedded in adipose tissue is the main disadvantage.

Recently, the LAVA Flex 3D FSPGR imaging technique has been introduced that generates water only, fat only, in phase and out of phase echoes in one single acquisition, that is typically completed in single breath hold. This technique provides excellent homogeneous fat suppression over the entire field of view, including areas that are difficult to image using conventional fat suppression due to magnetic susceptibility effect.

Fat suppression techniques have been combined with 3D gradient-echo imaging, resulting in superior delineation of articular cartilage. The main indication for fat suppression is the assessment of small amounts of bone marrow edema in the subchondral bone, often accompanying osteochondral pathology such as in osteochondral fractures, osteochondritis dissecans, or osteonecrosis.

TABLE 2.1 Fat Suppression Techniques

Methods	Advantages	Disadvantages
Frequency-selective (chemical) fat saturation	Lipid-specific Signal in nonfat tissue unaffected Excellent imaging of small anatomic detail Can be used with any imaging sequence	Occasionally inadequate fat suppression Water signal may be suppressed. Heterogeneities in areas of sharp variations in anatomic structures Increased imaging time
Short time inversion recovery (STIR)	Excellent contrast resolution Very good for tumor detection Can be used with low-field-strength magnets	Low signal-to-noise ratio Tissue with a short T1 and long T1 may produce the same signal intensity. Signal from mucoid tissue, hemorrhage, and proteinaceous fluid may be suppressed.
Opposed-phase	Ability to demonstrate small amounts of lipid tissue Simple, fast, and available on every magnetic resonance imaging (MRI) system	Fat signal only partially suppressed Suppresses water signal Difficult to detect small tumors imbedded in fat In postgadolinium studies, contrast material may be undetected.

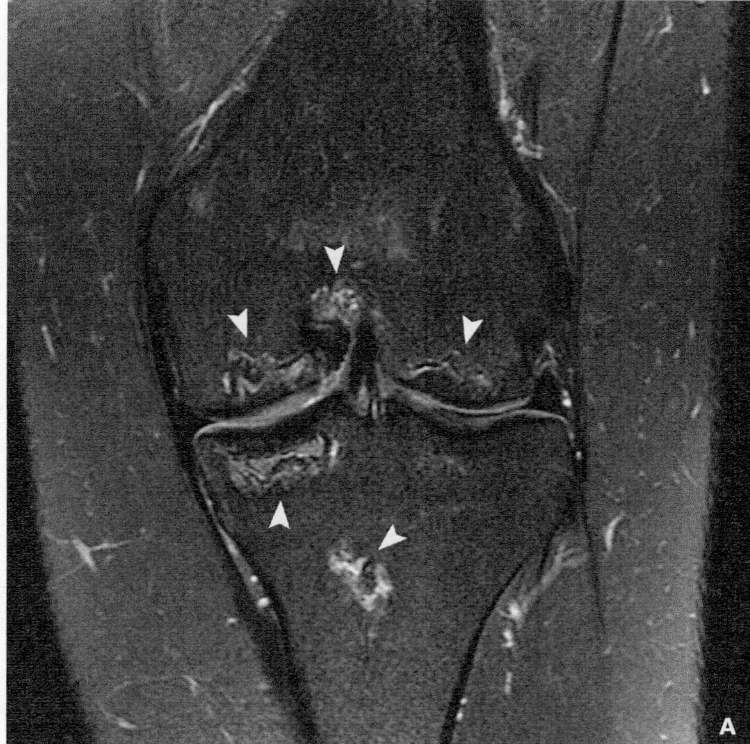

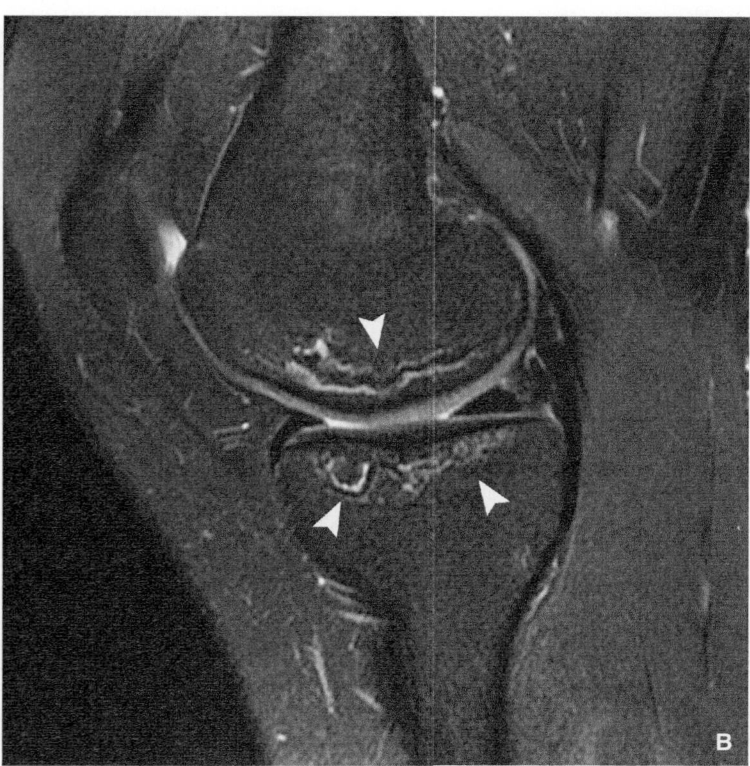

FIGURE 2.44 Fat-suppressed images. Coronal **(A)** and sagittal **(B)** PD-weighted fat-suppressed MR images of the left knee clearly demonstrate numerous medullary bone infarcts in the distal femur and proximal tibia *(arrowheads)*.

Fast imaging techniques have a number of advantages compared with much slower conventional SE imaging. *Gradient-recalled echo* (GRE) pulse sequences using variable flip angles (5 to 90 degrees) are frequently used in orthopaedic imaging because they represent a very effective means of performing fast MRI. The major advantage is the shortening of imaging time because the low flip angle rf pulses destroy only a small part of the longitudinal magnetization in each pulse cycle. In general, gradient-echo imaging can be performed using either a 2D technique or a 3D so-called *volume technique*. There are several different types of GRE methods in clinical use. Each of these methods relies on using a reduced flip angle to enhance signal with short TR. These techniques are known by a variety of acronyms such as FLASH (fast low-angle shot), FISP (fast imaging with steady procession), GRASS (gradient-recalled acquisition in the steady state), and MPGR (multiplanar gradient recalled) (see Fig. 2.52D). Gradient-echo sequences are particularly useful in imaging articular cartilage and loose bodies in the joint. The drawback of this technique is the so-called *susceptibility effect*, which results in artificial signal loss at the interface between tissues of different magnetic properties. This factor limits the use of gradient-echo sequences when imaging patients with metallic hardware. Another disadvantage of GRE techniques is their relatively low usefulness for the detection of bone marrow pathology due to the susceptibility artifacts created within the intertrabecular spaces.

When using MRI in the musculoskeletal system, one has to be aware of an important and very prevalent artifact known as *magic angle artifact*. This artifact occurs when imaging collagen-rich structures oriented approximately 55 degrees with main magnetic field and when using pulse sequences with TE of 20 msec or lower. Under these circumstances, there is an increase in signal intensity of the structure being imaged giving a false impression of an abnormality. Portions of tendon, ligaments, and articular cartilage in or around the joints are often oriented about 55 degrees to the magnetic field and when imaged using low TE sequences (T1-weighted, proton density [PD]-weighted, and GRE techniques) tears and tendinosis or cartilage pathology may be simulated (Figs. 2.45 and 2.46).

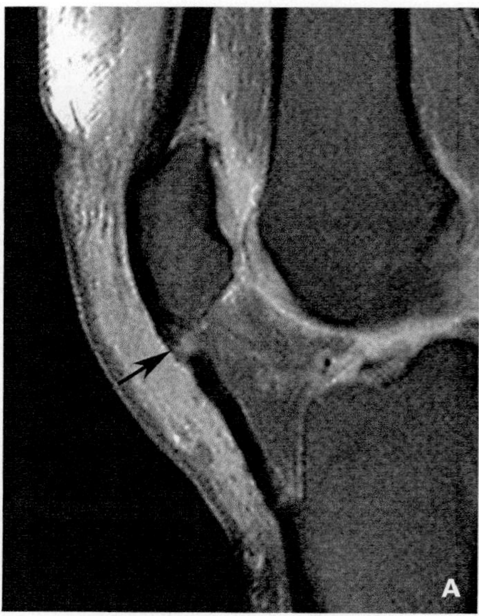

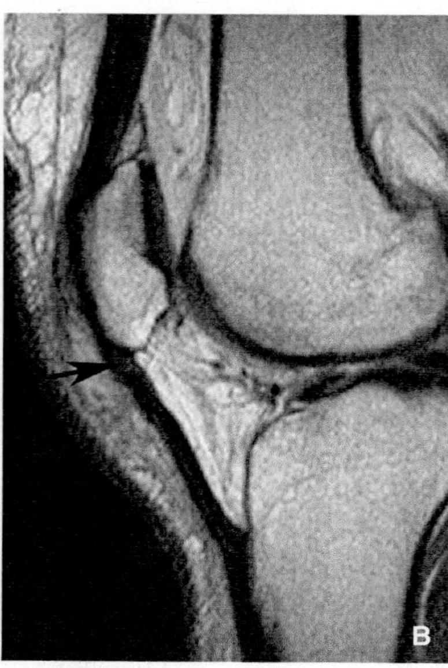

FIGURE 2.45 Magic angle artifact. **(A)** Sagittal PD-weighted fat-saturated MR image (TR 2,500 msec/TE 20 msec) of the knee demonstrates a focal area of increase signal intensity in the proximal patellar ligament *(arrow)* at the point where the ligament is oriented about 55 degrees with the B_0 axis of the magnetic field. **(B)** Sagittal T2-weighted MR image (TR 2,500 msec/TE 90 msec) demonstrates normal low signal intensity in the same area *(arrow)*, confirming a normal patellar ligament.

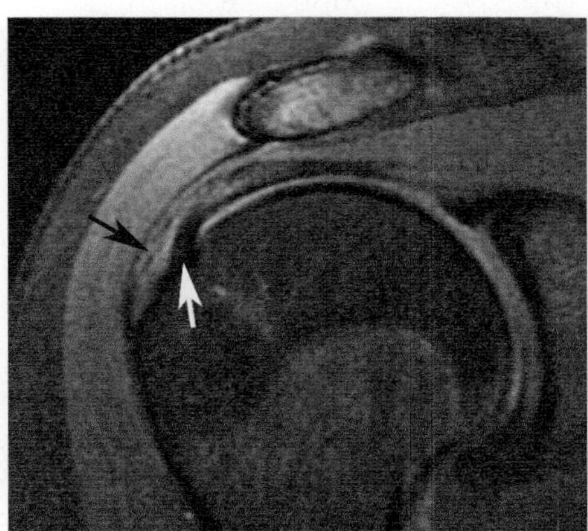

FIGURE 2.46 **Magic angle artifact.** Oblique coronal PD-weighted fat-saturated MR image (TR 2,450 msec/TE 20 msec) of the right shoulder demonstrates increased signal intensity of the superficial articular fibers of the supraspinatus tendon *(black arrow)* as they turn to a 55-degree angle with the B_0 axis of the magnetic field to insert into the greater tuberosity of the humerus. Note the normal low signal intensity of the deep fibers of the supraspinatus tendon *(white arrow)* oriented at less than 55-degree angulation.

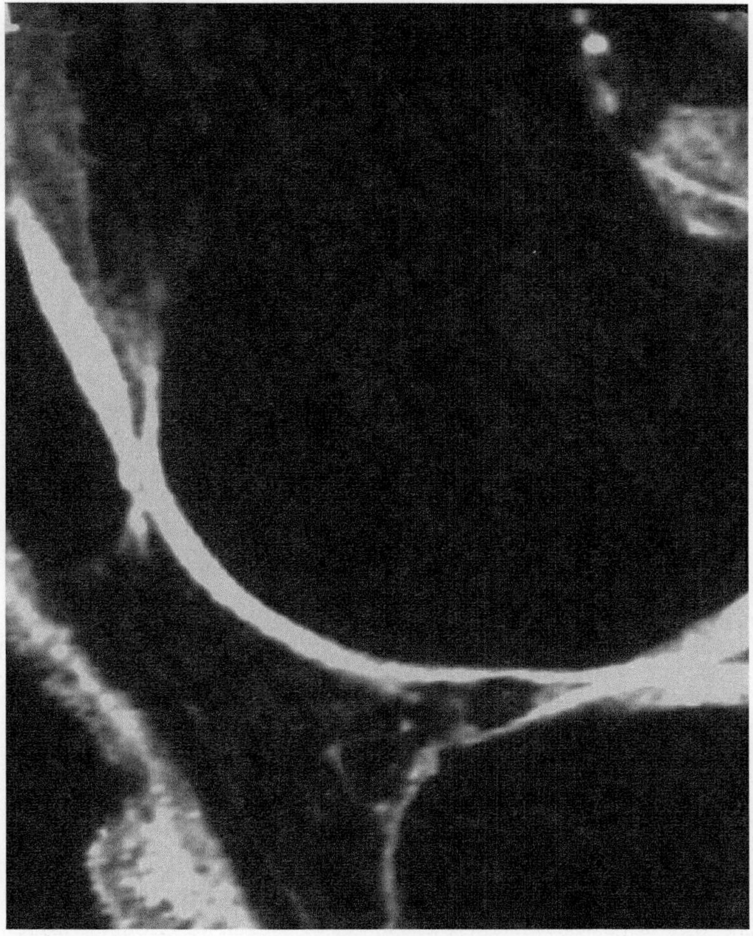

FIGURE 2.48 **MRI of cartilage.** Sagittal 3D Fourier transform fat-saturated FLASH image of the knee shows contrast between the bright articular cartilage and the adjacent infrapatellar fat, allowing excellent visualization of the articular cartilage.

MRI of articular cartilage has recently been recognized as an effective tool for the characterization of cartilage morphology, biochemistry, and function. Given the prevalence of cartilage pathology in humans (degeneration, trauma, arthritis), MRI researchers have focused their attention in developing optimal pulse sequences that would display accurately early degeneration and minor surface alterations of the articular cartilage in order to provide early therapy and/or intervention and to monitor noninvasively the effects of new therapies. A widely used pulse sequence for cartilage imaging is 2D or 3D spoiled gradient-echo (SPGR) (with fat saturation), also known as *FLASH*, depending on the manufacturer (Figs. 2.47 and 2.48). This pulse sequence provides high-resolution contiguous thin slices with excellent delineation of morphologic and subtle signal alterations. Disadvantages of this technique include long imaging time and sensitivity to susceptibility artifacts, as indicated earlier.

2D fast spin echo (FSE) imaging techniques with or without fat suppression allow high-resolution images in a relatively short time and have the advantage of being part of a standard protocol for joint imaging.

New pulse sequences for cartilage imaging are continuously evolving specially with the more extended use of 3 T magnetic resonance (MR) systems. Some of these new sequences include fast imaging employing steady-state acquisition (FIESTA) or its variants fast imaging with steady-state precession (true FISP) and balanced fast field echo and its variant, fluctuating equilibrium MR (FEMR) imaging; multiecho techniques such as dual echo in the steady state (DESS) (Fig. 2.49); driven equilibrium techniques such as driven equilibrium Fourier transform (DEFT) and fast-recovery FSE; echo-planar techniques such as 3D echo-planar imaging with fat suppression and 3D DEFT; and 3D FSE methods.

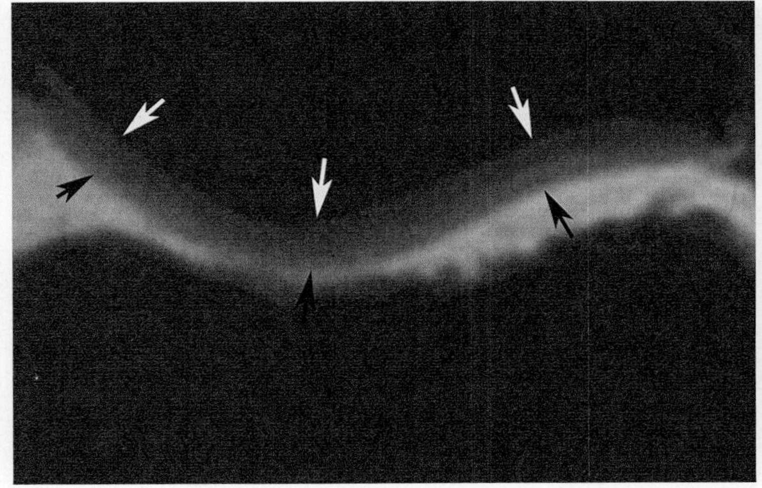

FIGURE 2.47 **MRI of cartilage.** Axial 2D Fourier transform FLASH image of the knee shows the hyaline articular cartilage of the patella *(arrows)* against the joint fluid.

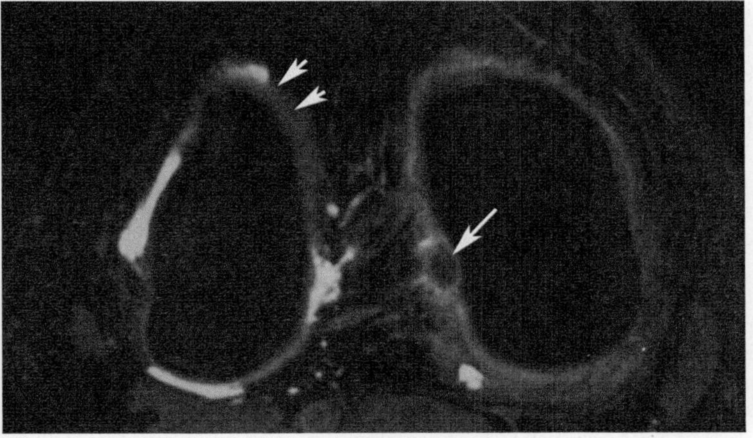

FIGURE 2.49 **MRI of cartilage.** Axial DESS pulse sequence of the knee demonstrates a displaced fragment of the medial meniscus *(long arrow)*. Note the contrast between the joint fluid and the articular hyaline cartilage in the lateral femoral condyle *(short arrows)*.

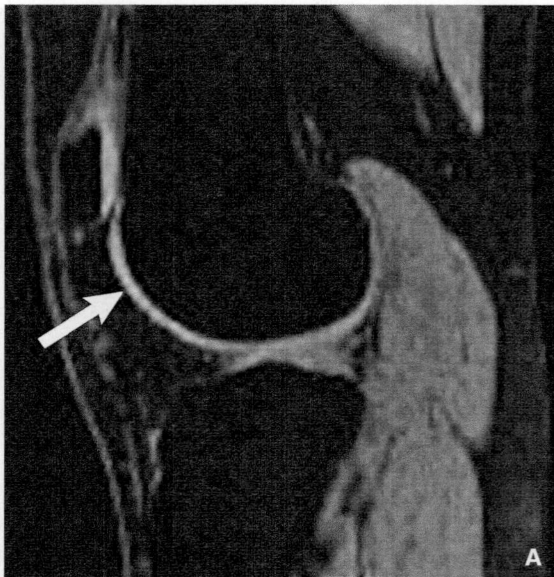

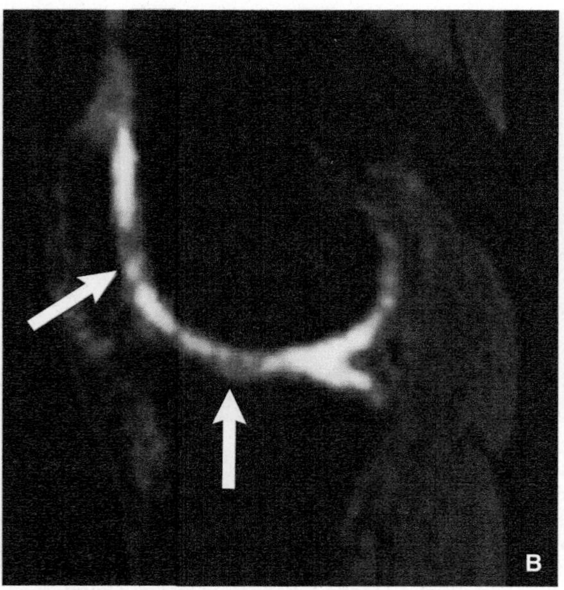

FIGURE 2.50 ^{23}Na MRI of the articular cartilage. **(A)** 2D sagittal PD-weighted FSE MR image of the knee shows normal articular cartilage of the distal femur *(arrow)*. **(B)** Same knee examined with ^{23}Na FLASH PD-weighted MRI demonstrates a focal loss of GAG *(arrows)* consistent with early osteoarthritis. (Courtesy of PZWL Wydawnictwo Lekarskie, Warsaw, Poland.)

Interest in measuring specific structural and biochemical components of the cartilage has led to techniques such as T2 mapping, ultrashort echo time (UTE) imaging, diffusion-weighted imaging (DWI), T1-rho (i.e., T1 in the rotating frame), and sodium-23 (^{23}Na) MRI. Because ^{23}Na atoms are associated with negatively charged glycosaminoglycan (GAG), loss of GAG due to cartilage degeneration results in loss of sodium ions from the tissue. That mechanism provides the basis for the latter technique, which proved to be effective in assessing the loss of proteoglycan (PG) molecules from the cartilage matrix in very early stages of osteoarthritis (Fig. 2.50). A novel approach to the assessment of biochemical changes within a morphologically intact cartilage is a contrast agent–based technique known as *delayed gadolinium-enhanced MRI of the cartilage* (d-GEMRIC). This technique measures the T1 variations within the cartilage following intravenous injection of Gd-DTPA negatively charged and provides information regarding cartilage GAG content (Fig. 2.51). The newest improvement in the evaluation of articular cartilage of the knee is the introduction of so-called *vastly undersampled isotropic projection steady-state free precession* (VIPR-SSFP) imaging pulse sequence, which combines balanced SSFP technique with 3D radial multiplayer image acquisition. In addition to providing important clinical information regarding the cartilage, this technique is also effective in the evaluation of the ligaments, menisci, and osseous structures of the knee in symptomatic patients. FEMR, mentioned already in the prior text, is a variant of SSFP, a technique that, by rendering a bright fluid signal while preserving cartilage signal, is also useful in cartilage imaging. Finally, it is worthy to mention the most recent trials of cartilage imaging using Fourier transform infrared microscopy (FTIR-MS), a method based on the absorption infrared light by molecules at characteristic frequencies, which yielded very promising results.

It is beyond the scope of this book to describe in detail these pulse sequences. The reader is referred to the excellent review article by Recht et al. (2007).

In most examinations, at least two orthogonal planes should be obtained (axial and either coronal or sagittal), and on many occasions, all three planes are necessary. Not infrequently, oblique planes need to be obtained in order to demonstrate the anatomy more accurately (i.e., shoulder). For adequate MRI, surface coils are necessary because they provide improved spatial resolution. Most surface coils are designed specifically for different areas of the body such as the knee, shoulder, wrist, and temporomandibular joints. Recently introduced is an eight-channel phased array extremity coil that tremendously increased the quality of MR image (see Fig. 7.40).

The use of MRI in orthopaedic radiology, previously confined to four areas (trauma, arthritides, tumors, and infections), has expanded to the evaluation of other types of pathology such as congenital disorders, vascular conditions, and avascular necrosis, just to name a few. The musculoskeletal system is ideally suited for the evaluation by MRI because different tissues display different signal intensities on T1- and T2-weighted images. The images displayed may have a low signal intensity, intermediate signal intensity, or high signal intensity. *Low signal intensity* may be subdivided into signal void (black) and signal lower than that of normal muscle (dark). *Intermediate signal intensity* may be subdivided into signal equal to that of normal muscle and signal higher than that of muscle but lower than that of subcutaneous fat (bright). *High signal intensity* may be subdivided into signal equal to that of normal subcutaneous fat (bright) and signal higher than that of subcutaneous fat (extremely bright). High signal intensity of fat planes and differences in the signal intensity of various structures allow the separation of the different tissue components including muscles, tendons, ligaments, vessels, nerves, hyaline cartilage, fibrocartilage, cortical bone, and trabecular bone (Fig. 2.52). For instance, fat and yellow (fatty) bone marrows display high signal intensity on T1-weighted images and intermediate signal on T2-weighted images; hematomas (acute or subacute) display relatively high signal intensity on T1 and T2 sequences. Cortical bone, air, ligaments, tendons, and fibrocartilage display low signal intensity on T1- and T2-weighted images; muscle, nerves, and hyaline cartilage display intermediate signal intensity on T1- and T2-weighted images. Red (hematopoietic) marrow displays low signal on T1-weighted images and low-to-intermediate signal on T2-weighted images. Fluid displays intermediate signal on T1-weighted images and high signal on T2-weighted images. Most tumors display low-to-intermediate signal intensity on T1-weighted images and high signal intensity on T2-weighted images. Lipomas display high signal intensity on T1-weighted images and intermediate signal on T2-weighted images (Table 2.2).

Traumatic conditions of the bones and soft tissues are particularly well suited to the diagnosis and evaluation by MRI. Some abnormalities, such as bone contusions or trabecular microfractures, not seen on radiography and CT are well demonstrated by this technique (Figs. 2.53 and 2.54). Occult fractures, which can be missed on conventional radiographs, become obvious on MRI (Figs. 2.55 and 2.56).

MRI proved to be successful in the diagnosis and evaluation of athletic pubalgia and so-called *sports hernia*, depicting abnormalities of pubic symphysis, of rectus abdominis insertional injury, and hip adductors tendon injury. The newest reports also revealed that MRI was effective in the diagnosis and evaluation of acute and subacute denervation of skeletal muscles.

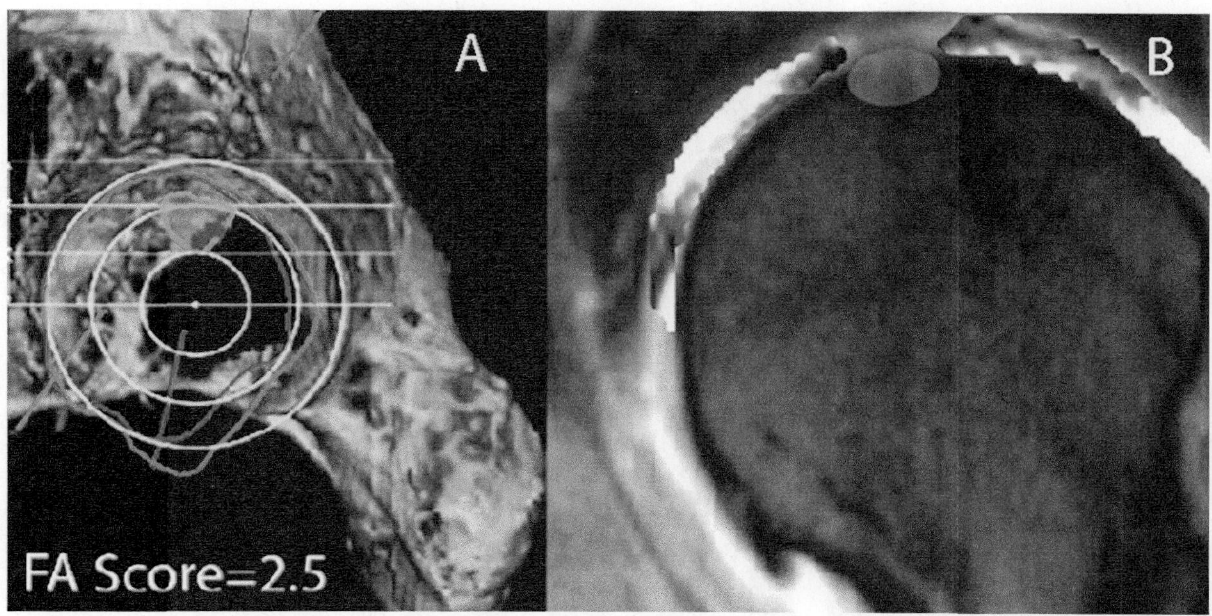

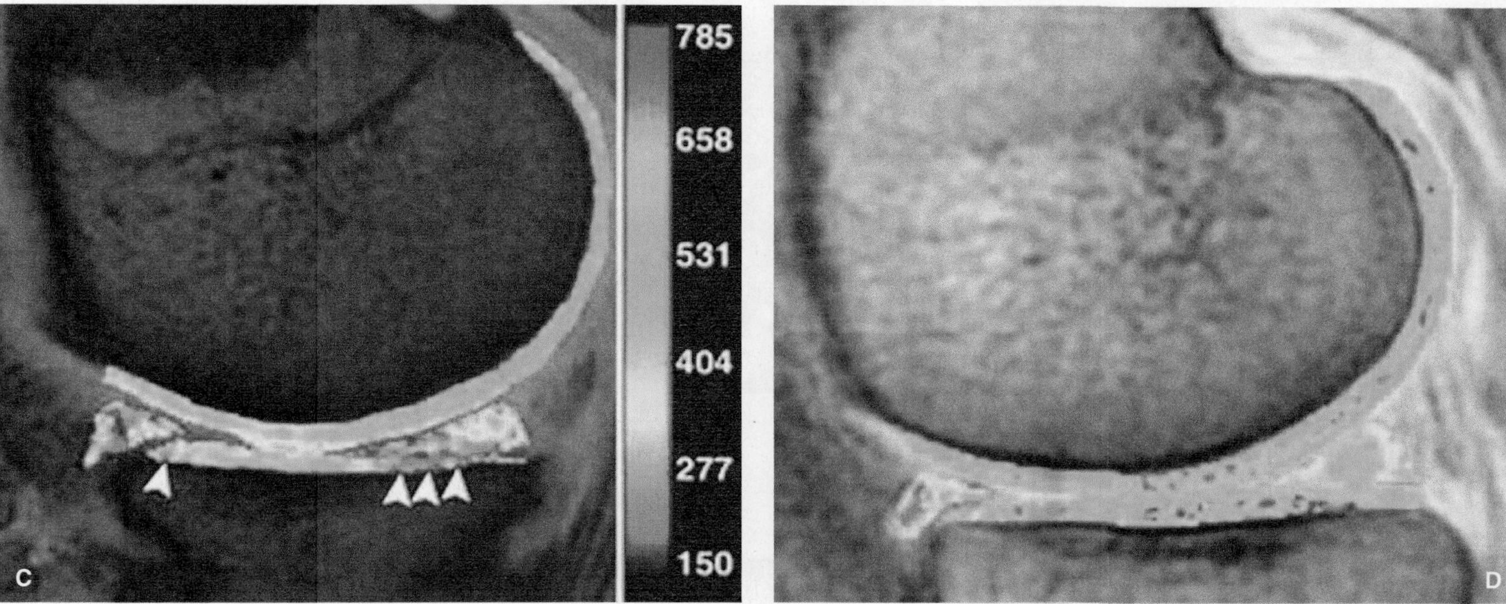

FIGURE 2.51 d-GEMRIC MRI of cartilage. 3D MR reconstructions of the hip **(A)** and d-GEMRIC MRI **(B)** in a patient with hip dysplasia. The 3D reconstructions are generated from MR data obtained during a conventional MRI of the hip. These 3D models are used to assess the osseous morphologic abnormalities and injuries that can occur along the surfaces of the acetabulum and femoral head in the setting of hip dysplasia. The d-GEMRIC parametric maps are generated from MR data obtained during intravenous administration of gadolinium contrast. These maps are used to assess biochemical abnormalities of cartilage in the hip joint that may occur in the setting of hip dysplasia. (Courtesy of Luis Beltran, MD and Jenny Bencardino, MD, New York.) **(C)** In another patient, sagittal MR image of the knee using d-GEMRIC technique shows cartilage changes typical of osteoarthritis *(arrowheads)*. **(D)** Normal appearance of the knee cartilage using the same technique is shown for comparison. (Courtesy of Prof. Herwig Imhof, Vienna, Austria.)

Occasionally, MR images may be enhanced by an intravenous injection of Gd-DTPA, known as *gadolinium*, a paramagnetic compound that demonstrates increased signal intensity on T1-weighted images. The mechanism by which gadolinium produces enhancement in MRI is fundamentally different from the mechanism of contrast enhancement occurring in CT. Unlike iodine in CT, gadolinium itself produces no MRI signal. Instead, it acts by shortening the T1 and T2 relaxation times of tissues into which it extravasates, resulting in an increase in signal intensity on T1-weighted (short TR/TE) imaging sequences.

MRa has become popular in recent years. The diagnostic accuracy of this technique may exceed that of conventional MRI because the intraarticular structures are better demonstrated if they are separated by means of capsular distention. Such distention can be achieved with an intraarticular injection of a contrast material such as diluted gadopentetate dimeglumine (gadolinium) or saline. Most commonly, a mixture of sterile saline, iodinated contrast agent, 1% lidocaine (or Xylocaine), and Gd-DTPA is injected into the joint under fluoroscopic guidance. The generated images are very similar to those obtained of the joint with preexisting joint fluid (joint effusion). In clinical practice, MRa is predominantly used in the evaluation of shoulder abnormalities, such as internal derangement, glenohumeral joint instability, rotator cuff disorders, or articular cartilage and cartilaginous labrum abnormalities (Fig. 2.57). This technique is equally effective in the evaluation of the fibrocartilaginous labrum of the acetabulum. In particular, femoroacetabular impingement (FAI) syndrome can be accurately diagnosed with MRa, especially when combined with radial reconstruction sequences (Fig. 2.58). The advantages of radial acquisitions are avoidance of partial volume averaging and the elimination of distorted anatomic details.

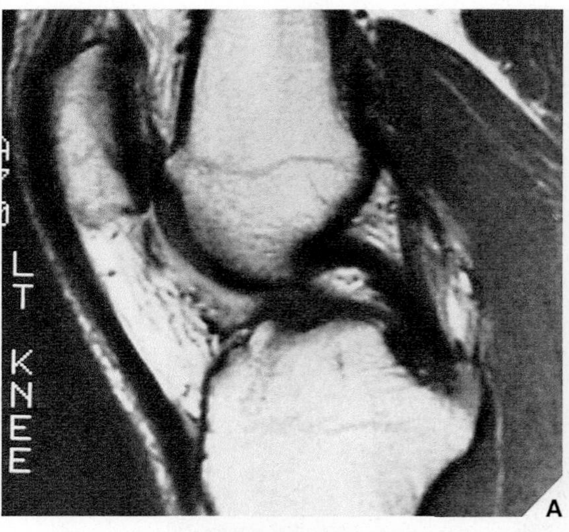

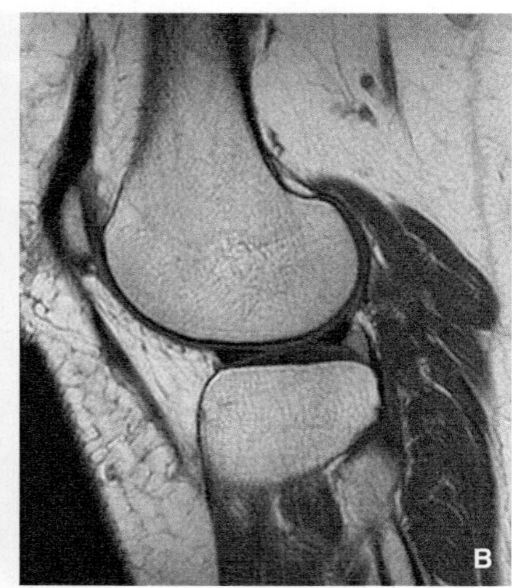

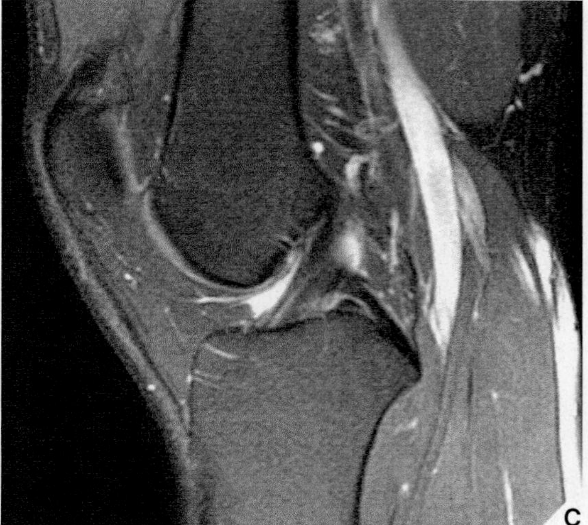

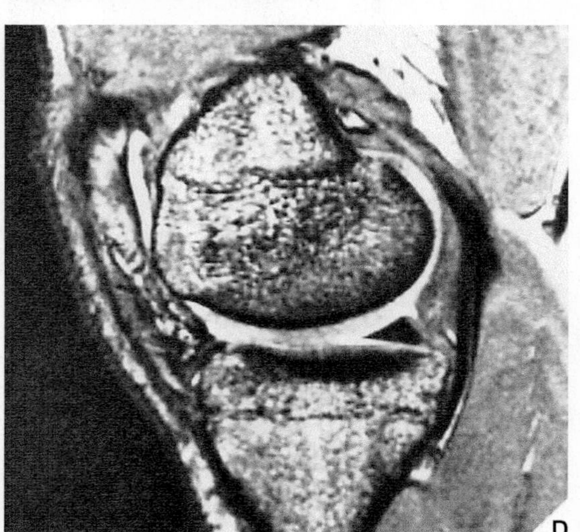

FIGURE 2.52 MRI of the knee. Sagittal SE T1-weighted image **(A)** (TR 600/TE 20 msec), sagittal PD-weighted image **(B)** (TR 2,366/TE 40 msec), sagittal PD-weighted fat-saturated image **(C)** (TR 3,300/TE 40 msec), and sagittal MPGR T2*-weighted image **(D)** (flip angle 30 degrees, TR 35/TE 15 msec) demonstrate various anatomic structures clearly depicted because of variations in signal intensity of bone, articular cartilage, fibrocartilage, ligaments, muscles, and fat.

TABLE 2.2 Magnetic Resonance Imaging Signal Intensities of Various Tissues

	Image	
Tissue	**T1 Weighted**	**T2 Weighted**
Hematoma, hemorrhage (acute, subacute)	Intermediate/high	High
Hematoma, hemorrhage (chronic)	Low	Low
Fat, fatty marrow	High	Intermediate
Muscle, nerves, hyaline cartilage	Intermediate	Intermediate
Cortical bone, tendons, ligaments, fibrocartilage, scar tissue	Low	Low
Hyaline cartilage	Intermediate	Intermediate
Red (hematopoietic) marrow	Low	Intermediate
Air	Low	Low
Fluid	Intermediate	High
Proteinaceous fluid	High	High
Tumors (generally)	Intermediate to low	High
Lipoma	High	Intermediate
Hemangioma	Intermediate (slightly higher than muscle)	High

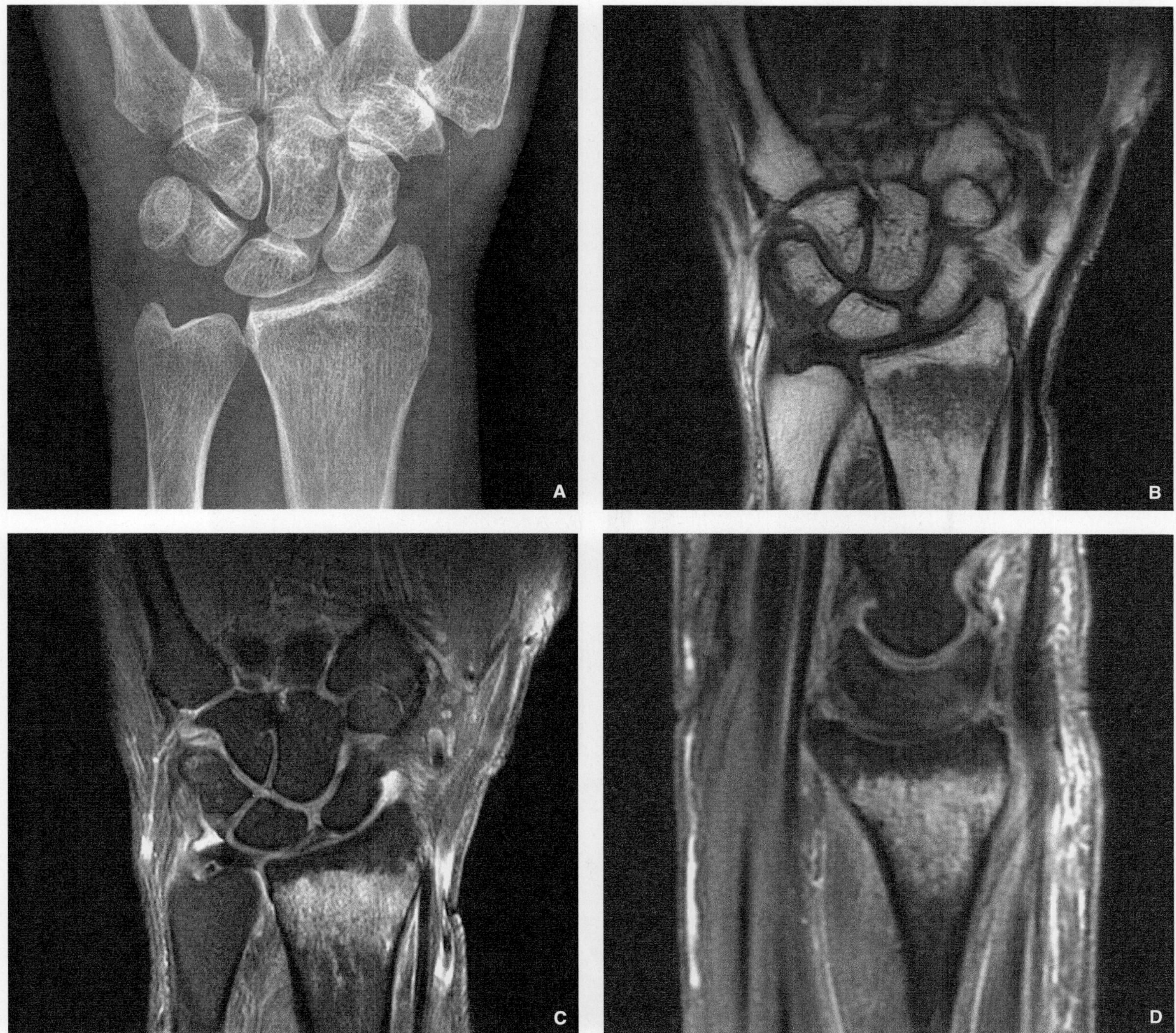

FIGURE 2.53 Bone contusion (trabecular injury). **(A)** Dorsovolar radiograph of the left wrist of a 40-year-old woman who presented with history of trauma to the distal forearm shows no traumatic abnormalities. **(B)** Coronal T1-weighted MR image shows a band of decreased signal intensity in the distal radius. Coronal **(C)** and sagittal **(D)** PD-weighted fat-suppressed MR images show band of increased signal intensity representing trabecular microfractures.

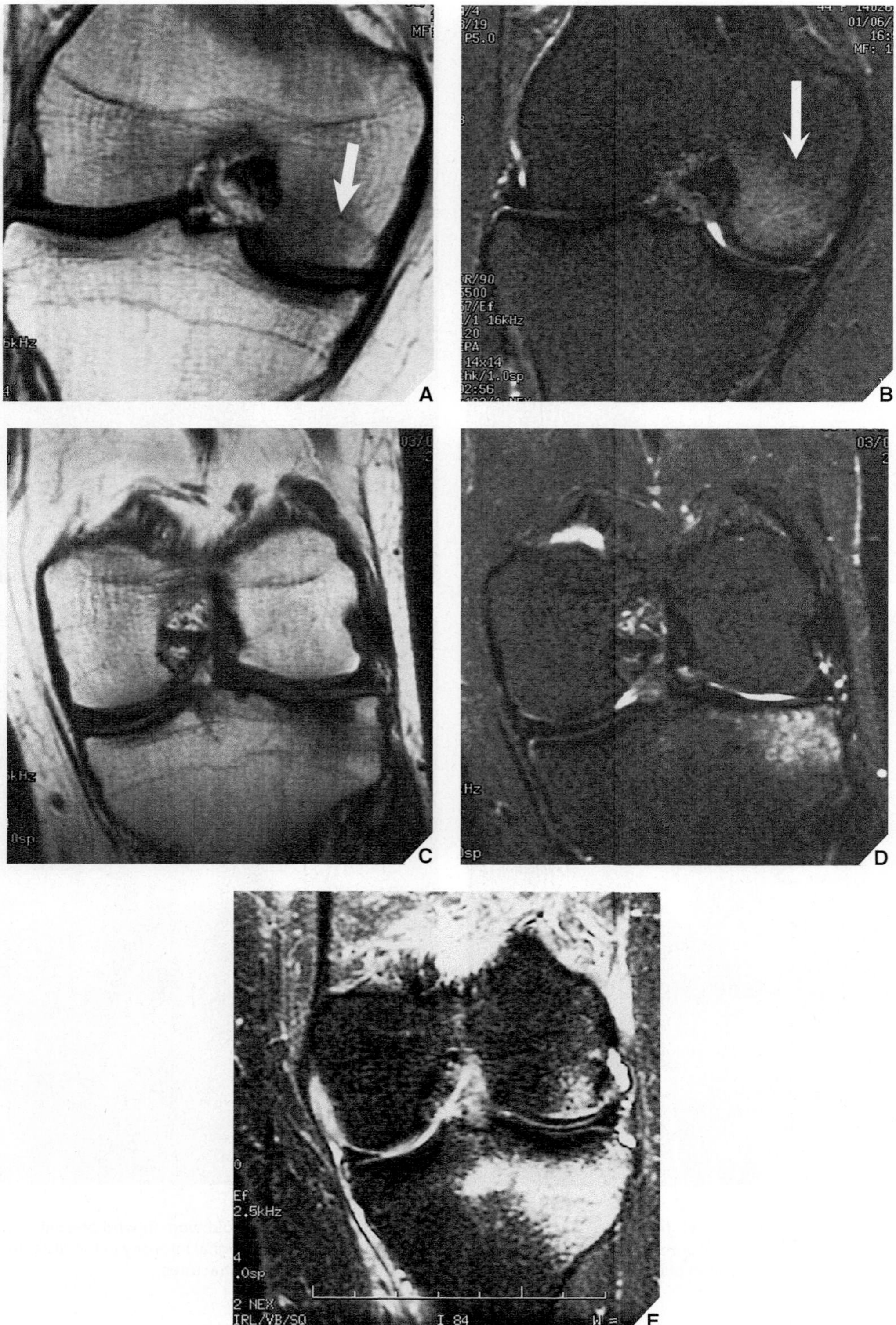

FIGURE 2.54 Bone contusion (trabecular injury). **(A)** Coronal T1-weighted MRI of a 44-year-old woman who sustained an injury to her right knee shows an area of low signal intensity in the medial femoral condyle *(arrow)*. **(B)** On the FSE-IR image, the trabecular injury becomes more conspicuous as a focus of high signal intensity against the low-intensity background of suppressed marrow fat *(arrow)*. In another patient, a 35-year-old man, T1-weighted **(C)** and FSE-IR **(D)** coronal MR images show a trabecular injury to the lateral aspect of tibial plateau of the left knee. In a 29-year-old woman, T2-weighted IR with fat saturation coronal MRI **(E)** shows a trabecular injury to the lateral femoral condyle and lateral aspect of the proximal tibia.

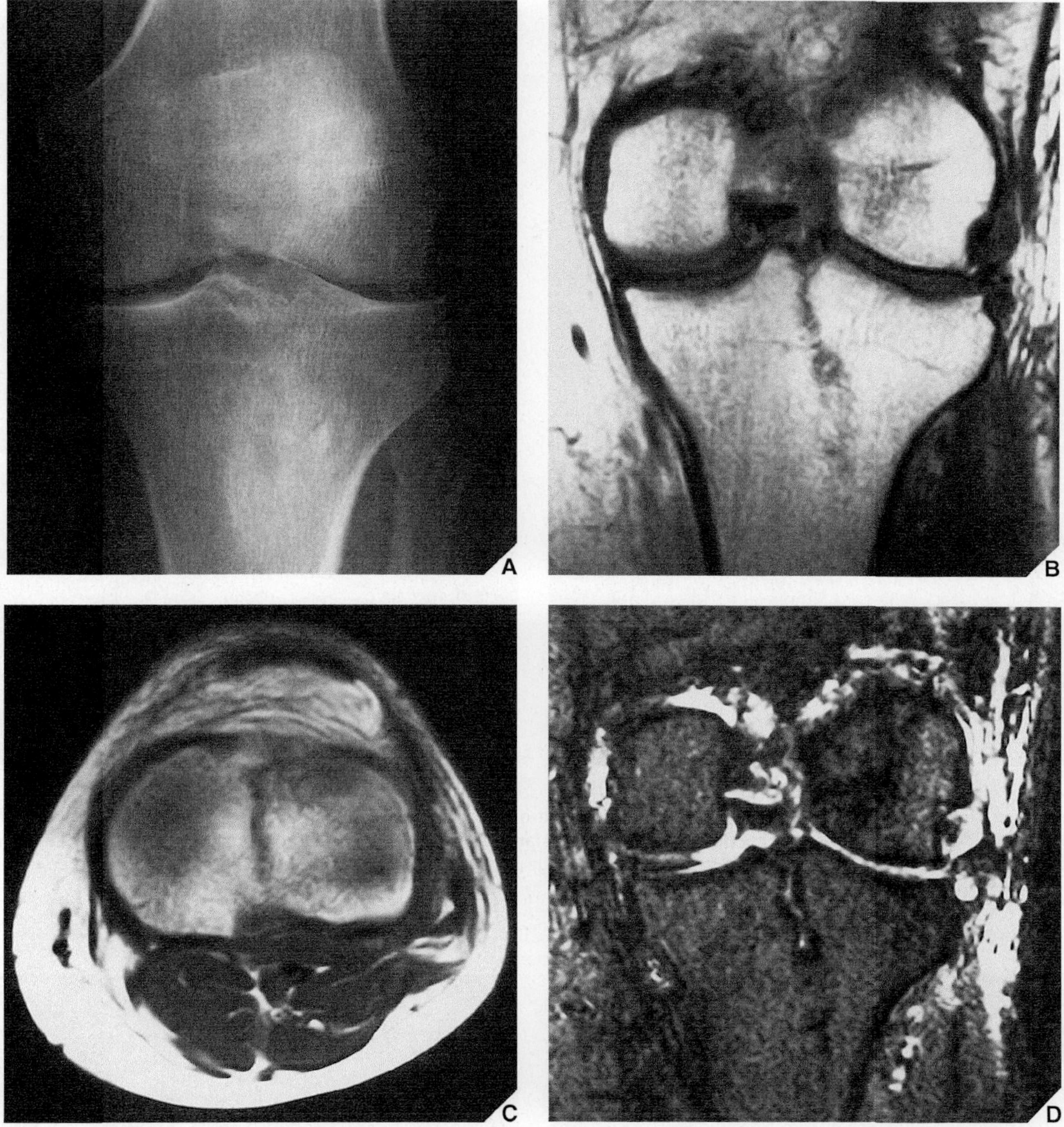

FIGURE 2.55 **Occult fracture of the tibia.** A 47-year-old woman sustained an injury to her left knee in a car accident. **(A)** Anteroposterior radiograph shows sclerotic area in the proximal tibia, but no definite fracture is apparent. Coronal **(B)** and axial **(C)** T1-weighted MR images demonstrate a vertical fracture line extending into the tibial spines. **(D)** A T2-weighted IR coronal MRI, in addition to the fracture line, shows the tears of the lateral meniscus and lateral collateral ligament, extensive soft-tissue edema and hemorrhage, and joint fluid.

Indirect MRa is a procedure in which an intravenous injection of gadolinium is administered before MRI examination of the joint. This technique, like direct MRa, may improve the detection of rotator cuff tears, labral pathology, and adhesive capsulitis.

The newest improvement in the evaluation of articular cartilage of the knee is the introduction of so-called *VIPR-SSFP* imaging pulse sequence that combines a balanced SSFP technique with a 3D radial multiplanar image acquisition (see the previous text). In addition to providing important clinical information regarding the cartilage, this technique is also effective in the evaluation of the ligaments, menisci, and osseous structures of the knee in symptomatic patients.

Magnetic resonance angiography (MRA) is a technique that helps to visualize blood vessels (Figs. 2.59 to 2.61). Unlike conventional contrast angiography, it does not visualize the blood volume itself but rather depicts a property of blood flow. One of its advantages is that after a 3D MRA data set is collected, one may choose any number of viewing directions. This feature also eliminates vascular overlapping. Numerous pulse sequences have been proposed to produce angiographic contrast. Some rely on the rapid inflow of relaxed blood into the region in which the stationary tissue is saturated. These methods are called *time of flight* (TOF) or *flow-related enhancement* (FRE). Others, which rely on the velocity-dependent change of phase of moving blood in the presence of a magnetic field gradient, are called the *phase-contrast methods*. Some methods involve the subtraction of flow-dephased images from flow-compensated images. Applications of MRA in orthopaedic radiology include the evaluation of the vascular structures in patients with trauma to the extremities and the assessment of vascularity of musculoskeletal neoplasms.

Although MRI has many advantages, disadvantages exist as well. These include the typical contraindications of scanning patients with cardiac pacemakers, cerebral aneurysm clips, and claustrophobia. The presence of metallic objects, such as ferromagnetic surgical clips, causes focal loss of signal with or without distortion of image. Metallic objects create "holes" in the image, but ferromagnetic objects cause more distortion. Similar to CT, an average volume effect may be observed in MR images, causing occasional pitfalls in interpretation.

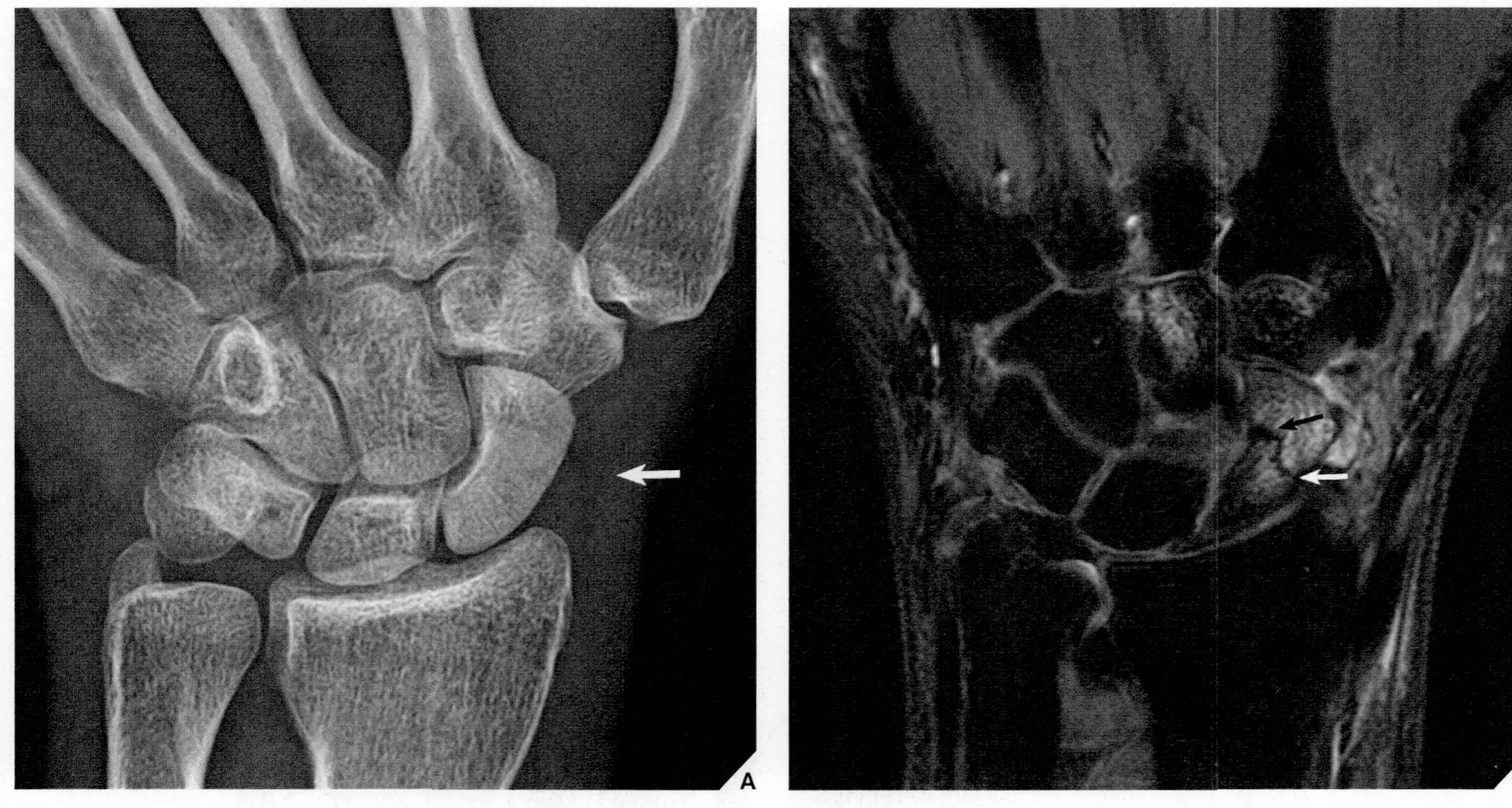

FIGURE 2.56 Occult fracture of scaphoid. A 46-year-old woman fell on the outstretched hand and presented with pain in the wrist and snuffbox tenderness. **(A)** Dorsovolar radiograph in ulnar deviation shows loss of the definition of scaphoid fat pad *(arrow)*, but no fracture line is evident on this view nor on the additional projections of the wrist (not shown here). **(B)** Coronal PD-weighted fat-suppressed MR image clearly shows scaphoid bone edema and a fracture line *(arrows)*.

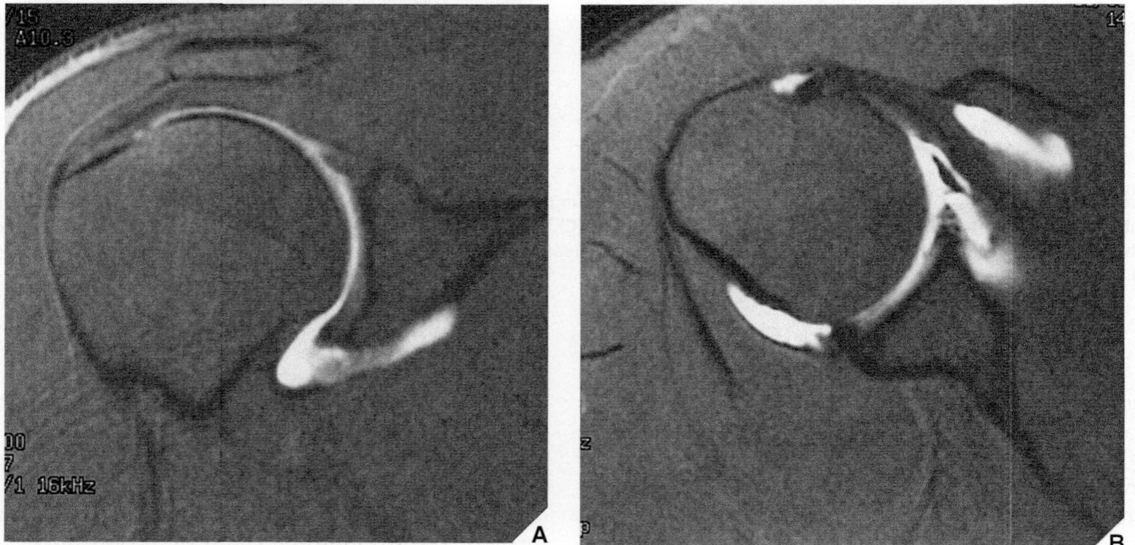

FIGURE 2.57 MRa of glenoid labrum tear. MRa of a 26-year-old man who sustained an injury to his right shoulder shows several abnormalities. **(A)** Coronal T1-weighted MR image with fat saturation shows a tear of the inferior cartilaginous labrum of the glenoid. **(B)** Axial T1-weighted MR image with fat saturation shows tears of the anterior and posterior cartilaginous labra associated with stripping of the anterior joint capsule.

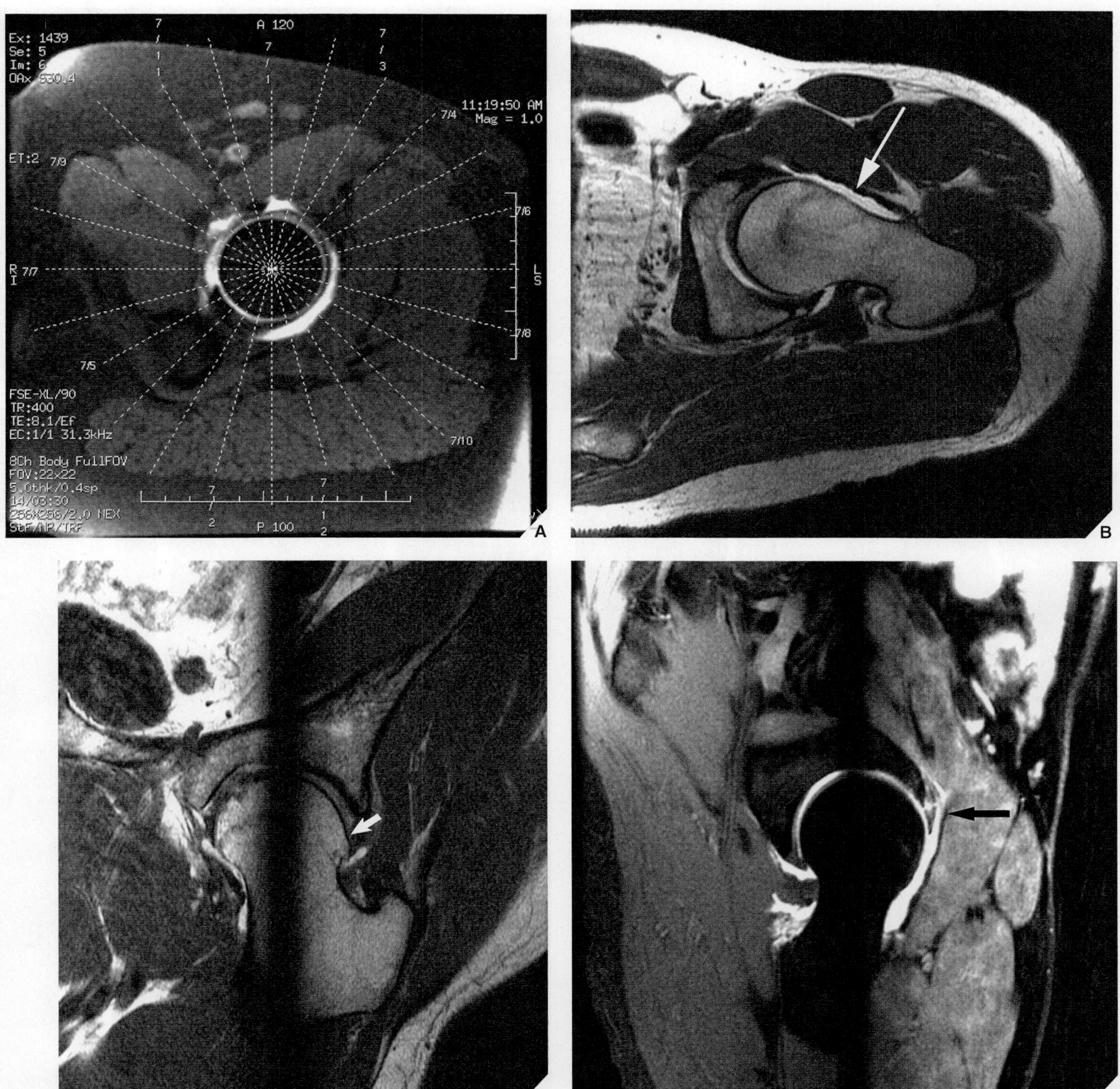

FIGURE 2.58 Radial MRa of a hip. A 28-year-old man presented with a left hip and groin pain for several months. Conventional radiographs (not shown here) were highly suggestive of a cam-type FAI syndrome, confirmed on radial MRa. **(A)** Prescription of the radial plane images off the oblique axial en face image of the acetabulum. **(B)** Transverse oblique FSE T1-weighted MR image obtained through the center of the femoral neck shows nonspherical shape of the femoral head and excessive bone formation at the anterosuperior aspect of the head/neck junction *(arrow)*. **(C)** The radial reformatted PD-weighted MR image shows a prominent osteophyte *(arrow)*. **(D)** Oblique axial PD-weighted fat-suppressed radial image shows a tear of the superior acetabular labrum *(arrow)*.

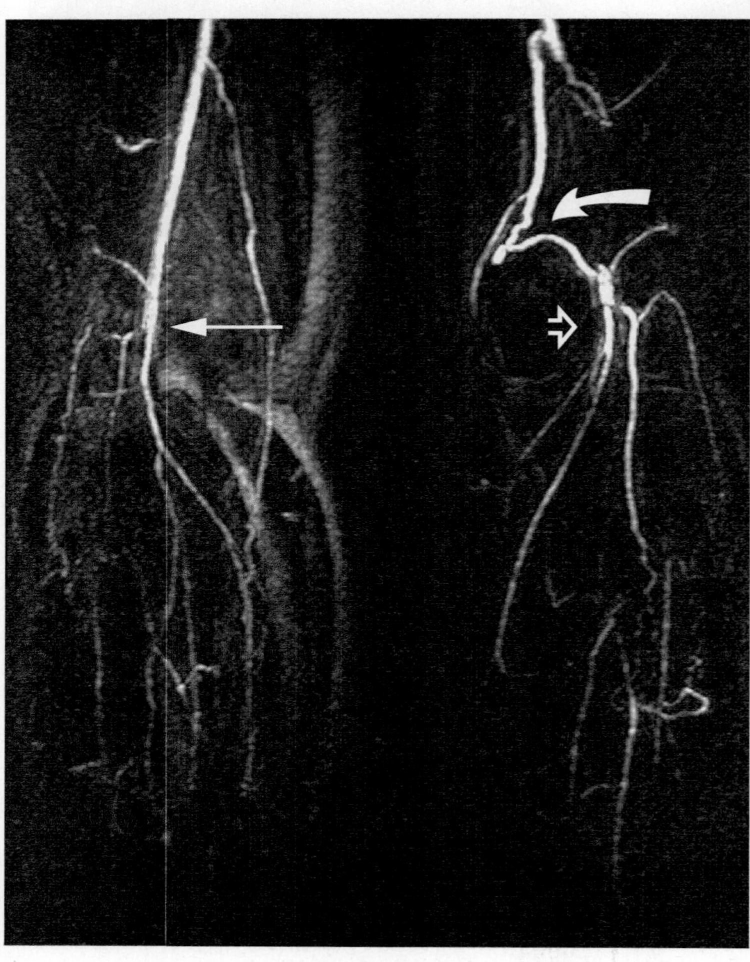

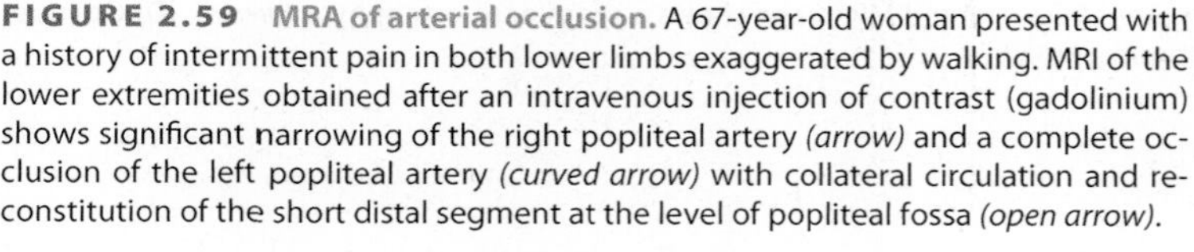

FIGURE 2.59 **MRA of arterial occlusion.** A 67-year-old woman presented with a history of intermittent pain in both lower limbs exaggerated by walking. MRI of the lower extremities obtained after an intravenous injection of contrast (gadolinium) shows significant narrowing of the right popliteal artery *(arrow)* and a complete occlusion of the left popliteal artery *(curved arrow)* with collateral circulation and reconstitution of the short distal segment at the level of popliteal fossa *(open arrow)*.

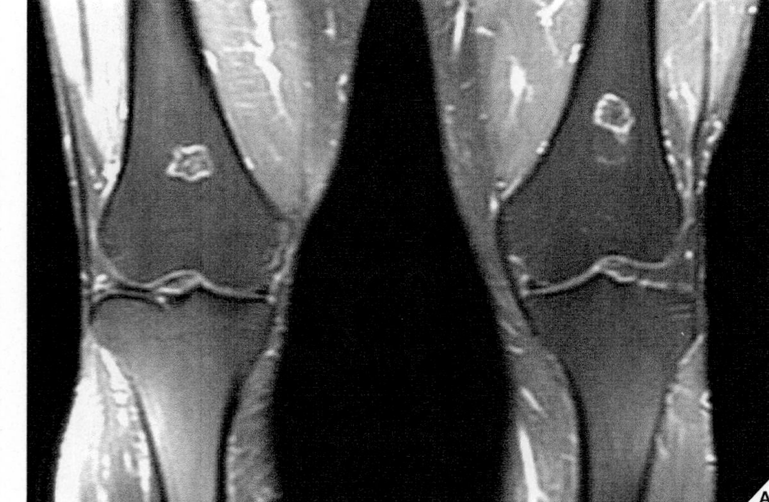

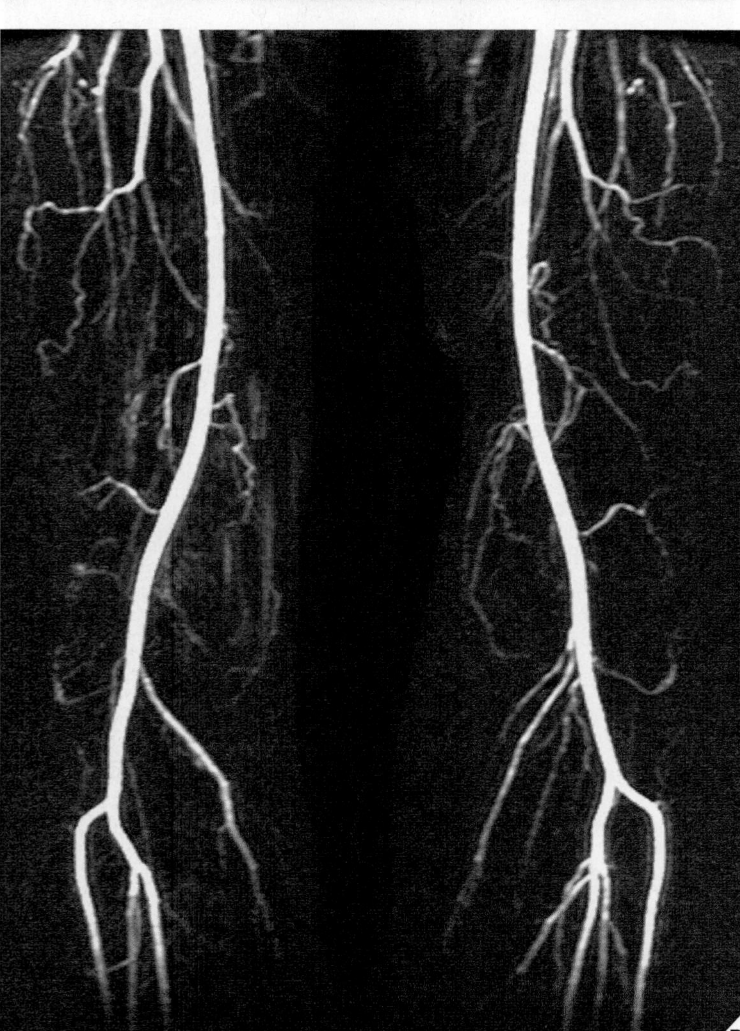

FIGURE 2.60 **MRA—normal findings.** A 27-year-old woman was diagnosed with mixed connective tissue disease. Because vasculitis and femoral artery occlusion were also clinically suspected, she underwent MRA. Coronal MR images of the knees **(A)** showed medullary bone infarction in the distal femora; however, MRA **(B)** demonstrated no abnormalities of the vessels.

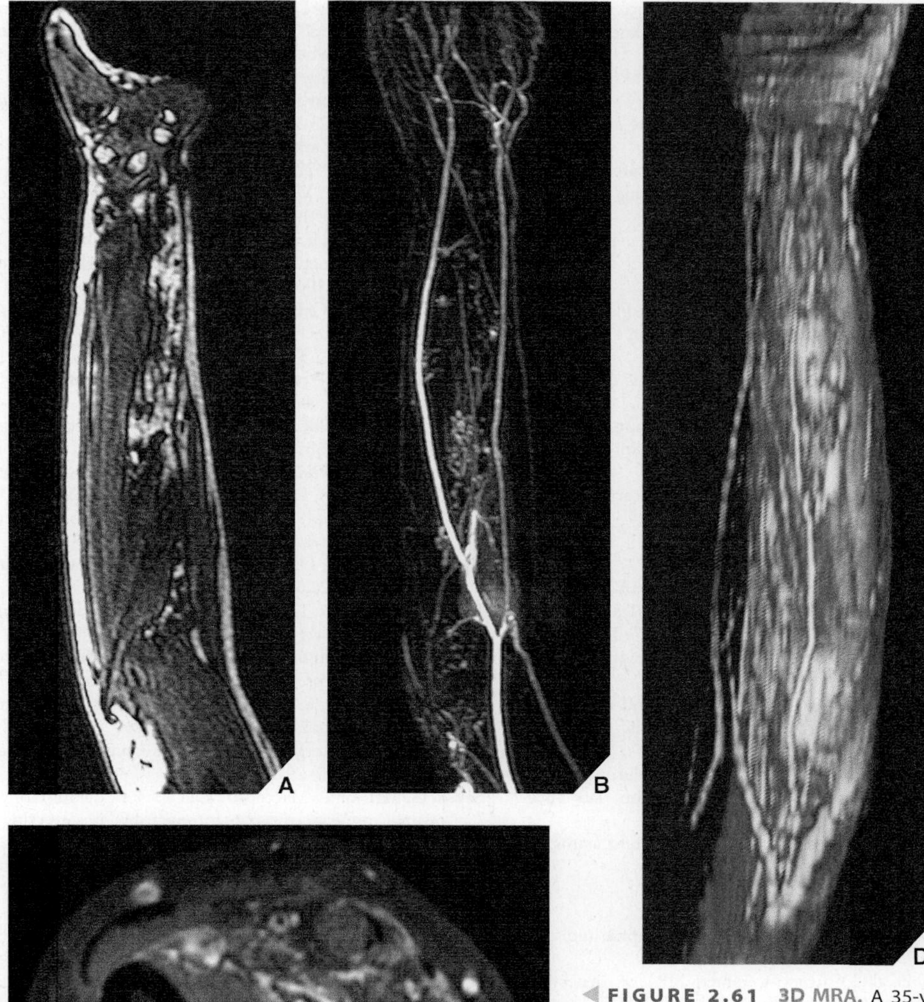

FIGURE 2.61 3D MRA. A 35-year-old woman presented with a history of swelling of the left forearm. Dynamic contrast MRI including arterial, venous, and delayed phases **(A–C)** shows multiple enhancing vascular spaces and areas of contrast puddling as well as large draining veins that empty into the antecubital artery. **(D)** 3D color volume MRA image shows simultaneous opacification of veins and arteries of the forearm, diagnostic of arteriovenous malformation.

SUGGESTED READINGS

Abdel-Dayem HM. The role of nuclear medicine in primary bone and soft tissue tumors. *Semin Nucl Med* 1997;27:355–363.

Abikhzer G, Srour S, Keidar Z, et al. Added value of SPECT/CT in the evaluation of benign bone diseases of the appendicular skeleton. *Clin Nucl Med* 2016;41:e195–e199.

Alazraki NP. Radionuclide imaging in the evaluation of infectious and inflammatory disease. *Radiol Clin North Am* 1993;31:783–794.

Alley MT, Shifrin RY, Pelc NJ, et al. Ultrafast contrast-enhanced three-dimensional MR angiography: state of the art. *Radiographics* 1998;18:273–285.

Allman K, Schafer O, Hauer M, et al. Indirect MR arthrography of the unexercised glenohumeral joint in patients with rotator cuff tears. *Invest Radiol* 1999;34:435–440.

Al Sheikh W, Sfakianakis GN, Mnaymneh W, et al. Subacute and chronic bone infections: diagnosis using In-111, Ga-67, and Tc-99m MDP bone scintigraphy, and radiography. *Radiology* 1985;155:501–506.

Anderson MW, Greenspan A. State of the art: stress fractures. *Radiology* 1996;199:1–12.

Aoki J, Watanabe H, Shinozaki T, et al. FDG PET of primary benign and malignant bone tumors: standardized uptake value in 52 lesions. *Radiology* 2001;219:774–777.

Aoki J, Watanabe H, Shinozaki T, et al. FDG-PET for preoperative differential diagnosis between benign and malignant soft tissue masses. *Skeletal Radiol* 2003;32:133–138.

Arndt WF III, Truax AL, Barnett FM, et al. MR diagnosis of bone contusions of the knee: comparison of coronal T2-weighted fast spin-echo with fat saturation and fast spin-echo STIR images with conventional STIR images. *Am J Roentgenol* 1996;166: 119–124.

Becker W, Goldenberg DM, Wolf F. The use of monoclonal antibodies and antibody fragments in the imaging of infectious lesions. *Semin Nucl Med* 1994;24:142–153.

Beltran J, Bencardino J, Mellado J, et al. MR arthrography of the shoulder: variants and pitfalls. *Radiographics* 1997;17:1403–1412.

Bhargava P, He G, Samarghandi A, et al. Pictorial review of SPECT/CT imaging application in clinical nuclear medicine. *Am J Nucl Med Mol Imaging* 2012;2:221–231.

Bianchi S, Martinoli C, Abdelwahab IF. Ultrasound of tendon tears. Part 1: general considerations and upper extremity. *Skeletal Radiol* 2005;34:500–512.

Breyer RJ III, Mulligan ME, Smith SE, et al. Comparison of imaging with FDG PET/CT with other imaging modalities in myeloma. *Skeletal Radiol* 2006;35:632–640.

Buckwalter KA, Braunstein EM. Digital skeletal radiography. *Am J Roentgenol* 1992;158: 1071–1080.

Bybel B, Brunken RC, DiFilippo FP, et al. SPECT/CT imaging: clinical utility of an emerging technology. *Radiographics* 2008;28:1097–1113.

Catana C, Procissi D, Wu Y, et al. Simultaneous in vivo positron emission tomography and magnetic resonance imaging. *Proc Natl Acad Sci U S A* 2008;105:3705–3710.

Chaudhari AJ, Ferrero A, Godinez F, et al. Characterization of an extremity PET/CT system for assessing early response to treatment in human inflammatory arthritis. *J Nucl Med* 2012;53(suppl 1):434.

Choi HK, Burns LC, Shojania K, et al. Dual energy CT in gout: a prospective validation study. *Ann Rheum Dis* 2012;71:1466–1471.

Choi J-A, Gold G. MR imaging of articular cartilage physiology. *Magn Reson Imaging Clin N Am* 2011;19:249–282.

Crema MD, Roemer FW, Marra MD, et al. Articular cartilage of the knee: current MR imaging techniques and applications in clinical practice and research. *Radiographics* 2011;31:37–61.

Crema MD, Watts VGJ, Guermazi A, et al. A narrative overview of the current status of MRI of the hip and its relevance for osteoarthritis research—what we know, what has changed, and where are we going? *Osteoarthritis Cartilage* 2017;25:1–13.
Delfaut EM, Beltran J, Johnson G, et al. Fat suppression in MR imaging: techniques and pitfalls. *Radiographics* 1999;19:373–382.
Erlemann R, Reiser MF, Peters PE, et al. Musculoskeletal neoplasms: static and dynamic Gd-DTPA-enhanced MR imaging. *Radiology* 1989;171:767–773.
Erlemann R, Sciuk J, Bosse A, et al. Response of osteosarcoma and Ewing sarcoma to preoperative chemotherapy: assessment with dynamic and static MR imaging and skeletal scintigraphy. *Radiology* 1990;175:791–796.
Fayad LM, Corl F, Fishman EK. Pediatric skeletal trauma: use of multiplanar reformatted and three-dimensional 64-row multidetector CT in the emergency department. *Radiographics* 2009;29:135–150.
Fishman EK. Spiral CT evaluation of the musculoskeletal system. In: Fishman EK, Jeffrey RB Jr, eds. *Spiral CT. Principles, techniques, and clinical applications.* Philadelphia: Lippincott-Raven; 1998:273–298.
Fox IM, Zeiger L. Tc-99m-HMPAO leukocyte scintigraphy for the diagnosis of osteomyelitis in diabetic foot infections. *J Foot Ankle Surg* 1993;32:591–594.
Gerscovich EO, Greenspan A, Cronan MS, et al. Three-dimensional sonographic evaluation of developmental dysplasia of the hip: preliminary findings. *Radiology* 1994;190:407–410.
Gold GE, Chen CA, Koo S, et al. Recent advances in MRI of articular cartilage. *Am J Roentgenol* 2009;193:628–638.
Gold GE, McCauley TR, Gray ML, et al. What's new in cartilage? *Radiographics* 2003;23:1227–1242.
Greenspan A. Imaging modalities in orthopaedics. In: Chapman MW, ed. *Chapman's orthopaedic surgery*, 3rd ed. Philadelphia: Lippincott Williams & Wilkins; 2001:53–74.
Greenspan A. Tumors of cartilage origin. *Orthop Clin North Am* 1989;20:347–366.
Greenspan A, Norman A. The radial head-capitellum view: useful technique in elbow trauma. *Am J Roentgenol* 1982;138:1186–1188.
Guhlmann A, Brecht Krauss D, Suger G, et al. Fluorine-18-FDG PET and technetium-99m antigranulocyte antibody scintigraphy in chronic osteomyelitis. *J Nucl Med* 1998;39:2145–2152.
Gupta R, Grasruck M, Suess C, et al. Ultra-high resolution flat-panel volume CT: fundamental principles, design architecture, and system characterization. *Eur Radiol* 2006;16:1191–1205.
Hartung MP, Grist TM, Francois J. Magnetic resonance angiography: current status and future directions. *J Cardiovasc Mag Res* 2011;13:19–40.
Harvey D. PET/MRI: new fusion. *Radiology Today* 2008;9:20–21.
Hodler J. Technical errors in MR arthrography. *Skeletal Radiol* 2008;37:9–18.
Hodler J, Fretz CJ, Terrier F, et al. Rotator cuff tears: correlation of sonographic and surgical findings. *Radiology* 1988;169:791–794.
Holl N, Enchaniz-Laguna A, Bierry G, et al. Diffusion-weighted MRI of denervated muscle: a clinical and experimental study. *Skeletal Radiol* 2008;247:797–807.
Huellner MV, Burkert A, Schleich FS, et al. SPECT/CT versus MRI in patients with nonspecific pain of the hand and wrist—a pilot study. *Eur J Nucl Med Mol Imaging* 2012;39:750–759.
Johnson RP. The role of bone imaging in orthopedic practice. *Semin Nucl Med* 1997;27:386–389.
Jung H-S, Jee W-H, McCauley TR, et al. Discrimination of metastatic from acute osteoporotic compression spinal fractures with MR imaging. *Radiographics* 2003;23:179–187.
Kaplan PA, Matamoros A Jr, Anderson JC. Sonography of the musculoskeletal system. *Am J Roentgenol* 1990;155:237–245.
Kertesz JL, Anderson SW, Murakami AM, et al. Detection of vascular injuries in patients with blunt pelvic trauma by using 64-channel multidetector CT. *Radiographics* 2009;29:154–164.
Kijowski R, Blankenbaker DG, Klaers JL, et al. Vastly undersampled isotropic projection steady-state free precession imaging of the knee: diagnostic performance compared with conventional MR. *Radiology* 2009;251:185–194.
König H, Sieper J, Wolf KJ. Rheumatoid arthritis: evaluation of hypervascular and fibrous pannus with dynamic MR imaging enhanced with Gd-DTPA. *Radiology* 1990;176:473–477.
Kowalska B. Ultrasound-guided joint and soft tissue interventions. *J Ultrasound* 2014;14:163–170.
Lee M-J, Kim S, Lee S-A, et al. Overcoming artifacts from metallic orthopedic implants at high-field-strength MR imaging and multidetector CT. *Radiographics* 2007;27:791–803.
Levinsohn EM, Palmer AK, Coren AB, et al. Wrist arthrography: the value of the three compartment injection technique. *Skeletal Radiol* 1987;16:539–544.
Li X, Ma CB, Link TM, et al. In vivo T1rho and T2 mapping of articular cartilage in osteoarthritis of the knee using 3 tesla MRI. *Osteoarthritis Cartilage* 2007;15:789–797.
Link TM, Stahl R, Woeltler K. Cartilage imaging: motivation, techniques, current and future significance. *Eur Radiol* 2007;17:1135–1146.
Love C, Din AS, Tomas MB, et al. Radionuclide bone imaging: an illustrative review. *Radiographics* 2003;23:341–358.
McCollough CH, Zink FE. Performance evaluation of a multi-slice CT system. *Med Phys* 1999;26:2223–2230.
Meuli RA, Wedeeen VJ, Geller SC, et al. MR gated subtraction angiography: evaluation of lower extremities. *Radiology* 1986;159:411–418.
Moon CH, Kim J-H, Zhao T, Bae KT. Quantitative 23Na MRI of human knee cartilage using dual-tuned 1H/23Na transceiver array radiofrequency coil at 7 tesla. *J Man Res Imag* 2013;38:1063–1072.
Omar IM, Zoga AC, Kavanagh EC, et al. Athletic pubalgia and "sports hernia": optimal MR imaging technique and findings. *Radiographics* 2008;28:1415–1438.
Palestro CJ, Love C, Tronco GG, et al. Combined labeled leukocyte and technetium 99m sulfur colloid bone marrow imaging for diagnosing musculoskeletal infections. *Radiographics* 2006;26:859–870.
Peh WC, Cassar-Pullicino VN. Magnetic resonance arthrography: current status. *Clin Radiol* 1999;54:575–587.
Pettersson H, Resnick D. Musculoskeletal imaging. *Radiology* 1998;208:561–562.
Ramdhian-Wihlm R, Le Minor J-M, Schmittbuhl M, et al. Cone-beam computed tomography arthrography: an innovative modality for evaluation of wrist ligament and cartilage injuries. *Skeletal Radiol* 2012;41:963–969.
Raya JG, Horng A, Dietrich O, et al. Articular cartilage in vivo diffusion-tensor imaging. *Radiology* 2012;262:550–559.
Pugh DG, Winkler TN. Scanography of leg-length measurement: an easy satisfactory method. *Radiology* 1966;87:130–133.
Recht MP, Goodwin GW, Winalski GS, et al. MRI of articular cartilage: revisiting current status and future directions. *Am J Roentgenol* 2007;185:899–915.
Reichardt B, Sarwar A, Bartling SH, et al. Musculoskeletal applications of flat-panel volume CT. *Skeletal Radiol* 2008;37:1069–1076.
Sabharwal S, Kumar A. Methods for assessing leg length discrepancy. *Clin Orthop Relat Res* 2008;466:2010–2922.
Savelli G, Maffioli L, Maccauro M, et al. Bone scintigraphy and the added value of SPECT (single photon emission tomography) in detecting skeletal lesions. *Q J Nucl Med* 2001;45:27–37.
Schmitt B, Zbyn S, Steizeneker D, et al. Cartilage quality assessment by using glycosaminoglycan chemical exchange saturation transfer and 23Na MR imaging at 7T. *Radiology* 2011;260:257–264.
Seo Y, Aparici CM, Hasegawa B. Technological development and advances in SPECT/CT. *Semin Nucl Med* 2008;38:177–198.
Sostman HD, Charles HC, Rockwell S, et al. Soft-tissue sarcomas: detection of metabolic heterogeneity with P-31 MR spectroscopy. *Radiology* 1990;176:837–843.
Steinbach LS, Palmer WE, Schweitzer ME. Special focus session. MR arthrography. *Radiographics* 2002;22:1223–1246.
Stumpe KD, Dazzi H, Schaffner A, et al. Infection imaging using whole-body FDG-PET. *Eur J Nucl Med* 2000;27:822–832.
Sundaram M, McLeod RA. MR imaging of tumor and tumorlike lesions of bones and soft tissues. *Am J Roentgenol* 1990;155:817–824.
Tang HR, DaSilva AJ, Matthay KK, et al. Neuroblastoma imaging using a combined CT scanner-scintillation camera and I-131MIBG. *J Nucl Med* 2001;42:237–247.
Tian R, Su M, Tian Y, et al. Dual-time point PET/CT with F-18 FDG for the differentiation of malignant and benign bone lesions. *Skeletal Radiol* 2009;38:451–458.
Widmann G, Riedl A, Schoepf D, et al. State-of-the-art HR-US imaging findings of the most frequent musculoskeletal soft-tissue tumors. *Skeletal Radiol* 2009;38:637–649.
Winalski CS, Prabhakar R. The evolution of articular cartilage imaging and its impact on clinical practice. *Skeletal Radiol* 2011;40:1197–1222.
Yagei B, Manisals M, Yilmaz E, et al. Indirect MR arthrography of the shoulder in detection of rotator cuff ruptures. *Eur Radiol* 2001;11:258–262.
Yoon LS, Palmer WE, Kassarjian A. Evaluation of radial-sequence imaging in detecting acetabular labral tears at hip MR arthrography. *Skeletal Radiol* 2007;36:1029–1033.
Zbyn S, Mlynarik V, Juras V, et al. Sodium MR imaging of articular cartilage pathologies. *Curr Radiol Rep* 2014;2:41–57.
Zoga AC, Kavanagh EC, Omar IM, et al. Athletic pubalgia and the "sport hernia": MR imaging findings. *Radiology* 2008;247:797–807.

3

Histology, Formation, and Growth of Bone and Articular Cartilage

Bone: Histology, Formation, and Growth

The skeleton is made of cortical and cancellous bones, which are highly specialized forms of connective tissue. Each type of bony tissue has the same basic histologic structure (Fig. 3.1), but the cortical component has a solid, compact architecture interrupted only by narrow canals containing blood vessels (Haversian systems), while the cancellous component consists of trabeculae separated by fatty or hematopoietic marrow. A bone is a rigid calcified material and grows by the addition of new tissues to existing surfaces. The removal of unwanted bones, called *simultaneous remodeling*, is also a necessary component of skeletal growth. Unlike most tissues, a bone grows only by apposition on the surface of an already existing substrate, such as a bone or calcified cartilage. Cartilages, however, grow by interstitial cellular proliferation and matrix formation.

A normal bone is formed through a combination of two processes: *endochondral (enchondral) ossification* and *intramembranous (membranous) ossification* (Fig. 3.2). In general, the spongiosa develops by endochondral ossification and the cortex by intramembranous ossification. Once formed, a living bone is never metabolically at rest. Beginning in the fetal period, it constantly remodels and reappropriates its minerals along lines of mechanical stress. This process continues throughout life, accelerating during infancy and adolescence. The factors controlling bone formation and resorption are still not well understood, but one fact is clear: Bone formation and bone resorption are exquisitely balanced, coupled processes that result in net bone formation equaling net bone resorption.

Most of the skeleton is formed by endochondral ossification (Fig. 3.3), a highly organized process that transforms a cartilage to a bone and contributes mainly to increasing the bone length. Endochondral ossification is responsible for the formation of all tubular and flat bones, vertebrae, the base of the skull, the ethmoid, and the medial and lateral ends of the clavicle. At approximately 5 weeks of embryonic life, cartilage cells (chondroblasts and chondrocytes) produce a hyaline cartilage model of the long tubular bones from the condensed mesenchymal aggregate (Fig. 3.4). The histologic events related to this process are first evident by changes in the condensation of undifferentiated mesenchymal cells, during which some of the cells inside the area of the future model become slightly larger and rounder and acquire noticeable cytoplasm. At the same time, the cells at the periphery of the models remain more spindle-shaped, less differentiated, and more condensed (Fig. 3.5). The mechanisms leading to the calcification of the cartilaginous matrix are not completely understood, but it is generally believed that the promoters of calcification are small membrane-bound vesicles known as *matrix vesicles*, which are present in the interstitial matrix between the cells (Fig. 3.6). At approximately the 9th week of embryonic life, peripheral capillaries penetrate the model, inducing the formation of osteoblasts. Osseous tissue is then deposited on the spicules of the calcified cartilage matrix that remain after osteoclastic resorption, thereby transforming the primary spongiosa into the secondary spongiosa (Fig. 3.7).

As this process moves rapidly toward the epiphyseal ends of the cartilage model, a loose network of bony trabeculae containing cores of calcified cartilage is left behind, creating a well-defined line of advance. This line represents the growth plate (physis) (Fig. 3.8) and the adjacent metaphysis to which the secondary spongiosa moves as it is formed. The many trabeculae of the secondary spongiosa that are resorbed soon after being formed become the marrow cavity, while other trabeculae enlarge and thicken through the apposition of a new bone, although these too eventually undergo resorption and remodeling. Others extend toward the shaft and become incorporated into the developing cortex of the bone, which is formed by intramembranous ossification. At the ends of tubular bones, a similar process is initiated. The cartilage at these sites expands by the interstitial accumulation of cartilage matrix. This appositional growth constitutes the main growth center that becomes vascularized by a network of invaginations from the perichondrium called *cartilage canals* (Fig. 3.9A). The cartilage surrounding these canals undergoes calcification and hypertrophy, followed by chondrocyte apoptosis, vascular invasion, and the formation of secondary ossification center in the epiphysis (Fig. 3.9B). This nucleus increases in size by the process of maturation and calcification of the cartilage surrounding the secondary center. The peripheral margin of epiphysis termed *acrophysis* is formed of zones of cell hypertrophy, degeneration, calcification, and ossification, similar to that of the growth plate. Endochondral bone formation is not normally observed after growth plate closure.

In intramembranous ossification, a bone is formed directly without an intervening cartilaginous stage (Fig. 3.10). Initially, condensed mesenchymal cells differentiate into osteoprogenitor cells, which then differentiate into fibroblasts that produce collagen and fibrous connective tissues and osteoblasts that produce osteoid (Fig. 3.11). Beginning at approximately the 9th week of fetal life, the fibrous membrane produced by the fibroblasts forms a periosteal collar and is replaced with osteoid by the action of the osteoblasts. Bones formed by this process include the frontal, parietal, and temporal bones and their squamae; bones of the upper face as well as the tympanic parts of the temporal bone; and the vomer and the medial pterygoid.

Intramembranous ossification also contributes to the appositional formation of periosteal bones around the shafts of the tubular bones, thus forming the cortex of the long and flat bones. This type of bone formation increases the bone width. In addition to the periosteal envelope on

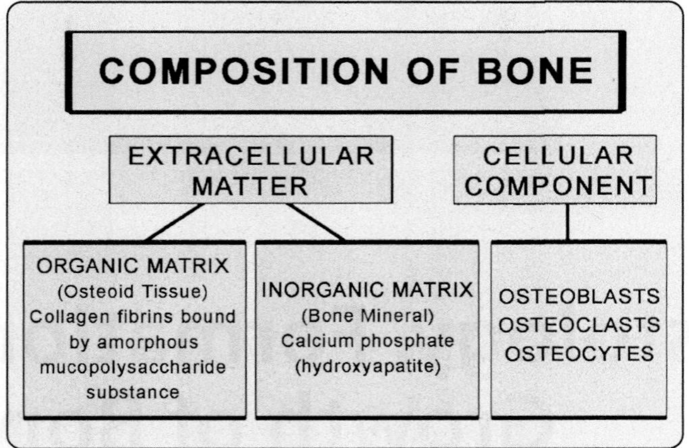

FIGURE 3.1 Composition of bone. A bone consists of extracellular matter and cellular component.

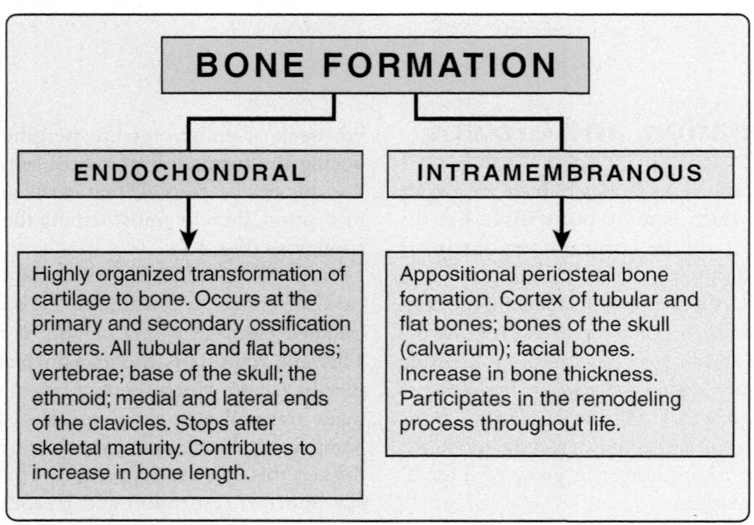

FIGURE 3.2 Processes of bone formation.

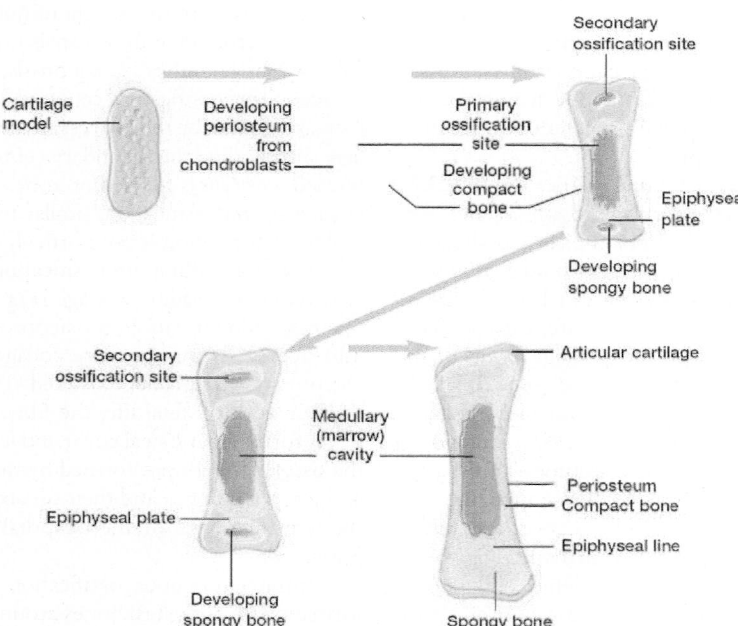

FIGURE 3.3 Endochondral bone formation. This process occurs at the ossification center, growth plate, and metaphysis. (Reprinted with permission from Anatomical Chart Company. *Rapid review anatomy reference guide*, 3rd ed. Philadelphia, PA: Wolters Kluwer Health; 2010, Fig. 1-11.)

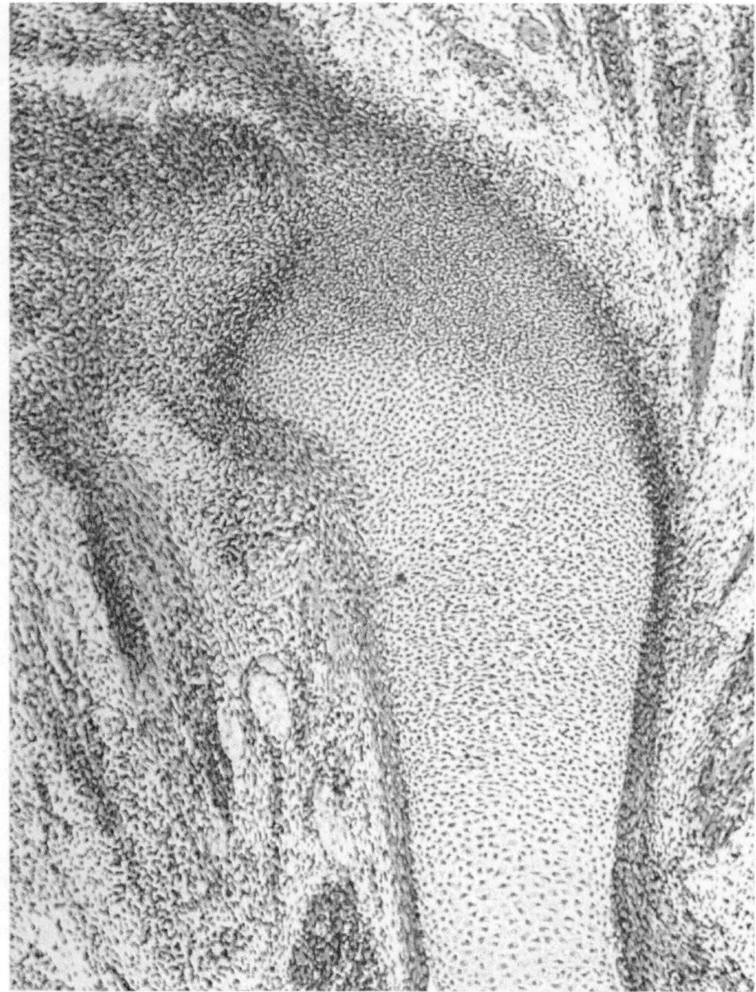

FIGURE 3.4 Endochondral bone formation. Photomicrograph of the proximal femur and hip joint in a 5-week-old fetus shows that the bone is already modeled in cartilage and it is covered by condensation of mesenchymal cells, which eventually will become the periosteum. Note that the cells in the diaphysis of the cartilage model of the bone are larger and paler than those at the articular end of the bone (H&E, ×4). (Reprinted from Bullough P. *Orthopaedic pathology*, 5th ed. Maryland Heights, MO: Mosby; 2009, with permission from Elsevier.)

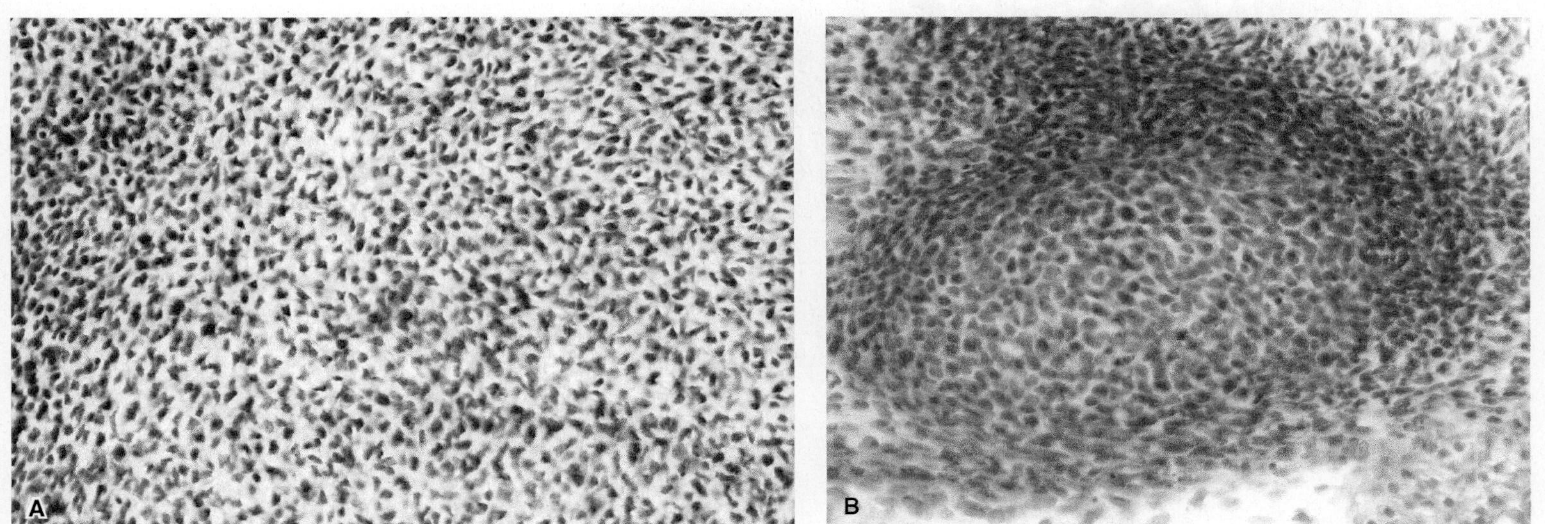

FIGURE 3.5 Histology of early endochondral bone formation. **(A)** Randomly arranged and with no discernible differentiating features, spindle-shaped and stellate cells are predating the formation of the cartilage model. No extracellular matrix is present. **(B)** The formation of cartilage is preceded by the condensation of mesenchymal cells. Their aggregation into rudimentary shapes is defined by a higher peripheral density due to appositional mitotic activity. The nuclei of the cell still contain dense chromatin. *(Continued)*

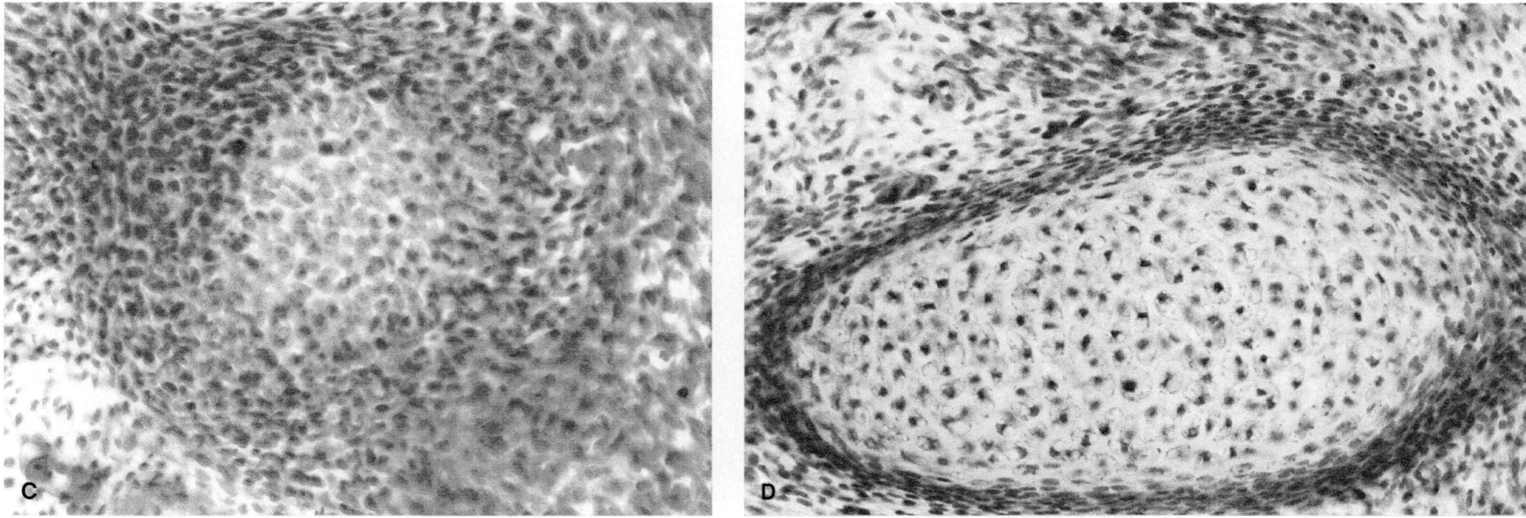

FIGURE 3.5 Histology of early endochondral bone formation. ***(Continued)*** **(C)** The first histologic evidence of cartilaginous differentiation is the formation of extracellular mucopolysaccharide matrix in the condensed areas of mesenchyme. Between the lightly basophilic matrix, the nuclei of the mesenchymal cells become round and their chromatin is more vascular than that of the surrounding spindle cells. **(D)** In the later stages, the cells acquire lacunae, which separate the cytoplasm from the interstitial matrix. The model become histologically identical to hyaline cartilage. (Reprinted with permission from American Registry of Pathology, from Klein MJ, Bonar SF, Freemont T, et al, eds. *Atlas of nontumor pathology. Non-neoplastic diseases of bones and joints*. Washington, DC: American Registry of Pathology and Armed Forces Institute of Pathology; 2011:5–6, Figs. 1.4A–C and 1.5C.)

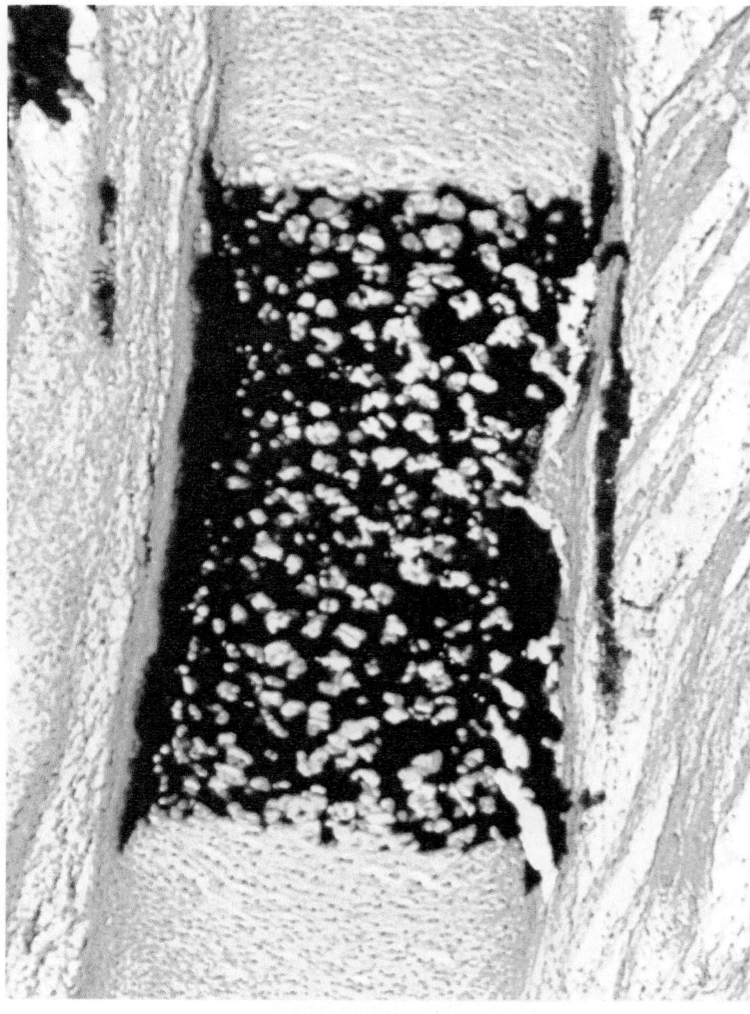

FIGURE 3.6 Histology of late endochondral bone formation. Photomicrograph of the diaphysis of the long bone in a 7-week-old fetus shows calcification of the cartilage matrix *(black)* (von Kossa stain, ×4). (Reprinted from Bullough P. *Orthopaedic pathology*, 5th ed. Maryland Heights, MO: Mosby; 2009, with permission from Elsevier.)

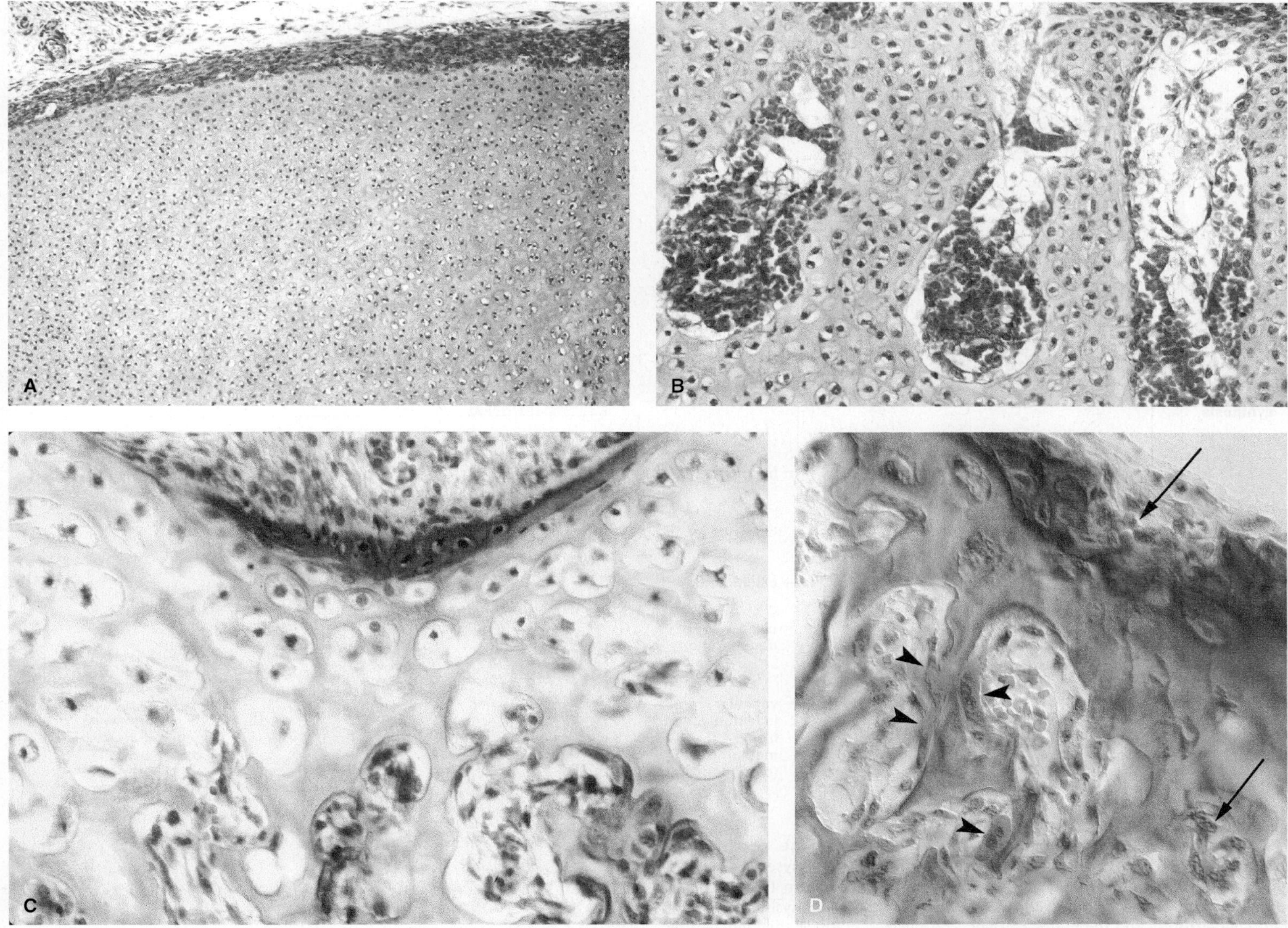

FIGURE 3.7 Endochondral bone formation: replacement of the cartilage model by bone. (A) The diaphysis of the fully developed cartilage model exhibits a solid cylinder composed of hyaline cartilage. There are no blood vessels. The outside part of the cylinder is covered by cellular perichondrium **(top)**. **(B)** Delicate neovascularization derived from the periosteum invades the cartilage. The capillaries from the overlying periosteum penetrate the empty lacunar spaces in the cartilage vacated by apoptotic chondrocytes. **(C)** The new blood vessels in the center of the cartilage model have brought with them osteoblasts, which have begun to form bone on the empty lacunar walls. **(D)** At higher magnification power, osteoclasts *(arrowheads)* are absorbing the mixed trabeculae of calcified cartilage and bone matrix (primary spongiosa). Osteoblasts also synthesize bone matrix *(long arrows)*. (Reprinted with permission from American Registry of Pathology, from Klein MJ, Bonar SF, Freemont T, et al, eds. *Atlas of nontumor pathology. Non-neoplastic diseases of bones and joints*. Washington, DC: American Registry of Pathology and Armed Forces Institute of Pathology; 2011:8, Fig. 1.7A,C–E.)

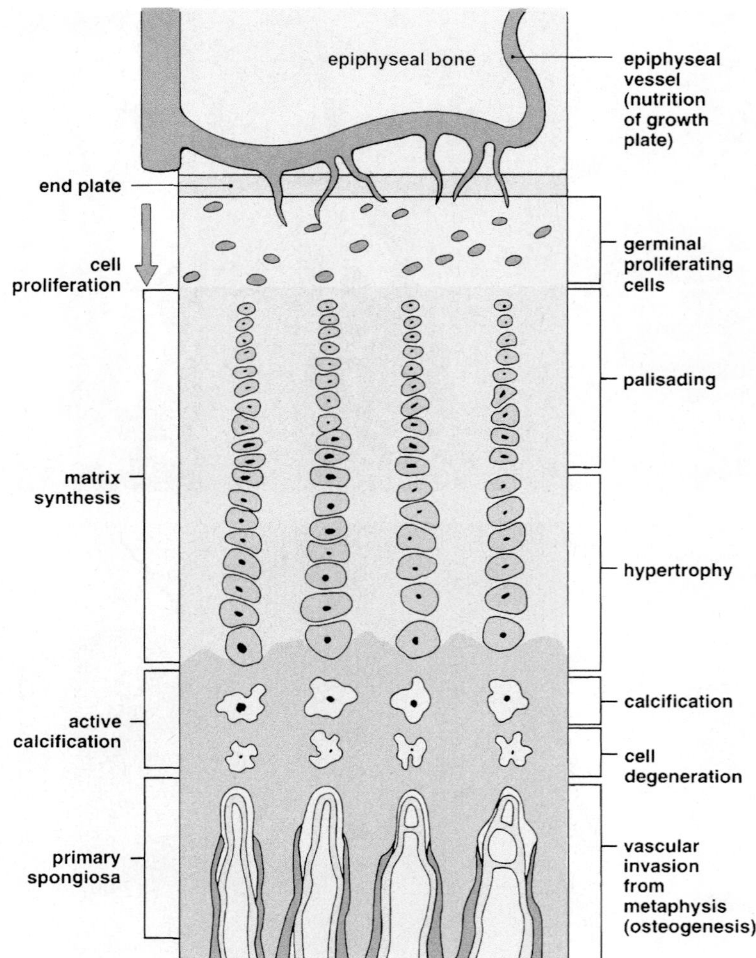

FIGURE 3.8 Schematic representation of the growth plate. Growth plate during active bone growth. At the top of the diagram, the epiphyseal vessels are supplying nutrition to the germinal proliferating cells. Further down, the cells begin to palisade into vertical columns, and as they approach the metaphysis, the cells undergo hypertrophy and the matrix calcifies. The calcified matrix is then invaded by blood vessels, and the primary spongiosa forms. (Reprinted from Bullough P. *Orthopaedic pathology*, 5th ed. Maryland Heights, MO: Mosby; 2009, with permission from Elsevier.)

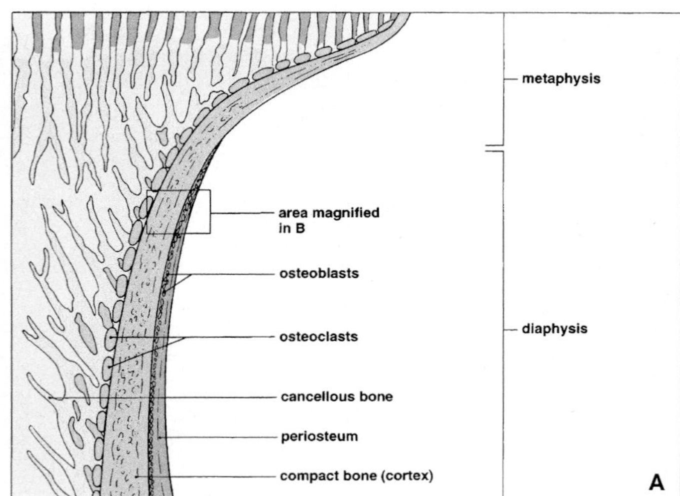

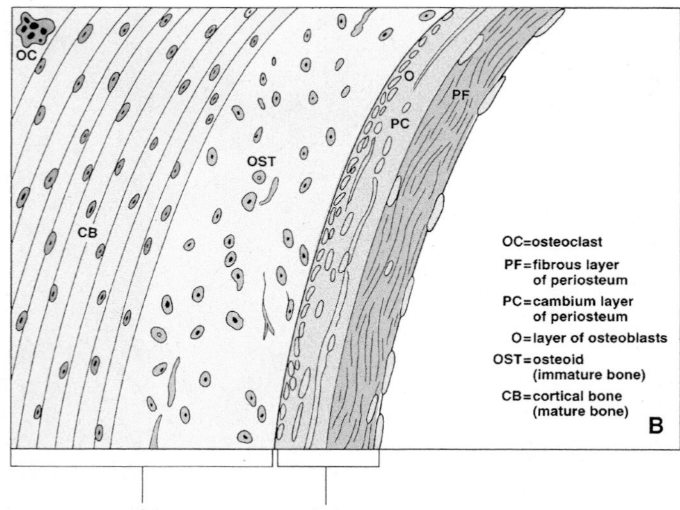

FIGURE 3.10 Schematic representation of intramembranous ossification. (A,B) Intramembranous bone formation at the junction of the periosteum and the cortex. Subperiosteal bone formation progresses from an immature (woven) to a more mature bone. (From Greenspan A, Beltran J. *Orthopedic imaging: a practical approach*, 6th ed. Philadelphia: Wolters Kluwer; 2015:51.)

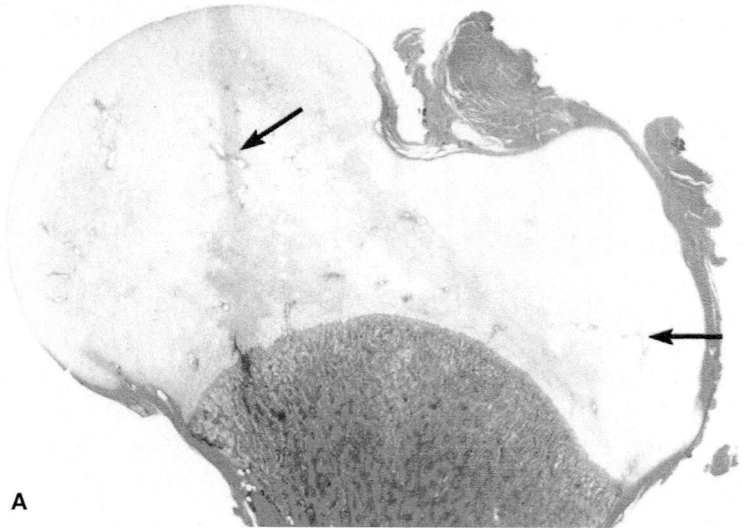

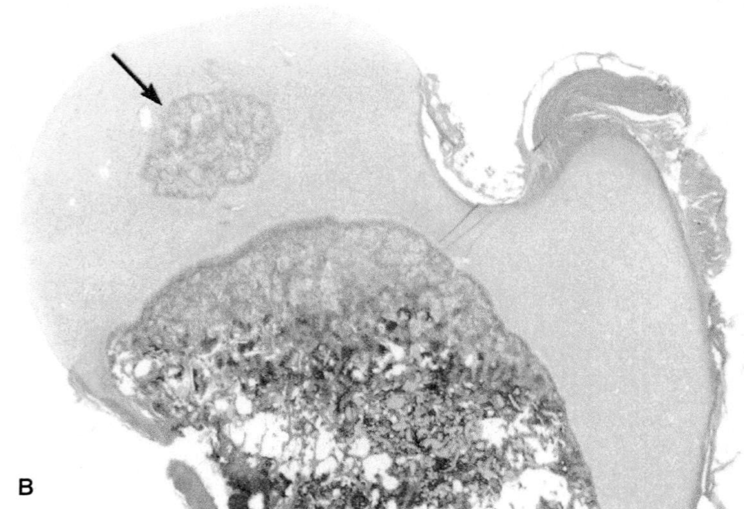

FIGURE 3.9 Histology of secondary ossification center. (A) Cartilage canals *(arrows)* in the articular end of the femur constitute the epiphysis of the femoral head and apophysis of the greater trochanter. **(B)** The secondary ossification center of the femoral head *(arrow)* is developed. Note lack of the secondary ossification center in the greater trochanter, which will develop later. (Reprinted with permission from American Registry of Pathology, from Klein MJ, Bonar SF, Freemont T, et al, eds. *Atlas of nontumor pathology. Non-neoplastic diseases of bones and joints*. Washington, DC: American Registry of Pathology and Armed Forces Institute of Pathology; 2011:10, Figs. 1.9 and 1.10.)

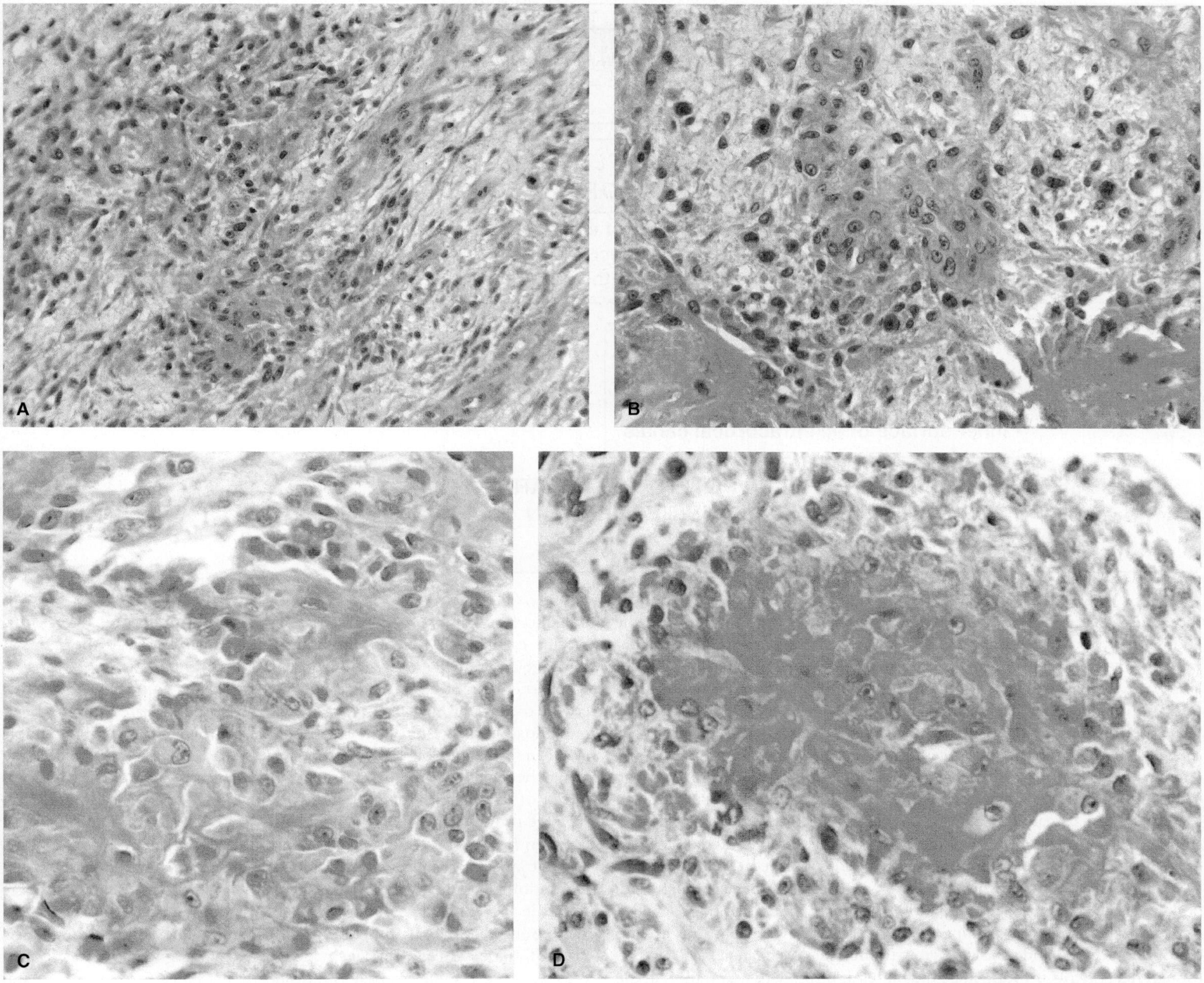

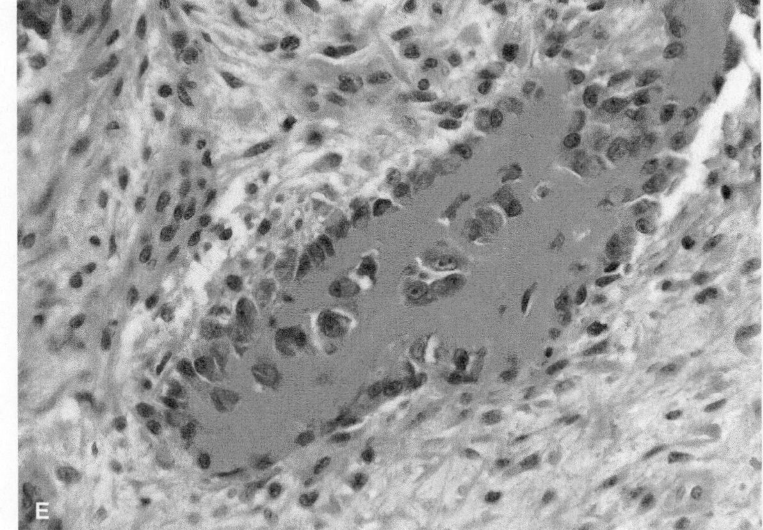

FIGURE 3.11 Histology of intramembranous bone formation. (A) The mesenchymal cells arranged in a loose fibrous background exhibit early cellular condensation *(center)*. A few of the cells in the condensed area are polyhedral and beginning to resemble osteoblasts. Elsewhere *(right)*, there is active mitotic activity reflecting less differentiation. **(B)** In the early osteoblast differentiation, the cells in the center have become polyhedral with basophilic cytoplasm and exhibit a few extracellular wisps of pink osteoid between them. **(C)** Further along in development, the cells vary from polyhedral to pear-shaped. Their cytoplasm is distinctly basophilic except for the cellular regions that contain paranuclear clear zones. Abundant intercellular lacelike osteoid separates the cells. Some are beginning to line up on the surface of the osteoid, and some are beginning to be incorporated. Mitotic activity is not seen in or around this early bone formation. **(D)** The lacelike osteoid has become bulkier in configuration. Osteoblasts are incorporated into the matrix as large osteocytes. **(E)** The osteoid is microtrabecular and lined on both sides by active osteoblasts. (Reprinted with permission from American Registry of Pathology, from Klein MJ, Bonar SF, Freemont T, et al, eds. *Atlas of nontumor pathology. Non-neoplastic diseases of bone and joints*. Washington, DC: American Registry of Pathology and Armed Forces Institute of Pathology; 2011:3, Fig. 1.1A–C,E.)

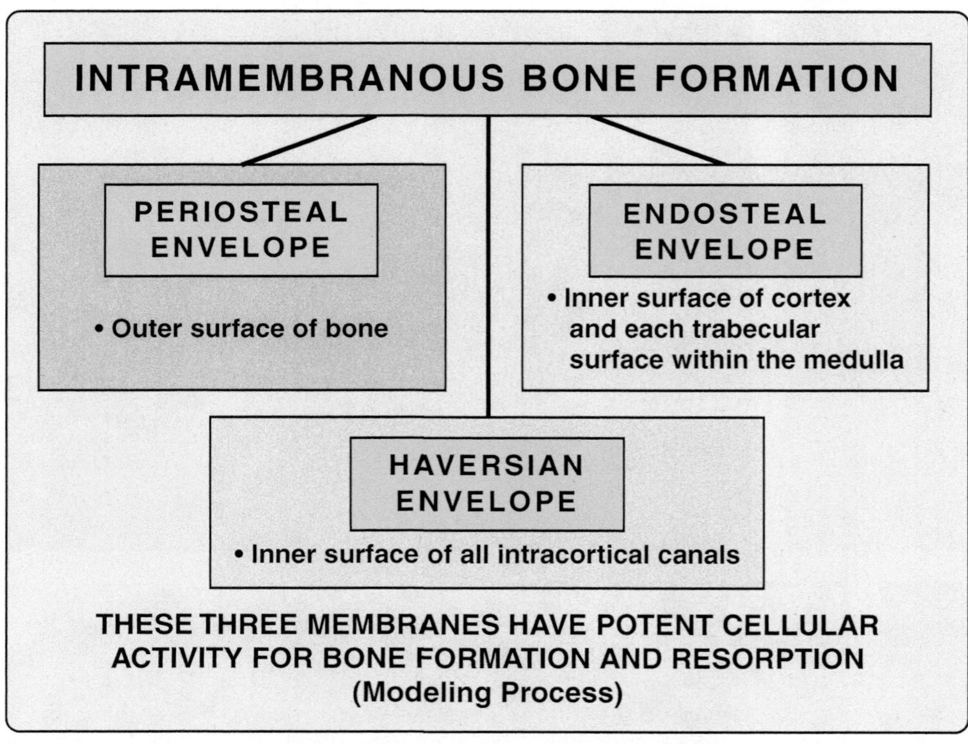

FIGURE 3.12 Process of intramembranous bone formation.

the outer surface of a bone, intramembranous ossification is active in the endosteal envelope covering the inner surface of the cortex and in the haversian envelope at the internal surface of all intracortical canals (Fig. 3.12). These three envelopes are sites of potent cellular activity involving resorption and formation of bones throughout life.

It is interesting to note that the mandible and middle portions of the clavicle are formed by a process that shares features of endochondral and intramembranous ossification. These bones are preformed in cartilage in embryonic life, but they do not undergo endochondral ossification in the conventional manner. Instead, the cartilage model simply serves as a surface for the deposition of bone by connective tissues. Eventually, the cartilage is resorbed, and the bones become fully ossified.

The spaces between the trabecular/cancellous bones are filled with bone marrow elements, a combination of hematopoietic red marrow (also referred to as *cellular* or *myeloid*) and fatty yellow marrow. The amount and distribution of red and yellow marrow in the skeleton change with age. Although red marrow is found in all the bones at birth, with maturation in the postnatal period, hematopoietic marrow becomes largely confined to the axial skeleton, being gradually replaced by fatty marrow in some areas of the skeleton, following a predictable pattern. In children, the conversion of red to yellow marrow starts in the long bones at the level of the middiaphysis and epiphysis, progressing to the distal metaphysis during adolescence and young adult life. Red marrow is present until late adulthood in the skull, sternum, pelvis, spine, ribs, and proximal metaphysis of the humeri and femora, with some degree of yellow marrow islands. Reconversion of yellow to red marrow occurs in situations where increased hematopoiesis is required, such as in chronic anemia, but it has also been recognized in obese individuals and smokers.

Articular Cartilage: Histology, Formation, and Growth

During the early stages of skeletal development, the location of joints is marked by a condensation of mesenchymal cells. After the 5th to 8th week of gestation, those cells undergo transformation to form a joint cleft (Fig. 3.13A–C). At some point during development, a secondary center of ossification is formed within the cartilaginous end of the bone (see Fig. 3.9). Calcification occurs initially at the middle of the secondary ossification center. This area is then invaded by blood vessels and the process of endochondral ossification begins. As maturation continues, the residual hyaline cartilage that covers the end of the bones becomes the articular cartilage and remains cartilaginous throughout life.

Articular hyaline cartilage is a highly specialized connective tissue that covers the diarthrodial joints. It provides a smooth lubricated surface facilitating load transmission with low frictional coefficient. It is highly durable and can withstand big loads. It is an avascular, aneural, and alymphatic tissue; hence, its capability of healing and repair is very limited. It is composed of 1% cellular matrix (chondrocytes), 60% to 80% of water, 15% of large protein aggregates (proteoglycans [PGs]) and 40% to 60% type II collagen fibers. These collagen fibers provide tensile strength to the tissue and entrap the PG aggregates. Type II collagen fibers have higher elasticity than another abundant type I collagen fibers which is the type of fibers found in tissue repair, tendons, ligaments, endomysium of myofibrils, organic bone, dermis, dentin, and organ capsules. The composition of articular hyaline cartilage changes with age as it undergoes degeneration. In young people, hyaline cartilage is translucent and bluish-white in color, and in older individuals, it is opaque and slightly yellowish (Fig. 3.14).

PG aggregates (aggrecans) are the major extracellular matrix components of the hyaline cartilage. They are attached to a central filament of hyaluronan molecule with glycosaminoglycans (GAGs) chains containing amino acids attached to it (Fig. 3.15). The GAGs are highly negatively charged (fixed charge density), attracting water (bound water). Sodium ions are attracted to the negatively charged GAGs and thus providing electronic neutrality (Fig. 3.16).

Articular hyaline cartilage is organized in several layers (zones) (Fig. 3.17). From surface to depth, the more superficial very thin layer is called *lamina splendens*, and it has a high water contents and low PG contents. This zone is in contact with the synovial fluid and is responsible for most of the tensile properties of the articular cartilage. The next layer is the transitional or intermediate layer containing a rich network of randomly organized collagen fibers, high water, and low PG concentration. The next layer is the radial region which contains vertically oriented collagen fibers, low water, and high PG concentration (Fig. 3.18). This zone provides the greatest resistance to compressive forces. Chondrocytes organized in columns are found in this radial layer. The next layer is the calcified cartilage and is separated from the radial layer by the so-called *tidemark* (Fig. 3.19). Few chondrocytes are present in this layer which is continuous with the subchondral end plate, which contains a capillary network.

Water is the most abundant component of articular cartilage. Approximately 10% of the water is bound to the collagen and PG chains, and

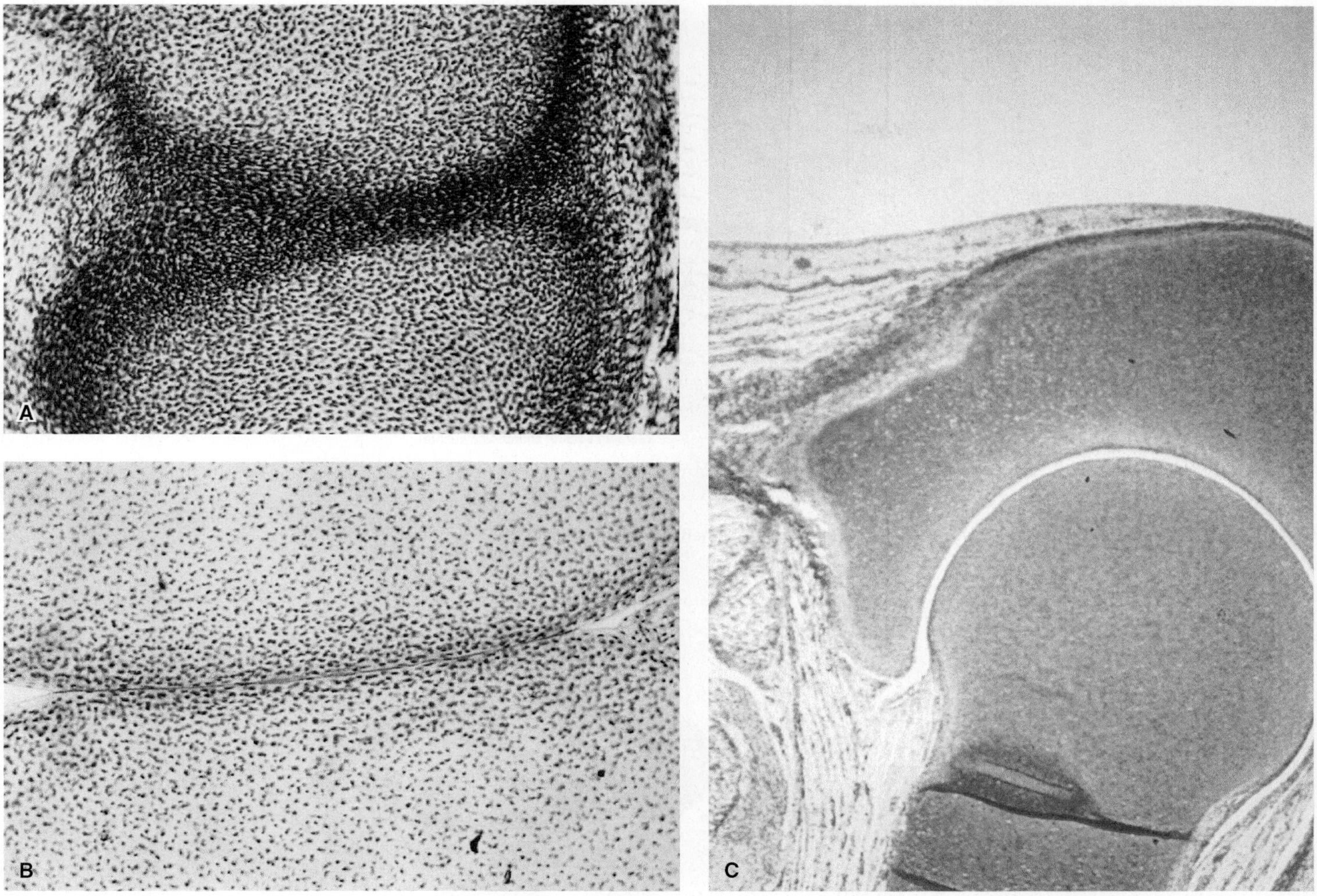

FIGURE 3.13 **Formation of joints.** **(A)** Photomicrograph of a sagittal section through the fetal knee joint at the 6th week of gestation shows the condensation of the mesenchyme, marking the future joint space (H&E, ×10). **(B)** Photomicrograph of a sagittal section through the knee joint at the 9th week of gestation shows the development of the joint space from the periphery to the center of the joint (H&E, ×10). **(C)** Photomicrograph of a section through the hip joint at the 10th week of gestation shows a fully developed joint space (H&E, ×4). (Modified from Bullough P. *Orthopaedic pathology*, 5th ed. Maryland Heights, MO: Mosby; 2009, with permission from Elsevier.)

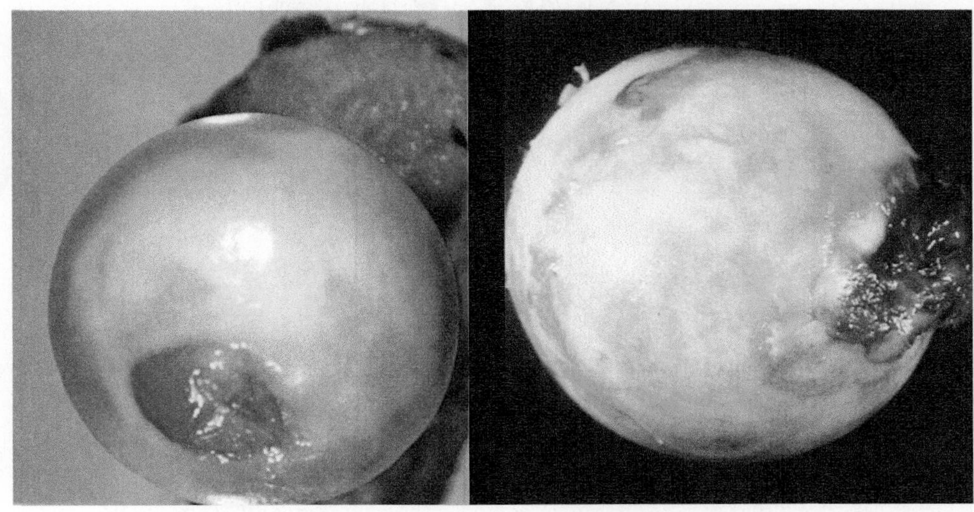

FIGURE 3.14 **Gross specimen of articular hyaline cartilage.** Femoral head of an 18-year-old man shows a translucent bluish-white cartilage *(left)*. Femoral head of a 65-year-old woman shows an opaque, slightly yellowish cartilage *(right)*. (Modified from Bullough P. *Orthopaedic pathology*, 5th ed. Maryland Heights, MO: Mosby; 2009, with permission from Elsevier.)

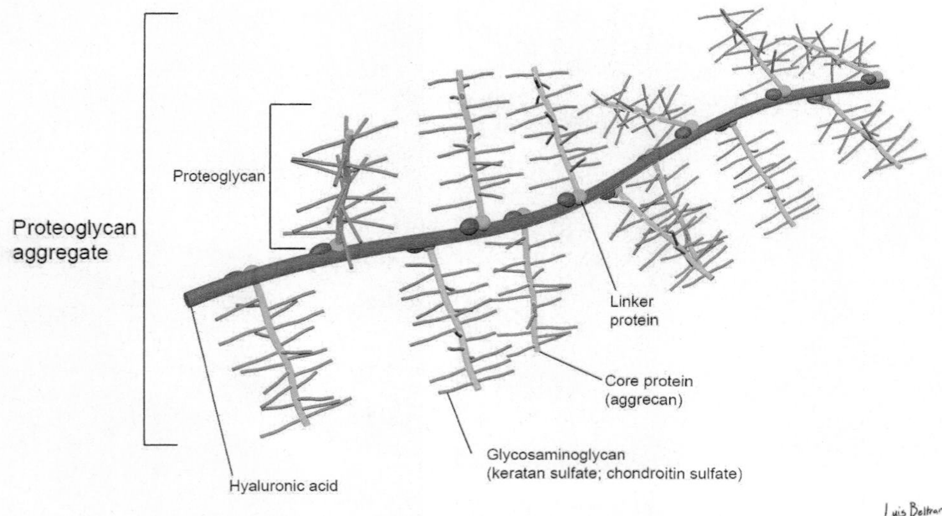

FIGURE 3.15 **Diagram of PG aggregate (aggrecan).** Note the central filament of hyaluronic acid with the side chains of GAGs.

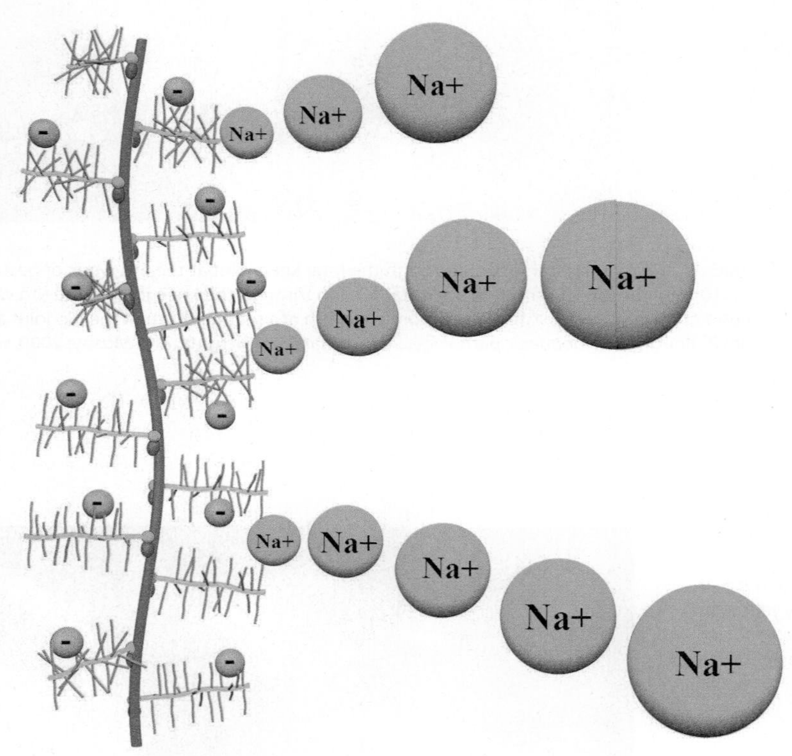

FIGURE 3.16 **Diagram of PG charges.** Note the negative charge of the PG aggregates, attracting positively charged ions such as sodium *(Na+)*.

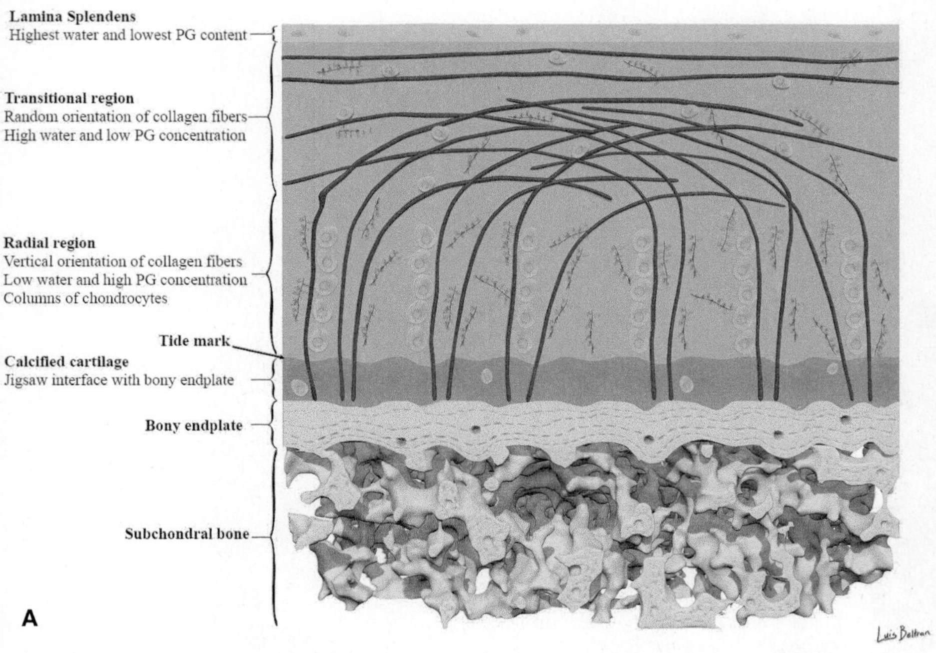

Lamina Splendens
Highest water and lowest PG content

Transitional region
Random orientation of collagen fibers
High water and low PG concentration

Radial region
Vertical orientation of collagen fibers
Low water and high PG concentration
Columns of chondrocytes

Tide mark

Calcified cartilage
Jigsaw interface with bony endplate

Bony endplate

Subchondral bone

A

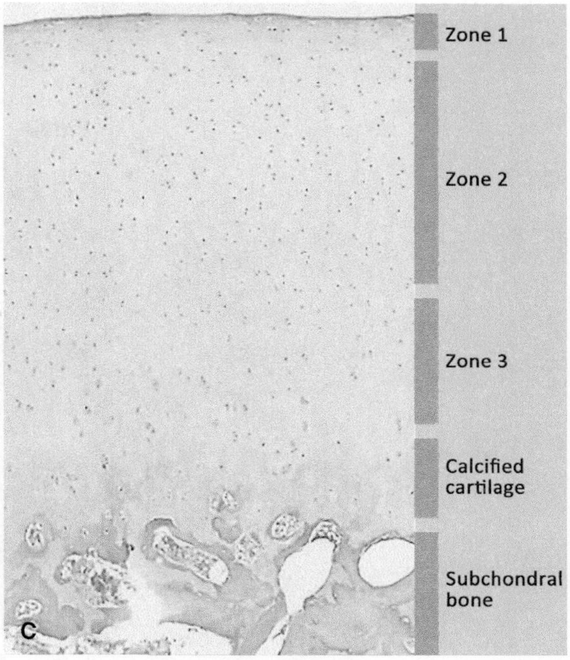

Zone 1
Zone 2
Zone 3
Calcified cartilage
Subchondral bone

C

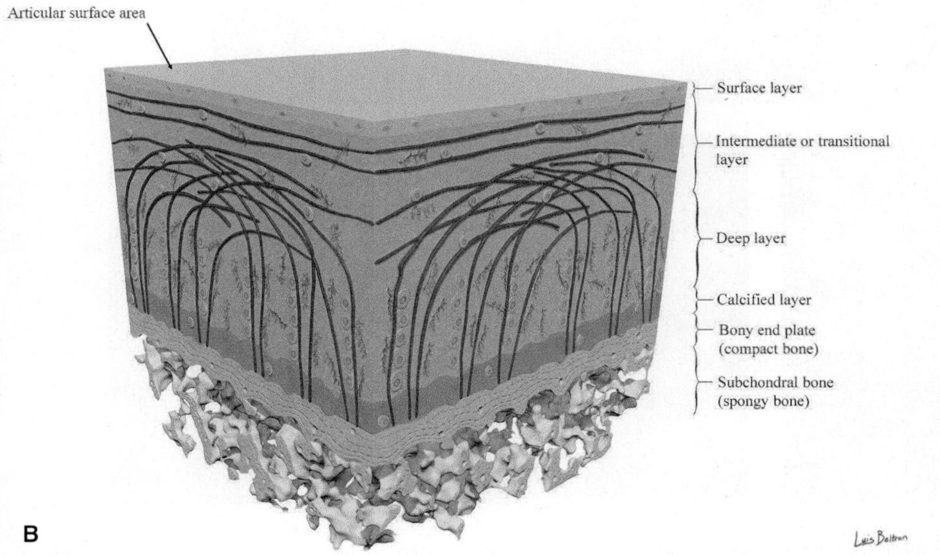

Articular surface area
Surface layer
Intermediate or transitional layer
Deep layer
Calcified layer
Bony end plate (compact bone)
Subchondral bone (spongy bone)

B

FIGURE 3.17 Histology of the articular cartilage. Two-dimensional **(A)** and three-dimensional **(B)** schematic representation of the layers of hyaline articular cartilage. Observe the different orientation of the collagen fibers as it changes from the superficial to the deep layers. Note also the higher PG concentration in the deep layers and the columnar distribution of the chondrocytes. **(C)** Photomicrograph of the articular cartilage depicting various zones (layers).

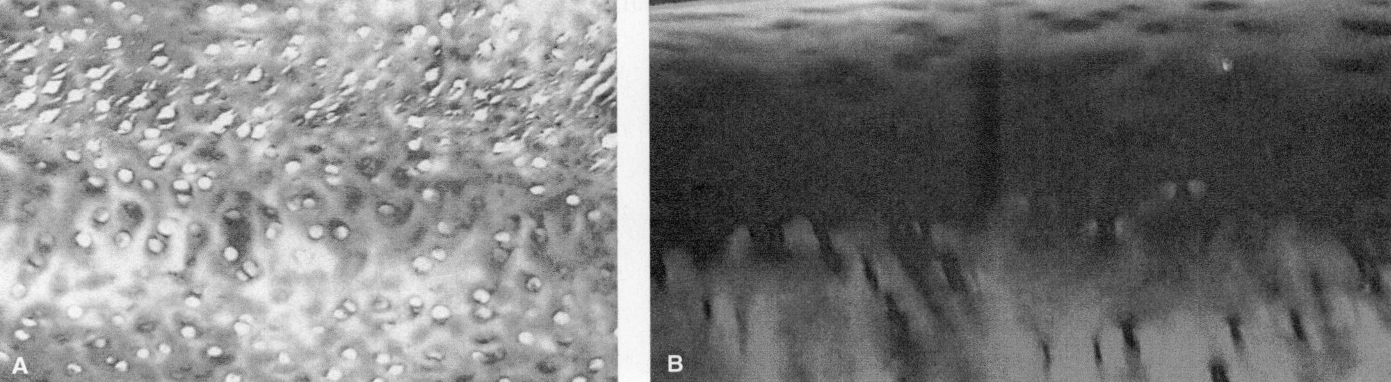

FIGURE 3.18 Histology of normal articular cartilage. **(A)** Photomicrograph of normal articular cartilage shows intense staining of PG. **(B)** Photomicrograph of the articular cartilage using polarized light and a first-order red compensator filter shows the fibers at the surface of the cartilage in blue color and the fibers in the deeper part of the cartilage in red color. Between the two layers, there is less polarization. These observations can be interpreted as demonstrating that at the surface the fibers are horizontally oriented, in the deep part of the cartilage they are vertically oriented, and in between there is a crossover of fibers (×10). (Modified from Bullough P. *Orthopaedic pathology*, 5th ed. Maryland Heights, MO: Mosby; 2009, with permission from Elsevier.)

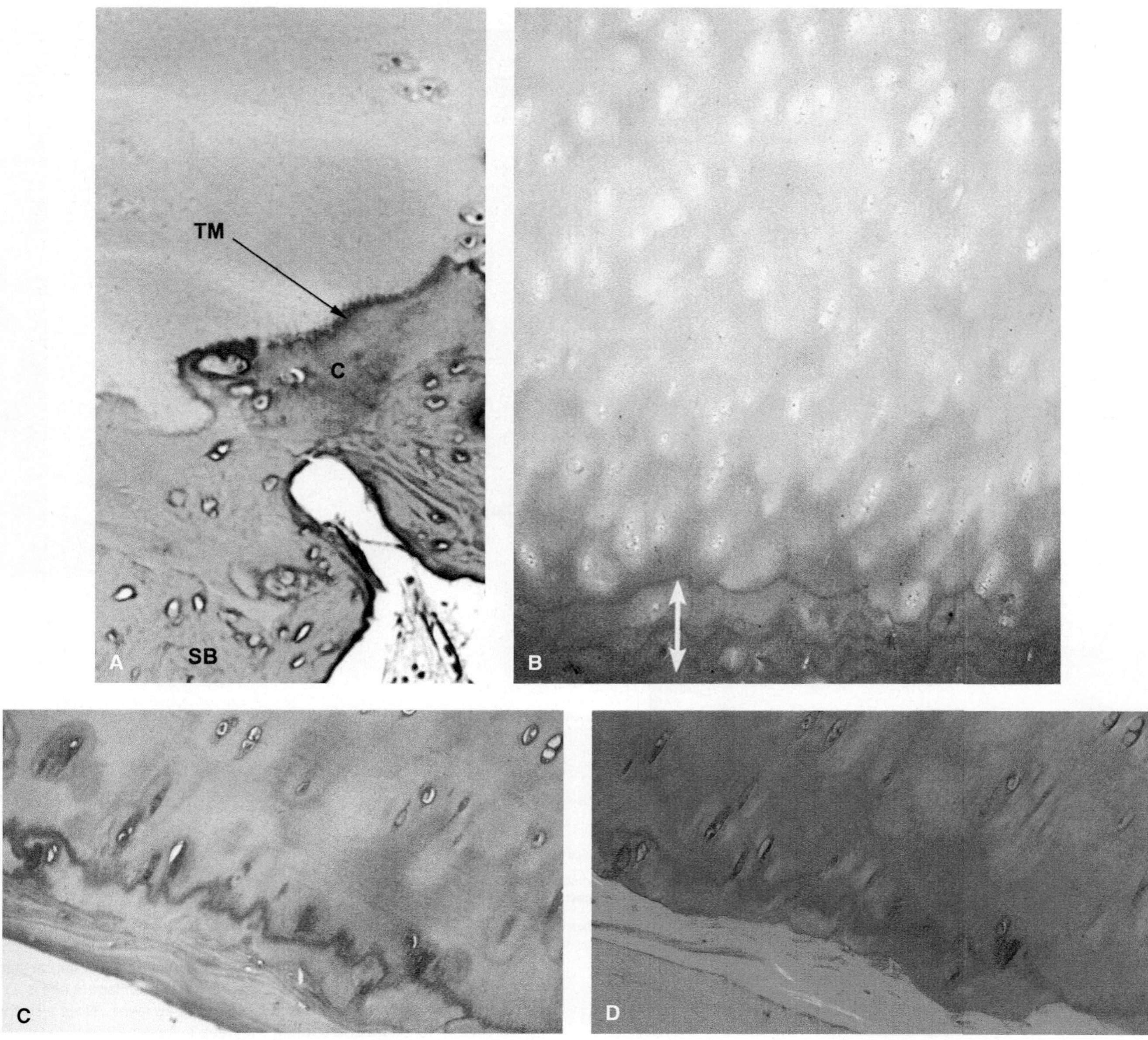

FIGURE 3.19 Histology of normal articular cartilage. **(A)** On this photomicrograph, the cartilage *(C)* immediately adjacent to the subchondral bone *(SB)* exhibits calcified matrix demarcated from the rest of the cartilage by a wavy interface known as the *tidemark (TM)*. **(B)** Mature articular cartilage at its base contains a calcified zone *(double-headed arrow)* into which anchored are the collagen arcades of the cartilage. Because this area resembles high and low tidemarks on a beach, it is referred to as *tidemark*. **(C)** Photomicrograph of the bone–cartilage interface demonstrate the tidemark, which is identified by a dark red wavy line (H&E, ×10). **(D)** When the same histologic field is viewed in a polarized light using a first-order red compensator filter, the bone–cartilage interface is depicted more clearly (H&E, ×10, polarized light). (**A** and **B**, Reprinted with permission from American Registry of Pathology, from Klein MJ, Bonar SF, Freemont T, et al, eds. *Atlas of nontumor pathology. Non-neoplastic diseases of bones and joints.* Washington, DC: American Registry of Pathology and Armed Forces Institute of Pathology; 2011:38, 552, Figs. 1.37 and 7.16. **C** and **D**, (Modified from Bullough P. *Orthopaedic pathology*, 5th ed. Maryland Heights, MO: Mosby; 2009, with permission from Elsevier.)

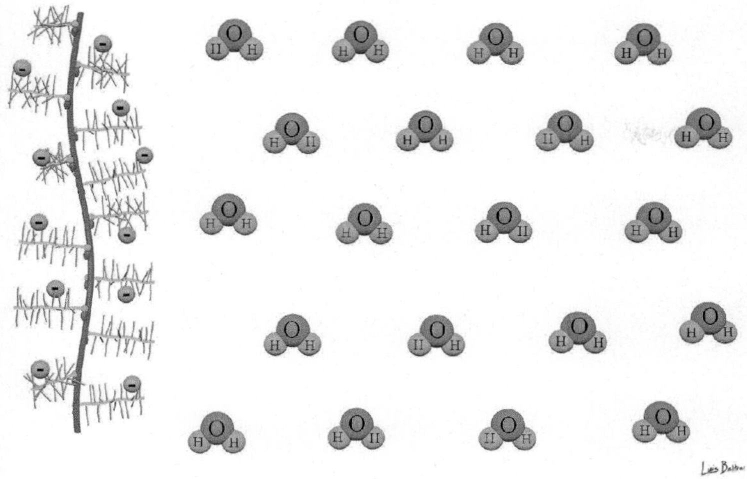

FIGURE 3.20 Diagram of water dynamics. Most of the water in articular cartilage exists as free water. Only about 10% of the water is bound to the PG aggregates.

the remainder free water is in pore spaces of the matrix existing as a gel (Fig. 3.20). Inorganic ions such as sodium, calcium, and potassium are dissolved it the water. Positively charged ions such as sodium are attracted to the negatively charged PGs, achieving electronic neutrality (see Fig. 3.16). Water molecules flow through the cartilage when pressure load is applied (Fig. 3.21). This movement of water helps to transport and distribute nutrients to chondrocytes and provide lubrication.

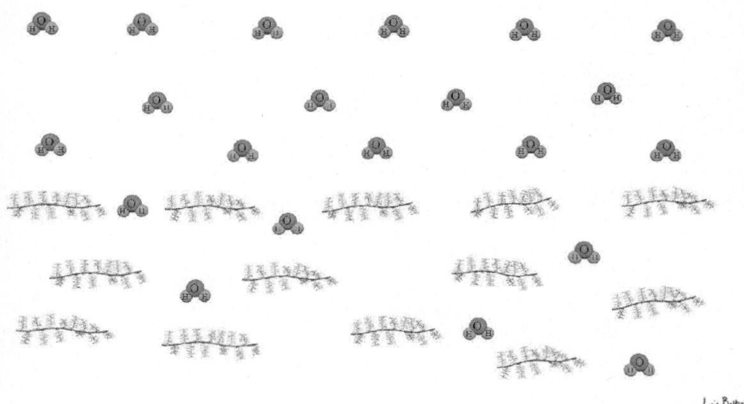

FIGURE 3.21 Diagram of water dynamics. The movement of free water is restricted by the concentration of macromolecules of PGs. In the early stages of cartilage degeneration, there is decreased concentration of PGs allowing increased free water movement.

SUGGESTED READINGS

Anderson HC. Mechanism of mineral formation in bone. *Lab Invest* 1989;60:320–330.

Aoki J, Yamamoto I, Hino M, et al. Reactive endosteal bone formation. *Skeletal Radiol* 1987;16:545–551.

Bernard GW, Pease DC. An electron microscopic study of initial intramembranous osteogenesis. *Am J Anat* 1969;125:271–290.

Bullough PG. *Atlas of orthopedic pathology: with clinical and radiologic correlations*, 2nd ed. New York: Gower Medical Publishing; 1992:1.2–1.35.

Canalis E, McCarthy T, Centrella M. Growth factors and the regulation of bone remodeling. *J Clin Invest* 1988;81:277–281.

Chan BY, Gill KG, Rebsamen SL, et al. MR imaging of pediatric bone marrow. *Radiographics* 2016;36:1911–1930.

Cohen NP, Foster RJ, Mow VC. Composition and dynamics of articular cartilage: structure, function, and maintaining healthy state. *J Orthop Sports Phys Ther* 1998;28:203–215.

Huber M, Trattnig S, Lintner F. Anatomy, biochemistry, and physiology of articular cartilage. *Invest Radiol* 2000;35:573–580.

Iannotti JP. Growth plate physiology and pathology. *Orthop Clin North Am* 1990;21:1–17.

Jaffe HL. *Metabolic, degenerative, and inflammatory diseases of bones and joints.* Philadelphia: Lea & Febiger; 1972.

Jaramillo D, Laor T, Hoffer FA, et al. Epiphyseal marrow in infancy: MR imaging. *Radiology* 1991;180:809–812.

Kirkpatrick JA Jr. Bone and joint growth—normal and in disease. *Clin Rheum Dis* 1981;7:671–688.

Klein MJ, Bonar SF, Freemont T, et al, eds. *Atlas of nontumor pathology. Non-neoplastic diseases of bones and joints.* Washington, DC: American Registry of Pathology and Armed Forces Institute of Pathology; 2011:1–53.

Lee WR, Marshall JH, Sissons HA. Calcium accretion and bone formation in dogs. *J Bone Joint Surg Br* 1965;47B:157–180.

Oestreich AE. The acrophysis: a unifying concept for enchondral bone growth and its disorders. *Skeletal Radiol* 2003;32:121–127.

Oestreich AE, Crawford AH. *Atlas of pediatric orthopedic radiology.* Stuttgart: Thieme; 1985:17–18.

Pearle AD, Warren RF, Rodeo SA. Basic science of articular cartilage and osteoarthritis. *Clin Sports Med* 2005;24:1–12.

Poulton TB, Murphy WD, Duerk JL, et al. Bone marrow reconversion in adults who are smokers: MR imaging findings. *Am J Roentgenol* 1993;161:1217–1221.

Raisz LG, Kream BE. Regulation of bone formation. *N Engl J Med* 1983;309:83–89.

Reddi AH, Anderson WA. Collagenous bone matrix-induced endochondral ossification and hemopoiesis. *J Cell Biol* 1976;69:557–572.

Reed MH. Normal and abnormal development. In: Reed MH, ed. *Pediatric skeletal radiology.* Baltimore: Williams & Wilkins; 1992:349–392.

Resnick D, Manolagas SC, Niwayama G. Histogenesis, anatomy, and physiology of bone. In: Resnick D, ed. *Bone and joint imaging.* Philadelphia: WB Saunders; 1989:16–28.

Rubin P. *Dynamic classification of bone dysplasias.* Chicago: Year Book Medical Publishers; 1964:1–23.

Sissons HA. Structure and growth of bones and joints. In: Taveras JM, Ferrucci JT, eds. *Radiology, diagnosis-imaging-intervention*, vol. 5. Philadelphia: JB Lippincott; 1986:1–11.

Sissons HA. The growth of bone. In: *The biochemistry and physiology of bone*, vol. 3, 2nd ed. New York: Academic Press; 1971.

Sophia Fox AJ, Bedi A, Rodeo SA. The basic science of articular cartilage: structure, composition, and function. *Sports Health* 2009;16:461–468.

Vande Berg BC, Lecouvet FE, Galant C, et al. Normal variants and frequent marrow alterations that simulate bone marrow lesions at MR imaging. *Radiol Clin of North Am* 2005;43:761–770.

Vande Berg BC, Malghem J, Lecouvet FE, et al. Magnetic resonance imaging of the normal bone marrow. *Skeletal Radiol* 1998;27:471–483.

Warshawsky H. Embryology and development of the skeletal system. In: Cruess RL, ed. *The musculoskeletal system. Embryology, biochemistry, physiology.* New York: Churchill Livingstone; 1982.

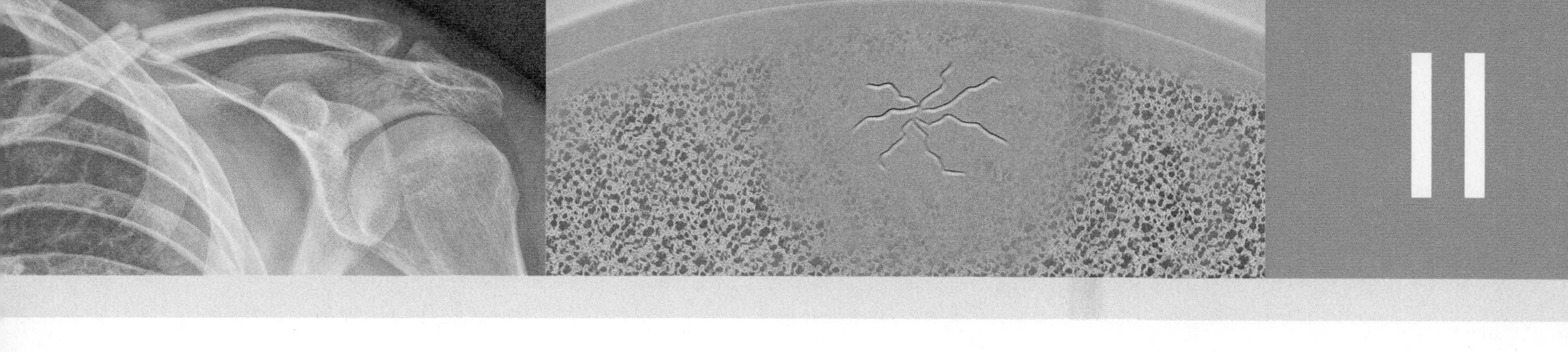

II

TRAUMA

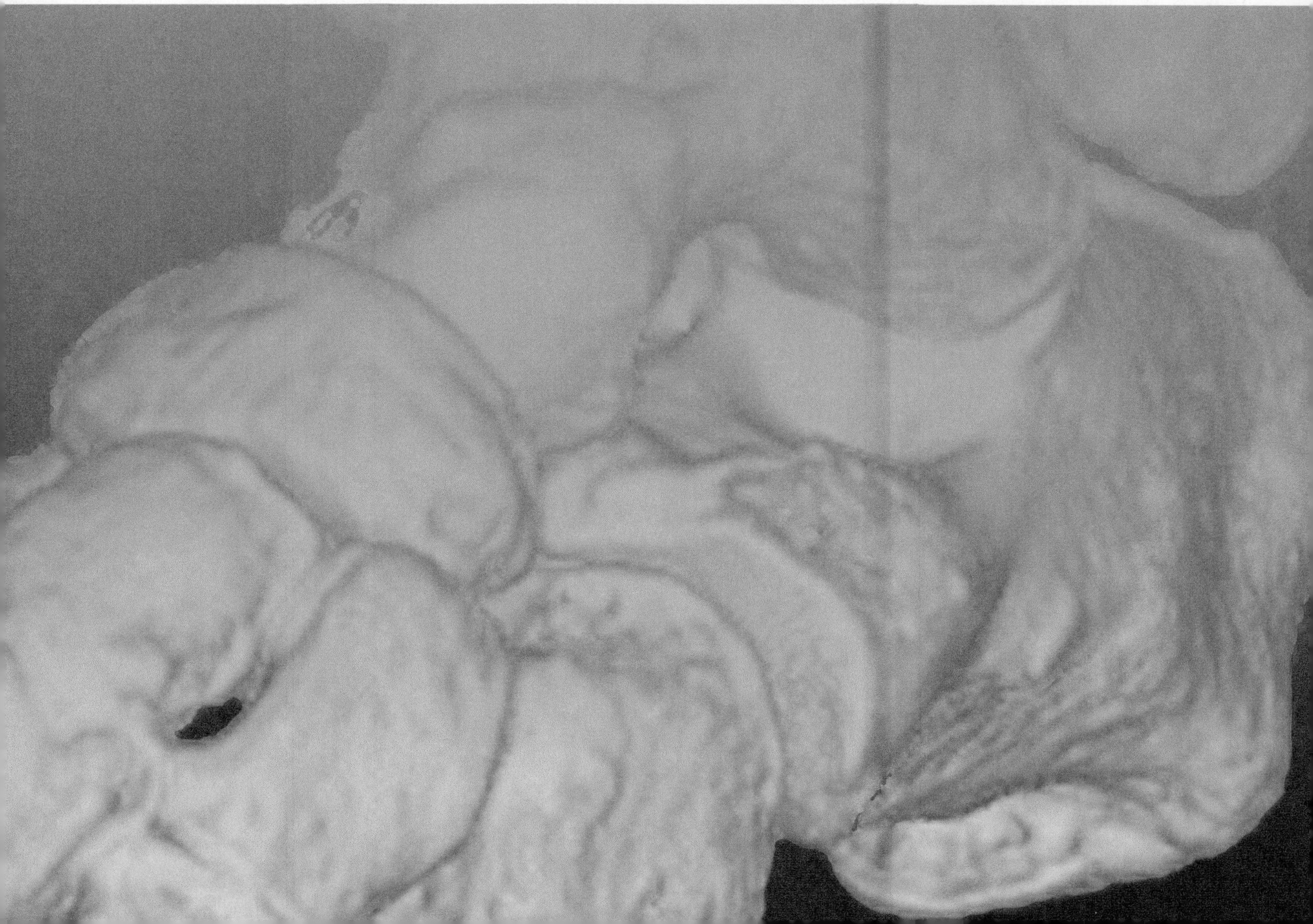

4

Imaging Evaluation of Trauma

Imaging Modalities

The imaging modalities used in analyzing an injury to the musculoskeletal system are as follows:

1. Conventional radiography, including routine views (specific for various body parts), special views, and stress views
2. Digital (computed) radiography, including digital subtraction arthrography (DSa) and digital subtraction angiography (DSA)
3. Fluoroscopy, alone or combined with videotaping
4. Computed tomography (CT), including three-dimensional (3D) CT
5. Arthrography
6. Myelography and diskography
7. Angiography (arteriography and venography)
8. Scintigraphy (radionuclide bone scan), including single-photon emission CT (SPECT) and SPECT/CT
9. Ultrasound (US)
10. Magnetic resonance imaging (MRI) including MR-arthrography (MRa)

Radiography and Fluoroscopy

In most instances, radiographs obtained in two orthogonal projections, usually the anteroposterior and lateral, at 90 degrees to each other are sufficient (Figs. 4.1 and 4.2). Occasionally, oblique and special views are necessary, particularly in evaluating fractures of complex structures such as the pelvis, elbow, wrist, and ankle (Figs. 4.3 and 4.4). Stress views are important in evaluating ligamentous tears and joint stability (Fig. 4.5).

Fluoroscopy and videotaping are useful in evaluating the kinematics of joints and fragments. It is also valuable in monitoring the progress of healing.

Computed Tomography

CT is essential in the evaluation of complex fractures, particularly of the spine, pelvis, and scapula, although this modality is useful in the assessment of any fracture near or extending into the joint (Figs. 4.6, to 4.8; see also Figs. 7.13B, 7.14B, and 7.15B). The advantage of CT over conventional radiography is its ability to provide excellent contrast resolution and accurate measurement of the tissue attenuation coefficient. The use of sagittal, coronal, and multiplanar reformation (see Figs. 9.26B,C, 9.27A, and 9.28A,B) as well as reconstruction to create the 3D CT images (Figs. 4.9 and 4.10; see also Figs. 2.9 to 2.11) provides an added advantage over other imaging modalities.

Scintigraphy

Radionuclide bone scanning can detect occult fractures or fractures too subtle to be seen on conventional radiographs (Fig. 4.11). This technique is also effective in the differentiation of tibial stress fractures from shin splints. Scintigraphy is also helpful in distinguishing noninfected fractures from infected ones. With osteomyelitis, scanning, using gallium-67 (^{67}Ga) citrate and indium-labeled white blood cells (indium-111 [^{111}In]), demonstrates a significant increase in the uptake of the tracer. Because ^{67}Ga is also actively taken up at the site of a normally healing fracture but significantly less than that encountered with technetium-99m (^{99m}Tc) scanning agents, the combination of ^{67}Ga and ^{99m}Tc methylene diphosphonate (MDP) has been suggested, using the ratio of uptake of ^{67}Ga to ^{99m}Tc to determine whether the fracture is infected. The ratio of ^{67}Ga to ^{99m}Tc MDP should be higher in infected fractures than in noninfected fractures.

Ultrasound

Ultrasound as a diagnostic procedure has a limited application in trauma, occasionally being used to evaluate the rotator cuff tears. More often, it is applied in form of ultrasound-guided interventional procedures (see discussion in Chapter 2).

Arthrography

Arthrography is still occasionally used in the evaluation of injuries to articular cartilage, menisci, joint capsules, tendons, and ligaments, although, in general, it has been replaced by MRI and MRa. Although virtually, every joint can be injected with a contrast agent, the examination is most frequently performed in the knee (Fig. 4.12), shoulder (Fig. 4.13), wrist (see Figs. 7.97 and 7.98), ankle (see Fig. 10.94C), and elbow (see Fig. 6.15) articulations..

Myelography and Diskography

Myelography, either alone or in conjunction with CT scan, is used to evaluate certain traumatic conditions of the spine (Fig. 4.14A). If a disk abnormality is suspected and a myelographic study is not diagnostic, diskography may yield information required for further patient management (Fig. 4.14B).

Angiography

Angiography is indicated if a concomitant injury to the vascular system is suspected (Fig. 4.15). DSA is preferred because subtraction of the overlying bones results in a clear delineation of vascular structures (see Fig. 2.3).

Magnetic Resonance Imaging

MRI plays a leading role in the evaluation of trauma to bone, cartilage, and soft tissue. MRI evaluation of trauma to the knee, particularly abnormalities of the menisci and ligaments, has a high negative predictive value. MRI can be used to screen patients before surgery so that unnecessary arthroscopies are avoided. MRI is probably the only imaging modality that can demonstrate so-called *bone contusions* (see Figs. 2.53 and 2.54). These abnormalities consist of posttraumatic marrow change resulting from a

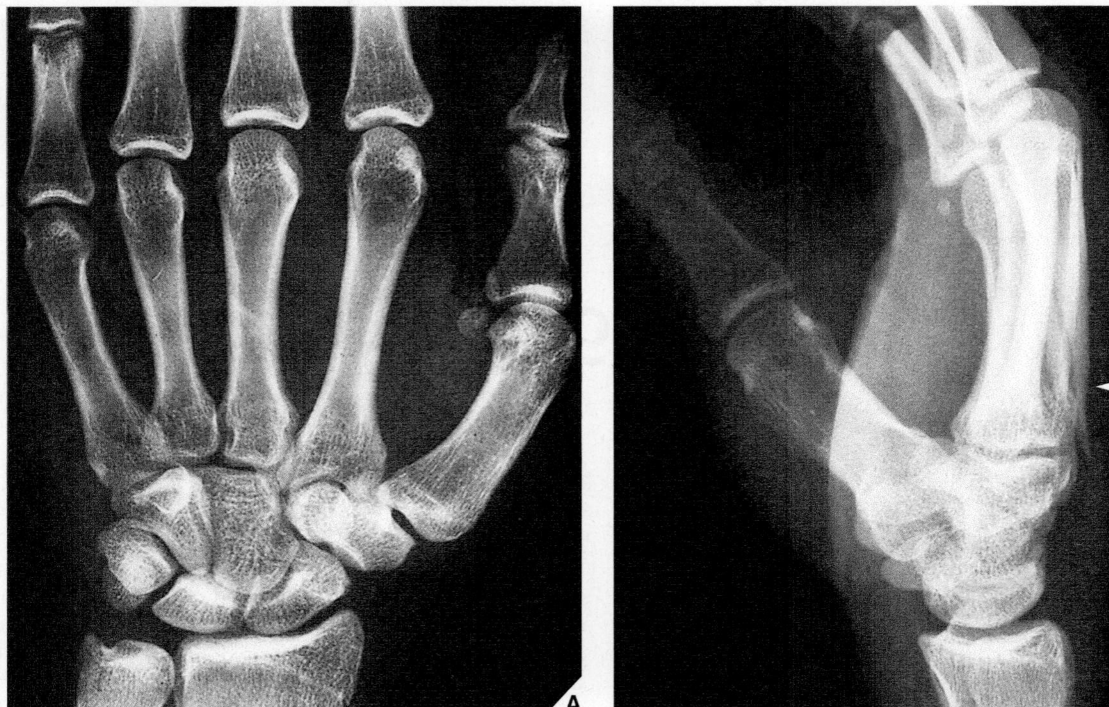

FIGURE 4.1 Fracture of the metacarpal bone in an adult. **(A)** Dorsovolar (posteroanterior) radiograph of the hand does not demonstrate a fracture. **(B)** The lateral radiograph reveals a fracture of the third metacarpal bone *(arrow)*.

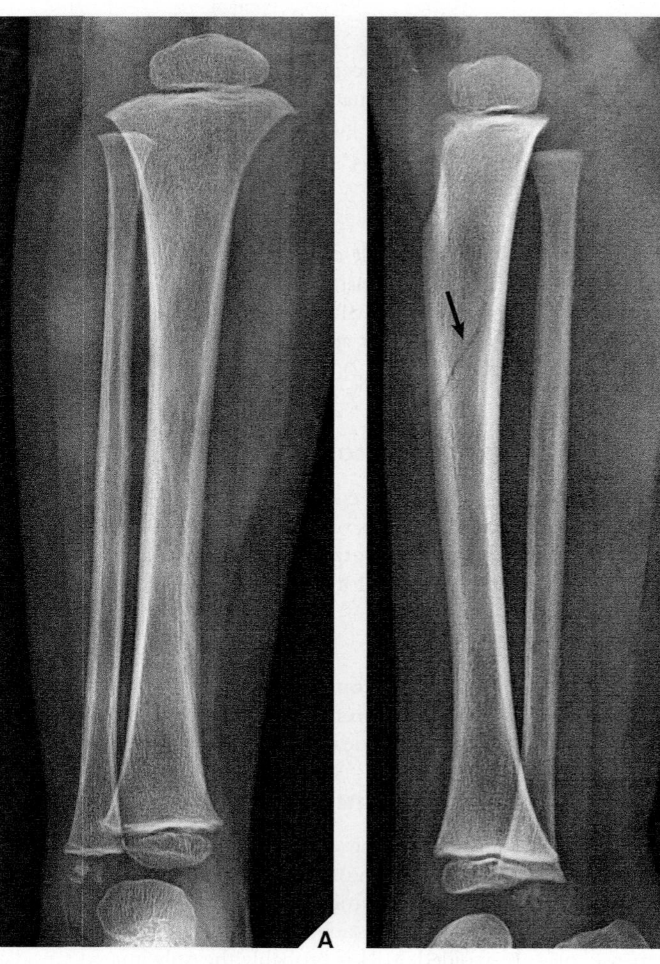

FIGURE 4.2 Fracture of the tibia in a child. **(A)** Anteroposterior radiograph of the leg of a 3-year-old boy shows no abnormalities. **(B)** The lateral radiograph demonstrates a nondisplaced oblique fracture of the tibial diaphysis *(arrow)*.

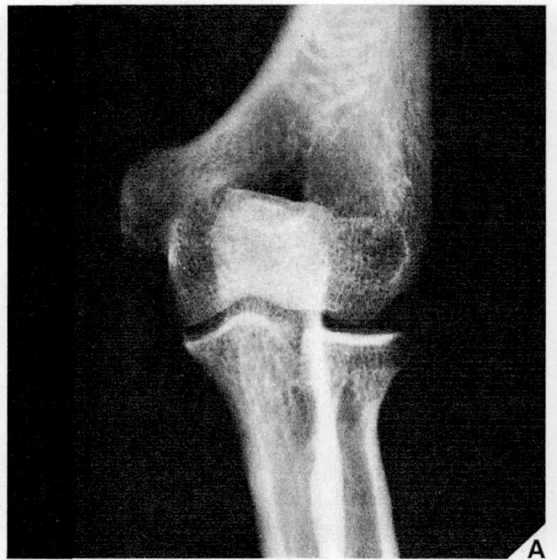

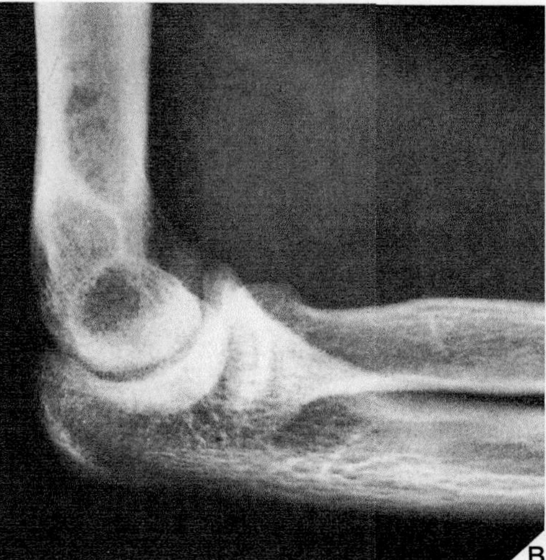

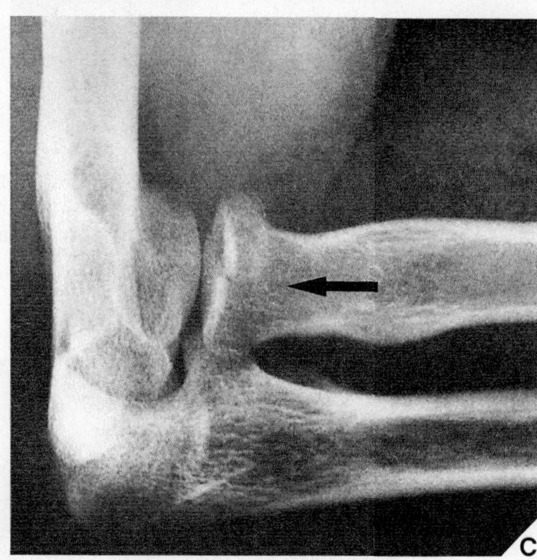

FIGURE 4.3 Fracture of the radial head. A patient presented with elbow pain after a fall. Anteroposterior **(A)** and lateral **(B)** radiographs are normal; however, the radial head and coronoid processes are not well demonstrated because of a bony overlap. A special 45-degree angle view of the elbow **(C)** is used to project the radial head ventrad, free of the overlap of other bones. A short, intraarticular fracture of the radial head is now clearly visible *(arrow)*.

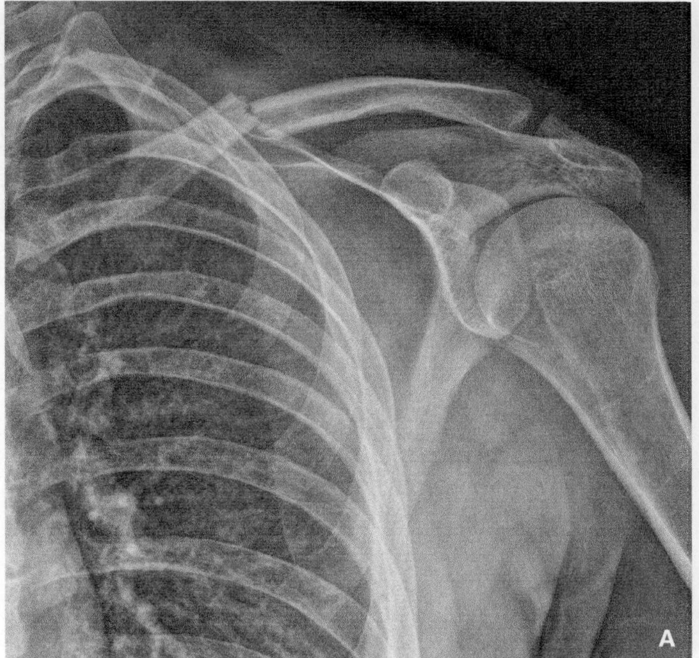

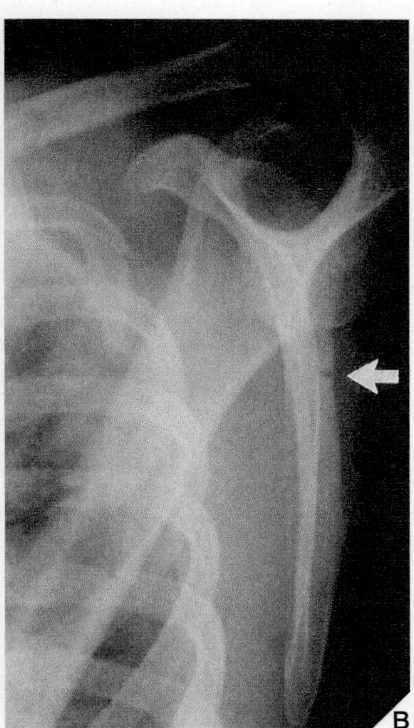

FIGURE 4.4 Fracture of the scapula. **(A)** Anteroposterior radiograph of the left shoulder shows a fracture of the clavicle. An injury to the scapula is not well demonstrated. **(B)** A special "Y" view of the scapula clearly shows the fracture *(arrow)*.

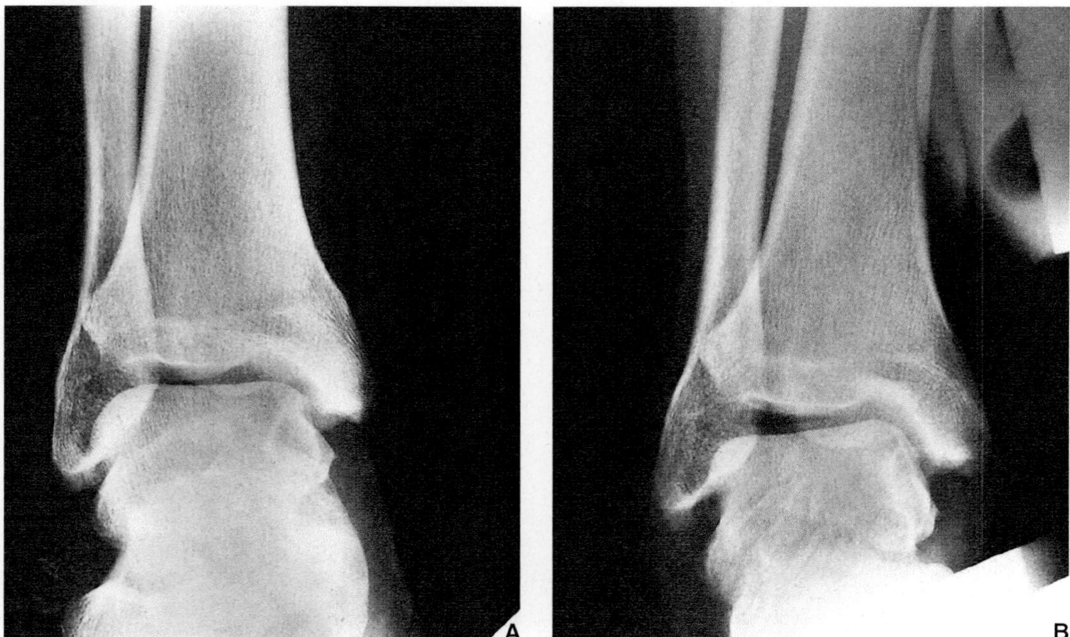

FIGURE 4.5 Tear of the lateral collateral ligament. In most ankle injuries, if a ligamentous tear is suspected, then conventional films may be supplemented by stress views. The standard anteroposterior radiograph of this ankle **(A)** is not remarkable. The same view after the application of adduction (inversion) stress **(B)** shows a widening of the lateral compartment of the tibiotalar (ankle) joint, indicating a tear of the lateral collateral ligament.

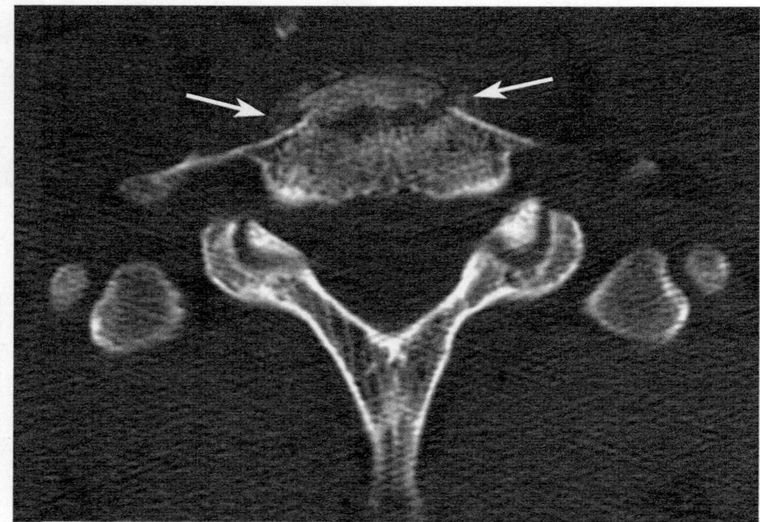

FIGURE 4.6 CT of fracture of the vertebra. Conventional radiographs of the cervical spine (not shown here) were suggestive but not conclusive of a fracture of C7 vertebral body, which is, however, clearly demonstrated on this axial CT image *(arrows)*.

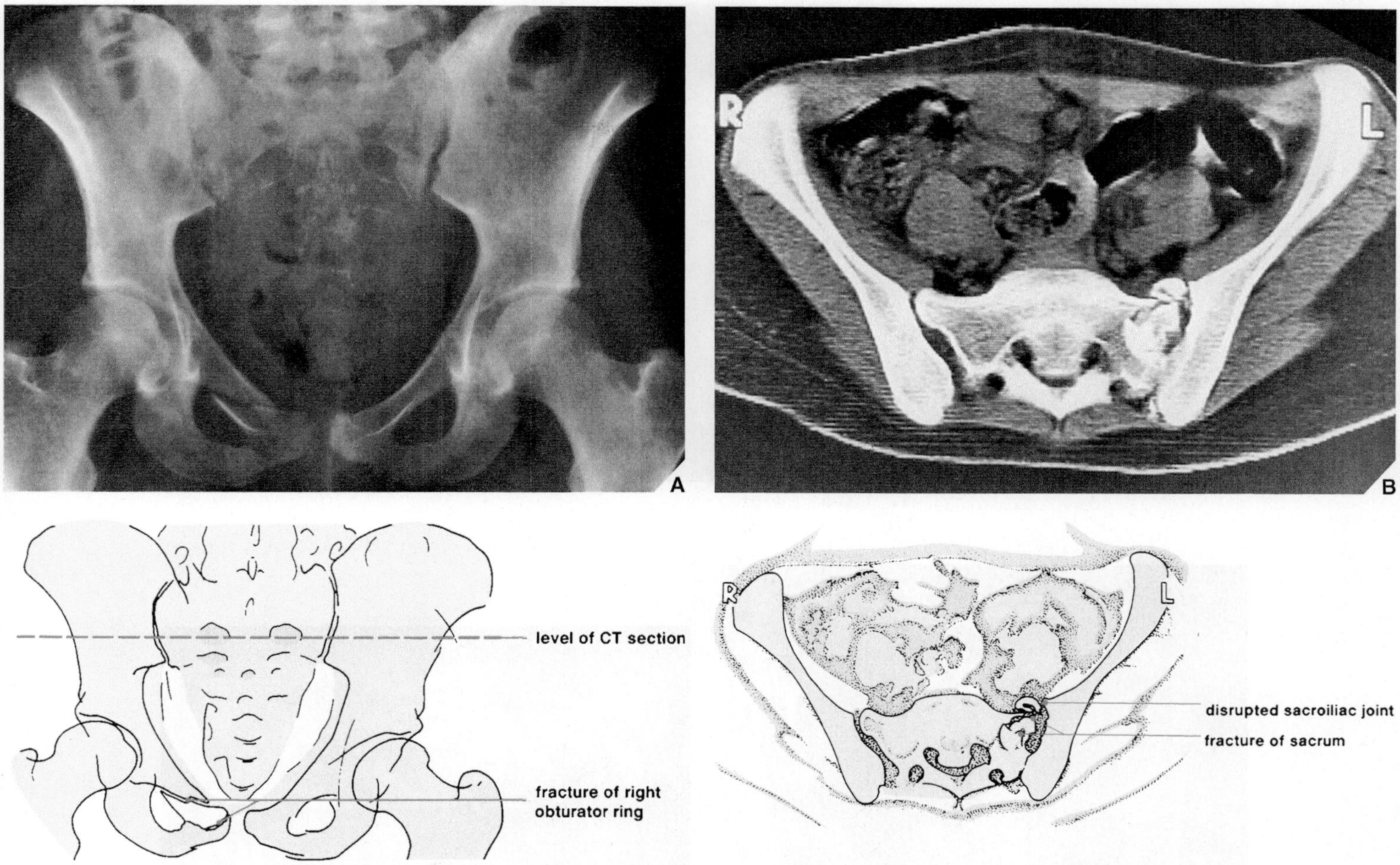

FIGURE 4.7 CT of fracture of the sacrum. **(A)** Standard anteroposterior radiograph of the pelvis shows obvious fractures of the right obturator ring. **(B)** CT section demonstrates an unsuspected fracture of the sacrum and disruption of the left sacroiliac joint.

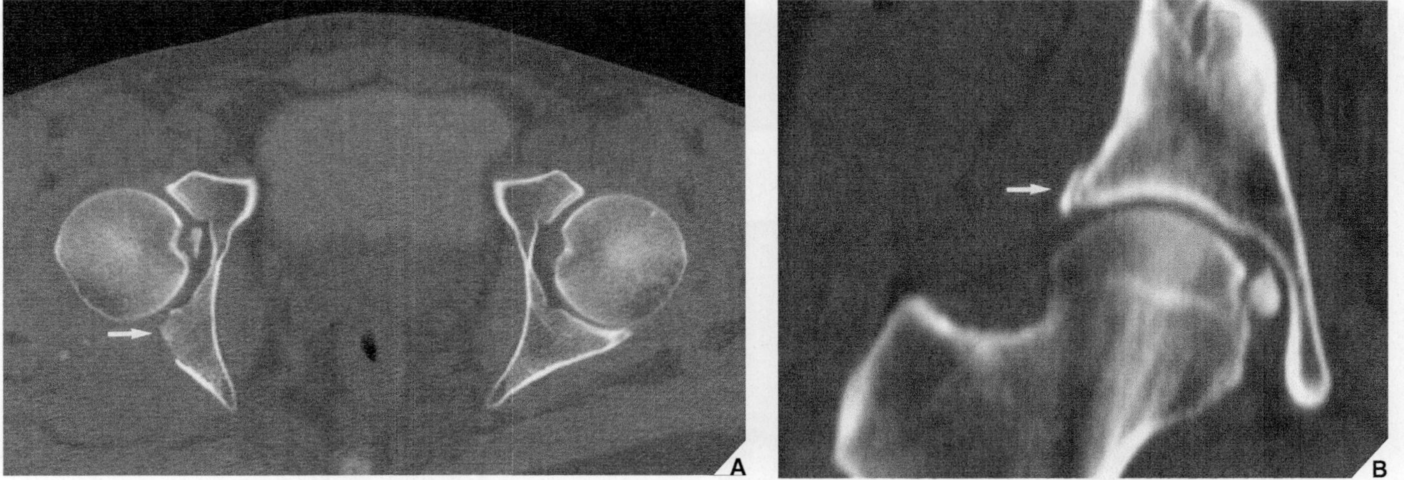

FIGURE 4.8 CT of fracture of the acetabulum. Axial **(A)** and coronal **(B)** CT reformatted images show a fractured fragment, unsuspected on conventional radiographs, displaced into the right hip joint. The *arrows* point to the fracture of the posterior column of the right acetabulum.

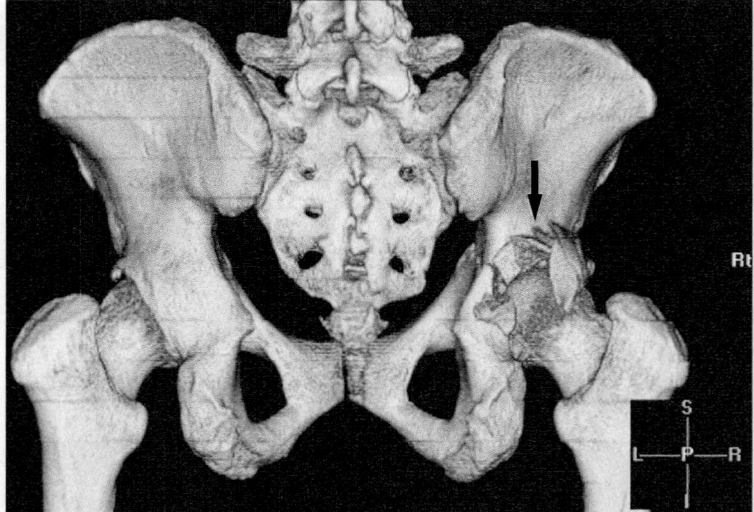

FIGURE 4.9 3D CT of fracture of the acetabulum. 3D CT reconstructed image shows distinctive features of a fracture of the posterior wall of the left acetabulum *(arrow)*.

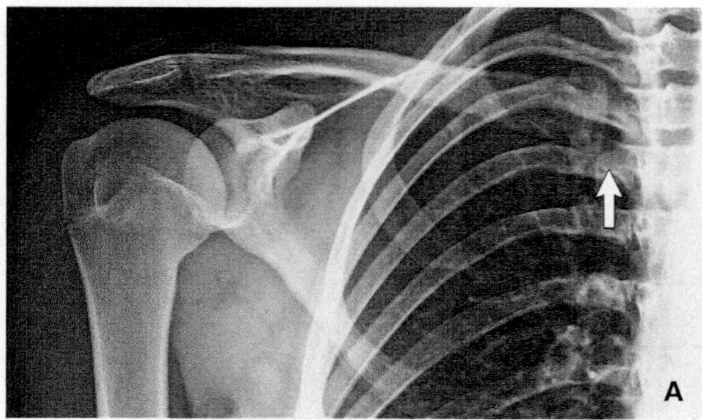

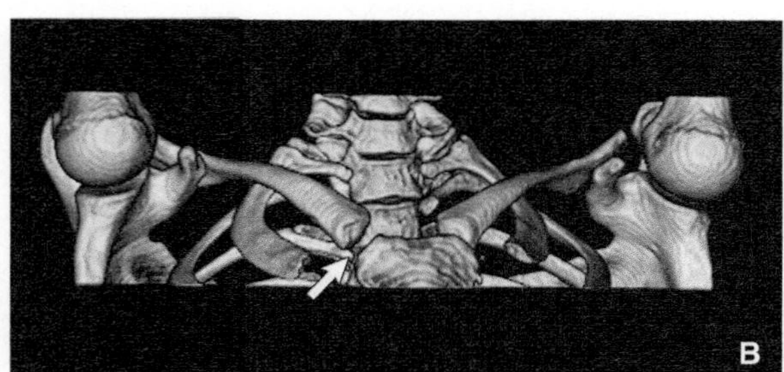

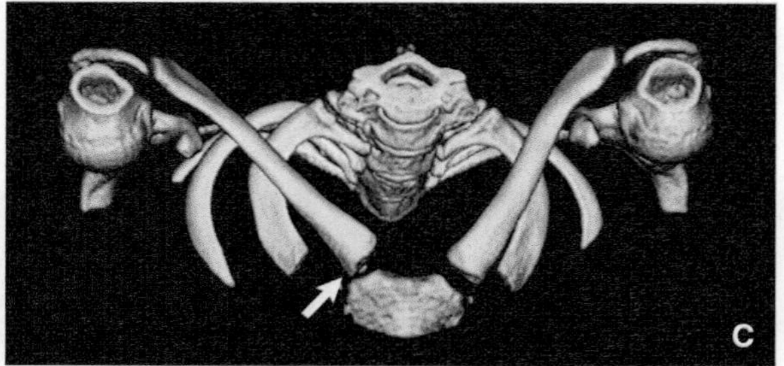

FIGURE 4.10 3D CT of subluxation in the sternoclavicular joint. A 19-year-old woman presented with history of trauma to the anterior chest wall and pain in the region of the right sternoclavicular joint. **(A)** Anteroposterior radiograph of the right shoulder shows no abnormalities. Sternoclavicular joint appears normal *(arrow)*. 3D CT reconstructed images in frontal **(B)** and craniocaudal **(C)** projection (bird's eye view) clearly demonstrate subluxation in the right sternoclavicular joint *(arrows)*.

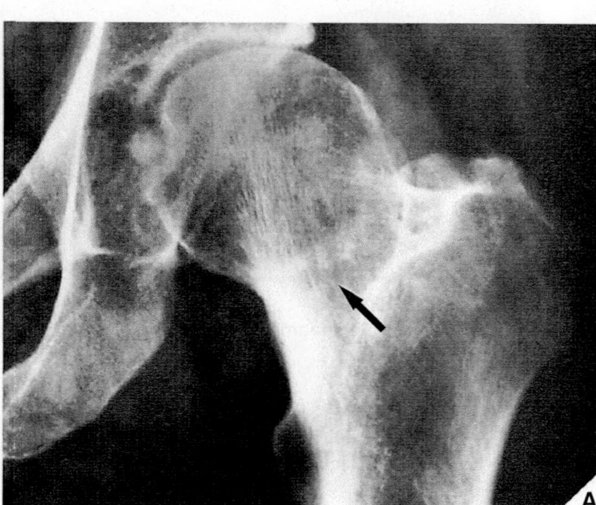

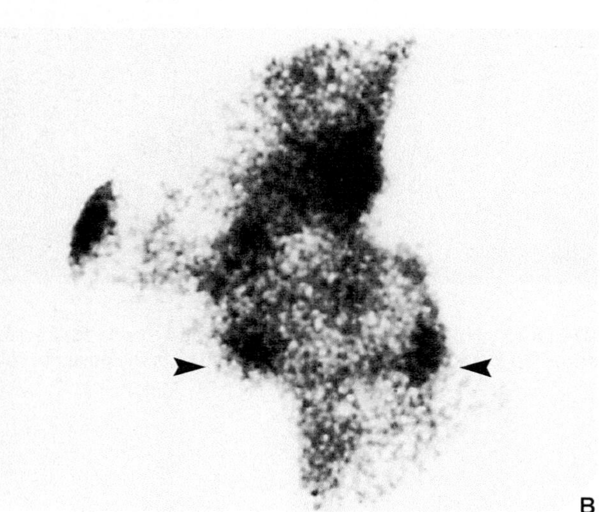

FIGURE 4.11 Scintigraphy of fracture of the femoral neck. **(A)** Anteroposterior view of the left hip reveals a band of increased density *(arrow)*, suggesting a fracture of the femoral neck. **(B)** A radionuclide bone scan performed after the administration of 15 mCi (555 MBq) of ^{99m}TC-labeled MDP shows increased uptake of isotope in the region of the femoral neck *(arrowheads)*, confirming the fracture.

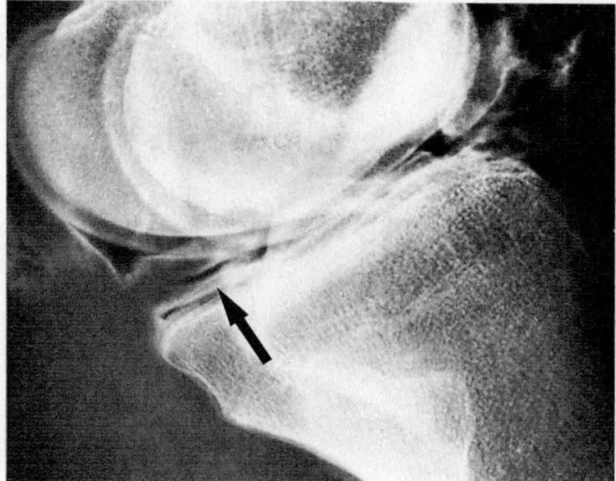

FIGURE 4.12 Arthrography of tear of the medial meniscus. In this patient, double-contrast arthrography of the knee shows a horizontal cleavage tear in the posterior horn of the medial meniscus *(arrow)*.

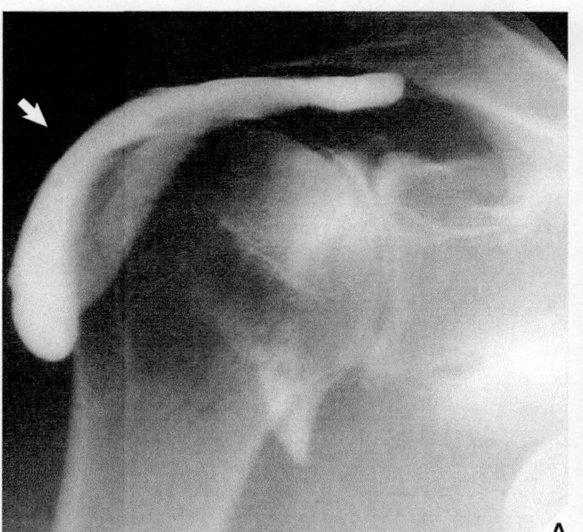

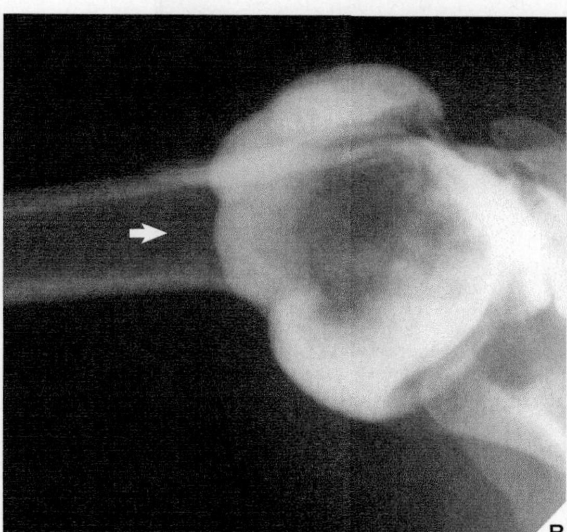

FIGURE 4.13 Tear of the rotator cuff. **(A)** Anteroposterior and **(B)** axillary radiographs, obtained after single-contrast arthrogram of the right shoulder was performed, show a leak of the contrast into the subacromial-subdeltoid bursae complex *(arrows)* diagnostic of a full-thickness tear of the supraspinatus tendon.

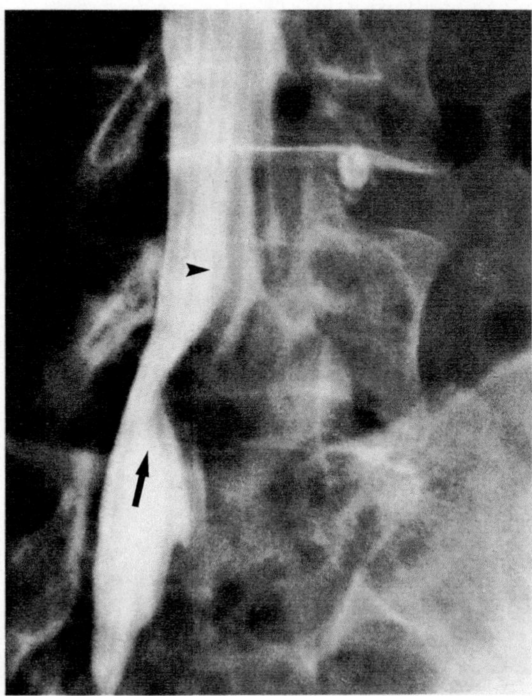

FIGURE 4.14A Myelography of herniation of the lumbar disk. A patient strained his back by lifting a heavy object. An oblique view of the lower lumbosacral spine after an injection of metrizamide contrast into the subarachnoid space shows an extradural pressure defect on the thecal sac at the L5-S1 intervertebral space *(arrow)* characteristic of disk herniation. Note the markedly swollen, displaced nerve root *(arrowhead)*.

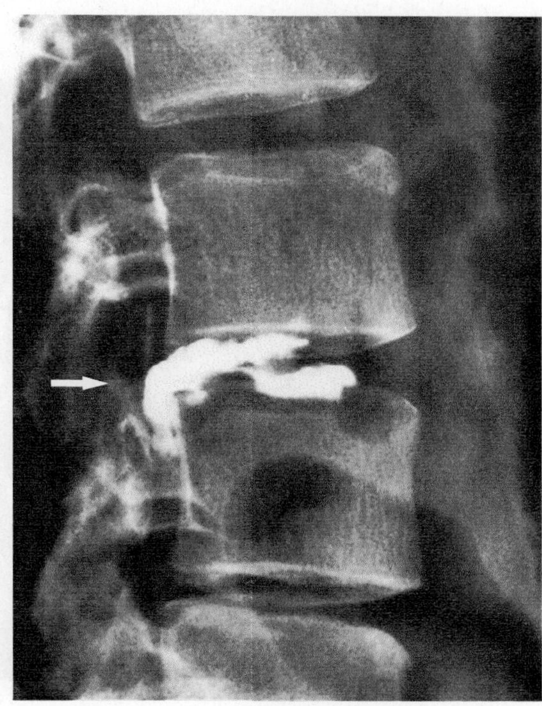

FIGURE 4.14B Diskography of rupture of the annulus fibrosus and disk herniation. A spinal needle was placed in the center of the nucleus pulposus and a few milliliters of metrizamide were injected. The leak of contrast into the extradural space *(arrow)* indicates a tear of the annulus fibrosus and posterior disk herniation.

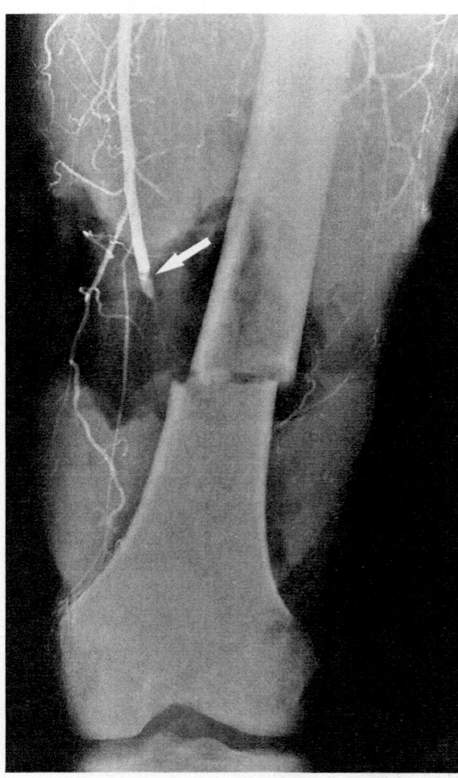

▲
FIGURE 4.15 **Angiography of tear of the femoral artery.** A femoral arteriogram was performed to rule out damage to vascular structures by a fractured femur. Transverse fracture of the distal femur resulted in transsection of the superficial femoral artery *(arrow)*.

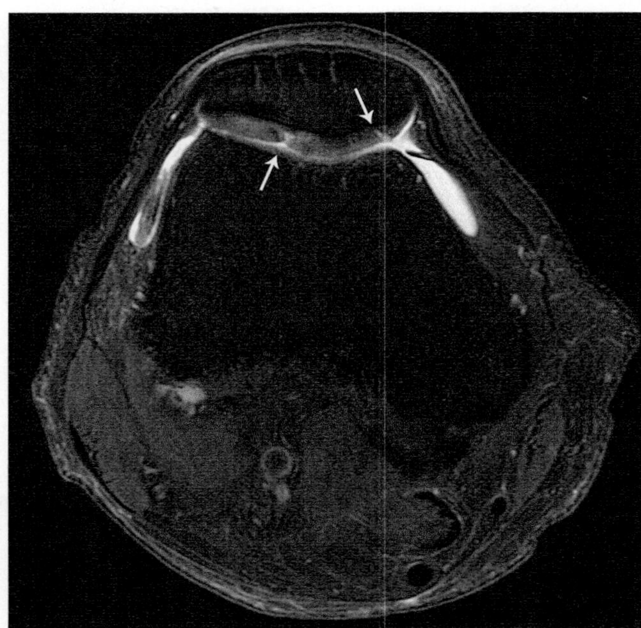

▲
FIGURE 4.16 **MRI of chondral defects.** Axial proton density–weighted fat-saturated MRI of the knee demonstrates subtle defects in the articular cartilage of the right patella *(arrows)*.

combination of hemorrhage, edema, and microtrabecular injury. Meniscal injuries, such as bucket-handle tears, tears of the free edge, and peripheral detachments, can be accurately diagnosed. Other subtle abnormalities of various structures, such as articular cartilage, and posttraumatic joint effusion can also be well visualized (Figs. 4.16 and 4.17). Similarly, the medial and lateral collateral ligaments, anterior and posterior cruciate ligaments, and tendons around the knee joint can be well demonstrated (see Figs. 9.12 and 9.13), and abnormalities of these structures can be diagnosed with high accuracy. In the shoulder, impingement syndrome and complete and incomplete rotator cuff tears may be effectively diagnosed most of the time (Fig. 4.18). Traumatic lesions of the tendons (such as biceps tendon rupture), traumatic joint effusions, and hematomas are easily diagnosed with MRI. Likewise, this modality is effective to diagnose a tear of the cartilaginous labrum. The changes of osteonecrosis at various sites, particularly in its early stage, may be detected by MRI when other modalities, such as conventional radiography and even radionuclide bone scan, may be normal. MRI of the ankle and foot has been used among others in diagnosing tendon ruptures and posttraumatic osteonecrosis of the talus. In the wrist and hand, MRI has been successfully used in the early diagnosis

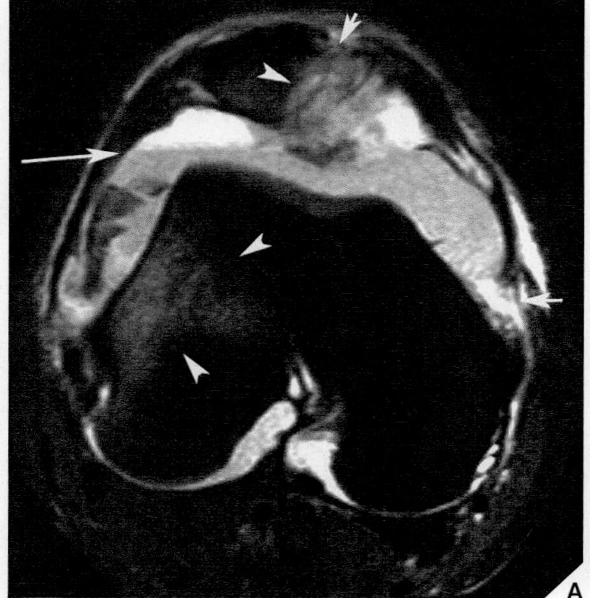

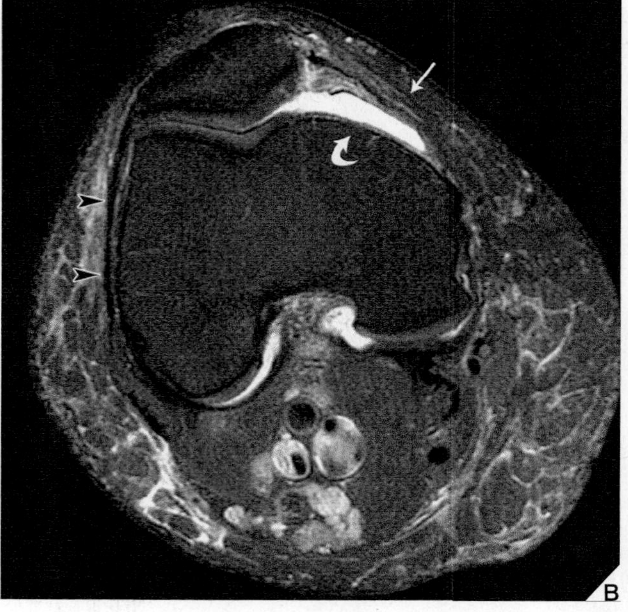

▲
FIGURE 4.17 **MRI of joint effusion and a tear of the patellar retinaculum.** **(A)** A young man sustained a twisting injury to the knee. Axial short time inversion recovery (STIR) pulse sequence MR image demonstrates hemarthrosis with a fluid–fluid level *(long arrow)*, bone contusion of the lateral femoral condyle *(arrowheads)*, osteochondral fracture of the medial facet of the patella *(arrowhead)*, and rupture of the medial patellofemoral ligament (a component of the medial patellar retinaculum) at the patellar and femoral insertions *(short arrows)*. **(B)** A 33-year-old woman injured her right knee in a ski accident. Axial proton density–weighted fat-suppressed MRI shows a tear of the medial retinaculum of the patella *(arrow)*. The lateral retinaculum is intact *(arrowheads)*. A *curved arrow* points to posttraumatic joint effusion.

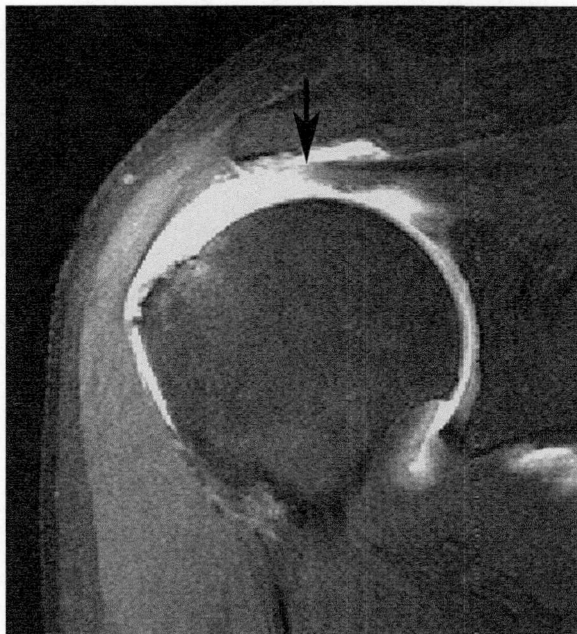

FIGURE 4.18 **MRa of tear of the rotator cuff.** A 56-year-old man presented with right shoulder pain. Oblique coronal T1-weighted fat-suppressed MRa demonstrates a full-thickness rotator cuff tear. The supraspinatus tendon is retracted medially *(arrow)* and no tendon tissue is present in the subacromial space.

of posttraumatic osteonecrosis of the scaphoid and Kienböck disease. MRI is strongly advocated as the technique of choice in the evaluation of abnormalities of the triangular fibrocartilage complex, although arthrography, particularly in conjunction with digital imaging and CT, is also a very effective modality. The greatest use of MRI is for evaluating trauma of the spine, the spinal cord, the thecal sac, and nerve roots as well as for evaluating disk herniation (see Figs. 11.105 to 11.107). MRI is also useful in the evaluation of spinal ligament injuries. The demonstration of the relationship of vertebral fragments to the spinal cord with direct sagittal imaging is extremely helpful, particularly to evaluate injuries in the cervical and thoracic areas.

Fractures and Dislocations

Fractures and dislocations are among the most common traumatic conditions encountered by radiologists. By definition, a *fracture* is a complete disruption in the continuity of a bone (Fig. 4.19). If only some of the bony trabeculae are completely severed while others are bent or remain intact, the fracture is incomplete (Figs. 4.20 and 4.21). A *dislocation* is a complete disruption of a joint; articular surfaces are no longer in contact (Fig. 4.22). A *subluxation*, however, is a minor disruption of a joint in which some articular contact remains (Fig. 4.23). Proper imaging evaluation of these conditions contributes greatly to successful treatment by the orthopaedic surgeon.

In dealing with trauma, the radiologist has two main tasks:

1. Diagnosing and evaluating the type of fracture or dislocation
2. Monitoring the results of treatment and looking for possible complications

Diagnosis

The important radiographic principle in diagnosing skeletal trauma is to obtain at least two views of the bone involved, with each view including two joints adjacent to the injured bone (Fig. 4.24). In so doing, the radiologist eliminates the risk of missing an associated fracture, subluxation, and/or dislocation at a site remote from the apparent primary injury. In children, it is frequently necessary to obtain a radiograph of the normal, unaffected limb for comparison.

Radiographic Evaluation of Fractures

The complete radiographic evaluation of fractures should include the following elements: (a) the anatomic *site* and *extent* of a fracture (Fig. 4.25); (b) the *type* of fracture, whether it is incomplete, as seen predominantly in children, or complete (Fig. 4.26); (c) the *alignment* of the fragments with regard to displacement, angulation, rotation, foreshortening, or distraction (Fig. 4.27); (d) the *direction* of the fracture line in relation to the longitudinal axis of the bone (Fig. 4.28); (e) the presence of *special features* such as impaction, depression, or compression (Fig. 4.29); (f) the presence of *associated abnormalities* such as a fracture with concomitant dislocation or diastasis (Fig. 4.30); and (g) *special types* of fractures that may occur as the result of abnormal stress or secondary to pathologic processes in the bone (Fig. 4.31). The distinction between an *open* (or *compound*) fracture, one in which the fractured bone communicates with the outside environment

FIGURE 4.19 **A complete fracture.** **(A)** The continuity of the bone (tibia) in this 11-year-old-boy is disrupted, and there is a narrow gap between the bone fragments. **(B)** A complete fracture of the femur in an adult patient.

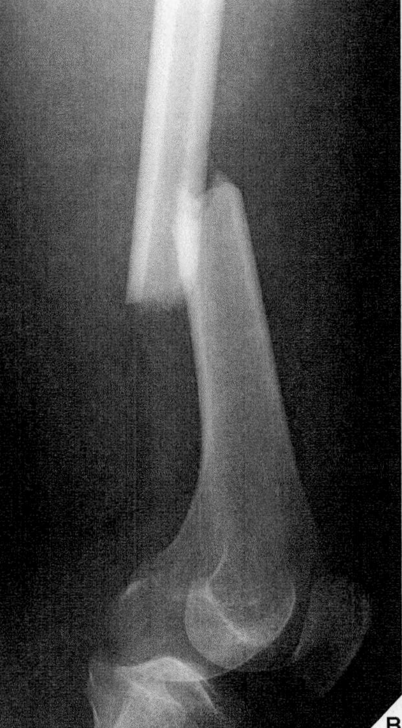

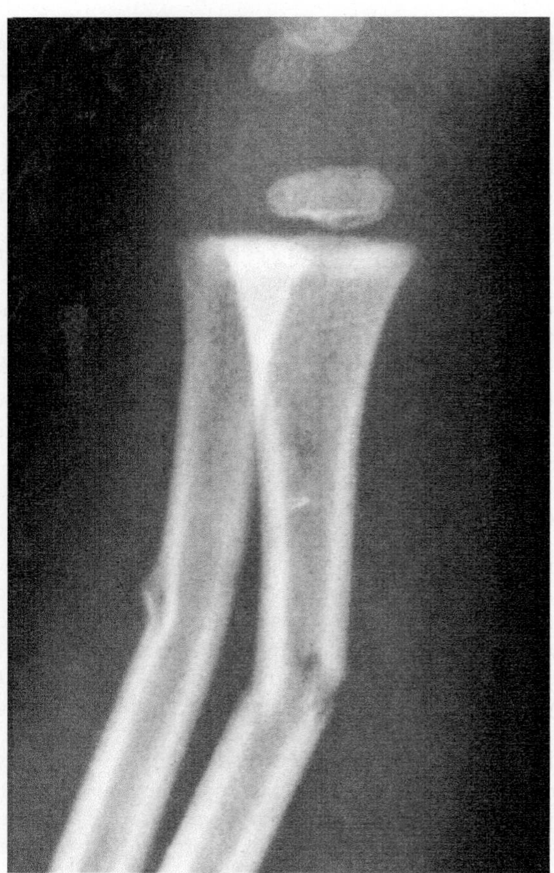

FIGURE 4.20 An incomplete (greenstick) fracture. The ulna is bent, and there is a fracture line extending only through the posterior cortex. In the fracture of the radius, some trabeculae remain intact.

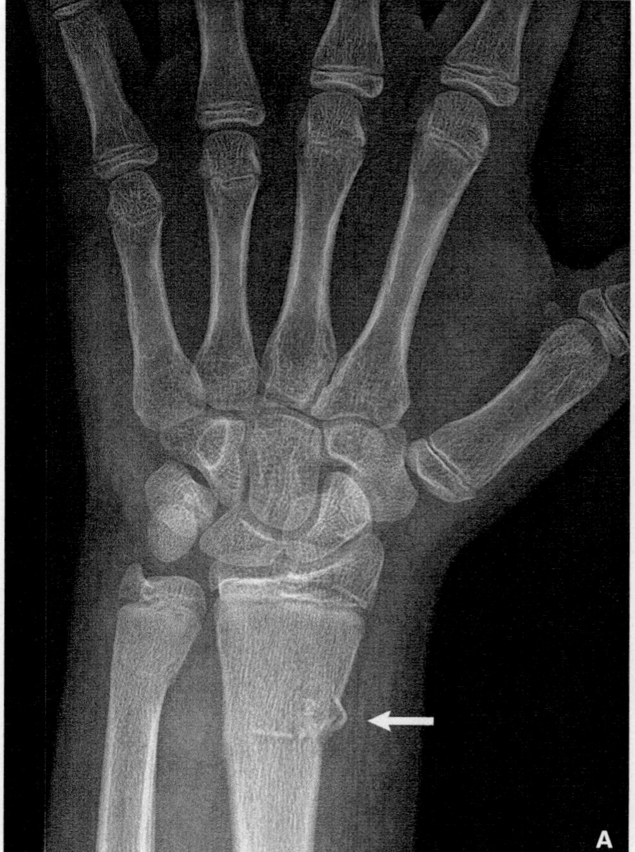

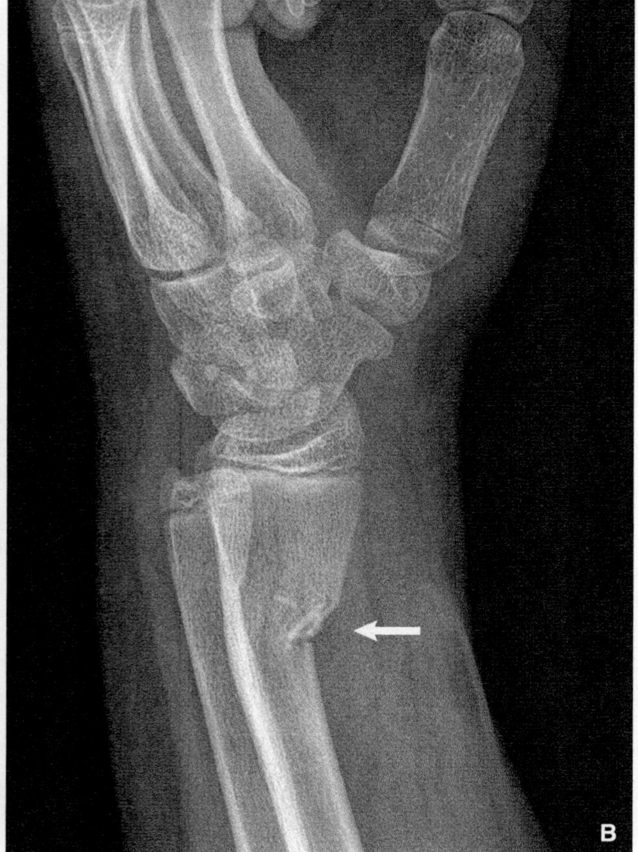

FIGURE 4.21 An incomplete (greenstick) fracture. Anteroposterior **(A)** and lateral **(B)** radiographs of the wrist of a 12-year-old boy show the fracture line extending only through the anterolateral cortex of the distal radial diaphysis *(arrows)*.

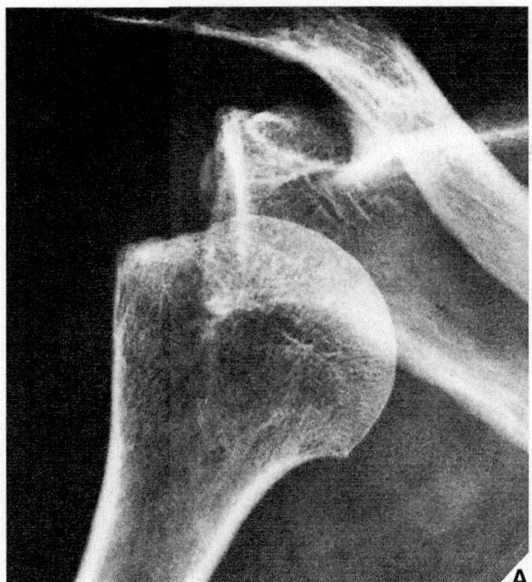

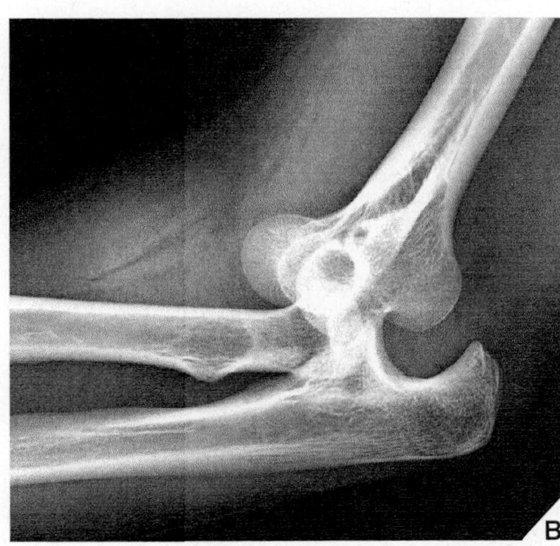

FIGURE 4.22 Dislocation. **(A)** Typical anterior dislocation of the humeral head. The articular surface of the humerus loses contact with the articular surface of the glenoid. **(B)** Typical posterior dislocation in the elbow joint.

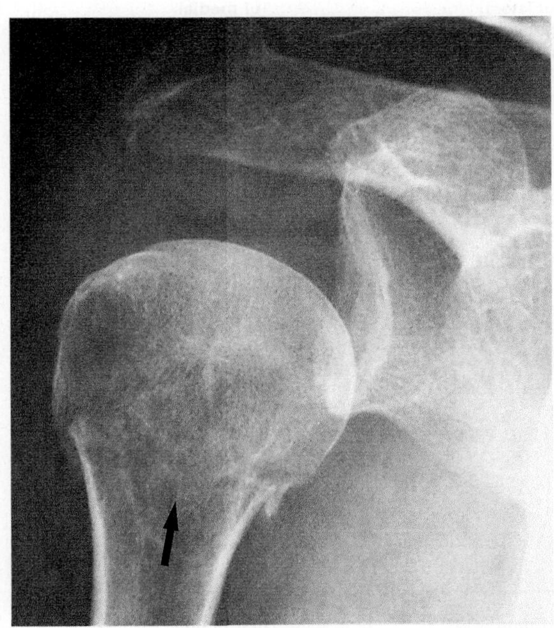

FIGURE 4.23 Subluxation. There is malalignment of the head of the humerus and the glenoid fossa, but some articular contact remains. Note the associated fracture of the surgical neck of the humerus *(arrow)*.

IMAGING ADJACENT JOINTS

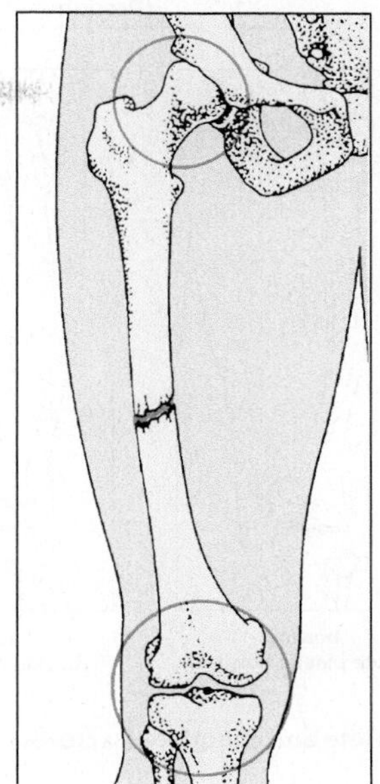

FIGURE 4.24 Adjacent joints. The radiograph of a suspected fracture of the femoral shaft should include the hip and knee articulations *(red circles)*.

through an open wound (Figs. 4.32 to 4.34), and a *closed* (or *simple*) fracture, one that does not produce an open wound in the skin, should preferably be made by clinical rather than radiographic examination.

In children, the radiographic evaluation of fractures, particularly of the ends of tubular bones, should also take into consideration the involvement of the growth plate (physis). Localization of the fracture line has implications with respect to the mechanism of injury and possible complications. A useful classification of injuries, that can be complete or incomplete, displaced or nondisplaced, affecting the physis, metaphysis, epiphysis, or all of these structures has been proposed by Salter and Harris (types I to V) and has been expanded by Rang (type VI) and Ogden (types VII to IX) to include four additional types of fractures (Fig. 4.35). Although the injuries described by Rang and Ogden do not directly involve the growth plate, the sequelae of such trauma affect the physis in the same way as the direct injuries described by Salter and Harris. In *type I*, the fracture affects the growth plate only. It is subdivided to incomplete, complete, nondisplaced, and displaced fractures (Figs. 4.36 to 4.39). These injuries

SITE AND EXTENT OF FRACTURE

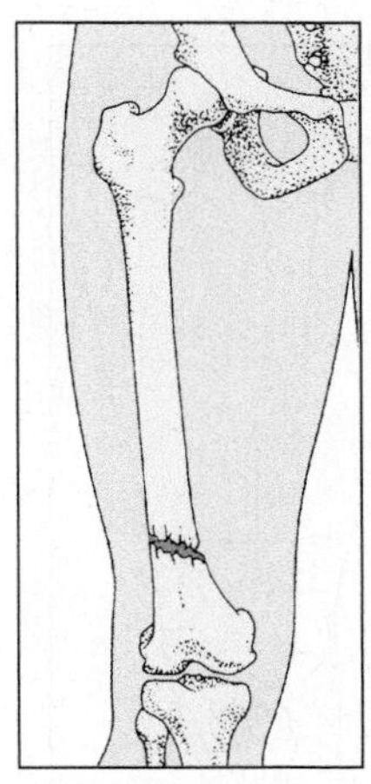

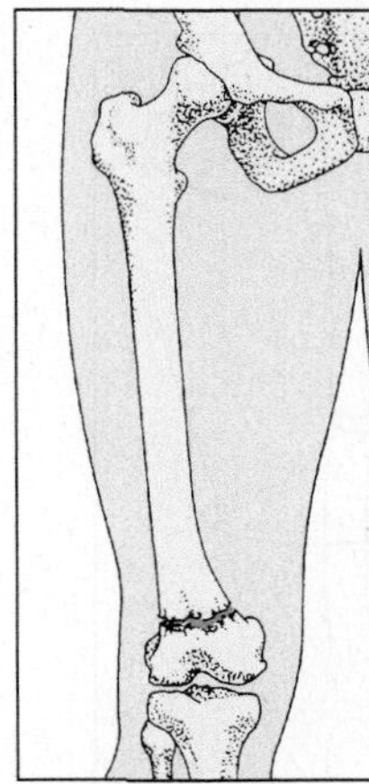

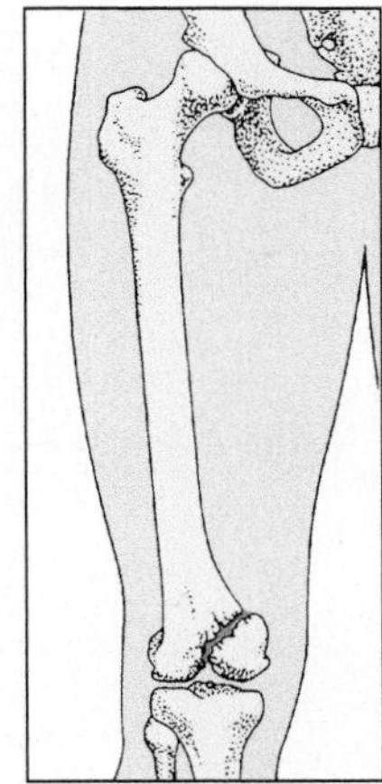

FIGURE 4.25 Site and extent of a fracture. Factors in the radiographic evaluation of a fracture: the anatomic site and extent.

TYPE OF FRACTURE

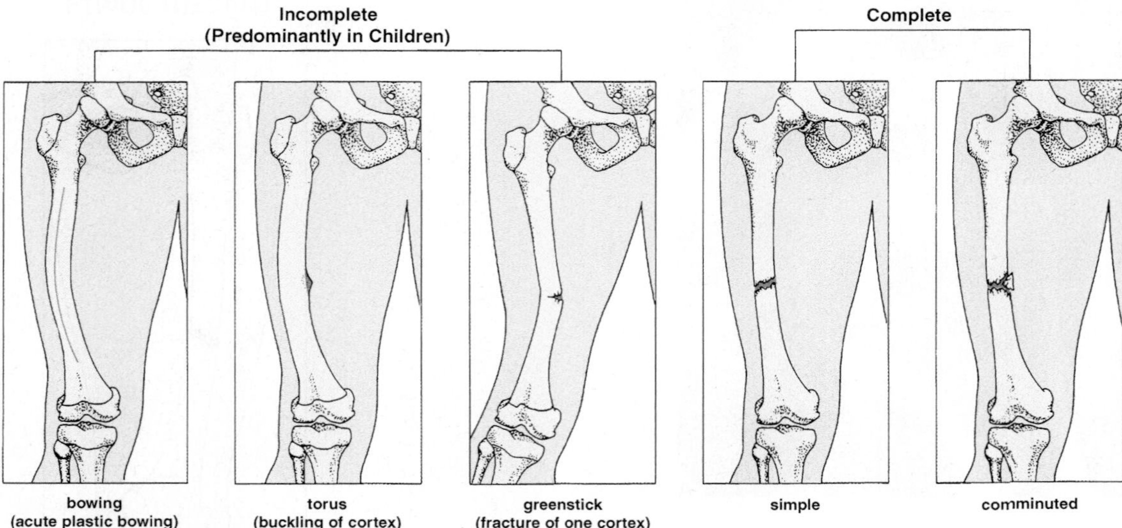

FIGURE 4.26 **Incomplete and complete fractures.** Factors in the radiographic evaluation of a fracture: the type of fracture—incomplete or complete.

ALIGNMENT OF FRAGMENTS

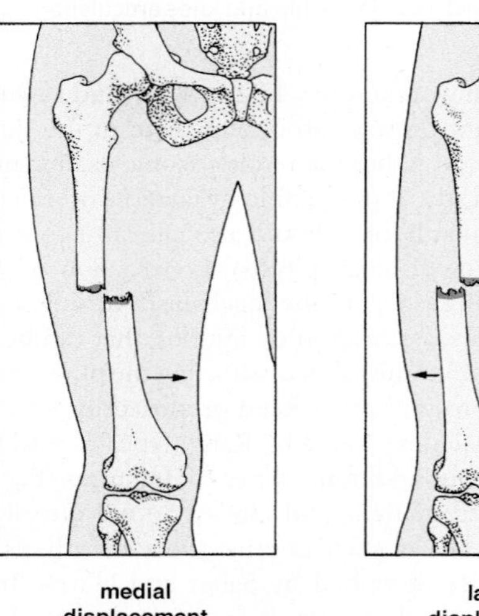

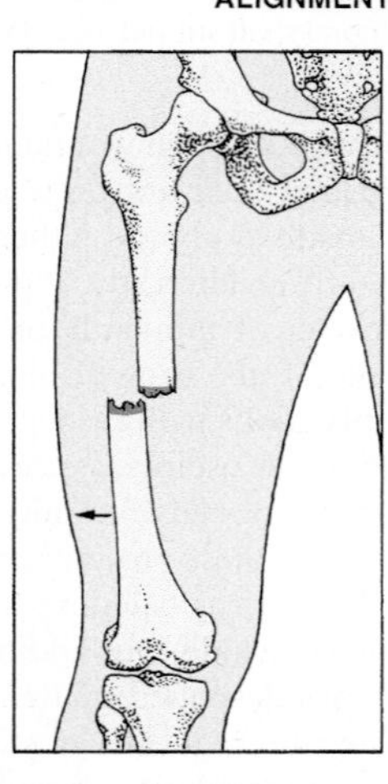

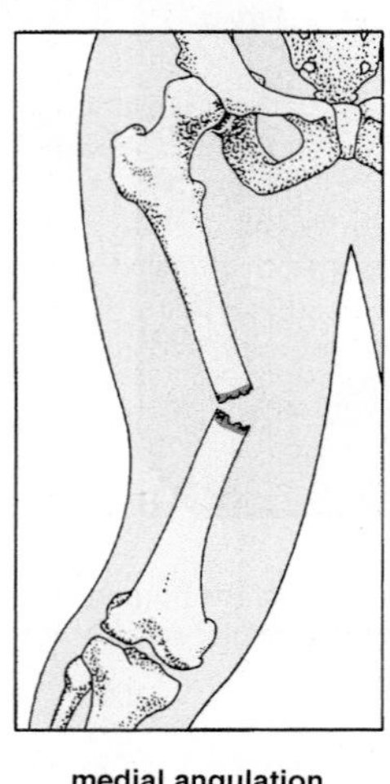

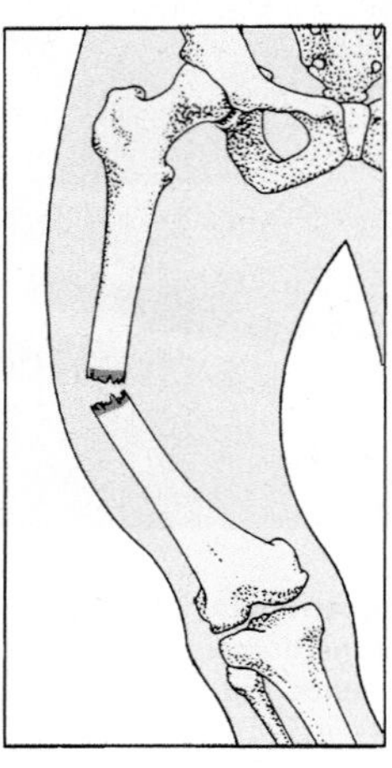

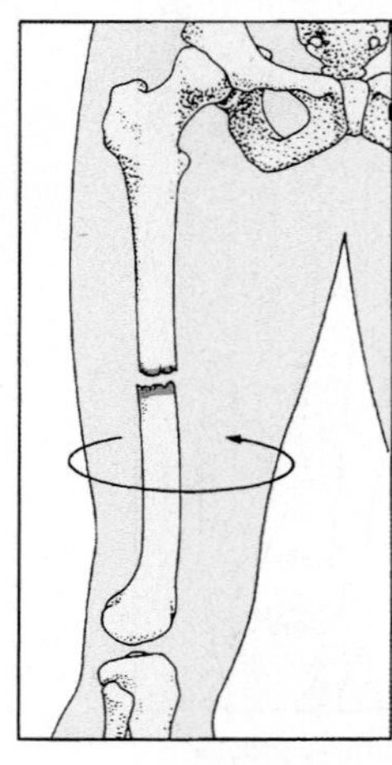

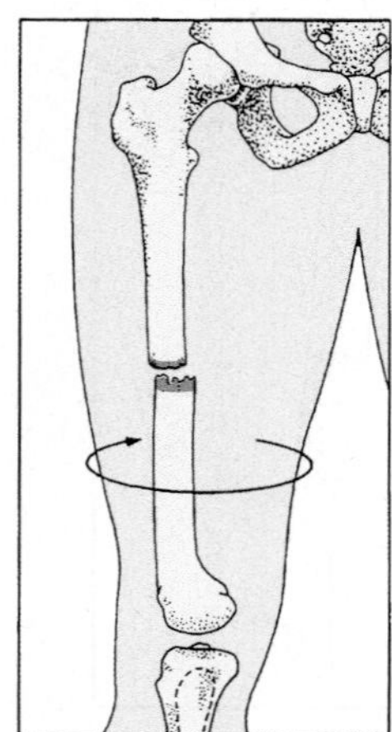

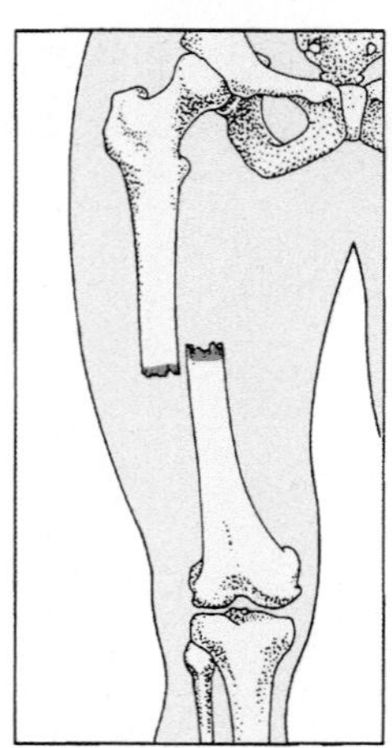

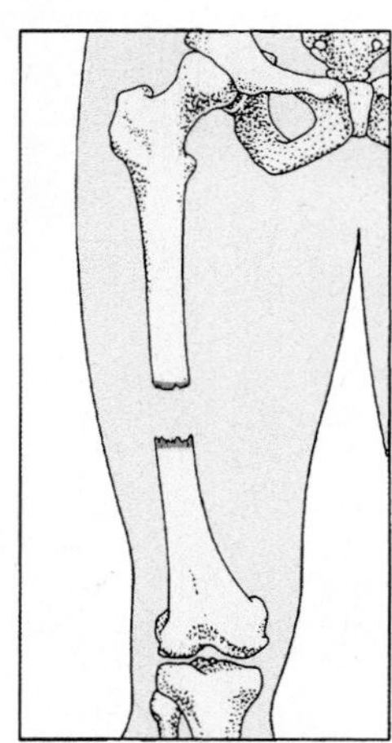

FIGURE 4.27 **Alignment of a fracture.** Factors in the radiographic evaluation of a fracture: the alignment of the fragments.

DIRECTION OF FRACTURE LINE

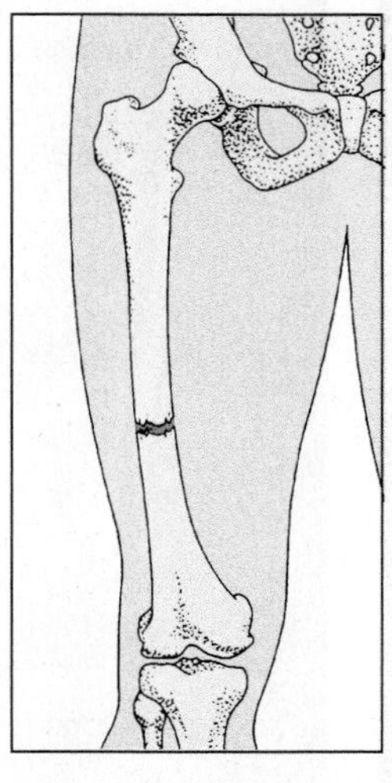

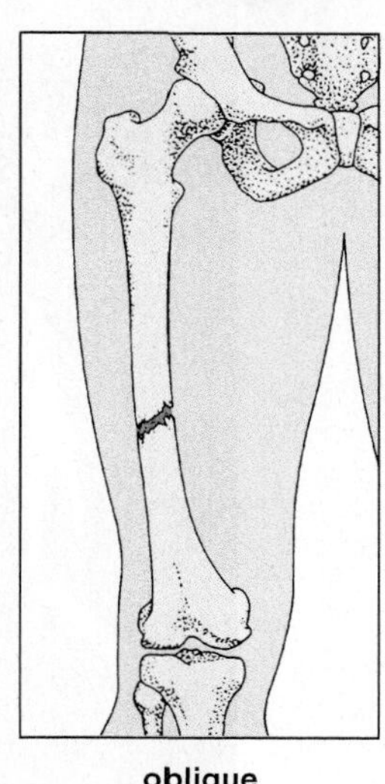

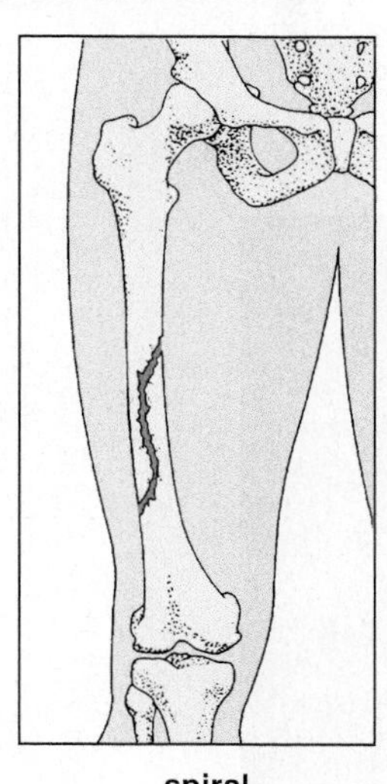

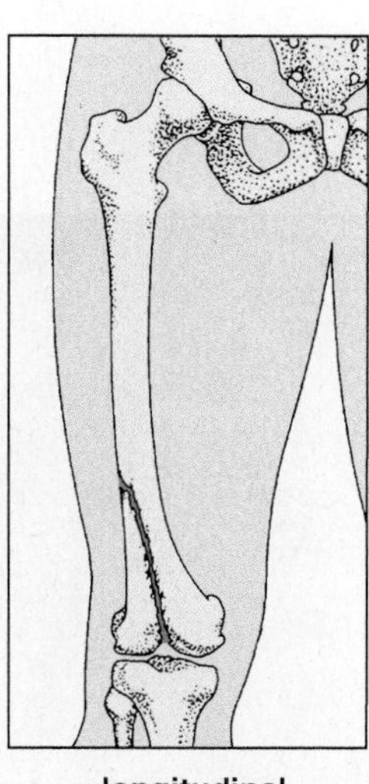

FIGURE 4.28 **Direction of a fracture line.** Factors in the radiographic evaluation of a fracture: the direction of the fracture line.

SPECIAL FEATURES

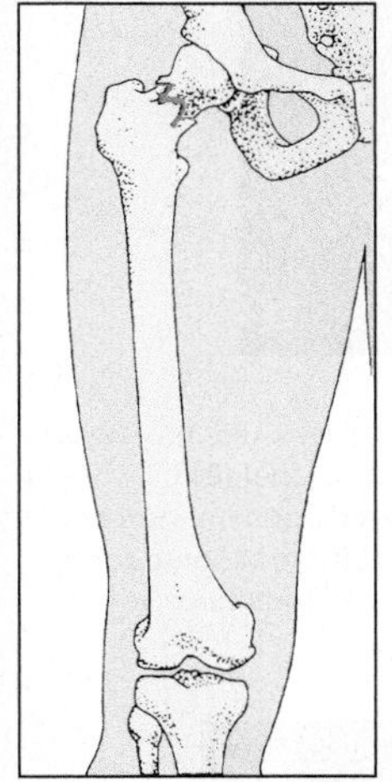

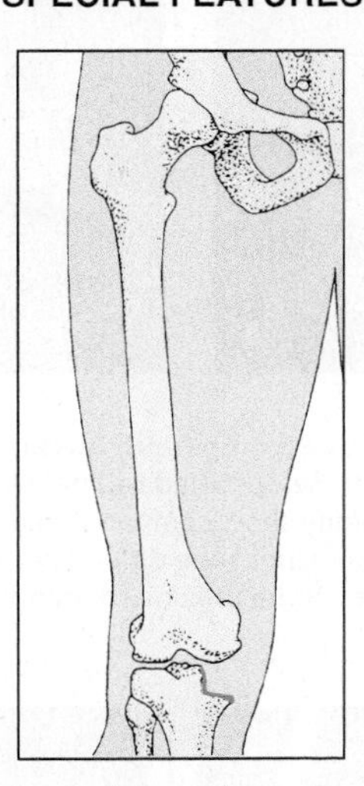

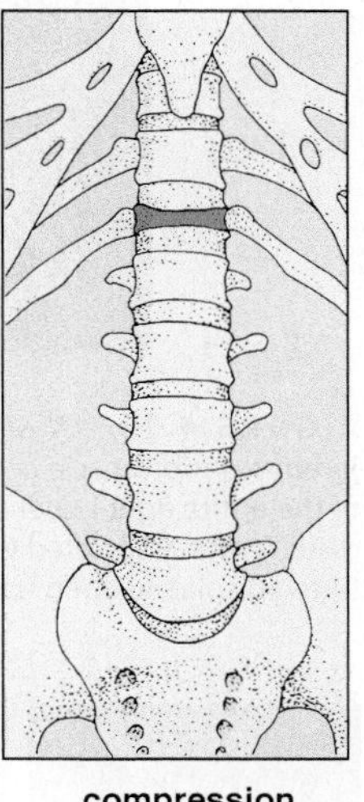

FIGURE 4.29 **Special features of a fracture.** Factors in the radiographic evaluation of a fracture: special features.

ASSOCIATED ABNORMALITIES

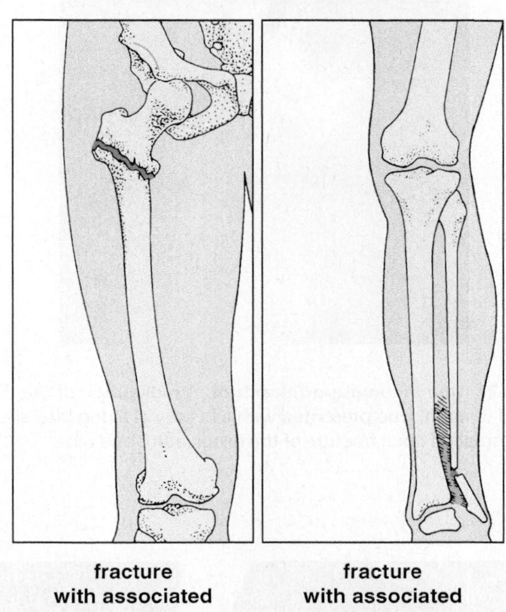

FIGURE 4.30 **Associated abnormalities.** Factors in the radiographic evaluation of a fracture: associated abnormalities.

SPECIAL TYPES OF FRACTURES

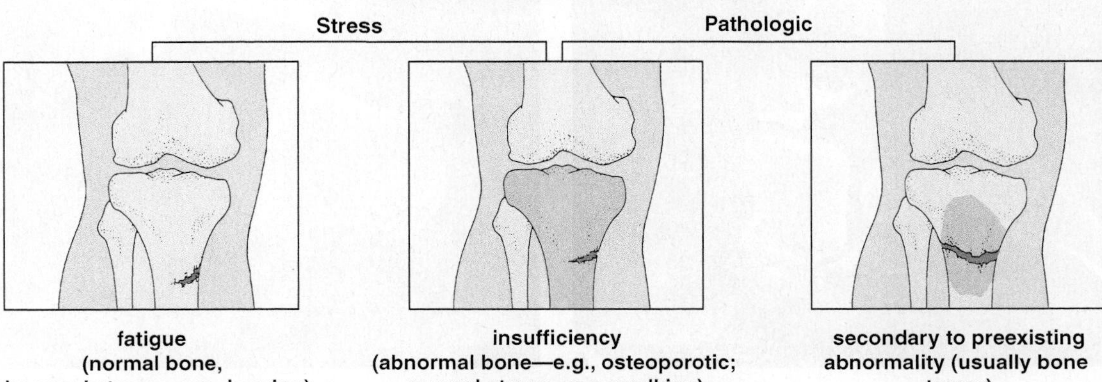

FIGURE 4.31 **Special types of fractures.** Factors in the radiographic evaluation of a fracture: special types of fractures.

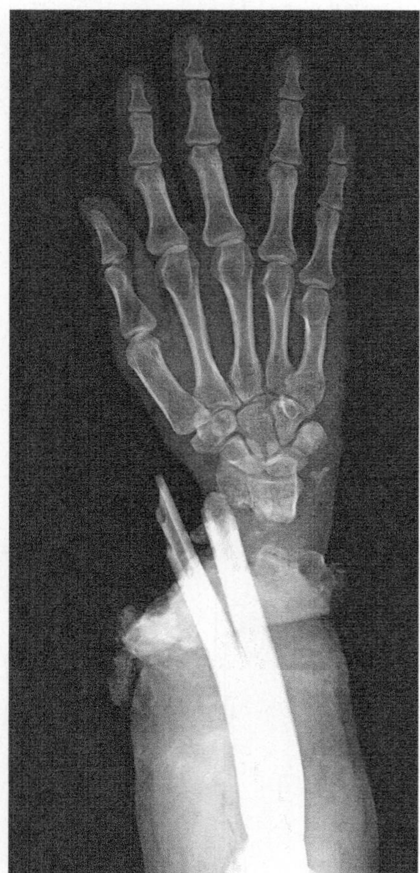

FIGURE 4.32 Open (compound) fracture. A radiograph of the distal forearm of a 29-year-old woman, who presented with a history of a dog bite, shows an acute comminuted displaced open fracture of the distal radius and ulna.

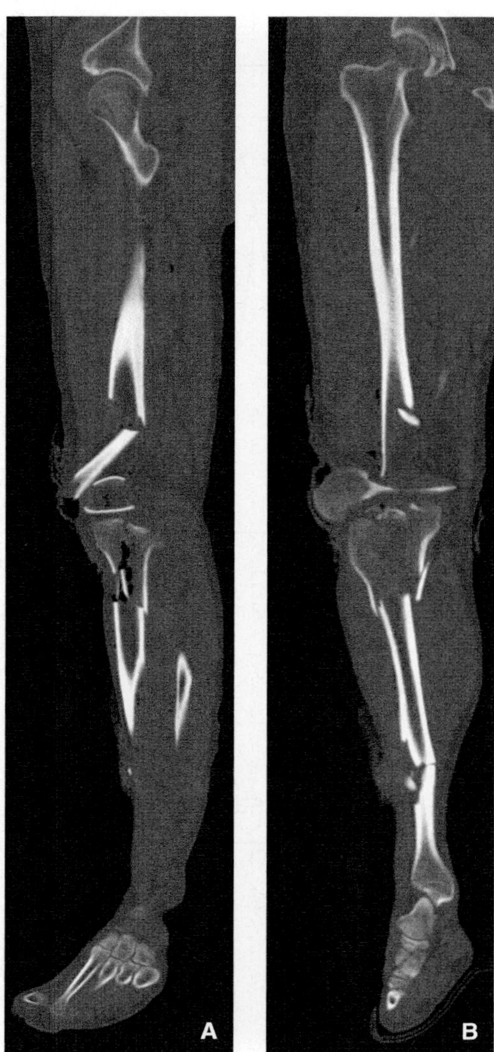

FIGURE 4.33 CT of an open (compound) fracture. A 61-year-old man was injured in a motorcycle accident. Reformatted sagittal **(A)** and coronal **(B)** CT images of the entire right lower extremity show comminuted displaced open fracture of the distal femur associated with posterior knee dislocation. In addition, observe comminuted displaced open fractures of the proximal in midportion of the tibia.

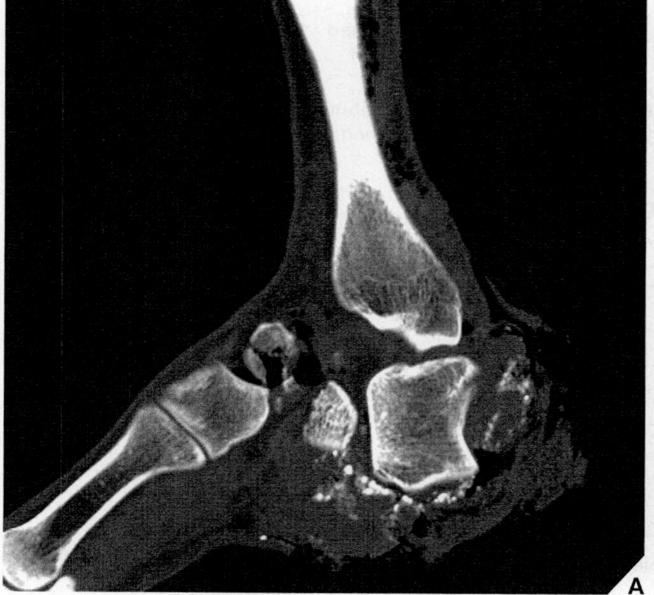

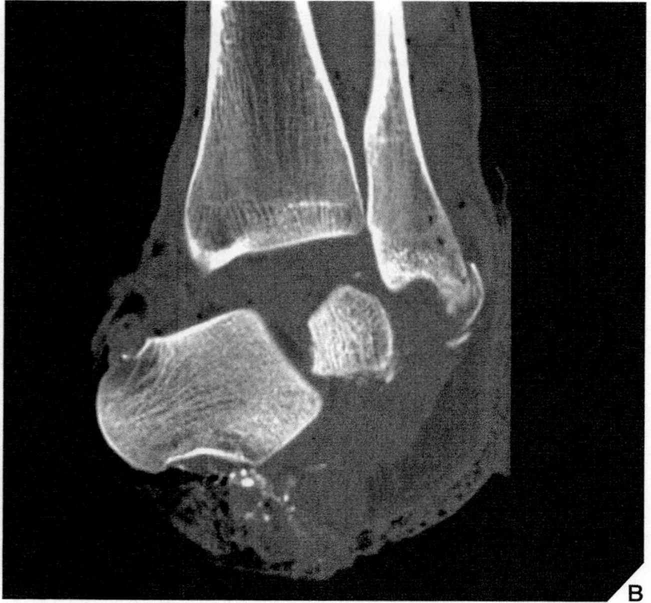

FIGURE 4.34 CT of an open (compound) fracture. Reformatted sagittal **(A)** and coronal **(B)** CT images show a fracture–dislocation in the ankle and subtalar joints. Note communication of the fracture fragments with outside environment.

INVOLVEMENT OF THE GROWTH PLATE

Salter-Harris Classification

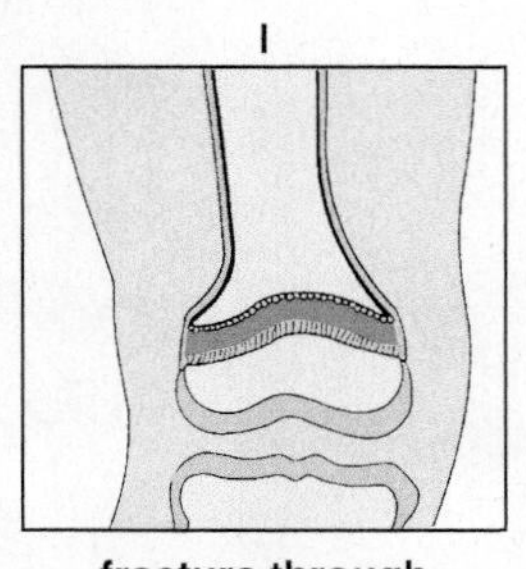

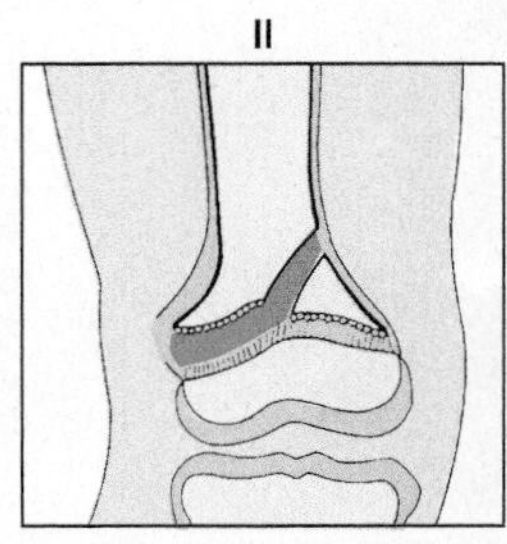

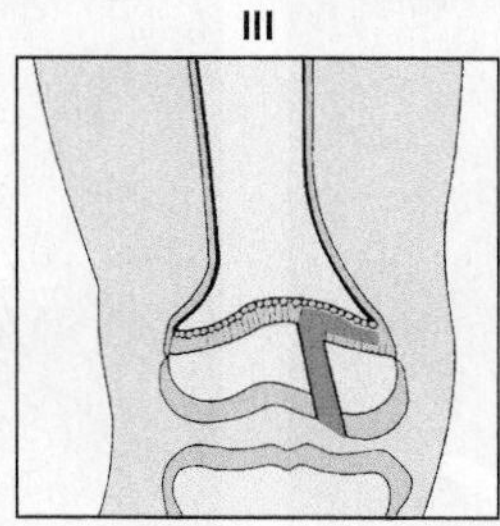

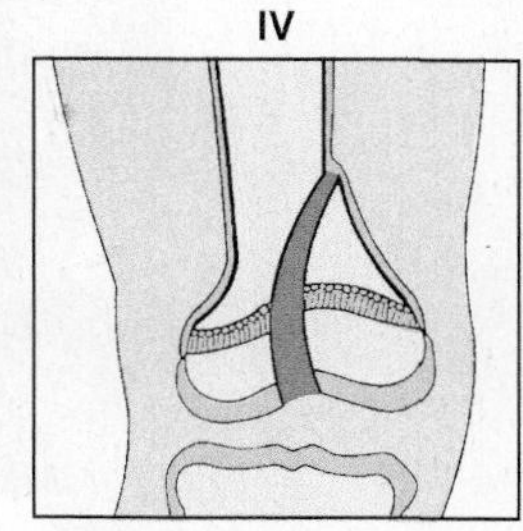

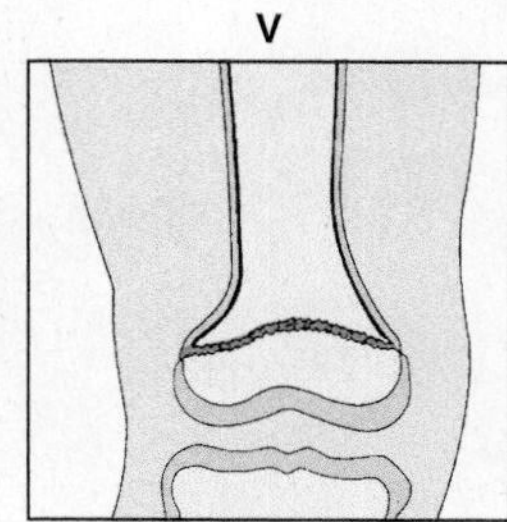

Rang and Ogden Additions to Salter-Harris

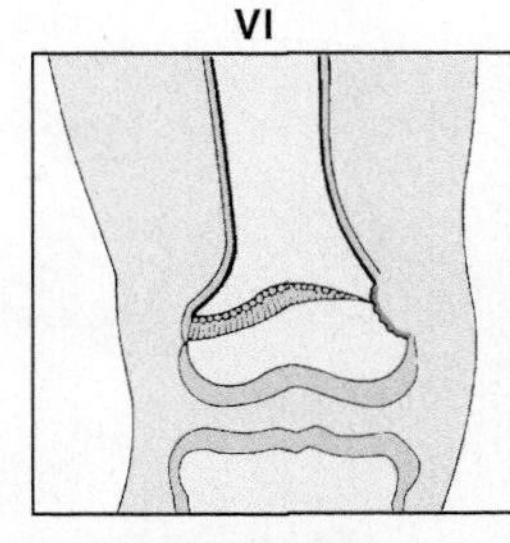

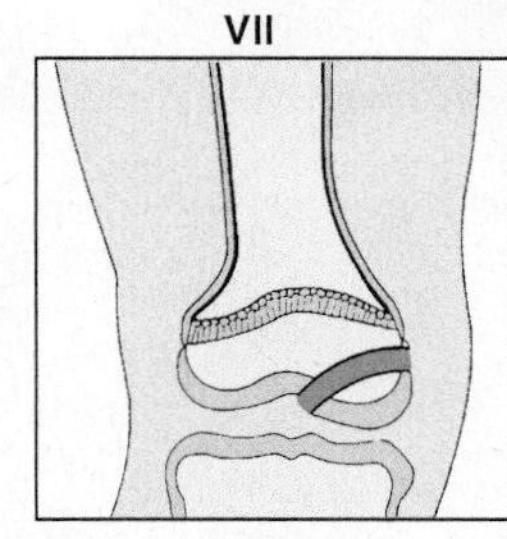

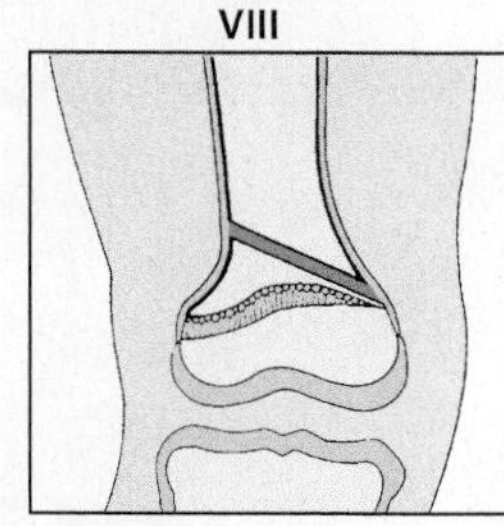

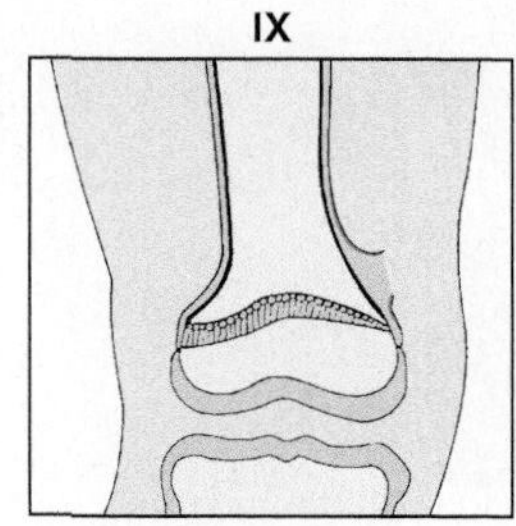

FIGURE 4.35 Classification of the growth plate injuries. The Salter-Harris classification of injuries involving the growth plate (physis) together with Rang and Ogden additions.

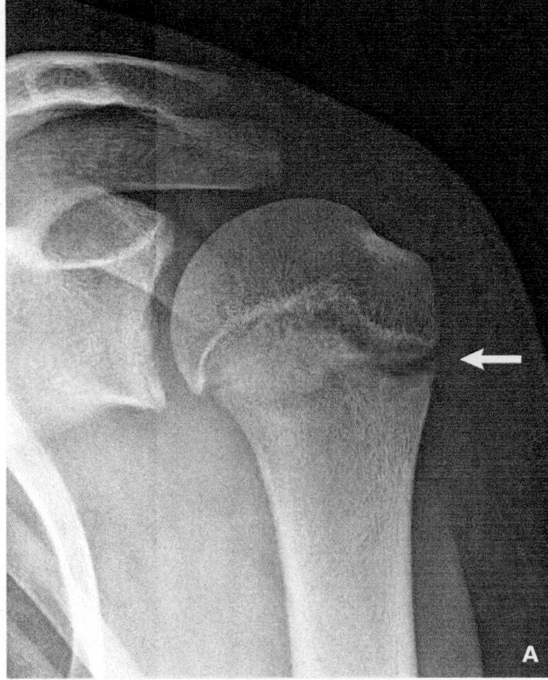

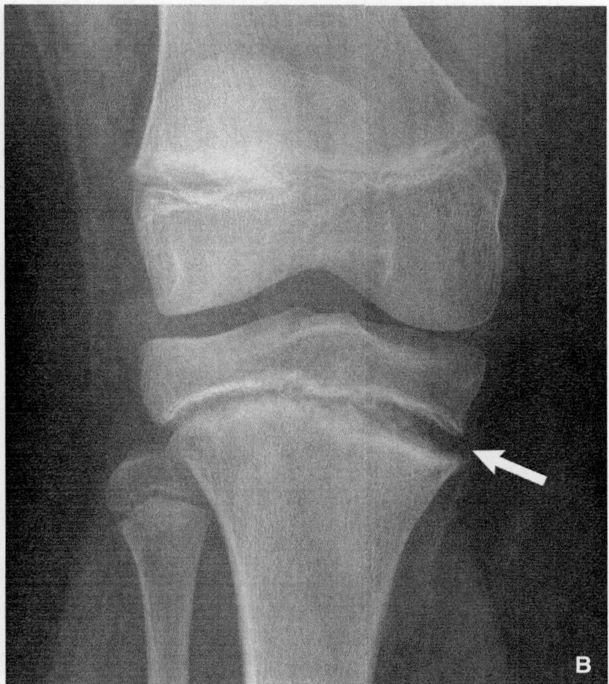

FIGURE 4.36 Type I Salter-Harris fracture (incomplete). (A) Anteroposterior radiograph of the left shoulder of a 14-year-old boy shows incomplete fracture through the growth plate of the proximal humerus affecting only the lateral aspect *(arrow)*. The medial aspect of the growth plate is intact. **(B)** Anteroposterior radiograph of the right knee of a 10-year-old girl shows incomplete fracture through the growth plate of the proximal tibia affecting only the medial aspect *(arrow)*.

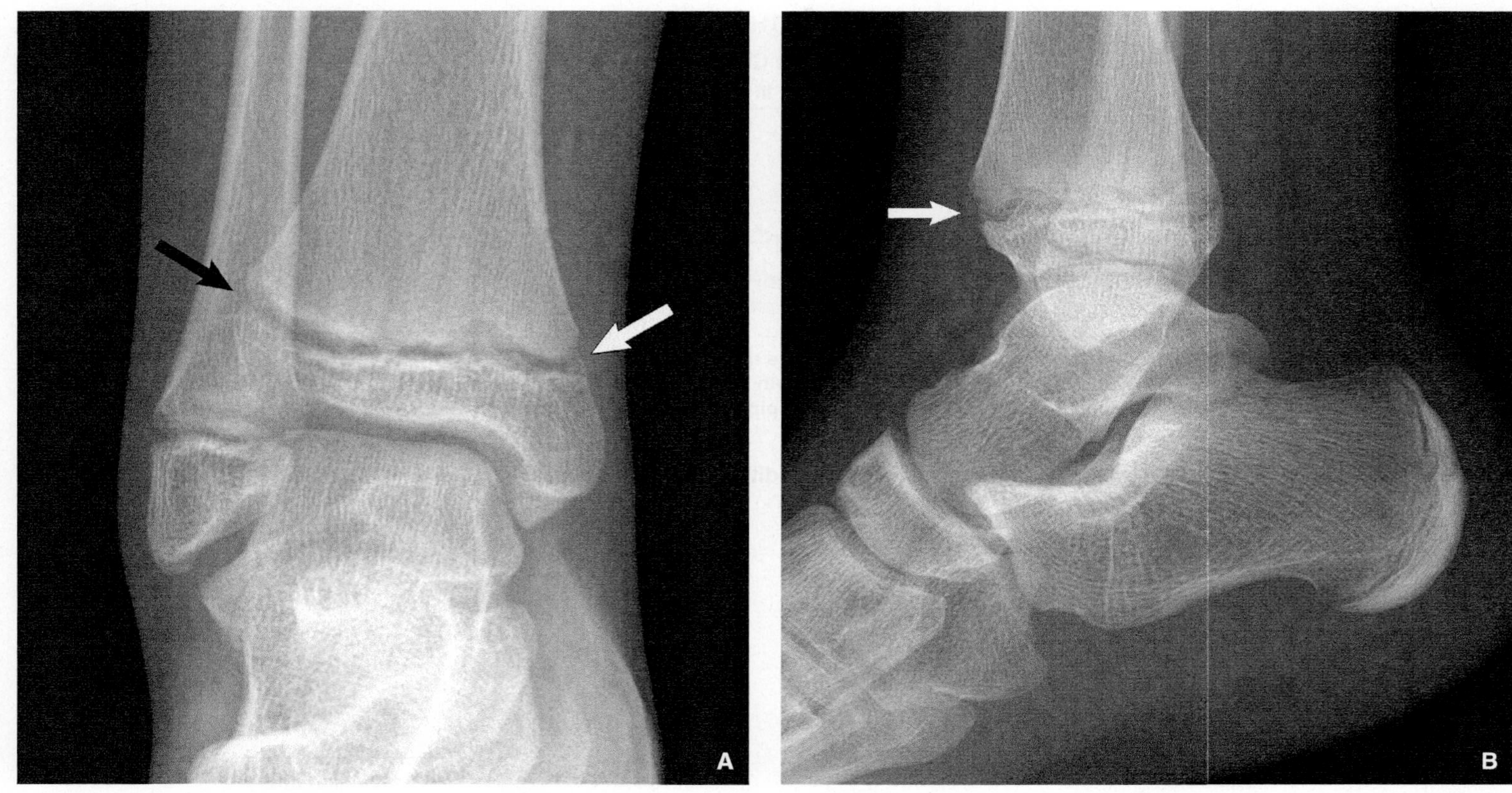

FIGURE 4.37 **Type I Salter-Harris fracture (complete).** Anteroposterior **(A)** and lateral **(B)** radiographs of the left ankle of a 13-year-old boy show a complete nondisplaced fracture through the growth plate of the distal tibia *(arrows)*.

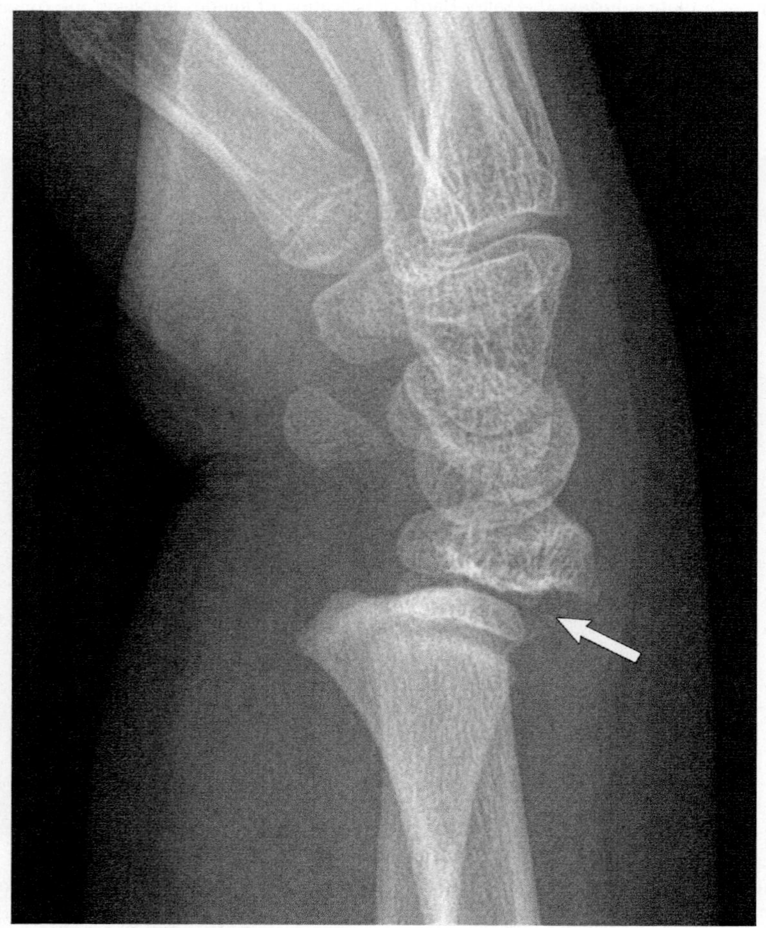

FIGURE 4.38 **Type I Salter-Harris fracture (displaced).** Lateral radiograph of the wrist of an 8-year-old girl shows a displaced fracture through the growth plate of the distal radius *(arrow)*.

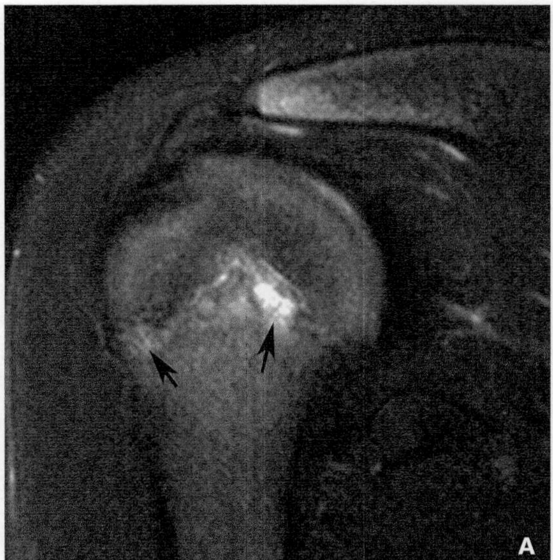

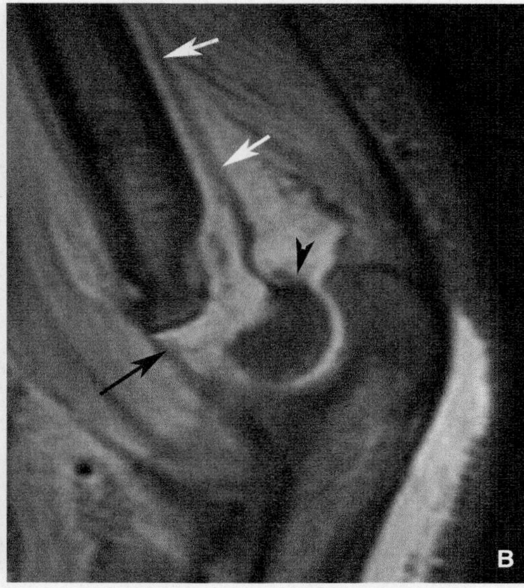

FIGURE 4.39 **MRI of type I Salter-Harris fracture.** **(A)** Coronal T2-weighted fat-saturated MR image of the right shoulder of a young baseball player shows widening and high signal intensity of the proximal growth plate of the humerus without displacement *(arrows)*, consistent with so-called *Little League shoulder*. **(B)** Sagittal gradient recalled echo (GRE) MR image of the elbow of a child who fell during playground activities shows complete displaced fracture through the distal humeral physis without involvement of the metaphysis or epiphysis *(black arrow)*. The trochlea is dorsally displaced *(arrowhead)*, and there is separation of the distal posterior periosteum from bone *(white arrows)*.

typically occur in children younger than 5 years old, and the most commonly affected sites are the proximal and distal humerus and proximal femur. The prognosis is usually very good. In *type II*, the fracture affects the growth plate and extends through the metaphysis (Figs. 4.40 and 4.41). This is the most common type, comprising about 75% of all growth plate injuries, and occurs in children between 10 and 16 years of age. The common sites of involvement in order of decreasing frequency are the distal radius, tibia, fibula, femur, and the ulna. The prognosis is generally favorable. In *type III*, the fracture affects the growth plate and extends through the epiphysis (Figs. 4.42 and 4.43). This type of fracture is common in

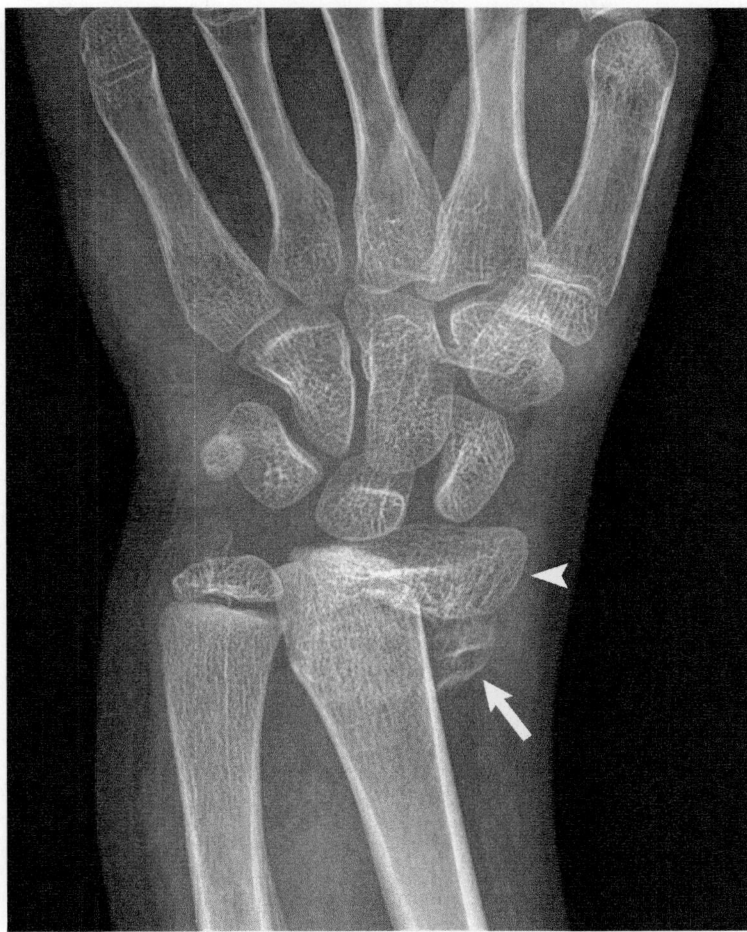

FIGURE 4.40 **Type II Salter-Harris fracture (displaced).** Dorsovolar radiograph of the left wrist of a 12-year-old boy shows a fracture through the growth plate of the distal radius affecting also the metaphysis *(arrow)*. The epiphysis is displaced laterally *(arrowhead)*.

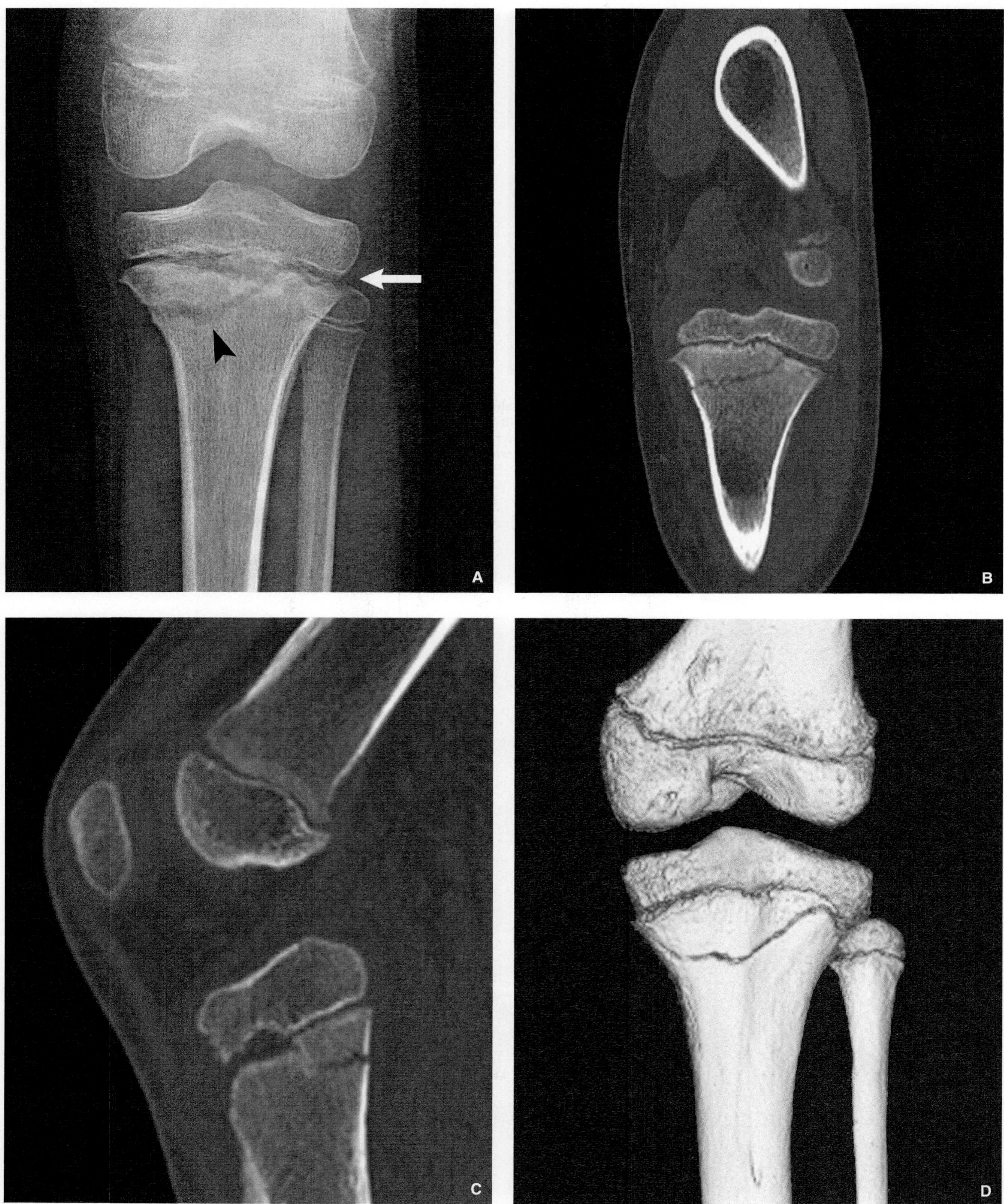

FIGURE 4.41 CT and 3D CT of type II Salter-Harris fracture. **(A)** Anteroposterior radiograph of the left knee of a 7-year-old girl shows a fracture through the growth plate of the proximal tibia *(arrow)* extending through the metaphysis *(arrowhead)*. Coronal **(B)** and sagittal **(C)** reformatted CT images of the left knee supplemented with 3D reconstructed CT image **(D)** show this type of injury more clearly.

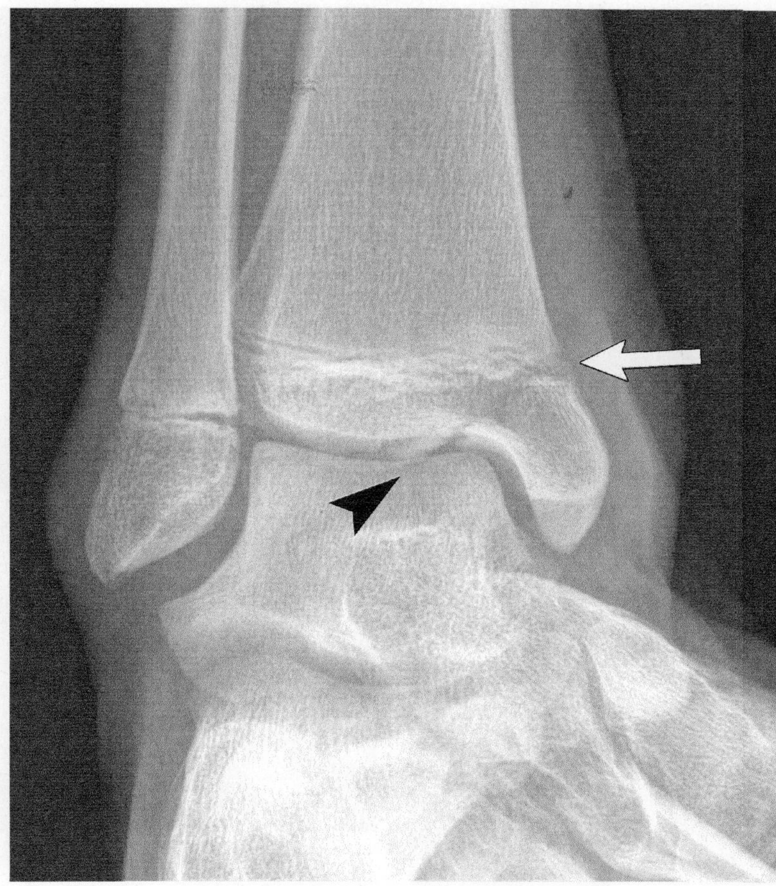

FIGURE 4.42 **Type III Salter-Harris fracture.** Anteroposterior radiograph of the right ankle of a 14-year-old boy shows a fracture through the growth plate of the distal tibia *(arrow)*, extending through the epiphysis *(arrowhead)*.

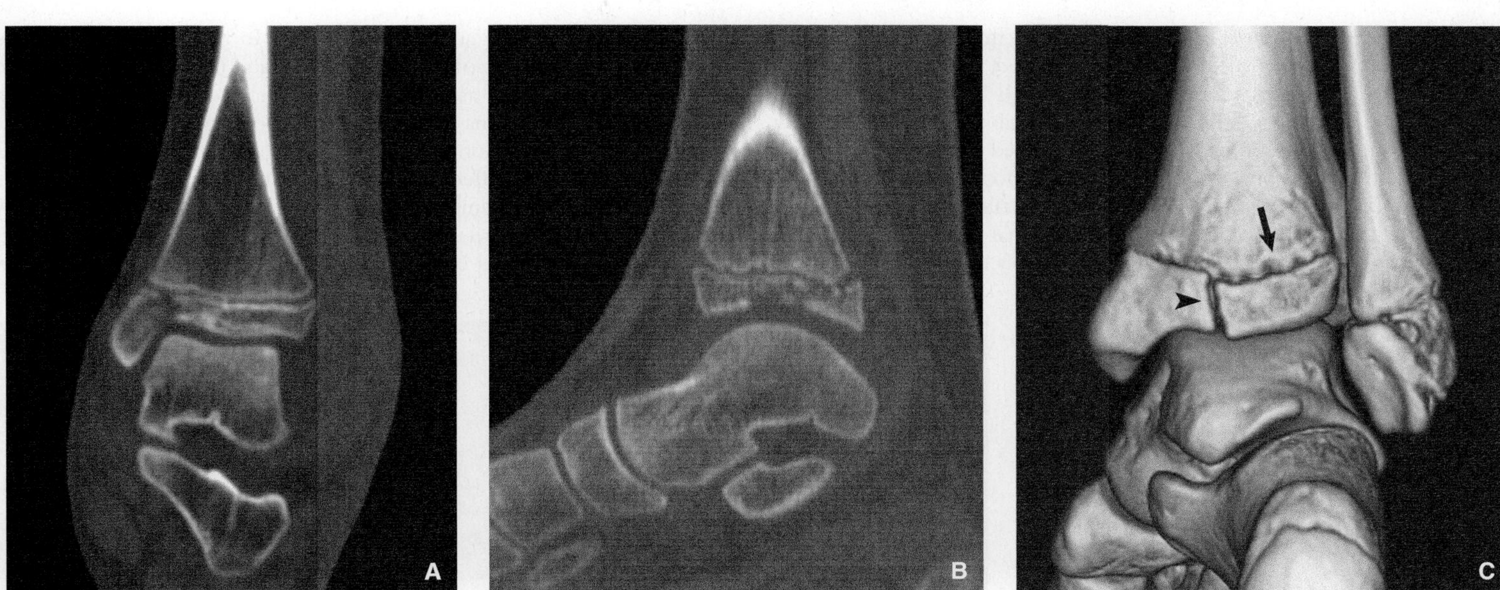

FIGURE 4.43 **CT and 3D CT of type III Salter-Harris fracture.** Coronal **(A)** and sagittal **(B)** reformatted CT images of the left ankle of an 11-year-old girl and 3D reconstructed CT image **(C)** show a fracture through the growth plate of the distal tibia *(arrow)* extending through the epiphysis *(arrowhead)*.

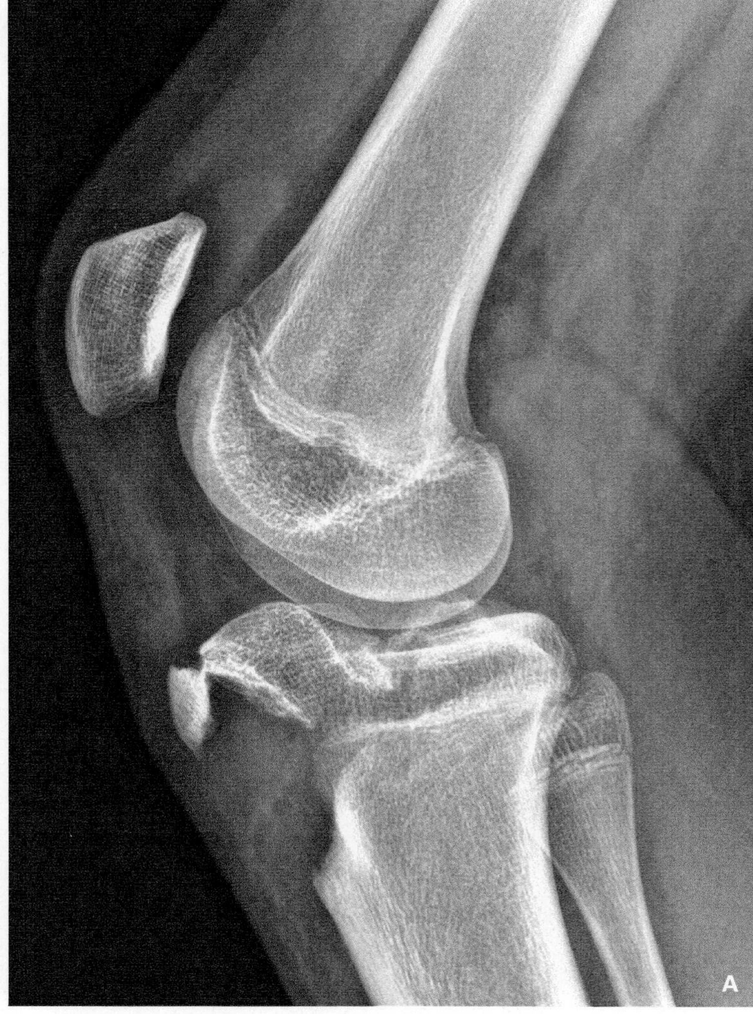

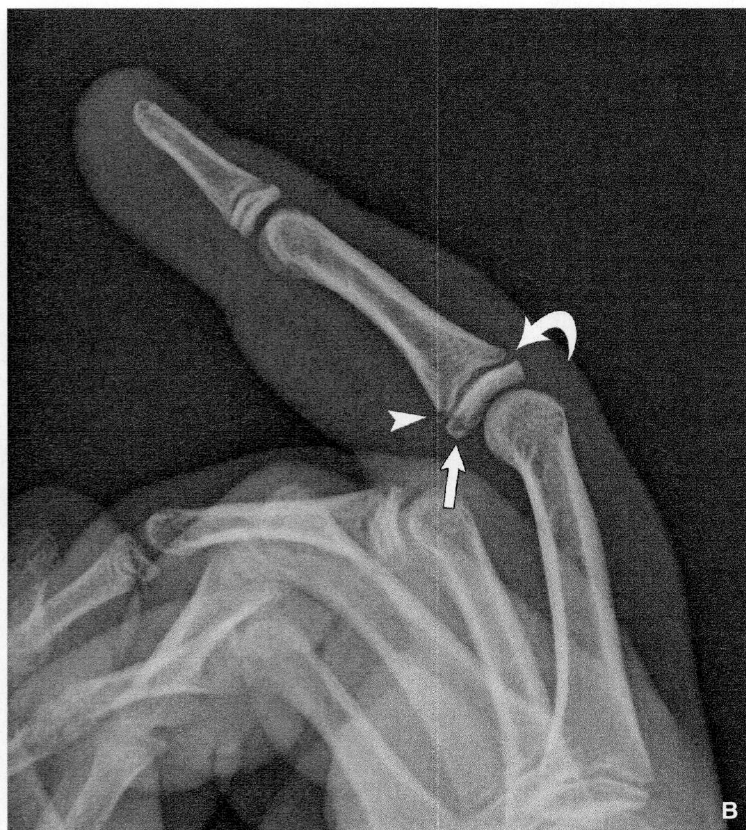

FIGURE 4.44 **Type IV Salter-Harris fracture.** **(A)** Lateral radiograph of the knee of a 15-year-old boy shows a fracture through the growth plate of the proximal tibia extending through the metaphysis and epiphysis. **(B)** Lateral radiograph of an index finger of a 10-year-old girl shows fracture through the growth plate of the middle phalanx *(curved arrow)*, fracture of the epiphysis *(arrow)*, and fracture of the metaphysis *(arrowhead)*.

children between the ages of 10 and 15 years, and the distal and proximal tibia and distal femur are most frequently affected. In *type IV*, the fracture affects the growth plate and extends through both metaphysis and epiphysis (Figs. 4.44 to 4.47). Distal humerus and tibia are most frequently affected, and this type of injury may be complicated by growth arrest and joint deformity. *Type V* consists of crushing injury to the growth plate (Fig. 4.48; see also Fig. 4.111B) and is more common in older children and adolescents. The growth plate of the proximal and distal tibia and distal femur are typically affected. This type of fracture invariably leads to growth arrest of the affected extremity and joint deformity. In *type VI*, which involves only the peripheral region of the growth plate and the perichondrium, the injury may not always be associated with a fracture. It may result from a localized contusion, trauma-induced infection, or severe burn. The resulting reactive bone formation and osseous bridging of the physis may lead to growth arrest of the affected bone and joint deformity. *Type VII* injury consists of a purely transepiphyseal fracture, which is divided to subtype A (when the fracture line extends to the growth plate) and subtype B (when the fracture line does not extend into the growth plate) (Figs. 4.49 and

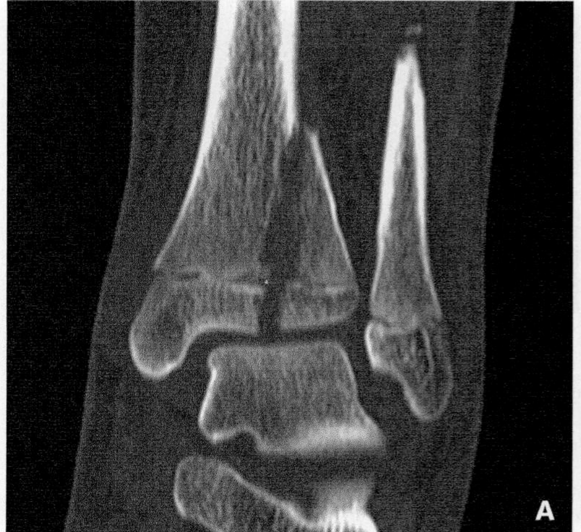

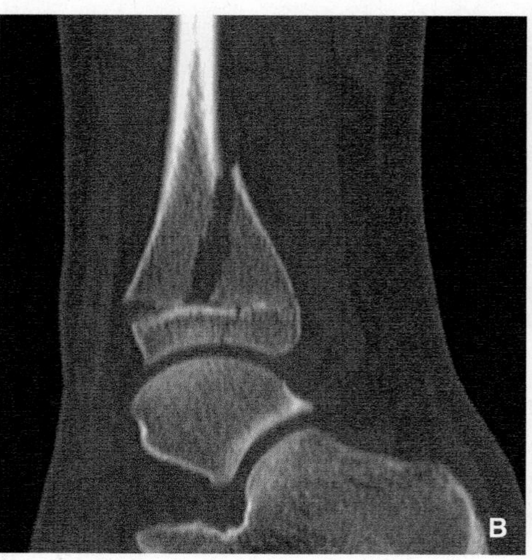

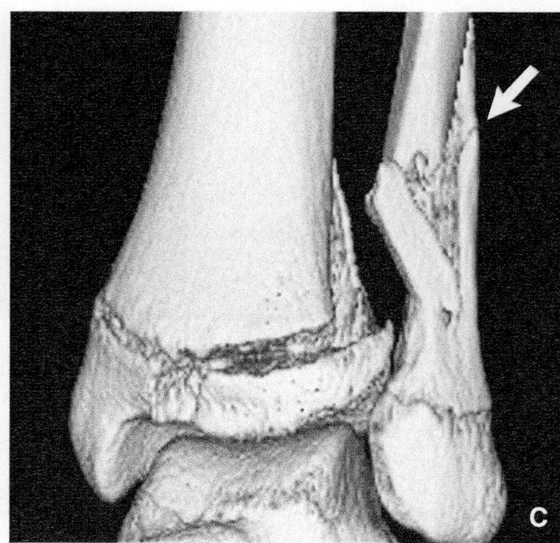

FIGURE 4.45 **CT and 3D CT of type IV Salter-Harris fracture.** Coronal **(A)** and sagittal **(B)** reformatted CT images and 3D reconstructed CT image **(C)** of the left ankle of a 16-year-old boy show a fracture through the growth plate of the distal tibia extending through the tibial metaphysis and epiphysis. Observe the normal-appearing growth plate of the distal fibula and associated fracture of the fibular diaphysis *(arrow)*.

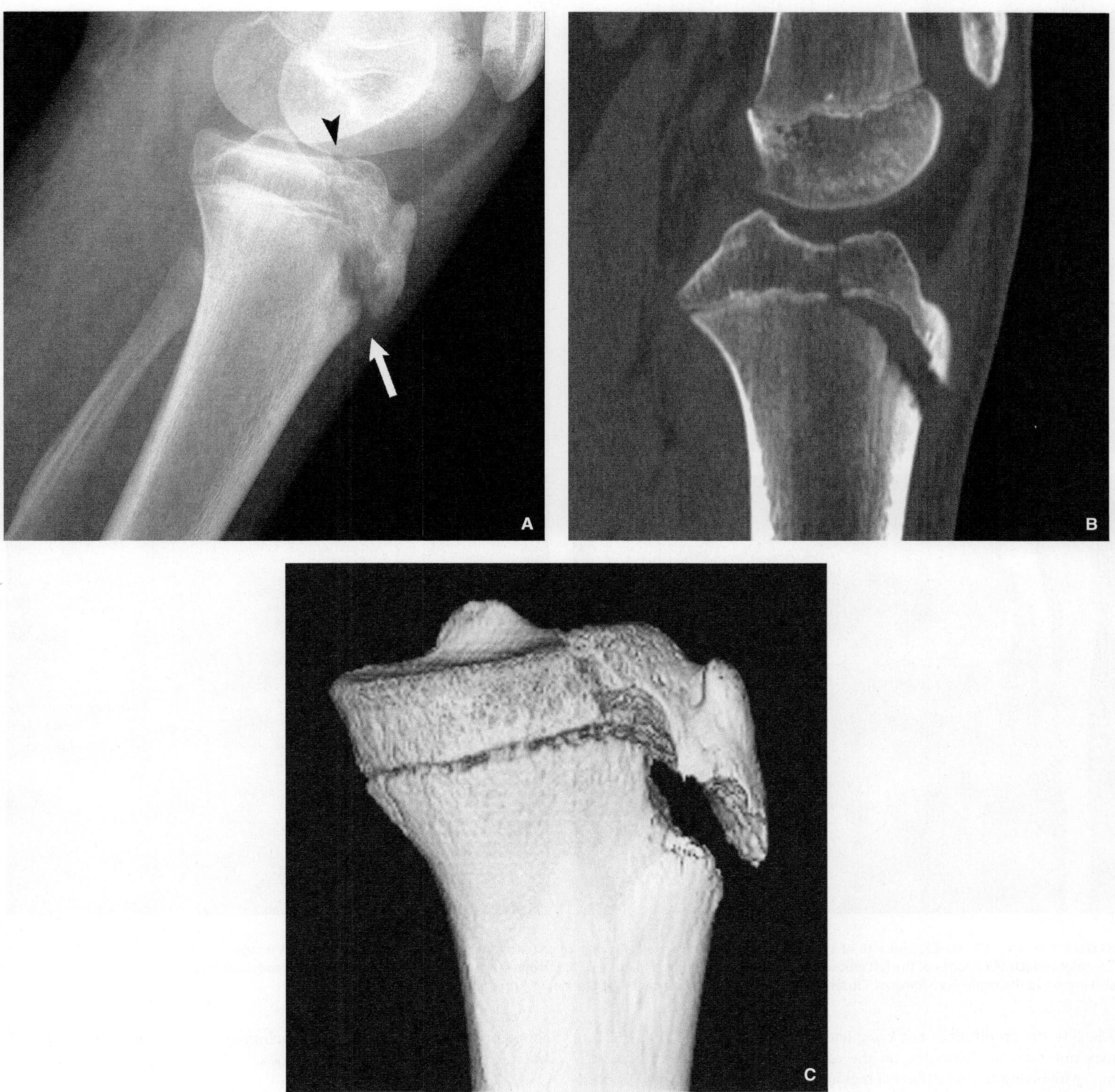

FIGURE 4.46 **CT and 3D CT of type IV Salter-Harris fracture.** **(A)** Lateral radiograph of the knee of a 16-year-old boy shows a fracture of the proximal tibial epiphysis *(arrowhead)* extending through the growth plate to the metaphysis *(arrow)*. These findings are confirmed by sagittal reformatted **(B)** and 3D reconstructed **(C)** CT images.

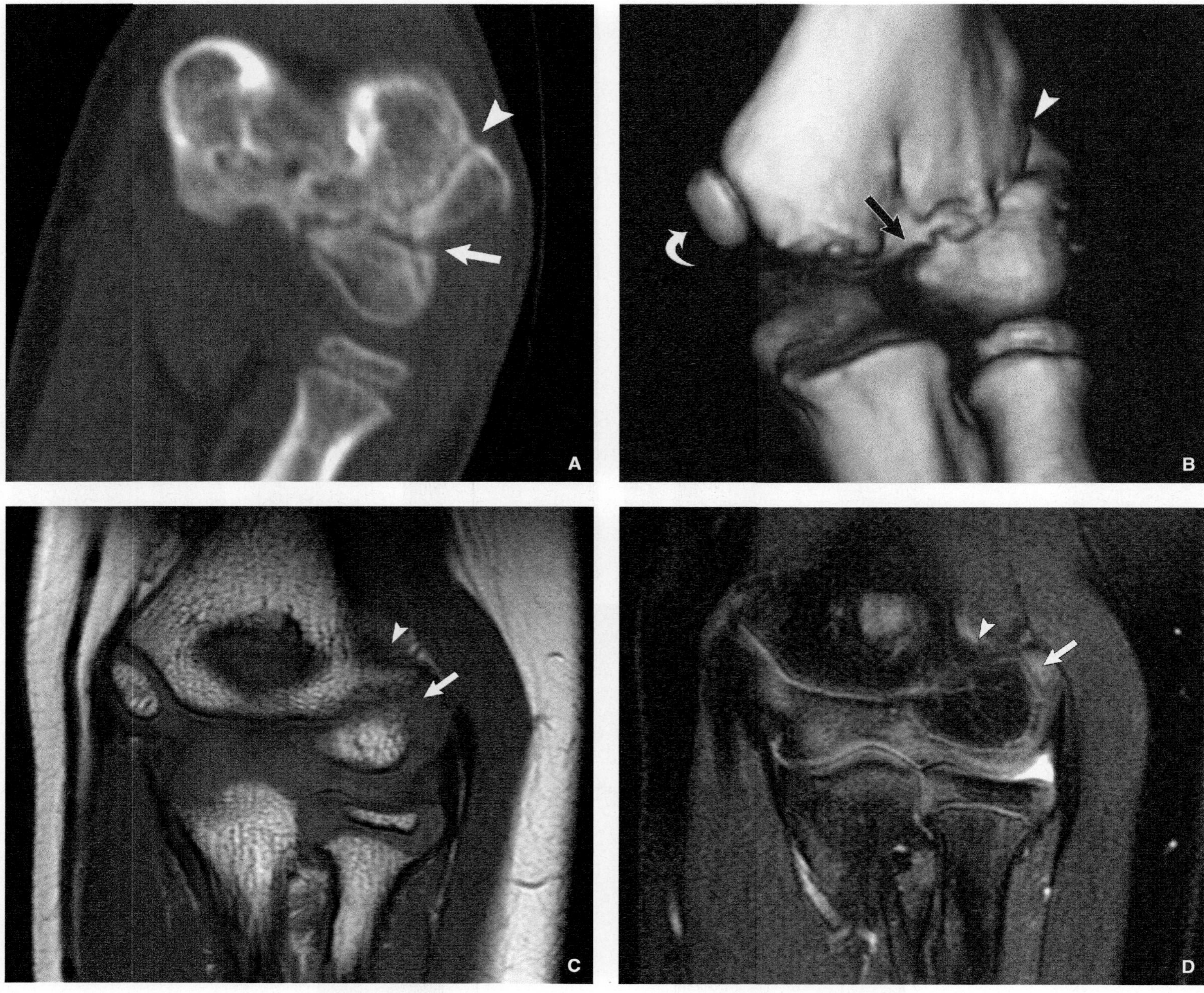

FIGURE 4.47 CT, 3D CT, and MRI of type IV Salter-Harris fracture. Coronal reformatted **(A)** and 3D reconstructed **(B)** CT images and coronal T1-weighted **(C)** and T2-weighted **(D)** MR images of the left elbow of a 7-year-old boy show a fracture of the lateral epicondyle of the humerus *(arrowheads)*, extending through the growth plate and involving the capitellum *(arrows)*. Observe the normal ossification center of the medial humeral epicondyle *(curved arrow)*.

4.50). If the epiphysis is not completely ossified, this kind of a fracture may not even be detectable on the conventional radiographs. *Type VIII* injury involving the metaphyseal region (Figs. 4.51 and 4.52) may be complicated by damage to the blood vessels supplying the growth plate, and in *type IX*, an injury to the periosteum may interfere with the membranous mechanism of bone formation. All such trauma, but particularly types IV and V (see Fig. 4.111), may lead to growth disturbance with consequent limb-length discrepancy.

Focal periphyseal edema (FOPE) is a recently described entity involving the areas surrounding the growth plate in the growing skeleton, more frequently in the knee, thought to be related to either a physiologic stage of growth plate closure or more likely related to microtrauma sustained during sports activities. This abnormality is seen only on MRI as focal areas of edema surrounding the growth plate. In most cases, the lesion is associated with pain in an adolescent patient with history of sports activities (Fig. 4.53).

Indirect Signs as Diagnostic Clues

Although the diagnosis of most fractures can be made from conventional radiographs, some subtle, nondisplaced, and hairline fractures may not be apparent at the time of injury. In such instances, certain indirect signs of fracture provide useful diagnostic clues.

Soft-Tissue Swelling

Skeletal trauma is always associated with an injury to the soft tissues, and in almost all cases of acute fracture, there is some radiographic evidence of soft-tissue swelling at the fracture site (Fig. 4.54A). The absence of soft-tissue swelling, however, virtually excludes the possibility of an acute fracture (Fig. 4.54B).

Obliteration or Displacement of Fat Stripes

Subtle fractures, particularly in the distal radius, carpal scaphoid, trapezium, and base of the first metacarpal, result in obliteration or displacement of fascial planes. On the lateral view of the wrist, one can detect a radiolucent stripe representing a collection of fat between the pronator quadratus (quadratipronator) and the tendons of the flexor digitorum profundus. A fracture of the distal radius results in a change in the appearance of the *pronator quadratus fat stripe*, which may be anteriorly (volarly) displaced, blurred, or obliterated (MacEwan sign) (Fig. 4.55).

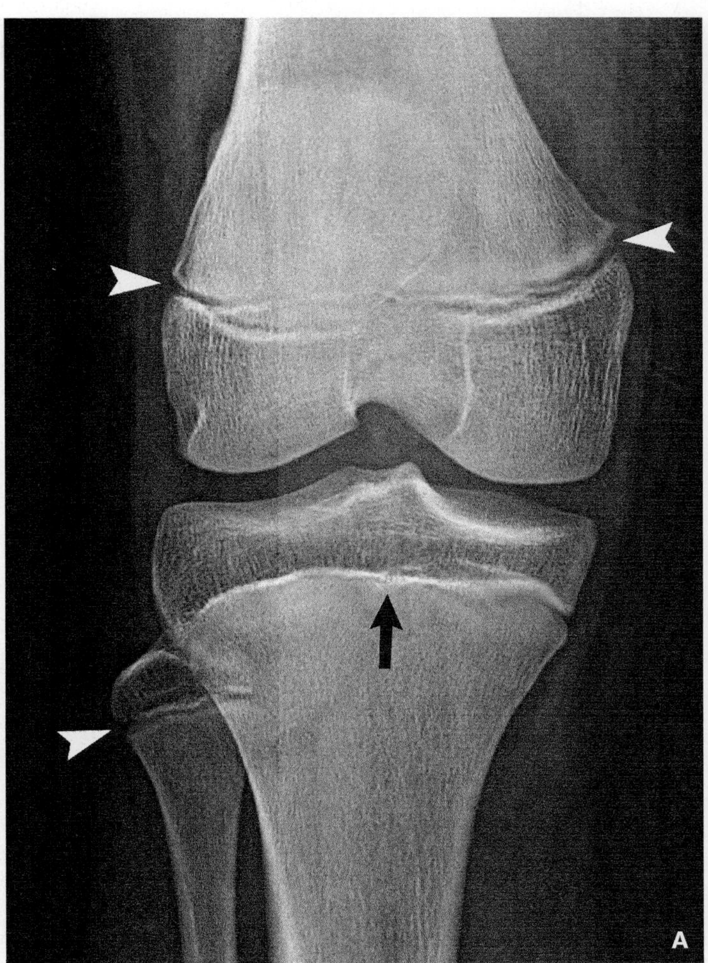

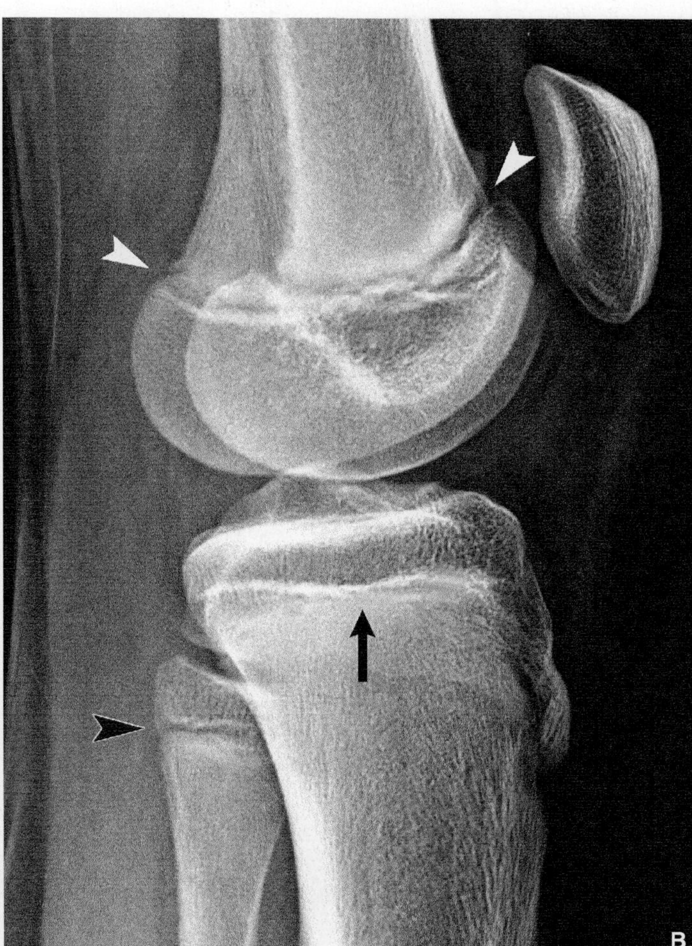

FIGURE 4.48 Type V Salter-Harris fracture. A 12-year-old boy injured his knee in a fall from a 15-feet-high ledge. Original radiographs were interpreted as "normal." Because of continued pain, the radiographs were repeated 4 weeks after the original injury. Anteroposterior **(A)** and lateral **(B)** radiographs of the right knee show narrowing and sclerosis of the proximal tibial growth plate *(arrows)* consistent with a crash injury to the physis. Observe normal appearance of the growth plates of the distal femur and proximal fibula *(arrowheads)*.

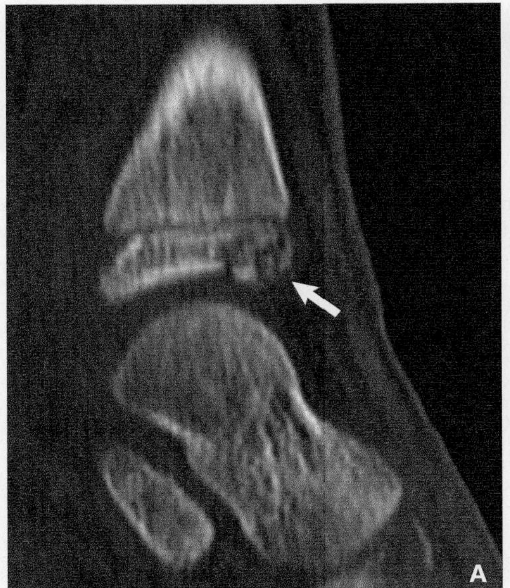

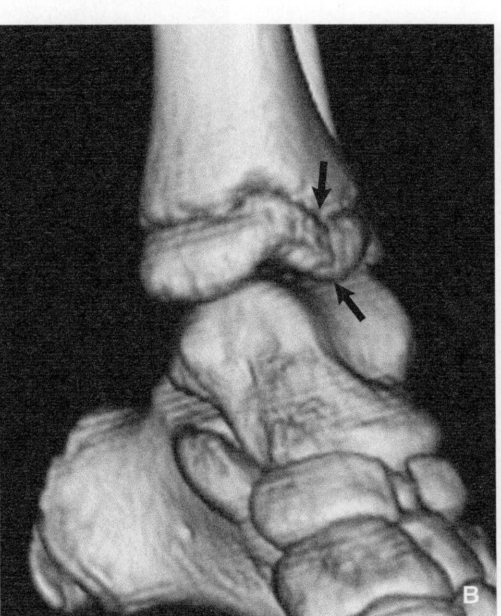

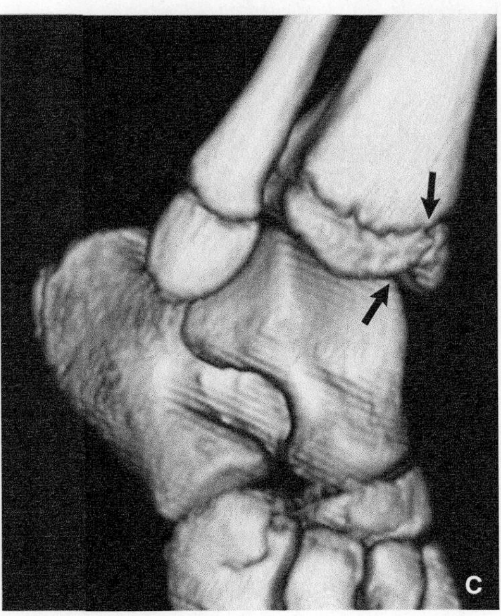

FIGURE 4.49 CT and 3D CT of type VII-A Ogden fracture. An 8-year-old boy was injured in the bike accident. Sagittal reformatted CT image **(A)** and two reconstructed 3D CT images **(B,C)** of the right ankle show a fracture through the epiphysis of the tibia extending to but not involving the distal growth plate (type A) *(arrows)*.

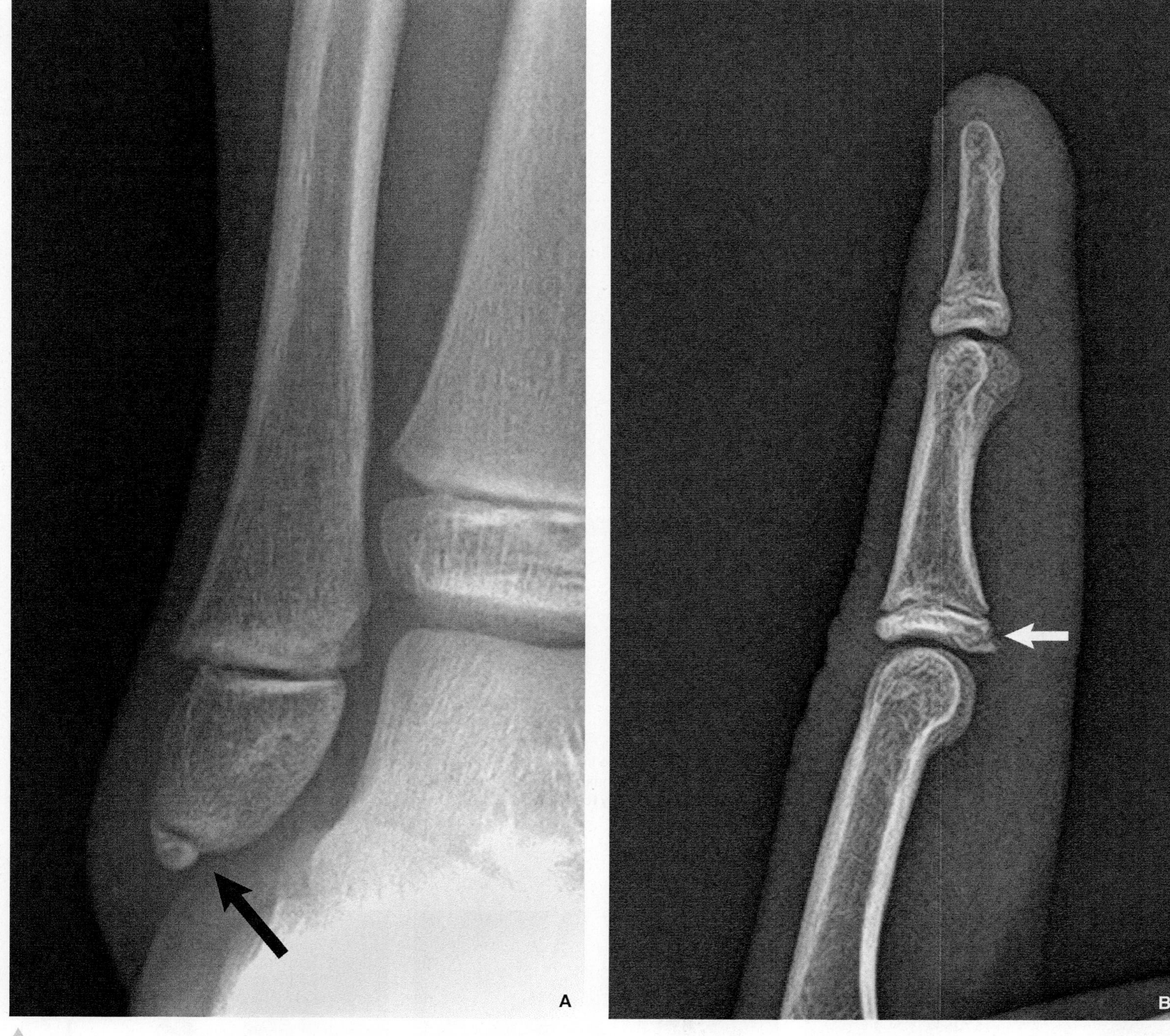

FIGURE 4.50 Type VII-B Ogden fracture. **(A)** An 11-year-old girl sustained a fracture through the fibular epiphysis that does not extend into the growth plate (type B) *(arrow)*. **(B)** A 12-year-old boy sustained a fracture through the epiphysis of the middle phalanx of the index finger (volar plate) that does not extend into the growth plate (type B) *(arrow)*.

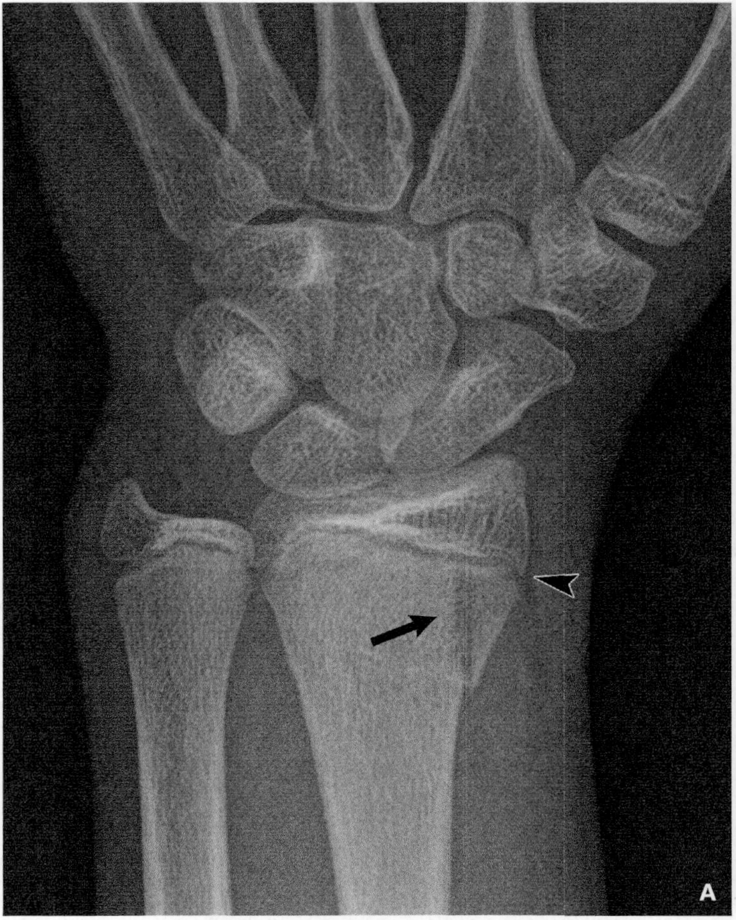

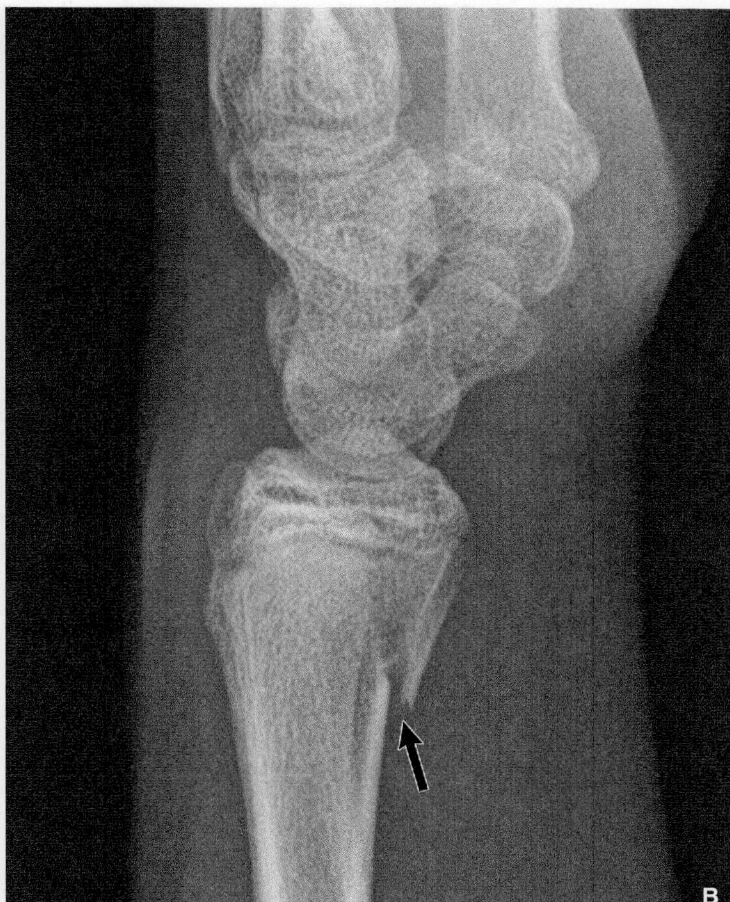

FIGURE 4.51 Type VIII Ogden fracture. Dorsovolar **(A)** and lateral **(B)** radiographs of the right wrist of a 14-year-old boy show a fracture through the distal radial metaphysis *(arrows)* that extends to but does not affect the growth plate, which is normal *(arrowhead)*.

Terry and Ramin have pointed out the usefulness of recognizing the *scaphoid fat stripe*, which is usually visible as a thin radiolucent line paralleling the lateral surface of the scaphoid bone between the radial collateral ligament and the synovial sheath of the abductor pollicis longus and the extensor pollicis brevis. In most fractures of the carpal scaphoid, radial styloid, trapezium, or base of the first metacarpal, the scaphoid fat stripe is obliterated or displaced. This finding is most apparent on the dorsovolar radiograph of the wrist (Fig. 4.56).

FIGURE 4.52 MRI of type VIII Ogden fracture. Coronal gradient recalled echo (GRE) MR image of the elbow demonstrates an oblique fracture of the distal humeral metaphysis *(arrows)* extending to but not involving the growth plate of the distal humerus.

Periosteal and Endosteal Reaction

The fracture line may not be visible, but the periosteal or endosteal response may be the first radiographic sign of a fracture (Fig. 4.57).

Joint Effusion

This finding, which results in the radiographic appearance of the fat-pad sign, is particularly useful in diagnosing elbow injuries. The posterior (dorsal) fat pad lies deep in the olecranon fossa and is not visible in the lateral projection. The anterior (ventral) fat pad occupies the shallower anterior coronoid and radial fossae and is usually seen as a flat radiolucent strip ventrad to the anterior cortex of the humerus. Distention of the articular capsule by synovial or hemorrhagic fluid causes the posterior fat pad to become visible and also displaces the anterior fat pad, yielding the *fat-pad sign* (Fig. 4.58). When there is a history of elbow trauma and the fat-pad sign is positive, there is usually an associated fracture and every effort should be made to demonstrate it. Even if the fracture line is not demonstrated on multiple radiographs, the patient should be treated for fracture.

Intracapsular Fat–Fluid Level

If a fracture involves the articular end of a bone (particularly a long bone such as the tibia, humerus, or femur), blood and bone marrow fat enter the joint (lipohemarthrosis) and produce a characteristic layering of these two substances on the radiograph: the fat–blood interface, or *FBI sign* (Fig. 4.59). A CT or an MRI study can also demonstrate this phenomenon (Figs. 4.60 and 4.61). When the fracture line cannot be demonstrated, the diagnosis should be made on the strength of this sign alone.

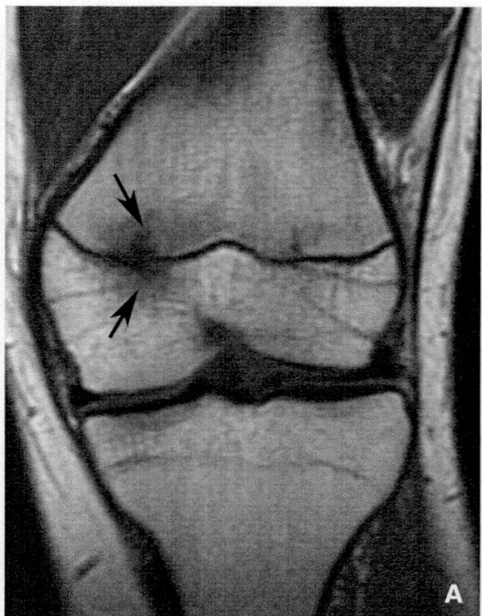

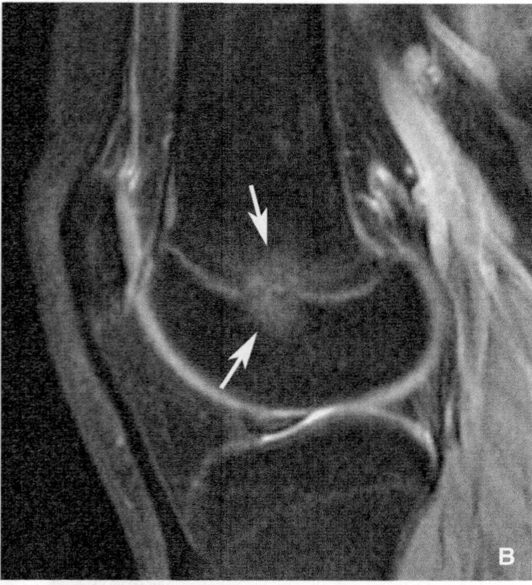

FIGURE 4.53 FOPE. **(A)** Coronal T1-weighted and **(B)** sagittal T2-weighted fat-saturated MR images of the knee of an adolescent patient demonstrate focal area of abnormal signal intensity around the distal femoral physis *(arrows)*. There was no clear history of trauma, but the patient was involved in contact sports.

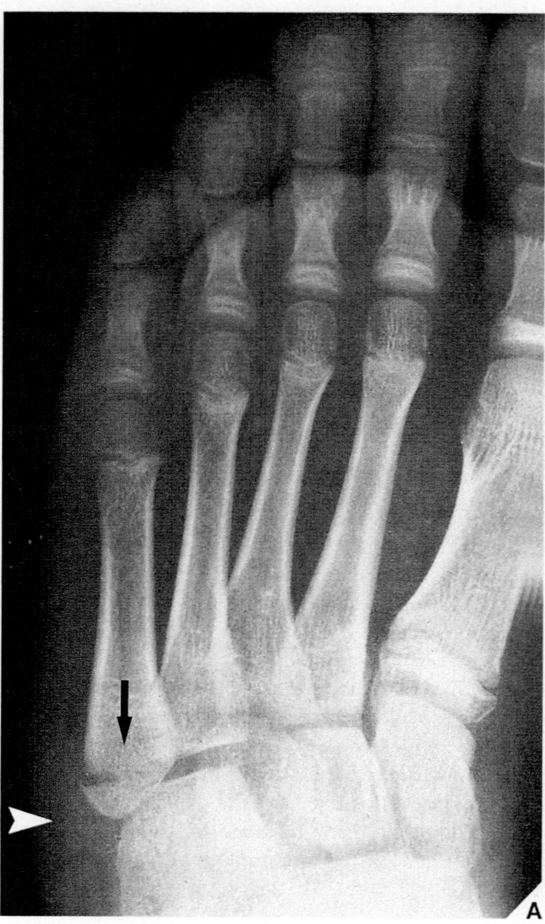

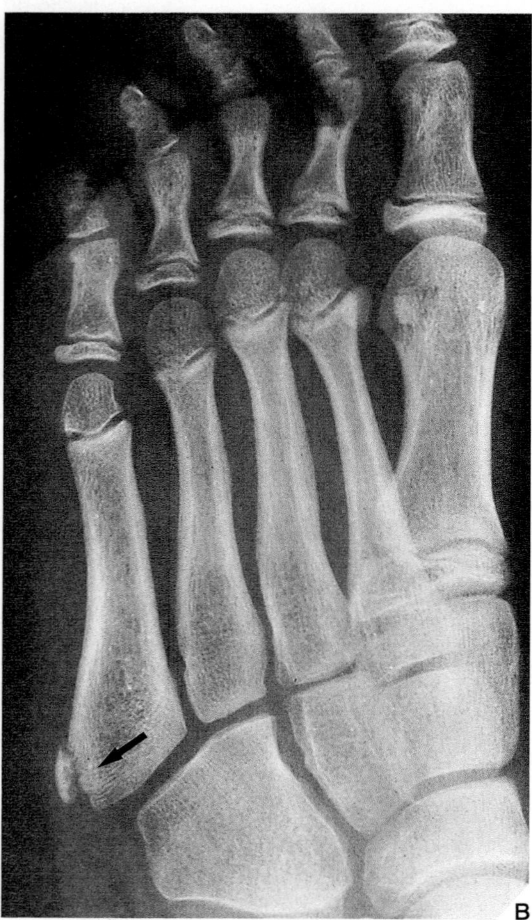

FIGURE 4.54 **Fracture versus ossification center.** **(A)** Dorsoplantar view of the foot reveals prominent soft-tissue swelling localized in the lateral aspect *(arrowhead)*. The radiolucent line at the base of the fifth metatarsal indicates a fracture *(arrow)*. **(B)** A similar radiolucent line *(arrow)* separates a bone fragment from the base of the fifth metatarsal in another patient who was suspected of sustaining a fracture of this bone. Note the complete lack of soft-tissue swelling. The finding represents a secondary ossification center, not a fracture.

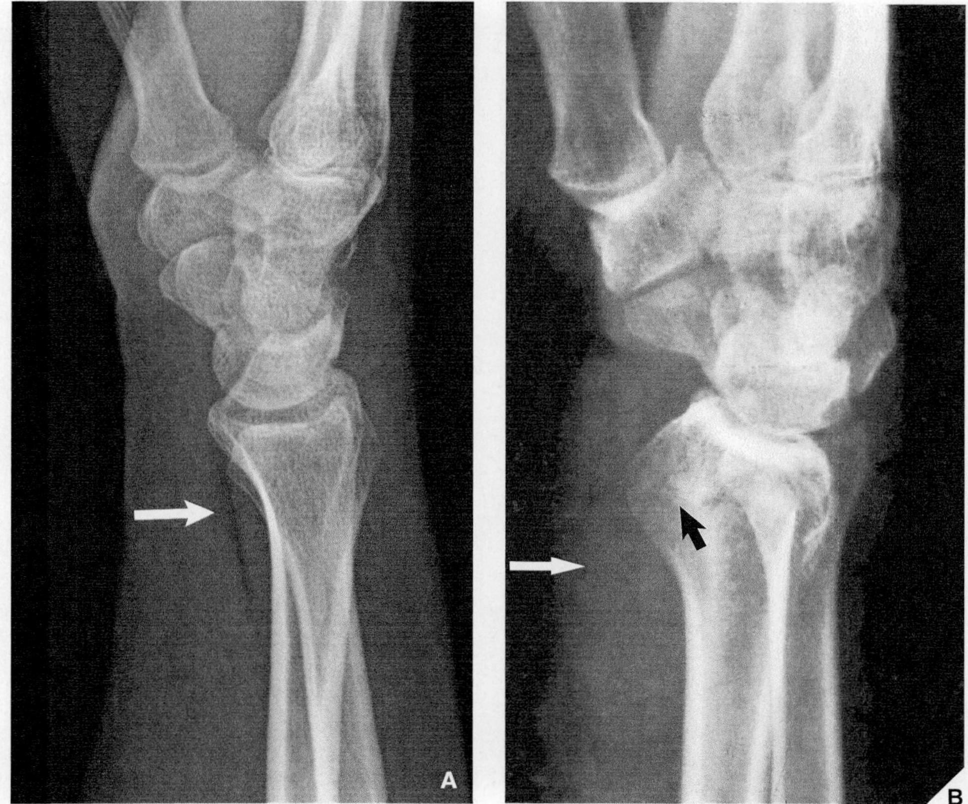

FIGURE 4.55 **Pronator quadratus fat stripe.** **(A)** The fascial plane of the pronator quadratus is demonstrated on the volar aspect of the distal forearm as a radiolucent stripe *(arrow)*. **(B)** With a fracture of the distal radius, the fat stripe is blurred and volarly displaced *(arrow)* secondary to local edema and periosteal hemorrhage. A *short black arrow* points to the subtle nondisplaced fracture of the distal radius.

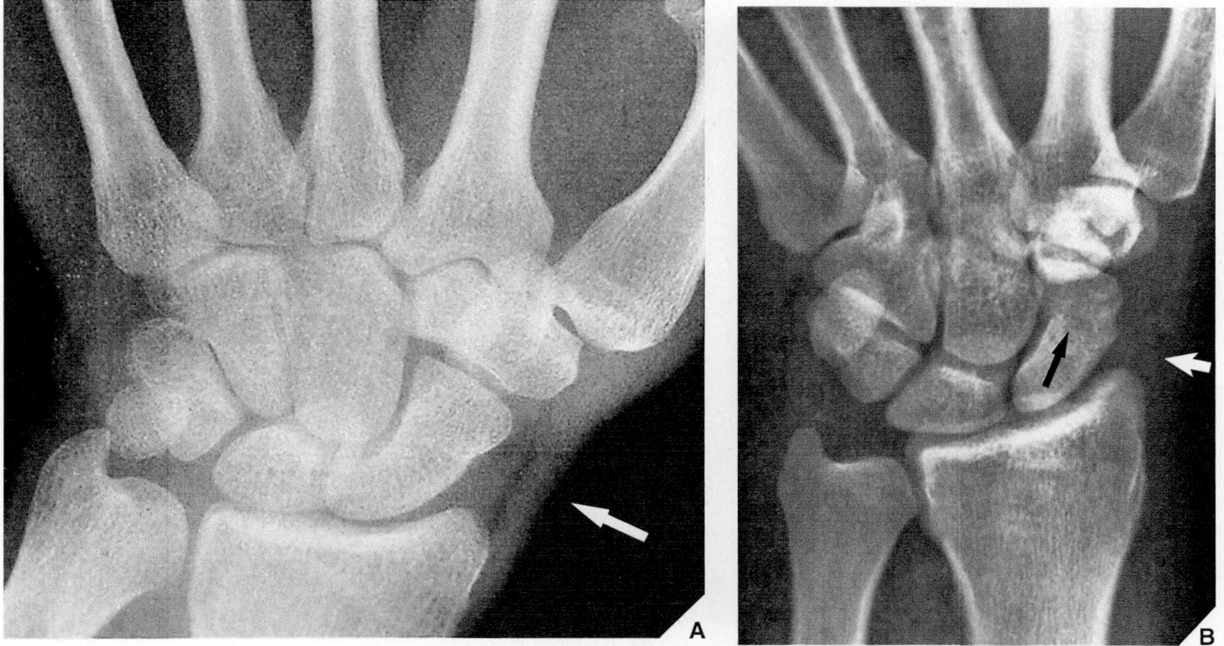

FIGURE 4.56 **Scaphoid fat stripe.** **(A)** Normal scaphoid fat stripe *(arrow)*. **(B)** A subtle fracture of the scaphoid *(black arrow)* resulted in obliteration and radial displacement of the fat stripe *(white arrow)*.

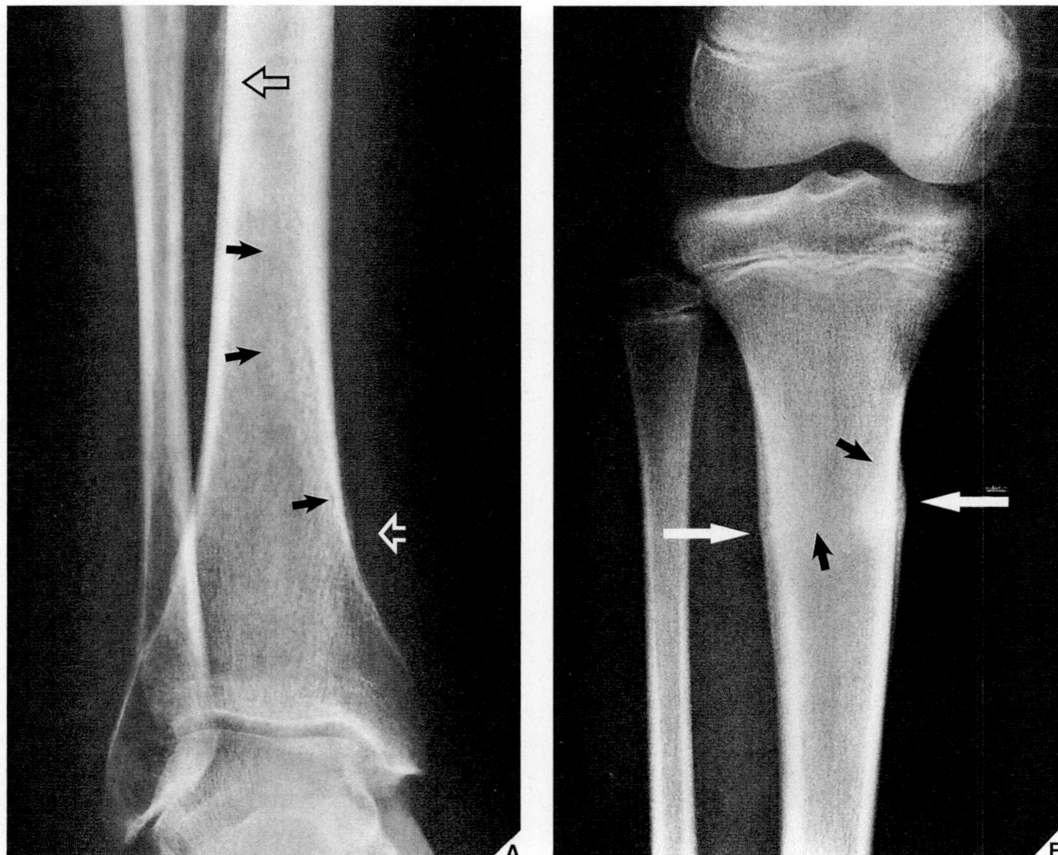

FIGURE 4.57 **Secondary signs of a fracture.** **(A)** A 49-year-old woman sustained an injury to the lower leg. Anteroposterior radiograph shows periosteal new bone at the medial cortex of the distal third of the tibia just above the malleolus and more proximally at the lateral aspect *(open arrows)*. This indirect sign of a fracture represents an early stage of external callus formation. The actual hairline spiral fracture line is barely discernible *(black arrows)*. **(B)** An example of periosteal callus formation at the medial and lateral cortices of the proximal tibial diaphysis *(white arrows)*. A transverse band of increased density, visible in the medullary portion of the bone *(black arrows)*, represents endosteal callus. The fracture line is practically invisible. These features are commonly seen in a stress fracture.

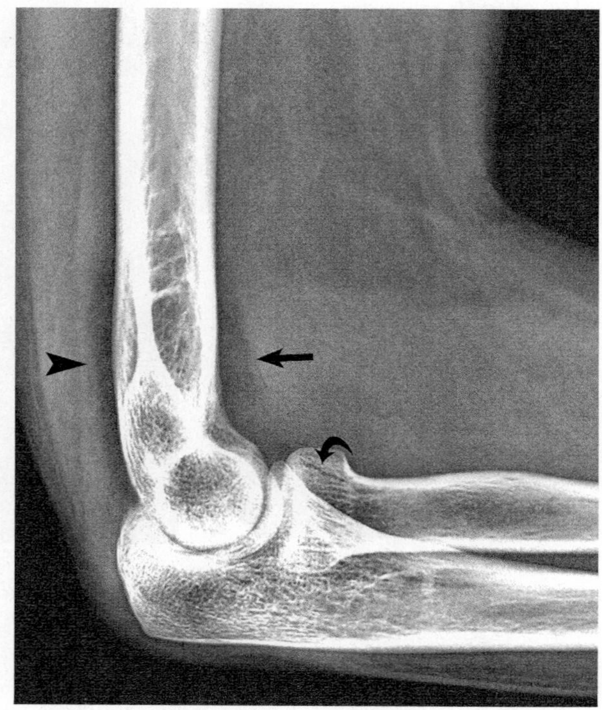

FIGURE 4.58 **Fracture of the radial head.** Lateral view of the elbow shows a positive fat-pad sign. The anterior fat pad is markedly elevated *(arrow)*, and the posterior fat pad *(arrowhead)* is clearly visible in this patient. There is a subtle, nondisplaced fracture of the radial head *(curved arrow)*.

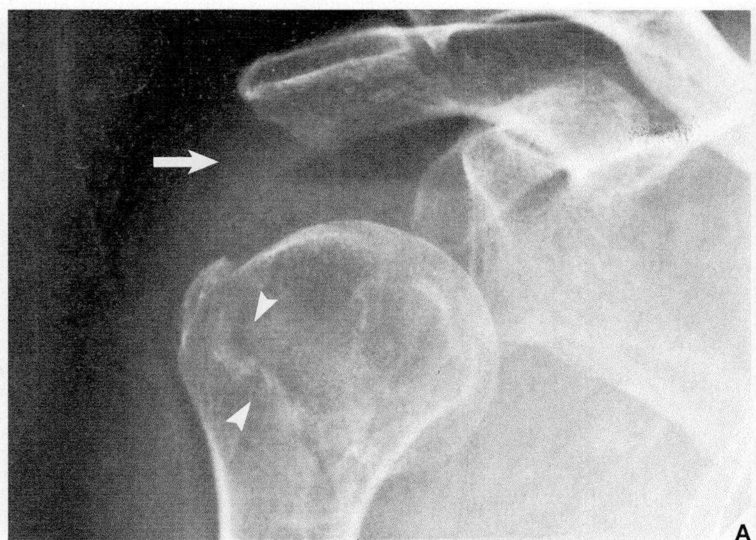

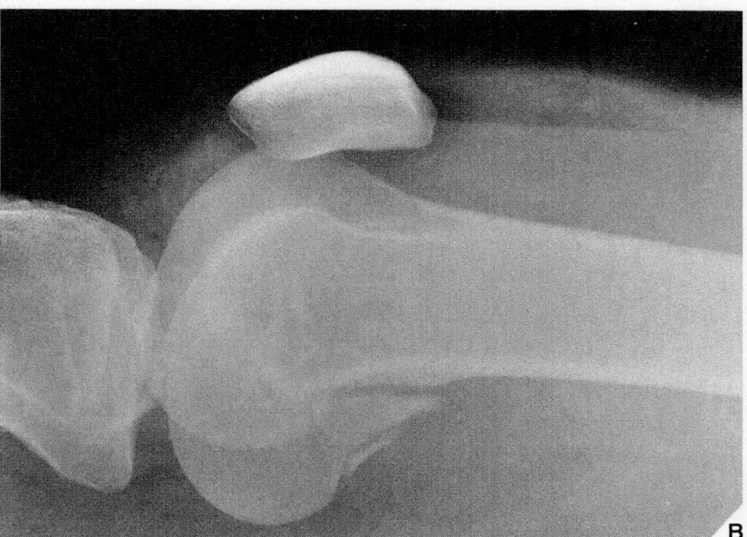

FIGURE 4.59 FBI sign. **(A)** Erect anteroposterior view of the shoulder demonstrates the fat–fluid level in the joint *(arrow)*, an example of the FBI sign. The fracture line extends from the humeral neck cephalad to the greater tuberosity *(arrowheads)*. To demonstrate the FBI sign, the cassette should be positioned perpendicular to the expected fat–fluid level with the central ray directed horizontally. For example, in the shoulder, an upright radiograph (patient standing or sitting) should be obtained. In the knee **(B)**, the patient must be supine, and a cross-table lateral view should be performed.

Lava Lamp Sign

Similar to the sign described earlier, this sign is produced when droplets of bone marrow fat enter the joint through the intraarticular fracture, which may not be apparent on the radiography, but may be demonstrated on MRI (Fig. 4.62). Even when fracture line cannot be seen, the presence of fat droplets within the joint is diagnostic.

Double Cortical Line

This finding indicates a subtle but depressed fracture. The actual fracture line may not be apparent, but the double contour of the cortex reflects impaction (Fig. 4.63).

Buckling of the Cortex

Known as the *torus fracture*, this may be the only sign of a tubular bone fracture in children (Figs. 4.64). This finding is sometimes identified more easily on the lateral than on the frontal projection.

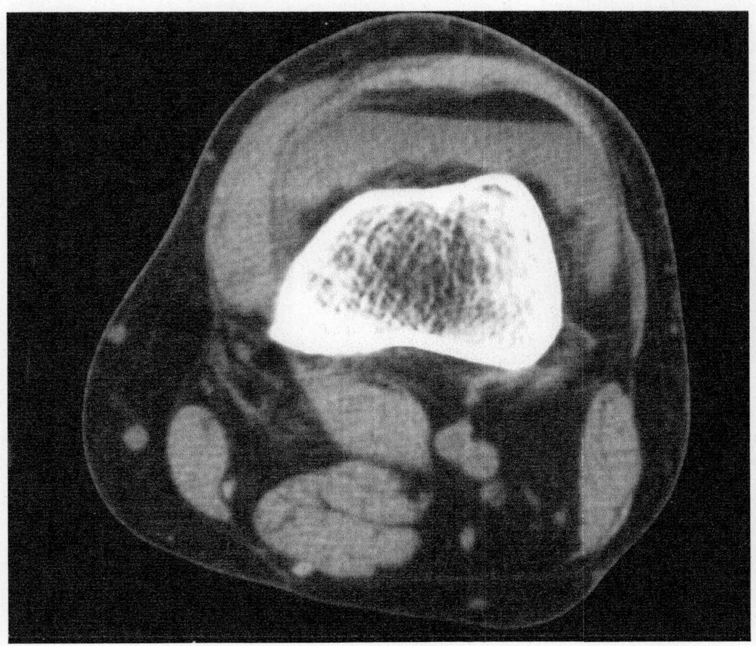

FIGURE 4.60 FBI sign on CT. Axial CT section through the knee joint shows an FBI sign in a patient with tibial plateau fracture (not seen on this image).

Irregular Metaphyseal Corners

This sign, which is secondary to small avulsion fractures of the metaphysis, indicates a subtle injury to the bone caused by a rapid rotary force exerted on the ligaments' insertion. As a result, small fragments of bone are separated from the metaphysis. These *corner fractures* are often present in infants and children who sustain skeletal trauma, and they should be looked for particularly if battered child syndrome, also known as *shaken baby syndrome* or *parent–infant trauma syndrome* (PITS), is suspected (Fig. 4.65).

Radiographic Evaluation of Dislocations

Dislocations are more obvious than fractures on conventional radiographs and, consequently, are more easily diagnosed (Fig. 4.66). Some display such a characteristic appearance on frontal projection (anteroposterior view) that this single examination suffices (Fig. 4.66C). However, the same principle of obtaining at least two projections oriented at 90 degrees to each other should apply. Supplemental radiographs are occasionally necessary, and in some instances, CT is required for the exact evaluation of a dislocation.

Monitoring the Results of Treatment

Radiography plays the leading role in monitoring the progress of fracture healing and in detecting any posttraumatic complications. Follow-up radiographs should be taken at regular intervals to evaluate the stage and

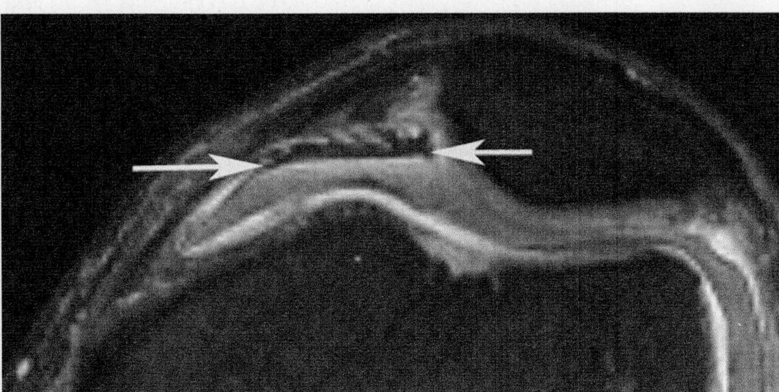

FIGURE 4.61 FBI sign on MRI. Axial proton density–weighted fat-saturated MR image of the knee with the patient in the supine position demonstrates an FBI sign secondary to differential layering of fat (low signal intensity) floating on top of blood (intermediate signal intensity) *(arrows)*, representing lipohemarthrosis.

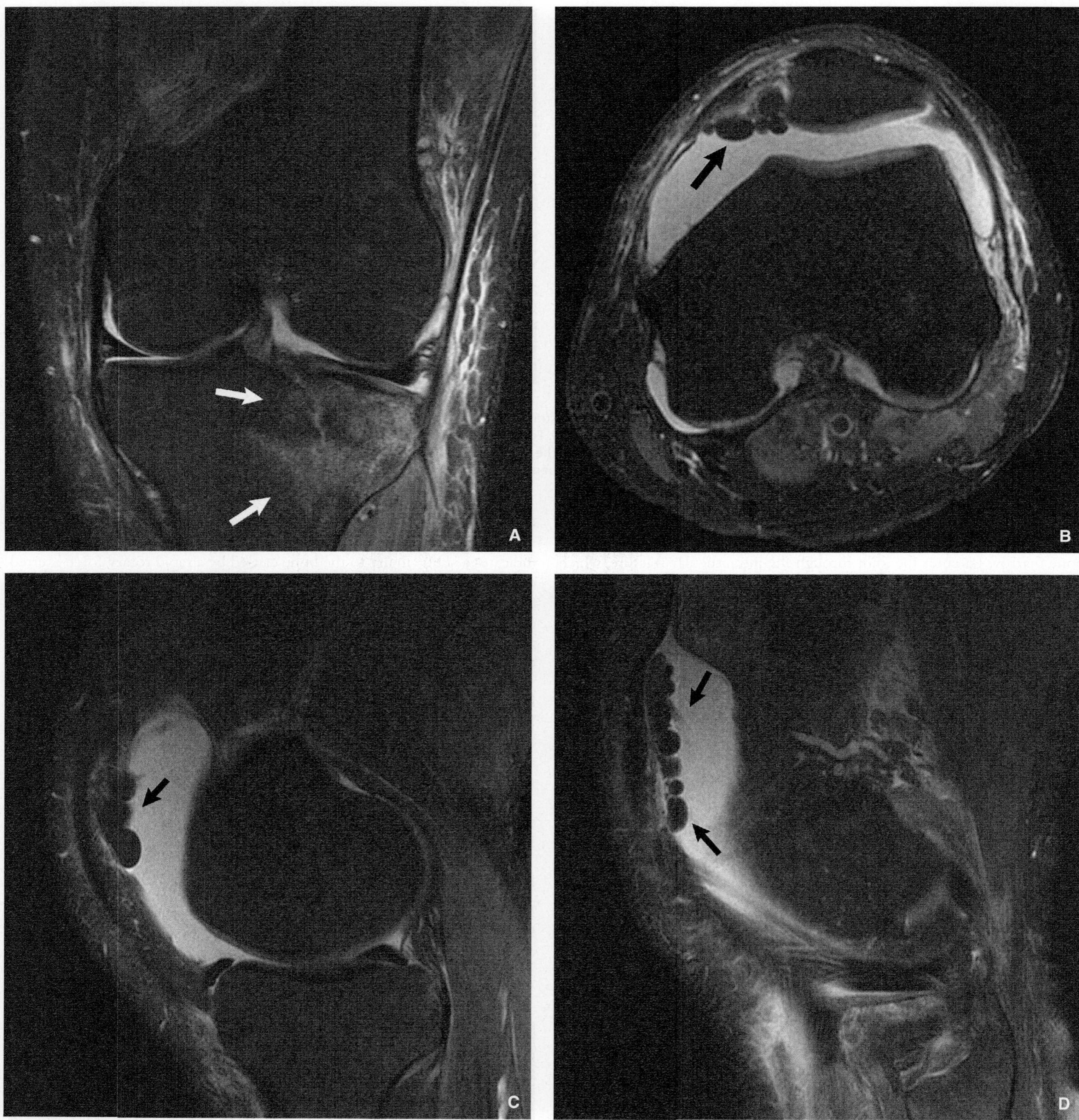

FIGURE 4.62 **Lava lamp sign of occult intraarticular facture.** A 36-year-old man injured his left knee in a fall. The radiographs (not shown here) revealed no fracture. **(A)** Coronal proton density–weighted fat-suppressed MR image shows an intraarticular fracture of the lateral tibial plateau *(white arrows)*. Axial **(B)**, sagittal through the medial part of the joint **(C)**, and sagittal through the lateral part of the joint **(D)** proton density–weighted fat-suppressed MR images show a lava lamp sign representing the droplets of bone marrow fat *(black arrows)* against high–signal intensity joint fluid.

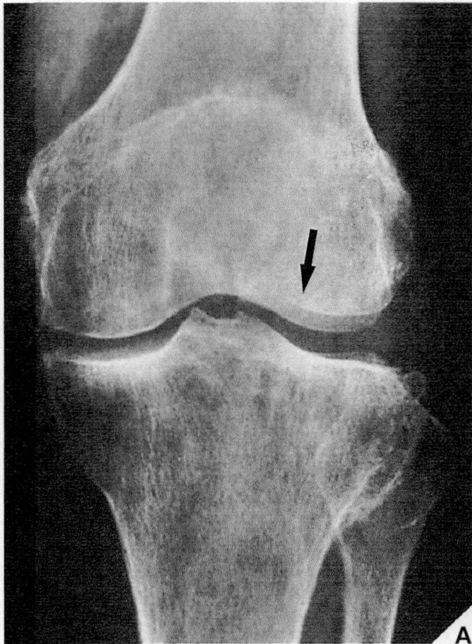

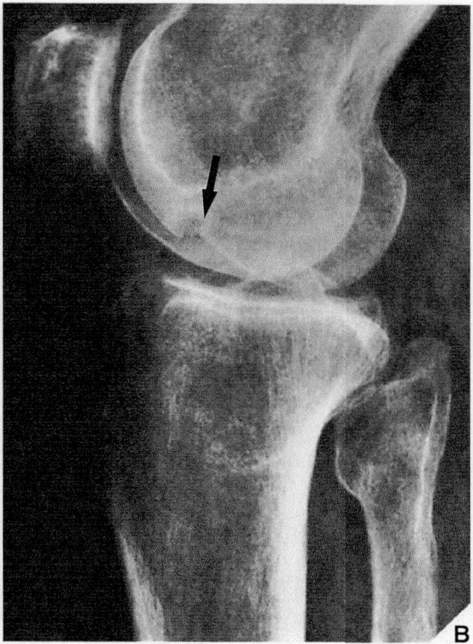

FIGURE 4.63 **Fracture of the femur.** **(A)** On the anteroposterior radiograph of the knee, the fracture line is not apparent, but a depressed articular cortex of the lateral femoral condyle projects proximally to the normal subchondral line of the intact segment, producing a double cortical line *(arrow)*. **(B)** Lateral radiograph confirms the presence of a depressed fracture of the femoral condyle *(arrow)*.

possible associated complications of fracture healing and other complications that may follow a fracture, dislocation, or other injury to the musculoskeletal system. If radiographs are ambiguous in this respect, CT is the next technique to apply.

Fracture Healing and Complications

The healing of a fracture can be divided into three phases: inflammatory (reactive), reparative, and remodeling. The *inflammatory phase* is characterized by vasodilatation, serum exudation, and infiltration by inflammatory cells. It lasts about 2 to 7 days. The *reparative phase* is characterized by the formation of periosteal and endosteal (medullary) calluses by the periosteal and bone marrow osteoblasts. Mesenchymal cell proliferation and differentiation are accompanied by intense vascular proliferation. The resulting osteoblasts produce collagen at a high rate. This phase lasts about a month. The *remodeling phase* is characterized by both modeling and remodeling at the site of a fracture to restore the original contours of the bone and its optimal internal structure. The endosteal and periosteal calluses are removed, and the woven immature bone is replaced by a secondary lamellar (cortical or trabecular) bone. If the fracture, particularly in the growing skeleton, has healed with incorrect angulation (malunion), this may be corrected by selectively removing bone from the convex side of the cortex by the process of osteoclastic resorption and adding bone to the concave side by the process of osteoblastic apposition. This phase may last from about 3 months to 1 year or even longer.

Fracture healing depends on many factors: the patient's age, the site and type of fracture, the position of the fragments, the status of the blood supply, the quality of immobilization or fixation, and the presence or absence of associated abnormalities such as infection or osteonecrosis (Table 4.1). An average healing time of some fractures is depicted in Table 4.2. Most fractures heal by some combination of endosteal and periosteal callus.

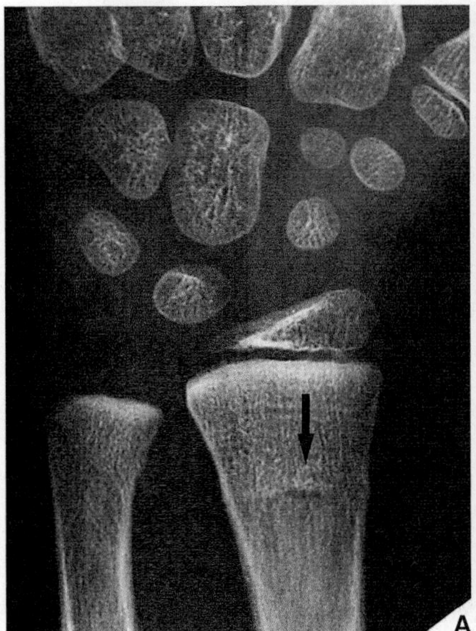

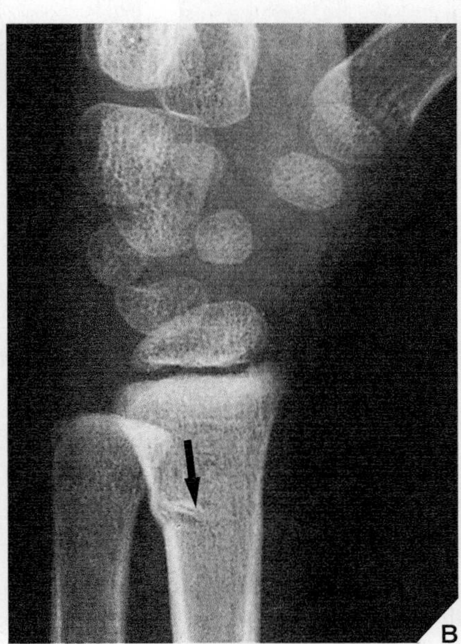

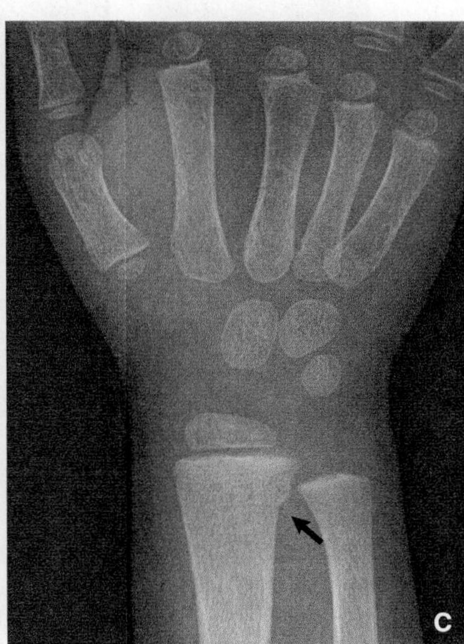

FIGURE 4.64 **Torus fracture.** Posteroanterior **(A)** and lateral **(B)** radiographs of the distal forearm demonstrate buckling of the dorsal cortex of the diaphysis of the distal radius *(arrows)*. This represents an incomplete torus fracture. Note that the lateral view is more revealing. **(C)** In another patient, a 4-year-old boy, a dorsovolar radiograph of the left wrist shows typical torus fracture manifesting by buckling of the medial cortex of the radial metaphysis *(arrow)*.

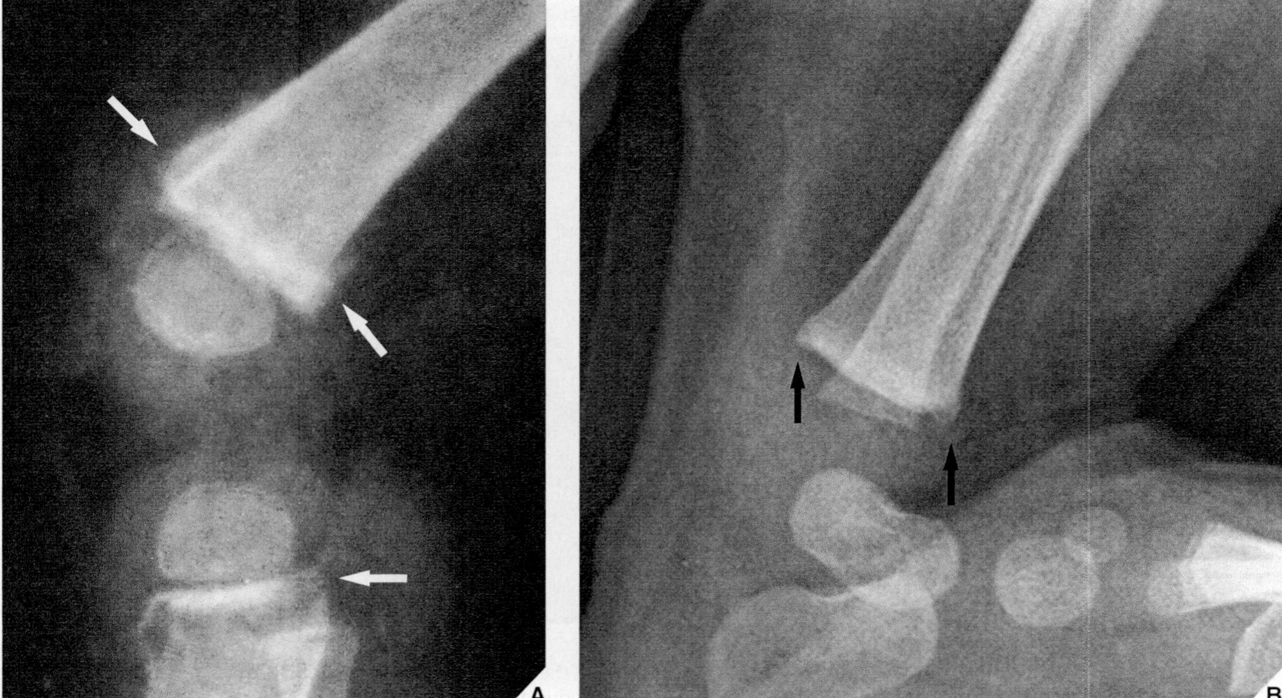

FIGURE 4.65 Battered child syndrome. **(A)** Lateral radiograph of the knee reveals irregular outlines of the metaphyses of the distal femur and the proximal tibia and subtle corner fractures *(arrows)* characteristic of the battered child syndrome. **(B)** In another infant, metaphyseal corner fractures are identified in the distal tibia *(arrows)*.

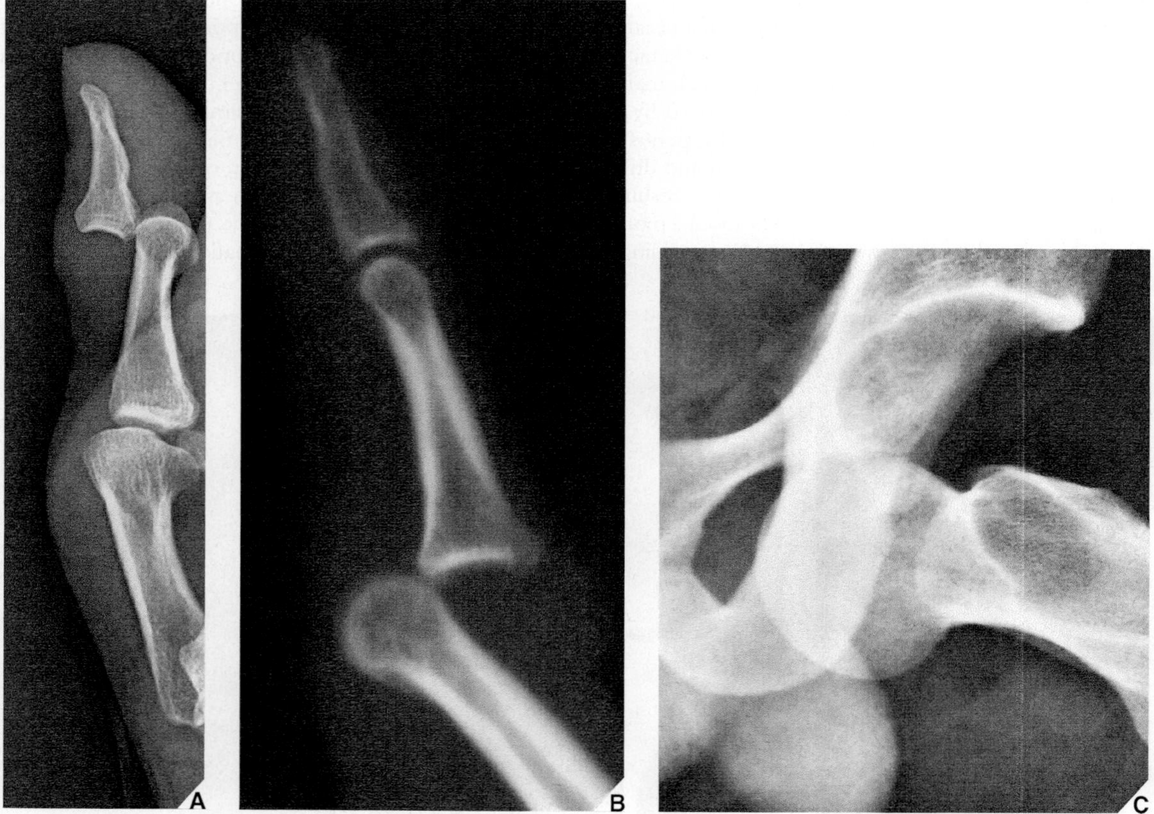

FIGURE 4.66 Dislocations. **(A)** Lateral radiograph of the thumb shows a dislocation in the interphalangeal joint. **(B)** Lateral radiograph shows a dislocation in the proximal interphalangeal joint of the index finger. **(C)** Anteroposterior radiograph of the left hip shows a typical anterior dislocation of the femoral head. The clue to this diagnosis is the presence of abduction and external rotation of the femur and the position of the femoral head, which is medial and inferior to the acetabulum.

TABLE 4.1 Factors Influencing Fracture Healing

Promoting	Retarding
Good immobilization	Motion
Growth hormone	Corticosteroids
Thyroid hormone	Anticoagulants
Calcitonin	Anemia
Insulin	Radiation
Vitamins A and D	Poor blood supply
Hyaluronidase	Infection
Electric currents	Osteoporosis
Oxygen	Osteonecrosis
Physical exercise	Comminution
Young age	Old age

TABLE 4.2 Fracture Healing

Bone	Average Healing Time (Weeks)
Metacarpal	4–6
Metatarsal	4–8
Distal radius (extraarticular)	6–8
Distal radius (intraarticular)	6–10
Humeral shaft	12
Femoral shaft	12
Radius and ulnar shaft	16
Tibial shaft	16–24
Femoral neck	24

Provided that blood supply is adequate, nondisplaced fractures and anatomically reduced fractures immobilized with adequate compression heal by *primary union*. In this type of healing, the fracture line becomes obliterated by endosteal (internal) callus. Displaced fractures, that is, those that are not anatomically aligned or with a gap between fragments, heal by *secondary union*. This type of healing is achieved mainly by excessive periosteal (external) callus, which undergoes full ossification through the stages of granulation tissue, fibrous tissue, fibrocartilage, woven bone, and compact bone. For the radiologist evaluating follow-up radiographs, the primary indication of bone repair is radiographic evidence of periosteal (external) and endosteal (internal) callus formation (Fig. 4.67). This process, however, may not be radiographically apparent in the early stage of healing. Periosteal response may not be visible on radiographs at sites where there is an anatomic lack of periosteum, for example, in the intracapsular portion of the femoral neck. Likewise, radiographs may not demonstrate endosteal callus formation because the callus contains only fibrous tissue and cartilage, which are radiolucent. At this early stage of healing, a fracture may be *clinically united*, that is, shows no evidence of motion under stress, yet radiographically, the radiolucent band between the fragments may persist (Fig. 4.68A). As the primary temporarily radiolucent callus is gradually converted by the process of endochondral ossification to more mature lamellar bone, it is seen on the film as a dense bridge (Fig. 4.68B). This constitutes *radiographic union*.

Although conventional radiographs are frequently sufficient to evaluate the progress of fracture healing, routine studies must, at times, be supplemented by CT. This modality with multiplanar reformation proves to be a good method to assess fracture healing. It is, in particular, effective in patients with remaining metallic hardware and those who had multiple surgical procedures including bone grafting. CT with reformation in the

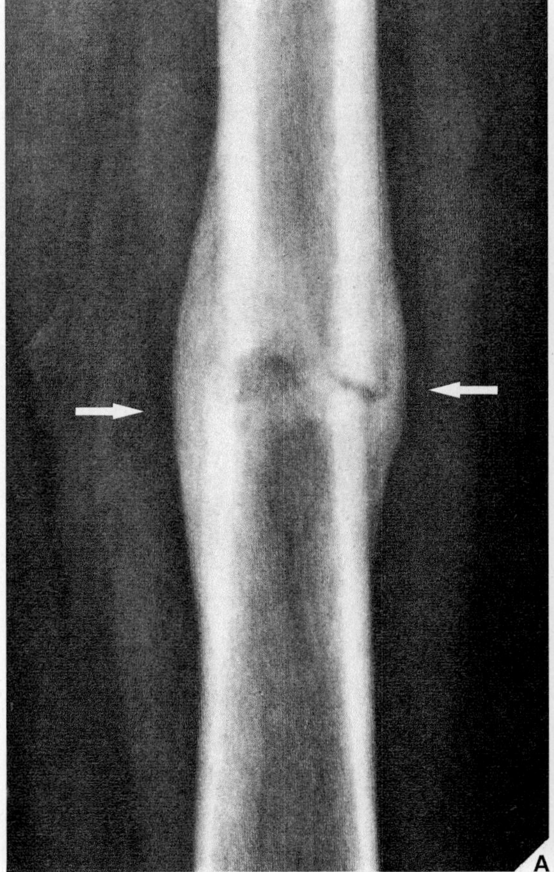

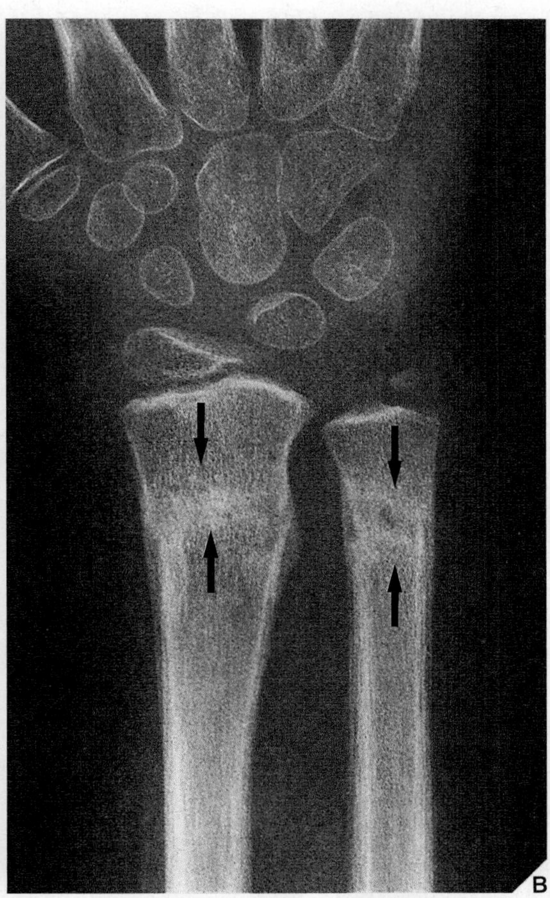

FIGURE 4.67 Fracture healing. (A) Anteroposterior radiograph of the femur shows a fracture healing predominantly by periosteal callus formation *(arrows)*. There is no radiographic evidence of endosteal callus, and the fracture line is still visible. **(B)** Posteroanterior radiograph of the distal forearm demonstrates healing fractures of the radius and ulna. The fracture lines are almost completely obliterated secondary to the formation of endosteal callus *(arrows)*. Note also the minimal amount of periosteal callus.

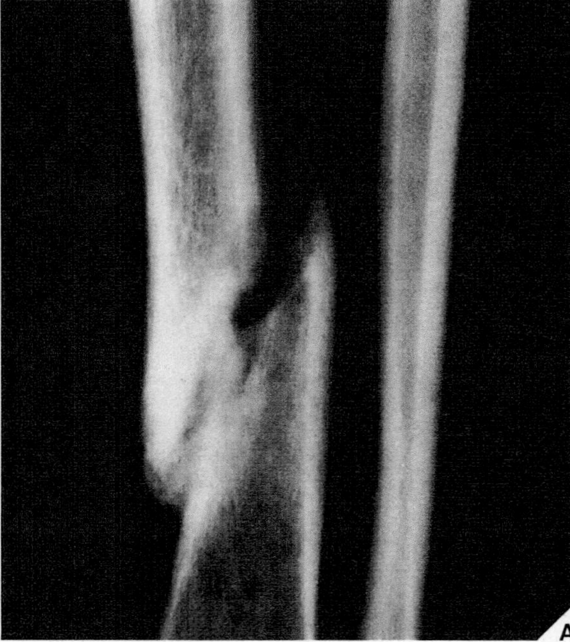

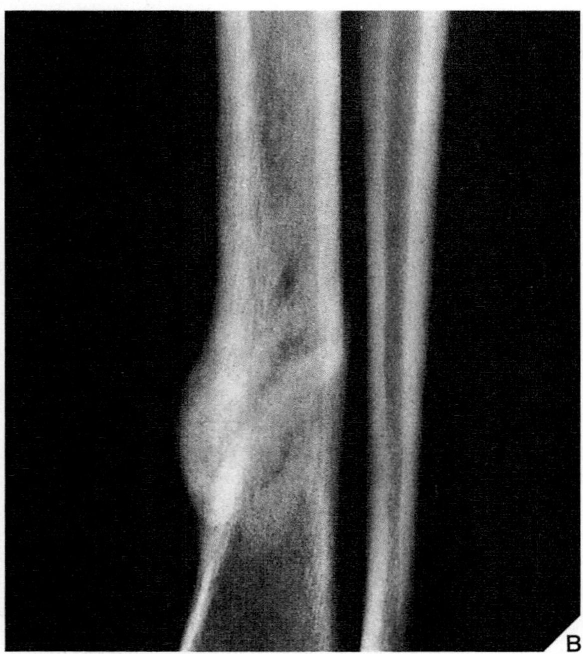

FIGURE 4.68 Clinical versus radiographic union. A 30-year-old woman sustained a fracture of the distal third of the tibia. **(A)** After 3 months of immobilization, the plaster cast was removed. The radiograph shows a unilateral periosteal callus from the medial aspect, but the fracture line is still clearly visible. Clinically, however, this fracture was fully united, and the patient was allowed to bear weight without a cast. **(B)** One and a half months later, there is evidence of a dense bridge of periosteal and endosteal callus, indicating radiographic union.

coronal and sagittal planes supplemented with 3D reconstruction aids surgical planning by providing a more detailed assessment of malalignment and angular deformities, the magnitude of the gap in the bone, and the integrity of the adjacent weight-bearing joints.

In addition to monitoring the progress of callus formation, the radiologist should be aware of radiographic evidence of associated complications of the healing process. These complications are delayed union, nonunion, and malunion. Of the three, *malunion* is the most apparent radiographically and is characterized by a union of the bone fragments in a faulty and unacceptable position (Fig. 4.69A); surgical intervention is usually the preferred method of treatment in this case (Fig. 4.69B).

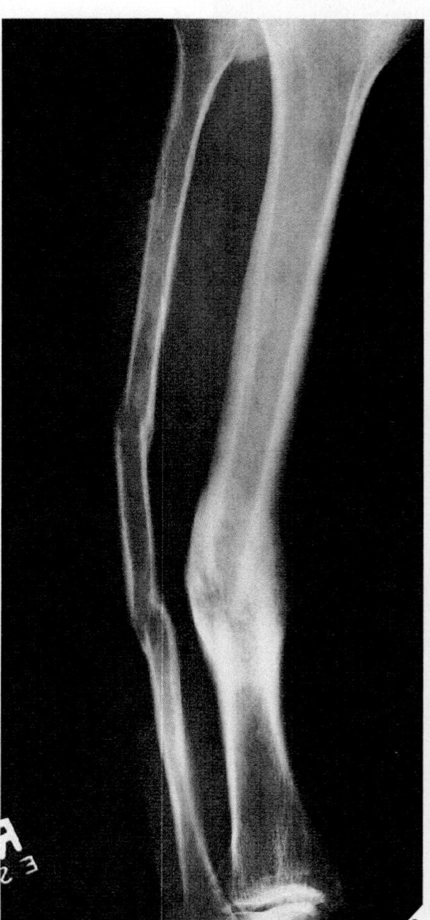

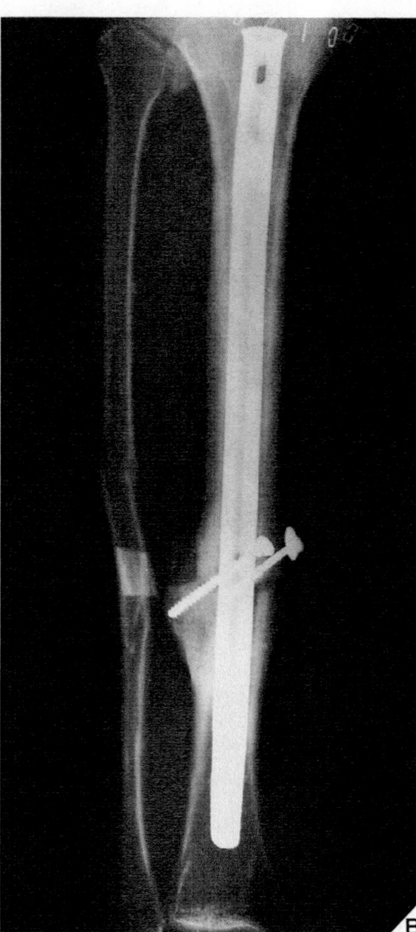

FIGURE 4.69 Malunion. **(A)** Anteroposterior radiograph of the leg demonstrates angular malunion. The fracture of the tibia and the segmental fracture of the fibula are solidly united. The distal part of the tibia, however, shows rotation and anterior angulation, and the fractures of the fibula have joined in a bowing deformity. **(B)** The malunion was surgically treated by double osteotomy and internal fixation of the tibia with an intramedullary rod to correct the longitudinal alignment and restore the anatomic axis.

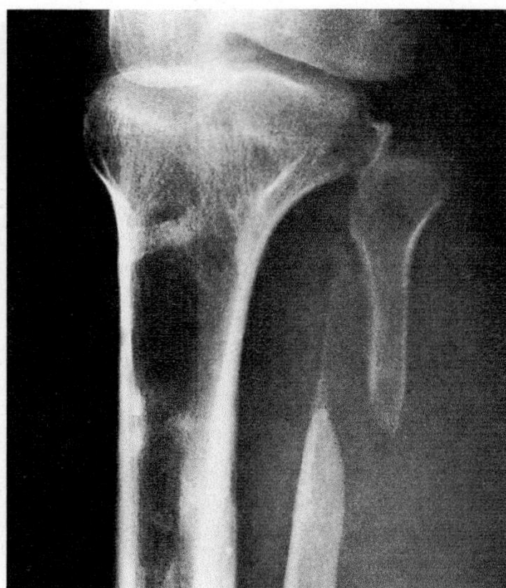

FIGURE 4.70 **Nonunion.** A fracture of the proximal fibula failed to unite. Note the gap between the fragments, the complete lack of callus formation, and the rounding of the fragment edges.

TABLE 4.3 Causes of Nonunion

I. *Excess Motion (Inadequate Immobilization)*
II. *Gap between Fragments*
  A. Soft-tissue interposition
  B. Distraction by traction or hardware
  C. Malposition, overriding, or displacement of fragments
  D. Loss of bone substance
III. *Loss of Blood Supply*
  A. Damage to nutrient vessels
  B. Excessive stripping or injury to periosteum and muscle
  C. Free fragments, severe comminution
  D. Avascularity caused by hardware placement
  E. Osteonecrosis
IV. *Infection*
  A. Osteomyelitis
  B. Extensive necrosis of fracture margins (gap)
  C. Bone death (sequestrum)
  D. Osteolysis (gap)
  E. Loosening of implants (motion)

Modified with permission from Rosen H. Treatment of nonunions: general principles. In: Chapman MW, ed. *Operative orthopaedics*, 2nd ed. Philadelphia: JB Lippincott; 1993:749–769.

Delayed union refers to a fracture that does not unite within a reasonable amount of time (16 to 24 weeks), depending on the patient's age and the fracture site. *Nonunion*, however, applies to a fracture that simply fails to unite (Fig. 4.70). Some of the causes of nonunion are listed in Table 4.3. A *pseudoarthrosis* is a variant of nonunion in which there is formation of a false joint cavity with a synovial-like capsule and even synovial fluid at the fracture site; however, some physicians refer to any fracture that fails to heal within 9 months as a *pseudoarthrosis* and use the term as a synonym for nonunion. Radiographically, nonunion is characterized by rounded edges; smoothness and sclerosis (eburnation) of the fragment ends, which are separated by a gap; and motion between the fragments (demonstrated under fluoroscopy or on consecutive stress films). To provide adequate evaluation of healing failure, the radiologist needs to distinguish between the three types of nonunion: reactive, nonreactive, and infected (Fig. 4.71).

Reactive (Hypertrophic and Oligotrophic) Nonunion

Radiographically, this type of nonunion is characterized by exuberant bone reaction and resultant flaring and sclerosis of bone ends, the elephant-foot or horse-hoof type (Fig. 4.72). The sclerotic areas do not represent dead bones but the apposition of well-vascularized new bones. Radionuclide bone scan shows a marked increase of isotope uptake at the fracture site. This type of nonunited fracture is usually treated by intramedullary nailing or compression plating.

Nonreactive (Atrophic) Nonunion

With this type of nonunion, the radiograph shows an absence of bone reaction at the fragment ends, and the blood supply is generally very scanty (Fig. 4.73). A radionuclide bone scan shows either minimal or no isotope uptake. In addition to stable internal fixation, such fractures often require extensive decortication and bone grafting.

Infected Nonunion

Radiographic presentation of infected nonunion depends on the infection's activity. Old, *inactive* osteomyelitis shows irregular thickening of the cortex, well-organized periosteal reaction, and reactive sclerosis of cancellous bone (Fig. 4.74), whereas the *active* form shows soft-tissue swelling,

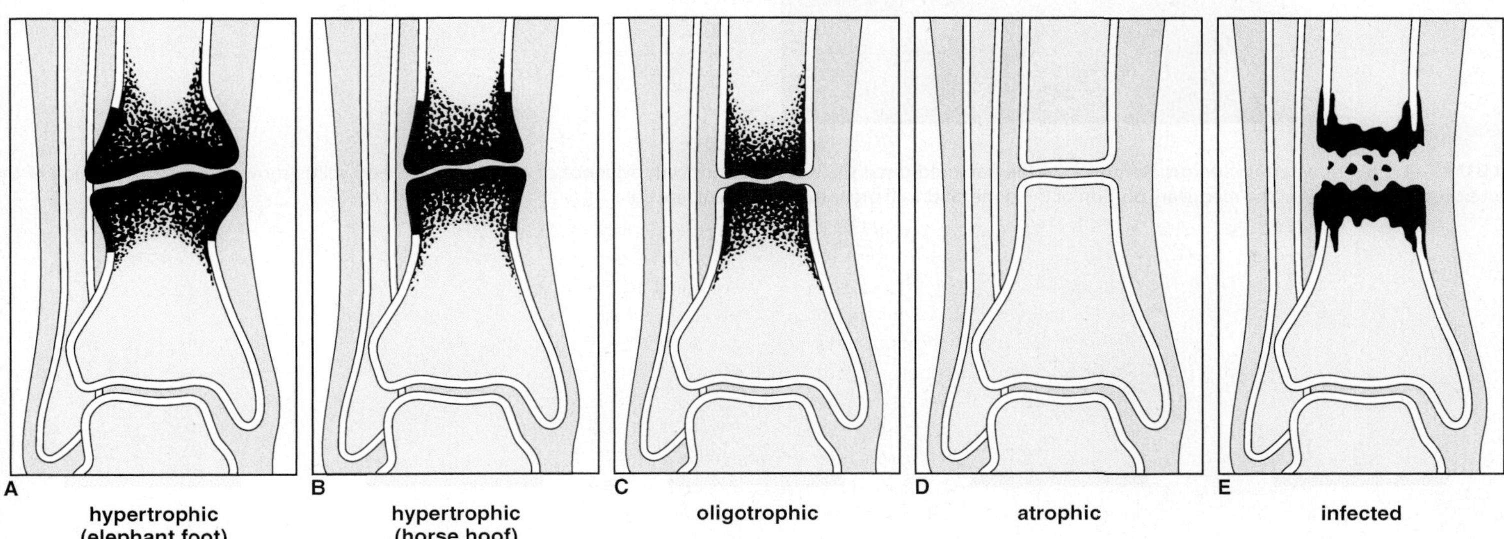

FIGURE 4.71 **Complications of a fracture.** Types of nonunion: reactive **(A–C)**, nonreactive **(D)**, and infected **(E)**.

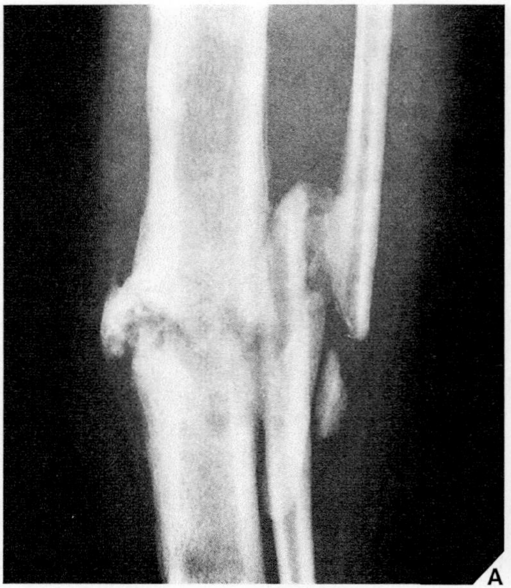
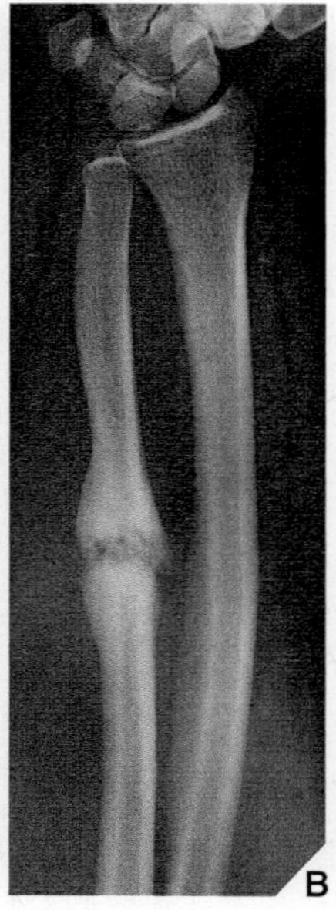

FIGURE 4.72 Reactive nonunion. **(A)** In hypertrophic nonunion, seen here in the shafts of the tibia and fibula, there is flaring of the bone ends, marked sclerosis, and periosteal response, but no evidence of endosteal callus formation. The gap between the bone fragments persists. **(B)** Similar hypertrophic nonunion is present in the shaft of the ulna.

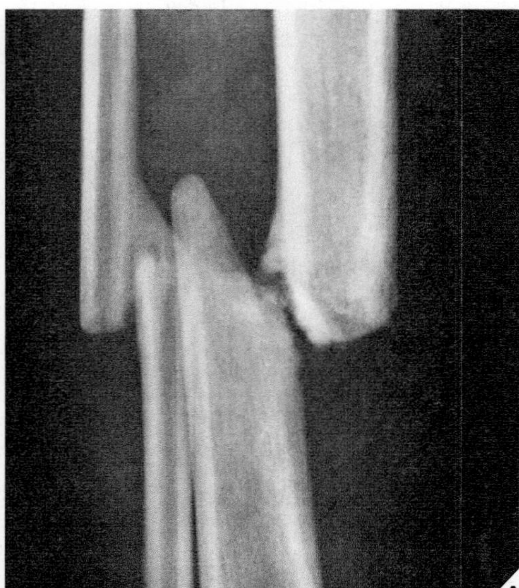
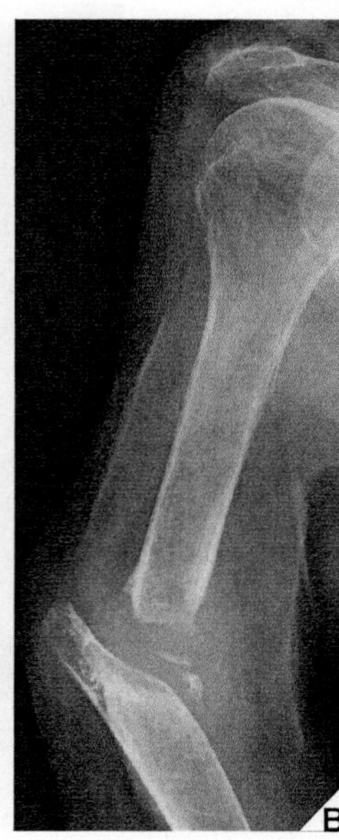

FIGURE 4.73 Nonreactive nonunion. **(A)** In atrophic nonunion, seen here at the junction of the middle and distal thirds of the tibia, there is a gap between the fragments, rounding of the edges, and an almost complete lack of bone reaction. Note the malunited fracture of the fibula. **(B)** Atrophic nonunion of the fracture of the right humerus.

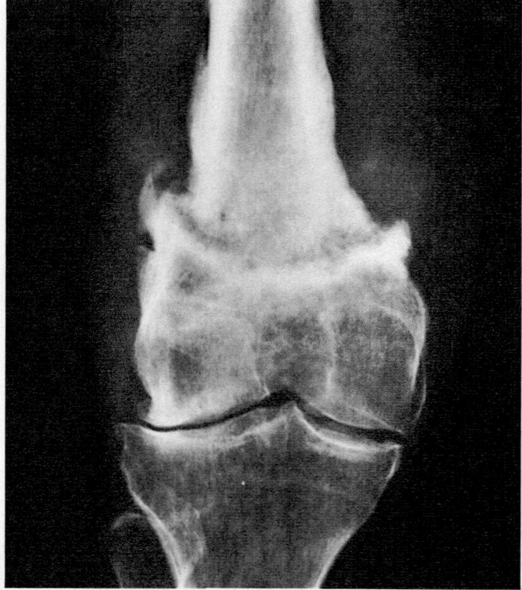
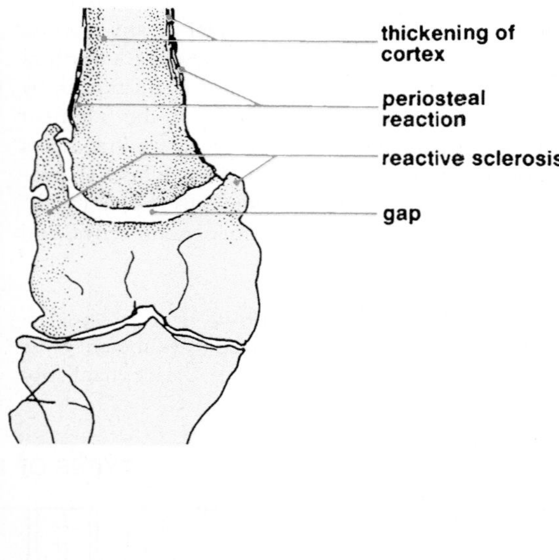

FIGURE 4.74 Infected nonunion. Nonunion of the fractured distal shaft of the femur with evidence of old, inactive osteomyelitis shows irregular thickening of the cortex, reactive sclerosis of the medullary portion of the bone, and well-organized periosteal reaction.

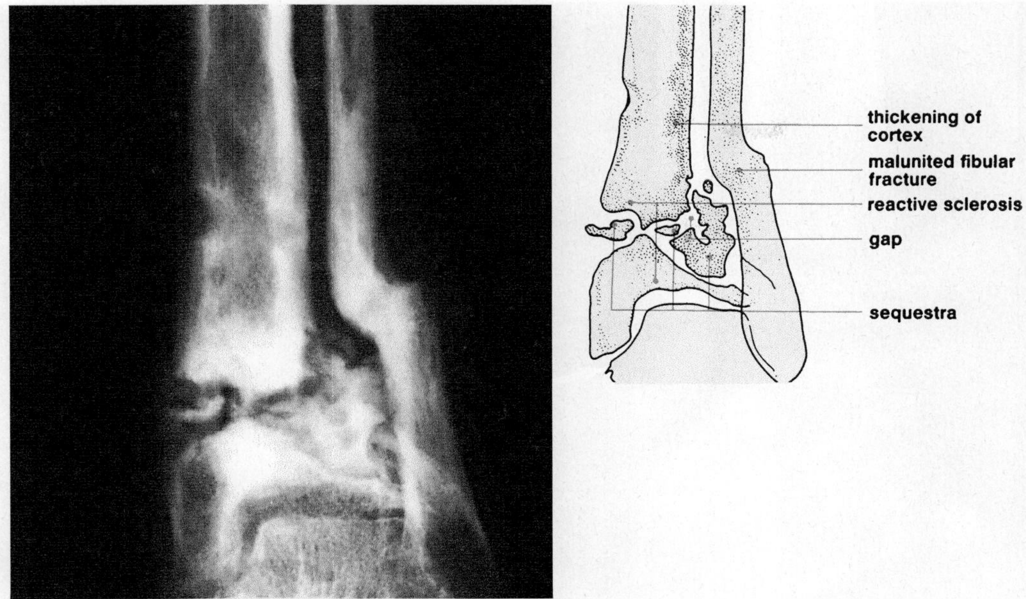

FIGURE 4.75 **Infected nonunion.** A radiograph of a nonunited fracture in the distal shaft of the tibia with associated active osteomyelitis shows thickening of the cortex, sclerosis of the cancellous bone, a gap between the bony fragments, and several sequestra.

destruction of the cortex and cancellous bone associated with periosteal new bone formation, and sequestration (Fig. 4.75). Treatment of infected nonunion depends on the stage of osteomyelitis. Decortication and bone grafting combined with compression plating are used if nonunion is accompanied by inactive osteomyelitis. Treatment of active osteomyelitis involves the application of antibiotics and sequestrectomy, usually followed by bone grafting and intramedullary stabilization. Different procedures are individually tailored, depending on the anatomic site and various general and local factors.

Other Complications of Fractures, Dislocations, and Traumatic Insults to the Bones and Soft Tissues

In addition to the possible complications associated with the process of fracture healing, the radiologist may encounter complications that are not related to that process. Radiographic evidence of the presence of such complications may not show up on immediate follow-up examination because they may occur weeks, months, or even years after the trauma and sometimes in a location distant from the original site of injury. Consequently, in dealing with patients presenting with a history of fracture or dislocation, radiologists should direct their investigation to areas where these associated complications may occur and should be aware of their radiologic characteristics and appearance.

Disuse Osteoporosis

Mild or moderate osteoporosis, which can be generally defined as a decrease in bone mass, frequently occurs after a fracture or dislocation as a result of disuse of the extremity caused by pain and immobilization in the plaster cast. Other terms often used to describe this condition are *demineralization, deossification, bone atrophy*, and *osteopenia*. The latter term is generally accepted as the best description of the nature of this complication. Radiographically, it is identified by radiolucent areas of decreased bone density secondary to thinning of the cortex and atrophy of the bone trabeculae. It may accompany united as well as nonunited fractures (Fig. 4.76).

Reflex Sympathetic Dystrophy Syndrome

Known also as *posttraumatic painful osteoporosis*, *complex regional pain syndrome* (CRPS), or *Sudeck atrophy*, reflex sympathetic dystrophy syndrome (RSDS), a severe form of osteoporosis, may occur subsequent to a fracture or even a milder form of injury. It has also been reported as resulting from neurologic or vascular abnormalities unrelated to trauma. Clinically, the patient presents with a painful, tender extremity with hyperesthesia, diffuse soft-tissue swelling, joint stiffness, vasomotor instability, and dystrophic skin changes. Three stages have been identified. The initial (or acute) inflammatory stage lasts from 1 to 7 weeks and is characterized by diffuse regional pain, inflammation, edema, and hypothermia or hyperthermia. In the second (or dystrophic) stage, which lasts from 3 to 24 months, the clinical findings include pain on exercise, increased sensitivity of the skin to pressure and temperature changes, and skin and muscle atrophy. In the final (or atrophic) stage, irreversible scleroderma-like skin changes and aponeurotic and tendinous retraction may occur. On the radiograph, RSDS is characterized by soft-tissue swelling and severe, patchy osteoporosis that progresses rapidly (Fig. 4.77). Three-phase technetium bone scan characteristically shows increased blood flow, blood pool, and periarticular increased uptake in the affected areas. These findings are seen in approximately 60% of affected patients.

Volkmann Ischemic Contracture

Developing usually after supracondylar fracture of the humerus, Volkmann contracture is caused by ischemia of the muscles followed by fibrosis. Clinically, it is characterized as the "five Ps" syndrome—pulselessness, pain, pallor, paresthesia, and paralysis. Radiographic examination usually reveals flexion–contracture in the wrist and in the interphalangeal joints of the fingers and hyperextension (or, rarely, flexion) of the metacarpophalangeal joints associated with soft-tissue atrophy (Fig. 4.78).

Posttraumatic Myositis Ossificans

Occasionally after a fracture, dislocation, or even minor trauma to the soft tissues, an enlarging, painful mass develops at the site of injury. Clinically, pain and swelling at this site persist for many days. The pain tends to become more localized and may increase in intensity for up to 4 to 6 weeks. The characteristic feature of this lesion includes the clearly recognizable pattern of its evolution, which correlates well with the lapse of time after the trauma. Thus, by the third or fourth week, calcifications and ossifications in the mass begin to develop (Fig. 4.79A,B), and by the sixth to eighth week, the periphery of the mass shows definite, well-organized cortical bone (Fig. 4.79C,D). The important radiographic hallmark of this complication is the presence of the so-called *zonal phenomenon*. On the radiograph, this phenomenon is characterized by a radiolucent area in the center of the lesion, indicating the formation of an immature bone, and by a dense zone of mature ossification at the periphery (myositis ossificans circumscripta). In addition, a thin radiolucent cleft separates the ossific mass from the adjacent cortex (Fig. 4.80). These important features help differentiate this condition from juxtacortical osteosarcoma, which may, at times, appear very similar. It must be stressed, however, that occasionally,

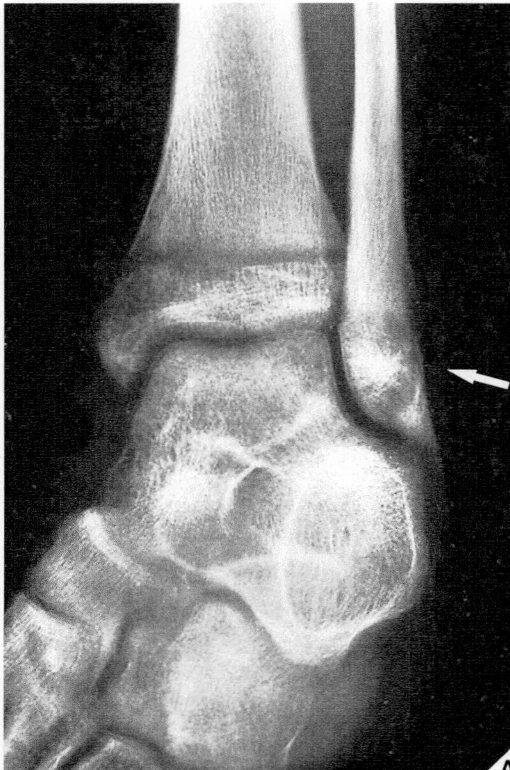

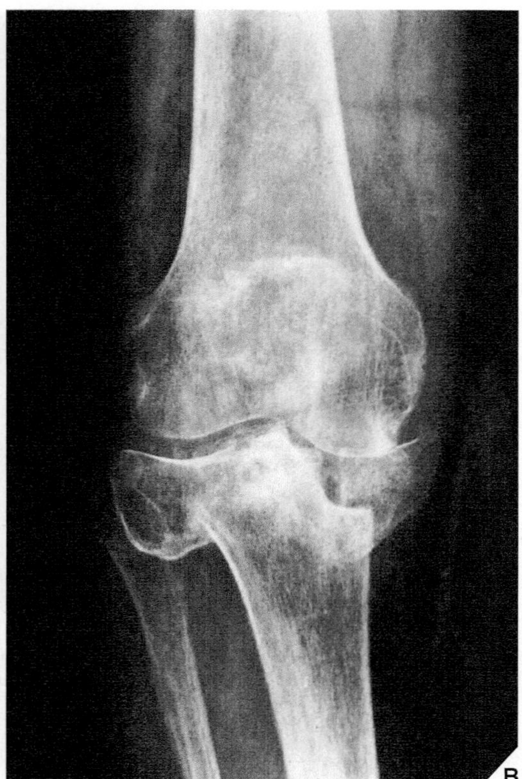

FIGURE 4.76 Disuse osteoporosis. **(A)** An oblique radiograph of the ankle shows a completely united fracture of the distal fibula *(arrow)*. Disuse juxtaarticular osteoporosis is evident from the thinning of the cortices associated with decreased bone density. **(B)** Anteroposterior radiograph of the knee shows a nonunited fracture of the tibial plateau, with a moderate degree of disuse osteoporosis.

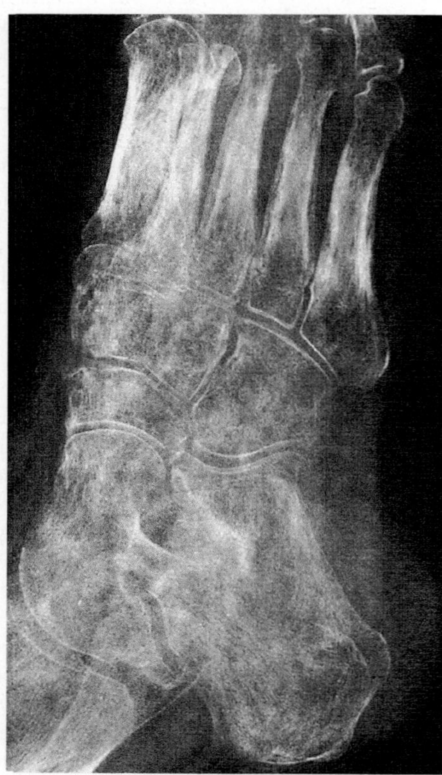

FIGURE 4.77 Sudeck atrophy. A 35-year-old man sustained fractures of the tibia and fibula, which eventually healed. Subsequently, however, he reported weakness, stiffness, and pain in his foot. Radiographic examination showed changes typical of RSDS in the foot: rapidly progressive, patchy osteoporosis associated with marked soft-tissue swelling.

the focus of myositis ossificans may adhere and fuse with the cortex, mimicking parosteal osteosarcoma on radiographs. In these cases, CT may provide additional information, such as the presence of the zonal phenomenon characteristic of myositis ossificans (Fig. 4.81).

The MRI appearance of myositis ossificans depends on the stage of maturation of the lesion. In the early stage, T1-weighted sequences usually show a mass that lacks definable borders with homogeneous intermediate signal intensity, slightly higher than that of adjacent muscle. T2-weighted images show the lesion to be of high signal intensity. After an intravenous injection of gadopentetate dimeglumine, T1-weighted images show a well-defined peripheral rim of contrast enhancement, but the center of the lesion does not enhance. The more mature lesions show intermediate signal intensity on T1-weighted sequences isointense with adjacent muscle, surrounded by a rim of low signal intensity, which corresponds to peripheral bone maturation. On T2 weighting, the lesion is generally of high signal intensity but may appear heterogenous. The rim of low signal is seen at the periphery (Fig. 4.82). Sometimes, the focus of myositis ossificans (whether immature or mature) may contain a fatty component, giving the lesion a high-intensity signal on T1-weighted images (Figs. 4.83 and 4.84).

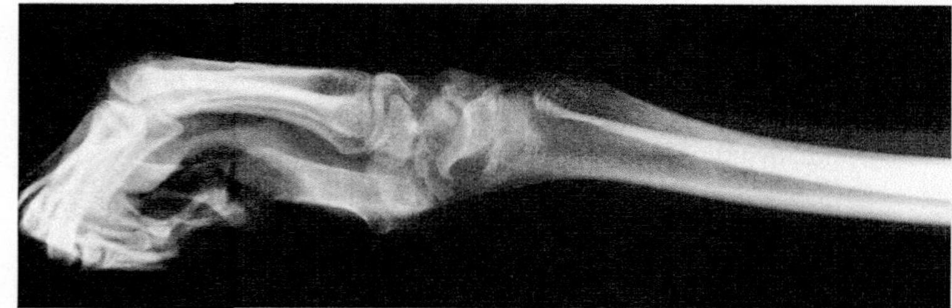

FIGURE 4.78 Volkmann contracture. Having sustained a supracondylar fracture of the humerus that united, a 23-year-old man presented with symptoms typical of Volkmann ischemic contracture. The lateral view of the distal forearm including the wrist and hand shows flexion–contracture in the metacarpophalangeal and the interphalangeal joints, together with a marked degree of soft-tissue atrophy.

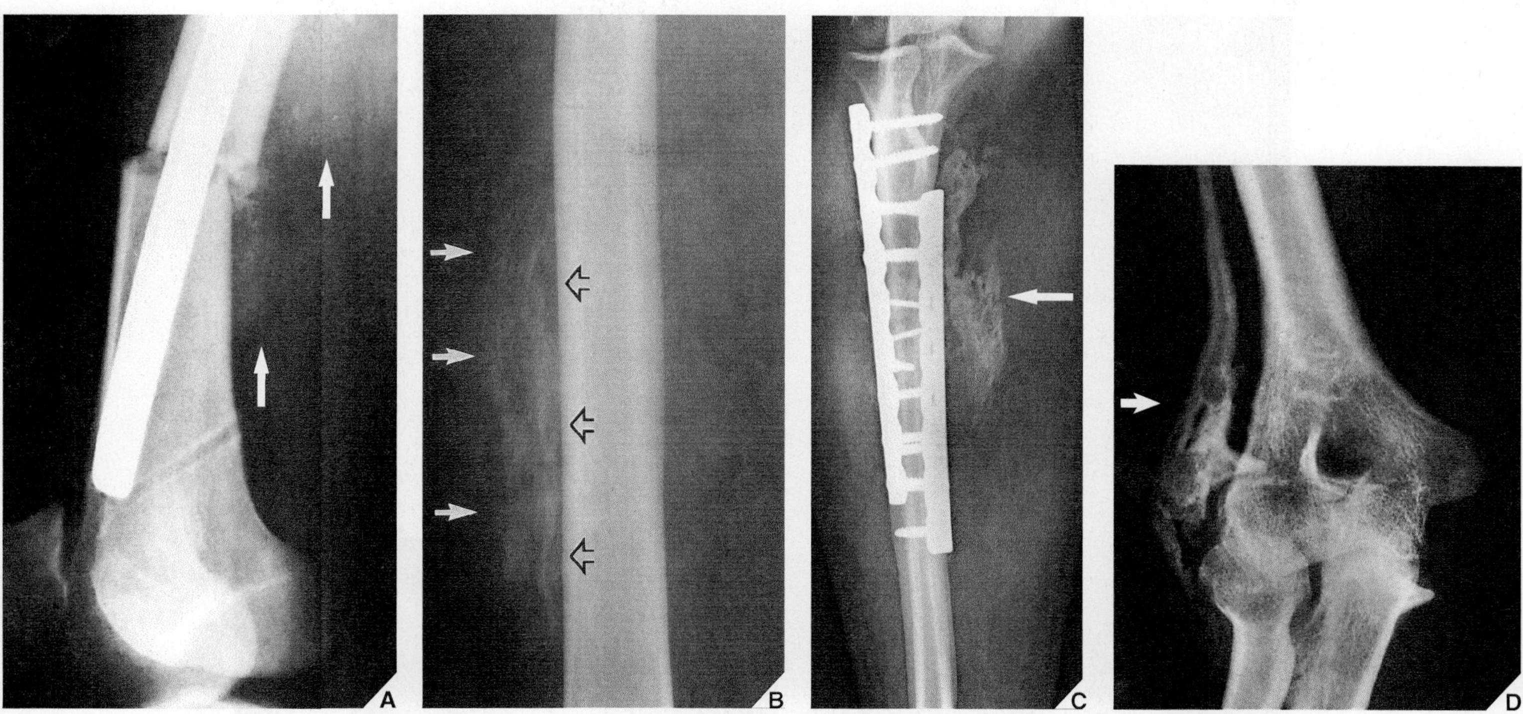

FIGURE 4.79 Posttraumatic myositis ossificans. (A) A 20-year-old man sustained a transverse fracture at the junction of the middle and distal thirds of the femur. The fracture was treated by open reduction and internal fixation with an intramedullary rod. On the lateral view, obtained 3.5 weeks after the injury, an immature focus of myositis ossificans with poorly defined densities in the soft-tissue mass is evident adjacent to the posterior cortex of the femur *(arrows)*. **(B)** Maturation of myositis ossificans in a 28-year-old woman who sustained an injury to the thigh 5 weeks before this radiograph was obtained. Note the formation of peripheral ossification *(arrows)* and the presence of a radiolucent cleft *(open arrows)*. **(C)** A mature focus of myositis ossificans *(arrow)* at the site of the fractures of the proximal radius and ulna, status post–open reduction and internal fixation in a 29-year-old woman. **(D)** This radiograph of a 27-year-old man who 1 year previously had sustained a fracture–dislocation in the elbow, which healed, shows a well-organized, mature focus of myositis ossificans circumscripta. Note the well-developed cortex at the periphery of the osseous mass *(arrow)* and the radiolucent gap separating the lesion from the cortex of the humerus.

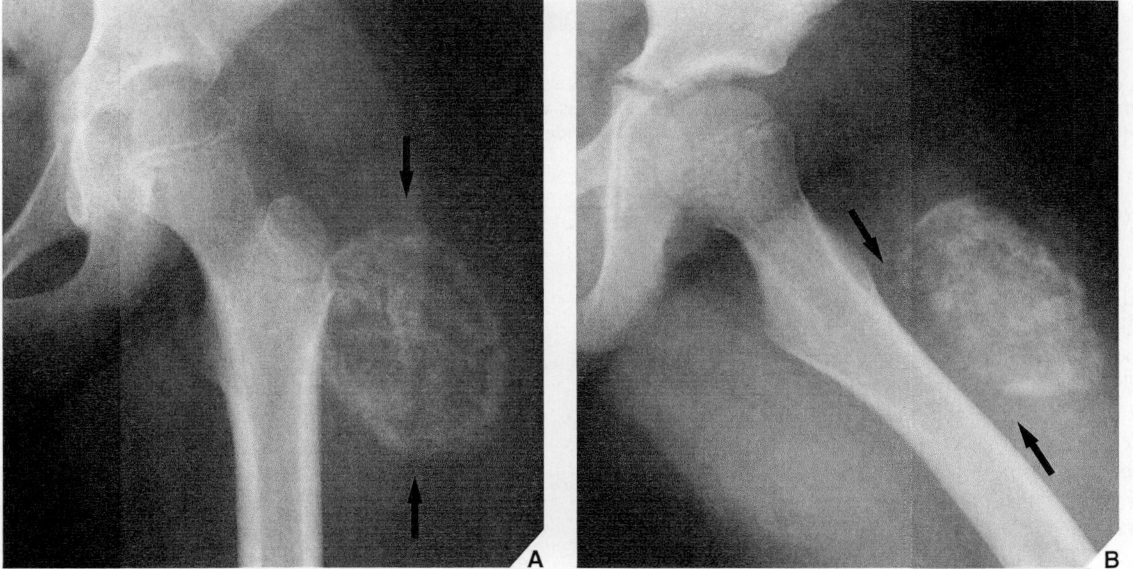

FIGURE 4.80 Posttraumatic myositis ossificans. A 7-year-old boy presented with a history of trauma 6 weeks before this radiographic examination. The anteroposterior radiograph of the left hip **(A)** demonstrates a lesion that exhibits features of zonal phenomenon characteristic of juxtacortical myositis ossificans *(arrows)*. On the frog-lateral projection **(B)**, note the cleft *(arrows)* separating the ossific mass from the posterolateral cortex.

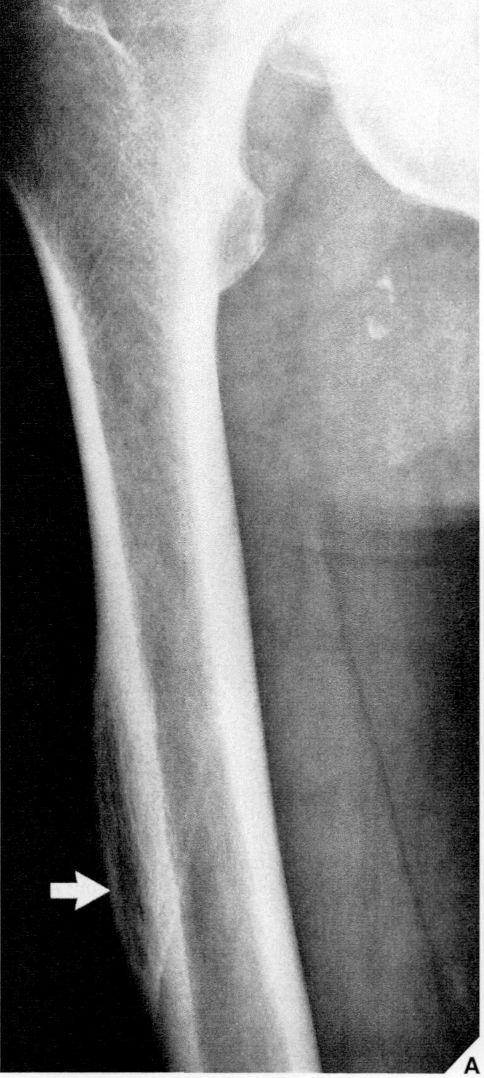

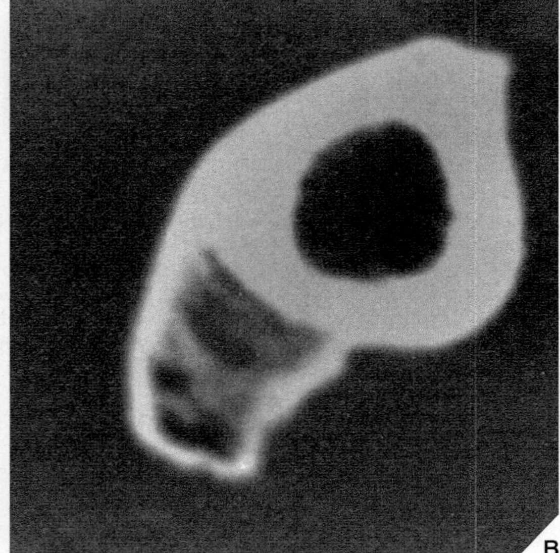

FIGURE 4.81 CT of posttraumatic myositis ossificans. A 52-year-old man sustained an injury to the lateral aspect of the left thigh 6 months previously. He was concerned about a hard mass he had palpated. **(A)** The radiograph shows an ossific mass adherent to the lateral cortex of the left femur *(arrow)*. **(B)** CT scan demonstrates the classic zonal phenomenon of myositis ossificans. Note the radiolucent center surrounded by mature cortex.

The histopathologic features are pathognomonic and consist of the least mature tissue in the center of the lesion and more mature at the periphery, corresponding to the radiographic zonal phenomenon. In the central portion of the lesion noted is increased cellularity and the presence of immature fibroblastic cells, whereas at the periphery, microtrabeculae with peripheral appositional osteoblasts are present (Fig. 4.85). Biopsy of the lesion in the early stage may lead to erroneous diagnosis of malignancy.

The treatment of myositis ossificans varies with each case. In most cases, so-called *wait and watch approach* is advisable because the lesion may shrink in time and become asymptomatic. Complete surgical excision may be performed after full maturation of the lesion. Nonsurgical treatment with shock waves has been occasionally tried.

Osteonecrosis (Ischemic or Avascular Necrosis)

Osteonecrosis, the cellular death of bone tissue, occurs after a fracture or dislocation when the bone is deprived of a sufficient supply of arterial blood, and delivery of oxygen is disrupted. However, it is important to recognize that this condition may also develop as a result of factors unrelated to mechanical trauma. Regardless of cause, the pathomechanism of osteonecrosis includes intraluminal vascular obstruction, vascular compression, or disruption of a blood vessel. Among the reported causes of osteonecrosis (other than a fracture or dislocation) are the following:

1. *Embolization of arteries*. This may occur in a variety of conditions. It is seen, for example, in certain hemoglobinopathies, such as sickle cell disease, in which arteries are occluded by abnormal red blood cells; in decompression states of dysbaric conditions, such as caisson disease, in which embolization by nitrogen bubbles occurs; or in chronic alcoholism and pancreatitis, when fat particles embolize arteries.
2. *Vasculitis*. Inflammation of the blood vessels may lead to interruption of the supply of arterial blood to the bone, as seen in collagen disorders such as systemic lupus erythematosus (SLE).
3. *Abnormal accumulation of cells*. In Gaucher disease, which is characterized by the abnormal accumulation of lipid-containing histiocytes in the bone marrow, or after steroid therapy, which can lead to an increase of fat cells, sinusoidal blood flow may be compromised, resulting in a deprivation of blood supply to the bone.
4. *Elevated intraosseous pressure*. This theory, championed by Hungerford and Lennox, suggests that any physiologic or pathologic process that results in increased pressure within the femoral head (which is essentially a sphere of cancellous bone, marrow, and fat surrounded by a cortical shell) may compromise the blood flow and lead to osteonecrosis.
5. *Inhibition of angiogenesis*. Osteonecrosis may result from compromise of normal angiogenesis that occurs consistently in bone tissue. This new hypothesis was introduced by Smith. It is supported by the fact that a number of drugs and mediators, including glucocorticoids, interferons, and other endogenously produced cytokines, inhibit angiogenesis. A similar effect was observed in the angiographic studies of the femoral head after the administration of steroids.

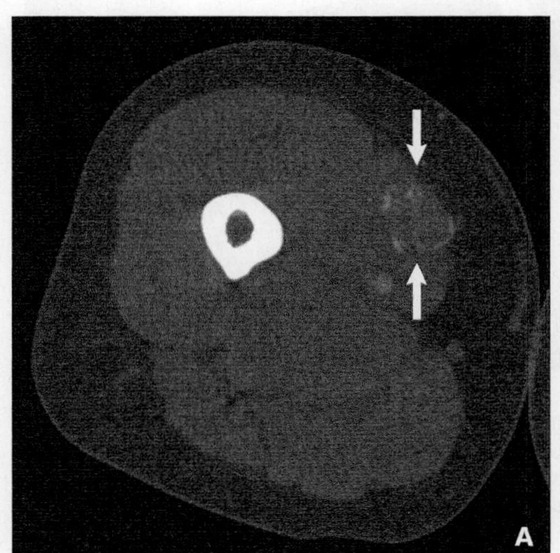

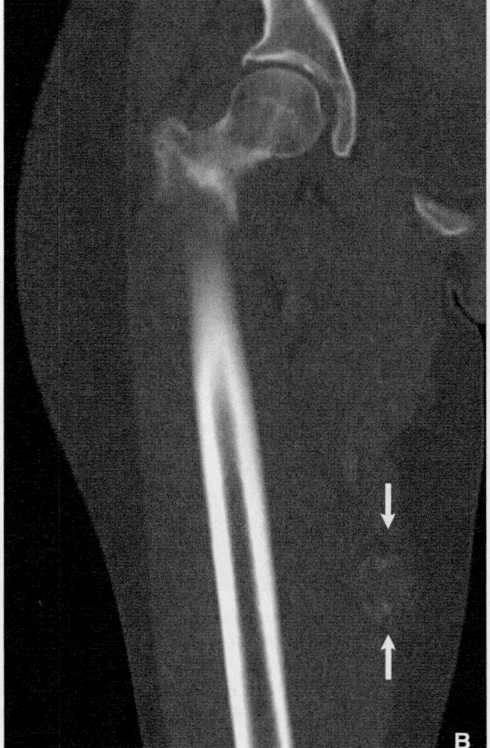

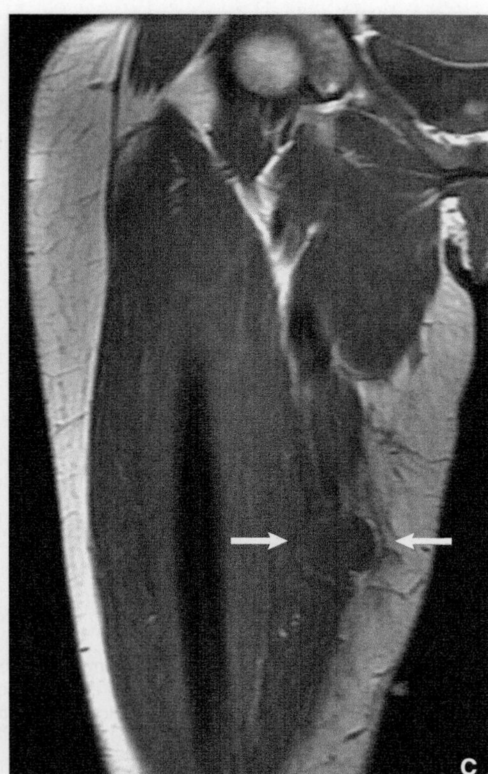

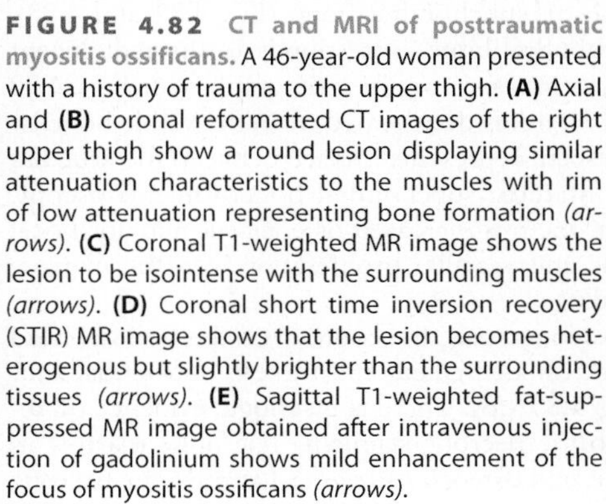

FIGURE 4.82 **CT and MRI of posttraumatic myositis ossificans.** A 46-year-old woman presented with a history of trauma to the upper thigh. **(A)** Axial and **(B)** coronal reformatted CT images of the right upper thigh show a round lesion displaying similar attenuation characteristics to the muscles with rim of low attenuation representing bone formation *(arrows)*. **(C)** Coronal T1-weighted MR image shows the lesion to be isointense with the surrounding muscles *(arrows)*. **(D)** Coronal short time inversion recovery (STIR) MR image shows that the lesion becomes heterogenous but slightly brighter than the surrounding tissues *(arrows)*. **(E)** Sagittal T1-weighted fat-suppressed MR image obtained after intravenous injection of gadolinium shows mild enhancement of the focus of myositis ossificans *(arrows)*.

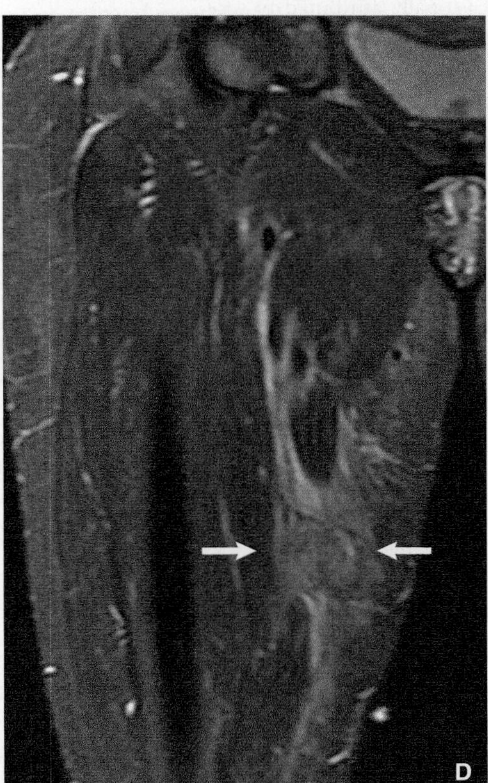

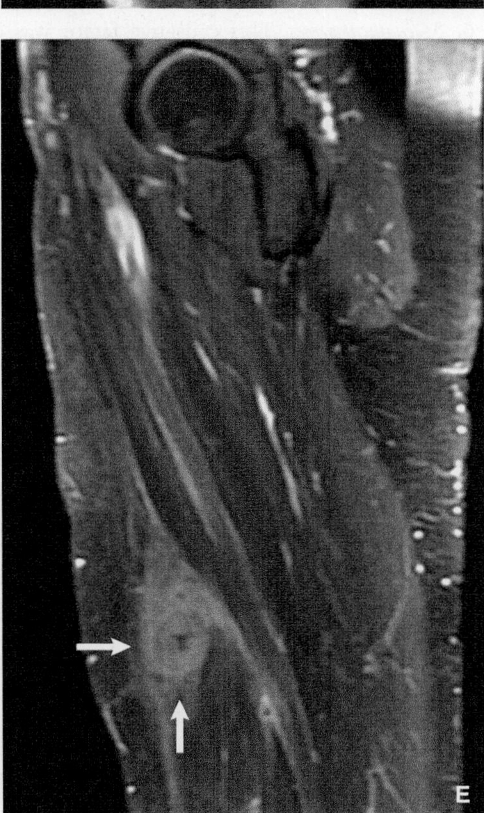

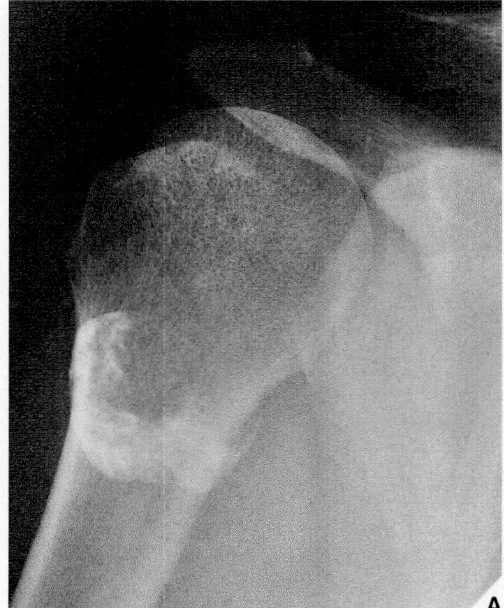

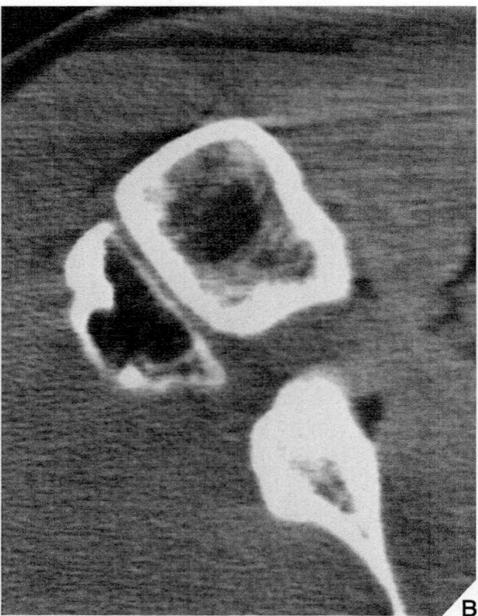

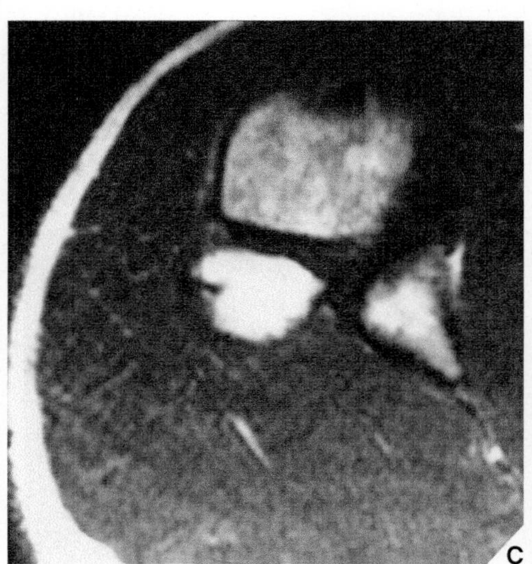

FIGURE 4.83 CT and MRI of posttraumatic myositis ossificans. A 41-year-old man presented with a palpable mass over the posterolateral aspect of the proximal right humerus. **(A)** Conventional anteroposterior radiograph of the right shoulder shows calcifications and ossifications overlaying the proximal humerus. **(B)** CT section demonstrates the zoning phenomenon typical of myositis ossificans. The center of the lesion shows a low-attenuation area caused by fatty changes. The cleft separates the mass from the cortex. **(C)** Axial T1-weighted (SE; TR 600/TE 20 msec) MRI shows the center of the lesion to be of high signal intensity, whereas the periphery exhibits low-to-intermediate signal.

6. *Mechanical stress.* This causative factor was occasionally attributed to nontraumatic osteonecrosis of the femoral head. The weight-bearing segment of the femoral head is the anterior–superior quadrant and, therefore, is under a large mechanical strain. Occlusion of the vessels in this region of the femoral head might be the result of cartilage breakdown secondary to excessive mechanical stress. Support for this hypothesis stems from experiments on rats by Iwasaki et al. and Suehiro et al.
7. *Radiation exposure.* Exposure to radiation may result in damage to the vascularity of a bone.
8. *Idiopathic.* Often, no definite cause can be established, as in the case of spontaneous osteonecrosis that predominantly affects the medial femoral condyle or in the case of certain osteochondroses such as Legg-Calvé-Perthes disease involving the femoral head or Freiberg disease affecting the head of the second metatarsal.

Diseases or conditions associated with or leading to osteonecrosis are listed in Table 4.4.

After trauma, osteonecrosis occurs most commonly in the femoral head, the carpal scaphoid, and the humeral head because of the precarious supply of blood to these bones. Less frequently osteonecrosis may affect femoral condyles, proximal tibia, talus, and vertebrae.

Osteonecrosis of the femoral head is a frequent complication after an intracapsular fracture of the femoral neck (60% to 75%), dislocation in the hip joint (25%), and slipped capital femoral epiphysis (15% to 40%). Pathologic findings of this process are very characteristic. In the early stage of osteonecrosis on the cut section of the gross specimen, the necrotic zone can be seen in subarticular location as wedge-shaped region in which bone marrow is dull-yellow, chalky, and opaque. This region is well demarcated and is separated from the surrounding unaffected bone marrow by a thin, red hyperemic border (Fig. 4.86A). At this stage, changes in the trabecular architecture are not appreciable (Fig. 4.86B). On microscopic examination, the subchondral bone is necrotic. The marrow elements are replaced by granular, eosinophilic material lacking cellular elements (Fig. 4.86C). In slightly more advanced stage of osteonecrosis, although the articular cartilage remains preserved and convex, the infarcted area becomes larger, and a small subchondral fracture may appear (Fig. 4.86D). Histopathologic examination shows necrotic bone trabeculae and necrotic bone marrow as well as the cysts of lipid material exhibiting extensive calcifications (Fig. 4.86E). The osteocytic lacunae in the bone may be empty, may contain cellular debris, or may have a pale-staining nucleus. In late stages of osteonecrosis, the gross pathologic specimen shows fracture and collapse of subchondral bone (Fig. 4.87 and 4.88). The linear fracture in subchondral bone corresponds to the radiolucent zone, referred to as the *crescent sign*, seen on the radiographs (see Figs. 4.90 and 4.91). The subchondral infarct is demarcated from the viable bone by zone of hyperemia. The crescent represents a space between the articular cartilage and the adjacent infarcted subchondral bone. On microscopy, at the margin of the infarct, there is increased osteoclastic activity. Focal fat necrosis and fibroblastic and vascular proliferation into the marrow spaces are the common findings.

With progression of osteonecrosis, the contour of the femoral head becomes flattened and markedly deformed, and there is substantial subchondral bone collapse (Fig. 4.89A,B). There is histologic evidence of repair in the bone adjacent to the necrotic segment. The bone marrow in this area becomes hyperemic, and osteoclasts begin to remove the necrotic bone at the interface between necrotic and viable bone. Accompanying this process of osteoclastic resorption is the deposition of new bone by osteoblasts on the surface of necrotic trabeculae. This process is known as "creeping substitution" (Fig. 4.89C, see also Fig. 4.89B). In addition, calcification of necrotic fat may be a prominent feature (Fig. 4.89C,D).

In its very early stages, radiographs may appear completely normal; however, radionuclide bone scan may show first decreased and later increased uptake of the radiopharmaceutical agent at the site of the lesion, which is a very valuable indication of abnormality. The earliest radiographic sign of this complication is the presence of a radiolucent crescent, which may be seen as early as 4 weeks after the initial injury. This phenomenon, as Norman and Bullough have pointed out, is secondary to the subchondral structural collapse of the necrotic segment and is visible as a narrow radiolucent line parallel to the articular surface of the bone. Radiographically, the sign is most easily demonstrated on the frog-lateral view of the hip (Figs. 4.90 and 4.91). Because the necrotic process most of the time does not affect the articular cartilage, the width of the joint space (i.e., the radiographic joint space: the width of the articular cartilage of adjoining bones plus the actual joint cavity) is preserved. Preservation of the joint space helps to differentiate this condition from osteoarthritis. In its later stage, osteonecrosis can be readily identified on the anteroposterior view of the hip by a flattening of the articular surface and the dense appearance of the femoral head (Figs. 4.92 and 4.93). The density is secondary to the compression of bony trabeculae after a microfracture of the nonviable bone, calcification of the detritic marrow, and repair of the necrotic area by the deposition of a new bone, the so-called *creeping substitution* (see text above). CT examination frequently helps to delineate the details of this condition (Figs. 4.94 and 4.95).

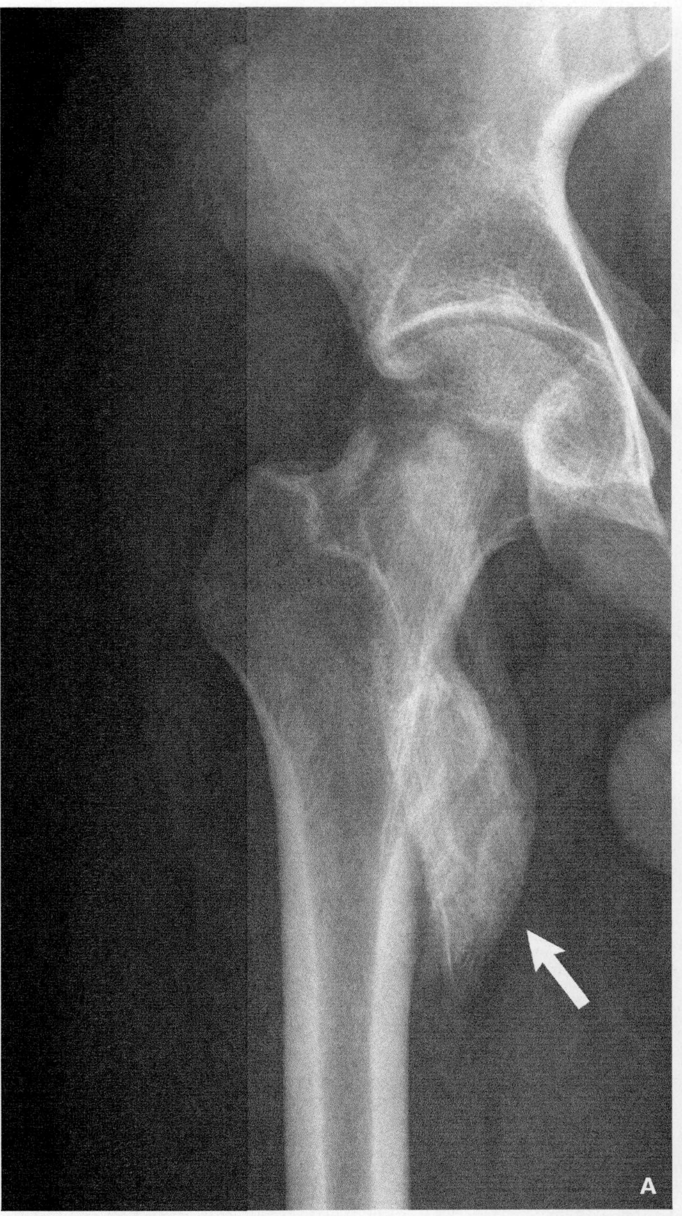

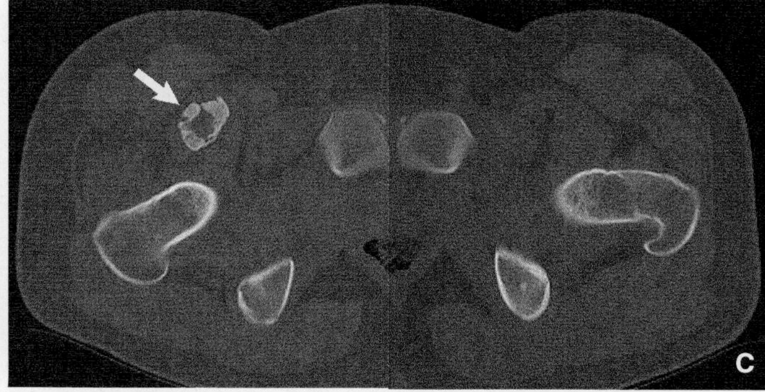

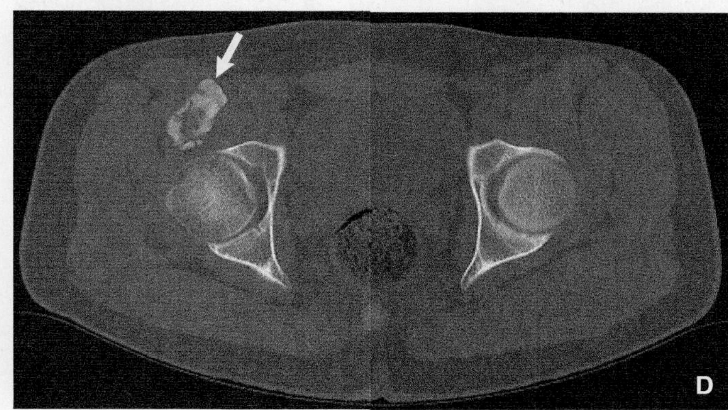

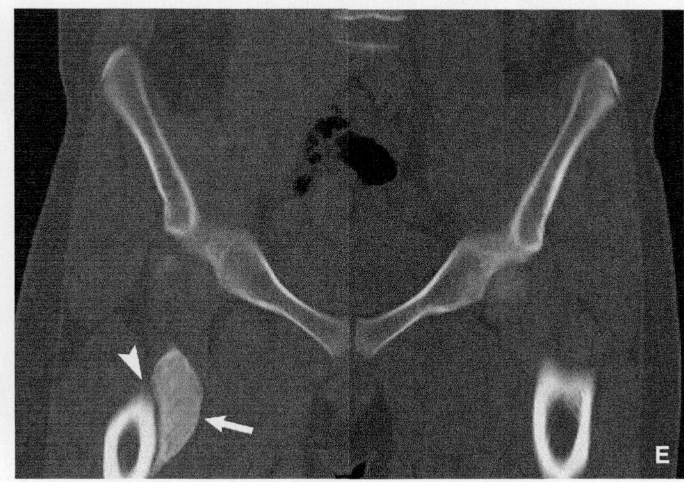

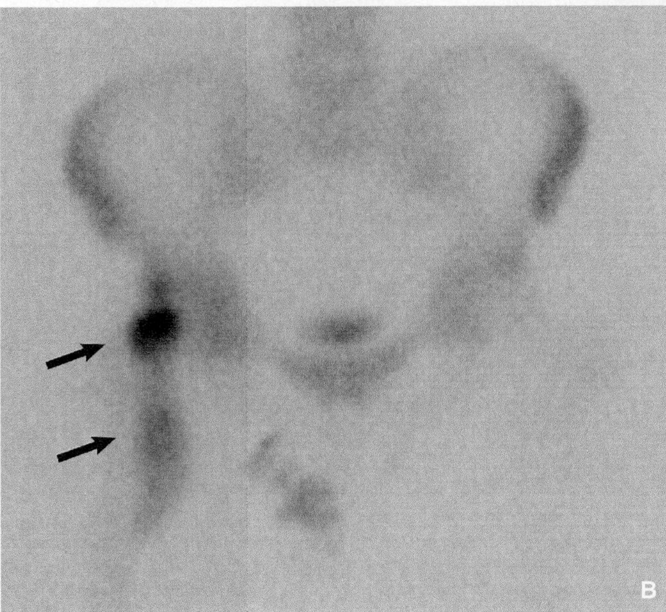

FIGURE 4.84 Scintigraphy, CT, 3D CT, SPECT/CT, and MRI of posttraumatic myositis ossificans. A 20-year-old man, who sustained trauma to the right upper thigh 6 months previously, presented with a hard mass in the soft tissues. **(A)** Anteroposterior radiograph of the right proximal femur shows an ossific mass adjacent to the medial femoral cortex *(arrow)*. **(B)** Delayed static image of the radionuclide bone scan shows accumulation of the radiopharmaceutical tracer in the region of the mass at the site of iliopsoas muscle *(arrows)*, with more increased uptake at the site of increased osteoblastic activity *(upper arrow)*. Axial CT images obtained at the level of greater trochanters **(C)** and hip joints **(D)** show the mass *(arrows)* displaying low-attenuation area in the center and high attenuation at the periphery, characteristic features of zonal phenomenon. **(E)** Coronal reformatted CT image shows the ossific mass *(arrow)* separated from the femoral cortex by a narrow cleft *(arrowhead)*, another characteristic feature of myositis ossificans. *(Continued)*

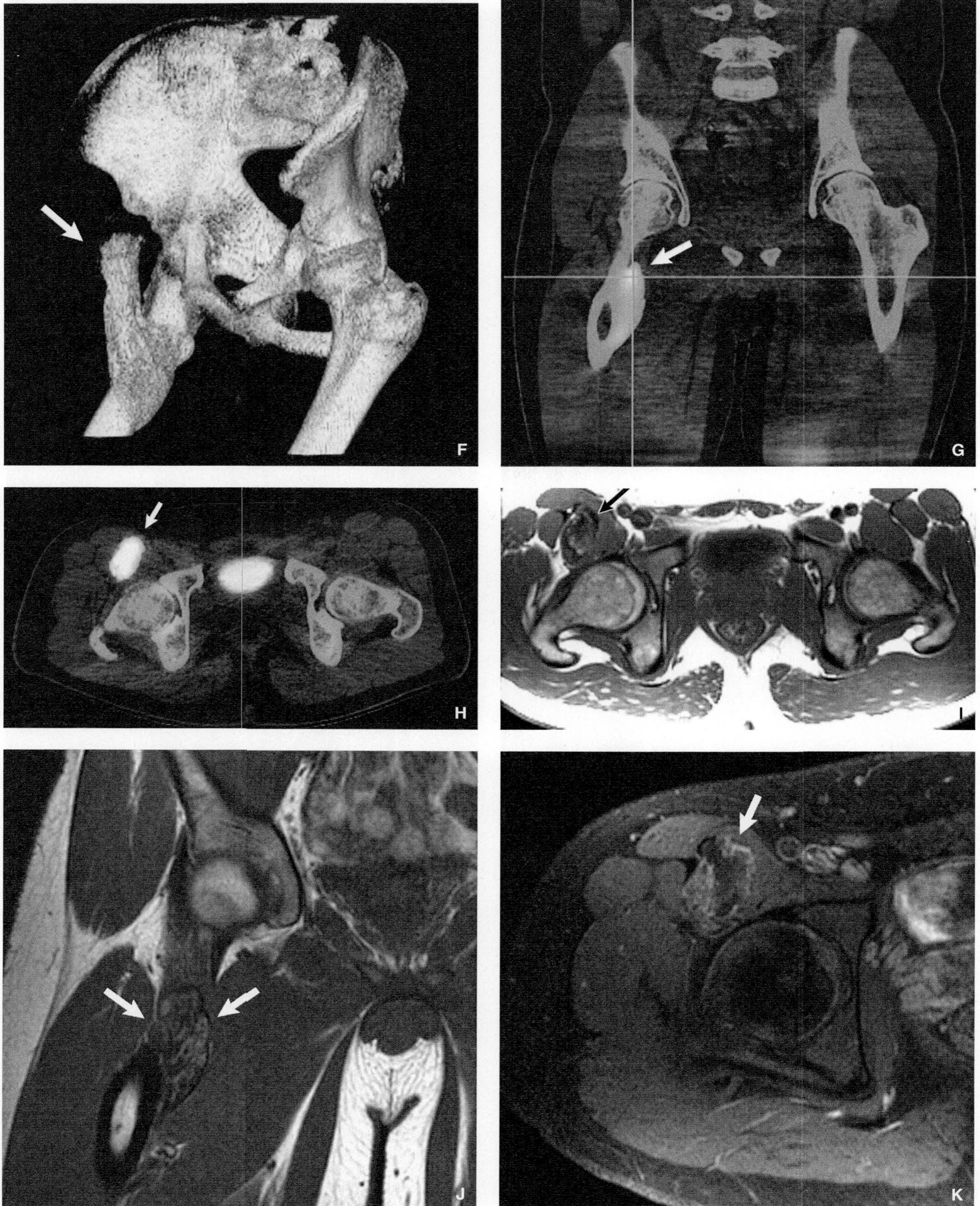

FIGURE 4.84 Scintigraphy, CT, 3D CT, SPECT/CT, and MRI of posttraumatic myositis ossificans. ***(Continued)*** **(F)** 3D CT image of the pelvis reconstructed in oblique projection shows ossific mass at the site of the right proximal femur *(arrow)*. SPECT/CT in coronal **(G)** and axial **(H)** planes show increased metabolic activity of the mass *(arrows)*. Axial **(I)** and coronal **(J)** T1-weighted MR images show the mass *(arrows)* displaying heterogeneous but predominantly low signal intensity. **(K)** Axial T1-weighted MR image obtained after intravenous administration of gadolinium shows mild peripheral enhancement of the mass *(arrow)*.

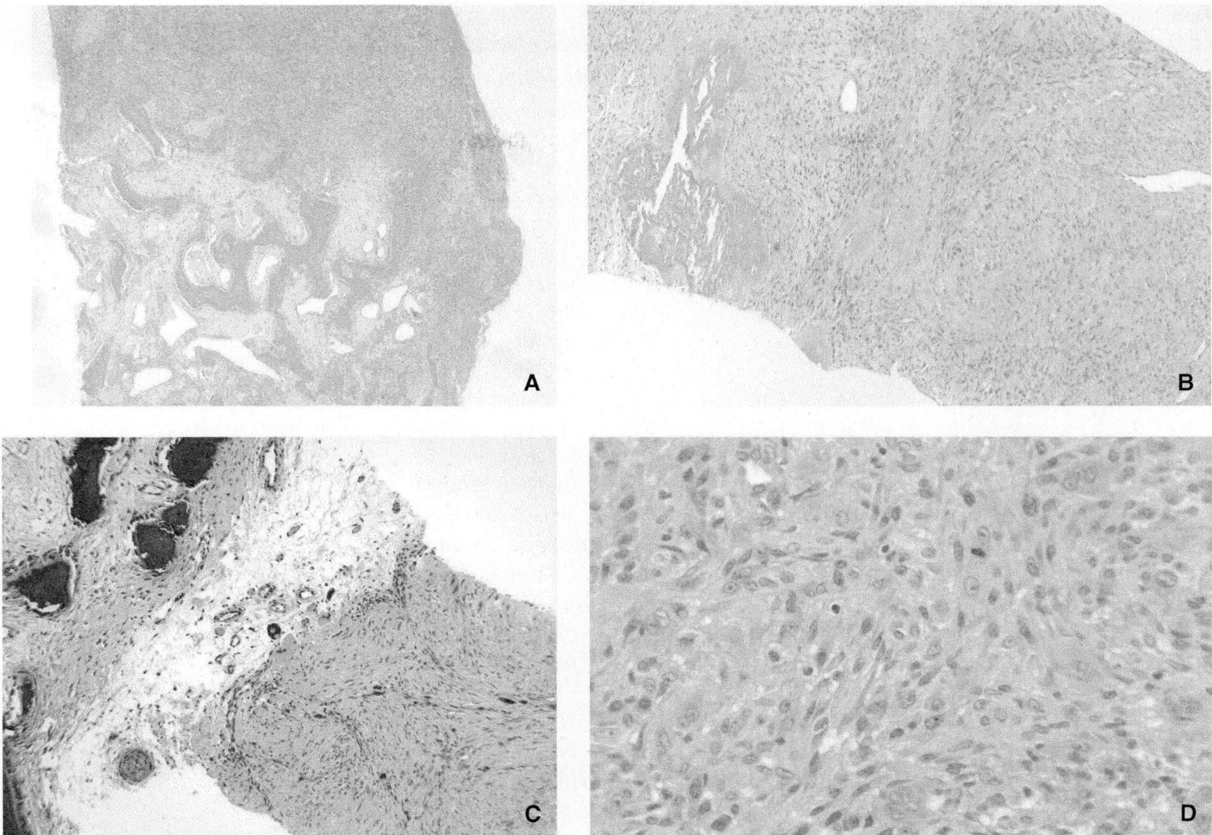

FIGURE 4.85 Histopathology of myositis ossificans. (A) Photomicrograph of the resected lesion shows the least mature portion, consisting of spindle cells *(top)*, whereas the most mature portion exhibits bone formation *(bottom)* (H&E, original magnification ×25). **(B)** Cellular area *(right)* shows separation of cells by osteoid matrix which becomes microtrabecular *(center)* and trabecular and osseous *(left)* (H&E, original magnification ×100). **(C)** At higher magnification observe central immature area with many spindle cells *(lower right)* and maturing trabecular bone at the periphery surrounded by active osteoblasts *(upper left)* (H&E, original magnification ×250). **(D)** The center of the lesion demonstrates a very cellular spindle-cell infiltrate in which mitotic activity can be identified (H&E, original magnification ×250). (Courtesy of Michael J. Klein, MD, New York.)

Ficat and Arlet proposed a classification system of osteonecrosis of the femoral head consisting of four stages, based on radiographic, hemodynamic, and symptomatic criteria (Table 4.5).

A significant breakthrough in identifying osteonecrosis in patients who had normal bone scan and normal conventional radiographs was achieved with MRI. Currently, this modality is considered the most sensitive and specific for the diagnosis and evaluation of osteonecrosis. Its characteristic MRI appearance consists of a serpentine band of low–signal intensity rim in the femoral head (Fig. 4.96A). This rim corresponds to the interface of repair between ischemic and normal bone consisting mainly of sclerosis and fibrosis. On T2-weighted images, a second inner rim of high signal has been observed (the double-line sign) (Fig. 4.96B). It is believed that this appearance represents fibrovascular tissue in the reparative zone. Many authors hypothesize that this finding is pathognomonic for osteonecrosis. Other authors have played down the importance of this finding, claiming that it may be largely artifactual, representing the so-called *chemical shift*. Bone marrow edema and joint effusion are frequently associated with osteonecrosis (Fig. 4.96C). Once the subchondral fracture occurs, the femoral head will collapse (Fig. 4.96D), and eventually, the hip joint will develop secondary osteoarthritis. Intravenous injection of gadolinium can help to delineate the extension of the osteonecrosis and determine if there are areas of residual viable tissue (Fig. 4.96E).

Several reports have established the diagnostic sensitivity of MRI in the early stages of osteonecrosis, when radiographic changes are not yet apparent or are nonspecific. MRI has been shown to have 97% sensitivity in differentiating osteonecrotic femoral head from normal femoral head and 85% sensitivity in differentiating osteonecrotic femoral head from other disorders of the femoral head, with an overall sensitivity of 91%. MRI appears to be a better predictive test for subsequent femoral head collapse than radionuclide bone scan. The narrow band-like area of low signal intensity that traverses the femoral head in midcoronal sections present on MRI was a significant indicator of subsequent collapses.

MRI is indispensable in the accurate staging of osteonecrosis because it reflects the size of the lesion and roughly the stage of the disease. Mitchell and colleagues have described a classification system of osteonecrosis based on alterations in the central region of magnetic resonance (MR) signal intensity in the osteonecrotic focus (Table 4.6). In early stages (class A or fat-like), there is preservation of a normal fat signal, except at the sclerotic reactive margin surrounding the lesion, that manifests as a central region of high signal intensity on short spin echo (SE) repetition time (TR)/echo time (TE) images (T1 weighted) and intermediate signal intensity on long TR/TE images (T2 weighted). Later, when there is sufficient inflammation or vascular engorgement, or if a subacute hemorrhage is present (class B or blood-like), a high signal intensity is noted on short and long TR/TE images. This signal is similar to that of a subacute hemorrhage. If there is enough inflammation, hyperemia, and fibrosis present to replace the fat content of the femoral head (class C or fluid-like), a low-intensity signal with short TR/TE and a high-intensity signal with long TR/TE are seen. Finally, in advanced stages, where fibrosis and sclerosis predominate (class D or fibrous-like), a low signal intensity is present on both short and long TR/TE images (see Table 4.6). It is of interest to mention here that in 2001 the Japanese Ministry of Health, Labor, and Welfare proposed revised criteria for the diagnosis and staging osteonecrosis of femoral head. Five diagnostic criteria that showed high specificity were selected for diagnosis: (a) collapse of the femoral head (including crescent sign) without joint space narrowing or acetabular abnormality as seen on radiography, (b) demarcating sclerosis of the femoral head without joint space narrowing or acetabular abnormality, (c) "cold in hot" areas on radionuclide bone scans, (d) a low-intensity band on T1-weighted MRI, and (e) histologic findings of trabecular and bone marrow necrosis. If a patient fulfills two of the five criteria, the diagnosis is established. MRI findings correlate well with histologic changes. The central region of high signal intensity corresponds to necrosis of the bone and marrow. The low signal of the peripheral band corresponds to the sclerotic margin of reactive tissue

TABLE 4.4 Diseases or Conditions Associated with or Leading to Osteonecrosis

Trauma	*Metabolic Conditions*
Fracture of femoral neck	Hypercortisolism
Dislocation of the femoral head	Corticosteroid medications
Proximal femoral epiphysiolysis	Cushing disease
Slipped capital femoral epiphysis	Gout and hyperuricemia
Epiphyseal compression	Hyperlipidemia
Fracture of proximal humerus (neck)	Hyperparathyroidism
Dislocation in shoulder joint	*Rheumatologic Conditions*
Fracture of talus	Rheumatoid arthritis
Fracture of scaphoid	Inflammatory bowel disease
Kienböck disease	Antiphospholipid antibody syndrome
Vascular injury	Systemic lupus erythematosus
Burns	Mixed connective tissue disease
Regional deep hyperthermia	Polymyositis
Radiation exposure	Giant cell arteritis
Hemoglobinopathies and Other Blood Disorders	Necrotizing arteritis
Sickle cell disease	*Dysbaric Disorders*
Hemophilia	Caisson disease
Hb S/C hemoglobinopathy	*Infectious and Inflammatory Conditions*
Hb S thalassemia	Osteomyelitis
Polycythemia	Pancreatitis
Acute lymphoblastic leukemia	Chronic liver disease
Congenital and Developmental Conditions	Thrombophlebitis
Congenital dysplasia of the hip	Acquired immunodeficiency syndrome
Ehlers-Danlos syndrome	Meningococcemia
Hereditary dysostosis	Severe acute respiratory syndrome
Legg-Calvé-Perthes disease	HIV
Local Infiltrative Lesions	*Miscellaneous Factors*
Gaucher disease	Alcohol consumption
Fabry disease	Cigarette smoking
Sarcoidosis	Chronic renal failure
Neoplastic conditions	Hemodialysis
Lymphoproliferative disorders	Bisphosphonate treatment
	Disseminated intravascular coagulation
	Organ transplantation
	Fat embolism
	Pregnancy
	Idiopathic

Hb, hemoglobin.

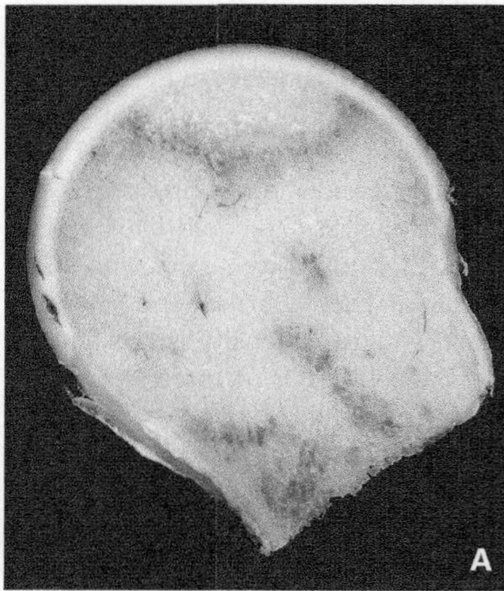

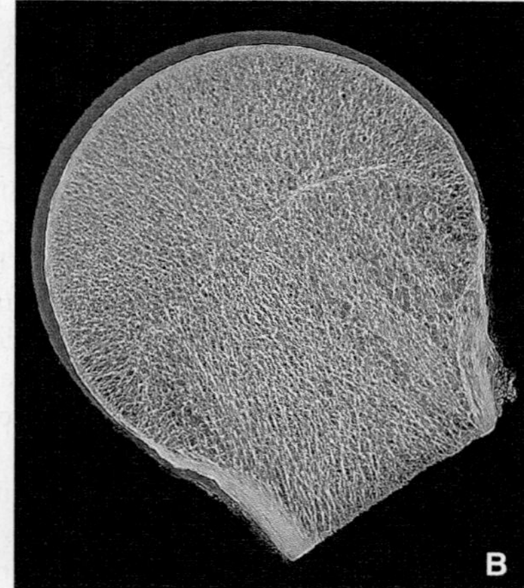

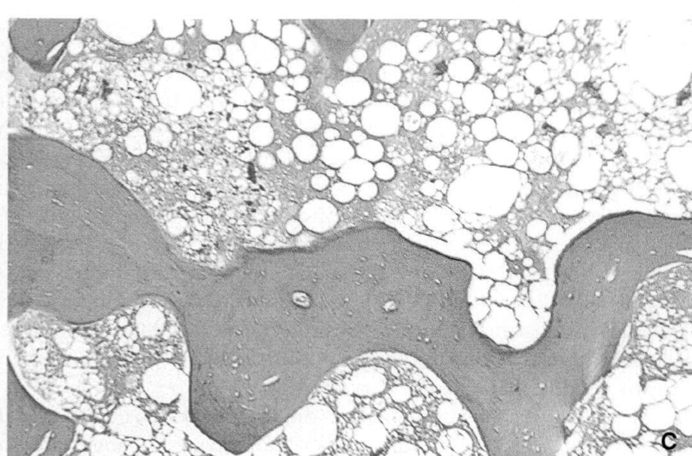

FIGURE 4.86 Pathology of osteonecrosis, early stage. (A) Photograph of a coronal section of the femoral head shows a well-demarcated wedge-shaped dull yellow necrotic region in subarticular location, separated from the normal bone marrow by a thin, red, hyperemic border. The articular cartilage is intact and convex. **(B)** Specimen radiograph shows no appreciable changes in the trabecular architecture. **(C)** Photomicrograph shows granular eosinophilic necrotic bone marrow lacking the cellular elements, with ghosts of disrupted fat cells (H&E, original magnification ×100). *(Continued)*

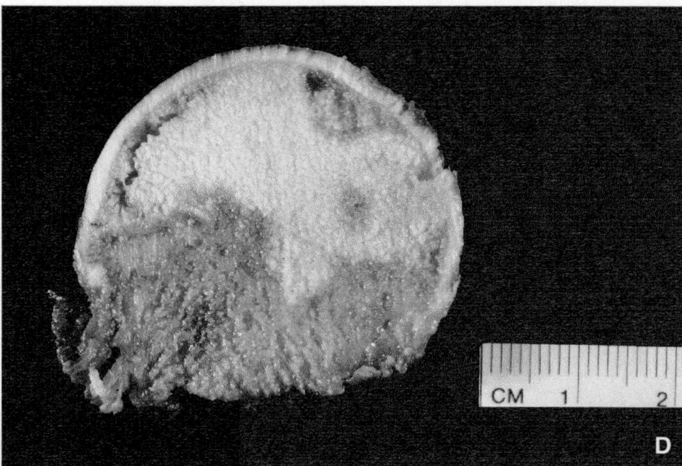

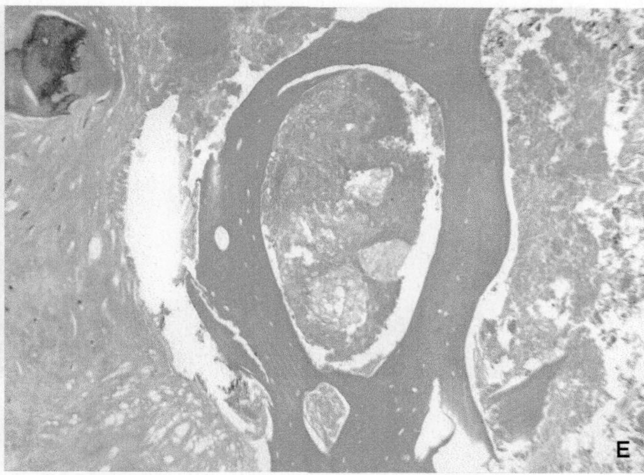

FIGURE 4.86 **Pathology of osteonecrosis, early stage.** ***(Continued)*** **(D)** In slightly more advanced stage of osteonecrosis, a photograph of coronal section of the femoral head specimen shows subchondral opaque-yellow area representing infarcted bone. The overlying articular cartilage is still preserved and convex, although there is subchondral fracture that separates the subarticular plate from the underlying necrotic bone (*upper left*). **(E)** Photomicrograph shows both the bone trabeculae and bone marrow being devoted of cellular elements. Observe saponified fat in the intertrabecular spaces with focal calcifications (H&E, original magnification ×100). (**A–C**, Reprinted from Bullough PG. *Orthopedic pathology*, 5th ed. Philadelphia: Elsevier; 2009, Figure 15.16 A, B, and C. Copyright © 2009 Elsevier. With permission; **D–E**, Courtesy of Michael J. Klein, MD, New York.)

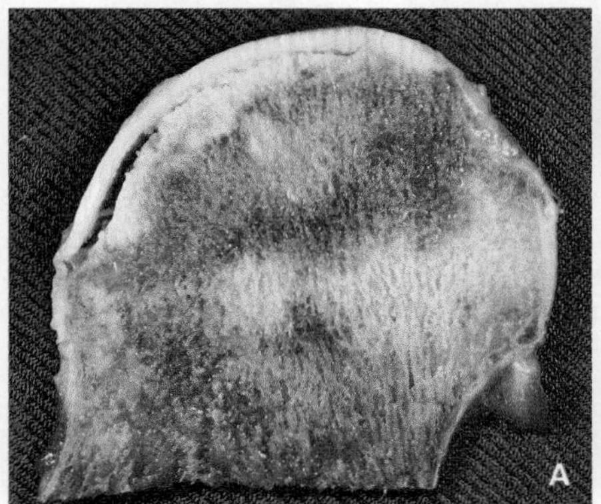

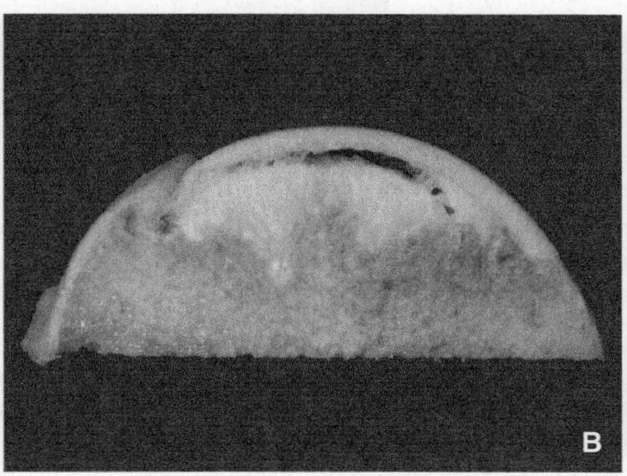

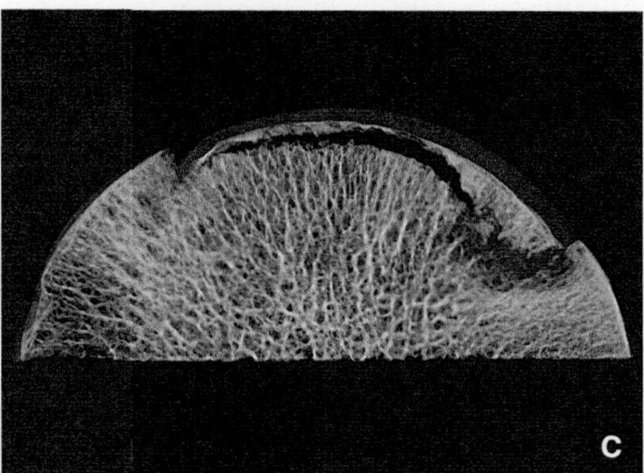

FIGURE 4.87 **Pathology of osteonecrosis, late stage.** **(A)** Photograph of a coronal section of the gross specimen of the resected femoral head shows the necrotic area confined to the superficial portion of the bone marrow with partially displaced fracture of the subarticular plate (*upper left*). Observe the second area of necrosis (*lower right*) separated from the subchondral fracture by red marrow. **(B)** A well-defined, wedge-shaped dull yellow area of infarction is present in subchondral area of the femoral head. The overlying articular cartilage and subchondral plate are separated from infarcted area by a fracture line. Observe focal area of folded cartilage (*upper left*) due to a localized collapse of the underlying bone. **(C)** The specimen radiograph demonstrates separation of the articular cartilage from the underlying bone by irregular fracture through the subarticular plate. There is no significant radiodensity of the necrotic area, probably because the underlying necrotic marrow fat has not yet saponified. (Courtesy of Michael J. Klein, MD, New York.)

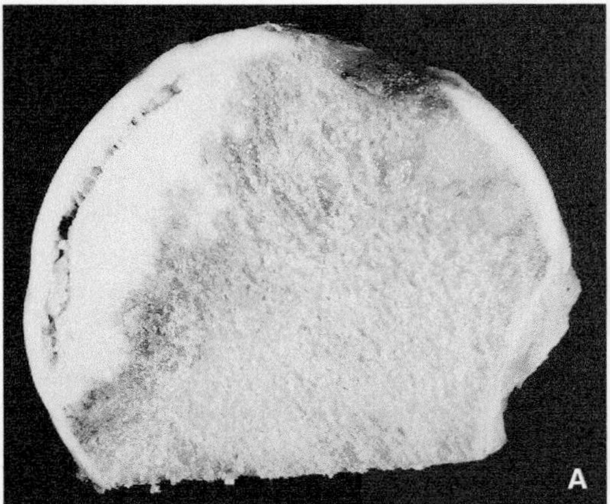

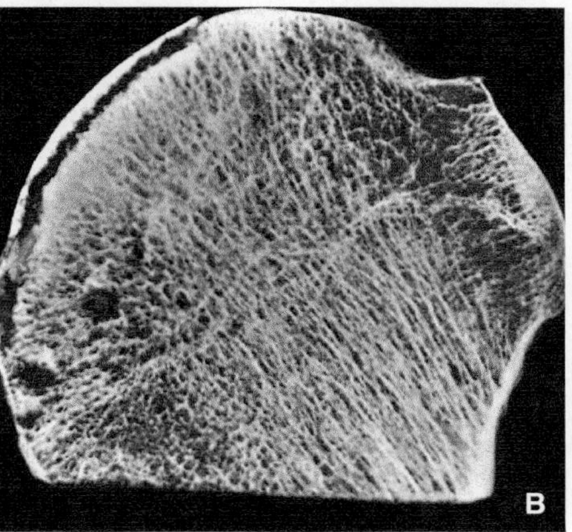

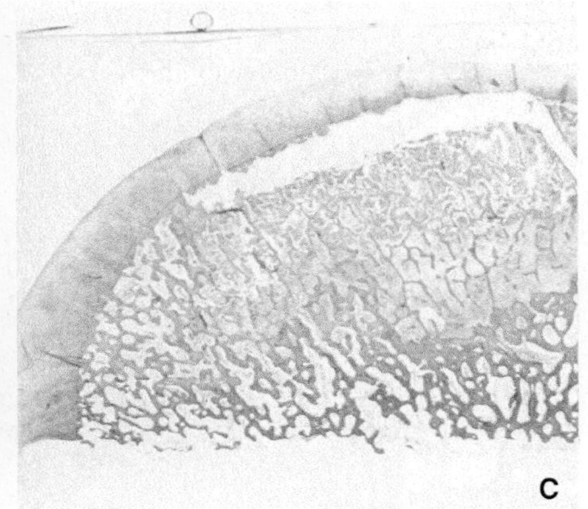

FIGURE 4.88 **Pathology of osteonecrosis, late stage.** **(A)** Photomicrograph of coronal section of the femoral head specimen shows the subchondral infarct *(yellow)* demarcated from the viable bone by a zone of hyperemia *(red)*. Note the crescent representing a fracture of subchondral bone. **(B)** Radiograph of the same specimen shows the crescent sign. **(C)** Photomicrograph of a histologic preparation of the femoral head shows space between the articular cartilage and subchondral bone. Observe the thickened trabeculae of the viable bone (H&E, ×1). (Reprinted with permission from Vigorita VJ. *Orthopaedic pathology*. Philadelphia: Wolters Kluwer Health; 2015.)

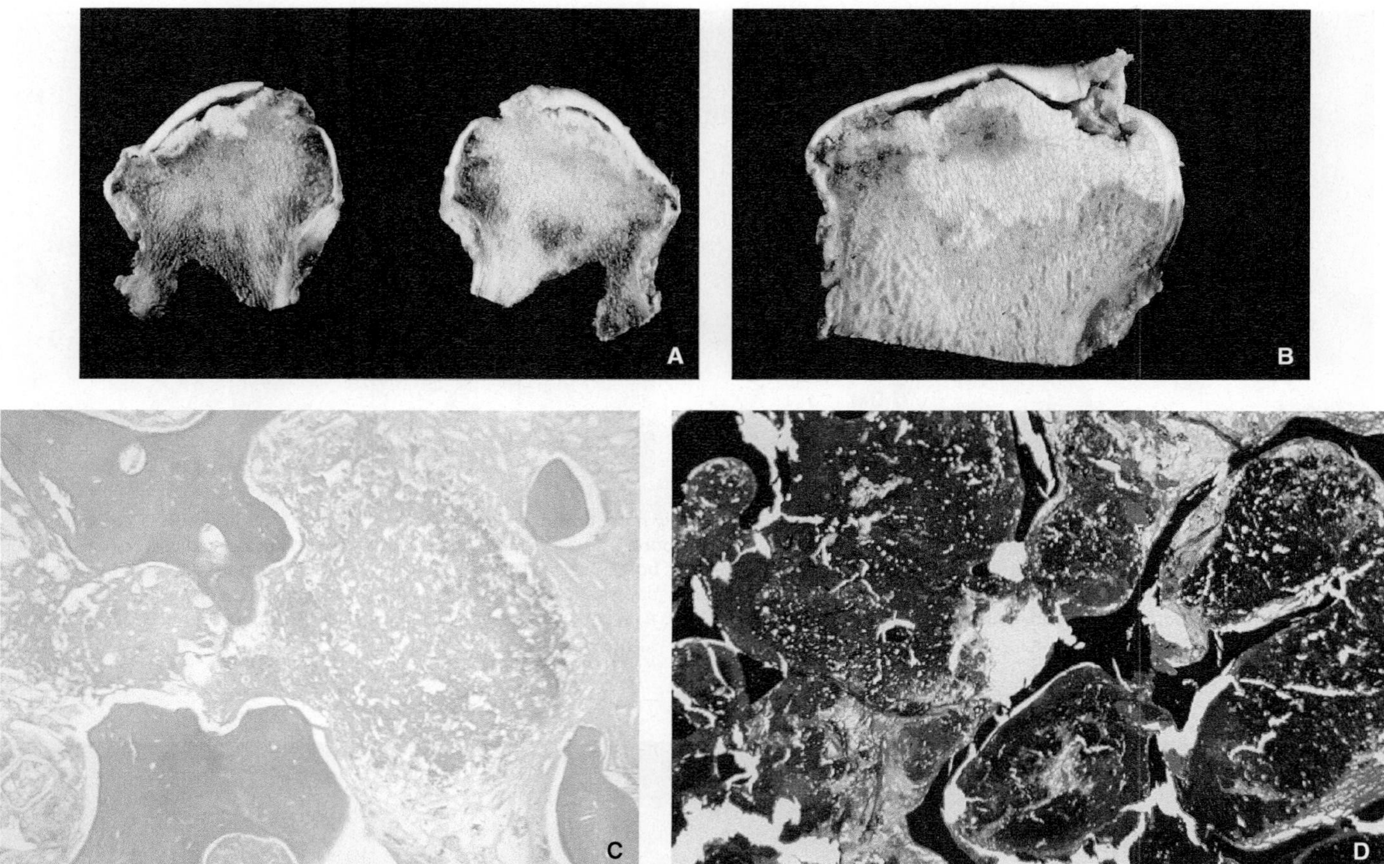

FIGURE 4.89 Pathology of osteonecrosis, late stage. **(A)** Photograph of bisected gross specimen of the femoral head shows marked flattening and deformity of the articular cartilage. Observe also subarticular fracture of the necrotic bone and subchondral collapse of the necrotic area. **(B)** In the femoral head resected from the different patient, the necrotic area comprises great portion of the bone covered by markedly deformed, flattened, and fractured articular cartilage. An area of cartilage repair is seen on the left side of the necrotic segment. In addition, on the right side observe a zone of osseous repair beneath the necrotic zone, known as a creeping substitution. Small marginal osteophytes indicate secondary osteoarthritis. **(C)** Photomicrograph shows necrotic trabeculae with empty osteocyte lacunae; a few arrest cement lines are present, indicating creeping substitution. The necrotic fat is replaced by grungy purple material representing calcium soaps (H&E, original magnification ×100). **(D)** An undecalcified section stained with the von Kossa method demonstrates marked dark staining of the intertrabecular spaces, indication of diffuse calcification of the fat released from broken down adipose tissue of the bone marrow (original magnification ×100). (Courtesy of Michael J. Klein, MD, New York.)

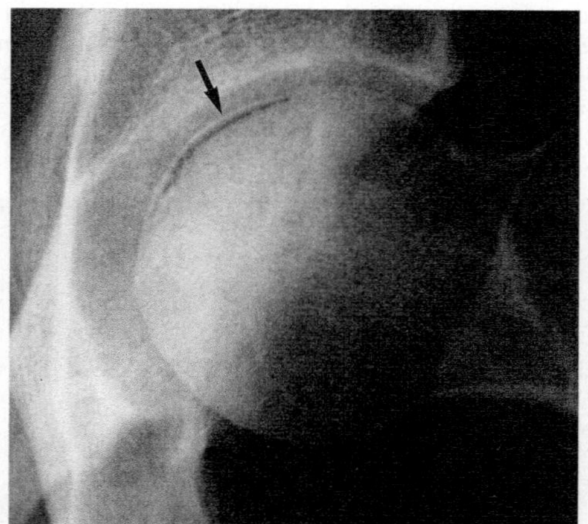

FIGURE 4.90 Osteonecrosis of the femoral head. The frog-lateral view of the left hip shows the crescent sign *(arrow)* in a 45-year-old woman who sustained a hip dislocation 5 weeks earlier.

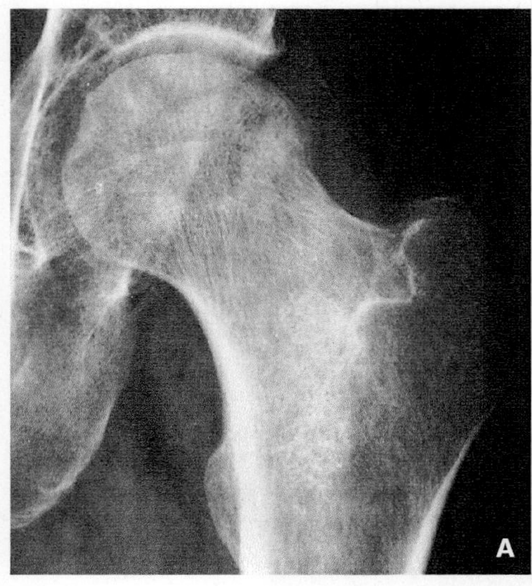
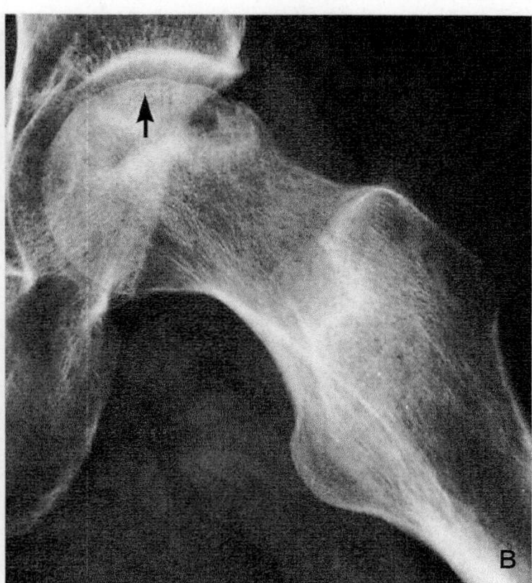

FIGURE 4.91 Osteonecrosis of the femoral head. **(A)** A 41-year-old man presented with a history of traumatic dislocation in the left hip joint. On frontal projection, the increased density of the femoral head suggests osteonecrosis, but a definite diagnosis cannot be made. **(B)** The frog-lateral view demonstrates a thin radiolucent line parallel to the articular surface of the femoral head *(arrow)*. This represents the crescent sign, a radiographic hallmark of osteonecrosis.

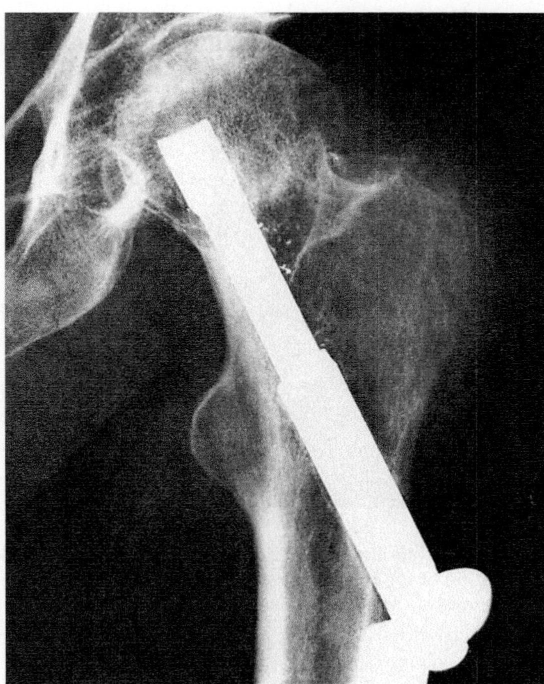

FIGURE 4.92 Osteonecrosis of the femoral head. A 56-year-old woman sustained an intracapsular fracture of the left femoral neck, which healed after surgical treatment by open reduction and internal fixation. The anteroposterior radiograph shows a Smith-Peterson nail inserted into the femoral neck and head. The fracture line is obliterated. The dense (sclerotic) appearance of the femoral head indicates the development of osteonecrosis.

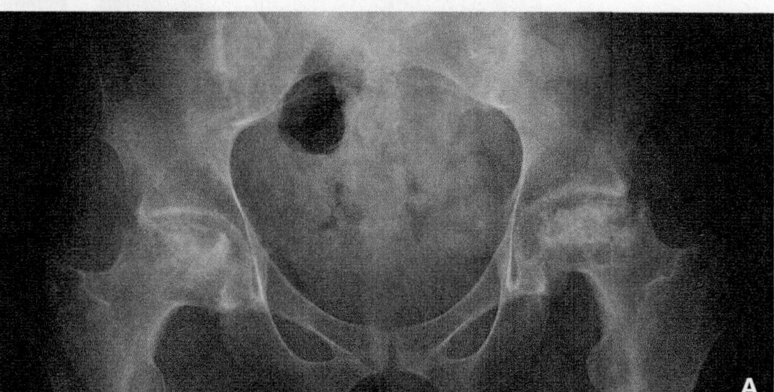
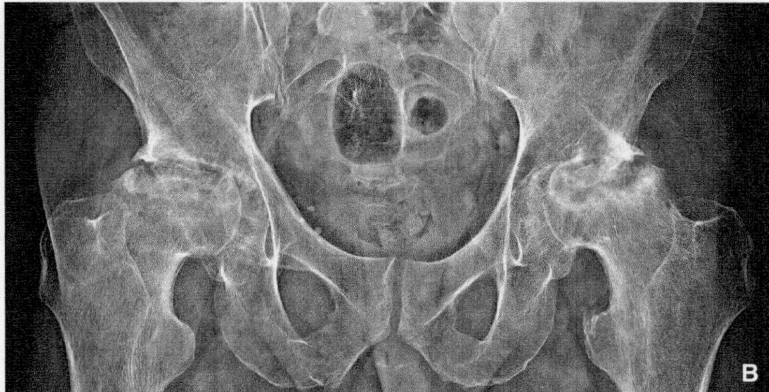

FIGURE 4.93 Osteonecrosis of both femoral heads. **(A)** Anteroposterior radiograph of the pelvis of a 40-year-old man with history of prior dislocation in both hip joints shows advanced stage of osteonecrosis of both femoral heads showing subchondral collapse. **(B)** Similar changes are seen affecting both femoral heads of a 50-year-old man.

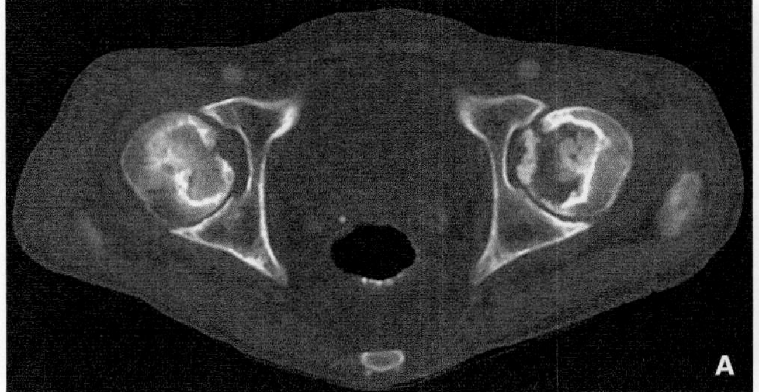
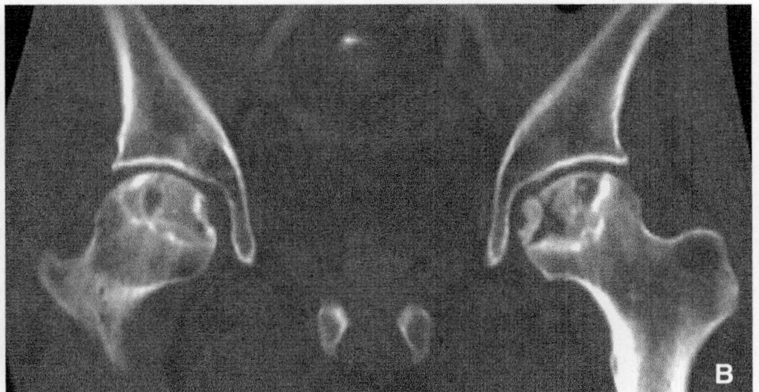

FIGURE 4.94 CT of osteonecrosis of the femoral head. **(A)** Axial and **(B)** coronal reformatted CT images of both hip joints of a 65-year-old man show subchondral sclerosis and fragmentation of the femoral heads. Note that despite advanced osteonecrotic changes, the hip joint spaces are well preserved. (Reprinted with permission from Greenspan A, Gershwin E. *Imaging in rheumatology*, 1st ed. Philadelphia: Wolters Kluwer; 2017, Figure 13.9.)

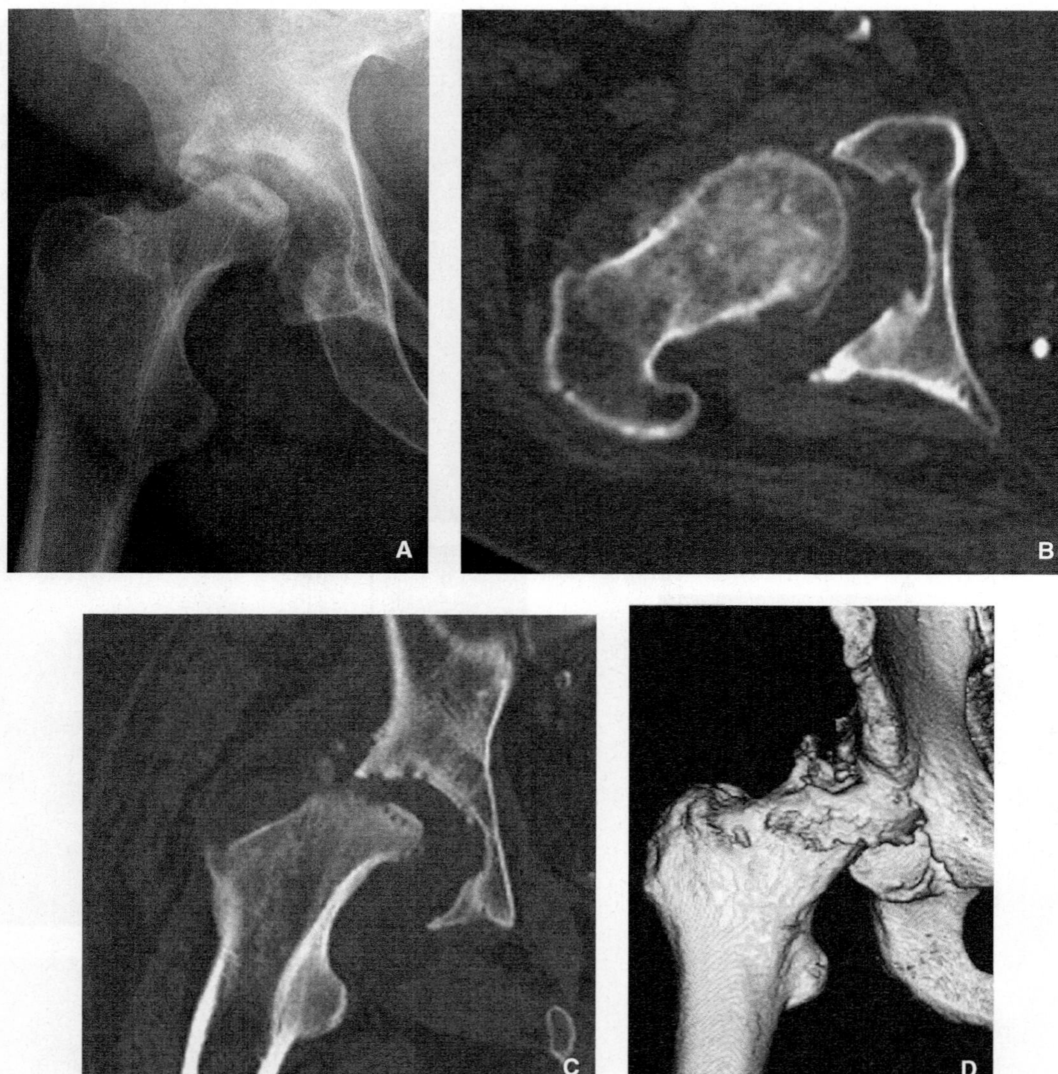

FIGURE 4.95 CT and 3D CT of osteonecrosis of femoral head. **(A)** Anteroposterior radiograph of the right hip shows sclerotic changes and subchondral radiolucency of the deformed femoral head, indicative of advanced osteonecrosis. Observe also superolateral subluxation of the femoral head. All these features are more effectively demonstrated on axial **(B)**, coronal reformatted **(C)**, and 3D reconstructed **(D)** CT images. (Reprinted with permission from Greenspan A, Gershwin E. *Imaging in rheumatology*, 1st ed. Philadelphia: Wolters Kluwer; 2017, Figure 13.10.)

TABLE 4.5 Osteonecrosis of Femoral Head: Correlation of Clinical Symptoms and Imaging Findings with Histopathologic Changes Based on Ficat and Arlet Classification

Stage	Clinical Symptoms	Radiographic Findings	Scintigraphy	Pathologic Changes	Biopsy
1	None	Normal	Normal	Infarction of weight-bearing segments	Necrotic marrow, osteoblasts
2	Mild pain	Increased density of femoral head, normal joint space	Increased uptake	Spontaneous repair	New bone deposition
3	Mild-to-moderate pain	Loss of sphericity and collapse of the femoral head, crescent sign	Increased uptake	Subchondral fracture with collapse, impaction and fragmentation of the necrotic segment	Dead bone trabeculae and dead marrow cells on both sides of the fracture line
4	Moderate pain, assistive devices needed	Joint space narrowing, acetabular changes	Increased uptake	Osteoarthritis	Degenerative changes in articular cartilage

Modified from Chang CC, Greenspan A, Gershwin ME. Osteonecrosis: current perspectives on pathogenesis and treatment. *Semin Arthritis Rheum* 1993;23(1):47–69.

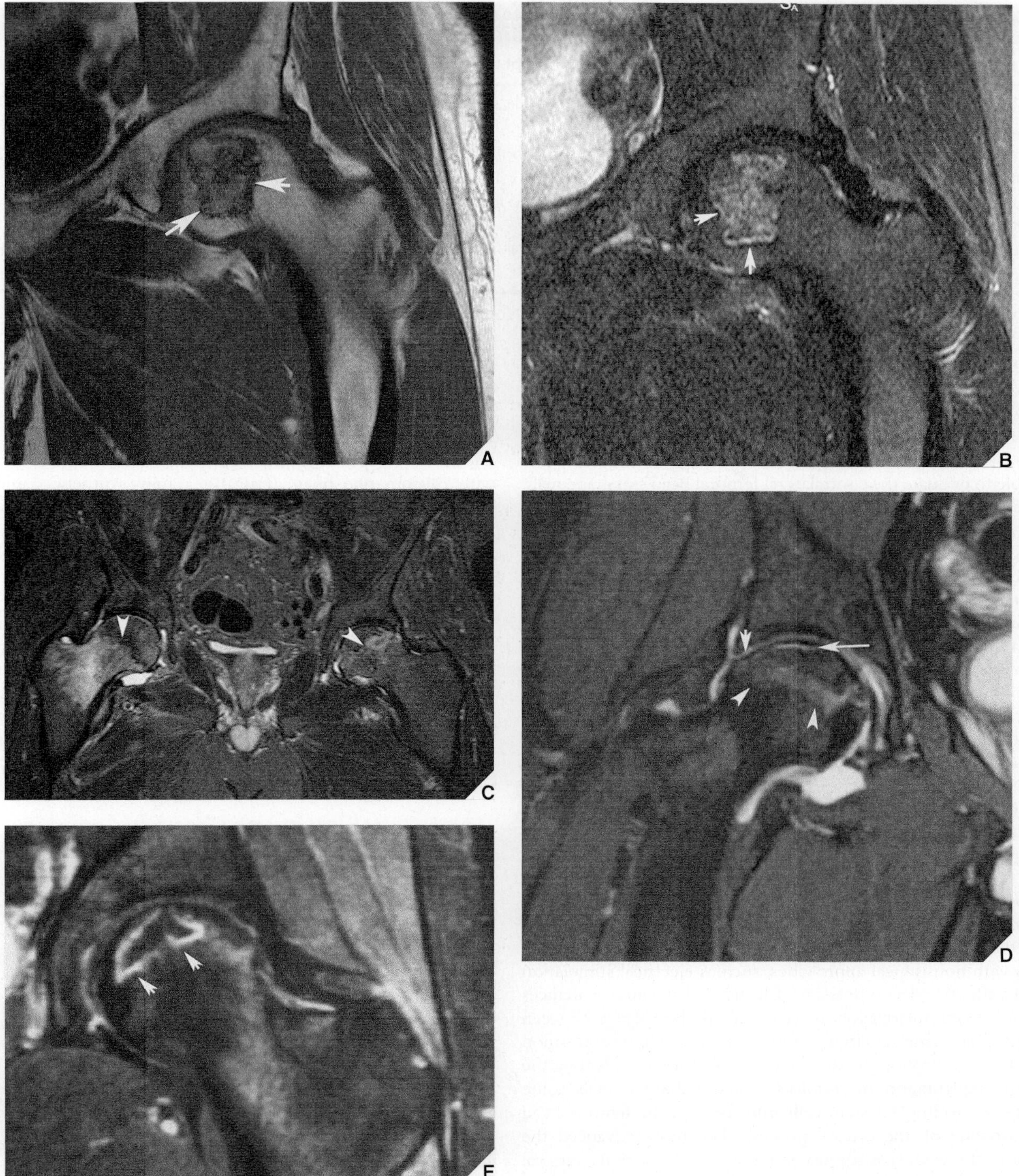

FIGURE 4.96 MRI of osteonecrosis of the femoral head. (A) Coronal T1-weighted image shows a serpentine band of low signal intensity *(short arrows)* representing the reactive interface surrounding the central area of bone necrosis. **(B)** Coronal short time inversion recovery (STIR) pulse sequence MR image shows a serpentine low-signal intensity line adjacent to a high-signal intensity line (so-called *double line sign*) *(short arrows)*. **(C)** Coronal T2-weighted fat-saturated MR image demonstrates osteonecrosis of both femoral heads *(arrowheads)*, with prominent bone marrow edema in the right femoral neck and joint effusions. The presence of bone marrow edema and joint effusion is frequently associated with osteonecrosis and correlates clinically with pain. **(D)** Coronal STIR pulse sequence MR image demonstrates osteonecrosis of the right femoral head *(arrowheads)* with a subchondral hyperintense line *(long arrow)* representing the subchondral fracture. This finding correlates with the crescent sign seen on the conventional radiographs (see Figs. 4.90 and 4.91B). Note the early collapse of the lateral aspect of the femoral head *(short arrow)* and the presence of a joint effusion. **(E)** T1-weighted fat-saturated coronal MR image following intravenous administration of gadolinium shows enhancement of the reactive interface *(short arrows)* but no enhancement of the necrotic area.

TABLE 4.6 Correlation of Magnetic Resonance Imaging Findings with Histologic Changes

Class	Magnetic Resonance Imaging Findings	Appearance	Histology
A	Normal fat signal except at the sclerotic margin surrounding the lesion	Fat-like	Premature conversion to fatty marrow within the femoral neck or intertrochanteric region
B	High signal intensity of the inner border and low signal intensity of the surrounding rim	Blood-like	Bone resorption and replacement by vascular granulation tissue
C	Diffusely decreased signal on T1 and high signal on T2 weighting	Fluid-like	Bone marrow edema
D	Decreased signal on T1- and T2-weighted images	Fibrous	Sclerosis from reinforcement of existing trabeculae at the margin of a live bone (i.e., repair tissue interface)

Modified from Chang CC, Greenspan A, Gershwin ME. Osteonecrosis: current perspectives on pathogenesis and treatment. *Semin Arthritis Rheum* 1993;23(1):47–69.

at the interface between necrotic and viable bones. As Seiler and coworkers have pointed out, MRI evaluation of osteonecrosis of the femoral head has several advantages: It is noninvasive, does not require ionizing radiation, provides multiplanar images, reflects physiologic changes in the bone marrow, provides excellent resolution of surrounding soft tissues, and makes it possible to evaluate the contralateral femoral head simultaneously.

A specific condition known as *bone marrow edema syndrome* was initially thought to be a precursor to osteonecrosis, but it is now considered to be a separate entity. Differentiation between bone marrow edema syndrome and osteonecrosis can be facilitated through analysis of perfusion patterns including mean transit times (MTTs) and plasma flow (PF) using a quantitative dynamic contrast material-enhanced (DCE) MRI. Bone marrow edema shows a subchondral elongated area of high PF and low MTT, surrounded by an area of low PF and long MTTs. In contrast, osteonecrosis shows a subchondral area with low or no detectable PF and MTT surrounded by a rim of high PF and intermediate MTT.

Treatment of Osteonecrosis of the Femoral Head. Most of the patients with osteonecrosis of the femoral head ultimately require surgical intervention. Nonsurgical approaches are effective only in the very early stages of osteonecrosis when the involved segment is smaller than 15% and is far from the weight-bearing region. They include refraining from weight bearing, use of analgesics and antiinflammatory medications, and physiotherapy. A number of newer pharmacologic therapeutic agents including growth and differentiation factors, cytokines, angiogenic factors, and bone morphogenic proteins have theoretical promise in the treatment of this condition. Sometimes, surgical procedures can be used in conjunction with nonsurgical approaches, such as electrical stimulation in conjunction with core decompression. Electrical stimulation enhances osteogenesis and neovascularization as well as alters the balance between osteoblastic and osteoclastic activity, resulting in increased bone deposition and decreased bone resorption. Most recently, a pilot study evaluating the effectiveness of implantation of autologous bone marrow cells using core decompression to implant stem cells into the necrotic femoral head demonstrated slowing of the disease process. The more advanced the disease, the more the extensive surgery is required. The various surgical procedures include core decompression, which involves the removal of a core of bone from the femoral neck and head, structural bone grafting, when the bone graft is inserted into the necrotic segment through the core tract, vascularized fibula grafting, in which procedure the core tract is used to insert corticocancellous bone graft into the femoral neck and head along with its vascular pedicle, osteotomy, resurfacing hip arthroplasty, hemiarthroplasty, and total hip replacement. Ficat in 1962 first introduced core decompression procedure (Fig. 4.97). The goal of this approach is to reduce the elevated intramedullary pressure within the femoral head resulting from venous congestion, promote vascular invasion, interrupt the cycle that results in worsening of the ischemia, and facilitate regeneration of the necrotic bone. This procedure also provides immediate and dramatic pain relief. Core decompression yields the best results when performed in the early stages of disease. Various types of bone graft procedures have been used to provide mechanical support for the affected joint and to delay the need for arthroplasty. These include autogenous and allogenous cortical bone grafts of ilium, fibula, or tibia, alone or in combination with core decompression (Fig. 4.98), osteochondral graft, demineralized bone matrix, muscle pedicle bone grafts, free vascularized bone grafts, bone marrow concentrate, bone morphogenetic protein, and porous tantalum implants. In all cases, the primary function of all these procedures is to provide a mechanical and structural support and to reinforce the necrotic segment until the lesion is restored biologically. In the past decade, injectable composite grafts—combination of calcium sulfate ($CaSO_4$) with calcium phosphate ($CaPO_4$), a fully synthetic composite material enhanced with autologous bone marrow concentrate, designed to be mixed intraoperatively and injected into the space created by core decompression (Fig. 4.99)—have been used with promising results. This treatment not only relieves hip pain but also prevents the progression of osteonecrotic process in the majority of cases (Fig. 4.100). Once the femoral head has collapsed, the treatment of choice is reconstruction surgery. The procedures most commonly performed are resurfacing (Fig. 4.101) or conventional (Fig. 4.102) hemiarthroplasty. Occasionally, particularly when the patient develops secondary osteoarthritis, the total hip arthroplasty is performed (Fig. 4.103). The decision to select one of these procedures over another depends on the stage and the extend of osteonecrosis.

Osteonecrosis of the humeral head may develop after a fracture of the humeral neck (Fig. 4.104), but this complication is seen in-

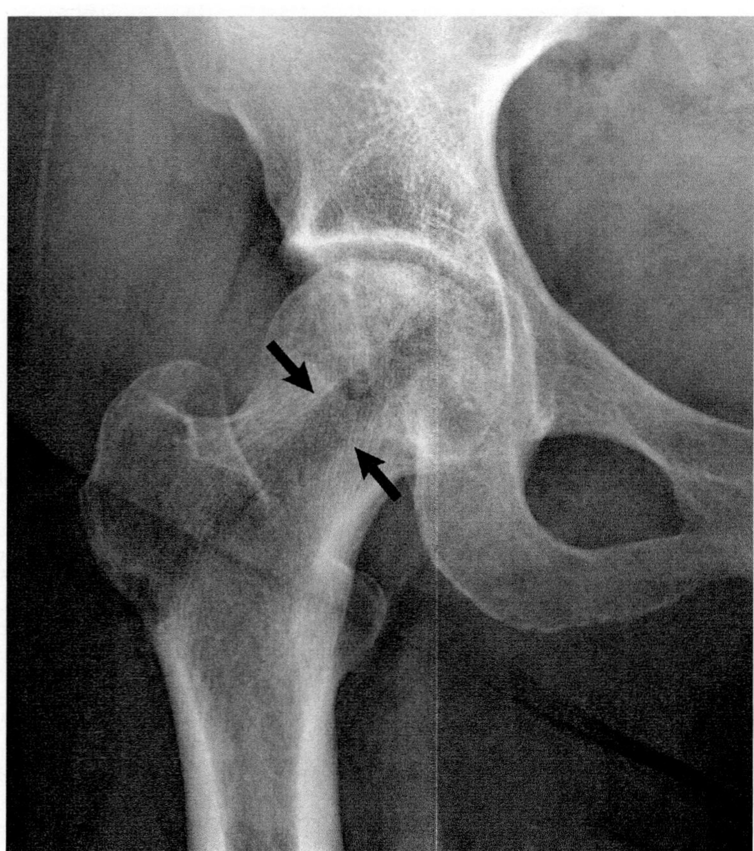

FIGURE 4.97 Treatment of osteonecrosis of the femoral head—core decompression procedure. A 46-year-old woman with osteonecrosis of the right femoral head was treated with core decompression procedure *(arrows)*.

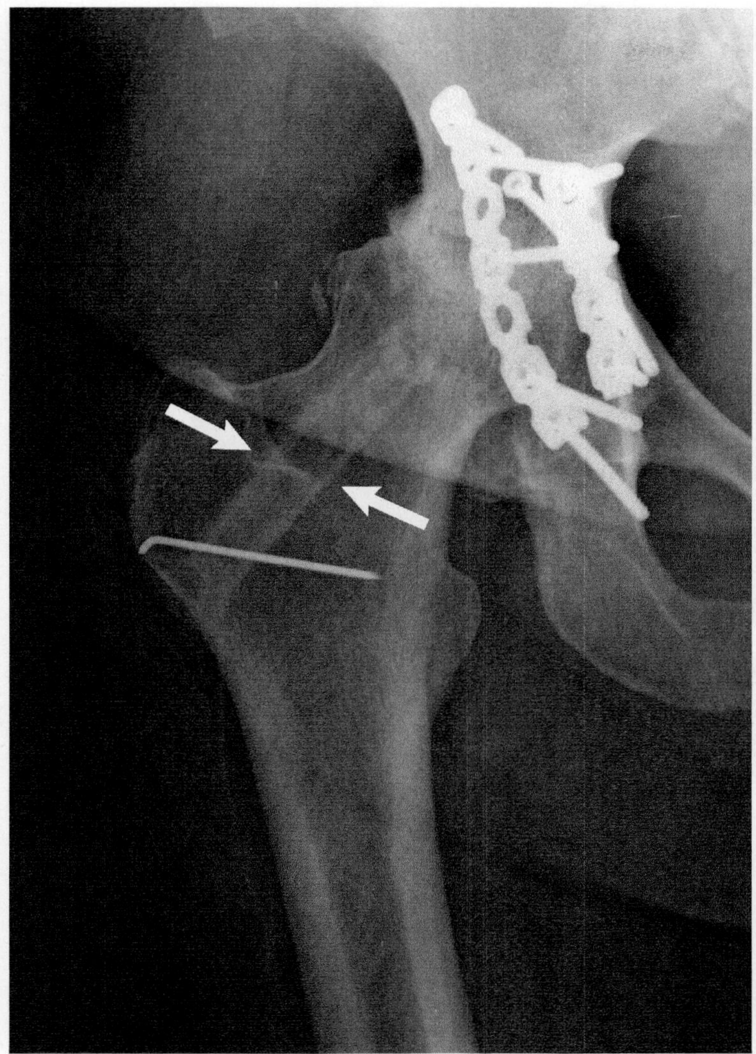

FIGURE 4.98 Treatment of osteonecrosis of the femoral head—fibular bone graft. A 69-year-old man sustained a fracture–dislocation in the right hip joint that was treated by open reduction and internal fixation. As a complication of this injury, he developed osteonecrosis of the femoral head. Anteroposterior radiograph shows osteonecrosis of the femoral head that was treated with application of the fibular bone graft *(arrows)*.

frequently. A majority of osteonecrosis of the humeral head is either related to connective tissue disorders (Fig. 4.105), treatment with steroids (Fig. 4.106), or idiopathic.

Osteonecrosis of the carpal scaphoid is a complication commonly seen in 10% to 15% of cases of carpal scaphoid fracture, increasing in incidence to 30% to 40% if there is nonunion. Necrosis generally involves the proximal bone fragment, but the distal fragment, although rarely, may also be affected. Evidence of this complication most frequently becomes apparent approximately 4 to 6 months after an injury, when radiographic examination shows an increased bone density. Although it is most often diagnosed on conventional radiographs, tomographic study (Fig. 4.107), CT (Fig. 4.108), and MRI (Fig. 4.109) are indicated when radiographic findings are equivocal.

Only exceptionally, a scaphoid bone may become osteonecrotic in the absence of a fracture. This abnormality is known as *Preiser disease*.

Osteonecrosis of the lunate (Kienböck disease) is discussed in Chapter 7.

Injury to Major Blood Vessels

A relatively infrequent complication of a fracture or dislocation, an injury to the major blood vessels occurs when bone fragments lacerate or completely transect an artery (see Figs. 2.3 and 4.15) or a vein, resulting in bleeding, the formation of hematoma, arteriovenous fistula, or a pseudoaneurysm. The latter complication may also occur without the fracture, after trauma to the soft tissues (Fig. 4.110). To demonstrate this abnormality, angiography may be performed (see Figs. 2.3 and 4.110B). This technique is invaluable in visualizing the site of laceration, ascertaining the exact extent of vascular damage, and assessing the status of collateral circulation. It may also be combined with an interventional procedure, such as embolization to control hemorrhage. At the present time, more often, CT-angiography is performed (see Figs. 2.12D,E and 2.13C–E).

Growth Disturbance

A common complication of Salter-Harris type IV and V fractures involving the physis, growth disturbance may result from an injury to the growth plate by the formation of an osseous bridge between the epiphysis and the metaphysis. As a result of this tethering of the growth plate, localized cessation of bone growth occurs. If the entire physis in a single long bone stops growing, a limb-length discrepancy will result (Fig. 4.111A). If only one growth plate at the articulations of parallel bones (the radius and ulna or the tibia and fibula) is damaged and ceases to grow, the uninjured bone continues to grow at the normal rate, leading to overgrowth and consequent joint deformity (Fig. 4.111B).

Posttraumatic Arthritis

If a fracture line extends into the joint, the articular surface may become irregular. Such incongruity in the articular surfaces results in abnormal stresses that lead to precocious degenerative changes recognized on the radiograph by narrowing of the joint space, subchondral sclerosis, and formation of marginal osteophytes (Fig. 4.112). A similar complication may also be seen after a dislocation (Fig. 4.113).

Stress Fractures

A bone is a dynamic tissue that requires stress for normal development. *Stress* is the force or absolute load applied to a bone that may arise from weight-bearing or muscular actions. The force may be of an axial, bending, or torsional nature, and the resulting change in shape of the bone is referred to as *strain*. *Tensile* forces are produced along the convex side of a bone, whereas *compressive* forces occur along its concave margin. According to Wolff law, intermittent forces applied to a bone stimulate remodeling of its architecture to withstand the new mechanical environment optimally. Stresses related to daily activities stimulate the remodeling process that, in a cortical bone, occurs at the level of the osteon, the basic unit of bone structure. The exact mechanism that activates this process is not known, but some evidence suggests that it may be related to the development of microfractures (Fig. 4.114A). Osteoclastic resorption leading to the formation of small resorption areas at the site of microfractures is the initial response to increased stresses; peak bone loss occurs after approximately 3 weeks. These resorption cavities are subsequently filled with lamellar bone, but if bone formation is slow, then the consequent imbalance between bone resorption and bone formation results in weakening of the bone. Periosteal proliferation, endosteal proliferation, or both may produce a new bone at the sites of stress in an apparent attempt to buttress the temporarily weakened cortex. Stresses in a cancellous bone may result in partial or complete trabecular microfractures (Fig. 4.114B). Microcallus is produced along the complete fractures, and these thickened trabeculae probably account for the sclerosis seen on radiographs when stress injuries occur in a cancellous bone. Although microdamage is a physiologic phenomenon, it becomes pathologic when its production greatly exceeds repair. If the inciting activity is not curtailed, repair mechanisms are overwhelmed, which results in the accumulation of microdamage and subsequent fatigue fracture of a trabecular or cortical bone (see Figs. 4.31 and 4.57B).

Diagnostic imaging has acquired a pivotal role in the assessment of stress injuries to bone because clinical evaluation alone is not definitive. If classic radiographic findings are present, then the diagnosis is straightforward. However, because the underlying pathophysiology is a continuing process rather than a single event, imaging findings are extremely variable and depend on such factors as the type of inciting activity, the bone involved, and the timing of the imaging procedure.

Conventional radiographs play an important role in the workup of a suspected stress fracture and should be the first imaging study obtained.

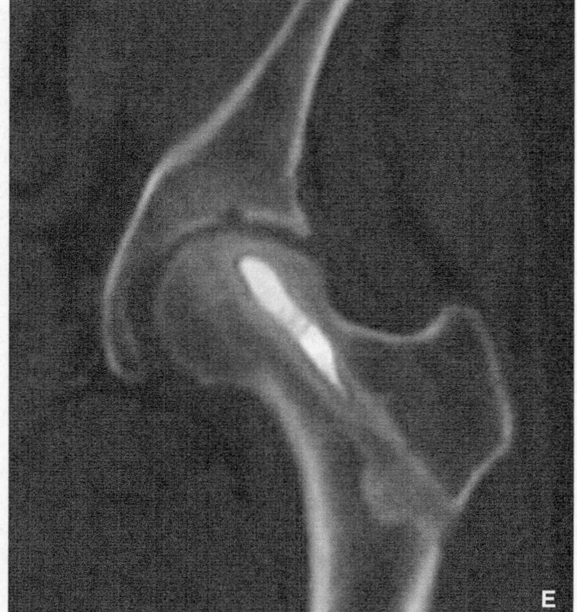

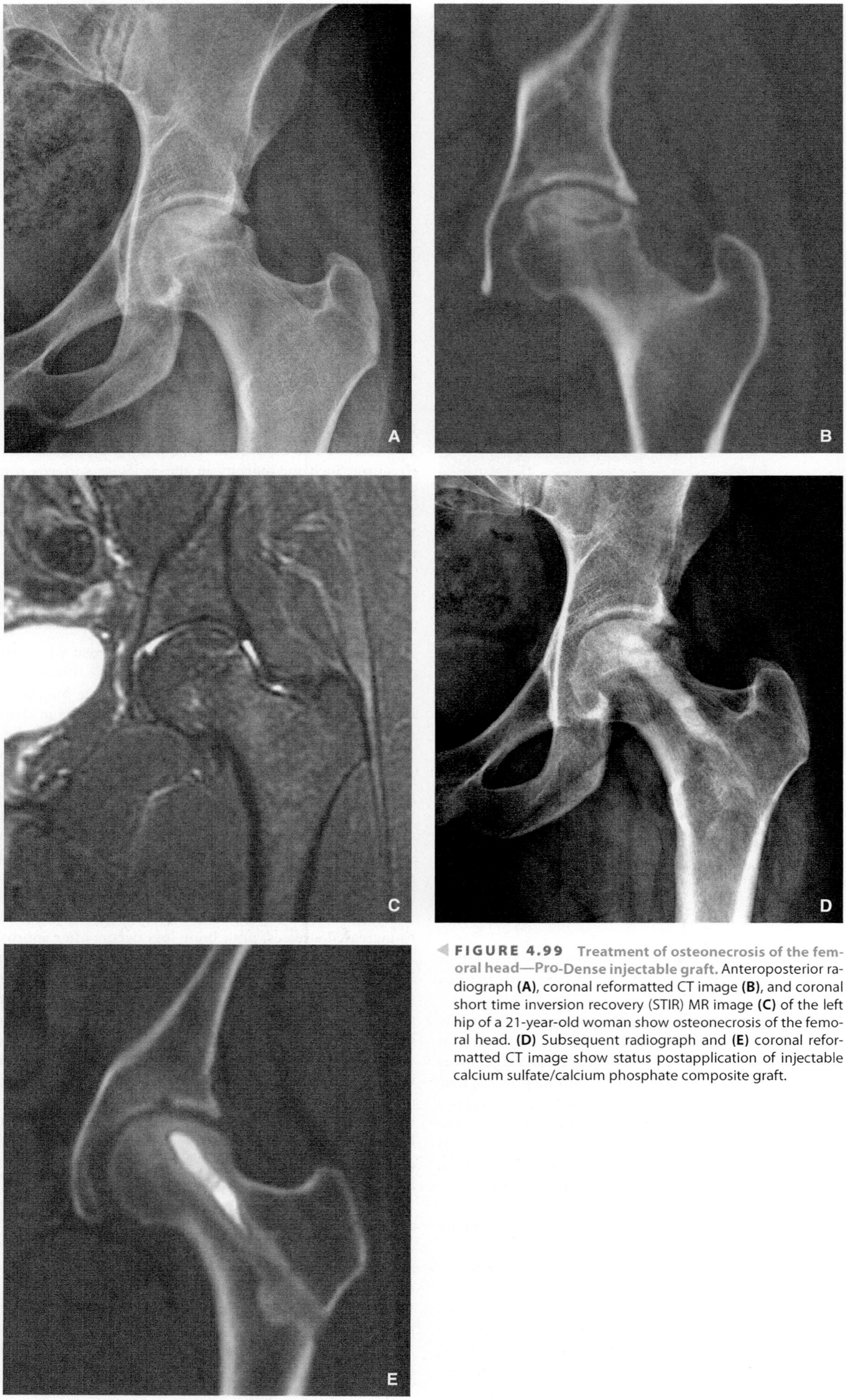

FIGURE 4.99 Treatment of osteonecrosis of the femoral head—Pro-Dense injectable graft. Anteroposterior radiograph **(A)**, coronal reformatted CT image **(B)**, and coronal short time inversion recovery (STIR) MR image **(C)** of the left hip of a 21-year-old woman show osteonecrosis of the femoral head. **(D)** Subsequent radiograph and **(E)** coronal reformatted CT image show status postapplication of injectable calcium sulfate/calcium phosphate composite graft.

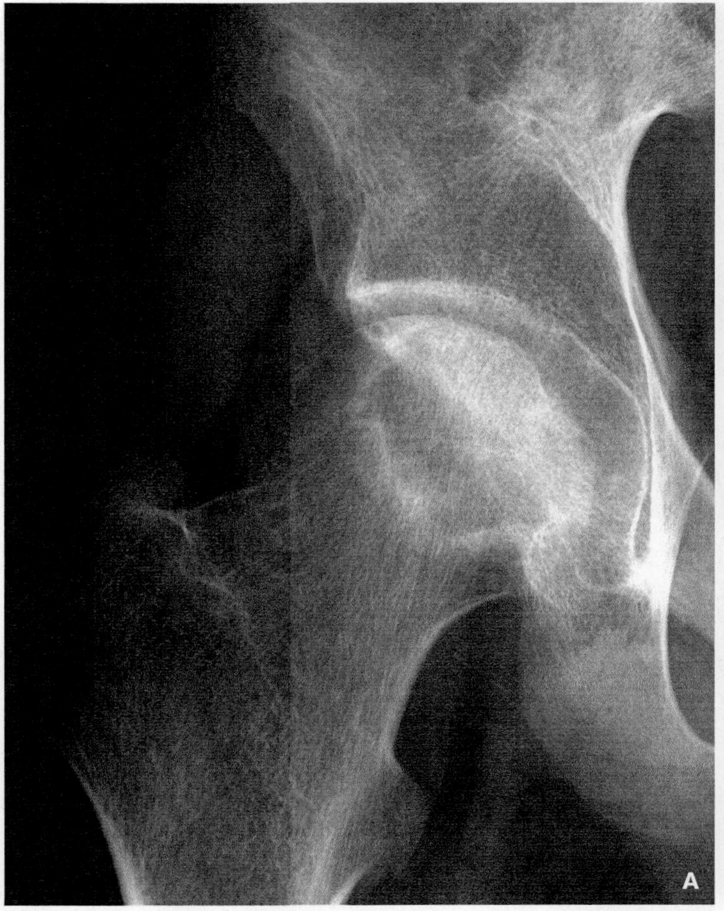

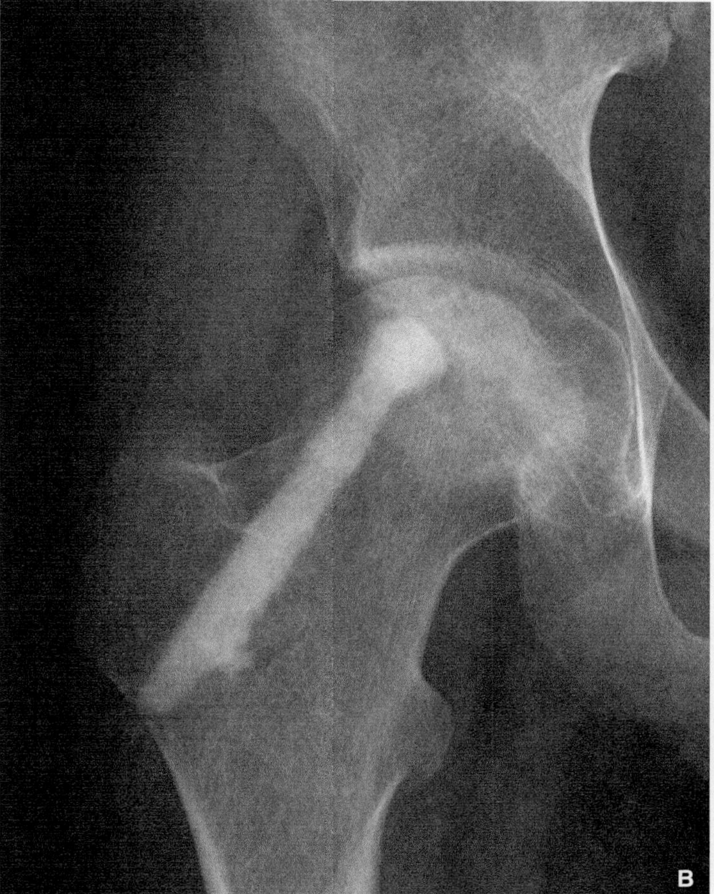

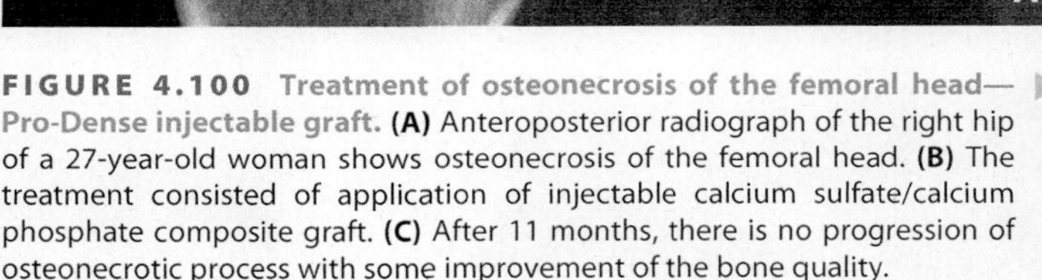

FIGURE 4.100 Treatment of osteonecrosis of the femoral head—Pro-Dense injectable graft. **(A)** Anteroposterior radiograph of the right hip of a 27-year-old woman shows osteonecrosis of the femoral head. **(B)** The treatment consisted of application of injectable calcium sulfate/calcium phosphate composite graft. **(C)** After 11 months, there is no progression of osteonecrotic process with some improvement of the bone quality.

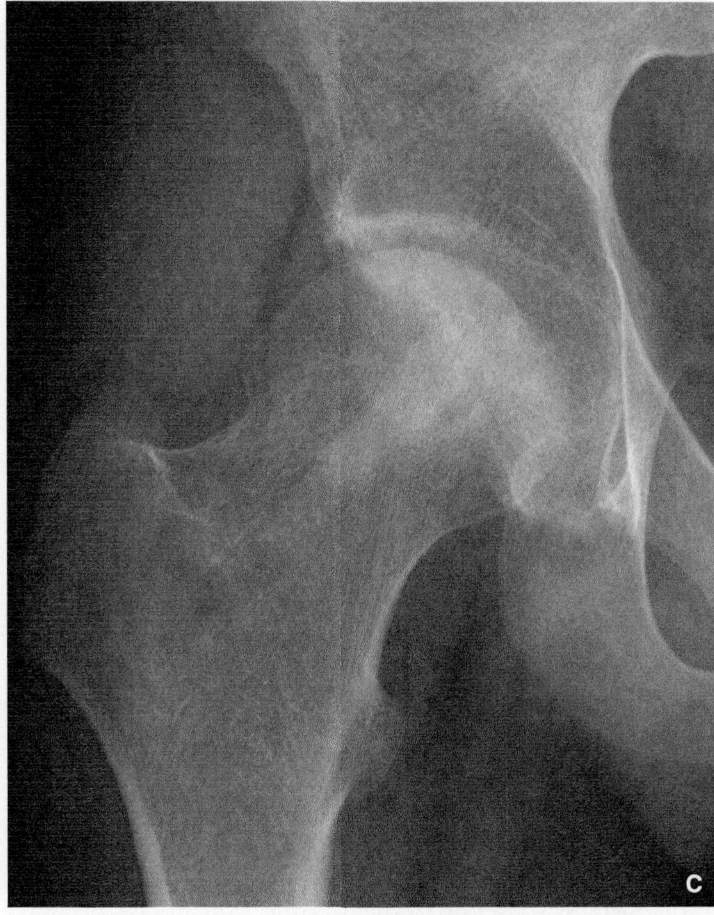

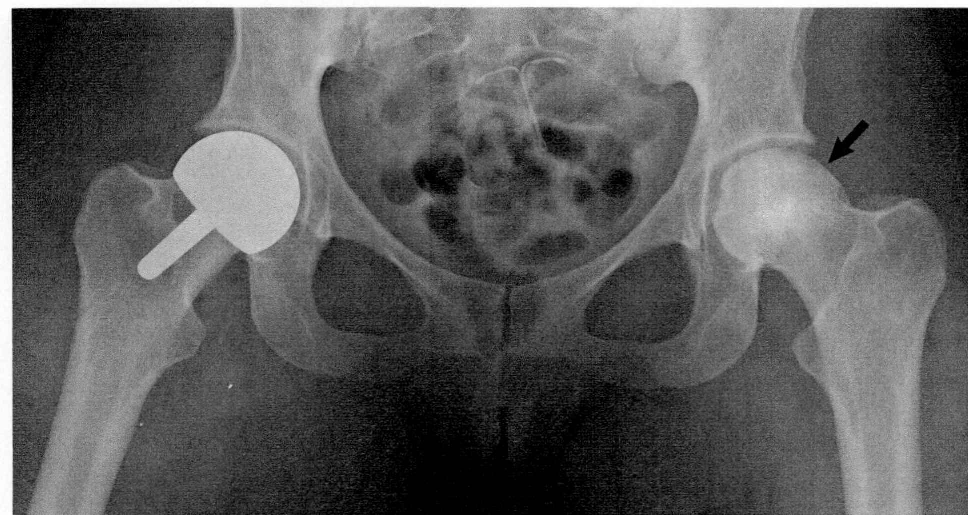

FIGURE 4.101 Treatment of osteonecrosis of the femoral head—resurfacing hemiarthroplasty. Anteroposterior radiograph of the pelvis of a 32-year-old woman shows osteonecrosis of the left femoral head *(arrow)*. Osteonecrosis of the right femoral head was treated with resurfacing hemiarthroplasty.

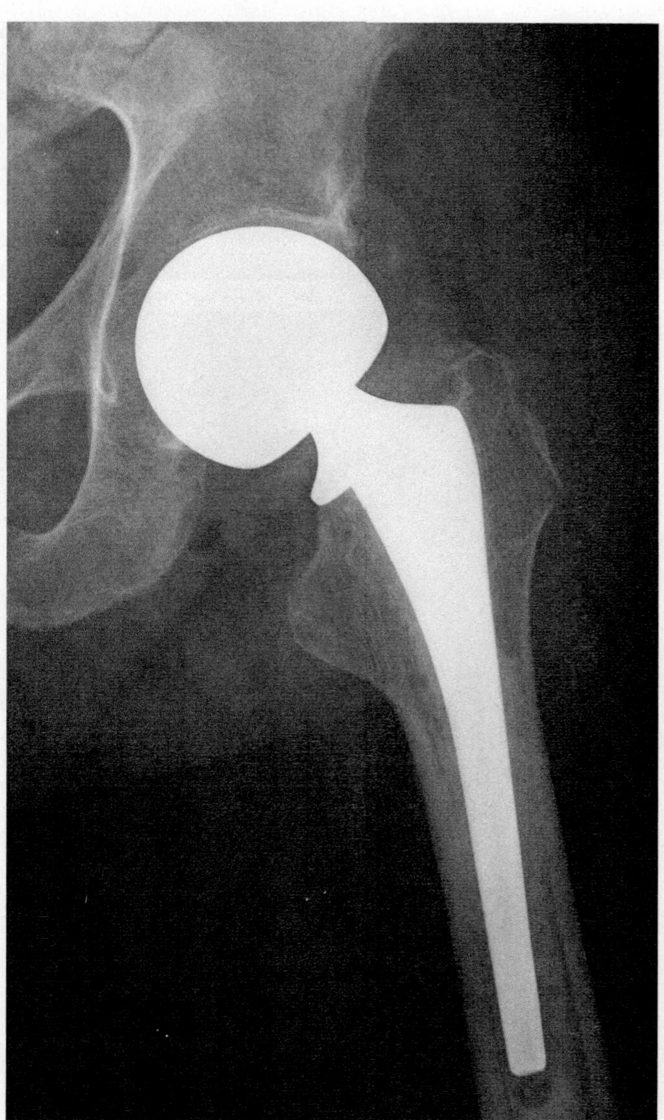

FIGURE 4.102 Treatment of osteonecrosis of the femoral head—bipolar hemiarthroplasty. A 75-year-old man, who was diagnosed with advanced osteonecrosis of the left femoral head, underwent hip hemiarthroplasty using bipolar type of the prosthesis. Tight-fitting cup of the prosthesis is symmetrically positioned within the native acetabulum, and the stem of the prosthesis is cemented in neutral position within the femoral shaft.

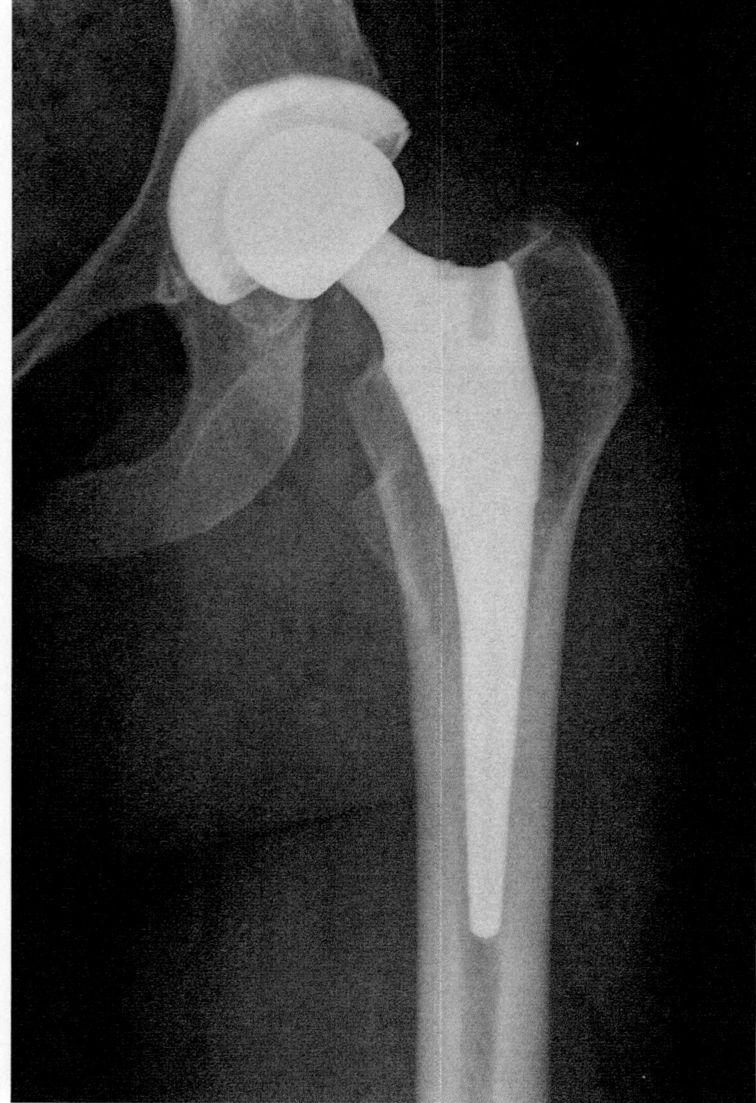

FIGURE 4.103 Treatment of the femoral head osteonecrosis—total hip arthroplasty. Anteroposterior radiograph of the left hip of a 35-year-old woman, who was diagnosed with osteonecrosis of the femoral head, shows status post–total hip arthroplasty using noncemented prosthetic components. Porous-coated acetabular component and partially coated femoral stem of the prosthesis are in anatomic alignment.

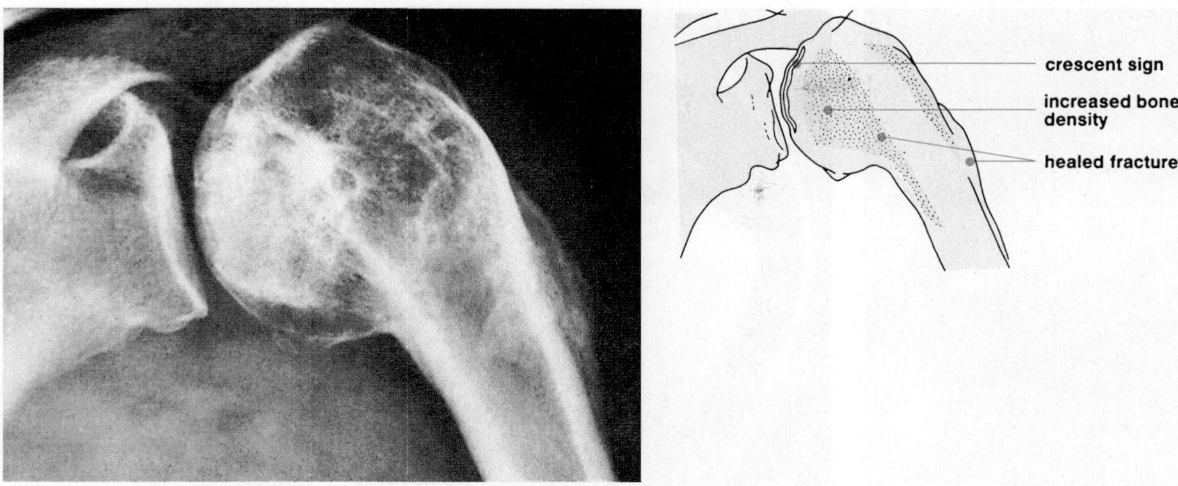

FIGURE 4.104 **Posttraumatic osteonecrosis of the humeral head.** Six months after sustaining a fracture of the left humeral neck that united, a 62-year-old man developed osteonecrosis of the humeral head, evident on this radiograph from the increased bone density and the collapse of the subchondral segment.

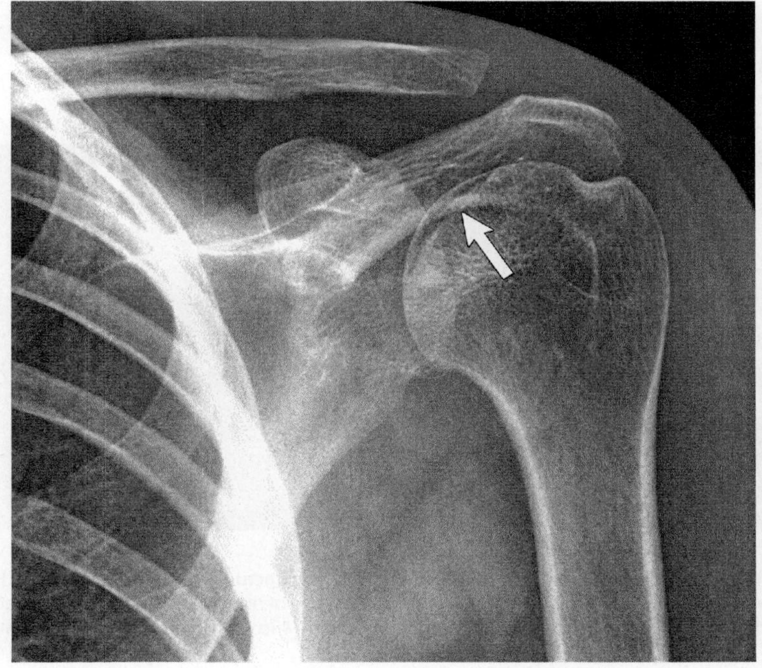

FIGURE 4.105 **Osteonecrosis of humeral head in SLE.** Anteroposterior radiograph of the left shoulder of a 28-year-old woman diagnosed with SLE shows a radiolucent crescent sign in subchondral bone of the humeral head *(arrow)* pathognomonic for osteonecrosis.

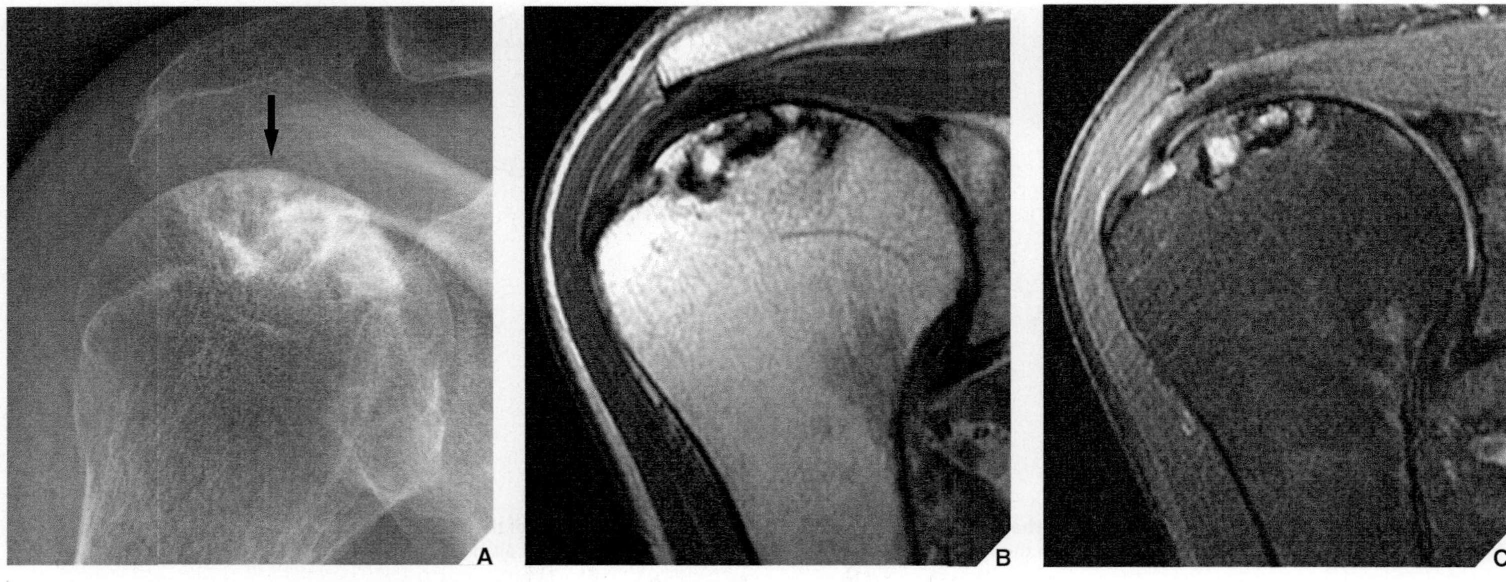

FIGURE 4.106 **Osteonecrosis of the humeral head.** A 58-year-old woman presented with right shoulder pain for several weeks after an apparent dislocation in the glenohumeral joint, which was spontaneously reduced. She also gives a history of SLE treated with corticosteroids. **(A)** Radiograph of the right shoulder shows a classic appearance of osteonecrosis of the humeral head *(arrow)*, a diagnosis that was confirmed on coronal proton density **(B)** and coronal proton density fat-suppressed **(C)** MR images. Osteonecrosis was more likely secondary to SLE and the treatment with steroids rather than due to traumatic event.

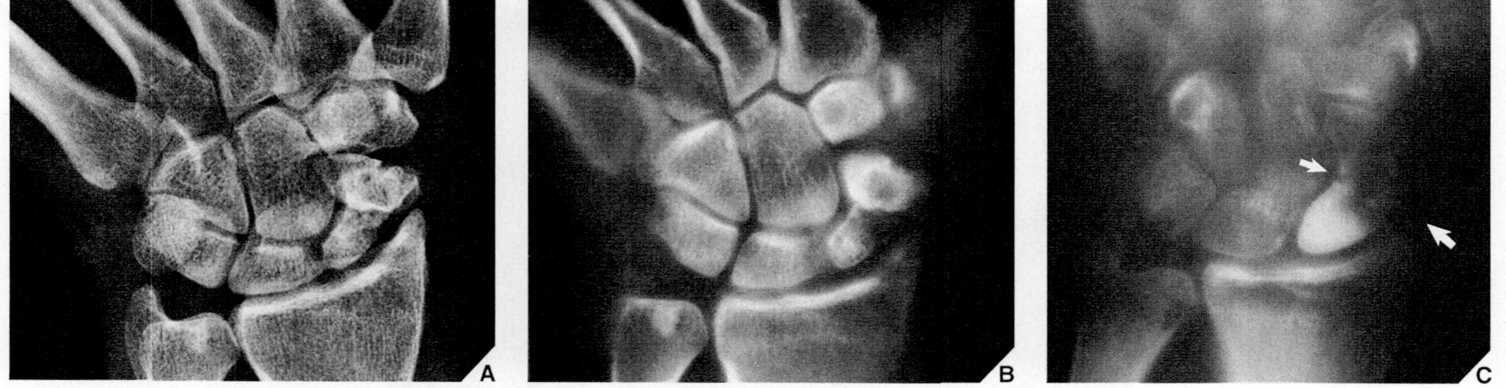

FIGURE 4.107 **Osteonecrosis of the scaphoid.** **(A)** Radiograph of the wrist demonstrates a fracture of the carpal scaphoid; however, it is unclear whether the fracture is complicated by osteonecrosis. **(B)** Trispiral tomogram clearly shows nonunion and the presence of osteonecrosis of the distal fragment, together with cystic degeneration. The dense spot in the articular end of the ulna represents a bone island. **(C)** In another patient, trispiral tomogram shows ununited fracture of the scaphoid *(arrows)* and osteonecrosis of the proximal fragment.

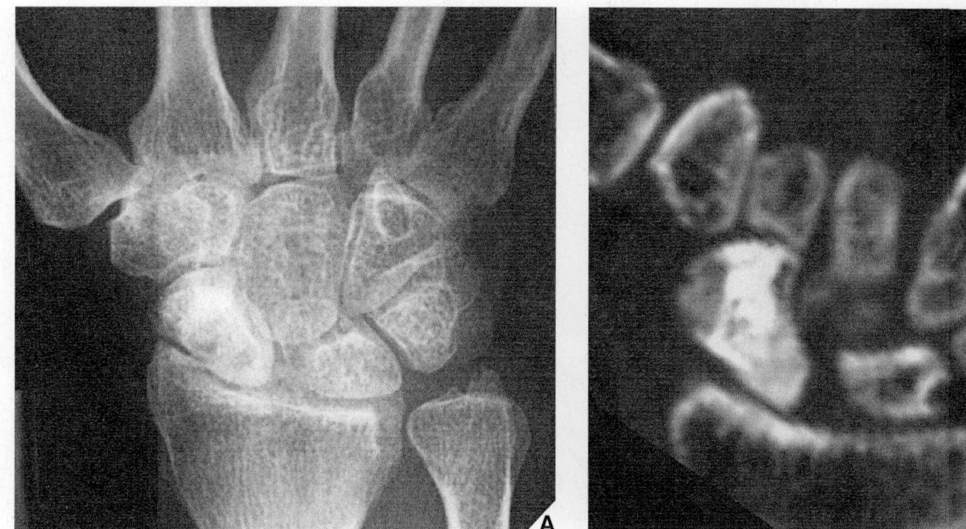

FIGURE 4.108 CT of scaphoid osteonecrosis. A 52-year-old woman sustained a fracture of the scaphoid bone, treated conservatively in a cast. **(A)** Conventional radiograph shows sclerotic changes in the scaphoid, which may be due to healing process or osteonecrosis. **(B)** Coronal reformatted CT shows an incompletely healed fracture of the scaphoid complicated by osteonecrosis.

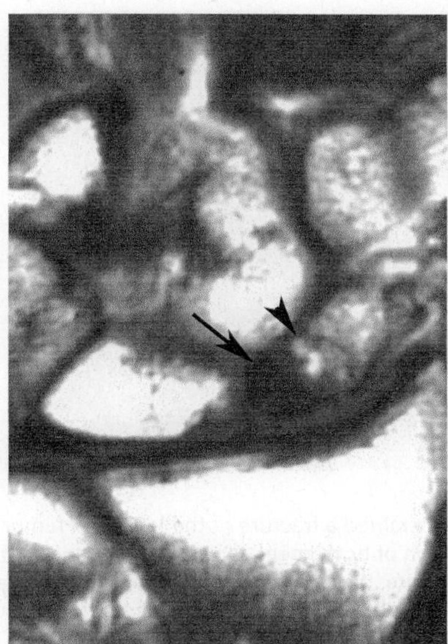

FIGURE 4.109 MRI of scaphoid osteonecrosis. A young man sustained a fracture of the waist of the scaphoid that was treated conservatively. T1-weighted postcontrast coronal MR image of the wrist obtained several months later demonstrates a nonunited fracture of the waist of the scaphoid *(arrowhead)* and low signal intensity of the proximal pole of the scaphoid without enhancement, consistent with osteonecrosis *(arrow)*.

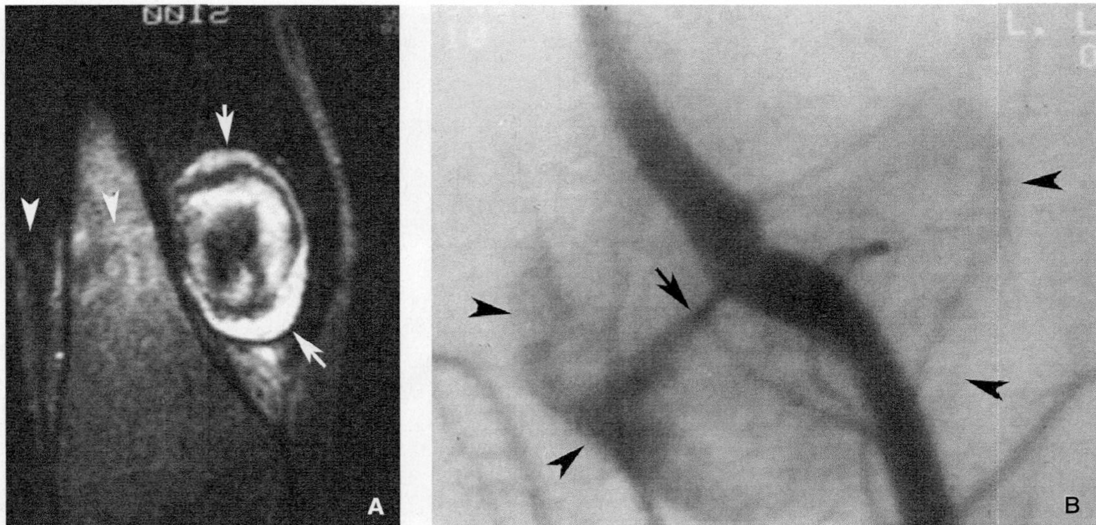

FIGURE 4.110 **Pseudoaneurysm of the popliteal artery. (A)** Coronal T2-weighted MR image of the knee of a young male with past history of trauma without a fracture and a palpable mass in the popliteal space demonstrates a fluid collection in the popliteal space (*arrows*) with characteristic "layering" within the lesion and pulsation artifact in the direction of the phase encoding gradient (*arrowheads*) consistent with pseudoaneurysm. **(B)** Digital subtraction arteriogram of the popliteal artery shows a small rupture and squirting of the contrast material (*arrow*) beginning to fill the pseudoaneurysm (*arrowheads*).

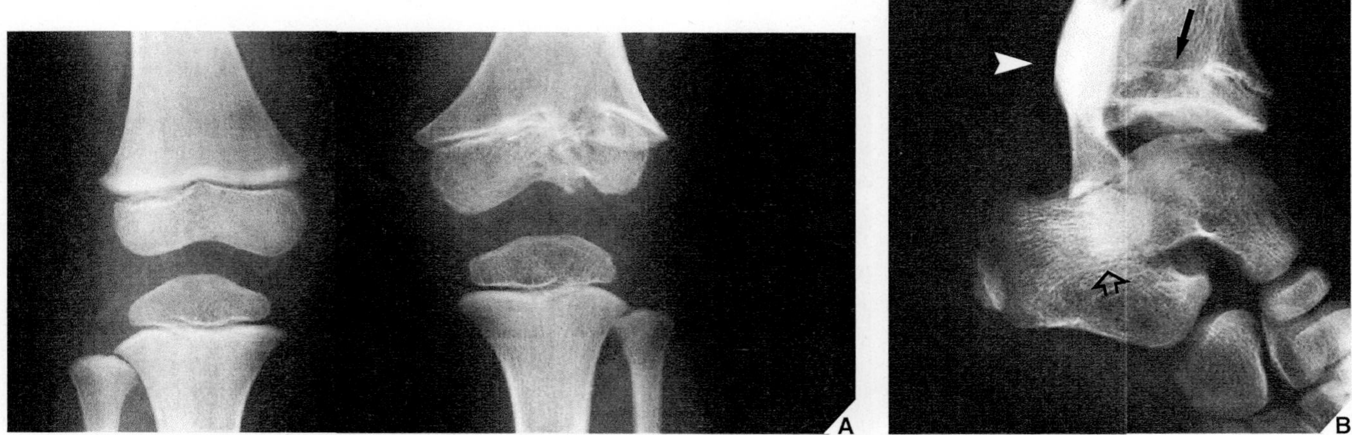

FIGURE 4.111 **Growth disturbance. (A)** A 3-year-old boy sustained a fracture of the left distal femur that extended through the growth plate. As a result, the bone at this end prematurely ceased to grow. Anteroposterior radiograph of both knees shows a discrepancy in the length of the femora associated with deformity of the distal epiphysis of the left femur secondary to tethering of the growth plate. **(B)** A 5-year-old girl sustained a Salter-Harris type V fracture of the distal tibia. On the lateral view, a joint deformity is evident as a result of the fusion of the physis of the tibia *(arrow)* and overgrowth of the distal fibula *(open arrow)*. Note also the posttraumatic synostosis of these two bones *(arrowhead)*.

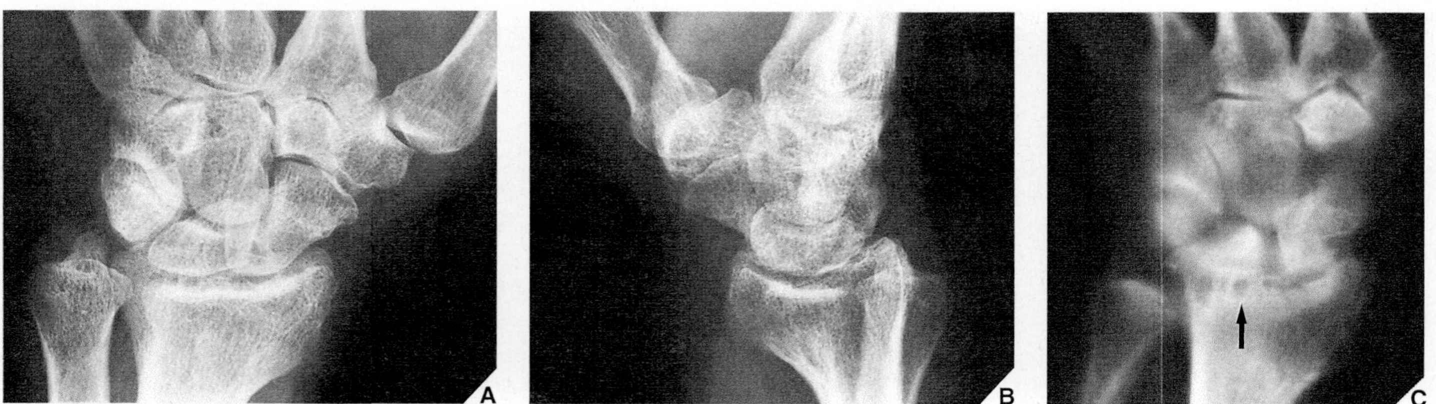

FIGURE 4.112 **Posttraumatic osteoarthritis.** Dorsovolar **(A)** and lateral **(B)** radiographs of the wrist of a 57-year-old man who had sustained an intraarticular fracture of the distal radius demonstrate residual deformity of this bone and narrowing of the radiocarpal articulation. Trispiral tomogram **(C)** shows, in addition, the multiple subchondral degenerative cysts *(arrow)* often seen in posttraumatic arthritis.

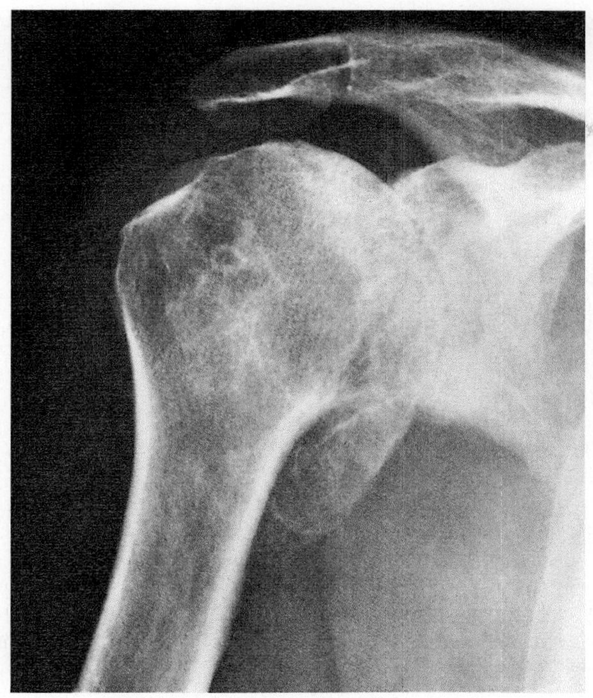

FIGURE 4.113 Posttraumatic osteoarthritis. The anteroposterior radiograph of the right shoulder of a 78-year-old man who presented with a history of several previous dislocations in that joint demonstrates the advanced osteoarthritis resulting from repeated trauma to the articular surfaces of the humeral head and glenoid.

Unfortunately, initial radiographs are often normal, which is not surprising given the degree of microscopic remodeling that occurs in the early stages of stress injury. The sensitivity of early radiographs can be as low as 15%, and follow-up radiographs will demonstrate diagnostic findings in only 50% of cases. The time that elapses between the manifestation of initial symptoms and the detection of radiographic findings ranges from 1 week to several months, and cessation of physical activity may prevent the development of any radiographic findings.

Initial changes in the cortical bone include subtle ill definition of the cortex (gray cortex sign) (Fig. 4.115) or faint intracortical radiolucent striations, which are presumably related to the osteoclastic tunneling found early in the remodeling process. These changes may be easily overlooked until periosteal new bone formation and/or endosteal thickening develops in an apparent attempt to buttress the temporarily weakened cortex. As damage increases, a true fracture line may appear (Fig. 4.116). These injuries typically involve the shaft of a long bone and are common in the anterior or posterior cortex of the tibia and in the medial cortex of the femur.

Stress injuries in cancellous bones are notoriously difficult to detect. Subtle blurring of trabecular margins and faint sclerotic radiopaque areas may be seen secondary to peritrabecular callus, but a 50% change in bone opacity is required for these changes to be radiographically detectable (Fig. 4.117). With progression of the pathologic process, a readily apparent sclerotic band is seen (Fig. 4.118).

Radionuclide bone scanning has become the gold standard for evaluating stress fractures owing in large part to its ability to demonstrate subtle changes in bone metabolism long before radiography can. The most widely used radiopharmaceuticals for imaging of a stress injury are the ^{99m}Tc phosphate analogs; these are taken up at sites of bone turnover, probably by means of chemisorption to the surface of the bone. The degree of

PATHOMECHANISM OF STRESS FRACTURE

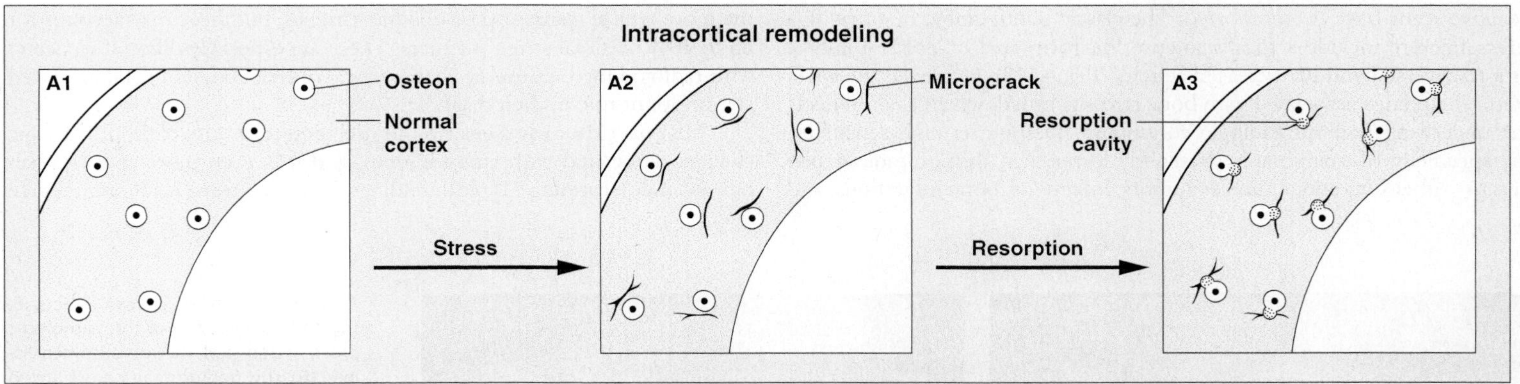

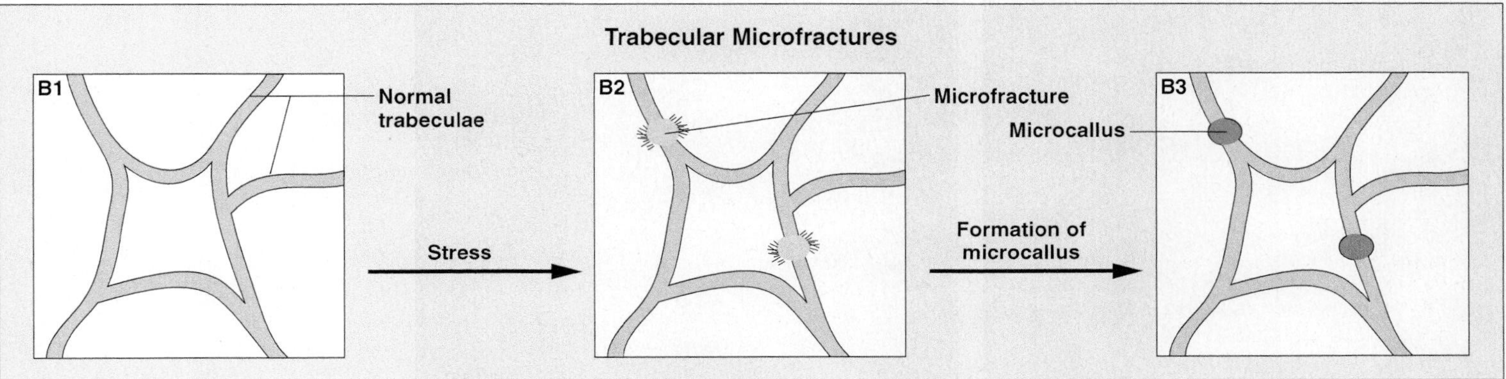

FIGURE 4.114 Pathomechanism of a stress fracture. **(A)** Intracortical remodeling. **(B)** Trabecular microfractures.

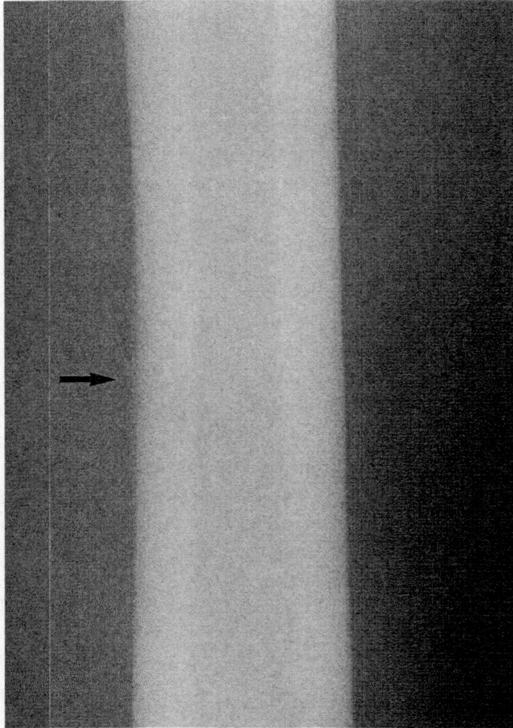

FIGURE 4.115 **Stress fracture.** The earliest radiographic changes of a stress fracture include "gray cortex" sign consisting of a subtle ill-defined cortical margin *(arrow)*. Compare with a normal definition of the contralateral cortex.

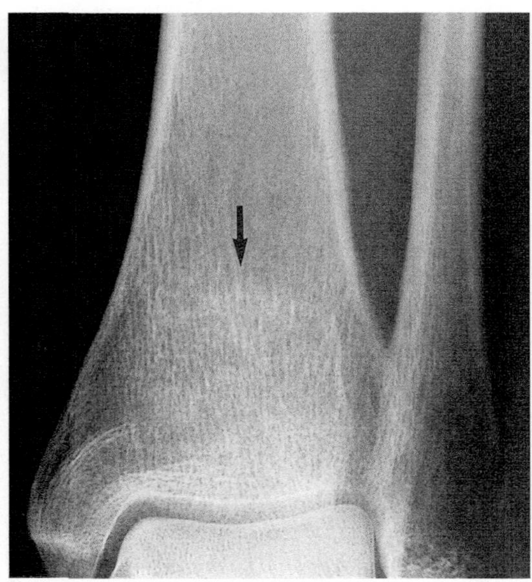

FIGURE 4.117 **Stress fracture.** The earliest radiographic changes of a stress fracture in cancellous bone include subtle blurring of the trabecular margins associated with faint sclerotic areas *(arrow)*.

uptake depends primarily on the rate of bone turnover and local blood flow, and abnormal uptake may be seen within 6 to 72 hours of injury. The sensitivity of scintigraphy approaches 100% because only a few false-negative scans have been reported. The classic scintigraphic findings of a stress fracture include a focally intense, fusiform area of cortical uptake or a transverse band of increased activity (Fig. 4.119). However, the spectrum of findings associated with bone stress is broad, which again reflects the underlying pathophysiologic continuum. Despite its high sensitivity, the specificity of scintigraphy is slightly lower than that of radiography because other conditions such as tumors, infections, bone infarctions, and shin splints or periostitis can produce a positive scan. In these instances, augmentation of scintigraphy with CT or MRI can be helpful in further diagnostic workup.

CT has a limited role in the diagnosis of stress injuries. It is less sensitive than scintigraphy and radiography in the diagnosis of stress fractures but can be quite useful for better defining an abnormality discovered with another modality (Figs. 4.120 and 4.121). It is well suited to delineate a fracture line in a location not well demonstrated on conventional radiography. Longitudinal stress fractures of the tibia occur less frequently than the more typical transverse or oblique varieties, but these may account for up to 10% of tibial stress fractures. These are especially difficult to detect with radiography because of their vertical orientation, and CT has played an important role in their diagnosis.

MRI is extremely sensitive in the detection of pathophysiologic changes associated with stress injuries, and it is even more specific than radionuclide scanning. Typical findings in early stress reactions include

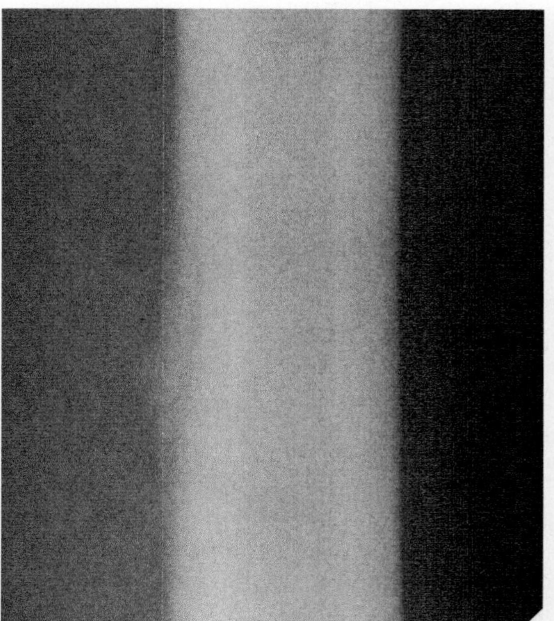

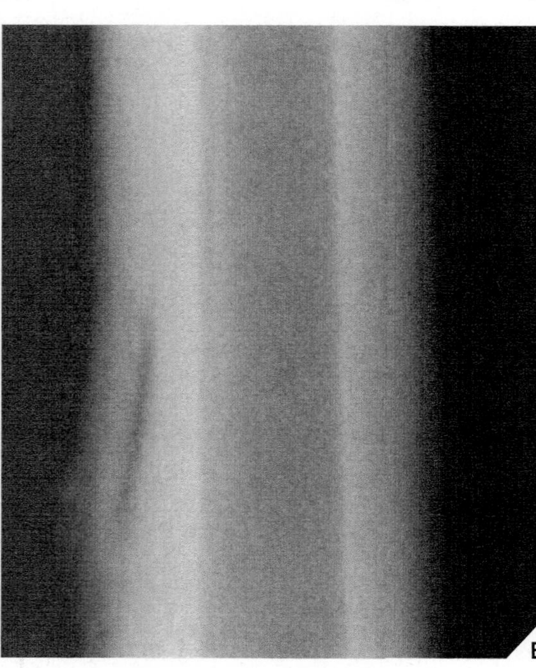

FIGURE 4.116 **Stress fracture.** **(A)** With progression of the pathologic process, a cortical fracture becomes visible. **(B)** This finding may be enhanced with a trispiral tomography.

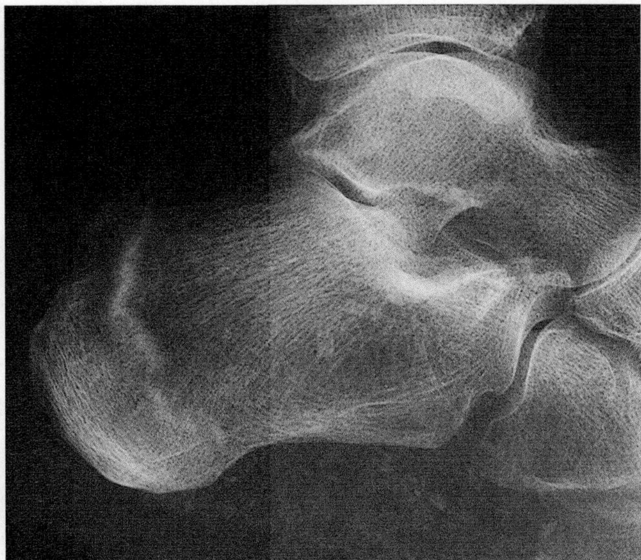

FIGURE 4.118 **Stress fracture.** Typical appearance of a stress fracture in the calcaneus: a vertical band of sclerosis in the posterior aspect of the bone is characteristic of this injury.

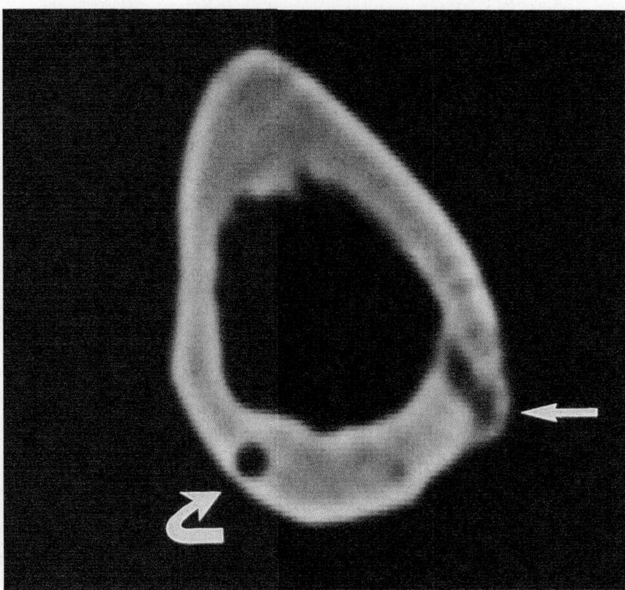

FIGURE 4.120 **CT of the stress fracture.** A stress fracture in the tibia *(arrow)* demonstrated by CT. The *curved arrow* points to the nutrient foramen.

areas of low signal intensity in the marrow on T1-weighted images that increase in signal intensity with T2 weighting. Fat saturation techniques, such as inversion recovery (IR) or fast SE (FSE) T2-weighted imaging with frequency-selective fat saturation, are especially useful for identifying these injuries. The increased water content of the associated medullary edema or hemorrhage results in high signal intensity against the dark background of suppressed fat such that these sequences should maximize sensitivity. On T2-weighted images of more advanced lesions, low-intensity bands, contiguous with the cortex, have been seen within the marrow edema; these presumably represent fracture lines (Figs. 4.122 and 4.123). The multiplanar capability of MRI provides a further advantage by allowing for optimal demonstration of the fracture line. In some cases, increased signal intensity has also been observed in juxtacortical and subperiosteal locations. MRI has been advocated as a problem-solving modality, such as in a patient with negative or confusing bone scan. It may secure the diagnosis if the fracture line is identified.

A subtype of stress fracture is the *insufficiency fracture*, which occurs in the osteoporotic bone. Classic stress fractures are produced by increased stress in an otherwise normal bone. Insufficiency fractures occur when normal stress is applied to an abnormal, osteoporotic bone. Typically, insufficiency fractures occur in the elderly and are more common in the sacrum, oriented parallel to the sacroiliac joints and occasionally transverse across the sacrum. They can be unilateral or bilateral, involving both sacral alae. When they are bilateral and are associated with a transverse fracture of the sacrum, the bone scan offers a characteristic "H"-shaped increased isotopic uptake (Fig. 4.124). Other common areas of insufficiency/osteoporotic fractures are in the vertebral bodies, pubic bones (parasymphyseal), femoral neck, and superior aspect of the acetabulum. Recently, a lot of attention was paid to the insufficiency fractures occurring in the distal femur and proximal tibia at the knee joint (Fig. 4.125). These subchondral insufficiency fractures of the knee, termed *SIFK*, originally were thought to represent spontaneous osteonecrosis (SONK) resulting

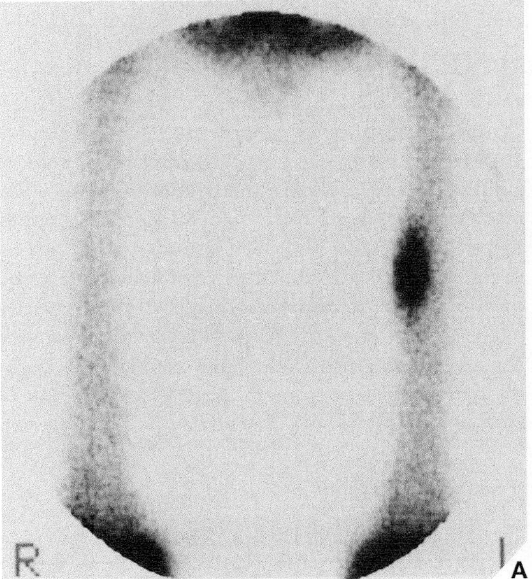

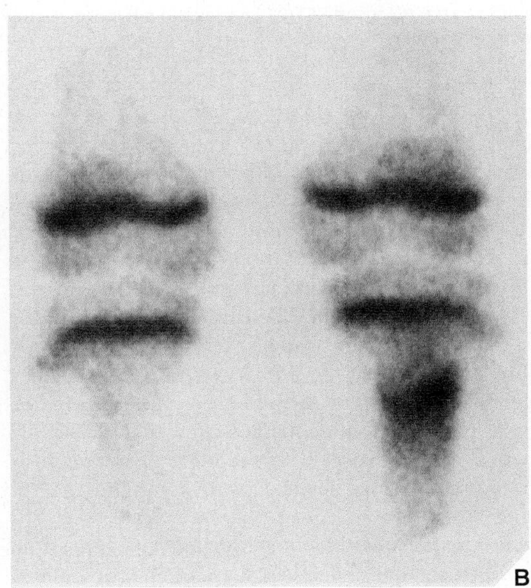

FIGURE 4.119 **Scintigraphic presentation of a stress fracture.** **(A)** Fusiform area of increased uptake in the medial cortex of the left femur. **(B)** A transverse band of increased uptake in the proximal diaphysis of the left tibia. Observe normal increased uptake of the radiopharmaceutical tracer within the growth plates.

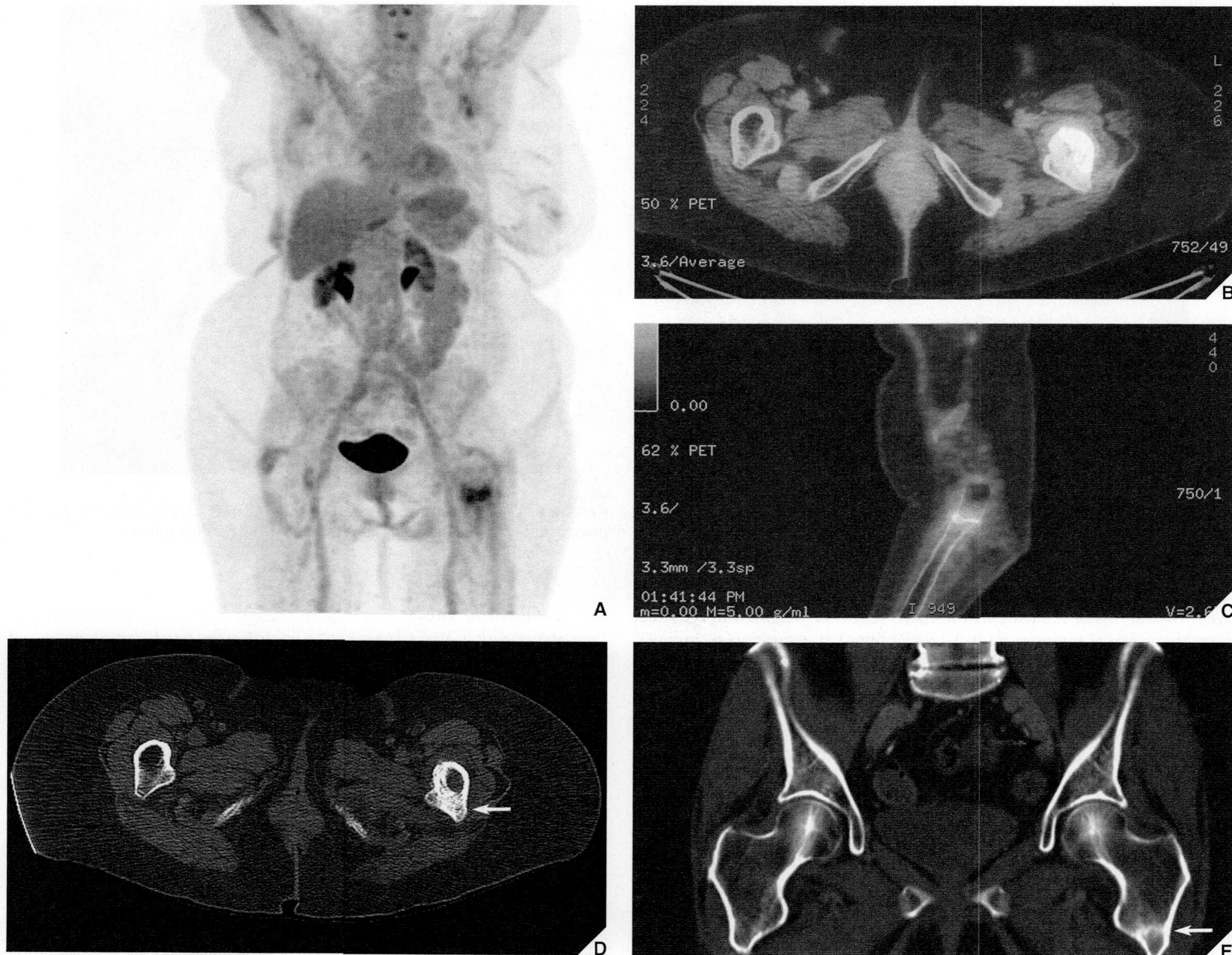

FIGURE 4.121 Stress fracture demonstrated by positron emission tomography (PET)/CT. A 45-year-old woman underwent mastectomy for a breast carcinoma. PET/CT study was performed to screen for possible skeletal metastases. **(A)** A whole-body PET scan shows transverse band of increased activity in the subtrochanteric region of the left femur. Axial **(B)** and sagittal **(C)** fused PET/CT images show hypermetabolic focus in the same location. **(D)** Axial and **(E)** coronal reformatted CT images confirmed the presence of a stress fracture *(arrows)*.

from vascular insufficiency with venous occlusion leading to venous hypertension and hypoxia. Although still not a fully understood condition, most cases of SIFK are seen within medial weight-bearing compartment of the knee due to the associated repetitive physiologic loading applied to weakened trabeculae, commonly in association with osteopenia and diminished protective function of the articular cartilage and meniscus. Despite the concurrent finding of low bone density, in majority of the patients, osteopenia is not the underlying cause of these fractures. A study by Yamamoto and Bullough showed that the primary event is insufficiency fracture followed by necrosis limited to the area between the fracture line and the subchondral bone plate. It is currently accepted that an SONK is an SIFK that progressed into collapse, with secondary osteonecrosis found within the collapsed tissues. More detailed discussion of these entities is provided in Chapter 9.

Osteoporotic patients treated with bisphosphonates have shown an increased incidence of subtrochanteric/diaphyseal transverse or oblique fractures of the femur. These fractures occur in the normal or slightly thickened cortex of the femur, in a younger population than the classic sacral or vertebral insufficiency fractures, and are dependent on the length of the bisphosphonate treatment (Figs. 4.126 and 4.127). Bisphosphonates are antiresorptive agents that act through inhibition of osteoclasts through apoptosis, thus reducing the overall bone turnover. Although this action results in increased bone mineral density, nonetheless suppressed bone turnover decreases remodeling and retards healing of cracks that occur in the cortex as a result of normal activity, referred to as *microdamage*. The prolonged use of bisphosphonates therapy causes an accumulation of this pathologic process and leads to reduced heterogeneity of the organic matrix and mineral properties, increased advanced glycation end products of the extracellular bone matrix, and deterioration of bone quality, which results in atypical femoral fractures.

Injury to Soft Tissues

Under normal physiologic circumstances, soft tissues such as muscles, tendons, ligaments, articular menisci, and intervertebral disks are only faintly outlined or not visible at all on conventional radiographs. As a result, only

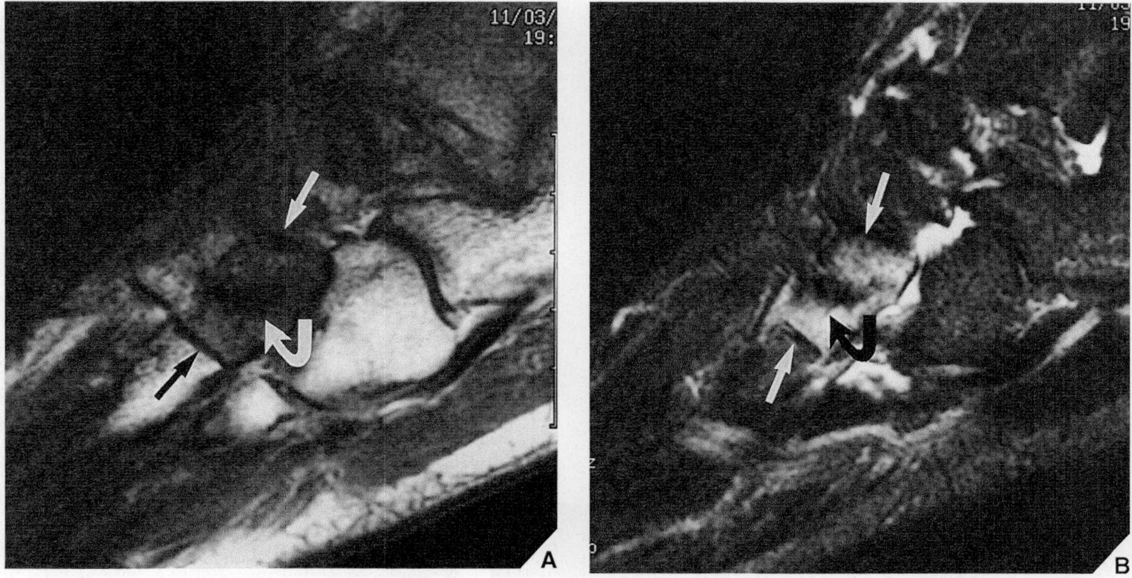

FIGURE 4.122 MRI of the stress fracture. **(A)** Sagittal T1-weighted image shows a diffusely decreased signal in the lateral cuneiform *(arrows)* and a band of signal void in the center of the bone *(curved arrow)*. **(B)** Sagittal FSE IR MR image shows increased signal in the cuneiform bone *(arrows)*, representing changes due to edema and hemorrhage. The stress fracture remains of low signal intensity *(curved arrow)*.

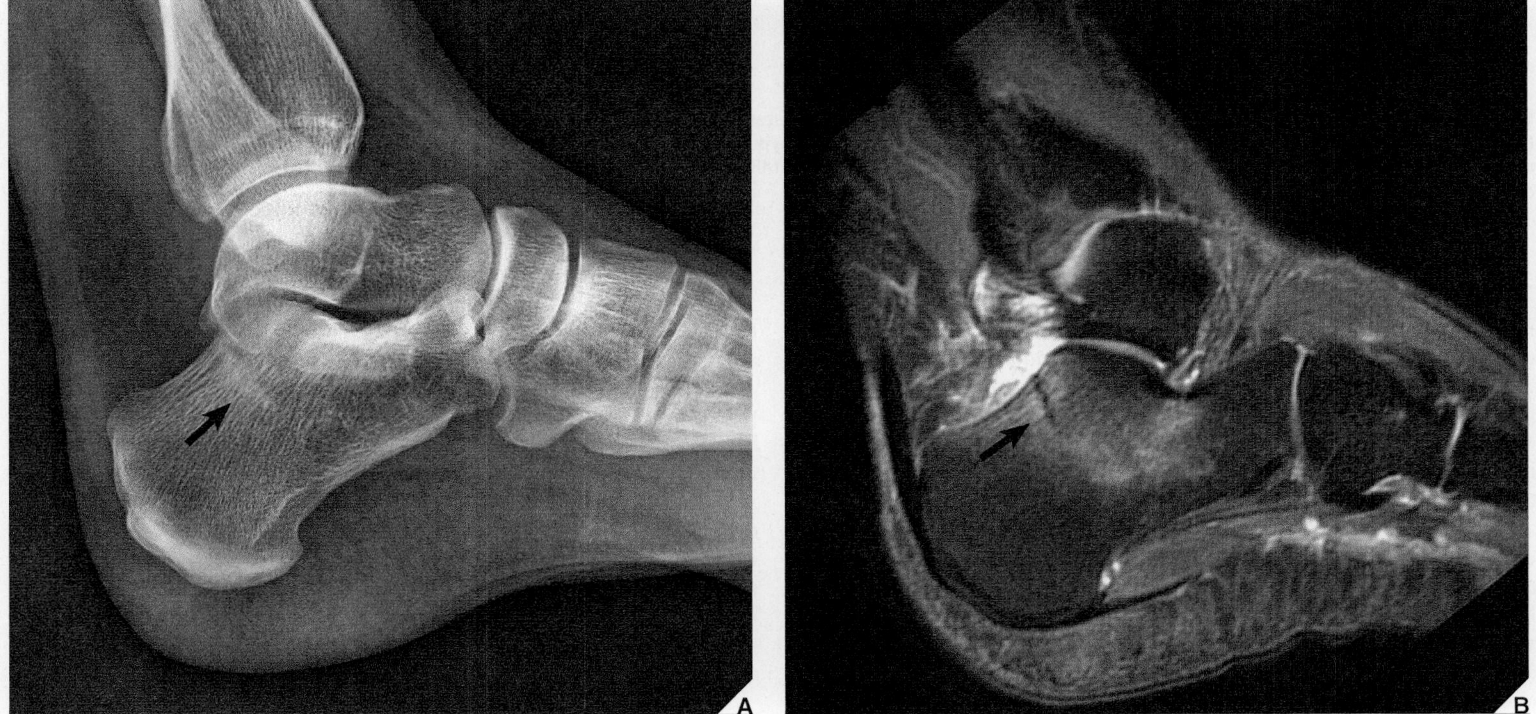

FIGURE 4.123 MRI of the stress fracture. A 44-year-old woman presented with a heel pain after completing a 10-km race. **(A)** Lateral radiograph of the ankle shows a vertically oriented sclerotic band in the calcaneus *(arrow)*. **(B)** Sagittal proton density–weighted fat-suppressed MR image shows diffuse area of high–signal intensity bone edema surrounding a linear zone of low signal, representing a stress fracture *(arrow)*.

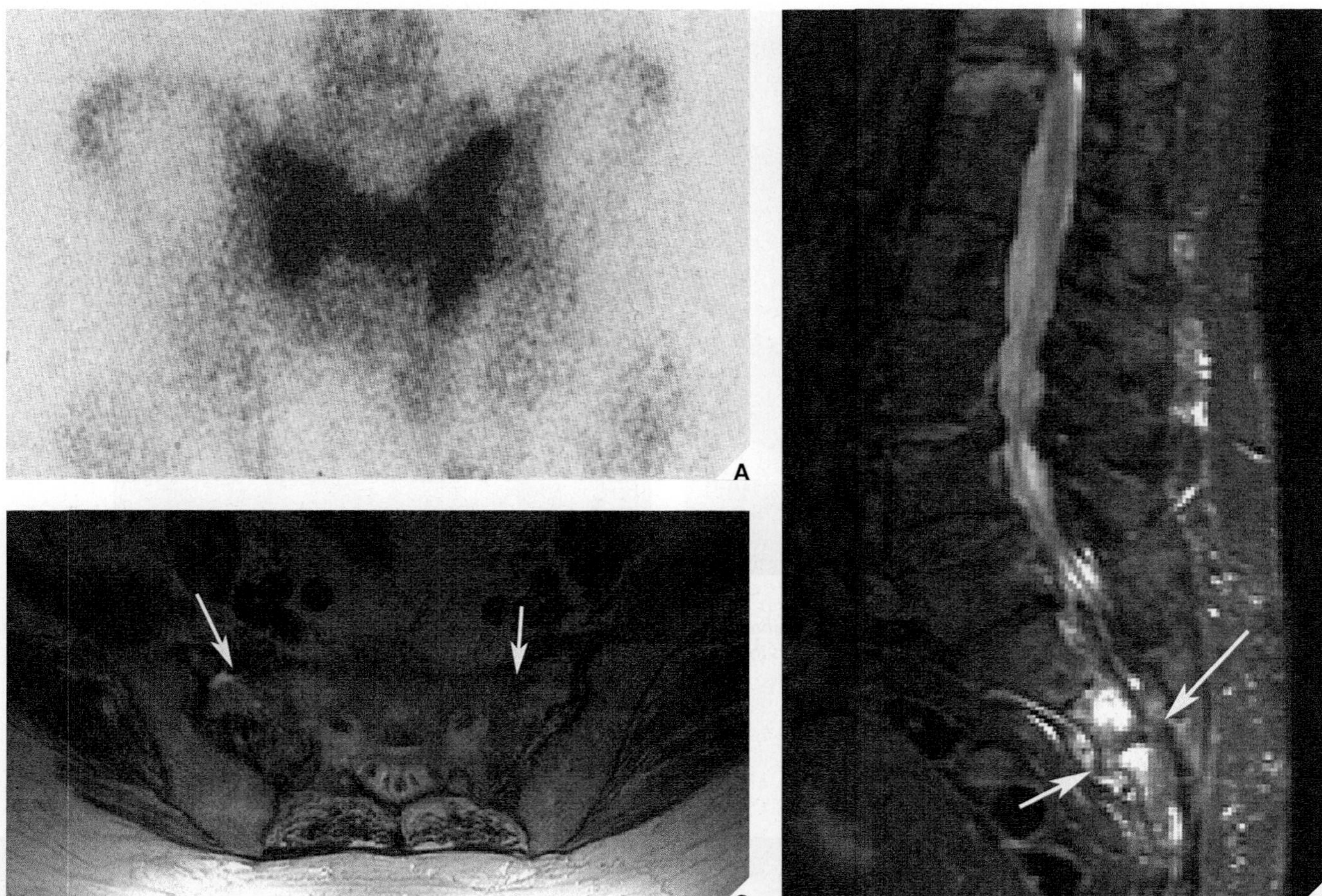

FIGURE 4.124 Insufficiency fractures of the sacrum. **(A)** Bone scan demonstrates classic H-shaped areas of increased activity in the sacrum, the so-called *Honda sign*. **(B)** Sagittal short time inversion recovery (STIR) pulse sequence MR image shows a hyperintensive band at the level of the S1-2 sacral segments *(arrows)*, corresponding to the horizontally oriented fracture line seen on the bone scan. **(C)** Axial T1-weighted MR image demonstrates irregular low–signal intensity bands in the sacral ala *(arrows)* corresponding to the vertically oriented fracture lines seen on the bone scan.

rarely, as in such traumatic conditions as myositis ossificans (see previous discussion) or certain tears of ligaments and tendons, does conventional radiography suffice to demonstrate trauma to the soft tissues (Fig. 4.128). Adequate evaluation of an injury to these structures and of the progress of treatment, consequently, requires supplemental studies, which may include stress radiography, arthrography, myelography, CT (Fig. 4.129), and MRI (Fig. 4.130).

MRI, in particular, is considered to be the best imaging modality for evaluating traumatic soft-tissue injuries. Differences in signal intensity enable abnormalities of the various structures (muscles, tendons, ligaments, fascias, vessels, and nerves) to be effectively demonstrated. Posttraumatic tenosynovitis, joint effusion, and soft-tissue hematomas are also seen well on MR images (see Fig. 4.130). Tears of various ligaments and tendons can be accurately diagnosed; for instance, when evaluating tendon injuries, MRI provides information regarding the location of the tear (whether it is within the tendon, at the tendon insertion, or at the musculotendinous interface), the size of the gap between both tendon ends, the size of the hematoma at the rupture site, and the presence of any inflammatory component (Fig. 4.131). MRI is also effective to demonstrate, characterize, and classify so-called *Morel-Lavallée lesion* (M-LL) (Fig. 4.132). M-LL is a posttraumatic, closed degloving soft-tissue injury occurring deep to subcutaneous plane, resulting in abrupt separation of the skin and subcutaneous tissue from the underlying fascia. The result is disruption of perforating vessels and lymphatics, thus creating a potential space filled with serosanguineous fluid, blood, hemolymph, and necrotic fat. An inflammatory reaction results in the formation of a peripheral pseudocapsule. The treatment depends on the size, location, and age of the lesion and ranges from percutaneous drainage to open debridement and irrigation.

MRI is invaluable in identifying various injuries to the muscles that may occur during traumatic hip dislocation (Figs. 4.133 and 4.134). Normal skeletal muscle exhibits an intermediate or slightly prolonged T1 relaxation time and a short T2 relaxation time relative to other soft tissues. When muscles are injured, MRI can effectively delineate the variable degrees of strain, contusion, tear, or hematoma and permits the quantification of these injuries. Acute muscle strain gives rise to increased T2 signal intensity, reflecting tissue edema. When an acute muscle tear occurs, muscle shape and architecture appear altered, and the signal within the muscle shows an abnormal increase because of intramuscular hemorrhage and edema.

Sports Injuries

An extensive number of sports-related injuries have been described—all related to the area of the body suffering the stress of a particular type of physical activity. Many of them are not specific of a particular sport and can be seen in an occasional trauma not related to a sport. For instance, although anterior cruciate ligament tears more commonly occur in soccer players and skiers, they are also very frequently seen in patients suffering a twisting injury to the knee not related to sports activities. Nevertheless, some other injuries are quite unique and seen very frequently in association with a particular sport, to the point they are named after that sport. In the

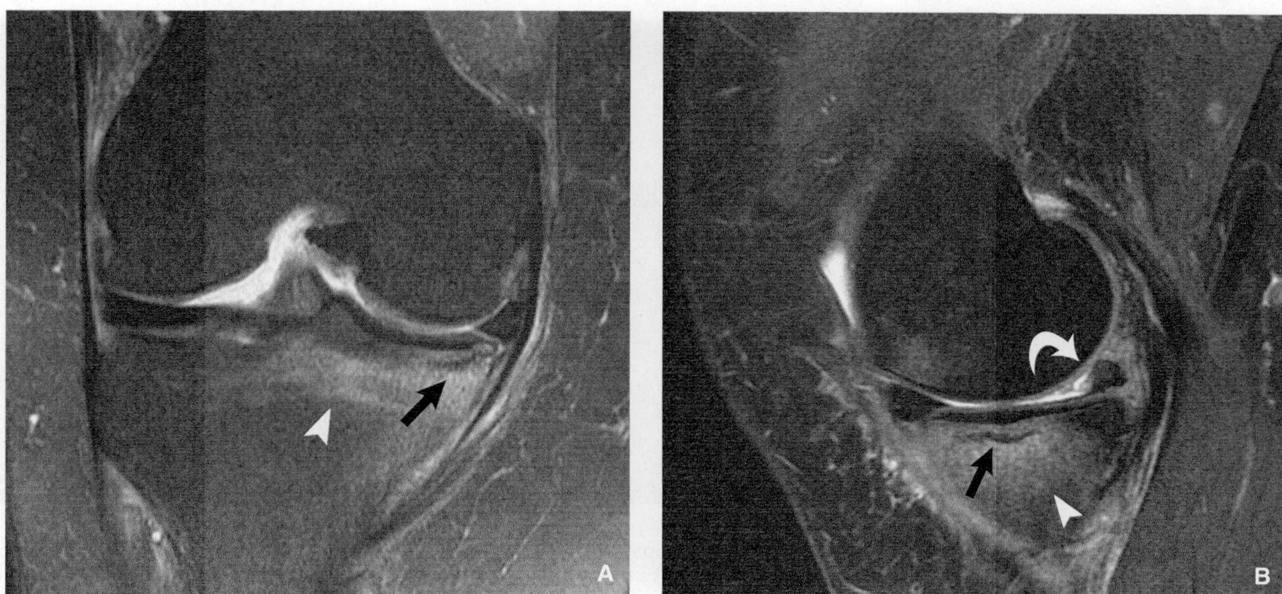

FIGURE 4.125 SIFK. A 77-year-old woman presented with pain in the right knee. The radiographs of the knee (not shown here) demonstrated no fracture. Coronal **(A)** and sagittal **(B)** proton density–weighted fat-suppressed MR images show low–signal intensity subchondral fracture line *(black arrows)* surrounded by high-intensity bone marrow edema *(arrowheads)*. Note also a tear of the posterior horn of the medial meniscus *(curved arrow)*.

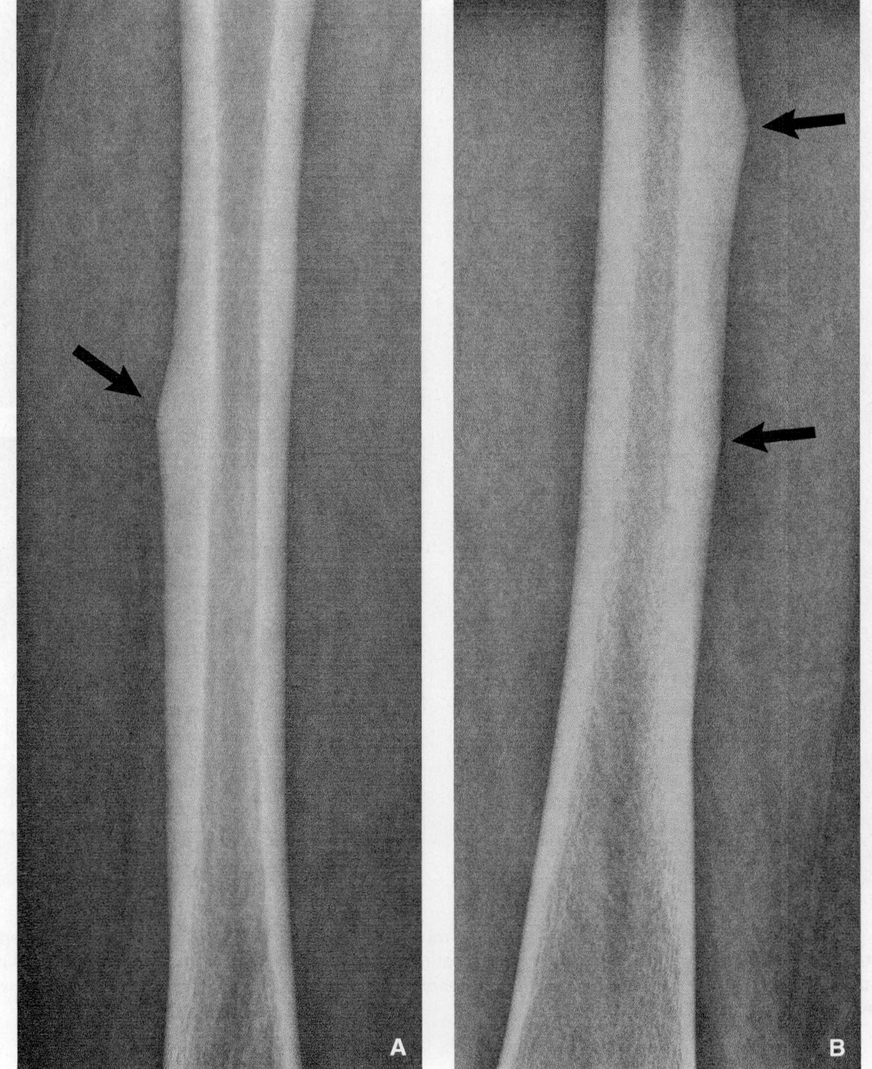

FIGURE 4.126 **Bisphosphonate insufficiency fractures.** A 67-year-old woman was treated for osteoporosis with alendronate for past 6 years. Anteroposterior radiographs of right **(A)** and left **(B)** femora show characteristic "nipple" or "wart" sign *(arrows)* representing insufficiency fractures.

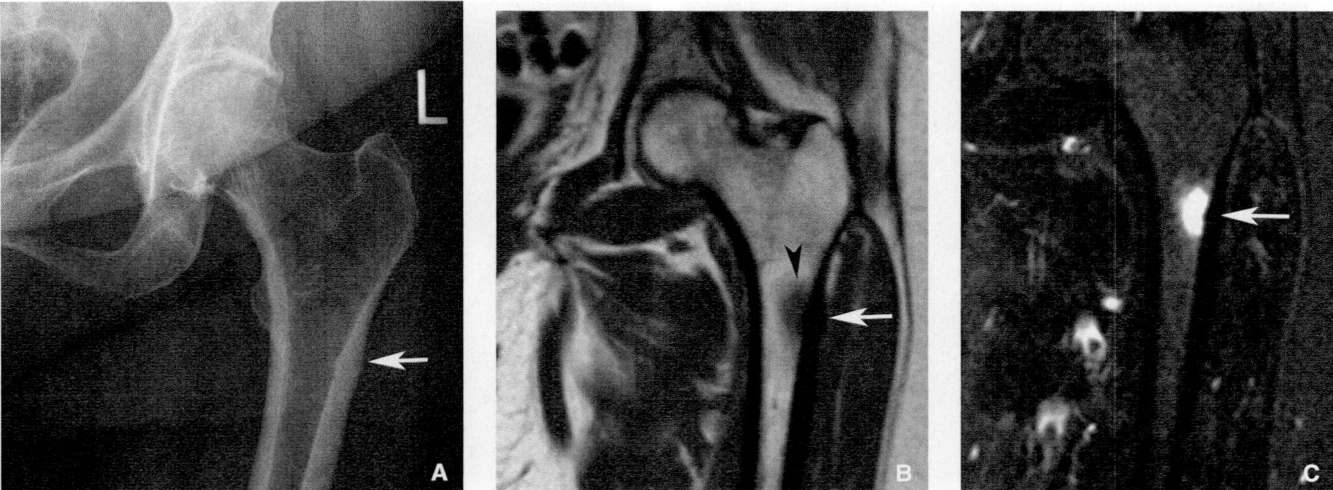

FIGURE 4.127 **Bisphosphonate insufficiency fracture.** An elderly postmenopausal woman with osteoporosis treated for several years with bisphosphonates presented with pain in the left hip. **(A)** Anteroposterior radiograph of the left hip shows a focal area of thickening in the lateral cortex of the left proximal femur *(white arrow)*. Coronal T1-weighted **(B)** and coronal T2-weighted **(C)** fat-suppressed MR images show an area of focal bone marrow edema *(black arrowhead)* adjacent to the focal area of cortical thickening *(white arrows)*. The location in the lateral cortex of the proximal femoral shaft, the focal area of cortical thickening with or without visualization of a fracture line, and the adjacent bone marrow edema are characteristic findings in bisphosphonate insufficiency fractures.

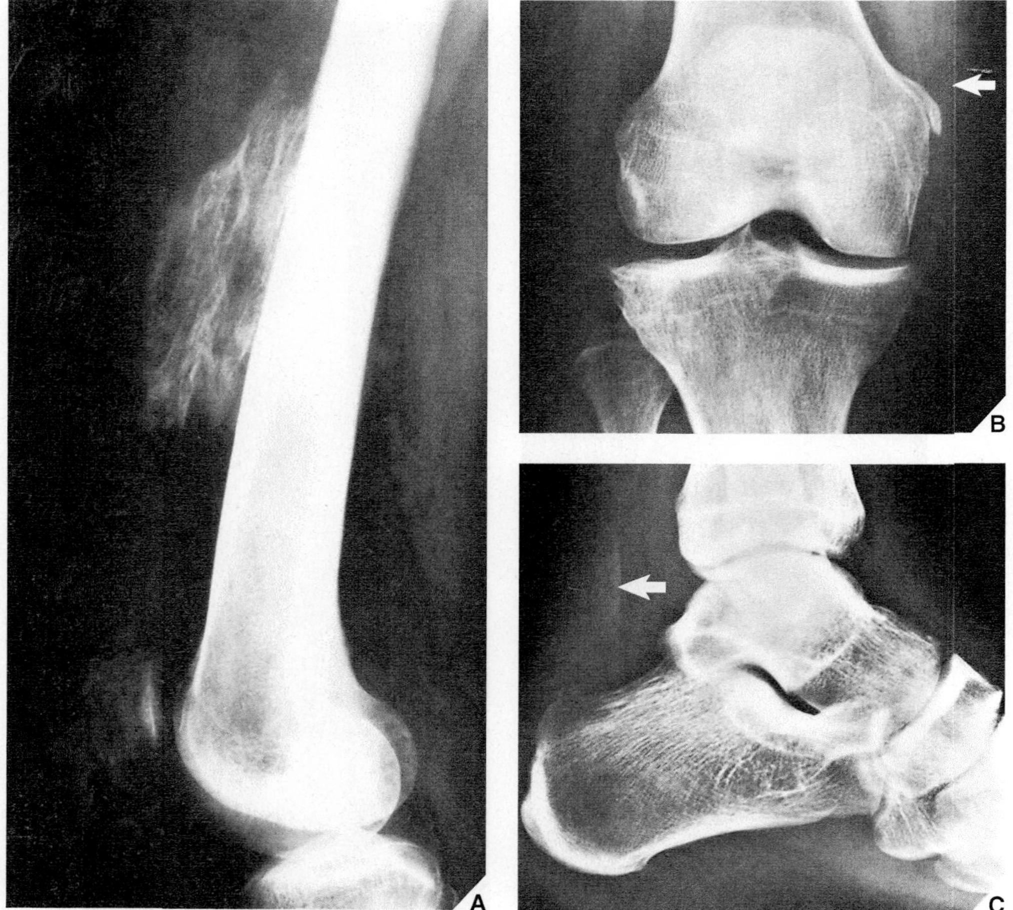

FIGURE 4.128 **Soft-tissue injury.** **(A)** A common complication of trauma to the muscular structures, myositis ossificans, is characterized by the formation of a bone in the injured muscle. This condition is apparent on conventional radiography. **(B)** The calcification of the medial collateral ligament of the knee, known as *Pellegrini-Stieda lesion (arrow)*, represents the sequela of traumatic tear of this ligament. **(C)** In certain instances, the tear of a tendon may be diagnosed on radiography. The lateral radiograph of the ankle shows the typical appearance of a torn Achilles tendon *(arrow)*.

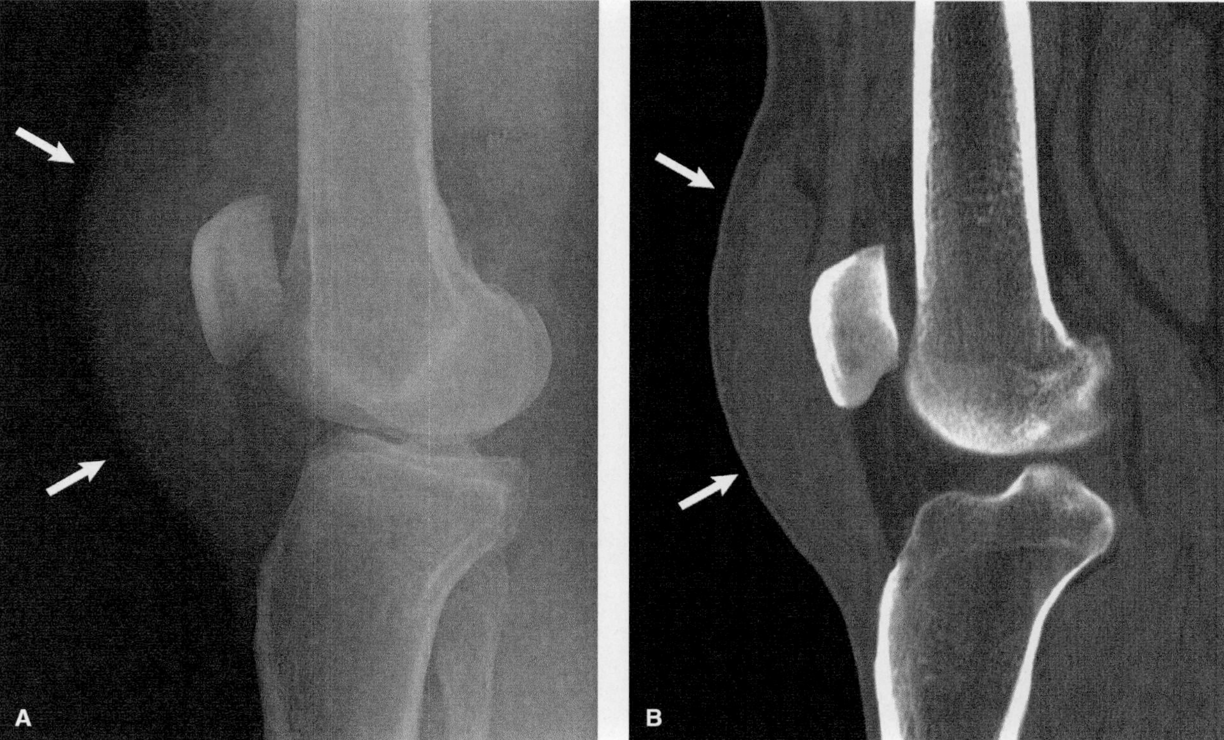

FIGURE 4.129 **Radiography and CT of soft-tissue hematoma.** Lateral radiograph **(A)** and sagittal reformatted CT image **(B)** of the knee of a 60-year-old man show a large prepatellar hematoma *(arrows)*.

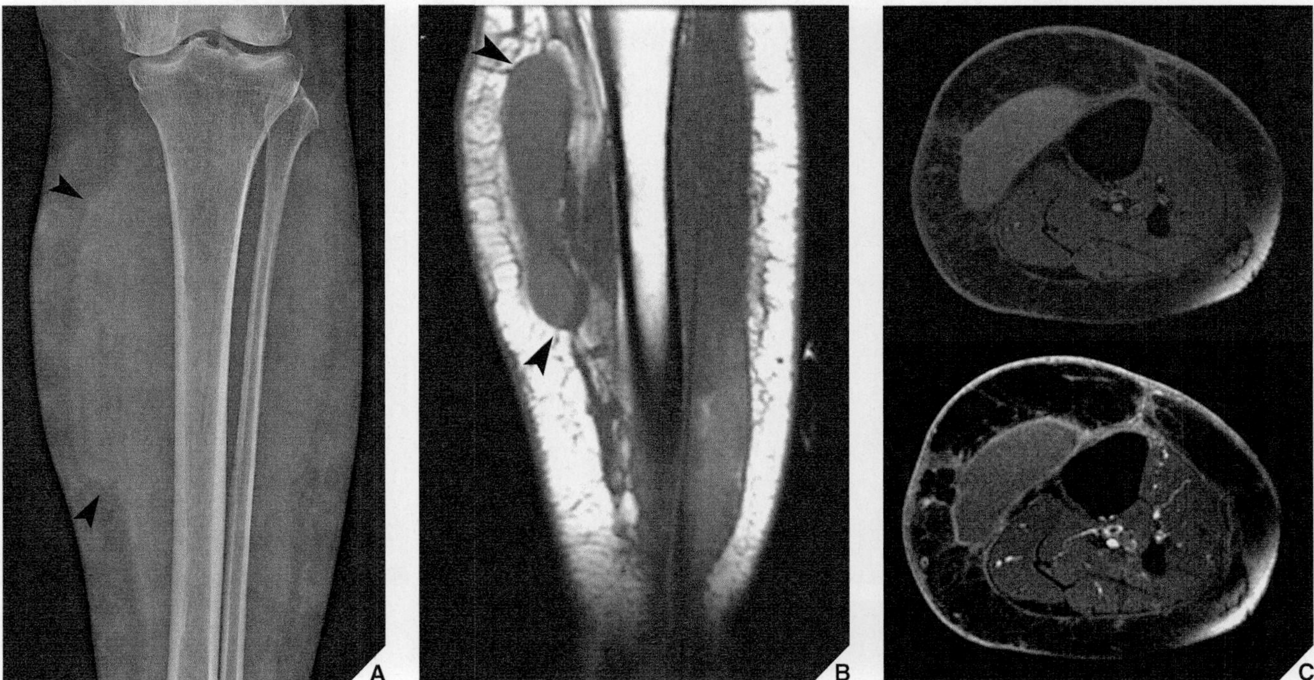

FIGURE 4.130 **MRI of soft-tissue hematoma.** A 64-year-old woman injured her left leg in a bicycle accident. **(A)** Anteroposterior radiograph of the leg shows an oval density adjacent to the soleus muscle *(arrowheads)*. **(B)** Coronal T1-weighted MR image reveals sharply demarcated homogeneous mass of intermediate signal intensity within the deep subcutaneous fat *(arrowheads)*. **(C)** Axial proton density–weighted fat-suppressed image *(top)* and one after intravenous administration of gadolinium *(bottom)* demonstrate only peripheral rim enhancement of the soft-tissue hematoma.

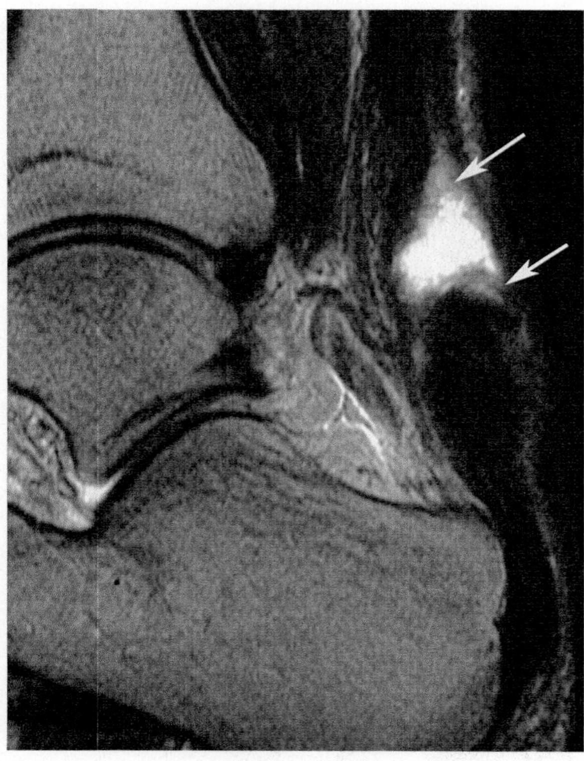

FIGURE 4.131 MRI of the tear of the Achilles tendon. Sagittal T2-weighted MRI of the ankle shows a discontinuity of the Achilles tendon near its insertion to the calcaneus *(arrows)*. A focal hematoma is seen at the rupture site.

following section, the most common injuries with names linked to a particular sport are discussed.

Upper Extremity

Weight Lifter Pectoralis

Bodybuilders and weight lifters can injure their pectoralis muscle when attempting to excessively stress their pectoralis muscles during bench press exercises. Ruptures can be partial (20%) or complete (80%), often unilateral, and are associated with acute pain and development of a focal hematoma at the site of the tear, which commonly occurs at the myotendinous junction (Fig. 4.135). The pectoralis major muscle is most often involved and rarely the pectoralis minor muscle.

Little League Shoulder

This injury is a Salter-Harris type I fracture of the proximal physis of the humerus produced by a rotational stress during baseball pitching. This injury occurs in children between the ages of 13 and 16 years old. Pain aggravated by throwing is the clinical manifestation. MRI shows widening of the growth plate with periphyseal edema (Fig. 4.136; see also Fig. 4.39A).

Golfer's Elbow

Also known as *medial epicondylitis*, it is a stress injury of the common flexor and pronator tendon origin in the medial epicondyle of the humerus. This lesion can also be related to improper golfing technique, hitting the ground instead of the ball, causing an abrupt deceleration that strains the medial elbow compartment. MRI typically depicts signal alteration of the common flexor–pronator group, occasionally with partial tears (Fig. 4.137).

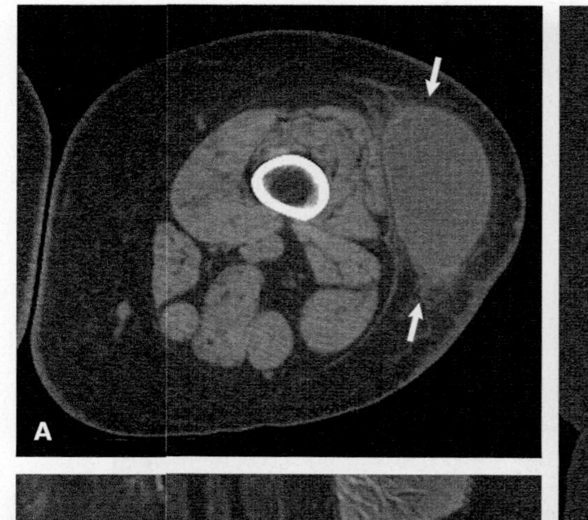

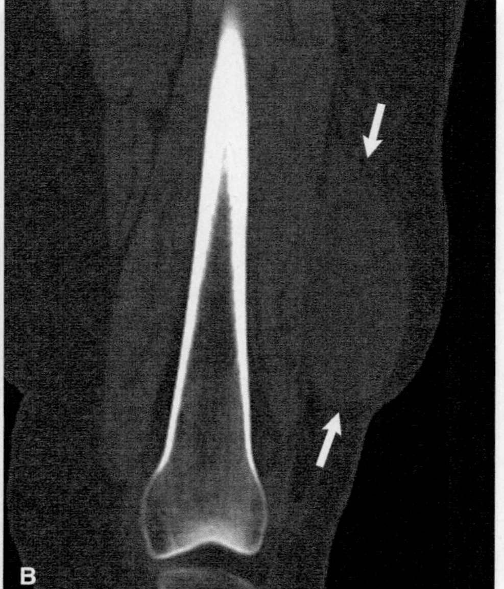

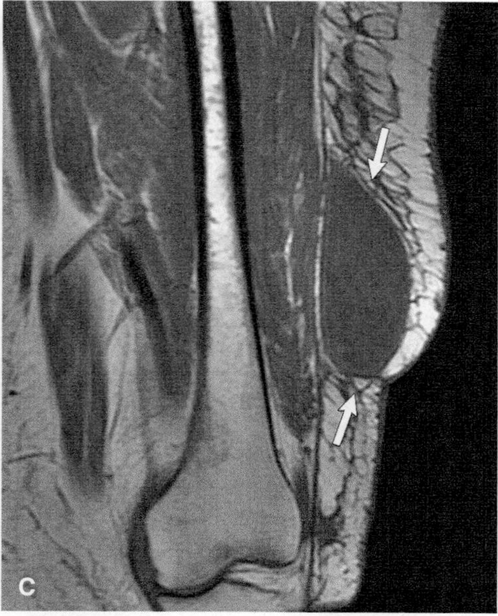

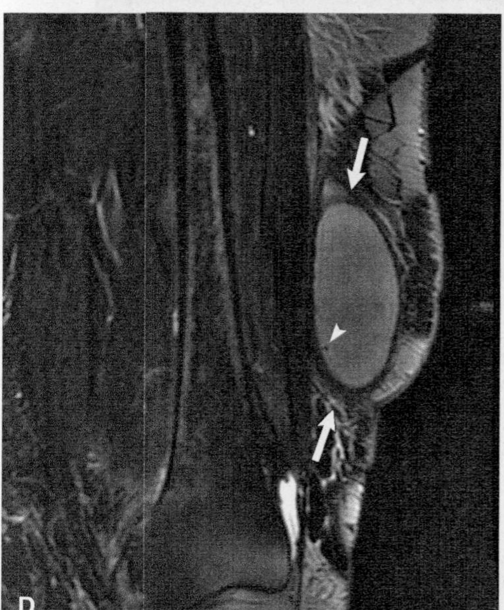

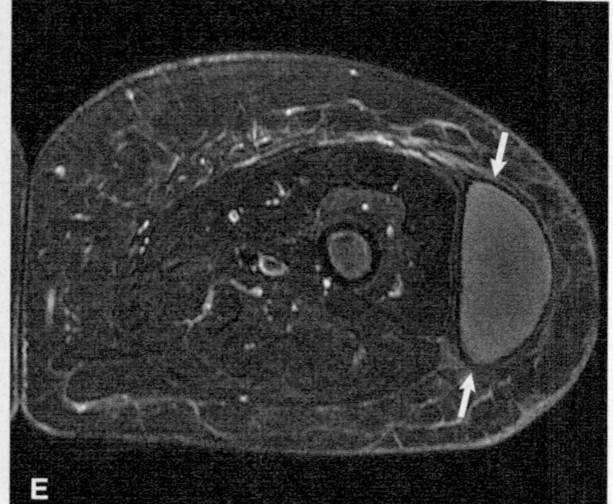

FIGURE 4.132 CT and MRI of M-LL. A 59-year-old woman presented with history of sudden violent shear-type injury to the anterolateral aspect of her right thigh. **(A)** Axial and **(B)** coronal reformatted CT images show a large, rounded, well-circumscribed lesion with smooth contours in the subcutaneous location compressing the vastus lateralis of the quadriceps muscle and exhibiting fluid-type attenuation *(arrows)*. **(C)** Coronal T1-weighted MR image shows homogeneous intermediate signal intensity lesion abutting the iliotibial band *(arrows)*. On coronal T2-weighted fat-suppressed **(D)** and axial T2 FSE **(E)** MR images, the lesion *(arrows)* shows higher signal when compared to the adjacent muscles, with low-intensity pseudocapsule and droplet of fat *(arrowhead)* (see also Fig. 8.76).

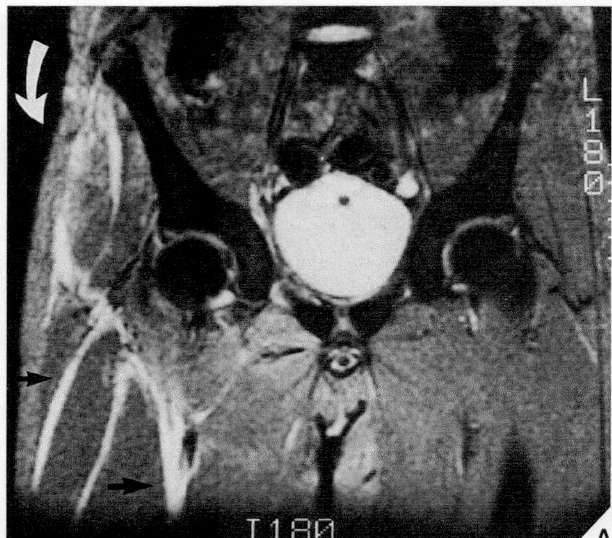

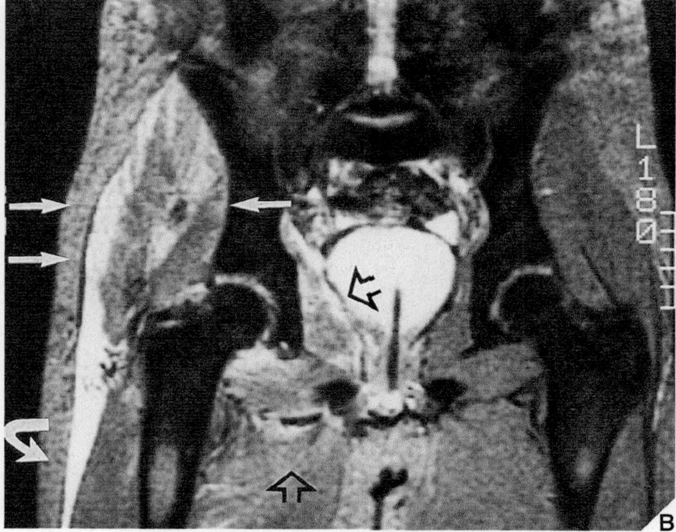

FIGURE 4.133 MRI of a soft-tissue injury. A 14-year-old boy presented with posterior dislocation of the right femoral head. After the dislocation was reduced, MRI was performed to assess the injury to the soft tissues. **(A)** Coronal T2*-weighted (multiplanar gradient recalled, TR 500/TE 15 msec, flip angle 15 degrees) sequence shows markedly increased signal surrounding the vastus lateralis and intermedius muscles *(straight arrows)*. Note also the injury involving the medial fascial compartment and gluteal region muscles *(curved arrow)*. **(B)** More posterior coronal section demonstrates increased signal in the gluteus medius and minimus muscles *(straight white arrows)* and the tensor fasciae latae *(curved arrow)*. There is also an injury of the obturator internus, obturator externus, and adductor brevis and magnus muscles *(open arrows)*. (Reprinted by permission from Springer: Laorr A, Greenspan A, Anderson MW, et al. Traumatic hip dislocation: early MRI findings. *Skeletal Radiol* 1995;24:239–245.)

Tennis Elbow

Also known as *lateral epicondylitis*, tennis elbow is related to overuse of the hand and wrist extensor muscles, most commonly the extensor carpi radialis brevis muscle. This lesion is related to improper backhand use, which causes excessive stress of the common extensor tendon, leading to tendinosis, peritendinitis, and partial tears, well demonstrated on MRI (Fig. 4.138). Improper hand and wrist positioning and eccentric ball impact in the tennis racket have also been incriminated as potential causes of tennis elbow.

Little League Elbow

This lesion is an avulsion fracture of the ossification center of the medial epicondyle in the immature skeleton produced by traction by the common flexor tendon during baseball pitching, using improper throwing technique with excessive valgus stress. MRI shows the displaced medial epicondyle and the surrounding soft-tissue edema (Fig. 4.139).

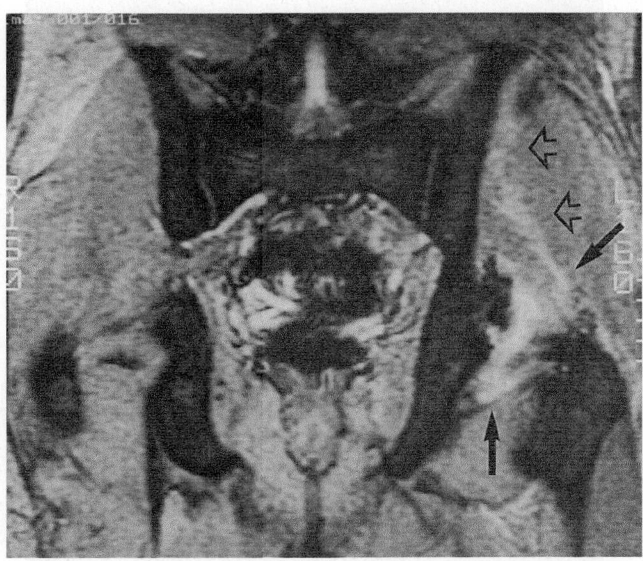

FIGURE 4.134 MRI of a soft-tissue injury. In another patient, a 20-year-old man who sustained posterior dislocation in the left hip, a coronal T2-weighted (multiplanar gradient recalled; TR 550/TE 15 msec, flip angle 15 degrees) MRI shows disruption and increased signal in the region of the superior and inferior gemelli muscles *(arrows)*. There is also an injury to the gluteal muscles *(open arrows)*. (Reprinted by permission from Springer: Laorr A, Greenspan A, Anderson MW, et al. Traumatic hip dislocation: early MRI findings. *Skeletal Radiol* 1995;24:239–245.)

Baseball Pitcher's Elbow

The essential lesion in this entity involves the anterior band of the ulnar collateral ligament of the elbow, which can be completely or partially torn. The lesion is produced by repetitive valgus stress during the early and late cocking phases of the throwing motion (valgus extension overload syndrome [VEOS]). It is often accompanied by other lesions in the elbow, including contusion of the capitellum and radial head, chondral lesions of the olecranon, and ulnar neuritis due to traction. These lesions are all well demonstrated with MRI (Fig. 4.140).

Goalkeeper's Elbow

Repetitive hyperextension trauma to the elbow during blocking of the ball by the goalkeeper leads to abutment of the olecranon in the olecranon fossa of the humerus, producing cartilage damage, osteophyte formation, and intraarticular loose bodies.

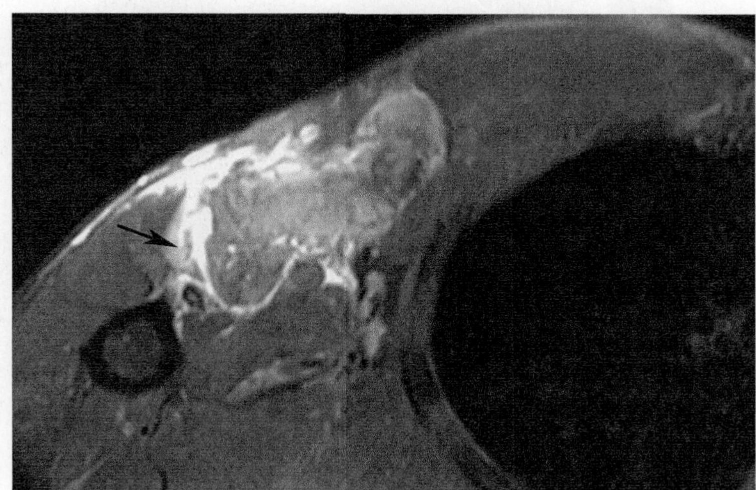

FIGURE 4.135 Weight lifter pectoralis. A 27-year-old bodybuilder presented with a sudden onset of pain in the right chest during weight lifting. Axial proton density–weighted fat-saturated MR image demonstrates a complete tear of the pectoralis major muscle with focal edema and hematoma *(arrow)*.

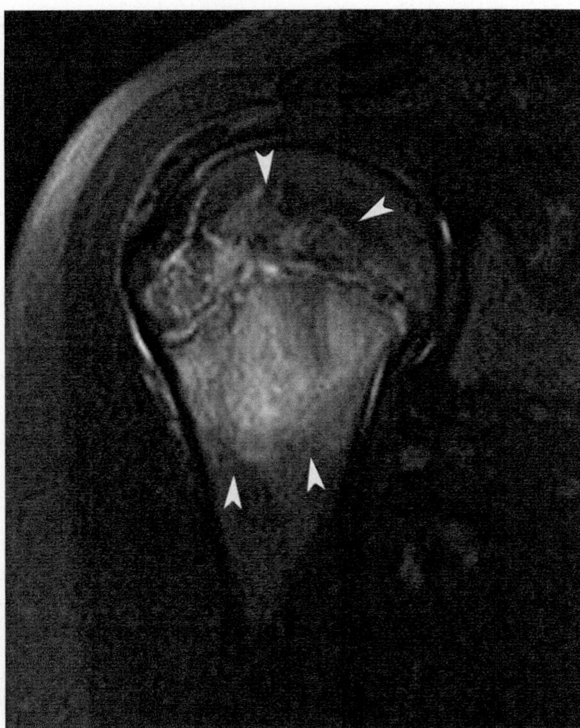

FIGURE 4.136 Little League shoulder. A 13-year-old boy, a baseball pitcher, presented with a chronic shoulder pain. Oblique coronal T2-weighted fat-saturated MR image demonstrates extensive metaphyseal stress edema extending into the epiphysis across the growth plate *(arrowheads)*.

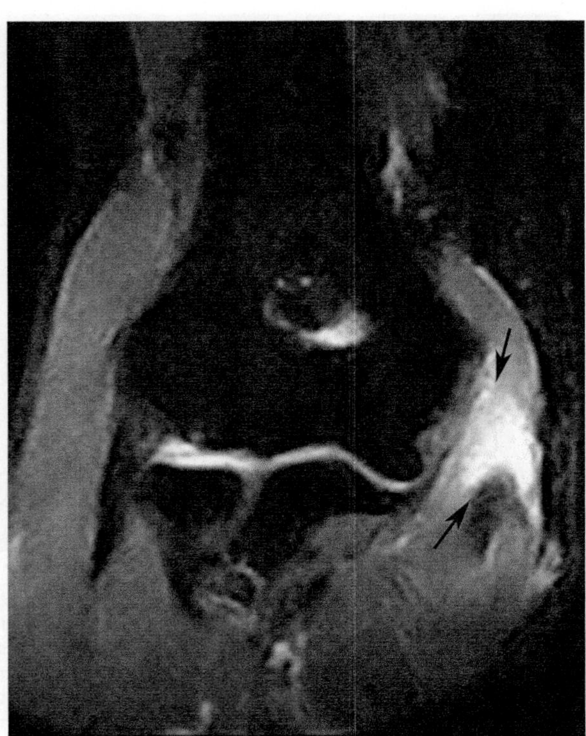

FIGURE 4.137 Golfer's elbow. A 67-year-old man presented with a medial elbow pain after golfing. Coronal short time inversion recovery (STIR) pulse sequence MR image demonstrates a tear of the common flexor tendon with focal edema and hematoma *(arrows)*.

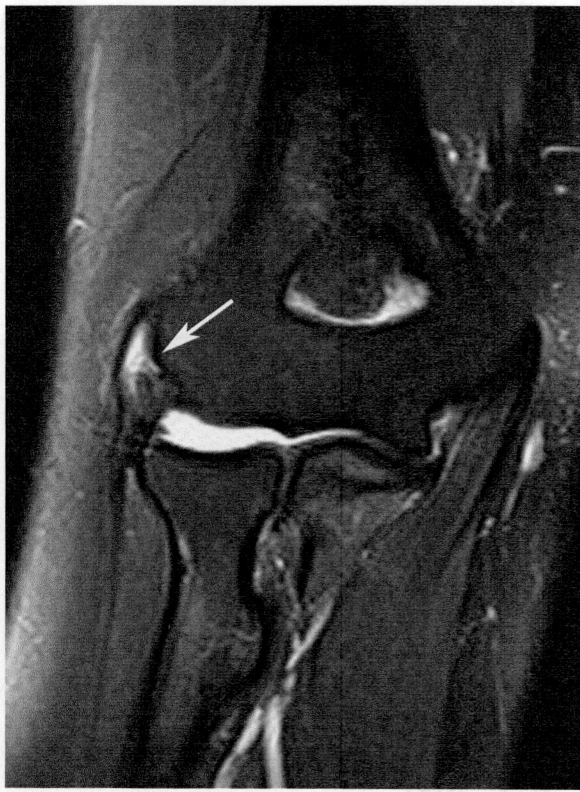

FIGURE 4.138 Tennis elbow. A 32-year-old man, an avid tennis player, presented with chronic, worsening right lateral elbow pain. Coronal short time inversion recovery (STIR) pulse sequence MR image demonstrates severe tendinosis and a high-grade partial tear of the common extensor tendon *(arrow)*. The radial collateral ligament is preserved.

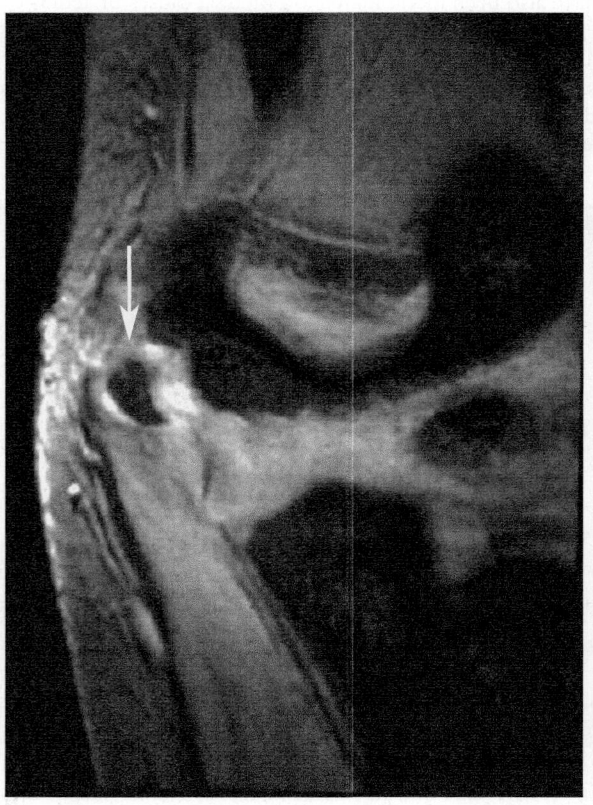

FIGURE 4.139 Little League elbow. A 10-year-old boy presented with acute onset of medial elbow pain after baseball pitching. Coronal short time inversion recovery (STIR) pulse sequence MR image demonstrates an avulsion fracture of the medial epicondyle *(arrow)* with increased signal intensity in the region of the avulsed growth plate. The common flexor tendon is intact.

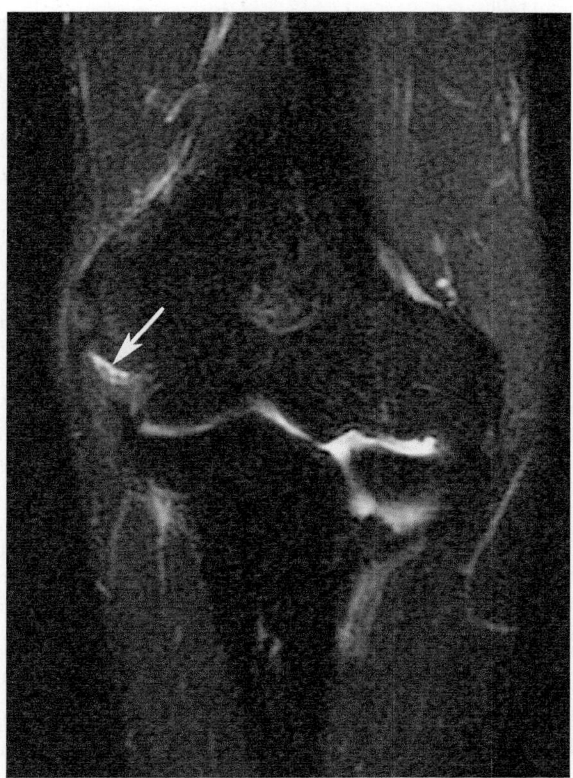

FIGURE 4.140 **Baseball pitcher's elbow.** A 20-year-old man, a professional baseball pitcher, presented with chronic medial elbow pain. Coronal short time inversion recovery (STIR) pulse sequence MR image demonstrates a partial tear of the humeral origin of the anterior band of the ulnar collateral ligament *(arrow)*. The common flexor tendon is intact.

Oarsman's Wrist

This lesion is produced by repetitive flexion and extension of the wrist, causing friction and tenosynovitis of the extensor carpi radialis brevis and longus tendons and the abductor pollicis longus and extensor pollicis brevis tendons. This entity is also known as *intersection syndrome*. Patients present with pain, swelling, and crepitus in the distal forearm. This syndrome

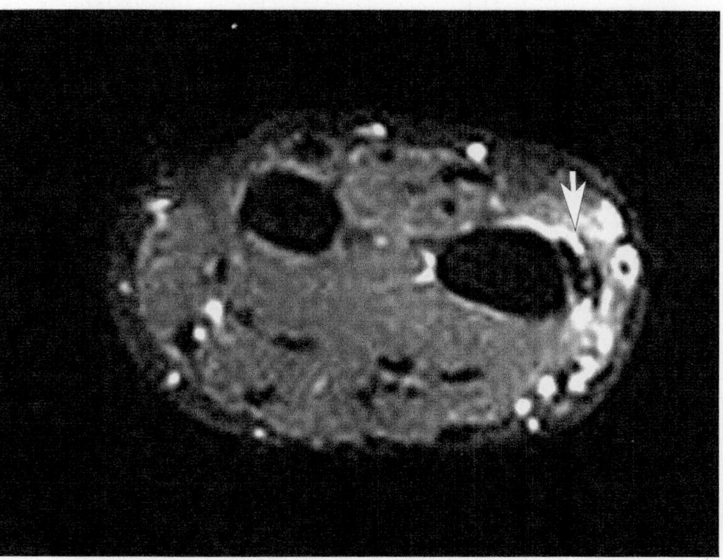

FIGURE 4.141 **Oarsman's wrist.** A 32-year-old man presented with pain, swelling, and crepitus in the radial aspect of the distal forearm, near the wrist. Axial short time inversion recovery (STIR) pulse sequence MR image shows peritendinous edema around the extensor carpi radialis longus and brevis tendons and the extensor pollicis brevis tendon *(arrow)*.

is very similar clinically to the *distal intersection syndrome* (tenosynovitis at the intersection of the extensor carpi radialis longus and brevis tendons and the extensor pollicis longus tendon) (Fig. 4.141).

Cyclist's Wrist

This lesion represents an ulnar neuropathy, known to cyclists as *handlebar palsy*, caused by compression of the ulnar nerve at the hand and wrist as a result of direct pressure on the nerve from the grip on the handlebars. Often, the nerve may be stretched or hyperextended when a drop-down handlebar is held in the lower position. The pressure placed on the ulnar nerve results in numbness and tingling in the ring and little fingers or hand weakness, or a combination of both. Occasionally, compression of the median nerve can also occur by pressure against the handlebar, with development of carpal tunnel syndrome (Fig. 4.142).

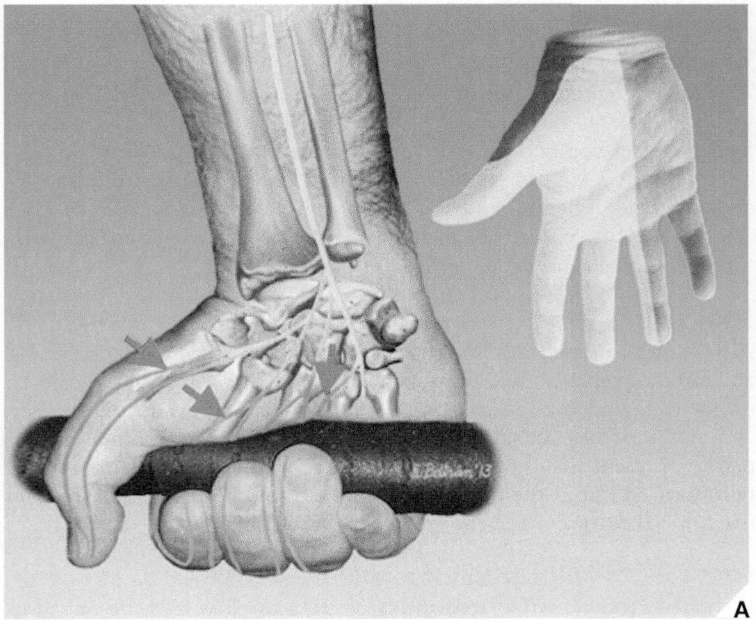

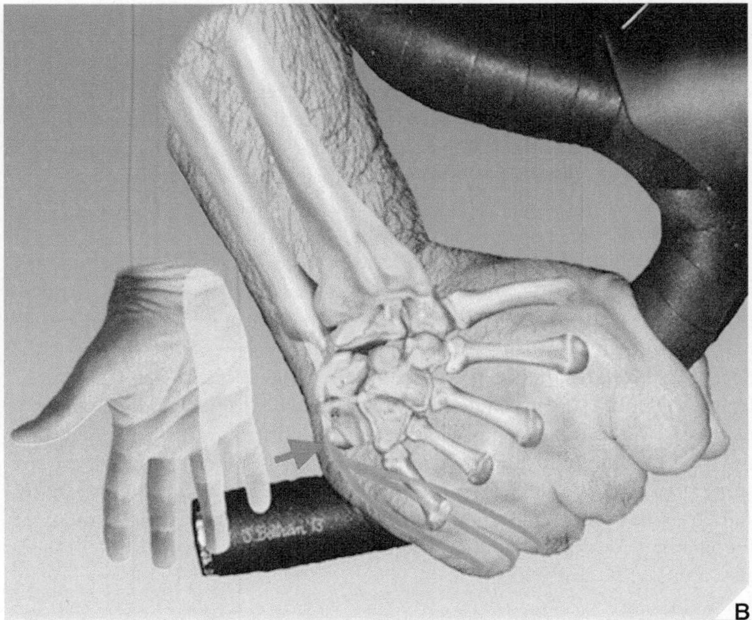

FIGURE 4.142 **Cyclist's wrist, mechanism of injury.** **(A)** Gripping of the drop-down handlebar held in upper position may produce compression of the digital branches of the median nerve *(arrows)* leading to sensory deficit of the innervated area (white region in the hand). **(B)** Gripping of the drop-down handlebar held in the lower position may produce compression of the sensory branch of the ulnar nerve *(arrow)*, leading to sensory deficit of the innervated area (white region in the hand). This is also known as *Guyon canal syndrome*.

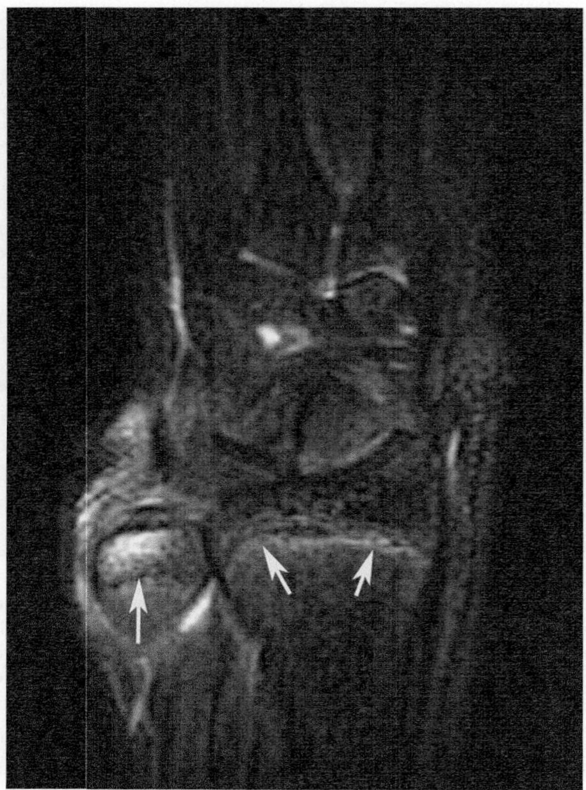

FIGURE 4.143 **Gymnast wrist.** A 13-year-old female gymnast was complaining of bilateral wrist pain during gymnastics. Coronal short time inversion recovery (STIR) pulse sequence MR image shows bone marrow stress edema of the distal ulna and around the physis of the distal radius *(arrows)*.

Gymnast's Wrist

This is an overuse injury that occurs in up to 40% of young gymnasts, before the growth plate of the distal radius and ulna is closed. Impact activities like tumbling and vaulting put a large amount of compressive force on the growth plate in the wrist, leading to a Salter-Harris type I lesion. Widening and irregularity of the growth plate of the distal radius may be seen on the radiographs and MRI (Fig. 4.143), simulating rickets; hence, the name of *pseudorickets* is also applied to this entity.

Boxer's Fracture

This common lesion is produced by hitting the head of the distal fifth metacarpal against a hard surface, such as the mandible of the opponent, causing a characteristic angulated fracture of the distal fifth metacarpal (metacarpal neck) easily diagnosed on conventional radiography (see Fig. 7.117).

Skier's Thumb

This lesion is caused by a fall on a hard surface with the ski pole in hand, producing valgus stress with injury of the ulnar (medial) collateral ligament of the thumb at the level of the metacarpophalangeal joint. This injury was first described in Scottish gamekeepers, related to repetitive twisting of the necks of the hares, hence the name of *gamekeeper's thumb* (see Chapter 7). In this injury, the ulnar collateral ligament may be displaced under the aponeurosis of the adductor pollicis (Stener lesion) or remain aligned with the joint capsule (non-Stener lesion). Typically, a Stener lesion will require surgery to replace the ligament in anatomic position and prevent joint instability. On MRI, the Stener lesion is demonstrated by displacement of the ligament under the adductor aponeurosis (yo-yo sign) (Fig. 4.144; see also Figs. 7.130 and 7.131).

Bowler's Thumb

This is a nerve compression syndrome due to pressure of the ulnar and radial digital nerves of the thumb on the edge of the bowling ball's thumb hole, resulting in paresthesias or hypesthesias of skin distal to the nerve. Continued pressure and friction may lead to perineural fibrosis and the formation of a painful nodule/neuroma, which can be demonstrated by MRI (Fig. 4.145).

Lower Extremity

Sports Hernia

Patients with the so-called *sports hernia* (which in fact is a misnomer) present with chronic hip and groin pain during hip extension, twisting, and turning. Pain usually radiates to the adductor muscle region and even the testicles, although it is often difficult for the patient to pinpoint the exact location. This entity is also known as *athletic pubalgia*, *hockey hernia*, *hockey groin*, and *Gilmore groin* and is more commonly seen in football and hockey players. The symptoms are related to a number of lesions, in isolation or combined, that include tear of the external oblique aponeurosis, partial tear of the adductor tendon from the pubic tubercle, or tear of the fascia transversalis, among others. MRI demonstrates stress edema in parasymphyseal location, with or without stress fractures or osteophytes (osteitis pubis), partial tear of the aponeurotic plate of the rectus abdominis and the adductors, and partial tears of the adductor longus–gracilis tendons at the pubic insertion (secondary cleft sign) (Fig. 4.146).

Runner's Knee (Iliotibial Band Friction Syndrome)

This syndrome is produced by continuous friction of the iliotibial band over the lateral femoral condyle. Patients complain of pain in the lateral aspect of the knee when the foot strikes the ground during running and may persist after the activity. Cycling and step aerobics can also produce this syndrome. MRI demonstrates thickening of the iliotibial band and peritendinous edema (Fig. 4.147). Occasionally, a frictional bursa may develop between the iliotibial band and the lateral femoral condyle.

Jumper's Knee

This is another overuse injury produced by constant jumping, landing, and changing direction, leading to strain of the patellar tendon with tendinosis of the proximal tendon. This entity is seen in basketball, volleyball, gymnastics, running, track and field, and soccer. Infrapatellar chronic pain is the most common clinical presentation. MRI demonstrates thickening of the proximal patellar ligament with signal alteration at its insertion in the inferior pole of the patella, most frequently involving the deep fibers (Fig. 4.148).

Tennis Leg

This entity typically is present in middle-aged patients, occurring acutely, with the knee in extension and forced dorsiflexion of the ankle, manifesting by development of pain and swelling in the calf. The symptoms are caused by a rupture of the medial head of the gastrocnemius at the myotendinous junction, and the lesion is well demonstrated with MRI (Fig. 4.149). A rupture of the plantaris tendon has been described as a possible occasional cause of tennis leg.

Shin Splints

Also known as *medial tibial stress syndrome*, it is an overuse injury of running and jumping athletes (basketball, tennis) involving the medial periosteum of the tibia and is considered a stress reaction. This syndrome is more common in female athletes and is bilateral in over 70% of the cases. The patients present with posteromedial tibial tenderness. MRI demonstrates periosteal edema in the posteromedial aspect of the tibia, without bone marrow edema or cortical abnormalities (Fig. 4.150).

Footballer's Ankle (Athlete's Ankle)

Increased incidence of osteoarthritis of the ankle has been described in former elite soccer players. This can be related to repetitive kicking, leading to degenerative changes that result in chronic anterior ankle pain aggravated in dorsiflexion (*anterior impingement syndrome*). MRI can demonstrate

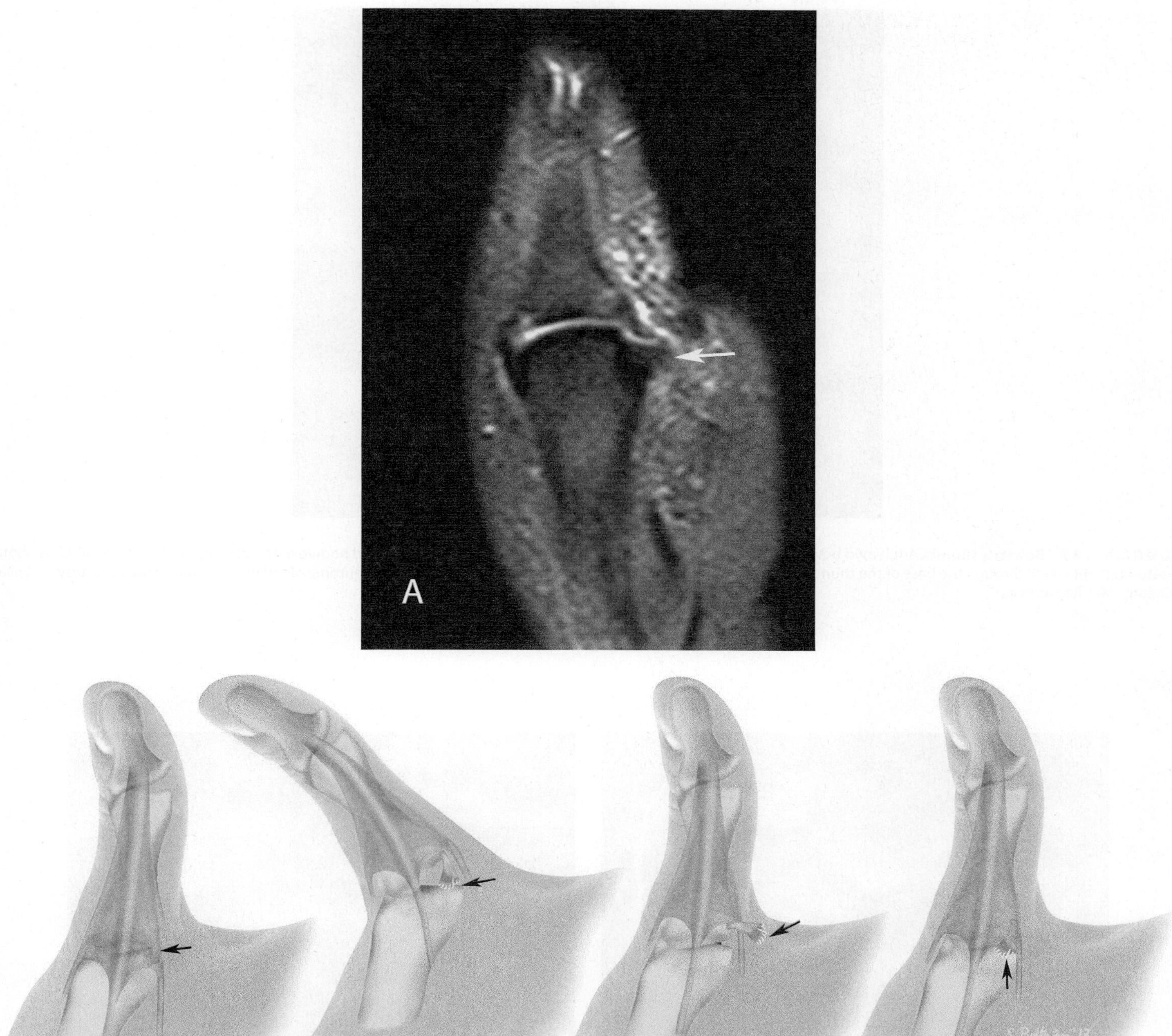

FIGURE 4.144 **Skier's thumb.** A 21-year-old man presented with pain and instability of the thumb after a skiing accident. **(A)** Coronal T2-weighted fat-saturated MR image through the first metacarpophalangeal joint shows a tear of the ulnar collateral ligament *(arrow)*, displaced under the aponeurotic hood of the adductor pollicis (Stener lesion). **(B)** Mechanism of injury: normal ulnar collateral ligament *(arrow)*. **(C)** Abduction injury: The ulnar collateral ligament is ruptured at the metacarpal insertion *(arrow)*. **(D)** Postreduction Stener lesion: The ruptured ulnar collateral ligament is displaced under the aponeurotic hood *(arrow)* (compare with **A**—MRI study). **(E)** Postreduction non-Stener lesion: The ruptured ulnar collateral ligament remains under the aponeurotic hood *(arrow)*.

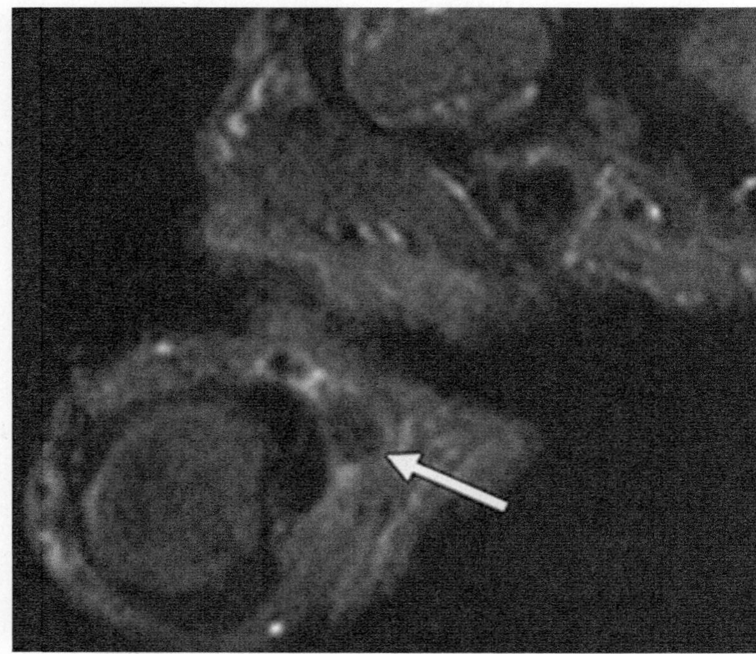

FIGURE 4.145 Bowler's thumb. Adult avid bowler presented with progressively developing skin paresthesia and nodule in the base of the thumb. Axial T2-weighted fat-saturated MR image through the base of the thumb shows hypointense nodular lesion *(arrow)* corresponding to a neuroma of the ulnar digital nerve. (Courtesy of William N. Snearly, MD, Radsource.)

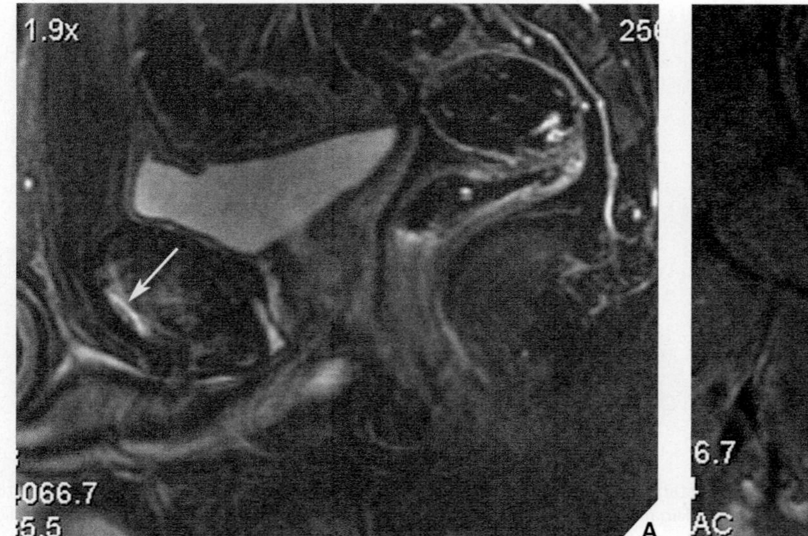

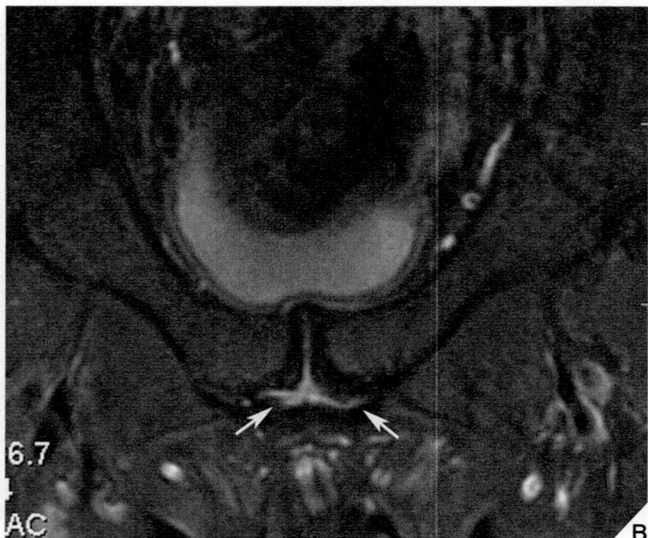

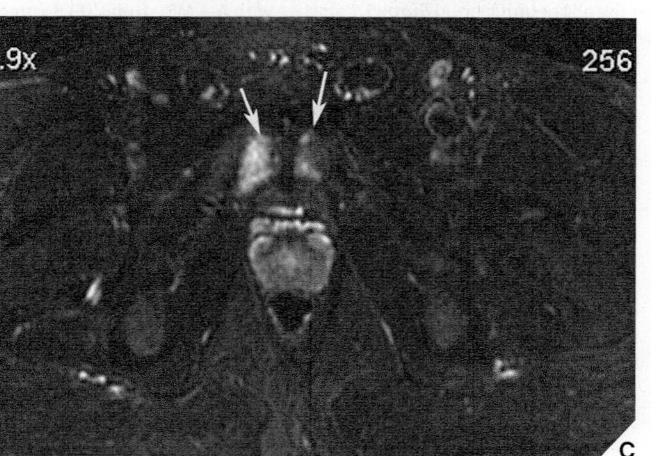

FIGURE 4.146 Sports hernia. Young soccer player presented with pain in the pubic area and groins. **(A)** Sagittal short time inversion recovery (STIR) pulse sequence MR image through the midline at the level of the pubic symphysis demonstrates separation of the rectus abdominis/adductor aponeurotic plate from the bone *(arrow)*. **(B)** Coronal T2-weighted MR image demonstrates the partial tear of the pubic insertion of the adductor tendons bilaterally *(arrows)* (double secondary cleft sign or "mustache sign"). **(C)** Axial T2-weighted fat-saturated MR image demonstrates parasymphyseal stress edema of the pubic bones *(arrows)*.

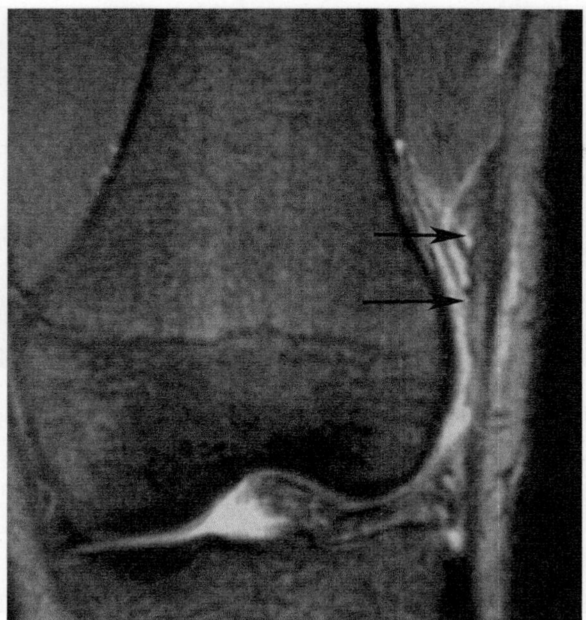

FIGURE 4.147 Runner's knee. A young woman, an avid runner, complained of pain in the lateral aspect of the knee. Coronal gradient recalled echo (GRE) MR image demonstrates thickening of the distal iliotibial band with surrounding edema at the level of the lateral femoral condyle *(arrows)*, consistent with iliotibial band friction syndrome.

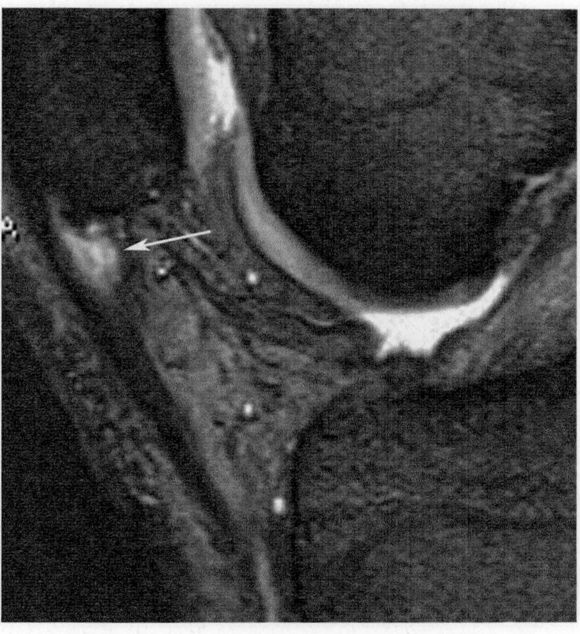

FIGURE 4.148 Jumper's knee. A young athletic man presented with anterior knee pain, localized inferiorly to the patella. Sagittal T2-weighted MR image shows a focal area of hyperintensity and thickening of the proximal patellar tendon *(arrow)* consistent with tendinosis and partial tear of the deep fibers.

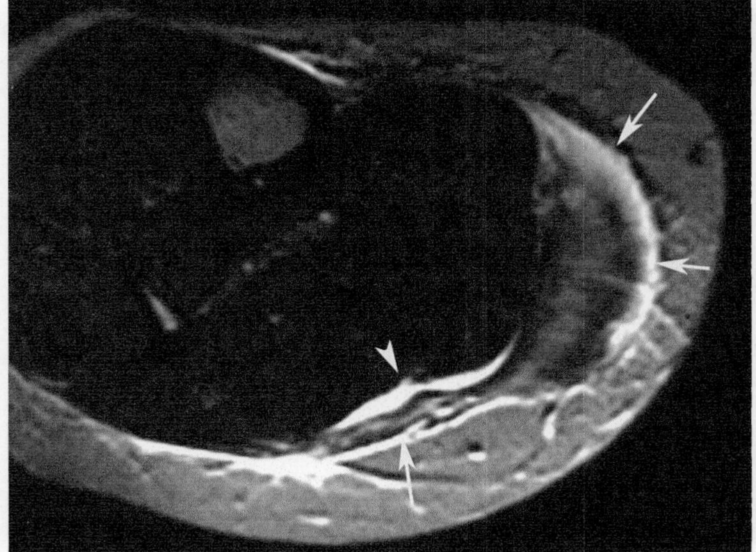

FIGURE 4.149 Tennis leg. A middle-aged man presented with acute onset of calf pain while playing tennis. Axial T2-weighted MR image shows perifascial edema and fluid involving the medial gastrocnemius muscle *(arrows)* and extending between the soleus and gastrocnemius muscles *(arrowhead)*, consistent with a myofascial strain.

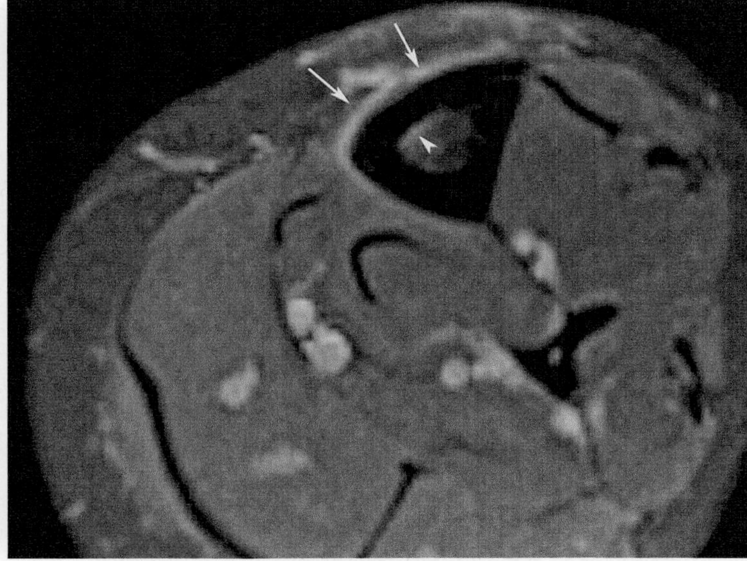

FIGURE 4.150 Shin splints. A young female runner presented with anterior leg pain. Axial T2-weighted MR image shows anterior pretibial soft-tissue edema *(arrows)* and minimal adjacent bone marrow edema *(arrowhead)*. (Courtesy of Luis Beltran, MD, Boston.)

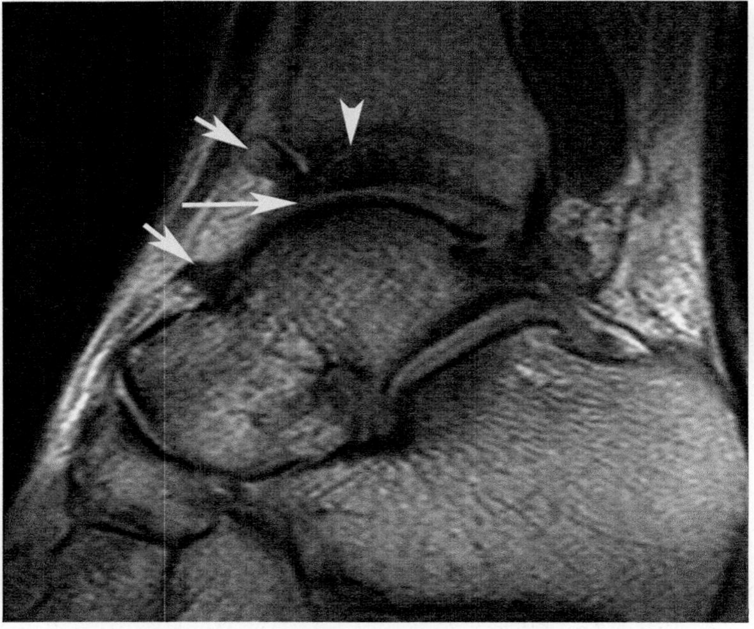

FIGURE 4.151 Footballer's ankle. A 32-year-old soccer player presented with a chronic anterior ankle pain aggravated with dorsiflexion of the ankle. Sagittal proton density–weighted MR image shows anterior osteophytes in the distal tibia and neck of the talus *(short arrows)*, associated with subchondral sclerosis of the distal tibia *(arrowhead)* and articular cartilage loss *(long arrow)*.

the degenerative changes of the ankle, including anterior osteophytes and cartilage loss (Fig. 4.151).

Snowboarder's Fracture

This is a fracture of the lateral process of the talus, not well demonstrated on the conventional radiographs. It is produced by inversion and dorsiflexion of the ankle. Patients present with acute onset of pain in the lateral aspect of the ankle, often misdiagnosed as ankle sprain. CT and MRI demonstrate the fracture clearly (Fig. 4.152).

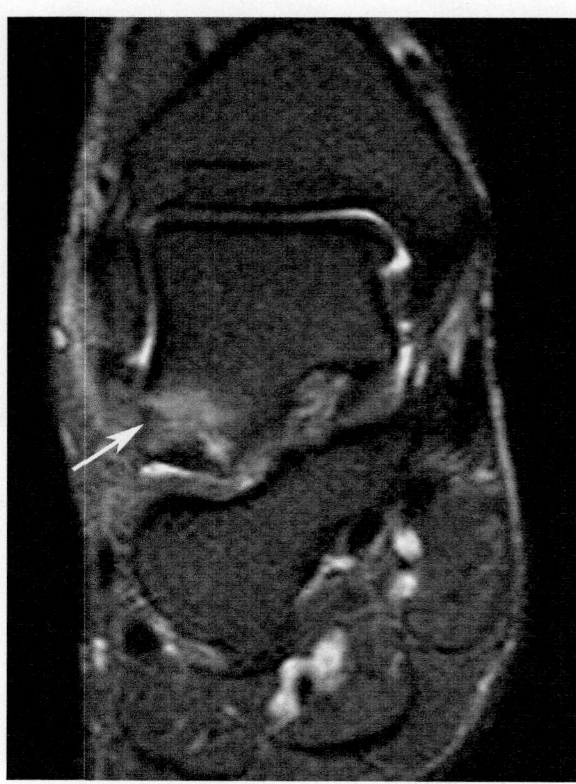

FIGURE 4.152 Snowboarder's fracture. A young man presented with acute onset of ankle pain following a snowboarding accident. Coronal T2-weighted MR image demonstrates a fracture of the lateral process of the talus *(arrow)*, with adjacent bone marrow edema.

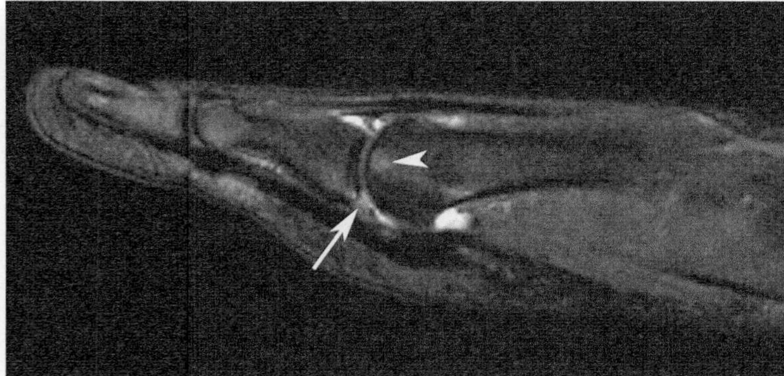

FIGURE 4.153 Turf toe. A young football player presented with pain in the plantar aspect of the great toe. Sagittal T2-weighted fat-saturated MR image shows a tear of the medial phalangeal sesamoid ligament, a component of the plantar plate, at the level of the phalangeal insertion *(arrow)*, with small focal area of bone contusion in the head of the first metatarsal *(arrowhead)*.

Turf Toe

This is a hyperextension injury of the first metatarsophalangeal joint against a hard turf surface leading to a lesion of the plantar plate and separation or fracture of the sesamoid bones. This lesion is typically seen in football players using light footwear. MRI demonstrates the injury to the plantar plate (Fig. 4.153).

PRACTICAL POINTS TO REMEMBER

1. When dealing with suspected fractures and dislocations, obtain radiographs in at least two projections at 90 degrees to each other.
2. To eliminate the risk of missing an associated injury, include the adjacent joints on the film.
3. When a fracture is suspected, look for associated abnormalities such as:
   - soft-tissue swelling
   - obliteration or displacement of fat stripes
   - periosteal and endosteal reaction
   - joint effusion
   - intracapsular fat–fluid level
   - double cortical line
   - buckling of the cortex
   - irregular metaphyseal corners.
4. When reporting a fracture, describe:
   - the site and extent
   - the type
   - the direction of the fracture line
   - the alignment of the fragments
   - the presence of impaction, depression, or compression
   - the presence of associated abnormalities
   - whether the fracture is a special type
   - whether the growth plate is involved. (In which case, the Salter-Harris classification, together with Rang and Ogden additions, provides a useful method of precise evaluation of the injury.)
5. FOPE is likely related to microtrauma sustained during sport activities and is identified on MRI as focal areas of edema surrounding the growth plate.
6. When a fracture fails to heal, distinguish between the three types of nonunion:
   - reactive (hypertrophic and oligotrophic)
   - nonreactive (atrophic)
   - infected.

7. In patients presenting with a history of skeletal trauma, be aware of such possible complications as:
    - disuse osteoporosis (mild or moderate)
    - RSDS
    - Volkmann ischemic contracture
    - posttraumatic myositis ossificans (The hallmarks of which are the clearly defined pattern of its evolution, the radiographic presence of the zonal phenomenon, and a radiolucent cleft.)
    - osteonecrosis (The earliest signs may be demonstrated by MRI or later may manifest as an increased uptake of a tracer on scintigraphy; the radiographic hallmark is the radiolucent crescent sign.)
    - injury to vessels (best demonstrated by DSA)
    - growth disturbance
    - posttraumatic arthritis.
8. Regarding juxtacortical myositis ossificans, remember that its MRI appearance depends on the stage of maturation of the lesion:
    - in the early stage, T1-weighted images will show a mass of intermediate signal intensity, whereas on T2-weighted images, the lesion will be of high signal intensity
    - in the mature stage, T1- and T2-weighted images will demonstrate a peripheral rim of low signal intensity corresponding to bone maturation
    - the fatty component of the lesion will image as high signal intensity on T1 weighting and as intermediate signal on T2 weighting.
9. Osteonecrosis can be best staged with MRI. Four classes of osteonecrosis (fat-like, blood-like, fluid-like, and fibrous) correlate well with histopathologic changes in the bone.
10. Stress fractures should be viewed as the endpoint of a spectrum along which a bone responds to a changing mechanical environment, ranging from excessive remodeling to a frank fracture.
11. In imaging these injuries, be aware that:
    - initial radiographs are often normal
    - the first radiographic abnormality to look for is a subtle poor definition of the cortex (gray cortex sign)
    - radionuclide bone scan is highly sensitive and frequently shows a characteristic fusiform area or transverse band of increased activity
    - MRI may show a typical finding of an area of low signal intensity in the bone marrow on T1 weighting that becomes of high signal on T2-weighted images, frequently showing a central low-signal band presumably representing the fracture line.
12. Insufficiency fracture is a subtype of a stress fracture that occurs in the osteoporotic bone. When it occurs in the sacrum and affects bilateral ala, the bone scan offers a characteristic H-shaped increased radiopharmaceutical uptake, referred to as a *Honda sign*.
13. SIFK refers to the subchondral insufficiency fracture of the knee, which should be distinguished from SONK, representing spontaneous osteonecrosis of the knee.
14. Patients with osteoporosis treated for a prolonged time with bisphosphonates commonly develop insufficiency fractures of the femur.
15. When dealing with an injury to soft tissues, consider using supplemental imaging modalities, including:
    - stress radiography
    - arthrography
    - CT
    - MRI.
16. MRI is an invaluable technique for identifying various injuries to the muscles, tendons, and ligaments. This modality can effectively delineate the variable degrees of strain, contusion, tear, or hematoma and permits the quantification of these injuries.
17. A great number of quite unique sport-related injuries are named after the particular sport. Learn the specific imaging characteristics of weight lifter pectoralis; Little League shoulder; golfer's and tennis elbow; Little League, baseball pitcher's, and goalkeeper's elbow; oarsman's, cyclist's, and gymnast's wrist; boxer's fracture; skier's and bowler's thumb; sports hernia; runner's and jumper's knee; tennis leg; shin splints; footballer's ankle; snowboarder's fracture; turf toe; and other injuries linked to the various sport activities.

SUGGESTED READINGS

Adelberg JS, Smith GH. Corticosteroid-induced avascular necrosis of the talus. *J Foot Surg* 1991;30:66–69.

An VVG, van den Broek M, Oussedik S. Subchondral insufficiency fracture in the lateral compartment of the knee in a 64-year-old marathon runner. *Knee Surg Relat Res* 2017;29:325–328.

Assouline-Dayan Y, Chang C, Greenspan A, et al. Pathogenesis and natural history of osteonecrosis. *Semin Arthritis Rheum* 2002;32:94–124.

Bassett LW, Grover JS, Seeger LL. Magnetic resonance imaging of knee trauma. *Skeletal Radiol* 1990;19:401–405.

Baumhauer JF. Anterior ankle impingement. *Orthopedics* 2011;34:789–790.

Beltran J, Herman LJ, Burk JM, et al. Femoral head avascular necrosis: MR imaging with clinical-pathologic and radionuclide correlation. *Radiology* 1988;166:215–220.

Boon AJ, Smith J, Zobitz ME, et al. Snowboarder's talus fracture. Mechanism of injury. *Am J Sports Med* 2001;29:333–338.

Bose VC, Baruach BD. Resurfacing arthroplasty of the hip for avascular necrosis of the femoral head: a minimum follow-up of four years. *J Bone Joint Surg Br* 2010;92B:922–928.

Brewer RB, Gregory AJ. Chronic lower leg pain in athletes: a guide for the differential diagnosis, evaluation, and treatment. *Sports Health* 2012;4:121–127.

Cao L, Guo C, Chen Z, et al. Free vascularized fibular grafting improves vascularity compared with core decompression in femoral head osteonecrosis: a randomized clinical trial. *Clin Orthop Relat Res* 2017;475:2230–2240.

Capeci CM, Tejwani NC. Bilateral low-energy simultaneous or sequential femoral fractures in patients on long-term alendronate therapy. *J Bone J Surg Am* 2009;91A:2556–2561.

Chadwick DJ, Bentley G. The classification and prognosis of epiphyseal injuries. *Injury* 1987;18:157–168.

Chan WP, Liu Y-J, Huang G-S, et al. MRI of joint fluid in femoral head osteonecrosis. *Skeletal Radiol* 2002;31:624–630.

Chang CC, Greenspan A, Gershwin ME. Osteonecrosis: current perspectives on pathogenesis and treatment. *Semin Arthritis Rheum* 1993;23:47–69.

Chapman C, Mattern C, Levine W. Arthroscopically assisted core decompression of the proximal humerus for avascular necrosis. *Arthroscopy* 2004;20:1003–1006.

Civinini R, De Biase P, Carulli C, et al. The use of an injectable calcium sulphate/calcium phosphate bioceramic in the treatment of osteonecrosis of the femoral head. *Int Orthop* 2012;36:1583–1588.

Colwell CW, Robinson C. Osteonecrosis of the femoral head in patients with inflammatory arthritis on asthma receiving corticosteroid therapy. *Orthopedics* 1996;19:941–946.

Crain JM, Phancao JP, Stidham K. MR imaging of turf toe. *Magn Reson Imaging Clin N Am* 2008;16:93–103.

Delgado GJ, Chung CB, Lektrakul N, et al. Tennis leg: clinical US study of 141 patients and anatomic investigation of four cadavers with MR imaging and US. *Radiology* 2002;224:112–119.

DeSmet AA. Magnetic resonance findings in skeletal muscle tears. *Skeletal Radiol* 1993;22:479–484.

Dudani B, Shyam AK, Arora P, et al. Bipolar hip arthroplasty for avascular necrosis of femoral head in young adults. *Indian J Orthop* 2015;49:329–335.

Ferlic OC, Morin P. Idiopathic avascular necrosis of the scaphoid—Preiser's disease? *J Hand Surg* 1989;14:13–16.

Ficat RP. Idiopathic bone necrosis of the femoral head: early diagnosis and treatment. *J Bone Joint Surg Br* 1985;67B:3–9.

Ficat RP. Treatment of avascular necrosis of the femoral head. In: Hungerford DS, ed. *The hip: Proceedings of the Eleventh Open Meeting of The Hip Society*. St. Louis: CV Mosby; 1983:279–295.

Ficat RP, Arlet J. Ischemia and necrosis of bone. In: Hungerford DS, ed. *Ischemia and necrosis of bone*. Baltimore: Williams & Wilkins; 1980:196.

Ficat RP, Arlet J. Treatment of bone ischemia and necrosis. In: Hungerford DS, ed. *Ischemia and necrosis of bone*. Baltimore: Williams & Wilkins; 1980:171–182.

Geith T, Niethammer T, Milz S, et al. Transient bone marrow edema syndrome versus osteonecrosis: perfusion patterns at dynamic contrast-enhanced MRI imaging with high temporal resolution can allow differentiation. *Radiology* 2017;283:478–485.

Gorbachova T, Melenevsky Y, Cohen M, et al. Osteochondral lesions of the knee: differentiating the most common entities at MRI. *Radiographics* 2018;38:1478–1495.

Gudena R, Werle J, Johnston K. Bilateral femoral insufficiency fractures likely related to long-term alendronate therapy. *J Osteoporosis* 2011;2011:810697. doi:10.4061/2011/810697.

Hendrix RW, Rogers LF. Diagnostic imaging of fracture complications. *Radiol Clin North Am* 1989;27:1023–1033.

Houdek MT, Wyles CC, Martin JR, et al. Stem cell treatment for avascular necrosis of the femoral head: current perspectives. *Stem Cells Cloning* 2014;7:65–70.

Hungerford DS, Lennox DW. The importance of increased intraosseous pressure in the development of osteonecrosis of the femoral head: implications for treatment. *Orthop Clin North Am* 1985;16:635–654.

Iannotti JP. Growth plate physiology and pathology. *Orthop Clin North Am* 1990;21:1–17.

Israelite C, Nelson CL, Ziarani CF, et al. Bilateral core decompression for osteonecrosis of the femoral head. *Clin Orthop Relat Res* 2005;441:285–290.

Iwasaki K, Hirano T, Sagara K, et al. Idiopathic necrosis of the femoral epiphyseal nucleus in rats. *Clin Orthop* 1992;277:31–40.

Jaramillo D, Hoffer FA, Shapiro F, et al. MR imaging of fractures of the growth plate. *Am J Roentgenol* 1990;155:1261–1265.

Jelinek JS, Kransdorf MJ. MR imaging of soft-tissue masses. Mass-like lesions that simulate neoplasms. *Magn Reson Imaging Clin N Am* 1995;3:727–741.

Jose J, Pasquotti G, Smith MK, et al. Subchondral insufficiency fractures of the knee: review of imaging findings. *Acta Radiol* 2015;56:714–719.

Khan W, Zoga AC, Meyers WC. Magnetic resonance imaging of athletic pubalgia and the sports hernia: current understanding and practice. *Magn Reson Imaging Clin N Am* 2013;21:97–110.

Kleinmann P. *Diagnostic imaging of child abuse.* St. Louis: Mosby; 1998.

Koo K-H, Ahn I-O, Kim R, et al. Bone marrow edema and associated pain in early stage osteonecrosis of the femoral head: prospective study with serial MR images. *Radiology* 1999;213:715–722.

Laorr A, Greenspan A, Anderson MW, et al. Traumatic hip dislocation: early MRI findings. *Skeletal Radiol* 1995;24:239–245.

Lonergan GJ, Baker AM, Morey MK, et al. From the archives of the AFIP. Child abuse: radiologic-pathologic correlation. *Radiographics* 2003;33:811–845.

Marciniak D, Furey C, Shaffer JW. Osteonecrosis of the femoral head. A study of 101 hips treated with vascularized fibular grafting. *J Bone Joint Surg Am* 2005;87A:742–747.

Merten DF, Carpenter BLM. Radiologic imaging of inflicted injury in the child abuse syndrome. *Ped Clin North Am* 1990;37:815–837.

Miller T, Reinius WR. Nerve entrapment syndromes of the elbow, forearm and wrist. *Am J Roentgenol* 2010;195:585–594.

Mink JH, Deutsch AL. Occult cartilage and bone injuries of the knee: detection, classification, and assessment with MR imaging. *Radiology* 1989;170:823–829.

Mirzai A, Chang CC, Greenspan A, et al. The pathogenesis of osteonecrosis and the relationship to corticosteroids. *J Asthma* 1999;36:77–95.

Mitchell DG, Rao VM, Dalinka MK, et al. Femoral head avascular necrosis: correlation of MR imaging, radiographic staging, radionuclide imaging, and clinical findings. *Radiology* 1987;162:709–715.

Nair AV, Nazar PK, Sekhar R, et al. Morel-Lavallee lesion: a closed degloving injury that requires real attention. *Indian J Radiol Imaging* 2014;24:288–290.

Norman A, Bullough P. The radiolucent crescent line—an early diagnostic sign of avascular necrosis of the femoral head. *Bull Hosp J Dis* 1963;24:99–104.

Norman A, Dorfman HD. Juxtacortical circumscribed myositis ossificans: evolution and radiographic features. *Radiology* 1970;96:301–306.

Nuovo MA, Norman A, Chumas J, et al. Myositis ossificans with atypical clinical, radiographic, or pathologic findings: a review of 23 cases. *Skeletal Radiol* 1992;21:87–101.

Ogden JA. Skeletal growth mechanism injury patterns. *J Pediatr Orthop* 1982;2:371–377.

Padmanabhan E, Rudrappa RK, Bhavishya T, et al. Morel-Lavallee lesion: case report with review of literature. *J Clin Diagn Res* 2017;11:TD05–TD07.

Pappas JN. The musculoskeletal crescent sign. *Radiology* 2000;217:213–214.

Peers KH, Lysens RJ. Patellar tendinopathy in athletes: current diagnostic and therapeutic recommendations. *Sports Med* 2005;35:71–78.

Porrino JA, Kohl CA, Taljanovic M, et al. Diagnosis of proximal femoral insufficiency fractures in patients receiving bisphosphonate therapy. *AJR Am J Roentgenol* 2010;194:1061–1064.

Ramnath RR, Kattapuram SV. MR appearance of SONK-like subchondral abnormalities in the adult knee: SONK redefined. *Skeletal Radiol* 2004;33:575–581.

Rockwood CA Jr, Green DP. *Fractures in adults*, vol. 1. Philadelphia: JB Lippincott; 1984.

Rockwood CA Jr, Wilkins KE, King RE. *Fractures in children*, vol. 3. Philadelphia: JB Lippincott; 1984.

Rogers LF. *Radiology of skeletal trauma.* New York: Churchill Livingstone; 1992.

Sagano N, Atsumi T, Ohzono K, et al. The 2001 revised criteria for diagnosis, classification, and staging of idiopathic osteonecrosis of the femoral head. *J Orthop Sci* 2002;7:601–605.

Saita Y, Ishijima M, Kaneko K. Atypical femoral fractures and bisphosphonate use: current evidence and clinical implications. *Ther Adv Chronic Dis* 2015;6:185–193.

Salter RB. *Textbook of disorders and injuries of the musculoskeletal system.* Baltimore: Williams & Wilkins; 1970.

Salter RB, Harris WR. Injuries involving the epiphyseal plate. *J Bone Joint Surg Am* 1963;45A:587–622.

Seiler JG III, Christie MJ, Homra I. Correlation of the findings of magnetic resonance imaging with those of bone biopsy in patients who have stage I or II ischemic necrosis of the femoral head. *J Bone Joint Surg Am* 1989;71A:28–32.

Seraphim A, Al-Hadithy N, Mordecai SC, et al. Do bisphosphonates cause femoral insufficiency fractures? *J Orthop Traumatol* 2012;13:171–177.

Sershon R, Balkissoon R, Della Vale CJ. Current indications for hip resurfacing arthroplasty in 2016. *Curr Rev Musculoskelet Med* 2016;9:84–92.

Smith DW. Is avascular necrosis of the femoral head the result of inhibition of angiogenesis? *Med Hypotheses* 1997;49:497–500.

Stevens K, Tao C, Lee S-V, et al. Subchondral fractures in osteonecrosis of the femoral head: comparison of radiography, CT, and MR imaging. *Am J Roentgenol* 2003;180: 363–368.

Suehiro M, Hirano T, Mihara K, et al. Etiologic factors in femoral head osteonecrosis in growing rats. *J Orthop Sci* 2000;5:52–56.

Sugimoto H, Okubu RS, Ohsawa T. Chemical shift and the double-line sign in MRI of early femoral avascular necrosis. *J Comput Assist Tomogr* 1992;16:727–730.

Szabo RM, Greenspan A. Diagnosis and clinical findings of Keinböck's disease. *Hand Clin* 1993;9:399–407.

Terry DW Jr, Ramin JE. The navicular fat stripe: a useful roentgen feature for evaluating wrist trauma. *Am J Roentgenol Radium Ther Nucl Med* 1975;124:25–28.

Trancik T, Lunceford E, Strum D. The effect of electrical stimulation on osteonecrosis of the femoral head. *Clin Orthop Relat Res* 1990;256:120–124.

Urban RM, Turner TM, Hall DJ, et al. Increased bone formation using calcium sulfate–calcium phosphate composite graft. *Clin Orthop* 2007;459:110–117.

Vande Berg B, Malghem J, Labaisse MA, et al. Avascular necrosis of the hip: comparison of contrast-enhanced and nonenhanced MR imaging with histologic correlation. *Radiology* 1992;182:445–450.

van der Worp MP, van der Horst N, de Wijer A, et al. Iliotibial band syndrome in runners: a systematic review. *Sports Med* 2012;42:969–992.

Vassalou EE, Zibis AH, Raoulis VA, et al. Morel-Lavallée lesions of the knee: MRI findings compared with cadaveric study findings. *AJR Am J Roentgenol* 2018;210: W234–W239.

Yamamoto T, Bullough PG. Spontaneous osteonecrosis of the knee: the result of subchondral insufficiency fracture. *J Bone Joint Surg Am* 2000;82(A):858–866.

Yu PA, Peng KT, Huang TW, et al. Injectable synthetic bone graft substitute combined with core decompression in the treatment of advanced osteonecrosis of the femoral head: a 5-year follow-up. *Biomed J* 2015;38:257–261.

Williams M, Laredo J-D, Setbon S, et al. Unusual longitudinal stress fractures of the femoral diaphysis: report of five cases. *Skeletal Radiol* 1999;27:81–85.

Wilmot AS, Ruutiainen AT, Bakhru PT, et al. Subchondral insufficiency fracture of the knee: a recognizable associated soft tissue edema pattern and similar distribution among men and women. *Eur J Radiol* 2016;85:2096–2103.

Zurlo JV. The double-line sign. *Radiology* 1999;212:541–542.

5

Upper Limb I

Shoulder Girdle

Trauma to the Shoulder Girdle

Trauma to the shoulder girdle is common throughout life, but the site of injury varies with age. In children and adolescents, fracture of the clavicle sustained during play or athletic activities is a frequent type of skeletal injury. Dislocations of the shoulder and acromioclavicular separation are often seen in the third and fourth decades of life, whereas fracture of the proximal humerus is commonly encountered in the elderly. Most of these traumatic conditions can be diagnosed on the basis of history and clinical examination, with radiographs obtained mainly to define the exact site, type, and extent of the injury. At times, however, as in posterior dislocation in the glenohumeral joint, for example, which is the most commonly missed diagnosis in shoulder trauma, only radiographic examination performed in the proper projections may reveal the abnormality.

Anatomic–Radiologic Considerations

The shoulder girdle consists of osseous components—proximal humerus, scapula, and clavicle, forming the glenohumeral and acromioclavicular joints (Fig. 5.1)—and various muscles, ligaments, and tendons reinforcing the joint capsule (Fig. 5.2). The joint capsule inserts along the anatomic neck of the humerus and along the neck of the glenoid. In front, it is reinforced by three glenohumeral ligaments (GHLs) (the superior, middle, and inferior), which converge from the humerus to be attached by the long head of the biceps tendon to the supraglenoid tubercle. The other important ligaments are the acromioclavicular, coracoacromial, and the coracoclavicular (including trapezoid and conoid portions) (Fig. 5.2A).

The essential muscles are those that form the rotator cuff (Fig. 5.3). The term *rotator cuff* is used to describe the group of muscles that envelops the glenohumeral joint, holding the head of the humerus firmly in the glenoid fossa. They consist of the subscapularis anteriorly, the infraspinatus posterosuperiorly, the teres minor posteriorly, and the supraspinatus superiorly (mnemonic SITS). The subscapularis muscle inserts on the lesser tuberosity anteriorly. The insertions of the supraspinatus, infraspinatus, and teres minor muscles are on the greater tuberosity, posteriorly. The supraspinatus tendon covers the superior aspect of the humeral head, inserting on the superior facet of the greater tuberosity. The infraspinatus tendon covers the superior and posterior aspects of the humeral head and inserts on the middle facet, located distal and more posterior to the superior facet. The teres minor is lower in position and inserts on the posteroinferior facet of the greater tuberosity (Fig. 5.3B). In addition, the long head of the biceps with its tendon, which in its intracapsular portion runs through the joint, and the triceps muscle, inserting on the infraglenoid tubercle inferiorly, provide additional support to the glenohumeral joint.

Most trauma to the shoulder area can be sufficiently evaluated on radiographs obtained in the *anteroposterior* projection with the arm in the *neutral* position (Fig. 5.4A) with the arm *internally* or *externally rotated* to visualize different aspects of the humeral head. The one limitation of these views is that the humeral head is seen overlapping the glenoid, thereby obscuring the glenohumeral joint space (Fig. 5.4B). Eliminating the overlap can be accomplished by rotating the patient approximately 40 degrees toward the affected side. This special posterior oblique view, known as the *Grashey projection*, permits the glenoid to be seen in profile (Fig. 5.5) and is thus particularly effective in demonstrating suspected posterior dislocation. Obliteration of the normally clear space between the humeral head and the glenoid margin on this view confirms the diagnosis (see Fig. 5.60). The Grashey view is also effective in demonstrating developmental variant of anterior portion of the acromion, so-called *os acromiale* (Fig. 5.6). It represents an unfused accessory center of ossification of the acromion and should not be mistaken for a fracture. It is believed that this anomaly increases the risk of subacromial impingement presumably due to increased mobility. Os acromiale can also be well seen on the axillary projection of the shoulder (see Fig. 5.8).

Other special views have proved to be useful in evaluating suspected trauma to various aspects of the shoulder. A superoinferior view of the shoulder, known as the *axillary projection*, is helpful in determining the exact relationship of the humeral head and the glenoid fossa (Fig. 5.7) as well as in detecting anterior or posterior dislocation. It also is proficient in showing the os acromiale (Fig. 5.8). This view, however, may at times be difficult to obtain, particularly if the patient is unable to abduct the arm, in which case a variant of the axillary projection known as the *West Point view* may be similarly effective. In addition to all the benefits of the axillary projection, the West Point view effectively demonstrates the anteroinferior rim of the glenoid (Fig. 5.9). Another useful variant of the axillary projection is the *Lawrence view*. The importance of this projection lies in the fact that it does not require full abduction of the arm because it can be compensated for by angulation of the radiographic tube (Fig. 5.10). Suspected trauma to the proximal humerus, which can also be demonstrated on the anteroposterior projection (see Fig. 5.4B), may require the *transthoracic lateral* view for sufficient evaluation (Fig. 5.11). Because this projection provides a true lateral view of the proximal humerus, it is particularly valuable in determining the degree of displacement or angulation of the osseous fragments (see Fig. 5.30B). When trauma to the bicipital groove is suspected, a *tangent* radiograph of this structure is required (Fig. 5.12). Injury to the acromioclavicular articulation is usually evaluated on the anteroposterior view obtained with a 15-degree cephalad tilt of the radiographic tube (Fig. 5.13). Stress views in this projection, for which weights are strapped to the patient's forearms, are often mandatory, especially in suspected occult acromioclavicular subluxation (see Fig. 5.93). Fracture of the scapula may require a *transscapular* (or *Y*) view for sufficient evaluation (Fig. 5.14). Fracture of the acromion can be adequately evaluated on the shoulder *outlet* view. This projection is obtained similarly to the Y view of the shoulder

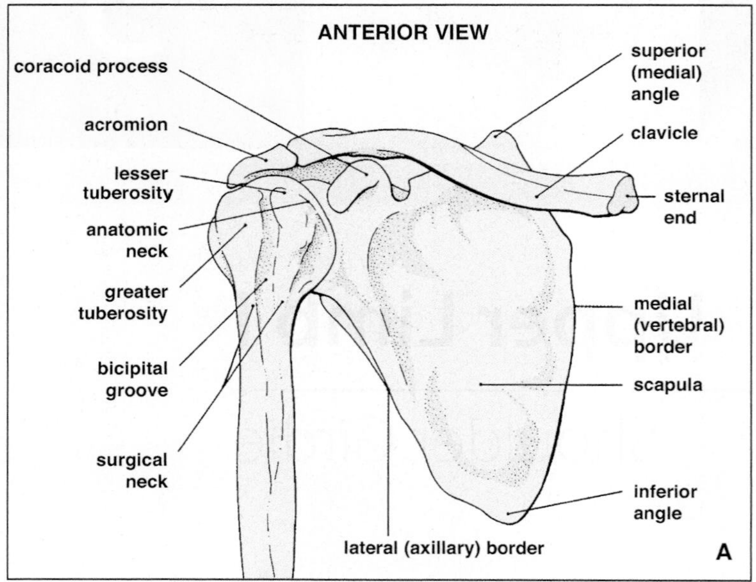

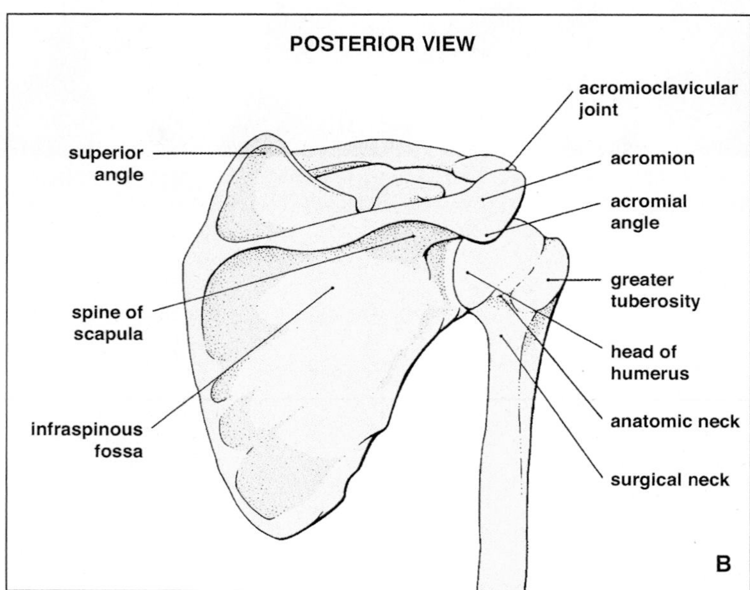

FIGURE 5.1 **Osseous structures of the shoulder.** Anterior **(A)** and posterior **(B)** views of the osseous components of the shoulder girdle.

girdle; however, the central beam is directed toward the superior aspect of the humeral head and is angled approximately 10 to 15 degrees caudad (Fig. 5.15). This view is also effective in demonstration of morphologic types of the acromion (Fig. 5.16; see also Fig. 5.28).

Ancillary imaging techniques are usually used to evaluate injury to the cartilage and soft tissues of the shoulder. The most frequently used modalities are arthrography and magnetic resonance imaging (MRI). Arthrography can be performed using a single- or double-contrast technique (Fig. 5.17). In cases of suspected tear of the rotator cuff, for example, a single-contrast arthrogram may reveal abnormal communication between the glenohumeral joint cavity and the subacromial–subdeltoid bursae complex, which is diagnostic of this abnormality (see Figs. 4.14 and 5.68). Although it is difficult to prescribe for which conditions a single-contrast as opposed to a double-contrast study should be chosen, the latter may be better suited to demonstrate abnormalities of the articular cartilage and capsule as well as the presence of osteochondral bodies in the joint. A double-contrast study, however, is always indicated when arthrography is to be combined with computed tomography (CT) scan (CT-arthrography) for evaluating suspected abnormalities of the fibrocartilaginous glenoid labrum (Fig. 5.18). The effectiveness of this combination lies in the fact that the injected air outlines the anterior and posterior labrum for better demonstration of subtle traumatic changes on CT images. For this study, the patient is placed supine in the CT scanner with the arm of the affected side in the neutral position to allow the air to rise and enhance the outline of the anterior labrum. To evaluate the posterior labrum, the arm is externally rotated (or the patient is positioned prone) to force the air to move posteriorly. CT-arthrography is also useful to evaluate the integrity of the rotator cuff, especially in patients who cannot tolerate an MRI (see Fig. 5.18).

Recent studies have shown the considerable advantage of MRI in the examination of the shoulder. This modality is particularly effective in demonstrating traumatic abnormalities of the soft tissues, such as impingement syndrome, partial and complete rotator cuff tears, biceps tendon rupture, glenoid labrum tears, and demonstration of the traumatic joint effusion. However, the shoulder presents unique difficulties for imaging. Because of

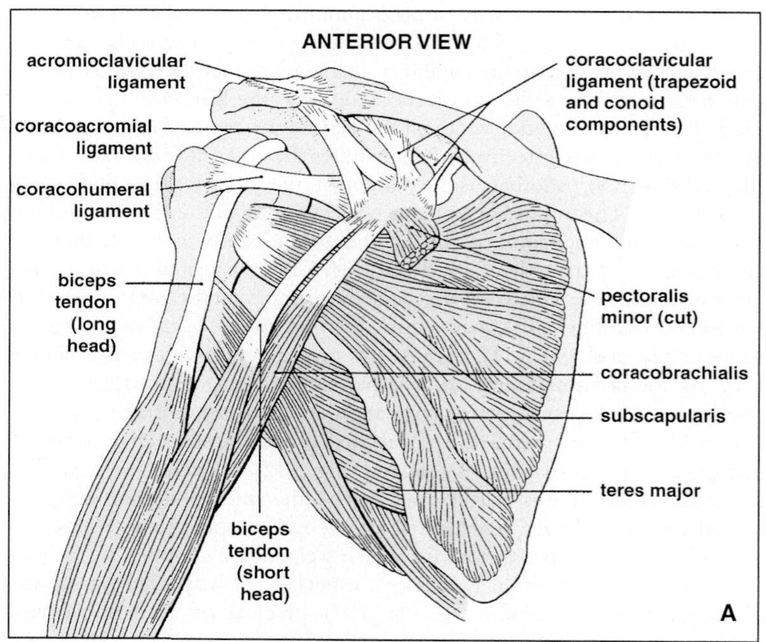

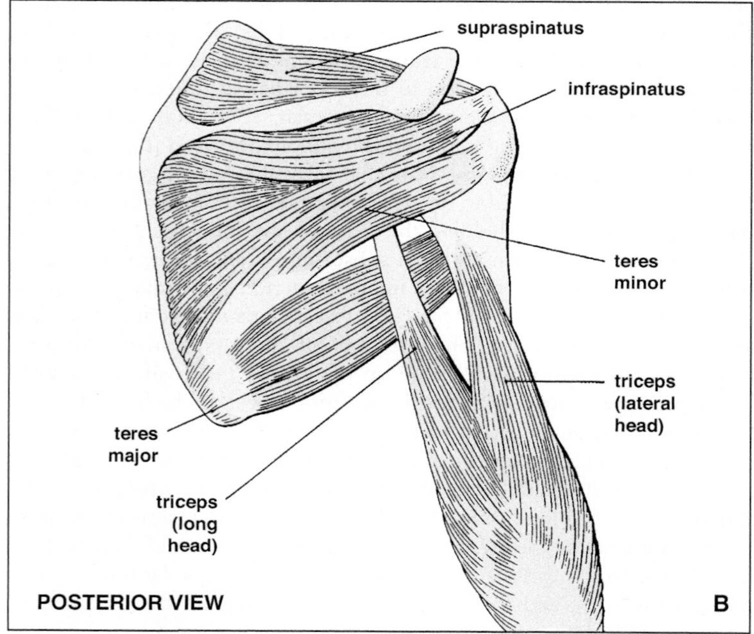

FIGURE 5.2 **Muscles, ligaments, and tendons of the shoulder.** Anterior **(A)** and posterior **(B)** views of the muscles, ligaments, and tendons of the shoulder girdle. (Modified with permission from Middleton WD, Lawson TL. *Anatomy and MRI of the joints*, 1st ed. New York: Raven Press; 1989.)

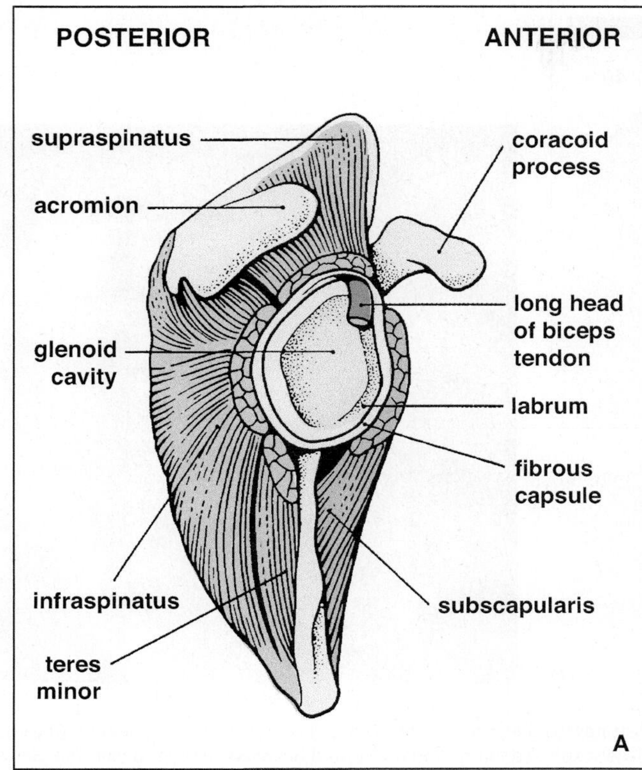

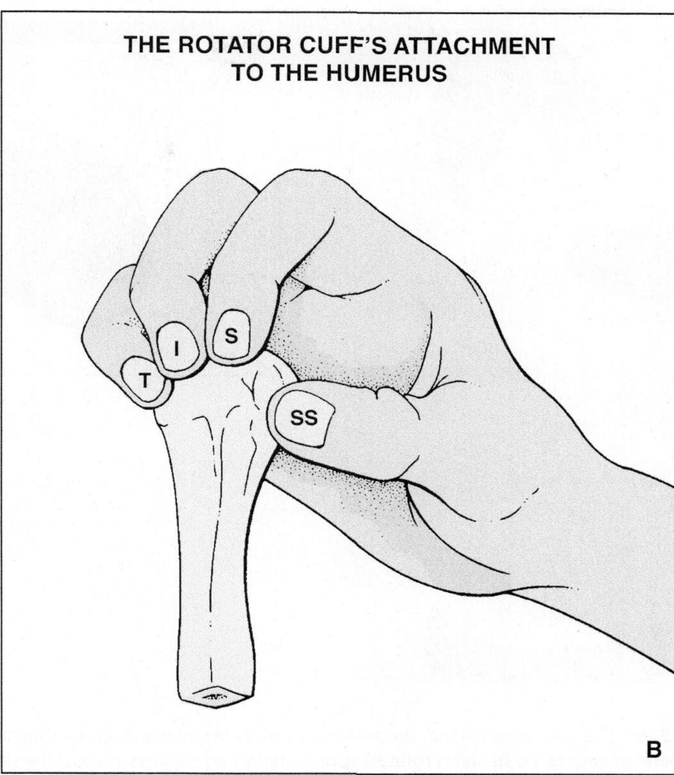

FIGURE 5.3 Rotator cuff. **(A)** Schematic of the glenoid fossa (with the humerus removed) shows the location of the muscles of the rotator cuff and the intracapsular portion of the long head of the biceps tendon. **(B)** Four muscles form the "rotator cuff": subscapularis *(SS)*, supraspinatus *(S)*, infraspinatus *(I)*, and teres minor *(T)*. They envelop the joint, blend with the capsule, and grasp their four points of attachment to the humerus, as does the hand in the figure, thus maintaining the integrity of the joint. (Modified with permission from Anderson JE. *Grant's atlas of anatomy*, 8th ed. Baltimore: Williams & Wilkins; 1983.)

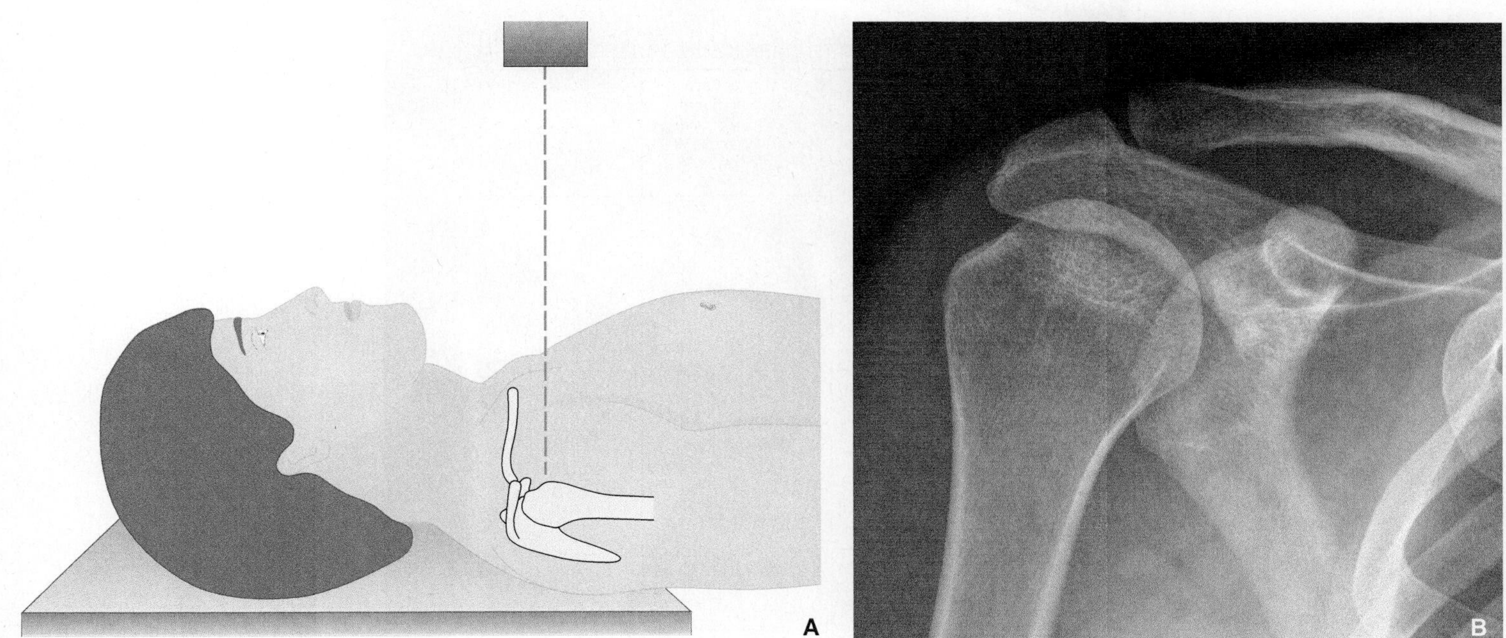

FIGURE 5.4 Anteroposterior view. **(A)** For the standard anteroposterior projection of the shoulder, the patient may be either supine, as shown here, or erect; the arm of the affected side is fully extended in the neutral position. The central beam is directed toward the humeral head. **(B)** On the radiograph obtained in this projection, the humeral head is seen overlapping the glenoid fossa. The glenohumeral joint is not well demonstrated, in contrast to the acromioclavicular joint. Observe the normal width of acromiohumeral (subacromial) space and coracoclavicular distance (interval).

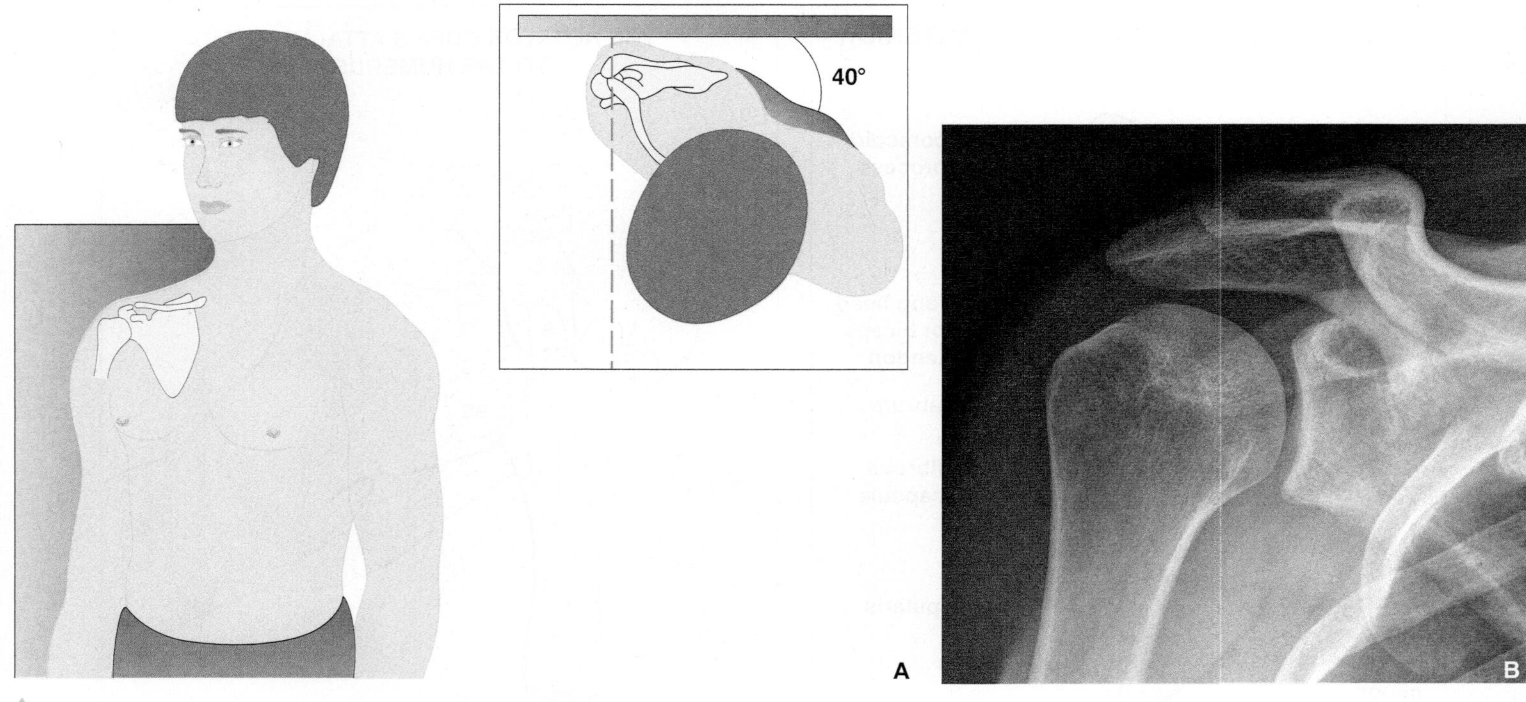

FIGURE 5.5 Grashey view. **(A)** For the anteroposterior view of the shoulder that demonstrates the glenoid in profile (Grashey projection), the patient may be either erect, as shown here, or supine. He or she is rotated approximately 40 degrees toward the side of the suspected injury, and the central beam is directed toward the glenohumeral joint. **(B)** The radiograph in this projection (posterior oblique view) shows the glenoid in true profile. Note that the glenohumeral joint space is now clearly visible in contrast to the acromioclavicular joint.

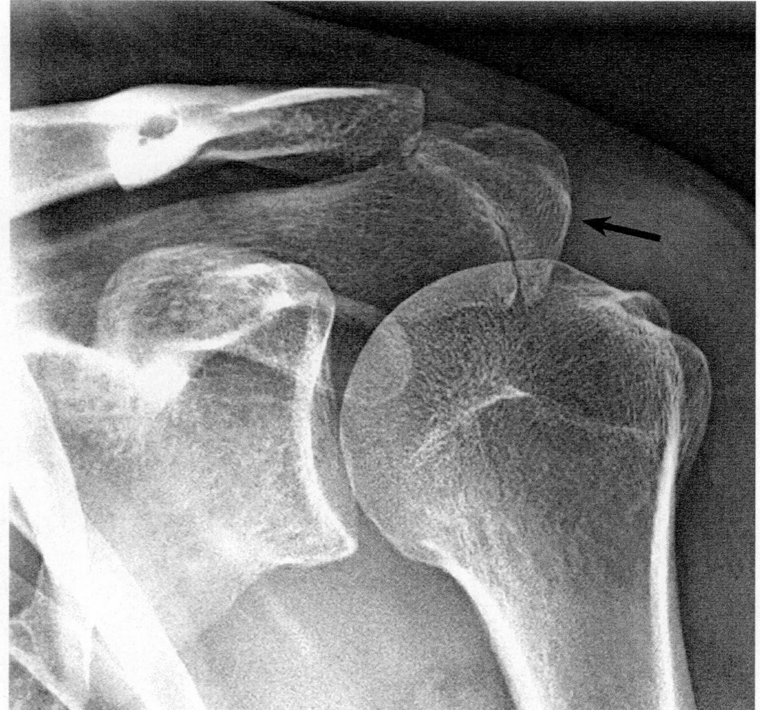

FIGURE 5.6 Grashey view of os acromiale. A 45-year-old man presented with clinical history of shoulder impingement. A Grashey projection shows an os acromiale *(arrow)*. This normal developmental variant should not be mistaken for a fracture.

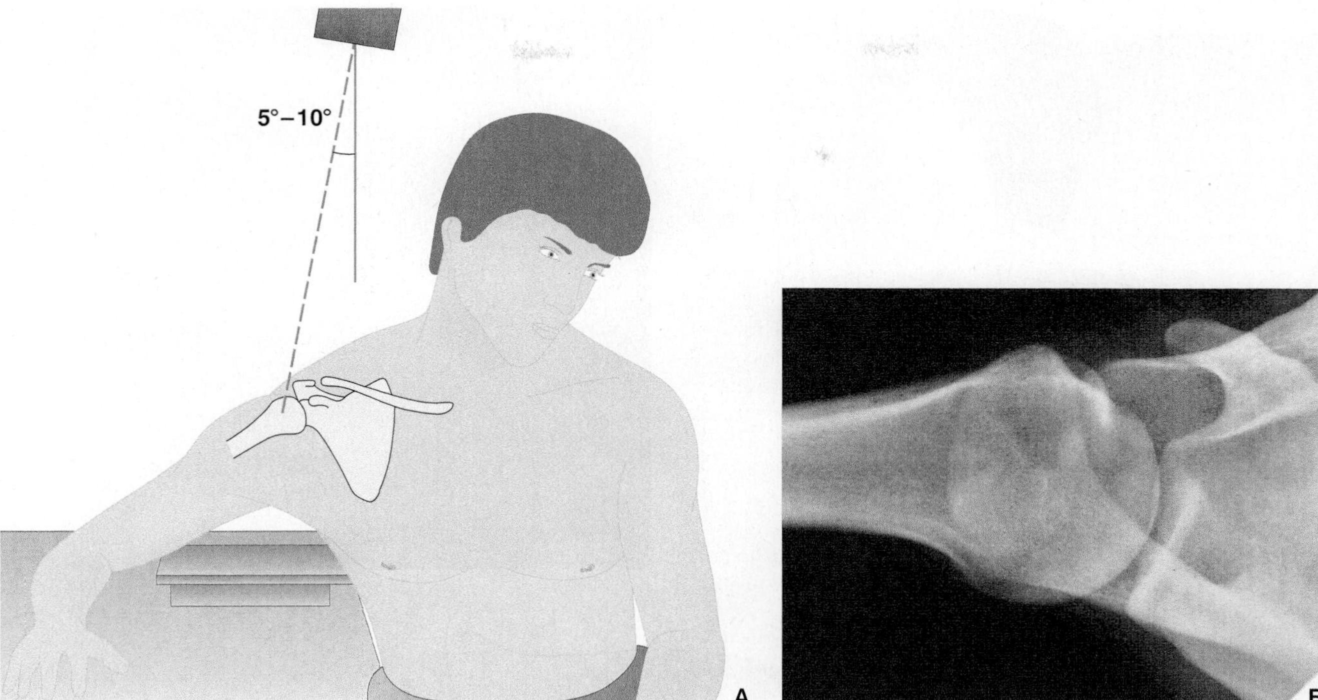

FIGURE 5.7 Axillary view. **(A)** For the axillary view of the shoulder, the patient is seated at the side of the radiographic table, with the arm abducted so that the axilla is positioned over the film cassette. The radiographic tube is angled approximately 5 to 10 degrees toward the elbow, and the central beam is directed through the shoulder joint. **(B)** The radiograph in this projection demonstrates the exact relationship of the humeral head and the glenoid.

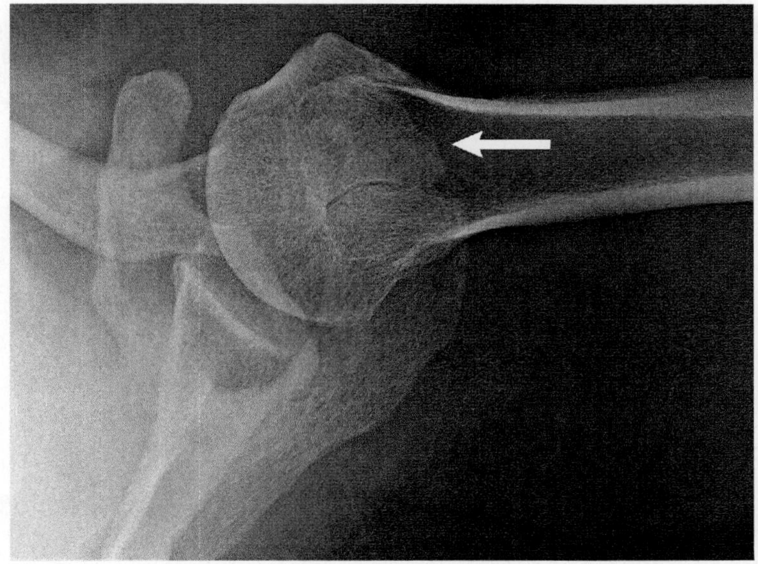

FIGURE 5.8 Axillary view of os acromiale. A 48-year-old woman presented with history of shoulder pain. An *arrow* points to os acromiale.

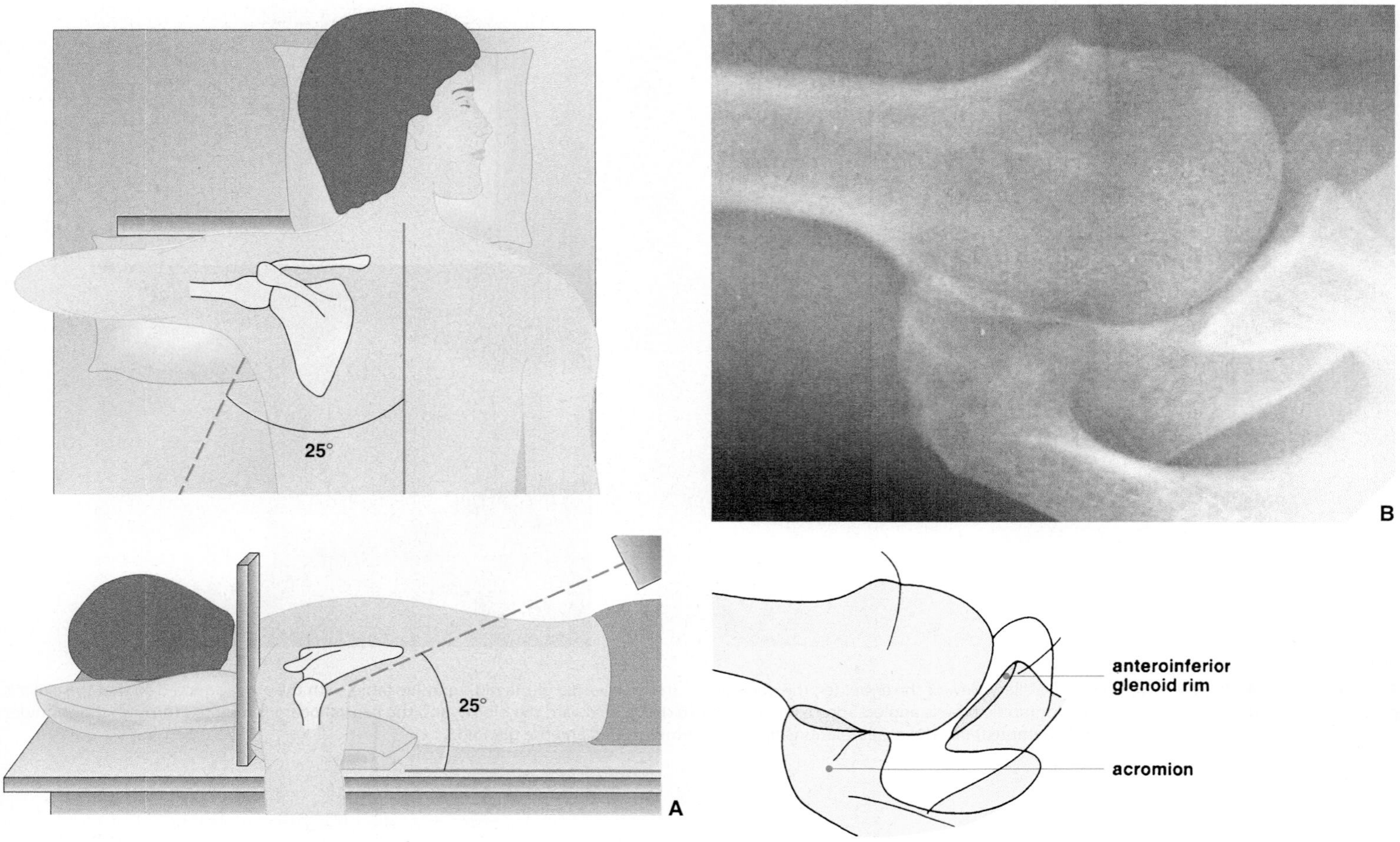

25°

B

25°

A

anteroinferior glenoid rim

acromion

FIGURE 5.9 West Point view. (A) For the West Point view of the shoulder, the patient lies prone on the radiographic table, with a pillow placed under the affected shoulder to raise it approximately 8 cm. The film cassette is positioned against the superior aspect of the shoulder. The radiographic tube is angled toward the axilla at 25 degrees to the patient's midline and 25 degrees to the table's surface. **(B)** On the radiograph in this projection, the relationship of the humeral head and the glenoid can be as sufficiently evaluated as on the axillary view, but the anteroinferior glenoid rim, which is seen tangentially, is better visualized.

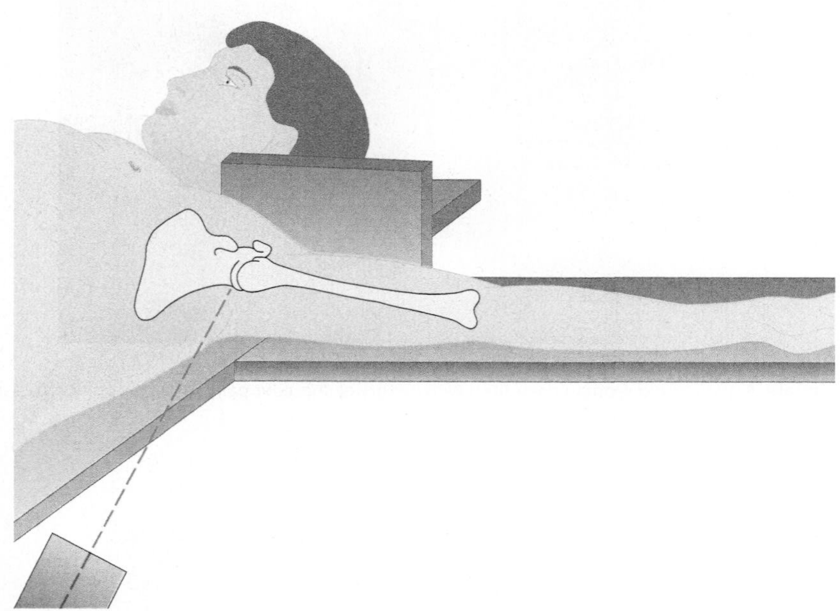

FIGURE 5.10 Lawrence view. For the Lawrence variant of the axillary view of the shoulder, the patient lies supine on the radiographic table, with the affected arm abducted up to 90 degrees. The film cassette is positioned against the superior aspect of the shoulder with the medial end against the neck, which places the midportion of the cassette level with the surgical neck of the humerus. The radiographic tube is at the level of the ipsilateral hip and is angled medially toward the axilla. The amount of angulation depends on the degree of abduction of the arm: Less abduction requires increased medial angulation. The central beam is directed horizontally slightly superior to the midportion of the axilla. The Lawrence view demonstrates the same structures as the standard axillary view.

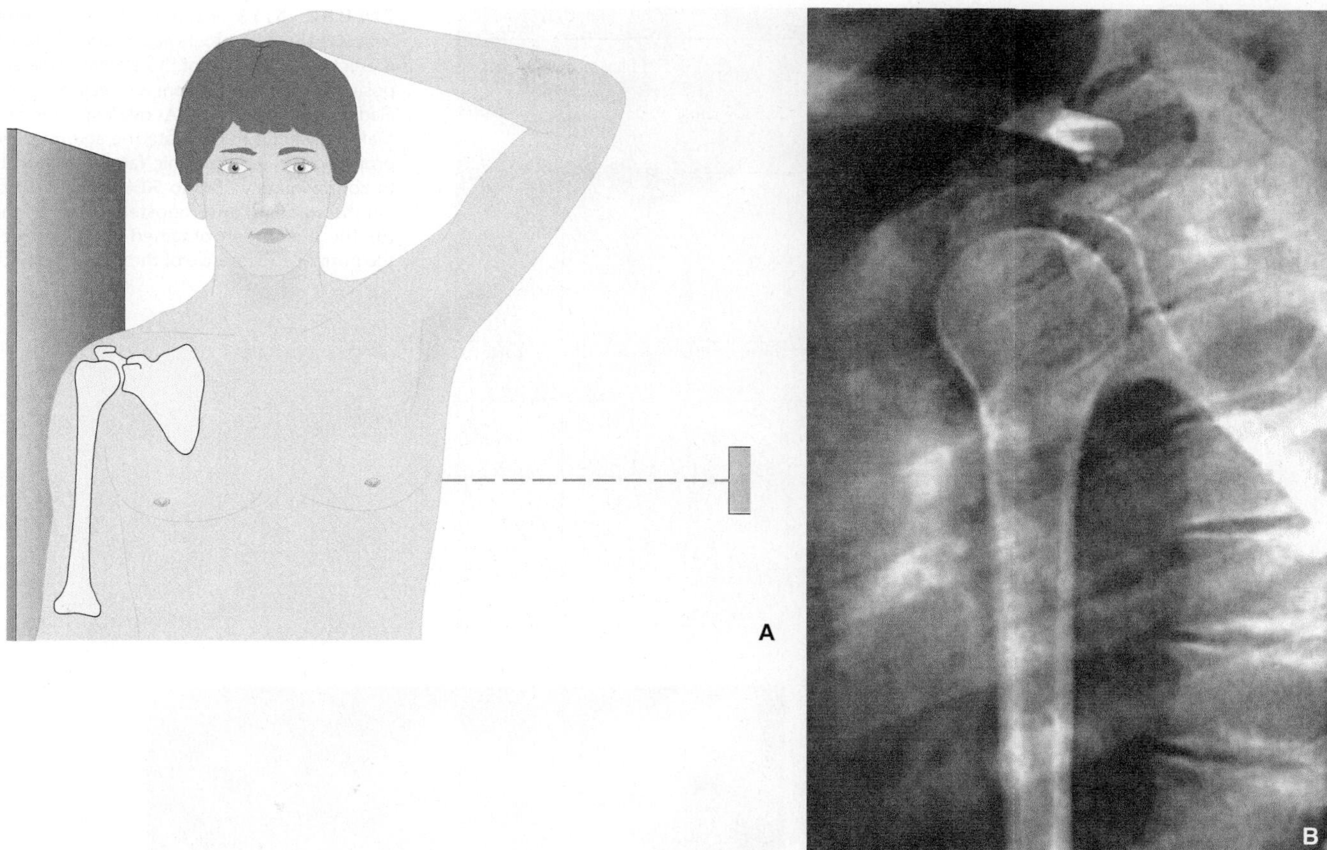

FIGURE 5.11 Transthoracic lateral view. **(A)** For the transthoracic lateral projection of the proximal humerus, the patient is erect with the injured arm against the radiographic table. The opposite arm is abducted so that the forearm rests on the head. The central beam is directed below the axilla, slightly above the level of the nipple. **(B)** The radiograph obtained in this projection demonstrates the true lateral view of the proximal humerus.

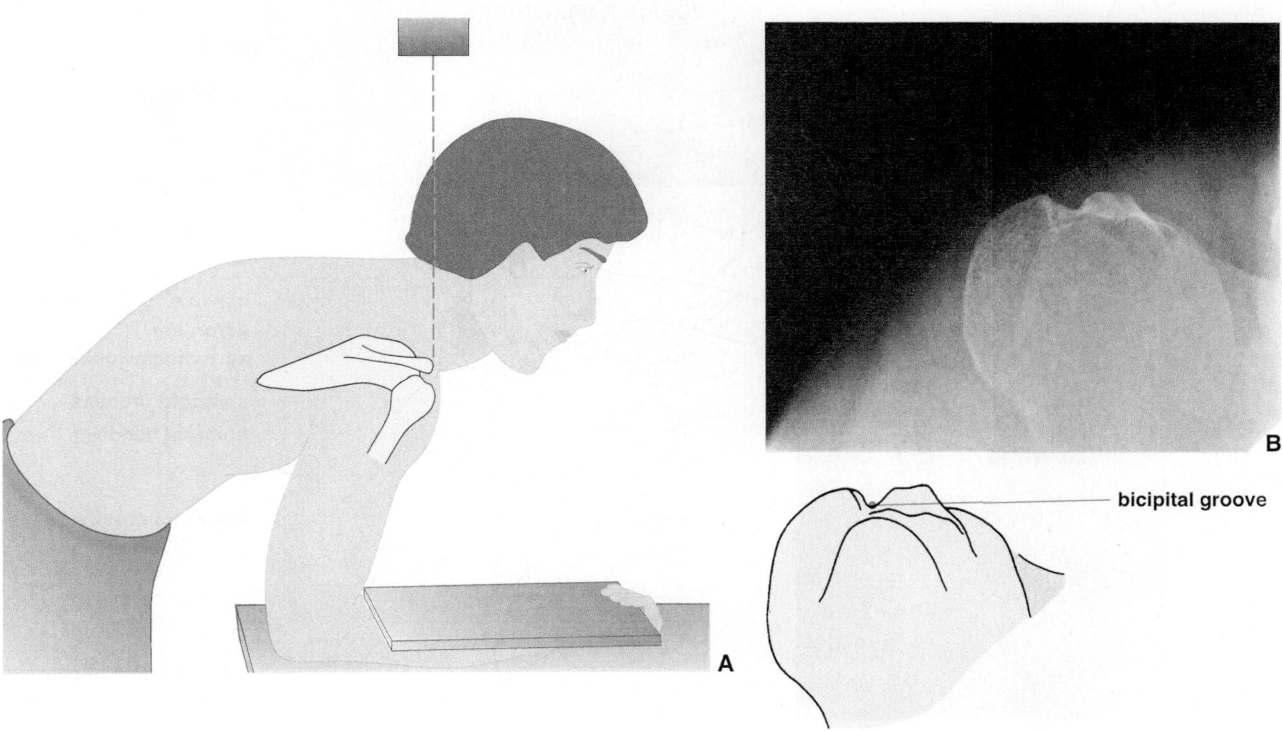

FIGURE 5.12 Bicipital groove view. **(A)** For a tangent film in the superoinferior (cephalocaudal) projection visualizing the bicipital groove (sulcus), the patient is standing and leaning forward, with the forearm resting on the table and the hand in supination. The film cassette rests on the patient's forearm. The central beam is directed vertically toward the bicipital groove, which has been marked on the skin. **(B)** On the radiograph obtained in this projection, the bicipital groove is clearly demonstrated.

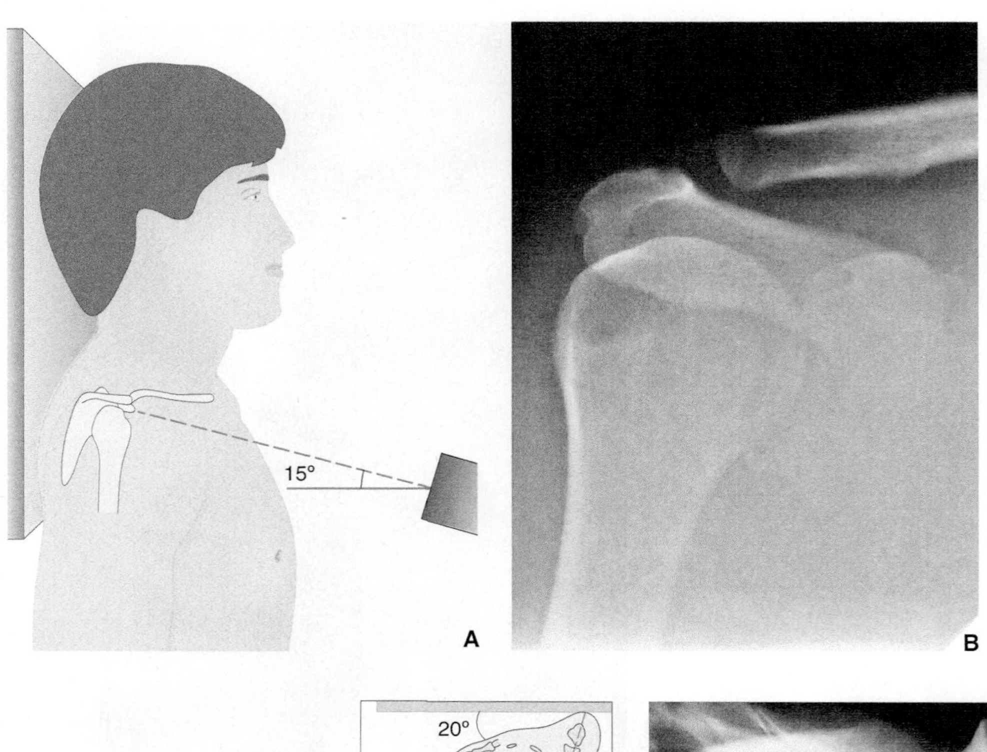

FIGURE 5.13 Acromioclavicular view. (A) To evaluate the acromioclavicular articulation, the patient is erect, with the arm of the affected side in the neutral position. The central beam is directed 15 degrees cephalad toward the clavicle. As overexposure of the film will make it difficult to evaluate the acromioclavicular joint properly, the radiographic factors should be reduced to approximately 33% to 50% of those used in obtaining the standard anteroposterior view of the shoulder. **(B)** The radiograph obtained in this projection shows the normal appearance of the acromioclavicular joint.

20°
A
B
C

clavicle
acromion
acromioclavicular joint
coracoid process
humeral head
lesser tuberosity
inferior angle of scapula

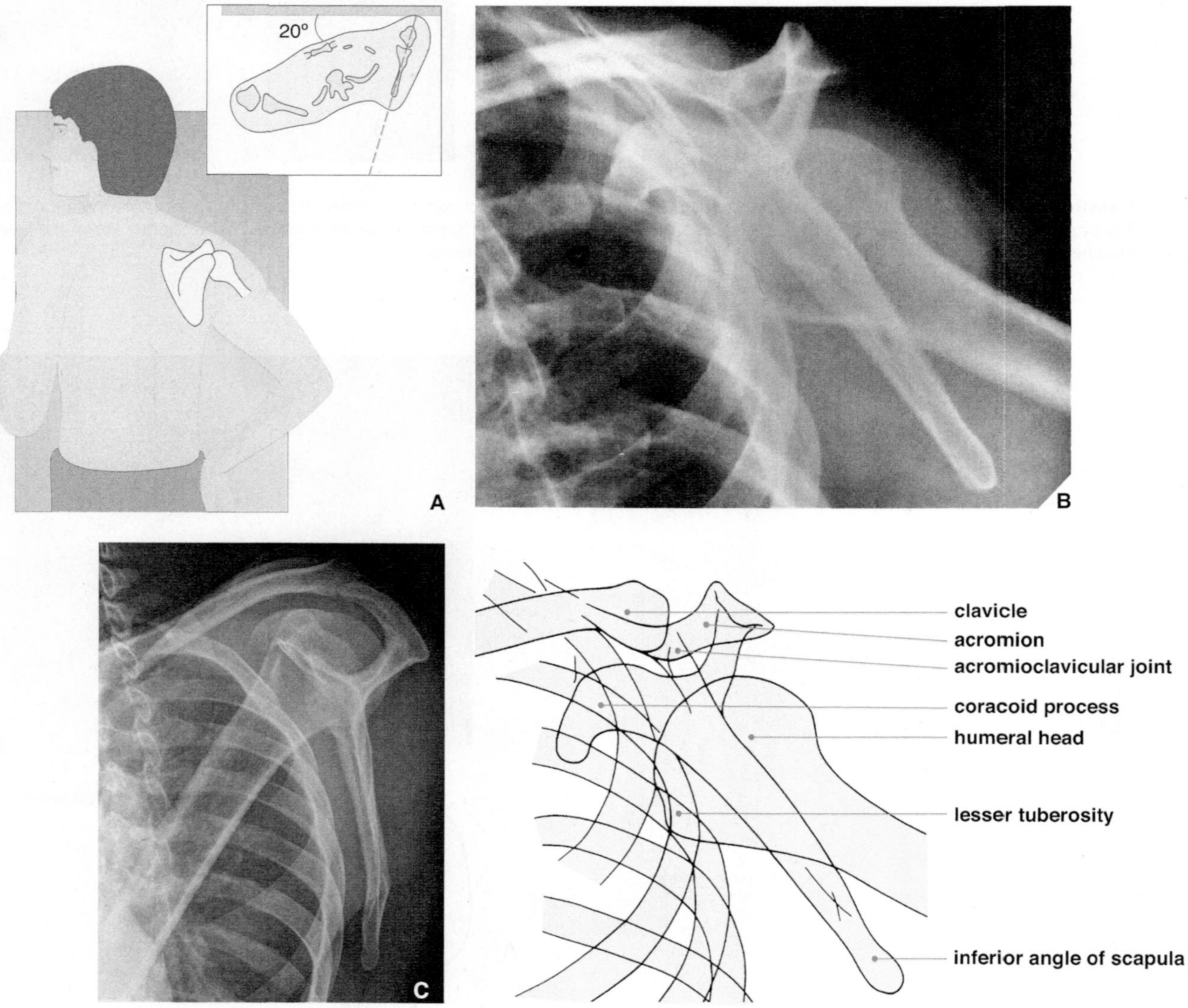

FIGURE 5.14 Transscapular view. (A) For the transscapular (or Y) projection of the shoulder girdle, the patient is erect, with the injured side against the radiographic table. The patient's trunk is rotated approximately 20 degrees from the table to allow for separation of the two shoulders *(inset)*. The arm on the injured side is slightly abducted and the elbow flexed, with the hand resting on the ipsilateral hip. The central beam is directed toward the medial border of the protruding scapula. (This view may also be obtained with the patient lying prone on the radiographic table and the uninjured arm elevated approximately 45 degrees.) **(B)** The radiograph obtained in this projection provides a true lateral view of the scapula as well as an oblique view of the proximal humerus. **(C)** Same structures can be visualized on the radiograph obtained without abduction of the arm.

FIGURE 5.15 Outlet view. This projection shows the same anatomic structures as demonstrated on the Y view of the shoulder girdle. In addition, coracoacromial arch and space occupied by the rotator cuff are well imaged.

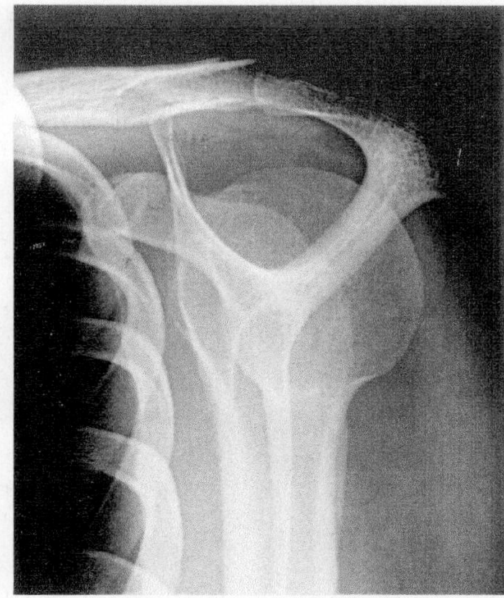

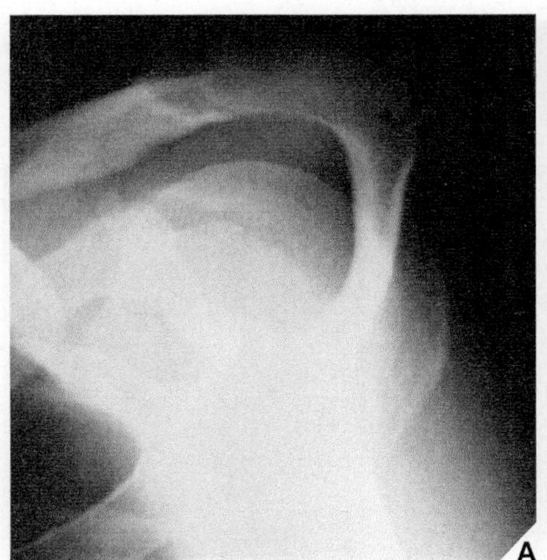

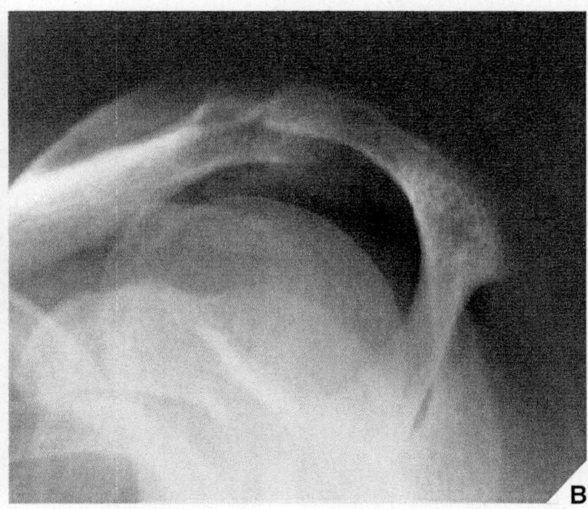

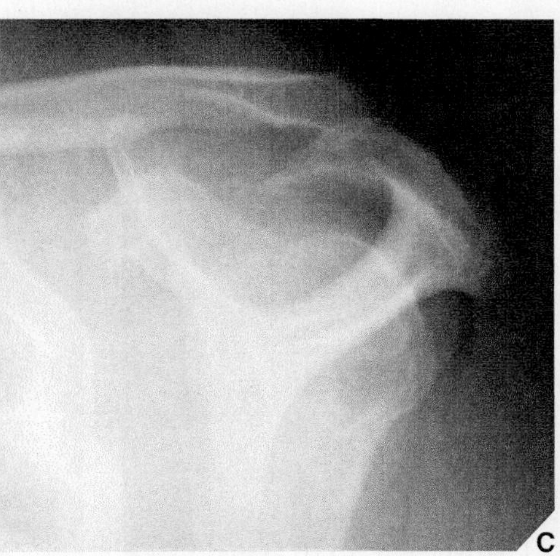

FIGURE 5.16 Types of the acromion. On the outlet view of the shoulder, three morphologic types of acromion are well demonstrated: type I (flat) **(A)**, type II (curved) **(B)**, and type III (hooked) **(C)**. Recently reported a very rare type IV (convex undersurface) is not shown here (see also Figs. 5.28 and 5.29).

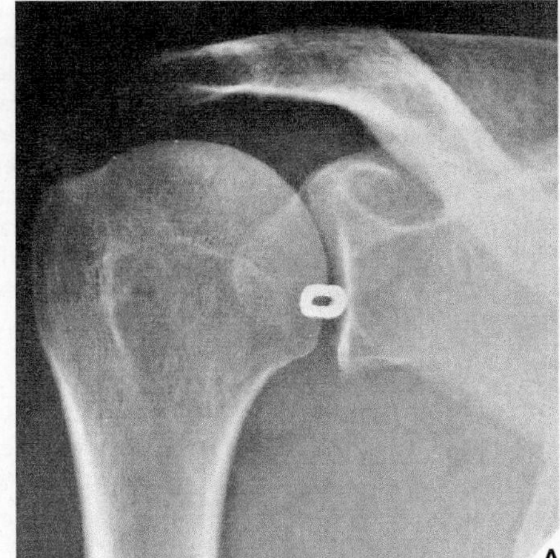

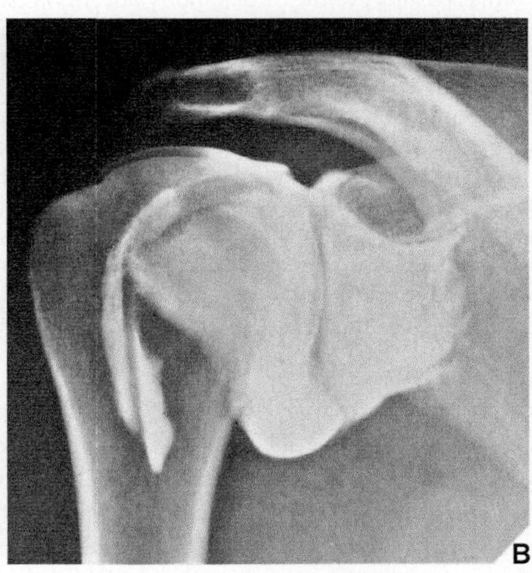

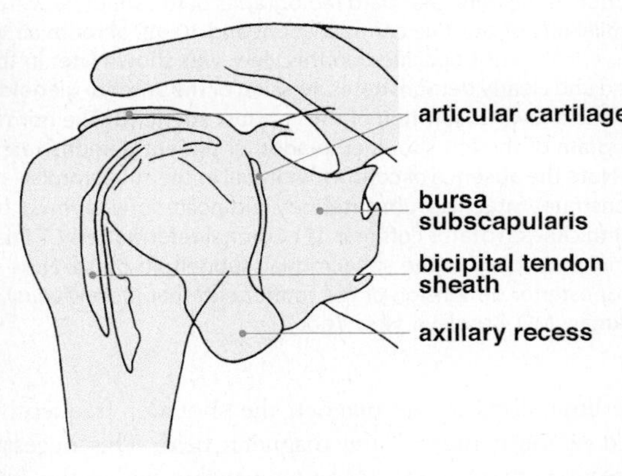

FIGURE 5.17 Technique for shoulder arthrography. The patient is positioned supine on the radiographic table, with the unaffected shoulder slightly elevated and the affected arm in external rotation with the palm up. **(A)** With the aid of fluoroscopy, a lead marker is placed near the lower third of the glenohumeral articulation to indicate the site of needle insertion. Under fluoroscopic control, 15 mL of positive contrast agent (60% diatrizoate meglumine or another meglumine-type contrast agent) is injected into the joint capsule. For MRa, 0.1 mL of gadolinium-based contrast material is diluted in 20 mL of saline and 3–5 mL of iodinated contrast material, and 10 mL of this solution is injected into the glenohumeral joint. The iodinated contrast material allows fluoroscopic confirmation of the proper intraarticular needle position. The usual study includes supine films of the shoulder in the standard anteroposterior (arm in the neutral position and in internal and external rotation) and the axillary projections. **(B)** A normal arthrogram of the shoulder shows contrast outlining the articular cartilage of the humerus and the glenoid and filling the axillary pouch, the subscapularis recess, and the bicipital tendon sheath. US-guided needle position into the glenohumeral joint can alternatively be used instead of fluoroscopic guidance, when the purpose is only to inject contrast prior to MRa. For MRa, a single fluoroscopic spot film demonstrating the flow of iodinated contrast material in the glenohumeral joint is sufficient. The patient is then taken to the MR suite for an MRI using the appropriate protocol, including T1-weighted fat-saturated images in the axial, oblique sagittal, and oblique coronal planes and T2-weighted fat-saturated images in the oblique coronal plane, followed by a T1-weighted fat-saturated image with the arm in the ABER position, if the patient can tolerate it (see Figs. 5.22F and 5.114B).

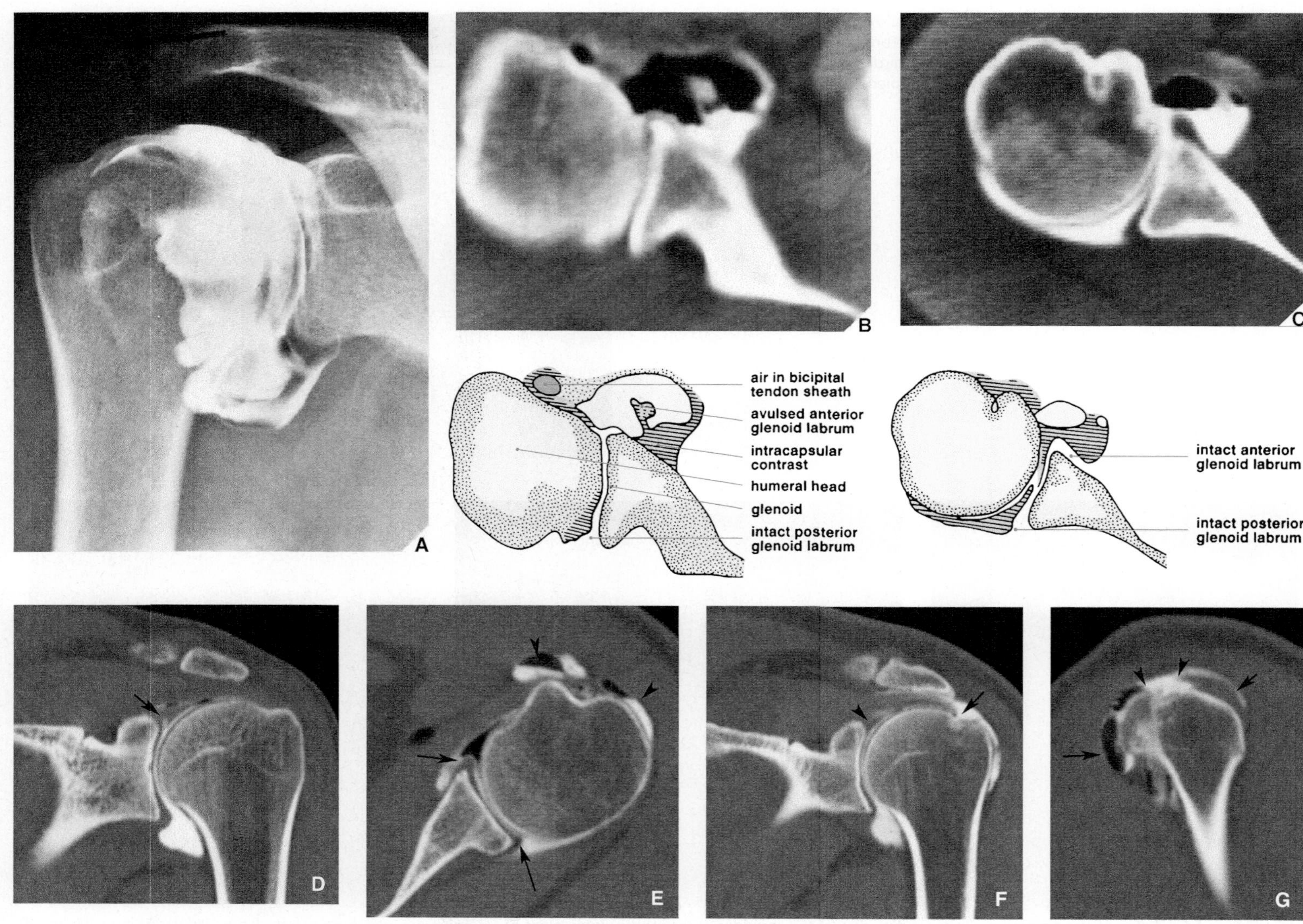

FIGURE 5.18 CT-arthrography. As the result of an auto accident, a 33-year-old woman sustained an injury to the right shoulder; she presented with pain and limitation of motion in the joint. Standard radiographs of the shoulder were normal. As injury to the cartilaginous labrum was suspected, double-contrast arthrography was performed. Five milliliters of positive contrast agent and 10 mL of room air were injected into the joint capsule. **(A)** This arthrogram shows no evident abnormalities. The subscapularis recess, which is not opacified on this view, was shown later in the study to fill with contrast. **(B)** In conjunction with arthrography, a CT scan of the same shoulder was performed and clearly demonstrates avulsion of the anterior glenoid labrum, a finding not appreciated on the arthrographic study. Note that the avulsed fragment is surrounded by air and shows absorption of the contrast agent. **(C)** The normal appearance of the glenoid labrum is shown for comparison. **(D)** Coronal reformatted CT double-contrast arthrogram of the left shoulder in another patient demonstrates a superior labral tear/SLAP lesion *(arrow)*. Iodinated contrast material and air distends the glenohumeral joint. Note the absence of contrast material in the subacromial–subdeltoid bursa, indicating an intact rotator cuff. **(E)** Axial CT double-contrast arthrogram in another patient demonstrates intact labrum anteriorly and posteriorly *(arrows)*, but there is contrast material and air in the subacromial–subdeltoid bursae complex *(arrowheads)* diagnostic of full-thickness rotator cuff tear. **(F)** Coronal reformatted CT image in the same patient shows a small full-thickness tear of the supraspinatus tendon *(arrow)* with contrast material extending to the subacromial–subdeltoid bursa. Note the intact superior labrum *(arrowhead)*. **(G)** Sagittal reformatted CT image in the same patient shows the anteroposterior dimension of the rotator cuff tear *(arrowheads)*, and the contrast material and air in the subacromial–subdeltoid bursa *(arrows)*. (**D** to **G**, Courtesy of Steve Shankman, MD, Brooklyn, New York.)

space limitations in the magnet, the shoulder frequently cannot be positioned in the center of the magnetic field. This necessitates lateral shift for image centering and scanning a region where the signal-to-noise ratio is relatively low. These problems have been overcome by combining high-resolution scanning with the use of special surface coils. Because the bones and muscles of the shoulder girdle are oriented along multiple nonorthogonal axes, scanning in oblique planes is more effective.

The patient should be positioned in the magnet supine with the arms along the thorax and the affected arm externally rotated. The scanning planes include oblique coronal (along the long axis of the belly of the supraspinatus muscle), oblique sagittal (perpendicular to the course of supraspinatus muscle), and axial (Fig. 5.19). The first two planes are ideal for evaluating all the structures of the rotator cuff; the axial plane is ideal for evaluating the glenoid labrum, bicipital groove, biceps tendon, and subscapularis tendon (Fig. 5.20). Appropriate pulse sequences are critical in displaying normal anatomy and traumatic abnormalities. T1-weighted pulse sequences sufficiently demonstrate the structural anatomy. Proton density– and T2-weighted pulse sequences provide the information necessary to evaluate pathology of rotator cuff, joint space, and bones. Magnetic resonance arthrography (MRa) provides excellent depiction of the undersurface of the rotator cuff and intracapsular structures (Fig. 5.21). For techniques of MRa, see discussion in the following section.

The demonstration of rotator cuff muscles and tendons is greatly facilitated by the use of MRI. The supraspinatus is best demonstrated on oblique coronal and sagittal images, preferably obtained on spin echo T1-weighted sequences. It is seen as a thick, intermediate-intensity structure, and its tendon inserts on the superolateral aspect of the greater tuberosity of the humerus (Fig. 5.22). The infraspinatus and subscapularis are best demonstrated on axial images as fusiform, intermediate-intensity structures (see Fig. 5.20). The infraspinatus tendon inserts distally and more posterior to the supraspinatus on the greater tuberosity, adjacent to the insertion of teres minor (Fig. 5.22B). The subscapularis muscle is located

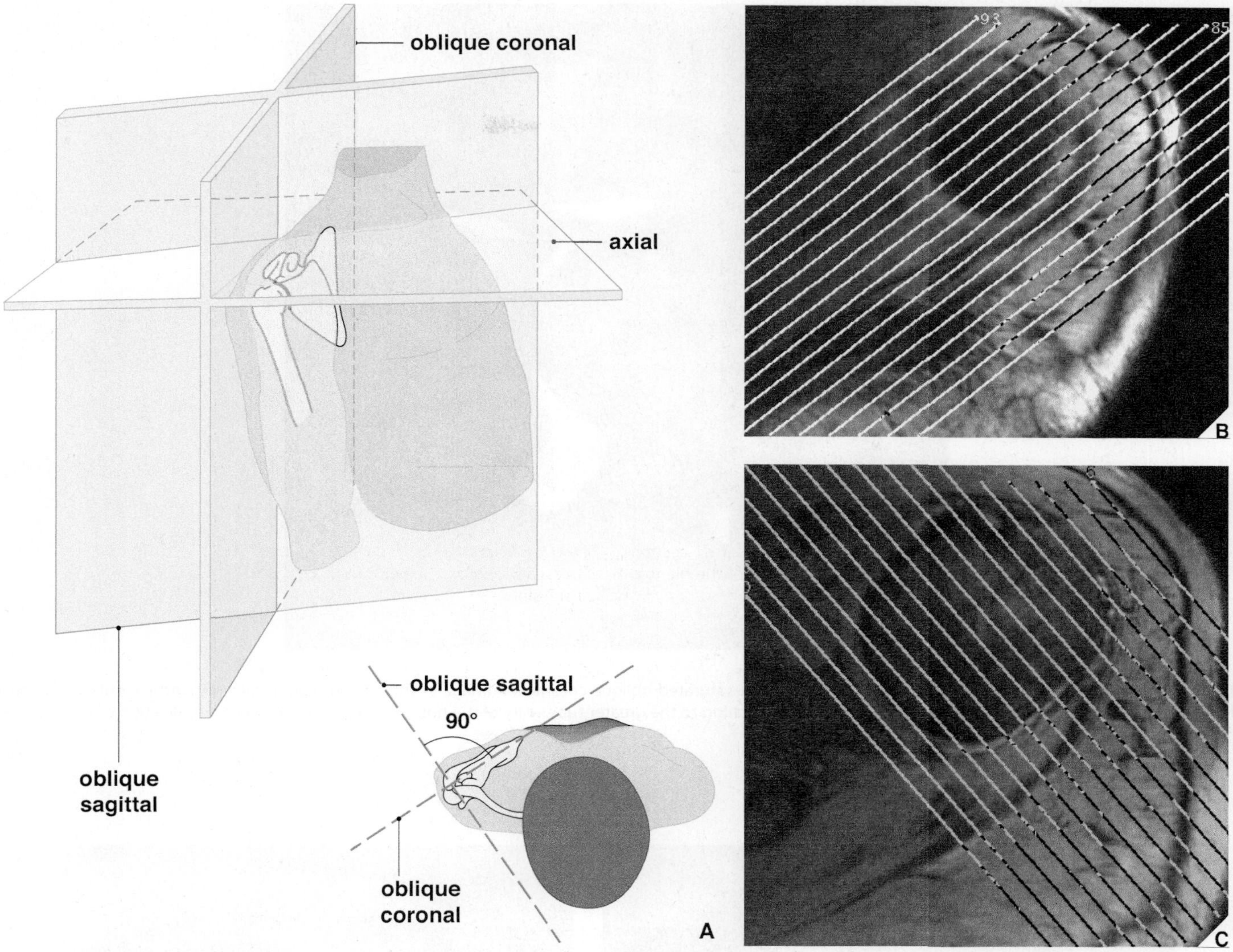

oblique coronal
axial
oblique sagittal
oblique sagittal
90°
oblique coronal
A
B
C

FIGURE 5.19 **MRI of the shoulder.** **(A)** Standard planes of MRI sections of the shoulder. **(B)** Oblique coronal sections are obtained parallel to the long axis of the scapula, perpendicular to the glenoid. **(C)** Oblique sagittal sections are obtained perpendicular to the oblique coronal sections, parallel to the glenoid.

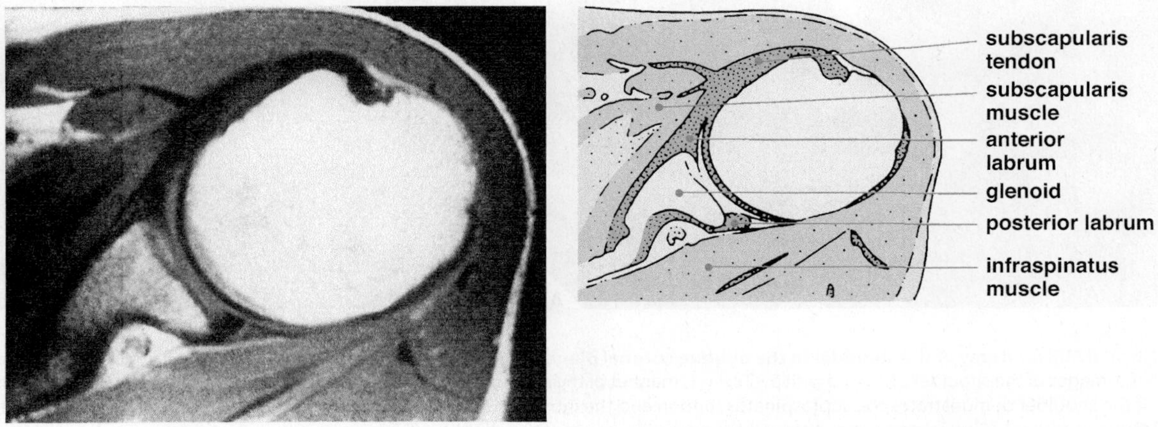

FIGURE 5.20 **MRI of the shoulder.** T1-weighted axial image of the left shoulder shows a normal subscapularis muscle and tendon and the infraspinatus muscle. The anterior and posterior glenoid labrum is also effectively demonstrated.

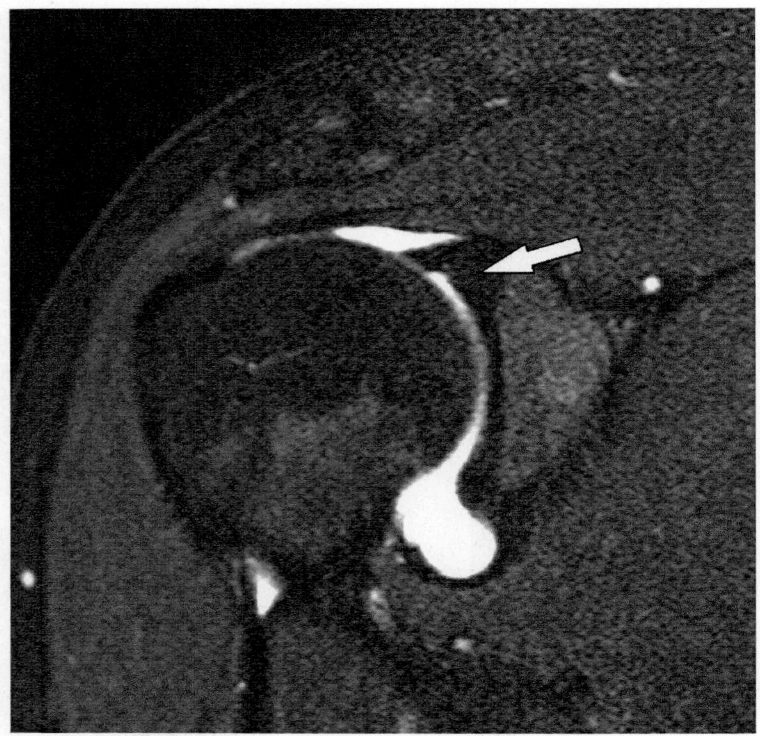

FIGURE 5.21 MR-arthrogram of the shoulder. T1-weighted fat-saturated oblique coronal MR image of the right shoulder following intraarticular injection of gadolinium demonstrates a normal supraspinatus muscle and tendon attaching to the greater tuberosity of the humerus. Note the excellent visualization of the superior labrum *(arrow)*.

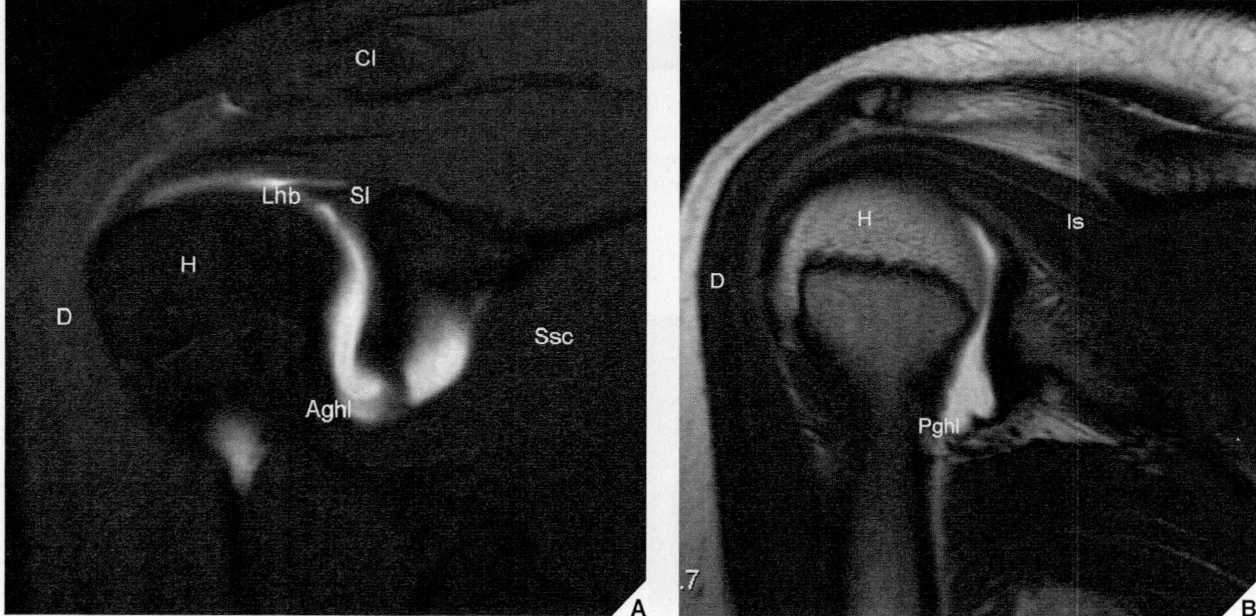

FIGURE 5.22 Normal MRI anatomy of the shoulder in the oblique coronal plane, oblique sagittal plane, and ABER position. Oblique coronal **(A,B)**, oblique sagittal **(C–E)**, and ABER **(F)** MRa images of the shoulder obtained with a 3 Tesla (T) magnet of the same patient. **(A)** Oblique coronal T1-weighted fat-saturated image obtained through the anterior aspect of the shoulder demonstrates the supraspinatus tendon and the intracapsular portion of the long biceps tendon at its junction with the superior labrum. Note the AIGHL. **(B)** Oblique coronal T2-weighted image through the posterior aspect of the shoulder demonstrates the infraspinatus tendon and the PIGHL. *(Continued)*

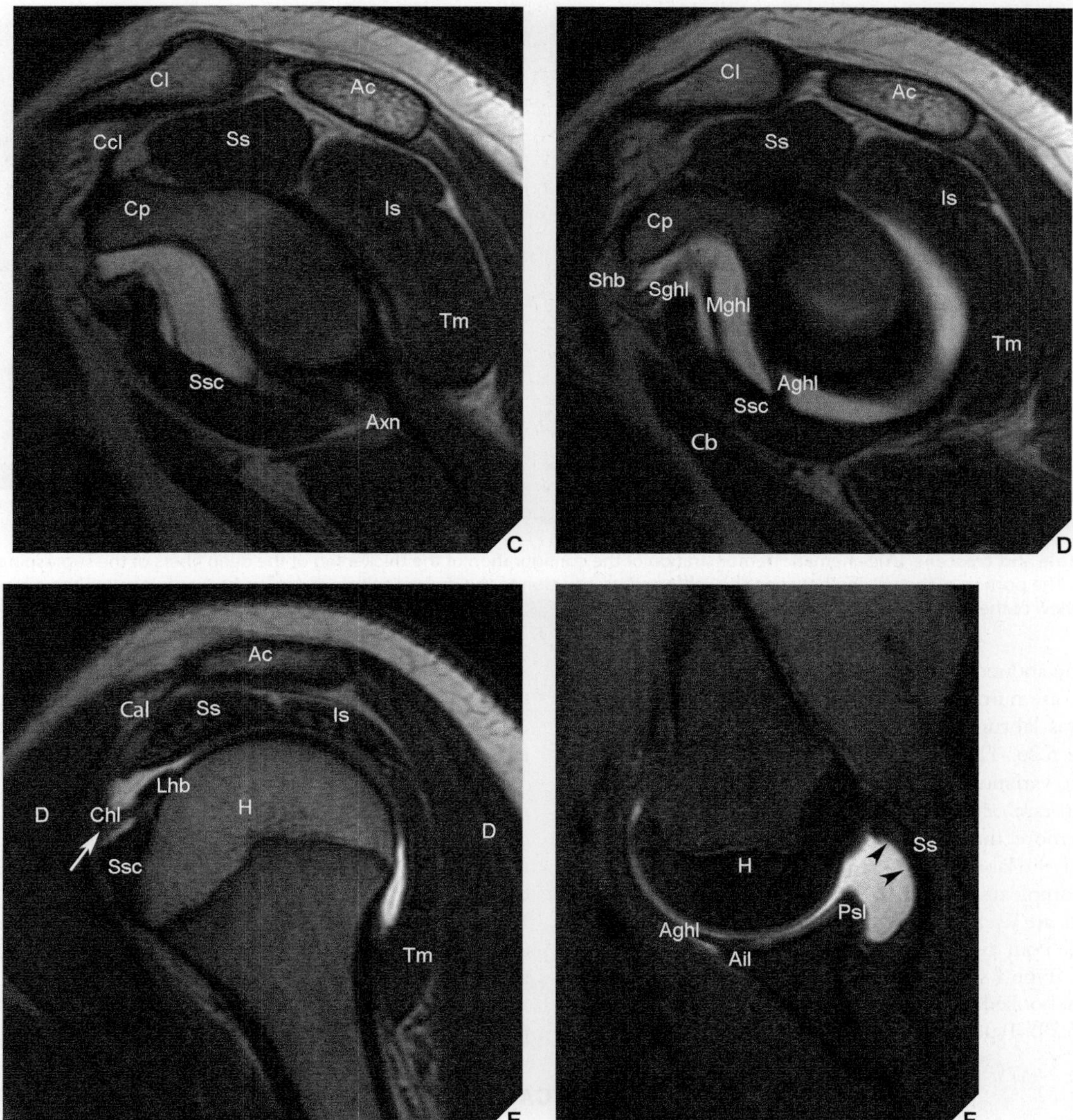

FIGURE 5.22 **Normal MRI anatomy of the shoulder in the oblique coronal plane, oblique sagittal plane, and ABER position.** ***(Continued)*** **(C)** Oblique sagittal T2-weighted image through the glenoid demonstrates the axillary nerve in the quadrilateral space. **(D)** Oblique sagittal T2-weighted image through the glenohumeral joint well depicts the SGHL and MGHL and the AIGHL. **(E)** Oblique sagittal T2-weighted image through the head of the humerus shows the relationship between the distal coracohumeral ligament and the long biceps tendon at the point where the tendon enters the joint capsule. The SGHL and the coracohumeral ligaments form the structure that surrounds the long biceps tendon *(arrow)* and provide stability of the tendon during arm motion. This structure is known as the *sling* or *reflective pulley*. **(F)** T1-weighted fat-saturated image in the ABER position shows the AIGHL and the anterior inferior labrum. Note the undersurface of the supraspinatus tendon *(arrowheads)*. H, humeral head; Ac, acromion; Cl, clavicle; Cp, coracoid process; D, deltoid; Ss, supraspinatus; Is, infraspinatus; Ssc, subscapularis; Tm, teres minor; Shb, short head of the biceps; Lhb, long head of the biceps; Cb, coracobrachialis; Aghl, anterior band of the glenohumeral ligament; Pghl, posterior band of the inferior glenohumeral ligament; Sl, superior labrum and bicipitolabral junction; Mghl, middle glenohumeral ligament; Sghl, superior glenohumeral ligament; Chl, coracohumeral ligament; Ail, anterior inferior labrum; Psl, posterior superior labrum; Ccl, coracoclavicular ligaments; Axn, axillary nerve in the quadrilateral space; Cal, coracoacromial ligament.

anterior to the body of the scapula. It appears on T1-weighted axial images as an intermediate-intensity structure that tapers anteriorly into a low-intensity tendon, where it merges with the anterior aspect of the capsule before inserting on the lesser tuberosity (see Fig. 5.20).

A variation of the normal anatomy of the supraspinatus tendon described by Burkhart et al. consists of a crescent-shaped thickening of the deep fibers of this tendon with a perpendicular orientation to the rest of the tendon fibers. This so-called *cable* attaches to the anterior and posterior aspects of the greater tuberosity of the humerus, and it acts as a restrain to proximal extension of a tear of the supraspinatus tendon. The portion of the tendon between the cable and the humeral insertion is called the *crescent* (Fig. 5.23).

The axial images are effective in demonstration of the joint capsule, which is anteriorly reinforced by the anterior GHLs. The capsular complex provides stabilization of the glenohumeral joint. The anterior capsular complex includes the fibrous capsule, the anterior GHLs, the synovial membrane and its recesses, the fibrous glenoid labrum, the subscapularis muscle and tendon, and the scapular periosteum. Three types of anterior capsular insertion have been identified by Zlatkin and colleagues. They are determined by the proximity of insertion to the glenoid margin (Fig. 5.24). In type I, the capsule inserts on the glenoid rim in close proximity to the glenoid labrum. In types II and III, the capsular insertion is further away from the glenoid rim and may reach the scapular neck (Fig. 5.25). The further the anterior capsule inserts from the glenoid margin, the more unstable the glenohumeral joint will be. The posterior portion of the capsule shows no variations and attaches directly to the labrum. The axial images are also effective in the demonstration of anterior and posterior cartilaginous labrum of the glenoid, which are seen as two small triangles of low signal intensity that are located anteriorly and posteriorly to the glenoid margin (Fig. 5.26). The superior and inferior aspects of the labrum are best demonstrated on the oblique coronal sections (Fig. 5.27). The anterior inferior aspect of the glenoid labrum and the anterior band of the inferior GHL (IGHL) can be

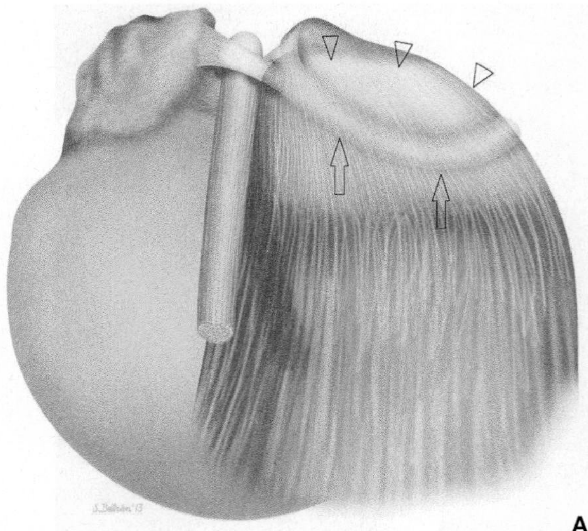

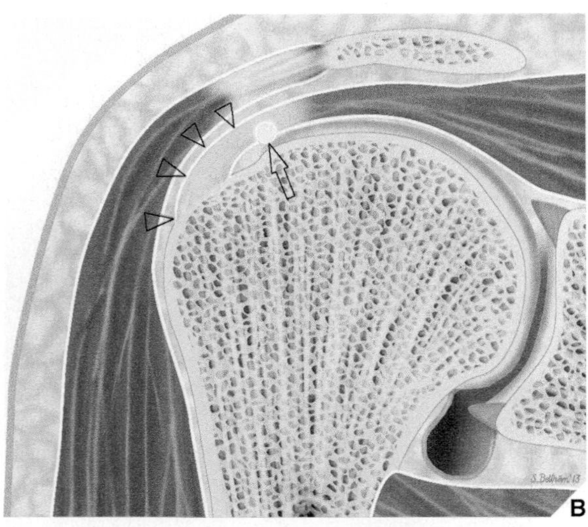

FIGURE 5.23 The cable and crescent. **(A)** Schematic demonstration of the configuration of the thickening of the deep fibers of the supraspinatus tendon or *cable (arrows)* viewed from above. The portion of the tendon between the cable and its insertion to the greater tuberosity of the humerus is called the *crescent* because of its shape *(arrowheads)*. **(B)** Frontal view of the cable *(arrow)* and crescent *(arrowheads)*.

seen with the arm in the abduction and external rotation (ABER) position (see Fig. 5.22F). There are numerous imaging variations of the morphology of the cartilaginous labrum. The most common shape is triangular as illustrated in Figure 5.26. The second most common shape is round. The other morphologic variations include the flat labrum and the cleaved or notched labrum. On rare occasions, the anterior and posterior labrum may be absent. Furthermore, there are appearances resembling labral tears, such as undercutting of the labrum by hyaline cartilage, sublabral holes or recesses, and Buford complexes (see Fig. 5.86).

The sagittal images are useful in demonstration of morphologic variations of the acromion. Four types of acromion have been identified by Bigliani and coworkers. Type I shows a flat undersurface; type II, a curved undersurface; type III, a hooked undersurface; and type IV, a convex undersurface (Figs. 5.28 and 5.29). Type III acromion is considered to be associated with tears of the rotator cuff proximal to the site of insertion of the supraspinatus tendon to the greater tuberosity of the humerus. The rare type IV exhibits convex undersurface. Sagittal images also effectively demonstrate the muscles of the rotator cuff and their respective tendons (see Fig. 5.22C,D).

In the past decade, direct MRa using injection of contrast solution into the shoulder joint gained worldwide acceptance. This technique is particularly effective for demonstrating labral–ligamentous abnormalities and distinguishing partial-thickness from full-thickness tears of the rotator cuff. A variety of concentrations and mixtures of solutions are used by different radiologists. In our institution, we follow the recommendation reported by Steinbach and colleagues. We add 0.8 mL of gadopentetate dimeglumine (gadolinium with strength 287 mg/mL) to 100 mL of normal saline solution. Subsequently, we mix 10 mL of this solution with 5 mL of 60% meglumine diatrizoate (iodinated contrast) and 5 mL of 1% lidocaine, which gives a final gadolinium

TYPES OF ANTERIOR CAPSULAR INSERTION

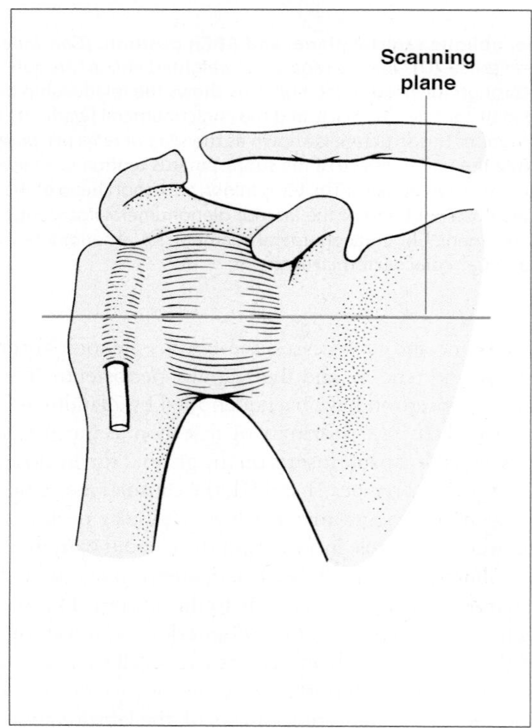

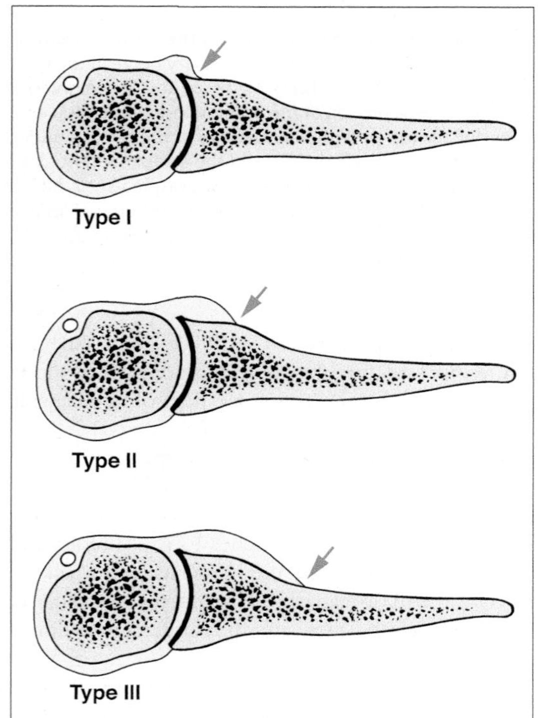

FIGURE 5.24 Capsule of the shoulder joint. Three types of anterior capsular insertion to the scapula.

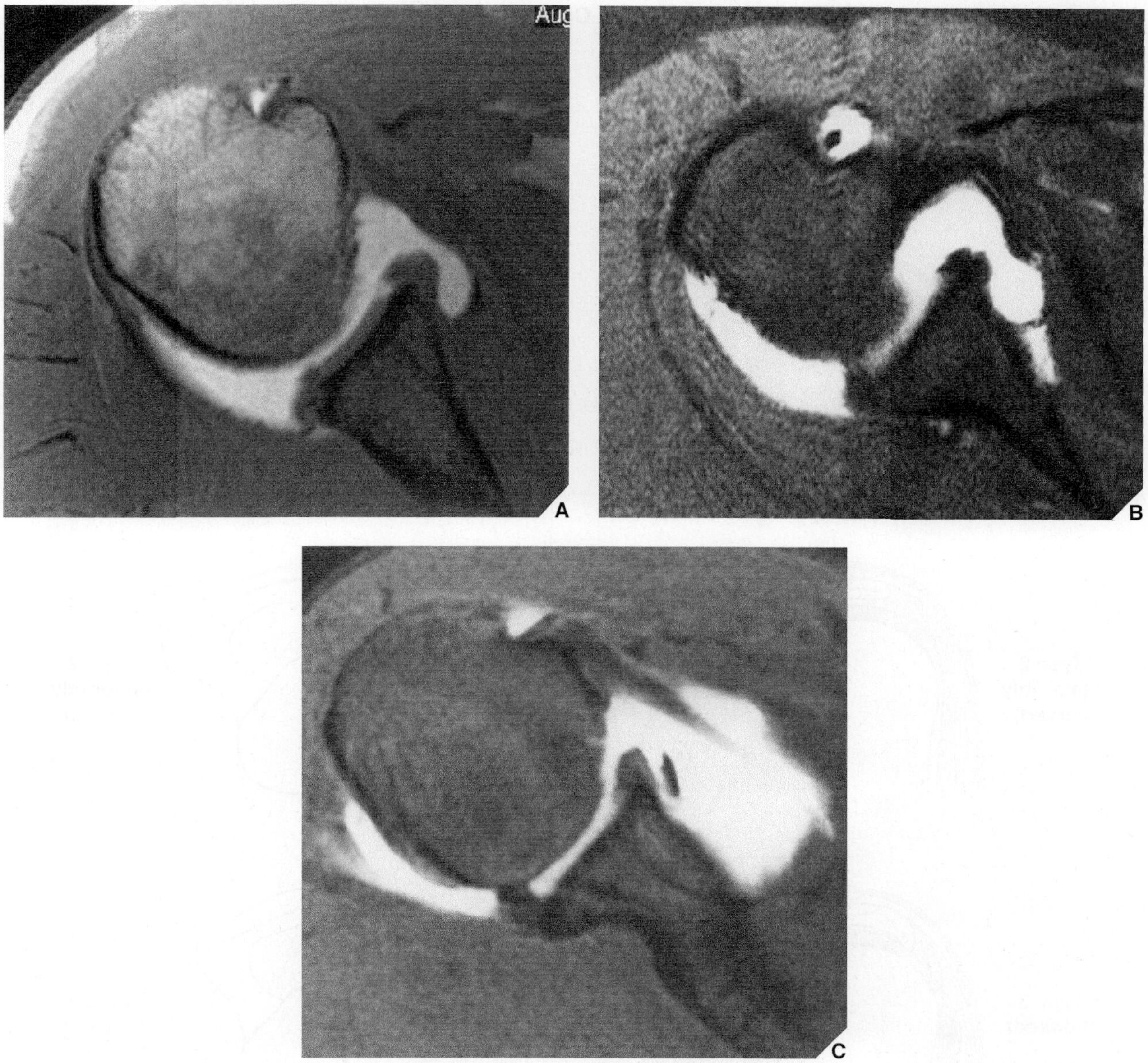

FIGURE 5.25 **Capsular insertion to glenoid margin.** **(A)** Axial T1-weighted MR image obtained after intraarticular injection of gadolinium shows type I of anterior capsular insertion. **(B)** Axial FSE MR image with fat saturation obtained after intraarticular injection of gadolinium shows type II of anterior capsular insertion. **(C)** Axial T1-weighted MR image with fat saturation obtained after intraarticular injection of gadolinium shows type III of anterior capsular insertion.

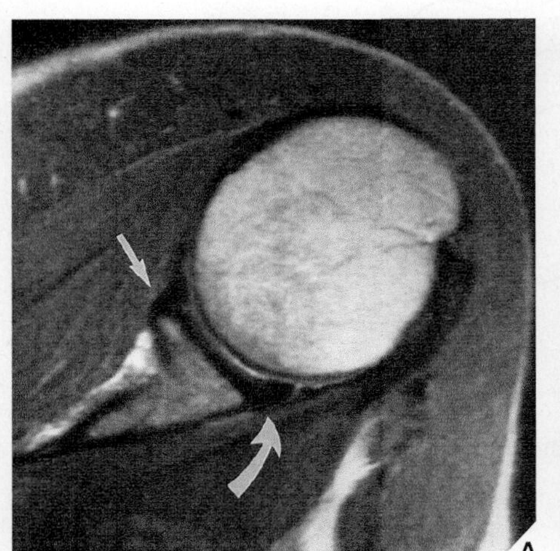

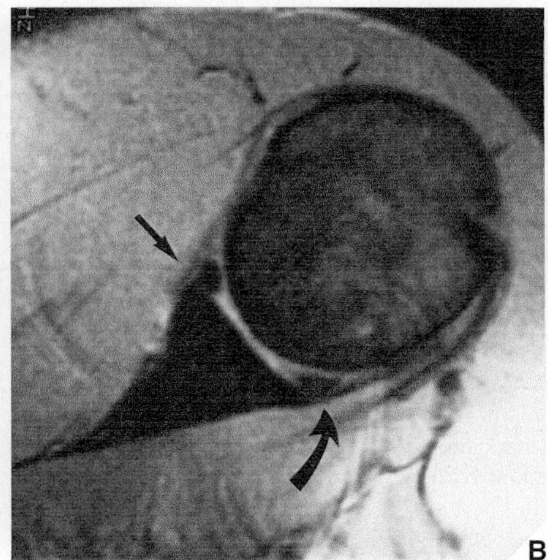

FIGURE 5.26 **Fibrocartilaginous labrum of the glenoid.** **(A)** Axial T1-weighted and **(B)** axial T2-weighted (multiplanar gradient-recalled [MPGR]) MR images show anterior *(arrows)* and posterior *(curved arrows)* labra as small triangles of low signal intensity.

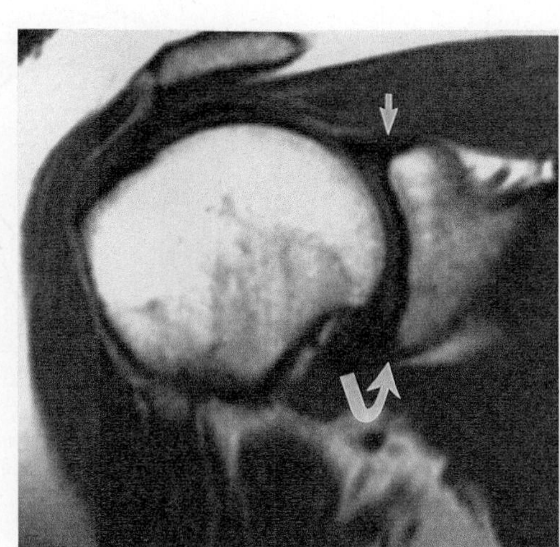

FIGURE 5.27 **Fibrocartilaginous labrum.** Oblique coronal T1-weighted fat-saturated MRI shows a superior labrum *(arrow)* and an inferior labrum *(curved arrow)*.

BIGLIANI CLASSIFICATION OF ACROMIAL MORPHOLOGY

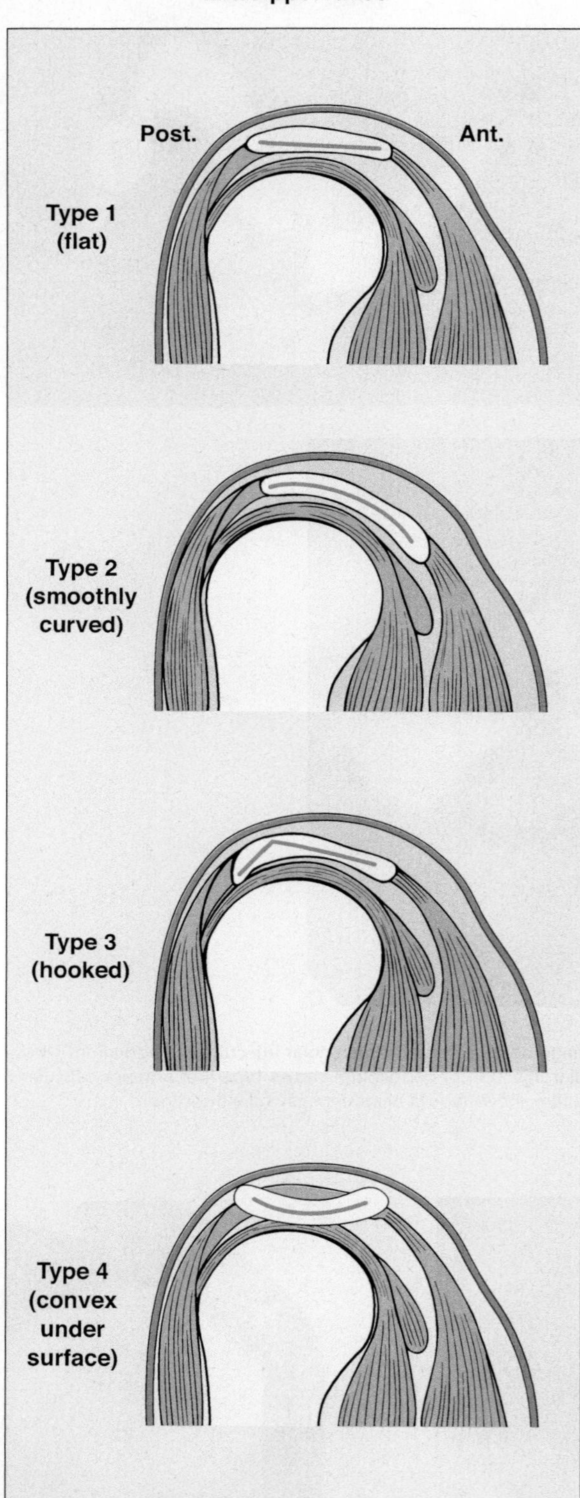

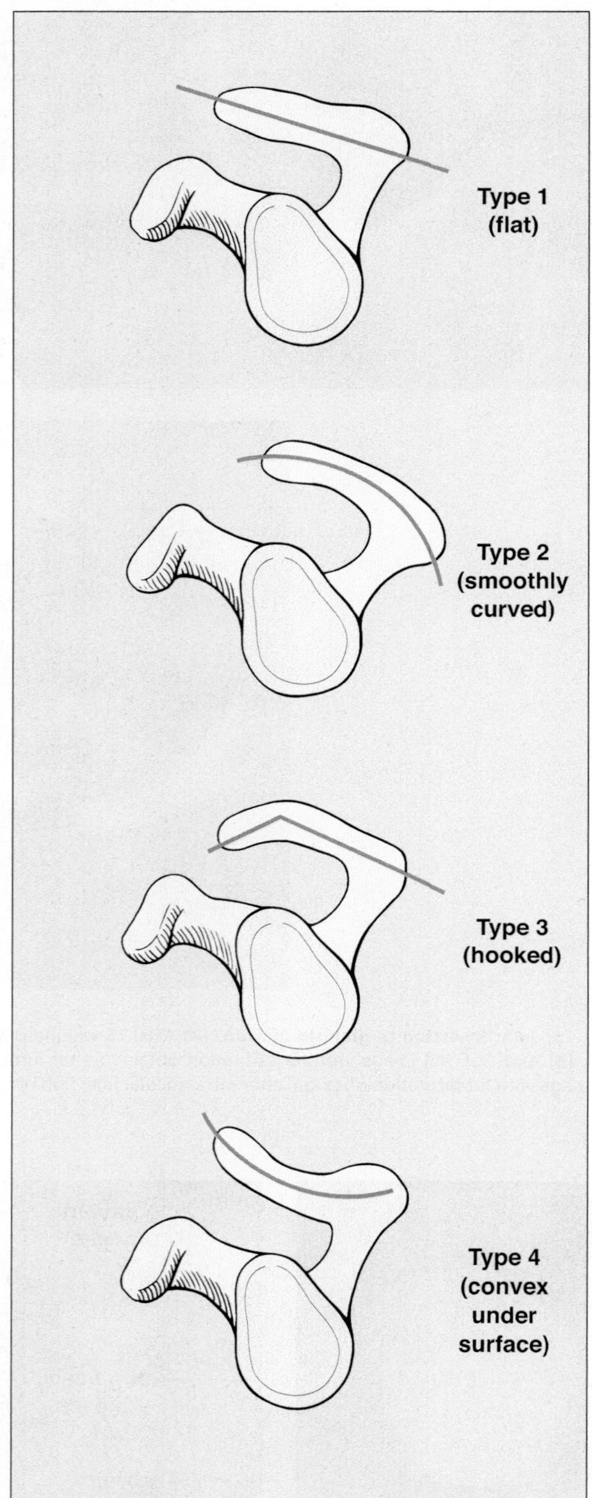

FIGURE 5.28 Variations of the acromial morphology. Schematic representation of morphologic variations of the acromion. **(A)** Magnetic resonance imaging (MRI) appearance on oblique sagittal sections. **(B)** Appearance on anatomic specimen.

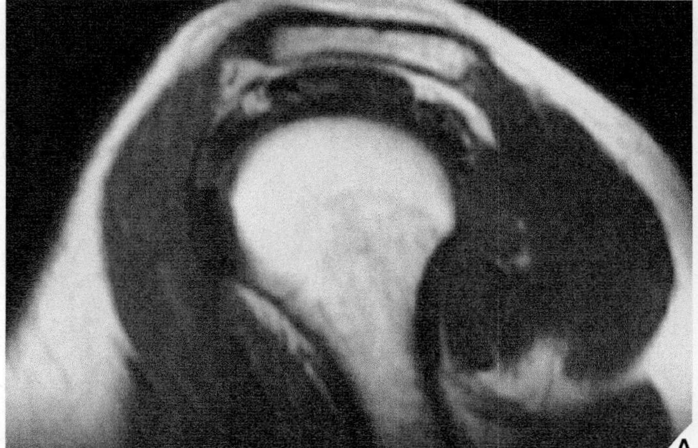

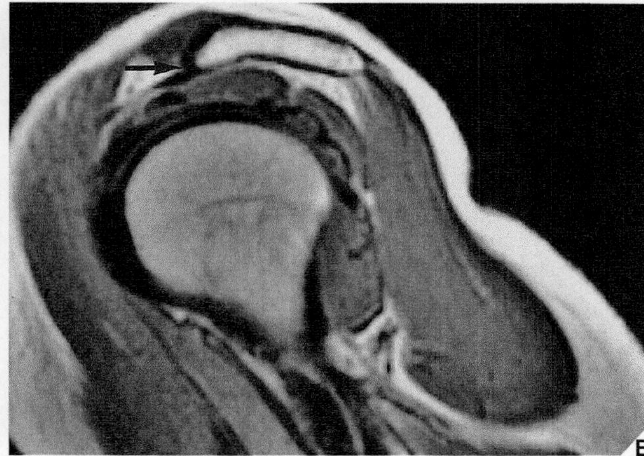

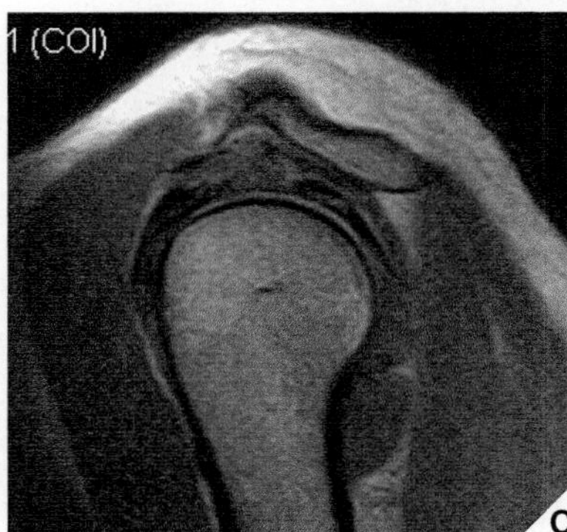

FIGURE 5.29 **Morphologic variations of the acromion.** **(A)** In the sagittal oblique plane, type II acromion shows a mild curved undersurface. **(B)** Type III acromion demonstrates a hooked undersurface *(arrow)*. **(C)** Type IV acromion demonstrates a convex undersurface.

dilution ratio of 1:250. From 12 to 15 mL of this mixture is then injected into the shoulder joint using fluoroscopic guidance in a similar fashion as for conventional shoulder arthrography (see Fig. 5.17). Multiple preexercise and postexercise radiographic spot images are obtained in neutral position and in external and internal rotation of the arm. Subsequently, without delay, the patient undergoes MRI examination using similar scanning planes as for a conventional magnetic resonance (MR) study. If glenoid labrum abnormalities are suspected, additional sequences are obtained in so-called *ABER position*.

During evaluation of MRI of the shoulder, it is helpful to use a checklist as provided in Table 5.1.

For a summary of the foregoing discussion in tabular form, see Tables 5.2 and 5.3.

Injury to the Shoulder Girdle

Fractures About the Shoulder

Fractures of the Proximal Humerus

Fractures of the upper humerus involving the head, the neck, and the proximal shaft usually result either from a direct blow to the humerus or, as is more often seen in elderly patients, from a fall on the outstretched arm.

TABLE 5.1 Checklist for Evaluation of Magnetic Resonance Imaging and Magnetic Resonance Arthrography of the Shoulder

Osseous Structures
Humeral head (c, s, a)
Glenoid (c, s, a)
Acromion (c, s)
Clavicle (c, s)
Coracoacromial arch (s)

Cartilaginous Structures
Articular cartilage (c, s, a)
Fibrocartilaginous labrum, anterior, posterior, superior, inferior (c, a)

Joints
Glenohumeral (c, a)
Acromioclavicular (c)

Capsule
Attachment (a)
Laxity (a)

Muscles and Their Tendons
Supraspinatus (c, s, a)
Infraspinatus (c, s, a)
Teres minor (c, s)

Muscles and Their Tendons (continued)
Subscapularis (s, a)
Biceps—long head (c, s, a)
Deltoid (c, a)

Ligaments
Superior glenohumeral (s, a)
Middle glenohumeral (s, a)
Inferior glenohumeral (s, a)
Coracohumeral (c)
Coracoclavicular—conoid and trapezoid (s)
Coracoacromial (s)
Acromioclavicular (c)

Bursae
Subacromial–subdeltoid (c)

Other Structures
Rotator interval—space between supraspinatus and subscapularis (s)
Quadrilateral space (s, a)
Suprascapular notch (c, a)
Spinoglenoid notch (c, a)

The best imaging planes for visualization of listed structures are given in parentheses: a, axial; c, coronal; s, sagittal.

TABLE 5.2 Standard and Special Radiographic Projections for Evaluating Injury to the Shoulder Girdle

Projection	Demonstration
Anteroposterior	
Arm in neutral position	Fracture of Humeral head and neck Clavicle Scapula Anterior dislocation Bankart lesion
Erect	FBI sign
Arm in internal rotation	Hill-Sachs lesion
Arm in external rotation	Compression fracture of humeral head (trough line impaction) secondary to posterior dislocation
40-degree posterior oblique (Grashey)	Glenohumeral joint space Glenoid in profile Posterior dislocation
15-degree cephalad tilt of radiographic tube	Acromioclavicular joint Acromioclavicular separation Fracture of clavicle
Stress	Occult acromioclavicular subluxation Acromioclavicular separation
Axillary	Relationship of humeral head and glenoid fossa Os acromiale Anterior and posterior dislocations Compression fractures secondary to anterior and posterior dislocations Fractures of Proximal humerus Scapula
West Point	Same structures and conditions as axillary projection Anteroinferior rim of glenoid
Lateral Transthoracic	Relationship of humeral head and glenoid fossa Fractures of proximal humerus
Tangent (Humeral Head)	Bicipital groove
Transscapular (Y)	Relationship of humeral head and glenoid fossa Fractures of Proximal humerus Body of scapula Coracoid process Acromion
Oblique (outlet)	Coracoacromial arch Rotator cuff outlet
Serendipity (cephalad 40 degrees)	Anterior and posterior sternoclavicular dislocation

FBI, fat–blood interface.

Nondisplaced fractures are the most common, representing approximately 85% of all such proximal humeral injuries.

The anteroposterior projection is usually sufficient to demonstrate the abnormality, but the transthoracic lateral or the transscapular (or Y) projection may be required to provide a fuller evaluation, particularly of the degree of displacement or angulation of the osseous fragments (Fig. 5.30). The erect anteroposterior radiograph may demonstrate the presence of fat and blood within the joint capsule (the fat–blood interface [FBI] sign of lipohemarthrosis; see Fig. 4.59A), indicating intraarticular extension of the fracture.

Traditional classifications of trauma to the proximal humerus, according to the level of the fracture or the mechanism of injury, have been inadequate to identify the various types of displaced fractures. The four-segment classification described by Neer in 1970 was complex and difficult to follow. He later modified this classification and simplified divisions to various groups. Classification of a displacement pattern depends on two main factors: the number of displaced segments and the key segment displaced. Fractures of the proximal humerus occur between one and all of four major segments: the articular segment (at the level of the anatomic neck), the greater tuberosity, the lesser tuberosity, and the humeral shaft (at the level of the surgical neck). One-part fracture occurs when there is minimal or no displacement between the segments. In two-part fractures, only one segment is displaced. In three-part fractures, two segments are displaced and one tuberosity remains in continuity with the humeral head. In four-part fractures, three segments are displaced, including both tuberosities. Two-part, three-part, and four-part fractures may or may not be associated with dislocation, either anterior or posterior. The involvement of the articular surface is classified separately into two groups: the anterior fracture–dislocation, termed by Neer *head splitting*, and posterior fracture–dislocation, termed *impression* (Fig. 5.31).

One-part fracture may involve any or all of the anatomic segments of the proximal humerus. There is no or minimal (less than 1 cm) displacement and no or minimal (less than 45 degrees) angulation; the fragments are being held together by the rotator cuff, the joint capsule, and the intact periosteum.

Two-part fracture indicates that only one segment is displaced in relation to the three that remain undisplaced. It may involve the anatomic neck, surgical neck, greater tuberosity, or lesser tuberosity. The two-part fracture involving the anatomic neck of the humerus with displacement of the articular end may be associated with tear of the rotator cuff, and complications such as malunion or osteonecrosis may develop. In two-part fractures involving the surgical neck of the humerus with displacement or angulation of the shaft, three types may be seen: impacted, unimpacted, and comminuted. These fractures may be associated with either anterior or posterior dislocation. With anterior dislocation, the fracture invariably

TABLE 5.3 Ancillary Imaging Techniques for Evaluating Injury to the Shoulder Girdle

Technique	Demonstration
Tomography (almost completely replaced by CT)	Position of fragments and extension of fracture line in complex fractures Healing process: Nonunion Secondary infection
CT	Relationship of humeral head and glenoid fossa Multiple fragments in complex fractures (particularly of scapula) Intraarticular displacement of bony fragments in fractures
MRI	Impingement syndrome Partial and complete rotator cuff tear[a] Biceps tendon rupture Glenoid labrum tears[a] Glenohumeral instability Traumatic joint effusion Subtle synovial abnormalities[a]
US	Rotator cuff tear Tear of biceps tendon
Arthrography Single or double contrast	Complete rotator cuff tear Partial rotator cuff tear Abnormalities of articular cartilage and joint capsule[b] Synovial abnormalities[b] Adhesive capsulitis Osteochondral bodies in joint[b] Abnormalities of bicipital tendon[b,c] Intraarticular portion of bicipital tendon[b,c] Inferior surface of rotator cuff[b,c]
Double contrast combined with CT	All of the above and in addition: Abnormalities of cartilaginous glenoid labrum Osteochondral bodies in joint Subtle synovial abnormalities

[a]These abnormalities are best demonstrated on MRa.
[b]These conditions are usually best demonstrated using double-contrast arthrography.
[c]These features are best demonstrated on erect films.
CT, computed tomography; MRI, magnetic resonance imaging; US, ultrasound.

involves the greater tuberosity; with posterior dislocation, the fracture invariably involves the lesser tuberosity.

Three-part fracture may involve either greater tuberosity or lesser tuberosity and may be associated with anterior or posterior dislocation. Two segments are displaced in relation to two other segments that are not displaced.

Four-part fracture involves the greater and lesser tuberosity in addition to the fracture of the surgical neck, and four major segments are displaced (Fig. 5.32). This may be associated with anterior or posterior dislocation. The four-part fracture is usually associated with impairment of the blood supply to the humeral head, and osteonecrosis of the humeral head is a frequent complication.

Fractures of the Clavicle

A common injury in infancy during delivery, in adolescence caused by a direct blow or fall, and in adulthood as the result of a motor vehicle accident is a fracture of the clavicle, which can be divided into three types according to the anatomic segment involved (Fig. 5.33A). The most common site of

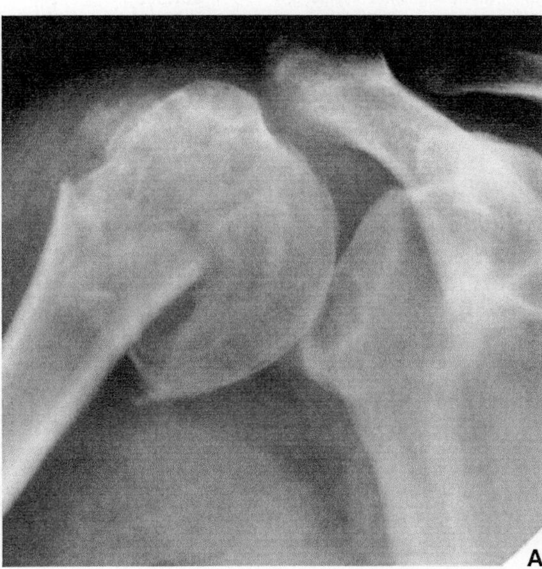

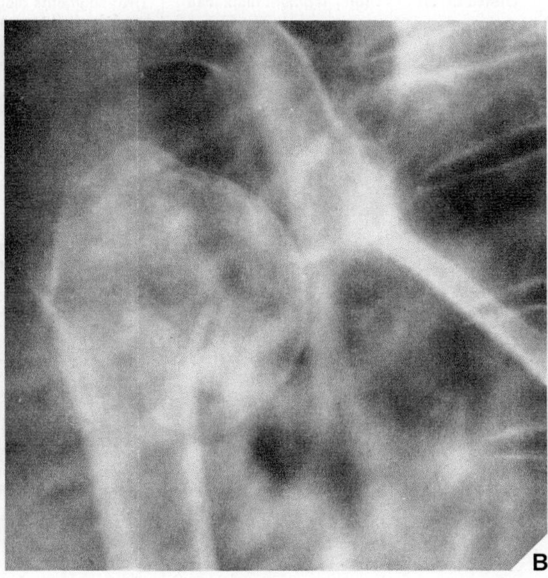

FIGURE 5.30 Fracture of the proximal humerus. A 60-year-old man fell on a staircase and injured his right arm. **(A)** Anteroposterior radiograph of the shoulder demonstrates a comminuted fracture through the surgical neck of the humerus. The greater tuberosity is fractured, too, but is not significantly displaced. To assess the degree of displacement of the various fragments better, the transthoracic lateral view **(B)** was obtained. It demonstrates slight anterior angulation of the humeral head, which in addition is inferiorly subluxed—a finding not well appreciated on the anteroposterior projection.

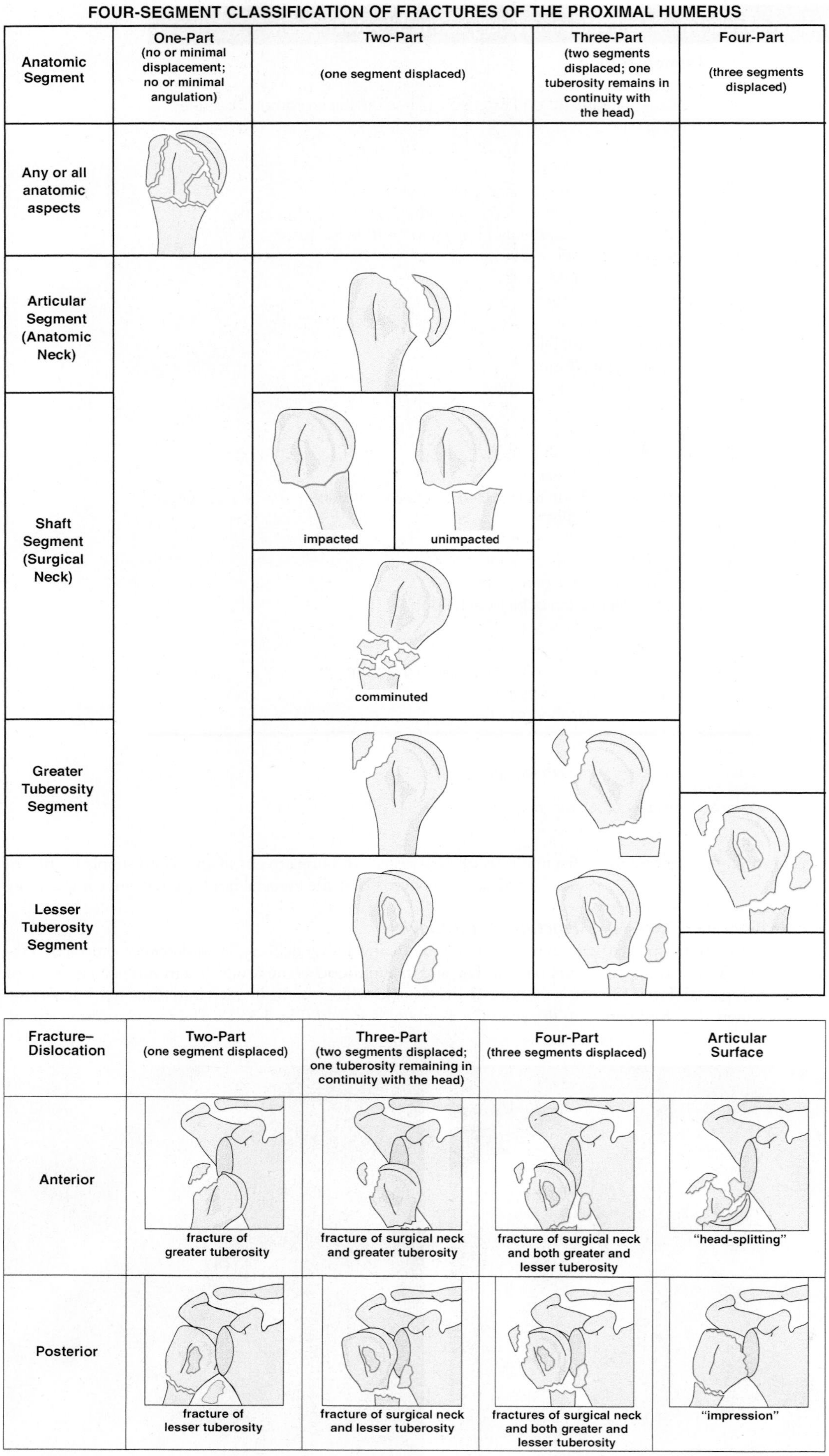

FOUR-SEGMENT CLASSIFICATION OF FRACTURES OF THE PROXIMAL HUMERUS

Anatomic Segment	One-Part (no or minimal displacement; no or minimal angulation)	Two-Part (one segment displaced)	Three-Part (two segments displaced; one tuberosity remains in continuity with the head)	Four-Part (three segments displaced)
Any or all anatomic aspects				
Articular Segment (Anatomic Neck)				
Shaft Segment (Surgical Neck)		impacted; unimpacted; comminuted		
Greater Tuberosity Segment				
Lesser Tuberosity Segment				

Fracture–Dislocation	Two-Part (one segment displaced)	Three-Part (two segments displaced; one tuberosity remaining in continuity with the head)	Four-Part (three segments displaced)	Articular Surface
Anterior	fracture of greater tuberosity	fracture of surgical neck and greater tuberosity	fracture of surgical neck and both greater and lesser tuberosity	"head-splitting"
Posterior	fracture of lesser tuberosity	fracture of surgical neck and lesser tuberosity	fractures of surgical neck and both greater and lesser tuberosity	"impression"

FIGURE 5.31 Neer classification. Fractures of the proximal humerus based on the presence or absence of displacement of the four major fragments that may result from fracture. (Modified with permission from Neer CS II. Displaced proximal humeral fractures. Part I. Classification and evaluation. *J Bone Joint Surg Am* 1970;52(6):1077–1089.)

FIGURE 5.32 **3D CT of four-part fracture of the proximal humerus.** 3D CT reconstructed images of the left shoulder viewed from the anterior **(A)** and posterior **(B)** sides show a complex markedly comminuted displaced and angulated gunshot wound fracture of the humeral head extending into the surgical neck and proximal shaft of the humerus. Note inferior displacement of the axillary artery due to a large soft-tissue hematoma.

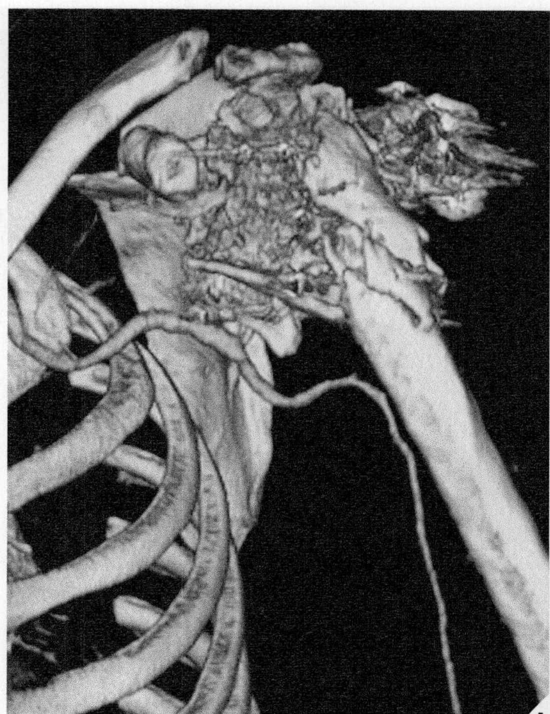

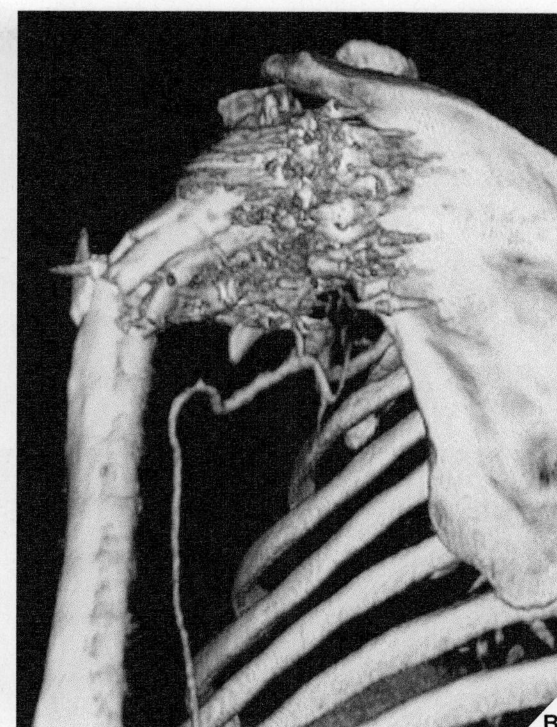

TYPES OF CLAVICLE FRACTURES

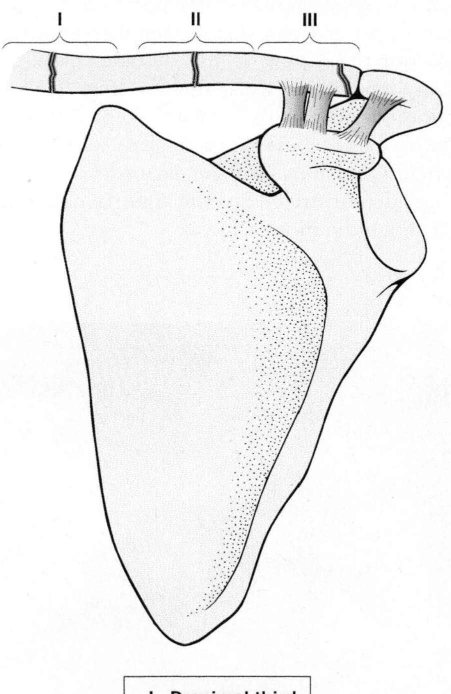

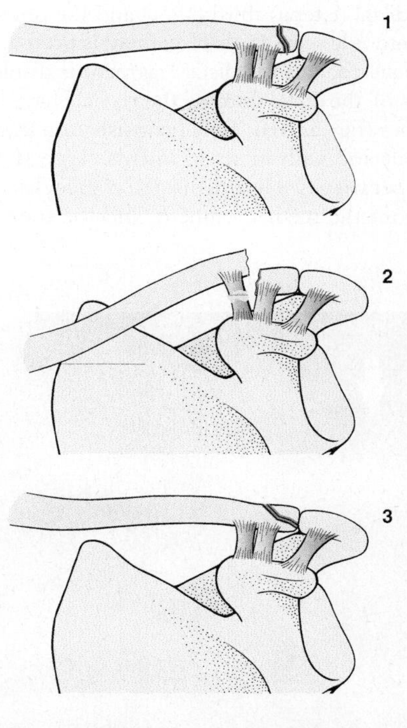

FIGURE 5.33 Classification of the fractures of the clavicle.

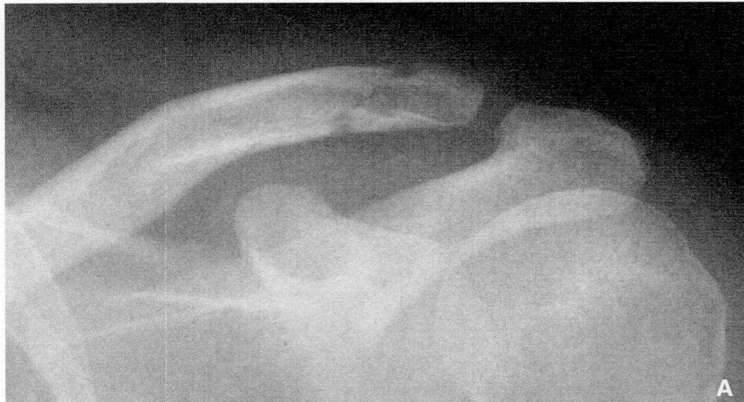

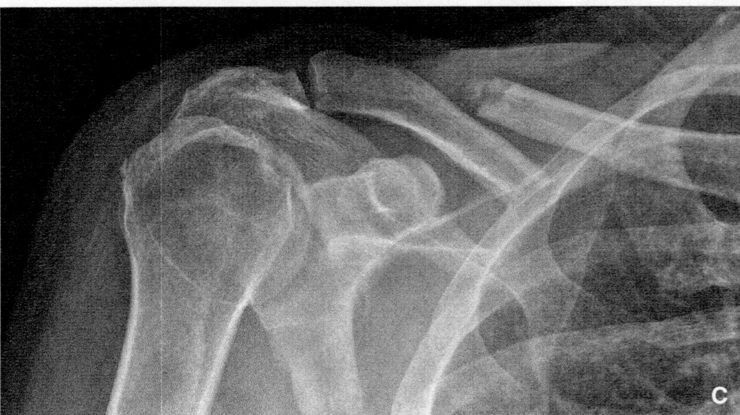

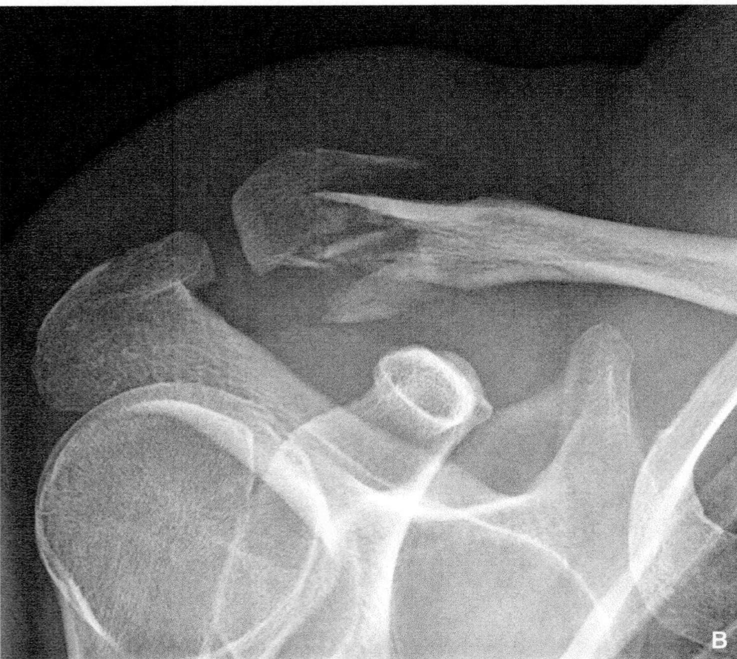

FIGURE 5.34 Fractures of the acromial end and middle third of the clavicle. **(A)** A simple fracture of the distal end of the clavicle without displacement of the fractured fragment. **(B)** A comminuted fracture of the distal end of the clavicle with displacement of the fractured fragments. **(C)** A markedly displaced fracture of the middle third of the clavicle.

injury is the middle third of the clavicle, representing 80% of all clavicular fractures. Fractures of the distal (lateral) third (15%) and the proximal (medial) third (5%) are less commonly seen. If displacement is present, the proximal fragment is usually elevated, and the distal fragment is displaced medially and caudally. Fractures of the distal third of the clavicle have been classified by Neer into three types (Fig. 5.33B). Type I consists of a fracture without significant displacement and with intact ligaments. Type II fractures are displaced and located between two ligaments: the coracoclavicular ligament, which is detached from the medial segment, and the trapezoid ligament, which remains attached to the distal segment. Type III fracture involves the articular surface, but the ligaments remain intact. The anteroposterior projection of the shoulder usually allows sufficient evaluation of any type of clavicular fracture (Figs. 5.34 and 5.35), but the same projection obtained with 15-degree cephalad angulation of the radiographic tube may also be useful, particularly in fractures of the middle third of the clavicle. Occasionally, if the diagnosis is in doubt, or if the fracture cannot be well demonstrated on conventional radiography, then CT (Figs. 5.36 and 5.37) might be more effective.

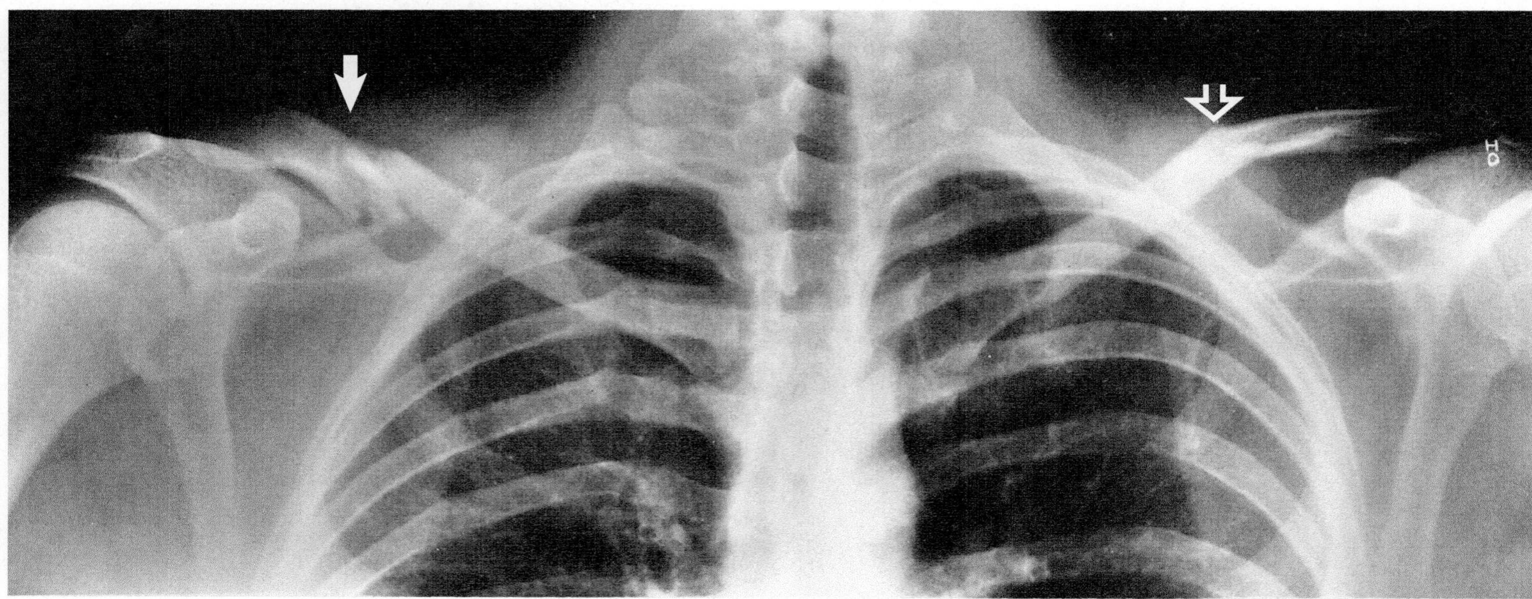

FIGURE 5.35 Fracture of both clavicles. A 22-year-old man sustained multiple traumas in a motorcycle accident. Anteroposterior radiograph of both shoulders demonstrates a comminuted fracture of the middle third of the right clavicle *(arrow)* and a simple fracture of the middle third of the left clavicle *(open arrow)*.

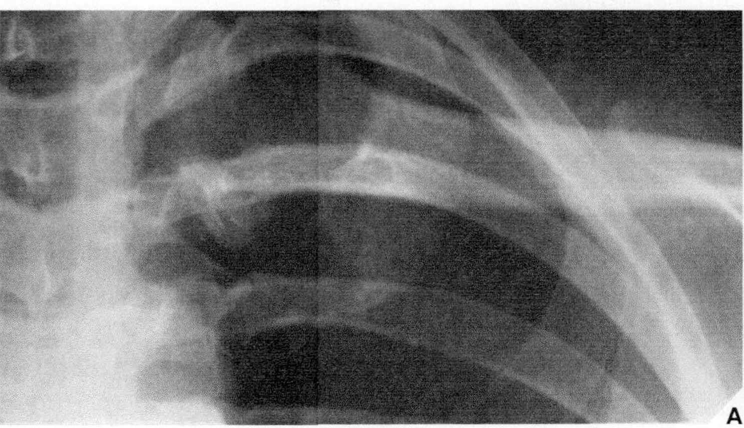

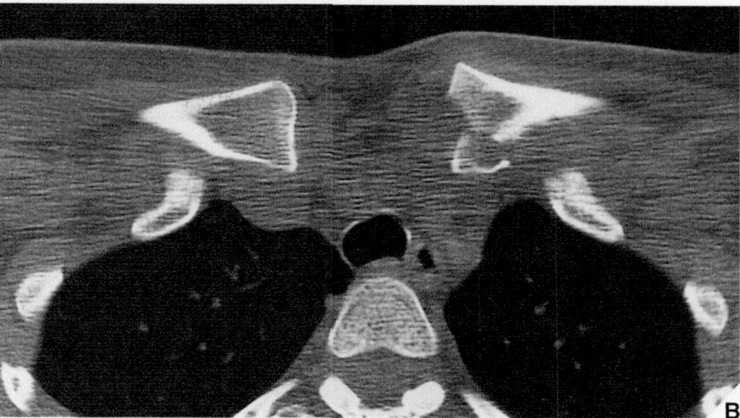

FIGURE 5.36 CT of fracture of the sternal end of the clavicle. A 21-year-old man was assaulted and sustained a direct injury to the left medial clavicle. **(A)** Anteroposterior radiograph is suggestive of a fracture of the medial end of the clavicle, but the fracture line is not well demonstrated. **(B)** Axial CT section shows a fracture of the sternal end of the clavicle and associated soft-tissue swelling.

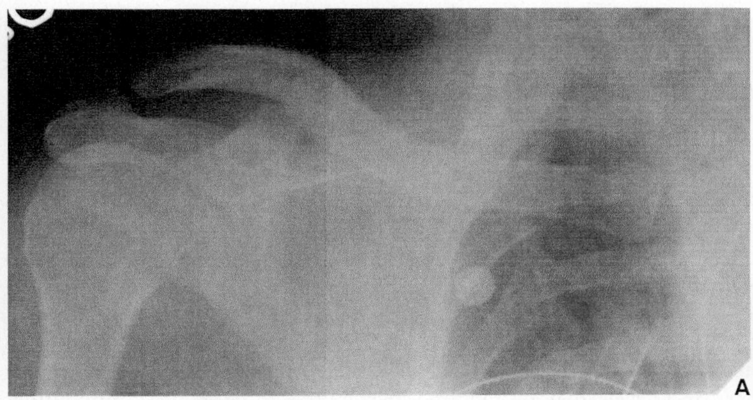

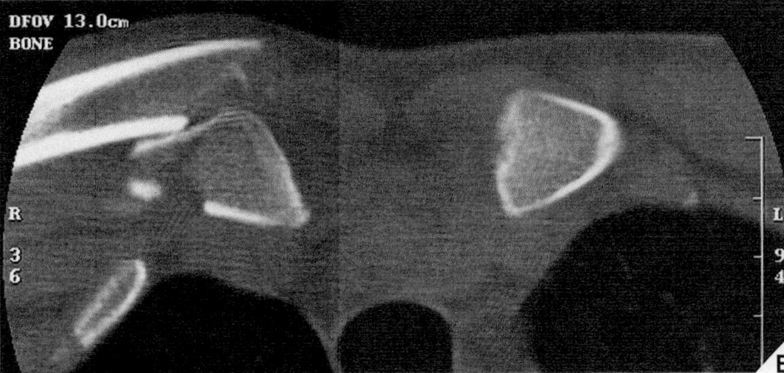

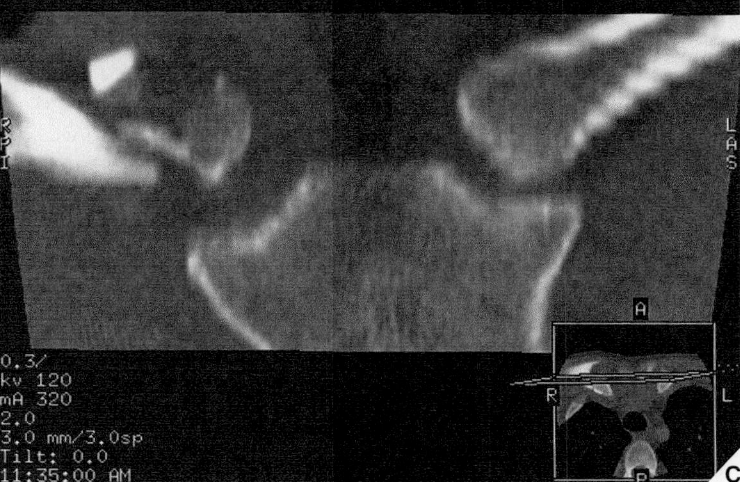

FIGURE 5.37 CT of fracture of the sternal end of the clavicle. A 34-year-old woman was severely injured in a car accident. **(A)** Anteroposterior radiograph of the right shoulder and upper chest shows multiple rib fractures. The medial portion of the clavicle is not adequately visualized. Axial CT scan **(B)** and coronal reformatted image **(C)** show a comminuted fracture of the sternal end of the right clavicle with anterior displacement and overriding of the fragments.

TYPES OF SCAPULA FRACTURES

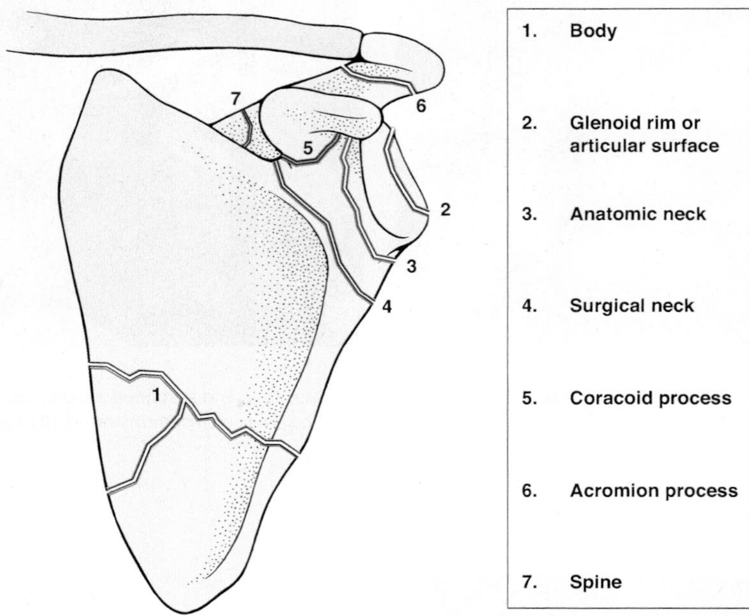

FIGURE 5.38 **Fractures of the scapula.** Classification of the fractures of the scapula according to anatomic location.

Fractures of the Scapula

Invariably resulting from direct trauma, commonly sustained in motor vehicle accidents or falls from heights, fractures of the scapula, which constitute approximately 1% of all fractures, 3% of shoulder girdle injuries, and 5% of all shoulder fractures, are classified according to their anatomic locations (Fig. 5.38). Because of their intraarticular extension, fractures of the glenoid rim and glenoid fossa are particularly important. They comprise 10% of all fractures of the scapula; however, fewer than 10% are significantly displaced. Fractures of the *glenoid rim* are subclassified into those involving the anterior portion and those affecting the posterior segment. Fractures of the *glenoid fossa* are subclassified into injuries involving the inferior segment; transverse disruption of the fossa extending into the vicinity of the suprascapular notch and the coracoid process; central fossa fractures extending across the entire scapula; and combination of the aforementioned fractures, frequently comminuted and displaced (Fig. 5.39).

Scapular fractures may occasionally be evaluated on the anteroposterior view of the shoulder (Fig. 5.40). More commonly, the transscapular (or Y) view may be required, particularly in cases of comminution, because this projection better demonstrates displacement of the fragments (Fig. 5.41). CT scan may also effectively demonstrate the displacement of various segments (Fig. 5.42), and three-dimensional (3D)

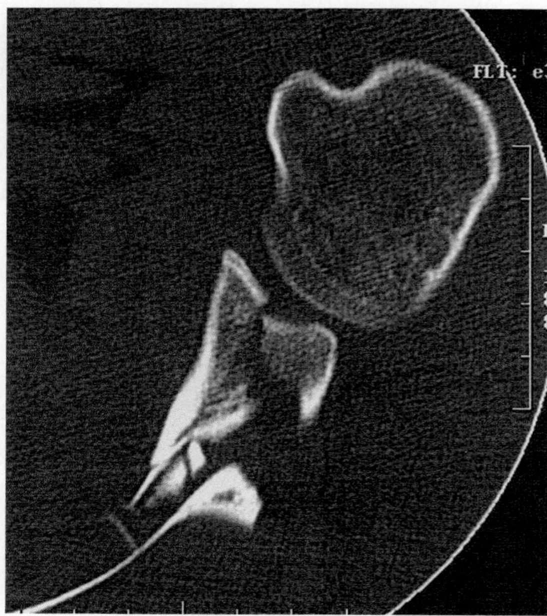

FIGURE 5.39 **CT of comminuted fracture of the glenoid.** Axial CT section through the shoulder joint shows a comminuted, displaced fracture of the glenoid fossa extending across the entire scapula.

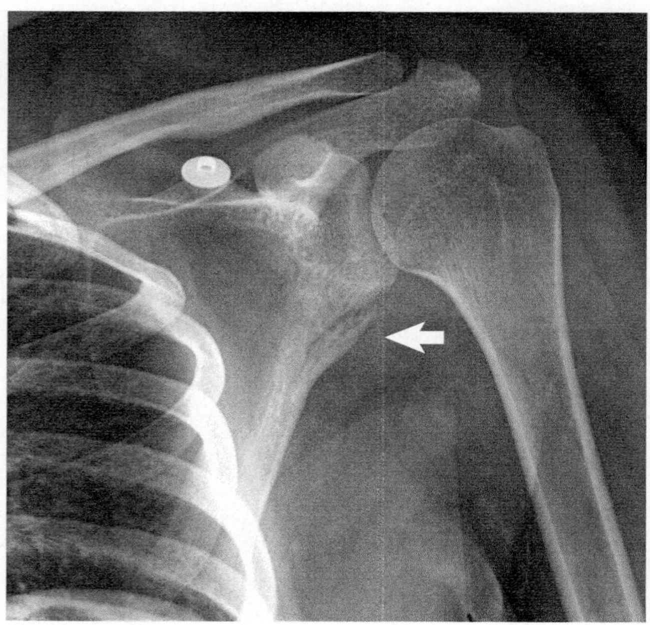

FIGURE 5.40 **Fracture of the scapula.** Minimally displaced subglenoid fracture of the scapula *(arrow)* is well demonstrated on this anteroposterior radiograph of the left shoulder.

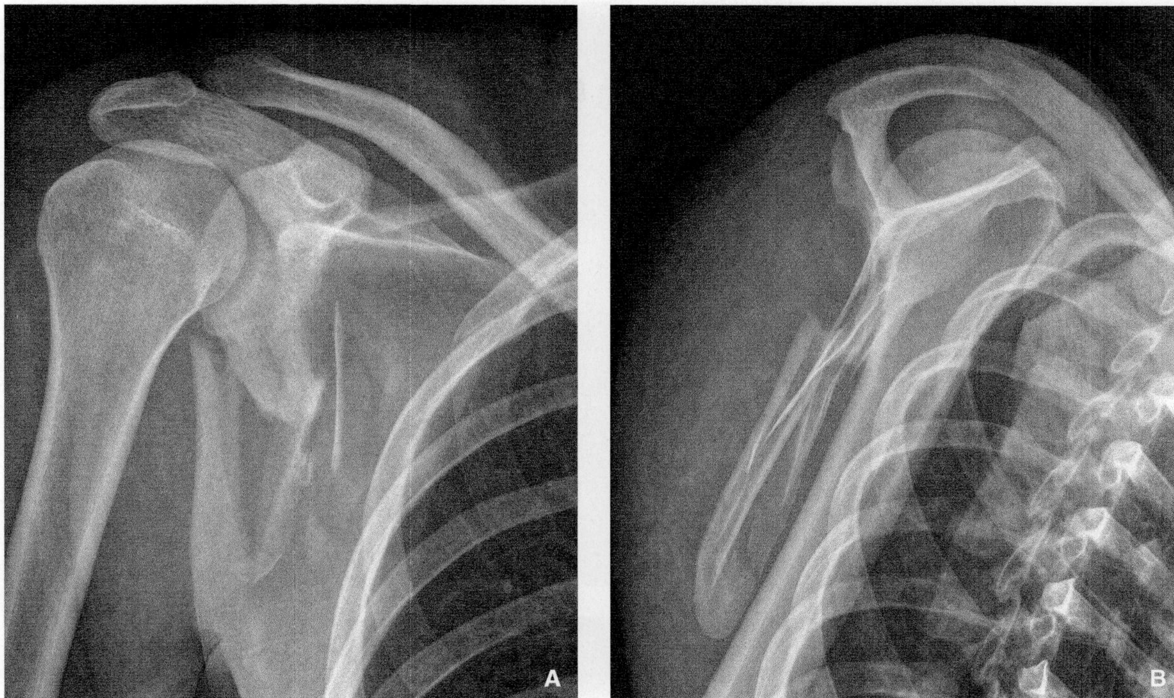

FIGURE 5.41 **Fracture of the scapula.** A 52-year-old man was injured in a motorcycle accident. **(A)** On the anteroposterior radiograph of the right shoulder, a comminuted fracture of the scapula is evident. Displacement of the fragments, however, cannot be evaluated. **(B)** Transscapular (or Y) view demonstrates lateral displacement of the body of the scapula.

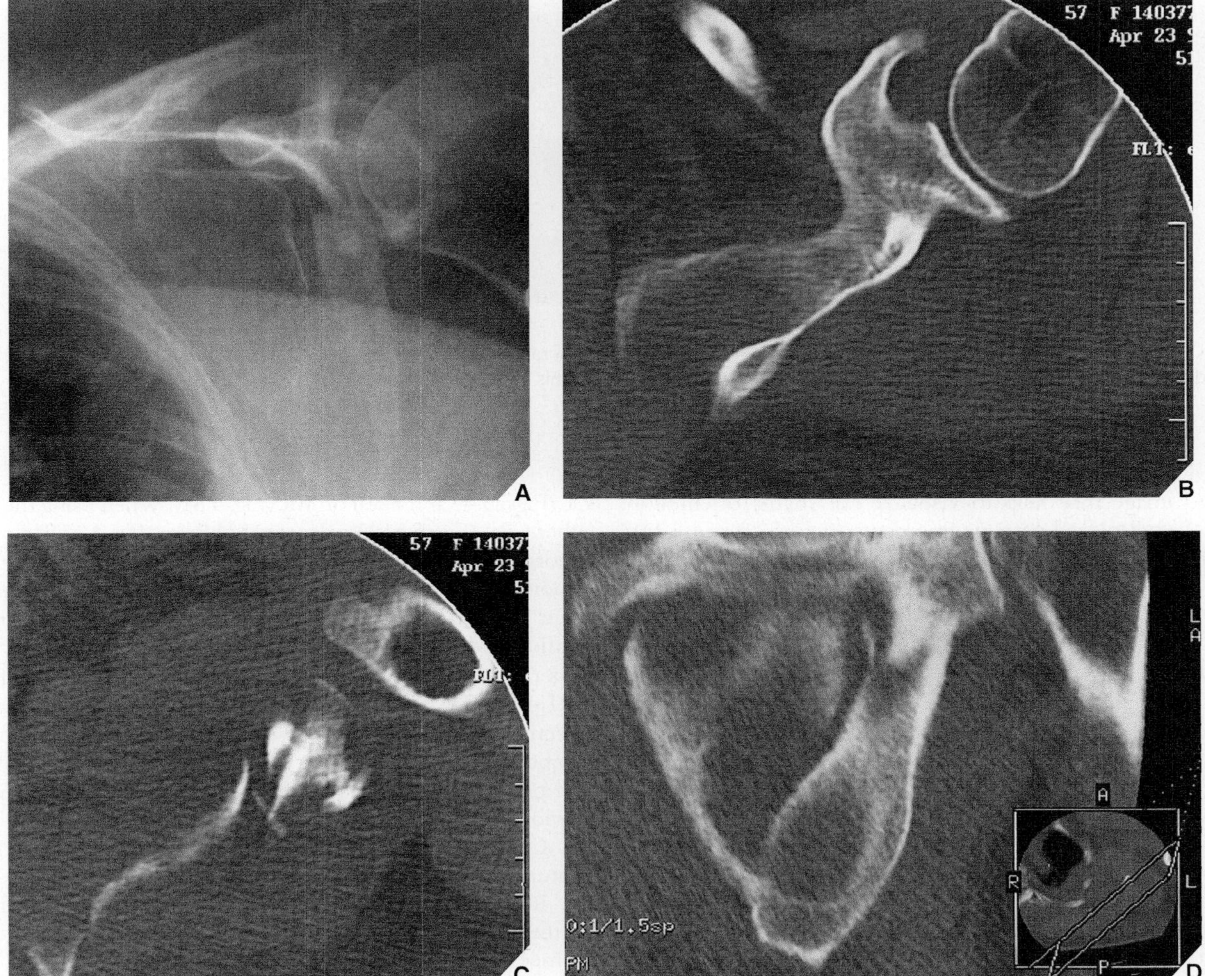

FIGURE 5.42 **CT of the fracture of the scapula.** A 57-year-old woman sustained an injury to the left shoulder in a motorcycle accident. **(A)** Anteroposterior radiograph shows a comminuted fracture of the left scapula. The glenohumeral joint cannot be properly assessed on this study. Two axial CT sections, one at the level of glenohumeral joint **(B)** and the other at the level of body of the scapula **(C)**, and reformatted coronal image **(D)** show to better advantage the configuration of various displaced fragments as well as an intact glenohumeral joint.

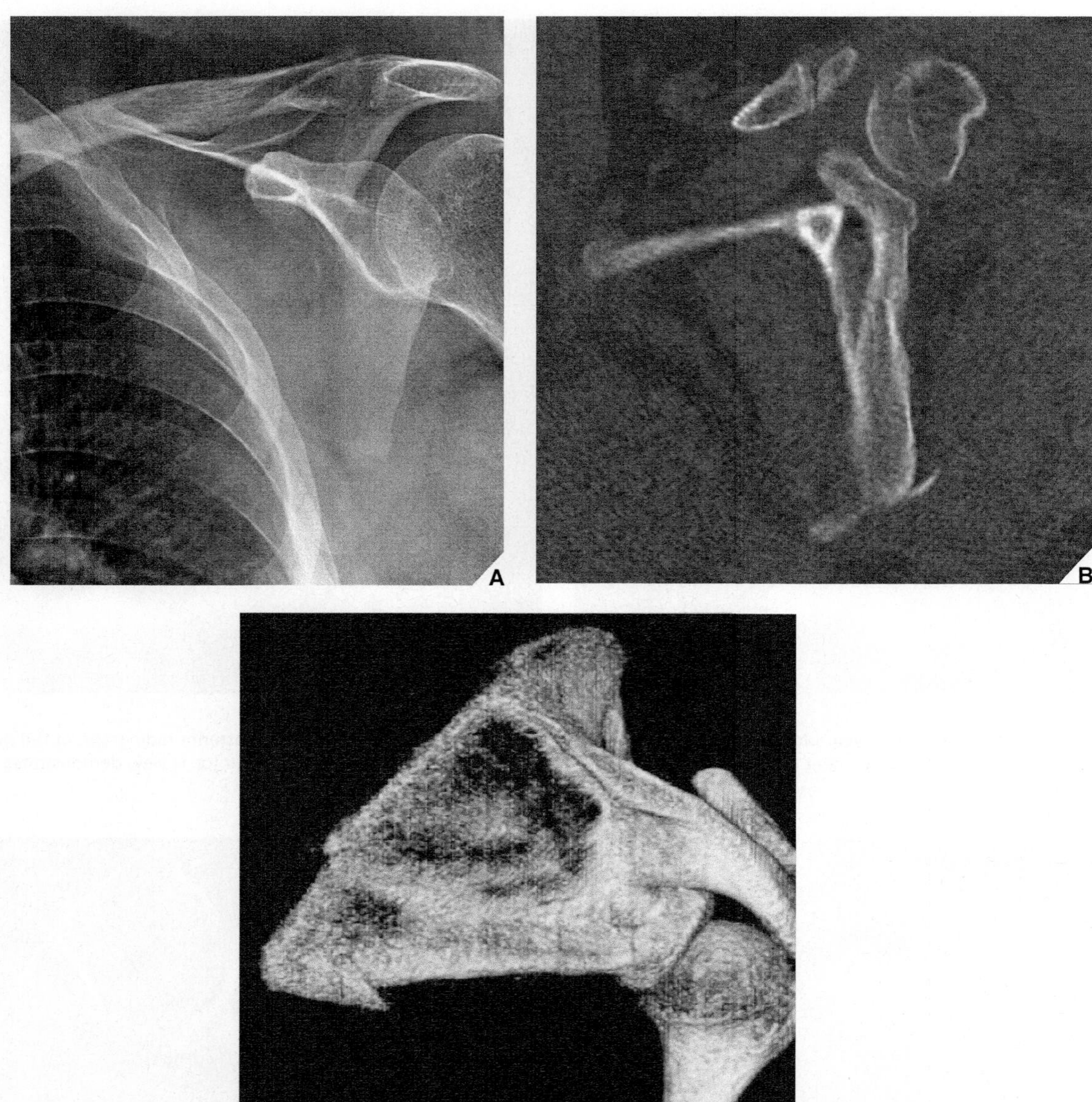

FIGURE 5.43 CT and 3D CT of the fracture of the scapula. **(A)** On this anteroposterior radiograph of the left shoulder, fracture of the scapula is barely visible. Coronal reformatted **(B)** and 3D reconstructed CT **(C)** images effectively demonstrate the details of this injury.

CT reconstructed image may help to visualize the spatial orientation of fracture lines and displaced osseous fragments (Figs. 5.43 and 5.44). Complications, such as injury to the axillary artery or the brachial plexus, are rare.

Dislocations in the Glenohumeral Joint

Anterior Dislocation

Displacement of the humeral head anterior to the glenoid fossa, which usually results from indirect force applied to the arm—a combination of abduction, extension, and external rotation—accounts for approximately 96% of cases of glenohumeral dislocation. It is readily diagnosed on the anteroposterior view of the shoulder (Fig. 5.45), although the Y view is effective as well (Fig. 5.46). CT or 3D CT is equally effective in demonstrating anterior dislocation (Fig. 5.47).

At the time of dislocation, the humeral head strikes the inferior margin of the glenoid, and this may result in compression fracture of one or both of these structures. Fracture most frequently occurs in the posterolateral aspect of the humeral head at the junction with the neck, producing a "hatchet" defect called the *Hill-Sachs lesion*; it is best demonstrated on the anteroposterior projection of the shoulder with the arm internally rotated (Fig. 5.48). Hill-Sachs lesion can also be imaged with CT (Figs. 5.49 and 5.50) or MR (Fig. 5.51). When using the latter modality, either axial (Fig. 5.51A) or coronal oblique (Fig. 5.51B) image reveals this abnormality. Fracture of the anterior aspect of the inferior rim of the glenoid, known as the *osseous Bankart lesion*, is less commonly seen. It may occur secondary to the anterior movement of the humeral head in dislocation and is readily demonstrated on the Grashey view or the anteroposterior radiograph of the shoulder (Fig. 5.52), by CT (Fig. 5.53) or by MRI (Fig. 5.54). When the site of the Bankart lesion is in the cartilaginous labrum, which at times may be detached, it may only be revealed by either computed arthrotomography (see Fig. 5.18) or MRI (Figs. 5.55 and 5.56). The presence of either of these abnormalities is virtually diagnostic of previous anterior dislocation.

Occasionally, the anterior shoulder dislocation may be complicated by fracture of the humeral neck (Figs. 5.57 and 5.58).

Recent studies indicated that recurrent instability and dislocations of the glenohumeral joint following arthroscopic repair of the labrum, ligaments, and capsule occur in about 35% of the cases, mostly related to bone loss of the glenoid (osseous Bankart lesion) or the humeral head (Hill-Sachs lesion). The coexistence of both lesions has been called *bipolar lesion*. It has been determined that the size of the osseous Bankart and the Hill-Sachs lesions have significant impact in causing recurrent instability

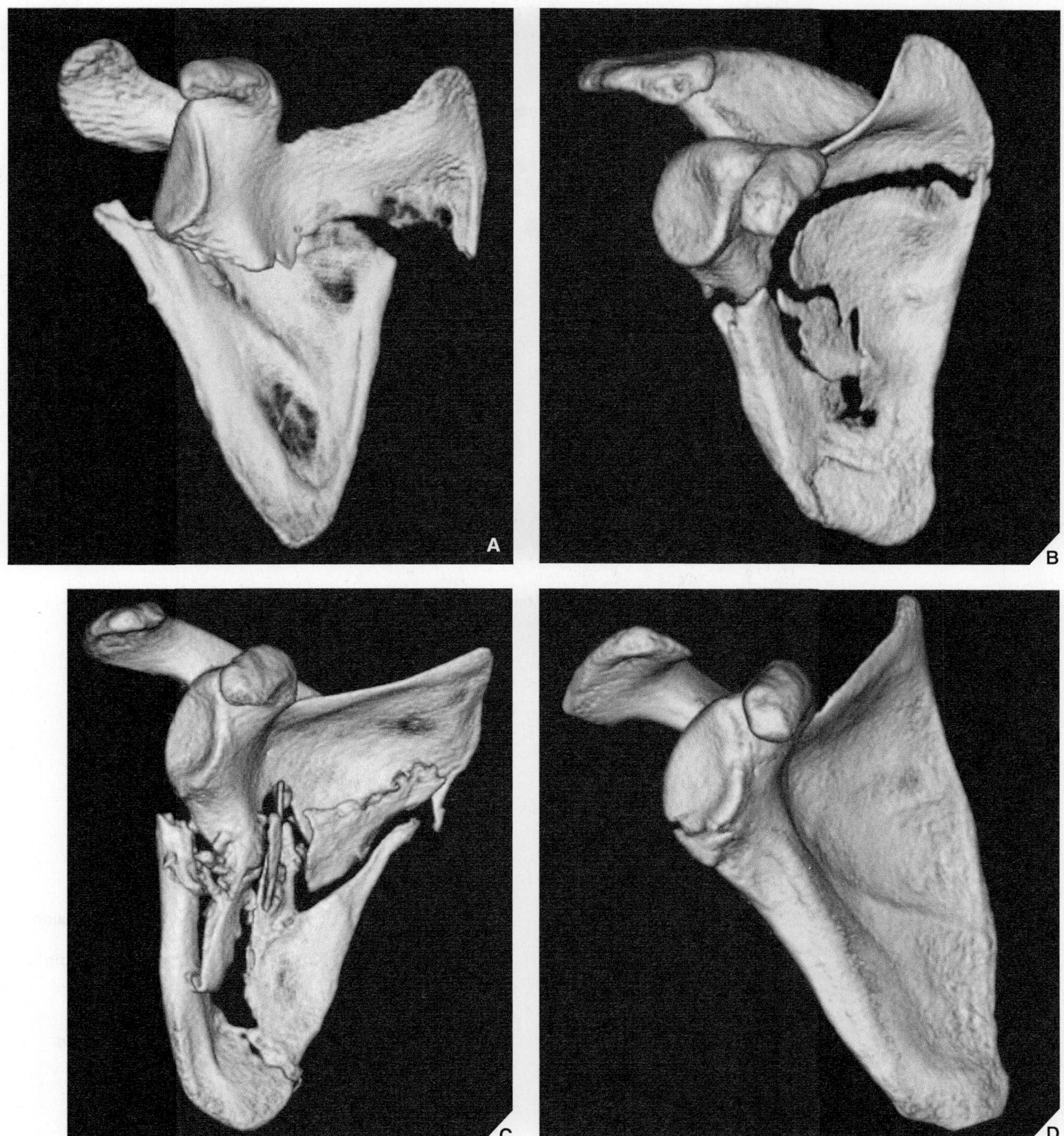

FIGURE 5.44 3D CT of the fractures of the scapula. **(A)** Simple transverse fracture of the body of the scapula not affecting the glenoid. **(B,C)** Comminuted fractures of the scapula not affecting the glenoid. **(D)** Fracture of the scapula extending to the inferior glenoid rim. *(Continued)*

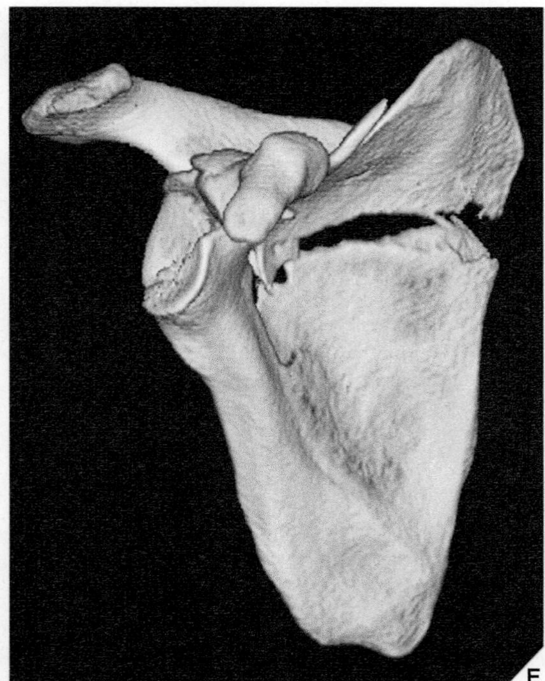

FIGURE 5.44 3D CT of the fractures of the scapula. ***(Continued)*** **(E)** Fracture of the body of the scapula extending to the glenoid fossa.

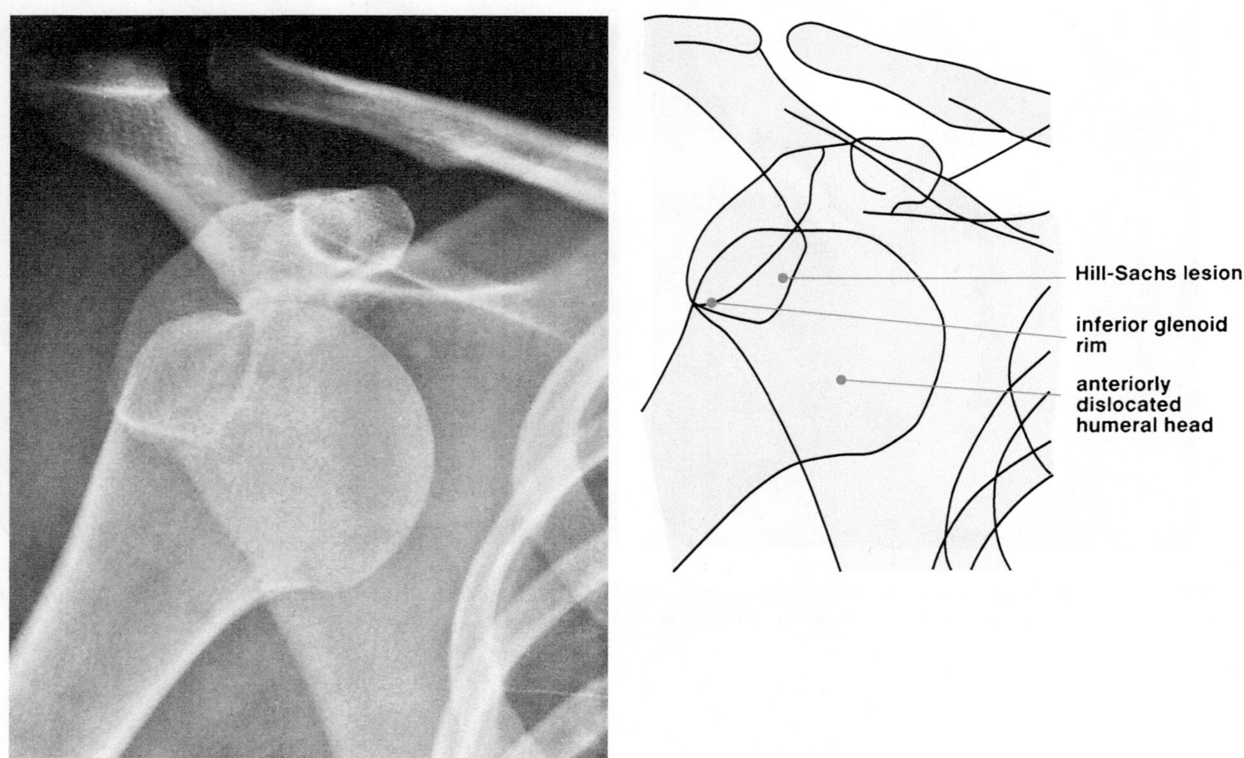

FIGURE 5.45 Anterior shoulder dislocation. Anteroposterior radiograph of the right shoulder shows the typical appearance of anterior dislocation. The humeral head lies beneath the inferior rim of the glenoid. Observe common complication of anterior dislocation - a compression fracture of the posterolateral aspect of the humeral head known as the *Hill-Sachs lesion*.

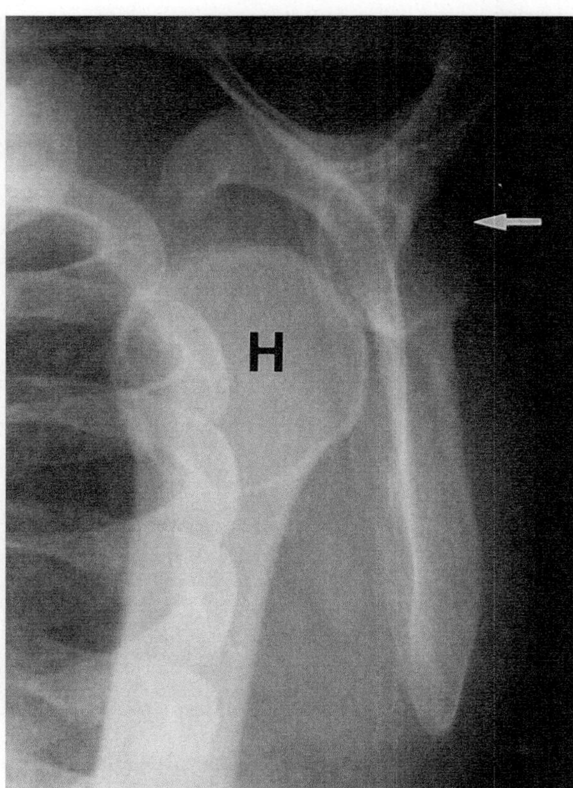

▲ **FIGURE 5.46 Anterior shoulder dislocation.** A dislocation is well demonstrated on this transscapular (or Y) projection of the left shoulder girdle. An *arrow* is pointing to the empty glenoid fossa. The humeral head *(H)* is medially and anteriorly displaced.

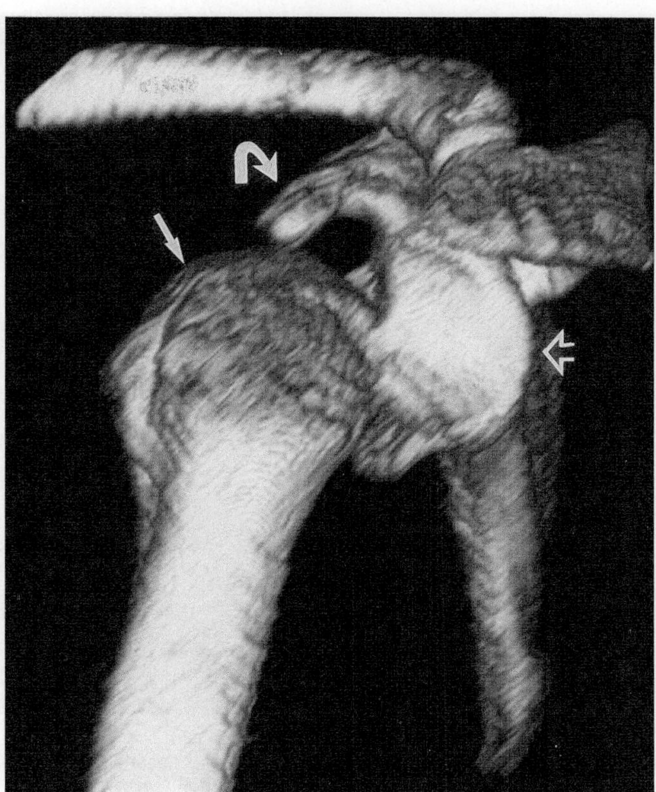

▲ **FIGURE 5.47 3D CT of the anterior shoulder dislocation.** A 3D shaded surface display CT reconstructed image (side view) demonstrates anterior dislocation of the right humeral head *(arrow)*. *Open arrow* points to the empty glenoid fossa, and a *curved arrow* points to the coracoid process.

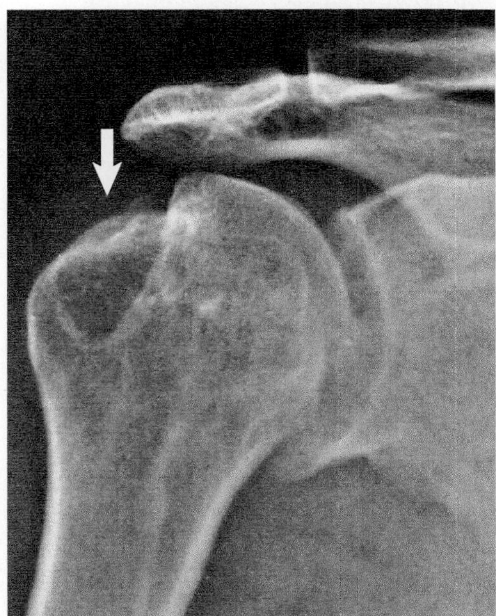

▲ **FIGURE 5.48 Hill-Sachs lesion.** Anteroposterior radiograph of the right shoulder with the arm internally rotated demonstrates a hatchet defect, known as the *Hill-Sachs lesion*, on the posterolateral aspect of the humeral head *(arrow)*.

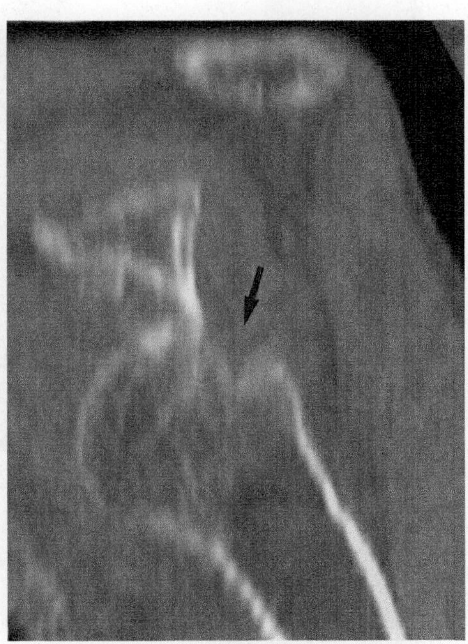

▲ **FIGURE 5.49 CT of Hill-Sachs lesion.** Coronal CT reformatted image shows anterior dislocation in the shoulder joint. The *arrow* points to the Hill-Sachs lesion.

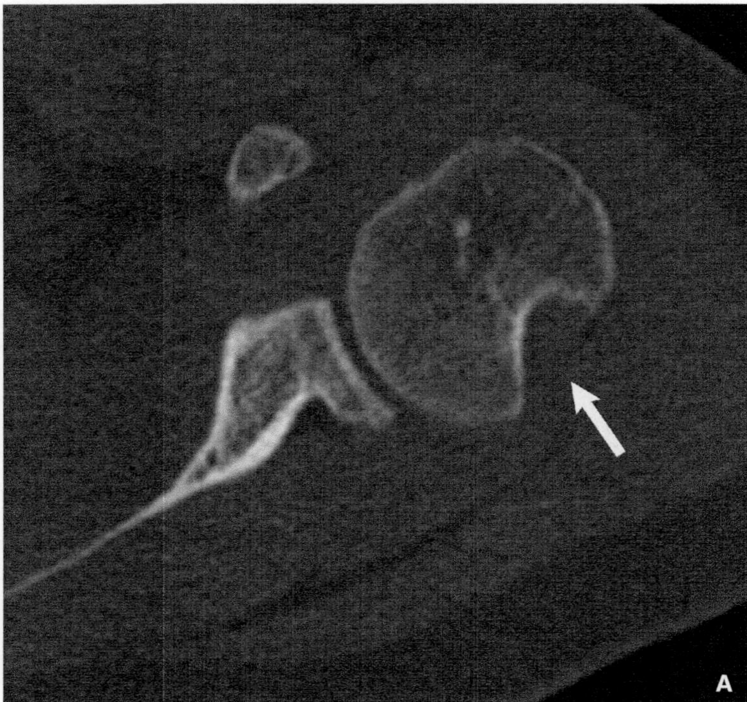

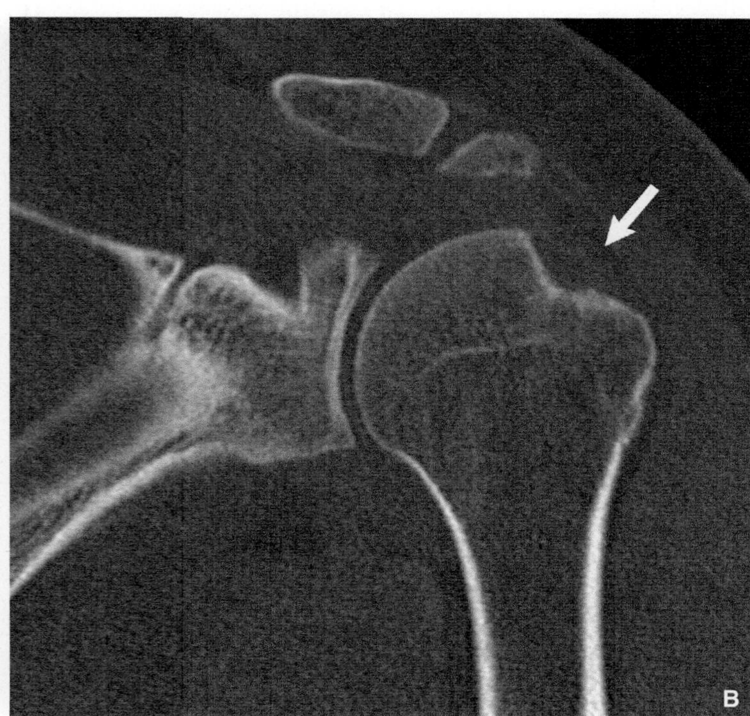

FIGURE 5.50 CT of Hill-Sachs lesion. After anterior dislocation has been relocated, **(A)** axial and **(B)** coronal reformatted CT images show a defect at the posterolateral aspect of the humeral head consistent with Hill-Sachs lesion *(arrows)*.

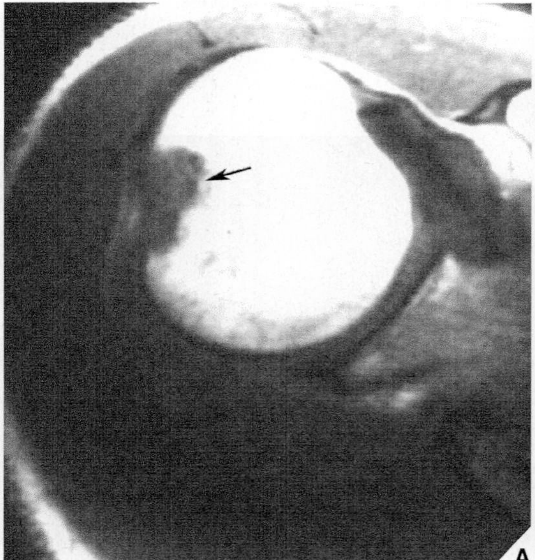

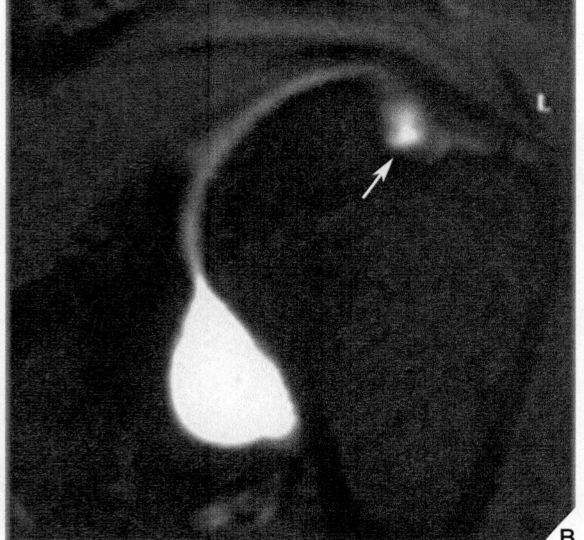

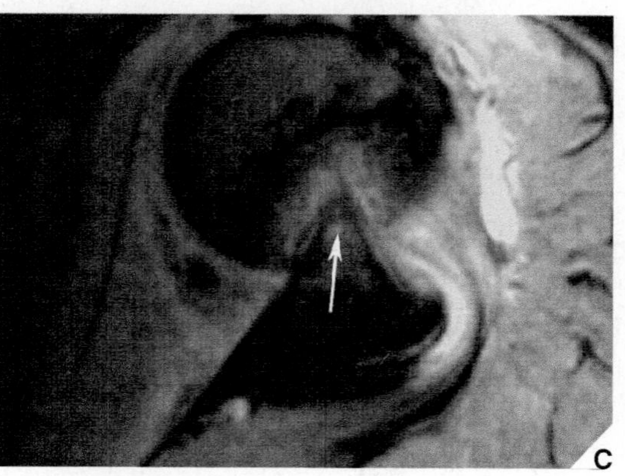

FIGURE 5.51 MRI of Hill-Sachs lesion. **(A)** Axial T1-weighted MR image demonstrates a deep Hill-Sachs lesion in the posterosuperior aspect of the humeral head *(arrow)*. **(B)** Coronal oblique MRa in another patient demonstrates a Hill-Sachs lesion at the insertion of the infraspinatus tendon *(arrow)*. **(C)** Axial GRE MR image in another patient with an engaged anterior dislocation demonstrates the mechanism of production of a Hill-Sachs lesion. Note the impaction of the humeral head against the anterior margin of the glenoid *(arrow)*.

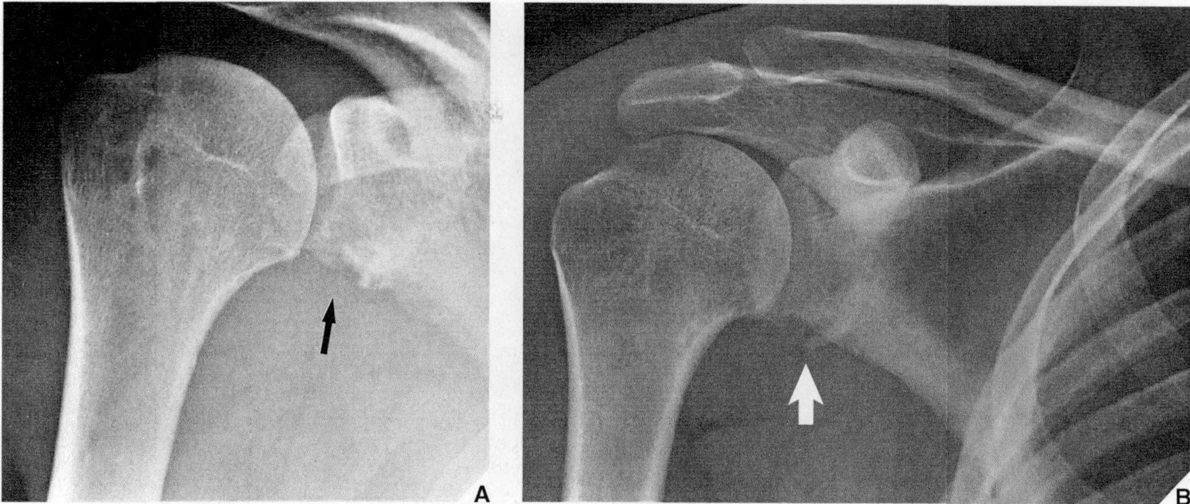

FIGURE 5.52 Osseous Bankart lesion. **(A)** Grashey view of the shoulder shows compression fracture of the anterior aspect of the inferior portion of the glenoid, known as the *osseous Bankart lesion (arrow)*. **(B)** In another patient, the anteroposterior radiograph of the right shoulder clearly demonstrates the osseous Bankart lesion *(arrow)*.

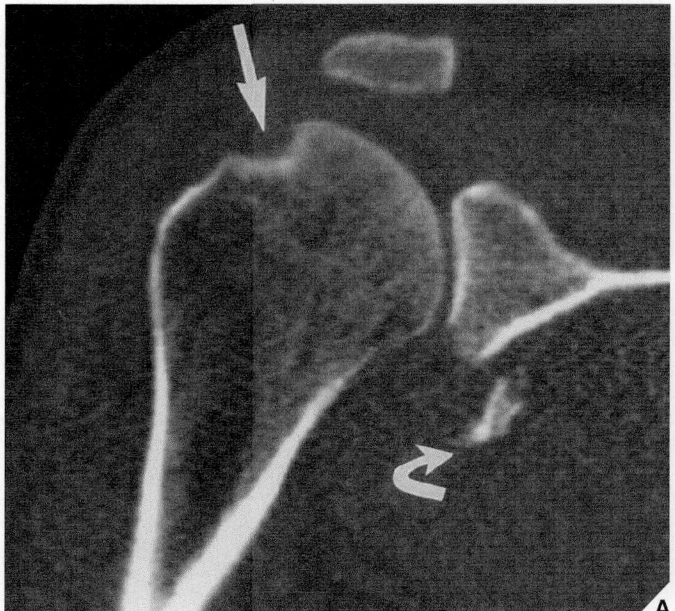

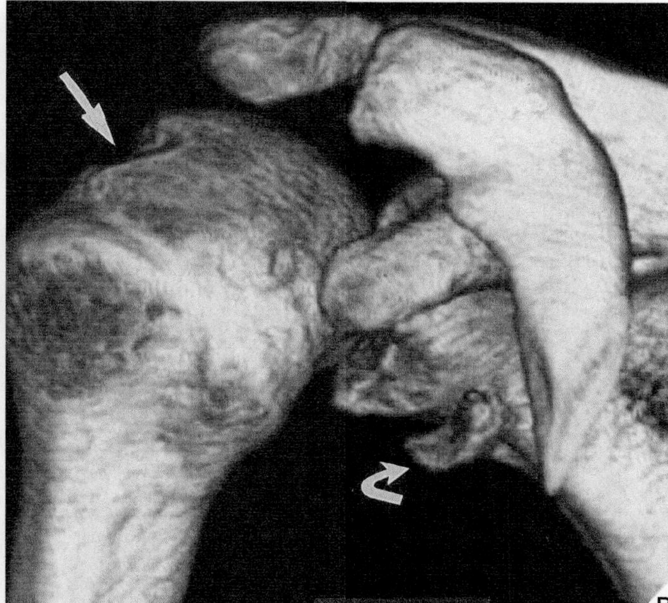

FIGURE 5.53 CT and 3D CT of Hill-Sachs and osseous Bankart lesions. Coronal CT reformatted **(A)** and 3D reconstructed **(B)** CT images show Hill-Sachs *(arrows)* and osseous Bankart *(curved arrows)* lesions in a 42-year-old woman with reduced anterior shoulder dislocation. **(C)** Axial CT image of the left shoulder in another patient demonstrates a large osseous Bankart lesion. The lesion involves over 50% of the anteroposterior diameter of the glenoid fossa *(arrow)*. *(Continued)*

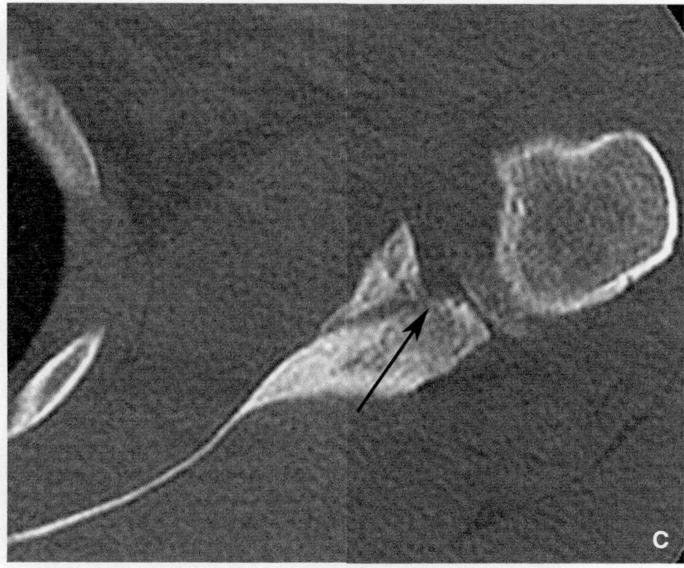

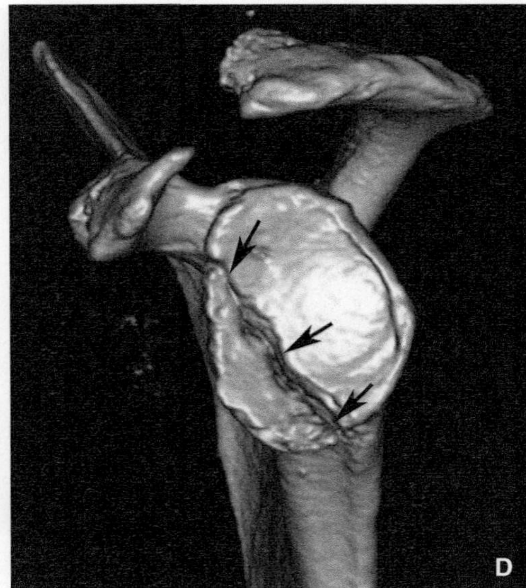

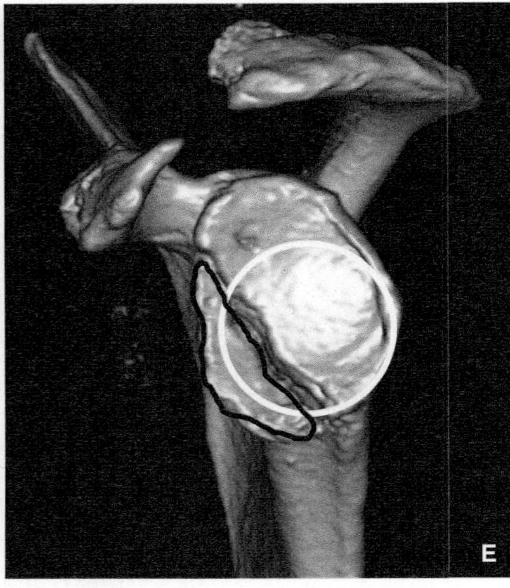

FIGURE 5.53 CT and 3D CT of Hill-Sachs and osseous Bankart lesions. ***(Continued)*** **(D)** Sagittal 3D reconstructed CT image of the same patient shows the large fracture of the anterior glenoid *(arrows)*. **(E)** On the same sagittal 3D reconstructed CT image, the white best fit circumference is placed on the inferior aspect of the glenoid, and it measures the expected surface area. The area of the osseous Bankart lesions is outlined in black. Dividing the area of the fracture fragment by the expected area of the glenoid and multiplying by 100 provides an accurate percentage of bone loss. The calculations of the areas are obtained with the region of interest (ROI) utilizing the appropriate software in the picture archive and communication system (PACS) workstation (see Fig. 5.59).

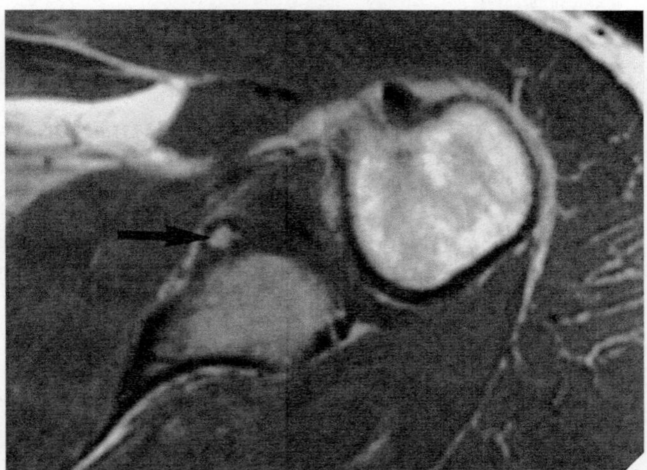

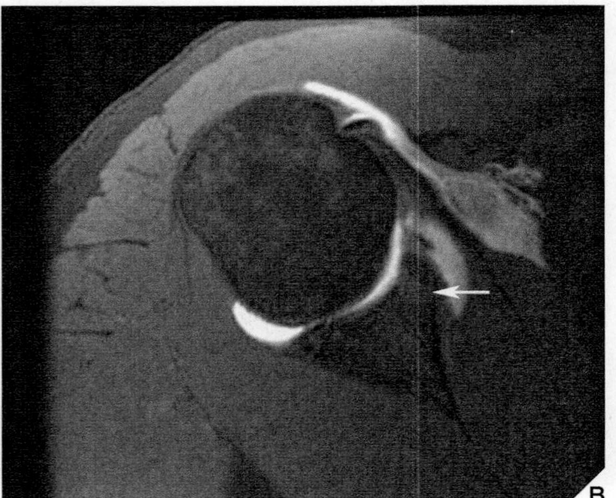

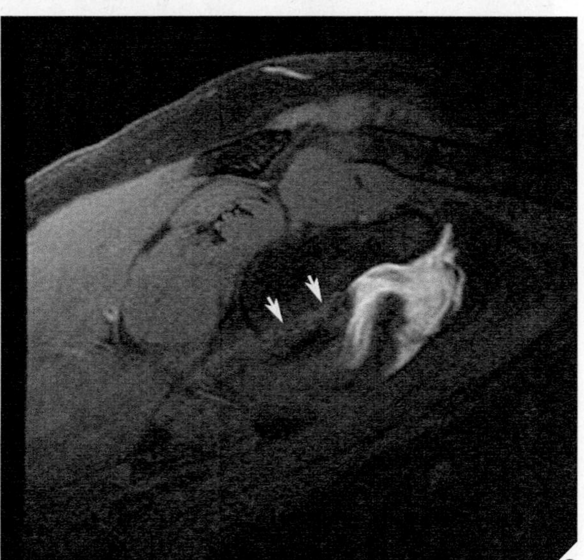

FIGURE 5.54 MRI of osseous Bankart lesion. **(A)** T1-weighted axial MR image shows a high signal of bone fragment adjacent to the anterior glenoid *(arrow)*, representing an osseous Bankart lesion. **(B)** Axial T1-weighted fat-saturated MRI in another patient shows an osseous Bankart lesion *(arrow)*. **(C)** Oblique sagittal T1-weighted fat-saturated MRI of the same patient as in **B** demonstrates the displaced osseous Bankart lesion *(arrows)*, producing a decreased transverse diameter of the inferior glenoid as compared with the superior glenoid, the so-called *inverted pear sign*. (**A**, Reprinted with permission from Steinbach LS, Tirman PFJ, Peterfy CG, et al, eds. *Shoulder magnetic resonance imaging*. Philadelphia: Lippincott-Raven; 1998.)

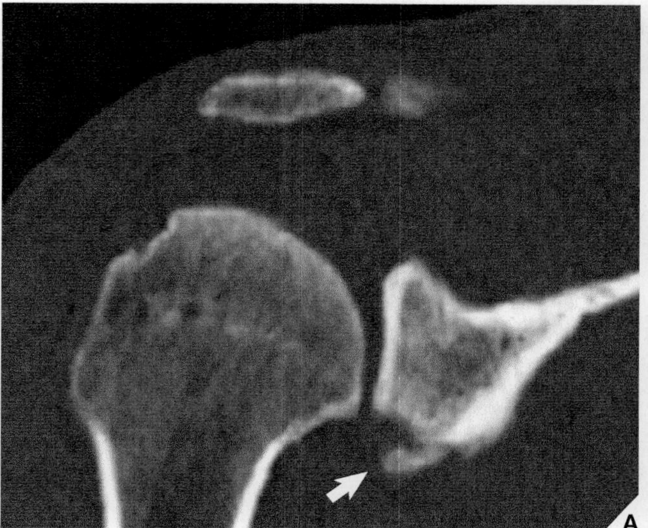

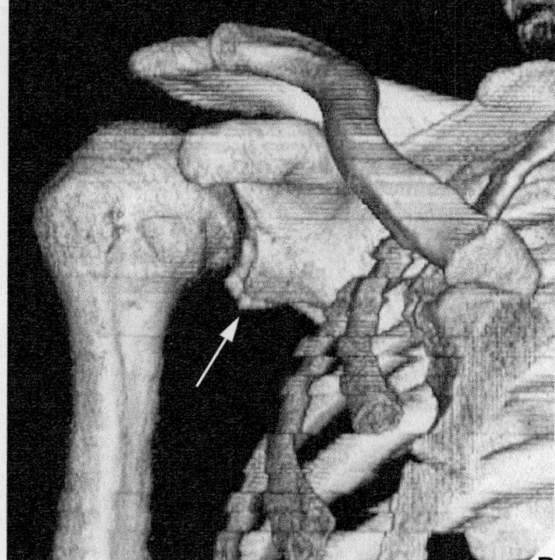

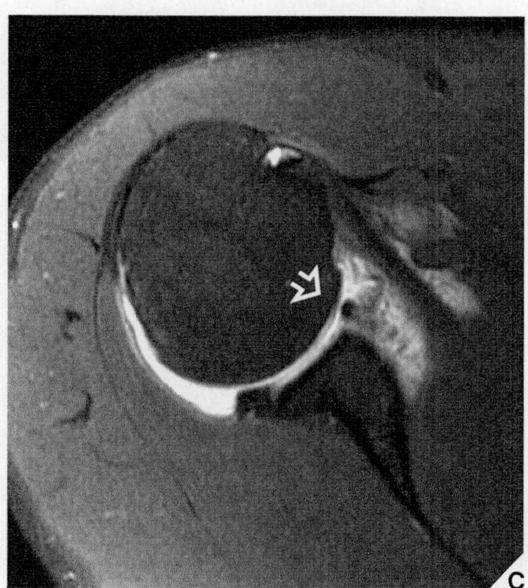

FIGURE 5.55 **CT, 3D CT, and MRI of osseous and cartilaginous Bankart lesion.** Coronal reformatted **(A)** and 3D reconstructed **(B)** CT images of the right shoulder show only osseous Bankart lesion *(arrows)*. **(C)** Axial T1-weighted fat-suppressed MR arthrographic image clearly demonstrate the cartilaginous Bankart lesion *(open arrow)*.

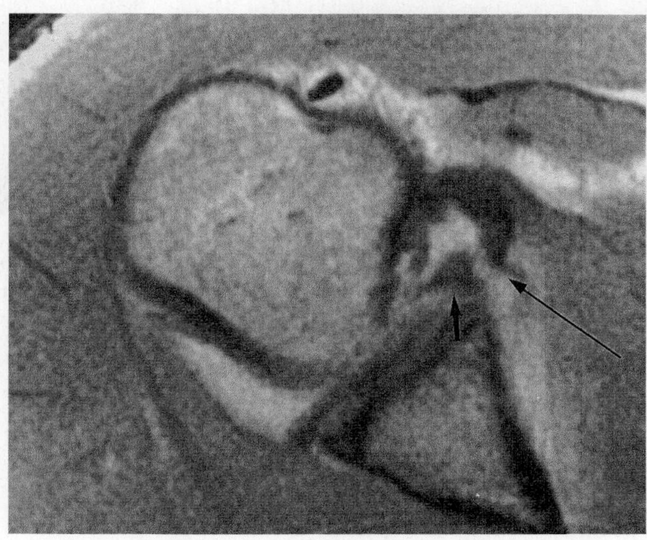

FIGURE 5.56 **MRI of cartilaginous Bankart lesion.** Axial proton density–weighted MR image shows a detachment of the anteroinferior labrum *(short arrow)* and a tear of the IGHL *(long arrow)*. (Reprinted with permission from Steinbach LS, Tirman PFJ, Peterfy CG, et al, eds. *Shoulder magnetic resonance imaging*. Philadelphia: Lippincott-Raven; 1998.)

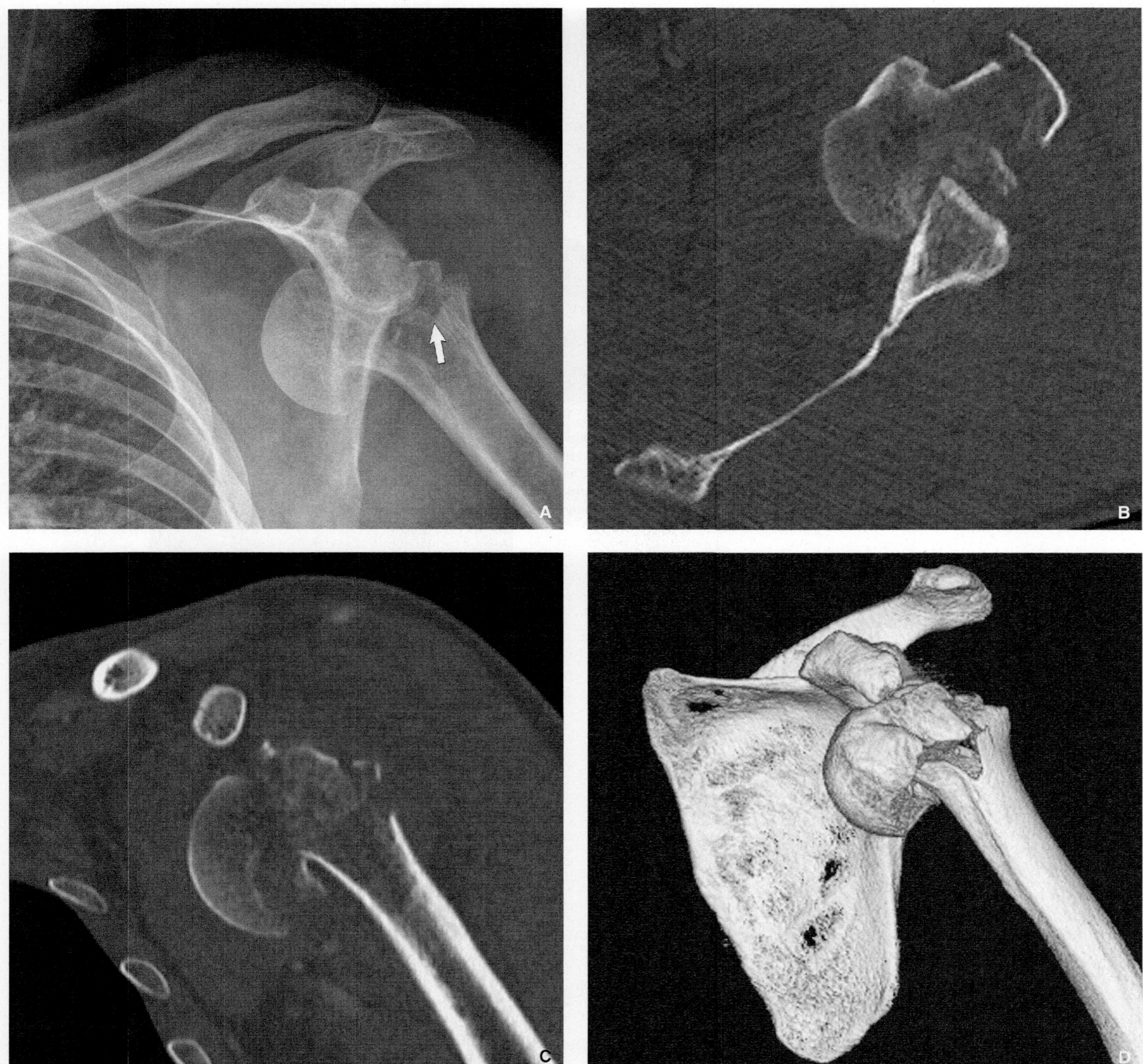

FIGURE 5.57 CT and 3D CT of anterior shoulder dislocation complicated by a fracture of the humerus. **(A)** Anteroposterior radiograph of the left shoulder of a 45-year-old woman shows anterior shoulder dislocation. Observe in addition a fracture of the neck of the humerus *(arrow)*. **(B)** Axial and **(C)** coronal reformatted CT images supplemented with 3D reconstructed CT image **(D)** show the details of the fracture more clearly.

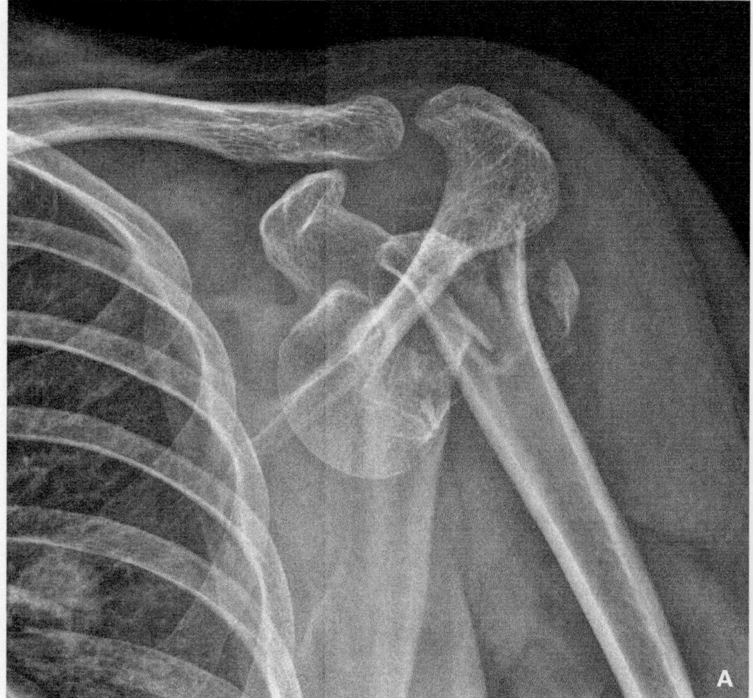

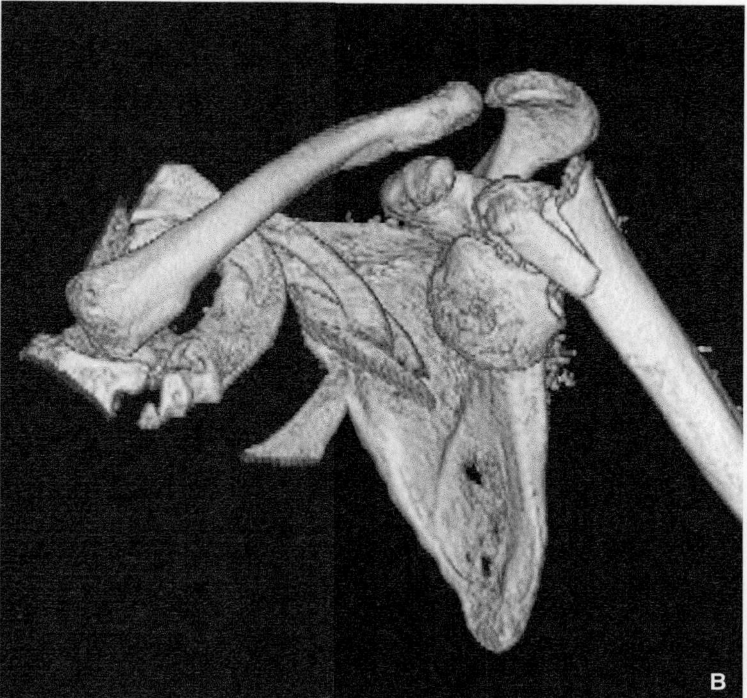

FIGURE 5.58 **3D CT of anterior shoulder dislocation complicated by a fracture of the humerus.** Anteroposterior radiograph **(A)** and 3D reconstructed CT **(B)** of the left shoulder of a 62-year-old man demonstrate anterior dislocation in the shoulder joint associated with a markedly comminuted and displaced fracture of the neck of the humerus.

following arthroscopic repair. Surgical reconstruction of the bone lesions has led to decreased rate of recurrent instability, and it has become evident that preoperative assessment of the degree of bipolar bone loss is important for surgical planning.

The osseous Bankart lesion refers to an osteochondral fracture of the anterior inferior margin of the glenoid. When the lesion involves more than 25% of the transverse diameter of the glenoid circumference, the shape of the glenoid fossa is altered giving the "inverted pear" sign on oblique sagittal CT or MR images, where the transverse diameter of the superior glenoid is larger than the inferior diameter (Fig. 5.59). A quantitative assessment of the bone loss can be made on CT or MRI, tracing the best fit circumference in the inferior aspect of the glenoid and measuring the transverse diameter of the circumference and the largest transverse diameter of the bone fragment. This allows to determine the percentage of bone loss (Griffith index). Alternatively, one can measure the area of the normal contralateral glenoid on sagittal CT images and compare with the injured glenoid, hence calculating the surface area of glenoid loss (PICO method). Another method is to measure the maximum transverse diameter of the glenoid in the axial CT or MRI planes and measure the maximum transverse diameter of the bony fragment thus calculating the percentage of bone loss.

Hill-Sachs lesions occur in about 93% of patients with recurrent glenohumeral instability. There is a relationship between recurrent dislocations and failure of arthroscopic Bankart repair and increasing size of the Hill-Sachs lesion. Concurrent osseous Bankart and Hill-Sachs lesions ("bipolar lesions") occur in about 62% of patients with glenohumeral instability. Vertical orientation of the Hill-Sachs lesions and lesions involving over 35% of the diameter of the humeral head are more prone to recurrent instability. Deep vertically oriented Hill-Sachs lesions lead to "engagement" of the humeral head against the posterior aspect of the glenoid on physical preoperative examination with the patient under anesthesia ("engaging Hill-Sachs lesion"). The reader is referred to the article by Saliken et al. for a comprehensive literature review of the different methods of quantitative evaluation of glenoid and humeral head bone loss.

Yamamoto et al. recently introduced the "glenoid track" concept. By measuring the location and distance of contact between the humeral head and the glenoid articular surface through a range of external rotation, horizontal extension, and abduction, they found that the zone of contact between the articular surfaces of the glenoid and humeral head (the glenoid track) was 84% ± 14% of the glenoid width. The calculation of the glenoid track using MRI has been found more predictive of continued instability after surgery than calculating bone loss alone. The glenoid track measurements are based on CT or MRI (see Fig. 5.59). The first step is to measure the width of the bone defect on oblique sagittal CT or MRI at the level of the glenoid using the best fit circle. This value is subtracted from the total diameter of the circle and multiplied by 0.83. This provides us with the glenoid track. The next step is the measuring of the "Hill-Sachs interval" on the axial plane by drawing a line between the anterior and posterior margins of the Hill-Sachs lesion and then a line from the most lateral margin of the lesion to the humeral attachment of the rotator cuff. This is known as the *bone ridge*. The Hill-Sachs lesion plus the bone ridge is termed the *Hill-Sachs interval*. If the Hill-Sachs interval is less than the glenoid track, the Hill-Sachs lesion is considered to be "on track," meaning that in extreme ABER, the Hill-Sachs lesion will not cross the anterior aspect of the glenoid and labrum and therefore will not "engage." On the contrary, if the Hill-Sachs interval is greater than the glenoid track, the lesion is considered to be "off track" and therefore engaging in extreme ABER, indicating that repair of the humeral and glenoid bone loss needs to be done to prevent recurrent glenohumeral instability.

Posterior Dislocation

This type of dislocation, which is much less commonly seen—accounting for only 2% to 3% of dislocations in the glenohumeral joint, results from either direct force, such as a blow to the anterior aspect of the shoulder, or indirect force applied to the arm combining adduction, flexion, and internal rotation. Posterior dislocation caused by indirect force most often occurs secondary to accidental electric shock or convulsive seizures. In this type of dislocation, the humeral head lies posterior to the glenoid fossa and usually impacts on the posterior rim of the glenoid.

Making a correct diagnosis is often problematic because the abnormality can easily be overlooked on the standard anteroposterior radiograph of the shoulder, where the overlapping humeral head and glenoid fossa may be interpreted as normal. It is imperative when dealing with suspected posterior dislocation to demonstrate radiographically the glenoid fossa in

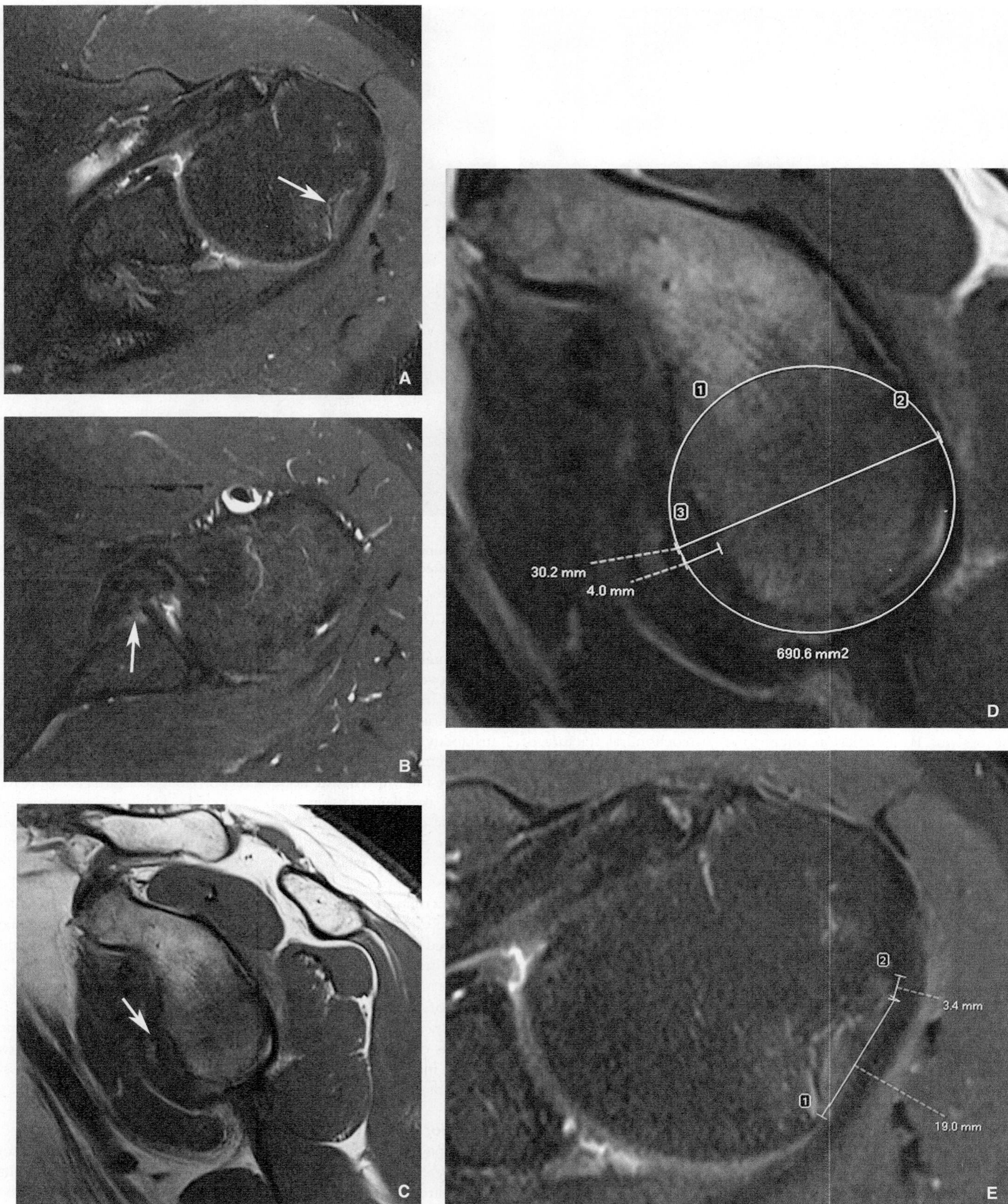

FIGURE 5.59 Measurement of glenoid track of bipolar lesion following anterior shoulder dislocation. (A) Axial T2-weighted fat-saturated MR image at the level of the superior humeral head demonstrates a prominent Hill-Sachs lesion *(arrow)*. **(B)** Axial T2-weighted fat-saturated MR image at the level of the lower glenoid demonstrates an osseous Bankart lesion *(arrow)*. The combination of both lesions represents a bipolar lesion. **(C)** Sagittal proton density–weighted MR image demonstrates the size of the osseous Bankart lesion *(arrow)*. **(D)** Same sagittal proton density–weighted MR image with the best fit circumference over the inferior glenoid measures the diameter of the circumference (30.2 mm) and the diameter of the bone loss (4.0 mm). Using the formula $30.2 - 4 \times 0.8 = 26.8$, we are getting the number that is termed the *glenoid track*. **(E)** On axial T2-weighted fat-saturated MR image, the anteroposterior dimension of the Hill-Sachs lesion measures 19 mm *(1)* and the distance between the anterior margin of the Hill-Sachs lesion and the posterior edge of the insertion of the rotator cuff measures 3.4 mm *(2)* ("bony ridge"). The Hill-Sachs interval (which represents the sum of the length of the Hill-Sachs lesion and the bony ridge) measures 22.4. This number is lower than the glenoid track (26.8); therefore, the bipolar lesion is on track, meaning that in extreme ABER, the Hill-Sachs lesion will not cross the anterior aspect of the glenoid and labrum and therefore will not engage.

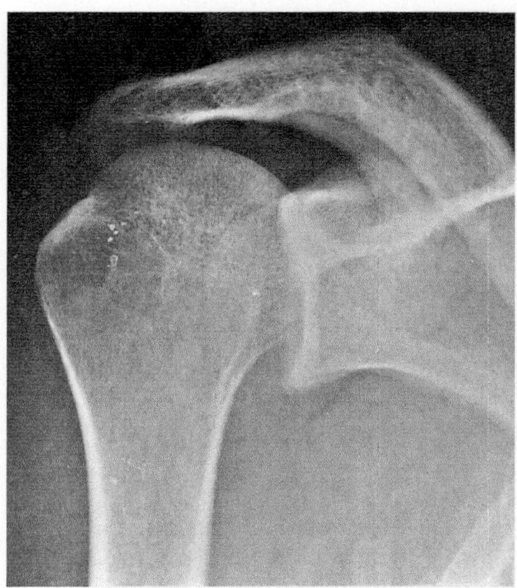

FIGURE 5.60 Posterior shoulder dislocation. On the anteroposterior radiograph of the right shoulder obtained by rotating the patient 40 degrees toward the affected side (Grashey view), overlap of the medially displaced humeral head with the glenoid is virtually diagnostic of posterior dislocation.

profile. This can be achieved on the anteroposterior projection by rotating the patient 40 degrees toward the affected side (see Fig. 5.5), known as the *Grashey projection*. Normally, the glenohumeral joint space is clear on this view. Obliteration of the space because of overlap of the humeral head with the glenoid is diagnostic of posterior dislocation (Fig. 5.60). Diagnosis can also be made on the axillary projection, although limited abduction of the arm may make it impossible to obtain this view (Fig. 5.61).

Compression fracture of the anteromedial aspect of the humeral head, known as *trough line impaction* (*trough sign*), commonly occurs in posterior dislocation secondary to the impaction of the humeral head on the posterior glenoid rim. This sign, also occasionally called a *reverse Hill-Sachs lesion*, refers to a vertical or arch-like line within the cortex of the humeral head that projects parallel and lateral to the articular end of this bone. The anteroposterior view of the shoulder with the arm externally rotated readily demonstrates this type of fracture (Fig. 5.62); it is also identifiable on the axillary projection (see Fig. 5.61) and on CT (Fig. 5.63).

MRI findings of posterior shoulder dislocation mirror those seen on the radiography and CT, but in addition, associated abnormalities of the articular cartilage, labrum, tendons, and ligaments can clearly be demonstrated (Fig. 5.64). In one study of 36 patients reported by Saupe et al., the reverse Hill-Sachs lesion was seen in 86% of patients, and posterocaudal labrocapsular lesion in nearly 60% of patients. In about 20% of patients, the associated abnormality included full-thickness rotator cuff tear.

Inferior Dislocation

Also known as *luxatio erecta humeri*, this is the rarest dislocation in the shoulder joint accounting for only 1%. The mechanism of this injury consists of either application of a direct axial force to a fully abducted arm or a severe hyperabduction of arm, resulting in the impingement of humeral head against the acromion. Rotator cuff tear and fracture of the greater tuberosity of the humerus are commonly associated abnormalities. The anteroposterior radiograph of the shoulder easily shows this dislocation (Fig. 5.65). Recently described MRI findings include injury to the glenoid labrum and injury to both the anterior and posterior bands of the IGHL.

Complications of Shoulder Dislocations

Dislocations in the glenohumeral joint may result in complications such as recurrent dislocations, posttraumatic arthritis, tear of the rotator cuff, and injury to the axillary nerve and axillary artery.

Impingement Syndrome

Impingement syndrome of the shoulder refers to a condition in which the supraspinatus tendon and subacromial bursa are chronically entrapped between the humeral head inferiorly and either the anterior acromion itself, spurs of the anterior acromion or acromioclavicular joint, or the coracoacromial ligament superiorly (coracoacromial arch). Early diagnosis and treatment of impingement syndrome are critical to prevent the progression of this condition and improve shoulder function. Frequently, however, clinical signs and symptoms are nonspecific, and the diagnosis is often delayed until a full-thickness defect in the rotator cuff has developed. Only rarely can it be definitely diagnosed based on the clinical findings, characterized by severe pain during ABER of the arm. More reliable are radiographic findings associated with this syndrome, including subacromial proliferation

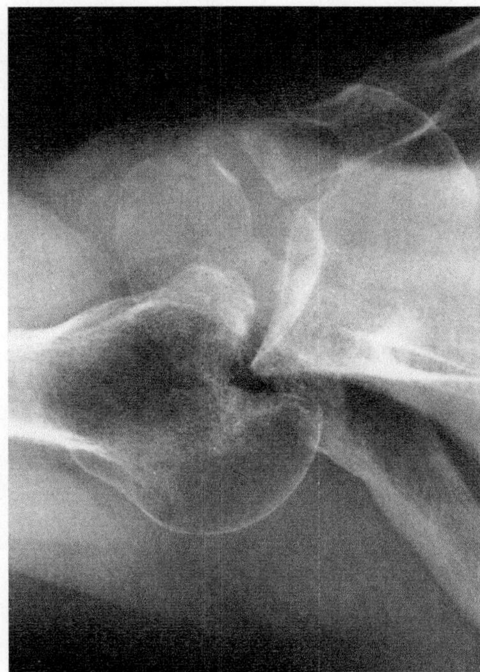

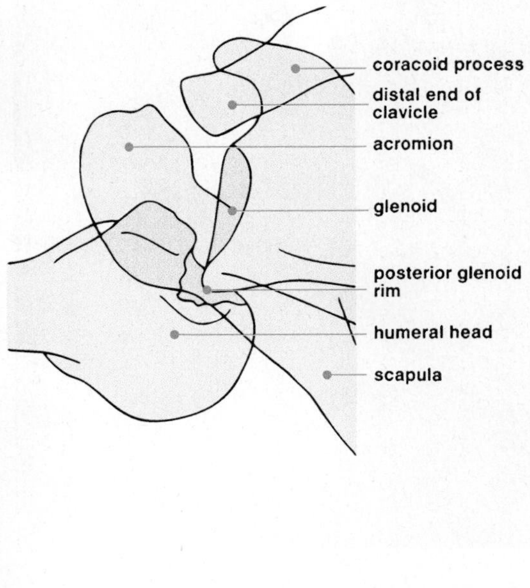

FIGURE 5.61 Posterior shoulder dislocation. Axillary projection of the shoulder demonstrates posterior dislocation. Note the associated compression fracture of the anteromedial aspect of the humeral head.

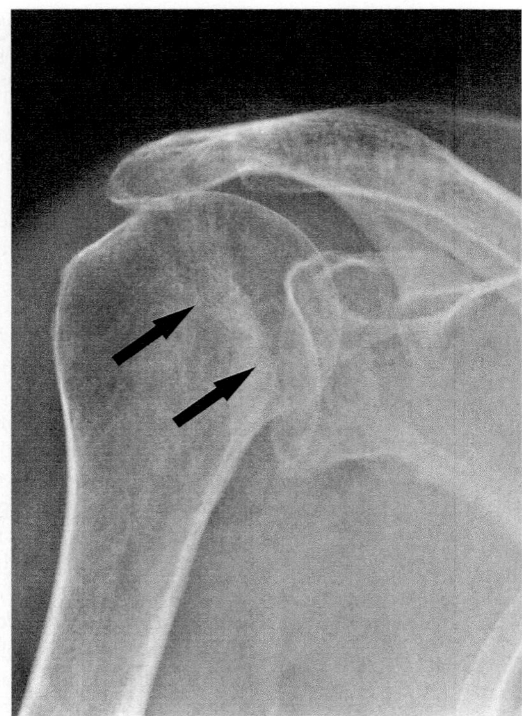

FIGURE 5.62 Posterior shoulder dislocation. Anteroposterior radiograph of the right shoulder demonstrates posterior dislocation in the glenohumeral joint. Note the trough line impaction on the anteromedial aspect of the humeral head *(arrows)*.

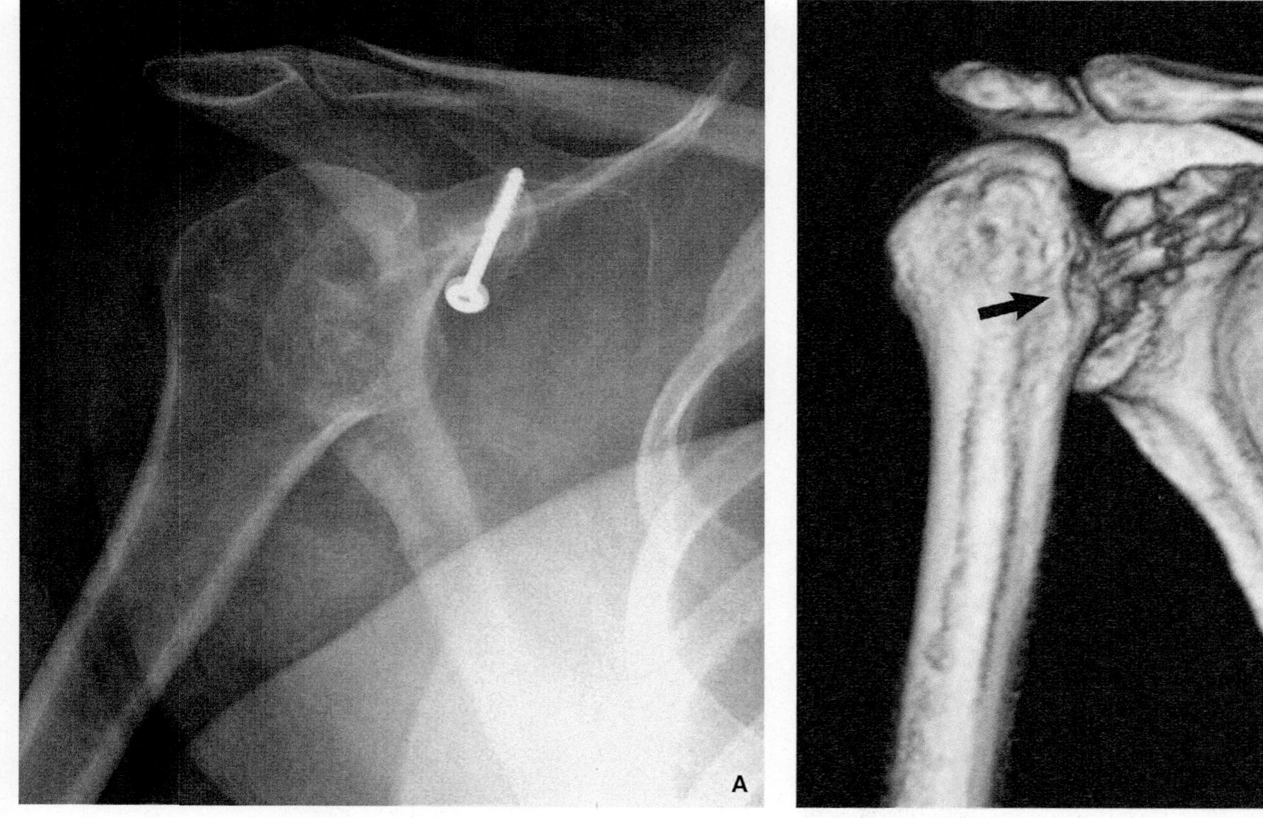

FIGURE 5.63 3D CT of posterior shoulder dislocation. Anteroposterior radiograph **(A)** and 3D CT reconstructed image **(B)** of the right shoulder show posterior dislocation. The *arrow* points to the trough sign.

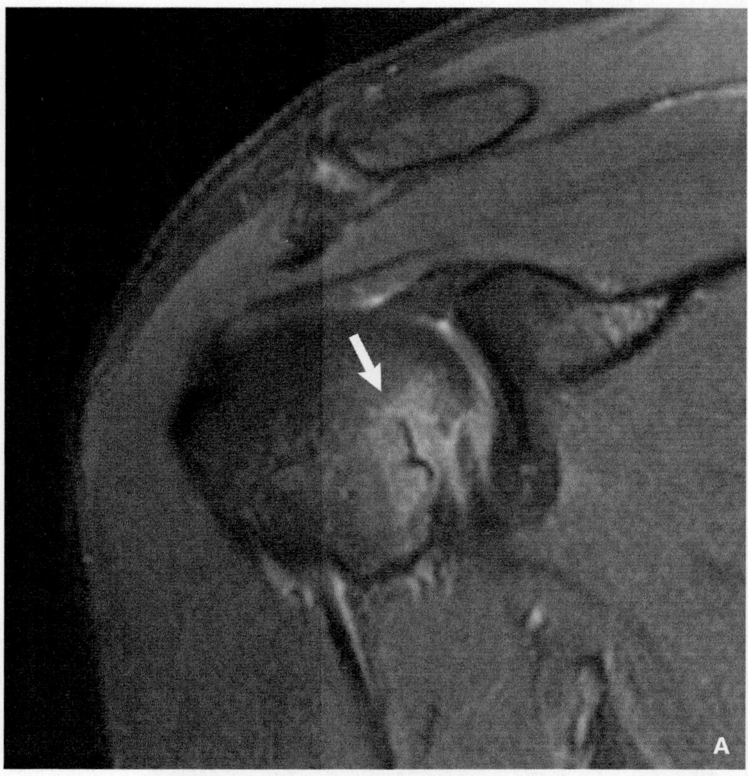

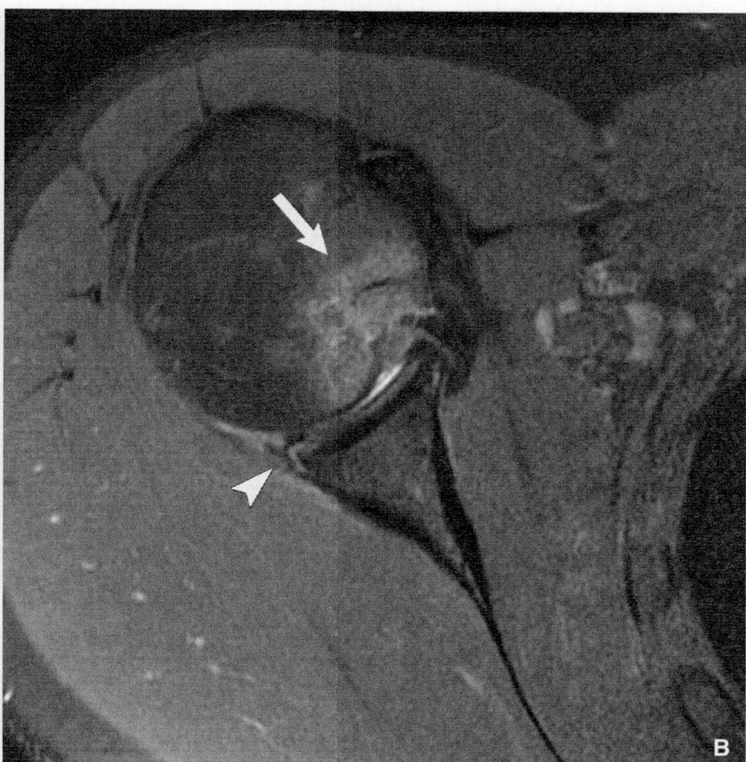

FIGURE 5.64 **MRI of posterior shoulder dislocation.** A 36-year-old man sustained a posterior shoulder dislocation that has been relocated. Coronal **(A)** and axial **(B)** proton density–weighted fat-suppressed MR images show a compression fracture at the anteromedial aspect of the humeral head *(arrows)*. In addition, observe a tear of the posterior labrum and stripping of the periosteum from the scapula *(arrowhead)*.

of bone, spurring at the inferior aspect of the acromion, and degenerative changes of the humeral tuberosities at the insertion of the rotator cuff.

Neer described three progressive stages of impingement syndrome apparent clinically and at surgery. Stage I consists of edema and hemorrhage and is reversible with conservative therapy. It typically occurs in young individuals engaged in sport activities requiring excessive use of the arm above the head (i.e., swimming). Stage II implies fibrosis and thickening of the subacromial soft tissue, rotator cuff tendinitis, and sometimes a partial tear of the rotator cuff. It is manifested clinically by recurrent pain and is often seen in patients 25 to 40 years old. Stage III represents complete rupture of the rotator cuff and is associated with progressive disability. It is usually seen in patients older than 40 years old. Arthrography aids little in the early diagnosis of impingement syndrome, and other ancillary imaging techniques are also unsatisfactory for demonstration of the lesion in the early stages. Because of its high soft-tissue contrast resolution and multiplanar imaging capabilities, MRI is the only technique that can accurately image the early changes of this condition, in particular bursal thickening and effusion (subacromial bursitis), edema, and inflammatory changes of the rotator cuff and its tendons (Fig. 5.66A,B), and later changes consisting of partial- and full-thickness tear of the rotator cuff (Fig. 5.66C,D).

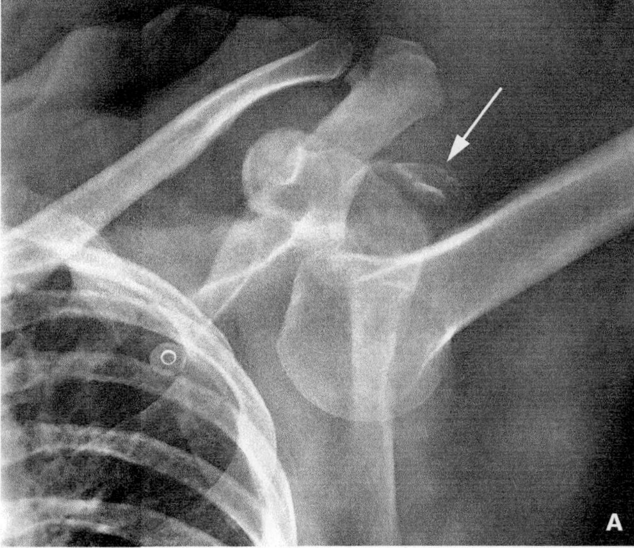

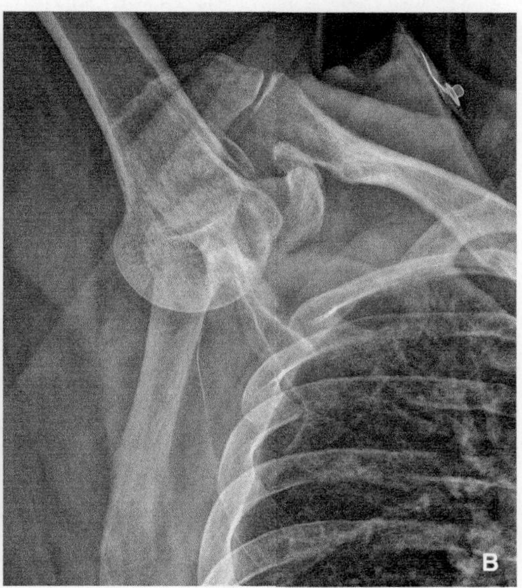

FIGURE 5.65 **Inferior shoulder dislocation.** **(A)** Anteroposterior radiograph of the left shoulder shows classic appearance of *luxatio erecta humeri*. Note that the humeral head faces inferiorly, and it is located below the rim of the glenoid. An *arrow* points to associated fracture of the glenoid. **(B)** In another patient, anteroposterior radiograph of the right shoulder shows typical appearance of this injury.

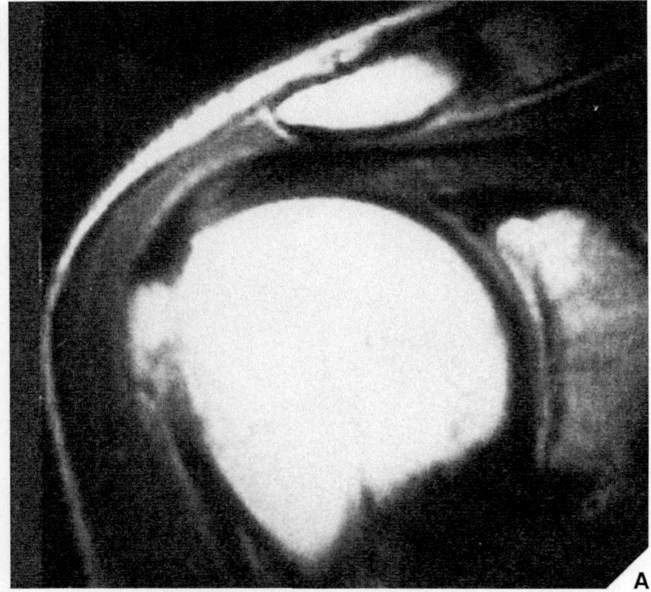

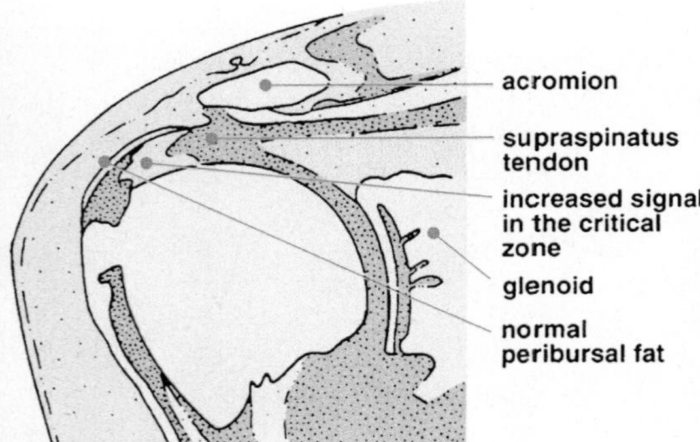

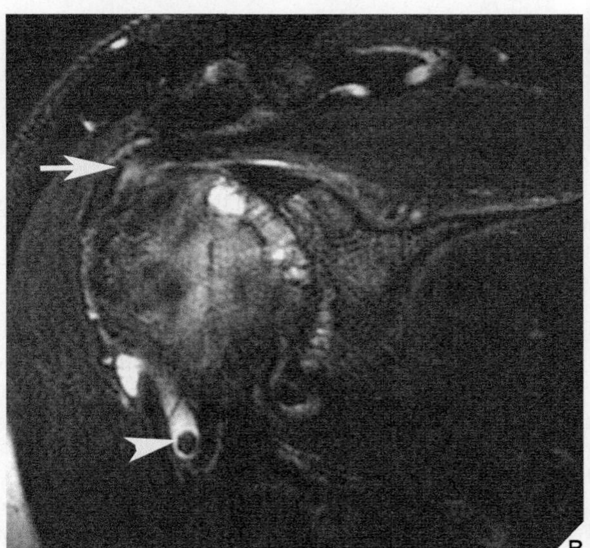

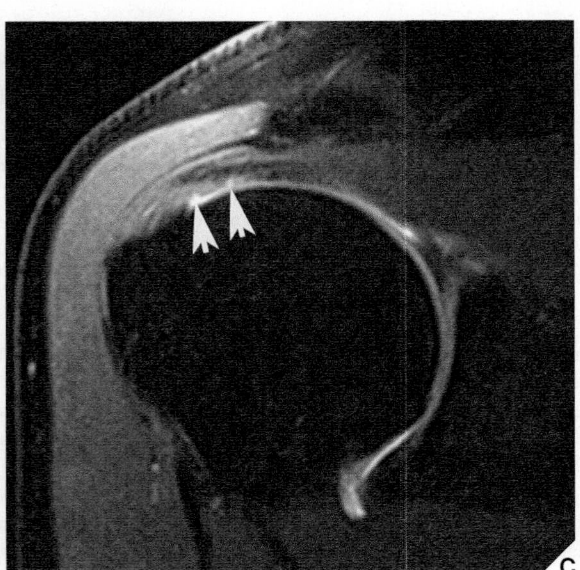

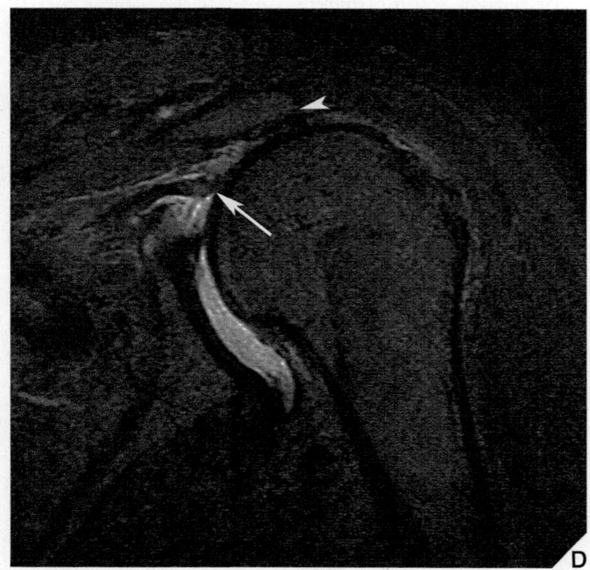

FIGURE 5.66 MRI of impingement syndrome. **(A)** Oblique coronal T1-weighted MR image of early stage of the impingement syndrome. There is slightly increased signal in the critical zone of the supraspinatus tendon. Peribursal fat demarcating the subacromial subdeltoid bursa complex is still intact. **(B)** Oblique coronal T2-weighted MR image of stage II impingement syndrome shows a focus of intermediate signal *(arrow)* of the supraspinatus tendon. Note the advanced degenerative changes of the glenohumeral joint and an intraarticular loose body *(arrowhead)*. **(C)** Oblique coronal T1-weighted fat-saturated MRa of stage II impingement syndrome demonstrates surface fibrillation of the articular fibers of the supraspinatus tendon *(arrows)*, representing a partial tear. **(D)** Oblique coronal T2-weighted fat-saturated MR image of the left shoulder demonstrates a full thickness retracted tear of the supraspinatus tendon *(arrow)*. Note the decreased acromiohumeral distance and the inferior acromial enthesophyte *(arrowhead)*. Findings correspond to a stage III impingement. (**A**, Reprinted by permission from Springer: Holt RG, Helms CA, Steinbach L, et al. Magnetic resonance imaging of the shoulder: rationale and current applications. *Skeletal Radiol* 1990;19:5–14.)

Rotator Cuff Tear

The rotator cuff of the shoulder, a musculotendinous structure about the joint capsule, consists of four intrinsic muscles: the subscapularis, the supraspinatus, the infraspinatus, and the teres minor (see Fig. 5.3). The tendinous portions of the cuff, which converge and fuse to form an envelope covering the humeral head, insert into the anatomic neck and tuberosities of the humerus. Tears may occur in the supraspinatus portion of the cuff, approximately 1 cm from the insertion into the greater tuberosity of the humerus (known as a *critical zone*), but more often, they occur at the insertion into the greater tuberosity.

Injury to the rotator cuff may occur secondary to dislocation in the glenohumeral joint or to sudden abduction of the arm against resistance. It is most commonly seen in patients older than 50 years of age because of normal degenerative changes in the cuff that predispose this structure to rupture after even minor shoulder injuries. Clinically, patients characteristically present with pain in the shoulder and inability to abduct the arm.

Although radiographs of the shoulder are usually insufficient to demonstrate the tear, certain radiographic features characteristic of chronic rotator cuff tear may be present on the anteroposterior view. These include (a) narrowing of the acromiohumeral space to less than 6 mm, (b) erosion of the inferior aspect of the acromion secondary to cephalad migration of the humeral head, and (c) flattening and atrophy of the greater tuberosity of the humeral head caused by the absence of traction stress by the rotator cuff (Fig. 5.67). Although these findings are usually diagnostic of chronic tear, contrast arthrography or MRa may be performed to confirm or exclude the suspected diagnosis. As the intact rotator cuff normally separates the subacromial–subdeltoid bursae complex from the joint cavity, only the glenohumeral joint, the axillary recess, the bursa subscapularis, and the bicipital tendon sheath should opacify on arthrographic or MRa examination (Fig. 5.68A; see also Fig. 5.17B). Opacification of the subacromial–subdeltoid bursae is diagnostic of rotator cuff tear (Fig. 5.68B–D). Occasionally, contrast is seen only in the substance of the rotator cuff, whereas the subacromial–subdeltoid bursae complex remains unopacified, indicating a partial tear of the cuff (Fig. 5.69).

Although arthrography of the shoulder remains the effective technique for evaluating a suspected rotator cuff tear, MRI and ultrasound (US) are being used more frequently as noninvasive methods to diagnose such a tear. The advantage of MRI over arthrography is not only that it is a noninvasive technique but also that it allows visualization of the osseous and periarticular soft tissue of the shoulder in the coronal, sagittal, axial, and oblique planes. It has proved to be highly sensitive (75% to 92%) and accurate (84% to 94%) for diagnosing full-thickness rotator cuff disruption. Moreover, there is excellent correlation between preoperative assessment of the size of rotator cuff tears by MRI and the measurement at surgery. The advantages of US include low cost, easy availability, and dynamic evaluation of the anatomic structures. Disadvantages include limited visualization of the deep structures such as the labrum and nonvisualization of the osseous structures.

Visualization of the rotator cuff is optimal when the MR images are obtained in all three planes: oblique coronal, oblique sagittal, and axial. The MRI findings for rotator cuff tear consist of focal discontinuity of the supraspinatus tendon, tendon and muscle retraction, abnormally increased signal within the tendon, and the presence of fluid in the subacromial–subdeltoid bursa complex (Fig. 5.70; see also Fig. 5.72). US has been shown to be highly accurate for the diagnosis of partial and complete rotator cuff tears. Images can be obtained in the short axis and long axis of the tendons (Figs. 5.71 and 5.72D). Power Doppler US images can also be effective (Fig. 5.72E).

It must be noted, however, that the complex MRI appearance of the rotator cuff can occasionally be confounding in the diagnosis of a tear; experience and total knowledge of normal anatomy are required for correct interpretation. Large tears are well visualized on MR images as areas of discontinuity and irregularity of the rotator cuff tendons, with joint fluid tracking through the cuff defect into the subacromial–subdeltoid bursa complex. With complete rotator cuff tears and retraction of the tendons, the corresponding muscle belly assumes a distorted globular shape that is easily recognized. Chronic tears may result in atrophy of the cuff musculature, manifested on T1-weighted images by a decrease in muscle size and bulk, and by infiltration of the muscle by a band of high–signal intensity fat. Partial tears, which can be characterized as affecting articular surface, bursal surface, or intrasubstance, may be seen as various foci of high signal within the homogeneous low signal intensity of the tendon or as irregularity or thinning of the tendon. Obliteration of the subacromial–subdeltoid fat line on T2-weighted images is a sensitive indicator of rotator cuff tears, and increased signal in the same region on T2-weighted sequences corresponds to the leakage of joint fluid into the subacromial–subdeltoid bursae complex.

MRI provides the surgeon with critical information regarding size and location of a tear, the specific tendons involved, the degree of musculature atrophy and tendon retraction, and the quality of the torn edges. Such information is invaluable for assessing the feasibility of surgery and the type of necessary repair.

Chronic, massive rotator cuff tears are often associated with complete or partial tears of the intracapsular portion of long biceps tendon, with distal retraction of the tendon. MRI and US demonstrate absence of the long biceps tendon within the bicipital groove.

FIGURE 5.67 Chronic rotator cuff tear. The characteristics of chronic rotator cuff tear are identifiable on the anteroposterior radiograph of the right shoulder.

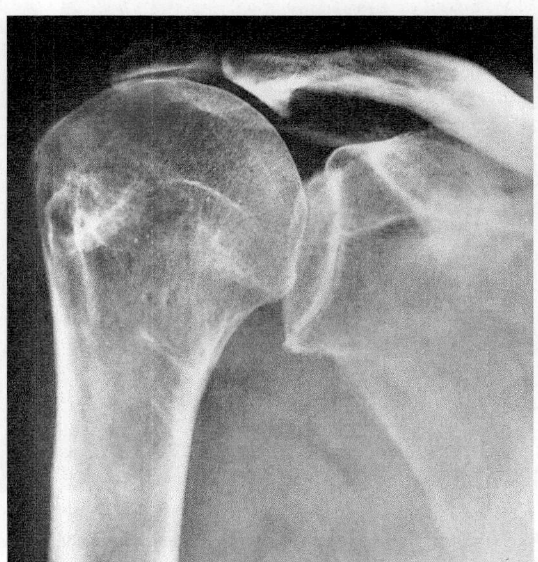

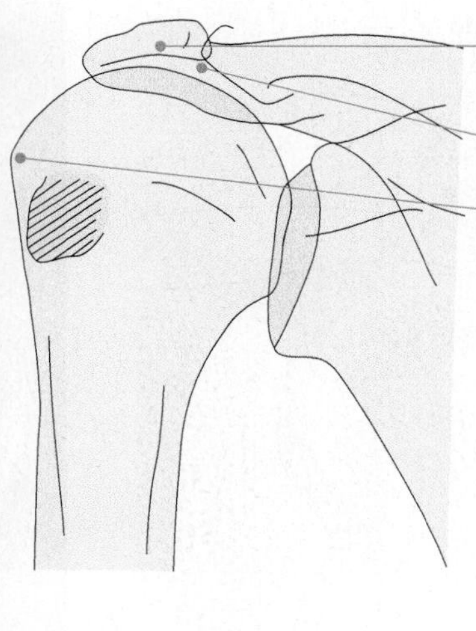

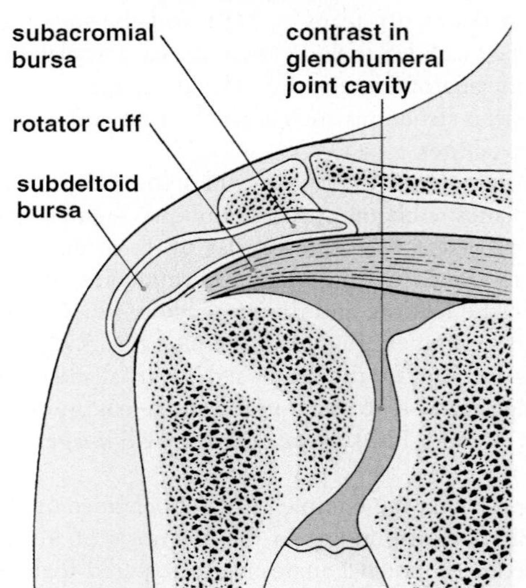

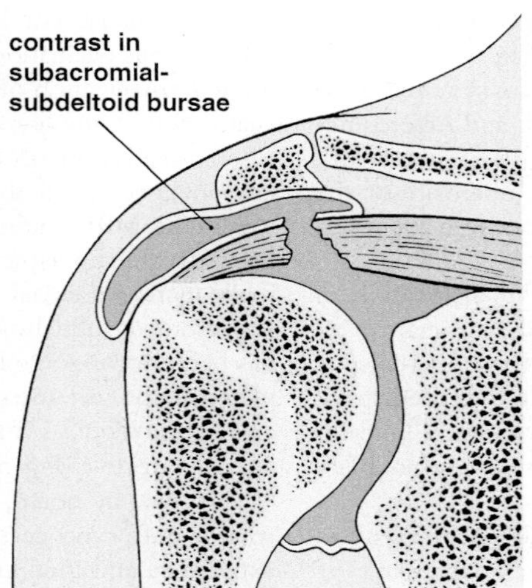

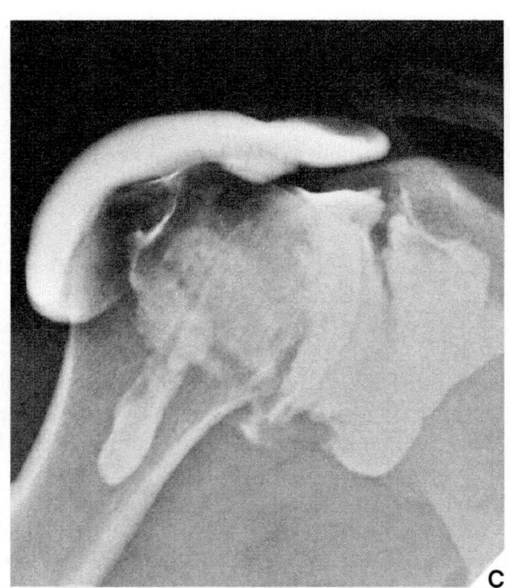

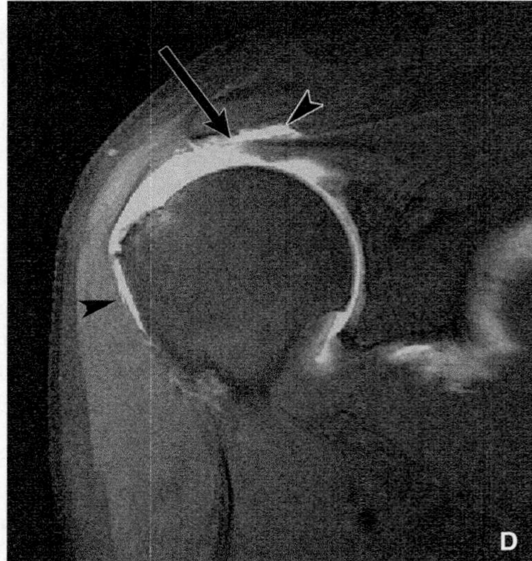

FIGURE 5.68 **Arthrography and MRa of the shoulder joint.** The intact rotator cuff **(A)** does not allow communication between the glenohumeral joint cavity and the subacromial–subdeltoid bursae complex. When arthrography or MRa is performed for suspected tear of the cuff, opacification of the bursa **(B,C)** indicates abnormal communication between the bursa and the joint cavity, confirming diagnosis. When MRa is performed **(D)** and contrast material (or native joint fluid) extends from the glenohumeral joint to the subacromial subdeltoid bursa complex *(arrowheads)*, this finding confirms the diagnosis of full-thickness tear (the *arrow* points to the tear associated with tendon retraction).

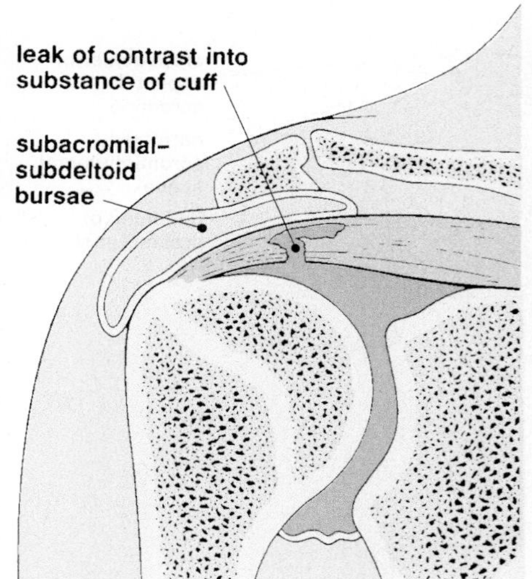

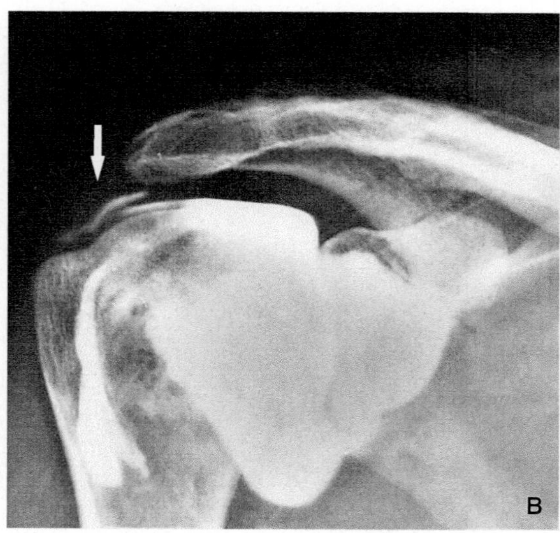

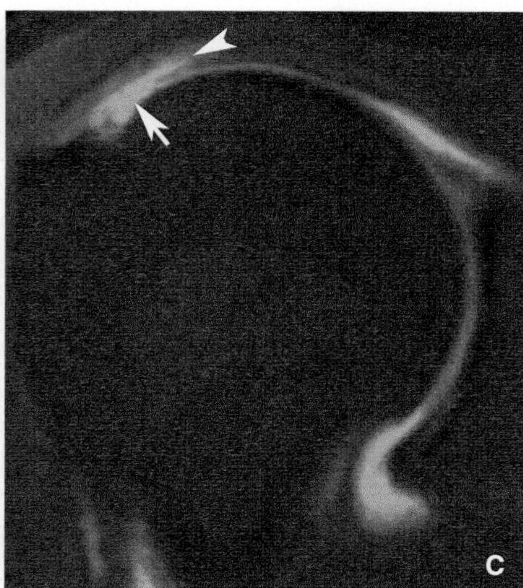

FIGURE 5.69 **Partial tear of the rotator cuff.** This injury **(A)** allows tracking of contrast into the substance of the cuff *(arrow)* **(B)**, whereas the subacromial–subdeltoid bursae remain free of contrast. **(C)** Oblique coronal T1-weighted fat-saturated image of MR-arthrogram in another patient demonstrates a high-grade partial tear of the articular fibers of the supraspinatus tendon *(arrow)* with proximal delamination *(arrowhead)*. Note the absence of contrast material in the subacromial subdeltoid bursa.

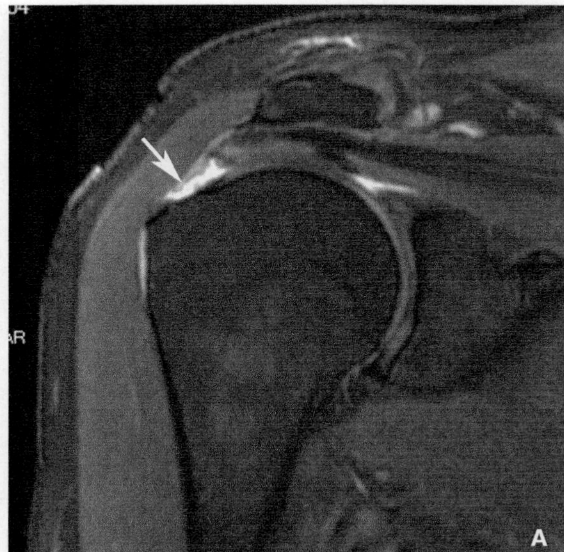

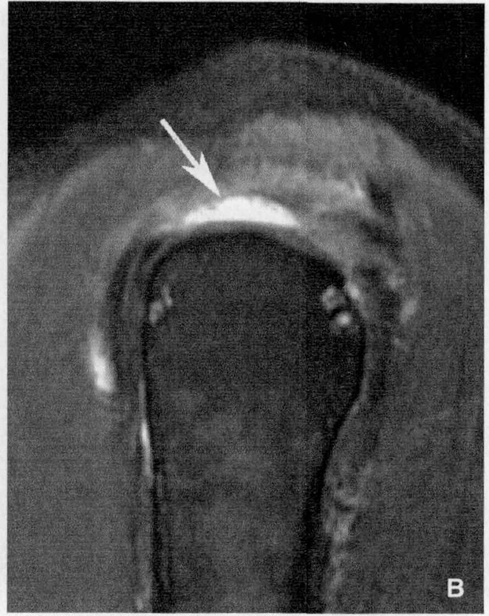

FIGURE 5.70 **MRI of full-thickness tear of the supraspinatus tendon.** **(A)** Oblique coronal T2-weighted fat-saturated MR image of the right shoulder demonstrates interruption of the supraspinatus tendon *(arrow)* and fluid in the subacromial–subdeltoid bursae diagnostic of complete rotator cuff tear. **(B)** Oblique sagittal T2-weighted fat-suppressed MR image in the same patient demonstrates the anteroposterior size of the tear *(arrow)*.

The presence of atrophy of the supraspinatus and infraspinatus muscles is important factor for surgical planning. It has been proven that patients with severe muscular atrophy have a higher rate of retear following surgical repair. The most frequently used grading of muscular atrophy is the Goutallier classification, which assesses the amount of muscular fatty infiltration. Although this classification was based on CT imaging, it has been validated for use with MRI (Fig. 5.73):

Stage 0: normal muscle
Stage 1: some fatty streaks
Stage 2: less than 50% fatty muscle atrophy
Stage 3: 50% fatty muscle atrophy
Stage 4: greater than 50% fatty muscle atrophy

Injury to the Cartilaginous Labrum

Bankart Lesion

Injury to the anterior–inferior cartilaginous labrum, which is usually associated with an avulsion of the IGHL from the anterior–inferior glenoid rim, occurs during anterior dislocation in the glenohumeral joint. It may affect only a fibrocartilaginous portion of the glenoid, or it may be associated with a fracture of the anterior aspect of the inferior osseous rim of the glenoid (see Figs. 5.52 to 5.56).

POLPSA Lesion

The POLPSA lesion, recently reported as the *posterior labrocapsular periosteal sleeve avulsion*, consists of avulsion of the attachment of the glenohumeral capsule and the periosteum to which it is attached sustained during posterior shoulder dislocation. Unlike the Bankart lesion, the posterior glenoid labrum is intact, although it is detached from the osseous glenoid (Fig. 5.74).

ALPSA Lesion

The ALPSA lesion is similar to the Bankart lesion. It is an avulsion injury of the anterior labroligamentous periosteal sleeve sustained during anterior dislocation in glenohumeral joint; however, the anterior scapular periosteum does not rupture as it does in the classic Bankart lesion. This results in medial displacement of the labroligamentous structures that also rotate inferiorly on the scapular neck. ALPSA lesion is best seen on axial MRI (Fig. 5.75).

Perthes Lesion

Perthes lesion, originally described by the German surgeon Perthes in 1905, is very similar to ALPSA lesion. The scapular periosteum is intact; however, it is stripped anteromedially causing incomplete avulsion of the anterior glenoid labrum. Because avulsed cartilaginous labrum is either not

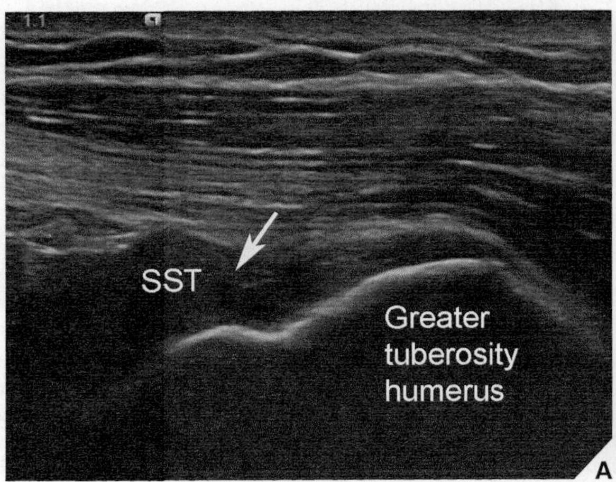

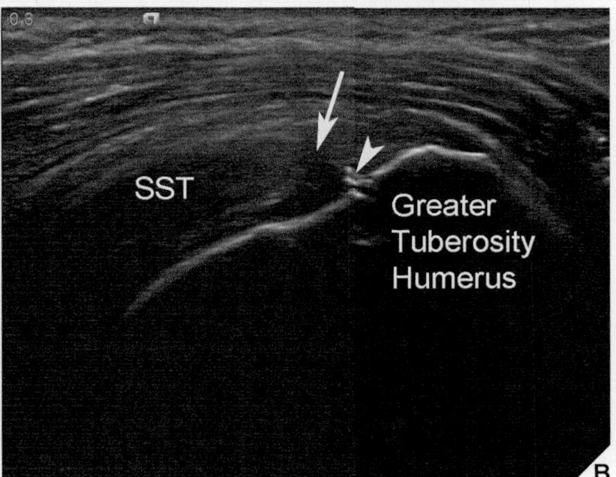

FIGURE 5.71 **US of rotator cuff tear.** **(A)** US examination in the long axis view shows a full-thickness tear of supraspinatus tendon (SST) with retraction of tendon fibers *(arrow)* away from the greater tuberosity. **(B)** US examination in the long axis view in another patient shows a partial articular sided tear of the SST. The tear is indicated by a hypoechoic defect in the tendon extending to articular surface *(arrow)*; calcific tendinopathy *(arrowhead)* is indicated by punctate echogenic foci of calcification in the tendon insertion *(arrowhead)*. (Courtesy of Luis Beltran, MD, Boston.)

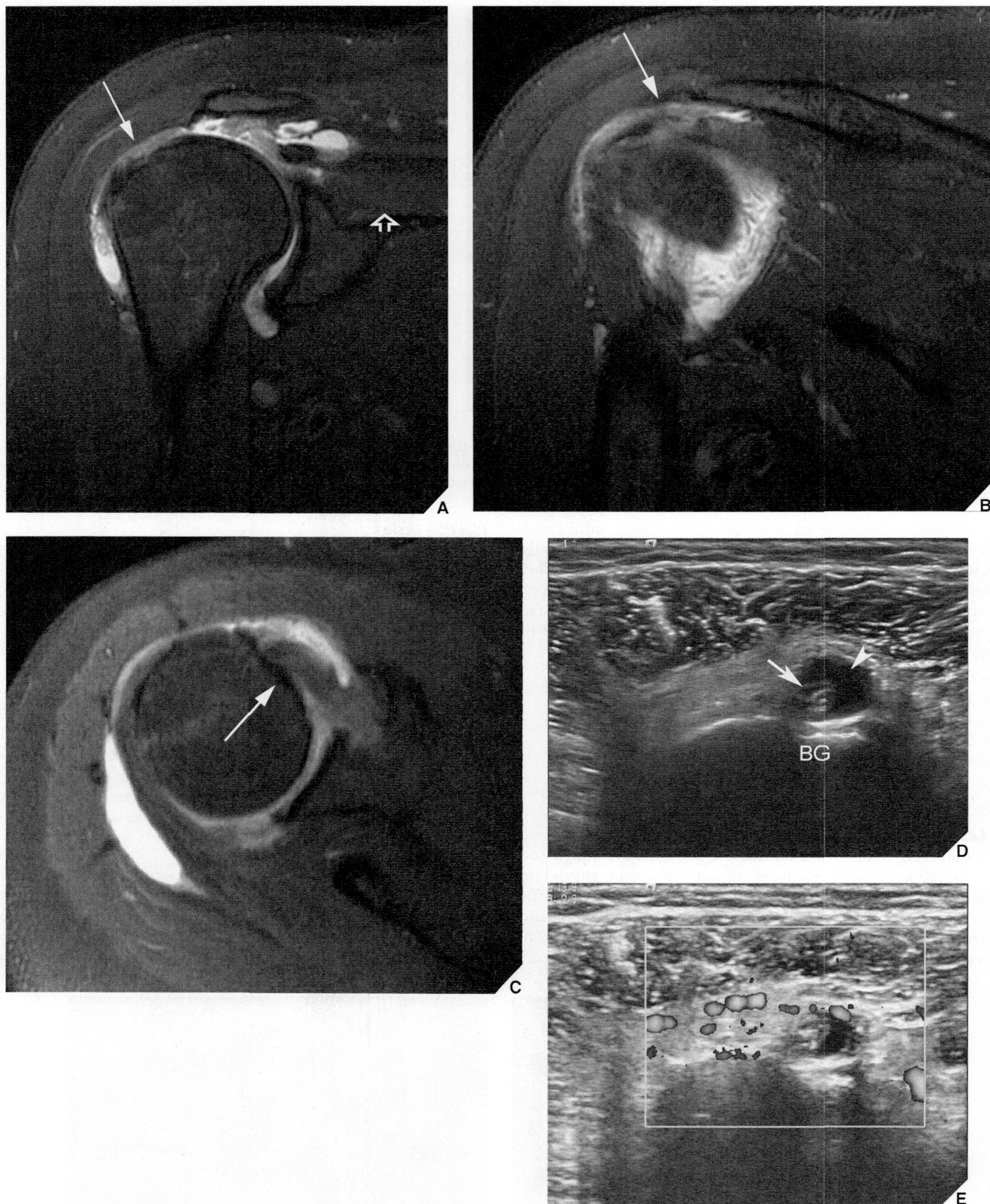

FIGURE 5.72 **MRI and US of massive rotator cuff tear.** **(A)** Coronal proton density–weighted fat-suppressed MR arthrographic image of the right shoulder shows a full-thickness tear of the supraspinatus tendon *(arrow)*. The supraspinatus muscle is medially retracted *(open arrow)*. **(B)** More posterior section shows a tear of the infraspinatus tendon *(arrow)*. **(C)** Axial sequence shows a tear of the subscapularis tendon *(arrow)*. **(D)** In another patient with chronic rotator cuff tear, transverse US images of the biceps tendon in the bicipital groove *(BG)* show partial intrasubstance split tear of this structure indicated by a hypoechoic defect within the tendon fibers *(arrow)*, associated with synovitis in the bicipital groove signified by hypoechoic fluid around the tendon *(arrowhead)* and hypervascularity *(red foci)* on power Doppler US **(E)**. (Courtesy of Luis Beltran, MD, Boston.)

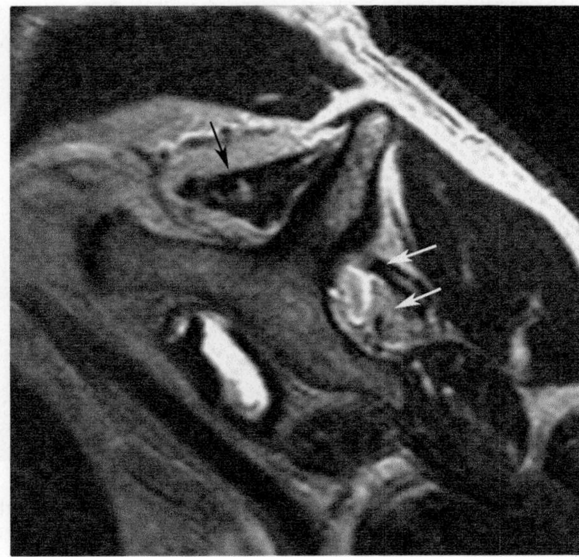

FIGURE 5.73 MRI of muscular atrophy. Sagittal T2-weighted MR image shows grade 2 atrophy of the supraspinatus muscle *(black arrow)* and grade 4 atrophy of the infraspinatus muscle *(white arrows)*.

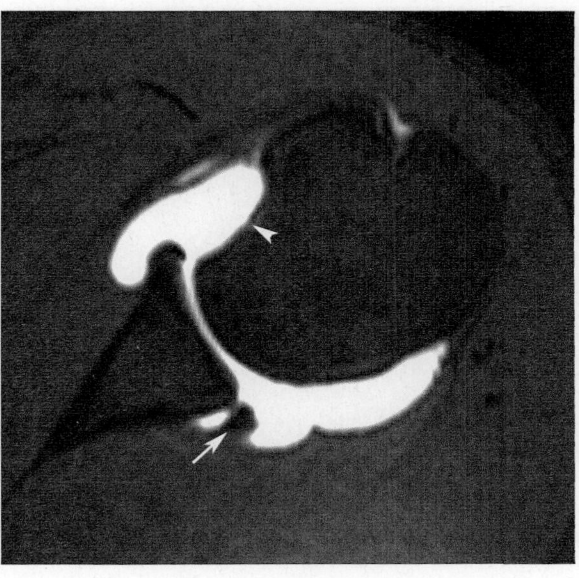

FIGURE 5.74 MRI of POLPSA lesion. Axial T1-weighted fat-saturated MRa demonstrates a detached and medially displaced posterior labrum *(arrow)*. Note the reverse Hill-Sachs lesion in the anterior aspect of the humeral head *(arrowhead)*.

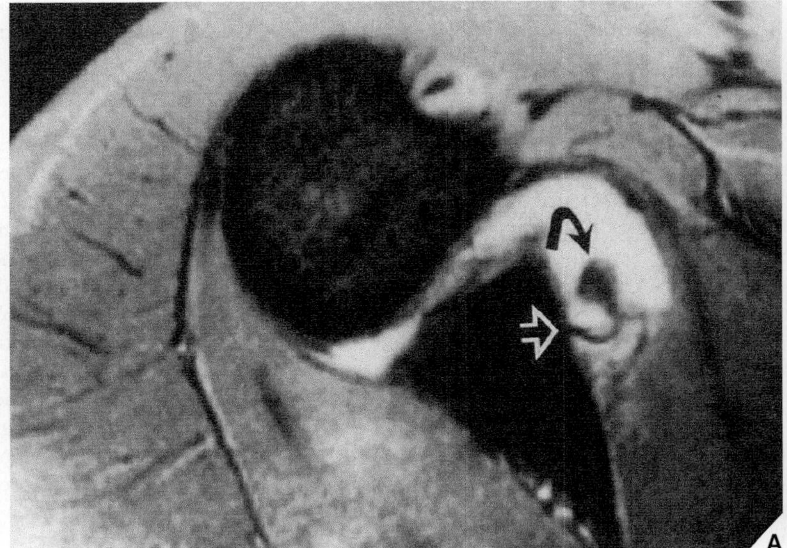

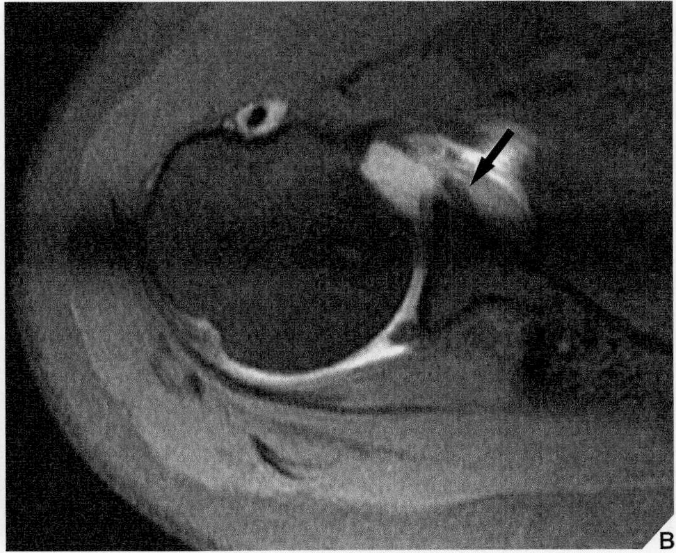

FIGURE 5.75 MRI of ALPSA lesion. **(A)** Axial gradient-echo T2*-weighted MR image shows avulsion of the anterior cartilaginous labrum *(curved arrow)*, but the anterior scapular periosteum, although stripped from the bone, remains attached to the labrum *(open arrow)*. **(B)** In another patient, T1-weighted fat-suppressed MR radial arthrographic image shows medial displacement of the torn anterior labrum and intact periosteal sleeve *(arrow)*.

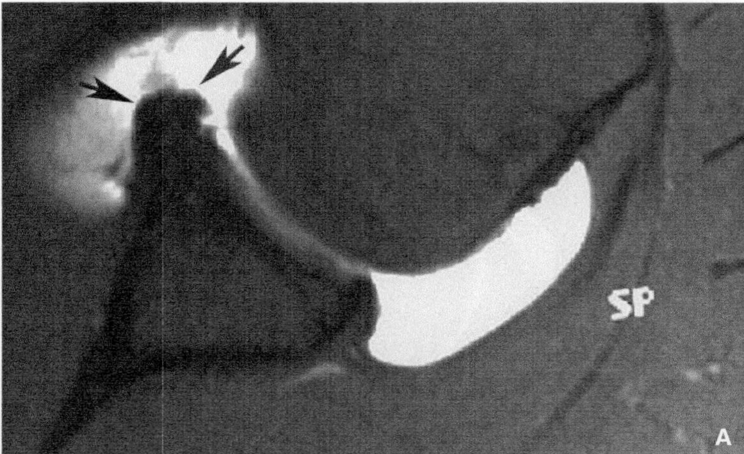

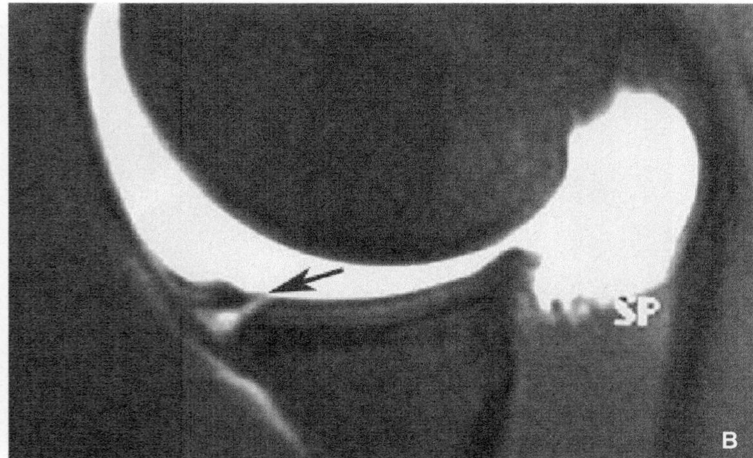

FIGURE 5.76 MRI of Perthes lesion. A young man had anterior shoulder instability after a fall on outstretched hand. **(A)** Axial T1-weighted fat-saturated MR-arthrogram shows thickened anterior labrum *(arrows)*, but no tear is demonstrated. **(B)** Oblique axial T1-weighted MR-arthrogram obtained in ABER position shows detachment of the anterior labrum from the glenoid *(arrow)*.

displaced or minimally displaced, conventional MRI may not detect this abnormality. The most effective technique to diagnose this lesion is MRa with patient's arm in abduction and external rotation (so-called *ABER position*) (Fig. 5.76).

SLAP Lesion

Injury to the superior portion of the cartilaginous glenoid labrum, on either side of the attachment of the long head of the biceps tendon into the labrum at the superior glenoid tubercle, is referred to as *SLAP lesion* (a superior labral, anterior, and posterior tear) and results from a sudden forced abduction of the arm. It is usually sustained in athletic activities such as tennis, volleyball, or baseball, although occasionally, the mechanism of this injury may be a fall on the outstretched arm with the shoulder in abduction and slight forward flexion at the time of impact. SLAP lesions have been classified into four types (Fig. 5.77). Type I is the least common (10%) and consists of a degenerative frayed irregular appearance of the superior portion of the cartilaginous labrum. In this type of injury, the labrum remains firmly attached to the glenoid rim. Type II is the most common (40%) and consists of separation of the superior portion of the cartilaginous labrum to the level of the middle GHL (MGHL) as well as separation of the tendon of the long head of the biceps from the glenoid rim. Type III (30%) consists of a bucket-handle tear of the superior portion of the labrum; however, the attachment site of the tendon of the long head of the biceps is intact. Type IV (15%) consists of the bucket-handle tear of the superior labrum extending into the long head of the biceps tendon. Several additional types of SLAP lesion have recently been described; however, as Helms et al. pointed out, from the practical point of view, it is only important to determine whether a SLAP lesion consists of a partial- or full-thickness (bucket-handle) tear of the superior labrum, whether the labrum is completely separated from the glenoid, and if the biceps tendon is torn at its labral anchor. MRI findings of SLAP lesion include linear increased signal intensity in the superior portion of the cartilaginous labrum on T2-weighted sequences (Fig. 5.78); on MRa, contrast extends into a detached superior portion of the labrum (Figs. 5.79 to 5.81). Distinction between a normal sublabral recess and a SLAP lesion may be challenging. The sublabral recess is a normal variant representing partial separation between the superior labrum and the glenoid margin. When present, it is oriented medially, toward the head of the patient, paralleling the glenoid margin, with smooth edges, and no more than 2 mm in width. It does not extend beyond the insertion of the long biceps tendon. Conversely, a SLAP lesion exhibits lateral orientation, toward the shoulder of the patient, with signal alteration extending inside the substance of the labrum, irregular margins, and wider than 2 mm. SLAP lesions often extend posteriorly, beyond the insertion of the long biceps tendon, and are associated with an anterior labral tear and often a paralabral cyst (Fig. 5.82).

SLAP lesions may be associated with other osseous and soft-tissue lesions of the shoulder, including partial- or full-thickness rotator cuff tears, Bankart lesions, glenohumeral chondromalacia, Buford complex (thickening of the MGHL and congenitally absent anterior superior labrum), and high-grade acromioclavicular separation.

GLAD Lesion

Injury to the anteroinferior portion of the cartilaginous glenoid labrum associated with glenolabral articular disruption is referred to as a *GLAD lesion*. The usual mechanism of this injury is a fall on an outstretched arm in ABER resulting in the forced adduction injury to the shoulder where the humeral head strikes against the adjacent articular cartilage of the glenoid. The lesion consists of a superficial tear of the anteroinferior portion of the labrum and is always associated with an inferior flap tear but without evidence of anterior glenohumeral joint instability on physical examination. The deep fibers of the IGHL remain attached to the labrum and glenoid rim. A GLAD lesion is effectively diagnosed on MRa. The findings include a nondisplaced tear of the anteroinferior labrum with an adjacent chondral injury, which can range from a cartilaginous flap tear to a depressed lesion of the articular cartilage (Figs. 5.83 and 5.84).

GLOM Lesion

GLOM lesion or GLOM sign (glenolabral ovoid mass) represents an avulsion of a portion of the anterior labrum seen on axial MR image.

Bennett Lesion

This lesion consists of a bony spur of the posterior glenoid margin, commonly seen in professional pitchers. It is best demonstrated on axial T1-weighted MR images (Fig. 5.85).

Buford Complex

A congenital variant of absence of the anterior superior labrum and marked thickening of the MGHL that can mimic a labral tear has been termed the *Buford complex* (Fig. 5.86). MRI appearance of this complex should be differentiated from other normal anatomic variants, such as an isolated detachment of the anterior superior labrum (also known as *sublabral foramen* or *sublabral hole*), undercutting of articular cartilage between the labrum and the glenoid cortex, or the presence of a synovial recess (sulcus) interposed between the glenoid rim and the cartilaginous labrum.

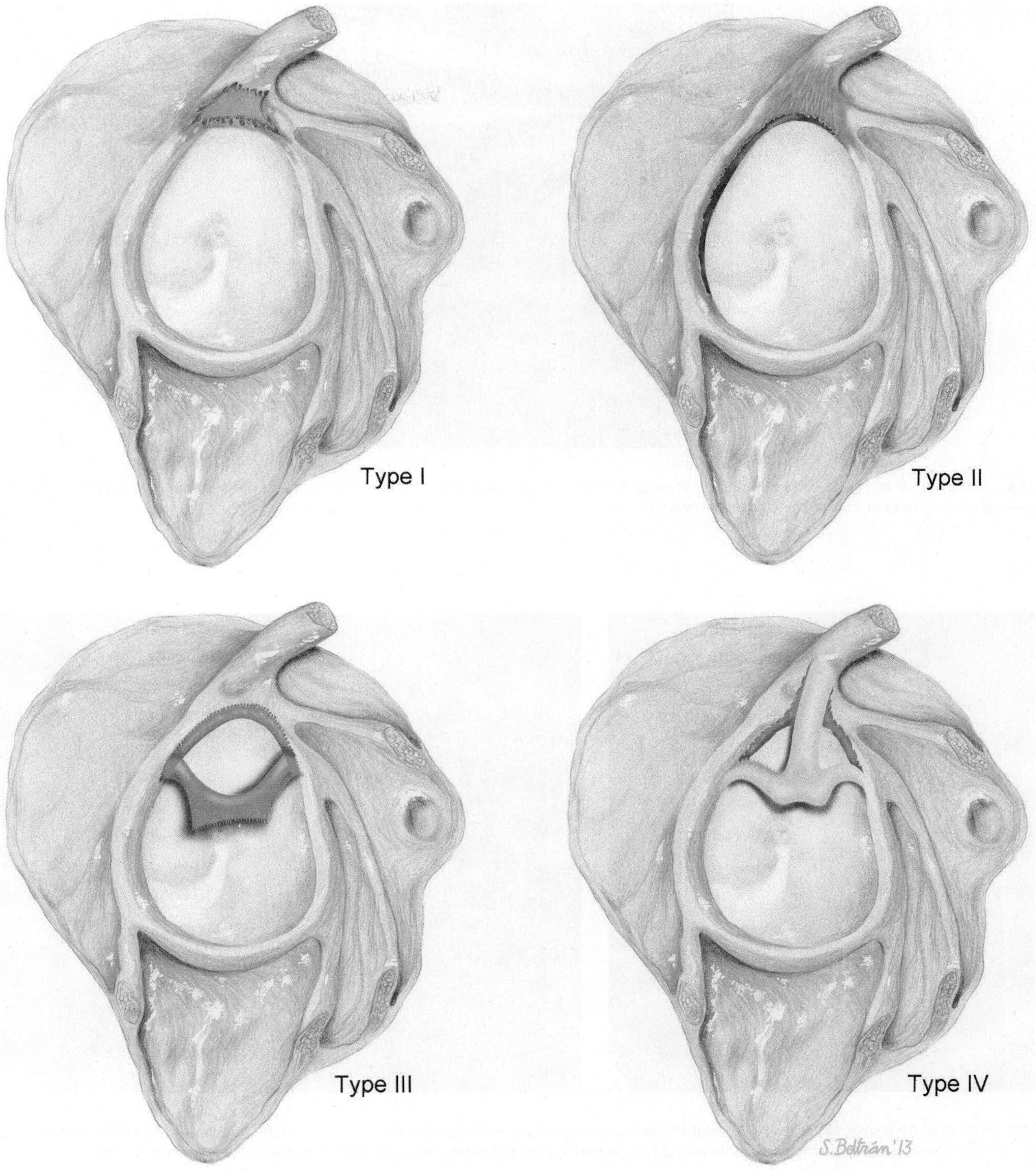

FIGURE 5.77 Types of SLAP lesions (as originally described by Schneider). Type I: degenerative fraying of the superior labrum. Type II: separation of the superior labrum from the glenoid margin. Type III: bucket-handle tear of the superior labrum. Type IV: bucket-handle tear of the superior labrum extending into the long head of the biceps tendon.

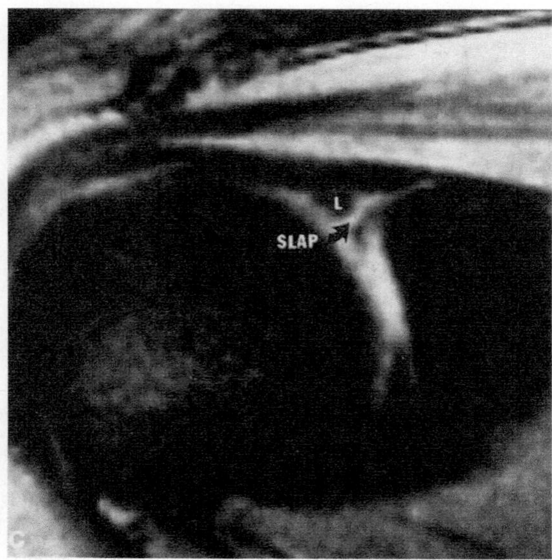

FIGURE 5.78 **MRI of SLAP lesion.** A coronal oblique T2*-weighted MRI shows a type II SLAP lesion involving anterior superior glenoid labrum *(L)*. Note linear high-intensity signal extending across the base of the labrum *(arrow)*.

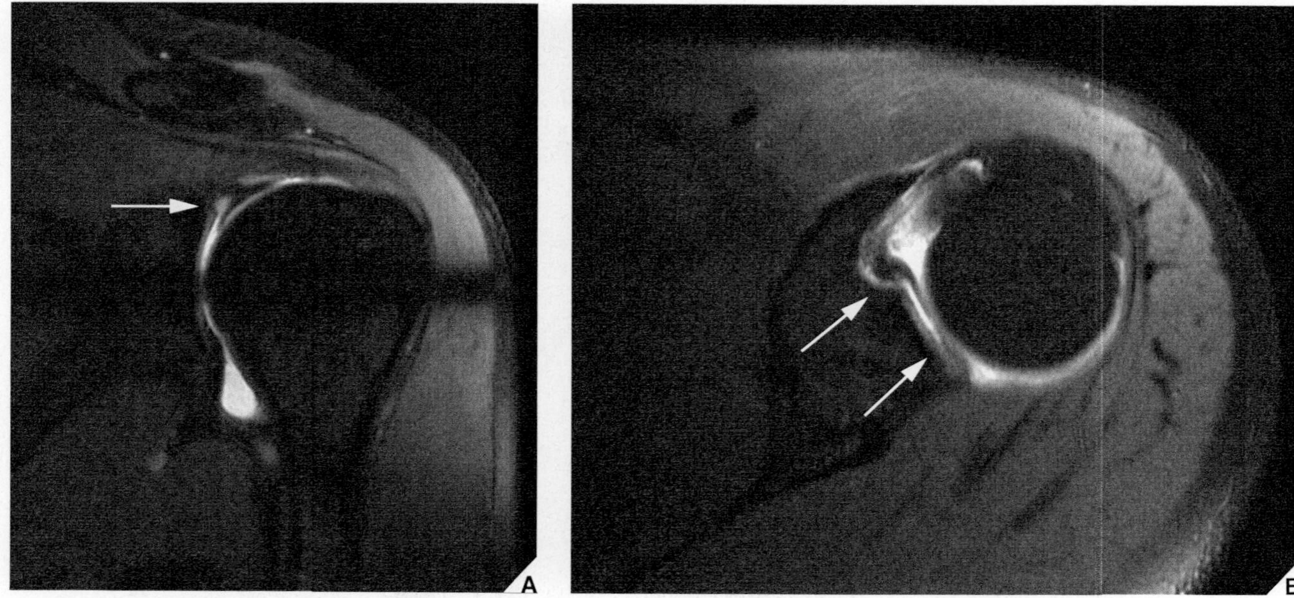

FIGURE 5.79 **MRa of SLAP lesion.** **(A)** Coronal T1-weighted fat-suppressed radial arthrographic MR image of the left shoulder shows a full-thickness tear of the superior labrum *(arrow)*. **(B)** Axial sequence shows a bucket-handle tear of the glenoid labrum extending from the anterior to the posterior aspect *(arrows)*.

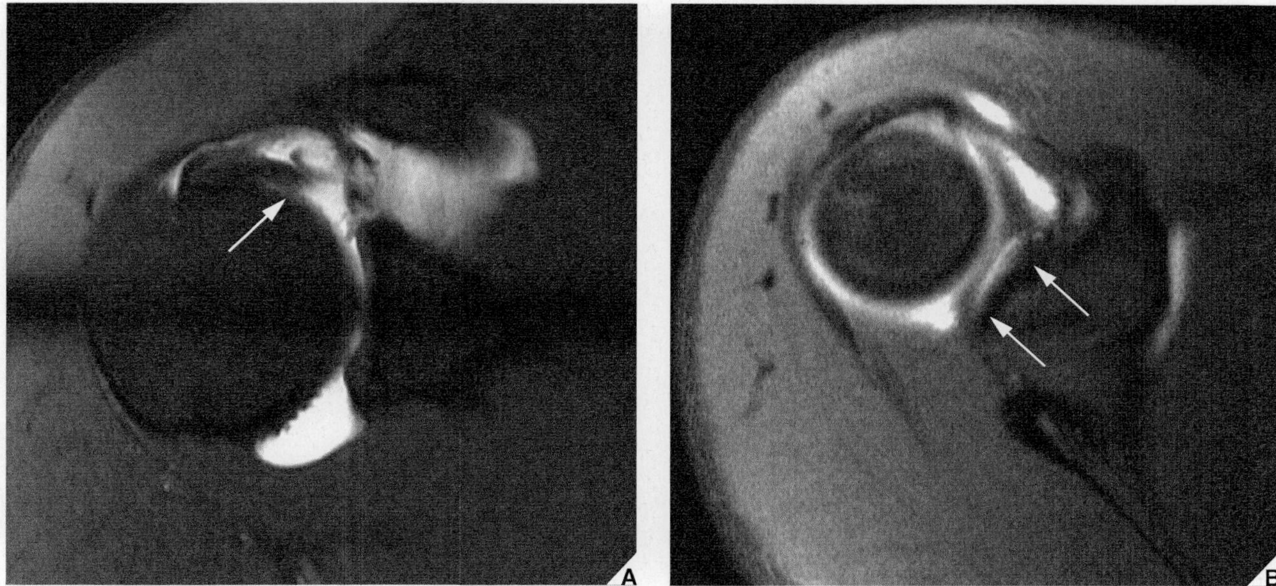

FIGURE 5.80 MRa of SLAP lesion. **(A)** Coronal T1-weighted fat-suppressed radial arthrographic MR image of the right shoulder shows a full-thickness tear of the superior labrum affecting the labral anchor of the long head of the biceps tendon *(arrow)*. **(B)** Axial sequence shows contrast tracking into the tear between the labrum and the glenoid from the anterior to the posterior aspect *(arrows)*.

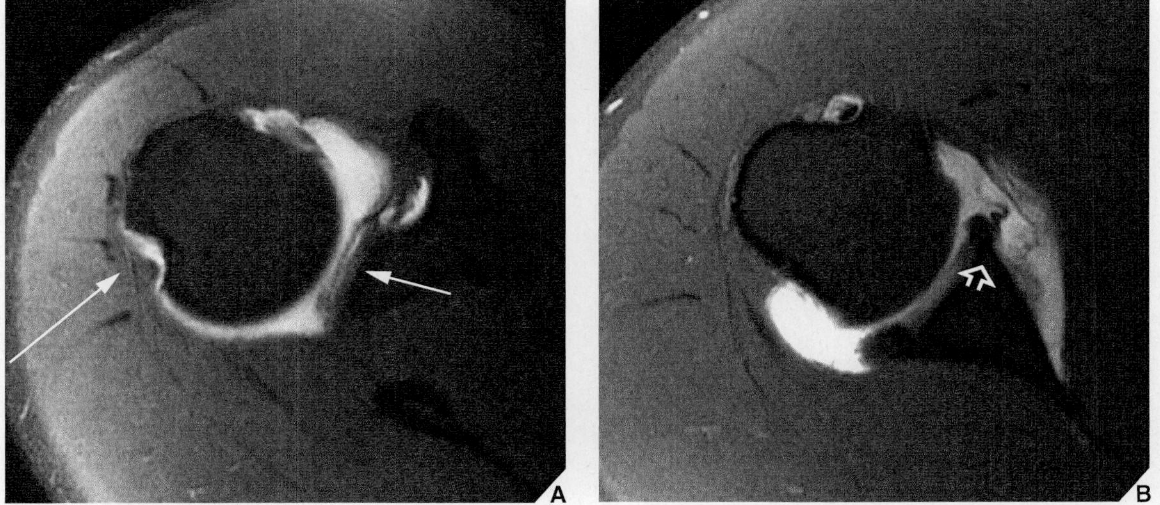

FIGURE 5.81 MRa of SLAP lesion. **(A,B)** Axial proton density–weighted fat-suppressed arthrographic MR images show an extensive tear of the posterosuperior aspect of the glenoid labrum *(short arrow)*, extending anteriorly through the torn MGHL *(open arrow)*. The *long arrow* points to the Hill-Sachs lesion.

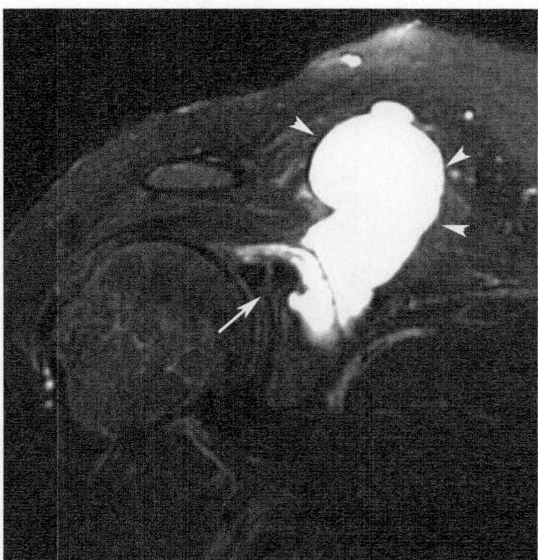

FIGURE 5.82 MRI of SLAP lesion with large paralabral cyst. Oblique coronal T2-weighted MR image demonstrates a superior labral tear *(arrow)* with a large superior paralabral cyst *(arrowheads)* extending into the suprascapular notch and superiorly.

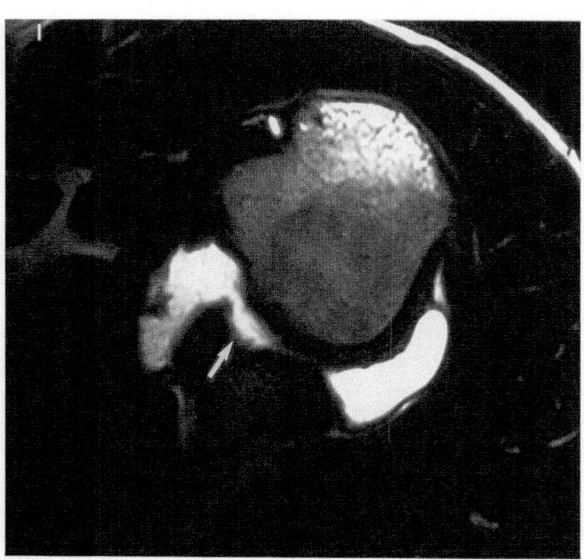

FIGURE 5.83 MRa of GLAD lesion. Axial T2-weighted MR arthrographic image of the left shoulder shows a nondisplaced tear of the anteroinferior labrum associated with an osteochondral defect *(arrow)* in a 21-year-old professional ice hockey player who sustained anterior shoulder dislocation. (Courtesy of J. Tehranzadeh, MD, Orange, California.)

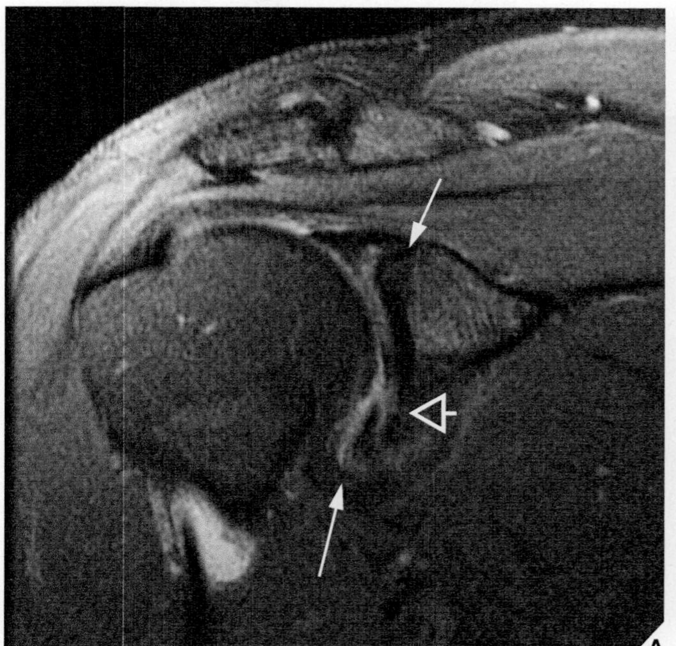

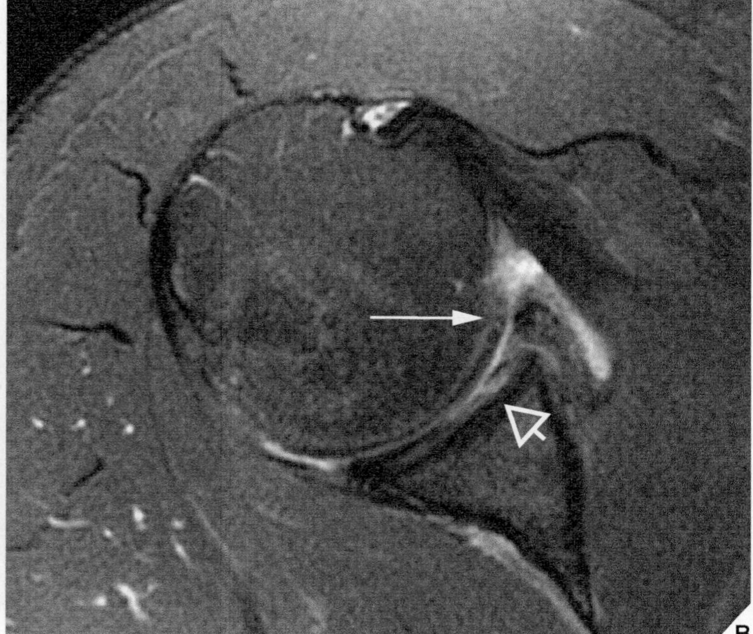

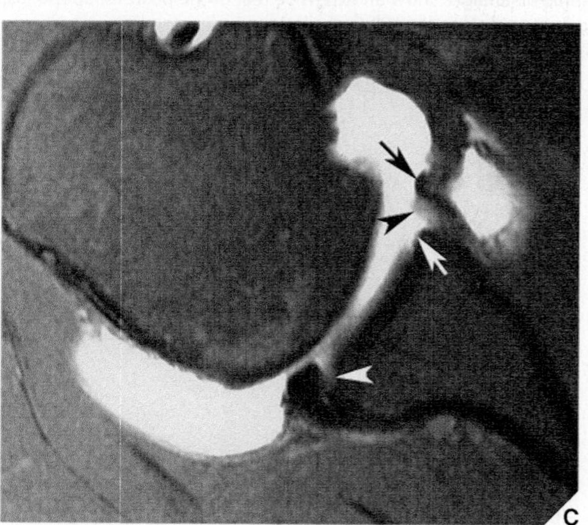

FIGURE 5.84 MRI of GLAD lesion. (A) Coronal T2-weighted fat-suppressed MR image of the right shoulder shows a tear of the anterior aspect of the superior and inferior glenoid labrum *(arrows)* associated with articular chondral defect *(open arrows)*, findings confirmed on the axial section **(B)**. **(C)** Axial T1-weighted fat-saturated MRa in another patient demonstrates a tear of the anterior labrum *(black arrow)* with a detached portion of the articular cartilage *(black arrowhead)*. Note the area of the glenoid denuded of articular cartilage *(white arrow)*. The patient also had a posterior labral tear *(white arrowhead)*.

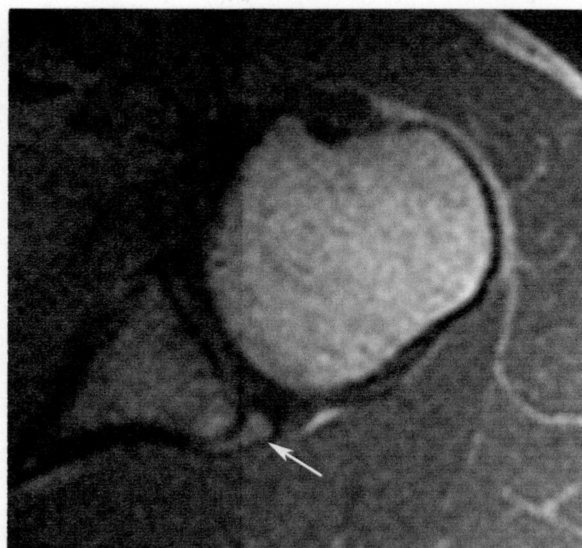

FIGURE 5.85 MRI of Bennett lesion. Axial T1-weighted image demonstrates a spur-like formation *(arrow)* in the posterior aspect of the glenoid at the capsular insertion.

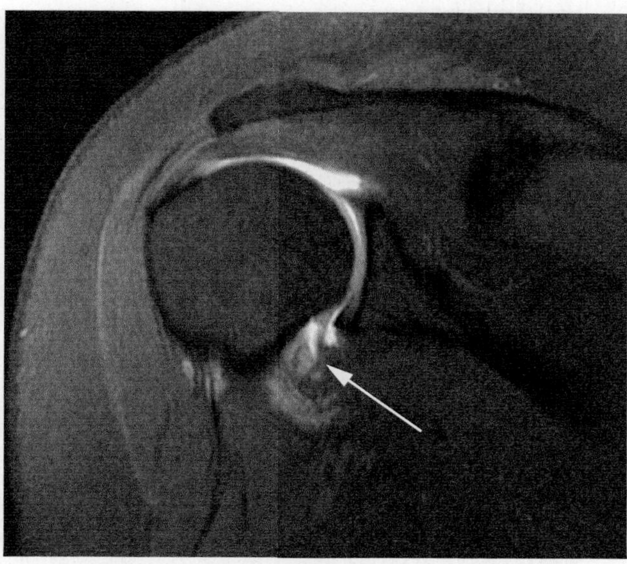

FIGURE 5.87 MRI of HAGL lesion. Coronal proton density–weighted fat-suppressed MR image shows evulsion of the IGHL from the humerus *(arrow)*.

Injury to the Glenohumeral Ligaments

There are three GHLs located within the anterior portion of the glenohumeral joint that contribute to anterior shoulder stability. The IGHL is the thickest structure and extends from the glenoid labrum to the anatomic neck of the humerus. The MGHL originates at the superior portion of the anterior labrum and attaches to the base of the lesser tuberosity of the humerus. The superior GHL (SGHL) originates from the superior–anterior labrum and attaches distally to the superior aspect of the lesser tuberosity of the humerus. All of these ligaments may be injured during a traumatic event to the shoulder joint; however, the IGHL, the most important stabilizer of the glenohumeral joint, is most commonly traumatized.

HAGL Lesion

Avulsion of the IGHL from the anatomic neck of the humerus is referred to as a *HAGL* (**h**umeral **a**vulsion of the **g**lenohumeral **l**igament) *lesion.* It may be caused by shoulder dislocation and is often associated with a tear of the subscapularis tendon. This abnormality can be seen on axial, oblique coronal, or sagittal MR images or on MRa (Figs. 5.87 and 5.88).

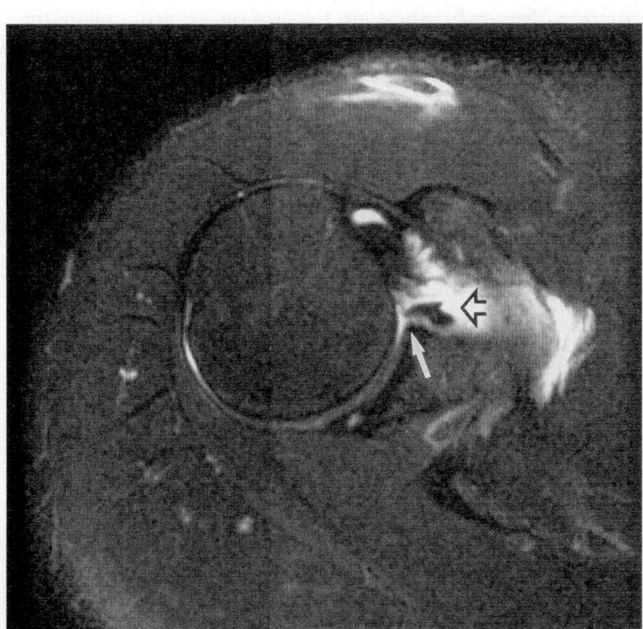

FIGURE 5.86 MRa of Buford complex. MR-arthrogram shows an absent anterior superior glenoid labrum *(arrow)* and markedly thickened MGHL *(open arrow)*, characteristic features of the Buford complex. This congenital variant can mimic a labral tear. (Courtesy of L. Steinbach, MD, San Francisco, California.)

BHAGL Lesion

Bony HAGL (BHAGL) is similar to HAGL, but it is associated with avulsion of a bone fragment from the humerus.

Floating AIGHL Lesion

This lesion represents a tear of the glenoid and humeral attachments of the anterior band of the IGHL.

GAGL Lesion

Glenoid avulsion of the anterior glenohumeral ligament (GAGL) from the glenoid represents a tear of the glenoid insertion of the anterior band of the IGHL better seen in the coronal images (Fig. 5.89).

Reverse GAGL Lesion

This lesion is referred to the glenoid avulsion of the posterior GHL.

PHAGL Lesion

Posterior humeral avulsion of the posterior band of the IGHL is known as a *PHAGL lesion* (Fig. 5.90).

Floating PIGHL Lesion

This lesion represents an avulsion of the humeral and glenoid attachments of the posterior band of the IGHL.

Miscellaneous Abnormalities

Adhesive Capsulitis

Adhesive capsulitis, also referred to as *frozen shoulder*, usually results from posttraumatic adhesive inflammation between the joint capsule and the peripheral articular cartilage of the shoulder. Clinically, it is characterized by progressive shoulder pain, stiffness, and limitation of passive and active motion in the shoulder joint.

Four stages of this condition have been initially described by Neviaser and later, based on arthroscopic criteria, modified by the same author. *Stage I* is characterized by pain with passive and active motion accompanied by limitation of forward flexion, abduction, and internal and external rotation; however, examination under anesthesia shows normal or only minimal loss of range of motion (ROM). Arthroscopic examination shows diffuse glenohumeral synovitis but normal underlying capsule. Pathologic examination shows hypertrophic synovitis and occasional inflammatory cell infiltrates. *Stage II* is characterized by pain with passive and

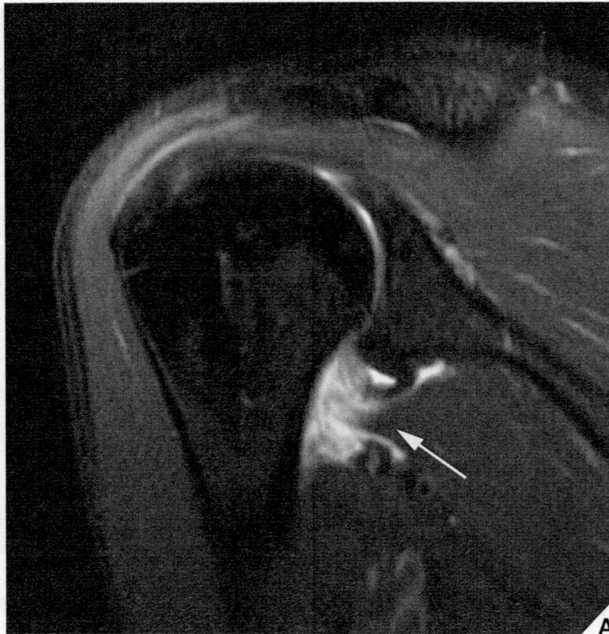

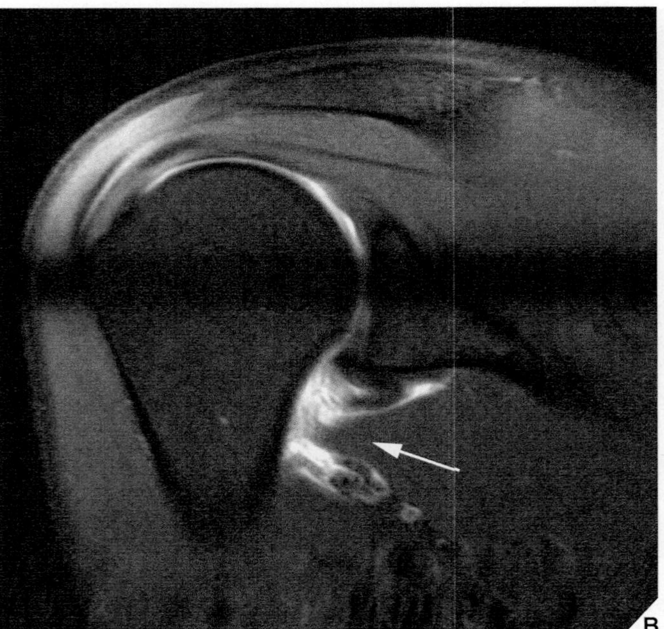

FIGURE 5.88 MRa of HAGL lesion. Coronal proton density–weighted fat-suppressed MR arthrographic image of the right shoulder **(A)** and T1-weighted fat-suppressed radial MR image **(B)** show complete disruption of the humeral attachment of the IGHL *(arrows)*.

active motion and limitation of ROM as in stage I, but examination under anesthesia shows no change in ROM compared with that when patient is awake. Arthroscopy shows diffuse, hypertrophic synovitis and capsular thickening. Pathology shows hypertrophic, hypervascular synovitis with subsynovial scars and fibroplasia. *Stage III* is characterized by minimal pain, but significant limitation of ROM, and no change on examination under anesthesia. Arthroscopy demonstrates lack of hypervascularity, but remnants of fibrotic synovium, and significantly diminished capsular volume. Pathology reveals "burned-out" atrophic synovitis and dense scar formation within the joint capsule. *Stage IV* is characterized by minimal pain and progressive improvement in ROM.

Because radiography, which may only reveal disuse periarticular osteoporosis secondary to this condition, is insufficient to make a diagnosis, single- or double-contrast arthrography is the technique of choice when this abnormality is suspected. The arthrogram usually reveals decreased capacity of the joint capsule, or even complete obliteration of the axillary and subscapular recesses, findings diagnostic of this condition (Fig. 5.91).

MRI has been advocated to diagnose adhesive capsulitis of the shoulder. Emig et al. reported that thickening of the capsule and synovium at the level of the axillary pouch greater than 4 mm detected on MR studies may be a useful criterion for the diagnosis of this condition. Additional MRI signs of adhesive capsulitis include thickening of the coracoacromial ligament and loss of the fat signal at the level of the rotator cuff interval (Fig. 5.92).

Acromioclavicular Separation

Injuries to the acromioclavicular joint, which are commonly sustained during athletic activities by individuals between the ages of 15 and 40 years, often result in acromioclavicular separation (dislocation). Various forces may cause injury to the acromioclavicular joint. The most common is a downward blow to the lateral aspect of the shoulder that drives the acromion inferiorly (caudad); others are traction on the arm pulling the shoulder away from the chest wall and a fall on the outstretched hand or on the flexed elbow with the arm flexed forward 90 degrees.

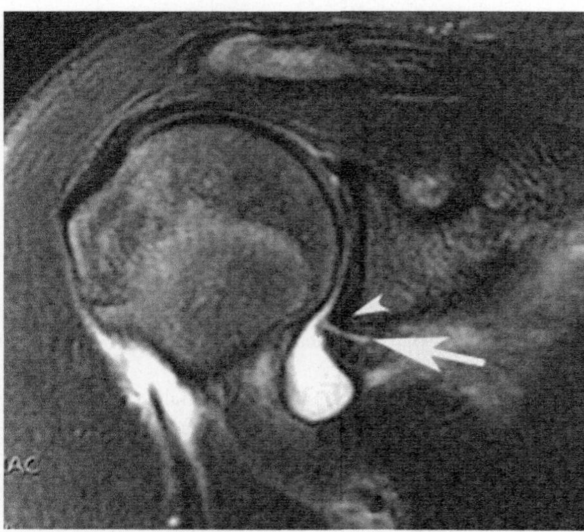

FIGURE 5.89 MRI of GAGL lesion. T2-weighted oblique coronal MR image demonstrates a tear of the glenoid attachment of the anterior band of the IGHL *(arrow)* with an intact inferior labrum *(arrowhead)*.

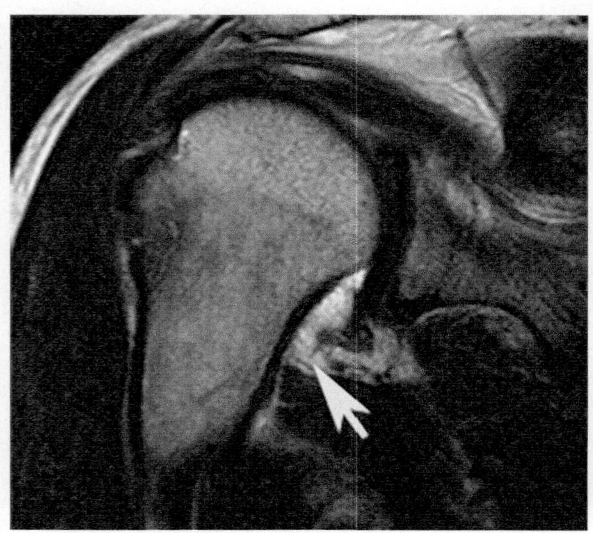

FIGURE 5.90 MRI of PHAGL lesion. T2-weighted oblique coronal MR image demonstrates a tear of the humeral insertion of the posterior band of the IGHL *(arrow)*.

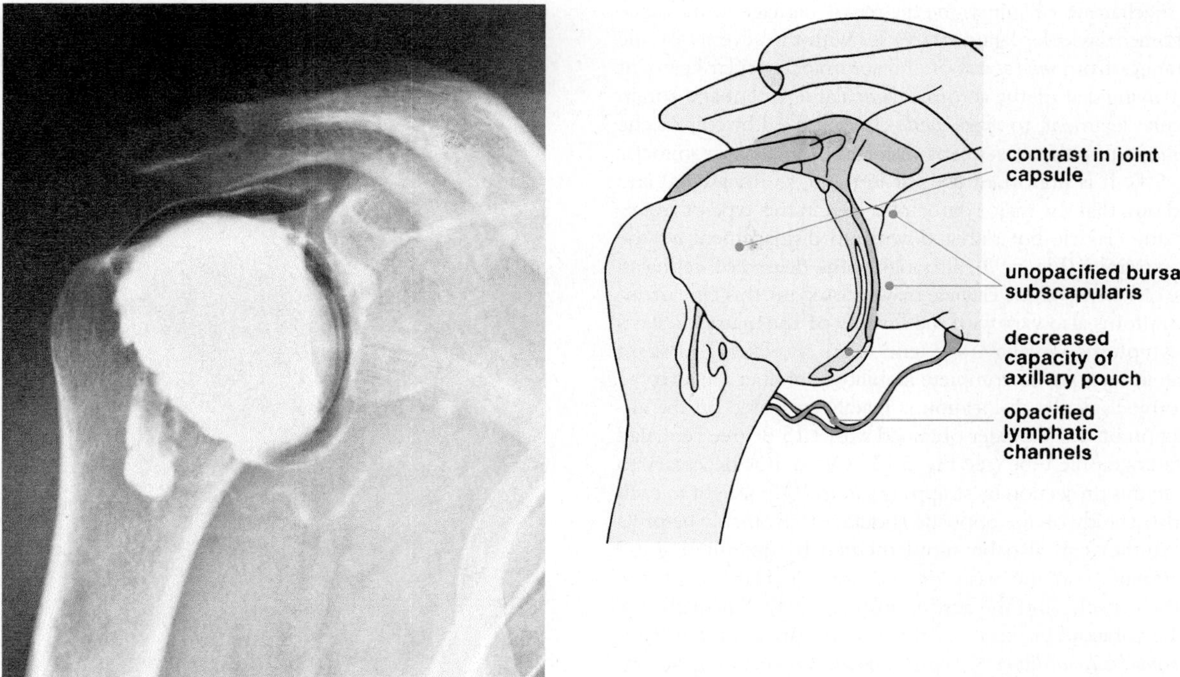

FIGURE 5.91 Arthrogram of adhesive capsulitis. Double-contrast arthrogram of the shoulder demonstrates the characteristic findings of frozen shoulder. The capacity of the axillary pouch is markedly decreased, and the subscapularis recess remains unopacified, whereas the lymphatic channels are filled with contrast secondary to increased intracapsular pressure.

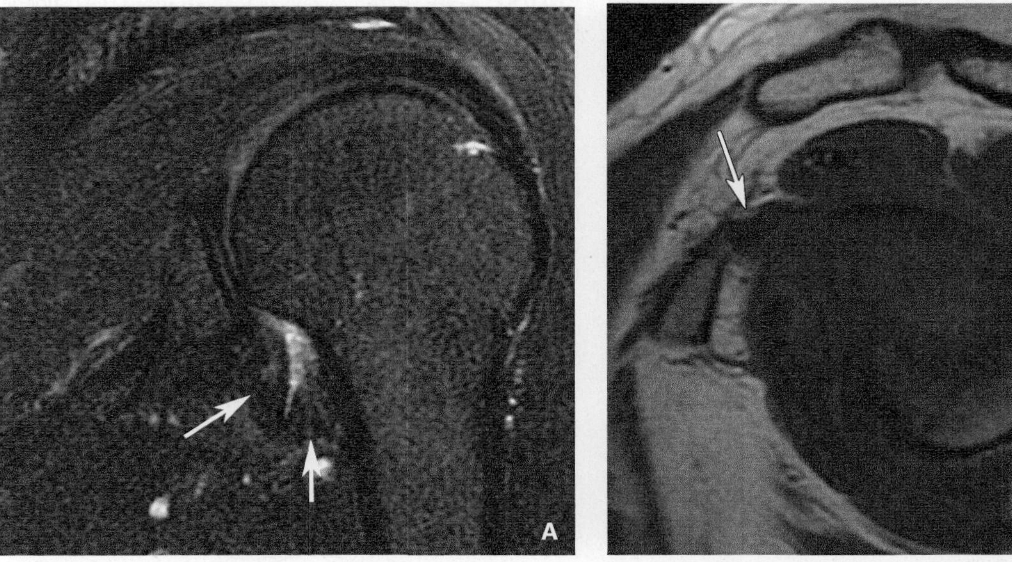

FIGURE 5.92 MRI of adhesive capsulitis. **(A)** Oblique coronal T2-weighted fat-saturated MR image of the left shoulder demonstrates thickening of the axillary recess of the joint capsule *(arrows)*, measuring over 4 mm in thickness. **(B)** Oblique sagittal proton density–weighted MR image shows loss of normal fat signal in the rotator cuff interval with thickening of the coracohumeral ligament *(arrow)*. **(C)** Oblique sagittal T2-weighted fat-saturated MR image shows marked thickening of the more distal segment of the coracohumeral ligament *(arrow)*.

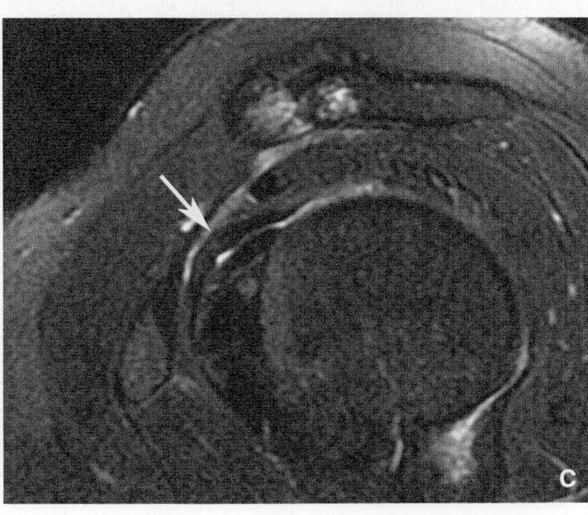

Whatever the mechanism of injury, the degree of damage to the acromioclavicular and coracoclavicular ligaments varies with the severity of the applied force and ranges from *mild sprain* of the acromioclavicular ligament to *moderate sprain* involving tear of the acromioclavicular ligament and sprain of the coracoclavicular ligament, to *severe sprain* characterized by tear of the coracoclavicular ligament, with consequent dislocation in the acromioclavicular joint (Table 5.4). It is important to bear in mind, as Rockwood and Green have pointed out, that the major deformity seen in this type of injury is not elevation of the clavicle but rather downward displacement of the scapula and upper extremity (Fig. 5.93), although some degree of cephalad displacement of the distal end of the clavicle may accompany this type of injury. The clinical symptoms also vary with the severity of the injury; patients may present with symptoms ranging from tenderness, swelling, and slight limitation of motion in the joint to complete inability to abduct the arm.

Suspected acromioclavicular dislocation is readily evaluated on the anteroposterior projection of the shoulder obtained with a 15-degree cephalad angulation of the radiographic tube (see Fig. 5.13). Often, it is necessary to obtain a stress view in this projection by strapping a 5- to 10-lb weight to each forearm. A comparison study of the opposite shoulder is invariably helpful.

Radiographic studies can also be supplemented by quantitating acromioclavicular separation on the basis of the normal relations of the coracoid process, the clavicle, and the acromion (Fig. 5.94). Normally, the distance between the coracoid process and the inferior aspect of the clavicle, known as the *coracoclavicular distance* or *coracoclavicular interval*, ranges from 1.0 to 1.3 cm; the joint space at the articulation of the clavicle with the acromion measures 0.3 to 0.8 cm. The degree of widening at these points helps to determine the severity of the injury. An increase, for example, of 0.5 cm in the coracoclavicular distance or a widening of the distance by 50% or more compared with that in the opposite shoulder is characteristic of grade III acromioclavicular separation (dislocation) (Fig. 5.95).

One of the useful from the practical point of view classification of acromioclavicular joint injury was offered by Tossy et al. *Grade 1* represents contusion or strain, without offset at the inferior margin of the acromioclavicular joint. *Grade 2* has less than 50% offset or overlap. It is subdivided to subtype 2A involving sprain or partial tear of the trapezoid segment, and 2B affecting both conoid and trapezoid segments of coracoclavicular ligament. *Grade 3* is diagnosed when there is more than 50% overlap. Coracoclavicular interval is significantly increased, and there is complete tear of the coracoclavicular ligament.

Antonio and colleagues introduced MRI classification of acromioclavicular joint injury (Fig. 5.96). In *type I injury*, there is a sprain of the acromioclavicular ligament, but the coracoclavicular ligaments are intact.

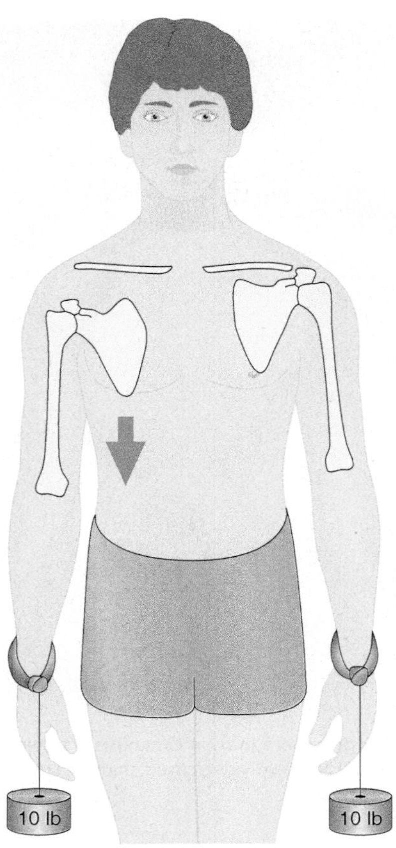

FIGURE 5.93 Acromioclavicular separation. The major deformity seen in acromioclavicular separation is the downward displacement of the scapula *(arrow)* and upper extremity, whereas the position of the clavicle in the affected side remains the same relative to the clavicle in the unaffected side. (Modified with permission from Rockwood CA Jr, Green DO, Bucholz RW. *Rockwood and Green's fractures in adults,* vol. 2, 3rd ed. Philadelphia: Lippincott; 1991.)

TABLE 5.4 Grades of Acromioclavicular Separation

Grade	Radiographic and Magnetic Resonance Imaging (MRI) Characteristics
I	Minimal widening of acromioclavicular joint space, which normally measures 0.3–0.8 cm Coracoclavicular distance within normal range of 1.0–1.3 cm MRI may show pericapsular edema.
II	Widening of acromioclavicular joint space to 1.0–1.5 cm Increase of 25%–50% in coracoclavicular distance MRI shows pericapsular edema, widening of the acromioclavicular distance, and edema of the coracoclavicular ligaments without tear. There may be bone marrow edema.
III	Marked widening of acromioclavicular joint space to 1.5 cm or more and of coracoclavicular distance by 50% or more Dislocation in acromioclavicular joint Apparent cephalad displacement of distal end of clavicle Additional MRI findings include disruption of the coracoclavicular ligaments and occasionally detachment of the deltoid and trapezius muscles from the distal end of the clavicle.
IV	The acromial end of the clavicle is posteriorly dislocated, and the scapula is displaced anteroinferiorly. The coracoclavicular ligaments and the joint capsule are torn.
V	The trapezius and deltoid muscle attachments on the clavicle and acromion are completely stripped, and the scapula droops inferiorly. The acromial end of the clavicle is displaced cephalad. The coracoclavicular ligaments and the joint capsule are torn.
VI	The acromial end of the clavicle is displaced inferiorly toward the acromion and coracoid processes. The coracoclavicular ligaments and the joint capsule are torn.

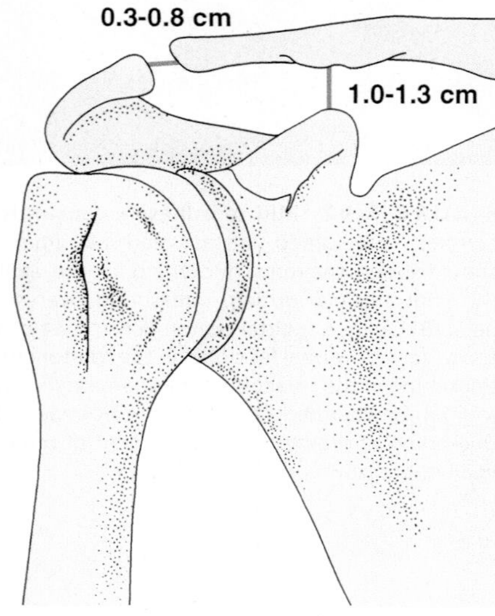

FIGURE 5.94 Normal measurements. Schematic diagram shows the normal relation of the coracoid process to the inferior aspect of the clavicle (known as coracoclavicular distance or coracoclavicular interval) and the normal width of the joint space at the acromioclavicular articulation.

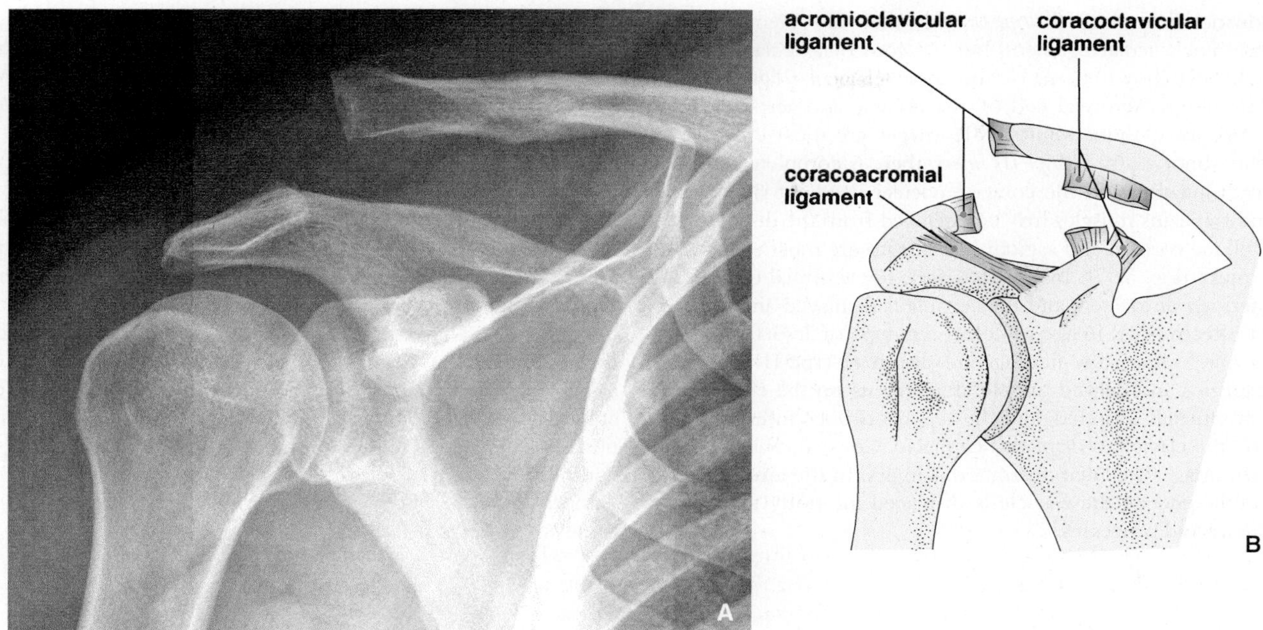

FIGURE 5.95 Acromioclavicular dislocation. **(A)** Anteroposterior radiograph of shoulder shows apparent cephalad displacement of the distal end of the clavicle and the widening of the acromioclavicular joint and the coracoclavicular distance. The marked deformities seen here, which are characteristic of grade III acromioclavicular separation (severe sprain), are the result of tear of the coracoclavicular and acromioclavicular ligaments with consequent dislocation in the acromioclavicular joint **(B)**.

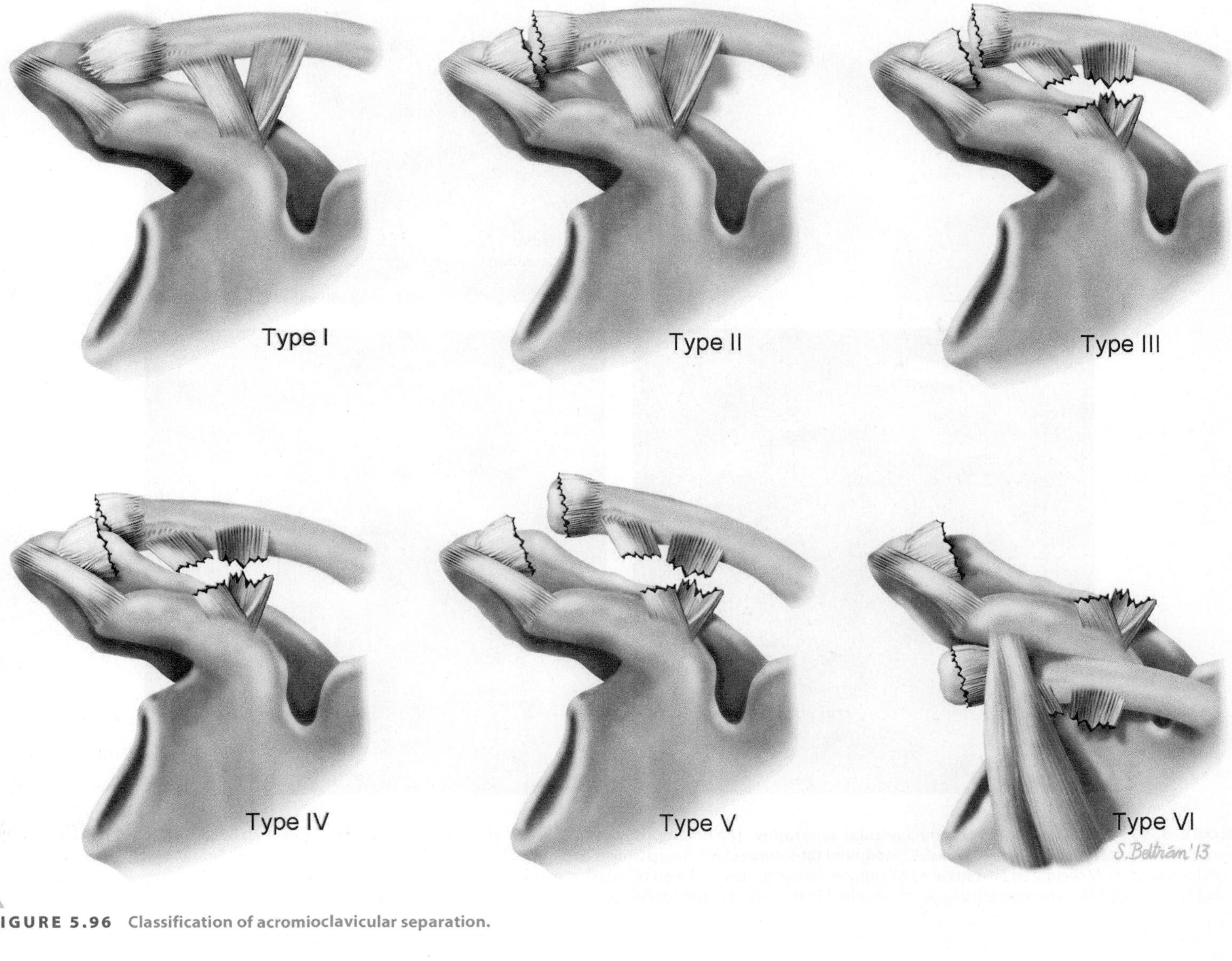

Type I

Type II

Type III

Type IV

Type V

Type VI

S.Beltrán'13

FIGURE 5.96 Classification of acromioclavicular separation.

MRI shows nonspecific findings. In *type II injury*, there is evidence of rupture of the acromioclavicular ligament, but the coracoclavicular ligament is only sprained. MRI shows edema of the coracoclavicular ligament and continuity of its fibers. Acromial end of the clavicle and acromion may show marrow edema. Oblique sagittal MR images are most effective to demonstrate this abnormality. In *type III injury*, there is complete acromioclavicular joint dislocation and the coracoclavicular ligament is ruptured. The deltoid and trapezius muscles may be detached from the distal end of the clavicle. Oblique coronal and sagittal MR images are most effective to diagnose this injury (Fig. 5.97). In *type IV injury*, the acromial end of the clavicle is posteriorly dislocated, and the scapula is displaced anteroinferiorly. The most effective MR image to detect this type of injury is in axial orientation. In *type V injury*, the findings are similar to type III but more severe. The trapezius and deltoid muscle attachments on the clavicle and acromion are completely stripped, and the scapula droops inferiorly. The acromial end of the clavicle is displaced cephalad. Coronal, oblique sagittal, and axial MR images well demonstrate this injury. In the rarest, *type VI injury*, the acromial end of the clavicle is displaced inferiorly toward the acromion and coracoid processes.

Sternoclavicular Dislocation

This injury usually is the result of direct or indirect blow to the shoulder, most commonly during motor vehicle collisions, athletic injuries, and a fall onto the shoulder. It may be either anterior or posterior. In the anterior dislocation, which is more common, and caused by a force that drives shoulder backward and sternal end of the clavicle forward, the medial (sternal) end of the clavicle is displaced in front of manubrium. The posterior (retrosternal) dislocation may create more problems because displaced clavicle may impinge on the vital organs such as the great vessels, the nerves in the superior mediastinum, the trachea, or the esophagus. Not infrequently, the posterior dislocation is associated with a fracture. Conventional radiography is usually not effective in the demonstration of this injury, although so-called *serendipity view* introduced by Rockwood occasionally may be helpful (Fig. 5.98). On this projection, if dislocation is anterior, the affected clavicle will project higher (cephalad) and if dislocation is posterior, it will project lower (caudal) in relation to the unaffected contralateral clavicle. However, the most effective imaging modality for demonstrating the sternoclavicular joints and traumatic abnormalities of these structures is CT and 3D CT (Figs. 5.99 and 5.100).

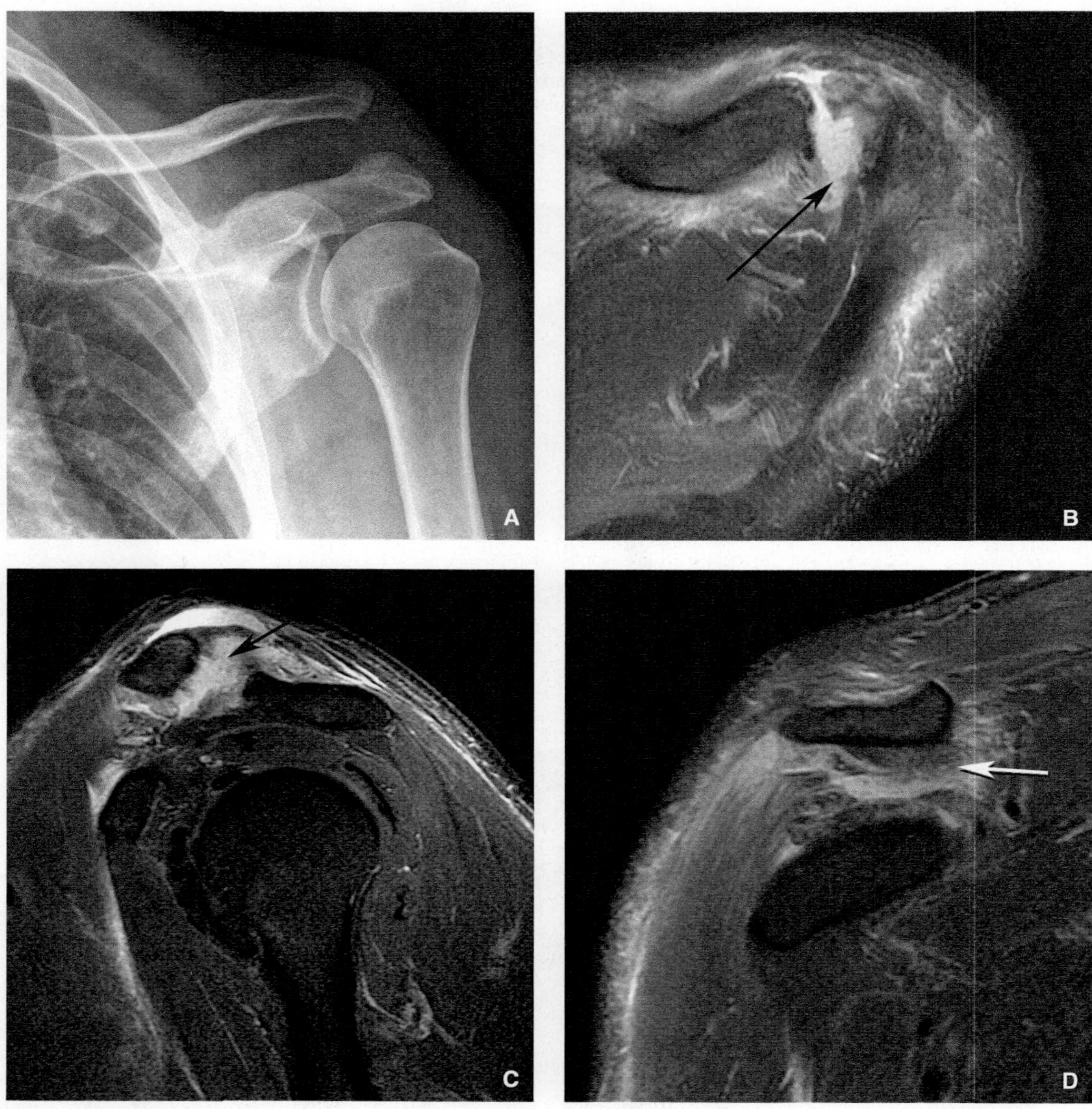

FIGURE 5.97 MRI of stage III acromioclavicular separation. **(A)** Anteroposterior radiograph of the left shoulder shows cephalad dislocation of the clavicle. Note increased coracoclavicular interval. **(B)** Axial T2-weighted fat-saturated MR image shows acromioclavicular separation with joint effusion *(arrow)* and pericapsular edema. **(C)** Oblique sagittal T2-weighted fat-saturated MR image demonstrates cephalad dislocation of the clavicle with joint effusion and pericapsular edema *(arrow)*. **(D)** Oblique coronal T2-weighted fat-saturated MR image shows a tear of the coracoclavicular ligaments with focal edema *(arrow)*.

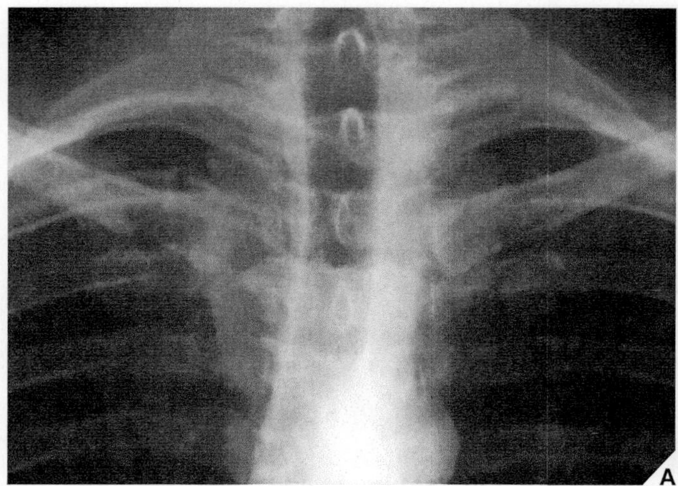

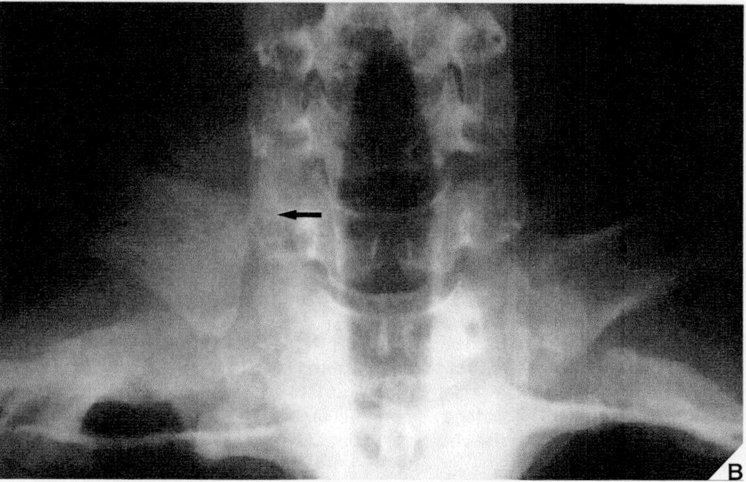

FIGURE 5.98 Sternoclavicular dislocation. **(A)** Anteroposterior radiograph of sternoclavicular joints shows no obvious abnormalities. **(B)** The serendipity view, which is obtained with the patient supine on the radiographic table and the central beam centered over manubrium sterni but directed cephalad with 40-degree angulation of the x-ray tube, shows that the sternal end of the right clavicle projects superiorly (cephalad) in relation to the contralateral clavicle *(arrow)*, a feature diagnostic of anterior dislocation.

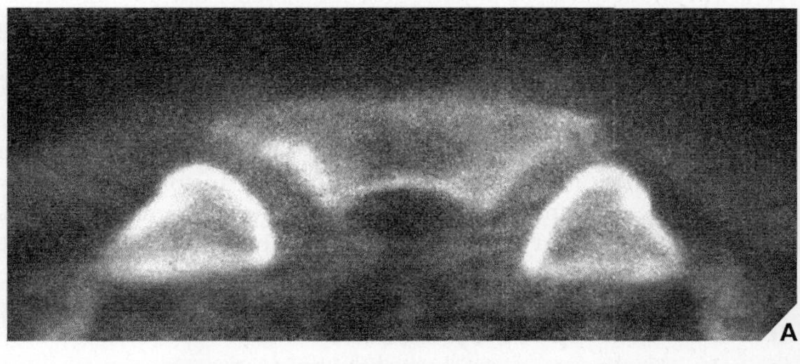

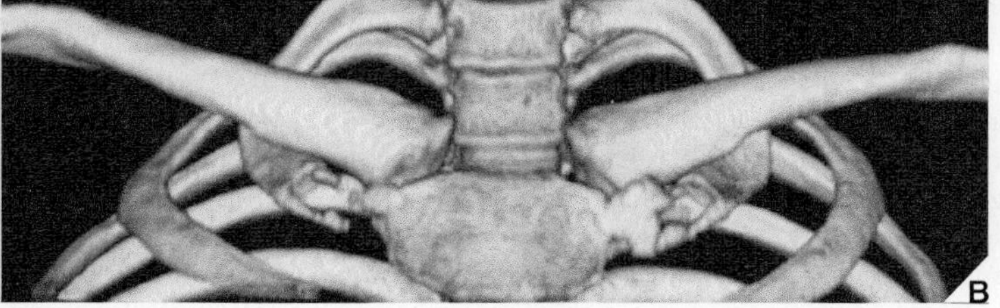

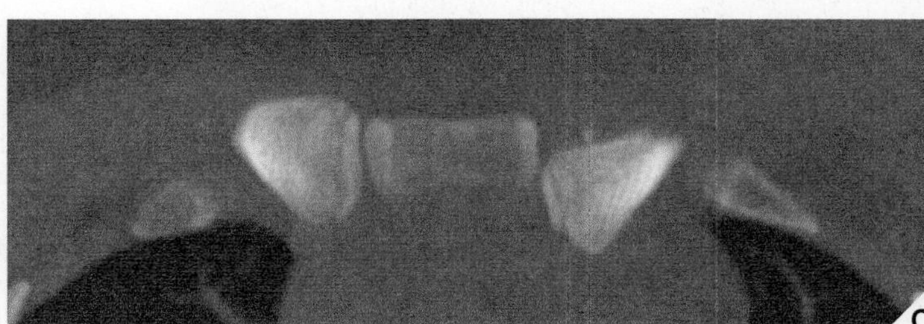

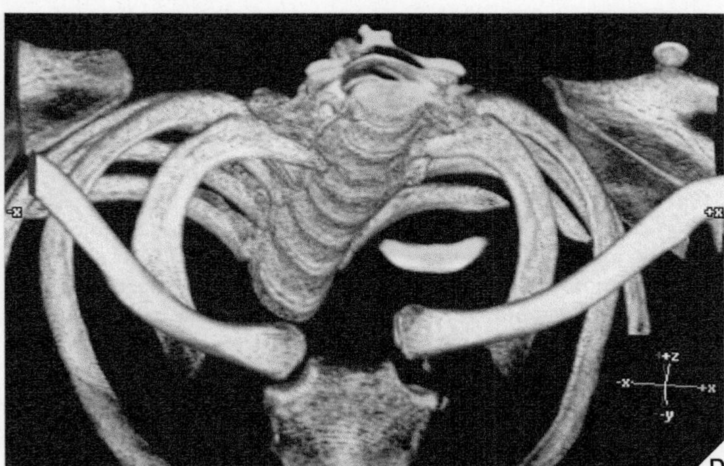

FIGURE 5.99 CT and 3D CT of sternoclavicular subluxation. **(A)** Axial CT section and **(B)** 3D shaded surface display CT reconstructed image show normal appearance of the sternoclavicular joints. **(C)** Axial CT and **(D)** 3D reconstructed CT images show posterior subluxation of the left sternoclavicular joint in a 20-year-old woman injured in a motorcycle accident.

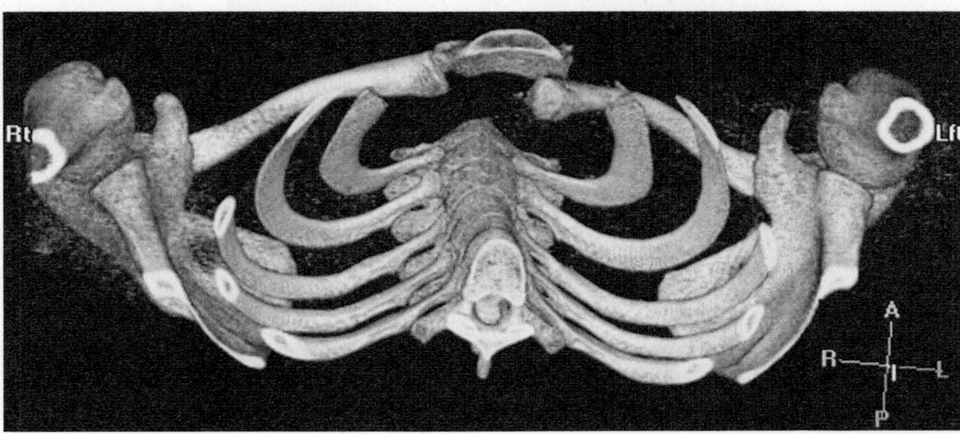

FIGURE 5.100 3D CT of sternoclavicular dislocation. 3D shaded surface display CT reconstructed image viewed from the caudal-cephalad direction shows posterior dislocation of the left sternoclavicular joint in a 26-year-old woman injured in a car accident.

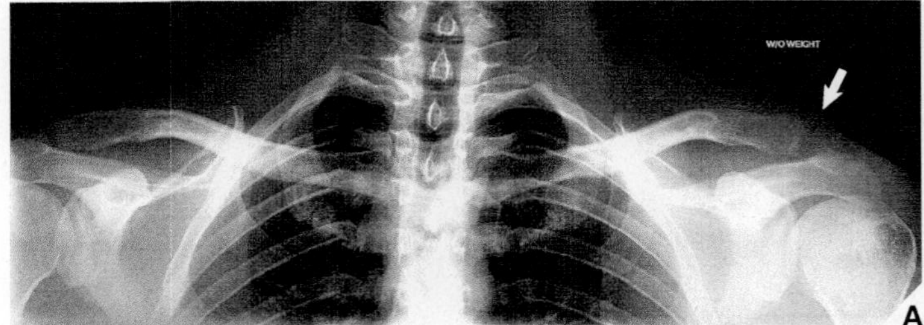

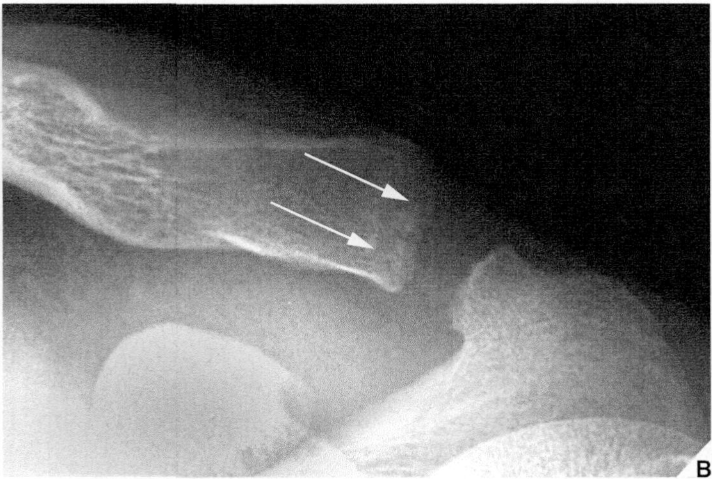

FIGURE 5.101 Posttraumatic osteolysis of the distal clavicle—early findings. **(A)** Anteroposterior radiograph of both clavicles shows slight widening of the left acromioclavicular joint *(arrow)*. **(B)** A coned-down view of the left acromioclavicular joint shows periarticular osteoporosis and irregular contour of acromial end of the clavicle associated with small radiolucent foci *(arrows)*.

Posttraumatic Osteolysis of the Distal Clavicle

After injury to the shoulder, such as sprain of the acromioclavicular joint, resorption of the distal (acromial) end of the clavicle may occasionally occur. The osteolytic process, which is associated with mild-to-moderate pain, usually begins within 2 months after the injury. The initial radiographic findings consist of soft-tissue swelling and periarticular osteoporosis associated with slightly irregular outline of acromial end of the clavicle (Fig. 5.101). Later, small erosions may develop (Fig. 5.102). MRI findings comprise increased signal intensity on water-sensitive sequences of the acromial end of the clavicle related to the bone marrow edema, marginal irregularity of the bone contour, and fluid within the acromioclavicular joint (Fig. 5.103). In its late stage, resorption of the distal end of the clavicle results in marked widening of the acromioclavicular joint (Fig. 5.104).

Compressive and Entrapment Neuropathies of the Shoulder

Suprascapular Nerve Syndrome

The suprascapular nerve runs within the suprascapular notch of the scapula extending into the spinoglenoid notch. It divides in branches for the supraspinatus and infraspinatus muscles. It is a mixed motor and sensory nerve that provides motor fibers to the supraspinatus and infraspinatus muscles and carries pain fibers from the glenohumeral and acromioclavicular joints. Suprascapular nerve syndrome results from entrapment or compromise of this nerve at some point in its path (Fig. 5.105). Most patients report nonspecific pain in the shoulder, neck, anterior chest, or in a combination in these anatomic sites. Later, severe weakness and atrophy of the supraspinatus and infraspinatus muscles may occur. A variety of causes of injury or entrapment of the suprascapular nerve have been reported, including fracture of the scapula or humerus, anterior shoulder dislocation, thickening of the transverse scapular ligament, rotator cuff tendonitis, and various malignant and benign tumors. Of the latter, the most commonly encountered mass is a ganglion located in the suprascapular and/or spinoglenoid notch (Fig. 5.106). The most effective technique to diagnose suprascapular nerve syndrome is MRI. This modality can distinguish different etiologic factors responsible for the syndrome and provide anatomic information and demonstrate atrophy of the supraspinatus or infraspinatus muscles in cases of compression of individual muscular branches or both muscles if the lesion involves the suprascapular nerve proximal to its bifurcation.

Quadrilateral Space Syndrome

The quadrilateral or quadrangular space is a space located just below the inferior glenohumeral joint capsule bound laterally by the medial cortex of the proximal humerus, superiorly by the teres minor muscle, medially by the long head of the triceps muscle, and inferiorly by the superior margin of the teres major muscle. The space contains the posterior circumflex artery and vein and the axillary nerve, which is a branch of the posterior division of the upper trunk of the brachial plexus containing fibers of the C5 and C6 nerve roots. The axillary nerve is a motor and sensory nerve providing innervation to the deltoid muscle and the teres minor muscle. A small articular branch provides innervation to the glenohumeral joint. The axillary nerve can be damaged as a result of trauma (anterior inferior

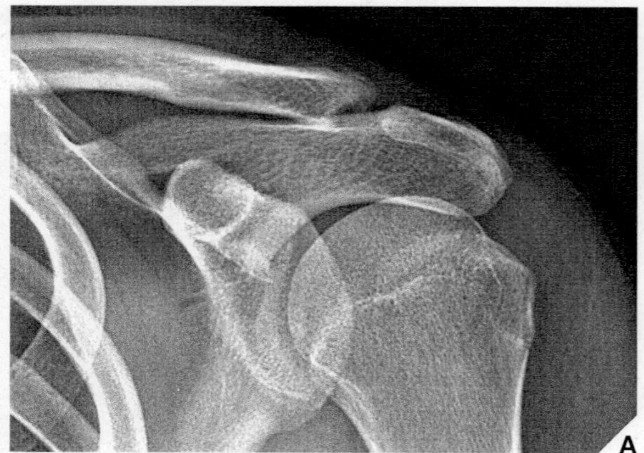

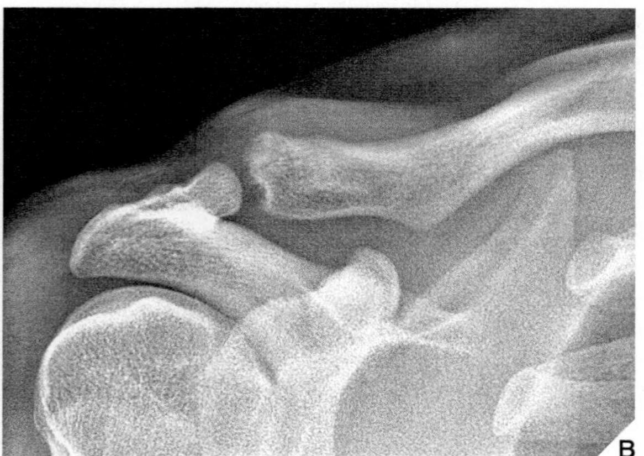

FIGURE 5.102 Posttraumatic osteolysis of the distal clavicle. **(A)** Anteroposterior radiograph of the left shoulder of a 20-year-old man who presented with shoulder pain following a football injury 5 months ago shows erosion of the acromial end of the clavicle. **(B)** Anteroposterior radiograph of the right acromioclavicular joint (obtained with a 15-degree cephalad angulation of the radiographic tube) of a 22-year-old rugby player who presented with shoulder pain of 6 months duration shows similar erosion of the distal clavicle.

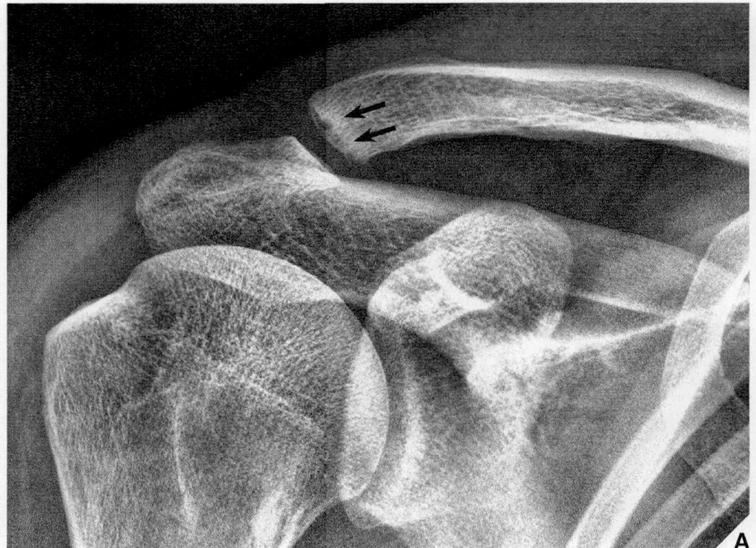

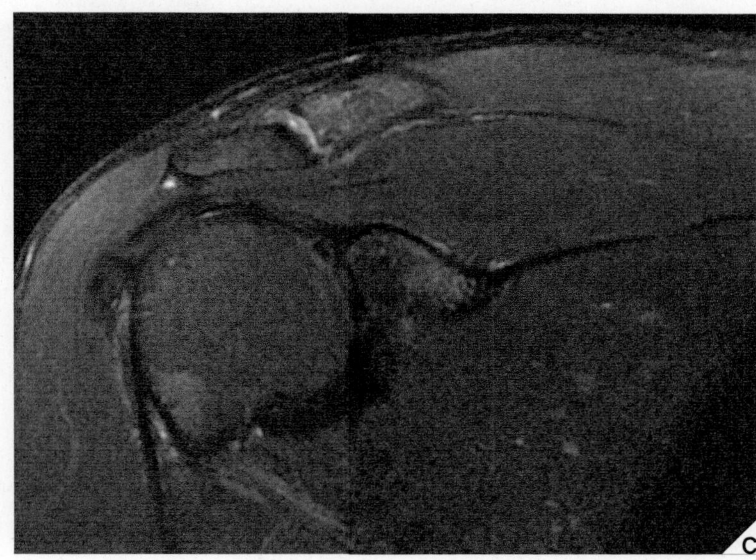

FIGURE 5.103 MRI of posttraumatic osteolysis of the distal clavicle. A 32-year-old weight lifter presented with right shoulder pain for past 4 months. **(A)** Anteroposterior radiograph shows subtle erosions in the acromial end of the clavicle *(arrows)*. **(B)** Coronal T1-weighted MR image shows irregular contour of the distal clavicle. **(C)** Coronal proton density–weighted fat-suppressed MR image shows in addition an increased signal within the distal end of the clavicle and fluid within the acromioclavicular joint.

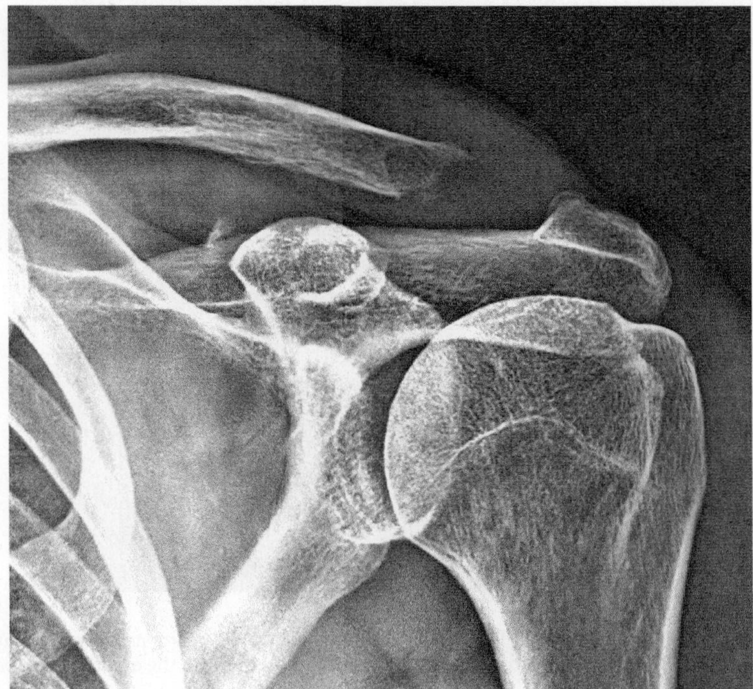

FIGURE 5.104 Posttraumatic osteolysis of the distal clavicle—late findings. A 59-year-old man who 12 months previously had injured the left shoulder in a fall presented with symptoms of pain while playing tennis. Anteroposterior radiograph of the left shoulder shows marked widening of the acromioclavicular joint secondary to resorption of the distal end of the clavicle—radiographic features typical of posttraumatic osteolysis.

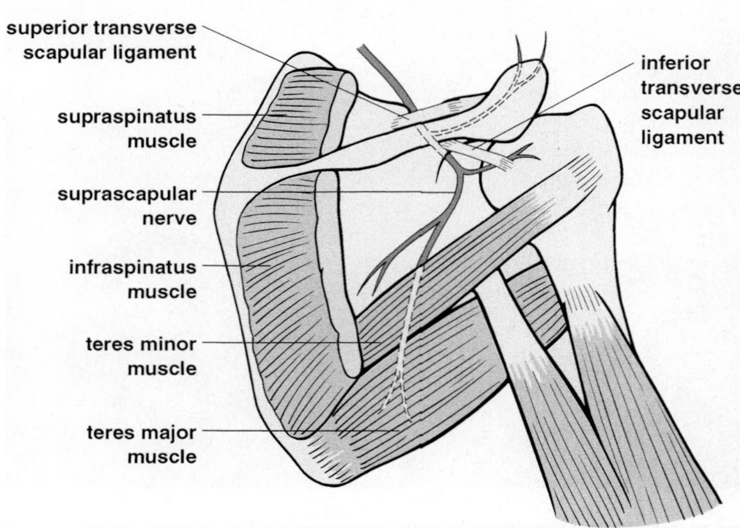

FIGURE 5.105 Suprascapular nerve. Pathway of the suprascapular nerve as seen from the posterior aspect of the right scapula.

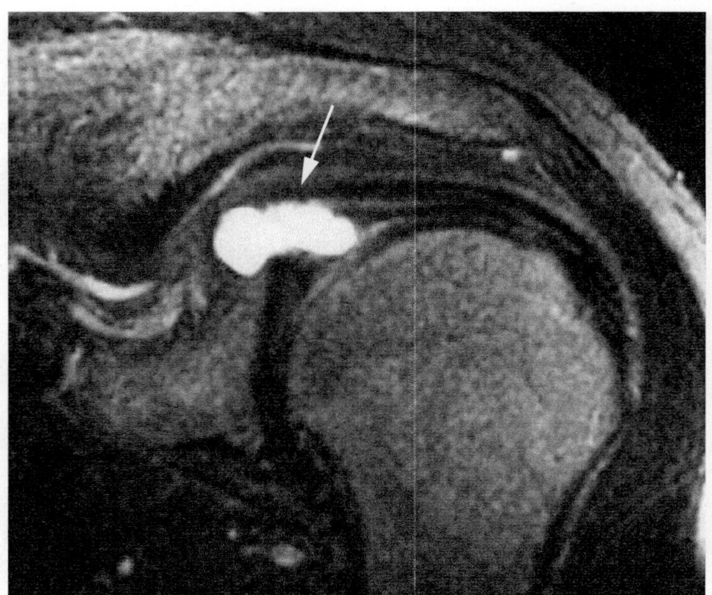

FIGURE 5.106 MRI of ganglion of the spinoglenoid notch. Coronal T2-weighted MR image of the left shoulder shows a bright lobulated mass *(arrow)* located within the spinoglenoid notch of scapula, causing a suprascapular nerve syndrome in this 50-year-old man. (Reprinted from Gerscovich EO, Greenspan A. Magnetic resonance imaging in the diagnosis of suprascapular nerve syndrome. *Can Assoc Radiol J* 1993;44:307–309. Copyright © 1993 Canadian Association of Radiologists. With permission.)

dislocation of the humeral head), or space-occupying lesions such as soft-tissue masses, large inferior humeral head osteophytes, or medial osteochondromas of the proximal humerus. Repetitive overhead activities like of the throwing athlete can also cause traction injuries to the axillary nerve. MRI can demonstrate the early effect of denervation of the teres minor muscle (edema) and late effects (atrophy). The deltoid branch is less frequently involved (Fig. 5.107).

Parsonage-Turner Syndrome (Idiopathic Brachial Plexopathy, Neuralgic Amyotrophy)

This is a rare disorder consisting of a constellation of symptoms with abrupt onset of shoulder pain (usually unilateral) followed by progressive motor weakness, dysesthesias, and numbness. It can be related to various etiologies, including viral infection, trauma, postoperative, and postvaccination. From the imaging point of view, MRI can demonstrate neuritis of the brachial plexus and edema or atrophy of the involved muscles, usually the deltoid, rotator cuff, and trapezius muscles, although other muscles groups may also be affected. Soft-tissue masses like neck lymphadenopathy can also cause compressive neuropathy of the brachial plexus leading to Parsonage-Turner syndrome (Fig. 5.108).

Serratus Anterior Paralysis (Scapular Winging)

The serratus anterior muscle is innervated by the long thoracic nerve, which originates from the C5 and C6 nerve roots. Paralysis of the serratus anterior muscle has been well documented among professional and amateur athletes of a variety of sports, including archery, baseball, basketball, body building/weight lifting, bowling, football, golf, gymnastics, hockey, soccer, tennis, and wrestling. It also has been reported in ballet dancers. Scapular winging is a rare debilitating condition that leads to limited functional activity of the upper extremity. It is the result of numerous causes, including traumatic, iatrogenic, and idiopathic processes that most often

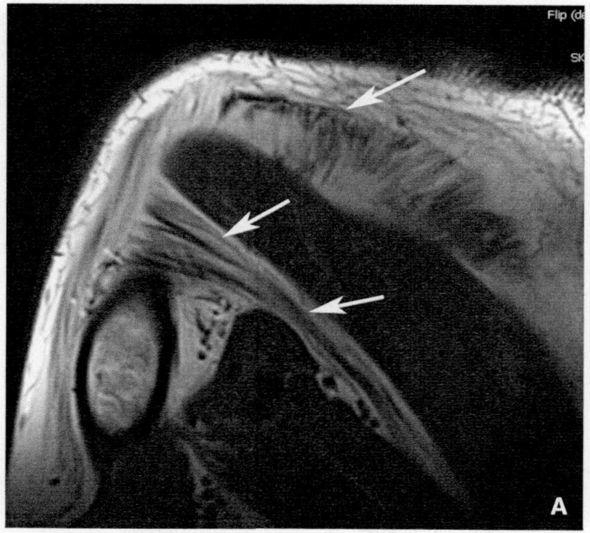

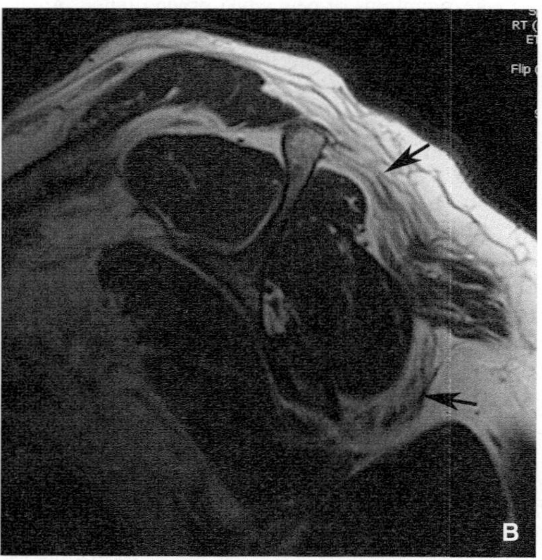

FIGURE 5.107 Quadrilateral space syndrome. Oblique coronal **(A)** and oblique sagittal **(B)** MR images of the right shoulder demonstrate fatty atrophy of the deltoid and teres minor muscles *(arrows)*. Although no lesions are seen in the quadrilateral space, the selective atrophy of the deltoid and teres minor muscles indicates axillary nerve damage.

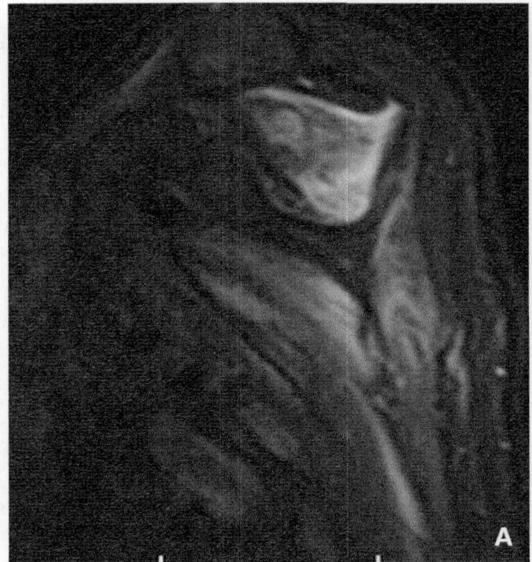

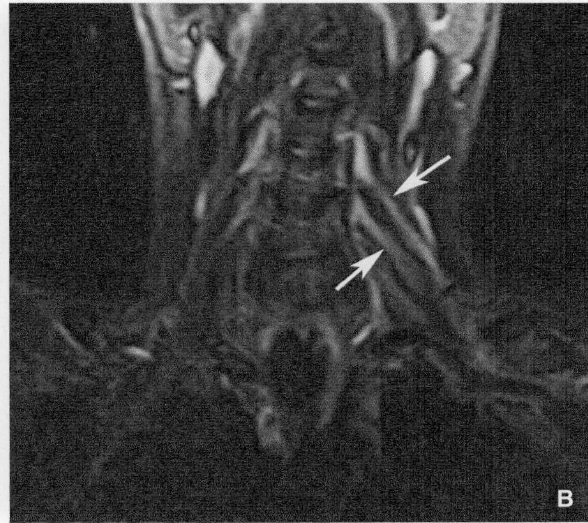

FIGURE 5.108 Parsonage-Turner syndrome. **(A)** Sagittal T2-weighted fat-saturated MR image of the left shoulder demonstrates edema of the supraspinatus, infraspinatus, and subscapularis muscles, without surrounding edema, indicating early denervation, which does not follow the pattern of a peripheral nerve lesion. **(B)** Coronal T2-weighted fat-saturated MR image of the brachial plexus shows increased size and signal intensity of the trunks and divisions of the left brachial plexus *(arrows)*, consistent with brachial plexopathy.

result in nerve injury and paralysis of either the serratus anterior, trapezius, or rhomboid muscles. Diagnosis is easily made upon visible inspection of the scapula, with serratus anterior paralysis resulting in medial winging of the scapula. This is in contrast to the lateral winging generated by trapezius and rhomboid paralysis. Most cases of serratus anterior paralysis spontaneously resolve within 24 months, whereas conservative treatment of trapezius paralysis is less effective. MRI can show early denervation edema or atrophy of the serratus anterior muscle (Fig. 5.109).

The Postoperative Shoulder

Frequently performed surgical procedures include rotator cuff repair, superior capsular reconstruction, subacromial decompression, biceps tenotomy and tenodesis, and labral repair, or a combination of these techniques, depending on the preoperative assessment. Shoulder surgery for these indications may be performed via open approach or via arthroscopic approach. Each technique has its indications and its own advantages and disadvantages. Advantages of open surgery include better long-term results, improved intraoperative visualization of the rotator cuff and subacromial space, and easy performance. Disadvantages of the open procedures include increased operative morbidity, longer rehabilitation, and requirement of detachment of the deltoid muscle. Advantages of arthroscopic surgery include fewer complications, performance through small incisions, better intraarticular visualization, and decreased operative morbidity and pain.

Surgical procedures for rotator cuff pathology include among the others subacromial decompression with or without resection of the distal end of the clavicle (Mumford procedure) (Fig. 5.110), and with or without resection or release of the coracoacromial ligament (Fig. 5.111), and

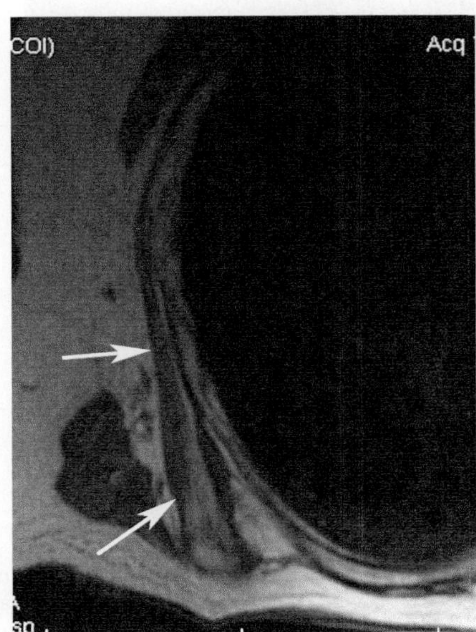

FIGURE 5.109 Serratus anterior paralysis. Axial T1-weighted MR image demonstrates atrophy of the serratus anterior muscle with fatty infiltration *(arrows)*.

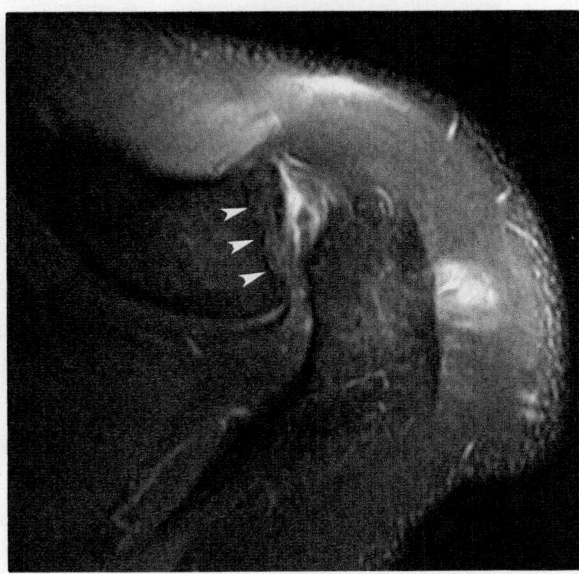

FIGURE 5.110 Resection of the distal end of the clavicle (Mumford procedure). Axial MR GRE image demonstrates surgical resection of the distal end of the clavicle *(arrowheads)*.

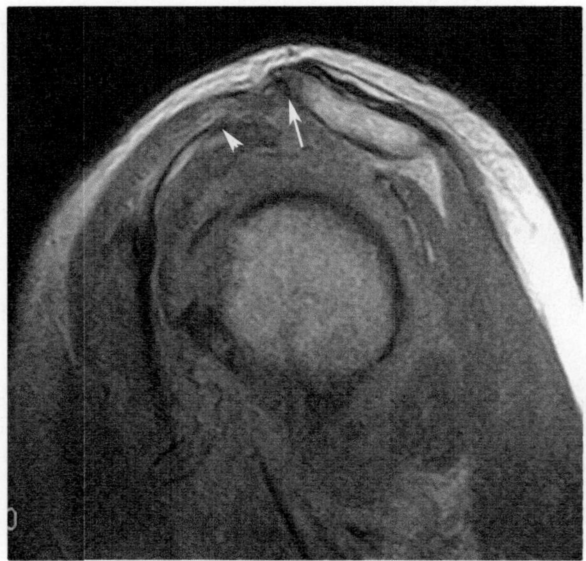

FIGURE 5.111 Acromioplasty with coracoacromial ligament release. Oblique sagittal proton density MR image demonstrates thinning of the anterior lateral portion of the acromion *(arrow)* related to acromioplasty and subacromial decompression. Note the discontinuity of the coracoacromial ligament related to the ligamentous release *(arrowhead)*.

rotator cuff debridement or tendon repair (Fig. 5.112). Simple rotator cuff debridement is preferred for young patients and for partial rotator cuff tears. Cuff repair is done arthroscopically for small tears, whereas open repair is preferred for large full-thickness tears and is often accompanied by subacromial decompression and acromioplasty. However, arthroscopic techniques for large rotator cuff repair have been developed by Burkhart et al. based on the shape of the tear ("U" shape, "C" shape, or "L" shape) (Fig. 5.113).

More recent surgical techniques for rotator cuff repair have been described. Patch augmentation of rotator cuff repair is based on the placement of a patch of autologous graft material (fascia lata), allograft material (acellular human dermis), xenograft (porcine dermis, bovine Achilles tendon), or synthetic graft (poly-L-lactide acid). These patch augmentation techniques may be indicated in reparable rotator cuff tears when there are concerns about healing, or when there is an irreparable defect in the rotator cuff by means of primary surgical repair.

Superior capsular reconstruction may be performed in young patients with irreparable massive rotator cuff tear, without significant arthrosis. This technique is based on the placement of a graft from the superior glenoid to the grater tuberosity of the humerus and side-to-side with adjacent intact rotator cuff muscle and tendon.

Other described techniques for large rotator cuff reconstruction in irreparable large teas include tendon/muscle transfer of the latissimus dorsi or pectoralis major and subacromial spacer implant with an inflatable biodegradable balloon that induces granulation tissue in the subacromial space, providing a "cushion-like" tissue between the humeral head and acromion.

Complications or failure of these procedures include inadequate decompression, leaving inferior clavicular osteophytes, failure to recognize an os acromiale, progression of rotator cuff disease, recurrent rotator cuff tear, deltoid detachment, and deltoid atrophy in open decompressions.

Surgical procedures for glenohumeral instability include Bankart repair (primary repair of the torn labrum with suture anchors) and procedures aimed to provide strength to the anterior soft-tissue structures of the shoulder, including Putti Platt procedure (shortening of the anterior capsule and subscapularis muscle, rarely performed), Magnuson-Stack procedure (transfer of the subscapularis tendon to the greater tuberosity), Bristow-Latarjet procedure (coracoid transfer to the anterior inferior glenoid margin through a split of the subscapularis tendon, rarely performed), and capsular plication procedures. Failure and complications of these procedures include recurrent instability (Fig. 5.114), nerve damage, overtight repair (Putti Platt procedure), with loss of sternal external rotation, posterior subluxation and development of degenerative disease, misplacement or detachment of anchors, adhesive capsulitis, reactive synovitis, and other complications related to any surgery such as infection and hematoma.

It has been demonstrated that recurrent rate of glenohumeral instability following arthroscopic repair may be in the range of 15% to 20% if preoperative imaging assessment demonstrates capsular laxity and bone lesions of the humerus (engaging Hill-Sachs lesion) or the glenoid fossa

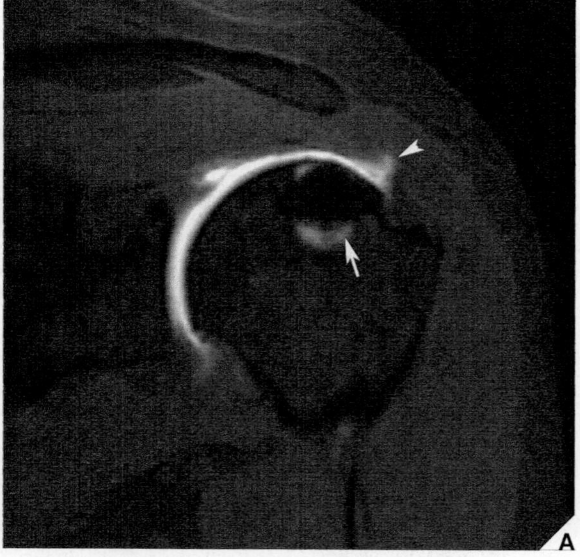

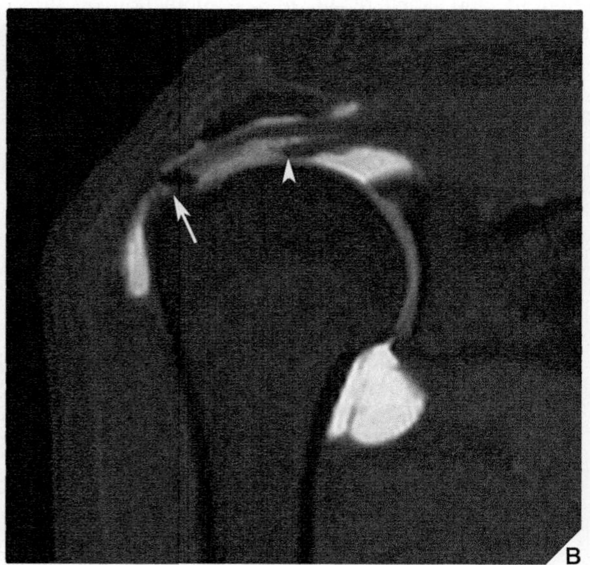

FIGURE 5.112 MRa of rotator cuff repair with recurrent tear. **(A)** Oblique coronal T1-weighted fat-saturated MRa image of the left shoulder shows metallic susceptibility artifact in the humeral head related to the presence of a suture anchor *(arrow)*. Note the high-grade partial articular surface recurrent tear of the supraspinatus tendon *(arrowhead)*. Intraarticular contrast material is noted penetrating into the partial tear; however, there is no extension of the contrast into the subacromial–subdeltoid bursae complex. **(B)** Oblique coronal T1-weighted fat-saturated MRa image of the right shoulder of another patient, who had rotator cuff repair, shows the recurrent tear of the distal superficial fibers of the supraspinatus tendon at the level of the insertion into the greater tuberosity of the humerus *(arrow)*. Note also the retraction of the deep fibers *(arrowhead)* and the delamination between the superficial and the deep fibers. There is extravasation of contrast material from the glenohumeral joint into the subacromial–subdeltoid bursae complex through the recurrent tear.

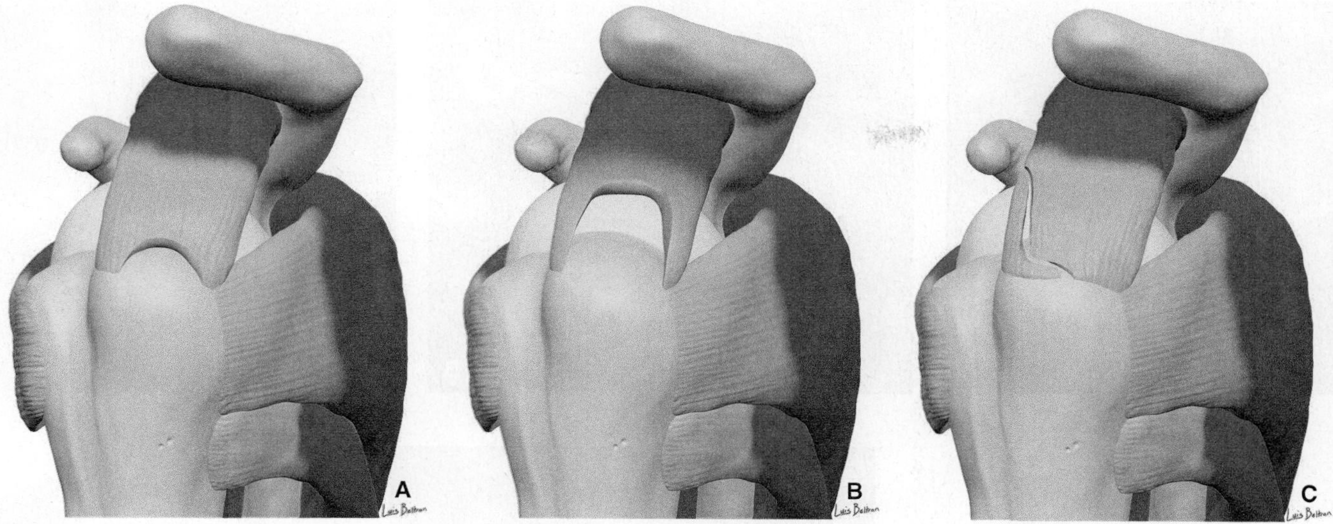

FIGURE 5.113 Classification of rotator cuff tears based on their shape. **(A)** C-shaped tear. The anteroposterior dimension is larger than the transverse dimension. The tear extends proximally to the level of the "cable," which prevents further proximal extension. **(B)** U-shaped tear. The anteroposterior dimension is shorter than the transverse dimension. **(C)** L-shaped tear. The tear has a longitudinal component that extends anteriorly or posteriorly.

(osseous Bankart lesion involving over 25% of the glenoid articular surface, the so-called *inverted pear sign*). Burkhart et al. demonstrated 4% recurrence rate of glenohumeral instability following arthroscopic repair if no bony deficiency was present but 67% recurrence if osseous deficiency was present, in which case, open surgical repair is recommended. Therefore, contraindications for arthroscopic surgical repair include engaging Hill-Sachs lesion, significant glenoid bone loss, attenuation of the AIGHL, and HAGL.

Different surgical techniques have been developed to address the bone deficiency caused by osseous Bankart lesions and Hills Sachs lesions. Simple open reduction and internal fixation of a noncomminuted osseous Bankart lesion with reattachment of the fracture fragment with screw provides a good chance for restoring normal articular surface congruity. In a chronic osseous Bankart lesion, the bone fragment may become resorbed leading to chronic deficiency of the anterior glenoid and chronic instability. In these cases, glenoid reconstruction techniques are available, including coracoid transfer (Bristow-Latarjet procedure) or autografts or cadaver allografts implants (Fig. 5.115).

Regarding significant bone loss in Hill-Sachs lesions, several techniques to address the bone defect in the humeral head have been proposed. For relatively shallow Hill-Sachs lesions, two procedures have been developed: humeroplasty with a bone tamp, or balloon osteoplasty to elevate the Hill-Sachs defect, often accompanied with cancellous bone graft and screw fixation, or remplissage procedure with transfer of the infraspinatus tendon filling the bone defect (Fig. 5.116). For large Hill-Sachs lesions in young patients, other procedures include osteochondral humeral allograft plug transfer and size-matched bulk humeral allograft. Shoulder arthroplasty is preferred in elderly patients.

Recurrent shoulder pain following shoulder surgery is a common complaint. MRI can provide a clue to the etiology of the patient's symptoms,

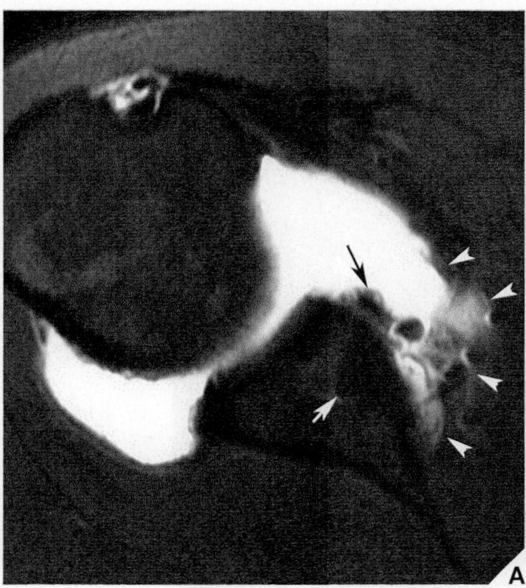

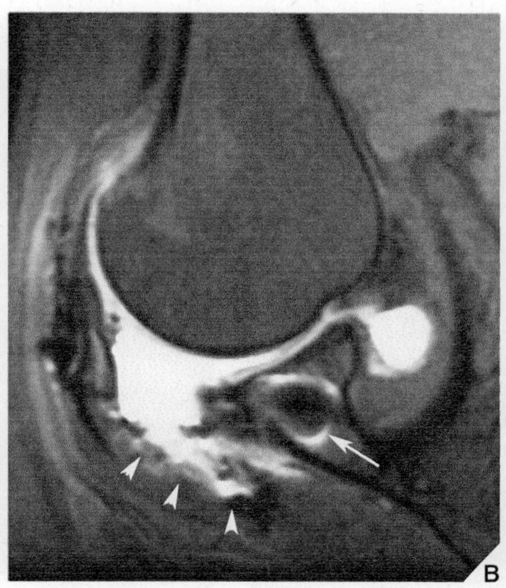

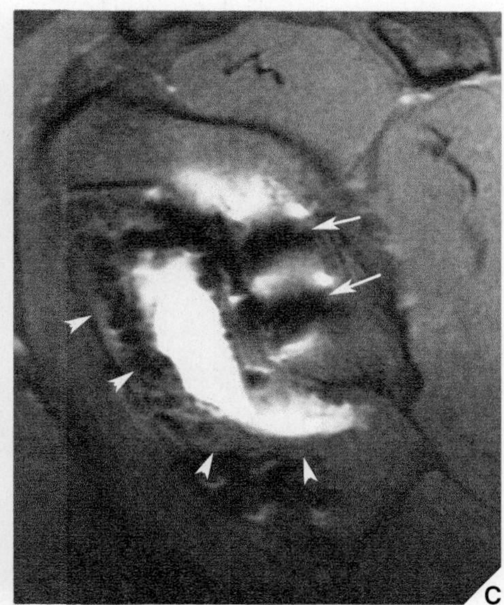

FIGURE 5.114 MRa of recurrent labral tear following arthroscopic repair. **(A)** Axial T1-weighted fat-saturated MRa demonstrates the postsurgical changes in the anterior capsule with focal areas of metallic susceptibility artifact. There is recurrent stripping of the capsule and periosteum *(arrowheads)*. Note also the suture anchor in the anterior glenoid *(white arrow)* and the recurrent tear of the anterior labrum *(black arrow)*. **(B)** T1-weighted fat-saturated MRa image in the ABER position in the same patient demonstrates the complete disruption of the anterior capsule and the AIGHL *(arrowheads)*. Note the suture anchor in the glenoid *(arrow)*. **(C)** Oblique sagittal T1-weighted MRa image in the same patient shows the disruption of the anterior capsule *(arrowheads)* and the suture anchors in the glenoid *(arrows)*.

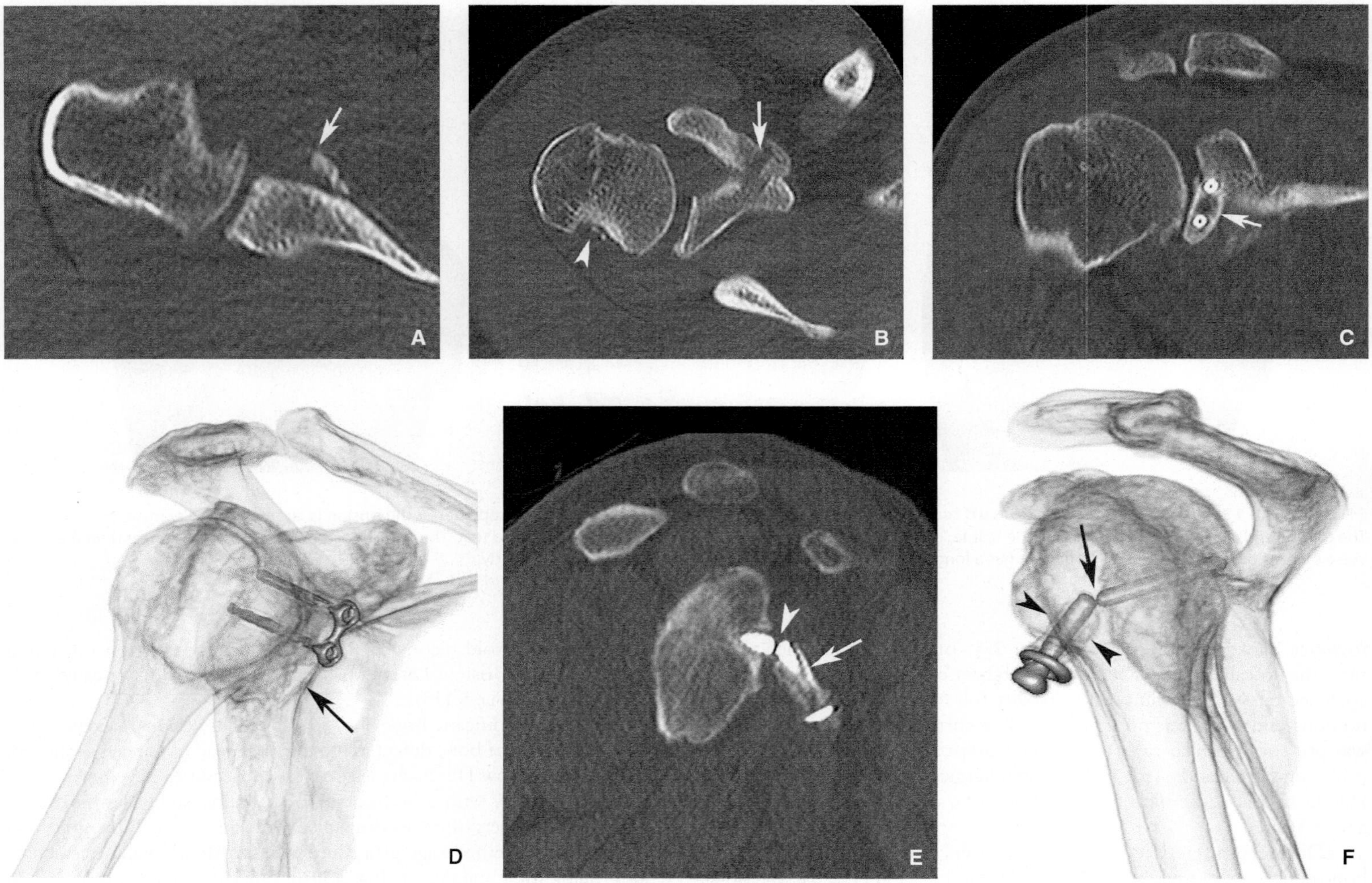

FIGURE 5.115 **Bristow-Latarjet procedure.** **(A)** Preoperative axial CT image shows a displaced osseous Bankart lesion *(arrow)*. **(B)** Preoperative axial CT image shows a Hill-Sachs lesion *(arrowhead)* and a fracture of the base of the coracoid process *(arrow)*. **(C)** Postoperative coronal reformatted CT image demonstrates the coracoid process transfer into the anterior margin of the glenoid, secured with two screws *(arrow)*. **(D)** 3D transparency rendering CT shows the coracoid process *(arrow)* attached into the anterior glenoid margin with two screws. **(E)** Sagittal CT reformatted image in another patient who underwent Bristow-Latarjet procedure shows a nonunited displaced coracoid process fracture *(arrow)* and a broken screw *(arrowhead)*. **(F)** 3D transparency rendering CT in the same patient also demonstrates the displaced nonunited coracoid fragment *(arrowheads)* and the broken screw *(arrow)*.

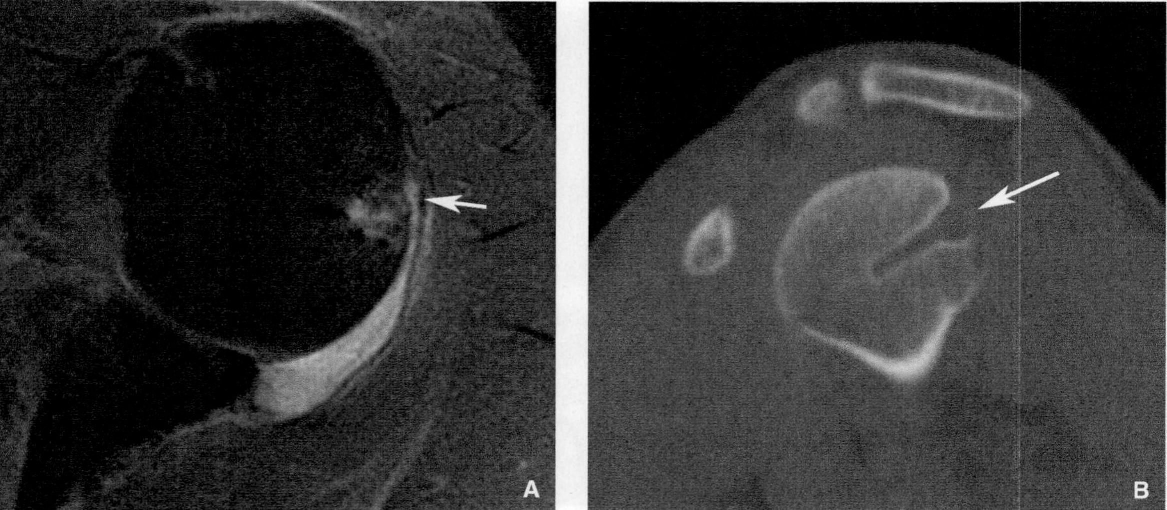

FIGURE 5.116 **Remplissage procedure for Hill-Sachs lesion.** **(A)** Axial T2-weighted fat-saturated MR image demonstrates transfer of the infraspinatus tendon over the posterosuperior aspect of the humeral head *(arrow)*. **(B)** Sagittal reformatted CT image shows the postsurgical changes *(arrow)*.

although it is often compromised by the presence of metallic artifacts produced by sutures and anchors. Imaging strategies that help in minimizing the metallic susceptibility artifacts include avoiding gradient recalled echo (GRE) pulse sequence; removing fat suppression; adding intraarticular or intravenous contrast (direct or indirect MRa); using short time inversion recovery (STIR) sequences instead of T2-weighted fat-saturated sequences; using fast spin echo (FSE) to acquire T1-weighted images instead of conventional spin echo; increasing bandwidth, field of view, and matrix size; and using lower echo time (TE) and swap phase/frequency encoding gradients to shift artifacts. MRI signs of recurrent rotator cuff tear include fluid within a defect of the rotator cuff with (greater than 1 cm) or without tendon retraction, large amount of fluid in the subacromial–subdeltoid bursae complex, and displaced or broken sutures. Other unwarranted findings that may be observed with MRI include muscle atrophy and development of glenohumeral osteoarthritis.

PRACTICAL POINTS TO REMEMBER

1. Fractures of the proximal humerus may be evaluated on the anteroposterior, transscapular, and transthoracic lateral projections. The latter view:
   - provides a true lateral image of the proximal humerus
   - allows sufficient evaluation of the degree of displacement or angulation of the fragments.
2. Four-segment Neer classification based on the presence or absence of displacement of the four major fragments is a practical and effective way to evaluate the fractures of the proximal humerus.
3. Fractures of the scapula, particularly if comminuted and displaced, are best evaluated on the transscapular (or Y) projection. If the diagnosis is in doubt, or the fracture cannot be well demonstrated on conventional radiography, CT should be performed.
4. Neer classification of fractures of the acromial end of the clavicle is based on the site and direction of the fracture line and integrity of the ligaments.
5. For precise evaluation of the shoulder joint and better demonstration of the glenohumeral articulation, the anteroposterior radiograph obtained with the patient rotated approximately 40 degrees toward the affected side (Grashey view):
   - eliminates the overlap of the humeral head and the glenoid fossa
   - allows visualization of the glenohumeral joint space and the glenoid in profile.
6. The Hill-Sachs lesion, which is best demonstrated on the anteroposterior radiograph obtained with the arm internally rotated, and the Bankart lesion are virtually diagnostic of previous anterior dislocation.
7. The coexistence of both the Hill-Sachs and Bankart lesions is known as *bipolar lesion*.
8. Compression fracture (trough line sign) of the anteromedial aspect of the humeral head is a common sequela of posterior dislocation. The anteroposterior radiograph obtained with the arm externally rotated readily demonstrates this finding.
9. MRI characteristics of impingement syndrome include:
   - cystic and sclerotic changes in the greater tuberosity
   - perimuscular and peritendinous edema
   - thickening of subacromial bursa (or effusion)
   - thinning of the supraspinatus tendon
   - increased signal intensity in the tendon (on T2 weighting)
   - subacromial spur.
10. Rotator cuff tear may effectively be evaluated by contrast arthrography or MRa. Opacification of the subacromial–subdeltoid bursae complex is diagnostic of this injury.
11. MRI characteristics of rotator cuff tear include:
    - discontinuity of the rotator cuff tendons
    - high signal within the tendon structure (on T2-weighted images)
    - retraction of the musculotendinous junction of supra- and infraspinatus muscles
    - atrophy of the supraspinatus muscle and infiltration by fat
    - obliteration of the subacromial–subdeltoid fat line (on T1-weighted images)
    - fluid in the subacromial–subdeltoid bursae complex.
12. US is also an effective modality to diagnose partial- and full-thickness rotator cuff tears and tears of the biceps tendon.
13. The presence of atrophy of the rotator cuff muscles is important information for surgical planning. Goutallier classification based on CT imaging and validated by MRI proved to be very effective in this respect.
14. Oblique sagittal MR images are useful to demonstrate four types of acromion: type I, flat; type II, smoothly curved; type III, hooked; and type IV, convex undersurface.
15. Axial MR images are useful to demonstrate three types of anterior capsular insertion to the scapula.
16. ABER position of the arm is effective to evaluate subtle abnormalities of cartilaginous labrum and labral ligamentous complex during MRa.
17. Acromioclavicular separation is best demonstrated on the stress anteroposterior projection obtained with a 15-degree cephalad angulation of the radiographic tube and weights strapped to the patient's forearms. The radiographic characteristics of this condition include:
    - increased width of the acromioclavicular joint space
    - increased width of the coracoclavicular distance
    - presence of apparent cephalad displacement of the distal end of the clavicle.
18. Learn to distinguish six types of acromioclavicular separation based on MRI.
19. Compressive and entrapment neuropathies of the shoulder include the following abnormalities: suprascapular nerve syndrome; quadrilateral space syndrome; Parsonage-Turner syndrome, also known as *idiopathic brachial plexopathy* or *neuralgic amyotrophy*; and serratus anterior paralysis, also known as *scapular winging*. All these conditions can be effectively diagnosed with MRI.
20. Suprascapular nerve syndrome results from the entrapment of this nerve caused by a variety of pathologic processes including fracture of the scapula or humerus, anterior shoulder dislocation, rotator cuff tendonitis, and benign or malignant tumors. MRI is the ideal technique to diagnose this syndrome.
21. Different surgical techniques have been developed to address the bone deficiency caused by osseous Hill-Sachs and Bankart lesions. Learn to recognize the postsurgical appearance of the shoulder such as after Bristow-Latarjet procedure or remplissage procedure on CT and MRI.
22. MRI of postoperative shoulder provides clues to possible postsurgical complications. For instance, the imaging signs of recurrent rotator cuff tear include the presence of fluid within a defect of the rotator cuff with or without tendon retraction, large amount of fluid in the subacromial–subdeltoid bursae complex, and displaced or broken sutures.

SUGGESTED READINGS

Anderson JE. *Grant's atlas of anatomy*, 8th ed. Baltimore: Williams & Wilkins; 1983.

Antonio GE, Cho JH, Chung CB, et al. MR imaging appearance and classification of acromioclavicular joint injury. *Am J Roentgenol* 2003;180:1103–1110.

Armitage MS, Faber KJ, Drosdowech DS, et al. Humeral head bone defects: remplissage, allograft, and arthroplasty. *Orthop Clin North Am* 2010;41:417–425.

Bankart A. The pathology and treatment of recurrent dislocation of the shoulder joint. *Br J Surg* 1938;26:23–29.

Baudi, Righi P, Bolognesi S, et al. How to identify and calculate glenoid bone deficit. *Chir Organi Mov* 2005;90:145–152.

Beltran J, Rosenberg ZS, Chandnani VP, et al. Glenohumeral instability: evaluation with MR arthrography. *Radiographics* 1997;17:657–673.

Beltran LS, Duarte A, Bencardino JT. Review. Postoperative imaging in anterior glenohumeral instability. *Am J Roentgenol* 2018;211:528–537.

Bencardino JT, Beltran J, Rosenberg ZS, et al. Superior labrum anterior-posterior lesions: diagnosis with MR arthrography of the shoulder. *Radiology* 2000;214:267–271.

Bergin D, Schweitzer ME. Indirect magnetic resonance arthrography. *Skeletal Radiol* 2003;10:551–558.

Bigliani LU, Ticker JB, Flatlow EL, et al. The relationship of acromial architecture to rotator cuff disease. *Clin Sports Med* 1991;10:823–838.

Brenner ML, Morrison WB, Carrino JA, et al. Direct MR arthrography of the shoulder: is exercise prior to imaging beneficial or detrimental? *Radiology* 2000;215:491–496.
Bryan HMN, Kumar VP. The arthroscopic Hill-Sachs remplissage: a technique using a PASTA repair kit. *Arthrosc Techn* 2016;5:573–578.
Burkhart SS, De Beer JF. Traumatic glenohumeral bone defects and their relationship to failure of arthroscopic Bankart repairs: significance of the inverted-pear glenoid and the humeral engaging Hill-Sachs lesion. *Arthroscopy* 2000;16:677–694.
Burkhart SS, Esch JC, Jolson RS. The rotator crescent and rotator cable: an anatomic description of the shoulder's "suspension bridge." *Arthroscopy* 1994;9:611–616.
Burkhart SS, Morgan CD, Kibler WB. The disabled throwing shoulder: spectrum of pathology part I: pathoanatomy and biomechanics. *Arthroscopy* 2003;19:404–420.
Burkhart SS, Morgan CD, Kibler WB. The disabled throwing shoulder: spectrum of pathology part III: the SICK scapula, scapular dyskinesis, the kinetic chain, and rehabilitation. *Arthroscopy* 2003;19:641–661.
Carroll KW, Helms CA. Magnetic resonance imaging of the shoulder: a review of potential sources of diagnostic errors. *Skeletal Radiol* 2002;31:373–383.
Carroll KW, Helms CA, Otte MT, et al. Enlarged spinoglenoid notch veins causing suprascapular nerve compression. *Skeletal Radiol* 2003;32:72–77.
Cartland JP, Crues JV III, Stauffer A, et al. MR imaging in the evaluation of SLAP injuries of the shoulder: findings in 10 patients. *Am J Roentgenol* 1992;159:787–792.
Chapovsky F, Kelly JD IV. Osteochondral allograft transplantation for treatment of glenohumeral instability. *Arthroscopy* 2005;21:1007.
Chung CB, Dwek JR, Feng S, et al. MR arthrography of the glenohumeral joint: a tailored approach. *Am J Roentgenol* 2001;177:217–219.
Cisternino SJ, Rogers LF, Stufflebam BC, et al. The trough line: a radiographic sign of posterior shoulder dislocation. *Am J Roentgenol* 1978;130:951–954.
Cothran RL, Helms C. Quadrilateral space syndrome: incidence of imaging findings in a population referred for MRI of the shoulder. *Am J Roentgenol* 2005;184:989–992.
de Jesus JO, Parker L, Frangos AJ, et al. Accuracy of MRI, MR arthrography, and ultrasound in the diagnosis of rotator cuff tears: a meta-analysis. *Am J Roentgenol* 2009;192:1701–1707.
Dépelteau H, Bureau NJ, Cardinal E, et al. Arthrography of the shoulder: a simple fluoroscopically guided approach for targeting the rotator cuff interval. *Am J Roentgenol* 2004;182:329–332.
El-Azab HM, Rott O, Irlenbusch U. Long-term follow-up after latissimus dorsi transfer for irreparable posterosuperior rotator cuff tears. *J Bone Joint Surg Am* 2015;97A:462–469.
Elkinson I, Giles J, Faber K, et al. The effect of the remplissage procedure on shoulder stability and range of motion: an in vitro biomechanical assessment. *J Bone Joint Surg* 2012;94:1003–1012.
Emig EW, Schweitzer D, Karasick D, et al. Adhesive capsulitis of the shoulder: MR diagnosis. *AJR Am J Roentgenol* 1995;164:1457–1459.
Flury M, Rickenbacher D, Jung C, et al. Porcine dermis patch augmentation of supraspinatus tendon repairs: a pilot study assessing tendon integrity and shoulder function 2 years after arthroscopic repair in patients aged 60 years or older. *Arthroscopy* 2018; 34:24–37.
Fritz RC, Helms CA, Steinbach LS, et al. Suprascapular nerve entrapment: evaluation with MR imaging. *Radiology* 1992;182:437–444.
Gerscovich EO, Greenspan A. Magnetic resonance imaging in the diagnosis of suprascapular nerve syndrome. *Can Assoc Radiol J* 1993;44:307–309.
Gobezie R, Warner JJP. SLAP lesion: what is it . . . really? *Skeletal Radiol* 2007;36:379.
Gor DM. The trough line sign. *Radiology* 2002;224:485–486.
Goss TP. Fractures of the scapula. In: Moehring HD, Greenspan A, eds. *Fractures—diagnosis and treatment.* New York: McGraw-Hill; 2000:207–216.
Goutallier D, Postel JM, Gleyze P, et al. Influence of cuff muscle fatty degeneration on anatomic and functional outcomes after simple suture of full-thickness tears. *J Shoulder Elbow Surg* 2003;12:550–554.
Greenspoon JA, Millett PJ, Moulton SG, et al. Irreparable rotator cuff tears: restoring joint kinematics by tendon transfers. *Open Orthop J* 2016; 10:266–276.
Griffith JF, Antonio GE, Tong CWC, et al. Anterior shoulder dislocation: quantification of glenoid bone loss with CT. *Am J Roentgenol* 2003;180:1423–1430.
Guntern DV, Pfirrmann CWA, Schmid MR, et al. Articular cartilage lesions of the glenohumeral joint: diagnostic effectiveness of MR arthrography and prevalence in patients with subacromial impingement syndrome. *Radiology* 2003;226:165–170.
Hamada J, Igarashi I, Akita K, et al. A cadaveric study of the serratus anterior muscle and the long thoracic nerve. *J Shoulder Elbow Surg* 2008;17:790–794.
Hangge PT. Breen I, Albadawi H, et al. Quadrilateral space syndrome: diagnosis and clinical management. *J Clin Med* 2018;7:86–89.
Hannafin JA, Chiaia TA. Adhesive capsulitis: a treatment approach. *Clin Orthop* 2000;372:95–109.
Haygood TM, Langlotz CP, Kneeland JB, et al. Categorization of acromial shape: interobserver variability with MR imaging and conventional radiography. *Am J Roentgenol* 1994;162:1377–1382.
Helms CA, Major NM, Anderson MW, et al. *Musculoskeletal MRI*, 2nd ed. Philadelphia: Saunders-Elsevier; 2009:177–221.
Hendrix RW. Imaging of fractures of the shoulder girdle and upper extremities. In: Moehring HD, Greenspan A, eds. *Fractures—diagnosis and treatment.* New York: McGraw-Hill; 2000:33–46.
Hill HA, Sachs MD. The grooved defect of the humeral head. A frequently unrecognized complication of dislocations of the shoulder joint. *Radiology* 1940;35:690–700.
Jacobson JA. Shoulder US: anatomy, technique and scanning pitfalls. *Radiology* 2011;260:6–16.
Jacobson JA, Lin J, Jamadar DA, et al. Aids to successful shoulder arthrography performed with a fluoroscopically guided anterior approach. *Radiographics* 2003;23:373–379.
Jee W-H, McCauley TR, Katz LD, et al. Superior labral anterior posterior (SLAP) lesions of the glenoid labrum: reliability and accuracy of MR arthrography for diagnosis. *Radiology* 2001;218:127–132.
Jin W, Ryu KN, Kwon SH, et al. MR arthrography in the differential diagnosis of type II superior labral anteroposterior lesion and sublabral recess. *Am J Roentgenol* 2006;187:887–983.
Kalia V, Freehill MT, Miller BS, et al. Review. Multimodality imaging review of normal appearance and complications of the postoperative rotator cuff. *Am J Roentgenol* 2018;211:538–547.
Kilcoyne RF, Shuman WP, Matsen FA III, et al. The Neer classification of displaced proximal humeral fractures: spectrum of findings on plain radiographs and CT scans. *Am J Roentgenol* 1990;154:1029–1033.
Kropf EJ, Sekiya JK. Osteoarticular allograft transplantation for large humeral head defects in glenohumeral instability. *Arthroscopy* 2007;23:322–325.
Krug DK, Vinson EN, Helms CA. MRI findings associated with luxatio erecta humeri. *Skeletal Radiol* 2010;39:27–33.
Kurokawa D, Yamamoto N, Nagamoto H, et al. The prevalence of a large Hill-Sachs lesion that needs to be treated. *J Shoulder Elb Surg* 2013;22:1285–1289.
Lee JHE, van Raalte V, Malian V. Diagnosis of SLAP lesions with Grashey-view arthrography. *Skeletal Radiol* 2003;32:388–395.
Lee MJ, Motamedi K, Chow K, et al. Gradient-recalled echo sequences in direct shoulder MR arthrography for evaluating the labrum. *Skeletal Radiol* 2008;37:19–25.
Lo IK, Parten PM, Burkhart SS. The inverted pear glenoid: an indicator of significant glenoid bone loss. *Arthroscopy* 2004;20(2):169–174.
Martin RM, Fish DE. Scapular winging: anatomical review, diagnosis, and treatments. *Curr Rev Musculoskelet Med* 2008;1: 1–11.
Matthew CDR, Provencher T, Bhatia S, et al. Recurrent shoulder instability: current concepts for evaluation and management of glenoid bone loss. *J Bone Joint Surg Am* 2010A;92:133–151.
McNally EG, Rees JL. Imaging in shoulder disorders. *Skeletal Radiol* 2007;36:1013–1016.
Melenevsky Y, Yablon CM, Ramappa A, et al. Clavicle and acromioclavicular joint injuries: a review of imaging, treatment, and complications. *Skeletal Radiol* 2011;40:831–842.
Mellado JM, Calmet J, Olona M, et al. Surgically repaired massive rotator cuff tears: MRI of tendon integrity, muscle fatty degeneration, and muscle atrophy correlated with intraoperative and clinical findings. *Am J Roentgenol* 2005;184:1456–1463.
Mengiardi B, Pfirmann CWA, Gerber C, et al. Frozen shoulder: MR arthrographic findings. *Radiology* 2004;233:486–492.
Mohana-Borges AVR, Chung CB, Resnick D. MR imaging and MR arthrography of the postoperative shoulder: spectrum of normal and abnormal findings. *Radiographics* 2004;24:69–85.
Mohana-Borges AVR, Chung CB, Resnick D. Superior labral anteroposterior tear: classification and diagnosis on MRI and MR arthrography. *Am J Roentgenol* 2003;181:1449–1462.
Morag Y, Jacobson JA, Lucas D, et al. US appearance of the rotator cable with histologic correlation: preliminary results. *Radiology* 2006;241:485–491.
Neer CS. Displaced proximal humeral fractures. I. Classification and evaluation. *J Bone Joint Surg Am* 1970;52A:1077–1089.
Neer CS II, Rockwood CA Jr. Fractures and dislocations of the shoulder. In: Rockwood CA, Green DP, eds. *Fractures in adults.* Philadelphia: JB Lippincott; 1983:677.
Neviaser TJ. The GLAD lesion: another cause of anterior shoulder pain. *Arthroscopy* 1993;9:22–23.
Omori Y, Yamamoto N, Koishi H, et al. Measurement of the glenoid track in vivo as investigated by 3-dimensional motion analysis using open MRI. *Am J Sports Med* 2014;42: 1290–1295.
Perthes G. Über Operationen bei habitueller Schulterluxation. *Dtsch Z Chir* 1906;85:199–227.
Petri M, Greenspoon JA, Moulton SG, et al. Patch-augmented rotator cuff repair and superior capsule reconstruction. *Open Orthop J* 2016;10:315–323.
Provencher MT, Ghodadra N, LeClere L, et al. Anatomic osteochondral glenoid reconstruction for recurrent glenohumeral instability with glenoid deficiency using a distal tibia allograft. *Arthroscopy* 2009;25:446–452.
Ramhamadany E, Modi CS. Current concepts in the management of recurrent anterior gleno-humeral joint instability with bone loss. *World J Orthop* 2016;7:343–354.
Resnick D. Internal derangements of joints. In: Resnick D, ed. *Diagnosis of bone and joint disorders*, vol. 5, 3rd ed. Philadelphia: WB Saunders; 1995:2899–3228.
Rockwood CA Jr, Green DO, Bucholz RW. *Rockwood and Green's fractures in adults*, vol. 2, 3rd ed. Philadelphia: JP Lippincott; 1991.
Sandmann GH, Ahrens P, Schaeffeler C, et al. Balloon osteoplasty—a new technique for minimally invasive reduction and stabilization of Hill-Sachs lesions of the humeral head: a cadaver study. *Int Orthop* 2012;36:2287–2291.
Saliken DJ, Bornes TD, Bouliane MJ, et al. Imaging methods for quantifying glenoid and Hill-Sachs bone loss in traumatic instability of the shoulder: a scoping review. *BMC Musculoskelet Disord* 2015;16:164–170.
Saupe N, White LM, Bleakney R, et al. Acute traumatic posterior shoulder dislocation: MR findings. *Radiology* 2008;248:185–193.
Scalf RE, Wenger DE, Frick MA. MRI findings of 26 patients with Parsonage-Turner syndrome. *Am J Roentgenol* 2007;189:39–44.
Senekovic V, Poberaj B, Kovacic L, et al. The bio-degradable spacer as a novel treatment modality for massive rotator cuff tears: a prospective study with 5-year follow-up. *Arch Orthop Trauma Surg* 2017; 137:95–103.
Shah N, Tung GA. Imaging signs of posterior glenohumeral instability. *Am J Roentgenol* 2009;192:730–735.
Sheehan SE, Gaviola G, Gordon R, et al. Traumatic shoulder injuries: a force mechanism analysis—glenohumeral dislocation and instability. *Am J Roentgenol* 2013;201:378–373.
Skupinski J, Piechota MZ, Wawrzynek W, et al. The bony Bankart lesion: how to measure the glenoid bone loss. *Pol J Radiol* 2017;82:58–63.
Sofka CM, Ciavarra GA, Hannafin JA, et al. Magnetic resonance imaging of adhesive capsulitis: correlation with clinical staging. *Hosp Spec Surg J* 2008;4:164–169.

Steinbach LS, Gunther SB. Magnetic resonance imaging of the rotator cuff. *Semin Roentgenol* 2000;35:200–216.

Torchia ME. Fractures of the humeral head and neck. In: Moehring HD, Greenspan A, eds. *Fractures—diagnosis and treatment.* New York: McGraw-Hill; 2000:217–224.

Tossy JD, Mead NC, Sigmond HM. Acromioclavicular separations: useful and practical classification for treatment. *Clin Orthop* 1963;28:111–119.

Wenzel WW. The FBI sign. *Rocky Mount Med J* 1972;69:71–72.

Wilson L, Sundaram M, Piraino DW, et al. Isolated teres minor atrophy: manifestation of quadrilateral space syndrome or traction injury to the axillary nerve? *Orthopedics* 2006;29:447–450.

Williams MM, Snyder SJ, Buford D. The Buford complex—the cordlike middle glenohumeral ligament and absent anterosuperior labrum complex: a normal anatomic capsulolabral variant. *Arthroscopy* 1994;10:241–247.

Wischer TK, Bradella MA, Genant HK, et al. Perthes lesion (a variant of the Bankart lesion): MR imaging and MR arthrographic findings with surgical correlation. *Am J Roentgenol* 2002;178:233–237.

Yamamoto N, Itoi E, Abe H, et al. Contact between the glenoid and the humeral head in abduction, external rotation, and horizontal extension: a new concept of glenoid track. *J Shoulder Elb Surg* 2007;16:649–656.

Yang HP, Ji YL, Sung HM, et al. MR arthrography of the labral capsular ligamentous complex in the shoulder: imaging variations and pitfalls. *Am J Roentgenol* 2000;175: 667–672.

Younan Y, Wong PH, Karas S, et al. The glenoid track: a review of the clinical relevance, method of calculation and current evidence behind this method. *Skeletal Radiol* 2017; 46: 1625–1634.

Yu JS, Ashman CJ, Jones G. The POLPSA lesion: MR imaging findings with arthroscopic correlation in patients with posterior instability. *Skeletal Radiol* 2002;31:396–399.

Zlatkin MB, Dalinka MK. The glenohumeral joint. *Top Magn Reson Imaging* 1989;1(3):1–13.

Zumstein MA, Schiessl P, Ambuehl B, et al. New quantitative radiographic parameters for vertical and horizontal instability in acromioclavicular joint dislocations. *Knee Surg Sports Traumatol Arthroscopy* 2018;26:125–135.

6

Upper Limb II

Elbow

Trauma to the Elbow

Trauma to the elbow is commonly encountered in all age groups but is particularly common in childhood when children, as toddlers, often sustain elbow injuries. Play and athletic activities in childhood and young adolescence are also frequent occasions of trauma. Although history and clinical examination usually provide clues to the correct diagnosis, radiologic examination is indispensable in determining the type of fracture or dislocation, the direction of the fracture line and the position of the fragments, and also in evaluating concomitant soft-tissue injuries.

Anatomic–Radiologic Considerations

The elbow articulation, a compound synovial joint, comprises the humeroulnar (ulnatrochlear), the humeroradial (radiocapitellar), and the proximal radioulnar joints (Fig. 6.1). It is a hinged articulation with approximately 150 degrees of flexion from a completely extended position. The flexion and extension movements in the elbow occur in the ulnatrochlear and radiocapitellar joints. The biceps, brachioradialis, and brachialis muscles are the primary elbow flexors, whereas the triceps is the extensor of the elbow joint (Fig. 6.2). Rotational movement occurs as the head of the radius, held tightly by the annular ligament of the ulna, rotates within the ulna's radial notch. The proximal and distal radioulnar joints allow 90 degrees of pronation and supination of the forearm. The stability of the joint is ascertained by the group of ulnar collateral ligaments (UCLs) medially and radial collateral ligaments (RCLs) laterally (Fig. 6.3). The UCL consists of the anterior bundle, which extends from the anteroinferior aspect of the medial epicondyle to the medial coronoid margin; the posterior bundle, which extends from the posteroinferior aspect of the medial epicondyle to the medial olecranon margin; and the transverse bundle, which extends over the notch between the coronoid process and the olecranon. The RCL is thinner than the UCL and inserts in the annular ligament, which in turn encircles the radial head and attaches to the anterior and posterior margins of the radial notch of the ulna. A fibrous capsule deep within the ligament structures surrounds the elbow joint. The anterior joint capsule and synovium insert proximally to the coronoid and radial fossae at the anterior aspect of the humerus. The posterior joint capsule attaches to the humerus just proximal to the olecranon fossa.

When trauma to the elbow is suspected, radiographs are routinely obtained in the anteroposterior and lateral projections, occasionally supplemented by internal and external oblique views.

The *anteroposterior* projection usually suffices to demonstrate an injury to the medial and the lateral epicondyles, the olecranon fossa, the capitellum, the trochlea, and the radial head (Fig. 6.4). It also reveals an important anatomic relation of the forearm to the central axis of the arm known as the *carrying angle* (Fig. 6.5). Normally, the long axis of the forearm forms a valgus angle of 15 degrees with the long axis of the arm; the forearm is thus angled laterally, that is, away from the central axis of the body.

On the anteroposterior view in children, it is essential to recognize the four secondary ossification centers of the distal humerus: those of the capitellum, the medial and the lateral epicondyles, and the trochlea. The usual order in which these centers appear and the age at which they become radiographically visible are important factors in the evaluation of injuries to the elbow (Fig. 6.6). The displacement of any of these centers serves as a diagnostic indicator of the type of fracture or dislocation. For example, the medial epicondyle always ossifies before the trochlea. If radiographic examination in a child between the age of 4 and 8 years reveals a bony structure in the region of the trochlea (i.e., before this center of ossification should appear) and shows no evidence of the ossification center of the medial epicondyle, then it must be assumed that the ossification center of the medial epicondyle has been avulsed and displaced into the joint (Fig. 6.7). Some radiologists prefer to use a mnemonic "CRITOE 1-3-5-7-9-11" to determine the sequence and age of appearance of the six ossification centers around elbow joint: the capitellum, the radial head, the internal (medial) epicondyle, the trochlea, the olecranon, and the external (lateral) epicondyle (Figs. 6.8 and 6.9).

The *lateral* view of the elbow allows sufficient evaluation of the olecranon process, the anterior aspect of the radial head, and the humeroradial articulation. It is limited, however, in the information it can provide, particularly with respect to the posterior half of the radial head and the coronoid process, because of the overlap of osseous structures (Fig. 6.10).

As with the anteroposterior projection, the lateral view in children reveals significant configurations and relations, which, if distorted, indicates the presence of an abnormality. The distal humerus in children has an angular appearance resembling a hockey stick, the angle of which normally measures approximately 140 degrees. Loss of this configuration occurs in supracondylar fracture (Fig. 6.11). Rogers has pointed out, in addition, the importance of the position of the capitellum relative to the distal humerus and the proximal radius. He found that a line drawn along the longitudinal axis of the proximal radius passes through the center of the capitellum and that a line drawn along the anterior cortex of the distal humerus and extended downward through the articulation intersects the middle third of the capitellum (Fig. 6.12). A disruption of this relation serves as an important indication of the possible presence of a fracture or dislocation. Finally, regardless of the patient's age, a displacement of the normal positions of the fat pads of the elbow also provides a useful diagnostic clue to the presence of a fracture. Normally, the posterior fat pad, which lies deep in the olecranon fossa, is not visible on the lateral view. When it becomes visible and the anterior fat pad appears displaced—the positive fat-pad sign (Fig. 6.13; see also Figs. 6.25B and 6.31A)—demonstration of the fracture line should be undertaken.

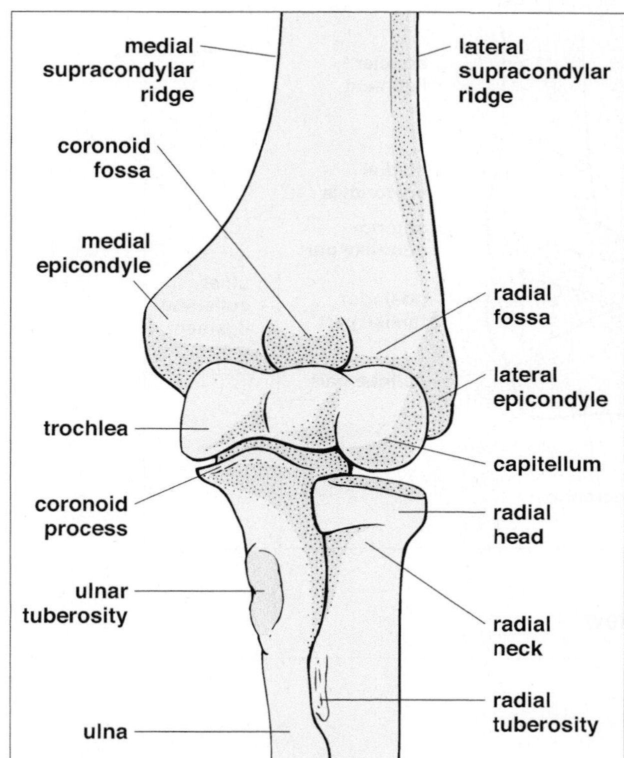

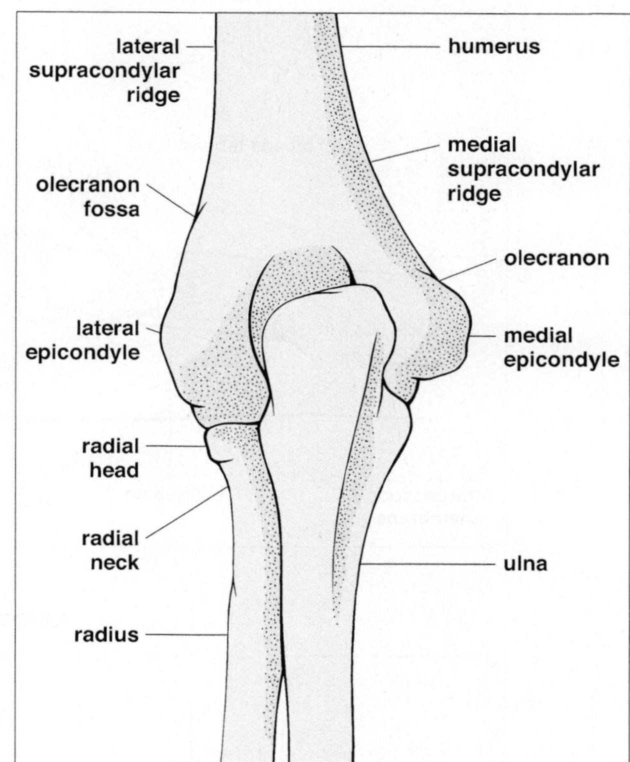

FIGURE 6.1 **Osseous structures of the elbow.** Anterior and posterior views of the distal humerus and the proximal radius and ulna.

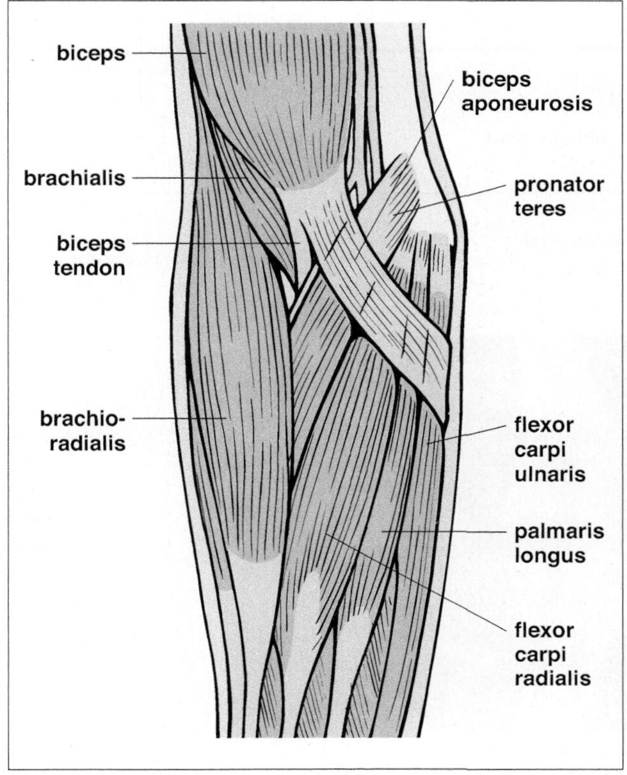

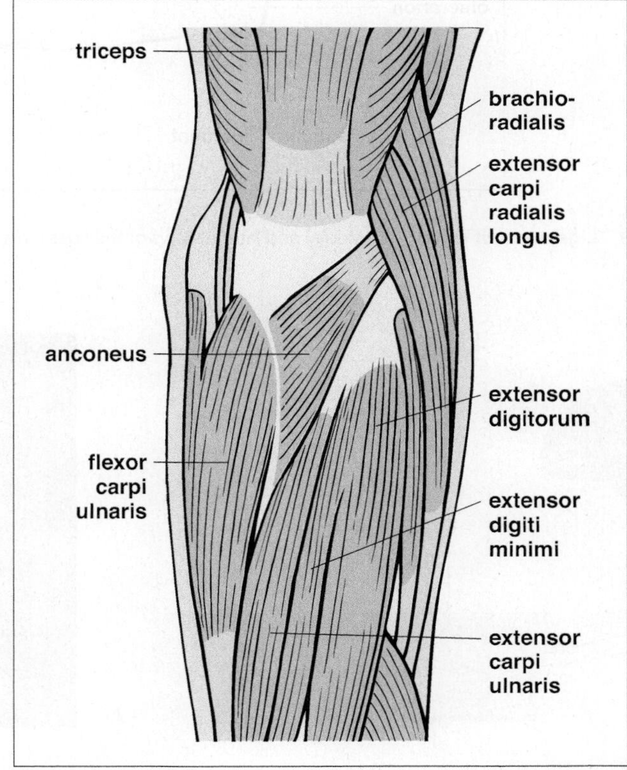

FIGURE 6.2 **Muscles of the elbow.** Anterior and posterior views of the muscles of the elbow joint.

Medial View

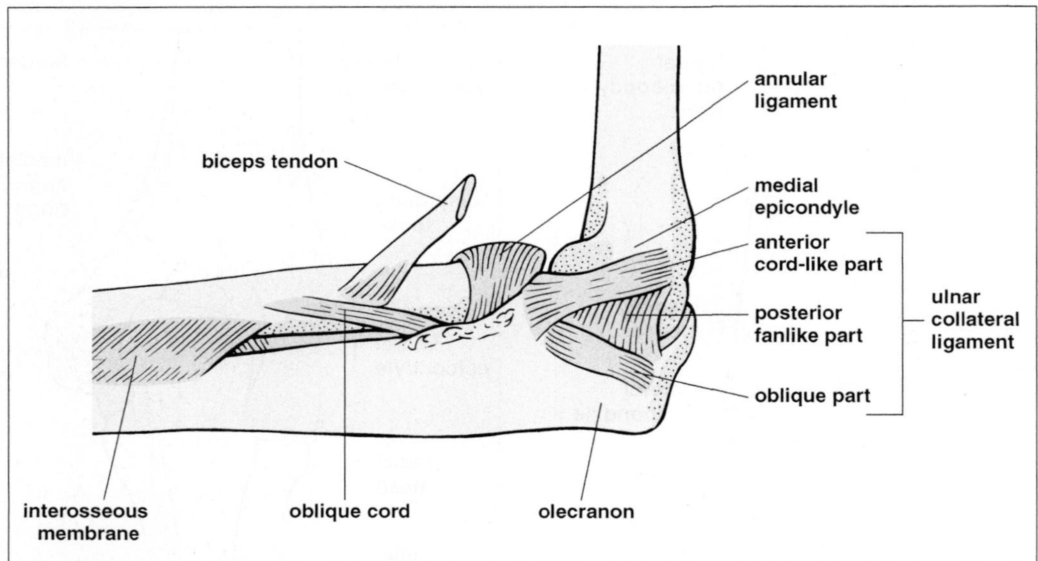

Lateral View

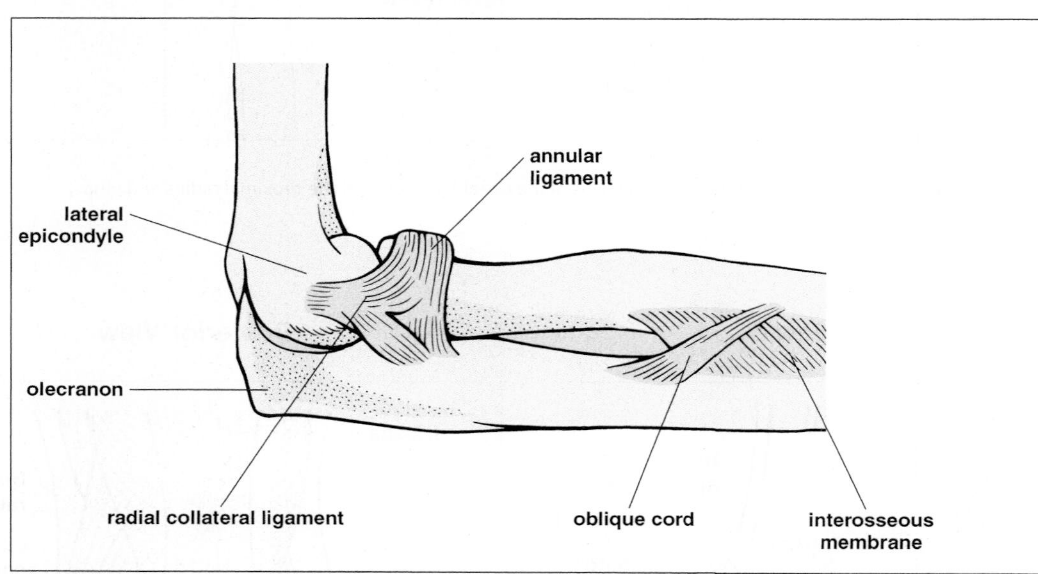

FIGURE 6.3 **Ligaments of the elbow.** Medial and lateral views of the ligaments of the elbow joint.

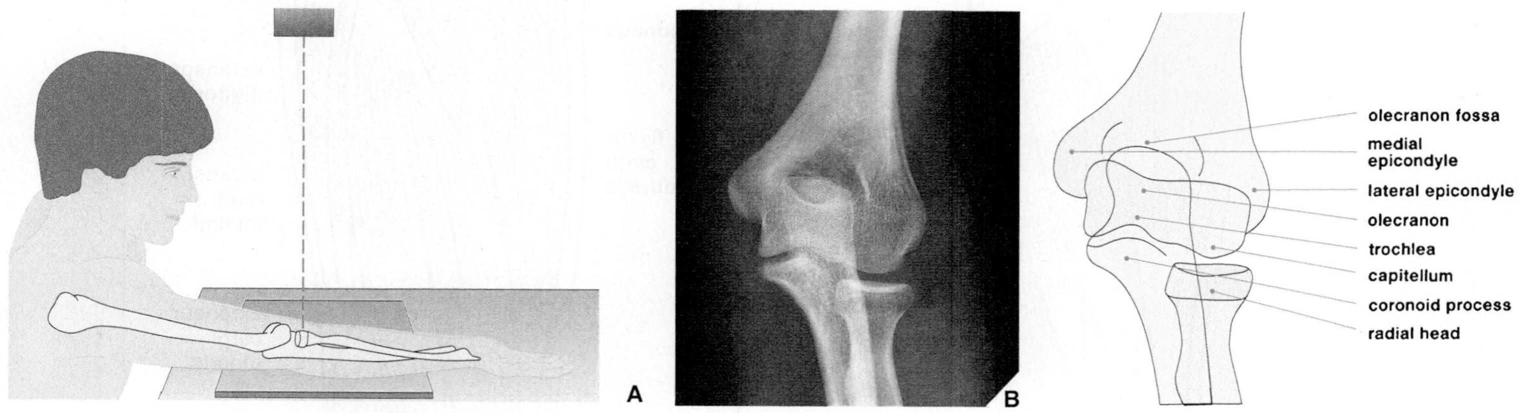

FIGURE 6.4 **Anteroposterior view.** **(A)** For the anteroposterior view of the elbow, the forearm is positioned supine (palm up) on the radiographic table, with the elbow joint fully extended and the fingers slightly flexed. The central beam *(red broken line)* is directed perpendicularly toward the elbow joint. **(B)** The radiograph obtained in this projection demonstrates the medial and the lateral epicondyles, the olecranon fossa, the capitellum, and the radial head. The coronoid process is seen en face, and the olecranon overlaps the trochlea.

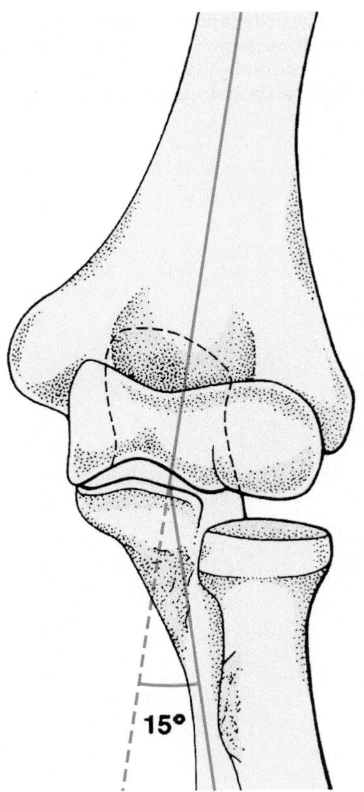

FIGURE 6.5 Carrying angle. The angle formed by the longitudinal axes of the distal humerus and the proximal ulna constitutes the carrying angle of the forearm. Normally, there is a valgus angle of 15 degrees.

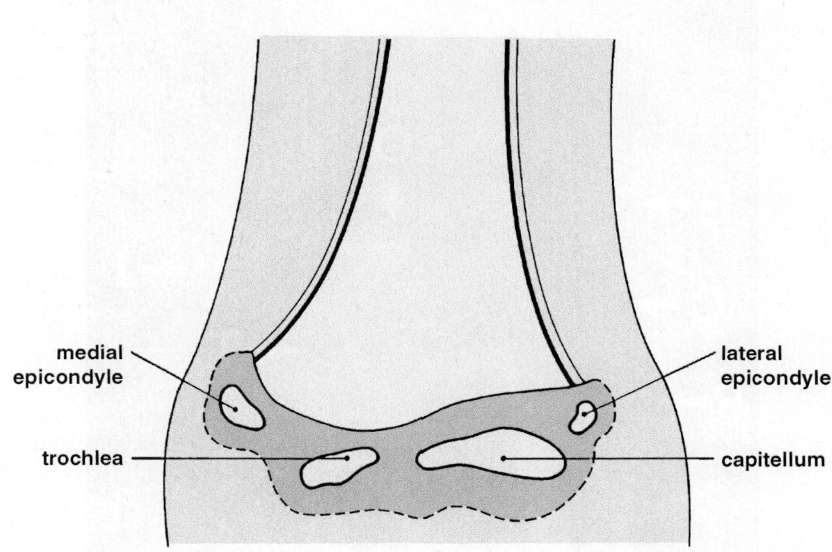

FIGURE 6.6 Ossification centers of the distal humerus. The secondary centers of ossification of the distal humerus usually appear in the following order: the capitellum at 1 to 2 years of age, the medial epicondyle at 4 to 5 years of age, the trochlea at 7 to 8 years of age, and the lateral epicondyle at 10 to 11 years of age.

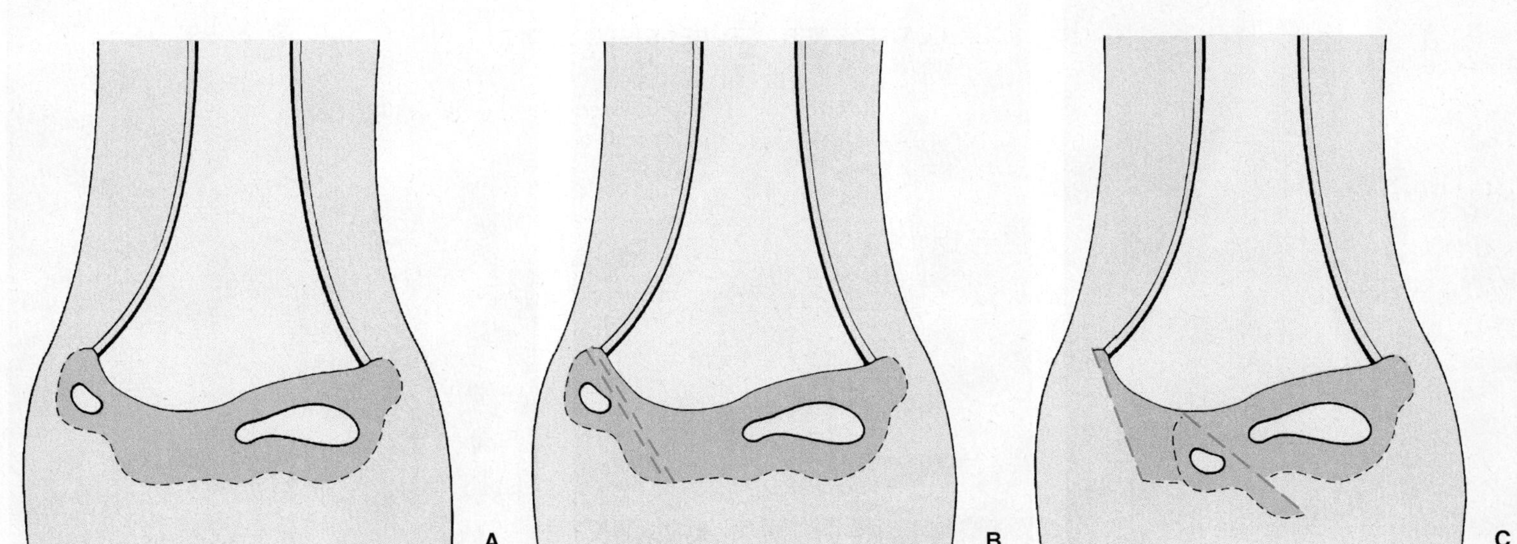

FIGURE 6.7 Fracture of the medial epicondyle. **(A,B)** Displacement of the ossification center of the medial epicondyle secondary to fracture may mimic the normal appearance of the ossification center of the trochlea **(C)**. The orange areas represent unossified cartilage, which is not visualized on the radiographs.

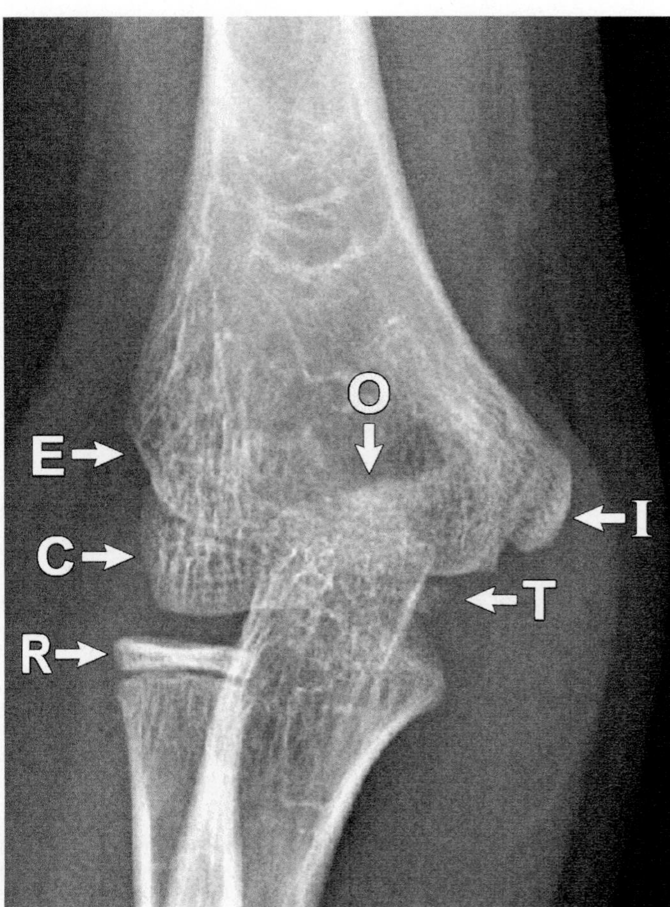

FIGURE 6.8 **CRITOE—the order and age of appearance of ossification centers around the elbow joint.** C, capitellum (1 year); R, radius (3 years); I, internal (medial) epicondyle (5 years); T, trochlea (7 years); O, olecranon (9 years); E, external (lateral) epicondyle (11 years).

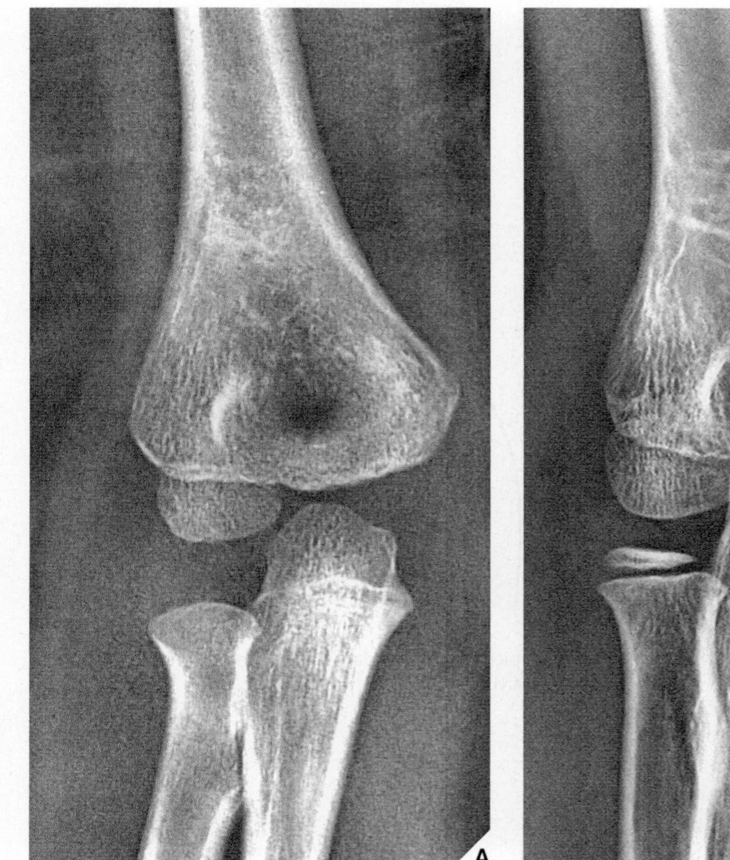

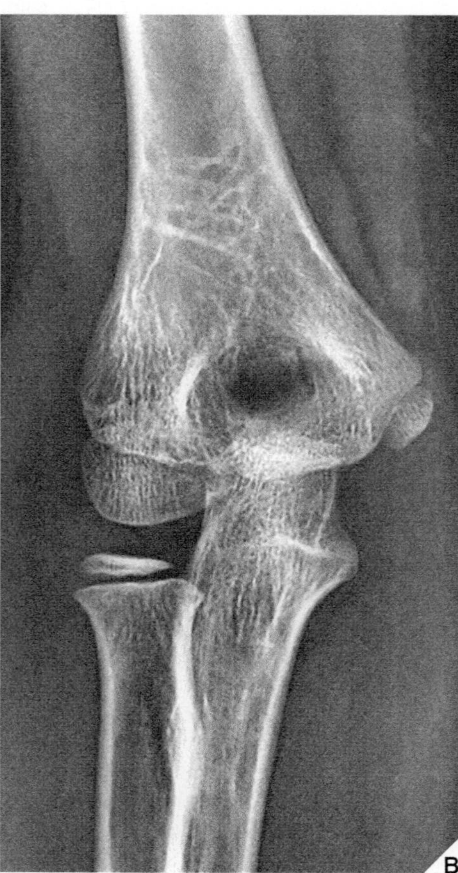

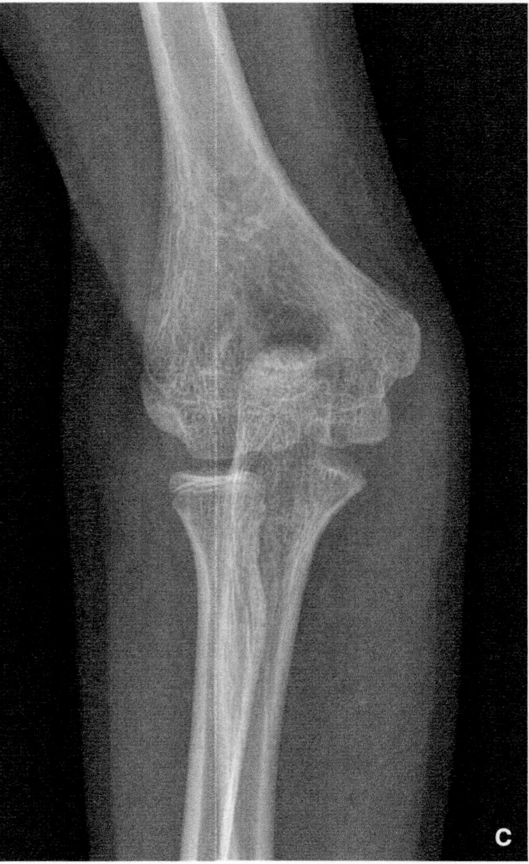

FIGURE 6.9 **Anteroposterior radiographs of the elbow in a child.** **(A)** A 2.5-year-old boy. Only ossification center for the capitellum is present. **(B)** A 6.5-year-old girl. Three centers of ossification are present: for the capitellum, for the radial head, and for the medial (internal) epicondyle of the humerus. **(C)** A 12.5-year-old girl. All six ossification centers are present.

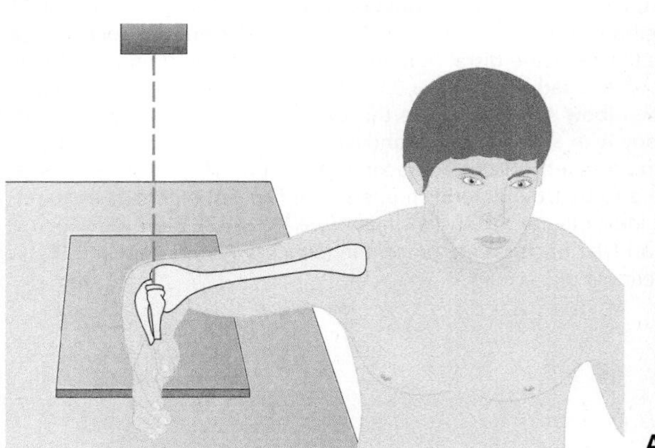

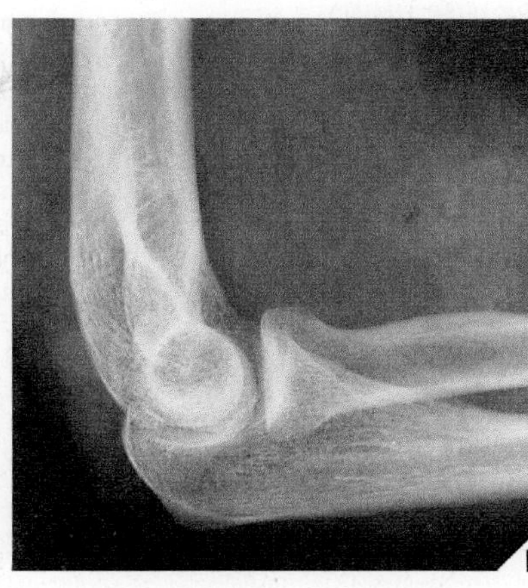

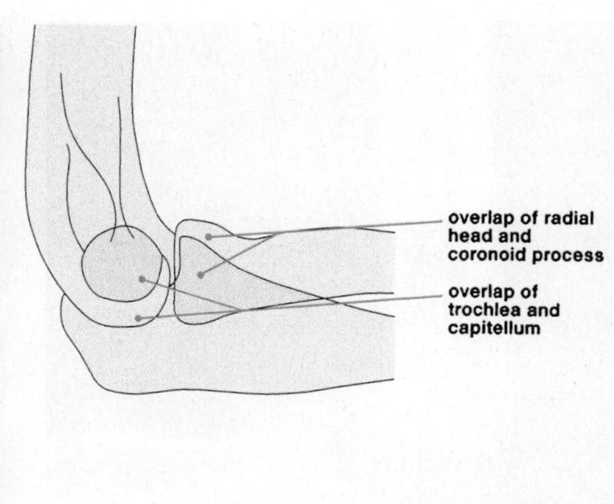

FIGURE 6.10 Lateral view. **(A)** For the lateral projection of the elbow, the forearm rests on its ulnar side on the radiographic cassette, with the joint flexed 90 degrees, the thumb pointing upward, and the fingers slightly flexed. The central beam *(red broken line)* is directed vertically toward the radial head. **(B)** The radiograph obtained in this projection demonstrates the distal shaft of the humerus, the supracondylar ridge, the olecranon process, and the anterior aspect of the radial head. The articular surface and posterior aspect of the radial head are not well demonstrated on this view because of overlap by the coronoid process. The capitellum is also obscured by the overlapping trochlea.

The *radial head–capitellum* view is a variant of the lateral projection, which was introduced by Greenspan in 1982. Because it overcomes the major limitation of the standard lateral view by projecting the radial head ventrad, free of overlap by the coronoid process, it has proved to be a particularly effective technique. In addition to the radial head, it also clearly demonstrates the capitellum, the coronoid process, the humeroradial and humeroulnar articulations (Fig. 6.14), and subtle fractures of these structures that may be obscure on other projections (see Figs. 6.27, 6.28, and 6.36).

Other modalities may also be necessary for sufficient evaluation of an injury to the elbow. Single-contrast or, preferably, double-contrast arthrography, combined (in the past) with tomography (*arthrotomography*) and presently with computed tomography (CT), has proved effective in visualizing subtle chondral fractures, osteochondritis dissecans, synovial and capsular abnormalities, and osteochondral bodies in the joint. In general, indications for elbow arthrography include detection of the presence, size, and number of intraarticular osteochondral bodies; determination of whether calcifications around the elbow joint are intraarticular or extraarticular; evaluation of the articular cartilage; evaluation of juxtaarticular cysts if they are communicating with the joint; evaluation of the joint capacity; and evaluation of various synovial and capsular abnormalities. Single-contrast arthrography is preferable when evaluating synovial abnormalities and intraarticular osteochondral bodies because double contrast may result in air bubbles in the joint. Double-contrast arthrography, however, provides more detailed information; in particular, the articular surface and synovial lining are better delineated, and the small details can be better visualized (Fig. 6.15). In the past, in conjunction with elbow arthrography, conventional tomography was used in a procedure called *arthrotomography*; however, currently, it has been substituted by CT examination (CT-arthrography) (Fig. 6.16).

Axial CT images of the extended elbow are occasionally effective in demonstrating traumatic abnormalities. They are, however, difficult to obtain in the traumatized patient, and except for the visualization of the proximal radioulnar joint and ulnatrochlear articulation, they are not frequently used. Occasionally, these sections can demonstrate osteochondral fractures of the radial head and assess the integrity of the proximal radioulnar joint. However, Franklin and colleagues noted that axial CT images of the flexed elbow (so-called *coronal sections*) provide an ideal plane for the evaluation of the olecranon fossa and the space between the trochlea and the olecranon process posteriorly, as well as the radius and the capitellum, and the trochlea and the coronoid process anteriorly. Axial scans through the flexed elbow also allow additional demonstration of the proximal radius in its long axis.

Magnetic resonance imaging (MRI) examination effectively demonstrates traumatic abnormalities of the elbow joint and surrounding soft tissues. Coronal, sagittal, and axial planes are routinely used for elbow imaging. On coronal images, the trochlea, capitellum, and radial head are well demonstrated as well as the various tendons, ligaments, and muscles around the elbow (Fig. 6.17A). On the sagittal images, the ulnatrochlear and radiocapitellar articulations are well seen, and the biceps, triceps, and brachialis muscle groups are well demonstrated in their long axis. The biceps tendon and anconeus muscles are also well imaged (Fig. 6.17B,C). The axial plane is ideal to display the anatomic relationship of the proximal radioulnar joint and the head of the radius. Various tendons, muscles, annular ligament, and neurovascular bundles are also effectively imaged (Fig. 6.17D–F).

MR-arthrography (MRa) is occasionally performed, mainly to evaluate synovial abnormalities and integrity of the joint capsule and ligaments. In addition, subtle intraarticular loose bodies can be detected with this technique, and the stability of osteochondral fracture or osteochondritis dissecans of the capitellum can be assessed. Similar to one used for shoulder MRa, a concentration of gadolinium mixed with normal saline, iodinated contrast agent, and lidocaine is prepared and a total of up to 10 mL of fluid is injected into the elbow joint. Lateral approach, identical to the technique for conventional elbow arthrography (see Fig. 6.15), is preferred. Coronal, sagittal, and axial images are obtained using fat-suppressed spin echo sequences (Fig. 6.18). During the evaluation of MRI of the elbow, it is helpful to use a checklist as provided in Table 6.1.

For a summary of the preceding discussion in tabular form, see Tables 6.2 and 6.3.

Injury to the Elbow

Fractures About the Elbow

Fractures of the Distal Humerus

Because the nomenclature of the various structures of the distal humerus used in different anatomy and surgery textbooks is not uniform, confusion has arisen regarding the classification of fractures of the distal humerus. To clarify the picture, a simplified anatomic division of the distal humerus is shown in Figure 6.19. The significance of the distinction between the articular and the extraarticular parts of the distal humerus lies in its importance to diagnosis, treatment, and prognosis. For example, as many orthopaedic surgeons contended, a fracture involving only the articular portion of the distal humerus usually results in a loss of motion, but not a loss of stability, whereas a fracture of an entire condyle—that is, both articular and extraarticular portions—usually leads to restriction of motion and instability.

Based on the structure involved, fractures of the distal humerus can be classified as supracondylar, transcondylar, and intercondylar as well as fractures of the medial and the lateral epicondyles, the capitellum, and the trochlea. The Müller classification is recommended because it is a practical one based on a distinction between intraarticular and extraarticular fractures (Fig. 6.20). Usually, such injuries pose no diagnostic problems in adults and are readily evaluated on the anteroposterior and lateral projections of the elbow (Figs. 6.21 and 6.22). In the past, tomographic examination was usually performed to localize comminuted fragments. Currently, CT is the modality of choice for this purpose (Fig. 6.23).

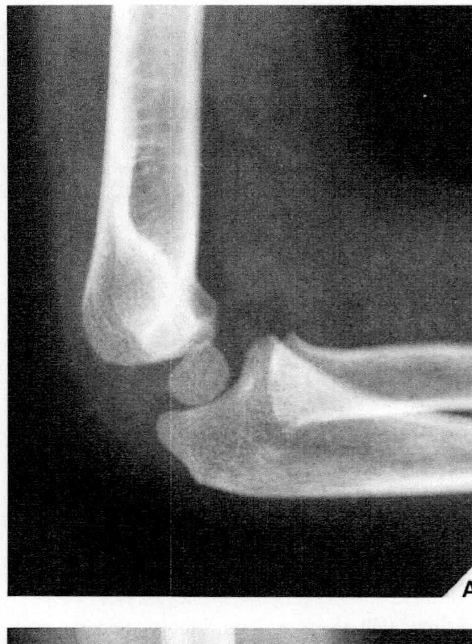

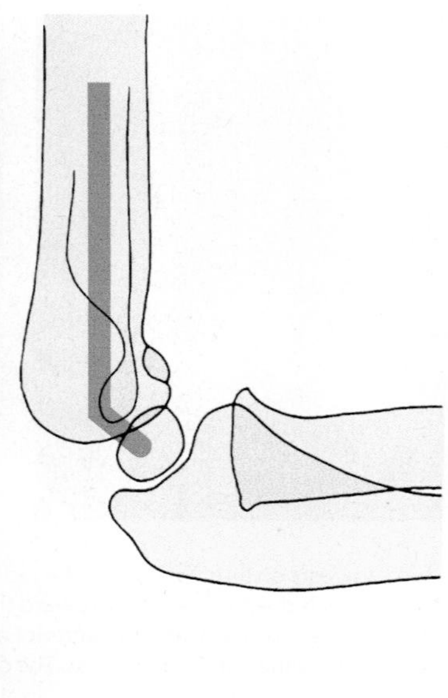

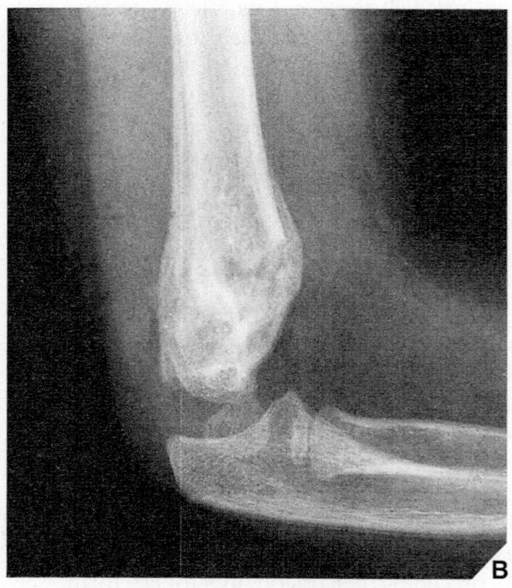

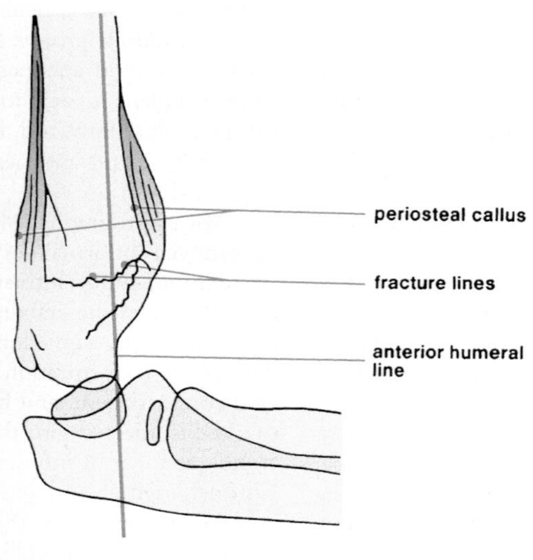

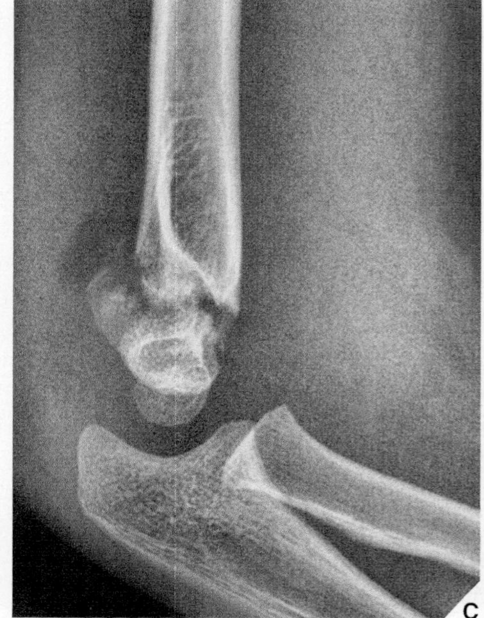

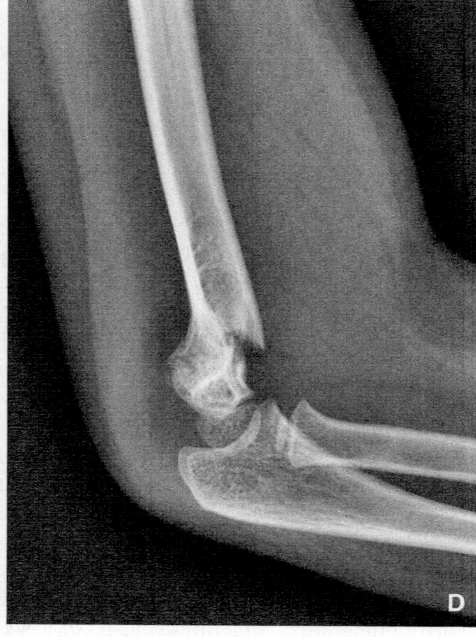

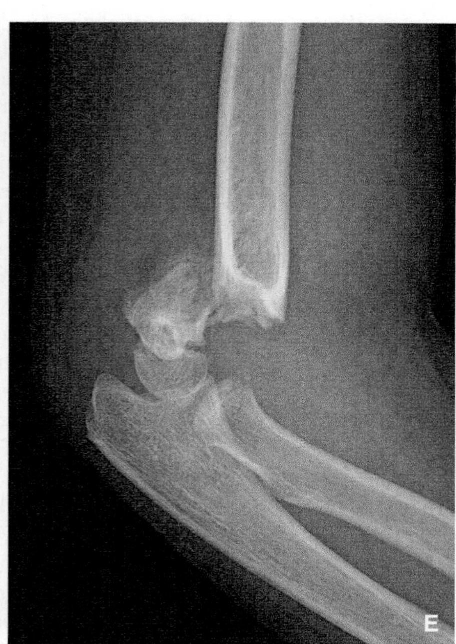

FIGURE 6.11 Supracondylar fracture. **(A)** Lateral radiograph of the elbow joint in a 3-year-old child shows the normal hockey-stick appearance of the distal humerus. **(B)** Loss of this configuration, as seen in this radiograph of a 3.5-year-old girl who sustained trauma to the elbow 4 weeks before this examination, and **(C)** of a 4-year-old boy with an acute supracondylar fracture, serves as an important landmark in recognizing supracondylar fracture of the distal humerus. Note also that the anterior humeral line falls anterior to the capitellum, indicating an extension injury (see Fig. 6.12). More obvious supracondylar fractures are present in **(D)** a 6.5-year-old girl and **(E)** an 11-year-old girl.

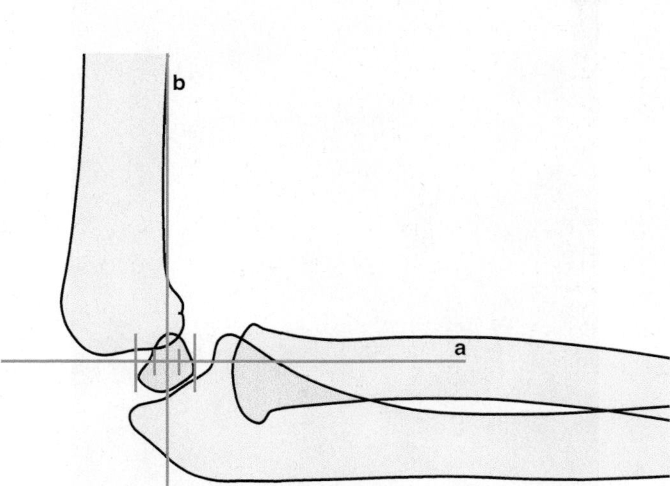

FIGURE 6.12 Landmarks of the elbow joint. In children, the normal position of the capitellum relative to the distal humerus and the proximal radius is determined by the portions of the capitellum intersected by two lines: Line *a* coincident with the longitudinal axis of the proximal radius passes through the center of the capitellum, and line *b* parallel to the anterior cortex of the distal humerus intersects the middle third of the capitellum. Disruption of this relation indicates the possible presence of an abnormality (see Figs. 6.11B,C and 6.25B).

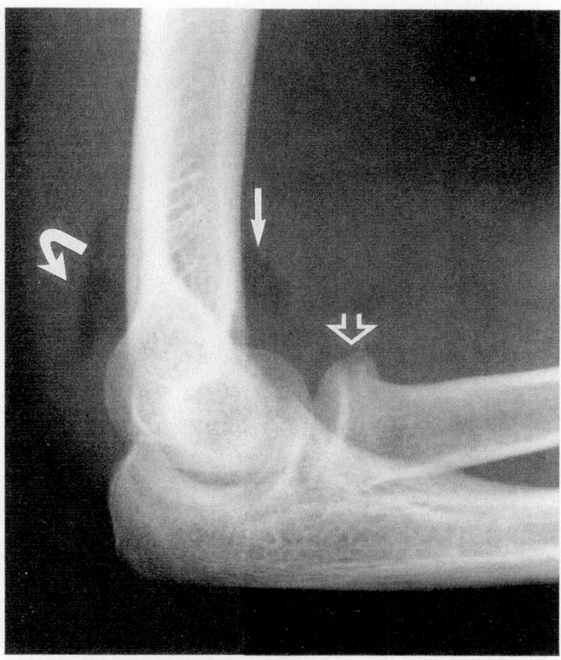

FIGURE 6.13 Fat-pad sign. Lateral radiograph of the elbow joint shows positive anterior *(arrow)* and posterior *(curved arrow)* fat-pad sign. *Open arrow* points to the subtle fracture of the radial head.

FIGURE 6.14 Radial head–capitellum view. **(A)** For the radial head–capitellum projection of the elbow, the patient is seated at the side of the radiographic table, with the forearm resting on its ulnar side, the elbow joint flexed 90 degrees and the thumb pointing upward. The central beam *(red broken line)* is directed toward the radial head at a 45-degree angle to the forearm. **(B)** The radiograph obtained in this projection shows the radial head projected ventrad, free of overlap by the coronoid process, which is also well demonstrated. This projection is also effective in evaluating the capitellum and the humeroradial and humeroulnar articulations. **(C)** Same view of the skeletally immature elbow.

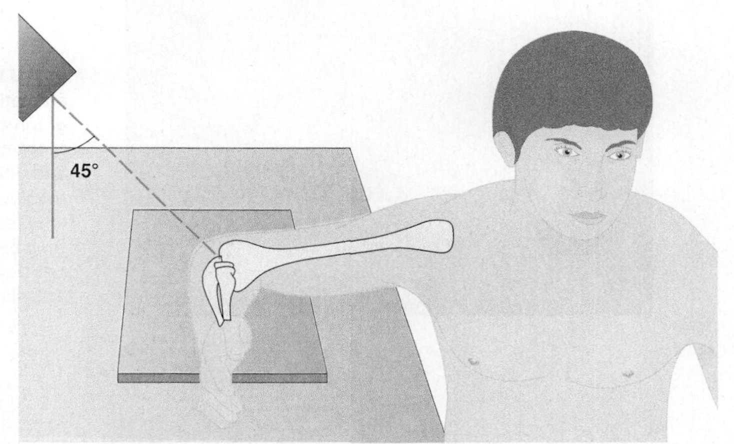

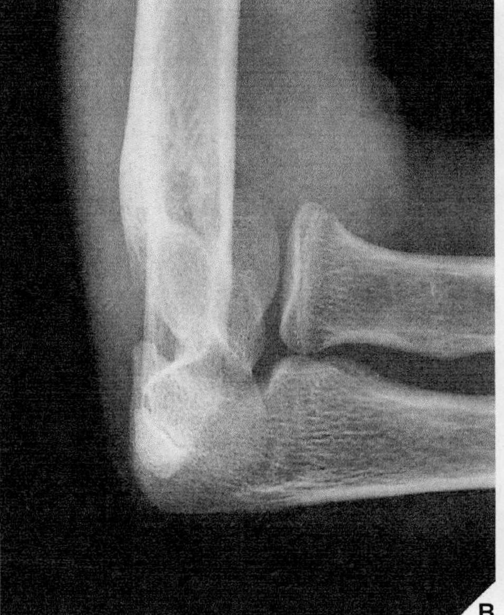

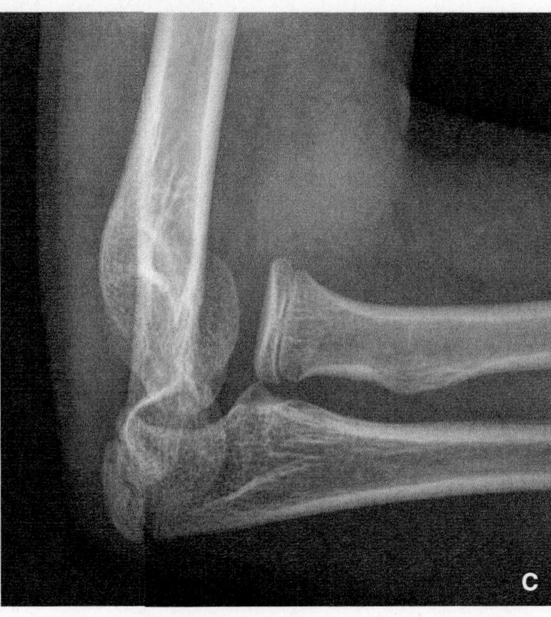

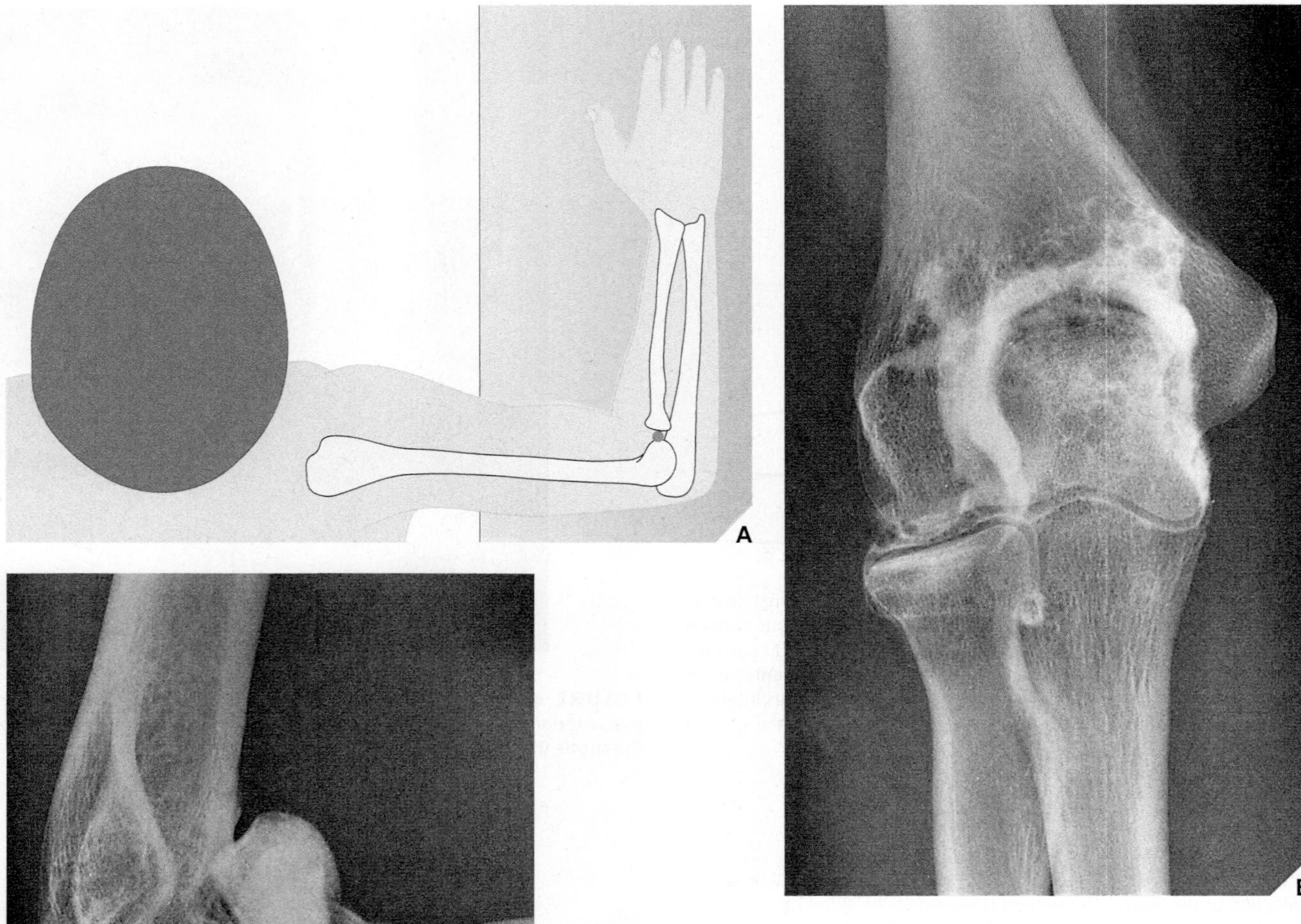

◀ **FIGURE 6.15** Arthrography of the elbow joint. **(A)** For arthrographic examination of the elbow, the patient's forearm is positioned prone on the radiographic table, with the joint flexed 90 degrees and the fingers lying flat. The joint is entered from the lateral aspect between the radial head and the capitellum, and under fluoroscopic control, 2 mL of positive contrast agent (60% diatrizoate meglumine) and 8 to 10 mL of room air are injected into the radiocapitellar joint. (The *red dot* marks the point of needle entrance.) Conventional radiographs may then be obtained in the standard projections. **(B,C)** On the elbow arthrogram, one can distinguish anterior, posterior, and annular recesses of the joint capsule. The articular cartilage of the radial head and capitellum is also well demonstrated.

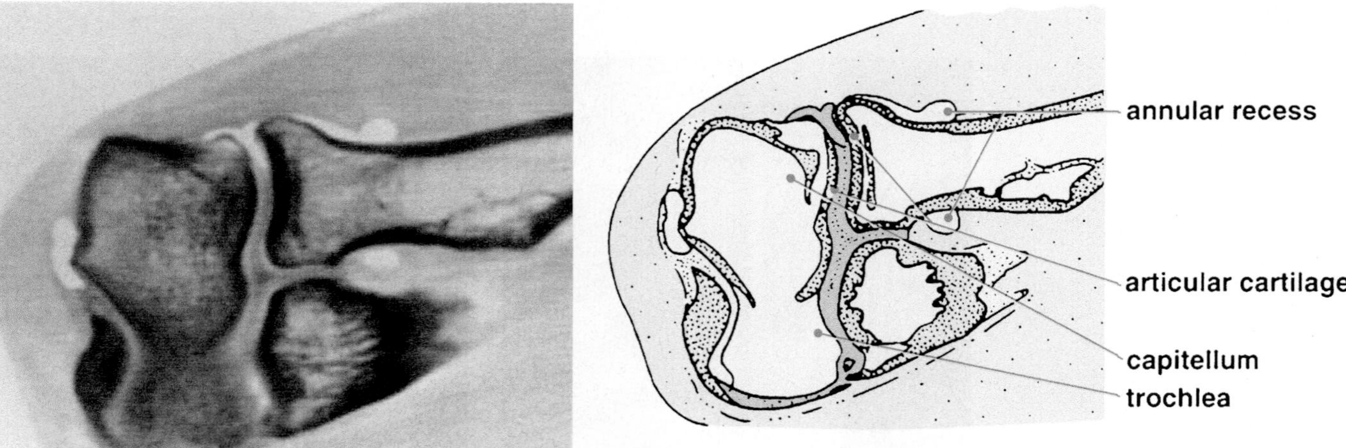

▲ **FIGURE 6.16** CT-arthrography of the elbow. Postarthrography coronal CT scan of the elbow joint clearly demonstrates the annular recess and the outline of the lateral extension of the joint capsule. The articular cartilage is also well demonstrated.

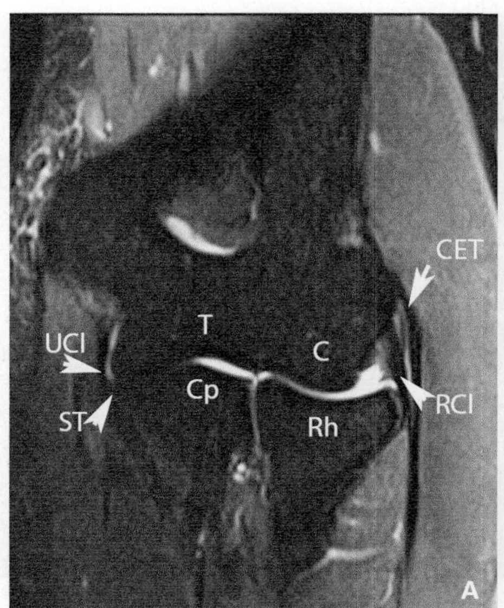

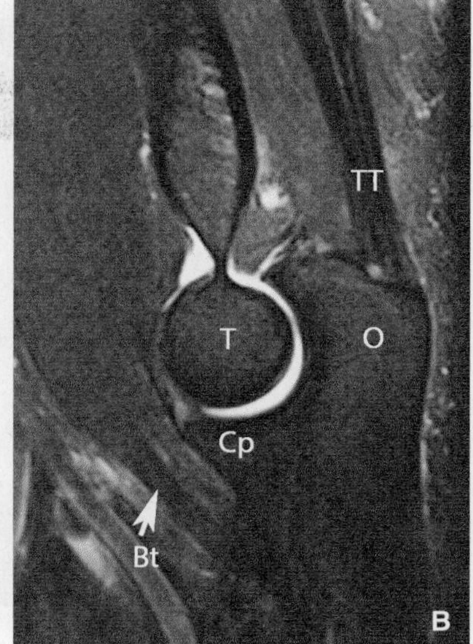

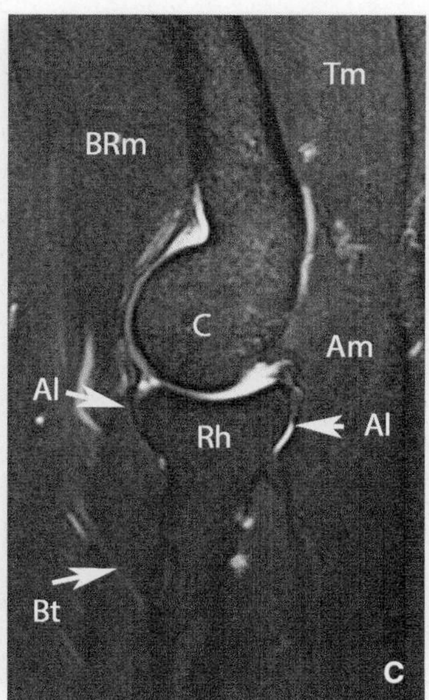

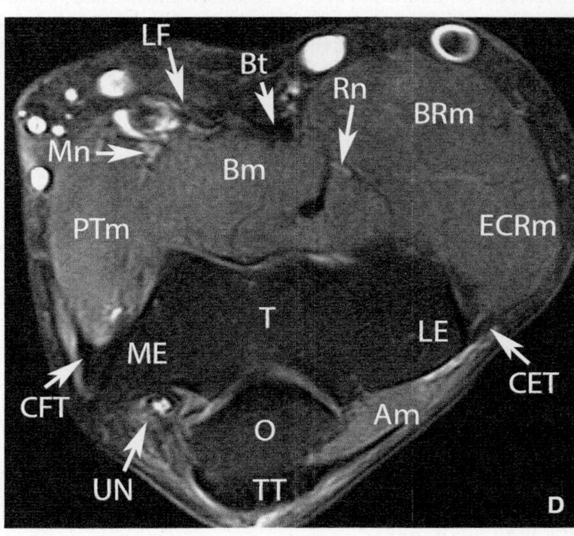

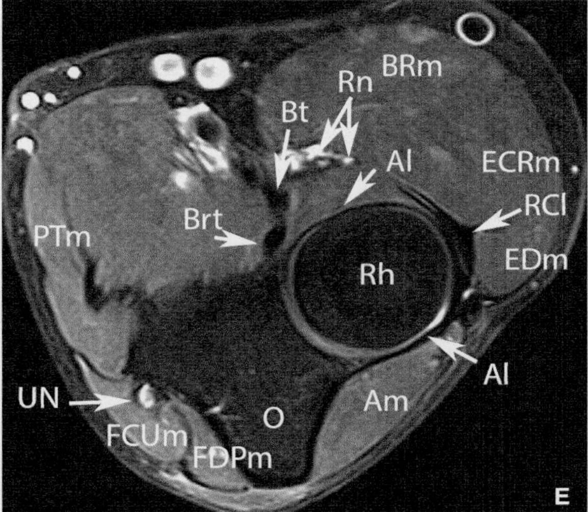

FIGURE 6.17 **Normal MRI anatomy of the elbow joint.** **(A–C)** T1-weighted fat-saturated MRa. On the coronal section **(A)**, note the anatomic relationship of osseous, muscular, and tendinous structures. On the sagittal sections, one through the trochlea **(B)** and the other through the capitellum **(C)**, the muscular structures (brachialis muscle, anconeus muscle), tendons (triceps tendon, biceps tendon), and bones (distal humerus, olecranon process, and radial head) are well demonstrated. **(D–F)** Axial proton density–weighted fat-saturated MR images in another patient, at the level of the distal humerus **(D)**, head of the radius **(E)**, and radial tuberosity **(F)**. UCl, ulnar collateral ligament; T, humeral trochlea; C, capitellum; CET, common extensor tendon; ST, sublime tubercle; Cp, coronoid process; Rh, radial head; RCl, radial collateral ligament; Bt, biceps tendon; TT, Triceps tendon; O, olecranon; BRm, brachioradialis muscle; Tm, triceps muscle; Al, annular ligament; Am, Anconeus muscle; LF, lacertus fibrosus; Rn, radial nerve (*double arrows* in **E** and **F** shows the superficial and deep branches of the radial nerve); Mn, median nerve; Bm, brachialis muscle; PTm, pronator teres muscle; ECRm, extensor carpi radialis muscle; CFT, common flexor tendon; ME, medial epicondyle; LE, lateral epicondyle; UN, ulnar nerve; Brt, brachialis tendon; EDm, extensor digitorum muscles; FCUm, flexor carpi ulnaris muscle; FDPm, flexor digitorum profundus muscle; Sm, supinator muscle; R, radius; U, ulna.

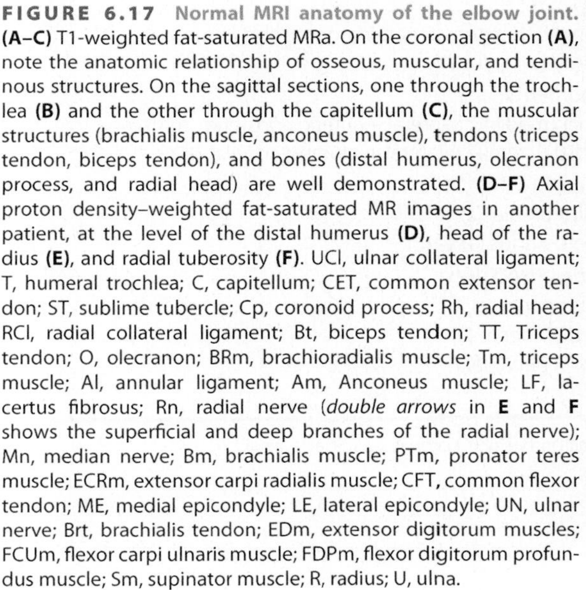

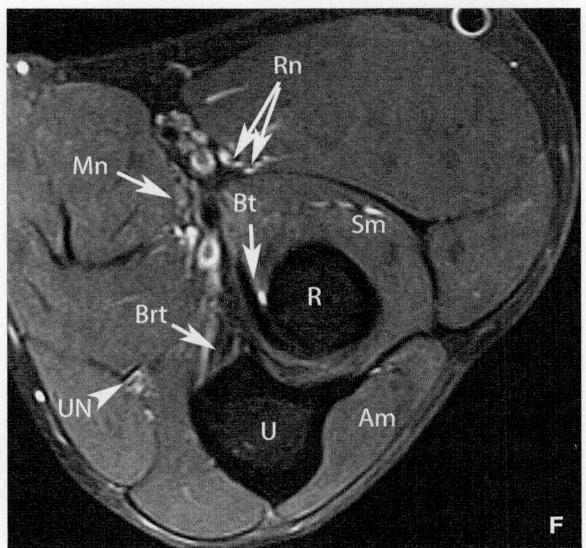

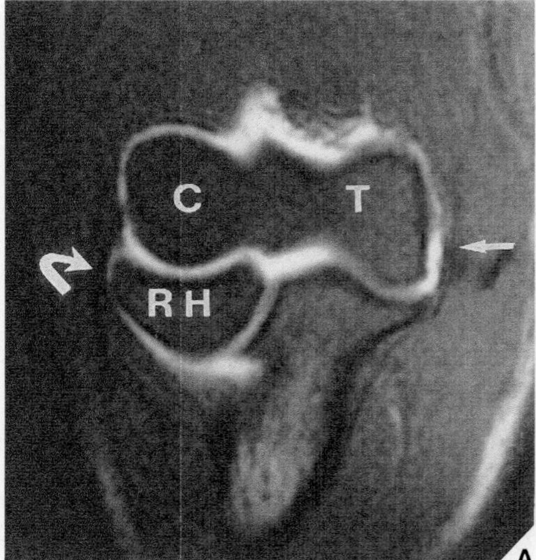

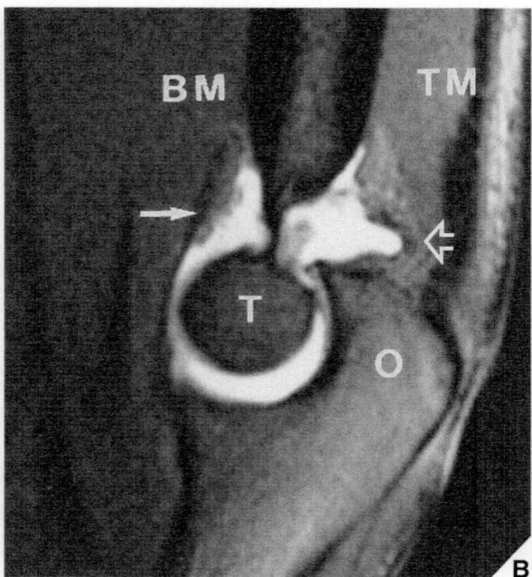

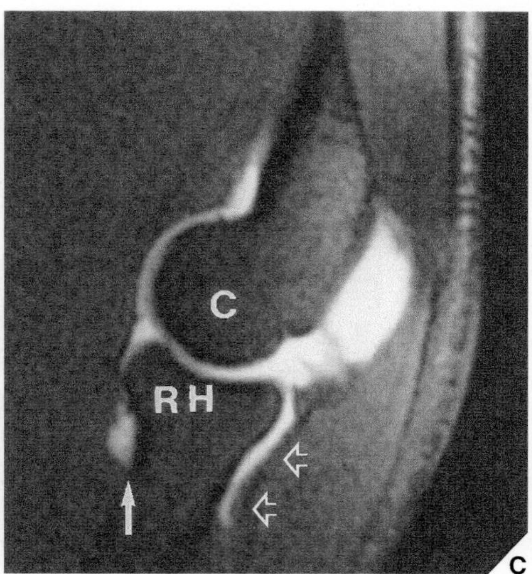

FIGURE 6.18 **MRa of the elbow.** **(A)** Coronal T1-weighted fat-suppressed MR image shows the anterior band of the UCL *(arrow)* and the RCL *(curved arrow)*. The joint is outlined by a bright contrast agent. C, capitellum; T, trochlea; RH, radial head. **(B)** Sagittal T1-weighted fat-suppressed image obtained through the medial part of the elbow joint shows anterior *(arrow)* and posterior *(open arrow)* recesses. T, trochlea; O, olecranon; BM, brachialis muscle; TM, triceps muscle. **(C)** Sagittal T1-weighted fat-suppressed image obtained through the lateral part of the elbow joint shows attachment of the joint capsule to the proximal radius *(arrow)* and its posterior extent *(open arrows)*. C, capitellum; RH, radial head.

TABLE 6.1 Checklist for Evaluation of Magnetic Resonance Imaging and Magnetic Resonance Arthrography of the Elbow

Osseous Structures	*Muscles and Their Tendons (continued)*
Medial epicondyle of the humerus (c, s, a)	Extensor carpi ulnaris (c, a)
Lateral epicondyle of the humerus (c, s, a)	Extensor digitorum (c, a)
Trochlea (c, s)	Flexor carpi ulnaris (c, a)
Capitellum (c, s)	Flexor carpi radialis (c, a)
Radial head (c, s)	Flexor digitorum—superficialis, profundus (c, a)
Radial neck (c, s)	Pronator teres (c, a)
Coronoid process (s)	Supinator (c, a)
Olecranon (s)	Conjoined extensor–supinator tendon (c, a)
Cartilaginous Structures	Palmaris longus (a)
Articular cartilage (c, s, a)	*Ligaments*
Joints	Ulnar (medial) collateral—anterior, posterior, transverse (c)
Radiocapitellar (c, s)	Radial (lateral) collateral, including annular (a, c)
Ulnatrochlear (c, s)	*Bursae*
Proximal radioulnar (c, s, a)	Bicipitoradial (a)
Muscles and Their Tendons	Interosseous (a)
Biceps (s, a)	*Other Structures*
Triceps (s, a)	Ulnar nerve (a)
Anconeus (s, a)	Median nerve (a)
Brachioradialis (c, s, a)	Radial nerve (a)
Extensor carpi radialis—brevis, longus (c, a)	

The best imaging planes for visualization of listed structures are given in parentheses: c, coronal; s, sagittal; a, axial.

TABLE 6.2 Standard and Special Radiographic Projections for Evaluating Injury to the Elbow

Projection	Demonstration
Anteroposterior	Supracondylar, transcondylar, and intercondylar fractures of the distal humerus Fractures of Medial and lateral epicondyles Lateral aspect of capitellum Medial aspect of trochlea Lateral aspect of radial head Valgus and varus deformities Secondary ossification centers of distal humerus
Lateral	Supracondylar fracture of the distal humerus Fractures of Anterior aspect of radial head Olecranon process Complex dislocations in elbow joint Dislocation of radial head Fat-pad sign
External oblique	Fractures of Lateral epicondyle Radial head
Internal oblique	Fractures of Medial epicondyle Coronoid process
Radial head–capitellum	Fractures of Radial head Capitellum Coronoid process Abnormalities of humeroradial and humeroulnar articulations

TABLE 6.3 Ancillary Imaging Techniques for Evaluating Injury to the Elbow

Technique	Demonstration
Tomography (presently replaced by CT)	Complex fractures about the elbow joint, particularly to assess the position of fragments in comminution Healing process: Nonunion Secondary infection
Arthrography (single or double contrast)	Subtle abnormalities of articular cartilage Capsular ruptures Synovial abnormalities Chondral and osteochondral fractures Osteochondritis dissecans Osteochondral bodies in joint
CT (alone or combined with double-contrast arthrography)	Same as for arthrography
MRI and MRa	Abnormalities of the ligaments,[a] tendons, muscles, and nerves, including compressive and entrapment neuropathies Capsular ruptures[a] Joint effusion Synovial cysts[a] Hematomas Subtle abnormalities of bones (e.g., bone contusion) Osteochondritis dissecans[a] Epiphyseal fractures (in children)

[a]These abnormalities are best demonstrated on magnetic resonance arthrography (MRa).
CT, computed tomography; MRI, magnetic resonance imaging.

FIGURE 6.19 Anatomic structures of the distal humerus. A simplified anatomic division of the structures of the distal humerus.

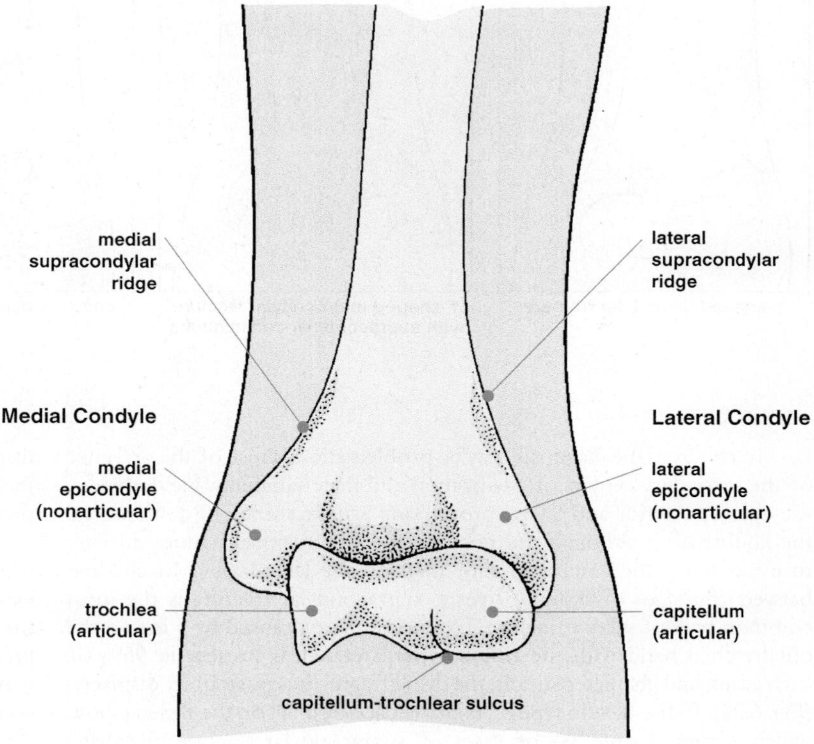

FRACTURES OF THE DISTAL HUMERUS

Extra-articular—Epicondylar, Supracondylar

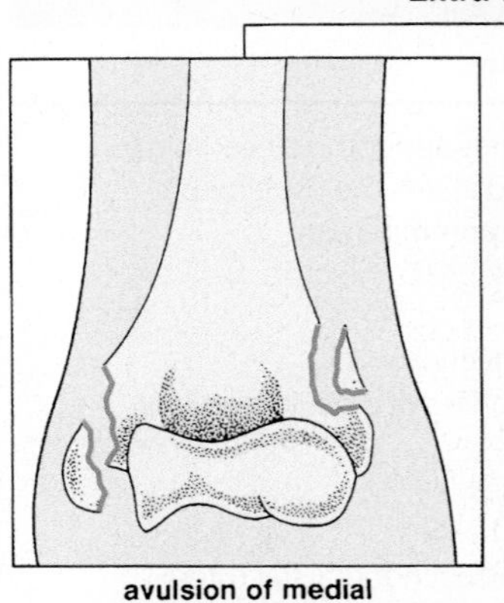

avulsion of medial and/or lateral epicondyle

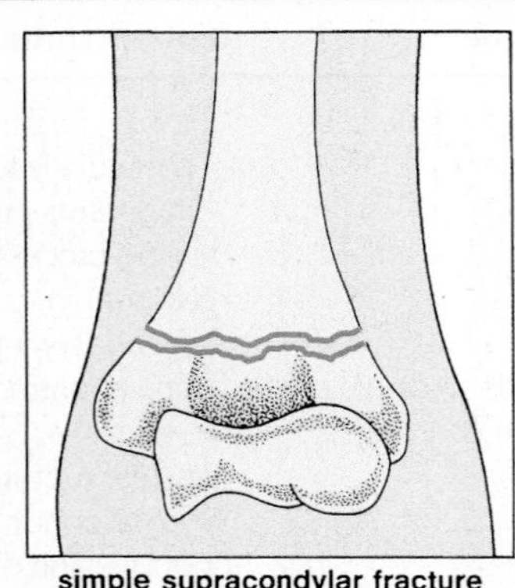

simple supracondylar fracture

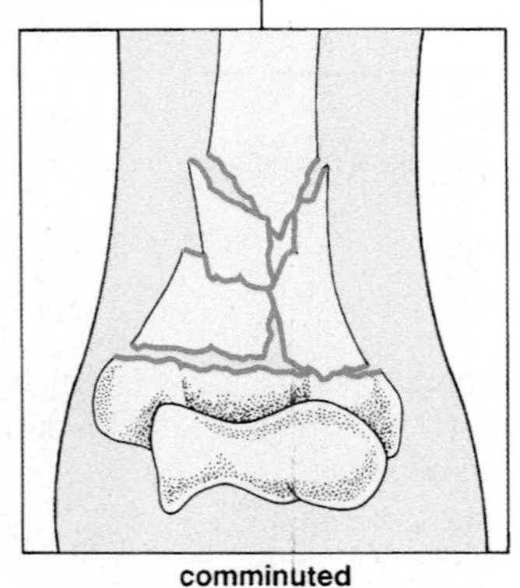

comminuted supracondylar fracture

Intra-articular—Transcondylar

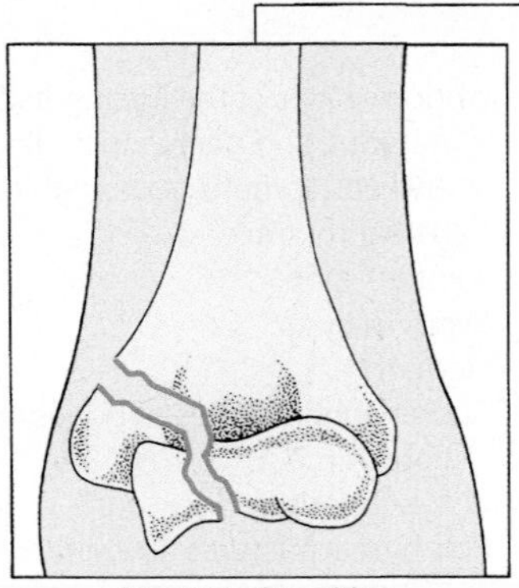

fracture of trochlea

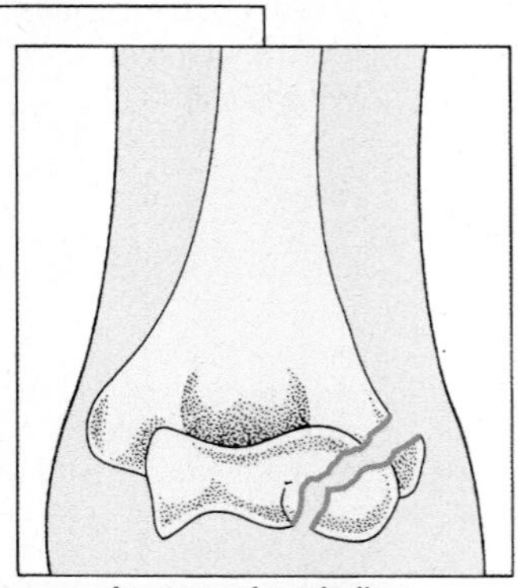

fracture of capitellum

Intra-articular—Bicondylar, Intercondylar

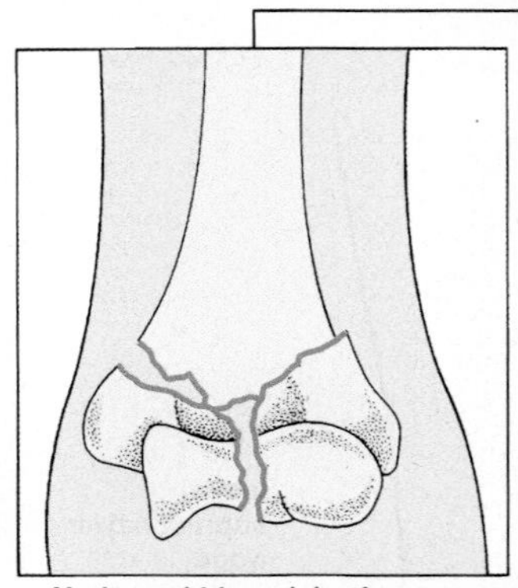

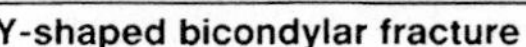

Y-shaped bicondylar fracture

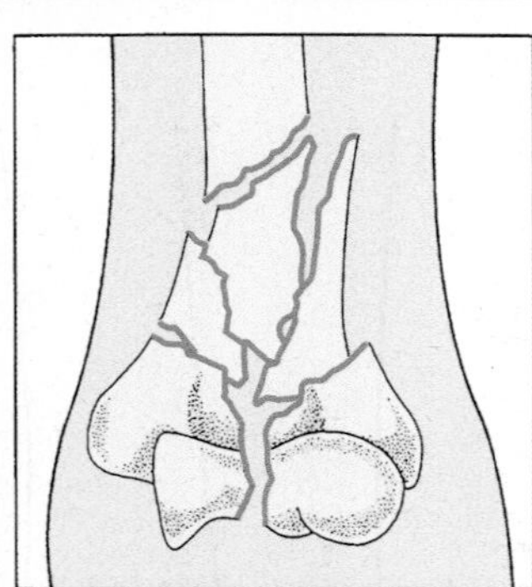

Y-shaped intercondylar fracture with supracondylar comminution

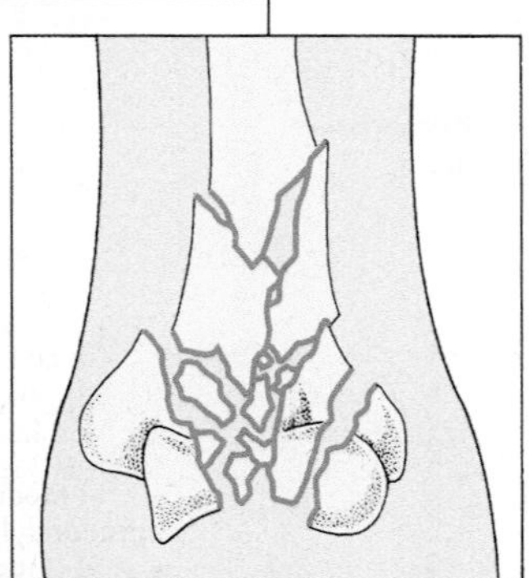

complex comminuted fracture

FIGURE 6.20 Fractures of the distal humerus. Classification of fractures of the distal humerus on the basis of extraarticular and intraarticular extension. (Modified by permission from Springer: Müller ME, Allgower M, Schneider R, et al. *Manual of internal fixation, techniques recommended by the AO Group*, 2nd ed. Berlin, Germany: Springer-Verlag; 1979.)

In children, the diagnosis may be problematic because of the presence of the secondary centers of ossification and their variability. Nevertheless, the anteroposterior and lateral projections usually suffice to demonstrate the abnormality, although the fracture line is occasionally more difficult to evaluate on the anteroposterior than on the lateral view. In children between the ages of 3 and 10 years, supracondylar fracture is the most common type of elbow fracture. Extension injury, caused by a fall on the outstretched hand with the elbow hyperextended, is present in 95% of such cases, and characteristically, the distal fragment is posteriorly displaced (Fig. 6.24). In the flexion type of injury caused by a fall on the flexed elbow, which occurs in only 5% of cases of supracondylar fracture, the distal fragment is anteriorly and upwardly displaced. Identifying supracondylar fracture on the lateral projection is usually facilitated by recognition of the loss of the normal hockey-stick appearance of the distal humerus and displacement of the capitellum relative to the line of the anterior cortex of the humerus (see Figs. 6.11 and 6.12). A positive fat-pad sign is invariably present (Fig. 6.25).

Whatever the age of the patient, it is important in a fracture of the distal humerus to demonstrate and evaluate fully the type of injury, the extension of the fracture line, and the degree of displacement because the method of treatment varies accordingly. When difficulties in interpretation of the type of fracture and the degree of displacement arise, it may be helpful to obtain films of the contralateral normal elbow for comparison.

Complications. The most serious complications of supracondylar fracture are Volkmann ischemic contracture (see Fig. 4.78) and malunion. The latter commonly results in a varus deformity of the elbow, known as *cubitus varus*.

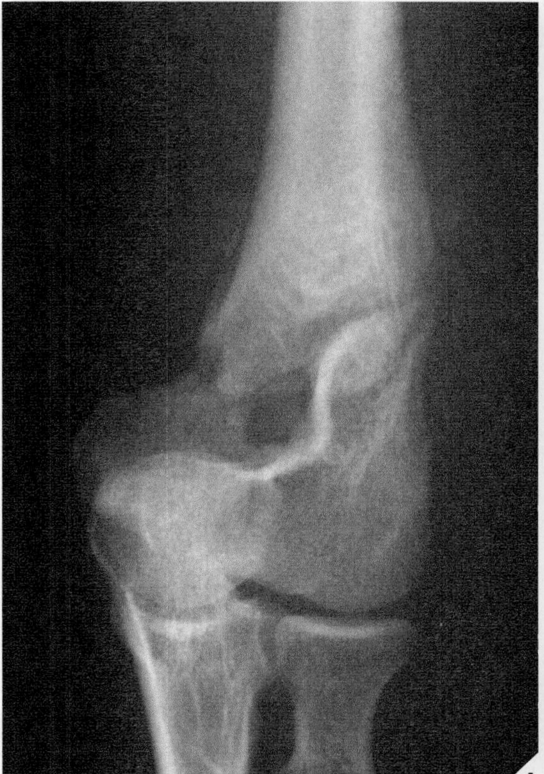

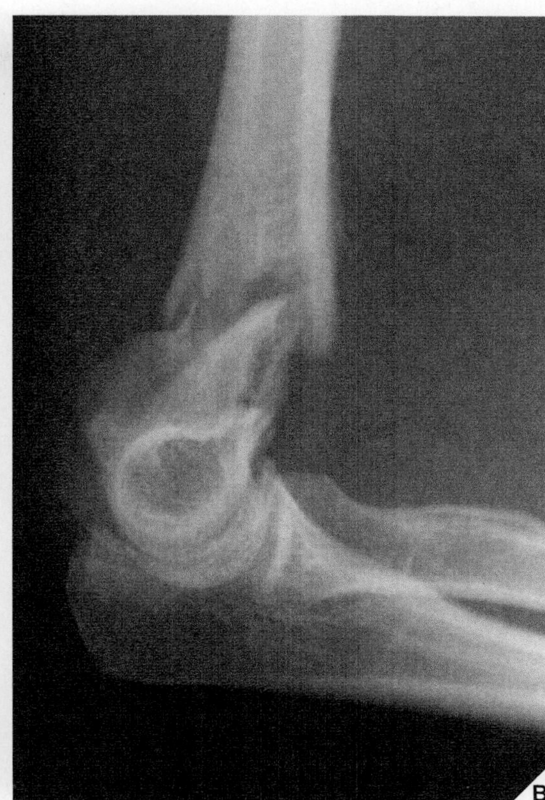

FIGURE 6.21 Supracondylar fracture. A 27-year-old man fell from the ladder onto his outstretched arm. **(A)** Anteroposterior and **(B)** lateral radiographs show a simple supracondylar fracture of the humerus with posterior displacement of the distal fragment.

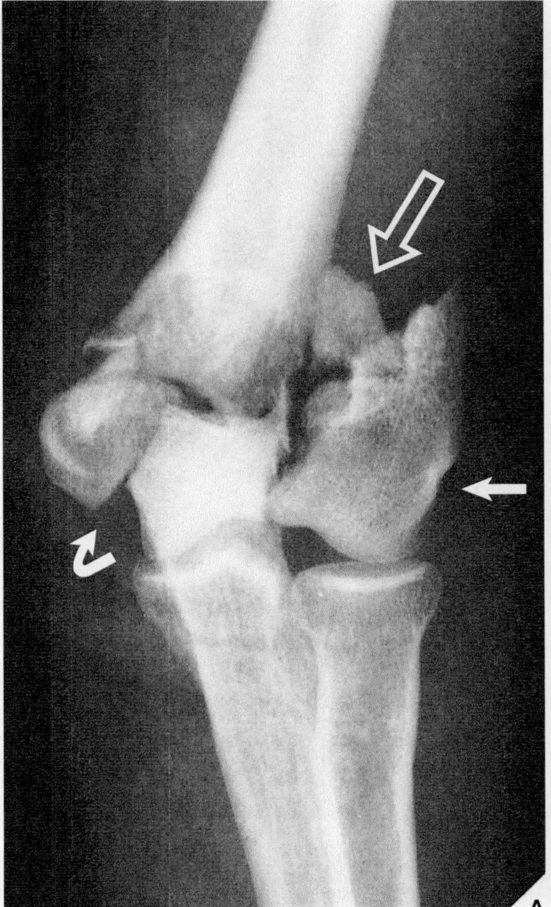

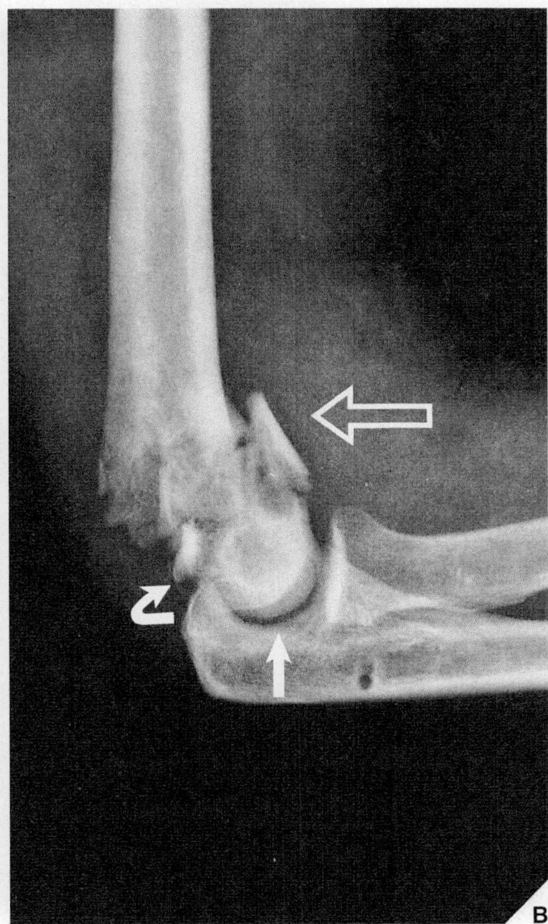

FIGURE 6.22 Fracture of the distal humerus. A 25-year-old man sustained a complex intraarticular fracture of the distal humerus in a motorcycle accident. **(A)** Anteroposterior and **(B)** lateral radiographs clearly demonstrate the extension of the fracture lines and the position of the various fragments. The capitellum is separated, laterally displaced, and subluxed *(arrow)*; the lateral supracondylar ridge is avulsed and anterolaterally displaced *(open arrow)*; and the medial epicondyle is externally rotated and medially displaced *(curved arrow)*.

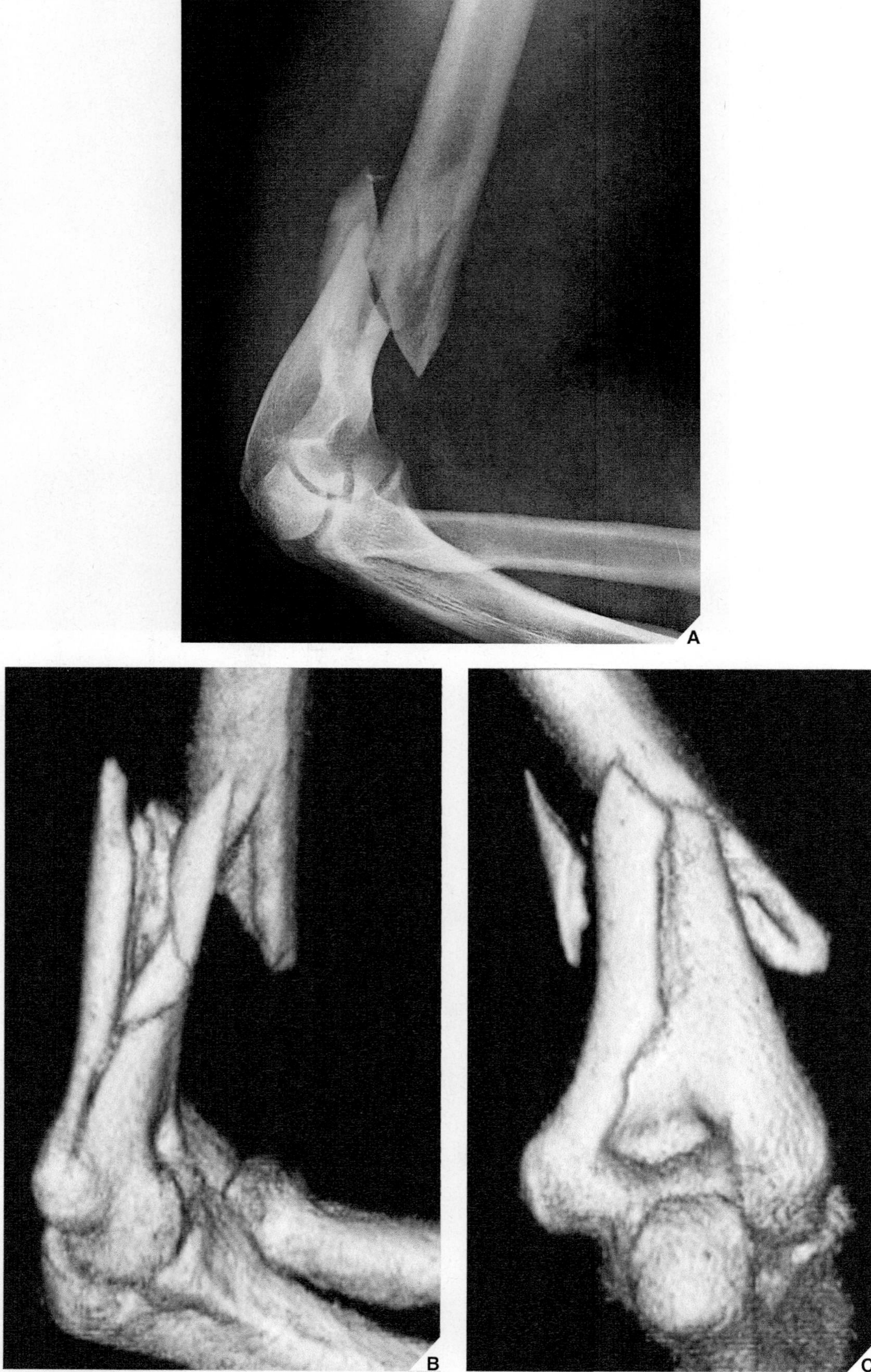

FIGURE 6.23 Three-dimensional (3D) CT of a fracture of the distal humerus. **(A)** A conventional radiograph shows a comminuted supracondylar fracture of the humerus. **(B,C)** 3D CT reconstructed images demonstrate the details of this injury, including displacement, angulation, and spatial orientation of various fragments.

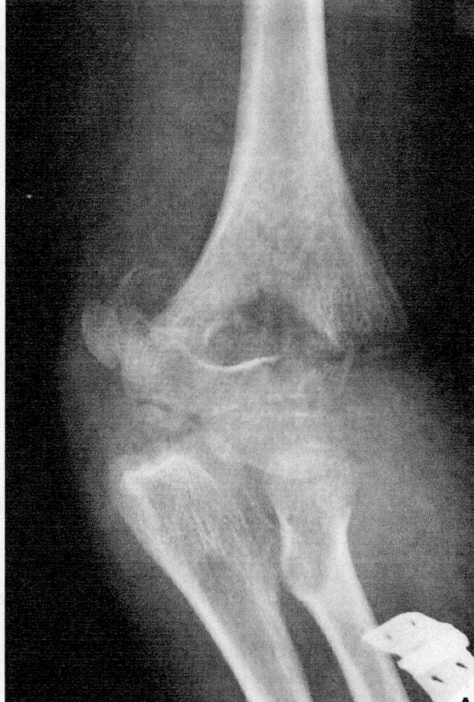
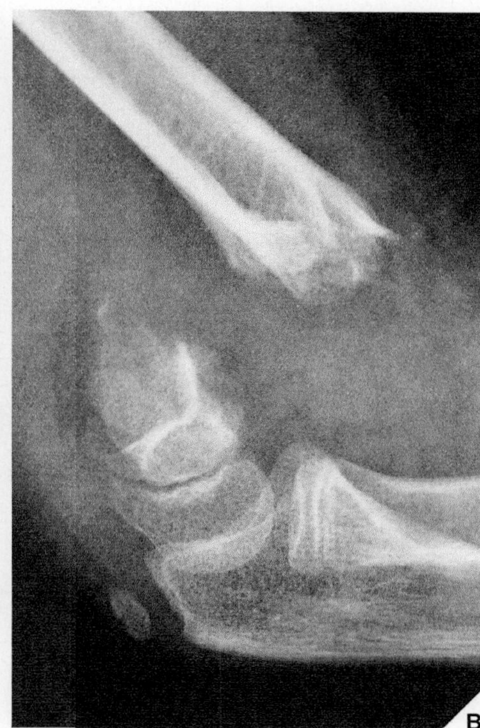

FIGURE 6.24 Displaced supracondylar fracture. A 9-year-old boy fell off his bicycle onto his outstretched hand. **(A)** Anteroposterior and **(B)** lateral radiographs of the elbow show supracondylar fracture of the distal humerus with posteromedial displacement of the distal fragment. Note the increase in the valgus angle of the forearm on the anteroposterior view (see also Fig. 6.11D,E).

Fractures of the Radial Head

A fracture of the radial head is a common injury that results, in most cases, from a fall on the outstretched arm and, only rarely, from a direct blow to the lateral aspect of the elbow.

Radial head fractures have been classified by Mason into three types: type I, undisplaced fractures; type II, marginal fractures with displacement (including impaction, depression, and angulation); and type III, comminuted fractures involving the entire head. Later, DeLee, Green, and Wilkins suggested adding type IV, fractures of the radial head in association with elbow dislocation (Fig. 6.26). All these fractures can be adequately demonstrated on the anteroposterior and lateral radiographs of the elbow. However, because nondisplaced or minimally displaced fractures may go undetected on these projections, the radial head–capitellum view should be included in the routine radiographic examination to detect occult injuries and to evaluate the degree of displacement (Figs. 6.27 to 6.29). Determination of the exact extension of the fracture line (i.e., whether it is extraarticular or intraarticular) and the degree of displacement is crucial to deciding the course of treatment. CT examination plays an important role in this assessment (Fig. 6.30), although MRI may be helpful in confirming the presence of a fracture not clearly shown on routine radiographs (Fig. 6.31). Nondisplaced or minimally displaced fractures are usually treated conservatively by the use of splints or casts, until healing allows active mobilization of the elbow. However, a cleavage fracture of the radial articular surface involving one third or one half of the head with displacement greater than 3 to 4 mm usually indicates the need for open reduction and internal fixation; this is particularly true in younger individuals. Excision of the radial head is the procedure of choice when comminution and displacement of the radial head are present (Fig. 6.32).

Essex-Lopresti Fracture–Dislocation

This complex injury comprises a comminuted fracture of the radial head and neck with or without distal extension of fracture line, tear of the

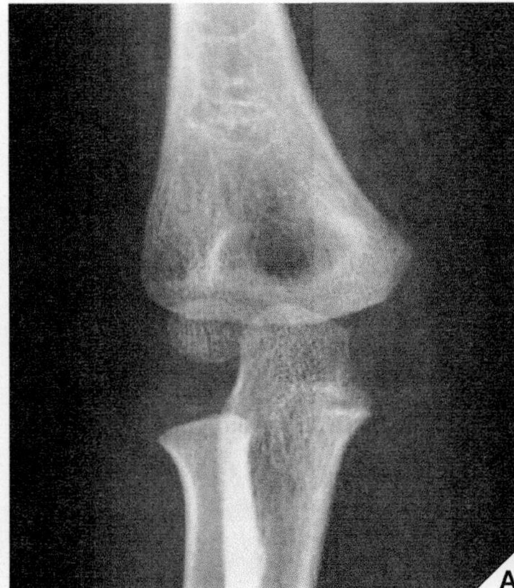
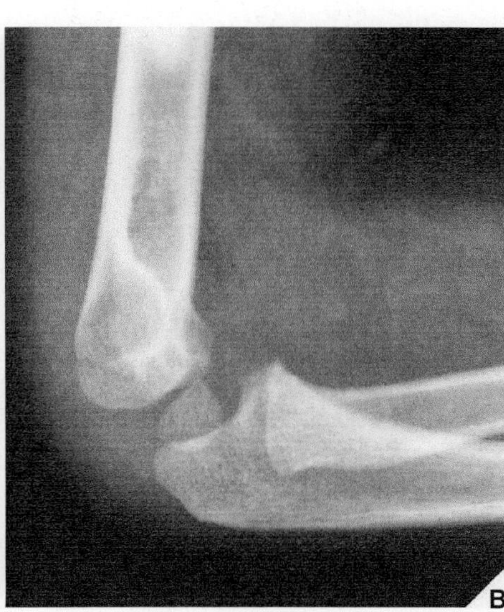
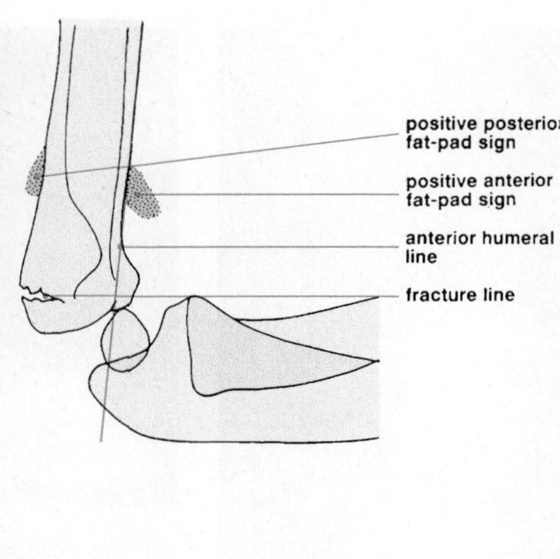

FIGURE 6.25 Nondisplaced supracondylar fracture. A 3-year-old girl fell on the street. On the anteroposterior radiograph **(A)**, the fracture line is practically invisible, whereas on the lateral view **(B)**, it is more obvious. There is a positive posterior fat-pad sign, and the anterior fat pad is also clearly displaced. Note that the anterior humeral line intersects the posterior third of the capitellum, indicating slight anterior angulation of the distal fragment.

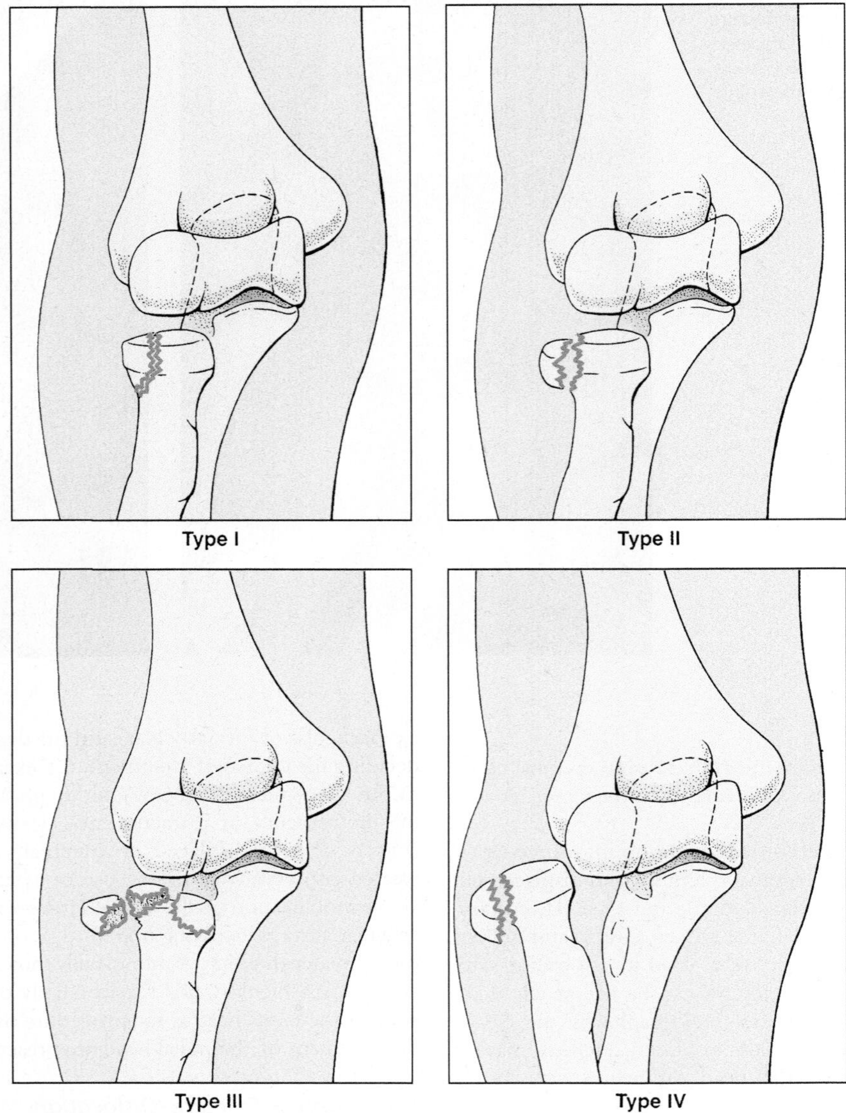

FIGURE 6.26 Mason classification of fractures of the radial head.

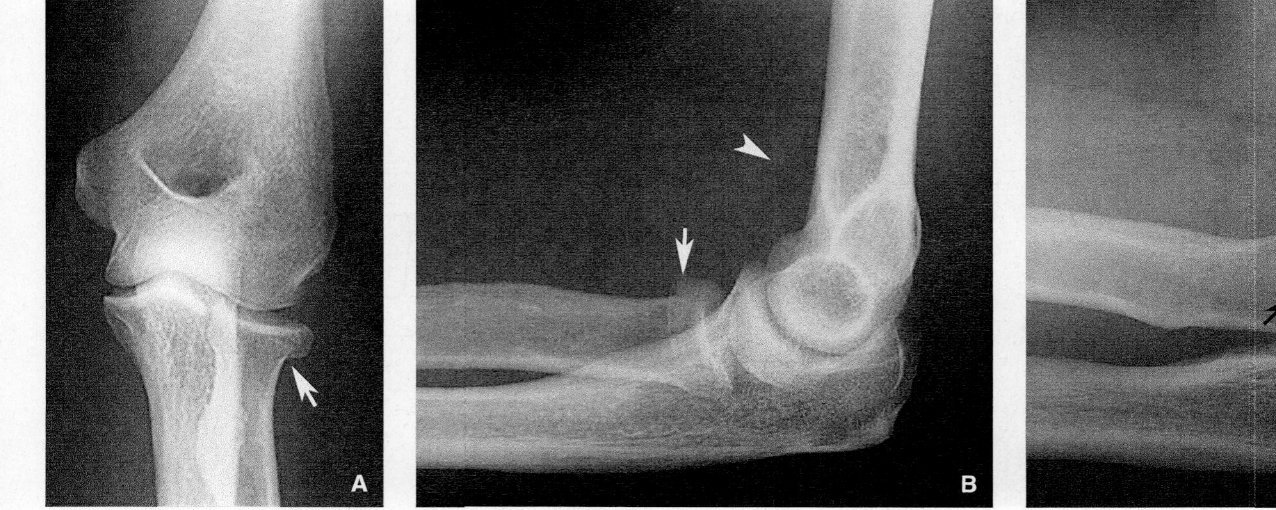

FIGURE 6.27 Fracture of the radial head. Anteroposterior **(A)** and lateral **(B)** radiographs of the elbow show what appears to be a nondisplaced fracture of the radial head *(arrows)*. Note the elevation of the anterior fat pad indicative of a joint effusion (*arrowhead*). On the radial head—capitellum view **(C)**, however, intraarticular extension of the fracture line and 2-mm depression of the subchondral fragment are clearly demonstrated *(arrow)*. (Courtesy of Oleg Opsha, MD, Brooklyn, New York.)

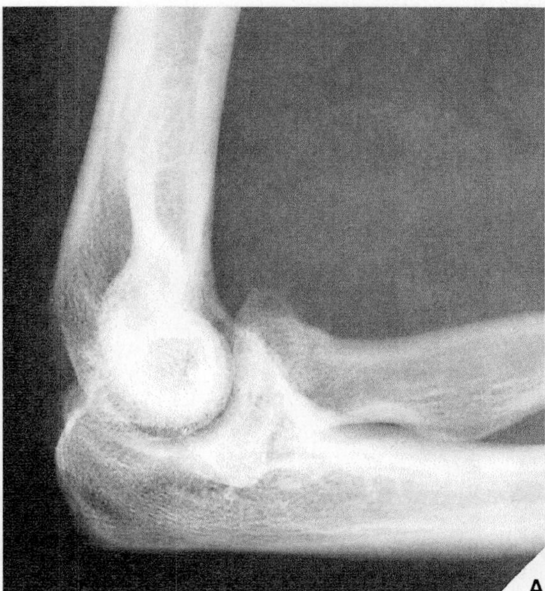

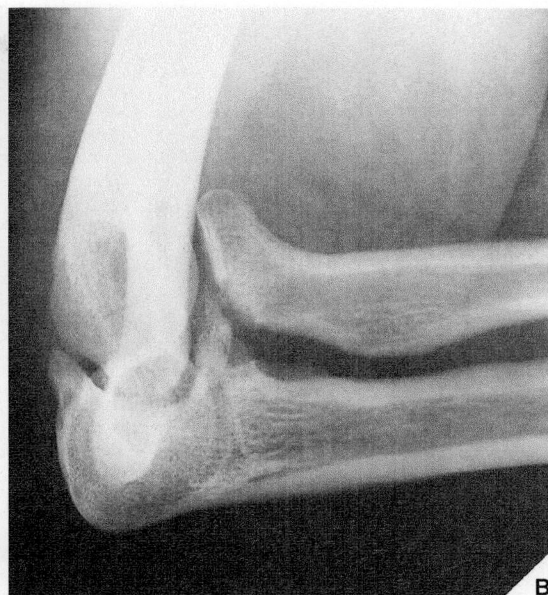

FIGURE 6.28 Fracture of the radial head. **(A)** Standard lateral radiograph of the elbow demonstrates a fracture of the radial head, but an overlap of the osseous structures prevents the exact evaluation of the extent of the fracture line and the degree of displacement. **(B)** Radial head–capitellum view reveals it to be a displaced articular fracture involving the posterior third of the radial head. (Reprinted from Greenspan A, Norman A, Rosen H. Radial head-capitellum view in elbow trauma: clinical application and radiographic-anatomic correlation. *Am J Roentgenol* 1984;143:355–359. Copyright © 1984 American Roentgen Ray Society.)

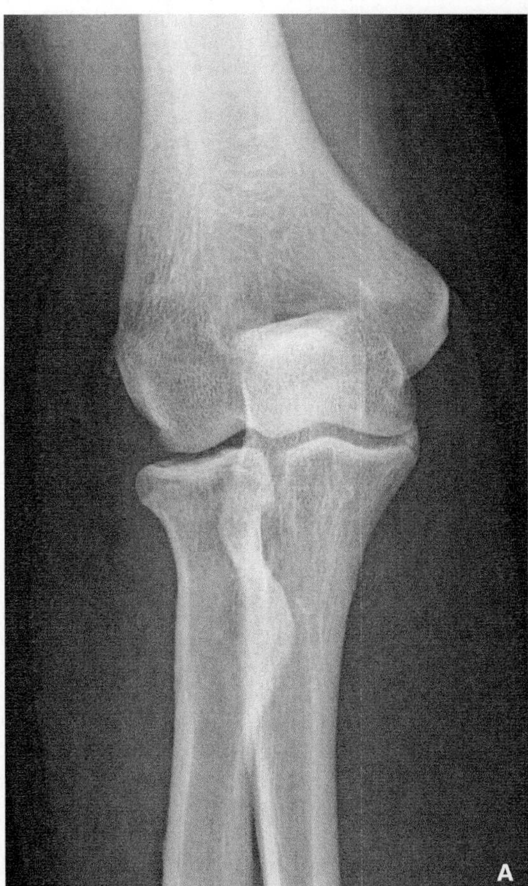

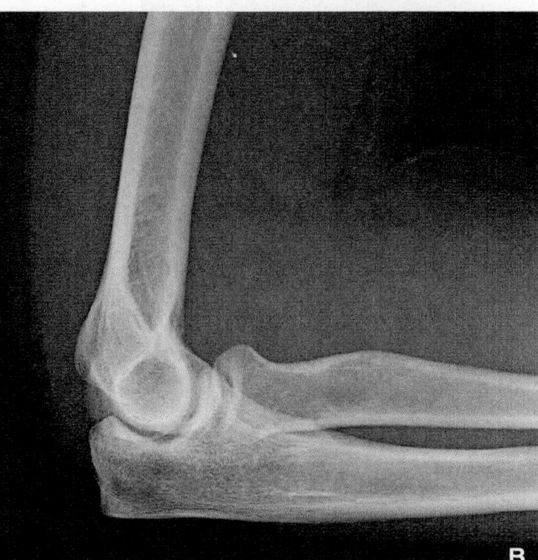

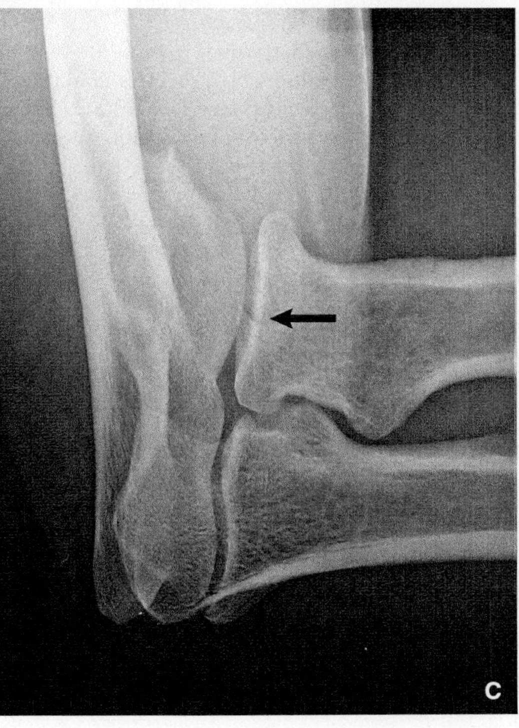

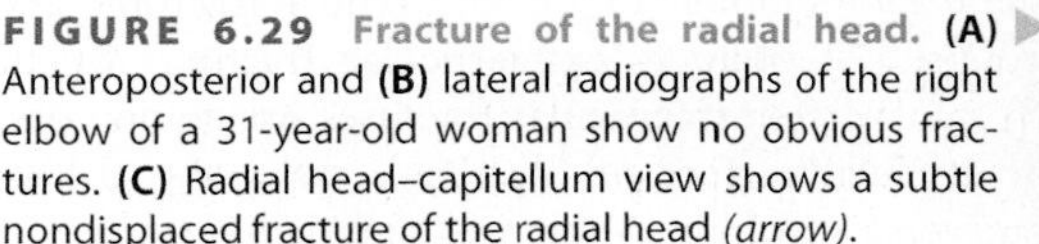

FIGURE 6.29 Fracture of the radial head. **(A)** Anteroposterior and **(B)** lateral radiographs of the right elbow of a 31-year-old woman show no obvious fractures. **(C)** Radial head–capitellum view shows a subtle nondisplaced fracture of the radial head *(arrow)*.

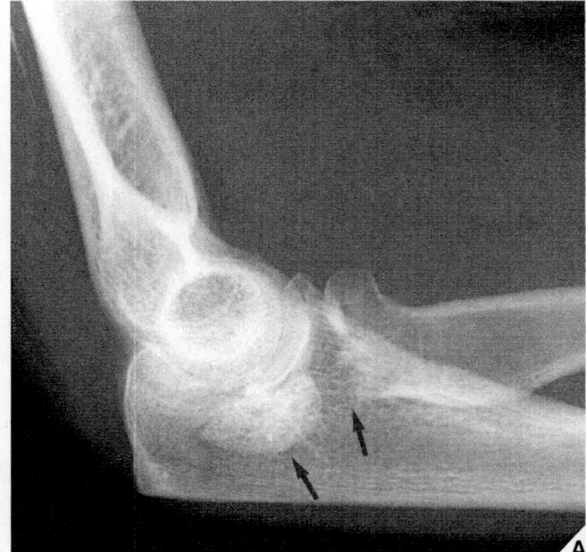

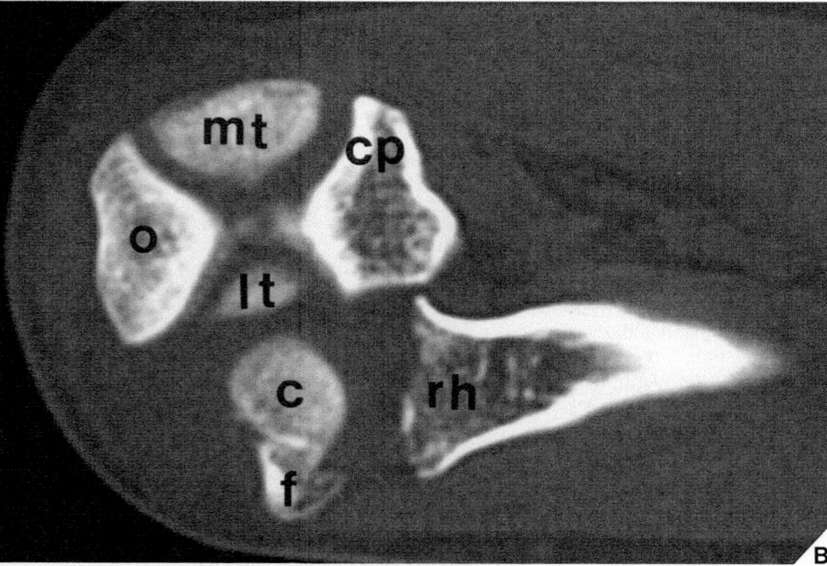

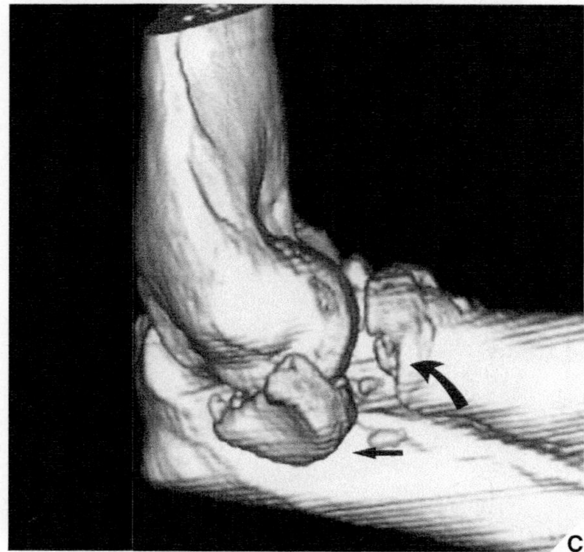

FIGURE 6.30 **CT and 3D CT of a fracture of the radial head. (A)** Conventional lateral radiograph of the elbow shows a displaced fracture of the radial head *(arrows)*. **(B)** Oblique coronal CT shows posterolateral displacement of the fractured fragment, although anatomic orientation is somewhat ambiguous on this image. o, olecranon; mt, medial trochlea; cp, coronoid process; lt, lateral trochlea; c, capitellum; rh, radial head; f, displaced fractured fragment. **(C)** Three-dimensional (3D) CT reconstruction image (viewed from the lateral aspect) demonstrates the spatial orientation of the fracture. The *arrow* points to the posterolaterally displaced fragment, and the *curved arrow* indicates a defect in the radial head.

interosseous membrane of the forearm, and dislocation in the distal radioulnar joint (Fig. 6.33). This is an unstable injury that, because of bipolar loss of radial support at both sites (elbow and wrist), requires unique and tailored treatment. In most patients, interfragmentary fixation of a radial head fracture is performed, or, in cases of severe comminution, silastic or metallic radial head prosthesis may be indicated to maintain length and stability. Chronic Essex-Lopresti injury with irreducible proximal migration of the radius may require ulnar shortening to restore neutral ulnar variance.

Fracture of the Coronoid Process

Rarely occurring as an isolated injury (Fig. 6.34), a fracture of the coronoid process is most often associated with posterior dislocation in the elbow joint (Fig. 6.35). It is, therefore, important in cases of elbow injury to exclude the possibility of a fracture of the coronoid process, because if undiagnosed, it may fail to unite, leading to instability and recurrent subluxation in the joint. The anteroposterior and lateral projections are usually insufficient to evaluate the coronoid process because of overlap of structures on these views. The demonstration of an injury can be made on the radial head–capitellum projection (Fig. 6.36) and, occasionally, on the internal oblique view; however, the best technique to show the coronoid process fracture is CT (Figs. 6.37 and 6.38).

Fracture of the Olecranon

Olecranon fractures usually result from a direct fall on the flexed elbow, and this mechanism frequently produces comminution and marked displacement of the major fragments. An indirect mechanism, such as a fall on the outstretched arm, produces an oblique or transverse fracture with minimal displacement. The fracture is usually well demonstrated on a lateral projection of the elbow.

A number of classifications have been developed to evaluate an olecranon fracture. Colton classified olecranon fractures as undisplaced and displaced, the latter group being subdivided into avulsion fractures, oblique and transverse fractures, comminuted fractures, and fracture–dislocations.

Another practical classification has been developed by Horne and Tanzer, who classified these fractures by their location apparent on the lateral radiographs (Fig. 6.39). Type I fractures are subdivided into two groups: (A) oblique, extraarticular fractures of the olecranon tip and (B) transverse intraarticular fractures originating on the proximal third of the articular surface of olecranon fossa (Fig. 6.40). Type II fractures are transverse or oblique fractures originating on the middle third of the articular surface of olecranon fossa. These fractures also are subdivided into two groups: (A) single fracture line and (B) two fracture lines, one proximal (transverse or oblique) and the second, more distal, extending posteriorly (Figs. 6.41 and 6.42). Type III fractures involve the distal third of the olecranon fossa and may be either transverse or oblique (Fig. 6.43). Most common fractures are of type II.

As far as treatment is concerned, nondisplaced fractures are usually treated conservatively, whereas displaced fractures are most often treated by open reduction and internal fixation.

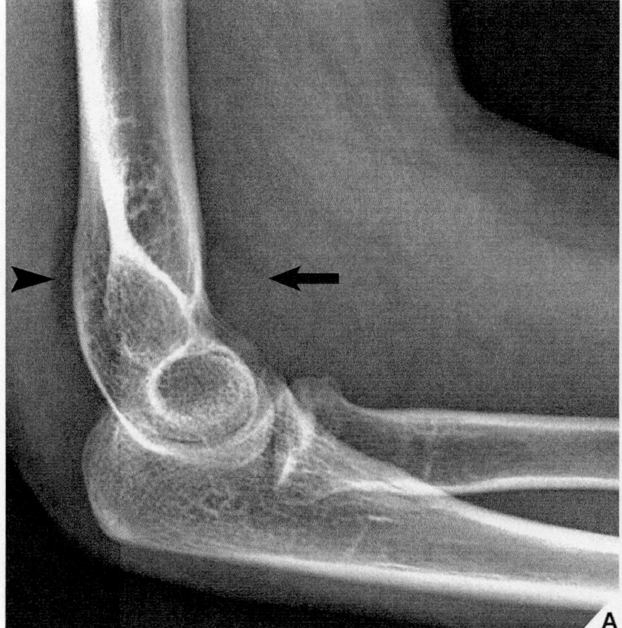

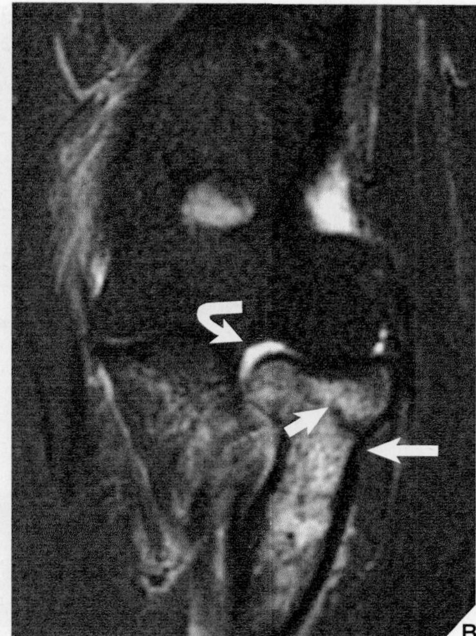

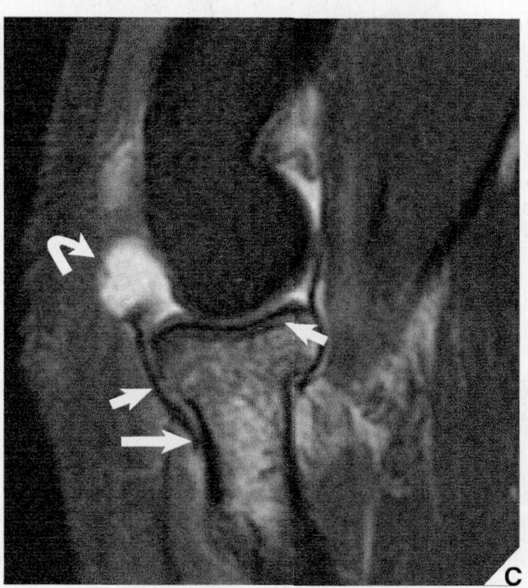

FIGURE 6.31 MRI of a fracture of the radial head. **(A)** Conventional lateral radiograph of an elbow shows a positive anterior *(arrow)* and posterior *(arrowhead)* fat-pad sign. The radial head is somewhat deformed, suggestive of an acute fracture. **(B)** Coronal and **(C)** sagittal T2-weighted MR images demonstrate bone marrow edema of the radial head and neck *(arrows)*, joint effusion *(curved arrows)*, and low–signal intensity linear areas representing fracture lines *(short arrows)*.

FIGURE 6.32 Fracture of the radial head. **(A)** Anteroposterior and **(B)** lateral radiographs of the elbow show a markedly comminuted and displaced fracture of the radial head. An excision of the entire radial head would most likely be necessary.

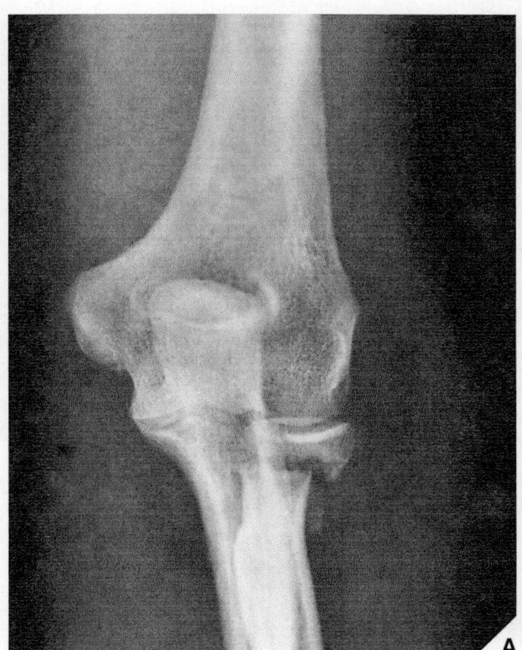

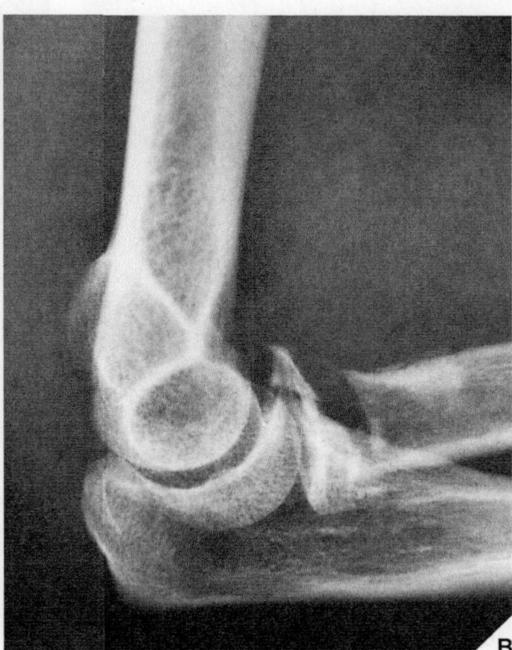

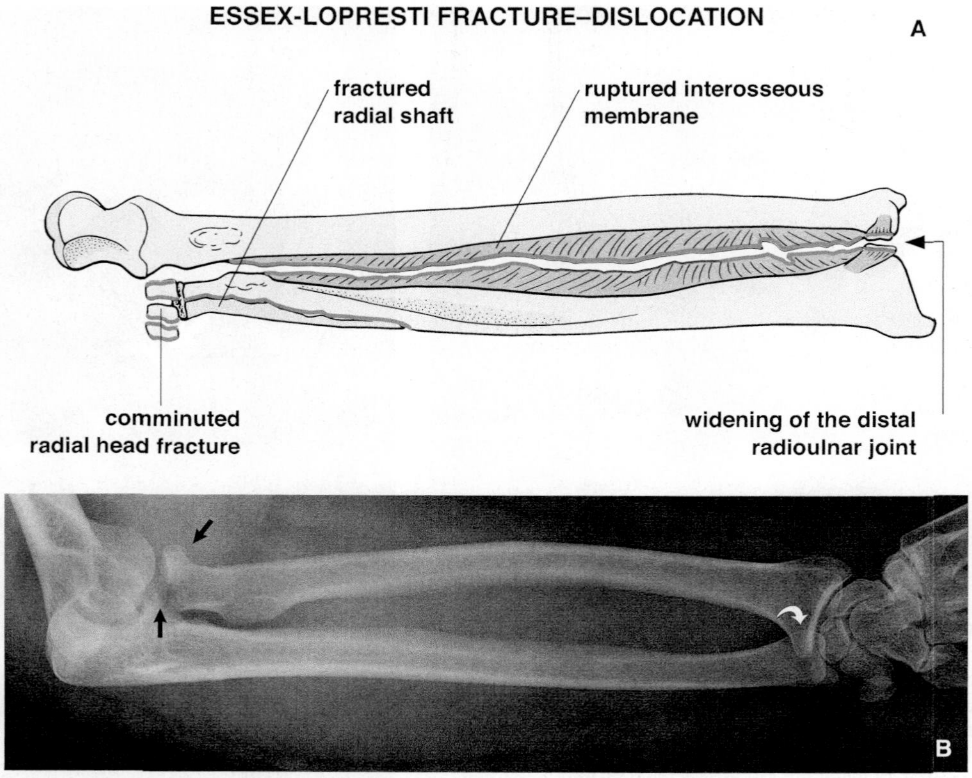

ESSEX-LOPRESTI FRACTURE–DISLOCATION

A

fractured radial shaft

ruptured interosseous membrane

comminuted radial head fracture

widening of the distal radioulnar joint

B

FIGURE 6.33 Essex-Lopresti fracture–dislocation. **(A)** The crucial elements of this injury comprise a comminuted fracture of the radial head, ruptured interosseous membrane, and dislocation in the distal radioulnar joint. **(B)** A 62-year-old man presented with injury to the right forearm sustained in a motorcycle accident. Note a comminuted fracture of the radial head *(arrows)* and dislocation in the distal radioulnar joint *(curved arrow)*.

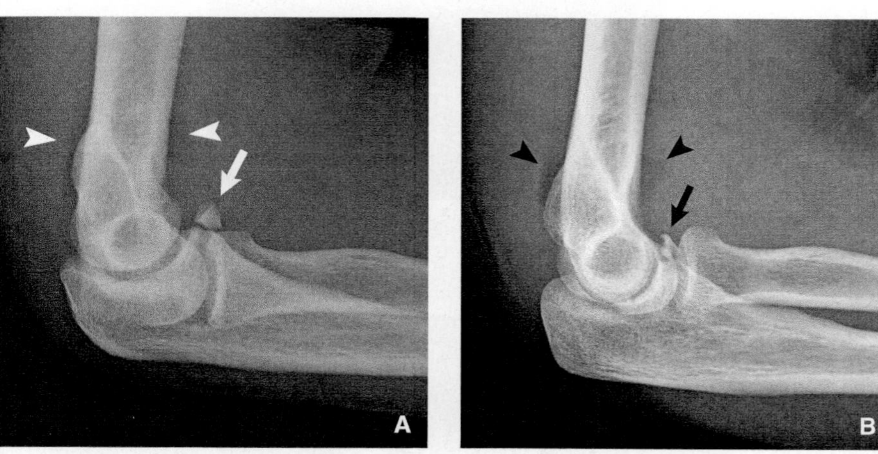

FIGURE 6.34 Fracture of the coronoid process. **(A)** Lateral radiograph of the elbow shows a fracture at the base of the coronoid process *(arrow)*. The *arrowheads* point to the positive anterior and posterior fat-pad sign. **(B)** Lateral radiograph of the elbow of another patient shows similar fracture of the coronoid process *(arrow)* and joint effusion *(arrowheads)*.

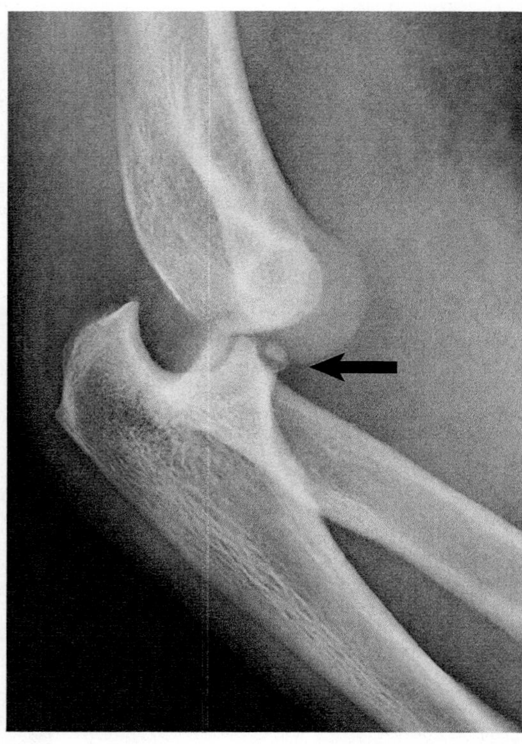

FIGURE 6.35 Fracture of the coronoid process. This injury *(arrow)* commonly occurs during a posterior dislocation in the elbow joint.

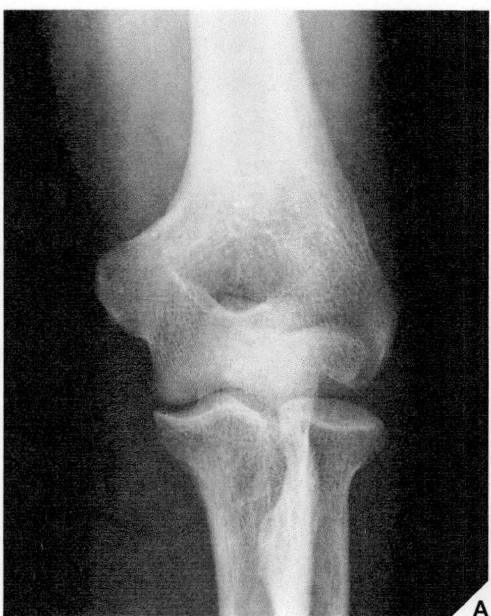

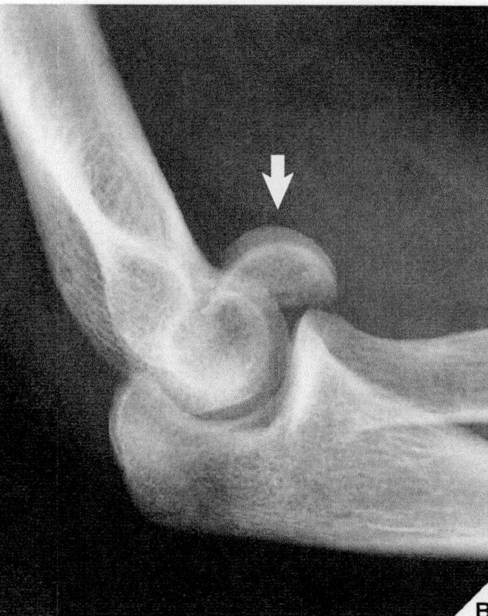

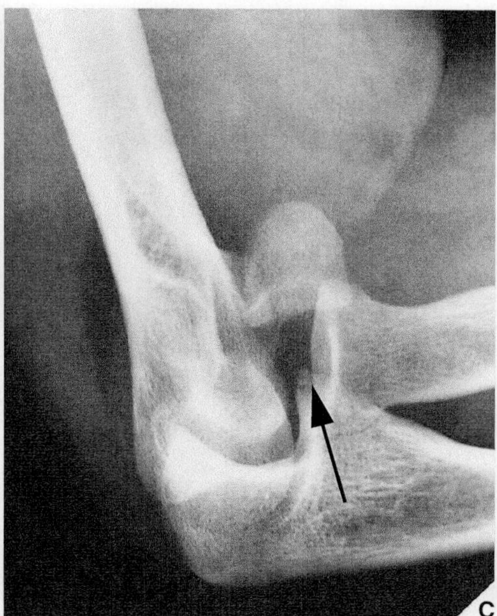

FIGURE 6.36 **Fractures of the capitellum and the coronoid process.** While playing ice hockey, a 37-year-old man injured his right elbow in a fall. The initial anteroposterior **(A)** and lateral **(B)** radiographs show a fracture of the capitellum with anterior rotation and displacement. Note the typical "half-moon" appearance of the displaced capitellum on the lateral view *(arrow)*. On the radial head–capitellum film **(C)**, an unsuspected, nondisplaced fracture of the coronoid process is evident *(long arrow)*.

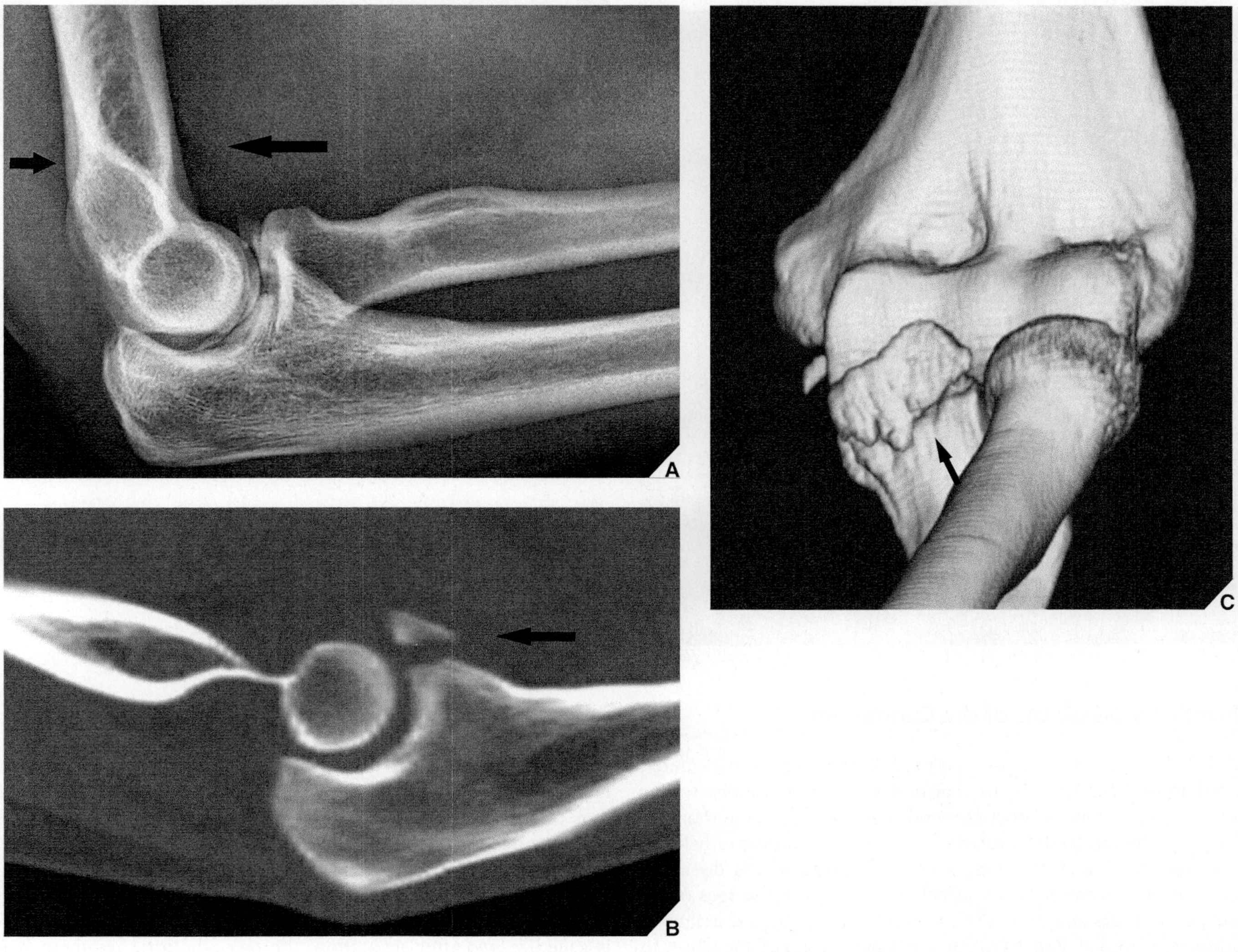

FIGURE 6.37 **CT and three-dimensional (3D) CT of a fracture of the coronoid process.** **(A)** Lateral radiograph of the elbow shows a positive posterior and anterior fat-pad sign *(arrows)*, but a fracture of the coronoid process is not well demonstrated. **(B)** Sagittal reformatted CT image and **(C)** 3D CT reconstructed image in shaded surface display are diagnostic for this injury *(arrows)*.

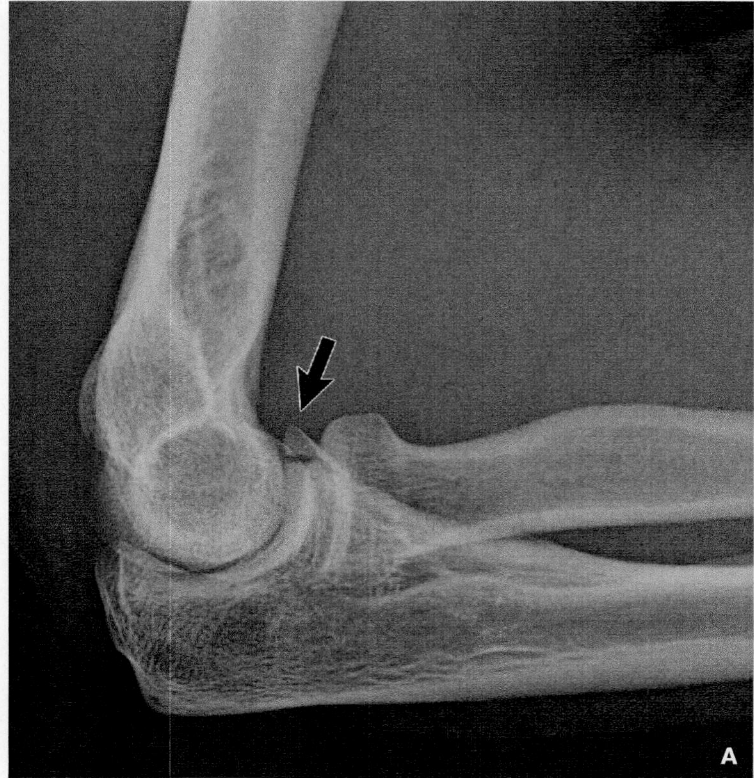

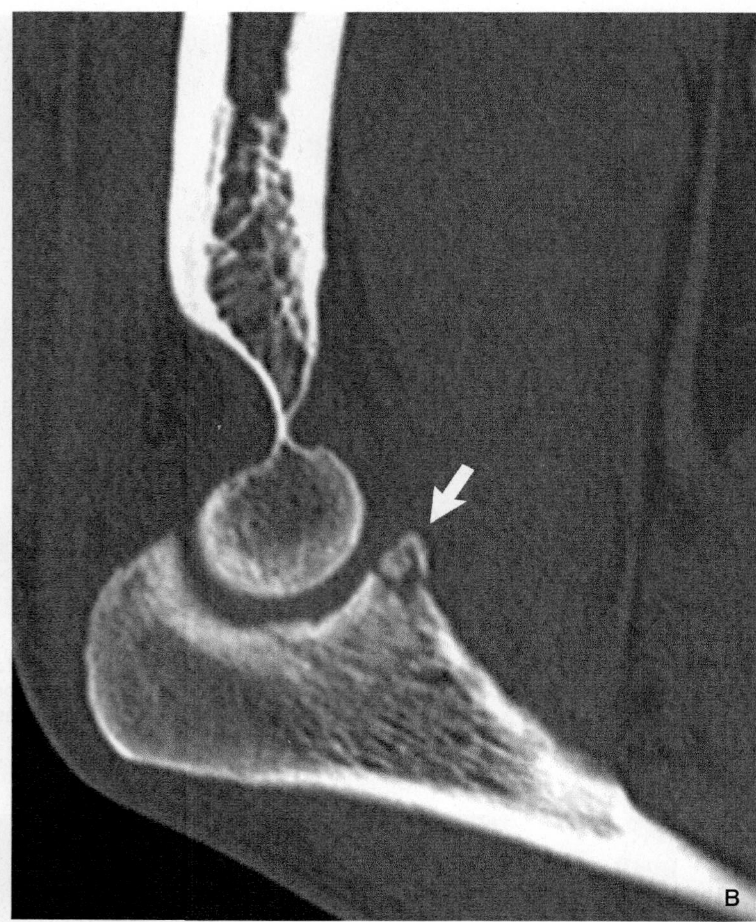

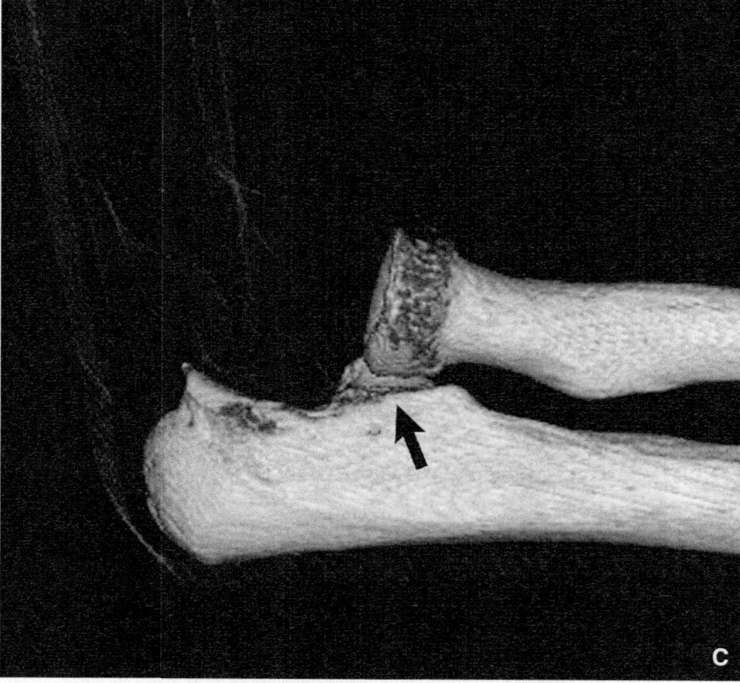

FIGURE 6.38 CT and three-dimensional (3D) CT of a fracture of the coronoid process. **(A)** Lateral radiograph of the elbow, **(B)** sagittal reformatted CT image, and **(C)** 3D reconstructed CT image viewed from the lateral aspect of the elbow joint demonstrate a fracture of the coronoid process *(arrows)*.

Osteochondritis Dissecans of the Capitellum

This condition, also occasionally referred to as *Panner disease*, is considered to be related to trauma, namely, to repeated exogenous injuries to the elbow. However, some investigators contend that Panner disease is an osteochondrosis of the capitellum and affects children (predominantly boys) between the ages of 7 and 12 years, whereas osteochondritis dissecans of the capitellum is a separate entity, affects boys between the ages of 12 and 15 years, and occurs at a time when the epiphysis of the capitellum is almost completely ossified. Regardless of age, valgus strain of the elbow in throwing sports such as baseball and football has been implicated as one causative factor. Apparently during the throwing motion, the capitellum is subjected to compression and to shear forces. It most frequently affects the right elbow in right-handed children and adolescents, the majority of whom are males.

In the early stage of the disease, anteroposterior and lateral films may show no significant abnormality (Fig. 6.44A,B); the only radiographic sign of early-stage Panner disease may become apparent on the radial head–capitellum view with the finding of subtle flattening of the capitellum (Fig. 6.44C). As the condition progresses, the lesion, consisting of a detached segment of subchondral bone with overlying cartilage, gradually separates from its bed in the capitellum. Before separation, the lesion is called *in situ*; after separation, the osteochondral fragment becomes a "loose" body in the joint (Fig. 6.45). Because sometimes more than one fragment is discharged into the joint, osteochondritis dissecans may be mistaken for idiopathic synovial (osteo)chondromatosis, a nontraumatic

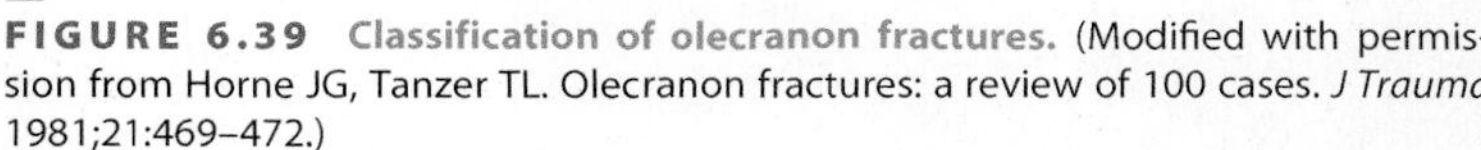

FIGURE 6.39 **Classification of olecranon fractures.** (Modified with permission from Horne JG, Tanzer TL. Olecranon fractures: a review of 100 cases. *J Trauma* 1981;21:469–472.)

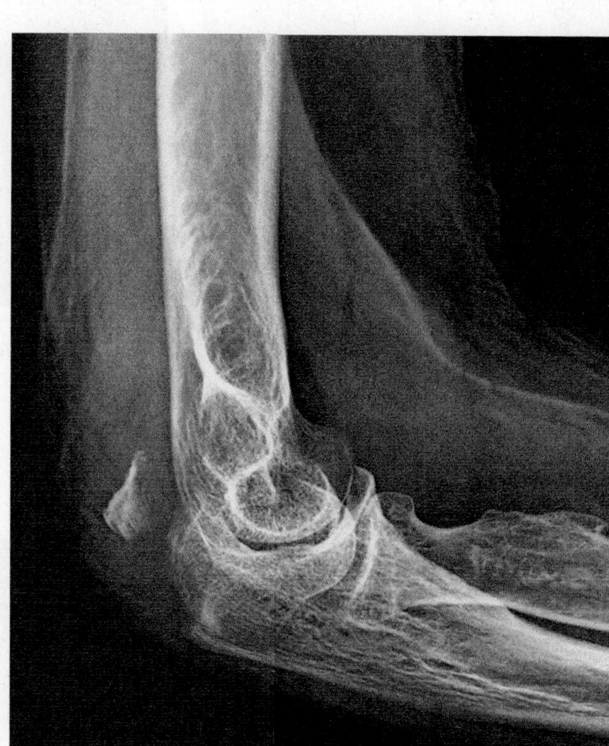

FIGURE 6.40 **Olecranon fracture.** A 76-year-old woman sustained a type I A olecranon fracture after a fall on the stairs.

condition that is a form of synovial metaplasia. In this condition, multiple cartilaginous bodies that are regular in outline and usually uniform in size are seen in the joint (see Fig. 23.2).

In the past, one of the radiologic procedures for evaluating osteochondritis dissecans was arthrotomography, which localized the defect in the cartilaginous surface of the capitellum and distinguished an *in situ* lesion from the more advanced stage of the disease. This information is crucial for the orthopaedic surgeon because the *in situ* lesion may be treated conservatively, whereas surgical intervention may be required if the osteochondral fragment has been partially separated from its bed or discharged into the joint. At the present time, CT-arthrography almost completely replaced arthrotomography, although MRI is also effective to demonstrate the lesion (Fig. 6.46) and to provide information about its stability (Fig. 6.47). Type I lesions are intact (*in situ*), with no fragment displacement; type II lesions are slightly displaced, and the articular surface is damaged; type III lesions show detachment of the osteochondral fragment (Fig. 6.48).

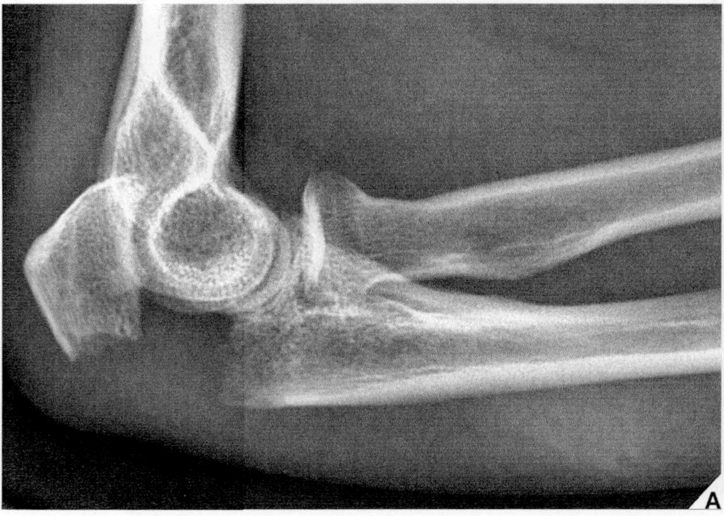

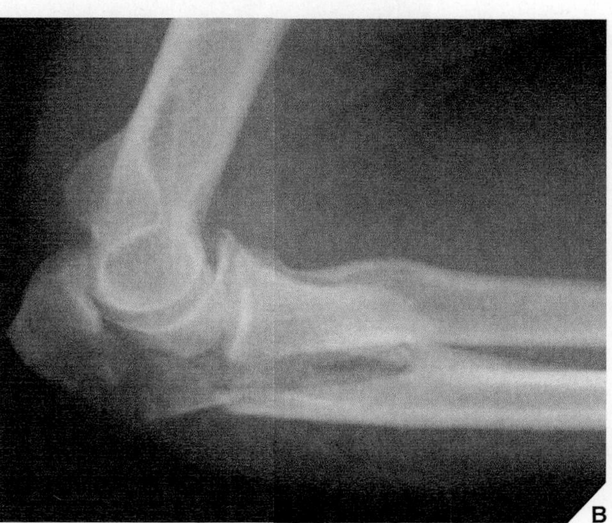

FIGURE 6.41 **Olecranon fracture.** **(A)** A 50-year-old woman fell from a ladder and sustained a type II A displaced olecranon fracture, well demonstrated on this lateral radiograph. **(B)** A 41-year-old man fell on his flexed elbow and sustained a type II B comminuted olecranon fracture.

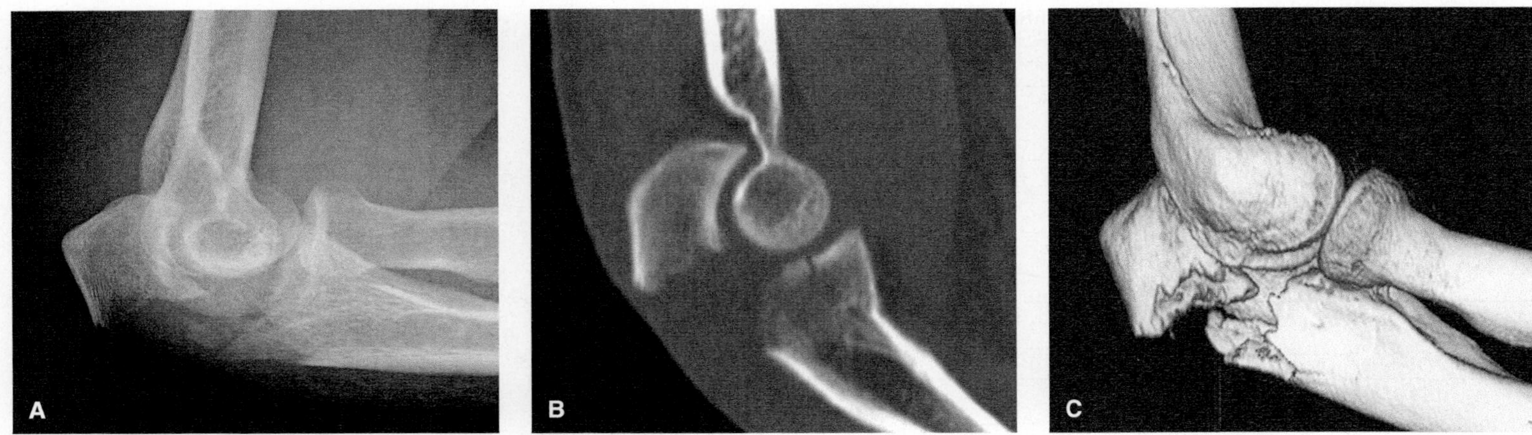

FIGURE 6.42 CT and three-dimensional (3D) CT of the olecranon fracture. **(A)** Lateral radiograph of the elbow, **(B)** sagittal reformatted CT image, and **(C)** 3D CT reconstructed image show type II B fracture of the olecranon.

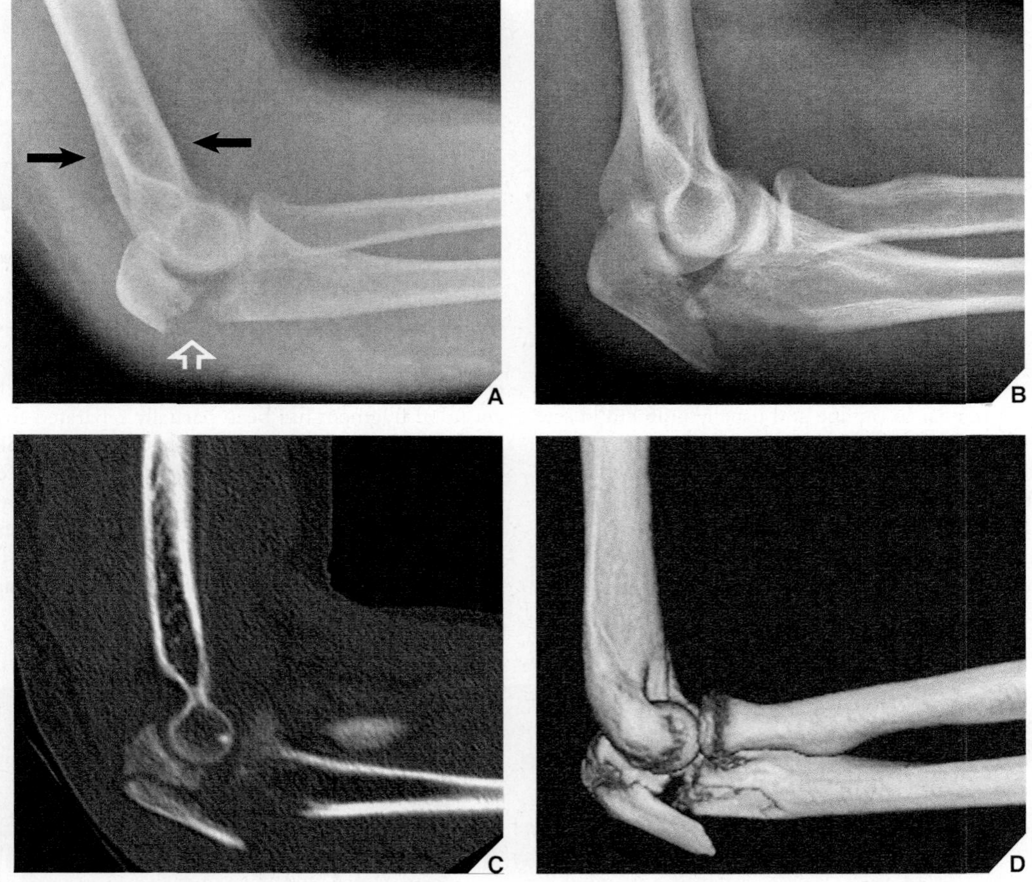

FIGURE 6.43 CT and three-dimensional (3D) CT of olecranon fracture. **(A)** A 52-year-old woman fell on her outstretched arm and sustained a type III olecranon fracture, effectively demonstrated on the lateral radiograph of the elbow. Note the transverse orientation of the fracture line *(open arrow)* and the positive anterior and posterior fat-pad sign *(arrows)*. **(B)** A variant of type III olecranon fracture, where a fracture line is oblique in orientation. **(C)** A sagittal reformatted CT image in another patient shows similar variant of type III fracture, more effectively demonstrated on the 3D CT reconstructed image **(D)**.

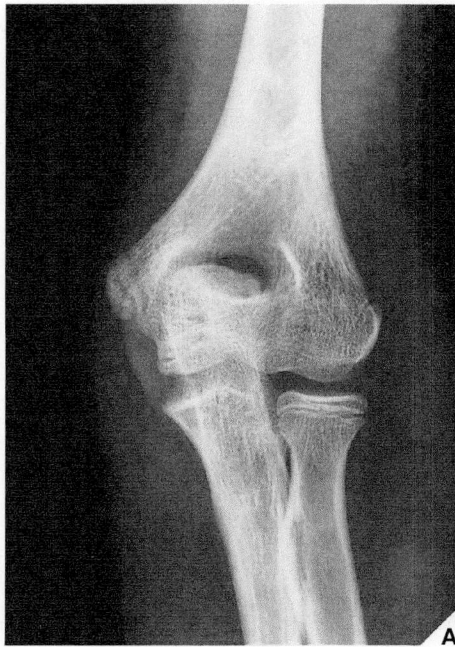

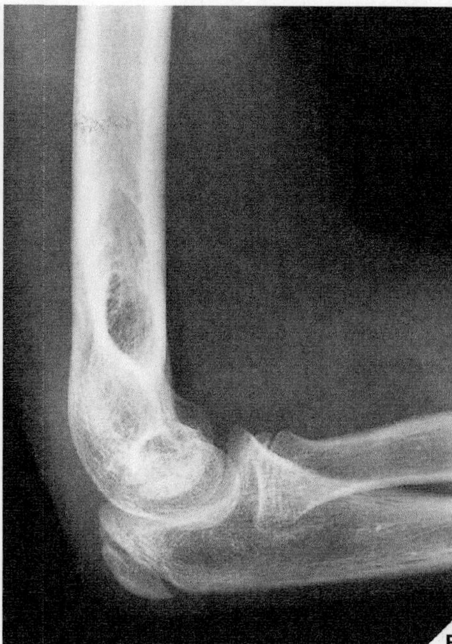

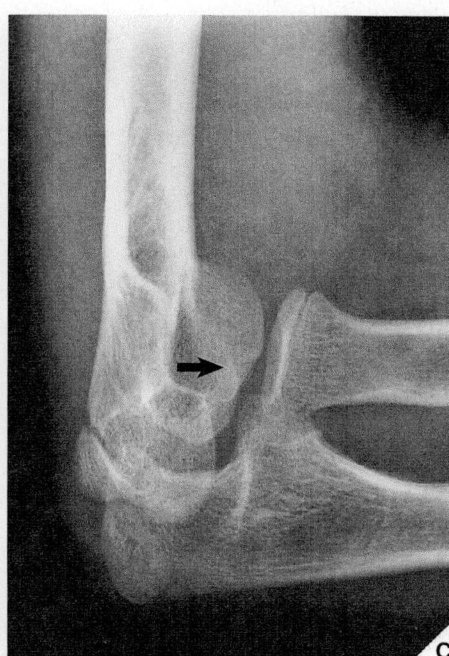

FIGURE 6.44 Osteochondritis dissecans of the capitellum. A 13-year-old boy who was very active in Little League baseball reported pain in his right elbow for several months. **(A)** Anteroposterior and **(B)** lateral radiographs of the elbow demonstrate no abnormalities. **(C)** On the radial head–capitellum view, subtle flattening of the capitellum *(arrow)* may indicate early-stage osteochondritis dissecans. (Reprinted from Greenspan A, Norman A. The radial head-capitellum view: useful technique in elbow trauma. *Am J Roentgenol* 1982;138:1186–1188. Copyright © 1982 American Roentgen Ray Society.)

Dislocations in the Elbow Joint

Simple Dislocations

The standard method of classifying elbow dislocations is based on the direction of displacement of the radius and the ulna in relation to the distal humerus. Three main types of dislocation can be distinguished as those affecting (a) both the radius and the ulna, which may be dislocated posteriorly, anteriorly, medially, or laterally (or in a manner combining posterior or anterior with medial or lateral displacement); (b) the ulna only, which may be anteriorly or posteriorly displaced; and (c) the radius only, which may be anteriorly, posteriorly, or laterally dislocated.

Posterior and posterolateral dislocations of the radius and the ulna are, by far, the most common types. They account for 80% to 90% of all dislocations in the joint (Fig. 6.49). Anterior dislocations are uncommon (Fig. 6.50). Isolated dislocation of the radial head, however, is a rare occurrence; it is more commonly associated with a fracture of the distal humerus (Fig. 6.51) or a fracture of the ulna (see "Monteggia Fracture–Dislocation"). Dislocations are easily diagnosed on the standard anteroposterior and lateral radiographs of the elbow.

The presence of a dislocation should signal the possibility of an associated fracture of the ulna, which may be overlooked when radiographic examination is focused only on the elbow. For this reason, if a dislocation

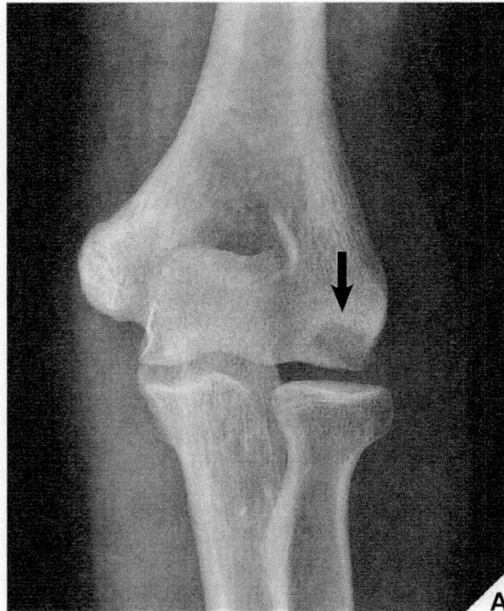

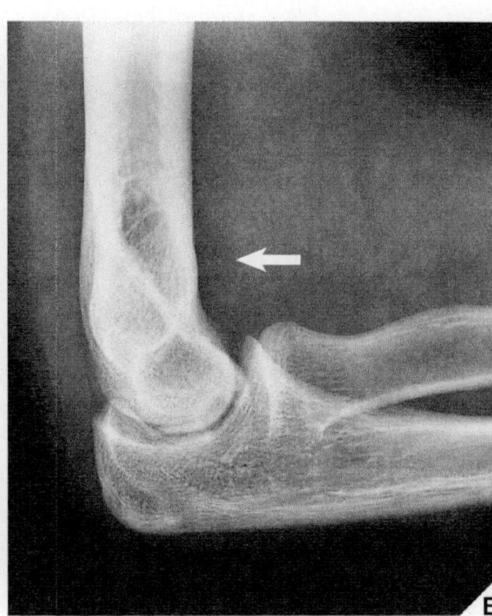

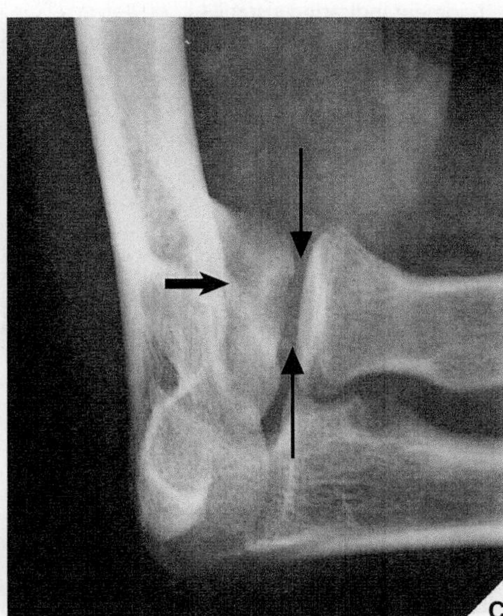

FIGURE 6.45 Osteochondritis dissecans of the capitellum. A 15-year-old boy, an active baseball player, reported pain in his right elbow for several months. **(A)** Anteroposterior radiograph of the elbow reveals a radiolucent defect in the capitellum *(arrow)* suggesting osteochondritis dissecans. **(B)** Lateral radiograph shows only positive anterior fat-pad sign *(arrow)*. **(C)** Radial head–capitellum projection demonstrates not only the full extent of the lesion in the capitellum *(thick arrow)* but also the osteochondral bodies in the joint *(thin arrows)*—a sign of advanced-stage osteochondritis dissecans. (Reprinted from Greenspan A, Norman A, Rosen H. Radial head-capitellum view in elbow trauma: clinical application and radiographic-anatomic correlation. *Am J Roentgenol* 1984;143:355–359. Copyright © 1984 American Roentgen Ray Society.)

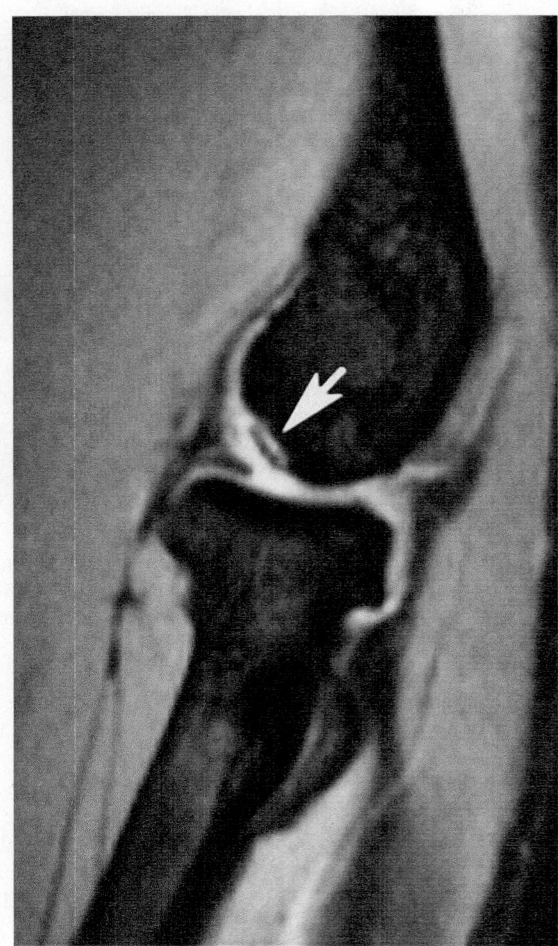

FIGURE 6.46 MRI of osteochondritis dissecans of the capitellum. A young baseball player presented with pain in the right elbow. The MR sagittal image demonstrates a focal osteochondral lesion in the anterior aspect of the capitellum *(arrow)*. The osteochondral fragment is *in situ*, but there is fluid signal between the donor site and the fragment indicating instability.

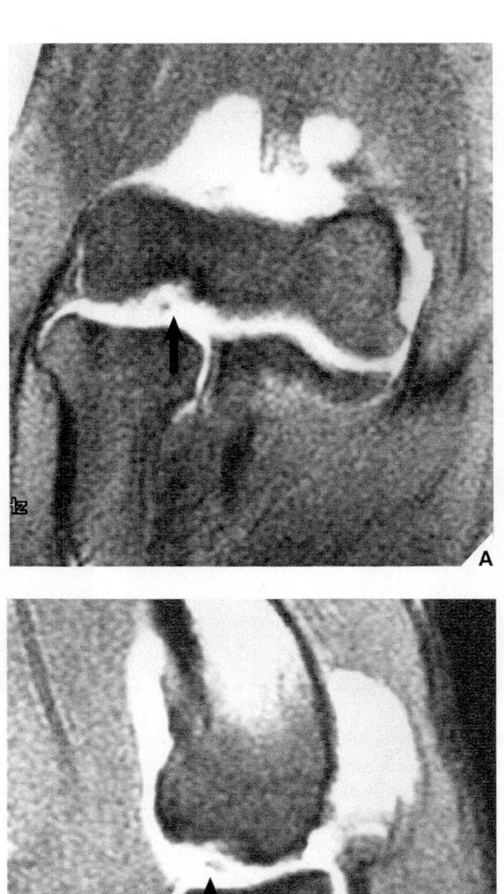

FIGURE 6.48 MRI of osteochondritis dissecans of the capitellum. A 16-year-old boy with chronic pain in the elbow underwent MRa. **(A)** Coronal and **(B)** sagittal fat-saturation T1-weighted (SE; TR 650/TE 17 msec) MRa demonstrates osteochondritis dissecans of the capitellum with completely separated, loose osteochondral body *(arrows)* (type III lesion).

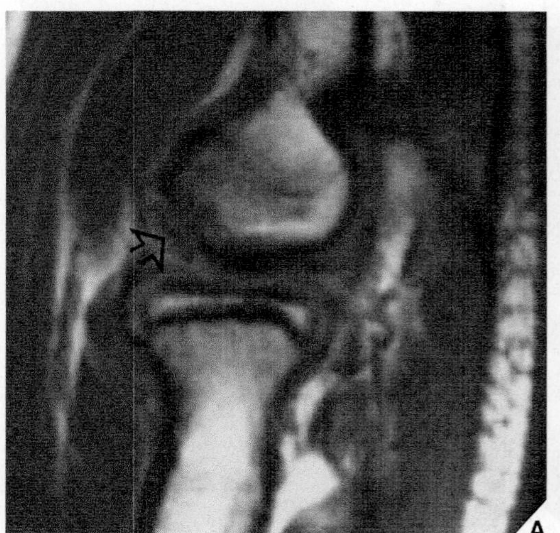

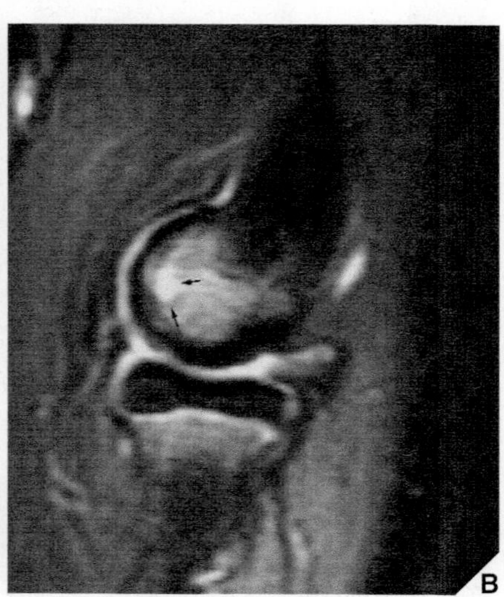

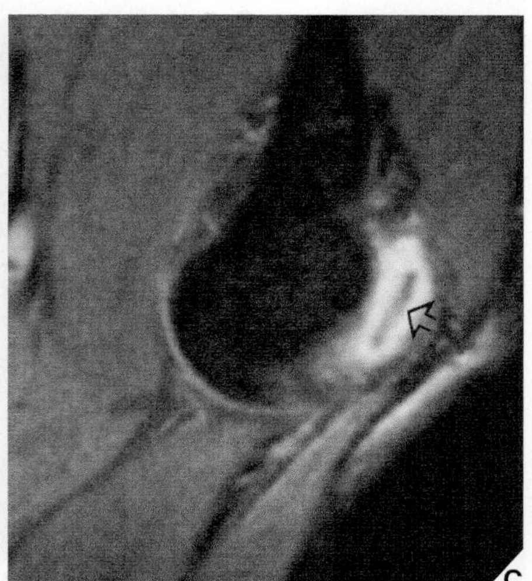

FIGURE 6.47 MRI of osteochondritis dissecans of the capitellum. **(A)** Sagittal T1-weighted MR image shows a linear focus of decreased signal *(open arrow)* at the anterior aspect of the capitellum. **(B)** Sagittal short time inversion recovery (STIR) image shows generalized increased signal surrounding a well-defined cystic-appearing focus *(arrows)* in the anterior aspect of the capitellum, consistent with osteochondritis dissecans. **(C)** Sagittal T2*-weighted gradient-echo image reveals a displaced osteochondral body *(open arrow)*. (Reprinted with permission from Deutsch AL, Mink JH, eds. *MRI of the musculoskeletal system: a teaching file*, 2nd ed. Philadelphia: Lippincott-Raven Publishers; 1997.)

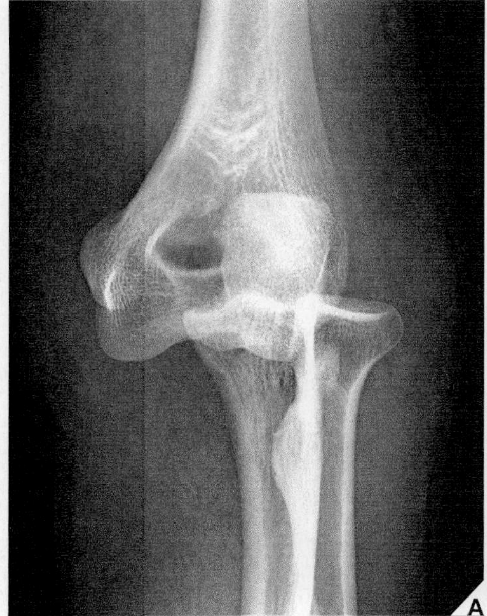

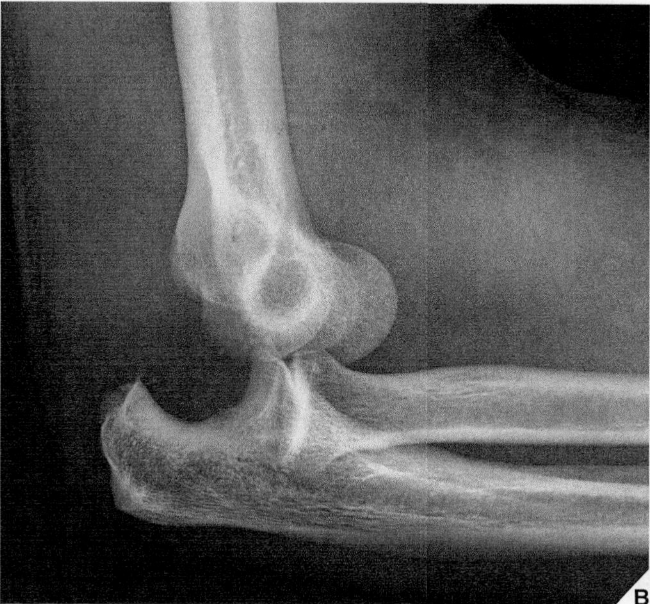

FIGURE 6.49 **Posterior elbow dislocation.** **(A)** Anteroposterior and **(B)** lateral radiographs show the most common type of dislocation in the elbow joint—both the radius and the ulna are posteriorly and laterally displaced. **(C)** In another patient, an oblique radiograph of the elbow shows posterolateral dislocation.

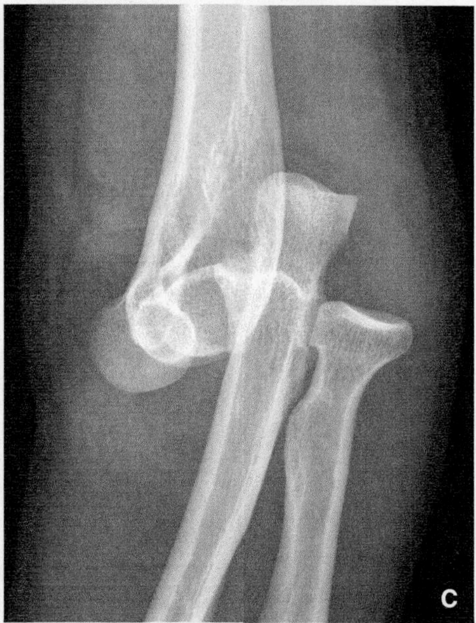

in the elbow joint is suspected, it is mandatory to include the entire forearm on the anteroposterior and lateral films; conversely, in cases of suspected ulnar fracture, radiographs should include the elbow joint. From a practical point of view, it is important, particularly in adults, to obtain two separate films, one centered over the elbow joint and the other over the site of the suspected fracture of the ulna. Care should be taken to center the films properly because a dislocation of the radial head can easily be missed on improperly centered films.

Monteggia Fracture–Dislocation

The association of a fracture of the ulna with a dislocation of the radial head is known by the eponym *Monteggia fracture–dislocation*. It usually results from forced pronation of the forearm during a fall or a direct blow to the posterior aspect of the ulna. The anteroposterior and lateral projections are sufficient to provide a full evaluation of these abnormalities.

Four types of this abnormality have been described (Fig. 6.52), but the features of the classic description are most commonly (in 60% to 70% of cases) seen as follows: a fracture at the junction of the proximal and middle thirds of the ulna, with anterior angulation associated with anterior dislocation of the radial head (type I) (Fig. 6.53). It is identifiable on physical examination by marked pain and tenderness about the elbow and displacement of the radial head into the antecubital fossa. The other types, which Bado has described, are as follows:

- Type II: a fracture of the proximal ulna with posterior angulation and posterior or posterolateral dislocation of the radial head
- Type III: a fracture of the proximal ulna with lateral or anterolateral dislocation of the radial head (Fig. 6.54); the variant of type III is an injury showing a comminution of ulnar fracture (Fig. 6.55). Type II and type III injuries account for approximately 30% to 40% of Monteggia fractures.
- Type IV: fractures of the proximal ends of the radius and the ulna, with anterior dislocation of the radial head (this is the least common type)

Injury to the Soft Tissues

Lateral Epicondylitis (Tennis Elbow)

Lateral epicondylitis, first described by Runge in 1878, affects approximately 3% of adults, usually between the ages of 35 and 55 years. The symptoms include pain of insidious onset, aggravated by activity, at the lateral aspect of the elbow joint. This condition is often diagnosed in tennis players, golfers, and carpenters. The pathomechanism of this abnormality is based on repetitive stress on muscles and tendons adjacent to the lateral aspect of

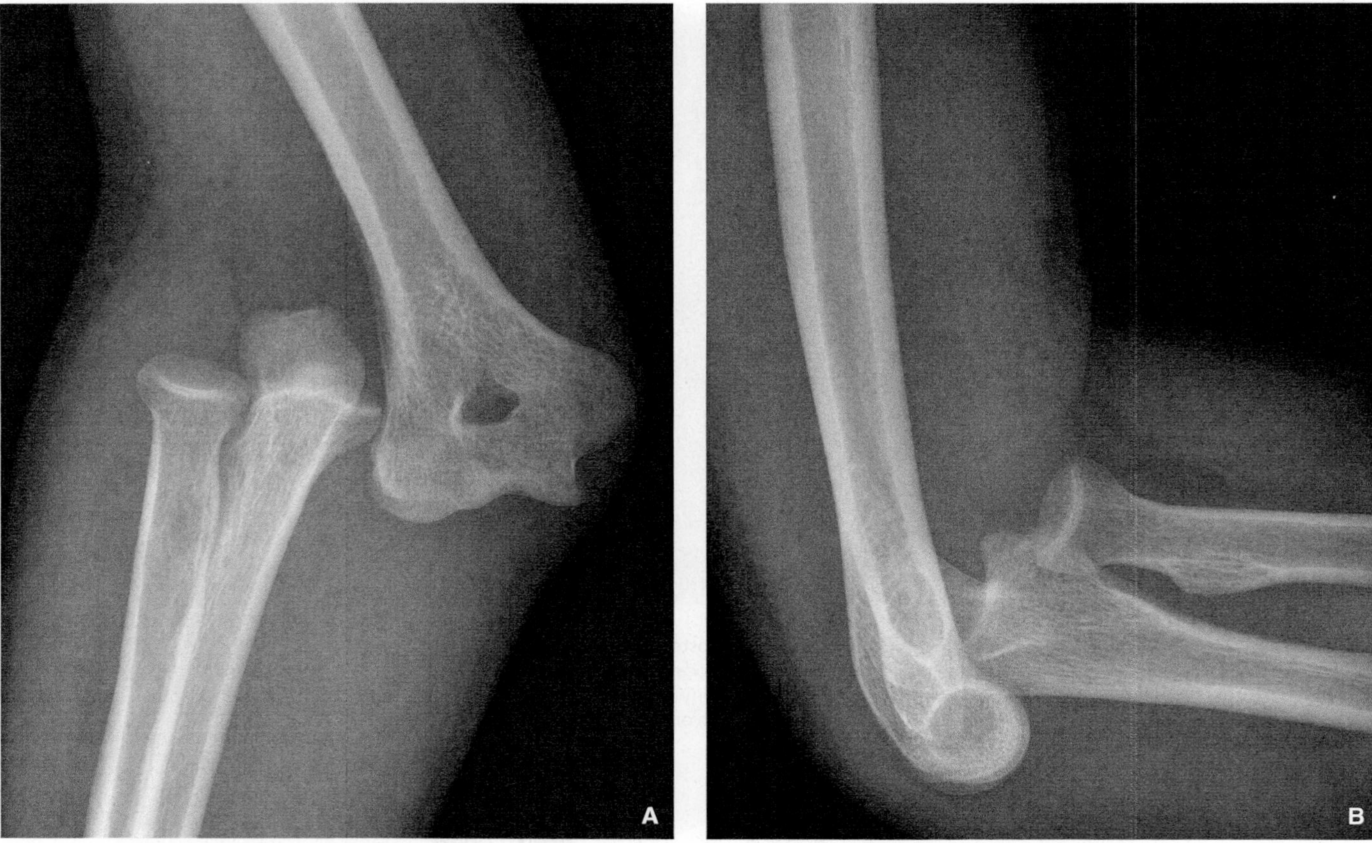

FIGURE 6.50 Anterior elbow dislocation. **(A)** Anteroposterior and **(B)** lateral radiographs show anterolateral elbow dislocation.

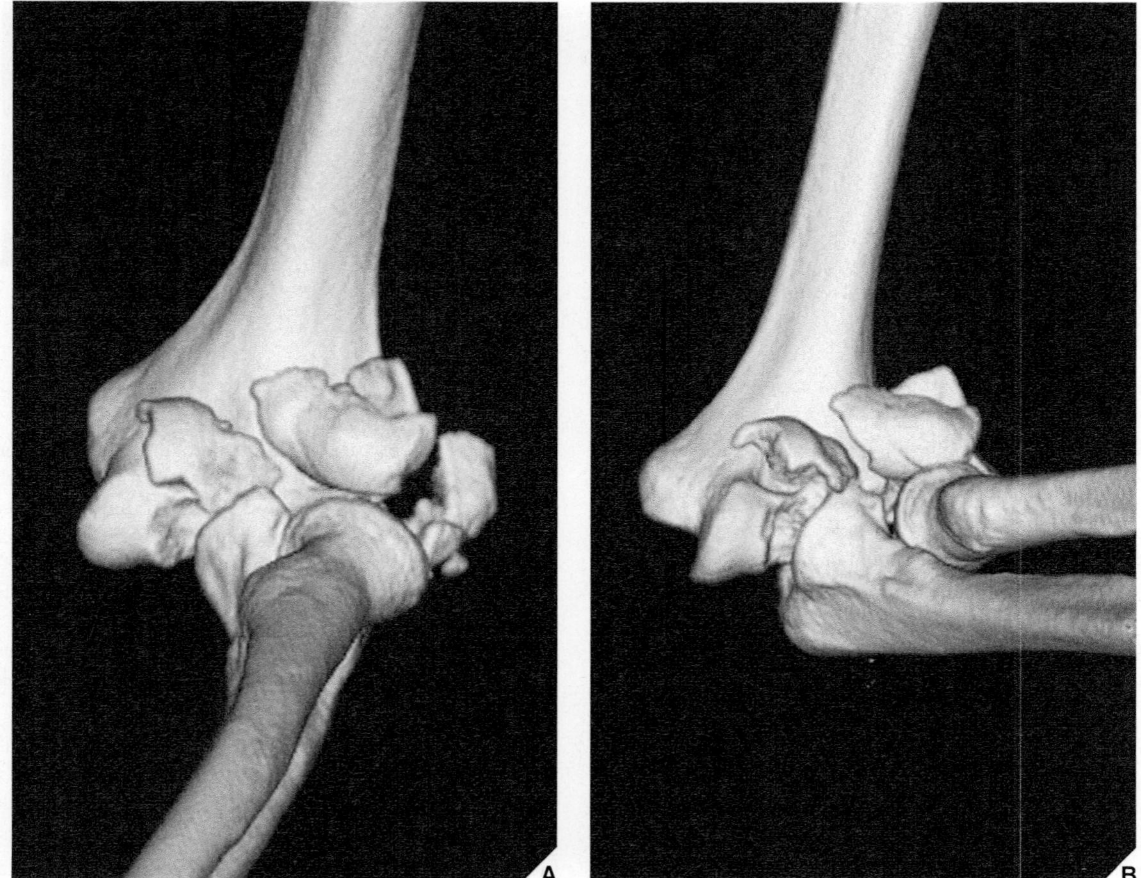

FIGURE 6.51 Three-dimensional (3D) CT of the fracture–dislocation in the elbow joint. A 59-year-old woman was injured in a car accident. 3D CT reconstructed images in anteroposterior **(A)** and lateral **(B)** projections show comminuted displaced fracture of the capitellum and lateral humeral condyle associated with lateral dislocation.

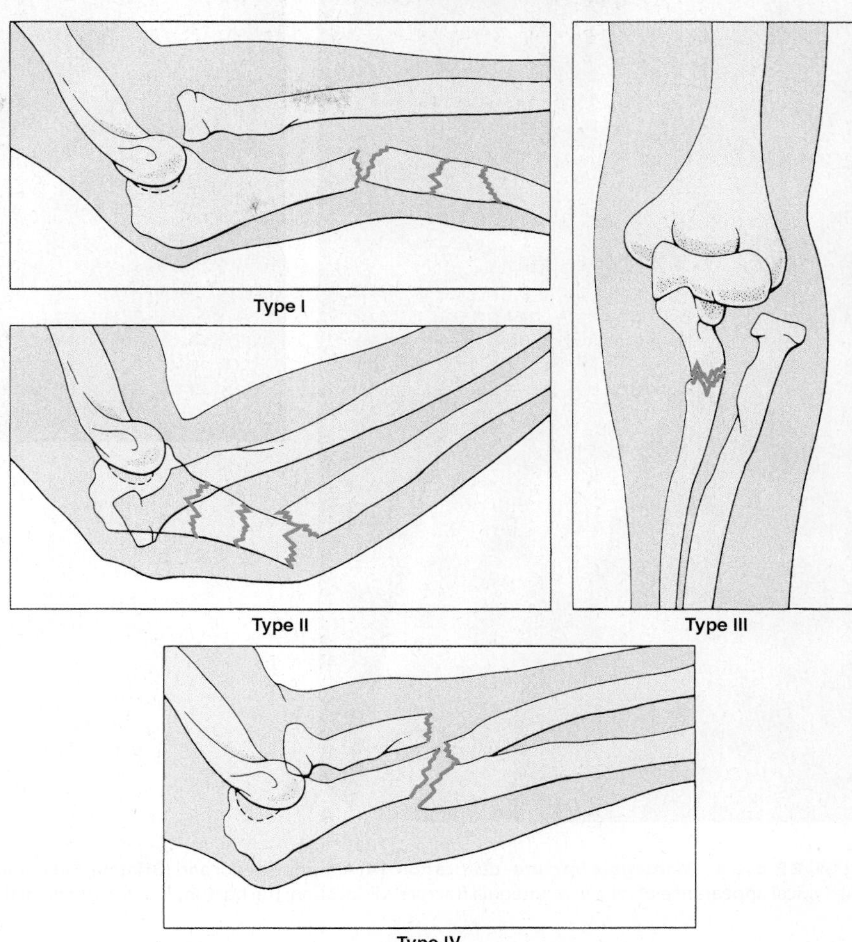

FIGURE 6.52 Monteggia fracture–dislocation. The Bado classification of Monteggia fracture–dislocation is based on the four types of abnormalities usually resulting from forced pronation of the forearm. These may occur during a fall or as a result of a direct blow to the posterior aspect of the ulna.

the distal humerus, particularly during excessive pronation and supination of the forearm when the wrist is extended. This results in mucoid degeneration and reactive granulation of the common extensor tendon, primarily the extensor carpi radialis brevis tendon, leading to avascularity and calcification of the tendon at its insertion on the lateral epicondyle.

Conventional radiographs are frequently normal, although soft-tissue swelling and calcification can sometimes be observed adjacent to the lateral epicondyle. MRI is useful for the assessment of damage to the tendons and the evaluation of associated abnormalities of the ligaments (Fig. 6.56; see also Fig. 4.138). Not uncommonly, MRI may show avulsion of the extensor carpi radialis brevis tendon from the lateral epicondyle and associated bone marrow edema. In some patients, MRI demonstrates increased signal within the anconeus muscle.

Medial Epicondylitis (Golfer's Elbow)

This condition affects the origin of tendons of the muscles flexor carpi radialis and pronator teres (common flexor tendon) at the attachment to the medial epicondyle of the humerus, and it is caused by overload of these structures due to repetitive valgus stresses. It is seen mainly in athletes such as golfers, tennis and racquetball players, baseball pitchers, javelin throwers, and occasionally in swimmers. The clinical symptoms include pain at the medial aspect of the elbow exacerbated by flexion of the wrist and pronation of the forearm. The diagnosis is made on the clinical basis but can be confirmed by MRI, which demonstrates thickening of the origin of the common flexor tendon associated with increased signal intensity on T2-weighted sequences and occasionally discontinuity of the fibers of the tendon when there is a complete rupture (see Fig. 4.137). Occasionally, the tear of adjacent UCL may coexist.

Rupture of the Distal Biceps Tendon

A tear of the distal biceps tendon may be either partial or complete and represents a common injury. It occurs usually in men between the ages of 40 and 50 years, and in most cases, the dominant arm is affected. The distal biceps tendon is composed of a long head and a short head. The long head is located more laterally, and it inserts in the proximal portion of the radial tuberosity. The short head is medial to the long head and it inserts in the distal part of the radial tuberosity. A rupture of the tendon is the result of a single traumatic event when a sudden extension force is applied to the arm with elbow flexed to 90 degrees and forearm in supination. The site of a rupture is invariably at the attachment of the tendon into the radial tuberosity. The patients present with an acute onset of pain and swelling in the antecubital fossa and local tenderness on palpation in this region. The most effective technique to demonstrate this injury is MRI. Partial tears exhibit

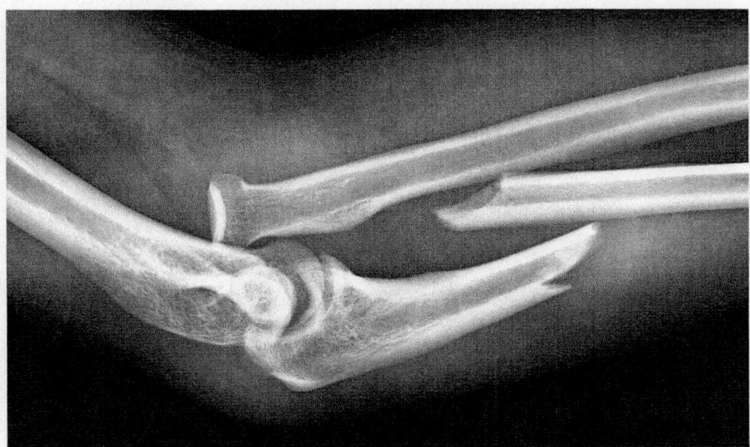

FIGURE 6.53 Monteggia fracture–dislocation. Lateral radiograph of the elbow joint and proximal third of the forearm shows type I Monteggia fracture–dislocation; the anteriorly angulated fracture is at the proximal third of the ulna, associated with anterior dislocation of the radial head.

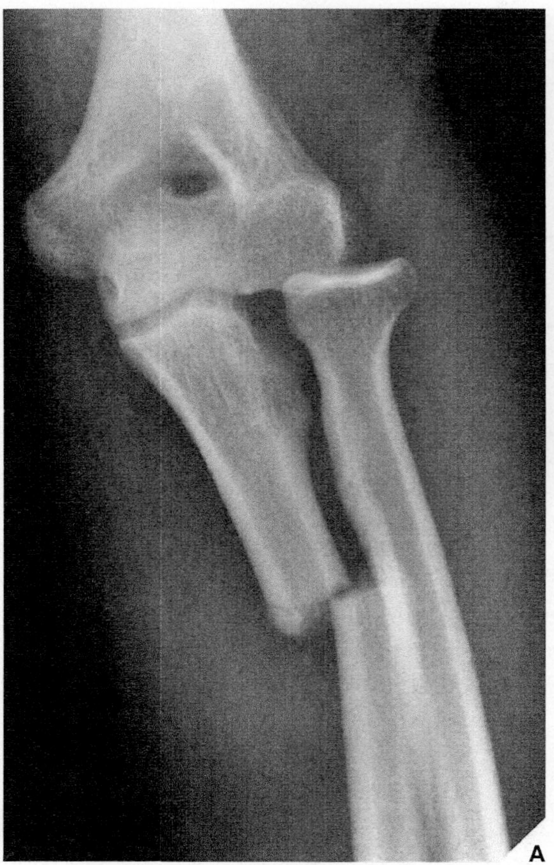

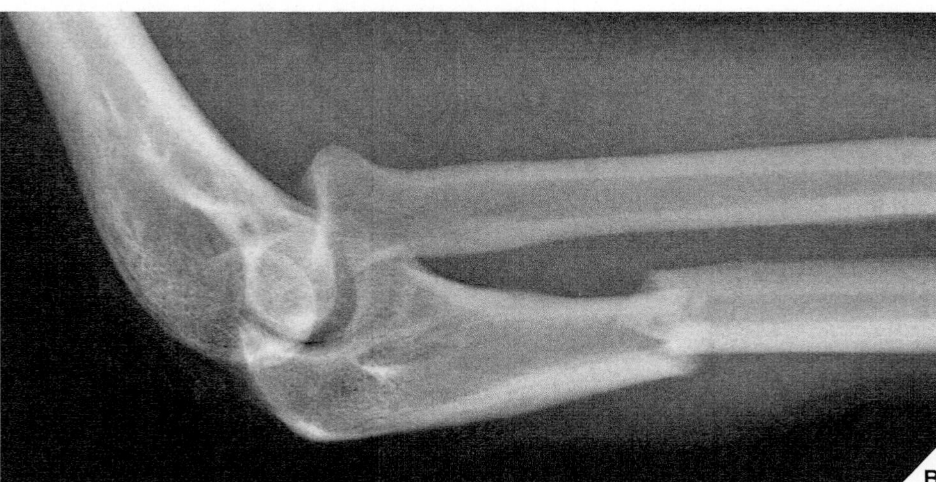

FIGURE 6.54 Monteggia fracture–dislocation. **(A)** Anteroposterior and **(B)** lateral radiographs of the elbow that include the proximal third of the forearm demonstrate the typical appearance of type III Monteggia fracture–dislocation; the fracture is at the proximal third of the ulna, associated with anterolateral dislocation of the radial head.

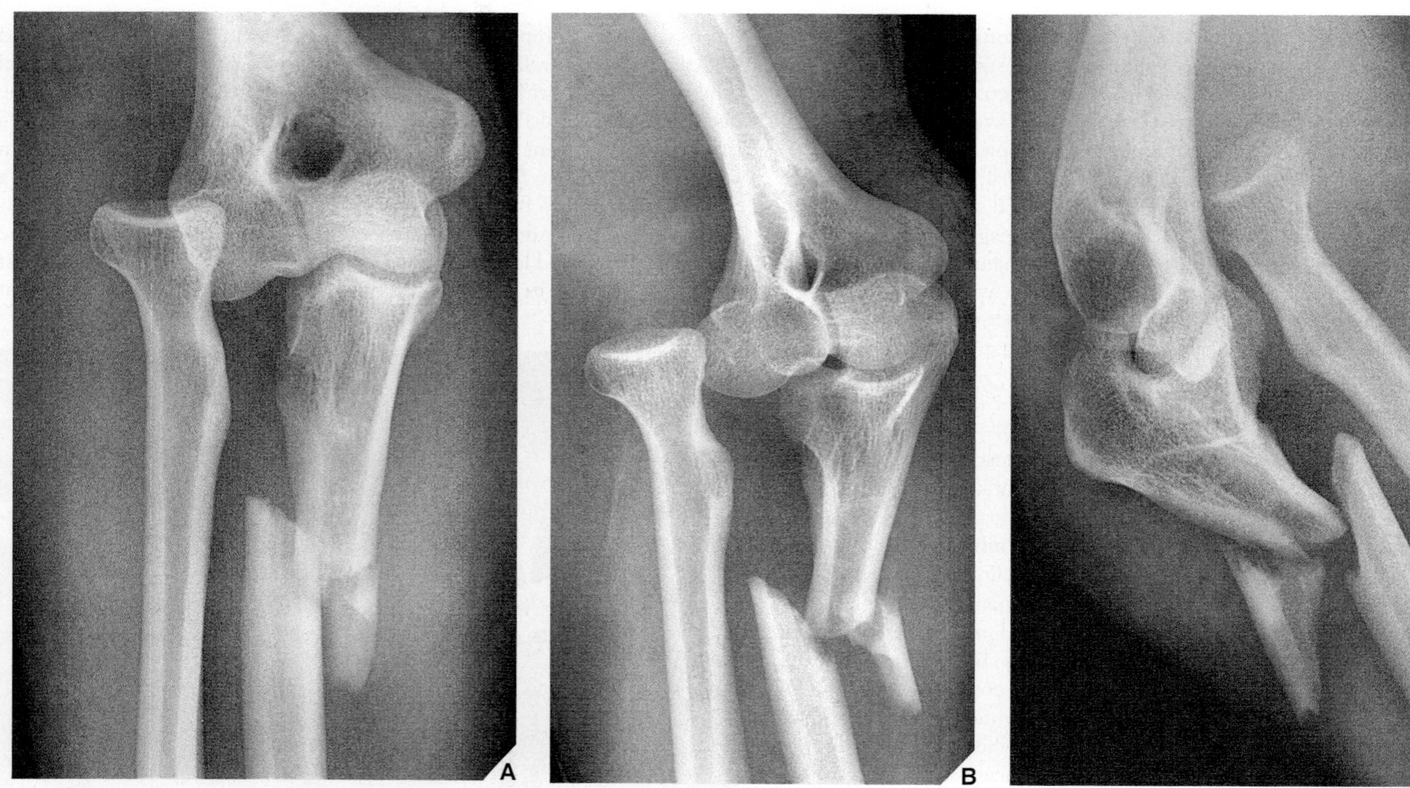

FIGURE 6.55 Monteggia fracture–dislocation. **(A)** Anteroposterior, **(B)** external oblique, and **(C)** lateral radiographs of the elbow joint show a variant of type III injury, where the fracture of the ulna is comminuted.

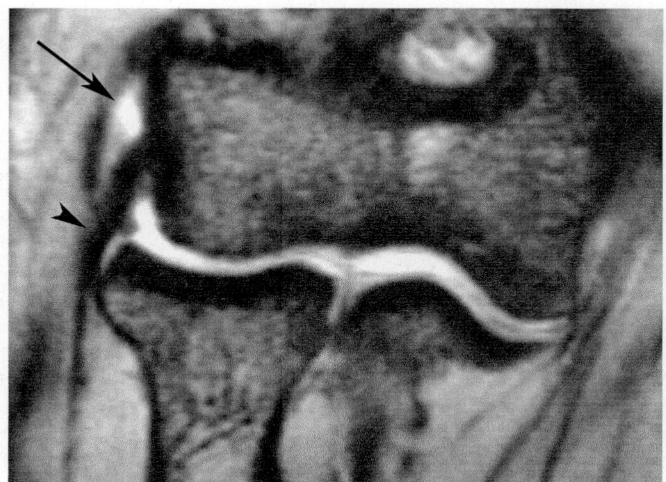

FIGURE 6.56 Lateral epicondylitis. A 35-year-old man presented with chronic pain at the lateral aspect of the elbow. Coronal gradient-echo MRI shows a severe tendinosis of the common extensor tendon with partial high-grade intrasubstance tear at the lateral epicondylar attachment *(arrow)*. Note the intact RCL *(arrowhead)*.

focal or diffuse alteration of signal intensity and size of the tendon. A full-thickness tear results in a gap within the tendon structure or proximal retraction of the distal part of the tendon and the biceps muscle. The best MRI planes for the demonstration of these injuries are sagittal and axial (Fig. 6.57), although some investigators recommend obtaining the MRI-modified coronal sections with the arm in abduction, elbow in flexion, and forearm in supination (FABS: flexion abduction supination). The images in this position clearly demonstrate the distal part of bicipital tendon from its musculotendinous junction to insertion into the radial tuberosity (Fig. 6.58). MRI is also effective in demonstrating the incomplete tears (Fig. 6.59).

Rupture of the Triceps Tendon

The rupture of this structure is the least common of all tendon tears, constituting approximately 2% of all tendon injuries and less than 1% of all upper extremity tendon ruptures. The mechanism of this injury is usually a direct blow to the tendon's attachment at the posterior aspect of the olecranon process of the ulna and, less commonly, after a fall on the outstretched hand. As with the ruptures of other tendons, MRI provides the best diagnostic evaluation. Imaging in axial and sagittal planes is most effective, showing discontinuity of the fibers and proximal retraction of the triceps muscle (Fig. 6.60).

Tears of the Radial (Lateral) Collateral Ligament Complex

The RCL complex (RCLC) consists of the RCL, the annular ligament, the accessory collateral ligament, and the posterolateral (lateral ulnar) collateral ligament. The first three ligaments provide lateral stability of the elbow joint and prevent varus deformation. The latter ligament provides posterolateral stabilization of the joint. Chronic repetitive microtrauma that results in varus stress may lead to a sprain or to disruption of the RCLC, both of which can be diagnosed with MRI. A sprain appears as a thinning or thickening of the ligament associated with high signal intensity within or adjacent to this structure. A complete tear manifests as a discontinuation of the fibers or a defect in the ligament. These abnormalities may also be seen in association with lateral epicondylitis (see previous text).

Posterolateral rotatory instability (PLRI) of the elbow is a clinical syndrome presenting with symptoms of clicking or locking and recurrent lateral instability in the elbow joint as a result of injury to the lateral collateral ligament complex. The typical mechanism of this injury is traumatic dislocation of the elbow, which was spontaneously reduced or was treated by closed reduction, but it has also been associated with chronic elbow sprains and fractures of the radial head and coronoid process (Fig. 6.61). In most cases, the injury is the result of a combination of axial compression, external rotation (supination), and valgus force applied to the elbow, which is seen in the setting of a fall on an outstretched hand.

Injury to the RCLC may result in instability in the setting of preexisting tennis elbow from chronic repetitive varus stress. Patients with insufficiency of the RCLC, particularly the lateral UCL (LUCL), experience laxity of the humeral-ulnar joint and secondary subluxation or dislocation of the humeral-radial joint.

Tears of the Ulnar (Medial) Collateral Ligament Complex

The UCL complex (UCLC) consists of the anterior, posterior, and transverse ligaments. These ligaments provide medial stability to the elbow joint and prevent valgus deformation. The most important of the three bands is the anterior portion, which originates on the inferior aspect of the medial epicondyle and inserts on the medial edge of the coronoid process at the sublime tubercle. UCLC injury commonly occurs in athletes, particularly in

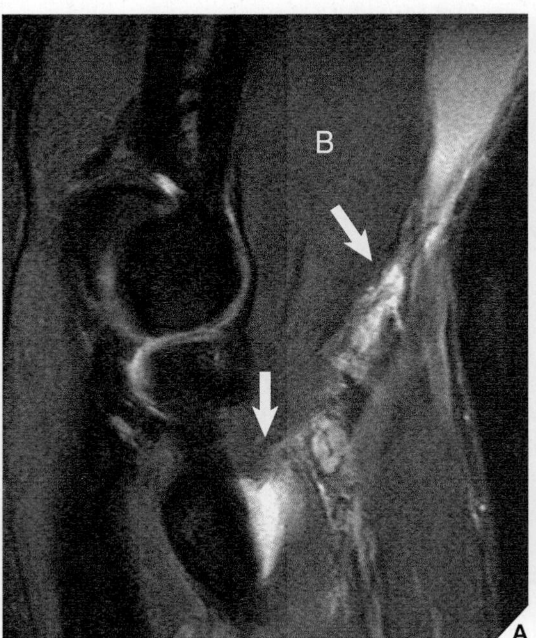

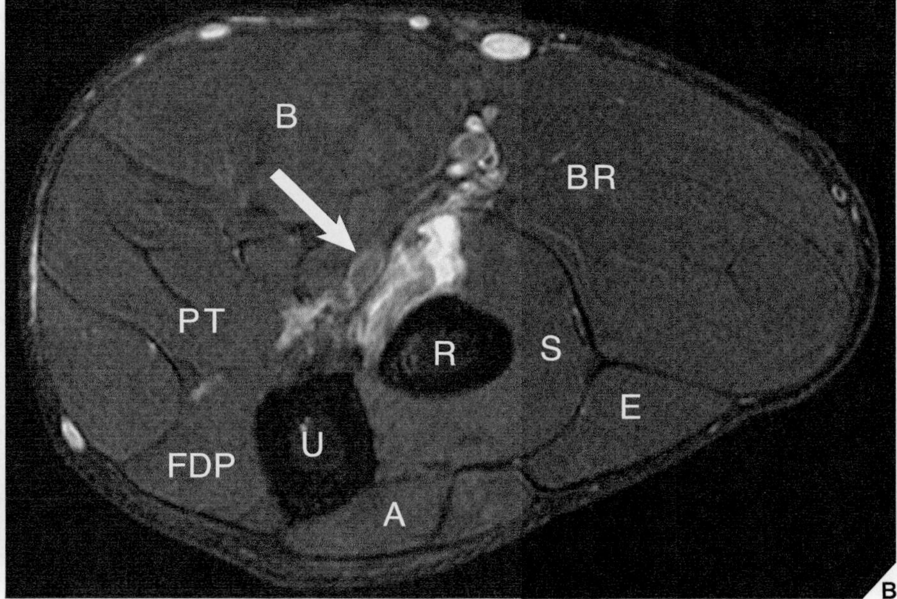

FIGURE 6.57 MRI of a complete tear of the distal biceps tendon. A 32-year-old man injured his right elbow in wrestling competition. **(A)** Sagittal and **(B)** axial proton density–weighted fat-suppressed MR images show a complete tear of the distal biceps tendon *(arrows)*. B, brachialis; PT, pronator teres; BR, brachioradialis; FDP, flexor digitorum profundus; U, ulna; R, radius; S, supinator; E, extensor carpi ulnaris; A, anconeus.

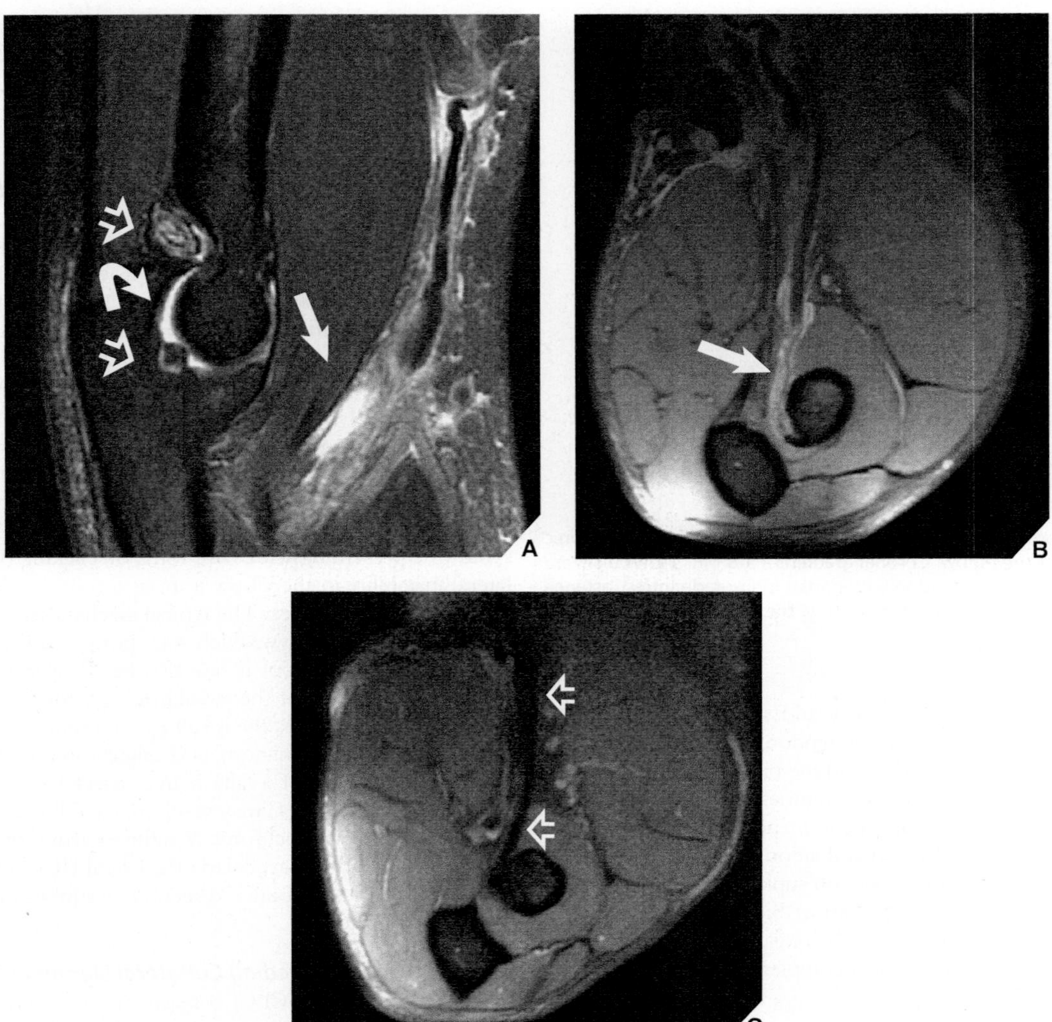

FIGURE 6.58 MRI of a tear of the biceps tendon. **(A)** Sagittal T2-weighted fat-suppressed and **(B)** modified (FABS) coronal proton density–weighted fat-suppressed MR images of the elbow show a complete rupture of the distal biceps tendon *(arrows)*. The *curved arrow* points to joint effusion, and *open arrows* point to the incidental finding of intraarticular osteochondral bodies. **(C)** Normal appearance of distal biceps tendon *(open arrows)* on modified coronal MR proton density–weighted fat-suppressed image is shown for comparison.

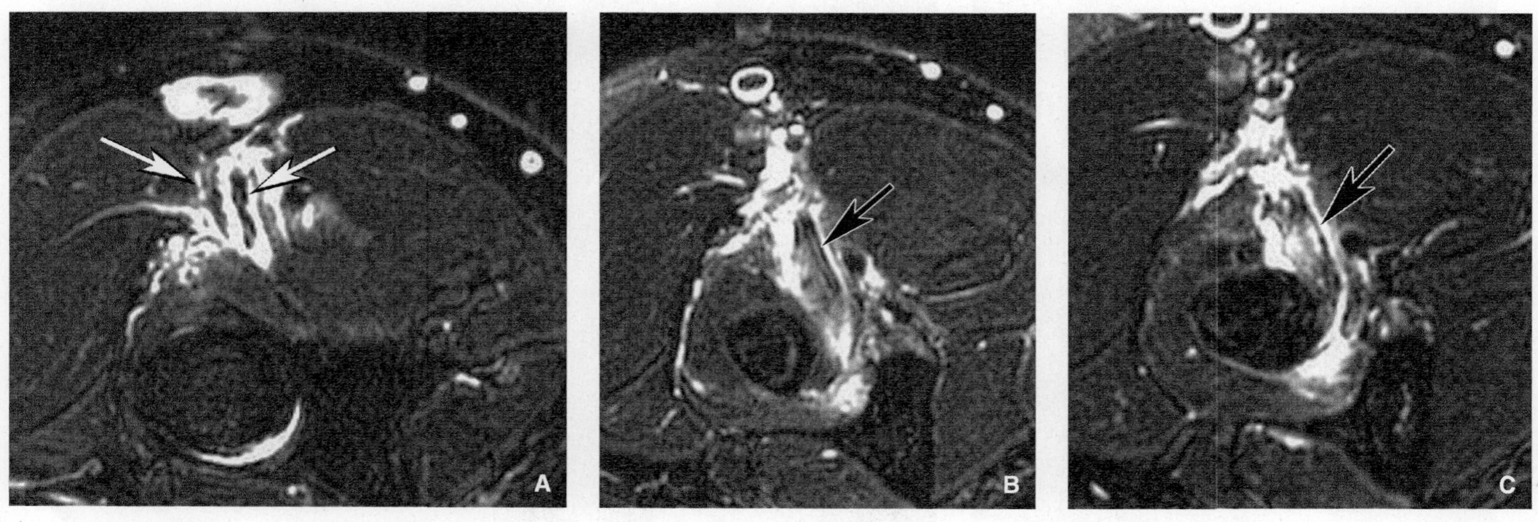

FIGURE 6.59 MRI of a partial tear of the long arm of the distal biceps tendon. **(A)** Axial T2-weighted fat-saturated MR image through the head of the radius and **(B)** more distally through the neck of the radius and **(C)** through the radial tuberosity shows irregularity and peritendinous edema of the long and short heads of the biceps (*arrows* in **A**). More distal axial images show the irregular but not torn short head of the distal biceps tendon (*arrows* in **B,C**). The long head is torn. Edema and hematoma are present at the rupture site.

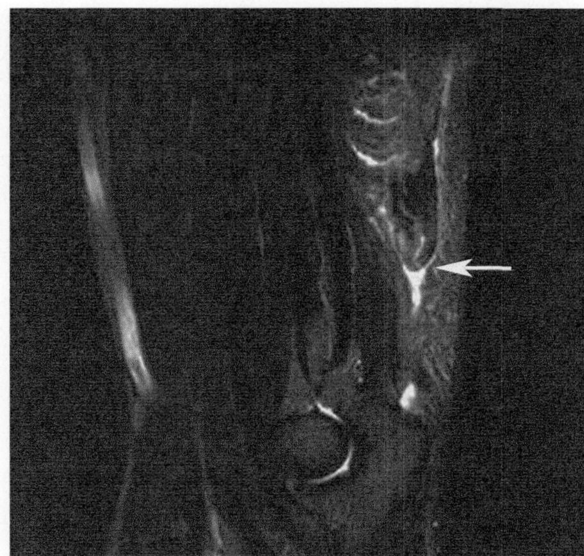

FIGURE 6.60 **MRI of a tear of the triceps tendon.** A 25-year-old man presented with acute posterior elbow pain after lifting a heavy object. Sagittal T2-weighted MR image of the elbow demonstrates a complete retracted tear of the triceps tendon *(arrow)* with focal edema and hematoma.

baseball pitchers and, less commonly, in javelin throwers, handball players, arm wrestlers, and tennis players. MRI findings include abnormal signal and interruption of the continuity of the fibers or defect in the ligament (in a complete rupture) or thickening of the ligament and foci of calcification or ossification (in a chronic injury).

The combination of a large valgus load and rapid elbow extension produces three forces of stress in the elbow: (a) tensile stress along the medial compartment structures including UCLC, flexor-pronator muscles, medial humeral epicondyle, and ulnar nerve; (b) shear stress along the osseous structures of the posterior elbow compartment at the posteromedial tip of the olecranon and trochlea/olecranon fossa; and (c) compression stress laterally along the radial head and capitellum. This combination of forces is the most common mechanism of elbow injury in the throwing athlete and it has been referred to as *valgus extension overload syndrome* (VEOS) (Fig. 6.62).

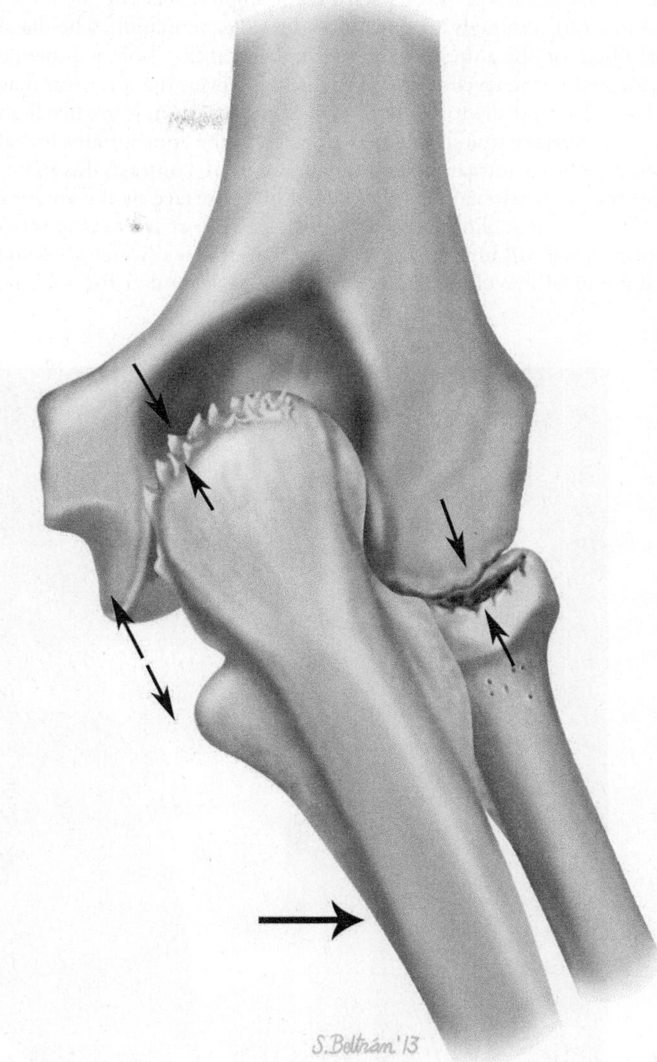

FIGURE 6.62 **VEOS.** Illustration of the different forces leading to VEOS *(arrows)*.

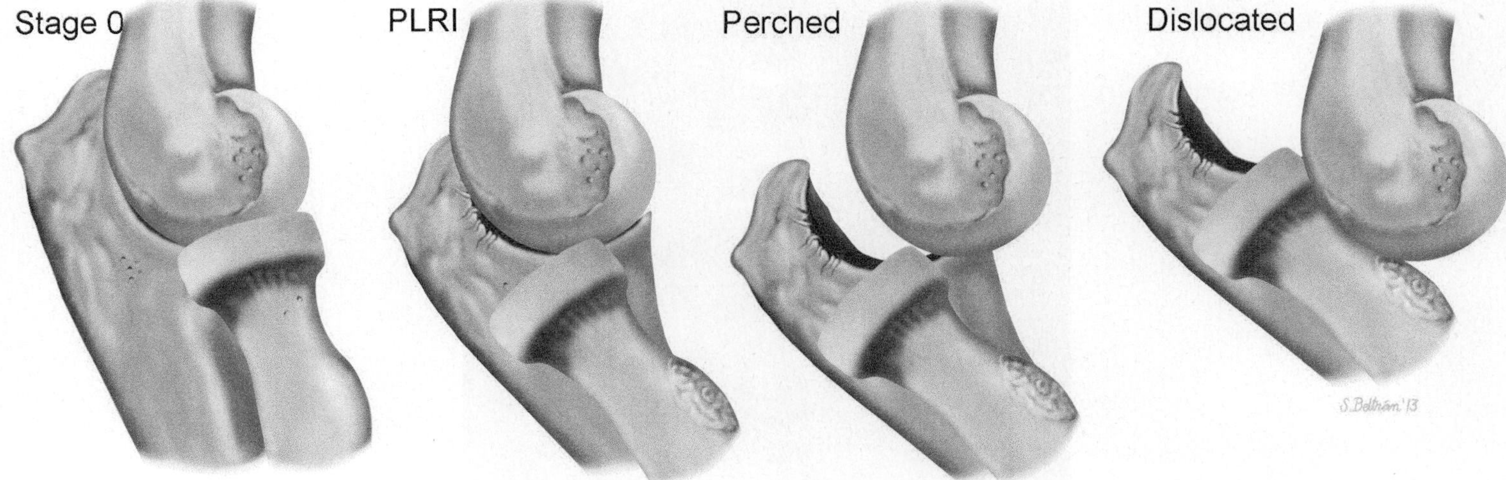

FIGURE 6.61 **Posterior lateral rotatory instability.** Illustration of the different stages of elbow instability. Stage 0: The elbow joint is reduced. PLRI: Axial compression, supination, and valgus lead to subluxation of the radius. Perched: The radius and ulna are subluxed posteriorly and laterally. Dislocated: The radius and ulna are dislocated posteriorly and laterally.

MRI can distinguish between partial and complete tears of the UCLs (Figs. 6.63 to 6.66), although MRa is the preferred examination. The distal insertional fibers of the anterior band of the UCL at the sublime tubercle are often located at the level of the joint line. However, the insertion may occur as far as 3 mm distal to the joint line. If the insertion is greater than 3 mm, an undersurface tear should be suspected in the appropriate clinical setting. On MRa after intraarticular administration of contrast, this manifests by contrast extension along the articular undersurface of the anterior band of UCL at the sublime tubercle, which has the characteristic morphology on coronal MR images of a "T" and therefore is referred to as the *T sign* (see Fig. 6.64). Avulsion injury of the anterior band at the sublime tubercle may also occur, which typically appears as an avulsed osseous fragment best seen on anteroposterior radiographs and on coronal MR images as a detached bone fragment that demonstrates continuity with the UCL (see Fig. 6.65). Recently, De Smet and colleagues have recommended the use of dynamic sonography with valgus stress to assess an injury to the UCL in baseball pitchers. This technique uniquely demonstrates the medial joint laxity and instability when measurements of the degree of joint widening during valgus stress of the elbow are obtained.

Surgical repair of UCL tears in professional baseball pitchers was originally performed by Dr. Frank Jobe and has been since referred to as the *Tommy John surgery* named after the former Major League baseball pitcher, who

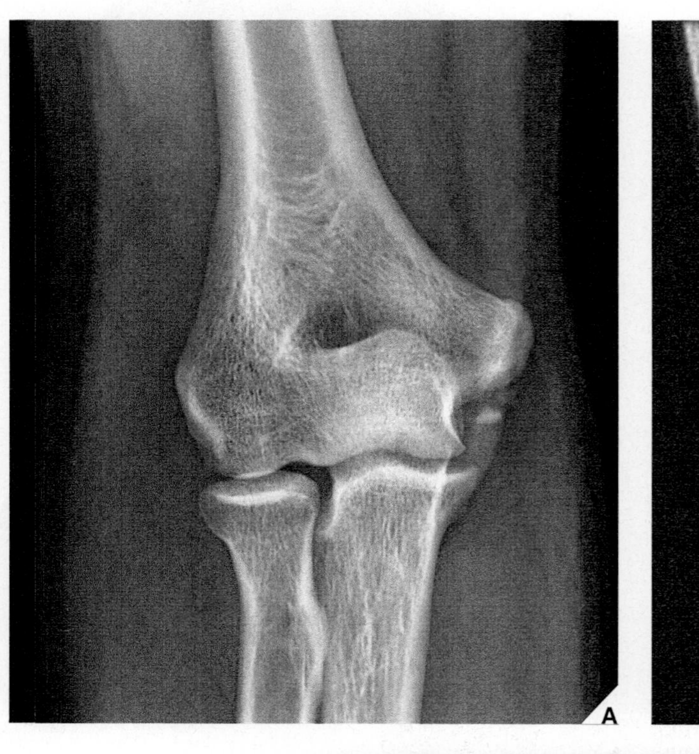

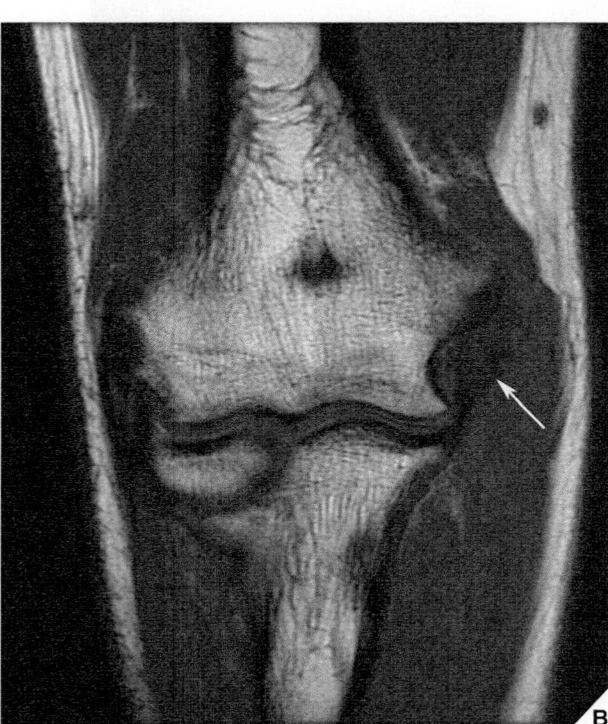

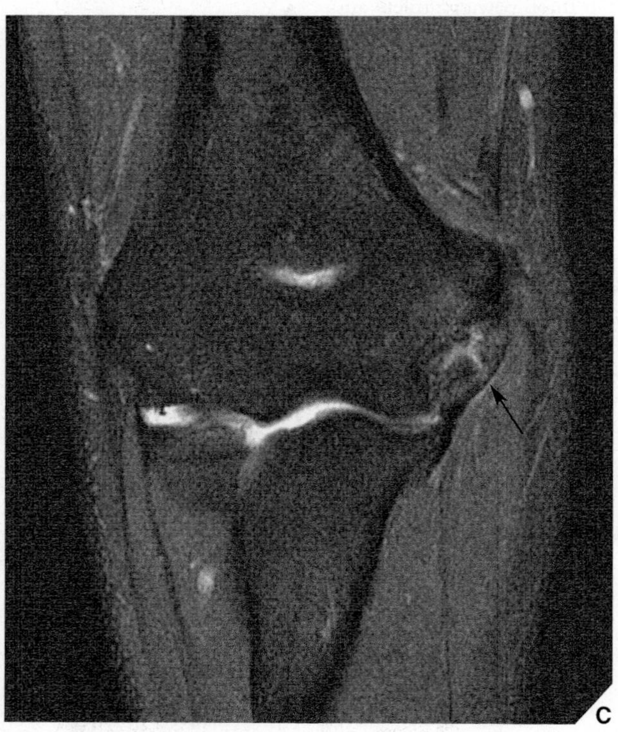

FIGURE 6.63 MRI of the partial tear of the UCL. A 15-year-old boy presented with pain in the medial aspect of the elbow. **(A)** Anteroposterior radiograph of the right elbow shows an avulsion fracture of the medial humeral epicondyle. **(B)** Coronal proton density–weighted and **(C)** T2-weighted fat-saturated MR images show the avulsion fracture of the medial epicondyle associated with a partial tear of the proximal UCL *(arrows)*.

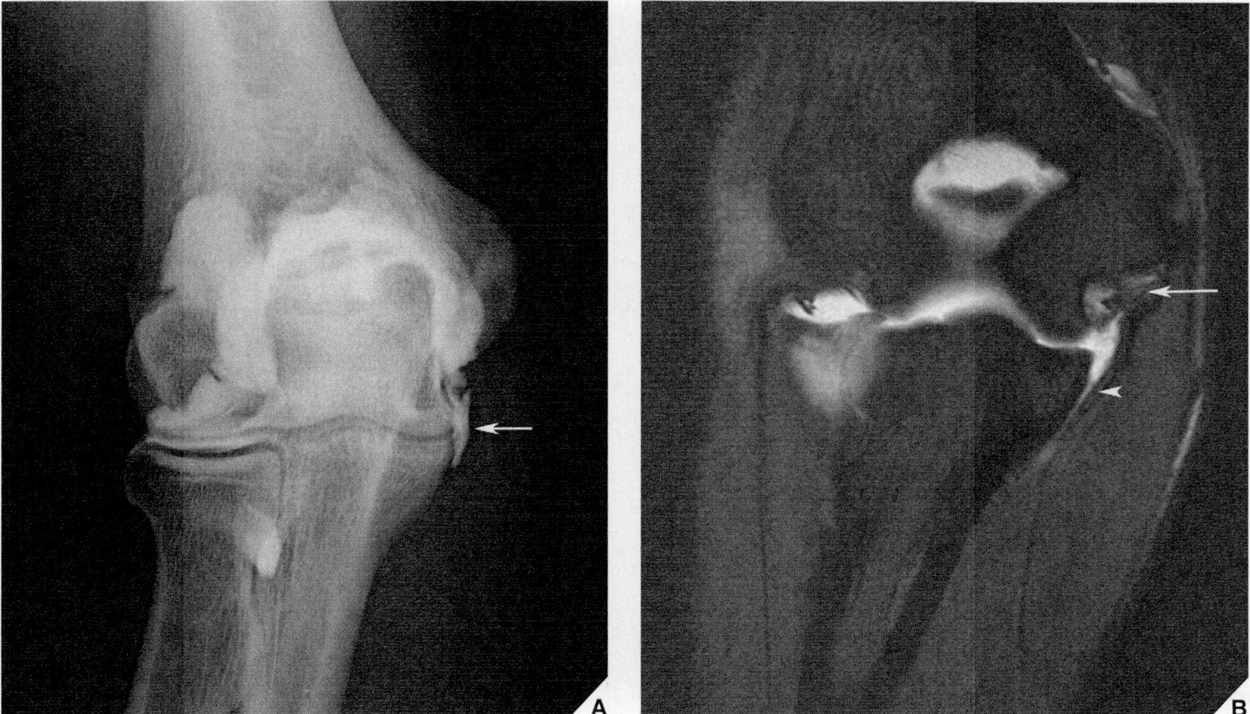

FIGURE 6.64 MRa of a full-thickness tear of the UCL. A 22-year-old professional baseball player presented with acute onset of elbow pain following a throw of a ball. **(A)** Arthrogram of the elbow shows leakage of the contrast agent at the site of the medial collateral ligament *(arrow)*. **(B)** T1-weighted fat-saturated MRa demonstrates the tear of the proximal UCL *(arrow)*. Note also a partial tear of the distal UCL, which is partially detached from its insertion in the sublime tubercle, the so-called *T sign (arrowhead)*.

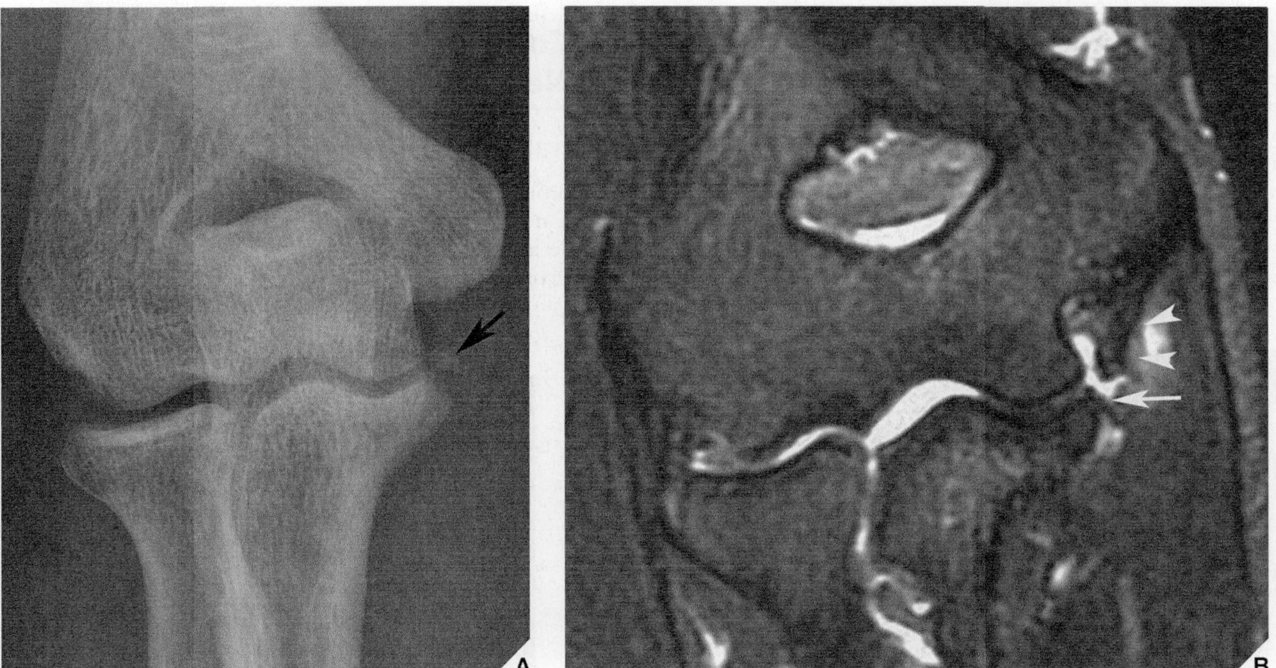

FIGURE 6.65 MRI of avulsion fracture of the sublime tubercle. **(A)** Anteroposterior radiograph of the elbow demonstrates an avulsion fracture of the sublime tubercle of the ulna *(arrow)*. **(B)** Coronal T2-weighted MRI demonstrates the avulsed fracture of the sublime tubercle *(arrow)* and the partial tear of the UCL, which is thickened, edematous, and partially torn *(arrowheads)*.

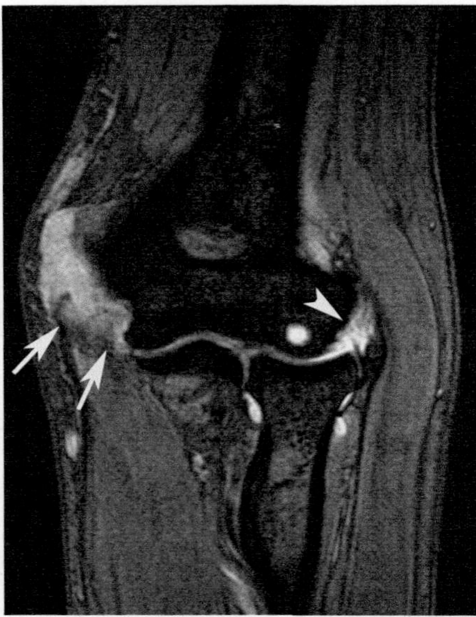

FIGURE 6.66 **MRI of a complete tear of the UCL and common flexor tendon.** A 26-year-old man suffered an elbow dislocation. MRI was obtained following reduction. Coronal gradient recalled echo (GRE) MR image demonstrates a complete tear of the UCL and common flexor tendon *(arrows)* with edema and hematoma. Note also the tear of the RCL and a partial tear of the common extensor tendon *(arrowhead)*.

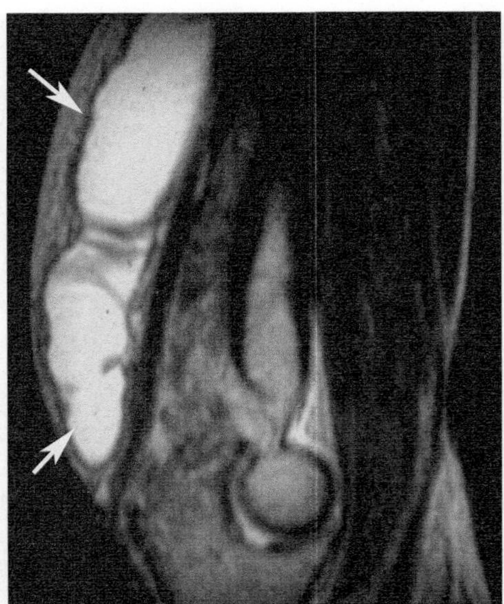

FIGURE 6.68 **MRI of olecranon bursitis.** Sagittal T2-weighted MR image demonstrates marked distension of the olecranon bursa in the dorsal aspect of the elbow in a patient with history of gout *(arrows)*. Very similar appearance may be seen in posttraumatic olecranon bursitis.

had the operation on his injured pitching arm in 1974, using a palmaris tendon graft to replace the torn UCL ligament. Subsequent variations of the technique have improved long-term results of this type of surgical repair. MRI obtained after surgery can confirm the integrity of the tendon graft (Fig. 6.67).

Bursitis

There are two bursae in the region of the elbow: the olecranon bursa and the bicipitoradialis bursa. The olecranon bursa is located between the skin of the posterior aspect of the elbow and the olecranon. Normally, the olecranon bursa does not contain sufficient fluid to be seen on MRI or ultrasound. However, it can become distended with fluid in patients with inflammatory arthritis such as rheumatoid arthritis or psoriasis, gout, trauma, and infection (Fig. 6.68).

The bicipitoradialis bursa is located between the distal biceps tendon at the insertion in the radial bicipital tuberosity and the radius. It can also become distended with fluid in cases of inflammatory arthritis, gout, infection, and trauma. When the bicipitoradialis bursa becomes distended with fluid, it is seen on MRI or ultrasound as a pear-shaped fluid collection adjacent to the distal biceps tendon (Fig. 6.69).

Compressive and Entrapment Neuropathies of the Elbow

Pronator Teres Muscle Syndrome

The pronator teres muscle syndrome is related to static or dynamic compression or entrapment of the median nerve between the pronator teres muscle and the two heads of the flexor digitorum superficialis muscle. Static compression of the median nerve can be due to myositis, a fibrous

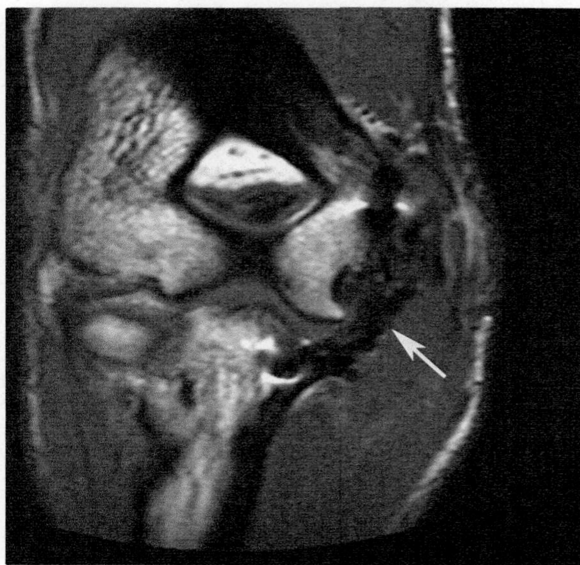

FIGURE 6.67 **MRI of Tommy John procedure.** Coronal T1-weighted MRI demonstrates the integrity of the tendon graft following UCL repair *(arrow)*.

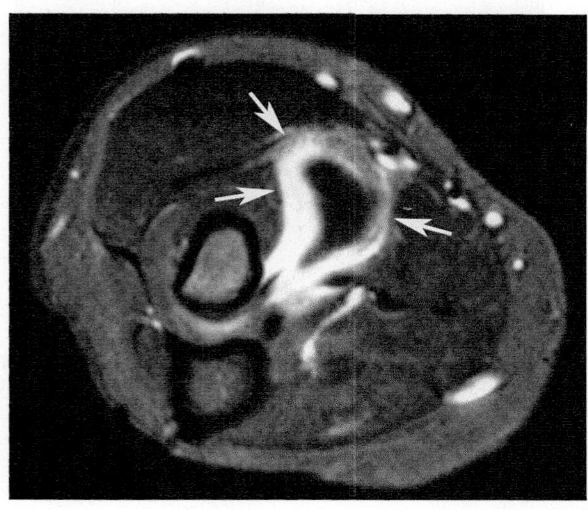

FIGURE 6.69 **MRI of bicipitoradialis bursitis.** Axial T1-weighted fat-saturated MRI following intravenous injection of gadolinium demonstrates distension of the bicipitoradialis bursa in the anterior aspect of the elbow *(arrows)* in this patient with tuberculosis (TB). Note the intense enhancement of the synovium.

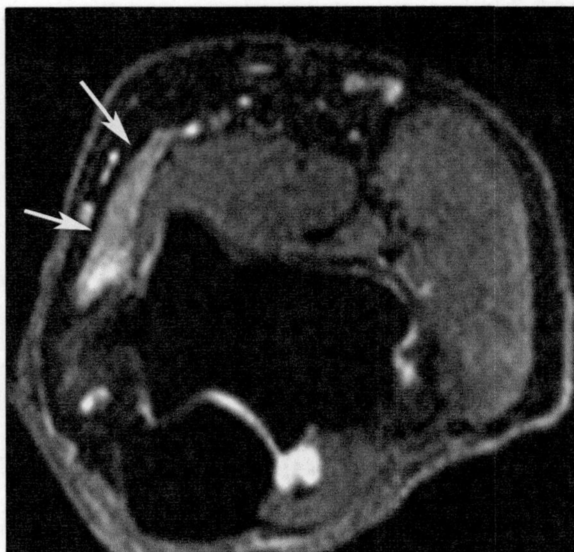

FIGURE 6.70 MRI of pronator teres syndrome. Axial sagittal short time inversion recovery (STIR) pulse sequence demonstrates edema of the teres muscle *(arrows)* indicating early denervation.

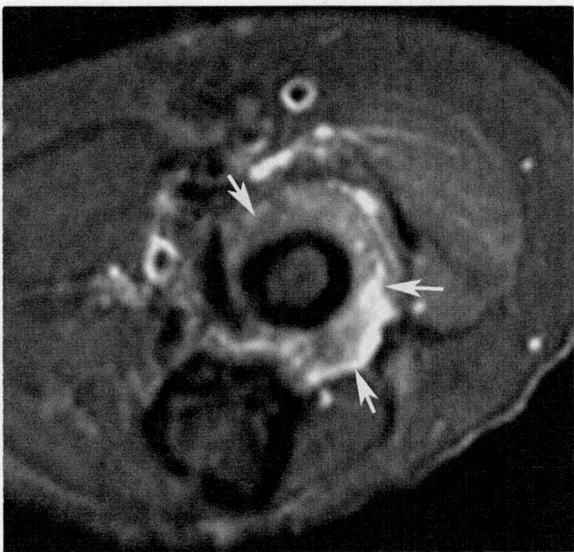

FIGURE 6.71 MRI of radial tunnel syndrome (posterior interosseous nerve syndrome). Axial T2-weighted MR image demonstrates edema of the supinator muscle *(arrows)*, one of the early signs of posterior interosseous nerve syndrome.

band, trauma with formation of a hematoma, or other soft-tissue masses. Dynamic compression can occur with repetitive alternating pronation and supination of the forearm. Other less common causes include compression by aponeurotic prolongation of the biceps brachii muscle, Volkmann contracture, and prolonged external compression ("honeymoon paralysis"). Patients with pronator teres muscle syndrome have motor disturbances of the first three fingers and sensory abnormalities of the palm of the hand.

With MRI, the normal median nerve can be seen as a structure of low signal intensity located between the brachialis artery and the pronator teres muscle. Additionally, denervation edema or atrophy of the teres muscle may be shown (Fig. 6.70). MR images obtained with the elbow in pronation can accentuate compression of the nerve by a hypertrophied pronator teres muscle.

Supinator Muscle Syndrome

The supinator muscle syndrome, also known as *radial tunnel syndrome* or *posterior interosseous nerve syndrome*, is produced by compression of the deep branch of the radial nerve, the posterior interosseous nerve, as it passes under the tendinous arch of the supinator muscle (arcade of Frohse). Trauma, tumors, bursitis, and cysts are frequently implicated as the cause of this syndrome. Dynamic compression of the posterior interosseous nerve occurs in activities involving overuse of the arm in pronation, forearm extension and wrist flexion, such as it happens in tennis players, violinists, and musical conductors. Often, this syndrome is mistaken for lateral epicondylitis or tennis elbow, and occasionally, both syndromes appear together.

On axial T1-weighted MR images, the superficial and deep branches of the radial nerve are normally seen within the sulcus nervi cubitalis radialis, the space between the brachialis and the brachioradialis muscles. MRI evidence of soft-tissue masses compressing the posterior interosseous nerve has been described as well as signs of denervation of the supinator muscle including edema in the early phase and atrophy in the late phase of denervation (Fig. 6.71).

Cubital Tunnel Syndrome

Compression of the ulnar nerve at the level of the distal part of the humerus is known as *cubital tunnel syndrome* and probably is the most common compressive and entrapment neuropathy (CEN) of the elbow. As the ulnar nerve approaches the elbow joint, it passes behind the medial humeral epicondyle. At this point, a fibroosseous tunnel is formed between the posterior fibers of the medial collateral ligament and the sulcus nervi ulnaris of the distal part of the humerus. Approximately 1 cm distally, the ulnar nerve crosses a second fibroosseous tunnel formed between the humerus and the ulnar and humeral heads of the flexor carpi ulnaris muscle, which are connected by a fibrous band called the *arcuate ligament*. Compression of the ulnar nerve can occur at the proximal or distal tunnel. However, as the clinical features and causes at the two locations are similar, they are discussed together.

Frequent causes of cubital tunnel syndrome include trauma, ganglion cysts, posttraumatic cubitus valgus, prolonged external compression with the arm in flexion ("sleep palsy"), repetitive microtrauma (e.g., from using jackhammers), and inflammatory arthritides. Thickening of the arcuate ligament can produce dynamic compression of the ulnar nerve. Among soft-tissue masses causing cubital tunnel syndrome, the most frequently encountered are ganglionic cysts and lipomas. Subluxation of the ulnar nerve related to tear or laxity of the arcuate ligament, shallow epicondylar groove, or cubitus valgus can cause similar signs and symptoms owing to friction neuritis. Asymptomatic ulnar nerve subluxation has been detected in 16% of healthy persons. Occasionally, an accessory anconeus epitrochlearis muscle can cause cubital tunnel syndrome (Figs. 6.72 and 6.73).

With MR images, the normal ulnar nerve is best seen on axial T1-weighted images. It is a round, hypointense structure within the cubital tunnel, surrounded by fat and accompanied by the ulnar recurrent artery and veins. Sagittal images obtained in the region of the medial epicondyle may also show the ulnar nerve. Dynamic compression and inflammation is seen on MR images as thickening and hyperintensity of the ulnar nerve. Soft-tissue masses compressing the ulnar nerve can also be well depicted with MRI. Detection of elbow nerve subluxation will be optimal with elbow flexion during MRI.

Surgical treatment of cubital tunnel syndrome with ulnar nerve transposition may be indicated in patients not responding to conservative measures. MRI can depict the transposed ulnar nerve and demonstrate the presence of excessive scar tissue around the nerve in patients with recurrent cubital tunnel syndrome following ulnar nerve transposition (Fig. 6.74).

PRACTICAL POINTS TO REMEMBER

1. On the anteroposterior projection of the elbow:
   - observe the normal 15-degree valgus carrying angle formed between the arm and the forearm
   - in the child, recognize the six secondary ossification centers around the elbow joint and the age at which they appear: capitellum at 1 year, radial head at 3 years, medial (internal) epicondyle at 5 years, trochlea at 7 years, olecranon at 9 years, and lateral (external) epicondyle at 11 years. The mnemonic CRITOE helps to remember this sequence of appearance.

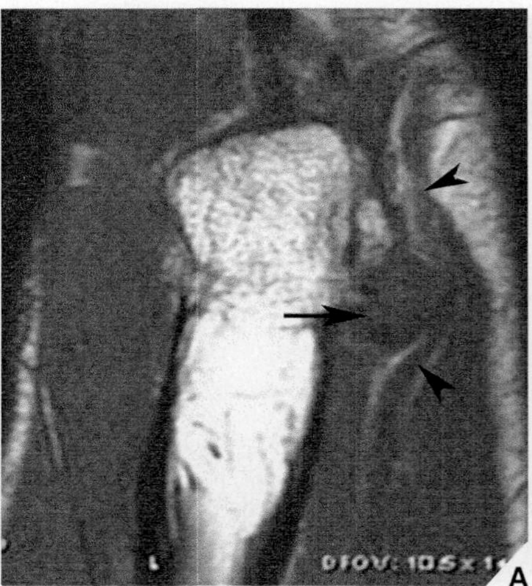

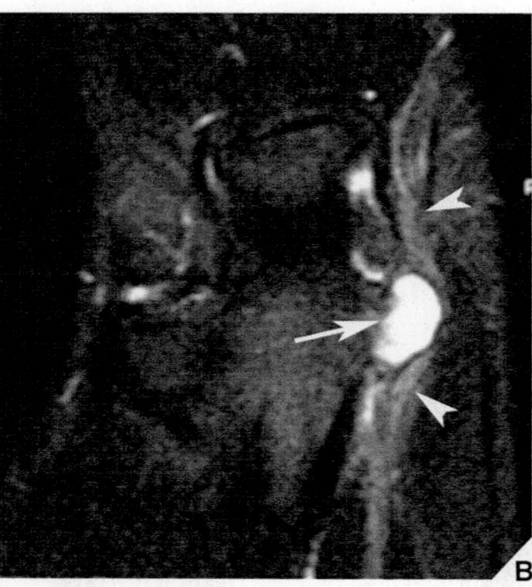

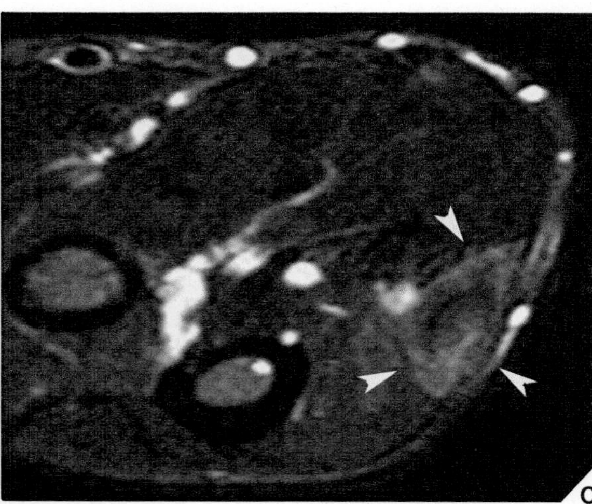

FIGURE 6.72 **MRI of cubital tunnel syndrome caused by a ganglion cyst.** **(A)** Coronal T1-weighted MRI of the elbow demonstrates a fluid collection in the posterior medial aspect of the elbow *(arrow)* producing compression and displacement of the ulnar nerve at the entrance into the cubital tunnel *(arrowheads)*. **(B)** Coronal STIR MRI demonstrates the fluid nature of the cyst *(arrow)* and the displaced, edematous ulnar nerve *(arrowheads)*. **(C)** Axial T2-weighted MRI shows early signs of denervation of the flexor carpi radialis muscle with edema *(arrowheads)*.

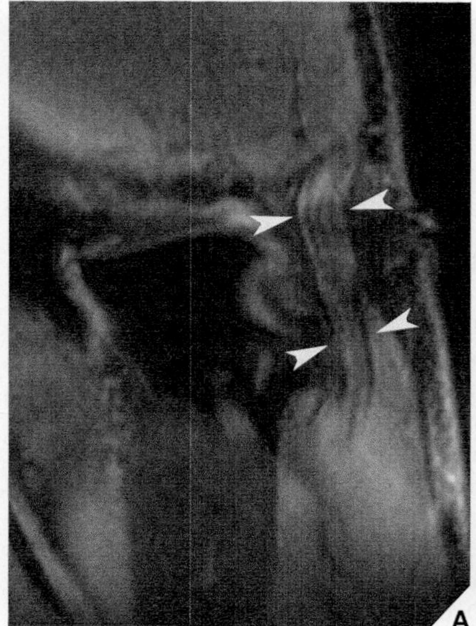

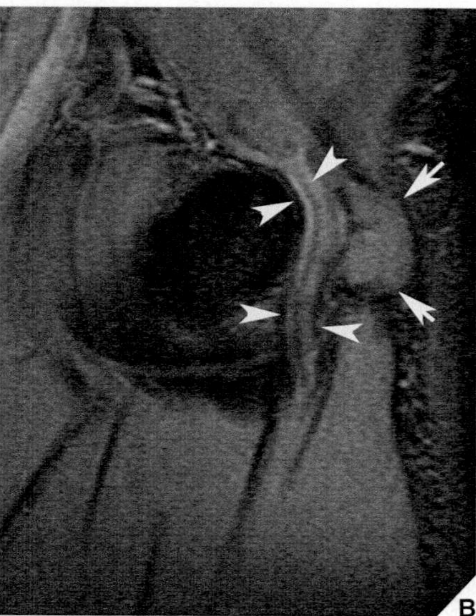

FIGURE 6.73 **MRI of cubital tunnel syndrome caused by an anconeus epitrochlearis muscle.** **(A)** Coronal STIR MRI demonstrates a thickened and hyperintense ulnar nerve proximal to the entrance into the cubital tunnel *(arrowheads)*, consistent with ulnar neuritis. **(B)** Sagittal STIR MRI through the medial aspect of the elbow shows the thickened and hyperintense ulnar nerve *(arrowheads)*. Dorsal to the ulnar nerve, there is a soft-tissue mass representing an anconeus epitrochlearis accessory muscle *(arrows)*.

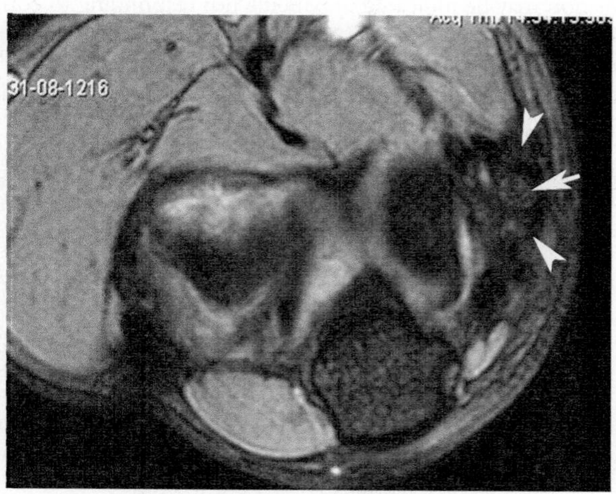

FIGURE 6.74 **MRI of failed ulnar nerve transposition.** Axial gradient recalled echo (GRE) MRI demonstrates the anteriorly transposed thickened ulnar nerve *(arrow)* surrounded by scar tissue *(arrowheads)* in this patient with recurrent signs of cubital tunnel syndrome following surgical nerve transposition.

2. On the lateral view of the elbow:
   - note the normal angular (hockey-stick) appearance of the distal humerus; the angle measures approximately 140 degrees; loss of this angle occurs in supracondylar fracture
   - evaluate the position of the capitellum relative to the longitudinal axis of the proximal radius and the anterior humeral line
   - pay attention to the presence or absence of the fat-pad sign; if this sign is positive in a patient with an elbow injury, then a fracture should always be considered.
3. The radial head–capitellum projection is very useful in evaluating elbow trauma and should always be obtained as part of a routine study.
4. Arthrotomography used to be an effective technique in selected cases of elbow injury. Currently it has been replaced by CT-arthrography. This procedure helps to visualize:
   - subtle chondral and osteochondral fractures
   - osteochondritis dissecans
   - synovial and capsular abnormalities
   - osteochondral bodies in the joint.
5. MRa of the elbow joint is useful to evaluate synovial abnormalities and the integrity of the joint capsule and ligaments and to detect intraarticular loose bodies.
6. Supracondylar fracture of the distal humerus (usually of the extension type) is very common in children. The lateral radiograph showing loss of the hockey-stick appearance of the distal humerus is diagnostic. If the lateral projection is equivocal, then obtain a radiograph of the contralateral (normal) elbow for comparison.
7. A fracture of the radial head is common in adults. It is important to demonstrate:
   - the type of fracture
   - the extension of the fracture line
   - the degree of articular displacement.

   This information determines whether a conservative or a surgical course of treatment is indicated.
8. A fracture of the coronoid process is usually occult and is most often associated with the posterior dislocation in the elbow joint. If unrecognized, it may fail to unite, leading to recurrent subluxation or dislocation in the joint. The radial head–capitellum view is best suited to demonstrate it.
9. Fractures of the olecranon are best demonstrated on the lateral view. They are classified into three types, according to the origin of the fracture line at the articular surface of the olecranon fossa.
10. The orthopaedic management of osteochondritis dissecans requires demonstrating the status of the articular cartilage of the capitellum and determining the stability of the osteochondral fragment. MRI or MRa is the procedure of choice.
11. In every case of ulnar fracture, look for associated dislocation of the radial head; conversely, in every case of dislocation, look for a fracture of the ulna (Monteggia fracture–dislocation). Proper radiographic technique for imaging these often-missed injuries requires, in adults, obtaining two separate radiographs that include the elbow joint and the forearm: one centered over the joint and the other over the midforearm. In children, a single film that includes the elbow joint and the entire forearm suffices.
12. Essex-Lopresti fracture–dislocation is a complex, unstable injury that comprises a comminuted fracture of the radial head and neck, tear of the interosseous membrane of the forearm, and dislocation in the distal radioulnar joint.
13. Lateral epicondylitis (or tennis elbow) is most effectively evaluated with MRI. This technique may show avulsion of the extensor carpi radialis brevis tendon from the lateral epicondyle and associated bone marrow edema.
14. PLRI of the elbow results from injury to the lateral collateral ligament complex.
15. VEOS is the most common mechanism of elbow injury in the throwing athlete and can be accurately diagnosed with MRI.
16. Medial epicondylitis (or golfer's elbow), a condition affecting the origin of the common flexor tendon at its attachment to the medial epicondyle of the humerus, shows on MRI thickening and increased signal of the affected tendons and discontinuity of the fibers with a complete rupture.
17. A rupture of the distal biceps tendon at its attachment to the radial tuberosity is most effectively demonstrated using MRI in sagittal and axial imaging planes. MRI-modified coronal section with the arm in abduction, elbow in flexion, and arm in supination (FABS position) is also very effective technique to demonstrate this injury.
18. CENs of the elbow include pronator teres muscle syndrome, supinator muscle syndrome, and cubital tunnel syndrome. All of these conditions have characteristic appearance on MRI.

SUGGESTED READINGS

Awaya H, Schweitzer ME, Feng SA, et al. Elbow synovial fold syndrome: MR imaging findings. *AJR Am J Roentgenol* 2001;177:1377–1381.

Bado JL. *The Monteggia lesion*. Springfield, IL: CC Thomas; 1962.

Beltran J, Rosenberg ZS. MR imaging of pediatric elbow fractures. *Magn Reson Imaging Clin N Am* 1997;5:567–578.

Bledsoe RC, Izenstark JL. Displacement of fat pads in diseases and injury of the elbow: a new radiographic sign. *Radiology* 1959;73:717–724.

Carrino JA, Morrison WB, Zou KH, et al. Noncontrast MR imaging and MR arthrography of the ulnar collateral ligament of the elbow: prospective evaluation of two-dimensional pulse sequences for detection of complete tears. *Skeletal Radiol* 2001;30:625–632.

Colton CL. Fractures of the olecranon in adults: classification and management. *Injury* 1973;5:121–129.

De Smet AA, Winter TC, Best TM, et al. Dynamic sonography with valgus stress to assess elbow ulnar collateral ligament injury in baseball pitchers. *Skeletal Radiol* 2002;31:671–676.

DeLee JC, Green DP, Wilkins KE. Fractures and dislocations of the elbow. In: Rockwood CA, Green DP, eds. *Fractures in adults*, 2nd ed. Philadelphia: Lippincott; 1984:559.

Deutsch AL, Mink JH, eds. *MRI of the musculoskeletal system: a teaching file*, 2nd ed. Philadelphia: Lippincott-Raven; 1997.

Dugas JR. Valgus extension overload: diagnosis and treatment. *Clin Sports Med* 2010;29:645–654.

Franklin PD, Dunlop RW, Whitelaw G, et al. Computed tomography of the normal and traumatized elbow. *J Comput Assist Tomogr* 1988;12:817–823.

Greenspan A, Norman A. Radial head-capitellum view in elbow trauma. Letter to the editor. *Am J Roentgenol* 1983;140:1273–1275.

Greenspan A, Norman A. The radial head-capitellum view: useful technique in elbow trauma. *Am J Roentgenol* 1982;138:1186–1188.

Greenspan A, Norman A, Rosen H. Radial head-capitellum view in elbow trauma: clinical application and radiographic-anatomic correlation. *Am J Roentgenol* 1984;143:355–359.

Horne JG, Tanzer TL. Olecranon fractures: a review of 100 cases. *J Trauma* 1981;21:469–472.

Hurd WJ, Eby E, Kaufman KR, et al. Magnetic resonance imaging of the throwing elbow in the uninjured, high school-aged baseball pitcher. *Am J Sports Med* 2011;39:722–728.

Jobe FW, Stark H, Lombardo SJ. Reconstruction of the ulnar collateral ligament in athletes. *J Bone Joint Surg Am* 1986;68:1158–1163.

Kijowski R, Tuite M, Sanford M. Magnetic resonance imaging of the elbow. Part I: normal anatomy, imaging technique, and osseous abnormalities. *Skeletal Radiol* 2004;33:685–697.

Kijowski R, Tuite M, Sanford M. Magnetic resonance imaging of the elbow. Part II: abnormalities of the ligaments, tendons, and nerves. *Skeletal Radiol* 2005;34:1–18.

Mak S, Beltran LS, Bencardino J, et al. MRI of the annular ligament of the elbow: review of anatomic considerations and pathologic findings in patients with posterolateral elbow instability. *AJR Am J Roentgenol* 2014;203:1272–1279.

Mason ML. Some observations on fractures of the head of the radius with a review of one hundred cases. *Br J Surg* 1959;42:123–132.

Müller ME, Allgower M, Schneider R, et al. *Manual of internal fixation, techniques recommended by the AO Group*, 2nd ed. Berlin, Germany: Springer-Verlag; 1979.

Ouellette H, Bredella M, Labis J, et al. MR imaging of the elbow in baseball pitchers. *Skeletal Radiol* 2008;37:115–121.

Poltawski L, Ali S, Jayaram V, et al. Reliability of sonographic assessment of tendinopathy in tennis elbow. *Skeletal Radiol* 2012;41:83–89.

Potter HGH, Weiland AJA, Schatz JAJ, et al. Posterolateral rotatory instability of the elbow: usefulness of MR imaging in diagnosis. *Radiology* 1997;204:185–189.

Reckling FW, Peltier LF. Riccardo Galeazzi and Galeazzi's fracture. *Surgery* 1965;58:453–459.

Rogers LF. Fractures and dislocations of the elbow. *Semin Roentgenol* 1978;13:97–107.

Rogers LF, Malave S Jr, White H, et al. Plastic bowing, torus and greenstick supracondylar fractures of the humerus: radiographic clues to obscure fractures of the elbow in children. *Radiology* 1978;128:145–150.

Sanchez-Sotelo J, Morrey BF, O'Driscoll SW. Ligamentous repair and reconstruction for posterolateral rotatory instability of the elbow. *J Bone Joint Surg Br* 2005;87:54–61.

Schueller-Weidekamm C, Kainberger F. The elbow joint—a diagnostic challenge: anatomy, biomechanics, and pathology. *Radiologe* 2008;48(12):1173–1185.

Sharma SC, Singh R, Goel T, et al. Missed diagnosis of triceps tendon rupture: a case report and review of literature. *J Orthop Surg (Hong Kong)* 2005;13:307–309.

Steinbach LS, Palmer WE, Schweitzer ME. Special focus session. MR arthrography. *Radiographics* 2002;22:1223–1246.

Takahara M, Ogino T, Takagi M, et al. Natural progression of osteochondritis dissecans of the humeral capitellum: initial observations. *Radiology* 2000;216:207–212.

7

Upper Limb III

Distal Forearm, Wrist, Hand, and Fingers

Distal Forearm

An injury to the distal forearm, caused predominantly (90% of cases) by a fall on the outstretched hand, is common throughout life but is most common in the elderly. The type of injury usually sustained is a fracture of the distal radius or ulna, the incidence of which substantially exceeds that of a dislocation in the distal radioulnar and radiocarpal articulations. Although history and physical examination usually provide important information regarding the type of injury, radiographs are indispensable in determining the exact site and extent; in several types of fractures, only adequate imaging examination can lead to a correct diagnosis.

Anatomic–Radiologic Considerations

Radiographs obtained in the posteroanterior and lateral projections are usually sufficient to evaluate most injuries to the distal forearm (Figs. 7.1 and 7.2). On each of these views, it is important to appreciate the normal anatomic relations of the radius and the ulna for a complete evaluation of trauma.

The posteroanterior view of the distal forearm reveals anatomic variations in the length of the radius and the ulna, known as *ulnar variance* or *Hulten variance*. As a rule, the radial styloid process exceeds the length of the articular end of the ulna by 9 to 12 mm. At the site of articulation with the lunate, however, the articular surfaces of the radius and the ulna are on the same level, yielding *neutral ulnar variance* (Fig. 7.3). Occasionally, the ulna projects more proximally—*negative ulnar variance* (or ulna minus variant)—or more distally—*positive ulnar variance* (or ulna plus variant) (Fig. 7.4). Wrist position is an important determinant of ulnar variance. The generally accepted standard position is a posteroanterior view obtained with the wrist flat on the radiographic table, neutral forearm rotation, and with the elbow flexed 90 degrees and the shoulder abducted 90 degrees. The posteroanterior radiograph also reveals an important anatomic feature of the radius known as the *radial angle* (also called the *ulnar slant* of the articular surface of the radius), which normally ranges from 15 to 25 degrees (Fig. 7.5).

The lateral view of the distal forearm demonstrates another significant feature, the *volar tilt* of the articular surface of the radius (known variously as the *dorsal angle*, *palmar facing*, or *palmar inclination*). The tilt normally ranges from 10 to 25 degrees (Fig. 7.6).

Both these measurements have practical importance to the orthopaedic surgeon in assessing the displacement and the position of fragments after a fracture of the distal radius. They can also help the surgeon to decide between closed and open reduction as well as assist in follow-up examinations.

Ancillary imaging techniques are commonly required for evaluating trauma to the distal forearm and wrist. Arthrographic examination (Fig. 7.7) may need to be performed in cases of suspected injury to the triangular fibrocartilage complex (TFCC), which consists of the triangular fibrocartilage (articular disk), the meniscus homolog, the dorsal and volar radioulnar ligaments, and the ulnar collateral ligament (Fig. 7.8). Because the radiocarpal cavity into which contrast is injected normally does not communicate with the distal radioulnar joint, opacification of this compartment indicates a tear of the triangular fibrocartilage (see Fig. 7.29B). In a small percentage of cases, a false-positive result may be caused by a normal anatomic variant allowing communication between the radiocarpal compartment and the distal radioulnar joint. Currently, computed tomography (CT) and magnetic resonance imaging (MRI) play an important role in evaluation of injuries to the distal forearm, wrist, and hand (see the text that follows).

For a summary in tabular form of the standard radiographic projections and ancillary imaging techniques used to evaluate trauma to the distal forearm, see Tables 7.1 and 7.2.

Injury to the Distal Forearm

Fractures of the Distal Radius

Colles Fracture

The most frequently encountered injury to the distal forearm, *Colles fracture*, usually results from a fall on the outstretched hand with the forearm pronated in dorsiflexion. It is most commonly seen in adults older than the age of 50 years and more often in women than in men. In the classic description of this injury, known in the European literature as the *Pouteau fracture*, the fracture line is extraarticular, usually occurring approximately 2 to 3 cm from the articular surface of the distal radius. In many cases, the distal fragment is radially and dorsally displaced and shows dorsal angulation, although other variants in the alignment of fragments may also be seen (Fig. 7.9). Commonly, there is an associated fracture of the ulnar styloid process. It should be noted that some authors (e.g., Frykman) include intraarticular extension of the fracture line, as well as an associated fracture of the distal end of the ulna, under this eponym (Fig. 7.10; Table 7.3).

Radiographs in the posteroanterior and lateral projections are usually sufficient to demonstrate Colles fracture. The complete evaluation on both views should take note of the status of the radial angle and the palmar inclination as well as the degree of foreshortening of the radius secondary to impaction or bayonet-type displacement (Figs. 7.11 and 7.12). CT scanning may provide additional information concerning the exact position of displaced fragments (Figs. 7.13 to 7.16). Occasionally, radiographs of the wrist may not show an acute nondisplaced fracture of the distal radius (occult fracture). In these cases, MRI is more effective in demonstrating the fracture line leading to appropriate treatment (Fig. 7.17).

Complications. At the time of fracture, a concomitant injury to the median and ulnar nerves may occur. A lack of stability of the fragments

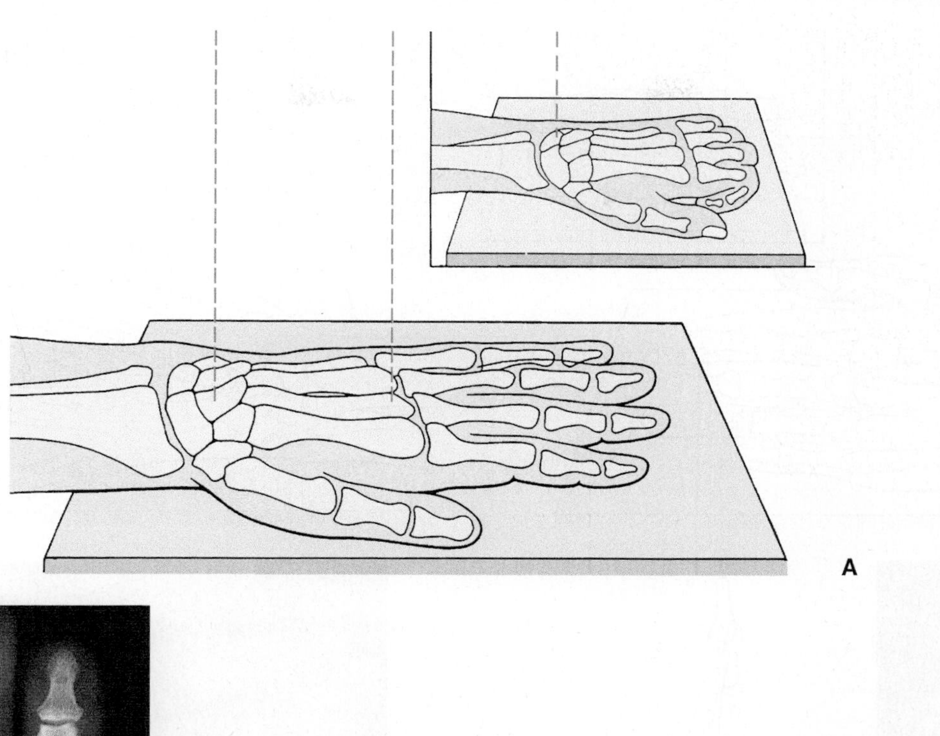

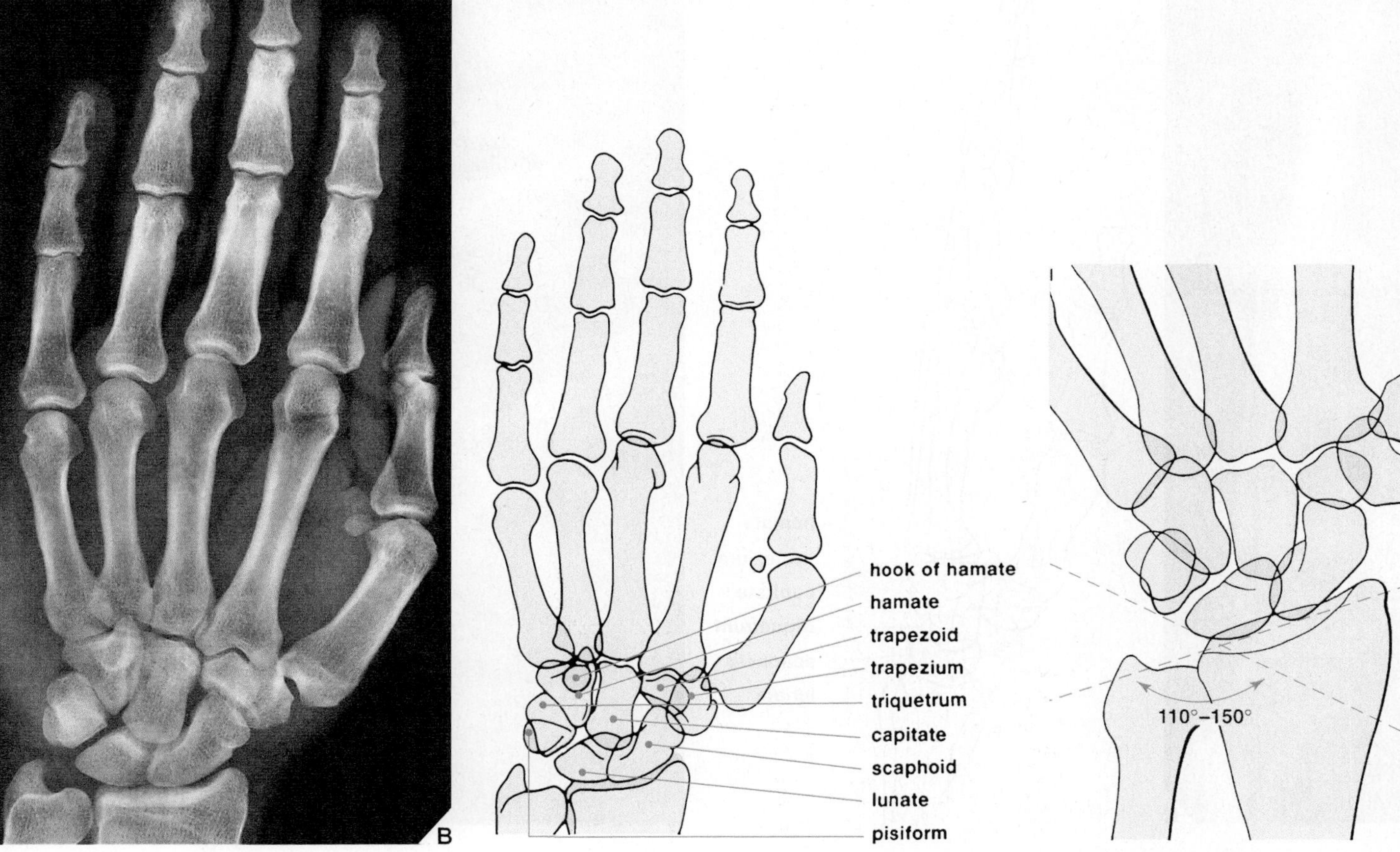

FIGURE 7.1 Dorsovolar (posteroanterior) view of the distal forearm, wrist, and hand. For the purpose of classification, a distinction is made between traumatic conditions involving the distal forearm, the wrist, and the hand. From a radiologic perspective, however, the positioning of the limb for posteroanterior and lateral films of the wrist area (i.e., the distal forearm and the carpus) and the hand is essentially the same. **(A)** For the posteroanterior (dorsovolar) view of the wrist and the hand, patients are seated with the arm fully extended on the radiographic table. The portion of the limb from the distal third of the forearm to the fingertips rests prone on the film cassette. Whether the wrist area or the hand is the focus of evaluation, the hand usually lies flat (palm down), with the fingers slightly spread. The point toward which the central beam *(red broken line)* is directed, however, varies. For the wrist, the beam is directed toward the center of the carpus; for the hand, the beam is directed toward the head of the third metacarpal bone. For better demonstration of the wrist area, the patient's fingers may be flexed to cause the carpus to lie flat on the film cassette *(inset)*. **(B)** On the radiograph obtained in this projection, the distal radius and the ulna, as well as the carpal and metacarpal bones and phalanges, are well demonstrated. The thumb, however, is seen in an oblique projection; the bases of the second to fifth metacarpals partially overlap. In the wrist, there is also overlap of the pisiform and the triquetrum, as well as the trapezium and trapezoid bones. **(C)** On this projection, a carpal angle can be determined. It is formed by two tangents, the first drawn against the proximal borders of the scaphoid and lunate *(1)* and the second drawn against the proximal borders of the triquetrum and lunate *(2)*. The angle measures normally between 110 and 150 degrees, showing considerable deviation with age, gender, and race.

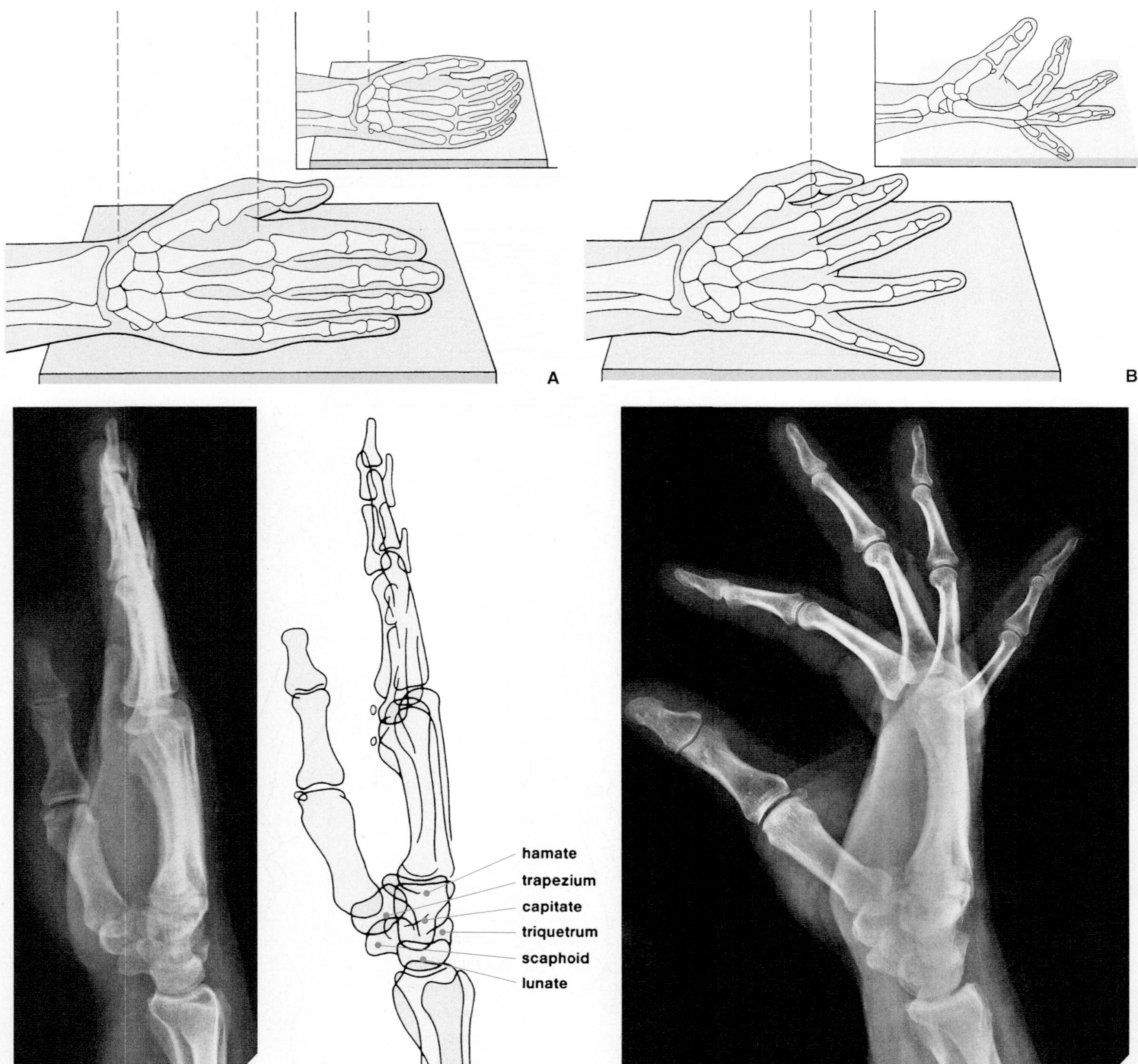

FIGURE 7.2 Lateral view of the wrist and hand. (A) For the lateral projection of the wrist area and the hand, the patient's arm is fully extended and resting on its ulnar side. The fingers may be fully extended or, preferably, slightly flexed *(inset)*, with the thumb slightly in front of the fingers. For the evaluation of the wrist area, the central beam *(red broken line)* is directed toward the center of the carpus, whereas for the hand, it is directed toward the head of the second metacarpal **(B)**. On the radiograph obtained in this projection **(C)**, the distal radius and the ulna overlap, but the relation of the longitudinal axes of the capitate, the lunate, and the radius can sufficiently be evaluated (see Fig. 7.92). Although the metacarpals and the phalanges also overlap, dorsal or volar displacement of a fracture of these bones can easily be detected (see Fig. 4.1). The thumb is imaged in true dorsovolar projection. A more effective way of imaging the fingers in the lateral projection is to have the patient spread the fingers in a fan-like manner, with the ulnar side of the fifth phalanx resting on the film cassette. The central beam *(red broken line)* is directed toward the heads of the metacarpals. **(D)** On the film in this projection, the overlap of the phalanges commonly seen on the standard lateral view is eliminated. The interphalangeal joints can readily be evaluated.

FIGURE 7.3 Neutral ulnar variance. **(A)** As a rule, the radial styloid process rises 9 to 12 mm above the articular surface of the distal ulna. This distance is also known as the *radial length.* **(B)** At the site of articulation with the lunate, the articular surfaces of the radius and the ulna are on the same level.

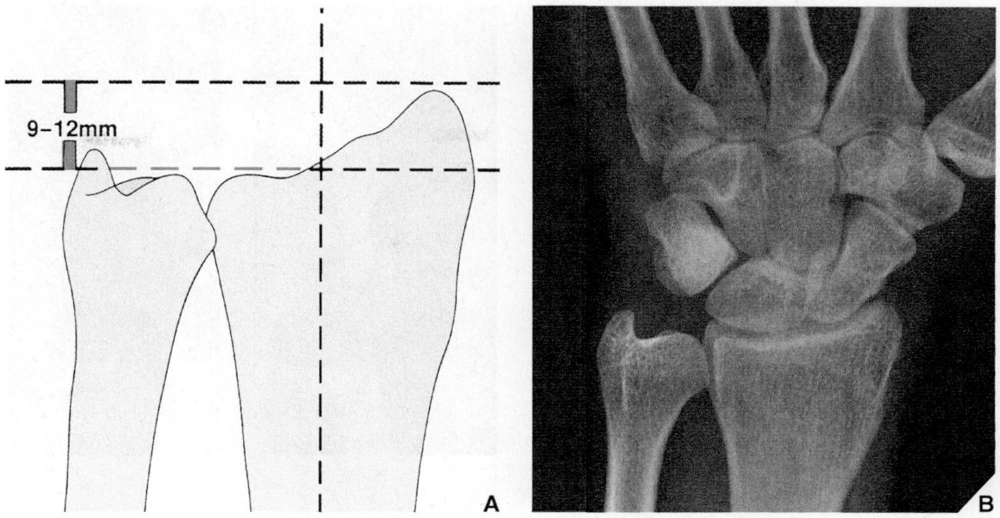

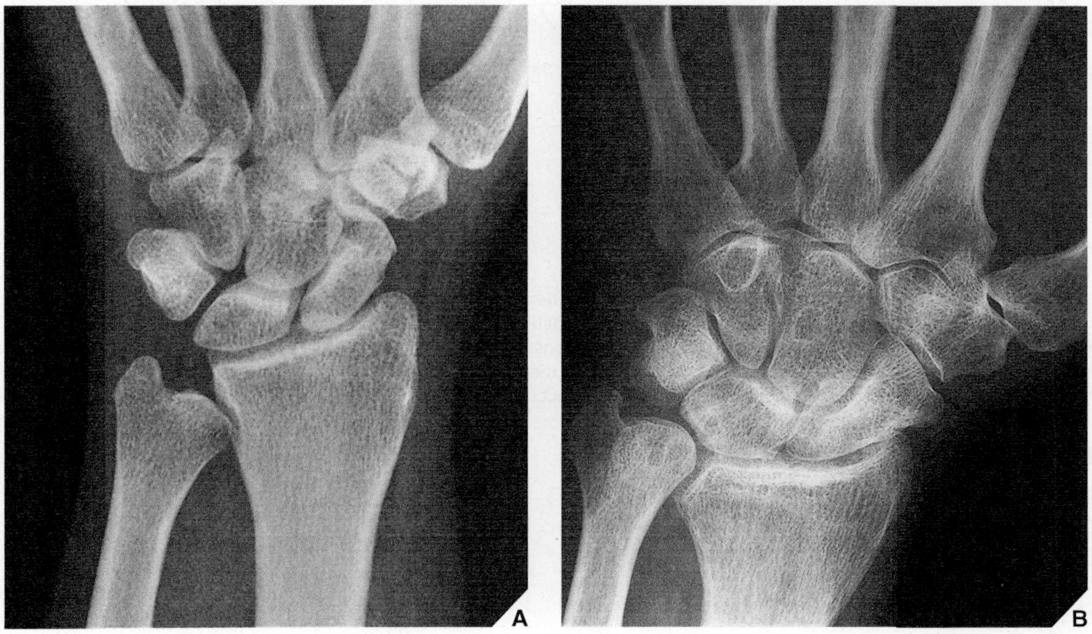

FIGURE 7.4 Negative and positive ulnar variance. **(A)** Negative ulnar variance. The articular surface of the ulna projects 5 mm proximal to the site of radiolunate articulation. Ulnar negative variance may be associated with avascular necrosis of the lunate. **(B)** Positive ulnar variance. The articular surface of the ulna projects 8 mm distal to the site of radiolunate articulation. Note the subchondral cysts in the head of the ulna and ulnar aspect of the lunate bone, consistent with ulnolunate abutment syndrome, often associated with ulnar positive variance (see discussion below).

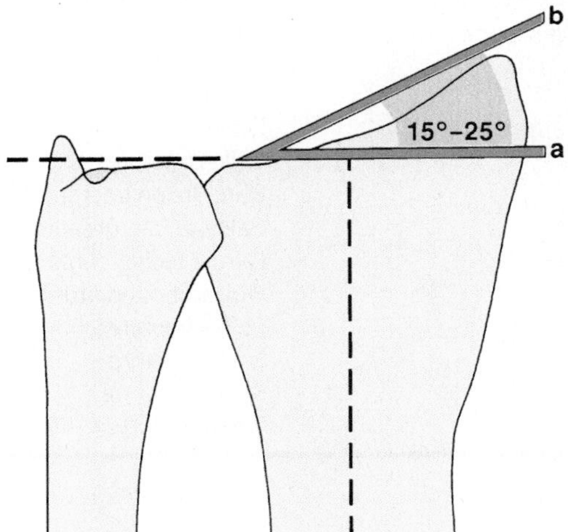

FIGURE 7.5 Ulnar slant. The ulnar slant of the articular surface of the radius is determined, with the wrist in the neutral position, by the angle formed by two lines: one perpendicular to the long axis of the radius at the level of the radioulnar articular surface *(a)* and a tangent connecting the radial styloid process and the ulnar aspect of the radius *(b)*.

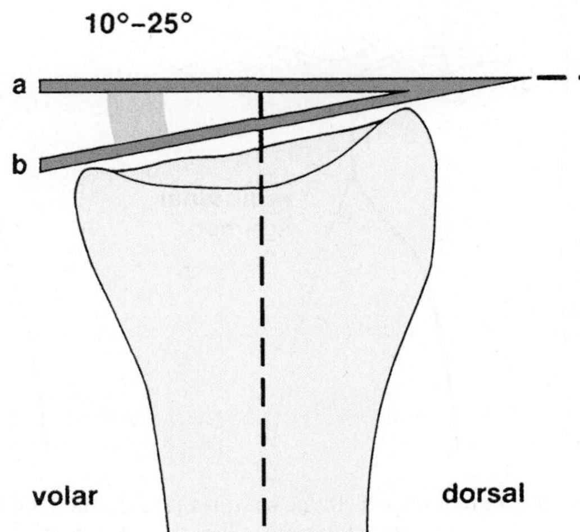

FIGURE 7.6 Palmar inclination. The palmar inclination of the radial articular surface is determined by measuring the angle formed by a line perpendicular to the long axis of the radius at the level of the styloid process *(a)* and a tangent connecting the dorsal and volar aspects of the radial articular surface *(b)*.

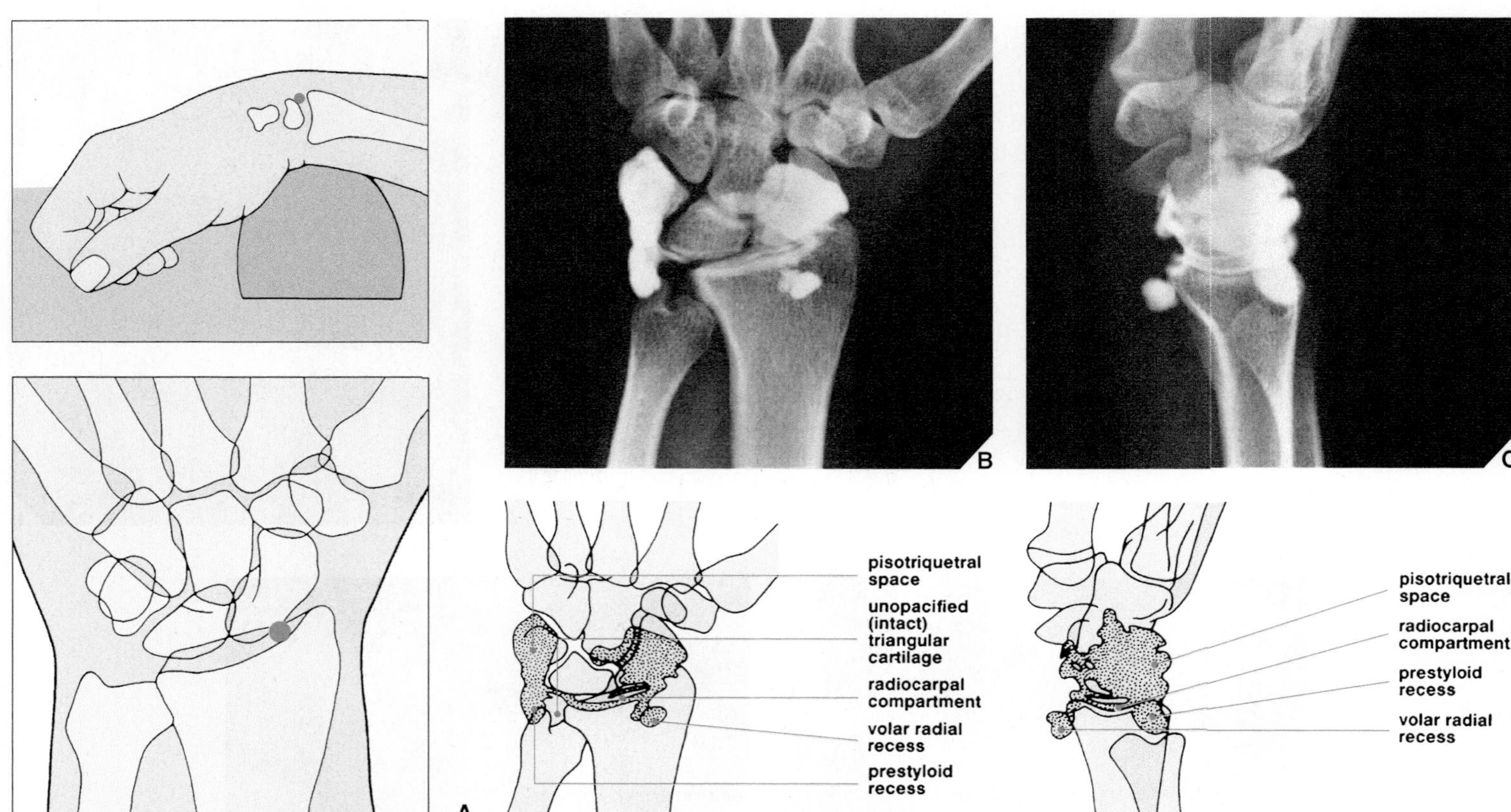

FIGURE 7.7 Arthrography of the wrist. (A) For arthrographic examination of the radiocarpal joint, the wrist is positioned prone on a radiolucent sponge to open the joint for needle insertion. Under fluoroscopic control, the joint is entered using a 22-gauge needle at a point lateral to the scapholunate ligament. (The *red dot* marks the site of puncture.) Two or 3 mL of contrast (60% diatrizoate meglumine) is injected, and posteroanterior (dorsovolar), lateral, and oblique films are obtained. **(B)** Posteroanterior and **(C)** lateral radiographs show the contrast filling the radiocarpal compartment, the prestyloid and volar radial recesses, and the pisotriquetral space. Intact triangular fibrocartilage does not allow the contrast to enter the distal radioulnar joint, and intact intercarpal ligaments prevent a leak of contrast into the intercarpal articulations.

TRIANGULAR FIBROCARTILAGE COMPLEX (TFCC)

extensor carpi ulnaris
ulnar collateral ligament
meniscus homologue
triangular fibrocartilage
radioulnar ligament

FIGURE 7.8 Triangular fibrocartilage complex (TFCC). The TFCC includes the triangular fibrocartilage, radioulnar ligament, ulnocarpal ligament, extensor carpi ulnaris tendon and tendon sheath, and meniscus homolog. It is located between the distal ulna and the proximal carpal row, stabilizes the distal radioulnar joint, and functions as a cushion of compressing axial forces. The triangular fibrocartilage attaches medially to the fovea of the ulna and laterally to the lunate fossa of the radius.

TABLE 7.1 Standard Radiographic Projections for Evaluating Injury to the Distal Forearm

Projection	Demonstration
Posteroanterior	Ulnar variance Carpal angle Radial angle Distal radioulnar joint Colles fracture Hutchinson fracture Galeazzi fracture–dislocation
Lateral	Palmar facing of radius Pronator quadratus fat stripe Colles fracture Smith fracture Barton fracture Galeazzi fracture–dislocation

TABLE 7.2 Ancillary Imaging Techniques for Evaluating Injury to the Distal Forearm

Technique	Demonstration
Arthrography	Radiocarpal articulation Tear of triangular fibrocartilage complex (TFCC)
Arteriography	Concomitant injury to the arteries of the forearm
Radionuclide imaging (scintigraphy, bone scan)	Subtle fractures of the radius and the ulna
Computed tomography (CT) (including three-dimensional [3D] CT)	Depression, displacement, and spatial orientation of fracture fragments of the radius and the ulna Fracture healing and complications of healing Soft-tissue injury (muscles)
Magnetic resonance imaging (MRI) and magnetic resonance arthrography (MRa)	Soft-tissue injury (muscles, tendons, ligaments) Subtle fractures and bone contusion of the radius and the ulna Tear of TFCC Injury to the interosseous membrane Abnormalities of various tendons, ligaments, muscles, and nerves

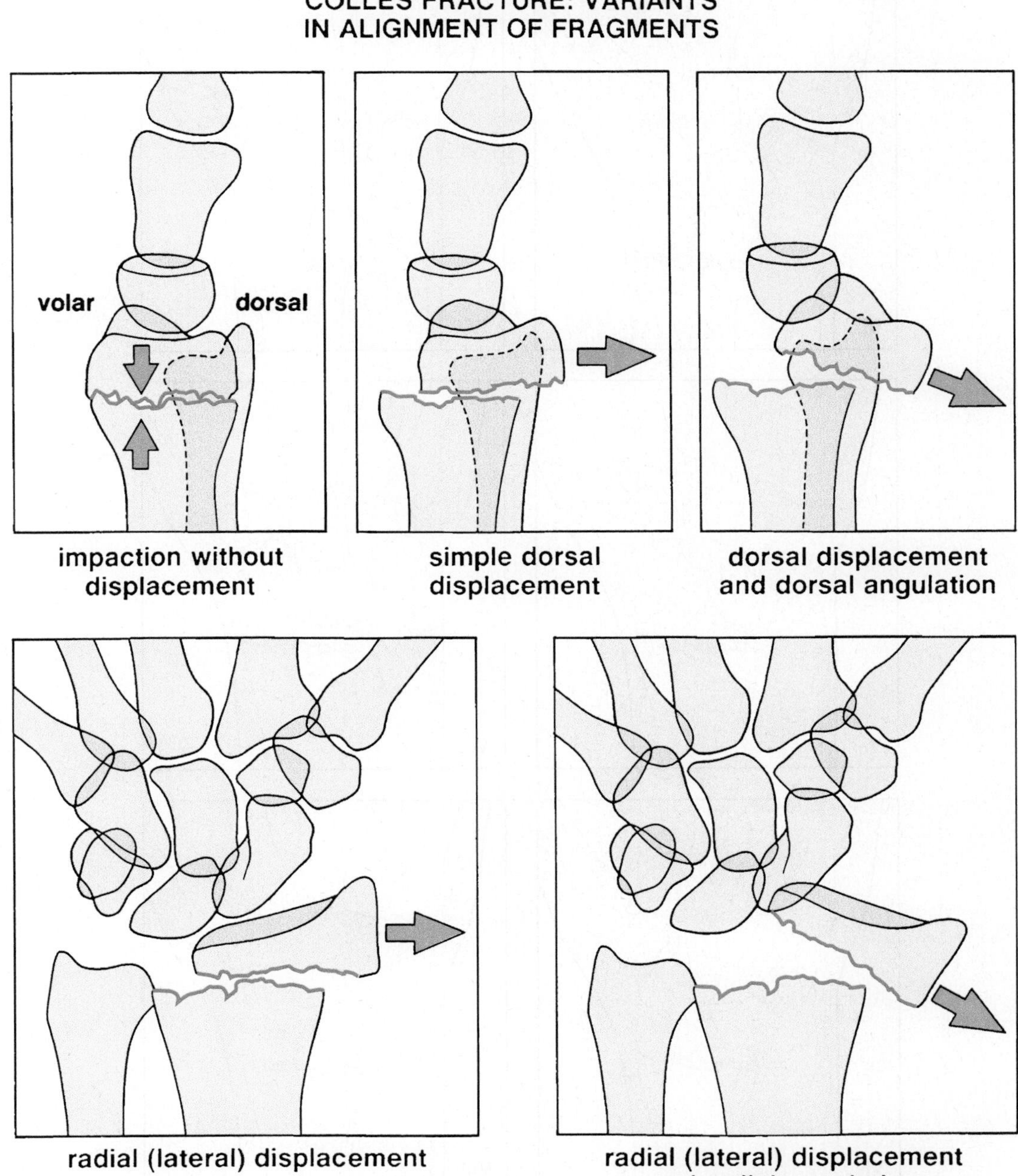

FIGURE 7.9 Colles fracture. Five variants of displacement and angulation of the distal fragment in Colles fracture. Some of these patterns may occur in combinations, yielding a complex deformity.

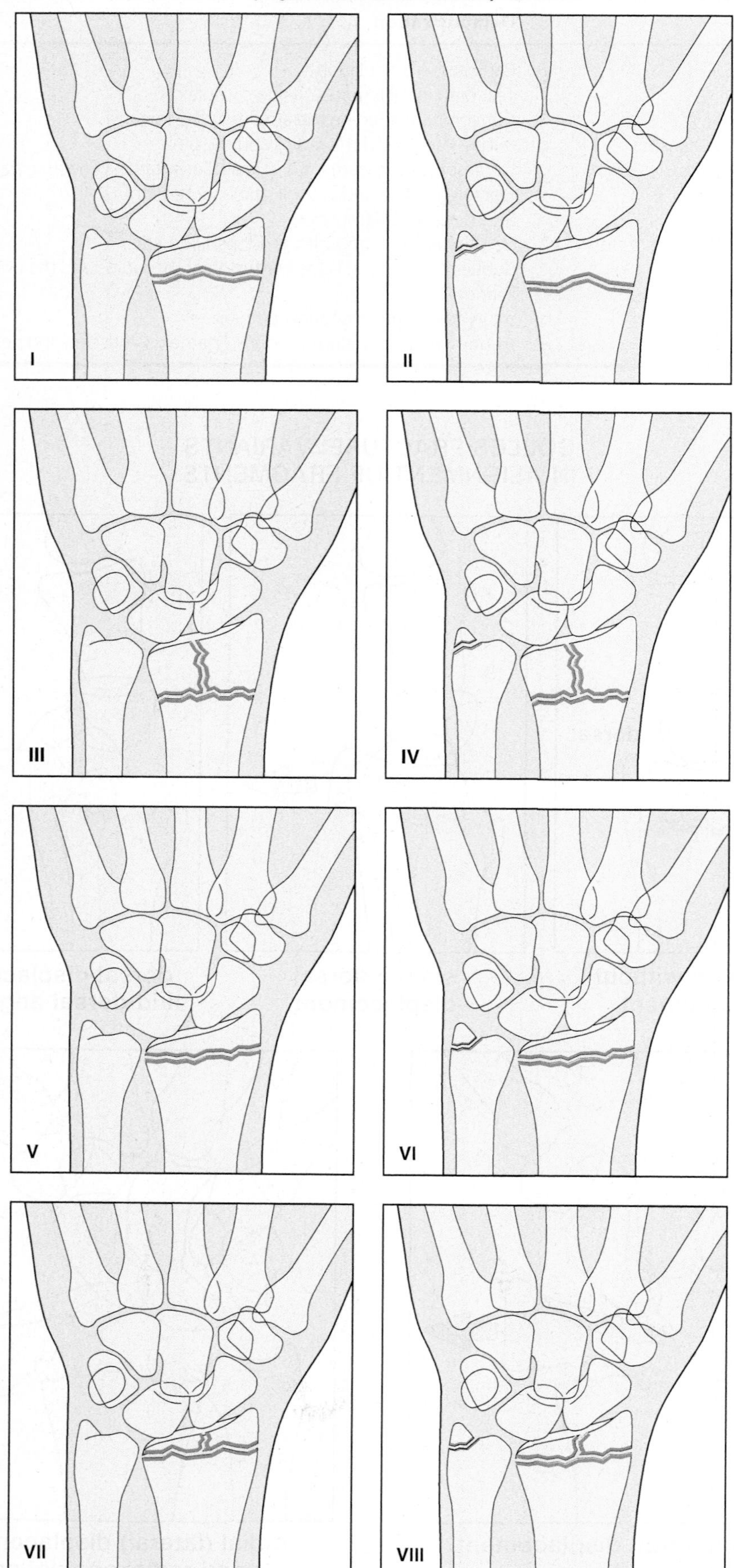

FIGURE 7.10 Distal radius fractures. Frykman classification of distal radius fractures according to the location of fracture line (intraarticular vs. extraarticular) and association of distal ulna fracture.

TABLE 7.3 Frykman Classification of Distal Radius Fractures

Radius Fracture	Distal Ulna Fracture	
Location	Absent	Present
Extraarticular	I	II
Intraarticular (radiocarpal joint)	III	IV
Intraarticular (radioulnar joint)	V	VI
Intraarticular (radiocarpal and radioulnar joints)	VII	VIII

during healing may result in a loss of reduction, but delayed union and nonunion are very rarely seen. As a sequela, posttraumatic arthritis may develop in the radiocarpal articulation.

Barton and Hutchinson Fractures

Both these fractures are intraarticular fractures of the distal radius. The classic *Barton fracture* affects the dorsal margin of the distal radius and extends into the radiocarpal articulation (Fig. 7.18); occasionally, there may also be an associated dislocation in the joint. When the fracture involves the volar margin of the distal radius with an intraarticular extension, it is known as a *reverse* (or *volar*) *Barton fracture* (Fig. 7.19). Because in both variants the fracture line is oriented in the coronal plane, it is best demonstrated on the lateral or oblique projections.

The *Hutchinson fracture* (also known as *chauffeur's fracture*—a name derived from the era of hand-cranked automobiles when direct trauma to the radial side of the wrist was often sustained from recoil of the crank) involves the radial (lateral) margin of the distal radius, extending through the radial styloid process into the radiocarpal articulation. Because of the sagittal orientation of the fracture line, the posteroanterior view is better suited to diagnose this type of injury (Fig. 7.20).

Smith Fracture

Usually resulting from a fall on the back of the hand or a direct blow to the dorsum of the hand in palmar flexion, a Smith fracture consists of a fracture of the distal radius, which sometimes extends into the radiocarpal joint, with volar displacement and angulation of the distal fragment (Fig. 7.21). Because the deformity in this fracture is the opposite of

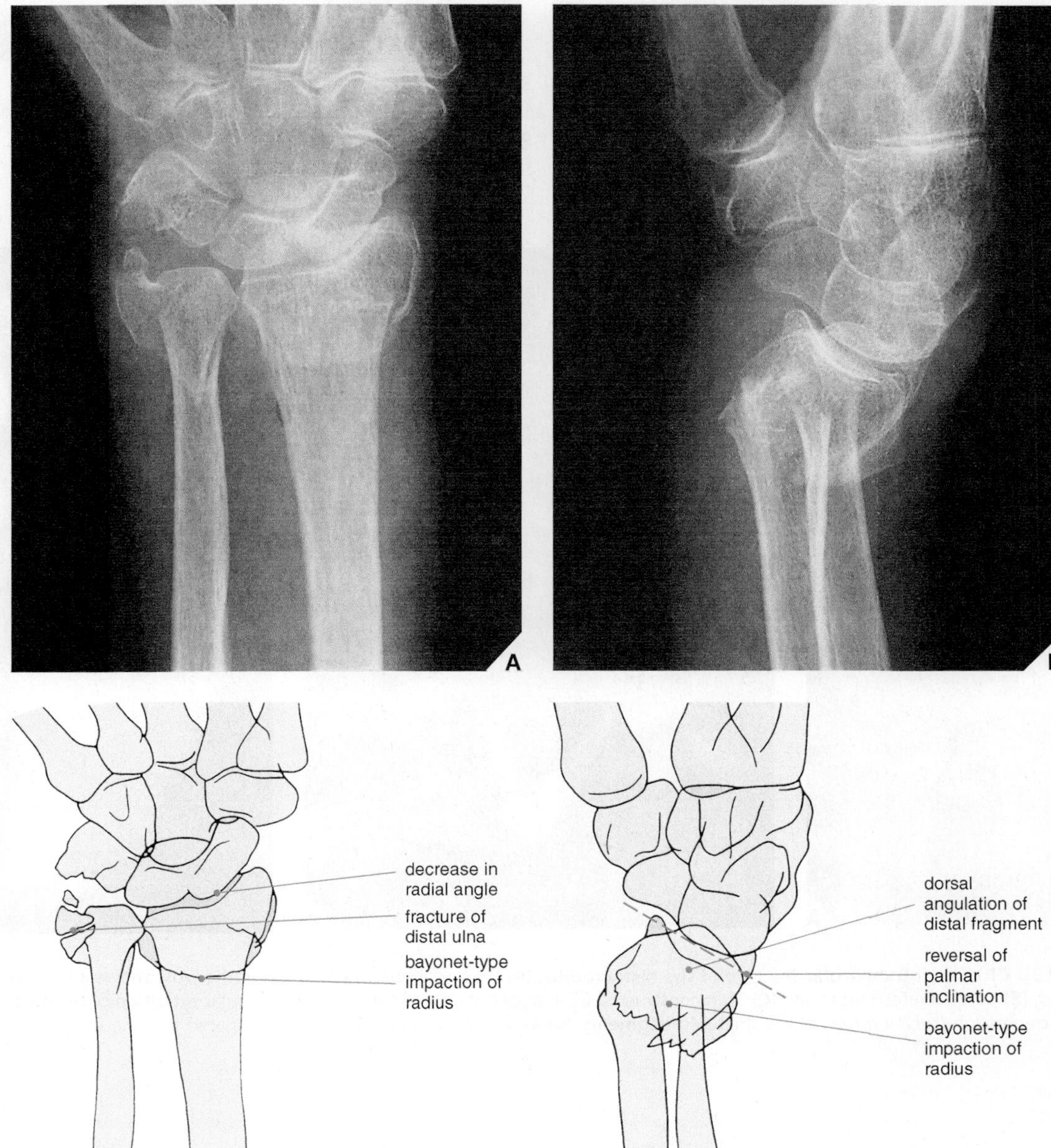

FIGURE 7.11 **Colles fracture.** **(A)** Posteroanterior and **(B)** lateral radiographs of the distal forearm demonstrate the features of Colles fracture. On the posteroanterior projection, a decrease in the radial angle and an associated fracture of the distal ulna are evident. The lateral view reveals the dorsal angulation of the distal radius as well as a reversal of the palmar inclination. On both views, the radius is foreshortened secondary to bayonet-type displacement. The fracture line does not extend to the joint (Frykman type II).

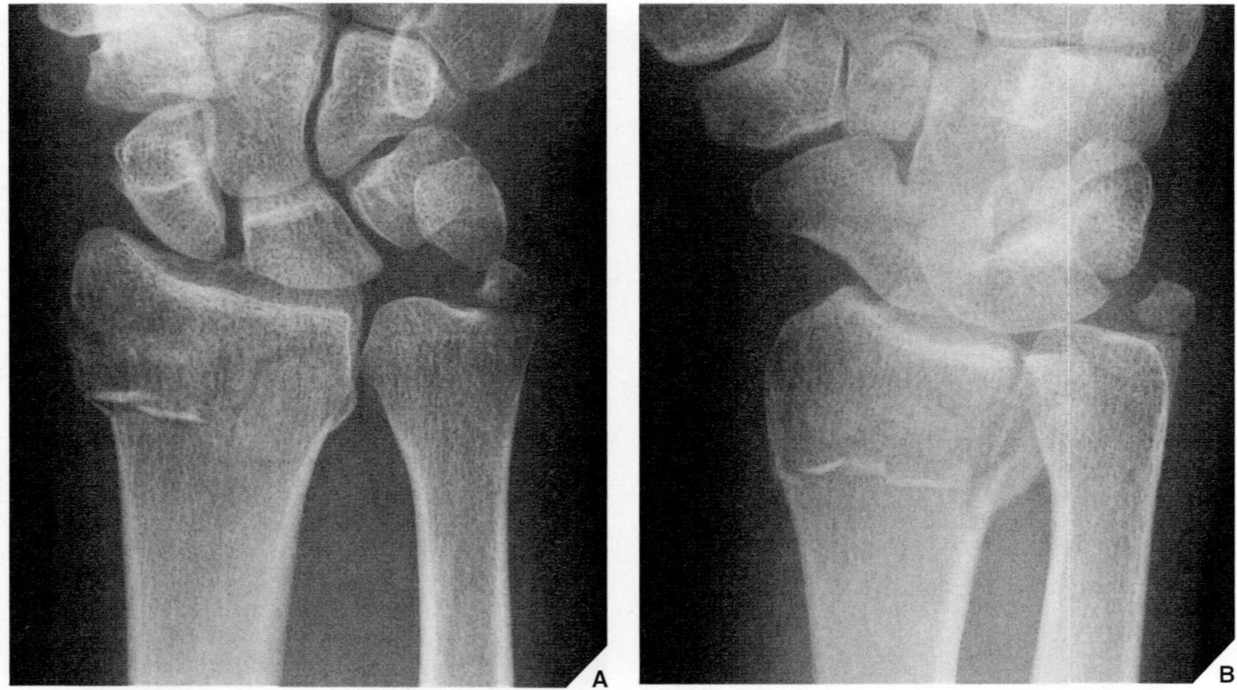

FIGURE 7.12 Intraarticular fracture of the distal radius. **(A)** Posteroanterior and **(B)** oblique radiographs of the distal forearm show Frykman type VI fracture. The fracture line extends into the distal radioulnar joint, and, in addition, there is a fracture of the ulnar styloid.

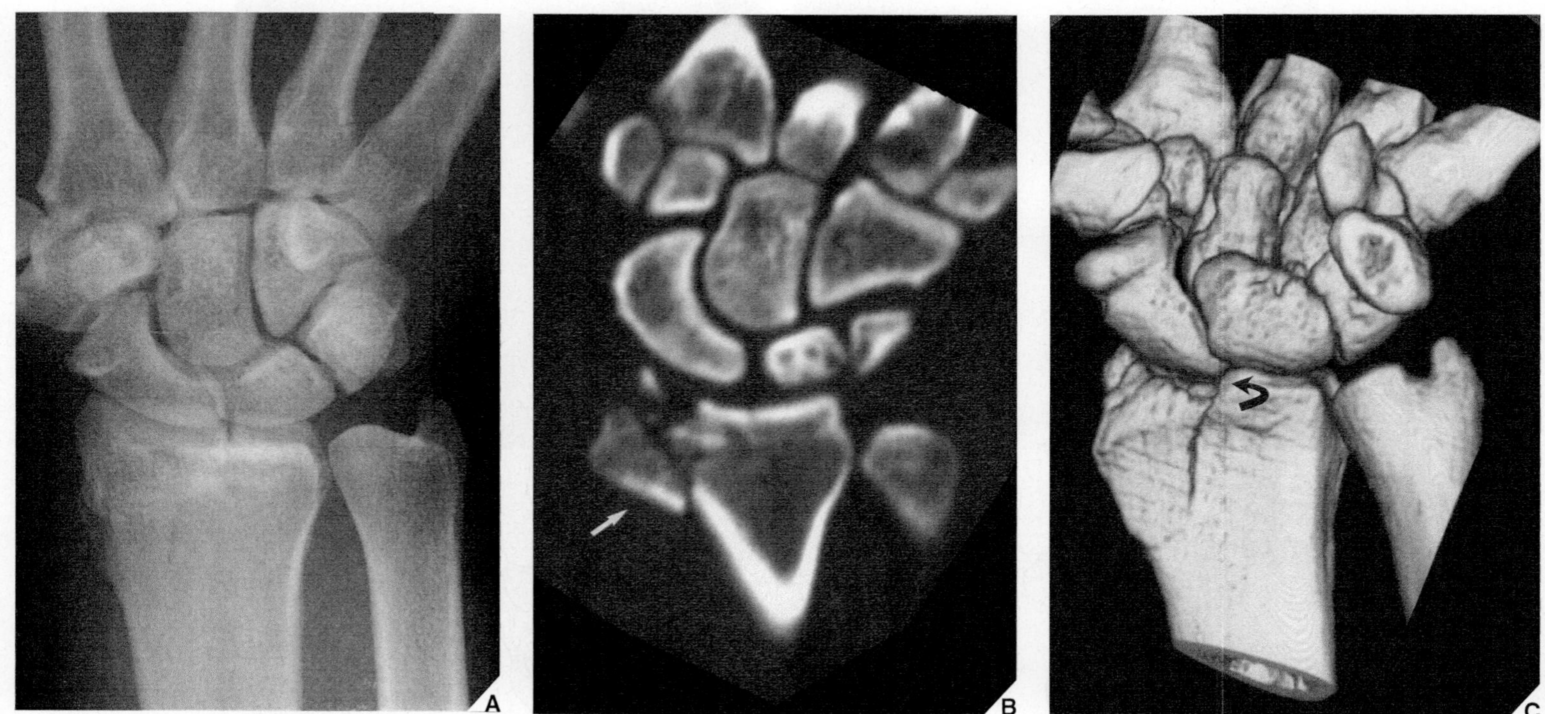

FIGURE 7.13 CT and 3D CT of an intraarticular fracture of the distal radius. **(A)** Posteroanterior radiograph of the wrist shows a fracture of the distal radius that appears to be nondisplaced. **(B)** Coronal reformatted and **(C)** 3D reconstructed CT images not only confirm the intraarticular extension of the fracture but also demonstrate displacement *(arrow)* and depression *(curved arrow)* of the fractured fragments. Because the distal radioulnar joint is spared and the ulna is intact, this injury represents Frykman type III fracture.

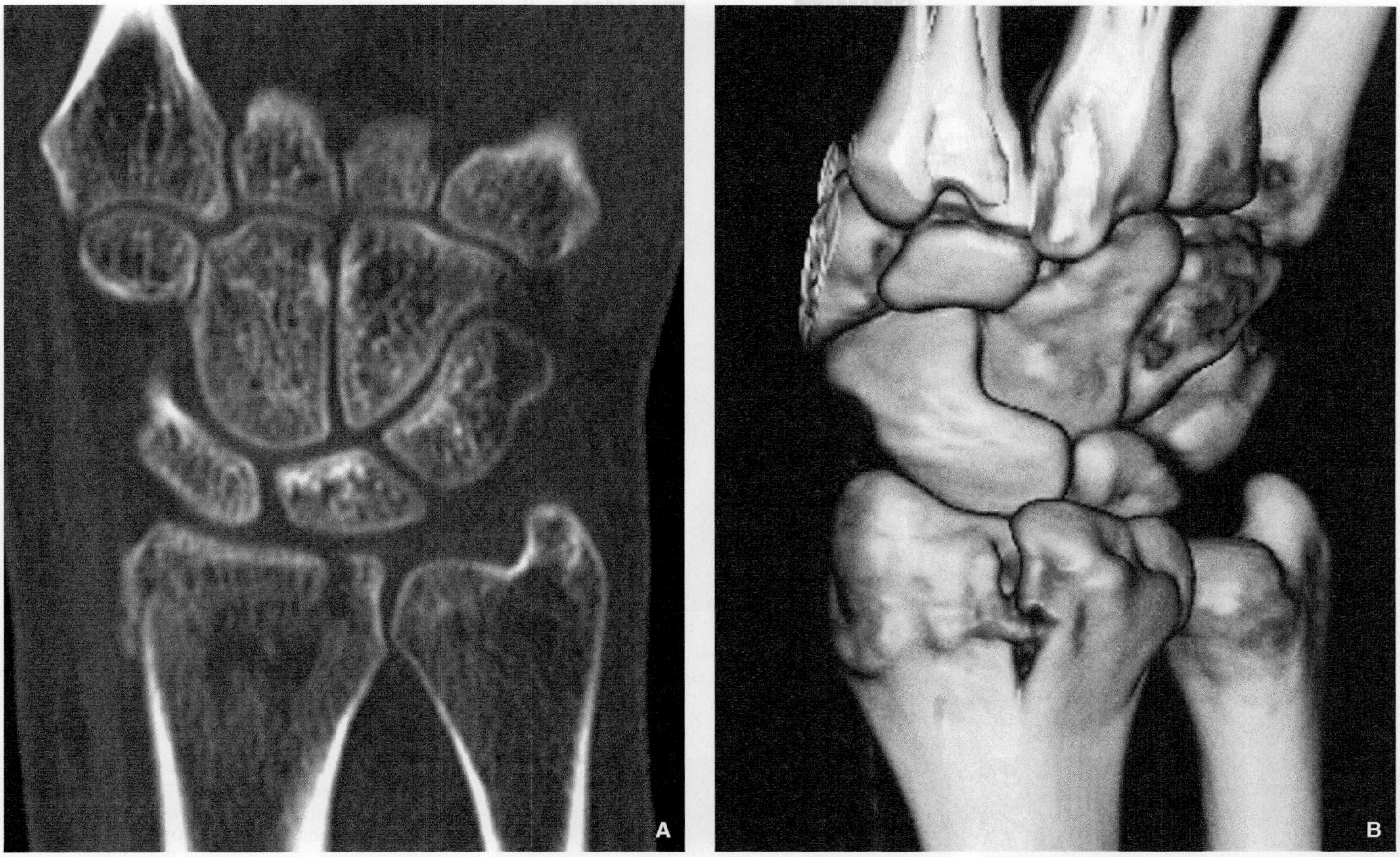

FIGURE 7.14 **CT and 3D CT of an intraarticular fracture of the distal radius.** **(A)** Coronal reformatted and **(B)** 3D reconstructed CT images of the left wrist of a 36-year-old woman show an intraarticular comminuted fracture of the distal radius extending into the radiocarpal joint. The fracture does not affect the distal radioulnar joint, consistent with Frykman type III fracture.

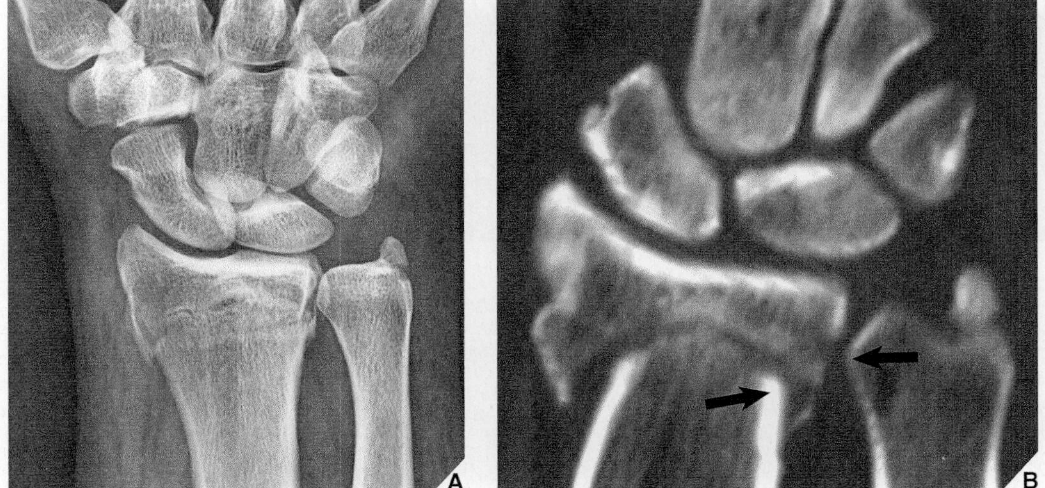

FIGURE 7.15 **CT of an intraarticular fracture of the distal radius.** **(A)** Dorsovolar radiograph of the wrist shows a fracture of the distal radius, but it is unclear if the fracture is extraarticular or intraarticular. In addition, there is a fracture of the styloid process of ulna. **(B)** Coronal reformatted CT image confirms that the fracture line extends into the distal radioulnar joint *(arrows)*, but the radiocarpal joint is spared, thus rendering the diagnosis of Frykman type VI fracture.

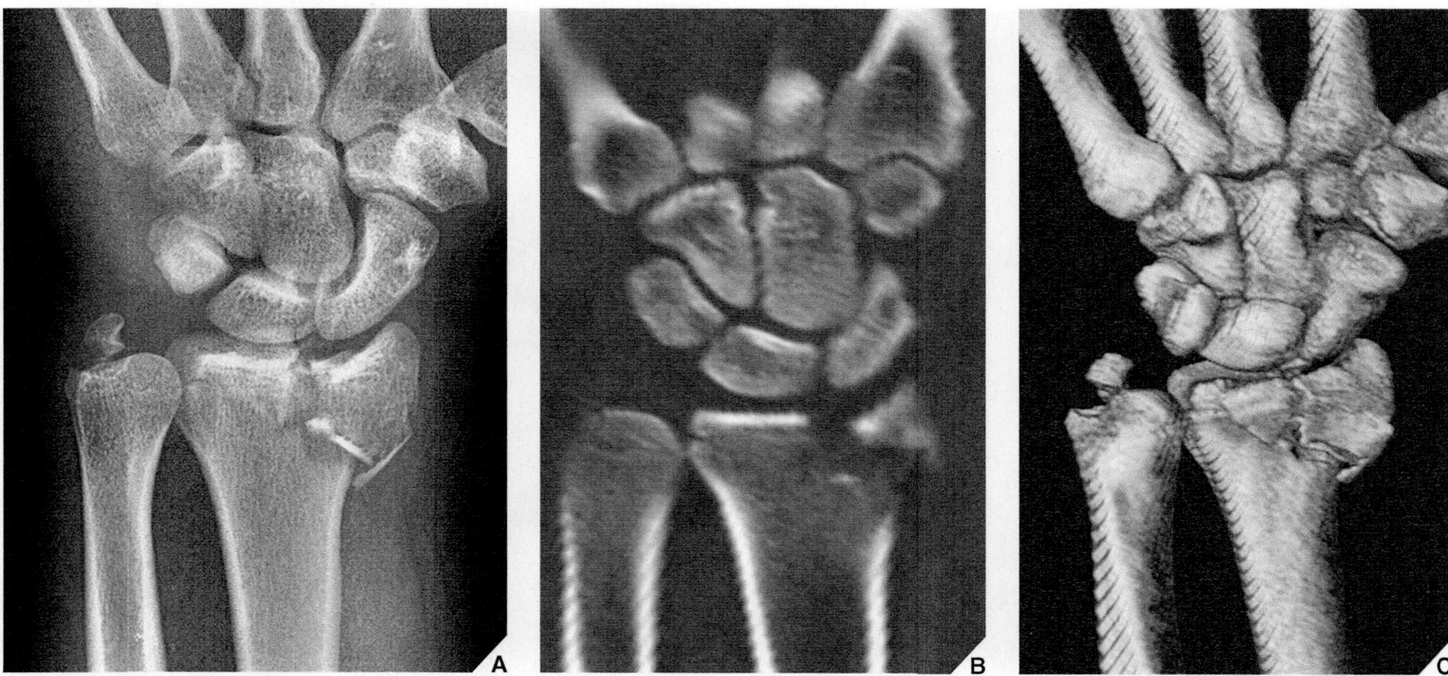

FIGURE 7.16 CT of an intraarticular fracture of the distal radius. **(A)** Dorsovolar radiograph of the wrist shows an intraarticular fracture of the distal radius and a fracture of the ulnar styloid. **(B)** Coronal reformatted and **(C)** 3D reconstructed CT images clearly show an extension of the fracture lines into both the radiocarpal and the distal radioulnar joint compartments, confirming Frykman type VIII fracture.

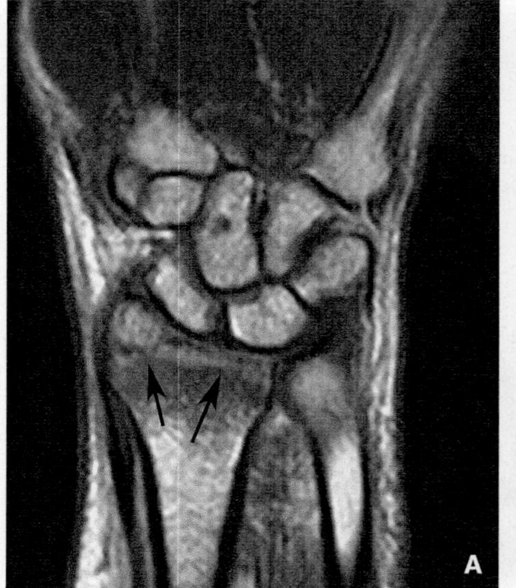

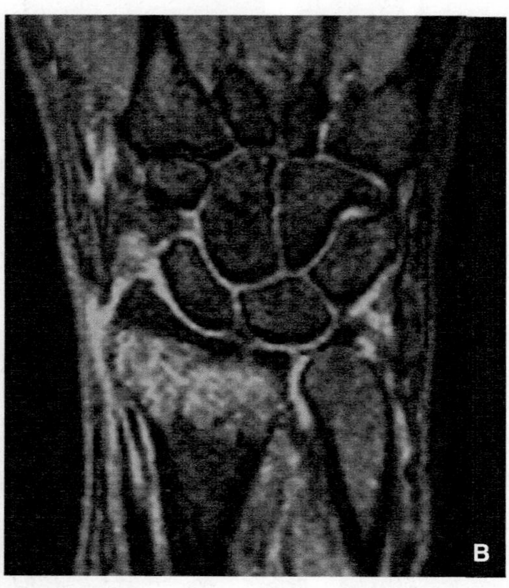

FIGURE 7.17 MRI of Colles fracture. **(A)** Coronal T1-weighted and **(B)** coronal T2-weighted MR images of the wrist show an acute nondisplaced fracture of the distal radius (*arrows* in **A**) with extensive surrounding bone marrow edema. The radiographs (not shown here) obtained prior to MRI were normal.

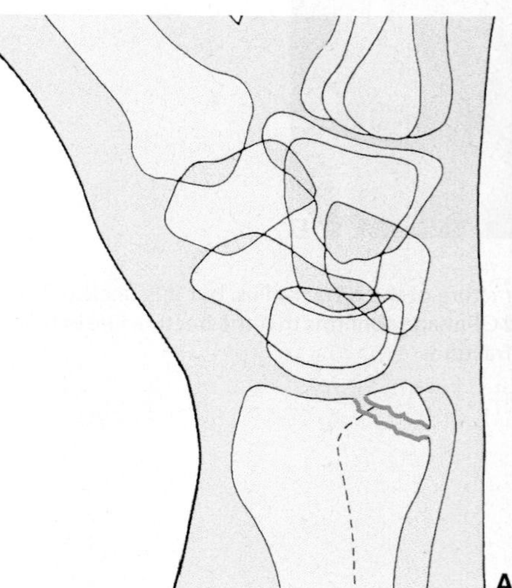

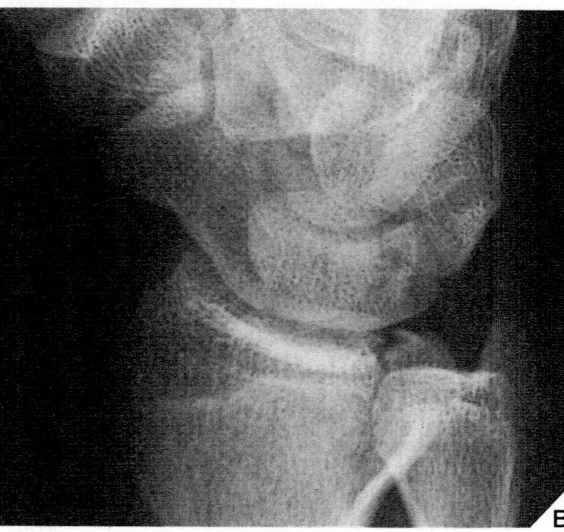

FIGURE 7.18 Barton fracture. **(A)** Schematic and **(B)** oblique radiographs show the typical appearance of Barton fracture. The fracture line in the coronal plane extends from the dorsal margin of the distal radius into the radiocarpal articulation.

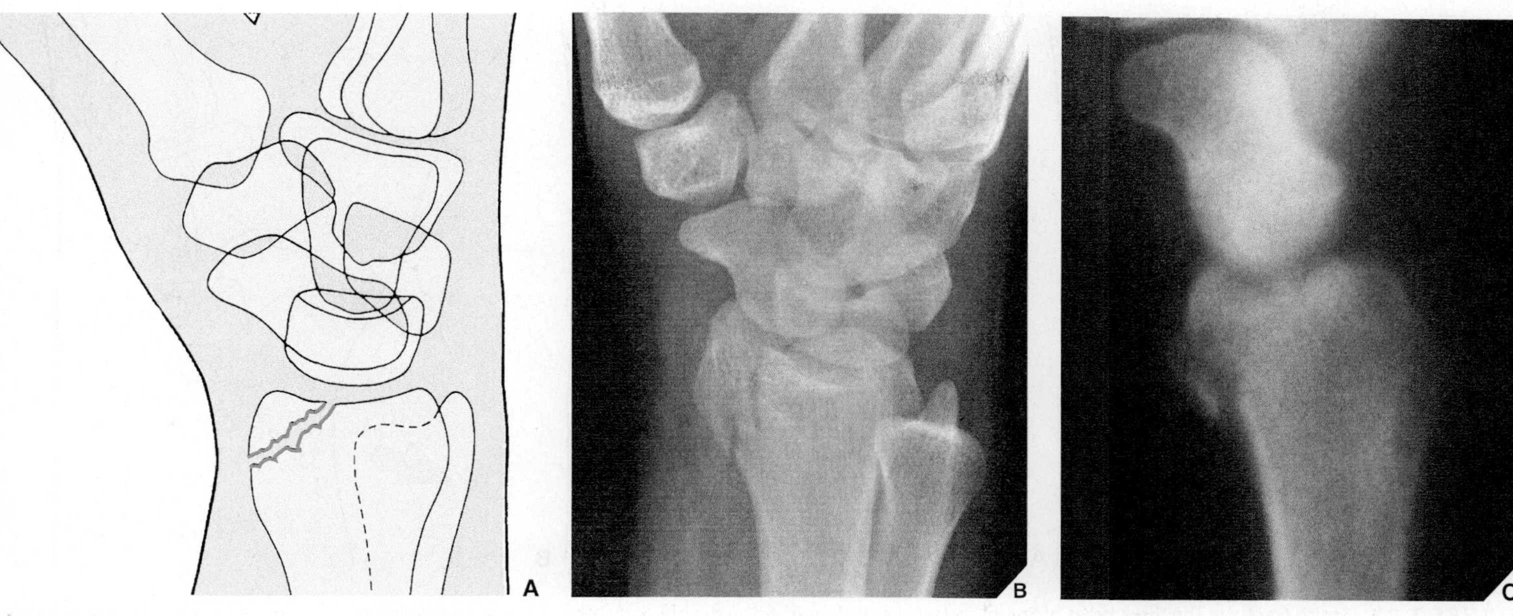

FIGURE 7.19 Reverse Barton fracture. **(A)** Schematic, **(B)** oblique radiographs and **(C)** lateral trispiral tomogram show the reverse (or volar) Barton fracture; the fracture line is also oriented in the coronal plane but extends from the volar margin of the radial styloid process into the radiocarpal joint.

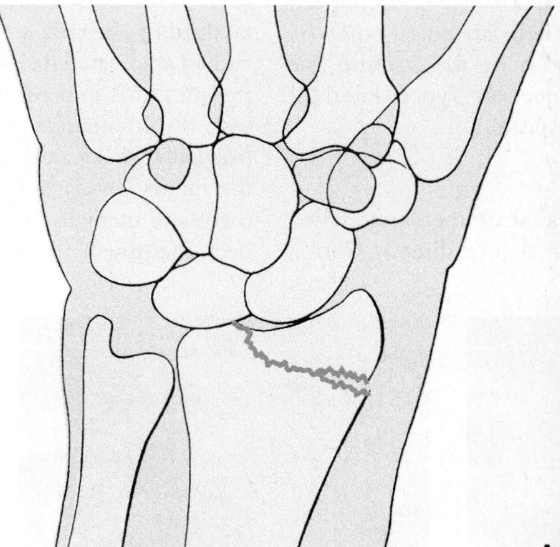

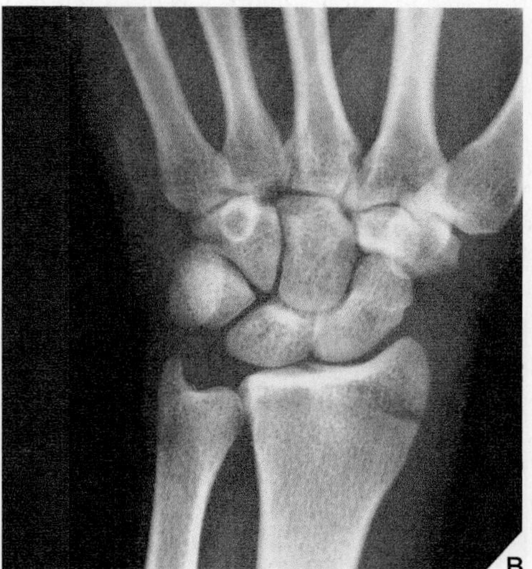

FIGURE 7.20 Hutchinson fracture. **(A)** Schematic and **(B)** dorsovolar radiographs show classic appearance of Hutchinson fracture. The fracture line in the sagittal plane extends through the radial margin of the radial styloid process into the radiocarpal articulation.

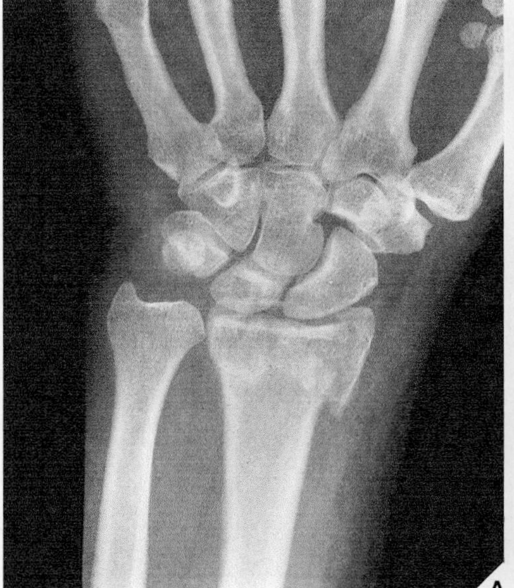

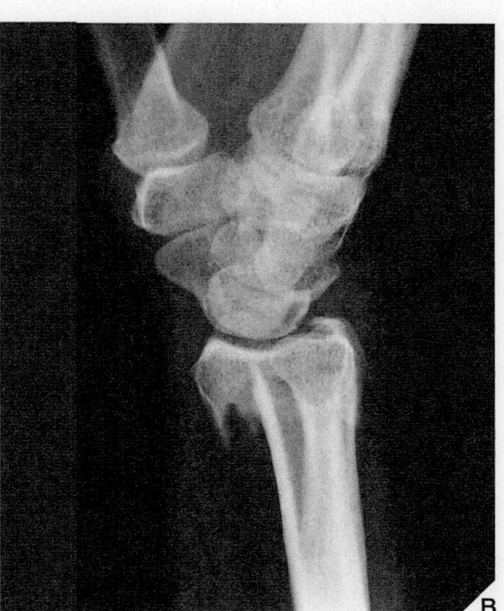

FIGURE 7.21 Smith fracture. **(A)** Posteroanterior and **(B)** lateral radiographs of the distal forearm show the typical appearance of Smith fracture. Volar displacement of the distal fragment is clearly evident on the lateral view.

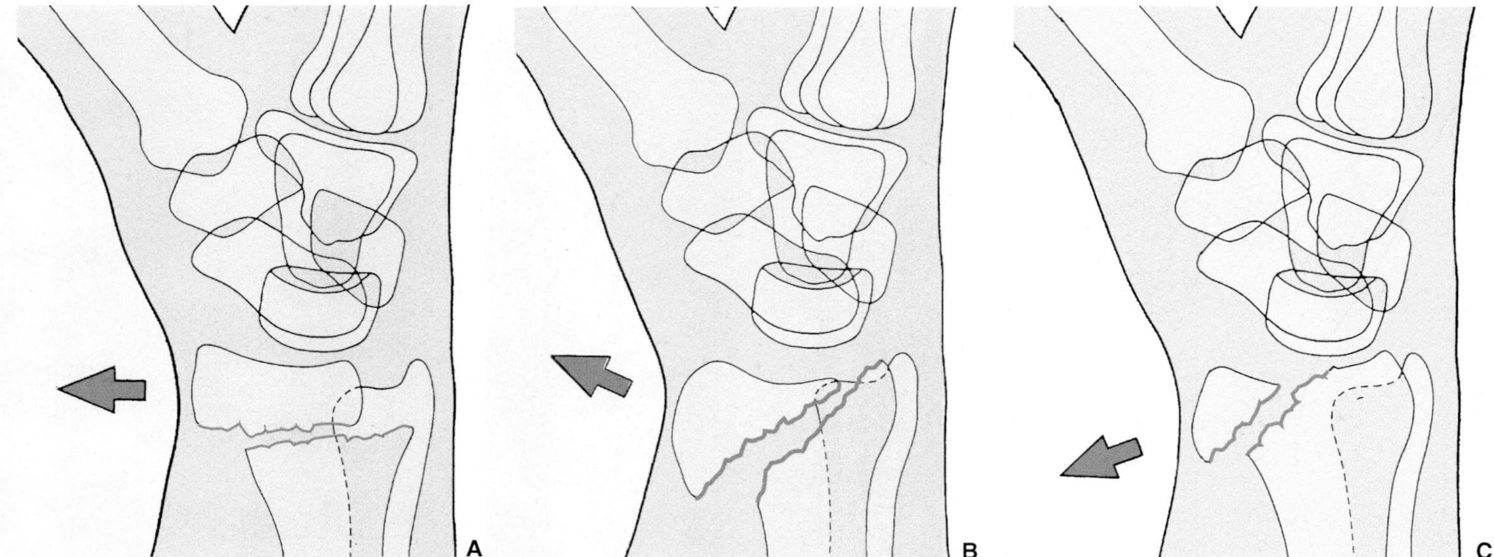

FIGURE 7.22 Smith fracture. The three types of Smith fracture are distinguished by the obliquity of the fracture line. Volar displacement of the distal fragment is characteristic of all three types. **(A)** In Smith type I, the fracture line is transverse, extending from the dorsal to the volar cortices of the radius. **(B)** The oblique fracture line in type II extends from the dorsal lip of the distal radius to the volar cortex. **(C)** Type III, which is almost identical to the reverse Barton fracture (see Fig. 7.19), is an intraarticular fracture with an extension to the volar cortex of the distal radius.

that seen in a Colles injury, it is often referred to as a *reverse Colles fracture*; it is, however, much less common than Colles. There are three types of Smith fracture, defined on the basis of the obliquity of the fracture line (Fig. 7.22), which is best assessed on the lateral projection. Types II and III are usually unstable and may require surgical intervention.

Galeazzi Fracture–Dislocation

This abnormality, which may result indirectly from a fall on the outstretched hand combined with marked pronation of the forearm or directly from a blow to the dorsolateral aspect of the wrist, consists of a fracture of the distal third of the radius, sometimes extending into the radiocarpal articulation and an associated dislocation in the distal radioulnar joint. Characteristically, the proximal end of the distal fragment is dorsally displaced, commonly with dorsal angulation at the fracture site; the ulna is dorsally and ulnarly (medially) dislocated (Fig. 7.23). On rare occasion, the distal fragment of the radius is volarly (anteriorly) displaced in relation to the proximal fragment and medially angulated (Fig. 7.24). Two types of Galeazzi injury have been identified. In type I, the fracture of the radius is extraarticular in the

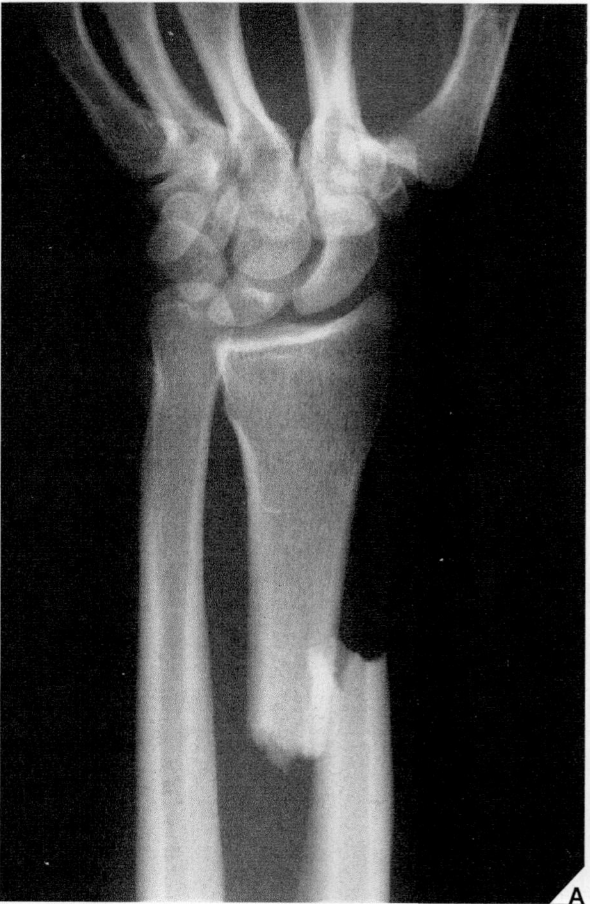

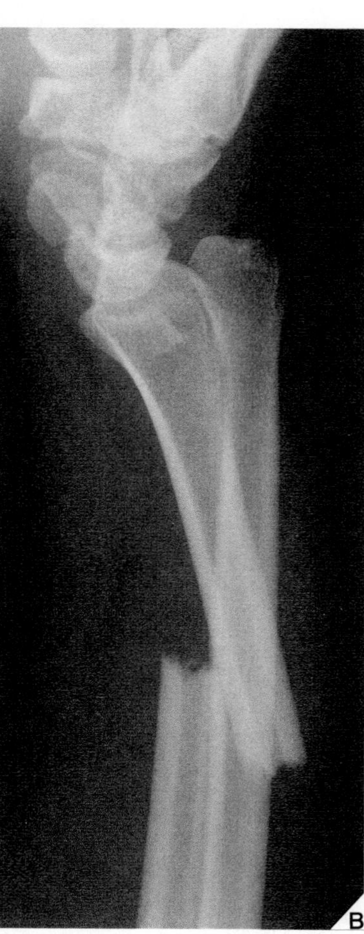

FIGURE 7.23 Galeazzi fracture–dislocation. **(A)** Posteroanterior and **(B)** lateral radiographs of the distal forearm show type I Galeazzi fracture–dislocation. The simple fracture of the radius affects the distal third of the bone, and the proximal end of the distal fragment is dorsally displaced and angulated. In addition, there is dislocation in the distal radioulnar joint.

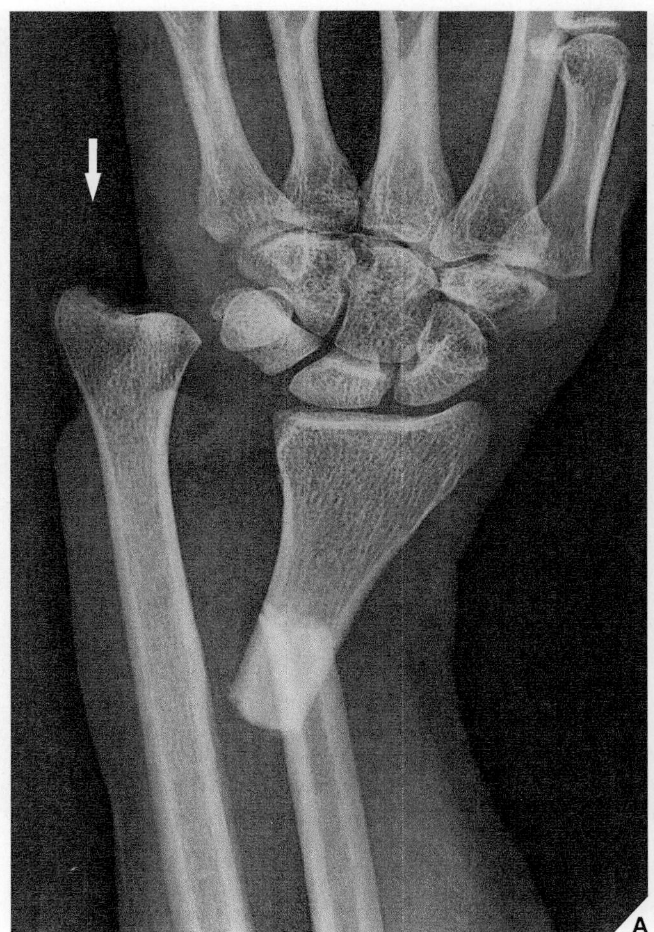

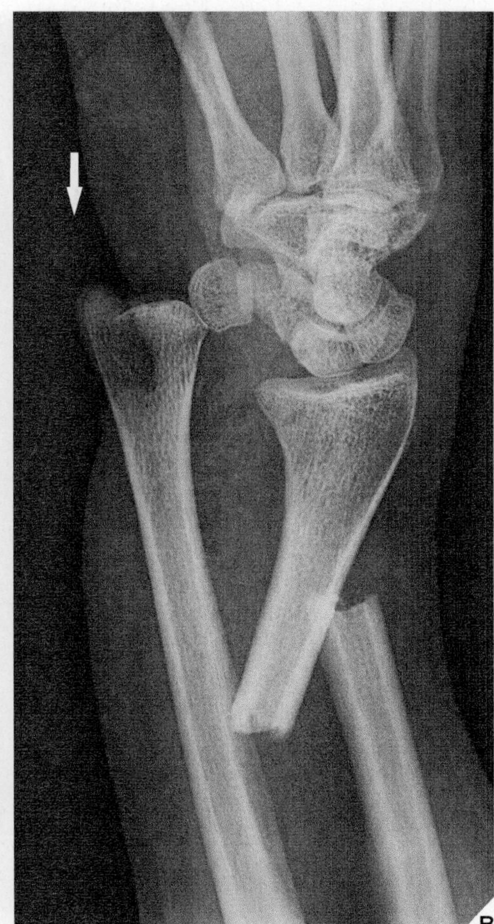

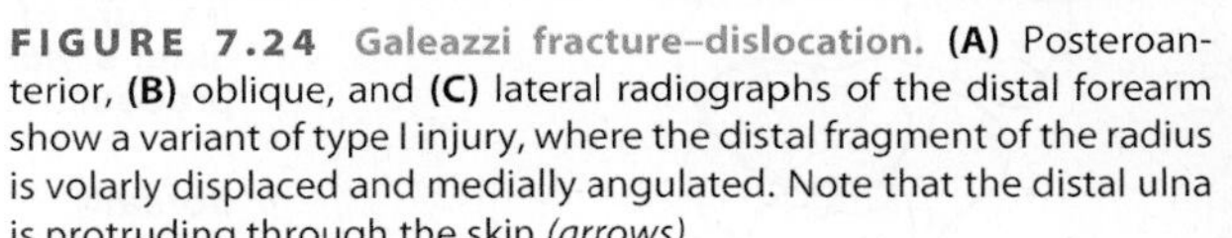

FIGURE 7.24 Galeazzi fracture–dislocation. (A) Posteroanterior, **(B)** oblique, and **(C)** lateral radiographs of the distal forearm show a variant of type I injury, where the distal fragment of the radius is volarly displaced and medially angulated. Note that the distal ulna is protruding through the skin *(arrows)*.

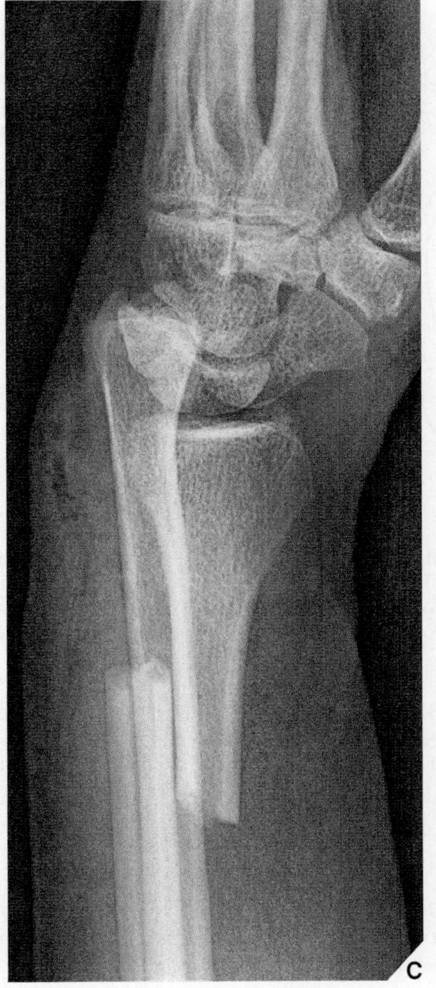

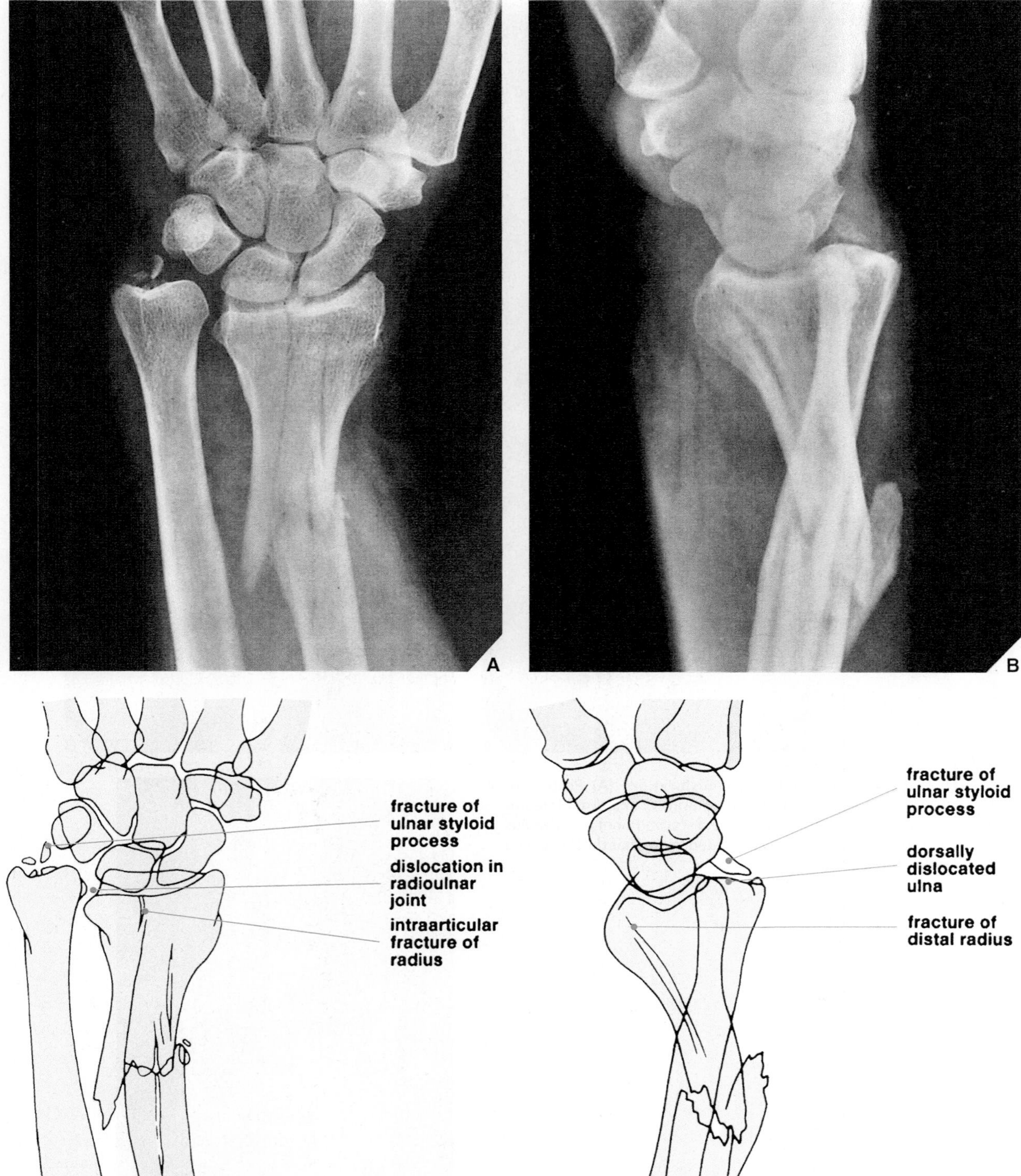

FIGURE 7.25 Galeazzi fracture–dislocation. (A) Posteroanterior and **(B)** lateral radiographs of the distal forearm demonstrate the two components of Galeazzi fracture–dislocation type II. The posteroanterior radiograph clearly reveals the fracture of the distal radius, which, in this case, is comminuted, extending into the radiocarpal joint. The distal fragment has a slight lateral angulation. Note also the associated comminuted fracture of the ulnar styloid process and the dislocation in the radioulnar joint. These features are also seen on the lateral projection, but this view provides in addition a better demonstration of the dorsal dislocation of the distal ulna.

distal third of the bone (see Figs. 7.23 and 7.24). In type II, the radius fracture is usually comminuted and extends into the radiocarpal joint (Fig. 7.25).

Posteroanterior and lateral radiographs are routinely obtained when this injury is suspected, but the lateral view clearly reveals its nature and extent (see Figs. 7.23B, 7.24C, and 7.25B).

Piedmont Fracture

An isolated fracture of the radius at the junction of the middle and distal thirds without an associated disruption of the distal radioulnar joint is known as the *Piedmont fracture* (Fig. 7.26A). This injury is also called *fracture of necessity* because open reduction and internal fixation are necessary to achieve an acceptable functional result (Fig. 7.26B). If this fracture is treated conservatively with closed reduction and cast application, then the interosseous space may be compromised because of muscle action, resulting in the loss of pronation and supination after the bone union is completed.

Essex-Lopresti Fracture–Dislocation

This fracture, which affects the radial head and is associated with a tear of the interosseous membrane of the forearm and dislocation in the distal radioulnar joint, was discussed in Chapter 6.

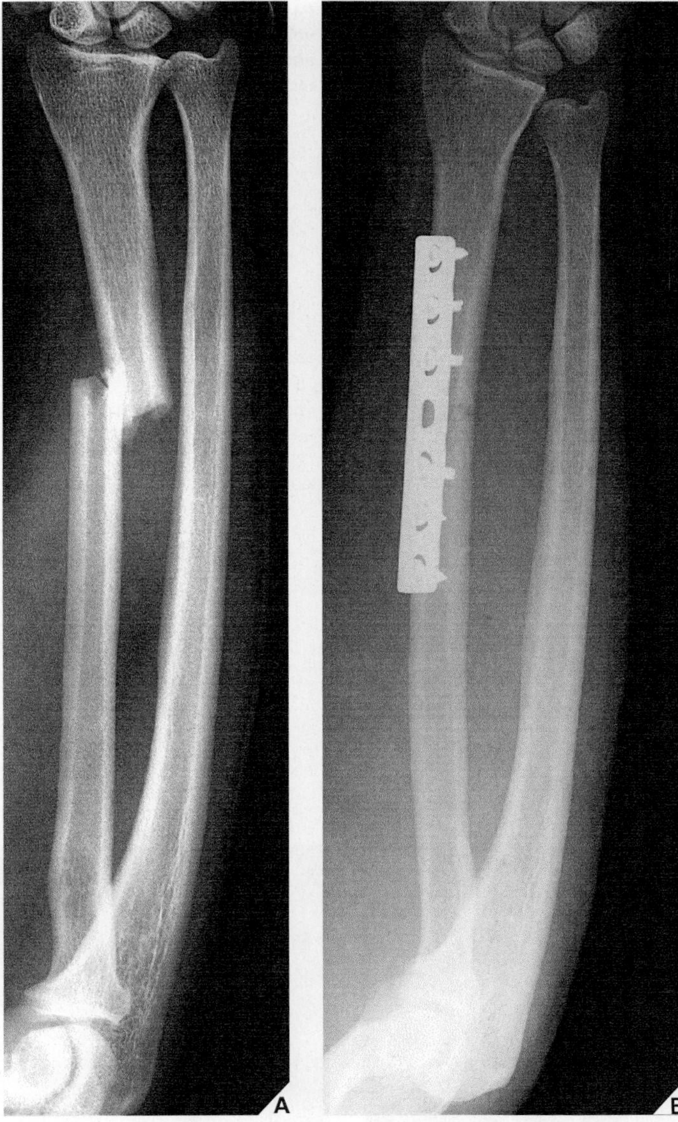

FIGURE 7.26 Piedmont fracture. **(A)** Anteroposterior radiograph of the forearm shows a typical appearance of the Piedmont fracture, an isolated fracture at the junction of the middle and distal thirds of the radius, necessitating an open reduction and internal fixation **(B)**.

Ulnar Impingement Syndrome

Ulnar impingement syndrome is caused by a short distal ulna that impinges on the distal radius proximal to the sigmoid notch. A short ulna may represent a congenital anomaly, such as negative ulnar variance, or may be the result of premature fusion of the distal ulnar growth plate secondary to previous trauma. In most cases, however, it is caused by surgical procedures that involve a resection of the distal ulna secondary to trauma, rheumatoid arthritis, or correction of a Madelung deformity. The clinical symptoms of the ulnar impingement syndrome consist of ulnar-sided wrist pain and limitation of motion in the radiocarpal joint. In addition, patients experience discomfort during pronation and supination of the forearm. On radiography, the characteristic changes of this abnormality include a short ulna and scalloping of the medial aspect of the distal radius, in cases of negative ulnar variance (Fig. 7.27) or premature fusion of the distal ulnar growth plate, or radial scalloping and radioulnar convergence, in cases of distal ulnar resection. Before these findings become obvious on conventional radiologic studies, MRI may be helpful in early recognition of this condition.

Ulnar Impaction Syndrome

Also known as the *ulnolunate abutment syndrome* or *ulnocarpal loading*, the ulnar impaction syndrome is a well-recognized entity clinically characterized by ulnar-sided wrist pain and limitation of motion in the radiocarpal joint. It is frequently associated with the positive ulnar variance. The pathologic mechanism of this syndrome is linked to altered and increased forces transmitted across the ulnar side of the wrist, leading to a compression of the distal ulna on the medial surface of the lunate bone. This causes the development of degenerative changes in the cartilage covering both bones. In addition, frequent association of the tear of the triangular fibrocartilage has been reported. In cases of excessive ulnar length, dorsal subluxation of the ulna is present compromising supination of the forearm. The conventional radiography shows a positive ulnar variance associated with significantly decreased ulnolunate interval and occasionally foci of sclerosis or cystic changes in the lunate (Fig. 7.28). MRI and MRa are the most effective technique for the diagnosis of this syndrome and demonstration of pathologic changes in the affected bones and surrounding soft tissues. Both these techniques reveal bone marrow edema of the distal ulna and lunate, subchondral sclerosis and cyst formation, and destruction of the cartilage. Associated abnormalities, such as tears of the triangular fibrocartilage and lunotriquetral ligament, are also well imaged (Figs. 7.29 to 7.31). Treatment of this condition includes TFCC debridement and ulnar shortening.

Injury to the Soft Tissue at the Distal Radioulnar Articulation

One of the most common sequelae of injury to the distal radioulnar articulation is a tear of the TFCC. A tear may occur as the result of fractures such as those described in the preceding sections or independently after an injury to the distal forearm and wrist.

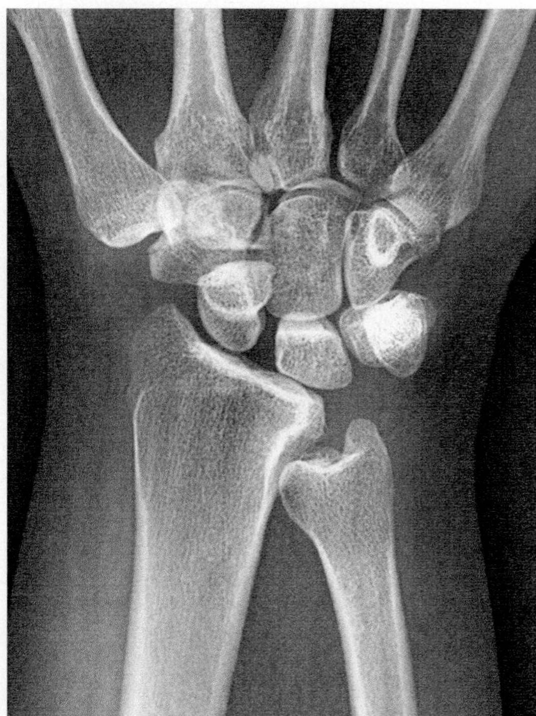

FIGURE 7.27 **Ulnar impingement syndrome.** Dorsovolar radiograph of the wrist shows a negative ulnar variance. The distal ulna impinges on the medial cortex of distal radius.

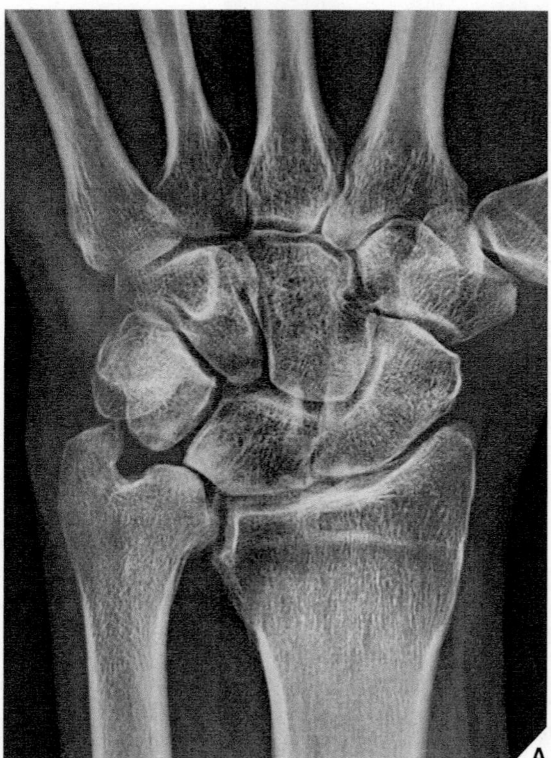

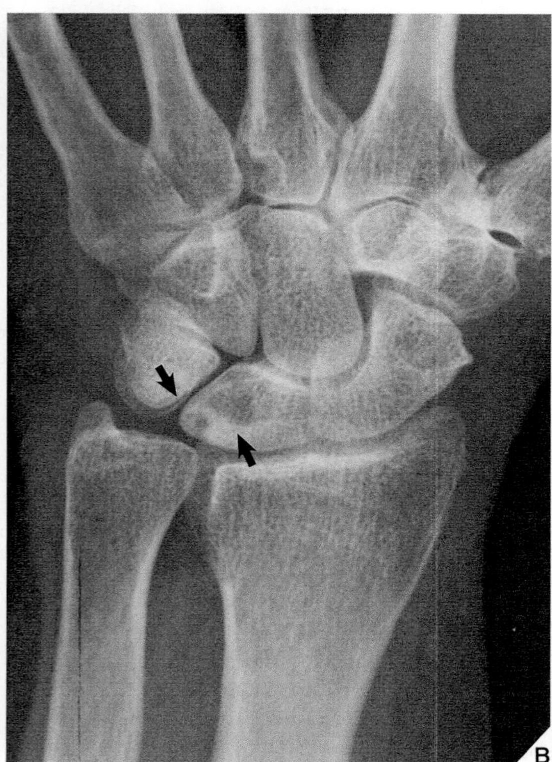

FIGURE 7.28 **Ulnar impaction syndrome.** **(A)** Dorsovolar radiograph of the wrist shows a positive ulnar variance. The ulnolunate interval is significantly decreased, and there is sclerosis of the distal ulna and medial aspect of the lunate. **(B)** In another patient, note the cystic changes in the lunate *(arrows)*.

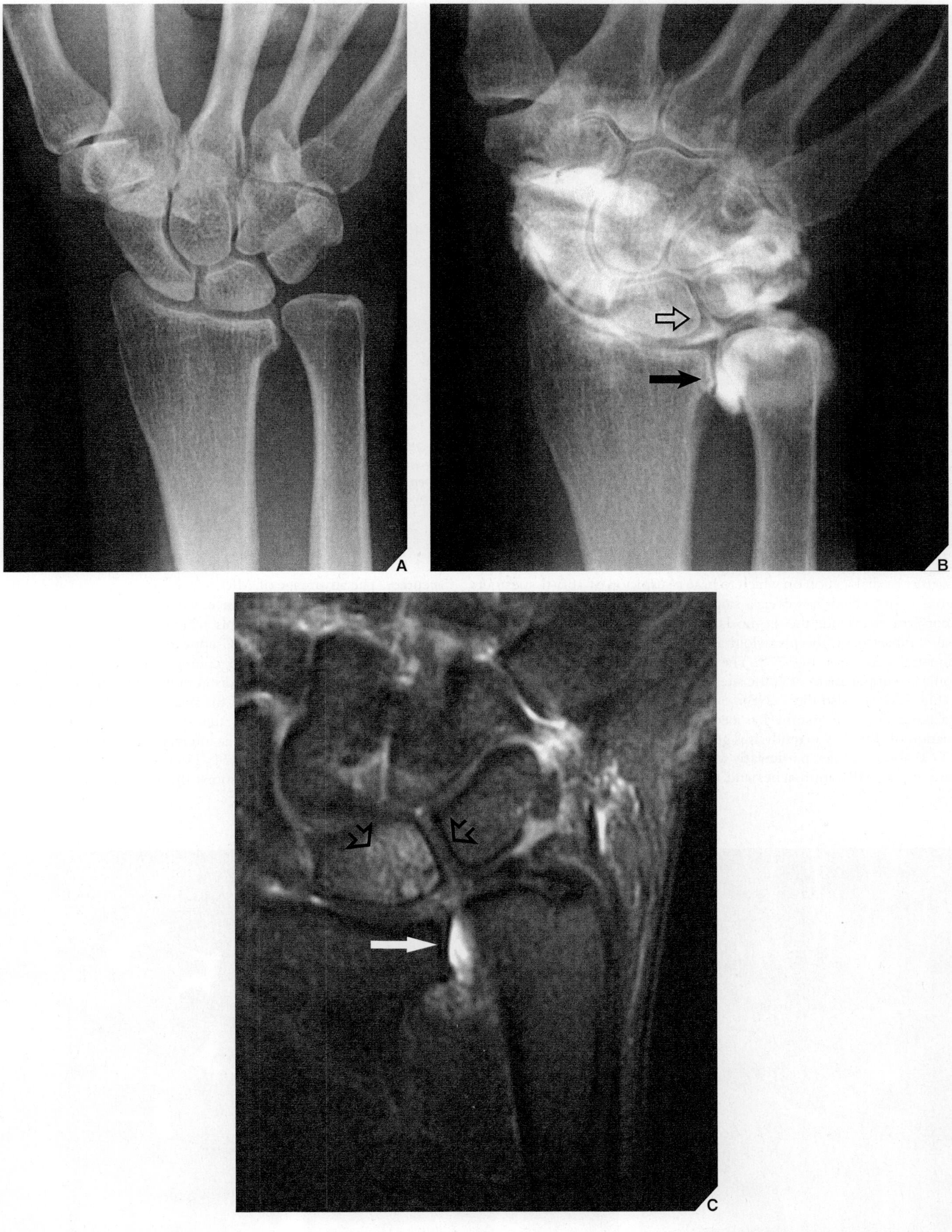

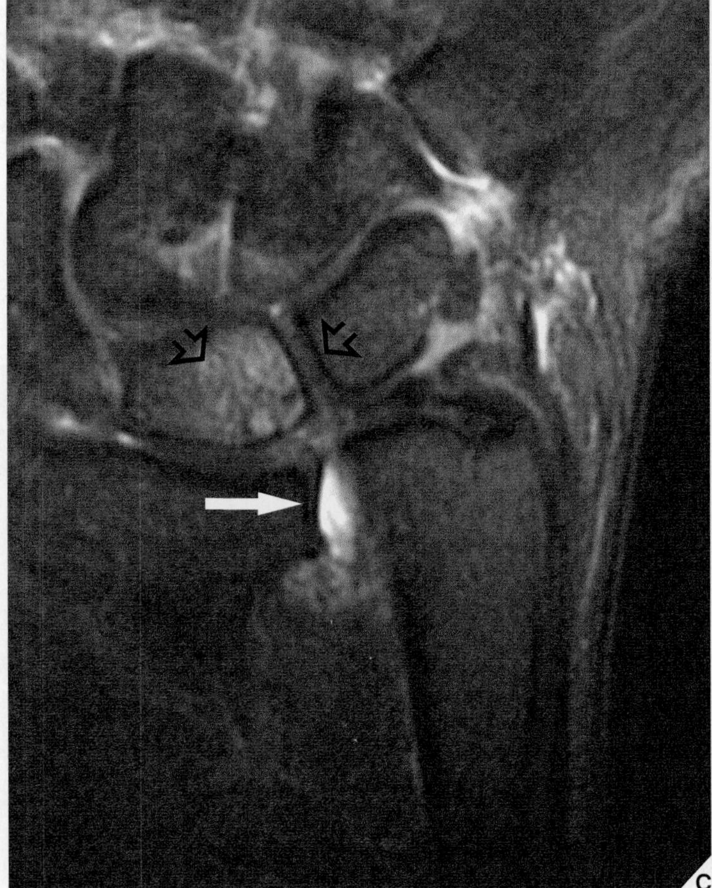

FIGURE 7.29 **Arthrography and MRa of the ulnar impaction syndrome.** **(A)** Conventional radiograph of the wrist shows a positive ulnar variance, but there are no other appreciated abnormalities seen. **(B)** Wrist arthrogram shows a tear of the TFCC *(black arrow)* and a tear of the lunotriquetral ligament *(open arrow)*. **(C)** Coronal T2-weighted fat-suppressed MR arthrographic image shows contrast in the distal radioulnar joint *(white arrow)*, confirming the diagnosis of a tear of TFCC, and cystic changes and edema of the lunate *(open arrows)*, confirming the diagnosis of ulnar impaction syndrome.

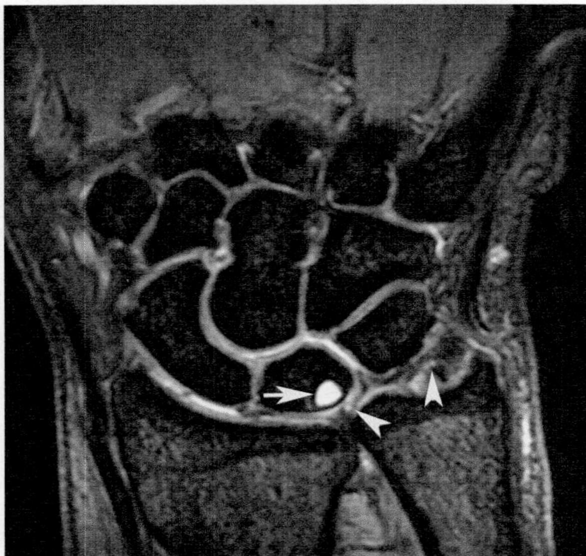

FIGURE 7.30 **MRI of the ulnar impaction syndrome.** Coronal gradient recalled echo (GRE) MR image demonstrates ulnar positive variance. There is a complete tear of the TFCC *(arrowheads)* and subchondral cyst in the ulnar aspect of the lunate *(arrow)*.

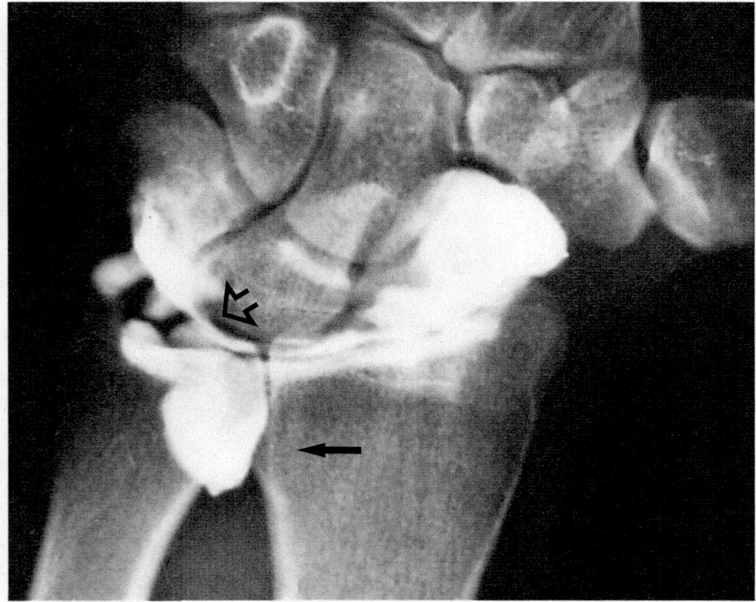

FIGURE 7.32 **Arthrography of a TFCC tear.** A single-contrast arthrogram of the wrist shows a leak of contrast into the space occupied by the triangular cartilage *(open arrow)*, with characteristic filling of the distal radioulnar compartment *(black arrow)*, confirming a tear of the TFCC (compare with Fig. 7.7B).

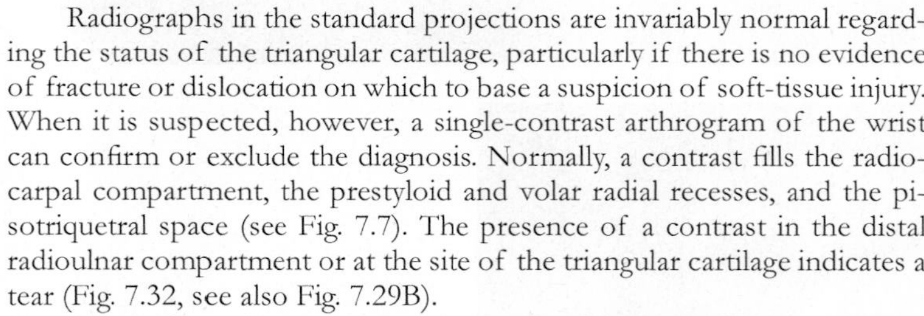

Radiographs in the standard projections are invariably normal regarding the status of the triangular cartilage, particularly if there is no evidence of fracture or dislocation on which to base a suspicion of soft-tissue injury. When it is suspected, however, a single-contrast arthrogram of the wrist can confirm or exclude the diagnosis. Normally, a contrast fills the radiocarpal compartment, the prestyloid and volar radial recesses, and the pisotriquetral space (see Fig. 7.7). The presence of a contrast in the distal radioulnar compartment or at the site of the triangular cartilage indicates a tear (Fig. 7.32, see also Fig. 7.29B).

Classically, arthrography has been the procedure of choice for the evaluation of TFCC. Currently, it is generally believed that in the diagnosis of TFCC abnormalities, particularly when using eight-channel phased array extremity coil, MRI approaches and frequently surpasses arthrography in accuracy. The advantage of MRI is its noninvasiveness and ability to image the entire fibrocartilage substance, whereas arthrography is limited to the evaluation of the surface of this structure only. On coronal T1-weighted MR images, the normal TFCC appears as a biconcave band of homogeneous low signal intensity extending across the space between the distal ulna, the medial aspect of distal radius, and the triquetrum and lunate bones (Fig. 7.33; see also Fig. 7.8). Tears of the TFCC manifest as discontinuities and fragmentation of this structure. The torn fibrocartilage becomes irregular in contour and is interrupted by high–signal intensity areas on T2-weighted images (Fig. 7.34). However, one of the studies published by Haims and colleagues questions the sensitivity of MRI in diagnosing

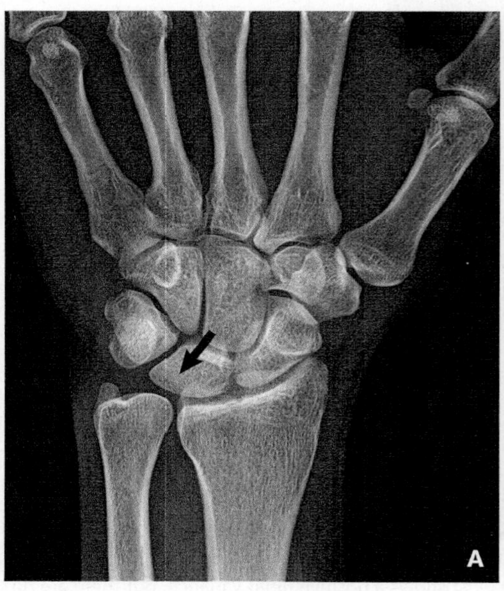

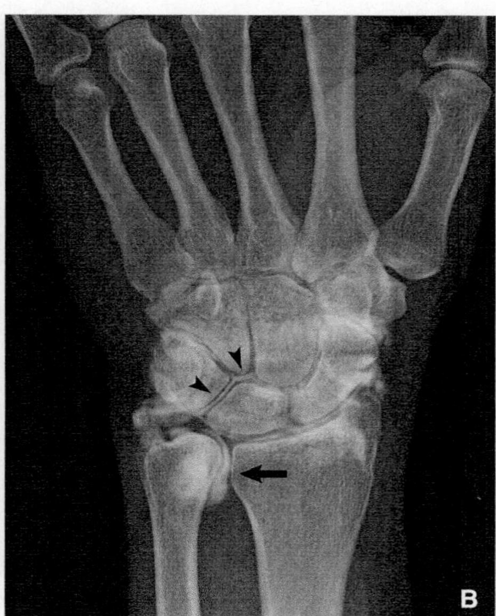

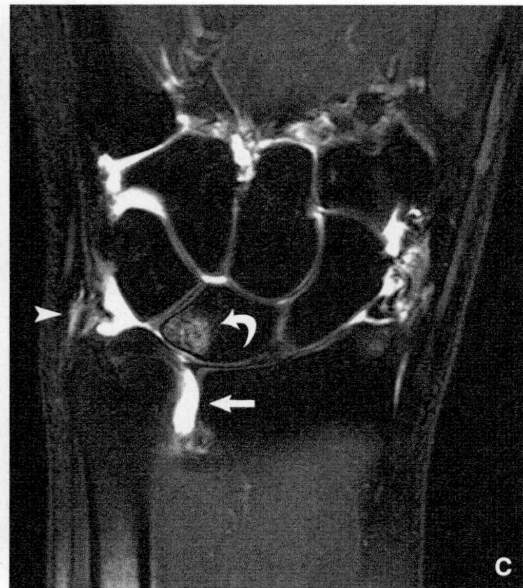

FIGURE 7.31 **MRa of the ulnar impaction syndrome.** **(A)** Dorsovolar radiograph of the right wrist of a 56-year-old man shows positive ulnar variance and subtle cystic changes within the lunate *(arrow)*. **(B)** After injection of contrast agent into the radiocarpal joint, there is a leak into the distal radioulnar joint *(arrow)* indicative of a tear of the TFCC. In addition, there is a leak into the midcarpal compartment *(arrowheads)* through the tear of the lunotriquetral ligament. **(C)** MRa demonstrates edematous changes within the lunate *(curved arrow)* and presence of contrast within the distal radioulnar joint *(arrow)* secondary to the tear of the TFCC *(arrowhead)*.

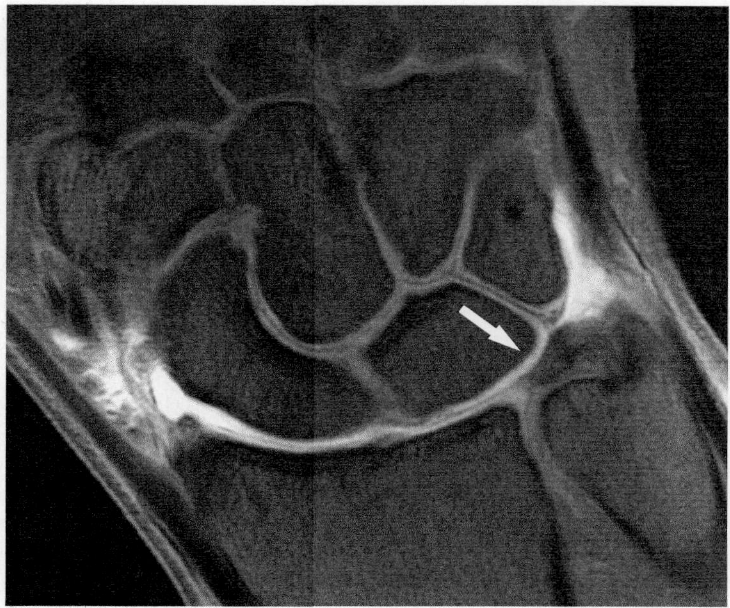

FIGURE 7.33 MRa of the wrist. Coronal T1-weighted fat-suppressed MR arthrographic image of the wrist shows a normal appearance of the TFCC *(arrow)*.

peripheral tears of the triangular fibrocartilage. In this respect, the authors reported the sensitivity of MRI of only 17%, with a specificity of 79%, and accuracy of 64%.

Wrist and Hand

Considered as a functional unit, the wrist and hand are the most common sites of injury in the skeletal system. Fractures of the metacarpals and phalanges, however, by far predominate in incidence over fractures and dislocations in the carpal bones and joints, which constitute approximately 6% of all such injuries. In most instances, history and physical examination provide valuable information on which to base a suspected diagnosis, but radiographic findings derived from films obtained in at least two projections at 90 degrees to each other are essential to determine a specific diagnosis of injury to these sites.

Anatomic–Radiologic Considerations

Trauma to the wrist and hand usually can be sufficiently evaluated on conventional radiographs in the dorsovolar (posteroanterior) and lateral projections (see Figs. 7.1 and 7.2). However, the determination of the exact extent of damage to the different carpal bones forming the complex structure of the wrist may require supplemental studies specific for the various anatomic sites. These special views include the following:

1. Dorsovolar obtained in ulnar deviation of the wrist for the evaluation of the scaphoid bone, which appears foreshortened on the standard dorsovolar projection as a result of its normal volar tilt (Fig. 7.35)
2. Supinated oblique for visualizing the pisiform bone and the pisotriquetral joint (Fig. 7.36)
3. Pronated oblique for imaging the triquetral bone, the radiovolar aspect of the scaphoid, and the radial styloid process (Fig. 7.37)
4. Carpal tunnel for demonstrating the hook of the hamate, the pisiform, and the volar aspect of the trapezium (Fig. 7.38)

A full assessment of traumatic conditions and their sequelae may also require ancillary imaging techniques. Among the most commonly performed in the past was conventional tomography, most often in the form of thin-section trispiral cuts for detecting occult fractures, currently almost completely replaced by CT. Fluoroscopy combined with videotaping is occasionally used for the evaluation of wrist kinematics and joint instability. Arthrography, MRI, and magnetic resonance arthrography (MRa) are effective for determining soft-tissue injuries, such as tears of various ligaments, as well as capsular and tendinous ruptures; and radionuclide bone scan is very sensitive for detecting subtle fractures and early complications of fracture healing. CT has evolved as a versatile tool and adjunctive procedure for imaging various traumatic abnormalities of the wrist. In many institutions, this technique virtually replaced conventional tomography because it is easier to perform, is faster, and has a lower radiation dose. After standard axial sections are obtained, reformation images in additional imaging planes can be acquired and three-dimensional (3D) reconstruction can be performed (see Fig. 2.8A,B). CT can be combined with arthrography (see Fig. 2.19) or can be enhanced by an intravenous contrast material. It is effective in demonstrating subluxation in the distal radioulnar joint and in evaluating the so-called *humpback deformity* of the scaphoid, osteonecrosis of the lunate (Kienböck disease), and fractures of the hook of the hamate, among other abnormalities. Axial sections are obtained after positioning the patient prone with the arm extended above the head. Contiguous sections of 1 or 2 mm are acquired, preferably using a spiral (helical) technique. Direct coronal sections can also be obtained with the wrist in maximal volar flexion or dorsal extension.

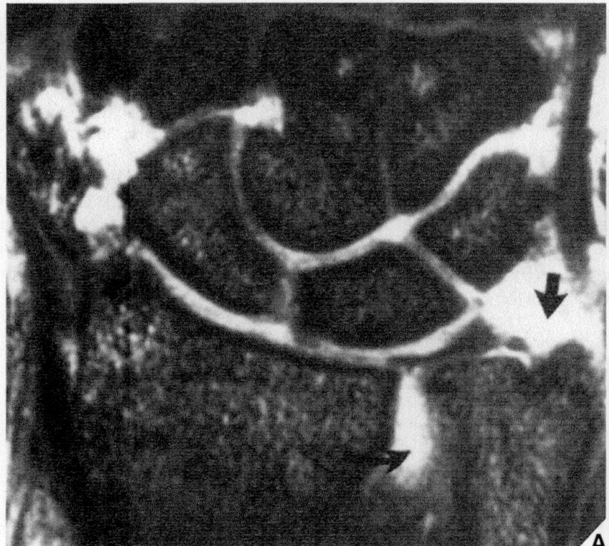

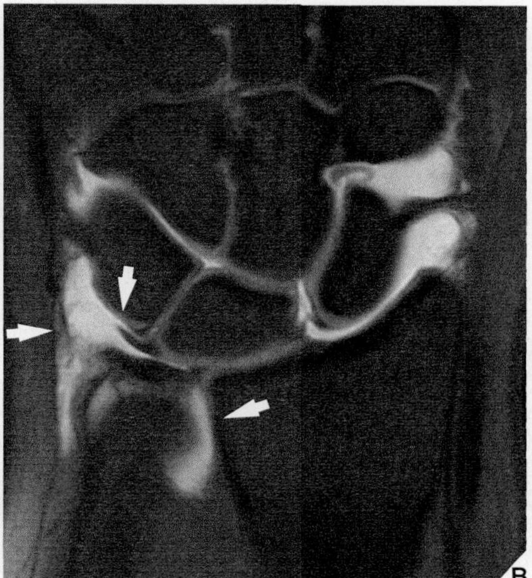

FIGURE 7.34 MRI of the tear of the TFCC. **(A)** Coronal T2*-weighted gradient-recalled acquisition in the steady state (GRASS) image of the left wrist shows a full-thickness tear of the TFCC. The triangular fibrocartilage is torn and displaced from the ulnar styloid *(arrow)*. Moderate amount of fluid is seen in the distal radioulnar joint *(curved arrow)*. **(B)** In another patient, coronal proton density–weighted fat-suppressed arthrographic MR image of the wrist shows a tear of the TFCC *(arrows)*. (**A**, Reprinted with permission from Deutsch AL, Mink JH, eds. *MRI of the musculoskeletal system: a teaching file*, 2nd ed. Philadelphia: Lippincott-Raven; 1997.)

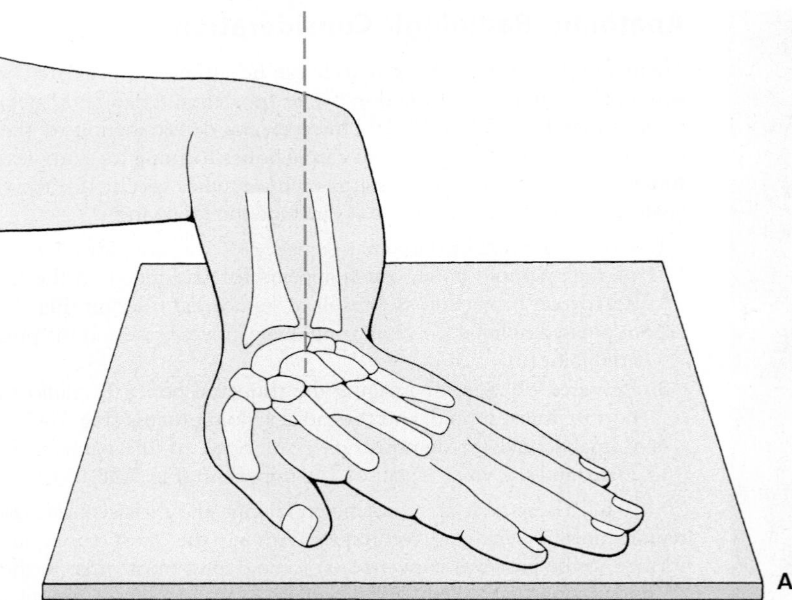

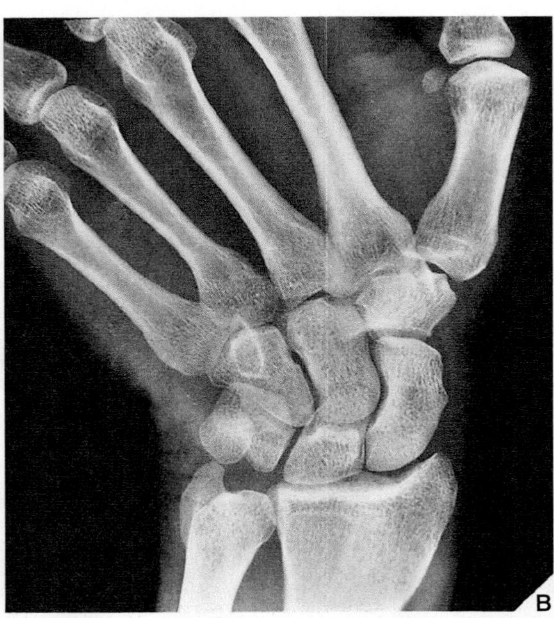

FIGURE 7.35 Ulnar deviation. **(A)** For the dorsovolar view of the wrist in ulnar deviation, the forearm rests flat on the radiographic table with the anterior surface down and the elbow flexed 90 degrees. The hand, lying flat on the film cassette, is ulnarly deviated. The central beam *(red broken line)* is directed toward the carpus. **(B)** The radiograph in this projection demonstrates the scaphoid free of the distortion because of its normal volar tilt when the wrist is in the neutral position.

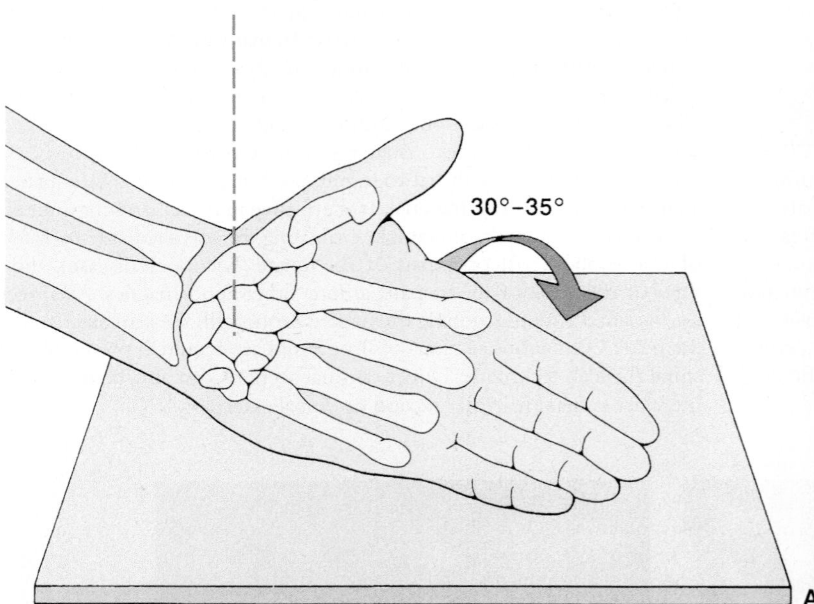

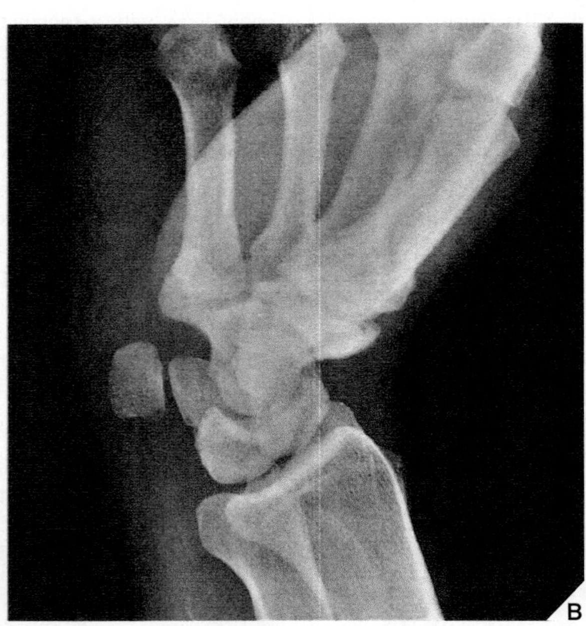

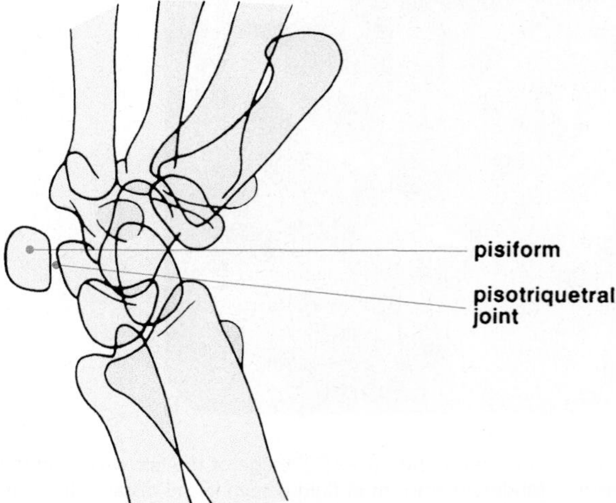

FIGURE 7.36 Supinated oblique view. **(A)** For the supinated oblique view of the wrist, the hand resting on its ulnar side on the film cassette is tilted approximately 30 to 35 degrees toward its dorsal surface. The outstretched fingers are held together, with the thumb slightly abducted. The central beam *(red broken line)* is directed toward the center of the wrist. **(B)** The radiograph in this projection demonstrates the pisiform bone and the pisotriquetral joint.

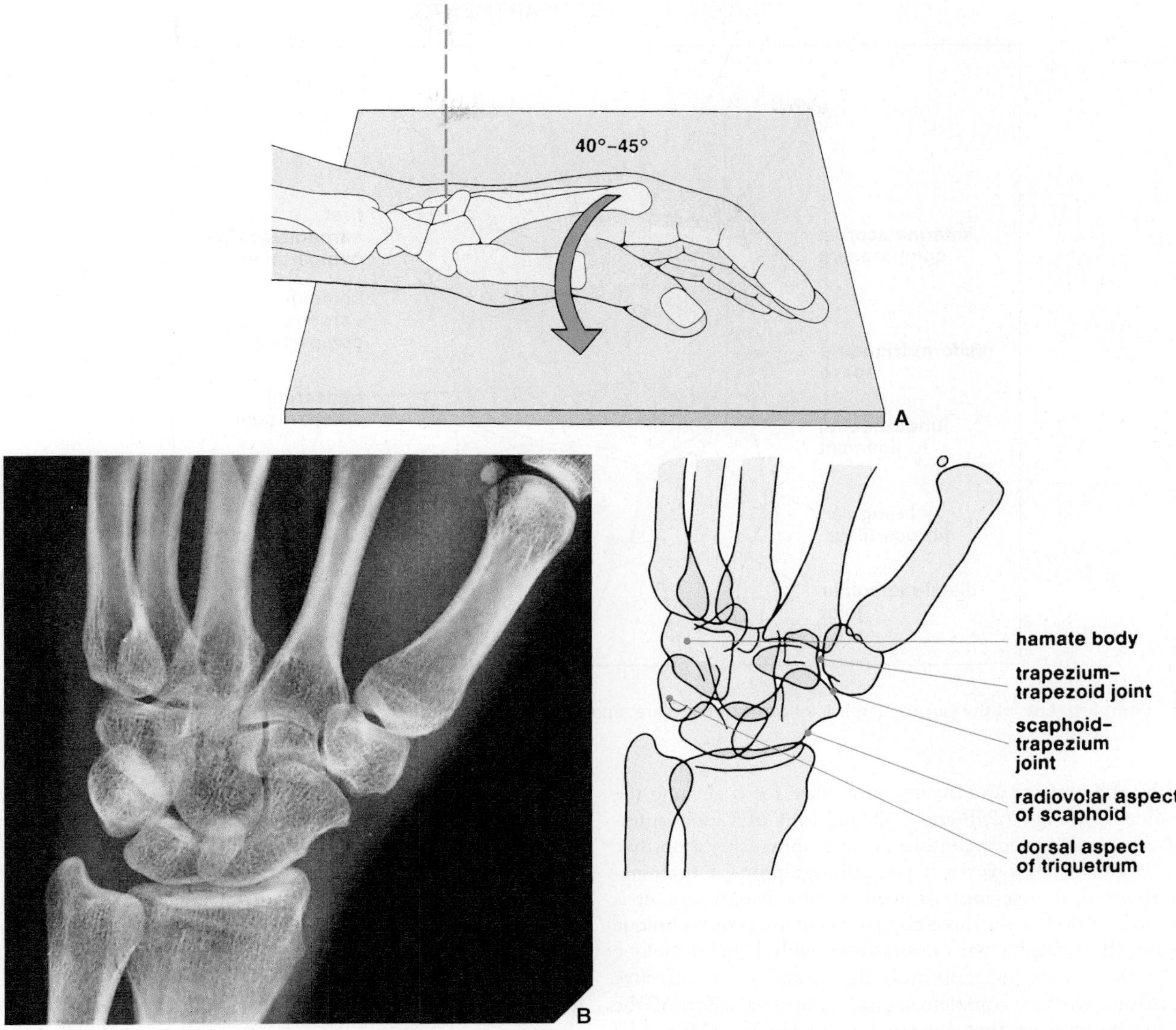

40°–45°

A

hamate body
trapezium–trapezoid joint
scaphoid–trapezium joint
radiovolar aspect of scaphoid
dorsal aspect of triquetrum

B

FIGURE 7.37 **Pronated oblique view.** **(A)** For the pronated oblique view of the wrist, the hand resting on its ulnar side on the film cassette is tilted approximately 40 to 45 degrees toward its palmar surface *(red curved arrow)*. The slightly flexed fingers are held together, with the thumb in front of them. The central beam *(red broken line)* is directed toward the center of the carpus. **(B)** The radiograph in this projection demonstrates the dorsal aspect of the triquetrum, the body of the hamate, the radiovolar aspect of the scaphoid, and the scaphoid–trapezium and trapezium–trapezoid articulations.

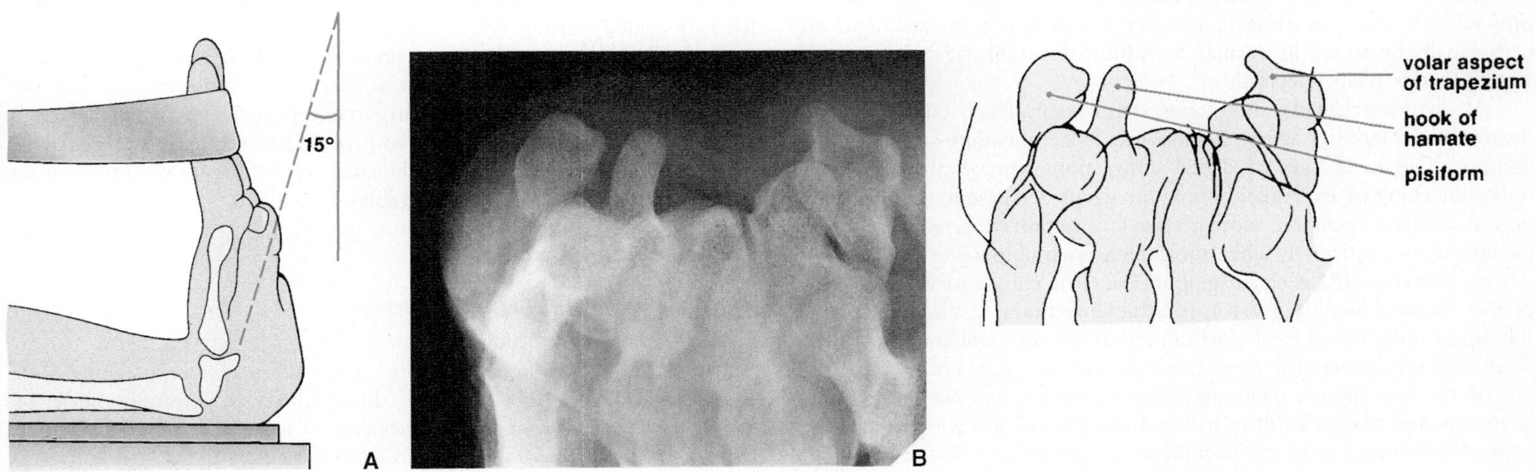

FIGURE 7.38 **Carpal tunnel view.** **(A)** For the carpal tunnel view of the wrist, the hand is maximally dorsiflexed by means of the patient's opposite hand or a strap, with the palmar surface of the wrist resting on the film cassette. The central beam *(red broken line)* is directed toward the cup of the palm at approximately an angle of 15 degrees. **(B)** The radiograph in this projection demonstrates an axial view of the hook of the hamate as well as the pisiform bone and the volar margin of the trapezium.

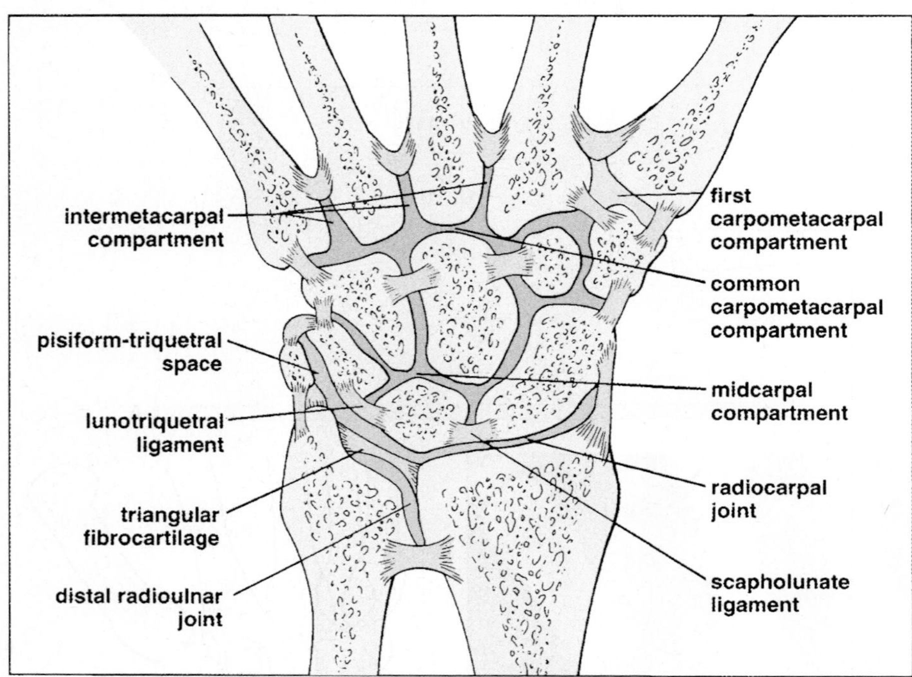

FIGURE 7.39 **Compartments of the carpus.** Carpal joint compartments are separated from one another by various interosseous ligaments.

Arthrography still remains an effective procedure for evaluating the TFCC abnormalities (see Figs. 7.29B and 7.32) and tears of various intercarpal ligaments. In general, single-contrast arthrography using a positive contrast agent is performed. However, if postarthrographic CT examination is to be performed, double-contrast arthrography using room air is preferable. The introduction of the three-compartment injection technique and combining the arthrographic wrist examination with digital technique and postarthrographic CT examination make this modality very effective in evaluating a painful wrist. A complete arthrographic evaluation of the wrist requires opacification of the midcarpal compartment, radiocarpal compartment, and distal radioulnar joint. These three compartments are normally separated from one another by various interosseous ligaments and, in the case of distal radioulnar joint, by the TFCC (Fig. 7.39). The flow of a contrast from one compartment to another indicates a defect in one of these ligaments. Unidirectional contrast flow through the ligament defects, associated with a small flap acting as a valve, has been reported and may be overlooked if the contrast is injected on only one side of the defect. For this reason, the separate injection of all three compartments is preferable. It has to be stressed, however, that defects in the ligaments may occasionally be found in normal, asymptomatic subjects; therefore, their significance remains uncertain.

More recently, digital subtraction arthrography has been advocated by Resnick and Manaster as an effective way to demonstrate subtle leaks of contrast. The advantages of digital subtraction arthrography include not only shortening of examination time but also a decrease in the concentration of contrast agent and more precise localization of defects in intercarpal ligaments, particularly when the defects are multiple (see Fig. 2.2).

At present, MRI is an imaging modality of choice for the evaluation of the wrist and hand (Fig. 7.40). To achieve optimum quality examination, the use of a dedicated local (surface) radiofrequency coil and limited field of view is recommended. This technique may image not only abnormalities of the soft tissues, including various muscles, tendons, interosseous ligaments, and triangular fibrocartilage but also osseous abnormalities such as occult fractures and early osteonecrosis, particularly of the lunate and scaphoid. It is also very useful in imaging the carpal tunnel and detecting the subtle abnormalities of carpal tunnel syndrome (Fig. 7.41, see also Fig. 7.118) and Guyon canal syndrome (see Fig. 7.120). Commonly, MRI is performed after an intraarticular injection of a contrast agent (diluted gadolinium) into the radiocarpal compartment (MRa) (see Figs. 2.20 and 7.33).

The coronal plane is the best to demonstrate the interosseous ligaments of the proximal carpal row (scapholunate and lunotriquetral ligaments) and the TFCC. These structures exhibit a low-intensity signal on T1- and T2-weighted sequences (see Fig. 7.40). In this plane, various intrinsic and extrinsic dorsal and volar ligaments of the wrist (Fig. 7.42) are also seen. In the sagittal plane, all flexor and extensor tendons with their respective insertions are clearly depicted, as well as some of the ligaments including the radioscaphocapitate, radiolunotriquetral, and dorsal radiolunate (Fig. 7.43). In the axial plane, various ligaments and tendons are shown in cross sections; their anatomic relationship to the bone structures, arteries, and nerves can be evaluated effectively (Fig. 7.44). This plane is also ideal for imaging of the Guyon canal. This anatomic structure is located on the volar aspect of the wrist, medially to the carpal tunnel, between the pisiform bone and the hook of the hamate. It is bounded by the flexor retinaculum from the dorsal aspect, hypothenar musculature from the medial aspect, and by fascia from the volar aspect. It contains the ulnar vein, ulnar artery, and ulnar nerve.

During the evaluation of MRI of the wrist, it is helpful to use a checklist as provided in Table 7.4.

Ancillary techniques such as stress films and arthrography may also need to be used for the evaluation of disruption or displacement of the ligaments of the hand, particularly in gamekeeper's thumb (see Figs. 7.127B and 7.128). For a summary in tabular form of the standard and special radiographic projections, as well as the ancillary techniques used to evaluate trauma to the wrist and hand, see Tables 7.5 and 7.6.

Injury to the Wrist

Fractures of the Carpal Bones

Fracture of the Scaphoid Bone

Fractures of the scaphoid (from the Greek word *skaphos*, meaning *boat*), sometimes called *carpal navicular*, are the second most common injuries of the upper limb, exceeded in frequency only by fractures of the distal radius, and they constitute 2% of all fractures. Of all fractures and dislocations in the carpus, these fractures are the most common, accounting for 50% to 60% of such injuries. They frequently occur in young adults (ages 15 to 30 years) after falls on the outstretched palm of the hand. Scaphoid fractures can be classified according to the direction of the fracture line (Fig. 7.45), the degree of stability of the fragments, and the location of the

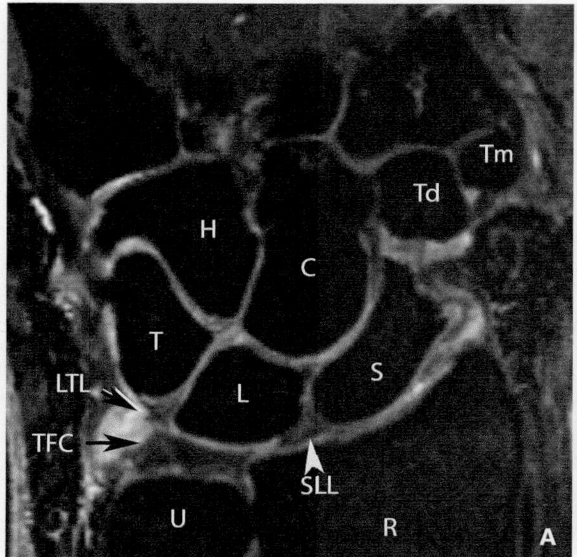

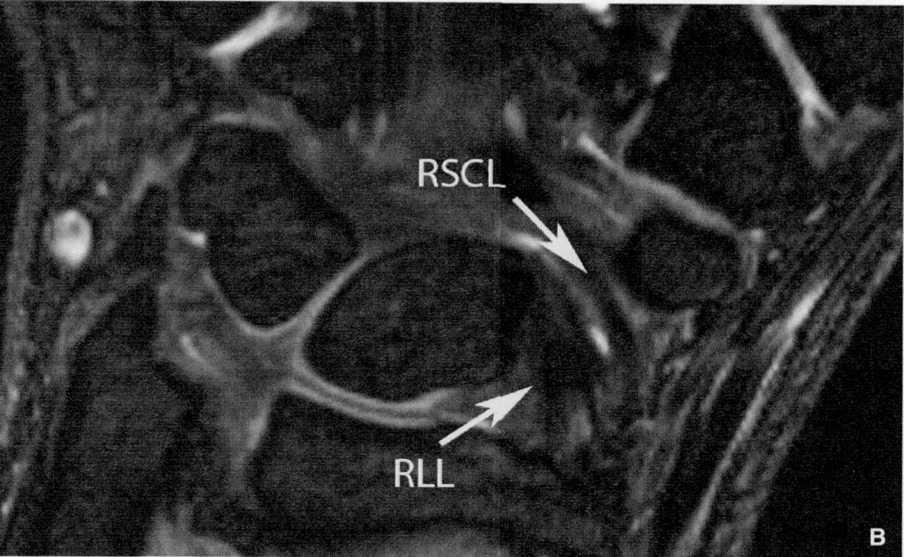

FIGURE 7.40 MRI of the wrist. **(A)** Coronal gradient-echo MR image of the wrist demonstrates distal radius and ulna and carpal bones. The proximal interosseous scapholunate ligament (SLL) and lunotriquetral ligament (LTL) and the triangular fibrocartilage (TFC) are clearly delineated. **(B)** Coronal gradient-echo MR image through the volar aspect of the wrist demonstrates the extrinsic radiolunate ligament (RLL) and radioscaphocapitate ligament (RSCL). R, radius; U, ulna; S, scaphoid; L, lunate; T, triquetrum; H, hamate; C, capitate; Td, trapezoid; Tm, trapezium.

fracture line. From a diagnostic perspective, the latter is a more practical way of classifying fractures of the scaphoid (5% to 10% of which occur in the tuberosity and distal pole, 15% to 20% in the proximal pole, and 70% to 80% in the waist) because it has prognostic value (Fig. 7.46). Fractures of the tuberosity (extraarticular) and distal pole usually result from a direct trauma and rarely cause any significant clinical problems. Fractures of the waist, if there is no displacement or carpal instability, display a good healing pattern in more than 90% of cases. Fractures involving the proximal pole have a high incidence of nonunion and osteonecrosis.

When a fracture of the scaphoid is suspected, standard radiographs are routinely obtained in the dorsovolar, dorsovolar in ulnar deviation, oblique, and lateral projections, and these conventional studies usually suffice to demonstrate the abnormality. When they failed to do so, in the past, thin-section trispiral tomography has proved very effective (Fig. 7.47). This technique was equally helpful in monitoring the progress of healing of scaphoid fractures and in detecting posttraumatic complications, especially when routine follow-up films were unconvincing. Currently, CT is the technique of choice in this respect (Figs. 7.48 to 7.50). In particular, the so-called *humpback deformity* of the scaphoid after a fracture (in which the proximal fragment dorsiflexes and the distal fragment undergoes palmar flexion, resulting in dorsal apical angulation of the scaphoid) can be well evaluated by this modality (Fig. 7.51). In the past decade, MRI became the technique of choice to diagnose subtle fractures of the carpal bones and to detect various complications, including osteonecrosis. In particular, MRI is very effective in demonstrating a fracture line that is not apparent on conventional radiographs (Fig. 7.52).

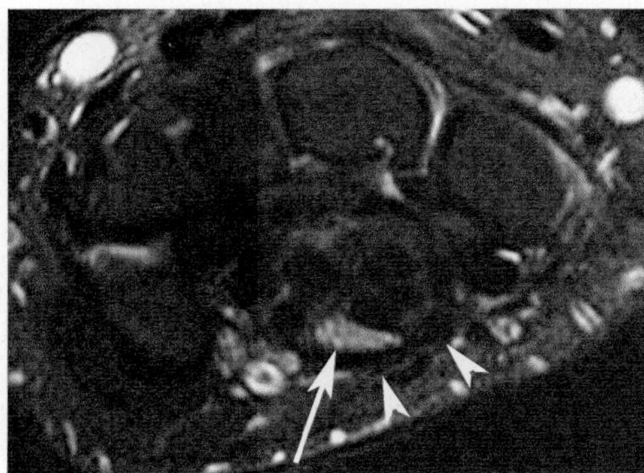

FIGURE 7.41 MRI of carpal tunnel syndrome. Axial short time inversion recovery (STIR) MR image in a patient with carpal tunnel syndrome demonstrates high signal intensity of the median nerve *(arrow)* and bowing of the flexor retinaculum *(arrowheads)*.

Complications. Delayed diagnosis and consequently delayed treatment of a scaphoid fracture may lead to complications such as nonunion, osteonecrosis, and posttraumatic arthritis, the first two of which are the most commonly seen. Although occasionally both fragments of the scaphoid may become necrotic, osteonecrosis usually affects the proximal fragment (see Fig. 7.54) and only rarely the distal pole (Fig. 7.53) because of the good supply of blood to this part of the bone. Osteonecrosis most frequently becomes apparent 3 to 6 months after the injury when the affected fragment shows evidence of increased density. Because conventional radiography may, at times, fail to demonstrate this feature, CT scanning that almost completely replaced conventional tomography is recommended as a valuable aid. Patients with delayed union or nonunion are more prone to osteonecrosis, but healing may sometimes occur despite it (Fig. 7.54). Delayed union and nonunion are usually treated surgically by bone grafting (Fig. 7.55). If this approach fails, then the scaphoid may be excised and replaced by prosthesis (Fig. 7.56). One of the more serious complications of chronic fracture of scaphoid is the development of scapholunate advanced collapse (SLAC) of the wrist. This condition comprises scapholunate ligament disruption and instability in lunocapitate joint associated with proximal migration of the capitate bone, eventually leading to osteoarthritis of the radiocarpal joint (Figs. 7.57 and 7.58). Similar condition where the fracture of the scaphoid is complicated by nonunion is termed *scaphoid nonunion advanced collapse* (SNAC) of the wrist (Fig. 7.59).

Treatment of those conditions includes proximal row carpectomy and/or limited carpal fusion (so-called *four-corner fusion*) consisting of arthrodesis of lunate, capitate, hamate, and triquetrum (Fig. 7.60). In cases of advanced osteoarthritis, a total wrist arthrodesis using rigid stabilization with a dorsal plate and bone grafting is usually required.

Fracture of the Triquetral Bone

Although a fracture of the triquetrum is not uncommon, it can easily be missed if proper radiographic examination is not performed. In most cases, a triquetral fracture is best demonstrated on the lateral and pronated oblique projections of the wrist. However, as overlapping bones on these views may, at times, obscure the fracture line, tomographic examination in the lateral projection used to be required to confirm the diagnosis. Radionuclide bone scan was also a valuable aid in localizing the site of trauma when a fracture was suspected and routine films were normal (Fig. 7.61).

A. Dorsal Ligaments of the Wrist

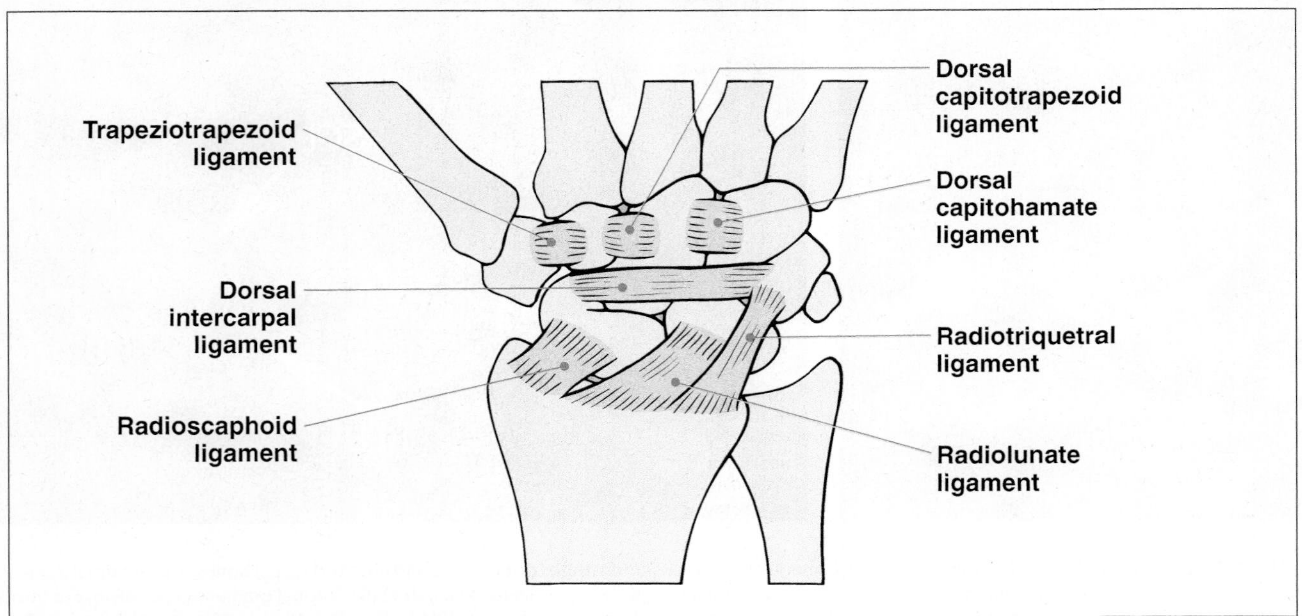

B. Volar Ligaments of the Wrist

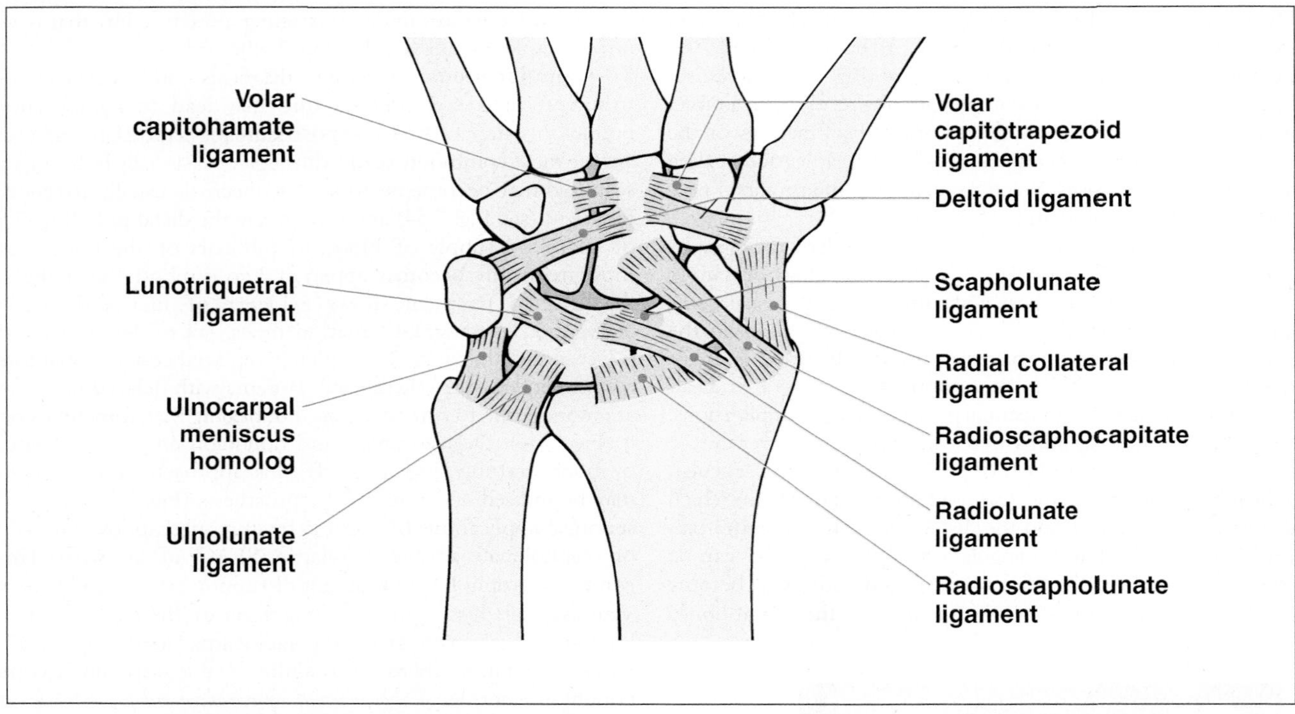

FIGURE 7.42 Ligaments of the wrist. A schematic representation of the dorsal **(A)** and volar **(B)** ligaments of the wrist.

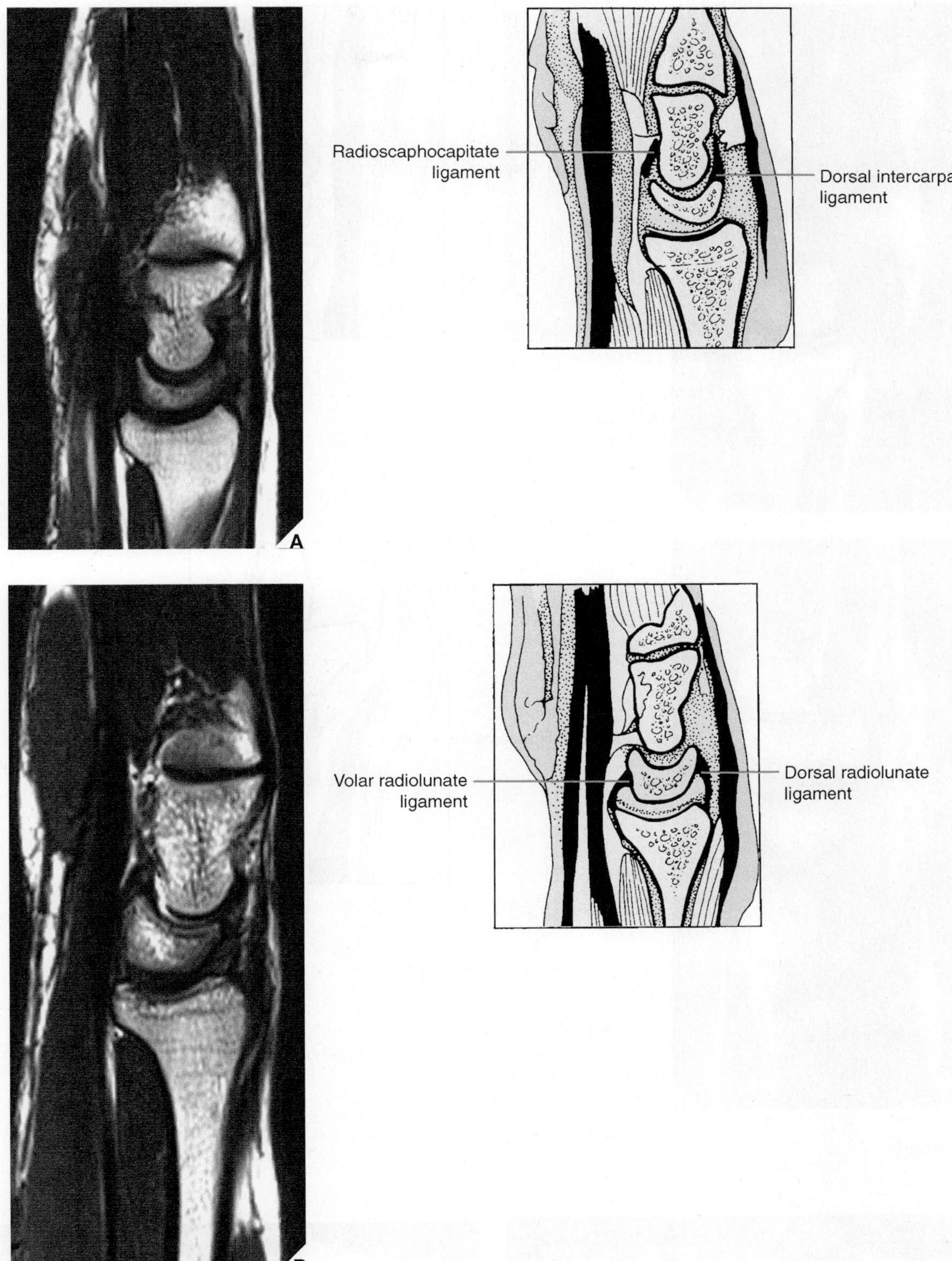

FIGURE 7.43 **MRI of the wrist.** Sagittal MRI through the wrist from the midaspect **(A,B)** to the ulnar aspect **(C,D)**. The volar and dorsal radiolunate components of the radioscapholunate ligaments are well demonstrated. The radiolunotriquetral ligament is seen volar to the capitate–lunate articulation. The radioscaphocapitate ligament is seen inserting at the volar and proximal one third of the capitate bone.

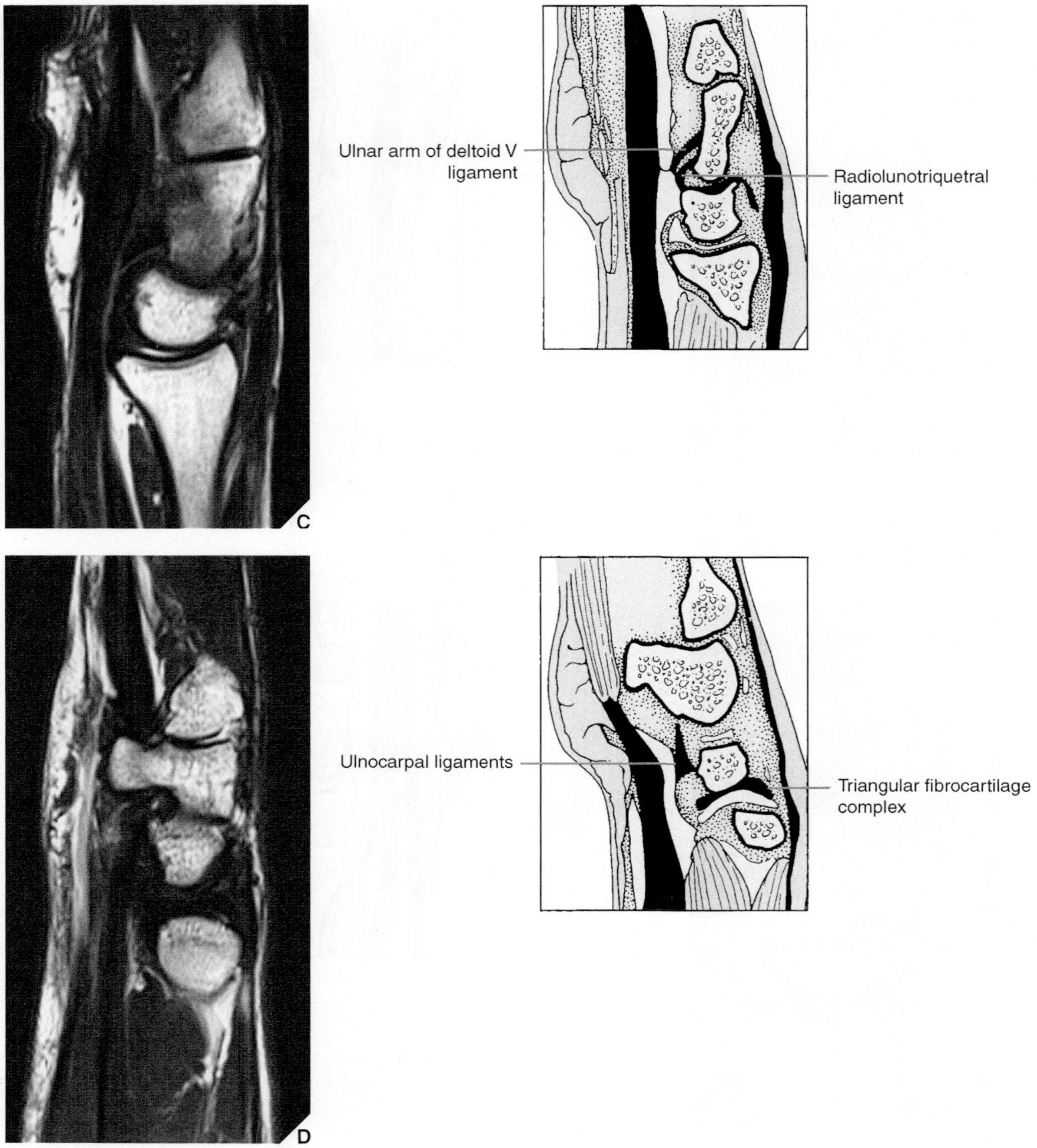

Ulnar arm of deltoid V ligament
Radiolunotriquetral ligament
C
Ulnocarpal ligaments
Triangular fibrocartilage complex
D

FIGURE 7.43 *(Continued).*

ER
ED
EDM
ECU
EPL
ECRB
ECRL
LT
EPB
APL
A
Td
C
H
MC1
T
Mn
Fr
Ua
Un
GC
B

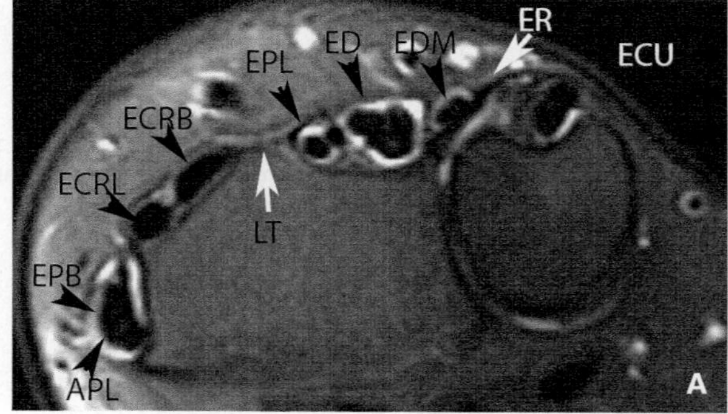

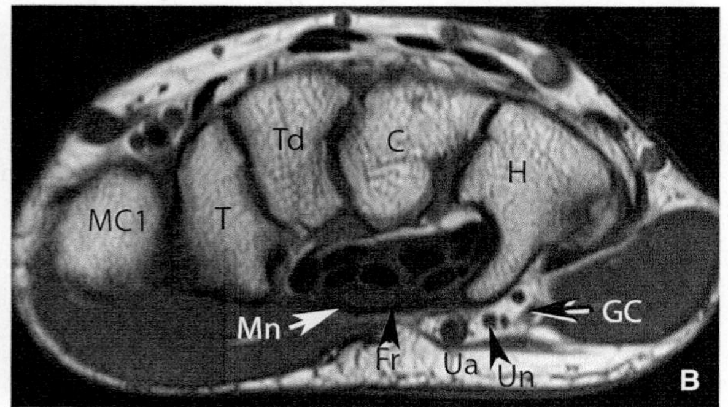

FIGURE 7.44 MRI of the wrist. Axial MR images through the proximal **(A)** and distal **(B)** carpus effectively demonstrate various atomic structures of the wrist including the extensor compartments at the level of the distal radius and ulna **(A)** and more distally at the level of the carpal tunnel and Guyon canal **(B)**. Note the extensor tendons **(A)** are separated in six different compartments by individual retinacula. Note the deep and superficial flexor tendons within the carpal tunnel **(B)**. APL, abductor pollicis longus tendon; EPB, extensor pollicis brevis tendon; ECRL, extensor carpi radialis longus tendon; ECRB, extensor carpi radialis brevis tendon; EPL, extensor pollicis longus tendon; LT, Lister tubercle; ED, extensor digitorum tendons; EDM, extensor digiti minimi tendon; ER, extensor retinaculum; ECU, extensor carpi ulnaris tendon; MC1, proximal first metacarpal; T, trapezium; Td, trapezoid. C, capitate; H, hamate; Mn, median nerve; Fr, flexor retinaculum; Ua, ulnar artery; Un, ulnar nerve; GC, Guyon canal.

TABLE 7.4 Checklist for Evaluation of Magnetic Resonance Imaging and Magnetic Resonance Arthrography of the Wrist

Osseous Structures
- Distal radius, lister tubercle (c, s, a)
- Distal ulna, styloid process (c, s, a)
- Scaphoid (c, s)
- Lunate (c, s)
- Triquetrum (c, s)
- Pisiform (c)
- Hamate, body, hook (c, s, a)
- Capitate (c, s)
- Trapezium (c)
- Trapezoid (c)

Triangular Fibrocartilage Complex
- Triangular fibrocartilage proper (c, a)
- Dorsal and volar radioulnar ligaments (c, a)
- Meniscus homolog (c)
- Extensor carpi ulnaris tendon (c, a)
- Ulnar collateral ligament (c)

Ligaments
- Intrinsic
  - Scapholunate
    - Volar (trapezoid shape) (c)
    - Middle (triangle shape) (c)
    - Dorsal (band-like) (c)
  - Lunotriquetral (c)

Ligaments (continued)
- Extrinsic
  - Volar
    - Radiocapitate (c, s)
    - Radiolunotriquetral (c, s)
    - Ulnocapitate (c, a)
    - Ulnotriquetral (c, a)
    - Ulnolunate (c, a)
  - Dorsal
    - Radioscaphoid (c)
    - Radiolunate (c)
    - Radiotriquetral (c)
    - Scaphotriquetral (c)
    - Intercarpal (c)

Tendons
- Flexors (a)
- Extensors (a)

Nerves
- Median, ulnar (a)

Other Structures
- Carpal tunnel (c)
- Guyon canal (c)
- (Ulnar nerve, ulnar artery, ulnar vein)

The best imaging planes for visualization of listed structures are given in parentheses: c, coronal; s, sagittal; a, axial.

TABLE 7.5 Standard and Special Radiographic Projections for Evaluating Injury to the Wrist, Hand, and Fingers

Projection	Demonstration

Dorsovolar	Carpal bones
	Three carpal arcs
	Eye of the hamate
	Scaphoid fat stripe
	Radiocarpal articulation
	Metacarpals
	Phalanges
	Carpometacarpal, metacarpophalangeal, and interphalangeal joints
	Scapholunate dissociation
	  Terry-Thomas sign
	  Scaphoid signet-ring sign
	Fractures of
	  Scaphoid
	  Capitate
	  Lunate
	  Hamate (body)
	  Metacarpals
	  Phalanges

In ulnar deviation	Bennett and Rolando fractures

Lateral	Scaphoid fractures
	Longitudinal axial alignment of third metacarpal, capitate, lunate, and radius
	Fractures of
	  Triquetrum
	  Metacarpals
	  Phalanges
	Carpal dislocations
	  Lunate
	  Perilunate
	  Midcarpal
	Volar intercalated segment instability
	Dorsal intercalated segment instability
	Dislocations of metacarpals and phalanges
	Fractures of the dorsal and volar plates of the phalanges

Oblique (hand)	Fractures of
	  Metacarpals
	  Phalanges
	Boxer's fracture

Supinated oblique (wrist)	Pisotriquetral joint Pisiform fractures

Pronated oblique (wrist)	Dorsal aspect of triquetrum and triquetral fractures
	Radiovolar aspect of scaphoid
	Articulations between
	  Scaphoid and trapezium
	  Trapezium and trapezoid

Carpal tunnel	Volar aspect of trapezium
	Fractures of
	  Hook of the hamate
	  Pisiform

Abduction–stress (thumb)	Gamekeeper's thumb

TABLE 7.6 Ancillary Imaging Techniques for Evaluating Injury to the Wrist, Hand, and Fingers

Technique	Demonstration
Fluoroscopy/videotaping	Kinematics of wrist and hand Carpal instability Transient carpal subluxations
Radionuclide imaging (scintigraphy, bone scan)	Subtle chondral and osteochondral fractures Fracture healing and complications (e.g., infection, osteonecrosis)
Arthrography (single contrast)	Tear of TFCC Intercarpal ligaments Ulnar collateral ligament (gamekeeper's thumb)
MRI and MRa	Same as for arthrography Guyon canal and its abnormalities Carpal tunnel syndrome AIN syndrome Injury to the soft tissues de Quervain syndrome Tendons and ligament tears of the fingers Subtle fractures Osteonecrosis Ulnar impaction (abutment) syndrome
Tomography, usually trispiral (currently replaced by CT)	Fractures of carpal bones, particularly scaphoid, hamate, and lunate Rolando fracture Bennett fracture Kienböck disease Fracture healing and complications (e.g., nonunion, osteonecrosis) Fractures of the hook of the hamate Stability of a scaphoid fracture
CT, MRI	Humpback deformity of scaphoid Subtle fractures, particularly of the hook of the hamate Fracture healing and complications

TFCC, triangular fibrocartilage complex; MRI, magnetic resonance imaging; MRa, magnetic resonance arthrography; AIN, anterior interosseous nerve; CT, computed tomography.

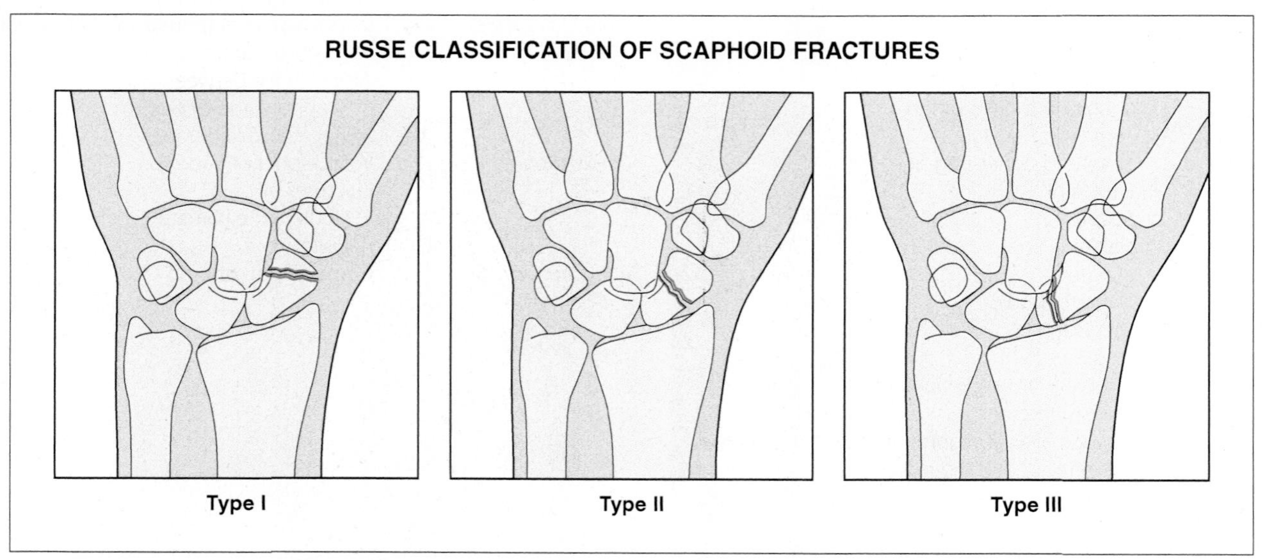

FIGURE 7.45 Scaphoid fractures. Russe classified fractures of the scaphoid bone according to the direction of the fracture line.

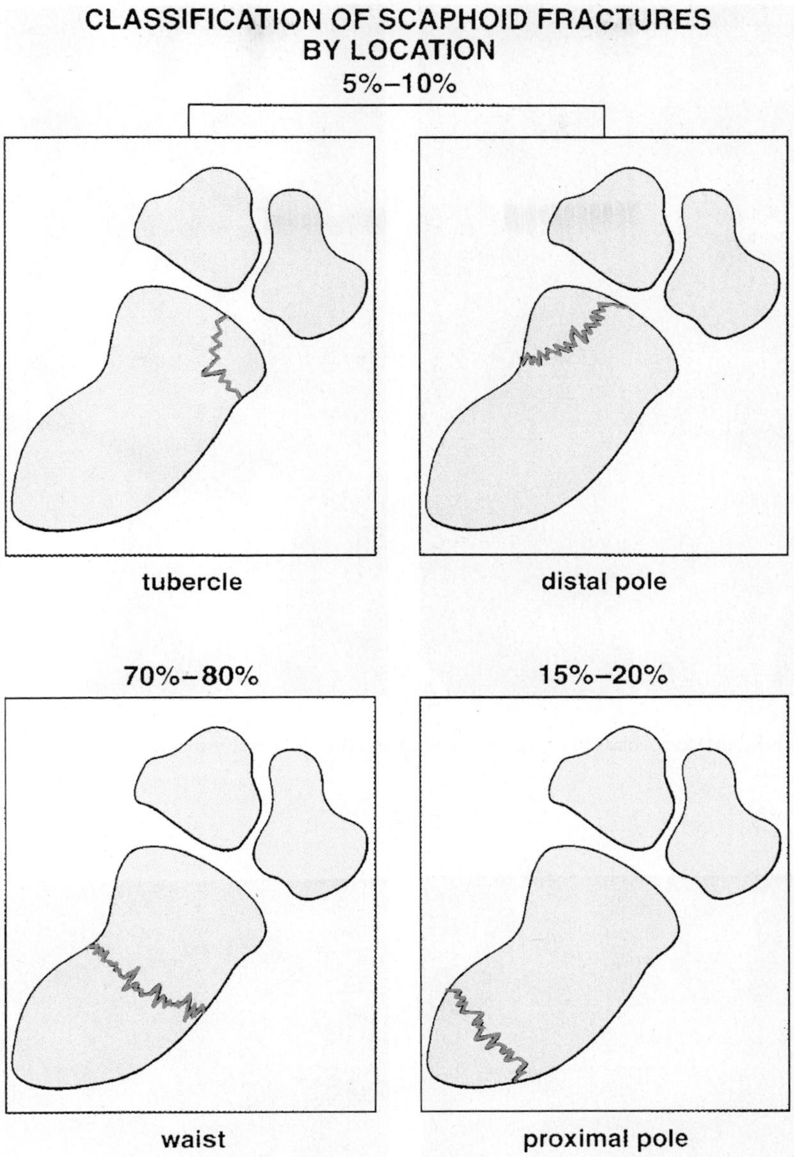

CLASSIFICATION OF SCAPHOID FRACTURES
BY LOCATION

5%–10%

tubercle

distal pole

70%–80%

15%–20%

waist

proximal pole

FIGURE 7.46 **Scaphoid fractures.** Classification of scaphoid fractures by the location of the fracture line.

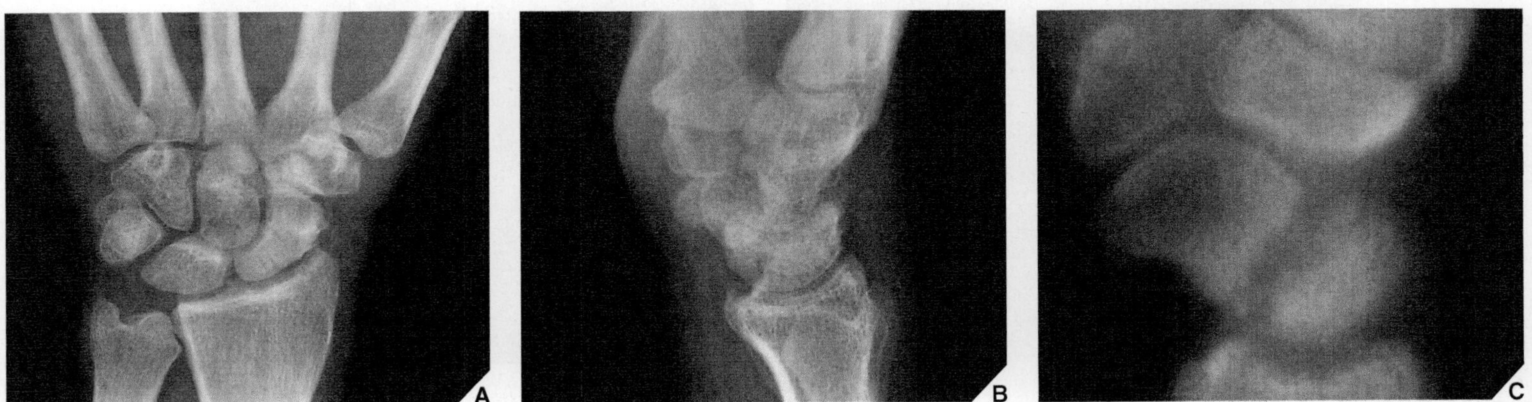

FIGURE 7.47 **Scaphoid fracture.** A 28-year-old man sustained an injury to his left wrist; pain persisted for 3 weeks. **(A)** Dorsovolar and **(B)** lateral radiographs show periarticular osteoporosis, but no fracture line is evident. **(C)** On a thin-section trispiral tomogram in the lateral projection, a fracture of the scaphoid becomes apparent.

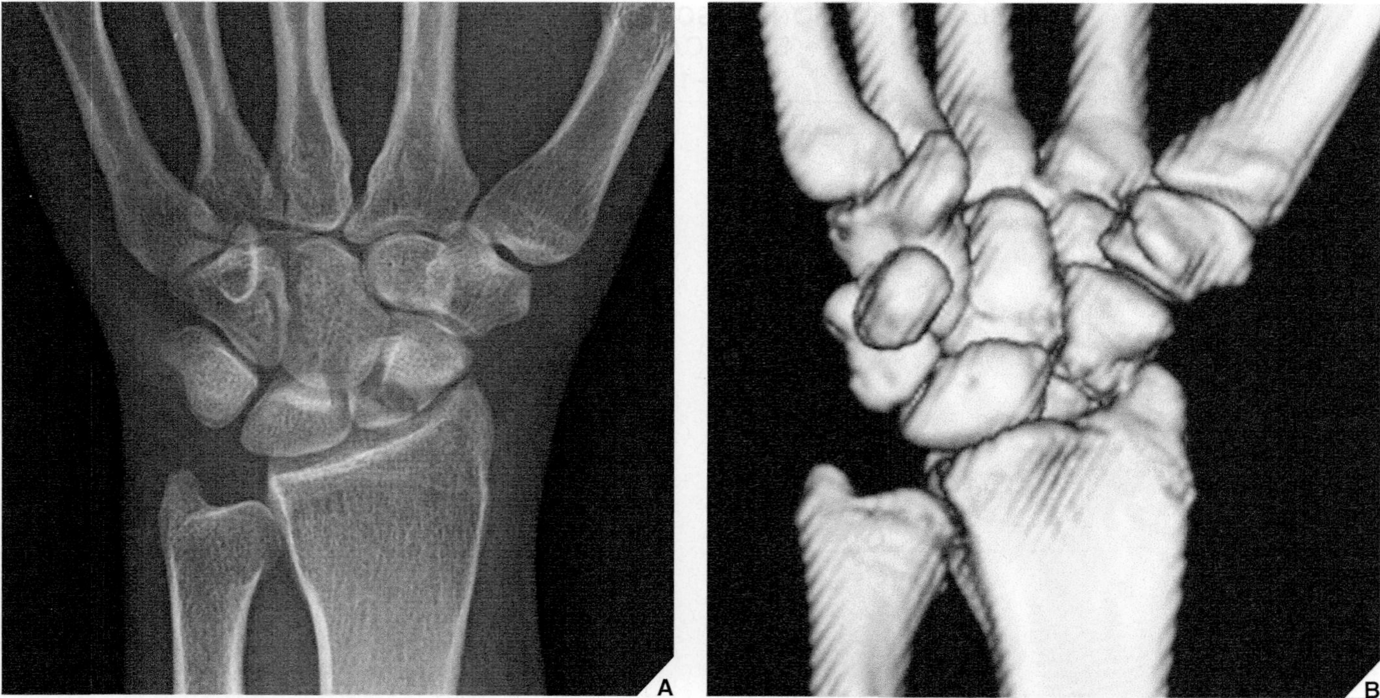

FIGURE 7.48 3D CT of scaphoid fracture. **(A)** Dorsovolar radiograph of the wrist and **(B)** 3D CT reconstructed image show type III acute scaphoid fracture.

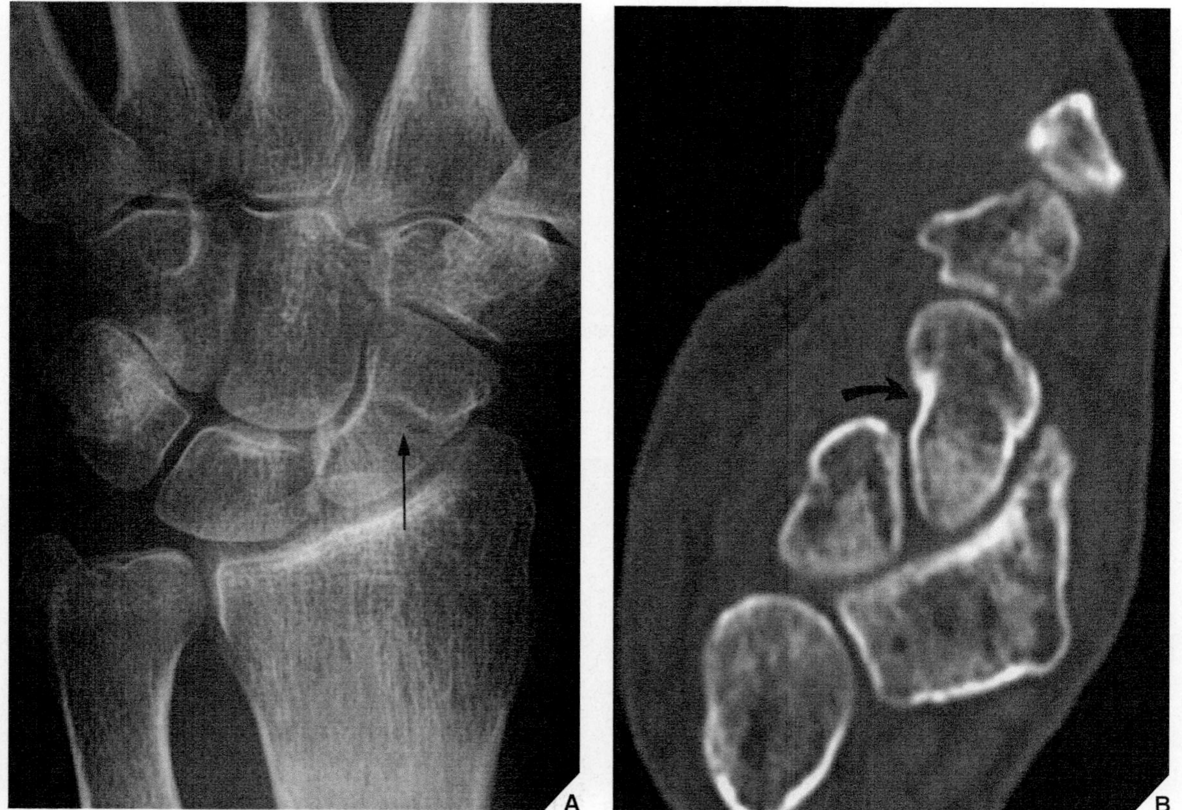

FIGURE 7.49 CT of a healed scaphoid fracture. A 56-year-old man was treated conservatively for a scaphoid fracture with closed reduction and cast application. **(A)** Dorsovolar radiograph of the wrist shows a radiolucent line *(arrow)* suggestive of a nonunion. **(B)** Oblique coronal CT image demonstrates, however, complete union *(curved arrow)*.

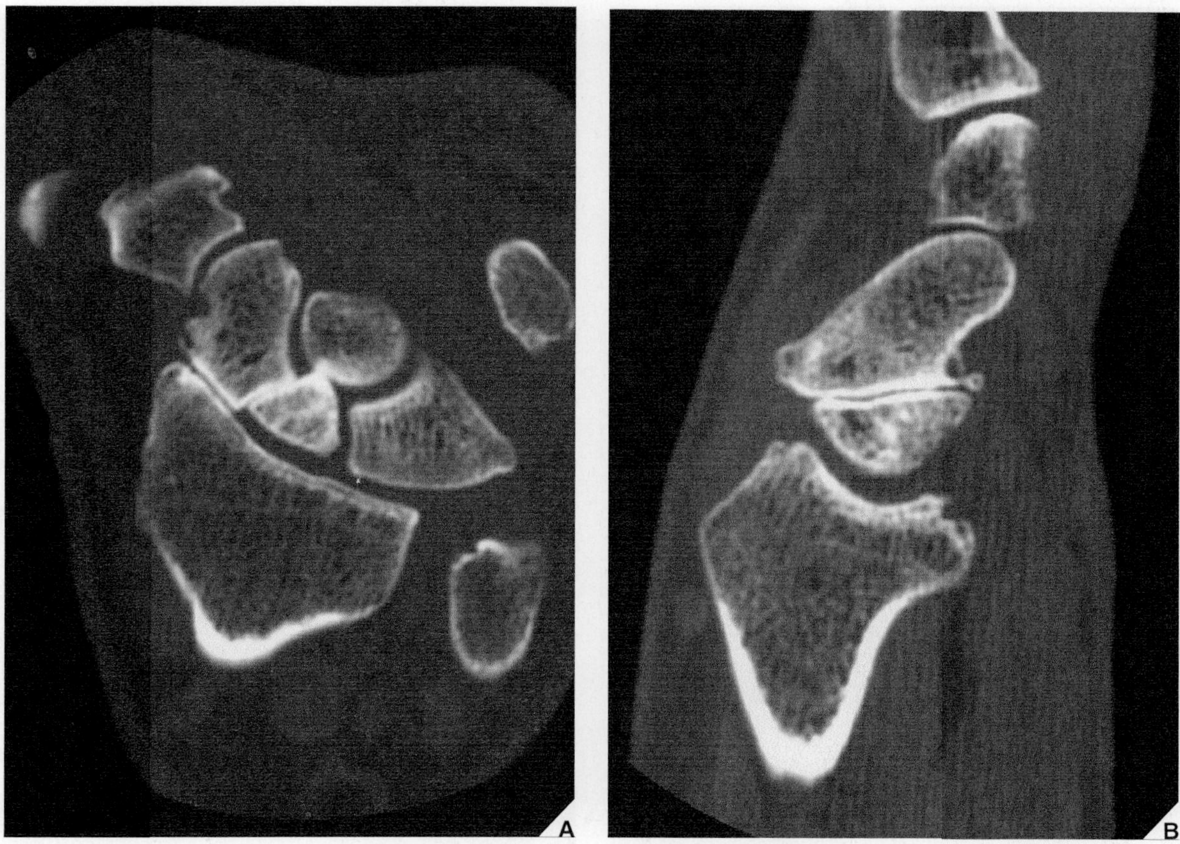

FIGURE 7.50 CT of an ununited scaphoid fracture. **(A)** Coronal and **(B)** sagittal reformatted CT images show nonunion of a scaphoid fracture. Note the sclerotic edges and gap between the fractured fragments.

FIGURE 7.51 Humpback deformity. A sagittal reformatted CT image shows a humpback deformity of a fractured scaphoid. Note the palmar flexion of the distal fragment *(arrow)* and the dorsal apex angulation *(curved arrow)*.

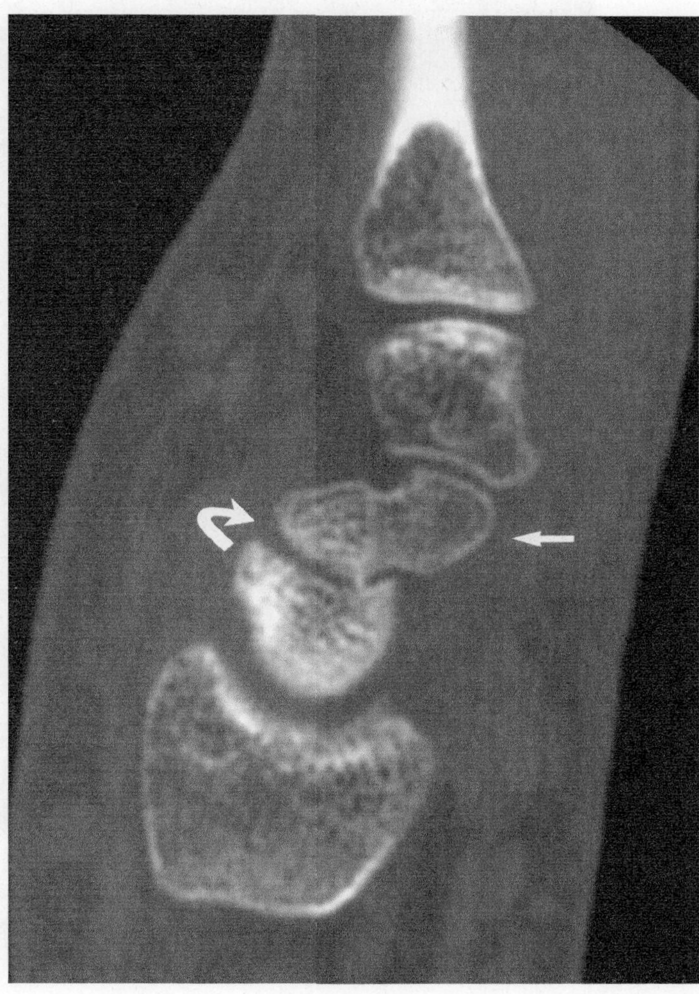

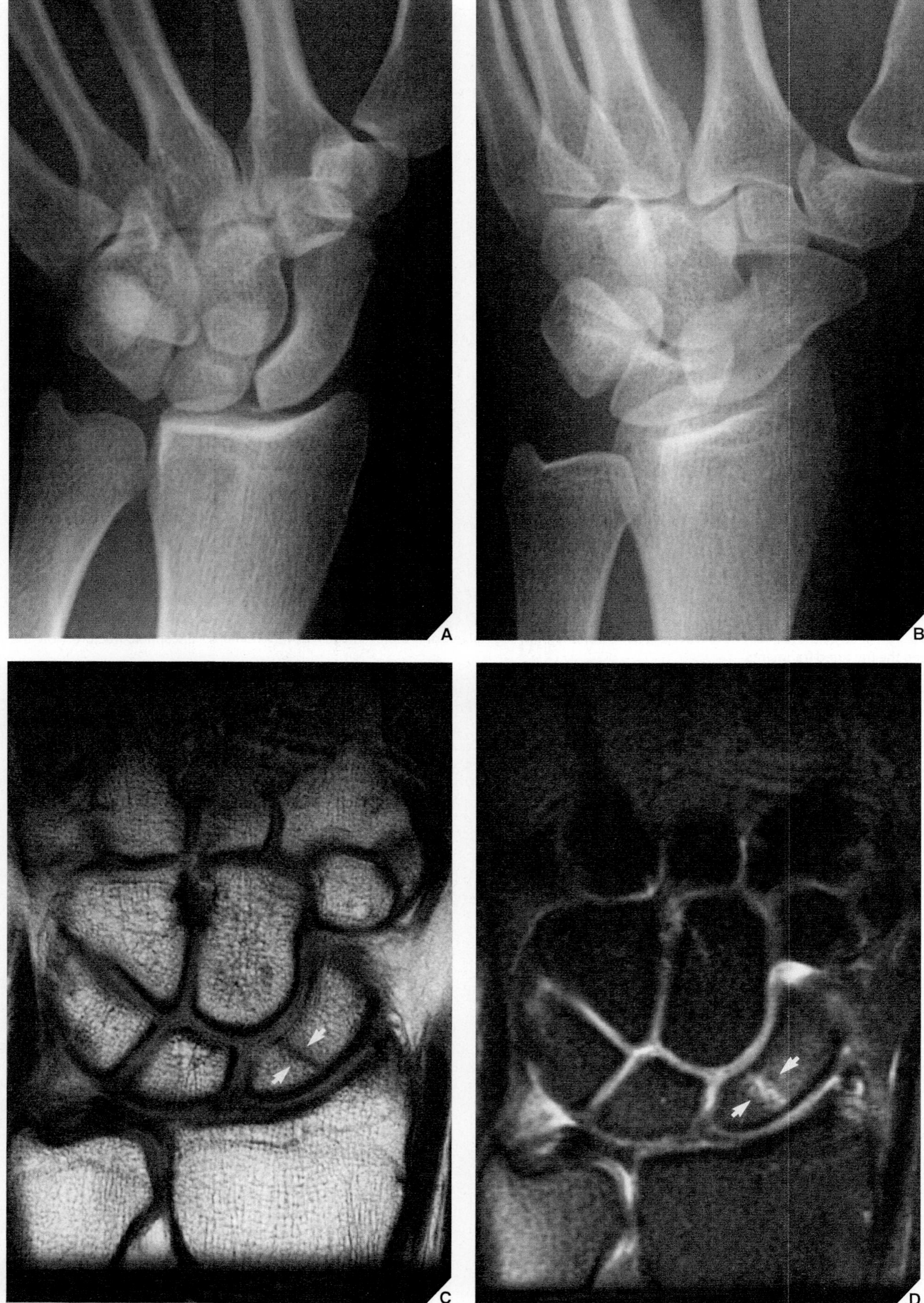

FIGURE 7.52 MRI of a scaphoid fracture. A 27-year-old man fell on ice and presented with snuffbox tenderness. **(A)** Dorsovolar in ulnar deviation and **(B)** oblique radiographs (as well as conventional dorsovolar and lateral views, not shown here) were normal. **(C)** Coronal T1-weighted and **(D)** coronal fat-suppressed T2-weighted MR images show a fracture of the proximal pole of the scaphoid *(arrows)*.

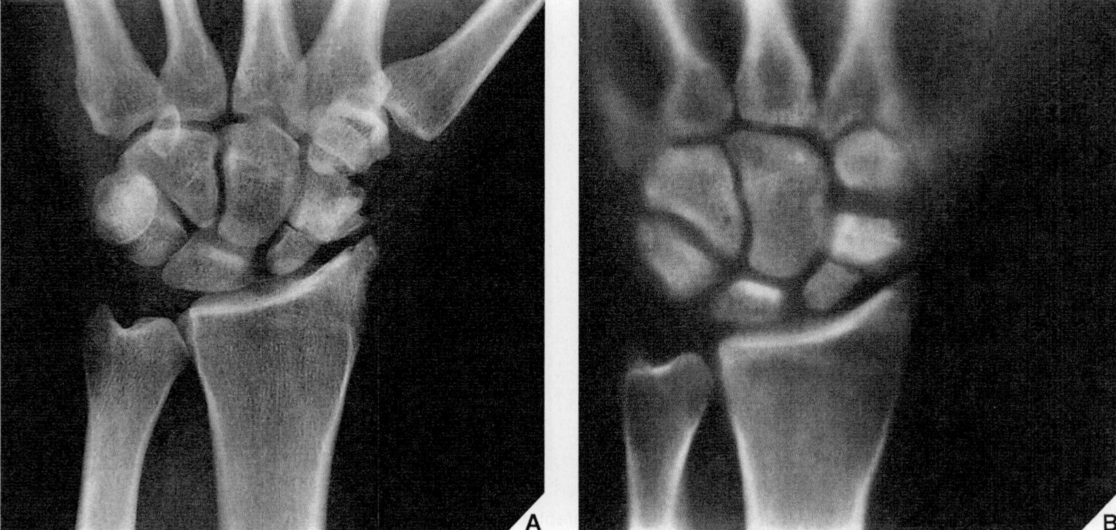

FIGURE 7.53 **Scaphoid fracture complicated by osteonecrosis.** On follow-up examination of a 40-year-old man who had sustained a fracture of the scaphoid treated by immobilization for 3 months, the dorsovolar radiograph **(A)** shows persistence of the fracture line and oddly shaped distal scaphoid pole. Trispiral tomography **(B)** revealed unsuspected osteonecrosis of the distal fragment. (Reprinted by permission from Springer: Sherman SB, Greenspan A, Norman A. Osteonecrosis of the distal pole of the carpal scaphoid following fracture—a rare complication. *Skeletal Radiol* 1983;9:189–191.)

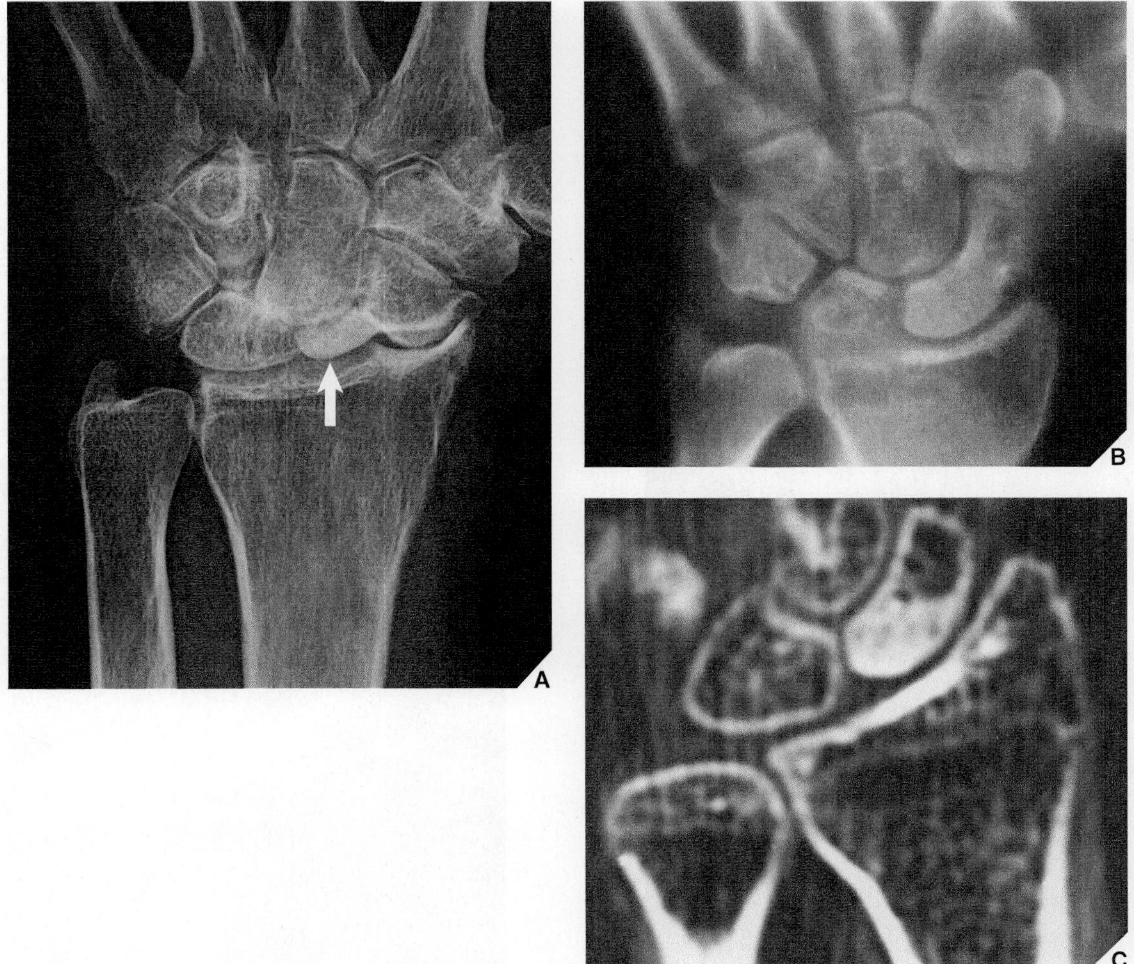

FIGURE 7.54 **Scaphoid fracture complicated by osteonecrosis.** **(A)** Dorsovolar radiograph of the wrist shows an ununited fracture of the scaphoid and osteonecrosis of the proximal fragment *(arrow)*. **(B)** In another patient, who sustained a scaphoid fracture treated conservatively for 4 months, trispiral tomogram shows a dense proximal segment of the scaphoid indicative of osteonecrosis, but the fracture is fully united. **(C)** Yet in another patient, a coronal CT reformatted image shows a healed fracture of the scaphoid with osteonecrosis of the proximal fragment.

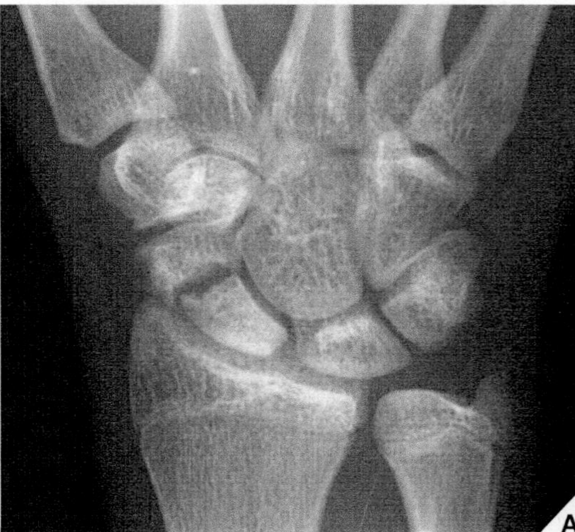

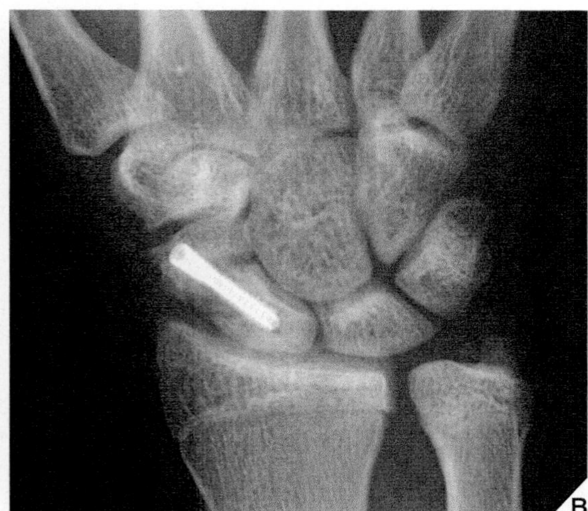

FIGURE 7.55 Surgical treatment of a scaphoid fracture. **(A)** Dorsovolar radiograph of the wrist shows a fracture of the scaphoid, treated by open reduction and internal fixation using a bone graft and an Acutrak screw **(B)**.

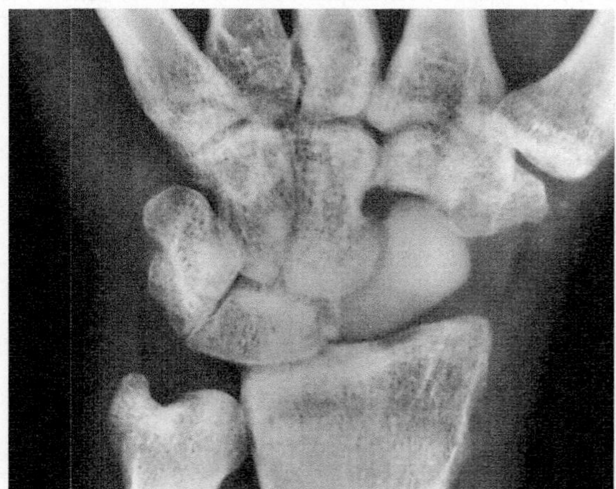

FIGURE 7.56 Scaphoid prosthesis. A 35-year-old man sustained a fracture of the scaphoid. Nonunion was complicated by osteonecrosis. The bone was excised and silastic prosthesis inserted. Note the smoothness of the margins of the prosthesis as well as its ivory-like homogeneous density and lack of trabecular pattern.

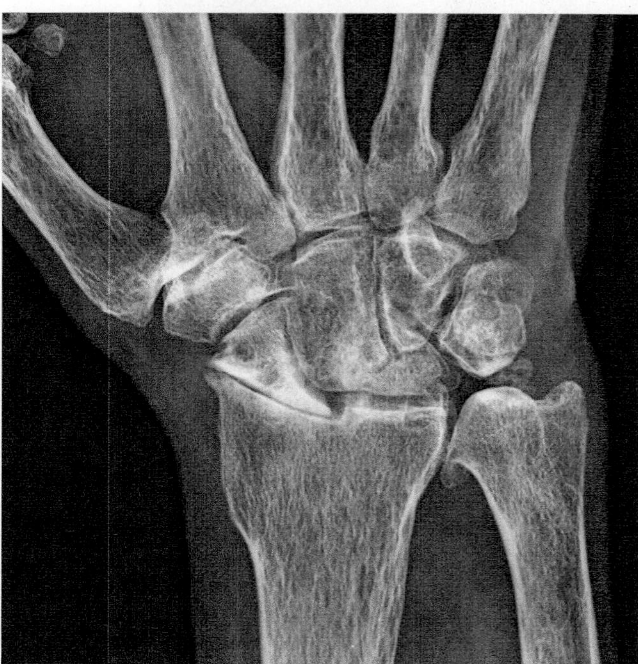

FIGURE 7.57 SLAC wrist. A 70-year-old woman presented with chronic wrist pain for past 15 years. Dorsovolar radiograph shows deformity of the scaphoid from the previous fracture associated with osteonecrosis. The scapholunate interval is widened, and there is proximal migration of the capitate. Osteoarthritis of the radiocarpal joint is apparent.

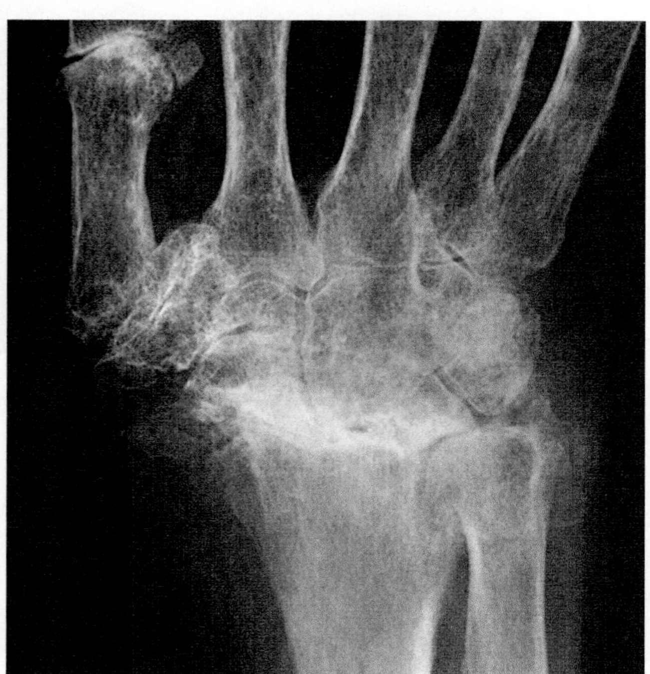

FIGURE 7.58 SLAC wrist (more advanced). A 72-year-old woman presented with chronic untreated scaphoid fracture complicated by osteonecrosis of the proximal fragment. Note the proximal migration of the capitate and advanced osteoarthritis of the radiocarpal joint, representing an SLAC wrist deformity.

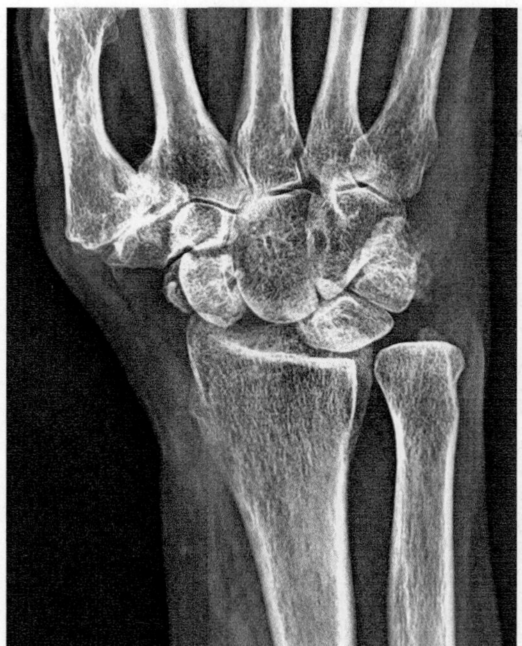

FIGURE 7.59 **SNAC wrist.** A 63-year-old woman sustained a fracture of the scaphoid that failed to unite. The lunate is medially displaced, and there is proximal migration of the capitate.

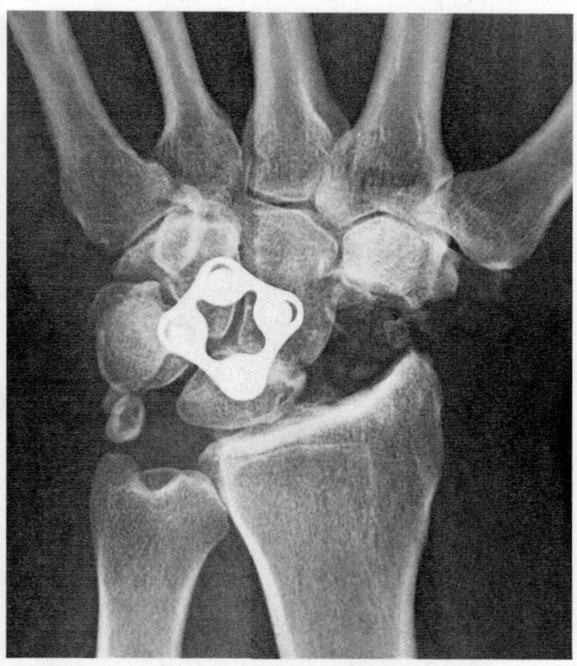

FIGURE 7.60 **Limited carpal fusion.** A 58-year-old man who sustained a scaphoid fracture complicated by nonunion and osteonecrosis was surgically treated with a resection of the scaphoid and four-corner carpal fusion.

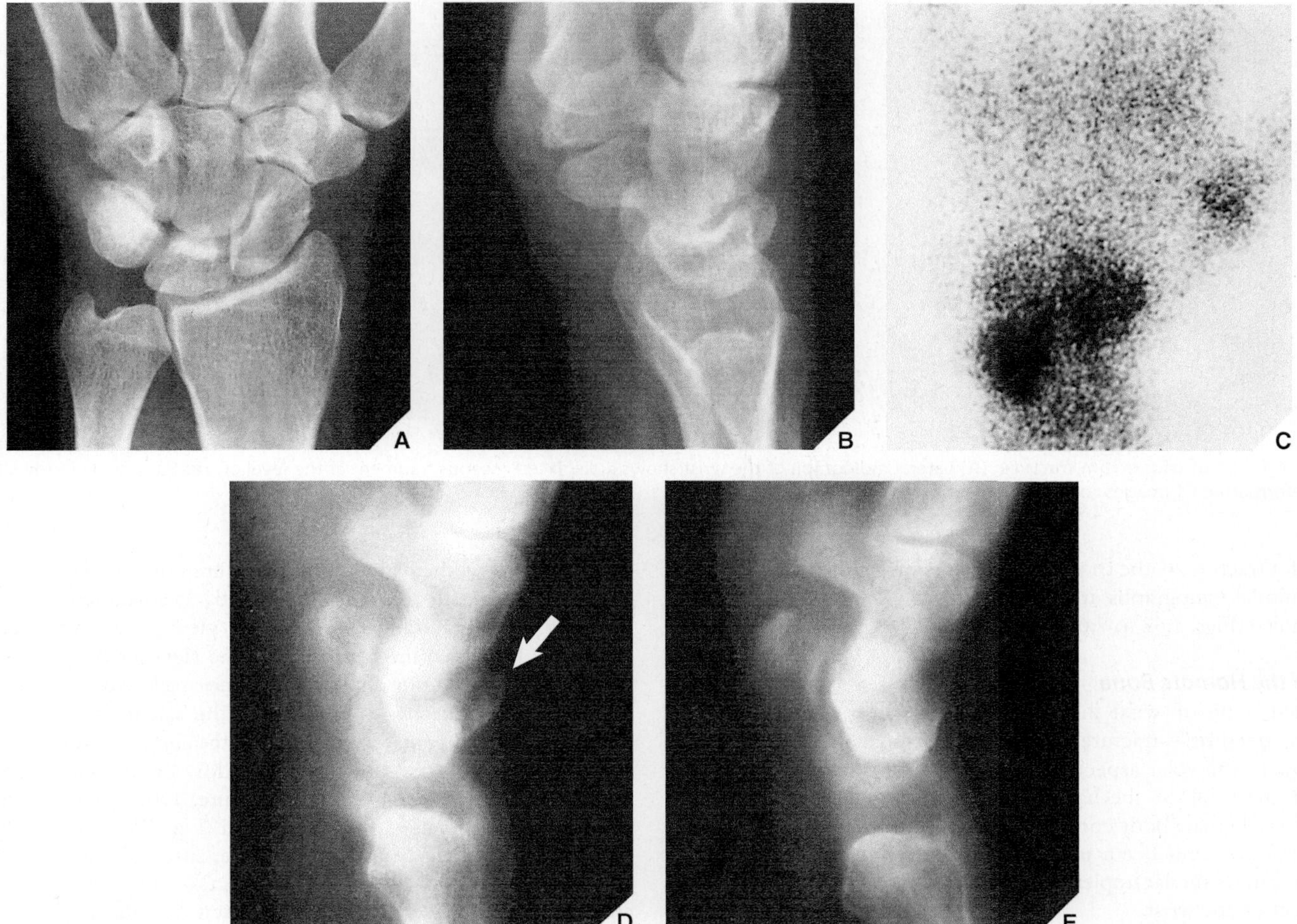

FIGURE 7.61 **Triquetrum fracture.** A 45-year-old man, having fallen on his outstretched hand, presented with localized tenderness on the dorsal aspect of the wrist. **(A)** Dorsovolar and **(B)** lateral radiographs of the wrist are normal. **(C)** Radionuclide bone scan, which was performed to localize the possible site of trauma, reveals an increased uptake of the tracer on the ulnar side of the carpus, suggesting a fracture. **(D)** Tomographic examination in the lateral projection unequivocally demonstrates triquetral fracture *(arrow)*. **(E)** The tomographic appearance of the normal triquetrum is shown for comparison.

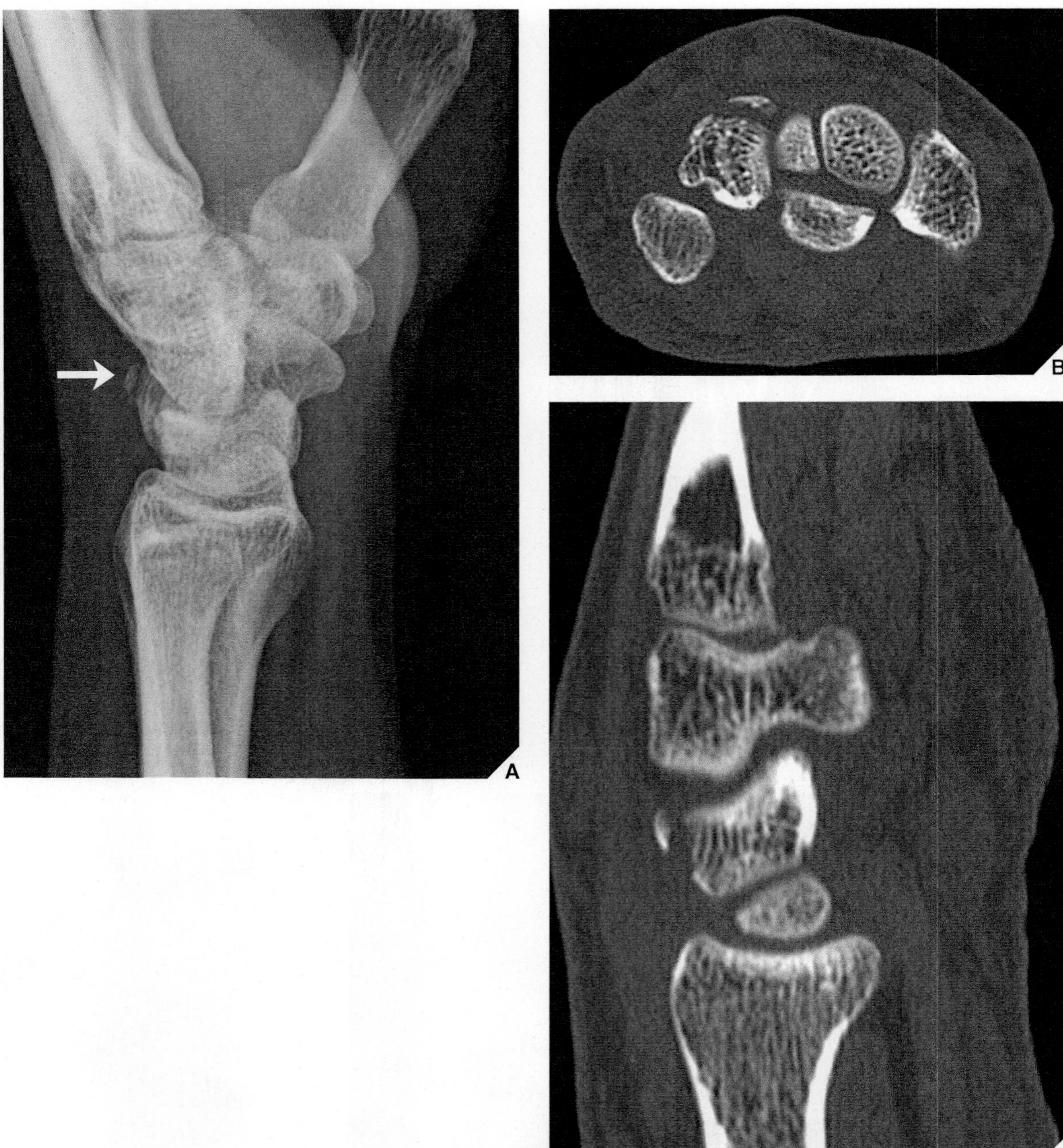

FIGURE 7.62 CT of triquetrum fracture. **(A)** Lateral radiograph of the wrist shows a displaced osseous fragment at the level of triquetral bone *(arrow)*. **(B)** Axial and **(C)** sagittal reformatted CT images confirm the diagnosis of triquetrum fracture.

Currently, if a fracture of the triquetral bone is clinically strongly suspected and conventional radiographs are not diagnostic, CT or MRI is the technique of choice (Figs. 7.62 to 7.64).

Fracture of the Hamate Bone

An infrequent type of wrist injury—accounting for approximately 2% of all carpal fractures—fracture of the hamate most often results from a direct blow to the volar aspect of the wrist. This is particularly true in fractures of the hook of the hamate (or hamulus), which together with fractures of the hamate body constitute the two groups of hamate injuries. Most hamulus fractures occur in sports activities requiring the use of a racket, club, bat, or similar implement that may cause a direct injury to the palmar aspect of the wrist.

Fractures of the hamate body, which may extend either ulnarly or radially to the hamulus, usually are readily demonstrated on the standard views of the wrist. The lateral and pronated oblique radiographs are preferable, particularly in detecting fractures that may be oriented in the coronal plane (Fig. 7.65).

Fractures of the hamulus, however, are not apparent on routine studies and consequently may go undiagnosed. As an aid to recognizing hamulus fracture on the standard dorsovolar view of the wrist, Norman and colleagues have identified the *eye sign*. The sign derives its name from the dense, oval, cortical ring shadow that is normally seen over the hamate on the dorsovolar projection. This "eye" of the hamate is actually the hook of the hamate seen on end (see Fig. 7.1). Although in most cases, the absence or indistinct outline of the cortical shadow or the presence of sclerosis suggests the diagnosis of hamulus fracture, a radiograph of the opposite wrist should be obtained for comparison (Fig. 7.66A,B). Confirmation of the diagnosis and evaluation of the type, site, and extent of the fracture may be made on the carpal tunnel projection (Fig. 7.66C). This view may also be effective when the suspected fracture is distal to the base of the hook and, as a result, the eye of the hamate may still be visible (Fig. 7.67). The carpal tunnel view, however, is not always definitively diagnostic because the degree of dorsiflexion of the wrist required for this projection (see Fig. 7.38) is often limited because of pain, particularly in patients with acute or subacute fractures. Limited dorsiflexion may cause the anterior

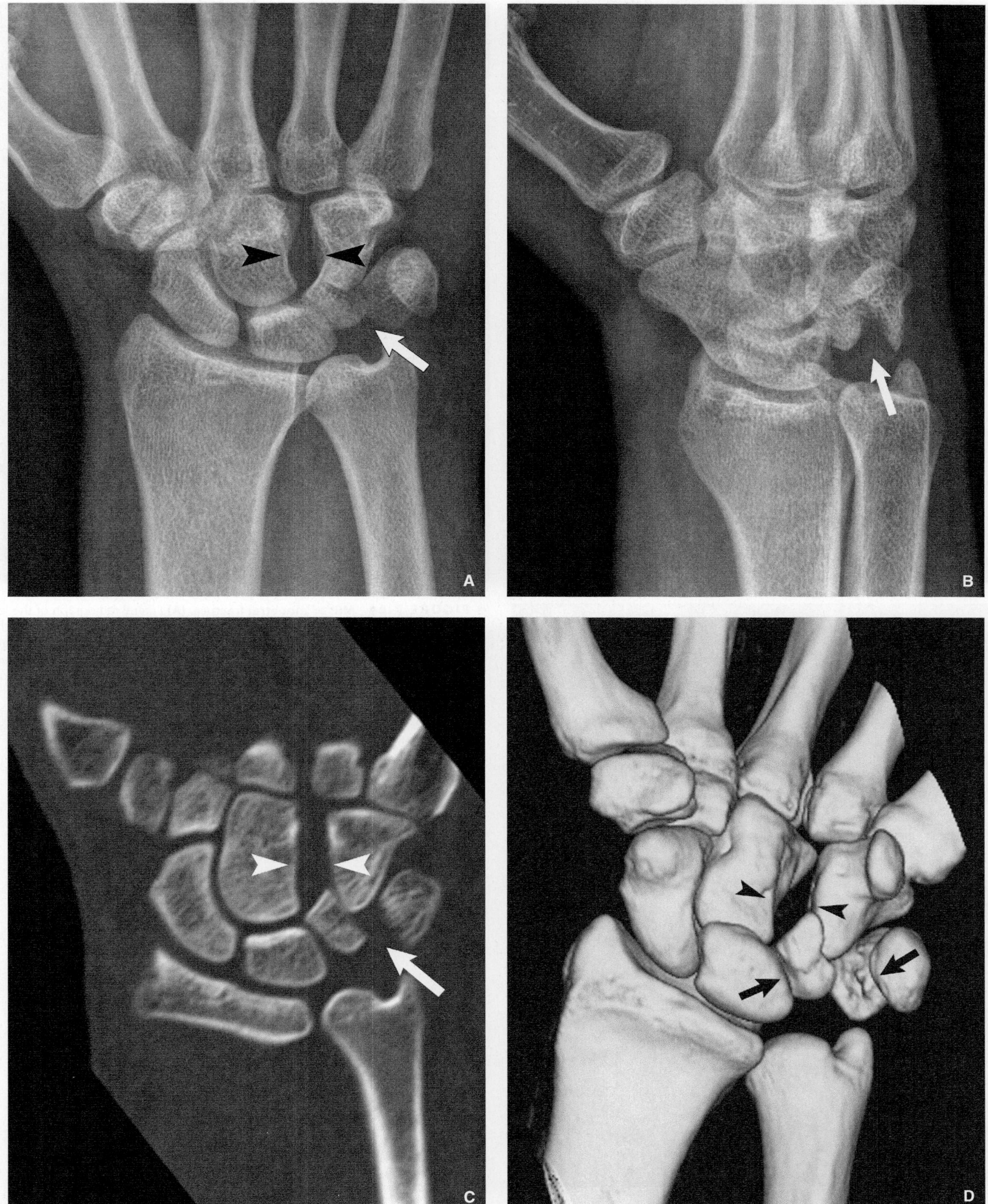

FIGURE 7.63 CT and 3D CT of triquetral fracture. **(A)** Dorsovolar and **(B)** oblique radiographs of the left wrist of a 21-year-old man show a comminuted fracture of the triquetrum *(arrow)*. Observe widening of the capitohamate interval *(arrowheads)* secondary to ligamentous tear. **(C)** Coronal reformatted and **(D)** 3D reconstructed CT images confirm the findings seen on the radiographs, namely comminuted fracture of the triquetrum *(arrows)* and widening of the capitohamate interval *(arrowheads)* due to the tear of the capitohamate ligaments.

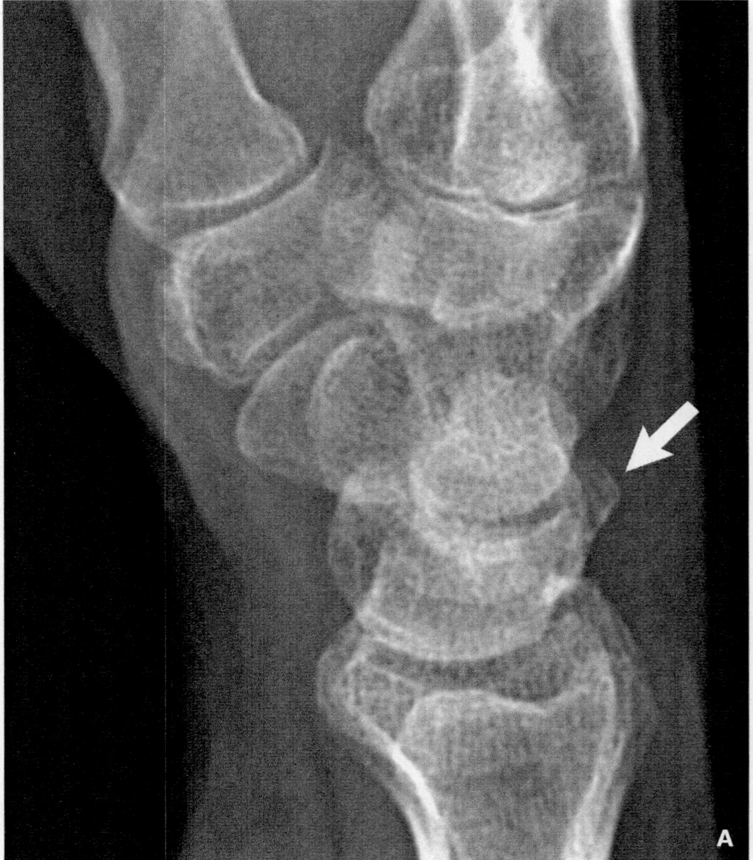

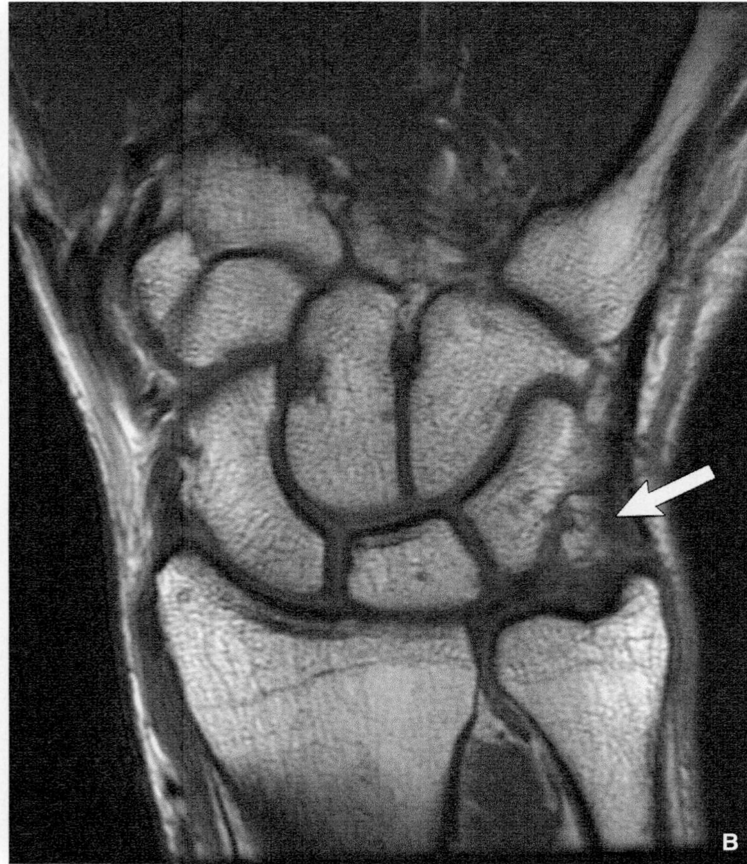

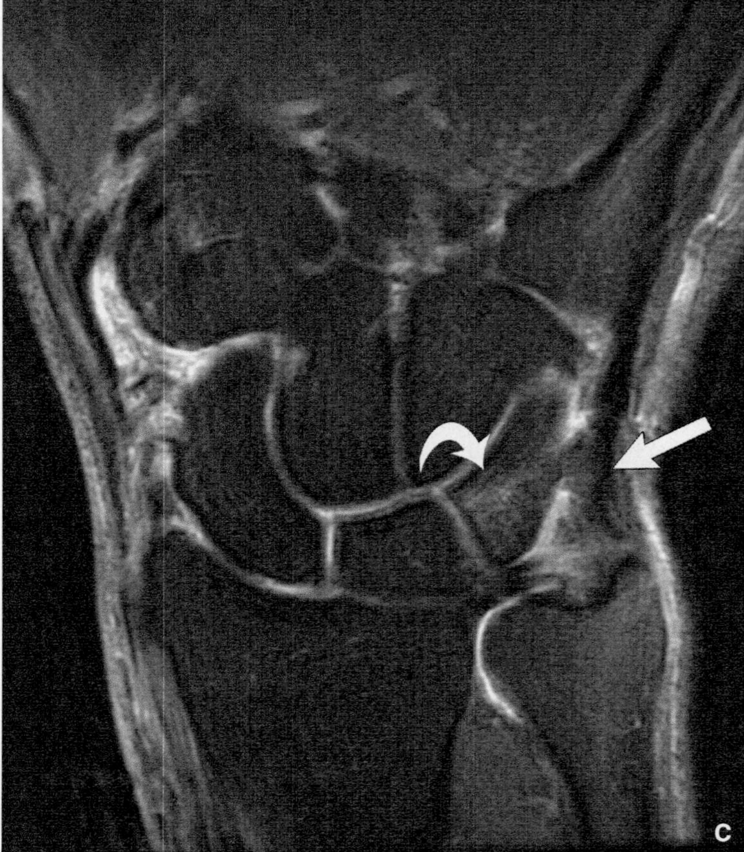

FIGURE 7.64 MRI of triquetral fracture. **(A)** Lateral radiograph of the left wrist of a 78-year-old shows slightly displaced fracture of the dorsal aspect of the triquetrum *(arrow)*. **(B)** Coronal proton density–weighted and **(C)** coronal proton density–weighted fat-suppressed MR images demonstrate that the fracture is comminuted *(arrow)*. The *curve arrow* points to high-intensity bone marrow edema.

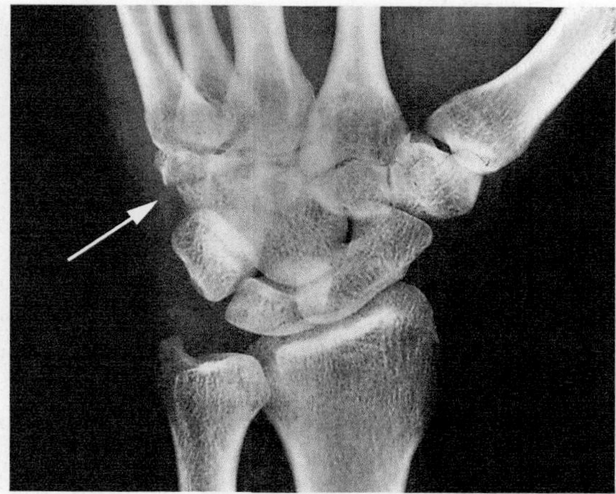

FIGURE 7.65 Hamate fracture. On the pronated oblique radiograph of the wrist, a fracture of the hamate body is clearly evident *(arrow)*.

margins of the capitate and the pisiform to overlap and obscure the fracture line (Fig. 7.67B). In such cases, trispiral tomographic studies in the lateral and carpal tunnel projections (Fig. 7.67C,D) were usually diagnostic. At the present time, CT axial sections of the wrist with sagittal reformation are routinely performed (Fig. 7.68). Although MRI is not indicated in the preliminary evaluation of patients with suspected fracture of the hook of the hamate, it can be helpful if the initial conventional radiographs failed to demonstrate this injury (Figs. 7.69 and 7.70).

Fracture of the Pisiform Bone

A fracture of the pisiform is rare. It usually results from a direct injury to the wrist as, for example, from a fall on the outstretched hand or use of the hand as a hammer to strike an object. It may be an isolated injury or may coexist with fractures of other bones. Although this injury may be seen on posteroanterior radiographs of the wrist (Fig. 7.71), radiographs in the supinated oblique and carpal tunnel projections are best suited to demonstrate the abnormality (Fig. 7.72).

Fracture of the Capitate Bone

An uncommon type of carpal injury, accounting for only 1% to 3% of carpal fractures, fracture of the capitate usually occurs in association with other injuries to the carpus, particularly a fracture of the scaphoid and perilunate dislocation. It usually results from a fall on the outstretched hand, with hyperdorsiflexion of the hand causing impingement of the bone against the distal radius; it may also result from a direct blow to the wrist. The waist (or neck) of the capitate is the most common site of fracture. The dorsovolar radiograph of the wrist usually demonstrates the abnormality (Fig. 7.73A), although the lateral view may be helpful in determining the rotation or displacement of the fragment. Trispiral tomography was useful in outlining the details of the fracture and determining the stage of healing (Fig. 7.73B), although currently this technique has been replaced by CT and MRI (Fig. 7.74).

Fracture of the Lunate Bone

Usually, the result of a fall on the dorsiflexed wrist or a strenuous push on the heel of the hand, a fracture of the lunate is a rare type of carpal injury, accounting for less than 3% of all carpal fractures. It is often seen in association with perilunate dislocation but more commonly occurs as a pathologic fracture of necrotic bone secondary to Kienböck disease (see in the following text). The standard radiographs of the wrist, particularly the dorsovolar and lateral projections, are usually sufficient to demonstrate the abnormality, although CT scanning may also be required for a full evaluation.

Kienböck Disease

Single or repeated trauma to the lunate or dislocation of the bone may impair its blood supply and cause it to become necrotic. However, the development of Kienböck disease, as this form of osteonecrosis affecting the lunate is known, may not be solely attributable to extrinsic trauma. Whether the natural history begins with a single simple transverse fracture or numerous compression fractures from repeated compressive strains is still the subject of speculation. An interesting but controversial hypothesis links this condition with negative ulnar variance in individuals whose ulna projects more proximally. They may be predisposed to Kienböck disease because of compression of the lunate against the irregular articular surface created by the discrepancy in radial and ulnar lengths.

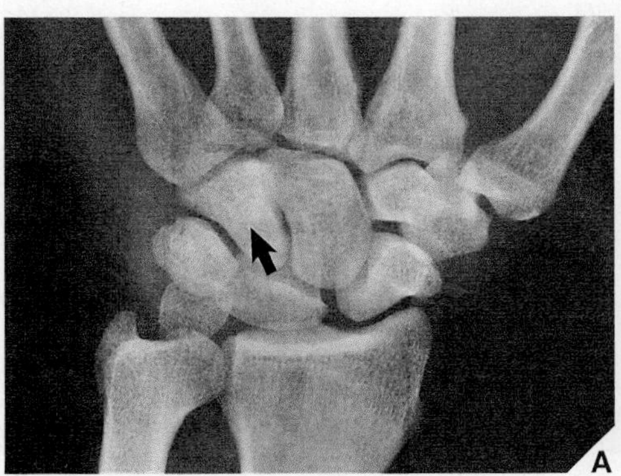

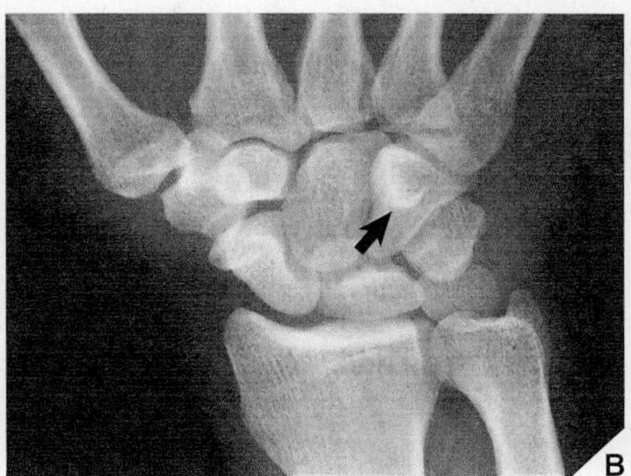

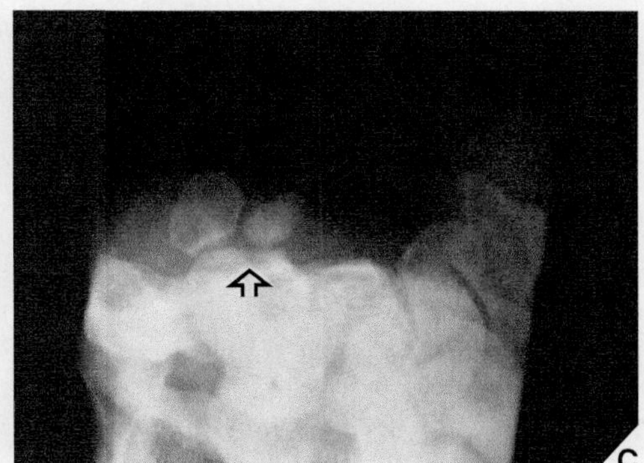

FIGURE 7.66 Fracture of the hook of the hamate. Having injured his right wrist while playing golf, a 36-year-old man presented with symptoms of pain in his palm on pressure, weakness of grasp, and occasional paresthesia of the little finger. The tenderness was limited to the area over the hook of the hamate. **(A)** On the dorsovolar radiograph of the wrist, the oval cortical shadow normally seen projecting over the hamate is not visible *(arrow)*, suggesting a fracture. **(B)** On a comparison study of the left wrist, the eye of the hamate is clearly seen *(arrow)*. **(C)** A fracture of the hook of the hamate *(open arrow)*, suggested by the disappearance of the cortical shadow of the hamate, is confirmed on the carpal tunnel projection.

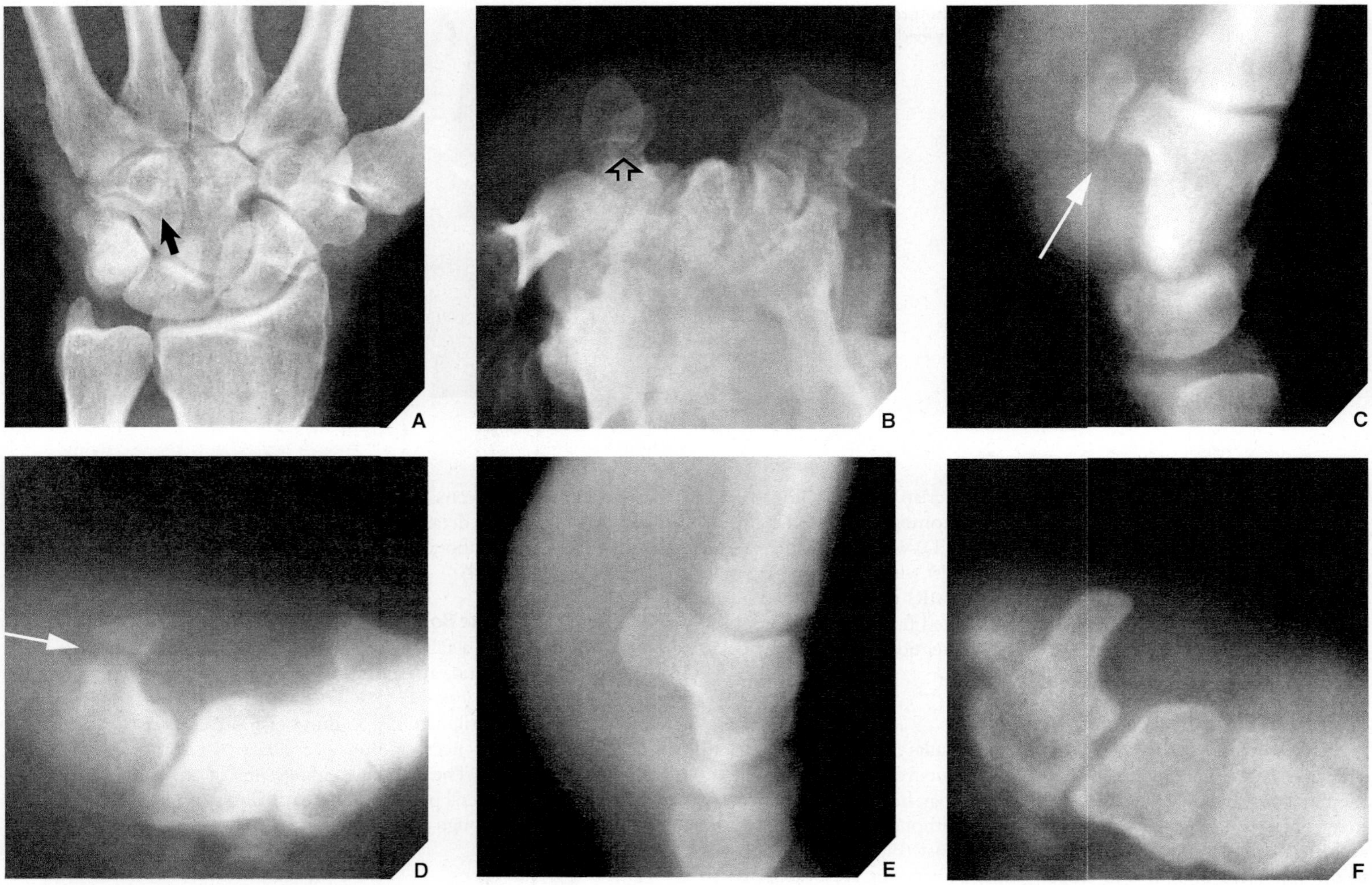

FIGURE 7.67 **Fracture of the hook of the hamate.** After falling on the palm of his right hand, a 66-year-old man reported pain in the palm, numbness, and weakness in the fingers innervated by the ulnar nerve. No obvious abnormalities are seen on the dorsovolar view of the wrist **(A)**; the eye of the hamate is clearly discernible *(arrow)*. On the conventional carpal tunnel view **(B)**, obtained without the maximum degree of dorsiflexion caused by pain, the pisiform partially overlaps the hamulus. A short radiolucent line is evident, however, at the base of the hamulus *(open arrow)*, but the diagnosis of a fracture cannot be made conclusively. Trispiral tomograms in the lateral **(C)** and carpal tunnel **(D)** projections unquestionably demonstrate a fracture of the hook of the hamate distal to the base *(arrows)*. The normal appearance of the hamulus on, respectively, the same projections **(E,F)** is shown for comparison. (**A**, **B**, and **D**, Reprinted with permission from NYU Grossman School of Medicine, from Greenspan A, Posner MA, Tucker M. The value of carpal tunnel trispiral tomography in the diagnosis of fracture of the hook of the hamate. *Bull Hosp Joint Dis Orthop Inst* 1985;45:74–79.)

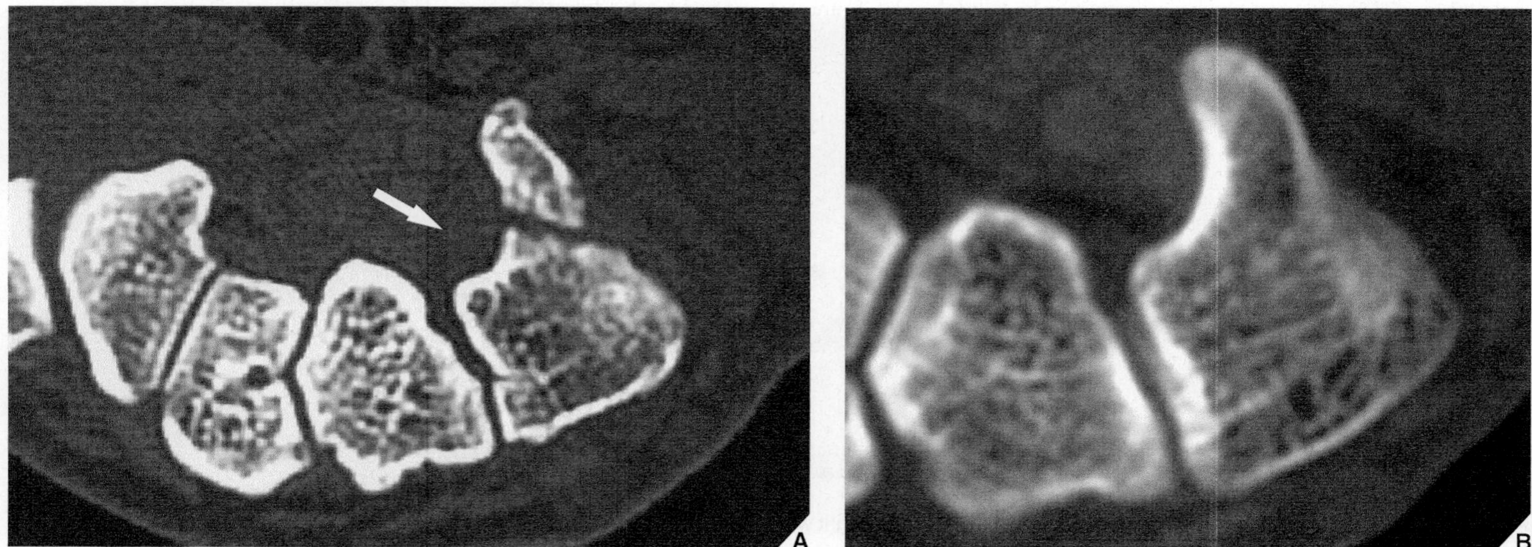

FIGURE 7.68 **CT of a fracture of the hook of the hamate.** **(A)** Axial CT image of the wrist shows a fracture of the hook of the hamate *(arrow)*. **(B)** Axial CT image of an intact hook is shown for comparison.

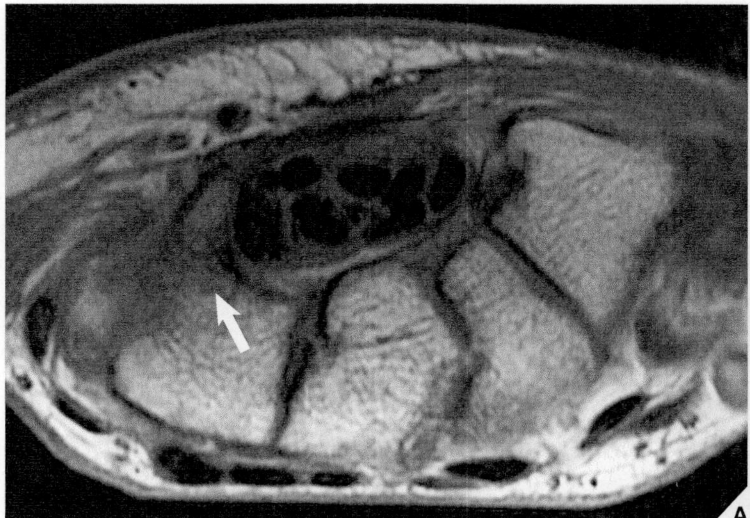

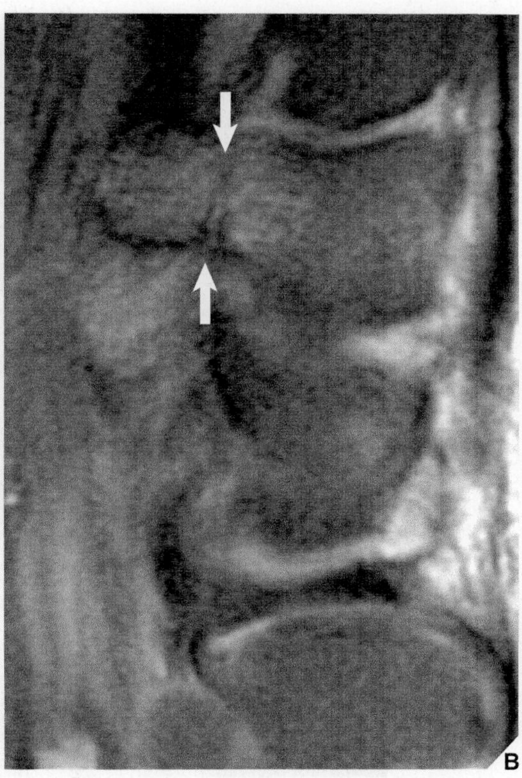

FIGURE 7.69 MRI of a fracture of the hook of the hamate. **(A)** Axial and **(B)** sagittal proton density–weighted fat-suppressed MR images of the wrist demonstrate a fracture of the hook of the hamate *(arrows)*.

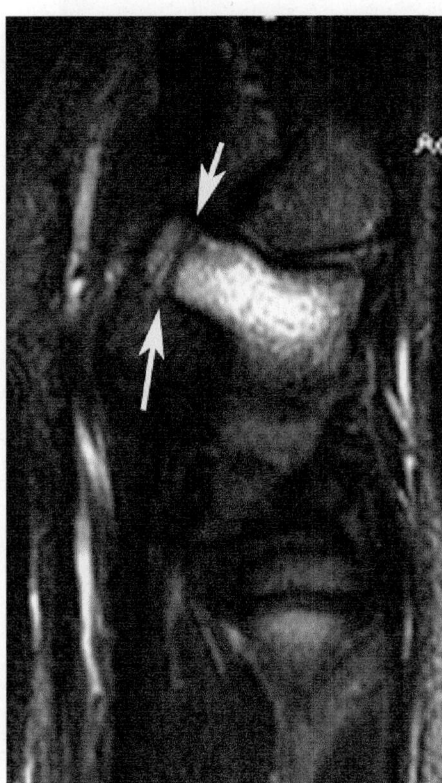

FIGURE 7.70 MRI of a fracture of the hook of the hamate. Sagittal T2-weighted MRI shows an acute nondisplaced fracture of the tip of the hook of the hamate. The fracture line *(arrows)* is surrounded by bone marrow edema. The radiographs (not shown here) obtained prior to MRI were normal.

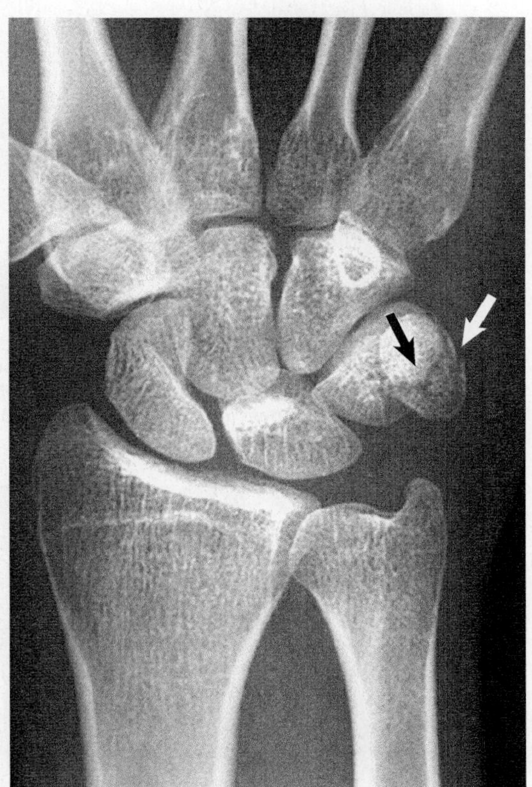

FIGURE 7.71 Pisiform fracture. Dorsovolar radiograph of the wrist shows a comminuted fracture of the pisiform bone *(arrows)*.

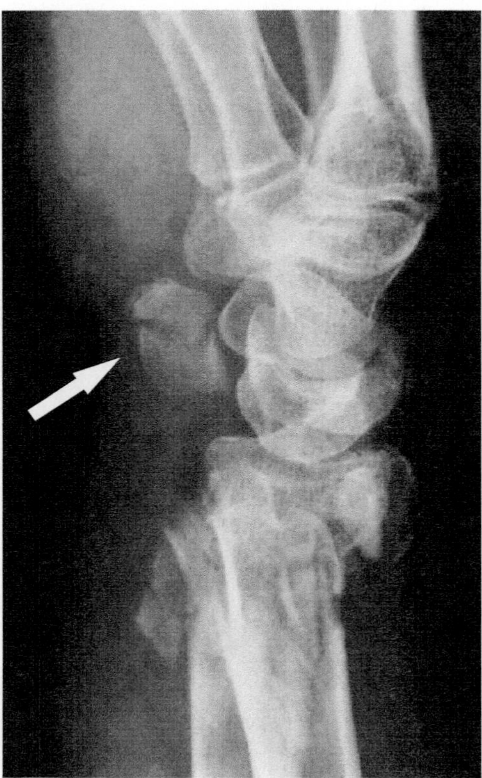

FIGURE 7.72 Pisiform fracture. A 66-year-old woman sustained a crush injury to the left wrist in a motor vehicle accident. Conventional radiographs in the dorsovolar, lateral, and oblique projections (not shown here) revealed comminuted fractures of the distal radius and the ulna. To exclude the possibility of associated carpal fractures, especially in view of the severity of the injury seen on the routine studies, a radiograph in the supinated oblique projection was obtained. This view clearly demonstrates, in addition, a fracture of the pisiform *(arrow)*.

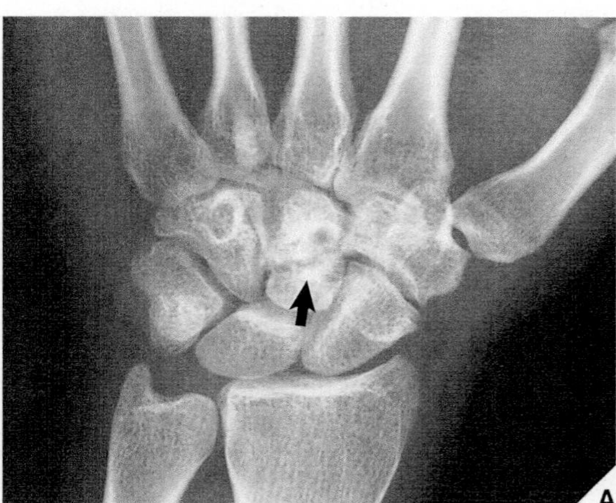

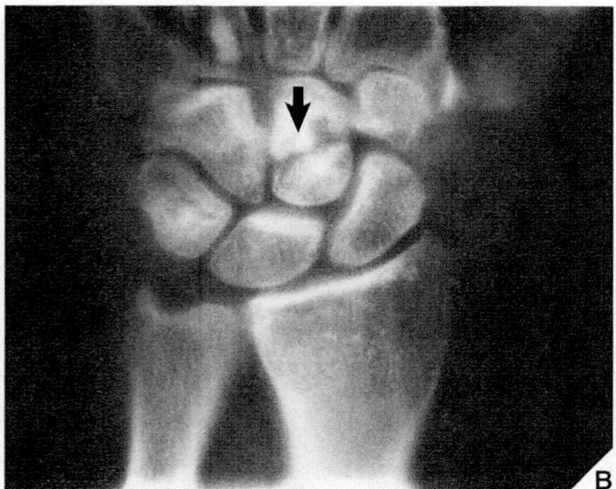

FIGURE 7.73 Capitate fracture. A 23-year-old man fell on his outstretched hand. **(A)** Dorsovolar radiograph of the wrist demonstrates a fracture through the neck of the capitate *(arrow)*. **(B)** After conservative treatment (3 months of immobilization in a plaster cast), trispiral tomography was performed. This technique clearly shows lack of union. Note the small necrotic bone fragment *(arrow)*, which was not too well demonstrated on the standard projection.

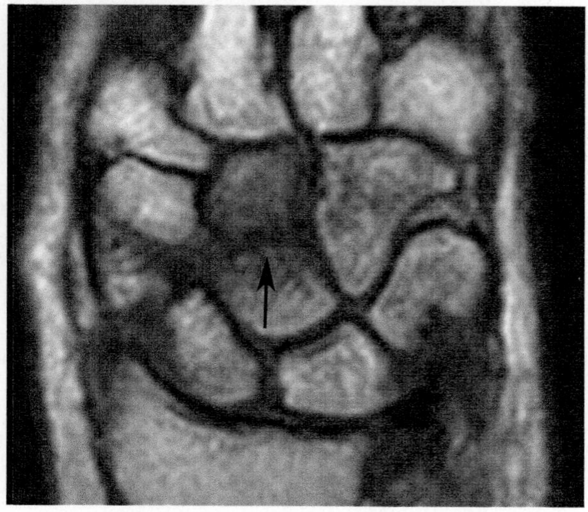

FIGURE 7.74 MRI of occult nondisplaced capitate fracture. Coronal T1-weighted MRI of the wrist shows fracture of the capitate *(arrow)*, not visualized on the originally obtained radiographs. Note the low signal intensity of the bone marrow edema surrounding the fracture line.

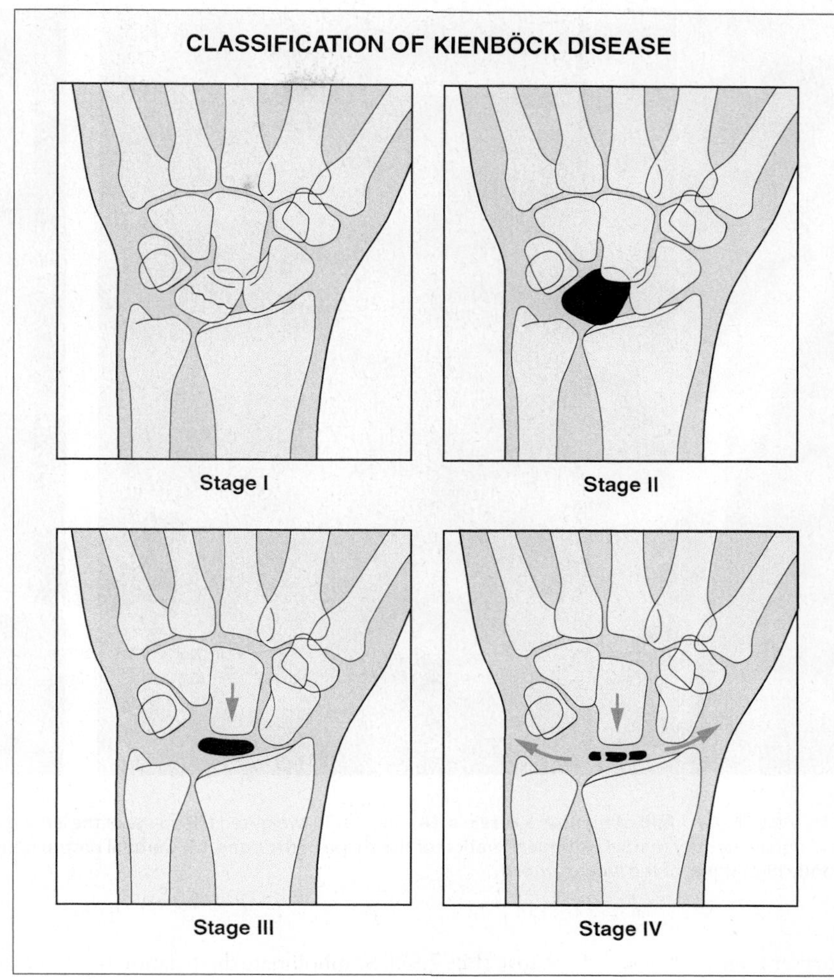

FIGURE 7.75 **The four stages of Kienböck disease.** Proximal migration of the capitate is seen in stages III and IV *(vertical arrows)*. Lateral and medial migration of the fractured fragments of the lunate is seen in stage IV *(curved horizontal arrows)*. (Modified from Gelberman RH, Szabo RM. Kienböck's disease. *Orthop Clin North Am* 1984;15:355–367. Copyright © 1984 Elsevier. With permission.)

Once lunate necrosis begins, an established progressive sequence of events is set in motion. This progression is marked by lunate flattening and elongation, proximal migration of the capitate, scapholunate dissociation, and, finally, osteoarthritis of the radiocarpal joint. This series of changes also forms the basis for the classification of Kienböck disease (Fig. 7.75). Clinically, stage I is indistinguishable from a wrist sprain. Wrist radiographs may be completely normal, and only CT may detect a subtle linear fracture. Skeletal scintigraphy may show an increased uptake of a radiopharmaceutical tracer by the lunate. MRI invariably demonstrates the abnormality, displaying decreased signal intensity of lunate on T1-weighted images (Fig. 7.76) and increased signal on water-sensitive sequences (Figs. 7.77 to 7.79). As the condition progresses (stage II), the conventional radiographs and trispiral tomographic studies in the dorsovolar and lateral projections show increased density of the lunate accompanied by some degree of flattening on the radial side of this bone (Fig. 7.80). The radionuclide bone scan is always positive in this stage. In stage III, the radiographs demonstrate marked decrease in the height of the lunate and proximal migration of the capitate (Fig. 7.81). Necrotic and cystic degeneration may lead to

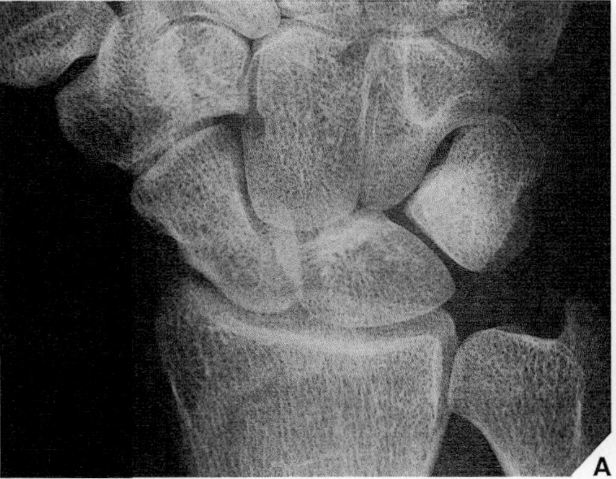

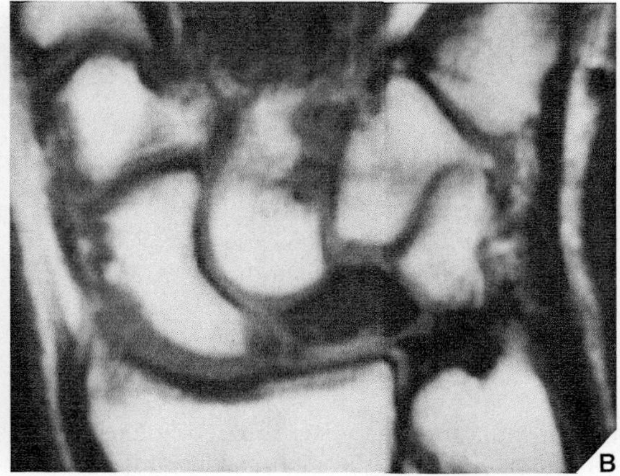

FIGURE 7.76 **MRI of Kienböck disease.** A 35-year-old man with wrist pain underwent radiologic investigation for possible Kienböck disease. **(A)** Conventional dorsovolar radiograph of the left wrist is normal. **(B)** Coronal T1-weighted MRI shows low signal intensity of the lunate consistent with osteonecrosis. (Courtesy of Dr. L. Steinbach, San Francisco, California.)

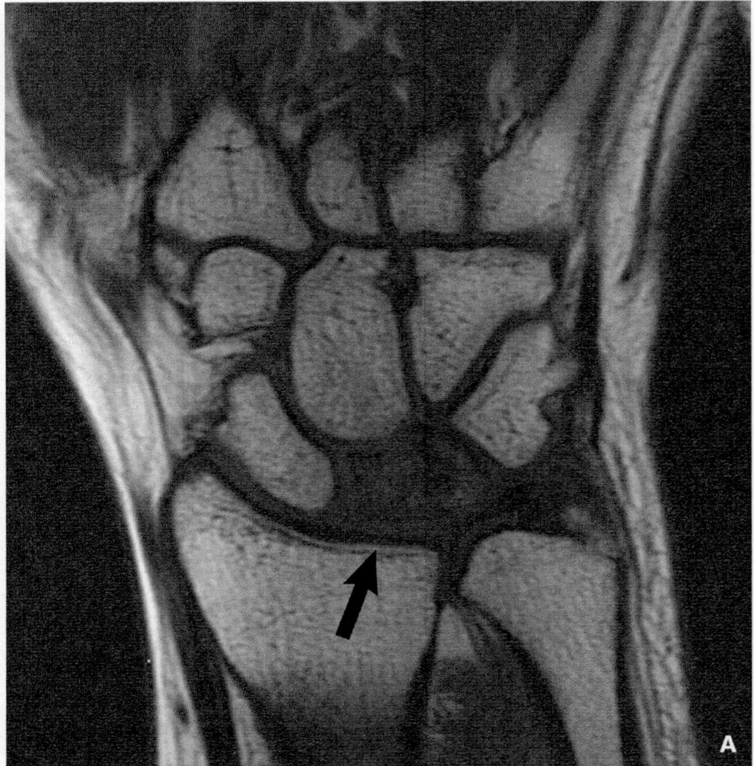

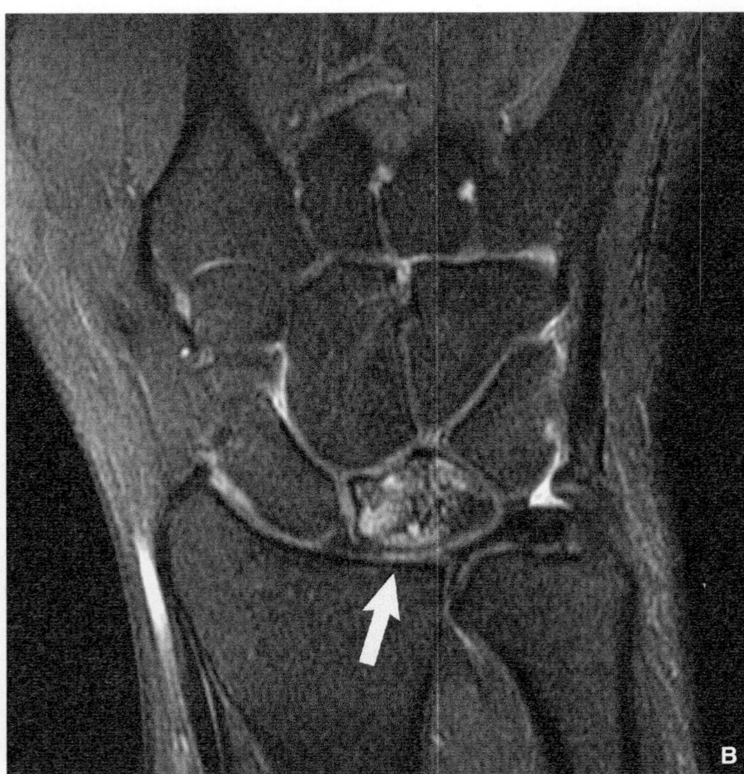

FIGURE 7.77 MRI of Kienböck disease. **(A)** Coronal T1-weighted MR image of the left wrist of an 18-year-old woman with stage I of the disease shows lunate exhibiting low signal intensity *(arrow)* without alteration of the shape of the bone. **(B)** Coronal proton density–weighted fat-suppressed MR image shows heterogeneous but predominantly high signal of the lunate *(arrow)*.

further fragmentation and collapse (Fig. 7.82). Scapholunate dissociation is a prominent feature of this stage. Stage IV is marked by almost complete disintegration of the lunate (Fig. 7.83) and the development of radiocarpal osteoarthritis with typical changes of joint space narrowing, osteophyte formation, subchondral sclerosis, and degenerative cysts (Fig. 7.84).

Merely, diagnosing Kienböck disease is not sufficient from the orthopaedic point of view; rather, it is essential for the radiologist to demonstrate the integrity of the bone. The reason for this is that at an early stage of the disease, in the absence of a fracture or fragmentation, a revascularization procedure aimed at restoring circulation to the lunate may prevent further progression of the necrotic process and eventual collapse of the bone (Fig. 7.85). In the event of a fracture (Fig. 7.86) or fragmentation (Fig. 7.87) of the lunate, which is best diagnosed on CT, alternatives to revascularization—such as silastic arthroplasty or, in the absence of a collapse deformity, ulnar lengthening or radial shortening—would then have to be considered. In some cases, the latter procedures restoring neutral ulnar variance may allow spontaneous healing of a lunate fracture.

Hamatolunate Impaction Syndrome

Hamatolunate impaction syndrome results from an anatomic variant of the lunate bone that has an "extra" facet articulating with the hamate bone (so-called *type II lunate bone*). The repeated contact of these two bones when the wrist is in ulnar deviation leads to bone marrow edema, chondromalacia, and, occasionally, erosive changes of the proximal pole of hamate, best demonstrated on MRI (Figs. 7.88 and 7.89).

Dislocations of the Carpal Bones

The most frequent types of dislocation in the wrist are scapholunate dislocation, perilunate dislocation, midcarpal dislocation, and lunate dislocation. To understand better the pattern of dislocation of the carpal bones, Johnson stressed the occurrence of the so-called *vulnerable zone*, the common site of wrist injuries (Fig. 7.90). Two major types of injury are recognized: the lesser arc and greater arc patterns. A lesser arc injury involves, in sequential stages, rotary subluxation of the scaphoid, perilunate dislocation, midcarpal dislocation, and lunate dislocation, whereas a greater arc injury involves a fracture of any of the bones adjacent to the lunate associated with dislocations. The wrist ligaments stabilize the carpus to the distal radius and ulna. The radiocapitate and capitotriquetral ligaments are the prime stabilizers of the distal carpal row. The proximal carpal row is stabilized by the volar radiotriquetral, the dorsal radiocarpal, the ulnolunate, the ulnotriquetral, and the ulnar collateral ligaments. The scaphoid is stabilized distally by the radiocapitate and radial collateral ligaments and proximally

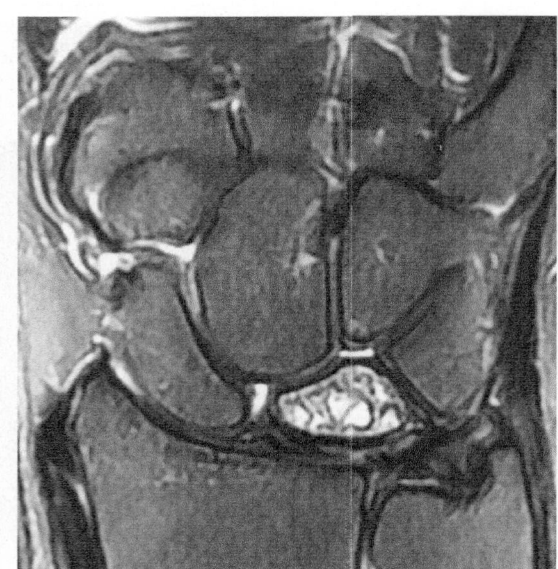

FIGURE 7.78 MRI of Kienböck disease. Coronal T2-weighted image of the left wrist of a patient with recent onset of wrist pain shows high signal intensity of the lunate with a serpentine pattern, consistent with avascular necrosis. There is no collapse of the bone.

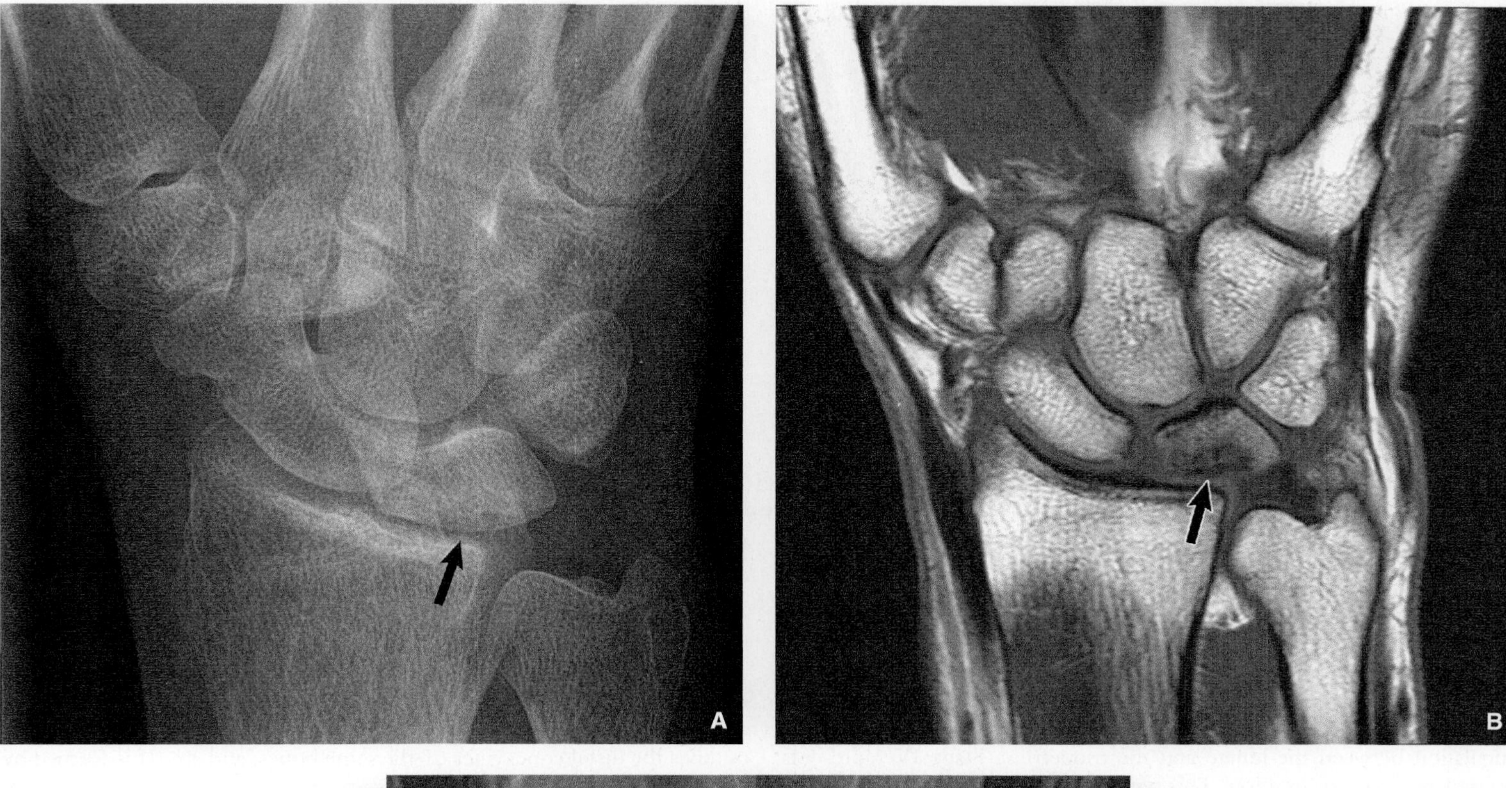

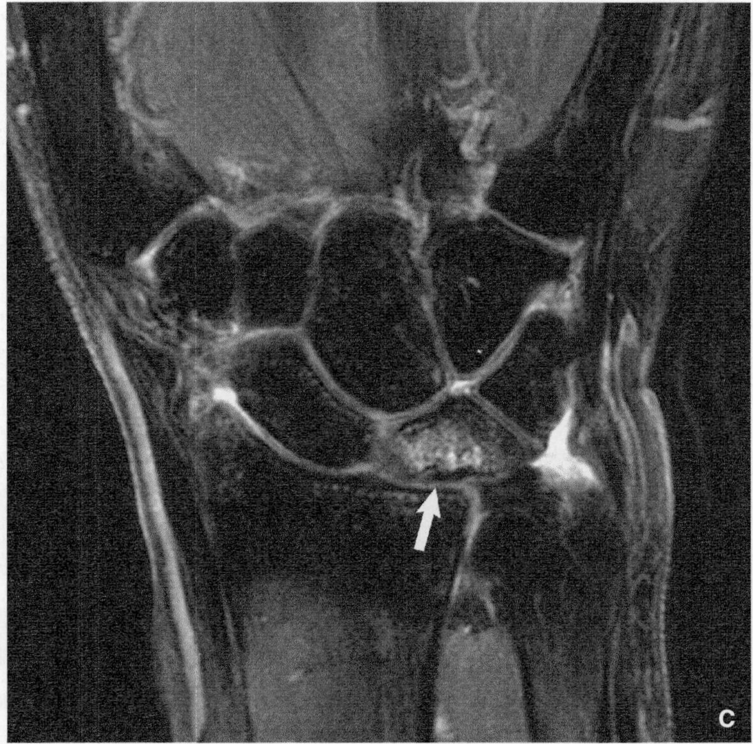

FIGURE 7.79 MRI of Kienböck disease. **(A)** Oblique radiograph of the left wrist of a 65-year-old man shows decreased height of the lunate and cortical irregularity of the radial aspect *(arrow)*. **(B)** Coronal T1-weighted MR image shows low signal intensity of the lunate and fracture at its proximal aspect *(arrow)*, better demonstrated on **(C)** coronal proton density–weighted fat-suppressed MR image *(arrow)*.

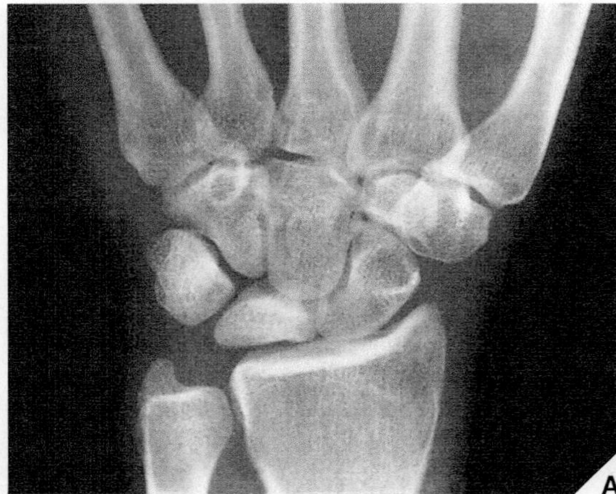

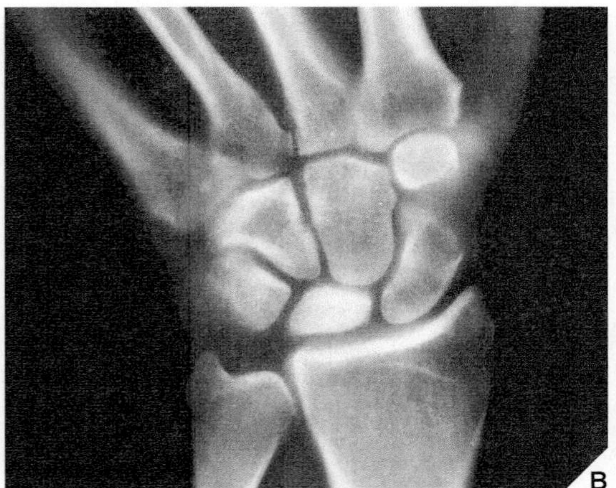

FIGURE 7.80 Tomography of Kienböck disease. **(A)** Dorsovolar radiograph and **(B)** tomogram of the wrist show the dense, flattened appearance of the lunate characteristic of Kienböck disease. Note the presence of negative ulnar variance, a possible predisposing factor in this condition.

by the radioscaphoid and scapholunate ligaments (see Figs. 7.42 and 7.43). Mayfield, and later Yeager, Dalinka, and Gilula, stressed the pattern of four sequential stages of lesser arc injury (Fig. 7.91). Stage I represents a scapholunate dissociation and rotary subluxation of the scaphoid. Stage II represents a dislocation of the capitate known also as *perilunate dislocation.* Stage III represents a midcarpal dislocation, the result of disruption of articulation between the lunate and the triquetrum. Stage IV represents a complete lunate dislocation. This pattern follows the progression from the least severe injury, *scapholunate dissociation* (rotary subluxation of the scaphoid), in which there is a tear of the radioscaphoid, palmar radiocapitate, and scapholunate ligaments; to a more severe *perilunate dislocation*, in which there is, in addition, a tear of the radiocapitate ligaments; to a still more severe injury, *midcarpal dislocation* (dislocation of the capitate dorsally to the lunate and subluxation, but not complete dislocation, of the lunate), with a tear of the volar and dorsal radiotriquetral and ulnotriquetral ligaments; to the severest injury, *lunate dislocation*, in which there is a tear of the radiolunate fascicle of the dorsal radiocarpal ligament and of the volar ligaments, leaving the lunate entirely without ligamentous attachments.

An appreciation of two important normal relations of the carpal bones—one seen on the lateral view and the other on the dorsovolar view of the wrist—should aid in recognizing the presence of abnormality. The lateral view obtained with the wrist in the neutral position reveals the alignment of the radius, the lunate, the capitate, and the third metacarpal along their longitudinal axes (Fig. 7.92). On the dorsovolar view of the wrist in the neutral position, Gilula has identified three smooth arcs outlining the proximal and distal carpal rows. Arc I joins the proximal articular surfaces of the scaphoid, the lunate, and the triquetrum; arc II outlines the distal concavities of the same bones; and arc III is formed by the proximal convexities of the capitate and the hamate (Fig. 7.93). The diagnostic significance of distortion in both these relations is discussed in the sections that follow.

Scapholunate Dissociation

An injury to the scapholunate ligament may result in intercarpal ligament instability that leads to rotary subluxation of the scaphoid, a type of scapholunate dissociation. On the dorsovolar radiograph of the wrist, which alone is sufficient to diagnose this condition, two signs can be seen that indicate its presence.

The first, known in the literature as the *Terry-Thomas sign*, is characterized by a widening of the space between the scaphoid and the lunate, which normally measures no more than 2 to 3 mm (Fig. 7.94). The sign is named after a distinctive British comedian, movie and TV personality

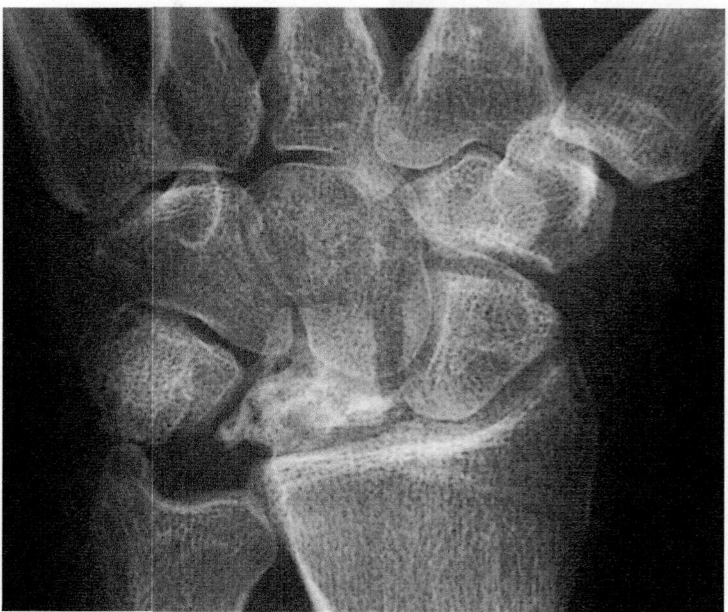

FIGURE 7.81 Kienböck disease. A 21-year-old man presented with longstanding wrist pain. A dorsovolar radiograph shows stage III of Kienböck disease. Note the collapse of osteonecrotic lunate and proximal migration of the capitate.

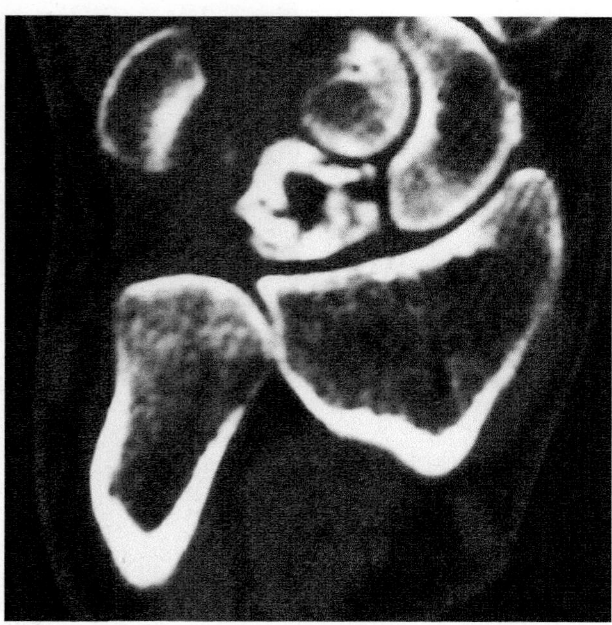

FIGURE 7.82 CT of Kienböck disease. Coronal reformatted CT image of the wrist reveals cystic changes of the osteonecrotic lunate associated with a pathologic fracture. (Courtesy of L. Friedman, MD, Hamilton, Canada.)

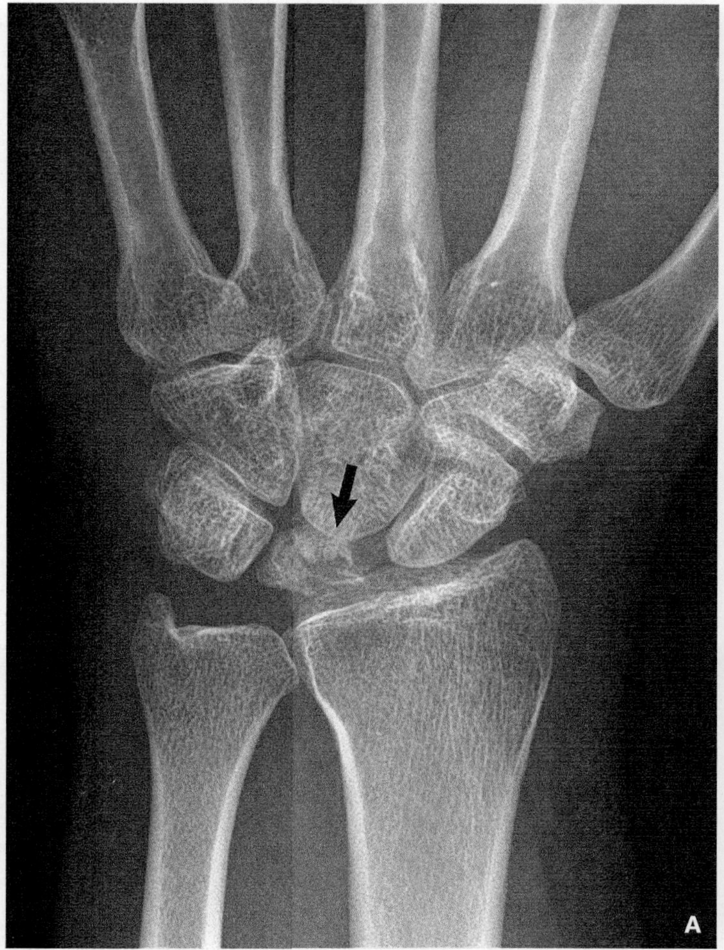

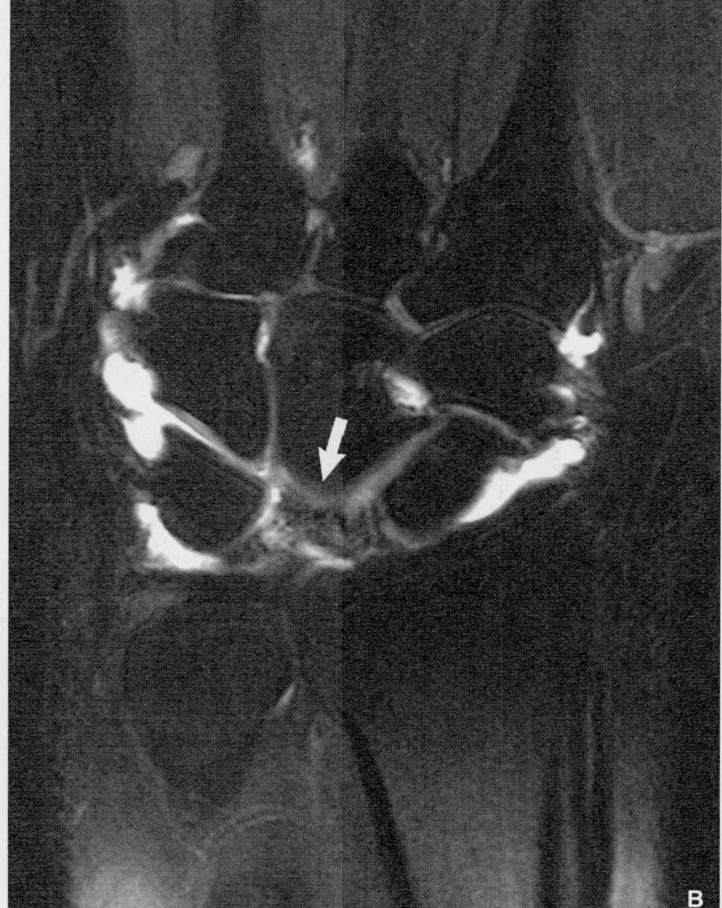

FIGURE 7.83 MRI of Kienböck disease. **(A)** Dorsovolar radiograph of the right wrist of a 33-year-old man shows deformity and fragmentation of the osteonecrotic lunate *(arrow)*. **(B)** Coronal proton density–weighted fat-suppressed and **(C)** coronal 3D GRE fat-saturated MR images show complete disintegration of the lunate *(arrows)* representing stage IV of the disease.

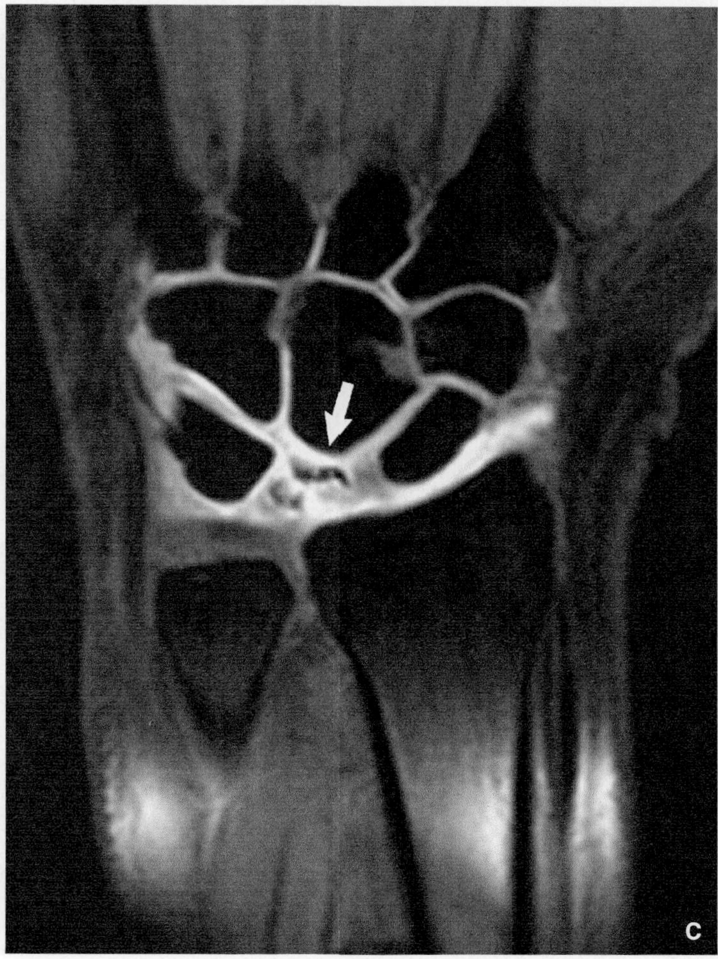

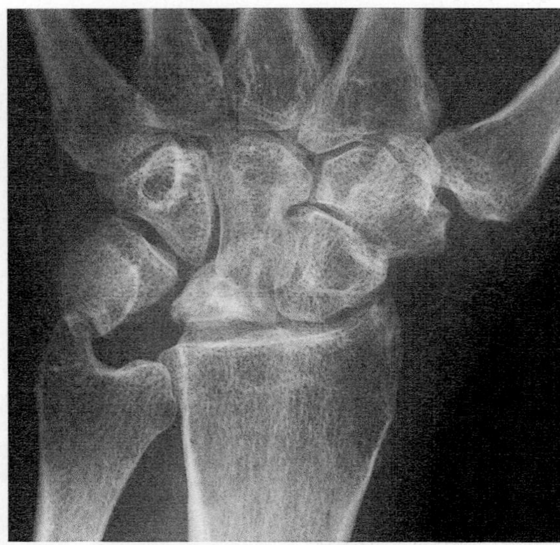

FIGURE 7.84 Kienböck disease. Stage IV of Kienböck disease is marked by fragmentation and collapse of the lunate, proximal migration of the capitate, rotary subluxation of the scaphoid, and osteoarthritis of the radiocarpal joint.

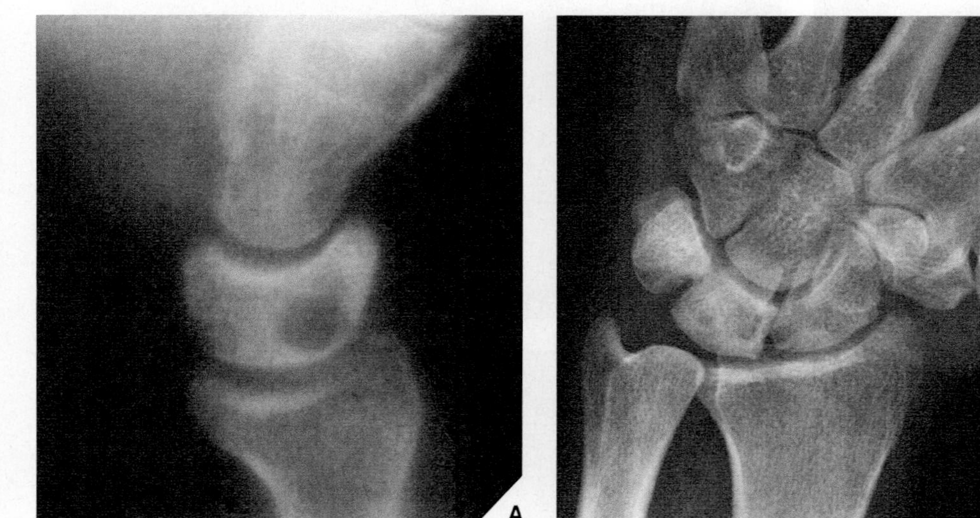

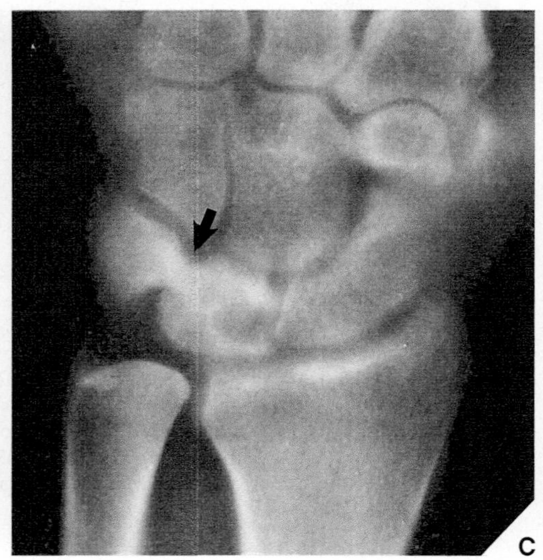

FIGURE 7.85 Kienböck disease. **(A)** Lateral tomogram of the wrist shows the dense appearance of the lunate characteristic of osteonecrosis; there is also clear evidence of cystic degeneration. Because no fracture line is present, the surgeon has the option of performing a revascularization procedure. After triquetrolunate arthrodesis, the dorsovolar view of the wrist in radial deviation **(B)** and a trispiral tomogram **(C)** demonstrate the vascular bone flap *(arrow)* bridging the triquetrum and the lunate.

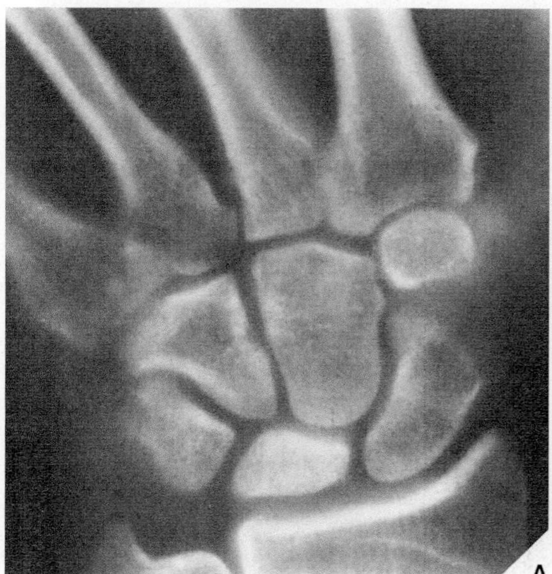

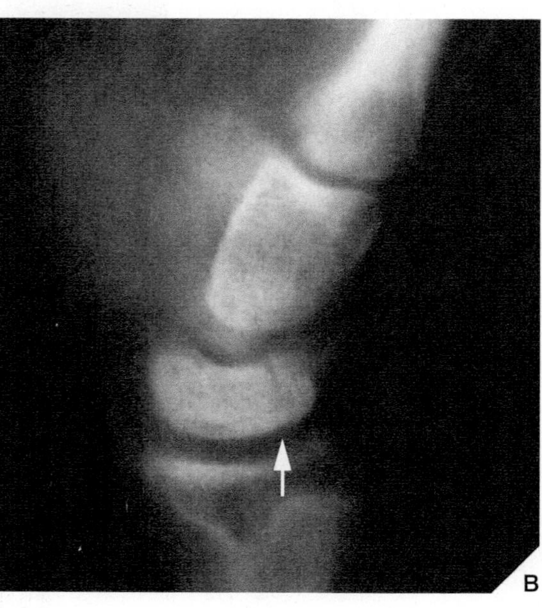

FIGURE 7.86 Kienböck disease. **(A)** On a trispiral tomogram in the dorsovolar projection with the wrist ulnarly deviated, there is no evidence of lunate fracture. **(B)** The lateral tomographic section, however, shows clear indication of a fracture line *(arrow)*.

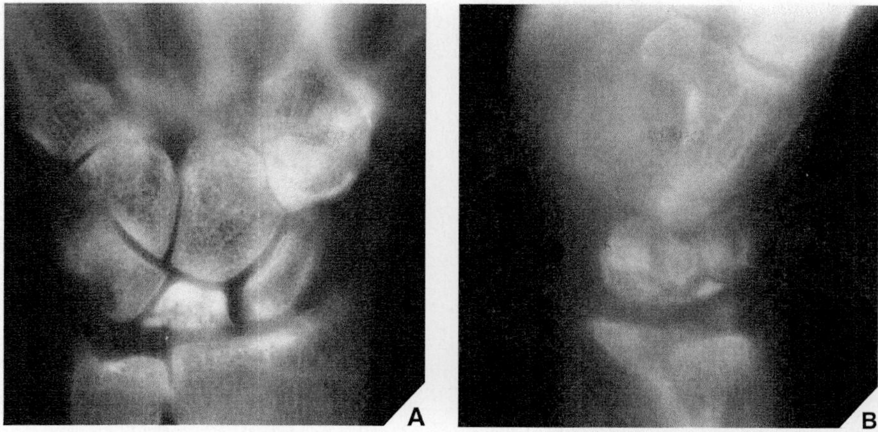

FIGURE 7.87 Kienböck disease. **(A)** Dorsovolar and **(B)** lateral trispiral tomograms of the wrist demonstrate fragmentation of the lunate seen in advanced stage of the disease.

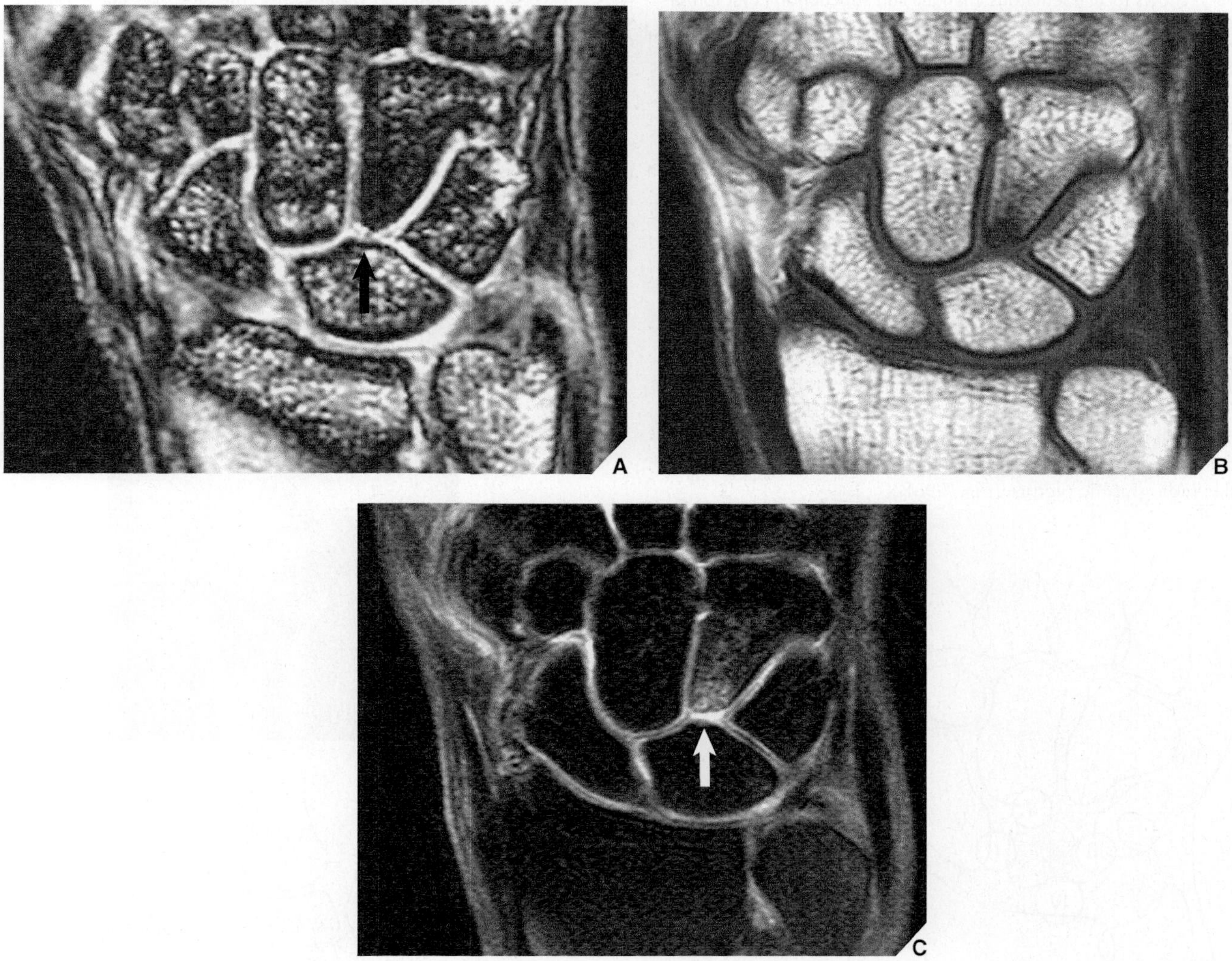

FIGURE 7.88 MRI of the hamatolunate impaction syndrome. **(A)** Coronal 3D gradient-echo MR image shows a type II lunate articulating with the hamate *(arrow)*. Note a decreased signal intensity within the most proximal aspect of the hamate bone. **(B)** Coronal T1-weighted and **(C)** coronal T2-weighted fat-suppressed MR images demonstrate the erosion of the cartilage *(arrow)* and edematous changes of the hamate, diagnostic of hamatolunate impaction syndrome.

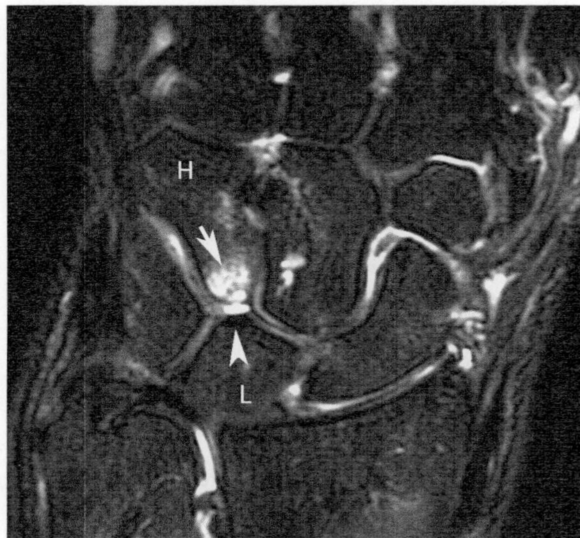

FIGURE 7.89 MRI of the hamatolunate impaction syndrome. Coronal T2-weighted MR image shows focal edematous changes and subchondral cyst formation in the proximal pole of the hamate *(H) (arrow)*. Note an additional facet of the lunate *(L) (arrowhead)*.

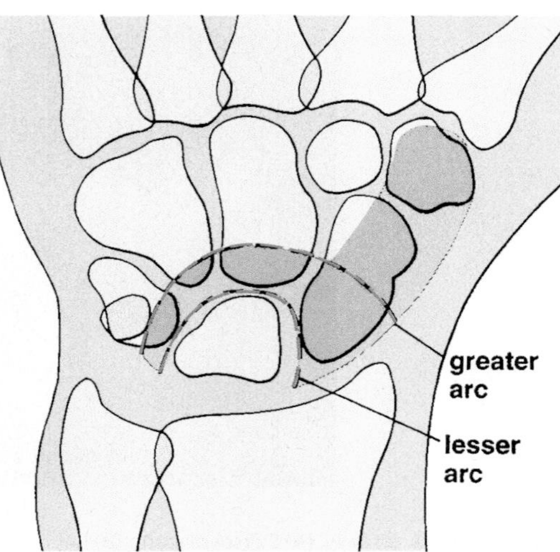

FIGURE 7.90 Vulnerable zone of the wrist. The "vulnerable zone" of the carpus is represented by shaded areas. Most fractures, fracture–dislocations, and dislocations of the carpal bones occur within it. The lesser arc outlines the "dislocation zone," whereas the greater arc outlines the "fracture–dislocation zone." (Modified with permission from Johnson RP. The acutely injured wrist and its residuals. *Clin Orthop* 1980;149:33–44.)

Terry Thomas, who had a large gap between his two frontal teeth (frontal dental diastema). For the same reason it is also called the *David Letterman sign*. Occasionally, this finding is not evident on the dorsovolar view of the wrist in the neutral position but becomes apparent when the wrist is ulnarly deviated (Fig. 7.95).

The other of these signs, the *signet-ring sign*, receives its name from a cortical ring shadow that is normally *not* seen on the scaphoid on the dorsovolar projection with the wrist in the neutral position (see Figs. 7.1B and 7.93). In rotary subluxation of the scaphoid, however, volar tilt and rotation of the scaphoid cause it to appear foreshortened and the bone's tuberosity to be seen on end, producing the characteristic ring shadow (Fig. 7.96A). To rely on this sign as a diagnostic indicator, dorsovolar films must be obtained with the wrist in the neutral position or in ulnar deviation because in radial deviation of the wrist, the scaphoid normally tilts volarly, creating a similar radiographic picture (Fig. 7.96B).

When radiographic findings are normal in cases of suspected injury to the intercarpal ligament complex, fluoroscopy combined with videotaping can sometimes contribute to an evaluation of wrist kinematics and to the diagnosis of carpal instability or transient subluxation. An arthrographic examination of the wrist (see Fig. 7.7) is effective when routine radiographic or videofluoroscopic findings are not conclusive.

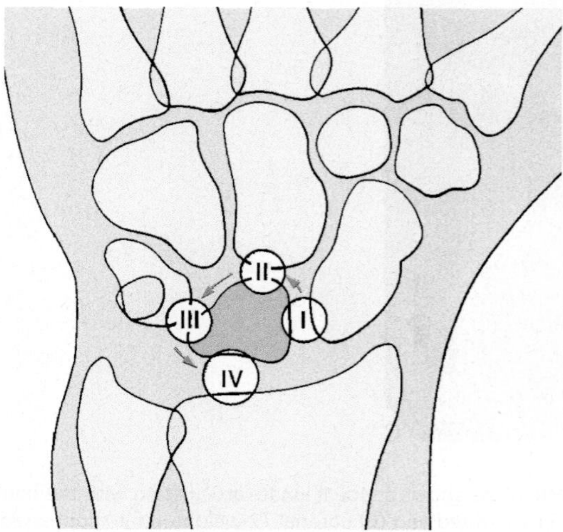

FIGURE 7.91 Injuries of the lesser arc. Sequential stages of lesser arc injury. Stage I represents a scapholunate failure that results in a scapholunate dissociation or rotary subluxation of the scaphoid. Stage II represents a capitolunate failure that results in a dislocation of the capitate (perilunate dislocation). Stage III represents a triquetrolunate failure because the articulation between the lunate and the triquetrum is disrupted, leading to a midcarpal dislocation. Stage IV represents a complete lunate disruption, caused by dorsal radiocarpal ligament failure. (Modified with permission from Mayfield JK. Mechanism of carpal injuries. *Clin Orthop* 1980;149:45–54.)

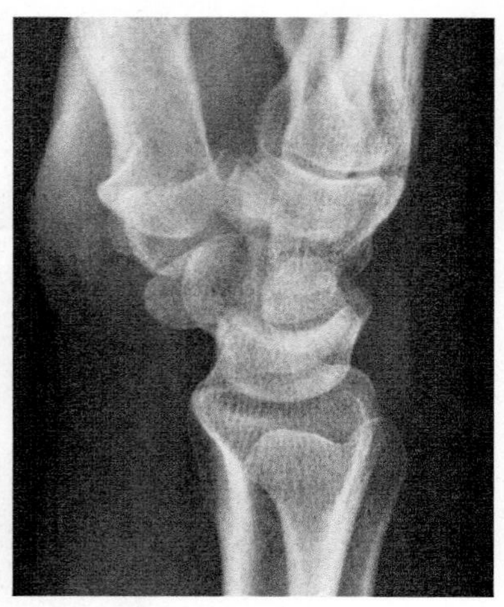

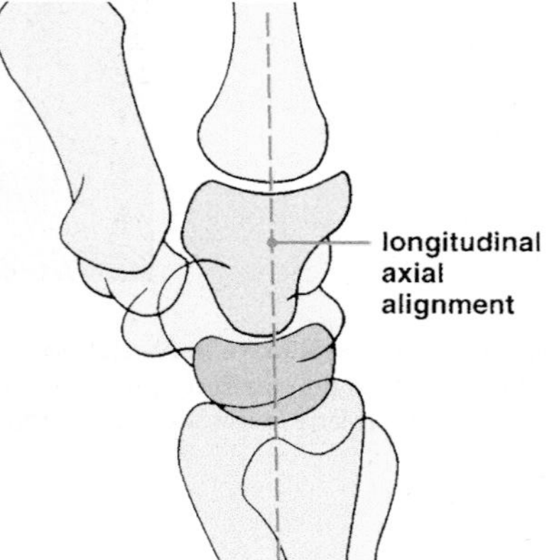

FIGURE 7.92 Longitudinal axial alignment. On the lateral radiograph of the wrist, the central axes of the radius, the lunate, the capitate, and the third metacarpal normally form a straight line.

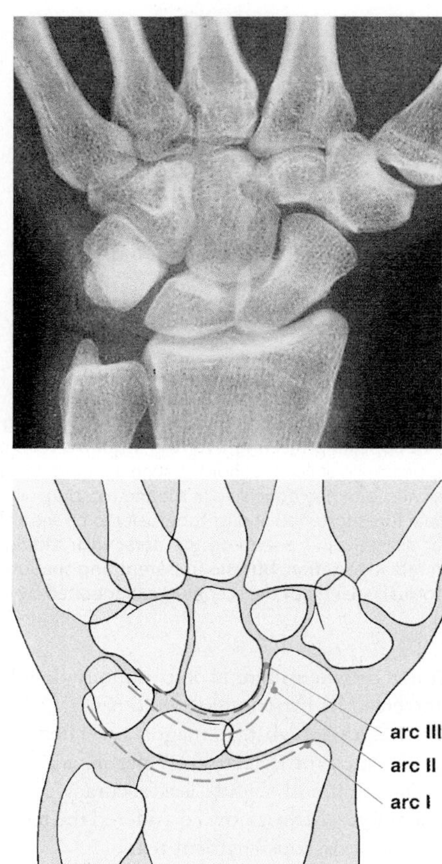

FIGURE 7.93 **Arcs of the carpus.** Three smooth arcs outlining the proximal and distal carpal rows are identifiable on the dorsovolar radiograph of the normal wrist.

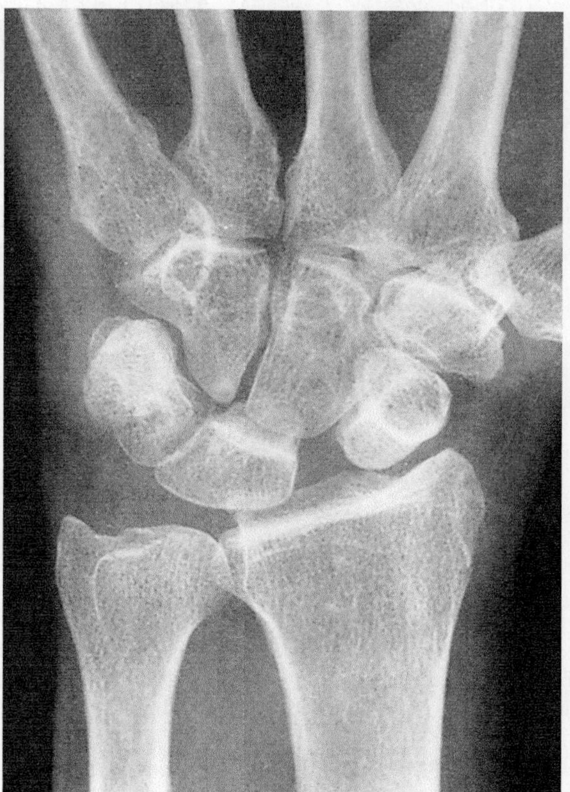

FIGURE 7.94 **Terry-Thomas sign.** Dorsovolar radiograph of the wrist shows an abnormally wide space between the scaphoid and the lunate—the Terry-Thomas sign—indicating scapholunate dissociation caused by a tear of the scapholunate ligament.

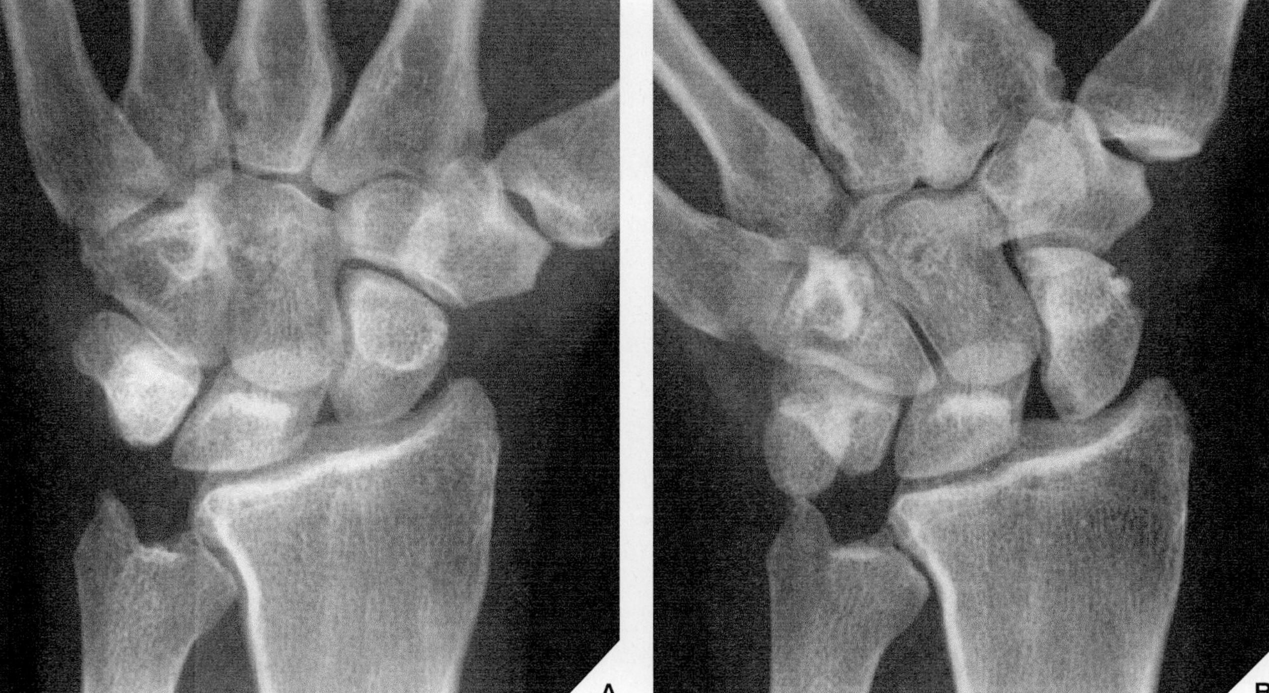

FIGURE 7.95 **Scapholunate dissociation.** **(A)** On the dorsovolar projection of the wrist in the neutral position, a gap between the scaphoid and the lunate is not well demonstrated. **(B)** On ulnar deviation, however, the gap becomes apparent, indicating scapholunate dissociation.

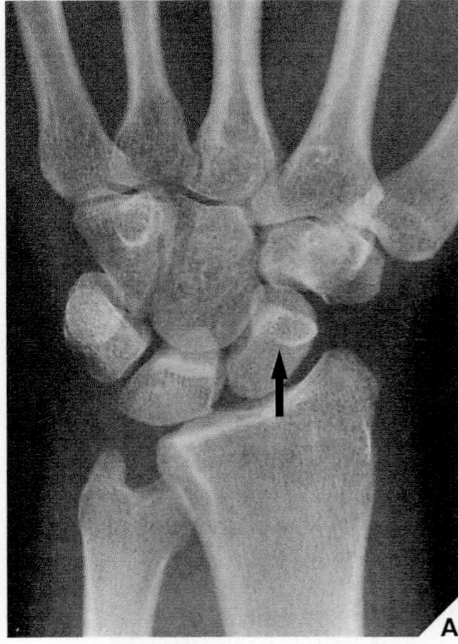

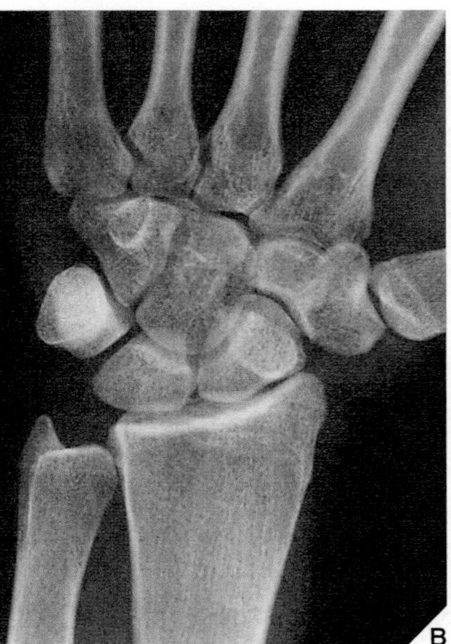

FIGURE 7.96 Signet-ring sign. **(A)** On the dorsovolar radiograph of the wrist in the neutral position, rotary subluxation of the scaphoid can be recognized by the cortical ring shadow *(arrow)* that appears projecting over the scaphoid (compare with normal appearance of the scaphoid as seen in Fig. 7.1B). This phenomenon is caused by the bone's volar tilt and rotation, which cause it to appear foreshortened and its tuberosity to be seen on end. **(B)** A similar picture can be seen on the dorsovolar radiograph of the wrist in radial deviation, but this apparent ring shadow is caused by the normal volar tilt of the scaphoid exaggerated by radial deviation.

A wrist arthrogram can reveal abnormal communication between the radiocarpal and the midcarpal compartments that indicates a tear in the scapholunate or lunotriquetral interosseous ligament complex (Figs. 7.97 and 7.98).

MRI may also demonstrate abnormalities of scapholunate and lunotriquetral ligaments. The scapholunate ligament connects the volar, proximal, and dorsal borders of the scaphoid bone to the lunate bone. On MRI, it appears as a structure of low signal intensity. The lunotriquetral ligament connects the volar, proximal, and dorsal borders of the lunate bone to the triquetral bone, also exhibiting low signal intensity. Both ligaments blend almost imperceptibly with the articular cartilage of the corresponding carpal bones. The tears of these ligaments are diagnosed on MRI when the single or scattered areas of high signal intensity are identified within the structures or when there is discontinuity of a ligament of low signal intensity traversed by hyperintense fluid (Fig. 7.99). Recent publications pertinent to MRI using high-field magnets and dedicated surface coils have shown high accuracy for detection of partial and complete tears of the scapholunate ligament and slightly less accuracy for detection of lunotriquetral ligament tears. MRa is now considered the technique of choice for the diagnosis of interosseous ligament tears.

Extrinsic ligament tears are more difficult to diagnose. Using high-field magnets, dedicated surface coils, and optimized pulse sequences with thin contiguous sections, the extrinsic ligaments, especially the volar radiolunate and radioscaphoid, can be effectively demonstrated (see Fig. 7.99E,F). The radioscaphoid ligament may have an extension inserting into the capitate, hence some authors call this ligament radioscaphocapitate ligament.

FIGURE 7.97 A tear of the scapholunate ligament. A 21-year-old man injured his right wrist during a wrestling competition. Standard views, including ulnar deviation of the wrist, were unremarkable. Likewise, videofluoroscopic examination did not reveal significant abnormalities. A wrist arthrogram, however, shows a leak of contrast into the midcarpal articulations, indicating a tear in the scapholunate interosseous ligament complex. Note also that the TFCC is intact because no contrast entered the distal radioulnar joint.

Lunate and Perilunate Dislocations

Dorsovolar and lateral radiographs of the wrist in the neutral position are usually sufficient to diagnose suspected lunate and perilunate dislocations.

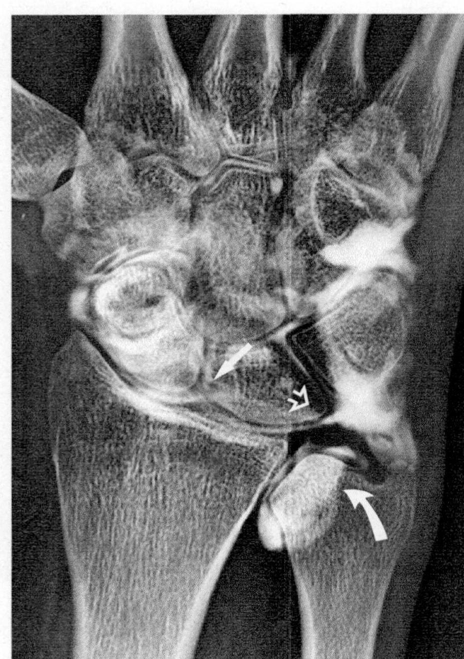

FIGURE 7.98 A tear of the scapholunate and lunotriquetral ligaments. Wrist arthrogram demonstrates tears of the scapholunate *(arrow)* and lunotriquetral *(open arrow)* ligaments. There is also a tear of TFCC *(curved arrow)*.

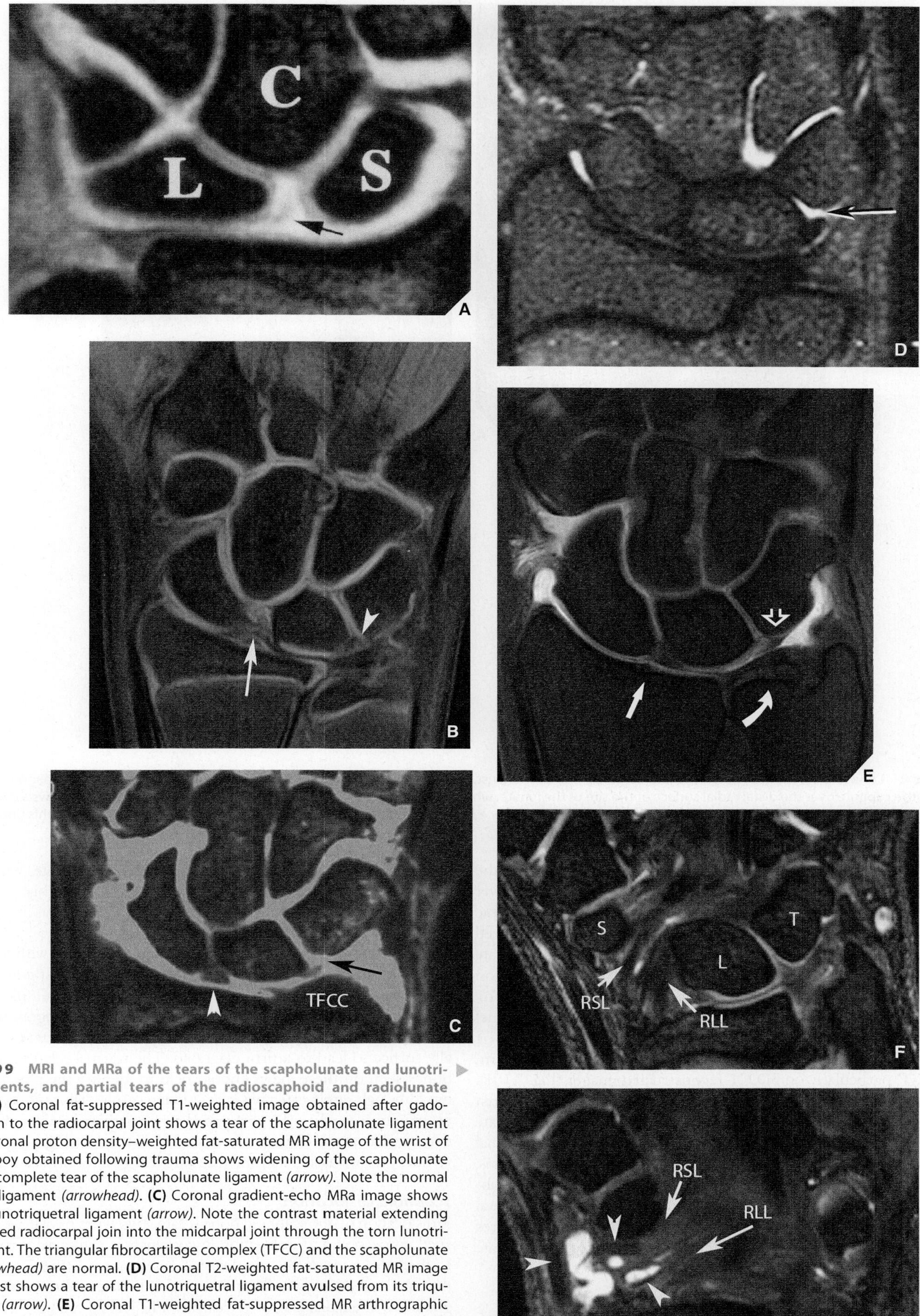

FIGURE 7.99 MRI and MRa of the tears of the scapholunate and lunotriquetral ligaments, and partial tears of the radioscaphoid and radiolunate ligaments. **(A)** Coronal fat-suppressed T1-weighted image obtained after gadolinium injection to the radiocarpal joint shows a tear of the scapholunate ligament *(arrow)*. **(B)** Coronal proton density–weighted fat-saturated MR image of the wrist of a 12-year-old boy obtained following trauma shows widening of the scapholunate interval and a complete tear of the scapholunate ligament *(arrow)*. Note the normal lunotriquetral ligament *(arrowhead)*. **(C)** Coronal gradient-echo MRa image shows a tear of the lunotriquetral ligament *(arrow)*. Note the contrast material extending from the injected radiocarpal join into the midcarpal joint through the torn lunotriquetral ligament. The triangular fibrocartilage complex (TFCC) and the scapholunate ligament *(arrowhead)* are normal. **(D)** Coronal T2-weighted fat-saturated MR image without contrast shows a tear of the lunotriquetral ligament avulsed from its triquetral insertion *(arrow)*. **(E)** Coronal T1-weighted fat-suppressed MR arthrographic image of a normal wrist is shown for comparison. *Arrow* points to intact scapholunate ligament, *open arrow* to lunotriquetral ligament, and *curved arrow* to TFCC. **(F)** Coronal gradient-echo pulse sequence through the volar aspect of the wrist demonstrates the normal radioscaphoid ligament *(RSL)* and radiolunate ligament *(RLL)*. **(G)** Coronal gradient-echo MR image in another patient shows partial tears of the radioscaphoid ligament and radiolunate ligament with synovial joint fluid extending into the lateral aspect of the wrist through the small tears, forming a multilocular ganglion cyst *(arrowheads)*. L, lunate; C, capitate; S, scaphoid; T, triquetrum.

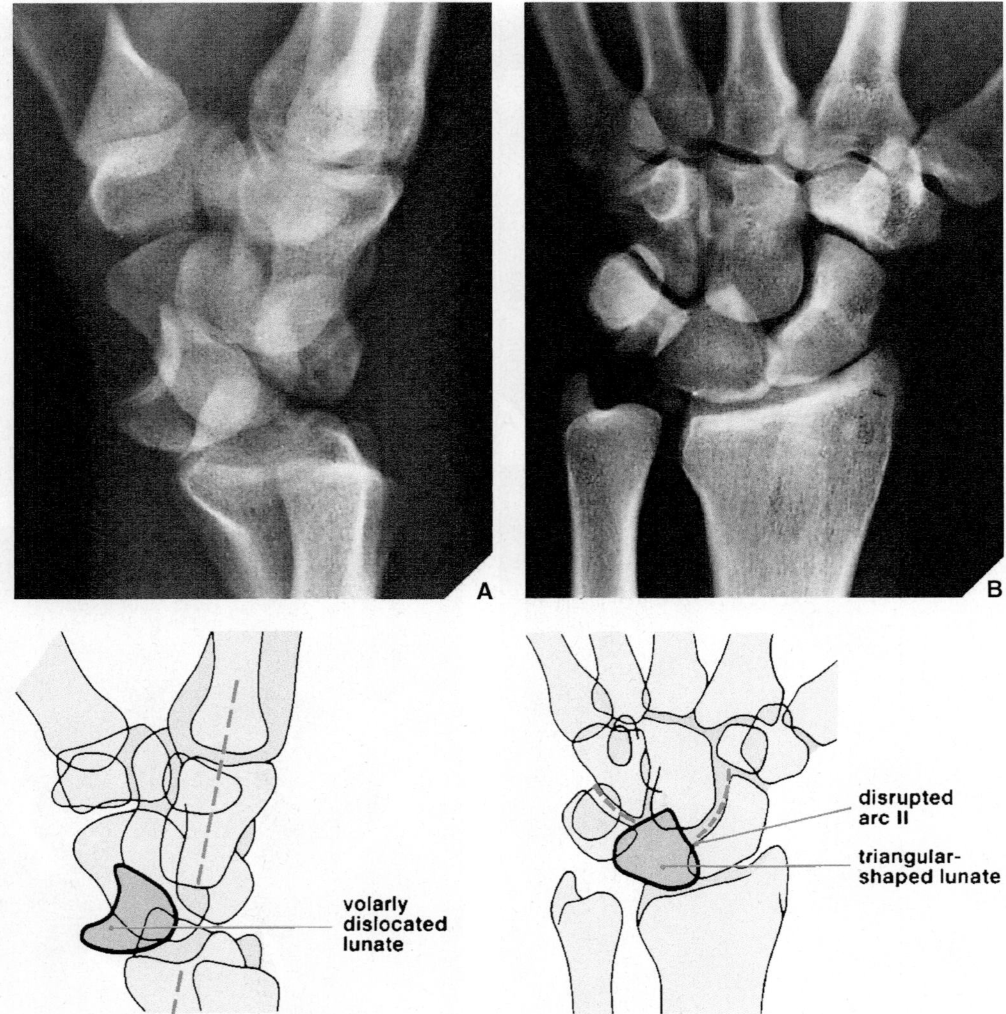

FIGURE 7.100 Lunate dislocation. **(A)** On the lateral radiograph of the wrist, lunate dislocation is evident from the break in the longitudinal alignment of the third metacarpal and the capitate over the distal radial surface at the site of the lunate, which is volarly rotated and displaced. **(B)** Dorsovolar projection shows a disrupted arc II at the site of the lunate, indicating malalignment. Note also the triangular appearance of the lunate, a finding virtually pathognomonic of dislocation of this bone.

As the lateral view clearly demonstrates the normal alignment of the longitudinal axes of the lunate, the capitate, and the third metacarpal over the distal radial surface, a break at any point in this line is pathognomonic of subluxation or dislocation. A *lunate dislocation* can thus be recognized when its axis is angled away from the distal radial surface, while the capitate remains in its normal alignment (Fig. 7.100A). Similarly, lunate dislocation can also be identified on the dorsovolar projection by the disruption of arc II described by the distal concave surfaces of the scaphoid, the lunate, and the triquetrum as well as the concomitant triangular appearance of the lunate (Fig. 7.100B). Lunate dislocation can also be effectively demonstrated on CT, particularly on 3D CT reconstructed images (Fig. 7.101).

A *perilunate dislocation* can be recognized on the lateral view of the wrist by the dorsal or volar angulation of the longitudinal axis of the capitate away from its normal central alignment with the lunate and the distal radial surface. The lunate, in this case, remains in articulation with the radius, although there may be some degree of tilt of the lunate because of subluxation associated with perilunate dislocation. On the dorsovolar view, the overlapping of the proximal and distal carpal rows and a break in arcs II and III at the site of the capitate indicate the presence of a perilunate dislocation (Figs. 7.102 and 7.103).

Midcarpal Dislocation

This injury is the result of disruption of articulation between the lunate and the triquetrum, secondary to tears of the volar and dorsal radiotriquetral and ulnotriquetral ligaments in addition to the tears of the radiolunotriquetral and lunotriquetral ligaments. Although this abnormality can be diagnosed on the conventional radiography (Fig. 7.104A), CT is usually better suited to demonstrate the position of the lunate, which is volarly subluxed, and the capitate, which is dorsally subluxed (Fig. 7.104B).

Transscaphoid Perilunate Dislocation

When a dislocation of the carpal bones is associated with a fracture, the prefix *trans* indicates which bone is fractured. The most common fracture associated with carpal dislocation is transscaphoid perilunate dislocation. As in the preceding types of carpal dislocations, radiographs in the standard dorsovolar, dorsovolar in ulnar deviation, and lateral projections usually suffice to lead to a firm diagnosis. The normal relations of the carpal bones seen on these views should help to identify the type of abnormality. Although rarely effective in evaluating carpal dislocations, tomographic examination used to be performed when radiographs of the wrist were equivocal as to which carpal bones were dislocated (Figs. 7.105 and 7.106). Other types of associated fractures are less commonly seen (Fig. 7.107).

Scaphoid Dislocation

A dislocation of the scaphoid bone is rare. Two types have been reported: isolated dislocation and dislocation in conjunction with axial carpal disruption. In the former injury, the distal carpal row is normal (Fig. 7.108), whereas in the latter type, there is a disruption of the distal carpal row and proximal migration of the radial half of the carpus (Fig. 7.109). A common factor of this injury is dorsiflexion and ulnar deviation of the wrist when a sudden force causes a distraction effect on the radial aspect of the wrist, with subsequent ejection of the scaphoid. Isolated dislocations of the scaphoid are generally treated with closed reduction. Dislocations associated with axial carpal disruption mandate open reduction and internal fixation to stabilize the carpus.

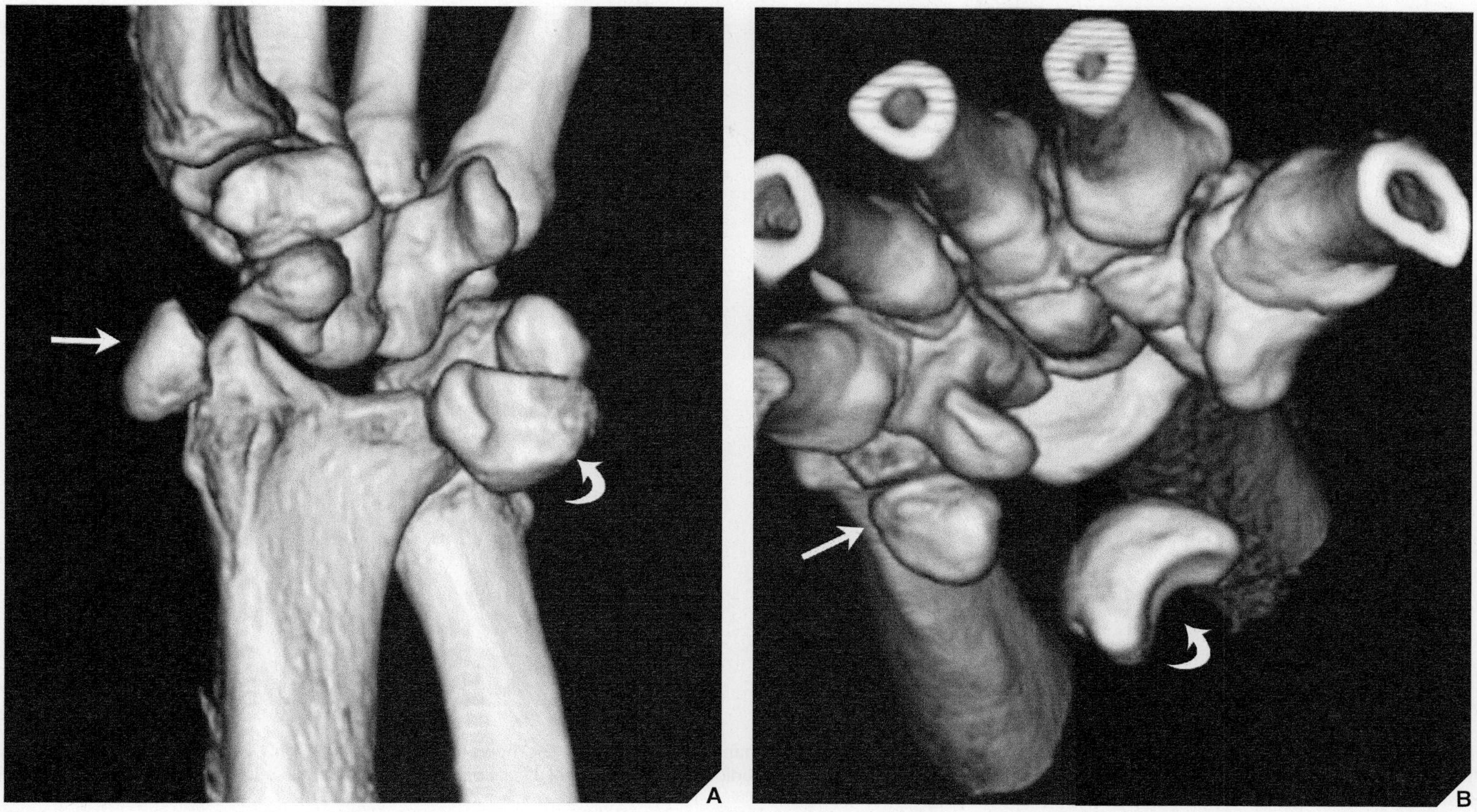

FIGURE 7.101 **3D CT of transscaphoid lunate dislocation.** 3D CT reconstructed images of the wrist in the frontal **(A)** and axial **(B)** projections show a fracture of the scaphoid *(arrows)* and volarly dislocated lunate *(curved arrows)*.

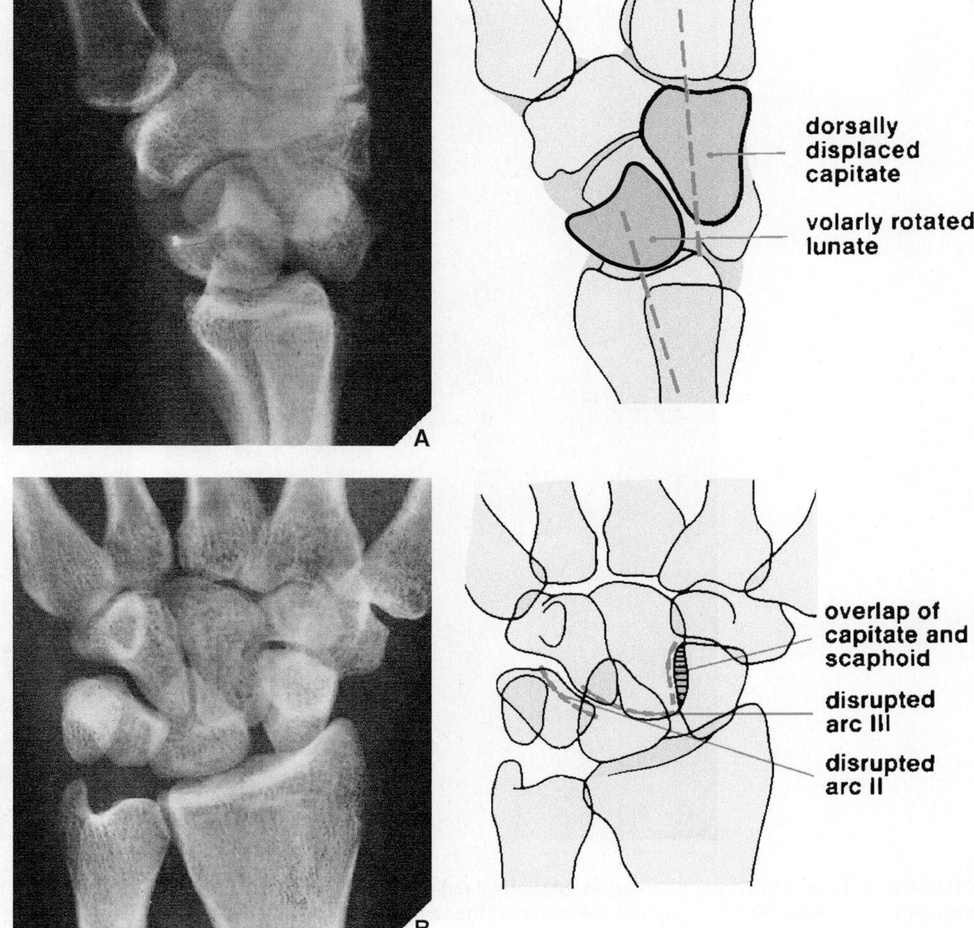

FIGURE 7.102 **Perilunate dislocation.** **(A)** Lateral radiograph of the wrist demonstrates perilunate dislocation characterized by displacement of the capitate dorsal to the lunate, which, although slightly volarly rotated, remains in articulation with the distal radius. Note the break in the longitudinal alignment of the third metacarpal and the capitate with the lunate and the distal radial surface. **(B)** On the dorsovolar projection, perilunate dislocation is evident from the overlapping proximal and distal carpal rows and the resulting disruption of arcs II and III.

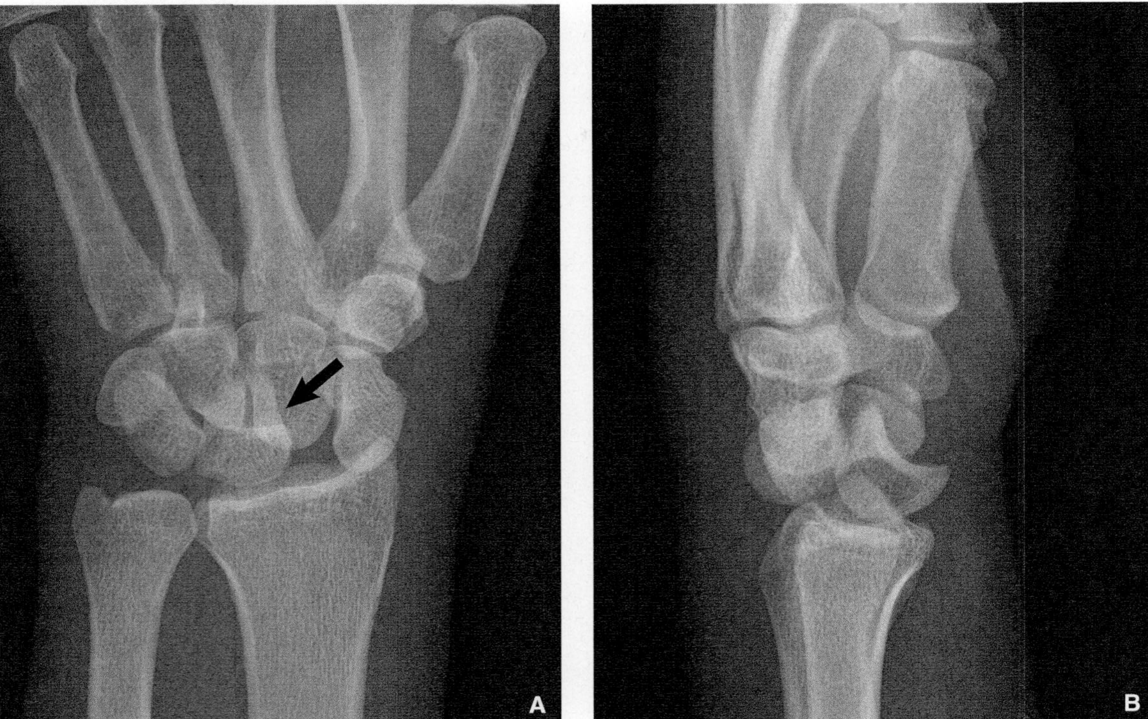

FIGURE 7.103 Perilunate dislocation. **(A)** Dorsovolar radiograph of the right hand of a 33-year-old man shows disruption of carpal arcs II and III, overlap of the lunate, hamate, and capitate *(arrow)*, and widening of the scapholunate interval. **(B)** Lateral radiograph shows dorsal displacement of the capitate in relation to the radius. The lunate is slightly tilted volarly but articulates with the radius.

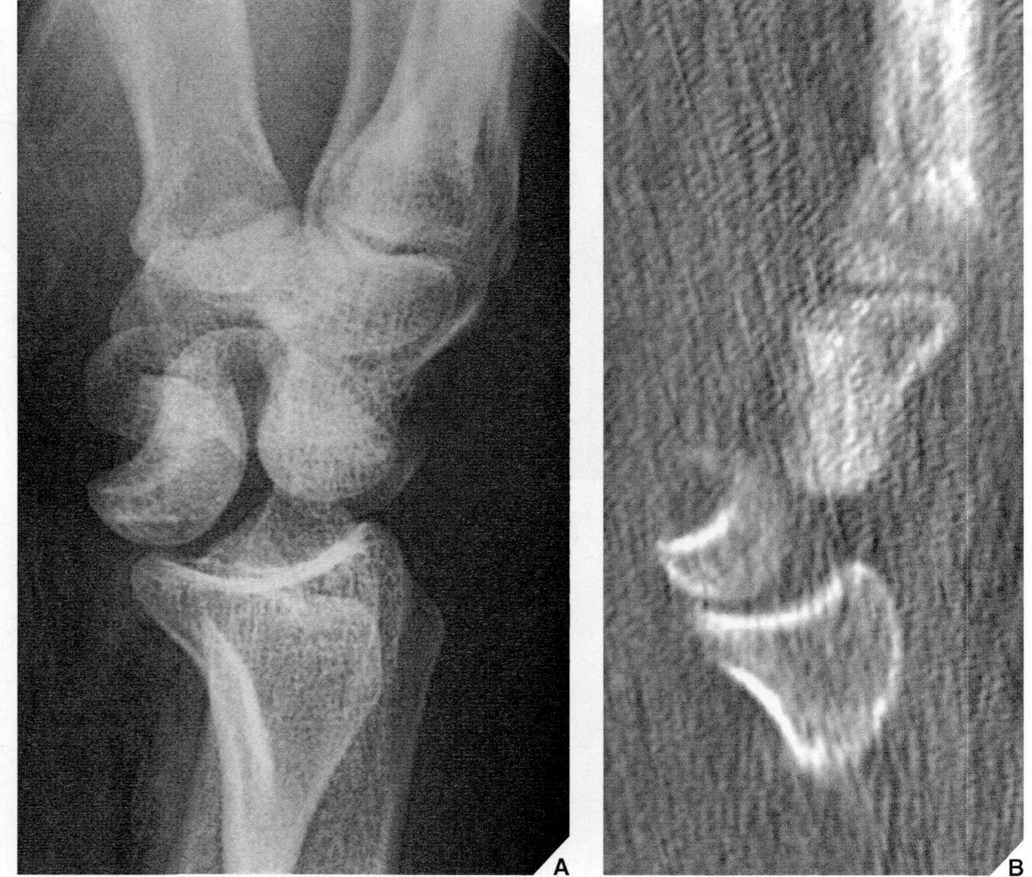

FIGURE 7.104 Midcarpal dislocation. **(A)** Lateral radiograph of the wrist shows volar subluxation of the lunate and dorsal subluxation of the capitate, features of midcarpal dislocation. **(B)** This injury was confirmed on the sagittal reformatted CT image.

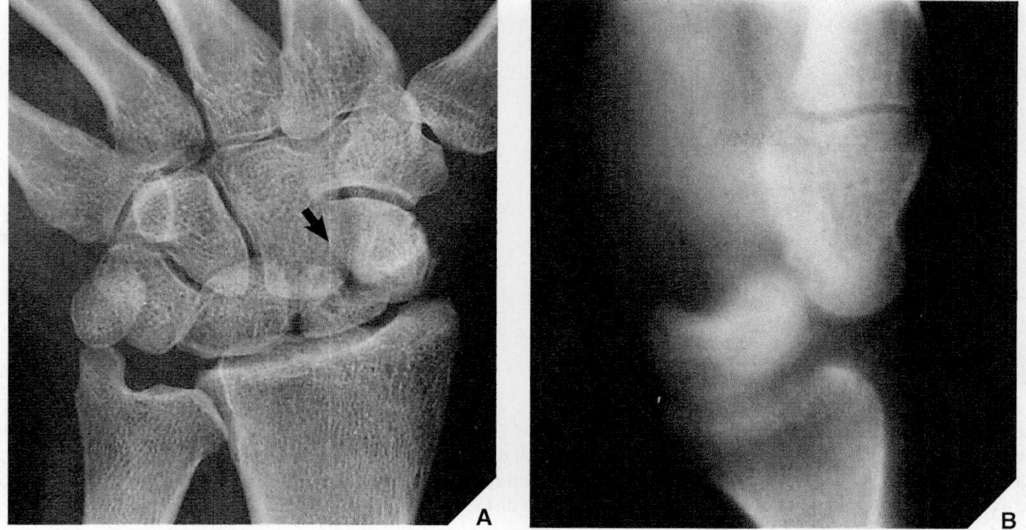

FIGURE 7.105 Transscaphoid perilunate dislocation. **(A)** Dorsovolar radiograph of the wrist in ulnar deviation clearly shows a scaphoid fracture *(arrow)*, but the disruptions in the distal carpal arcs are unclear as to the type of dislocation. The lateral view was also inconclusive. **(B)** Lateral tomogram demonstrates that the capitate is displaced dorsal to the lunate, which remains in articulation with the distal radius—the classic appearance of perilunate dislocation.

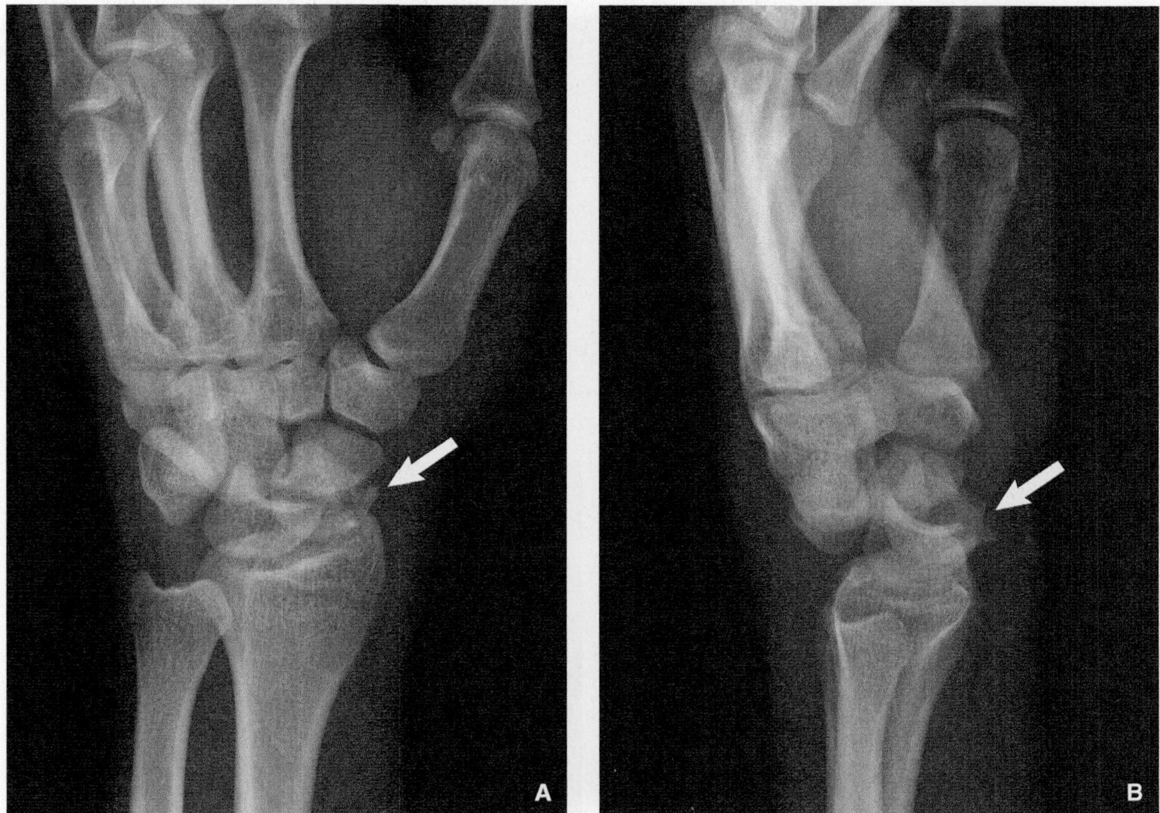

FIGURE 7.106 Transscaphoid perilunate dislocation. **(A)** Oblique and **(B)** lateral radiographs of the right hand of a 24-year-old man shows typical perilunate dislocation associated with a fracture of the scaphoid bone *(arrows)*.

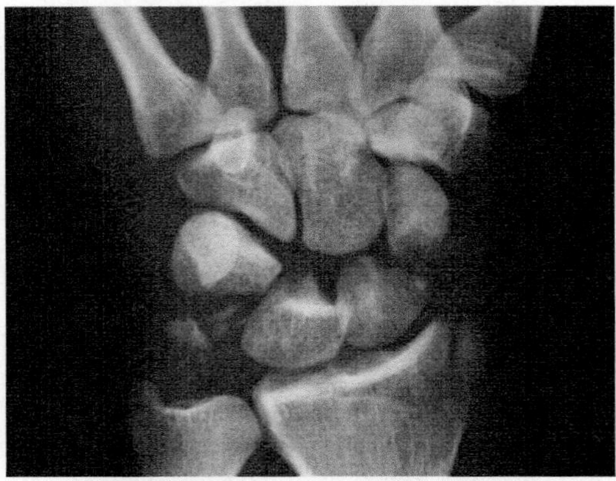
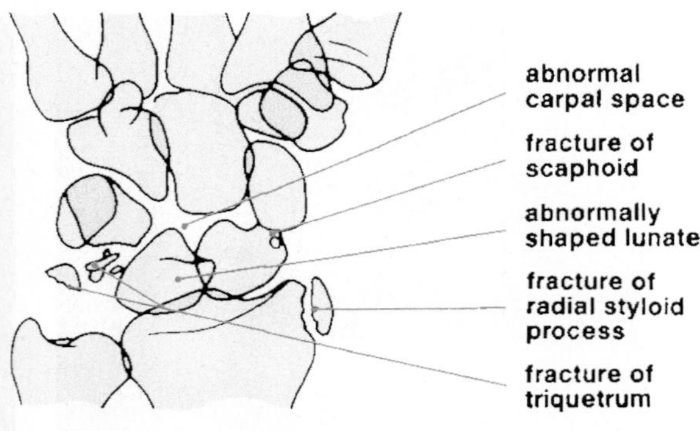

FIGURE 7.107 **Transradial, transscaphoid, transtriquetral lunate dislocation.** Dorsovolar view of the wrist clearly reveals fractures of the radial styloid process, the scaphoid, and the triquetrum. The wide space separating the proximal and the distal carpal rows and the triangular shape of the lunate indicate the possibility of lunate dislocation. Note the disruption in arcs I and II. The lateral view (not shown here) confirmed volar displacement of the lunate and the normal position of the capitate. This abnormality can be described as transradial, transscaphoid, and transtriquetral lunate dislocation.

Carpal Instability

Various carpal instabilities have been described. The most common include dorsal intercalated segment instability (DISI) and volar intercalated segment instability (VISI).

To explain the carpal instability, Lichtman and colleagues developed the carpal ring theory. The proximal carpal row, which represents the intercalated segment, moves as a unit firmly stabilized by interosseous ligaments. Controlled mobility occurs at the scaphotrapezium (radial link) and triquetrohamate (ulnar link) joints (Fig. 7.110). With a break in the ring, either within bony structures or within ligaments, the proximal carpal row no longer moves as a unit. The lunate will then tilt either dorsally or volarly in response to this uncontrolled mobility, manifested by either DISI or VISI (Fig. 7.111). DISI is the most common deformity. It is recognized on the true lateral view of the wrist by dorsal tilt of the lunate, frequently associated with volar (palmar) tilt of the scaphoid (the capitolunate angle measures more than 30 degrees, and the scapholunate angle more than 60 degrees) (Fig. 7.111C). It may be caused by either bony or ligamentous disruption in the ring on the radial side of the wrist. Most commonly, a scaphoid fracture with or without nonunion and scapholunate ligamentous dissociation may be the cause of this deformity. VISI is recognized when a volar tilt of the lunate is noted on the true lateral view frequently accompanied by a dorsal tilt of the capitate (the capitolunate angle measures more than 30 degrees and the scapholunate angle less than 30 degrees) (Fig. 7.111D). It is caused by a break in the ring on the ulnar side of the wrist. Most frequently, it is the ligamentous dissociation and triquetrohamate joint disruption that lead to this deformity. When breaks in the ring occur on the radial and ulnar sides as, for instance, in concurrent scapholunate and lunotriquetral ligamentous dissociation, the VISI pattern predominates (Fig. 7.112).

Injury to the Bones of the Hand

Bennett and Rolando Fractures

Bennett and Rolando fractures are *intraarticular* fractures that occur at the base of the first metacarpal bone. From the perspective of orthopaedic management, it is important to distinguish these from the *extraarticular* types, which are transverse or oblique fractures of the first metacarpal just distal to the carpometacarpal joint (Fig. 7.113). Failure to diagnose and treat properly intraarticular metacarpal fractures may result in protracted pain, stiffness, and posttraumatic arthritis caused by incongruity of articular surfaces.

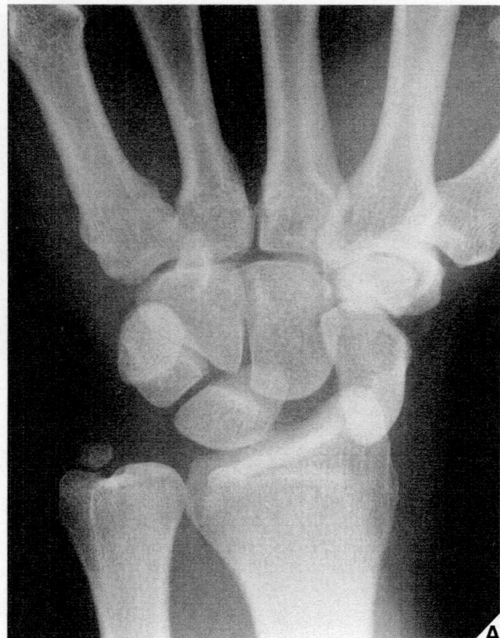

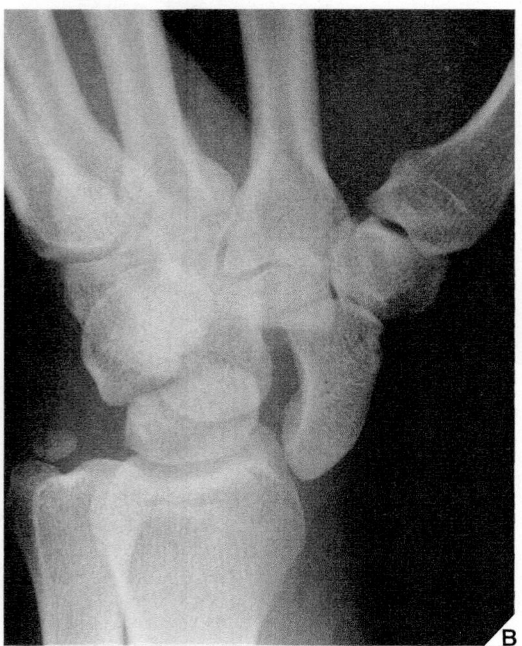

FIGURE 7.108 **Isolated scaphoid dislocation.** **(A)** Dorsovolar and **(B)** oblique radiographs show volar dislocation of the scaphoid. The distal carpal row is not affected, and the capitate bone is in anatomic position.

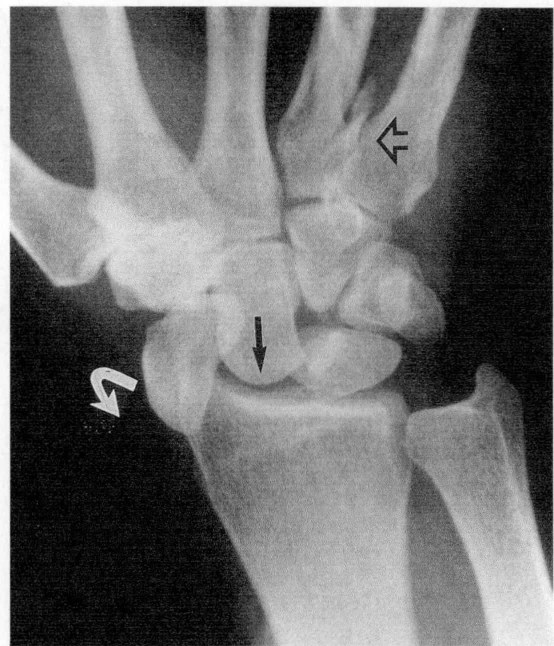

FIGURE 7.109 **Scaphoid dislocation with axial carpal disruption.** Dorsovolar radiograph of the wrist shows radial volar dislocation of the scaphoid bone *(curved arrow)* associated with the proximal migration of the capitate *(arrow)*. Note the interruption of the third arc of the carpus (compare with Fig. 7.93). An *open arrow* points to the associated fracture of the fourth metacarpal bone. (Courtesy of Robert M. Szabo, MD, Sacramento, California.)

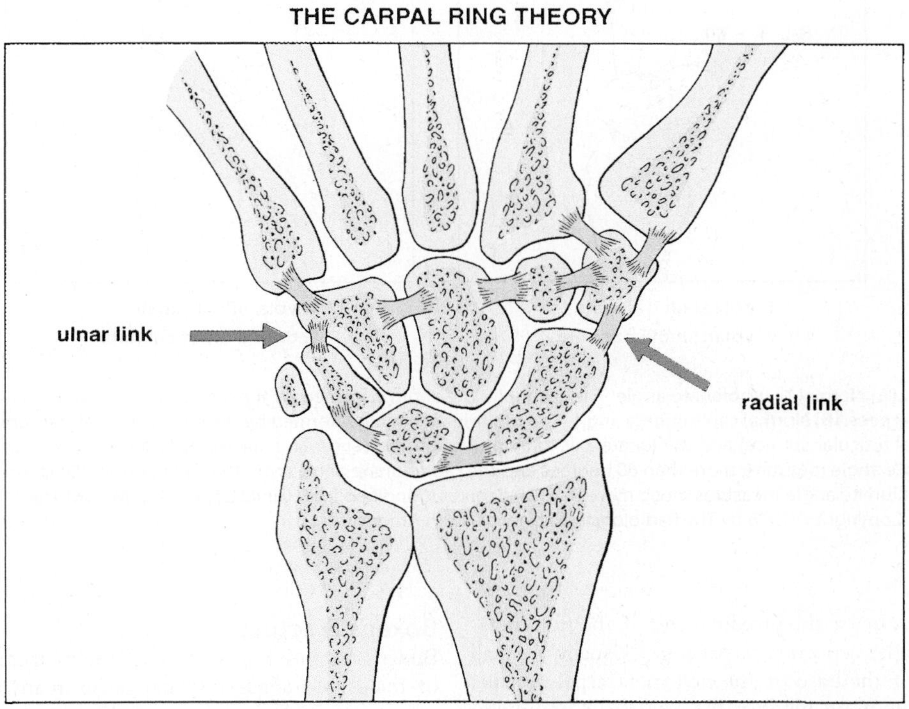

FIGURE 7.110 **The carpal ring theory.** The proximal carpal row (intercalated segment) moves as a unit firmly stabilized by interosseous ligaments. *Controlled* mobility occurs at the scaphotrapezium (radial link) and triquetrohamate (ulnar link) joints. A break in the ring, either bony or ligamentous, can produce *uncontrolled* mobility, manifested by either DISI or VISI. (Modified from Lichtman DM, Schneider JR, Swafford AF, et al. Ulnar midcarpal instability—clinical and laboratory analysis. *J Hand Surg Am* 1981;6A:515–523. Copyright © 1981 American Society for Surgery of the Hand. With permission.)

SCAPHOLUNATE ANGLE

CAPITOLUNATE ANGLE

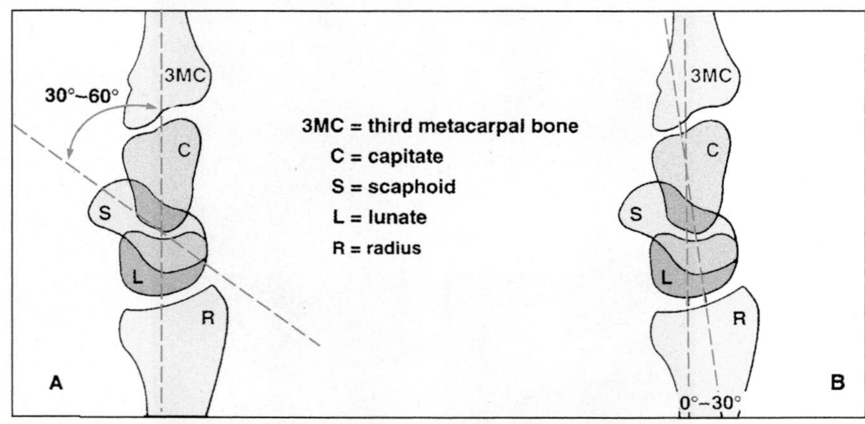

in normal wrist the scapholunate angle is between 30°–60°

in normal wrist the capitolunate angle is between 0°–30°

DISI AND VISI DEFORMITIES

DISI

Dorsal Intercalated Segment Instability (Dorsiflexion Carpal Instability)

VISI

Volar Intercalated Segment Instability (Volarflexion Carpal Instability)

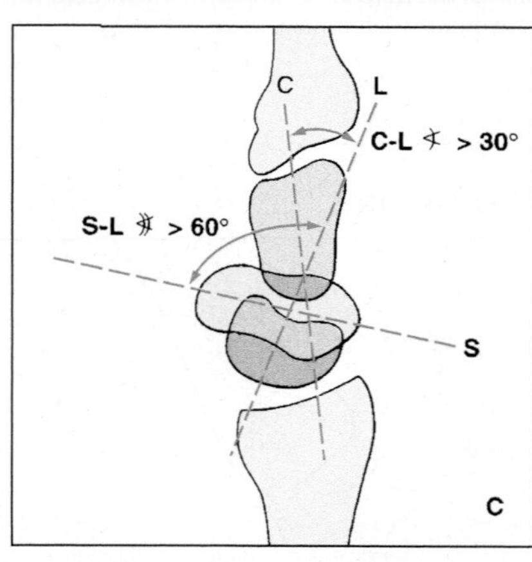

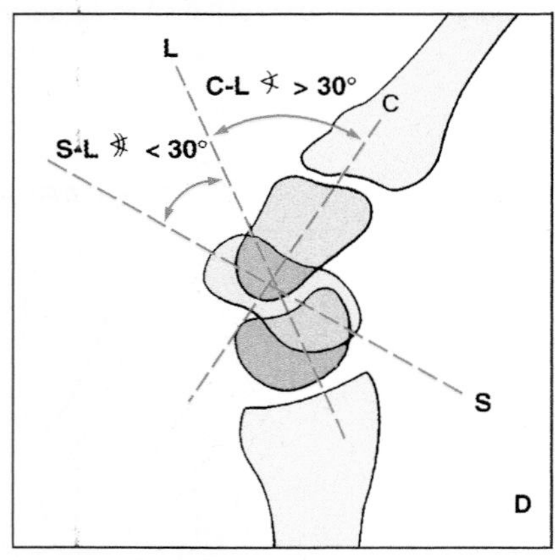

1. dorsal tilt of lunate
2. volar tilt of scaphoid

1. volar tilt of lunate
2. dorsal tilt of capitate

FIGURE 7.111 DISI and VISI. **(A)** Normal scapholunate angle. The scapholunate angle is formed by the intersection of longitudinal axes of scaphoid and lunate and normally measures from 30 to 60 degrees. **(B)** Normal capitolunate angle. The capitolunate angle is formed by the intersection of the capitate axis (drawn from the midpoint of its head to the center of its distal articular surface) and the lunate axis (drawn through the center of its proximal and distal poles) and normally measures from 0 to 30 degrees. **(C)** In DISI, the scapholunate angle measures more than 60 degrees and the capitolunate angle more than 30 degrees. **(D)** In VISI, the scapholunate angle measures less than 30 degrees, and the capitolunate angle measures much more than 30 degrees. (Modified from Gilula LA, Weeks PM. Post-traumatic ligamentous instabilities of the wrist. *Radiology* 1978;129:641–651. Copyright © 1978 by The Radiological Society of North America, Inc.)

The *Bennett fracture* is a fracture of the proximal end of the first metacarpal that extends into the first carpometacarpal joint. Usually, a small fragment on the volar aspect of the base of the first metacarpal remains in articulation with the trapezium bone, whereas the rest of the first metacarpal is dorsally and radially dislocated as the result of pull of the abductor pollicis longus (Fig. 7.114). For this reason, the injury should properly be called a *fracture–dislocation*. The diagnosis and evaluation of the Bennett fracture are readily made on conventional radiographs of the hand in the dorsovolar, oblique, and lateral projections.

The *Rolando fracture* is a comminuted Bennett fracture; the fracture line may have a Y, V, or T configuration (Figs. 7.115 and 7.116). Because there may be multiple fragments, the routine radiographic projections used to diagnose the Bennett fracture occasionally need to be supplemented by CT to localize comminuted fragments and to exclude the possibility of entrapment of a small osseous fragment in the first carpometacarpal joint.

Boxer's Fracture

Boxer's fracture is a fracture of the metacarpal neck with volar angulation of the distal fragment. It may occur in any of the metacarpal bones but is most commonly seen in the fifth metacarpal. The fracture and deformity are sufficiently demonstrated on conventional radiographs of the hand in the dorsovolar and oblique projections (Fig. 7.117). Because comminution frequently accompanies this type of fracture, it is important to determine its extent. Comminution may predispose the fracture after reduction to settle into an angular deformation. The oblique projection usually suffices to determine the extent of comminution (see Fig. 7.117B).

Injury to the Soft Tissue of the Hand

Carpal Tunnel Syndrome

Carpal tunnel syndrome is a compressive neuropathy of the median nerve within the carpal tunnel. Frequently, the syndrome is related to

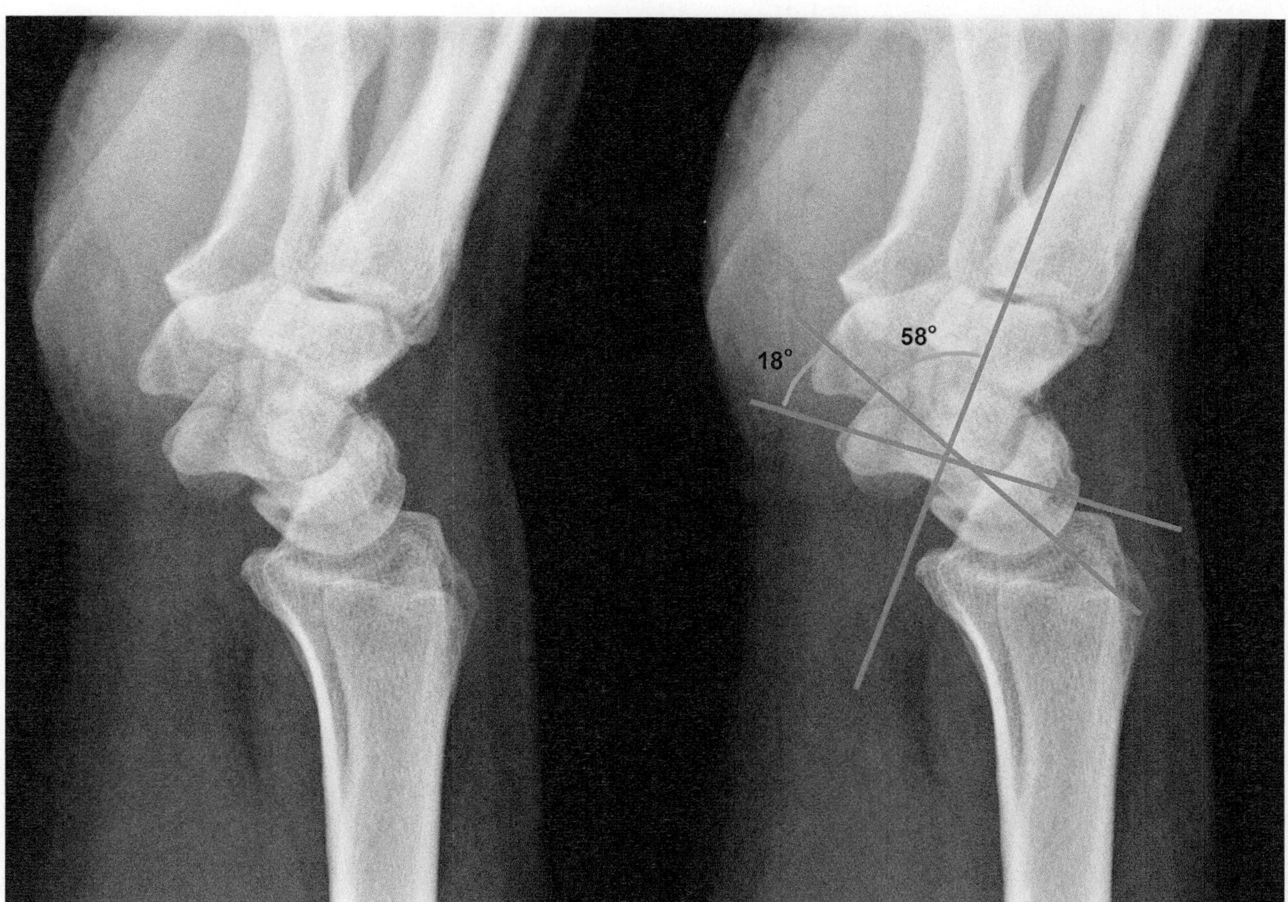

FIGURE 7.112 **VISI deformity.** A 42-year-old man presented with a wrist pain for past 2 years. MRI demonstrated tears of the scapholunate and lunotriquetral ligaments. The lateral radiograph shows decreased scapholunate angle and increased capitolunate angle, confirming the diagnosis of VISI.

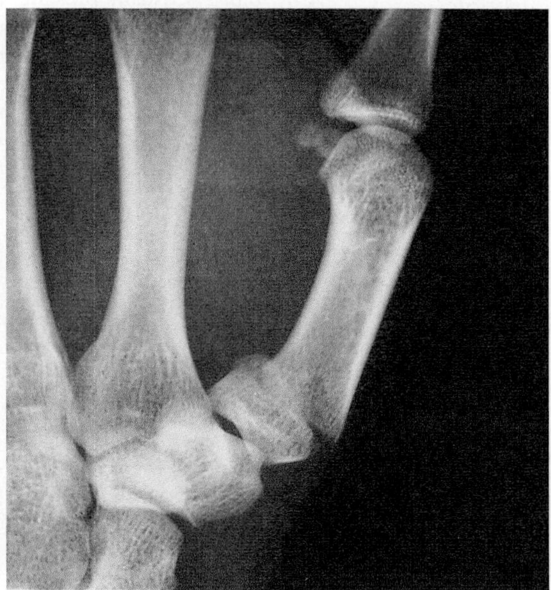

FIGURE 7.113 **Extraarticular fracture.** An extraarticular fracture at the base of the first metacarpal should not be confused with Bennett and Rolando fractures, which are intraarticular.

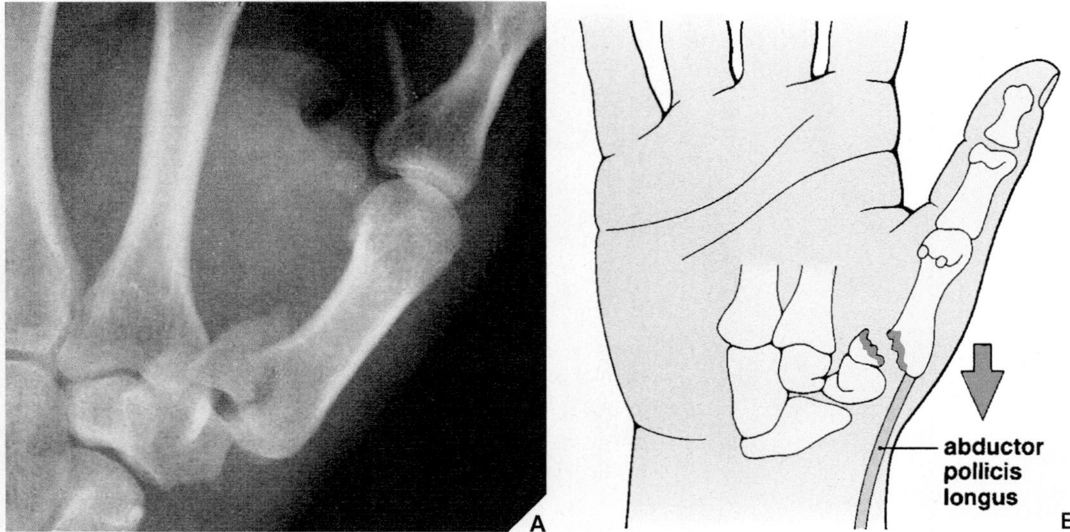

FIGURE 7.114 Bennett fracture. A 27-year-old man who was involved in a fistfight presented with pain localized in the right thenar. **(A)** Coned-down dorsovolar radiograph of the thumb shows a typical appearance of Bennett fracture. A small fragment at the base of the first metacarpal remains in articulation with the trapezium, whereas the rest of the bone is dorsally and radially dislocated. The accompanying schematic diagram **(B)** shows the pathomechanics of this injury.

tenosynovitis of the flexor tendons, but mass lesions such as ganglion cysts, amyloid tissue, and vascular anomalies, among others, have been described as potential etiologies. In most cases, electromyographic changes are sufficient for the diagnosis of this condition.

The most common MRI findings in patients with carpal tunnel syndrome include thickening of the median nerve proximal to the carpal tunnel, flattening of the median nerve in the distal portion of the tunnel, anterior bowing of the flexor retinaculum, and increased signal intensity of the median nerve on T2-weighted images (Fig. 7.118). Additional findings include the presence of fluid surrounding the flexor tendons in cases of tenosynovitis or visualization of solid or cystic masses. MRI has also been used to evaluate patients with recurrent symptoms after carpal tunnel release (Fig. 7.119).

Guyon Canal Syndrome

Guyon canal syndrome represents a compressive neuropathy of the ulnar nerve within the Guyon canal. If the compression occurs proximal to the division of the ulnar nerve, sensory and motor neuropathy in the corresponding territories of innervation will be present clinically. If the compression occurs more distally, sensory or motor deficits will take place, depending on the site of the compression.

The most common etiologies of Guyon canal syndrome include trauma (fracture of the hook of the hamate), external compression (bicycle riding), and anatomic variants such as passing of the fourth flexor tendon through the canal and aberrant muscles. Less common causes include ganglion cysts (Fig. 7.120), giant cell tumors of the tendon sheaths, soft-tissue masses, inflammatory arthritis, and soft-tissue edema.

Anterior Interosseous Nerve Syndrome

Anterior interosseous nerve (AIN) syndrome, also referred to as the *Kiloh-Nevin syndrome*, is a rare clinical complex describing defect in the pincer grasp of the thumb and the index finger and inability to make a fist, due to loss of flexion of distal interphalangeal joints of the index finger and the thumb. Patients often present with pain and paresthesias. A history of injury is usually present. The AIN branches from the median nerve just distal to the neck of the radius and proximal to median nerve's dive under the pronator teres. It is in this location that the compression of the AIN is thought to occur. AIN then follows the interosseous vasculature onto the interosseous membrane and runs between the flexor pollicis longus and the flexor digitorum profundus muscles; it then proceeds into the pronator quadratus muscle, innervating all three.

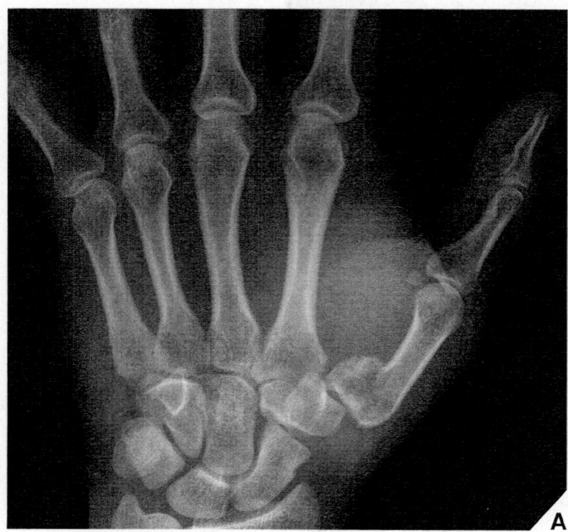

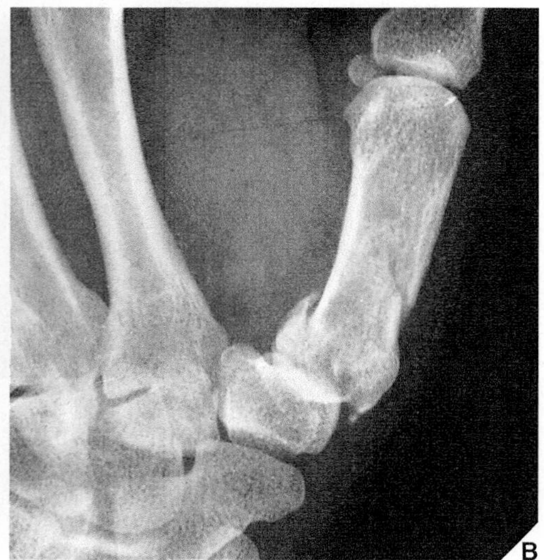

FIGURE 7.115 Rolando fracture. **(A)** Dorsovolar radiograph of the right hand shows a comminuted intraarticular fracture of the first metacarpal bone. **(B)** Coned-down oblique radiograph of the right thumb in another patient shows a classic appearance of this injury.

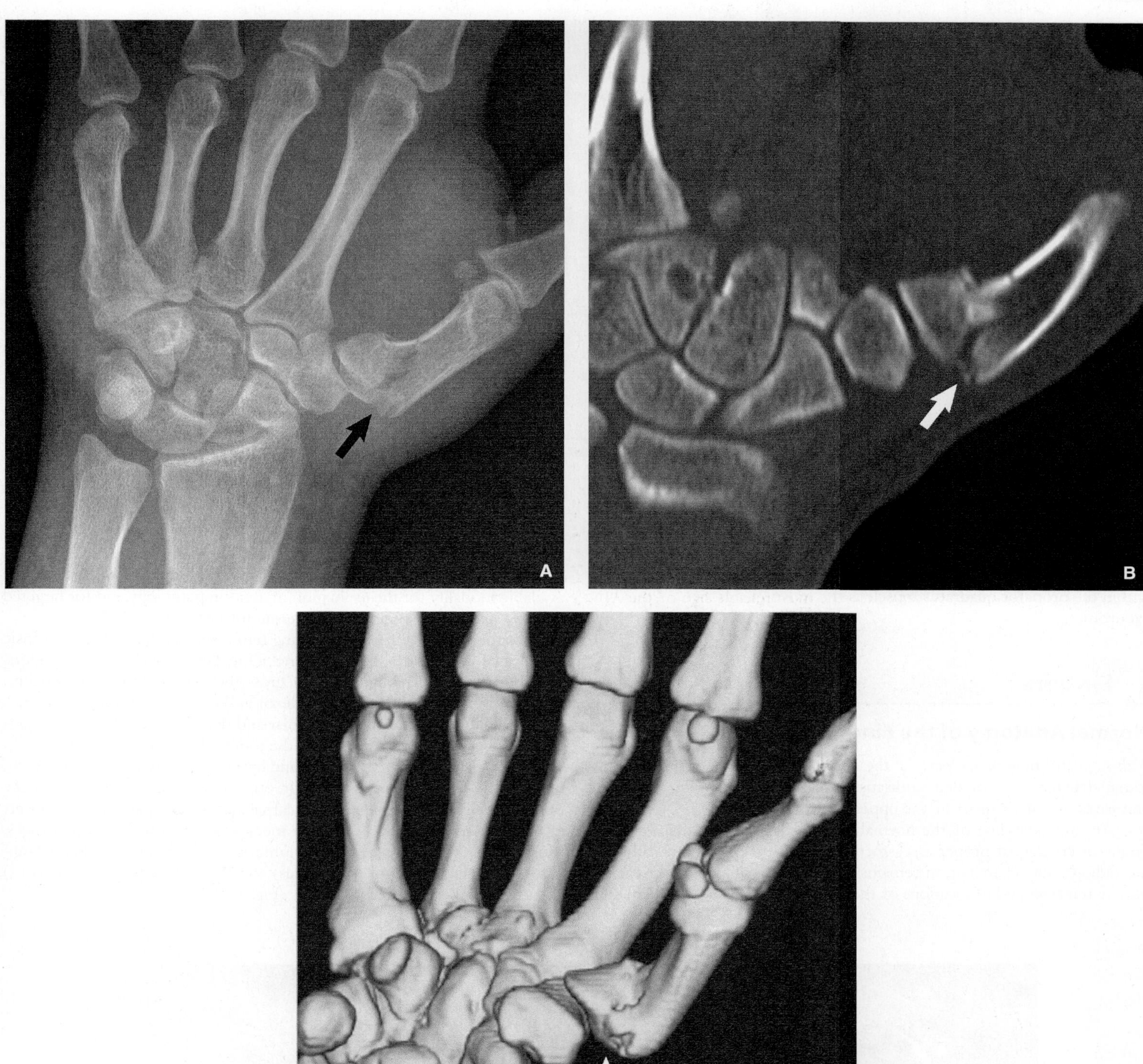

FIGURE 7.116 CT and 3D CT of Rolando fracture. **(A)** Dorsovolar radiograph of the right hand of a 33-year-old man shows comminuted intraarticular fracture at the base of the first metacarpal bone *(arrow)*, confirmed on the **(B)** coronal reformatted and **(C)** 3D reconstructed CT images *(arrows)*.

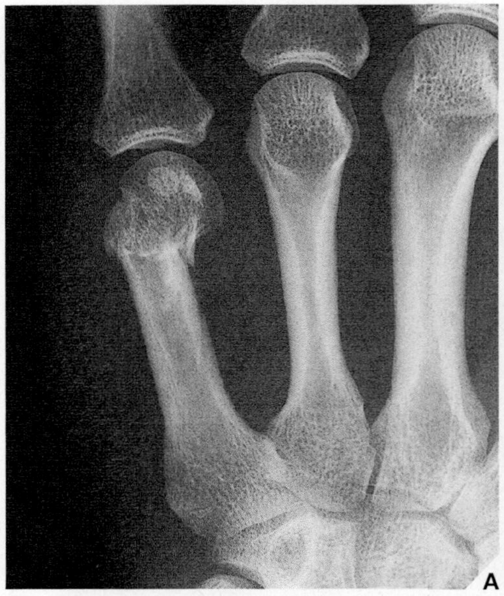

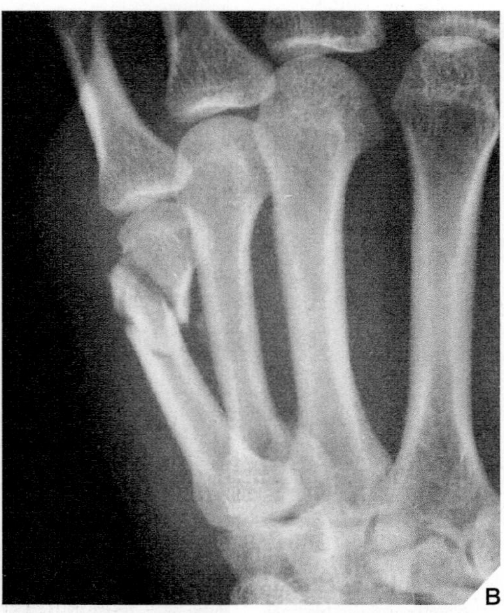

FIGURE 7.117 **Boxer's fracture.** **(A)** Dorsovolar radiograph of the right hand demonstrates a fracture of the fifth metacarpal with volar angulation of the distal fragment—a simple boxer's fracture. When comminution is present, it is essential for its prognostic value to demonstrate the extent of fracture lines because such fractures are frequently unstable. The oblique projection **(B)** usually suffices to determine the extent of comminution.

MRI findings of the AIN syndrome include edema or atrophy within the pronator quadratus muscle (Fig. 7.121), edema of the radial half of the flexor digitorum profundus, or edema of the flexor carpi radialis. Edema within the pronator quadratus muscle is the most reliable sign of the AIN syndrome.

Fingers

Normal Anatomy of the Fingers

Although the fingers are part of the hand because of their unique anatomic structure, we decided to discuss separately some of the traumatic abnormalities of this part of the upper extremity.

An understanding of the normal anatomy of the soft tissues of the fingers is crucial for proper assessment of potential pathology. Although the radiographic examination remains the modality of choice for evaluation of fractures and dislocations of the fingers, MRI provides information about the normal anatomy of the soft tissues (Figs. 7.122), and consequently about traumatic abnormalities (see text that follows). Ultrasound (US) has also been proven to be a very effective, inexpensive, and readily available modality for the evaluation of tendon pathology and for targeted needle placement, aspiration, and steroid injection (Fig. 7.123).

Surrounded by the corresponding retinacula, tendons of the extrinsic muscles of the hand and fingers, including flexor and extensor tendons and abductor pollicis longus tendon, cross the wrist and insert distally into the corresponding phalanges. The flexor and extensor tendons of the fingers are held in position along the volar and dorsal aspect of the phalanges by the pulley system (volar) and by the sagittal bands (dorsal) (Fig. 7.124). The intrinsic muscles of the thenar and hypothenar eminences of the hand include flexor, abductor and adductor, opponens muscles, and the palmaris brevis muscle. They originate in the carpal and metacarpal bones and insert in the corresponding first and fifth metacarpals and proximal phalanges. More distally the interosseous and lumbricals muscles of the hand originate in the flexor tendons (lumbricals) and the metacarpals (interosseous) and insert in the proximal phalanges (Fig. 7.125).

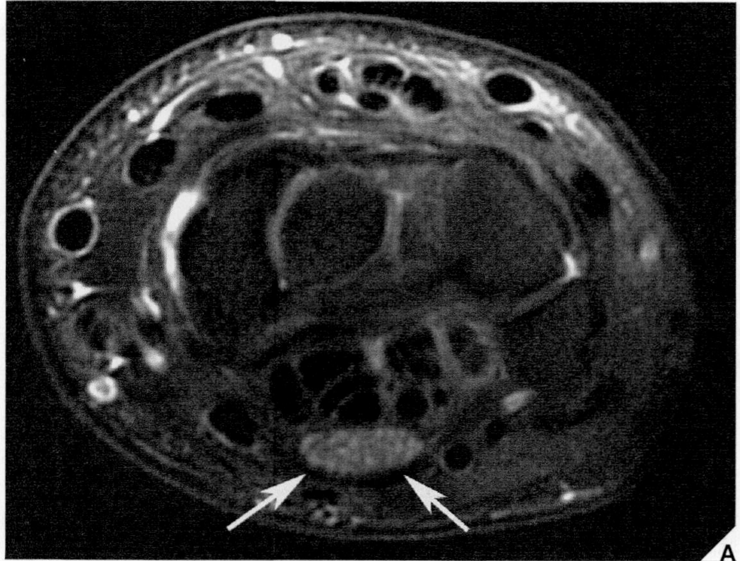

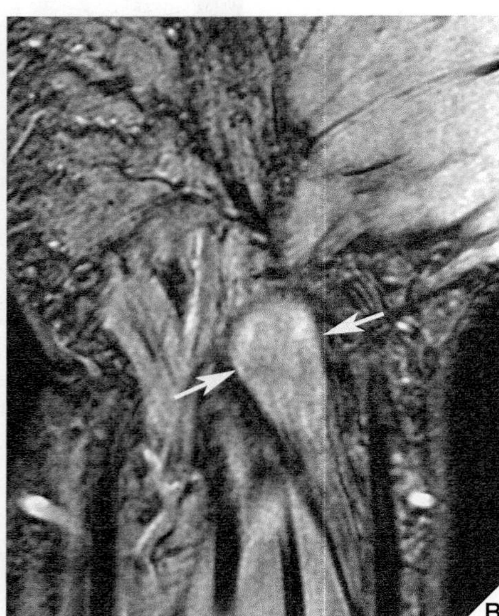

FIGURE 7.118 **MRI of carpal tunnel syndrome.** Young woman presented with signs of median neuritis. **(A)** Axial STIR MRI demonstrates increased signal intensity of the median nerve just proximal to the carpal tunnel, with a "granular" pattern and increased thickness, consistent with severe median neuritis and carpal tunnel syndrome *(arrows)*. **(B)** Coronal GRE image demonstrates the thickened median nerve *(arrows)* proximal to the carpal tunnel.

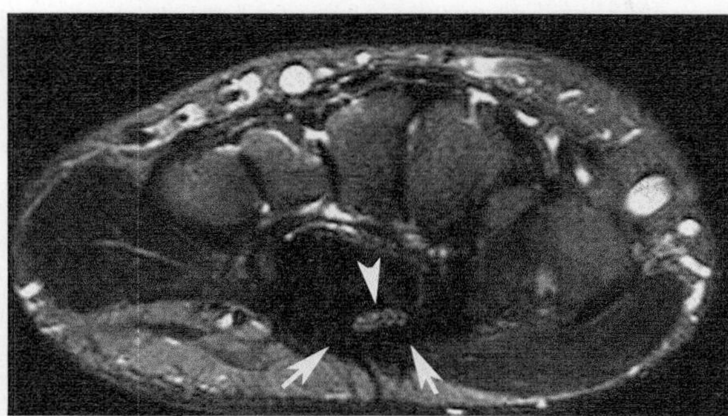

FIGURE 7.119 MRI of recurrent carpal tunnel syndrome. Middle-aged woman presented with recurrent signs of carpal tunnel syndrome, 6 months following carpal tunnel release. Axial T2-weighted MRI demonstrates scar tissue *(arrows)* surrounding the median nerve, which appears hyperintense, thickened, and with the characteristic "granular" appearance *(arrowhead)*.

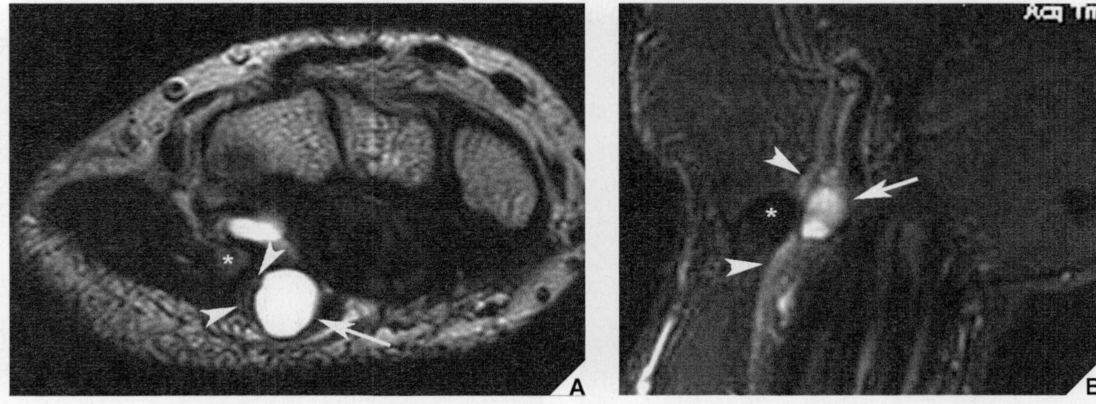

FIGURE 7.120 MRI of Guyon canal syndrome. A 48-year-old man presented with sensory deficit in the territory of the sensory branch of the ulnar nerve. **(A)** Axial T2-weighted MR image demonstrates a ganglion cyst in the Guyon canal *(arrow)* compressing the ulnar nerve *(arrowheads)* against the pisiform *(asterisk)*. **(B)** Coronal STIR image demonstrates the ganglion cyst *(arrow)* compressing the ulnar nerve *(arrowheads)* against the pisiform *(asterisk)*.

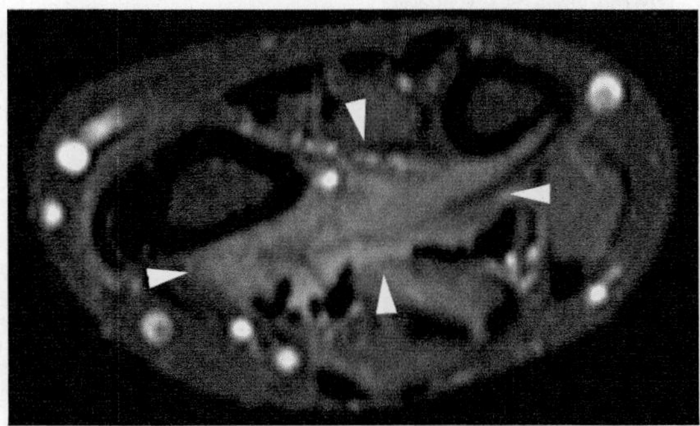

FIGURE 7.121 MRI of AIN syndrome. Young woman presented with a history of inability to pick up small objects with the thumb and the index finger. Axial STIR MR image demonstrates increased signal intensity of the pronator quadratus muscle *(arrowheads)* consistent with early signs of denervation secondary to compression of the AIN. Surgical release was performed, with improvement of the patient's symptoms.

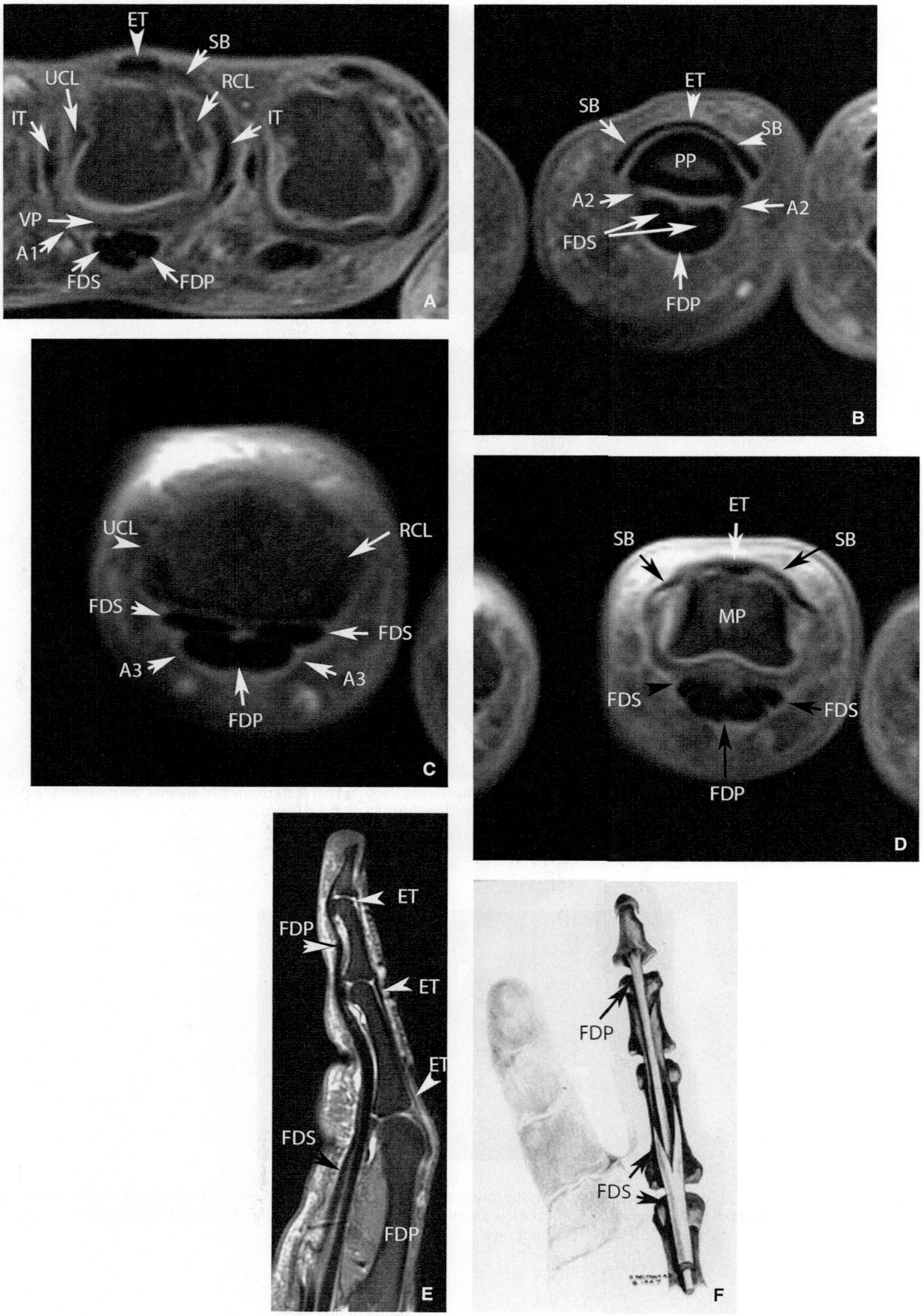

FIGURE 7.122 Normal MRI anatomy of the fingers. **(A)** Axial T1-weighted fat-saturated MR image of the fingers obtained through the metacarpophalangeal (MCP) joint, **(B)** through the proximal phalanx, **(C)** through the PIP joint, and **(D)** through the base of the middle phalanx. **(E)** Sagittal T2-weighted image of the finger. **(F)** Schematic representation of the normal anatomy of the flexor digitorum superficialis and profundus. Observe the normal split of the FDS at the level of the proximal phalanx **(D,F)**, where it becomes deep to the FDP. Note the thinning of the ET at the level of the middle phalanx **(D)**. FDS, flexor auditoriumuperficialis tendon; FDP, flexor diauditoriumfpro-foundn; A1, A1 pulley; A2, A2 pulley; A3, A3 pulley; VP, volar plate; IT, interointer-osseous; UCL, ulnar collateral ligament; RCL, radial collateral ligament; ET, extensor tendon; SB, sagittal band; PP, proximal phalanx; MP, middle phalanx.

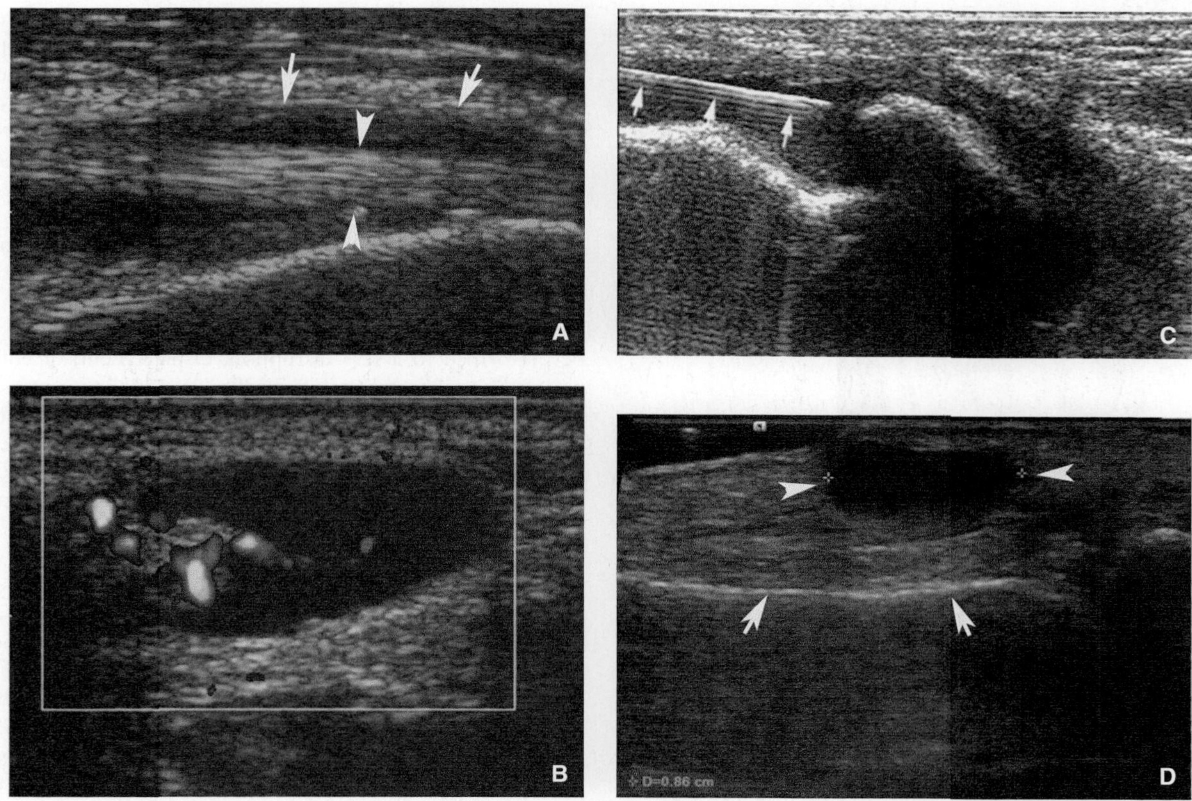

FIGURE 7.123 **US of tenosynovitis of the flexor pollicis longus.** **(A)** US image along the longitudinal axis of the flexor pollicis longus shows the tendon sheath distended by hypoechoic fluid *(arrows)*. Note the normal fibrillar structure of the tendon *(arrowheads)*. **(B)** Color Doppler US demonstrates hypervascularity of the synovium indicating an active inflammatory process. **(C)** US obtained during needle placement in the tendon sheath *(arrows)* for the purpose of fluid aspiration and steroid injection. (Courtesy of Luis Cerezal, MD, Santander, Spain.) **(D)** US evaluation of a ganglion cyst *(arrowheads)* adjacent to the normal appearing extensor pollicis longus tendon *(arrows)* in another patient. (Courtesy of Christopher Burke, MD, New York, NY.)

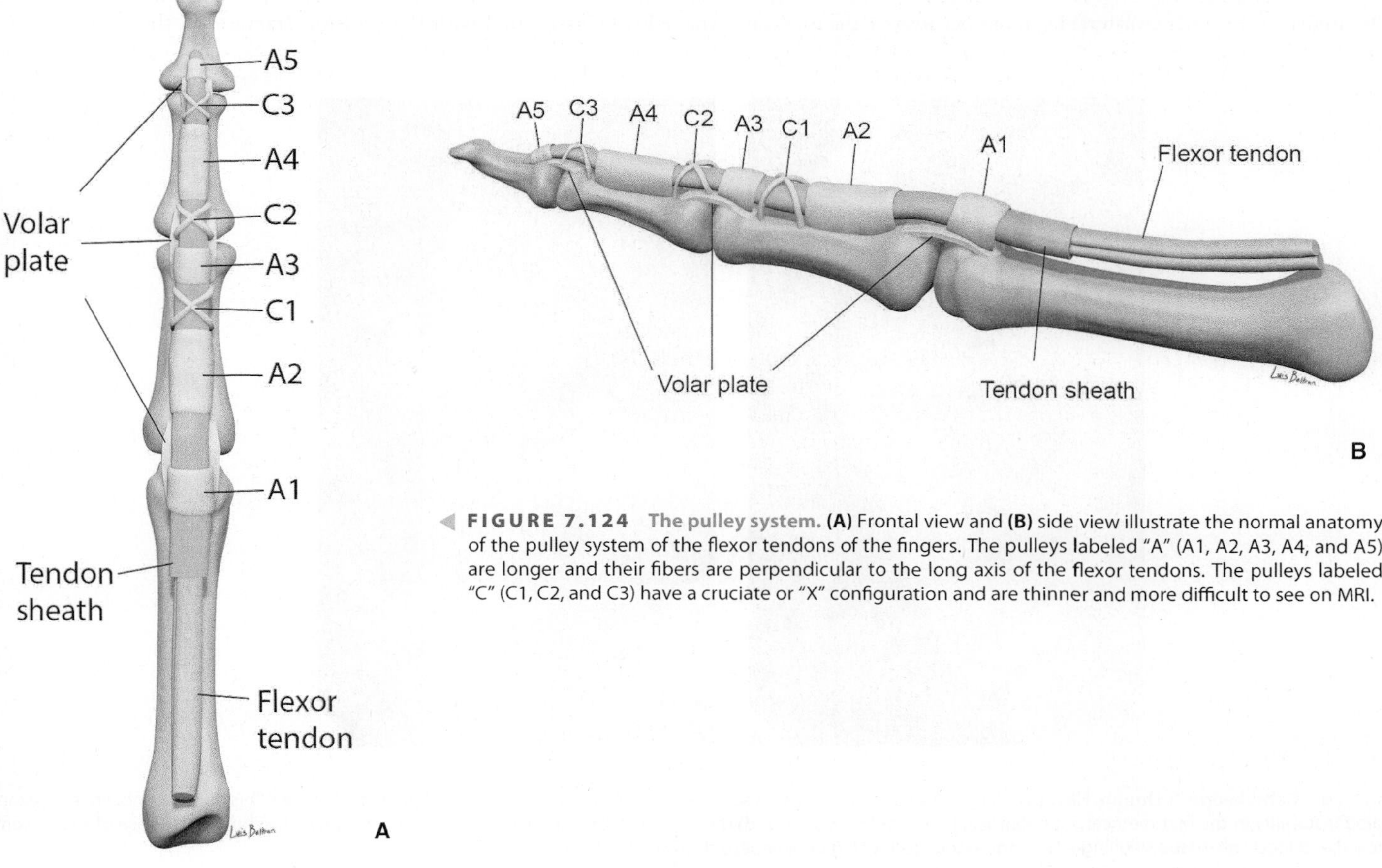

FIGURE 7.124 **The pulley system.** **(A)** Frontal view and **(B)** side view illustrate the normal anatomy of the pulley system of the flexor tendons of the fingers. The pulleys labeled "A" (A1, A2, A3, A4, and A5) are longer and their fibers are perpendicular to the long axis of the flexor tendons. The pulleys labeled "C" (C1, C2, and C3) have a cruciate or "X" configuration and are thinner and more difficult to see on MRI.

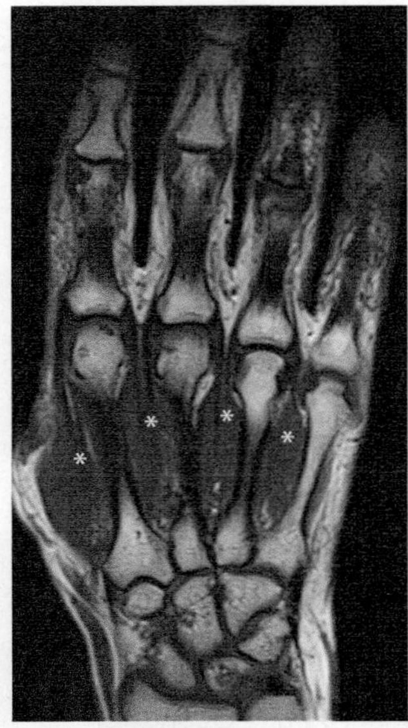

FIGURE 7.125 Normal anatomy of the hand and fingers. Coronal T1-weighted MR image shows the normal osseous and soft-tissue anatomy. Note the interosseous muscles and tendons *(asterisks)*.

The metacarpophalangeal and interphalangeal articulations are stabilized by the joint capsules, collateral ligaments, and the fibrocartilaginous volar plates.

Injury to the Bones and Soft Tissues of the Fingers

Gamekeeper's Thumb

Gamekeeper's thumb results from a disruption of the ulnar collateral ligament of the first metacarpophalangeal joint, often accompanied by a fracture of the base of the proximal phalanx. The abnormality is termed *gamekeeper's thumb* because it was originally seen affecting Scottish game wardens who injured their ulnar collateral ligament because of the method they used to kill rabbits. Currently, because it is more frequently seen in skiing accidents, the term *skier's thumb* is applied. This type of injury can also occur in break-dancers (break-dancer's thumb). When ruptured, the torn end of the ulnar collateral ligament can become displaced superficially to the adductor pollicis aponeurosis. This is known as the *Stener lesion* (see Figs. 7.130 and 7.131). Standard dorsovolar and oblique radiographs of the thumb usually suffice to demonstrate the associated fracture (Fig. 7.126A,B), but the full evaluation requires an abduction–stress film of the thumb when this condition is suspected. An increase to more than 30 degrees in the angle between the first metacarpal and the proximal phalanx is a characteristic finding in gamekeeper's thumb, indicating subluxation (Fig. 7.127A,B). Arthrographic examination of the thumb may also be performed to assess disruption, displacement, or entrapment of the ulnar collateral ligament (Fig. 7.128).

Currently, MRI is the procedure of choice to investigate this injury (Fig. 7.129), particularly to detect a displaced tear of the ulnar collateral ligament (Figs. 7.130 and 7.131). Likewise, US has proved to be a simple, reliable, and cost-effective tool for recognition of the Stener lesion.

Avulsion Fractures of the Fingers

Avulsion fractures of the fingers are frequent injuries sustained during sports activities. Typically, they occur at the level of extensor tendon insertion in the dorsal aspect of the distal phalange when a ball strikes the tip of the finger, resulting in a hyperflexion injury of the distal interphalangeal joint. A flexion deformity in the distal interphalangeal joint is noticeable clinically, with inability to straighten the finger (mallet finger, baseball finger). The avulsed bone fragment is easily recognizable on lateral radiographs of the finger (Fig. 7.132). Occasionally, the extensor tendon is ruptured, without associate osseous avulsion fracture. The nail bed may also be avulsed during the traumatic event. Conservative treatment with application of a splint and physical therapy are the treatment of choice for small fractures or isolated tendon lesions; however, surgery with pinning and tendon repair may be required in larger fractures with deformity of the articular surface.

Volar plate injuries are the result of a hyperextension injury of the finger with aftermath of an avulsion fracture of the volar aspect of the base of the middle phalanx (volar plate), readily recognizable on lateral radiographs of the finger (Fig. 7.133). Lateral collateral ligament injuries may also be associated with the avulsion fracture. In these cases, side to

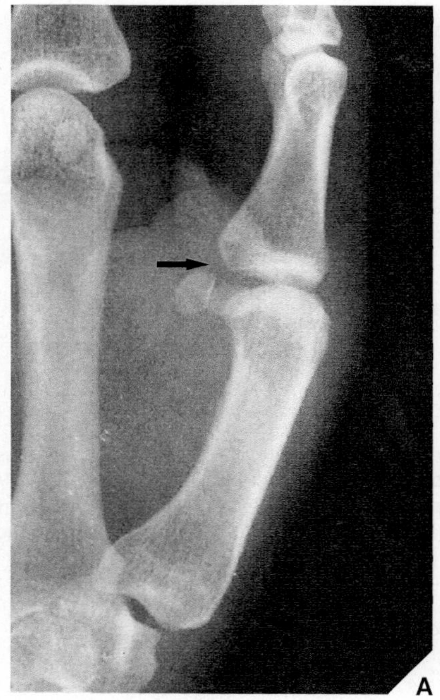

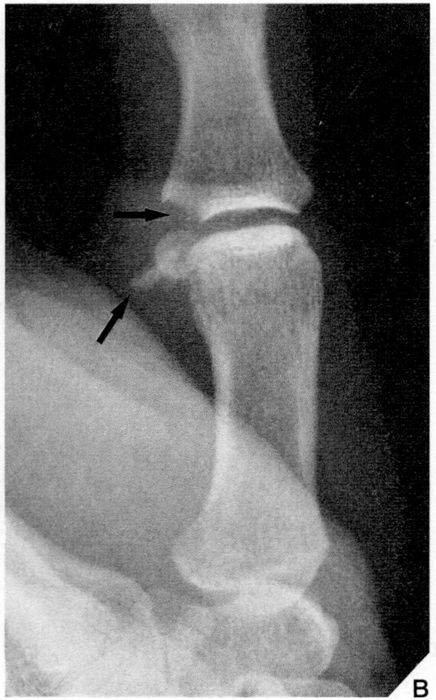

FIGURE 7.126 Gamekeeper's thumb. Having fallen on his hand on the ski slopes, a 38-year-old man presented with pain at the base of his right thumb. Physical examination revealed instability in the first metacarpophalangeal joint. **(A)** Oblique and **(B)** dorsovolar radiographs of the right thumb show a fracture of the base of the proximal phalanx *(arrows)* and local soft-tissue swelling—findings associated with gamekeeper's thumb.

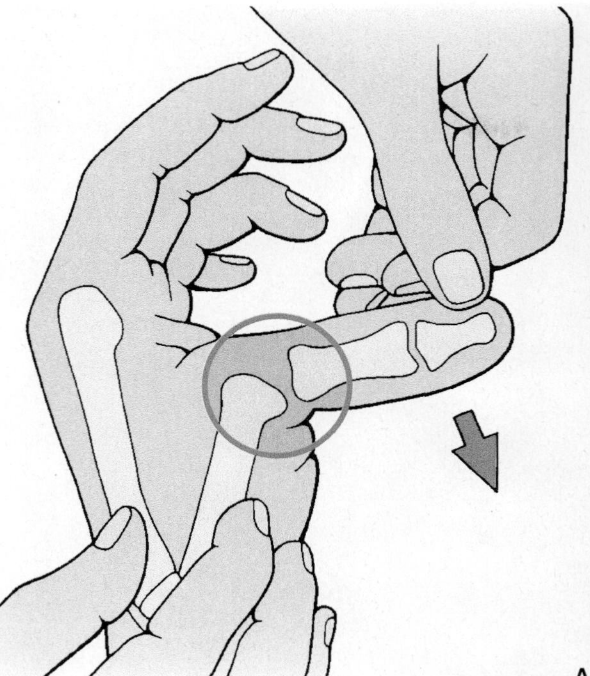

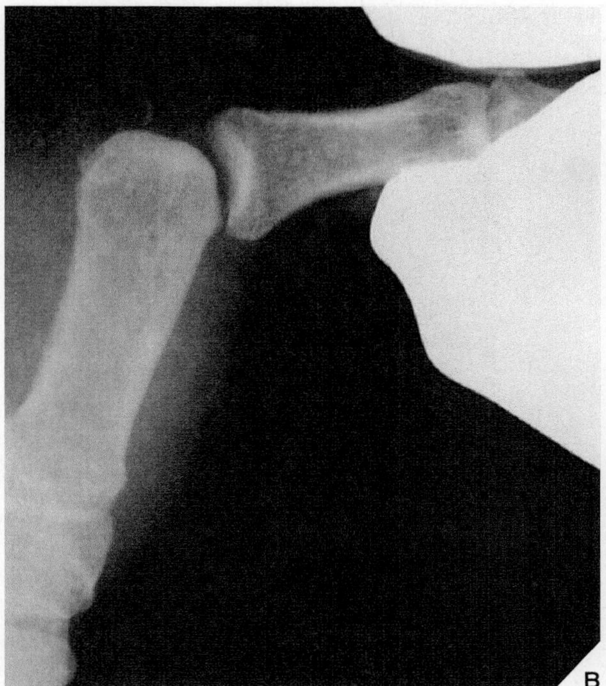

FIGURE 7.127 **Gamekeeper's thumb.** In another patient, dorsovolar and lateral radiographs of the first phalanx (not shown here) did not show a fracture, but because instability of the first metacarpophalangeal joint was indicated on physical examination **(A)**, an abduction–stress film of the thumb was obtained. The stress radiograph **(B)** demonstrates subluxation of the joint by an increase to more than 30 degrees in the angle between the first metacarpal and the proximal phalanx of the thumb, confirming gamekeeper's thumb.

side instability of the joint is noted clinically. These injuries respond well to conservative treatment which consists of taping the injured finger with the adjacent normal finger ("buddy taping").

Flexor Pulley System Rupture (Climber's Finger)

Rock climbing places a significant stress on the flexor tendons and pulley system of the fingers, especially the middle and ring fingers, when the climber is trying to support the entire weight of the body the fingers. This is an overuse injury leading to rupture of the pulley system of the flexor tendons, most frequently the A2 and A3 pulleys. MRI of the fingers provides unique visualization of these injuries. In order to assess properly these pulley lesions, the images should be obtained in extension and flexion of the interphalangeal joints. The images in extension demonstrate the tear of the corresponding pulleys, and the flexion images demonstrate the "bowstringing" of the flexor tendons with increased distance between the phalanges and the tendons (Fig. 7.134).

de Quervain Syndrome

Also known as *de Quervain tenosynovitis*, this abnormality refers to tenosynovitis of the abductor pollicis longus and extensor pollicis brevis tendons in the first dorsal extensor compartment of the wrist. This syndrome is caused by chronic overuse, with gradual onset of symptoms of pain and swelling at

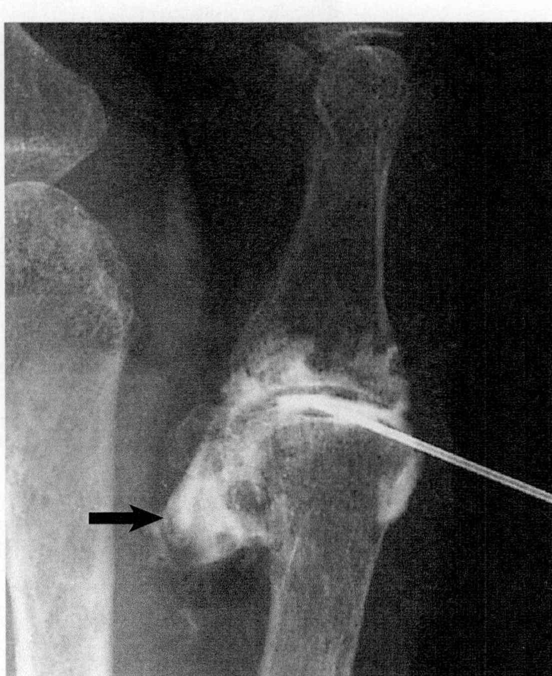

FIGURE 7.128 **Arthrogram of the gamekeeper's thumb.** An arthrogram of the first metacarpophalangeal joint demonstrates the characteristic findings in gamekeeper's thumb. The leak of contrast along the ulnar side of the head of the first metacarpal *(arrow)* indicates a tear of the ulnar collateral ligament. (Courtesy of Donald Resnick, MD, San Diego, California.)

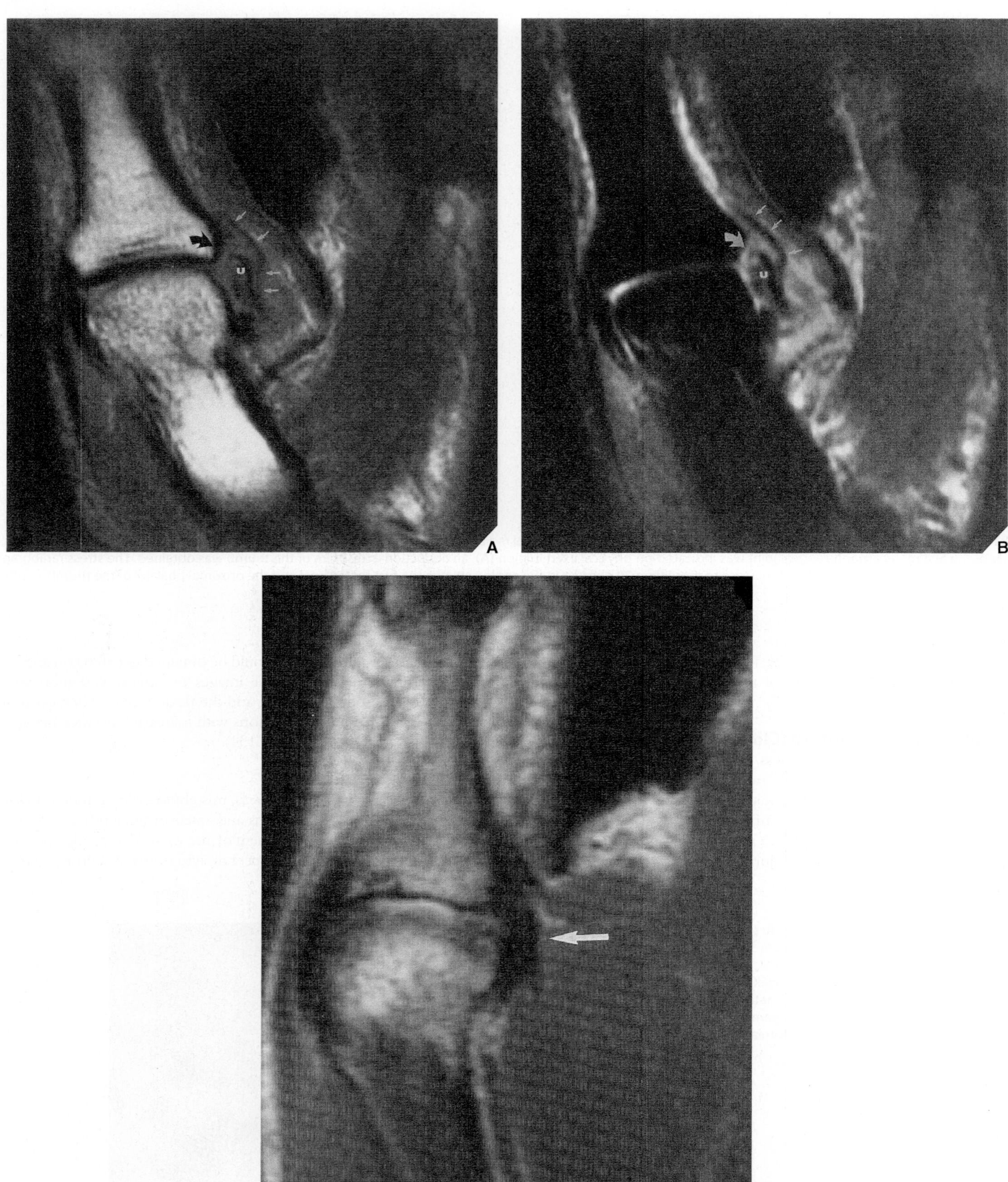

FIGURE 7.129 MRI of the gamekeeper's thumb. **(A)** Coronal T1-weighted and **(B)** coronal STIR images show a tear of the ulnar collateral ligament *(u)* of the first metacarpophalangeal joint *(curved arrows)*. The torn ligament is not displaced, maintaining its longitudinal orientation *(small arrows)*. **(C)** Coronal fat-suppressed T2-weighted image shows a normal appearance of intact ulnar collateral ligament *(arrow)*. (Reprinted with permission from Stoller DW. *MRI in orthopaedics and sports medicine.* Philadelphia: JB Lippincott; 1993.)

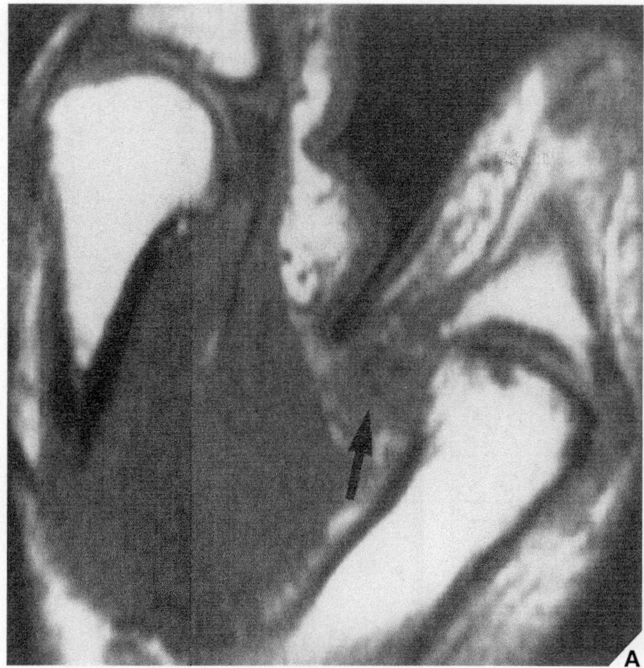

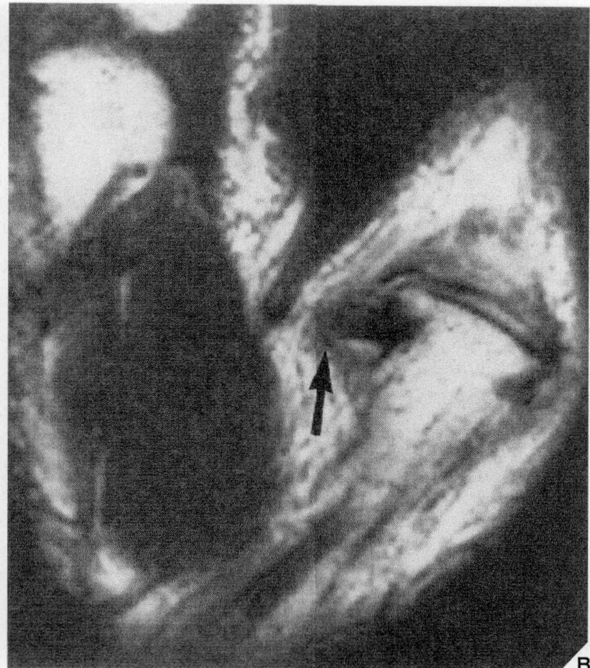

FIGURE 7.130 **MRI of the Stener lesion.** **(A)** Coronal T1-weighted MR image shows a disruption of the ulnar collateral ligament *(arrow)*. The normal low-intensity signal of this structure is not present. **(B)** Coronal T2-weighted MR image shows displacement of the proximal fragment of this ligament away from the joint and its perpendicular rather than longitudinal orientation *(arrow)*, characteristic of the Stener lesion. (**A**, Reprinted with permission from Deutsch AL, Mink JH, eds. *MRI of the musculoskeletal system: a teaching file,* 2nd ed. Philadelphia: Lippincott-Raven; 1997.)

the base of the thumb. The symptoms can be alleviated with antiinflammatory medications, splint therapy, physical therapy and/or steroid injection into the tendon sheath. Rarely, this condition requires surgery. MRI or US shows tenosynovitis often accompanied by tendinosis and tearing of the tendons of the first extensor compartment of the wrist (Fig. 7.135).

Tendon and Ligament Tears

Tears of the flexor and extensor tendons are common traumatic injuries to the fingers. The value of US or MRI is not to diagnose the tendon rupture, which is generally done based on clinical grounds, but to diagnose the exact location of the tear and the size of the gap between the proximal and distal ends of the tendons (Fig. 7.136).

Tears of the sagittal bands especially at the level of the third knuckle are seen in patients with history of hitting a hard object with the fist. The sagittal band at the level of the third metacarpophalangeal joint ruptures on the radial side more frequently and consequently the extensor tendon becomes unstable and dislocates toward the ulnar aspect (Fig. 7.137).

Dislocations and subluxations of the interphalangeal joints can lead to fractures, but often only soft-tissue injuries are present, especially involving the collateral ligaments (Fig. 7.138).

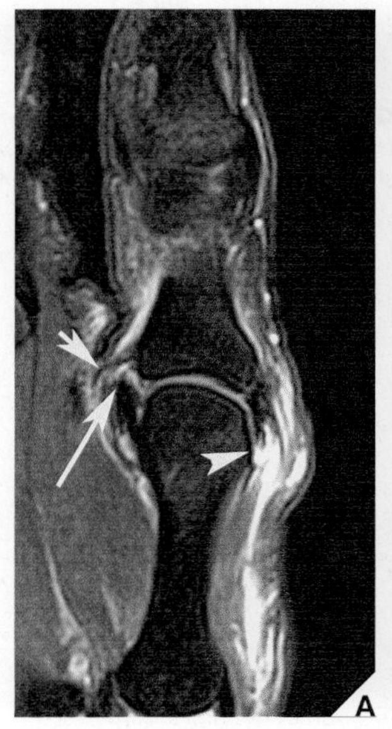

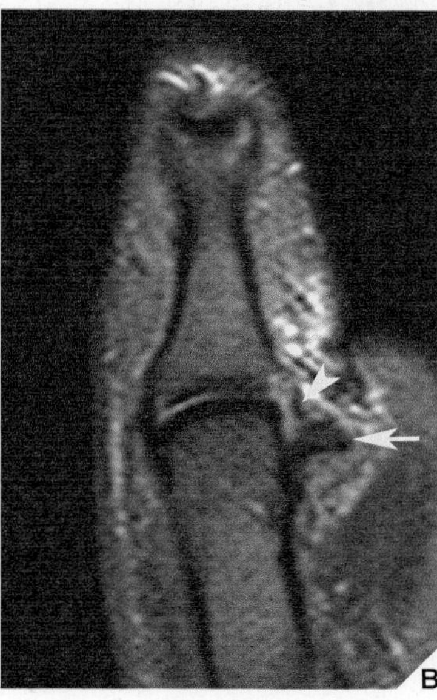

FIGURE 7.131 **MRI of the non-Stener and Stener lesions.** **(A)** ***Non-Stener lesion.*** Coronal STIR MR image demonstrates a tear of the phalangeal insertion of the ulnar collateral ligament *(long arrow)*, which remains under the adductor pollicis aponeurosis *(short arrow)*. Additionally, there is a tear of the metacarpal insertion of the radial collateral ligament *(arrowhead)*. **(B)** ***Stener lesion.*** Note the displaced ulnar collateral ligament oriented perpendicular to the distal first metacarpal *(arrow)*, displaced under the adductor pollicis aponeurosis *(arrowhead)*.

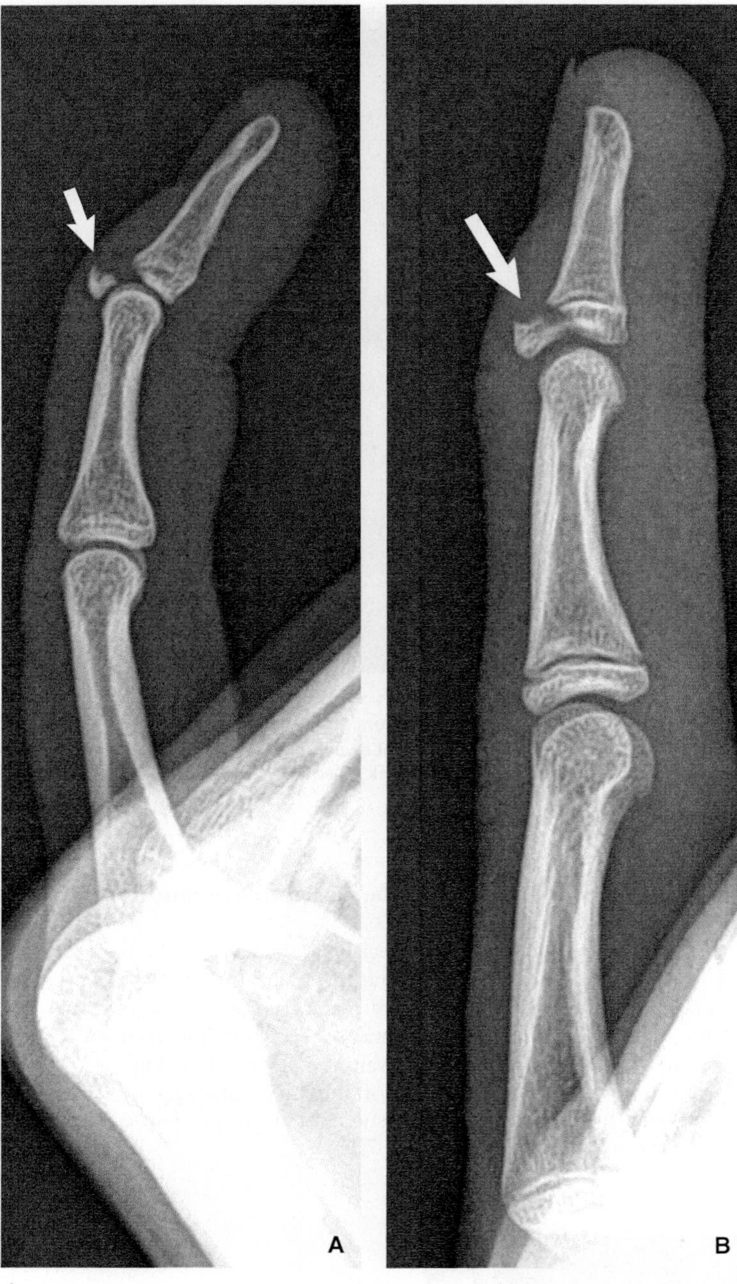

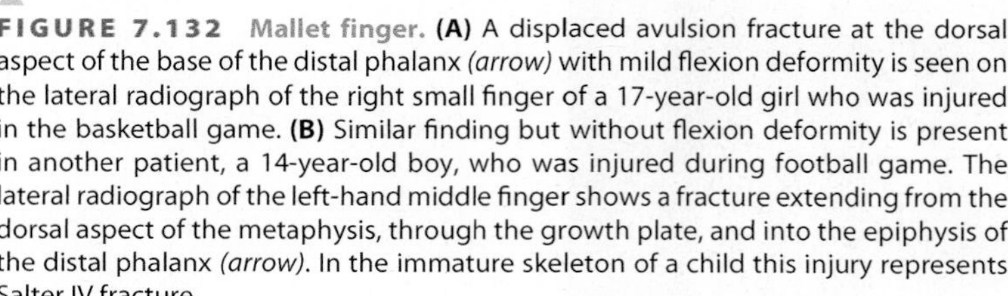

FIGURE 7.132 Mallet finger. **(A)** A displaced avulsion fracture at the dorsal aspect of the base of the distal phalanx *(arrow)* with mild flexion deformity is seen on the lateral radiograph of the right small finger of a 17-year-old girl who was injured in the basketball game. **(B)** Similar finding but without flexion deformity is present in another patient, a 14-year-old boy, who was injured during football game. The lateral radiograph of the left-hand middle finger shows a fracture extending from the dorsal aspect of the metaphysis, through the growth plate, and into the epiphysis of the distal phalanx *(arrow)*. In the immature skeleton of a child this injury represents Salter IV fracture.

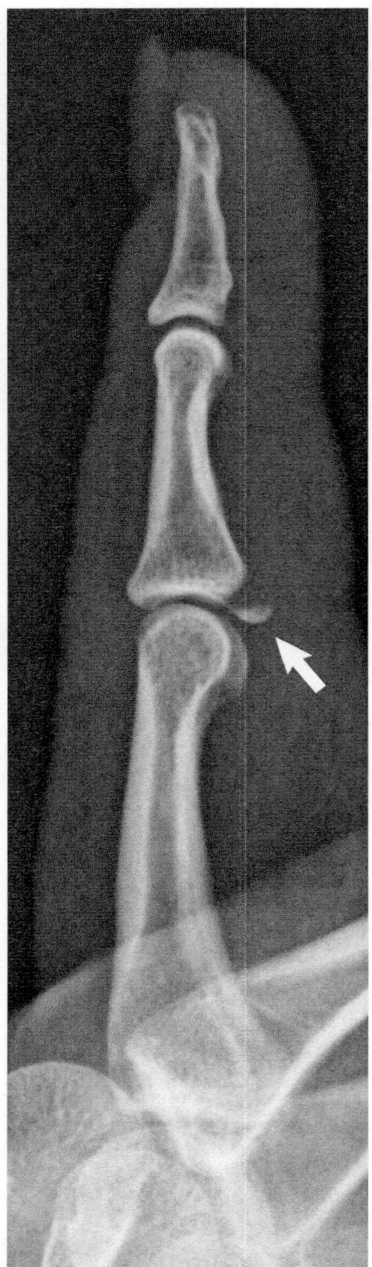

FIGURE 7.133 Volar plate injury. A 54-year-old woman fell to the ground on outstretched hand. Lateral radiograph of the right index finger shows a displaced avulsion fracture of the volar aspect of the base of the middle phalanx *(arrow)*.

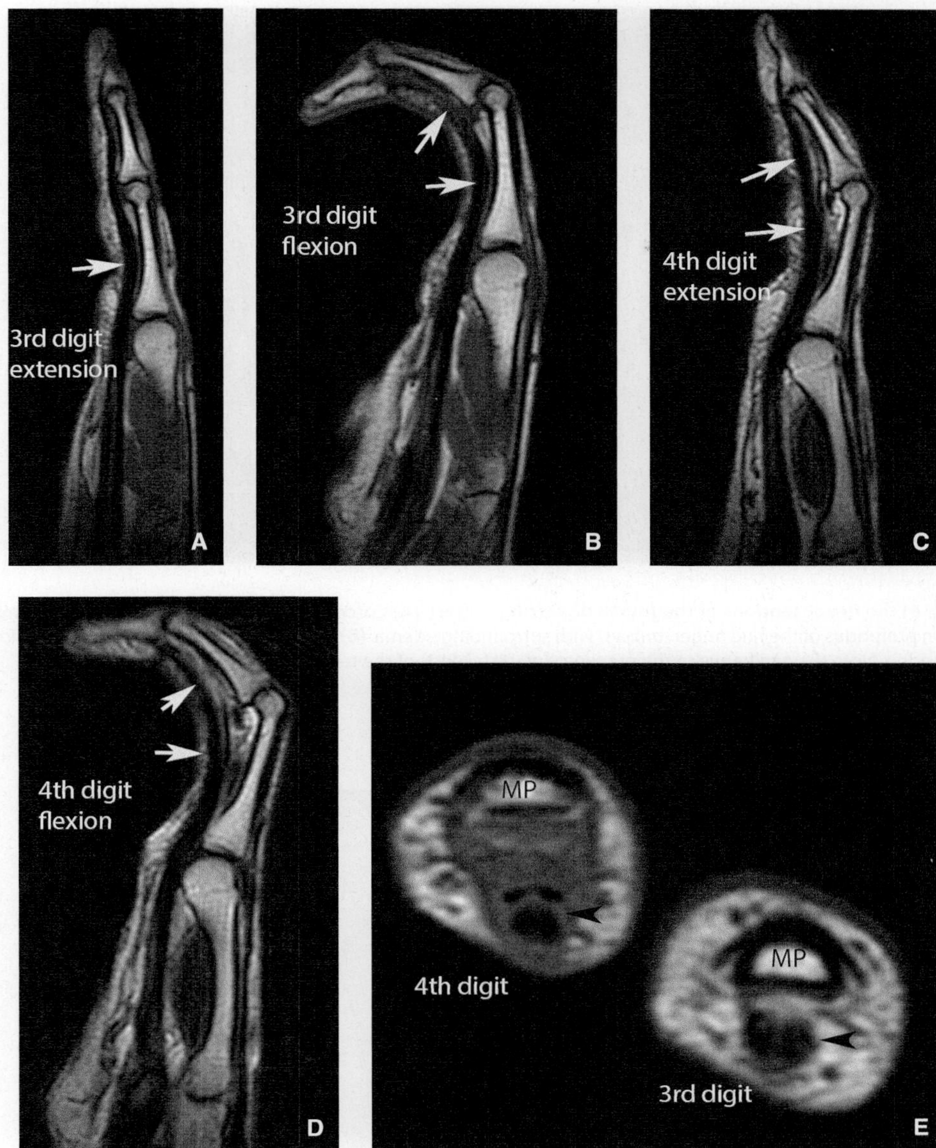

FIGURE 7.134 **Pulley rupture of the flexor tendons (climber's finger).** **(A)** Sagittal T2-weighted MR image of the normal third (middle) finger in extension. Note the normal close distance between the flexor tendons *(arrow)* and the proximal and middle phalanges (MP). **(B)** Sagittal T2-weighted MR image of the same normal third digit in flexion shows the normal distance between the flexor tendons *(arrows)* and the proximal and MP. **(C)** Sagittal T2-weighted MR image of the fourth digit (ring finger) of the same patient on attempted extension. Note the mild flexion at the level of proximal interphalangeal (PIP) joint and increased distance between the flexor tendons *(arrows)* and the proximal and MP. **(D)** Sagittal T2-weighted MR image of the fourth digit of the same patient, in flexion. Note the further increase distance between the flexor tendons *(arrows)* and the proximal and MP ("bowstringing"), reflecting disruption of the A2, A3, A4, C1, and C2 pulleys. **(E)** Axial T1-weighted MR image through the MP of the third and fourth digits demonstrate the increase distance between the flexor tendons *(arrowheads)* and the MP of the fourth digit as compared with the third digit.

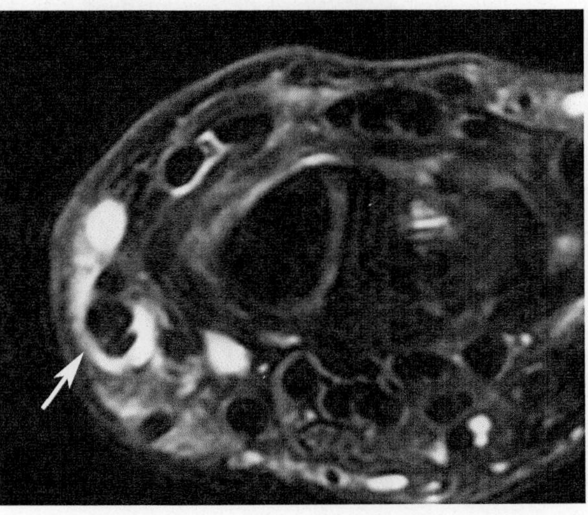

FIGURE 7.135 **de Quervain syndrome.** Axial T2-weighted MRI of the wrist shows tendinosis and tenosynovitis of the abductor pollicis longus and extensor pollicis brevis tendons in the first extensor compartment of the wrist *(arrow)*.

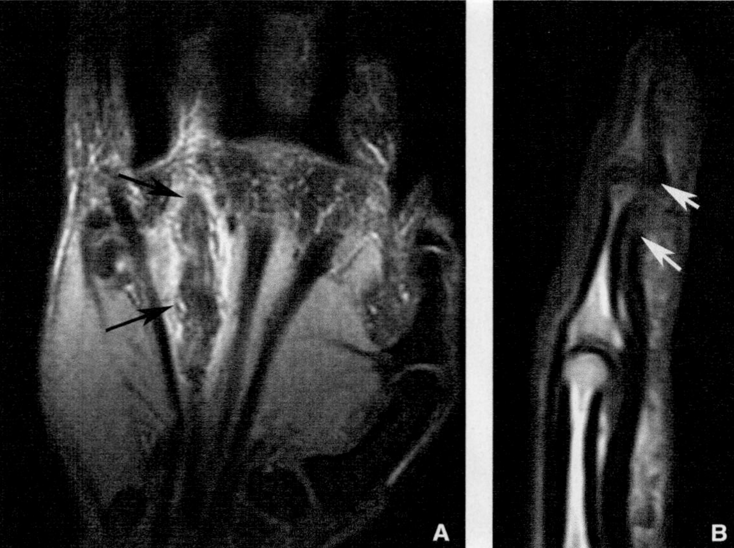

FIGURE 7.136 MRI of the tear of the flexor tendons of the fourth digit (ring finger). **(A)** Coronal T2-weighted fat-suppressed MR image demonstrates the torn and proximally retracted flexor digitorum profundus of the ring finger *(arrows)* with surrounding edema. **(B)** Sagittal T2-weighted MR image in another patient shows a tear of the distal flexor digitorum profundus tendon. Note the gap between the proximal and distal ends of the tendons *(arrows)*.

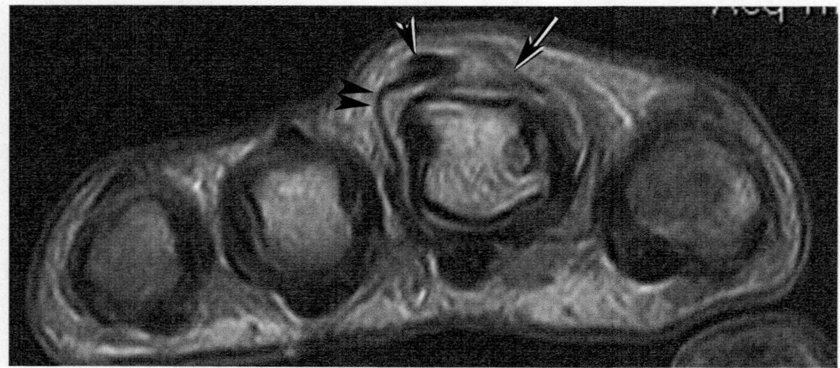

FIGURE 7.137 MRI of the tear of the sagittal band of the third digit (middle finger). Axial T2-weighted MR image shows a tear of the radial aspect of the sagittal band of the middle finger at the level of the head of the third metacarpal *(arrow)*, with ulnar dislocation of the extensor tendon *(arrowheads)*. This injury is characteristic in patients hitting a hard surface with the fist.

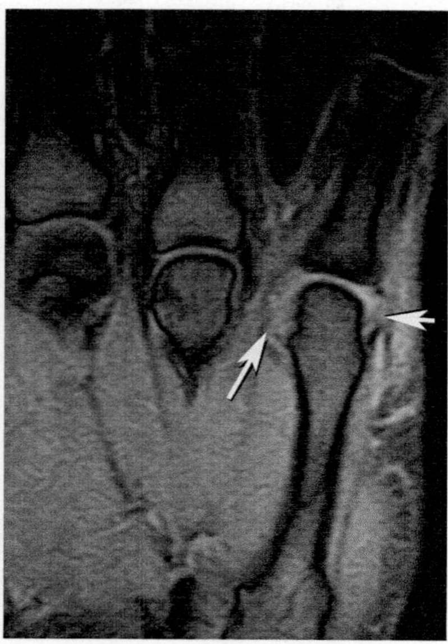

FIGURE 7.138 MRI of the tear of the ulnar and radial collateral ligaments of the fifth digit (small finger). Coronal proton density–weighted fat-suppressed MR image at the level of the metacarpophalangeal (MCP) joint shows a tear of both ulnar and radial collateral ligaments *(arrows)*. Compare with the normal collateral ligaments of the fourth digit (ring finger).

PRACTICAL POINTS TO REMEMBER

Distal Forearm

1. For a full evaluation of trauma on the posteroanterior radiograph of the distal forearm, it is important to recognize:
   - ulnar variance: neutral, negative, and positive
   - the radial angle, which normally ranges from 15 to 25 degrees
   - the radial length.
2. For a full evaluation of trauma on the lateral radiograph of the distal forearm, it is important to recognize the volar tilt of the articular surface of the radius, which normally ranges from 10 to 25 degrees.
3. A complete evaluation of the Colles fracture should take into consideration:
   - the degree of foreshortening of the radius
   - the direction of displacement of the distal fragment
   - intraarticular extension of the fracture line
   - associated fracture of the ulna.
4. Learn to distinguish the Colles fracture from the:
   - Barton fracture, dorsal and volar types, which are best demonstrated on the lateral projection
   - Hutchinson (or chauffeur's) fracture, which is best seen on the posteroanterior view
   - Smith fracture, which is best evaluated on the lateral projection.
5. Frykman classification of distal radius fractures according to the location of the fracture line (intraarticular vs. extraarticular) and association of distal ulna fracture has a practical prognostic value and serves as a guide to orthopaedic management.
6. With the finding of a dislocation in the distal radioulnar articulation, look for an associated fracture of the radius—Galeazzi fracture–dislocation.
7. Learn to distinguish ulnar impingement syndrome from ulnar impaction (ulnolunate abutment) syndrome. The former is caused by short distal ulna that impinges on the distal radius. The latter, frequently associated with positive ulnar variance, leads to compression of the distal ulna on the medial surface of the lunate bone.
8. A common sequela of trauma to the distal radioulnar joint, a tear of the TFCC can be confirmed or excluded by a single-contrast arthrogram of the wrist or MRI examination.

Wrist

1. If clinical history and physical examination are consistent with a scaphoid fracture and routine radiographs appear normal, then either CT or MRI is the next logical step.
2. CT examination is effective in demonstrating and evaluating the so-called *humpback deformity* of the scaphoid.
3. Delayed diagnosis and treatment of a scaphoid fracture may result in nonunion, osteonecrosis, and posttraumatic arthritis (SLAC and SNAC wrist deformity).
4. Triquetral fracture is best diagnosed on the lateral and pronated oblique views of the wrist. If conventional radiographs appear normal, then CT can confirm or exclude the diagnosis.
5. Fractures of the hamate body are best demonstrated on the lateral and pronated oblique projections.
6. In a suspected fracture of the hook of the hamate, look for the oval cortical ring shadow projecting over the hamate on the dorsovolar view of the wrist. If this eye of the hamate is absent, indistinctly outlined, or sclerotic, then hamulus fracture is highly probable.
7. A fracture of the pisiform is best demonstrated on the supinated oblique and carpal tunnel projections.
8. In Kienböck disease, the choice of surgical procedures depends on a demonstration of the integrity of the lunate. MRI may reveal osteonecrosis in the early stages.
9. Hamatolunate impaction syndrome results from an anatomic variant of the lunate bone that has an "extra" facet articulating with the hamate bone. Repeated contact of these bones leads to bone marrow edema and chondromalacia, best demonstrated on MRI.
10. Lunate, perilunate, and midcarpal dislocations are readily identified on the lateral radiographs by disruption of the normal central alignment of the longitudinal axes of the capitate and lunate over the distal radial surface:
    - in lunate dislocation, disruption of the alignment occurs at the lunate
    - in perilunate dislocation, it occurs at the capitate
    - in midcarpal dislocation, it occurs at the site of both bones.
11. In any type of carpal dislocation, look for an associated fracture.
12. If intercarpal instability is suspected and routine radiographs are normal, then fluoroscopy combined with videotaping should be the next examination. If a ligament tear is suspected, then arthrography or MRI should be performed.
13. There are two main types of carpal instability: DISI and VISI.
14. Carpal tunnel syndrome is a compressive neuropathy of the median nerve within the carpal tunnel. MRI will show thickening of the median nerve proximal to the carpal tunnel, flattening of the median nerve in the distal portion of the tunnel, anterior bowing of the flexor retinaculum, and increased signal of the median nerve on T2-weighted images.
15. Guyon canal syndrome is a compressive neuropathy of the ulnar nerve within this canal.
16. Most reliable sign of the AIN syndrome, a clinical complex of defect in the pincer grasp of the thumb and index finger and inability to make a fist, is the edema or atrophy within pronator quadratus muscle demonstrated by MRI.

Hand

1. Learn to distinguish the Bennett and Rolando fractures—intraarticular fractures occurring at the base of the first metacarpal bone—from extraarticular fractures.
2. The Bennett fracture involves a dislocation of most of the first metacarpal and is, therefore, a fracture–dislocation.
3. When evaluating the Rolando fracture—really a comminuted Bennett fracture—exclude the possibility of entrapment of an osseous fragment in the first carpometacarpal joint.
4. In the boxer's fracture, comminution of the volar cortex is often present. It is essential to demonstrate its presence radiographically.
5. In suspected gamekeeper's thumb, obtain an abduction–stress film of the thumb.
6. Disruption, displacement, or entrapment of the ulnar collateral ligament in gamekeeper's thumb can be evaluated on an arthrogram of the first metacarpophalangeal joint.
7. MRI is an effective technique to distinguish between a nondisplaced and a displaced tear (Stener lesion) of the ulnar collateral ligament of the first metacarpophalangeal joint.

Fingers

1. Avulsion fractures of the fingers are common injuries sustained during sports activities. They include fractures of the dorsal plate of the distal phalanx associated with a flexion in the distal interphalangeal joint (mallet finger) and fractures of the volar plate as a result of hyperextension injury.
2. Rock climbers commonly sustain a flexor pulley system rupture (so-called *climber's finger*). MRI provides unique visualization of these injuries.
3. de Quervain syndrome refers to tenosynovitis of the abductor pollicis longus and extensor pollicis brevis tendons caused by chronic overuse. MRI and US are imaging modalities of choice to diagnose this abnormality.

SUGGESTED READINGS

Ali M, Ali M, Mohamed A, et al. The role of ultrasonography in the diagnosis of occult scaphoid fractures. *J Ultrason* 2018;18:325–331.

Andreisek G, Crook DW, Burg D, et al. Peripheral neuropathies of the median, radial, and ulnar nerves: MR imaging features. *Radiographics* 2006;26:1267–1287.

Bado JL. The Monteggia lesion. *Clin Orthop Relat Res* 1967;50:71–86.

Bateni CP, Bartolotta RJ, Richardson ML, et al. Imaging key wrist ligaments: what the surgeon needs the radiologist to know. *AJR Am J Roentgenol* 2013;200:1089–1095.
Bencardino JT, Rosenberg ZS. Entrapment neuropathies of the upper extremity. In: Stoller DW, ed. *Magnetic resonance imaging in orthopaedics and sports medicine*, 3rd ed. Baltimore: Lippincott Williams & Wilkins; 2007:1933–1976.
Bordalo-Rodrigues M, Amin P, Rosenberg ZS. MR imaging of common entrapment neuropathies at the wrist. *Magn Reson Imaging Clin N Am* 2004;12:265–279.
Buck FM, Gheno R, Nico MAC, et al. Ulnomeniscal homologue of the wrist: correlation of anatomic and MR imaging findings. *Radiology* 2009;253:771–779.
Cerezal L, del Piñal F, Abascal F, et al. Imaging findings in ulnar-sided wrist impaction syndromes. *Radiographics* 2002;22:105–121.
Crema MD, Zentner J, Guermazi A, et al. Scapholunate advanced collapse and scaphoid nonunion advanced collapse: MDCT arthrography features. *AJR Am J Roentgenol* 2012;199:W202–W207.
Draghi F, Bortolotto C. Intersection syndrome: ultrasound imaging. *Skeletal Radiol* 2014;43:283–287.
Faccioli N, Foti G, Barillari M, et al. Finger fractures imaging: accuracy of cone-beam computed tomography and multislice computed tomography. *Skeletal Radiol* 2010;39:1087–1095.
Gilula LA. Roentgenographic evaluation of the hand and wrist. In: Weeks PM, ed. *Acute bone and joint injuries of the hand and wrist*. St. Louis: Mosby; 1981:3.
Gilula LA, Weeks PM. Post-traumatic ligamentous instabilities of the wrist. *Radiology* 1978;129:641–651.
Goldfarb CA, Yin Y, Gilula LA, et al. Wrist fractures: what the clinician wants to know. *Radiology* 2001;219:11–28.
Goyal A, Srivastava DN, Ansari T. MRI in de Quervain tenosynovitis: is making the diagnosis sufficient? *AJR Am J Roentgenol* 2018;210:W133–W134.
Gupta P, Lenchik L, Wuertzer SD, et al. High-resolution 3-T MRI of the fingers: review of anatomy and common tendon and ligament injuries. *AJR Am J Roentgenol* 2015;204:W314–W323.
Haims AH, Schweitzer ME, Morrison WB, et al. Limitations of MR imaging in the diagnosis of peripheral tears of the triangular fibrocartilage of the wrist. *AJR Am J Roentgenol* 2002;178:419–422.
Henrichon SS, Foster BH, Shaw C, et al. Dynamic MRI of the wrist in less than 20 seconds: normal midcarpal motion and reader reliability. *Skeletal Radiol* 2020;49:241–248.
Hunter TB, Peltier LF, Lund PJ. Radiologic history exhibit. Musculoskeletal eponyms: who are those guys? *Radiographics* 2000;20:819–836.
Johnson PG, Szabo RM. Angle measurements of the distal radius: a cadaver study. *Skeletal Radiol* 1993;22:243–246.
Johnson RP. The acutely injured wrist and its residuals. *Clin Orthop Relat Res* 1980;(149):33–44.
Kienböck R. Über traumatische Malazie des Mondbeins, und ihre Folgezustande: Entartungsformen und Kompressionsfrakturen. *Fortschr Roentgenstr* 1910;16:77–103.
Lamaris GA, Matthew MK. The diagnosis and management of mallet finger injuries. *Hand (N Y)* 2017;12:223–228.
Lee RKL, Griffith JF, Ng AWH, et al. Imaging of radial wrist pain. I. Imaging modalities and anatomy. *Skeletal Radiol* 2014;43:713–724.
Lee RKL, Ng AWH, Tong CSL, et al. Intrinsic ligament and triangular fibrocartilage complex tears of the wrist: comparison of MDCT arthrography, conventional 3-T MRI, and MRI arthrography. *Skeletal Radiol* 2013;42:1277–1285.
Lichtman DM, Schneider JR, Swafford AF, et al. Ulnar midcarpal instability—clinical and laboratory analysis. *J Hand Surg Am* 1991;6A:515–523.
Lok RLK, Griffith JF, Ng AWH, et al. Imaging of radial wrist pain. Part II: pathology. *Skeletal Radiol* 2014;43:725–743.
Magee T. Comparison of 3-T MRI and arthroscopy of intrinsic wrist ligament and TFCC tears. *AJR Am J Roentgenol* 2009;192:80–85.
Maizlin ZV, Brown JA, Clement JJ, et al. MR arthrography of the wrist: controversies and concepts. *Hand (N Y)* 2009;4:66–73.
Mak WH, Szabo RM, Myo GK. Assessment of volar radiocarpal ligaments: MR arthrographic and arthroscopic correlation. *AJR Am J Roentgenol* 2012;198:423–427.
Manaster BJ. Digital wrist arthrography: precision in determining the size of radiocarpal-midcarpal communication. *AJR Am J Roentgenol* 1986;147:563–566.
Manaster BJ. The clinical efficacy of triple-injection wrist arthrography. *Radiology* 1991;178:267–270.
Martinoli C, Bianchi S, Cotten A. Imaging of rock climbing injuries. *Semin Musculoskelet Radiol* 2005;9:334–345.
Mayfield JK. Mechanism of carpal injuries. *Clin Orthop Relat Res* 1980;(149):45–54.
Milner CS, Manon-Matos Y, Thirkannad SM. Gamekeeper's thumb—a treatment-oriented magnetic resonance imaging classification. *J Hand Surg Am* 2015;40:90–95.
Mitsuyasu H, Patterson RM, Shah MA, et al. The role of the dorsal intercarpal ligament in dynamic and static scapholunate instability. *J Hand Surg Am* 2004;29:279–288.
Norman A, Nelson JM, Green SM. Fractures of the hook of the hamate: radiographic signs. *Radiology* 1985;154:49–53.
Ragheb D, Stanley A, Gentili A, et al. MR imaging of the finger tendons: normal anatomy and commonly encountered pathology. *Eur J Radiol* 2005;56:296–306.
Resnick D. Arthrography and tenography of the hand and wrist. In: Dalinka MK, ed. *Arthrography*. New York: Springer-Verlag; 1980:
Resnick D, Danzig LA. Arthrographic evaluation of injuries of the first metacarpophalangeal joint: gamekeeper's thumb. *AJR Am J Roentgenol* 1976;126:1046–1052.
Scalcione LR, Pathria MN, Chung CB. The athlete's hand: ligament and tendon injury. *Semin Musculoskelet Radiol* 2010;16:338–349.
Shahabpour M, Staelens B, Van Overstraeten L, et al. Advanced imaging of the scapholunate ligamentous complex. *Skeletal Radiol* 2015;44:1709–1725.
Theumann NH, Pessis E, Lecompte M, et al. MR imaging of the metacarpophalangeal joints of the fingers: evaluation of 38 patients with chronic joint disability. *Skeletal Radiol* 2005;34:210–216.
Theumann NH, Pfirrmann CWA, Antonio GE, et al. Extrinsic carpal ligaments: normal MR arthrographic appearance in cadavers. *Radiology* 2003;226:171–179.
Tresley J, Singer AD, Ouellette EA, et al. Multimodality approach to a Stener lesion: radiographic, ultrasound, magnetic resonance imaging, and surgical correlation. *Am J Orthop (Belle Mead NJ)* 2017;46:E195–E199.
Yeager BA, Dalinka MK. Radiology of trauma to the wrist: dislocations, fracture dislocations, and instability patterns. *Skeletal Radiol* 1985;13:120–130.
Yoshioka H, Tanaka T, Ueno T, et al. High-resolution MR imaging of the proximal zone of the lunotriquetral ligament. *Skeletal Radiol* 2006;35:288–294.
Zanetti M, Hodler J, Gilula LA. Assessment of dorsal or ventral intercalated segmental instability configurations of the wrist: reliability of sagittal MR images. *Radiology* 1998;206:339–345.
Zanetti M, Linkous MD, Gilula LA. Characteristics of triangular fibrocartilage defects in symptomatic and contralateral asymptomatic wrists. *Radiology* 2000;216:840–845.

8

Lower Limb I

Pelvic Girdle, Sacrum, and Proximal Femur

Trauma to the Pelvic Girdle

Fractures involving the structures of the pelvic girdle, which are usually sustained in motor vehicle accidents or falls from heights, represent only a small percentage of all skeletal injuries. Their importance, however, lies in the significant morbidity and mortality associated with them, which is usually caused by accompanying injury to the major blood vessels, nerves, and lower urinary tract. Because the clinical signs of pelvic trauma may not always be obvious, radiologic examination is essential to establish a correct diagnosis. Fractures of the acetabulum constitute approximately 20% of all pelvic fractures, and they may or may not be associated with dislocation in the hip joint. Fractures of the proximal (upper) femur, occasionally referred to as *hip fractures*, occur commonly in the elderly, often as a result of minimal injury. They are seen more frequently in women than in men (2:1), with intracapsular fractures of the proximal femur having an even higher female-to-male ratio (5:1).

Anatomic–Radiologic Considerations

The main imaging modalities used in the evaluation of traumatic conditions of the pelvic girdle, acetabulum, and proximal femur include conventional radiography and computed tomography (CT). Other ancillary techniques are also essential for a complete evaluation of concomitant soft-tissue and pelvic–organ injuries: angiography for the pelvic blood vessels and cystourethrography for the lower urinary tract. Radionuclide bone scan and magnetic resonance imaging (MRI) may also be necessary to disclose subtle fractures of the femoral neck and early stages of posttraumatic osteonecrosis of the femoral head.

The standard and special radiographic projections used to evaluate injury to the pelvic girdle and proximal femur include the anteroposterior view of the pelvis, the anterior and posterior oblique views of the pelvis, the anteroposterior view of the hip, and the frog-lateral view of the hip. At times, the groin-lateral or other special projections may also be required.

Most traumatic conditions involving the sacral wings, the iliac bones, the ischium, the pubis, and the femoral head and neck can be evaluated sufficiently on the *anteroposterior* projection of the pelvis and hip (Fig. 8.1). This view also demonstrates an important anatomic relation of the longitudinal axes of the femoral neck and shaft. Normally, the angle formed by these axes ranges from 125 to 135 degrees. This measurement is valuable in determining displacement in femoral neck fractures. A varus configuration is characterized by a decrease in this angle, and a valgus configuration by an increase in this angle (Fig. 8.2). The anteroposterior view, however, is frequently not sufficient to provide adequate evaluation of the entire sacral bone, the sacroiliac joints, and the acetabulum. Demonstration of the sacroiliac joints requires either a posteroanterior projection, which is obtained to greater advantage with 25 to 30 degrees caudal angulation of the radiographic tube, or an anteroposterior view with 30 to 35 degrees cephalad angulation. The latter projection, known as the *Ferguson view*, is also helpful in more effectively evaluating injury to the sacral bone and the pubic and ischial rami (Fig. 8.3). Oblique projections, known as *Judet views*, are necessary to evaluate the acetabulum. The *anterior (internal) oblique* projection helps delineate the iliopubic (anterior) column and the posterior lip (rim) of the acetabulum (Fig. 8.4). The *posterior (external) oblique* projection delineates the ilioischial (posterior) column and the anterior acetabular rim (Fig. 8.5). Of value in demonstrating the structures of the proximal femur and hip, the *frog-lateral* projection allows adequate evaluation of fractures of the femoral head and the greater and the lesser trochanters (Fig. 8.6). Demonstration of the anterior and posterior aspects of the femoral head as well as the anterior rim of the acetabulum may require a *groin-lateral* projection of the hip, which is particularly useful in evaluating anterior or posterior displacement of fragments in proximal femoral fractures and the degree of rotation of the femoral head. This projection, by providing an almost true lateral image of the proximal femur, also demonstrates an important anatomic feature, the angle of anteversion of the femoral neck, which normally ranges from 25 to 30 degrees (Fig. 8.7). *The Dunn-lateral* view of the hip (Fig. 8.8) and *false-profile* view (Fig. 8.9) are occasionally obtained to analyze morphology of the femoral head/neck junction in the setting of femoroacetabular impingement (FAI) and to assess acetabular coverage of the femoral head.

Ancillary imaging techniques play a crucial role in the evaluation of traumatic conditions of the pelvis and acetabulum, providing essential and often otherwise unobtainable information that helps the orthopaedic surgeon determine the method of treatment and assess the prognosis of pelvic and acetabular fractures. Because the surgical management of such fractures is based on the stability of the fragments and the presence or absence of intraarticular extension of the fracture line and intraarticular fragments, CT examination is necessary to provide information that is not available from the standard and special projections of conventional radiography (Fig. 8.10; see also Figs. 8.23 to 8.25). In addition to ascertaining the size, number, and position of the major fragments and data about the condition of the weight-bearing parts of the joint and the configuration of the fracture fragments, CT can delineate soft-tissue and concomitant injury to soft-tissue structures. However, in cases of severe injury when immediate surgical intervention is required, obtaining CT scans may be time-consuming and impractical. In such cases, conventional radiographs can be obtained more quickly, allowing more rapid recognition of the type of injury. CT is particularly effective in the postsurgical assessment of the alignment of fragments and fracture healing.

MRI and magnetic resonance arthrography (MRa) are the modalities of choice for the evaluation of multiple intracapsular and extracapsular conditions of the hip. Knowledge of the normal anatomy is important for proper understanding of the pathologic processes that may involve the hip (Fig 8.11).

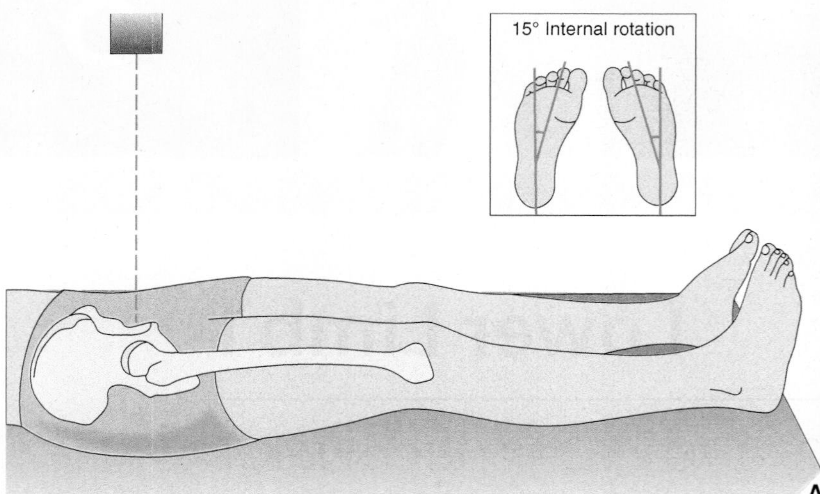

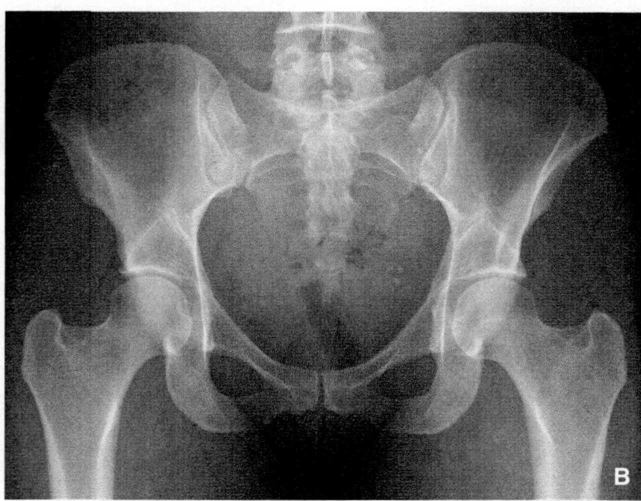

FIGURE 8.1 **Anteroposterior view.** **(A)** For the anteroposterior view of the pelvis and hip, the patient is supine with the feet in slight (15 degrees) internal rotation *(inset)*, which compensates for the normal anteversion of the femoral neck (see Fig. 8.7B), elongating its image. For a view of the entire pelvis, the central beam *(red broken line)* is directed vertically toward the midportion of the pelvis; for selective examination of either hip joint, it is directed toward the affected femoral head. **(B)** The radiograph in this projection demonstrates the iliac bones, the sacrum, the pubis, and the ischium as well as the femoral heads and necks and both the greater and the lesser trochanters. The acetabula are partially obscured by the overlying femoral heads, and the sacroiliac joints are seen *en face*.

MRI offers superior capabilities for evaluating traumatic conditions of the hip. In particular, it has been shown to provide a rapid, precise, and cost-effective diagnosis of radiographically occult hip fractures and may help reveal traumatic lesions such as bone contusions (trabecular microfractures) as the cause of hip pain when the history of trauma is unknown. MRI is also effective in the diagnosis of posttraumatic osteonecrosis of the femoral head and can identify and quantify the muscle injury and joint effusion/hemarthrosis that invariably accompany traumatic anterior and posterior dislocation in the hip joint (see Figs. 4.133 and 4.134).

The urinary system is frequently at risk in pelvic fractures. Bladder injuries have been reported in 6% and urethral injuries in 10% of patients with pelvic fractures. The evaluation of such conditions requires contrast examination of the urinary system by means of CT, intravenous urography (intravenous pyelogram [IVP]), and cystourethrography. Pelvic arteriography and venography may also be required to evaluate injury to the vascular system. In addition to its diagnostic value, arteriography can be combined with an interventional procedure, such as embolization, to control hemorrhage.

For a summary of the preceding discussion in tabular form, see Tables 8.1 and 8.2.

Injury to the Pelvis and Acetabulum

The pelvis is a nearly rigid ring essentially comprising three elements: the sacrum and two paired lateral components, each composed of the ilium, the ischium, and the pubis. Because of this configuration and the interrelationship of its components, identification of an apparently solitary fracture should not end the process of radiographic examination. The pelvis should be scrutinized carefully for other fractures of the ring or diastasis in the sacroiliac joints or the pubic symphysis (see Fig. 4.7).

Classification of Pelvic Fractures

Various classification systems have been proposed not only to identify the distinctive appearances of pelvic injuries as an aid to radiographic recognition and diagnosis but also to categorize such injuries as an aid to orthopaedic management and prognosis. The latter point is particularly important in pelvic fractures because of the inherent instability of the structures composing the pelvic girdle, their integrity depending entirely on ligamentous support, and the stabilizing influence of the sacroiliac joints. Thus, pelvic fractures can be grouped according to whether they significantly detract from the stability of the pelvic ring, with the orthopaedic

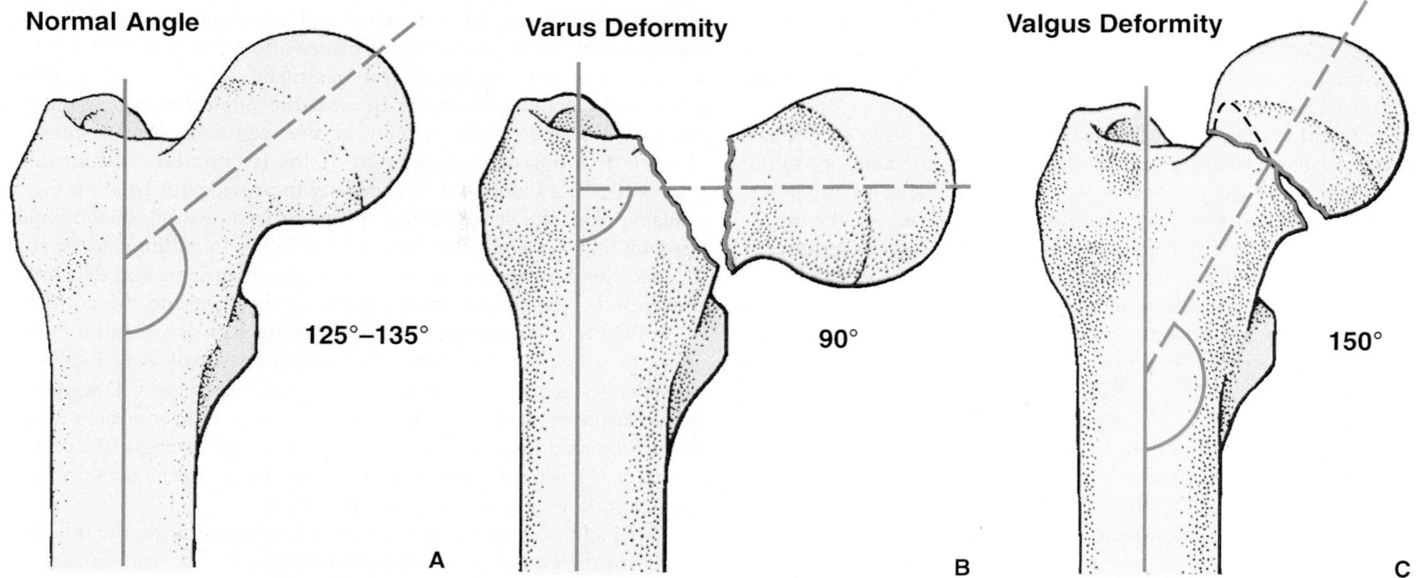

FIGURE 8.2 **Femoral shaft and neck angles.** **(A)** The angle formed by the longitudinal axes of the femoral shaft and neck normally ranges from 125 to 135 degrees. In the evaluation of displacement in femoral neck fractures, a decrease in this angle **(B)** is known as a *varus deformity*, whereas an increase **(C)** characterizes a *valgus deformity*.

FIGURE 8.3 Ferguson view. **(A)** For the angled anteroposterior (Ferguson) view of the pelvis, the patient is in the same position as for the standard anteroposterior projection. The radiographic tube, however, is angled approximately 30 to 35 degrees cephalad, and the central beam *(red broken line)* is directed toward the midportion of the pelvis. **(B)** The radiograph in this projection provides a tangential view of the sacroiliac joints and the sacral bone. The pubic and ischial rami are also well demonstrated.

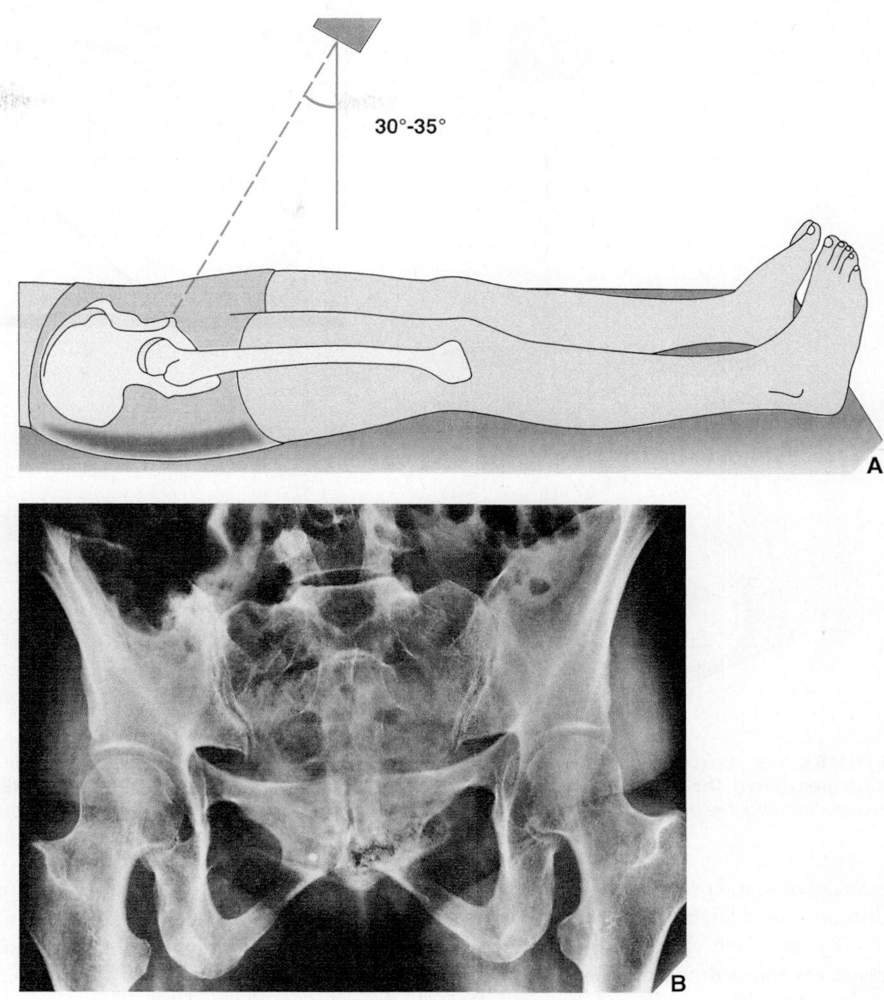

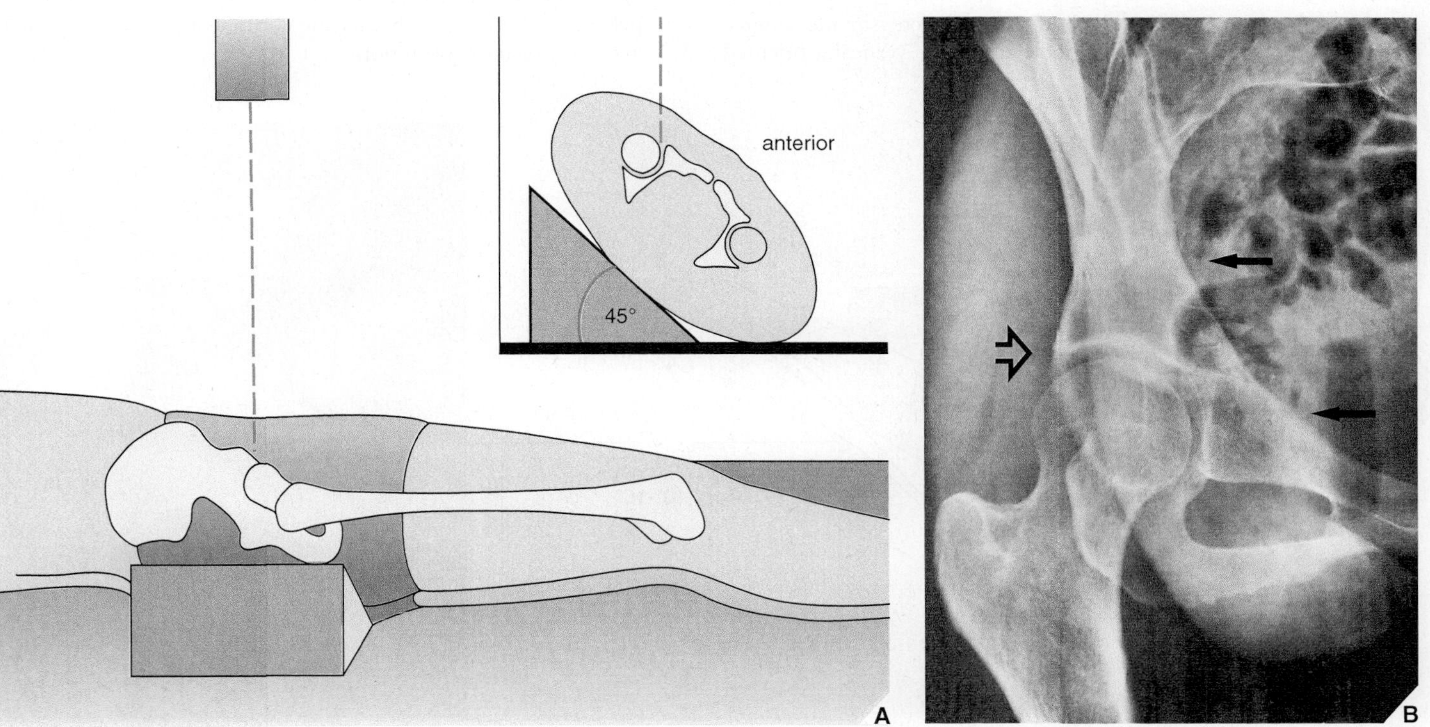

FIGURE 8.4 Anterior oblique view. **(A)** For the anterior oblique (Judet) view of the pelvis, the patient is supine and anteriorly rotated, with the affected hip elevated 45 degrees *(inset)*. The central beam *(red broken line)* is directed vertically toward the affected hip. **(B)** On the radiograph in this projection, the iliopubic (anterior) column *(arrows)* (see Fig. 8.20B) and the posterior lip (rim) of the acetabulum *(open arrow)* are well delineated.

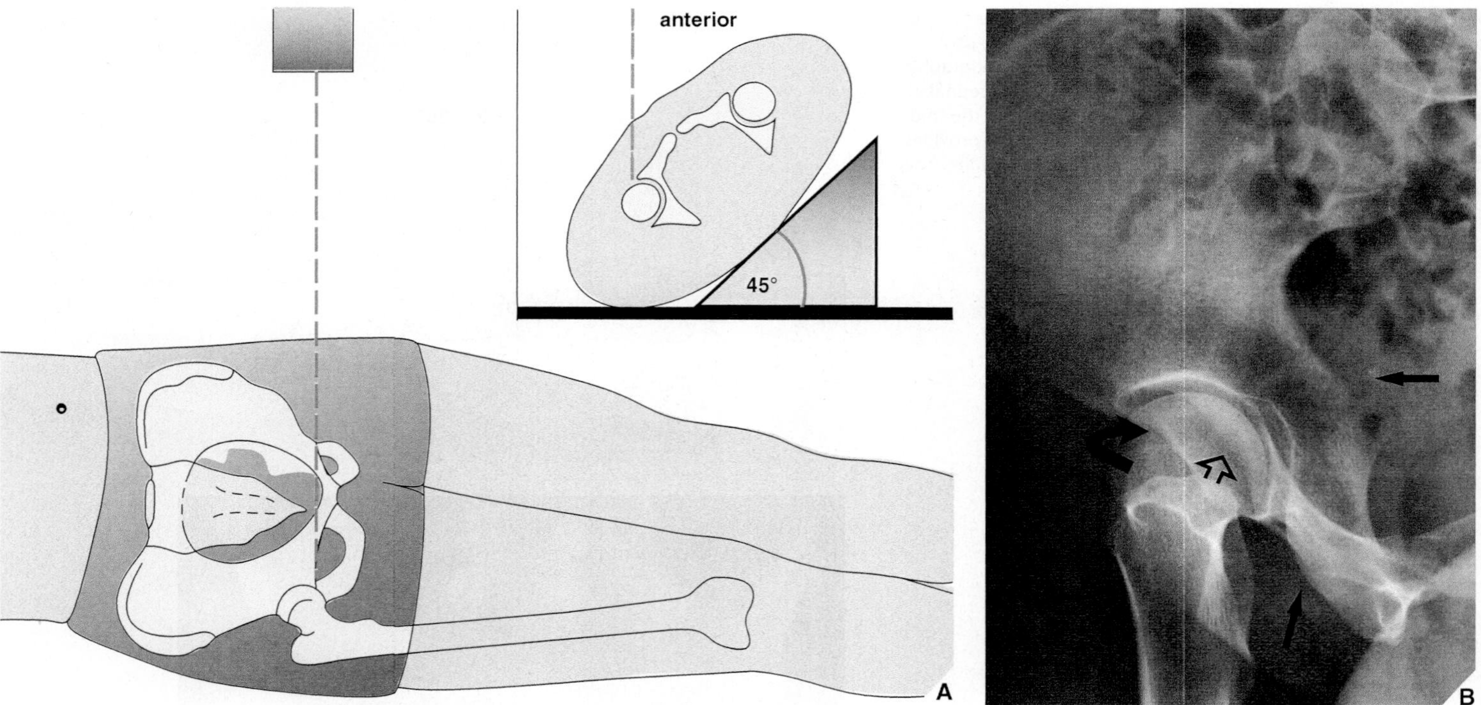

FIGURE 8.5 Posterior oblique view. **(A)** For the posterior oblique (Judet) view of the pelvis, the patient is supine and anteriorly rotated, with the unaffected hip elevated 45 degrees *(inset)*. The central beam *(red broken line)* is directed vertically through the affected hip. **(B)** On the radiograph obtained in this projection, the ilioischial (posterior) column *(arrows)*, the posterior acetabular lip *(open arrow)*, and the anterior acetabular rim *(curved arrow)* are well demonstrated.

management and prognosis of those fractures identified as stable (Fig. 8.12), differing considerably from that of unstable fractures (Fig. 8.13).

Systems that classify pelvic injuries for the purpose of radiographic diagnosis and orthopaedic management using categories other than stable and unstable have also been suggested. Pennal and colleagues have elaborated a system based on the direction of the force that produces pelvic injuries. They identified four patterns of force as underlying mechanisms of injury that produce distinctive radiographic appearances:

1. *Anteroposterior compression*, in which the force vector in the anteroposterior or posteroanterior direction produces vertically oriented fractures of the pubic rami and disruption of the pubic symphysis and sacroiliac joints, which often results in bilateral pelvic "dislocation" (sprung pelvis, "open book" injury)
2. *Lateral compression*, in which the lateral force vector often results in horizontally or coronally oriented fractures of the pubic rami, compression fractures of the sacrum, fractures of the iliac wings, and central dislocation in the hip joint as well as varying degrees of pelvic instability caused by displacement or rotation of one or both hemipelves, depending on whether the compressive force is applied more anteriorly or more posteriorly

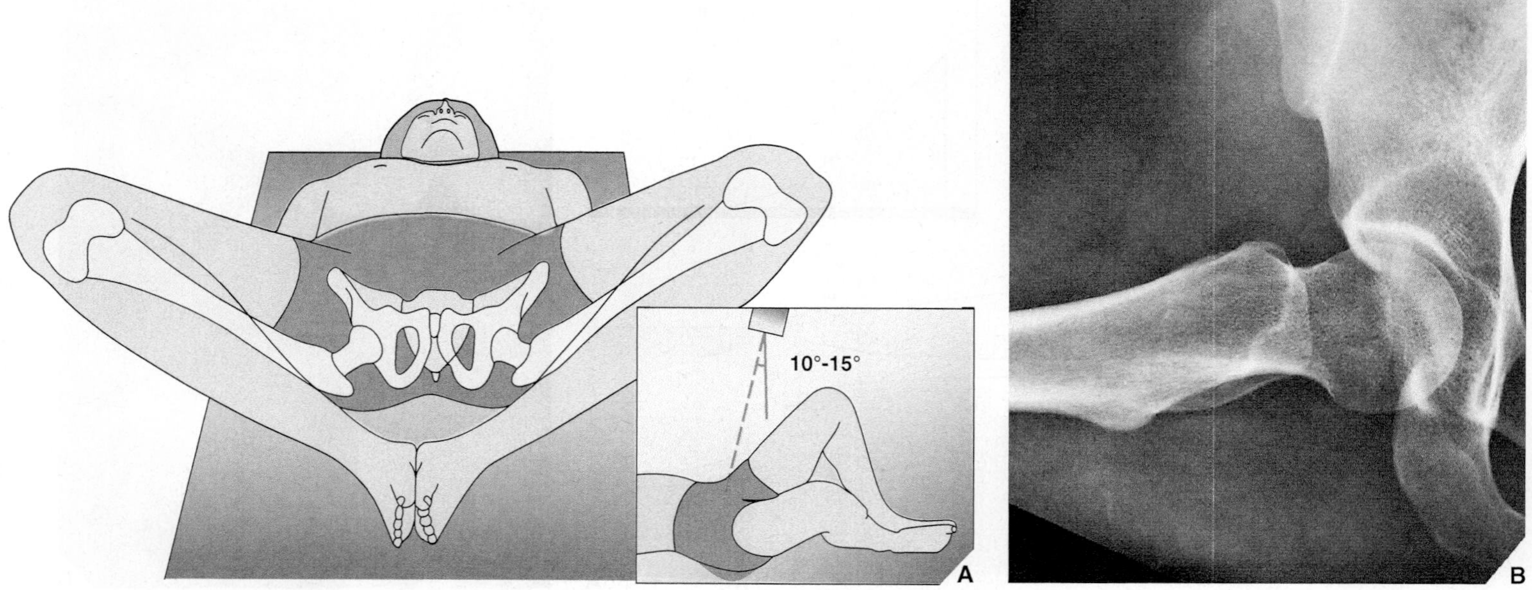

FIGURE 8.6 Frog-lateral view. **(A)** For the frog-lateral view of the proximal femur and hip, the patient is supine with the knees flexed, the soles of the feet together, and the thighs maximally abducted. For simultaneous imaging of both hips, the central beam *(red broken line)* is directed vertically or with 10 to 15 degrees cephalad angulation to a point slightly above the pubic symphysis *(inset)*; for selective examination of one hip, it is directed toward the affected hip joint. **(B)** The radiograph obtained in this projection demonstrates the lateral aspect of the femoral head and both trochanters.

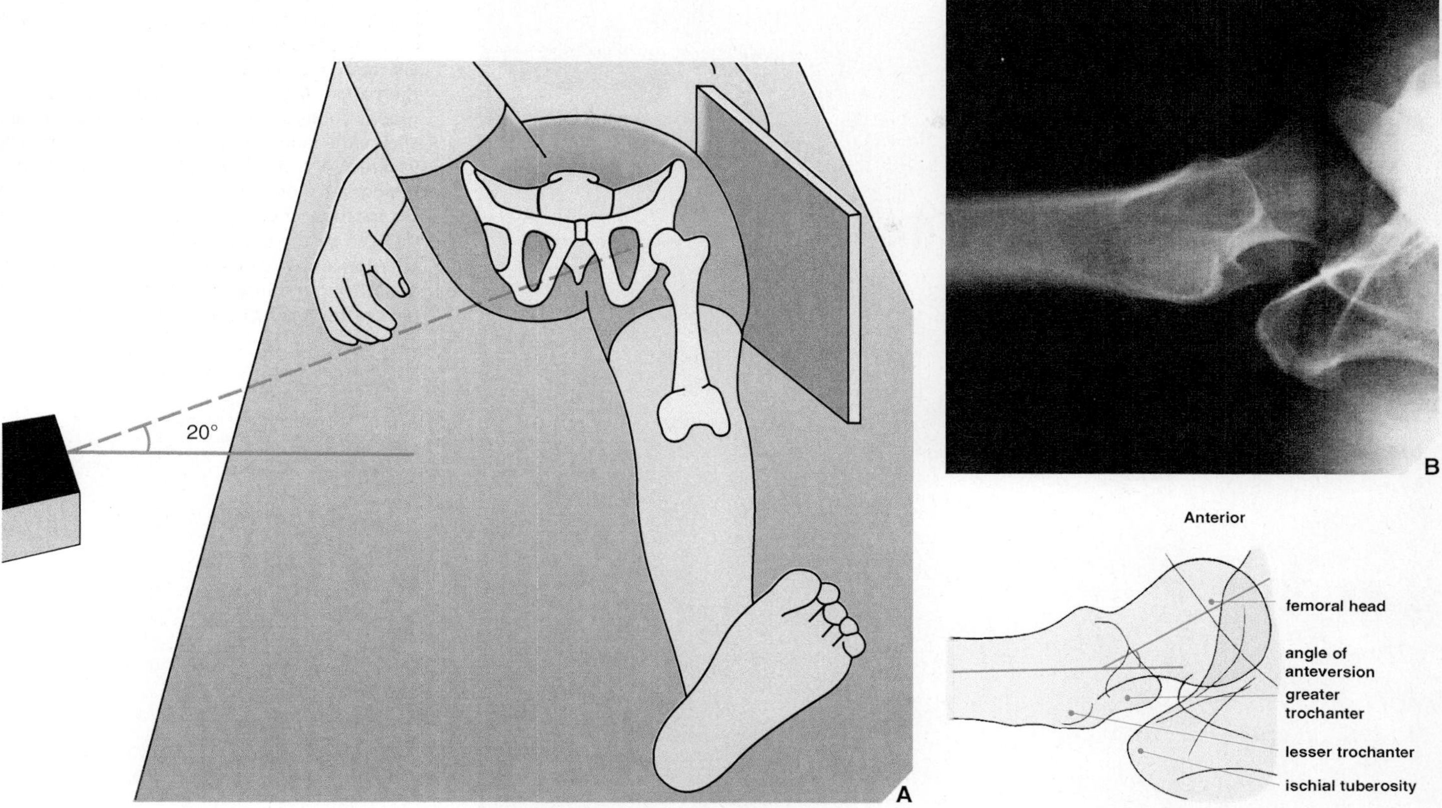

FIGURE 8.7 Groin-lateral view. **(A)** For the groin-lateral view of the hip, the patient is supine with the affected extremity extended and the opposite leg elevated and abducted. The cassette is placed against the affected hip on the lateral aspect, and the central beam *(red broken line)* is directed horizontally toward the groin with approximately 20 degrees cephalad angulation. **(B)** The radiograph obtained in this projection provides almost a true lateral image of the femoral head, thereby allowing evaluation of its anterior and posterior aspects. It also demonstrates the anteversion of the femoral neck, which normally ranges from 25 to 30 degrees.

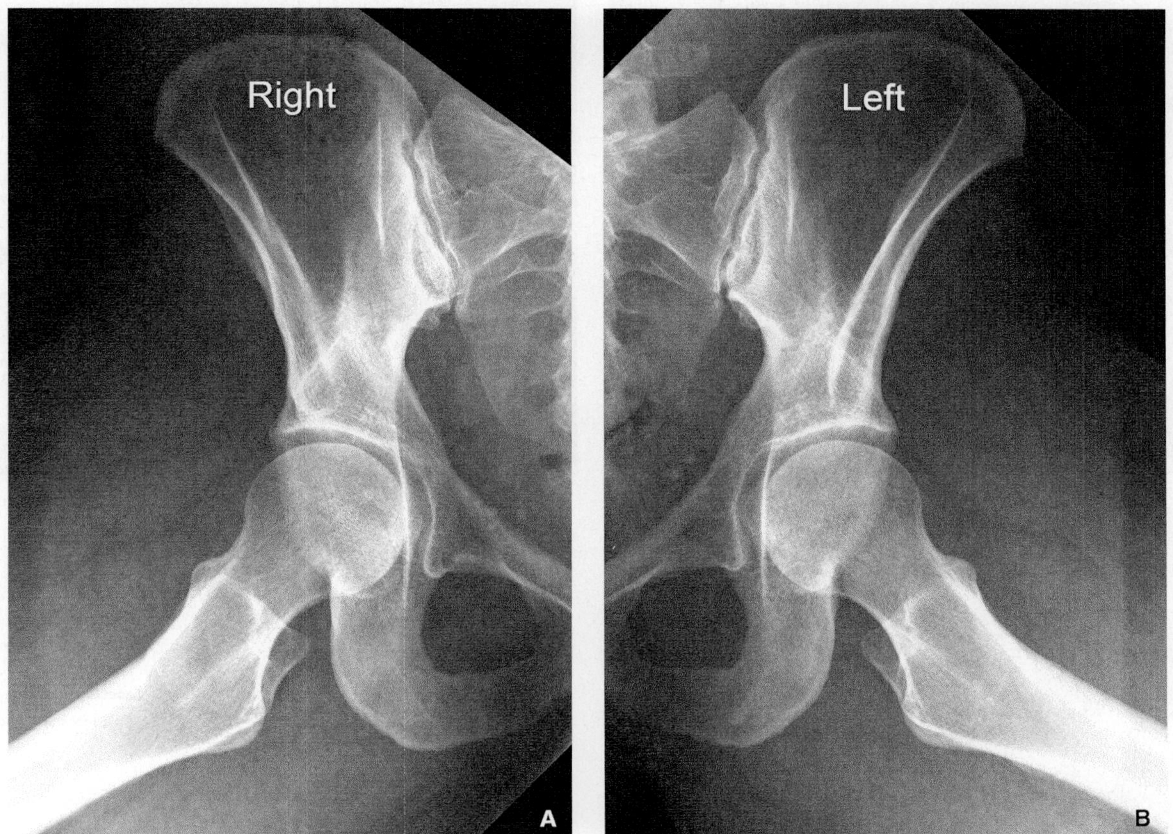

FIGURE 8.8 Dunn-lateral view. For this projection of the hip, the patient is supine with the radiographed hip flexed 90 degrees and abducted 20 degrees. The central beam is directed at a point midway between the anterior superior iliac spine and the symphysis pubis. The similar radiograph may be obtained with hip flexed only to 45 degrees. **(A,B)** The radiographs obtained in this projection clearly demonstrate the femoral head/neck junction and the shape of the femoral head (spherical or aspherical).

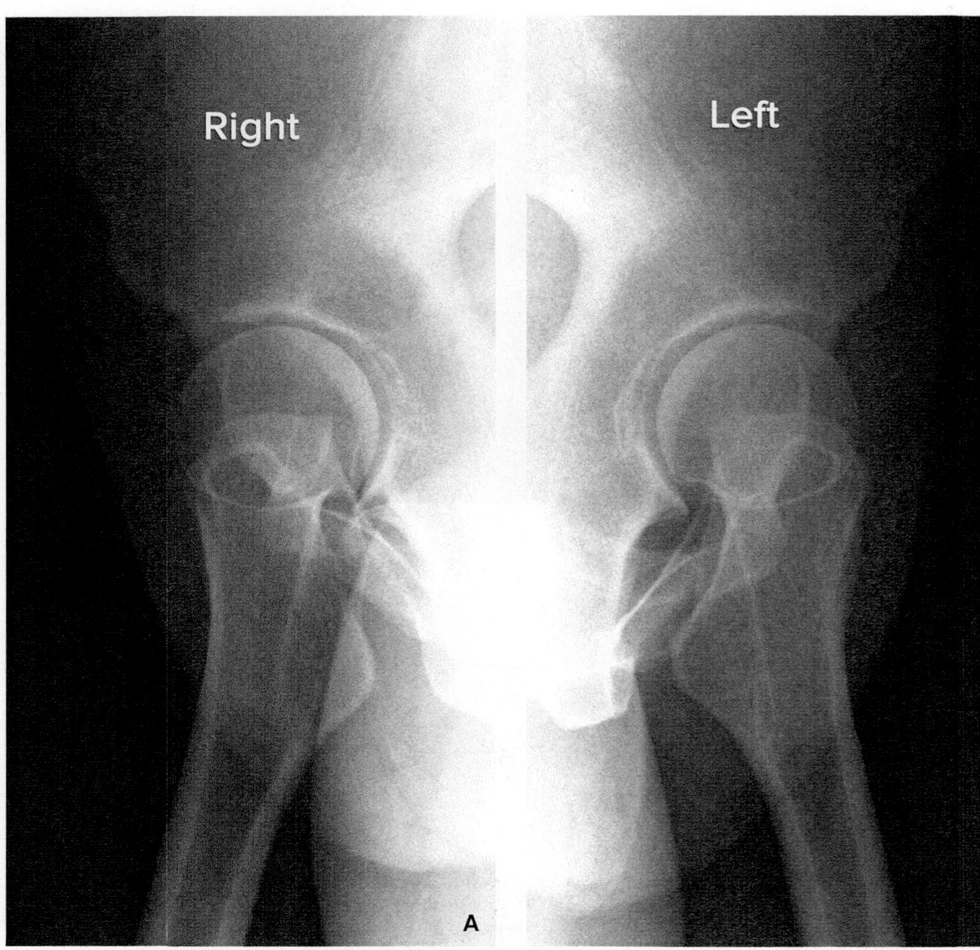

FIGURE 8.9 False-profile view. This view is obtained with the patient in a standing position with the affected hip against the cassette, the pelvis rotated 25 degrees backward, so the back of the patient is at 65 degrees angle with the radiographic table, and the foot on the affected side parallel to the radiographic cassette. The central beam is directed toward the femoral head. **(A,B)** The radiographs obtained in this projection clearly demonstrate the degree of coverage of the femoral head by the bony acetabulum. In addition, the anterior center-edge angle (or angle of Lequesne) quantifying the anterior acetabular coverage of the femoral head can be calculated.

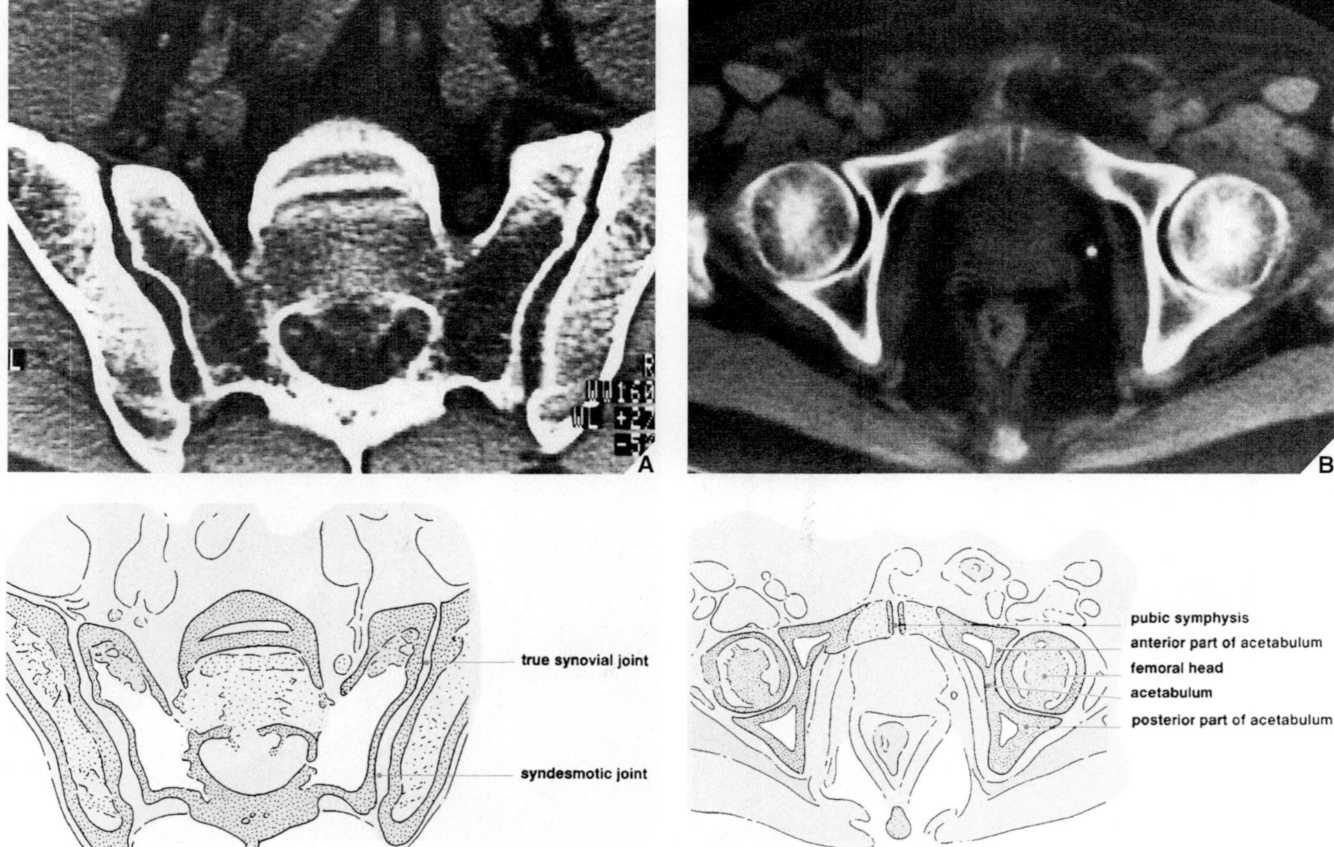

FIGURE 8.10 CT of the sacroiliac and hip joints. **(A)** CT section at the level of S2 demonstrates the true (synovial) sacroiliac joints. **(B)** In this section through the hip joints, the relation of the femoral heads to the acetabula can be evaluated sufficiently. The pubic bone and the pubic symphysis are also well delineated.

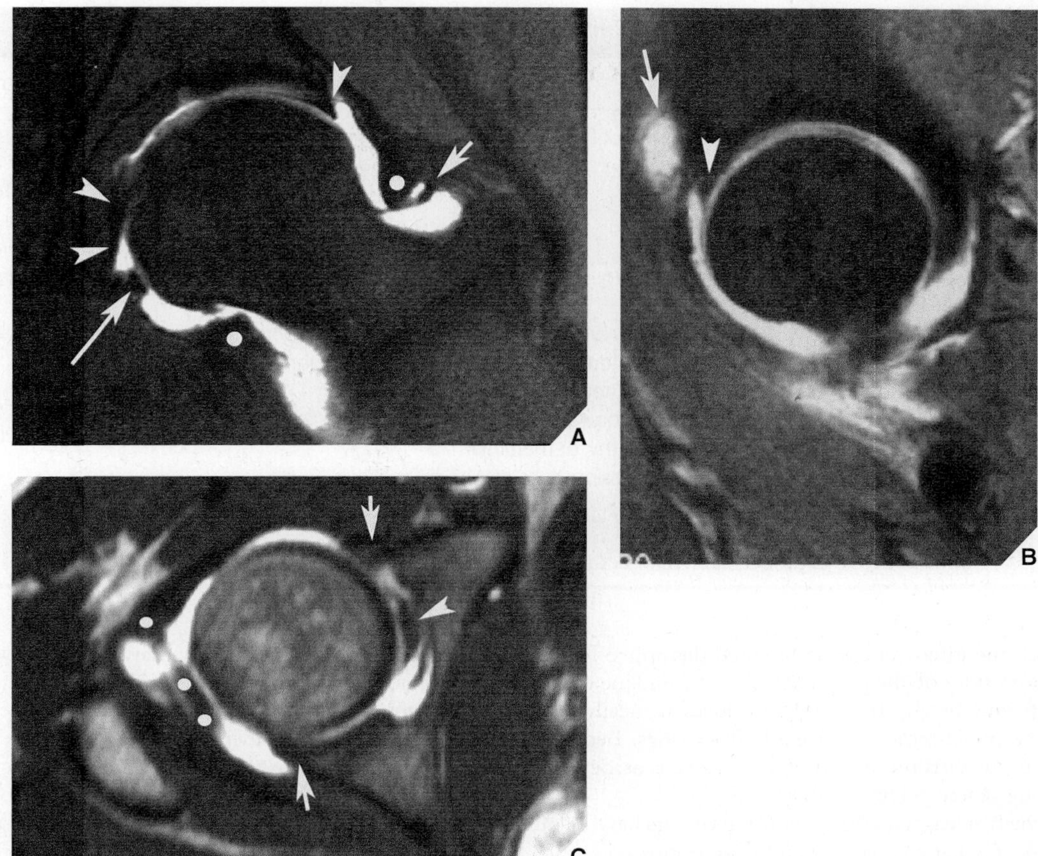

FIGURE 8.11 **Normal MRa of the hip. (A)** Coronal T1-weighted fat-saturated MRa demonstrates the normal superior labrum *(single arrowhead)*, the ligamentum teres *(double arrowheads)*, the orbicular zone *(white dots)*, the transverse ligament *(long arrow)*, and the superior retinaculum *(short arrow)*. **(B)** Sagittal T1-weighted fat-saturated MRa demonstrates the superior labrum *(arrowhead)* and a small amount of contrast material in the iliopsoas bursa *(arrow)*, a feature seen in about 15% of the normal population. **(C)** Axial T1-weighted MRa demonstrates the ligamentum teres *(arrowhead)*, the orbicular zone *(white dots)*, and the anterior and posterior labrum *(arrows)*.

TABLE 8.1 Standard and Special Radiographic Projections for Evaluating Injury to the Pelvis, Acetabulum, Sacrum, and Proximal Femur

Projection	Demonstration	Projection	Demonstration
Anteroposterior	Angle of femoral neck	*Oblique* (Judet views)	
	Radiographic landmarks (lines) relating to acetabulum:	Anterior (internal)	Iliopubic line
	Iliopubic (iliopectineal)		Fractures of
	Ilioischial		Anterior (iliopubic) column
			Posterior acetabular rim
	Teardrop	Posterior (external)	Quadrilateral plate
	Acetabular roof		Fractures of
	Anterior acetabular rim		Posterior (ilioischial) column
	Posterior acetabular rim		Anterior acetabular rim
	Varus and valgus deformities	*Frog-lateral*	Fractures of
	Avulsion fractures		Femoral head and neck
	Malgaigne fracture		Greater and lesser trochanters
	Fractures of	*Groin-lateral*	Angle of anteversion of femoral head
	Ilium (Duverney)		Anterior and posterior cortices of femoral neck
	Ischium		
	Pubis		Ischial tuberosity
	Sacrum (in some cases)		Rotation and displacement of femoral head in subcapital fractures
	Femoral head and neck		
	Dislocations in hip joint		
With 30–35 degrees cephalad angulation (Ferguson) (or posteroanterior with or without 25–30 degrees caudal angulation)	Fractures of		
	Sacrum		
	Pubis ramus		
	Ischium		
	Injury to sacroiliac joints		

TABLE 8.2 Ancillary Imaging Techniques for Evaluating Injury to the Pelvis, Acetabulum, and Proximal Femur

Technique	Demonstration	Technique	Demonstration
Computed tomography (CT) including three-dimensional (3D) CT	Position of fragments and extension of fracture line in complex fractures, particularly of pelvis, acetabulum, and sacrum Weight-bearing parts of joints Sacroiliac joints Intraarticular fragments Soft-tissue injuries Concomitant injury to ureters, urinary bladder, and urethra	*CT-angiography* *Radionuclide imaging* (scintigraphy, bone scan) *Intravenous pyelogram, intravenous urography* *Cystourethrography* *Angiography* (arteriography, venography)	Injury to the vascular system Occult fractures Stress fractures Posttraumatic osteonecrosis Concomitant injury to ureters, urinary bladder, and urethra Injury to vascular system
Magnetic resonance imaging (MRI)	Soft-tissue injuries, including various tendon abnormalities, compressive and entrapment neuropathies (piriformis syndrome, iliacus syndrome, obturator neuropathy, lateral femoral cutaneous neuropathy, or meralgia paresthetica), and Morel-Lavallée lesion Posttraumatic osteonecrosis Occult fractures Bone contusions (trabecular microfractures)		

3. *Vertical shear*, in which the inferosuperiorly oriented disruptive force, delivered to one or both sides of the pelvis lateral to the midline often as a result of a fall from a height, frequently produces vertically oriented fractures of the pubic rami, sacrum, and iliac wings. Because of significant ligamentous disruption, this type of force is associated with injuries producing severe pelvic instability.
4. *Complex patterns*, in which at least two different force vectors have been delivered to the pelvis, the patterns produced by anteroposterior and lateral compression being the most commonly encountered

This system, which corresponds to the more traditional categorization of pelvic fractures into stable and unstable, has practical value in allowing sufficient evaluation of pelvic injuries to be made on the anteroposterior projection in patients requiring immediate surgical intervention when CT scans would be impractical to obtain. It also provides correlations between the type of force delivered to the pelvis and the concomitant ligamentous and pelvic–organ injury that can be expected. In anteroposterior compression-type injuries, for example, the anterior sacroiliac ligaments, the sacrotuberous–sacroiliac ligament complex, and the symphysis ligaments are damaged. This type of injury may also be associated with urethral and urinary bladder rupture and damage to the pelvic blood vessels. In lateral compression injuries, rupture of the posterior sacroiliac ligament and/or the sacrospinous–sacrotuberous ligament complex may result. Injury to the urinary tract may or may not be present. In vertical shear injuries, the ipsilateral posterior and anterior sacroiliac, the sacrospinous–sacrotuberous, and the anterior symphysis ligaments are usually ruptured. Vertical shear injuries are frequently accompanied by damage to the sciatic nerve and pelvic blood vessels, often resulting in massive hemorrhage. The discussion that follows, however, focuses on the more traditional pedagogic categories of pelvic trauma.

Fractures of the Pelvis

Avulsion Fractures

Usually involving the anterosuperior or anteroinferior iliac spine or the ischial tuberosity, avulsion fractures, which are classified as stable fractures (Fig. 8.14; see also Fig. 8.12), most commonly occur in athletes as a result of forcible muscular contraction: the *sartorius* muscle and *tensor*

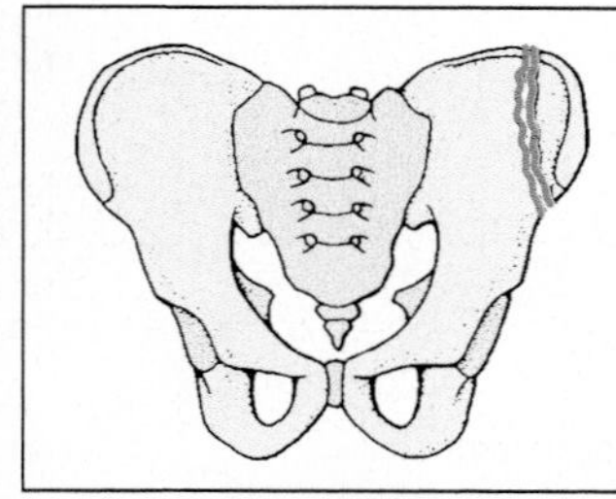

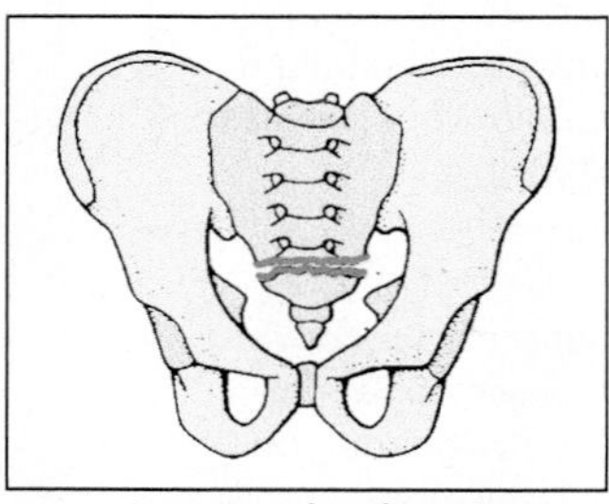

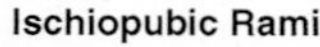

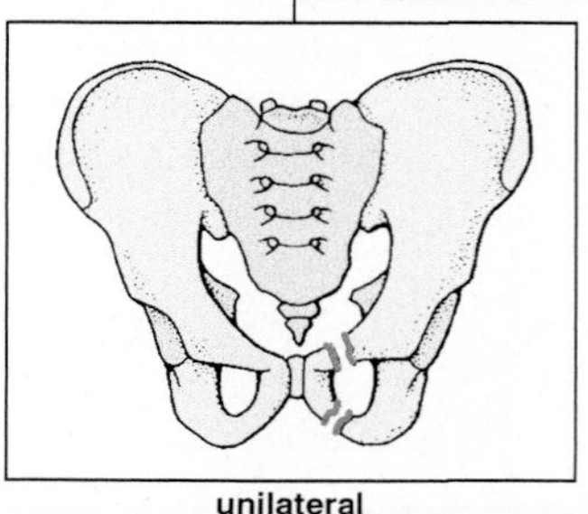

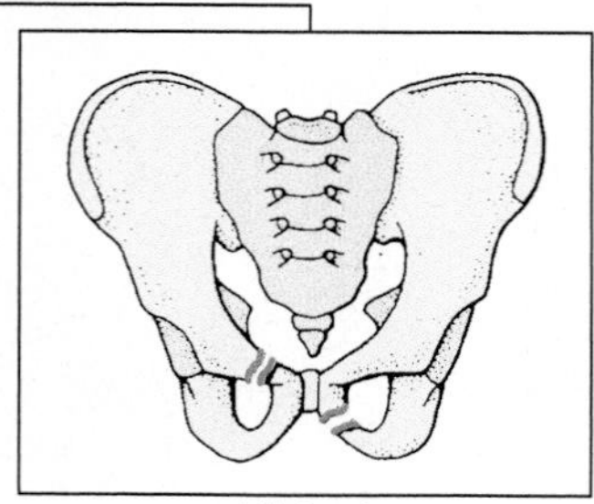

FIGURE 8.12 Stable pelvic fractures. (Modified with permission from Dunn AW, Morris HD. Fractures and dislocations of the pelvis. *J Bone Joint Surg Am* 1968;50:1639–1648.)

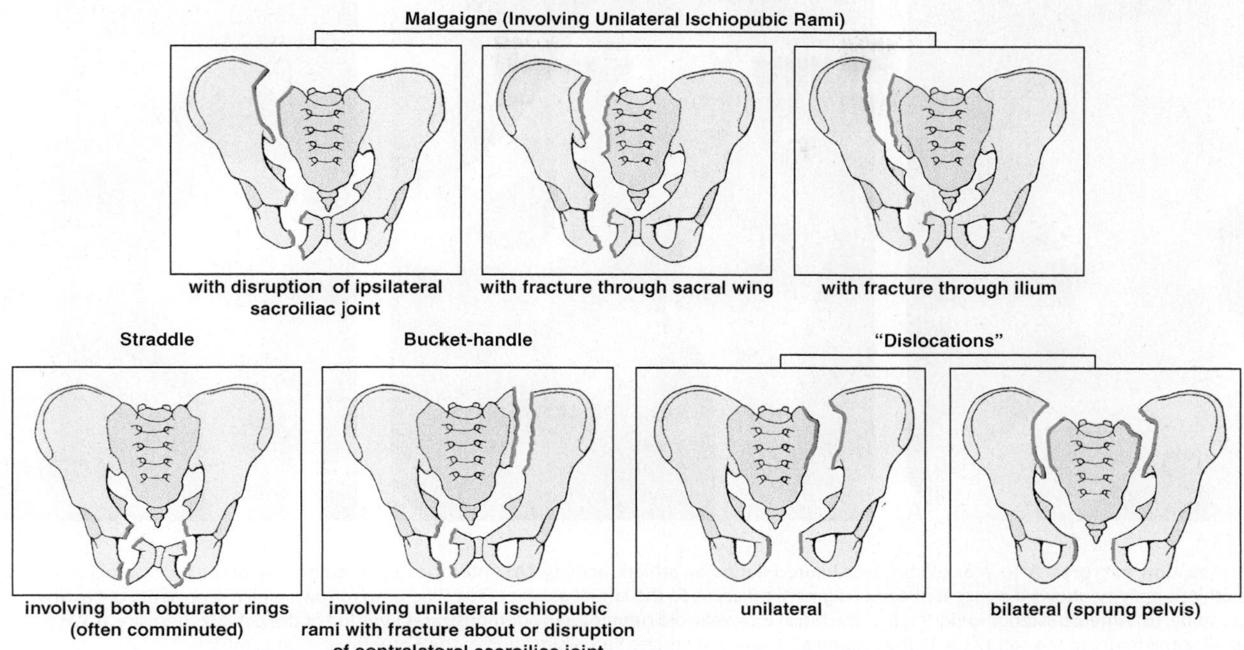

FIGURE 8.13 Unstable pelvic fractures. (Modified with permission from Dunn AW, Morris HD. Fractures and dislocations of the pelvis. *J Bone Joint Surg Am* 1968;50:1639–1648.)

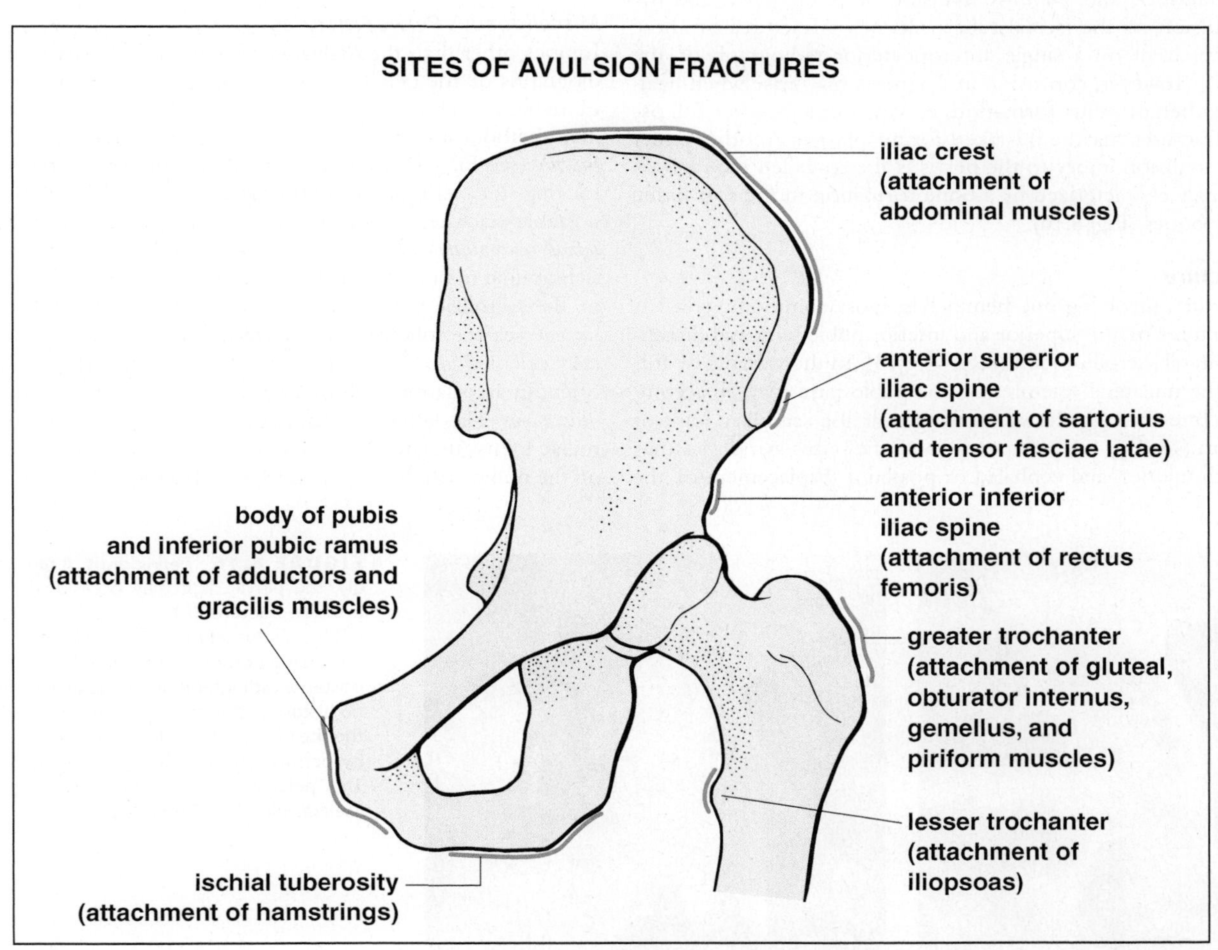

FIGURE 8.14 Sites of avulsion fractures.

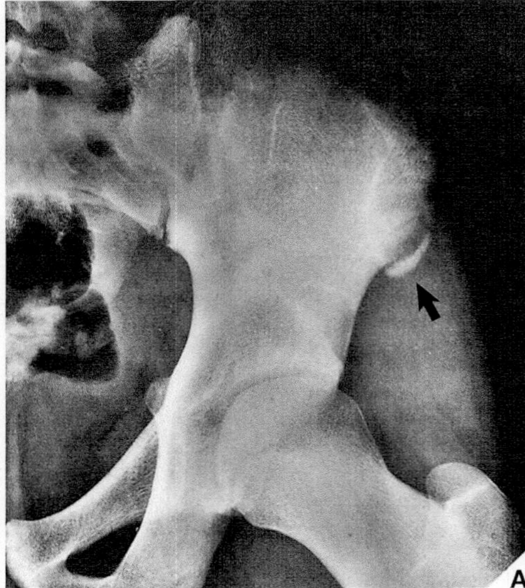
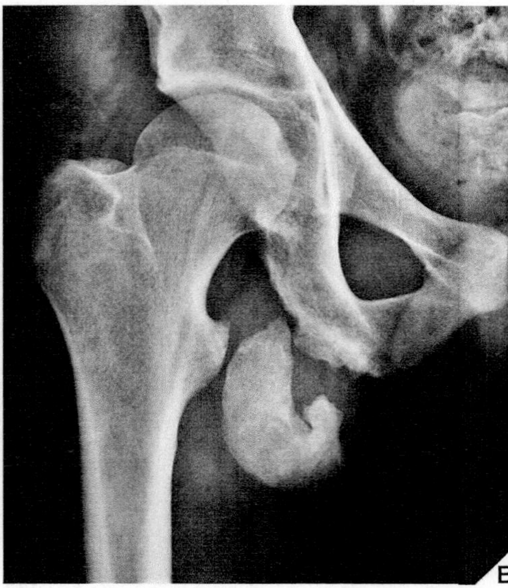
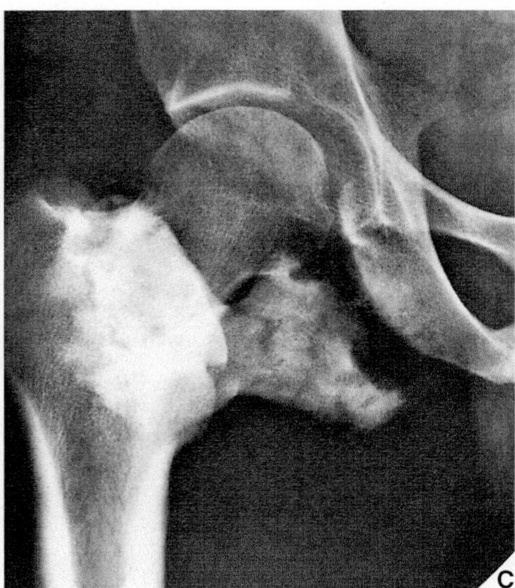

FIGURE 8.15 Avulsion fractures. A 16-year-old boy was injured during an athletic activity. **(A)** Anteroposterior radiograph of the pelvis of a 16-year-old boy, who was injured during an athletic activity, shows a crescent-shaped fragment adjacent to the lateral aspect of the iliac wing *(arrow)*, which represents the avulsed apophysis of the anterosuperior iliac spine. **(B)** Anteroposterior radiograph of the hip in a 26-year-old runner clearly demonstrates avulsion of the ischial tuberosity. **(C)** As a sequela of avulsion of the ischial tuberosity and injury to the soft tissue in the region, a 28-year-old athlete had ossification of the obturator externus muscle.

fasciae latae in avulsion of the anterosuperior iliac spine, the *rectus femoris* muscle in avulsion of the anteroinferior iliac spine, the *hip rotators* in avulsion of greater trochanter, the *iliopsoas* in avulsion of the lesser trochanter, the *adductors* and *gracilis* in avulsion of pubic bone, and the *hamstrings* in avulsion of the ischial tuberosity. Most fractures of these structures are apparent on a single anteroposterior radiograph of the pelvis (Fig. 8.15). However, confusion in diagnosis may arise when healing occurs by exuberant callus formation, at which time or after full ossification such fractures may be mistaken for neoplasms. Another entity that may mimic avulsion injury to the pelvis is the so-called *pelvic digit*, a congenital anomaly characterized by a bone formation in the soft tissue about the pelvic bones (Fig. 8.16).

Malgaigne Fracture

This unstable injury, involving one hemipelvis, most commonly consists of unilateral fractures of the superior and inferior pubic rami and disruption of the ipsilateral sacroiliac joint (see Fig. 8.13). In the variants of this type of injury, the unilateral fractures of the pubic rami may be accompanied by a fracture through the sacral wing near the sacroiliac joint or through the ilium (see Fig. 8.13). Separation of the pubic symphysis may coexist with such injuries, and cephalad or posterior displacement of the entire hemipelvis may occur. The Malgaigne fracture, which is recognized clinically by shortening of the lower extremity, is readily demonstrated on the anteroposterior radiograph of the pelvis (Fig. 8.17).

Miscellaneous Pelvic Fractures

Injuries other than the Malgaigne fracture are also easily evaluated on radiographs of the pelvis in the standard and special projections or on CT examination. The *Duverney fracture* is a stable fracture of the wing of the ilium without interruption of the pelvic ring (see Fig. 8.12). The *straddle fracture* (see Fig. 8.13) consists of comminuted fractures of both obturator rings (i.e., all four ischiopubic rami). In one third of patients with this unstable fracture, bladder rupture or urethral injuries occur. The *bucket-handle* or *contralateral double vertical fracture* involves the superior and inferior ischiopubic rami on one side combined with fracture about or disruption of the sacroiliac joint on the opposite side (see Fig. 8.13). *Fractures of the sacrum* (see the following text), which may be either transversely or vertically oriented (see Figs. 8.12 and 8.28 to 8.31), may occur alone or, more often, in association with other pelvic injuries, such as the so-called *pelvic dislocations*. The latter are characterized by disruption in one or both sacroiliac joints (unilateral or bilateral dislocation) associated with separation of the pubic symphysis (Fig. 8.18; see also Fig. 8.13). The anteroposterior

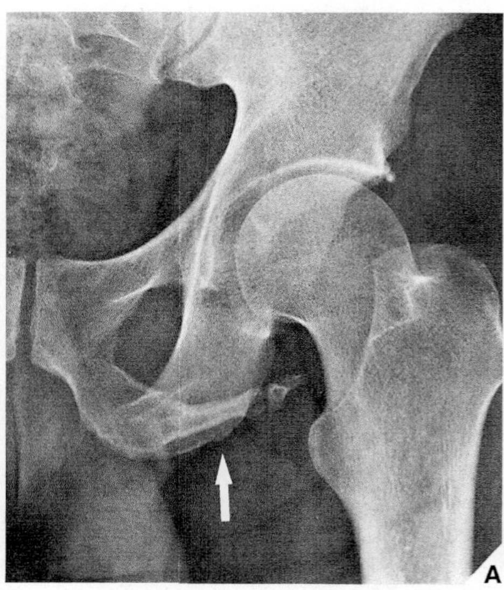
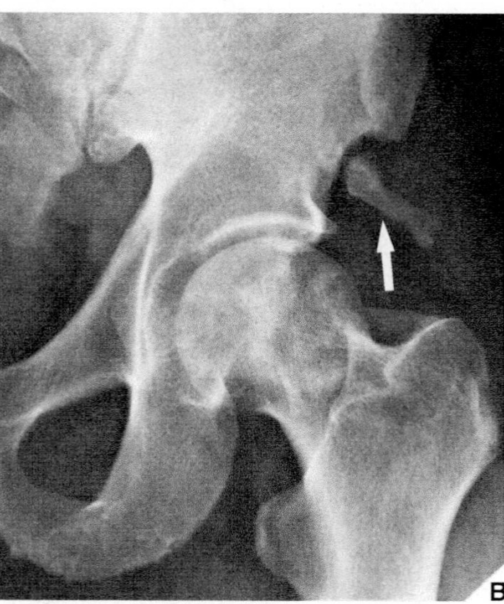

FIGURE 8.16 Pelvic digit. A rare congenital anomaly, the pelvic digit may occasionally be mistaken for avulsion fracture. **(A)** Anteroposterior radiograph of the left hip shows a finger-like, jointed structure attached to the caudal portion of the left ischium *(arrow)*. **(B)** Anteroposterior radiograph of the hip in a 55-year-old man with no history of trauma demonstrates a well-formed digit at the site of the anteroinferior iliac spine *(arrow)*. (Reprinted by permission from Springer: Greenspan A, Norman A. The "pelvic digit"—an unusual developmental anomaly. *Skeletal Radiol* 1982;9:118–122.)

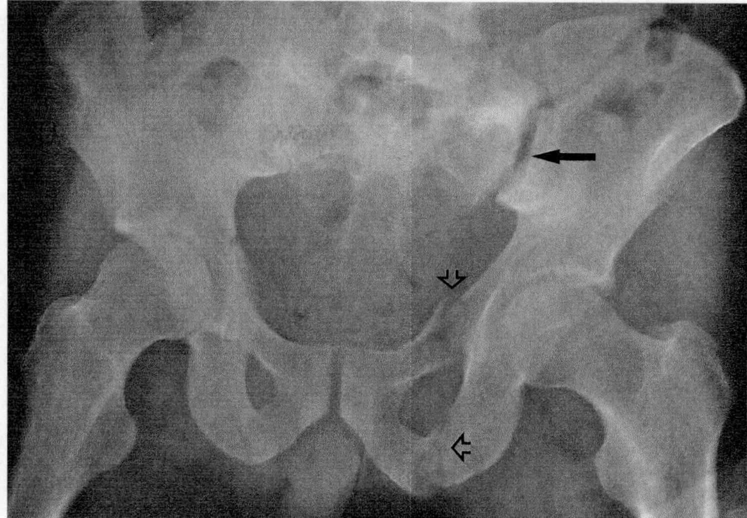

FIGURE 8.17 **Malgaigne fracture.** A 35-year-old man who was involved in an automobile accident sustained vertical fractures of the left obturator ring *(open arrows)* and fracture of the ipsilateral iliac bone *(arrow)*—a typical Malgaigne injury.

projection obtained with 30 degrees cephalad angulation or CT is helpful in disclosing sacral fractures, which are frequently overlooked.

Fractures of the Acetabulum

Evaluation of the acetabulum on conventional radiographs may be difficult because of obscuring overlying structures. If acetabular fracture is suspected, then radiographs in at least four projections should be obtained: the anteroposterior view of the pelvis, the anteroposterior view of the hip, and the anterior and posterior oblique (Judet) views. Radiography may also need to be supplemented by CT, as discussed previously.

As an aid in recognizing the presence of abnormality on the anteroposterior projection of the pelvis and hip, Judet, Judet, and Letournel have identified six lines relating to the acetabulum and its immediately surrounding structures (Fig. 8.19). Fracture of the acetabulum usually distorts these radiographic landmarks, allowing a diagnosis to be made on the anteroposterior projection, but an accurate and complete evaluation of the fracture requires that oblique views be obtained (Fig. 8.20). As mentioned, the anterior (internal) oblique projection demonstrates the iliopubic column and the posterior lip of the acetabulum (see Fig. 8.4), and the posterior (external) oblique view images the ilioischial column and the anterior

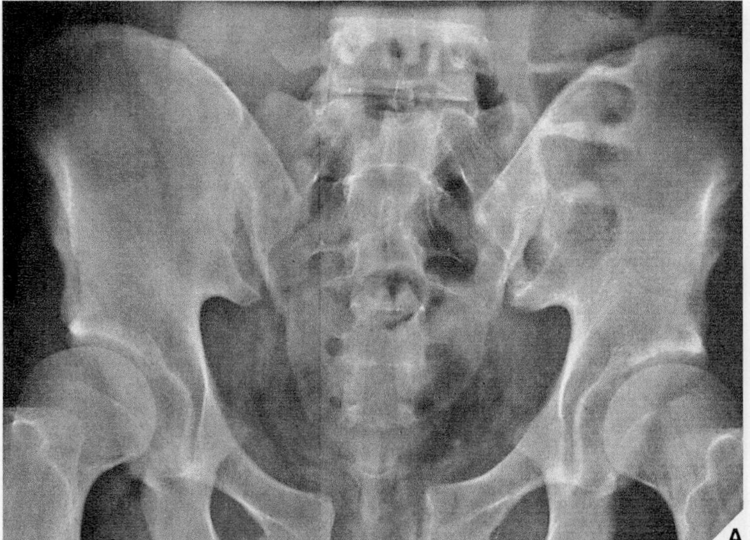

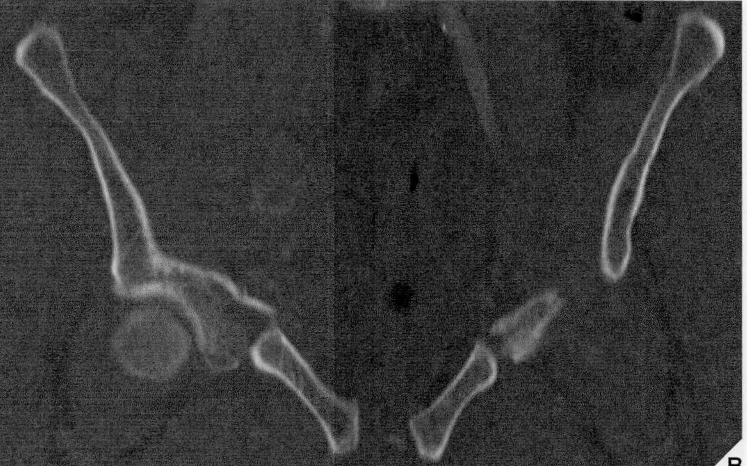

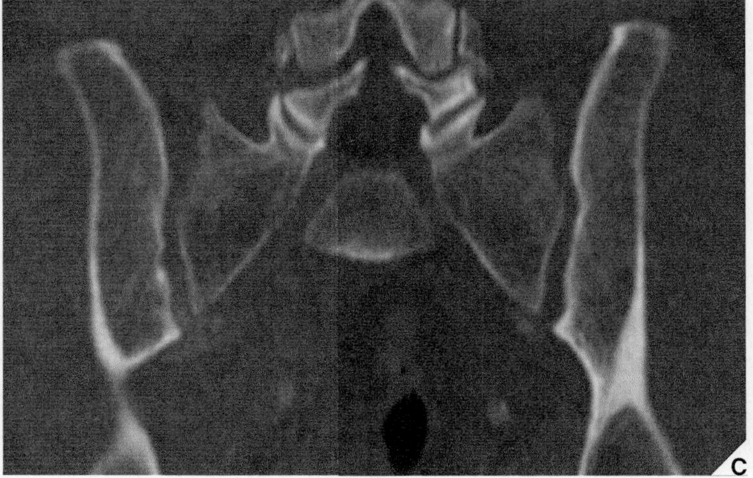

FIGURE 8.18 **Sprung pelvis (bilateral dislocation).** **(A)** Anteroposterior radiograph of the pelvis of a 25-year-old man who was injured in a motorcycle accident reveals the typical appearance of pelvic dislocation. The pubic symphysis is disrupted and markedly widened, and there is widening of both sacroiliac joints. **(B,C)** In another patient, two coronal reformatted CT images show similar injury. Note the widening of the symphysis pubis and both sacroiliac joints.

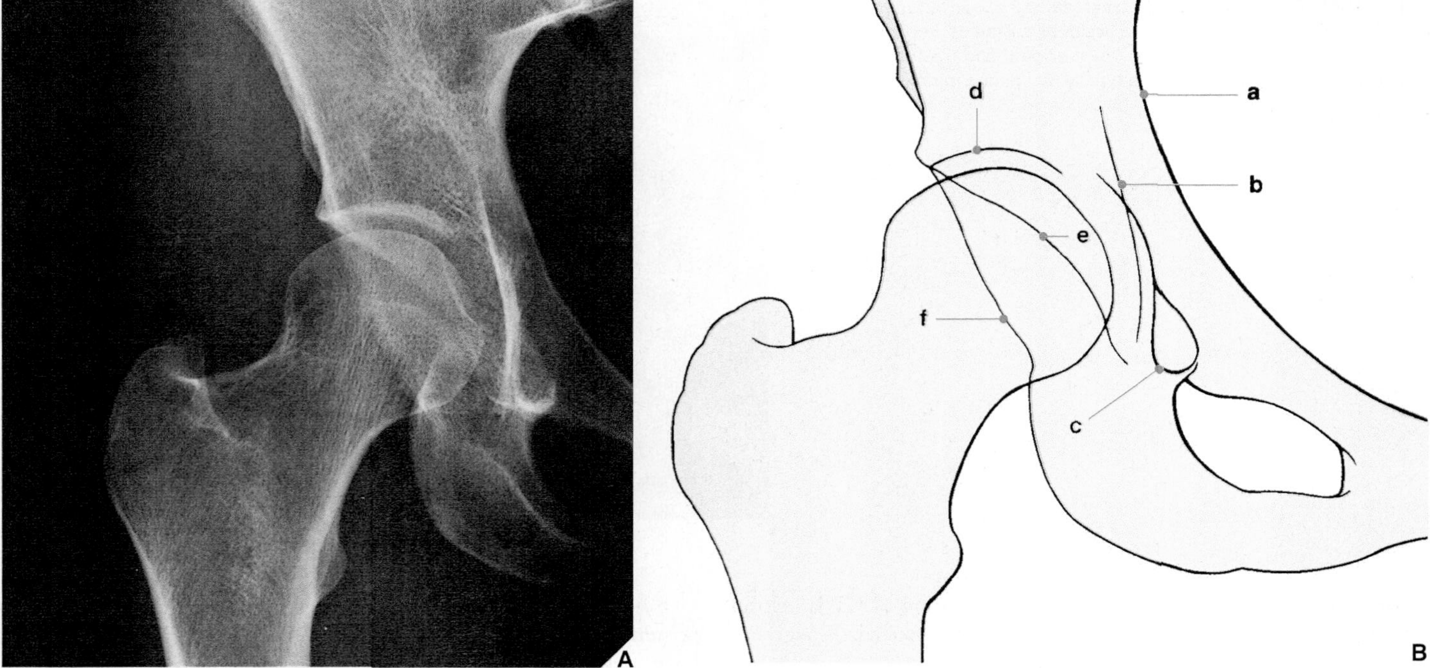

FIGURE 8.19 **Radiographic landmarks of the hip.** **(A,B)** On the anteroposterior radiograph of the hip, six lines relating to the acetabulum and its surrounding structures can be distinguished: *(a)* iliopubic or iliopectineal (arcuate) line; *(b)* ilioischial line, formed by the posterior portion of the quadrilateral plate (surface) of the iliac bone; *(c)* teardrop, formed by the medial acetabular wall, the acetabular notch, and the anterior portion of the quadrilateral plate; *(d)* roof of the acetabulum; *(e)* anterior rim of the acetabulum; and *(f)* posterior rim of the acetabulum. Distortion of any of these normal radiographic landmarks indicates the possible presence of abnormality.

rim of the acetabulum (see Fig. 8.5). These projections, together with the division of the pelvic bone into anterior and posterior columns (Fig. 8.21), provide the basis for the traditional classification of acetabular fractures. This classification has been modified by Letournel to include the following types of fractures (Fig. 8.22):

1. Fracture of the iliopubic (anterior) column (rare type of fracture)
2. Fracture of the ilioischial (posterior) column (common type of fracture)
3. Transverse fracture through the acetabulum involving both pelvic columns (common type of fracture)
4. Complex fractures, including T-shaped and stellate fractures, in which the acetabulum is broken into three or more fragment (the most common type of fracture)

CT plays a leading role in the evaluation of acetabular and pelvic fractures because of its capability of demonstrating the exact position of displaced fragments, which may be trapped within the hip joint, as well as

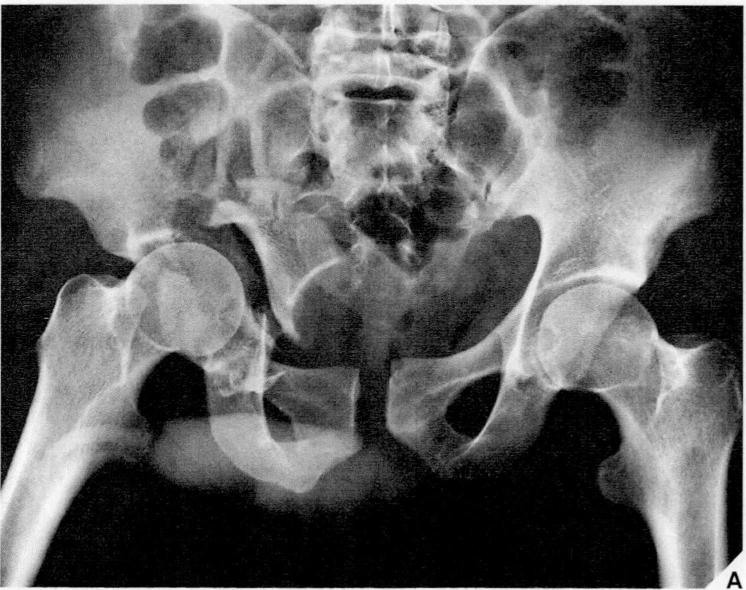

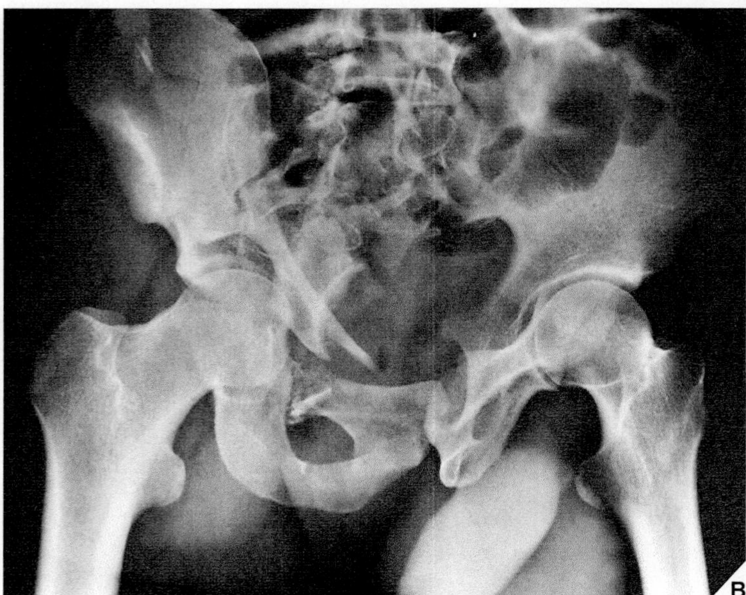

FIGURE 8.20 **Acetabular fracture.** A 32-year-old drug-addicted man was hit by a car. **(A)** Anteroposterior radiograph of the pelvis shows a comminuted fracture of the right acetabulum, fracture of the right ilium, and diastasis of the pubic symphysis. There is also a fracture of the sacrum with diastasis of the left sacroiliac joint. **(B)** On the anterior oblique projection, the acetabular fracture is seen to involve mainly the anterior pelvic column.

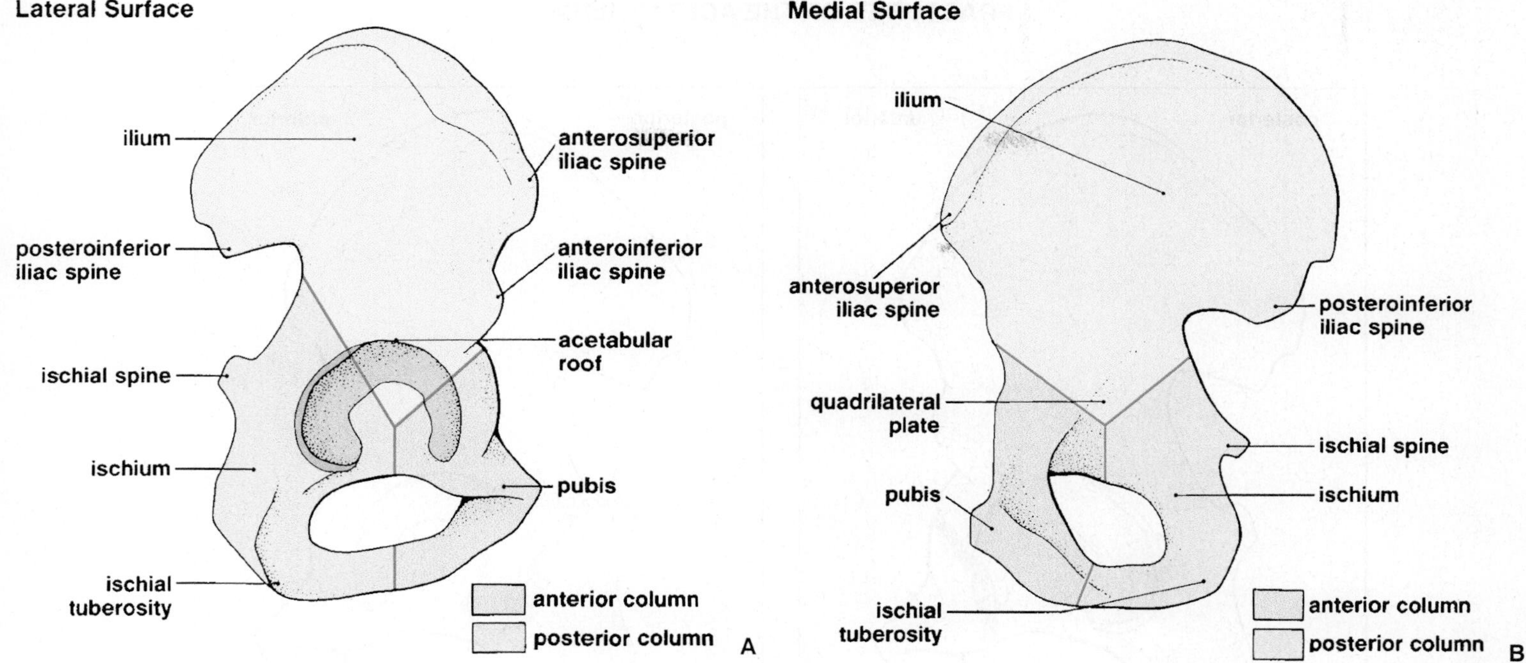

FIGURE 8.21 Columns of the pelvis. **(A)** Lateral and **(B)** medial views of the pelvis show the division of the bone into anterior and posterior columns, which provide the basis for the traditional classification of acetabular fractures. (Modified with permission from Judet R, Judet J, Letournel E. Fractures of the acetabulum: classification and surgical approaches for open reduction—preliminary report. *J Bone Joint Surg Am* 1964;46:1615–1646.)

allowing adequate assessment of concomitant soft-tissue injury (Figs. 8.23 to 8.25). It also requires less manipulation of the patient than the standard radiographic views—a fact especially important in patients with multiple injuries.

Injuries of the Acetabular Labrum

The fibrocartilaginous labrum is directly attached to the osseous rim of the acetabulum. It blends with the transverse ligament at the margins of the acetabular notch. Because the labrum is thicker posterosuperiorly and thinner anteroinferiorly, on cross section it appears as a triangular structure, similar to the labrum of the scapular glenoid. The acetabular labrum can be injured in conjunction with acetabular fracture, hip dislocation, or even minor trauma to the hip joint. In the latter situation, the clinical symptoms include anterior inguinal pain, limitation of motion in the hip joint, painful clicking, transient locking, and "giving way" of the hip. Onset of pain may be linked to sports activities or to twisting or slipping injury. Conventional radiographs, unless obvious fracture or dislocation is present, are invariably normal. The most effective technique for diagnosis of a pathologic labral condition is MRa. Czerny and colleagues have recently reported a sensitivity of 90% and accuracy of 91% of MRa for the detection of labral tears and detachments. The normal labrum appears on axial and coronal images as a triangular structure with low signal intensity on all imaging sequences (Fig. 8.26). A tear of the labrum is diagnosed either when deformity of its contour is present or when a linear diffuse high signal is present. In the most severe cases, the labrum is detached from the acetabulum (Fig. 8.27). Based on MRa findings that included labral morphology, intralabral signal, presence of tear or labral detachment, and the presence or absence of adjacent perilabral recess, Czerny classified labral tears into the three groups (six subgroups). In general, these groupings take into consideration only either the presence of labrum substance tear or peripheral detachment. Another classification introduced by Lage et al. is based on arthroscopic findings, reflecting morphology of the labrum and functional stability of the tear. Because some investigators found no correlation between these two grading systems, Blankenbaker and colleagues proposed instead to use a description of the labral abnormalities seen at MRa that can be outlined as follows: (a) *frayed labrum*—irregular margins of the labrum without a discrete tear, (b) *flap tear*—contrast extending into or through the labral substance, (c) *peripheral longitudinal tear*—contrast partially or completely extending between the labral base and acetabulum, and (d) *thickened and distorted labrum*—most likely unstable lesion.

Treatment of labral tears includes arthroscopic resection of the injured labrum or repair of a tear.

Femoroacetabular Impingement Syndrome

This condition results from incongruity of the femoral head and acetabulum and leads to injury of the fibrocartilaginous labrum and subsequent development of precocious osteoarthritis of the hip joint. FAI syndrome is discussed in detail in Chapter 13.

During evaluation of MRI and MRa of the hip and pelvis, it is helpful to use the checklist as provided in Table 8.3.

Injury to the Sacrum

Sacral fractures most commonly occur in conjunction with pelvic ring injuries but may also occur as isolated fractures. They occur in approximately 45% of all pelvic fractures and typically result from high-energy injuries sustained in motor vehicle accidents or fall from the heights. According to Denis classification, they are categorized into three types: zone I—fracture across sacral ala, lateral to the neural foramina; zone II—fracture through the neural foramina; and zone III—fracture through the body of the sacrum, medial to the neural foramina, and involving the spinal canal. Transverse sacral fractures are classified as Denis zone III fractures because they extend into the spinal canal, although they commonly traverse all three zones. These fractures are uncommon (less than 5% of all sacral fractures) and have been described, based on the morphologic pattern of the fracture line, as H, U, lambda, and T-shaped fractures.

Sacral fractures are difficult to visualize on the conventional radiographs, and the modality of choice is CT. A thin 2-mm section with coronal and sagittal reformation, supplemented with three-dimensional (3D) CT reconstructed images, provides the optimal solution for their identification and evaluation (Figs. 8.28 to 8.31). MRI occasionally may be required to evaluate associated neurologic complications.

FRACTURES OF THE ACETABULUM

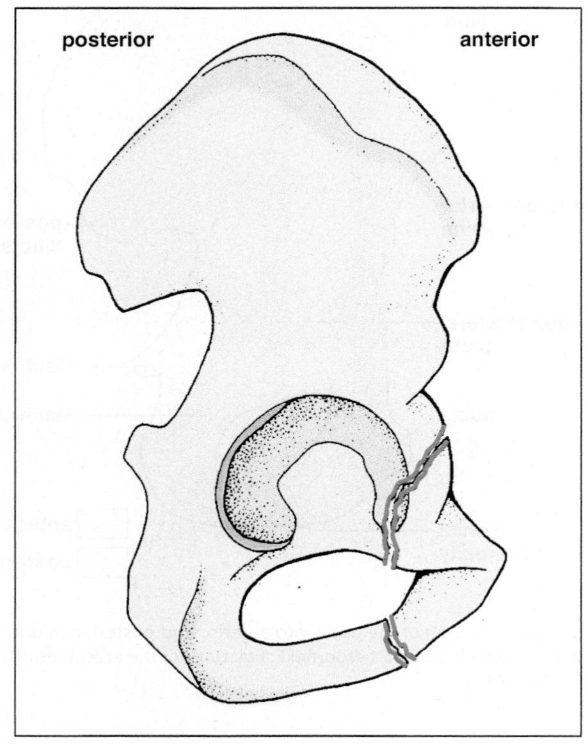

involving anterior (iliopubic) column

posterior
anterior

involving posterior (ilioischial) column

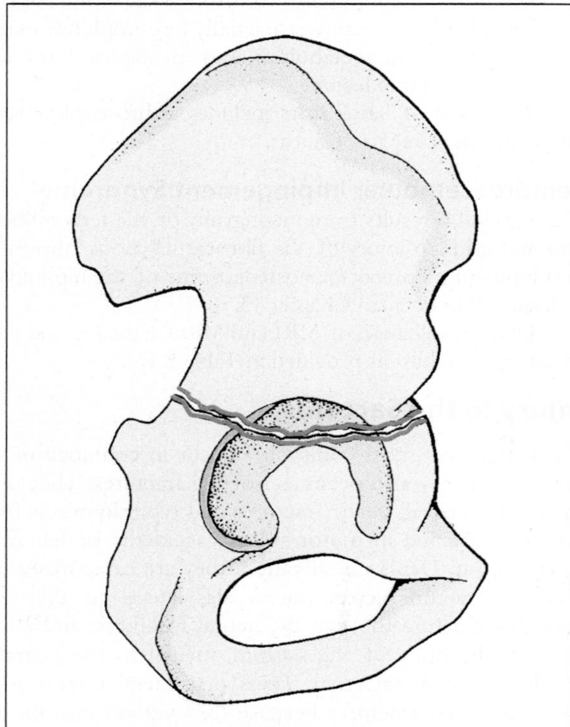

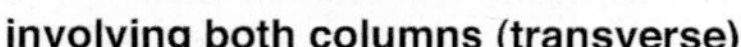

involving both columns (transverse)

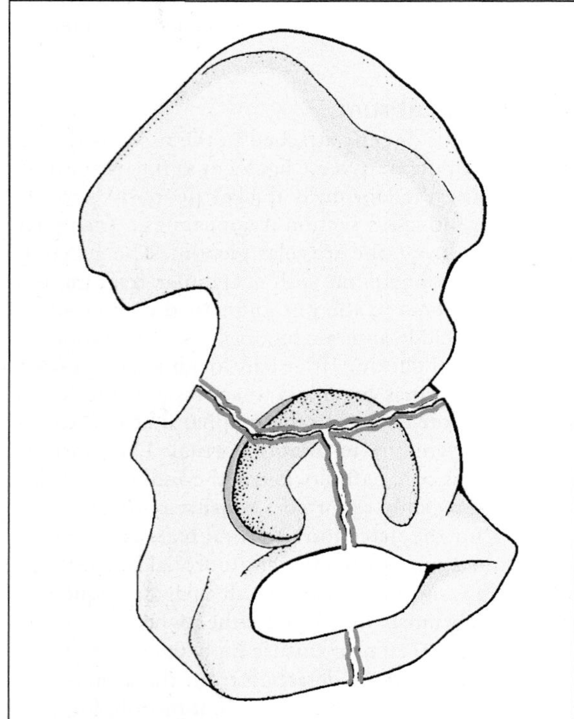

complex fractures (T-shaped or stellate)

FIGURE 8.22 Classification of acetabular fractures. In the traditional classification of acetabular fractures, the fracture may involve the anterior column, the posterior column, or both columns. In complex acetabular fractures, both columns are involved, and the fracture line may be T-shaped or stellate. (Modified with permission from Letournel E. Acetabulum fractures: classification and management. *Clin Orthop Relat Res* 1980;151:81–106.)

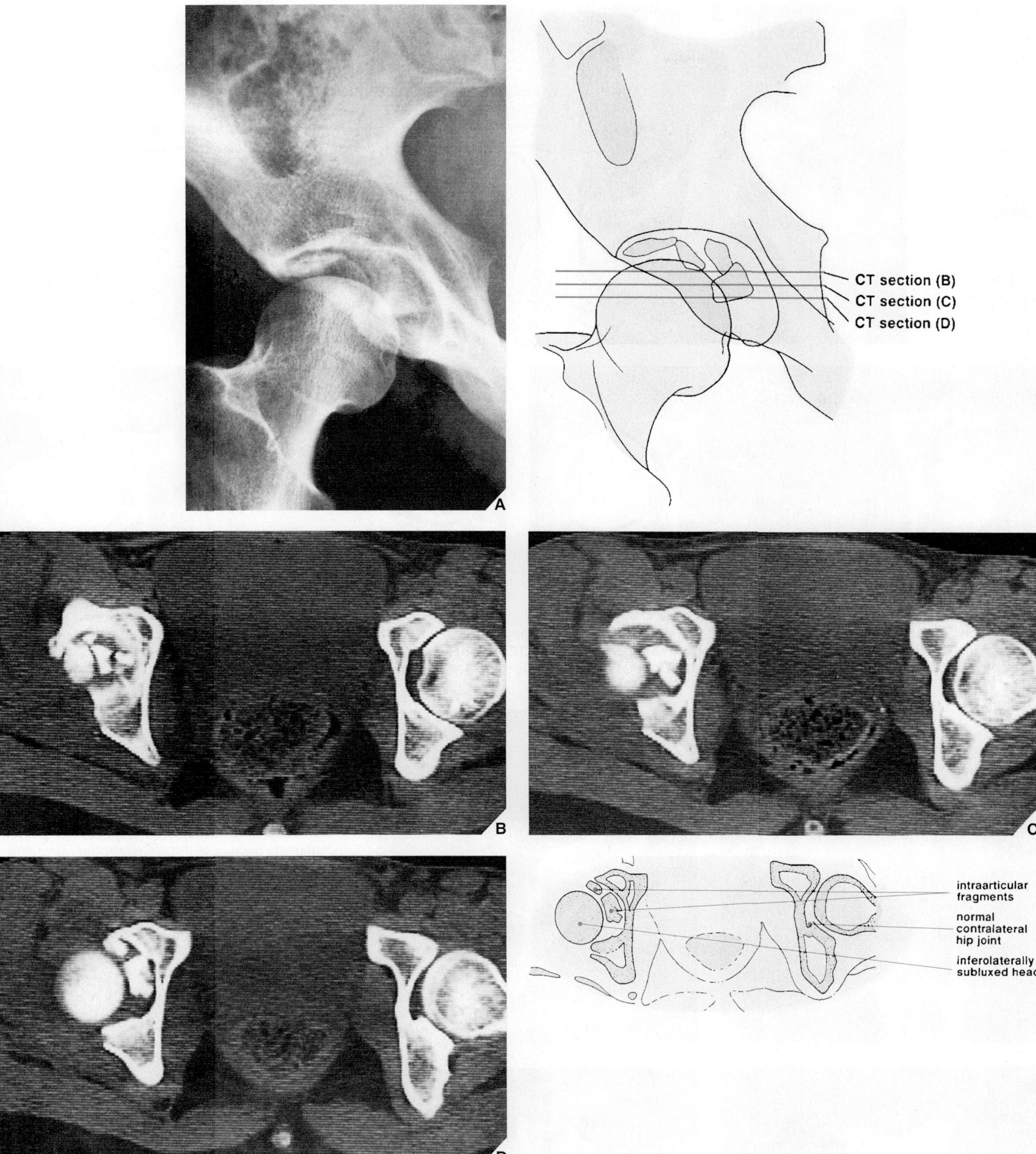

FIGURE 8.23 CT of the acetabular fracture. As a result of an automobile accident, a 30-year-old woman sustained an injury that was diagnosed on the standard projections as a fracture of the acetabular roof. **(A)** On the posterior oblique projection, the fracture is shown to be comminuted. CT examination was performed, and sections **B**, **C**, and **D** show the topographic orientation of the various intraarticular fragments and evidence of inferolateral subluxation of the femoral head—important information not appreciated on the standard projections.

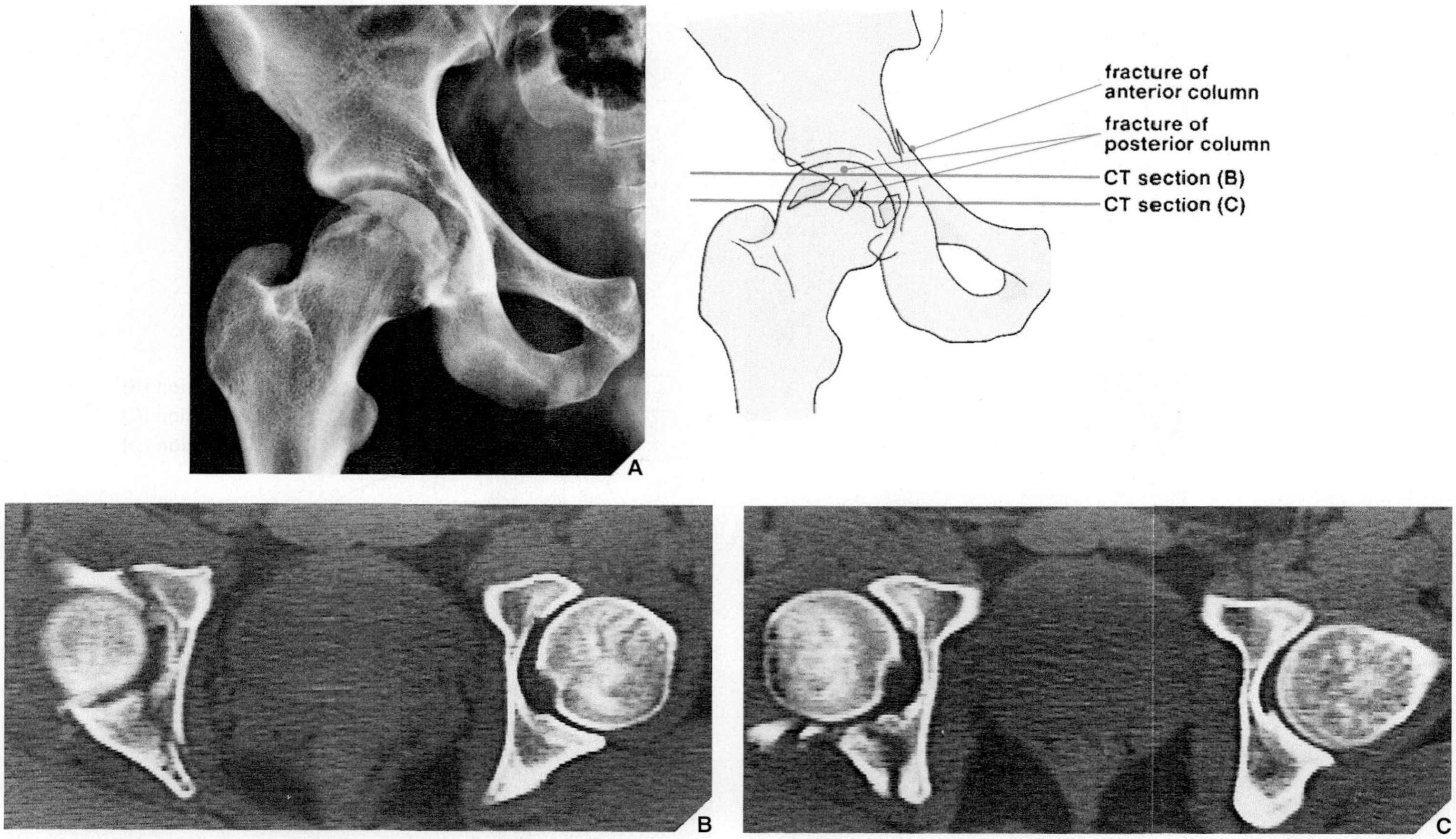

fracture of anterior column
fracture of posterior column
CT section (B)
CT section (C)

FIGURE 8.24 CT of the acetabular fracture. A 22-year-old man sustained an injury caused by the dashboard during an automobile accident. **(A)** Standard anteroposterior radiograph of the hip shows fractures of the anterior and posterior columns. **(B,C)** CT sections demonstrate the exact extent of the fracture lines and the spatial relationships between the fragments and provide crucial information for the orthopaedic surgeon in planning open reduction and internal fixation.

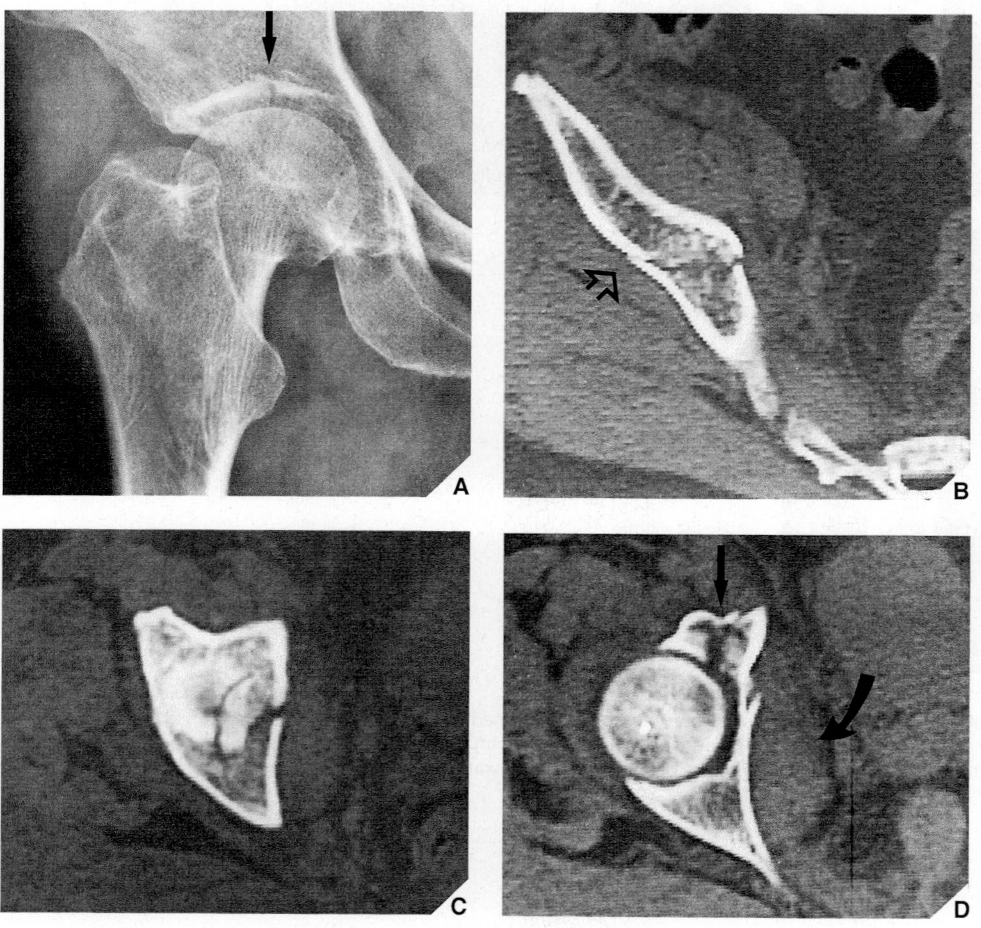

FIGURE 8.25 CT of the acetabular fracture. After a fall on the street, a 63-year-old man experienced discomfort while walking. **(A)** Standard anteroposterior radiograph of the right hip shows a radiolucent line in the acetabular roof *(arrow)* but no other findings indicative of abnormality. Other views of the pelvis were not obtained because the patient refused. With his consent the next day, multiple CT sections **(B–D)** were obtained, confirming fracture of the acetabular roof. They reveal, in addition, completely unsuspected fractures of the anterior column *(arrow)* and iliac bone *(open arrow)*, with marked thickening of the obturator internus muscle *(curved arrow)* secondary to hemorrhage and edema.

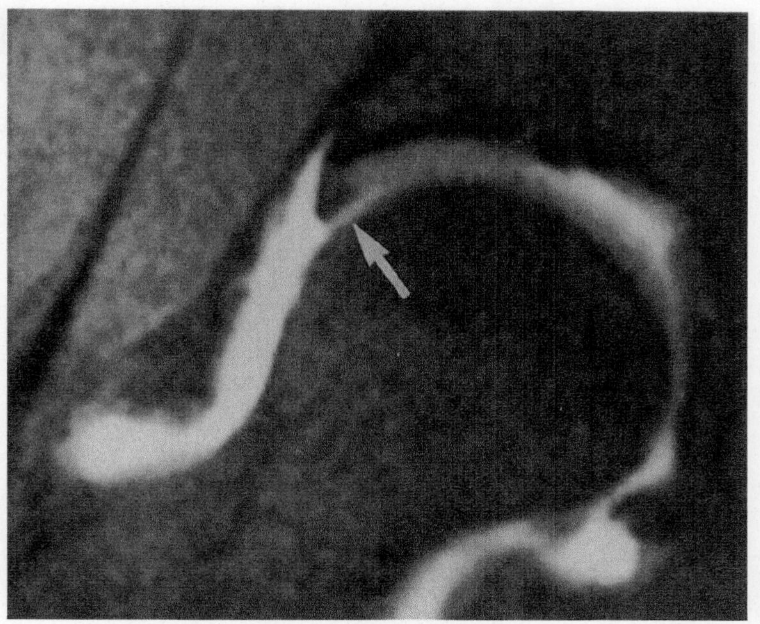

FIGURE 8.26 **MRa of normal acetabular labrum.** Coronal fat-suppressed T1-weighted MR arthrographic image of the right hip shows a normal appearance of the acetabular labrum *(arrow)*. Note the triangular shape, smooth contour, and low signal intensity of this structure. (Reprinted from Steinbach LS, Palmer WE, Schweitzer ME. Special focus session. MR arthrography. *Radiographics* 2002;22:1223–1246. Copyright © 2002 by The Radiological Society of North America, Inc.)

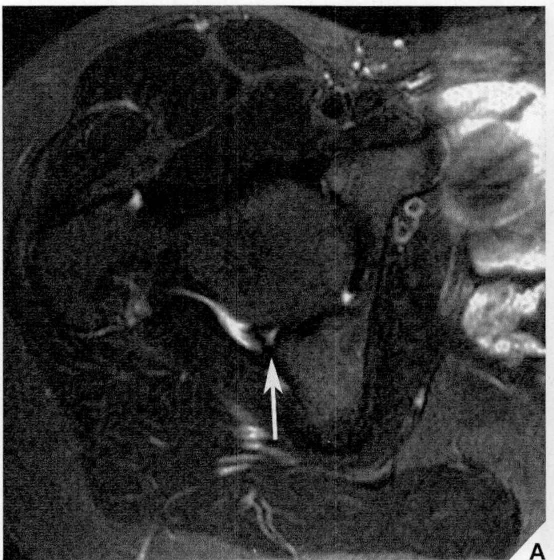

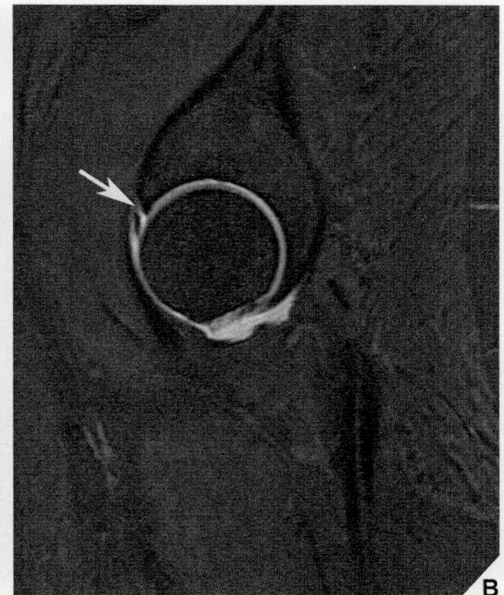

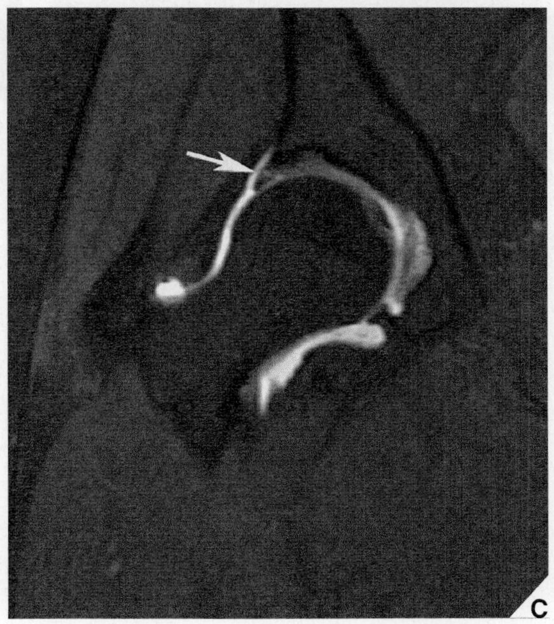

FIGURE 8.27 **MRI and MRa of torn acetabular labrum.** **(A)** Axial T2-weighted image demonstrates a tear of the posterior labrum *(arrow)*. **(B)** Sagittal T1-weighted fat-saturated MRa in another patient demonstrates a tear of the anterior superior labrum *(arrow)*. **(C)** Yet in another patient, coronal T1-weighted fat-saturated MRa demonstrates a superior labral tear *(arrow)*.

TABLE 8.3 Checklist for Evaluation of Magnetic Resonance Imaging and Magnetic Resonance Arthrography of the Hip and Pelvis

Osseous Structures	***Muscles and Their Tendons (continued)***
Femoral head (c, s, a)	Piriformis (a)
Femoral neck (c, a)	Obturators—internus, externus (a)
Greater and lesser trochanters (c, a)	Gemelli—superior, inferior (a)
Acetabulum (c, a)	Quadratus femoris—vastus lateralis, medialis, intermedius (a)
Cartilaginous Structures	Biceps femoris (c, a)
Articular cartilage (c, a)	Semimembranosus (c, a)
Fibrocartilaginous labrum (c, s, a)	Semitendinosus (c, a)
Joints	***Ligaments***
Hip (c, s, a)	Iliofemoral (c, a)
Sacroiliac (c, a)	Pubofemoral (c, a)
Muscles and Their Tendons	Ischiofemoral (c, a)
Gluteus—maximus, medius, minimus (c, a)	Teres (a)
Adductors—magnus, longus, brevis (c, a)	***Bursae***
Iliopsoas (c, a)	Iliopsoas (c, a)
Sartorius (a)	Greater trochanteric (c, a)
Rectus femoris (a)	***Other Structures***
Gracilis (a)	Pulvinar (a)
Pectineus (a)	Sciatic nerve (c, a)
Tensor fasciae latae (a)	Arteries and veins (a)

The best imaging planes for visualization of listed structures are given in parentheses: c, coronal; s, sagittal; a, axial.

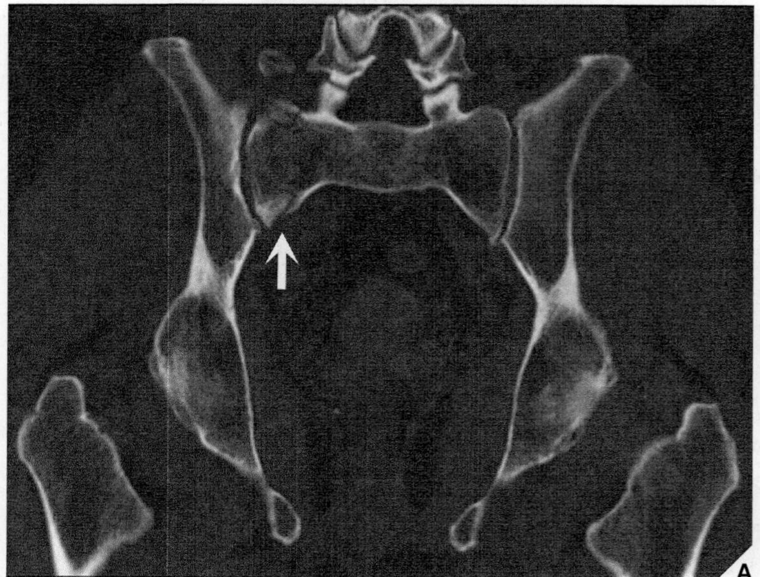

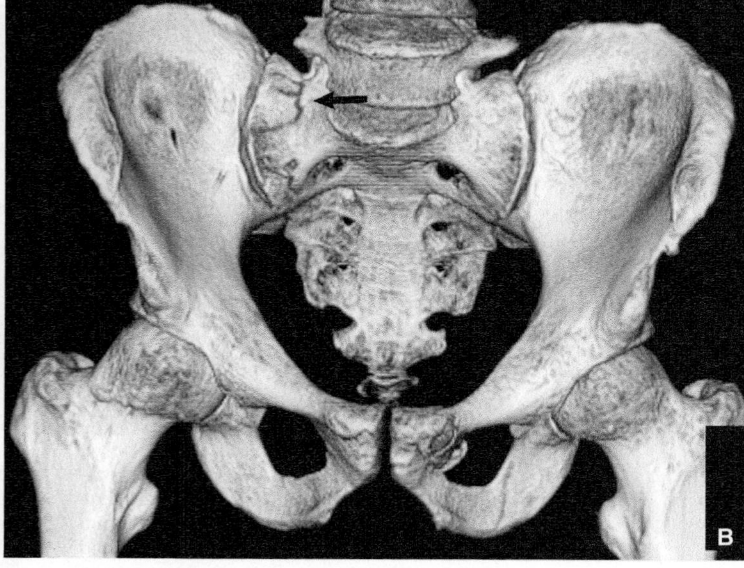

FIGURE 8.28 Sacral fracture not affecting the neural foramina (zone I). A 62-year-old man was injured in the motorcycle accident. **(A)** Coronal reformatted CT image and **(B)** 3D CT reconstruction show a fracture of the right sacrum not affecting the neural foramina *(arrow)*.

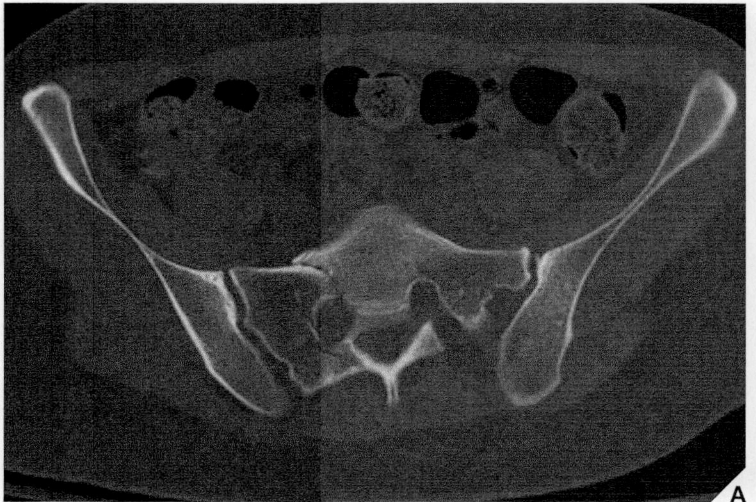

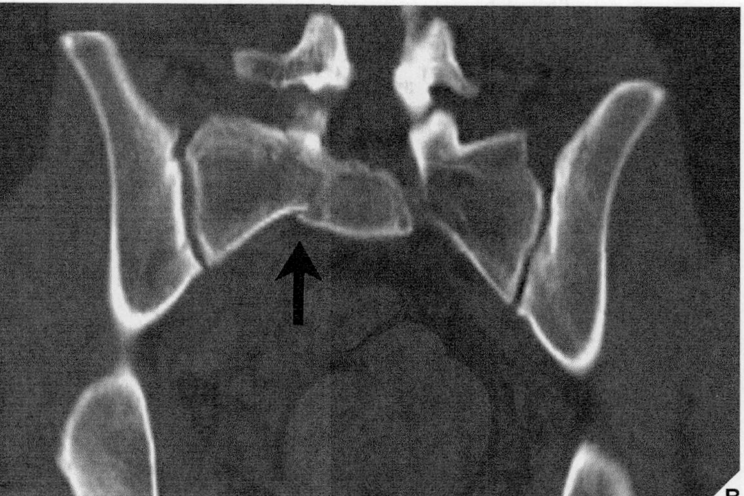

FIGURE 8.29 **Sacral fracture affecting the neural foramina (zone II).** **(A)** Axial, **(B)** coronal reformatted, and **(C)** 3D reconstructed CT images show a fracture of the right side of the sacral bone *(arrows)* extending to the neural foramina.

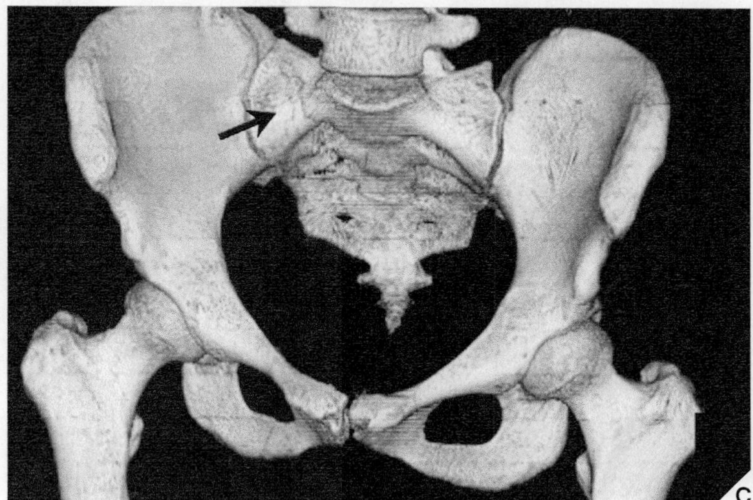

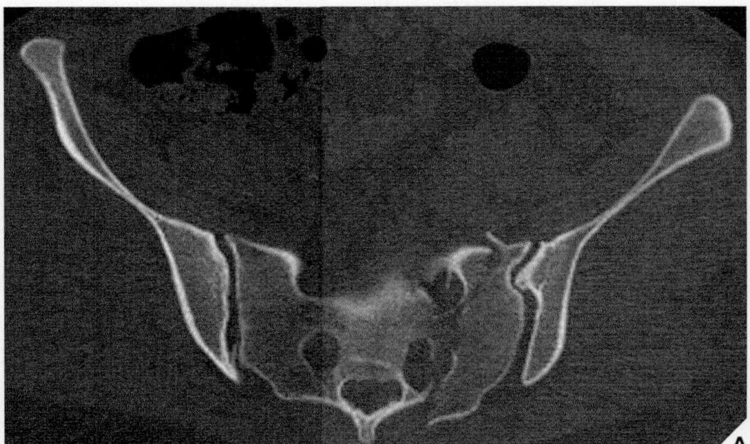

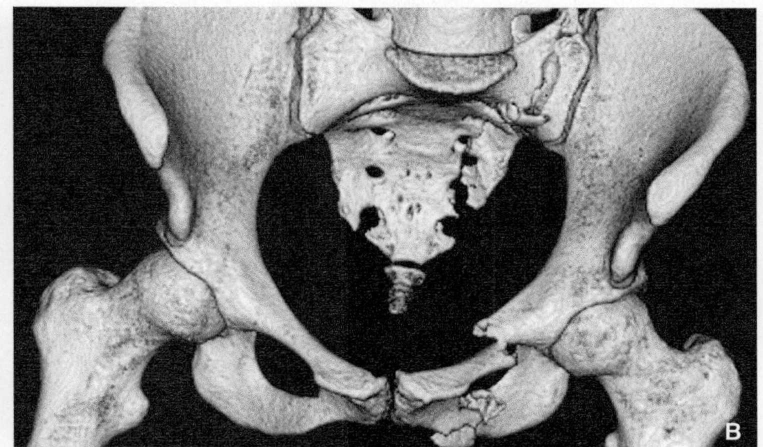

FIGURE 8.30 **Sacral fracture through the neural foramina (zone II) associated with fracture of the obturator foramen.** A 26-year-old man fell from the scaffold. **(A)** Axial and **(B)** 3D reconstructed CT images show a fracture of the sacrum extending to the left-sided neural foramina. In addition, there is displaced comminuted fracture of the superior and inferior pubic rami.

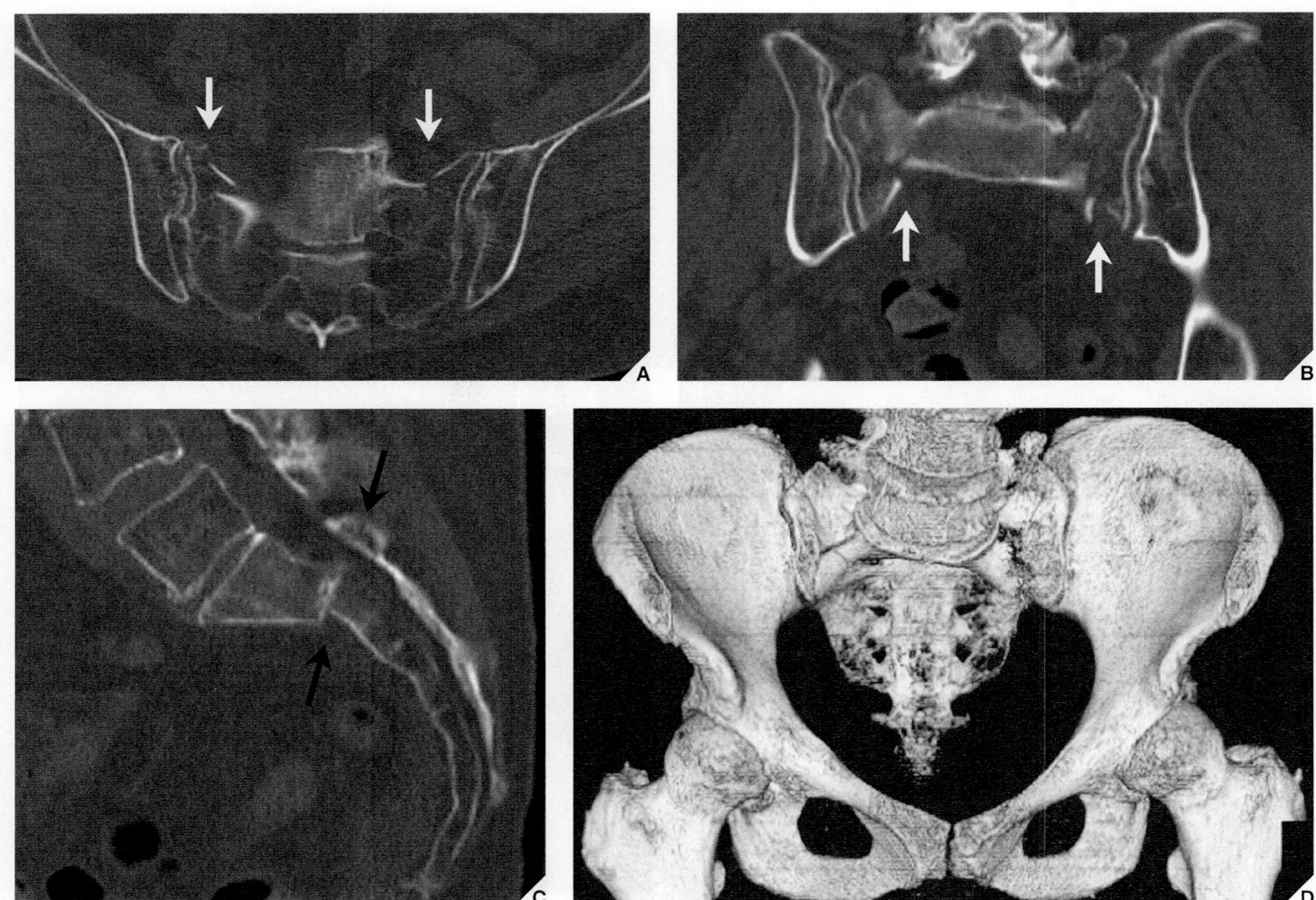

FIGURE 8.31 Transverse sacral fracture (zone III). A 65-year-old woman was hit by the car while crossing the street. **(A)** Axial, **(B)** coronal reformatted, **(C)** sagittal reformatted, and **(D)** 3D reconstructed CT images show an H-type sacral fracture *(white arrows)*. Note the extension of the fracture line through the spinal canal *(black arrows)*.

Trauma to the Proximal Femur

Fractures of the Proximal Femur

When fracture of the proximal femur is suspected, the standard radiographic examination should include at least two projections: the anteroposterior and the frog-lateral views of the hip (see Figs. 8.1 and 8.6); the groin-lateral radiograph of the hip is also frequently required (see Fig. 8.7). For many nondisplaced and displaced fractures, however, a single anteroposterior radiograph of the hip may suffice (Figs. 8.32 and 8.33). CT or MRI may occasionally be necessary, particularly to determine the type of the fracture and degree of displacement (Figs. 8.34 to 8.37). Radionuclide bone scan may also need to be called on in questionable cases (see Fig. 4.11B).

Traditionally, fractures of the proximal femur (so-called *hip fractures*) are divided into two groups: (a) *intracapsular fractures* involving the femoral head or neck, which may be capital, subcapital, transcervical, or basicervical, and (b) *extracapsular fractures* involving the trochanters, which may be intertrochanteric or subtrochanteric (Fig. 8.38). The significance of this distinction lies in the greater incidence of posttraumatic complications after intracapsular fracture of the upper femur. The most common complication, osteonecrosis (ischemic or avascular necrosis), occurs in 15% to 35% of patients sustaining intracapsular fractures, but the percentage varies according to the reported series.

The reason for the high incidence of the development of osteonecrosis after fracture of the femoral neck lies in the nature of the blood supply to the proximal femur. The capsule of the hip joint arises from the acetabulum and attaches to the anterior aspect of the femur along the intertrochanteric line at the base of the femoral neck. Posteriorly, the capsule envelops the femoral head and proximal two thirds of the neck. Most of the blood supply to the femoral head is derived from the circumflex femoral arteries, which form a ring at the base of the neck, sending off branches that ascend subcapsularly along the femoral neck to the femoral head. Only a very small portion of the femoral head is supplied by arteries in the ligamentum teres (ligamentum capitis femoris) (Fig. 8.39). Because of this vascular configuration, intracapsular fractures tend to tear the vessels, interrupting the blood supply and leading eventually to osteonecrosis. The trochanteric region, however, is extracapsular and receives an excellent supply of blood from branches of the circumflex femoral arteries and from muscles that attach around both trochanters. Thus, as a rule, intertrochanteric fractures do not lead to osteonecrosis of the femoral head.

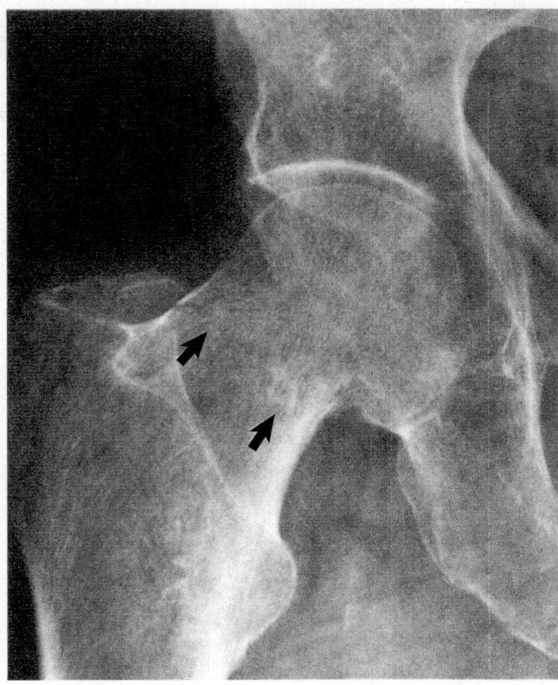

FIGURE 8.32 Midcervical fracture. In a fall in her bathroom, an 83-year-old woman sustained a typical nondisplaced midcervical fracture of the femoral neck *(arrows)*, as demonstrated on this anteroposterior radiograph of the right hip.

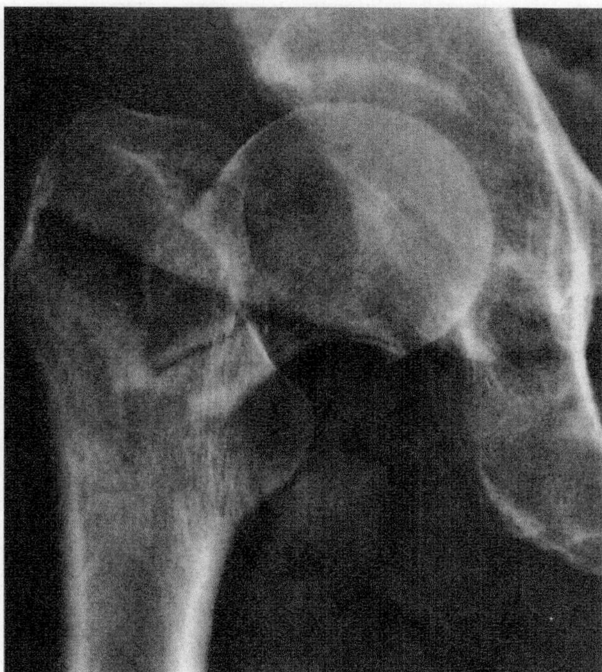

FIGURE 8.33 Basicervical fracture. A 37-year-old man fell from a ladder. On the anteroposterior radiograph of the right hip, a displaced basicervical fracture of the femoral neck is evident.

Nonunion is also a common complication following fracture of the femoral neck, occurring in 10% to 44% of patients with such fractures. According to Pauwels, the obliquity of the fracture line determines the prognosis. The more oblique the fracture line is, the more likely nonunion will occur (Fig. 8.40).

Intracapsular Fractures

Of the many classifications of femoral neck fractures that have been proposed, the Pauwels and Garden classifications are useful from a practical point of view because they take into consideration the stability of the fracture—an important factor in orthopaedic management and prognosis.

Pauwels classifies femoral neck fractures according to the degree of angulation of the fracture line from the horizontal plane on the postreduction anteroposterior radiograph, stressing that the closer the fracture line approximates the horizontal, the more stable the fracture and the better the prognosis (see Fig. 8.40). Garden, however, proposed a staging system of femoral neck fractures based on displacement of the femoral head before reduction. Displacement in the Garden system is graded according to the position of the principal (medial) compressive trabeculae (Fig. 8.41). His classification of such fractures is divided into four stages (Fig. 8.42):

Stage I: Incomplete subcapital fracture. In this so-called *impacted* or *abducted fracture*, the femoral shaft is externally rotated and the femoral head is in valgus. The medial trabeculae of the femoral head and neck form an angle greater than 180 degrees (Fig. 8.43). This is a stable fracture with a good prognosis.

Stage II: Complete subcapital fracture without displacement. In this complete fracture through the neck, the femoral shaft

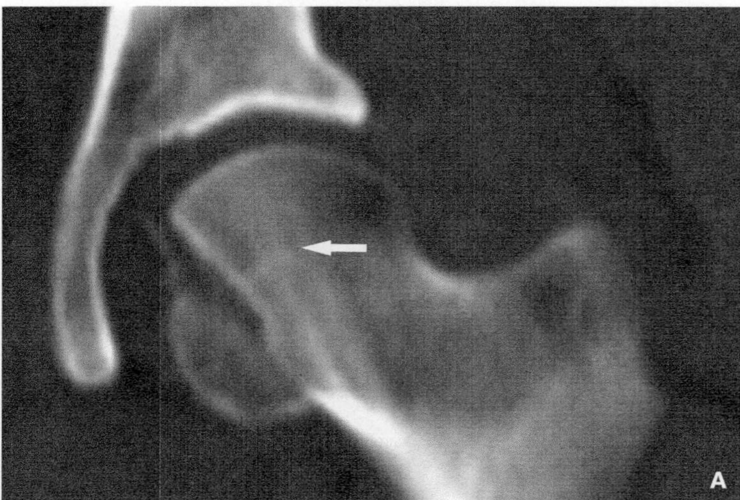

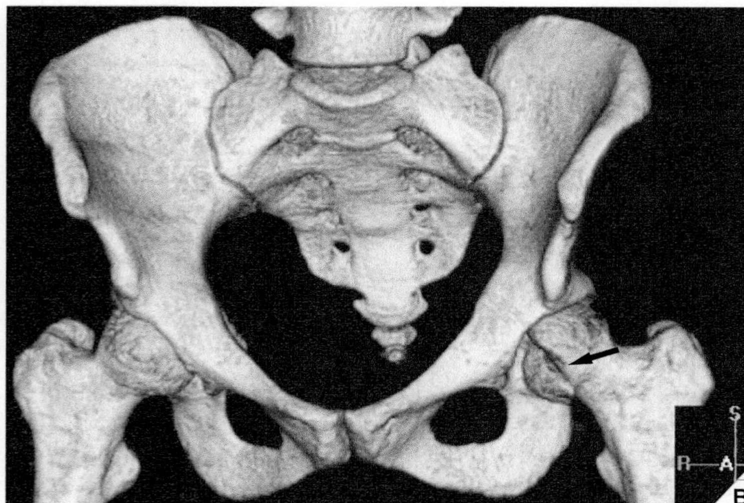

FIGURE 8.34 **CT and 3D CT of the fracture of the femoral head.** A 20-year-old woman sustained a posterior dislocation of the left hip. The dislocation was successfully relocated. **(A)** Coronal reformatted CT of the left hip and **(B)** 3D reconstructed CT image of the pelvis show one of the complications of posterior hip dislocation—a fracture of the femoral head *(arrows)*.

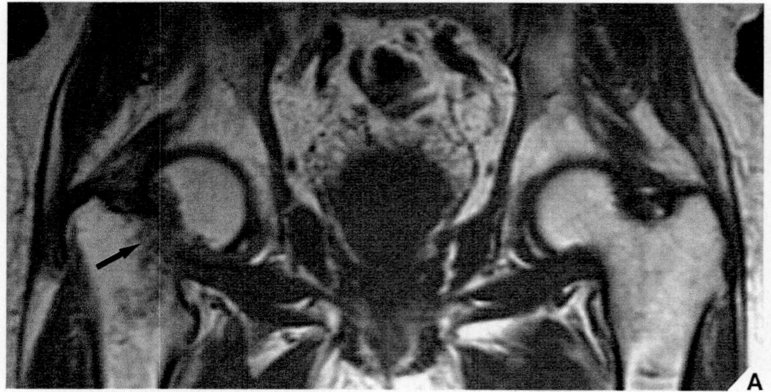

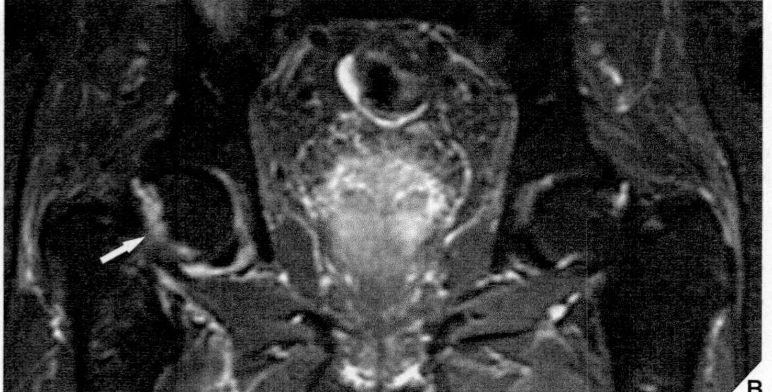

FIGURE 8.35 **MRI of the subcapital fracture.** A 77-year-old woman presented with right hip pain after a fall on the street. **(A)** Coronal proton density–weighted and **(B)** coronal inversion recovery MR images of the pelvis show a subcapital fracture of the right femur *(arrows)*.

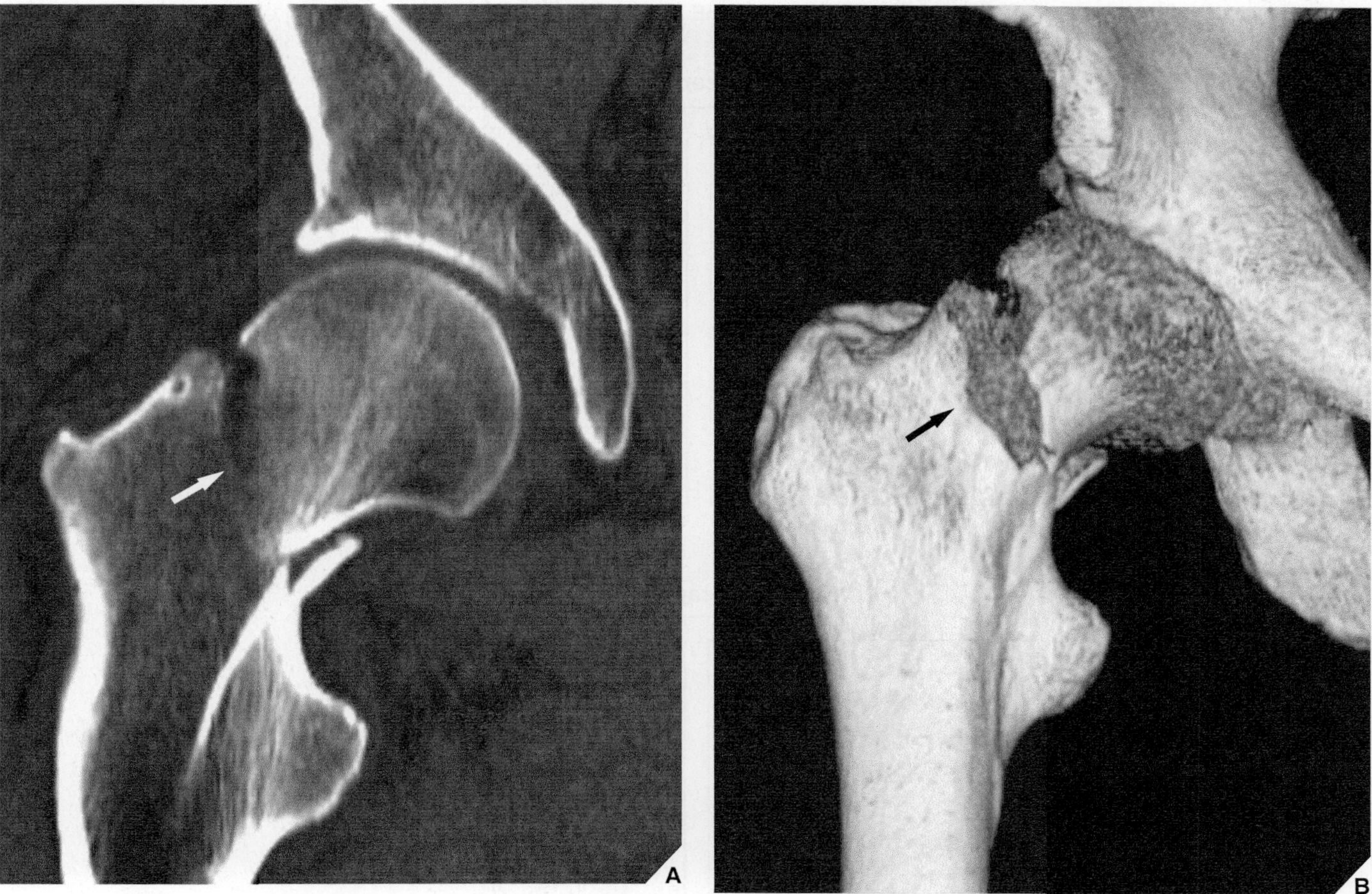

FIGURE 8.36 CT and 3D CT of midcervical fracture. **(A)** Coronal reformatted and **(B)** 3D reconstructed CT images of the right hip demonstrate a midcervical fracture of the femur *(arrows)*.

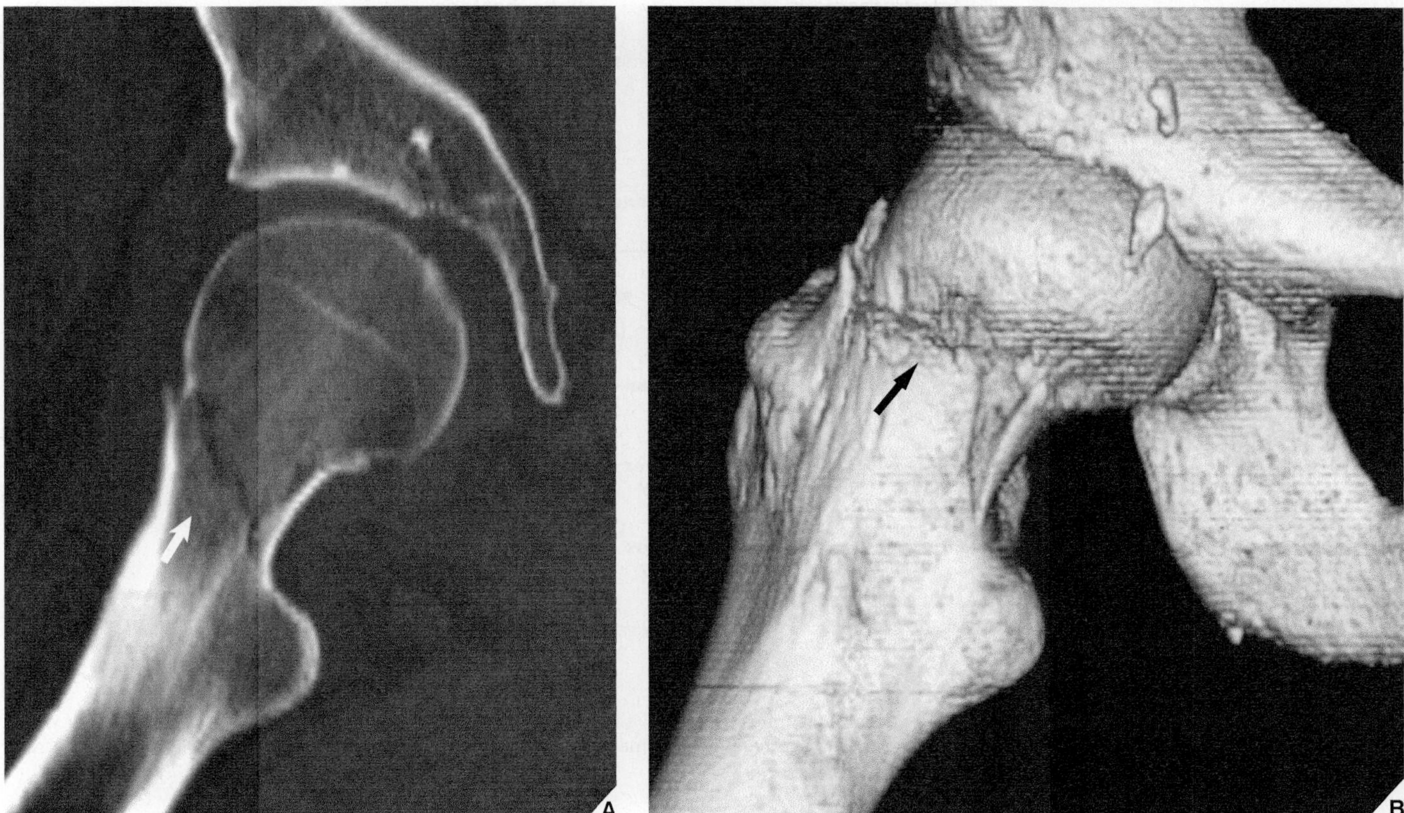

FIGURE 8.37 CT and 3D CT of basicervical fracture. **(A)** Coronal reformatted and **(B)** 3D reconstructed CT images of the right hip show a basicervical fracture *(arrows)* in this 60-year-old woman who fell from the stairs.

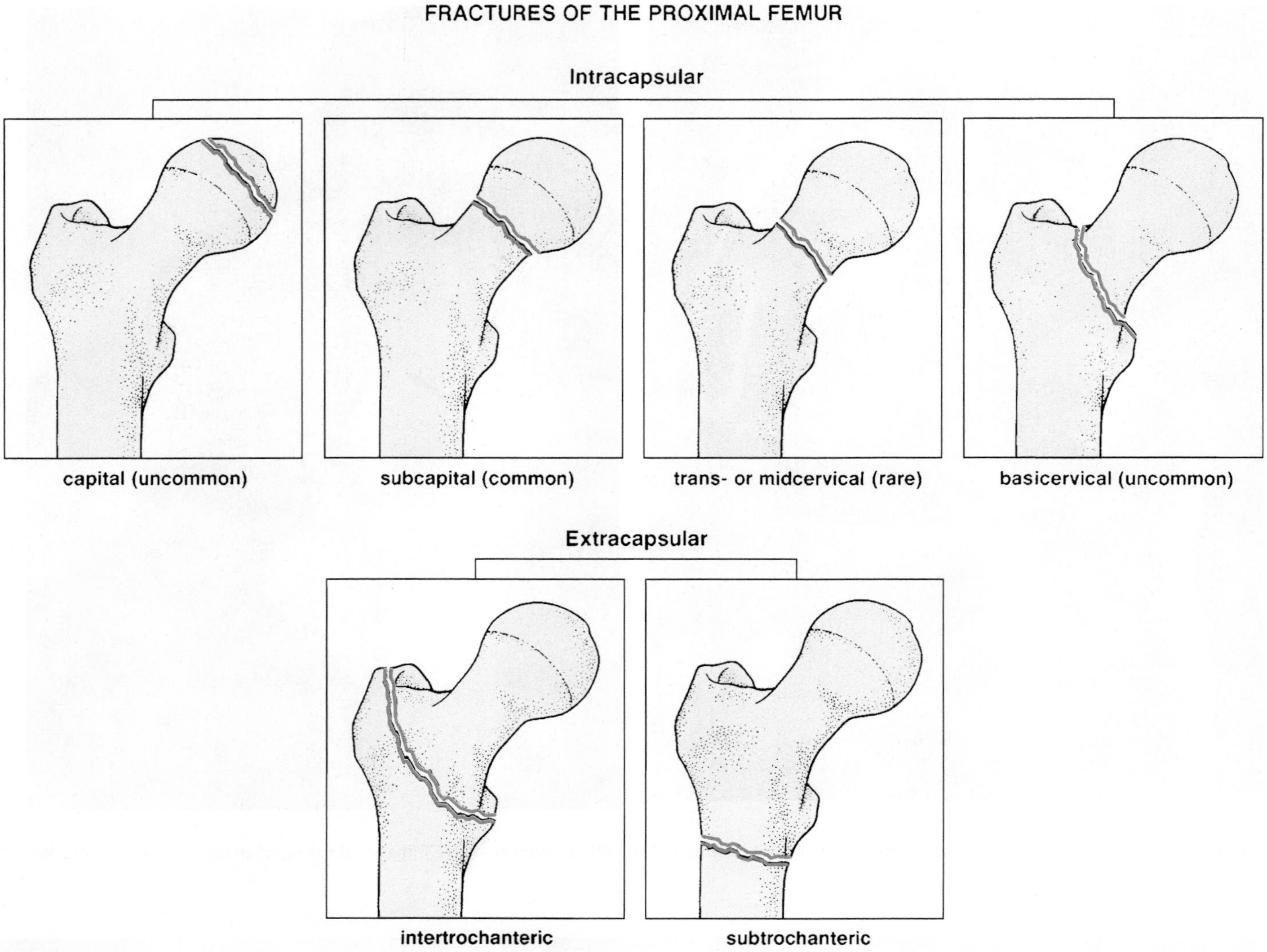

FRACTURES OF THE PROXIMAL FEMUR

Intracapsular

capital (uncommon)

subcapital (common)

trans- or midcervical (rare)

basicervical (uncommon)

Extracapsular

intertrochanteric

subtrochanteric

FIGURE 8.38 **Fractures of the proximal femur.** Fractures of the proximal femur are traditionally classified as intracapsular and extracapsular.

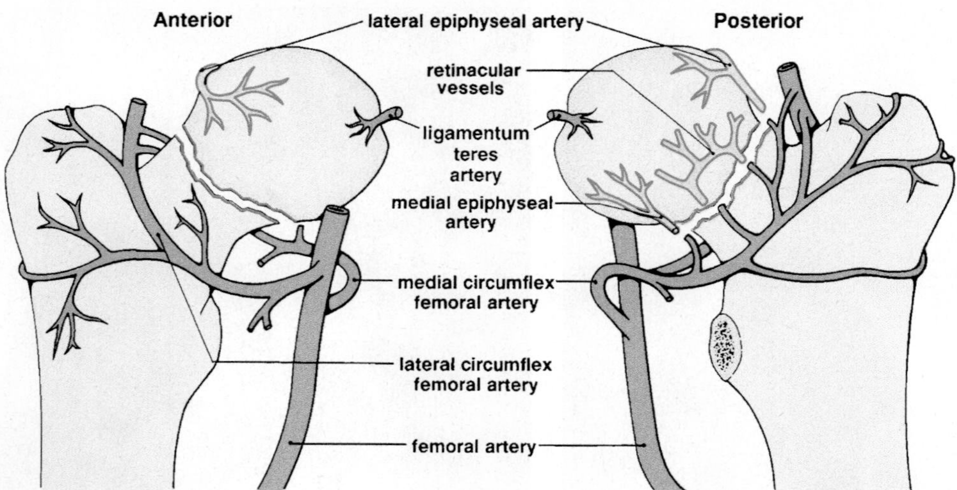

FIGURE 8.39 **Blood supply to the proximal femur.** The proximal femur is supplied with blood mainly by the circumflex femoral arteries, branches of which ascend subcapsularly along the femoral neck to the femoral head. Intracapsular fracture of the proximal femur may so severely interrupt the blood supply that osteonecrosis results.

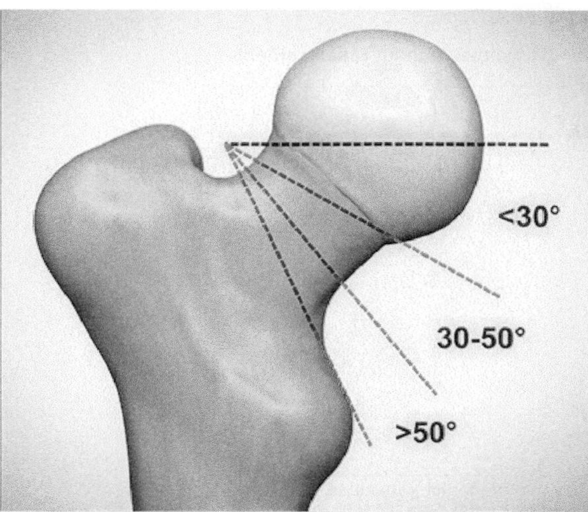

FIGURE 8.40 **The Pauwels classification of intracapsular fractures.** The classification is based on the obliquity of the fracture line: The more the fracture line approaches the vertical, the less stable is the fracture and consequently the greater are the chances for nonunion.

remains in normal alignment with the femoral head, which is not displaced but rather tilted in a varus deformity so that its medial trabeculae do not align with those of the pelvis. The medial trabeculae of the head form an angle of approximately 160 degrees with those of the femoral neck. This is also a stable fracture with a good prognosis.

Stage III: Complete subcapital fracture with partial displacement. In this category, the femoral shaft is externally rotated. The femoral head is medially rotated, abducted, and tilted in a varus deformity. The medial trabeculae of the head are out of alignment with those of the pelvis. This fracture is usually unstable, but it may be converted to a stable fracture by proper reduction. The prognosis is not as good as that for stage I and stage II fractures.

Stage IV: Complete subcapital fracture with full displacement. In this type, the femoral shaft, in addition to being externally rotated, is upwardly displaced and lies anterior to the femoral head. Although the head is completely detached from the shaft, it remains in its normal position in the acetabulum. The medial trabeculae are in alignment with those of the pelvis (Fig. 8.44). This is an unstable fracture with a poor prognosis.

This staging of femoral neck fractures has important prognostic value. In following up 80 patients over 1 year, Garden found complete union in all those graded stages I and II, 93% in those graded stage III, and only 57% in those graded stage IV. Osteonecrosis occurred in only 8% of nondisplaced stage I or stage II fractures but in 30% of displaced stage III or IV fractures.

Extracapsular Fractures

Frequently resulting from direct injury in a fall, extracapsular fractures occur in an even older age group than do intracapsular fractures. Most of these fractures are intertrochanteric, the major fracture line extending from the greater to the lesser trochanter, and they are usually comminuted. Radiographic diagnosis can usually be made on a single anteroposterior view of the hip (Fig. 8.45). Rarely, the fracture line may be obscure, requiring oblique projections for its demonstration. For the purpose of surgical planning, CT and 3D CT are commonly requested by the orthopaedic surgeon (Figs. 8.46 and 8.47).

As mentioned, extracapsular fractures of the proximal femur, for which several classifications have been developed, can generally be divided into two major subgroups: intertrochanteric and subtrochanteric. Intertrochanteric fractures can be further subdivided according to the number of fragments or the extension of the fracture line. A simple classification of such fractures has been proposed that considers the number of fragments (Fig. 8.48). The two-part fracture in this system is stable, whereas the four-part and multipart fractures are unstable. Boyd and Griffin have proposed a classification of intertrochanteric fractures according to the presence or absence of comminution and involvement

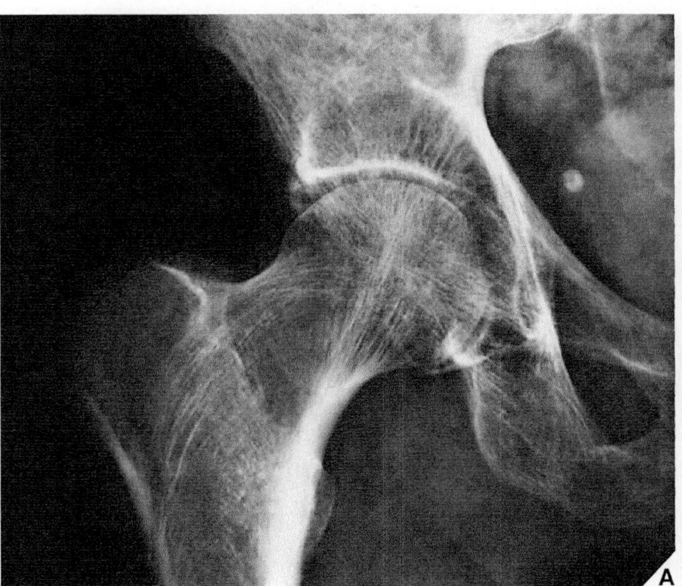

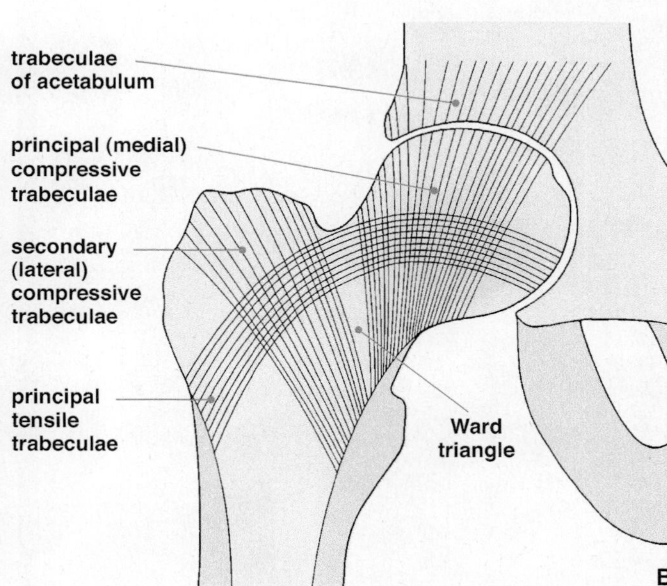

FIGURE 8.41 **Trabeculae of the hip.** The Garden staging system of femoral neck fractures is based on the three groups of trabeculae that are demonstrable within the femoral head and neck. The principal tensile trabeculae form an arc, extending from the lateral margin of the greater trochanter, through the superior cortex of the neck and across the femoral head, ending at its inferior aspect below the fovea. The principal (medial) compressive trabeculae are vertically oriented, extending from the medial cortex of the neck into the femoral head in a triangular configuration. They are normally aligned with the trabeculae seen in the acetabulum. The secondary (lateral) compressive trabeculae extend from the calcar and lesser trochanter to the greater trochanter in a fan-like pattern. The central area bounded by this trabecular system is known as *Ward triangle*.

GARDEN STAGING OF SUBCAPITAL FEMORAL FRACTURES

Stage I—Incomplete (Abducted or Impacted)

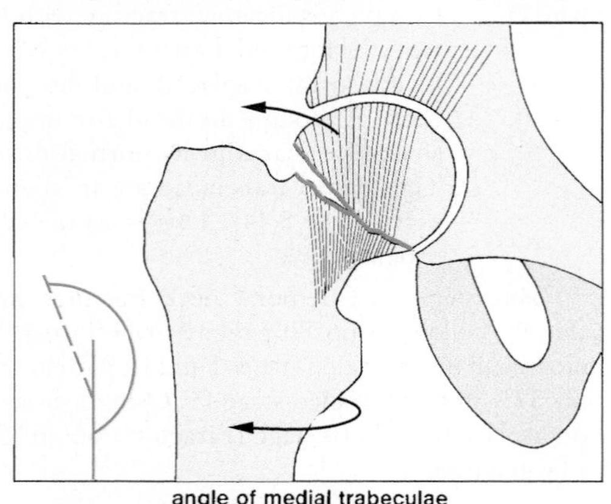

angle of medial trabeculae of head and neck > 180°

Stage II—Complete, without Displacement

angle of medial trabeculae of head and neck ≈ 160°

Stage III—Complete, with Partial Displacement

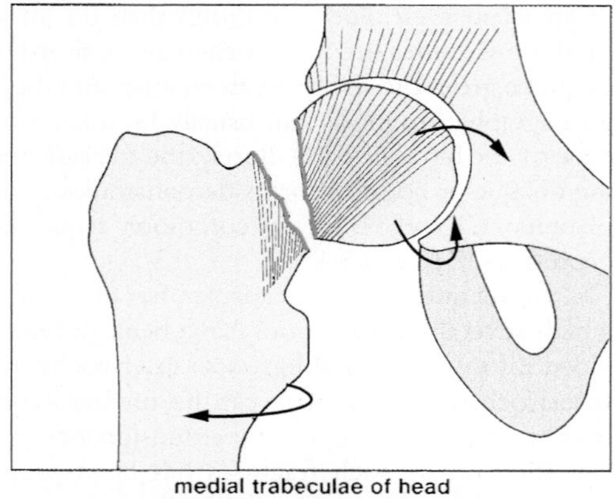

medial trabeculae of head not aligned with pelvic trabeculae

Stage IV—Complete, with Full Displacement

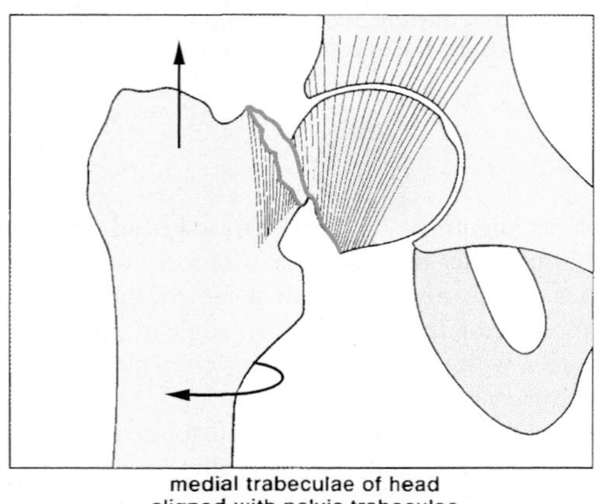

medial trabeculae of head aligned with pelvic trabeculae

FIGURE 8.42 The Garden classification of subcapital fractures. The Garden staging of subcapital femoral fractures is based on displacement of the femoral head before reduction. Displacement is graded according to the position of the medial compressive trabeculae. (Modified from Garden RS. Reduction and fixation of subcapital fractures of the femur. *Orthop Clin North Am* 1974;5(4):683–712. Copyright © 1974 Elsevier. With permission.)

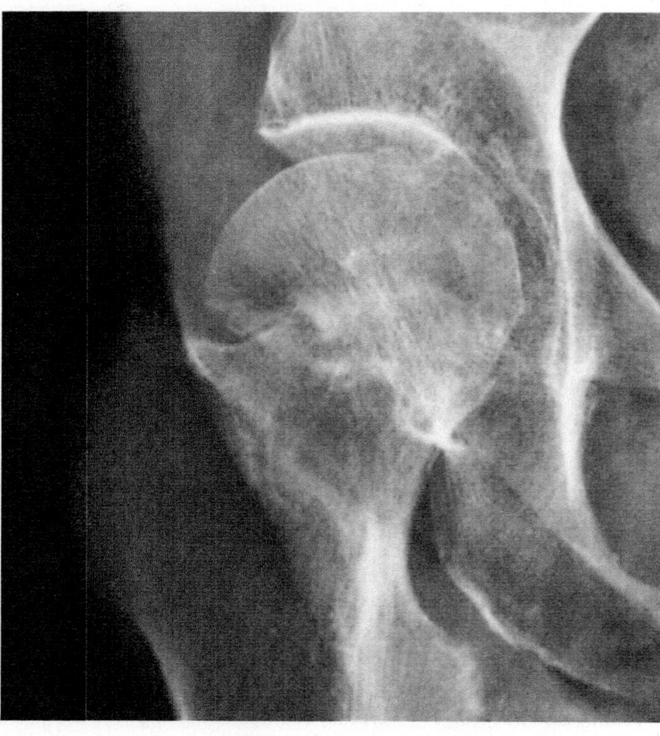

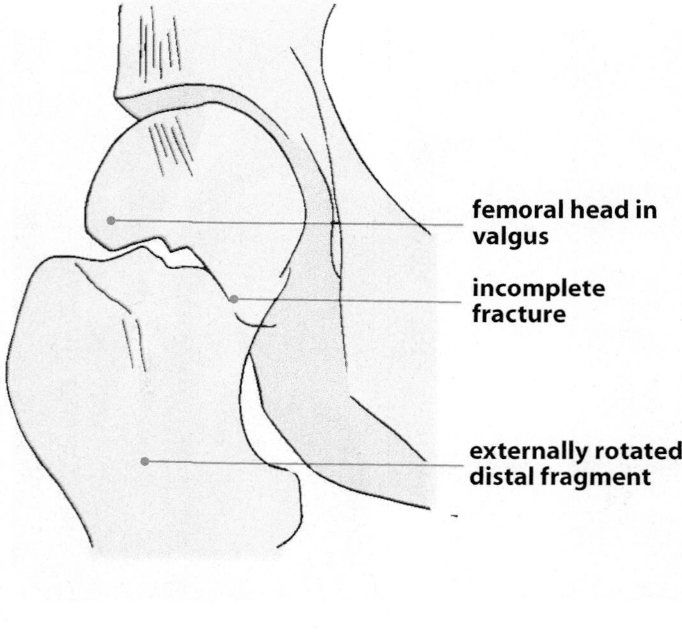

FIGURE 8.43 Subcapital fracture. After a fall to the floor, a 72-year-old woman sustained a fracture of the right femoral neck. Anteroposterior radiograph demonstrates a subcapital fracture, which appears to be impacted. The femoral head is in valgus, the distal fragment is externally rotated, and the medial trabeculae of the femoral head and neck form an angle greater than 180 degrees. These features characterize a Garden stage I fracture.

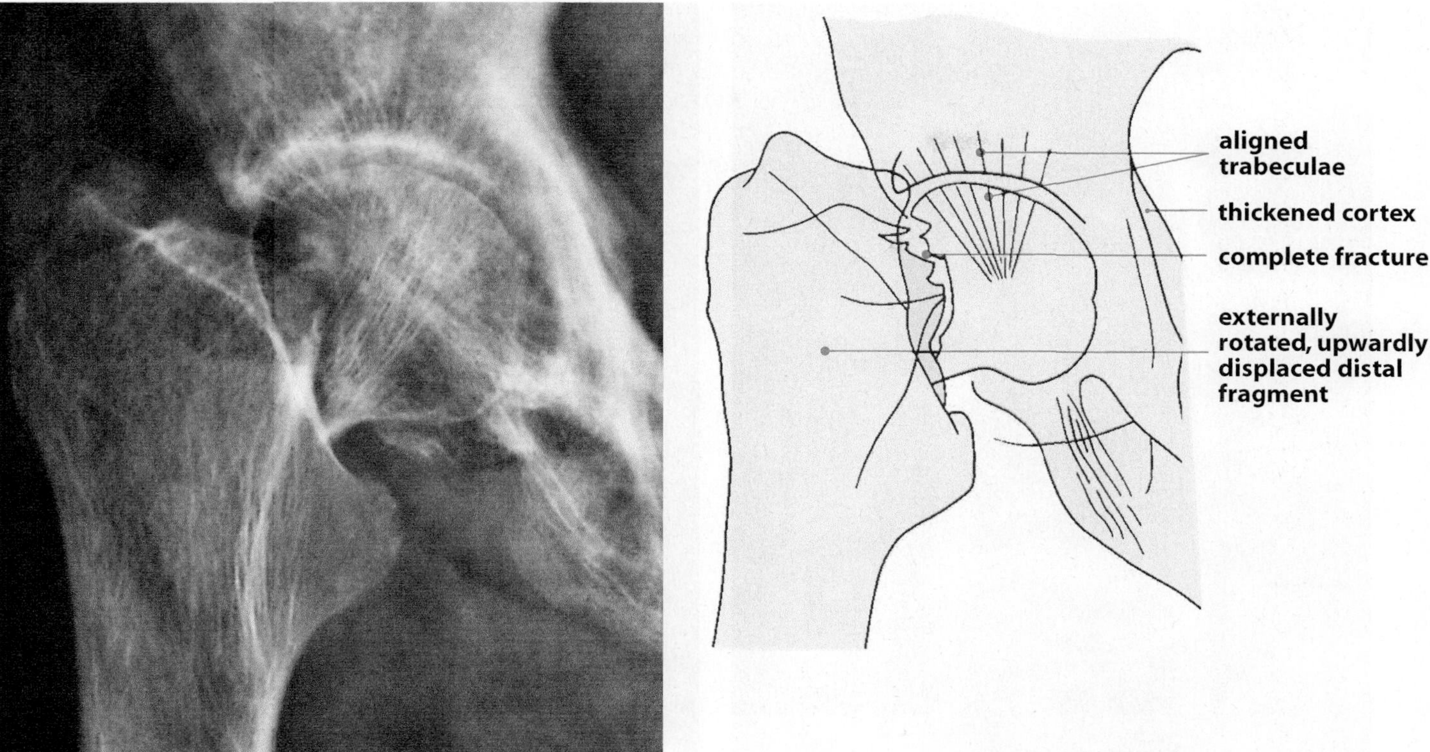

FIGURE 8.44 Subcapital fracture. After a fall on a subway platform, a 77-year-old woman sustained a fracture of the right femoral neck. Anteroposterior radiograph of the hip shows a complete subcapital fracture with full displacement. The femoral head, which is detached from the neck, is in its normal position in the acetabulum. Note the alignment of the trabeculae in the head and acetabulum. The femoral shaft is upwardly displaced and externally rotated. These features identify this injury as a Garden stage IV fracture.

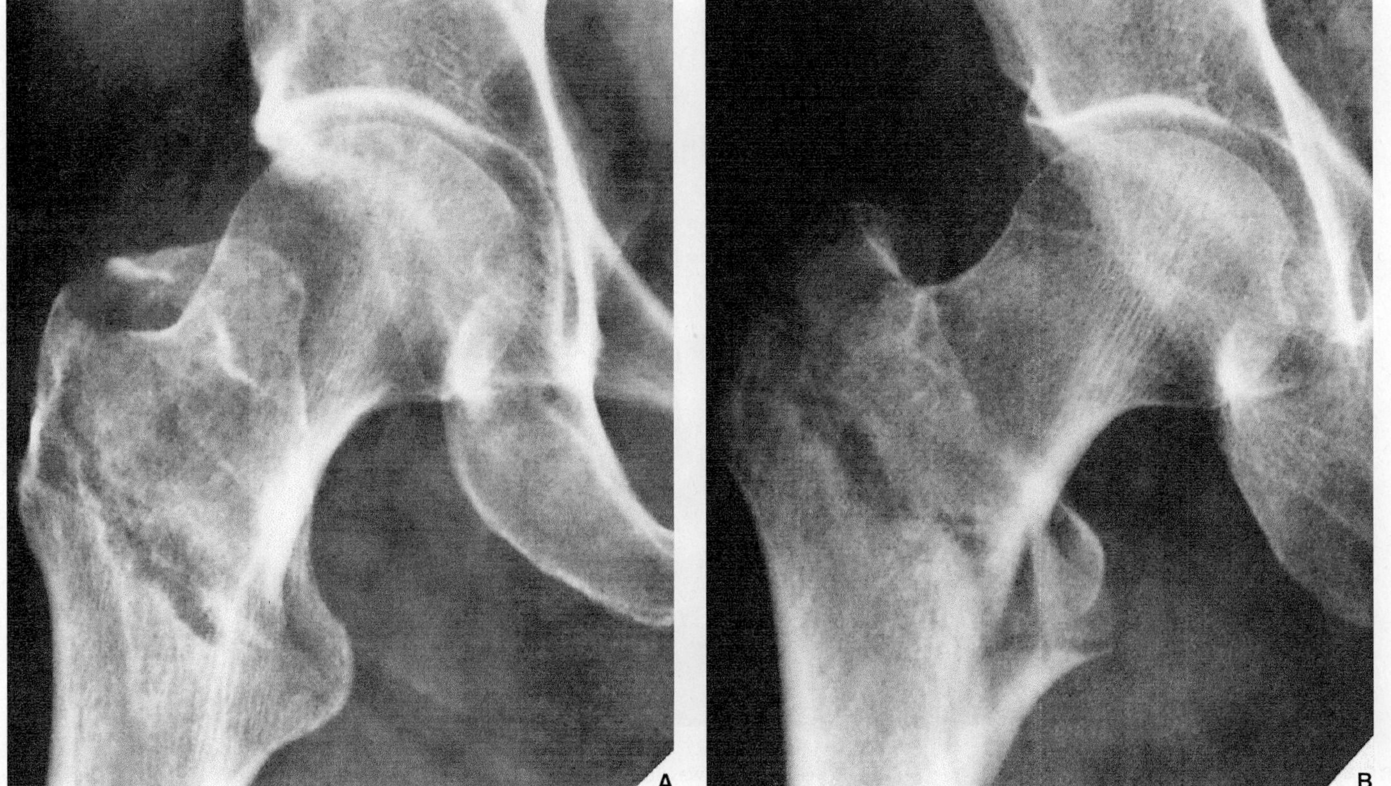

FIGURE 8.45 Intertrochanteric fracture. **(A)** Anteroposterior radiograph of the right hip demonstrates a comminuted, three-part intertrochanteric fracture, which can be classified as a Boyd-Griffin type II fracture. **(B)** Anteroposterior radiograph of the right hip shows a comminuted, multipart intertrochanteric fracture associated with a subtrochanteric component. This fracture can be classified as a Boyd-Griffin type III fracture. (For the Boyd-Griffin classification of intertrochanteric fractures, see Fig. 8.49.)

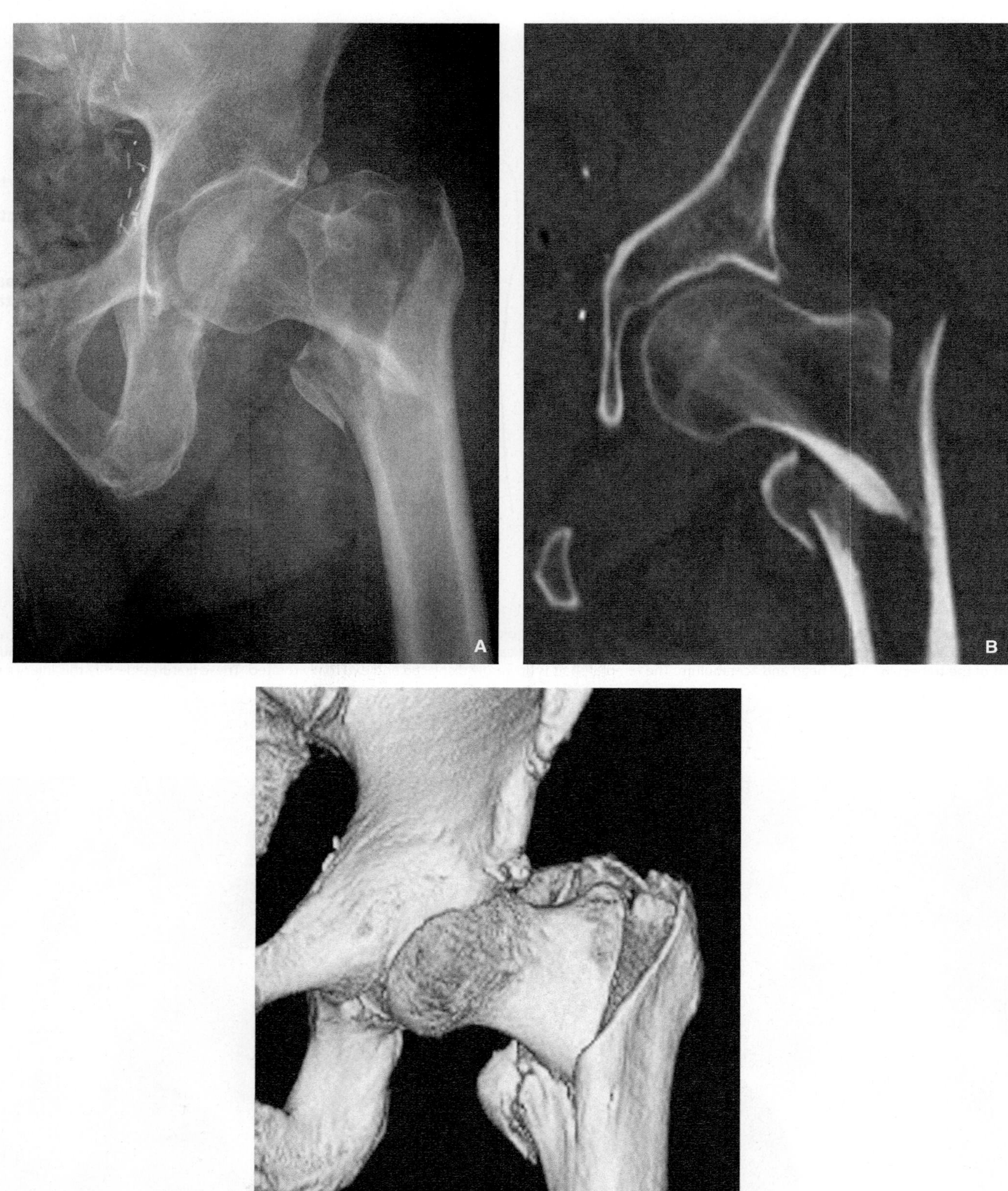

FIGURE 8.46 **CT and 3D CT of intertrochanteric fracture.** An 86-year-old man was injured in a fall from the stairs. **(A)** Anteroposterior radiograph of the left hip, **(B)** coronal reformatted, and **(C)** 3D reconstructed CT images show comminuted intertrochanteric fracture with varus deformity, which can be classified as a Kyle type III fracture.

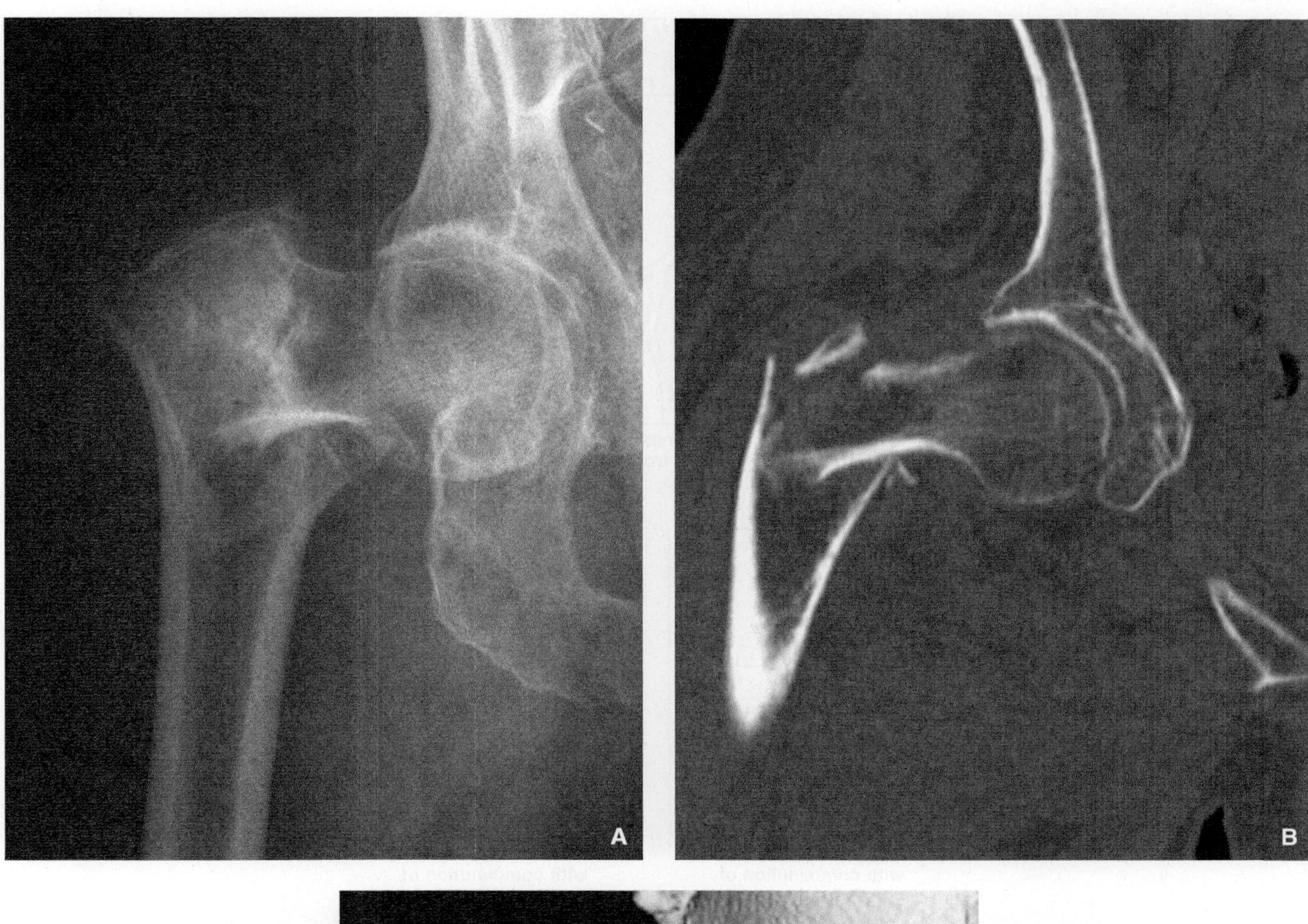

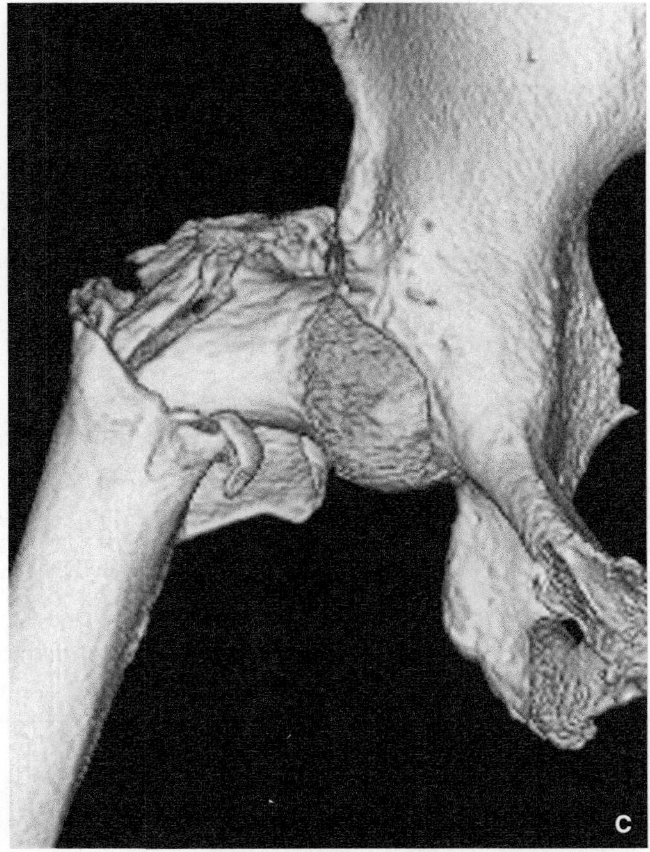

FIGURE 8.47 CT and 3D CT of intertrochanteric fracture. An 89-year-old woman fell on the street. **(A)** Anteroposterior radiograph of the right hip, **(B)** coronal reformatted, and **(C)** 3D reconstructed CT images show a comminuted intertrochanteric fracture with varus deformity extending into the femoral neck, which can be classified as a Kyle type V fracture.

SIMPLE CLASSIFICATION OF INTERTROCHANTERIC FRACTURES

Two-Part | Three-Part

linear intertrochanteric | with comminution of lesser trochanter | with comminution of greater trochanter

Four-Part | Multipart

with comminution of both trochanters | with comminution of both trochanters and intertrochanteric region

FIGURE 8.48 **Classification of intertrochanteric fractures.** The simple classification of intertrochanteric fractures is based on the number of osseous fragments.

of the subtrochanteric region (Fig. 8.49). Comminution of the posterior and medial cortices has important prognostic value. If comminuted, the fracture is unstable and may require a displacement osteotomy, a procedure particularly important in the treatment of four-part fractures when both trochanters are involved. If there is no comminution, then the fracture is stable and treatment involves fixation with a compression screw.

Classification introduced by Kyle is very effective from the practical point of view because it is based on the stability of various fractured fragments. Types I and II are stable fractures; and types III, IV, and V are unstable (Fig. 8.50; see also Figs. 8.46 and 8.47). Stability of the fracture is the crucial information for the orthopaedic surgeon and key to successful treatment. It also permits to render a more accurate prognosis.

Subtrochanteric fractures have been classified by Fielding according to the level of the fracture line and by Zickel according to their level, obliquity, and comminution (Fig. 8.51). An important fact about subtrochanteric fractures is their relatively benign course caused by the good supply of blood and adequate collateral circulation to this region of the femur. The occurrence of osteonecrosis of the femoral head and the incidence of nonunion as a result of intertrochanteric and subtrochanteric fractures are very low. The only serious complication to watch for is postoperative infection.

Dislocations in the Hip Joint

Traumatic dislocation of the femoral head is an uncommon injury resulting from a high-energy force and often accompanied by other significant injuries. The injury is caused by a substantial axial force, such as a knee impacting against the dashboard in a motor vehicle accident.

BOYD–GRIFFIN CLASSIFICATION OF INTERTROCHANTERIC FRACTURES

Type I | Type II | Type III | Type IV

linear intertrochanteric | with comminution of trochanteric region

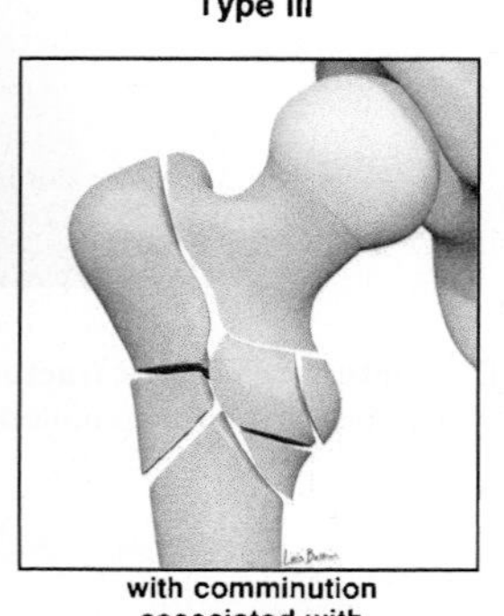

with comminution associated with subtrochanteric component

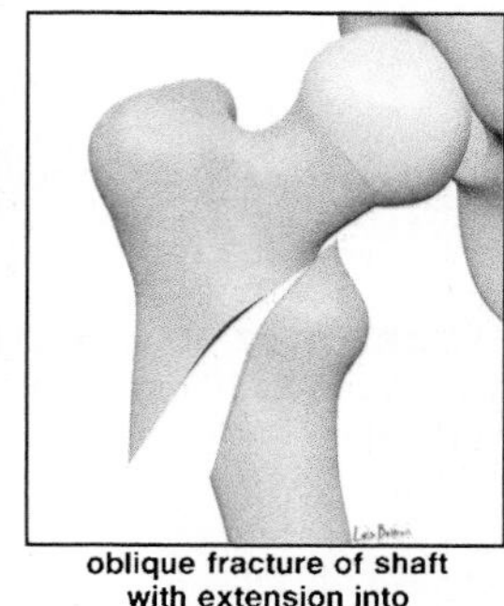

oblique fracture of shaft with extension into subtrochanteric region

FIGURE 8.49 **The Boyd-Griffin classification of intertrochanteric fractures.** This classification is based on the presence or absence of comminution and the involvement of the subtrochanteric region.

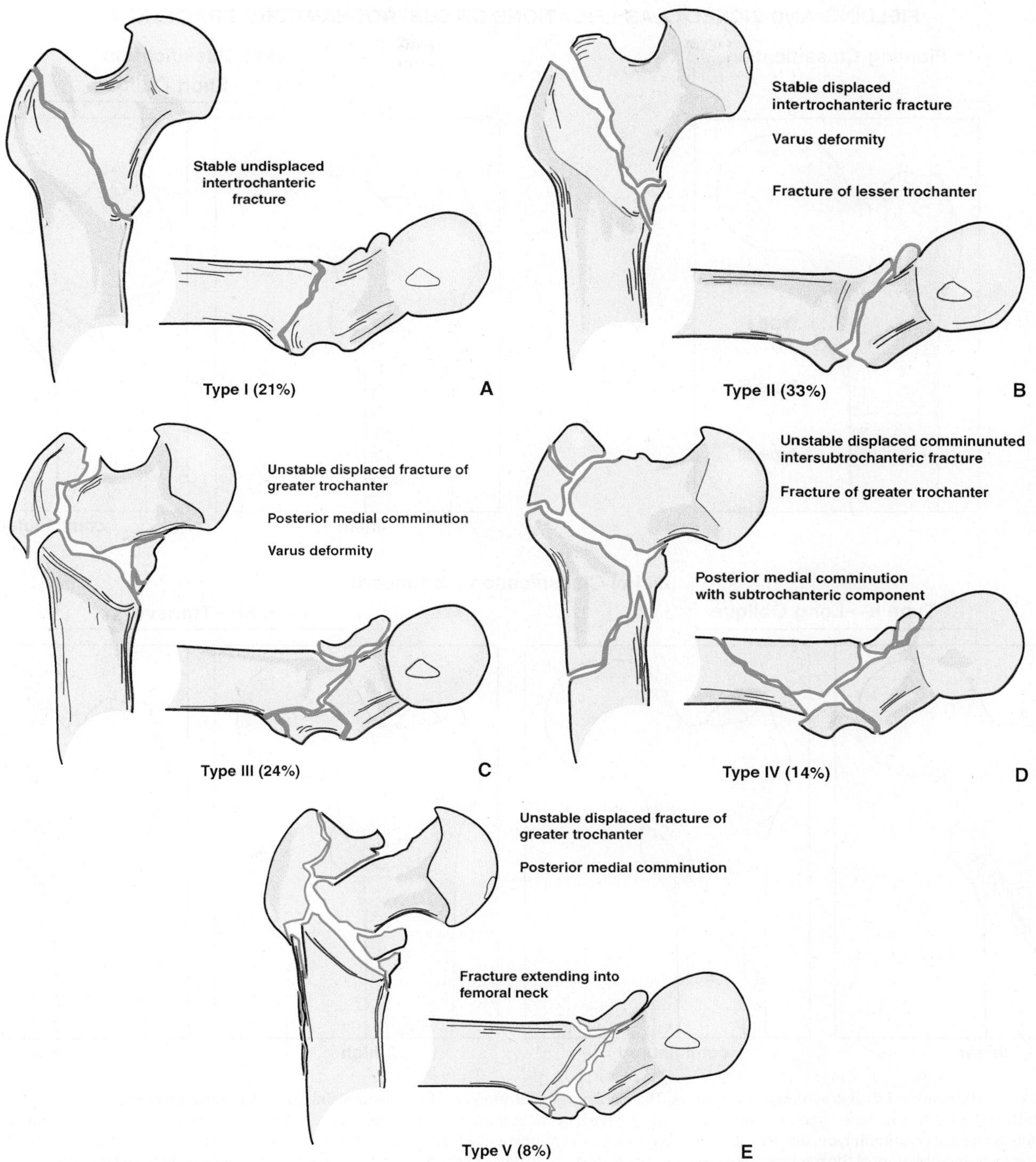

FIGURE 8.50 The Kyle classification of intertrochanteric fractures. This classification is based on stability of the fracture fragments and permits a more accurate prognosis of this injury. (Modified with permission by McGraw-Hill, from Moehring HD, Greenspan A, eds. *Fractures—diagnosis and treatment.* New York: McGraw-Hill; 2000:99–105.)

Generally, dislocations in the hip joint can be classified as anterior, posterior, or central (medial). The position of the hip at the moment of impact determines the direction of dislocation: hip flexion, adduction, and internal rotation result in posterior dislocation; and hip abduction and external rotation yield anterior dislocation. Posterior dislocation of the femoral head is far more common than anterior dislocation, which constitutes only 5% to 18% of all hip dislocations. It is also more frequently associated with fractures, particularly involving the posterior acetabular rim; anterior dislocation, in contrast, tends to be simple, without associated fracture. A predisposition to traumatic posterior hip dislocation has been suggested for individuals with retroversion or decreased anteversion of the femoral neck. Similarly, increased femoral neck anteversion may predispose to traumatic anterior hip dislocation. Dislocations are readily identified on radiographs of the hip in the anteroposterior projection. In *anterior dislocation*, which accounts for only 13% of all hip dislocations, the femoral head is displaced into the obturator, pubic, or iliac region. On the anteroposterior film, the femur is abducted and externally rotated, and the femoral head lies medial and inferior to the acetabulum (Fig. 8.52). In *posterior dislocation*, which is the most common type of dislocation, the anteroposterior view reveals the femur to be internally rotated and adducted, whereas the femoral head lies lateral and superior to the acetabulum (Fig. 8.53). Posterior dislocations are occasionally complicated by the presence of the acetabular or femoral head fractures (Figs. 8.54 and 8.55). *Central dislocation* (or *central protrusio*) is always associated with an acetabular fracture, with the femoral head protruding into the pelvic cavity (Figs. 8.56 and 8.57).

Dislocation of the femoral head is often accompanied by significant injuries involving the bone and cartilage and the muscles and ligaments

FIELDING AND ZICKEL CLASSIFICATIONS OF SUBTROCHANTERIC FRACTURES

Fielding Classification

type I

type II

type III

Zickel Classification

Type I—Short Oblique

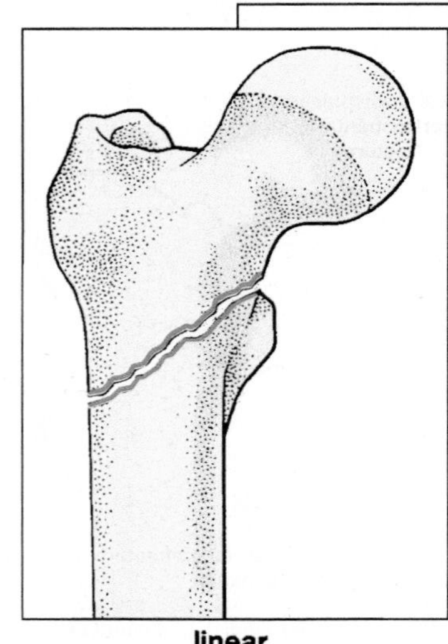

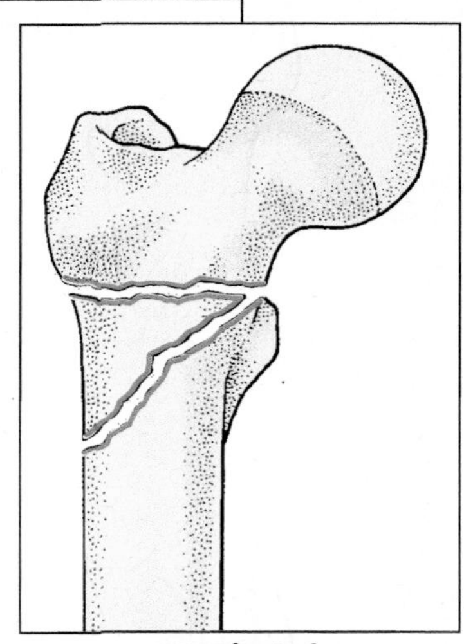

Zickel Classification (continued)

Type II—Long Oblique

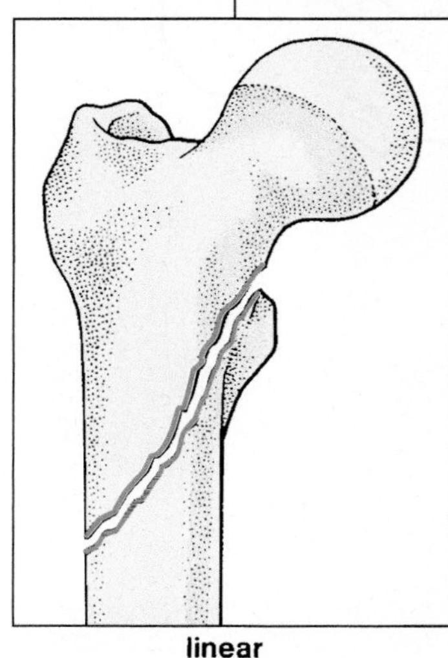

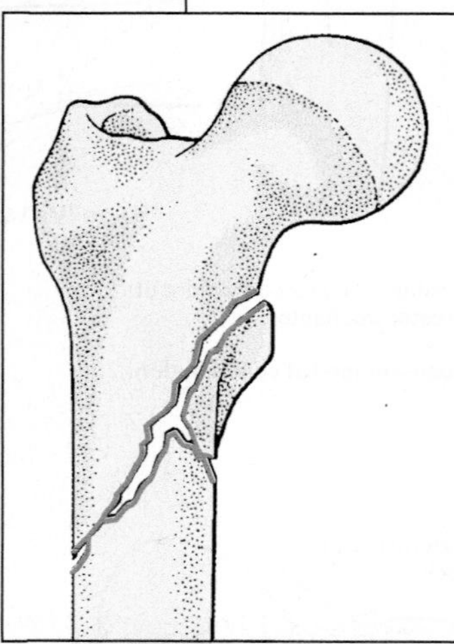

Type III—Transverse

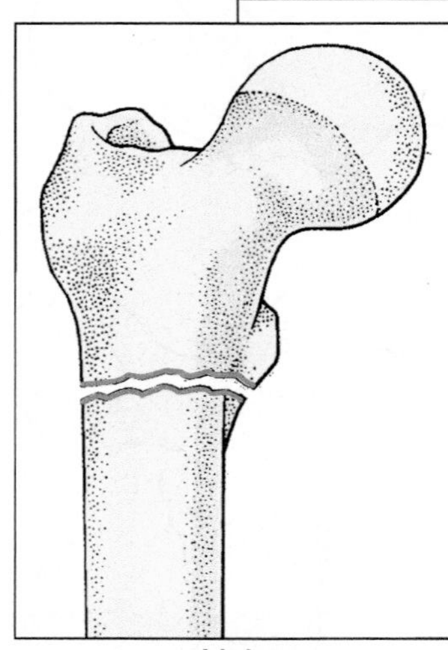

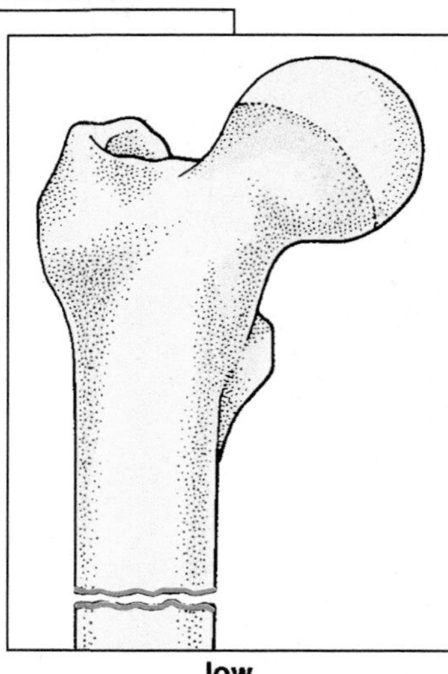

FIGURE 8.51 Classification of subtrochanteric fractures. The Fielding classification of subtrochanteric fractures **(top left)** is based on the level of the subtrochanteric region in which the fracture occurs. Type I fractures, the most common type, occur at the level of the lesser trochanter; type II, within the region 2.5 cm below the lesser trochanter; and type III, the least common type, occurs within the region 2.5 to 5 cm below the lesser trochanter. The Zickel classification of subtrochanteric fractures takes into consideration the level and obliquity of the fracture line as well as the presence or absence of comminution. (Modified with permission from Fielding JW. Subtrochanteric fractures. *Clin Orthop* 1973;92:86–99; Zickel RE. An intramedullary fixation device for the proximal part of the femur. Nine years' experience. *J Bone Joint Surg Am* 1976;58:866–872.)

surrounding the joint. CT has proved indispensable for identifying fractures associated with hip dislocations, and it remains the best means of detecting cortical disruption (see Figs. 8.54 and 8.55). MRI has assumed a highly significant role among imaging modalities, especially because of its superior capabilities in comparison with CT in evaluating cancellous bone, cartilage, muscle, ligaments, and intraarticular fluid. MRI can effectively identify and quantify the muscle injury and joint effusion/hemarthrosis that invariably accompany traumatic anterior and posterior dislocation of the hip (see Figs. 4.133 and 4.134). It is also useful for demonstrating bone contusions, which occur commonly in both types of dislocation, as well as the less common sequelae of acute hip dislocation, including cortical infraction, osteochondral fracture, and tear of the acetabular labrum. It may also be helpful in identifying soft-tissue interposition in the joint space. The real importance of performing MRI after hip dislocation is to identify possible complications such as osteonecrosis of the femoral head.

Traumatic hip dislocations are treated with immediate closed reduction, preferably within 6 hours of injury. Such attention is required to lower the risk of osteonecrosis, one of the two main complications related to hip dislocation; the other is posttraumatic osteoarthritis.

A recent study found that osteonecrosis developed in only 4.8% of patients whose hip dislocation was reduced within 6 hours, compared with 58.8% of patients whose reduction occurred more than 6 hours after injury. The early detection of osteonecrosis is critical because the initial period offers the greatest chance of preserving joint function with surgical procedures such as drilling, rotational osteotomy, or core decompression with or without vascularized grafting. Posttraumatic osteoarthritis, with an incidence ranging from 17% to 48.8% in different series, has been attributed to the severity of the initial injury, intraarticular loose bodies, and continued heavy work after injury. Simple dislocations have a better prognosis than those with an associated fracture.

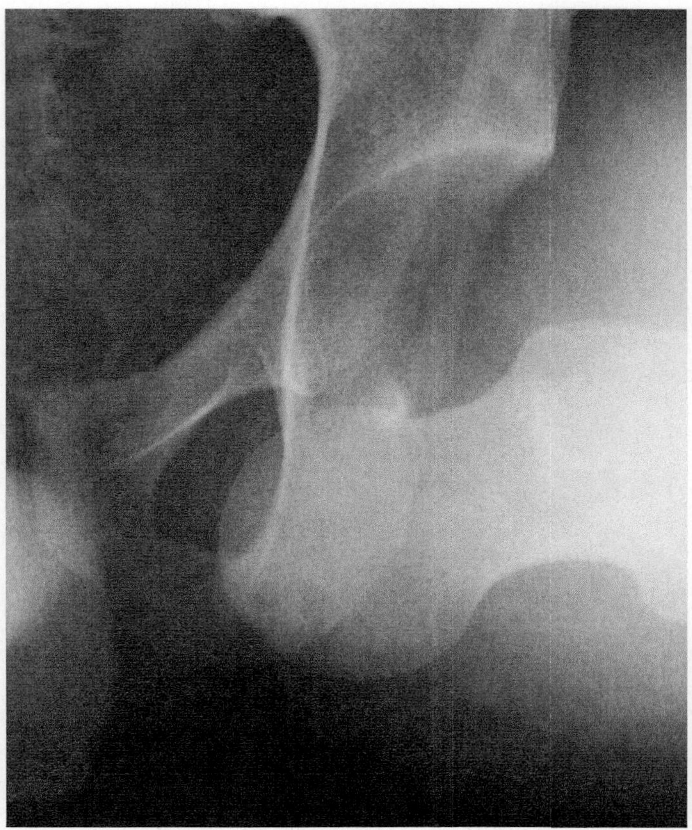

FIGURE 8.52 Anterior hip dislocation. A 19-year-old man sustained an anterior hip dislocation. Note on this anteroposterior radiograph a typical position of the femoral head, which lies inferior and medial to the acetabulum.

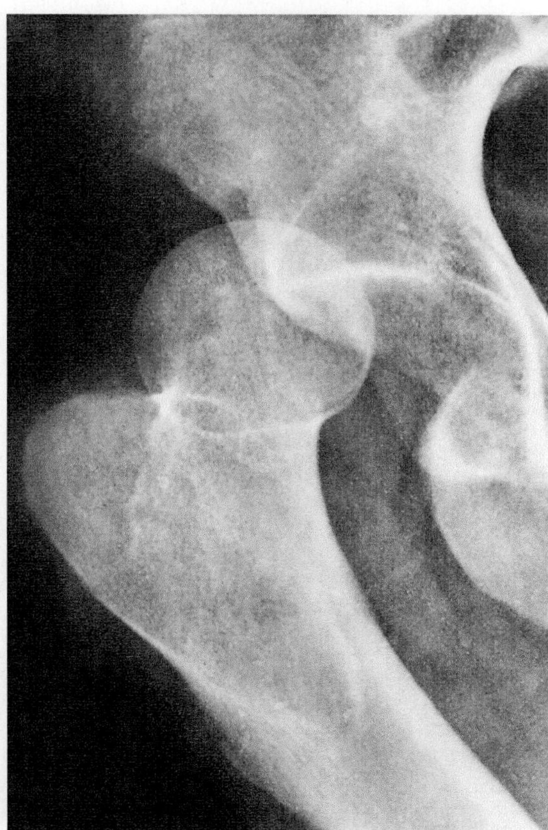

FIGURE 8.53 Posterior hip dislocation. A 30-year-old woman sustained a typical posterior hip dislocation in an automobile accident. Note on this anteroposterior radiograph that the extremity is adducted, and the femoral head overlaps the posterior acetabular rim.

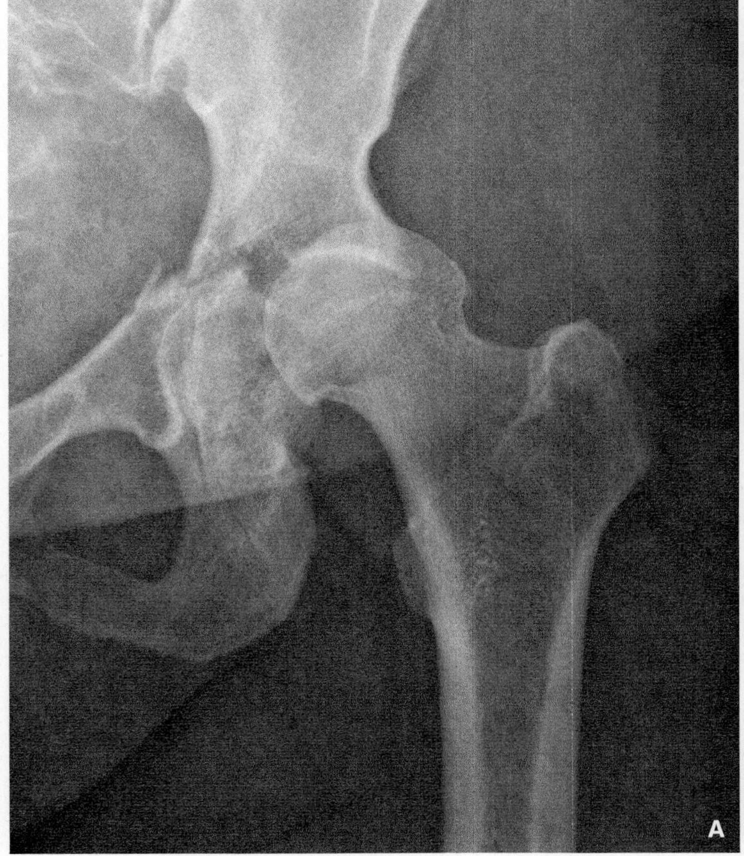

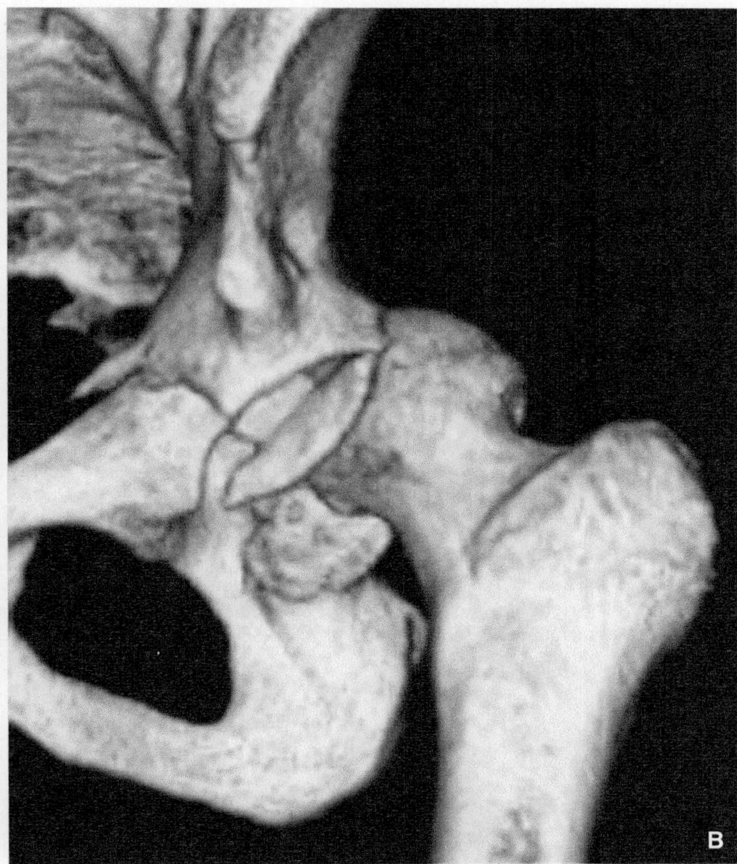

FIGURE 8.54 3D CT of posterior hip dislocation complicated by acetabular fracture. A 39-year-old woman was injured in a car accident. **(A)** Anteroposterior radiograph of the left hip and **(B)** 3D reconstructed CT image show posterior hip dislocation complicated by acetabular fracture.

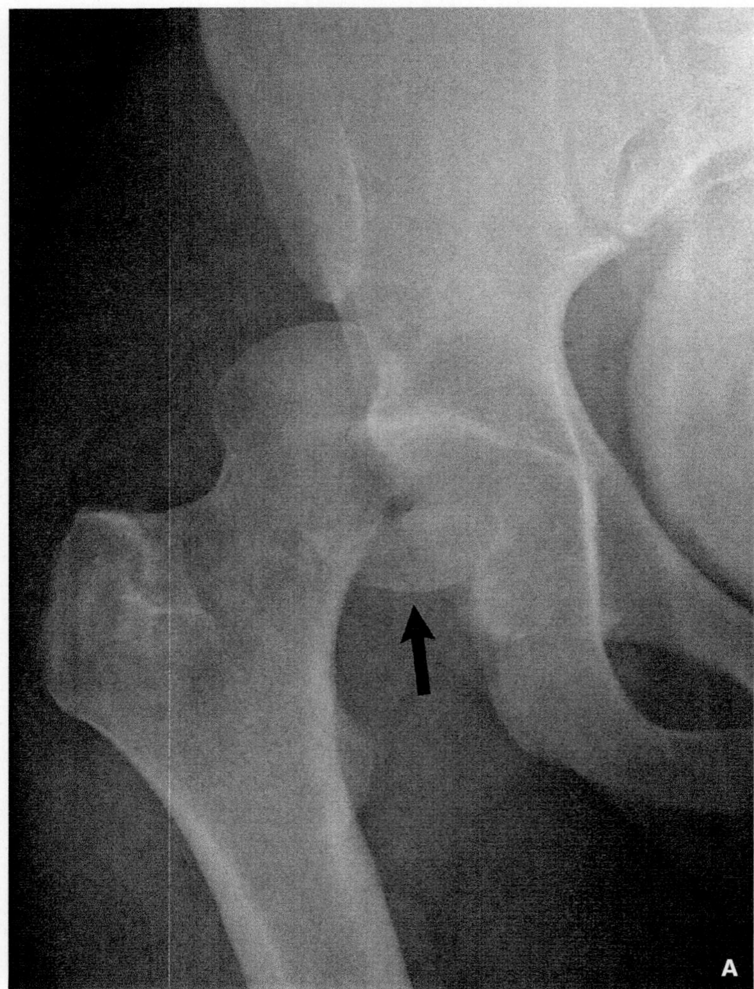

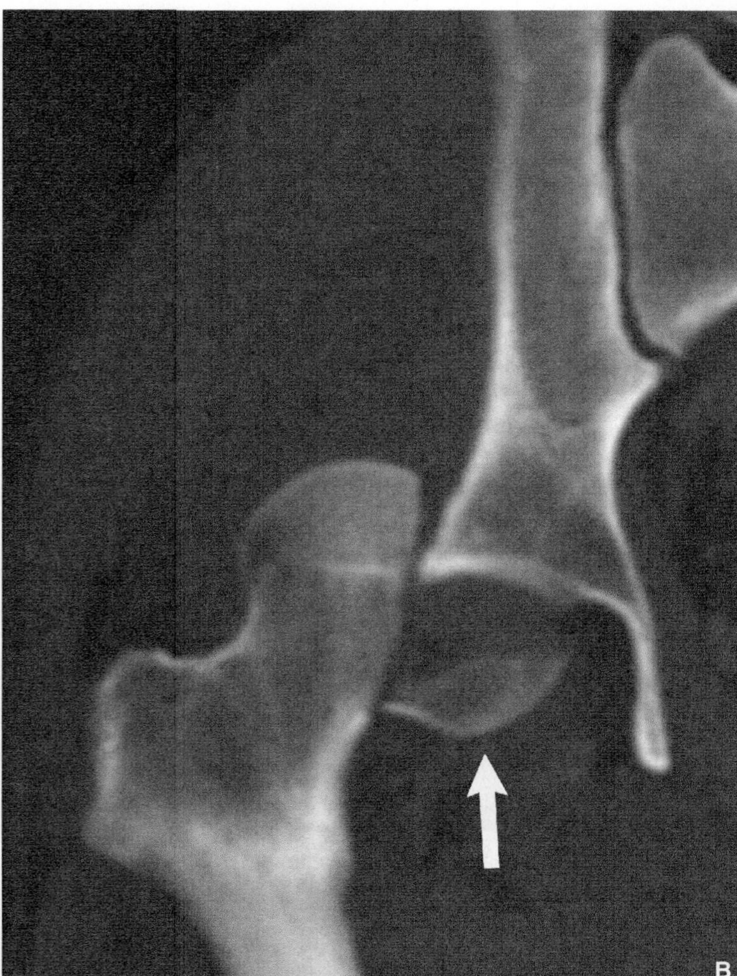

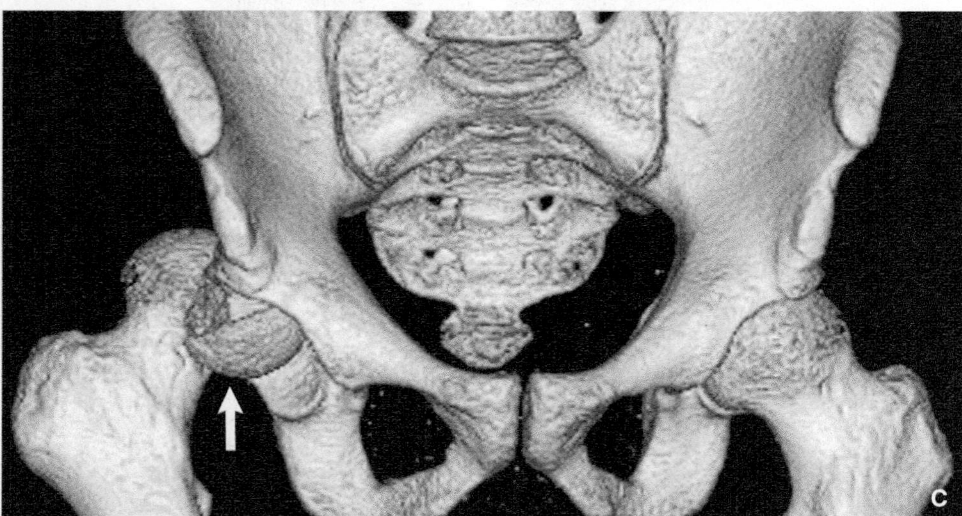

FIGURE 8.55 CT and 3D CT of posterior hip dislocation complicated by femoral head fracture. **(A)** Anteroposterior radiograph of the right hip, **(B)** coronal reformatted CT image of the right hip, and **(C)** 3D reconstructed image of the pelvis of a 37-year-old man who was injured in a motorcycle accident show posterior hip dislocation complicated by a fracture of the femoral head *(arrows)*. (See also Fig. 8.34.)

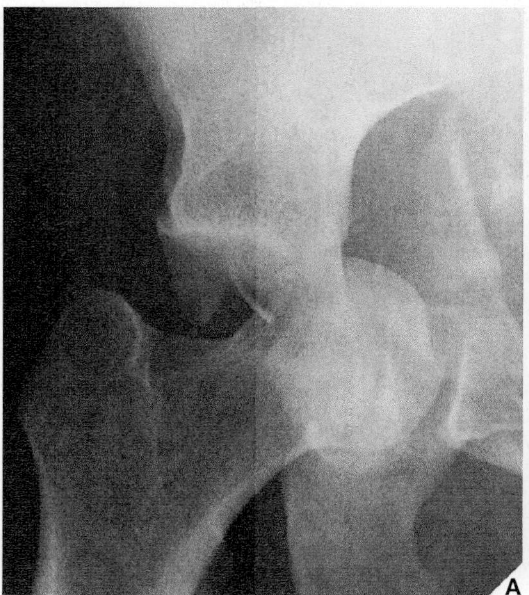

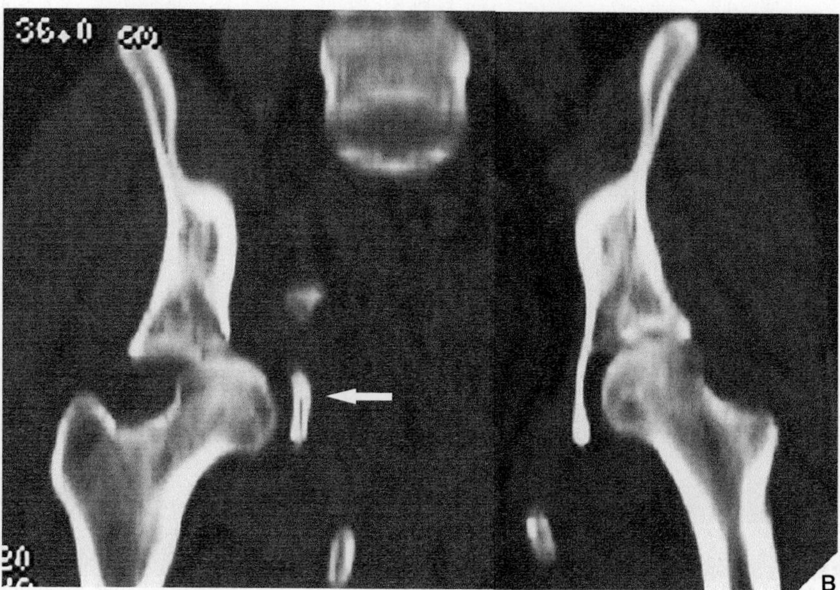

FIGURE 8.56 Central hip dislocation. A 22-year-old woman was injured in a car accident. **(A)** Anteroposterior radiograph of the right hip shows a complex acetabular fracture associated with a central displacement of the femoral head. **(B)** A coronal CT reformatted image shows medial displacement of the medial acetabular wall *(arrow)* and central hip dislocation.

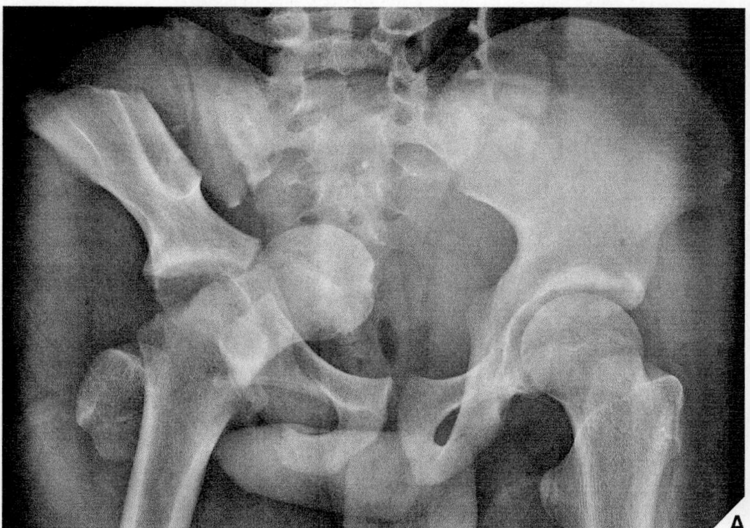

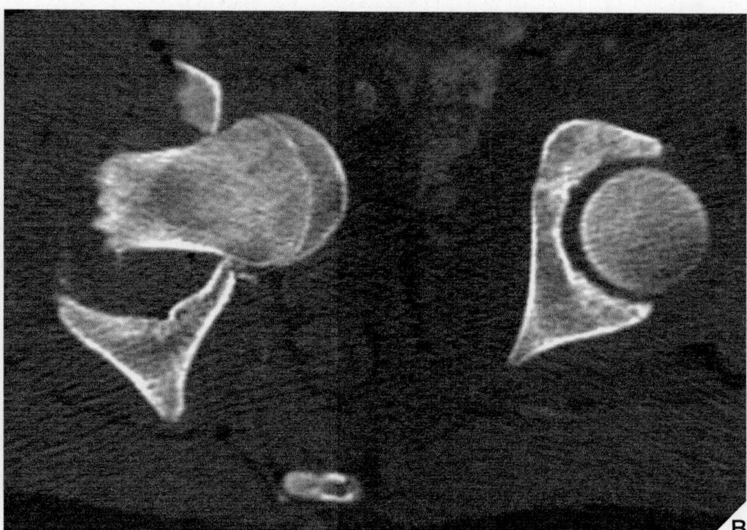

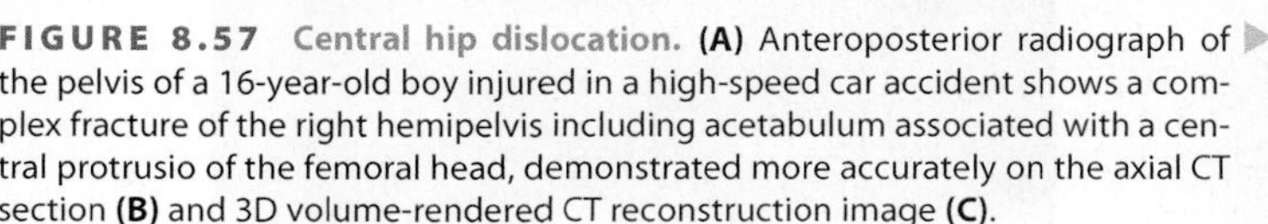

FIGURE 8.57 Central hip dislocation. (A) Anteroposterior radiograph of the pelvis of a 16-year-old boy injured in a high-speed car accident shows a complex fracture of the right hemipelvis including acetabulum associated with a central protrusio of the femoral head, demonstrated more accurately on the axial CT section **(B)** and 3D volume-rendered CT reconstruction image **(C)**.

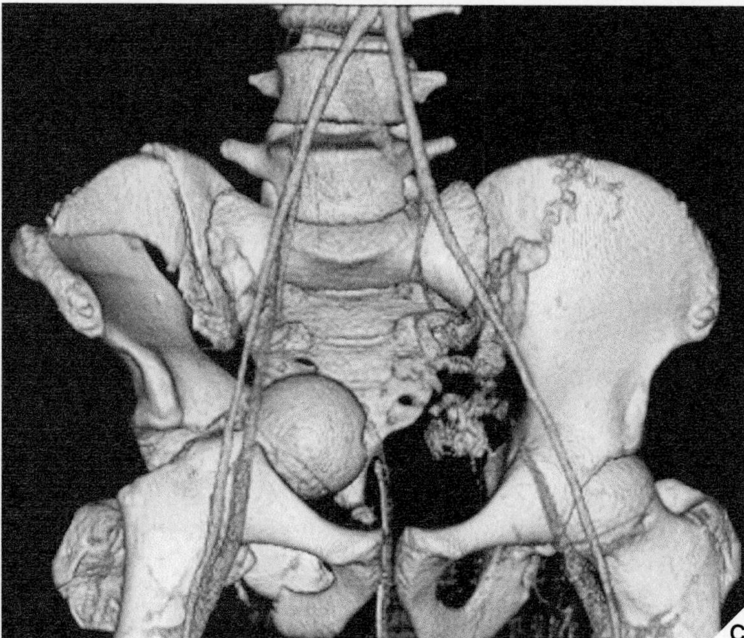

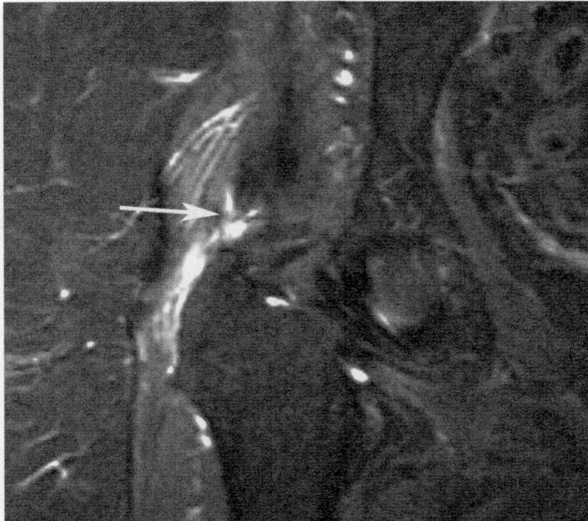

FIGURE 8.58 **Gluteus medius tendon tear.** Coronal short time inversion recovery (STIR) MR image demonstrates a complete tear of the right gluteus medius tendon *(arrow)* at the level of the greater trochanter, with focal edema.

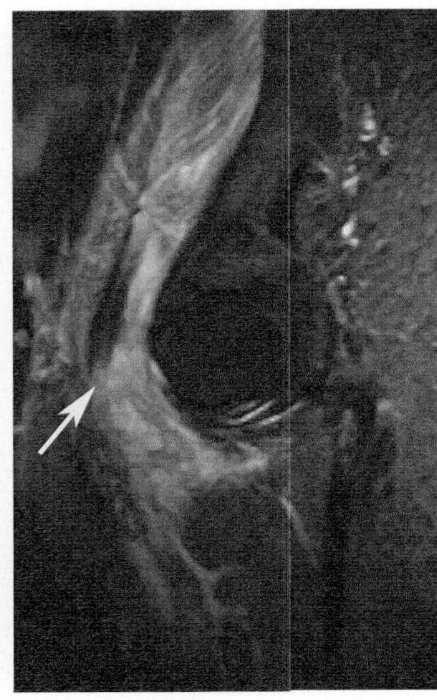

FIGURE 8.60 **Iliopsoas tendon tear.** Sagittal STIR MR image demonstrates a tear of the iliopsoas tendon at the level of the insertion to the lesser trochanter with proximal retraction *(arrow)*. There is surrounding edema and hematoma.

Tendon and Muscle Lesions

Lesions of the tendons about the hip are frequent in the elderly with involvement of the gluteus minimus and medius tendons, causing greater trochanteric pain syndrome related to peritendinitis, tendinosis, tears, and bursitis (Figs. 8.58 and 8.59), in a similar manner as in the shoulder, to the point that these tendons have been named the *rotator cuff of the hip*. Tears of the iliopsoas tendon can be seen in the elderly as well as in the young athletic population (Fig. 8.60). Other tendon lesions frequently seen in the young athletes include rectus femoris, sartorius, and hamstring tendon injuries (Figs. 8.61 and 8.62).

Additional etiologies for lateral hip pain/greater trochanteric pain syndrome include calcific peritendinitis (Fig. 8.63), ischiofemoral impingement, and snapping hip syndrome. Ischiofemoral impingement syndrome occurs when the distance between the ischial tuberosity and the lesser trochanter is decreased, causing compression of the quadratus femoris muscle. MRI demonstrates edema of the quadratus femoris muscle with decreased space between the ischial tuberosity and the lesser trochanter (Fig. 8.64). Snapping hip syndrome, also called *coxa saltans* or *dancer's hip* is a clinical syndrome presenting with pain and snapping sensation and/or popping noise and pain in the hip with certain movements, such as flexion, extension, abduction, and external rotation. It occurs more frequently in dancers and athletes. The etiology of snapping hip syndrome is more often related to external causes such as iliopsoas tendinitis and thickening of the iliotibial band in the region of the greater trochanter (Fig. 8.65). Internal causes of snapping hip syndrome include labral tear (Fig. 8.66), ligamentum teres pathology (Fig. 8.67), loose bodies, and synovial (osteo)chondromatosis (Fig. 8.68). Dynamic ultrasound of the hip provides a good assessment of the abnormal motion of the iliopsoas tendon when the patient is scanned during the hip movements that elicit the snapping sensation. MRI provides morphologic assessment of other potential etiologies for hip pain.

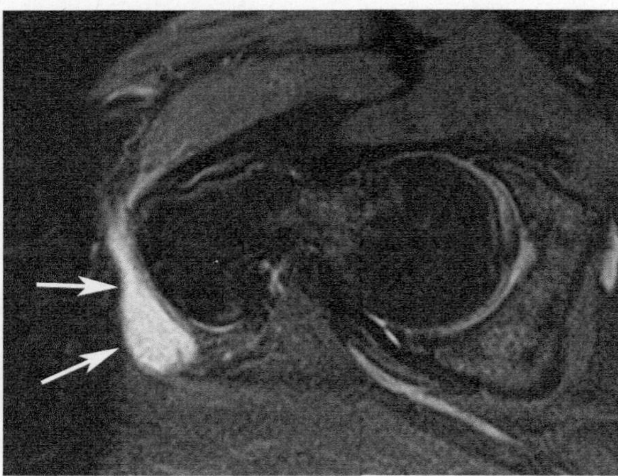

FIGURE 8.59 **Greater trochanteric bursitis.** Axial STIR MR image of the right hip of a middle age woman with chronic lateral hip pain demonstrates fluid distension of the greater trochanteric bursa *(arrows)*, consistent with bursitis.

Compressive and Entrapment Neuropathies

Compressive and entrapment neuropathies of the pelvis and hips are relatively infrequent and include piriformis syndrome, iliacus syndrome,

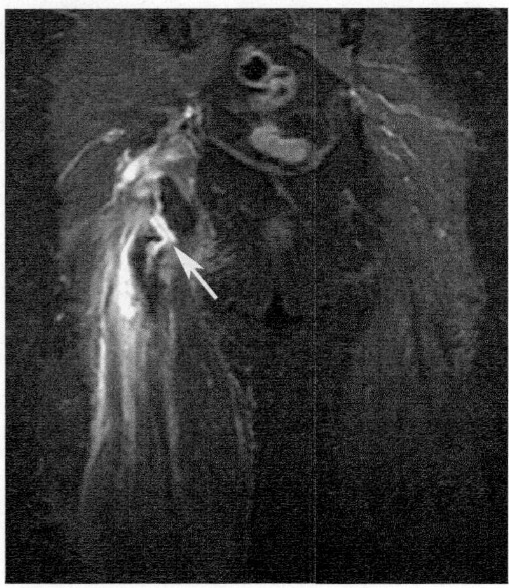

FIGURE 8.61 **Hamstring tendon tear.** Coronal STIR MR image demonstrates a complete tear of the right hamstring tendons with minimal retraction *(arrow)*. There is extensive soft-tissue edema and hematoma extending to the posterior thigh.

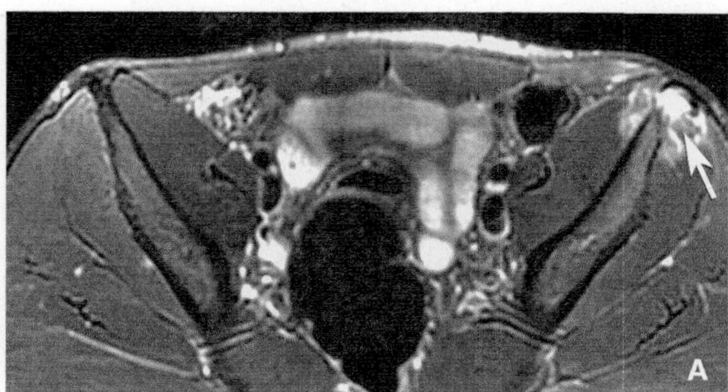

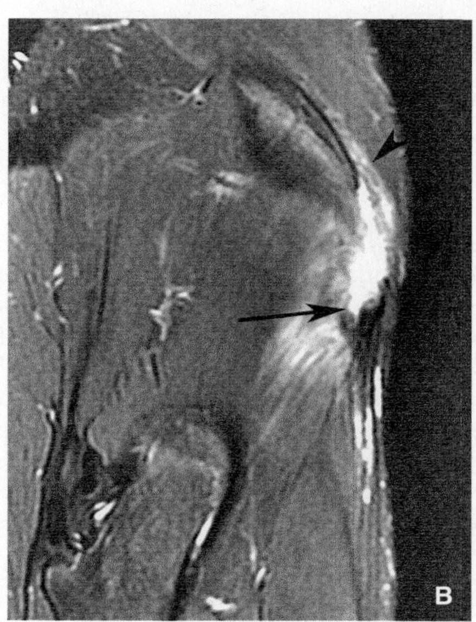

FIGURE 8.62 **Avulsion of the left sartorius tendon.** **(A)** Axial and **(B)** sagittal T2-weighted MR images in a young athlete demonstrate avulsion of the sartorius tendon *(arrows)* at the origin in the anterior superior iliac spine *(arrowhead)*, with focal edema and hematoma.

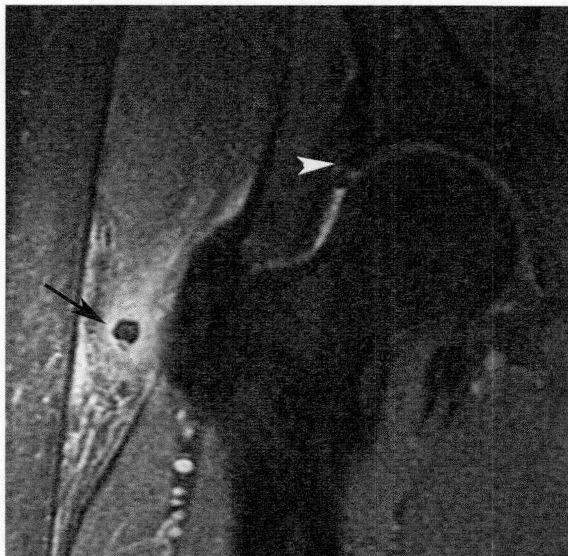

FIGURE 8.63 **Calcific peritendinitis as a cause of greater trochanteric pain syndrome.** Coronal STIR MR image of the right hip of a young adult with pain in the region of the greater trochanter shows a focal area of calcium deposit adjacent to the greater trochanter *(arrow)*, with prominent inflammatory changes and surrounding edema. Note the incidental finding of a superior labral tear *(arrowhead)*.

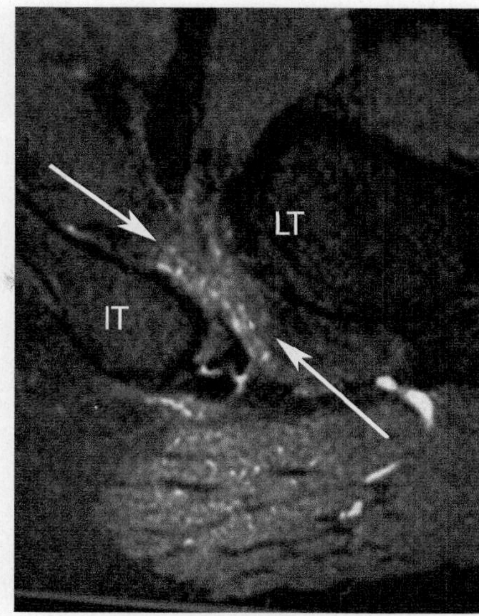

FIGURE 8.64 **Ischiofemoral impingement syndrome.** Axial STIR MR image in an adult patient with chronic hip pain shows decreased space between the lesser trochanter *(LT)* and the ischial tuberosity *(IT)* with edema of the quadratus femoris muscle *(arrows)*, which is impinged between the two osseous structures.

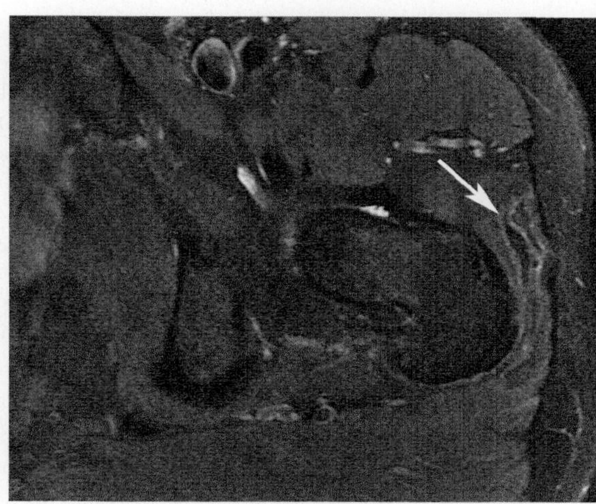

FIGURE 8.65 **Coxa saltans externa or external snapping hip syndrome.** Axial STIR MR image in a young woman with painful symptoms in the left hip shows fibrotic thickening and mild edema medial to the iliotibial band adjacent the greater trochanter *(arrow)*.

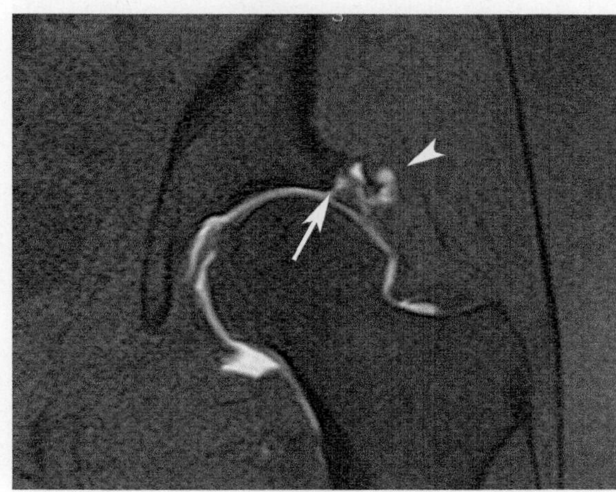

FIGURE 8.66 **Internal snapping syndrome due to labral tear.** Coronal T1-weighted fat-saturated MRa in a young female with chronic left hip pain and occasional snapping sensation shows a superior labral tear at the chondrolabral junction *(arrow)* associated with a small adjacent paralabral cyst *(arrowhead)*.

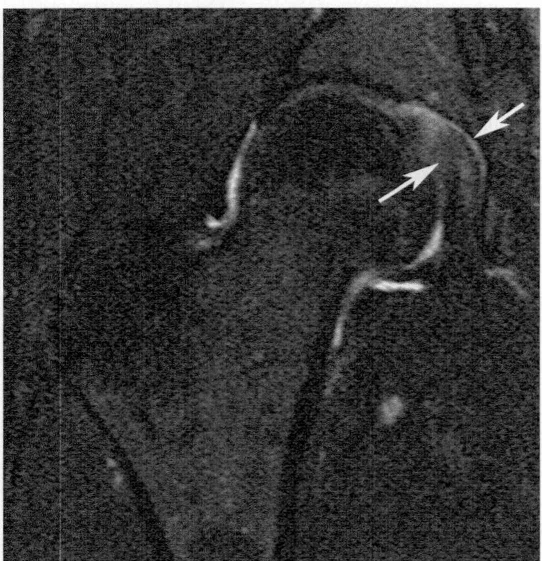

FIGURE 8.67 Internal snapping hip syndrome due to teres ligament degeneration. Coronal T2-weighted fat-saturated MR image in a young adult with painful right hip and snapping sensations demonstrates thickening and degeneration of the teres ligament *(arrows)*.

obturator neuropathy, motor deficits of the thigh muscle due to compression or entrapment of the obturator nerve at the level of the obturator foramen (secondary to trauma, surgery, myositis ossificans, or soft-tissue masses), and lateral femoral cutaneous neuropathy also known as *meralgia paresthetica* (entrapment or compression of the lateral femorocutaneous nerve, producing sensory deficit in the anterior thigh due to trauma, masses, and congenital or developmental anomalies, such as leg length discrepancy or scoliosis, among others). The role of MRI, as in other compressive neuropathies, is to detect the cause of the compression and identify the morphologic and signal changes of the affected nerve.

Piriformis Syndrome

The sciatic nerve descends anterior to the piriformis muscle in the pelvis and courses downward in the thigh. In the distal third of the thigh, the tibial and peroneal divisions separate into the tibial nerve and the common peroneal nerve. The sciatic nerve supplies the posterior thigh muscles (hamstrings) and provides all sensory and motor functions below the knee, except for the sensory innervation of the medial leg. As the sciatic nerve exits the pelvis, it contacts the piriformis muscle. At this level, the nerve may be compressed by hypertrophy of the piriformis muscle giving symptoms similar to lumbar disc herniation. Inflammation of the piriformis muscle secondary to infectious or inflammatory process of the adjacent lower lumbar spine, sacroiliac joint, or iliopsoas muscle; spasticity of the piriformis muscles due to cerebral palsy, posttraumatic hematoma, or fibrous adhesions of the piriformis muscle; and intramuscular course of the sciatic nerve or peroneal division of the sciatic nerve are associated etiologies of piriformis syndrome (Fig. 8.69).

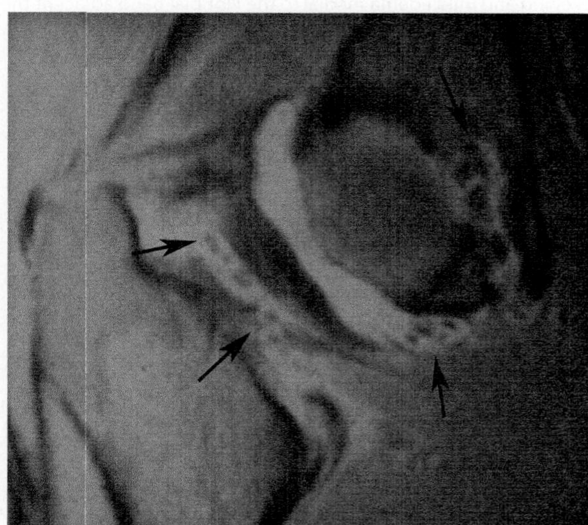

FIGURE 8.68 Internal snapping hip syndrome due to synovial chondromatosis. Coronal T2-weighted MR image in a middle-age man with chronic right hip pain associated with grinding sensation and occasional snapping feeling shows multiple small cartilaginous bodies lodged in the recesses of the joint capsule *(arrows)*.

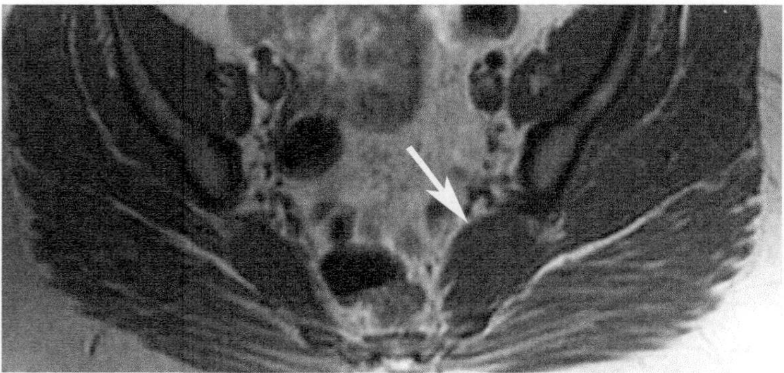

FIGURE 8.69 Piriformis syndrome. Axial T1-weighted MR image demonstrates hypertrophy of the left piriformis muscle *(arrow)* in this patient with chronic sciatic symptoms.

Iliacus Syndrome

The iliacus syndrome is caused by entrapment of the femoral nerve at the level of the pelvis and groin. The femoral nerve emerges from the sacral plexus under the psoas muscles coursing in the pelvis between the iliacus and psoas muscles and exits the pelvis underneath the inguinal ligament. Entrapment of the femoral nerve at the level of the pelvis occurs as the nerve passes underneath the inguinal ligament, where there is a rigid tunnel called the *lacuna musculorum* (Fig. 8.70). The roof of this tunnel is formed by the iliopectineal arch and the inguinal ligament. The floor of this tunnel is formed by the iliac bone and iliopsoas muscle. The femoral nerve supplies

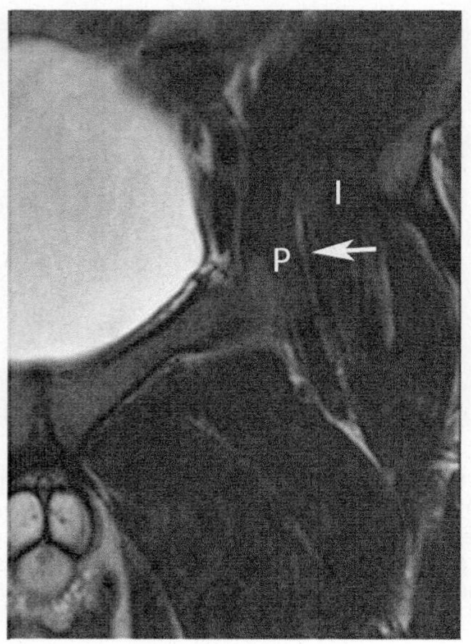

FIGURE 8.70 Normal femoral nerve. Coronal T2-weighted fat-saturated MR image demonstrates the normal femoral nerve *(arrow)* at the level of the lacuna musculorum, between the psoas *(P)* and iliacus *(I)* muscles.

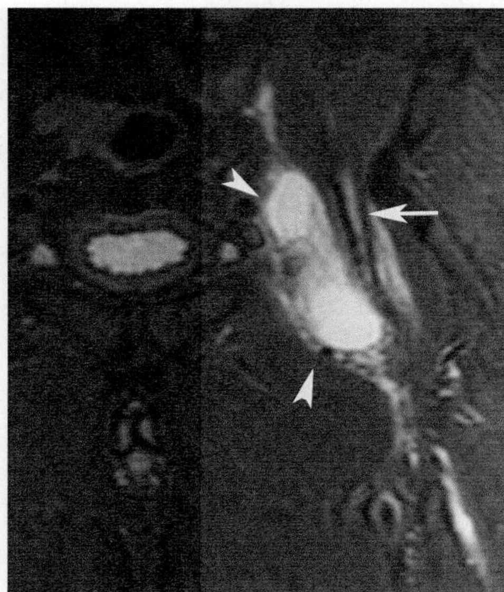

FIGURE 8.71 Iliacus syndrome. Coronal T2-weighted fat-saturated MR image demonstrates iliopsoas bursitis *(arrowheads)* causing thickening and hyperintensity of the adjacent femoral nerve *(arrow)*.

all anterior thigh muscles except for the *tensor fasciae latae*. It provides sensory innervation to the anterior and distal medial thigh, anteromedial knee, and medial leg and foot. Clinical manifestations include knee weakness with frequent falls, anterior thigh muscle atrophy, as well as numbness and paresthesias in the anterior thigh, medial calf, medial foot, and great toe. Causes for iliacus syndrome include iatrogenic injury from pelvic surgery, hip surgery, hysterectomy, femoral artery catheterization, and arterial bypass procedures; traumatic injury as a result of hip/pelvic fractures, gunshot wounds, and lacerations; enlargement of the iliopsoas muscles secondary to tear, hematoma, or mass; distended iliopsoas bursa (Fig. 8.71); and pseudoaneurysm of the iliac vessels. Magnetic resonance (MR) findings include swelling and/or mass effect from the iliacus or iliopsoas muscle, hematomas, and posttraumatic pseudoaneurysm of the iliac vessels. Denervation edema of the quadriceps femoris muscle may also be seen.

Obturator Neuropathy

Obturator neuropathy may occur within the obturator foramen where the obturator nerve exits the pelvis and can become injured or compressed. The obturator nerve is formed within the substance of the psoas major muscle by the ventral divisions of the L2, L3, and L4 nerve roots. The course of the obturator nerve in the pelvis is more medial than that of the femoral nerve. The obturator nerve descends through the psoas muscle to emerge from its medial border at the pelvic brim (Fig. 8.72). The nerve descends inferiorly and anteriorly along the iliopectineal line into the lesser pelvis. It exits the pelvis at the obturator foramen in which it divides into anterior and posterior branches; the anterior branch enters the thigh over the obturator externus muscle and the posterior branch through the fibers of that muscle. The anterior division provides motor innervation to the gracilis, adductor longus, adductor brevis, and pectineus muscles as well as sensory innervation to the hip joint and medial thigh. The posterior division provides motor innervation to the obturator externus, adductor magnus, and adductor brevis muscles as well as sensory innervation to the knee joint. The following are causes of obturator neuropathy: (a) penetrating/iatrogenic trauma; (b) pelvic and acetabular fractures; (c) posttraumatic hematomas; (d) myositis ossificans, pelvic tumors, obturator hernia; and (e) obturator neuropathy in athletes with formation of fibrous bands secondary to chronic adductor tendinopathy/osteitis pubis. Clinical manifestations include groin or medial thigh pain associated with weakness of the adductor musculature, which may result in a wide gate. MR findings include alterations in size and signal of the obturator nerve, mass effect from soft-tissue or osseous pelvic tumors, and denervation injury of the medial thigh muscles (Fig. 8.73).

Lateral Femoral Cutaneous Neuropathy (Meralgia Paresthetica)

Lateral femoral cutaneous neuropathy (also known as *meralgia paresthetica*) is caused by entrapment of the lateral femoral cutaneous nerve as it travels under the inguinal ligament or as it pierces the fascia lata (Fig. 8.74). The lateral femoral cutaneous nerve is formed by contributions of the L2 and L3 nerve roots. It travels laterally under the psoas muscle and across the iliacus muscle. The nerve exits the pelvis under the inguinal ligament just medial to the anterosuperior iliac spine and then it pierces the fascia lata. The following are causes of meralgia paresthetica: (a) peritendinitis and avulsion fracture of the anterosuperior iliac spine at the sartorius origin (Fig. 8.75); (b) pelvic and retroperitoneal tumors; (c) stretching of the nerve due to prolong leg and trunk hyperextension; (d) leg length discrepancy; (e) iatrogenic; (f) prolonged standing; and (g) external compression by belts, weight gain, or tight clothing. Clinical manifestations include burning pain, numbness, and tingling sensation located to the lateral aspect of the thigh. The symptoms are aggravated by local pressure over the anterosuperior iliac spine. Hip flexion relieves the symptoms. MR findings include alteration in size and signal of the entrapped nerve, avulsion injuries of the anterosuperior iliac spine, and mass effect from

FIGURE 8.72 Normal obturator nerve. **(A)** Coronal T1-weighted and **(B)** sagittal T2-weighted fat-saturated MR images show the normal obturator nerves *(arrows)*.

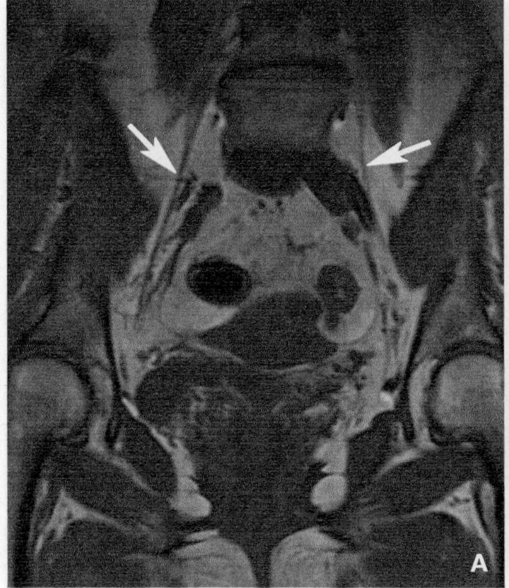

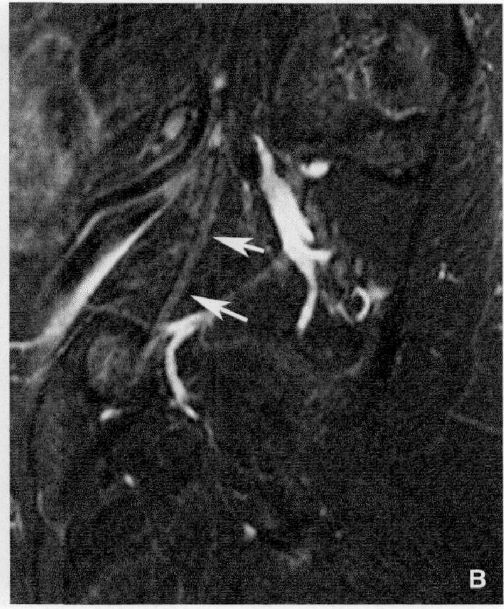

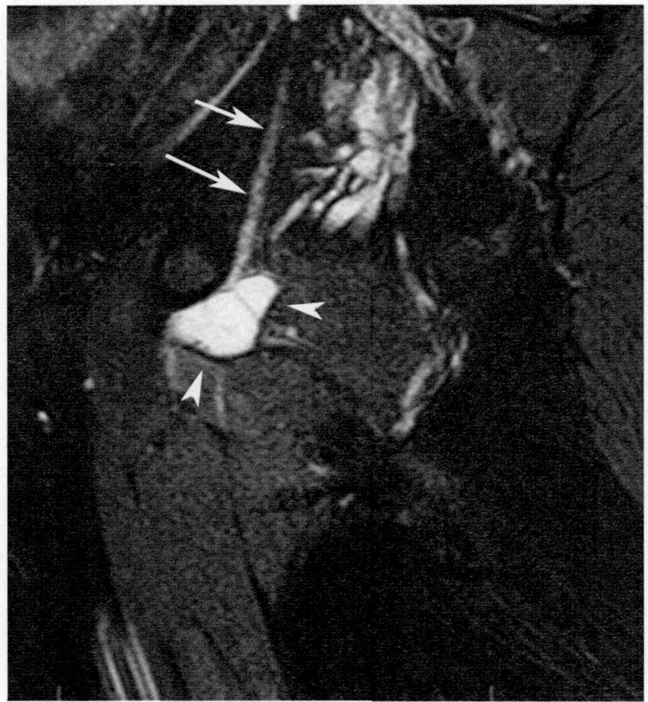

FIGURE 8.73 Obturator bursitis causing obturator neuropathy. Sagittal T2-weighted MR image demonstrates obturator bursitis *(arrowheads)* contacting the obturator nerve *(arrows)*, which is thickened and hyperintense.

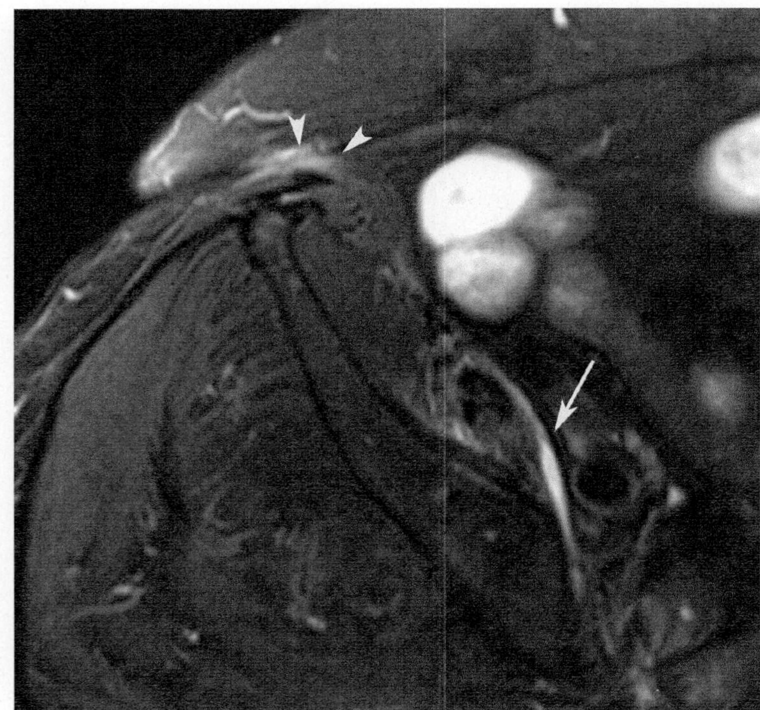

FIGURE 8.75 Peritendinitis of the sartorius tendon causing meralgia paresthetica. Axial T2-weighted fat-saturated MR image demonstrates peritendinous edema surrounding the sartorius tendon origin *(arrowheads)* and thickening and hyperintense intrapelvic segment of the lateral femorocutaneous nerve *(arrow)* indicating neuritis.

space-occupying lesions. The differential diagnosis includes lumbar diskogenic disease.

Morel-Lavallée Lesion (Closed Degloving Injury)

Shear stress forces at the interface between the subcutaneous fat and the crural fascia cause this relatively frequent condition around the hip and knee. Most typically, this injury occurs during a fall on the hip, such as in motorcycle accidents, resulting in a hematoma between the fat and the fascia adjacent to the greater trochanter, and is well demonstrated on MRI or ultrasound (Fig. 8.76, see also Fig. 4.132). This fluid collection may heal spontaneously but more often becomes encapsulated and persistent. It may extend to the subcutaneous fat with entrapment of lacerated fat tissue. Treatment is conservative with compressive dressing, but occasionally, it may require surgical or percutaneous drainage.

Sports Hernia

This lesion is produced by twisting injuries around the lower abdomen and pelvis, leading to characteristic symptoms in the groin and exhibiting well-described MRI findings. Sports hernia is discussed in more detail in Chapter 4.

Stress and Insufficiency Fractures

Stress and insufficiency fractures are common in the pelvis and proximal femora. They occur in the sacral ala, body of the sacrum, acetabula, subchondral region of the femoral heads, femoral neck, and in the parasymphyseal areas. These lesions are described in more detail in Chapters 4 and 9.

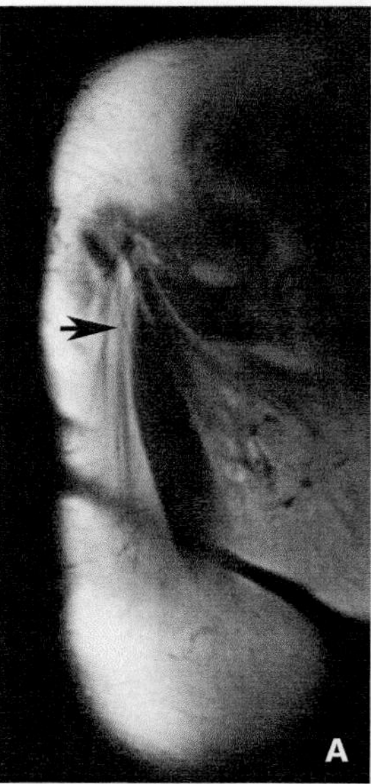

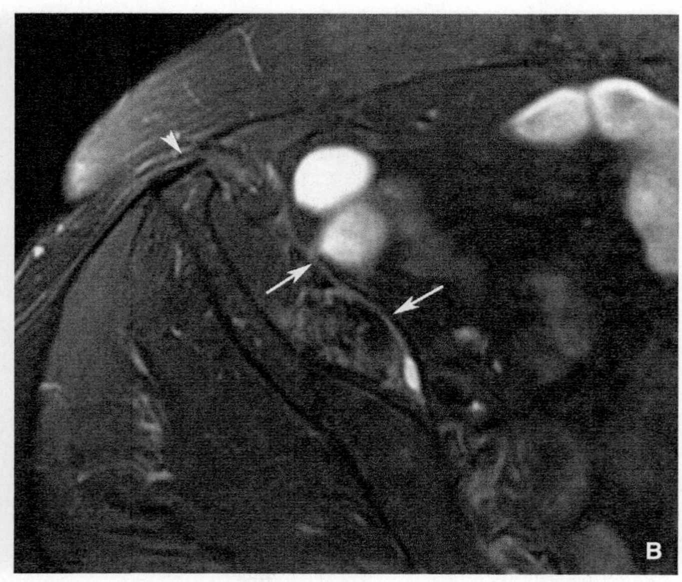

FIGURE 8.74 Normal lateral femorocutaneous nerve. (A) Coronal T1-weighted MR image shows the normal superficial subcutaneous lateral femorocutaneous nerve *(arrow)* as it exits medial to the anterior superior iliac spine. **(B)** Axial T2-weighted fat-saturated MR image demonstrates the intrapelvic segment of the lateral femorocutaneous nerve *(arrows)*. Note the normal origin of the sartorius tendon in the anterior superior iliac spine *(arrowhead)*, adjacent to the pelvic exit point of the lateral femorocutaneous nerve.

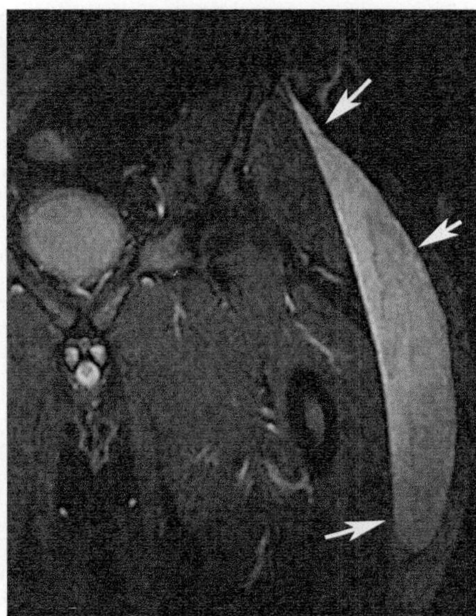

FIGURE 8.76 **Morel-Lavallée lesion.** Coronal STIR MR image demonstrates a large, fusiform encapsulated hematoma between the subcutaneous fat and the crural fascia *(arrows).* The patient relates a history of a fall several months ago. Note the absence of soft-tissue edema around the hematoma.

PRACTICAL POINTS TO REMEMBER

Pelvis and Acetabulum

1. Fractures of the pelvis are important because of the high incidence of concomitant injury to:
   - major blood vessels
   - nerves
   - lower urinary tract.
2. Pelvic fractures can be classified for the purposes of radiographic diagnosis and orthopaedic management:
   - into stable and unstable injuries on the basis of the stability of the fragments
   - according to the direction of the force delivered to the pelvis as injuries resulting from anteroposterior compression, lateral compression, vertical shear, or complex pattern.
3. Fractures of the acetabulum are best demonstrated on the anterior and posterior oblique projections (Judet views).
4. In acetabular fractures, it is important to distinguish between:
   - fractures of the anterior pelvic column
   - fractures of the posterior pelvic column.
5. CT plays an important role in the evaluation of fractures of both the pelvis and acetabulum because of its capability in demonstrating:
   - the exact position and configuration of comminuted fragments
   - the presence or absence of intraarticular fragments
   - injury to the soft tissues.
6. MRI offers superior capabilities for evaluating traumatic conditions of the hip, in particular:
   - to diagnose occult fractures and bone contusions (trabecular microfractures)
   - to identify and quantify effectively the muscle injury and joint effusion that accompany traumatic hip dislocations
   - to identify the emergence of such complications as osteonecrosis of the femoral head
   - to diagnose the variety of compressive and entrapment neuropathies
   - to diagnose Morel-Lavallée lesion—a closed degloving injury of the soft tissues.
7. MRa is effective to evaluate injuries to the acetabular labrum, such as tears and detachments.
8. IVP and cystourethrography are essential in the evaluation of concomitant injury to the lower urinary system.

Sacrum

1. Sacral fractures are classified by Denis into three groups: those occurring across sacral ala, lateral to the neural foramina (zone I); fractures through the neural foramina (zone II); and fractures through the body of the sacrum involving the spinal canal (zone III).
2. CT and 3D CT are the best imaging modalities to identify and evaluate these injuries.

Proximal Femur

1. The importance of distinguishing between intracapsular and extracapsular fractures of the proximal femur (hip fractures) lies in the possible complications. Intracapsular fractures of the femoral neck are associated with a higher incidence of nonunion and osteonecrosis of the femoral head.
2. The Garden staging of intracapsular fractures of the femoral neck has practical value in determining stability and prognosis.
3. The Boyd-Griffin classification of intertrochanteric fractures according to the presence or absence of comminution and involvement of the subtrochanteric region has important prognostic value and serves as a guide to operative management.
4. The Kyle classification is very effective from the practical point of view because it is based on the stability of various fractured fragments and allows more accurate determination of prognosis of this injury.
5. Subtrochanteric fractures are classified by:
   - Fielding, according to the level of the fracture line
   - Zickel, according to the level, obliquity, and comminution of the fracture.
6. MRI is the ideal modality to detect and evaluate early changes of posttraumatic osteonecrosis of the femoral head.

Dislocations in the Hip Joint

1. Dislocations in the hip joint are classified as anterior, posterior, and central (medial).
2. Posterior dislocations are more common and are frequently associated with fractures involving the posterior acetabular rim.
3. Anterior dislocations are rare. On the anteroposterior radiograph, the femur is abducted and externally rotated, and the femoral head lies medial and inferior to the acetabulum.

Tendon and Muscle Lesions

1. Lesions of the tendons about the hip joint are common in the elderly patients and are related to peritendinitis, tendinosis, tears, and bursitis. They include among others a snapping hip syndrome (coxa saltans or dancer's hip), ischiofemoral impingement, and calcific peritendinitis.
2. MRI is the modality of choice to diagnose those lesions.

Compression and Entrapment Neuropathies

1. Those conditions include piriformis syndrome, iliacus syndrome, obturator neuropathy, and lateral femoral cutaneous neuropathy (meralgia paresthetica).
2. MRI findings are diagnostic for all these abnormalities.

SUGGESTED READINGS

Allen WC, Cope R. Coxa saltans: the snapping hip revisited. *J Am Acad Orthop Surg* 1995;3:303–308.

Aly AR, Rajasekaran S, Obaid H. MRI morphometric hip comparison analysis of anterior acetabular labral tears. *Skeletal Radiol* 2013;42:1245–1252.

Banks KP, Grayson DE. Retroversion of the acetabulum as a rare cause of chronic hip pain: recognition of the "figure-eight" sign. *Skeletal Radiol* 2007;36(suppl 1):108–111.

Bencardino JT, Mellado JM. Hamstring injuries of the hip. *Magn Reson Imaging Clin N Am* 2005;13:677–690.

Blankenbaker DG, De Smet AA, Keene JS, et al. Classification and localization of acetabular labral tears. *Skeletal Radiol* 2007;36:391–397.

Blundell CM, Parker MJ, Pryor GA, et al. Assessment of the AO classification of intracapsular fractures of the proximal femur. *J Bone Joint Surg Br* 1998;80:679–683.

Boyd HB, Griffin LL. Classification and treatment of trochanteric fractures. *Arch Surg* 1949;58:853–866.

Brandser E, Marsh JL. Acetabular fractures: easier classification with a systematic approach. *AJR Am J Roentgenol* 1998;171:1217–1228.

Bray TJ. Acetabular fractures: classification and diagnosis. In: Chapman MW, ed. *Operative orthopaedics*, vol. 11, 2nd ed. Philadelphia: JB Lippincott; 1993:539–553.

Bray TJ, Templeman DC. Fractures of the femoral neck. In: Chapman MW, ed. *Operative orthopaedics*, vol. 1, 2nd ed. Philadelphia: JB Lippincott; 1993:583–594.

Burgess AR, Tile M. Fractures of the pelvis. In: Rockwood CA Jr, Green DP, Bucholz RW, eds. *Rockwood and Green's fractures in adults*, vol. 2, 3rd ed. Philadelphia: JB Lippincott; 1991:1399–1479.

Clohisy JC, Carlisle JC, Beaulé PE, et al. A systematic approach to the plain radiographic evaluation of the young adult hip. *J Bone Joint Surg Am* 2008;90(suppl 4):47–66.

Cvitanic O, Henzie G, Skezas N, et al. MRI diagnosis of tears of the hip abductor tendons (gluteus medius and gluteus minimus). *Am J Roentgenol* 2004;182:137–143.

Czerny C, Hofmann S, Urban M, et al. MR arthrography of the adult acetabular capsular-labral complex: correlation with surgery and anatomy. *AJR Am J Roentgenol* 1999; 173:345–349.

Davies AG, Clarke AW, Gilmore J, et al. Review: imaging of groin pain in the athlete. *Skeletal Radiol* 2010;39:629–644.

DeLee JC. Fractures and dislocations of the hip. In: Rockwood CA Jr, Green DP, Bucholz RW, eds. *Rockwood and Green's fractures in adults*, vol. 2, 3rd ed. Philadelphia: JB Lippincott; 1991:1481–1651.

Denis F, Davis S, Comfort T. Sacral fractures: an important problem. Retrospective analysis of 236 cases. *Clin Orthop Relat Res* 1988;227:67–81.

Dunn AW, Morris HD. Fractures and dislocations of the pelvis. *J Bone Joint Surg Am* 1968;50:1639–1648.

Erbay H. Meralgia paresthetica in differential diagnosis of low-back pain. *Clin J Pain* 2002;18:132–135.

Fielding JW. Subtrochanteric fractures. *Clin Orthop Relat Res* 1973;92:86–99.

Garden RS. Reduction and fixation of subcapital fractures of the femur. *Orthop Clin North Am* 1974;5:683–712.

Garden RS. The structure and function of the proximal end of the femur. *J Bone Joint Surg Br* 1961;43B:576–589.

Greenspan A, Norman A. The "pelvic digit"—an unusual developmental anomaly. *Skeletal Radiol* 1982;9:118–122.

Grothaus MC, Holt M, Mekhail AO, et al. Lateral femoral cutaneous nerve: an anatomic study. *Clin Orthop Relat Res* 2005;(437):164–168.

Hashemi SA, Dehghani J, Vasoughi AR. Can the crossover sign be a reliable marker of global retroversion of the acetabulum? *Skeletal Radiol* 2017;46:17–21.

Hochman MG, Zilberfarb JL. Nerves in a pinch: imaging of nerve compression syndromes. *Radiol Clin North Am* 2004;42:221–245.

Judet R, Judet J, Letournel E. Fractures of the acetabulum: classification and surgical approaches for open reduction. Preliminary report. *J Bone Joint Surg Am* 1964;46:1615–1646.

Khoury AN, Brooke K, Helal A, et al. Proximal iliotibial band thickness as a cause for recalcitrant greater trochanteric pain syndrome. *J Hip Preserv Surg* 2018;5:296–300.

Kim S, Choi JY, Huh YM, et al. Role of magnetic resonance imaging in entrapment and compressive neuropathy—what, where, and how to see the peripheral nerves on the musculoskeletal magnetic resonance image: part 1. Overview and lower extremity. *Eur Radiol* 2007;17:139–149.

Kricun ME. Fractures of the pelvis. *Orthop Clin North Am* 1990;21:573–590.

Kyle RF, Campbell SJ. Intertrochanteric fractures. In: Chapman MW, ed. *Operative orthopaedics*, vol. 1, 2nd ed. Philadelphia: JB Lippincott; 1993:595–604.

Kyle RF. Intertrochanteric fractures. In: Chapman MW, ed. *Operative orthopaedics*. Philadelphia: JB Lippincott; 1988:353–359.

Lacour-Petic MC, Lozeron P, Ducreux D. MRI of peripheral nerve lesions of the lower limbs. *Neuroradiology* 2003;45:166–170.

Lage LA, Patel JV, Villar RN. The acetabular labral tear: an arthroscopic classification. *Arthroscopy* 1996;12:269–272.

Letournel E. Acetabulum fractures: classification and management. *Clin Orthop Relat Res* 1980;151:81–106.

Lewis CL. Extra-articular snapping hip: a literature review. *Sports Health* 2010;2:186–190.

Mellado JM, Pérez del Palomar L, Díaz L, et al. Long-standing Morel-Lavallée lesions of the trochanteric region and proximal thigh: MRI features in five patients. *AJR Am J Roentgenol* 2004;182:1289–1294.

Moehring HD, Greenspan A, eds. *Fractures: diagnosis and treatment*. New York: McGraw-Hill; 2000:99–105.

Oka M, Monu JUV. Prevalence and patterns of occult hip fractures and mimics revealed by MRI. *AJR Am J Roentgenol* 2004;182:283–288.

Pauwels F. *Biomechanics of the normal and diseased hip*. New York: Springer; 1976.

Pennal GF, Tile M, Waddell JP, et al. Pelvic disruption: assessment and classification. *Clin Orthop Relat Res* 1980;151:12–21.

Rosenberg ZS, Cavalcanti C. Entrapment neuropathies of the lower extremity. In: Stoller DW, ed. *Magnetic resonance imaging in orthopaedics and sports medicine*. Philadelphia: Lippincott Williams & Wilkins; 2007:1051–1098.

Samim M, Eftekhary N, Vigdorchick JM, et al. 3D-MRI versus 3D-CT in the evaluation of osseous anatomy in femoroacetabular impingement using Dixon 3D FLASH sequence. *Skeletal Radiol* 2019;48:429–436.

Sapkas GS, Mavrogenis AF, Papagelopoulos PJ. Transverse sacral fractures with anterior displacement. *Eur Spine J* 2008;17:342–347.

Schmid MR, Nötzli HP, Zanetti M, et al. Cartilage lesions in the hip: diagnostic effectiveness of MR arthrography. *Radiology* 2003;226:382–386.

Schultz E, Miller TT, Boruchov SD, et al. Incomplete intertrochanteric fractures: imaging features and clinical management. *Radiology* 1999;211:237–240.

Steinbach LS, Palmer WE, Schweitzer ME. Special focus session. MR arthrography. *Radiographics* 2002;22:1223–1246.

Sutter R, Zanetti M, Pfirrmann CWA. New developments in hip imaging. *Radiology* 2012;264:651–667.

Windisch G, Braun E, Anderhuber F. Piriformis muscle: clinical anatomy and consideration of the piriformis syndrome. *Surg Radiol Anat* 2007;29:37–45.

Yen Y-M, Lewis CL, Kim Y-J. Understanding and treating the snapping hip. *Sports Med Arthrosc Rev* 2015;23:194–199.

Zickel RE. An intramedullary fixation device for the proximal part of the femur. Nine years' experience. *J Bone Joint Surg Am* 1976;58:866–872.

Zingg PO, Werner VM, Sukthankar A, et al. The anterior center edge angle in Lequesne's false profile view: interrater correlation, dependence on pelvic tilt and correlation to anterior acetabular coverage in the sagital plane. A cadaver study. *Arch Orthop Trauma Surg* 2009;129:787–791.

9

Lower Limb II

Knee

Trauma to the Knee

The vulnerability of the knee, the largest joint in the body, to direct trauma makes knee injuries very common throughout life. Most acute injury to the knee is sustained during adolescence and adulthood, with motor vehicle accidents and athletic activities being the major causing factors. Fractures are much more common than dislocations, but injuries to the cartilaginous and soft-tissue structures, such as tears of the menisci and ligaments, are the most common types of injuries, particularly in older adolescents and younger adults. The symptoms accompanying knee trauma vary according to the specific site of injury and thus constitute important indications of the type of injury. However, clinical history and physical examination are rarely sufficient for making a precise diagnosis. Radiologic examination plays a determining role in diagnosing the various traumatic conditions involving the knee joint.

Anatomic–Radiologic Considerations

Conventional radiographs are the first-line approach to the traumatized knee, and often they are sufficient for evaluating many traumatic conditions of the joint. However, the great incidence of cartilaginous and soft-tissue injuries, occurring either as isolated conditions or in association with fractures, requires the use of ancillary imaging techniques for adequate evaluation of the joint capsule, articular cartilage, menisci, and ligaments.

The standard radiographic examination usually consists of obtaining radiographs of the knee in four projections: the anteroposterior, the lateral, and the tunnel projections as well as an axial view of the patella. The *anteroposterior* radiograph of the knee allows sufficient evaluation of many of the most important aspects of the distal femur and proximal tibia: the medial and lateral femoral and tibial condyles, the medial and lateral tibial plateaus and tibial spines, and the medial and lateral joint compartments and the head of the fibula (Fig. 9.1). However, the patella is not well demonstrated on this view because it is superimposed on the distal femur. Proper evaluation of this structure requires a *lateral* projection (Fig. 9.2) on which the relationship of the patella and femur can also be assessed. Proximal (superior, cephalad) displacement of the patella is called *patella alta*; distal (inferior, caudad) displacement is called *patella baja*. The length of the patella is measured from its upper pole (base) to the lower pole (apex). The length of the patellar ligament is measured from its proximal attachment, just above the apex, to the notch on the proximal margin of the tibial tubercle. These two measurements are approximately equal, and the normal variation does not exceed 20% (Fig. 9.3). In addition to imaging the patella in profile, the lateral radiograph of the knee allows evaluation of the femoropatellar compartment, the suprapatellar recess (pouch), and the quadriceps tendon. The femoral condyles overlap on this projection, and the tibial plateaus are demonstrated in profile. Occasionally, a cross-table lateral view of the knee—obtained with the patient supine, the affected leg extended, and the central beam directed horizontally—may be required to demonstrate the intracapsular fat–fluid level (fat–blood interface [FBI] sign of lipohemarthrosis; see Fig. 4.59B). An angled posteroanterior projection of the knee, known as the *tunnel* (or *notch*) *view*, is also obtained as part of the standard radiographic examination (Fig. 9.4). This view is useful in visualizing the posterior aspect of the femoral condyles, the intercondylar notch, and the intercondylar eminence of the tibia.

To demonstrate an *axial* view of the patella, various techniques are available. The one most commonly used provides what has been called the *sunrise view* (Fig. 9.5). However, the degree of flexion required to obtain this view results in depressing the patella more deeply within the intercondylar fossa; consequently, the articular surfaces of the femoropatellar joint are not well demonstrated, and subtle subluxations of the patella may not be detected. To overcome this limitation, Merchant and colleagues have described a technique for obtaining an axial view of the patella that demonstrates the femoropatellar joint to better advantage (Fig. 9.6). It is particularly effective in detecting subluxations of the patella because it allows specific measurements to be made of the normal relations of the patella to the femoral condyles. Subtle abnormalities in these relations may not be seen on the standard axial view because of the degree of knee flexion required for that view, which prevents the patella from subluxing.

The measurements of the femoropatellar relations obtainable from Merchant axial projection concern the sulcus angle and the congruence angle (Fig. 9.7). Normally, the *sulcus angle*, which is described by the highest points of the femoral condyles and the deepest point of the intercondylar sulcus, measures approximately 138 degrees. By dissecting this angle with two lines—a reference line drawn from the apex of the patella to the deepest point of the sulcus and a second line from the lowest point of the patellar articular ridge to the deepest point of the sulcus—Merchant and colleagues were able to determine the degree of congruence, or the *congruence angle*, of the femoropatellar joint. When the deepest point of the patellar articular ridge fell medial to the reference line, the angle formed was assigned a negative value; when it fell lateral to the reference line, the angle was designated with a positive value. In 100 normal subjects included in their study, the average congruence angle was −6 degrees. An angle of +16 degrees or greater was found to be associated with various patellofemoral disorders, particularly lateral patellar subluxation (see Fig. 9.45). On occasion, patellofemoral disorders that are more difficult to diagnose may require, as Ficat and Hungerford recommended, additional tangential views obtained with 30, 60, and 90 degrees of knee flexion.

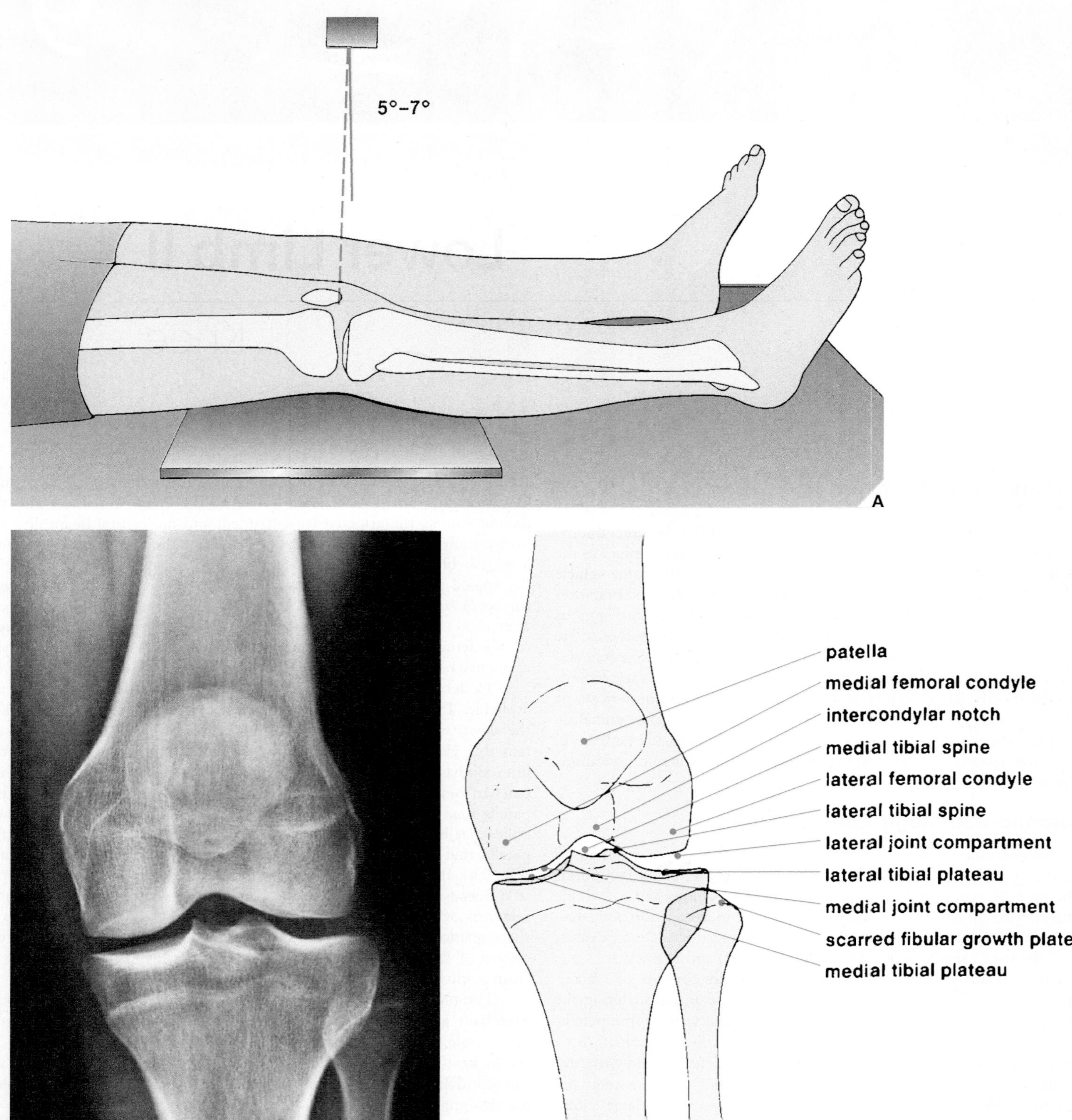

FIGURE 9.1 Anteroposterior view. **(A)** For the anteroposterior view of the knee, the patient is supine, with the knee fully extended and the leg in the neutral position. The central beam *(red broken line)* is directed vertically to the knee with a 5- to 7-degree cephalad angulation. **(B)** The radiograph in this projection sufficiently demonstrates the medial and lateral femoral and tibial condyles, the tibial plateaus and spines, and both the medial and lateral joint compartments. The patella is seen en face as an oval structure between the femoral condyles.

FIGURE 9.2 Lateral view. (A) For the lateral view of the knee, the patient is lying flat on the same side as the affected knee, which is flexed approximately 25 to 30 degrees. The central beam *(red broken line)* is directed vertically toward the medial aspect of the knee joint with an approximately 5- to 7-degree cephalad angulation. **(B)** The radiograph in this projection demonstrates the patella in profile as well as the femoropatellar joint compartment and a faint outline of the quadriceps tendon. The femoral condyles are seen overlapping, and the tibial plateaus are imaged in profile. Note the slight posterior tilt of the tibial plateaus, which normally measures approximately 10 degrees.

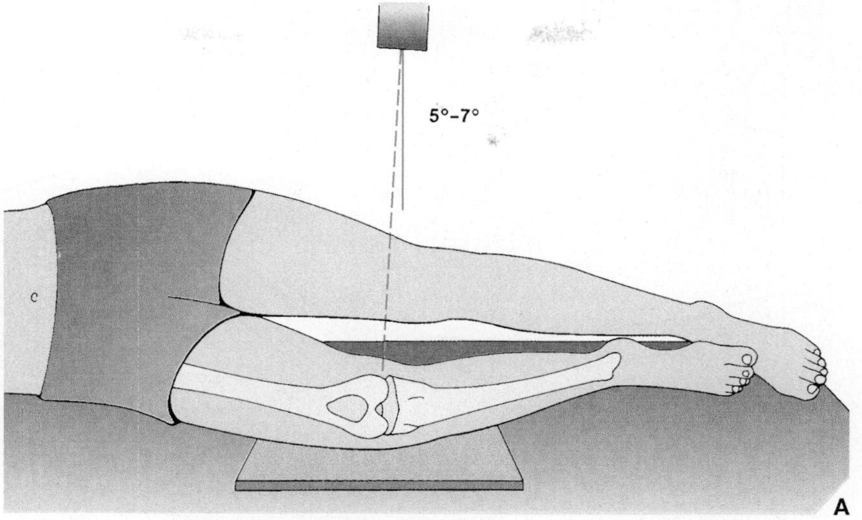

5°–7°

A

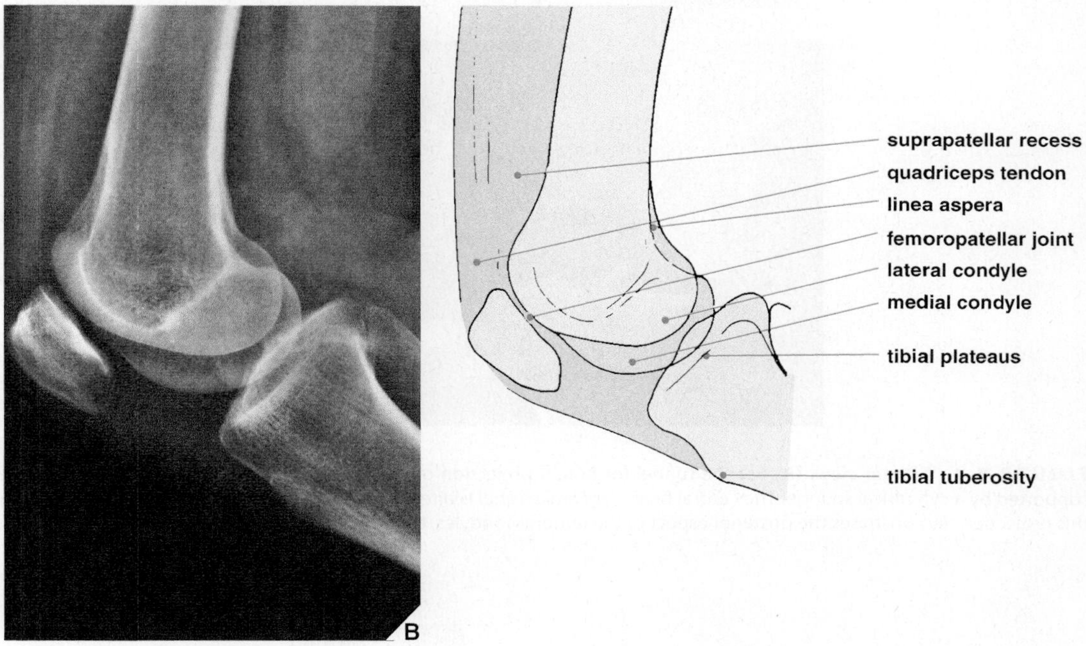

suprapatellar recess
quadriceps tendon
linea aspera
femoropatellar joint
lateral condyle
medial condyle
tibial plateaus
tibial tuberosity

B

FIGURE 9.3 Femoropatellar relationship. The length of the patella and the patellar ligament are approximately equal; normal variability does not exceed 20%.

FEMOROPATELLAR RELATIONSHIP

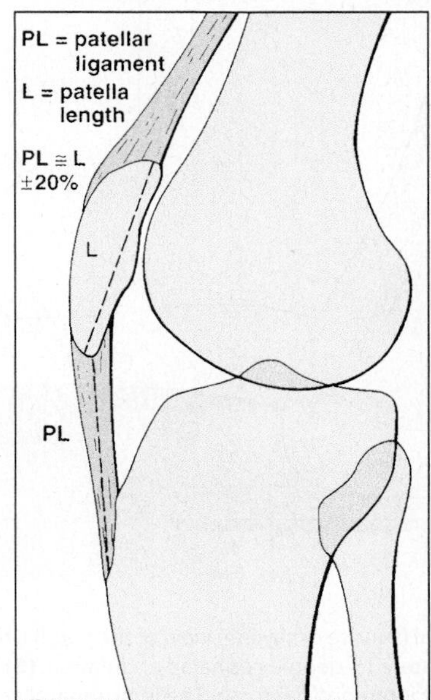

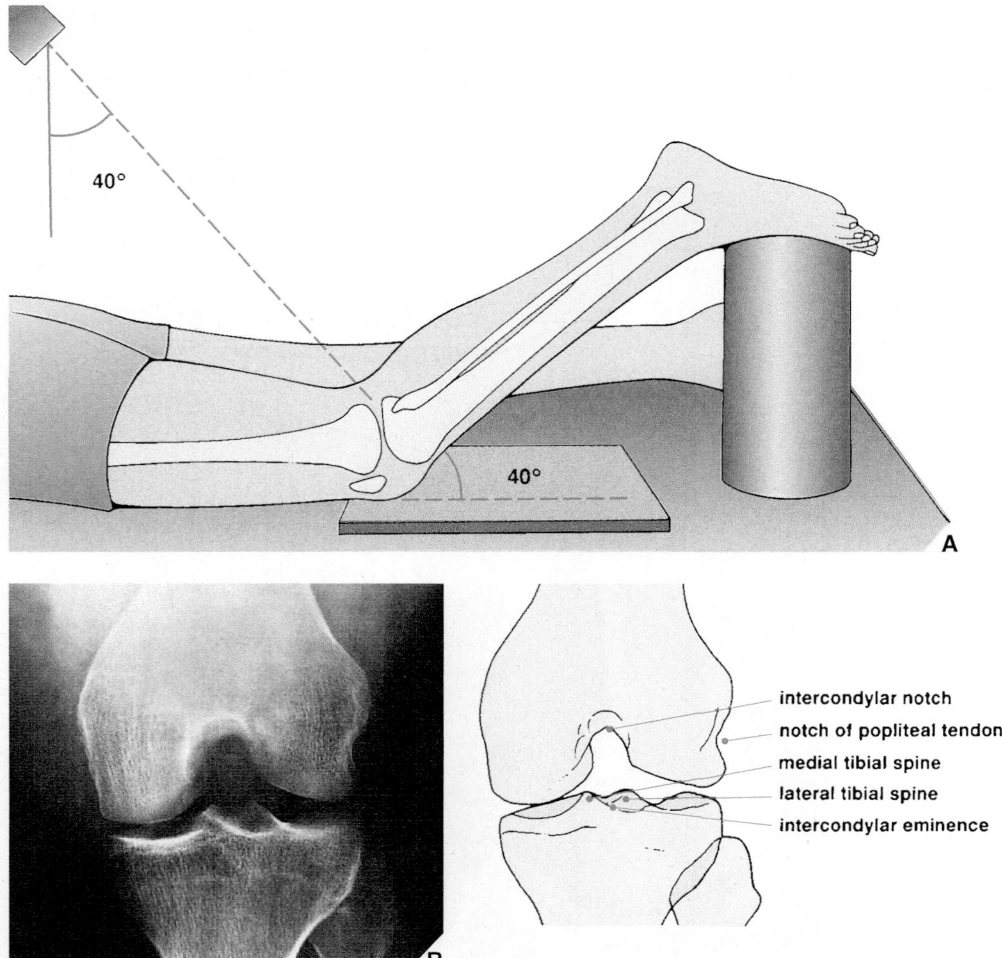

FIGURE 9.4 Tunnel view. **(A)** For the tunnel (or notch) projection of the knee, the patient is prone with the knee flexed approximately 40 degrees, with the foot supported by a cylindrical sponge. The central beam *(red broken line)* is directed caudally toward the knee joint at a 40-degree angle from the vertical. **(B)** The radiograph in this projection demonstrates the posterior aspect of the femoral condyles, the intercondylar notch, and the intercondylar eminence of the tibia.

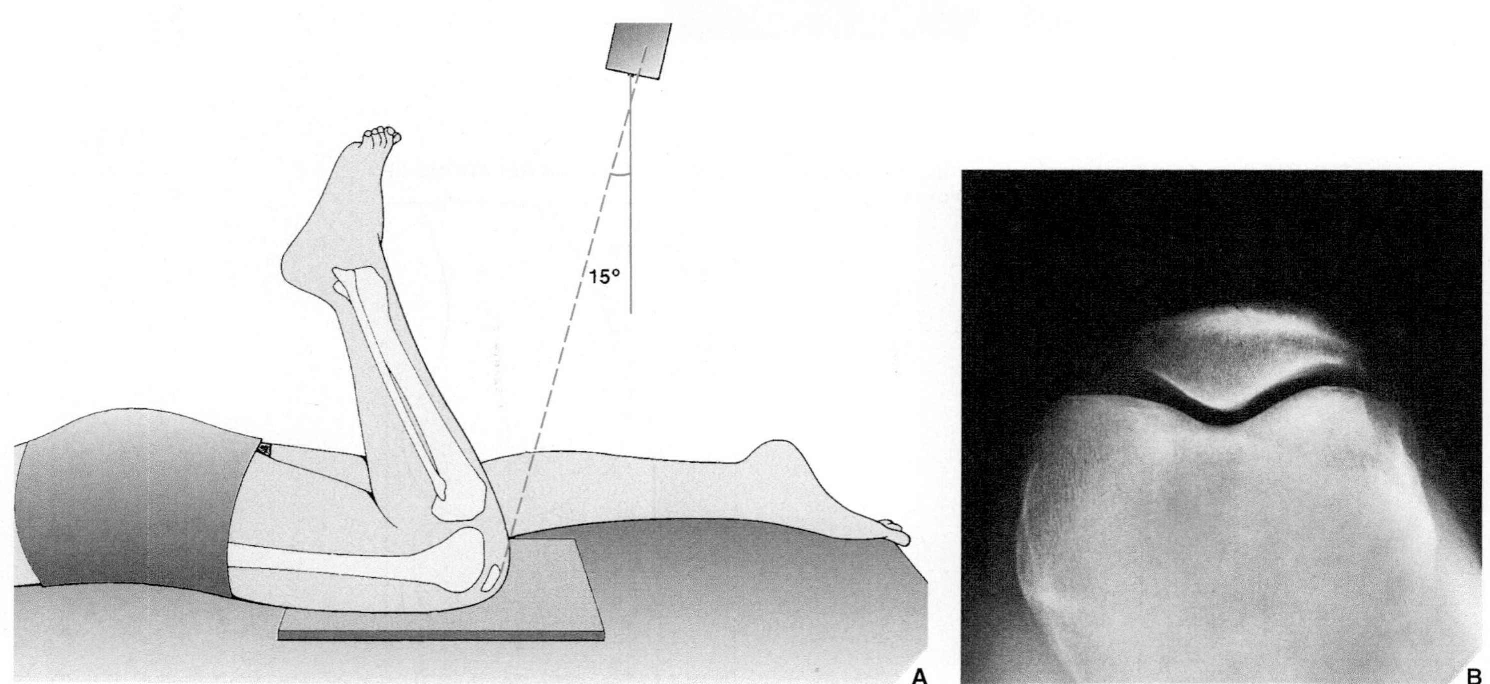

FIGURE 9.5 Sunrise view. **(A)** For an axial (sunrise or skyline) view of the patella, the patient is prone, with the knee flexed 115 degrees. The central beam *(red broken line)* is directed toward the patella with approximately 15-degree cephalad angulation. **(B)** The radiograph in this projection demonstrates a tangential (axial) view of the patella. Note the deep position of this structure in the intercondylar fossa. The femoropatellar joint compartment is well demonstrated.

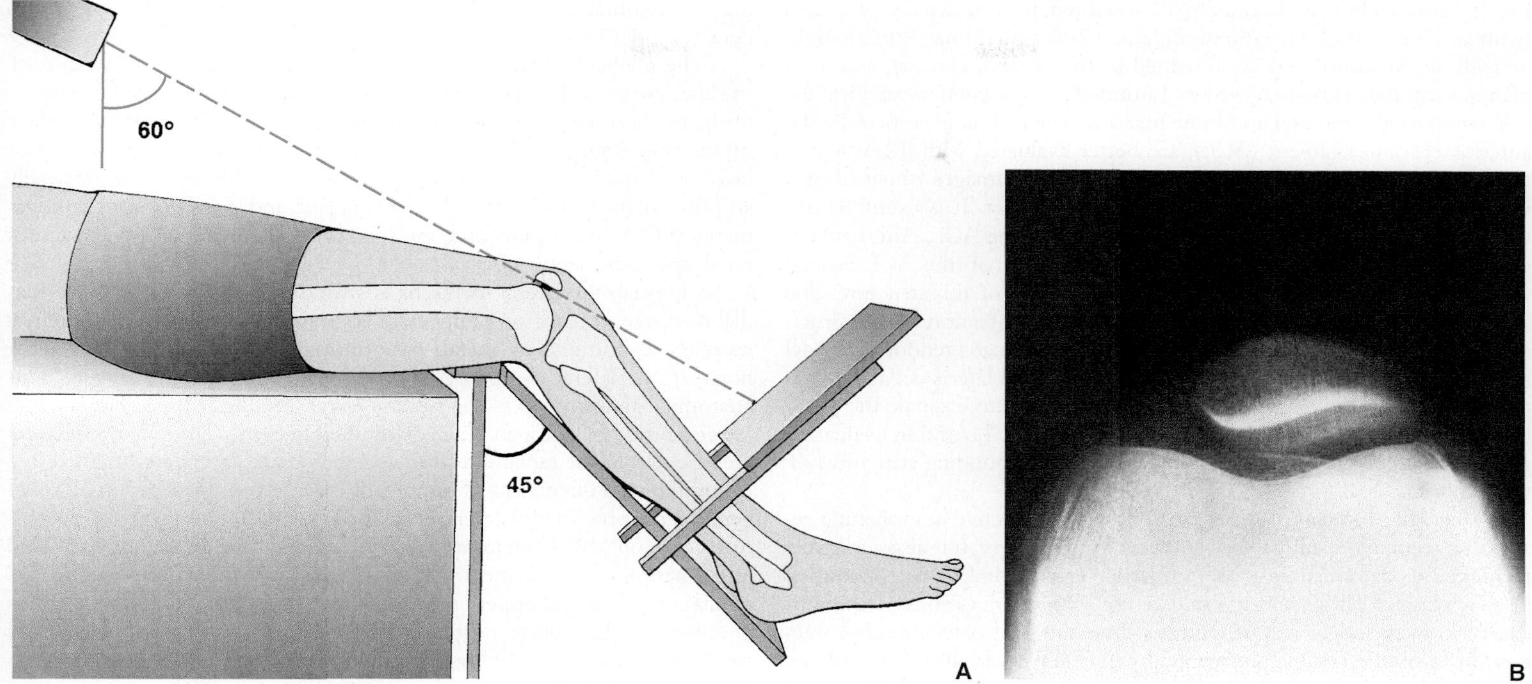

FIGURE 9.6 Merchant view. **(A)** For the Merchant axial view of the patella, the patient is supine on the table, with the knee flexed approximately 45 degrees at the table's edge. A device keeping the knee at this angle also holds the film cassette. The central beam *(red broken line)* is directed caudally through the patella at a 60-degree angle from the vertical. **(B)** On the radiograph obtained in this projection, the articular facets of the patella and femur are well demonstrated.

Among the ancillary techniques available for the evaluation of injuries to the knee, computed tomography (CT), and magnetic resonance imaging (MRI) provide crucial information. CT is especially useful in the evaluation of complex fractures of the distal femur, the tibial plateaus, and the patella. In fractures of the tibial plateaus, it is effective in determining the amount of depression of the articular surface and in identifying small comminuted fragments that may be displaced into the joint, as well as comminution about the tibial spines, which may indicate avulsion of the cruciate ligaments.

MRI of the knee has become the method of choice in evaluating various knee structures, including extracapsular structures (tendons, collateral ligaments, muscles, subcutaneous tissues, and bones) as well as intracapsular structures (menisci, cruciate ligaments, cartilage, and synovium). CT-arthrography is a useful substitute to MRI in patients with contraindication

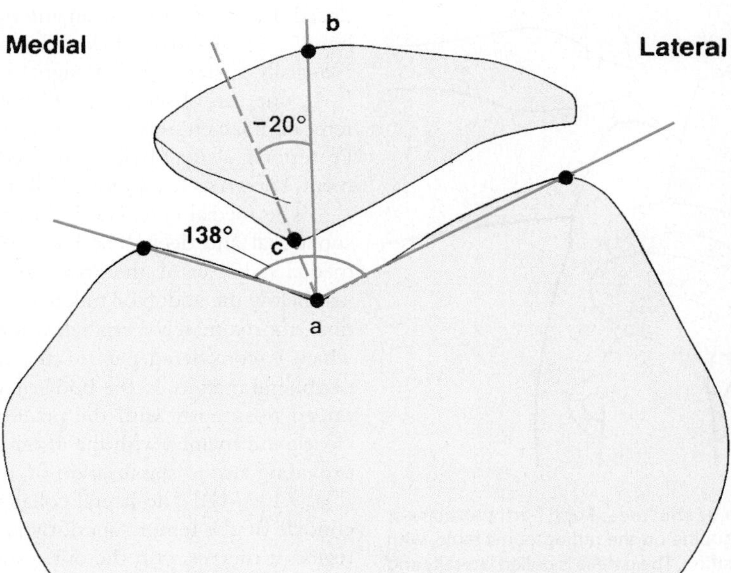

FIGURE 9.7 Sulcus and congruence angles. Two specific measurements can be obtained from the Merchant axial view: the sulcus angle and the congruence angle. The sulcus angle, formed by lines extending from the deepest point of the intercondylar sulcus *(a)* medially and laterally to the tops of the femoral condyles, normally measures approximately 138 degrees. To determine the congruence angle, the sulcus angle is bisected to establish a reference line *(ba)*, which is drawn to connect the apex of the patella *(b)* with the deepest point of the sulcus *(a)*. In normal subjects, this line is close to vertical. A second line *(ca)* is then drawn from the lowest point on the articular ridge of the patella *(c)* to the deepest point of the sulcus *(a)*. The angle formed by this line and the reference line is the congruence angle. If the lowest point on the patellar articular ridge is lateral to the reference line, then the congruence angle has a positive value; if it is medial to the reference line, as in the present example, then the angle has a negative value. In Merchant's study, the average congruence angle in normal subjects was −6 degrees (standard deviation [SD], ±11 degrees). (Modified with permission from Merchant AC, Mercer RL, Jacobsen RH, et al. Roentgenographic analysis of patello-femoral congruence. *J Bone Joint Surg Am* 1974;56[7]:1391–1396.)

for the latter technique. Routinely, T1-weighted, proton density–weighted (with and/or without fat saturation), and T2-weighted images (with and/or without fat saturation) are obtained in the sagittal, coronal, and axial planes. Proton density–weighted fat saturated pulse sequences are ideal for evaluation of the menisci and bone marrow. The ligaments, especially the anterior cruciate ligament (ACL), are better evaluated with T2-weighted pulse sequences because proton density–weighted images obtained at a low echo time (TE) can provide magic angle artifact. It is useful to obtain the sagittal images oriented along the axis of the ACL. Alternatively, oblique coronal images along the longitudinal axis of the ACL can be added to the imaging protocol for better assessment of this structure. The sagittal plane is generally the most effective for evaluation of the cruciate ligaments, menisci, patellar ligament, and quadriceps tendon. Coronal sections are needed for evaluation of the medial and lateral collateral ligaments, as well as the menisci. The axial plane is best to evaluate the patellofemoral joint compartment. The axial plane is also helpful in evaluating the popliteal cysts and their relationship to the surrounding structures of the popliteal fossa.

Magnetic resonance arthrography (MRa) is effective in evaluating residual or recurrent meniscal tears after meniscal surgery. It is also a valuable technique to demonstrate loose intraarticular chondral or osteochondral bodies, synovial plicae, and to evaluate the stability of various osteochondral lesions, including osteochondritis dissecans and osteochondral fracture. MRa of the knee is performed by injecting up to 40 mL of diluted gadolinium solution into the joint using the same technique as described for conventional knee arthrography (Fig. 9.8). Coronal, sagittal, and axial images are obtained, most commonly with fat-suppressed T1- (or proton density) and T2-weighted sequences.

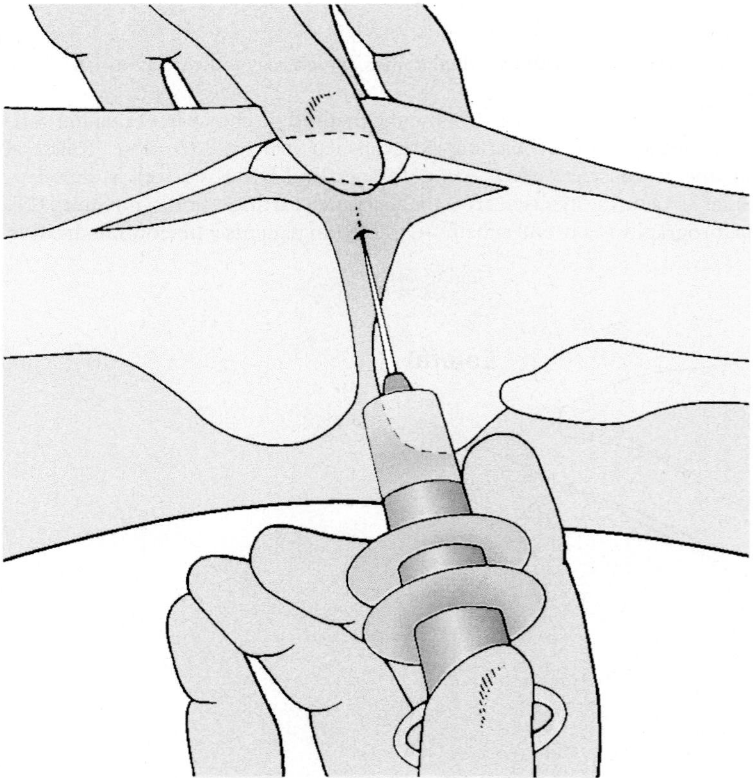

FIGURE 9.8 CT-arthrography and MRa of the knee. For CT-arthrography or MRa examination of the knee, the patient is supine on the radiographic table, with both legs fully extended and in the neutral position. The patella is pulled laterally and rotated anteriorly, and the joint is entered from the lateral aspect at the midpoint of the patella. Before injection of contrast, the joint should be aspirated to avoid dilution of the contrast agent by joint fluid. For CT-arthrography, diluted iodinated contrast material mixed with 0.3 mL of epinephrine 1:1,000 is then injected into the joint. If a double-contrast CT-arthrography is preferred, additional 50 to 60 mL of room air are also injected. In order to properly distribute the contrast material around the knee recesses, CT images are then obtained with the patient in the supine and prone position. For MRa, 40 mL of diluted gadolinium-based contrast material (0.2 mL of gadolinium diluted in 40 mL of saline) with 0.3 mL of epinephrine 1:1,000 are injected.

The medial and lateral menisci (also known as *semilunar cartilages*) of the knee are crescent-shaped fibrocartilaginous structures attached, respectively, to the medial and lateral aspects of the superior articular surface of the tibia (Fig. 9.9). The menisci are seen on MRI as wedge-shaped or bow tie–shaped structures of uniformly low signal intensity in practically all pulse sequences (Fig. 9.10). The anterior and posterior cruciate ligaments (PCL), like the menisci, are seen as low–signal intensity structures on all spin echo sequences.

Although the lateral meniscus is structurally very similar to the medial meniscus, it has a very important distinguishing feature. The popliteal muscle's tendon and its sheath pass through a portion of the posterior horn of the lateral meniscus, separating it from the joint capsule. This anatomic site is known as the *popliteal hiatus* (see Fig. 9.10C). The menisci are composed of collagen fibers distributed in layers. The superficial layers are oriented in the radial direction and the deeper layers are oriented in a circumferential direction. A horizontally oriented compact group of collagen fibers is present in the periphery of the menisci. This group of fibers is often seen on MRI as an intrasubstance intermediate–signal intensity band in the periphery of the meniscus, most often in the posterior horn of the medial meniscus and appear more prominent in younger individuals. The periphery of the menisci near the meniscocapsular junction has a capillary vascular bed, whereas the more central portion of the meniscus is avascular. The peripheral irrigated portion of the meniscus has a pink appearance on arthroscopic observation, and it has been termed the *red zone*. The central avascular portion is termed the *white zone*. This zonal distribution of the vascularity is important because tears involving the red zone may be amenable to surgical repair with subsequent healing, whereas the tears involving the white zone cannot be repaired and partial meniscectomy is the procedure of choice. The free edge of the medial meniscus occasionally has an undulating appearance called the *meniscus flounce*. This is a normal variant not associated with a meniscal tear (see Fig. 9.10E).

The crucial ligaments of the knee are also commonly subjected to injury. The topography of the cruciate ligaments is depicted in Figure 9.11. On MRI, the ACL is straight and fan shaped (slightly wider at its femoral attachment) and demonstrates low-to-intermediate signal intensity (Fig. 9.12A). The ACL is composed of an anterior medial bundle and a posterior lateral bundle. The PCL is arcuate in shape when the knee is in extension or mild flexion and becomes increasingly taut as the knee is flexed. It is composed of an anterior lateral bundle and a posterior medial bundle. These two PCL bundles may be seen as independent structures. Normally, it has very low signal intensity (Fig. 9.12B). Anteriorly to the PCL, one can observe a small bulge produced by the anterior meniscofemoral ligament, also known as the *ligament of Humphrey* (Fig. 9.12B,C). Posteriorly, a small bulge is created by the posterior meniscofemoral ligament, known as the *ligament of Wrisberg* (Fig. 9.12D,E).

The medial collateral ligament (MCL) consists of two components: superficial and deep. The superficial component, which is the principal medial stabilizer of the knee, arises from the medial femoral epicondyle just below the adductor tubercle and inserts into the medial aspect of the tibia, approximately 5 cm below the joint line. The deep layer of the MCL, which is considered part of the fibrous capsule, attaches loosely to the peripheral margin of the body of the medial meniscus. The MCL is continued posteriorly with the posterior oblique ligament. This ligament is closely intertwined with the distal arms of the semimembranosus tendon, providing strong stabilization of the posterior medial corner of the knee (Fig. 9.13A–D). The lateral collateral ligament attaches to the lateral epicondyle of the femur superiorly just above the popliteus groove, in which region it merges with the outer surface of the capsule. From here, it extends inferiorly and posteriorly to attach to the anterior portion of the apex of the fibular head (Fig. 9.13E,F). Both collateral ligaments are best demonstrated on the images obtained in the coronal plane. Like the menisci and cruciate ligaments, they also display low signal intensity

During evaluation of MRI of the knee, it is helpful to use a checklist as provided in Table 9.1.

Evaluation of knee instability caused by ligament injuries may require obtaining stress views. These techniques are most commonly performed in

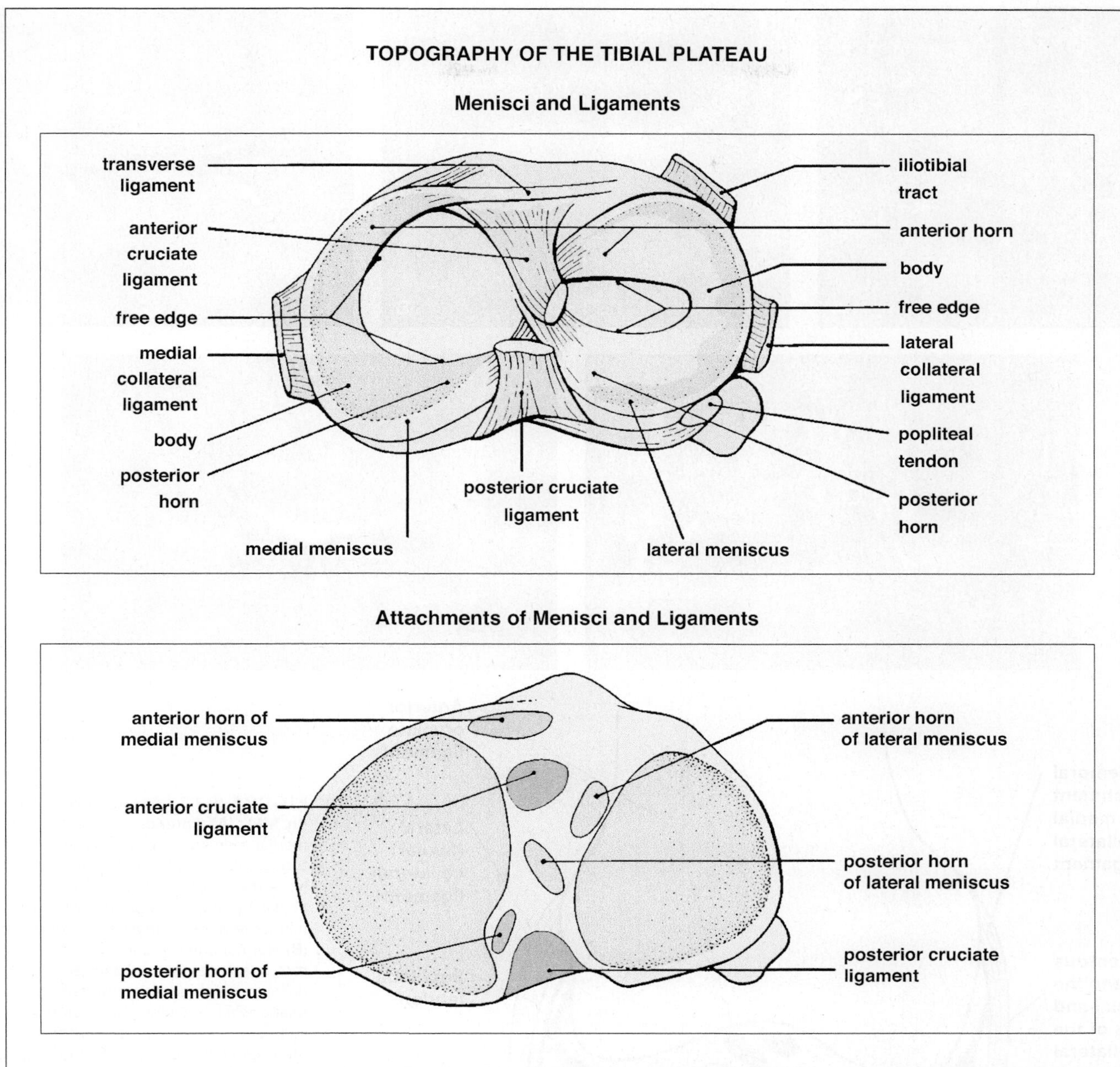

FIGURE 9.9 **Tibial plateau.** In the topography of the tibial plateau, the medial meniscus is a C-shaped fibrocartilaginous structure with anterior horn attached anteriorly to the intercondylar eminence of the tibia and with posterior horn inserted into the intercondylar area in front of the attachment of the PCL. The anterior horn of the lateral meniscus, which is an O-shaped structure, is attached in front of the lateral intercondylar tubercle, and the posterior horn inserts medially into the lateral intercondylar tubercle, in front of the attachment of the posterior horn of the medial meniscus.

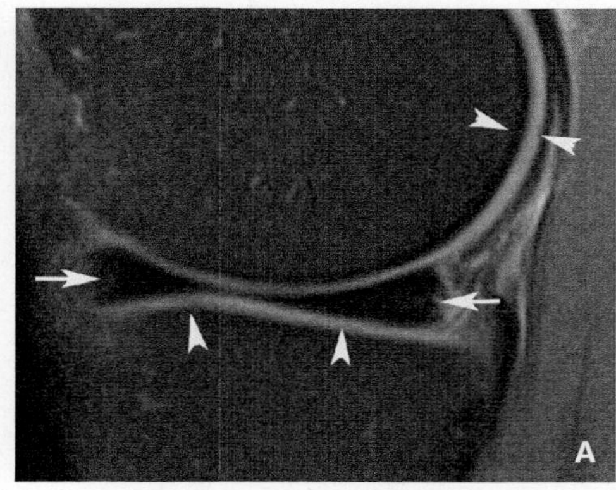

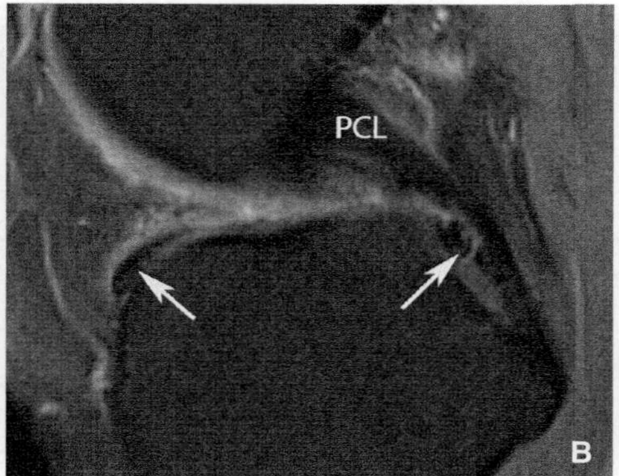

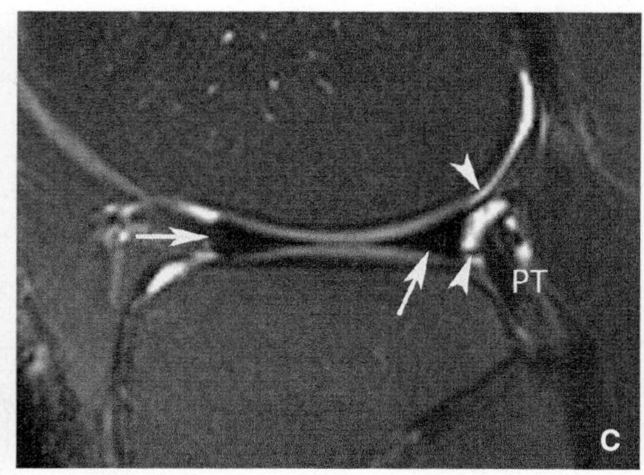

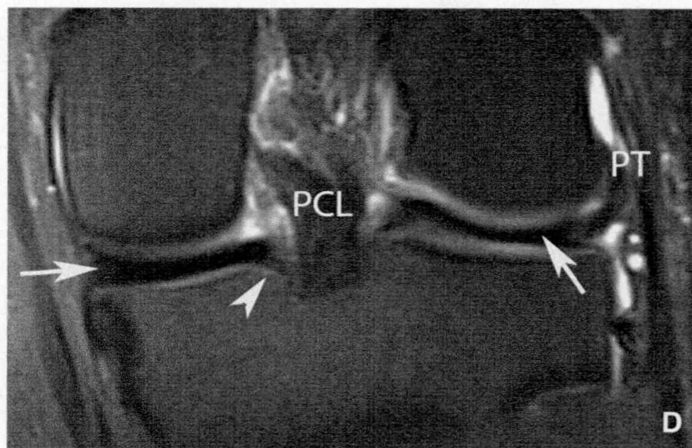

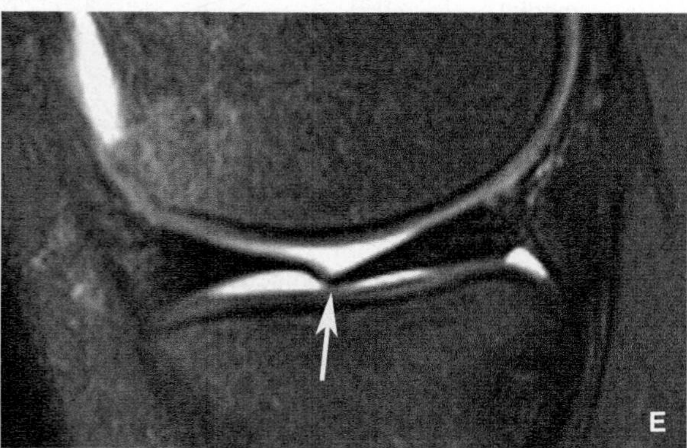

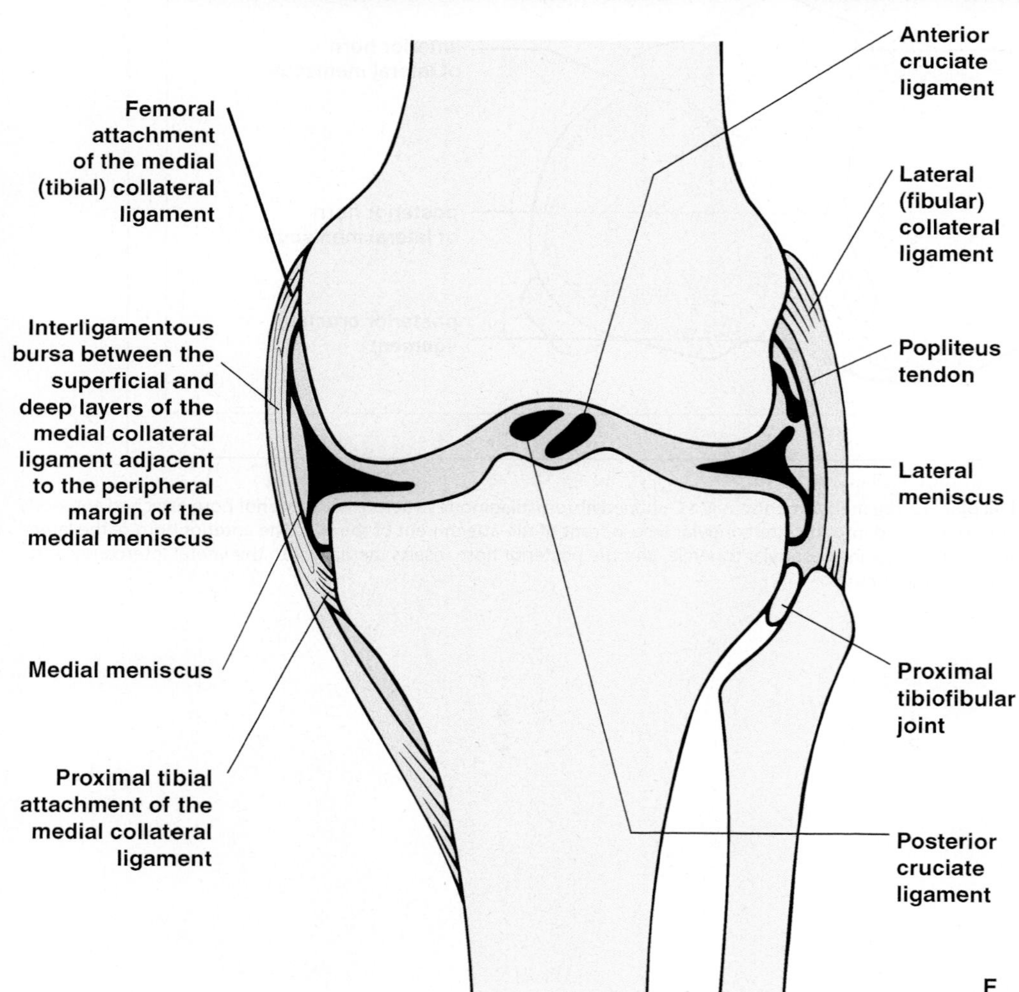

FIGURE 9.10 Appearance of normal menisci on MRI. **(A)** Anterior and posterior horns of the medial meniscus *(arrows)* as seen on sagittal proton density–weighted fat-saturated MR sequence. Note the smooth surface of the hyperintense articular hyaline cartilage *(arrowheads)* covering the medial femoral condyle and medial tibial plateau. **(B)** Normal anterior and posterior medial meniscal root ligaments *(arrows)* as seen on sagittal proton density–weighted fat-saturated image. Note the relationship between the posterior meniscal root ligament and the distal posterior cruciate ligament *(PCL)* at the tibial insertion. **(C)** Anterior and posterior horns of the lateral meniscus as seen on sagittal proton density–weighted fat-saturated MR image *(arrows)*. Note the posterior superior and inferior meniscal fascicles *(arrowheads)* delineating the popliteal hiatus that allows the passage of the popliteus tendon *(PT)*. **(D)** Posterior horns of the medial and lateral menisci *(arrows)* as seen on a coronal proton density–weighted fat-saturated pulse sequence obtained through the posterior aspect of the femoral condyles. Observe the posterior medial meniscal root ligament *(arrowhead)* adjacent to the tibial insertion of the PCL. Note the PT at the origin in the lateral femoral condyle. **(E)** Sagittal T2-weighted MR image demonstrates an undulating appearance of the medial meniscus or meniscal "flounce" *(arrow)*, a normal variant. **(F)** Schematic representation of topography of the medial and lateral menisci and surrounding structures as seen in the midplane of the coronal MRI. (**F**, Modified from Firooznia H, Golimbu C, Rafii M. MR imaging of the menisci: fundamentals of anatomy and pathology. *Magn Reson Imaging Clin N Am* 1994;2(3):325–347. Copyright © 1994 Elsevier. With permission.)

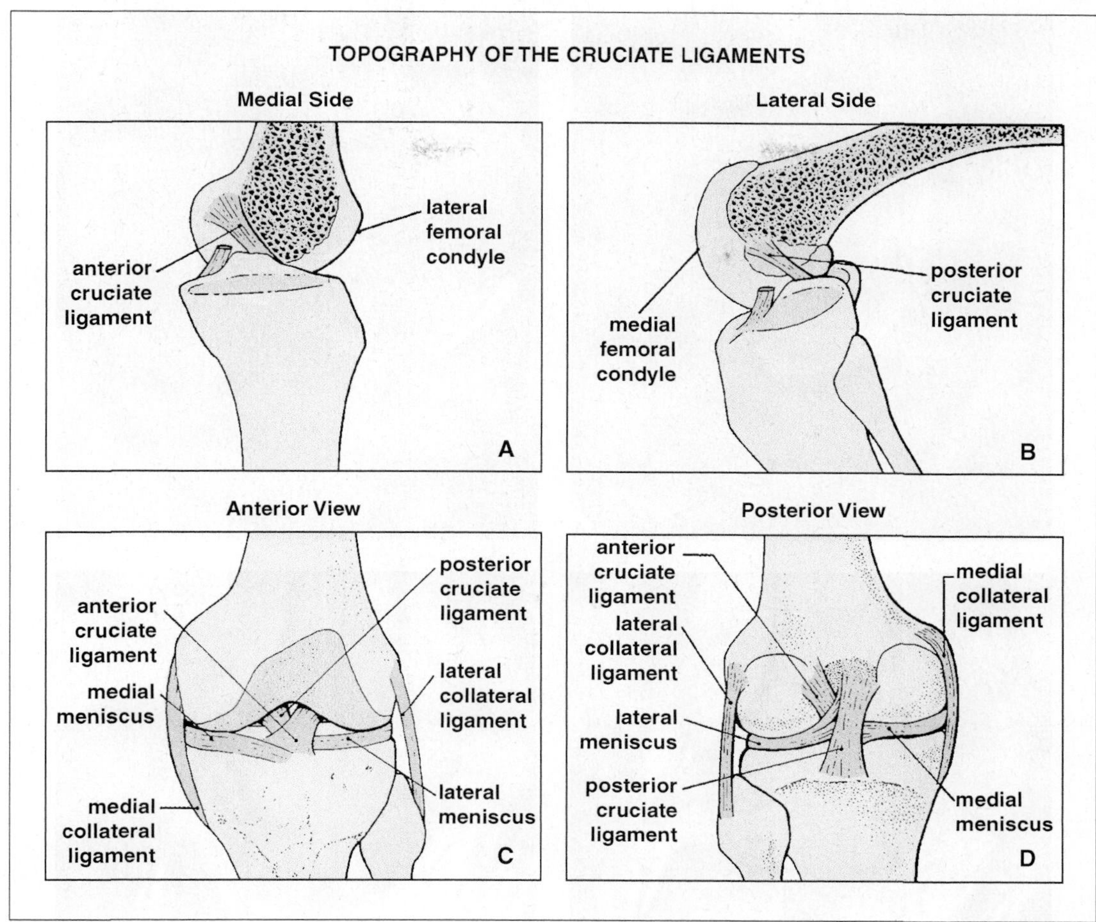

FIGURE 9.11 **The cruciate ligaments.** In the topography of the cruciate ligaments of the knee, the ACL arises on the medial surface of the lateral femoral condyle at the intercondylar notch **(A)** and attaches on the anterior portion of the intercondylar eminence of the tibia **(C)** (see also Fig. 9.9). The PCL originates on the lateral surface of the medial femoral condyle within the intercondylar notch **(B)** and inserts on the posterior surface of the intercondylar eminence **(D)** (see also Fig. 9.9). Neither cruciate ligament is attached to the tibial tubercles.

cases of suspected injury to the MCL (Fig. 9.14). They are less frequently performed during the evaluation of insufficiency of the anterior and PCL (Fig. 9.15). These examinations should preferably be performed under local anesthesia.

Arteriography and venography may need to be used in the evaluation of concomitant injury to the vascular system, although recently more often magnetic resonance angiography (MRA) is performed for this purpose. CT is effective in the evaluation of tibial plateau fractures, and it is occasionally used to evaluate injury to the cartilage and soft tissues, particularly the menisci and cruciate ligaments. CT used in conjunction with arthrography (computed arthrotomography) is useful in the evaluation of osteochondritis dissecans (see Fig. 9.61C,D) and in detecting nonopaque osteochondral bodies in the knee joint.

For a summary of the preceding discussion in tabular form, see Tables 9.2 and 9.3.

Injury to the Knee

Fractures About the Knee

Fractures of the Distal Femur

Most often sustained in motor vehicle accidents or falls from heights, fractures of the distal femur are classified according to the site and extension of the fracture line as supracondylar, condylar, and intercondylar. Supracondylar fractures can be further classified as nondisplaced, impacted, displaced, and comminuted (Fig. 9.16). These injuries are usually well demonstrated on the standard anteroposterior and lateral radiographs of the knee (Fig. 9.17); however, in rare instances, an oblique view of the knee may be needed to evaluate an obliquely oriented fracture line. In the past, tomography used to be required in cases of comminution for a full evaluation of the fracture lines and localization of the fragments (Fig. 9.18), although currently helical CT with multiplanar reformation and three-dimensional (3D) reconstruction has surpassed conventional tomographic technique (Fig. 9.19).

Fractures of the Proximal Tibia

The medial and lateral tibial plateaus are the most common sites of fractures of the proximal tibia. Because they usually result when the knee is struck by a moving vehicle, they are also called *fender* or *bumper fractures*; some, however, may be the result of twisting falls. The Hohl classification gives an overview of six different types of tibial plateau fractures and is useful in correlating the various types of injuries with the applied forces causing them (Fig. 9.20). In the Hohl classification, pure abduction injury results in a nondisplaced split fracture of the lateral tibial plateau (type I) (Fig. 9.21). When axial compression is combined with abduction force, local central depression (type II) and local split depression (type III) fractures occur (Fig. 9.22). Total depression fractures (type IV), which are more commonly seen in the medial tibial plateau because of its anatomic configuration (absence of the fibula), are characterized by the lack of comminution of the articular surface. Type V fractures in the Hohl classification, which are infrequently encountered, are local split fractures without central depression involving the anterior or posterior aspects of the tibial plateau. Comminuted fractures involving both tibial plateaus and having a Y or T configuration (type VI) usually result from vertical compression, such as a fall on the extended leg (Fig. 9.23). Types III and VI are frequently

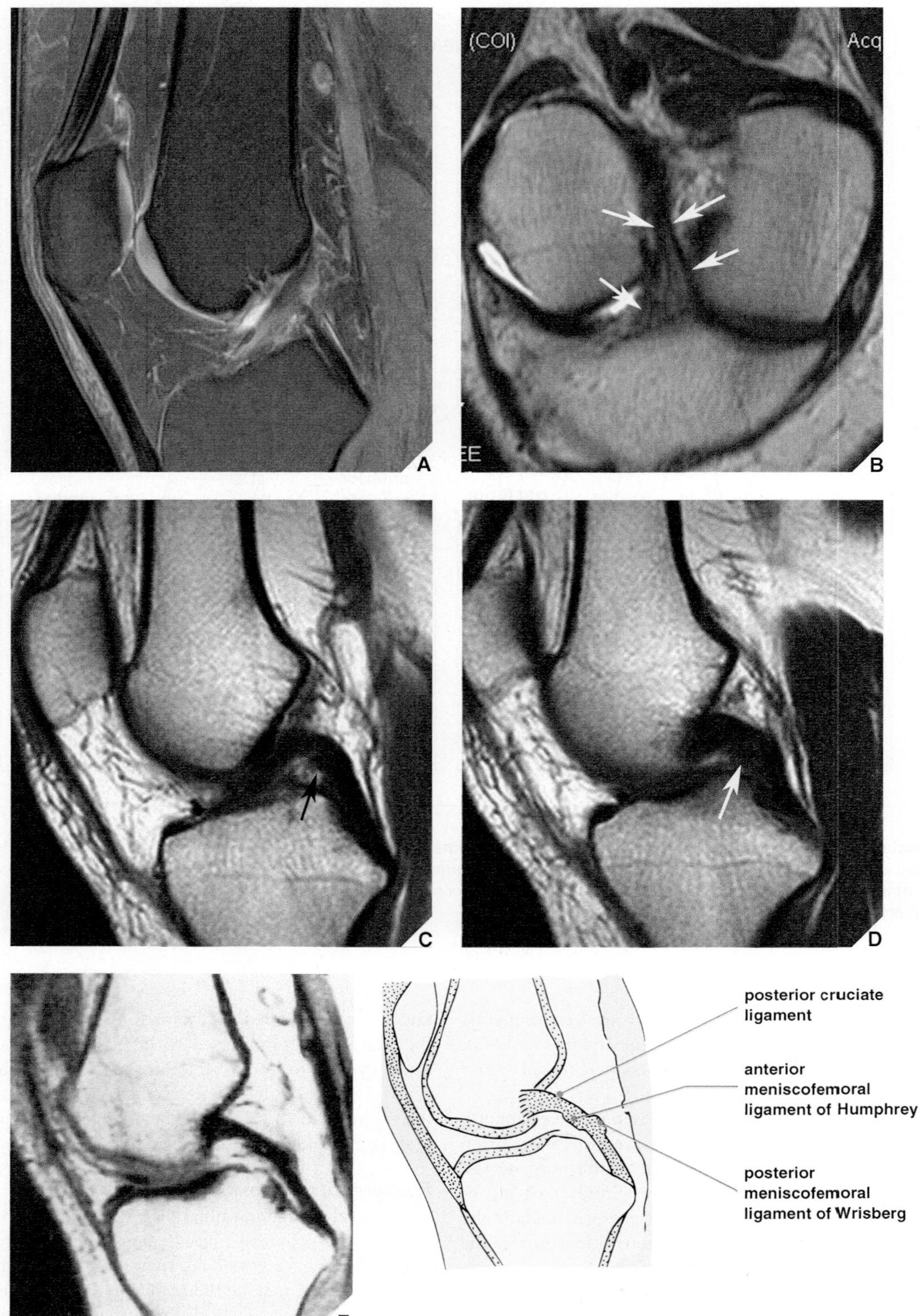

FIGURE 9.12 Spin echo MR images of the normal cruciate ligaments. **(A)** Sagittal proton density–weighted MR image demonstrates the anterior margin of the ACL, straight and well defined, representing the anteromedial bundle; the posterior margin is ill-defined because of the oblique orientation of the ligament, and it represents the posterolateral bundle. **(B)** Oblique coronal T2-weighted MR image depicts the ACL from the origin in the lateral femoral condyle to the insertion in the tibia *(arrows)*. **(C)** The PCL is seen in its entirety, in one sagittal image, from the femoral to the tibial attachments. Observe the small bulge anteriorly produced by the anterior meniscofemoral ligament *(arrow)*. **(D)** In this sagittal section, the anterior meniscofemoral ligament of Humphrey is very prominent, simulating a loose body or meniscal fragment *(arrow)*. **(E)** Sagittal T1-weighted MR image depicts both anterior (Humphrey) and posterior (Wrisberg) meniscofemoral ligaments to be prominent.

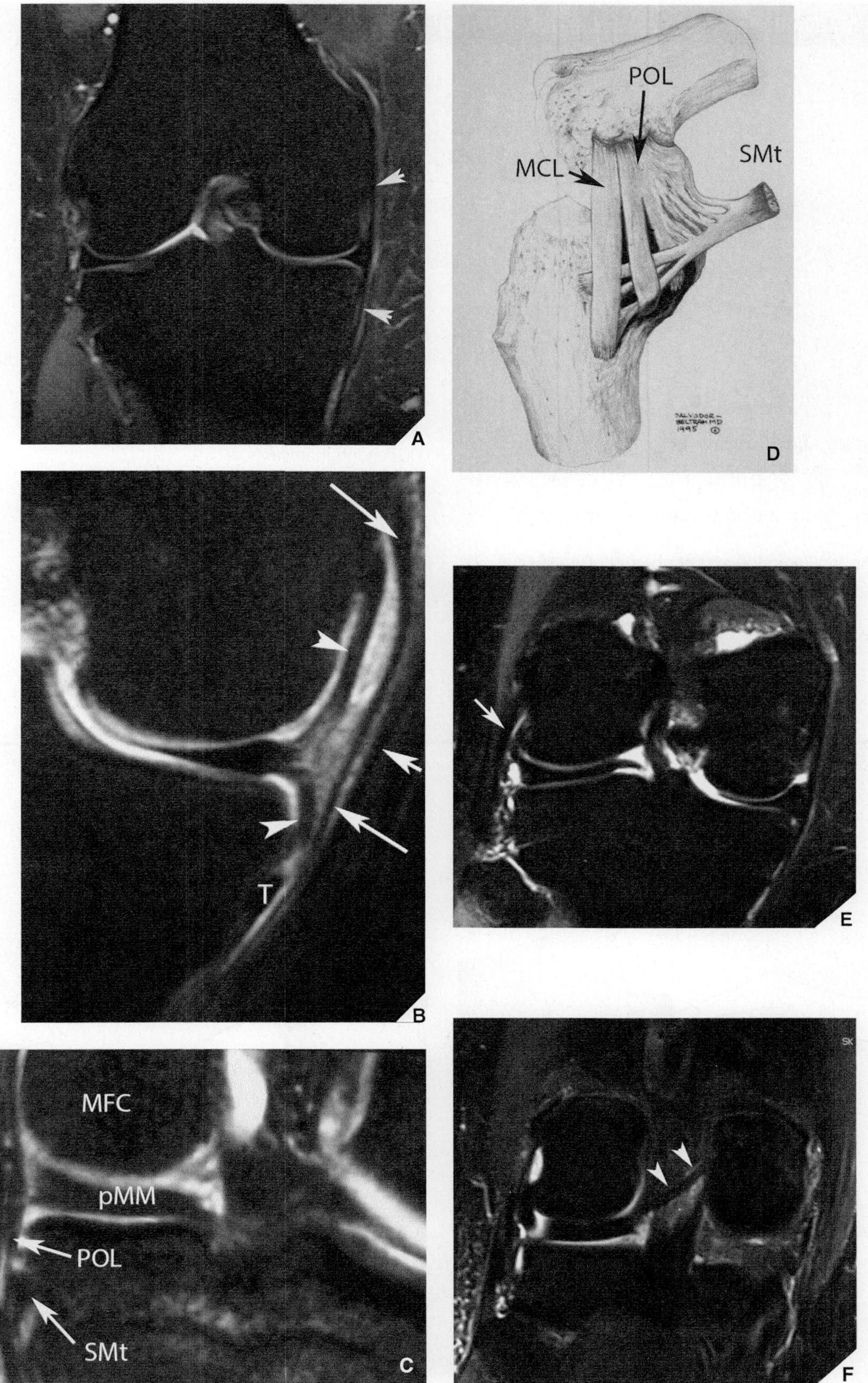

FIGURE 9.13 MRI of the collateral ligaments. **(A)** Coronal T2-weighted fat-saturated MR image of the normal MCL. The superficial fibers of the MCL are well defined in this section through the intercondylar notch *(arrows)*. The insertion of the PCL in the inner aspect of the medial femoral condyle (MFC) is well demonstrated. The menisci are seen as small triangles of low signal intensity. **(B)** Coronal T2-weighted fat-saturated image demonstrates the superficial *(long arrows)* and deep *(arrowheads)* fibers of the MCL. Note the deep crural fascia *(short arrow)* and the tibial arm (T) of the semimembranosus tendon *(SMt)*. **(C)** Coronal gradient echo MR image through the posterior aspect of the MFC and posterior horn of the medial meniscus *(pMM)* demonstrates the relationship between the posterior oblique ligament *(POL)* and the anterior arm of the SMt. **(D)** Schematic illustration of the posterior medial corner of the knee showing the relationship between the MCL, the POL, and the arms of the distal SMt. **(E,F)** Coronal T2-weighted fat-saturated MR images of the lateral (fibular) collateral ligament *(arrow)*. On this posterior section, note the meniscofemoral ligament, which extends from the posterior horn of the lateral meniscus to the inner surface of the MFC *(arrowheads)*. The lateral and medial menisci and PCL are well demonstrated.

TABLE 9.1 Checklist for Evaluation of Magnetic Resonance Imaging of the Knee

Osseous Structures
- Femoral condyles (c, s, a)
- Tibial plateau (c, s)
- Gerdy tubercle (s, a)
- Patella (c, s, a)
- Proximal fibula (c, s, a)

Cartilaginous Structures
- Articular cartilage (c, s, a)

Joints
- Femorotibial (c, s)
- Femoropatellar (s, a)

Menisci
- Medial (c, s)
- Lateral (c, s)

Ligaments
- Medial collateral—deep and superficial fibers (c)
- Lateral collateral complex—biceps femoris tendon, lateral collateral ligament proper, iliotibial band (c)
- Anterior cruciate—anteromedial and posterolateral bundles (c, s)
- Posterior cruciate (c, s)
- Meniscofemoral—Humphrey (anterior) and Wrisberg (posterior) (c, s)
- Transverse (s)
- Patellar ("tendon") (s)
- Patellar retinacula—medial and lateral (a)
- Arcuate (c, a)
- Popliteofibular (c, s)
- Fabellofibular (c)

Muscles and Their Tendons
- Quadriceps (s, a)
- Popliteus (c, s)
- Plantaris (a)
- Biceps femoris (c)
- Semimembranosus (s, a)
- Semitendinosus (s, a)
- Gracilis (s, a)
- Sartorius (s, a)
- Gastrocnemius (s, a)
- Soleus (s, a)

Bursae
- Popliteal (Baker) between the tendons of the medial head of gastrocnemius and semimembranosus (s, a)
- Prepatellar (s, a)
- Superficial infrapatellar (s, a)
- Deep infrapatellar (s, a)
- Pes anserinus (c)
- Semimembranosus—tibial collateral ligament (c)

Other Structures
- Suprapatellar recess (s)
- Synovial plicae (c, a)
- Infrapatellar plica (s)
- Hoffa (infrapatellar) fat pad (s, a)
- Popliteus hiatus (c)
- Popliteal artery and vein (a)
- Lateral geniculate artery (c)
- Tibial and peroneal nerves (a)

The best imaging planes for visualization of listed structures are given in parentheses: c, coronal; s, sagittal; a, axial.

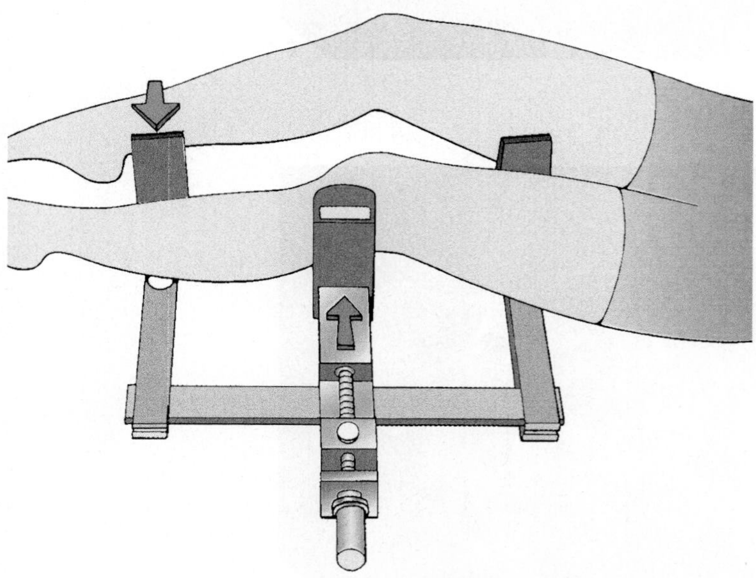

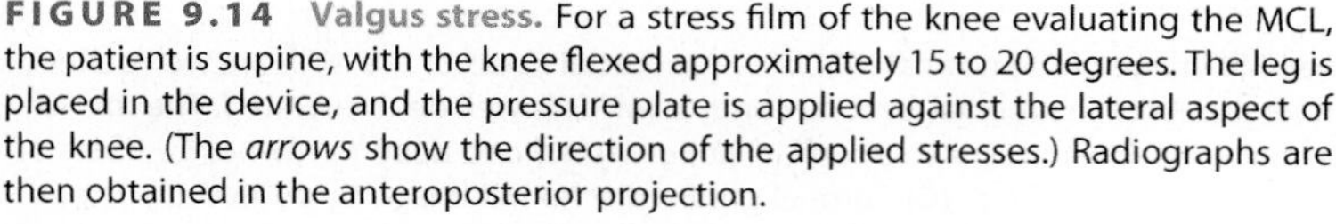

FIGURE 9.14 **Valgus stress.** For a stress film of the knee evaluating the MCL, the patient is supine, with the knee flexed approximately 15 to 20 degrees. The leg is placed in the device, and the pressure plate is applied against the lateral aspect of the knee. (The *arrows* show the direction of the applied stresses.) Radiographs are then obtained in the anteroposterior projection.

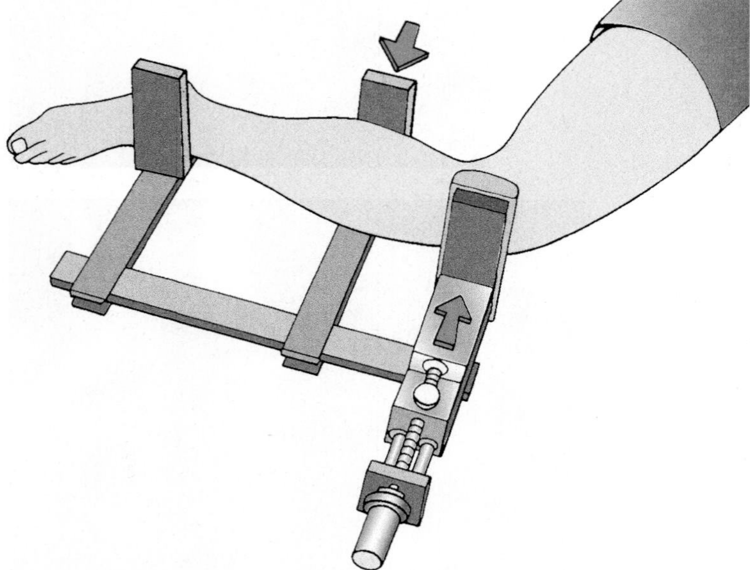

FIGURE 9.15 **Anterior-draw stress.** For a stress film of the knee evaluating the ACL, the patient is placed in the device on his or her side, with the knee flexed 90 degrees. The pressure plate is applied against the anterior aspect of the knee. (The *arrows* show the direction of the applied stresses.) Radiographs are then obtained in the lateral projection.

TABLE 9.2 Standard and Special Radiographic Projections for Evaluating Injury to the Knee

Projection	Demonstration
Anteroposterior	Medial and lateral joint compartments Varus and valgus deformities Fractures of: Medial and lateral femoral condyles Medial and lateral tibial plateaus Tibial spines Proximal fibula Osteochondral fracture Osteochondritis dissecans (late stage) Spontaneous osteonecrosis Pellegrini-Stieda lesion
Overpenetrated	Bipartite or multipartite patella Fractures of patella
Stress	Tear of collateral ligaments
Lateral	Femoropatellar joint compartment Patella in profile Suprapatellar recess Fractures of: Distal femur Proximal tibia Patella Dislocations
Lateral (continued)	Sinding-Larsen-Johansson disease[a] Osgood-Schlatter disease[a] Osteochondral fracture Osteochondritis dissecans (late stage) Spontaneous osteonecrosis Joint effusion Bursitis of: Prepatellar bursa Superficial and deep infrapatellar bursae Tears of: Quadriceps tendon Patellar ligament
Stress	Tears of cruciate ligaments
Cross-table	Fat-blood interface (FBI sign) of lipohemarthrosis
Tunnel (posteroanterior)	Posterior aspect of femoral condyles Intercondylar notch Intercondylar eminence of tibia
Axial (sunrise and Merchant)	Articular facets of patella[b] Sulcus angle[b] Congruence angle[b] Fractures of patella Subluxation and dislocation of patella[b]

[a]These conditions are best demonstrated using a low-kilovoltage/soft-tissue technique.

[b]These features are better demonstrated on Merchant axial view.

TABLE 9.3 Ancillary Imaging Techniques for Evaluating Injury to the Knee

Technique	Demonstration
Arthrography (usually double-contrast; occasionally single-contrast using air only); currently replaced by MRI and MRa (see the following text)	Meniscal tears Injuries to: Cruciate ligaments Medial collateral ligament Quadriceps tendon Patellar ligament Joint capsule Chondral and osteochondral fractures Osteochondritis dissecans (early and late stages) Osteochondral bodies in joint Subtle abnormalities of articular cartilage
CT and computed arthrotomography	Spontaneous osteonecrosis Injuries to: Articular cartilage Cruciate ligaments Menisci Osteochondral bodies in joint Osteochondritis dissecans
Radionuclide imaging (scintigraphy, bone scan)	Subtle fractures not demonstrated on standard studies Early and late stages of: Osteochondritis dissecans Spontaneous osteonecrosis
Angiography (arteriography, venography	Concomitant injury to arteries and veins
MRI	Same as arthrography, CT, and radionuclide imaging
MRa	Residual or recurrent meniscal tears Complications after meniscal surgery Loose intraarticular bodies Synovial plicae Stability of osteochondral lesions Tears of collateral ligaments Tears of cruciate ligaments
MR angiography	Same as angiography

MRI, magnetic resonance imaging; MRa, magnetic resonance arthrography; CT, computed tomography; MR, magnetic resonance.

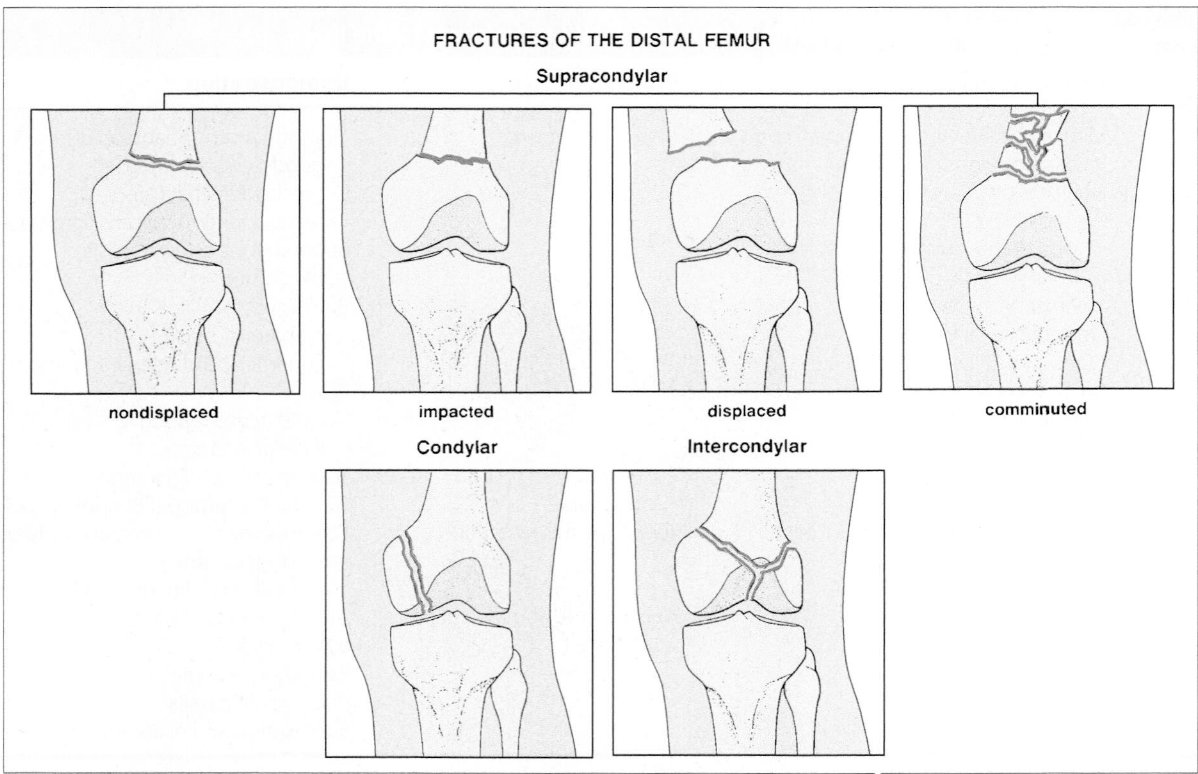

FIGURE 9.16 Classification of distal femur fractures. Fractures of the distal femur can be classified according to the site and extension of the injury as supracondylar, condylar, and intercondylar fractures.

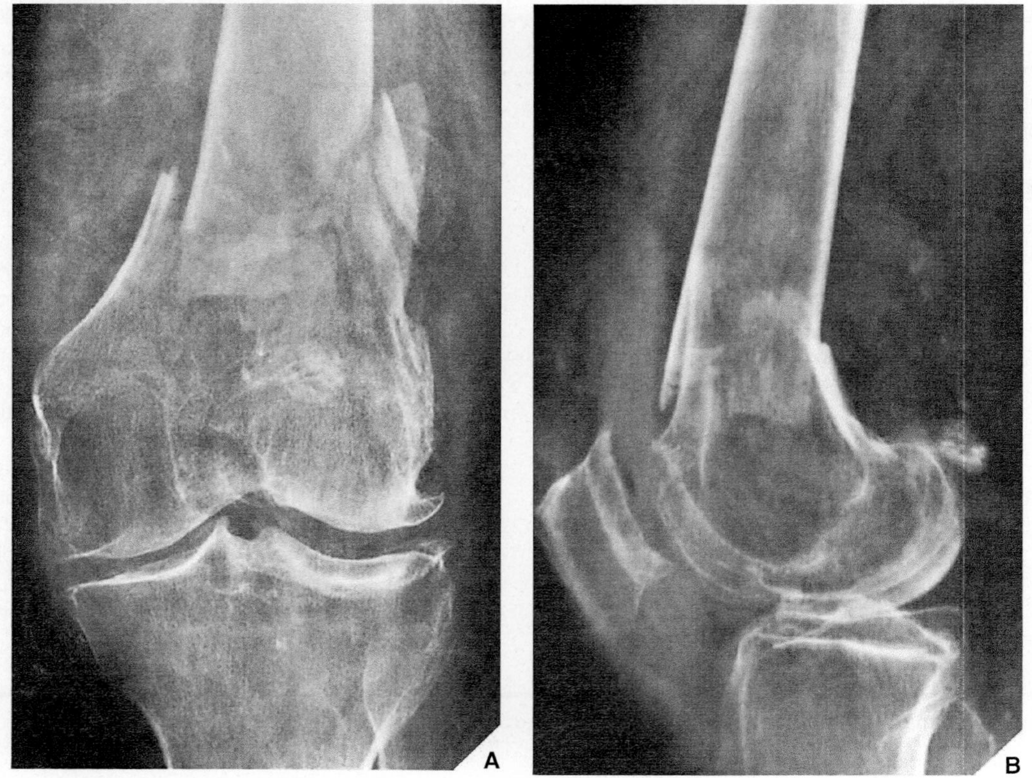

FIGURE 9.17 Supracondylar fracture. A 58-year-old man was injured in a motorcycle accident. **(A)** Anteroposterior and **(B)** lateral radiographs of the knee demonstrate a comminuted supracondylar fracture of the distal femur. The extension of the fracture lines and the position of the fragments can be assessed adequately on these standard studies.

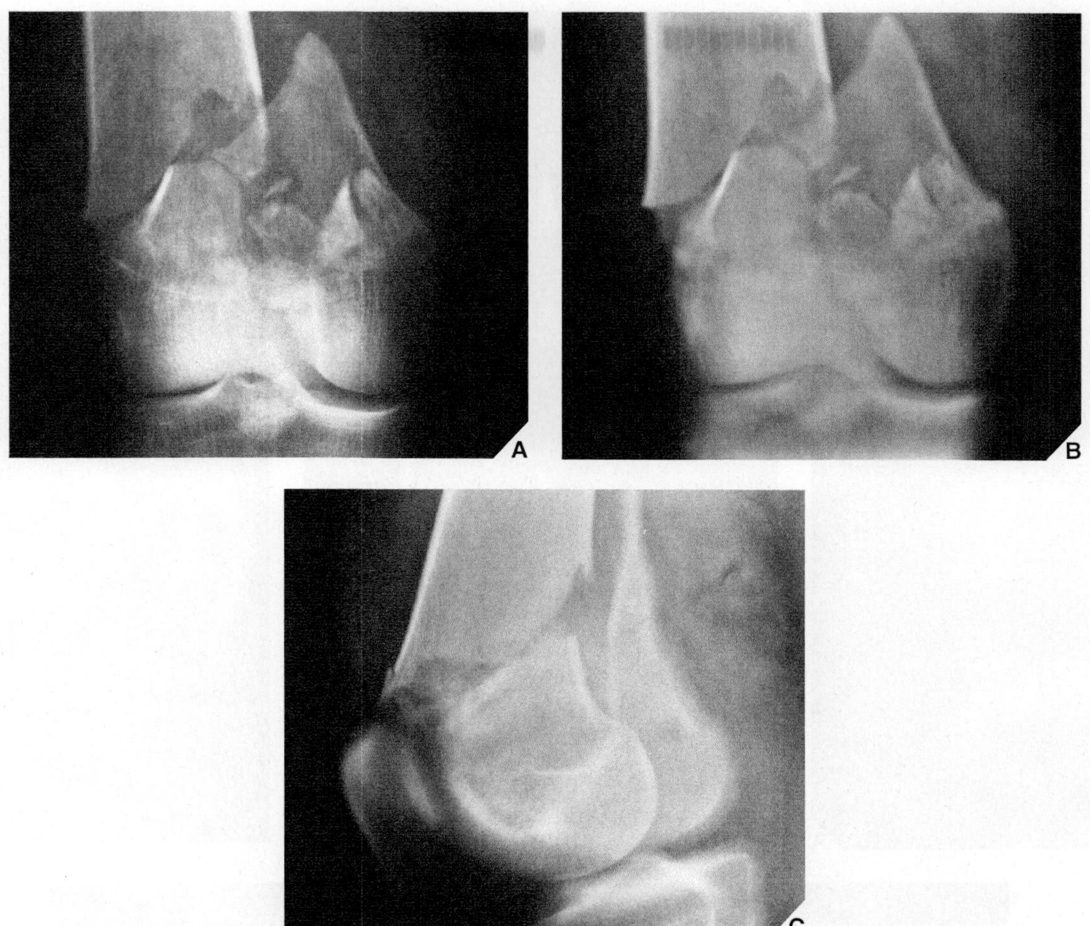

FIGURE 9.18 Supracondylar fracture. A 22-year-old racing car driver was injured in an accident on the track. **(A)** Anteroposterior radiograph of the right knee shows a comminuted fracture of the distal femur. Tomography was performed, and sections in the anteroposterior **(B)** and lateral **(C)** projections demonstrate intraarticular extension of the fracture lines, with split of the condyles and posterior displacement of the distal fragments. The multiple comminuted fragments can be localized.

associated with fracture of the proximal fibula. In our institution, we use the Schatzker classification of tibial plateau fractures, which, similar to the Hohl classification, arranges tibial plateau fractures into six types but according to involvement of the medial or lateral plateau (Fig. 9.24).

Fractures of the tibial plateau may not be obvious on the routine radiographic examination of the knee, particularly if there is no depression (Fig. 9.25A,B). In such cases, however, the cross-table lateral projection often reveals the FBI sign, which indicates the presence of an intraarticular fracture (Fig. 9.25C). Demonstration of an obscure fracture line may require oblique projections.

The role of CT in evaluation of tibial plateau fractures has been well established. CT provides optimal visualization of the plateau depression, defects, and split fragments. It also proved to be accurate in assessing depressed and split fractures when they involved the anterior and posterior border of the plateau and in demonstrating the extent of fracture comminution. Particularly useful are reformatted images in various planes and 3D reconstruction (Figs. 9.26 to 9.28). Kode and coworkers suggested that MRI was equivalent or superior to two-dimensional (2D) CT reformation for the depiction of tibial plateau fracture configuration (Figs. 9.29 and 9.30). The multiplanar capabilities of MRI may facilitate 3D perception, and in addition, this technique permits assessment of the associated injuries to the ligaments and menisci that are not visible on CT scans (Fig. 9.31).

An important feature of tibial plateau fractures is their association with injury to ligaments and the menisci. The structures most at risk are the MCL and the ACL (see Fig. 9.11) and the lateral meniscus (see Fig. 9.9) because lateral tibial plateau fractures usually result from valgus stress (Fig. 9.32). Moreover, damage to the ACL may be associated with avulsion of the lateral tibial spine or the anterior intercondylar eminence. Stress views and MRI usually reveal these associated abnormalities. If clinical examination and imaging studies, including stress views, show ligamentous structures to be intact, then nondisplaced fractures of the tibial plateau can be treated conservatively. In depression-type fractures, however, some orthopaedic surgeons recommend open reduction in patients whose fractures show 8 mm of articular depression. Generally, surgery is indicated for fractures of the tibial plateau showing articular depression of 10 mm or more.

Complications. The most frequent complications of fractures of the distal femur and the proximal tibia are malunion and posttraumatic arthritis.

Segond Fracture

The Segond fracture consists of a small-fragment avulsion fracture from the lateral aspect of the proximal tibia just below the level of the tibial plateau, best demonstrated on anteroposterior radiograph of the knee (Fig. 9.33). The mechanism of this injury is internal rotation of the leg associated with varus stress on a flexed knee that creates tension on the lateral capsule and lateral capsular ligament. This, in turn, causes an avulsion fracture at the insertion of this ligament on the lateral tibial plateau. This injury may be associated with capsular tear, a tear of the ACL, and lateral meniscus tear, resulting in chronic anterolateral knee instability (Fig. 9.34).

Hall and Hochman described a reverse Segond-type fracture affecting medial tibial plateau, associated with tears of the PCL, MCL, and medial meniscus (Fig. 9.35). The mechanism of this injury and the constellation of radiographic findings are the reverse of that seen with the classic Segond

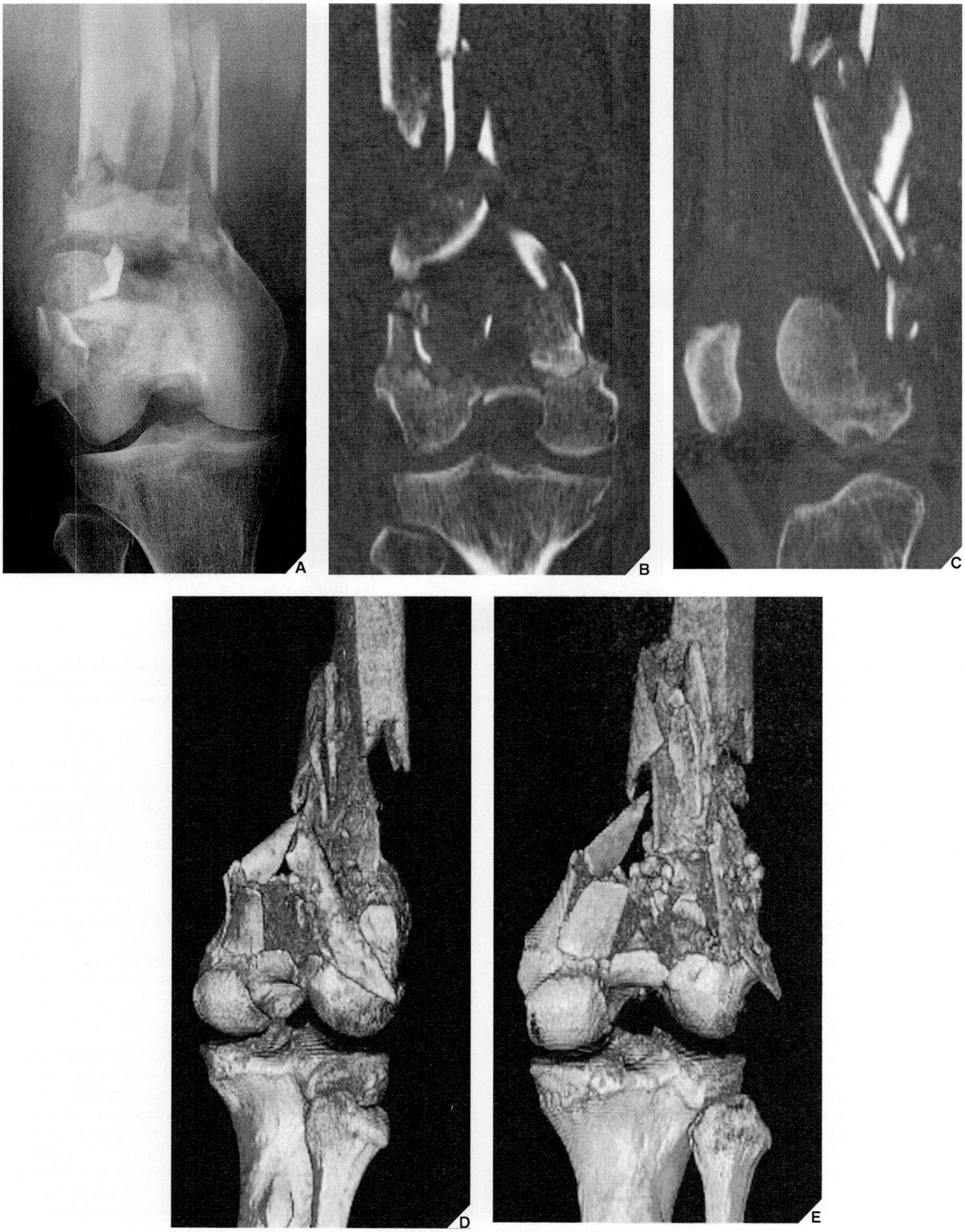

FIGURE 9.19 CT and 3D CT of supracondylar fracture. A 54-year-old woman was injured in a motor vehicle accident. **(A)** Anteroposterior radiograph of the right knee shows markedly comminuted supracondylar fracture of the femur. **(B)** Coronal and **(C)** sagittal reformatted CT images show displacement of various fracture fragments. 3D CT reconstructed images, **(D)** oblique and **(E)** viewed from the posterior aspect, depict the position and orientation of displaced fracture fragments in more comprehensive fashion.

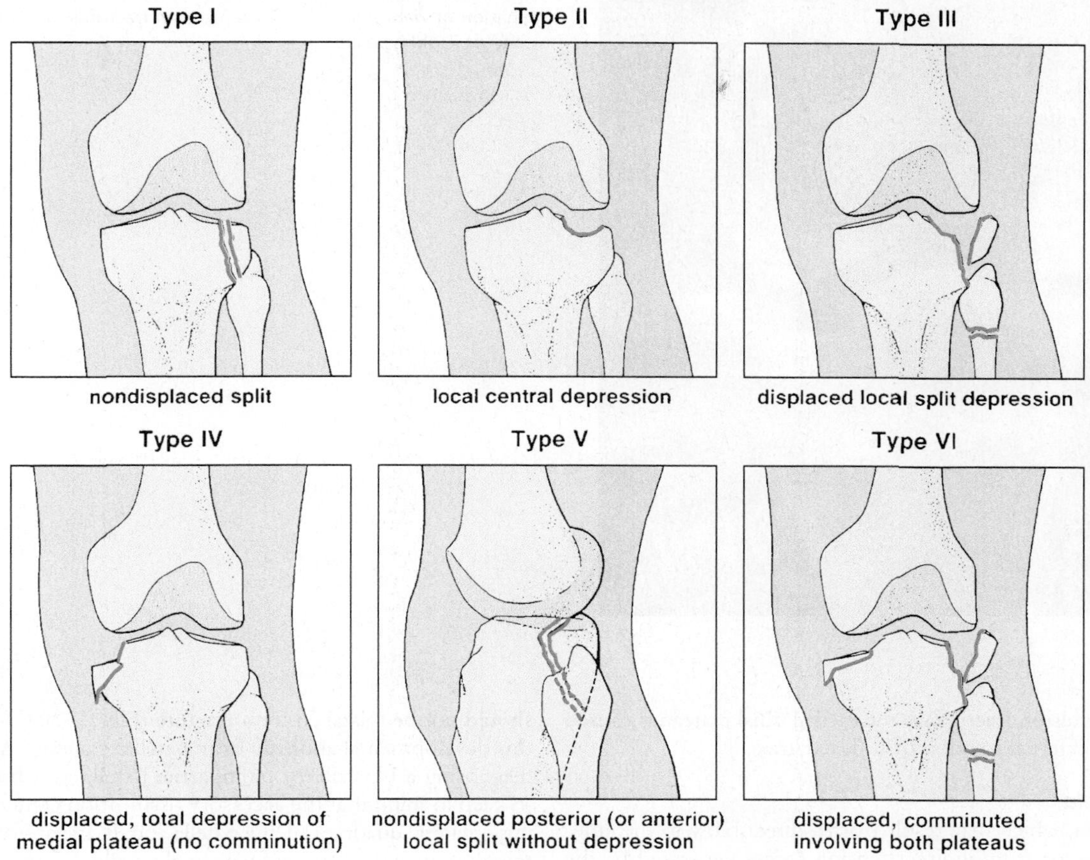

FIGURE 9.20 **The Hohl classification of fractures of the tibial plateau.** (Modified with permission from Hohl M. Tibial condylar fractures. *J Bone Joint Surg Am* 1967;49A:1455–1467.)

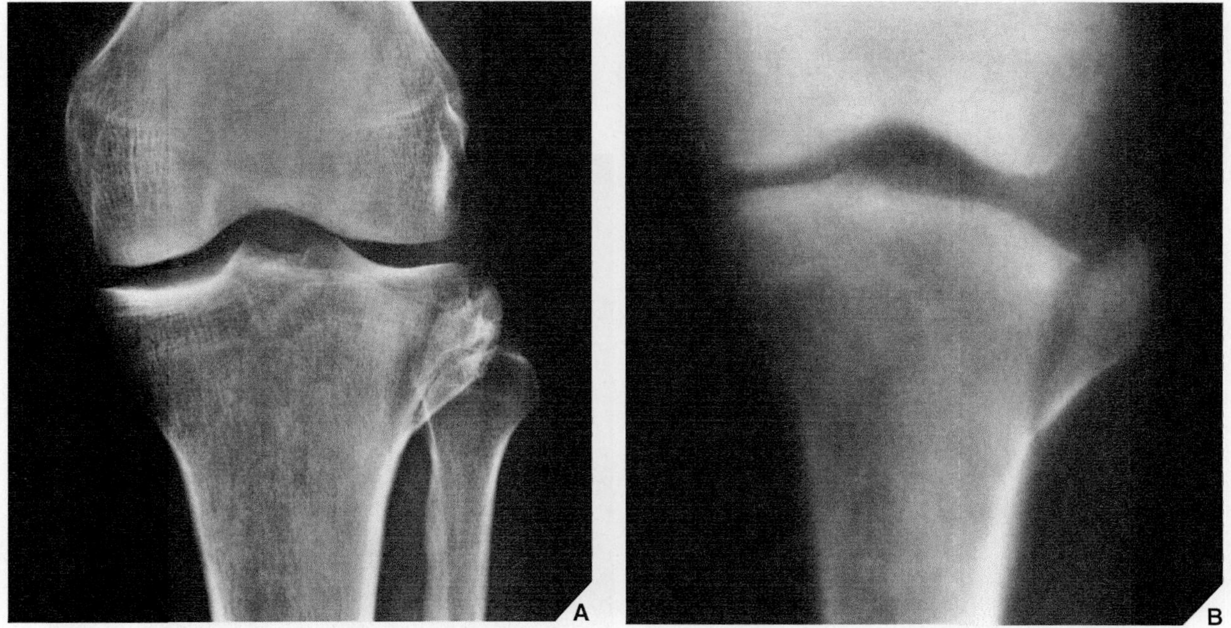

FIGURE 9.21 **Fracture of the tibial plateau.** A 30-year-old man was hit by a car while he was crossing the street. **(A)** Anteroposterior radiograph and **(B)** tomogram show a split fracture of the lateral tibial plateau (Hohl type I).

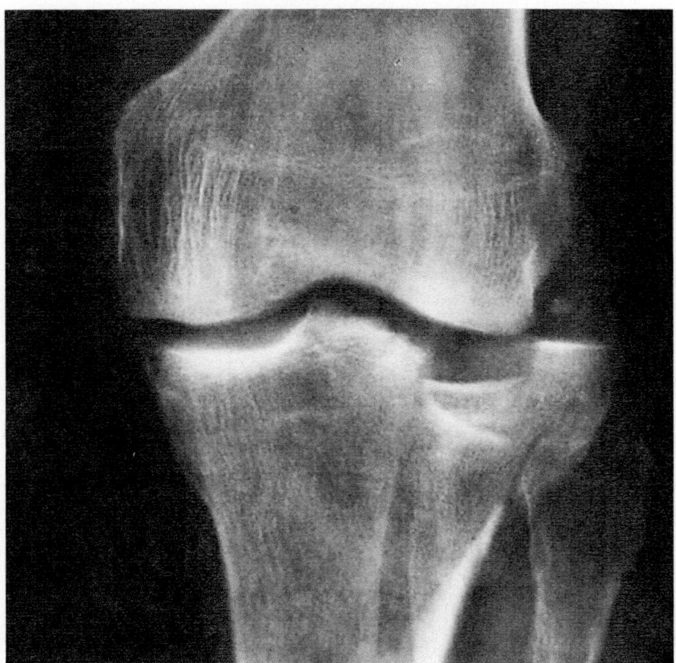

FIGURE 9.22 Fracture of the tibial plateau. Anteroposterior radiograph of the knee shows the appearance of a tibial plateau fracture, which is a combination of wedge and central depression fractures involving the lateral tibial condyle (Hohl type III).

injury complex. The avulsion fracture of the medial tibial plateau is caused by a valgus stress and external rotation of a flexed knee.

Fractures of the Patella

Fractures of the patella, which may result from a direct blow to the anterior aspect of the knee or from indirect tension forces generated by the quadriceps tendon, constitute approximately 1% of all skeletal injuries. Generally, patellar fractures may be longitudinal (vertical), transverse, or comminuted (Fig. 9.36). In the most commonly encountered patellar injury, seen in 60% of cases, the fracture line is transverse or slightly oblique, involving the midportion of the patella. In evaluation of such injury, it is important to recognize what has been called the *bipartite* or *multipartite patella*. This anomaly represents a developmental variant of the accessory ossification center or centers of the superolateral margin of the patella and should not be mistaken for a fracture (Fig. 9.37). CT may help distinguish this developmental anomaly from patellar fracture. As an aid to avoid misdiagnosing a bipartite or multipartite patella as a fracture, it is important to keep in mind that the accessory ossification centers are invariably in the upper lateral quadrant of the patella and, if the apparent fragments are put together, they do not form a normal patella. Fracture fragments, however, form a normal patella if they are replaced. Injury to the patella is usually sufficiently demonstrated on the overpenetrated anteroposterior and lateral radiographs of the knee or CT (Figs. 9.38 to 9.41), although MRI may also be effective.

Dislocations of the Patella

Dislocations of the patella, which are usually lateral, result from acute injury and are easily diagnosed on the standard projections of the knee (Fig. 9.42).

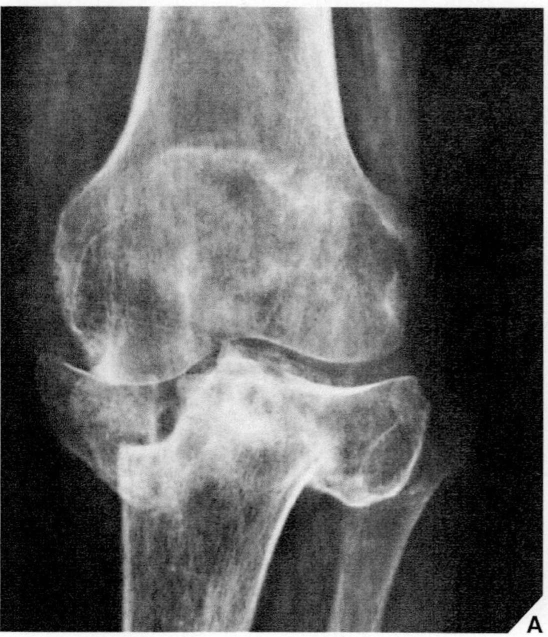

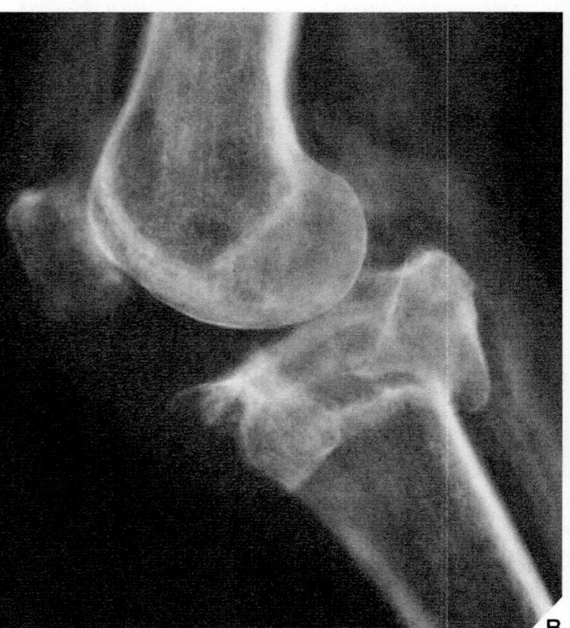

FIGURE 9.23 Fracture of the tibial plateau. **(A)** Anteroposterior radiograph and **(B)** lateral tomogram demonstrate the characteristic appearance of the Y-type bicondylar tibial fracture (Hohl type VI).

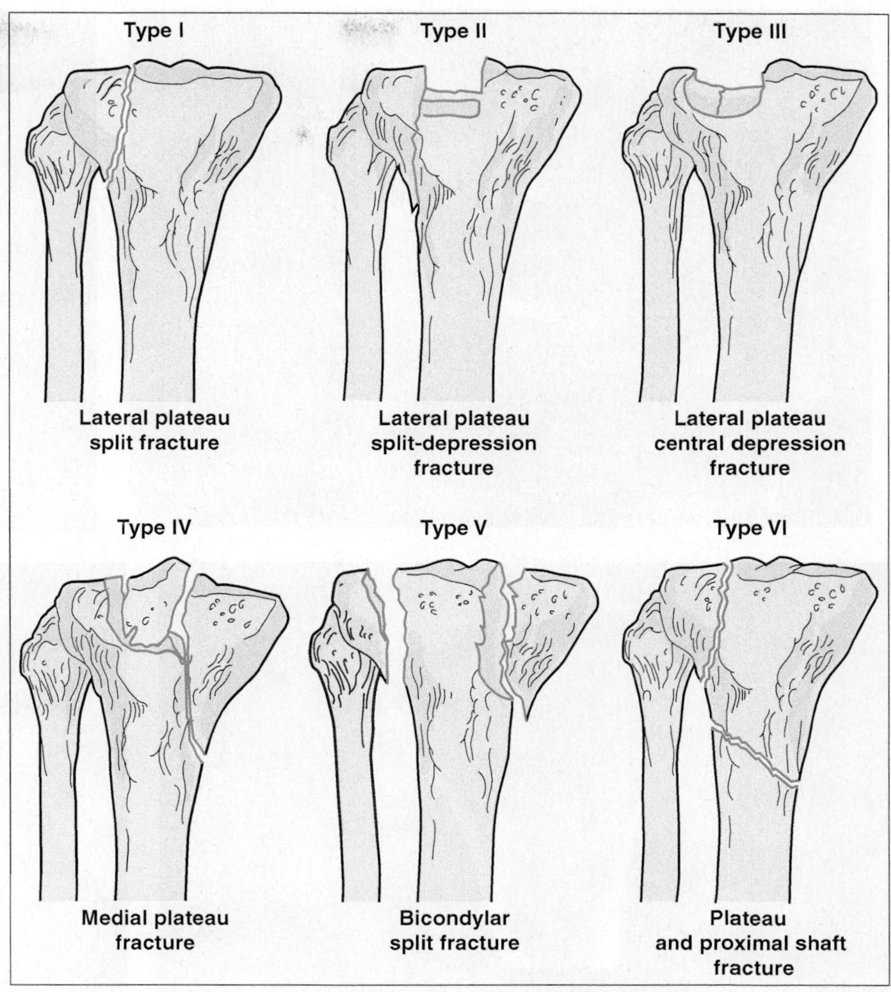

FIGURE 9.24 The Schatzker classification of fractures of the tibial plateau. (Modified with permission from Koval JK, Helfet DI. Tibial plateau fractures: evaluation and treatment. *J Am Acad Orthop Surg* 1995;3:86–93.)

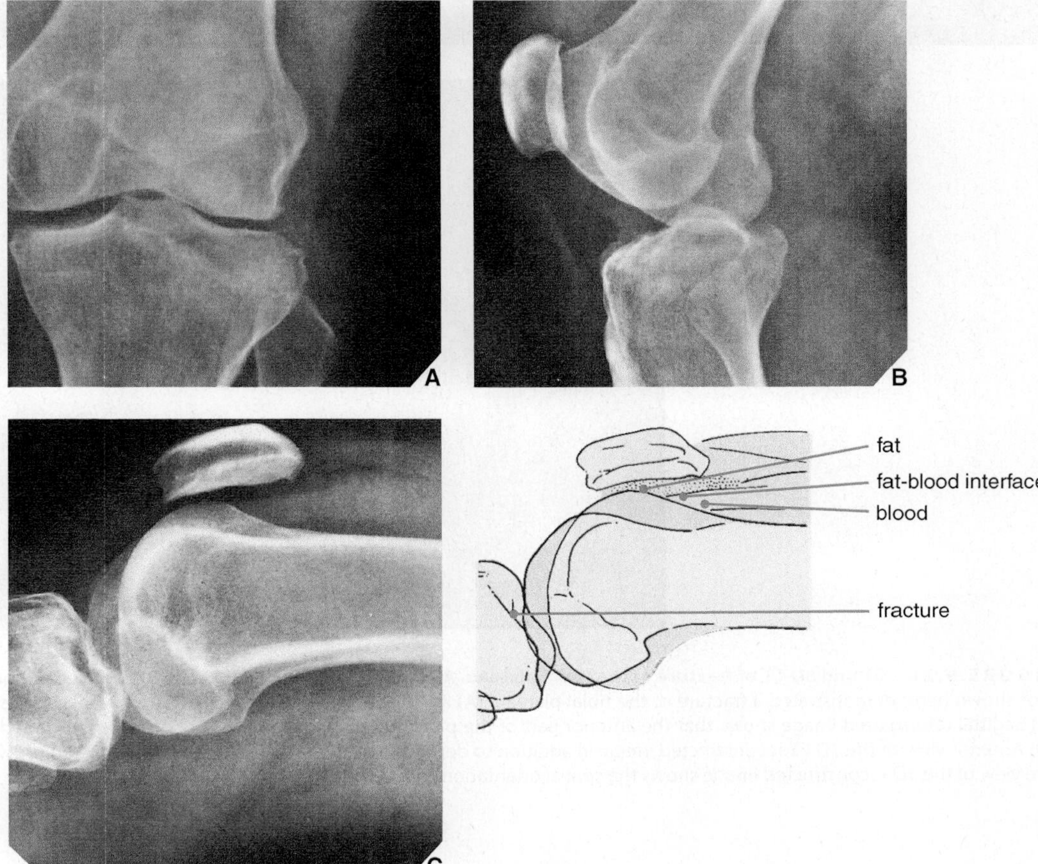

FIGURE 9.25 Fracture of the tibial plateau. While crossing the street, a 38-year-old woman was struck by a car. **(A)** Anteroposterior and **(B)** lateral radiographs show substantial joint effusion, but the fracture line is not clearly seen. **(C)** Cross-table lateral view demonstrates the FBI sign, indicating intraarticular extension of the fracture.

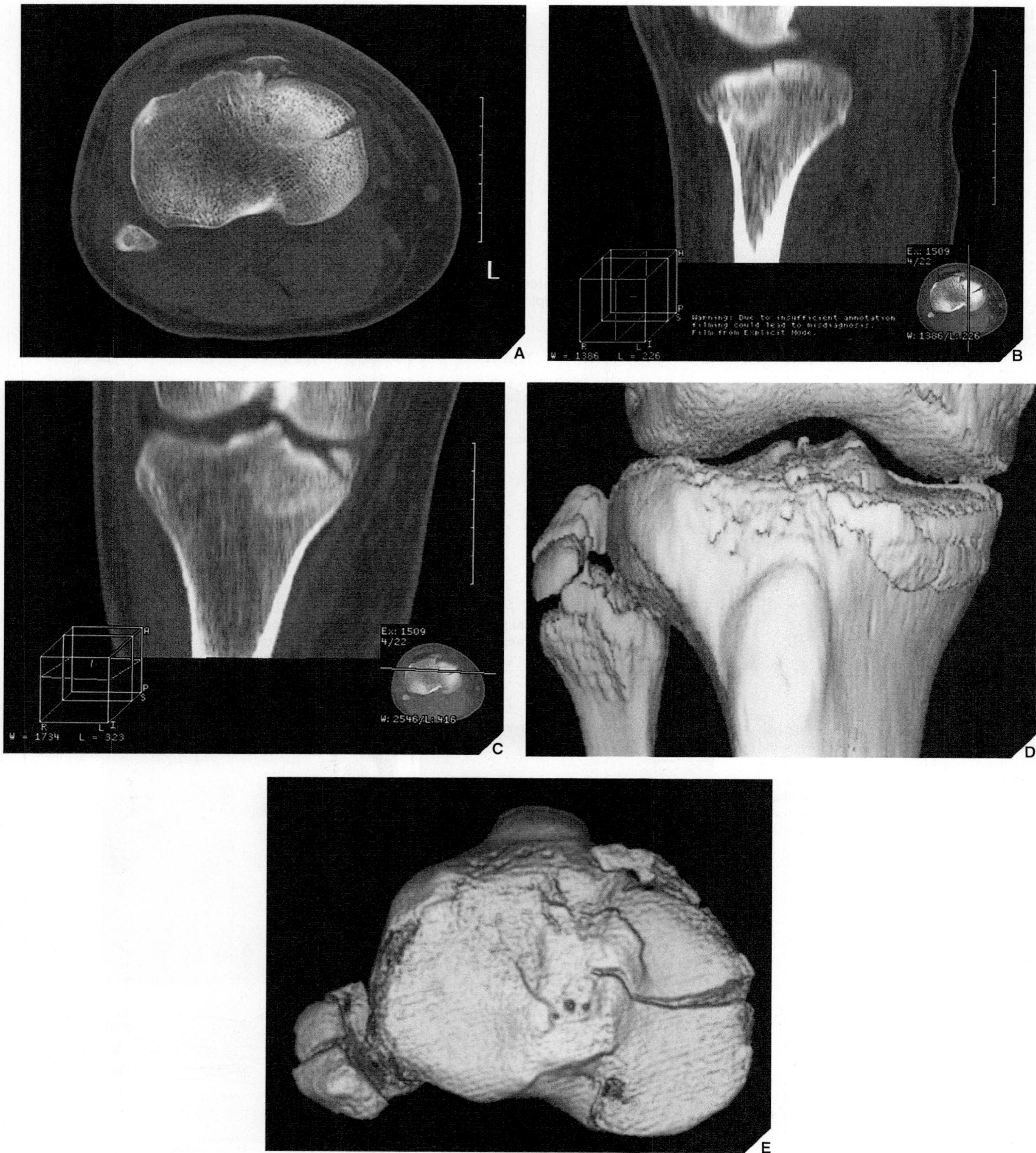

FIGURE 9.26 CT and 3D CT of fracture of the tibial plateau. A 23-year-old man was injured in a motorcycle accident. The conventional radiographs of the right knee (not shown here) demonstrated a fracture of the tibial plateau. **(A)** Axial CT section through the proximal tibia shows a comminuted fracture of the medial tibial plateau. **(B)** Sagittal reformatted image shows that the anterior part of the plateau is mainly affected. **(C)** Coronal reformatted image demonstrates comminution and depression. **(D)** Anterior view of the 3D CT reconstructed image in addition to depression of the medial anterior tibial plateau shows associated fracture of the proximal fibula. **(E)** Bird's eye view of the 3D reconstructed image shows the spatial orientation of the fracture lines.

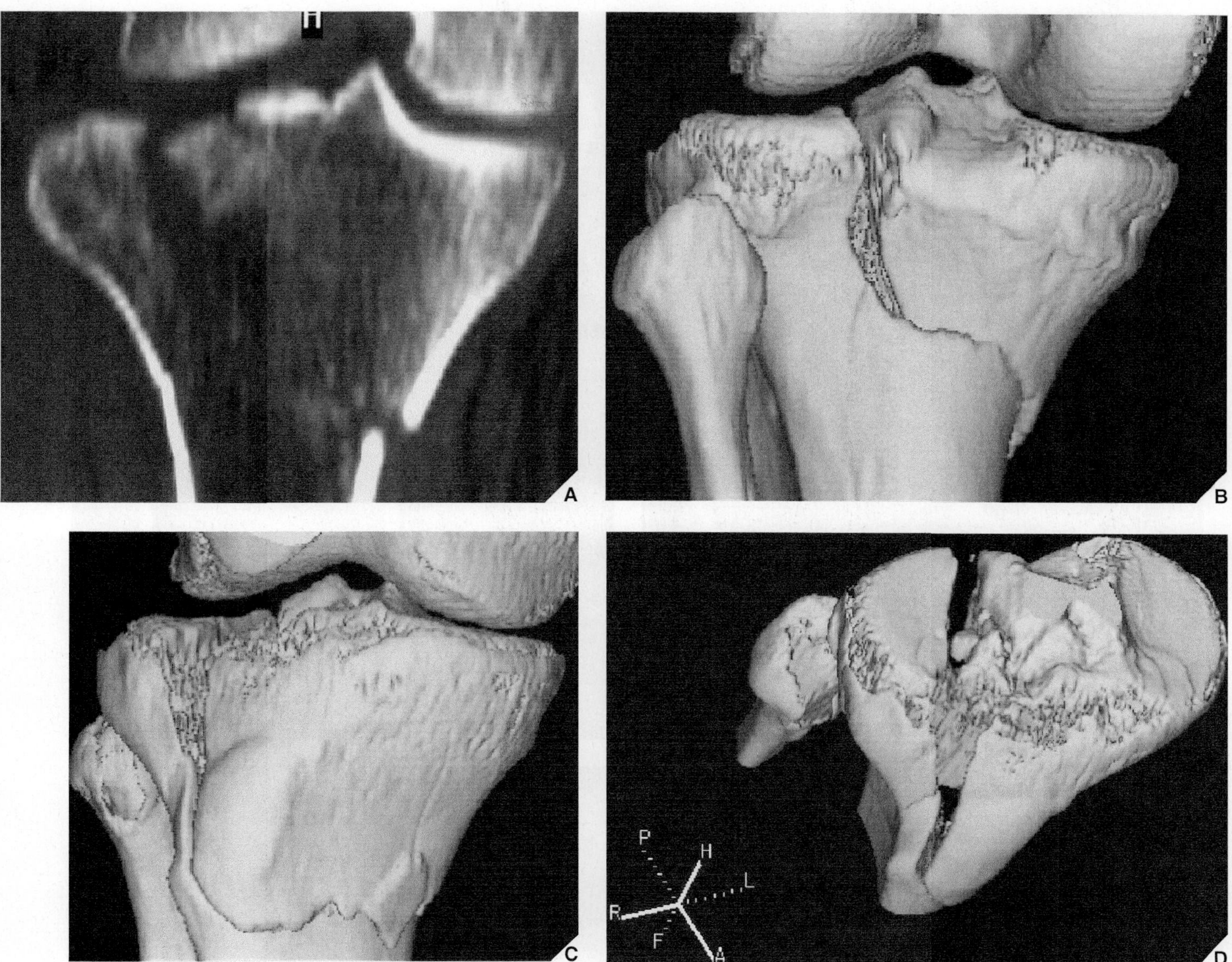

FIGURE 9.27 **CT and 3D CT of fracture of the tibial plateau.** A 22-year-old man fell down from a tall ladder and injured his right knee. The conventional radiographs demonstrated fracture of the tibial plateau. **(A)** Coronal reformatted CT scan shows extension of the lateral tibial plateau fracture into the tibial shaft. **(B)** Posterior view of the 3D CT reconstruction shows the fracture line, but the interfragmental split is not well demonstrated. **(C)** Anterior view of the 3D reconstruction shows the split better. **(D)** Bird's eye view of the 3D CT scan effectively demonstrates the details of the split and comminution of the tibial plateau.

It is much more difficult to diagnose so-called *transient dislocation*, referred to as the traumatic condition when dislocated patella reduces on its own. Transient dislocation may be associated with hypoplastic trochlear notch of the femur and increased distance between the tibial tubercle and trochlear groove. This is known as the *Tt–Tg distance*, and it can be measured on MRI (Fig 9.43). Although clinical symptoms are helpful, the most accurate diagnostic modality in this respect is MRI. It shows a characteristic pattern of "bone contusion" or trabecular injury on the medial aspect of the patella and anterior lateral femoral condyle (Fig. 9.44). The medial retinaculum, most often the medial patellofemoral ligament component of the retinaculum, is invariably injured, but medial patellar cartilage may or may not show abnormalities. Subluxations of the patella are much more common than true dislocations and usually result from chronic injury. The best radiographic examination for demonstrating patellar subluxation, particularly in subtle cases, is the Merchant axial view (Fig. 9.45).

Dislocations of the Knee

Dislocations in the knee joint are rare. They usually are the result of high-energy traumatic injuries such as sustained in automobile accidents, severe falls, and contact sports. They are classified as anterior, posterior, medial, lateral, and rotary. More than 50% of all dislocations are either anterior or posterior. They invariably are associated with tears of the ACL and PCL, and either medial or lateral collateral ligament. Common complication is the coexistence of vascular injuries (particularly to the popliteal artery), peroneal nerve injury, and compartment syndrome. Conventional radiography is effective in diagnosis (Fig. 9.46A), but MRI is required to demonstrate the ligamentous and menisci abnormalities (Fig. 9.46B–D). CT angiography is the modality of choice to diagnose vascular complications (Fig. 9.47).

Sinding-Larsen-Johansson Disease

Sinding-Larsen-Johansson disease is a condition that is seen predominantly in active adolescent boys and is now considered to be related to trauma. It is caused by repetitive avulsion injury at the patellar ligament attachment to the lower pole (apex) of the patella and shares clinical, histopathologic, and imaging features with Osgood-Schlatter disease. Sinding-Larsen-Johansson disease is characterized clinically by local pain and tenderness on palpation and radiographically by separation and fragmentation of the lower pole of the patella, associated with soft-tissue swelling and, occasionally, calcifications at the site of the patellar ligament. This condition is believed to be

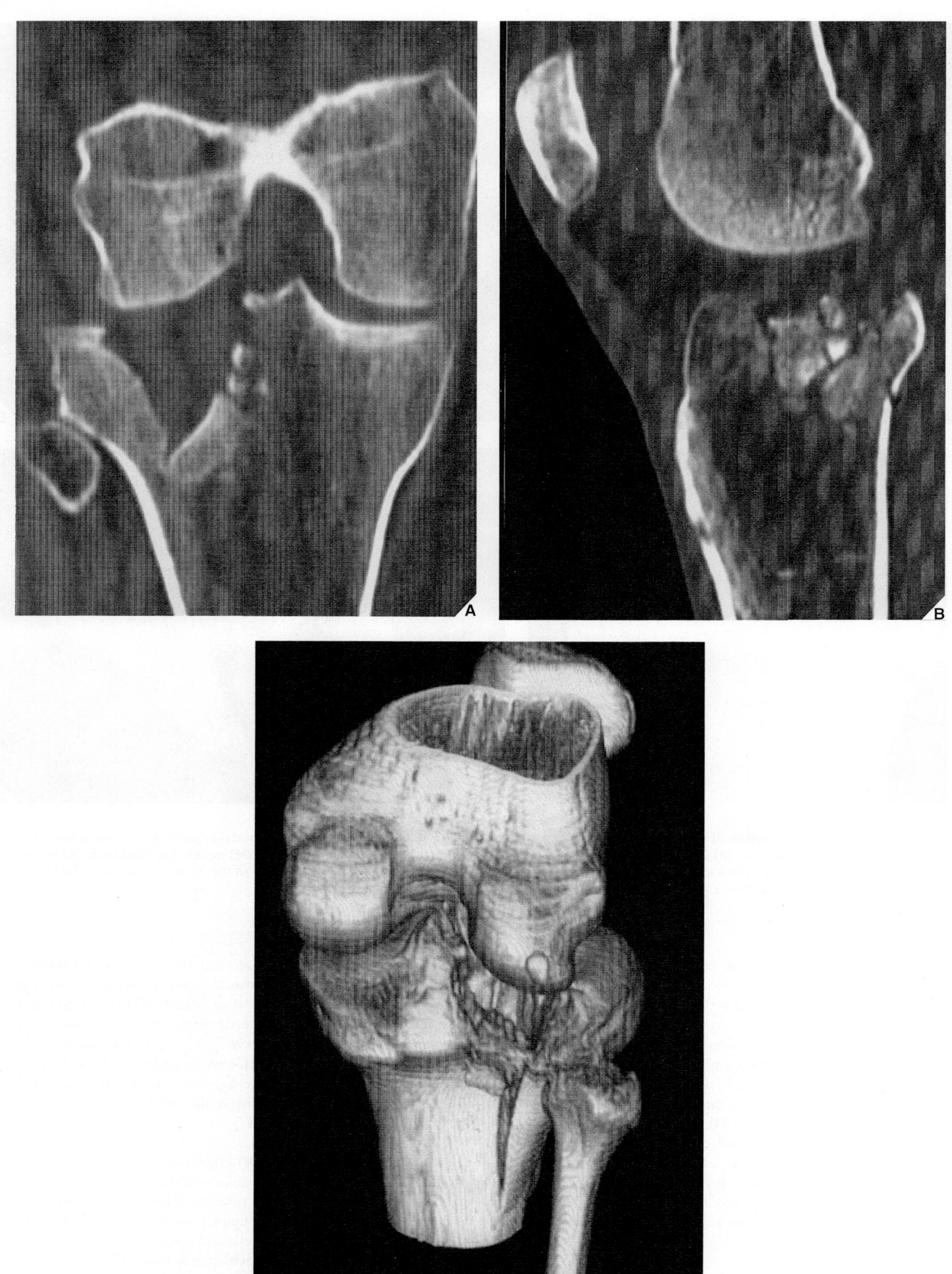

FIGURE 9.28 CT and 3D CT of fracture of the tibial plateau. (A) Coronal and **(B)** sagittal CT reformatted images show a Hohl type III (displaced, local spit depression) fracture of the lateral tibial plateau. **(C)** 3D CT reconstructed image (posterior view) more realistically depicts the features of this injury.

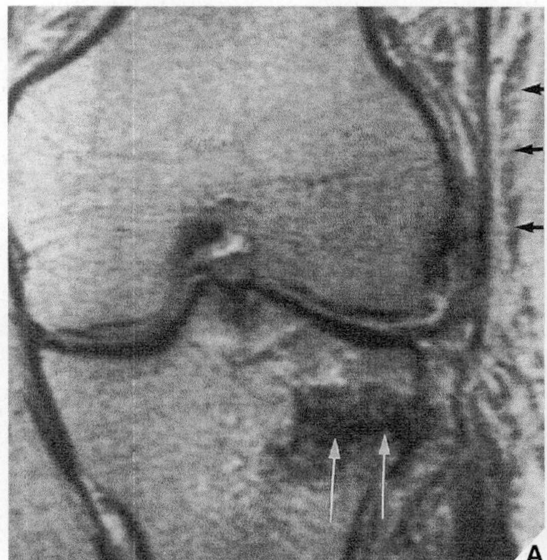

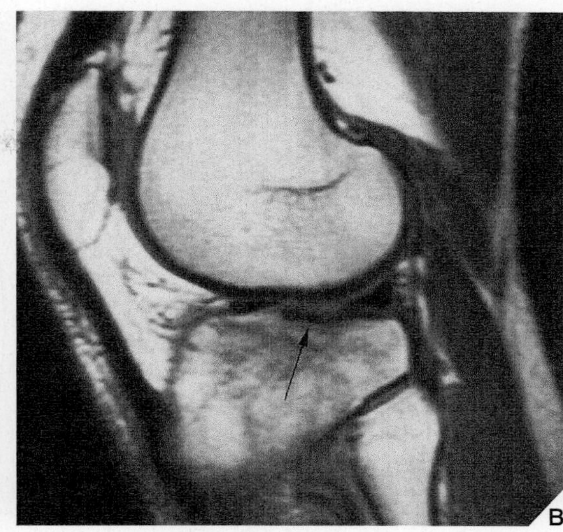

FIGURE 9.29 **MRI of fracture of the tibial plateau.** **(A)** T2-weighted (spin echo, repetition time [TR] 2000/TE 80 msec) coronal image shows a broad-based band of low signal intensity traversing the lateral tibial plateau *(long arrows)*. Extensive soft-tissue edema is seen superficial to the iliotibial band *(small arrows)*. **(B)** Proton density–weighted (spin echo, TR 2000/TE 20 msec) sagittal image shows central localized depression of the tibial plateau *(arrow)*. The degree of comminution and depression is well depicted. (Reprinted with permission from Bloem JL, Sartoris DJ, eds. *MRI and CT of the musculoskeletal system. A text-atlas*. Baltimore: Williams Wilkins; 1992.)

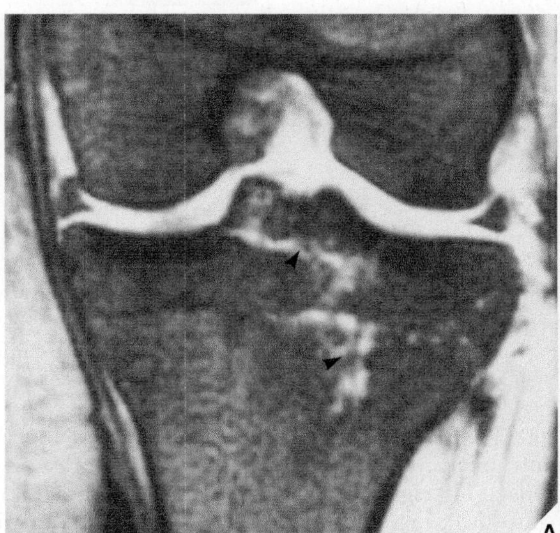

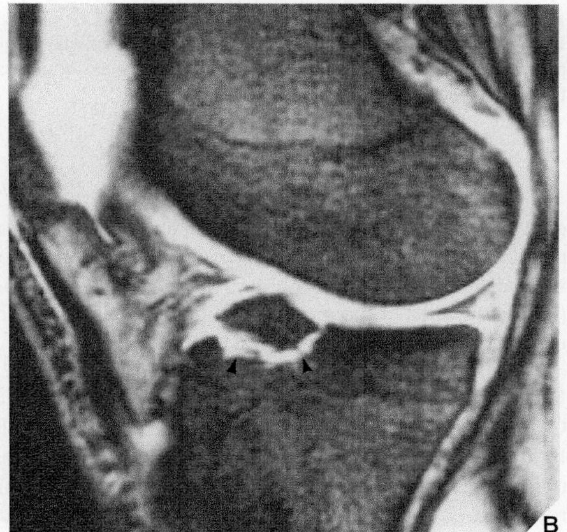

FIGURE 9.30 **MRI of fracture of the tibial plateau.** **(A)** Coronal gradient echo (MGPR) image shows a tibial plateau fracture *(arrowheads)*. **(B)** Sagittal gradient echo (MGPR) image demonstrates the anterior extension of the fracture and evulsion of the tibial spines *(arrowheads)*. (Reprinted with permission from Berquist TH, ed. *MRI of the musculoskeletal system*, 3rd ed. Philadelphia: Lippincott-Raven; 1997.)

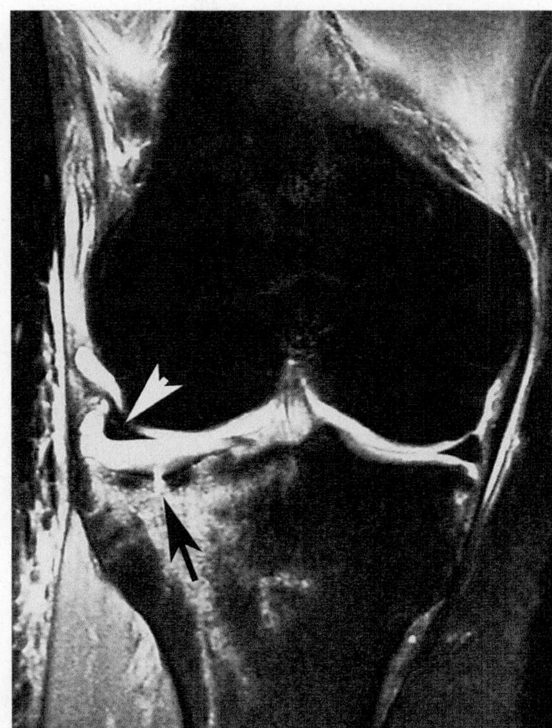

FIGURE 9.31 **MRI of fracture of the tibial plateau.** Coronal T2-weighted fat-saturated MRI shows a slightly depressed fracture of the lateral tibial plateau *(black arrow)* with extensive bone contusion. Note the superiorly displaced lateral meniscus *(white arrowhead)* due to a tear of the inferior meniscal fascicle ("floating meniscus").

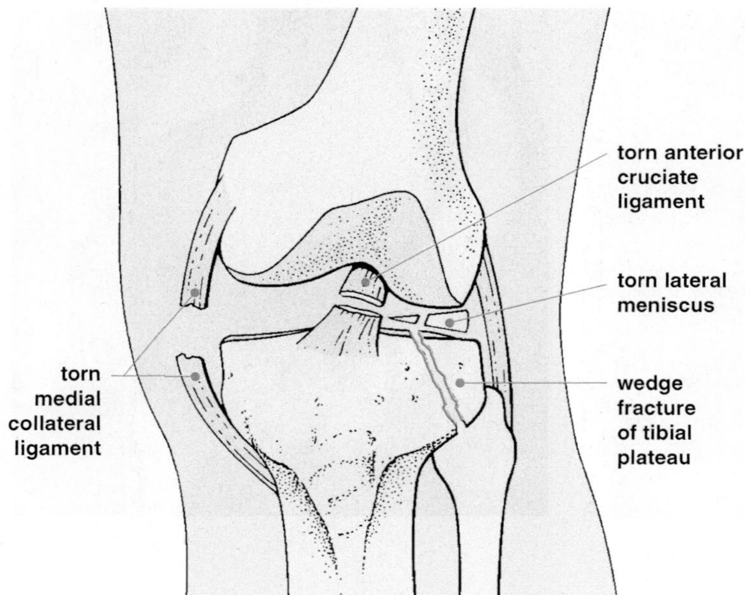

FIGURE 9.32 Tibial plateau fracture–associated injuries. Lateral tibial plateau fractures, which result from valgus stress, are often associated with tears of the lateral meniscus and the MCL and ACL.

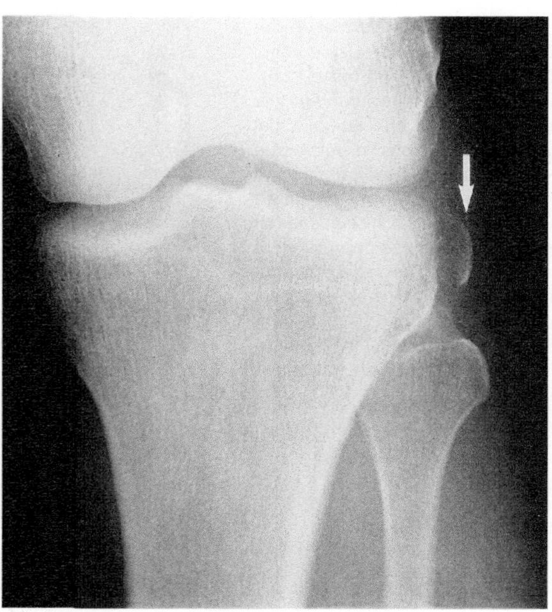

FIGURE 9.33 Segond fracture. A 27-year-old woman sustained an injury to her left knee in a skiing accident. Anteroposterior radiograph shows a small fragment of bone evulsed from the lateral aspect of the tibia *(arrow)*, characteristic of Segond fracture.

caused by persistent traction at the cartilaginous junction of the patella and patellar ligament. The lateral radiograph, preferably obtained with a low-kilovoltage/soft-tissue technique, is the single most important examination (Fig. 9.48); in combination with a positive clinical examination, it usually establishes the diagnosis.

Osgood-Schlatter Disease

Osgood-Schlatter disease, first described in 1903 by Robert Osgood of Boston and Carl Schlatter of Zurich, occurs 3 times more frequently in adolescent boys than in adolescent girls and is characterized by fragmentation of the tibial tuberosity, soft-tissue swelling and thickening at the insertion of the patellar ligament, and inflammation of the deep infrapatellar bursa. In 25% to 33% of all reported cases, the condition is bilateral. As in Sinding-Larsen-Johansson disease, the lateral radiograph, obtained using a soft-tissue technique, is most effective in demonstrating this condition (Fig. 9.49). However, an accurate diagnosis is based on both imaging and clinical findings. Soft-tissue swelling and deep infrapatellar bursitis and/or fibrosis are fundamental diagnostic features. Ultrasound (US) of the tibial tuberosity complex is an effective method to demonstrate all features of the Osgood-Schlatter disease because it provides excellent visualization of the fine structures of the patellar ligament, the superficial and deep infrapatellar bursae, and the status of the cartilage of the ossification center of the tibial tuberosity (Fig. 9.50). On MRI, T1-weighted images show replacement of the

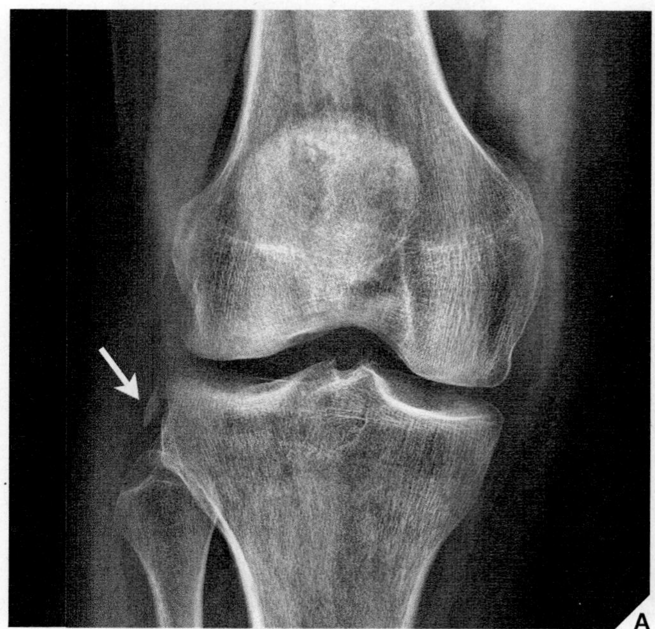

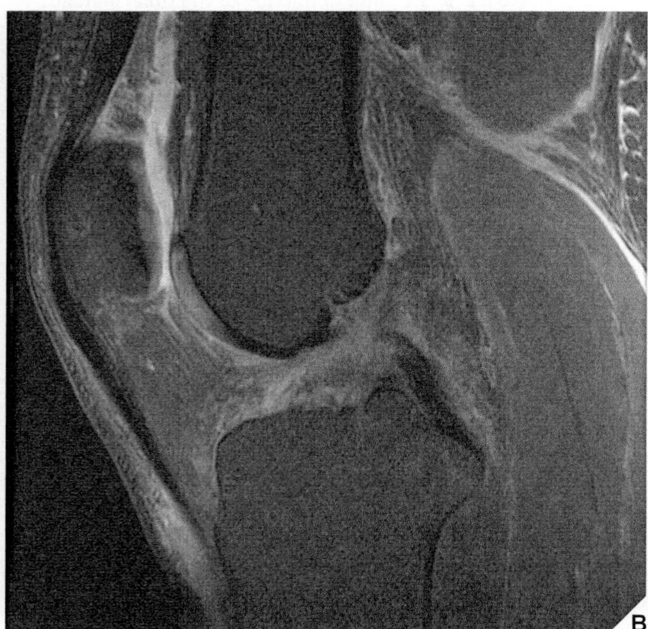

FIGURE 9.34 MRI of the Segond fracture. **(A)** Anteroposterior radiograph of the right knee shows avulsed osseous fragment from the lateral aspect of the tibia *(arrow)*. **(B)** Sagittal proton density–weighted fat-suppressed MR image shows a tear of the ACL.

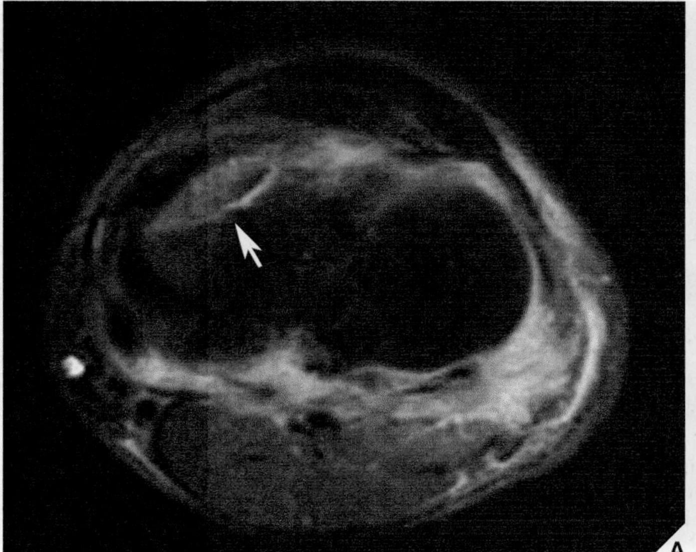

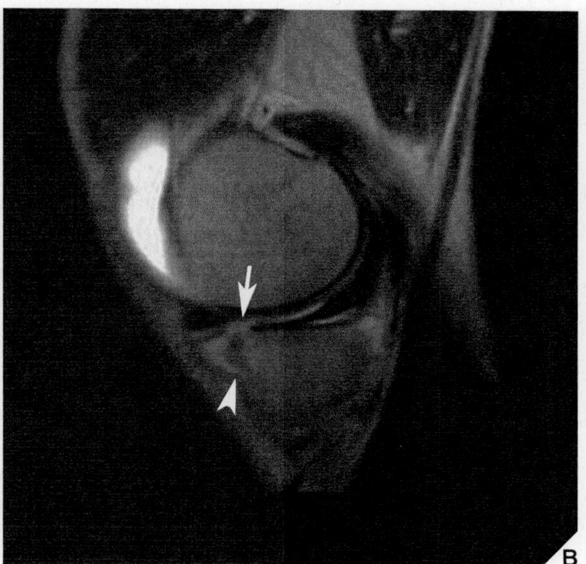

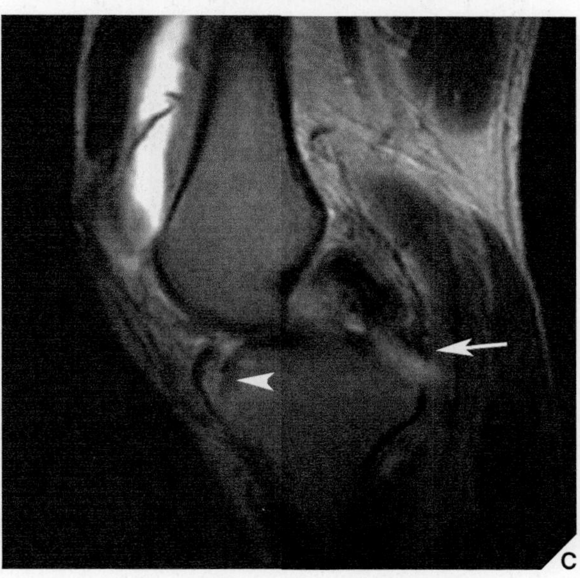

FIGURE 9.35 **MRI of the reverse Segond fracture.** **(A)** Axial short time inversion recovery (STIR) MR image demonstrates a fracture of the anterior medial tibial plateau *(arrow)*. **(B)** Sagittal T2-weighted MR image shows a tear of the medial meniscus *(arrow)* and the medial tibial plateau fracture *(arrowhead)*. **(C)** Sagittal T2-weighted MR image demonstrates an avulsion of the tibial insertion of the PCL *(arrow)* and the medial tibial plateau fracture *(arrowhead)*.

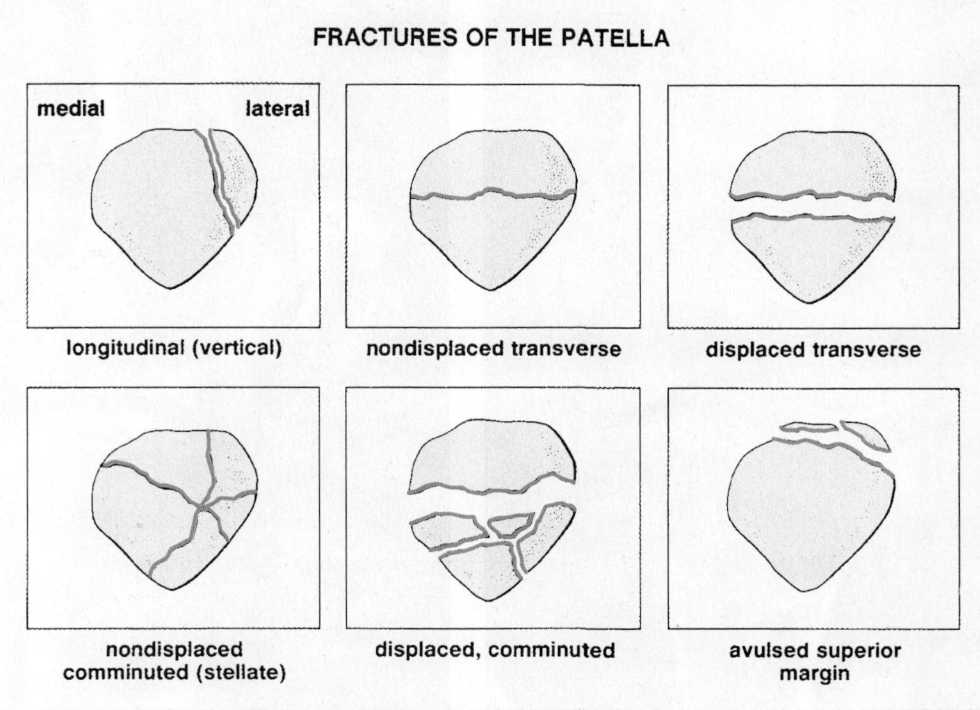

FIGURE 9.36 **Classification of patellar fractures.** (Modified with permission from Hohl M, Larson RL. Fractures and dislocations of the knee. In: Rockwood CA Jr, Green DP, eds. *Fractures*. Philadelphia: Lippincott; 1975.)

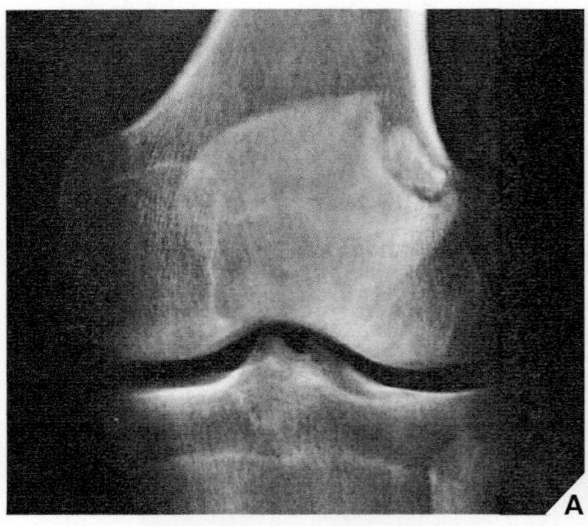
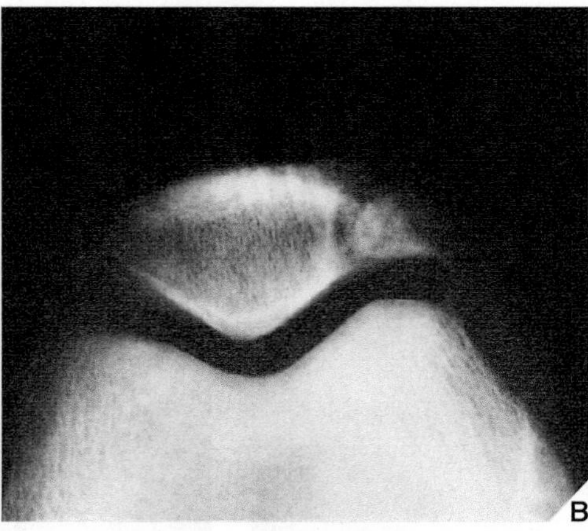
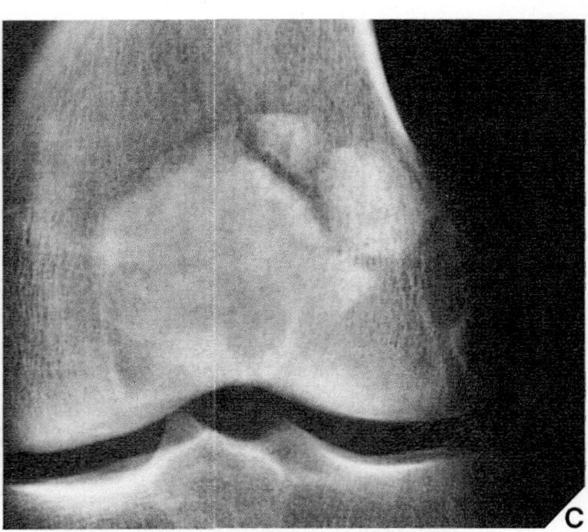

FIGURE 9.37 **Bipartite and multipartite patella.** **(A)** Anteroposterior and **(B)** axial radiographs of the knee demonstrate the typical appearance of a bipartite patella. Note the position of the accessory ossification center at the superolateral margin of the patella. **(C)** A tripartite patella was an incidental finding on this overpenetrated anteroposterior radiograph, which was obtained to exclude the possibility of gouty arthritis.

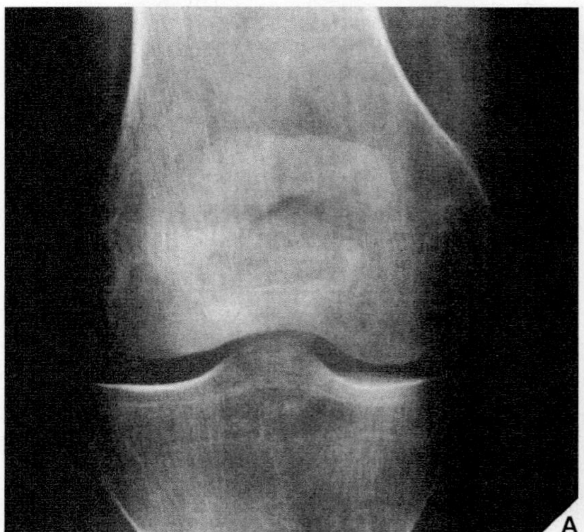
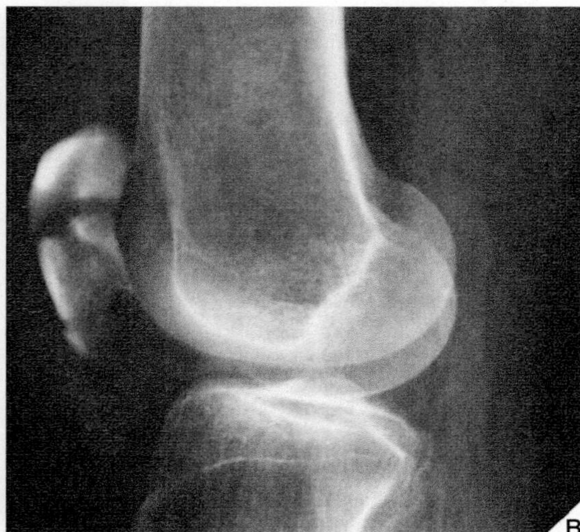

FIGURE 9.38 **Fracture of the patella.** After a fall on the stairs, a 63-year-old man presented with severe pain in the anterior aspect of the right knee. **(A)** Anteroposterior and **(B)** lateral radiographs show the typical appearance of comminuted fracture of the patella.

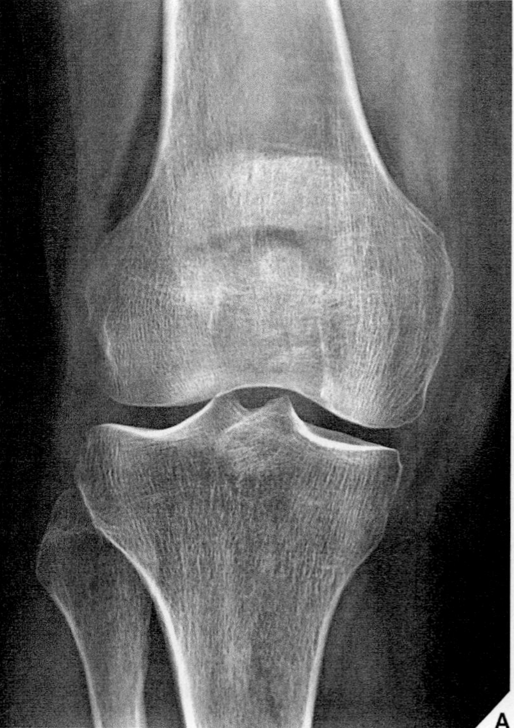
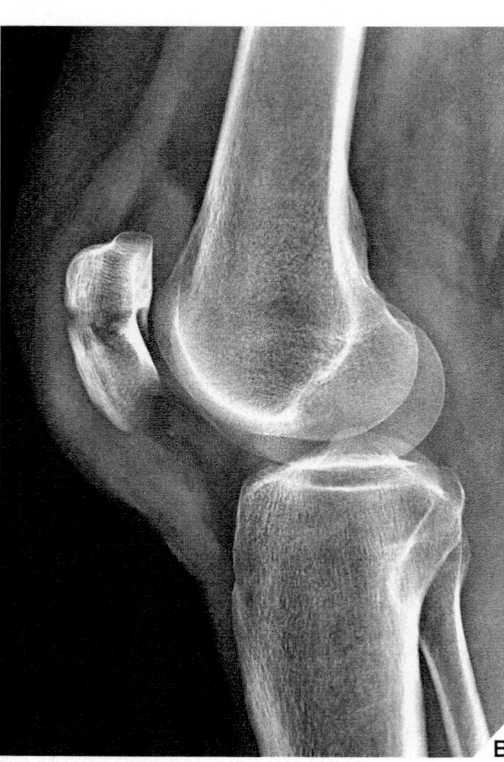

FIGURE 9.39 **Transverse fracture of the patella.** **(A)** Anteroposterior and **(B)** lateral radiographs of the knee demonstrate a transverse fracture of the patella. Note the prepatellar soft-tissue swelling and joint effusion.

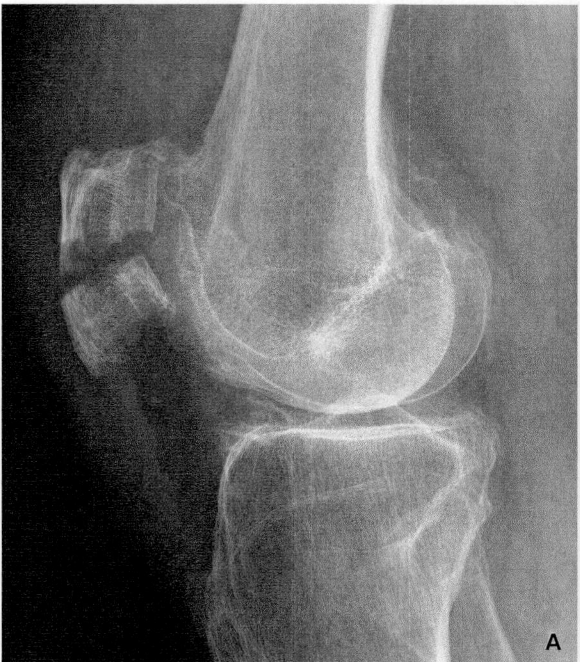

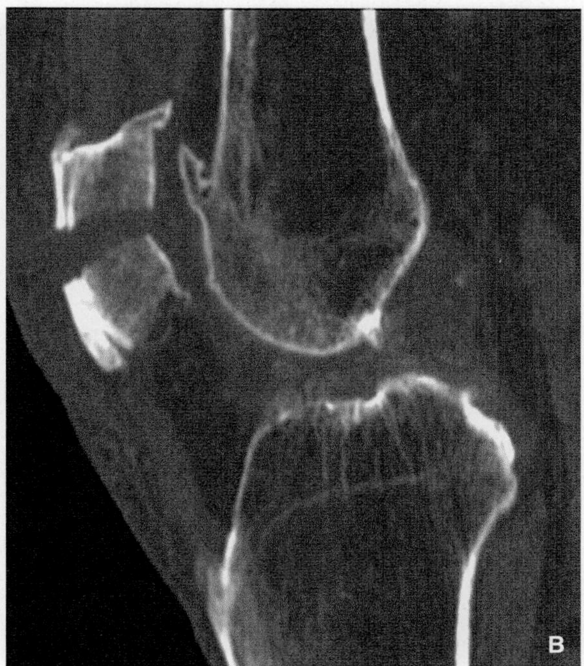

FIGURE 9.40 CT of transverse fracture of the patella. **(A)** Lateral radiograph and **(B)** sagittal reformatted CT image of the knee of an 80-year-old man who fell on the street show a transverse displaced fracture of the patella.

normal high-signal infrapatellar fat with an area of decreased signal adjacent to the patellar ligament insertion. The ligament itself may show focal areas of increased signal, depending on the degree of associated tendinitis (Figs. 9.51 and 9.52).

Occasionally, Sinding-Larsen-Johansson and Osgood-Schlatter diseases may coexist. It is important to remember that the presence of multiple ossification centers in the tibial tuberosity and lower pole of the patella may at times mimic these conditions. However, the absence of soft-tissue swelling in such cases allows the distinction to be made (see Fig. 9.49C).

Injuries to the Cartilage of the Knee

Chondral, Subchondral, and Osteochondral Lesions

Several pathologic conditions may manifest as an osteochondral lesion of the knee including localized abnormalities involving subchondral bone, articular cartilage, or both. These lesions are often confused with each other, and in many instances, the terms are used interchangeably. They represent, however, separate orthopaedic entities, each with a specific cause and each requiring a specific treatment. Usually, history, physical examination, and particularly magnetic resonance (MR) imaging presentation can help to distinguish these conditions from one another.

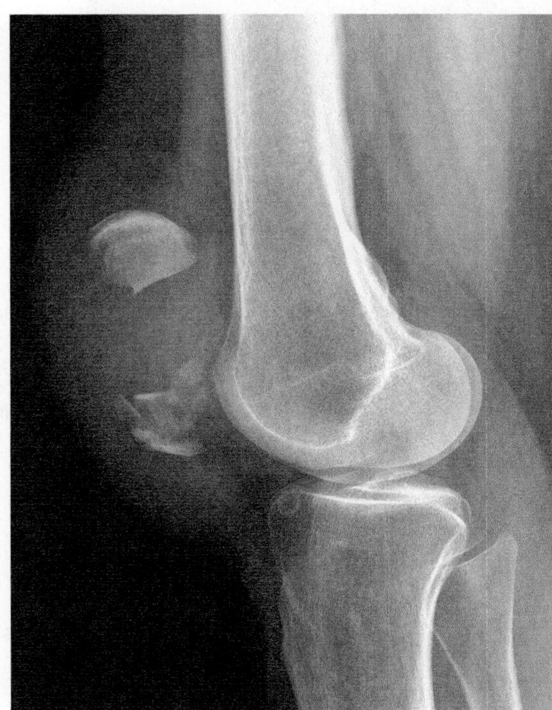

FIGURE 9.41 Comminuted fracture of the patella. A lateral radiograph of the knee shows markedly comminuted and displaced fracture of the patella.

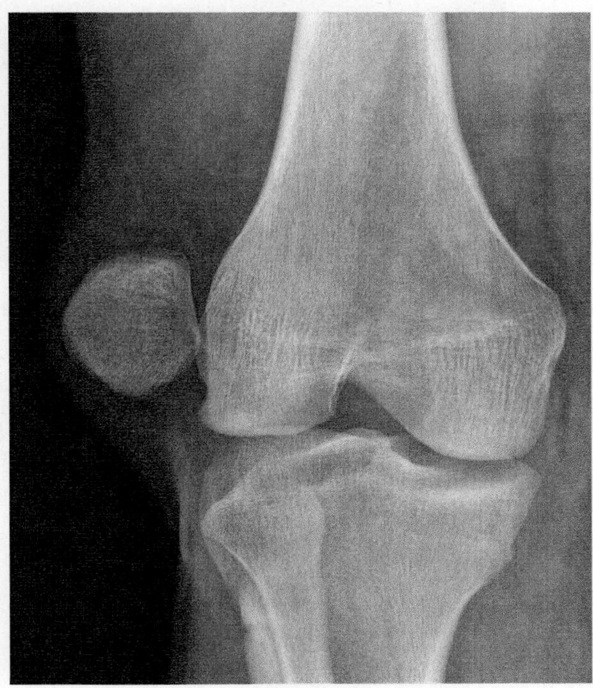

FIGURE 9.42 Lateral dislocation of the patella. Anteroposterior radiograph of the right knee of an 18-year-old man who was injured in a ski accident shows lateral dislocation of the patella.

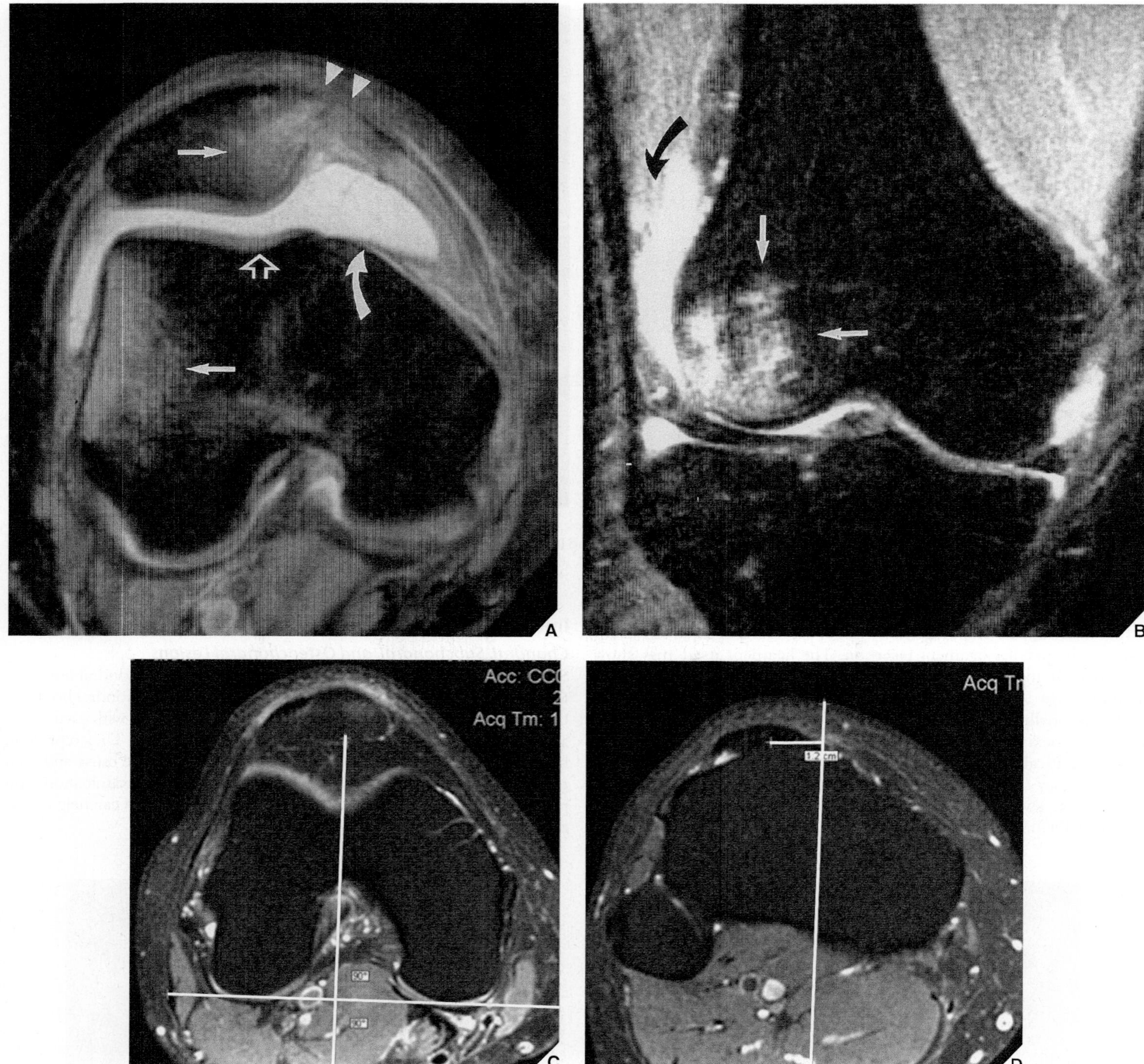

FIGURE 9.43 Transient lateral dislocation of the patella. **(A)** Axial and **(B)** coronal reformatted T2-weighted fat-suppressed MR images of the right knee of a 38-year-old woman show characteristic abnormalities of this injury: "bone contusion" on the medial aspect of the patella and lateral femoral condyle *(arrows)* associated with hypoplastic trochlear notch *(open arrow)* and joint effusion *(curved arrows)*. *Arrowheads* are indicating a tear of the medial retinaculum. The Tt–Tg distance is measured as follows: The axial section through the femoral condyles showing the deepest femoral trochlea is selected **(C)**, and a bicondylar line is traced through the posterior aspects of the condyles. A perpendicular line at the level of the deepest point of the trochlea is obtained. This line is then transferred to the axial section through the tibia showing the tibial tubercle **(D)**. The distance between the most prominent central point of the tibial tubercle and the trochlear line is the Tt–Tg distance. The normal values are 10 mm +/− 1 mm in males and females, although values of up to 15–20 mm have been reported as being within the upper limits of normal.

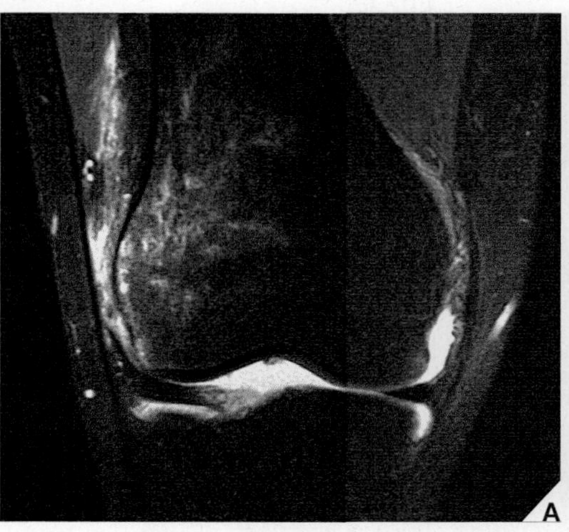
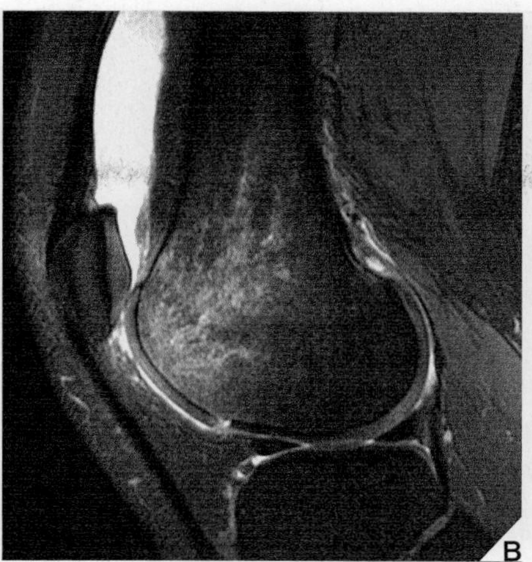
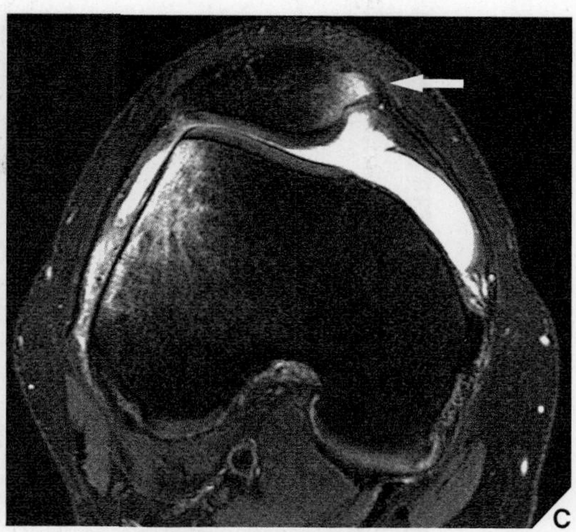

FIGURE 9.44 **Transient lateral dislocation of the patella.** **(A)** Coronal and **(B)** sagittal proton density–weighted fat-suppressed MR images of the right knee of a 22-year-old woman show large areas of high signal intensity within anterior aspect of the lateral femoral condyle. Large joint effusion is also present. **(C)** An axial proton density–weighted fat-suppressed MR image, in addition to bone marrow edema within the lateral femoral condyle, shows a focus of high signal intensity at the medial aspect of the patella *(arrow)*, characteristic features of transient dislocation.

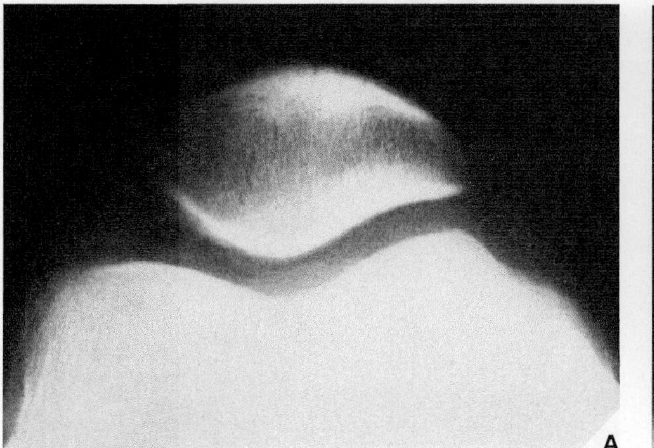
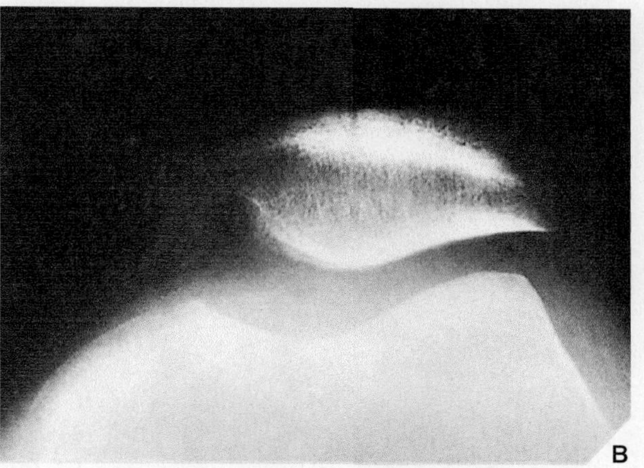

FIGURE 9.45 **Subluxation of the patella.** A 23-year-old woman experienced occasional knee pain and buckling, particularly while jogging. **(A)** Standard axial (sunrise) view of the patella shows no apparent abnormalities. **(B)** Merchant axial view, however, demonstrates lateral subluxation of the patella. Note the positive congruence angle (see Fig. 9.7).

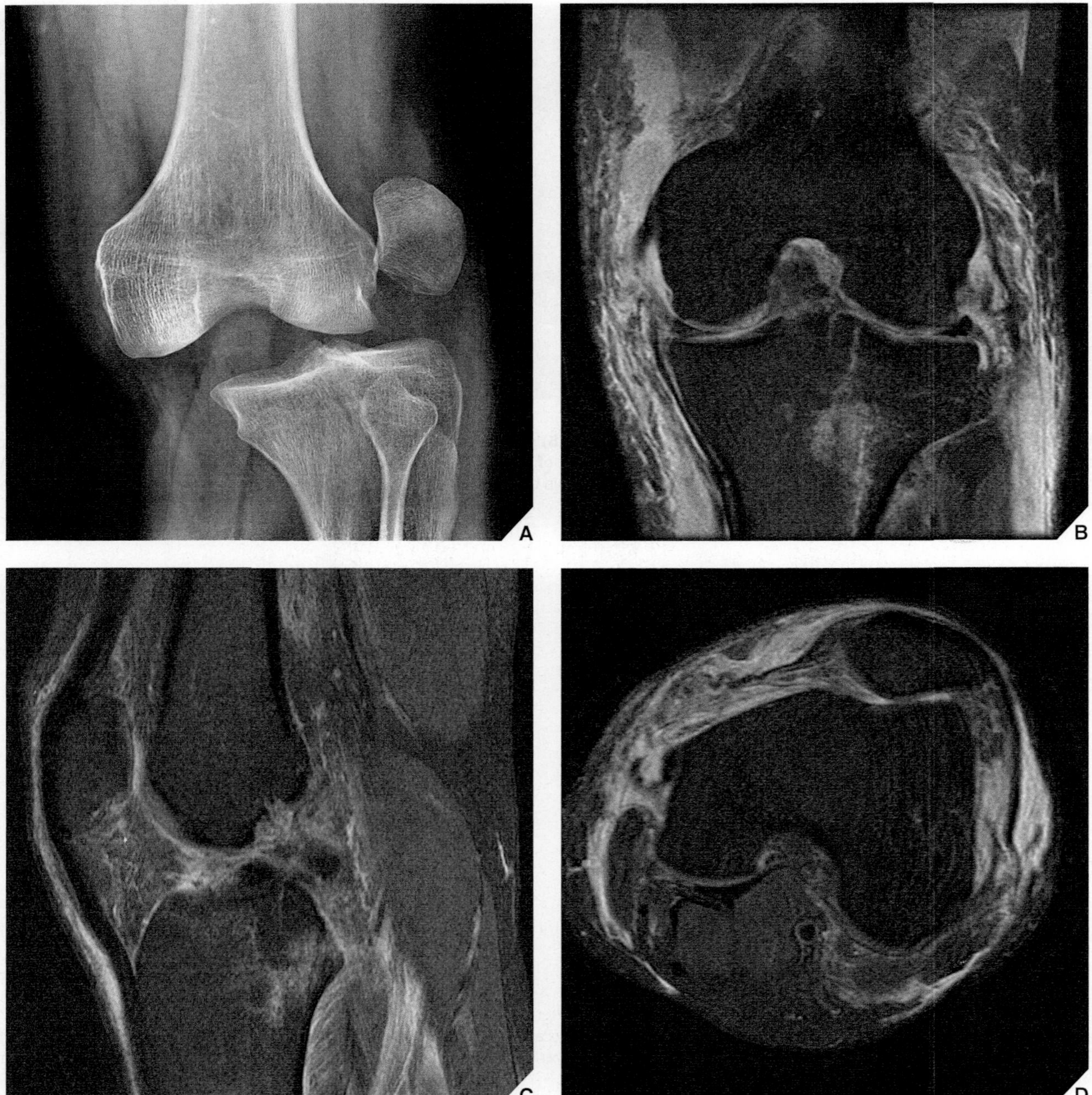

FIGURE 9.46 **Knee dislocation.** A 46-year-old man was injured in a motorcycle accident. **(A)** Anteroposterior radiograph of the left knee shows lateral dislocation with rotary component and dislocation of the patella. After knee dislocation was relocated, MRI was performed. **(B)** Coronal proton density–weighted fat-suppressed MR image shows tears of the medial and lateral collateral ligaments and a tear of the medial meniscus. In addition, noted is trabecular injury to the lateral tibia. **(C)** Sagittal MR image shows a tear of the ACL, fracture of the inferior pole of the patella, and trabecular injury of the posterior tibia. **(D)** Axial MR image shows a tear of the medial patellar retinaculum and lateral subluxation of the patella.

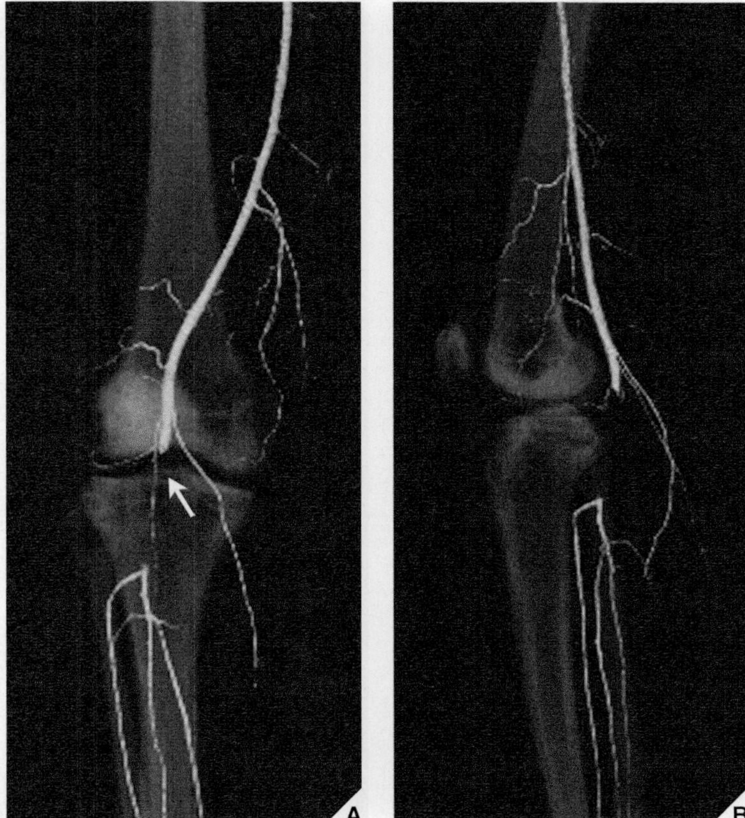

FIGURE 9.47 **Complication of knee dislocation.** Vascular 3D reconstructed CT images in **(A)** frontal and **(B)** lateral projections show an occlusion of popliteal artery *(arrow)* in a 32-year-old man who sustained a posterior knee dislocation in a skiing accident, spontaneously reduced.

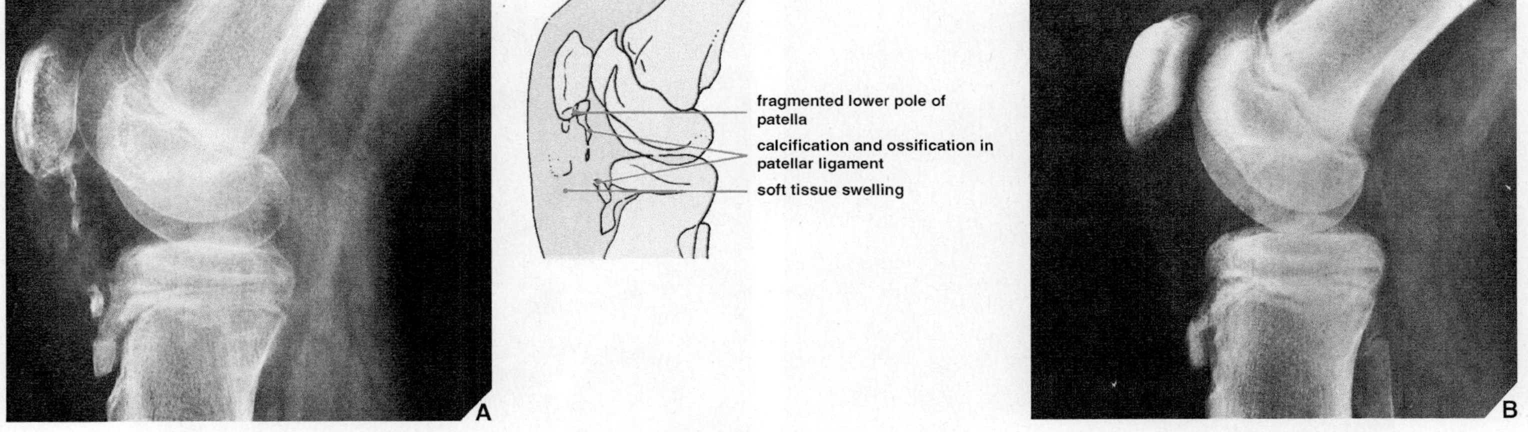

FIGURE 9.48 **Sinding-Larsen-Johansson disease.** A 13-year-old boy experienced pain and swelling at the site of the patellar ligament. He had no history of acute trauma. **(A)** Lateral radiograph of the right knee shows fragmentation of the lower pole of the patella and significant soft-tissue swelling associated with calcifications and ossifications of the patellar ligament—findings characteristic of Sinding-Larsen-Johansson disease. **(B)** The normal left knee is shown for comparison.

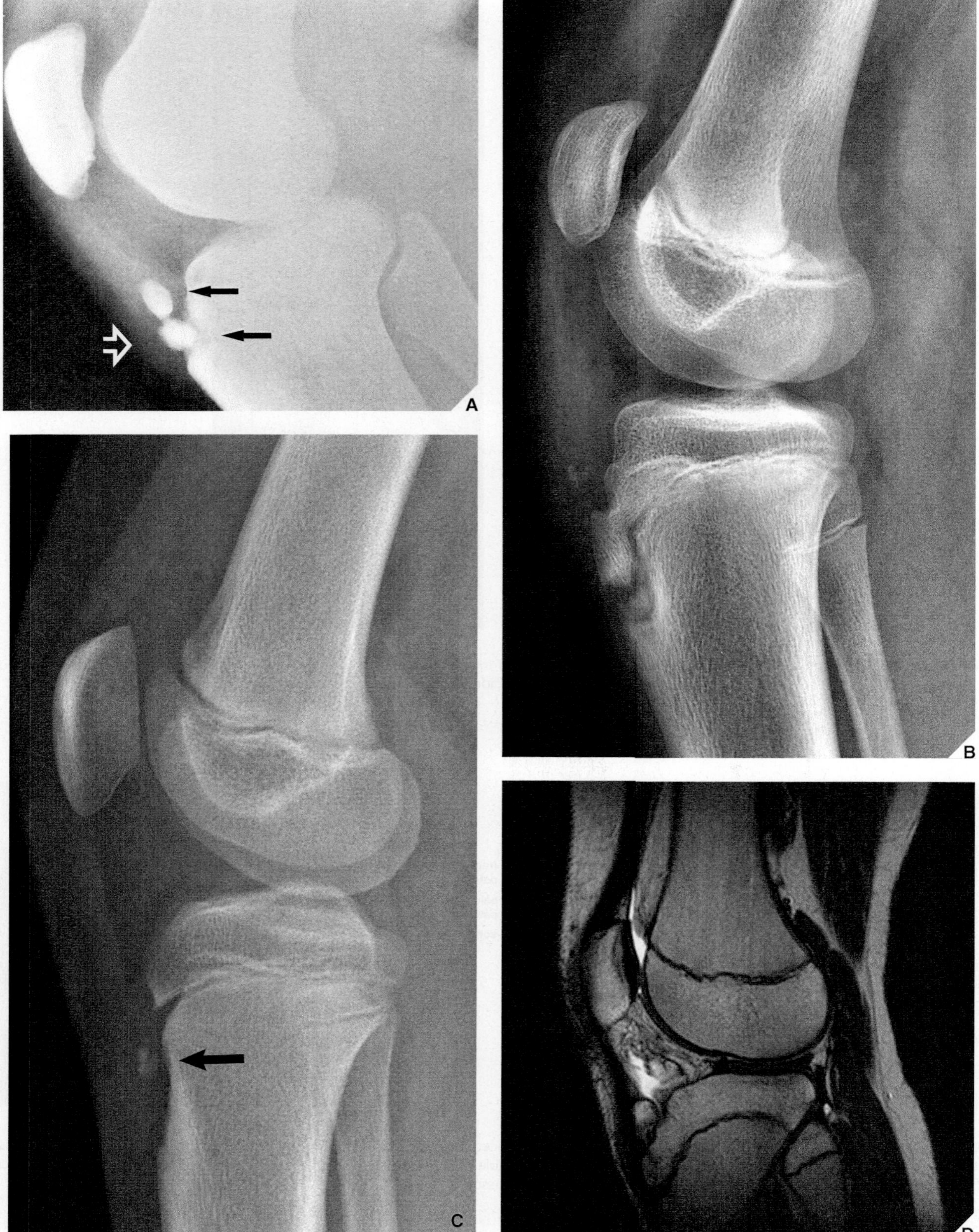

FIGURE 9.49 Osgood-Schlatter disease. **(A)** A 12-year-old boy had severe tenderness over the left tibial tuberosity. The lateral radiograph, obtained with a low-kilovoltage/soft-tissue technique, reveals fragmentation of the tibial tuberosity *(arrows)* in association with soft-tissue swelling *(open arrow)* characteristic findings in Osgood-Schlatter disease. **(B)** In another patient, a 15-year-old girl, the lateral radiograph of the knee shows fragmentation of the tibial tuberosity and soft-tissue swelling at the site of the patellar ligament. **(C)** It has to be pointed out that occasionally normal fragmented ossification center for tibial tuberosity *(arrow)* may mimic Osgood-Schlatter disease. Note, however, lack of soft-tissue abnormalities. **(D)** In a patient with acute Osgood-Schlatter disease, sagittal T2-weighted MR image demonstrates tendinosis of the distal patellar ligament with fragmentation of the tibial tubercle and associated deep infrapatellar bursitis.

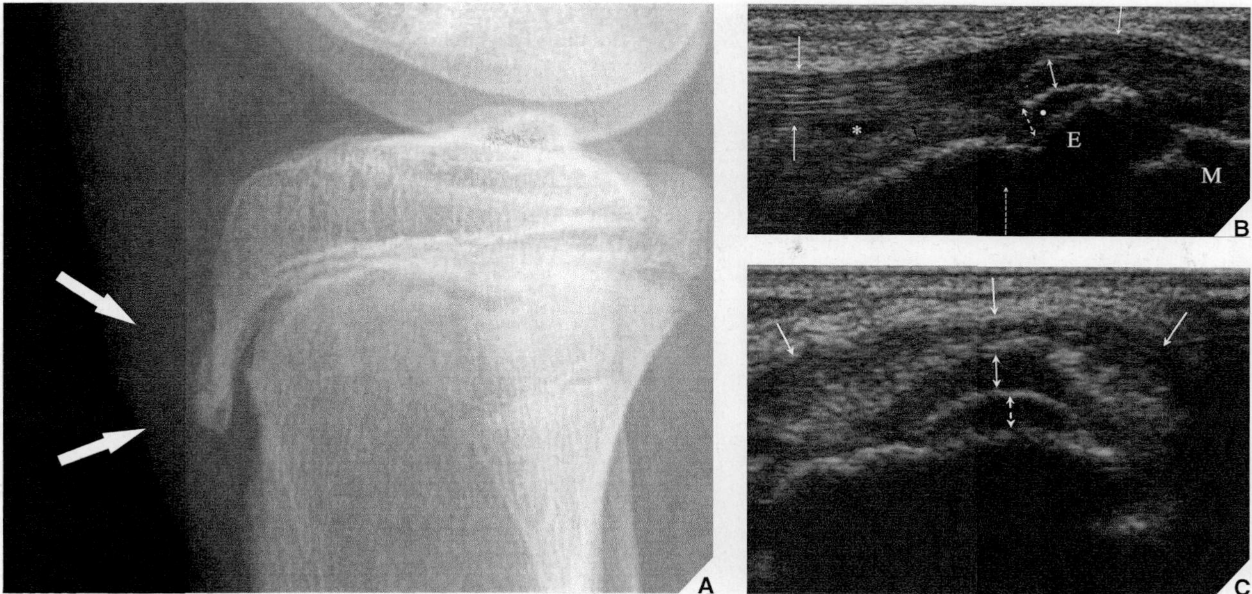

FIGURE 9.50 US of Osgood-Schlatter disease. An 11-year-old boy presented with pain and swelling for several weeks in the region of tibial tuberosity. **(A)** Lateral radiograph shows soft-tissue swelling and small calcifications at the site of ossification center of tibial tuberosity *(arrows)*. **(B)** Longitudinal and **(C)** transverse US images show a fracture and delamination of the cartilaginous portion of ossification center of tibial tuberosity, characteristic of Osgood-Schlatter disease. *Arrows* point to the margins of the patellar ligament; *double solid arrow* indicates the thickness of cartilage between the ossification center and patellar ligament insertion; *double dashed arrow* indicates delamination thickness within the ossification center; *double black arrow* indicates fibrosis within deep infrapatellar bursa; *asterisk*, effusion within deep infrapatellar bursa; *dot*, ossification center; E, epiphysis; M, metaphysis. (Courtesy of Dr. Zbigniew Czyrny, Warsaw, Poland.)

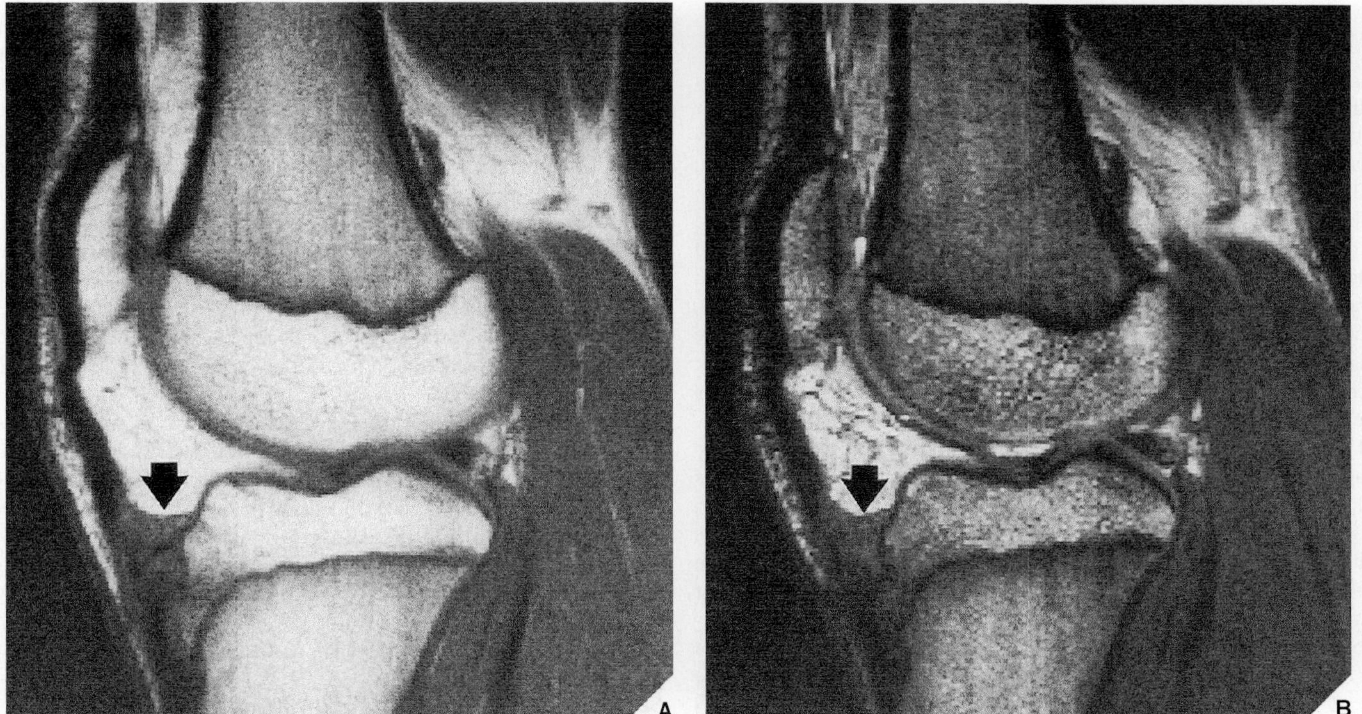

FIGURE 9.51 MRI of Osgood-Schlatter disease. **(A)** T1-weighted (spin echo, repetition time [TR] 700/TE 20 msec) and **(B)** T2*-weighted sagittal MR images demonstrate focus of decreased signal within normal sharp V-shaped area formed by the patellar ligament and anterior tibia *(arrows)*. (Reprinted with permission from Bloem JL, Sartoris DJ, eds. *MRI and CT of the musculoskeletal system. A text-atlas*. Baltimore: Williams Wilkins; 1992.)

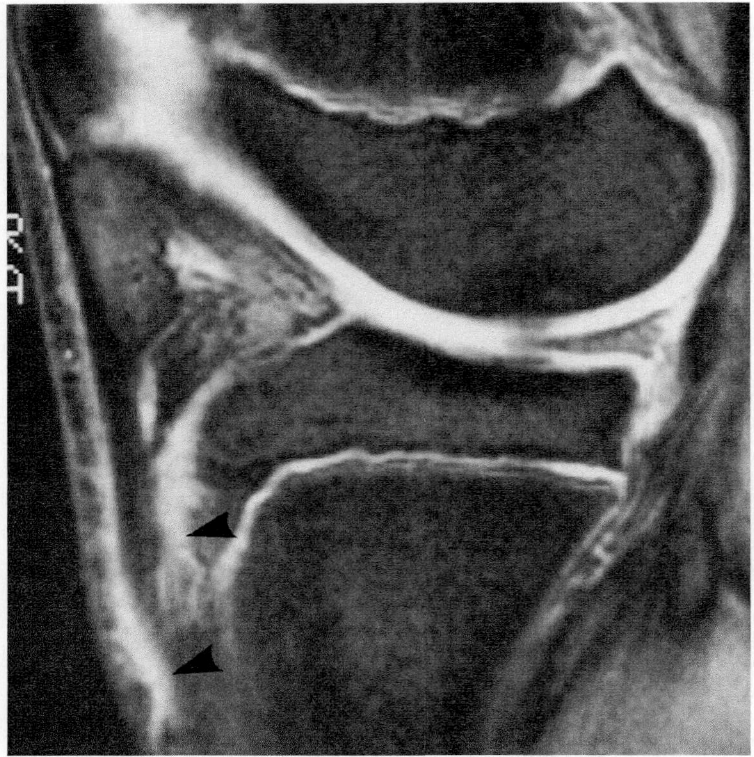

FIGURE 9.52 MRI of Osgood-Schlatter disease. A sagittal T2-weighted MR image of the knee of a 14-year-old boy demonstrates inflammatory changes along the distal patellar ligament *(arrowheads)*. (Reprinted with permission from Berquist TH, ed. *MRI of the musculoskeletal system*, 3rd ed. Philadelphia: Lippincott-Raven; 1997.)

Chondral Lesions. Shearing, rotary, or tangentially aligned impaction forces directed to the knee joint may result in acute injury to the articular end of the femur or tibia. The resulting lesion may involve cartilage only (chondral lesion), the subchondral bone only (subchondral lesion) or both, the cartilage and subchondral bone (osteochondral lesion).

Isolated posttraumatic chondral lesions may involve only a portion of the articular cartilage resulting in a "flap tear (Fig. 9.53A,B), can extend deep into the articular cartilage reaching the subchondral bone plate and extending along the deep chondral layer with delamination (Fig. 9.53C,D), or involve only the deep cartilage layer adjacent to the subchondral bone plate (Fig. 9.53E,F). In this case, the lesion is called *concealed* because it is not seen on superficial arthroscopic examination. Additionally, a full-thickness or partial-thickness chondral lesion may be seen, with complete detachment of a fragment of cartilage, resulting in a chondral defect. In the acute stage, the full-thickness chondral defects exhibit acute sharp margins oriented perpendicular to the subchondral bone plate known as *shouldering* (Fig. 9.54A). With time, the margins of the chondral defect become more blunted and are oriented obliquely to the subchondral bone plate (Fig. 9.54B). Isolated chondral lesions are not identified on radiography but are easily demonstrated on high-quality MRI examinations.

Subchondral Lesions. The hyaline articular cartilage is more resilient than the more rigid subchondral bone and trabecular bone because of its elastic properties, which allow for vertical compression without altering significantly its integrity. Therefore, it is not infrequent that under compression load stresses over articular surface, the cartilage is not damaged, but the subchondral bone may exhibit contusion and microtrabecular fracture (Fig. 9.55), which can evolve into a well-defined subchondral fracture. When a subchondral fracture occurs, it may weaken the subchondral bone plate that eventually may collapse, leading to an incongruent articular surface and into secondary osteoarthritis. This situation is seen often in the elderly (see next section for discussion on spontaneous osteonecrosis of the knee [SONK]). Although in the elderly the subchondral fracture is related to osteoporosis and thinning of the trabecula (insufficiency fracture), and not related to a direct impact, the imaging findings and evolution are often similar. A subchondral lesion is not detected on routine radiographic examination, unless there is a well-established subchondral fracture and/or collapse of the subchondral bone.

Osteochondral Lesions. Fractures involving the articular cartilage and the subchondral bone may be related to repetitive stress and trauma. Osteochondritis dissecans is the term often used to describe a specific type of osteochondral fractures. This is a relatively common condition, seen predominantly in adolescents and young adults, more often in males than in females, and is more frequently seen in the knee and ankle joints. As in acute osteochondral fractures, shearing or rotary forces applied to the articular surface of the femur result in detachment of a fragment of articular cartilage, often together with a segment of subchondral bone.

Aichroth has pointed out that the separated segment is avascular, and this feature distinguishes osteochondritis dissecans from acute osteochondral fracture. In a clinical survey of osteochondritis dissecans in 200 patients, he also determined the distribution of the lesion. The most common location was the lateral aspect of the medial femoral condyle, a non–weight-bearing segment; other sites were less commonly affected (Fig. 9.56). The degree of damage to the articular cartilage, as in acute osteochondral fractures, varies from an in situ osteochondral body, to an osteocartilaginous flap, to complete detachment of an osteochondral segment (Fig. 9.57). In the early stages of the disease, conventional radiographs in the standard projections usually show no abnormality. The only positive finding may be joint effusion. In more advanced stages of the disease, a radiolucent line is seen separating the osteochondral body from the femoral condyle (Fig. 9.58). In the past, arthrography was routinely performed for evaluation of osteochondral lesions (Figs. 9.59 and 9.60), currently replaced by CT and MRI. CT, CT-arthrography, or MRI may in addition demonstrate the presence and distribution of the osteochondral bodies (Figs. 9.61 and 9.62). T1-weighted and T2-weighted images in coronal and sagittal planes are most effective (Fig. 9.63). The lesion usually displays intermediate signal intensity on all sequences and is separated by a narrow zone of low signal intensity from the viable bone. The disruption of articular cartilage is best seen on T2-weighted or T2*-weighted (gradient echo) images (Fig. 9.64). When osteochondral body is separated from the host bone by a rim of a high signal intensity on T2-weighted images (a phenomenon that denotes a fluid or granulation tissue), it usually signifies loosening or complete detachment of the necrotic fragment (Fig. 9.65).

Occasionally, a small, disk-shaped secondary ossification center is present at the posterior portion of the femoral condyle; this normal variant should not be mistaken for osteochondritis dissecans. Similarly, during normal ossification of the distal femoral epiphysis, developmental changes may appear as irregularities in the outline of the condyle. The appearance of these irregularities, which are usually posteriorly located and hence best seen on the tunnel projection, may mimic osteochondritis dissecans (see Fig. 9.58). This normal variant is usually seen between the ages of 2 and 12 years.

Besides osteochondritis dissecans, there are a variety of lesions involving the cartilage and subchondral bone, which may be traumatic or degenerative in nature. In order to stage and clarify the nature of these lesions, various types of classifications have been proposed, based on the degree and size of cartilage damage and involvement of the subchondral bone. Some of these classifications are based on arthroscopic observations. A useful classification was created by the International Cartilage Repair Society (ICRS), based on MRI and arthroscopic correlation, with emphasis on the depth of cartilage damage (Fig. 9.66).

Spontaneous Osteonecrosis of the Knee/Subchondral Insufficiency Fracture

Characterized by acute onset of pain, SONK is a distinct clinicopathologic entity with a predilection for the weight-bearing segment of the medial femoral condyle. It occurs in older adults, frequently in their sixth and seventh decades of life, and should not be mistaken for adult onset of osteochondritis dissecans. Although the cause is obscure, certain factors such as trauma, intraarticular injection of steroids, and possibly tear of the meniscus, as Norman and Baker have pointed out, may play a role in the pathogenesis of this condition. They postulated that the concentration of stress of the torn meniscus on the articular cartilage may result in local ischemia, thus predisposing to development of osteonecrosis. Current concepts indicate that this condition represents a subchondral insufficiency fracture.

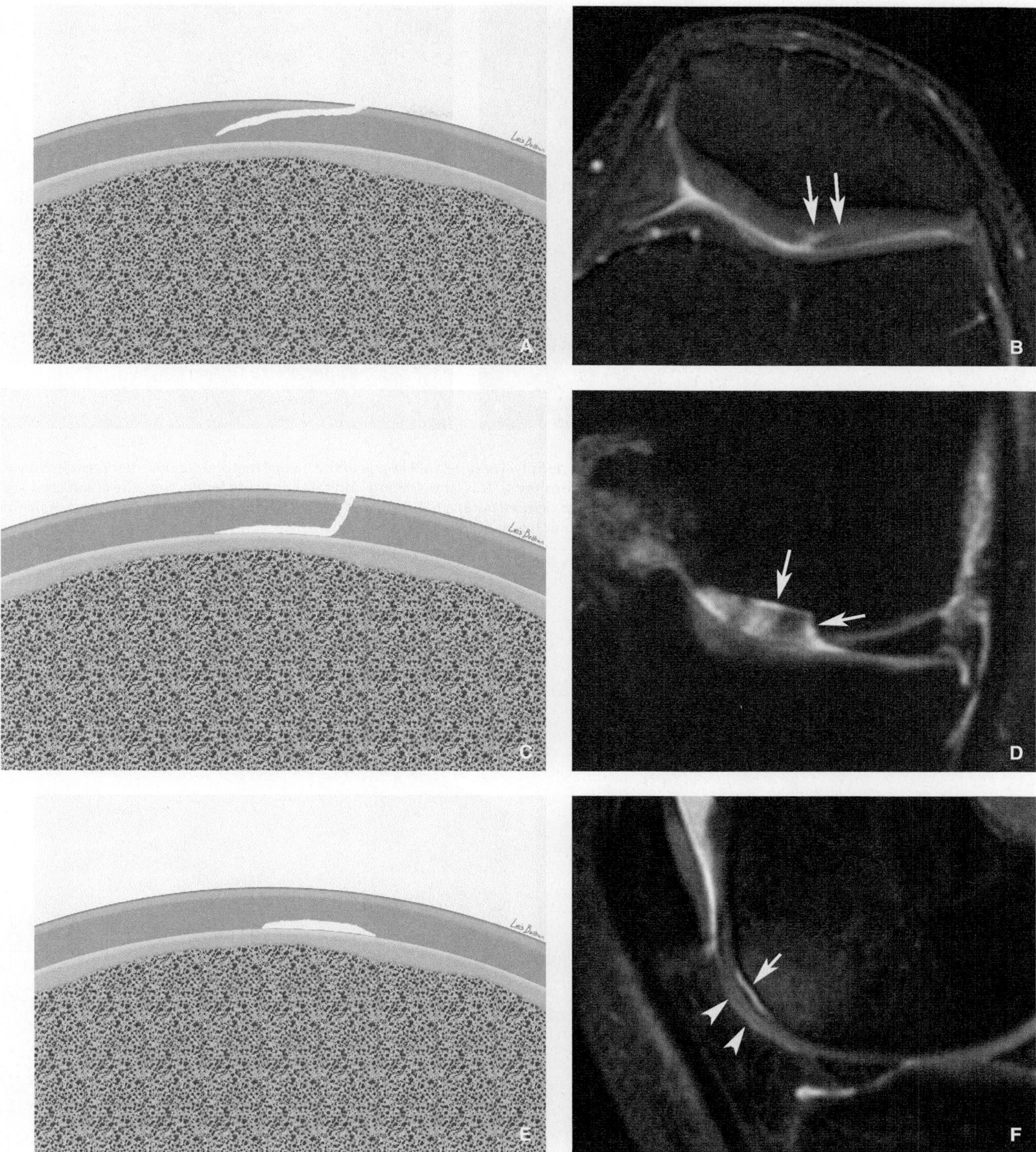

FIGURE 9.53 Chondral lesions. **(A)** A schematic of a partial, oblique chondral flap tear with delamination and **(B)** MRI demonstration of the same lesion in the lateral facet of the patella *(arrows)*. **(C)** A schematic of a deep vertical chondral tear delaminating along the subchondral bone plate and **(D)** MRI demonstration of the same lesion in the medial femoral condyle *(arrows)*. **(E)** A schematic of a concealed chondral lesion and **(F)** MRI demonstration of the same lesion in the femoral trochlea *(arrow)*. Note the intact surface of the articular cartilage *(arrowheads)*.

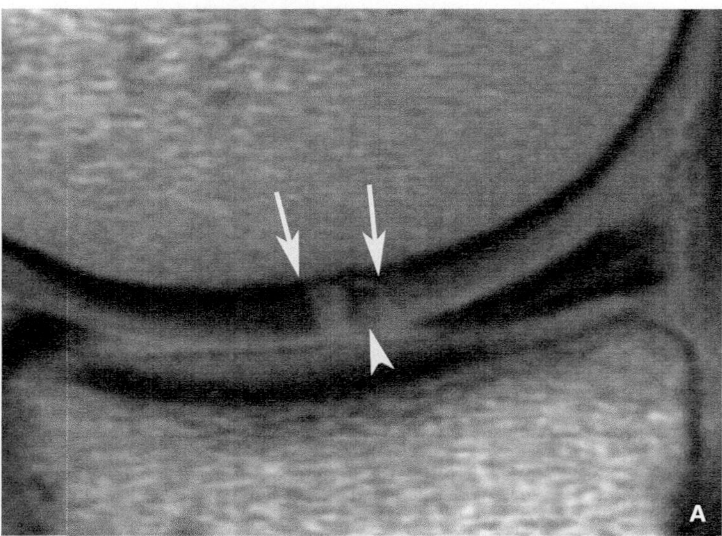

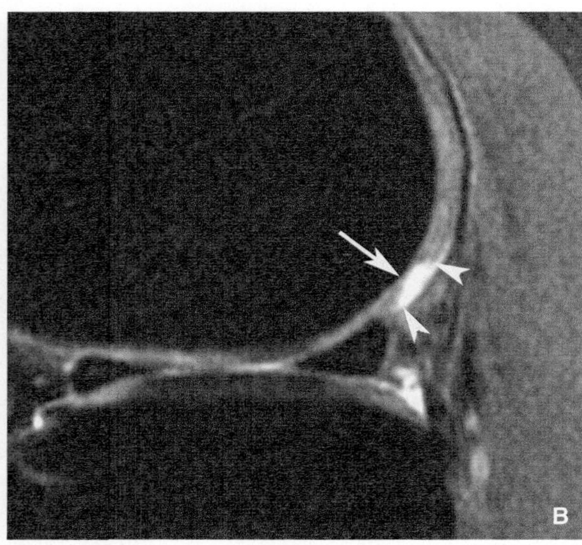

FIGURE 9.54 Chondral lesions, acute versus chronic. **(A)** Sagittal proton density–weighted MR image of the medial femoral condyle demonstrates an acute chondral lesion with sharp margins oriented perpendicular to the subchondral bone plate *(arrows)*. This "shouldering" indicates an acute lesion. Note the completely separated *in situ* chondral fragment *(arrowhead)*. **(B)** Sagittal T2-weighted fat-saturated MR image demonstrates a full-thickness chondral lesion in the posterior aspect of the medial femoral condyle *(arrow)*, with obliquely oriented margins *(arrowheads)*, indicating a chronic lesion.

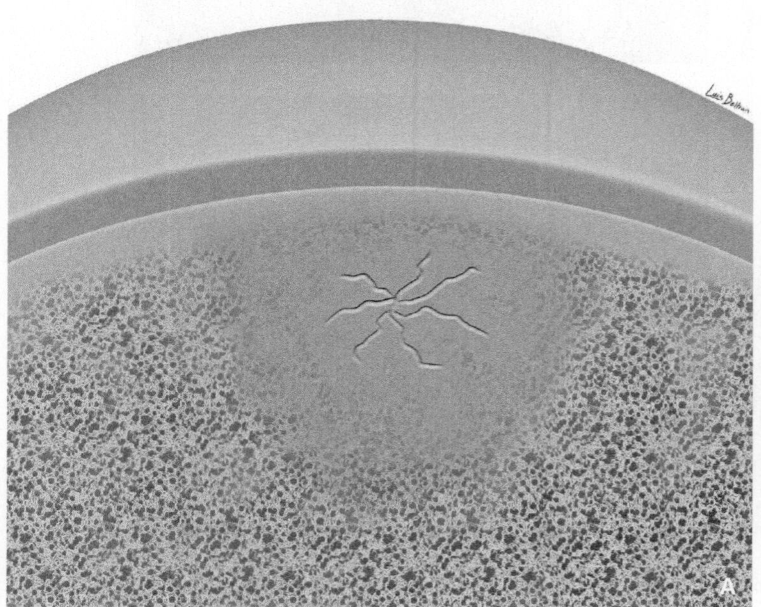

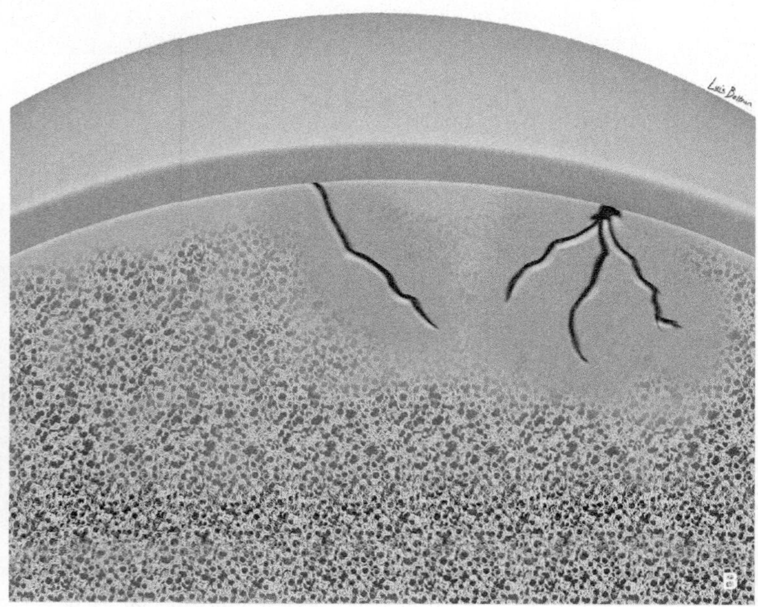

FIGURE 9.55 Subchondral lesions. Illustrations of **(A)** subchondral bone contusion also known as *bone bruise* and **(B)** better defined subchondral microtrabecular fracture. Note the coverage of subchondral bone by intact articular cartilage.

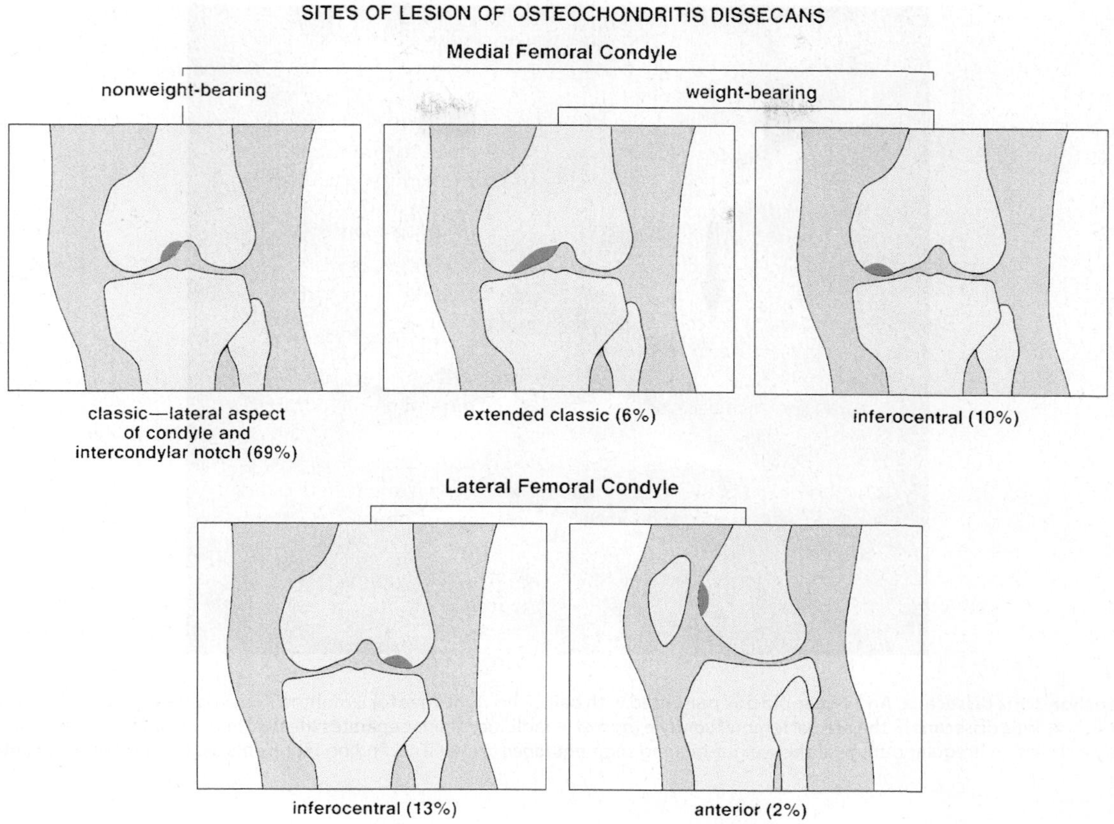

SITES OF LESION OF OSTEOCHONDRITIS DISSECANS

Medial Femoral Condyle

nonweight-bearing

weight-bearing

classic—lateral aspect of condyle and intercondylar notch (69%)

extended classic (6%)

inferocentral (10%)

Lateral Femoral Condyle

inferocentral (13%)

anterior (2%)

FIGURE 9.56 Osteochondritis dissecans—site of the lesion. Osteochondritis dissecans most frequently affects the medial femoral condyle, the non–weight-bearing portion (the lateral aspect of the condyle and the intercondylar notch), which is the most common site of the lesion. The lateral femoral condyle is much less commonly involved. (Republished with permission of British Editorial Society of Bone and Joint Surgery, from Aichroth P. Osteochondritis dissecans of the knee: a clinical survey. *J Bone Joint Surg Br* 1971;53B:440–447; permission conveyed through Copyright Clearance Center, Inc.)

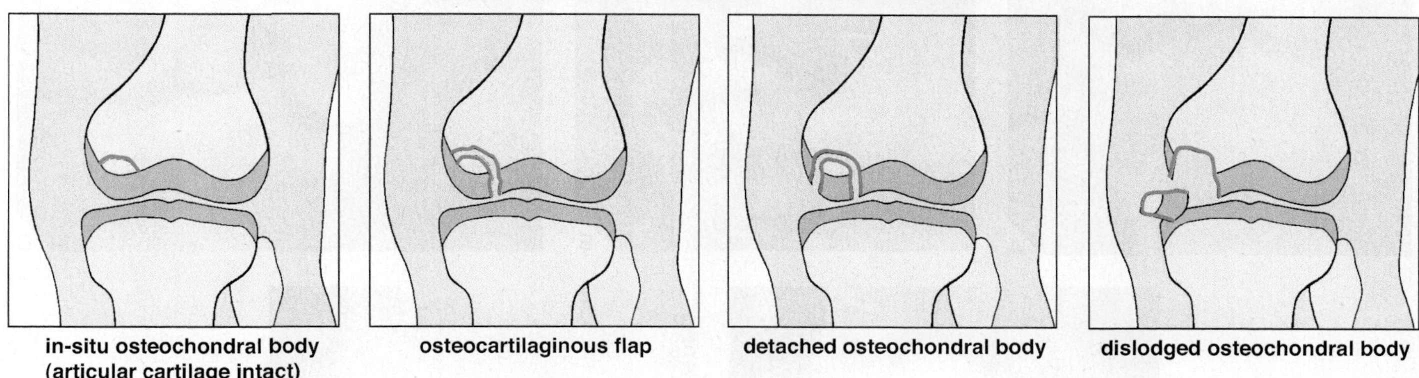

FIGURE 9.57 Stages of osteochondritis dissecans. The spectrum of chronic injury to the articular end of the distal femur (osteochondritis dissecans) ranges from an *in situ* lesion to a defect in the subchondral bone associated with a dislodged osteochondral body.

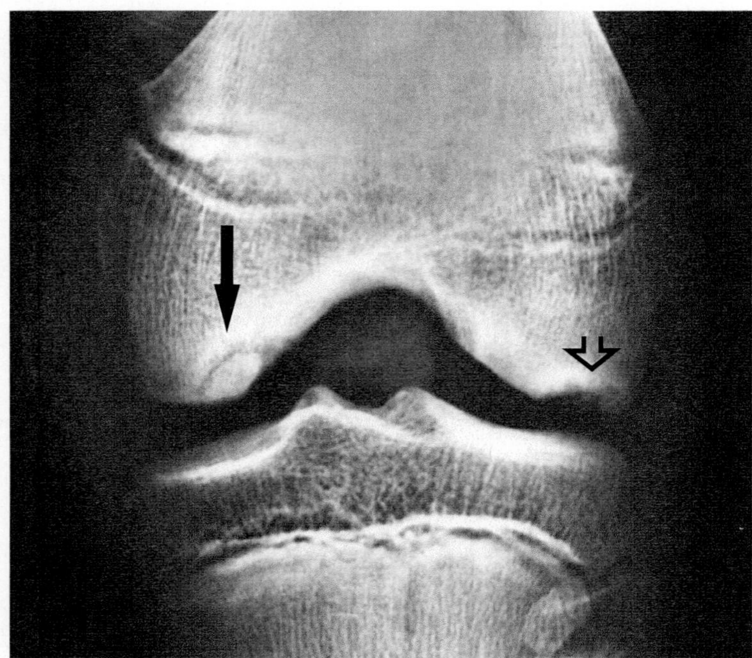

FIGURE 9.58 **Osteochondritis dissecans.** An 11-year-old boy presented with pain in his right knee for 3 months. Posteroanterior (tunnel) radiograph of the knee shows the typical lesion of osteochondritis dissecans in the medial femoral condyle *(arrow)*. A radiolucent line separates the oval *in situ* body from the femoral condyle. Incidentally, the lateral femoral condyle shows an irregular outline of the weight-bearing segment *(open arrow)*. This finding represents a developmental variant in ossification and is of no further consequence.

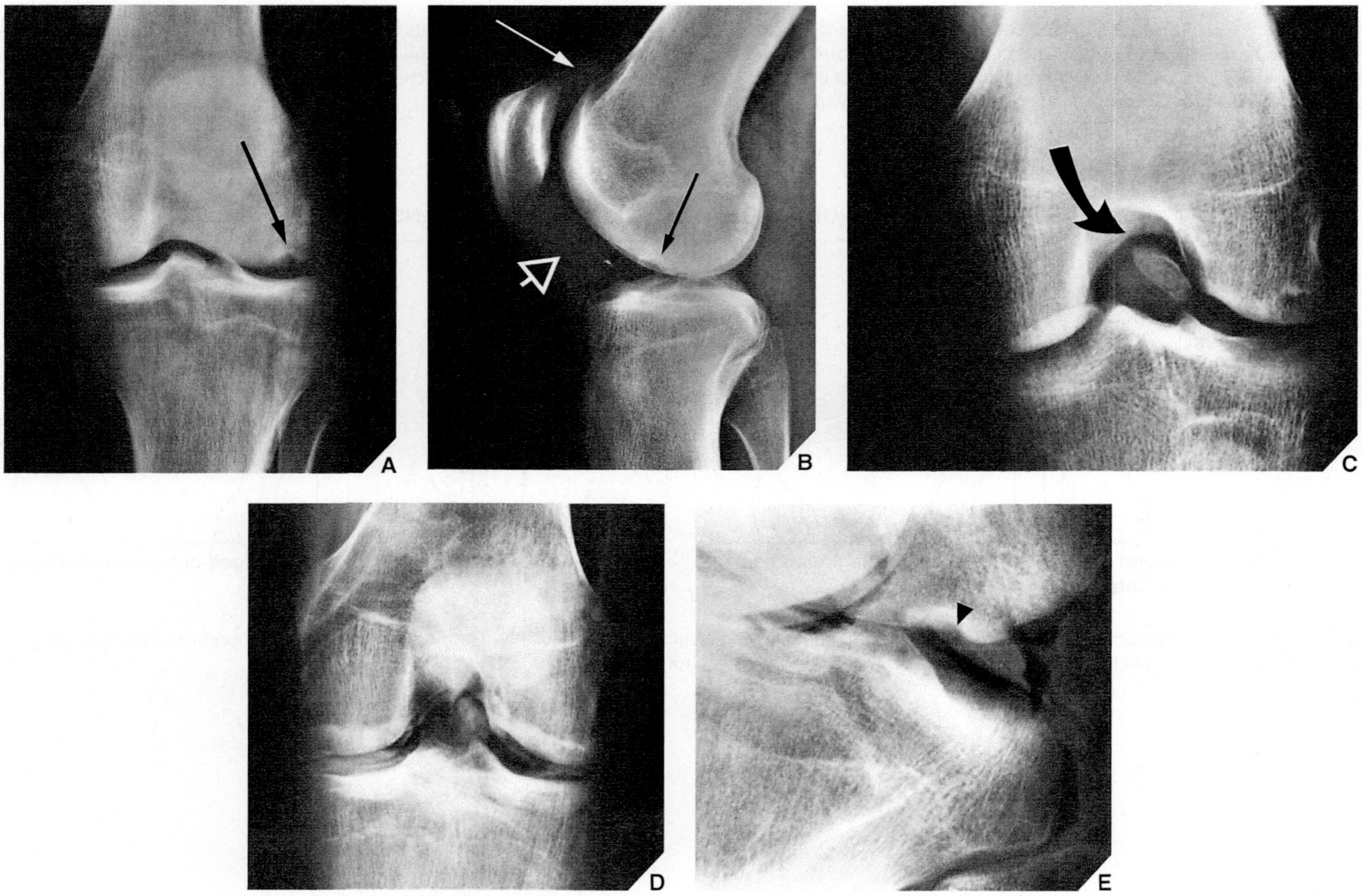

FIGURE 9.59 **Arthrography of osteochondral fracture.** A 22-year-old man dislocated his left patella in a skiing accident. The dislocation was spontaneously reduced, and he did not seek medical attention. Eight months later, he was seen by an orthopaedic surgeon for chronic joint effusion and locking of the knee. The standard radiographic examination in the anteroposterior **(A)**, lateral **(B)**, and tunnel **(C)** projections reveal joint fluid *(white arrow)*, infrapatellar soft-tissue swelling *(open arrow)*, a defect in the lateral femoral condyle *(black arrows)*, and a large osteochondral body *(curved arrow)*, representing an osteochondral fracture, in the area of the intercondylar notch. Double-contrast arthrography **(D)** confirmed the intraarticular osteochondral body and also showed a defect in the articular cartilage covering the posterolateral aspect of the lateral femoral condyle *(arrowhead)* **(E)**. Note the similarity between this condition and osteochondritis dissecans (see Fig. 9.58).

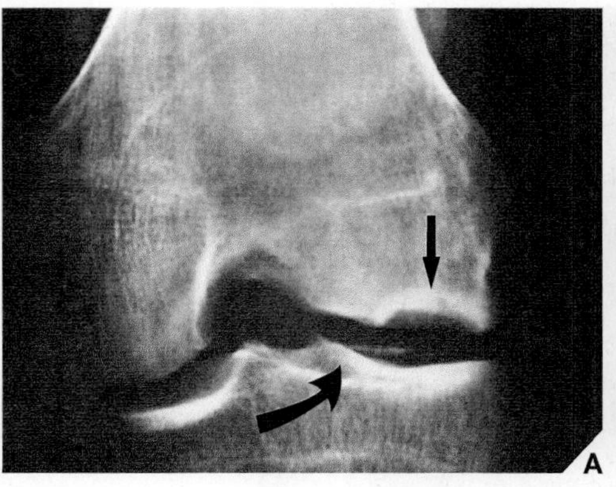

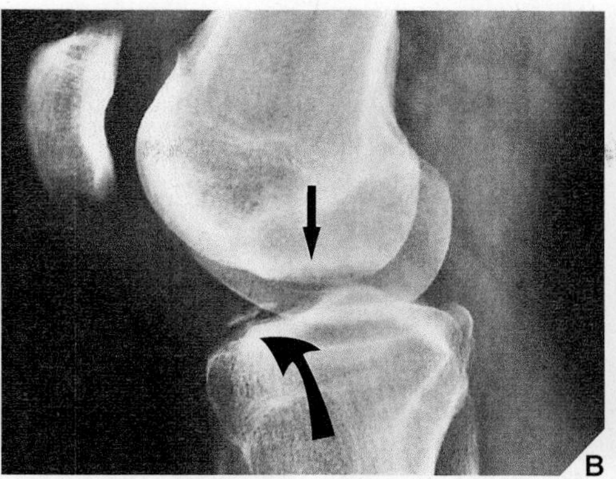

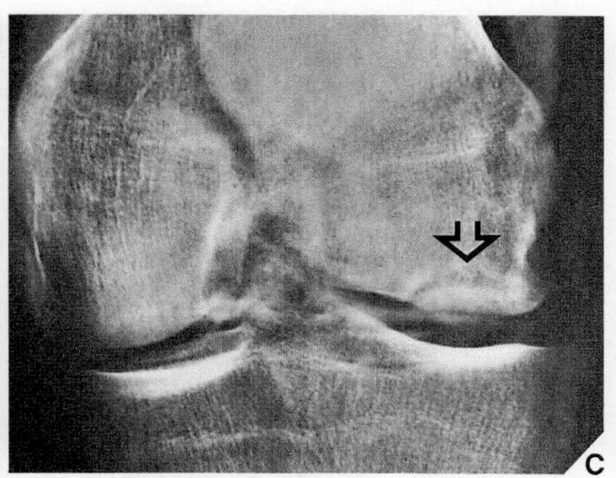

FIGURE 9.60 **Arthrography of osteochondritis dissecans.** A 23-year-old man presented with chronic pain in the knee for 4 months. He had no history of acute trauma in recent years. **(A)** Tunnel and **(B)** lateral radiographs of the left knee show a defect in the subchondral bone at the inferocentral aspect of the lateral femoral condyle *(arrows)* and an osteochondral fragment that has been discharged into the joint *(curved arrows)*. Arthrography was performed to evaluate the articular cartilage. The arthrogram **(C)** shows contrast filling the subchondral defect (*open arrow*), indicating damage to the articular cartilage.

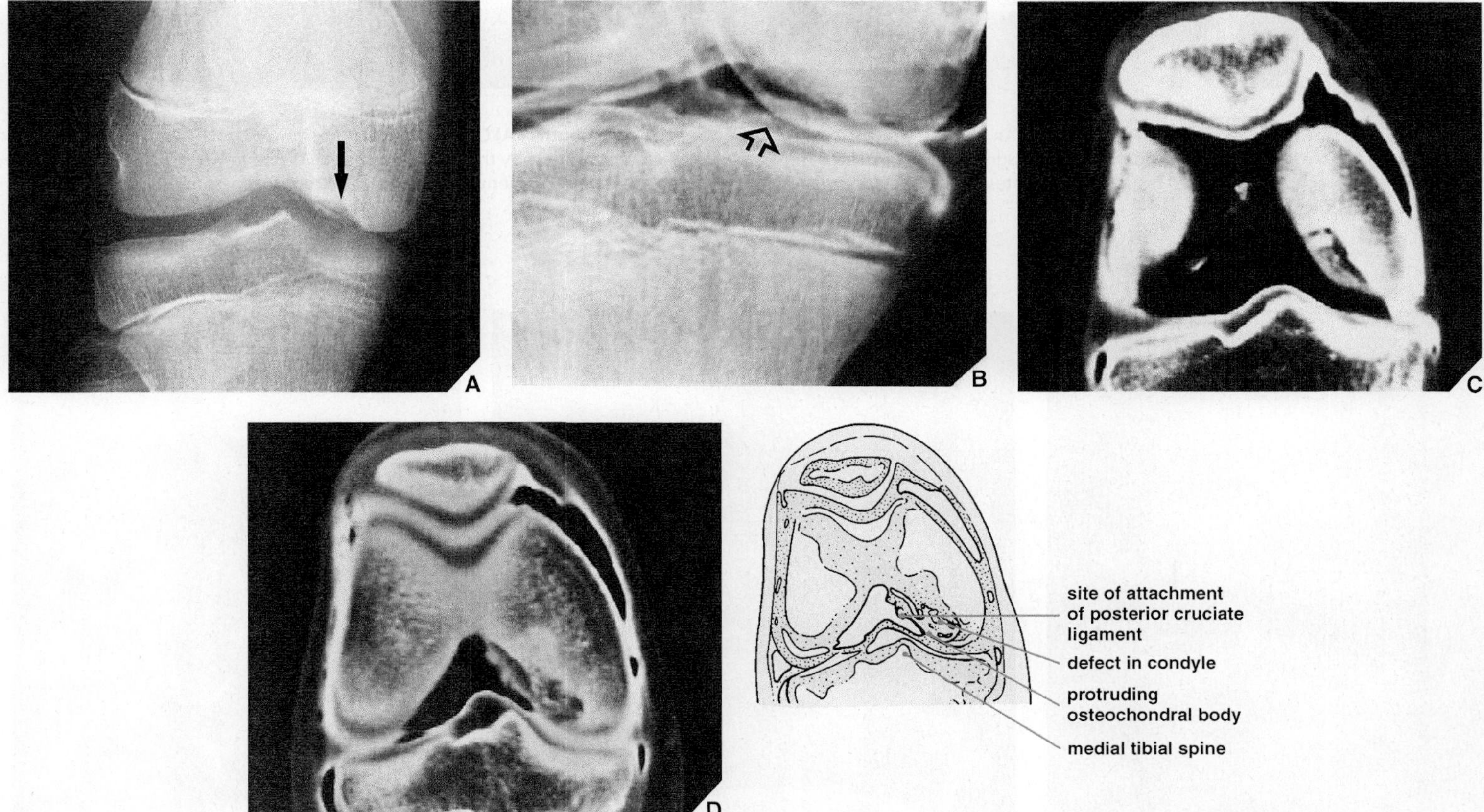

FIGURE 9.61 **CT-arthrography of osteochondritis dissecans.** A 13-year-old boy presented with pain in his right knee for 8 months. **(A)** Anteroposterior radiograph shows the lesion of osteochondritis dissecans in its classic location: the lateral aspect of the medial femoral condyle *(arrow)*. The lesion appears to be still *in situ*. **(B)** On contrast arthrography, the lesion is shown to be covered by intact articular cartilage from the inferior aspect of the femoral condyle *(open arrow)*, but **(C,D)** computed arthrotomographic sections demonstrate that the lesion, located in the anterolateral aspect of the femoral condyle (a portion not protected by articular cartilage), is partially discharged into the joint at the site of the attachment of the PCL.

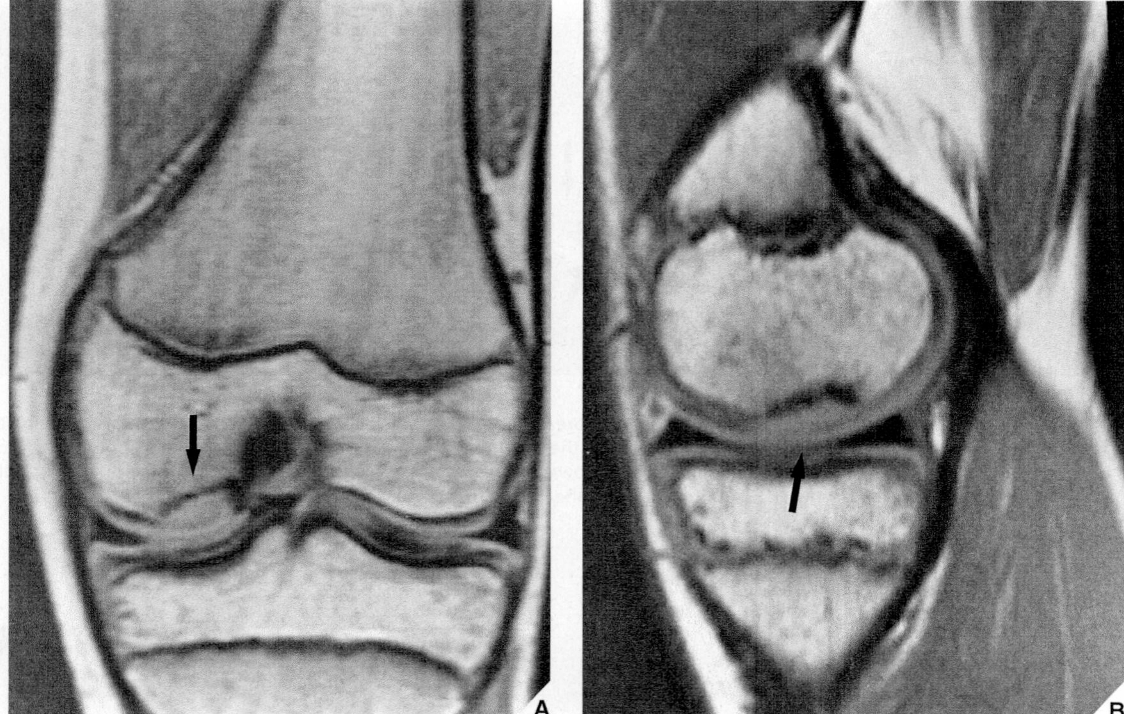

FIGURE 9.62 **MRI of osteochondritis dissecans.** An 11-year-old boy experienced knee pain for 3 months. **(A)** Coronal proton density–weighted (spin echo, repetition time [TR] 1800/TE 20 msec) MR image shows osseous fragment well separated from the medial femoral condyle by the low–signal intensity line *(arrow)*. **(B)** MR image in the sagittal plane (spin echo TR 800/TE 20 msec) demonstrates intact articular cartilage overlying the separated fragment *(arrow)*, indicating an *in situ* lesion.

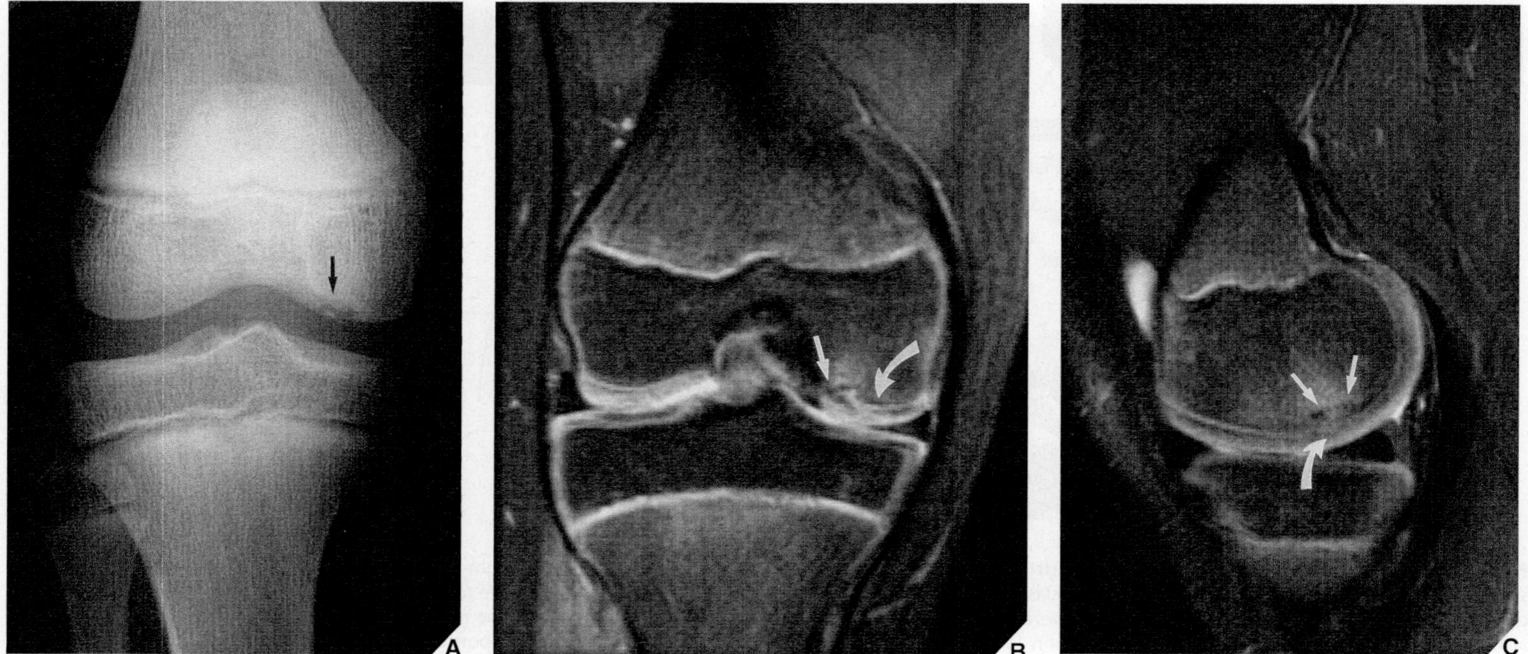

FIGURE 9.63 **MRI of osteochondritis dissecans.** **(A)** Anteroposterior radiograph of the right knee shows a lesion of osteochondritis dissecans in the medial femoral condyle *(arrow)*. **(B)** Coronal and **(C)** sagittal T2-weighted fat-suppressed MR images demonstrate the osteochondral body being still *in situ (arrows)*, although the articular cartilage is already damaged *(curved arrows)*.

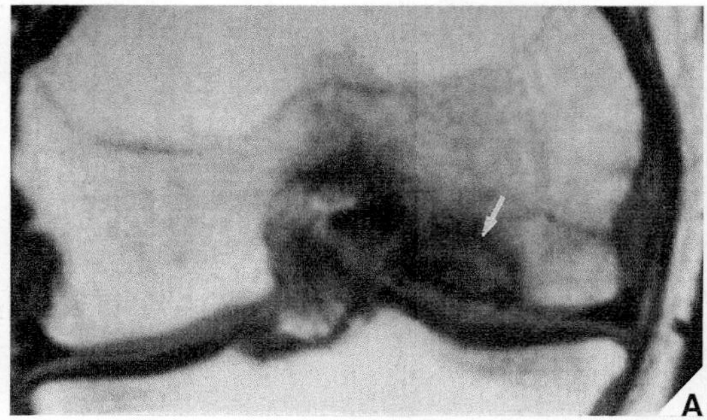

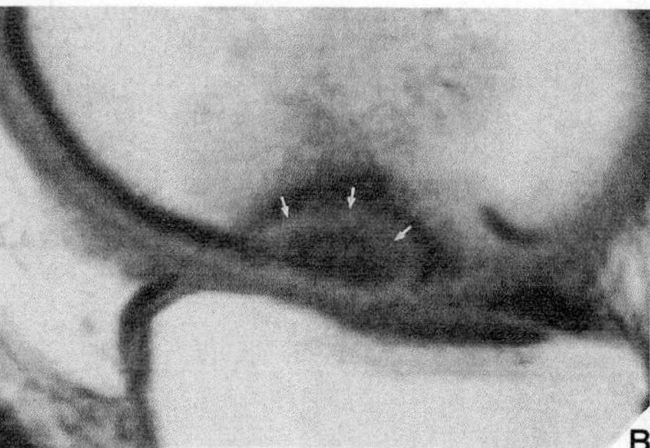

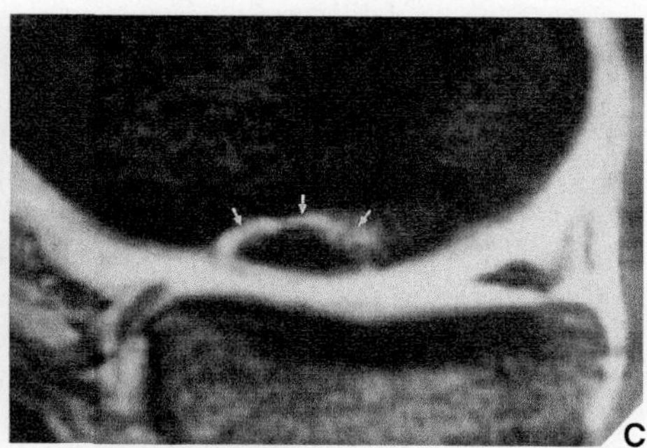

FIGURE 9.64 MRI of osteochondritis dissecans. A loose osteochondral body in the medial femoral condyle is seen on **(A)** T1-weighted coronal and **(B)** sagittal MR images *(white arrows)*. **(C)** On the sagittal T2*-weighted sequence, high–signal intensity fluid *(small arrows)* separates the loose fragment from the viable bone. (Reprinted with permission from Stoller DW. *Magnetic resonance imaging in orthopaedics and sports medicine*. Philadelphia: JB Lippincott; 1993.)

The earliest radiologic sign of this condition is an increased uptake of radiopharmaceutical on radionuclide bone scan; radiographically, the earliest indication is a minimal degree of flattening of the femoral condyle (Fig. 9.67). Later, usually 1 to 3 months after the sudden onset of symptoms, radiographs may show a subchondral focus of radiolucency. As the condition progresses, the lesion may be seen radiographically as a subchondral osteolytic (necrotic) focus surrounded by a sclerotic margin representing a zone of repair (Fig. 9.68). Frequently, these lesions are accompanied by meniscal tears (Fig. 9.69). In the early stages, before collapse of the subchondral bone plate, MRI demonstrates the subchondral insufficiency fracture with surrounding edema (Fig. 9.70). Unless the knee is protected from weight bearing, the lesion will progress, and the subchondral bone plate will collapse.

Injury to the Soft Tissues About the Knee

Knee Joint Effusion

Normally, the suprapatellar recess is apparent on a radiograph of the knee in the lateral projection as a thin, radiodense strip just posterior to the quadriceps tendon (Fig. 9.71). In knee joint effusion, which often occurs secondary to injury elsewhere in the knee, the suprapatellar recess fills with fluid. Distention of the recess is evident radiographically as an oval density that obliterates the fat space anterior to the femoral cortex (Fig. 9.72). If there is an associated intraarticular fracture of either the distal femur or the proximal tibia, then a cross-table lateral view may demonstrate the FBI sign.

Bursae of the Knee

The anterior aspect of the knee contains a number of synovial-lined bursae (Fig. 9.73) that can become distended by fluid under variety of clinical circumstances, including overuse, trauma, infection, inflammatory arthropathies, chronic glucocorticoid use, or gout (see Fig. 15.39A,B), and less commonly as a result of other synovial conditions such as pigmented villonodular synovitis or synovial chondromatosis (see Fig. 23.4). In some instances, the cause is unknown. The prepatellar bursa, which is located between the patella and the overlying anteriorly subcutaneous tissues, is the one most commonly affected. Prepatellar bursitis typically occurs in patients that spent long hours on their knees (conditions known as *nun's knee*, *tiler's knee*, *carpet layer's knee*, or *housemaid's knee*). Clinically, patients present with pain and swelling over the patella, redness of the skin, and limited range of motion in the knee joint. The fluid-distended prepatellar bursa is readily seen on MRI (Fig. 9.74) or US. Conventional lateral radiographs of the knee can show a focal area of water density in the prepatellar space. Repetitive shearing forces over the anterior aspect of the knee can lead to fibrosis and thickening of the wall of the prepatellar bursa. This has been described in long-time surfers who paddle while kneeling ("surfer's knobs"), elite bicyclists, football linemen, and wrestlers (Fig. 9.75). Infected bursitis characteristically will show on MRI a distended bursa with extensive surrounding soft-tissue edema/cellulitis with enhancement following intravenous administration of gadolinium (Fig. 9.76).

The second most common bursitis around the knee involves the deep infrapatellar bursa, a wedge-shaped synovium-lined structure located between the tibial tubercle and the tibial insertion of the patellar ligament, and superiorly bounded by infrapatellar (Hoffa) fat pad. A small amount of fluid distending the deep infrapatellar bursa is often seen in asymptomatic patients, but it can become significantly distended in repetitive trauma and overuse (also known as *clergyman's knee*) (Fig. 9.77). Deep infrapatellar bursitis may also be present in patients with Osgood-Schlatter disease (see Fig. 9.49D).

The prepatellar bursa may or may not communicate with another synovial-lined bursa located inferior to the prepatellar bursa, called *superficial infrapatellar bursa*. The same conditions causing prepatellar bursitis may also affect this bursa (Figs. 9.78 and 9.79). Occasionally, both prepatellar and superficial infrapatellar bursae may be simultaneously affected (Fig. 9.80).

Two additional bursae related to the tendons are described: the semimembranosus bursa and the pes anserine bursa. Both bursae are found in the medial aspect of the knee at the level of the medial tibial plateau (semimembranosus bursa), or more distally at the level of the proximal tibial shaft, deep to the osseous insertion of the pes anserine tendons consisting of the distal sartorius, gracilis, and semitendinosus tendons (pes anserine bursa). The pes anserine bursitis commonly results from overuse, particularly in runners. Under normal circumstances, these bursae, like all bursae in the body, are not distended by fluid, and therefore are not seen on different imaging techniques, but when distended by fluid secondary to any of the aforementioned circumstances, they can be readily visualized on MRI or US.

Meniscal Injury

Similar to the other fibrocartilaginous structures, the menisci of the knee (see Fig. 9.9) are not visible on conventional radiographs. MRI has become a standard procedure for evaluating these structures. Normal menisci are seen as triangular- or bow tie–shaped structures in the medial and lateral knee compartments, mostly hypointense on all pulse sequences (see Fig. 9.11). Areas of hyperintensity within the substance of the menisci without extension to the surface most likely represent intrasubstance myxoid degeneration, if they are globular, longitudinal, or linear in shape and seen in the periphery of the meniscus (see normal MRI meniscal anatomy). Meniscal "lesions" were originally classified into four types (Fig. 9.81), depending on their morphology and surface extension. Some of these abnormalities, known as *type I* (round focus) and *type II* (linear area) *meniscal lesions* (Fig. 9.81A,B), are not seen on arthroscopic examination of the knee. The true tears are designated as type III and type IV lesions (Fig. 9.81C; see also Fig. 9.83). Occasionally, when tears extend to the periphery of the meniscus, they may be associated with meniscal or parameniscal cysts (Fig. 9.82). Horizontal oblique tears of the posterior horn of the medial meniscus extending to the inferior articular surface are the most common tears (see Fig. 9.90).

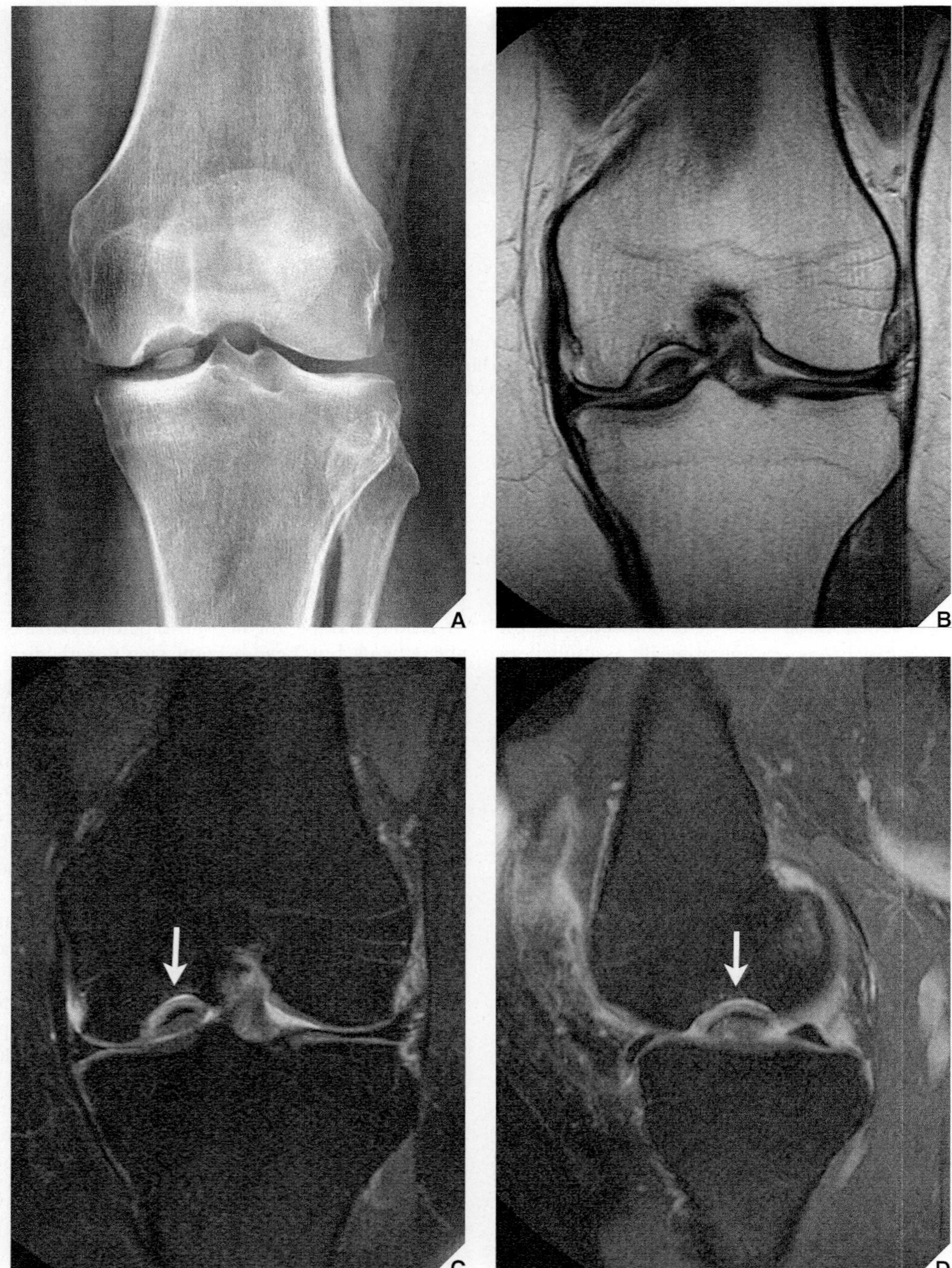

FIGURE 9.65 MRI of osteochondritis dissecans. **(A)** Anteroposterior radiograph of the left knee of a 23-year-old man shows an osteochondral body within the subchondral defect in the medial femoral condyle. **(B)** Coronal proton density–weighted, **(C)** coronal proton density–weighted fat-suppressed, and **(D)** sagittal proton density–weighted fat-suppressed MR images show that the osteochondral fragment is separated from the host bone by fluid *(arrows)*, a diagnostic sign of instability. In addition, the osteochondral fragment is flipped vertically with the articular cartilage and subchondral bone plate in the superior aspect of the fragment, confirming instability.

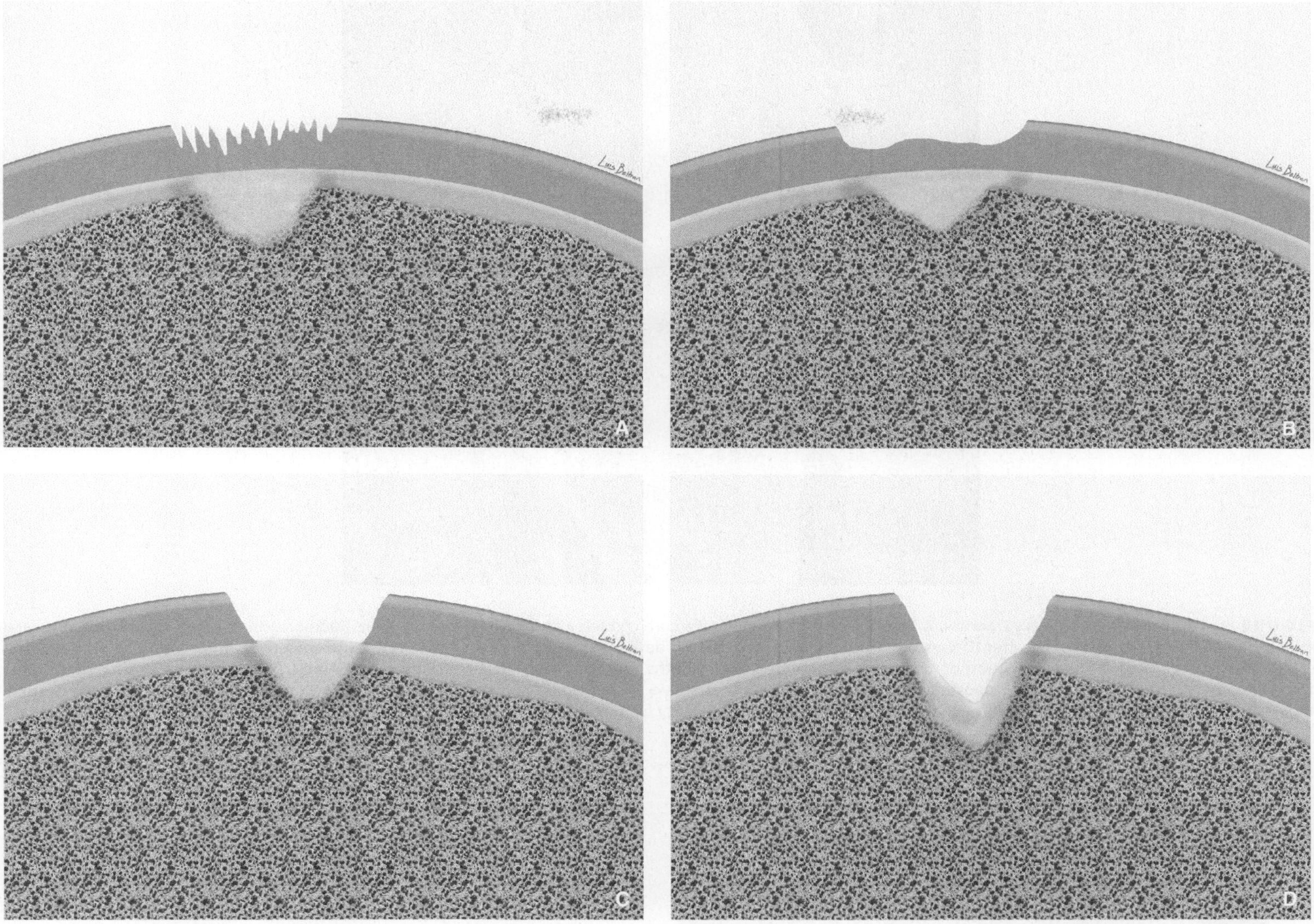

FIGURE 9.66 ICRS classification of osteochondral lesions. **(A)** Stage I: articular cartilage surface fibrillation and fissuring with subchondral contusion without depression. **(B)** Stage II: partial-thickness chondral defect with underlying bone contusion without depression. **(C)** Stage III: full-thickness chondral defect with subchondral contusion. **(D)** Stage IV: full-thickness chondral defect with underlying bone defect.

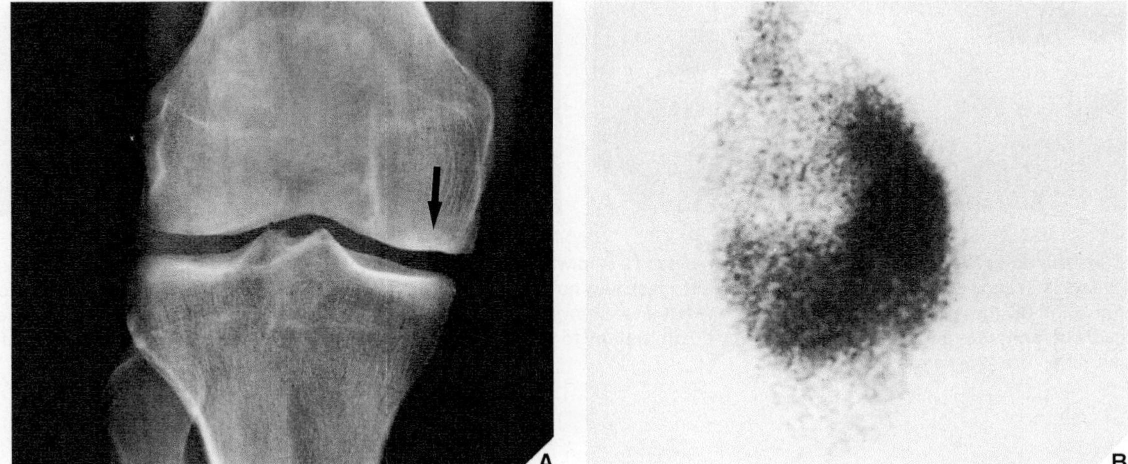

FIGURE 9.67 SONK also known as *insufficiency fracture*. Four weeks before this radiographic examination, a 58-year-old man felt a sharp pain in the right knee when he stepped off a curb. The pain subsided after 1 week but recurred soon afterward. **(A)** Anteroposterior radiograph of the right knee shows flattening of the medial aspect of the medial femoral condyle *(arrow)*. **(B)** Radionuclide bone scan was performed, and it shows a marked increase in uptake of the tracer in the area of the medial femoral condyle. The features seen in both studies characterize an early stage of SONK or insufficiency fracture.

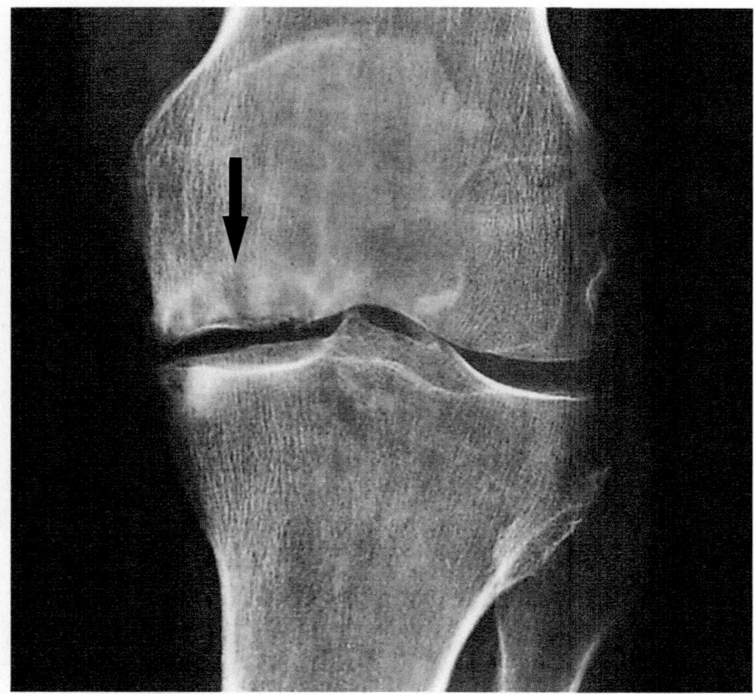

FIGURE 9.68 **SONK/insufficiency fracture.** A 74-year-old man stepped off a curb and felt a sharp pain in the left knee. Radiographs obtained on the next day were normal. The pain in the knee subsided after 10 days, but 2 months later, joint effusion developed, which was aspirated. He was given a series of three intraarticular injections of steroids (hydrocortisone), after which most of the symptoms subsided. Four months after the initial injury, the symptoms recurred, and at this time, the standard radiographic examination was repeated. Anteroposterior radiograph of the left knee shows a large radiolucent defect surrounded by a zone of sclerosis in the weight-bearing segment of the medial femoral condyle *(arrow)*. The lesion represents an insufficiency fracture.

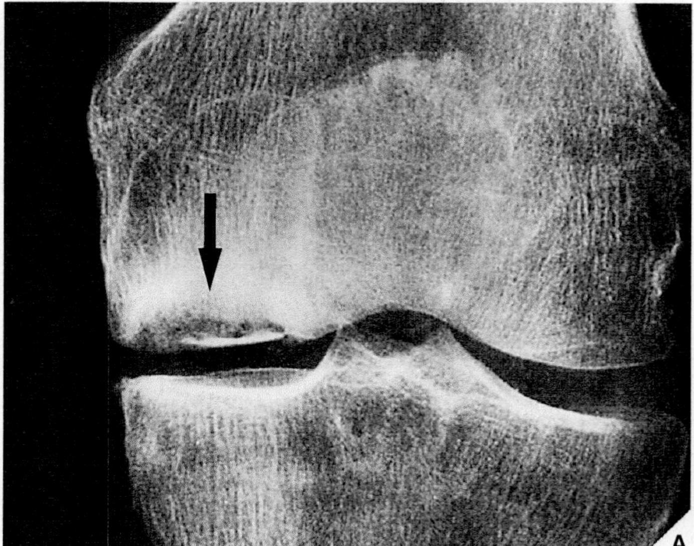

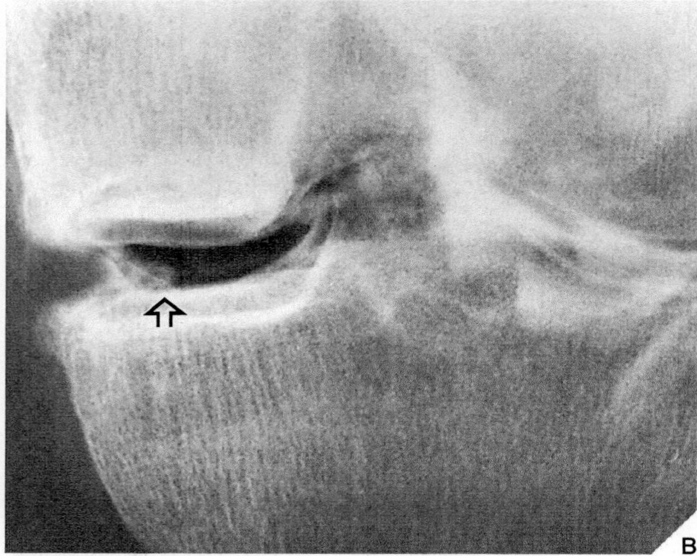

FIGURE 9.69 **SONK/insufficiency fracture.** A 63-year-old woman missed a step while descending the staircase and felt a sharp pain in the left knee. The radiographic examination performed 3 days later showed only moderate osteoporosis, which was not related to trauma. Three months later, she was reexamined for persistent pain and accumulation of fluid in the joint. **(A)** Anteroposterior radiograph of the left knee shows insufficiency fracture in the weight-bearing portion of the medial femoral condyle *(arrow)*. Double-contrast arthrography was performed to evaluate any possible injury to the menisci. **(B)** The arthrogram demonstrates a vertical tear of the medial meniscus at the site of the insufficiency fracture *(open arrow)*.

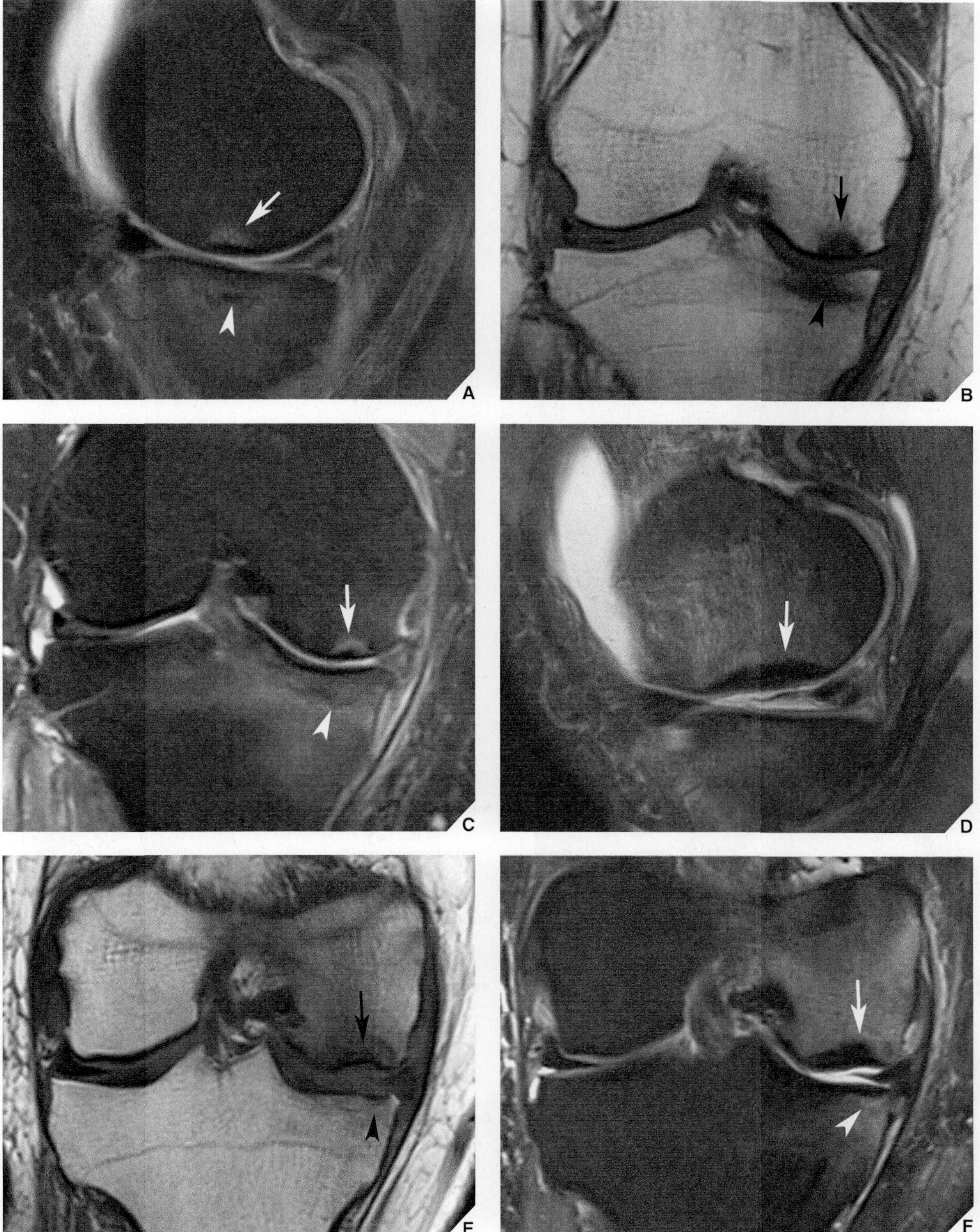

FIGURE 9.70 MRI of SONK/insufficiency fracture. **(A–C)** Subchondral insufficiency fractures without depression. **(A)** Sagittal proton density–weighted fat-saturated, **(B)** coronal T1-weighted, and **(C)** coronal proton density–weighted fat-saturated MR images of the knee in an 85-year-old man with acute onset of knee pain demonstrate a nondepressed subchondral insufficiency fracture in the medial femoral condyle with a halo of surrounding bone marrow edema *(arrows)*. Also present is the second insufficiency fracture of the proximal medial tibia with surrounding bone marrow edema *(arrowheads)*. Note also the presence of a horizontal tear of the posterior horn of the medial meniscus. **(D–F)** Subchondral insufficiency fracture with depression. **(D)** Sagittal proton density–weighted fat-saturated, **(E)** coronal T1-weighted, and **(F)** coronal proton density–weighted fat-saturated images of the knee of a 63-year-old man with acute onset of knee pain demonstrate a depressed subchondral insufficiency fracture in the medial femoral condyle *(arrows)* with extensive surrounding bone marrow edema. There is also a smaller subchondral insufficiency fracture of the medial tibial plateau with minimal depression *(arrowheads)*. Note in addition the presence of a tear of the posterior horn of the medial meniscus.

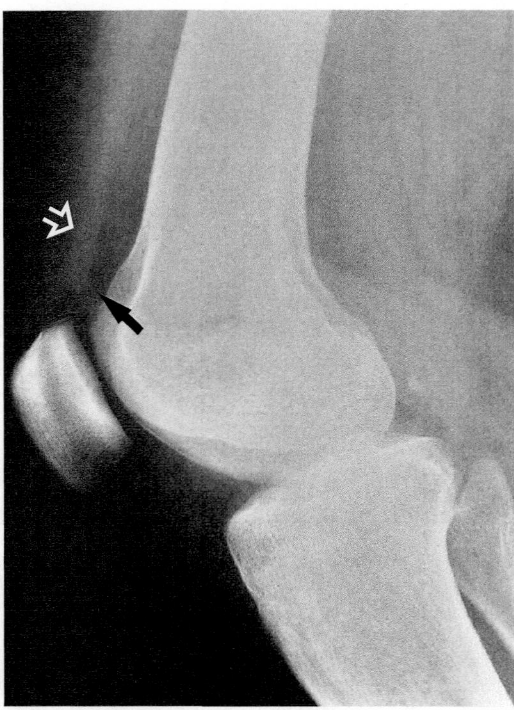

FIGURE 9.71 **Normal appearance of suprapatellar recess.** The suprapatellar recess normally appears on the lateral radiograph of the knee as a radiodense strip *(arrow)* just posterior to the quadriceps tendon *(open arrow)*.

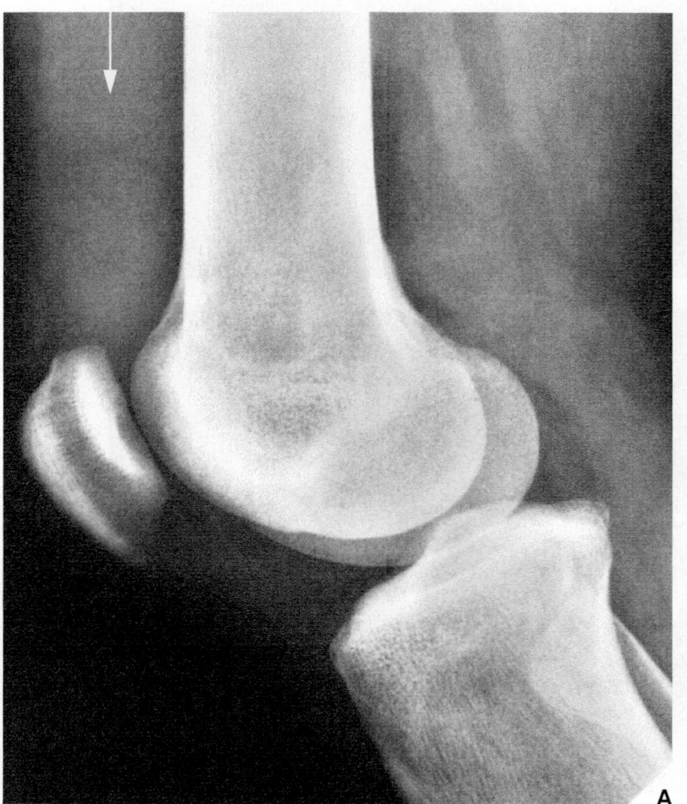

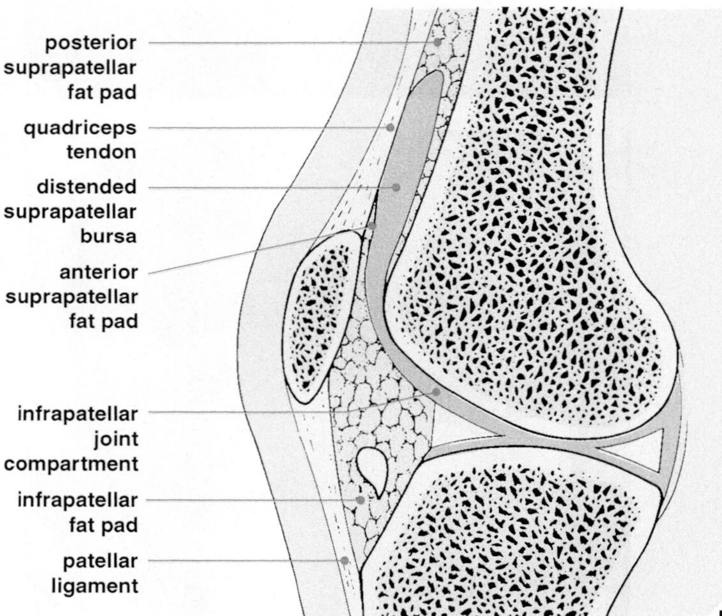

FIGURE 9.72 **Knee joint effusion.** **(A,B)** In knee joint effusion, the suprapatellar recess distends with fluid, thus obliterating the fat space posterior to the quadriceps tendon *(arrow)*. (**B**, Modified from Hall FM. Radiographic diagnosis and accuracy in knee joint effusions. *Radiology* 1975;115:49–54. Copyright © 1975 by The Radiological Society of North America, Inc.)

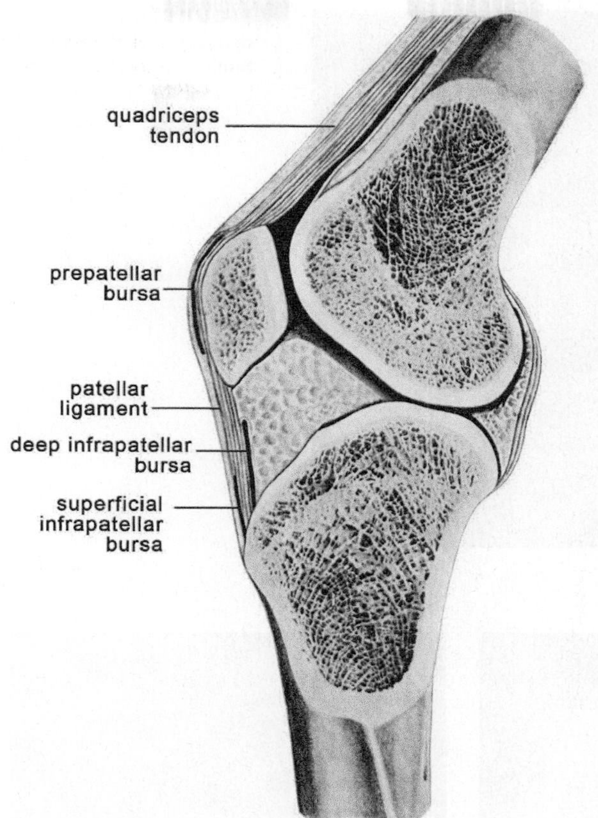

FIGURE 9.73 Prepatellar and infrapatellar bursae of the knee.

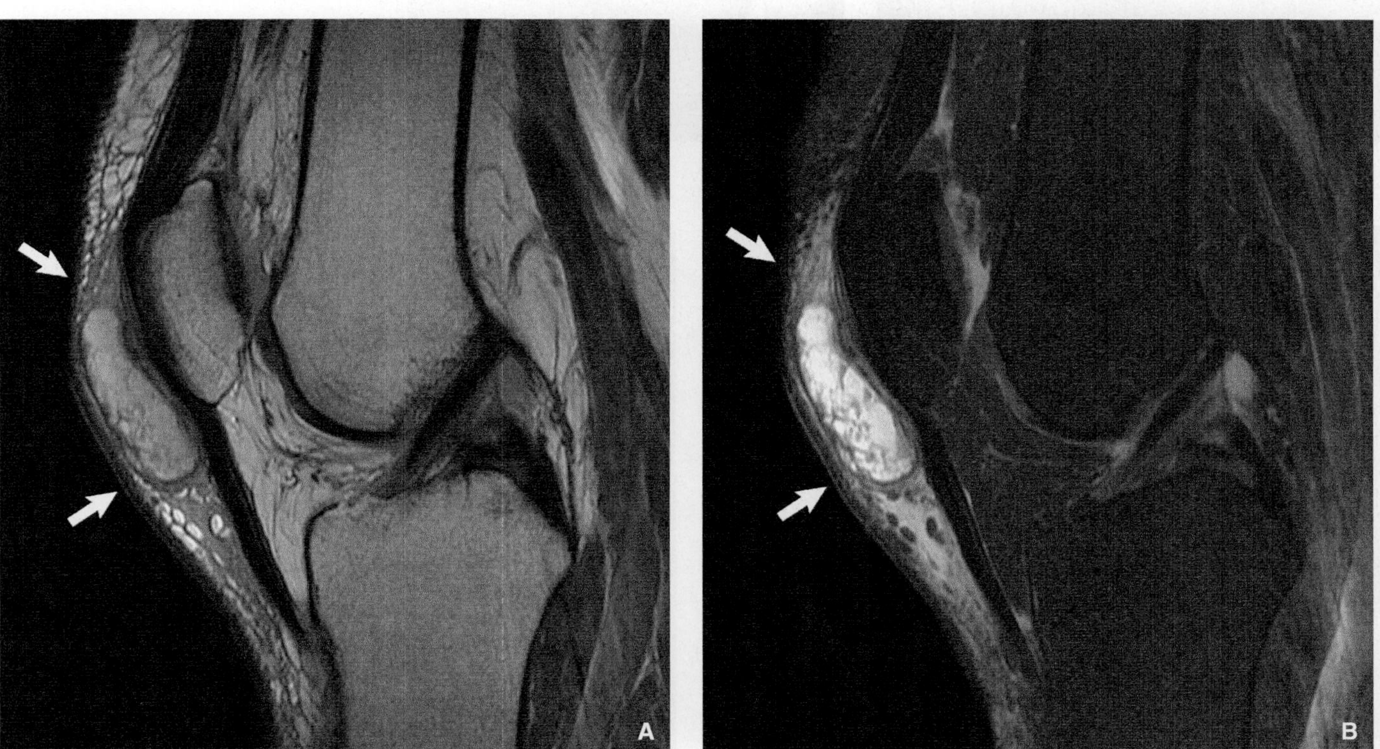

FIGURE 9.74 **MRI of prepatellar bursitis.** A 58-year-old carpet-layer worker presented with painful swelling over the patella. **(A)** Sagittal proton density–weighted and **(B)** sagittal proton density–weighted fat-suppressed MR images of the knee show prepatellar bursa distended with fluid (*arrows*) associated with peripheral swelling and edema.

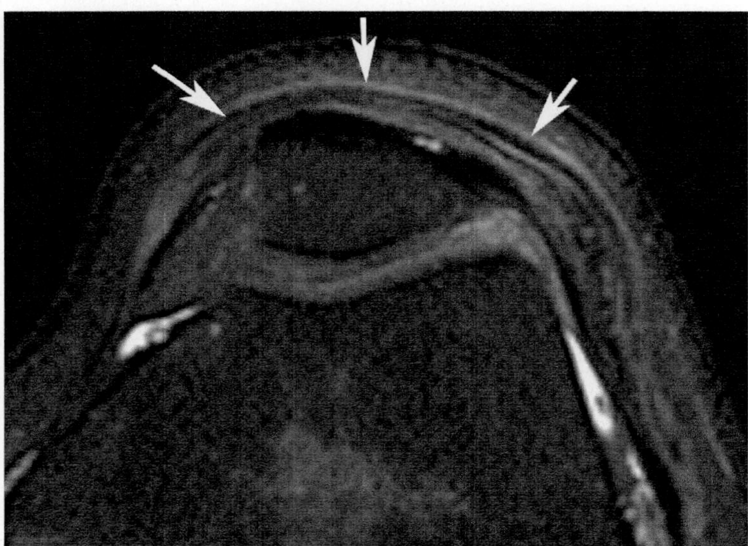

FIGURE 9.75 MRI of the "wrestler's knee." Axial T2-weighted MR image demonstrates thickening and fibrosis of the prepatellar bursa without fluid distention *(arrows)* in a young wrestler.

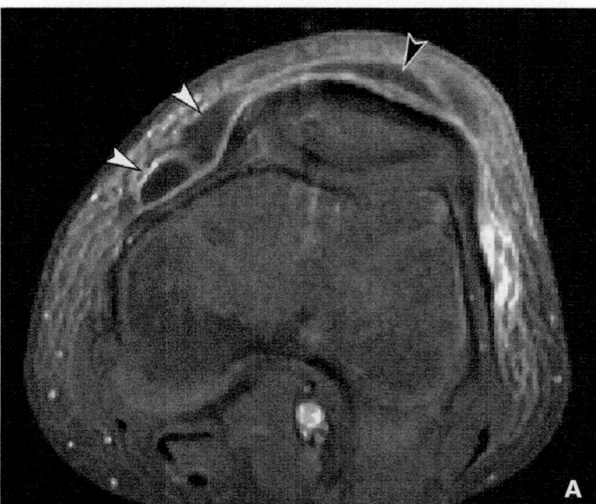

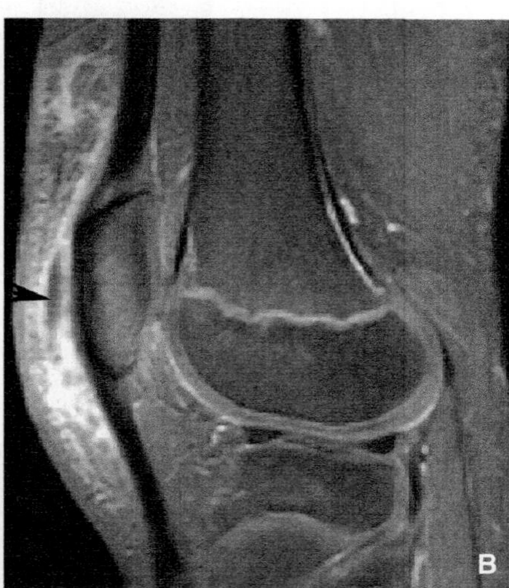

FIGURE 9.76 MRI of infected bursitis. A young child was presented with anterior knee swelling and skin redness. **(A)** Axial and **(B)** sagittal T1-weighted fat-saturated MR images of the knee obtained following intravenous administration of gadolinium show prepatellar bursitis with rim enhancement *(arrowheads)* accompanied by extensive surrounding soft-tissue edema/cellulitis.

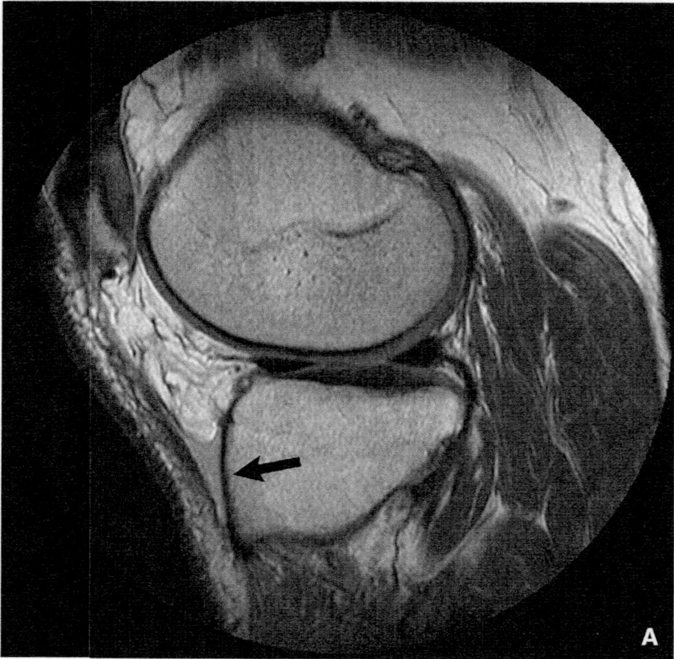

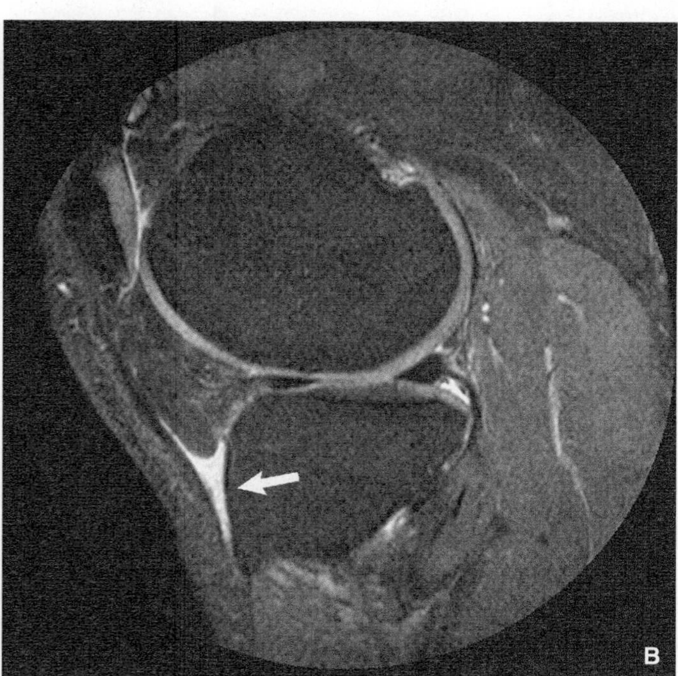

FIGURE 9.77 MRI of deep infrapatellar bursitis. **(A)** Sagittal T1-weighted and **(B)** sagittal T2-weighted MR images of the knee of a 51-year-old man who presented with a long-standing infrapatellar pain show fluid-filled deep infrapatellar bursa *(arrows)*.

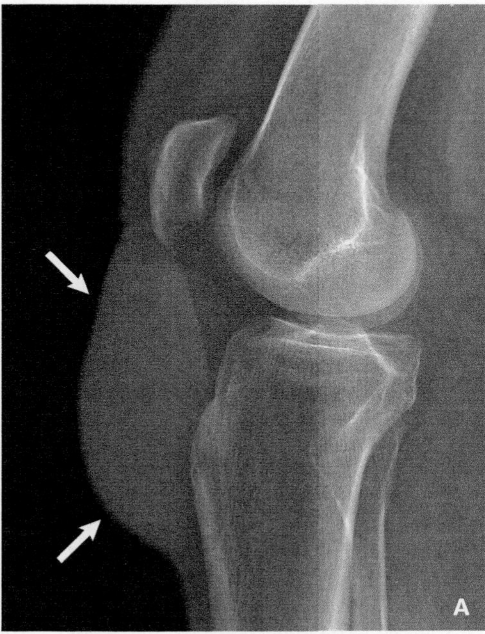

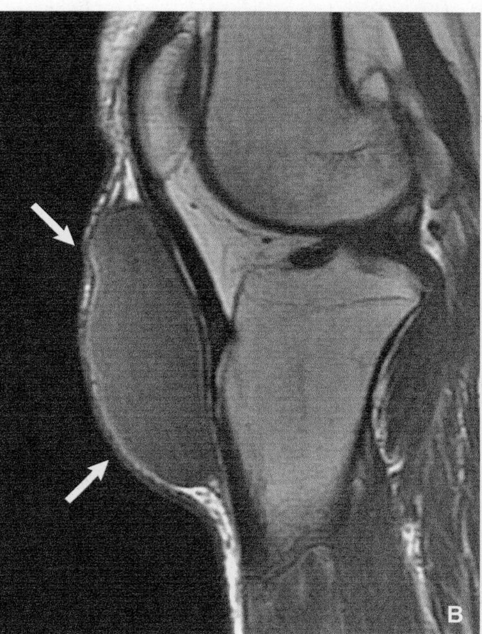

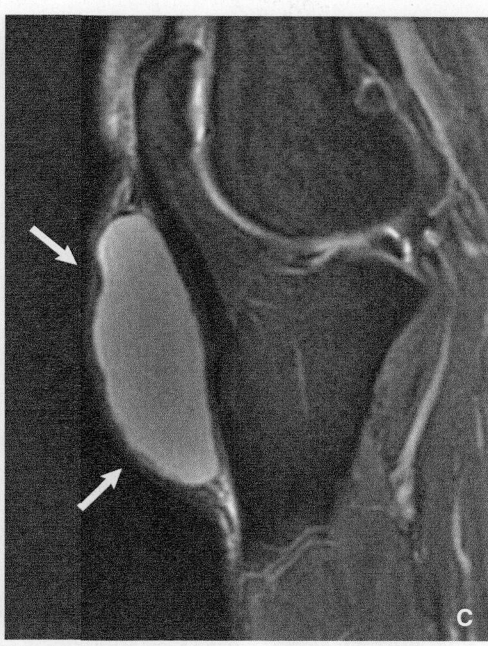

FIGURE 9.78 **MRI of superficial infrapatellar bursitis.** A 51-year-old man presented with a huge soft-tissue mass below the patella. **(A)** Lateral radiograph of the knee shows a water-density soft-tissue mass extending from the lower pole of the patella to the area just below the tibial tuberosity *(arrows)*. **(B)** Sagittal T1-weighted and **(C)** sagittal T2-weighted MR images of the knee show the superficial infrapatellar bursa distended with fluid *(arrows)*.

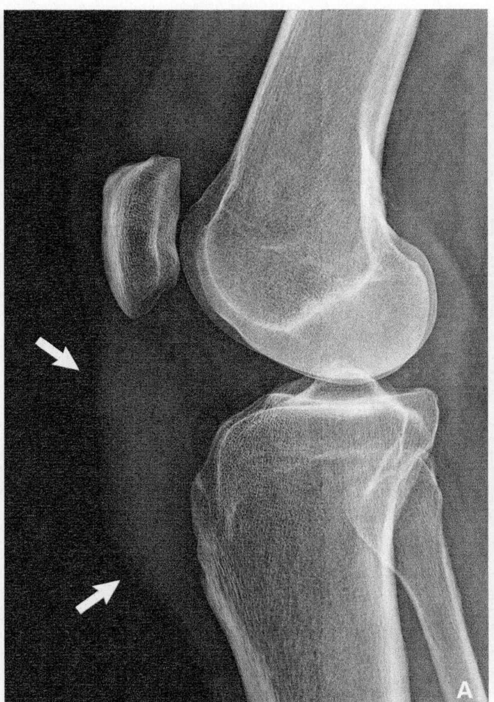

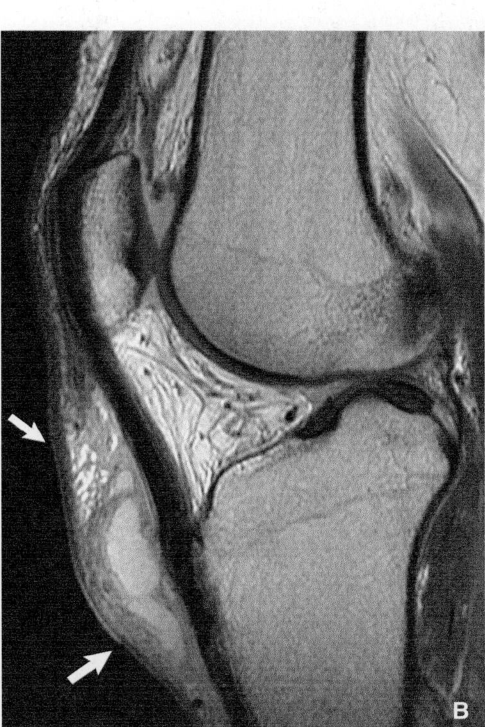

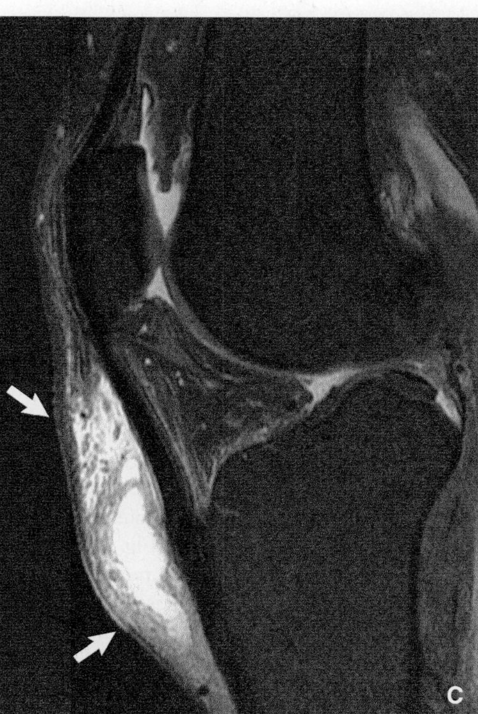

FIGURE 9.79 **MRI of superficial infrapatellar bursitis.** **(A)** Lateral radiograph of the knee of a 70-year-old woman shows a water-density soft-tissue mass extending from the inferior pole of the patella to the tibial tuberosity *(arrows)*. **(B)** Sagittal proton density–weighted and **(C)** sagittal proton density–weighted fat-saturated MR images of the knee show heterogenous-appearing fluid within distended superficial infrapatellar bursa *(arrows)*.

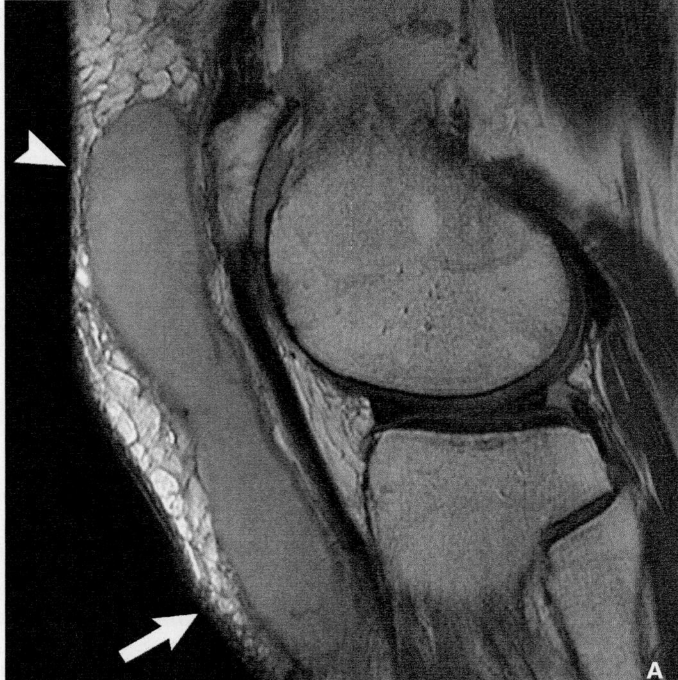

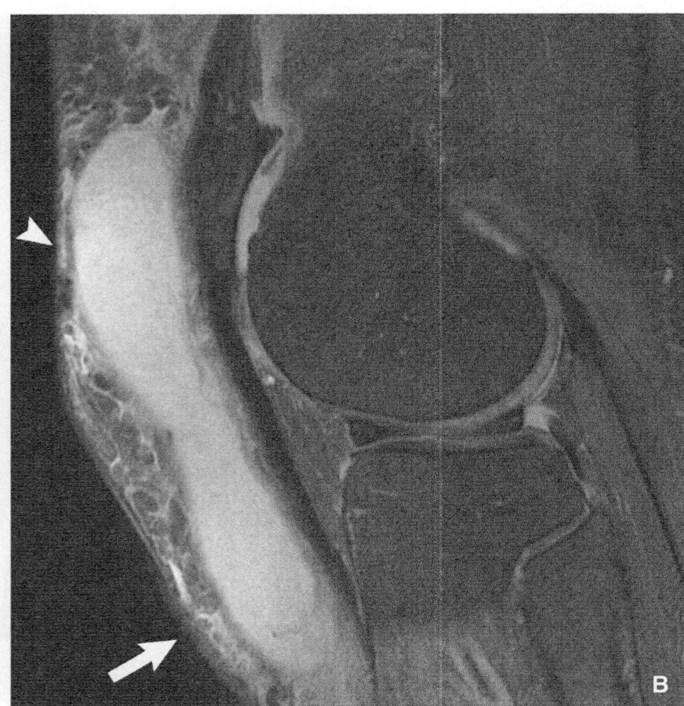

FIGURE 9.80 MRI of prepatellar and superficial infrapatellar bursitis. **(A)** Sagittal proton density–weighted and **(B)** sagittal proton density–weighted fat-suppressed MR images of the knee of a 78-year-old woman show fluid-filled connected and enlarged prepatellar *(arrowheads)* and superficial infrapatellar *(arrows)* bursae.

From the practical point of view, it is useful to use more specific descriptions of the morphology and extension of the tear. Figure 9.83 illustrates a classification based on the orientation and distribution of the meniscal tears and, perhaps more importantly, the presence of displaced meniscal fragments, which indicates instability and requires surgery.

The sensitivity and specificity of MRI for the diagnosis of meniscal tears are high, ranging from 90% to 95% in most studies. A number of signs related to specific types of meniscal tears have been identified. Among the most accurate secondary signs of the bucket-handle tear of the medial meniscus are absence of two consecutive "bow-tie" appearances of this meniscus on sagittal images and the so-called *double posterior cruciate ligament sign*. The normal body of the medial meniscus, which is usually approximately 9 to 12 mm in width, should appear at least on two sections on the peripheral sagittal images as a bow tie. The presence of only a single bow-tie configuration indicates a displaced bucket-handle tear into the middle part of the knee joint. On more central sagittal sections, the displaced part of the meniscus assumes a PCL-like configuration, projecting more anteriorly to the PCL (Fig. 9.84).

Another type of displaced meniscal tear is the "flap" tear. In these tears, a fragment of meniscal tissue is displaced superiorly, inferiorly, or into the intercondylar notch, while still retaining central continuation with the rest of the meniscus (Figs. 9.85 and 9.86).

Radial tears are vertical tears oriented perpendicular to the meniscus in the radial plane. They can be complete, reaching the periphery of the meniscus, or partial, preserving the most peripheral circumferential fibers of the meniscus (Fig. 9.87). A variant of an incomplete radial tear is an oblique radial tear also called *a parrot beak* tear because of its resemblance to a parrot beak on arthroscopic examination (Fig. 9.88). Another variant of a radial tear is the one that occurs at the level of the posterior medial meniscal root ligament (Fig. 9.89). This type of tear is frequently seen in the elderly population, without history of trauma and it may be associated with insufficiency fractures of the medial femoral condyle and intrasubstance degeneration of the meniscus, with meniscal extrusion.

Although meniscal tears are best diagnosed on coronal and sagittal MR images (Fig. 9.90), Lee and colleagues pointed out the effectiveness of axial fat-saturated fast spin echo imaging in demonstrating some tears (Fig. 9.91). In particular, vertical radial and bucket-handle tears and displaced meniscal fragments can be well demonstrated with this technique (see Fig. 9.91; see also Figs. 9.87 and 9.88).

Tears of the lateral meniscus are less common (Fig. 9.92). This has been attributed to the greater degree of mobility of the lateral meniscus because of its rather loose peripheral attachment to the synovium and lack of attachment to the fibular (lateral) collateral ligament. Lateral meniscal tears, however, commonly accompany a developmental anomaly, the so-called *discoid meniscus*, which according to Kaplan is probably related to an abnormal attachment of its posterior horn to the tibial plateau and repetitive abnormal movements, with subsequent enlargement and thickening of meniscal tissue. The discoid meniscus is recognized clinically by a loud clicking sound on flexion and extension of the knee joint and radiographically on the anteroposterior radiograph by an abnormally wide lateral joint compartment (Fig. 9.93). On MRI, the discoid meniscus is similar in appearance to the arthrographic image with a lack of normal triangular shape and deep extension into the interior of the joint. On sagittal images, the normal bow-tie configuration of the body of the lateral meniscus is seen on more than two sections when the discoid variant is present (Figs. 9.94 and 9.95). Because of its abnormal shape and thickness, the lateral discoid meniscus is prone to tears (Figs. 9.96 and 9.97).

Meniscal tears may also be associated with fractures of the tibial plateau resulting from direct trauma. In this case, both menisci are equally subject to injury.

Ligament and Tendon Injuries

Tears of the Medial and Lateral Collateral Ligaments. The most common injury to the ligaments of the knee is tear of the MCL (tibial collateral ligament). It is diagnosed clinically by instability of the medial joint compartment and radiographically on a stress film of the knee by widening of the medial tibiofemoral joint compartment (Fig. 9.98). It is important to remember that partial or total tear of the MCL is almost always associated with tear of the joint capsule because these two structures are intimately attached to each other.

As the ligament heals, the fibrous tissue may calcify and later ossify, giving a characteristic appearance on the anteroposterior radiograph of the knee known as the *Pellegrini-Stieda lesion/disease*. The presence of this abnormality is virtually diagnostic of previous tear of the MCL (Fig. 9.99;

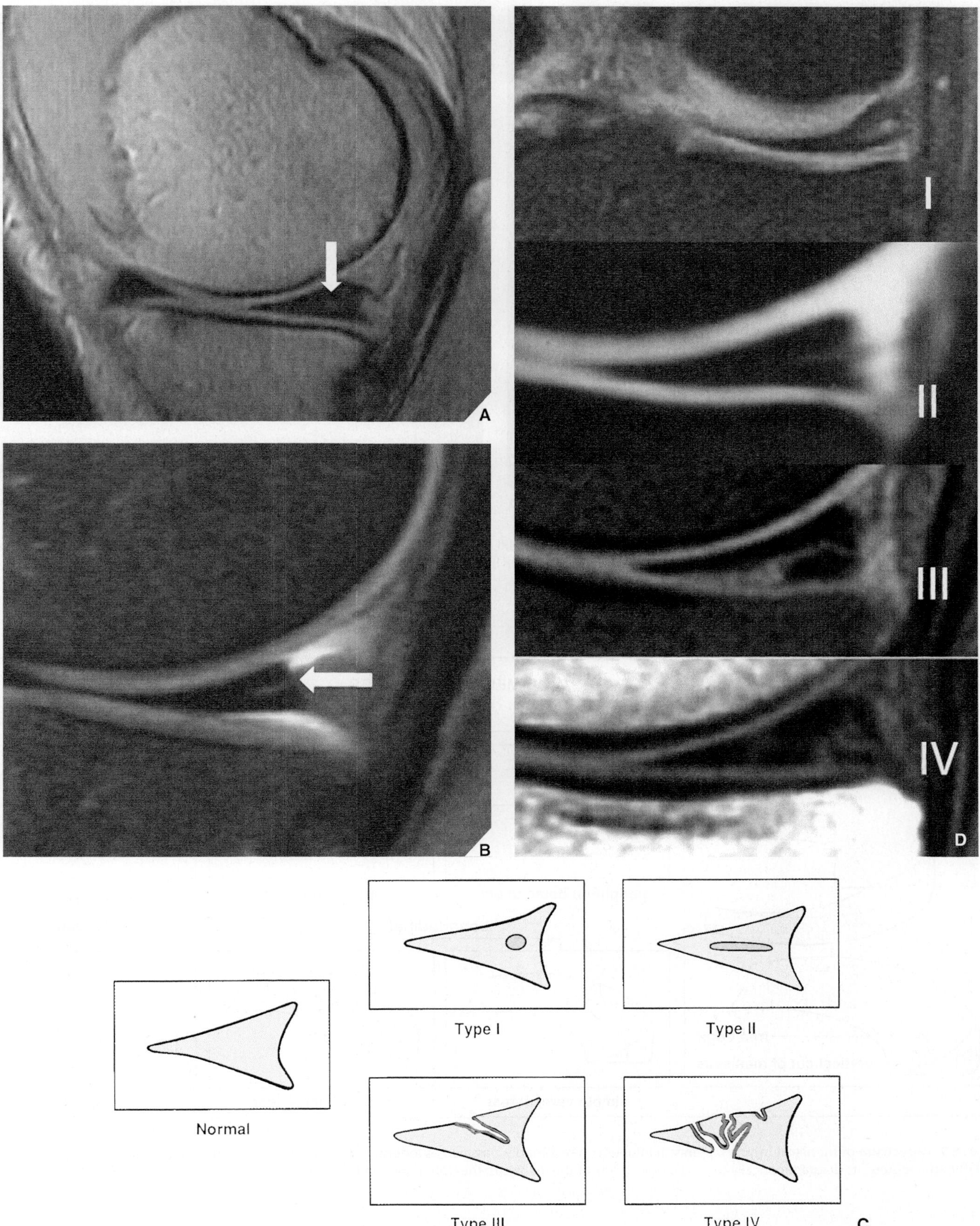

FIGURE 9.81 Classification of meniscal lesions. (A) Sagittal spin echo MR image (SE; repetition time [TR] 2000/TE 20 msec) shows a type I lesion of the posterior horn of the medial meniscus *(arrow)*, most likely representing intrasubstance degeneration. The intrameniscal round lesion does not extend to the articular surface. **(B)** In a type II lesion of the posterior horn of the medial meniscus *(arrow)*, the configuration is linear, most likely represents a longitudinal bundle of collagen fibers, and as with a type I, the lesion does not extend into the articular surface. **(C)** Schematic representation of various types of meniscal lesions. Types I and II do not correlate with arthroscopic demonstration of meniscal tears, whereas types III and IV have high correlation with meniscal tears demonstrated at arthroscopic surgery. **(D)** MRI demonstration of the four types of meniscal lesions.

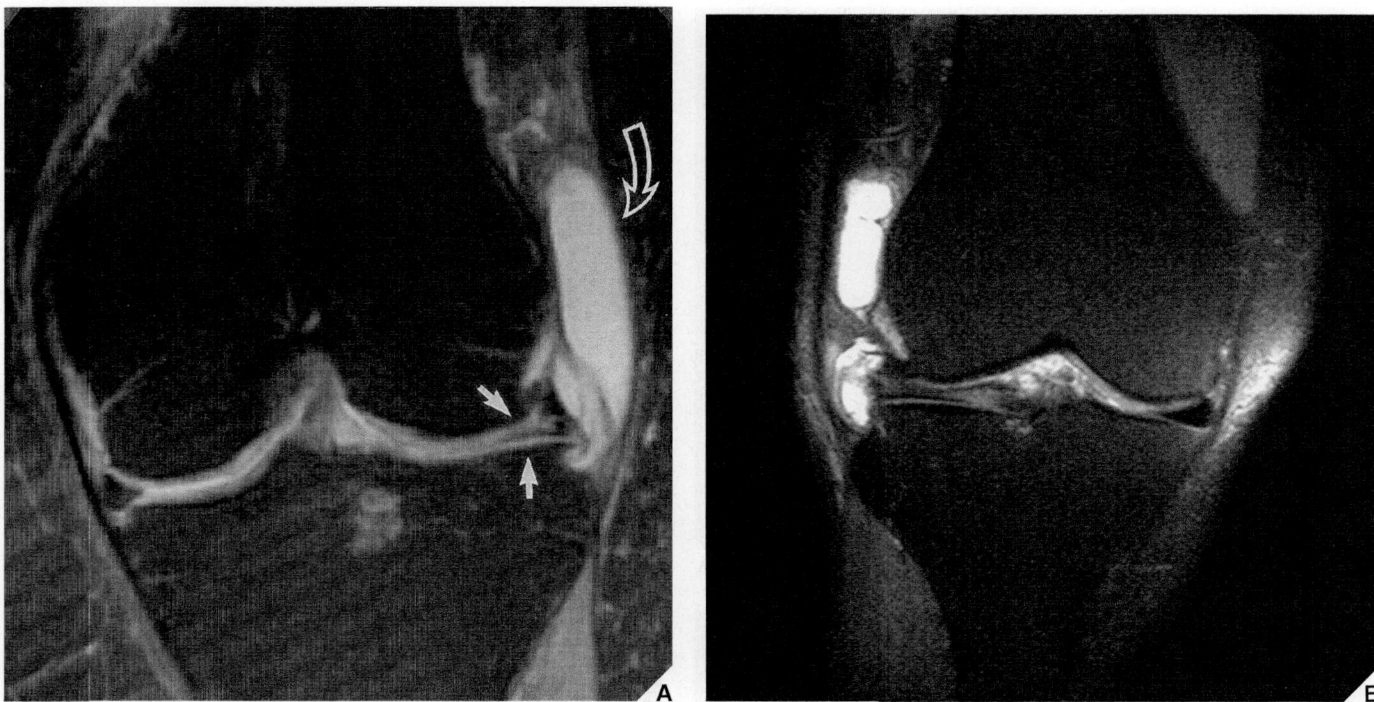

FIGURE 9.82 Parameniscal cyst. **(A)** Coronal T2-weighted fat-suppressed MRI shows a tear of the medial meniscus *(arrows)* and a large parameniscal cyst *(curved arrow)*. **(B)** In another patient, a coronal proton density–weighted fat-suppressed MR image demonstrates a tear of the lateral meniscus and a large parameniscal cyst.

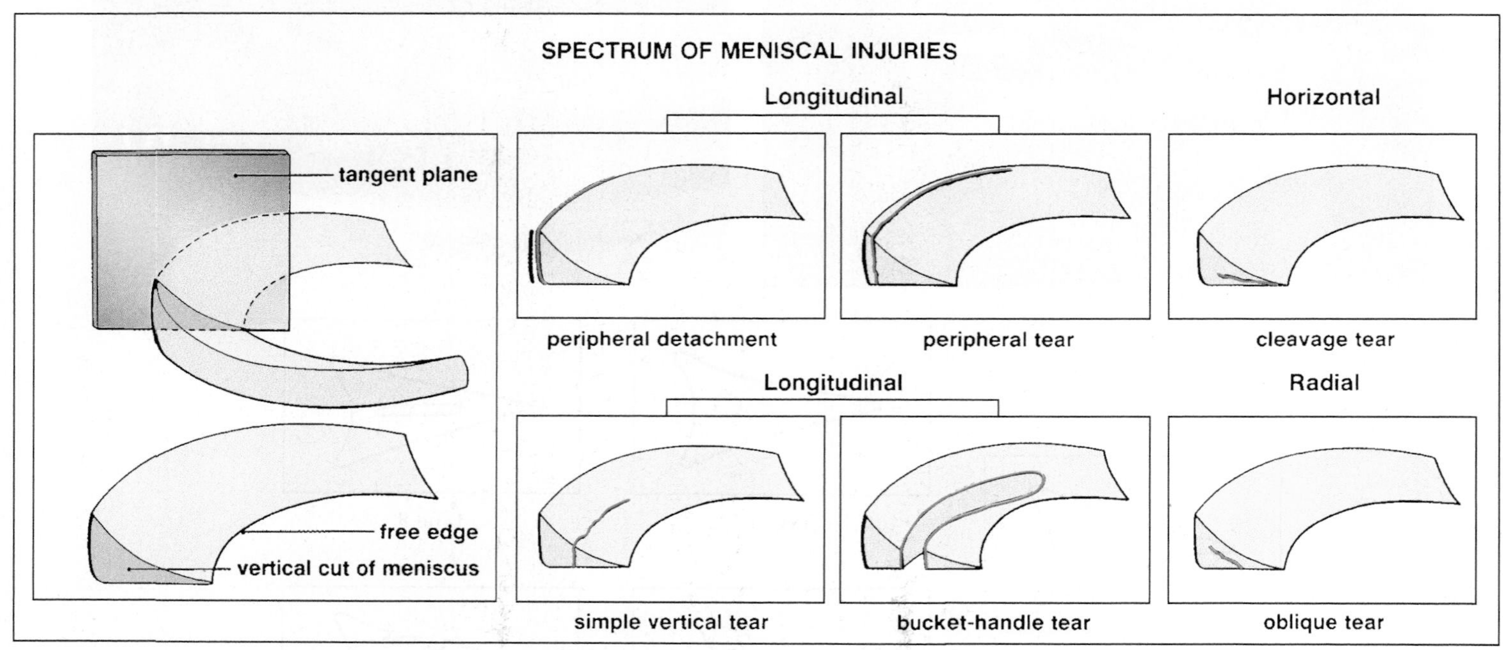

FIGURE 9.83 Spectrum of meniscal injuries. Meniscal injuries can be broadly classified as longitudinal, horizontal, and radial, depending on the plane in which they occur. The left panel represents diagrammatically the radiologic image of the meniscus; the right panel, various tears.

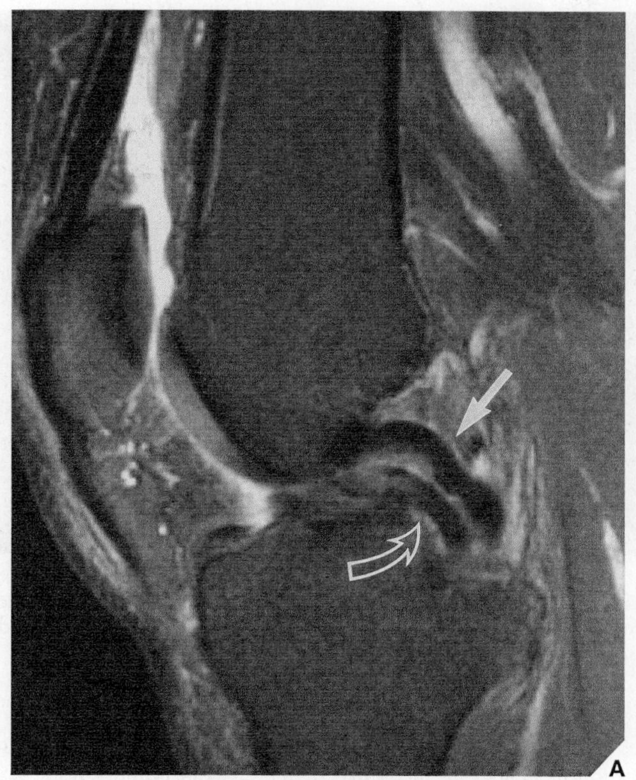

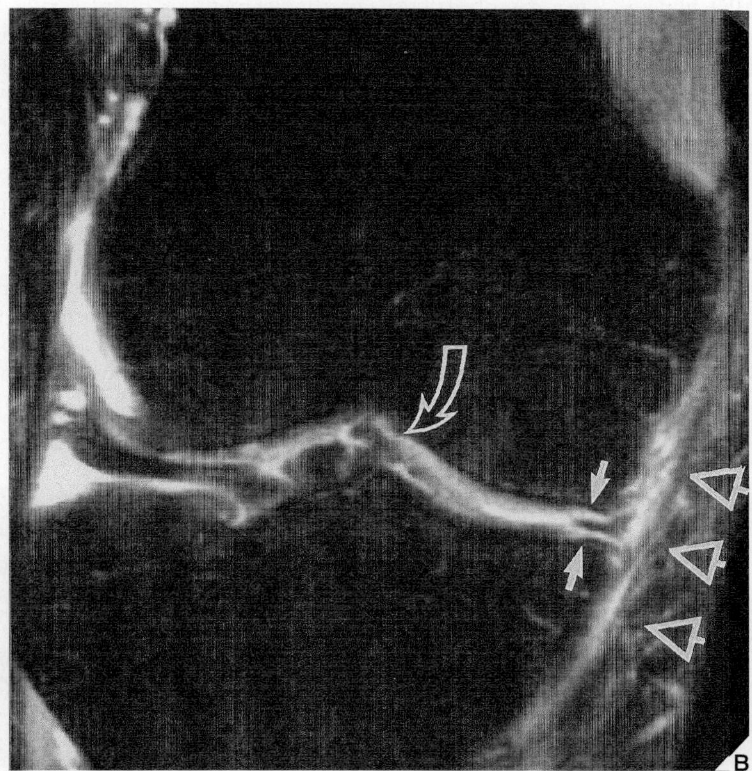

FIGURE 9.84 Bucket-handle tear of the medial meniscus. **(A)** Sagittal T2-weighted fat-suppressed MRI shows a double PCL sign. An *arrow* points to the normal PCL and a *curved arrow* points to the displaced fragment of the medial meniscus that assumed configuration of the PCL. **(B)** Coronal T2-weighted fat-saturated MR image confirms the presence of a bucket-handle tear of the medial meniscus *(arrows)*. A *curved arrow* points to the medially displaced part of the meniscus. Note also a tear of the MCL *(open arrowheads)*.

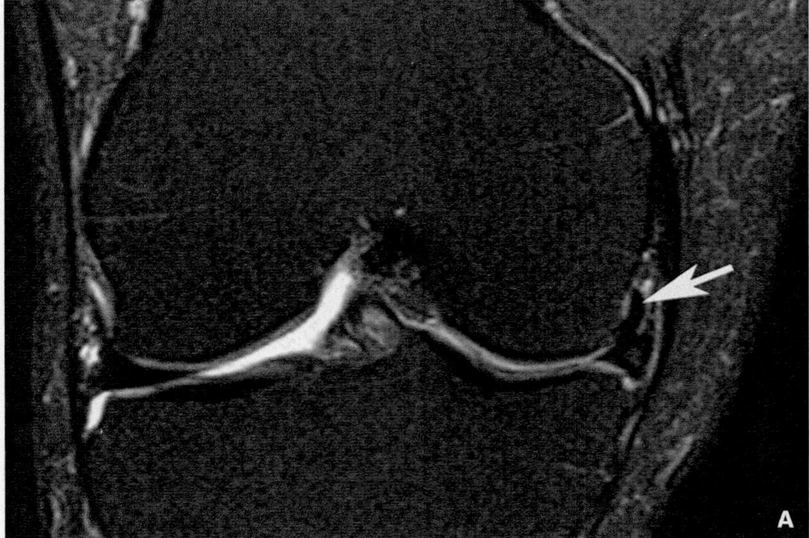

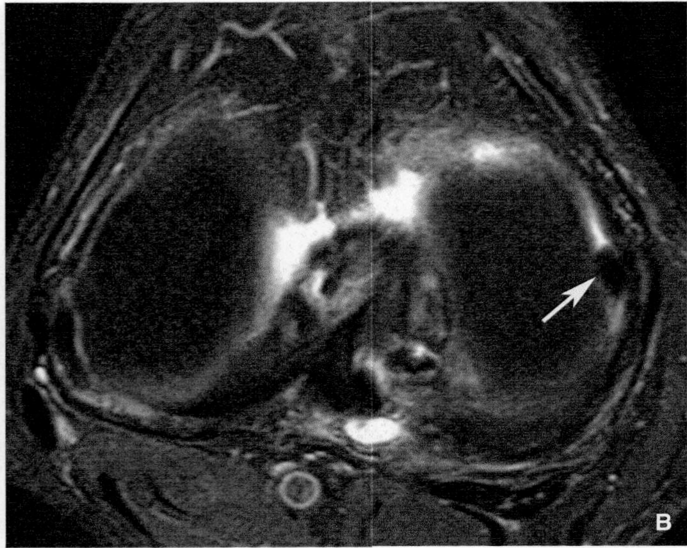

FIGURE 9.85 Flap tear of the medial meniscus. **(A)** Coronal and **(B)** axial T2-weighted fat-saturated MR images demonstrate a superiorly displaced flap of meniscal tissue *(arrows)*. These types of displaced tears may not be easily identified during arthroscopy; therefore, it is important to describe the location of the "flap" of meniscal tissue on the MRI report.

see also Fig. 4.128B). Mendes and colleagues have undertaken a study to determine the nature of ossification/calcification in Pellegrini-Stieda disease, based on the radiographic and MRI findings. They described four distinctive patterns: (a) a beak-like appearance with an inferior orientation, parallel to the femur; (b) a drop-like appearance with an inferior orientation, parallel to the femur; (c) an elongated appearance with a superior orientation, parallel to the femur; and (d) a beak-like appearance with an inferior and superior orientation, attached to the femur. The ossification was present either within the MCL, within the adductor magnus tendon, or in both of these structures. McAnally and colleagues contended that in addition to the previously reported sites of ossification, this abnormality may also be secondary to associated medial femoral epicondylar periosteal stripping, proximal to the femoral attachment of MCL. Furthermore, this condition appears to be associated with a complete tear of the PCL.

Abnormalities of the medial and lateral collateral ligaments can be demonstrated effectively with MRI, with coronal T2-weighted sequences being most revealing. These ligamentous injuries are commonly subclassified into three grades. Grade 1 is diagnosed if only a few fibers are disrupted. Grade 2 is diagnosed with disruption of up to 50% of the ligamentous fibers. Grade 3 is a complete tear of the ligament. Sprain of the MCL is depicted on MRI as thickening of this structure associated with slightly increased internal signal caused by intraligamentous edema and hemorrhage. Fluid may be present on both sides of the ligament. Partial tear is diagnosed when abnormal increased signal intensity is identified within the ligament substance, extending into the superficial or deep surface. A complete tear exhibits discontinuity of the normally low–signal intensity ligament structure. It is usually associated with marked thickening and serpentine contours of the affected ligament (Figs. 9.100 and 9.101). The injury to the lateral collateral ligament is best demonstrated on the posterior coronal images. Edema and hemorrhage are seen as ligamentous thickening associated with increased signal intensity on T2-weighted or T2*-weighted images. A complete tear exhibits a wavy contour of the ligament and loss of its continuity (Fig. 9.102).

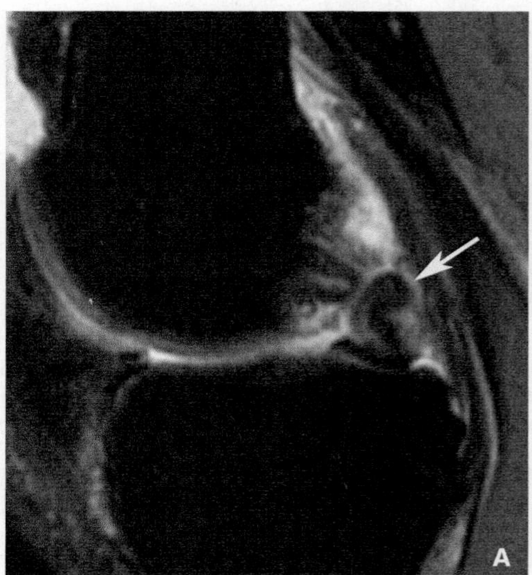

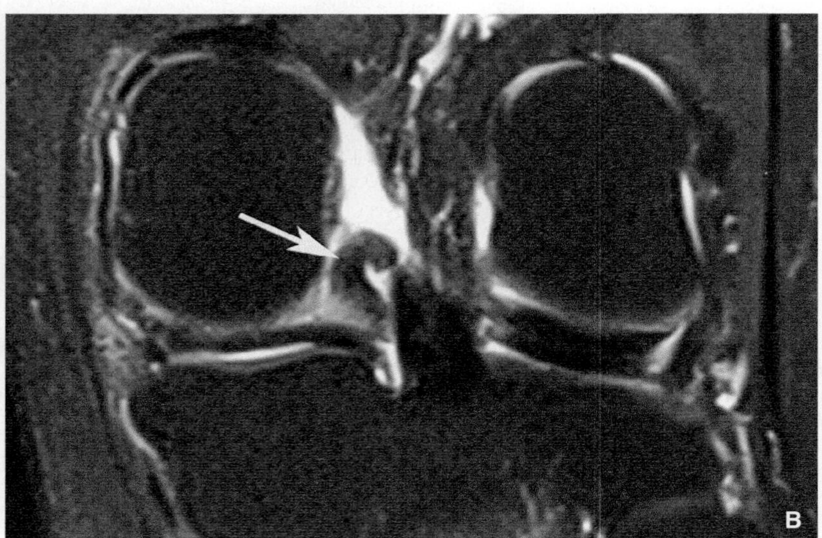

FIGURE 9.86 Flap tear of the medial meniscus. **(A)** Sagittal and **(B)** coronal T2-weighted fat-saturated MR images demonstrate a displaced fragment of meniscal tissue into the intercondylar notch *(arrows)*. The displaced fragment maintains its connection with the posterior horn of the medial meniscus. In fact, this type of "flap" tear displaced to the intercondylar notch represents a variant of a bucket-handle tear, where the anterior junction with the meniscus has become detached allowing the medial fragment to move freely, but still "hinged" with the posterior horn.

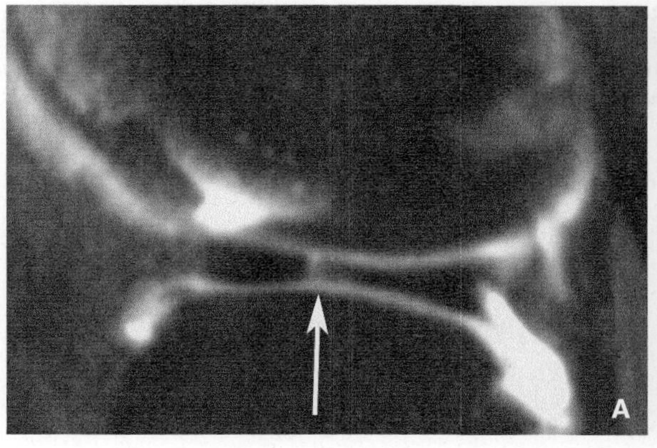

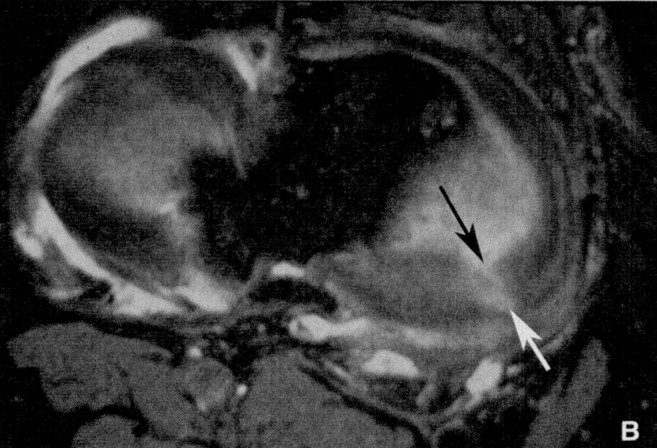

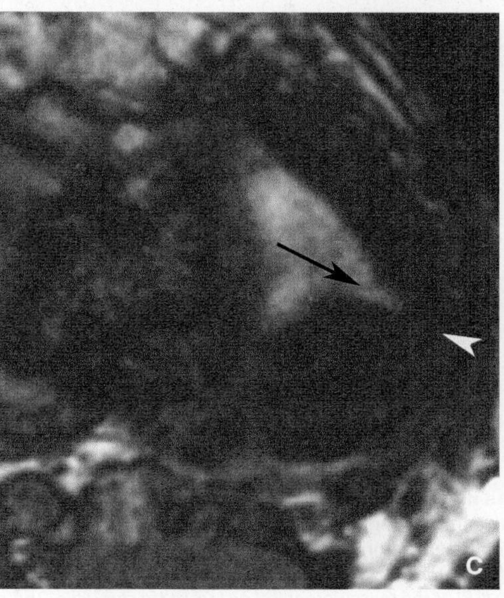

FIGURE 9.87 **Radial tear of the lateral and medial menisci.** **(A)** Sagittal T1-weighted fat-saturated MRa image shows a radial tear of the body of the lateral meniscus *(arrow)*. **(B)** Axial T2-weighted fat-saturated MR image in another patient shows a complete radial tear of the posterior horn of the medial meniscus *(arrows)*, extending to the most peripheral circumferential fibers. **(C)** Axial gradient recalled echo (GRE) MR image in another patient shows an incomplete radial tear of the posterior horn of the medial meniscus *(arrow)*, with preservation of the peripheral circumferential fibers *(arrowhead)*.

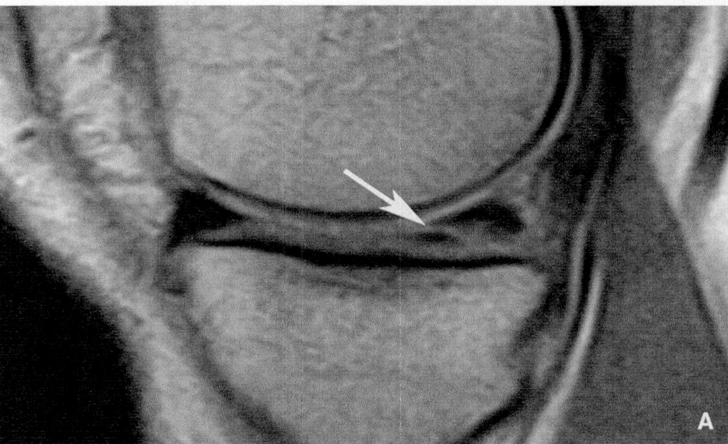

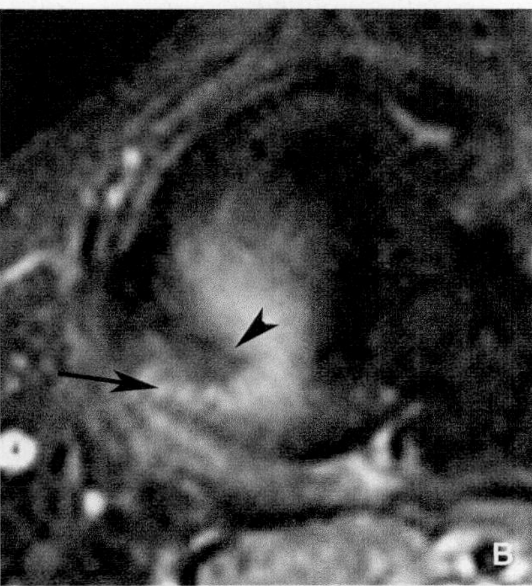

FIGURE 9.88 **Parrot beak tear.** **(A)** Sagittal proton density–weighted image and **(B)** axial T2-weighted fat-saturated MR image of the knee demonstrate an oblique tear of the posterior horn of the medial meniscus *(arrows)*. Note the "parrot beak" shape on the axial image *(arrowhead)*.

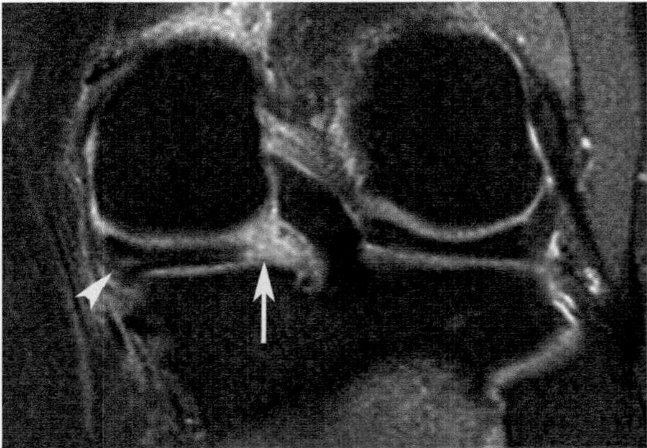

FIGURE 9.89 **Medial meniscal posterior root ligament tear.** Coronal proton density–weighted fat-saturated MR image through the posterior horns of the menisci demonstrates a tear of the medial meniscal posterior root ligament *(arrow)* with intrasubstance degeneration of the posterior horn *(arrowhead)*.

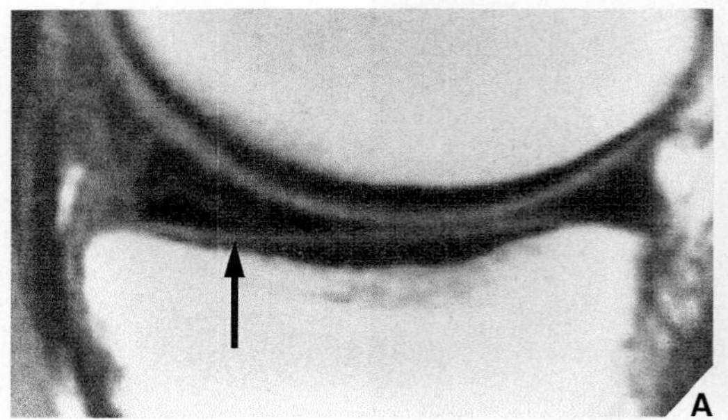

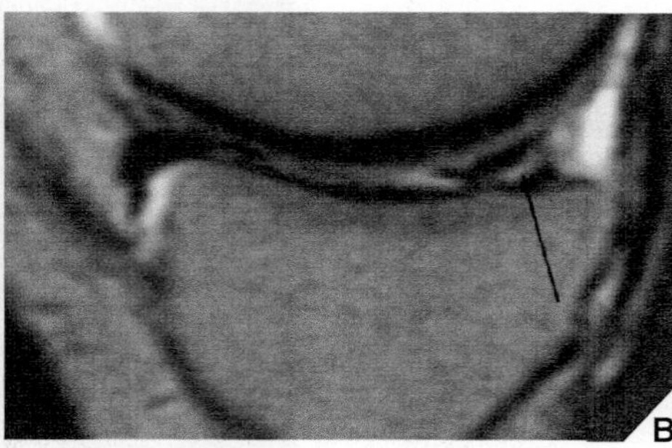

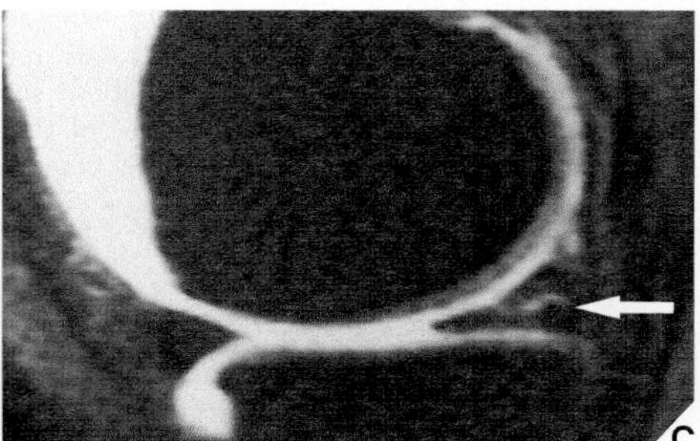

FIGURE 9.90 **Tears of the medial meniscus.** **(A)** Sagittal spin echo T1-weighted MR image (spin echo [SE]; repetition time [TR] 700/TE 20 msec) shows a tear of the medial meniscus. Note the high-intensity signal of the tear, which extends into the inferior surface of the meniscus *(arrow)*. **(B)** Sagittal T2-weighted MR image (SE; TR 2300/TE 80 msec) shows a tear of the posterior horn of the medial meniscus *(arrow)* extending into the tibial articular surface. **(C)** Sagittal fat-suppressed MR image obtained after intraarticular administration of a dilute solution of gadopentetate dimeglumine shows a tear of the posterior horn of the medial meniscus *(arrow)*. (Reprinted with permission from Deutsch AL, Mink JH, eds. *MRI of the musculoskeletal system: a teaching file*, 2nd ed. Philadelphia: Lippincott-Raven; 1997.)

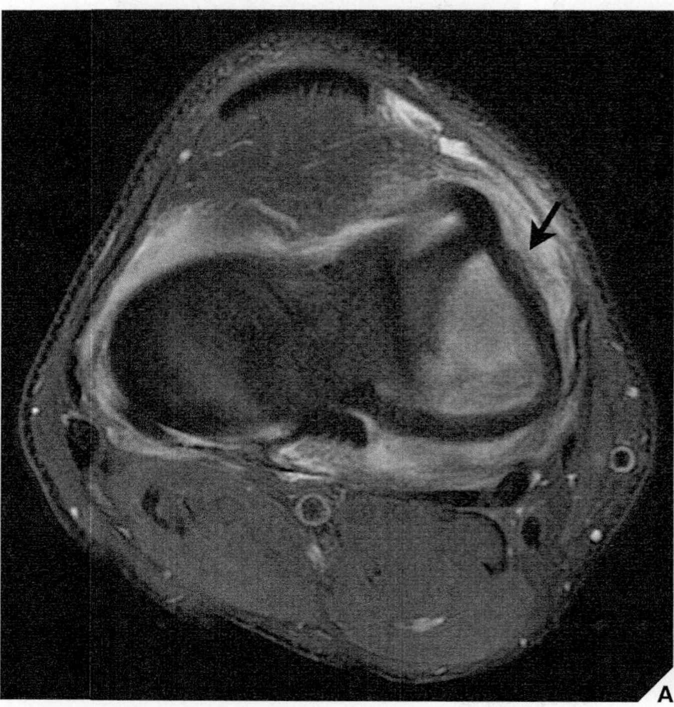

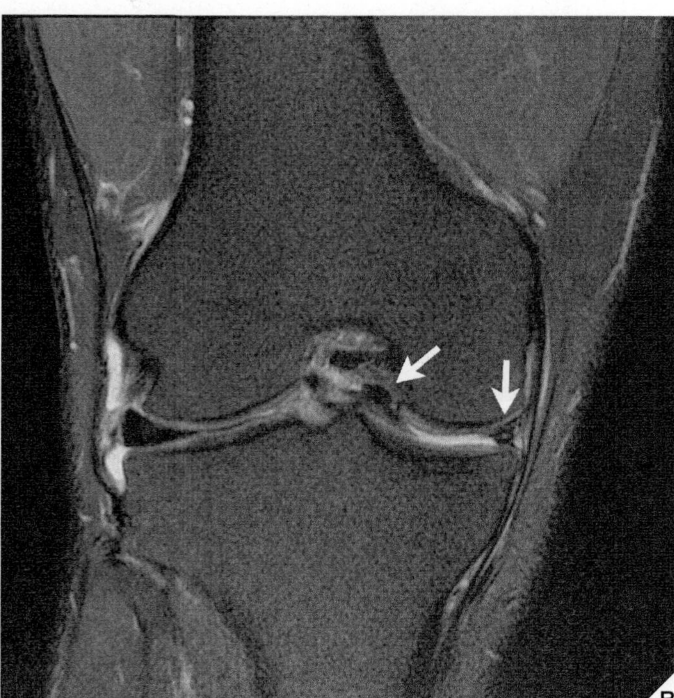

FIGURE 9.91 **Tear of the medial meniscus.** **(A)** Axial proton density–weighted fat-suppressed MR image shows a bucket-handle tear of the medial meniscus *(arrow)* confirmed on the coronal proton density–weighted fat-suppressed MRI *(arrows)* **(B)**.

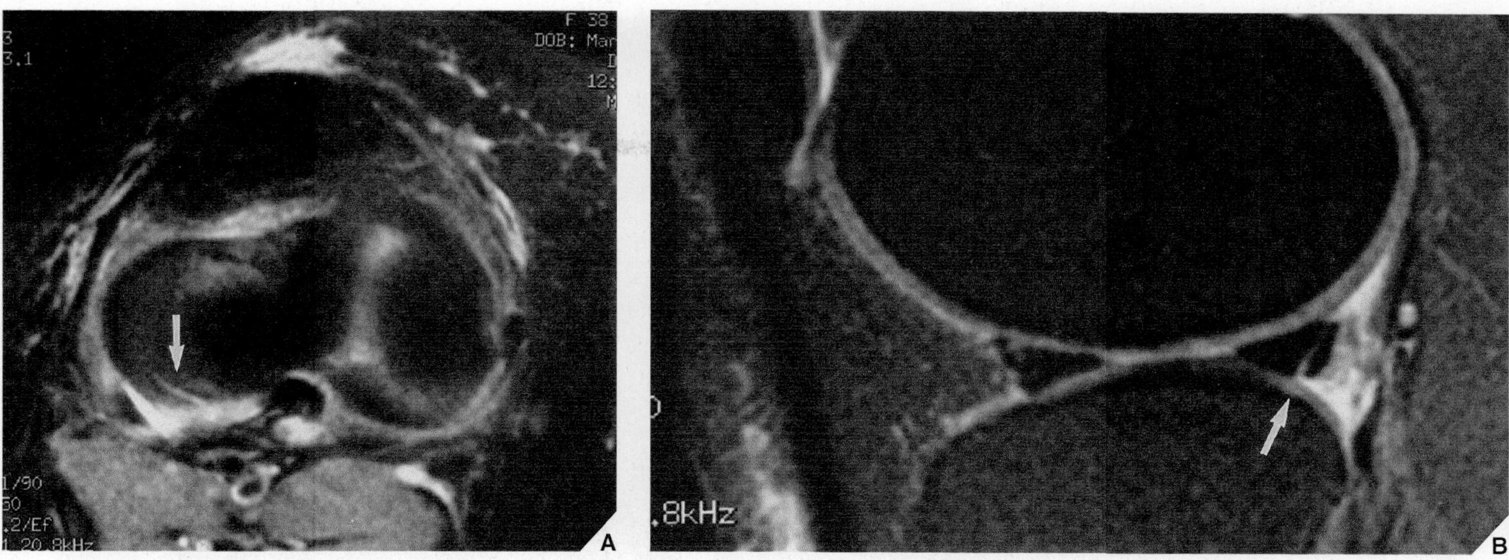

FIGURE 9.92 **Tear of the lateral meniscus.** **(A)** Axial fast spin echo MRI shows a tear of the posterior horn of the lateral meniscus *(arrow)* in a 38-year-old woman. **(B)** Sagittal MR image confirms the presence of a tear *(arrow)*.

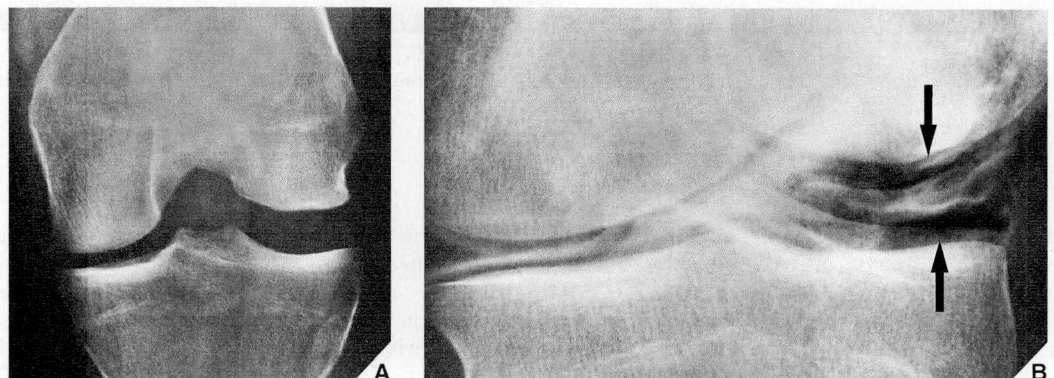

FIGURE 9.93 **Discoid meniscus.** A 20-year-old competition ice skater sustained an injury to her left knee. On physical examination, there was a loud click during movement of the knee joint. **(A)** Anteroposterior radiograph of the knee shows an abnormally wide lateral joint compartment. **(B)** Double-contrast arthrogram demonstrates a discoid meniscus *(arrows)*. Note the absence of the normal triangular shape of this structure and its extension deep into the interior of the joint. No tear is apparent.

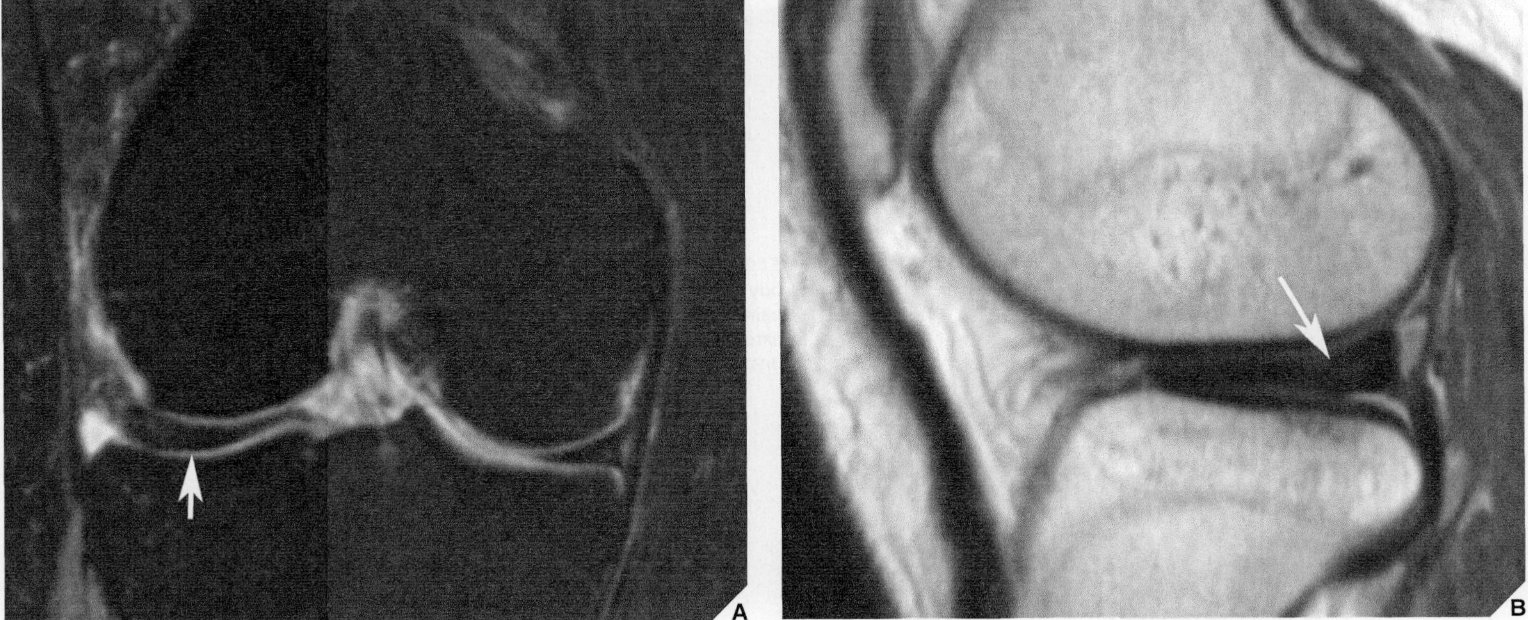

FIGURE 9.94 **MRI of the discoid meniscus.** **(A)** Coronal T2-weighted fat-saturated and **(B)** sagittal proton density–weighted MR images demonstrate thickening of the body of the lateral meniscus *(arrows)*. Note the lack of normal triangular shape of the meniscus.

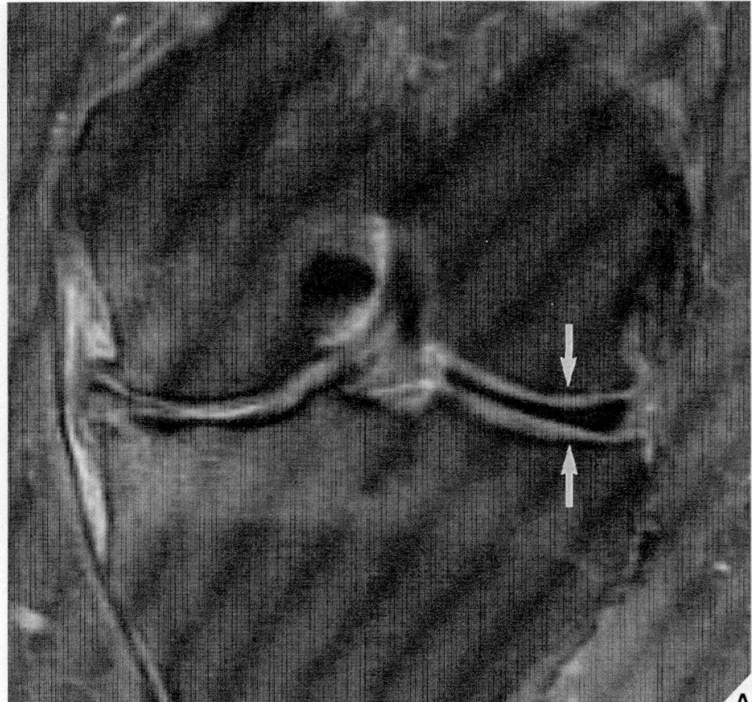

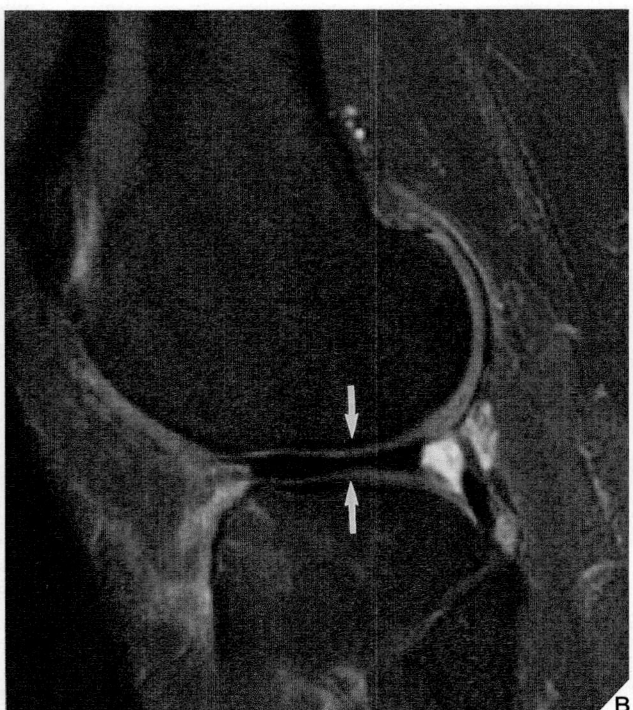

FIGURE 9.95 MRI of the discoid meniscus. **(A)** Coronal and **(B)** sagittal T2-weighted fat-suppressed MR images show a lateral discoid meniscus *(arrows)* in an 18-year-old woman.

Tears of the Cruciate Ligaments. Isolated injuries to the cruciate ligaments, which are usually the result of internal rotation of the leg combined with hyperextension, are uncommon. They are more often associated with another ligament injury (usually to the MCL) and meniscal tears (usually of the medial meniscus). This association of injuries has been called the unhappy O'Donoghue triad. Valgus stress on the knee joint opens the medial joint compartment and may result in tear of the posterior joint capsule as well as the PCL or ACL. This stress is also responsible for tear of the medial meniscus and MCL (Fig. 9.103).

The accuracy of radiographic examinations with respect to injury to the cruciate ligaments has not been completely determined. The standard anteroposterior and lateral radiographs may show a bone fragment, representing the avulsed intercondylar eminence of the tibia, at the site of cruciate insertion (Fig. 9.104).

For MR examination of the ACL, the knee should be placed in 10 to 15 degrees of external rotation to orient the ligament with the sagittal imaging plane. Either 3- or 5-mm thin contiguous sections are routinely obtained in axial, sagittal, and coronal planes. Alternatively, oblique coronal T2-weighted images along the longitudinal axis of the ACL can be obtained (see Fig. 9.12B). A torn ACL is demonstrated on MR images by the absence or abnormal course of this structure (Fig. 9.105), abnormal signal intensity within the ligamentous substance (Fig. 9.106), or the presence of an edematous focus (Fig. 9.107). The buckling of the PCL is an indirect sign of ACL tear. The best plane to demonstrate these findings is the sagittal plane, and the best pulse sequence is spin-echo T2 weighting with fat saturation.

Tears of the PCL are identified on sagittal T1-weighted images by disruption of the integrity of the ligament or by abnormal shape. On T2-weighted images, the tear is demonstrated by the presence of high signal intensity within the ligament, which represents fluid within the tear (Fig. 9.108). As Bassett and coworkers have pointed out, avulsion of the ligament from its tibial attachment is identified on MR images by bone fracture of the posterior tibial plateau and redundancy of the ligament.

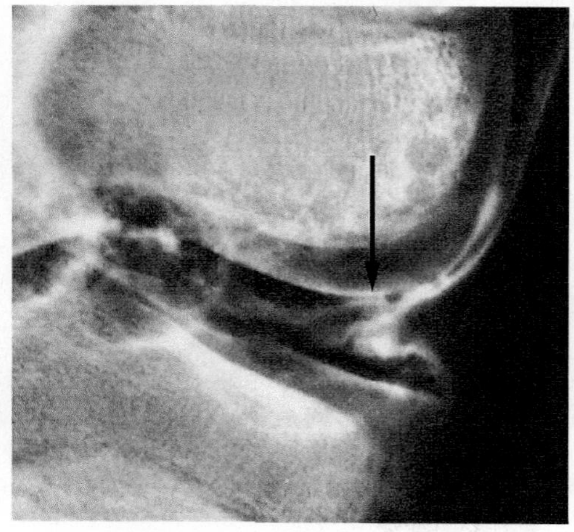

FIGURE 9.96 Tear of the discoid meniscus. A 10-year-old boy twisted his right knee during play and experienced severe pain. On physical examination, there was a loud click on flexion–extension of the knee joint. Double-contrast arthrogram demonstrates a tear of the body of a lateral discoid meniscus *(arrow)*.

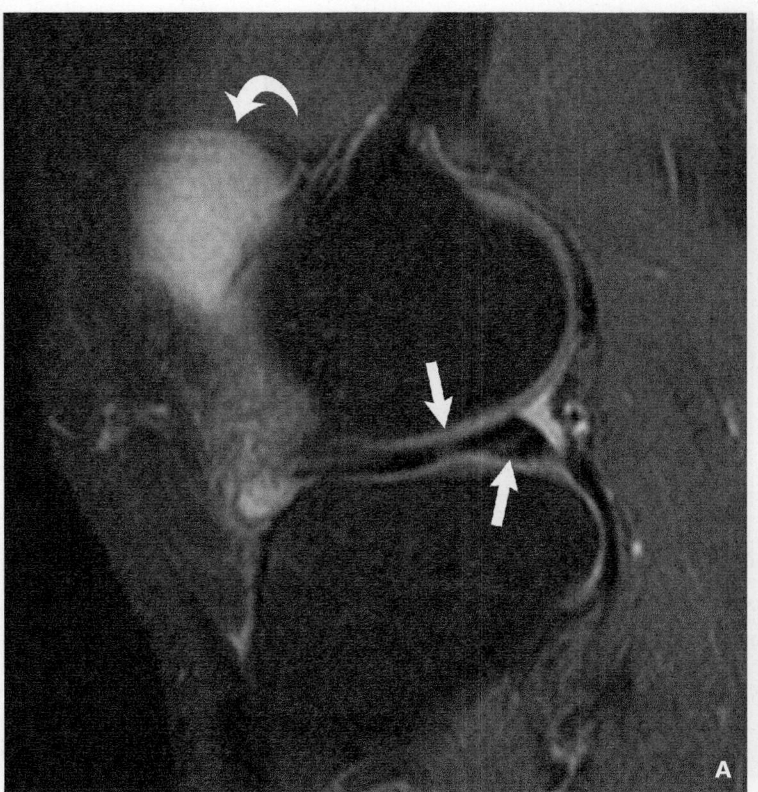

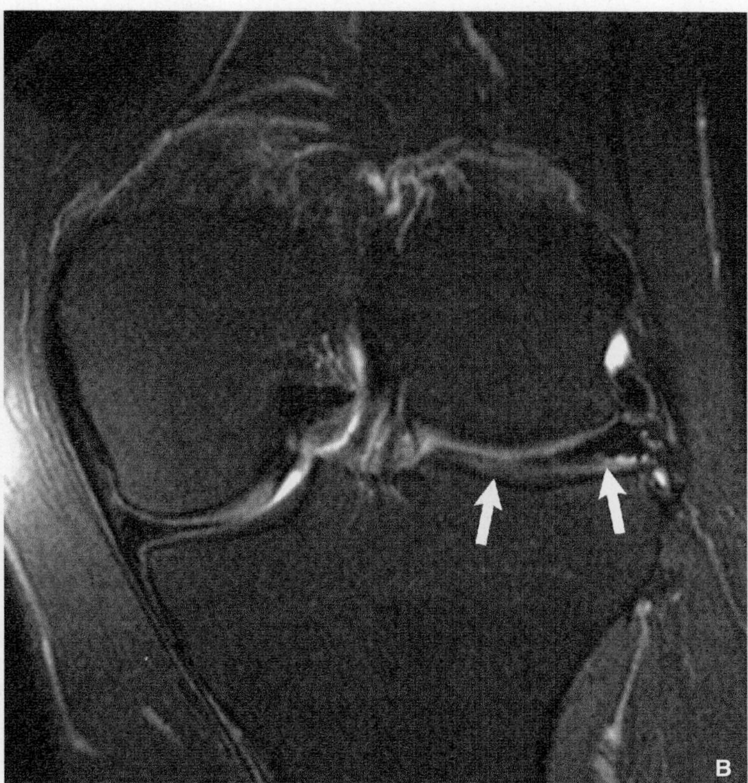

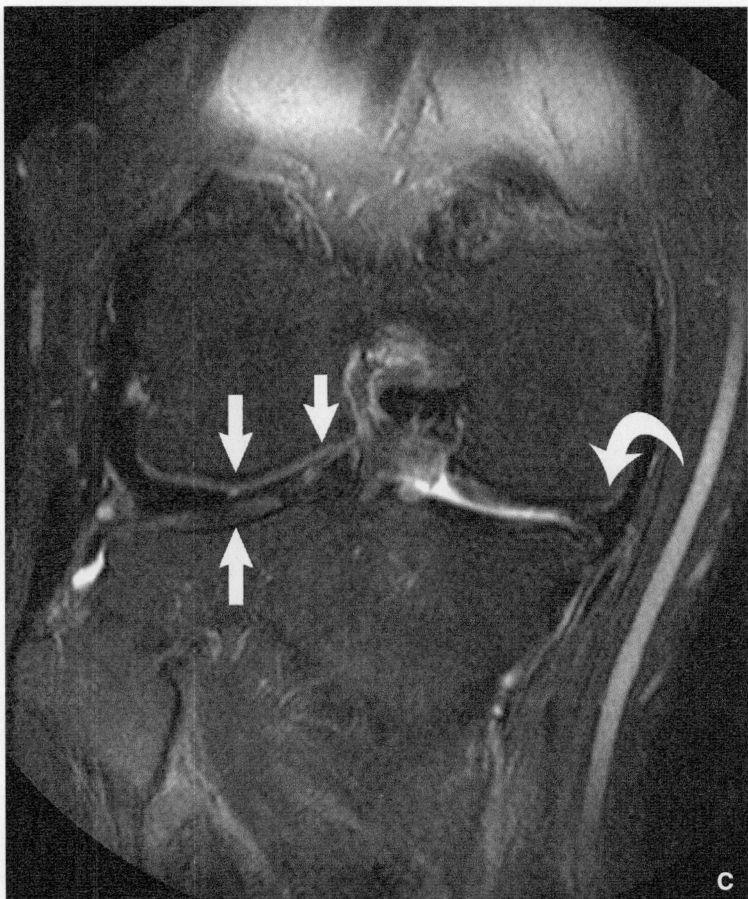

FIGURE 9.97 **MRI of the tear of the discoid meniscus.** A 28-year-old woman twisted her left knee during a dancing competition. **(A)** Sagittal and **(B)** coronal proton density–weighted fat-saturated MR images show a complex tear of the lateral discoid meniscus *(arrows)*. A *curved arrow* points to the joint effusion. **(C)** In another patient, a 24-year-old man, who presented with sudden onset of pain in his right knee, coronal proton-weighted fat-saturated MR image shows a tear of the lateral discoid meniscus *(arrows)*. Note also tear of the body of the medial meniscus *(curved arrow)*.

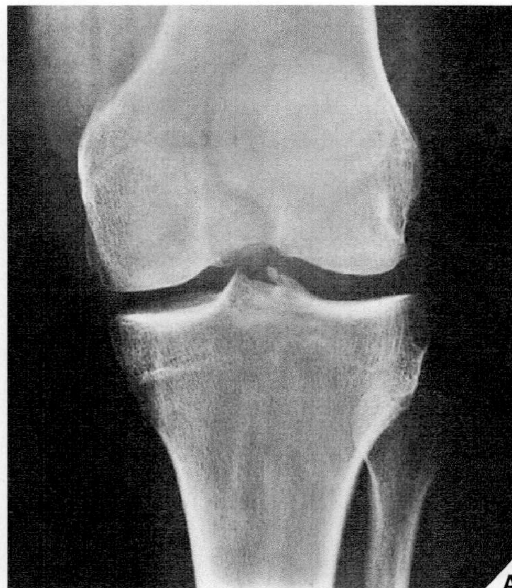

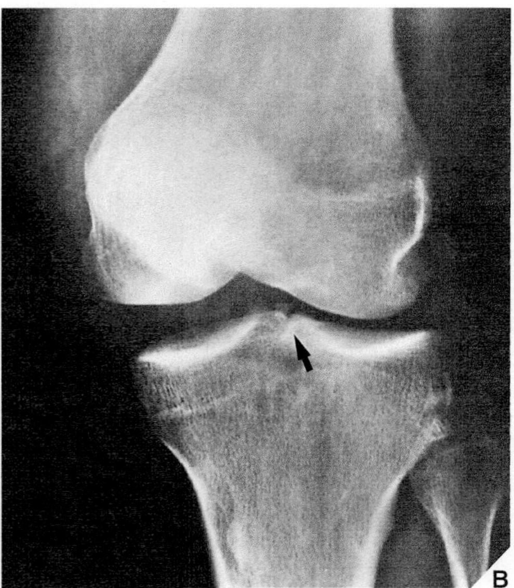

FIGURE 9.98 Tear of the MCL. A 24-year-old athlete twisted his knee while throwing the discus during field competition. Physical examination revealed tenderness in the medial aspect of the knee joint and medial instability. **(A)** Anteroposterior radiograph of the left knee shows the width of the medial and lateral joint compartments to be normal. **(B)** The same projection obtained after application of valgus stress shows widening of the medial joint compartment, a finding consistent with the clinical diagnosis of tear of the MCL. Note also the avulsion of the lateral tibial tubercle *(arrow)*, which is occasionally associated with tear of the ACL.

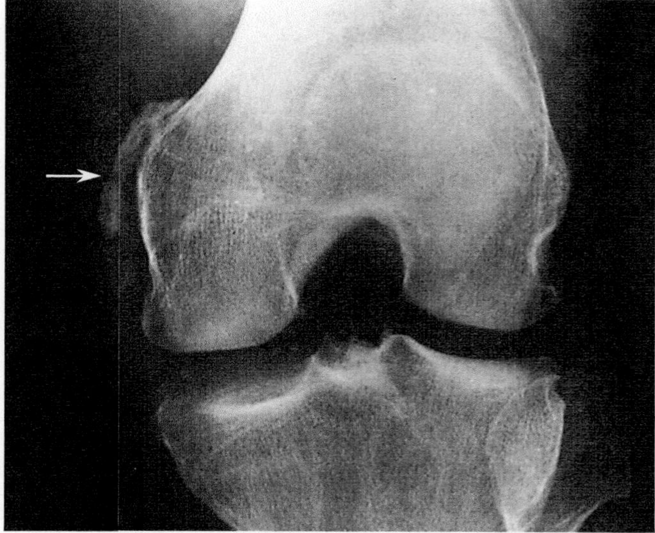

FIGURE 9.99 Pellegrini-Stieda lesion. A 50-year-old man presented with a history of injury, including tear of the MCL 3 years previously. Tunnel view of the left knee shows the typical appearance of the Pellegrini-Stieda lesion—calcification and ossification at the site of the femoral attachment of the MCL *(arrow)* (see also Fig. 4.128B).

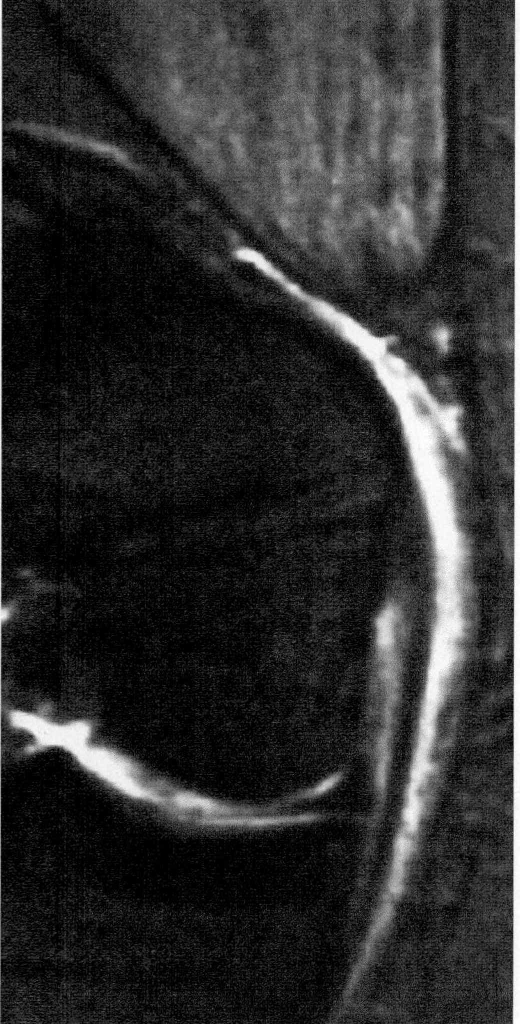

FIGURE 9.100 Grade 1 MCL injury. A coronal gradient recalled echo (GRE) MR image of the right knee shows fluid surrounding the superficial fibers of the MCL with an otherwise intact ligament.

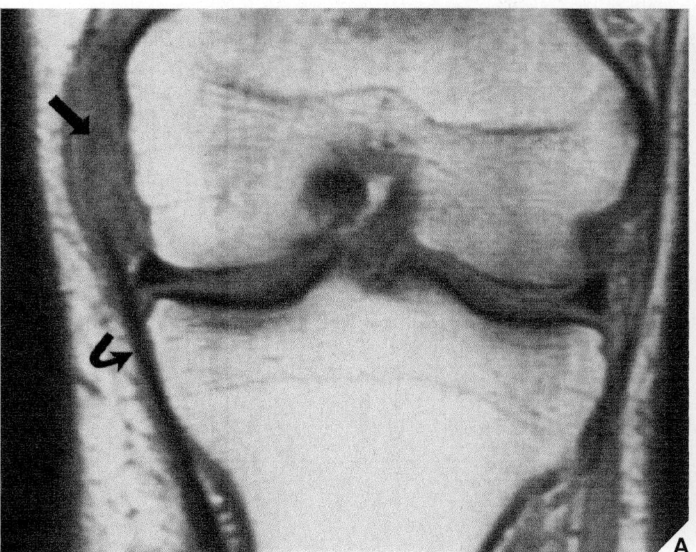

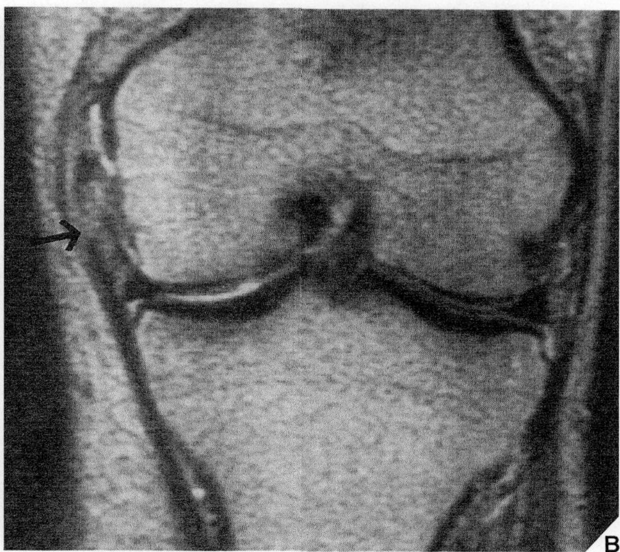

FIGURE 9.101 Grade 3 MCL injury. **(A)** Coronal proton density–weighted (spin echo [SE]; TR 2000/TE 20 msec) MR image of the left knee shows amorphous structure of intermediate signal intensity replacing the proximal attachment of the MCL *(arrow)*. The distal part of the ligament is intact *(curved arrow)*. **(B)** Coronal T2-weighted (SE; TR 2000/TE 80 msec) MR image shows mildly increased signal intensity within the region of the proximal segment of the MCL, representing a combination of edema and hemorrhage *(arrow)*. The underlying ligament cannot be defined. (Reprinted with permission from Bloem JL, Sartoris DJ, eds. *MRI and CT of the musculoskeletal system. A text-atlas*. Baltimore: Williams Wilkins; 1992.)

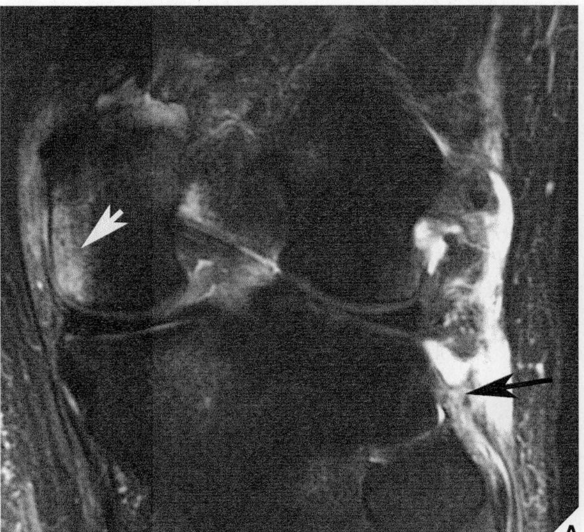

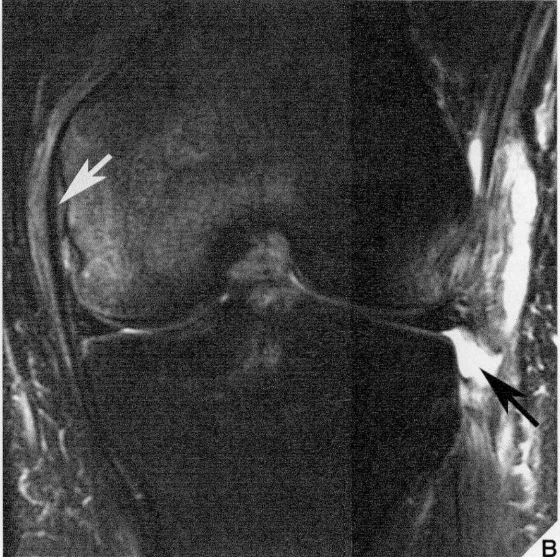

FIGURE 9.102 Tear of the lateral collateral ligament. A 23-year-old man presented with history of acute, severe sports-related injury. **(A)** Coronal proton density–weighted fat-saturated MRI of the left knee demonstrates complete rupture of the lateral collateral ligament *(black arrow)* with focal hematoma in the lateral posterior aspect of the knee. There is no associated meniscal tear. Note the bone contusion of the medial femoral condyle *(short white arrow)* and the absence of the cruciate ligaments in the intercondylar notch indicating rupture of the ACL and PCL. **(B)** More anteriorly obtained coronal MR image demonstrates a tear of the iliotibial band *(black arrow)* and a low-grade sprain of the MCL *(white arrow)*. Note again the absence of the ACL and PCL in the intercondylar notch.

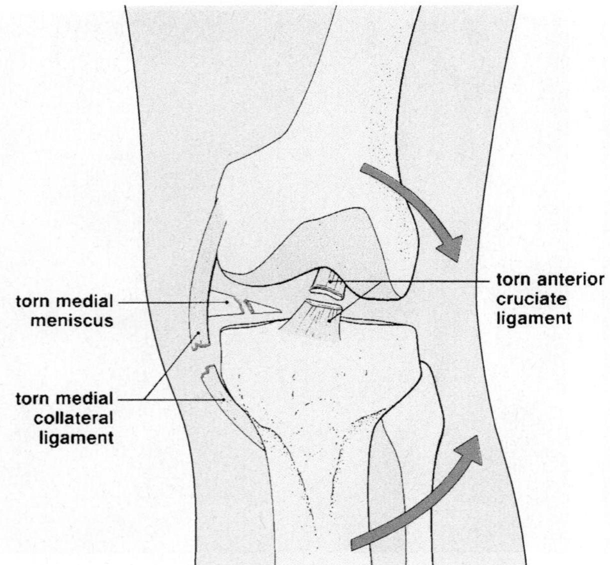

FIGURE 9.103 Triad of meniscoligamentous injury. The unhappy O'Donoghue triad results from valgus stress on the knee joint that causes the medial joint compartment to open. The triad comprises tears of the medial meniscus and the ACL and the MCL. (Modified from O'Donoghue DH. *Treatment of injuries to athletes,* 4th ed. Philadelphia: Saunders; 1984. Copyright © 1984 Elsevier. With permission.)

Posterolateral Corner Injuries. The posterolateral corner (PLC) of the knee is a complex unit consisting of several anatomic structures responsible for knee joint stabilization. They include popliteal tendon, the lateral collateral ligament, the PFL, and the posterolateral capsule, which is reinforced by the arcuate and fabellofibular ligaments. The most common mechanisms of injury to the PLC are a hyperextension injury (contact and noncontact), external rotation direct trauma to the anteromedial aspect of the knee, and noncontact varus force to the knee. Trauma to PLC, in addition to tears of the previously listed structures, usually is associated with injuries to the cruciate ligaments, both menisci, and MCL. MRI is the technique of choice when the PLC injuries are clinically suspected (Fig. 9.109). The popliteofibular ligament is significant for the stability of the posterolateral aspect of the knee and its integrity should be assessed with MRI in those patients presenting with signs of PLC injury. The normal popliteofibular ligament is seen on MRI as a hypointense linear or curvilinear structure extending from the popliteal tendon to the head of the fibula. This is well seen on the coronal or sagittal images (see Fig. 9.109).

Tears of the Quadriceps Tendon and Patellar Ligament. Under normal conditions, the balance of forces on the patellar ligamentous-tendinous attachments maintains the patella in proper position. Tear of the quadriceps tendon (which is a conjoint tendon formed by tendinous contributions from the rectus femoris, vastus lateralis, vastus medialis, and vastus intermedius muscles) or patellar ligament changes this balance (Fig. 9.110). Complete quadriceps tears are more common in men than in women. Although these ruptures usually occur in the elderly, they may at times be seen in athletes. A lateral radiograph of the knee may show lack of definition of the quadriceps tendon and widening of its anteroposterior diameter secondary to hemorrhage and edema (Fig. 9.111). Occasionally, the lateral radiograph may also show the patella in a lower-than-normal position secondary to an imbalance in forces on the patellar ligamentous attachments (Fig. 9.112); in tear of the patellar ligament (occasionally referred to as a *tendon,* because some of its fibers are derived from and continuous with those of the rectus femoris), which may occur either at its attachment to the patella or to the tibial tuberosity, the reverse of this mechanism occurs

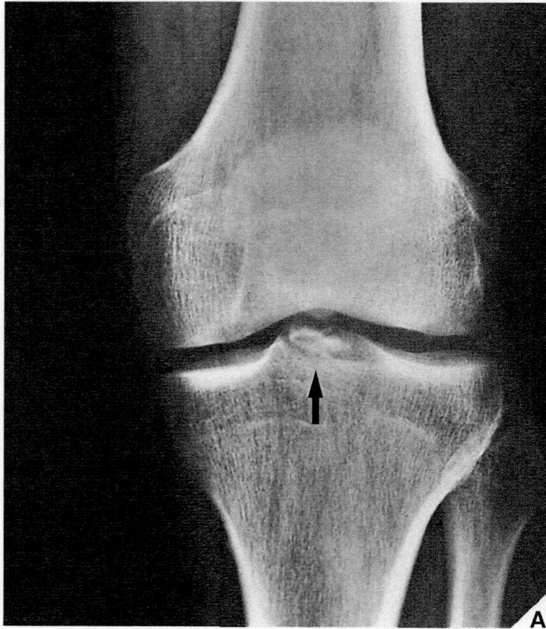

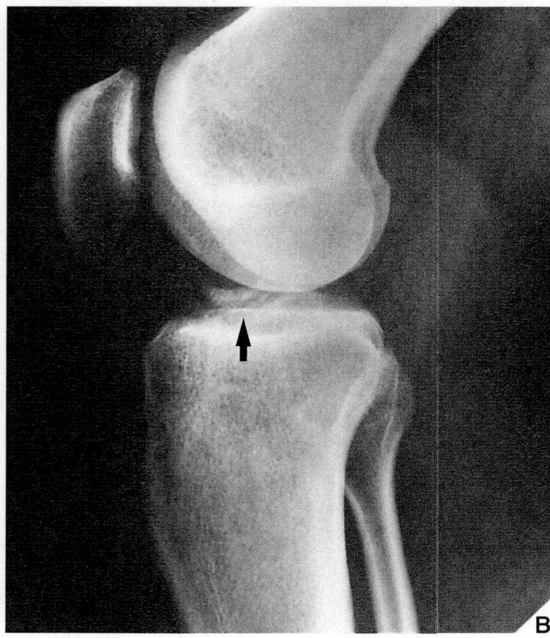

FIGURE 9.104 Tear of the ACL. **(A)** Anteroposterior and **(B)** lateral radiographs of the left knee in a 38-year-old soccer player show avulsion of the tibial eminence *(arrows),* suggesting tear of the ACL. The diagnosis was confirmed by arthroscopy.

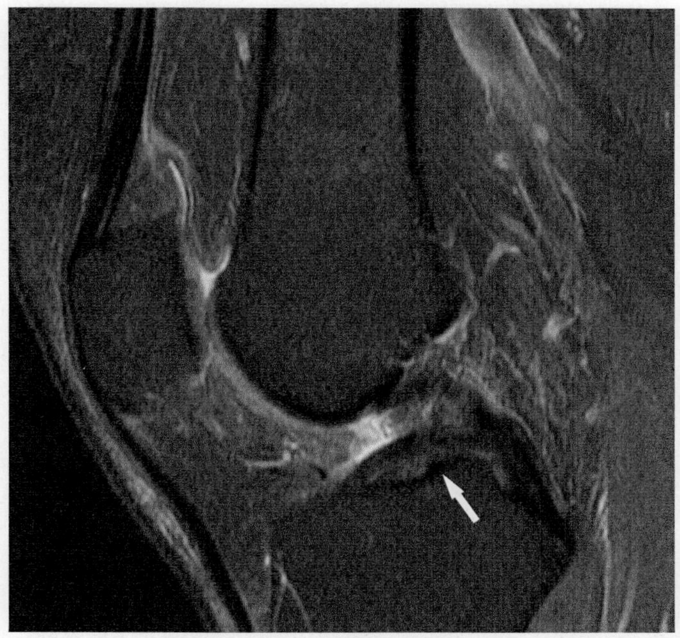

FIGURE 9.105 **MRI of tear of the ACL.** A 56-year-old woman twisted her right knee in a fall from the rock. Sagittal proton density–weighted fat-suppressed MR image shows a displaced tear of the ACL *(arrow)*.

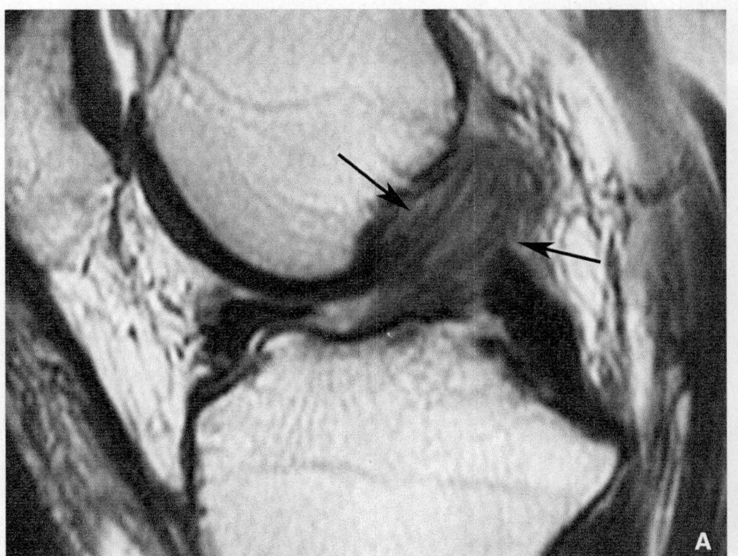

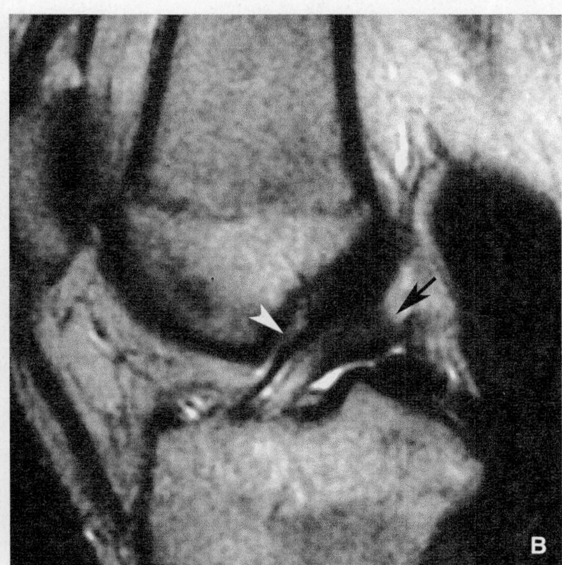

FIGURE 9.106 **MRI of partial tear of the ACL.** **(A)** Sagittal spin-echo T2-weighted MR image of the knee of a 15-year-old boy who was injured during soccer game shows swelling of the ACL *(arrows)* without discontinuation of the fibers. This represents an interstitial tear. **(B)** Sagittal T2-weighted MR image of the knee of another patient demonstrates a partial tear of the posterolateral bundle on the ACL displaced in top of the tibial spine *(arrow)*. Note the intact anteromedial bundle *(arrowhead)*.

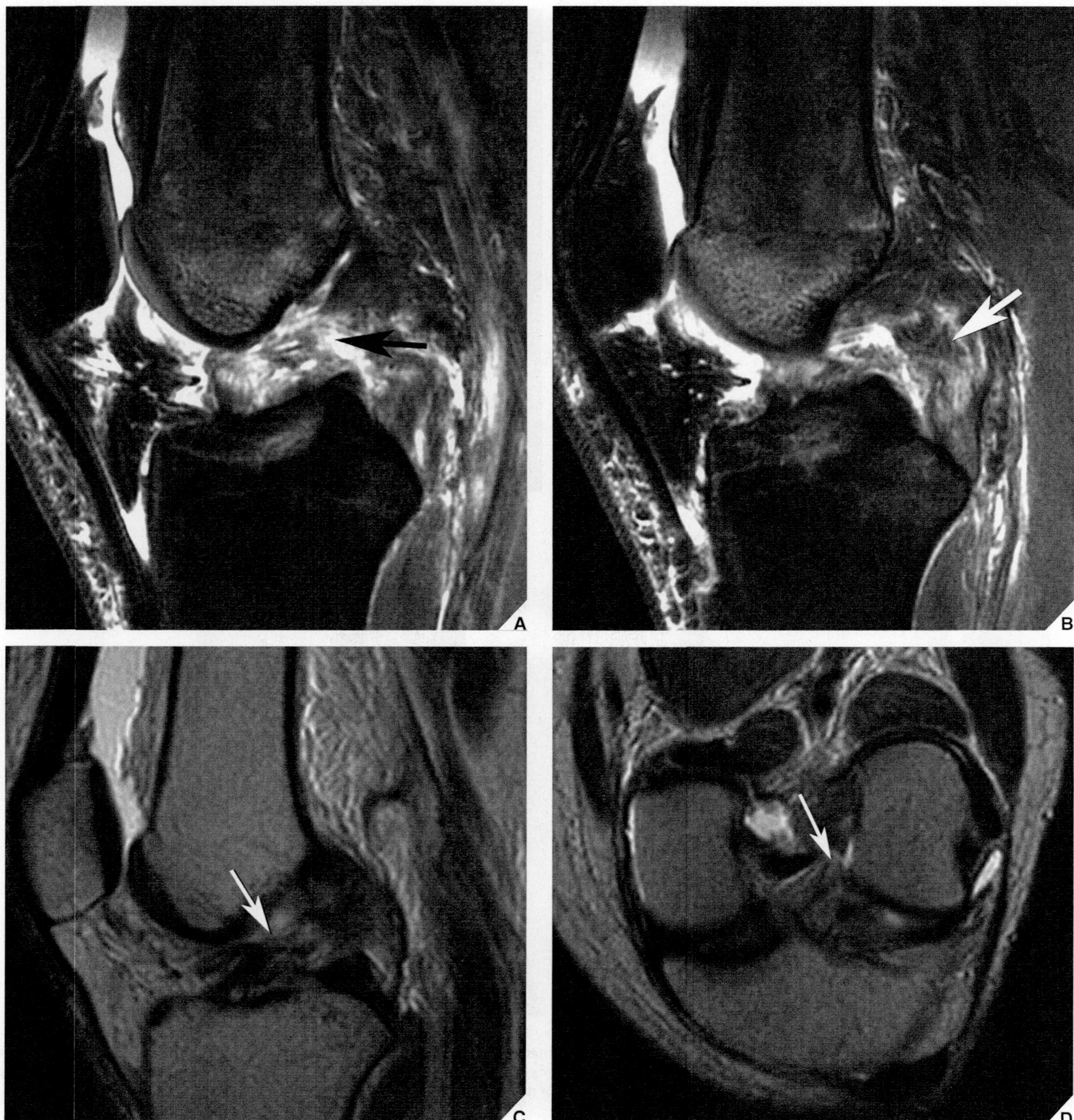

FIGURE 9.107 MRI of full-thickness tear of the ACL. **(A)** Sagittal T2-weighted fat-saturated MR image of the knee shows an acute complete tear of the ACL *(arrow)*, with edema and hematoma in the intercondylar notch. Note the bone contusion of the femoral condyle and tibial plateau. **(B)** Sagittal T2-weighted fat-saturated MR image shows an associated complete tear of the PCL *(arrow)*. **(C)** Sagittal T2-weighted MR image in another patient shows a complete disruption of the fibers of the ACL *(arrow)* with focal edema. **(D)** Oblique coronal T2-weighted image in the same patient shows the absence of the ACL in the intercondylar notch *(arrow)*.

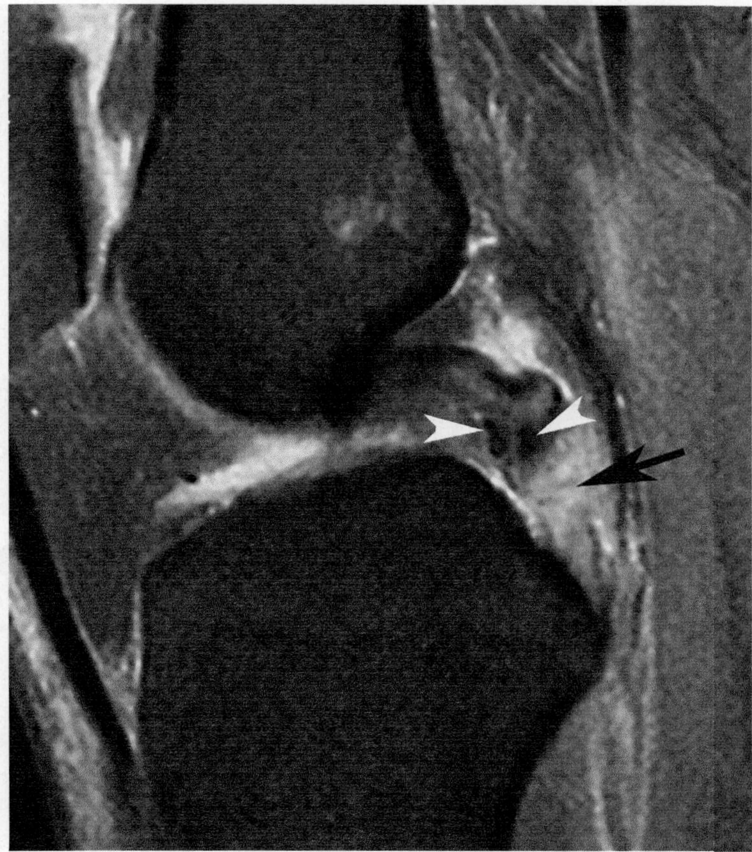

FIGURE 9.108 MRI of tear of the PCL. Sagittal T2-weighted MRI of the knee shows a complete tear of the distal fibers of the PCL *(arrow)*, with focal edema and hematoma. Note the preserved anterior and posterior meniscofemoral ligaments entrapped within the fibers of the ruptured PCL *(arrowheads)*.

(Figs. 9.113 and 9.114). MRI is the procedure of choice for demonstrating and evaluating those two types of injury (Figs. 9.115 to 9.121).

The Postoperative Knee

The most commonly performed procedures in the knee include meniscal and ligamentous surgery, mostly ACL and cartilage repair procedures. Today, these procedures are performed arthroscopically. MRI is the imaging modality of choice to assess patients with suspected meniscal or ligamentous re-tear or potential complications after surgery.

Surgical Management of Meniscal Tears

Three procedures may be performed to repair a torn meniscus: (a) **Partial meniscectomy**—in this procedure, the portion of the meniscus with a tear is removed and the meniscus is recontoured (Fig. 9.122). (b) **Meniscal repair**—this procedure is performed when the tear is located in the peripheral portion of the meniscus, in the meniscocapsular junction, the so-called *red zone*, where some capillary blood supply exists. Sutures between the capsule and the meniscus are arthroscopically placed, securing the stability of the meniscus and promoting healing, without meniscal resection (Fig. 9.123). (c) **Meniscal transplant**—in this procedure, the torn meniscus is completely excised and is replaced with a cadaver meniscus allograft (Fig. 9.124). The meniscal graft used for meniscal transplant is composed of meniscus and its tibial bony attachments. The tibial bony attachments can be obtained from the donor cadaveric knee as small plugs at the insertion of the anterior and posterior meniscal root ligaments, or as a bridge or bar of donor bone connected to the meniscus. The plugs or the bony bars are secured in place along with the cadaveric meniscus in the tibia of the recipient by means of sutures or by drilling a slot in the tibial plateau.

Complications of these procedures include meniscal retear and development of early osteoarthritis.

Anterior Cruciate Ligament Reconstruction

ACL tears are typically treated with tendon autographs more frequently using a patellar tendon graft (bone-tendon-bone repair) or the distal hamstring tendon graft (Fig. 9.125). Complications include recurrent tear, graft impingement due to faulty surgical technique, interference screw migration, anterior arthrofibrosis ("cyclops" lesion or sign), and cyst formation within the tibial or less frequently in the femoral tunnel (Fig. 9.126).

Cartilage Repair

Multiple arthroscopic procedures have been developed for repairing focal chondral lesions, including debridement of the damaged cartilage, microfracture (Fig. 9.127), autologous osteochondral transplantation (also known as *osteoarticular transplant system* [OATS] *procedure* or *mosaicplasty*) (Fig. 9.128), and autologous chondrocyte transplant. Microfracture is an arthroscopic procedure aimed at producing tiny fractures in the area of a chondral defect, in order to produce focal bleeding and formation of a clot with multipotential mesenchymal cells capable to regenerate fibrous cartilage and fill the defect. Mosaicplasty involves procurement of cylindrical osteochondral plugs from non–weight-bearing areas of the knee, typically in the outer margins of the femoral trochlea and transplant them into the chondral defect. Autologous chondrocyte transplantation is also an arthroscopic technique that involves procurement of healthy cartilage cells from the patient's knee from a non–weight-bearing area of the cartilage, follow-up with culture, and implantation into the chondral defect. The cultured material contains large number of autologous chondrocytes capable of regenerate hyaline cartilage. This material is injected into the original chondral defect into a matrix (matrix-assisted autologous chondrocyte implantation or MACI) and covered with a patch of autologous periosteum (Fig. 9.129). MRI is the most effective modality to assess the postoperative results and complications of these procedures (Fig. 9.130).

Less frequently performed surgical reconstructive procedures in the knee include PCL repair, MCL repair, and patellar realignment procedures.

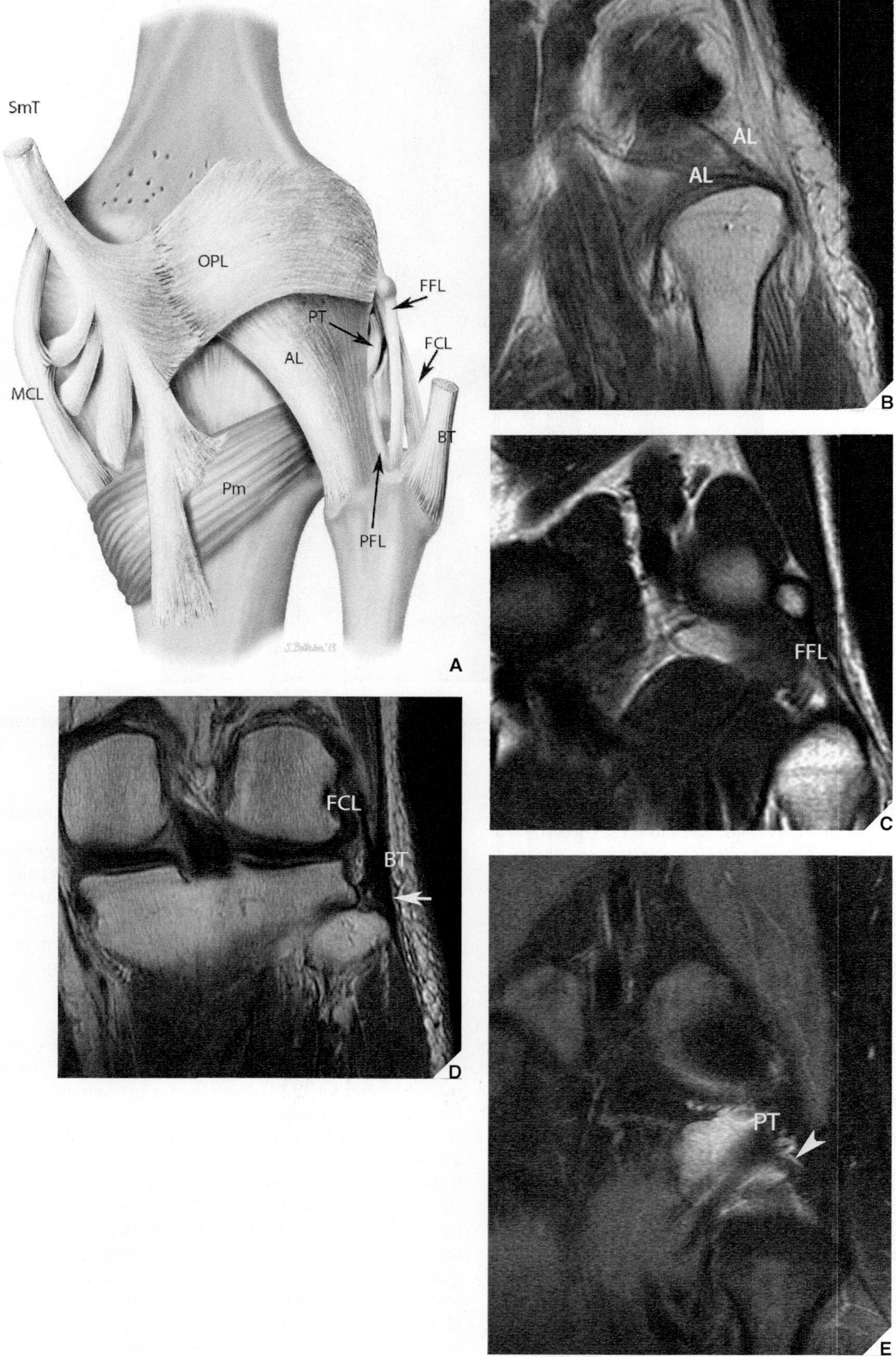

FIGURE 9.109 MRI of the posterolateral corner. **(A–F)** ***Normal anatomy***. **(A)** Artist rendering of the posterior aspect of the knee demonstrates the semimembranosus tendon *(SmT)* and its distal arms including the oblique popliteal ligament *(OPL)* crossing over to the posterolateral aspect of the knee and merging its fibers with the arcuate ligament *(AL)*. Note the medial and lateral bundles of the AL, the fabellofibular ligament *(FFL)*, the fibular collateral ligament *(FCL)*, the biceps femoris tendon *(BT)*, the popliteofibular ligament *(PFL)*, popliteus muscle *(Pm)*, and medial collateral ligament *(MCL)*. **(B)** Coronal proton density–weighted MR image shows the AL with the media land lateral bundles. **(C)** Coronal proton density–weighted MRI shows the FFL. **(D)** Coronal proton density–weighted MRI demonstrates the conjoined tendon of the FCL and BT at the insertion in the lateral aspect of the head of the fibula *(arrow)*. **(E)** Coronal T2-weighted MRI shows the PFL oriented perpendicular to the popliteus tendon *(PT)* *(arrowhead)*. *(Continued)*

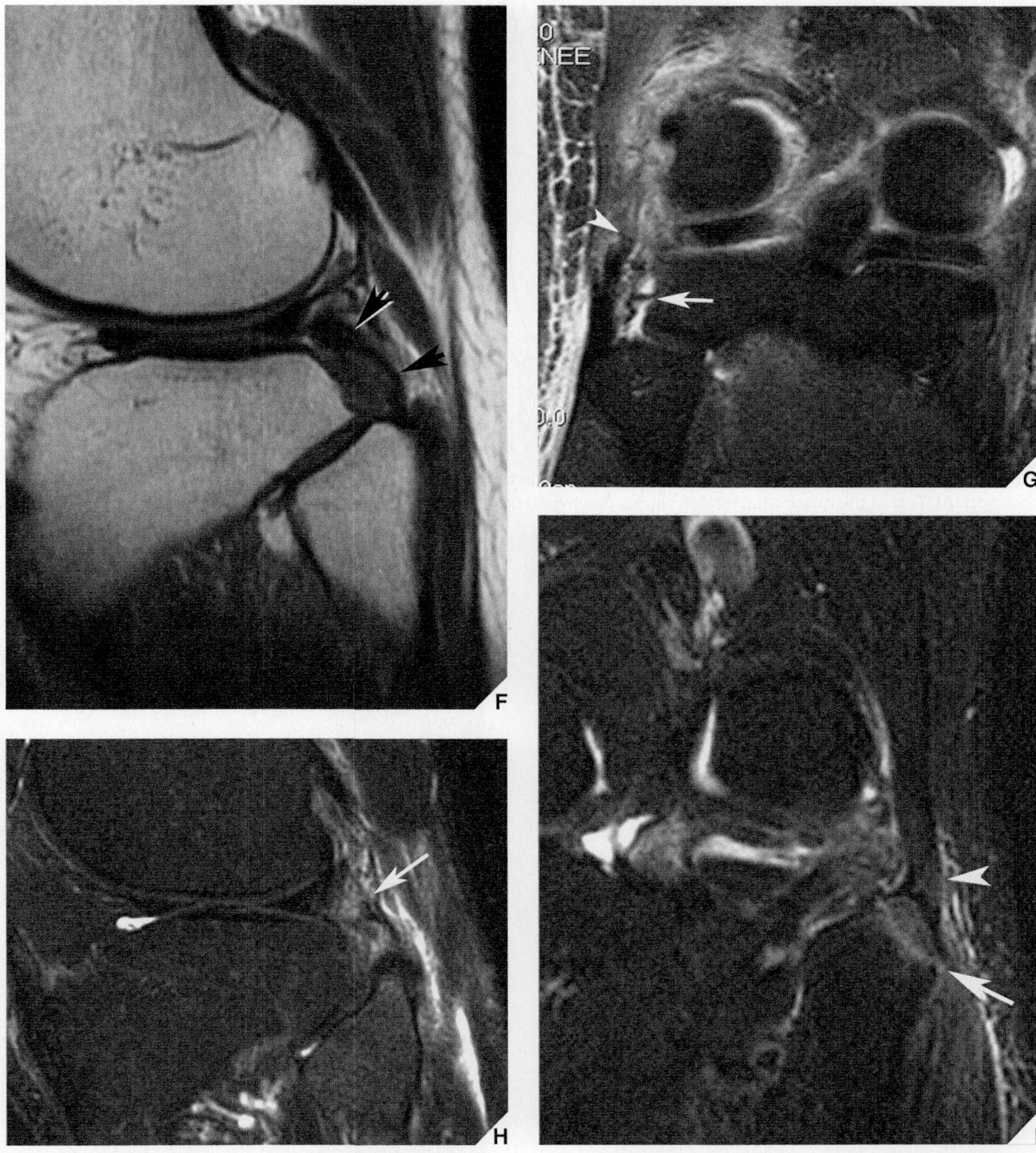

FIGURE 9.109 MRI of the posterolateral corner. ***(Continued)*** **(F)** Sagittal T1-weighted MRI demonstrates a coma-shaped structure *(arrows)* corresponding to the popliteus tendon and the PFL. **(G–I)** ***PLC injuries*.** **(G)** Coronal short time inversion recovery (STIR) MR image demonstrates tears of the PFL *(arrow)* and FCL *(arrowhead)*. **(H)** Sagittal T2-weighted fat-saturated MR image in another patient demonstrates a tear of the PFL *(arrow)*. **(I)** The "arcuate sign" is demonstrated on the coronal STIR MR image that shows an avulsion fracture *(arrow)* of the lateral aspect of the head of the fibula at the insertion of the conjoined tendon of the FCL and BT *(arrowhead)*.

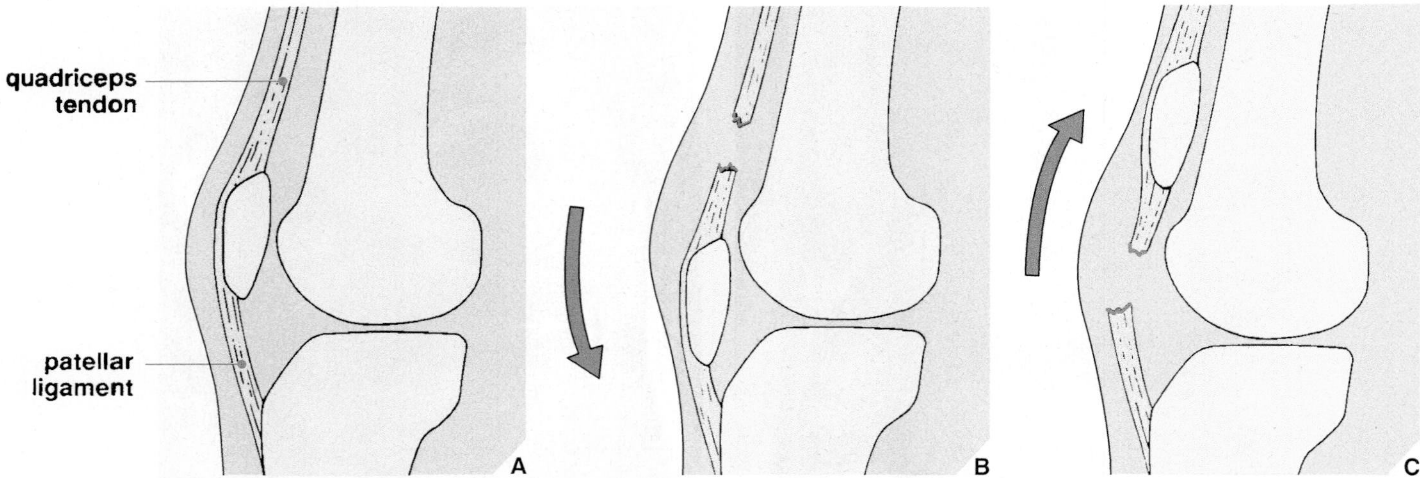

▲
FIGURE 9.110 **Patellar ligamentous-tendinous attachments.** Under normal circumstances, the balance of forces on the patellar ligamentous-tendinous attachments maintains the patella in position **(A)**. Tear of the quadriceps tendon causes downward displacement of the patella (*red curved arrow*) **(B)**. In tear of the patellar ligament, the reverse mechanism occurs (*red curved arrow*) **(C)** (see also Fig. 9.3).

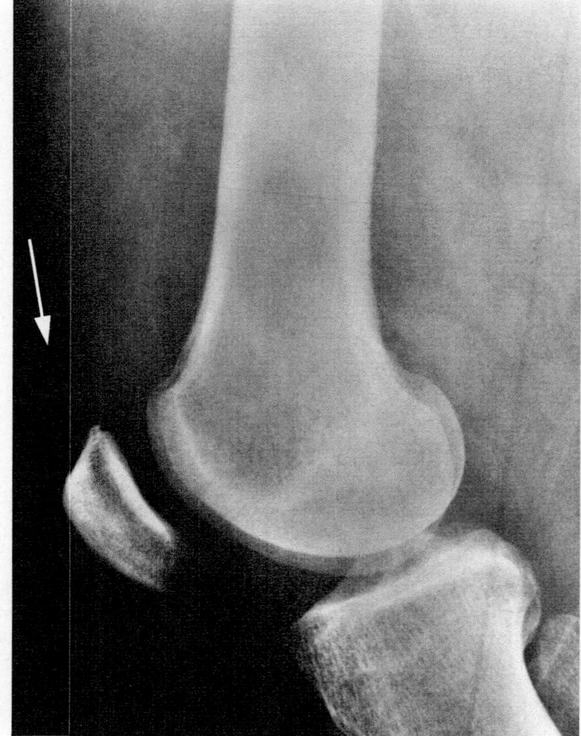

▲
FIGURE 9.111 **Tear of the quadriceps tendon.** A 30-year-old man was injured during a football game. Lateral radiograph of the knee shows lack of definition of the quadriceps tendon *(arrow)* and the presence of a soft-tissue mass in the suprapatellar region—findings characteristic of quadriceps tendon rupture.

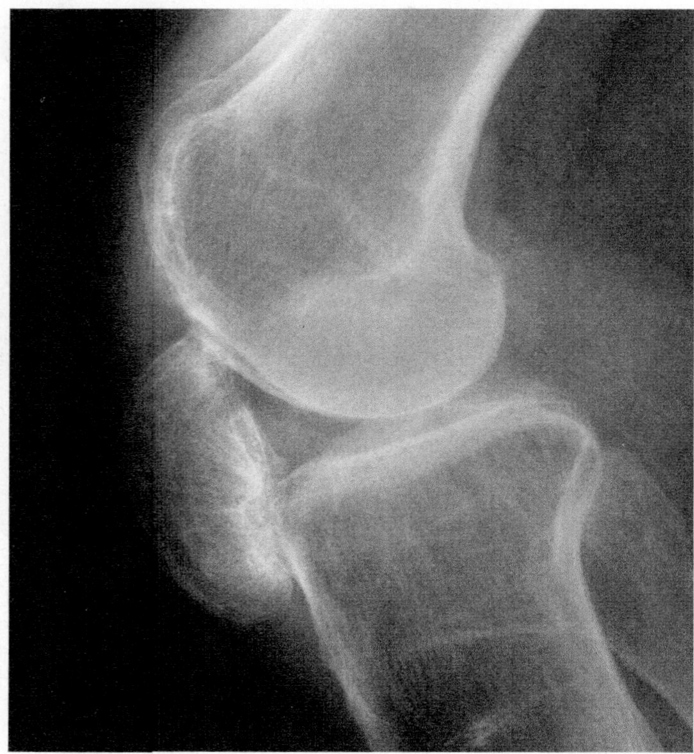

▲
FIGURE 9.112 **Tear of the quadriceps tendon.** A lateral radiograph of the knee shows low position of the patella (patella infera, patella baja) secondary to chronic tear of the quadriceps tendon.

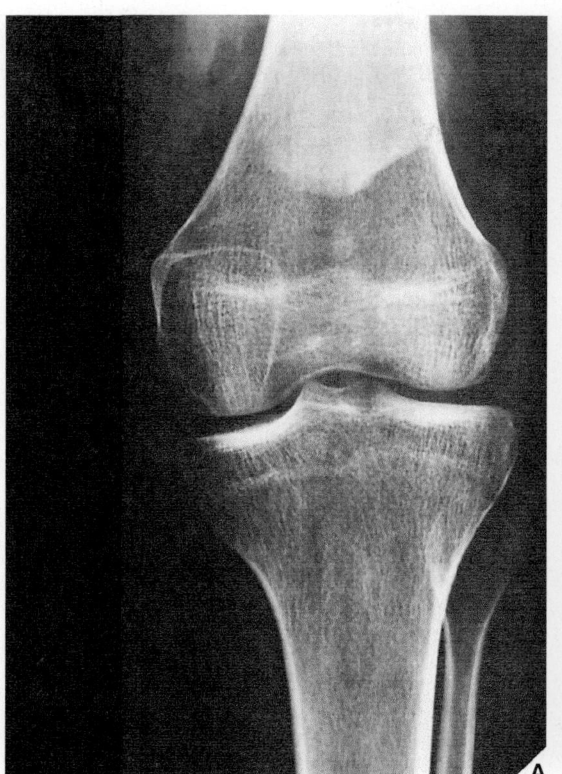

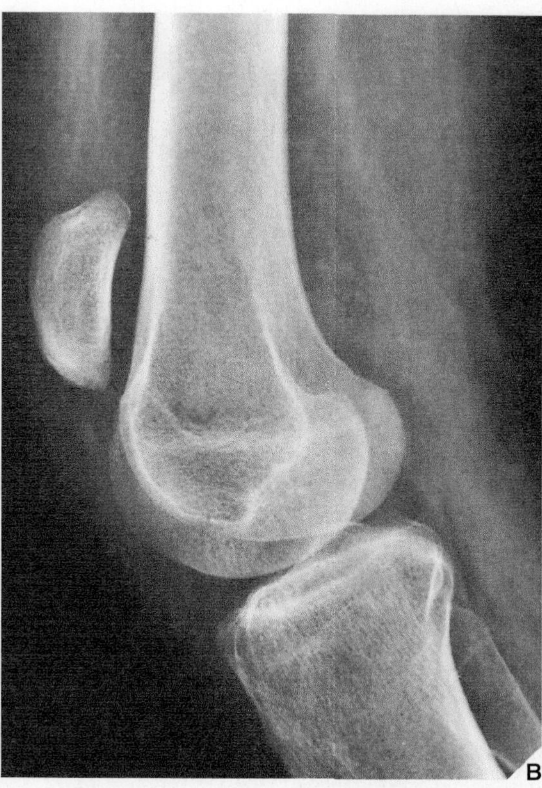

FIGURE 9.113 **Tear of the patellar ligament.** A 38-year-old woman athlete was injured during a running competition. **(A)** Anteroposterior and **(B)** lateral radiographs of the knee demonstrate an abnormally high position of the patella (patella alta), a finding suggesting tear of the patellar ligament. The diagnosis was confirmed on surgical exploration.

FIGURE 9.114 **Tear of the patellar ligament.** A 60-year-old man was injured in a car accident. Lateral radiograph of the knee shows a high position of the patella due to a complete rupture of the patellar ligament. Observe a large hematoma within the soft tissues anteriorly to the distal femur and proximal tibia.

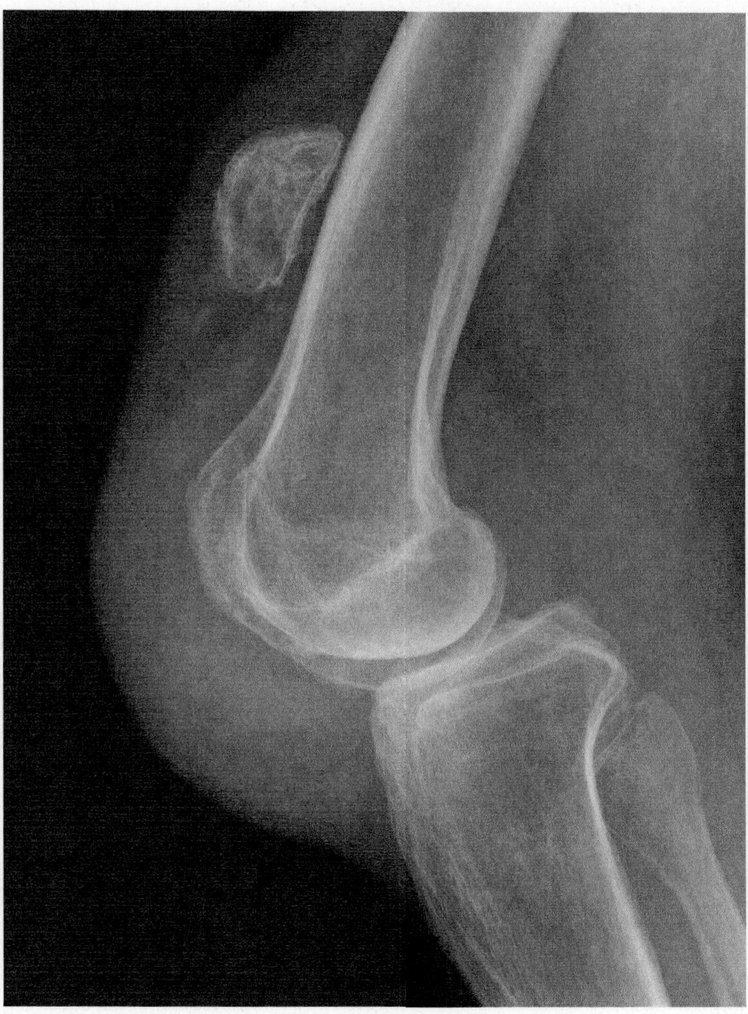

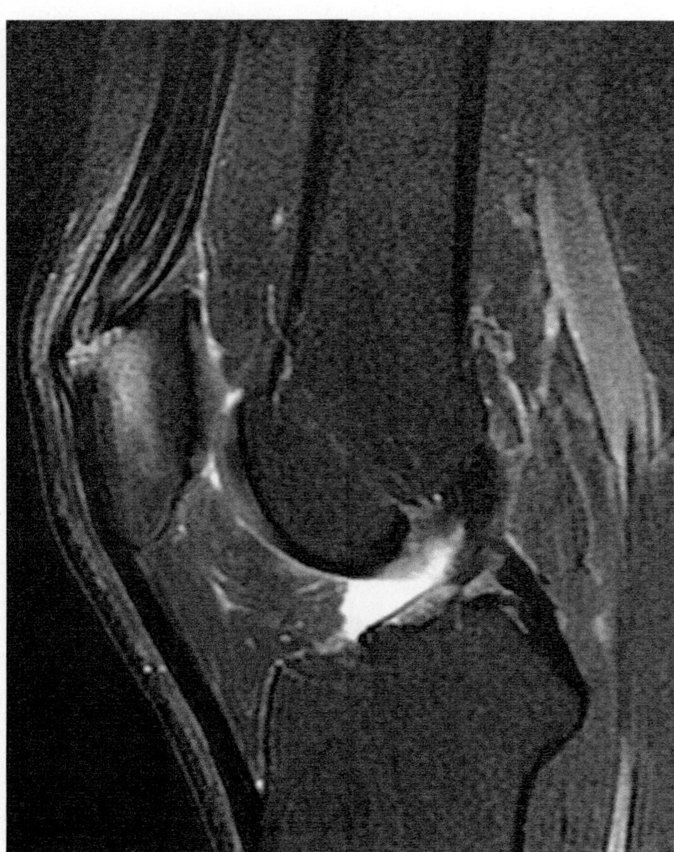

FIGURE 9.115 MRI of tear of the quadriceps tendon. A 38-year-old man injured left knee in a ski accident. Sagittal T2-weighted fat-suppressed MR image shows a high-grade partial tear of the quadriceps tendon at its insertion to the patella.

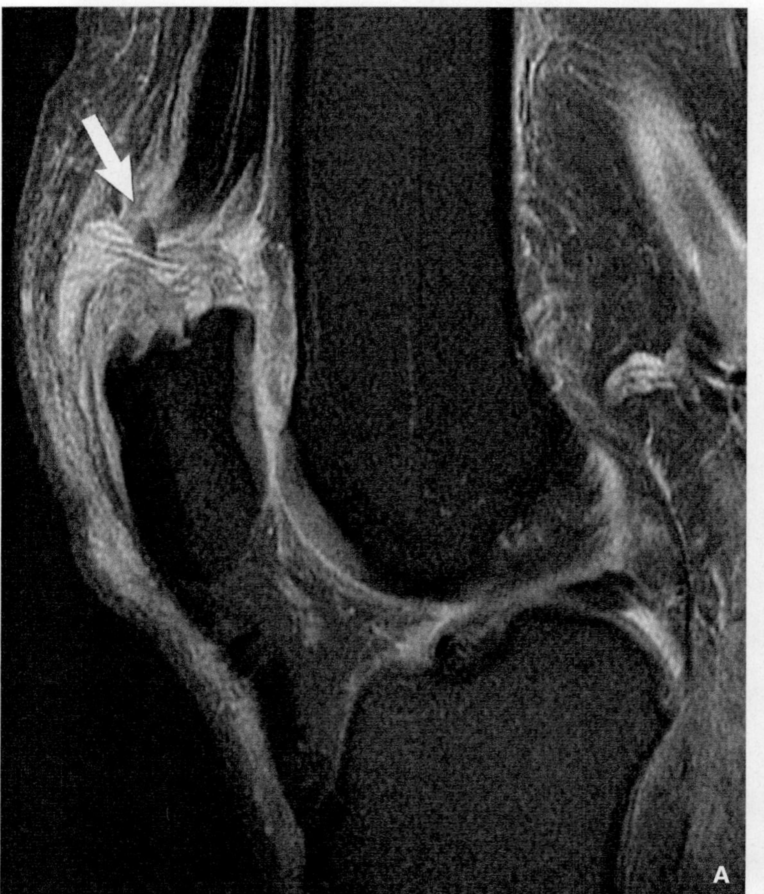

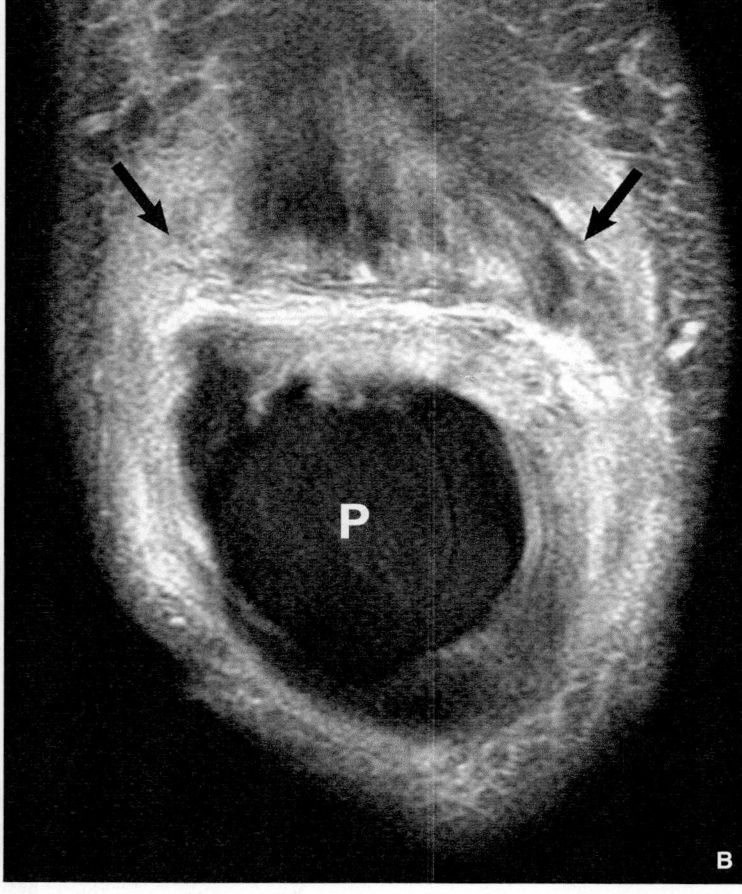

FIGURE 9.116 MRI of tear of the quadriceps tendon. **(A)** Sagittal T2-weighted fat-saturated and **(B)** coronal proton density–weighted fat-saturated MR images of the knee of a 78-year-old man who fell down the stairs show full-thickness tear of the quadriceps tendon at its attachment to the upper pole of the patella *(P) (arrows)*.

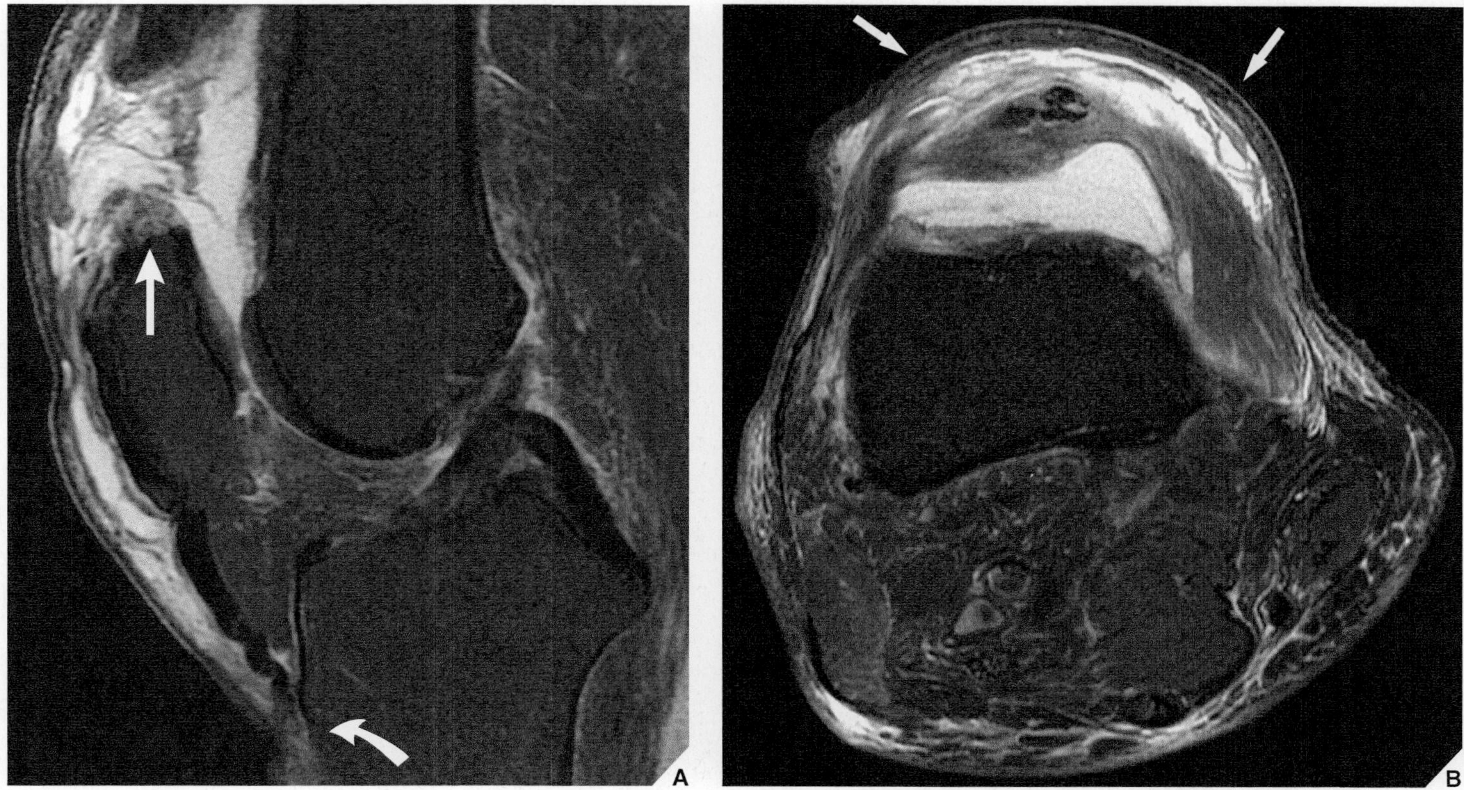

FIGURE 9.117 MRI of tear of the quadriceps tendon. **(A)** Sagittal T2-weighted and **(B)** axial proton density–weighted fat-suppressed MR images of the knee show a complete, full-thickness tear of the quadriceps tendon *(arrows)*. A *curved arrow* points to the associated tear of the patellar ligament.

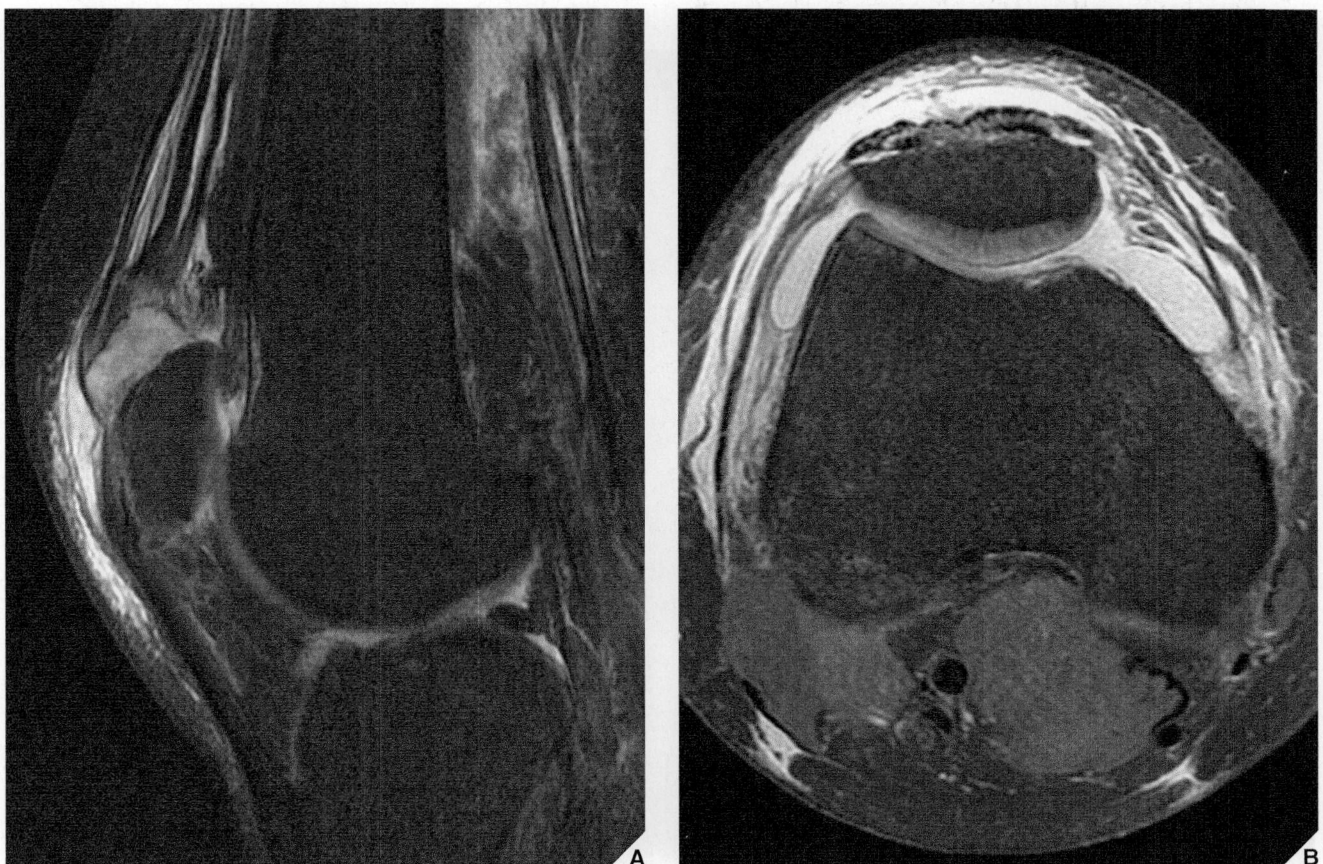

FIGURE 9.118 MRI of tear of the quadriceps tendon. **(A)** Coronal and **(B)** axial proton density–weighted fat-suppressed MR images of the knee show a complete tear of the quadriceps tendon in this 27-year-old man injured in an industrial accident.

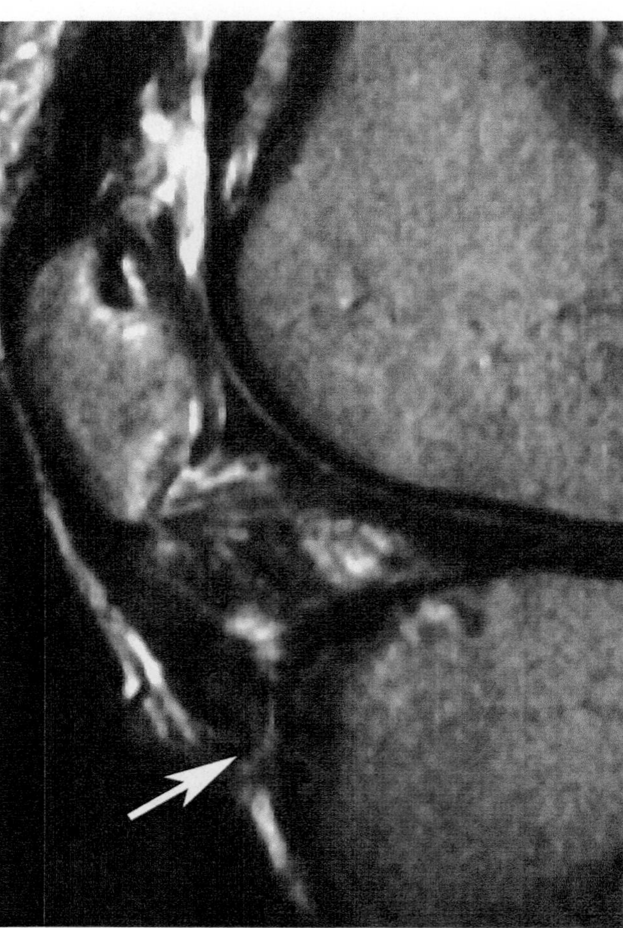

FIGURE 9.119 **MRI of tear of the patellar ligament.** Sagittal T2-weighted MR image demonstrates avulsion of the patellar ligament at the insertion into the tibial tuberosity *(arrow)*.

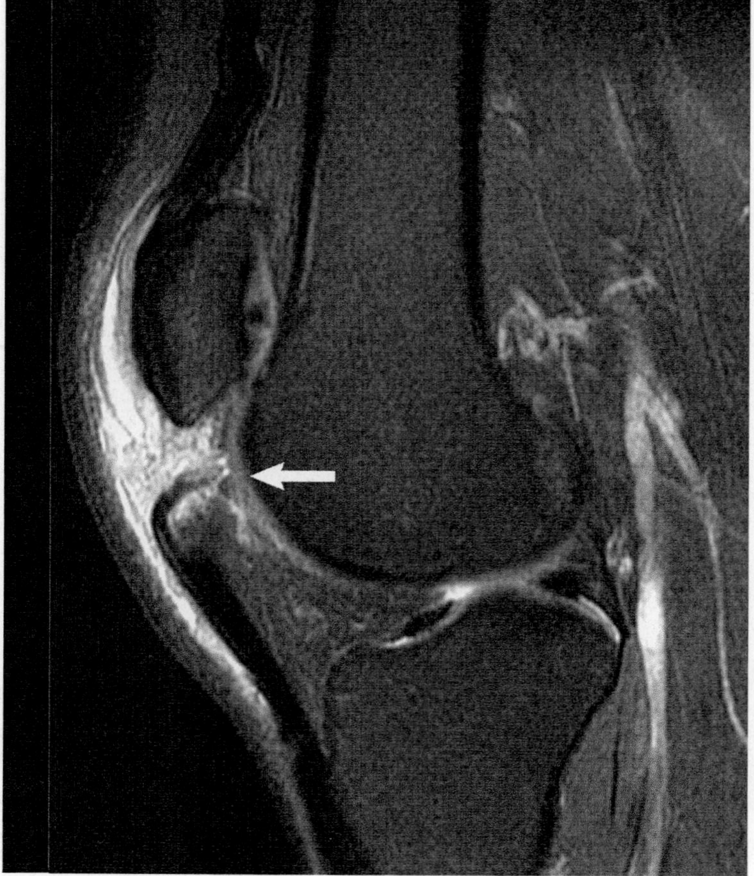

FIGURE 9.120 **MRI of tear of the patellar ligament.** A 45-year-old man was injured in a motorcycle accident. Sagittal T2-weighted fat-saturated MR image of the knee shows full-thickness tear of the patellar ligament at the site of its attachment to the lower pole of the patella *(arrow)*.

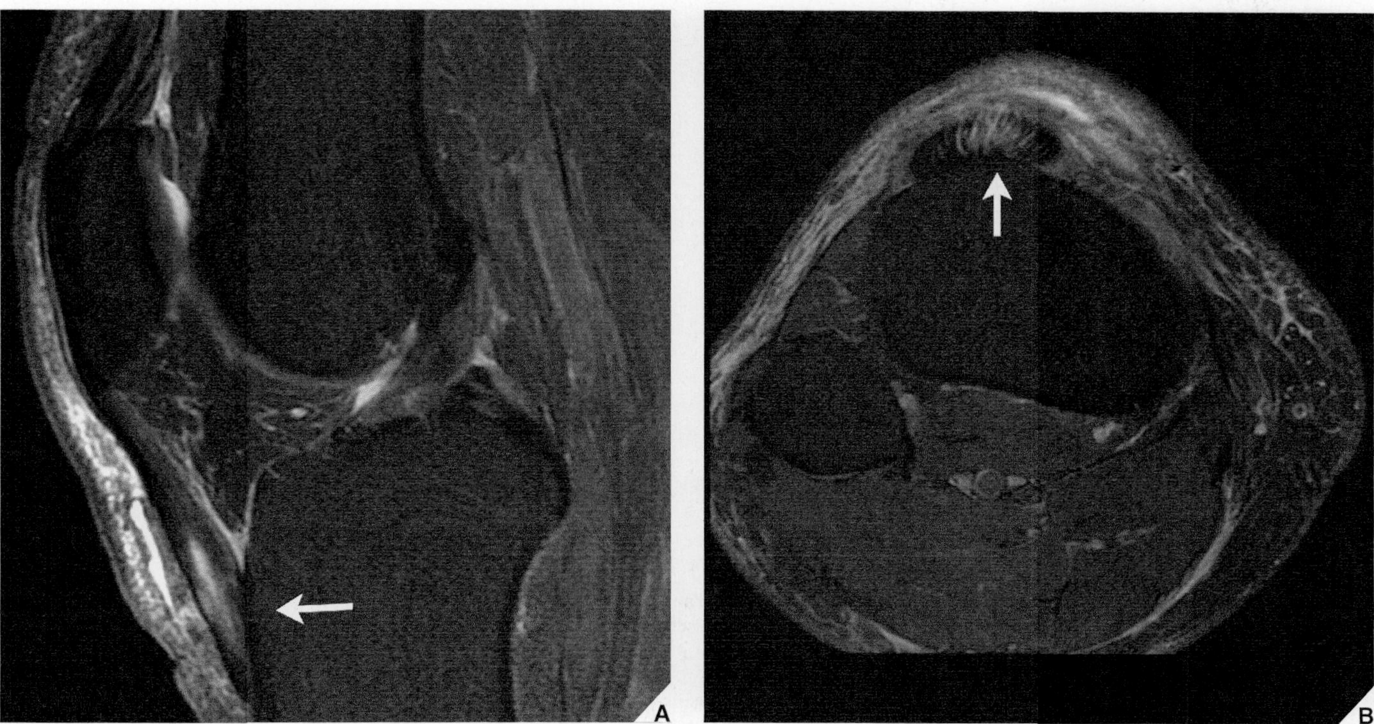

FIGURE 9.121 MRI of split tear of the patellar ligament. **(A)** Sagittal and **(B)** axial proton density–weighted fat-suppressed MR images show a split tear of the patellar ligament *(arrows)*.

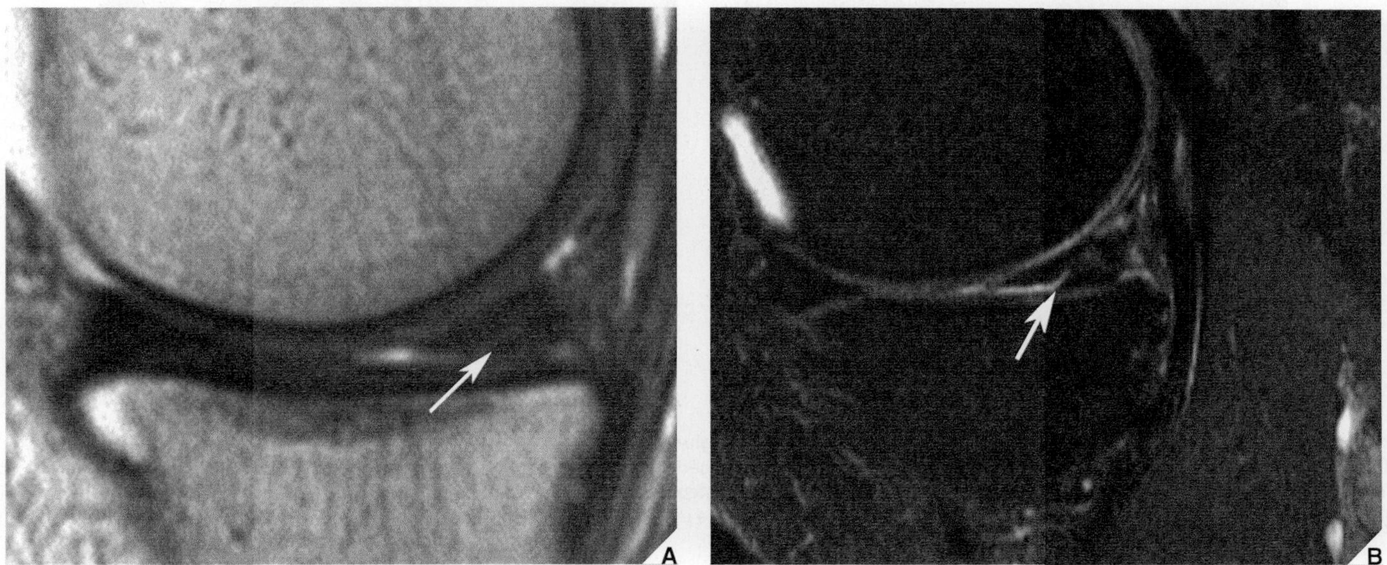

FIGURE 9.122 MRI of partial meniscectomy. **(A)** Sagittal T2-weighted MR image of the knee demonstrates irregularity of the posterior horn of the medial meniscus with linear signal abnormality *(arrow)*. Note that the signal intensity within the meniscus is intermediate as compared with the normal fluid signal in the joint. These findings are consistent with postmeniscectomy changes without recurrent tear. **(B)** Sagittal T2-weighted MR image in another patient with history of prior medial meniscectomy shows the linear fluid signal entering into the posterior horn of the medial meniscus *(arrow)*, consistent with recurrent meniscal tear.

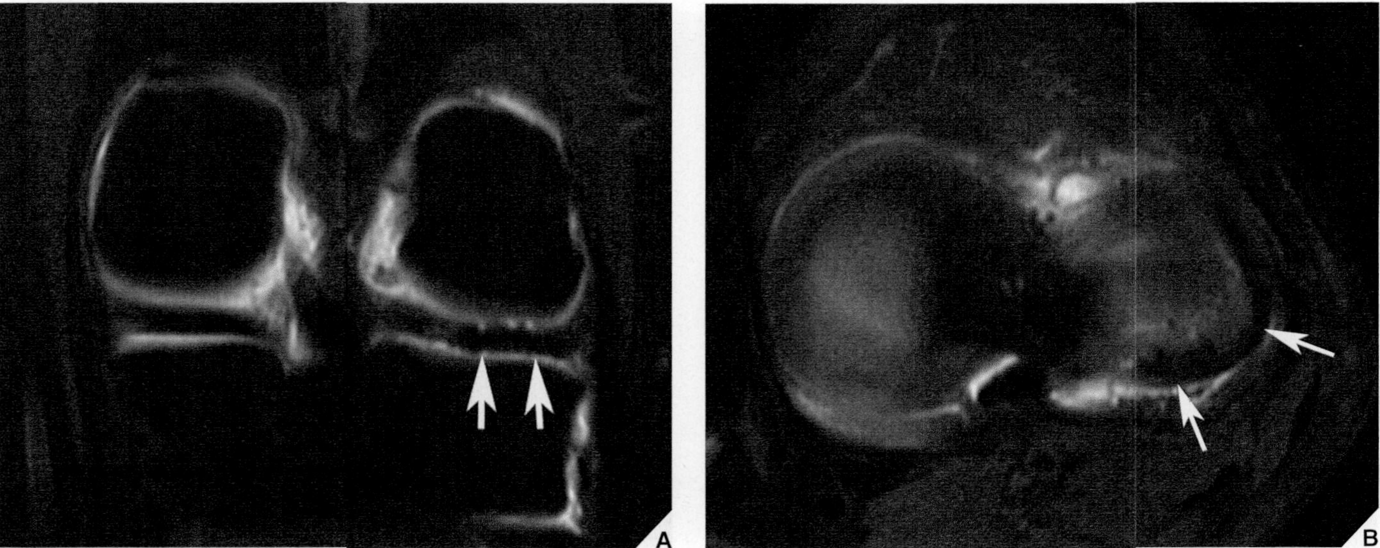

FIGURE 9.123 **MRI of meniscal repair.** **(A)** Coronal T2-weighted fat-saturated and **(B)** axial T2-weighted fat-saturated MR images demonstrate the artifact related to the presence of peripheral sutures in the posterior horn and body of the medial meniscus *(arrows)*.

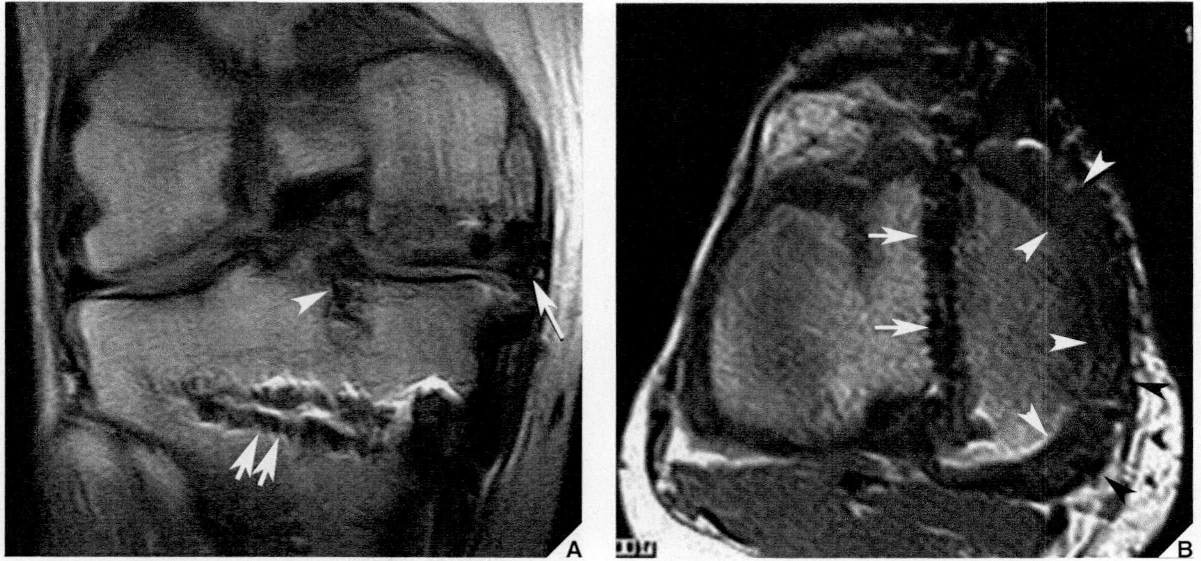

FIGURE 9.124 **MRI of meniscal transplant.** **(A)** Coronal proton density–weighted MR image of the knee demonstrates the transplanted medial meniscus *(arrow)*. The graft is degenerated and extruded, and there are degenerative changes in the medial compartment. Note the slot adjacent to the tibial spine where the bony bridge is placed *(arrowhead)*. This technique is called *bridge on slot*. This patient had also an osteotomy of the proximal tibia *(double arrows)* for correction of varus deformity. **(B)** Axial T1-weighted MR image demonstrates the bridge on slot in the tibia *(arrows)*. Note the extruded meniscus *(arrowheads)*.

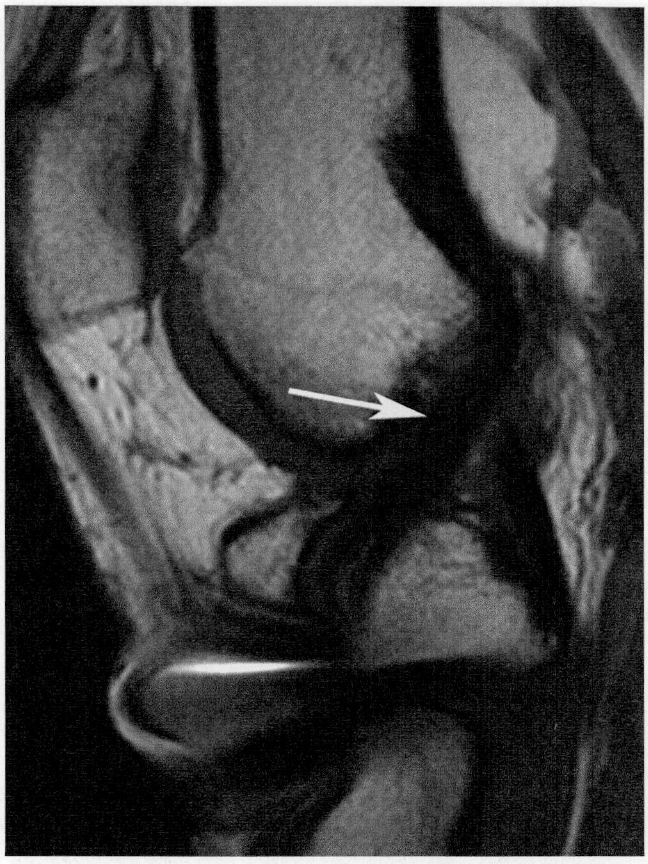

FIGURE 9.125 **MRI of ACL reconstruction.** T2-weighted sagittal MR image of the knee demonstrates the intact ACL graft (arrow). The metallic artifact in the tibia is produced by the hardware used to secure the graft in place.

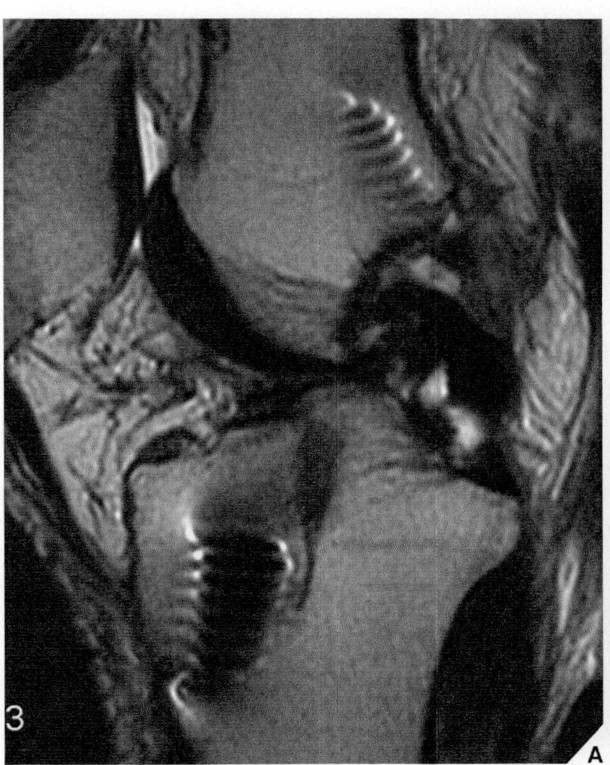

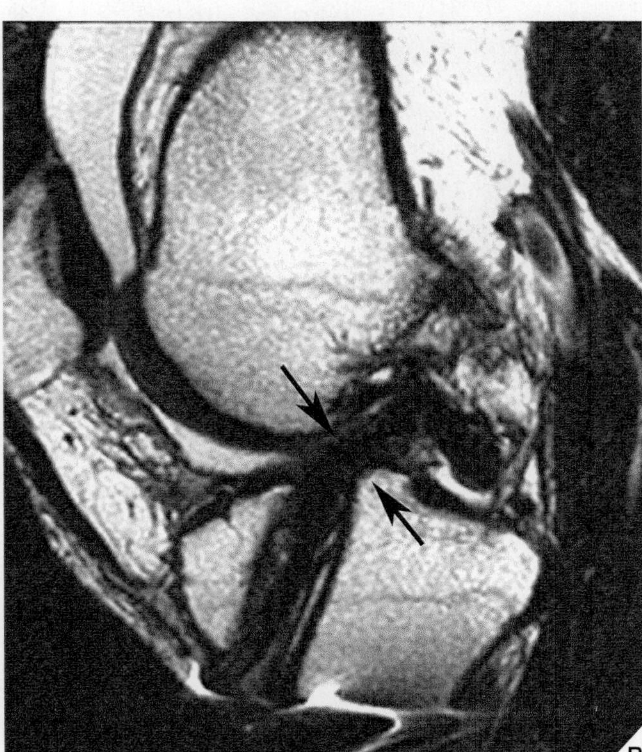

FIGURE 9.126 **MRI of ACL reconstruction.** **(A)** T2-weighted sagittal MR image in another patient demonstrates a recurrent tear of the graft. Note the interference screws in the proximal tibia and distal femur. **(B)** T2-weighted sagittal MR image in another patient demonstrates impingement of the graft between the intercondylar notch and the tibial spine *(arrows)*. The graft is still intact. *(Continued)*

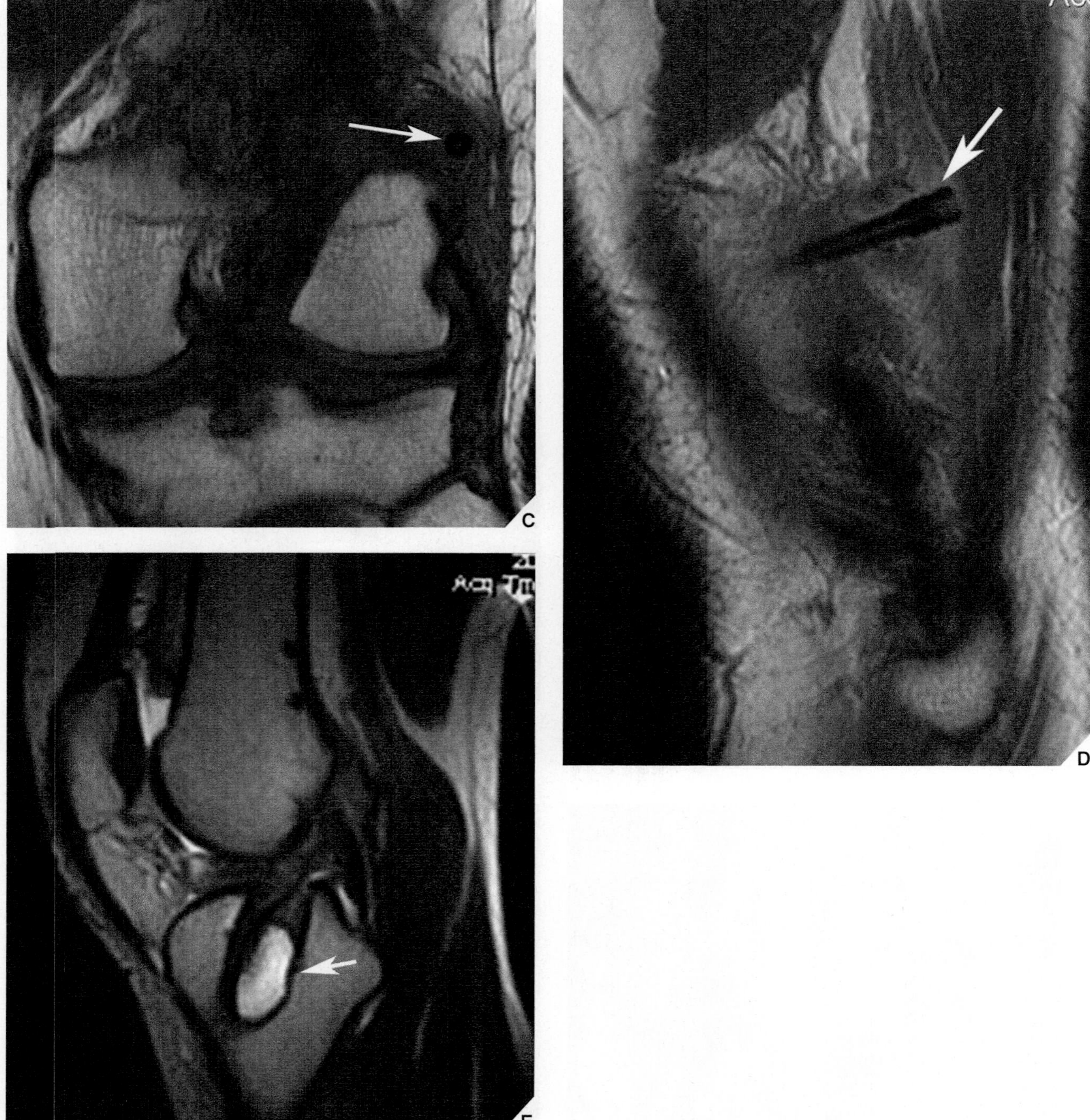

FIGURE 9.126 MRI of ACL reconstruction. ***(Continued)*** **(C,D)** Coronal T1-weighted and sagittal T2-weighted MR images of the knee in another patient demonstrate migration of the screw into the soft tissue adjacent to the lateral aspect of the knee *(arrows)*. **(E)** Sagittal T2-weighted MR image in another patient demonstrates the presence of a cyst within the enlarged tibial tunnel *(arrow)*. *(Continued)*

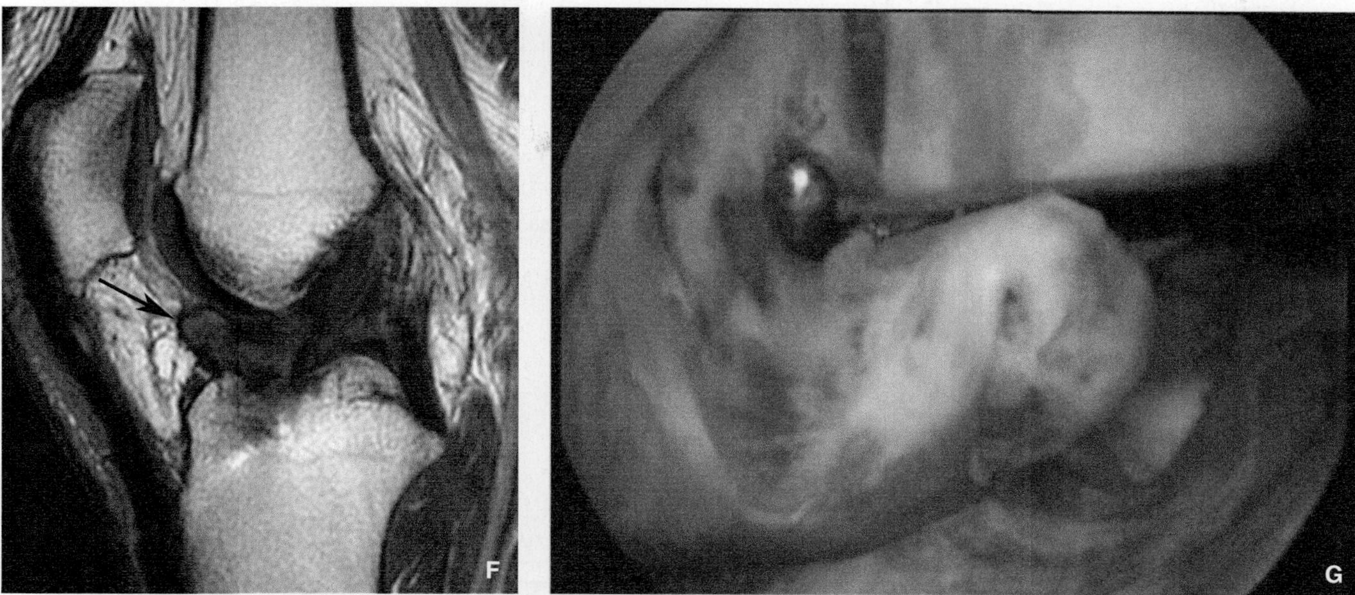

FIGURE 9.126 MRI of arthrofibrosis. ***(Continued)*** **(F)** Sagittal proton density–weighted MR image demonstrates a hypointense nodular lesion in the anterior aspect of the joint at the level of the joint line *(arrow)*, corresponding to a focal area of fibrosis, the so-called *cyclops sign*. **(G)** Arthroscopic image of a cyclops sign through an anterior portal. This lesion can produce pain on extension of the knee, and it may require surgical excision.

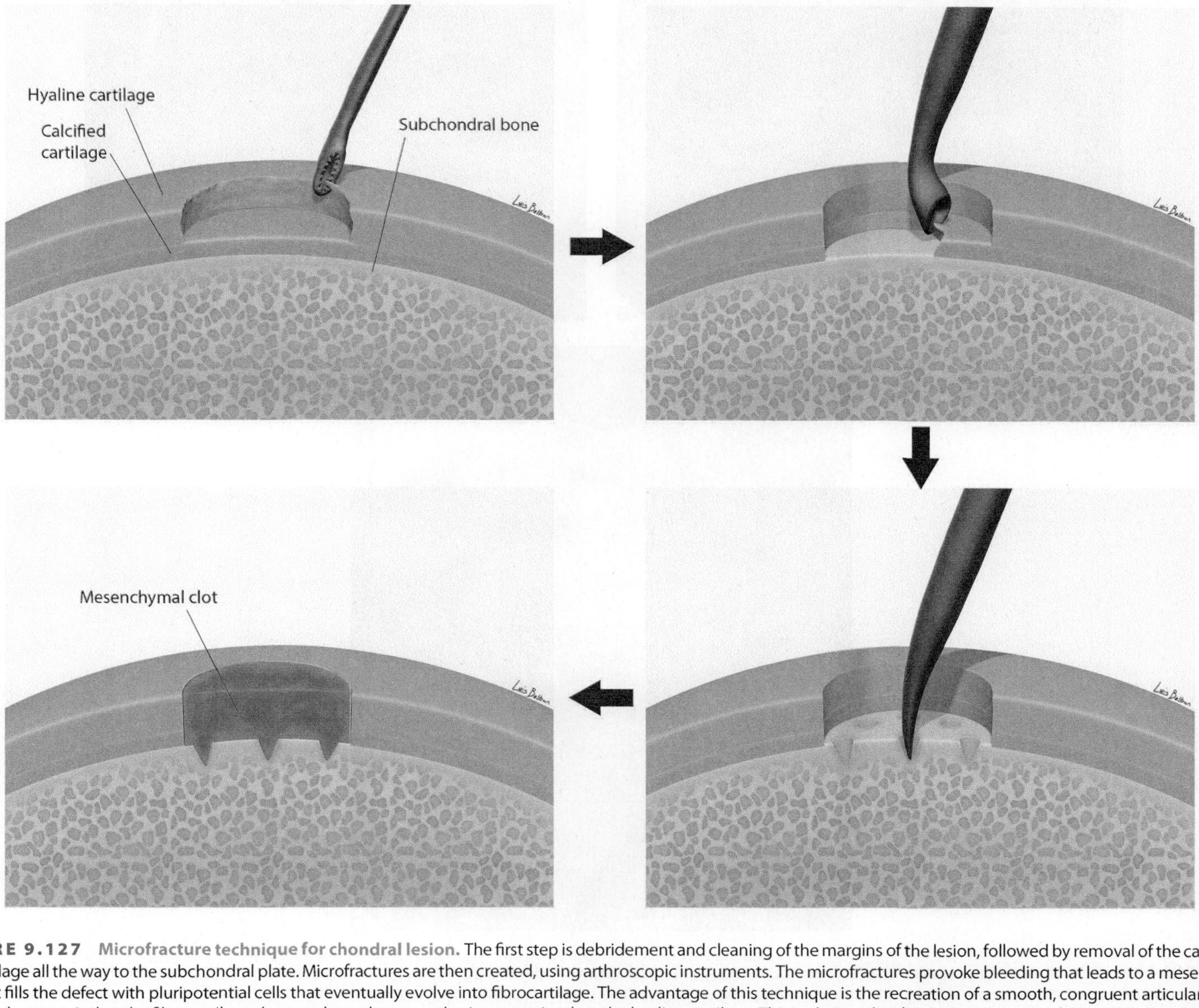

FIGURE 9.127 Microfracture technique for chondral lesion. The first step is debridement and cleaning of the margins of the lesion, followed by removal of the calcified fibrocartilage all the way to the subchondral plate. Microfractures are then created, using arthroscopic instruments. The microfractures provoke bleeding that leads to a mesenchymal clot that fills the defect with pluripotential cells that eventually evolve into fibrocartilage. The advantage of this technique is the recreation of a smooth, congruent articular surface. The disadvantage is that the fibrocartilage does not have the same elastic properties than the hyaline cartilage. This technique has been proven successful in small chondral lesions.

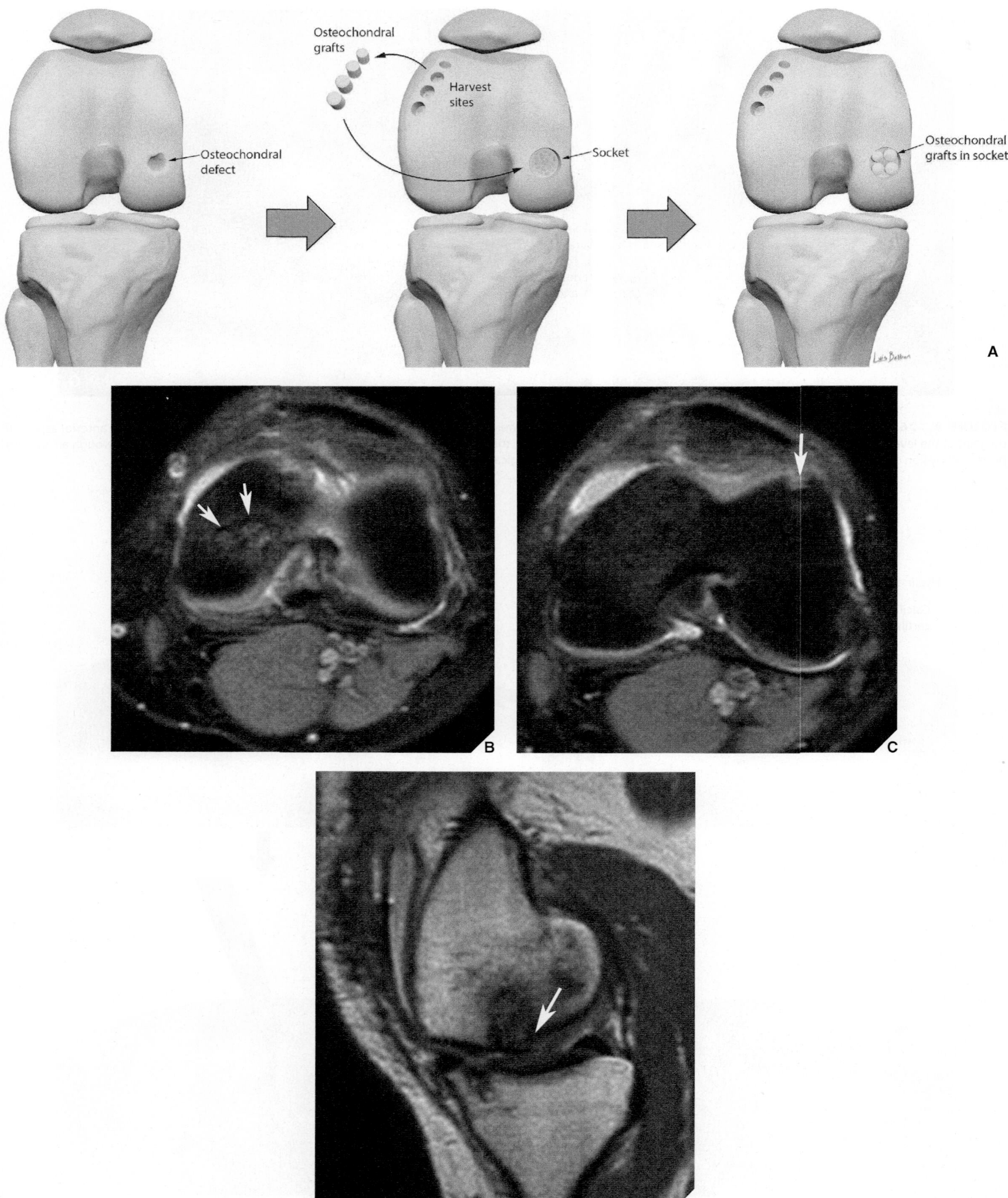

FIGURE 9.128 MRI of cartilage repair—OATS procedure. (A) A schematic drawing describing the steps for arthroscopic OATS procedure. **(B)** Axial T2-weighted image demonstrates two osteochondral plugs in the weight-bearing portion of the medial femoral condyle *(arrows)*. The distribution of the plugs resembles a mosaic, hence the term *mosaicplasty*. **(C)** Axial T2-weighted image demonstrates the donor site for the osteochondral plugs in the anterior aspect of the lateral femoral condyle, a non–weight-bearing area *(arrow)*. **(D)** Sagittal proton density–weighted image in the same patient demonstrates partial extrusion of one of the osteochondral plugs *(arrow)*.

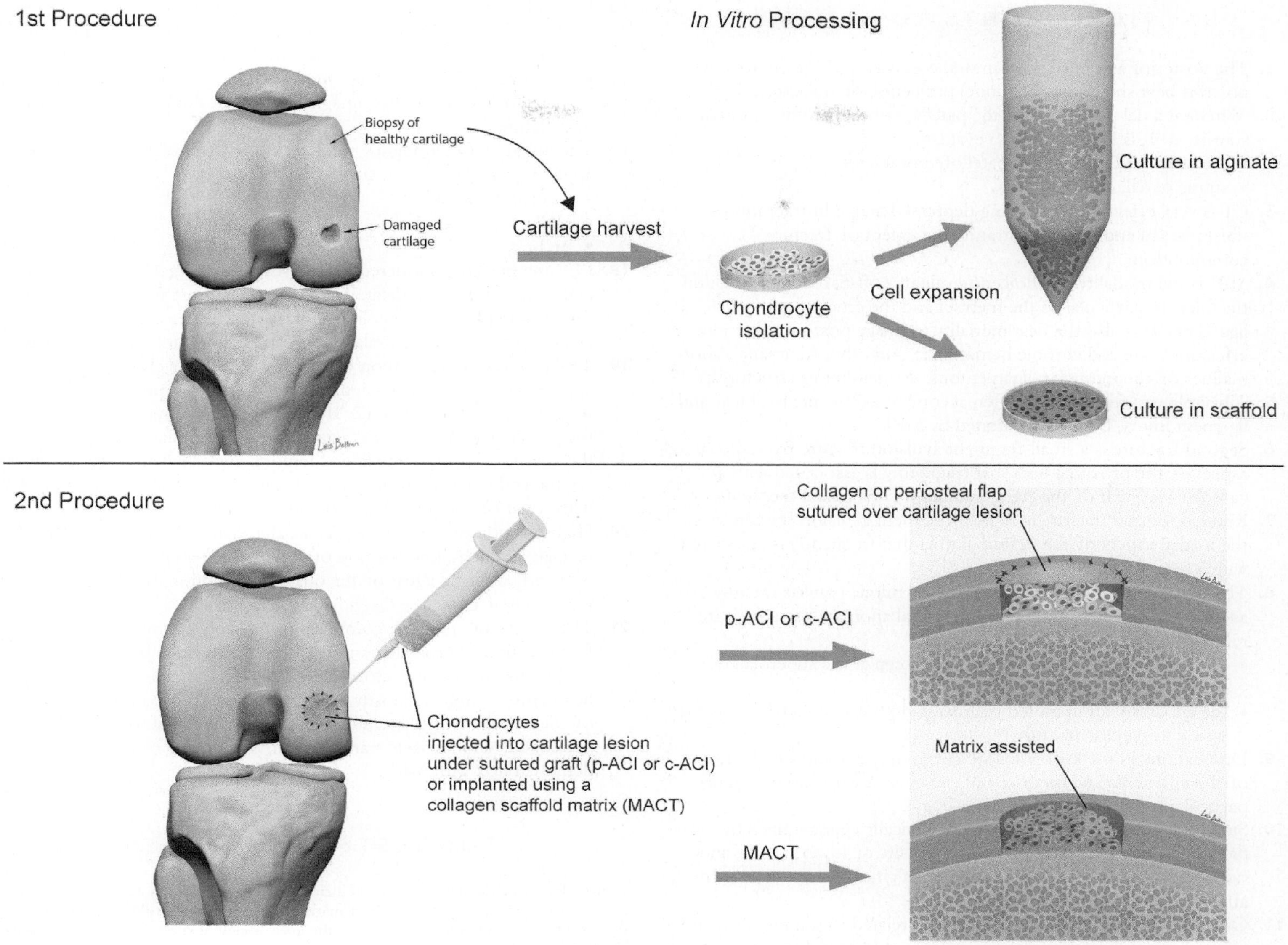

1st Procedure

In Vitro Processing

Biopsy of healthy cartilage

Damaged cartilage

Cartilage harvest

Chondrocyte isolation

Cell expansion

Culture in alginate

Culture in scaffold

2nd Procedure

Chondrocytes injected into cartilage lesion under sutured graft (p-ACI or c-ACI) or implanted using a collagen scaffold matrix (MACT)

p-ACI or c-ACI

Collagen or periosteal flap sutured over cartilage lesion

MACT

Matrix assisted

FIGURE 9.129 Autologous chondrocyte transplantation. This procedure is indicated for focal chondral lesions. It is done in two phases. During the *first phase*, a biopsy of a healthy part of the cartilage is obtained. The harvested cartilage is processed to isolate chondrocytes, which are then cultured and grown in a cell alginate suspension or are cultured in a collagen scaffold. In the *second phase*, the cultured chondrocytes are injected into the cartilage lesion under a sutured periosteal graft (p-ACI) or a collagen flap (c-ACI). Injection of the cartilage cells in a collagen scaffold matrix (matrix-assisted chondrocyte transplant [MACT]) has gained more interest because it does not require the step of collagen or periosteal flap. The injected chondrocytes are capable to generate hyaline cartilage, and this is the major advantage of this procedure, as opposed to the microfracture technique where the regenerated cartilage is fibrocartilage with decreased elastic properties.

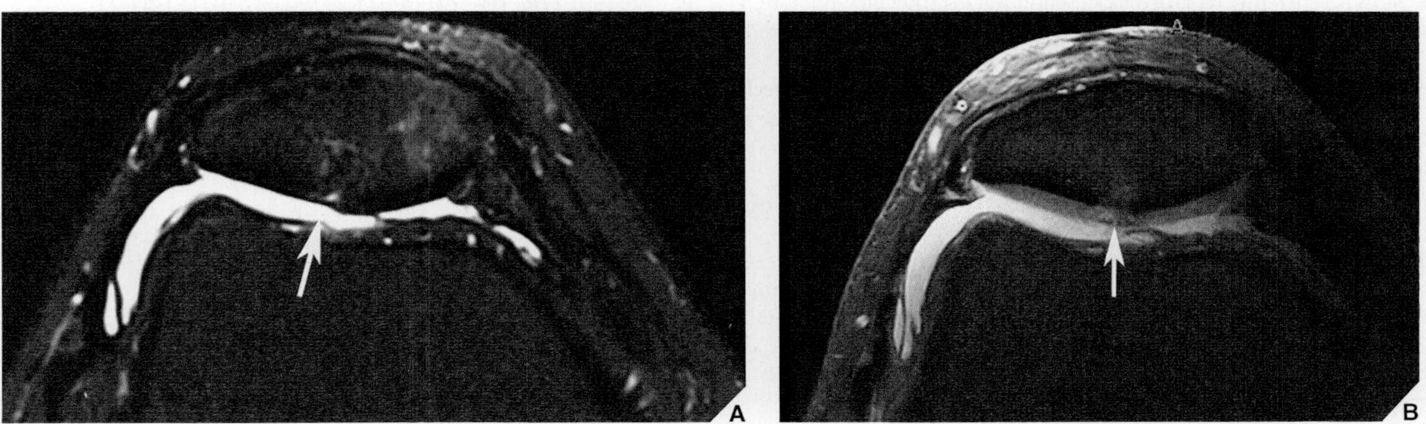

FIGURE 9.130 MRI of autologous chondrocyte transplantation. (A) Preoperative axial T2-weighted MR image shows the osteochondral lesion in the apex of the patella *(arrow)*. **(B)** Postoperative axial T2-weighted MR image obtained a year later demonstrates filling of the defect with hyaline cartilage *(arrow)*. This image was obtained with a research 7 Tesla magnet. (Courtesy of Greg Chang, MD, and Jenny Bencardino, MD, New York University Hospital for Joint Diseases, New York.)

PRACTICAL POINTS TO REMEMBER

1. The posterior aspect of the femoral condyles and the intercondylar notch is best shown on the tunnel projection of the knee.
2. Merchant axial projection of the patella, rather than the standard sunrise view, is better suited to evaluate:
   - the articular facets of the patellofemoral joint
   - subtle patellar subluxations.
3. CT is very effective in assessing depressed and split fractures of tibial plateau and in demonstrating the extent of fracture comminution.
4. MRI is the modality of choice to evaluate soft-tissue injury around the knee, in particular to the menisci and the cruciate and collateral ligaments. It is also the best modality to image posttraumatic joint effusion, acute and chronic hematomas, and other traumatic abnormalities of the muscular, ligamentous, and tendinous structures.
5. Tibial plateau fractures are often accompanied by meniscal tear and ligament injury, best demonstrated by MRI.
6. Segond fracture is a small-fragment avulsion fracture from the lateral aspect of the proximal tibia that frequently is associated with a capsular tear, tear of the ACL, and tear of the lateral meniscus.
7. Reverse Segond fracture is a small-fragment avulsion fracture from the medial aspect of the proximal tibia that frequently is associated with a tear of the PCL.
8. The bipartite or multipartite patella may mimic patellar fracture. To avoid misdiagnosing these developmental anomalies as a fracture, remember that:
   - the bipartite or multipartite patella is seen at the superolateral margin of the patella
   - the apparent comminuted fragments do not form a whole, as they would in patellar fracture.
9. Dislocations in the knee joint are commonly complicated by tears of the ligaments and menisci and can coexist with vascular injury, particularly to the popliteal artery.
10. Sinding-Larsen-Johansson disease is clinically characterized by local pain and tenderness on palpation at the site of lower patella, and radiographically by fragmentation and calcification at the proximal attachment of patellar ligament.
11. Osgood-Schlatter disease is a condition related to trauma. Pain and soft-tissue swelling on clinical examination and fragmentation of the ossification center of tibial tuberosity and fibrosis and fluid within the deep infrapatellar bursa on imaging studies (conventional radiography, US, and MRI) are fundamental diagnostic features.
12. Learn to distinguish three conditions that have very similar imaging presentations:
    - osteochondral fracture, which is an acute injury to the articular cartilage and subchondral bone
    - osteochondritis dissecans, which is the result of chronic injury
    - SONK, currently regarded as subchondral insufficiency fracture, which is characterized by acute onset of pain and has been linked to trauma, corticosteroid injections, and meniscal tear.

    Computed arthrotomography, MRI, and MRa are essential techniques in the evaluation of the status of the articular cartilage in each of these conditions.
13. The anterior aspect of the knee contains three synovial bursae: prepatellar, superficial infrapatellar, and deep infrapatellar, which can become distended by fluid (bursitis).
14. Tears of the menisci and ligaments of the knee are best demonstrated by MRI. Tears of the medial meniscus are much more common than tears of the lateral semilunar cartilage. The discoid lateral meniscus predisposes this structure to injury.
15. Bucket-handle tear of the medial meniscus has characteristic MRI appearance:
    - on sagittal sections through the body of the medial meniscus, there is only one image of the bow-tie sign
    - on more lateral sagittal sections obtained closer to the interior of the knee joint, a double PCL sign may be seen.
16. Discoid meniscus has characteristic MRI appearance:
    - on coronal sections, there is lack of normal triangular shape and deep extension of the meniscus into the interior of the joint
    - on sagittal sections through the body of the lateral meniscus, there are more than two images of bow-tie configuration of this structure.
17. The unhappy O'Donoghue triad, resulting from valgus stress forces applied to the knee joint, consists of tears of the:
    - medial meniscus
    - MCL
    - ACL.
18. PLC injuries are considered to be a surgical emergency, requiring operative repair without delay. The injured anatomic structures include popliteal tendon, lateral collateral ligament, posterolateral capsule, arcuate ligament, fabellofibular ligament, and popliteofibular ligament.
19. Transient lateral dislocation of the patella exhibits characteristic appearance on MR: high–signal intensity focus on proton density–weighted fat-saturated or T2/IR sequences in the medial aspect of the patella demonstrated on axial images and similar high signal in the anterior aspect of the lateral femoral condyle demonstrated on sagittal and coronal images of the knee. It is invariably associated with a tear of the medial patellar retinaculum.
20. High position of the patella (patella alta) may indicate a tear of the patellar ligament; low position of the patella (patella infera, patella baja) may indicate a tear of the quadriceps tendon, but MRI is the technique of choice to diagnose these injuries.
21. The results and possible complications of most commonly performed surgical procedures in the knee that include meniscal surgery (partial meniscectomy, meniscal repair, meniscal transplant), ligamentous surgery (mostly ACL), and cartilage repair (debridement of the damaged cartilage, autologous osteochondral transplantation, autologous chondrocyte transplant) among others, can effectively be demonstrated with MRI.

SUGGESTED READINGS

Aichroth P. Osteochondral fractures and their relationship to osteochondritis dissecans of the knee. An experimental study in animals. *J Bone Joint Surg Br* 1971;53B:448–454.

Aichroth P. Osteochondritis dissecans of the knee: a clinical survey. *J Bone Joint Surg Br* 1971;53B:440–447.

Alizai H, Virayavanich W, Joseph GB, et al. Cartilage lesion score: comparison of a quantitative assessment score with established semiquantitative MR scoring systems. *Radiology* 2014;271:479–487.

Bassett LW, Grover JS, Seeger LL. Magnetic resonance imaging of knee trauma. *Skeletal Radiol* 1990;19:401–405.

Blankenbaker DG, De Smet AA, Smith JD. Usefulness of two indirect MR imaging signs to diagnose lateral meniscal tears. *AJR Am J Roentgenol* 2002;178:579–582.

Bolog N, Hodler J. MR imaging of the posterolateral corner of the knee. *Skeletal Radiol* 2007;36:715–728.

Brown WE, Potter HG, Marx RG, et al. Magnetic resonance imaging appearance of cartilage repair in the knee. *Clin Orthop Relat Research* 2004;(422):214–223.

Campos JC, Chung CB, Lektrakul N, et al. Pathogenesis of the Segond fracture: anatomic and MR imaging evidence of an iliotibial tract or anterior band avulsion. *Radiology* 2001;219:381–386.

Chapin R. Imaging of the postoperative meniscus. *Radiol Clin North Am* 2018;56:953–964.

Chatra PS. Bursae around the knee joint. *Indian J Radiol Imaging* 2012;22:27–30.

de Abreu MR, Chung CB, Trudell D, et al. Meniscofemoral ligaments: patterns of tears and pseudotears of the menisci using cadaveric and clinical material. *Skeletal Radiol* 2007;36:729–735.

De Smet AA. MR imaging and MR arthrography for diagnosis of recurrent tears in the postoperative meniscus. *Semin Musculoskelet Radiol* 2005;9:116–124.

Dhanda S, Sanghvi D, Pardivala D. Case series: cyclops lesion—extension loss after ACL reconstruction. *Indian J Radiol Imaging* 2010;20:206–210.

Escobedo EM, Mills WJ, Hunter JC. The "reverse Segond" fracture: association with a tear of the posterior cruciate ligament and medial meniscus. *AJR Am J Roentgenol* 2002;178:979–983.

Ficat RP, Hungerford DS. *Disorders of the patellofemoral joint.* Baltimore: Williams & Wilkins; 1977.

Flores DV, Mejía Gómez CM, Pathria MN. Layered approach to the anterior knee: normal anatomy and disorders associated with anterior knee pain. *Radiographics* 2018;38:2069–2101.

Fox AJS, Bedi A, Rodeo SA. The basic science of human knee menisci: structure, composition, and function. *Sports Health* 2012;4:340–351.

Gorbachova T, Melenevsky Y, Cohen M, et al. Osteochondral lesions of the knee: differentiating the most common entities at MRI. *Radiographics* 2018;38:1478–1495.

Grelsamer RP, Meadows S. The modified Insall-Salvati ratio for assessment of patellar height. *Clin Orthop Relat Res* 1992;282:170–176.

Haims AH, Medvecky MJ, Pavlovich R Jr, et al. MR imaging of the anatomy of and injuries to the lateral and posterolateral aspects of the knee. *AJR Am J Roentgenol* 2003;180:647–653.

Hall FM, Hochman MG. Medial Segond-type fracture: cortical avulsion of the medial tibial plateau associated with tears of the posterior cruciate ligament and medial meniscus. *Skeletal Radiol* 1997;26:553–555.

Hangody L, Füles P. Autologous osteochondral mosaicplasty for the treatment of full-thickness defects of weight-bearing joints: ten years of experimental and clinical experience. *J Bone Joint Surg Am* 2003;85A(suppl 2):25–32.

Helms CA. The meniscus: recent advances in MR imaging of the knee. *AJR Am J Roentgenol* 2002;179:1115–1122.

Henrichs A. Review of knee dislocations. *J Athl Train* 2004;39:365–369.

Hohl M. Tibial condylar fractures. *J Bone Joint Surg Am* 1967;49A:1455–1467.

Inaba K, Potzman J, Munera F, et al. Multi-slice CT angiography for arterial evaluation in the injured lower extremity. *J Trauma* 2006;60:502–506.

Insall J, Salvati E. Patella position in the normal knee joint. *Radiology* 1971;101:101–104.

Jee W-H, McCauley TR, Kim J-M, et al. Meniscal tear configurations: categorization with MR imaging. *AJR Am J Roentgenol* 2003;180:93–97.

Kaplan PA, Nelson NL, Garvin KL, et al. MR of the knee: the significance of high signal in the meniscus that does not clearly extend to the surface. *AJR Am J Roentgenol* 1991;156:333–336.

Kijowski R, Rosas H, Williams A, et al. MRI characteristics of torn and untorn post-operative menisci. *Skeletal Radiol* 2018;46:1353–1360.

Klineberg EO, Crites BM, Flinn WR, et al. The role of arteriography in assessing popliteal artery injury in knee dislocations. *J Trauma* 2004;56:786–790.

Kode L, Lieberman JM, Motta AO, et al. Evaluation of tibial plateau fractures: efficacy of MR imaging compared with CT. *AJR Am J Roentgenol* 1994;163:141–147.

Lee J, Papakonstantinou O, Brookenthal KR, et al. Arcuate sign of posterolateral knee injuries: anatomic, radiographic, and MR imaging data related to patterns of injury. *Skeletal Radiol* 2003;32:619–627.

Lee JH, Singh TT, Bolton G. Axial fat-saturated FSE imaging of the knee: appearance of meniscal tears. *Skeletal Radiol* 2002;31:384–395.

Liu YW, Skalski MR, Patel DB, et al. The anterior knee: normal variants, common pathologies, and diagnostic pitfalls on MRI. *Skeletal Radiol* 2018;47:1069–1086.

Lu W, Yang J, Chen S, et al. Abnormal patella height based on Insall-Salvati ratio and its correlation with patellar cartilage lesions: an extremity-dedicated low-field magnetic resonance imaging analysis of 1703 Chinese cases. *Scand J Surg* 2016;105:197–203.

McAnally JL, Southam SL, Mlady GW. New thoughts on the origin of Pellegrini-Stieda: the association of PCL injury and medial femoral epicondylar periosteal stripping. *Skeletal Radiol* 2009;38:193–198.

McKnight A, Southgate J, Price A, et al. Meniscal tears with displaced fragments: common patterns on magnetic resonance imaging. *Skeletal Radiol* 2010;39:279–283.

Mendes LF, Pretterklieber ML, Cho JH, et al. Pellegrini-Stieda disease: a heterogeneous disorder not synonymous with ossification/calcification of the tibial collateral ligament—anatomic and imaging investigation. *Skeletal Radiol* 2006;35:916–922.

Merchant AC, Mercer RL, Jacobsen RH, et al. Roentgenographic analysis of patellofemoral congruence. *J Bone Joint Surg Am* 1974;56(7):1391–1396.

Norman A, Baker ND. Spontaneous osteonecrosis of the knee and medial meniscal tears. *Radiology* 1978;129:653–660.

O'Donoghue DH. Chondral and osteochondral fractures. *J Trauma* 1966;6:469–481.

Osgood RB. Lesions of the tibial tubercle occurring during adolescence. *Boston Med Surg J* 1903;148:114–117.

Pandit S, Frampton C, Stoddart J, et al. Magnetic resonance imaging assessment of tibial tuberosity-trochlear groove distance: normal values for males and females. *Int Orthop* 2011;35:1799–1803.

Rao N, Patel Y, Opsha O, et al. Use of the V-sign in the diagnosis of bucket-handle meniscal tear of the knee. *Skeletal Radiol* 2012;41:293–297.

Recht MP, Goodwin DW, Winalski CS, et al. MRI of articular cartilage: revisiting current status and future directions. *AJR Am J Roentgenol* 2005;185:899–914.

Recht MP, Kramer J. MRI Imaging of the postoperative knee: a pictorial essay. *Radiographics* 2002;22:765–774.

Recondo JA, Salvador E, Villanúa JA, et al. Lateral stabilizing structures of the knee: functional anatomy and injuries assessed with MR imaging. *Radiographics* 2000;20:91–102.

Redmond JM, Levy BA, Dajani KA, et al. Detecting vascular injury in lower-extremity orthopedic trauma: the role of CT angiography. *Orthopedics* 2008;31:761–767.

Robertson A, Nutton RW, Keating JF. Dislocation of the knee. *J Bone Joint Surg Br* 2006;88:706–711.

Rogers LF. *Radiology of skeletal trauma*, 2nd ed. New York: Churchill Livingstone; 1992:1199–1317.

Schatzker J, McBroom R, Bruce D. The tibial plateau fracture. The Toronto experience 1968–1975. *Clin Orthop Relat Res* 1979;138:94–104.

Schwaiger BJ, Gersing AS, Wamba JM, et al. Can signal abnormalities detected with MR imaging in knee articular cartilage be used to predict development of morphologic cartilage defects? 48-month data from the Osteoarthritis Initiative. *Radiology* 2016;281:58–116.

Shybut T, Strauss EJ. Surgical management of meniscal tears. *Bull NYU Hosp Jt Dis* 2011;69:56–62.

Sinding-Larsen MF. A hitherto unknown affection of the patella in children. *Acta Radiol* 1921;1:171–173.

Steadman JR, Briggs KK, Rodrigo J, et al. Outcomes of microfracture for traumatic chondral defects of the knee: average 11-year follow-up. *Arthroscopy* 2003;19:477–484.

Stoller DW. *Magnetic resonance imaging in orthopaedics and sports medicine*. Philadelphia: JB Lippincott; 1993.

Tokarsky G, Drescher M. Bilateral popliteal artery thrombosis from traumatic knee dislocation. *Israeli J Emer Med* 2006;6:37–39.

Venkatanarasimha N, Kamath A, Mukherjee K, et al. Potential pitfalls of a double PCL sign. *Skeletal Radiol* 2009;38:735–739.

Vinson EN, Major NM, Helms CA. The posterolateral corner of the knee. *AJR Am J Roentgenol* 2008;190:449–458.

Wilcox JJ, Snow BJ, Aoki SK, et al. Does landmark selection affect the reliability of tibial tubercle-trochlear groove measurements using MRI? *Clin Orthop Relat Res* 2012;470:2253–2260.

Yao L, Gai N, Boutin RD. Axial scan orientation and the tibial tubercle-trochlear groove distance: error analysis and correction. *AJR Am J Roentgenol* 2014;202:1291–1296.

Yilmaz B, Ozdemir G, Sirin E, et al. Evaluation of patella alta using MRI measurements in adolescents. *Indian J Radiol Imaging* 2017;27:181–186.

10

Lower Limb III

Ankle and Foot

Trauma to the Ankle and Foot

The ankle is the most frequently injured of all the major weight-bearing joints in the body. Most victims are young adults injured while participating in athletic activities such as running, skiing, and soccer. Ankle structures susceptible to injury include bones, ligaments, tendons, and syndesmoses; ligaments can be damaged in the absence of fractures. When this occurs, damage to ligaments may go unrecognized on conventional radiographs, with the result that the patient is not properly treated.

The type of fracture usually indicates the mechanism of injury determined, as Kleiger has pointed out, by the position of the foot, the direction and intensity of the applied force, and the resistance of the structures making up the joint. The mechanism of injury may in turn serve as an indicator of which ligament structures are damaged.

Although occasionally meticulous history taking and clinical examination can help determine the mechanism of trauma and predict damage to the various structures, radiologic examination is the key to reliable evaluation of the site and extent of injury. There are two basic types of ankle trauma: inversion injuries and eversion injuries. These, however, may be complicated by internal or external rotation, hyperflexion or hyperextension, and vertical compression forces.

Foot injuries are also common and usually result from direct trauma, such as a blow or a fall from a height; only rarely do such injuries result from indirect forces such as abnormal stress or strain of muscles or tendons. Foot fractures, accounting for 10% of all fractures, are more common than dislocations, which usually are associated with fractures, and occur at the midtarsal, tarsometatarsal, and metatarsophalangeal articulations.

Anatomic–Radiologic Considerations

The ankle joint proper consists of the tibiotalar and distal tibiofibular articulations, the latter a syndesmotic joint rather than a true synarthrodial one. In matters of injury, however, one must consider that the ankle joint acts as a unit with other joints of the foot, particularly the talocalcaneal (subtalar) articulation, where application of stress can have great impact on ankle injuries.

The ankle joint is formed by three bones—the distal tibia and fibula and the talus—and three principal sets of ligaments—the medial collateral (deltoid) ligament; the lateral collateral ligament, consisting of the anterior talofibular, posterior talofibular, and calcaneofibular ligaments; and the syndesmotic complex, a fibrous joint between the distal tibia and the fibula (Fig. 10.1). The distal tibiofibular syndesmotic complex, one of the most important anatomic structures in maintaining ankle integrity and stability, consists of three elements: the distal anterior tibiofibular ligament, the distal posterior tibiofibular ligament, and the interosseous membrane.

From the viewpoint of anatomy and kinetics, the foot is divided into three distinct sections: hindfoot, midfoot, and forefoot. The hindfoot, separated from the midfoot by the midtarsal (or Chopart) joint, includes the talus and calcaneus; the midfoot, separated from the forefoot by the tarsometatarsal (Lisfranc) joint, includes the navicular, cuboid, and three cuneiform bones; and the forefoot includes the metatarsals and phalanges (Fig. 10.2). The muscles attached to the tibia and fibula end in tendons proximal to or at the level of the ankle joint. These tendons insert into the foot (Fig. 10.3).

A word about terminology is in order because the terminology describing motion of the ankle and foot in the literature is not uniform and confusion has been created about the various mechanisms of ankle and foot injuries. Frequently, but incorrectly, the terms *adduction*, *inversion*, *varus*, and *supination* have been used interchangeably, as have their counterparts *abduction*, *eversion*, *valgus*, and *pronation*. However, supination and pronation are more appropriately applied to compound motion. *Supination* consists of adduction and inversion of the forefoot (motion in the tarsometatarsal and midtarsal joints) and inversion of the heel, which assumes a varus configuration (motion in subtalar joint), as well as slight plantar flexion of the ankle (tibiotalar) joint. In *pronation*, compound motion consists of abduction and eversion of the forefoot (motion in the tarsometatarsal and midtarsal joints) and eversion of the heel, which assumes a valgus configuration (motion in the subtalar joint), together with slight dorsiflexion (or dorsal extension) of the ankle (Fig. 10.4).

Adduction properly applies to medial deviation of the forefoot, and *abduction* to lateral deviation of the forefoot, both motions occurring in the tarsometatarsal (Lisfranc) joint; *adduction of the heel* refers to inversion of the calcaneus; and *abduction of the heel* refers to eversion of the calcaneus, both motions occurring in the subtalar joint. *Plantar flexion* refers to caudad (downward) foot motion, *dorsiflexion* to cephalad (upward) foot motion—motions occurring in the ankle (tibiotalar) joint. Varus and valgus should not be used to describe motion but should be reserved for the description of ankle or foot position in case of deformity. Occasionally, varus and valgus are used interchangeably with inversion and eversion to describe the applied stress.

Imaging of the Ankle and Foot

Ankle

The standard radiographic examination of the ankle, as a rule, includes the anteroposterior (including the mortise), lateral, and oblique projections. Stress views are also frequently obtained for evaluating ankle injuries. These may also need to be supplemented with special projections.

PRINCIPAL GROUPS OF ANKLE LIGAMENTS

Medial Collateral (Deltoid) Ligament

medial view
tibiotalar band
tibionavicular band
tibiocalcaneal band

Lateral Collateral Ligament

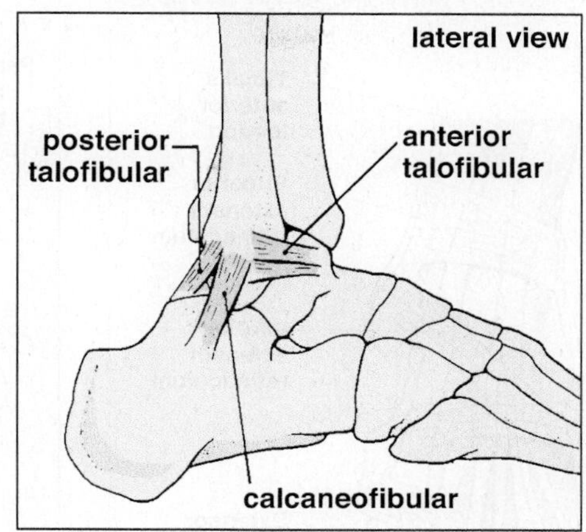

Distal Tibiofibular Syndesmotic Complex

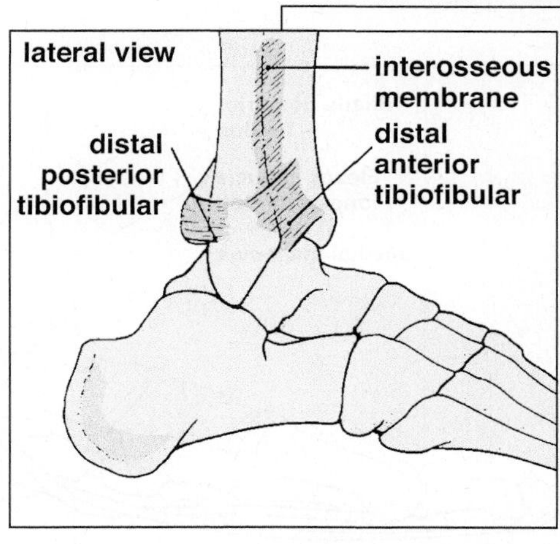

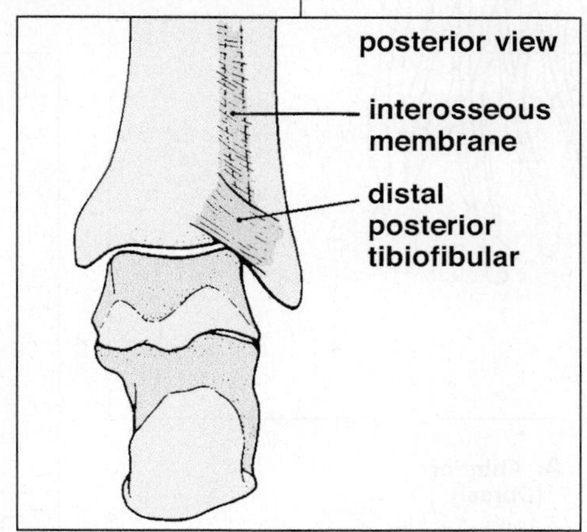

FIGURE 10.1 Ligaments of the ankle. Three principal sets of ligaments form the ankle joint: the medial collateral (deltoid) ligament, the lateral collateral ligament, and the distal tibiofibular syndesmotic complex, which is important for maintaining ankle integrity and stability.

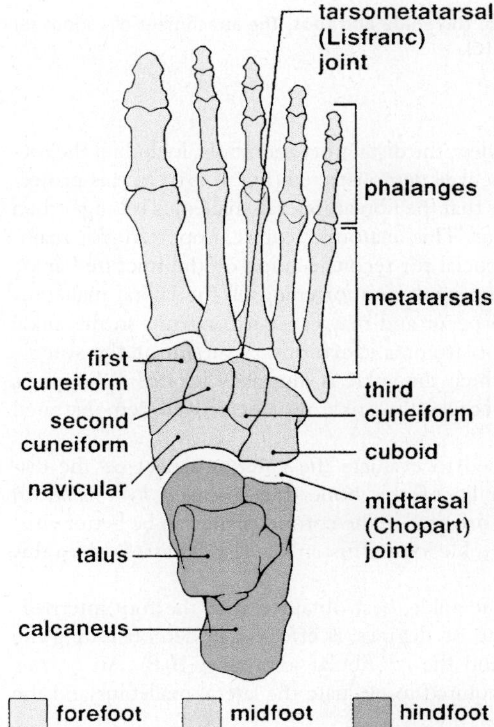

FIGURE 10.2 Anatomic divisions of the foot. The foot can be viewed as comprising three anatomic parts: the hindfoot, midfoot, and forefoot, separated, respectively, by the midtarsal (Chopart) and tarsometatarsal (Lisfranc) joints.

TENDONS OF THE ANKLE AND FOOT

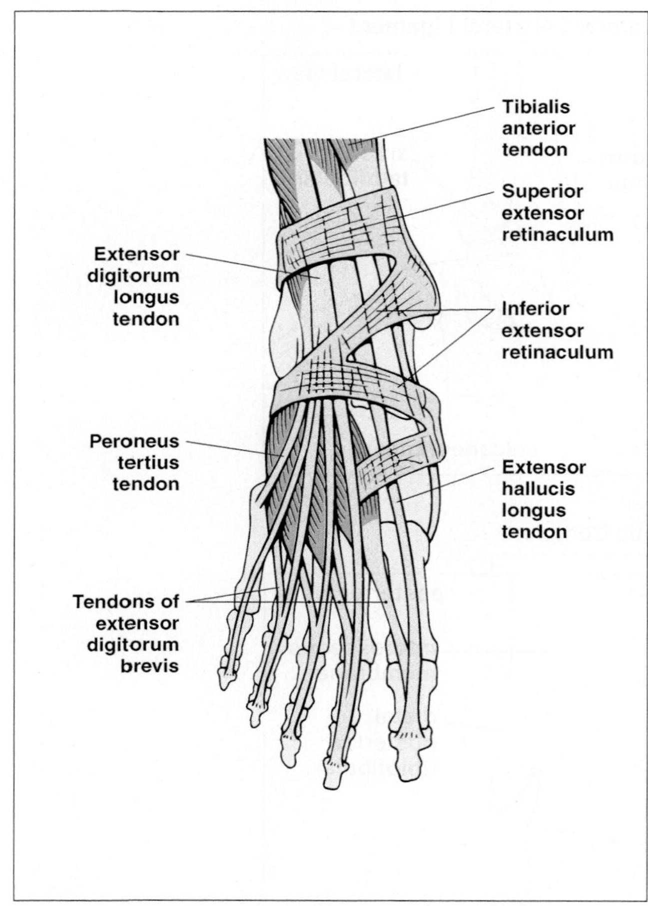

A. Anterior (Dorsal)

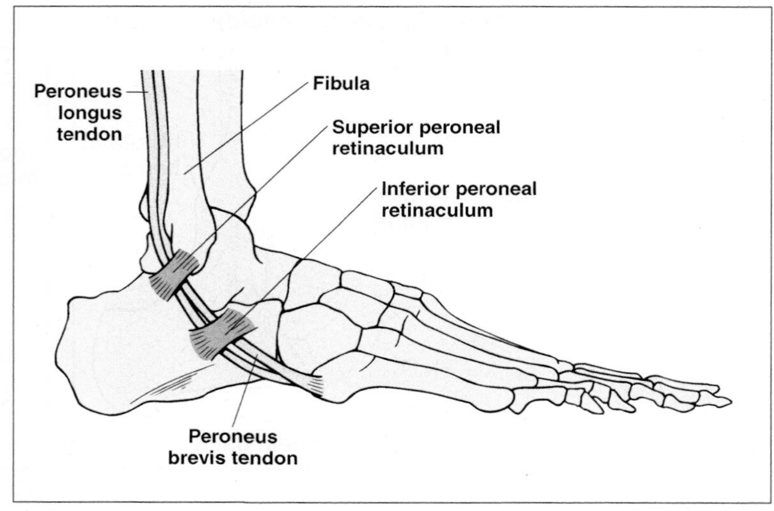

B. Lateral

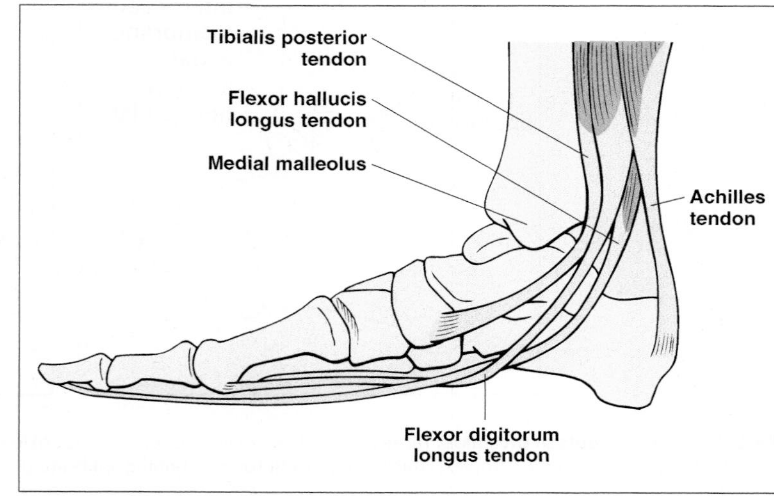

C. Medial

FIGURE 10.3 Tendons of the ankle and foot. The attachment of various tendons of the ankle and foot are depicted, as viewed from the dorsal aspect **(A)**, lateral aspect **(B)**, and medial aspect **(C)**.

On the *anteroposterior* view, the distal tibia and fibula, including the medial and lateral malleoli, are well demonstrated (Fig. 10.5). On this projection, it is important to note that the fibular (lateral) malleolus is longer than the tibial (medial) malleolus. This anatomic feature, important for maintaining ankle stability, is crucial for reconstruction of the fractured ankle joint. Even minimal displacement or shortening of the lateral malleolus allows lateral talar shift to occur and may cause incongruity in the ankle joint, possibly leading to posttraumatic arthritis. A variant of the anteroposterior projection, in which the ankle is internally rotated 10 degrees, is called the *mortise view* because the ankle mortise is well demonstrated on it (Fig. 10.6).

The *lateral* view is used to evaluate the anterior aspect of the distal tibia and the posterior lip of this bone (the so-called *third malleolus*) (Fig. 10.7). Some fractures oriented in the coronal plane can be better visualized on this projection. Ankle joint effusion can also be assessed on this view (see Fig. 10.69).

The *oblique* view of the ankle, best obtained with the foot internally rotated approximately 30 to 35 degrees, is effective in demonstrating the tibiofibular syndesmosis and the talofibular joint (Fig. 10.8). An *external oblique* view may also be required to evaluate the lateral malleolus and the anterior tibial tubercle (Fig. 10.9).

Most ankle ligament injuries require stress radiography, ankle joint arthrography, computed tomography (CT), or magnetic resonance imaging (MRI) (see the text that follows) for demonstration and sufficient evaluation. Some, however, can be deduced from the site and extension of fractures on the standard radiographic examination. A thorough knowledge of the skeletal and soft-tissue topographic anatomy of the ankle, together with an understanding of the kinematics and mechanism of ankle injuries, will aid the radiologist in correctly diagnosing traumatic conditions and predicting ligament injuries. With such understanding, the radiologist can even determine the sequence of injury to the various structures.

Some ligament injuries may be diagnosed on the basis of disruption of the ankle mortise and displacement of the talus; others can be deduced from the appearance of fractured bones. For example, fibular fracture above the level of the ankle joint indicates that the distal anterior tibiofibular ligament is torn. Fracture of the fibula above its anterior tubercle strongly suggests that the tibiofibular syndesmosis is completely disrupted. Fracture of the fibula above the level of the ankle joint without accompanying fracture of the medial malleolus indicates rupture of the deltoid ligament. Transverse fracture of the medial malleolus indicates that the deltoid ligament is intact. High fracture of the fibula associated with a

FIGURE 10.4 Motion in the ankle and foot. Supination is a compound motion consisting of adduction and inversion of the forefoot, together with inversion of the heel and slight plantar flexion in the ankle joint. In pronation, the compound motion involves abduction and eversion of the forefoot with eversion of the heel and slight dorsiflexion in the ankle joint.

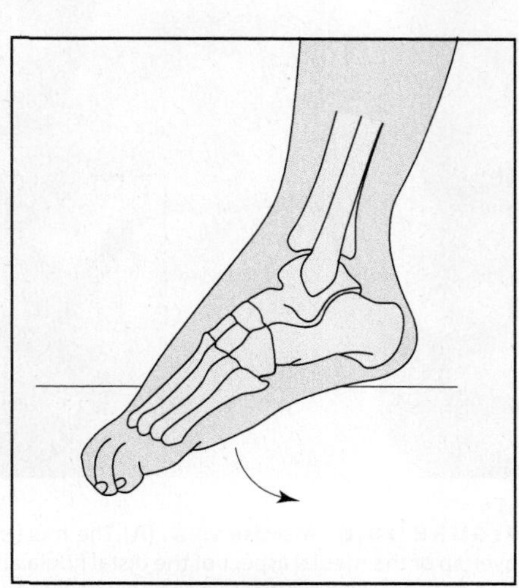

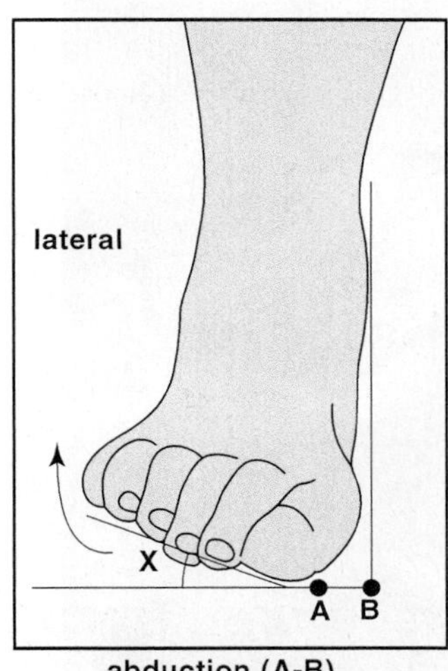

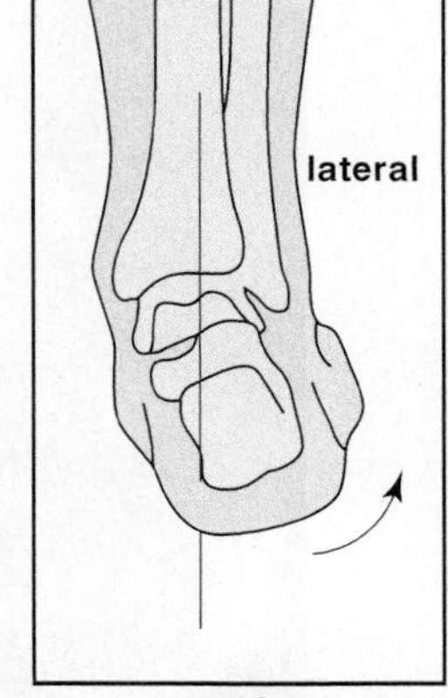

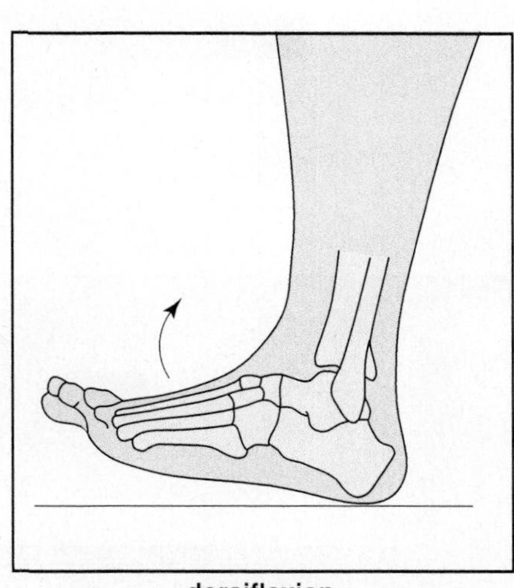

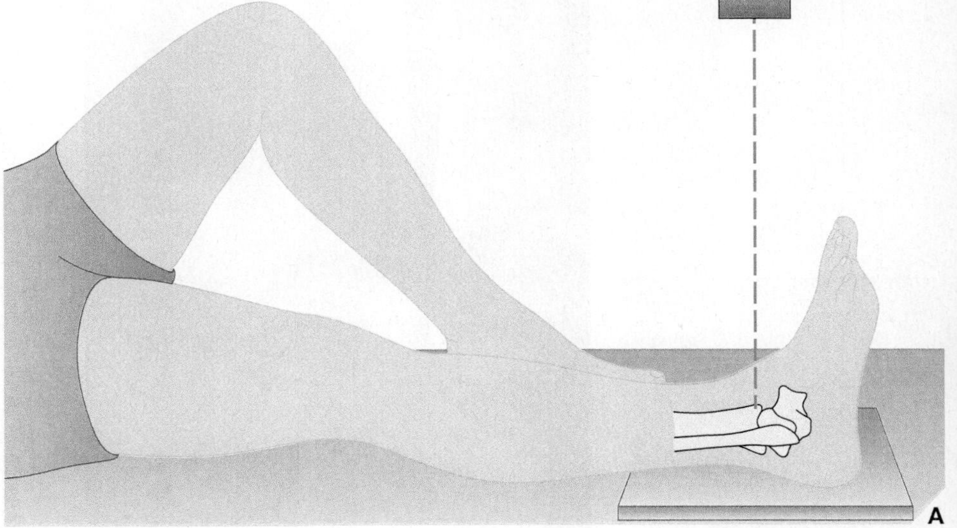

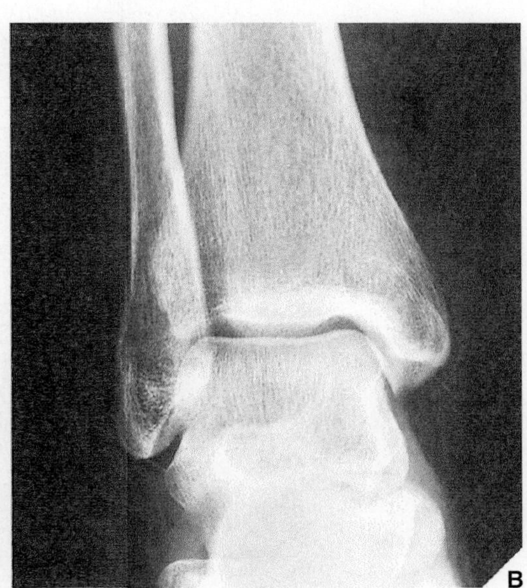

FIGURE 10.5 Anteroposterior view. (A) For the anteroposterior view of the ankle, the patient is supine on the radiographic table with the heel resting on the film cassette. The foot is in neutral position, with the sole perpendicular to the leg and the cassette. The central beam *(red broken line)* is directed vertically to the ankle joint at the midpoint between both malleoli. **(B)** The radiograph in this projection demonstrates the distal tibia, particularly the medial malleolus, the body of the talus, and the tibiotalar joint. Note, however, the overlap of the distal fibula and the lateral aspect of the tibia. The tibiofibular syndesmosis is not clearly demonstrated.

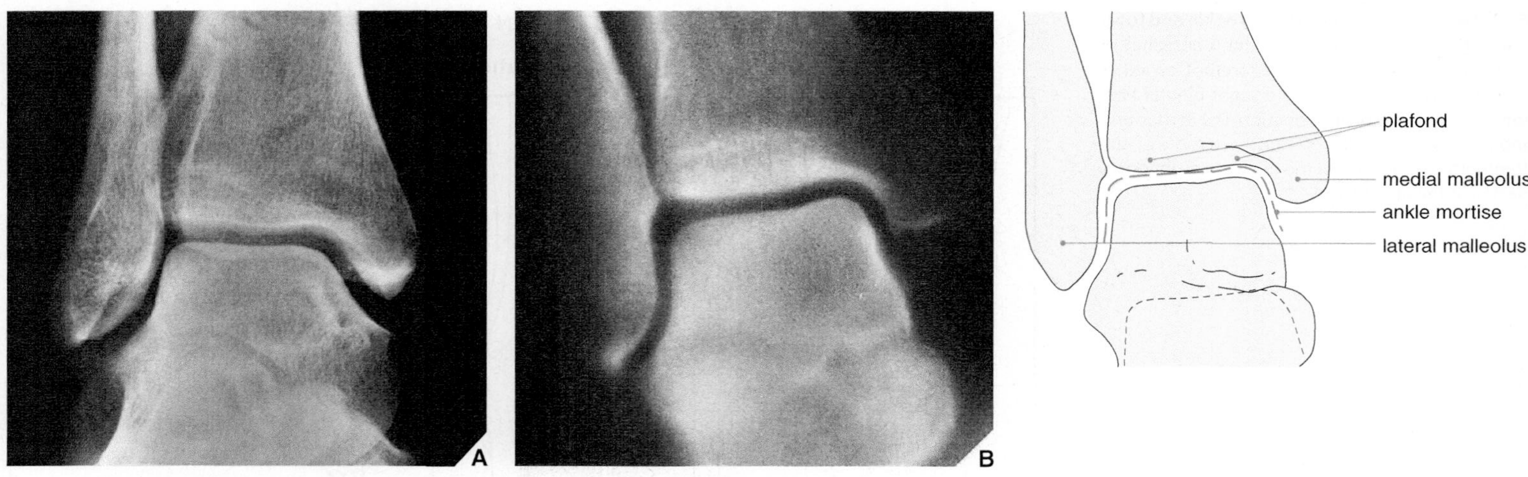

FIGURE 10.6 Mortise view. **(A)** The mortise view, a variant of the anteroposterior projection obtained with 10-degree internal rotation of the ankle, eliminates the overlap of the medial aspect of the distal fibula and the lateral aspect of the talus, so the space between these bones is well demonstrated. **(B)** The ankle mortise, shown here on a tomographic cut through the ankle joint, is formed by the medial malleolus, the articular surface of the distal tibia (the ceiling or plafond), and the lateral malleolus; it is shaped like an inverted U.

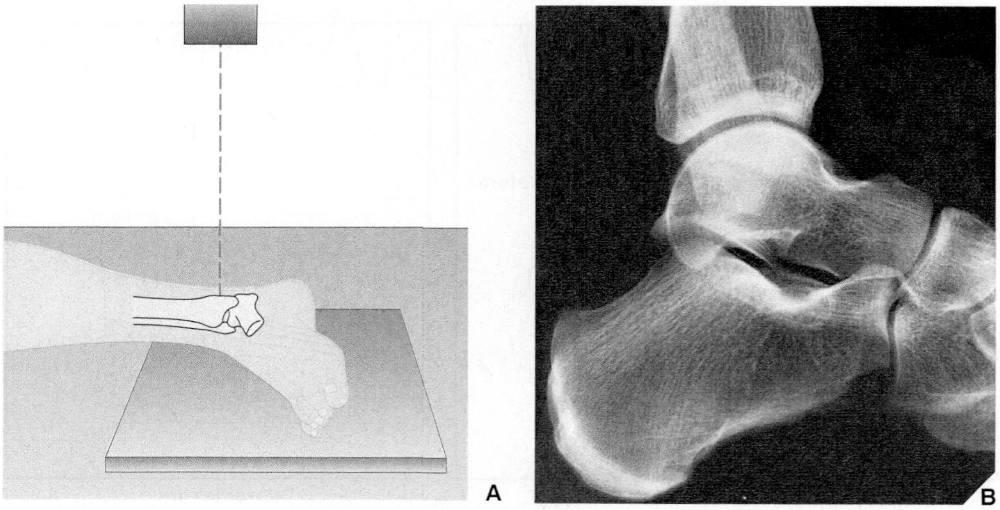

FIGURE 10.7 Lateral view. **(A)** For the lateral projection of the ankle, the patient is placed on his or her side with the fibula resting on the film cassette and the foot in the neutral position. The central beam *(red broken line)* is directed vertically to the medial malleolus. (The lateral view can also be obtained by placing the medial side of the ankle against the cassette.) **(B)** On the radiograph obtained in this projection, the distal tibia, talus, and calcaneus are seen in profile, and the fibula overlaps the posterior aspect of the tibia and the posterior aspect of the talus. The tibiotalar and subtalar joints are well demonstrated. Note the posterior lip of the tibia, also known as the *third malleolus*.

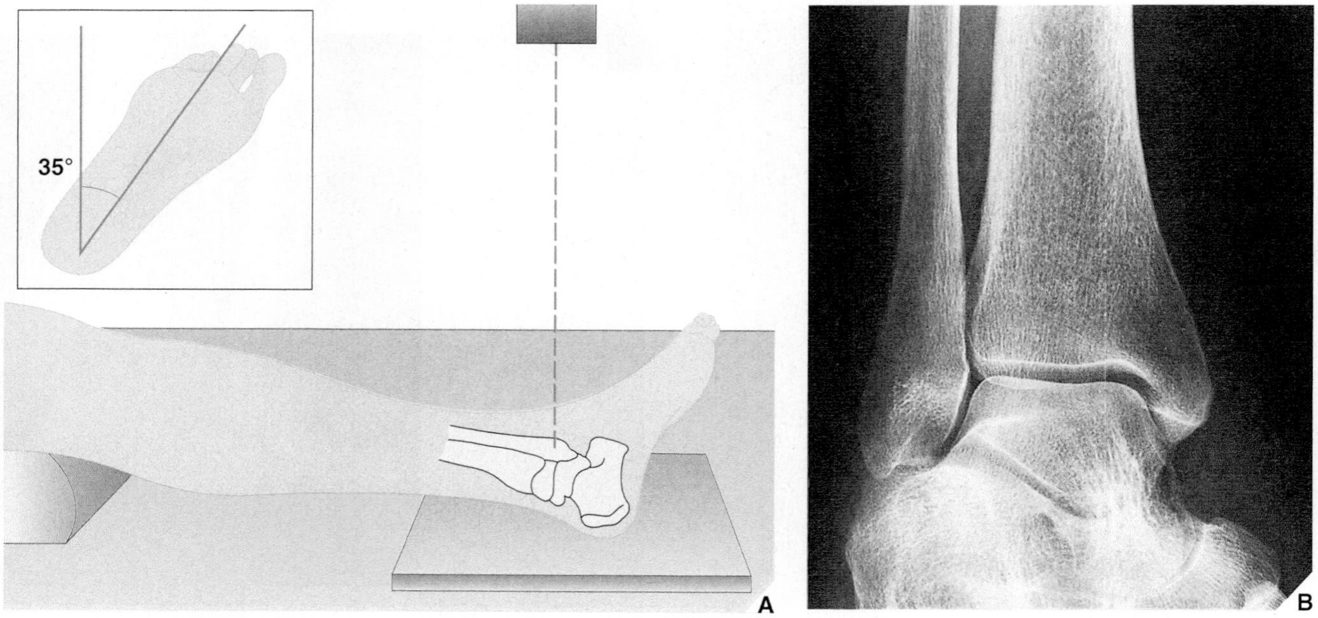

FIGURE 10.8 Internal oblique view. **(A)** For the internal oblique view of the ankle, the patient is supine, and the leg and foot are rotated medially approximately 35 degrees *(inset)*. The foot is in the neutral position, forming a 90-degree angle with the distal leg. The central beam *(red broken line)* is directed perpendicular to the lateral malleolus. **(B)** On the radiograph, the medial and lateral malleoli, the tibial plafond, the dome of the talus, the tibiotalar joint, and the tibiofibular syndesmosis are well demonstrated.

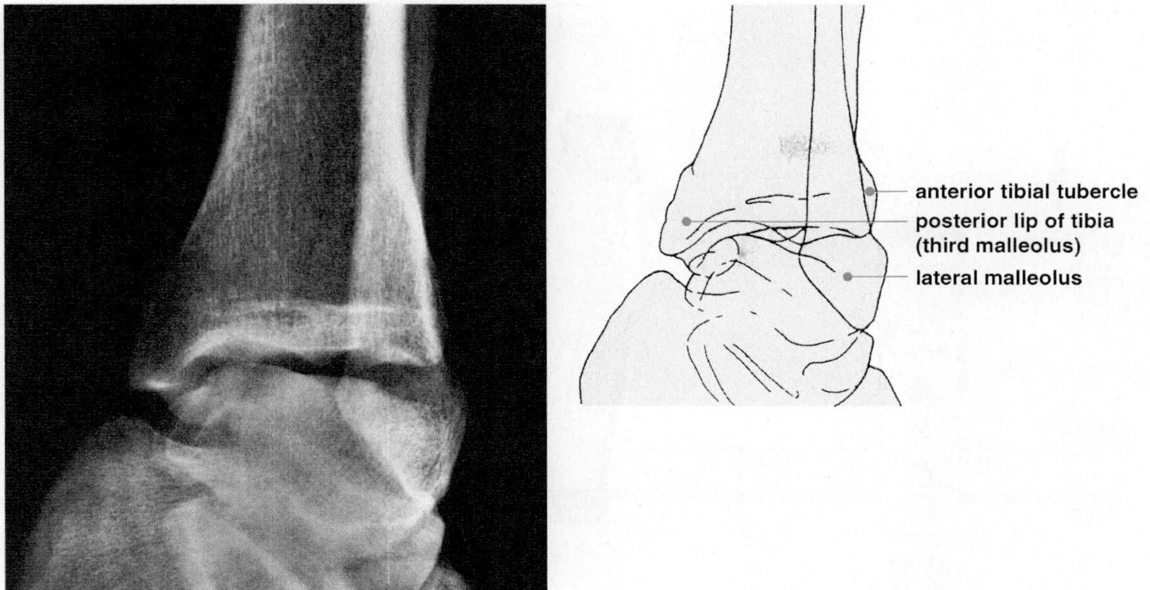

FIGURE 10.9 External oblique view. On the external oblique view, for which the patient is positioned as for the internal oblique view but with the limb rotated laterally approximately 40 to 45 degrees, the lateral malleolus and the anterior tibial tubercle are well demonstrated.

fracture of the medial malleolus or tear of the tibiofibular ligament, the so-called *Maisonneuve fracture* (see later), indicates rupture of the interosseous membrane up to the level of the fibular fracture.

When radiographs of the ankle are normal, however, stress views are extremely important in evaluating ligament injuries (see Fig. 4.5). Inversion (adduction) and anterior-draw stress films are most frequently obtained; only rarely is an eversion (abduction)-stress examination required.

On the *inversion-stress* radiograph, obtained in the anteroposterior projection, the degree of talar tilt can be measured by the angle formed by lines drawn along the tibial plafond and the dome of the talus (Fig. 10.10). This angle helps diagnose tears of the lateral collateral ligament. However, the wide range of normal values for these measurements can make interpretation difficult, and thus comparison studies of the contralateral ankle should be obtained. Even this method is not always accurate; up to

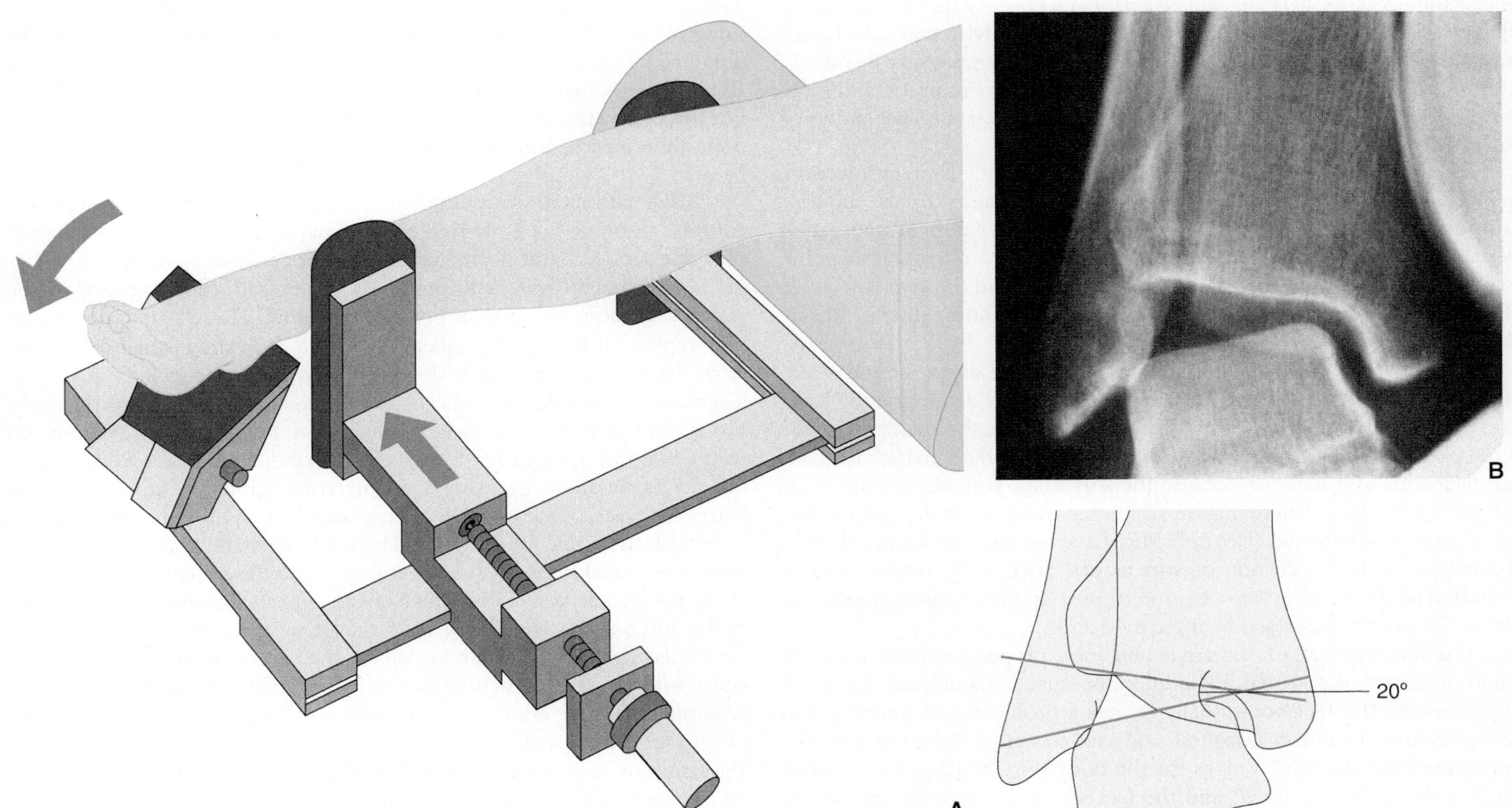

FIGURE 10.10 Inversion stress view. **(A)** For inversion (adduction)-stress examination of the ankle, the foot is fixed in the device while the patient is supine. The pressure plate, positioned approximately 2 cm above the ankle joint, applies varus stress *(red arrows)* adducting the heel. (If the examination is painful, 5 to 10 mL of 1% lidocaine or a similar local anesthetic is injected at the site of maximum pain.) **(B)** On the anteroposterior radiograph, the degree of talar tilt is measured by the angle formed by lines drawn along the tibial plafond and the dome of the talus. The contralateral ankle is subjected to the same procedure for comparison.

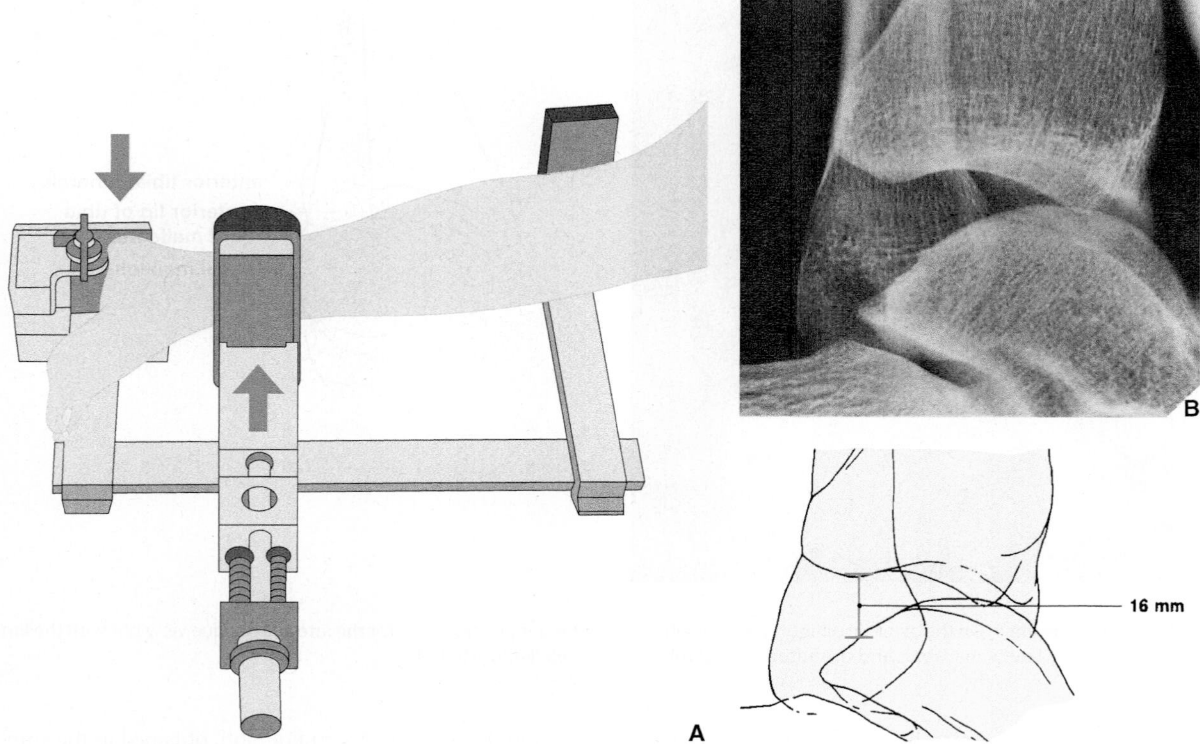

FIGURE 10.11 Anterior-draw stress view. **(A)** For anterior-draw stress examination, the patient is placed on his or her side, with the foot in the device. The pressure plate, positioned anteriorly approximately 2 cm above the ankle, applies posterior stress *(red arrows)* on the heel. During the examination, the amount of pressure is monitored on a light-emitting diode digital reader. **(B)** On the lateral stress radiograph, the amount of transposition of the talus in relation to the distal tibia can be determined.

25 degrees of talar tilt has been reported in people with no history of injury, and occasionally, there will be a patient whose ankles exhibit considerable variation in measurement. Many authorities advise that with forced inversion, tilt less than 5 degrees is normal, 5 to 15 degrees may be normal or abnormal, 15 to 25 degrees strongly suggests ligament injury, and more than 25 degrees is always abnormal. With forced eversion, talar tilting of more than 10 degrees is probably pathologic.

The *anterior-draw* stress radiograph, obtained in the lateral projection, provides a useful measurement for determining injury to the anterior talofibular ligament (Fig. 10.11). Values of up to 5 mm of separation between the talus and the distal tibia are considered normal; values between 5 and 10 mm may be normal or abnormal, and the opposite ankle should be stressed for comparison. Values above 10 mm always indicate abnormality.

Ancillary imaging techniques are essential to the diagnosis and evaluation of many ankle injuries. CT may be required to determine the position of comminuted fragments in complex fractures, for example, of the distal tibia, talus, and calcaneus. In addition, CT may demonstrate the various ligaments and tendons because the soft-tissue contrast resolution of CT allows the easy differentiation of these structures from surrounding fat. However, ultrasound (US) and MRI have become the more accepted techniques for the evaluation of soft tissues. Specifically, tendon injuries including tendinitis, tenosynovitis, and rupture and dislocation of tendons can be effectively diagnosed by these modalities.

For adequate CT of the ankle and foot, proper positioning of the leg in the gantry is essential. In addition, because nomenclature for imaging planes of the feet occasionally creates a problem, it is important to recognize that the coronal, sagittal, and axial planes of the ankle and foot are determined the same way as for the body (Fig. 10.12A). For coronal images, the knees are flexed and the feet are positioned flat against the gantry table. The coronal sections are obtained with the beam directed to the dorsum of the foot. More commonly modified coronal images are obtained by angling the gantry or by using a foot wedge (Fig. 10.12B). A lateral scanogram helps to establish the degree of necessary gantry tilt. Axial images are obtained with the feet perpendicular to the gantry table, great toes together, and the knees fully extended. The beam is directed parallel to the soles of the feet. Sagittal images are usually generated by using reformation technique, although direct sagittal sections can also be obtained by placing the patient in the lateral decubitus position. Images in all planes are usually acquired using 3- or 5-mm thin contiguous sections. For three-dimensional (3D) reconstruction, 1.5- or 2-mm contiguous sections are required, although 5-mm sections with a 3-mm overlap can also be used.

MRI, with its direct multiplanar capabilities and excellent soft-tissue contrast resolution, has proved to be superior to CT for the evaluation of ankle tendons and ligaments. The tendons show uniformly low signal intensity in all spin echo pulse sequences, with the exception of the Achilles tendon and tibialis posterior tendon. These two tendons, on long repetition time (TR) sequences, occasionally show small foci of intermediate signal intensity within their substance, particularly near their insertions to the calcaneal tuberosity and the navicular bone, respectively. From a practical point of view, it is helpful to memorize the location and relationship of various tendons seen on axial magnetic resonance (MR) image of the ankle by using the mnemonic phrase, "Tom, Dick, and Harry" for the posteromedial aspect, and "TED" for the anterolateral aspect of the ankle (Fig. 10.13). The ankle ligaments, likewise, demonstrate low signal intensity on MR images, with the exception of the posterior talofibular ligaments, which often appears heterogeneous, similar to the anterior cruciate ligament of the knee. The anterior and posterior talofibular ligaments can be visualized over their entire length on axial scans with the foot in neutral position (Fig. 10.14) because they are approximately in the same plane of section. The calcaneofibular ligament can be similarly visualized when the foot is in 40-degree plantar flexion. The anterior and posterior tibiofibular ligaments can be demonstrated on the axial images in more proximal sections (Fig. 10.15). Many of the ligamentous and tendon structures around the ankle are oriented in an angle with respect to the main magnetic field, creating a magic angle artifact on short echo time (TE) pulse sequences. This can be avoided by reorienting the position of the foot or using pulse sequences with a TE longer than 20 msec.

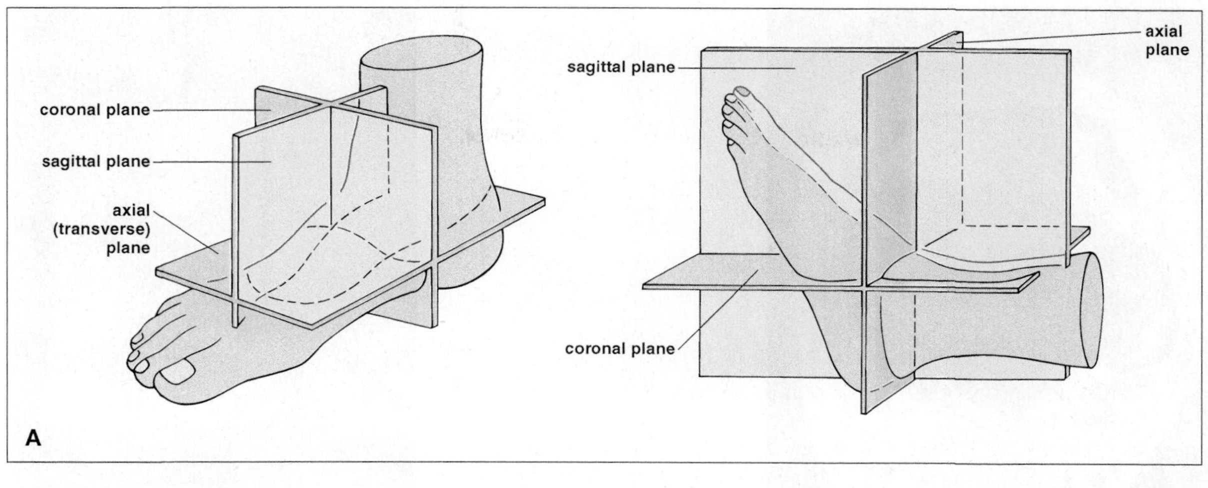

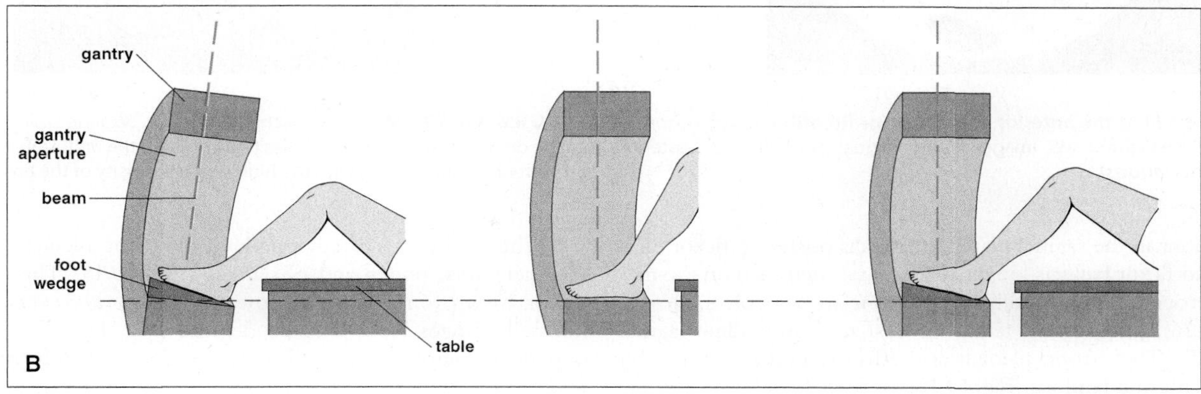

FIGURE 10.12 Anatomic and imaging planes. (A) Anatomic planes of the ankle and **(B)**foot and CT imaging planes. (**B**, Modified with permission from Berquist TH, ed. *Radiology of the foot and ankle*. New York: Raven Press; 1989.)

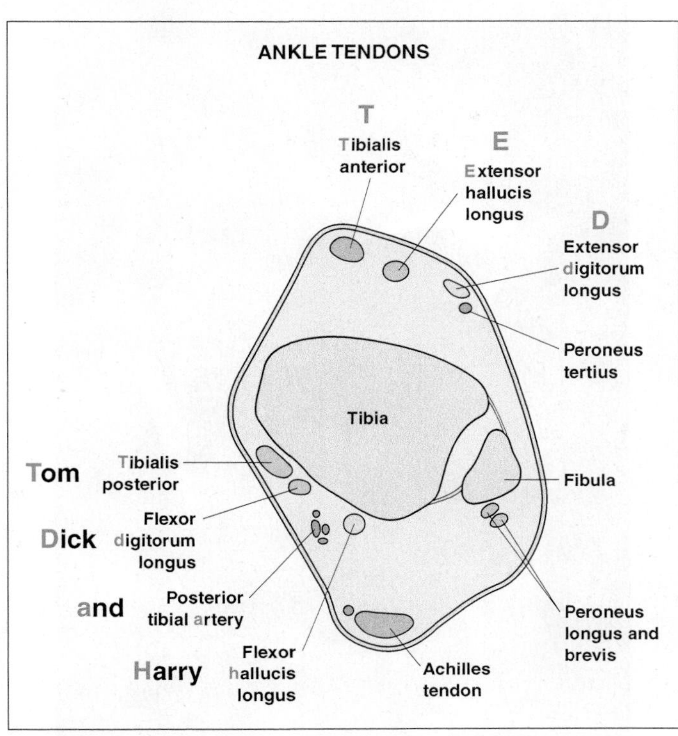

FIGURE 10.13 Schematic representation of ankle tendons on axial MRI. (Modified from Helms CA, Major NM, Anderson MW, et al. *Musculoskeletal MRI*, 2nd ed. Philadelphia: Saunders/Elsevier; 2009:384–429. Copyright © 2009 Elsevier. With permission.)

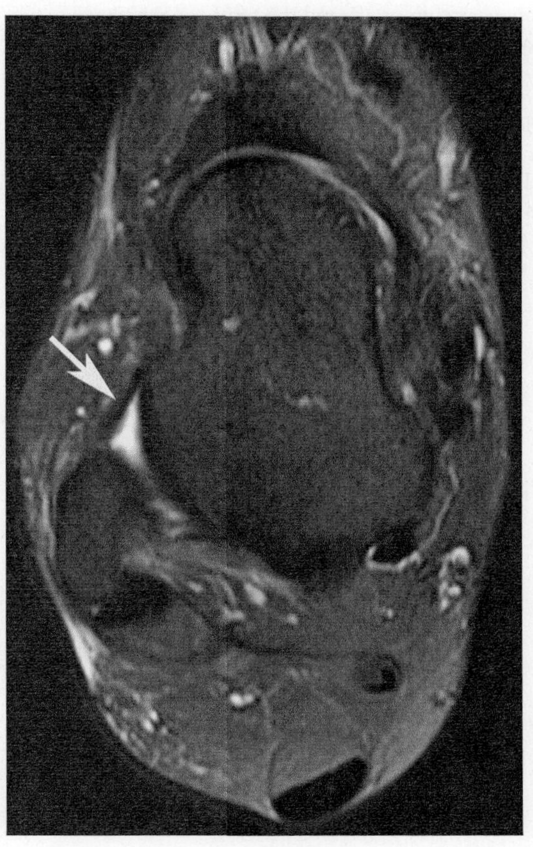

FIGURE 10.14 MRI of the anterior talofibular ligament. Axial T2-weighted MR image through the lateral malleolus and talus demonstrates normal anterior talofibular ligament *(arrow)*.

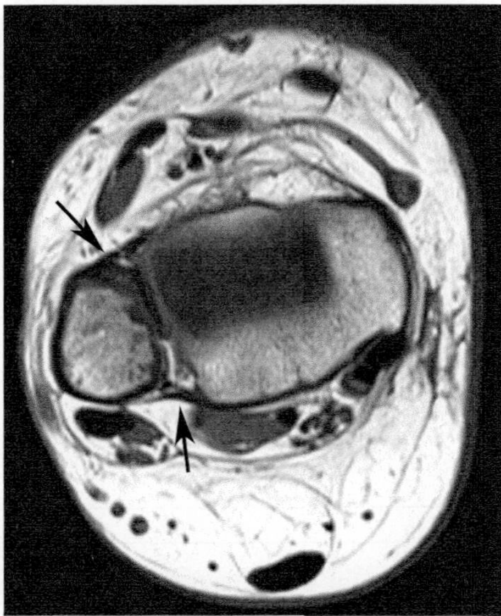

FIGURE 10.15 **MRI of the anterior and posterior tibiofibular syndesmotic ligaments.** Axial T1-weighted MR image shows normal anterior and posterior tibiofibular ligaments *(arrows)*.

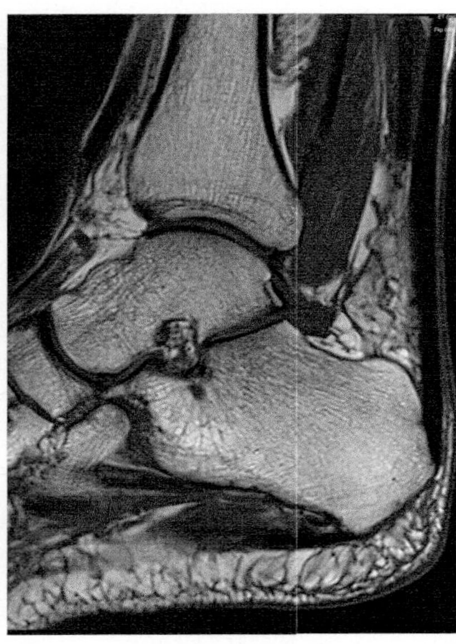

FIGURE 10.17 **MRI of the Achilles tendon.** Midline sagittal T1-weighted MR image demonstrates normal Achilles tendon. Note the uniformly low signal intensity of the tendon contrasting with the high signal intensity of the anterior fat pad.

On the sections in the sagittal plane, the tibialis posterior, flexor digitorum longus, and flexor hallucis longus tendons are identified on the medial cuts. The peroneus longus and brevis tendons are seen on the lateral sections (Fig. 10.16). The Achilles tendon is best seen on midline sagittal section (Fig. 10.17). The coronal plane is also effective in the visualization of various ligaments and tendons (Fig. 10.18).

The pathologic conditions of tendons and ligaments are demonstrated by discontinuity of the anatomic structure, the presence of high signal intensity within the tendon substance on T2-weighted images, and inflammatory changes within or around the tendons, which again can be demonstrated by a change in the normal signal intensity.

Foot

Most injuries to the foot can be sufficiently evaluated on the standard radiographic examination of the foot, which includes the anteroposterior, lateral, and oblique projections. Only occasionally are special tangential projections required.

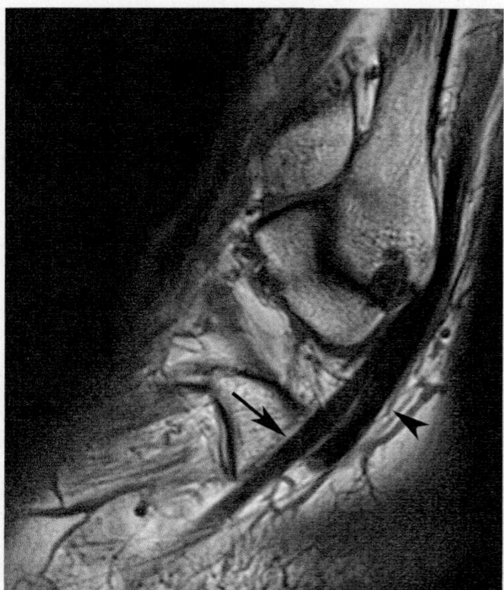

FIGURE 10.16 **MRI of the peroneus longus and brevis tendons.** Sagittal T1-weighted MR image through the lateral malleolus shows normal appearance of peroneus brevis *(arrow)* and longus *(arrowhead)* tendons as they curve around the lateral malleolus.

The *anteroposterior* radiograph of the foot adequately demonstrates the metatarsal bones and phalanges (Fig. 10.19) This view reveals an important anatomic feature known as the *first intermetatarsal angle*, which normally ranges from 5 to 10 degrees (Fig. 10.19C). This angle is an important factor in the evaluation of forefoot deformities because it

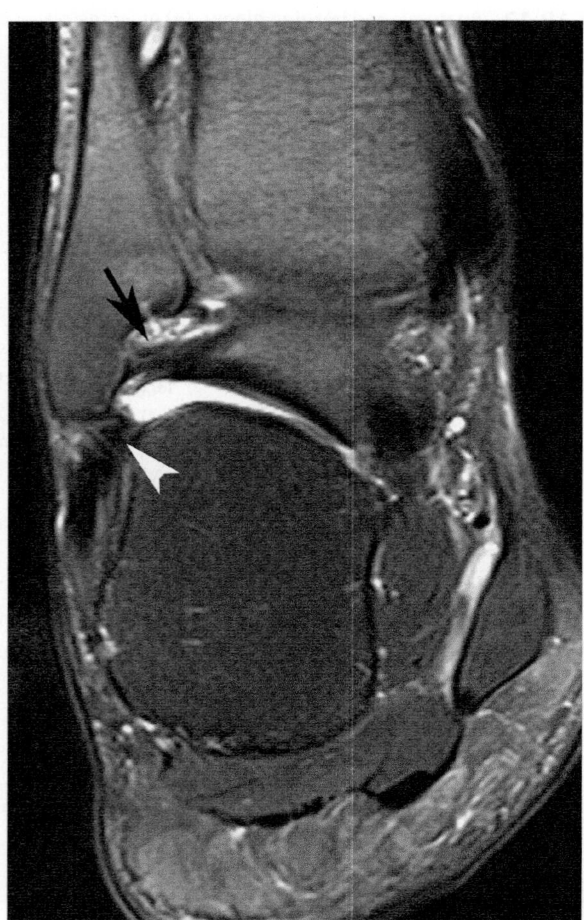

FIGURE 10.18 **MRI of the posterior talofibular and calcaneofibular ligaments.** Coronal T2-weighted MR image of the ankle shows normal posterior talofibular *(arrow)* and calcaneofibular *(arrowhead)* ligaments.

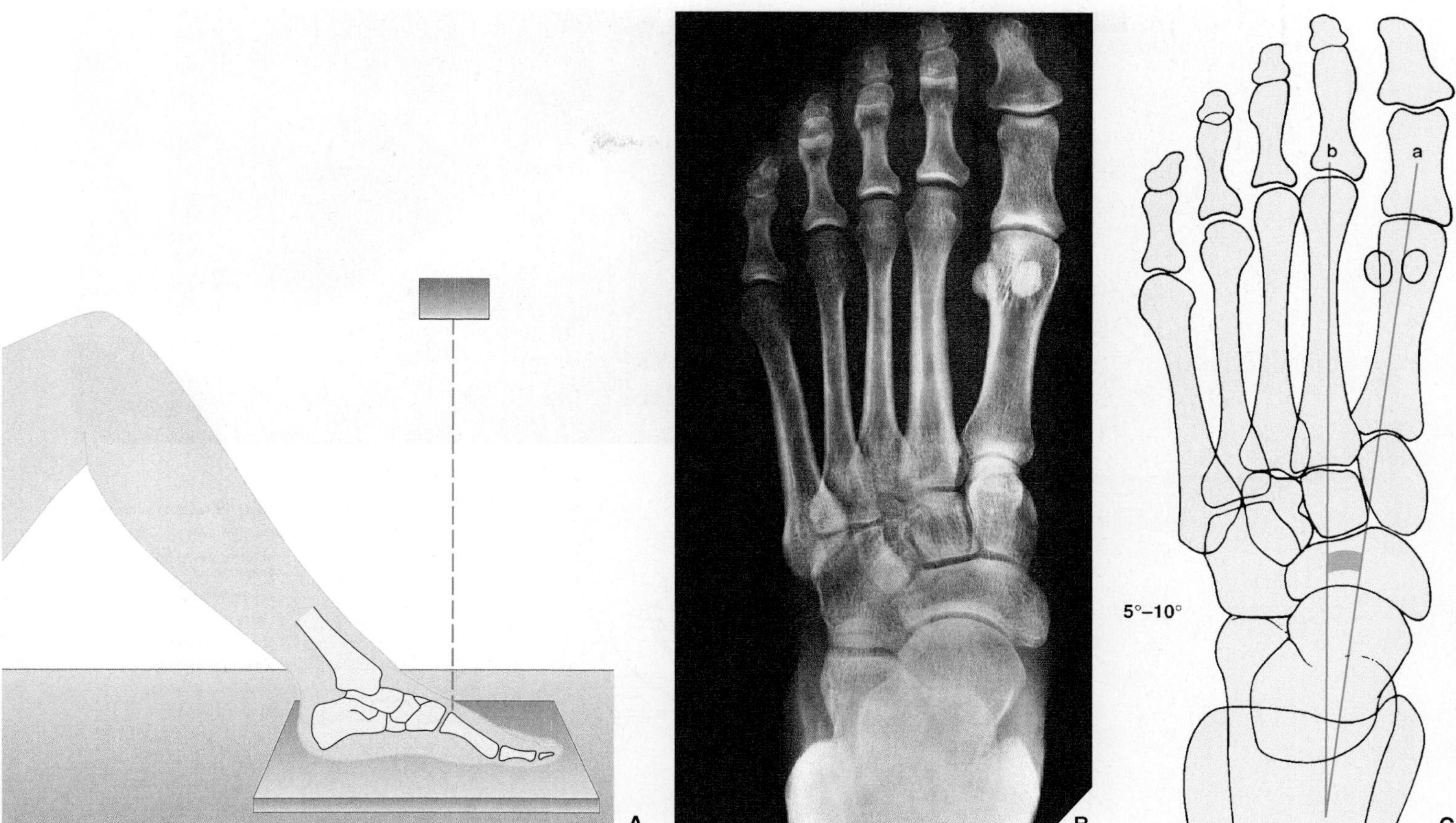

FIGURE 10.19 Anteroposterior view. **(A)** For the anteroposterior (dorsoplantar) view of the foot, the patient is supine, with the knee flexed and the sole placed firmly on the film cassette. The central beam *(red broken line)* is directed vertically to the base of the first metatarsal bone. **(B)** On the radiograph obtained in this projection, injury to the metatarsal bones and phalanges can be adequately assessed. Note that 75% of the talar head articulates with the navicular bone. (For identification of the bones of the foot, see Fig. 10.2.) **(C)** The first intermetatarsal angle is formed by the intersection of the lines bisecting the shafts of the first *(a)* and second *(b)* metatarsals.

represents a way to quantify the amount of metatarsus primus varus associated with hallux valgus. On the *lateral* radiograph (Fig. 10.20A,B), *Boehler angle* (also known as a *tuber angle*), an important anatomic relation of the talus and the calcaneus, can be appreciated (Fig. 10.20C). In fractures of the calcaneus, this angle, which normally ranges from 20 to 40 degrees, is decreased because of compression of the superior aspect of the bone. This measurement also aids in the evaluation of depression of the posterior facet of the subtalar joint. On the lateral view, calcaneal pitch can also be evaluated. This measurement is an indication of the height of the foot and normally ranges from 20 to 30 degrees (Fig. 10.20D). Higher values indicate a cavus foot deformity (*pes cavus*), and lower values indicate a flat foot deformity (*pes planus*). The other important measurement obtained on the lateral foot radiograph is the *angle of Gissane* (also known as a *critical angle*), which is formed by the downward and upward slopes of the calcaneal dorsal surface (Fig. 10.21). The normal values of this angle are 125 to 140 degrees. The greater values suggest a fracture of the posterior facet of the subtalar joint. An *oblique* radiograph of the foot is also obtained as part of the standard radiographic examination (Fig. 10.22). Injuries to the subtalar joint occasionally require special, tangential projections such as the posterior tangential (*Harris-Beath*) view (Fig. 10.23) or oblique tangential (*Broden*) view (Fig. 10.24). A tangential view of the sesamoid bones of the great toe (Fig. 10.25) may also be necessary.

Radiographic evaluation of foot injuries is complicated by the presence of multiple accessory ossicles, which are considered secondary centers of ossification, and the sesamoid bones, which may mimic a fracture (Fig. 10.26A,B); conversely, a chip fracture can be misinterpreted as a mere ossicle (Fig. 10.26C,D). Thus, it is important to recognize these structures on conventional radiographs.

In addition to radiography, ancillary imaging techniques may need to be used in the evaluation of injury to the foot. Radionuclide imaging (bone scan) is a valuable means of detecting stress fractures, common foot injuries that are not always obvious on the standard radiographic examination. CT is especially effective in assessing complex fractures, particularly of the calcaneus. MRI is now frequently used to evaluate trauma to the foot. During evaluation of MRI of the ankle and foot, it is helpful to use checklist as provided in Table 10.1.

For a tabular summary of the preceding discussion, see Tables 10.2 and 10.3.

Injury to the Ankle

All ankle injuries can be broadly classified, according to the mechanism of injury, as resulting from inversion (Fig. 10.27) or eversion (Fig. 10.28) stress forces. Inversion injuries are much more common, accounting for 85% of all traumatic conditions involving the ankle. These groupings apply to both fractures and injuries to the ligament complexes of the ankle. However, it is in the latter type of injuries that they are particularly helpful in determining and evaluating the specific type of ligament injury, especially in the presence of certain fractures about the ankle.

Fractures About the Ankle Joint

In addition to being classified by mechanism of injury, fractures about the ankle joint can also be classified by the anatomic structure involved (Fig. 10.29) and designated as:

1. *Unimalleolar*, when the fracture involves the medial (tibial), lateral (fibular), or posterior (tibial) malleolus (Figs. 10.30 to 10.32)
2. *Bimalleolar*, when two malleoli are fractured (Figs. 10.33 and 10.34)

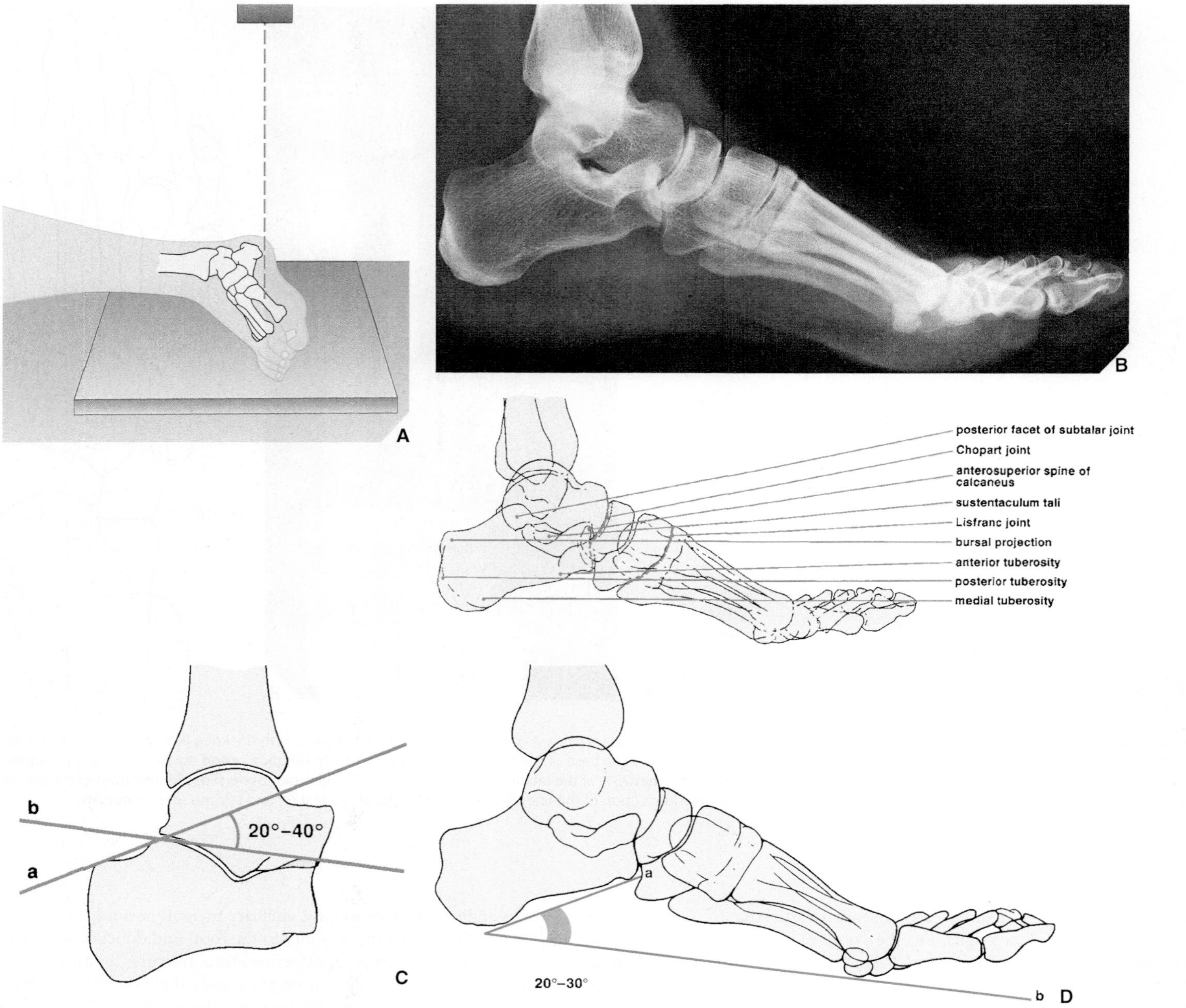

FIGURE 10.20 Lateral view. **(A)** For the lateral view of the foot, the patient lies on his or her side with the knee slightly flexed and the lateral aspect of the foot against the film cassette. The central beam *(red broken line)* is directed vertically to the midtarsus. **(B)** The lateral radiograph demonstrates the bursal projection, the most prominent feature on the posterior aspect of the calcaneus; the posterior tuberosity where the Achilles tendon inserts; the medial tuberosity on the plantar surface where the plantar fascia inserts; the anterior tuberosity; the anterosuperior spine of the calcaneus; the posterior facet of the subtalar joint; the sustentaculum tali; and the talonavicular and calcaneocuboid articulations. The Chopart and Lisfranc joints are also well visualized. **(C)** The lateral view also allows evaluation of the angular relationship between the talus and the calcaneus—Boehler angle. This feature is determined by the intersection of a line *(a)* drawn from the posterosuperior margin of the calcaneal tuberosity (bursal projection) through the tip of the posterior facet of the subtalar joint, and a second line *(b)* drawn from the tip of the posterior facet through the superior margin of the anterior process of the calcaneus. Normally, this angle ranges between 20 and 40 degrees. **(D)** Calcaneal pitch is described by the intersection of a line drawn tangentially to the inferior surface of the calcaneus and one drawn along the plantar surface of the foot.

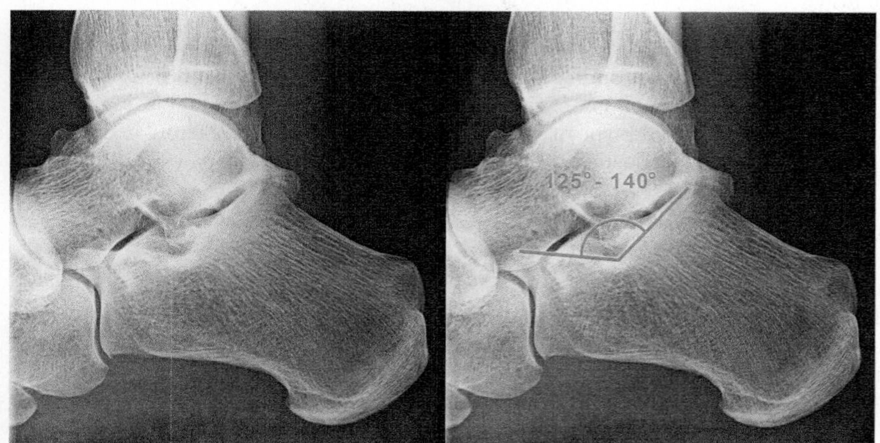

FIGURE 10.21 The angle of Gissane. This measurement is obtained on the lateral radiograph of the hindfoot. The angle is formed by intersection of the lines drawn along the downward and upward slopes of the calcaneal dorsal surfaces, with normal values between 125 and 140 degrees.

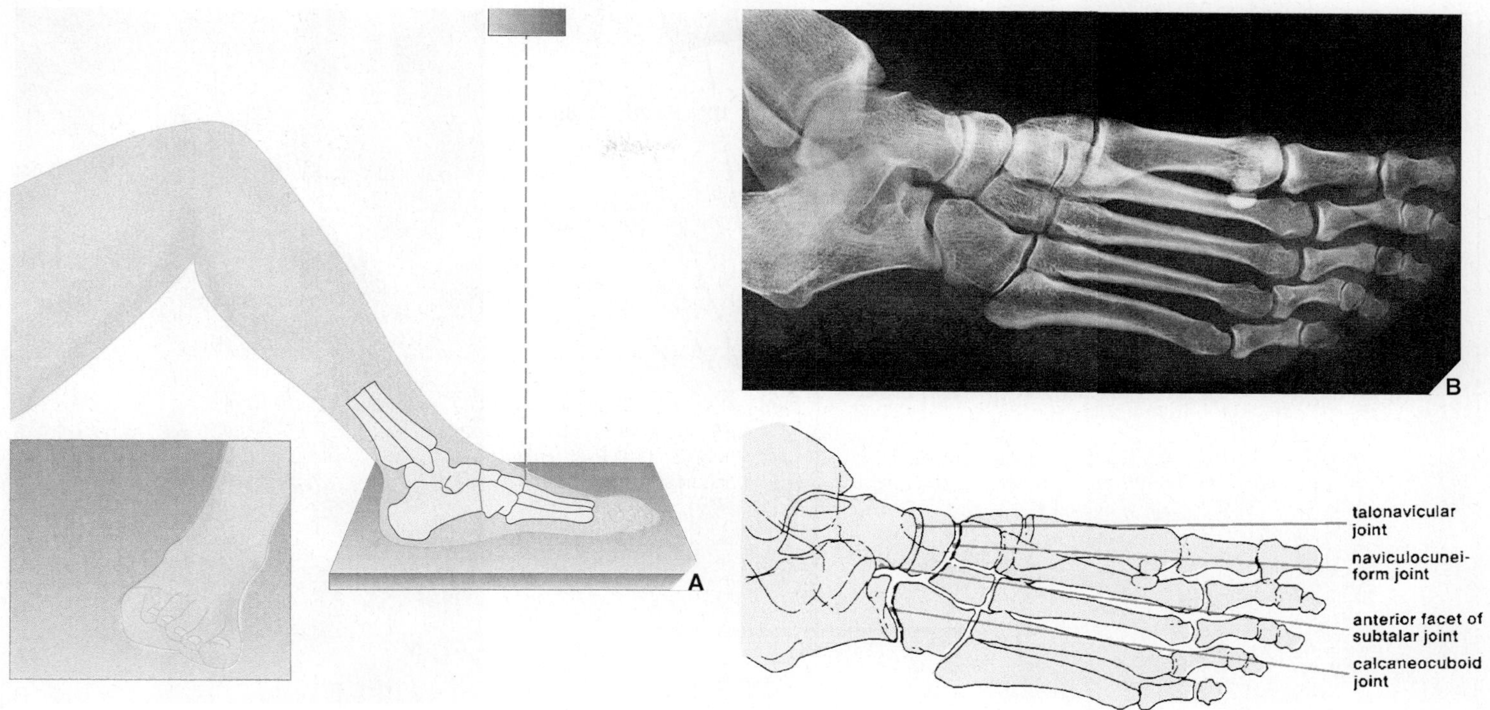

FIGURE 10.22 Oblique view. **(A)** For the oblique view of the foot, the patient is supine on the table with the knee flexed. The lateral border of the foot is elevated about 40 to 45 degrees *(inset)* so that the medial border of the foot is forced against the film cassette. The central beam *(red broken line)* is directed vertically to the base of the third metatarsal. **(B)** On the oblique radiograph of the foot, the phalanges and metatarsals are well demonstrated, as are the anterior part of the subtalar joint and the talonavicular, naviculocuneiform, and calcaneocuboid joints.

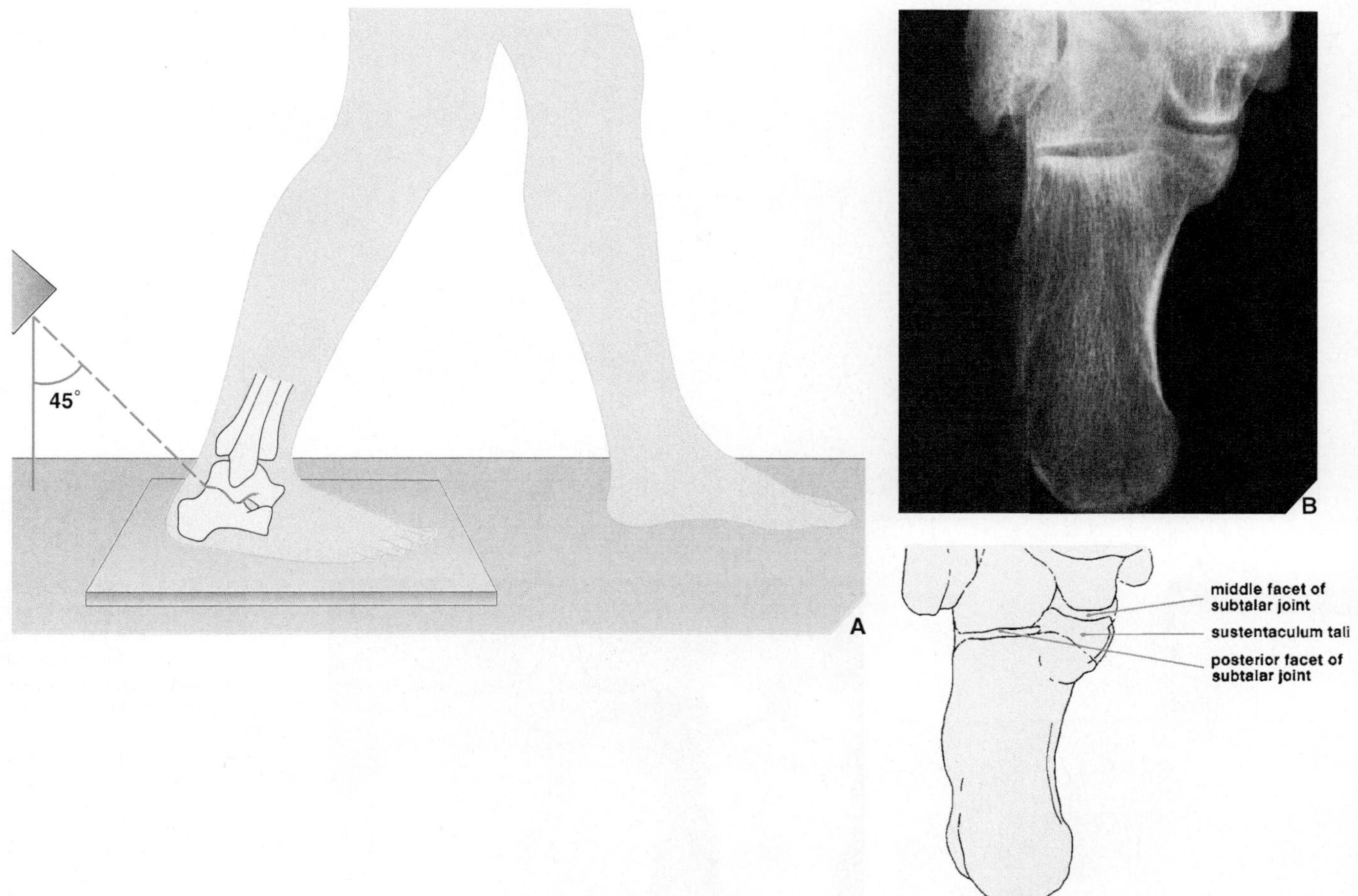

FIGURE 10.23 Harris-Beath view. **(A)** For the posterior tangential (Harris-Beath) view of the foot, the patient is erect, with the sole of the foot flat on the film cassette. The central beam *(red broken line)* is usually angled 45 degrees toward the midline of the heel, but 35 or 55 degrees of angulation may also be used. **(B)** On the radiograph in this projection, the middle facet of the subtalar joint is seen, oriented horizontally; the sustentaculum tali projects medially. The posterior facet projects laterally and is parallel to the middle facet. The body of the calcaneus is well demonstrated.

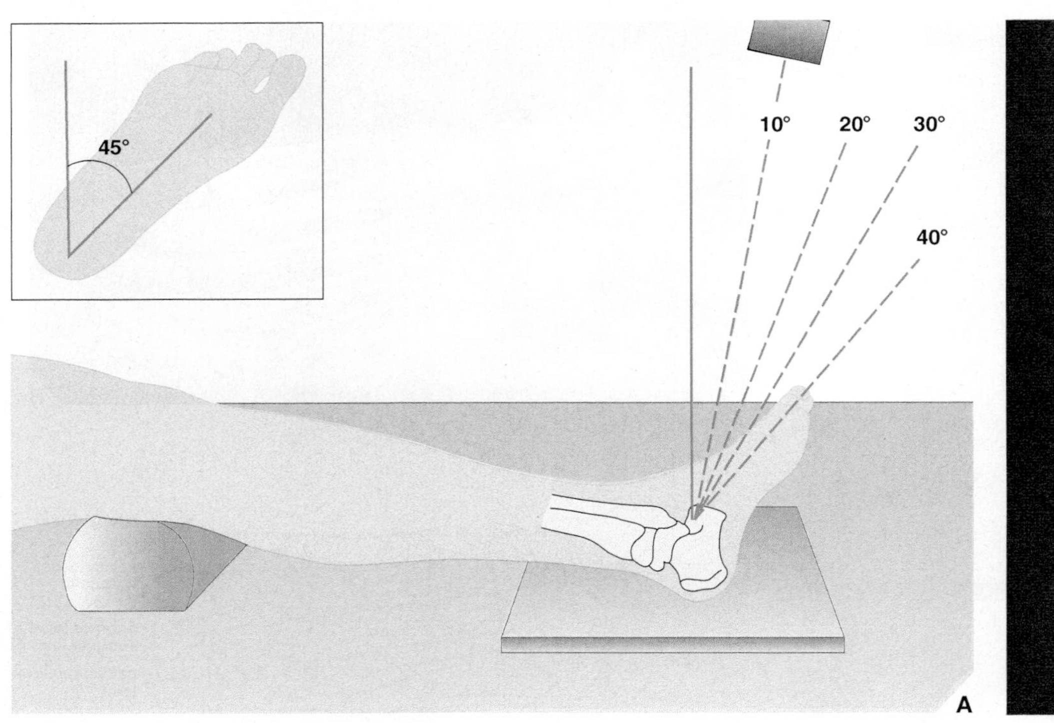

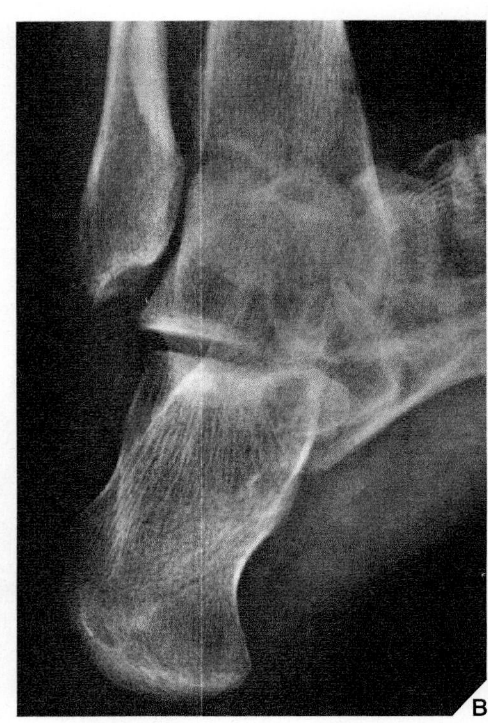

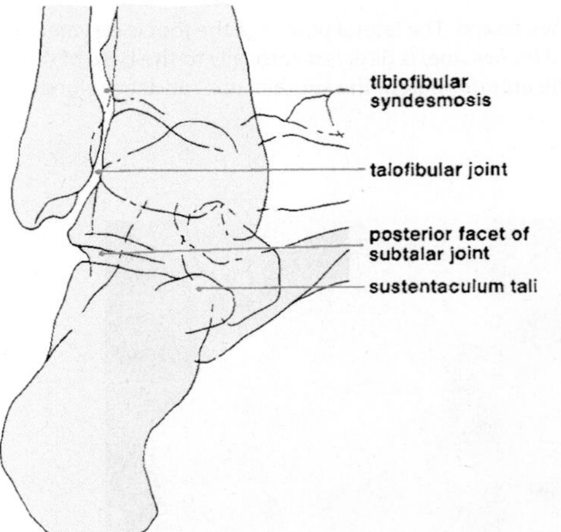

FIGURE 10.24 Broden view. **(A)** For the Broden view of the foot, the patient is supine, with the knee slightly flexed and supported by a small sandbag. The foot rests on the film cassette, dorsiflexed to 90 degrees, and, together with the leg, rotated medially approximately 45 degrees *(inset)*. The central beam *(red broken line)* is directed toward the lateral malleolus. Radiographs may be obtained at 10, 20, 30, and 40 degrees of cephalad angulation of the tube. **(B)** A radiograph obtained at 30-degree cephalad angulation demonstrates the posterior facet of the subtalar joint. Note also the good demonstration of the sustentaculum tali and the excellent visualization of the talofibular joint and the tibiofibular syndesmosis.

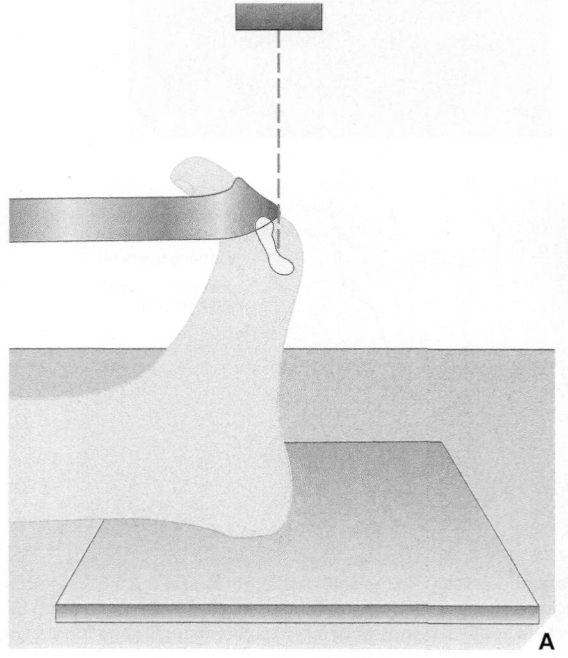

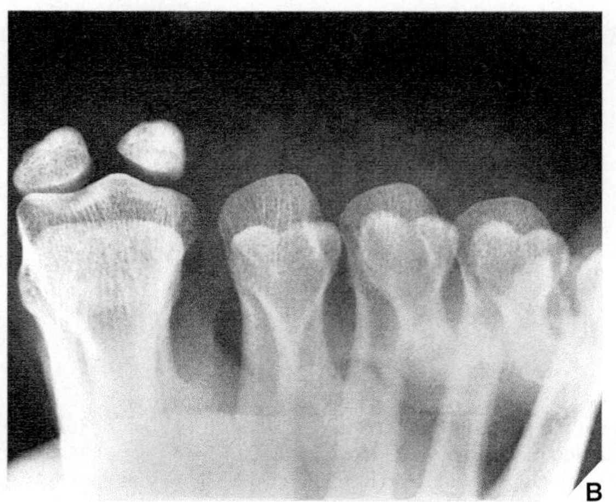

FIGURE 10.25 Tangential view. **(A)** For a tangential view of the sesamoid bones, the patient is seated on the table, with the foot dorsiflexed on the cassette, holding the toes in a dorsiflexed position with a strip of gauze. The central beam *(red broken line)* is directed vertically to the head of the first metatarsal bone. **(B)** This sesamoid view demonstrates the metatarsal heads and the sesamoid bones of the first metatarsal.

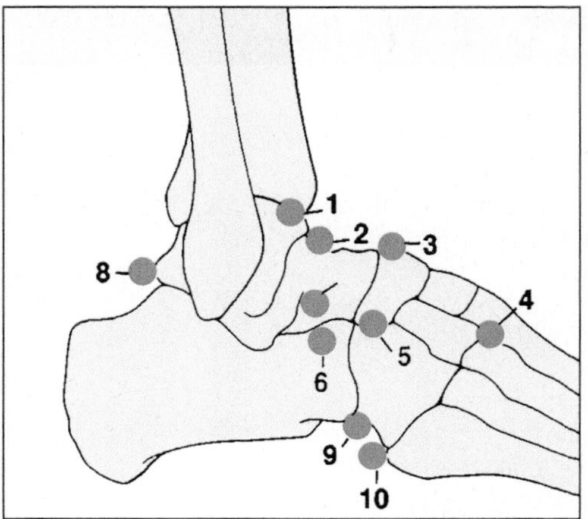

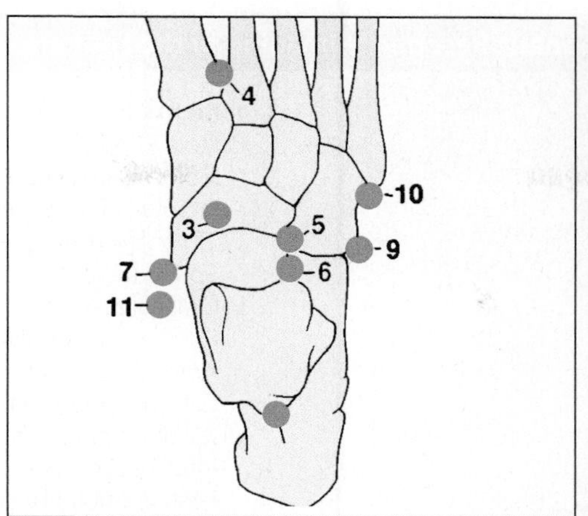

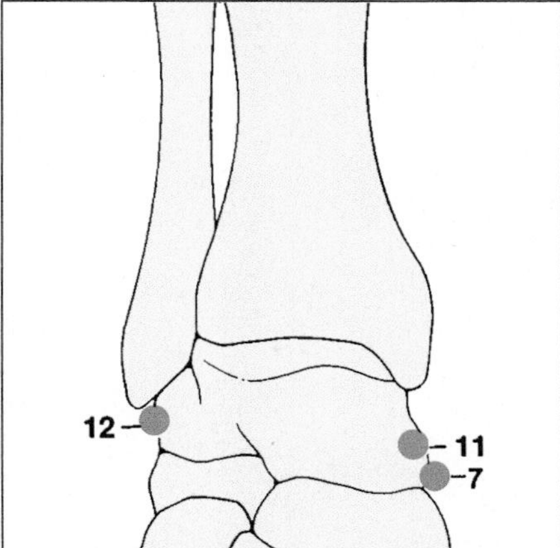

1 talotibial ossicle (os talotibiale)
2 supratalar ossicle (os supratalare)
3 supranavicular ossicle (os supranaviculare)
4 intermetatarsal ossicle (os intermetatarsale)
5 secondary cuboid (cuboides secundarium)
6 secondary calcaneus (calcaneus secundarius)
7 external tibial ossicle (os tibiale externum)
8 trigone ossicle (os trigonum)
9 peroneal ossicle (os peroneum)
10 vesalian ossicle (os vesalianum)
11 accessory talus (talus accessorius)
12 secondary talus (talus secundarius)

A

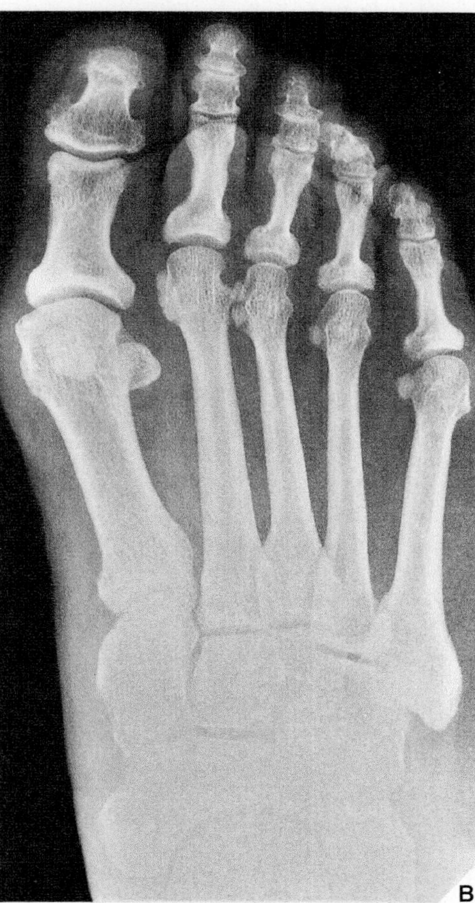

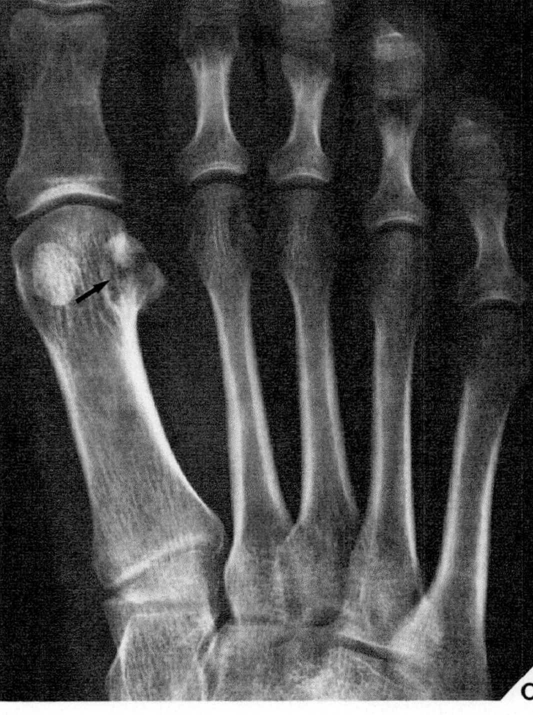

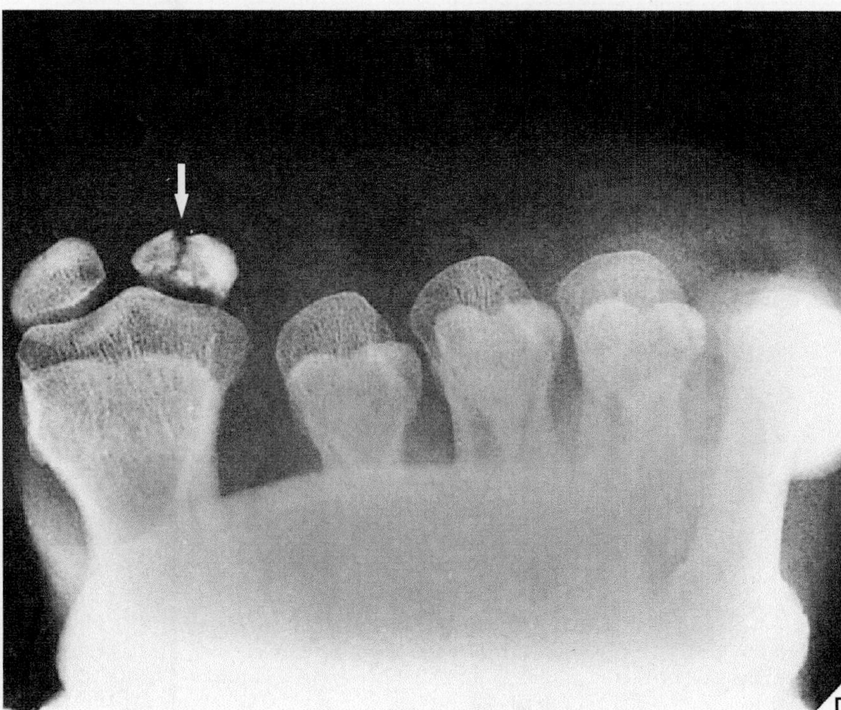

FIGURE 10.26 Accessory ossicles. **(A,B)** The numerous accessory ossicles of the foot and ankle *(red dots)* can complicate the evaluation of foot injuries by mimicking fracture. Fractures, however, may go undetected when misinterpreted as ossicles, as seen here on the anteroposterior **(C)** and sesamoid **(D)** views of the foot, which demonstrate a fracture of the lateral (fibular) sesamoid *(arrows)*.

TABLE 10.1 Checklist for Evaluation of Magnetic Resonance Imaging of the Foot and Ankle

Osseous Structures
- Distal tibia (c, s)
- Distal fibula (c, s)
- Talus (c, s, a)
- Calcaneus (c, s, a)
- Cuboid (s, a)
- Navicular (s, a)
- Cuneiform—medial, middle, lateral (c, a)
- Sesamoid bones (c, a)
- Os naviculare (external tibial ossicle) (a)
- Peroneal ossicle (c, s)

Joints and Articular Cartilage
- Tibiotalar (c, s)
- Chopart (s)
- Lisfranc (s)
- Subtalar (c, s)

Muscles and Their Tendons
- Achilles (s, a)
- Tibialis anterior (a)
- Tibialis posterior (a)
- Peroneus—longus, brevis, tertius (a)
- Flexor hallucis longus (s, a)
- Flexor hallucis brevis (s, a)
- Extensor hallucis longus (s, a)
- Extensor hallucis brevis (s, a)
- Flexor digitorum—longus, brevis (s, a)
- Extensor digitorum—longus, brevis (s, a)
- Plantaris (a)
- Abductor hallucis (a)
- Adductor hallucis (a)

Ligaments
- Deltoid
  - Tibiocalcaneal band (c)
  - Tibiotalar band—anterior, posterior (c, a)
  - Tibionavicular band (s, a)
  - Spring (tibio-spring) (c, a)
- Lateral collateral
  - Posterior talofibular (a)
  - Anterior talofibular (a)
  - Calcaneofibular (c)
- Distal tibiofibular syndesmosis
  - Interosseous membrane (c, a)
  - Posterior tibiofibular (c, a)
  - Anterior tibiofibular (c, a)
  - Inferior transverse (a)
  - Lisfranc (a)

Bursae
- Retrocalcaneal (s)
- Retro-Achilles (s, a)

Other Structures
- Fascia plantaris (s)
- Plantar plate (s)
- Sinus tarsi (c, s, a)
- Tarsal tunnel (c, s, a)
- Anterolateral gutter (a)
- Kager fat pad (s)
- Tibial artery, vein, nerve (a)
- Greater saphenous vein (a)

The best imaging planes for visualization of listed structures are given in parentheses: c, coronal (coronal of ankle, short-axis axial of foot); s, sagittal; a, axial (axial of ankle, long-axis axial of foot).

TABLE 10.2 Standard and Special Radiographic Projections for Evaluating Injury to the Ankle and Foot

Projection	Demonstration
Anteroposterior (ankle)	Fractures of Distal tibia Distal fibula Medial malleolus Lateral malleolus Pilon fractures (extension into tibiotalar joint)
Anteroposterior (foot)	Fractures of Talus (particularly dome) Navicular, cuboid, and cuneiform bones Metatarsals and phalanges (including stress fractures and accessory ossicles) Dislocations in Subtalar joint Peritalar (anterior and posterior types) Total talar Tarsometatarsal (Lisfranc) joint
With 10 degrees of internal ankle rotation (mortise view)	Same structures and abnormalities as anteroposterior but better demonstration of tibial plafond
Stress (inversion, eversion)	Tear of lateral collateral ligament Tear of deltoid ligament Ankle instability
Lateral (ankle and foot)	Boehler angle Angle of Gissane Fractures of Distal tibia Anterior aspect Posterior lip (third malleolus) Tibiotalar joint
Lateral (continued) (ankle and foot)	Talus (particularly neck) Calcaneus (particularly in coronal plane) Posterior facet of subtalar joint Sustentaculum tali Accessory ossicles Cuboid bone Dislocations in Ankle joint Subtalar joint Peritalar (anterior and posterior types) Tarsometatarsal (Lisfranc) joint Ankle joint effusion
Stress (anterior-draw)	Tear of anterior talofibular ligament Ankle instability
Oblique Internal External	Fractures of Medial malleolus Talus Tuberosity of calcaneus Metatarsals Phalanges
Posterior tangential (Harris-Beath)	Fractures involving Middle and posterior facets of subtalar joint Calcaneus (in axial plane)
Oblique tangential (Broden)	Fractures involving Posterior facet of subtalar joint Calcaneus Sustentaculum tali
Axial (sesamoid view)	Fractures of sesamoid bones

TABLE 10.3 Ancillary Imaging Techniques for Evaluating Injury to the Ankle and Foot

Technique	Demonstration
Radionuclide imaging (scintigraphy, bone scan)	Stress fractures Healing process
Arthrography (single-contrast or double-contrast, usually combined with CT), currently replaced by MRa	Tears of ligament structures of ankle joint Osteochondral fractures OCD of talus Osteochondral bodies in joint
CT and 3D CT	Complex fractures (particularly of os calcis) Intraarticular extension of fracture line Injuries to tendons (particularly peroneal, tibialis, and Achilles) and ligaments
MRI and MRa	Same as arthrography and CT Tarsal tunnel syndrome Sinus tarsi syndrome Mueller-Weis syndrome Wolin lesion Anteromedial impingement syndrome Os trigonum impingement syndrome Calcaneofibular entrapment
US	Traumatic injuries of tendons and ligaments Posttraumatic hematomas and fluid accumulation in the soft tissues Tarsal tunnel syndrome Sinus tarsi syndrome

CT, computed tomography; MRa, magnetic resonance arthrography; OCD, osteochondritis dissecans; 3D, three-dimensional; MRI, magnetic resonance imaging; US, ultrasound.

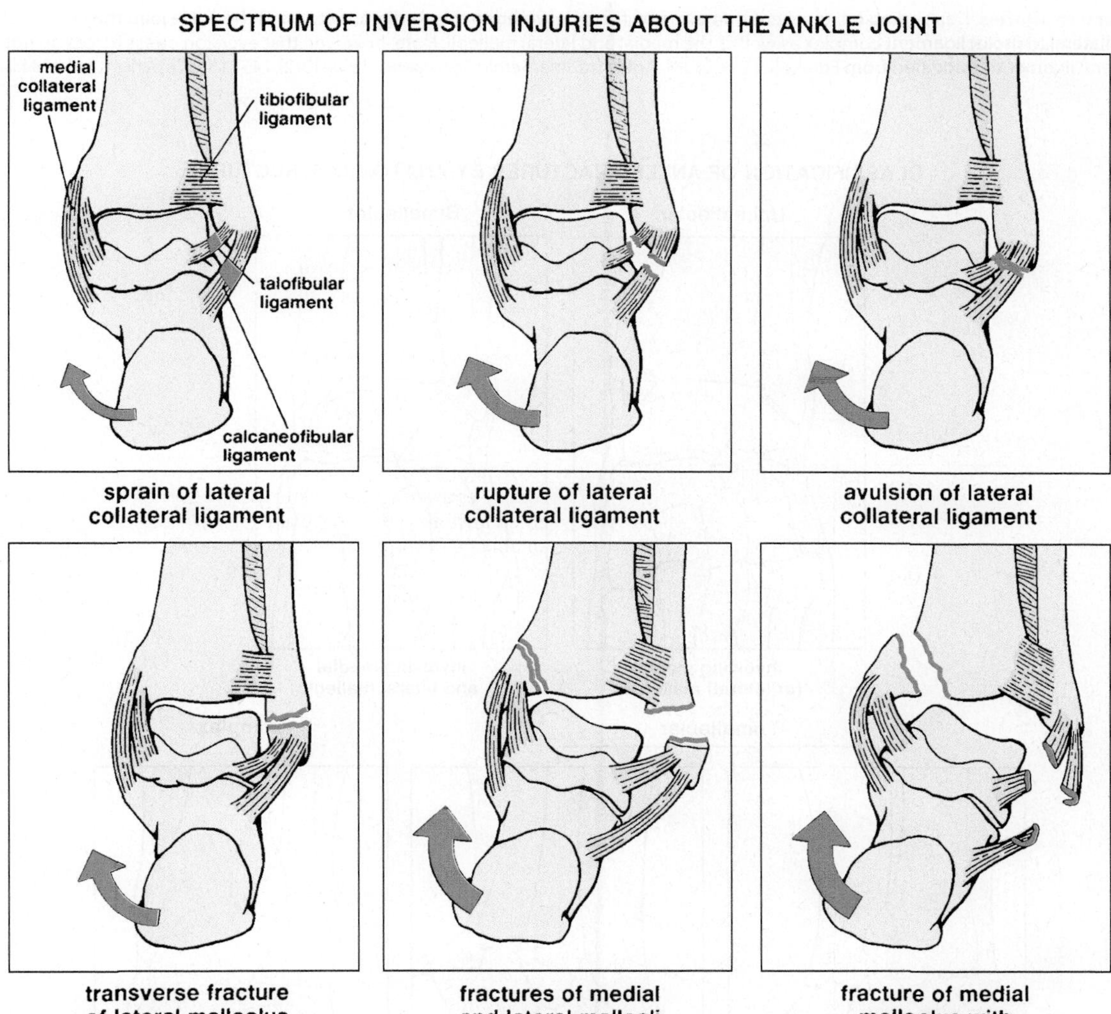

FIGURE 10.27 **Inversion injuries.** Depending on its severity, an inversion force *(red arrows)* delivered to the lateral structures of the ankle joint may manifest in a broad spectrum of injuries of the lateral collateral ligament complex as well as the lateral and medial malleoli. Note, however, that inversion-stress forces do not affect the posterior tibiofibular or medial collateral ligaments. (Modified from Edeiken J, Cotler JM. Ankle trauma. *Semin Roentgenol* 1978;13(2):145–155. Copyright © 1978 Elsevier. With permission.)

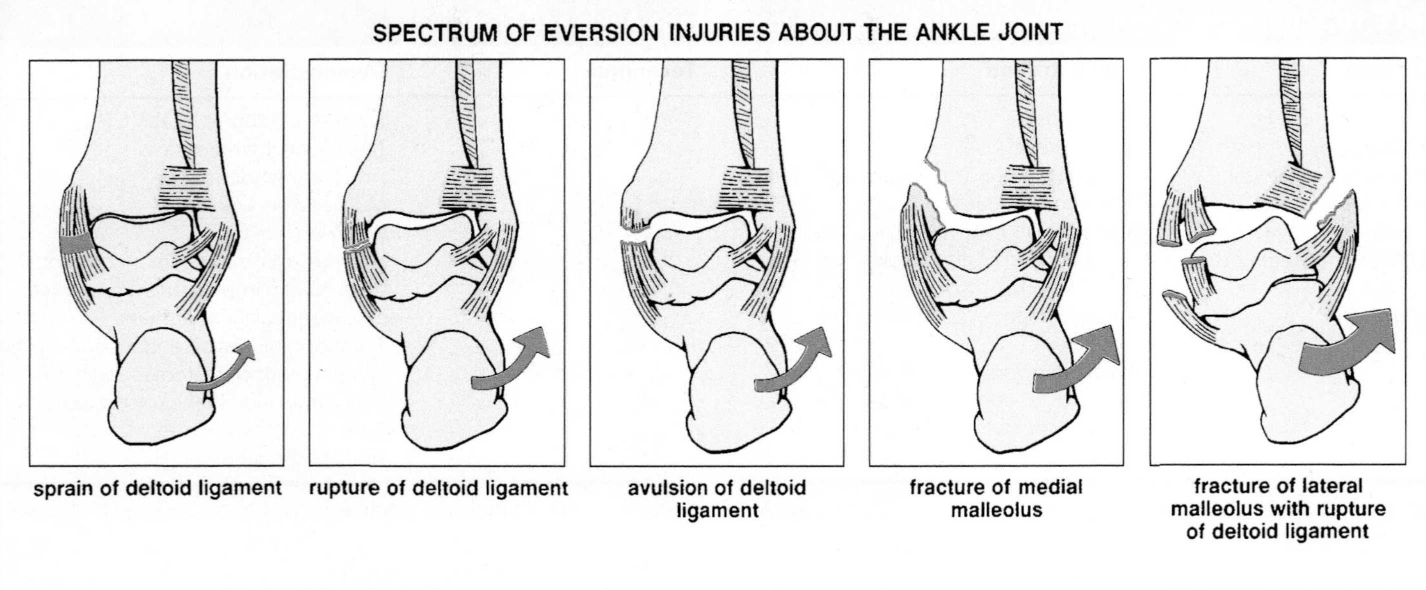

FIGURE 10.28 **Eversion injuries.** Depending on its severity, an eversion force delivered to the medial structures of the ankle joint may manifest in a broad spectrum of injuries of the medial collateral (deltoid) ligament complex as well as the medial and lateral malleoli. Note, however, that eversion-stress forces do not affect the posterior tibiofibular or lateral collateral ligaments. (Modified from Edeiken J, Cotler JM. Ankle trauma. *Semin Roentgenol* 1978;13(2):145–155. Copyright © 1978 Elsevier. With permission.)

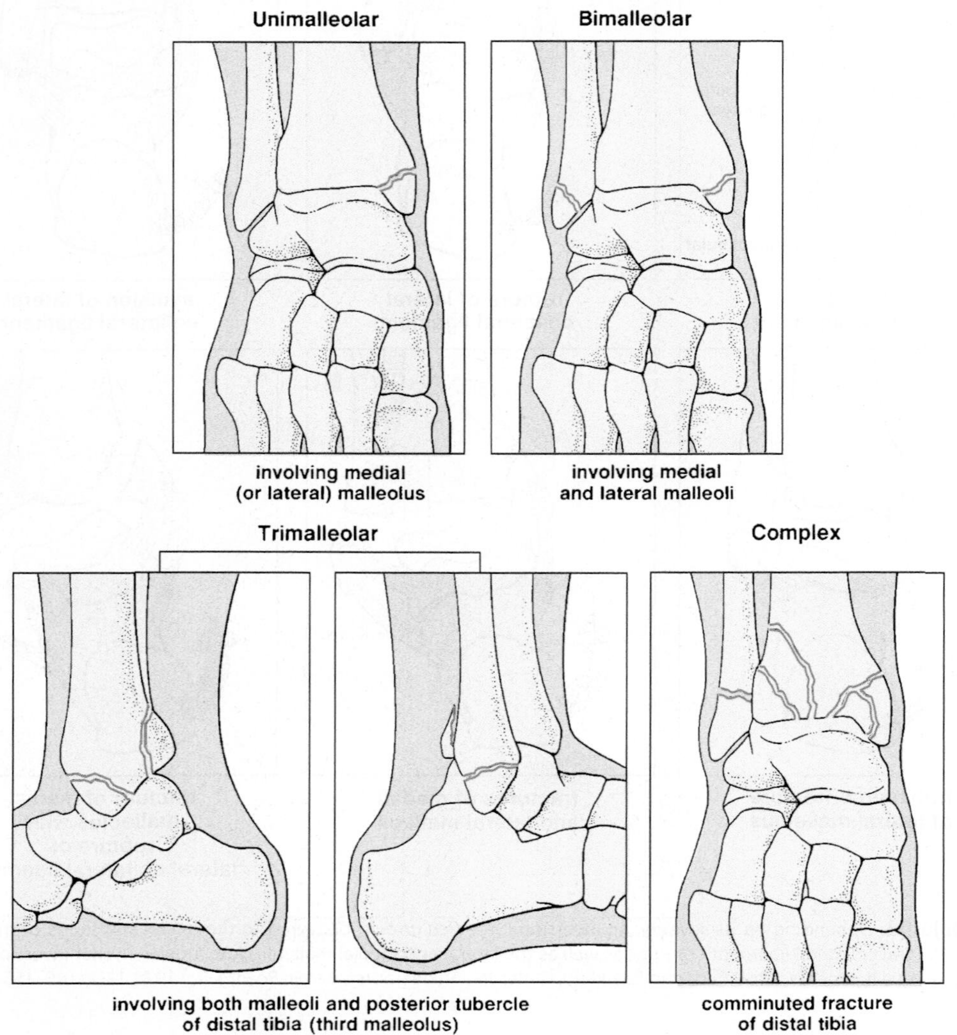

FIGURE 10.29 **Classification of ankle fractures.** Ankle fractures can be classified according to the anatomic structure as unimalleolar, bimalleolar, trimalleolar, or complex.

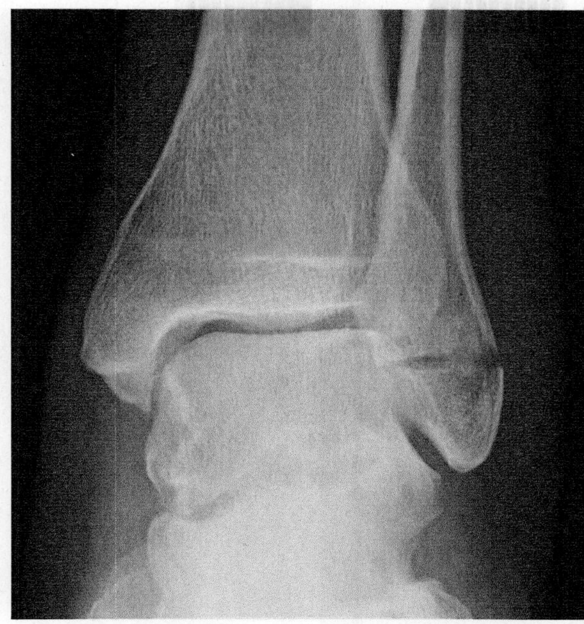

FIGURE 10.30 Unimalleolar fracture. Anteroposterior radiograph of the left ankle shows a transverse fracture of the lateral malleolus.

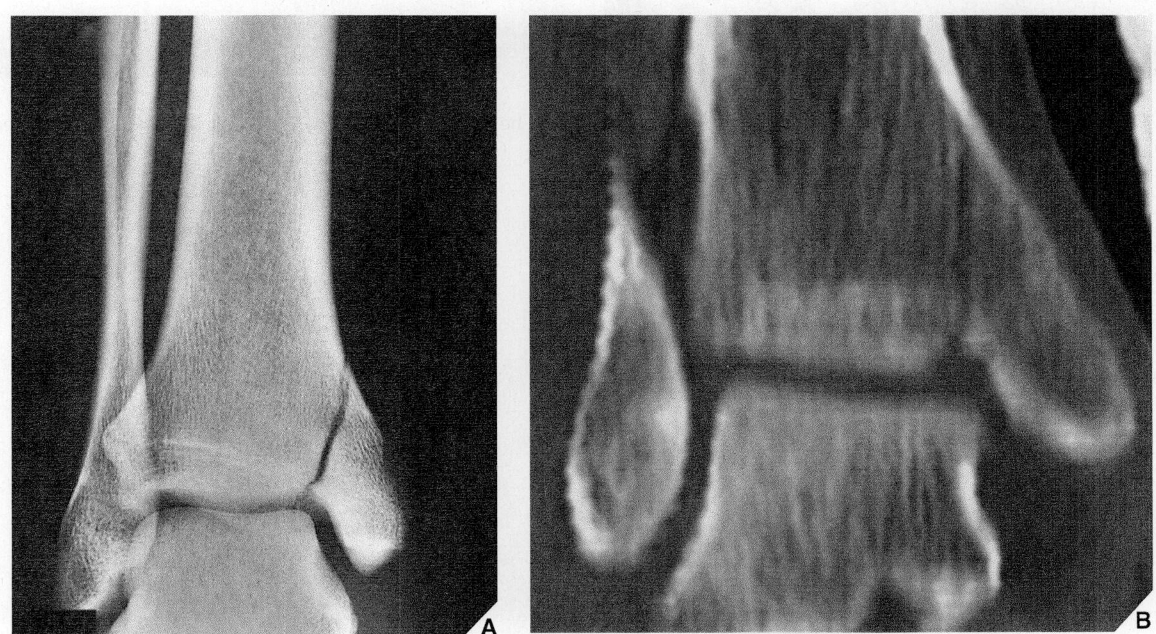

FIGURE 10.31 CT of unimalleolar fracture. **(A)** Anteroposterior radiograph of the ankle and **(B)** coronal reformatted CT image demonstrate the typical appearance of a unimalleolar fracture involving the medial malleolus.

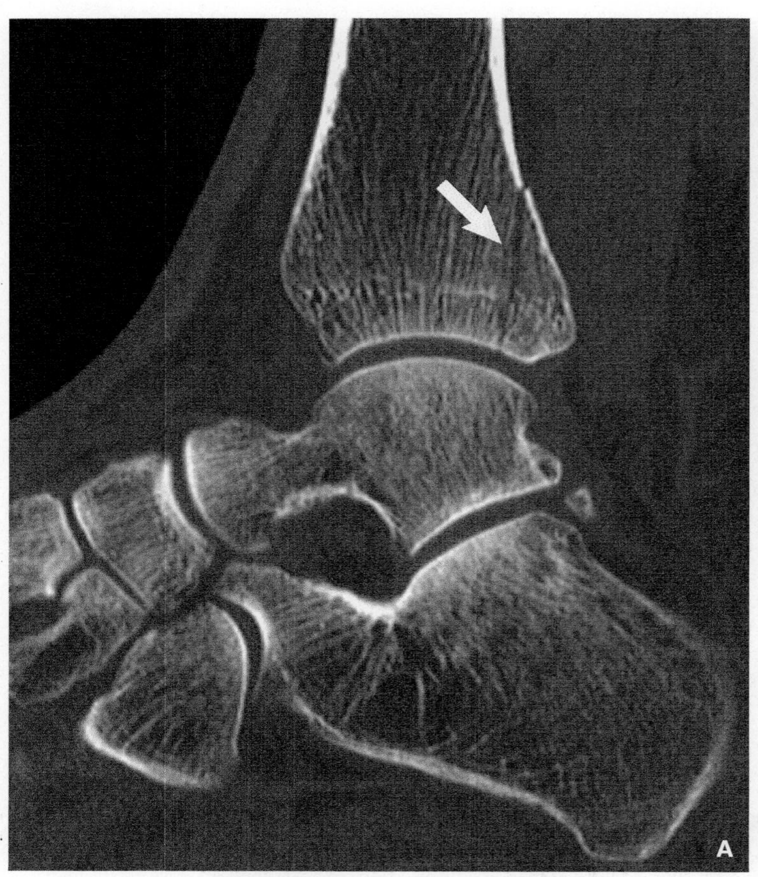

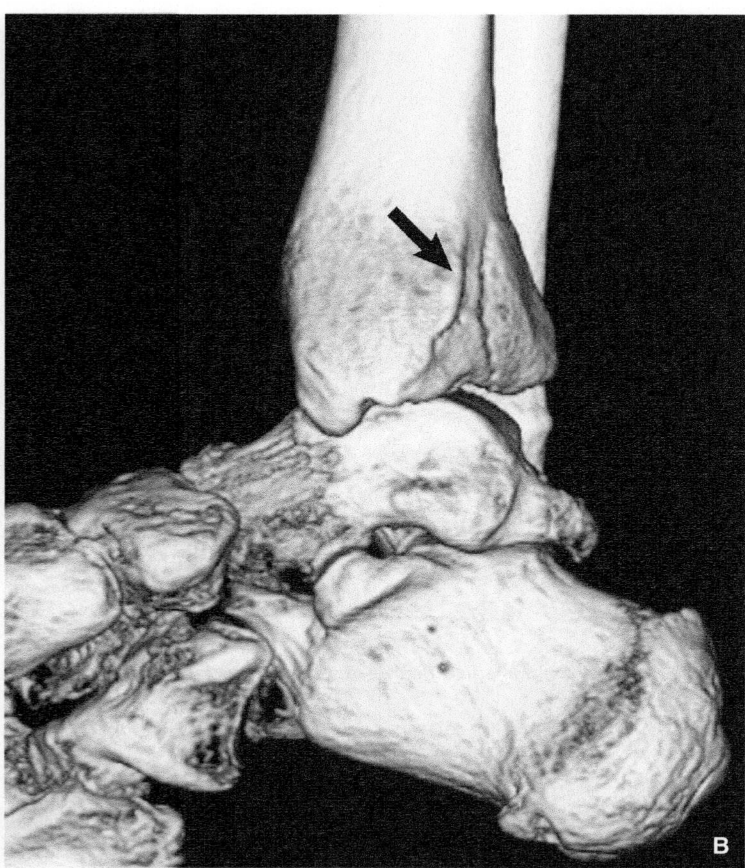

FIGURE 10.32 CT and 3D CT of unimalleolar fracture. A 68-year-old woman twisted her ankle while crossing the street. **(A)** Sagittal reformatted and **(B)** 3D reconstructed CT images show a fracture of the posterior (tibial) malleolus *(arrows)*.

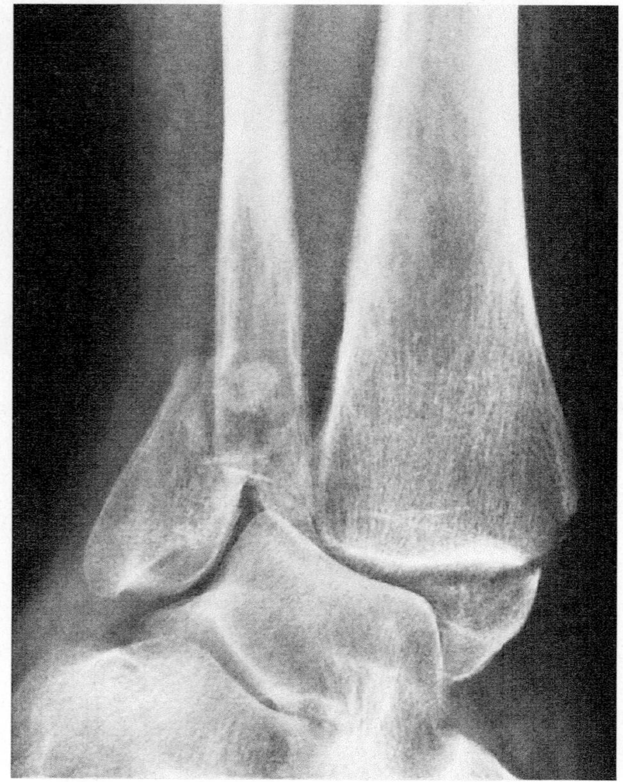

FIGURE 10.33 Bimalleolar fracture. Oblique radiograph of the ankle shows a bimalleolar fracture involving the tibial and fibular malleoli.

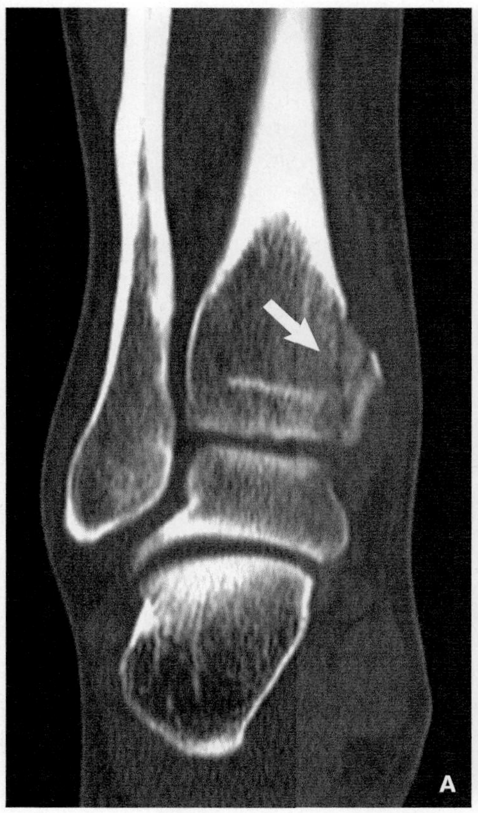

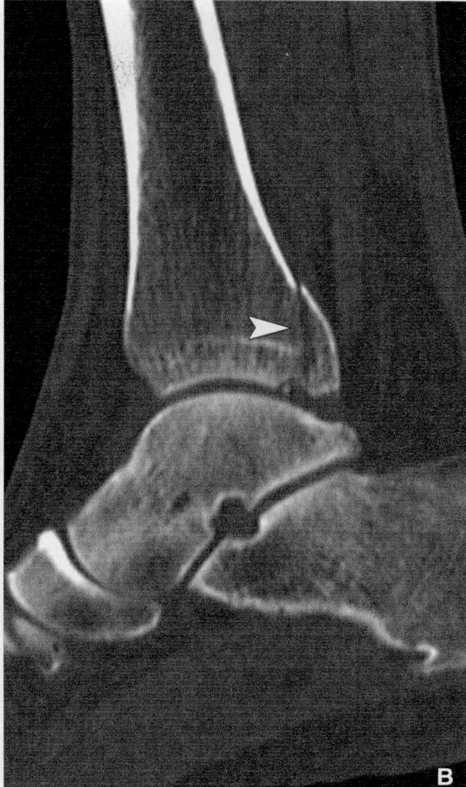

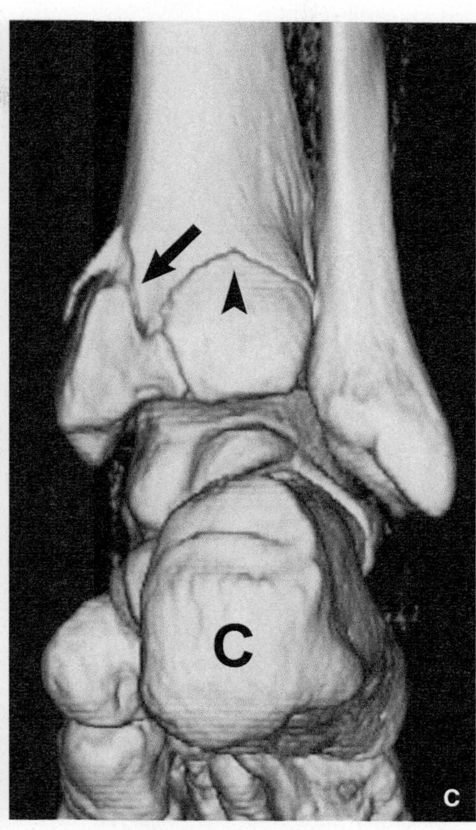

FIGURE 10.34 CT and 3D CT of bimalleolar fracture. **(A)** Coronal reformatted, **(B)** sagittal reformatted, and **(C)** 3D reconstructed CT image of the right ankle (viewed from the posterior direction) of a 47-year-old man show a fracture of the medial *(arrows)* and posterior *(arrowheads)* malleoli. C, calcaneus.

3. *Trimalleolar*, when fractures involve the medial and lateral malleoli as well as the posterior lip (or tubercle) of the distal tibia (the third malleolus) (Figs. 10.35 and 10.36)
4. *Complex fractures*, known also as *pilon fractures*, when comminuted fractures of the distal tibia and fibula occur (Figs. 10.37 to 10.40)
5. Fractures–dislocations (Figs. 10.41 and 10.42)

These fractures, when viewed from the standpoint of pathomechanics, may be either inversion or eversion injuries or a combination of both. The various types of eversion fractures are best known by their eponyms, including the Pott, Maisonneuve, Dupuytren, and Tillaux fractures (see later).

All of the following ankle fractures involving the distal tibia and fibula can be diagnosed on the standard radiographic projections. However, CT may be useful in delineating the extent of the fracture line, and this modality is particularly effective in evaluating lateral displacement in the juvenile Tillaux fracture. To evaluate associated ligament injuries, MRI is the technique of choice.

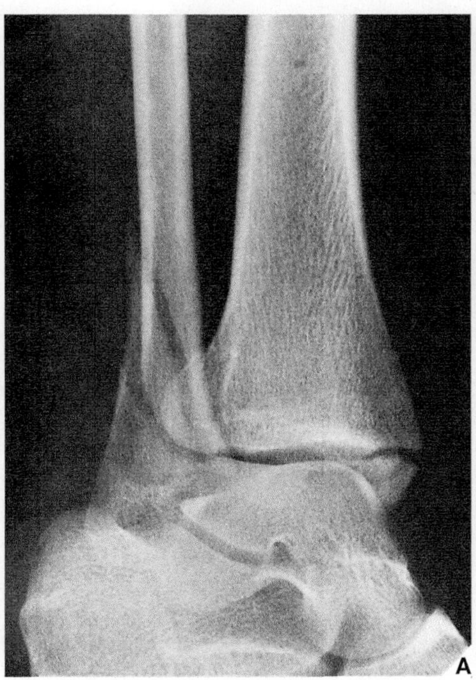

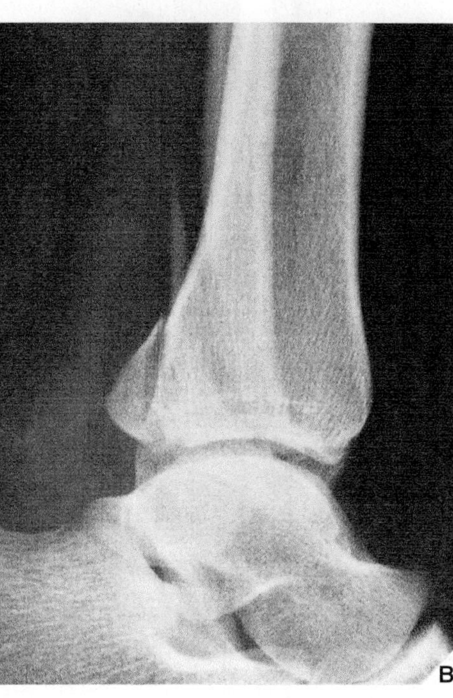

FIGURE 10.35 Trimalleolar fracture. **(A)** Oblique and **(B)** lateral radiographs of the ankle show a trimalleolar fracture affecting both malleoli and the posterior lip of the distal tibia. The latter feature is better seen on the lateral projection.

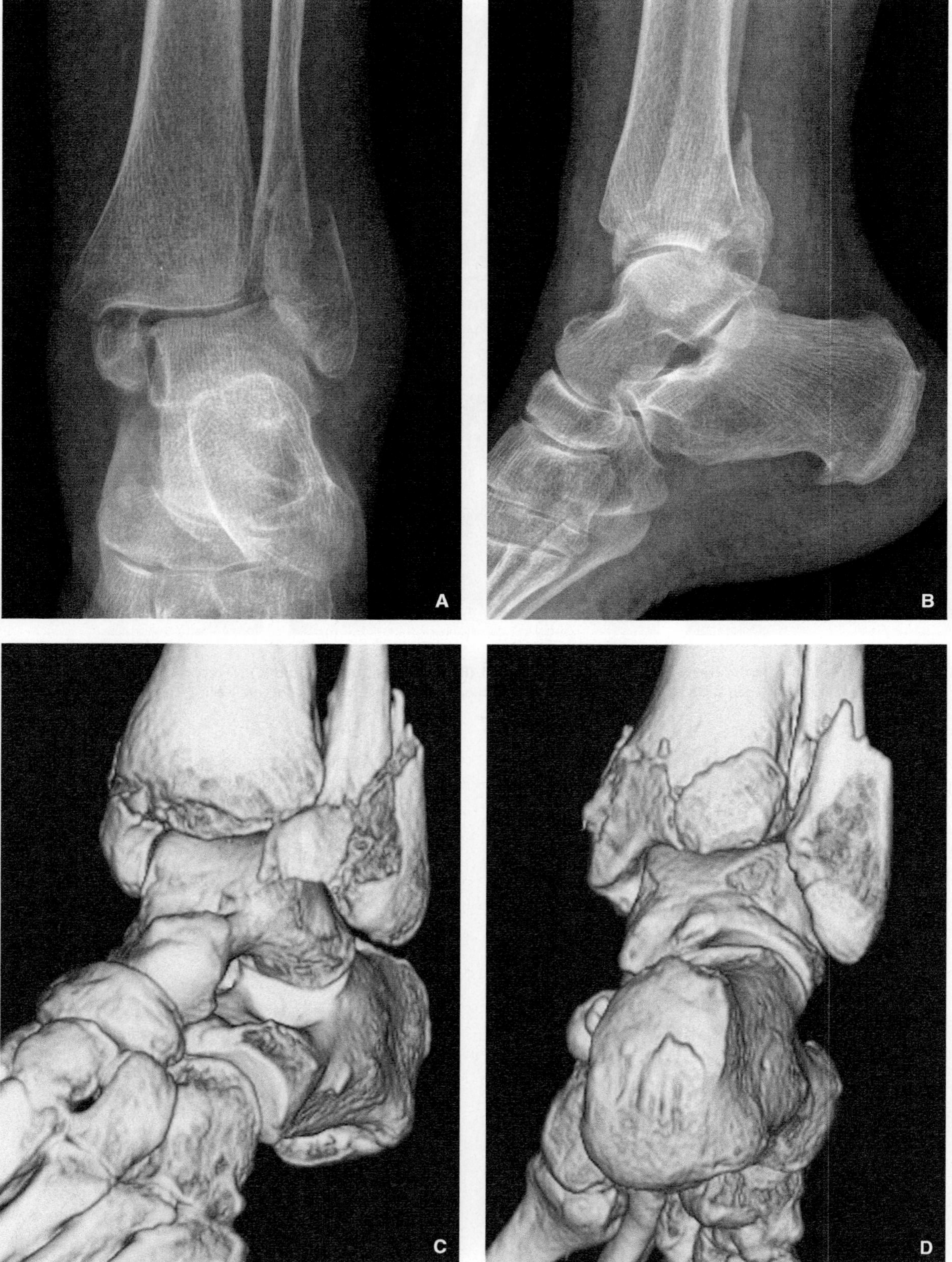

FIGURE 10.36 3D CT of trimalleolar fracture. **(A)** Anteroposterior and **(B)** lateral radiographs of the left ankle of the 69-year-old woman show fractures of the medial, lateral, and posterior malleoli. The fractures are also demonstrated on the 3D reconstructed CT images viewed from the **(C)** lateral and **(D)** posterior directions.

Fractures of the Distal Tibia

Pilon (Pylon) Fracture. Fracture of the distal tibia is called a pilon (pylon) fracture when the comminuted fracture lines extend into the tibiotalar joint (see Figs. 10.37 to 10.40). These injuries comprise approximately 5% of all lower leg fractures. Most pilon fractures occur during fall from a height, motor vehicle accidents, snow or water-skiing accidents, or are caused by a forward fall on a level surface with the foot entrapped. Although the pathomechanics of this injury may be complex, the predominant force is vertical compression. Not infrequently, there is associated fracture of the distal fibula, talus, and subluxation in the ankle joint (see Fig. 10.40) in addition to severe damage to the soft-tissue sleeve of the distal leg. Pilon fractures are a distinct clinical and radiologic entity and should not be confused with trimalleolar fractures. The following features distinguish pilon fractures from the trimalleolar fractures: the presence of profound comminution of the distal tibia, intraarticular extension of tibial fracture through the dome of the plafond, usual association of fracture of the talus, and usual preservation of tibiofibular syndesmosis. This fracture's significance comprises the intraarticular extension of the fracture line and its consequent potential to cause late complications of posttraumatic arthritis as well as nonunion and malunion.

There are several widely accepted classifications of the pilon fractures. Rüedi and Allgöwer classification divides these injuries into three groups, depending on the comminution, displacement of the fragments, and incongruity of the joint (Fig. 10.43).

Tillaux Fracture. In 1872, Tillaux described an ankle fracture resulting from abduction and external-rotation injury and consisting of avulsion of the lateral margin of the distal tibia. The fracture line is vertical and extends from the distal articular surface of the tibia upward to the lateral cortex (Figs. 10.44 to 10.48). In children, a similar type of fracture, referred to as juvenile Tillaux fracture, is actually a Salter-Harris type III injury to the distal tibial growth plate (Figs. 10.49 to 10.51). This injury probably occurs because the growth plate fuses from medial to lateral, making the medial side stronger than the lateral.

The imaging evaluation of a Tillaux fracture is critical for establishing whether surgery will be necessary. If the fracture fragment is laterally displaced more than 2 mm or if there is an irregularity of the articular surface of the distal tibia (a step-off), then surgical rather than conservative treatment is indicated. CT is the best method for obtaining this information (see Figs. 10.45 to 10.48 and 10.50).

If, instead of avulsion of the lateral margin of the tibia, the medial portion of the fibula becomes detached and the anterior tibiofibular ligament remains intact, then the fracture is called a *Wagstaffe-LeFort fracture* (Figs. 10.52 and 10.53).

Triplanar (Marmor-Lynn) Fracture. Fractures involving the lateral aspect of the distal tibial epiphysis may be complicated by extension of the fracture line into two other planes, hence the term triplanar fracture. The mechanism of this type of injury is usually plantar flexion and external rotation. The three planes involved are the sagittal plane, in which there is a vertical fracture through the epiphysis; the axial plane, in which a horizontally oriented fracture extends through the lateral aspect of the growth plate; and the coronal plane, in which there is an oblique fracture through the metaphysis into the diaphysis, extending superiorly (cephalad) from the anterior aspect of the growth plate to the posterior cortex of the tibia (Fig. 10.54).

The epiphyseal component of this fracture is best seen on the anteroposterior view, the axial component on both the anteroposterior and lateral views, and the diaphyseal extension on the lateral view. The typical triplanar fracture thus consists of a combination of the juvenile Tillaux fracture and a Salter-Harris type II fracture (Figs. 10.55 and 10.56) and should not be mistaken for a Salter-Harris type IV fracture (Fig. 10.57). Occasionally, metadiaphyseal component of the triplanar fracture may cross the growth plate and extend into the epiphysis, thus making the distinction from Salter-Harris type IV fracture more difficult (Fig. 10.58). CT is an effective technique to demonstrate the details of this injury (Figs. 10.59 and 10.60).

Fractures of the Fibula

Pott Fracture. After sustaining a fracture of his own leg, Sir Percivall Pott described in 1769 what he believed to be the most common type of ankle fracture, a fracture of the distal third of the fibula (Fig. 10.61). It is

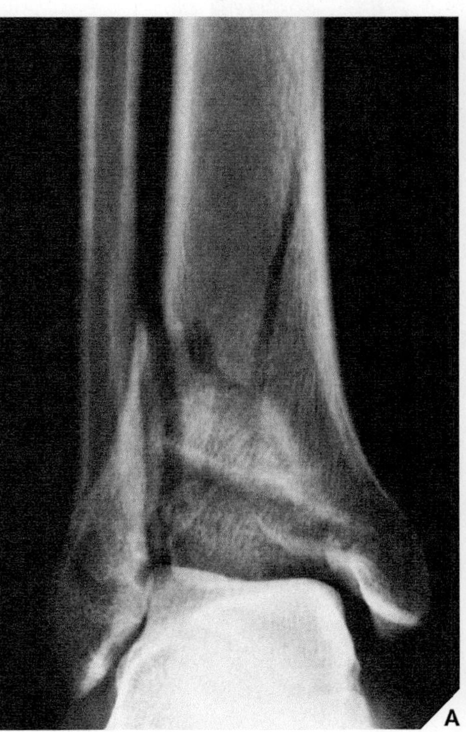

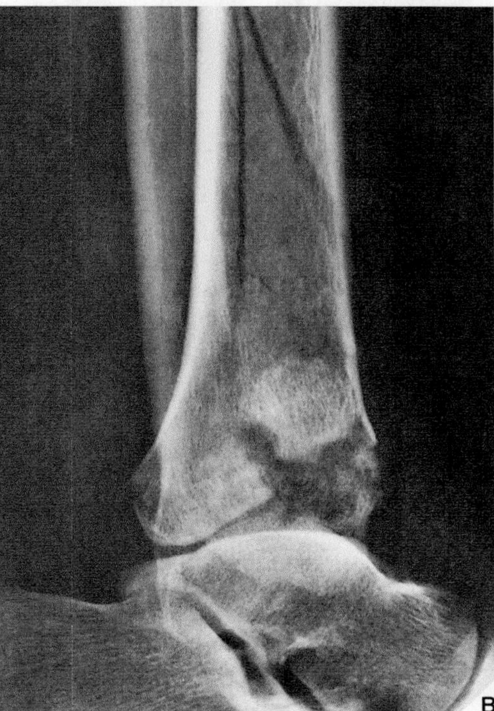

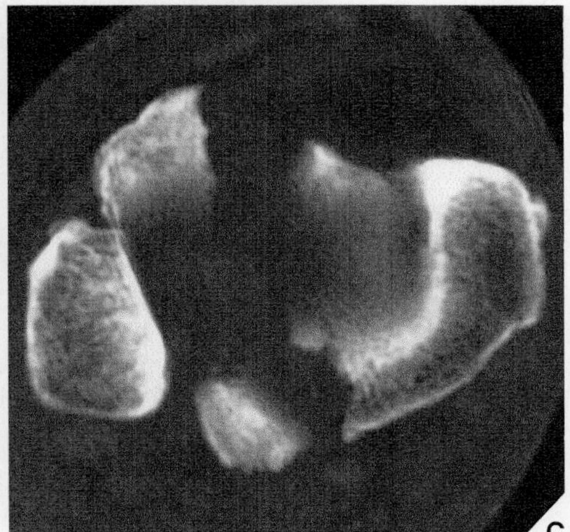

FIGURE 10.37 Pilon fracture. **(A)** Anteroposterior and **(B)** lateral radiographs of the right ankle demonstrate a complex, comminuted fracture of the distal tibia and fibula in a 30-year-old man who fell from a third-floor window. **(C)** Axial CT section through the tibial plafond shows typical appearance of pilon fracture.

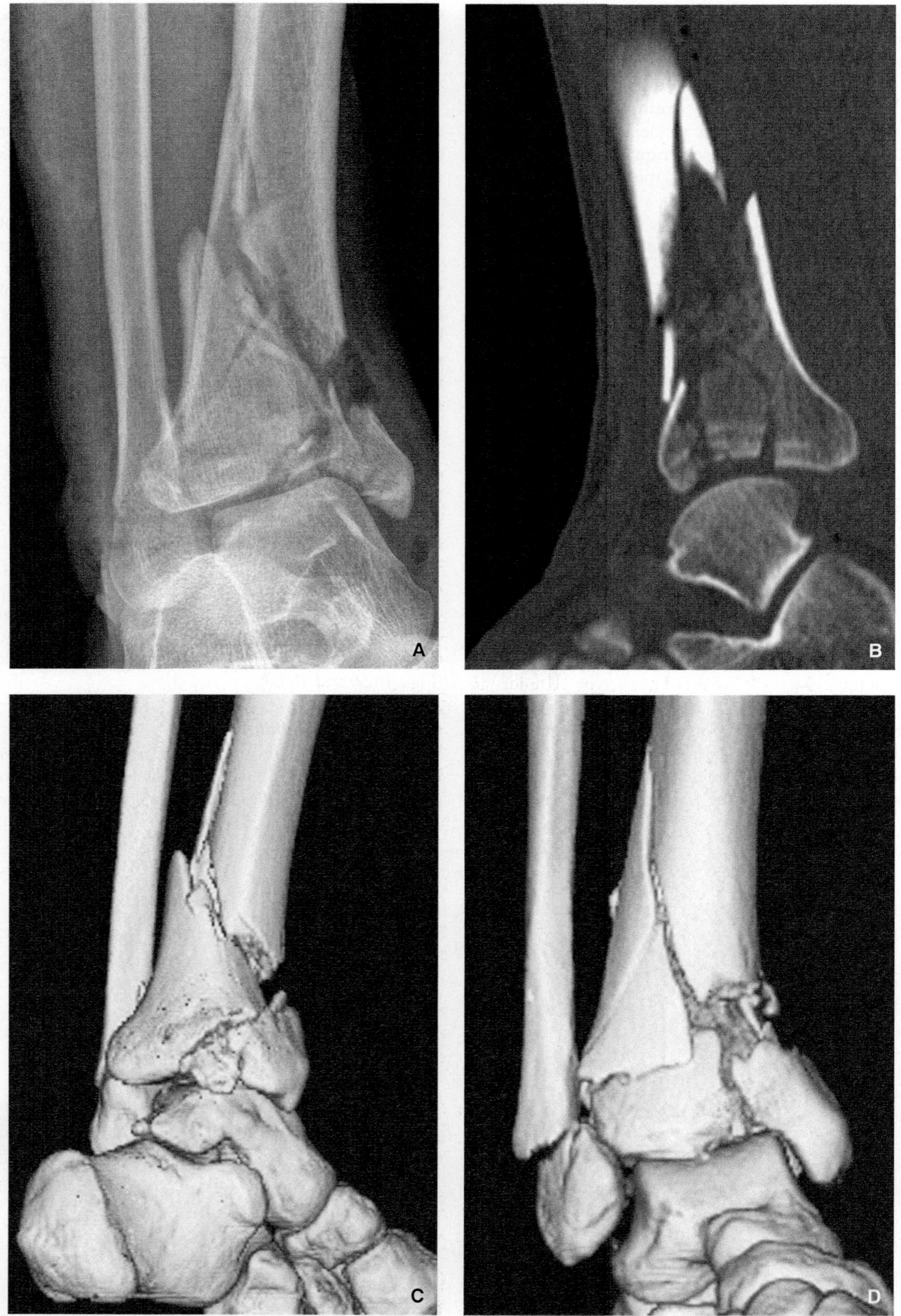

FIGURE 10.38 CT and 3D CT of the pilon fracture. **(A)** Oblique radiograph, **(B)** sagittal reformatted CT image, and **(C,D)** two 3D reconstructed CT images of the right ankle of a 29-year-old man show a pilon fracture. Note also fracture of the lateral malleolus.

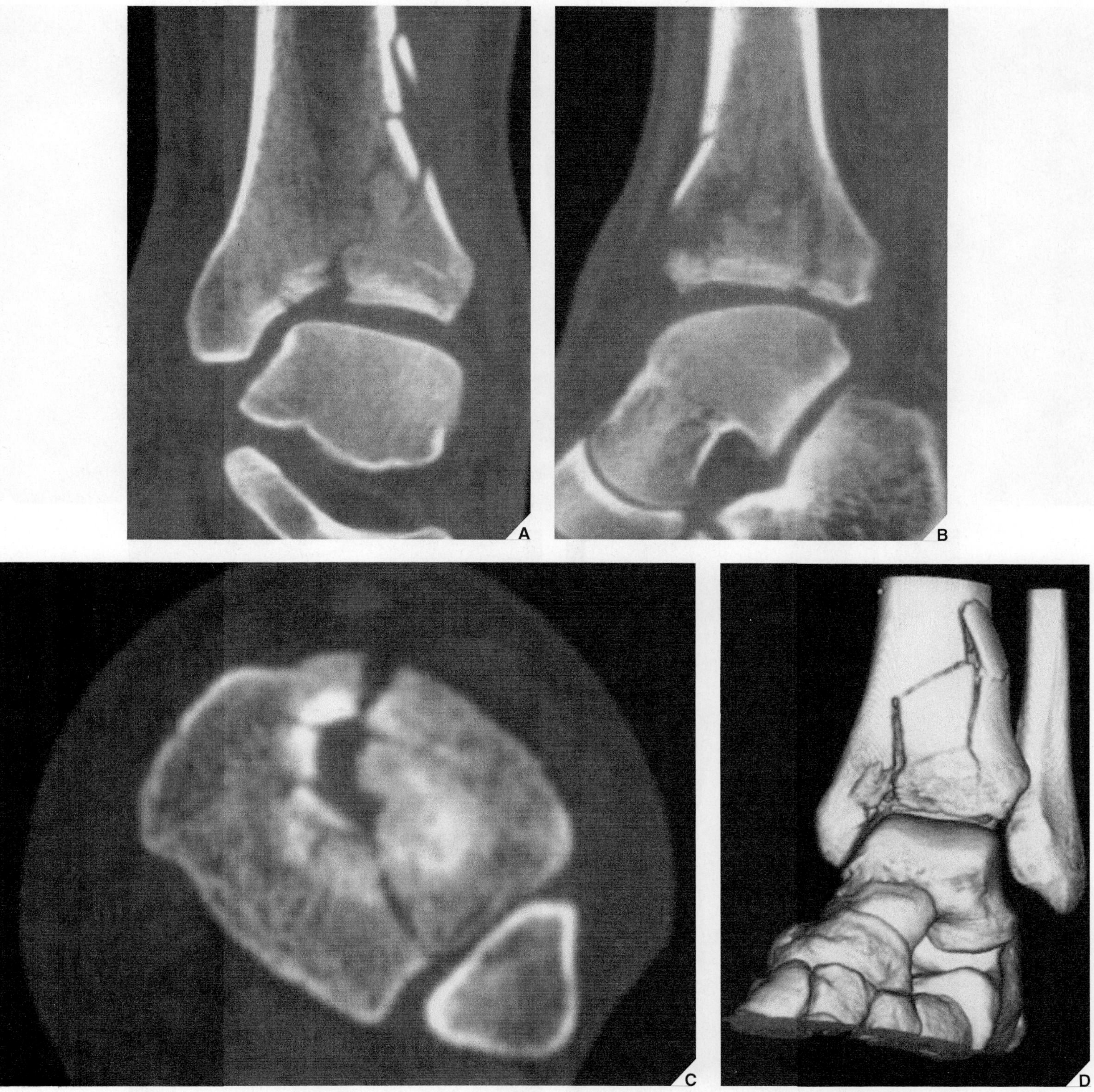

FIGURE 10.39 CT and 3D CT of pilon fracture. **(A)** Coronal, **(B)** sagittal, **(C)** axial, and **(D)** 3D reconstructed CT images show characteristic features of pilon fracture in a 30-year-old man who was injured in a motorcycle accident.

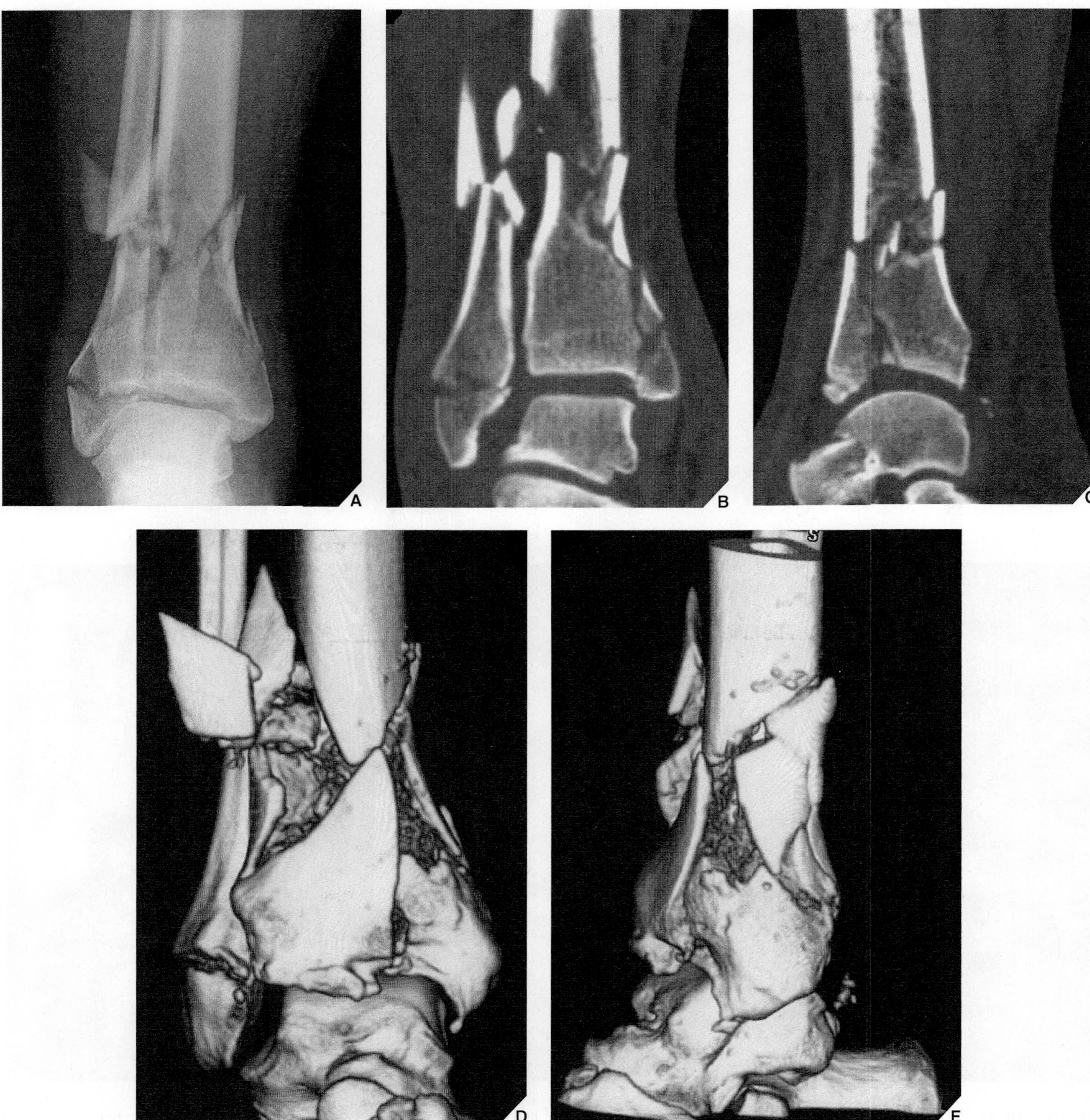

FIGURE 10.40 CT and 3D CT of pilon fracture. A 36-year-old man was injured in a motor vehicle accident and sustained a complex fracture of the distal tibia and fibula. **(A)** Conventional radiograph shows markedly comminuted intraarticular fracture of the distal tibia and segmental fracture of the distal fibula. **(B)** Coronal and **(C)** sagittal CT reformatted images demonstrate the number and direction of displaced fragments. **(D,E)** 3D reconstructed CT images viewed from anterior and medial directions display spatial orientation of various fractured fragments, thus providing an orthopaedic surgeon with a "road map" for successful open reduction and internal fixation of this complex fracture.

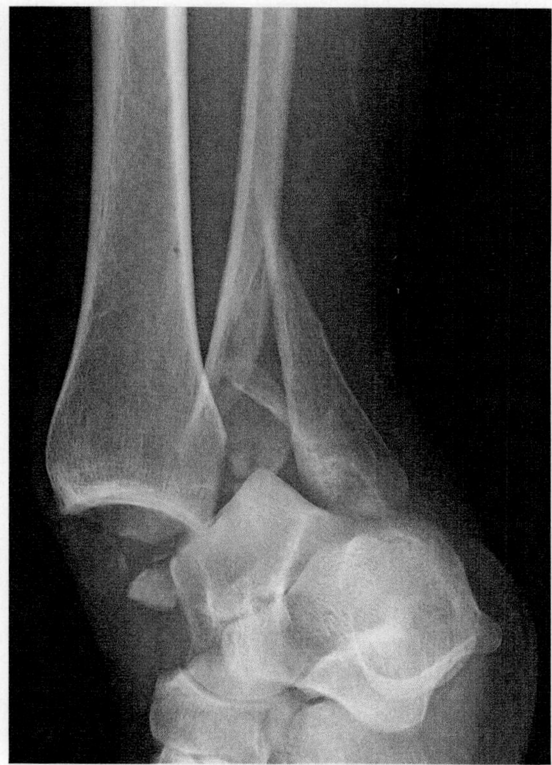

FIGURE 10.41 Fracture–dislocation of the ankle. A 28-year-old woman injured her right ankle in a skiing accident. Note comminuted fractures of the distal fibula and medial malleolus associated with posterior dislocation in the ankle joint.

now recognized that this type of fracture usually occurs as a result of the disruption of the tibiofibular syndesmosis. In fact, many authorities believe that the type of fracture Pott described does not exist as a primary fracture.

Dupuytren Fracture. Dupuytren fracture is the name given to a fracture of the fibula occurring 2 to 7 cm above the distal tibiofibular syndesmosis and including disruption of the medial collateral ligament (Fig. 10.62). The associated tear of the syndesmosis leads to ankle instability.

Maisonneuve Fracture. Like the Dupuytren fracture, the Maisonneuve fracture is an eversion-type injury of the fibula. The fracture, however, occurs in the proximal half of the bone, commonly at the junction of the proximal and middle thirds of the shaft (Fig. 10.63). If the fibula fracture is located in the distal half of the bone, the term low Maisonneuve fracture is applied (Fig. 10.64). The tibiofibular syndesmosis is always disrupted, and either tear of the tibiofibular ligament or fracture of the medial malleolus is also present (Fig. 10.65). The more proximal the location of the fibular fracture, the more is the damage to the interosseous membrane between the tibia and the fibula, which is always disrupted up to the point of the fibular fracture.

Injury to the Soft Tissues About the Ankle Joint and Foot

As mentioned, all ankle injuries can be grossly classified as resulting from inversion-stress or eversion-stress forces (see Figs. 10.27 and 10.28). However, the forces delivered to the ankle are rarely pure inversion or pure eversion. A combination of forces is usually at work to produce ligament and tendon injuries that may occur secondary to fractures or as primary injuries. Several classifications have been developed to reflect the complexity of these forces. Lauge-Hansen classified ankle injuries based on the mechanism of injury by combining the position of the foot (supination or pronation) with the direction of the deforming force vector (external rotation, adduction, or abduction) (Table 10.4). He emphasized the close relationship between bone and ligament injuries, but the complexity of his classification diminishes its value in treatment.

From the practical orthopaedic point of view, the Weber classification, based on the level of fibular fracture and therefore on the type of syndesmotic ligament injury, is much more useful (Fig. 10.66):

Type A: The fibular fracture may be a transverse avulsion fracture at the level of or just distal to the ankle joint. There may be an associated fracture of the medial malleolus. Alternatively, the fibula is intact, but the lateral collateral ligament is disrupted. In either case, the tibiofibular syndesmosis, the interosseous membrane, and the deltoid ligament are intact.

Type B: There is a spiral fracture of the distal fibula, beginning at the level of the tibiofibular syndesmosis, with partial disruption of mainly the posterior tibiofibular ligament. It may also be associated with an avulsion fracture of the medial malleolus below the level of the ankle joint (Fig. 10.67). Alternatively, the medial malleolus may be intact, and the deltoid ligament may be disrupted.

Type C: Fracture of the fibula occurs at a level higher than the ankle joint, with associated tear of the posterior tibiofibular ligament and resultant lateral talar instability. If the fibular fracture is high (Maisonneuve type), the interosseous membrane is torn to the level of the fracture. There is also an avulsion fracture of the medial malleolus, in which case the deltoid ligament is intact. Alternatively, the medial malleolus is intact, but the deltoid ligament is disrupted (Fig. 10.68).

The likelihood of injury to the distal tibiofibular syndesmosis can be inferred from the nature and level of the fibular fracture: The higher the fibular fracture, the more extensive the damage to the tibiofibular ligaments and, thus, the greater the risk of ankle instability. The greatest value of this classification lies in the fact that it emphasizes the lateral syndesmotic-malleolar complex as an important factor in congruence and stability in the ankle joint.

Posttraumatic Joint Effusion

This can be assessed on the lateral radiograph of the ankle by appearance of focal soft-tissue density anteriorly to the joint, and encroachment of the Kager triangle, also known as *pre-Achilles fat pad*—a radiolucent triangle bounded anteriorly by the flexor hallucis longus muscle and tendon, posteriorly by Achilles tendon, and inferiorly by the calcaneus (Fig. 10.69).

Tear of the Medial Collateral Ligament

Depending on the severity of the eversion force, injury to the medial collateral ligament ranges from sprain to complete rupture (see Fig. 10.28). Tear may occur either in the body of the ligament or at its attachment to the medial malleolus. Rupture of the medial collateral ligament is typically associated with a tear of the tibiofibular ligament and lateral subluxation of the talus. On clinical examination, soft-tissue swelling is prominent, distal to the tip of the medial malleolus. If the standard radiographic examination of the ankle reveals lateral shift of the talus in the absence of a

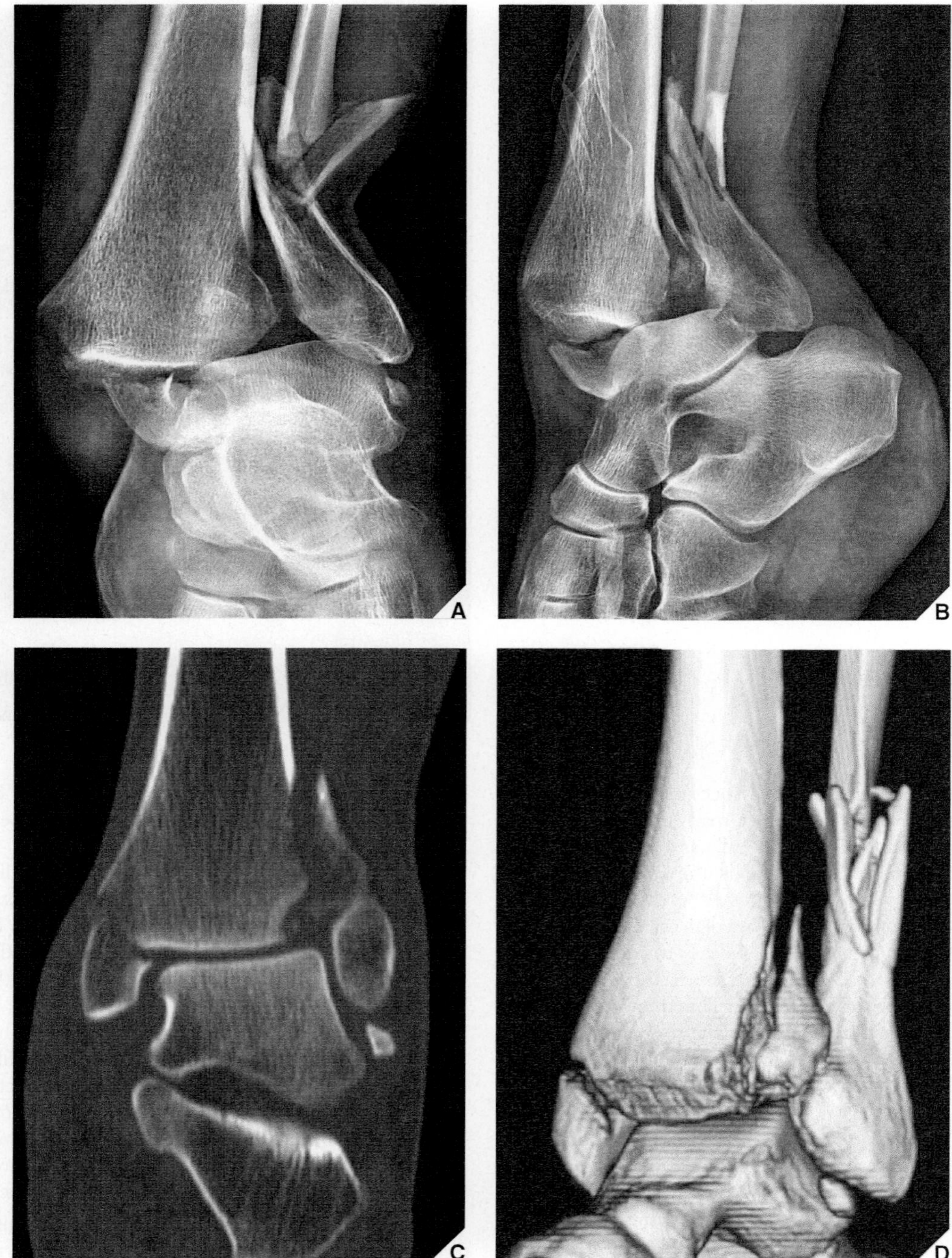

FIGURE 10.42 **CT and 3D CT of fracture–dislocation of the ankle.** **(A)** Anteroposterior and **(B)** cross-table lateral radiographs of the left ankle show trimalleolar fracture associated with posterior dislocation in the ankle joint. **(C)** Coronal reformatted and **(D)** 3D reconstructed CT images were obtained after the dislocation was relocated.

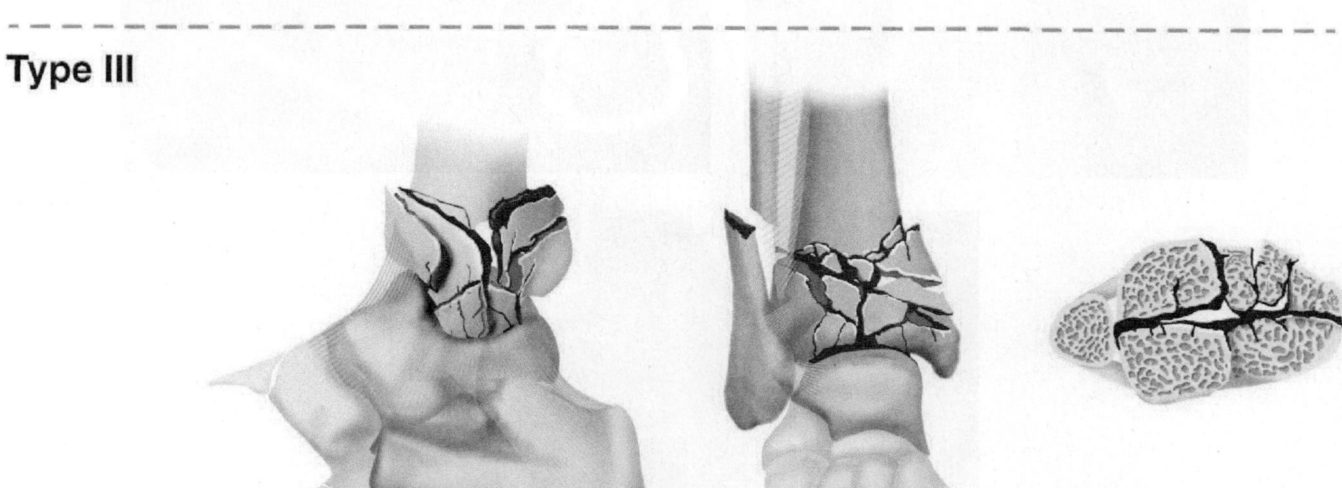

FIGURE 10.43 **Classification of pilon fractures.** The Rüedi and Allgöwer classification of intraarticular fractures of the distal tibia (pilon fractures) is based on the amount of displacement of the fragments and the consequent degree of incongruity of the joint. (Reprinted with permission from Brinker MR. *Review of orthopaedic trauma*, 2nd ed. Philadelphia, PA: Wolters Kluwer Health; 2013, Fig. 12.2.)

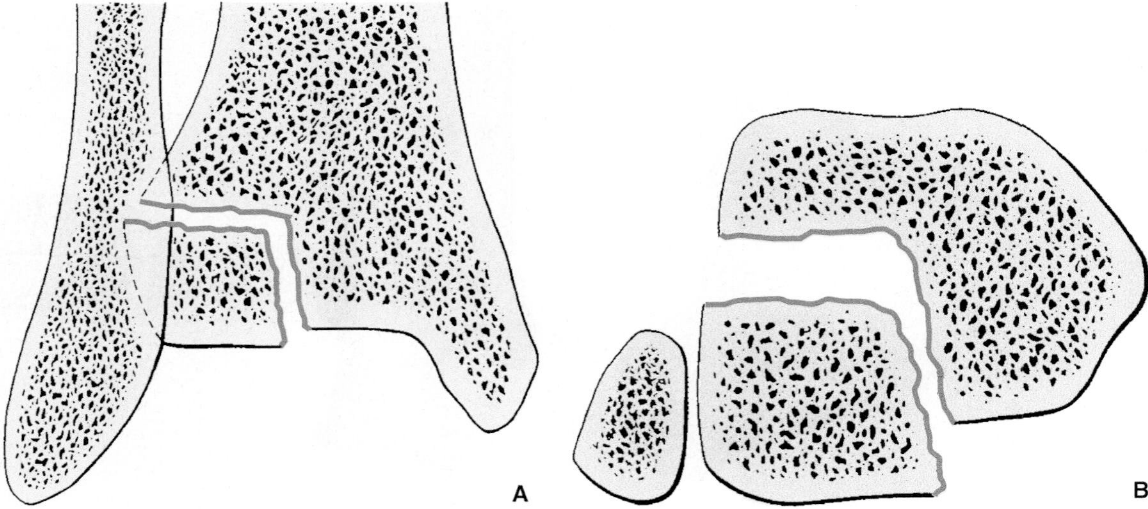

FIGURE 10.44 Tillaux fracture. In the classic Tillaux fracture, shown here schematically in coronal **(A)** and transverse **(B)** sections through the distal tibia, the fracture line extends from the distal articular surface of the tibia upward to the lateral cortex.

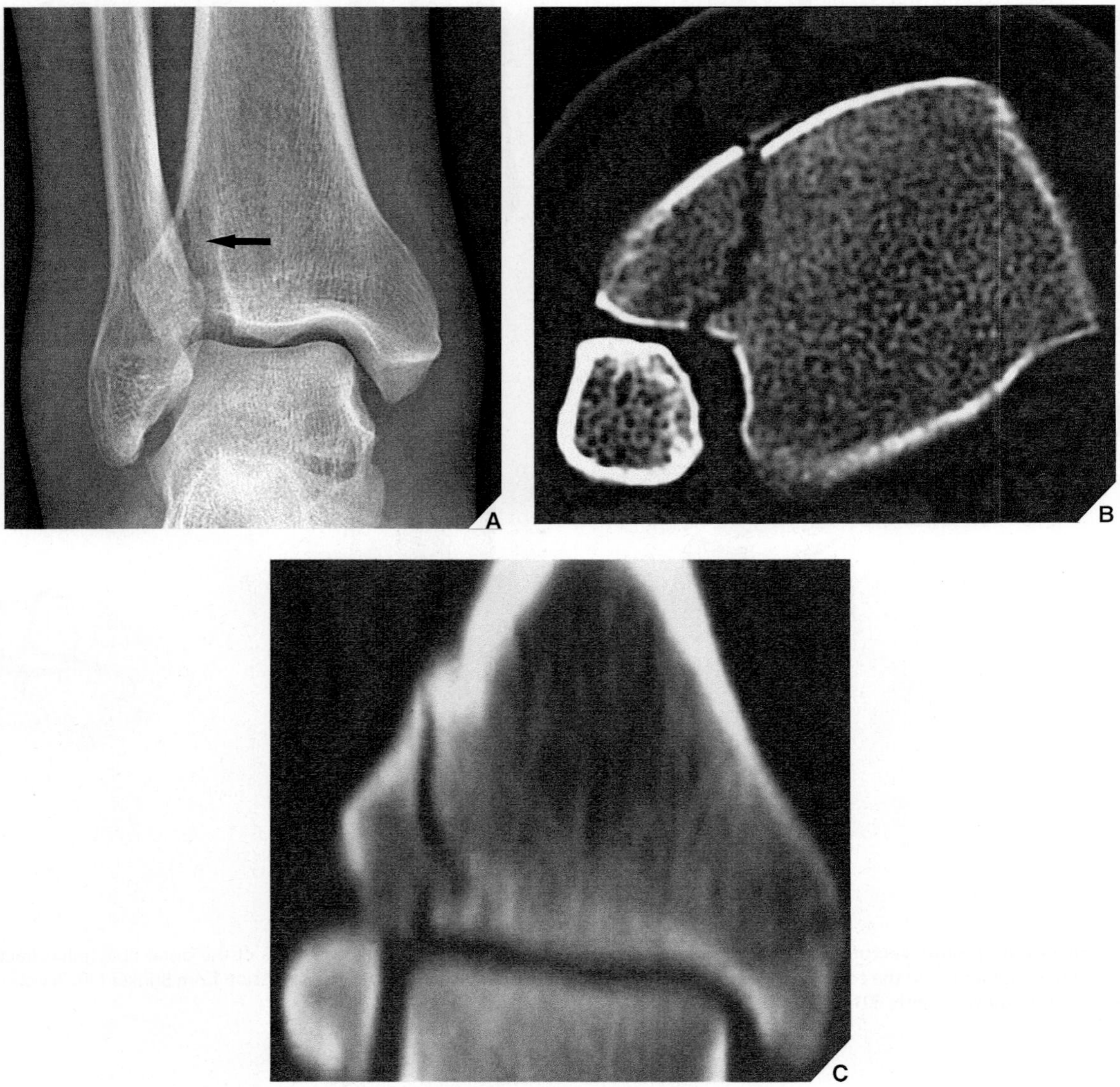

FIGURE 10.45 CT of Tillaux fracture. A 39-year-old man sustained a nondisplaced Tillaux fracture, demonstrated on **(A)** anteroposterior radiograph of the ankle *(arrow)*, **(B)** axial CT, and **(C)** coronal reformatted CT image.

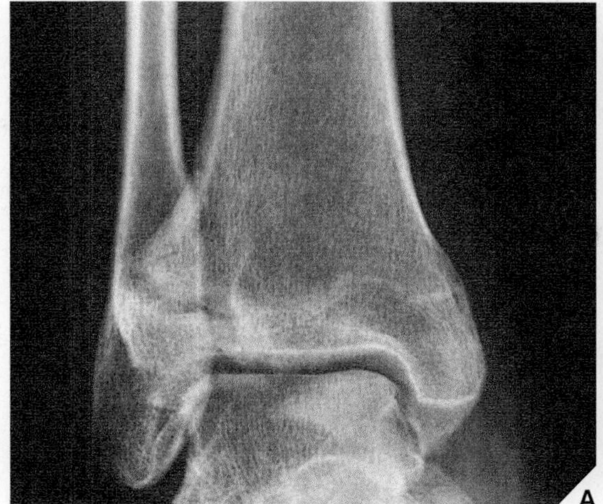

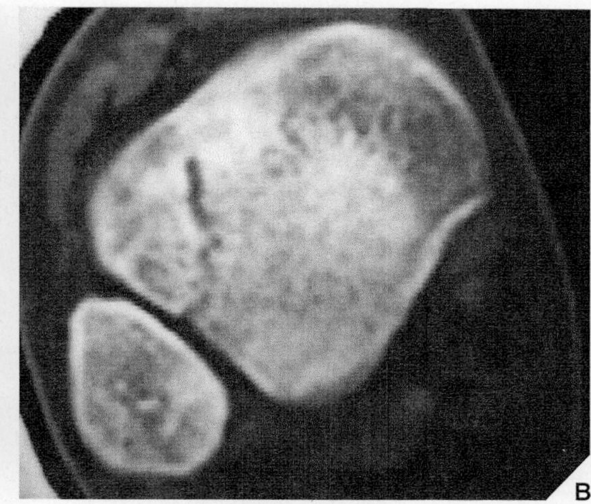

FIGURE 10.46 CT of Tillaux fracture. A 24-year-old woman twisted her ankle while ice skating. **(A)** Anteroposterior radiograph of the ankle and **(B)** axial CT section show a marginal fracture of the lateral aspect of the tibia, a characteristic Tillaux fracture. The minimal amount of displacement seen here would mandate only conservative treatment.

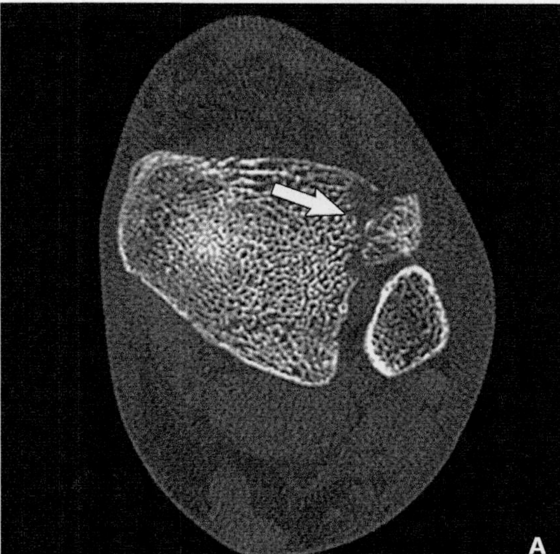

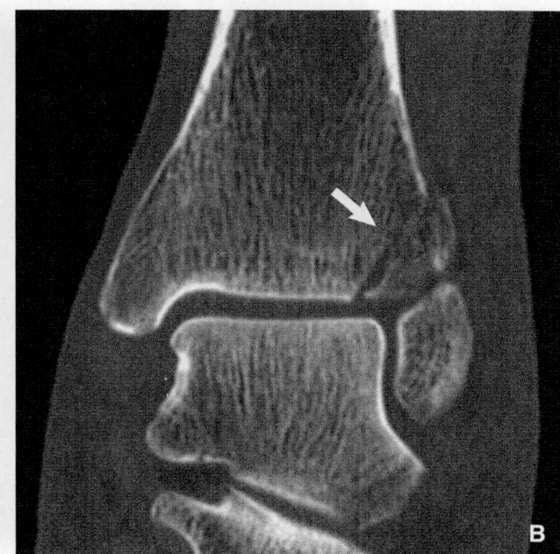

FIGURE 10.47 CT of Tillaux fracture. **(A)** Axial and **(B)** coronal reformatted CT images of the left ankle show a slightly displaced Tillaux fracture *(arrows)*.

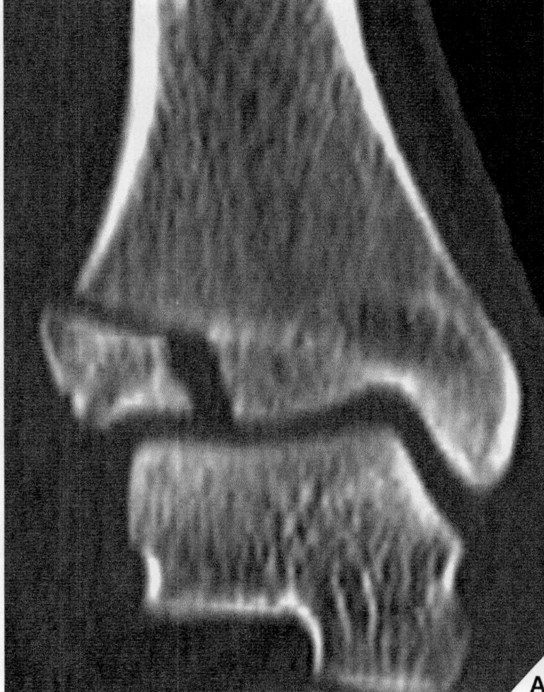

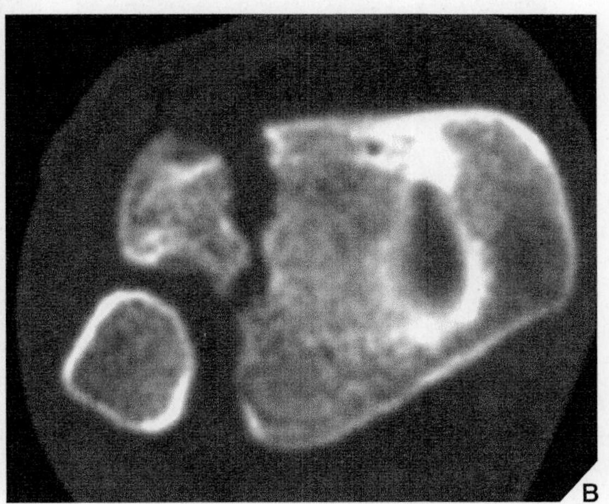

FIGURE 10.48 CT of Tillaux fracture. A 28-year-old woman injured right ankle during skiing competition. **(A)** Coronal reformatted and **(B)** axial CT images show a displaced Tillaux fracture that was later treated with open reduction and internal fixation.

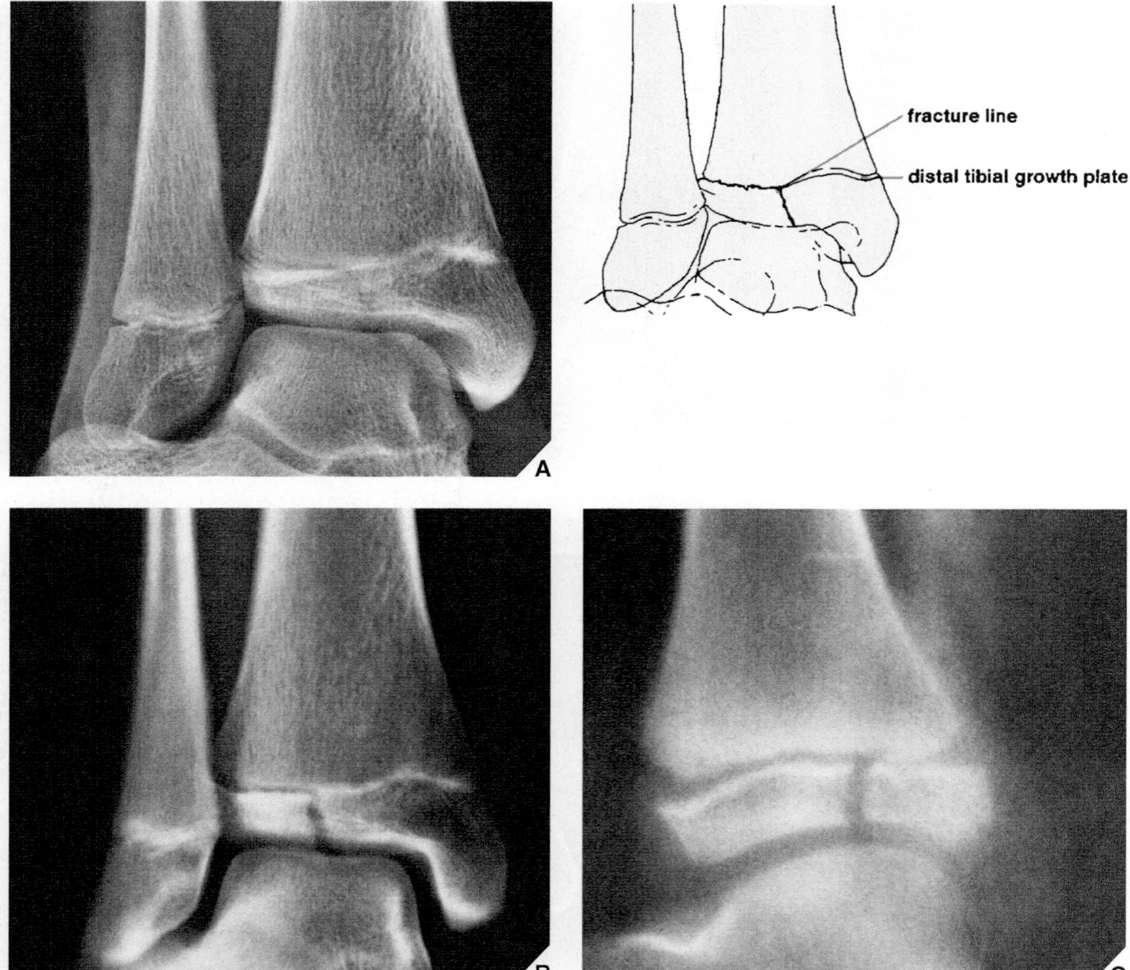

FIGURE 10.49 Juvenile Tillaux fracture. A 13-year-old girl injured her right ankle during a basketball game. **(A)** Oblique radiograph of the ankle and tomographic sections in the oblique **(B)** and lateral **(C)** projections demonstrate a typical Salter-Harris type III injury to the growth plate, also called *juvenile Tillaux fracture.*

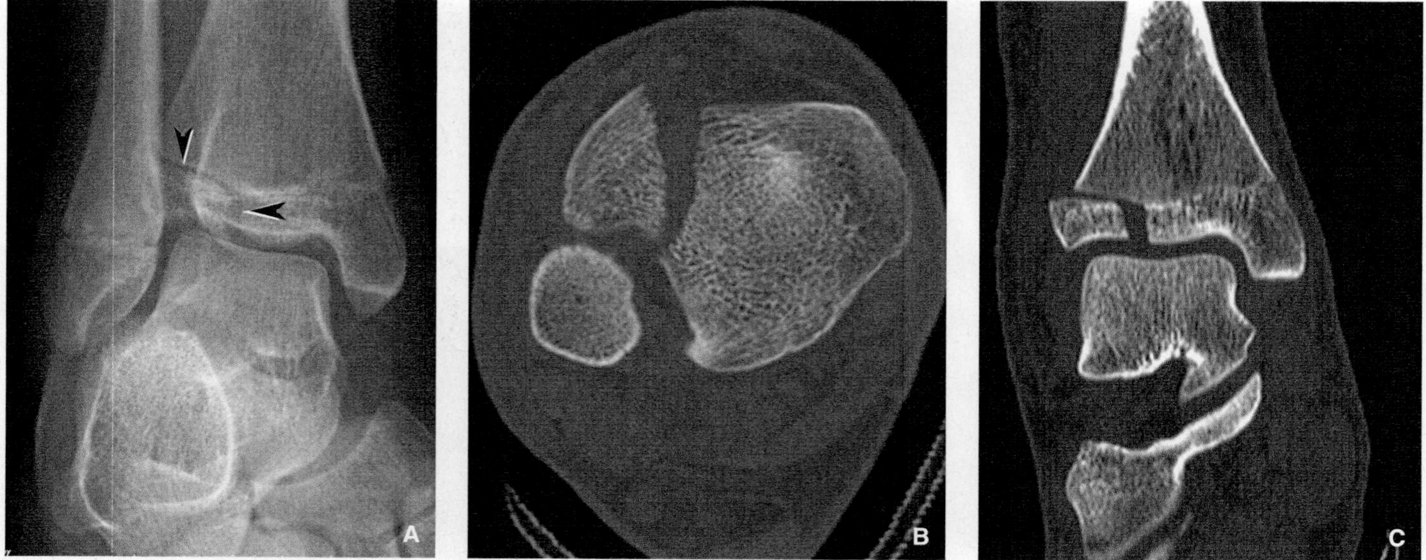

FIGURE 10.50 CT of juvenile Tillaux fracture. **(A)** Anteroposterior radiograph of the right ankle, and **(B)** axial and **(C)** coronal reformatted CT images show slightly displaced fracture of the distal lateral tibial metaphysis and epiphysis *(arrowheads).*

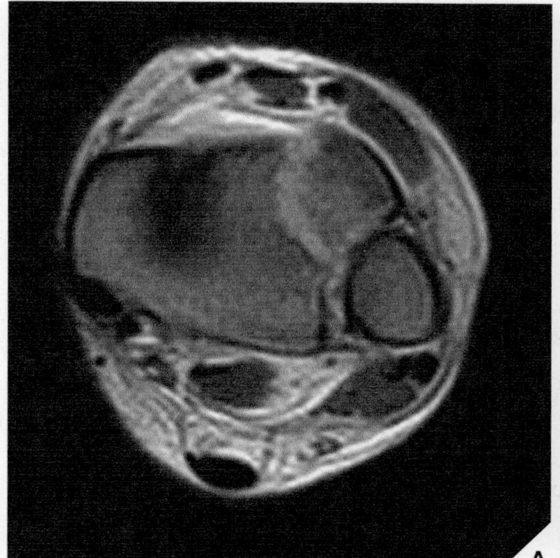
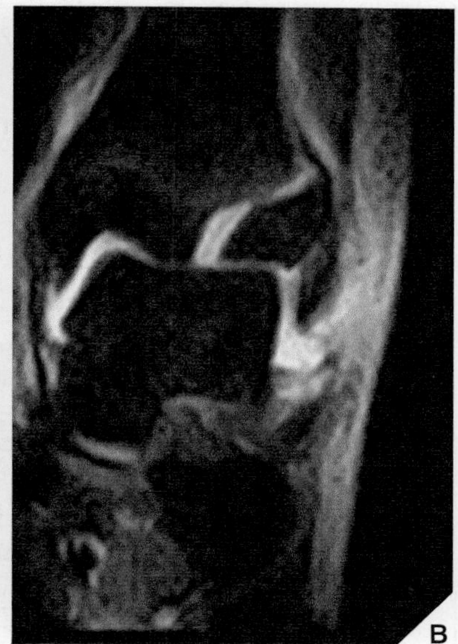

FIGURE 10.51 **MRI of juvenile Tillaux fracture.** **(A)** Axial T2-weighted and **(B)** coronal short time inversion recovery (STIR) MR images of the left ankle of a 12-year-old boy demonstrate the fracture of the anterior lateral aspect of the distal tibial epiphysis, the characteristic feature of this injury.

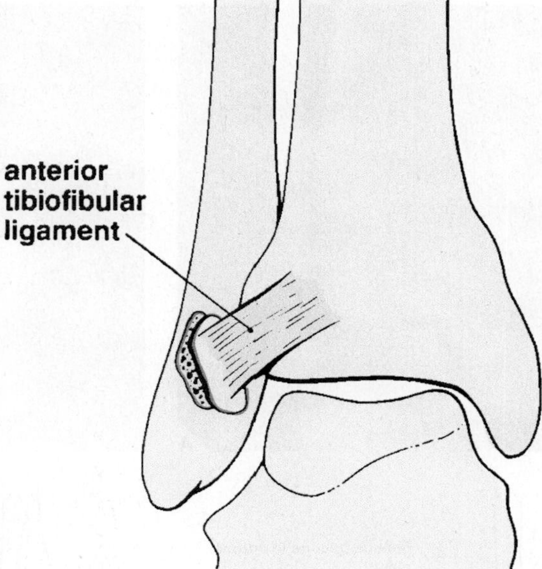

FIGURE 10.52 **Wagstaffe-LeFort fracture.** In the Wagstaffe-LeFort fracture, seen here schematically on the anteroposterior view, the medial portion of the fibula is avulsed at the insertion of the anterior tibiofibular ligament. The ligament, however, remains intact.

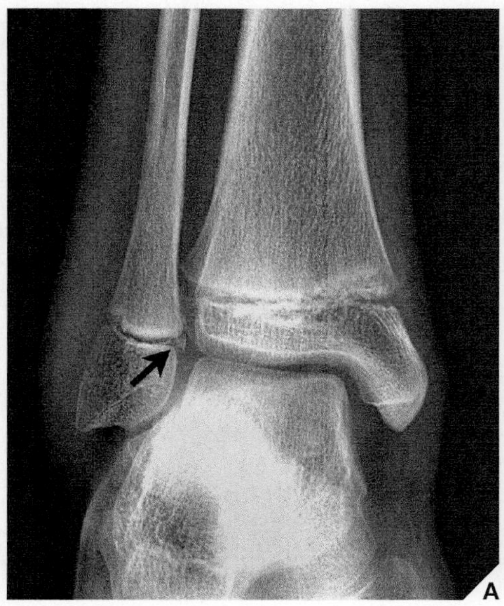
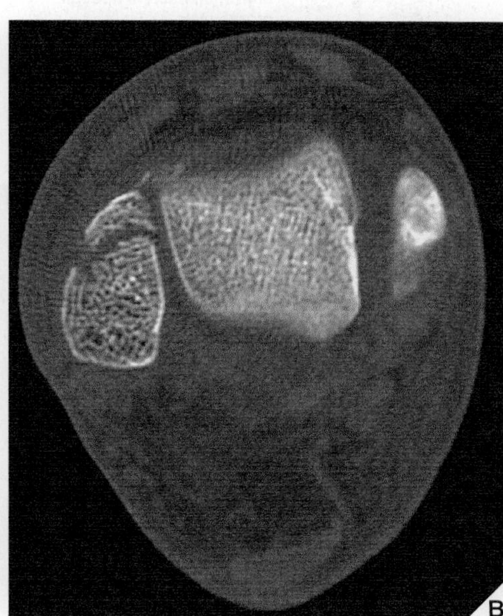
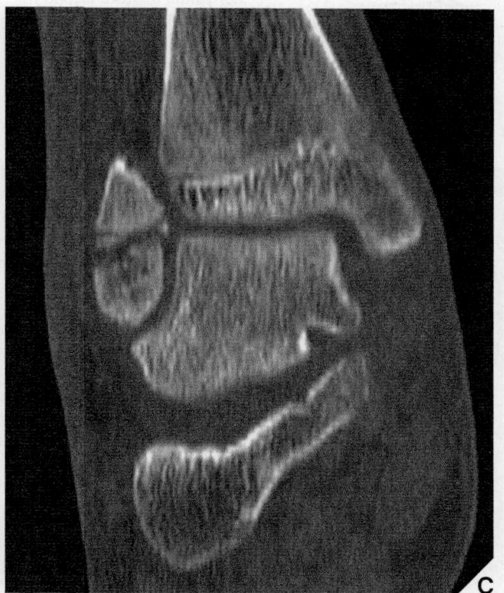

FIGURE 10.53 **CT of Wagstaffe-LeFort fracture.** **(A)** Anteroposterior radiograph of the right ankle shows evulsion of the osseous fragment from the fibula *(arrow)* at the site of insertion of the anterior tibiofibular ligament, better demonstrated on the axial **(B)** and coronal reformatted **(C)** CT images.

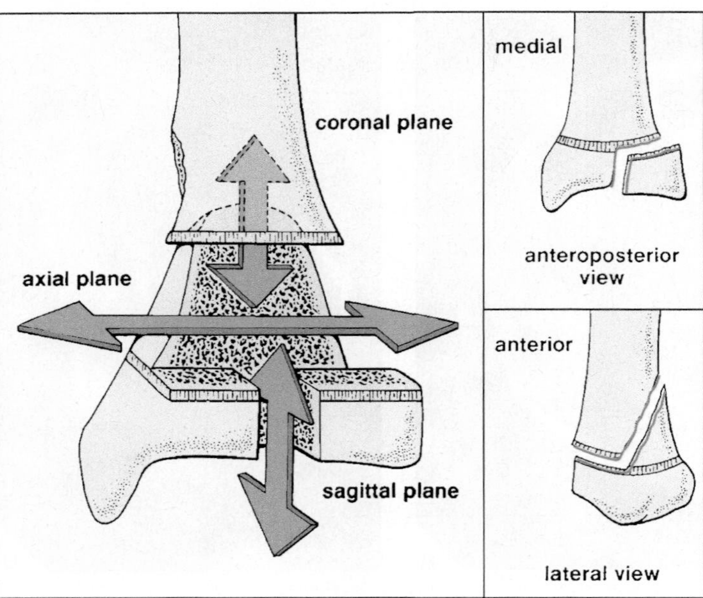

FIGURE 10.54 **Triplanar fracture.** The Marmor-Lynn (or triplanar) fracture comprises a vertical fracture of the epiphysis in the sagittal plane, a horizontally oriented fracture in the axial plane through the lateral aspect of the growth plate, and an oblique fracture through the metaphysis into the diaphysis in the coronal plane, extending superiorly from the anterior aspect of the growth plate to the posterior cortex of the tibia.

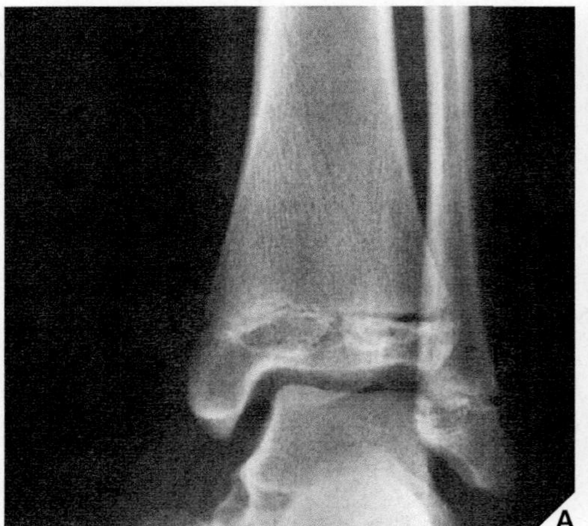

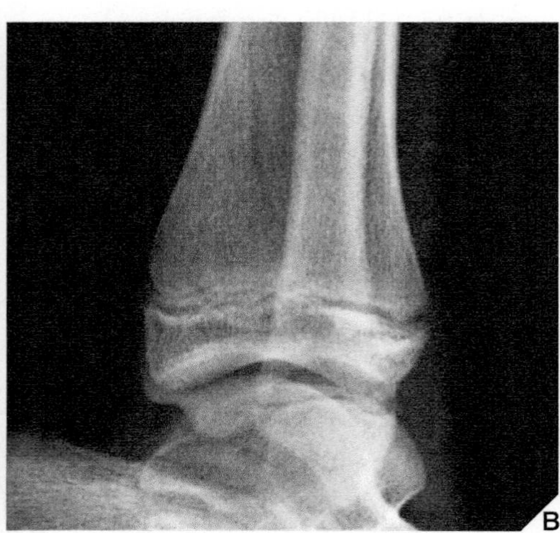

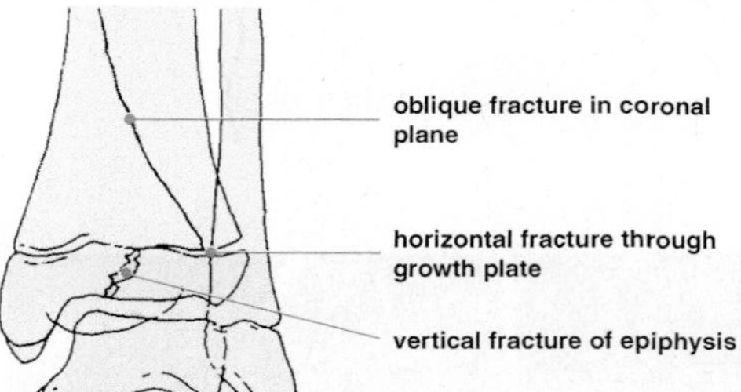

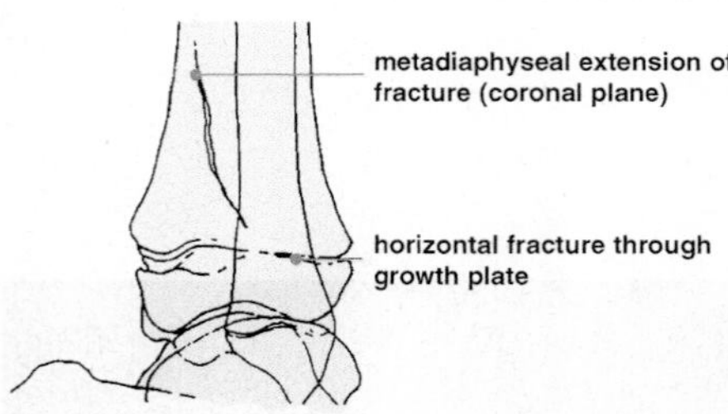

FIGURE 10.55 **Triplanar fracture.** A 12-year-old girl fell on ice and sustained a typical triplanar fracture. **(A)** Anteroposterior radiograph of the left ankle shows a vertical fracture of the epiphysis and horizontal extension through the lateral aspect of the growth plate. The metaphyseal and diaphyseal components of the fracture are barely seen. **(B)** Lateral radiograph clearly demonstrates the posteriorly directed fracture line in the coronal plane, the third component of a triplanar fracture.

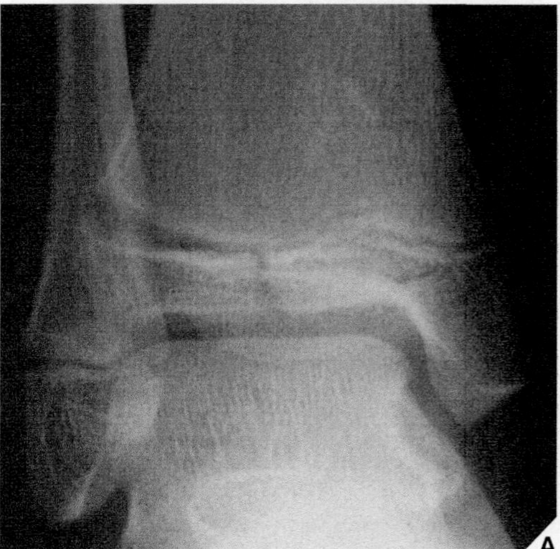

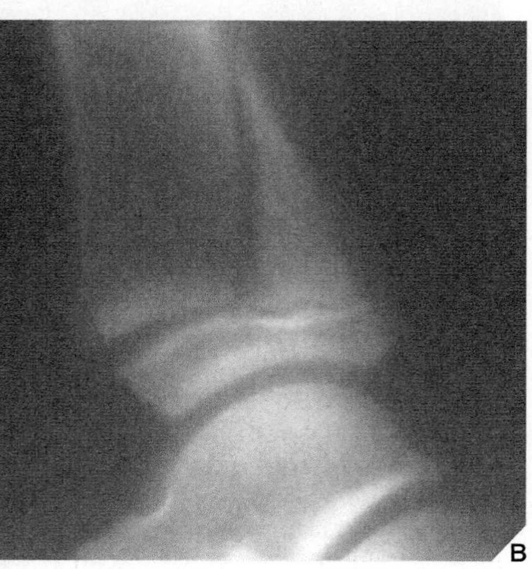

FIGURE 10.56 **Triplanar fracture.** A 13-year-old boy presented with a triplanar fracture. **(A)** Anteroposterior radiograph shows only horizontal and vertical components. **(B)** A trispiral lateral tomogram shows horizontal and oblique components.

FIGURE 10.57 **Salter-Harris type IV fracture.** Anteroposterior radiograph of the ankle in an 8-year-old boy demonstrates that the fracture line traverses the epiphysis and metaphysis of the distal tibia, but there is no horizontal extension through the growth plate. Note the associated Salter-Harris type I fracture of the distal fibula (see also Fig. 4.45).

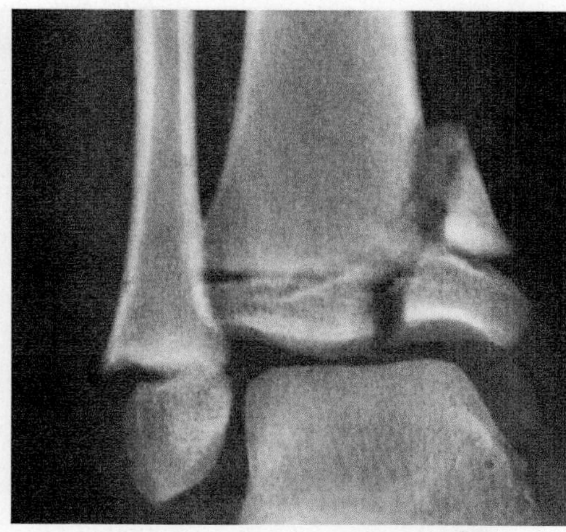

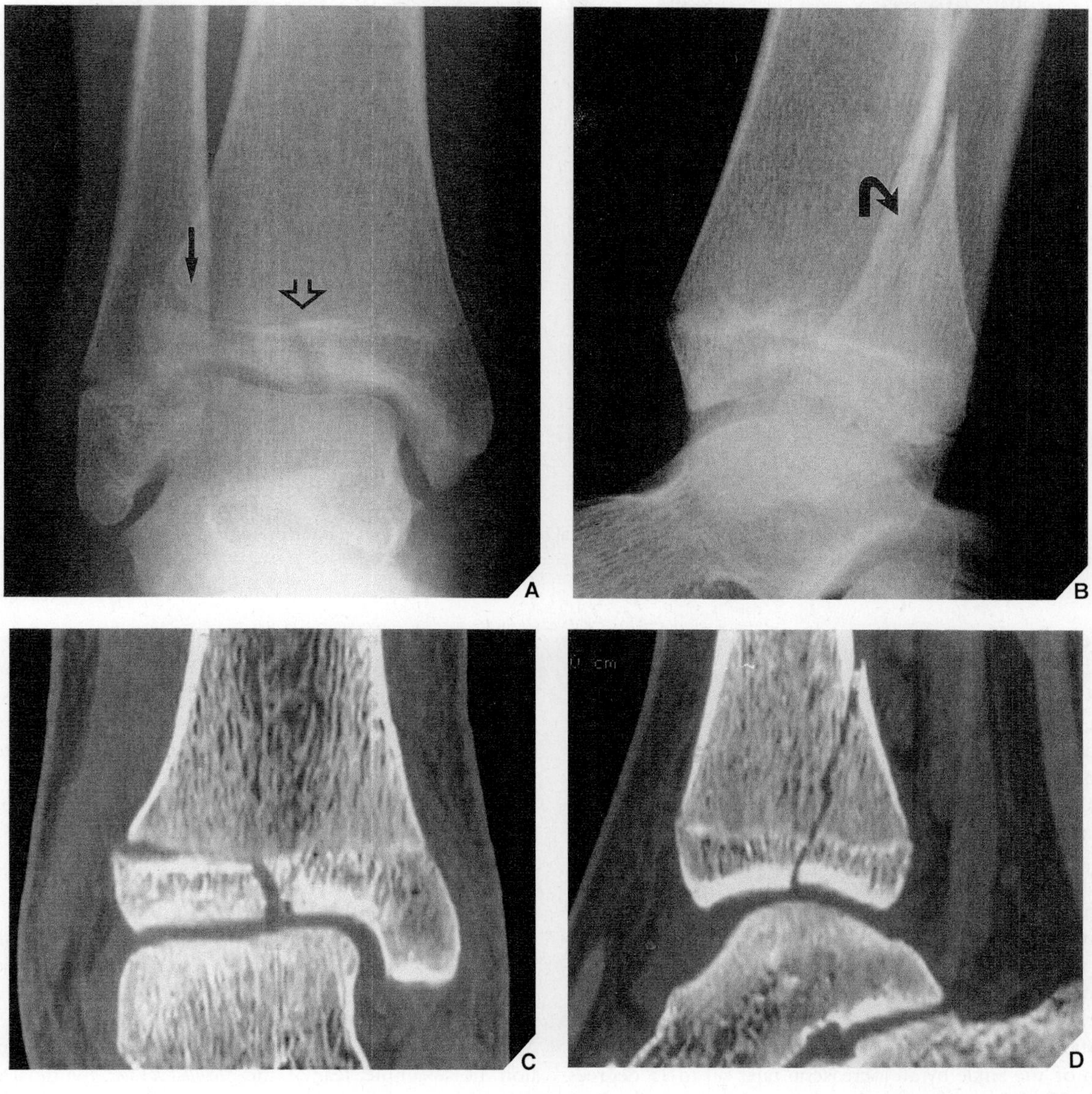

FIGURE 10.58 **CT of triplanar fracture.** **(A)** Anteroposterior radiograph of the right ankle shows horizontal *(arrow)* and vertical *(open arrow)* components of this injury. **(B)** Lateral radiograph shows the oblique component *(curved arrow)*, but the distal extent of the fracture line is not well demonstrated. **(C)** Coronal and **(D)** sagittal CT reformatted images confirm the diagnosis of triplanar fracture. Note that the obliquely oriented fracture line extends into the epiphysis.

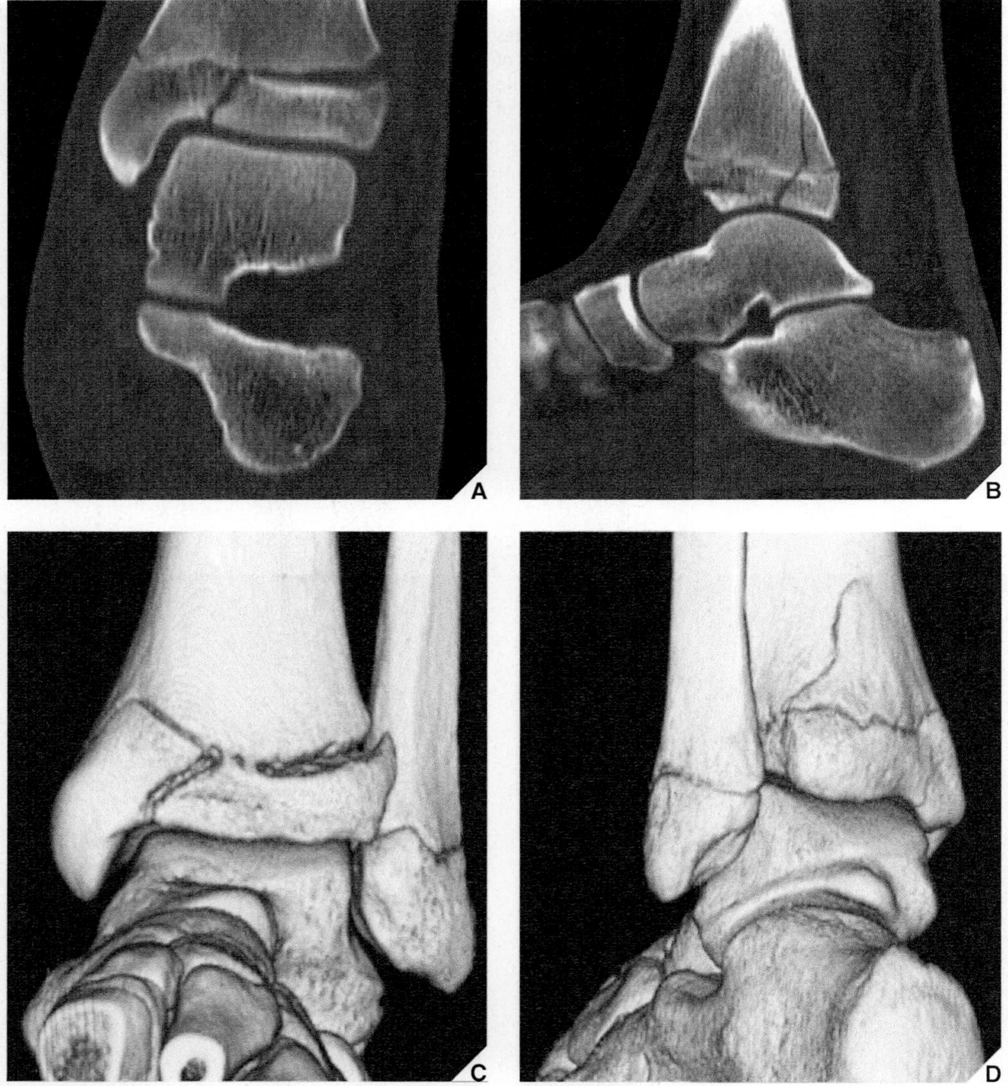

FIGURE 10.59 CT and 3D CT of triplanar fracture. **(A)** Coronal and **(B)** sagittal reformatted CT images demonstrate three components of this injury. **(C,D)** 3D reconstructed CT images show the spatial orientation of the fracture lines.

spiral fracture of the fibula, one must assume that both the tibiofibular and the medial collateral ligaments are torn.

Although tears of the ligaments of the ankle can be demonstrated on CT examination, more commonly these injuries are evaluated by MRI. Acute tear of the medial collateral ligament appears as disruption of continuity or absence of the low-intensity ligamentous fibers surrounded by edema or hemorrhage (Fig. 10.70). Chronic or healed ligamentous disruption shows generalized thickening of the ligament.

Tear of the Lateral Collateral Ligament

Inversion-stress forces delivered to the lateral ankle structures may cause a spectrum of injuries to the lateral collateral ligament, ranging from sprain to complete rupture (see Fig. 10.27). The body of the ligament or its attachment to the fibular malleolus may be the site of injury. In the absence of fracture of the fibular malleolus on the standard radiographic examination, disruption of the ligament complex can be recognized on the inversion-stress film of the ankle by an increase in talar tilt to 15 degrees or more (see Fig. 10.10B). The component ligaments of this complex may also be injured independently. The *anterior talofibular ligament* is the most frequently injured ankle ligament. It can be diagnosed on the inversion-stress film of the ankle (see Fig. 10.10), but MRI examination may be required for confirmation (Fig. 10.71).

This modality is equally effective in evaluating injury to the lateral collateral ligament. The diagnosis of a tear is based on lack of visualization of the one or more components of this ligament. The tears of the calcaneofibular ligament are best demonstrated either in the coronal or axial planes (Fig. 10.72), whereas the tears of the anterior and posterior talofibular ligaments are best seen on the axial sections (see Fig. 10.71B). Repetitive ankle sprains with injuries to the anterior talofibular ligament may lead to focal synovial thickening in the anterolateral aspect of the ankle, known as *Wolin lesion* or *meniscoid lesion*. Patients present with pain in the anterolateral aspect of the ankle on dorsiflexion. This syndrome is known as *anterolateral impingement syndrome* or *anterolateral gutter syndrome* (see Fig. 10.71C, see also Fig. 10.123).

Tear of the Distal Anterior Tibiofibular Ligament

Commonly associated with other ligament injuries, tear of the anterior tibiofibular syndesmotic ligament may also occur as an isolated injury (see Fig. 10.71).

Tendinosis and Tendon Ruptures

Most tendon ruptures can be diagnosed by history and clinical examination. For example, tear of the *Achilles tendon*, the most common injury to the soft tissues of the foot, is often indicated by severe tenderness at the tendon's insertion, together with limitation of plantar flexion. Avulsion of this tendon from its calcaneal insertion (Fig. 10.73) can be recognized on the lateral radiograph of the foot obtained with a low-kilovoltage/soft-tissue technique (Fig. 10.74). However, the best technique to diagnose the acute tears is MRI (Figs. 10.75 and 10.76A,B). Tendinosis is a precursor of tendon tears. The imaging manifestations of tendinosis include thickening of the tendon and focal or linear areas of intrasubstance degeneration,

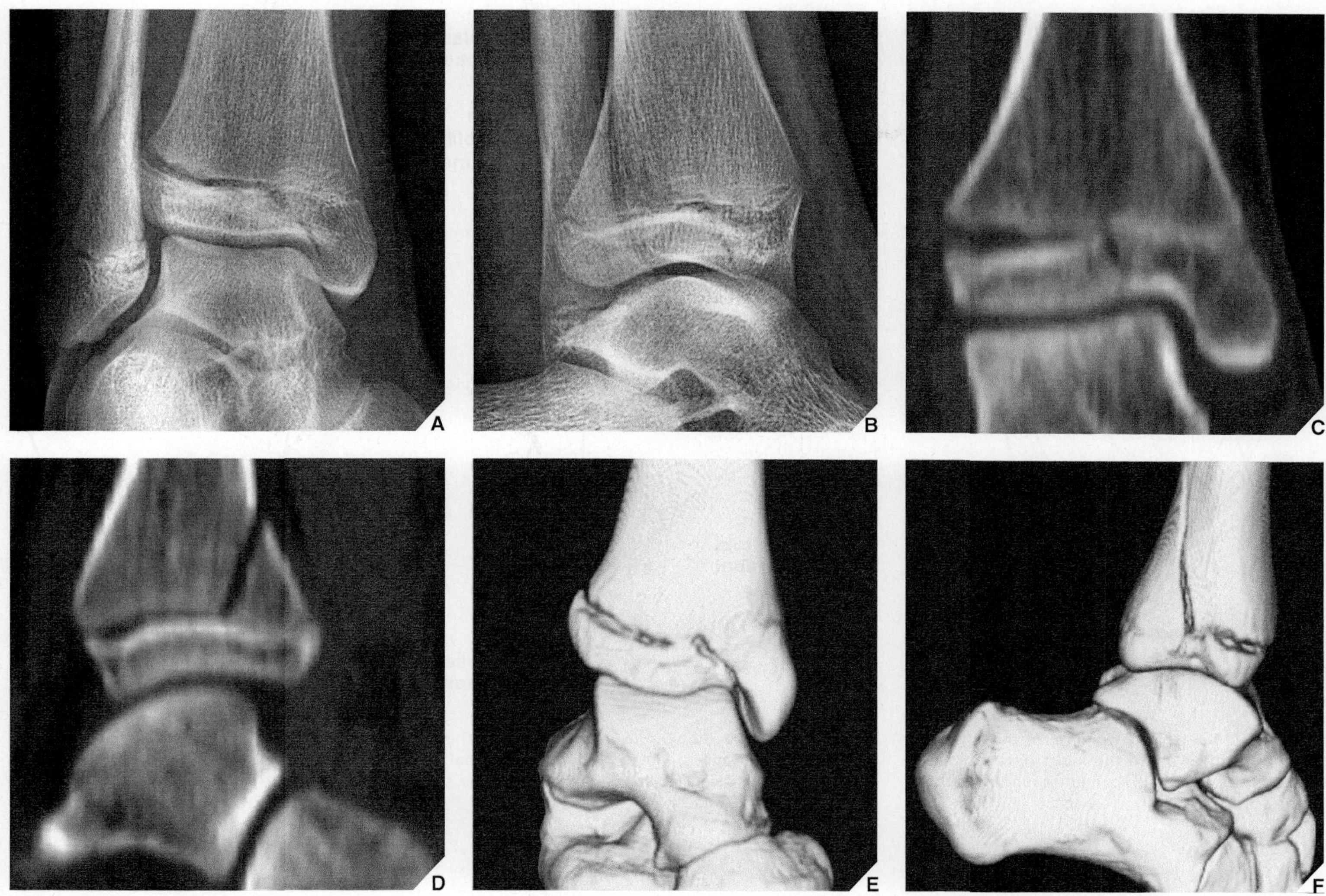

FIGURE 10.60 CT and 3D CT of triplanar fracture. **(A)** Anteroposterior and **(B)** lateral radiographs of the right ankle show all three components of the triplanar fracture that are more vividly demonstrated on **(C)** coronal and **(D)** sagittal reformatted CT images and on 3D CT reconstruction **(E,F)**.

which can be seen on US or MRI (Fig. 10.76C). Tendinosis of the Achilles tendon most often is manifested by fusiform thickening of the tendon at the watershed zone, proximal to the calcaneal insertion. However, in some cases, tendinosis and partial or complete tears occur at the insertion (insertional tendinosis) (Fig. 10.76D). Insertional tendinosis is associated with Haglund deformity (prominent superior posterior process of the calcaneus), retrocalcaneal bursitis, peritendinitis, and inflammatory arthritis.

Injury to the Foot

Fractures of the Foot

Fractures of the Calcaneus

Commonly sustained in falls from heights, fractures of the calcaneus are sometimes called *lover's fractures*; in 10% of cases, they are seen bilaterally. According to Cave, fractures of the calcaneus account for 60% of all major tarsal injuries.

In the evaluation of such injuries, it is critical to determine whether the fracture line involves the subtalar joint and, if so, to assess the degree of depression of the posterior facet. Determination of the Boehler angle (see Fig. 10.20C) and angle of Gissane (see Fig. 10.21) helps evaluate depression, but CT is usually essential (Fig. 10.77). The CT examination should include coronal and axial sections. Sagittal reformatted images and 3D reconstruction may enhance depiction and characterization of calcaneal fractures (Figs. 10.78 to 10.81) and may be helpful in the assessment of adequacy of postsurgical reduction. In all calcaneal fractures sustained in a fall from a height, a radiograph of the thoracolumbar spine is essential because of the commonly associated finding of compression fracture of one of the vertebral bodies (Fig. 10.82).

Several classifications of the intraarticular fractures of the calcaneus have been developed.

Essex-Lopresti classified calcaneal fractures into two main categories: those sparing the subtalar joint (25%) and those extending into it (75%), with the latter subdivided into joint-depression fractures and tongue-type fractures. Rowe and coworkers classified calcaneal fractures into five types (Fig. 10.83):

- Type I: fractures of the tuberosity, sustentaculum tali, or anterior process (21%)
- Type II: beak fractures and avulsion fractures of the Achilles tendon insertion (3.8%)
- Type III: oblique fractures not extending into the subtalar joint (19.5%)
- Type IV: fractures involving the subtalar joint (24.7%)
- Type V: fractures with central depression and varying degrees of comminution (31%).

Sanders classified intraarticular fractures of the calcaneus into four types, based on fracture line extension into the posterior facet of the subtalar joint:

- Type 1: nondisplaced fractures, regardless of the number of fracture fragments
- Type 2: two-part fractures
  - A. Affecting lateral third of the bone
  - B. Affecting central third of the bone
  - C. Affecting medial third of the bone
- Type 3: three-part fractures, affecting two of the earlier listed parts
- Type 4: highly comminuted fracture.

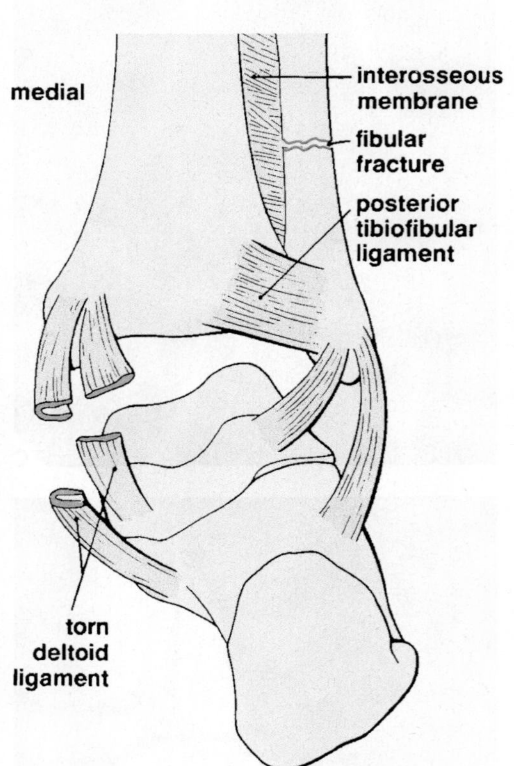

FIGURE 10.61 Pott fracture. In this injury, the fibula is fractured above the intact distal tibiofibular syndesmosis, the deltoid ligament is ruptured, and the talus is subluxed laterally.

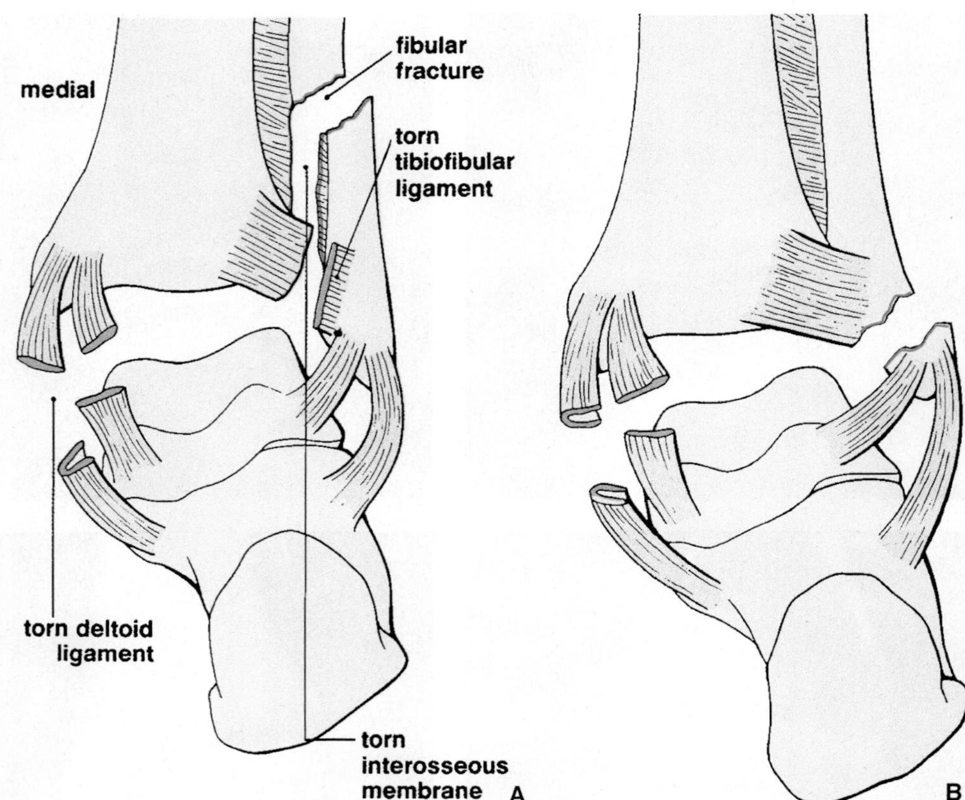

FIGURE 10.62 Dupuytren fracture. **(A)** This fracture usually occurs 2 to 7 cm above the distal tibiofibular syndesmosis, with disruption of the medial collateral ligament and, typically, tear of the syndesmosis leading to ankle instability. **(B)** In the low variant, the fracture occurs more distally, and the tibiofibular ligament remains intact.

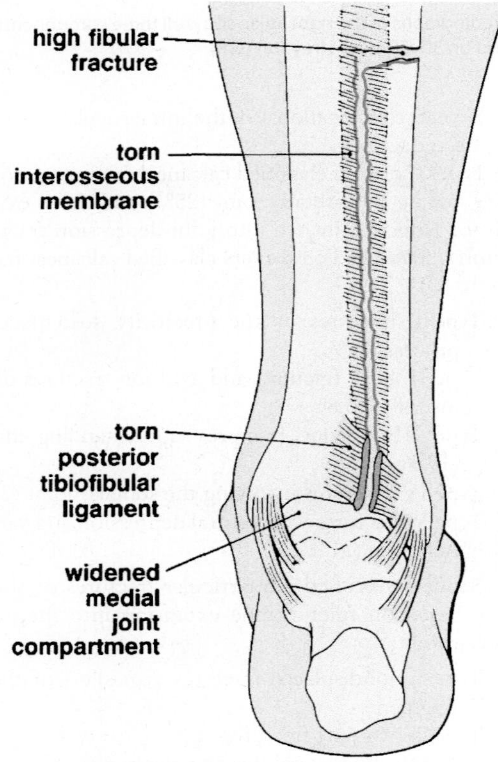

FIGURE 10.63 Maisonneuve fracture. The classic Maisonneuve fracture commonly occurs at the junction of the middle and distal thirds of the fibula. The tibiofibular syndesmosis is disrupted, and the interosseous membrane is torn up to the level of the fracture. The tibiotalar (medial) joint compartment is widened because of lateral subluxation of the talus.

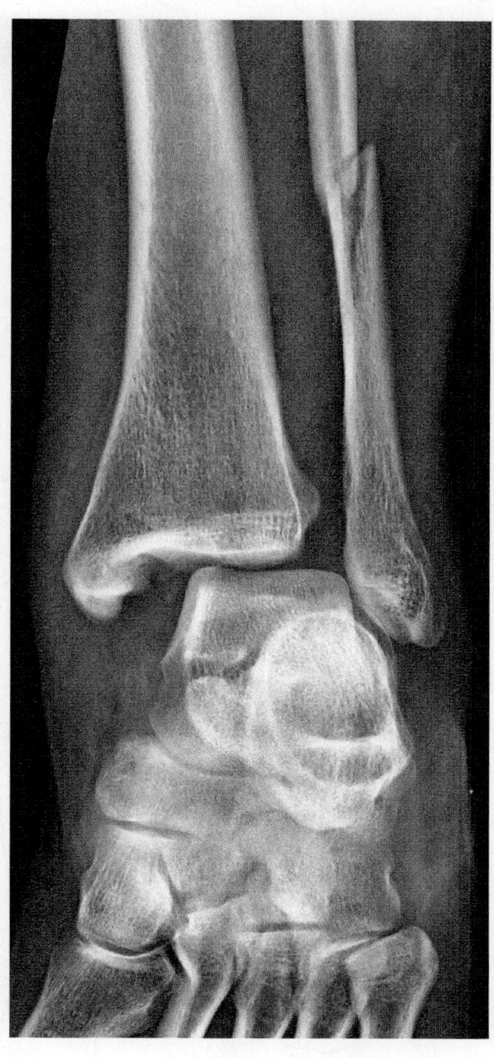

FIGURE 10.64 Maisonneuve fracture (low variant). Anteroposterior radiograph shows subluxation in the ankle joint secondary to the tear of the deltoid ligament, and a fracture of the distal third of the fibula.

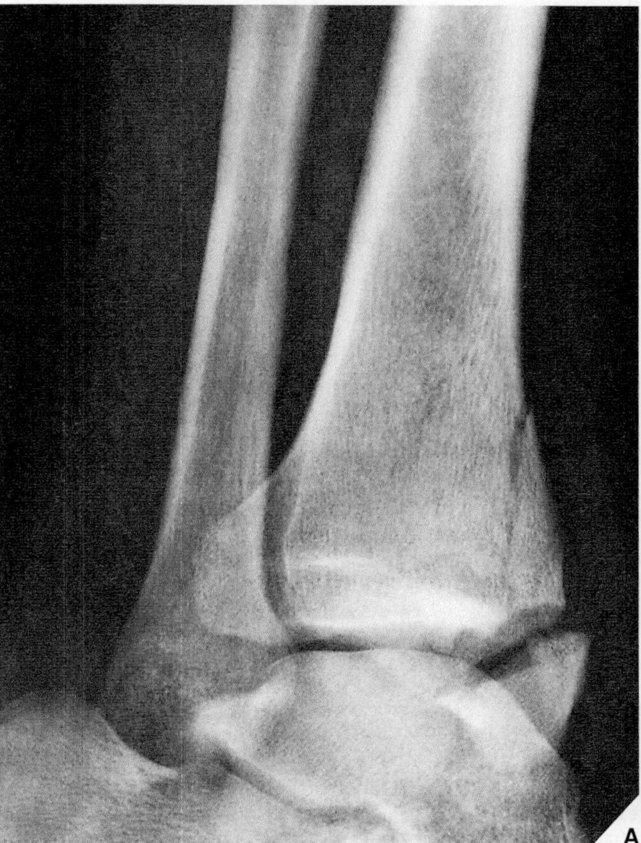

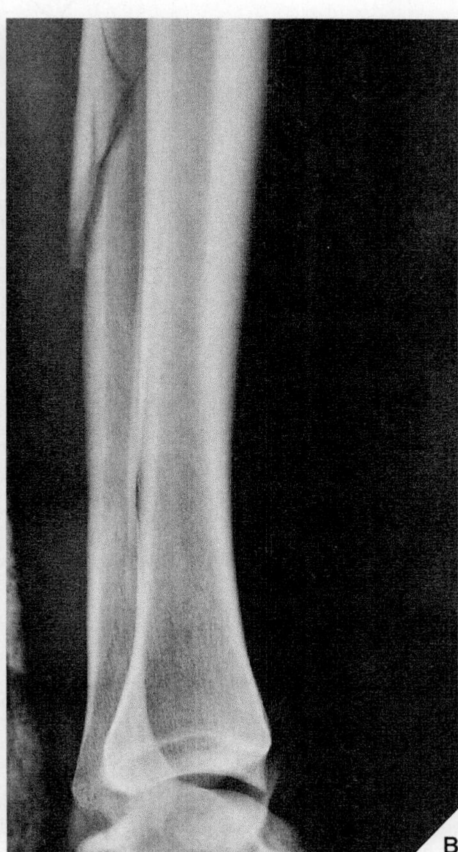

FIGURE 10.65 Maisonneuve fracture. A 22-year-old man injured his right ankle in a skiing accident. **(A)** Oblique radiograph of the ankle shows a comminuted fracture of the medial malleolus, with extension into the anterior lip of the tibia. **(B)** On the lateral view, a comminuted fracture of the fibula is apparent.

TABLE 10.4 Lauge-Hansen Classification of Ankle Injuries

Injury	Stage	Description
Pronation—Abduction Injuries		
	Stage I	Rupture of the deltoid ligament or transverse fracture of the medial malleolus
	Stage II	Disruption of the distal anterior and posterior tibiofibular ligaments
	Stage III	Oblique fracture of the fibula at the level of the joint[a] (best seen on the anteroposterior projection)
Pronation—Lateral (External) Rotation Injuries		
	Stage I	Rupture of the deltoid ligament or transverse fracture of the medial malleolus
	Stage II	Disruption of the anterior tibiofibular ligament and interosseous membrane
	Stage III	Fracture of the fibula usually 6 cm or more above the level of the joint[a]
	Stage IV	Chip fracture of the posterior tibia or rupture of the posterior tibiofibular ligament
Supination—Adduction Injuries		
	Stage I	Injury to the lateral collateral ligament or transverse fracture of the lateral malleolus below the level of the joint[a]
	Stage II	Steep oblique fracture of the medial malleolus
Supination—Lateral (External) Rotation Injuries		
	Stage I	Disruption of the anterior tibiofibular ligament
	Stage II	Spiral fracture of the distal fibula near the joint[a] (best seen on the lateral projection)
	Stage III	Rupture of the posterior tibiofibular ligament
	Stage IV	Transverse fracture of the medial malleolus

[a]The appearance of the fibular fracture is the key to determining the mechanism of injury. Reproduced with permission from Lauge-Hansen N. Fractures of the ankle. II. Combined experimental-surgical and experimental-roentgenologic investigations. *Arch Surg* 1950;60(5):957–985. Copyright © 1950 American Medical Association. All rights reserved.

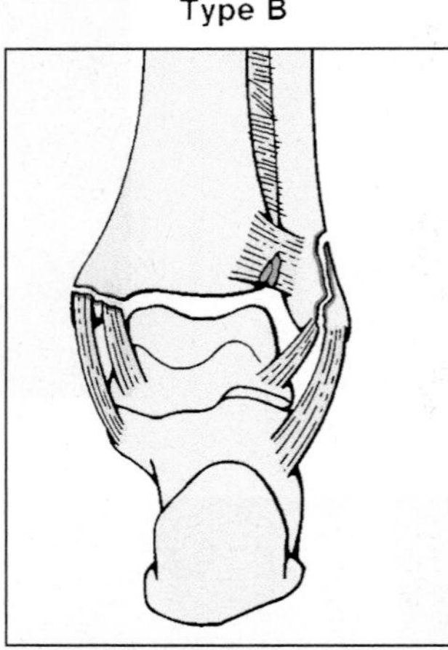

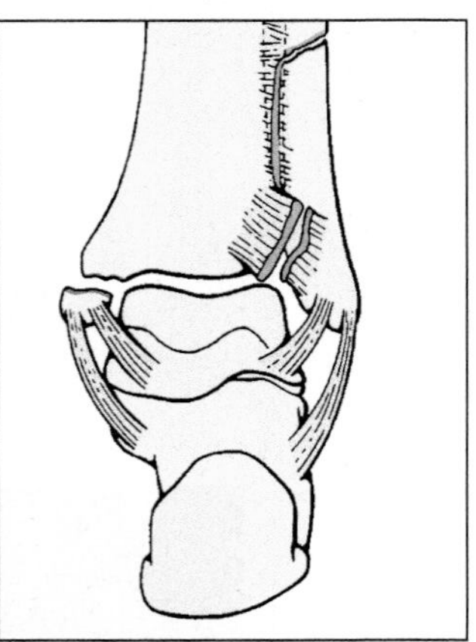

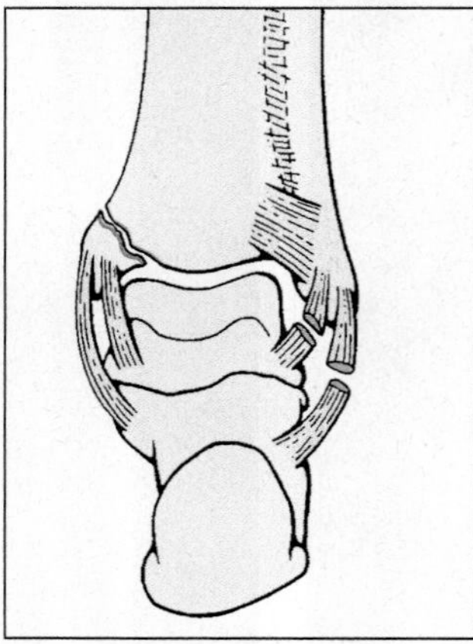

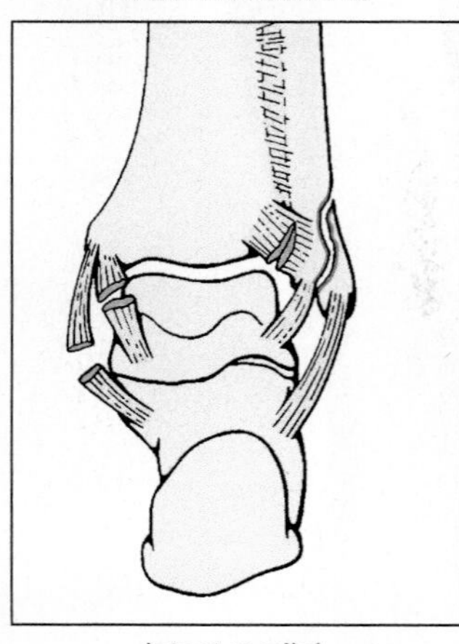

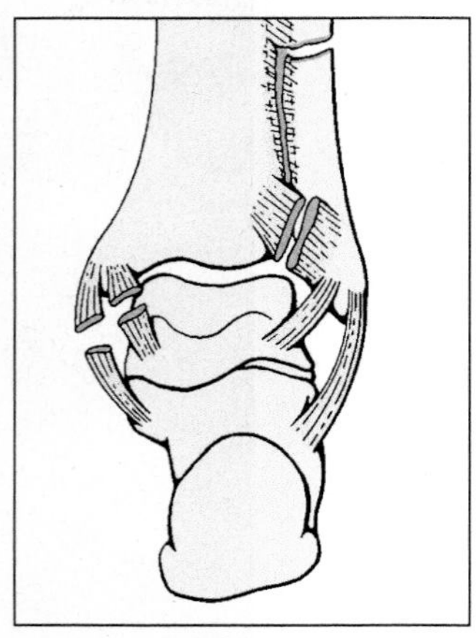

FIGURE 10.66 Weber classification. The Weber classification of injuries to the structures about the ankle joint is based on the level at which fibular fracture occurs as well as the presence or absence of an associated fracture of the medial malleolus. Disruption of the medial and lateral ligament complexes can be deduced from the level of the fibular fracture as well as that of the medial malleolar fracture. (Modified from Weber BG. *Die Verletzungen des Oberen Sprunggelenkes*. Stuttgart: Verlag Hans Huber; 1972. By courtesy of Hogrefe AG Bern.)

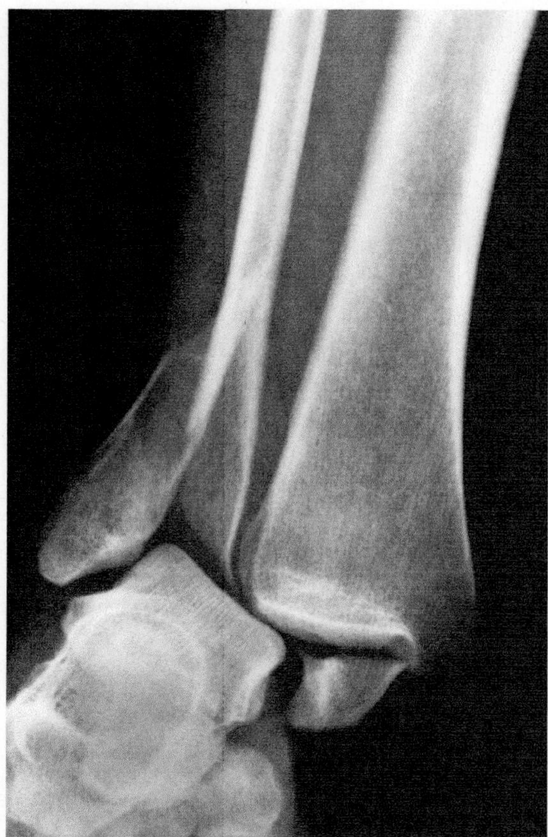

FIGURE 10.67 Weber type B fracture. A 24-year-old woman injured her right ankle in a skiing accident. Anteroposterior radiograph of the ankle demonstrates a spiral fracture of the fibula beginning at the level of the tibiofibular syndesmosis with consequent tear of the inferoposterior portion of the syndesmotic complex; the interosseous membrane is intact. The site of the fracture of the medial malleolus suggests that the deltoid ligament may be intact. According to the Weber classification, this is a type B fracture.

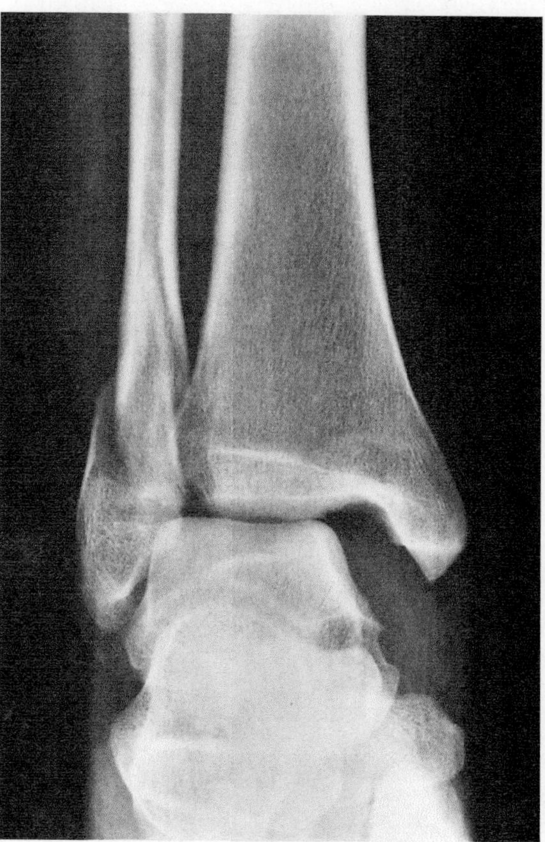

FIGURE 10.68 Weber type C fracture. A 32-year-old woman stepped into a pothole and injured her right ankle. Anteroposterior view of the ankle demonstrates a fracture of the fibula above the level of the ankle joint, indicating disruption of the interosseous membrane. The intact medial malleolus indicates a tear of the deltoid ligament. This type of fracture is classified as a Weber type C. The risk of ankle mortise instability due to disruption of the medial and lateral ligament complexes gives this type of injury a worse prognosis than type A or B.

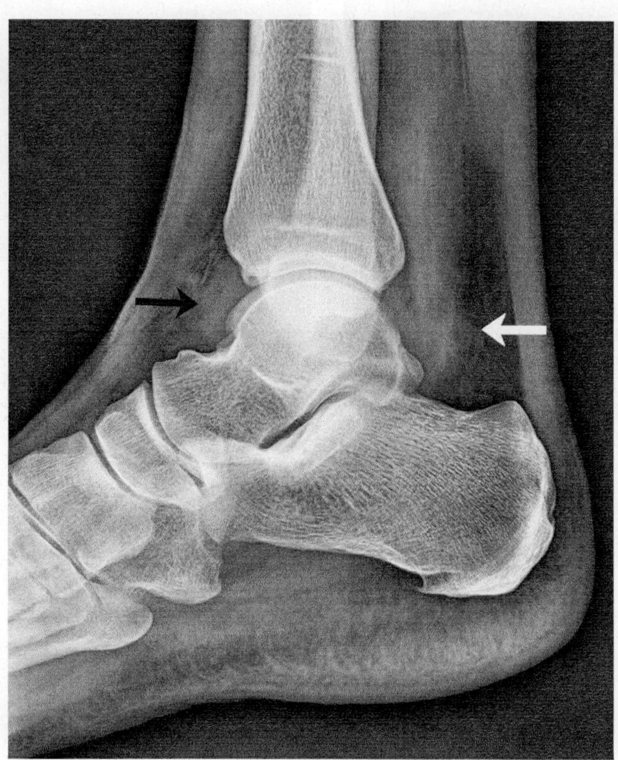

FIGURE 10.69 Posttraumatic ankle joint effusion. On the lateral radiograph of the ankle, the joint effusion is manifested by focal increased density anteriorly *(black arrow)* and encroachment of Kager triangle posteriorly *(white arrow)*.

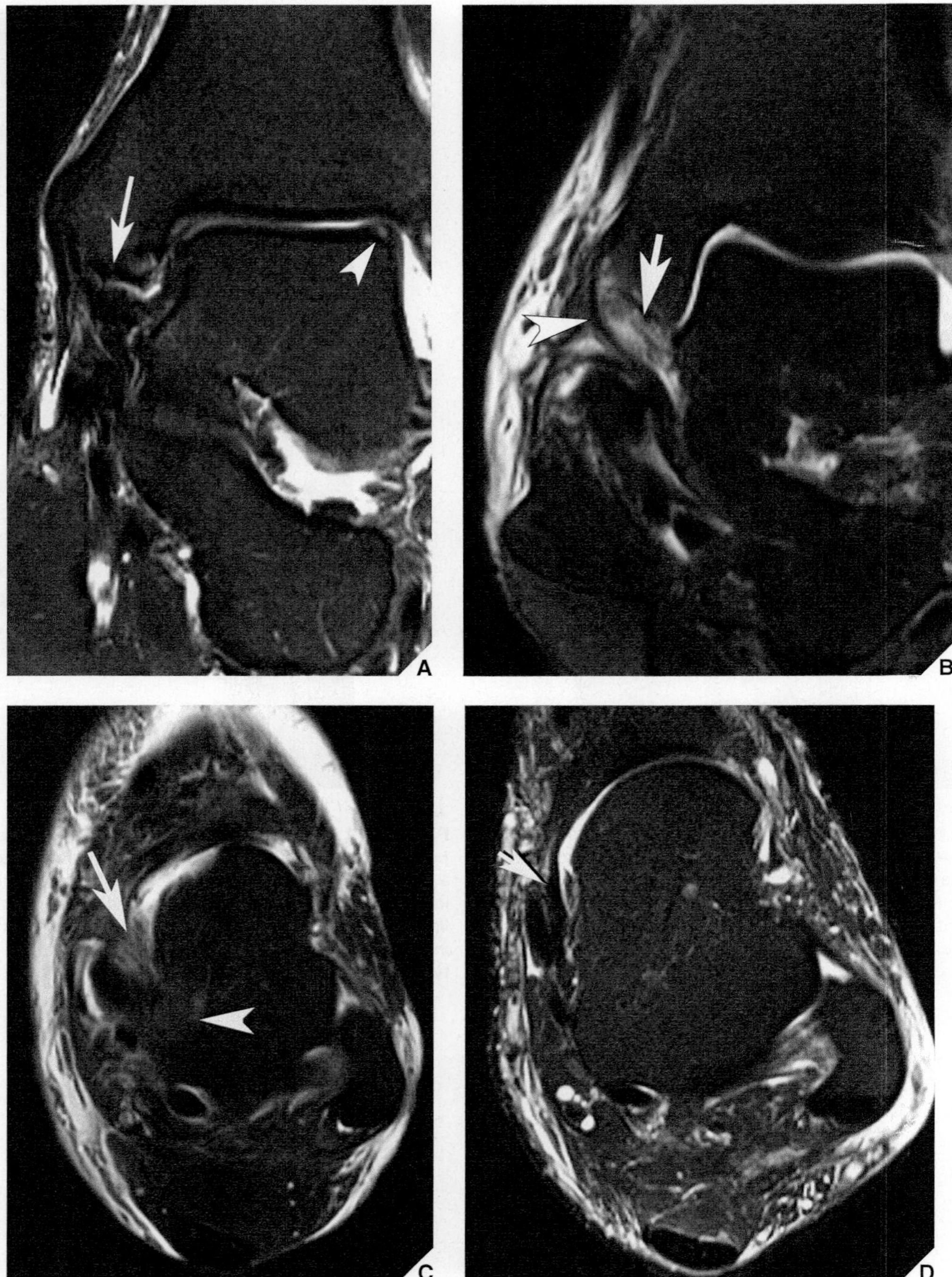

FIGURE 10.70 **MRI of the tear of the deltoid ligament. (A)** Coronal T2-weighted MR image demonstrates a tear of the tibial insertion of the deltoid ligament *(white arrow)*. Note the chondral lesion of the lateral talar dome *(white arrowhead)*. **(B)** T2-weighted MR image in another patient shows a partial tear of the deep fibers of the deltoid ligament *(arrow)* with high–signal intensity hemorrhage in the tibiotalar ligament. The tibiocalcaneal ligament is intact *(arrowhead)*. **(C)** Axial T2-weighted MR image demonstrates the tear of the deep fibers of the deltoid ligament *(arrow)*. There is bone contusion of the medial aspect of the talus *(arrowhead)*. **(D)** Axial T2-weighted MR image of a normal deltoid ligament that demonstrates low signal intensity of its intact fibers *(arrow)* is shown for comparison.

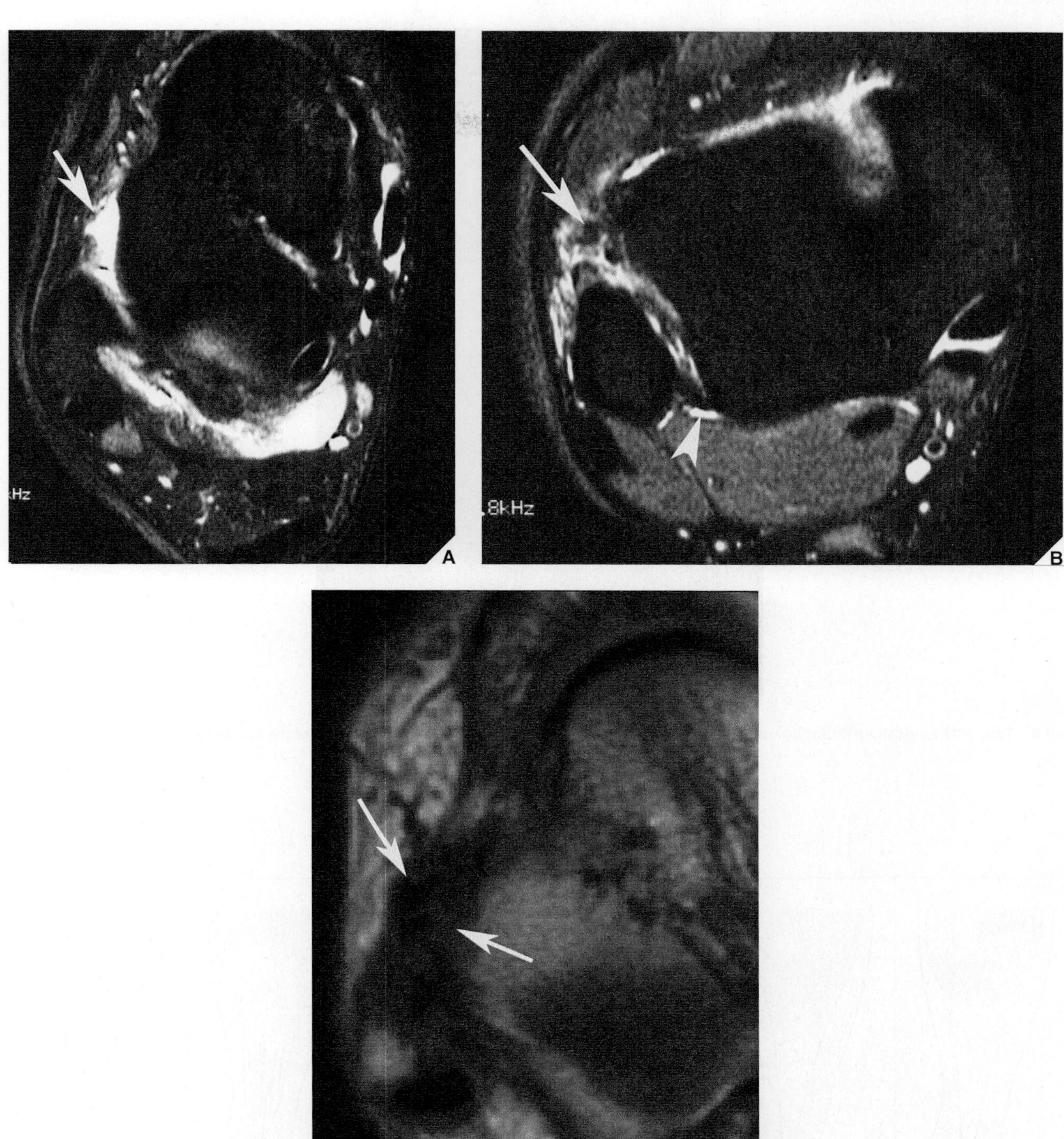

FIGURE 10.71 **MRI of the tear of the anterior talofibular ligament.** **(A)** Axial T2-weighted MRI shows disruption of the anterior talofibular ligament resulting in its replacement by high–signal intensity fluid *(arrow)*. **(B)** Axial T2-weighted MRI of the same patient at the level of the distal tibiofibular syndesmosis shows a tear of the anterior tibiofibular ligament *(arrow)*. The posterior tibiofibular ligament is normal *(arrowhead)*. **(C)** Axial T2-weighted MRI shows marked thickening of the anterior talofibular ligament *(arrows)* occupying the space between the lateral malleolus and the talus (lateral gutter). The thickening is in part due to ligamentous scarring and in part due to synovial proliferation (Wolin lesion) secondary to repetitive injuries to the anterior talofibular ligament. This is known as *anterolateral impingement syndrome* (see Fig. 10.123).

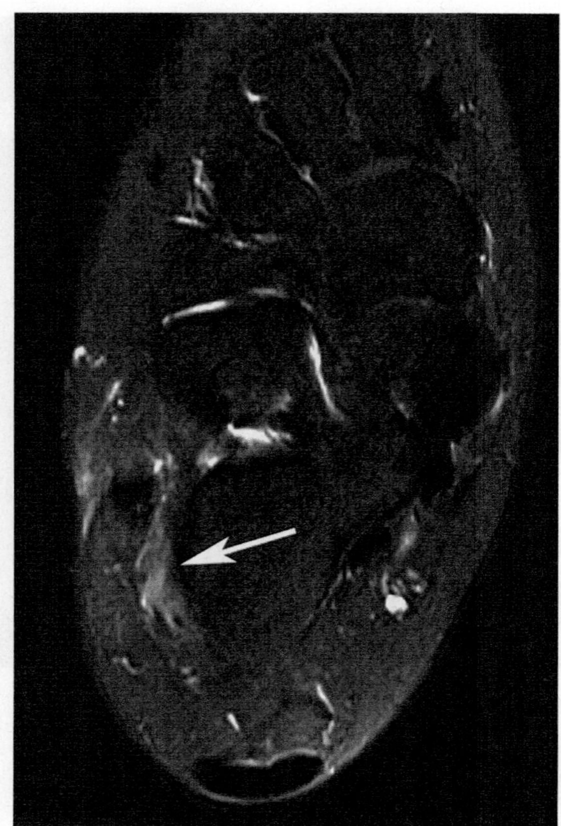

FIGURE 10.72 **Tear of the calcaneofibular ligament.** T2-weighted axial MR image demonstrates an acute tear of the calcaneofibular ligament *(arrow)*.

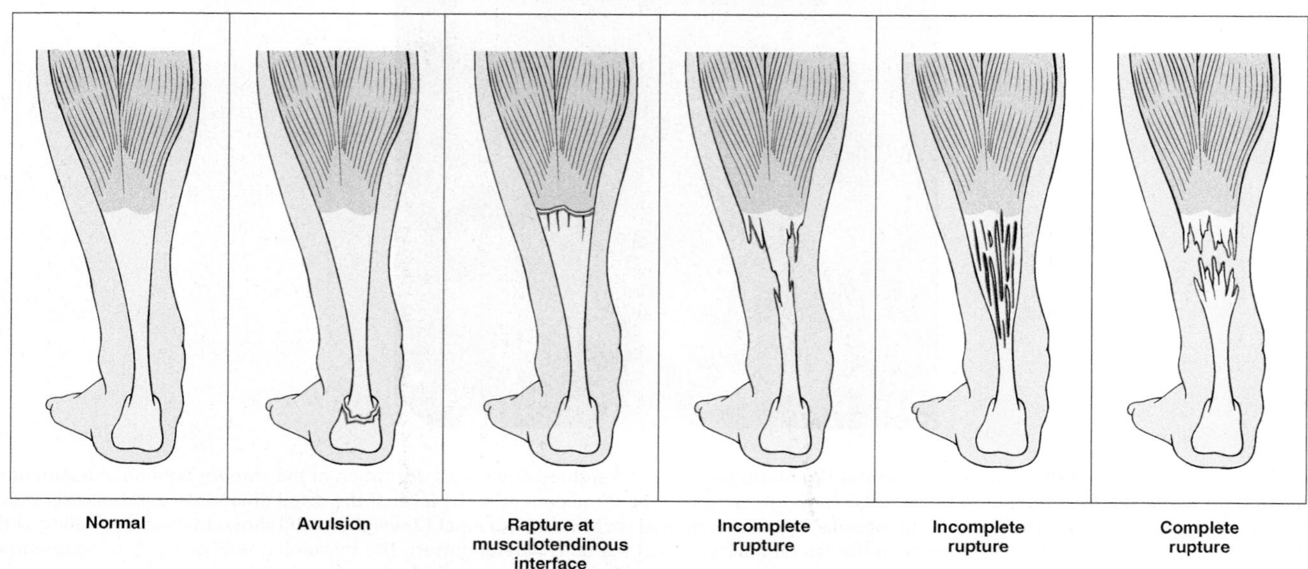

FIGURE 10.73 **Achilles tendon injury.** Schematic representation of various types of Achilles tendon injury.

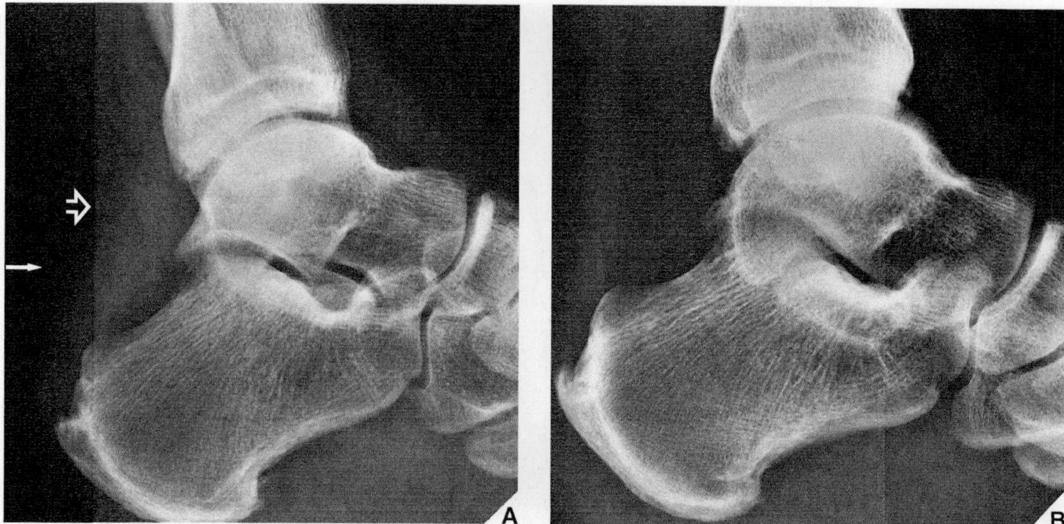

FIGURE 10.74 **Tear of the Achilles tendon.** A 54-year-old man stumbled into a pothole. Physical examination revealed severe tenderness at the insertion of the Achilles tendon and marked limitation of plantar flexion. **(A)** Lateral radiograph shows a lack of definition of the tendon and a lumpy soft-tissue mass *(arrow)* as well as faint calcifications within injured tendon *(open arrow)*. **(B)** The other, normal ankle is shown for comparison.

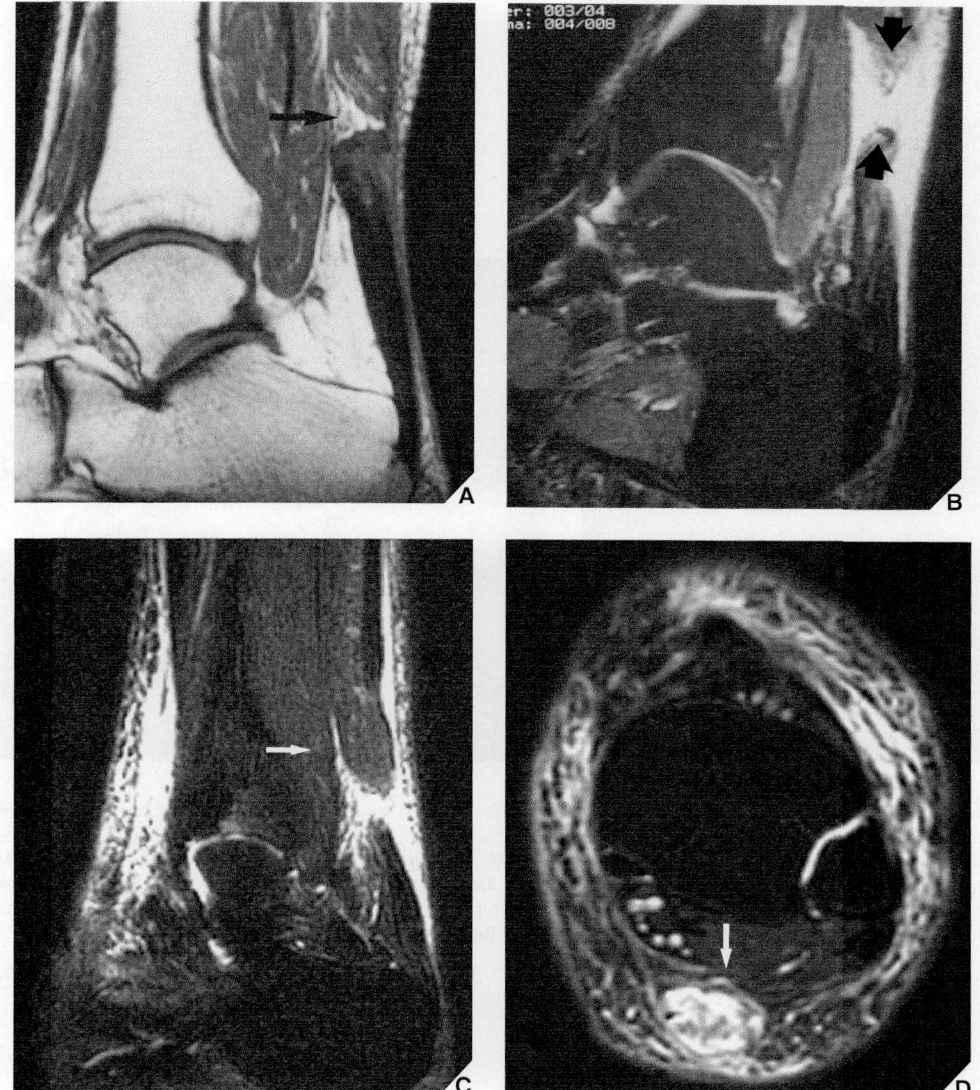

FIGURE 10.75 **MRI of the Achilles tendon tear.** **(A)** Sagittal T1-weighted MRI shows a complete rupture of the Achilles tendon near the musculotendinous junction *(arrow)*. **(B)** In another patient, a complete Achilles tendon tear with a large 3-cm gap *(arrows)* is seen on this sagittal STIR MR image. There is massive edema and hemorrhage subcutaneously and deep to the Achilles tendon. Yet, in another patient, sagittal inversion recovery **(C)** and axial T2-weighted fat-suppressed **(D)** MR images show a complete full-thickness tear of the Achilles tendon *(arrows)*. (**A**, Reprinted with permission from Deutsch AL, Mink JH, Kerr R, eds. *MRI of the foot and ankle*. New York: Raven Press; 1992.)

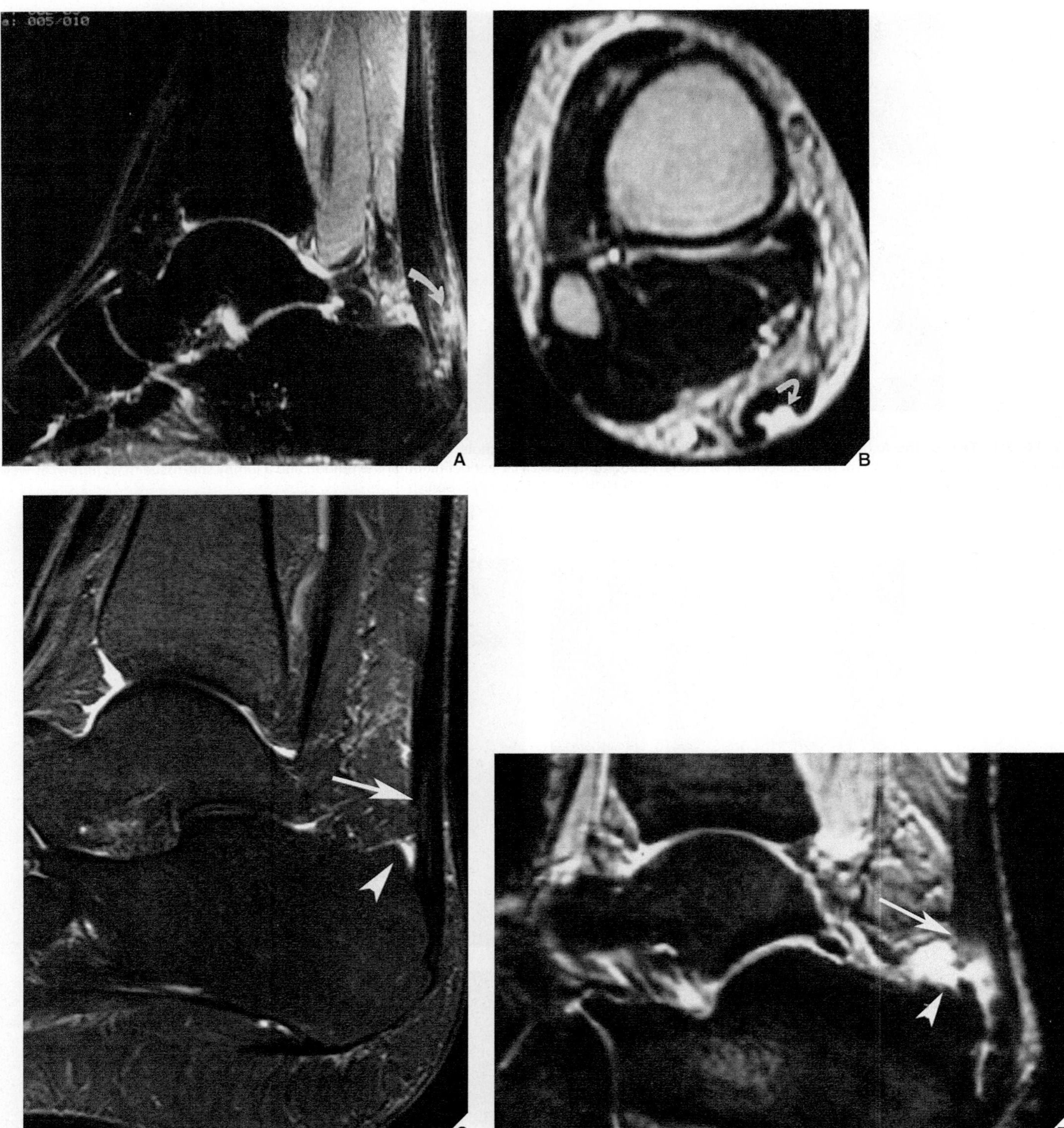

FIGURE 10.76 MRI of the Achilles tendon tear. **(A)** Sagittal STIR and **(B)** axial T2-weighted MR images show a focus of high signal intensity within the posterior part of the Achilles tendon *(curved arrows)*, indicating an acute partial tear. Edema is present within the fat pad and in the subcutaneous tissue. Note the thickening of the Achilles tendon proximal to the tear indicating chronic tendinosis. **(C)** Sagittal T2-weighted MR image in another patient demonstrates thickening of the distal Achilles tendon with linear areas of increased signal intensity *(arrow)* consistent with insertional tendinosis. Note the presence of mild retrocalcaneal bursitis *(arrowhead)*. **(D)** Sagittal T2-weighted MR image in another patient shows insertional tendinosis of the Achilles tendon with partial tear *(arrow)* and retrocalcaneal bursitis *(arrowhead)*. (**A** and **B**, Reprinted with permission from Deutsch AL, Mink JH, Kerr R, eds. *MRI of the foot and ankle*. New York: Raven Press; 1992.)

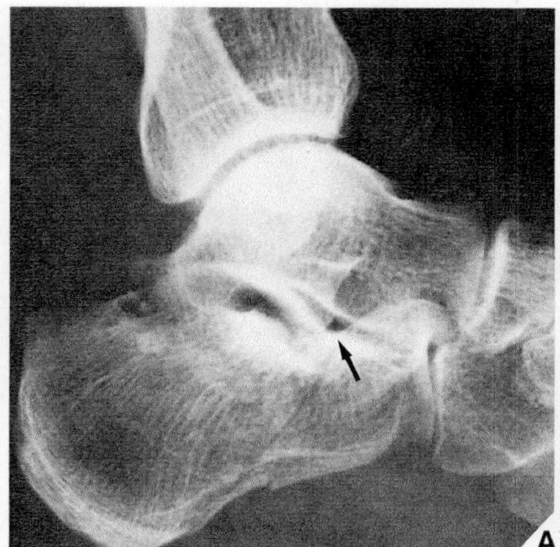
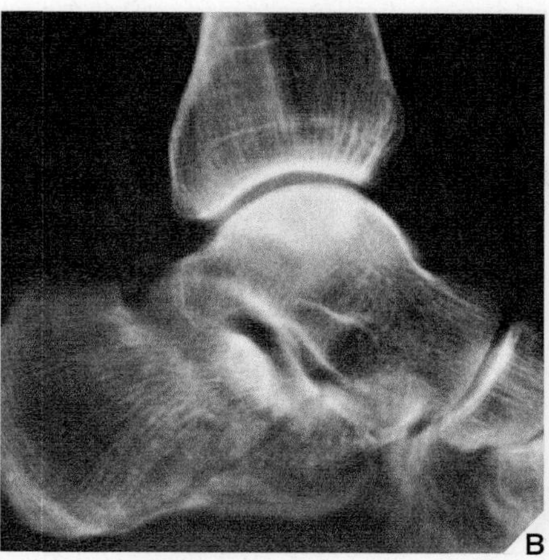
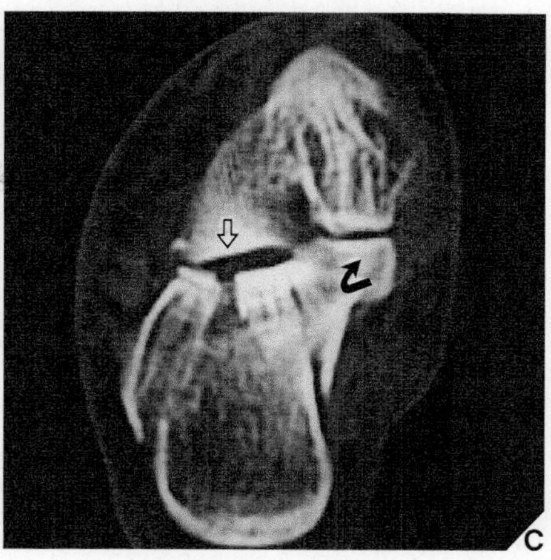

FIGURE 10.77 **Fracture of the calcaneus.** A 54-year-old man fell from a scaffold and injured his left foot. **(A)** Lateral radiograph shows a comminuted fracture of the calcaneus. There is a suggestion of extension of the fracture line into the subtalar joint *(arrow)*. **(B)** Tomographic examination in the lateral projection confirms intraarticular extension of the fracture line. The amount of depression of the articular surface, however, cannot be definitely assessed. **(C)** CT section precisely demonstrates the position of the comminuted fragments and depression at the posterior facet of the subtalar joint *(open arrow)*. It also shows that the middle facet is intact *(curved arrow)*, important information that the conventional and tomographic studies could not provide.

FIGURE 10.78 **CT of the calcaneus fracture.** A 34-year-old man sustained a comminuted fracture of the right calcaneus. **(A)** Coronal CT section shows extension of the fracture line to the subtalar joint. **(B)** Sagittal reformatted CT image shows, in addition, a fracture of the anterior process of the calcaneus with extension into the anterior facet of subtalar joint *(arrow)*.

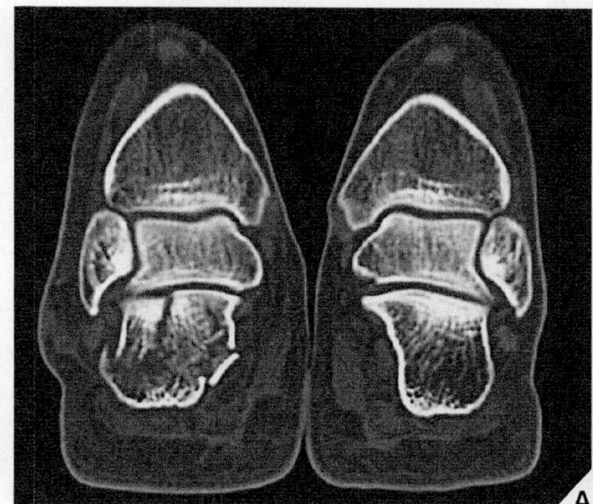
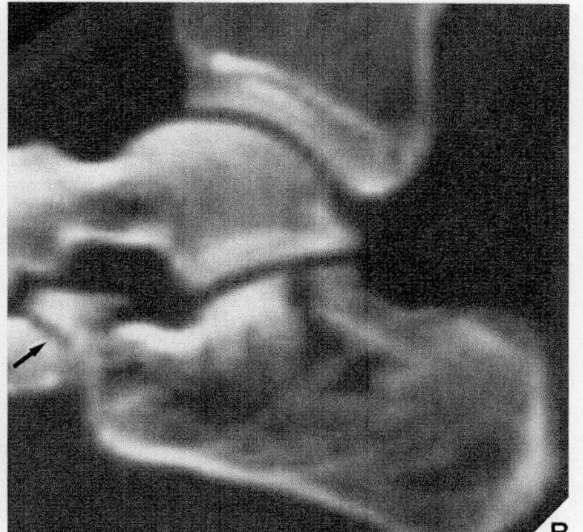

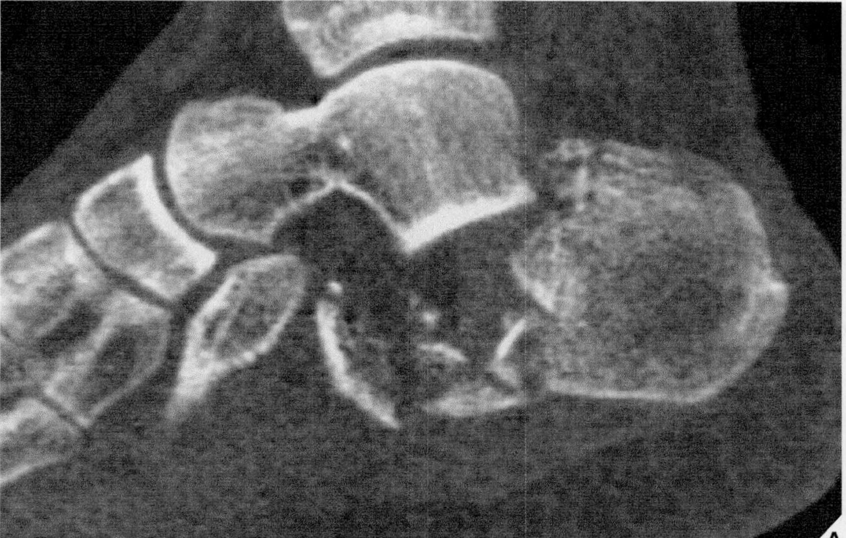
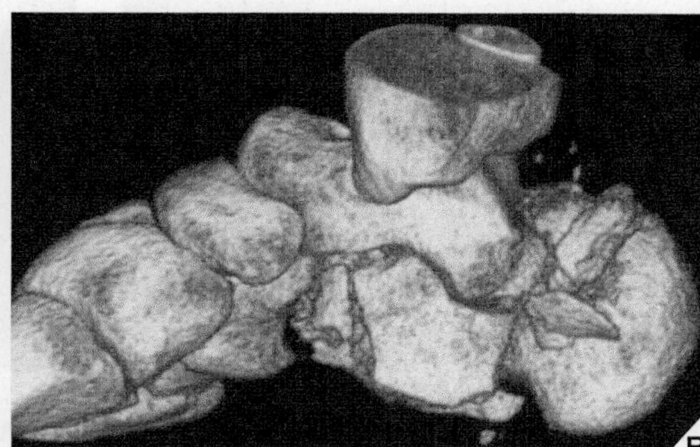
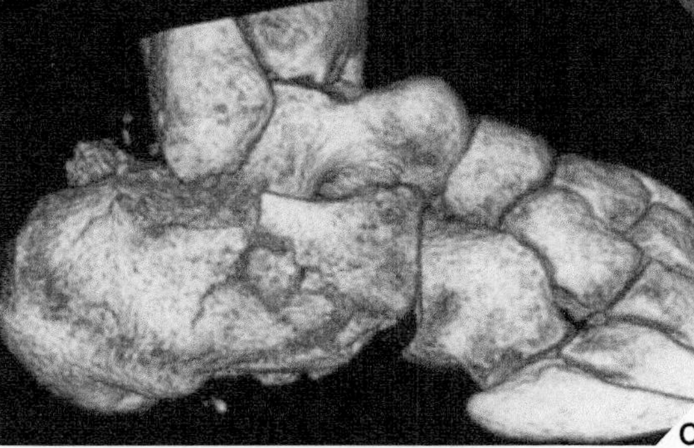

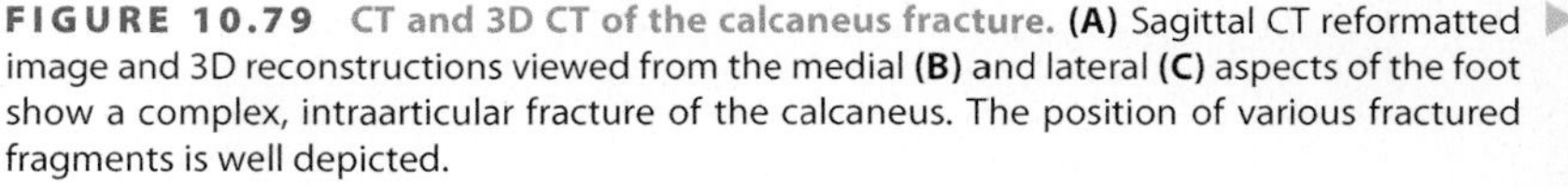

FIGURE 10.79 **CT and 3D CT of the calcaneus fracture.** **(A)** Sagittal CT reformatted image and 3D reconstructions viewed from the medial **(B)** and lateral **(C)** aspects of the foot show a complex, intraarticular fracture of the calcaneus. The position of various fractured fragments is well depicted.

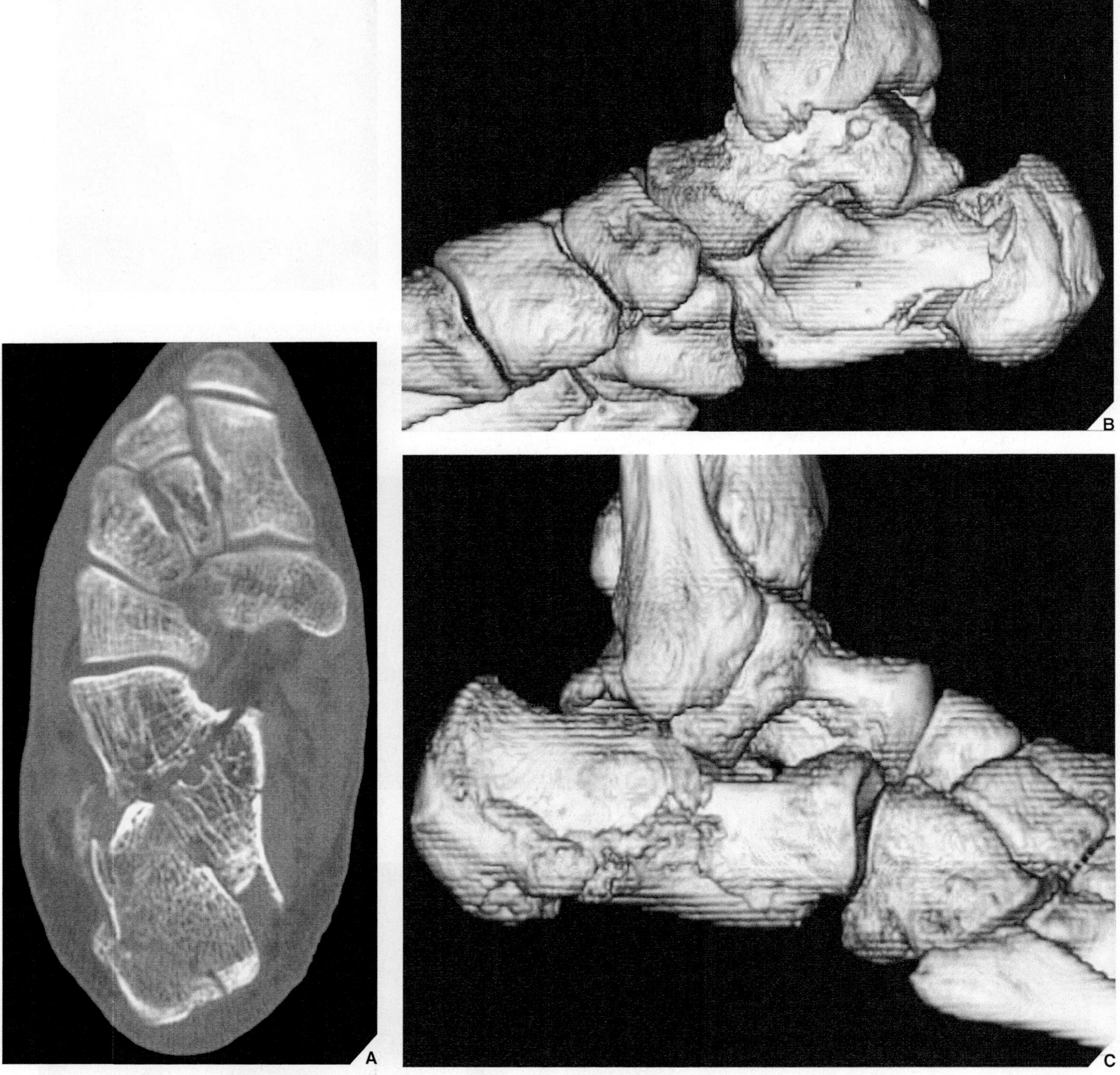

FIGURE 10.80 CT and 3D CT of the calcaneus fracture. **(A)** Axial CT image shows a comminuted fracture of the calcaneus. 3D reconstructed CT images of the foot viewed from the medial **(B)** and lateral **(C)** aspects show the various fracture lines and intraarticular extension to the better advantage.

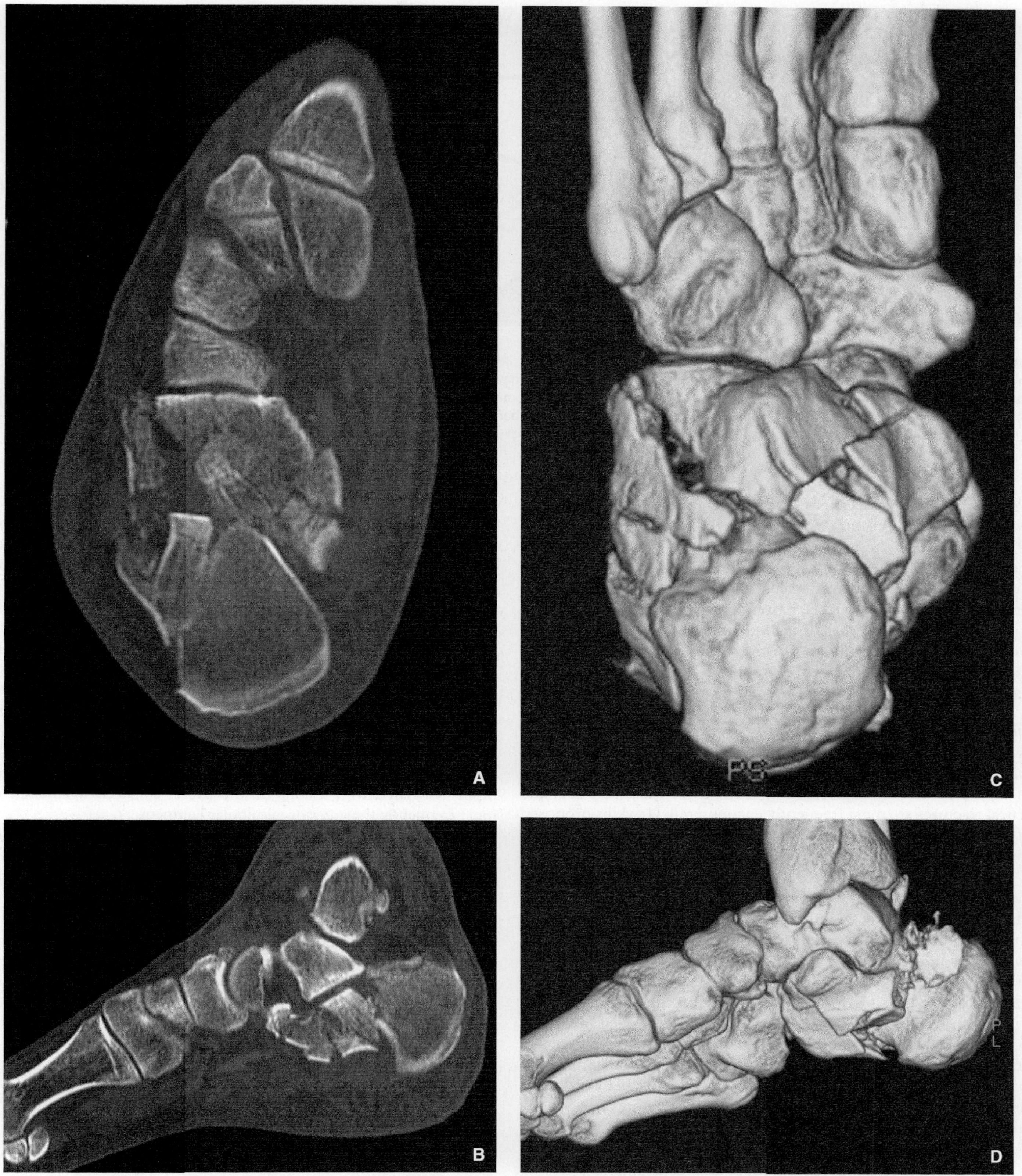

FIGURE 10.81 CT and 3D CT of the calcaneus fracture. **(A)** Axial (short axis) CT, **(B)** sagittal reformatted CT image, and **(C,D)** 3D reconstructed CT images of the foot show markedly comminuted intraarticular fracture of the calcaneus.

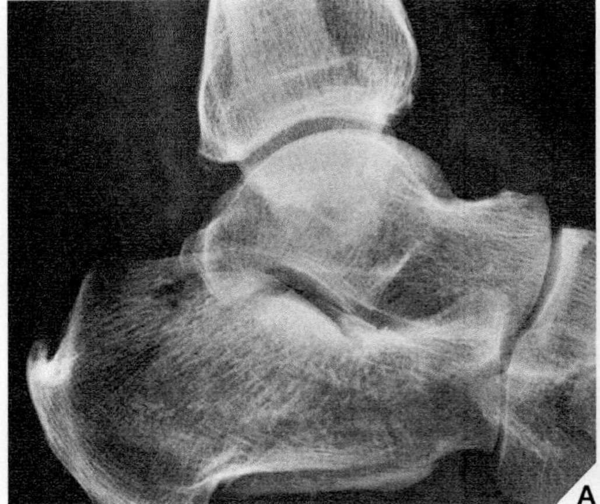

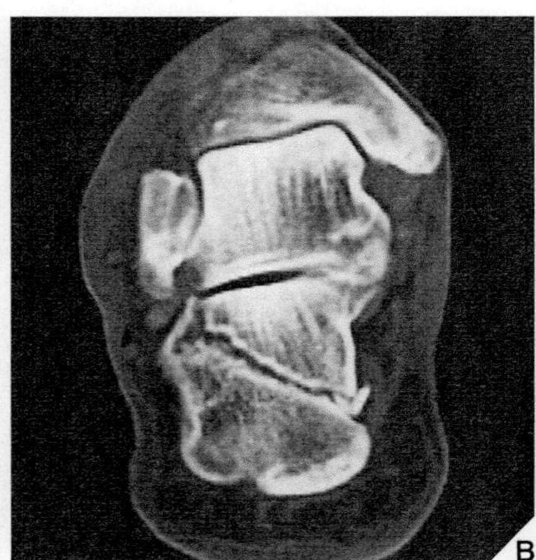

FIGURE 10.82 Fractures of the calcaneus and the thoracic vertebra. A 48-year-old man jumped from a second-floor window. **(A)** Lateral radiograph of the ankle demonstrates a comminuted fracture of the calcaneus. **(B)** Coronal CT section demonstrates the position of multiple, small, comminuted fragments and involvement of the sustentaculum tali. **(C)** Lateral radiograph of the thoracolumbar spine shows compression fracture of the T12 vertebral body.

Stress fractures of the calcaneus occur in joggers and runners but do not spare the older population when bones are weakened by osteoporosis (Fig. 10.84). Like stress fractures in long bones, these fractures are not immediately evident but typically become obvious approximately 10 to 14 days after the precipitating incident. They can be recognized on radiographs by a band of sclerosis, representing formation of endosteal callus. The fracture line is usually oriented either vertically or parallel to the posterior contour of the bone. If stress fractures are suspected but radiographs are normal, a bone scan may validate the diagnosis, although MRI examination is preferred (Fig. 10.85).

Fractures of the Talus

Fractures of the talus are the second most common tarsal bone fractures, after the calcaneus. Fracture may involve the head, neck, body, or posterior process. The neck of the talus is the most vulnerable site, and the vertical fractures are most frequently encountered. Hawkins proposed three types of vertical fractures of the neck of the talus (Fig. 10.86). His classification, based on the damage to the blood supply of the talus, serves as a guide to prognosis for healing of the fracture, incidence of osteonecrosis, and indication for open reduction. Canale and Kelly modified this classification to include a fourth, rare type of a displaced fracture with subtalar or tibiotalar dislocation and subluxation or dislocation in the talonavicular joint.

Whether vertical or comminuted, fractures of the talus most often result from forced dorsiflexion of the foot, as may occur in automobile accidents. Accompanying dislocation in the subtalar and talonavicular joints is common. Talar fractures are usually obvious on the standard radiographic projections, although CT is usually required for demonstration and quantification of displacement (Figs. 10.87 and 10.88). MRI may be of value for detecting various complications such as avascular necrosis in cases of talar neck fracture (Fig. 10.89).

The knowledge of the osseous anatomy of the posterior talus (Fig. 10.90) is crucial for diagnosis of various traumatic abnormalities of this part of the bone. There are specific fractures of the posterior aspect of the talus that involve the posterolateral process (known as *Shepherd fracture*) (Fig. 10.91) and the posteromedial process (known as *Cedell fracture*) (Fig. 10.92). An isolated fracture of the lateral process of the talus can be seen in cases of sudden vertical lateral loading forces applied to the ankle and hindfoot. This type of injury is known as the *snowboarder's fracture* (Fig. 10.93; see also Fig. 4.152).

Osteochondritis Dissecans of the Talus

Osteochondritis dissecans (OCD) of the talus is a relatively common lesion involving the talar dome. Originally, it was thought that OCD lesions were the result of ischemic necrosis of the subchondral bone leading to separation/dissection of a fragment of bone and cartilage. The current concept is that the vast majority of these lesions are related to a traumatic event because there is a history of injury in over 80% of the cases. The possibility of a primary ischemic event has not been completely excluded because no history of trauma is elicited in some patients. Furthermore, this entity can be familial. Multiple lesions can occur in the same patient and identical talar lesions in medial location have been described in identical twins, suggesting a congenital predisposition to cartilage and underlying bone damage.

OCD lesions may be located in the anterolateral or in the posteromedial aspect of the talar dome. Anterolateral lesions occur as a result of an inversion and dorsiflexion injury. Posteromedial lesions are related to an inversion injury with plantar flexion and external rotation (Fig. 10.94). Because of the common mechanism of inversion injury, OCD lesions are often associated with lesions of the lateral collateral ligament complex, most frequently the anterior talofibular ligament.

Although CT is effective in demonstrating OCD of the talus (Figs. 10.95 and 10.96A), MRI is widely used for the diagnosis and staging of OCD lesions of this bone (Fig. 10.96B,C). MRI can be used to assess not only the presence of the lesion but also its size, location, stability, and viability. The presence of fluid in the interface between the osteochondral fragment and the donor site in stage III lesions is considered a sign of instability, which may require surgical stabilization. The presence of cyst formation indicates chronicity of the lesion. Decreased signal intensity of the osseous fragment in all pulse sequences is an indicator of nonviable bone.

OCD lesions of the talus can be staged according to the Berndt and Harty classification (Fig. 10.97):

Stage I: subchondral lesion with no involvement of the subchondral bone plate or articular cartilage
Stage II: partial osteochondral lesion with one side of the lesion remaining attached to the adjacent bone
Stage III: completely separated osteochondral lesion with the fragment in situ
Stage IV: completely separated osteochondral lesion with a displaced fragment.

Anderson and associates developed a classification of OCD lesions similar to the Berndt and Harty classification but based on the MRI findings (Fig. 10.98).

Navicular Fractures

Navicular fractures are rare and are usually sustained along with fractures of other bones of the foot. Occasionally, navicular fracture may be caused by a fall from a height. Sangeorzan and colleagues classified navicular fractures into three types based on the orientation of the fracture line and the

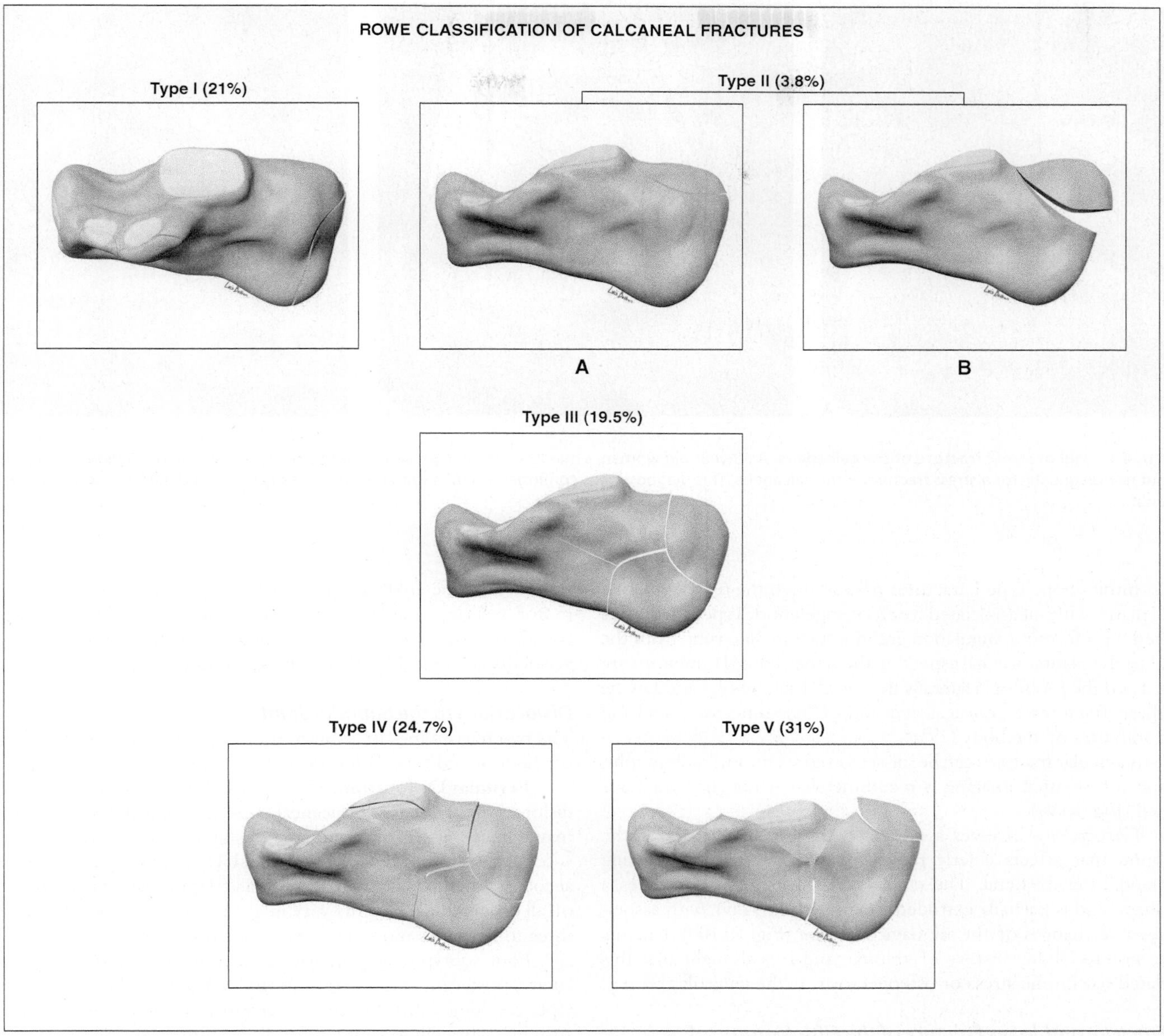

ROWE CLASSIFICATION OF CALCANEAL FRACTURES

Type I (21%)

Type II (3.8%)

A

B

Type III (19.5%)

Type IV (24.7%)

Type V (31%)

FIGURE 10.83 The Rowe classification of calcaneal fractures. Type I (21%)—fractures of the tuberosity, sustentaculum tali, or anterior process; type II (3.8%)—beak fractures **(A)** and avulsion fractures of the Achilles tendon insertion **(B)**; type III (19.5%)—oblique fractures not extending into the subtalar joint; type IV (24.7%)—fractures involving the subtalar joint; and type V (31%)—fractures with central depression and varying degrees of comminution.

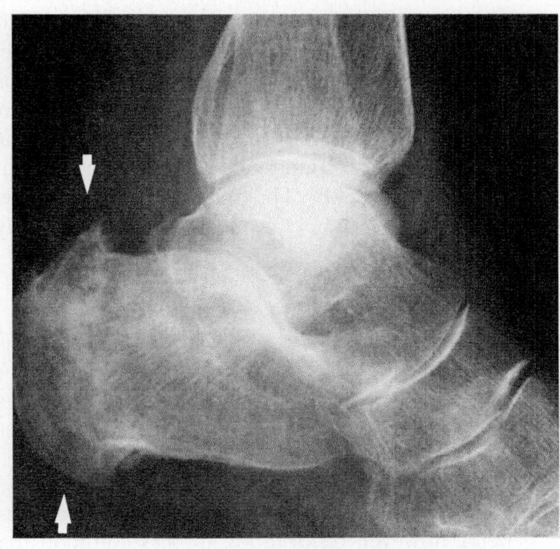

FIGURE 10.84 Stress fracture of the calcaneus. A 75-year-old woman reported pain in the left heel; she had no history of trauma. She walked about a mile to the supermarket every day. Lateral radiograph of the right ankle shows a typical stress fracture of the os calcis *(arrows)*.

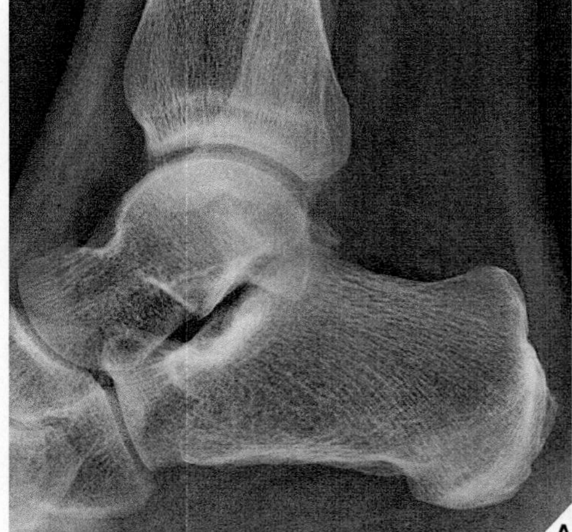

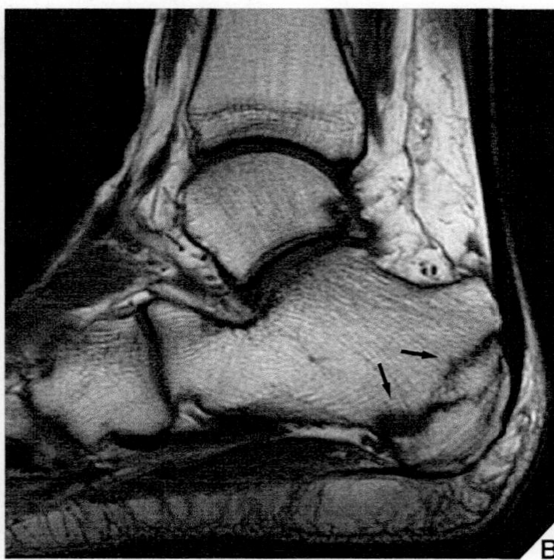

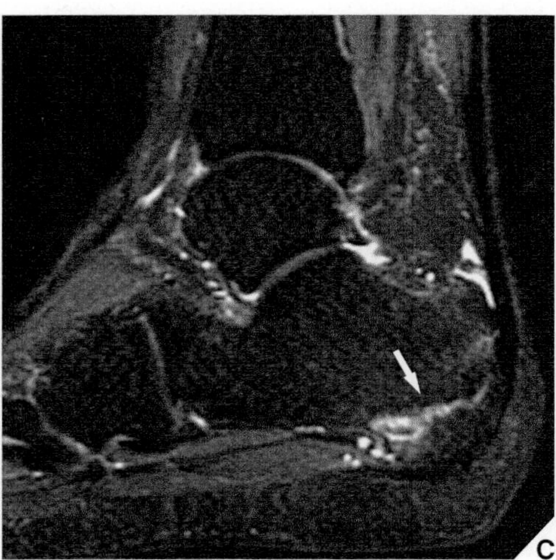

FIGURE 10.85 MRI of stress fracture of the calcaneus. A 30-year-old woman, a marathon runner, presented with a heel pain. **(A)** Lateral radiograph of the ankle was suspicious but not diagnostic for a stress fracture of the calcaneus. This diagnosis was confirmed on **(B)** sagittal proton density–weighted and **(C)** sagittal T2-weighted MR images *(arrows)*.

degree of comminution. Type I fractures pass through the navicular bone in a coronal plane, without associated forefoot angulation. Type II fractures are associated with forefoot angulation and the fracture line runs from the dorsolateral to the plantar-medial aspect of the bone. Type III fractures are comminuted and the forefoot is laterally displaced. Eichenholtz and Levine classified these fractures as cortical avulsion (47%), tuberosity avulsion (24%), and fractures of the body (29%).

Because navicular fractures can be missed on conventional radiography, CT including reformatted imaging is recommended when such fractures are suspected (Fig. 10.99).

Mueller-Weis syndrome involves a specific compression fracture of the navicular bone that affects elderly patients, more frequently occurring in females and often bilateral. The collapsed navicular bone acquires a triangular shape and is partially extruded superiorly (dorsally), with associated degenerative changes of the talonavicular joint (Fig. 10.100). Patients do not give nor recall any history of trauma, and it is thought that this lesion is related to chronic stress or osteonecrosis of the navicular bone.

Avulsion Fracture and Jones Fracture of the Fifth Metatarsal

Avulsion fracture of the base of the fifth metatarsal results from inversion stress placed on the peroneus brevis tendon, which is attached to the fifth metatarsal (Figs. 10.101 and 10.102). From a historical point of view, however, the term *Jones fracture* that occasionally is given for this type of fracture is used incorrectly because the original fracture described by Robert Jones in 1902 was extraarticular, at the site of approximately three fourths of 1 inch from the base of the fifth metatarsal (Fig. 10.103). The distinction between a "true" Jones fracture and an avulsion fracture of the base of the fifth metatarsal is also of prognostic value: avulsion fractures generally heal quickly, whereas fractures through the proximal metatarsal shaft, because of poor blood supply, have a significant incidence of delayed union and fibrous union. In children, it is important not to confuse this fracture with the normal (and frequently present) secondary ossification center of the base of the fifth metatarsal (see Fig. 4.54B). The fracture line is transversely oriented, whereas the gap separating the ossification center from the fifth metatarsal is oblique.

Complications

The most common complications of ankle and foot fractures are nonunion and posttraumatic arthritis. Although conventional radiography can usually demonstrate the features of these complications, CT is the better technique for delineating their details.

Dislocations in the Foot

The most common dislocation in the foot occurs in the tarsometatarsal (Lisfranc) joint. In general, however, dislocations are less common than fractures of the ankle and foot. They are occasionally seen as a result of motor vehicle or aircraft accidents, as in dislocation of the talus—the so-called *aviator's astragalus*. According to Shelton and Pedowitz, aircraft accidents account for 43% of all talar injuries.

Dislocations in the Subtalar Joint

The two major types of subtalar joint dislocations are peritalar dislocation of the foot and total dislocation of the talus.

Peritalar Dislocation. This type of abnormality involves simultaneous dislocations in the talocalcaneal and talonavicular joints with normal maintenance of the tibiotalar relationship. Often referred to as subtalar or subastragalar dislocation, peritalar dislocation, as Pennal has pointed out, accounts for approximately 15% of all talar injuries and approximately 1% of all dislocations. Patients vary in age from 10 to older than 60 years, but three to ten times more men than women sustain these injuries.

Four subtypes of peritalar dislocation have been identified: medial, lateral, posterior, and anterior. *Medial dislocation* is the most common subtype, resulting from a violent inversion force acting as a fulcrum for the sustentaculum tali to cause initial dislocation of the talonavicular joint, together with rotary subluxation of the talocalcaneal joint. A greater force may cause complete dislocation. The dorsoplantar (anteroposterior) view of the foot is recommended to demonstrate this abnormality. The radiographs should be scrutinized carefully for associated fractures, particularly of both malleoli, the articular margin of the talus, and the navicular and fifth metatarsal bones.

Lateral dislocation is the next most common subtype, accounting for approximately 20% of all peritalar dislocations. At the time of injury, the foot is everted and, with the anterior calcaneal process acting as a fulcrum, the head of the talus is forced out of the talonavicular joint; the calcaneus is dislocated laterally. As in medial dislocation, the dorsoplantar radiograph of the foot is diagnostic.

Posterior and *anterior dislocations* are the rarest subtypes, occurring as a result of a fall from a height onto the plantar-flexed foot (posterior dislocation) or the dorsiflexed foot (anterior dislocation). In either case, the lateral radiograph of the foot and ankle is best for demonstrating the abnormality (Fig. 10.104).

Total Talar Dislocation. Characterized by complete disruption of both the ankle (tibiotalar) and the subtalar joints, total talar dislocation is the most serious of all talar injuries (Fig. 10.105). It is frequently complicated by osteonecrosis of the astragalus.

Tarsometatarsal Dislocation

Also termed *Lisfranc fracture–dislocation* (named after Napoleonic army field surgeon Jacques Lisfranc de St. Martin), this is the most common dislocation in the foot. It also frequently occurs in association with various types

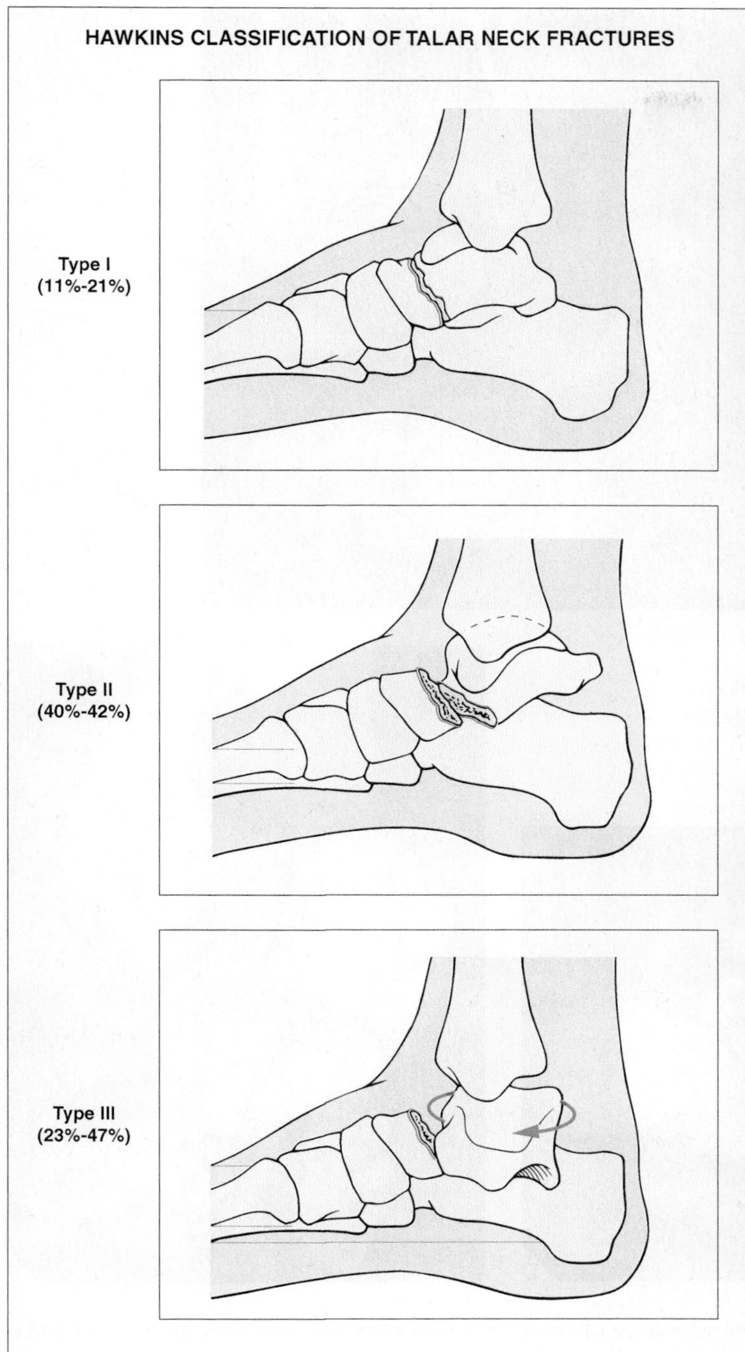

FIGURE 10.86 **The Hawkins classification of vertical talar neck fractures.** Type I fracture shows no displacement of the talus in relation to the subtalar joint. Type II fracture exhibits subluxation or dislocation of the talus in the subtalar joint. Type III fracture is characterized by the displacement of the body of the talus, which is locked behind the sustentaculum tali, so that the fracture surface is pointing laterally.

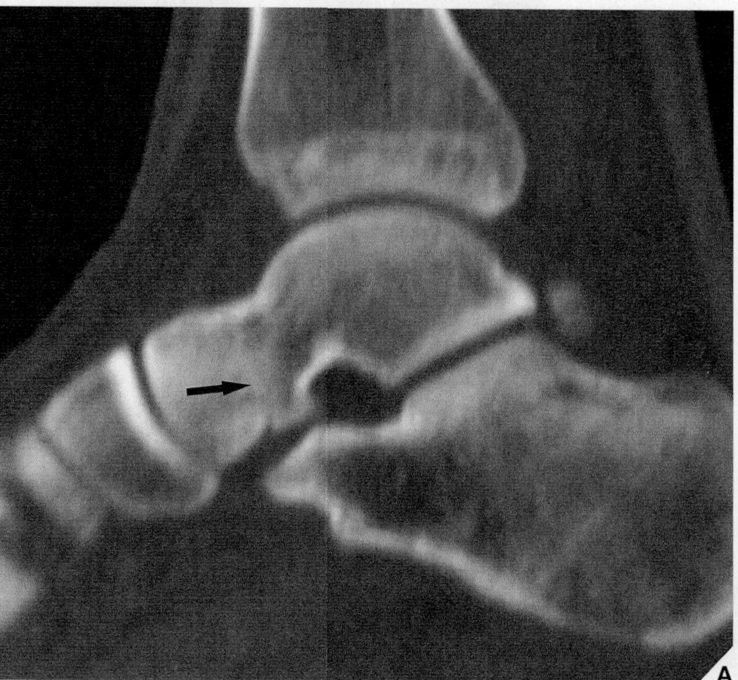

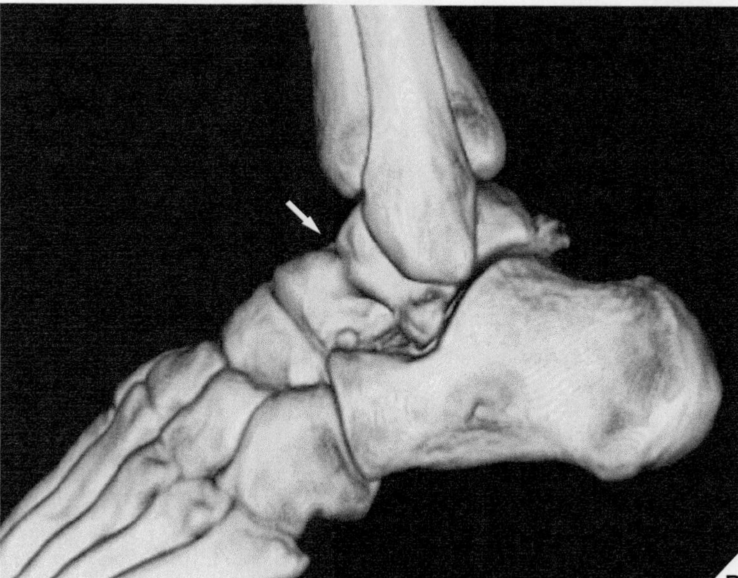

FIGURE 10.87 **CT and 3D CT of fracture of the talus.** **(A)** Sagittal reformatted CT image of the ankle and **(B)** 3D CT reconstruction in shaded surface display (SSD) show a nondisplaced fracture of the talus *(arrows)*.

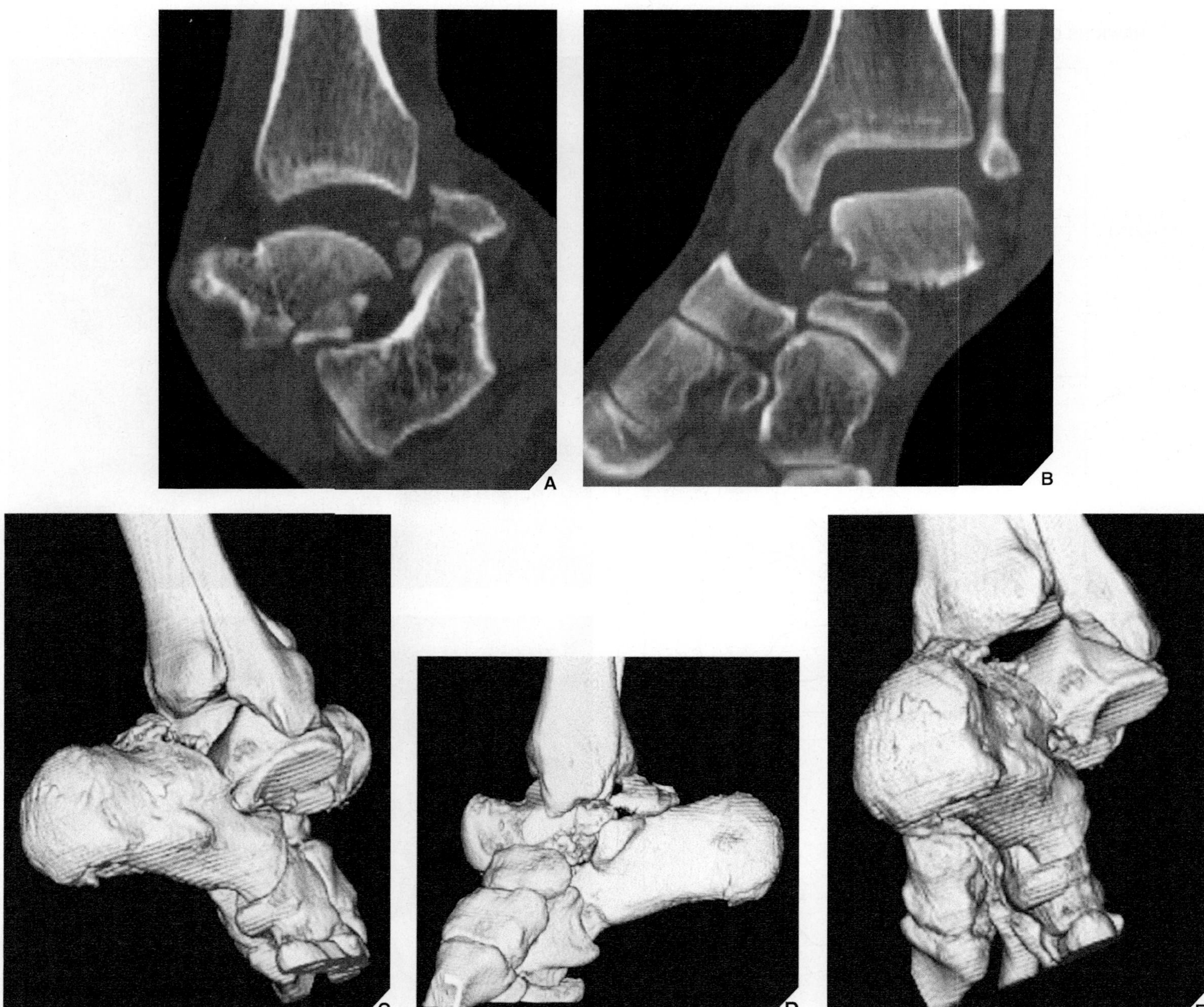

FIGURE 10.88 CT and 3D CT of fracture of the talus. **(A)** Coronal and **(B)** sagittal reformatted CT images of the ankle show a comminuted, displaced fracture of the talus. **(C–E)** 3D CT reconstructed images viewed from various angles depict the details of this injury.

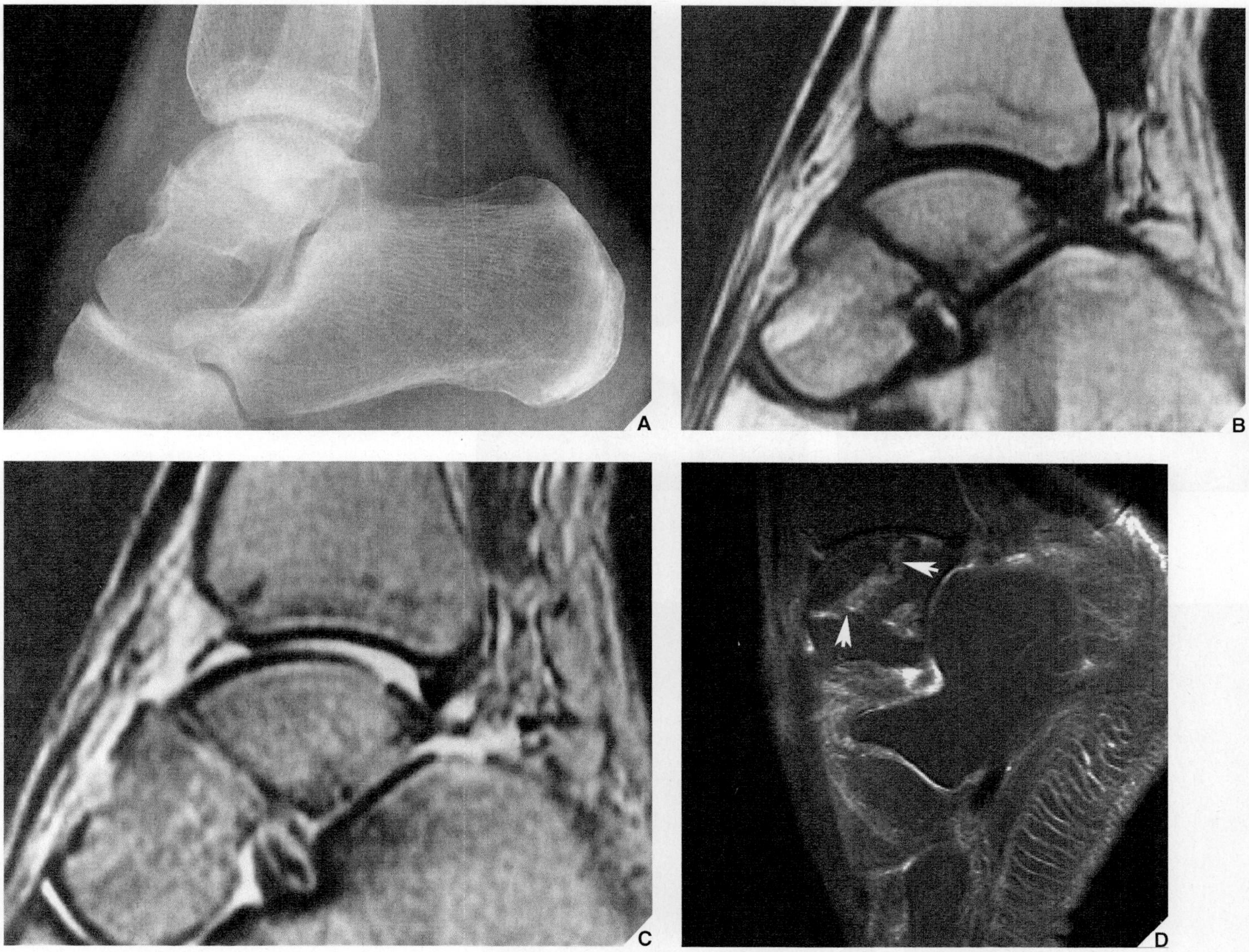

FIGURE 10.89 **MRI of fracture of the talus.** A 41-year-old woman injured her right foot in an automobile accident. **(A)** Lateral radiograph of the ankle demonstrates a vertical fracture of the talus. **(B)** T1-weighted and **(C)** T2-weighted sagittal spin echo MR images demonstrate lack of union and persistent joint effusion. In another patient who sustained a talar neck fracture, a sagittal T1-weighted fat-saturated image obtained after intravenous injection of gadolinium **(D)** demonstrates osteonecrosis of the body of the talus *(arrows)*. Note the low signal intensity of the necrotic area and the peripheral enhancement due to the granulation tissue in the reactive interface.

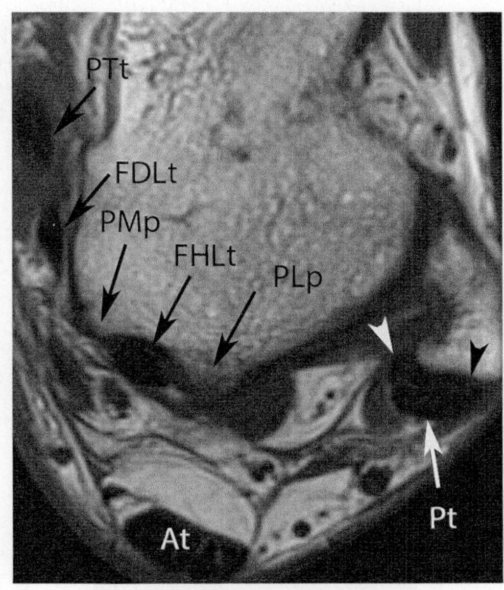

FIGURE 10.90 **Osseous anatomy of the posterior talus.** Axial T1-weighted MR image shows the posterior osseous anatomy of the talus and its relationship with the adjacent tendon structures. Note the thickening of the posterior tibialis tendon *(PTt)* consistent with tendinopathy. Note the split tear of the peroneus brevis tendon in the posterior aspect of the lateral malleolus *(arrowheads)* and the abnormal appearance of the peroneus longus tendon located posteriorly, consistent with tendinosis. FDLt, flexor digitorum longus tendon; PMp, posterior medial process; FHLt, flexor hallucis longus tendon, located in the grove between the two posterior talar processes; PLp, posterior lateral process (Stieda process); Pt, peroneal tendons.

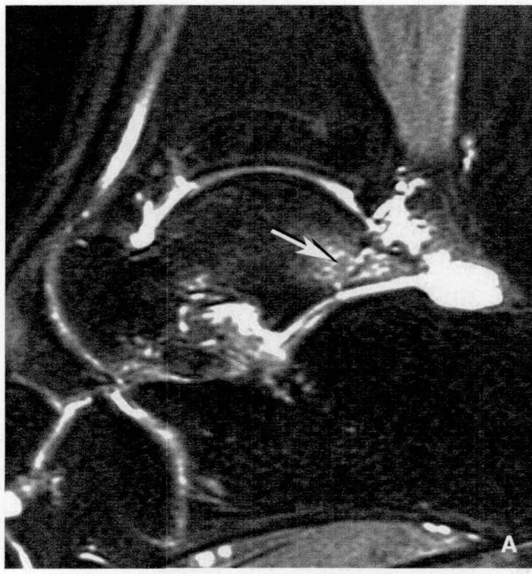

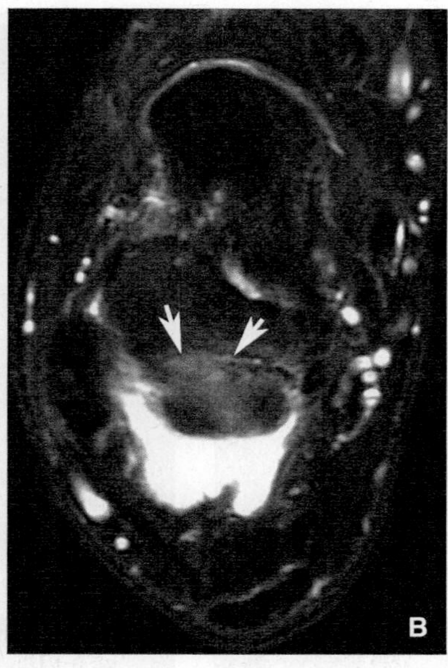

FIGURE 10.91 Shepherd fracture of the posterolateral process of the talus. **(A)** Sagittal and **(B)** axial STIR MR images demonstrate an acute fracture of the posterolateral process of the talus *(arrows)*. This fracture should not be confused with an os trigonum which occurs in the same location.

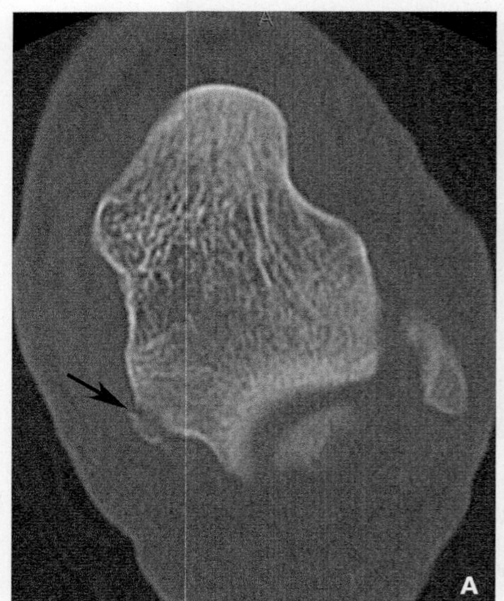

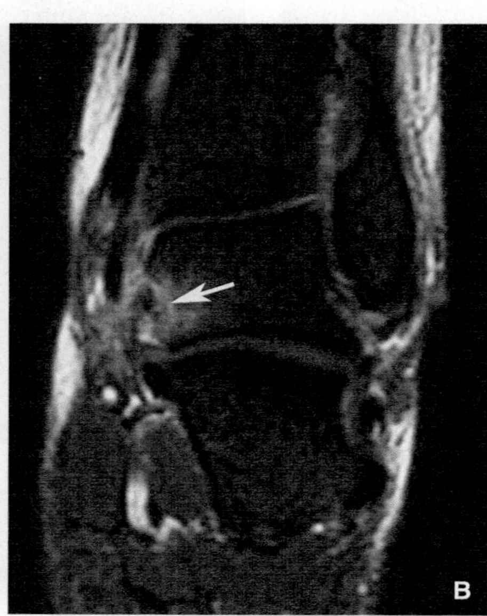

FIGURE 10.92 Cedell fracture of the posteromedial process of the talus. **(A)** Axial CT image demonstrates a fracture of the posteromedial process of the talus *(arrow)*. **(B)** Coronal STIR MR image shows also the fracture of the posterior medial process of the talus *(arrow)* with surrounding bone marrow edema.

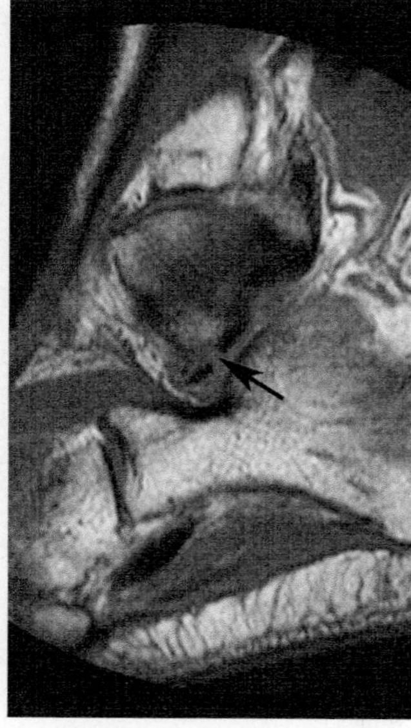

FIGURE 10.93 Snowboarder's fracture. Sagittal T1-weighted MR image shows a minimally displaced fracture of the lateral process of the talus *(arrow)*.

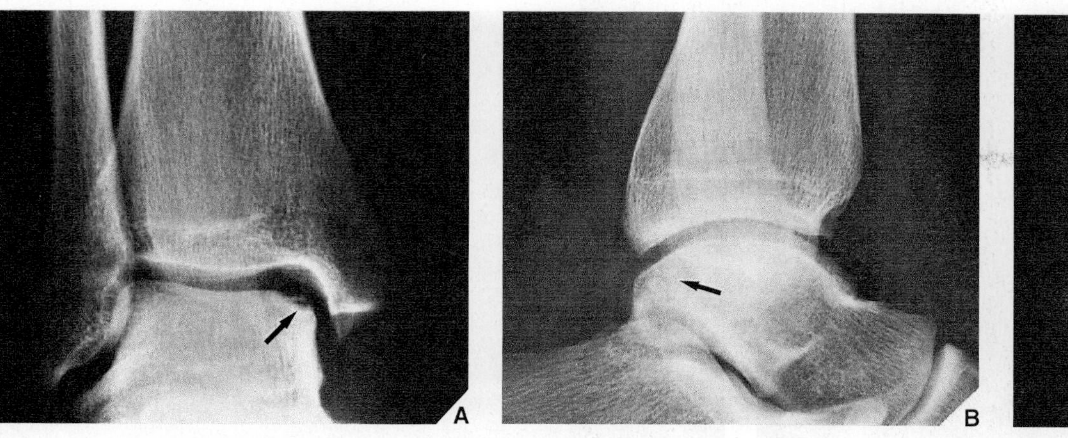

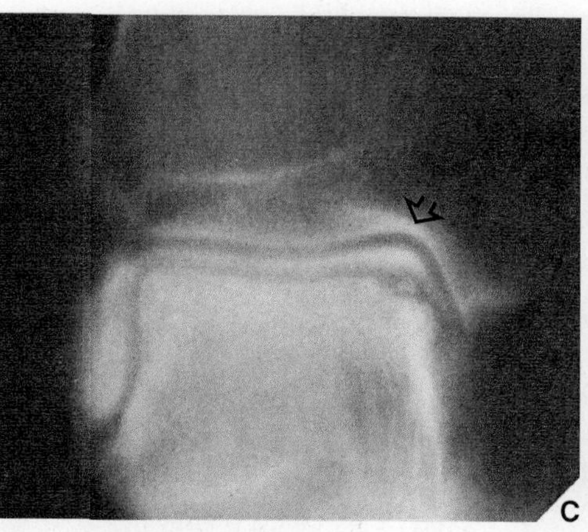

FIGURE 10.94 OCD of the talus. A 29-year-old man, a professional ballet dancer, reported pain in the ankle over the preceding 8 months. **(A)** Anteroposterior and **(B)** lateral radiographs demonstrate a radiolucent defect in the medial aspect of the dome of the talus and a small osteochondral body within the defect *(arrows)*, characteristic findings in OCD. **(C)** Arthrotomography demonstrates the intact articular cartilage over the lesion *(open arrow)*, distinguishing it as an *in situ* lesion.

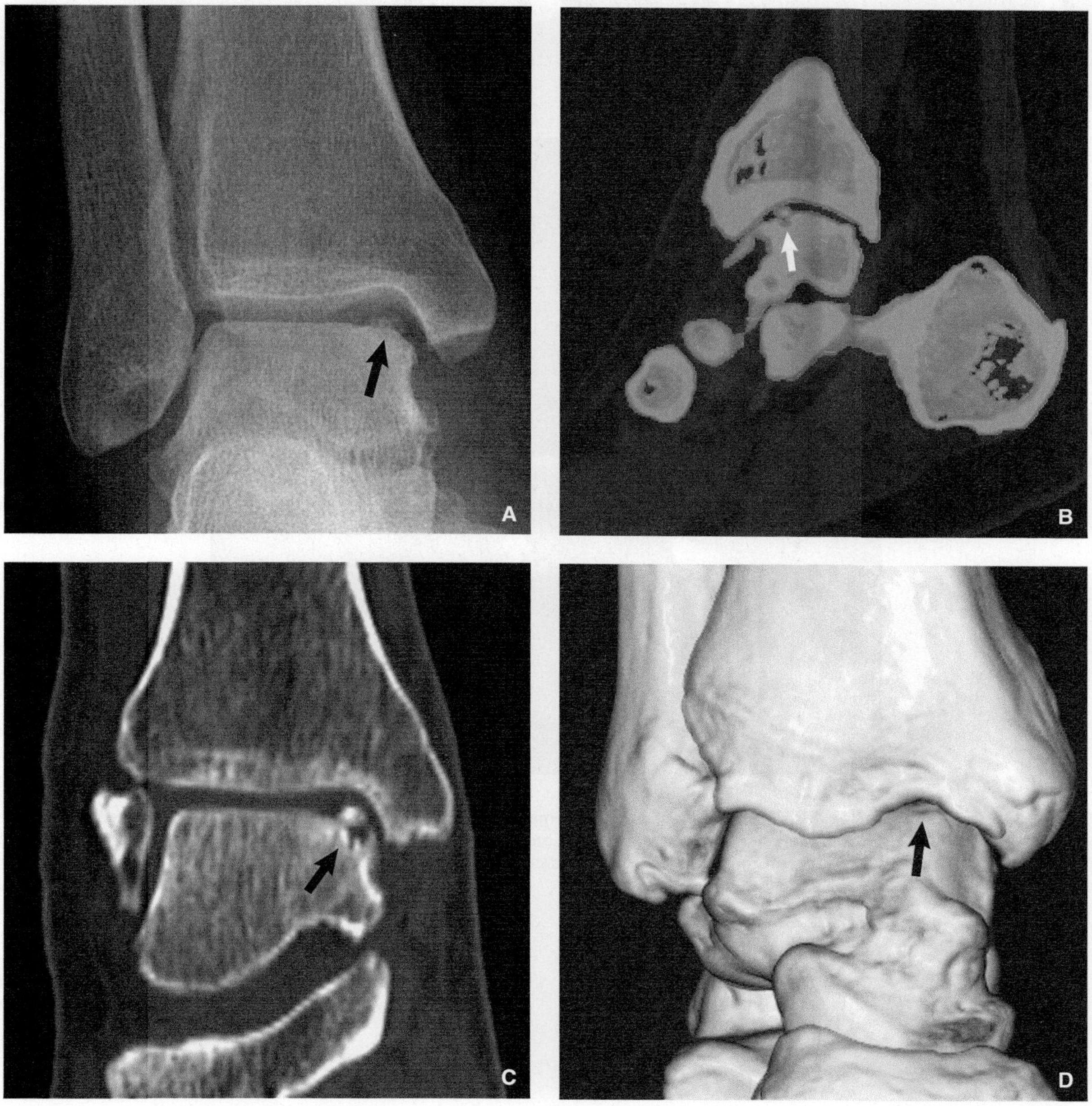

FIGURE 10.95 CT and 3D CT of OCD of the talus. A 36-year-old professional ice figure skater presented with chronic pain in his right ankle. **(A)** Anteroposterior radiograph of the ankle shows typical lesion of OCD in the medial dome of the talus *(arrow)*. **(B)** Sagittal reformatted dual-energy CT, performed to exclude gouty arthritis, confirmed the presence of osteochondral defect associated with displaced osteochondral fragment *(arrow)*, also demonstrated on **(C)** coronal reformatted CT section *(arrow)* and **(D)** 3D reconstructed CT image *(arrow)*. Arthroscopic examination revealed that the osteochondral body was discharged into the ankle joint space.

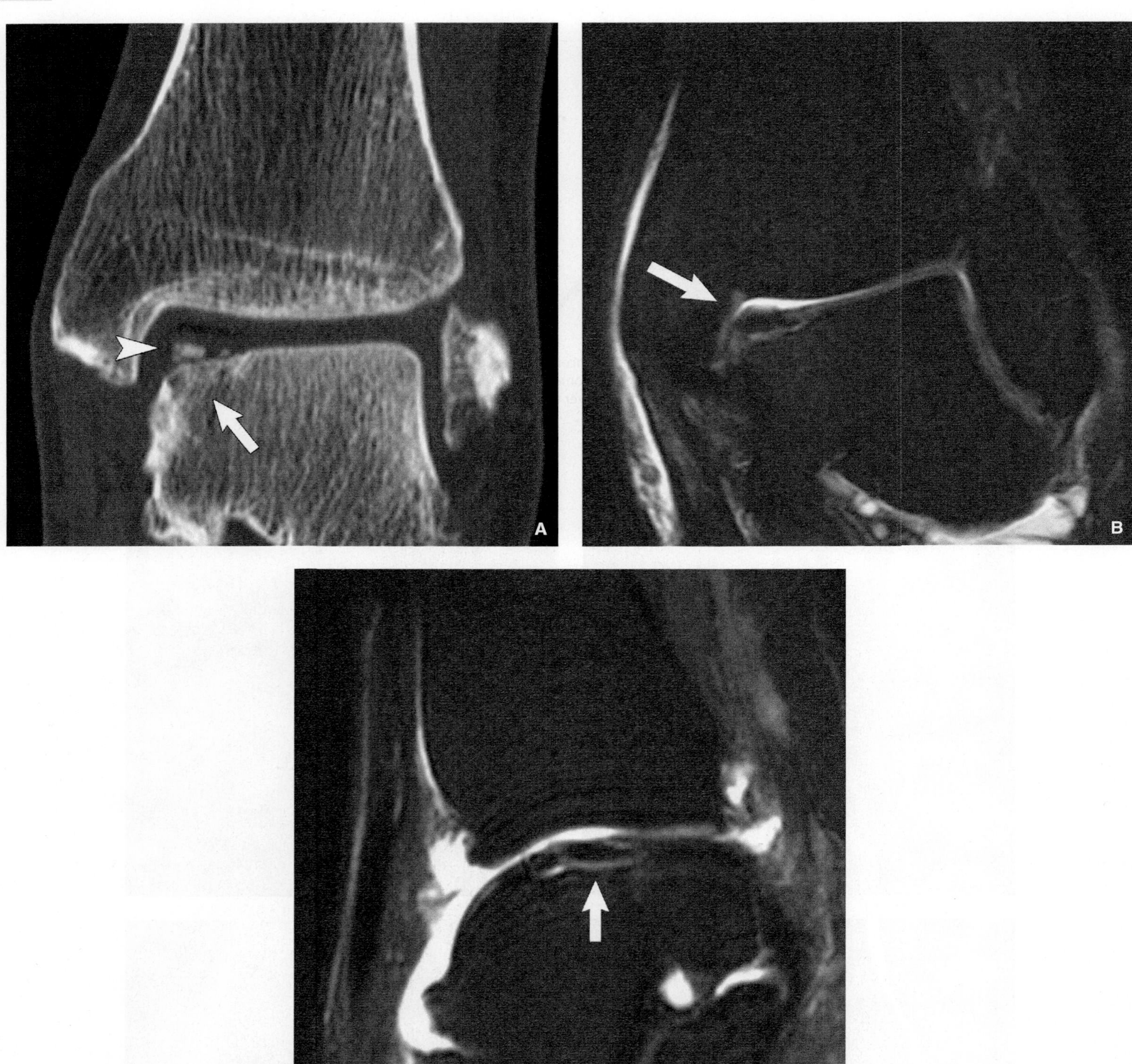

FIGURE 10.96 **CT and MRa of OCD of the talus.** **(A)** Coronal reformatted CT image of the left ankle of a 27-year-old man shows osteochondral defect in the medial dome of the talus *(arrow)* and displaced osteochondral fragment *(arrowhead)*. **(B)** Coronal and **(C)** sagittal proton density–weighted fat-suppressed MR images, obtained after intraarticular injection of 5 mL of diluted gadolinium contrast agent, show fluid/contrast undermining the osteochondral fragment *(arrows)* indicating that the lesion is unstable.

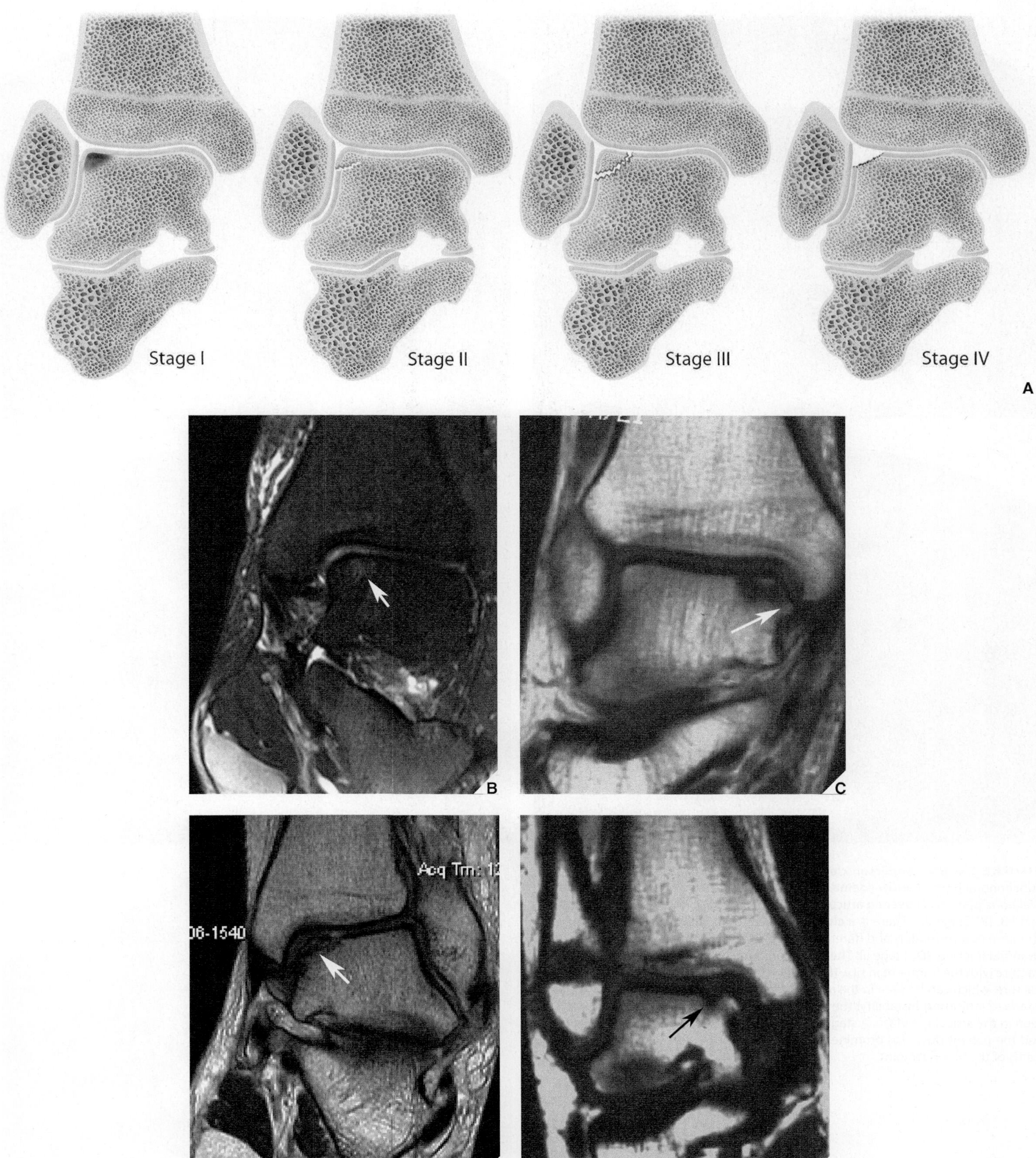

FIGURE 10.97 MRI of OCD of the talus. **(A)** Berndt and Harty classification of OCD lesions of the talus. **(B)** Coronal T2-weighted MR image demonstrates stage I subchondral lesion in the medial talar dome *(arrow)*. **(C)** Coronal T1-weighted MR image demonstrates stage II osteochondral lesion of the medial aspect of the talus. Note the osseous fragment remains partially united with the medial aspect of the talus *(arrow)*. **(D)** Coronal T2-weighted image demonstrates stage III OCD of the talus with the osteochondral fragment in situ *(arrow)*. **(E)** Coronal T1-weighted MR image demonstrates a stage IV OCD lesion of the medial talar dome. The fragment is no longer *in situ*, and there is an osteochondral defect in the talar dome *(arrow)*.

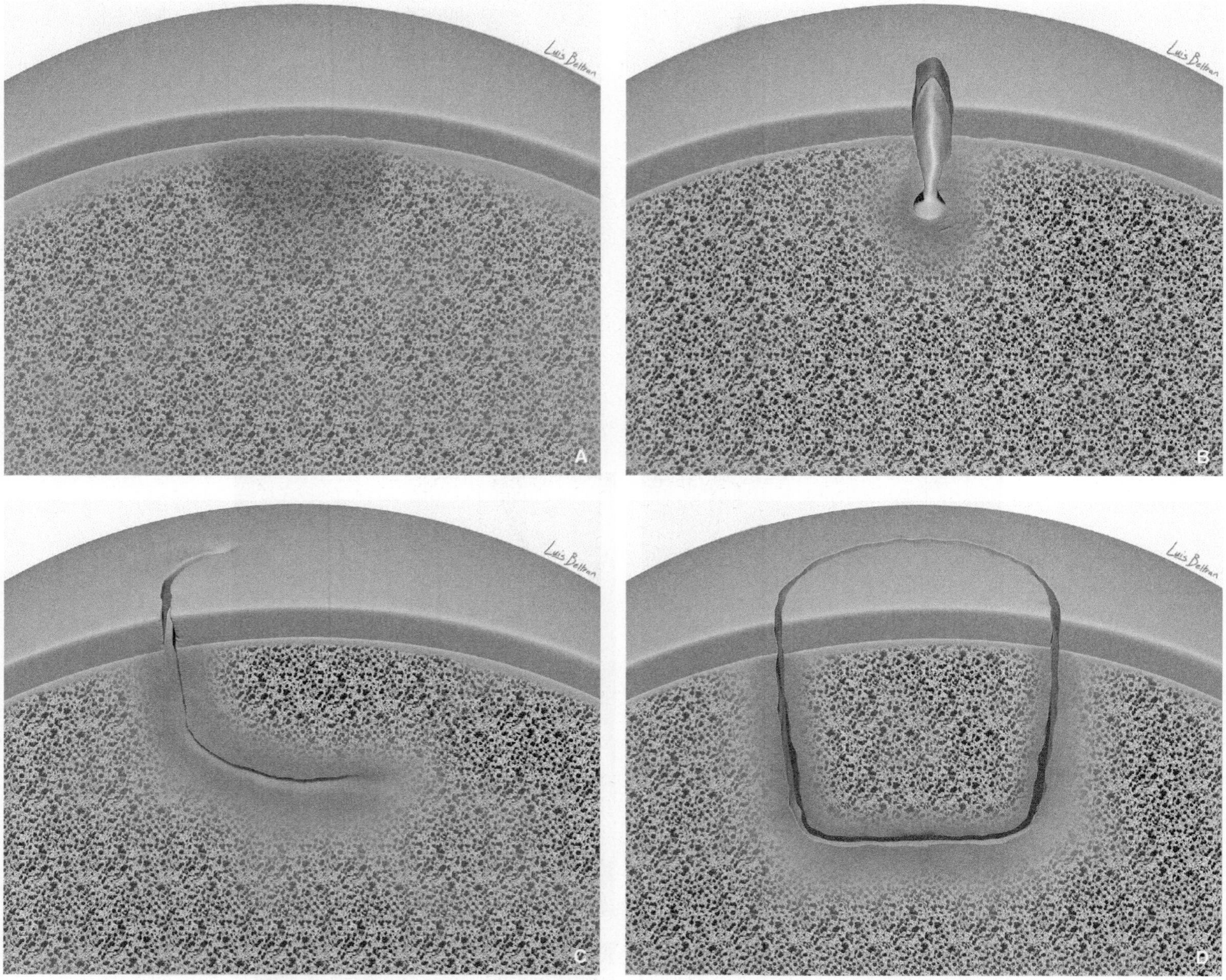

FIGURE 10.98 **Anderson classification of OCD of the talus.** **(A)** Stage I: Subchondral bone marrow edema/contusion with preservation of the subchondral bone plate and covering articular cartilage. Stage II is divided into stages IIA and IIB. **(B)** Stage IIA: There is a chondral defect or fissure associated with subchondral cyst formation of different sizes. **(C)** Stage IIB: There is a partial osteochondral fracture. **(D)** Stage III: There is a complete nondisplaced osteochondral fracture with the fragment in situ. **(E)** Stage IV: There is a displaced osteochondral fracture, which can be seen in the region of the donor site with fluid signal at the interface indicating instability; the fragment is no longer in situ, and a crater is seen in the articular surface. A stage V can be added when the OCD lesion is old, and the patient develops prominent subchondral cysts and secondary osteoarthritis of the tibiotalar joint.

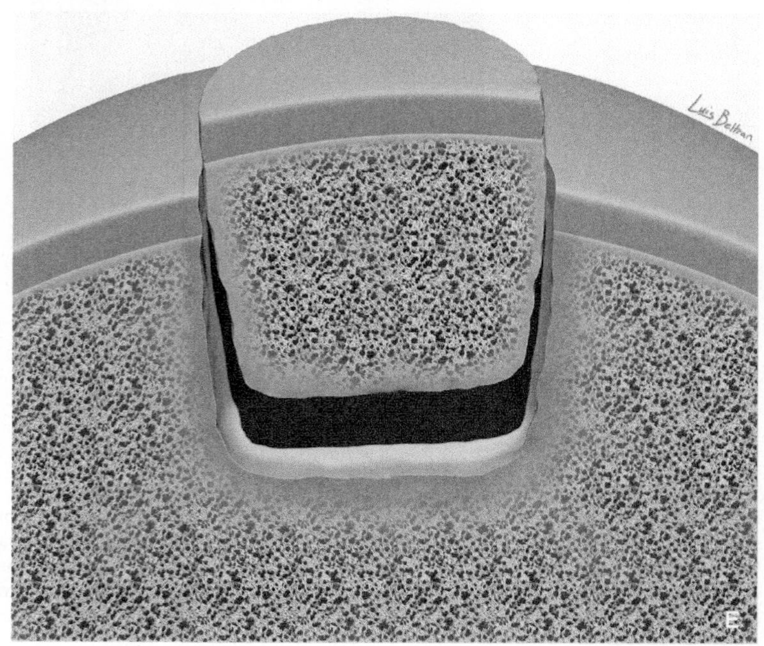

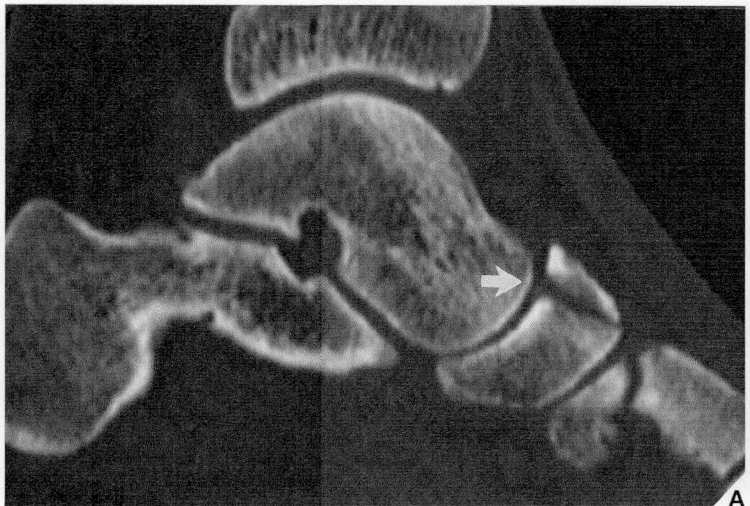

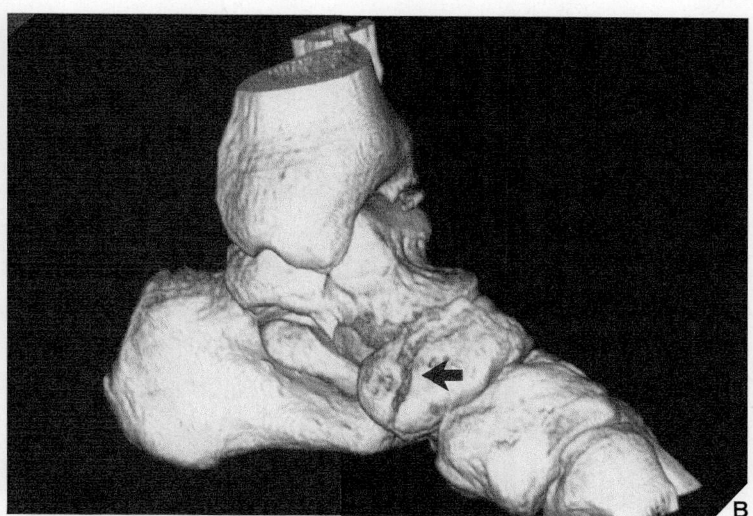

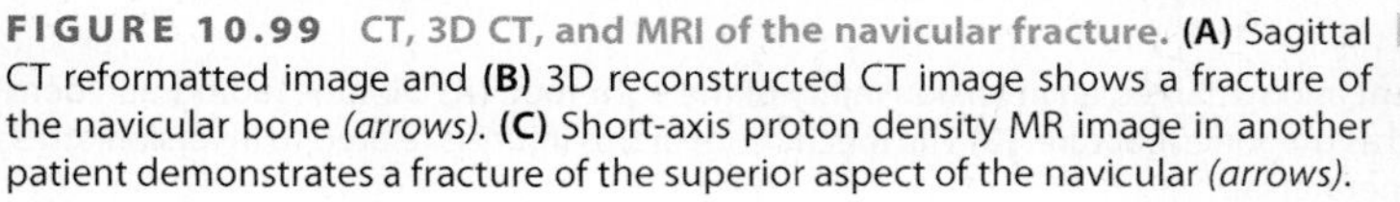

FIGURE 10.99 **CT, 3D CT, and MRI of the navicular fracture.** **(A)** Sagittal CT reformatted image and **(B)** 3D reconstructed CT image shows a fracture of the navicular bone *(arrows)*. **(C)** Short-axis proton density MR image in another patient demonstrates a fracture of the superior aspect of the navicular *(arrows)*.

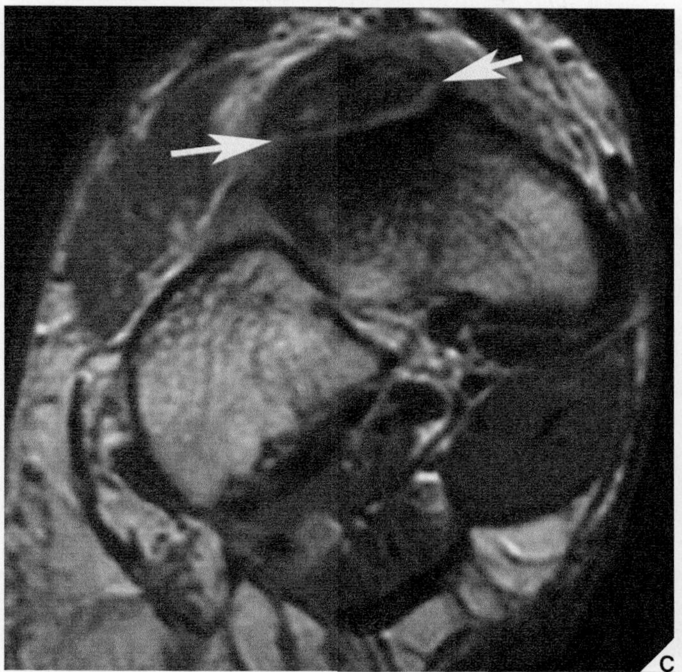

FIGURE 10.100 **Mueller-Weis syndrome.** **(A)** Lateral radiograph of the foot and **(B)** sagittal gradient recalled echo (GRE) MR image in two different patients with chronic midfoot pain show the collapse of the navicular bone *(arrows)* and the dorsal extrusion of the navicular. There is secondary osteoarthritis of the talonavicular joint *(arrowheads)*.

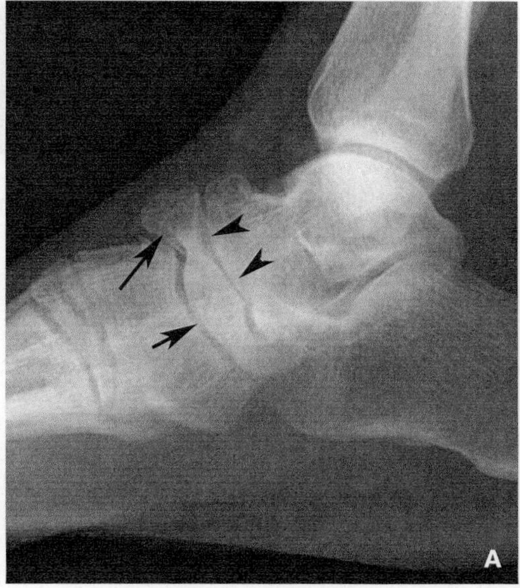

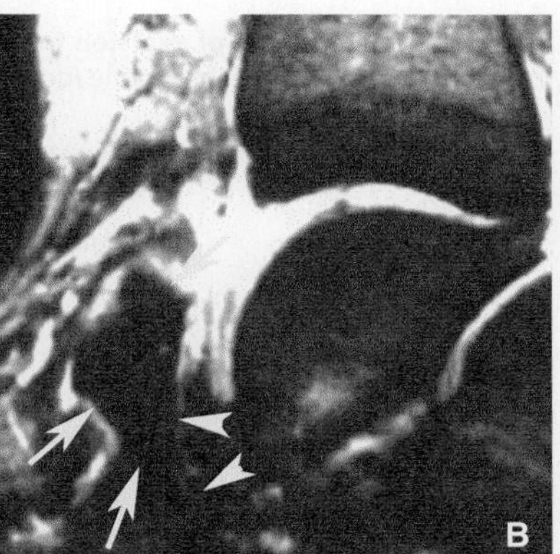

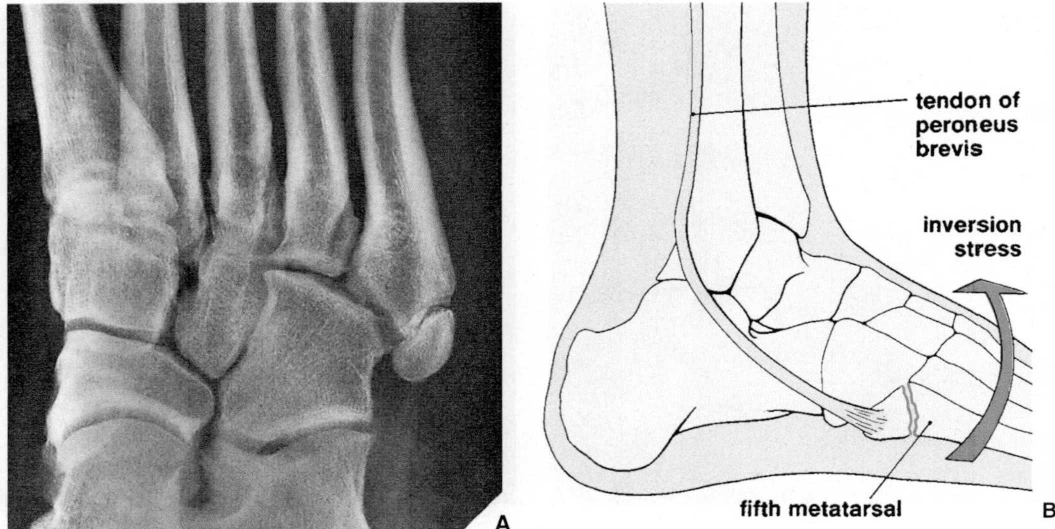

FIGURE 10.101 Avulsion fracture. A 28-year-old man stumbled on uneven pavement and sustained an inversion injury of the right foot. **(A)** Oblique radiograph demonstrates a fracture of the base of the fifth metatarsal, frequently but incorrectly interpreted as the Jones fracture. **(B)** The mechanism of this injury is related to inversion-stress forces on the peroneus brevis tendon that cause avulsion fracture of the base of the fifth metatarsal.

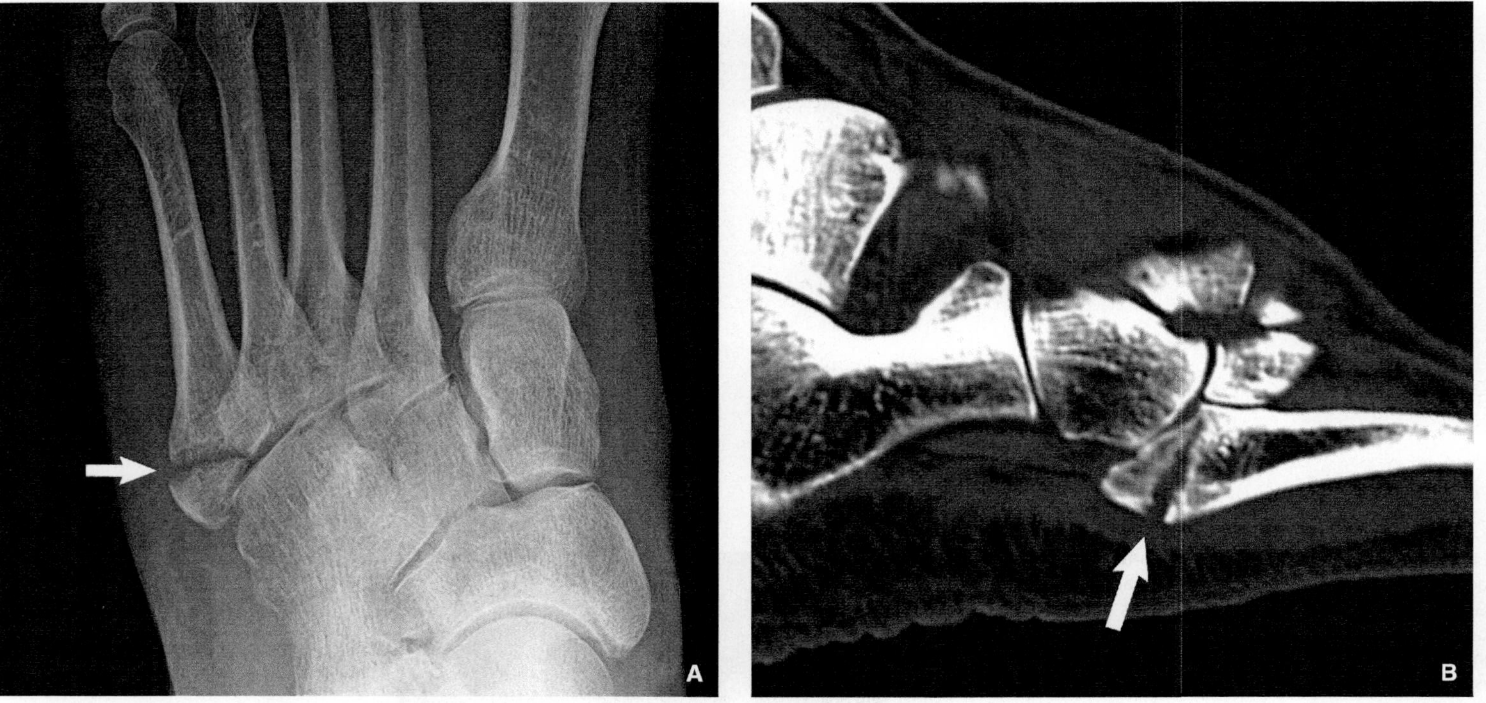

FIGURE 10.102 CT of avulsion fracture. **(A)** Dorsovolar radiograph of the right foot and **(B)** sagittal reformatted CT image show an intraarticular evulsion fracture at the base of the fifth metatarsal bone *(arrow)*.

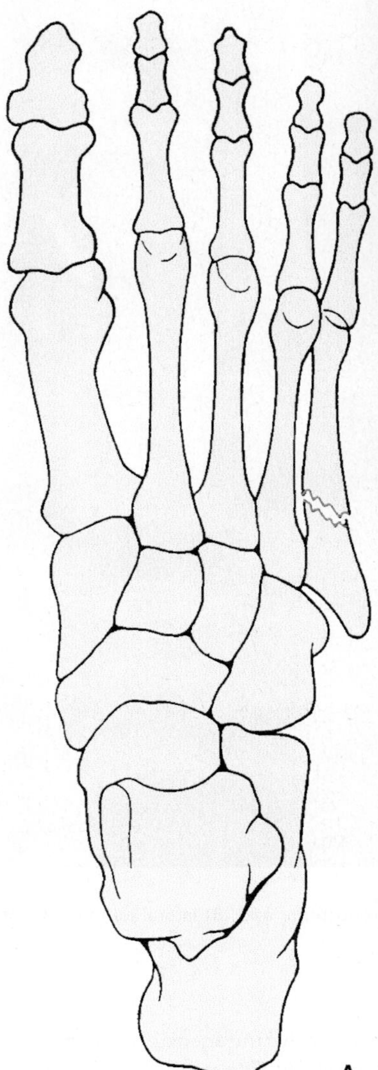

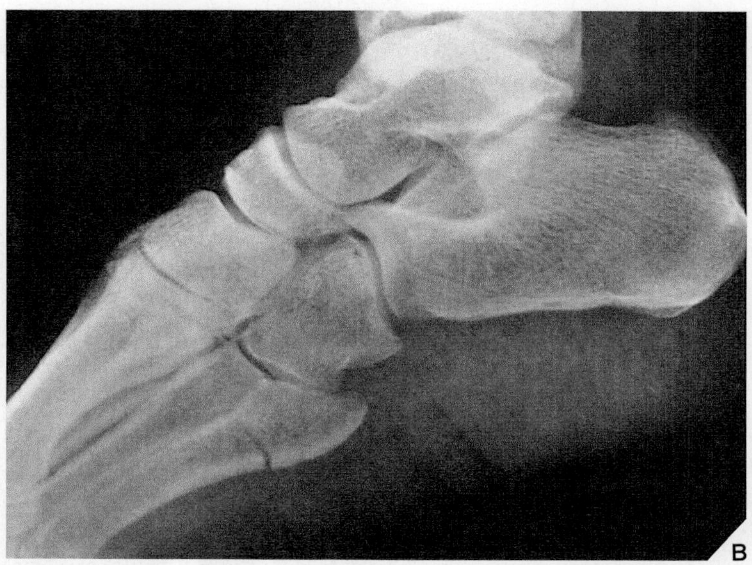

FIGURE 10.103 Jones fracture. **(A)** A "true" Jones fracture is located about an inch distally to the base of the fifth metatarsal. **(B)** A 43-year-old woman, while dancing, twisted her left foot and sustained a true Jones fracture of the fifth metatarsal.

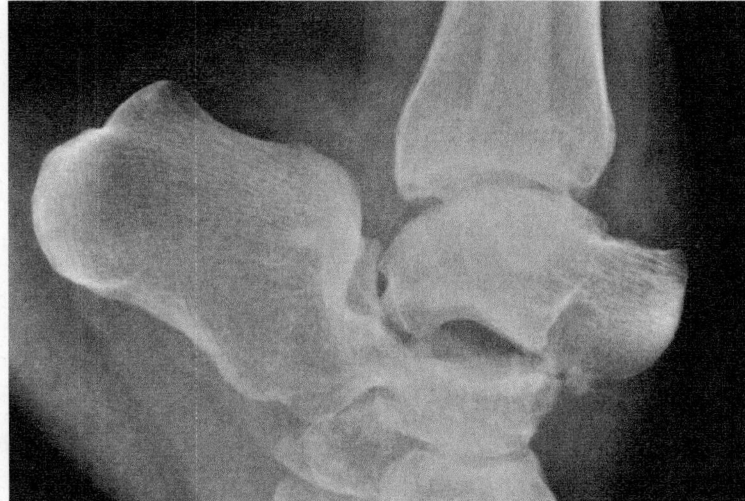

FIGURE 10.104 Peritalar dislocation. A 25-year-old man fell from a ladder and landed on his plantar-flexed left foot. Lateral radiograph demonstrates posterior peritalar dislocation. Note that the talus articulates normally with the tibia, but there are simultaneous dislocations in the talocalcaneal and talonavicular joints. The entire foot (except for the talus) is posteriorly displaced. Associated fractures of the navicular and cuboid bones are evident.

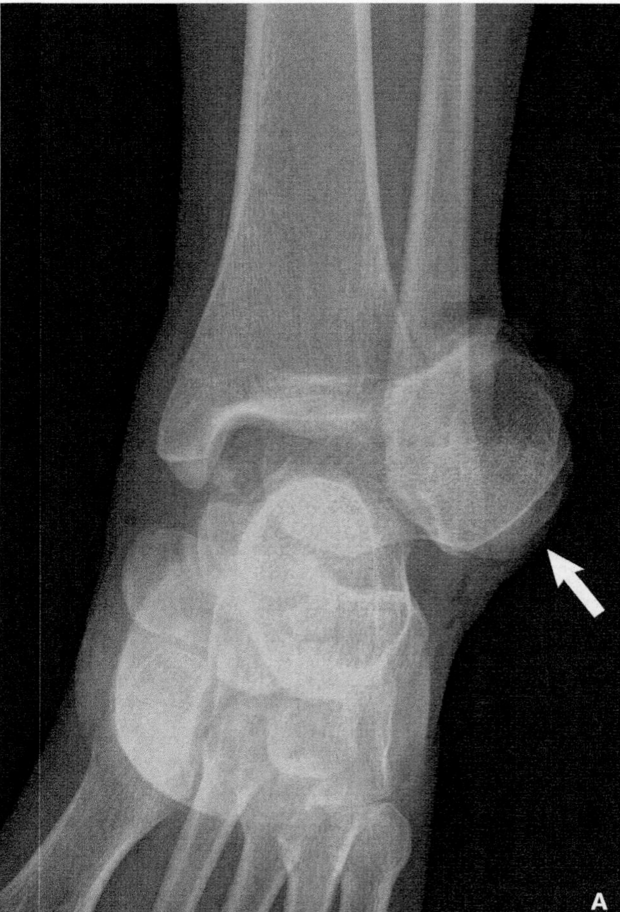

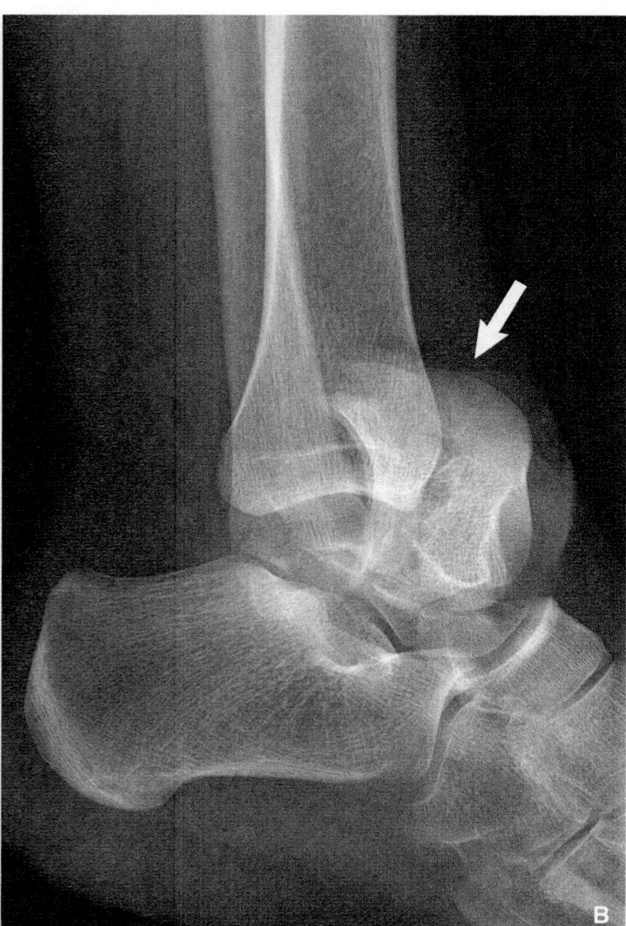

FIGURE 10.105 **Dislocation of the talus.** A 14-year-old girl was injured in a bike accident. **(A)** Anteroposterior and **(B)** lateral radiographs of the left ankle show anterolateral dislocation of the talus *(arrows)*.

of fractures. Basically, this is a dorsal dislocation, often occurring as the result of a fall from a height or down a flight of stairs or even of stepping off a curb. There are two basic forms of injury: *homolateral*—dislocation of the first to the fifth metatarsal—and *divergent*—lateral displacement of the second to the fifth metatarsals with medial or dorsal shift of the first metatarsal (Fig. 10.106). Associated fractures most often occur at the base of the second metatarsal bone; they may also be seen in the third metatarsal, first or second cuneiform, or navicular bones. The divergent form of tarsometatarsal dislocation is most frequently associated with such fractures. Although these injuries are well demonstrated on the standard radiographs of the foot (Figs. 10.107 and 10.108A), ancillary imaging techniques are frequently required. CT examination demonstrates the details of this injury (Figs. 10.108A and 10.109) and unsuspected additional fractures (see Fig. 10.109B,C), and MRI may disclose not seen otherwise associated tear of the Lisfranc ligament (Fig. 10.110).

The most common complications of ankle and foot fractures are nonunion and posttraumatic arthritis. Although conventional radiography can usually demonstrate the features of these complications, CT is the better technique for delineating their characteristic features.

Miscellaneous Painful Soft-Tissue Abnormalities of the Ankle and Foot

Tarsal Tunnel Syndrome

The tarsal tunnel is a fibroosseous structure located in the medial side of the ankle and hindfoot, extending from the medial malleolus to the navicular bone. The roof of the tunnel is formed by the flexor retinaculum; the lateral side is formed by the medial aspect of the talus and sustentaculum tali; and the medial side is bordered by the flexor retinaculum, abductor hallucis muscle, and the medial wall of the calcaneus. The tarsal tunnel contains the posterior tibial nerve, the posterior tibial artery and vein, the posterior tibial tendon, the flexor digitorum longus tendon, and the flexor hallucis longus tendon. The term *tarsal tunnel syndrome* was originally and independently coined by Keck and Lam in 1962. The syndrome is caused by the compression of the posterior tibial nerve or its branches as they pass deep to the flexor retinaculum, either by extrinsic masses or posttraumatic fibrosis. The clinical symptoms include pain, a burning sensation, and paresthesias in the sole of the foot and the toes. MRI is very effective in demonstrating the cause of nerve impingement (Fig. 10.111).

Sinus Tarsi Syndrome

The sinus tarsi (or tarsal sinus) is a cone-shaped space located in the lateral aspect of the foot between the neck of the talus and the anteroposterior surface of the calcaneus. The sinus tarsi contains fat, talocalcaneal ligaments, interosseous ligaments, portions of the joint capsule of the posterior subtalar joint, and neurovascular structures. The sinus tarsi syndrome is caused by abnormalities of one or more structures contained in the sinus and is characterized by pain in the lateral portion of the foot and a feeling of instability of the hindfoot. Pain relief can be achieved by injection of anesthetic agents into the tarsal sinus. In 70% of reported cases, the causing factor responsible for the sinus tarsi syndrome was trauma, usually involving inversion injury to the foot. MRI may show obliteration of sinus tarsi fat, tear of calcaneofibular and anterior talofibular ligaments, and tear of the posterior tibial tendon (Fig. 10.112).

Posterior Tibialis Tendon Dysfunction

Chronic Tendinosis of the Posterior Tibialis Tendon

This condition may lead to tear and subsequent loss of the arch of the foot, resulting in adult onset of pes planus and hindfoot valgus. This is more commonly seen in middle-aged women. Obesity, diabetes, and hypertension are considered contributing factors.

Tears of the Posterior Tibialis Tendon

This abnormality also can be the result of acute injuries or repetitive injuries in athletes. Patients present with pain in the medial aspect of the foot, at the level of the insertion of the tendon to the medial pole of the navicular bone. MRI demonstrates diffuse thickening and partial tearing of the posterior tibialis tendon in the early stages of tendon dysfunction and tear in the advanced stage of the disease (Fig. 10.113).

Painful Accessory Navicular Bone Syndrome

A large, triangular-shaped accessory navicular bone (also known as *os navicularis* or *os tibiale externum*) is present in about 10% of the population. This accessory bone is united to the medial aspect of the navicular bone with a synchondrosis. The posterior tibialis tendon attaches to the accessory navicular bone when present. Athletic activities may lead to inflammation of this accessory ossicle and associated tendinosis of the posterior tibialis tendon. MRI is the imaging technique of choice to demonstrate the signal alterations of the bone and the morphologic changes of the posterior tibialis tendon (Fig. 10.114).

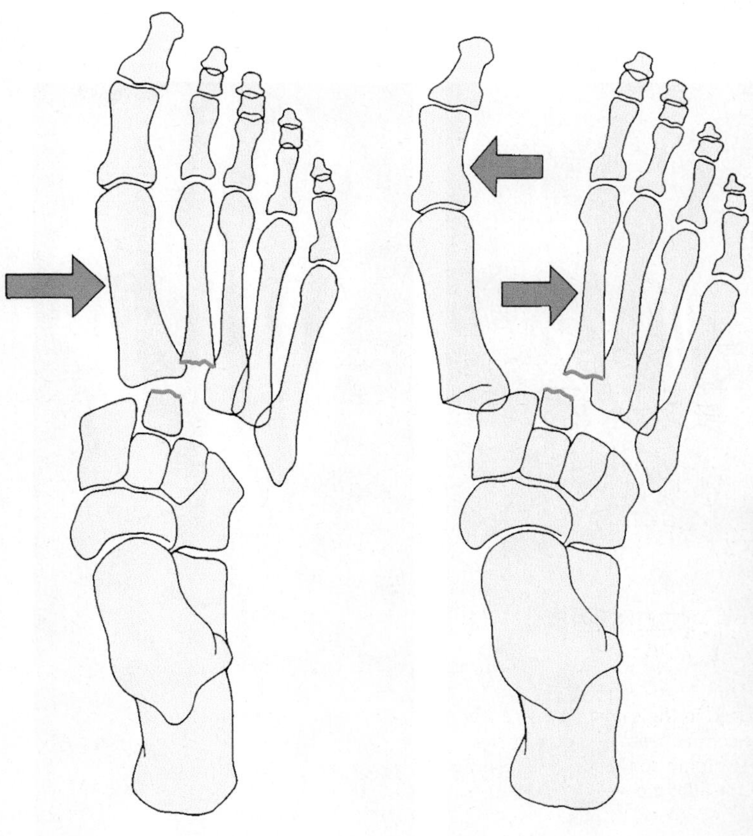

FIGURE 10.106 Types of the Lisfranc fracture–dislocation. Tarsometatarsal dislocation (Lisfranc fracture–dislocation) may be seen in two variants. In the homolateral form, the first to the fifth metatarsals are dislocated laterally. In the divergent form, the first metatarsal is medially dislocated. Both types are often associated with fracture of the base of the second metatarsal bone.

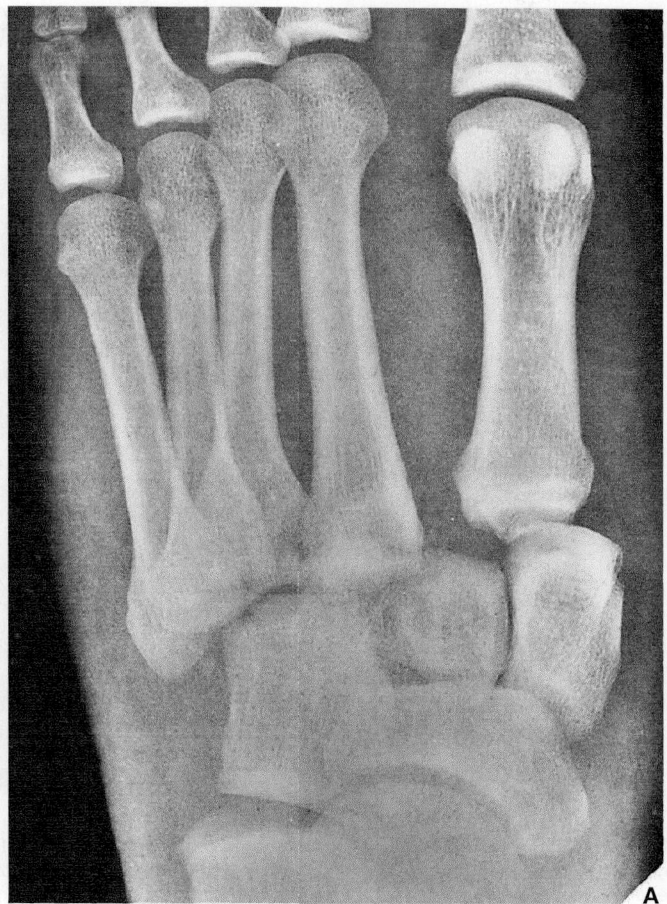

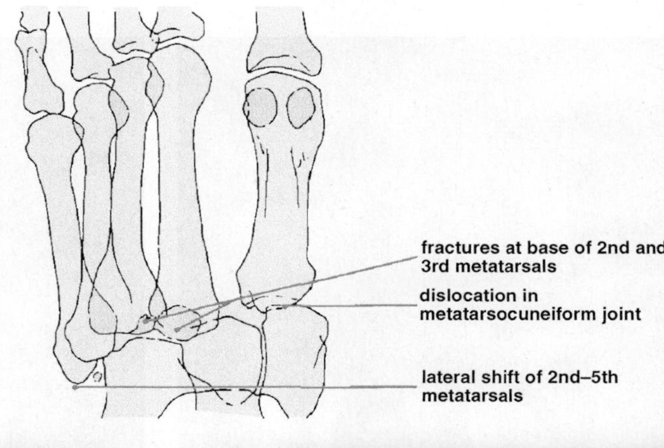

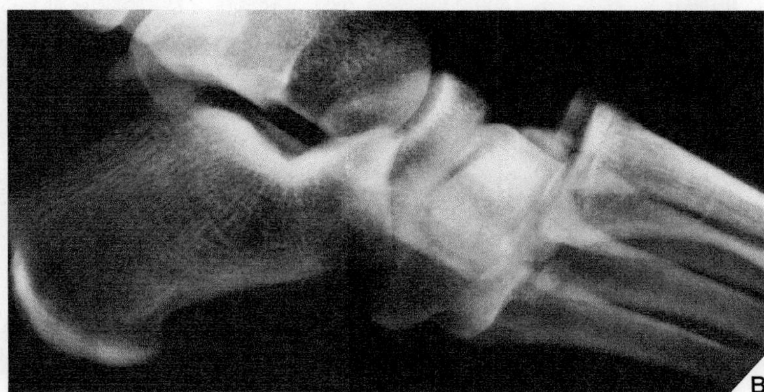

FIGURE 10.107 Divergent Lisfranc fracture–dislocation. A 39-year-old man fell down a flight of stairs. **(A)** Dorsoplantar and **(B)** lateral weight-bearing radiographs of the right foot show the divergent type of the Lisfranc fracture–dislocation. There is lateral shift of the second to fifth metatarsals as well as dislocation, and dorsal shift in the first metatarsocuneiform joint, which is better appreciated on the lateral radiograph. Note the fractures at the base of the second and third metatarsals.

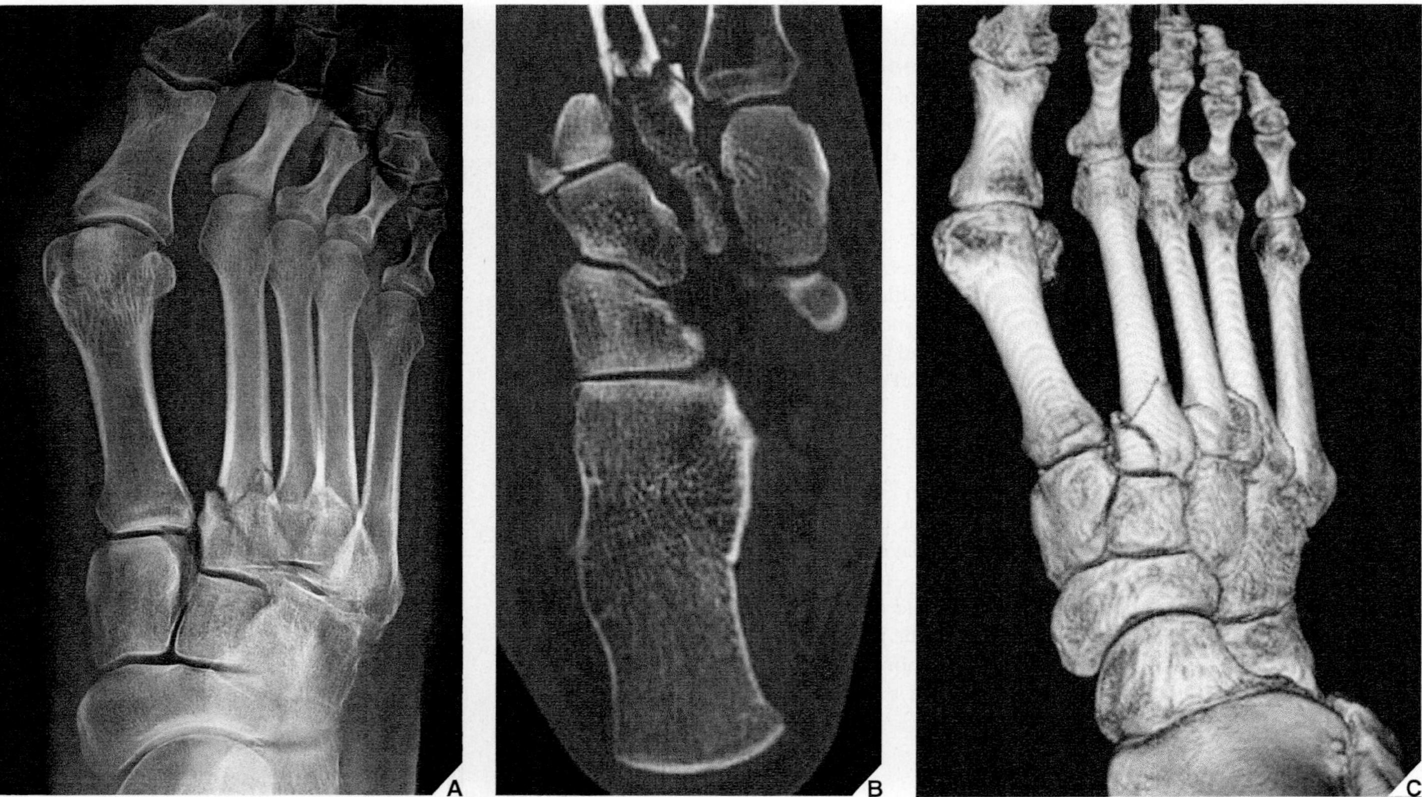

FIGURE 10.108 CT and 3D CT of the Lisfranc fracture–dislocation. **(A)** Dorsoplantar weight-bearing radiograph of the left foot shows a typical Lisfranc injury, more accurately displayed on the **(B)** axial CT image and **(C)** 3D CT reconstruction. Observe widening between the first and second metatarsal bones and a fracture at the base of the second metatarsal.

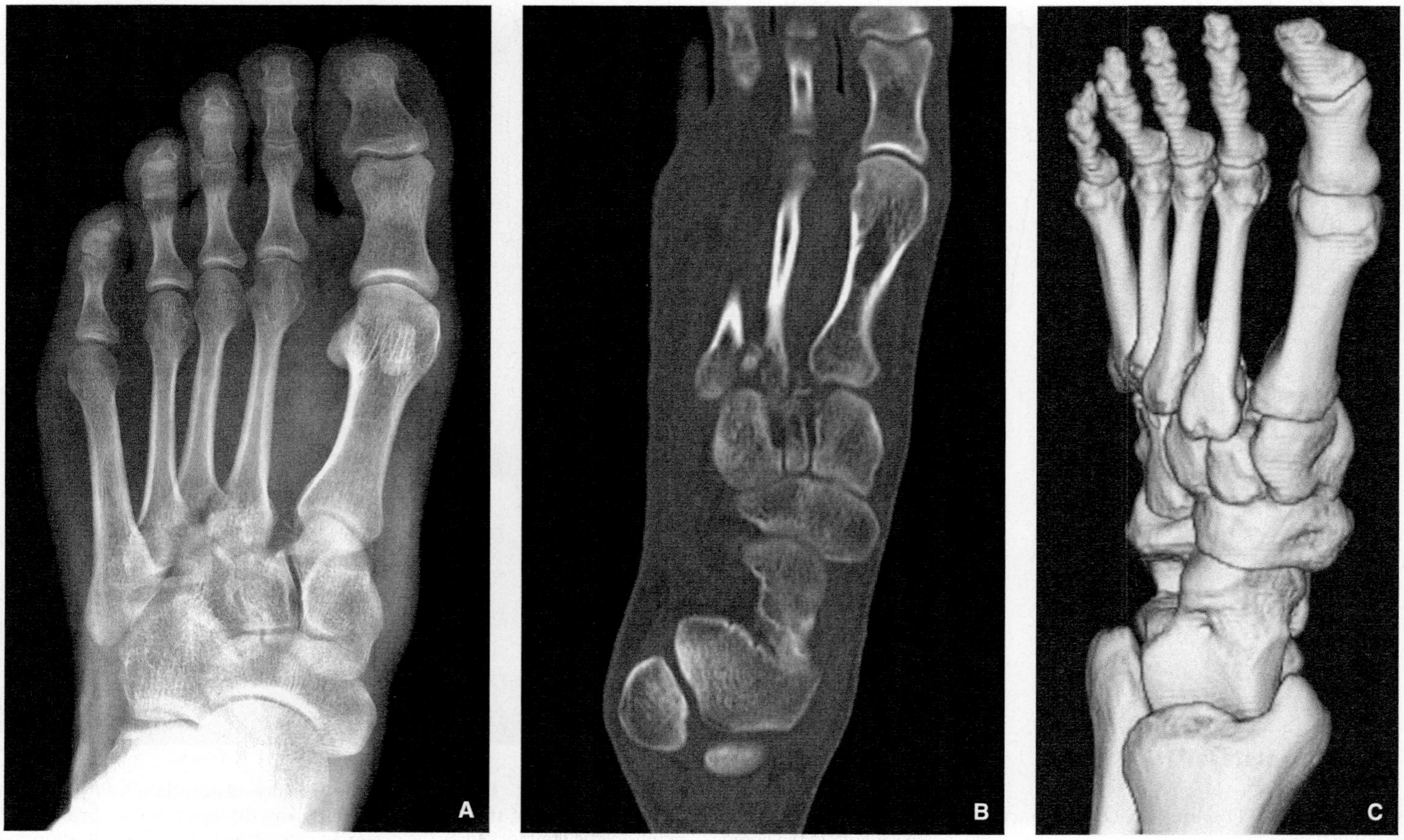

FIGURE 10.109 CT and 3D CT of the Lisfranc fracture-dislocation. A 24-year-old woman was injured in a ski accident. **(A)** Dorsoplantar weight-bearing radiograph of the right foot shows widening between the first and second metatarsal bones and several small osseous fragments wedged between the bases of these bones. It is not clear what bones have been fractures. **(B)** Coronal reformatted CT image and **(C)** 3D reconstructed CT clearly demonstrate fractures at the base of the second and third metatarsal bones and of the middle cuneiform bone.

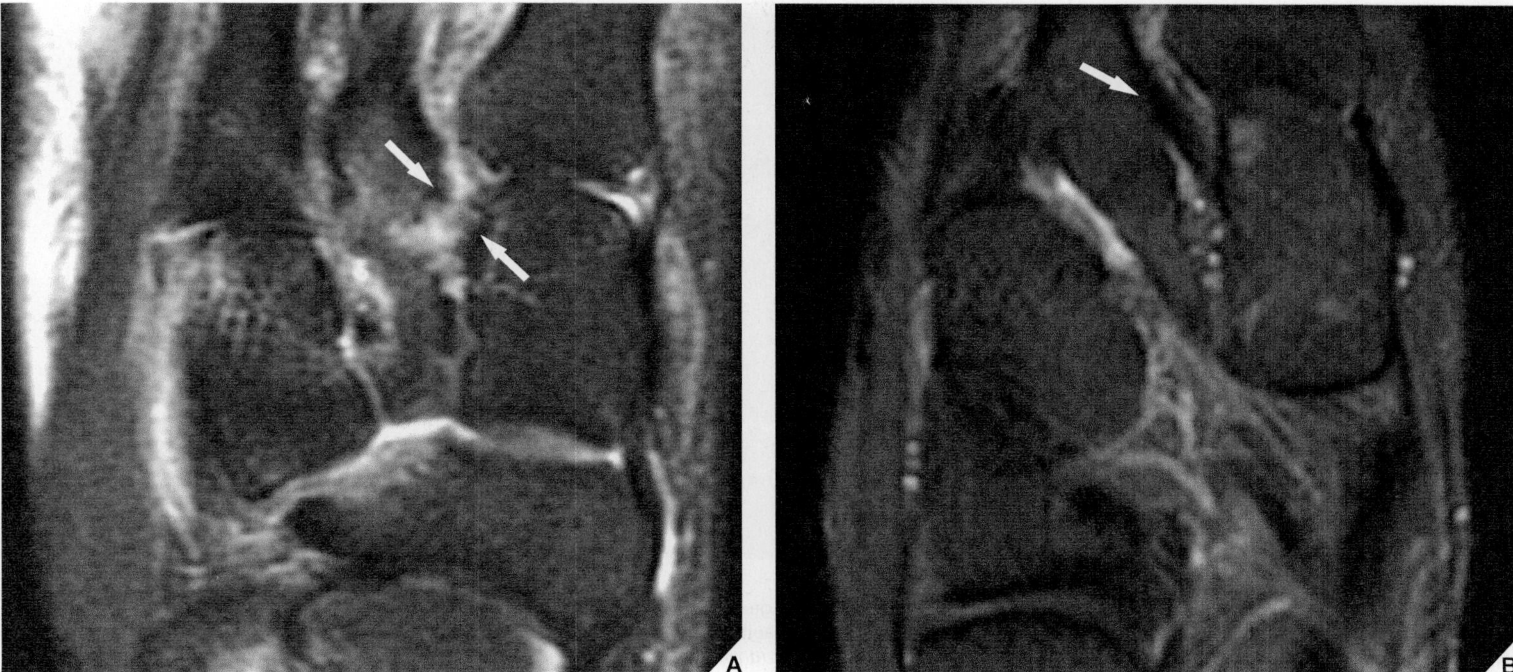

FIGURE 10.110 MRI of tear of the Lisfranc ligament. **(A)** Proton density–weighted fat-suppressed axial MR image shows a tear of the Lisfranc ligament *(arrows)*. **(B)** Normal appearance of Lisfranc ligament *(arrow)* is shown for comparison.

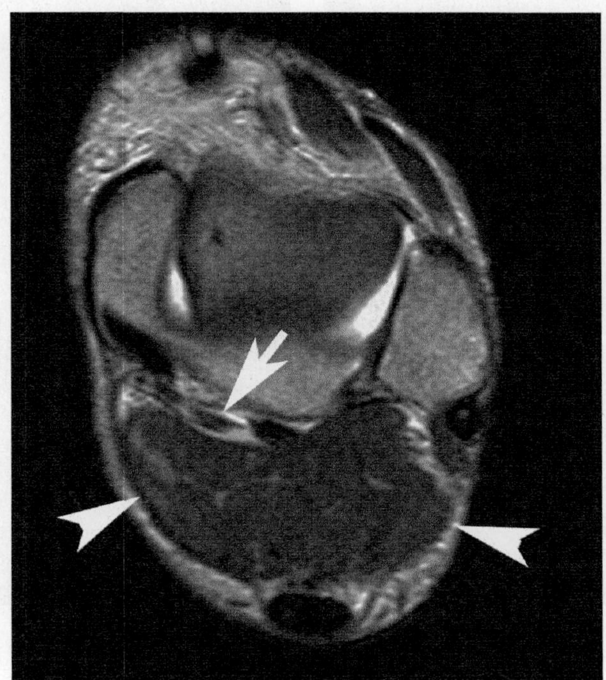

FIGURE 10.111 MRI of tarsal tunnel syndrome. Axial T2-weighted MR image of the ankle demonstrates an accessory soleus muscle *(arrowheads)* producing compression of the tibial nerve *(arrow)* in the tarsal tunnel.

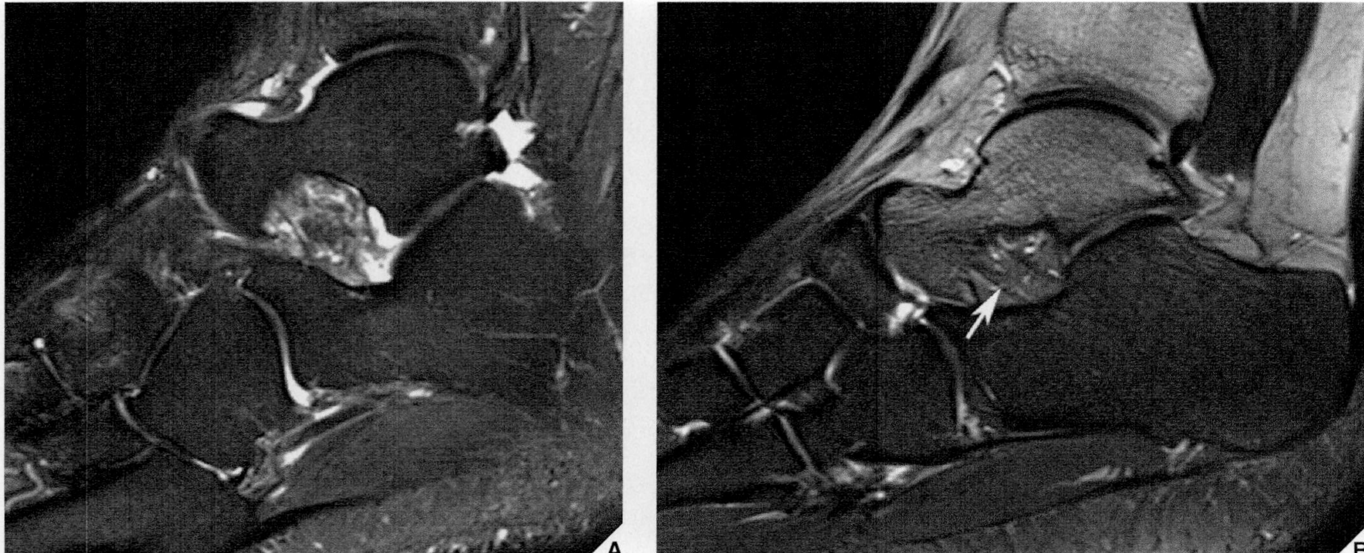

FIGURE 10.112 MRI of sinus tarsi syndrome. **(A)** Sagittal T2-weighted MR image shows edematous changes in the region of the sinus tarsi, with loss of the normal visualization of the interosseus ligaments, characteristic features of this syndrome. **(B)** Sagittal T2-weighted MR image demonstrating normal sinus tarsi with fat signal intensity is shown for comparison. Note the cervical ligament between the talus and calcaneus *(arrow)*.

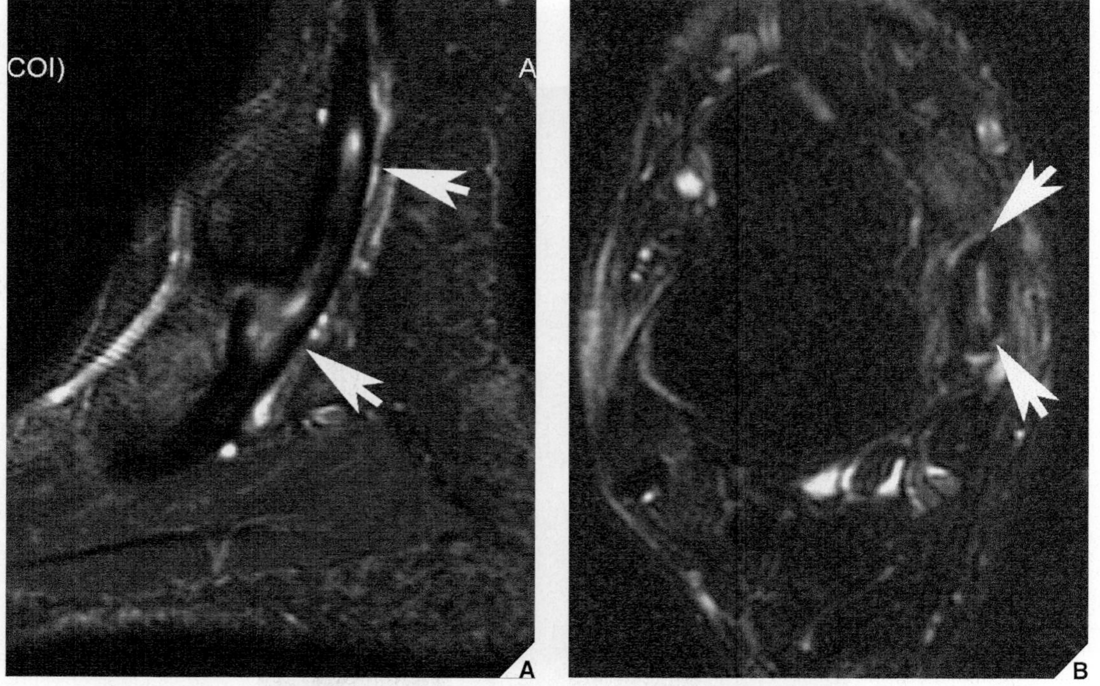

FIGURE 10.113 MRI of posterior tibialis tendon dysfunction. **(A)** Sagittal T2-weighted fat-saturated and **(B)** axial T2-weighted MR images demonstrate thickening of the posterior tibialis tendon with abnormal intrasubstance signal *(arrows)* consistent with severe tendinosis and intrasubstance tear.

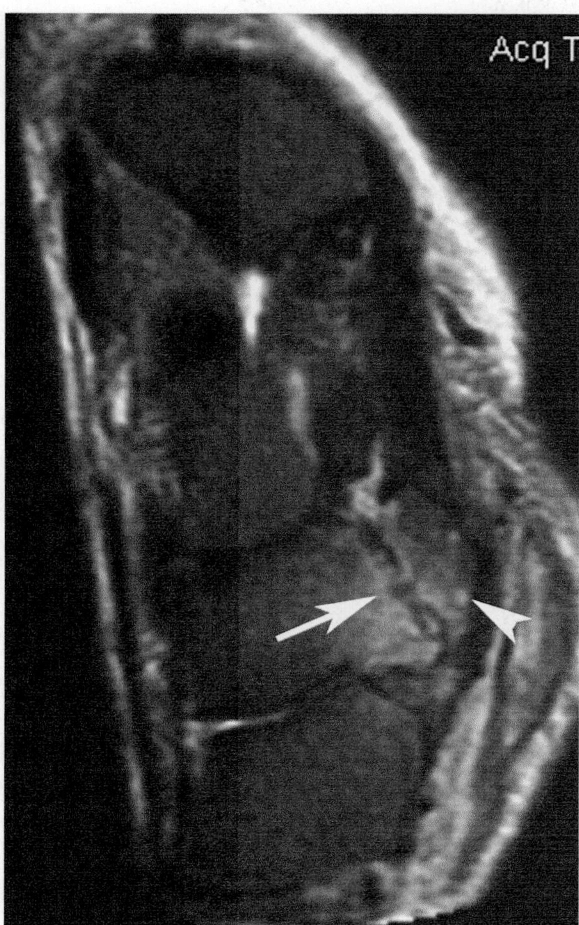

FIGURE 10.114 **MRI of painful accessory navicular bone syndrome.** Sagittal T2-weighted MRI demonstrates a type II triangular-shaped accessory navicular bone *(arrowhead)* with bone marrow edema in the ossicle and in the medial pole of the navicular bone *(arrow)*. Note the distal portion of the posterior tibialis tendon attached to the accessory ossicle.

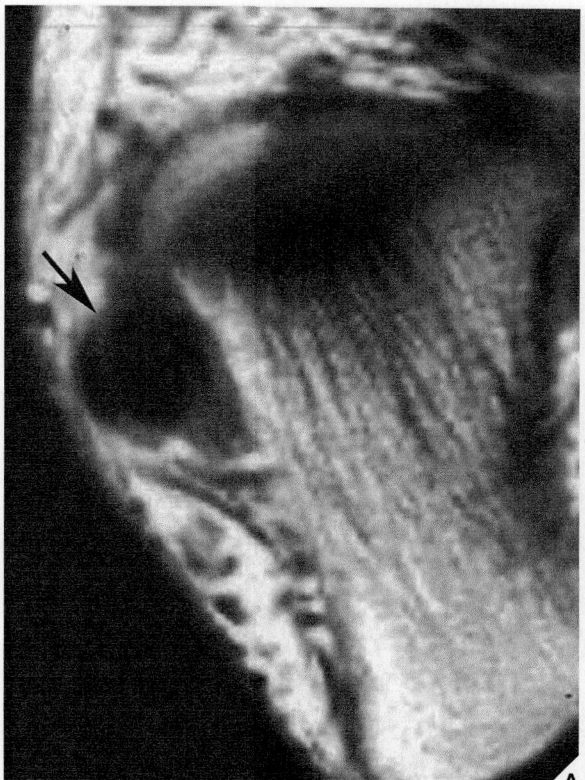

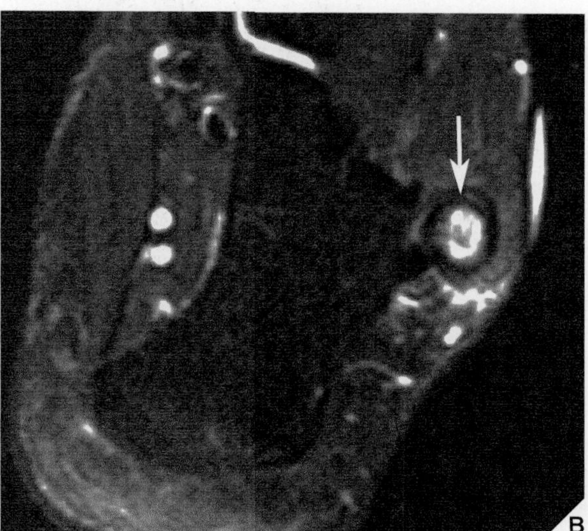

FIGURE 10.115 **MRI of peroneus brevis tears.** **(A)** Axial T1-weighted MR image demonstrates a longitudinal split tear of the peroneus brevis tendon *(arrow)*. **(B)** Axial T2-weighted MR image in another patient demonstrates a complete tear of the peroneus brevis tendon. Note the empty, fluid-distended tendon sheath *(arrow)*.

Peroneal Tendinopathies

Lesions of the peroneus brevis and longus tendons are a frequent cause of posterolateral and lateral ankle and foot pain. Common pathology seen on MRI and US are as follows.

Peroneus Brevis Split Tear

This abnormality is often accompanied with lateral ankle ligamentous instability related to inversion injuries. However sometimes, it is asymptomatic, without history of trauma, and can evolve into a complete tear (Fig. 10.115).

Peroneus Longus Tendinosis and Tear

Patients with this injury present with acute lateral foot pain, but the symptoms can be related to preexisting chronic tendinosis leading to partial and complete tears. Typically, tears of the peroneus longus tendon occur at the entrance of the tendon into the cuboid tunnel and MRI or US can depict the extent of the tear (Fig. 10.116).

Peroneal Tendon Dislocation

Dislocation of the peroneal tendon most commonly occurs as a result of injury during athletic activities. Rapid dorsiflexion with the foot inverted and rapid contraction of the peroneus muscles are the typical mechanisms of this injury. These lesions are often associated with tendinosis and longitudinal tears of the peroneal tendon and tear of the superior peroneal retinaculum. MRI or US can demonstrate the dislocation of the tendons and the underlying tendon damage (Fig. 10.117).

Painful Os Peroneum Syndrome

The os peroneum is a sesamoid bone located within the peroneus longus tendon just proximal to the entrance of the tendon into the cuboid tunnel and is well seen on conventional radiography. Pain in the lateral aspect of the foot can be related to acute or chronic fracture or diastasis of a bipartite or multipartite os peroneum; tendinosis or tear of the peroneus longus

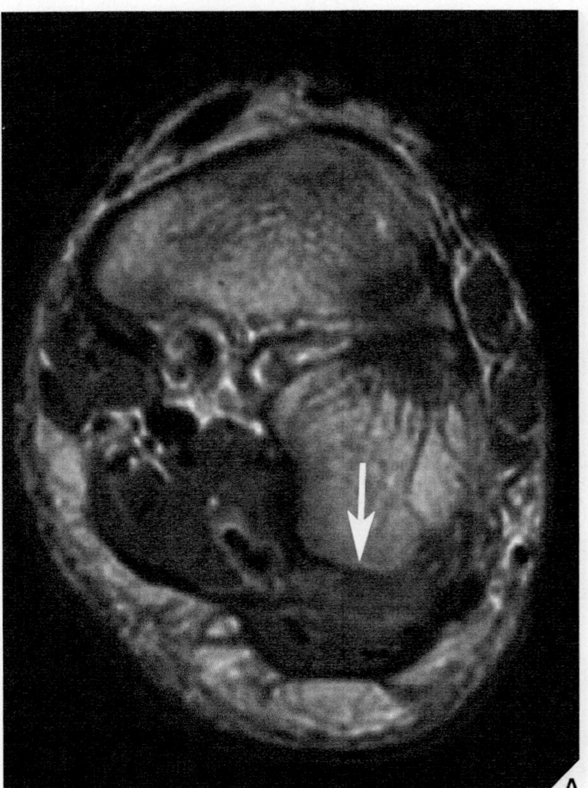

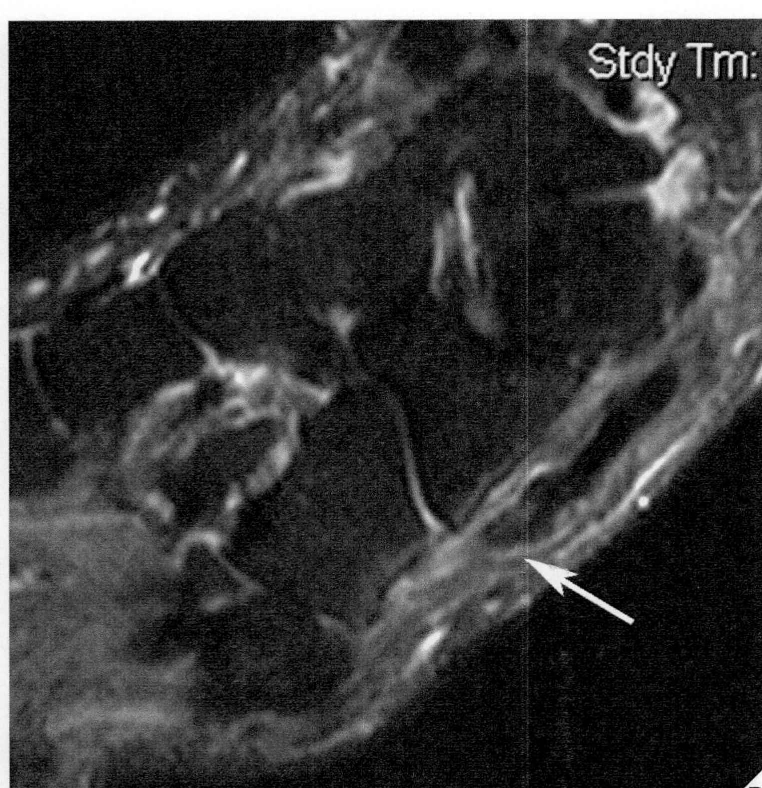

FIGURE 10.116 MRI of peroneus longus tear. **(A)** Short-axis T2-weighted and **(B)** sagittal T2-weighted MR images demonstrate a complete tear of the peroneus longus tendon at the level of the cuboid tunnel, with proximal tendon retraction *(arrows)*.

tendon (as discussed in the preceding section); and presence of a large peroneal tubercle in the lateral aspect of the calcaneus, which can entrap the peroneus longus tendon and the os peroneum during tendon excursion. MRI can demonstrate fragmentation and edema of the os peroneum and associated pathology of the peroneus longus tendon (Fig. 10.118).

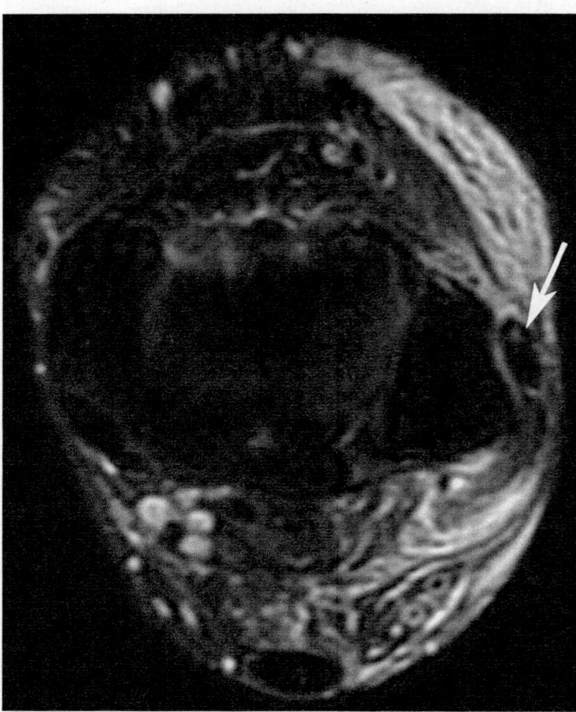

FIGURE 10.117 MRI of dislocation of the peroneal tendons. Axial T2-weighted MRI in a patient with acute lateral ankle pain demonstrates rupture of the peroneal retinaculum and dislocation of the peroneal tendons *(arrow)*, with surrounding soft-tissue edema.

Baxter Neuropathy

Baxter neuropathy is caused by compression of the inferior calcaneal nerve (known as *Baxter nerve*). The most common causes of compression of this nerve include entrapment by a hypertrophied abductor hallucis muscle particularly in runners, compression by inferior calcaneal enthesophyte/thickened plantar fascia, and stretching secondary to a hypermobile pronated foot. MR imaging findings include denervation edema or fatty atrophy of the abductor digiti minimi muscle (Fig. 10.119).

Morton Neuroma

Morton neuroma is caused by chronic entrapment of the plantar interdigital nerve and is more commonly found at the second and third intermetatarsal spaces. Patients present with intermetatarsal pain and numbness exacerbated by walking/standing and relieved by rest and shoe removal. MRI findings include a teardrop-shaped soft-tissue mass in the plantar aspect of the intermetatarsal space. The mass typically demonstrates low signal intensity on T1-weighted and T2-weighted images with enhancement following intravenous injection of gadolinium (Fig. 10.120).

Plantar Fasciitis

The plantar fascia originates on the plantar aspect of the calcaneus, and it extends over the intrinsic muscles of the foot, the abductor digiti minimi (lateral cord), the flexor digitorum brevis (central cord), and the abductor hallucis (medial cord). The most common pathology involving the plantar fascia is plantar fasciitis. Other less common conditions include infection (especially in the diabetic foot) and plantar fibromas. Plantar fasciitis can be acute or chronic. The patients present with pain in the plantar aspect of the heel on weight bearing. Predisposing factors include obesity, enthesopathy, pes cavus, systemic disease (inflammatory arthritis), overuse, altered gait, and trauma. MRI demonstrates thickening and perifascial edema, occasionally associated with plantar spurring and edema of the calcaneus. Occasionally, a tear of the plantar fascia may develop (Fig. 10.121).

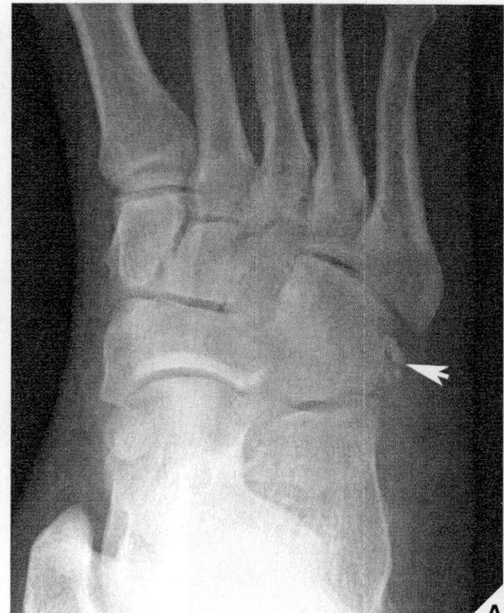

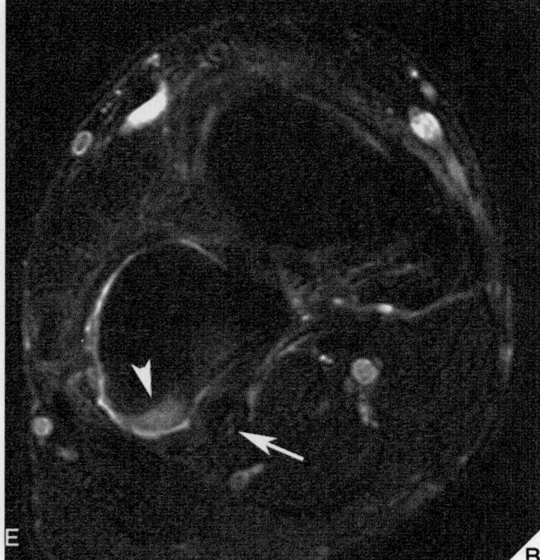

FIGURE 10.118 MRI of POPS. **(A)** Radiograph of the foot of a young man who presented with a lateral foot pain demonstrates fragmentation of the os peroneum *(arrow)*. **(B)** Short-axis T2-weighted fat-saturated MR image demonstrates tendinosis of the peroneus longus tendon within the cuboid tunnel *(arrow)* and associated reactive edema of the cuboid bone *(arrowhead)*.

Impingement Syndromes

Impingement syndromes can produce localized pain in different areas of the ankle and may be related to chronic, repetitive trauma. There are six described impingement syndromes around the ankle:

1. Anterior impingement syndrome, also called *footballer's ankle*, already discussed in chapter 4 (see Fig. 4.151)
2. Anterolateral impingement syndrome, caused by repetitive lateral ankle sprains and synovial proliferation in the anterior lateral gutter, also called *Wolin lesion* (Fig. 10.122; see also Fig. 10.71)
3. Anteromedial impingement syndrome, caused by repetitive anteromedial inversion injuries causing thickening of the deep fibers of the deltoid ligament, chondral lesions, and medial osteophyte formation (Fig. 10.123)
4. Posterior impingement syndrome, also called *os trigonum syndrome*, seen in patients with prominent os trigonum, doing frequent forced plantar flexion of their foot. The os trigonum is impinged between the posterior tibia and the calcaneus in a nutcracker mechanism, leading to focal inflammatory changes, often associated with tenosynovitis of the flexor hallucis longus tendon (Fig. 10.124)
5. Posterior medial impingement syndrome. This syndrome is related to inversion injuries of the ankle leading to hypertrophy and fibrosis of the deltoid ligament and posterior medial capsule. The MRI findings are similar to the anterior medial impingement but extending posteriorly.
6. Calcaneofibular entrapment. Patients with severe hindfoot valgus secondary to entities such as pes planus, posterior tibialis tendon dysfunction, or tarsal coalition may develop bony impingement between the calcaneus and the talus or between the calcaneus and the fibula, in which case the calcaneofibular ligament and/or the peroneal tendons can become entrapped between the osseous structures (Fig. 10.125).

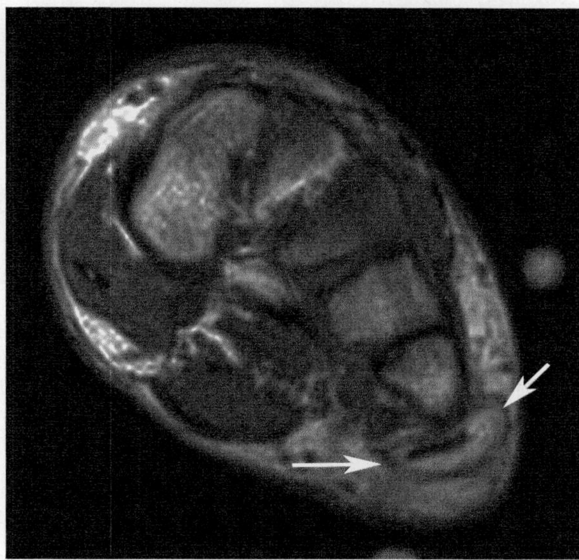

FIGURE 10.119 MRI of Baxter neuropathy. Short-axis T1-weighted MR image demonstrates complete fatty replacement of the abductor digiti minimi *(arrows)*.

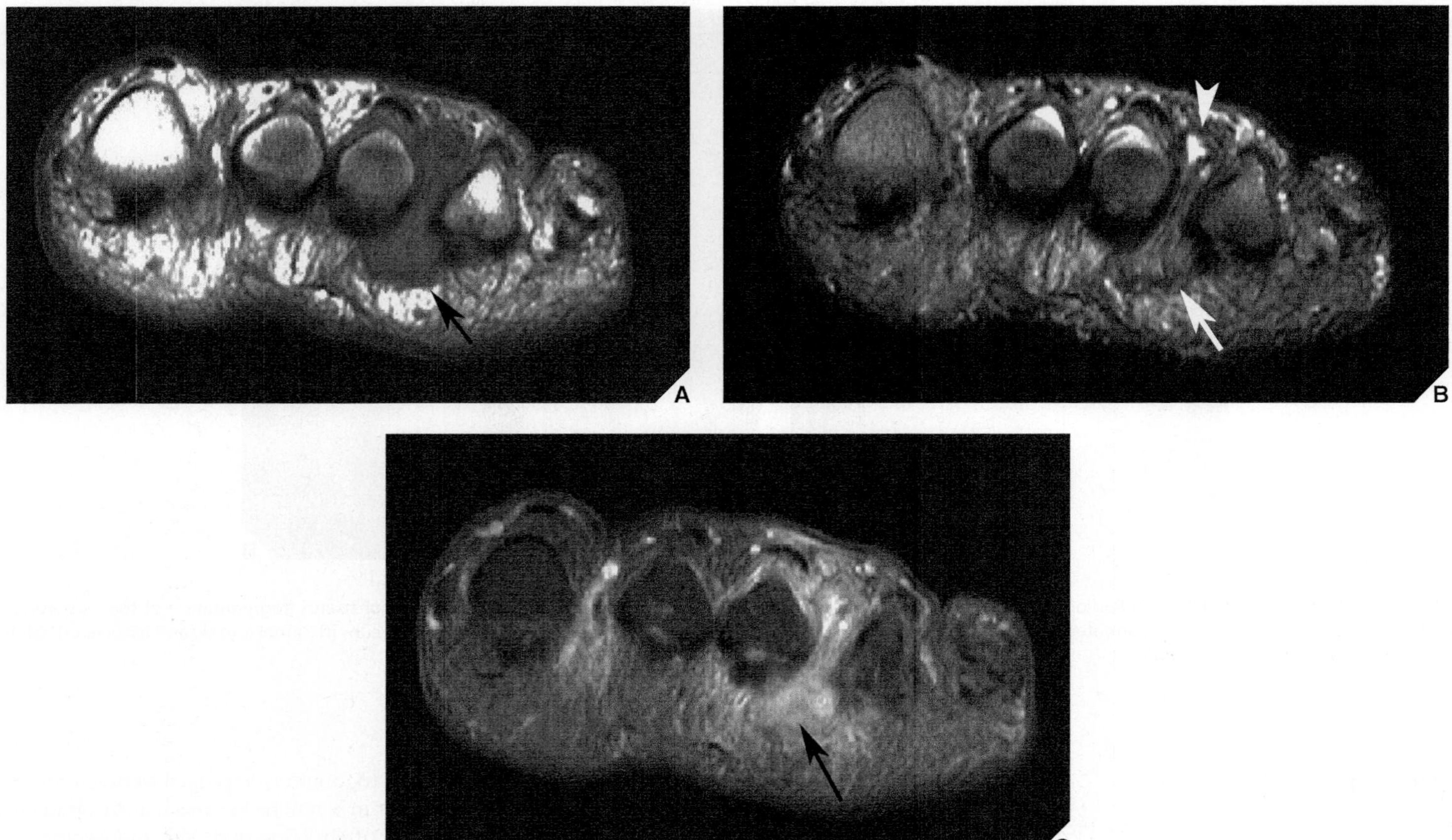

FIGURE 10.120 **MRI of Morton neuroma.** **(A)** Short-axis T1-weighted MR image of the forefoot demonstrates a hypointense mass in the plantar aspect of the third intermetatarsal space *(arrow)*. **(B)** Short-axis T2-weighted MR image demonstrates the neuroma as a hypointense mass similar to the surrounding fat and more difficult to see than on the T1-weighted image *(arrow)*. Note the presence of a small fluid collection in the superior aspect of the third intermetatarsal space, representing bursitis *(arrowhead)*. **(C)** Short-axis T1-weighted fat-saturated MR image obtained at the same level after intravenous administration of gadolinium demonstrates strong enhancement of the neuroma *(arrow)*.

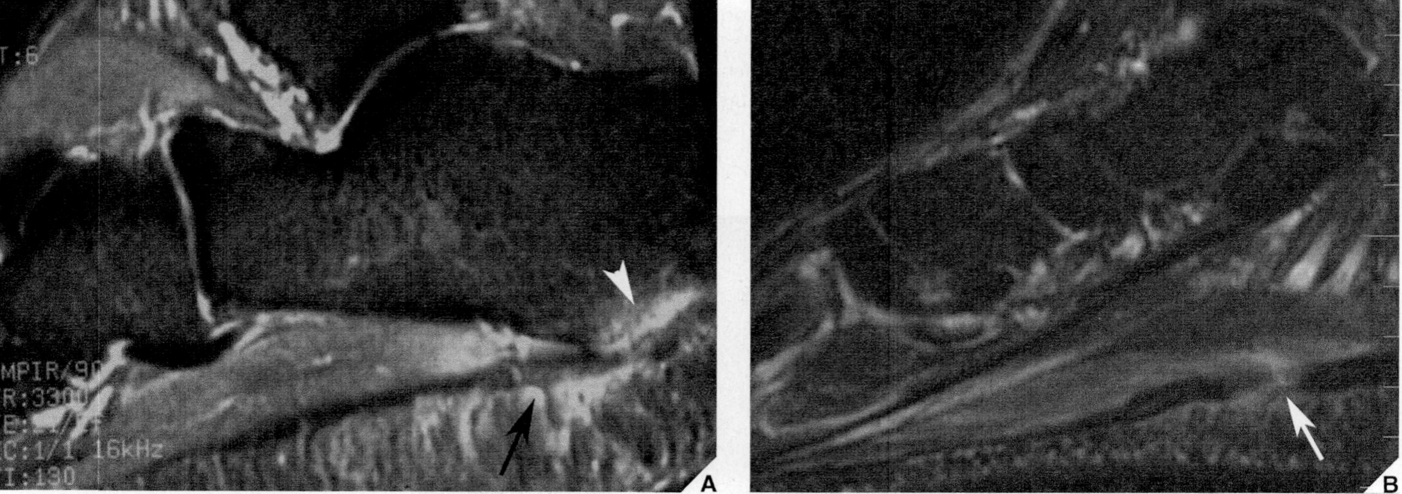

FIGURE 10.121 **MRI of plantar fasciitis.** **(A)** Sagittal T2-weighted MR image of the hindfoot demonstrates thickening and perifascial edema involving the central cord of the plantar fascia *(arrow)*. Note the reactive bone marrow edema of the calcaneus *(arrowhead)*. **(B)** Sagittal T2-weighted MR image in another patient who presented with acute heel pain shows the tear of the central cord of the plantar fascia *(arrow)* with surrounding soft-tissue edema.

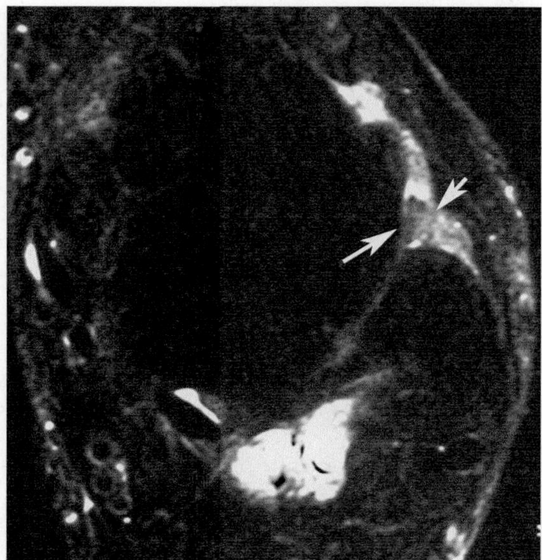

FIGURE 10.122 Anterolateral impingement (Wolin lesion). Axial T2-weighted fat-saturated MR image of the ankle of a patient with history of repetitive ankle sprains. Patient complained of selective pain in the anterolateral aspect of the ankle, especially during eversion and dorsiflexion of the foot (anterolateral impingement). Note the intermediate–signal intensity triangular-shaped lesion in the anterolateral gutter *(arrows)*, corresponding to synovial proliferation (see also Fig. 10.71C).

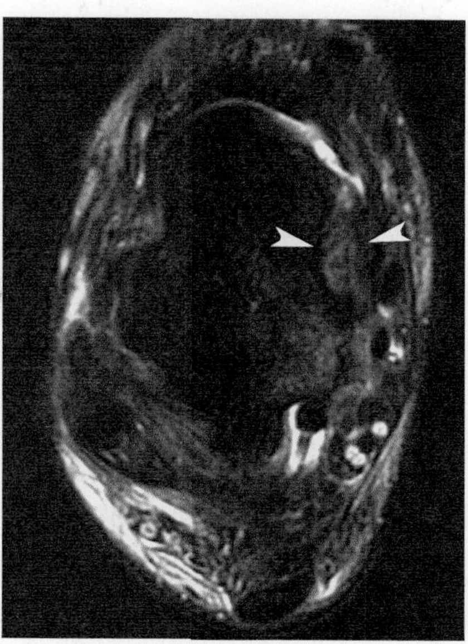

FIGURE 10.123 Anteromedial impingement syndrome. Axial T2-weighted fat-saturated MR image demonstrates thickening of the deep fibers of the deltoid ligament *(arrowheads)*.

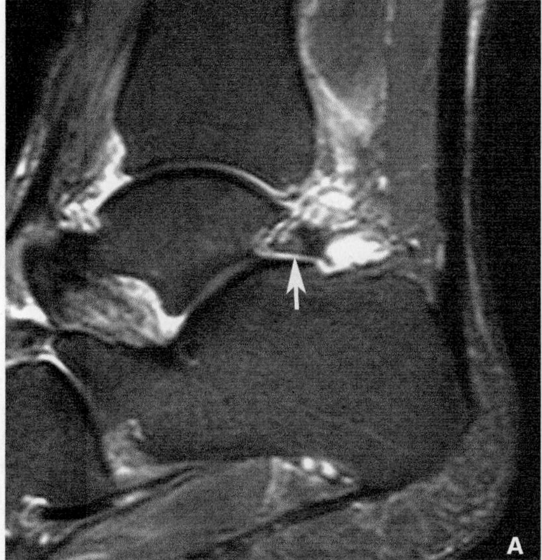

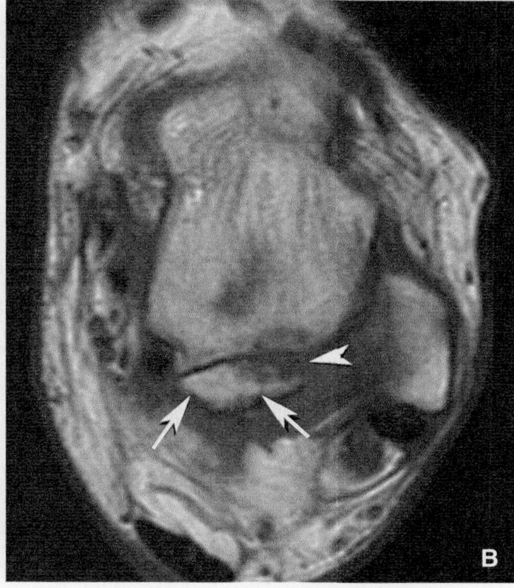

FIGURE 10.124 Os trigonum syndrome/posterior impingement syndrome. **(A)** Sagittal T2-weighted fat-saturated MR image of the ankle demonstrates a prominent os trigonum *(arrow)* with surrounding inflammatory changes. **(B)** Axial T1-weighted MR image shows the prominent os trigonum *(arrows)* with irregularity at the level of the synchondrosis *(arrowhead)*.

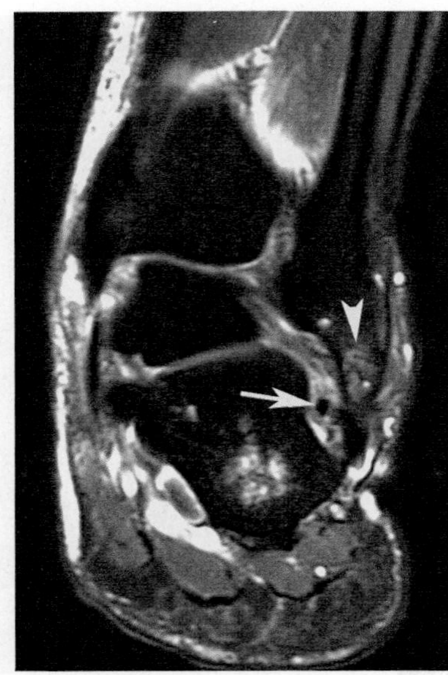

FIGURE 10.125 Calcaneofibular entrapment. Coronal T2-weighted fat-saturated MR image in a patient with subtalar coalition demonstrates hindfoot valgus with edematous changes of the lateral malleolus *(arrowhead)* and entrapment of the calcaneofibular ligament between the lateral malleolus and the calcaneus *(arrow)*.

PRACTICAL POINTS TO REMEMBER

Ankle

1. There are three principal sets of ligaments around the ankle joint:
   - the medial collateral (deltoid) ligament
   - the lateral collateral ligament
   - the distal tibiofibular syndesmotic complex.
2. Traumatic conditions of the ankle should be evaluated according to the mechanism that caused the injury, including:
   - inversion-stress forces
   - eversion-stress forces
   - complex stresses combining supination or pronation with rotation, abduction, or adduction.
3. Inversion-stress forces may manifest in a spectrum of injuries to the lateral collateral ligament as well as in associated fractures of the distal tip of the fibula and occasionally the medial malleolus.
4. Eversion-stress forces may manifest in a range of injuries to the medial collateral (deltoid) ligament as well as fracture of the medial malleolus. Pott, Maisonneuve, and Dupuytren fractures are all eversion injuries.
5. Pilon (pylon) fracture is a comminuted fracture of the distal tibia with extension into the tibiotalar joint.
6. Tillaux fracture consists of avulsion of the lateral margin of distal tibia resulting from abduction and external rotation injury.
7. Juvenile Tillaux fracture is a Salter-Harris type III injury to the distal tibial growth plate.
8. Triplanar Marmor-Lynn fracture consists of a vertical fracture through the distal tibial epiphysis (in the sagittal plane), horizontal fracture through the lateral aspect of the distal tibial growth plate (in the axial plane), and oblique fracture through the distal metaphysis extending into the diaphysis (in the coronal plane).
9. Traumatic conditions of the structures about the ankle joint may not be obvious on the standard radiographic examination when only damage of soft-tissue structures is present. Correct management of such injuries may be much more important to a successful orthopaedic outcome than correct management of a simple fracture. For this reason, stress views and MRI are of paramount importance for full evaluation of the extent of damage to the complex structures about the joint.
10. The ligament structure most important for congruence of the joint and ankle stability is the distal tibiofibular syndesmotic complex.
11. Lauge-Hansen classification of ankle trauma is based on the mechanism of injury, combining the position of the foot with the direction of deforming force vector.
12. The Weber classification of ankle fractures—based on the level of fibular fracture—is practical for assessing the risk of future ankle instability because of its emphasis on the lateral syndesmotic–malleolar complex as an important factor in ankle joint stability.
13. MRI is a noninvasive modality capable of demonstrating pathologic conditions of tendons and ligaments by displaying discontinuity of the anatomic structures, the presence of abnormal signal within them, and the presence of inflammatory changes.

Foot

1. It is important to recognize the multiple accessory ossicles of the foot:
   - the normal appearance of these secondary ossification centers may mimic fractures
   - conversely, an avulsion fracture may be misinterpreted as a normal ossicle.
2. Harris-Beath and Broden views, both tangential projections, are important techniques for evaluating injury to the subtalar joint.
3. The Boehler angle demonstrates an important anatomic relation of the calcaneus and subtalar joint. It is useful for evaluating compression fracture of the calcaneus, particularly with extension into the subtalar joint.
4. The angle of Gissane is helpful to diagnose the fractures of the dorsal aspect of calcaneus extending to the posterior facet of the subtalar joint.
5. In fracture of the calcaneus (so-called *lover's fracture*), look for an associated compression fracture of the vertebral body in the thoracic or lumbar spine.
6. Hawkins classification of talar neck fractures is based on the damage to the blood supply of the talus and serves as a prognostic guide for healing of the fracture, incidence of osteonecrosis, and indication for open reduction.
7. MRI is effective modality to demonstrate Shepherd fracture of the posterior medial process of talus, Cedell fracture of the posterior lateral process of talus, and snowboarder fracture (fracture of the lateral process of talus).
8. Learn to diagnose the OCD of the talus based on Berndt and Harty as well as Anderson classification of this abnormality.
9. In Lisfranc fracture–dislocation in the tarsometatarsal articulation, always look for an associated fracture either:
   - at the base of the metatarsals
   - or in the cuneiform bones.
10. Several painful conditions of the foot can be effectively diagnosed with MRI or US. Among them are the following abnormalities: chronic tendinosis of the posterior tibialis tendon, painful accessory navicular bone syndrome, peroneus longus tendinosis and tear, peroneal tendon dislocation, painful os peroneum syndrome (POPS), Baxter neuropathy, Morton neuroma, plantar fasciitis, anterolateral impingement syndrome (Wolin lesion), anteromedial impingement syndrome, os trigonum syndrome, and calcaneal entrapment.

SUGGESTED READINGS

Ala-Ketola L, Puranen J, Koivisto E, et al. Arthrography in the diagnosis of ligament injuries and classification of ankle injuries. *Radiology* 1977;125:63–68.

Anderson IF, Crichton KJ, Grattan-Smith T, et al. Osteochondral fractures of the dome of the talus. *J Bone Joint Surg Am* 1989;71:1143–1152.

Arimoto HK, Forrester DM. Classification of ankle fractures: an algorithm. *AJR Am J Roentgenol* 1980;135:1057–1063.

Beltran J. Magnetic resonance imaging of the ankle and foot. *Orthopedics* 1994;17:1075–1082.

Beltran J, Munchow AM, Khabiri H, et al. Ligaments of the lateral aspect of the ankle and sinus tarsi: an MR imaging study. *Radiology* 1990;177:455–458.

Bencardino J, Rosenberg ZS. MR imaging and CT in the assessment of osseous abnormalities of the ankle and foot. *Magn Reson Imaging Clin N Am* 2001;9:567–577.

Berndt AL, Harty M. Transchondral fractures (osteochondritis dissecans) of the talus. *J Bone Joint Surg Am* 1959;41A:988–1020.

Berquist TM. Foot, ankle, and calf. In: Berquist TM, ed. *MRI of the musculoskeletal system*. New York: Raven Press; 1990:253–311.

Boruta PM, Bishop JO, Braly WG, et al. Acute lateral ankle ligament injuries: a literature review. *Foot Ankle* 1990;11:107–113.

Brown KW, Morrison WB, Schweitzer ME, et al. MRI findings associated with distal tibiofibular syndesmosis injury. *AJR Am J Roentgenol* 2004;182:131–136.

Canale ST, Kelly FB Jr. Fractures of the neck of the talus. Long-term evaluation of seventy-one cases. *J Bone Joint Surg Am* 1978;60(2):143–156.

Cave EF. Fracture of the calcis—the problem in general. *Clin Orthop Relat Res* 1963;30: 64–66.

Cheung Y, Rosenberg ZS, Magee T, et al. Normal anatomy and pathologic conditions of ankle tendons: current imaging techniques. *Radiographics* 1992;12:429–444.

Chundru U, Liebeskind A, Seidelmann F, et al. Plantar fasciitis and calcaneal spur formation are associated with abductor digiti minimi atrophy on MRI of the foot. *Skeletal Radiol* 2008;37:505–510.

Cone RO III, Nguyen V, Flournoy JG, et al. Triplane fracture of the distal tibial epiphysis: radiographic and CT studies. *Radiology* 1984;153:763–767.

Corbett M, Levy A, Abramowitz AJ, et al. A computer tomographic classification system for the displaced intraarticular fracture of the os calcis. *Orthopedics* 1995;18:705–710.

Daffner RH. Ankle trauma. *Radiol Clin North Am* 1990;28:395–421.

De Smet AA, Fisher DR, Burnstein MI, et al. Value of MR imaging in staging osteochondral lesions of the talus (osteochondritis dissecans): results in 14 patients. *AJR Am J Roentgenol* 1990;154:555–558.

Donnelly EF. The Hawkins sign. *Radiology* 1999;210:195–196.

Donovan A, Rosenberg ZS. MRI of ankle and lateral hindfoot impingement syndromes. *AJR Am J Roentgenol* 2010;195:595–604.

Doyle T, Napier RJ, Wong-Chung J. Recognition and management of Müller-Weiss disease. *Foot Ankle Int* 2012;33:275–281.

Eichenholtz S, Levine DB. Fractures of the tarsal navicular bone. *Clin Orthop Relat Res* 1964;34:142.

Erickson SJ, Quinn SF, Kneeland JB, et al. MR imaging of the tarsal tunnel and related spaces: normal and abnormal findings with anatomic correlation. *AJR Am J Roentgenol* 1990;155:323–328.

Essex-Lopresti P. The mechanism, reduction technique, and results in fracture of the os calcis. *Br J Surg* 1952;39:395–419.

Farooki S, Yao L, Seeger LL. Anterolateral impingement of the ankle: effectiveness of MR imaging. *Radiology* 1998;207:357–360.

Finkel JE. Tarsal tunnel syndrome. *Magn Reson Imaging Clin N Am* 1994;2:67–78.

Gallo RA, Kolman BH, Daffner RH, et al. MRI of tibialis anterior tendon rupture. *Skeletal Radiol* 2004;33:102–106.

Geissler WB, Tsao AK, Hughes JL. Fractures and injuries of the ankle. In: Rockwood CA, Green DP, Bucholz RW, et al, eds. *Rockwood and Green's fractures in adults*, 4th ed. Philadelphia: Lippincott-Raven Publishers; 1996:2236–2242.

Goss CM, Gray H, eds. *Anatomy of the human body*, 29th ed. Philadelphia: Lea & Febiger; 1973:355–359.

Greenspan A. Imaging of the foot and ankle. *Curr Opin Orthop* 1996;7:61–68.

Greenspan A, Anderson MW. Imaging of the foot and ankle. *Curr Opin Orthop* 1993;4: 68–75.

Hawkins LG. Fractures of the lateral process of the talus. *J Bone Joint Surg Am* 1965;47: 1170–1175.

Hawkins LG. Fractures of the neck of the talus. *J Bone Joint Surg Am* 1970;52(5):991–1002.

Heckman JD. Fractures and dislocations of the foot. In: Rockwood CA Jr, Green DP, Bucholz RW, et al, eds. *Rockwood and Green's fractures in adults*, 4th ed. Philadelphia: Lippincott-Raven; 1996:2295–2308.

Higashiyama I, Kumai T, Takakura Y, et al. Follow-up study of MRI for osteochondral lesion of the talus. *Foot Ankle Int* 2000;21:127–133.

Jeong MS, Choi YS, Kim YJ, et al. Deltoid ligament in acute ankle injury: MR imaging analysis. *Skeletal Radiol* 2014;43:655–663.

Jones R. I. Fracture of the base of the fifth metatarsal by direct violence. *Ann Surg* 1902;35:697.

Kalia V, Fishman EK, Carrino JA, et al. Epidemiology, imaging, and treatment of Lisfranc fracture-dislocation revisited. *Skeletal Radiol* 2012;41:129–136.

Keck C. The tarsal-tunnel syndrome. *J Bone Joint Surg Am* 1962;44:180–182.

Kleiger B. Mechanisms of ankle injury. *Orthop Clin North Am* 1974;5:127–146.

Kleiger B. Review of ankle fractures due to lateral strains. *Bull Hosp Joint Dis* 1968;29:138–186.

Klein MA, Spreitzer AM. MR imaging of the tarsal sinus and canal: normal anatomy, pathologic findings, and features of the sinus tarsi syndrome. *Radiology* 1993;186:233–240.

Lam SJ. A tarsal-tunnel syndrome. *Lancet* 1962;2:1354–1355.

Lau JTC, Daniels TR. Tarsal tunnel syndrome: a review of the literature. *Foot Ankle Int* 1999;20:201–209.

Lauge-Hansen N. Fractures of the ankle: analytical survey as the basis of new experimental, roentgenologic and clinical investigations. *Arch Surg* 1948;56:259–317.

Lauge-Hansen N. Fractures of the ankle. II. Combined experimental-surgical and experimental-roentgenologic investigations. *Arch Surg* 1950;60:957–985.

Lauge-Hansen N. Ligamentous ankle fractures: diagnosis and treatment. *Acta Chir Scand* 1949;97:544–550.

Lee SH, Jacobson J, Trudell D, et al. Ligaments of the ankle: normal anatomy with MR arthrography. *J Comput Assist Tomogr* 1998;22:807–813.

Lee SJ, Jacobson JA, Kim S-M, et al. Ultrasound and MRI of the peroneal tendons and associated pathology. *Skeletal Radiol* 2013;42:1191–1200.

Leitch JM, Cundy PJ, Paterson DC. Three-dimensional imaging of a juvenile Tillaux fracture. *J Pediatr Orthop* 1989;9:602–603.

Lynn MD. The triplane distal tibial epiphyseal fracture. *Clin Orthop Relat Res* 1972;86: 187–190.

Magid D, Michelson JD, Ney DR, et al. Adult ankle fractures: comparison of plain films and interactive two- and three-dimensional CT scans. *AJR Am J Roentgenol* 1990;154:1017–1023.

Mainwaring BL, Daffner RH, Riemer BL. Pylon fractures of the ankle: a distinct clinical and radiologic entity. *Radiology* 1988;168:215–218.

Marmor L. An unusual fracture of the tibial epiphysis. *Clin Orthop Relat Res* 1970;73:132–135.

Mast J. Pilon fractures of the tibia. In: Chapman MW, ed. *Operative orthopaedics*, 2nd ed. Philadelphia: JB Lippincott; 1993:711–729.

Mehlhorn AT, Zwingmann J, Hirschmüller A, et al. Radiographic classification for fractures of the fifth metatarsal base. *Skeletal Radiol* 2014;43:467–474.

Müller ME, Allgower M, Schneider R, et al. *Manual of internal fixation techniques recommended by AO Group*, 2nd ed. New York: Springer; 1979.

Müller ME, Nazarian S, Koch P. *The AO classification of fractures*. New York: Springer; 1979.

Norman A, Kleiger B, Greenspan A, et al. Roentgenographic examination of the normal foot and ankle. In: Jahss MM, ed. *Disorders of the foot and ankle: Medical and surgical management*, vol. 1, 2nd ed. Philadelphia: WB Saunders; 1991:64–90.

Oae K, Takao M, Naito K, et al. Injury of the tibiofibular syndesmosis: value of MR imaging for diagnosis. *Radiology* 2003;227:155–161.

Peltier LF. Eponymic fractures: Robert Jones and Jones's fracture. *Surgery* 1972;71:522–526.

Peltier LF. Guillaume Dupuytren and Dupuytren's fracture. *Surgery* 1958;43:868–874.

Peltier LF. Percival Pott and Pott's fracture. *Surgery* 1962;51:280–286.

Pennal GF. Fractures of the talus. *Clin Orthop Relat Res* 1963;30:53–63.

Protas JM, Kornblatt BA. Fractures of the lateral margin of the distal tibia. The Tillaux fracture. *Radiology* 1981;138:55–57.

Rademaker J, Rosenber Z, Delfaut EM, et al. Tear of the peroneus longus tendon: MR imaging features in nine patients. *Radiology* 2000;214:700–704.

Robinson P, White LM. Soft-tissue and osseous impingement syndromes of the ankle: role of imaging in diagnosis and management. *Radiographics* 2002;22:1457–1471.

Rosenberg ZS, Beltran J, Bencardino JT. MR imaging of the ankle and foot. *Radiographics* 2000;20:S153–S179.

Rosenberg ZS, Bencardino J, Astion D, et al. MRI features of chronic injuries of the superior peroneal retinaculum. *AJR Am J Roentgenol* 2003;181:1551–1557.

Rowe CR, Sakellarides HT, Freeman PA, et al. Fracture of the os calcis: a long-term follow-up study of 146 patients. *JAMA* 1963;184:920.

Sanders R, Fortin P, DiPasquale T, et al. Operative treatment in 120 displaced intraarticular calcaneal fractures. Results using a prognostic computed tomography scan classification. *Clin Orthop Relat Res* 1993;290:87–95.

Sangeorzan BJ, Benirschke SK, Mosca V, et al. Displaced intra-articular fractures of the tarsal navicular. *J Bone Joint Surg Am* 1989;71:1504–1510.

Serbest S, Tiftikçi U, Tosun HB, et al. Isolated posterior malleolus fracture: a rare injury mechanism. *Pan Afr Med J* 2015;20:123.

Sharif B, Welck M, Saifuddin A. MRI of the distal tibiofibular joint. *Skeletal Radiol* 2020;49:1–17.

Shelton ML, Pedowitz WJ. Injuries to the talus and midfoot. In: Jahs MH, ed. *Disorders of the foot & ankle*, vol. 2. Philadelphia: WB Saunders; 1982:1463.

Smeeing DPJ, Houwert RM, Kruyt MC, et al. The isolated posterior malleolar fracture and syndesmotic instability: a case report and review of the literature. *Int J Surg Case Rep* 2017;41:360–365.

Sripanich Y, Weinberg MW, Krähenbühl N, et al. Imaging in Lisfranc injury: a systematic literature review. *Skeletal Radiol* 2020;49:31–53.

Stewart I. Jones' fracture: fracture of the base of the fifth metatarsal. *Clin Orthop* 1960;16:190–198.

Swanson TV. Fractures and dislocations of the talus. In: Chapman MW, ed. *Operative orthopaedics*, 2nd ed. Philadelphia: JB Lippincott; 1993:2143–2145.

Tehranzadeh J, Stuffman E, Ross SDK. Partial Hawkins sign in fractures of the talus: a report of three cases. *AJR Am J Roentgenol* 2003;181:1559–1563.

Theodorou DJ, Theodorou SJ, Kakitsubata Y, et al. Fractures of proximal portion of fifth metatarsal bone: anatomic and imaging evidence of a pathogenesis of avulsion of the plantar aponeurosis and the short peroneal muscle tendon. *Radiology* 2003;226:857–865.

Theodorou DJ, Theodorou SJ, Resnick D. Proximal fifth metatarsal bone: not everything is a Jones' fracture [abstract]. *Radiology* 2001;221(P):667.

Weber BG. *Die Verletzungen des Oberen Sprunggelenkes*. Stuttgart: Verlag Hans Huber; 1972.

Weber MJ. Ankle fractures and dislocations. In: Chapman MW, ed. *Operative orthopaedics*, 2nd ed. Philadelphia: JB Lippincott; 1993:731–745.

Wright PR, Fox MG, Alford B, et al. An alternative injection technique for performing MR ankle arthrography: the lateral mortise approach. *Skeletal Radiol* 2014;43:27–33.

Yablon CM. Ultrasound-guided interventions of the foot and ankle. *Semin Musculoskeletal Radiol* 2013;17:60–68.

Zanetti M, Weishaupt D. MR imaging of the forefoot: Morton neuroma and differential diagnoses. *Semin Musculoskelet Radiol* 2005;3:175–186.

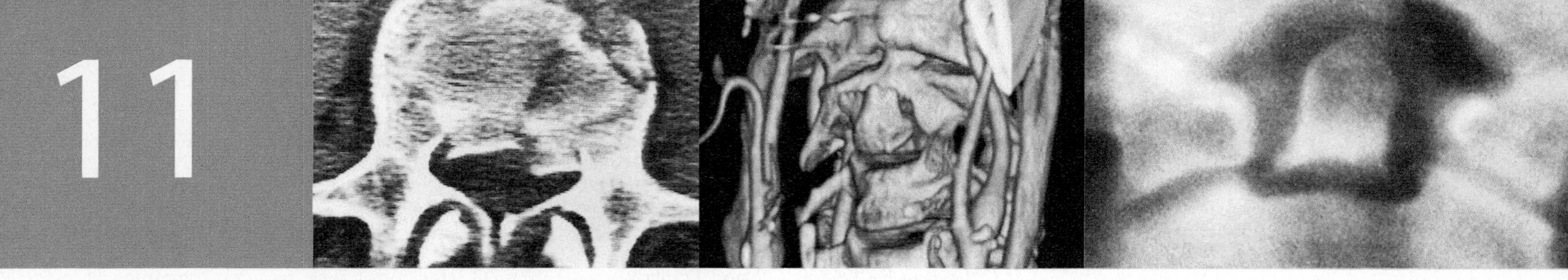

Spine

Introduction

Fractures of the vertebral column are important not only because of the structures involved but also because of the complications that may arise affecting the spinal cord. Constituting approximately 3% to 6% of all skeletal injuries, fractures of the vertebral column are most commonly encountered in people between the ages of 20 and 50 years, with the majority of cases (80%) being seen in males. Most spinal fractures occur at the thoracic and lumbar levels, but injury to the cervical area has a greater potential risk for spinal cord damage. Automobile accidents, sports-related activities (e.g., diving, skiing), and falls from heights are usually the circumstances in which spinal injuries are sustained.

The spine is composed of 33 vertebrae: 7 cervical, 12 thoracic, 5 lumbar, a sacrum of 5 fused segments, and a coccyx of 4 fused segments. With the exception of the first and second cervical vertebrae (C1 and C2), the vertebral bodies are separated from each other by intervertebral disks.

Cervical Spine

Anatomic–Radiologic Considerations

Structurally, the first and second cervical vertebrae possess anatomic features distinct from those of the remaining five cervical vertebrae (Fig. 11.1). The first cervical vertebra, C1 or atlas, is an osseous ring consisting of anterior and posterior arches connected by two lateral masses. The atlas has no body; its main structures are the lateral masses, also called *articular pillars*. The second vertebra, C2 or axis, is a more complex structure whose distinguishing feature is the odontoid process, also known as the *dens* (tooth), projecting cephalad from the anterior surface of the body. The space between the odontoid process and the anterior arch of the atlas, called the *atlantal–dens interval*, should not exceed 3 mm in adults, whether the head is flexed or extended. In children younger than age 8 years, this distance has been reported to be as much as 4 mm, particularly in flexion, secondary to greater ligamentous laxity.

The vertebrae C3-7 exhibit identical anatomic features and are more uniform in appearance, consisting of a vertebral body and a posterior neural arch, including the right and left pedicles and laminae, which together with the posterior aspect of the body enclose the spinal canal (Fig. 11.2). Extending caudad and cephalad from the junction of the pedicle and lamina on each side are superior and inferior articular processes, which form the apophyseal joints between the successive vertebrae. Extending laterally from the pedicle on each side is a transverse process and, in the posterior portion, a spinous process extends from the junction of the laminae in the midline. The vertebra C7, in addition, is distinguished by its long spinous process and large transverse processes.

Radiographic examination of a patient with cervical spine trauma may be difficult and is usually limited to one or two projections; because frequently, the patient is unconscious, there are associated injuries and unnecessary movement risks damage to the cervical cord. The single most valuable projection in these instances is the lateral view, which may be obtained in the standard fashion or with the patient supine, depending on the condition (Fig. 11.3). This projection suffices to demonstrate most traumatic conditions of the cervical spine, including injuries involving the anterior and posterior arches of C1; the odontoid process, which is seen in profile; and the anterior atlantal–dens interval. The bodies and spinous processes of C2-7 are fully visualized, and the intervertebral disk spaces and prevertebral soft tissues can be adequately evaluated. The lateral radiograph may also be obtained in flexion of the neck, which is particularly effective in demonstrating suspected instability at C1-2 by allowing evaluation of the atlanto–odontoid distance; an increase in this distance to more than 3 mm indicates atlantoaxial subluxation. It is of the utmost importance on the lateral projection of the cervical spine that the C7 vertebra be visualized because this is the most commonly overlooked site of injuries.

The lateral view of the cervical spine, including the lower part of the skull, is extremely important to evaluate the vertical subluxation involving the atlantoaxial articulation and the migration of the odontoid process into the foramen magnum. Several measurements are helpful to determine atlantoaxial impaction or cranial settling resulting in cephalad migration of the odontoid process (Figs. 11.4 to 11.7).

On the anteroposterior radiograph of the cervical spine (Fig. 11.8), the bodies of the C3-7 vertebrae (and occasionally in young persons, even the C1 and C2 vertebrae) are well demonstrated, as are the uncovertebral (Luschka) joints and the intervertebral disk spaces. The spinous processes are seen almost on end, casting oval shadows resembling teardrops. A variant of the anteroposterior projection known as the *open-mouth view* (Fig. 11.9) may also be obtained as part of the standard examination. This view provides effective visualization of the structures of the first two cervical vertebrae. The body of C2 is clearly imaged, as are the atlantoaxial joints, the odontoid process, and the lateral spaces between the odontoid process and the articular pillars of C1. If the open-mouth view is difficult to obtain or the odontoid process is not clearly visualized, particularly its upper half, then the Fuchs view may be helpful (Fig. 11.10). Oblique projections of the cervical spine (Fig. 11.11) are not routinely obtained, although at times they help visualize obscure fractures of the neural arch and abnormalities of the neural foramina and apophyseal joints. Special projections may occasionally be required for sufficient evaluation of the structures of the cervical spine. The pillar view (Fig. 11.12), which may be obtained in the anteroposterior or oblique projection, serves to demonstrate the lateral masses of the cervical vertebrae, and the swimmer's view (Fig. 11.13) may be used for better demonstration of the C7, T1, and T2 vertebrae, which on the standard lateral or oblique projection are obscured by the overlapping clavicle and soft tissues of the shoulder girdle. Fluoroscopy and videotaping are usually of little help in acute injuries because pain may prevent the necessary movement for positioning.

In order to not overlook an abnormality during evaluation of the conventional radiographs of the cervical spine, systematic approach to the imaging study is of paramount importance. "JOB LIST" such as provided in Figure 11.14 may be of help to methodically analyze the various anatomic structures.

TOPOGRAPHIC ANATOMY OF THE C-1 AND C-2 VERTEBRAE

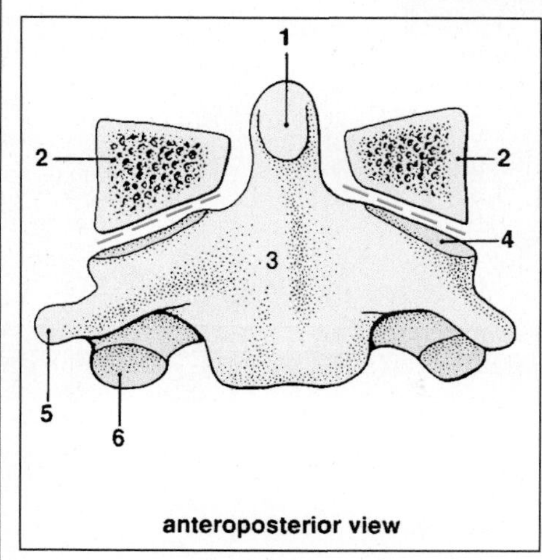

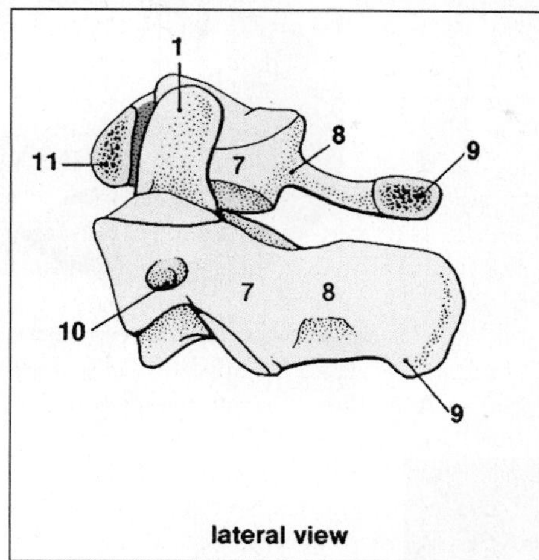

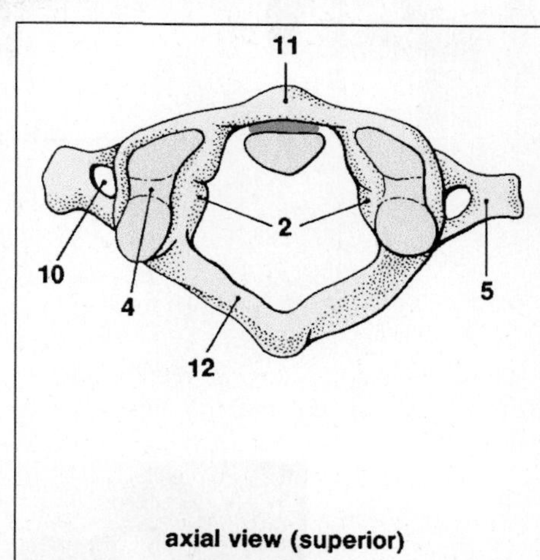

atlantoaxial joint
atlantal-dens interval

1 odontoid process of axis (dens)
2 lateral masses of atlas
3 body of axis
4 superior articular facet
5 transverse process
6 inferior articular facet
7 pedicle
8 lamina
9 spinous process
10 transverse foramen
11 anterior arch of atlas
12 posterior arch of atlas

FIGURE 11.1 Topographic anatomy of the C1 and C2 vertebrae.

TOPOGRAPHIC ANATOMY OF THE C-4 AND C-5 VERTEBRAE

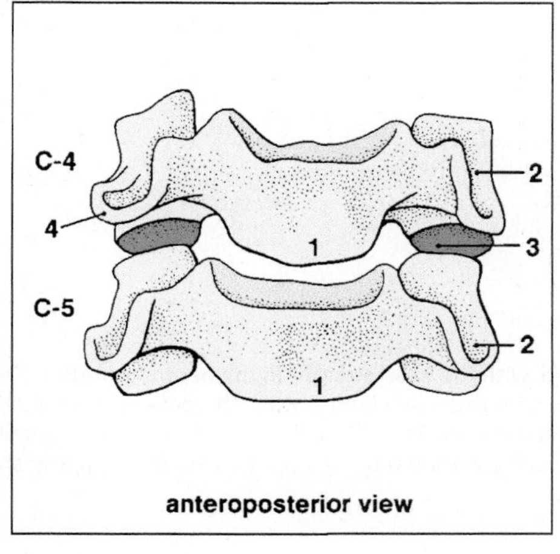

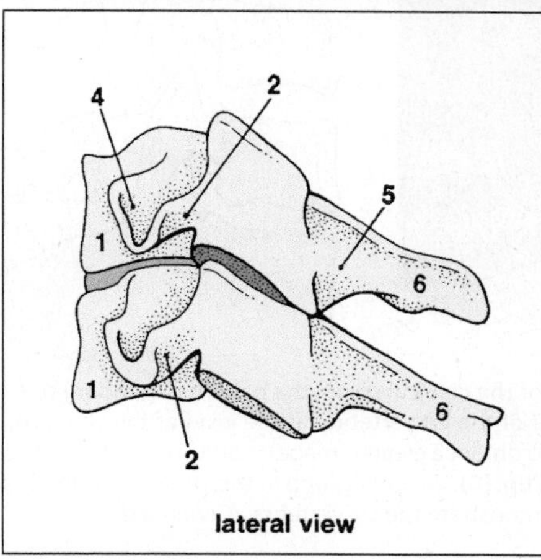

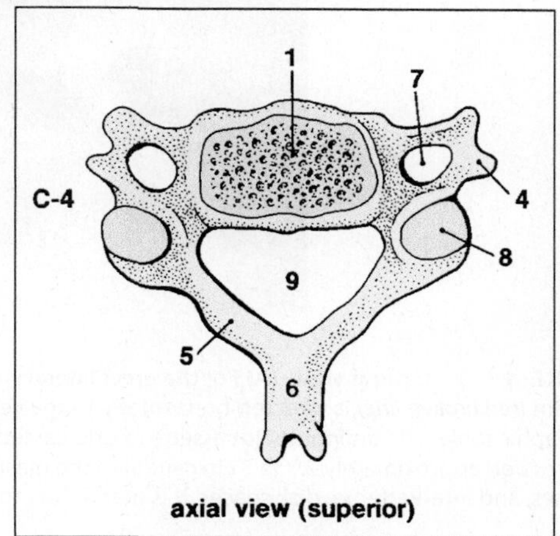

intervertebral disk
apophyseal joint

1 vertebral body
2 pedicle
3 inferior articular process
4 transverse process
5 lamina
6 spinous process
7 transverse foramen
8 superior articular process
9 spinal canal

FIGURE 11.2 Topographic anatomy of the C4 and C5 vertebrae, representing the midcervical and lower cervical vertebrae.

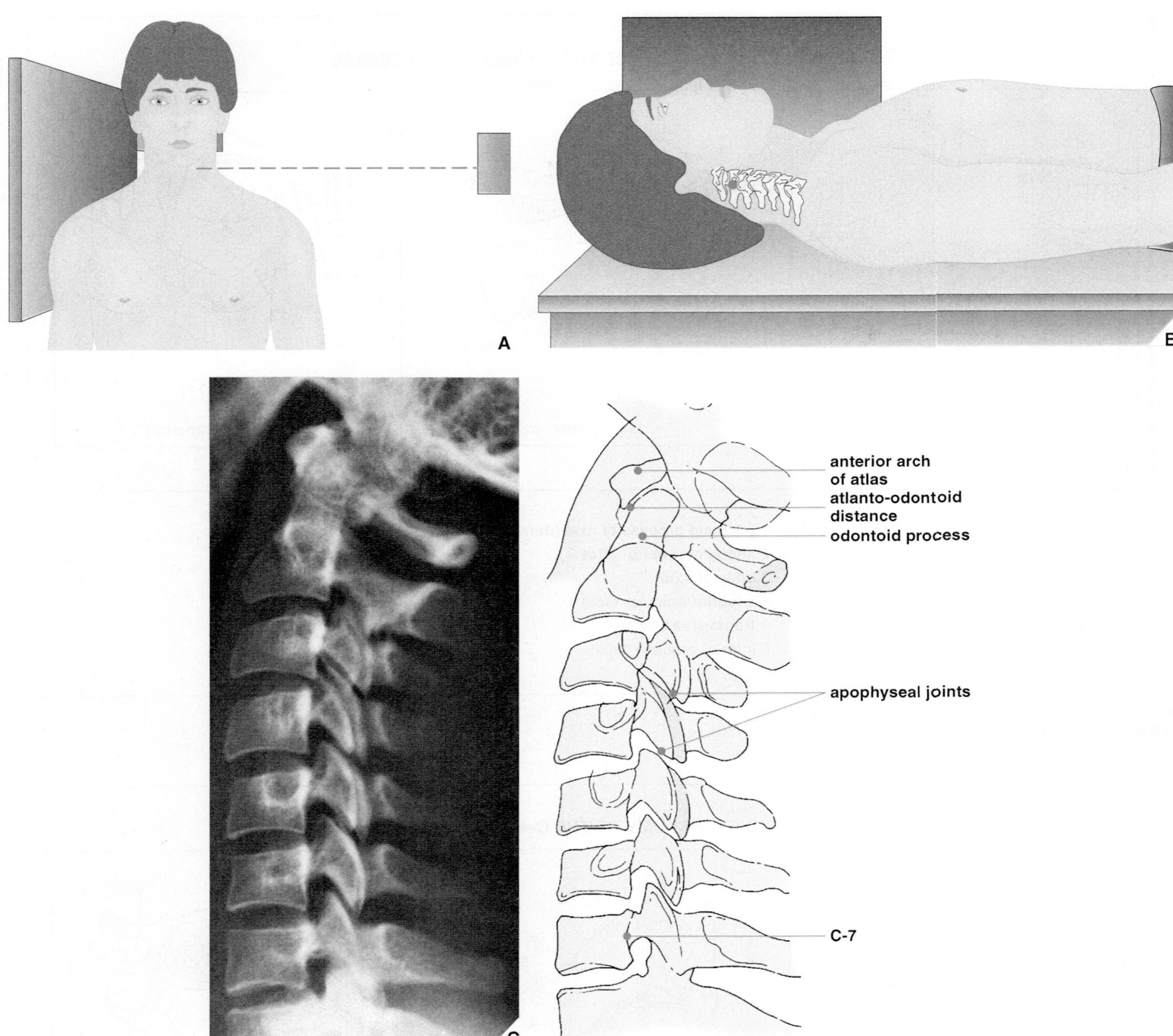

FIGURE 11.3 Lateral view. **(A)** For the erect lateral view of the cervical spine, the patient is standing or seated, with the head straight in the neutral position. The central beam *(red broken line)* is directed horizontally to the center of the C4 vertebra (at the level of the chin). **(B)** For the cross-table lateral view, the patient is supine on the radiographic table. The radiographic cassette (a grid cassette to obtain a clearer image) is adjusted to the side of the neck, and the central beam is directed horizontally to a point *(red dot)* approximately 2.5 to 3 cm caudal to the mastoid tip. **(C)** The radiograph in this projection clearly shows the vertebral bodies, apophyseal (facet) joints, spinous processes, and intervertebral disk spaces. It is mandatory to demonstrate the C7 vertebra. *(Continued)*

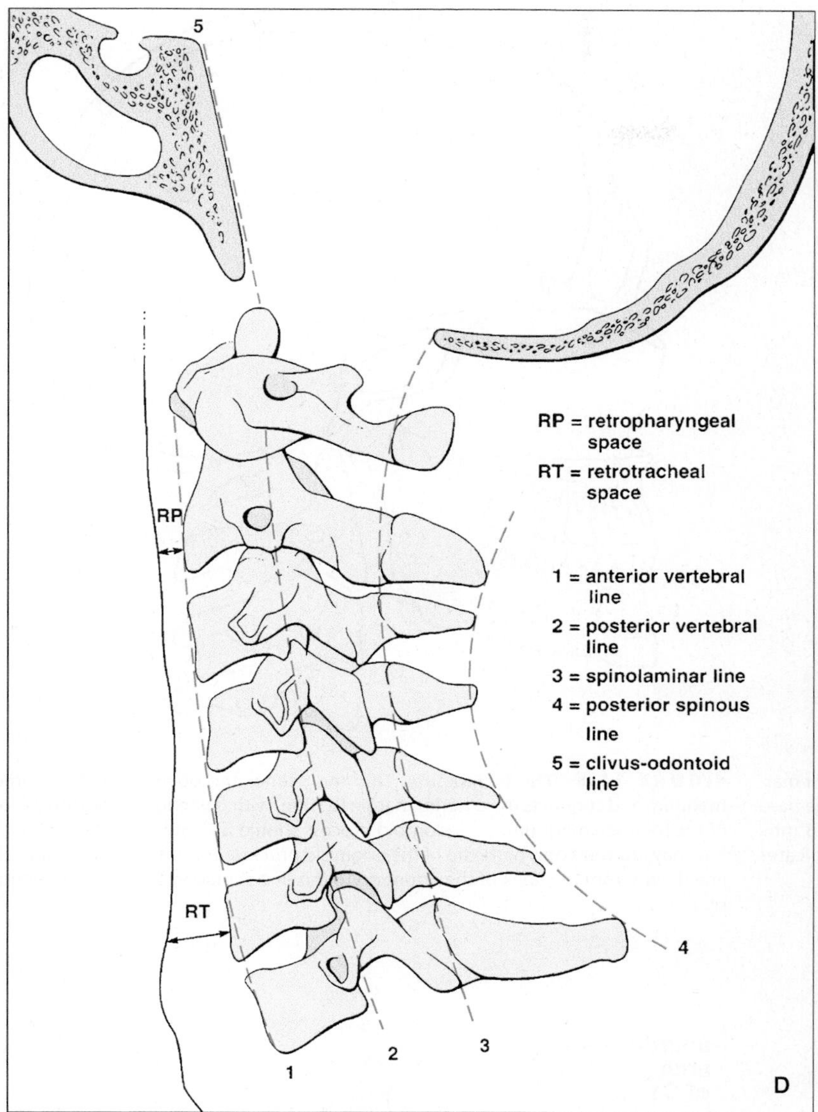

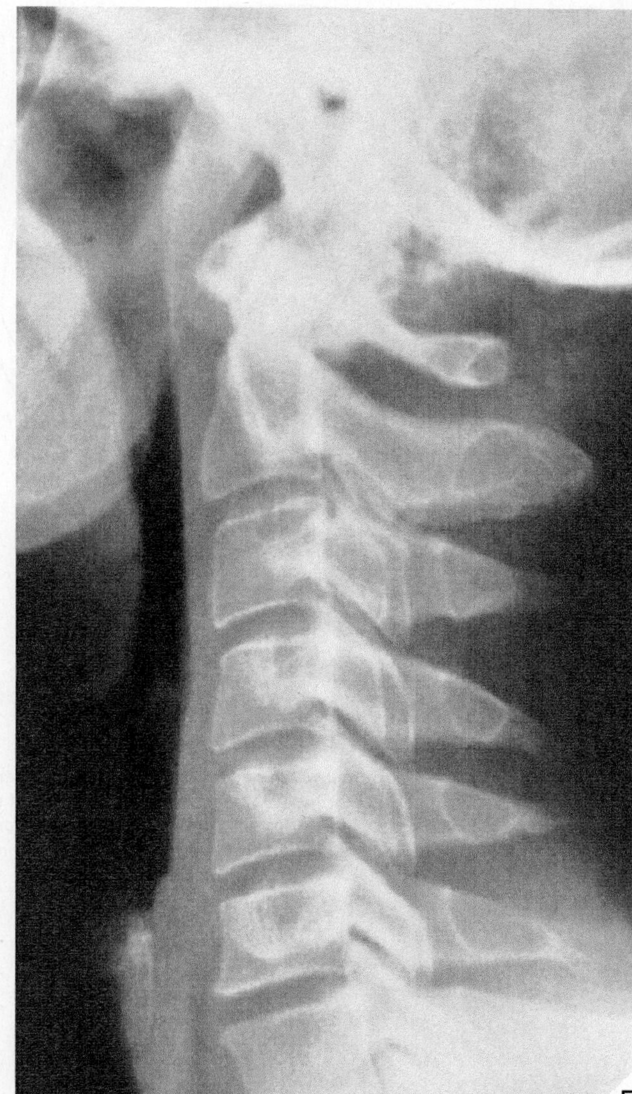

FIGURE 11.3 Lateral view. ***(Continued)*** **(D)** With this view, the five contour lines of the normal cervical spine can be demonstrated: anterior vertebral line, drawn along anterior margins of the vertebral bodies; posterior vertebral line (outlines anterior margin of spinal canal), drawn along posterior margins of the vertebral bodies; spinolaminar line (outlines posterior margin of the spinal canal), drawn along the anterior margins of the bases of the spinous processes at the junction with lamina; posterior spinous line, drawn along the tips of the spinous processes from C2-7, which should be running smoothly, without angulation or interruption; and the clivus-odontoid line, drawn from the dorsum sellae along the clivus to the anterior margin of the foramen magnum, which should point to the tip of the odontoid process at the junction of the anterior and middle thirds. The retropharyngeal space (distance from the posterior pharyngeal wall to the anteroinferior aspect of C2) should measure 7 mm or less; the retrotracheal space (distance from the posterior wall of the trachea to the anteroinferior aspect of C6) should measure no more than 22 mm in adults and 14 mm in children. **(E)** Radiograph obtained with low-kilovoltage technique demonstrates prevertebral soft tissues to better advantage.

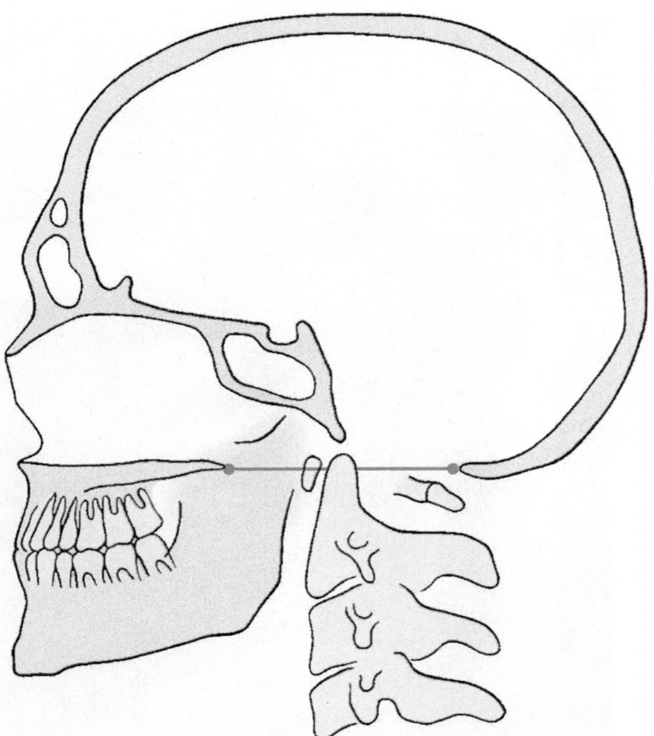

FIGURE 11.4 The Chamberlain line. This line is drawn from the posterior margin of the foramen magnum (opisthion) to the dorsal (posterior) margin of the hard palate. The odontoid process should not project above this line more than 3 mm; a projection of 6.6 mm (±2 standard deviation [SD]) above this line strongly indicates cranial settling.

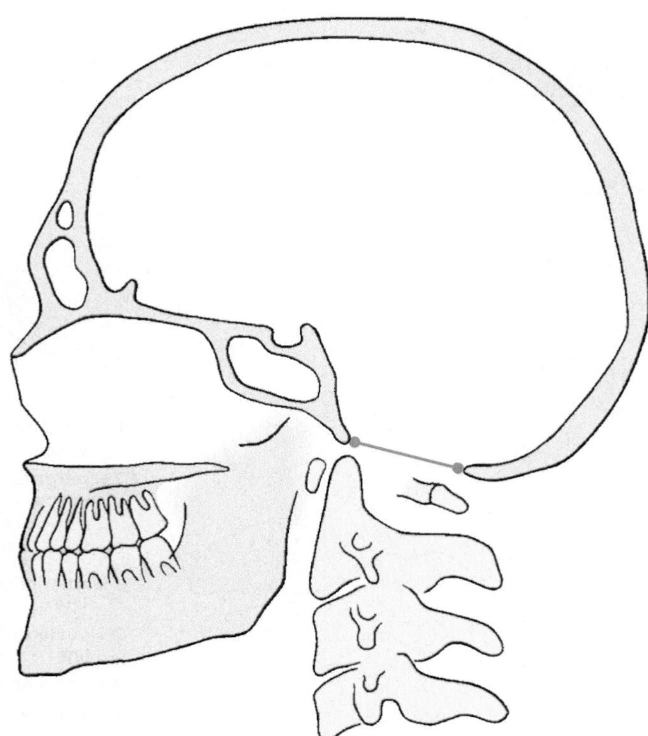

FIGURE 11.5 The McRae line. This line defines the opening of the foramen magnum and connects the anterior margin (basion) with posterior margin (opisthion) of the foramen magnum. The odontoid process should be just below this line or the line may intersect only at the tip of the odontoid process. In addition, a perpendicular line drawn from the apex of the odontoid to this line should intersect it in its ventral quarter.

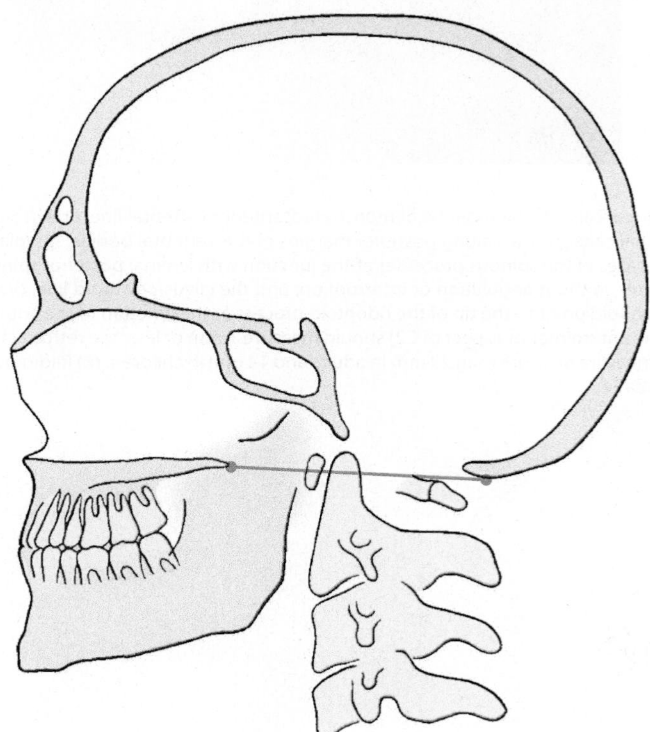

FIGURE 11.6 The McGregor line. This line connects the posterosuperior margin of the hard palate to the most caudal part of the occipital curve of the skull. The tip of the odontoid normally does not extend more than 4.5 mm above the line.

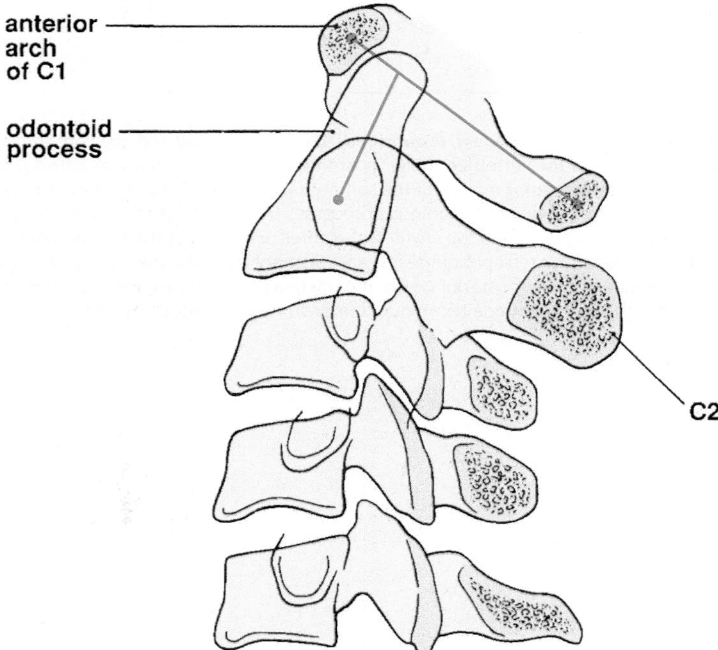

FIGURE 11.7 The Ranawat method. Ranawat and associates developed a method for determining the extent of the superior margin of the odontoid process because the hard palate often is not identifiable on radiographs of the cervical spine. The coronal axis of C1 is determined by connecting the center of the anterior arch of the first cervical vertebra with its posterior ring. The center of the sclerotic ring in C2, representing the pedicles, is marked. The line is drawn along the axis of the odontoid process to the first line. The normal distance between C1 and C2 in men averages 17 mm (± 2 mm standard deviation [SD]) and in women, 15 mm (± 2 mm SD). A decrease in this distance indicates cephalad migration of C2.

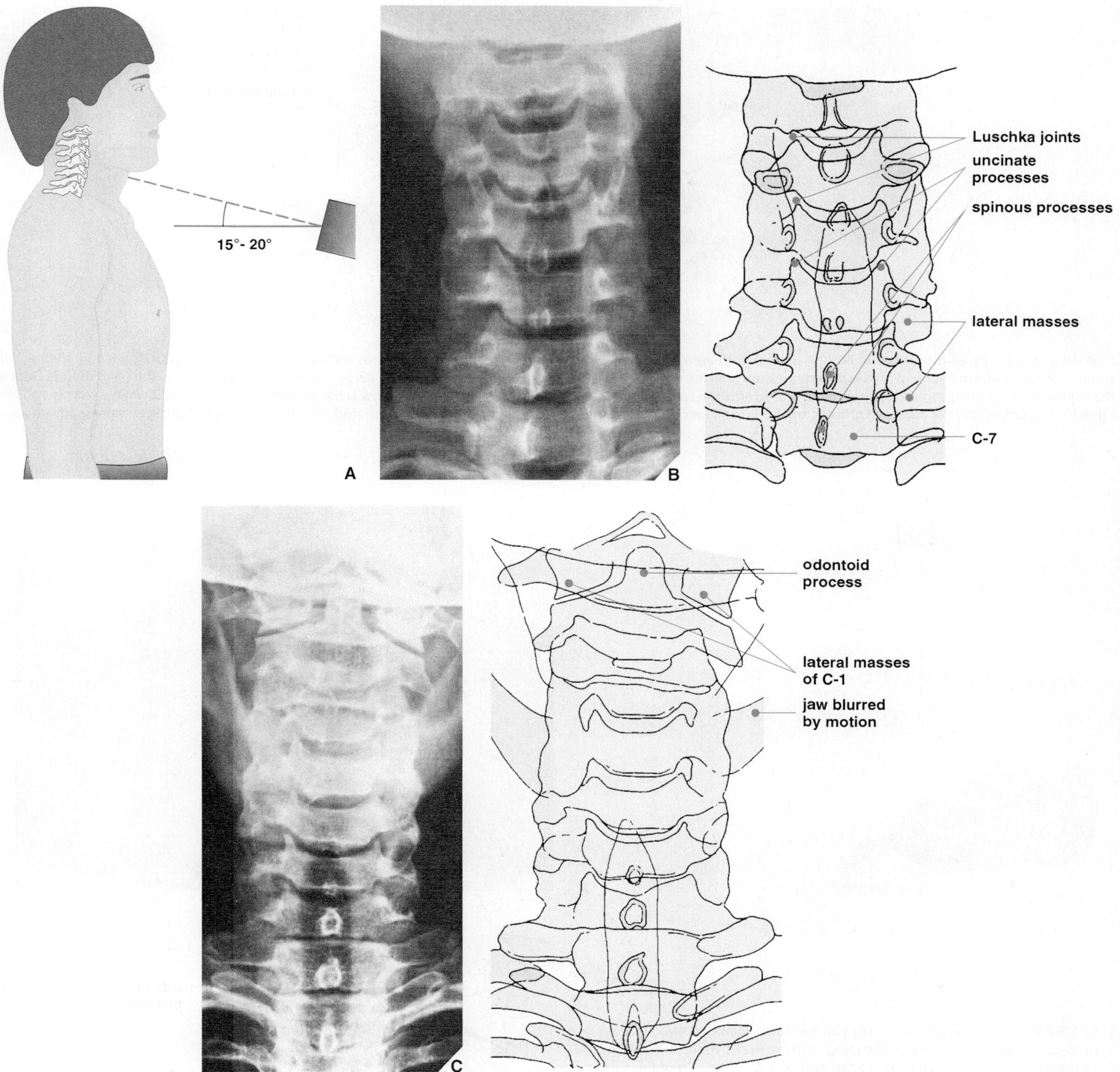

FIGURE 11.8 Anteroposterior view. **(A)** For the anteroposterior view of the cervical spine, the patient is either erect or supine. The central beam is directed toward the C4 vertebra (at the point of the Adam's apple) at an angle of 15 to 20 degrees cephalad. **(B)** The radiograph in this projection demonstrates the C3-7 vertebral bodies and the intervertebral disk spaces. The spinous processes are seen superimposed on the bodies, resembling teardrops. The C1 and C2 vertebrae are not adequately seen. For their visualization, the patient is instructed to open and close the mouth rapidly. Motion of the mandible blurs this structure, and C1 and C2 become visible **(C)**.

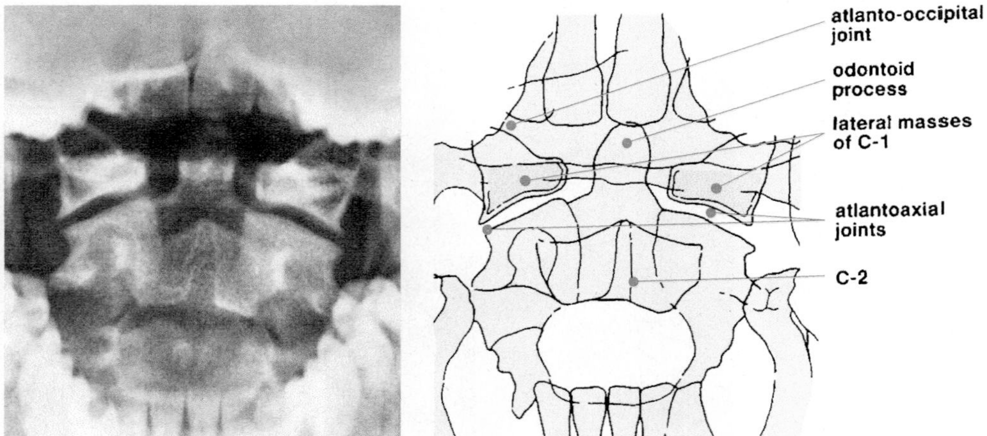

FIGURE 11.9 Open-mouth view. For the open-mouth view, the patient is positioned in the same manner as for the supine anteroposterior projection; the head is straight, in the neutral position. With the patient's mouth open as widely as possible, the central beam is directed perpendicular to the midpoint of the open mouth. During the exposure, the patient should softly phonate "ah" to affix the tongue to the floor of the mouth so that its shadow is not projected over C1 and C2. On the radiograph obtained in this projection, the odontoid process, the body of C2, and the lateral masses of the atlas are well demonstrated; the atlantoaxial joints are seen to best advantage.

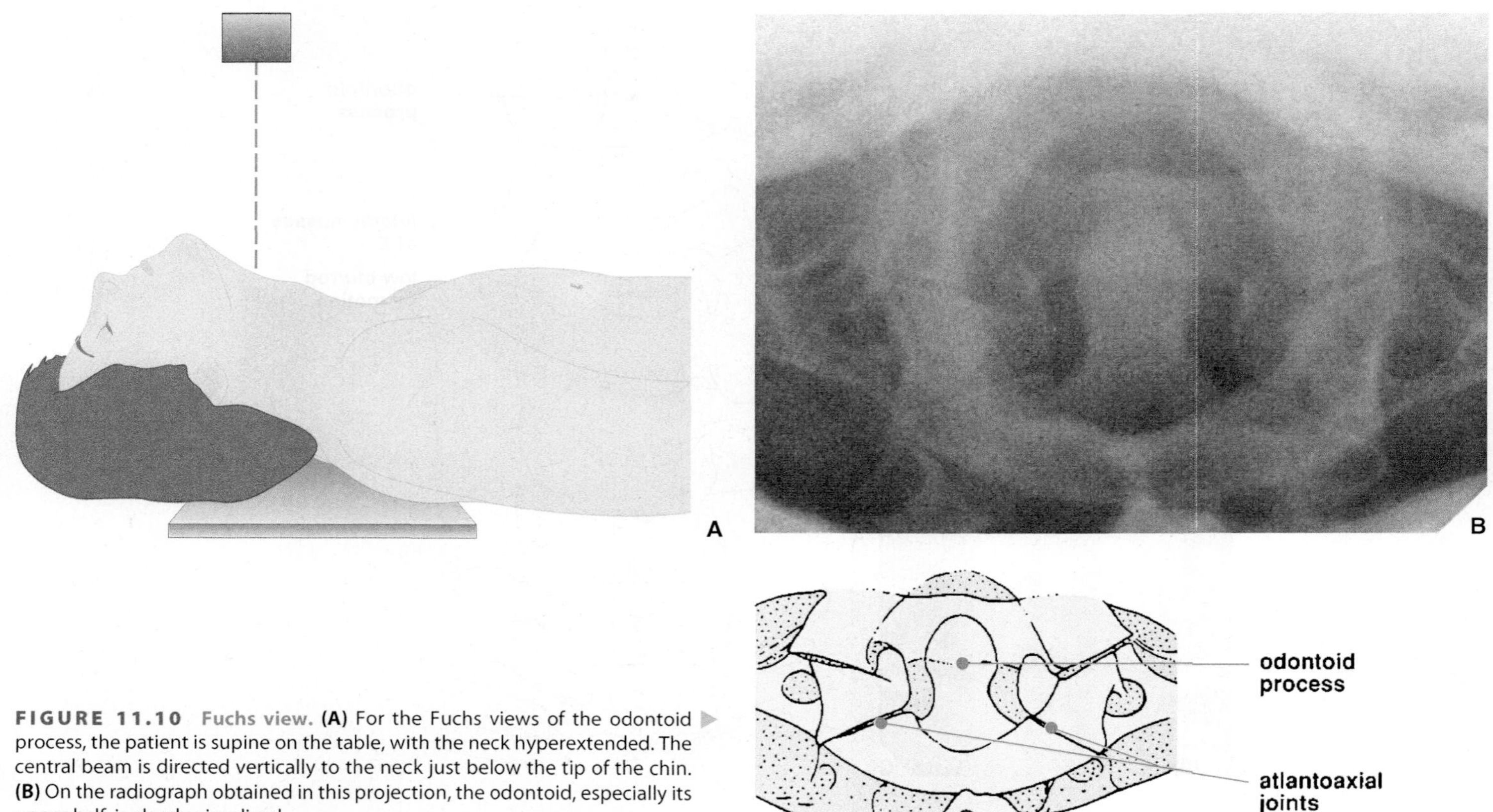

FIGURE 11.10 Fuchs view. **(A)** For the Fuchs views of the odontoid process, the patient is supine on the table, with the neck hyperextended. The central beam is directed vertically to the neck just below the tip of the chin. **(B)** On the radiograph obtained in this projection, the odontoid, especially its upper half, is clearly visualized.

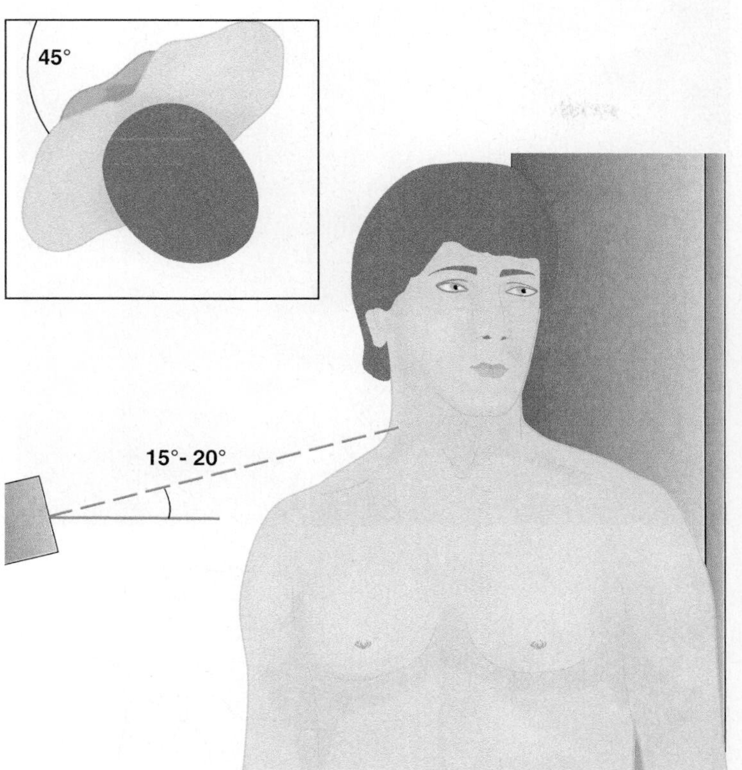

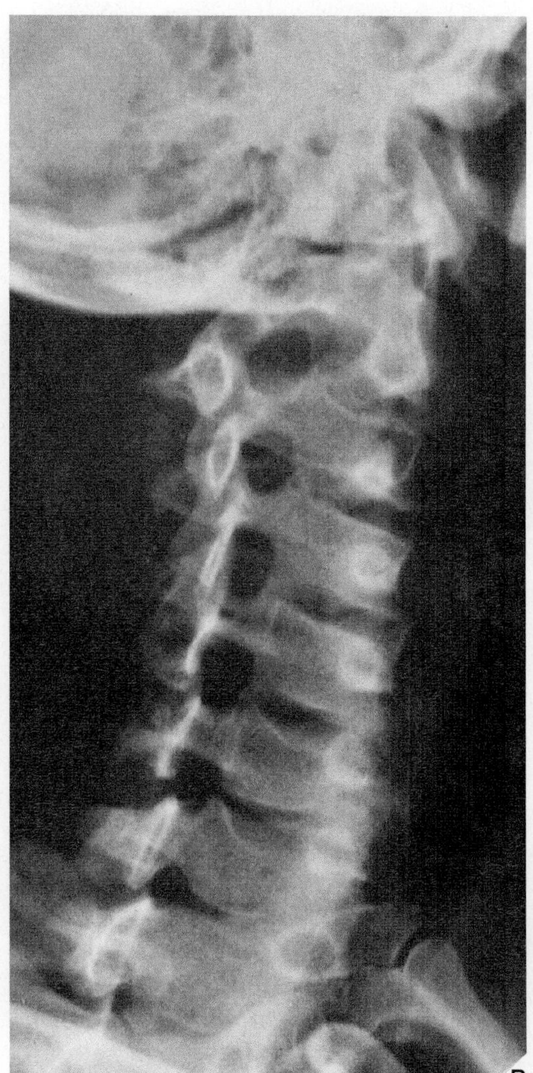

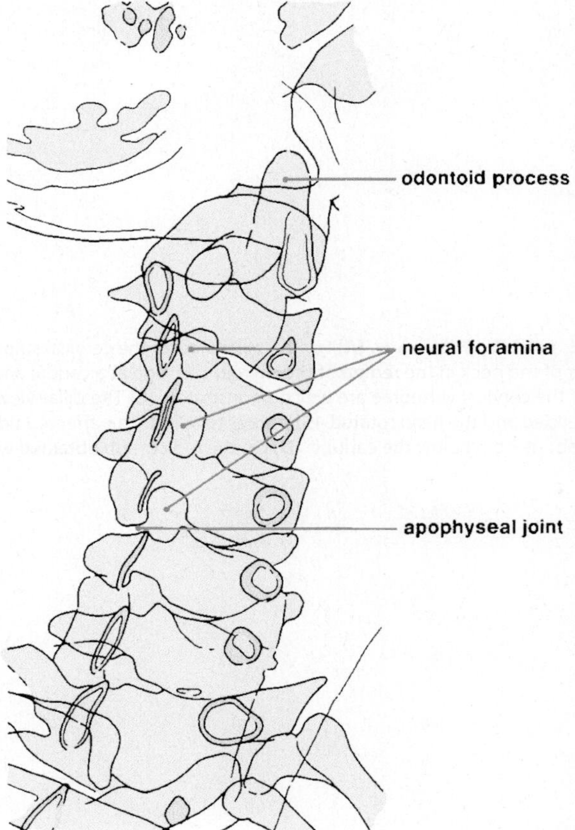

FIGURE 11.11 Oblique view. **(A)** An oblique view of the cervical spine may be obtained in the anteroposterior (as shown here) or posteroanterior projection. The patient may be erect or recumbent, but the erect position (seated or standing) is more comfortable. The patient is rotated 45 degrees to one side—to the left (as shown here) to demonstrate the right-sided neural foramina and to the right to demonstrate the left-sided neural foramina. The central beam is directed to the C4 vertebra with 15- to 20-degree cephalad angulation. **(B)** The radiograph obtained in this projection is effective primarily for demonstrating the intervertebral neural foramina.

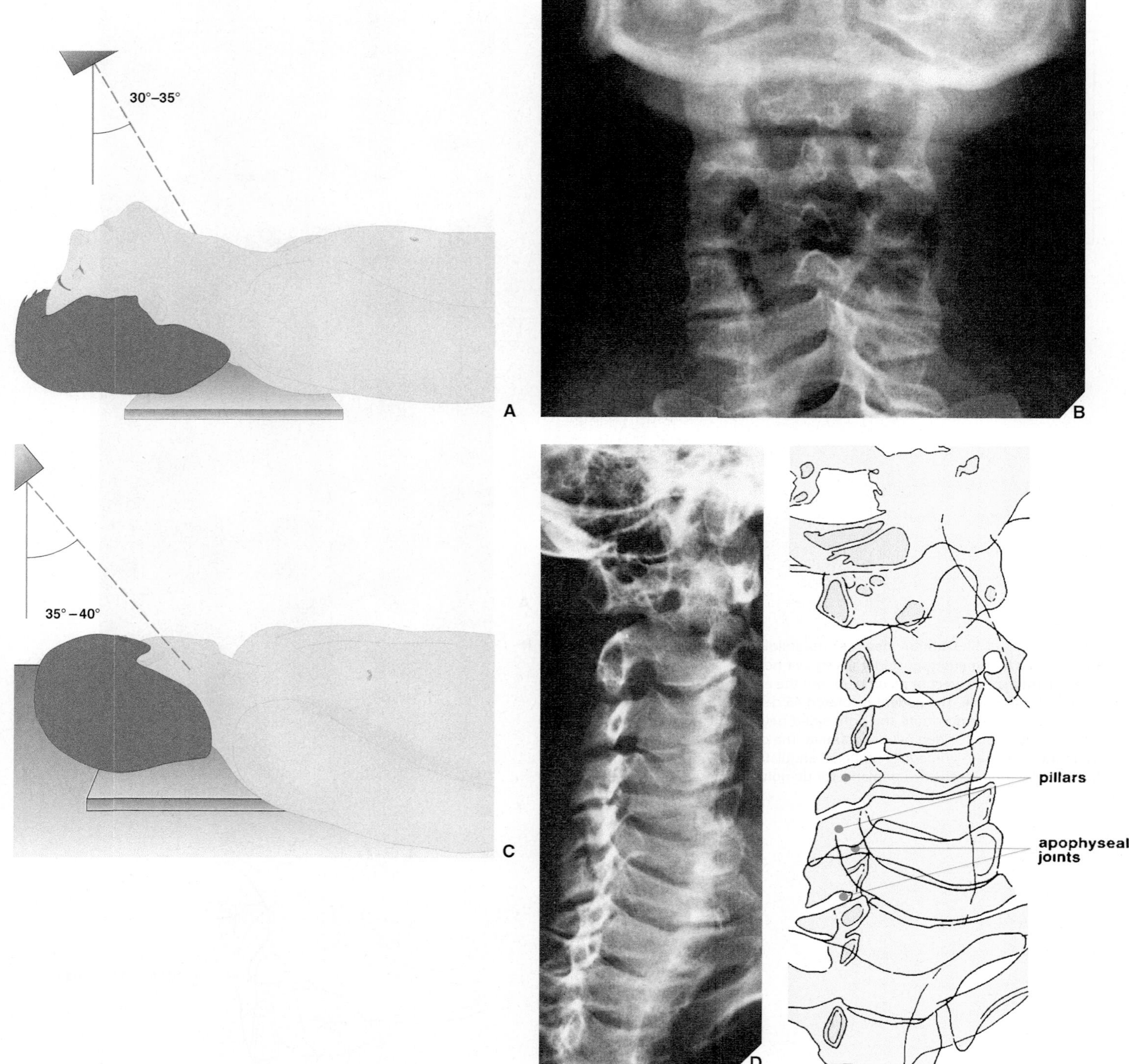

FIGURE 11.12 Pillar view. **(A)** For the pillar view of the cervical spine, the patient is supine on the table, with the neck hyperextended. The central beam is directed to the center of the neck in the region of the thyroid cartilage at a caudal angulation of 30 to 35 degrees. **(B)** On the radiograph obtained in this projection, the lateral masses (pillars) of the cervical vertebrae are well demonstrated. **(C)** The pillar view can also be obtained in the oblique projection. The patient is supine on the table, with the neck hyperextended and the head rotated 45 degrees toward the unaffected side. The central beam is directed with about 35- to 40-degree caudal angulation to the lateral side of the neck about 3 cm below the earlobe. **(D)** On the radiograph obtained with leftward rotation of the head, an oblique view of the right pillars is achieved.

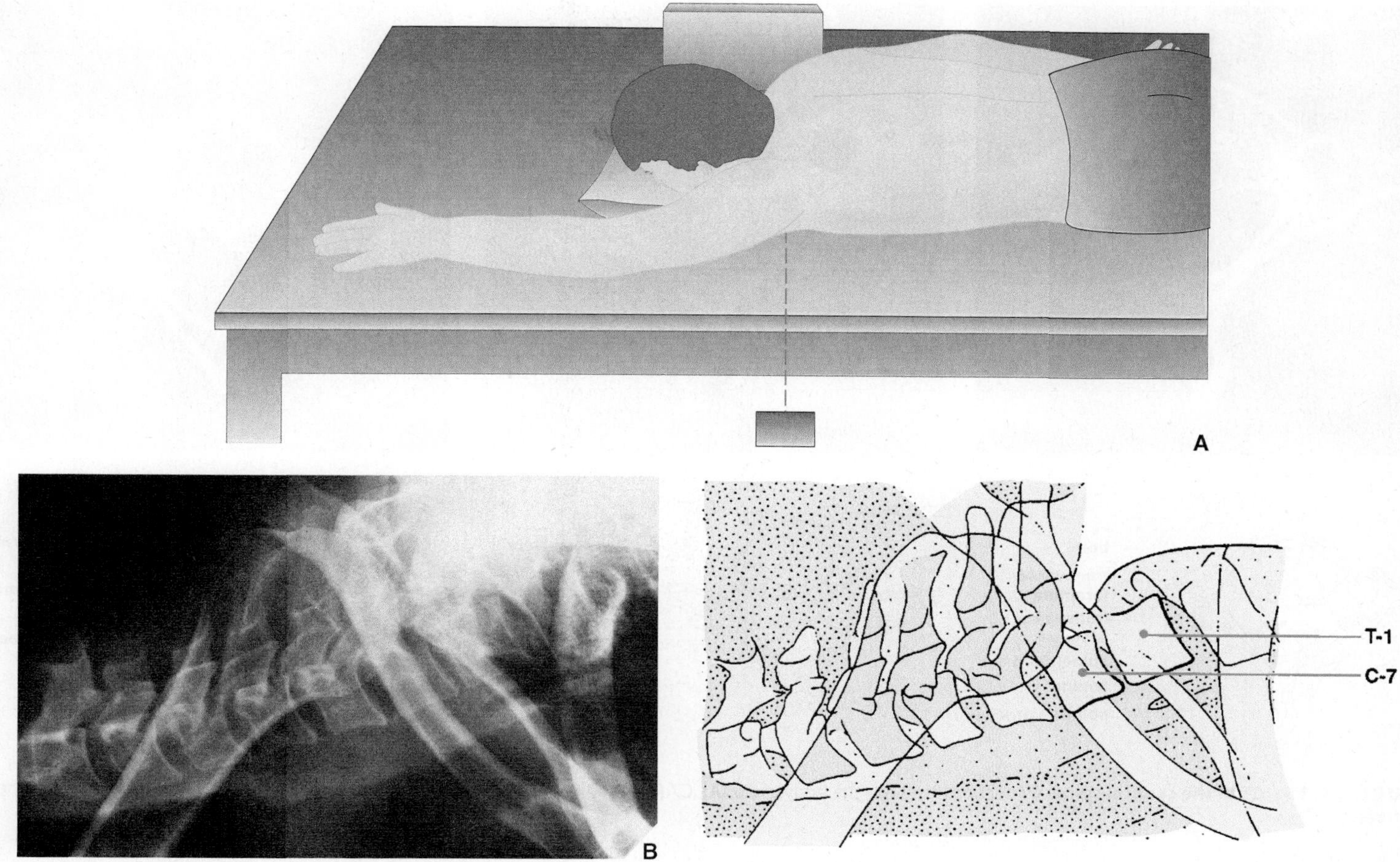

FIGURE 11.13 Swimmer's view. **(A)** For the swimmer's view of the cervical spine, the patient is placed prone on the table with the left arm abducted 180 degrees and the right arm by the side, as if swimming the crawl. The central beam is directed horizontally toward the left axilla. The radiographic cassette is against the right side of the neck, as for the standard cross-table lateral view. **(B)** The radiograph obtained in this projection provides adequate visualization of the C7, T1, and T2 vertebrae, which would otherwise be obscured by the shoulders.

Ancillary imaging techniques play an important role in the evaluation of suspected spinal trauma. Computed tomography (CT) is commonly used modality (Fig. 11.15). In the evaluation of fractures of the odontoid process, for example, CT is particularly helpful. In determining the extent of cervical spine injuries in general, including soft-tissue trauma, this technique provides valuable information regarding the integrity of the spinal canal and the localization of fracture fragments within the canal. With the advent of multidetector CT technology, images of the entire spine can be obtained quickly. Although there is significant radiation exposure, this technique is very useful in the emergency room when evaluating patient with multiple trauma.

JOB LIST

JO - JOINTS
occipitocervical, atlantoaxial, apophyseal (facet),
uncovertebral (Luschka),
intervertebral disks (not "true" joints)

B - BONES
occipital condyles, atlas,
odontoid and dens,
vertebrae C-3 - T-1, hyoid
} shape, density, texture

LI - LIGAMENTS (alignment)
ant. longitudinal, post. longitudinal,
interspinous, supraspinous, nuchae
} ant. vertebral line, post. vertebral line, spinolaminar line, post. spinous line

ST - SOFT TISSUES
retropharyngeal, retrotracheal

FIGURE 11.14 JOB LIST for evaluation of the cervical spine.

Magnetic resonance imaging (MRI) has become the most effective modality to evaluate vertebral trauma because of the impressive quality of its images and its multiplanar capabilities, which allow the examination of acutely traumatized patients without moving them. In evaluating fractures, MRI is useful not only to determine the relationship of bony fragments that may be displaced in the vertebral canal but also to demonstrate the full extent of injury, especially to the soft tissues and the spinal cord. The effect of the trauma on the spinal cord can be directly imaged, and spinal cord compression can be diagnosed. The superior soft-tissue contrast resolution of MRI can reveal even minimal edema and small quantities of hemorrhage within the spinal cord. Injury to ligamentous structures and extradural pathology also may be readily identified. In the cervical spine, 3-mm-thick sagittal sections and 5-mm-thick axial sections are routinely obtained. The most effective are spin echo T1- and T2- or T2*-weighted images obtained in the sagittal plane. Sagittal MR images permit the evaluation of vertebral body alignment and integrity, along with the size of the spinal canal (Fig. 11.16A). On the parasagittal section, the articular facets are well demonstrated (Fig. 11.16B). More recently, fast scans (fast spin echo [FSE]) have been advocated for demonstrating injuries in the sagittal and axial planes. These fast gradient-echo pulse sequences have become a popular addition to, or a replacement for, spin echo T2-weighted sequences. Gradient-echo sequences have short acquisition times and adequate resolution and show a satisfactory "myelographic effect" between cerebrospinal fluid and adjacent structures (Fig. 11.16C,D).

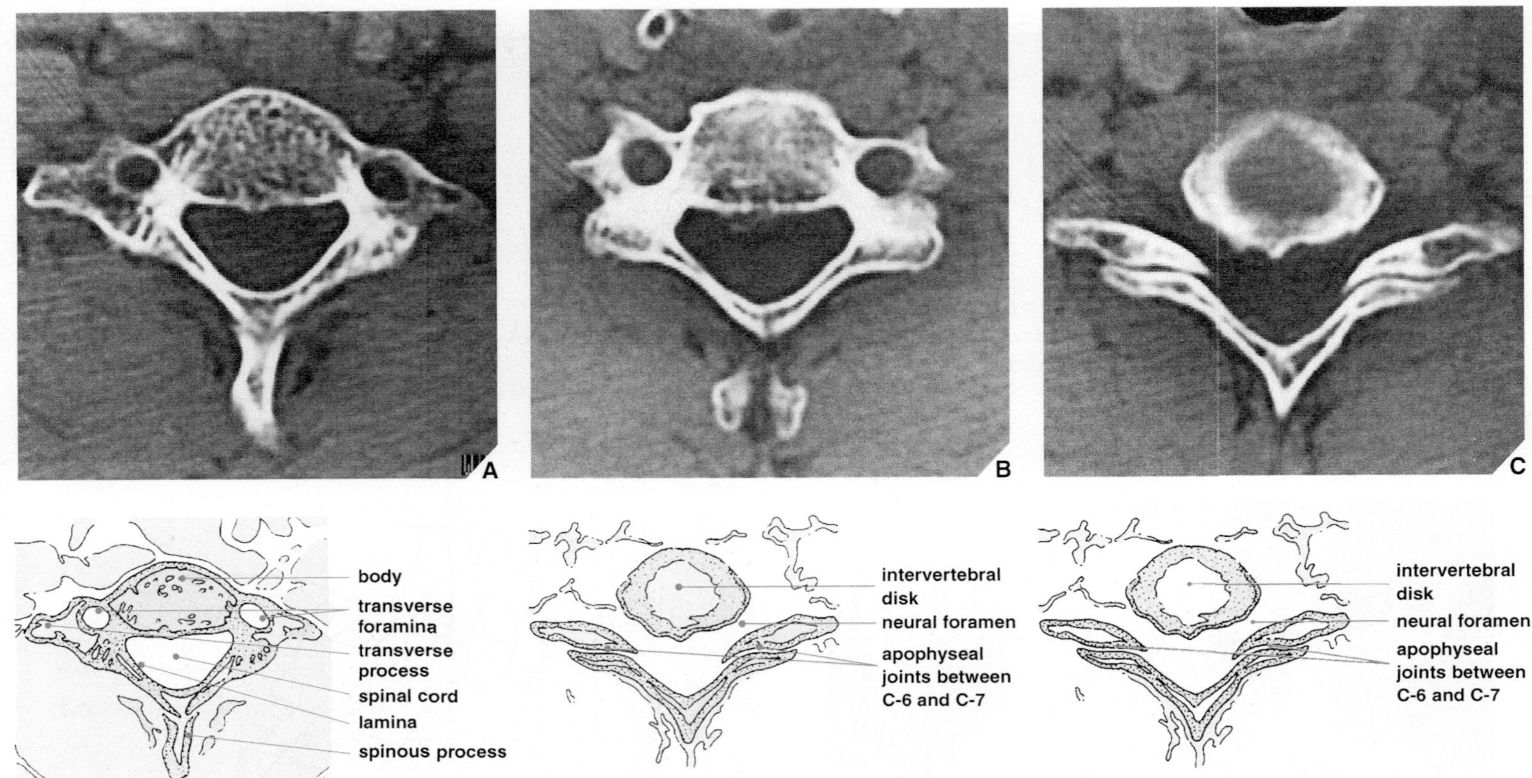

FIGURE 11.15 CT of the cervical spine. CT sections through the body of C6 **(A)**, C7 **(B)**, and the C6-7 intervertebral space **(C)** show the normal appearance of these structures.

On T1-weighted sagittal images of the cervical spine, the vertebral bodies that contain yellow (or fatty) marrow are imaged as high–signal intensity structures (see Fig. 11.16A). The intervertebral disks and the cord demonstrate intermediate signal intensity, whereas cerebrospinal fluid demonstrates low signal intensity.

On T2-weighted sagittal images, the vertebral bodies are imaged with low signal intensity, the intervertebral disks and cerebrospinal fluid demonstrate high signal intensity, and the cord demonstrates intermediate-to-low signal intensity.

On the axial images obtained in T1 weighting, the disk demonstrates intermediate signal intensity, the spinal fluid has low signal intensity, and the cord has high-to-intermediate signal intensity.

On the axial images obtained in T2* weighting, multiplanar gradient recalled (MPGR), the disk is of high signal intensity and the spinal fluid is also of high signal intensity, in contrast to the spinal cord, which images as an intermediate–signal intensity structure. The osseous structures demonstrate low signal intensity (see Fig. 11.16C,D).

In addition to its imaging capabilities, MR also has, according to some investigators, a prognostic value when attempting to predict the degree of neurologic recovery following trauma.

It has to be stressed, however, that CT alone or combined with myelography remains the better choice for evaluating vertebral fractures, especially when they are nondisplaced or involve the posterior elements (lateral masses, facets, laminae, spinous processes), largely because of the limitations of spatial resolution of MRI. In addition, imaging the acutely injured patient is difficult. The patient may be unstable or immobilized with either a halo or traction device unsuitable for the magnetic environment. For this reason, radiographs, CT, and myelography continue to play a significant role in the evaluation of the acutely traumatized spine. However, as Hyman and Gorey noted, chronic injury to the spinal cord is most accurately evaluated with MRI.

Since the advent of CT and MRI, myelography alone (Fig. 11.17A–C) is now rarely indicated in the evaluation of cervical injuries; if needed, this examination is usually performed in conjunction with CT (Fig. 11.17D).

For a summary of the preceding discussion in tabular form, see Tables 11.1 to 11.3.

Injury to the Cervical Spine

Traumatic conditions involving the cervical spine are almost always the result of indirect stress forces acting on the head and neck, the position of which at the time of impact determines the site and type of damage. As Daffner stressed, vertebral fractures occur in predictable and reproducible patterns that are related to the type of force applied to the vertebral column. The same force applied to the cervical, thoracic, or lumbar spine will result in injuries that appear quite similar, producing a pattern of recognizable signs that span the spectrum from mild soft-tissue damage to severe skeletal and ligamentous disruption. Daffner termed these patterns *fingerprints* of spinal injury; they depend on the mechanism of injury, which may be an excessive movement in any direction: flexion, extension, rotation, vertical compression, shearing, distraction—or a combination of these.

Of the greatest initial importance in suspected cervical injuries, however, is the question of stability of a fracture or dislocation (Table 11.4). Stability of the vertebral column depends on the integrity of the major skeletal components, the intervertebral disks, the apophyseal joints, and the ligamentous structures. One of the most important factors is the integrity of the ligaments of the spine: the supraspinous and interspinous ligaments, the posterior longitudinal ligament, and the ligamenta flava, which together with the capsule of the apophyseal joints constitute the so-called *posterior ligament complex of Holdsworth* (Fig. 11.18). Injuries are stable by virtue of intact ligamentous structures; the more severe the damage to these structures, the more liable they are to further displacement, with greater risk of sequelae involving the spinal cord. Radiographic findings that indicate instability, according to Daffner, are displacement of vertebrae, widening of the interspinous or interlaminar spaces, widening of the apophyseal joints, widening and elongation of the vertebral canal manifesting as widening of the interpedicular distance in transverse and vertical planes, and disruption of the posterior vertebral body line. Only one of these features needs to be present to make a radiographic assumption of an unstable injury. These remarks on stability also apply to injuries of the thoracic and lumbar segments.

Daffner and colleagues modified the classification of cervical vertebral injuries on the basis of CT findings, introducing "major" injuries and

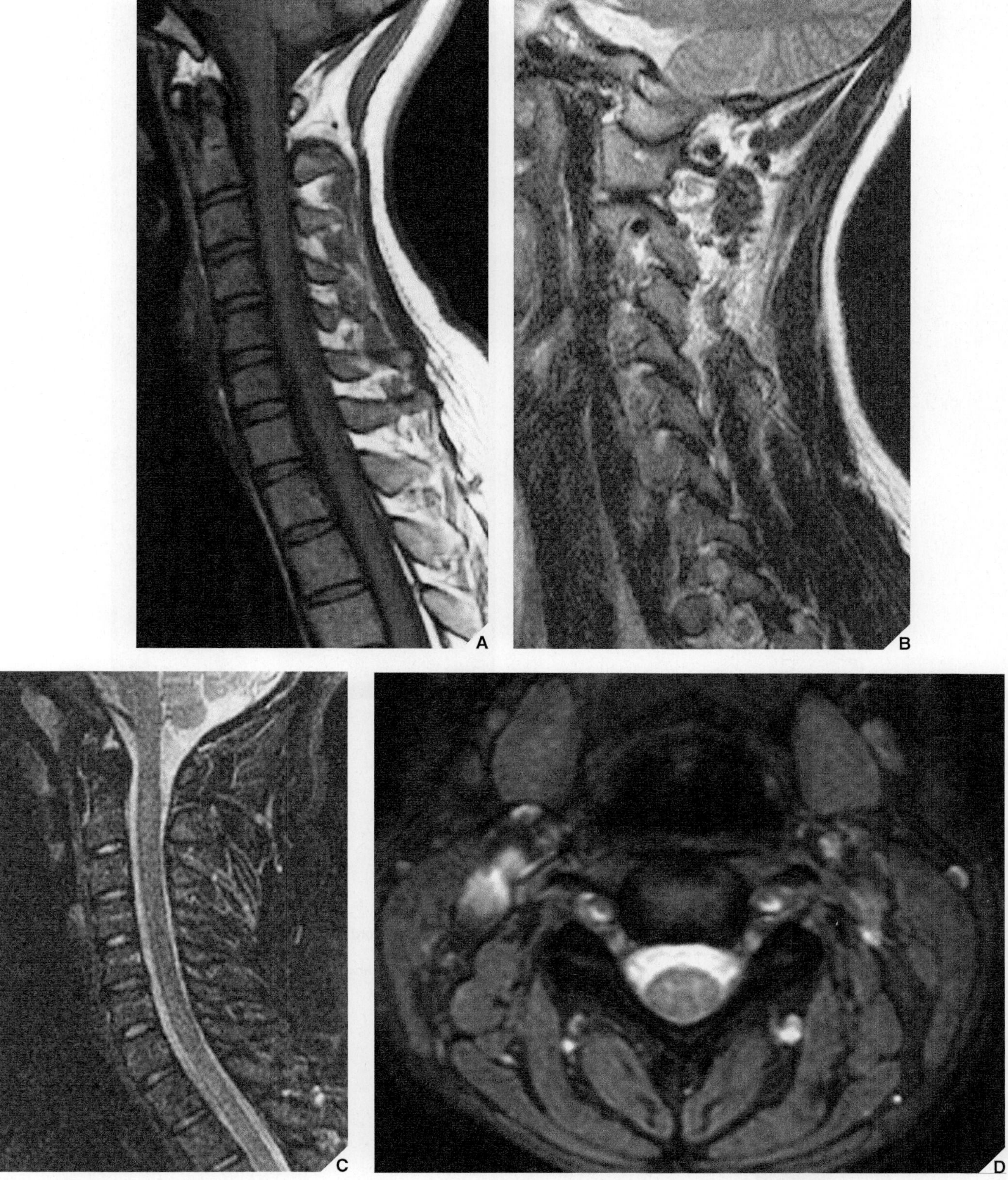

FIGURE 11.16 MRI of normal cervical spine. **(A)** T1-weighted spin echo sagittal midline section demonstrates anatomic details of the bones and soft tissues. The craniocervical junction is well outlined. The foramen magnum is defined by the fat within the occipital bone and clivus. The anterior and posterior arches of C1 appear as small oval marrow-containing structures at the upper cervical spine. The spinal cord is of an intermediate signal intensity outlined by lower signal of cerebrospinal fluid. The intervertebral disks are imaged with low signal intensity. **(B)** Parasagittal T2-weighted section demonstrates the apophyseal joints. **(C)** Short time inversion recovery (STIR) sagittal image shows vertebral bodies and spinous processes to be of low signal intensity. The high-water content of the intervertebral disks produces a very high signal similar to that of cerebrospinal fluid. The cord is imaged as an intermediate–signal intensity structure. **(D)** Axial GRE section demonstrates neural foramina and nerve roots. The cervical cord is well outlined.

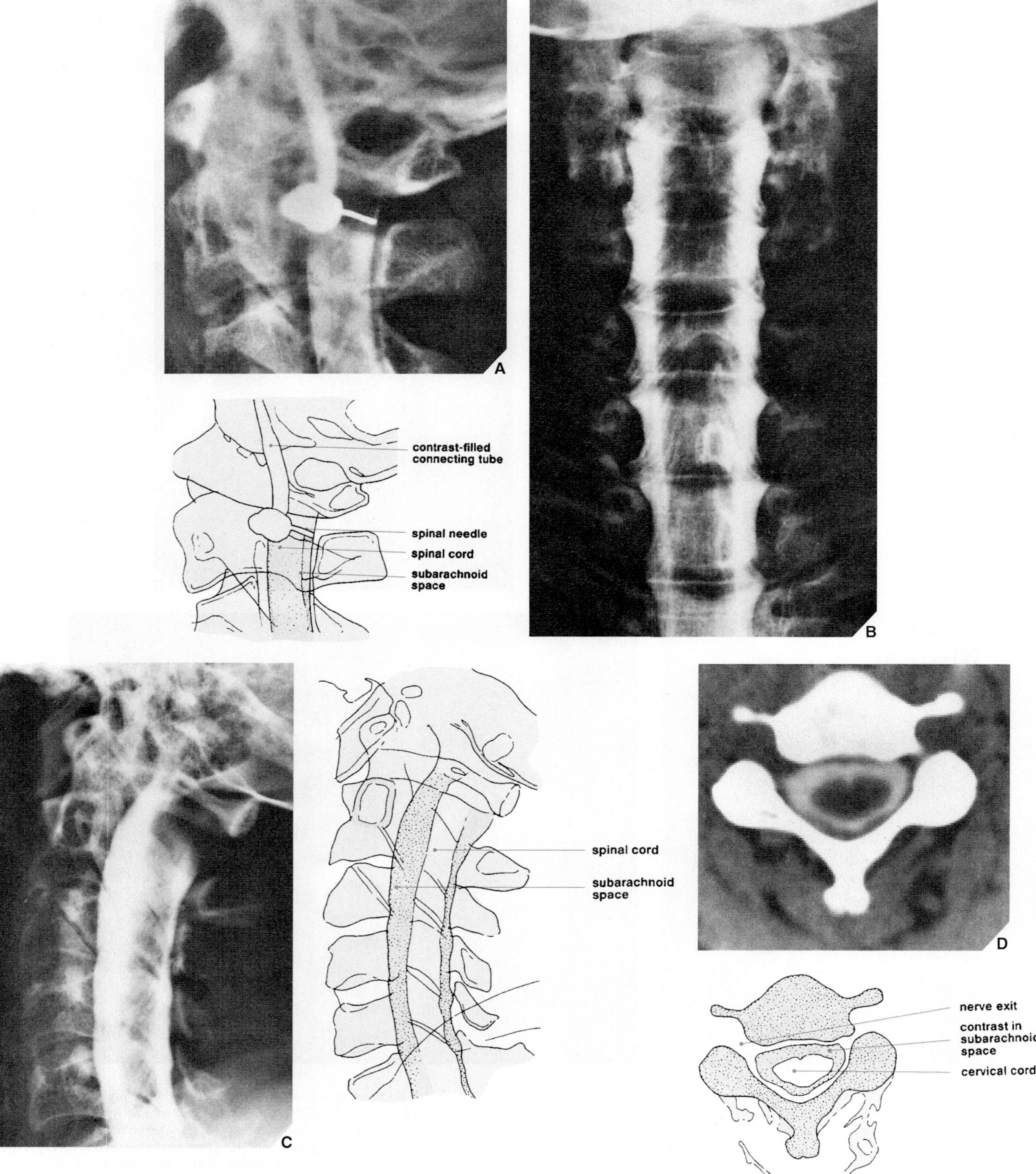

FIGURE 11.17 Myelography of the cervical spine. For myelographic examination of the cervical spine, the patient is recumbent on the table, lying on the left side. Using fluoroscopy, the point of entrance of the needle is marked at the C1-2 level, and a 22-gauge needle is inserted vertically, the tip being directed to the dorsal aspect of the subarachnoid space, above the lamina of C2. Free flow of spinal fluid indicates the correct position of the needle. **(A)** Approximately 10 mL of iohexol or iopamidol, water-soluble nonionic iodinated contrast agents, at a concentration of 240 mg iodine per mL, is slowly injected. Radiographs are obtained in the posteroanterior **(B)**, cross-table lateral **(C)**, and oblique projections. (Oblique projections, however, are obtained not by rotating the patient but by angling the radiographic tube 45 degrees.) If the lower segment of the cervical spine is not satisfactorily demonstrated or if the upper thoracic segment needs to be visualized, a radiograph may also be obtained in the swimmer's position. Myelography demonstrates the thecal sac filled with contrast and the outline of the normal nerve roots and nerve root sleeves. **(D)** CT section at the level C3-4 obtained following myelography demonstrates the normal appearance of contrast in the subarachnoid space.

TABLE 11.1 Tissue Magnetic Resonance Imaging Signal Characteristics

Signal Intensity	T1 Weighting	T2 Weighting	Gradient Echo (T2*)
Low signal	Cortical bone Vertebral end plates Degenerated disks Osteophytes Spinal vessels Cerebrospinal fluid	Cortical bone Vertebral end plates Ligaments Degenerated disks Osteophytes Spinal vessels Nerve roots	Bone marrow Vertebral bodies Vertebral end plates Ligaments Osteophytes
Intermediate signal	Spinal cord Paraspinal soft tissue Intervertebral disks Nerve roots Osteophytes	Paraspinal soft tissue Osteophytes Spinal cord Facet cartilage Bone marrow Vertebral bodies	Annulus fibrosus Spinal cord Nerve roots
High signal	Epidural venous plexus Hyaline cartilage Epidural and paraspinal fat Bone marrow Vertebral bodies	Well-hydrated nucleus pulposus Cerebrospinal fluid	Well-hydrated nucleus pulposus Cerebrospinal fluid Facet cartilage Epidural venous plexus Arteries

Republished with permission of British Editorial Society of Bone and Joint Surgery, from Kaiser MC, Ramos L. *MRI of the spine: a guide to clinical applications.* Stuttgart, Germany: Thieme; 1990; permission conveyed through Copyright Clearance Center.

TABLE 11.2 Standard and Special Radiographic Projections for Evaluating Injury to the Cervical Spine

Projection	Demonstration
Anteroposterior	Fractures of the bodies of C3-7 Abnormalities of the Intervertebral disk spaces Uncovertebral (Luschka) joints
Open-mouth	Fractures of Lateral masses of C1 Odontoid process Body of C2 Jefferson fracture Abnormalities of atlantoaxial joints
Fuchs	Fractures of odontoid process
Lateral	Occipitocervical dislocation Fractures of Anterior and posterior arches of C1 Odontoid process Bodies of C2-7 Spinous processes Hangman's fracture Burst fracture Teardrop fracture Clay shoveler's fracture Simple wedge (compression) fracture Unilateral and bilateral locked facets Abnormalities of Intervertebral disk spaces Prevertebral soft tissues Atlanto-odontoid space
In flexion	Atlantoaxial subluxation
Oblique	Abnormalities of Intervertebral (neural) foramina Apophyseal (facet) joints
Pillar (anteroposterior or oblique)	Fractures of lateral masses (pillars)
Swimmer's	Fractures of C7, T1, and T2

TABLE 11.3 Ancillary Imaging Techniques for Evaluating Injury to the Cervical, Thoracic, and Lumbar Spine

Technique	Demonstration
Tomography (almost completely replaced by computed tomography [CT])	Fractures, particularly of the odontoid process Localization of displaced fracture fragments Progress of treatment Fracture healing Status of spinal fusion
Myelography	Obstruction or compression of the dural (thecal) sac Displacement or compression of the spinal cord Abnormalities of Spinal nerve root sleeves (sheaths) Subarachnoid space Herniated disk
Diskography	Limbus vertebra Schmorl node Herniated disk
Computed tomography (CT) (alone or combined with myelography and/or diskography)	Fractures of the occipital condyles Abnormalities of Lateral recesses and neural foramina Spinal cord Complex fractures of the vertebrae Localization of displaced fracture fragments in spinal canal Spondylolysis Disk herniation Paraspinal soft-tissue injury (e.g., hematoma) Progress of treatment Fracture healing Status of spinal fusion
Radionuclide imaging (scintigraphy, bone scan)	Subtle or obscure fractures Recent versus old fractures Fracture healing
Magnetic resonance imaging (MRI)	Same as myelography and CT combined Annular tears

TABLE 11.4 Classification of Injuries to the Cervical Spine by Mechanism of Injury and Stability

Condition	Stability
Flexion Injuries	
Occipitocervical dislocation	Unstable
Subluxation	Stable
Dislocation in facet joints (locked facets)	
Unilateral	Stable
Bilateral	Unstable
Odontoid fractures	
Type I	Stable
Type II	Unstable
Type III	Stable
Wedge (compression) fracture	Stable
Clay shoveler's fracture	Stable
Teardrop fracture	Unstable
Burst fracture	Stable or unstable
Extension Injuries	
Occipitocervical dislocation	Unstable
Fracture of posterior arch of C1	Stable
Hangman's fracture	Unstable
Extension teardrop fracture	Stable
Hyperextension fracture–dislocation	Unstable
Compression Injuries	
Occipital condyle fracture (types I and II)	Stable
Jefferson fracture	Unstable
Burst fracture	Stable or unstable
Laminar fracture	Stable
Compression fracture	Stable
Shearing Injuries	
Lateral vertebral compression	Stable
Lateral dislocation	Unstable
Transverse process fracture	Stable
Lateral mass fracture	Stable
Rotation Injuries	
Occipital condyle fracture (type III)	Unstable
Rotary subluxation C1-2	Stable
Fracture–dislocation	Unstable
Facet and pillar fractures	Stable or unstable
Transverse process fracture	Stable
Distraction Injuries	
Occipitocervical dislocation	Unstable
Hangman's fracture	Unstable
Atlantoaxial subluxation	Stable or unstable

"minor" injuries. The former are defined as having either radiographic or CT evidence of instability, with or without associated localized or central neurologic findings. The latter injuries have no radiographic or CT evidence of instability and do not produce or have no potential to cause neurologic findings. According to these authors, cervical injury should be classified as major if the following radiographic and CT criteria are present: displacement of more than 2 mm in any plane, widening of the vertebral body in any plane, widening of the interspinous or interlaminar space, widening of the facet joints, disruption of the posterior vertebral body line, widening of the disk space, vertebral burst fracture, locked or perched facets either unilateral or bilateral, "hanged man" fracture of C2, fracture of the odontoid process, and type III occipital condyle fracture. All other types of fractures are considered to be minor.

Fractures of the Occipital Condyles

Fractures of the occipital condyles are rare. This injury is often overlooked and is not obvious on the conventional radiography. Instead, the diagnosis requires a high index of suspicion, after which confirmation can easily be obtained by CT with coronal reformation. A classification system of occipital condyle fractures was devised by Anderson and Montesano in 1988 based on fracture morphology, pertinent anatomy, and biomechanics (Fig. 11.19).

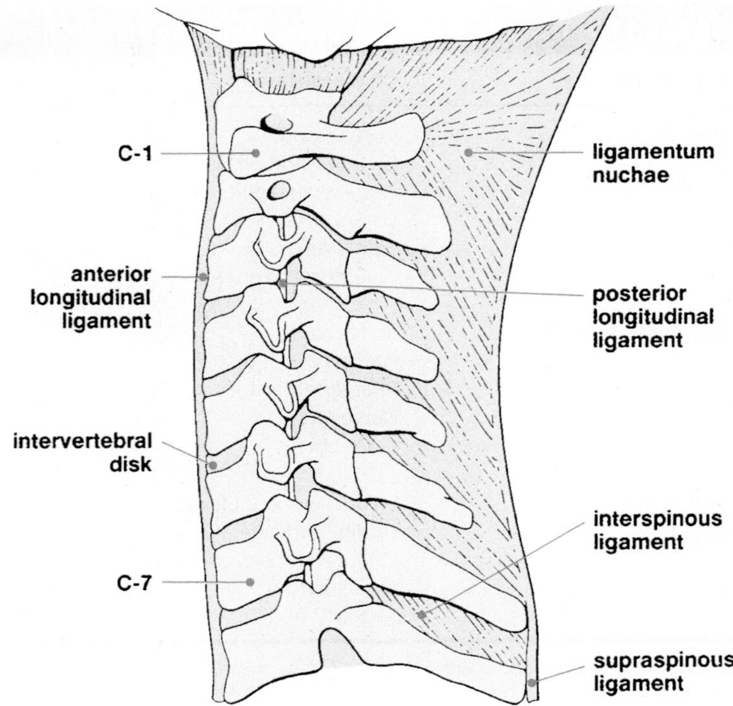

FIGURE 11.18 Anatomy of the principal ligaments of the cervical spine.

Type I is an impacted occipital condyle fracture occurring as the result of axial loading force on the skull, similar to the mechanism for a Jefferson fracture. CT shows comminution of the occipital condyle with minimal or no displacement of fragments into the foramen magnum (Fig. 11.20). Although the ipsilateral alar ligament may be functionally inadequate, spinal stability is ensured by the intact tectorial membrane and contralateral alar ligament.

Type II occipital condyle fracture occurs as a component of a basilar skull fracture. On axial CT sections of the base of the skull, a fracture line can be seen exiting the occipital condyle and entering the foramen magnum. The mechanism of injury is a direct blow to the skull. Stability is maintained by intact alar ligaments and tectorial membrane.

Type III is an avulsion fracture of the medial aspect of occipital condyle by the alar ligament: A small fragment of the condyle is displaced toward the tip of odontoid process (Figs. 11.21 and 11.22). The alar ligaments are primary restraints of occipitocervical rotation and lateral bending. Therefore, the mechanism of injury in this type is rotation, lateral bending, or a combination of the two. After avulsion of the occipital condyle, the contralateral alar ligament and tectorial membrane are loaded. Therefore, this type of occipital condyle fracture is a potentially unstable injury.

Occipitocervical Dislocations

Traumatic occipitocervical dislocations are usually fatal and therefore rarely present a clinical problem. With the improvement in trauma care, which now includes on-site intubation and immediate resuscitation as well as early hospital transport, more and more victims of this injury are presenting for definitive care. The radiographic diagnosis, however, still remains somewhat difficult because of the overlapping shadows of the base of the cranium and the mastoid processes. Traynelis and colleagues have classified occipital cervical dislocations according to the direction of displacement of the occiput: anterior, vertical, or posterior. Anderson and Montesano have modified this classification as follows.

Type I injuries are characterized by anterior translation of both occipital condyles on their corresponding atlantal facets (Fig. 11.23A). Biomechanical studies have demonstrated that for this injury to occur, all major

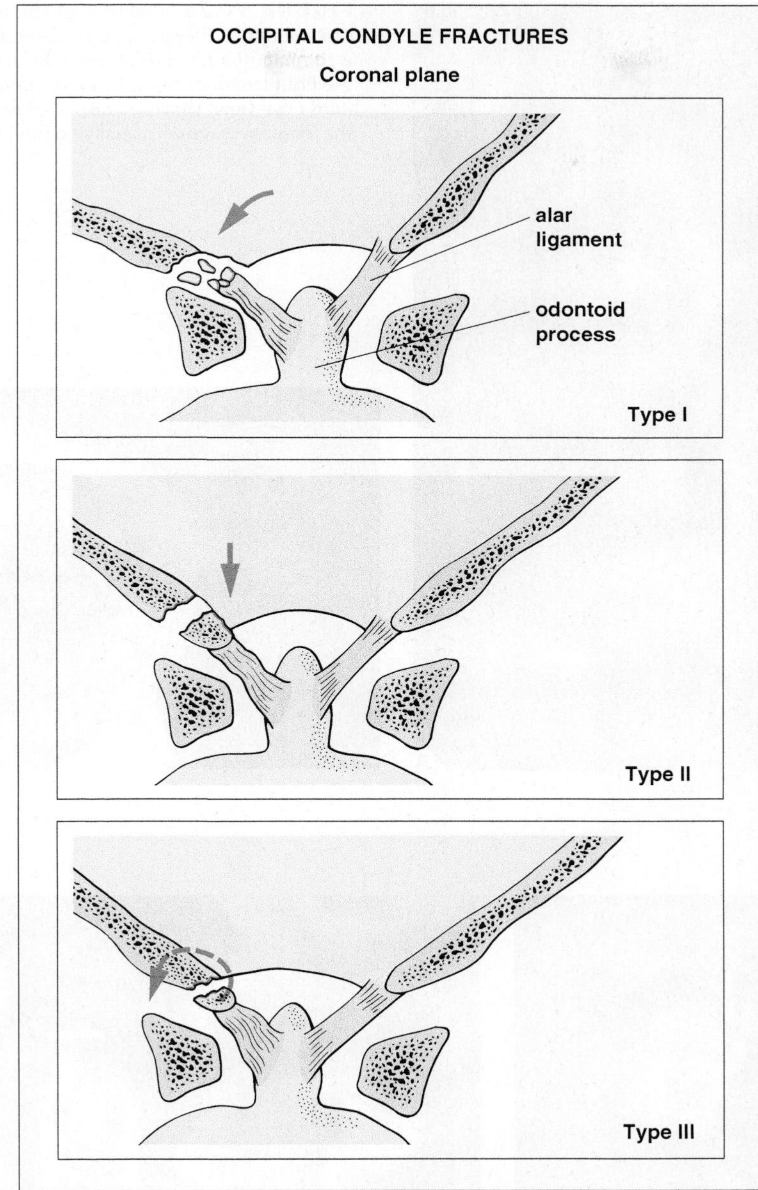

FIGURE 11.19 **Anderson and Montesano classification of the occipital condyle fractures.** (Modified with permission from Anderson PA, Montesano PX. Morphology and treatment of occipital condyle fractures. *Spine [Phila Pa 1976]* 1988;13:731–736.)

structures (alar ligaments, tectorial membrane, and occipital atlantal facet joint capsules) crossing the occipitocervical junction must be ruptured. This type of injury is seen more commonly in patients who survive transport to the hospital.

Type II injuries are associated with a vertical translation of the occiput on the cervical spine, secondary to the rupture of all occipitocervical ligaments. In type IIA, there is distraction between the occiput and C1, and vertical translation of the occiput on C1 is usually less than 2 mm. Vertical displacement greater than this represents failure of the tectorial membrane, alar ligaments, and occipitoatlantal facet joint capsules (Fig. 11.23B). If, conversely, the occipitoatlantal facet joint capsules remain intact and failure occurs at a more distal level of the tectorial membrane (i.e., at the level of the atlantoaxial facet joint ligaments), a type IIB injury results. In this type, there is also a vertical displacement of the spine, which occurs, however, between C1 and C2 rather than at the atlantooccipital level.

Type III injuries consist of posterior displacement of the occiput that is translated posteriorly to the atlas.

In all types of occipitocervical instability, associated injury to the transverse ligament and C1-2 instability should be suspected. Radiologic examination should include a standard lateral radiograph of the cervical spine that demonstrates the region from the occiput to the cervicothoracic junction. The articulations between occipital condyles and the atlanto-lateral masses must always be included and the clivus clearly visualized. In type III injuries, the clivus-odontoid line, which normally points into the tip of the odontoid process (see Fig. 11.3D), points posteriorly to the odontoid. Other suggestive findings on the lateral radiograph of the cervical spine are the absence of the projection of the mastoid processes over the odontoid and retropharyngeal soft-tissue swelling. CT is more effective for evaluating the occipitocervical junction. Using 1-mm-thin contiguous sections with multiplanar reformation, the alignment of the occiput-C1 and C1-2 articulations can be readily discerned.

Fractures of the C1 and C2 Vertebrae

Jefferson Fracture

This fracture results from a blow to the vertex of the head. The axial forces transmitted symmetrically through the cranium and occipital condyles into the superior surfaces of the lateral masses of the atlas drive the lateral masses outward, resulting in bilateral, symmetrical fractures of the anterior and posterior arches of C1, which are invariably associated with disruption of the transverse ligaments (Fig. 11.24). Neck pain and unilateral occipital headache are characteristic clinical features of Jefferson fracture.

The best radiographic projections for demonstrating this injury is the open-mouth anteroposterior view and lateral projection (Fig. 11.25A,B).

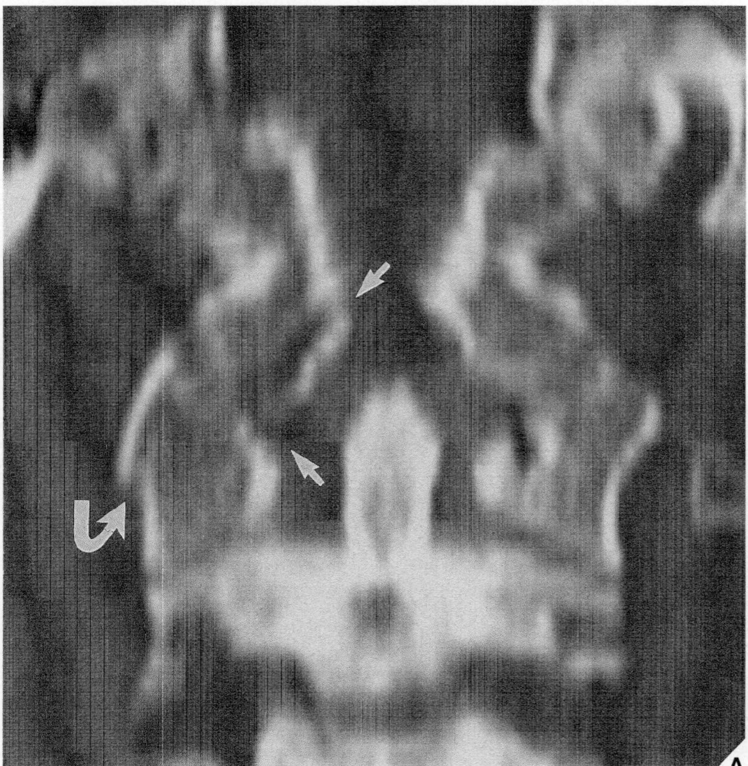

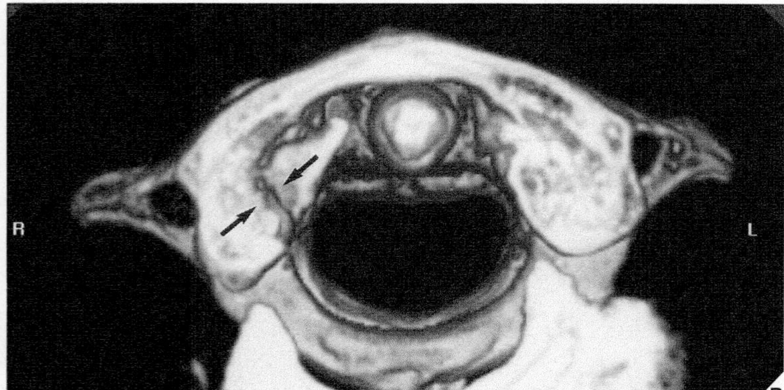

FIGURE 11.20 **Fracture of the occipital condyle.** A 23-year-old woman was injured in a motorcycle accident. **(A)** Coronal reformatted CT image shows a comminuted fracture of the right occipital condyle *(arrows)* and a fracture of the right lateral mass of the atlas *(curved arrow)*. **(B)** 3D CT reconstructed image (bird's eye view) shows no displacement of the fractured fragments *(arrows)* into the foramen magnum, classifying this injury as a type I.

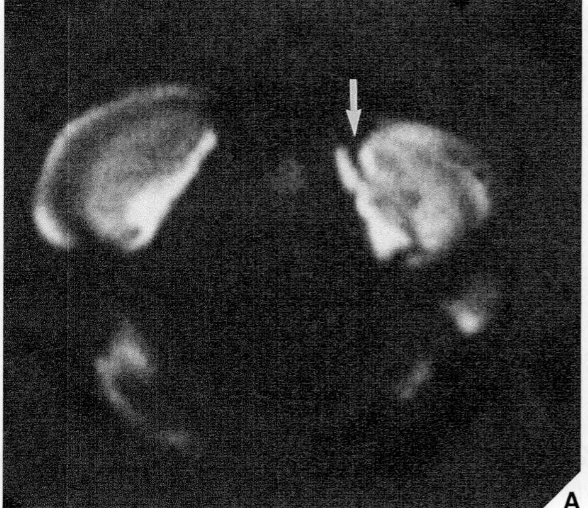

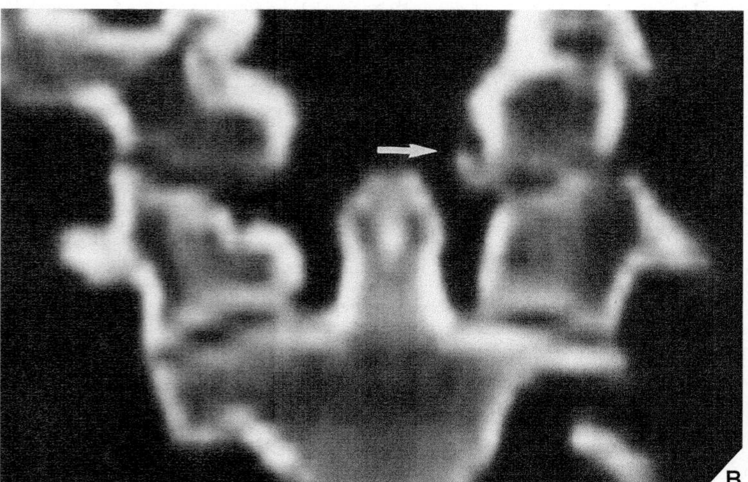

FIGURE 11.21 **Fracture of the occipital condyle.** A 16-year-old girl was assaulted and sustained a blow injury to the head. Conventional radiographs of the skull and upper cervical spine were interpreted as normal. **(A)** Axial CT section through the base of the skull shows a type III fracture of the left occipital condyle *(arrow)*. **(B)** Coronal reformatted CT image confirms the presence of an evulsion fracture *(arrow)*.

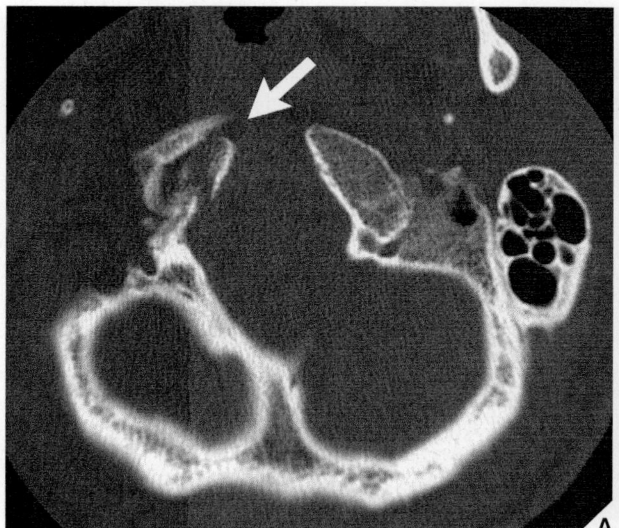
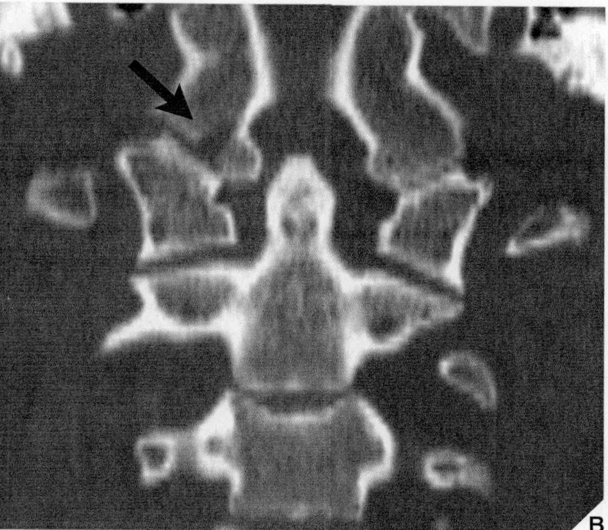

FIGURE 11.22 **Fracture of the occipital condyle.** An 18-year-old man was ejected from the convertible car during the accident. **(A)** Axial CT section through the base of the skull and **(B)** coronal reformatted CT image show a type III fracture of the right occipital condyle *(arrows)*. Note displaced fragment of the occipital condyle toward the odontoid process.

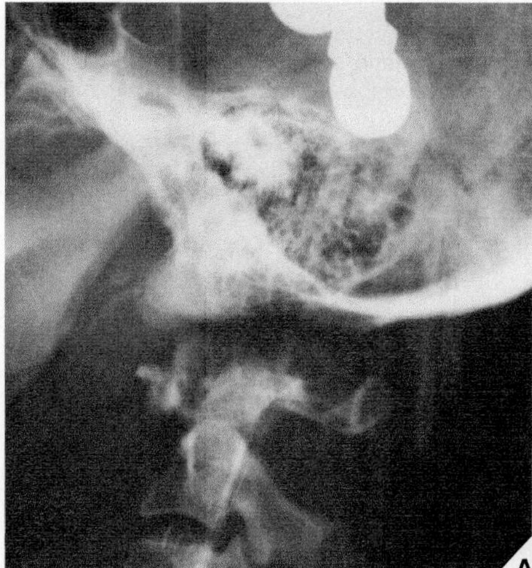
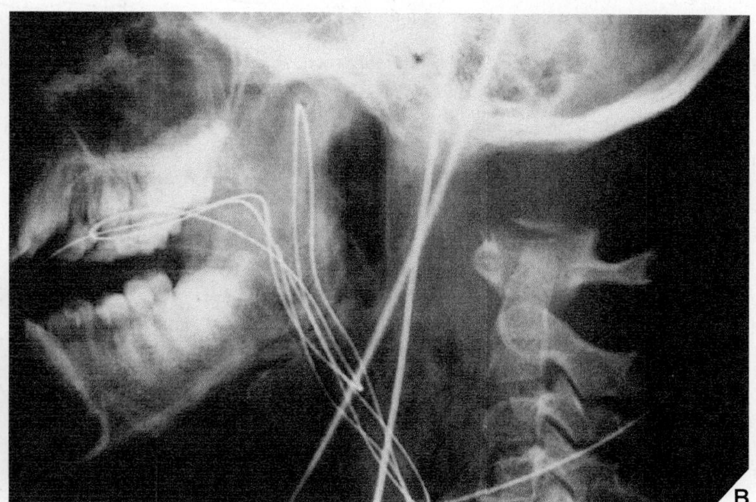

FIGURE 11.23 **Occipitocervical dislocation.** **(A)** Lateral radiograph of the cervical spine in a 24-year-old man, who injured his head and neck in a motorcycle accident that resulted in complete quadriplegia, shows type I of occipitocervical dislocation: The occipital condyles are anteriorly displaced in relation to C1 vertebra. **(B)** In another patient, lateral radiograph demonstrates a type IIA vertical occipitocervical dislocation. (**A**, Reprinted from Greenspan A, Montesano PX. *Imaging of the spine in clinical practice*. London, United Kingdom: Wolfe-Mosby-Gower Publishers; 1993:2.19, Fig. 2.23. Copyright © 1993 Elsevier. With permission; **B**, Reprinted with permission from Anderson PA, Montesano PX. Injuries to the occipitocervical articulation. In: Chapman MW, ed. *Operative orthopaedics*, vol. 4, 2nd ed. Philadelphia: JB Lippincott; 1993:2631–2640.)

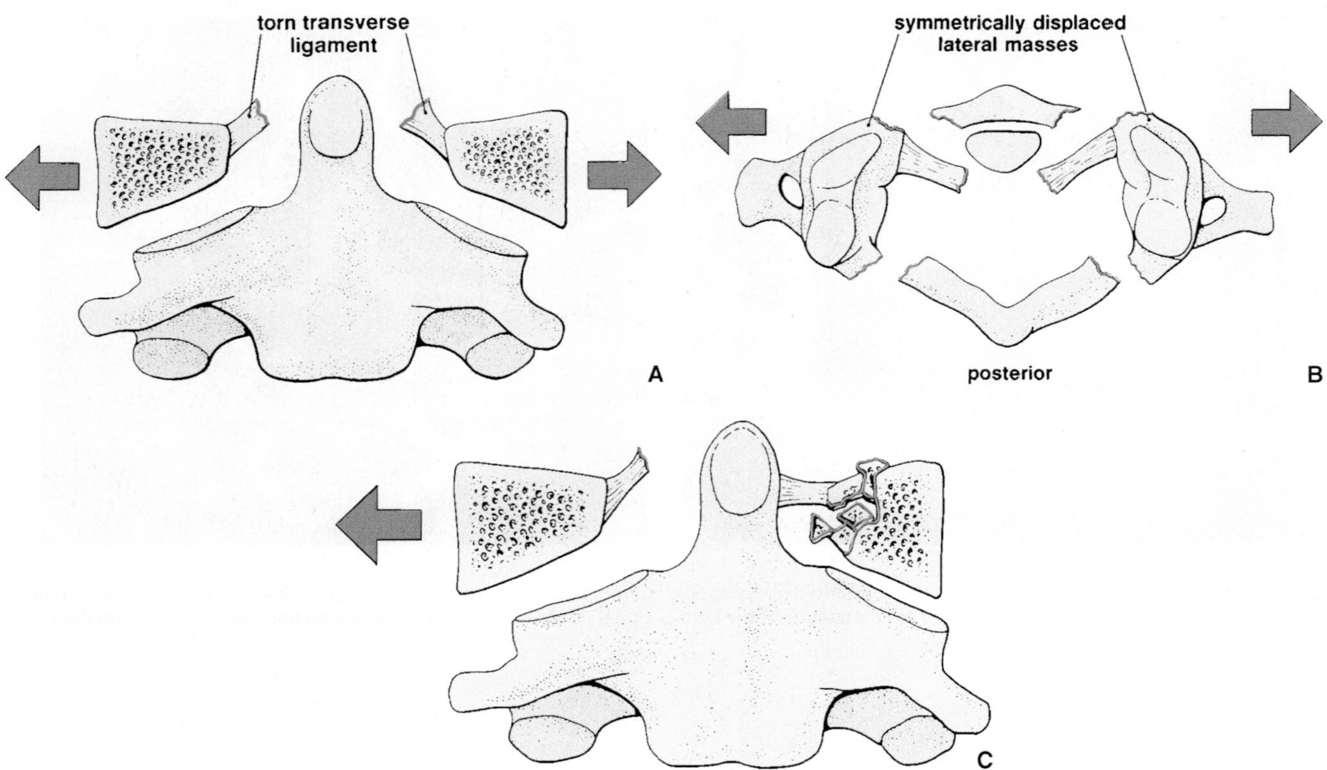

FIGURE 11.24 Jefferson fracture. The classic Jefferson fracture, seen here schematically on the **(A)** anteroposterior and **(B)** axial views, exhibits a characteristic symmetric overhang of the lateral masses of C1 over those of C2. Lateral displacement of the articular pillars results in disruption of the transverse ligaments. **(C)** On occasion, only unilateral lateral displacement of an articular pillar may be present.

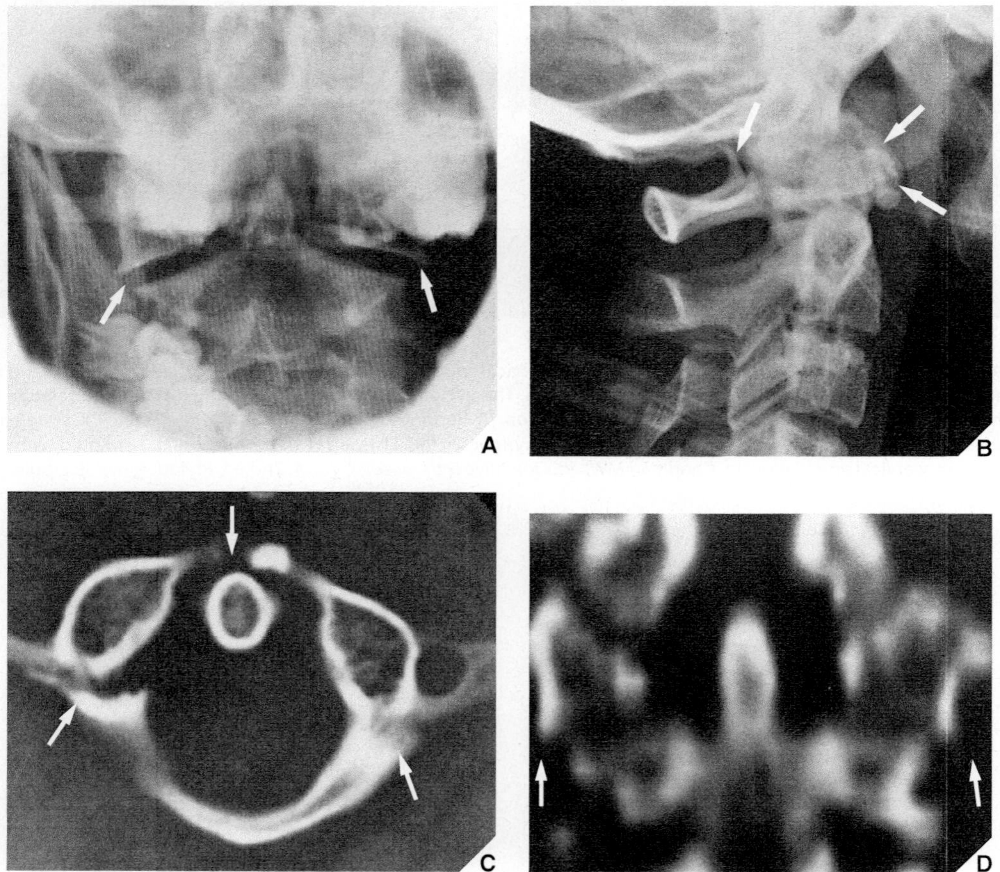

FIGURE 11.25 Jefferson fracture. A 19-year-old man sustained a neck injury while being mugged. **(A)** Open-mouth anteroposterior radiograph of the cervical spine shows lateral displacement of the lateral masses of the atlas *(arrows)*, suggesting a ring fracture of C1. **(B)** Lateral radiograph demonstrates fracture lines of the posterior and anterior arch of C1 *(arrows)*. **(C)** Axial CT section demonstrates two fracture lines of the posterior arch and a fracture of the anterior arch *(arrows)*. **(D)** CT coronal reformation confirms lateral displacement of the lateral masses *(arrows)*.

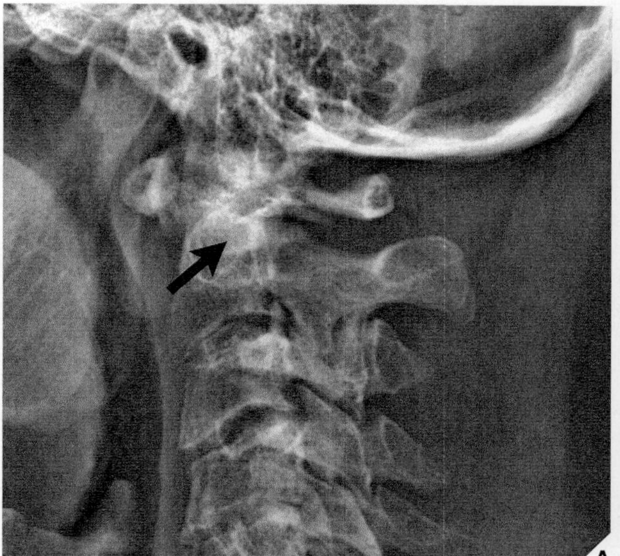

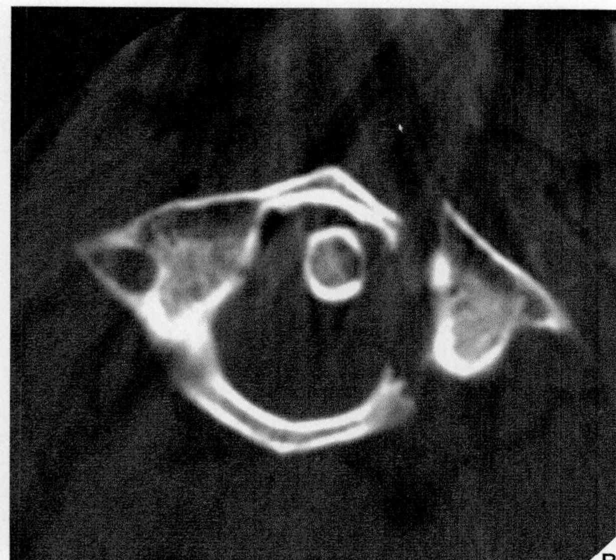

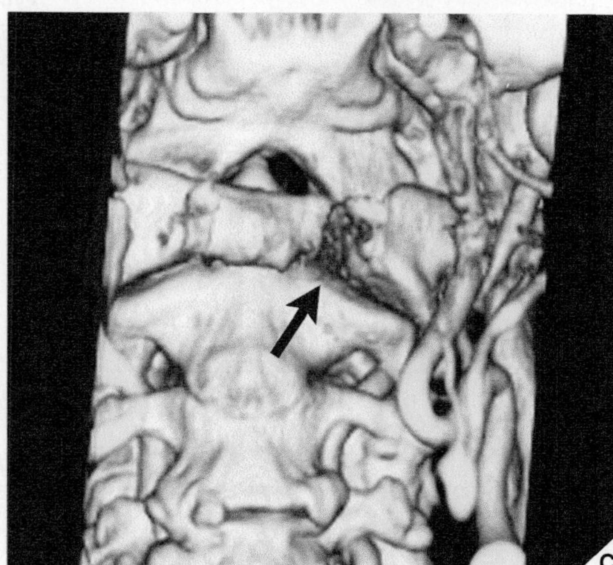

FIGURE 11.26 Jefferson fracture. A 56-year-old man was hit on the top of the head during the industrial accident. **(A)** Later radiograph of the cervical spine shows a fracture of C1 *(arrow)*. **(B)** Axial CT section and **(C)** 3D CT reconstructed image confirm unilateral fracture of the left anterior and posterior arches of C1 *(arrow)*.

CT may also be required in the evaluation of complex fractures (Fig. 11.25C,D and 11.26). MRI only occasionally is performed.

Fractures of the Odontoid Process

Fractures of the dens belong to the group of flexion injuries, although at times forces causing hyperextension of the cervical spine may also result in damage to the odontoid process. In hyperflexion injuries, the odontoid process is usually displaced anteriorly, and there may be associated forward subluxation of C1 or C2. Hyperextension injuries, however, usually cause the odontoid to be displaced posteriorly, with posterior subluxation of C1 or C2.

Several classifications of odontoid fractures have been proposed, based on the site and amount of displacement of a fracture. The system suggested by Anderson and D'Alonzo, however, is practical and has gained wide acceptance because of its emphasis on the most important feature of such fractures—their stability (Fig. 11.27):

Type I: fractures of the body of the dens distal (cephalad) to the base. They are usually obliquely oriented and are considered stable injuries. Conservative treatment usually suffices for healing. Some authorities do not recognize type I fractures, postulating that these "injuries" in fact represent a nonunited secondary ossification center (ossiculum terminale of Bergman) or os odontoideum.

Type II: Transverse fractures through the base of the odontoid are unstable injuries (Fig. 11.28). Conservative treatment has been complicated by nonunion in approximately 35% of cases; therefore, surgical fusion is the usual method of treatment.

Type III: Fractures through the base of the odontoid extending into the body of the axis are stable injuries (Figs. 11.29 and 11.30). Conservative treatment is usually sufficient.

The best techniques for demonstrating fractures of the dens are the anteroposterior view, including the open-mouth variant, or Fuchs projection, and the lateral projection; in the past, thin-section trispiral tomography (at present time almost completely abandoned) used to be effective in delineating ambiguous or subtle features (see Figs. 11.28C,D and 11.29C).

CT detection of the dens fractures, particularly type II, may be difficult if the axial sections are obtained parallel to the usually horizontally oriented fracture line. For this reason, it is essential to obtain routinely reformatted images in coronal and sagittal planes (see Fig. 11.30).

Hangman's Fracture

In 1912, Wood-Jones described the pathomechanism associated with execution by hanging. He found that hyperextension and distraction resulted in bilateral fractures through the pedicles of the axis, with anterior dislocation of the body and subsequent tearing of the spinal cord. A similar

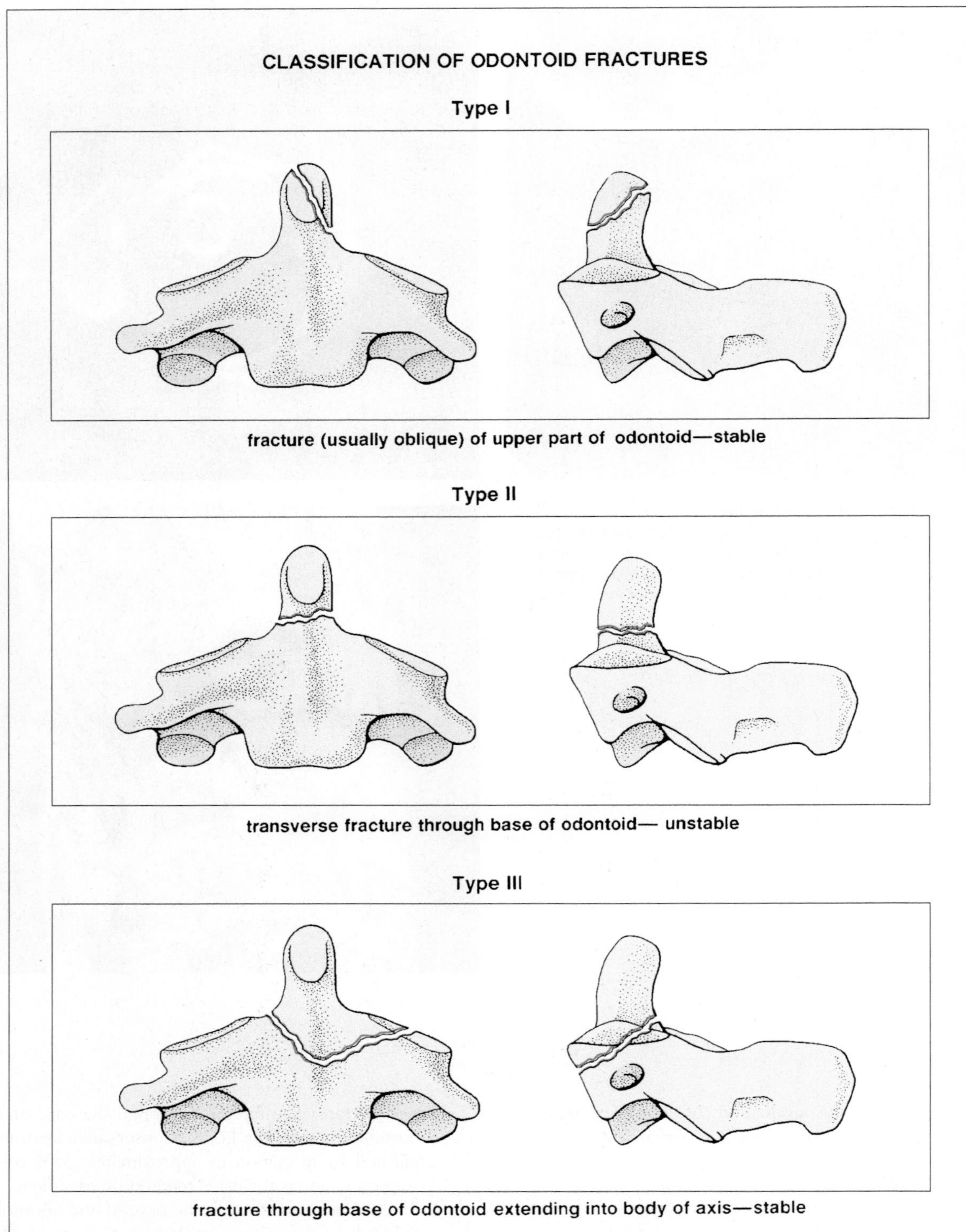

FIGURE 11.27 Classification of odontoid fractures. (Modified with permission from Anderson LD, D'Alonzo RT. Fractures of the odontoid process of the axis. *J Bone Joint Surg Am* 1974;56:1663–1674.)

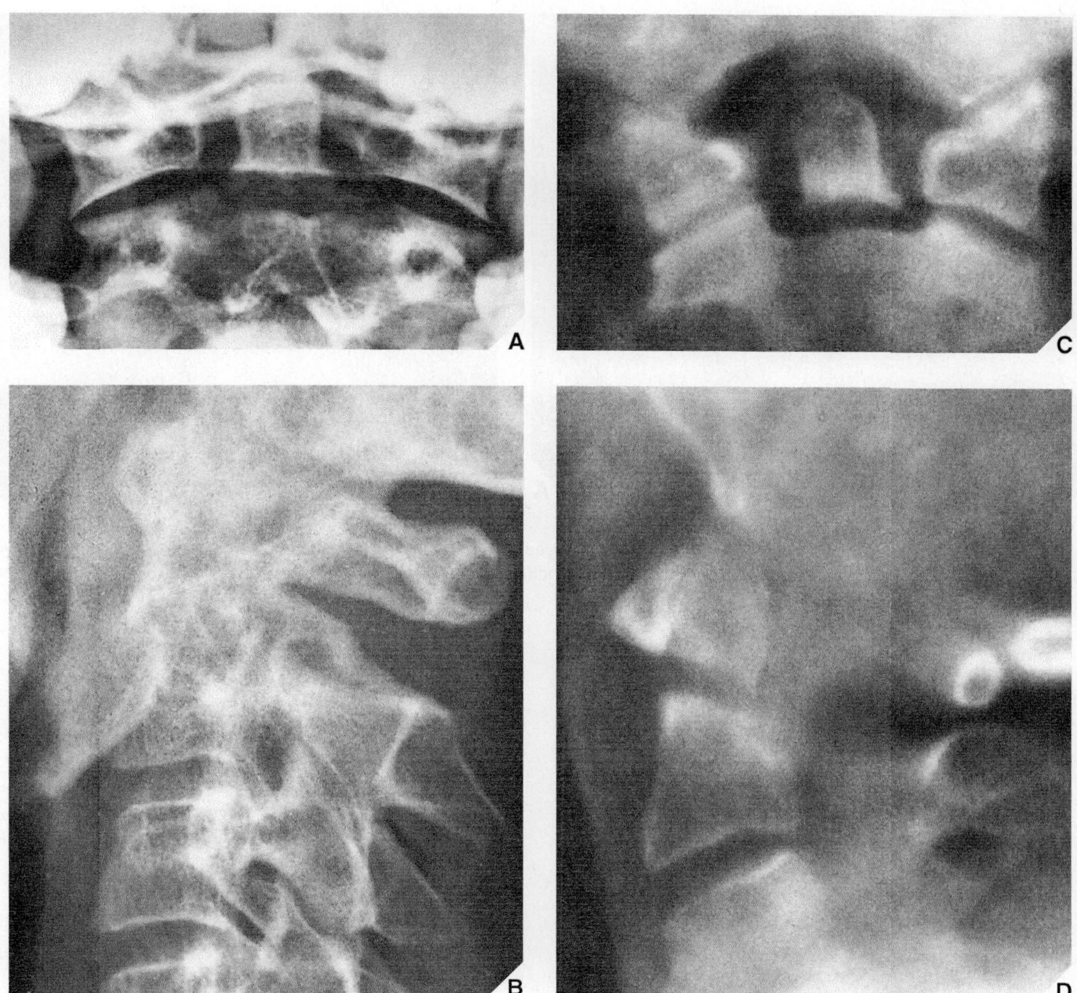

FIGURE 11.28 **Fracture of the odontoid process.** A 62-year-old man sustained a flexion injury of the cervical spine in an automobile accident. **(A)** Anteroposterior open-mouth and **(B)** lateral radiographs of the cervical spine demonstrate a fracture line at the base of the odontoid process, but the details of this injury cannot be well appreciated. Thin-section trispiral tomographic sections in the anteroposterior **(C)** and lateral **(D)** projections confirm the fracture at the base of the dens. This is a type II (unstable) fracture.

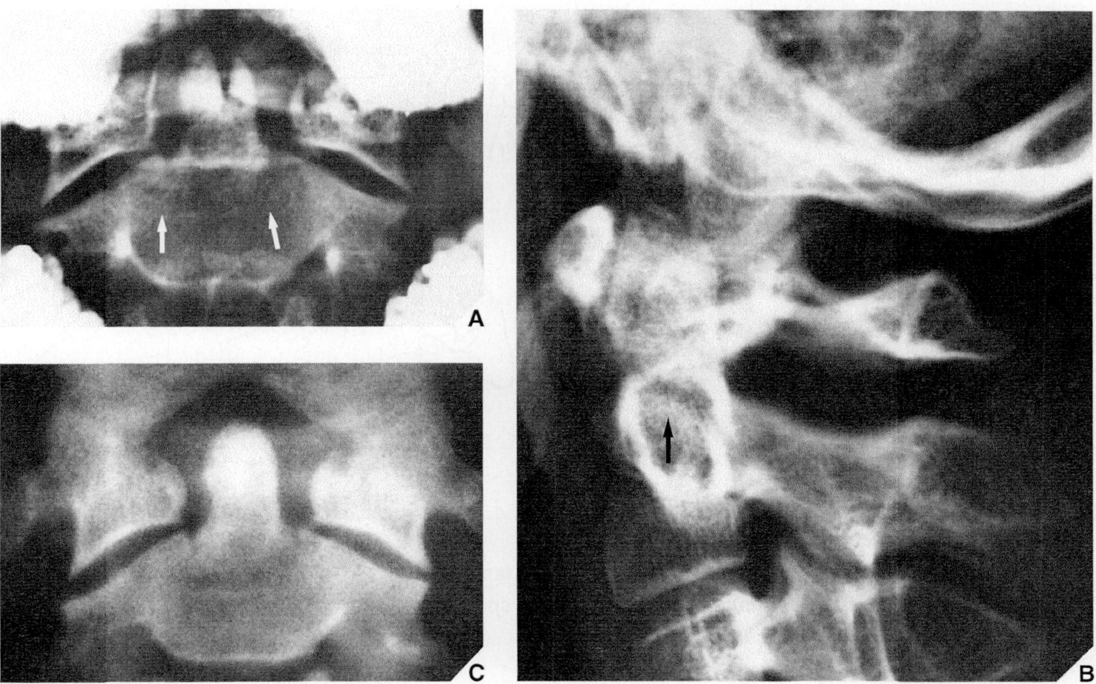

FIGURE 11.29 **Fracture of the odontoid process.** A 24-year-old man fell on his head in a skiing accident. **(A)** Anteroposterior open-mouth and **(B)** lateral radiographs of the cervical spine demonstrate a fracture of the odontoid process extending into the body of C2 *(arrows)*—a type III stable fracture. The diagnosis was confirmed by **(C)** trispiral tomography in the anteroposterior projection.

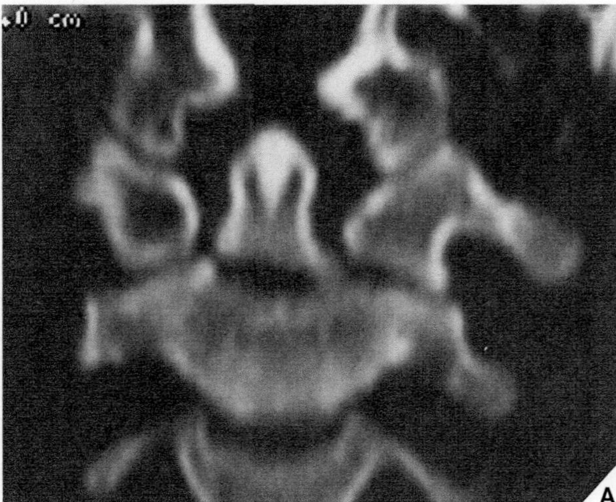

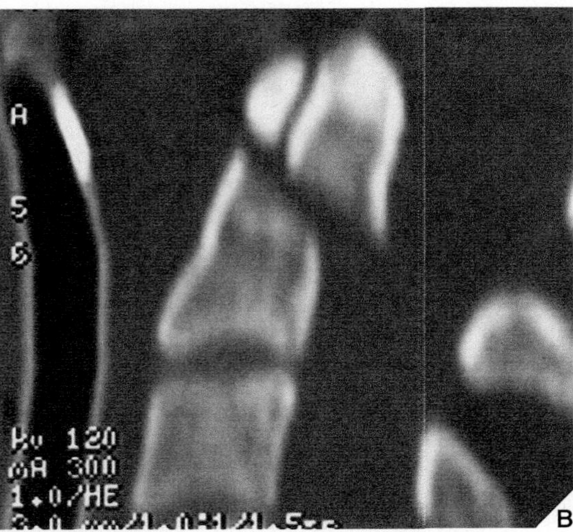

FIGURE 11.30 **CT demonstration of fracture of the odontoid process.** A 50-year-old man sustained a flexion neck injury during a motorcycle accident. The conventional radiographs of the cervical spine suggested odontoid fracture but were not conclusive. **(A)** Coronal and **(B)** sagittal reformatted CT images clearly demonstrate a type II odontoid fracture.

fracture, which in fact constitutes traumatic spondylolisthesis of C2, is common in automobile accidents, when the face strikes the windshield before the vertex of the head, forcing the neck into hyperextension. This injury, which accounts for 4% to 7% of all cervical spine fractures and dislocations, may present as simple, nondisplaced fractures through the pedicles of the axis or as fractures through the arches with anterior subluxation and angulation of C2 onto C3 (Fig. 11.31). The fracture line usually lies anterior to the inferior articular facet of C2 in both variants, but displaced fractures are more often associated with ligament disruption and intervertebral disk injuries. The best projection for demonstrating this injury is the lateral radiograph (Fig. 11.32).

Hangman's fractures (which probably should be correctly called *hanged man fractures*) have been classified into three types (Fig. 11.33). Type I injury is characterized by the fracture through the pedicle of C2 extending between the superior and inferior facets. Type II injury constitutes a type I fracture with concomitant disruption of intervertebral disk C2-3. Type III injury consists of a type II fracture associated with a C2-3 facet dislocation.

Fracture of the Body of C2

Fracture of the body of C2 (Fig. 11.34) is rare, usually presented as a stable "extension teardrop" injury (see later). It may occasionally be complicated by trauma to the vessels.

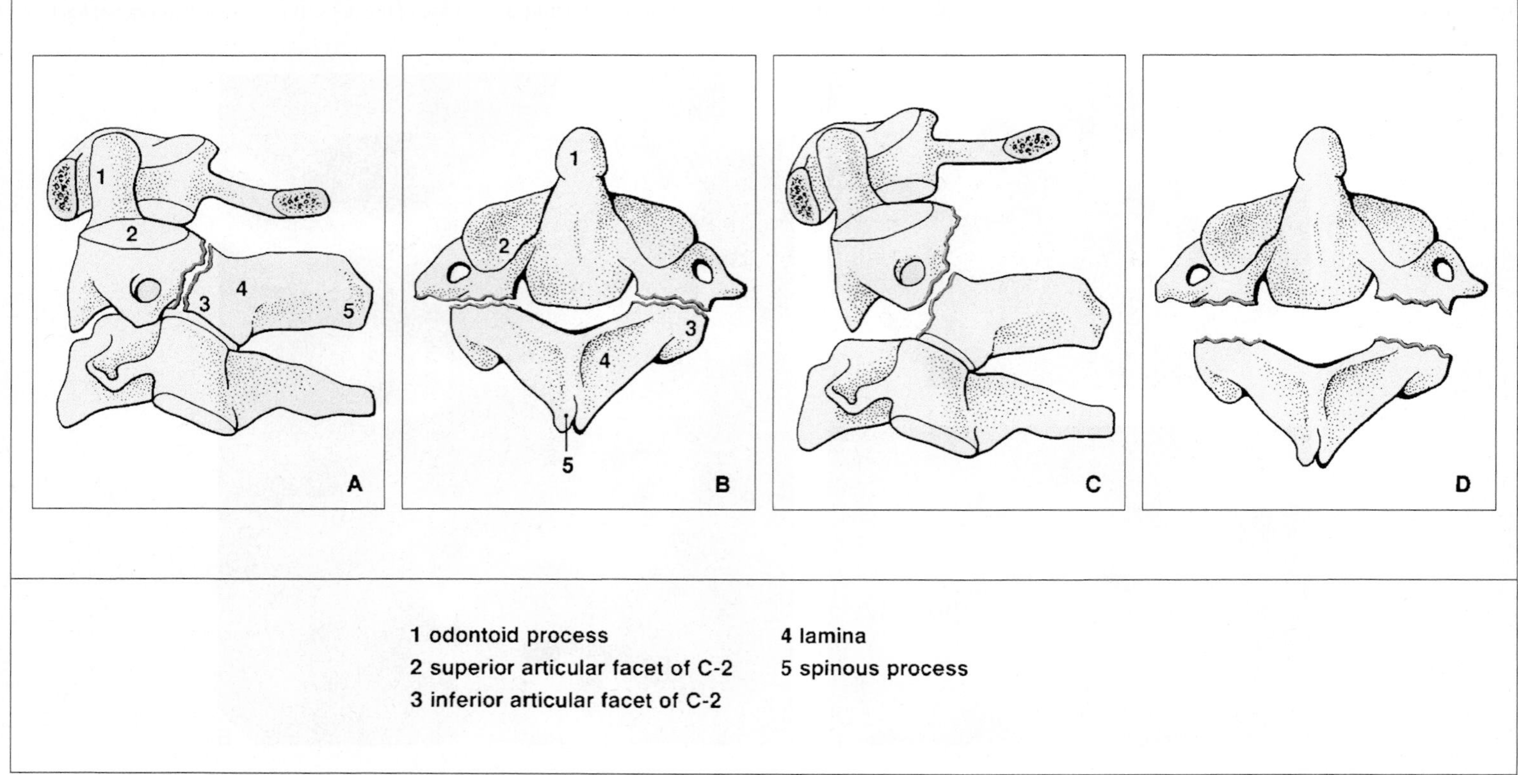

FIGURE 11.31 **Hangman's fracture.** This injury may present as nondisplaced fractures through the arches of C2, as seen here schematically on the **(A)** lateral and **(B)** axial views, or as displaced fractures with anterior angulation **(C)** and **(D)** associated with disruption of ligaments, the intervertebral disk, or articular facets.

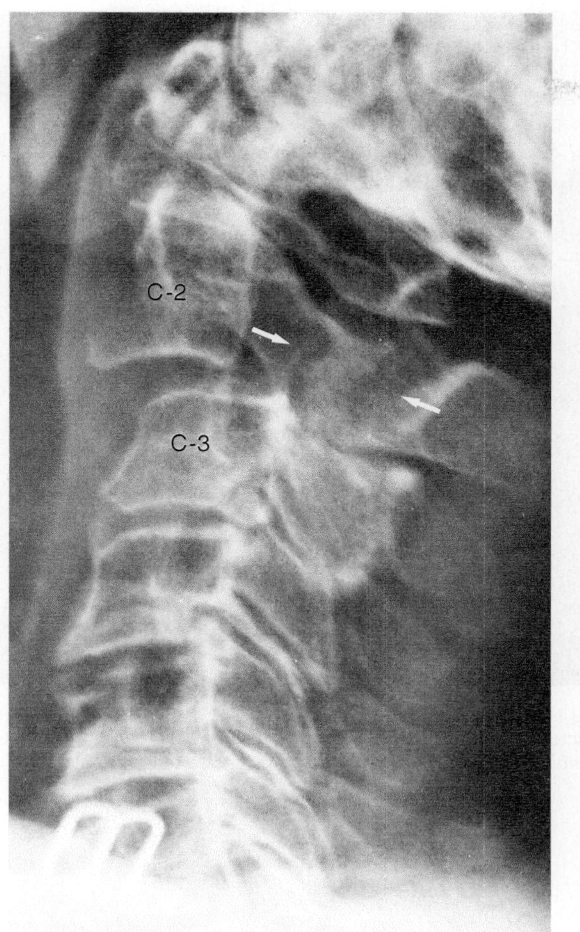

FIGURE 11.32 Hangman's fracture. A 62-year-old man sustained a severe hyperextension injury to the cervical spine in an automobile accident. Lateral radiograph shows a fracture through the pedicles of C2 *(arrows)* associated with C2-3 subluxation, a typical finding in hangman's fracture.

Fractures of the Mid and Lower Cervical Spine

Burst Fracture

The mechanism of this fracture is identical to that of Jefferson fractures involving C1, but burst fractures are seen in the lower cervical vertebrae (C3-7). When the nucleus pulposus, which is normally contained within the intervertebral disk, is driven through the fractured vertebral end plates into the vertebral body, the body explodes from within, resulting in a comminuted fracture. Typically, the posterior fragment is posteriorly displaced and may cause injury to the spinal cord. If the posterior ligament complex is not disrupted, a burst fracture is stable. Occasionally, with ligamentous disruption, a burst fracture becomes unstable. Radiographically, it is characterized by a vertical split in the vertebral body, as seen on the anteroposterior view, but the lateral projection better demonstrates the extent of comminution and posterior displacement (Fig. 11.35A). The most revealing modality in the case of burst fracture is CT because it demonstrates the details of fracture of the posterior part of the vertebral body in the axial plane (Fig. 11.35B).

Teardrop Fracture

The most severe and most unstable of injuries of the cervical spine, teardrop fracture, is characterized by posterior displacement of the involved vertebra into the spinal canal, fracture of its posterior elements, and disruption of the soft tissues, including the ligamentum flavum and the spinal cord, at the level of injury. In addition, stress applied to the anterior longitudinal ligament causes it either to rupture or to avulse from the vertebral body, taking along a piece of the anterior surface of the body. This small, triangular or teardrop-shaped fragment is usually anteriorly and inferiorly displaced (Fig. 11.36). Associated spinal cord injury results in the acute anterior cervical cord syndrome, consisting of abrupt quadriplegia and loss of pain and temperature distinction; however, posterior column senses—position, vibration, and motion—are usually preserved.

The lateral view is the best radiographic projection for demonstrating this injury, but CT is superior technique for this purpose (Figs. 11.37 and 11.38). The evaluation of spinal cord compression requires MRI (Fig. 11.39).

It should be kept in mind in the evaluation of this fracture that occasionally a triangular fragment of bone similar in shape and location to that seen in the classic teardrop fracture may be noted in an extension

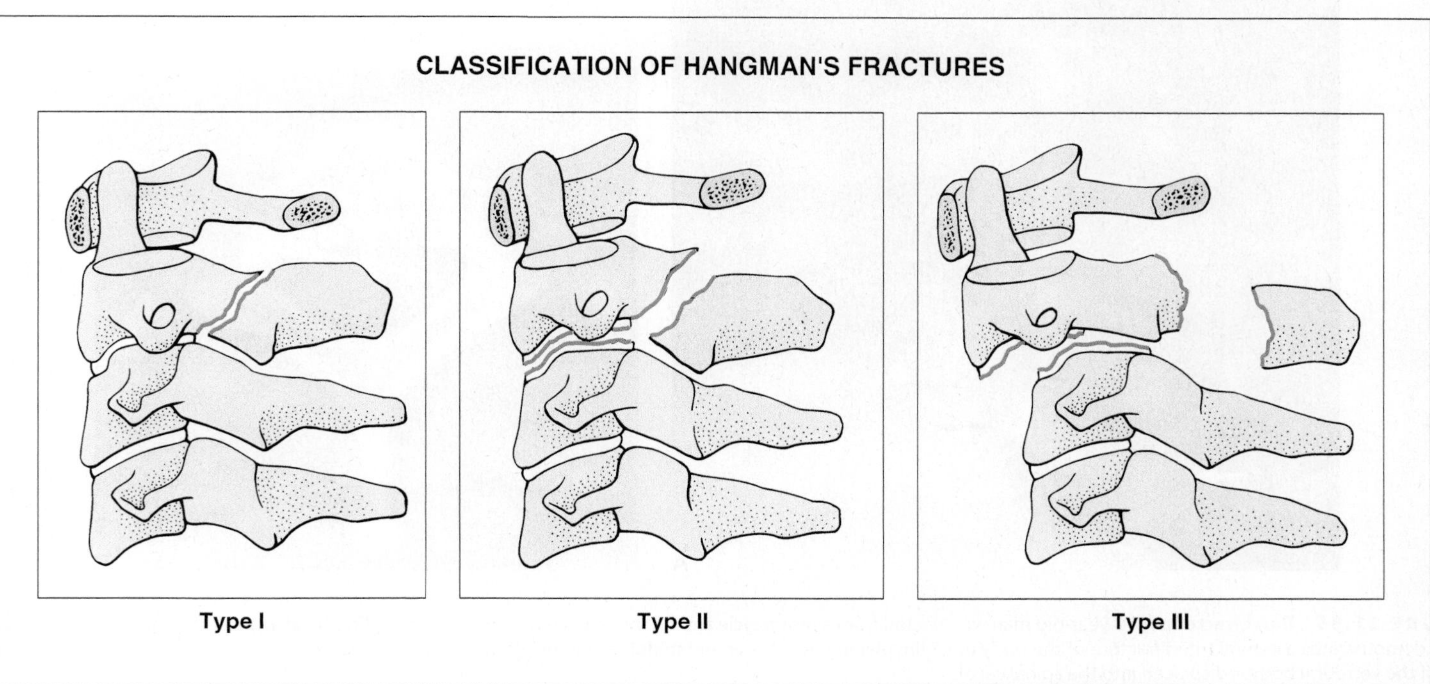

FIGURE 11.33 Classification of hangman's fractures. (Modified from Levine AM, Edwards CC. The management of traumatic spondylolisthesis of the axis. *J Bone Joint Surg Am* 1985;67:217–226.)

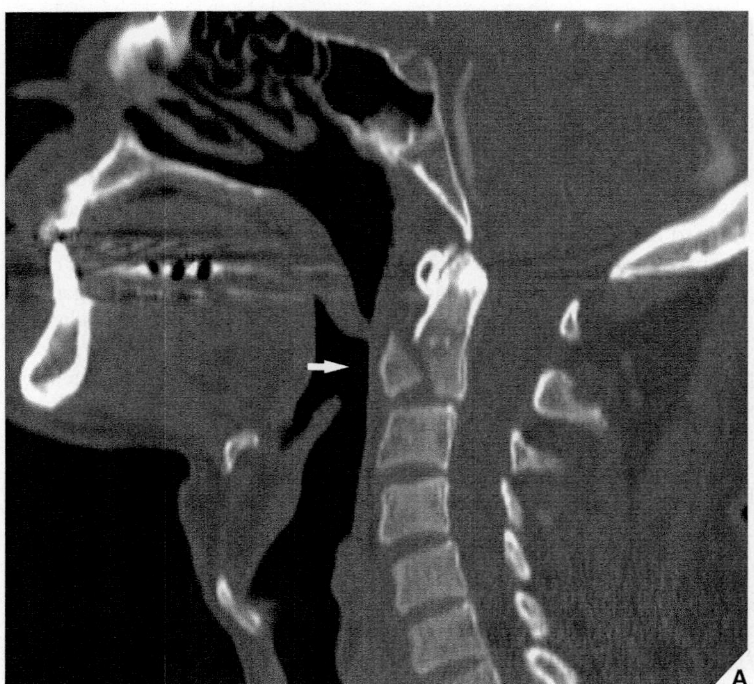
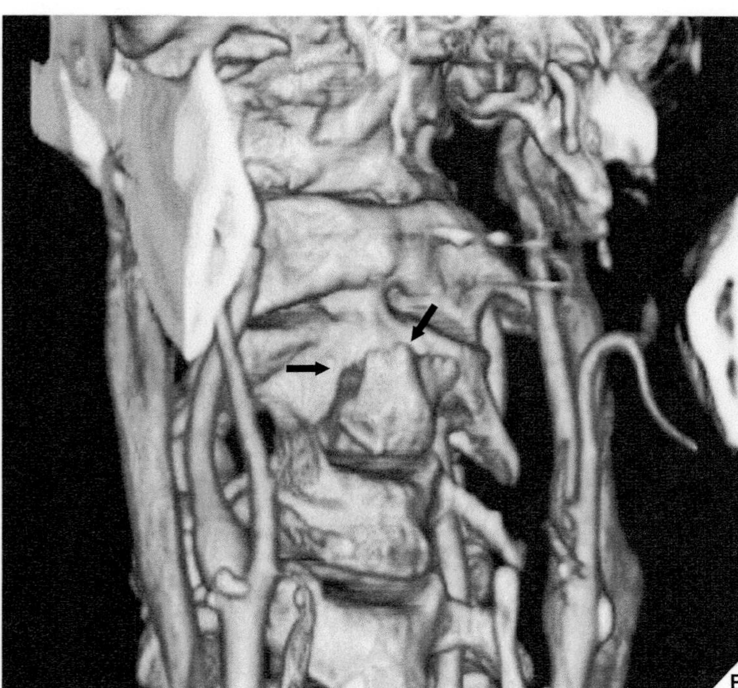

FIGURE 11.34 CT of fracture of the body C2. **(A)** Sagittal CT reformatted image shows a fracture of the body of C2 vertebra *(arrow)*. Because clinically injury to the neck vessels was suspected, 3D CT angiographic study was performed. **(B)** 3D reconstructed image confirmed the fracture *(arrows)*, but the neck arteries were intact.

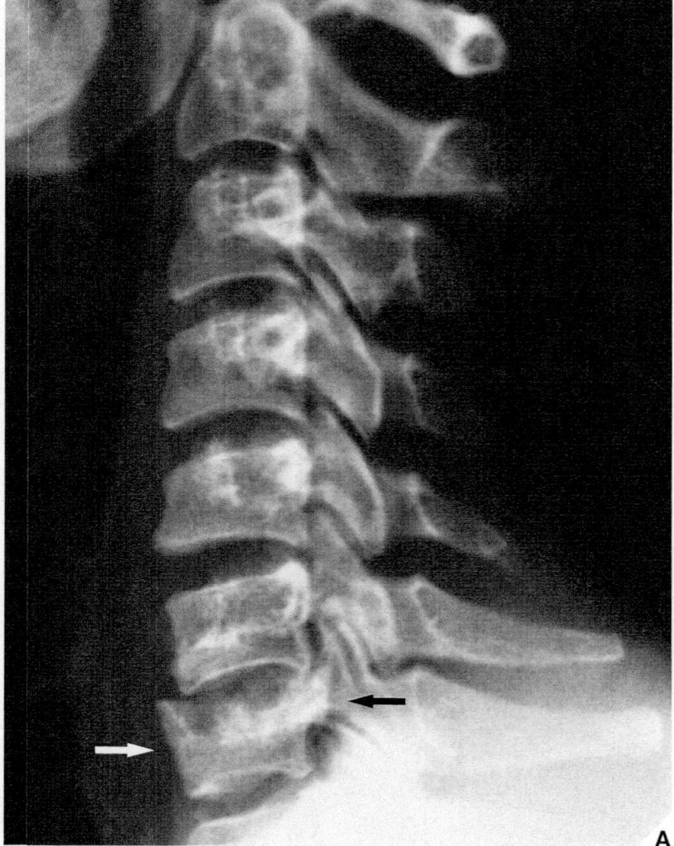
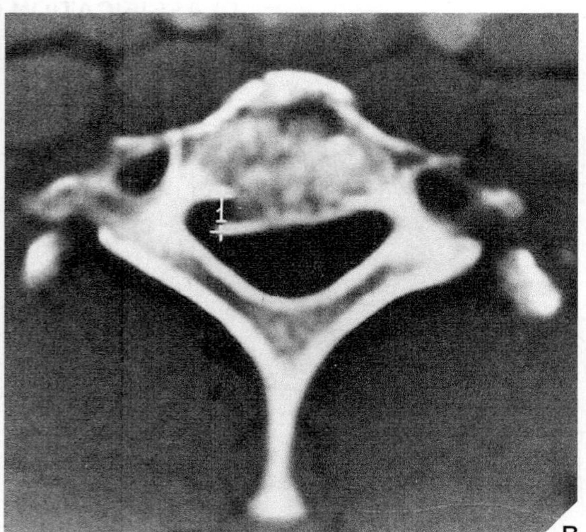

FIGURE 11.35 Burst fracture. A 40-year-old man was ejected from a motorcycle and hit the pavement with the vertex of his head. **(A)** Lateral radiograph of the cervical spine demonstrates a comminuted fracture of the body of C7, involving the anterior and middle columns *(arrows)*. **(B)** CT section confirms the burst fracture. The posterior part of the vertebral body is displaced into the spinal canal.

FIGURE 11.36 **Teardrop fracture.** Teardrop fracture, seen here schematically in a sagittal section of the lower cervical spine, is the most serious and unstable of cervical spine injuries. Disruption of the anterior longitudinal ligament may cause avulsion of a teardrop-shaped fragment of the anterior surface of the body of C5. This fracture is also typified by posterior displacement of the involved vertebra and fracture of its posterior elements. Depending on the severity of the injury, varying degrees of spinal cord damage may result.

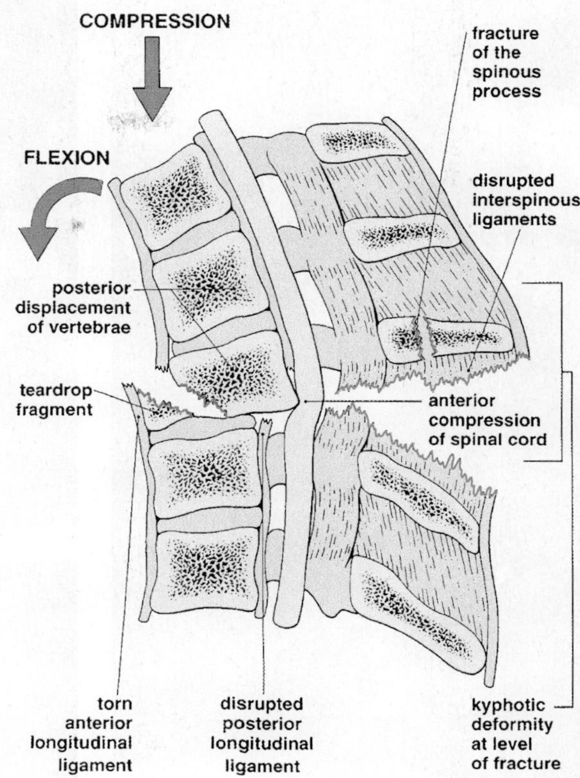

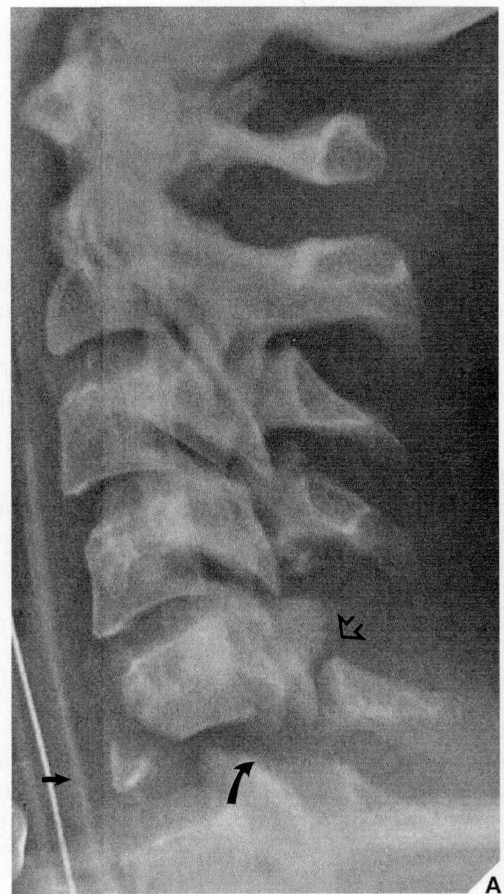

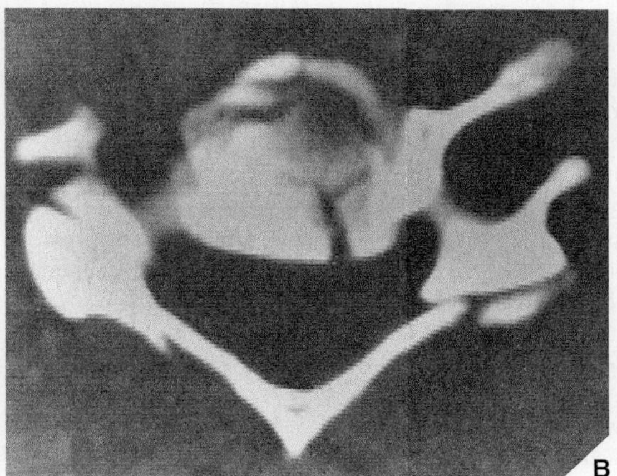

FIGURE 11.37 **Teardrop fracture.** A 38-year-old man sustained an injury of the neck in a motorcycle accident. **(A)** Lateral radiograph of the cervical spine demonstrates an avulsion fracture of the anteroinferior aspect of the body of C5 *(arrow)* and a fracture of its spinous process *(open arrow)*. The lamina of C4 is fractured as well. There is disruption of the facets at the level of C5-6 with marked widening *(curved arrow)*. There is posterior displacement of all vertebrae including and above C5. **(B)** Axial CT section demonstrates in addition a markedly comminuted fracture of the body of C5.

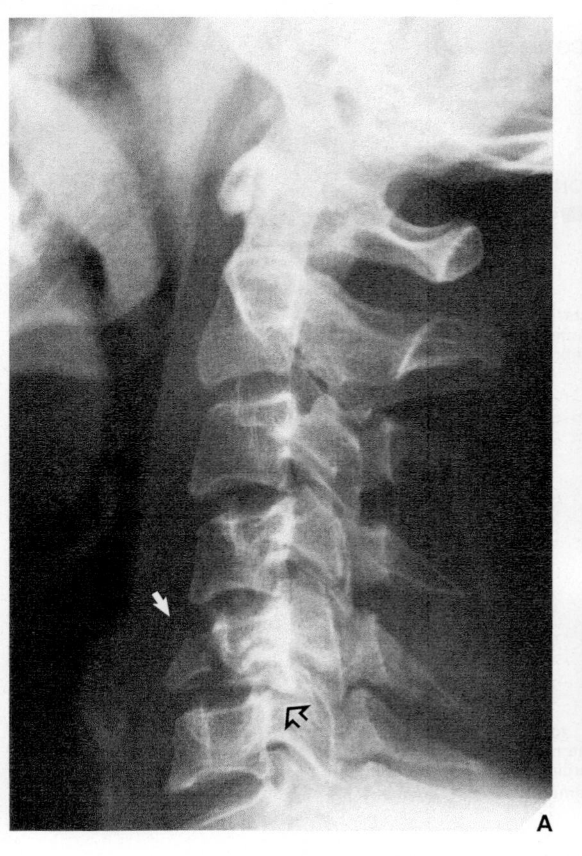

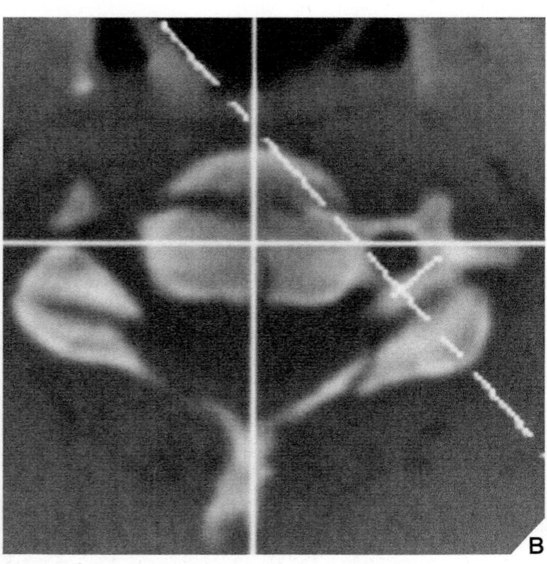

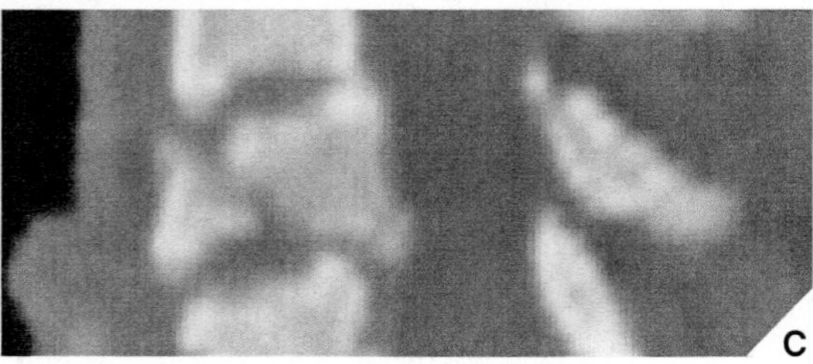

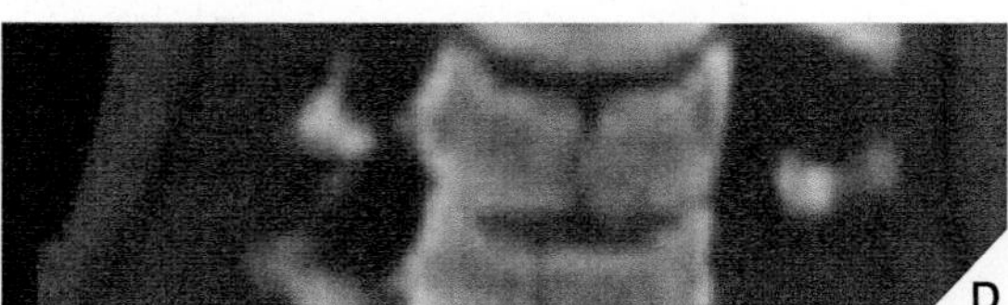

FIGURE 11.38 Teardrop fracture. A 36-year-old man sustained a neck injury in a motorcycle accident. **(A)** Lateral radiograph of the cervical spine shows a typical teardrop fracture of C5 *(arrow)* associated with C5-6 subluxation *(open arrow)*. **(B)** CT axial section and **(C)** sagittal reformatted image demonstrate the details of this injury. **(D)** CT coronal reformatted image shows the vertical fracture of the body of C5 oriented in the sagittal plane.

type of injury. This "extension teardrop" fracture, however, is completely different; it is a stable fracture without the potentially dangerous complications of the flexion type of injury and usually occurs at the level of C2 or C3 (Fig. 11.40; see also Fig. 11.34).

Clay Shoveler's Fracture

This oblique or vertical fracture of the spinous process of C6 or C7 is caused by an acute powerful flexion, such as that produced by shoveling. Deriving its name from its common occurrence in Australian clay miners in the 1930s, *clay shoveler's fracture* was simultaneously labeled with the same name in Germany, where it was seen among workers building the Autobahn. A direct blow to the cervical spine or indirect trauma to the neck in automobile accidents can result in similar injury.

Clay shoveler's fracture is a stable fracture, the posterior ligament complex remaining intact and is thus not associated with neurologic damage. The best radiographic projection for demonstrating this injury is the lateral view of the cervical spine (Fig. 11.41A). If C7 cannot be visualized despite good positioning and technique, for example, because of a short, thick neck or wide shoulders, then the swimmer's view should be obtained. This fracture can also be identified on the anteroposterior view by the so-called *ghost sign* (Fig. 11.41B) produced by displacement of the fractured spinous process. CT or MRI is rarely indicated (Figs. 11.42 and 11.43).

Simple Wedge (Compression) Fracture

Resulting from hyperflexion of the cervical spine, a simple wedge fracture generally occurs in the midcervical or lower cervical segment. There is anterior compression (wedging) of the vertebral body, and although the posterior ligament complex is stretched, it remains intact, making this a stable fracture. The lateral projection of the cervical spine adequately demonstrates this injury (Fig. 11.44), although CT is commonly required (Fig. 11.45).

Locked Facets

Unilateral Locked Facets

This type of injury is secondary to the flexion-rotation force with subsequent tearing of the joint capsule of one facet and posterior ligamentous complex. In the absence of disk space widening or subluxation, unilateral facet locking is a relatively stable injury. Frequently, however, there is approximately 25% anterior subluxation. These patients are at risk for sustaining nerve root injury or, rarely, a Brown-Sequard type spinal cord injury.

Bilateral Perched Facets

This type of vertebral subluxation occurs as a result of a flexion injury. There is disruption of the posterior ligamentous complex, and the inferior and superior articular processes of the involved vertebrae are in apposition. The shingled appearance of the facet joints is changed to a configuration in which the laminar cortices intersect at one point (Figs. 11.46 and 11.47A). This injury is best diagnosed on the lateral and oblique projections of the cervical spine or CT with sagittal and oblique reformation.

Bilateral Locked Facets

Bilateral dislocation of the cervical spine in the facet joints is the result of extreme flexion of the head and neck; it is an unstable condition caused by extensive disruption of the posterior ligament complex. Interlocking of the articular facets is initiated by the forward movement of the inferior articular facet of the upper vertebra over the superior articular facet of the underlying vertebra (Fig. 11.47). This causes the lamina and spinous process of the two adjacent vertebrae to spread apart and the vertebral bodies to sublux. In the later stage of dislocation, the inferior articular facet of the upper vertebra locks in front of the superior articular facet of the lower vertebra, which results in complete anterior dislocation. The configuration of this injury leads to complete disruption of the posterior ligament

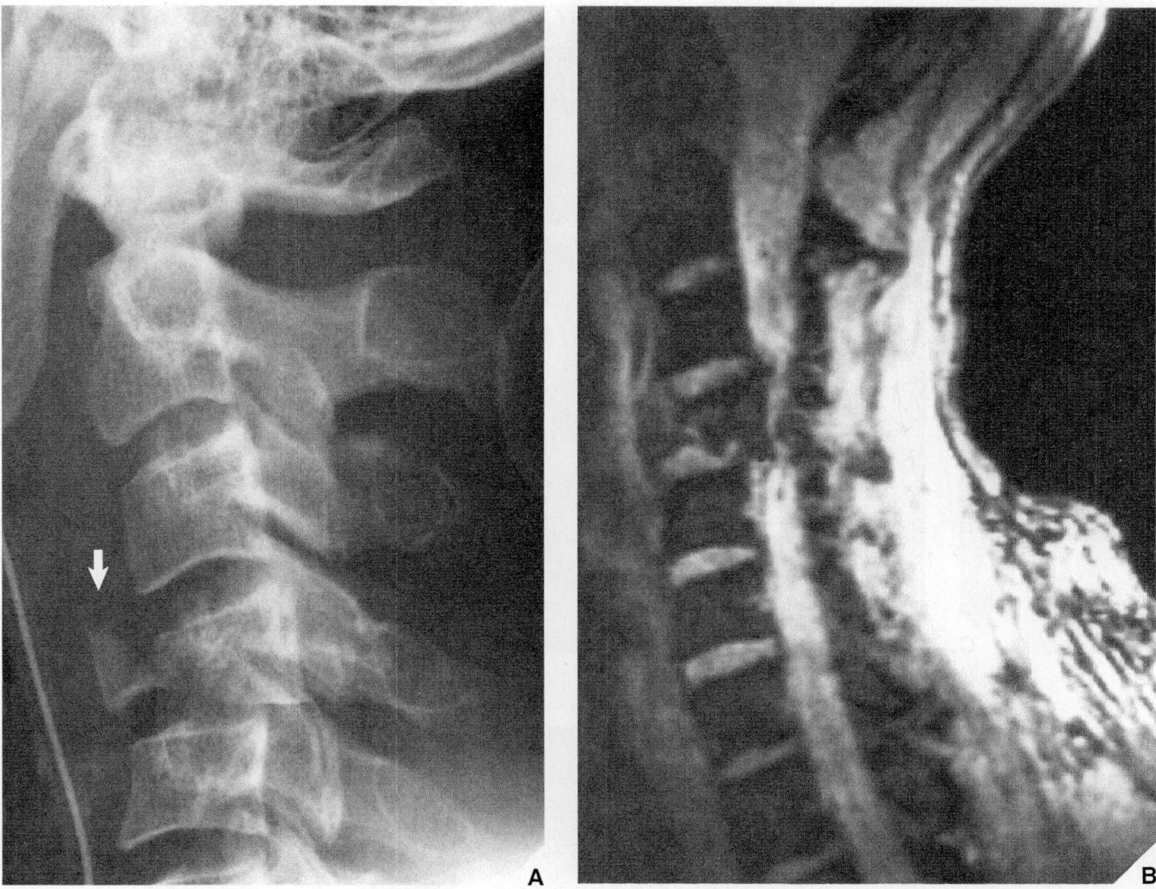

FIGURE 11.39 MRI of teardrop fracture. A 38-year-old man, an unrestrained passenger, was injured in a car accident. **(A)** Lateral radiograph of the cervical spine shows a teardrop fracture of C4 *(arrow)*. **(B)** Sagittal gradient-echo (MPGR) MR image shows posterior displacement of the C4 vertebral body compromising the spinal canal and almost complete transection of the cervical cord. Extensive high-signal soft-tissue edema and hemorrhage are evident.

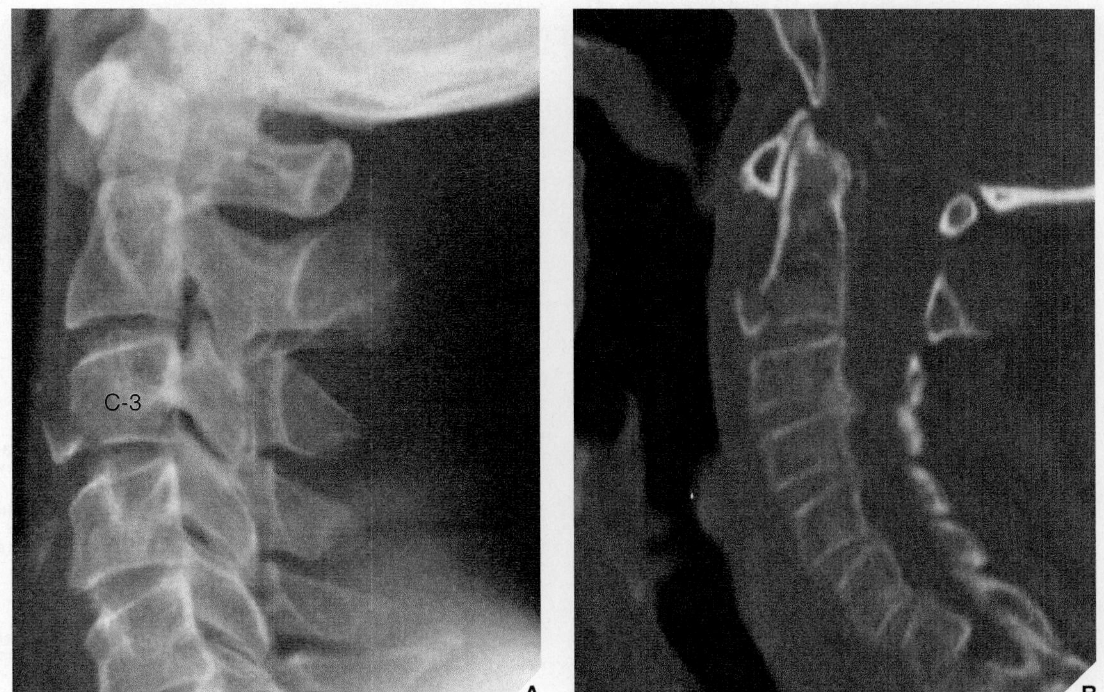

FIGURE 11.40 Extension teardrop fracture. **(A)** A 37-year-old man sustained an extension injury to the cervical spine in a fall. Lateral radiograph of the spine demonstrates an extension teardrop fracture of the vertebral body of C3. Note that, in contrast to a flexion-type injury, there is no subluxation, and the posterior vertebral and spinolaminar lines are not disrupted. **(B)** In another patient, a 63-year-old man who presented with neck pain following a car accident 3 weeks prior, a sagittal CT scan demonstrates a teardrop fracture of the C2 vertebral body. *(Continued)*

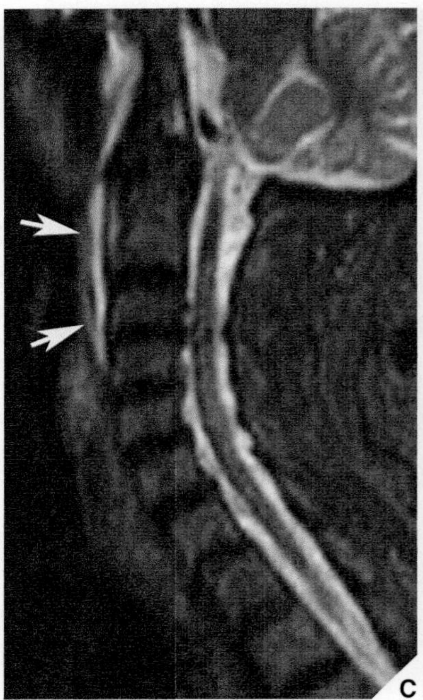

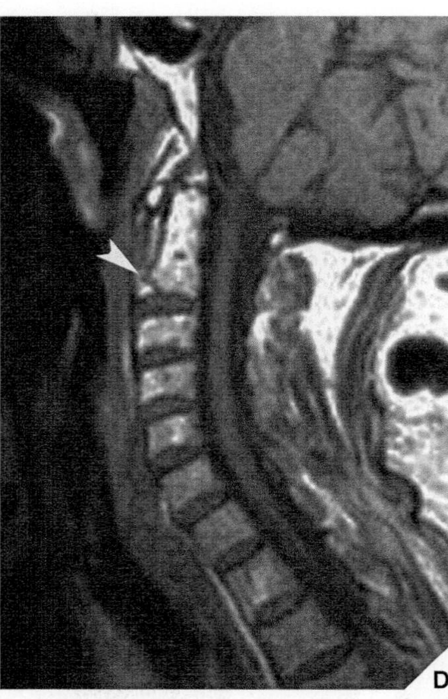

FIGURE 11.40 Extension teardrop fracture. ***(Continued)*** **(C)** Sagittal T2-weighted MR image displays the prevertebral soft-tissue edema *(arrows)*. The fracture of C2 is not well demonstrated. **(D)** Sagittal T1-weighted MR image clearly shows the fracture *(arrowhead)*. (**B**, **C**, and **D**, Courtesy of Evan Stein, MD, Brooklyn, New York.)

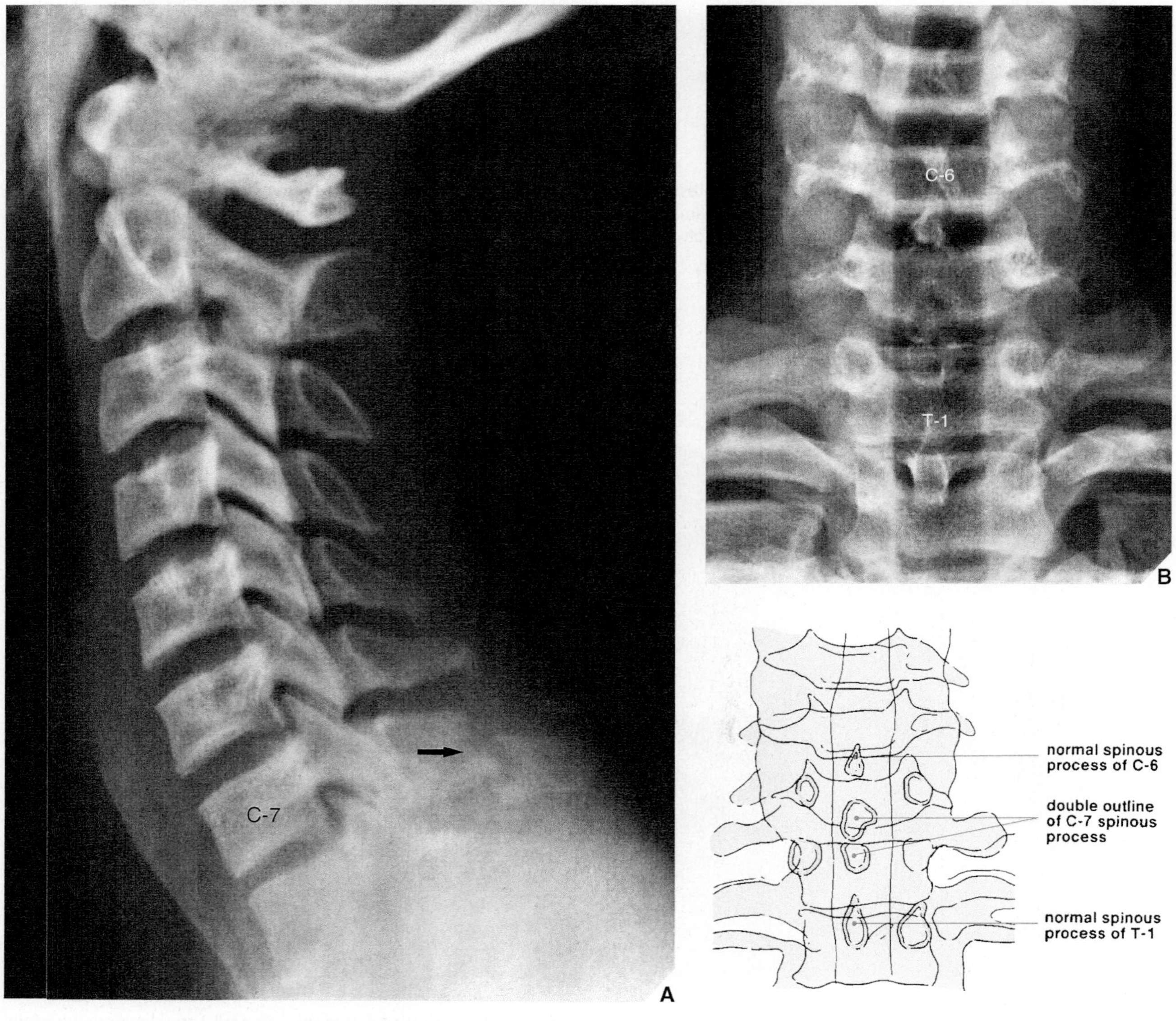

C-7

C-6

T-1

normal spinous process of C-6

double outline of C-7 spinous process

normal spinous process of T-1

FIGURE 11.41 Clay shoveler's fracture. A 22-year-old man sustained a neck injury in an automobile accident. **(A)** Lateral radiograph of the cervical spine shows a fracture of the spinous process of C7 *(arrow)*, identifying this injury as a clay shoveler's fracture. **(B)** On the anteroposterior view, clay shoveler's fracture can be identified by the appearance of a double spinous process for C7. This ghost sign is secondary to slight caudal displacement of the fractured tip of the spinous process.

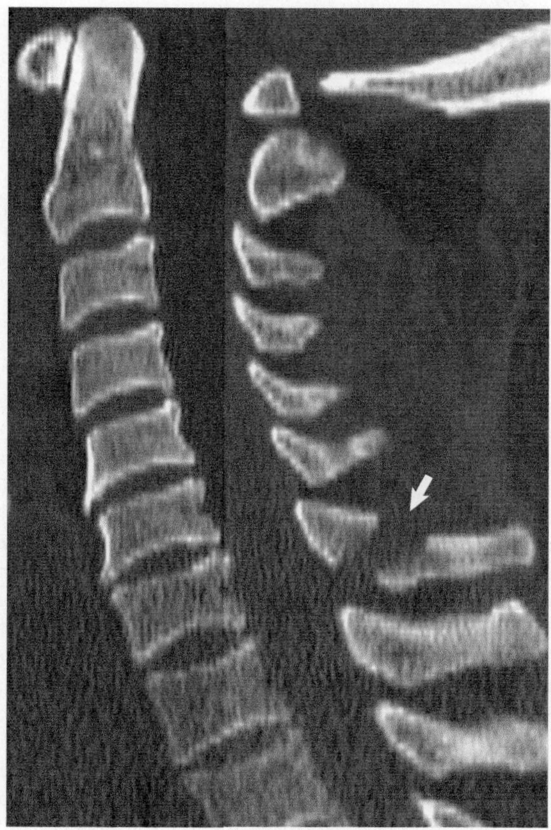

FIGURE 11.42 **CT of the clay shoveler's fracture.** A 33-year-old man injured his neck in wrestling competition. Conventional radiographs were not diagnostic because of excessive neck musculature. Sagittal CT reformatted image of the cervical spine shows a displaced fracture of the spinous process of C7 *(arrow)*.

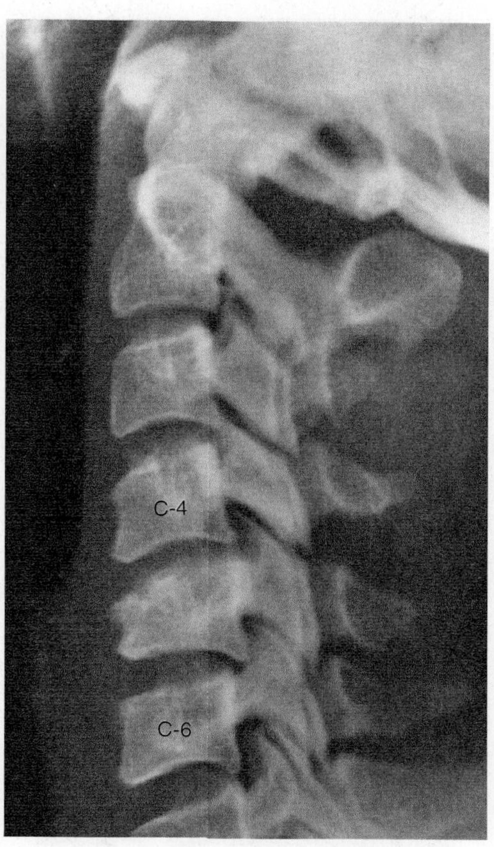

FIGURE 11.44 **Compression (wedge) fracture.** A 30-year-old woman sustained a neck injury in an automobile accident. Lateral radiograph of the cervical spine demonstrates a simple wedge fracture of C5.

complex, the posterior longitudinal ligament, the annulus fibrosus, and frequently the anterior longitudinal ligament. It is also associated with a high incidence of cervical spinal cord damage.

The lateral radiograph of the cervical spine, preferably a cross-table lateral, is sufficient to demonstrate bilaterally locked facets. The key to the correct diagnosis is the presence of malalignment of the affected vertebrae associated with disruption of all lateral cervical spine landmarks (see Fig. 11.3D) and position of the dislocated facets posteriorly and cephalad in relation to the facets of the vertebra above (Fig. 11.47C).

MRI is the modality of choice to demonstrate nonosseous lesions of the cervical spine following a traumatic event, such as ligamentous ruptures and epidural hematomas (Fig. 11.48).

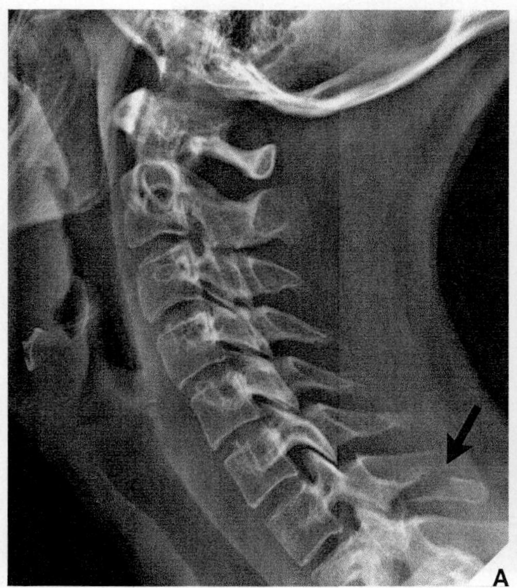

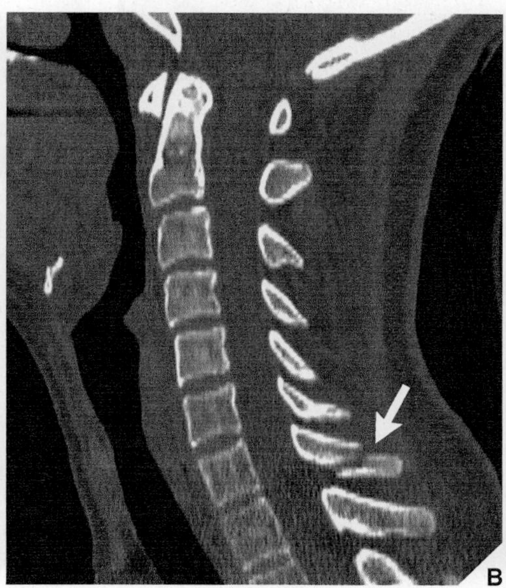

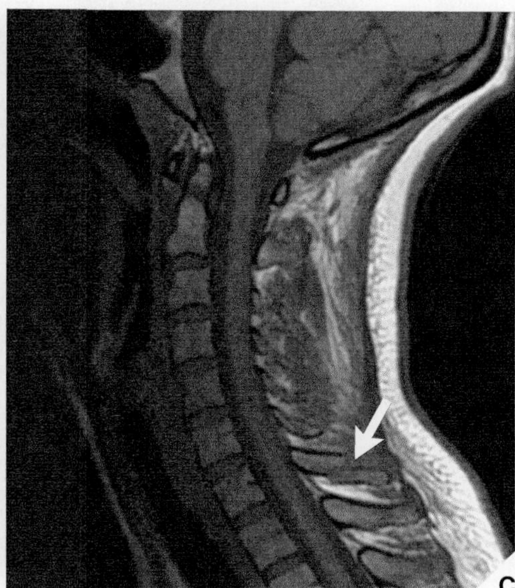

FIGURE 11.43 **CT and MRI of the clay shoveler's fracture.** A 22-year-old man injured his neck in a diving accident. **(A)** Lateral radiograph, **(B)** sagittal CT reformatted image, and **(C)** sagittal proton density-weighted MR image demonstrate slightly caudally displaced fracture of the spinous process of C7 *(arrows)*.

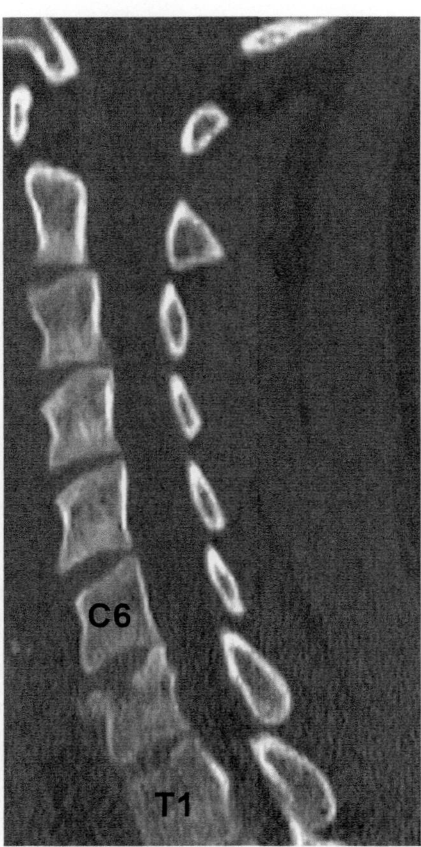

FIGURE 11.45 CT of the compression fracture. An 18-year-old man was injured in a diving accident. Sagittal CT reformatted image shows a compression fracture of C7. Note anatomic alignment of the posterior aspects of the vertebral bodies and intact posterior vertebral line.

Thoracolumbar Spine

Anatomic–Radiologic Considerations

The standard radiographic projections for evaluating an injury to the *thoracic spine* are the anteroposterior (Fig. 11.49) and lateral (Fig. 11.50) views. The lateral projection is obtained using a technique called *autotomography*, which requires shallow breathing by the patient to blur the structures involved in respiratory motion and give a clear view of the thoracic vertebral column.

As in cervical spine injuries, CT and MRI play leading roles in the evaluation of fractures of the thoracic spine, particularly in defining the extent of injury. Axial CT images provide an excellent means of evaluating not only osseous abnormalities but also soft-tissue injuries, and reformatted sagittal, coronal, and three-dimensional (3D) reconstructed images, in addition, allow to demonstrate axially oriented fracture lines that can be missed on axial sections. MR images are ideal for evaluating concomitant soft-tissue injury, particularly to the spinal cord and thecal sac. Sagittal images are obtained with T1 and T2 weighting, and T2-weighted axial sections are supplemented with gradient recalled echo (GRE) images.

The standard radiographic examination for evaluating injuries of the *lumbar spine* includes the anteroposterior, lateral, and oblique projections, supplemented by coned-down lateral spot films of the lumbosacral junction (L5-S1). The anteroposterior view is usually sufficient for evaluating traumatic conditions involving the vertebral bodies and transverse processes; the intervertebral disk spaces are also well demonstrated, except for the lowest (L5-S1) (Fig. 11.51). The spinous processes, seen as teardrops, and the articular facets, however, are not well demonstrated on this projection. A characteristic configuration of the end plates of the L3-5 vertebral bodies can be observed on the anteroposterior projection. Normally, the inferior aspects of these vertebrae form what is called a *Cupid's bow contour* (Fig. 11.52), which is lost in cases of compression fractures affecting this part of the vertebral column.

On the lateral projection of the lumbar spine, the vertebral bodies are seen in profile, and the superior and inferior end plates are well demonstrated (Fig. 11.53). Fractures of the spinous processes can be

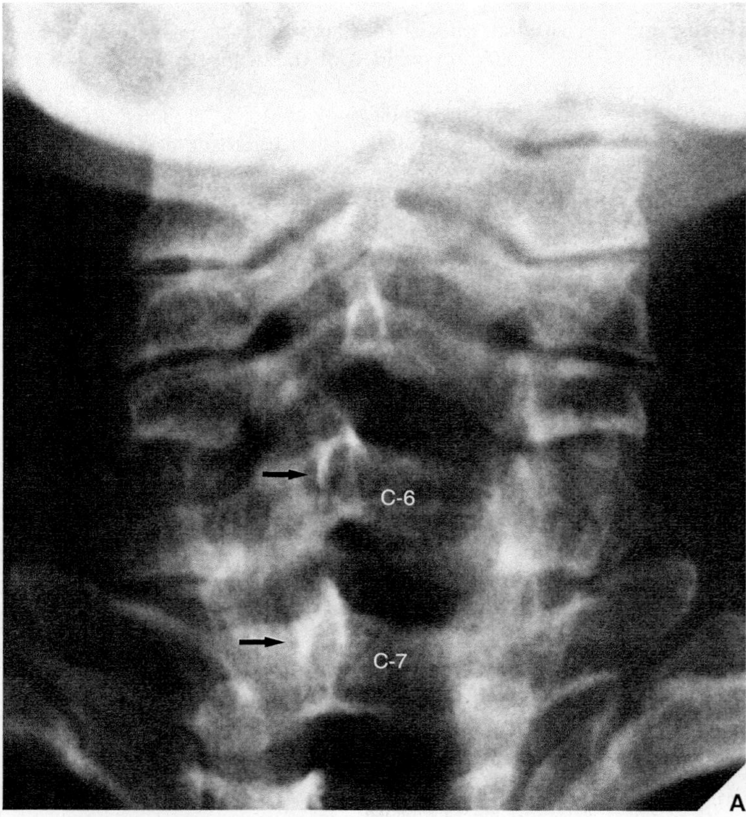

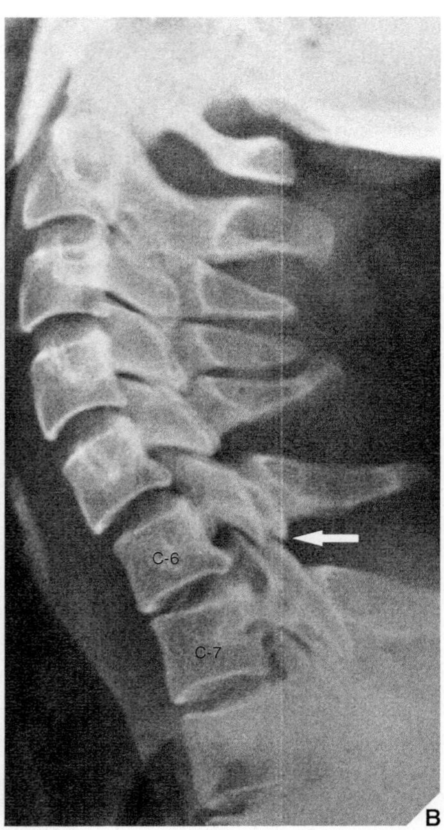

FIGURE 11.46 Perched facets. A 34-year-old woman injured her neck in a skiing accident. **(A)** Pillar view of the cervical spine demonstrates bilateral obliteration of the facet joints at the C6-7 level. The joints above appear normal. Displacement of the spinous processes to the right *(arrows)* is the result of rotation. **(B)** Lateral radiograph shows perched facets of vertebrae C6 and C7 *(arrow)*.

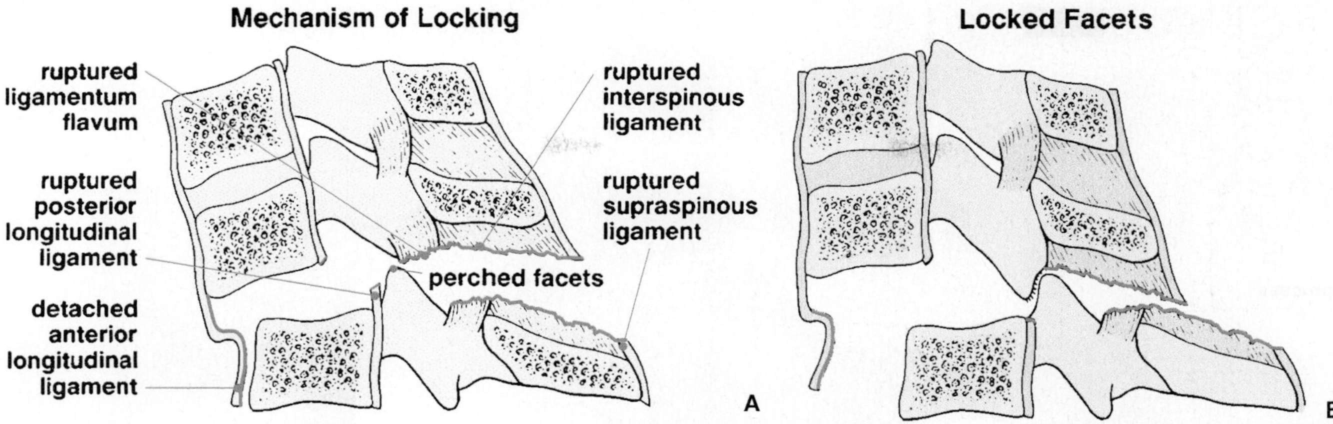

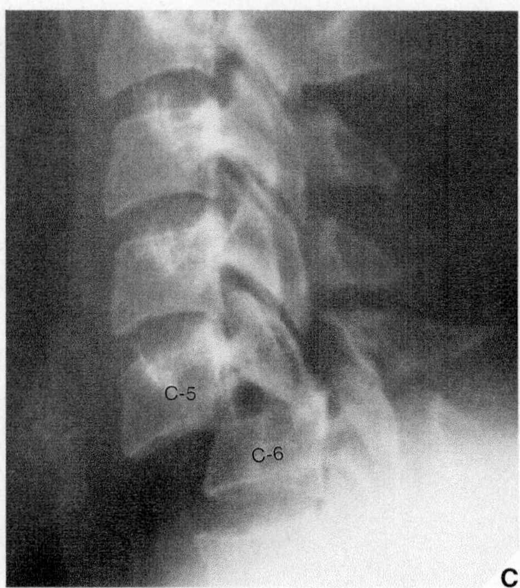

FIGURE 11.47 Locked facets. **(A,B)** Bilateral locked facets is a hyperflexion injury characterized by complete anterior dislocation of the affected vertebra. It is always associated with extensive ligament disruption and carries a great risk of cervical spinal cord damage. **(C)** A 36-year-old man injured his neck in a motor vehicle accident that resulted in quadriplegia. Lateral radiograph of the cervical spine shows bilateral locked facets at the C5-6 level.

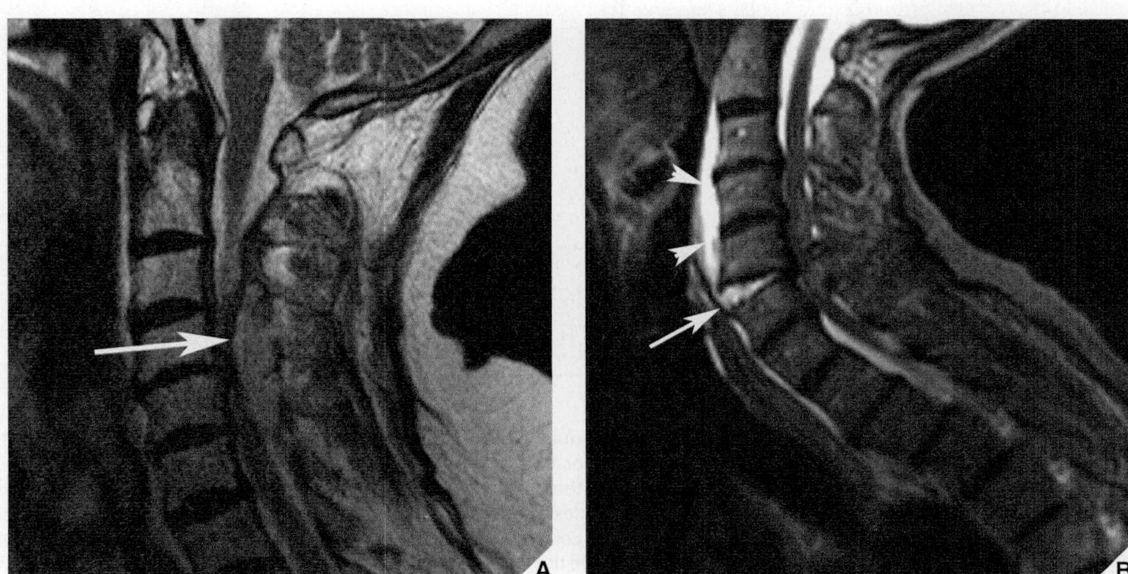

FIGURE 11.48 MRI of soft-tissue injuries of the cervical spine. **(A)** Sagittal T2-weighted MRI of a 53-year-old patient presenting with acute onset of paraplegia following an industrial accident, shows the hyperintense epidural hematoma at the level of C4 and C5 located posteriorly, with compression of the cord *(arrow)*. **(B)** Sagittal T2-weighted MR image of a 70-year-old man, who presented with severe neck pain after a hyperextension injury but without focal neurologic signs, shows the tear of the anterior longitudinal ligament with widening of the anterior aspect of the C5-6 disk space *(arrow)* and the anterior prevertebral hematoma *(arrowheads)*. (Courtesy of Evan Stein, MD, Brooklyn, New York.)

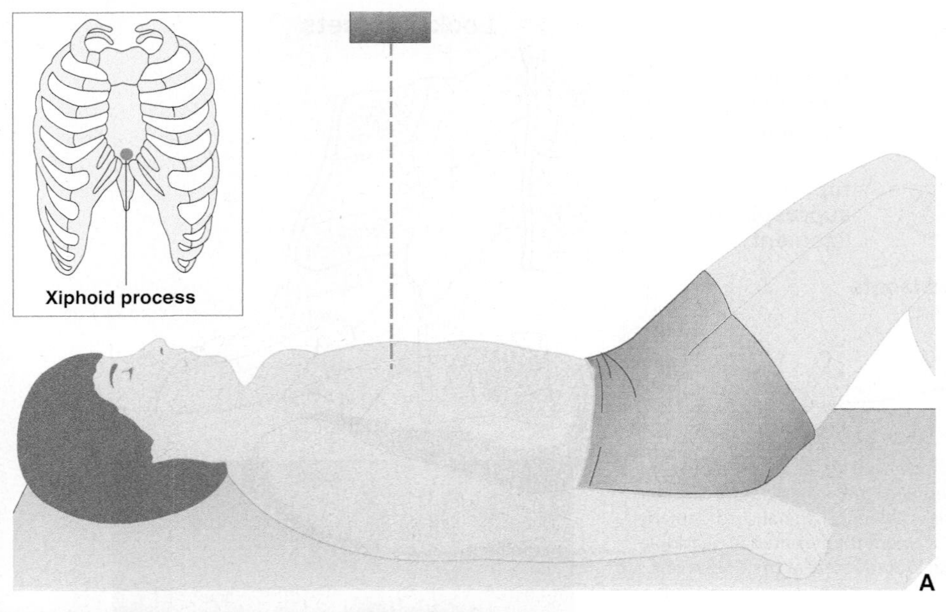

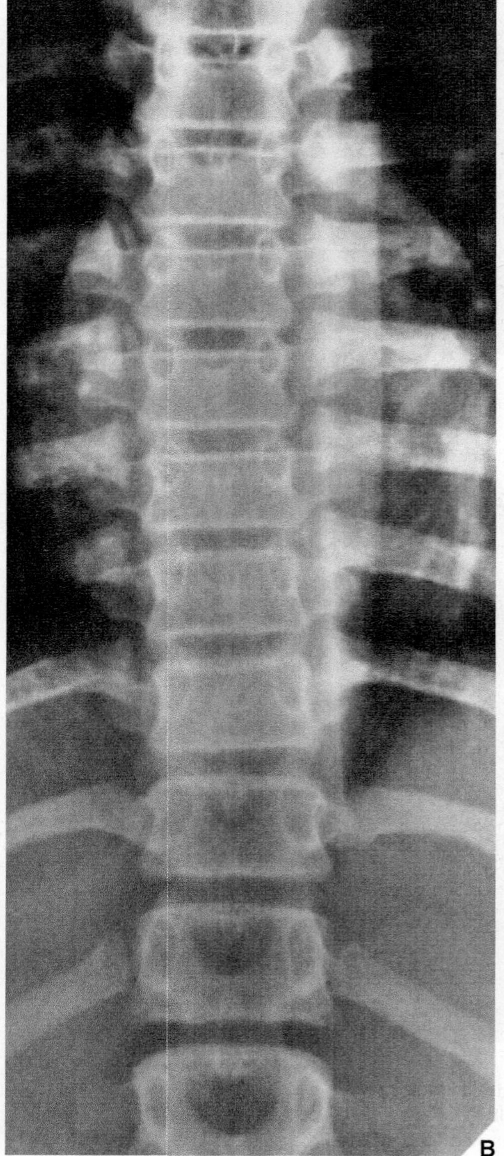

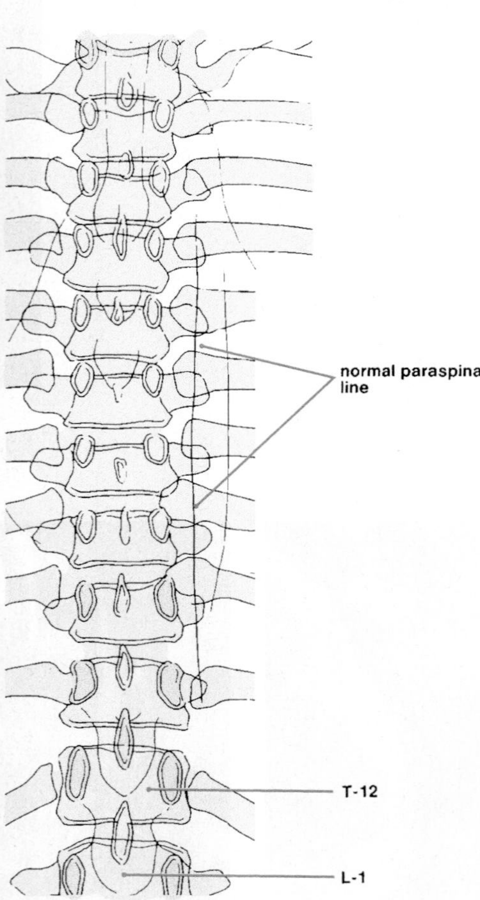

FIGURE 11.49 Anteroposterior view of the thoracic spine. **(A)** For the anteroposterior view of the thoracic spine, the patient is supine on the table, with the knees flexed to correct the normal thoracic kyphosis. The central beam is directed vertically about 3 cm above the xiphoid process. **(B)** On the radiograph in this projection, the vertebral end plates and pedicles and the intervertebral disk spaces are seen. The height of the vertebrae can be determined, and changes in the paraspinal line can be evaluated.

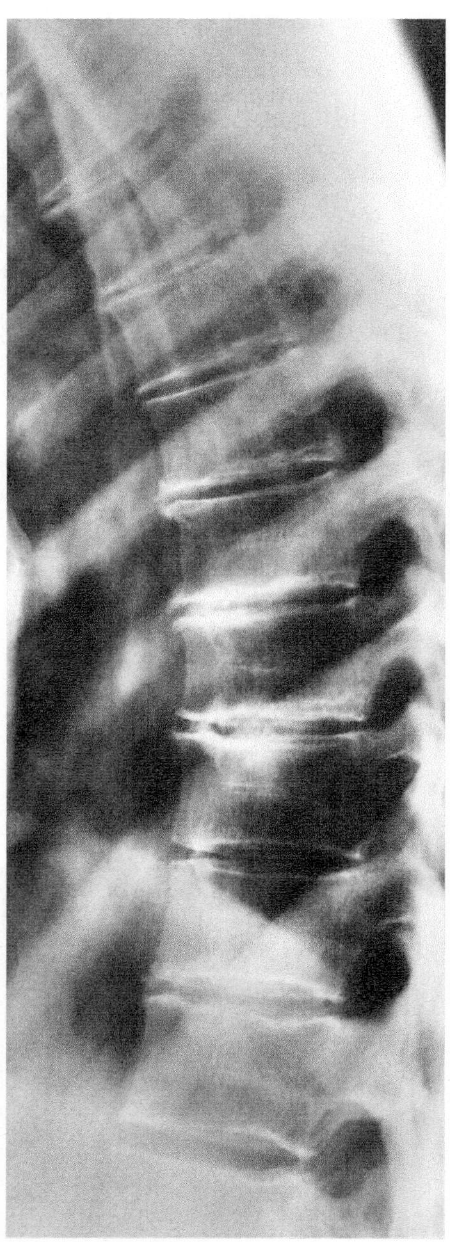

FIGURE 11.50 Lateral view of the thoracic spine. For the lateral view of the thoracic spine, the patient is erect with the arms elevated. To eliminate structures that would obscure the bony elements of the thoracic spine, the patient is instructed to breathe shallowly during the exposure. The central beam is directed horizontally to the level of the T6 vertebra with about 10-degree cephalad angulation. The radiograph in this projection demonstrates a lateral image of the vertebral bodies and intervertebral disk spaces.

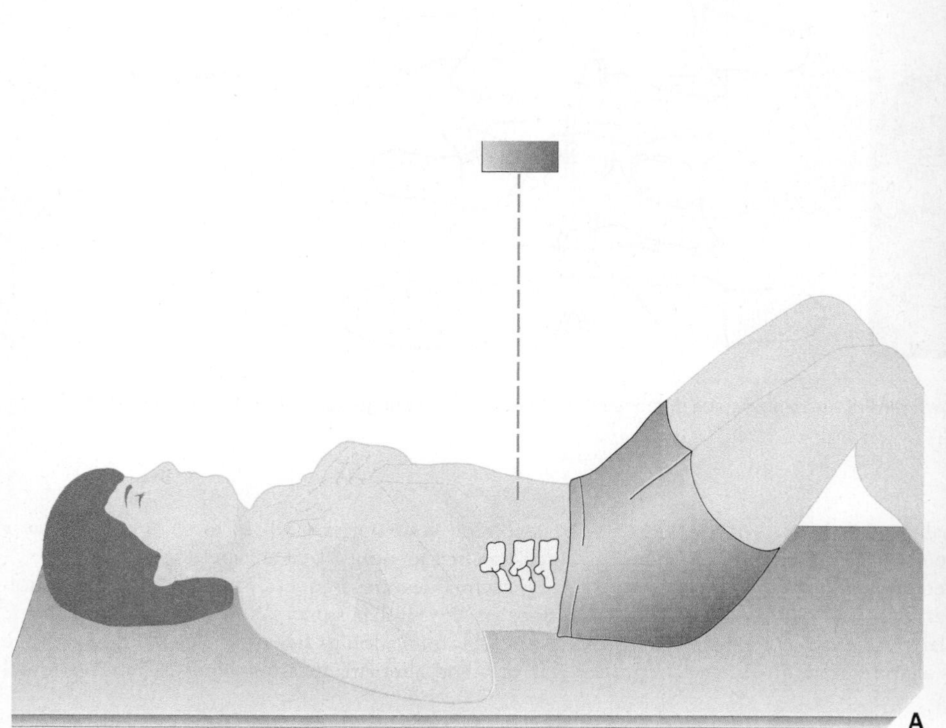

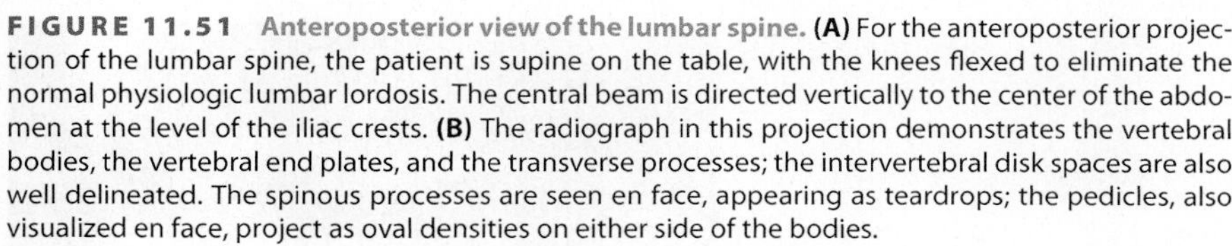

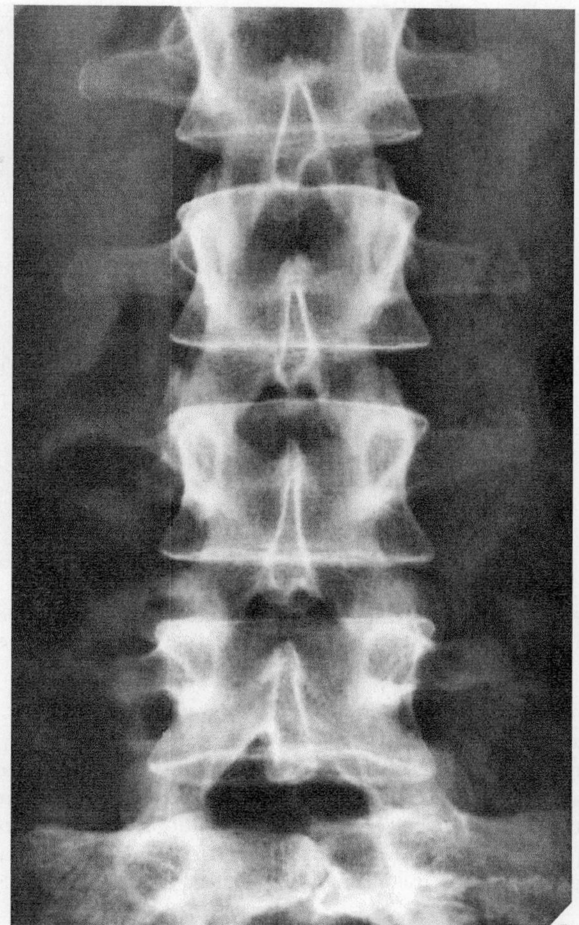

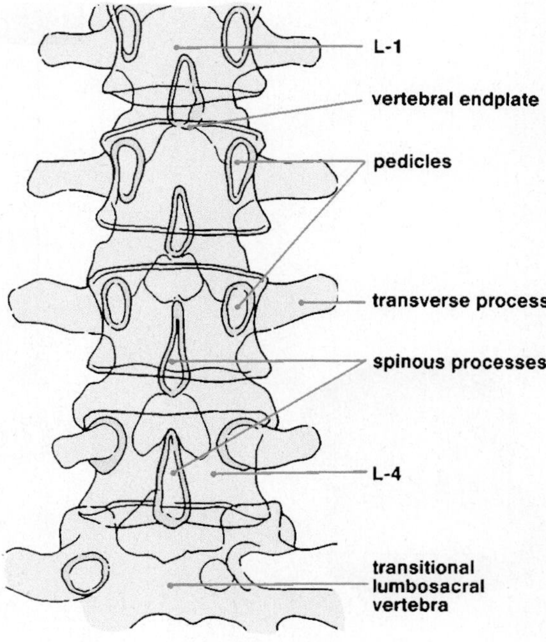

FIGURE 11.51 **Anteroposterior view of the lumbar spine.** **(A)** For the anteroposterior projection of the lumbar spine, the patient is supine on the table, with the knees flexed to eliminate the normal physiologic lumbar lordosis. The central beam is directed vertically to the center of the abdomen at the level of the iliac crests. **(B)** The radiograph in this projection demonstrates the vertebral bodies, the vertebral end plates, and the transverse processes; the intervertebral disk spaces are also well delineated. The spinous processes are seen en face, appearing as teardrops; the pedicles, also visualized en face, project as oval densities on either side of the bodies.

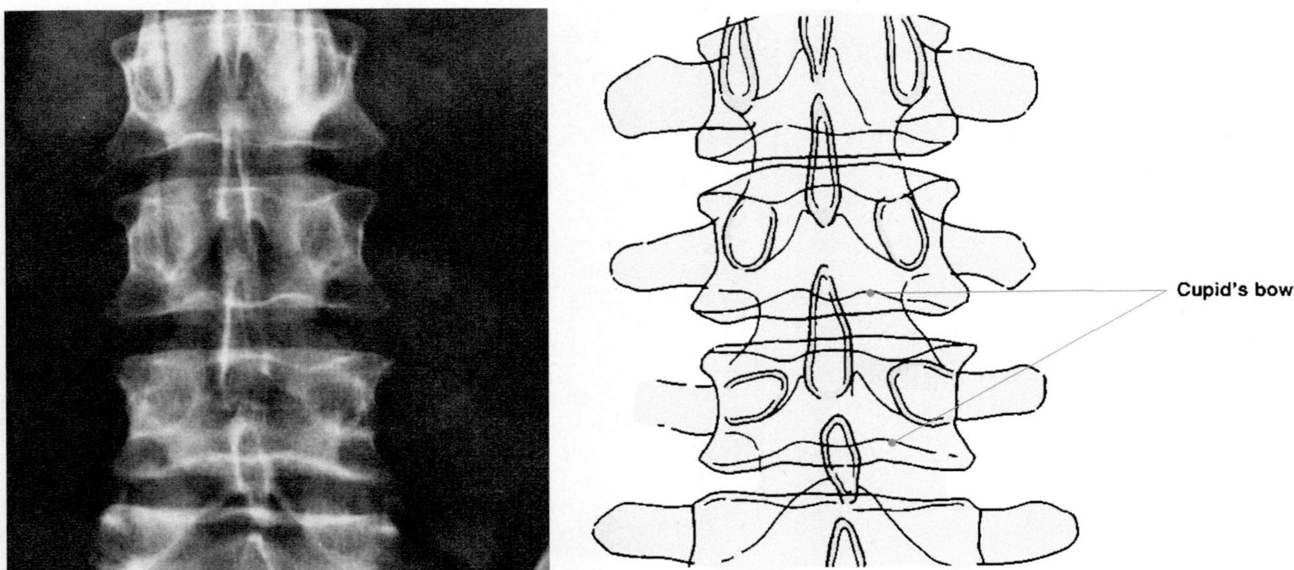

FIGURE 11.52 Cupid's bow sign. Anteroposterior coned-down view of the lumbar spine demonstrates a characteristic configuration of the lower aspects of L3 and L4. This "Cupid's bow" contour is lost in cases of compression fracture.

adequately evaluated on this projection, as can abnormalities involving the intervertebral disk spaces, including L5-S1. As in the cervical spine, an oblique projection of the lumbar spine can be obtained from the patient's anterior or posterior aspect, although the posteroanterior oblique projection is preferable (Fig. 11.54). This view is particularly effective in demonstrating the facet joints (articular facets) and reveals a configuration of the elements of adjoining vertebrae, known as the *Scotty dog formation* (Fig. 11.54C,D), which was first identified by Lachapele.

Ancillary imaging techniques are frequently used in the evaluation of traumatic conditions of the lumbar spine. As in cervical and thoracic injuries, CT provides useful information in assessing the extent of damage in vertebral body fractures and abnormalities involving the intervertebral

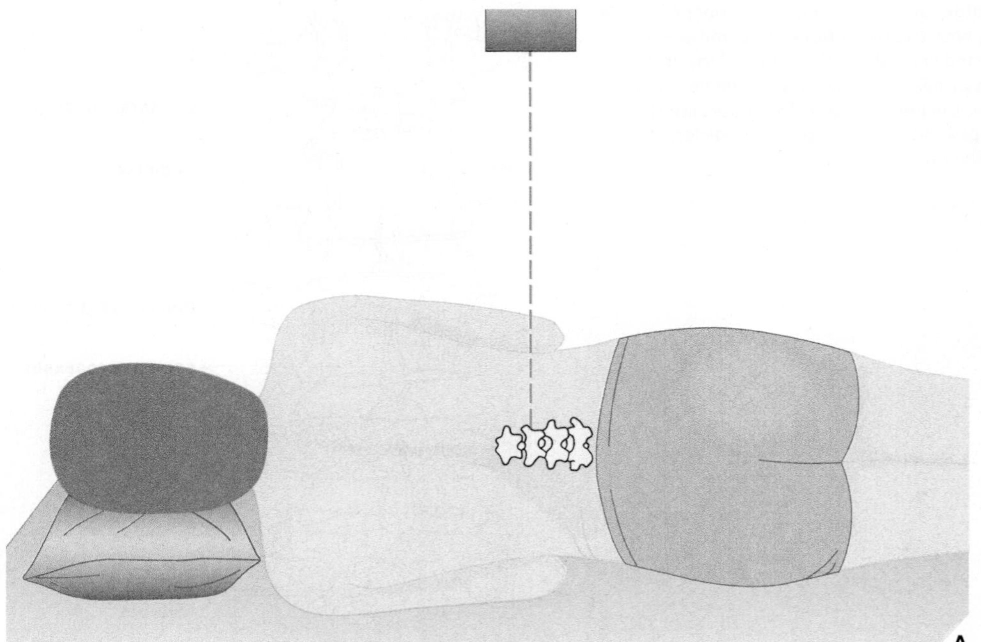

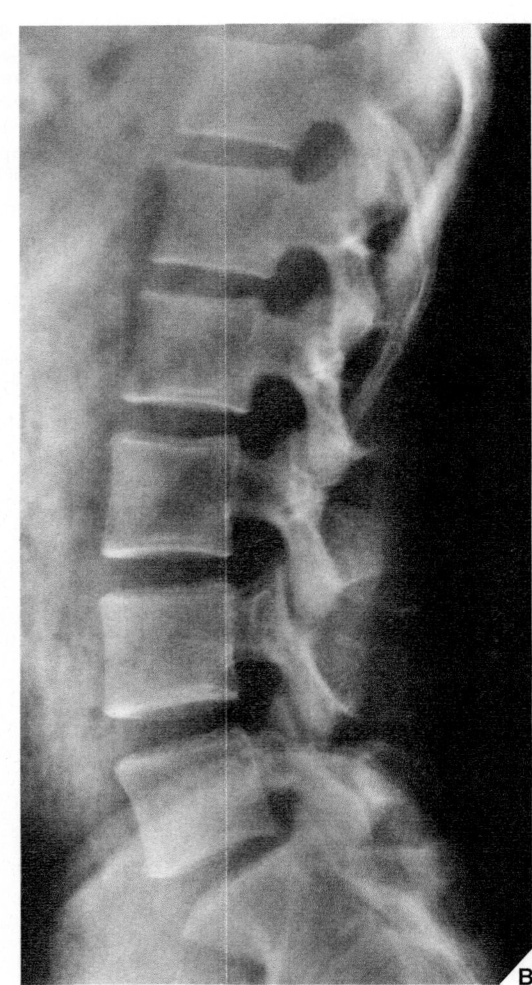

FIGURE 11.53 Lateral view of the lumbar spine. **(A)** For the lateral projection of the lumbar spine, the patient is recumbent on the radiographic table on either the left or right side; the knees and hips are flexed to eliminate the lordotic curve. The central beam is directed vertically to the center of the body of L3, at the level of the patient's waist. **(B)** The lateral radiograph of the lumbar spine allows adequate evaluation of the vertebral bodies, pedicles, and spinous processes as well as the intervertebral foramina and disk spaces.

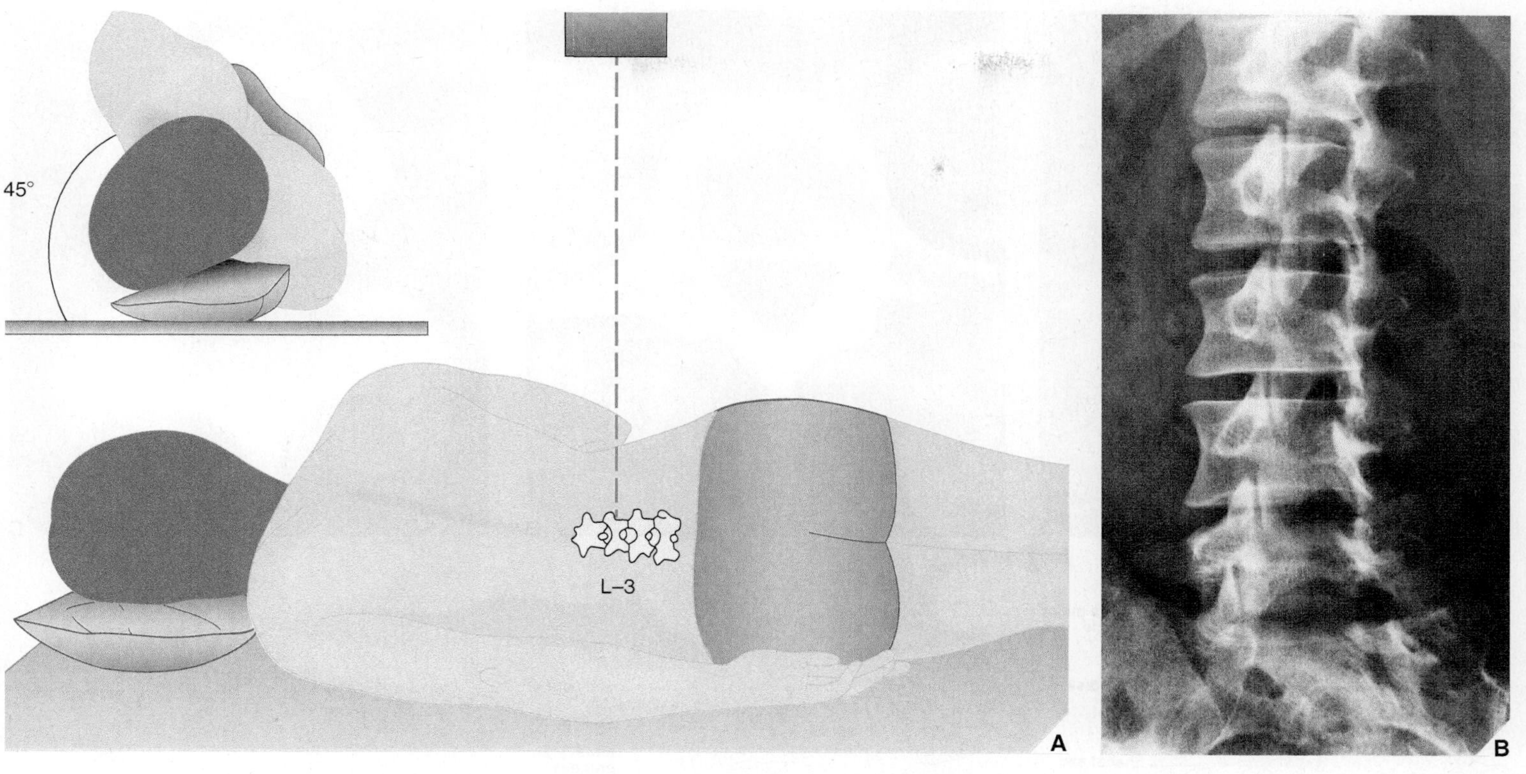

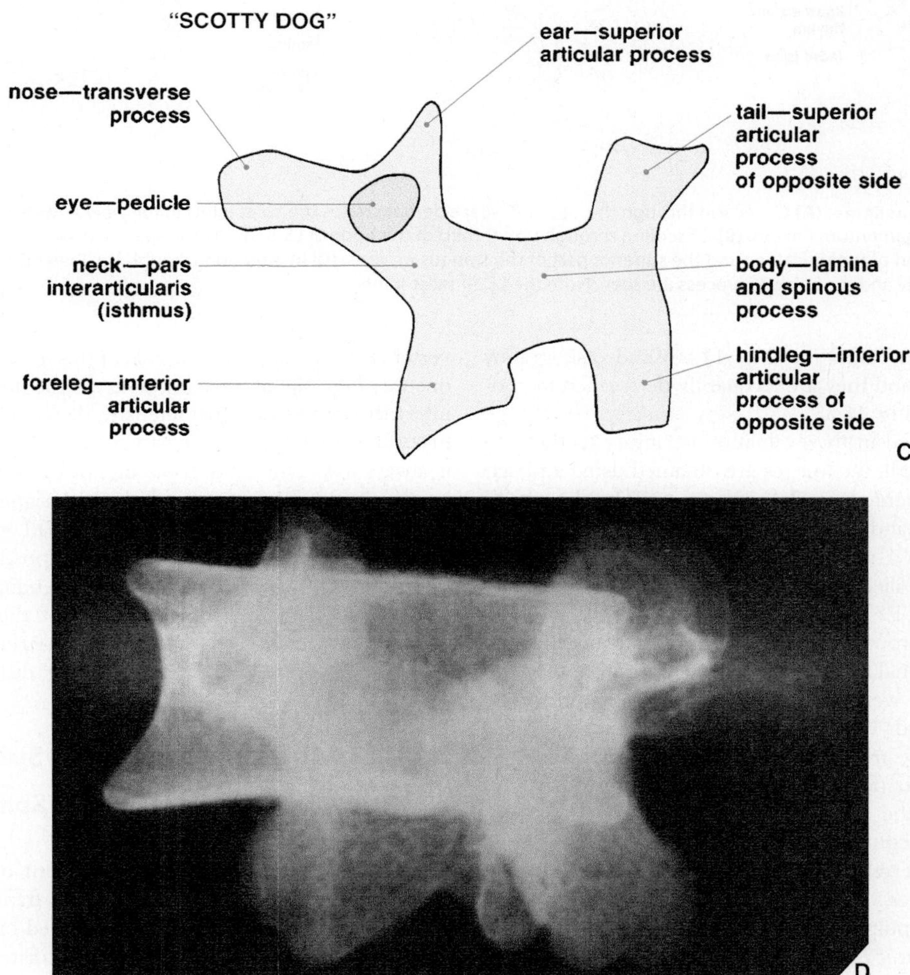

FIGURE 11.54 **Oblique view of the lumbar spine.** **(A)** For the posteroanterior oblique projection of the lumbar spine, the patient is recumbent on the table, with the right side rotated 45 degrees to demonstrate the right-sided articular facets. (Elevation of the left side allows demonstration of the left-sided articular facets.) The central beam is directed vertically toward the center of L3. **(B)** The posteroanterior oblique radiograph demonstrates the facet joints, the superior and inferior articular process, the pedicles, and the pars interarticularis. **(C,D)** The oblique radiograph also demonstrates a characteristic configuration of the elements of adjacent lumbar vertebrae known as the *Scotty dog*.

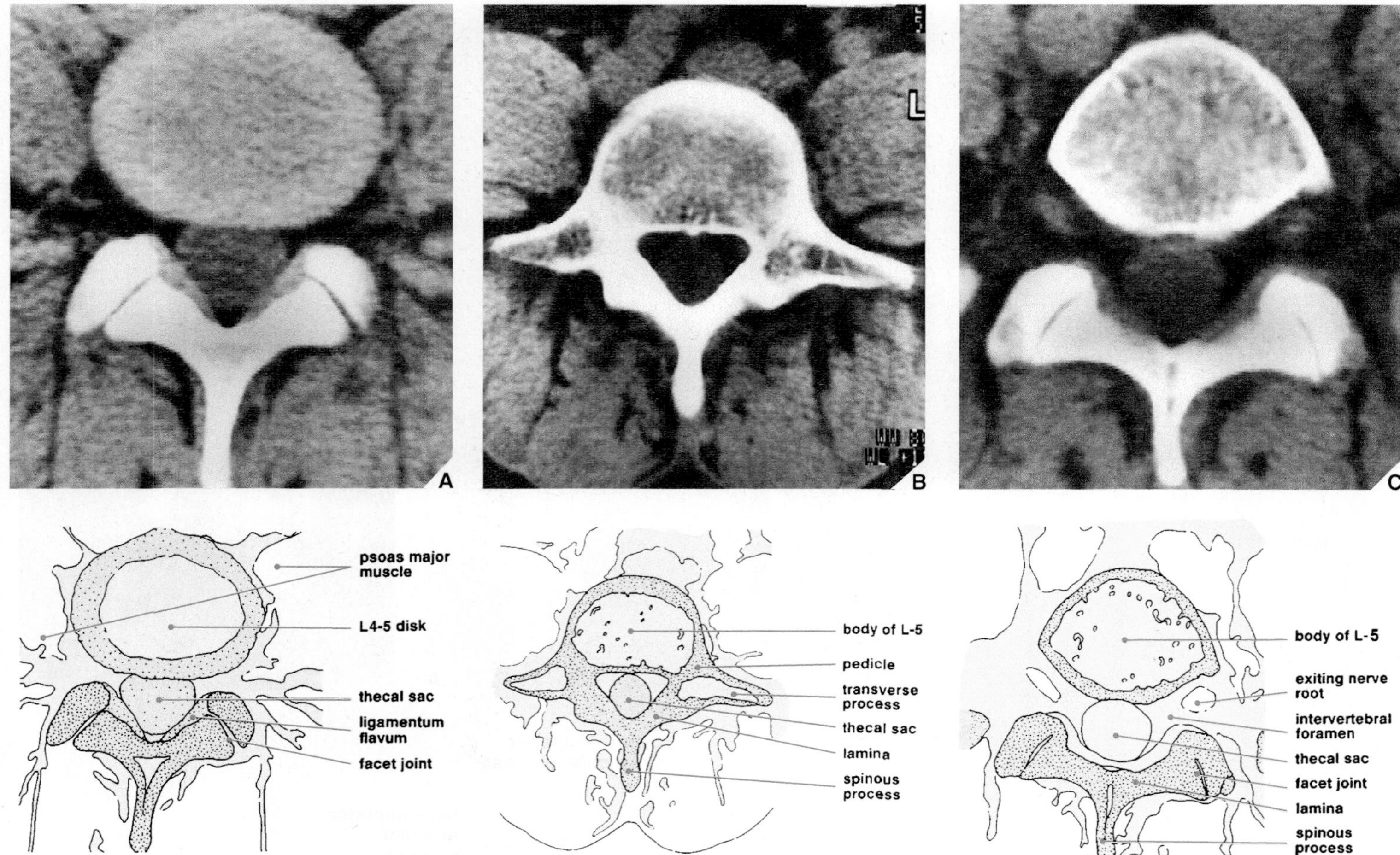

FIGURE 11.55 CT of the lumbar spine. **(A)** CT section through the L4-5 disk space demonstrates the facet joints in full view as well as the spinous process and laminae of L4. Note the appearance of the ligamentum flavum. **(B)** CT section through upper third of the body of L5 demonstrates an axial view of the pedicles, transverse processes, and laminae as well as a cross section of the thecal sac and the superior part of the spinous process. **(C)** In a section through the lower third of the body of L5 intervertebral foramina, the caudal part of the body and the spinous process are seen. Note the L5-S1 facet joints.

disks (Fig. 11.55). Moreover, myelography (Fig. 11.56) and diskography (Fig. 11.57) are often required, and they are frequently performed in conjunction with CT examination (Fig. 11.58).

MRI is now commonly used in the evaluation of injury to the thoracic and lumbar spine. In general, the images are obtained using a planar surface coil with its long axis oriented parallel to the spine. The slice thickness used to image the thoracic and lumbar spine in both sagittal and axial planes is usually 5 mm, with a 1-mm gap between slices to reduce the artifactual signal from adjacent slices. Sagittal images of the thoracic and lumbar spine are obtained with T1 and T2 weighting, whereas in the axial plane, T2-weighted images are routinely obtained. Similar to the imaging of the cervical spine, cerebrospinal fluid is visualized with low signal intensity on the sagittal images in T1 weighting, in contrast to the intermediate signal intensity of the spinal cord. The marrow within the vertebral bodies is seen as a high signal intensity, in contrast to the intermediate signal intensity of the intervertebral disks (Fig. 11.59A).

On T2-weighted images, the thoracic cord is visualized as low-to-intermediate signal intensity, in contrast to the high signal intensity of the cerebrospinal fluid. The intervertebral disks demonstrate variable signal intensity on T2-weighted images depending on the age of the patient. In young patients, the nucleus pulposus is highly hydrated and therefore exhibits high signal intensity on T2-weighted images. As the age of the patients' increases, hydration decreases and the signal intensity becomes intermediate to low. The vertebral body marrow is imaged as intermediate signal intensity on T1- and T2-weighted images, but the signal intensity of the bone marrow is highly dependent on the amount of red and yellow marrow, which also changes with age (Fig. 11.59B).

The axial images effectively demonstrate the relation of the intervertebral disk spaces to the thecal sac. On axial T1-weighted images, the vertebral body, pedicles, laminae, transverse, and spinous processes demonstrate high signal intensity, whereas the nucleus pulposus yields high-to-intermediate or low signal intensity, depending on the degree of hydration, in contrast to the signal intensity peripherally of the annulus fibrosus, which is always low. The nerve roots demonstrate low-to-intermediate signal intensity and are in contrast with the high signal intensity of the surrounding fat, better demonstrated on parasagittal T1-weighted images (Fig. 11.59C). On T2-weighted images, the nucleus pulposus again demonstrates high-to-intermediate or low signal intensity, depending on the degree of hydration, in contrast to the low signal intensity of the annulus fibrosus. The nerve roots are imaged as low–signal intensity structures (Fig. 11.59D).

For a summary of the preceding discussion in tabular form, see Tables 11.1, 11.3, and 11.5.

Injury to the Thoracolumbar Spine

Fractures of the Thoracolumbar Spine

Classification

Fractures of the thoracolumbar segment of the spine may involve the vertebral body and arch as well as the transverse, spinous, and articular processes. They can generally be grouped by the mechanism of injury as compression fractures, burst fractures, distraction fractures (Chance and other seat-belt injuries), and fracture–dislocations.

Because different classifications of thoracolumbar spine fractures have been used in the past by numerous authors, reports concerning the stability or lack of stability of a particular fracture pattern have varied. In 1983, Denis introduced the concept of the three-column spine classification of acute injuries to the thoracic and lumbar segments (Fig. 11.60). The significance of this system is its usefulness in determining the stability of

FIGURE 11.56 Myelography of the lumbar spine. For myelographic examination of the lumbar spine, the patient is prone on the table. The puncture site, usually at the L3-4 or L2-3 level, is marked under fluoroscopic control. A 22-gauge needle is inserted into the subarachnoid space, and free flow of spinal fluid indicates proper placement. Iohexol or iopamidol (15 mL), in a concentration of 180 mg iodine per milliliter, is slowly injected, and the radiographs are obtained in the posteroanterior **(A)**, left and right oblique **(B)**, and cross-table lateral **(C)** projections. In these normal studies, contrast is seen outlining the subarachnoid spaces of the thecal sac as well as the cul-de-sac or most caudal part of the subarachnoid space. The nerve roots appear symmetric on both sides of the contrast column. A linear filling defect represents a nerve root in its contrast-filled sleeve. The length of the root pocket may vary from one patient to another, but in each patient, all roots are approximately equal in length. It is imperative during myelographic examination of the lumbar segment to obtain one spot film of the thoracic segment at the level T10-12 **(D)** because tumors localized in the conus medullaris may mimic the clinical symptoms of a herniated lumbar disk.

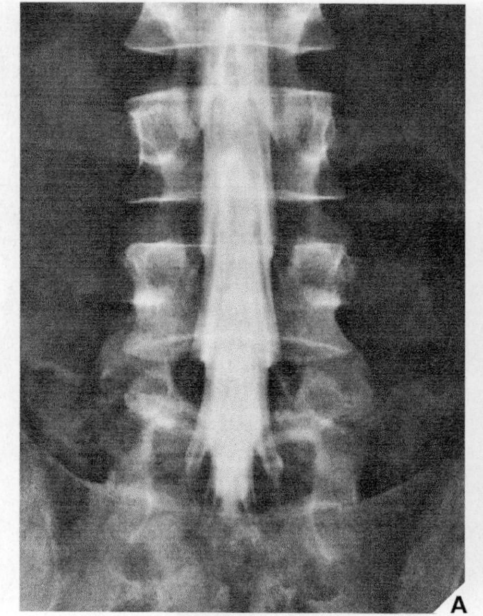

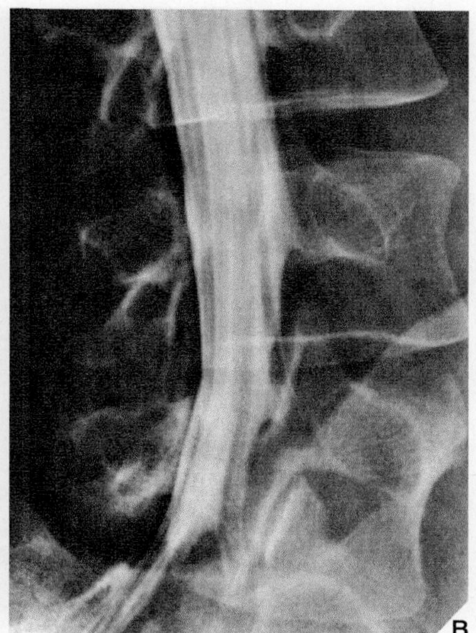

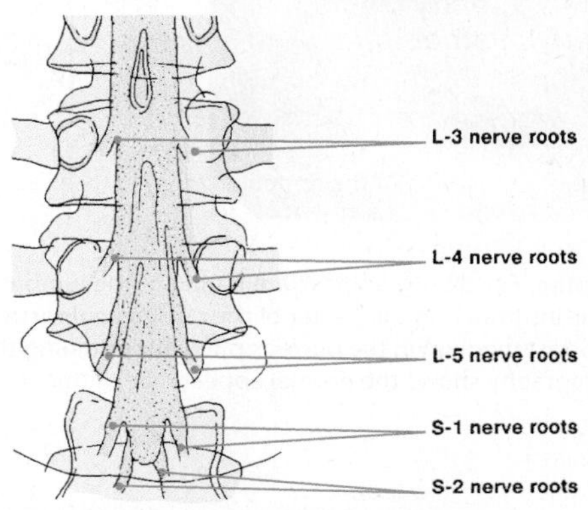

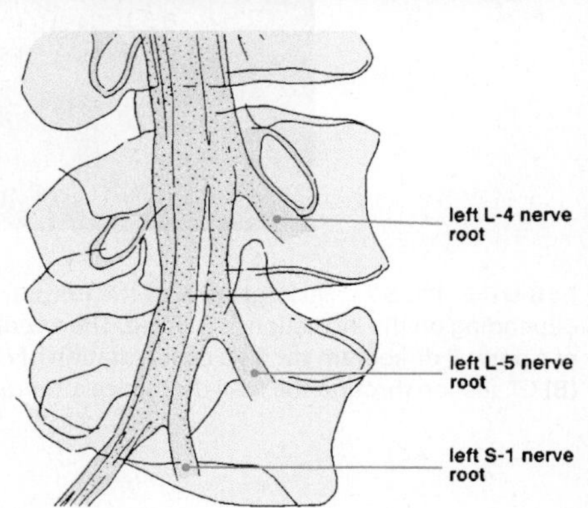

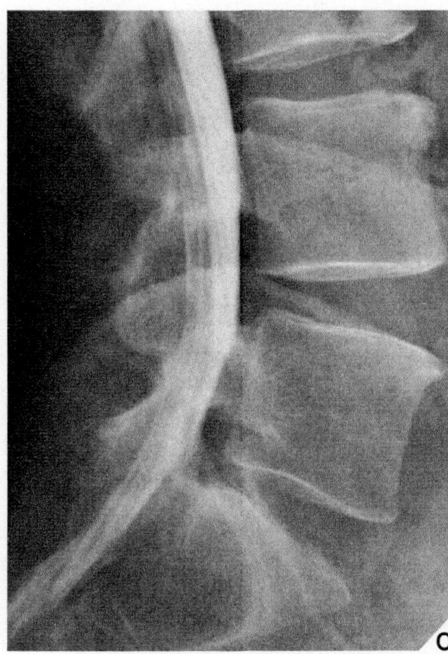

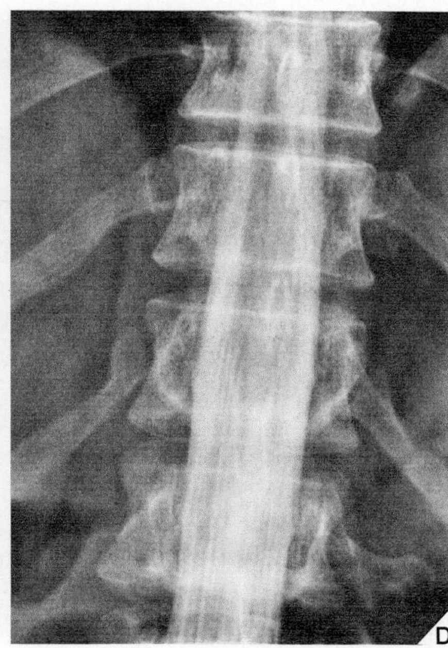

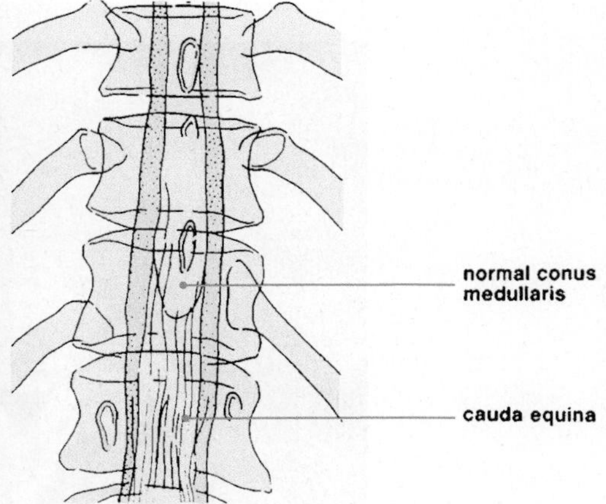

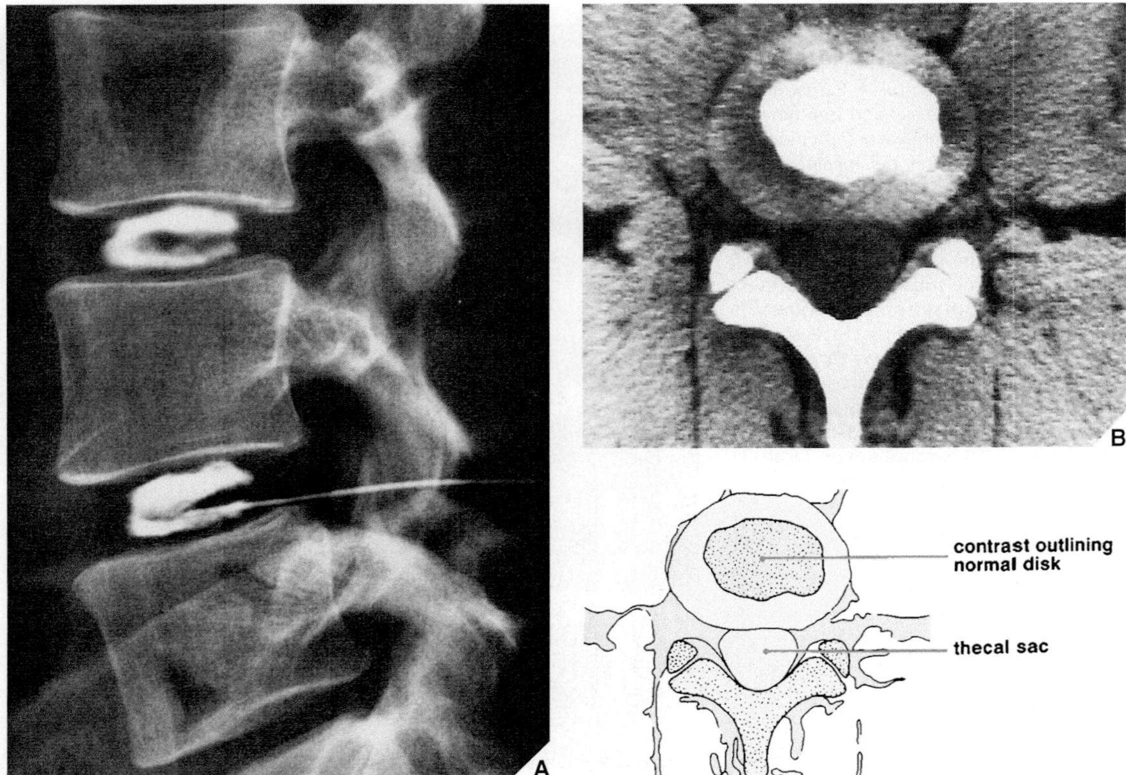

FIGURE 11.57 Diskography of the lumbar spine. For diskographic examination of the lumbar spine, the patient is prone on the table, and the level of the injection, depending on the indication, is marked. The needle is inserted into the center of the nucleus pulposus, and about 2 to 3 mL of metrizamide is injected. **(A)** Lateral radiograph of a normal diskogram shows a concentration of contrast medium in the nucleus pulposus outlining the disk; there should be no leak of contrast while the needle is in place. **(B)** CT section through the L3-4 disk space after diskography shows the normal appearance of this structure.

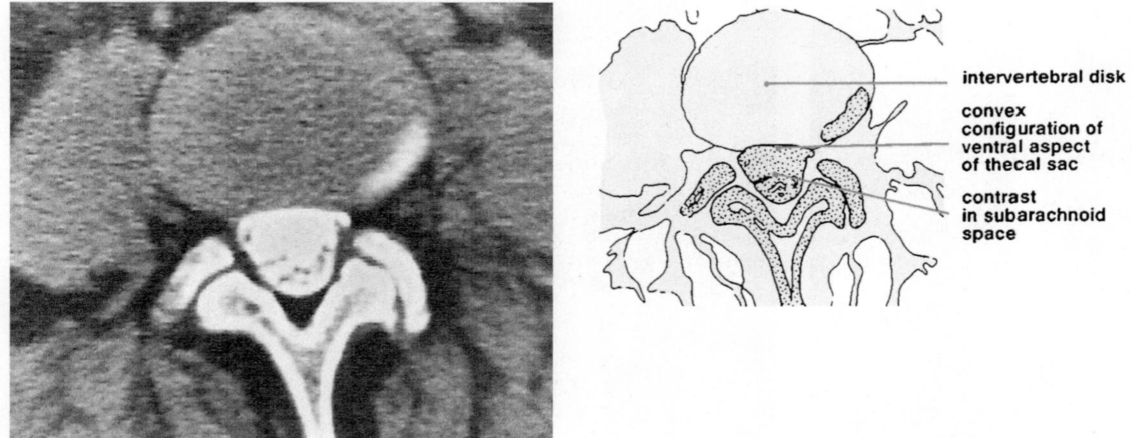

FIGURE 11.58 CT myelography of the lumbar spine. CT section obtained after myelography shows the normal appearance of contrast agent in the subarachnoid space. Note that the disk does not encroach on the ventral aspect of the thecal sac.

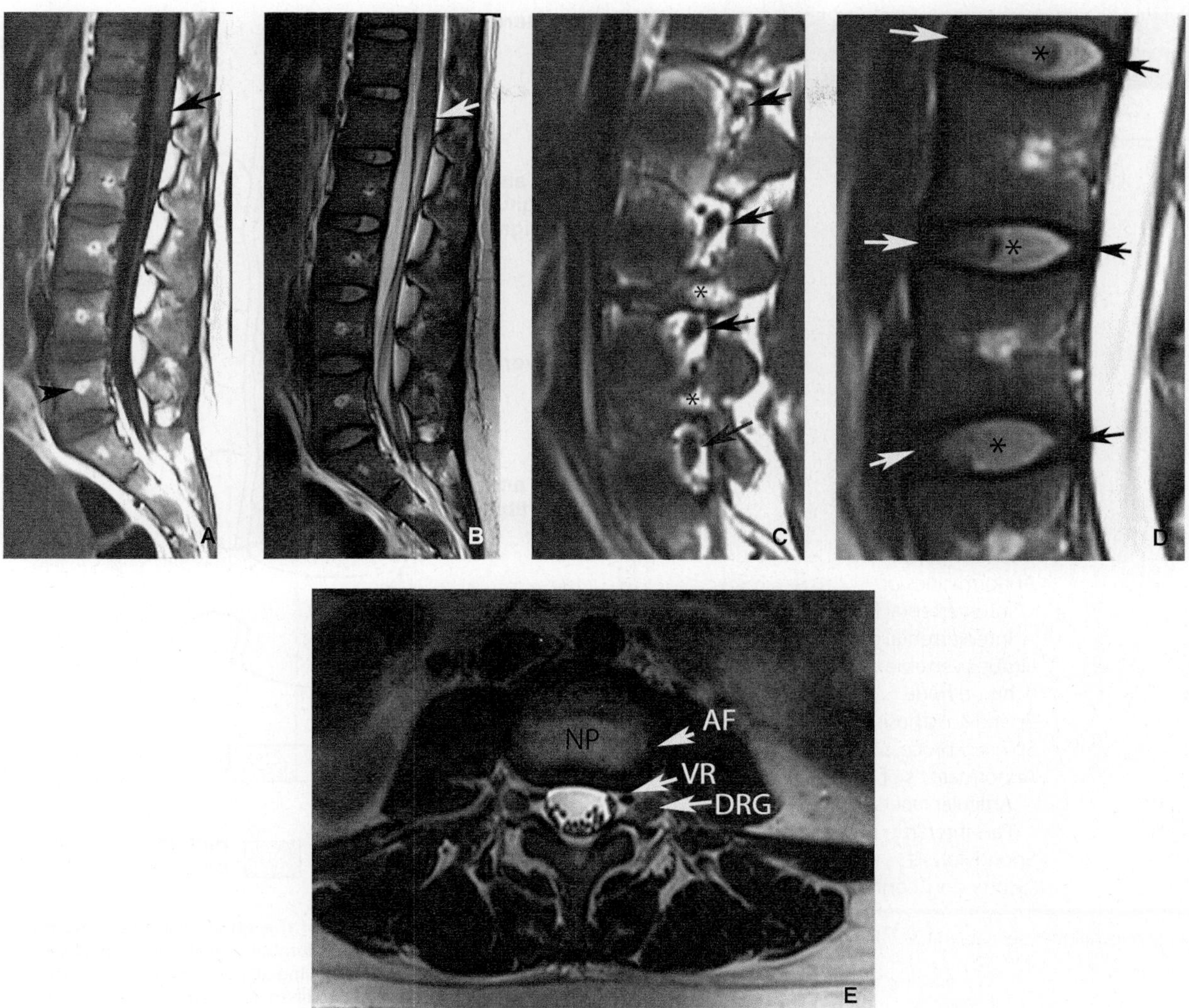

FIGURE 11.59 **MRI appearance of the normal lumbar spine in a young adult.** **(A)** Sagittal T1-weighted MR image. Note the intermediate-to-low signal intensity of the bone marrow in the vertebral bodies, reflecting predominantly red marrow, with the exception of high signal intensity corresponding to fatty tissue surrounding the basivertebral veins in the center of the vertebral bodies *(arrowhead)*. The conus medullaris *(arrow)* and the cauda equina are well identified, surrounded with low–signal intensity cerebrospinal fluid (CSF). Note the posterior epidural fat. **(B)** Sagittal T2-weighted MR image demonstrates again the low signal intensity of the red marrow, appropriate for the young age of the patient. Note the conus medullaris *(arrow)* and the cauda equina, surrounded by high–signal intensity CSF. **(C)** Right parasagittal T1-weighted MR image shows the normal exiting nerve roots surrounded by fat *(arrows)* within the corresponding neural foramina. Note the normal right pedicles *(asterisks)* with a small amount of fatty marrow. **(D)** Magnified sagittal T2-weighted MR image demonstrates the normal well-hydrated hyperintense nucleus pulposus *(asterisks)* and the peripheral anterior and posterior hypointense annulus fibrosus *(arrows)*. **(E)** Axial T2-weighted MR image through a normal intervertebral disk shows hyperintense nucleus pulposus (NP) and the hypointense anulus fibrosus (AF). The normal disk is slightly concave posteriorly. Low–signal intensity nerve roots of the cauda equina are well identified within the thecal sac, which has a normal rounded appearance in the central portion and in the lateral recesses. Note the ventral nerve root (VR) and the dorsal root ganglion (DRG). (Courtesy of Oleg Opsha, MD, Brooklyn, New York.)

various fractures, based on the site of injury in one or more of the spinal columns or elements:

The *anterior column* comprises the anterior two thirds of the annulus fibrosus and vertebral body and the anterior longitudinal ligament. The *middle column* includes the posterior longitudinal ligament and the posterior third of the vertebral body and annulus fibrosus. The *posterior column* consists of the posterior ligament complex, which has been defined by Holdsworth and associates to include the supraspinous and infraspinous ligaments, the capsule of the intervertebral joints, and the ligamentum flavum (or interlaminar ligament) as well as the posterior portion of the neural arch. Generally, one-column fractures are stable and three-column unstable; two-column fractures may be stable or unstable, depending on the extent of injury (Table 11.6).

Compression Fractures

Usually resulting from anterior or lateral flexion, compression fracture is a failure of the anterior column under compression forces; the middle column remains intact, acting as a hinge, even in severe cases in which there may also be partial failure of the posterior column. The standard radiographic examination of the thoracic and lumbar segments is usually sufficient to demonstrate this injury (Fig. 11.61), although CT or MRI may be required to delineate the extent of the fracture or demonstrate obscure features (Figs. 11.62 to 11.64). The anteroposterior radiograph reveals buckling of the lateral cortices of the vertebral body close to the involved end plates, together with a decrease in the height of the vertebral body. In lateral-flexion injuries, compression forces may result in a wedge-shaped deformity of the vertebral body. In subtle cases, a clue to the diagnosis may be seen in a localized bulge of the paraspinal line secondary to hemorrhage and edema. However, it should be kept in mind that this finding may also be seen in pathologic fractures secondary to skeletal metastases to the spine (see Fig. 22.81). On the lateral projection, a simple vertebral compression fracture can be identified by a decrease in the height of the anterior part of the body while the height of the posterior part and posterior cortex is maintained.

Burst Fractures

A burst fracture results from a failure of the anterior and middle columns secondary to axial-compression forces or a combination of axial compression with rotation or anterior or lateral flexion. The anteroposterior and

TABLE 11.5 Standard and Special Radiographic Projections for Evaluating Injury to the Thoracic and Lumbar Spine[a]

Projection	Demonstration
Anteroposterior	Fractures of Vertebral bodies Vertebral end plates Pedicles Transverse processes Fracture–dislocations Abnormalities of intervertebral disks Paraspinal bulge Inverted Napoleon's hat sign
Lateral	Fractures of Vertebral bodies Vertebral end plates Pedicles Spinous processes Chance fracture (seat-belt fractures) Abnormalities of Intervertebral foramina Intervertebral disk spaces Limbus vertebra Schmorl node Spondylolisthesis Spinous-process sign
Oblique	Abnormalities of Articular facets Pars interarticularis Spondylolysis "Scotty dog" configuration

[a]For the ancillary imaging techniques, see Table 11.3.

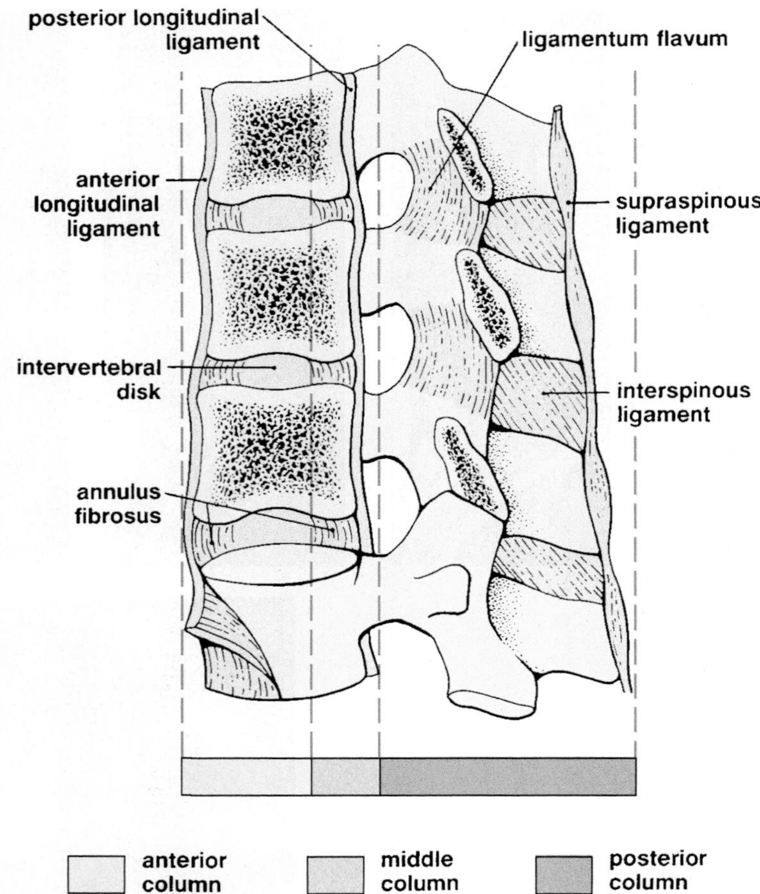

FIGURE 11.60 **Division of the spine into three columns.** The three-column concept in viewing the thoracolumbar spine is helpful in determining the stability of various injuries. Fractures involving all three columns are unstable, and those affecting one column are stable. (Modified with permission from Denis F. The three column spine and its significance in the classification of acute thoracolumbar spinal injuries. *Spine [Phila Pa 1976]* 1983;8:817–831.)

lateral projections of the thoracic and lumbar spine are usually adequate to demonstrate these fractures. The anteroposterior radiograph characteristically reveals a vertical fracture of the lamina, together with an increase in the interpedicular distance and splaying of the posterior facet joints (Fig. 11.65A). On the lateral radiograph, fracture of the posterior part of the vertebral body results in a decrease in the height of this portion of the bone (Fig. 11.65B). Comminution is often present, and fragments are retropulsed into the spinal canal, leading to compression of the thecal sac. For this reason, CT is an essential technique in the evaluation of burst fractures (Figs. 11.65C and 11.66A–C), and MRI (Figs. 11.67 and 11.68) or myelography (Fig. 11.69) may be required to localize the site and demonstrate the degree of compression on the thecal sac.

Chance Fractures

Originally described by G. Q. Chance, this type of distraction injury of the lumbar spine has also come to be called a *seat-belt fracture* because of the frequency of its occurrence in automobile accidents in individuals wearing only lap seat belts. Acute forward flexion of the spine across a restraining lap seat belt during sudden deceleration causes the spine above the belt to be pushed forward and distracted from the lower, fixed part of the spine. The classic Chance fracture involves a horizontal splitting of the vertebra, beginning in the spinous process or lamina and extending through the pedicles and the vertebral body without damage to ligament structures. Its constant feature is a transverse fracture without dislocation or subluxation (Figs. 11.70 and 11.71). The transverse process may be horizontally fractured as well, and at times, there is compression of the anterior aspect of the vertebral body. Chance fracture tends to be stable because the upper half of the neural arch remains firmly attached to the vertebra above and the lower half to the vertebra below. Since the original description of this fracture, three more types of seat-belt fractures have been reported, which involve varying degrees of ligament and intervertebral disk disruption (Figs. 11.72 and 11.73).

TABLE 11.6 Basic Types of Spinal Fractures and the Columns Involved in Each

	Column Involvement		
Type of Fracture	Anterior	Middle	Posterior
Compression	Compression	None	None or distraction (in severe fractures)
Burst	Compression	Compression	None or distraction
Seat belt	None or compression	Distraction	Distraction
Fracture–dislocation	Compression and/or rotation, shear	Distraction and/or rotation, shear	Distraction and/or rotation, shear

Reprinted with permission from Montesano PX, Benson DR. The thoracocolumbar spine. In: Rockwood CA, Green DP, Bucholz RW, eds. *Rockwood and Green's fractures in adults*, 3rd ed. Philadelphia: JB Lippincott; 1991:1359–1397.

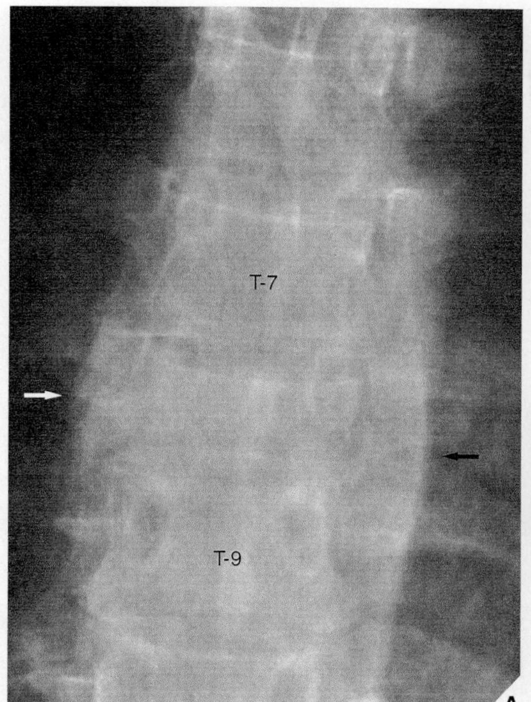

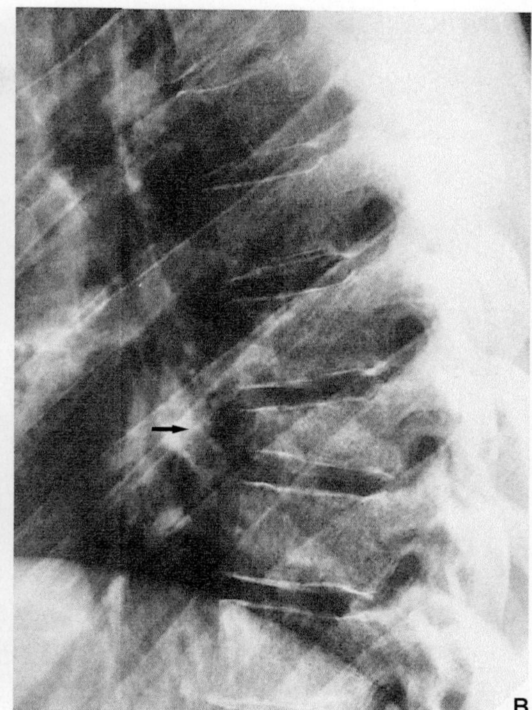

FIGURE 11.61 **Compression fracture.** A 48-year-old woman fell from a ladder and hurt her back. **(A)** Anteroposterior radiograph of the thoracic spine demonstrates a decrease in the height of the vertebral body of T8, secondary to compression fracture. Note the localized widening of the paraspinal line secondary to hemorrhage and edema *(arrows)*. **(B)** The lateral radiograph demonstrates anterior wedging of T8 *(arrow)*. Note the intact posterior vertebral body line. These are the features of simple compression fracture affecting only the anterior column.

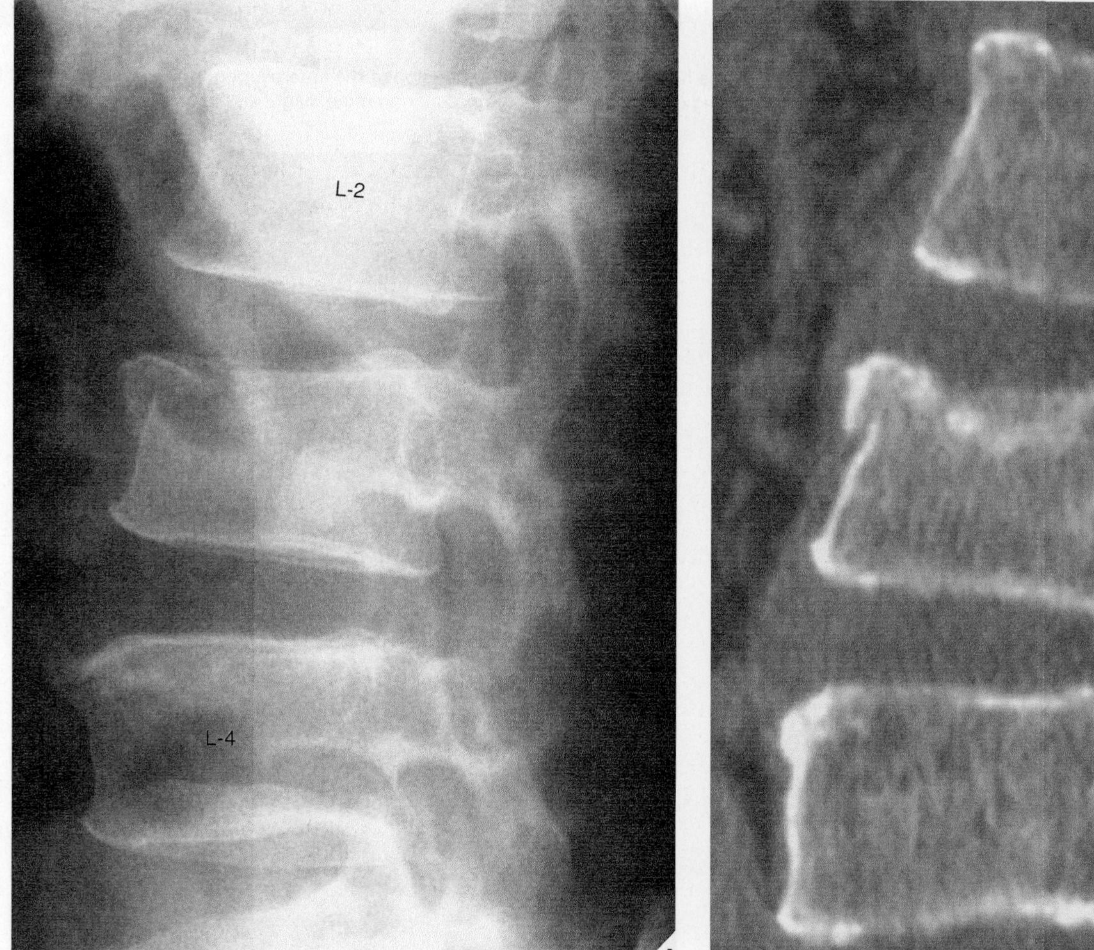

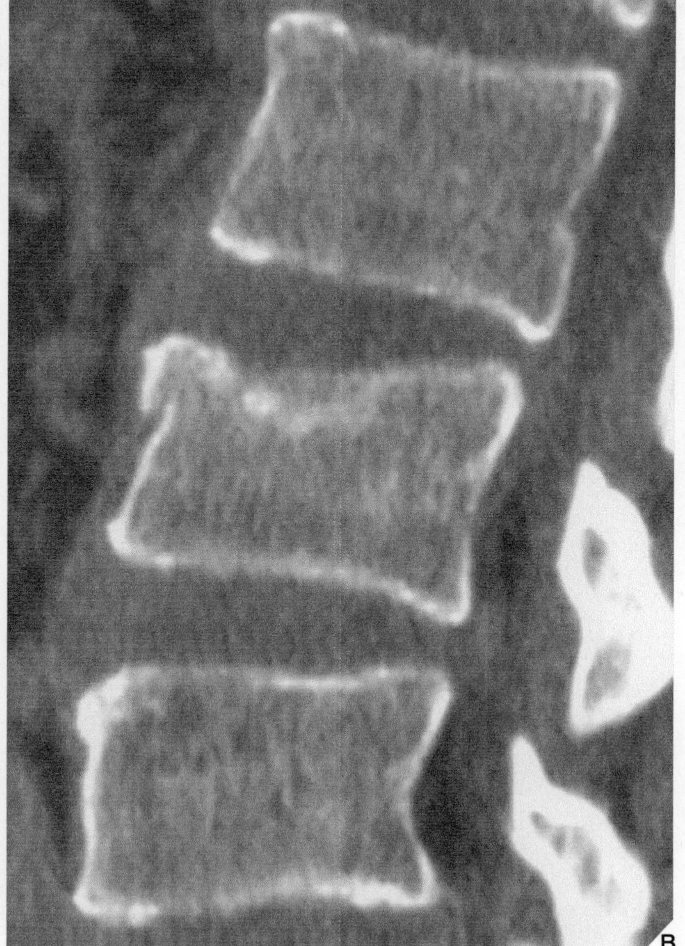

FIGURE 11.62 **CT of the compression fracture.** **(A)** Lateral radiograph of the lumbar spine shows compression of the anterior part of the vertebral body of L3, although the posterior part is not well demonstrated. **(B)** Sagittal CT reformatted image clearly shows intact middle column, confirming the presence of the compression and not the burst fracture.

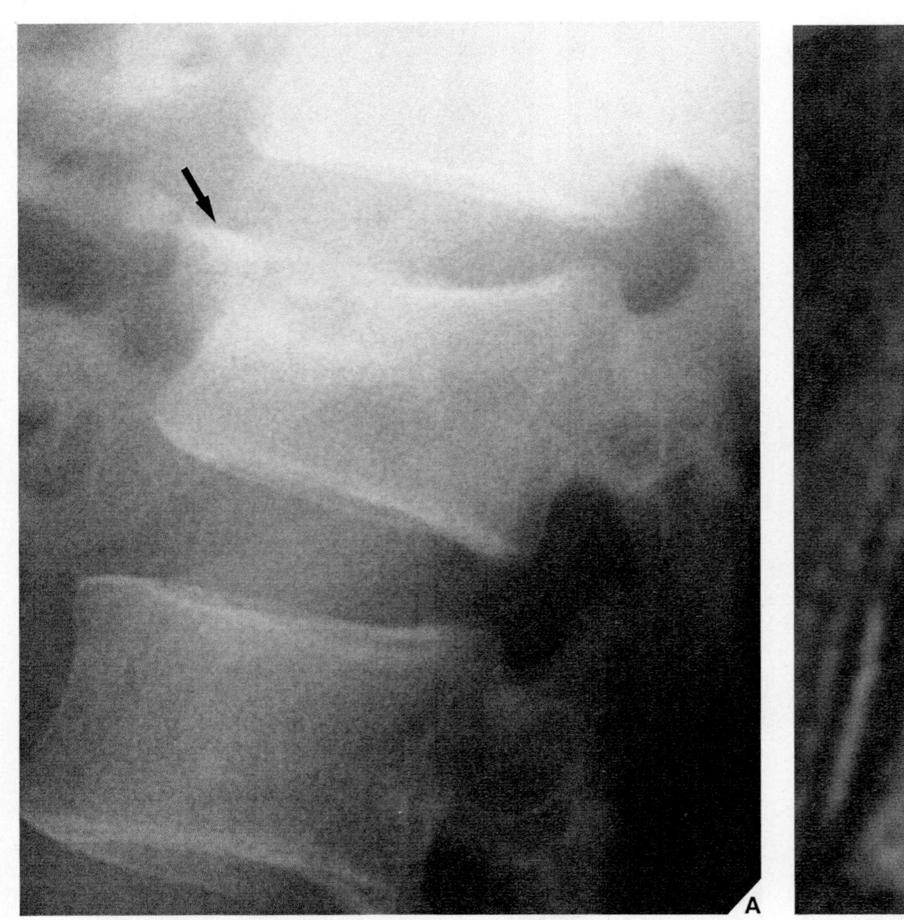

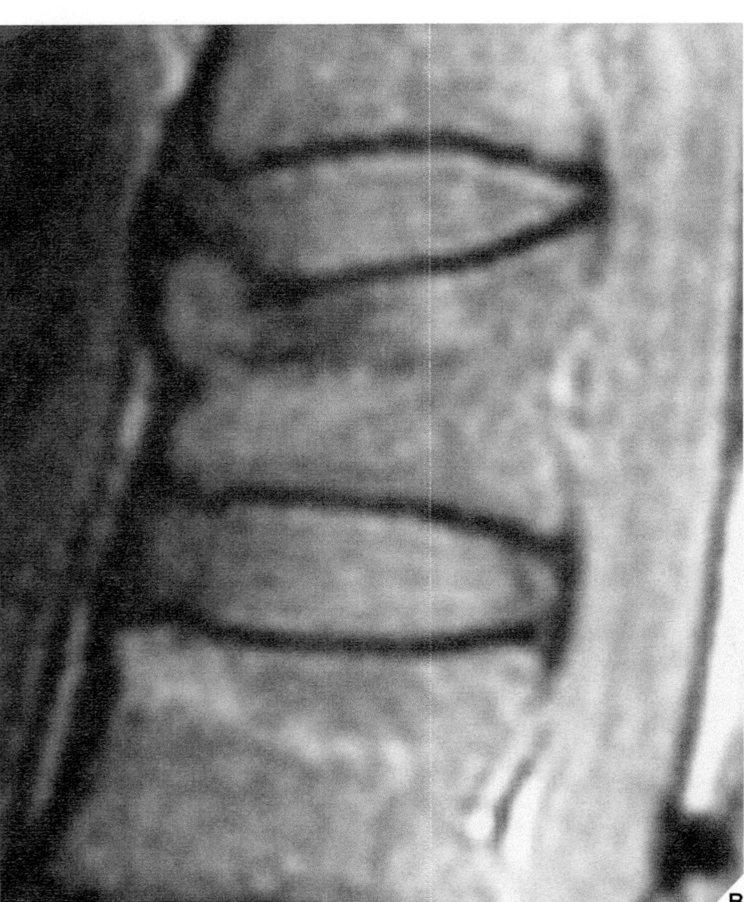

FIGURE 11.63 MRI of the compression fracture. **(A)** Lateral radiograph of the lumbar spine shows compression of the anterosuperior part of the vertebral body of L1 *(arrow)*. **(B)** Sagittal proton density-weighted MRI demonstrates a fracture involving only the anterior column, confirming the diagnosis of compression fracture.

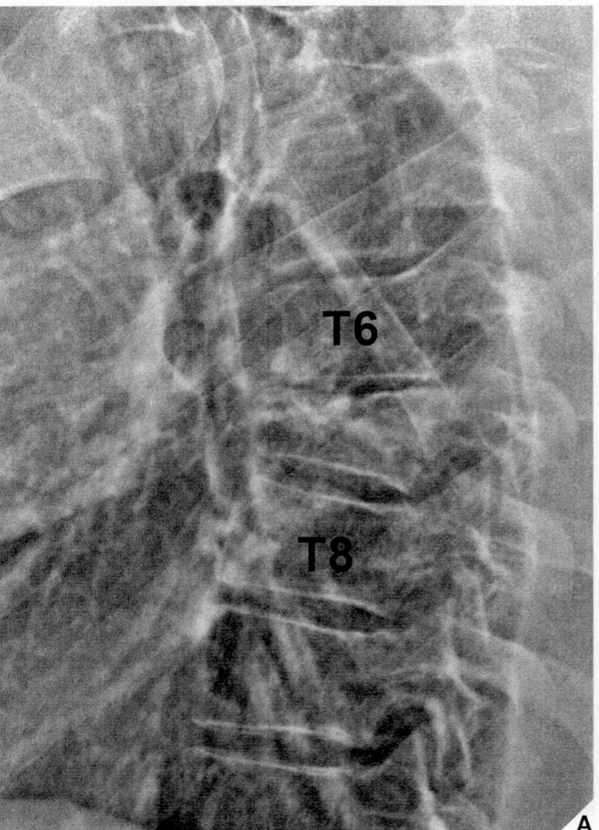

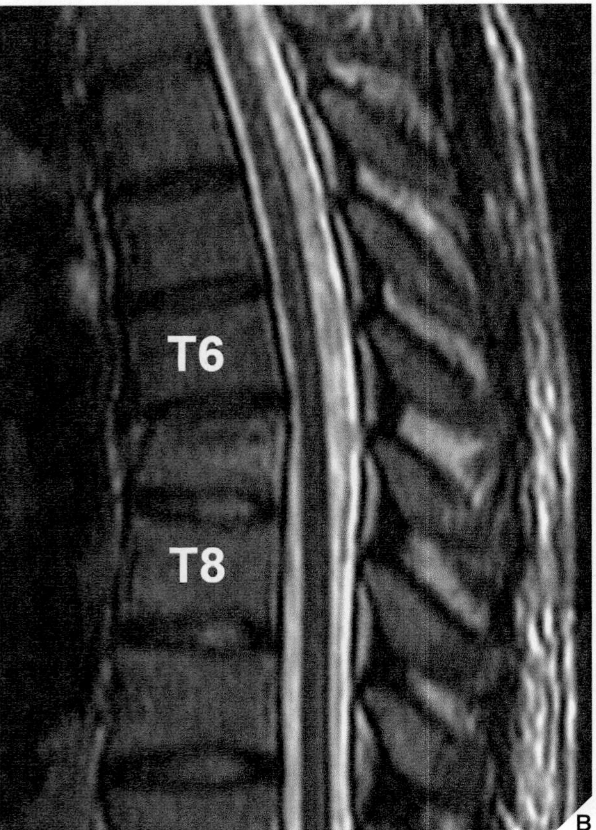

FIGURE 11.64 MRI of the compression fracture. A 44-year-old man was injured in the motor vehicle accident. **(A)** Lateral radiograph of the thoracic spine shows a compression fracture of T7. **(B)** Sagittal T2-weighted MR image shows lack of involvement of the middle column, intact posterior longitudinal ligament, and intact subarachnoid space at the level of fractured vertebra.

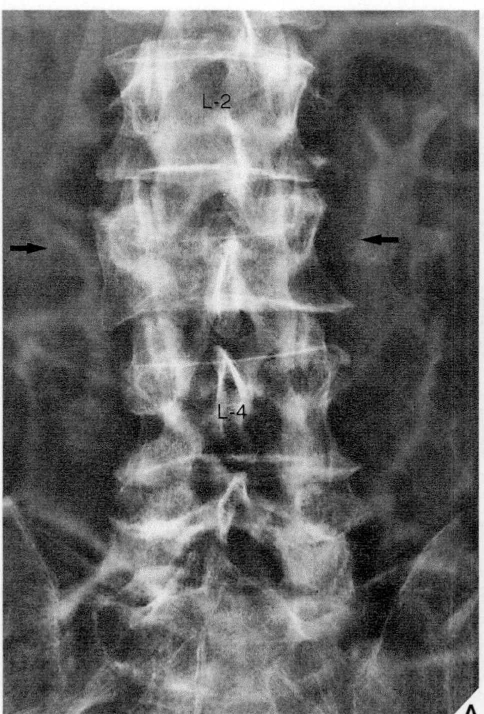

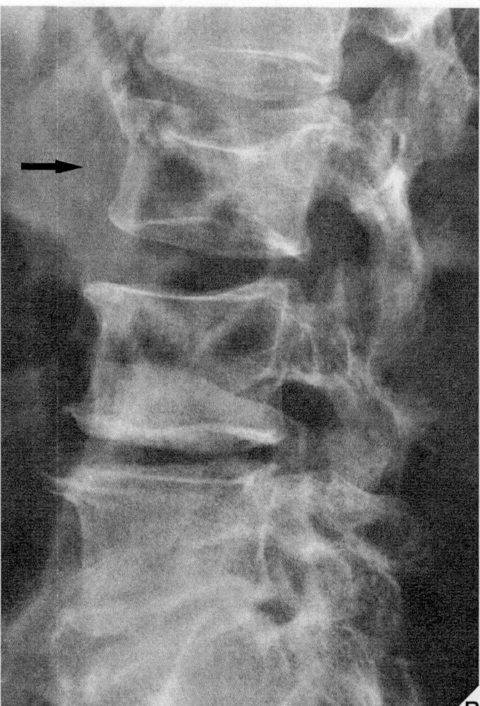

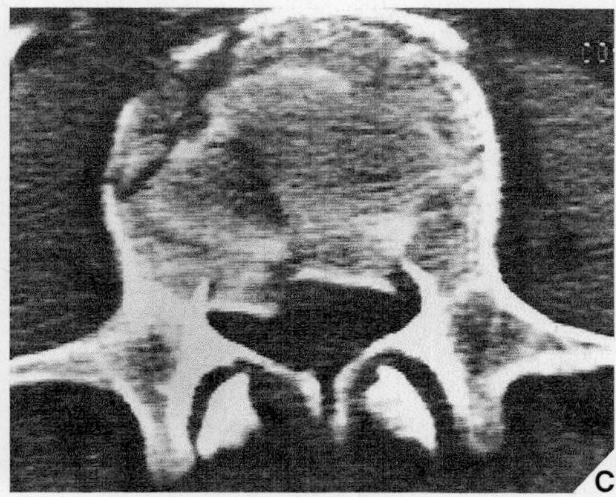

FIGURE 11.65 **Burst fracture.** A 56-year-old merchant seaman fell from a 60-foot-high ladder on a ship. **(A)** Anteroposterior and **(B)** lateral radiographs of the lumbar spine show a burst fracture of the body of L3 *(arrows)*. Note widening of the interpediculate distance on the anteroposterior radiograph, the hallmark of burst fracture. The severity of the injury, however, is better appreciated on a CT section **(C)** through the body of L3. There is comminution of the vertebral fracture and displacement of two osseous fragments into the spinal canal, with compression of the thecal sac, indicating involvement of anterior and middle columns.

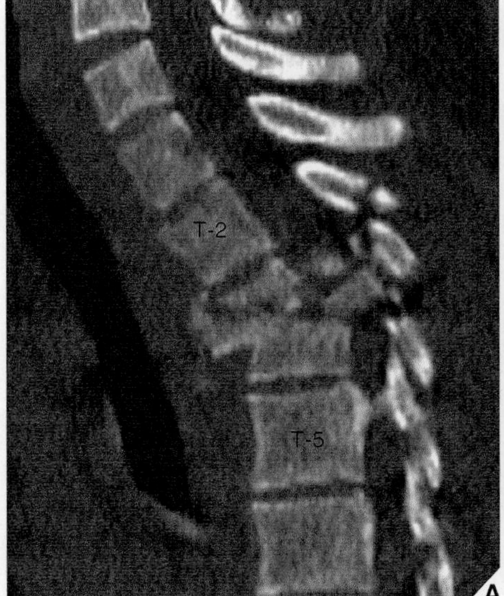

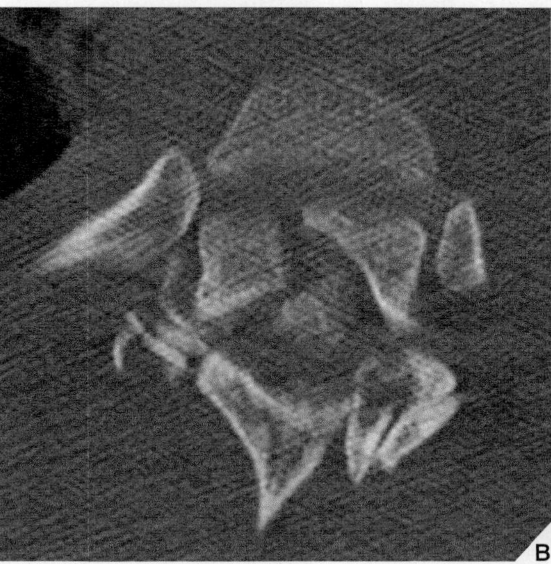

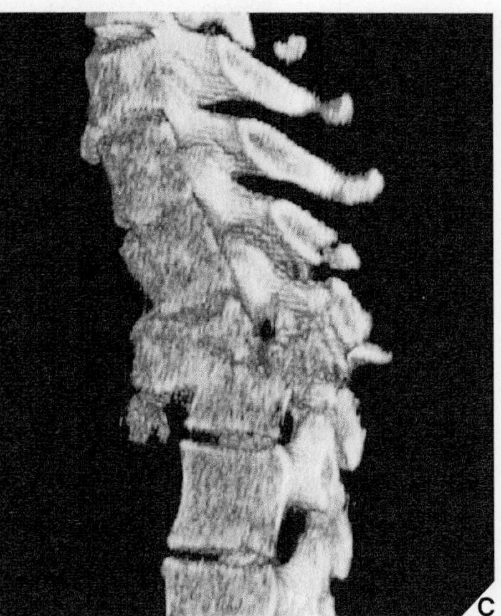

FIGURE 11.66 **CT and 3D CT of the burst fracture.** **(A)** Sagittal CT reformatted image shows the burst fractures of T3 and T4 vertebrae. **(B)** Axial CT image of T3 shows comminution and displacement of osseous fragments into the spinal canal. **(C)** 3D CT reconstructed image delivers more comprehensive picture of this injury.

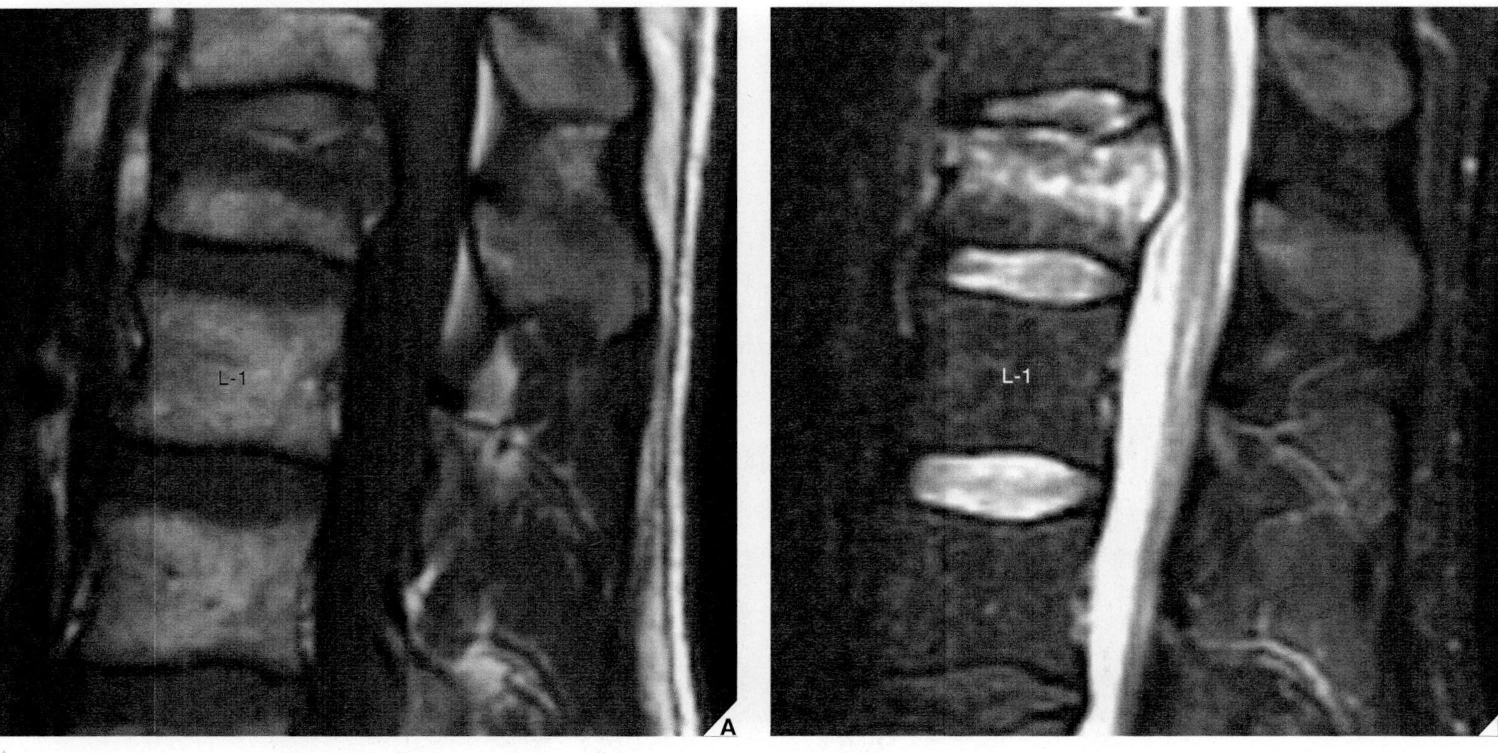

FIGURE 11.67 MRI of the burst fracture. **(A)** Sagittal T1-weighted and **(B)** T2-weighted MR images demonstrate a burst fracture of T12 vertebra. Note compression of the ventral aspect of the thecal sac, but the posterior longitudinal ligament remains intact.

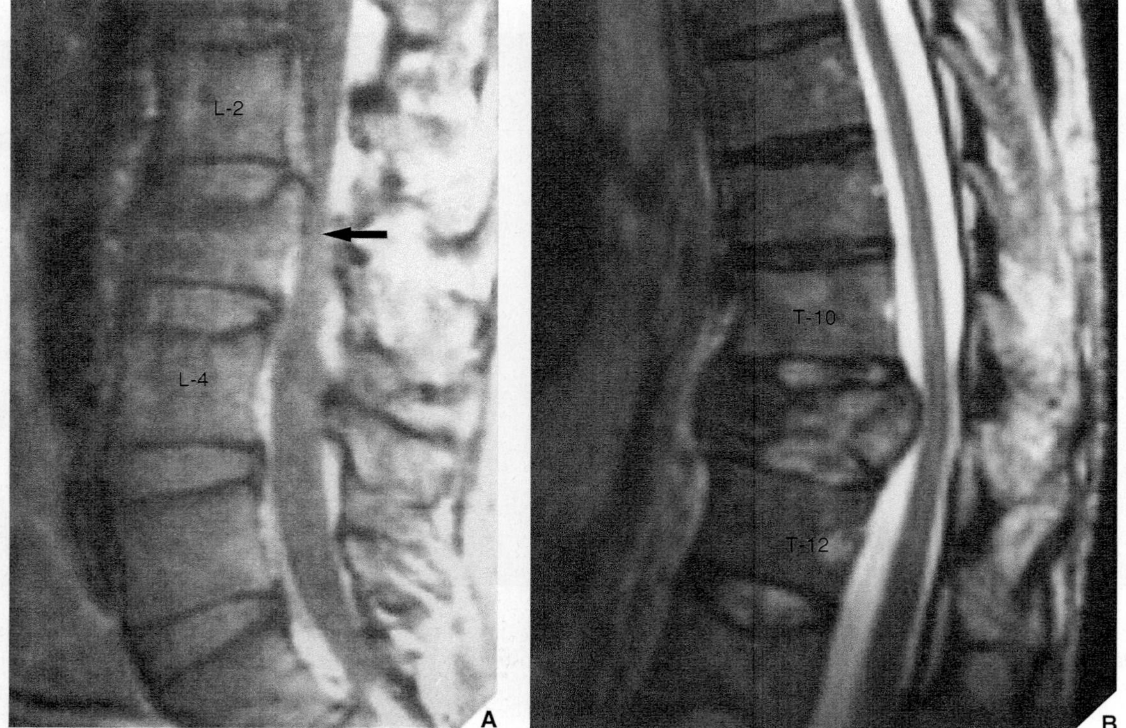

FIGURE 11.68 MRI of burst fracture. **(A)** In a 26-year-old man with a burst fracture of L3, sagittal T1-weighted MR image (spin echo [SE]; repetition time [TR] 800/echo time [TE] 20 msec) demonstrates posterior displacement of the middle column with compression of the thecal sac *(arrow)*. **(B)** A sagittal T2-weighted MR image of a 58-year-old man who fell from the roof of a three-story building shows a typical appearance of a burst fracture of T11. Note compression of the thecal sac.

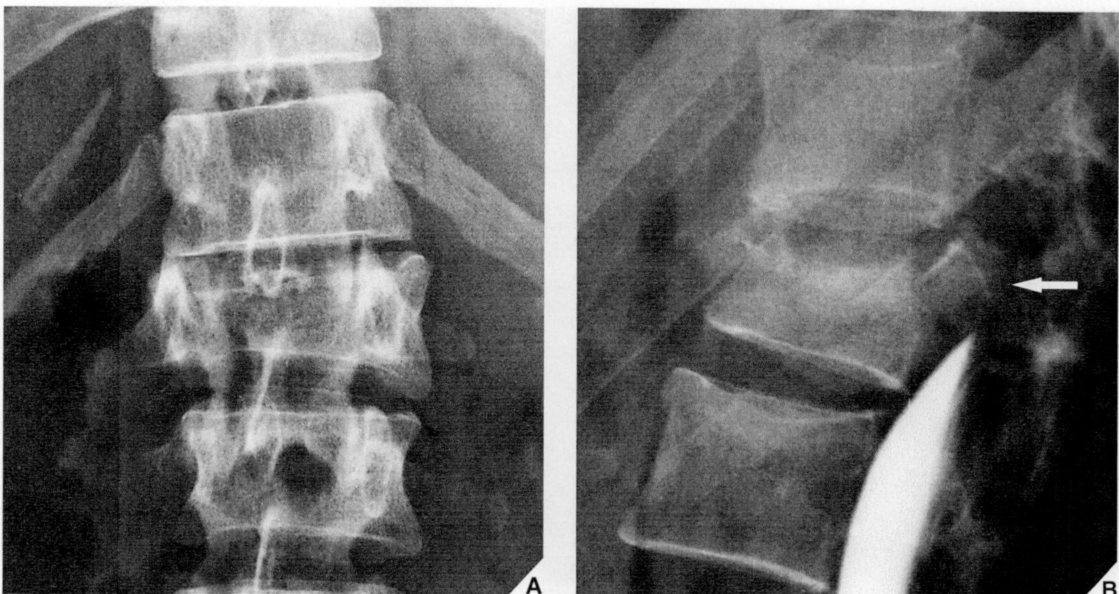

FIGURE 11.69 **Myelography of the burst fracture.** A 28-year-old woman made a parachute jump and landed on her back. Hemiplegia and incontinence developed thereafter. **(A)** Anteroposterior radiograph of the lumbar spine shows a burst fracture of L1. **(B)** Lateral radiograph as part of a myelogram shows complete obstruction of the flow of contrast agent at the level of fracture caused by a small osseous fragment impinging on the thecal sac *(arrow)*.

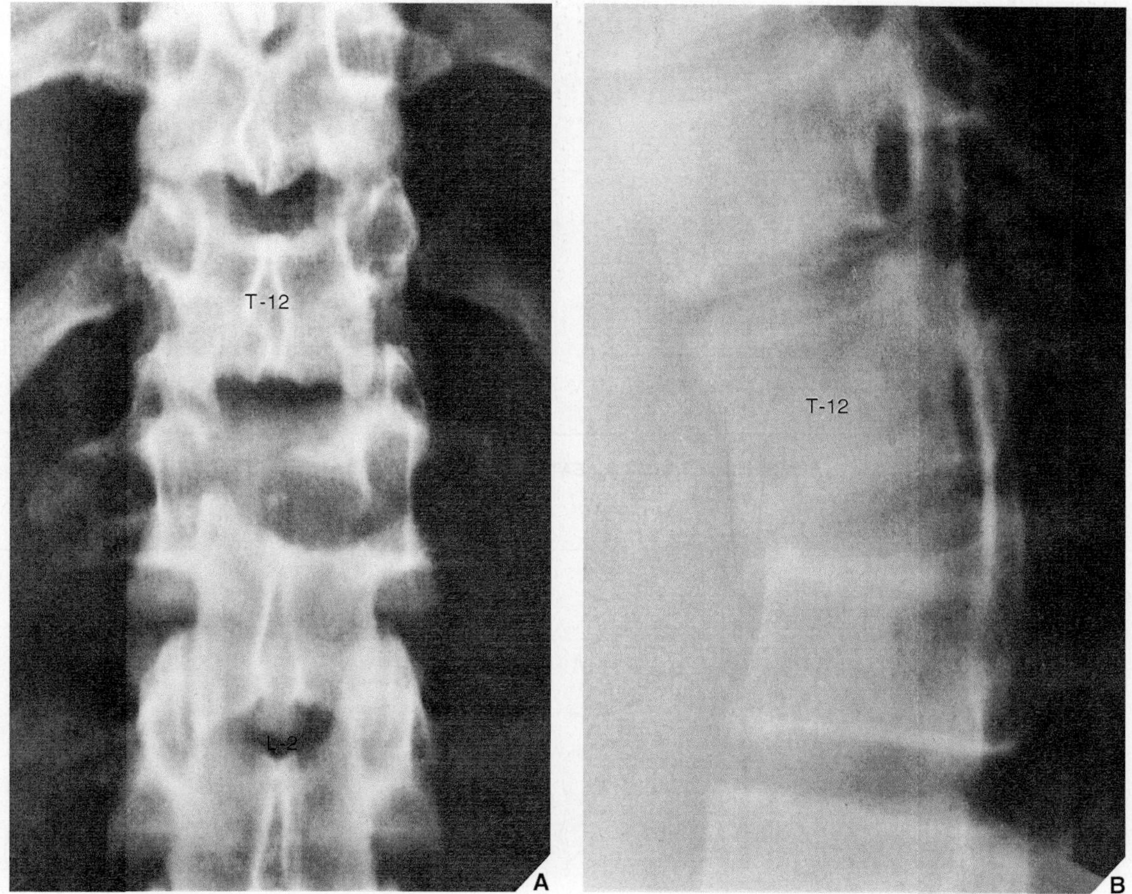

FIGURE 11.70 **Chance fracture.** A 30-year-old woman sustained an injury to the lower back in a car collision; she had been wearing a lap seat belt. **(A)** Anteroposterior and **(B)** lateral tomograms of the lumbar spine show a fracture of the vertebral body of L1 extending into the lamina and spinous process. (Courtesy of D. Faegenburg, MD, Mineola, New York.)

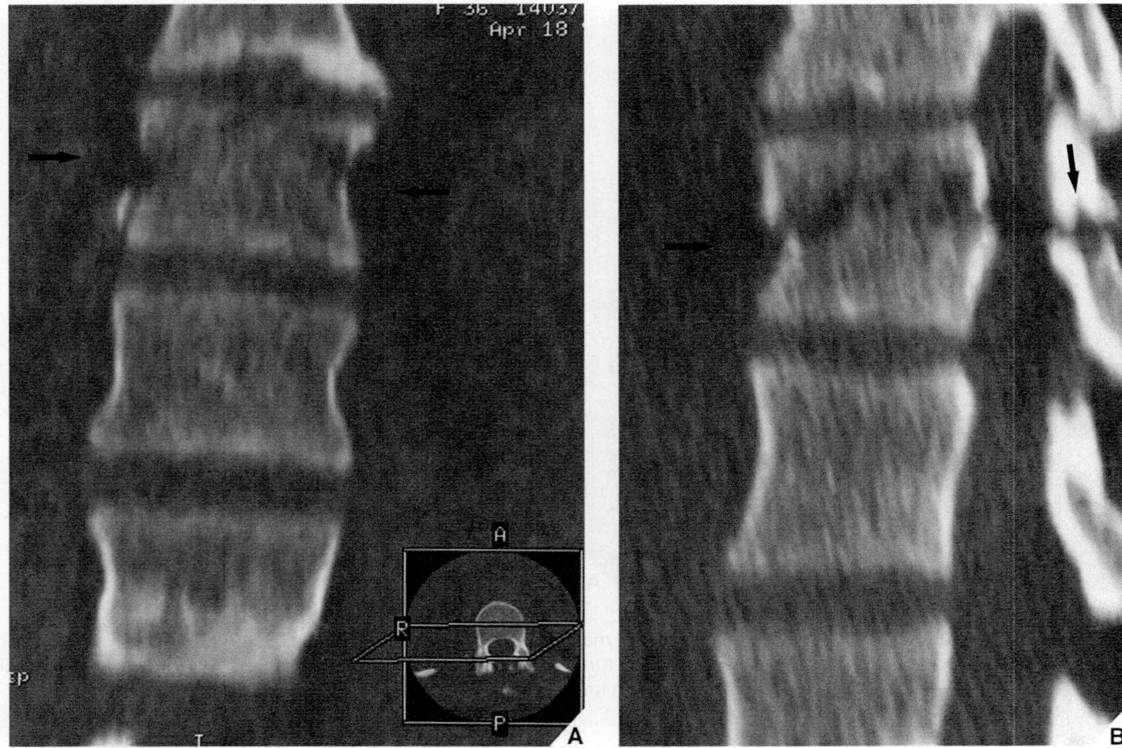

FIGURE 11.71 CT of the Chance fracture. A 36-year-old woman was injured in a car accident. She had been wearing a lap seat belt but not a restraining shoulder belt. Reformatted CT images in coronal **(A)** and sagittal **(B)** planes show a typical one-level Chance fracture through the L2 vertebra *(arrows)*.

According to the Denis three-column concept of thoracolumbar spine injuries, these latter types of fractures are essentially the result of failure of the posterior and middle columns, with the intact anterior element acting as a hinge. These injuries may be stable or unstable, depending on their extent and severity.

Fracture–Dislocations

Resulting from various forces—flexion, rotation, distraction, or anteroposterior or posteroanterior shear—acting on the thoracolumbar segment either alone or in combination, fracture–dislocations result in the failure of all three columns of the spine (Fig. 11.74); hence, such injuries are unstable and are usually associated with severe neurologic complications.

In the *flexion-rotation type* of injury, the posterior and middle columns are completely disrupted, and the anterior column may show on the lateral radiograph anterior wedging of the vertebral body. The lateral film also demonstrates subluxation or dislocation, together with an increase in the interspinous distance (Fig. 11.75). The posterior wall of the vertebral body may be intact if the dislocation occurs at the level of the intervertebral disk. The anteroposterior projection may not be diagnostic, but it occasionally reveals a displaced fracture of the superior articular process

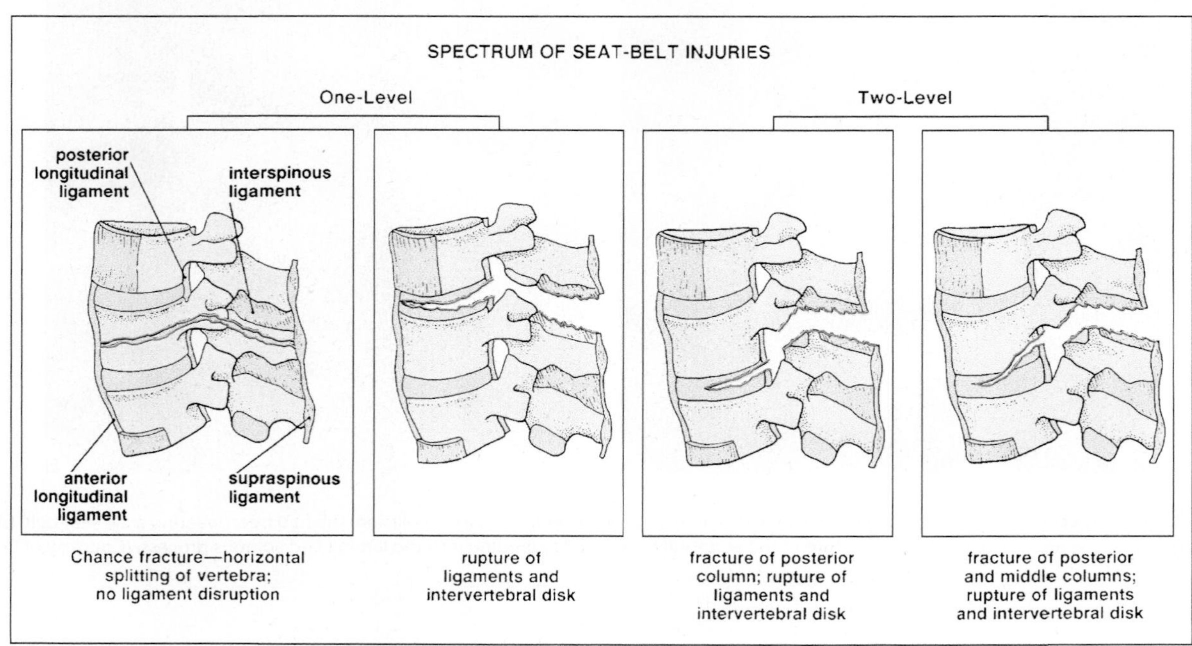

FIGURE 11.72 The spectrum of seat-belt injuries involving the lumbar spine.

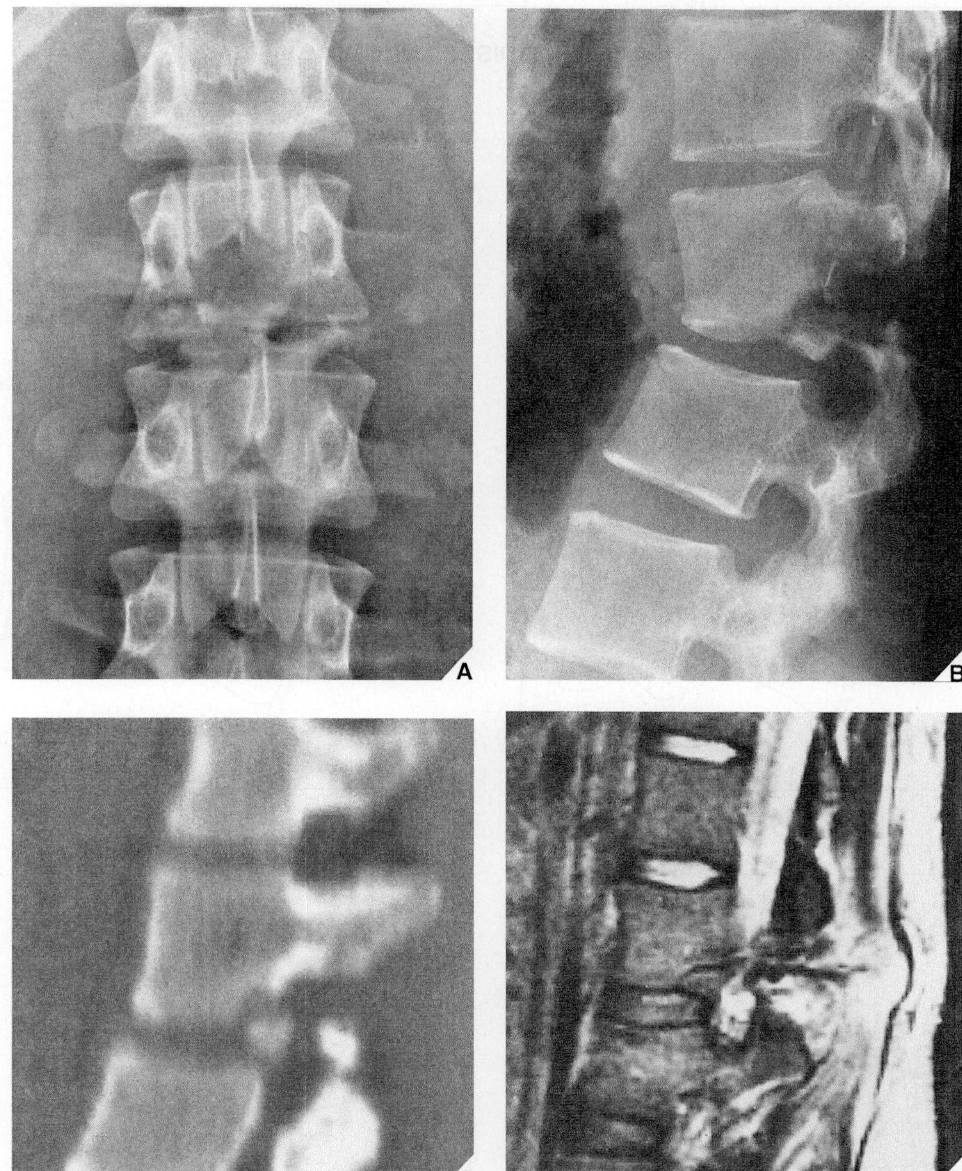

FIGURE 11.73 Two-level seat-belt injury. A 21-year-old woman sustained an injury to the lower back in a car accident. **(A)** Anteroposterior radiograph of the lumbar spine demonstrates a horizontal cleft in the L2 vertebral body. Note increased distance between the pedicles of L2 and L3 and fractures of several transverse processes. **(B)** Lateral radiograph shows posterior angulation at the L2-3 level and an oblique fracture extending from the inferoposterior part of the L2 vertebral body to the lamina and posterior elements. **(C)** Sagittal CT reformation demonstrates the fracture of posterior elements to better advantage. **(D)** Parasagittal MR image demonstrates disruption of the posterior ligaments and a large soft-tissue hematoma. The findings are typical of a two-level seat-belt injury.

on one side, representing failure of the posterior column secondary to rotational forces.

In the *shear types* of fracture–dislocation, all three columns are disrupted, including the anterior longitudinal ligament. The *posteroanterior shear variant* is characterized by forward displacement of the spinal segment onto the vertebra below at the point of shear; the vertebral bodies are intact without any decrease in their anterior or posterior height. However, the posterior elements of the dislocated vertebral segment, including the laminae, articular facets, and spinous processes, are usually fractured at several levels (Fig. 11.76). In *anteroposterior shear*, the spinal segment above the point of shear is dislocated posterior to the segment below (Fig. 11.77). It may be accompanied by a fracture of the spinous process.

Fracture–dislocation of the *flexion-distraction type* resembles seat-belt injuries involving failure of the posterior and middle columns (Fig. 11.78; see also Fig. 11.71). However, unlike seat-belt injuries, the entire annulus fibrosus is torn, which allows the vertebra above to dislocate or sublux onto the vertebra below.

Spondylolysis and Spondylolisthesis

Spondylolysis, a defect in the pars interarticularis (the junction of the pedicle, articular facets, and lamina) of a vertebra (neck of the "Scotty dog"), may be an acquired abnormality, secondary to an acute fracture, or, as is more commonly the case, it may result from chronic stress (stress fracture). Rarely, it is seen as a result of a congenital defect in the isthmus. The term derives from the Greek words *spondylos* (vertebra) and *lysis* (defect). It is encountered more commonly in the lower lumbar spine and has a high prevalence among athletes.

Spondylolisthesis, a term introduced by Killian in 1854, is defined as ventral slipping or gliding of all or part of one vertebra on a stationary vertebra beneath it. These abnormalities are seen predominantly in the lumbar spine (90% of cases) and most commonly at the L4-5 and L5-S1 levels. It is important to distinguish spondylolisthesis associated with spondylolysis from spondylolisthesis occurring without an associated defect in the pars interarticularis (Fig. 11.79). As a rule, this latter form, designated "pseudospondylolisthesis" by Junghanns in 1931, is associated with degenerative

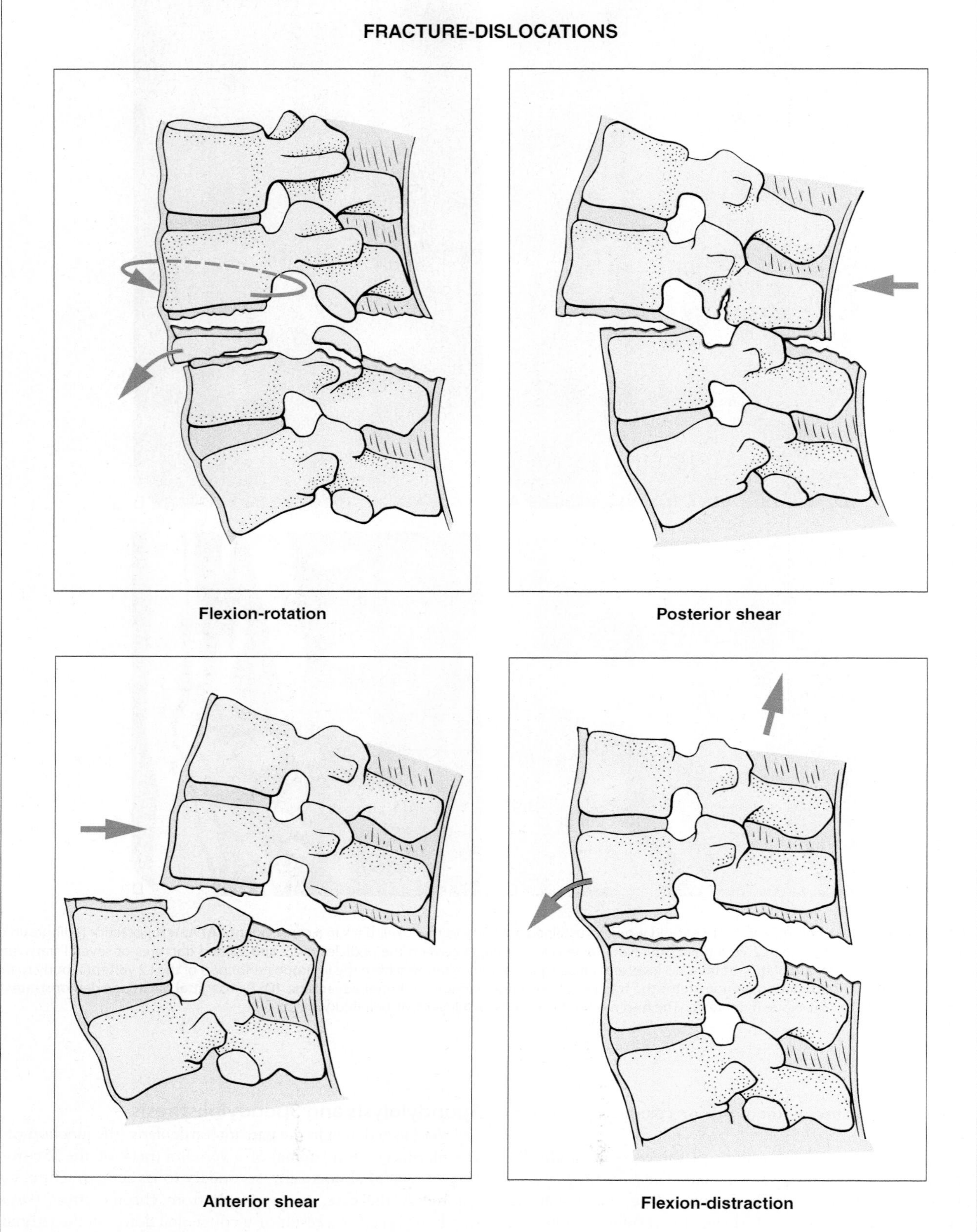

FIGURE 11.74 **Types of fracture–dislocations.** Schematic representation of various types of fracture–dislocation of the thoracolumbar spine (*red arrows* show the direction of acting forces).

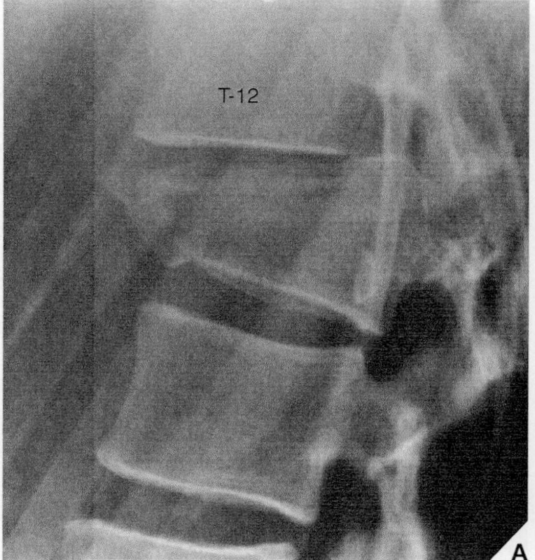

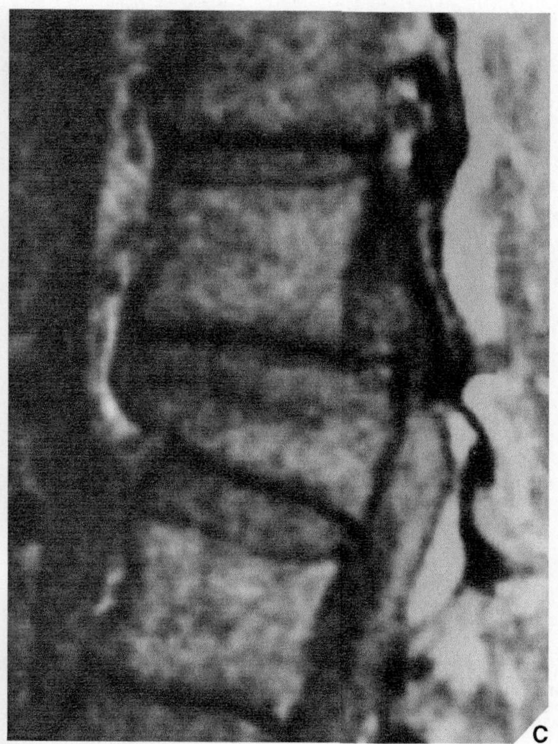

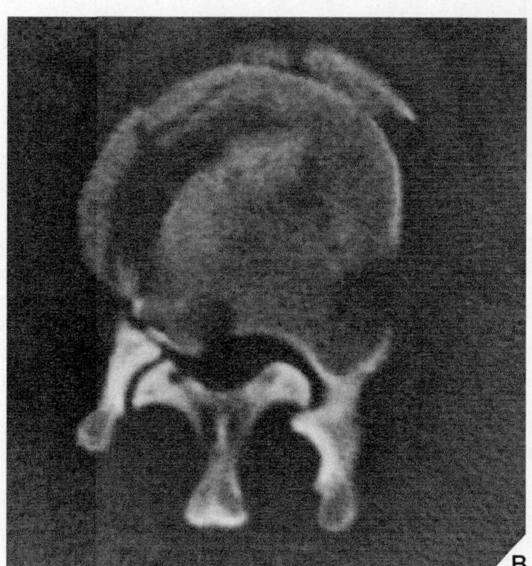

FIGURE 11.75 **CT and MRI of fracture–dislocation.** A 27-year-old man was injured in a motorcycle accident and sustained a flexion-rotation type of fracture–dislocation at the T12-L1 level. **(A)** Lateral radiograph shows anterior wedging of the body of L1 and disruption of the middle column. There is also slight anterior displacement of vertebra T12. **(B)** CT section through the vertebra L1 shows fracture of the middle column associated with retropulsion of the fractured fragment into the spinal canal, similar to that in the burst fracture. **(C)** Sagittal T2-weighted MR image shows in addition disruption of the posterior column, tear of the posterior longitudinal ligament, and compression of the thecal sac.

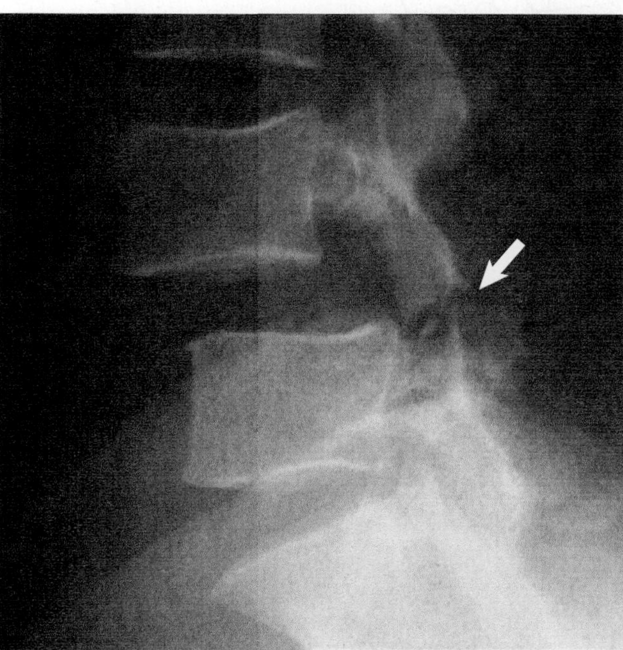

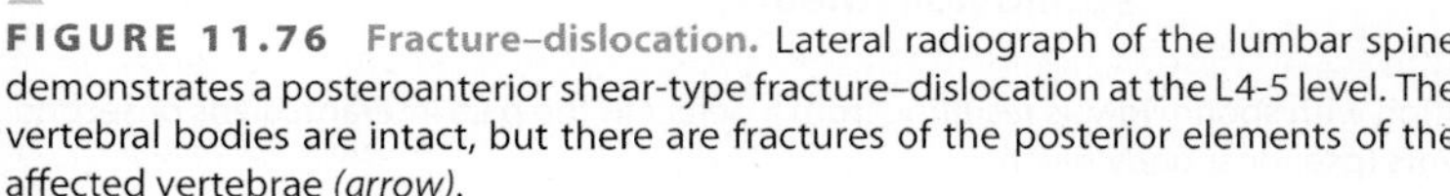

FIGURE 11.76 **Fracture–dislocation.** Lateral radiograph of the lumbar spine demonstrates a posteroanterior shear-type fracture–dislocation at the L4-5 level. The vertebral bodies are intact, but there are fractures of the posterior elements of the affected vertebrae *(arrow)*.

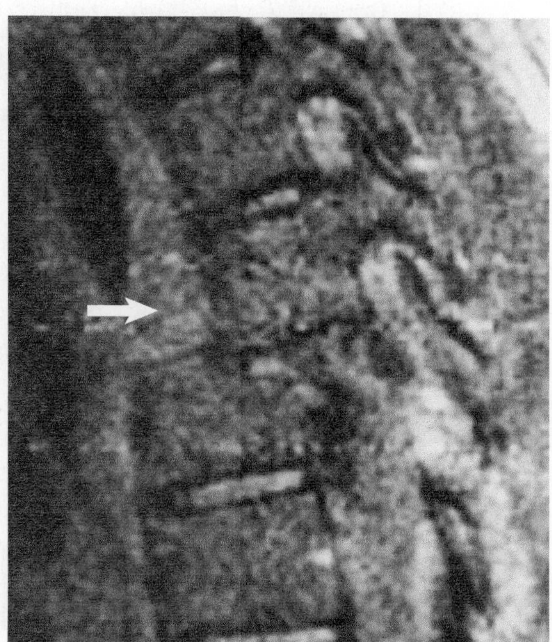

FIGURE 11.77 **MRI of fracture–dislocation.** Sagittal T2-weighted MR image demonstrates an anteroposterior shear-type fracture–dislocation at the lower thoracic level *(arrow)*.

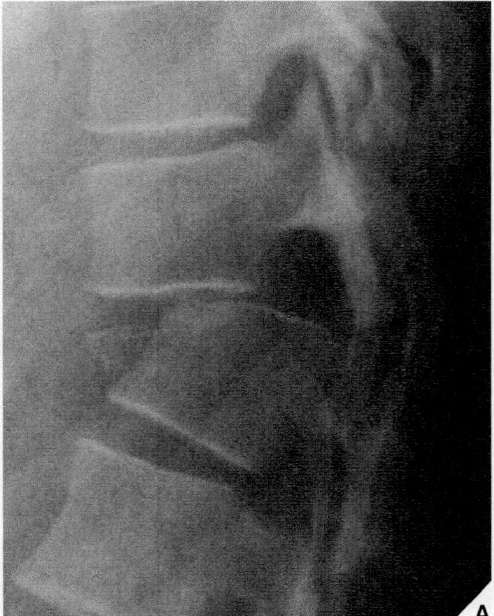

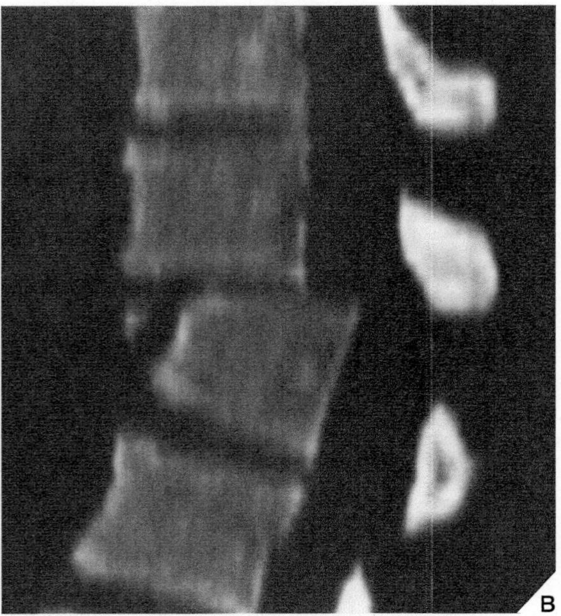

FIGURE 11.78 CT of fracture–dislocation. **(A)** Lateral radiograph of the thoracolumbar spine and **(B)** sagittal reformatted CT image demonstrate characteristic features of a flexion-distraction type of fracture–dislocation.

disk disease and degeneration and subluxation in the apophyseal joints, and it is often referred to as *degenerative spondylolisthesis* (see Chapter 13). Although the defect in the pars interarticularis cannot always be demonstrated on conventional radiographs, true spondylolisthesis can be differentiated from pseudospondylolisthesis by the spinous-process sign introduced by Bryk and Rosenkranz (Fig. 11.80). The sign is a logical outgrowth of the different processes at work in the two conditions. In true spondylolisthesis, a bilateral defect in the pars interarticularis leads to forward (ventral) slippage of the body, pedicles, and superior articular process of the involved vertebra, whereas the spinous process, laminae, and inferior articular process remain in normal position. Therefore, study of the most dorsal aspects of the spinous processes reveals a step-off at the interspace *above the level* of the slip (Fig. 11.81A). In pseudospondylolisthesis, however, the entire vertebra, including the spinous process, moves forward; in this situation, the most dorsal aspects of the spinous processes exhibit a step-off at the interspace *below the level* of the slipped vertebra (Fig. 11.81B). Application of this

Spondylolisthesis

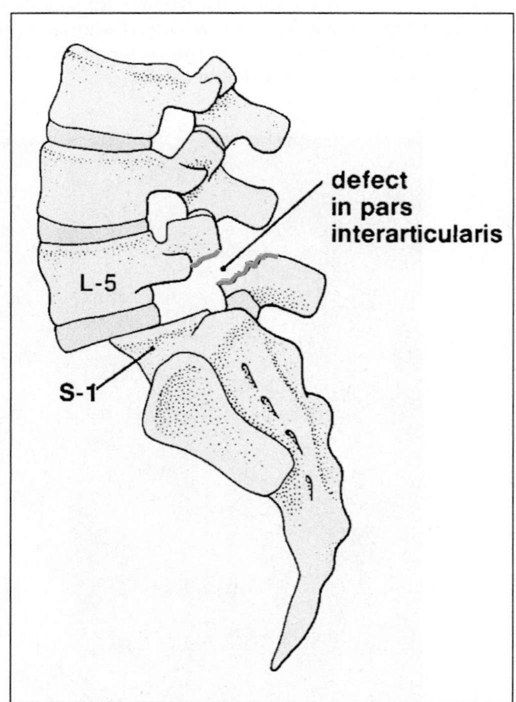

associated with spondylolysis (true spondylolisthesis)

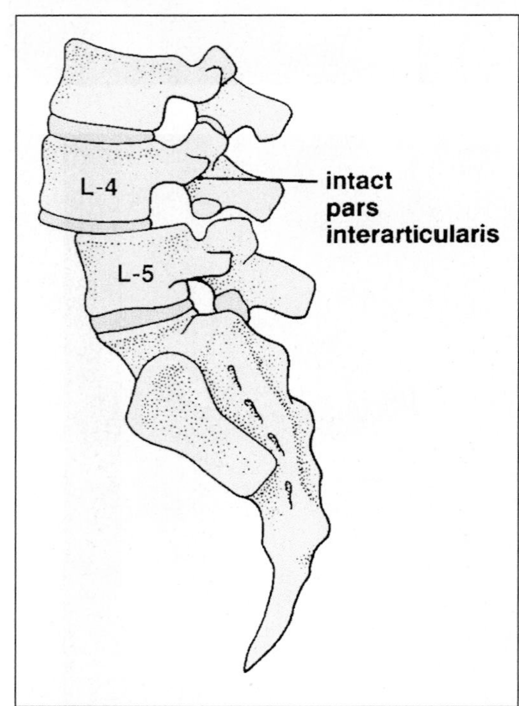

without spondylolysis (pseudo- or degenerative spondylolisthesis)

FIGURE 11.79 Types of spondylolisthesis. Spondylolisthesis may occur in association with spondylolysis resulting from a defect in the pars interarticularis or secondary to degenerative disk disease and degeneration and subluxation of the apophyseal joints (pseudospondylolisthesis).

Spinous-Process Sign

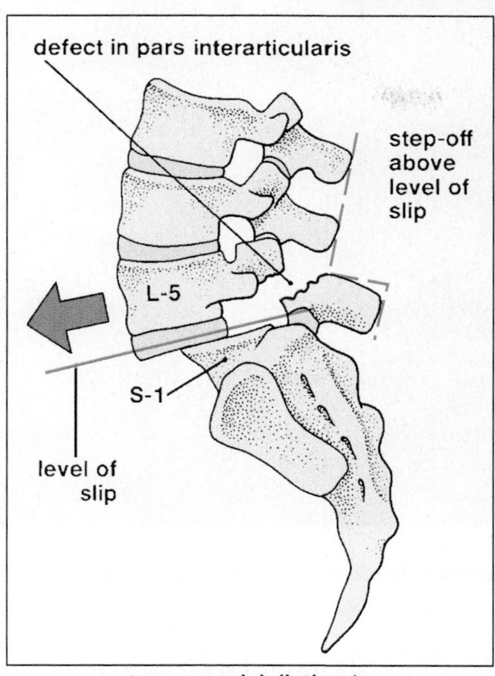

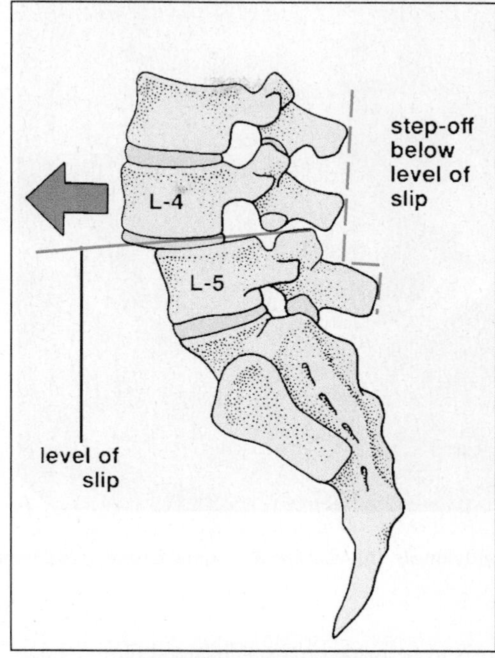

FIGURE 11.80 The spinous-process sign. The spinous-process sign can help differentiate true spondylolisthesis from pseudospondylolisthesis by the appearance of a step-off in the spinous processes above the level of vertebral slip in the former and below that level in the latter *(red arrows* indicate the direction of slip*)*.

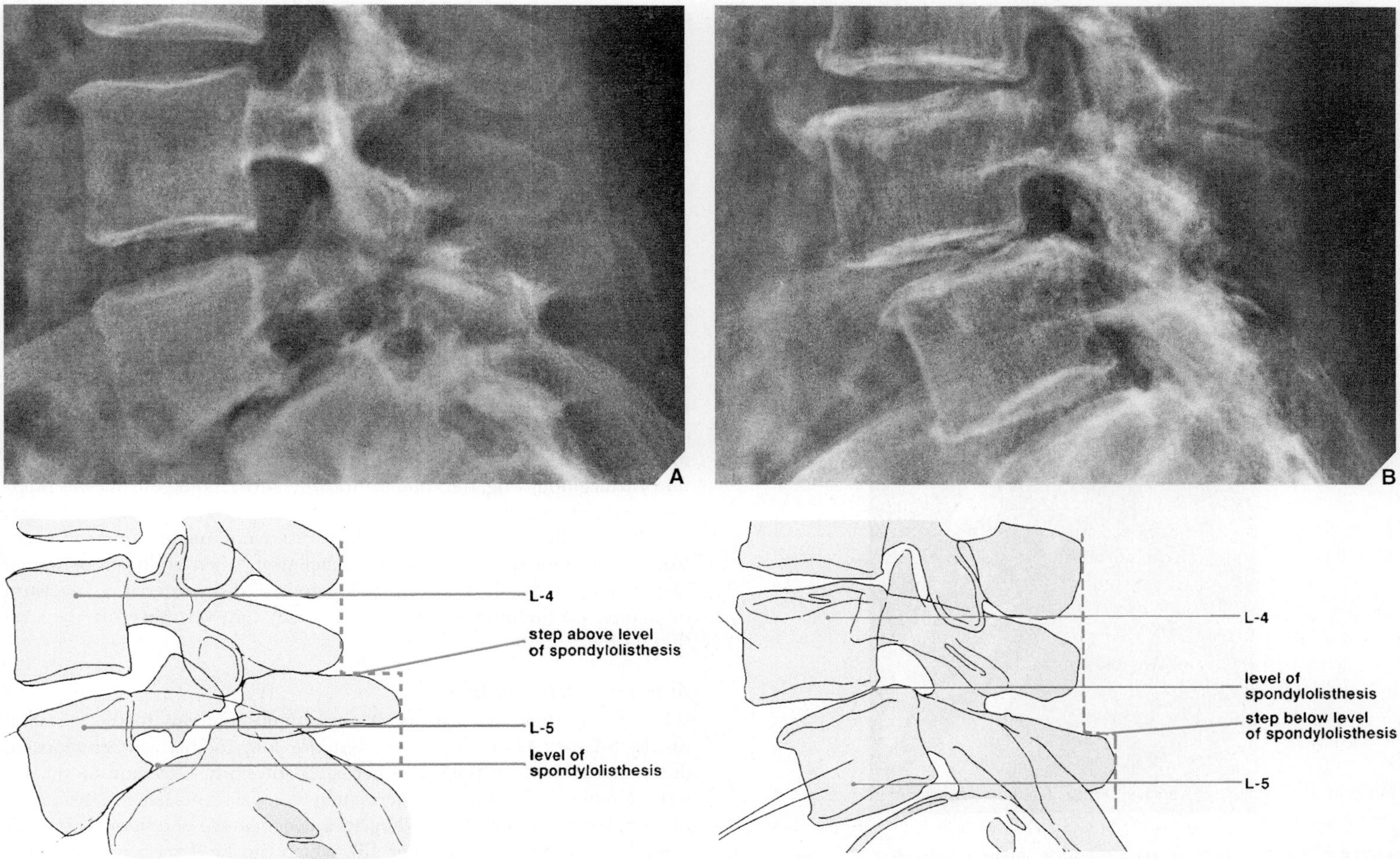

A

L-4
step above level of spondylolisthesis
L-5
level of spondylolisthesis

B

L-4
level of spondylolisthesis
step below level of spondylolisthesis
L-5

FIGURE 11.81 Spondylolisthesis and pseudospondylolisthesis. (A) Lateral radiograph of the lumbar spine demonstrates the typical appearance of spondylolisthesis secondary to a defect in the pars interarticularis. Note that the most dorsal aspect of the spinous process of L5 forms a step with that of L4 *above the level* of slippage of L5. **(B)** In spondylolisthesis without spondylolysis (degenerative spondylolisthesis), a step-off in the spinous processes *below the level* of vertebral slippage is an identifying feature.

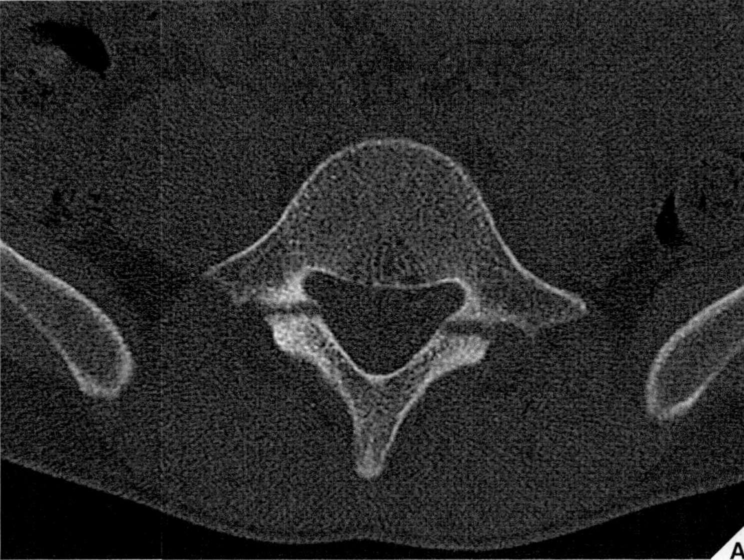

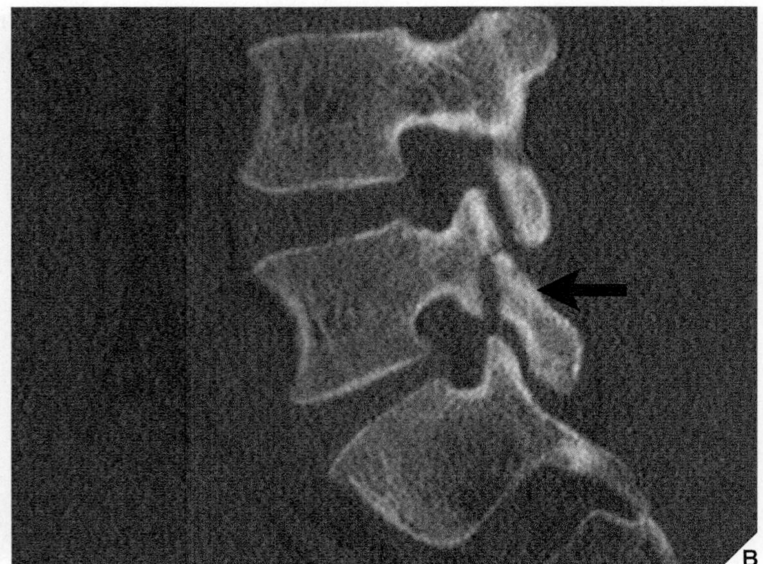

FIGURE 11.82 CT of spondylolysis. **(A)** Axial and **(B)** sagittal reformatted CT images show bilateral defect in the pars interarticularis of L5 vertebra *(arrow)*.

sign allows a correct diagnosis to be made on a single lateral film; oblique projections are not necessary. In obtaining the radiographs, however, it is important to avoid overexposure, which may obscure the posterior margins of the spinous processes.

The defect in the pars interarticularis precipitating spondylolisthesis can be demonstrated on the standard oblique projection of the lumbar spine, which in the past used to be supplemented by conventional tomography and currently by CT and MRI (Figs. 11.82, 11.83, and 11.84A–C); myelography on the lateral view may show an extradural defect on the ventral aspect of the thecal sac, similar to that created by disk herniation (Fig. 11.84D). A severe degree of spondylolisthesis at the L5-S1 level can be identified on the anteroposterior radiograph by the ventrocaudal displacement of L5 over the sacrum. This configuration creates curvilinear densities forming what is called the *inverted Napoleon's hat sign* (Figs. 11.85 and 11.86). The simple grading of spondylolisthesis proposed by Myerding is based on the amount of forward slipping (Fig. 11.87).

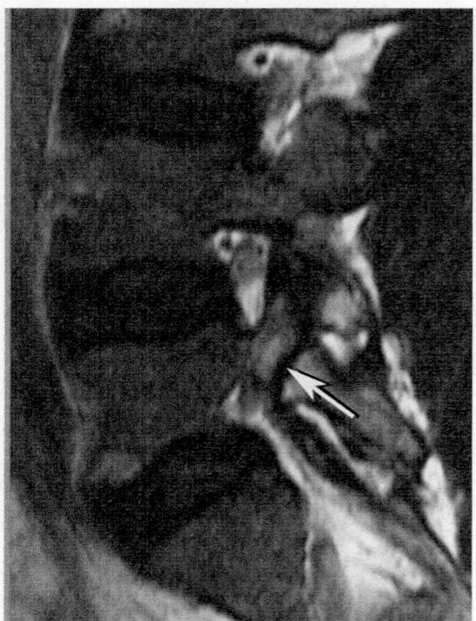

FIGURE 11.83 MRI of spondylolysis. Right parasagittal T2-weighted MRI shows a pars defect *(arrow)* with mild surrounding edema. (Courtesy of Steve Shankman, MD, Brooklyn, New York.)

Transitional Lumbosacral Vertebra

Transitional lumbosacral vertebrae are very common congenital variants. They can present as six lumbar type vertebra (lumbarization of S1) or four lumbar type vertebra (sacralization of L5). This can be difficult to assess unless the vertebrae are counted from C1 down. For practical purposes and for preoperative assessment, it is acceptable to indicate that a transitional lumbosacral vertebra is present and to identify which vertebra is labeled L5 or S1 based on morphologic features, for example, the presence of an inferior rudimentary disk. A further complication of accurate assessment of transitional lumbosacral vertebra is the presence of unilateral or bilateral widened transverse process creating a pseudoarthrosis (pseudoarticulation) or fusion with the sacral ala (Fig. 11.88). In these cases, the patients may experience low back pain and they are amenable to treatment with percutaneous injections of local anesthetic and steroids. Surgical resection may be necessary if conservative measures fail. This condition is called *Bertolotti syndrome* and is an important cause of low back pain in young patients. The diagnosis is usually made based on radiographs or CT of the pelvis and lumbosacral spine.

Injury to the Diskovertebral Junction

One of the most frequent conditions affecting the diskovertebral junction is herniation of an intervertebral disk. The chief structural unit between adjacent vertebral bodies, the intervertebral disk, comprises a soft central portion, the nucleus pulposus, composed of collagen fibrils and mucoprotein gel, lying eccentrically and somewhat posteriorly, and a firm fibrocartilaginous ring, the annulus fibrosus, surrounding the nucleus pulposus and reinforced by the anterior and posterior longitudinal ligaments. Injury to the intervertebral disk and the diskovertebral junction can result from acute trauma or from subtle subclinical, often endogenous injury. Depending on the direction of herniation of disk material, a spectrum of injuries of the intervertebral disk and adjacent vertebrae may be seen (Fig. 11.89).

Anterior Disk Herniation

When the normal attachments of the annulus fibrosus to the vertebral rim by Sharpey fibers and to the anterior longitudinal ligament loosen, disk material (nucleus pulposus) herniates anteriorly. Elevation of the anterior longitudinal ligament by herniating material stimulates the formation of peripheral osteophytes, leading to a degenerative condition known as *spondylosis deformans* (see Chapter 13), which can be demonstrated on the lateral radiograph of the lumbar spine (Fig 11.90A). Anterior herniation can also be demonstrated on diskography (Fig. 11.90B) and MRI.

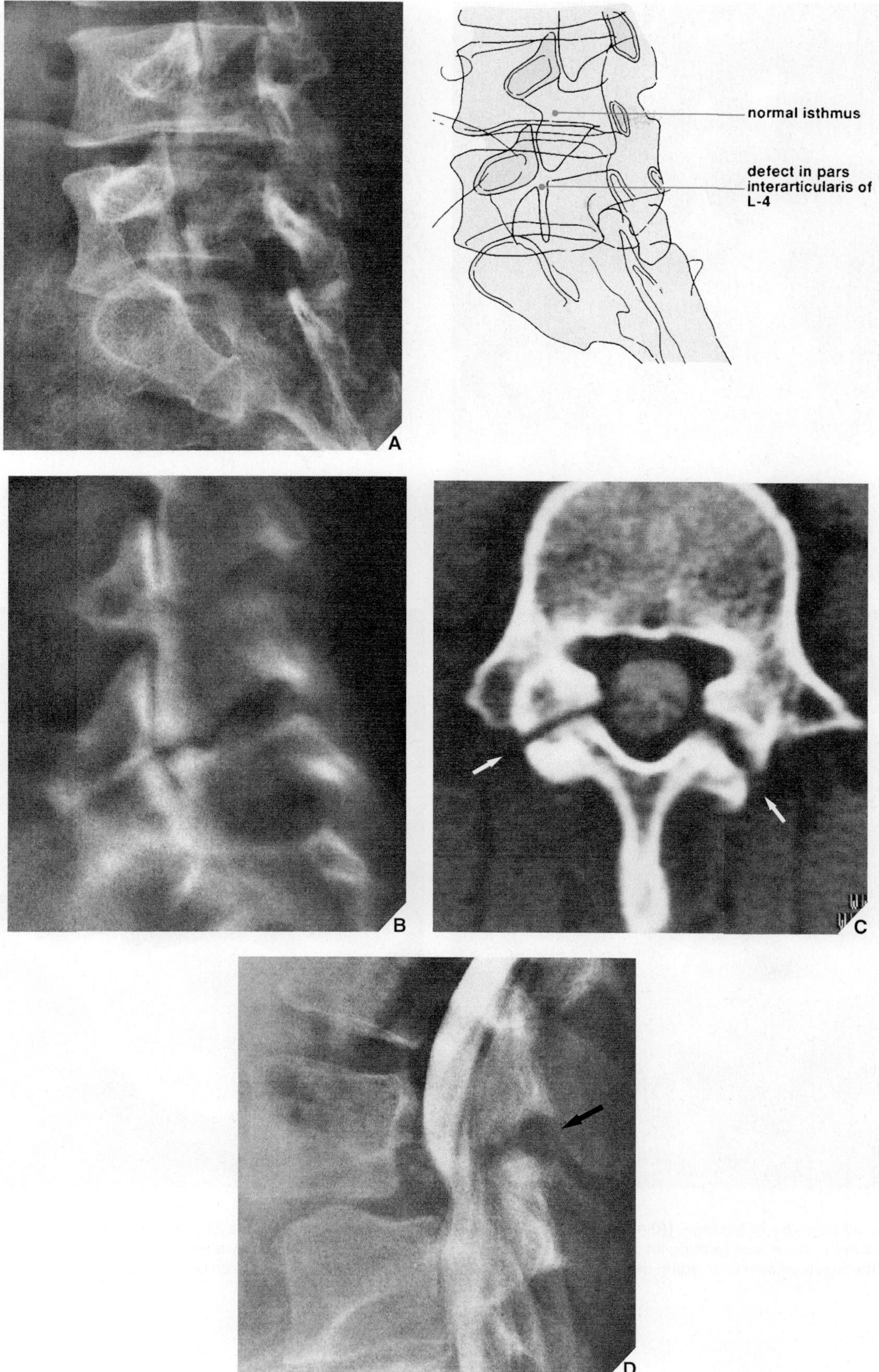

FIGURE 11.84 Spondylolysis and spondylolisthesis. (A) Oblique radiograph and **(B)** trispiral tomogram of the lumbar spine in a 28-year-old man show a defect in the pars interarticularis (neck of the "Scotty dog") of L4 typical of spondylolysis. **(C)** CT section through the vertebral body clearly demonstrates defects in the left and right pars interarticularis *(arrows)*. **(D)** Lateral spot film obtained during myelography shows an extradural defect on the ventral aspect of the thecal sac, similar to that of disk herniation, caused by grade 2 spondylolisthesis at L4-5. The defect in the pars interarticularis is also clearly seen *(arrow)*.

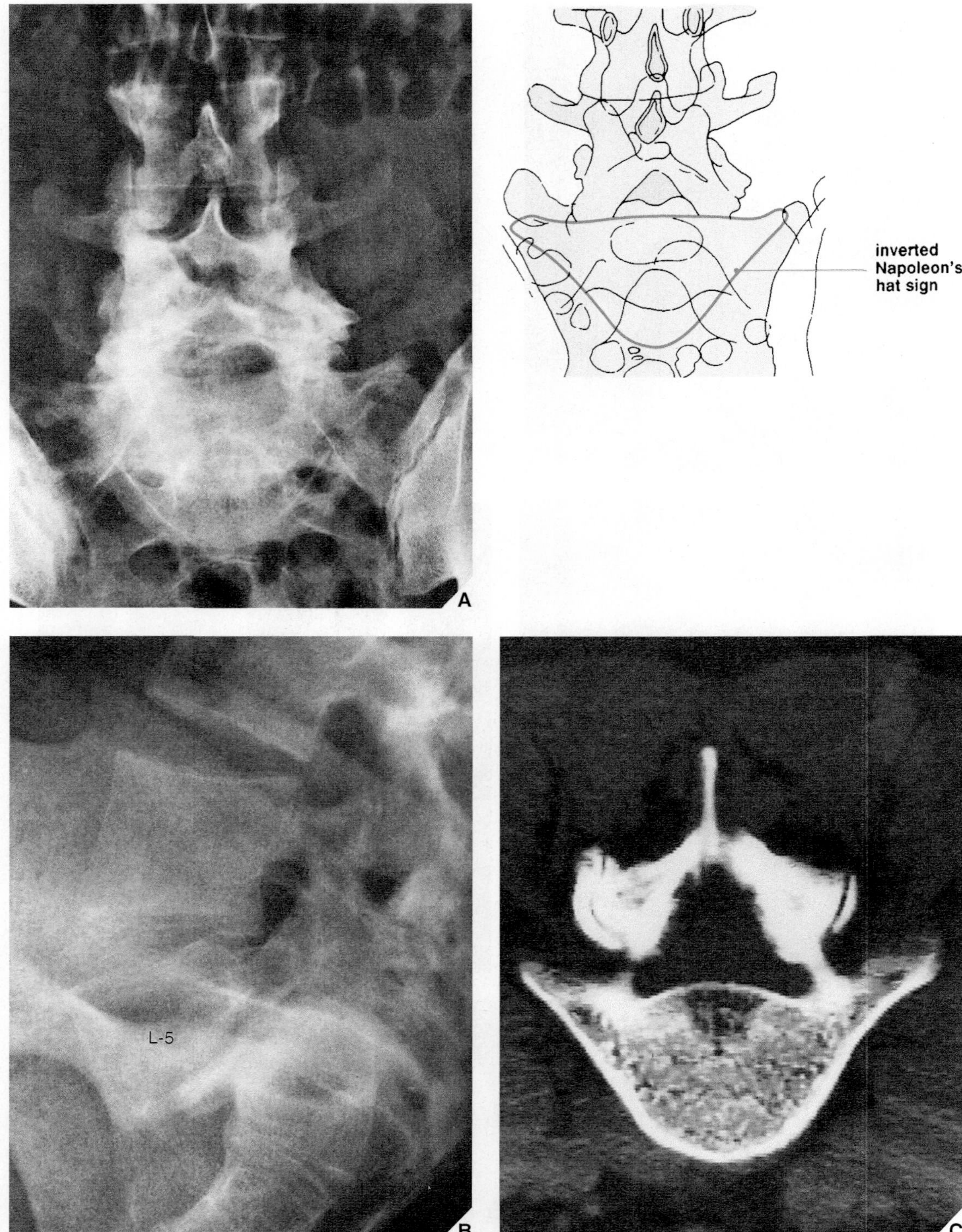

FIGURE 11.85 Inverted Napoleon's hat sign. **(A)** Anteroposterior radiograph of the lumbosacral spine in a 21-year-old man with severe (grade 4) spondylolisthesis shows curvilinear densities in the sacral area forming an inverted Napoleon's hat. This configuration is caused by a severe degree of slip at the L5-S1 level as seen on the lateral projection **(B)**. **(C)** The sign is created by imaging the vertebral body in the axial projection, similar to that seen on a CT section of a normal vertebra.

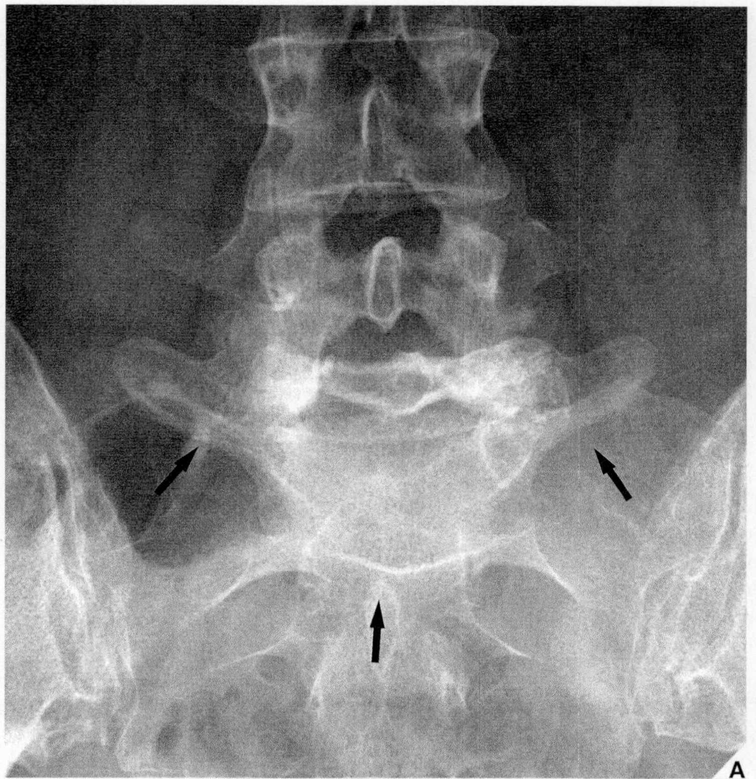

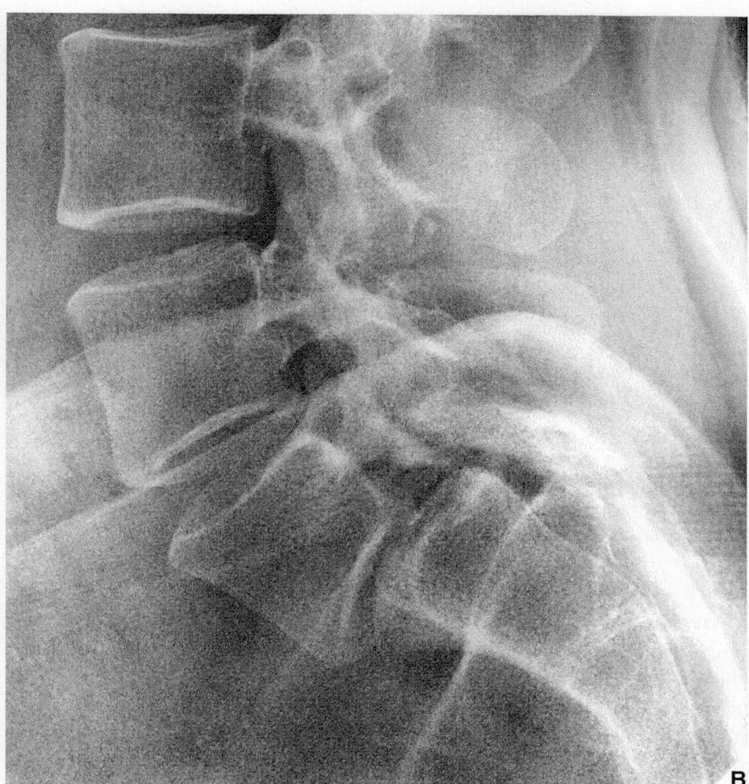

FIGURE 11.86 Inverted Napoleon's hat sign. **(A)** Anteroposterior radiograph shows an inverted Napoleon's hat sign *(arrows)*. **(B)** The lateral radiograph shows spondylolisthesis at L5-S1 level.

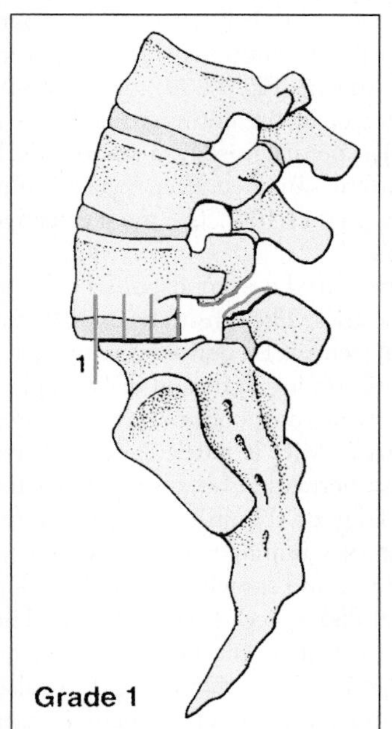

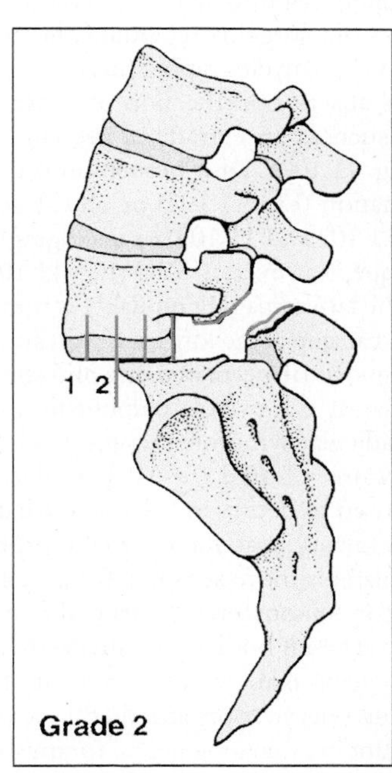

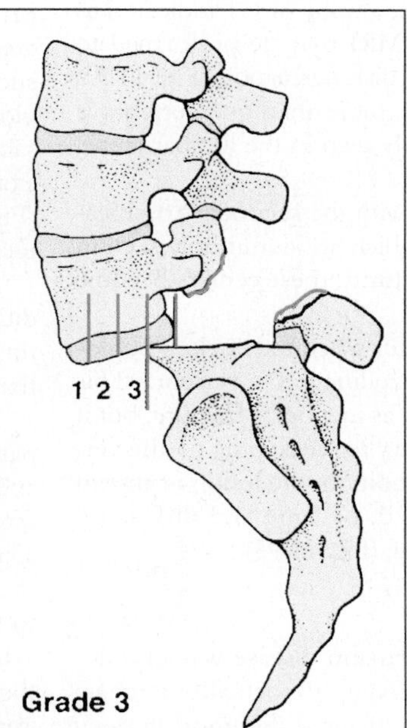

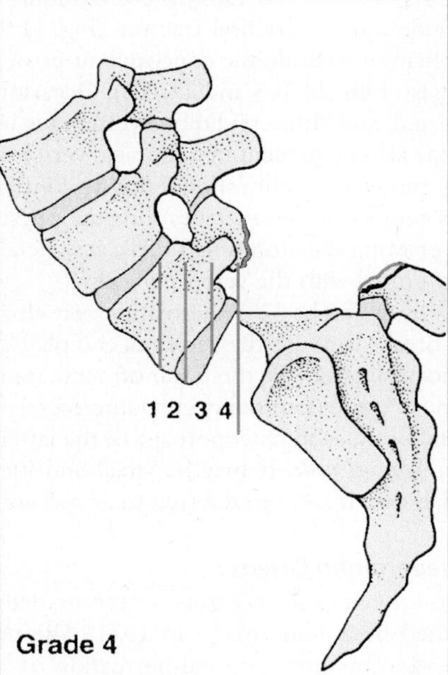

FIGURE 11.87 Grades of spondylolisthesis. The grading of spondylolisthesis, as proposed by Meyerding, is based on the amount of forward displacement of L5 on S1.

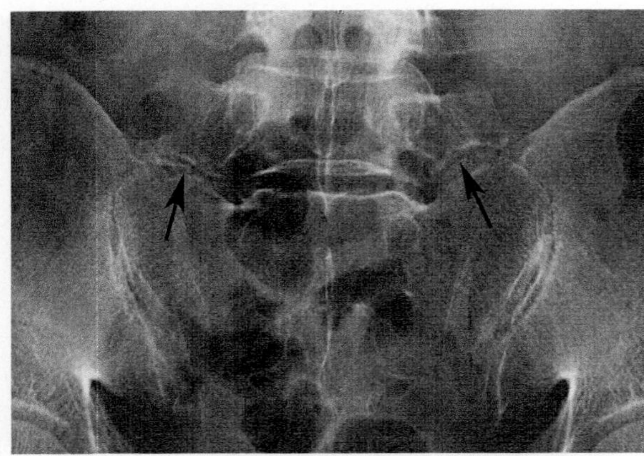

FIGURE 11.88 Bertolotti syndrome. Anteroposterior radiograph of the sacrum of a young adult, who presented with low back pain, reveals a transitional lumbosacral vertebra with bilateral wide transverse processes that pseudoarticulate with bilateral sacral ala *(arrows)*.

Intravertebral Disk Herniation

Ventrocaudal disk herniation, as well as ventrocephalad herniation, which is much less commonly seen, produces an abnormality known as *limbus vertebra*. Herniation of disk material into a vertebral body at the site of attachment of the annulus fibrosus to the body's rim separates a small, triangular fragment of bone, which is commonly mistaken for an acute fracture or infectious spondylitis. Reactive bone sclerosis adjacent to the defect, however, indicates a chronic process. The adjacent disk space is invariably narrowed, and a radiolucent cleft known as the *vacuum phenomenon* may be seen in the disk space, representing degeneration of the disk (Fig. 11.91). This abnormality, which is invariably asymptomatic, is the product of chronic, endogenous trauma. The characteristic radiographic changes are best seen on the lateral projection of the lumbar spine (see Fig. 11.91); only rarely is conventional tomography or CT indicated to exclude a true vertebral fracture (Fig. 11.92). MRI may be performed to confirm or exclude the concomitant posterior disk herniation (Fig. 11.93; see also Figs. 11.105 and 11.106). Occasionally, more than one vertebra is affected, and although limbus vertebra is usually seen in the lumbar spine, it may also be present in a thoracic vertebra.

Limbus vertebra should not be confused with the secondary ossification centers of the vertebral ring apophysis, which are commonly seen in the growing skeleton (Fig. 11.94); at skeletal maturity, these centers become fully united with the vertebral body.

Intravertebral disk herniation may also occur when the nucleus pulposus breaks through the vertebral end plates, extruding into a vertebra. This abnormality may be the result of acute trauma, as in a burst fracture, but it is much more commonly encountered secondary to weakening of the vertebral body, as in osteoporosis. In the latter condition, the lesion is known as a *Schmorl node*. It may be small and localized, or large and diffuse, in which case it is often referred to as *ballooned disk* (Fig. 11.95).

Scheuermann Disease

Also known as *juvenile thoracic kyphosis*, Scheuermann disease was first described by Scheuermann in 1921. The underlying abnormality is characterized by intravertebral herniation of disk material (Schmorl nodes), associated with anterior wedging (of 5 degrees or more) of at least three contiguous vertebral bodies. There is a wavy appearance of vertebral end plates and narrowing of the intervertebral disk spaces. Thoracic kyphosis is often present (Fig. 11.96). This condition usually affects adolescent boys and young adults. The clinical manifestations are variable. Some patients are completely asymptomatic, whereas others may experience fatigue and thoracic pain aggravated by physical exertion. Neurologic findings are rare. Although the thoracic spine is predominantly affected (Fig. 11.97), involvement of the lumbar spine has also been reported. This condition is called *Scheuermann disease type II* (in contrast to type I, which involves the upper thoracic spine), although some investigators prefer the term *juvenile lumbar osteochondrosis*. Imaging studies demonstrate changes almost identical to those seen in Scheuermann disease type I, including prominent Schmorl nodes, irregularity of the end plates, and narrowing of the disk spaces (Fig. 11.98). However, anterior vertebral wedging is not a constant feature of this variant.

Posterior and Posterolateral Disk Herniation

Intraspinal herniation or "herniated disk" is the most serious of the three variants of diskovertebral junction injury. It is most commonly seen in the lumbar spine, particularly L4-5 and L5-S1, although it may be seen in the cervical region. It is commonly associated with clinical symptoms such as sciatic pain and weakening of the lower extremity, especially when herniation in the lumbar segment causes compression on an exiting nerve root or the thecal sac. A predisposing factor in some patients may be the loss of elasticity of the annulus fibrosus caused by degenerative changes, with subsequent rupture of the annulus or even the posterior longitudinal ligament and retropulsion of the nucleus pulposus into the spinal canal. Typically, the patient, usually a young adult man, gives a history of straining his back by lifting a heavy object. The subsequent pain in the lumbar region radiates to the posterior aspect of the thigh and buttock and the lateral aspect of the leg and is aggravated by coughing and sneezing; sometimes, there is associated paresthesia or numbness in the foot. Physical examination reveals muscular spasm, limitation of forward bending, and restriction of straight-leg raising on the affected side. Various other symptoms and physical findings may be present depending on the level and degree of injury.

The standard radiographic examination in herniated disks is usually normal, and ancillary radiologic techniques including myelography and CT, either alone or in conjunction with one another, as well as diskography, and now MRI, are required to make a diagnosis. It has to be pointed out, however, that diskography is not only an imaging modality. Perhaps even more effective application of this technique is so-called *provocative diskography*, when during the procedure, the patient is asked if the increased pressure within the disk, while the contrast is being injected, causes much discomfort and whether this discomfort is the exact reproduction in quality and location of the patient's typical back pain. This functional information serves as an important diagnostic clue to the orthopaedic surgeon regarding the selection of disk levels to be operated on. The myelographic findings in disk herniation may be very subtle, such as absent opacification of a nerve sheath (Fig. 11.99), or more obvious, such as an extradural pressure defect in the contrast-filled thecal sac (Fig. 11.100). Disk herniation can also be diagnosed on standard CT examination (Fig. 11.101) or on CT sections obtained after myelography (Figs. 11.102 and 11.103) or diskography (Fig. 11.104). The most effective technique, however, is MRI (Fig. 11.105).

The latter imaging modality is routinely used for the diagnosis of conditions causing acute low back pain and sciatica. The sensitivity of MRI for the diagnosis of herniated disk and spinal stenosis is equivalent to or better than that of CT, even in combination with myelography and diskography.

Radicular symptoms represent one of the most common reasons why patients are referred for MRI of the spine. MRI is particularly sensitive and is used to detect and characterize disk herniation because it allows for direct evaluation of the internal morphology of the disk. The sagittal imaging plane is more sensitive for defining disk impingement on the thecal sac or for demonstrating extruded fragments and showing the relationship to the vertebral bodies and intervertebral disk spaces (Fig. 11.105A). The axial imaging plane can demonstrate the effect of the herniated disk on the exiting nerve roots and thecal sac (Fig. 11.105B). Axial images are also important in evaluating neural foramina and nerve root effacement in cases of lateral and posterolateral disk herniation. Free disk fragments can be easily identified (Fig. 11.106).

The use of T1-weighted images in the axial plane provides excellent contrast between high signal fat and low signal thecal sac, nerve roots, and disk fragments. Fast-scan techniques provide increased cerebrospinal fluid signal and allow enhanced contrast between herniated fragments and cerebrospinal fluid. Some advantages of MRI in comparison with myelography and CT of lumbar disk disease are evident. MRI is sensitive to the water content of the nucleus pulposus. As the water content of this structure decreases with aging or degeneration, decreased signal appears, particularly on T2-weighted images. In addition, the myelographic effect provided with heavily T2-weighted images and fast-scan techniques allows the visualization of nerve roots within the thecal sac. Anomalies such as conjoint nerve

SPECTRUM OF INTERVERTEBRAL DISK HERNIATION

Normal

Anterior Herniation

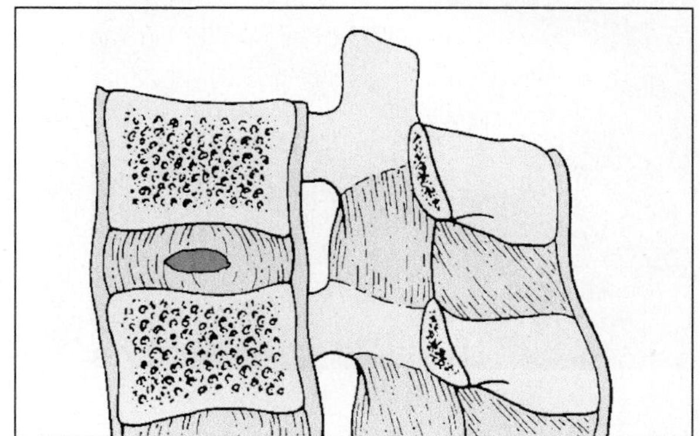

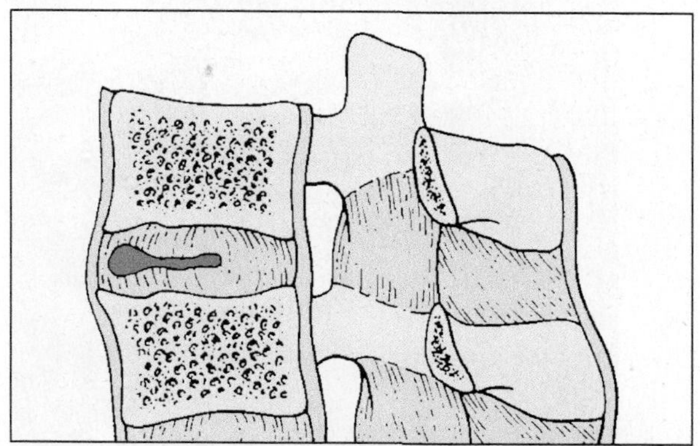

ventrad extrusion leading to elevation of anterior longitudinal ligament and osteophyte formation— spondylosis deformans

Intravertebral Herniation

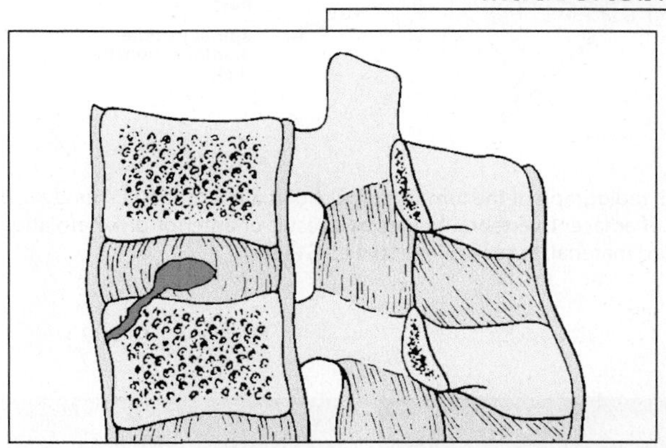

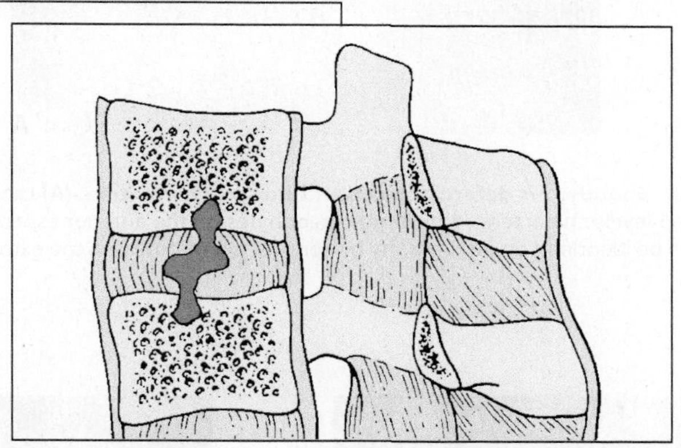

anterocaudad extrusion separating a triangular fragment from adjacent vertebra—limbus vertebra

cephalad or caudad extrusion through end plate into adjacent vertebra—Schmorl node

Intraspinal Herniation

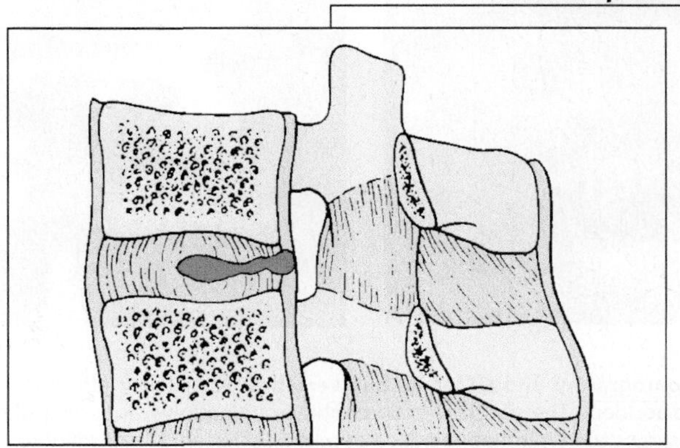

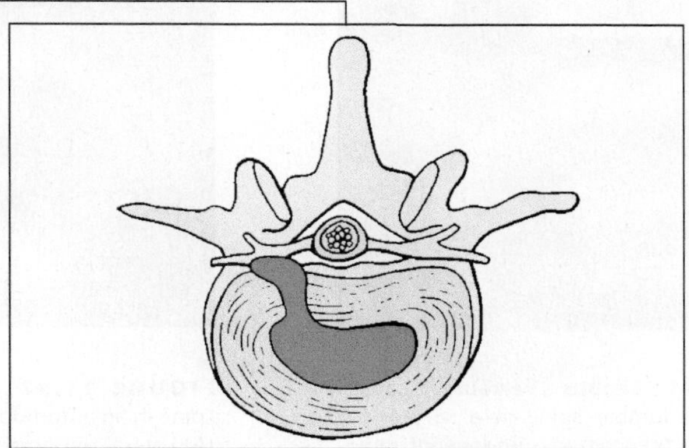

posterior or posterolateral extrusion into spinal canal—herniated disk

FIGURE 11.89 The spectrum of intervertebral disk herniation.

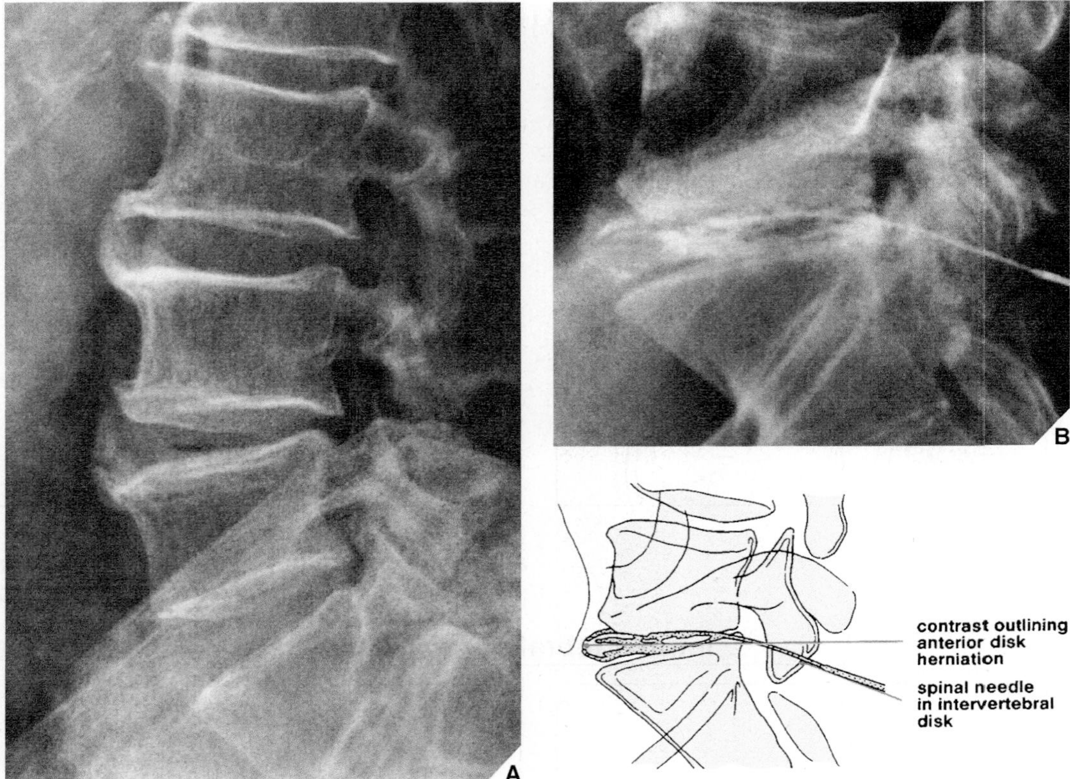

FIGURE 11.90 Spondylosis deformans and anterior disk herniation. **(A)** Lateral radiograph of the lumbar spine shows a late stage of spondylosis deformans at the L2-3, L3-4, and L4-5 levels characterized by large osteophytes on the anterior aspects of adjacent vertebral bodies as a result of anterior disk herniation. **(B)** Anterior disk herniation can also be identified on diskography by contrast agent outlining the extruded material, as seen here at the L5-S1 level.

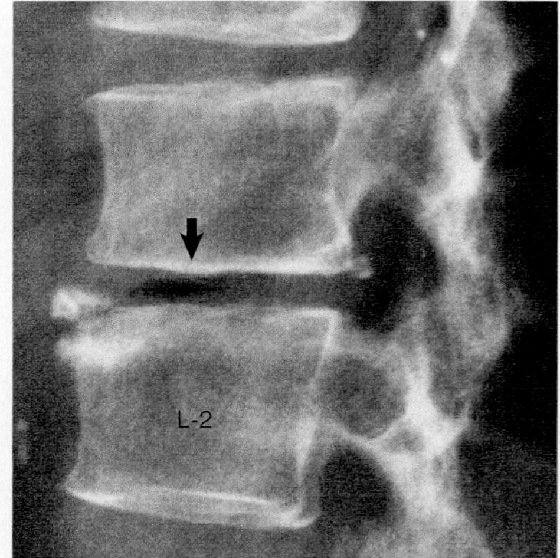

FIGURE 11.91 Limbus vertebra. Lateral radiograph of the lumbar spine in a 55-year-old woman with breast cancer, who underwent radiographic examination to exclude bone metastases shows anterior intravertebral disk herniation into the body of L2 (limbus vertebra). Note the vacuum phenomenon *(arrow)*, indicating disk degeneration.

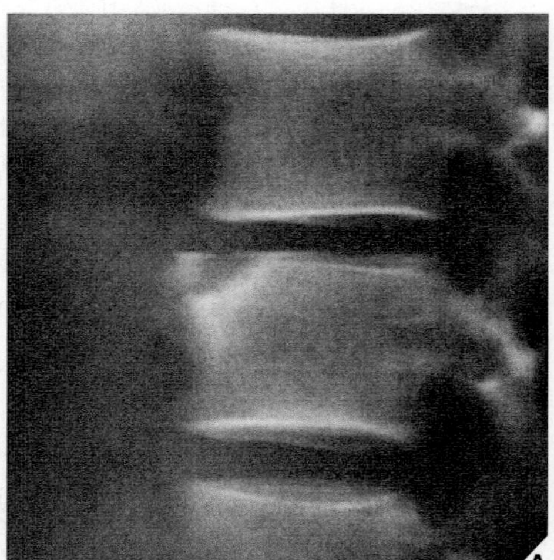

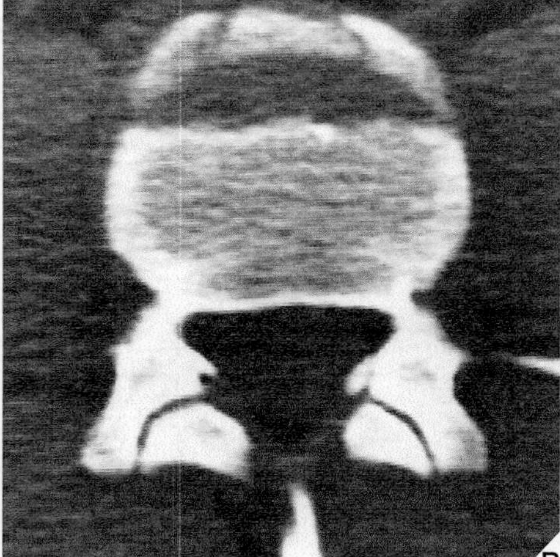

FIGURE 11.92 Tomography and CT of limbus vertebra. An 18-year-old man injured his lumbar spine in an automobile accident. The standard radiographic examination was equivocal regarding fracture. **(A)** Lateral tomogram shows the typical appearance of a limbus vertebra secondary to anterior herniation of the nucleus pulposus. The small triangular segment is separated from the body of L4 by a rim of reactive sclerosis, indicating a chronic process. Note the characteristic disk space narrowing. **(B)** CT examination was performed to investigate the possibility of concomitant posterior disk herniation into the spinal canal. The examination was negative for posterior herniation but confirmed the anterior herniation into the vertebral body, as seen in this more upper section through L4 vertebra.

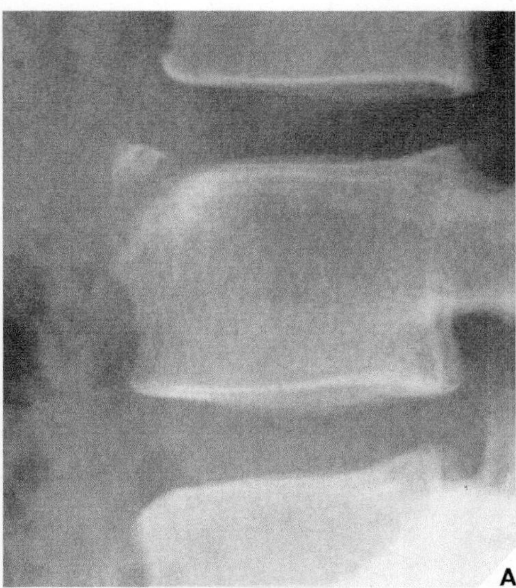

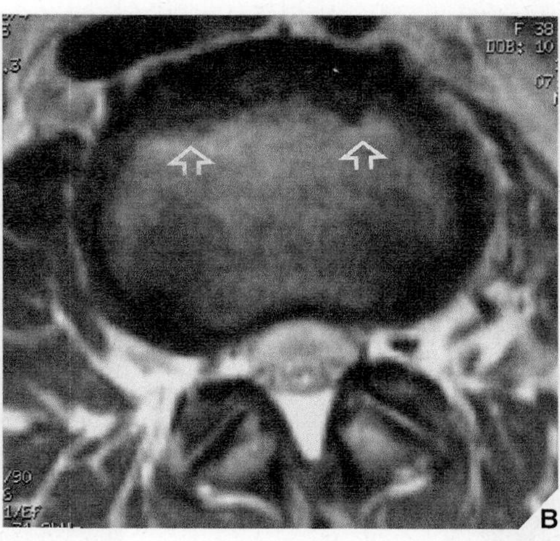

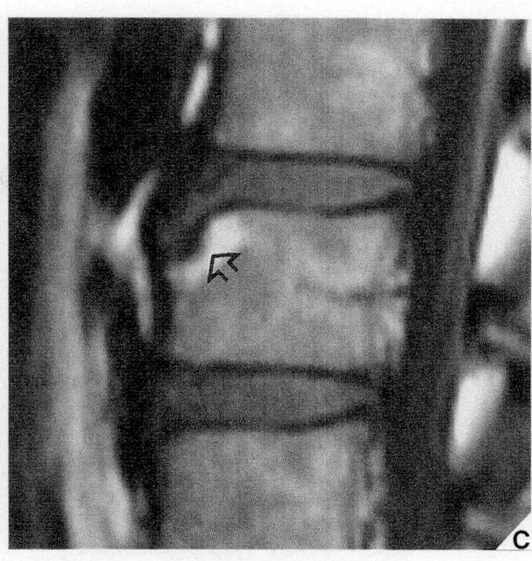

FIGURE 11.93 MRI of anterior intravertebral disk herniation (limbus vertebra). A 39-year-old woman presented with radicular pain after lifting a heavy object. **(A)** Lateral radiograph of the lumbar spine shows a typical appearance of limbus vertebra. **(B)** Axial and **(C)** sagittal MR images demonstrate anterior intravertebral disk herniation *(open arrows)*, but there is no evidence of posterior disk herniation.

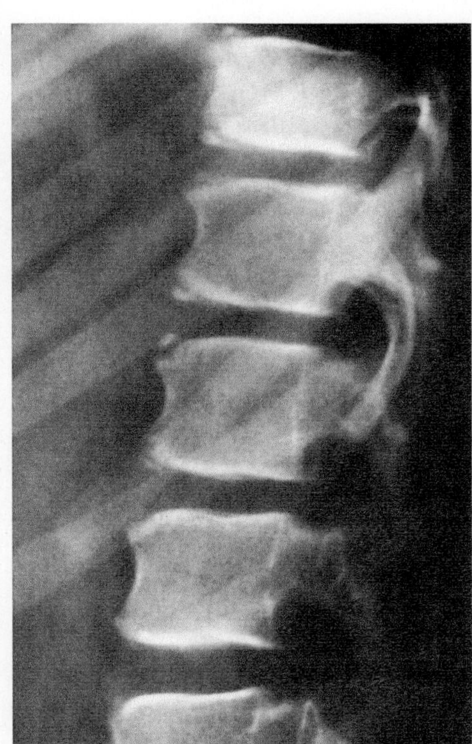

FIGURE 11.94 Secondary ossification centers. The secondary ossification centers of the vertebral ring apophysis in the growing skeleton, as seen here in a 5-year-old girl, should not be mistaken for limbus vertebrae.

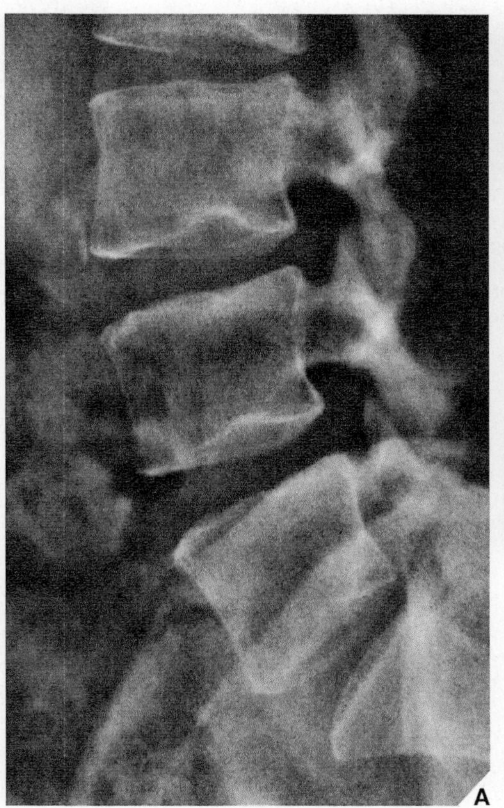

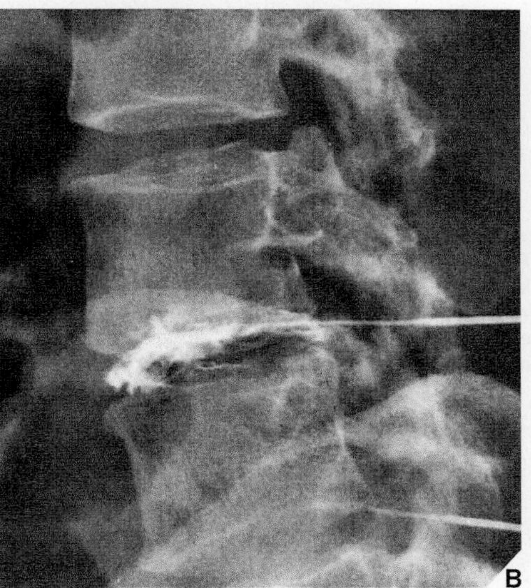

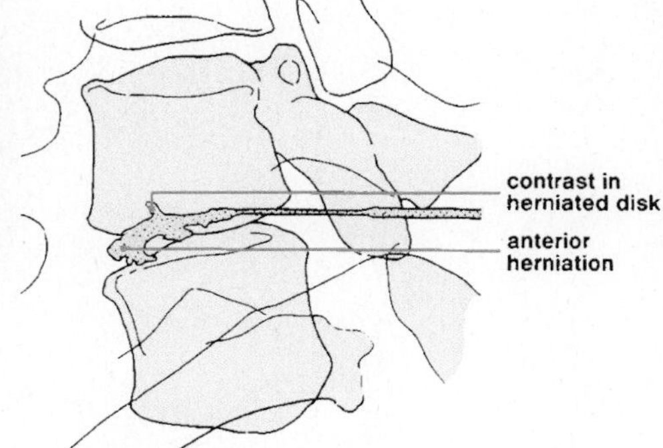

FIGURE 11.95 Schmorl nodes. **(A)** Lateral radiograph of the lumbar spine in an asymptomatic 77-year-old woman with osteoporosis of the spine shows multiple indentations particularly of the inferior end plates, representing the Schmorl nodes, secondary to intravertebral disk herniation caused by weakening of the vertebral end plates. **(B)** In another patient, a small Schmorl node is demonstrated on diskography by opacification of extruded disk material in the body of L4. Some anterior herniation is also evident.

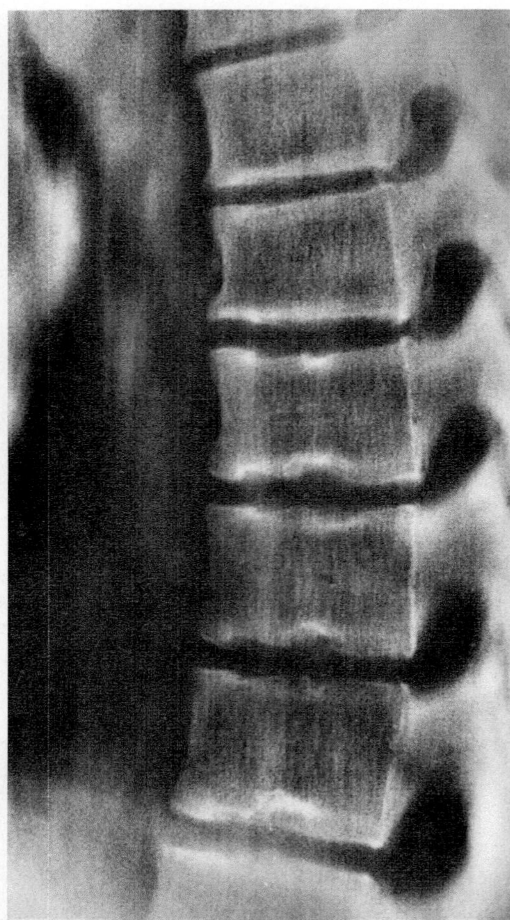

FIGURE 11.96 Scheuermann disease. Lateral tomogram of the thoracic spine in a 23-year-old man demonstrates several Schmorl nodes in T5-8 and slight anterior wedging of the vertebral bodies. Note the wavy outline of the superior and inferior end plates and the mild kyphotic curve of the thoracic spine in this patient, an abnormality also called *juvenile thoracic kyphosis*.

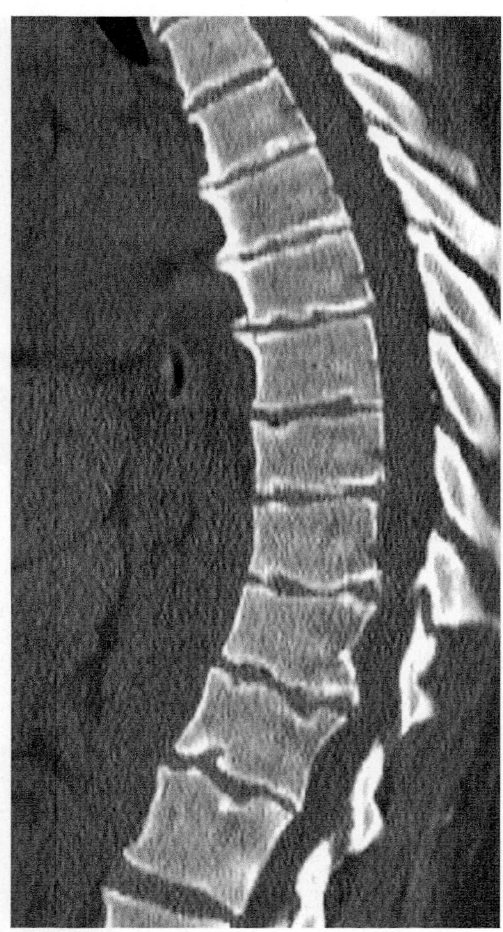

FIGURE 11.97 CT of Scheuermann disease. Sagittal reformatted CT image of the thoracic spine shows lower thoracic kyphosis and classic appearance of type I Scheuermann disease in 24-year-old man.

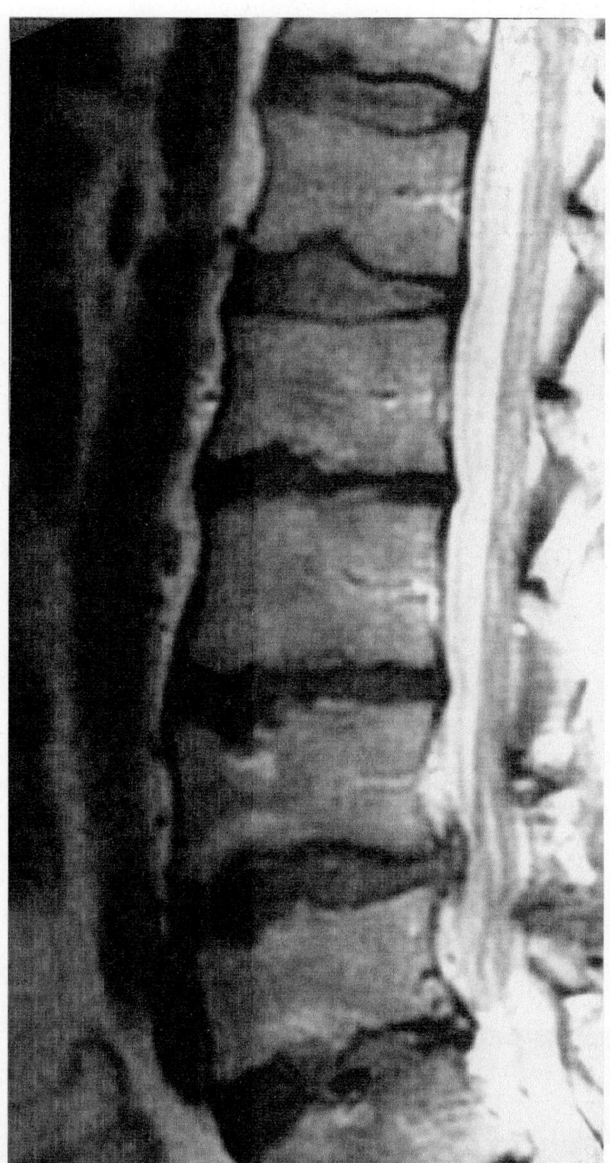

FIGURE 11.98 **MRI of Scheuermann disease.** A 28-year-old man presented with low back pain lasting several months. Sagittal MRI of the lumbar spine demonstrates characteristic features of Scheuermann disease, type II. Note prominent Schmorl nodes involving all five vertebral bodies, decreased height of the vertebral bodies, and narrowing of the intervertebral disk spaces.

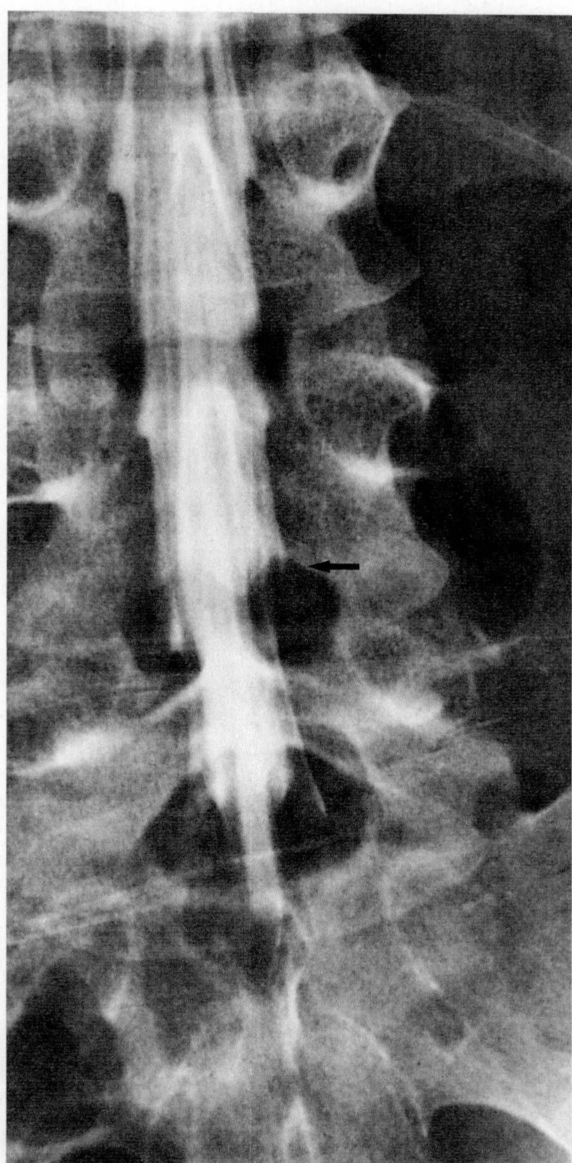

FIGURE 11.99 **Lateral disk herniation.** In lifting a heavy object, a 27-year-old man felt sudden, sharp pain in the lower back radiating to the left lower extremity. The standard radiographs of the lumbosacral spine were normal. Anteroposterior view of a myelogram demonstrates a subtle lack of filling of the left L5 nerve sheath *(arrow)*, which at surgery was found to be compressed by a lateral herniation of the L4-5 disk.

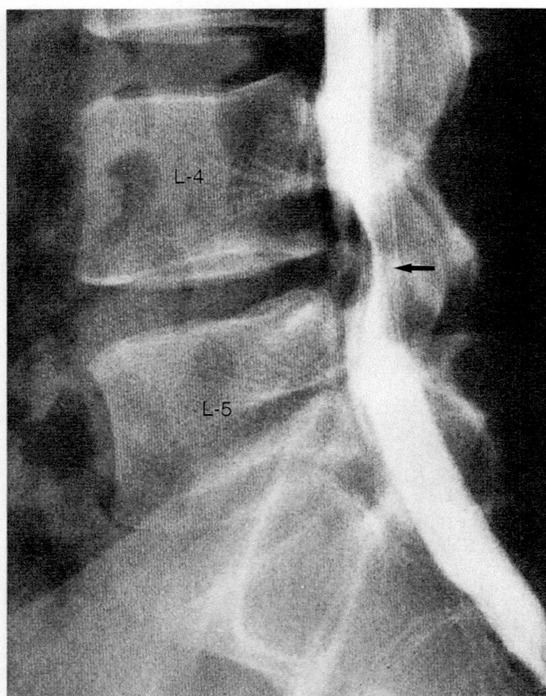

FIGURE 11.100 Myelography of herniated disk. Lateral spot film obtained during myelography in a 38-year-old man demonstrates a large posterior herniation of the intervertebral disk at L4-5 *(arrow)*. Note also narrowing of the intervertebral disk space L4-5.

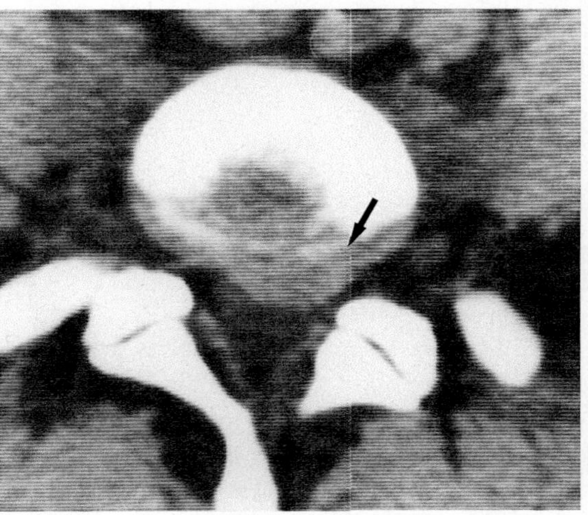

FIGURE 11.101 CT of herniated disk. Axial CT section of the lumbar spine at the L5-S1 level demonstrates a large centrolateral disk herniation encroaching on the left intervertebral foramen *(arrow)*.

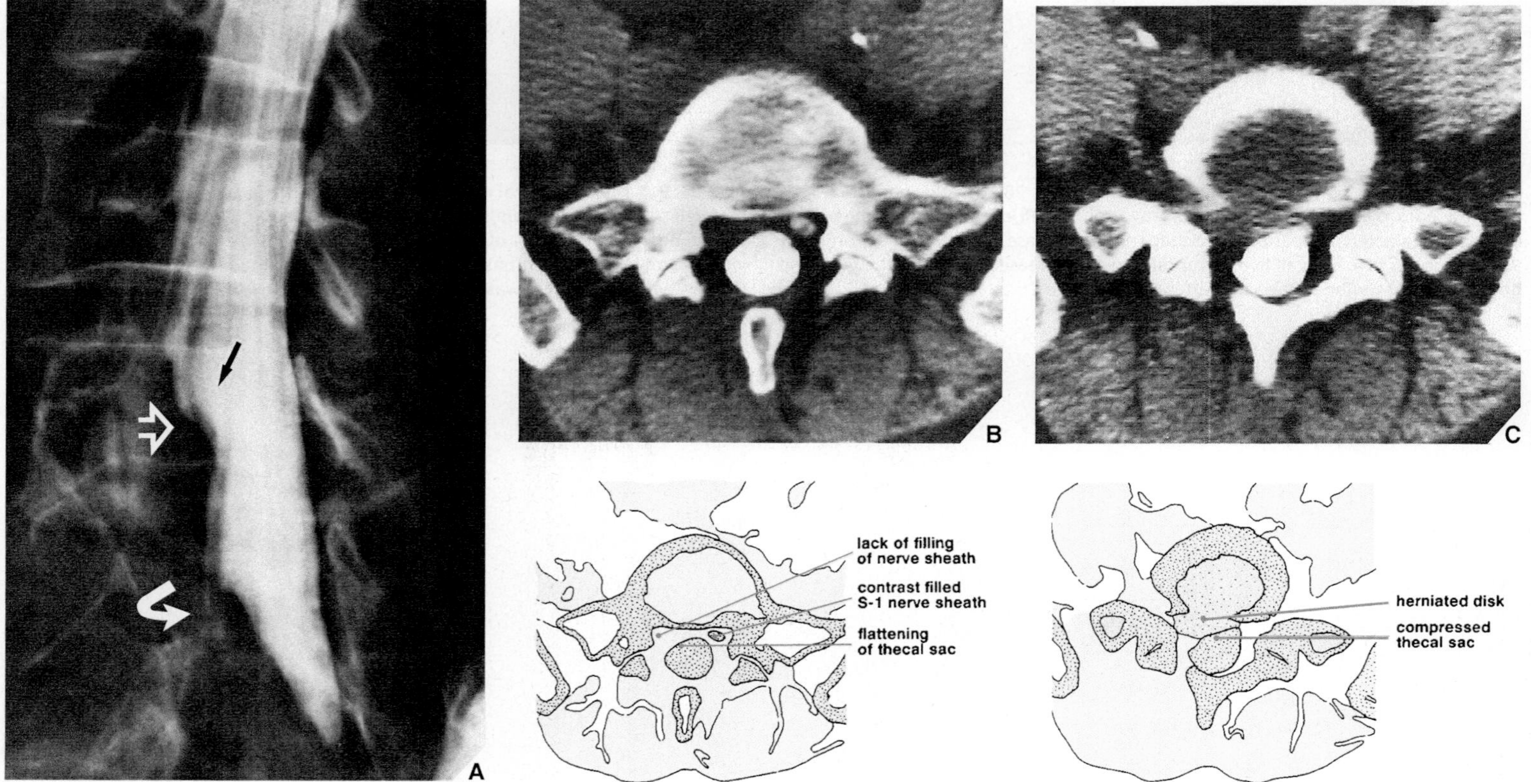

FIGURE 11.102 CT-myelography of herniated disk. A 47-year-old man presented with severe back pain radiating to the right buttock and leg. **(A)** Spot film in the oblique projection obtained during myelography shows an extradural defect on the right side of the thecal sac at the L5-S1 disk space *(arrow)* involving the right S1 nerve root, which is cut off *(open arrow)*. The S2 nerve root is normally outlined *(curved arrow)*. **(B,C)** CT sections also obtained during myelography demonstrate the lack of opacification of the S1 nerve root on the right side and a large herniation of the L5-S1 disk compressing the thecal sac from the right.

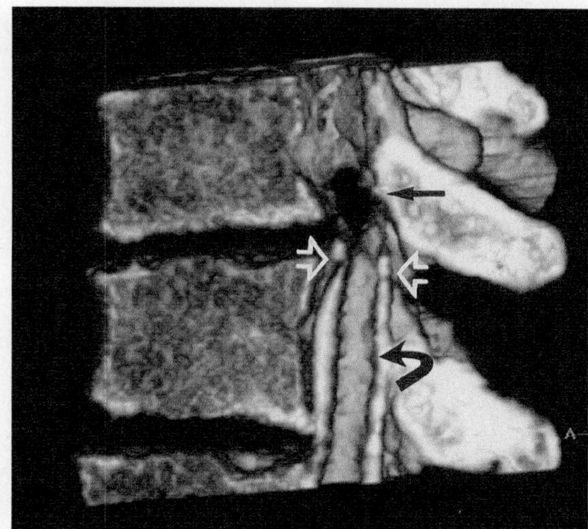

FIGURE 11.103 **3D CT-myelography of herniated disk.** A 3D CT reconstructed image in maximum intensity projection (MIP) of the lower thoracic spine was obtained after contrast agent was injected into the thecal sac (CT-myelography). There is disk herniation at the level of T7-8 *(arrow)* associated with complete obstruction of contrast flow *(open arrows)*. The *curved arrow* points to the spinal cord.

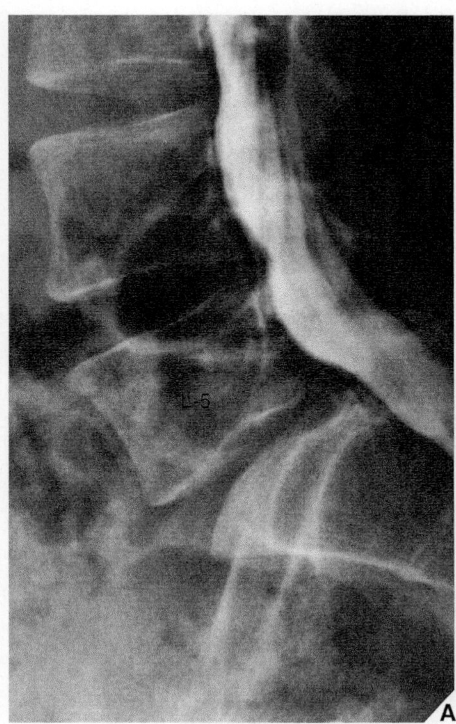

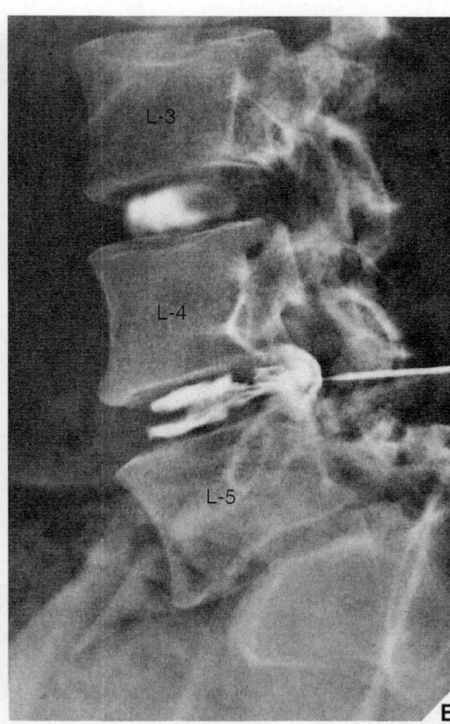

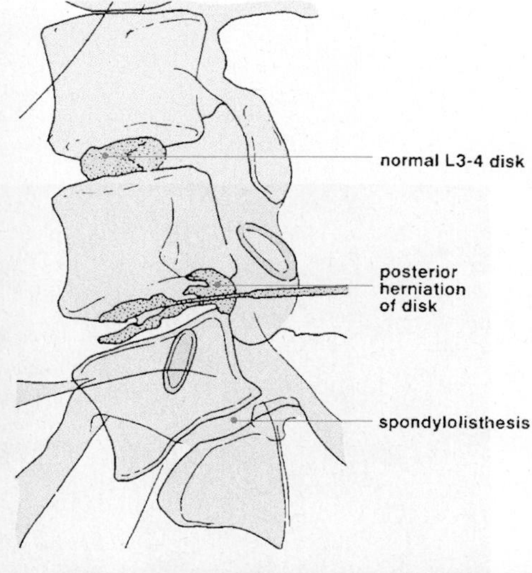

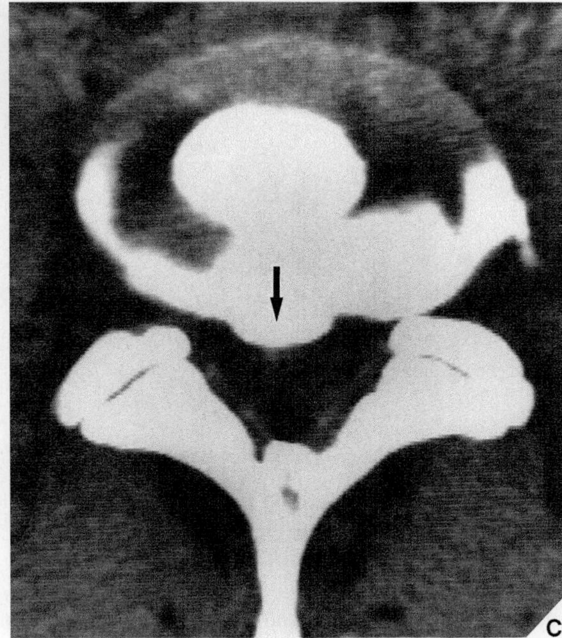

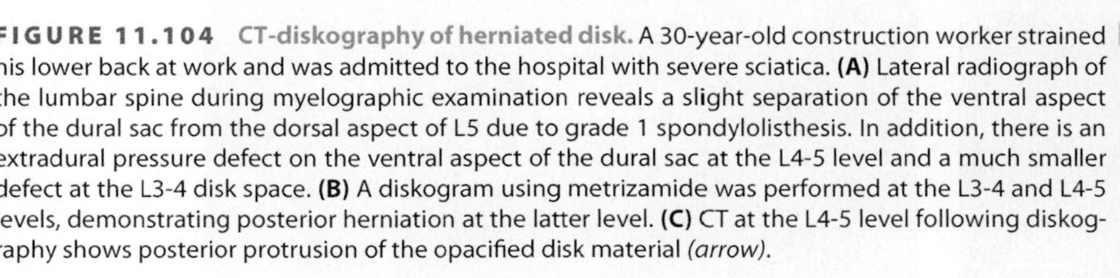

FIGURE 11.104 **CT-diskography of herniated disk.** A 30-year-old construction worker strained his lower back at work and was admitted to the hospital with severe sciatica. **(A)** Lateral radiograph of the lumbar spine during myelographic examination reveals a slight separation of the ventral aspect of the dural sac from the dorsal aspect of L5 due to grade 1 spondylolisthesis. In addition, there is an extradural pressure defect on the ventral aspect of the dural sac at the L4-5 level and a much smaller defect at the L3-4 disk space. **(B)** A diskogram using metrizamide was performed at the L3-4 and L4-5 levels, demonstrating posterior herniation at the latter level. **(C)** CT at the L4-5 level following diskography shows posterior protrusion of the opacified disk material *(arrow)*.

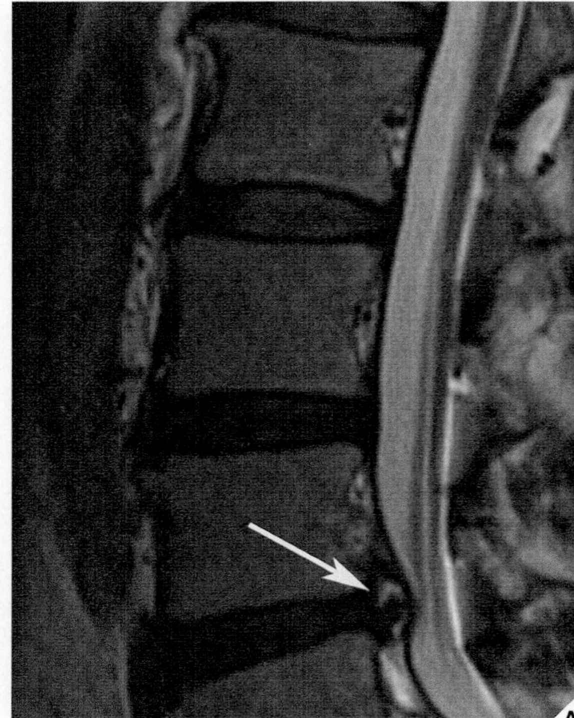

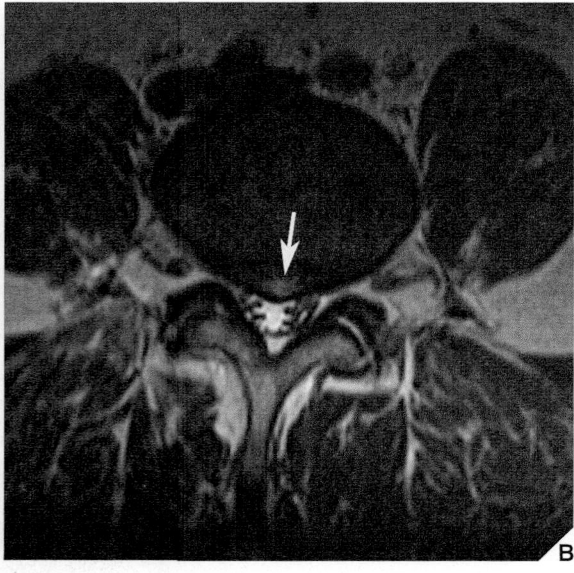

FIGURE 11.105 MRI of disk protrusion. A 59-year-old man presented with low back pain. **(A)** Sagittal T2-weighted MRI demonstrates a posterior herniation of the protrusion type of disk L4-5 *(arrow)*. Note the subligamentous position of the herniated disk. **(B)** Axial T2-weighted MRI shows posterior disk protrusion with marked compression of the thecal sac *(arrow)*.

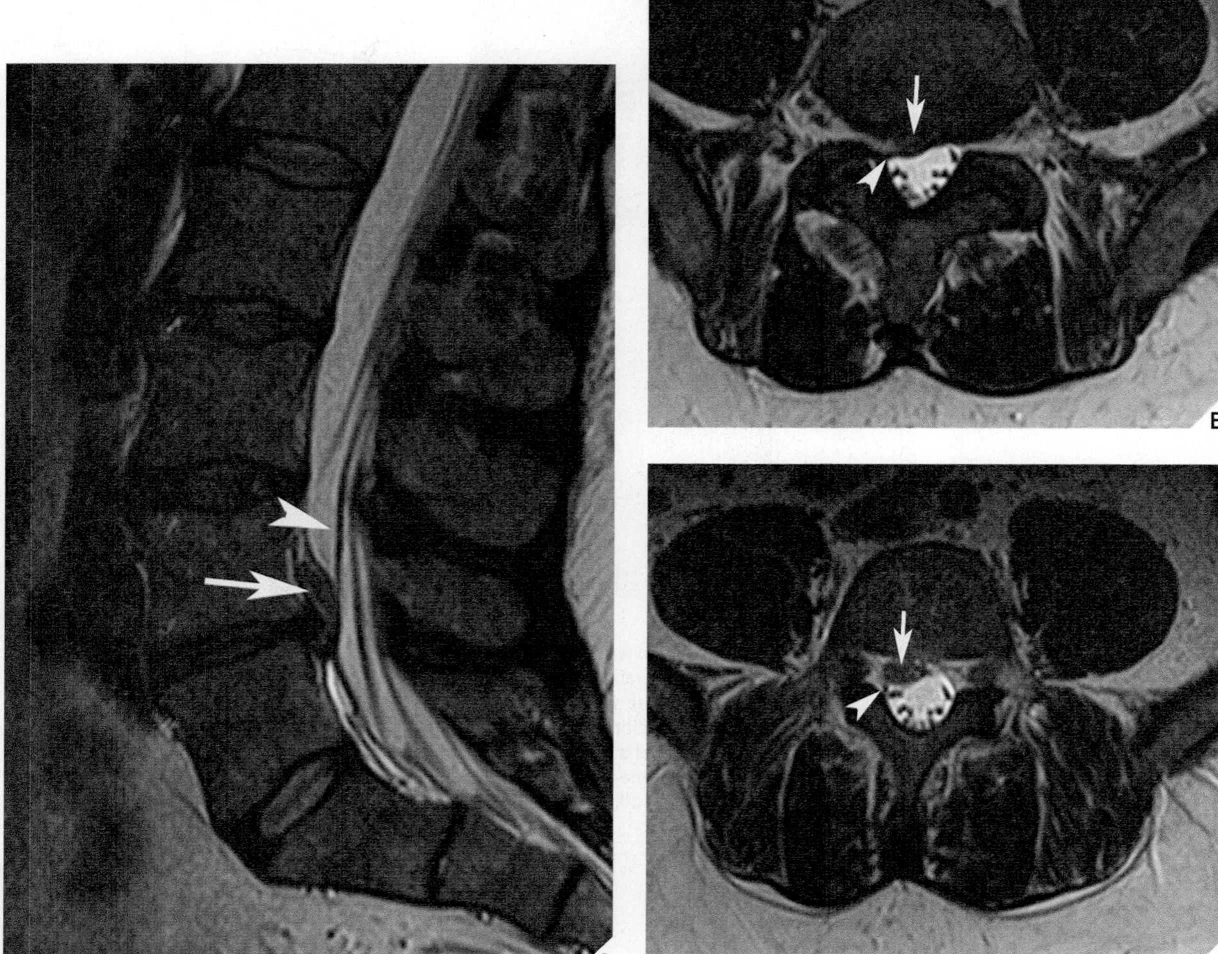

FIGURE 11.106 MRI of disk extrusion. A 46-year-old man presented with right radiculopathy. **(A)** Sagittal T2-weighted MRI demonstrates a central and right paracentral disk herniation of the extrusion type at the L4-5 level, extending cephalad *(arrow)*, with impingement of the right L5 nerve root *(arrowhead)*. **(B)** Axial T2-weighted MRI at the level of the L4-5 disk space demonstrates the extruded disk material *(arrow)* and the posterior displacement of the L5 nerve root *(arrowhead)*. **(C)** Axial T2-weighted MRI above the disk space L4-5 at the level of the L4 vertebra demonstrates the superiorly displaced disk material *(arrow)*, compressing the ventral aspect of the thecal sac and impinging on the L4 nerve root *(arrowhead)*.

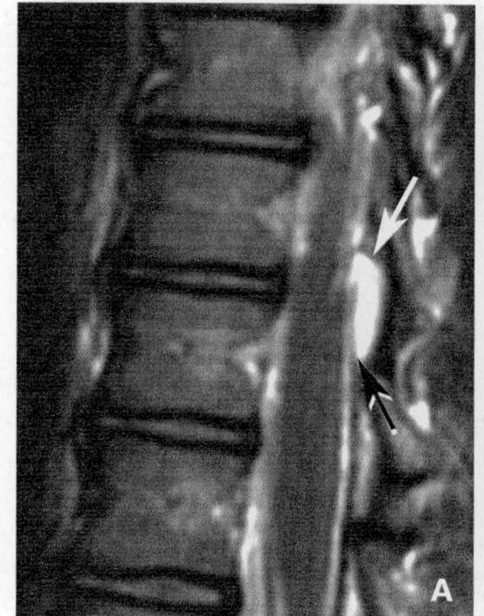
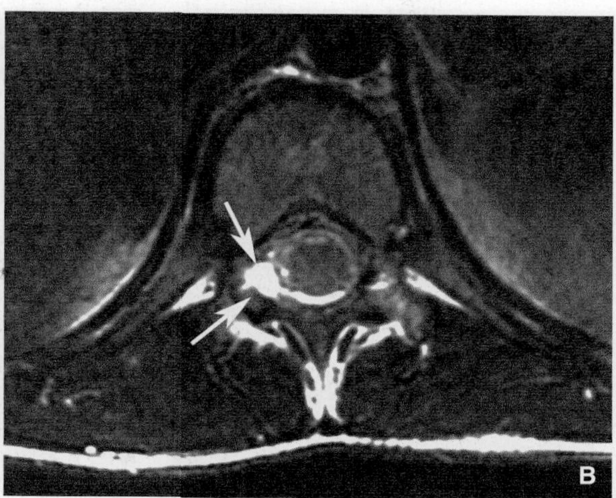

FIGURE 11.107 MRI of sequestered cystic disk herniation. **(A)** Right parasagittal T2-weighted MR image and **(B)** axial T2-weighted MR image of the lumbar spine of a young woman, who presented with acute right radicular pain, show a cystic structure in the right posterior epidural space *(arrows)* representing a cystic, sequestered acute disk herniation. (Courtesy of Evan Stein, MD, Brooklyn, New York.)

roots, which may simulate a herniated nucleus pulposus on CT studies, can be visualized directly with MRI. It has to be stressed, however, that evaluating patients with radiculopathy and herniated disk is an area in which both MRI and CT can be complementary. When an extradural defect is identified with MRI, it may be difficult to ascertain whether the lesion represents a herniated nucleus pulposus or an osteophyte; in these situations, CT can make the distinction easily by identifying the increased mineralization within the osteophyte. When the herniated fragment is clearly in continuity with the intervertebral disk and is of the same signal intensity, the diagnosis is suggested by MRI alone.

Rare manifestations of disk herniations include unusual locations such as epidural, intradural, and extreme lateral. Occasionally, disk herniations may present such atypical imaging features as diskal cyst (Fig. 11.107), or calcified disk, better identified with CT.

Annular Tears

Tears or fissures of the annulus fibrosus of lumbar intervertebral disks may occur secondary to trauma and may also be caused by degenerative changes of the disk related to normal aging. According to Munter and associates, these tears represent separations between annular fibers, separations of annular fibers from their vertebral insertions, or breaks through these fibers in any orientation, involving one or more layers of the annular lamellae. Annular tears are found in both symptomatic and asymptomatic individuals. In a cadaver study, Yu and colleagues identified three types of annular tears. Type I is a concentric tear that is characterized by rupture of the transverse fibers connecting adjacent lamellae in the annulus, without disruption of the longitudinal fibers. Type II is a radial tear that represents fissures extending from the periphery of the annulus to the nucleus pulposus associated with disruption of the longitudinal fibers. Type III is a transverse tear caused by the disruption of Sharpey fibers at the periphery of the annulus fibrosus. Type II and III tears can be seen on T2-weighted MRI as hyperintense foci within the annulus. These tears can also be occasionally demonstrated by CT-diskography.

Orthopaedic Management

Lumbar spine surgery with instrumentation is done for multiple reasons, including among others stabilization of scoliosis and fractures, decompression of the spinal canal in patients with spinal canal stenosis, and treatment of disk herniations. Among the most frequent surgeries performed in the lumbar spine are partial laminectomy and discectomy for herniated disk (Figs. 11.108 and 11.109) and laminectomy followed by posterior fusion using transpedicular screws and rods for spinal canal stenosis and for stabilization of spondylolisthesis (Figs. 11.110 and 11.111).

It is beyond the scope of this book to discuss the multiple techniques and instrumentations that have been developed throughout the years.

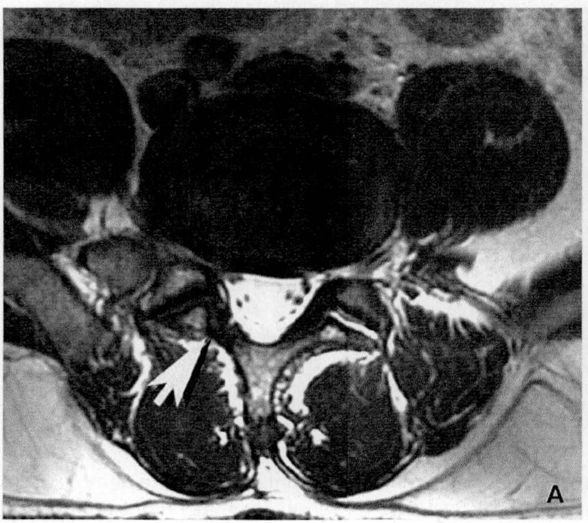
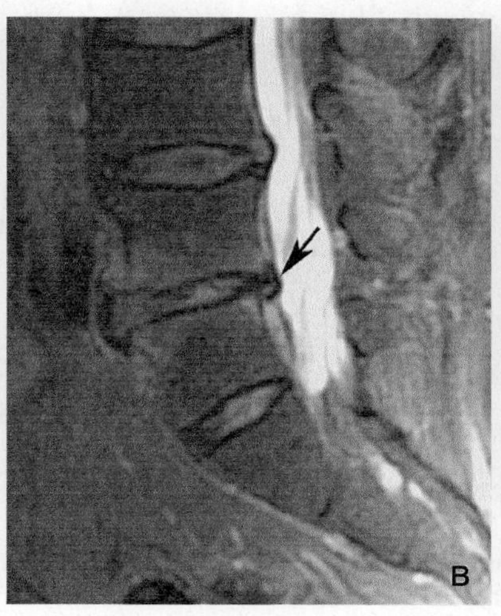
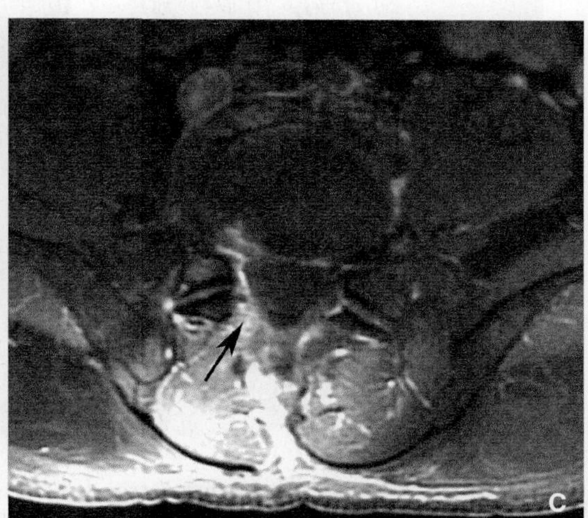

FIGURE 11.108 MRI of posthemilaminectomy and diskectomy with no recurrent disk herniation. Young adult patient presented with recurrent right radiculopathy, status post prior right L4 hemilaminectomy and diskectomy. **(A)** Axial T2-weighted MR image at the level of L4-5 shows no evidence of recurrent disk herniation. Note the right hemilaminectomy site *(arrow)*. **(B)** Right parasagittal T2-weighted MR image shows a possible small recurrent disk herniation at L4-5 *(arrow)*. **(C)** Axial T1-weighted fat saturated MR image obtained following intravenous administration of gadolinium confirms the absence of recurrent disk herniation. There is enhancing scar tissue in the right epidural space and in the area of the right hemilaminectomy *(arrow)*.

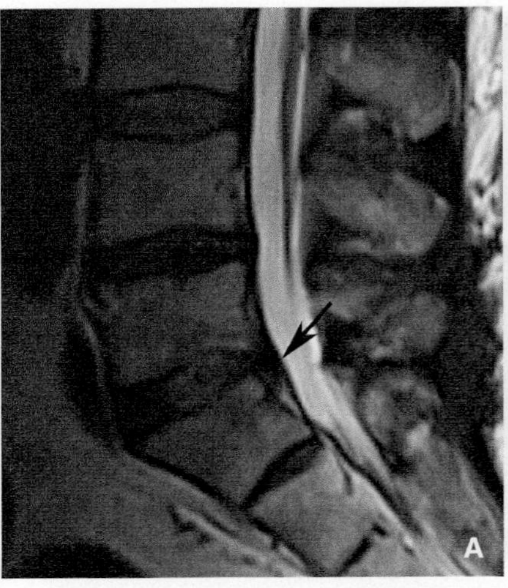

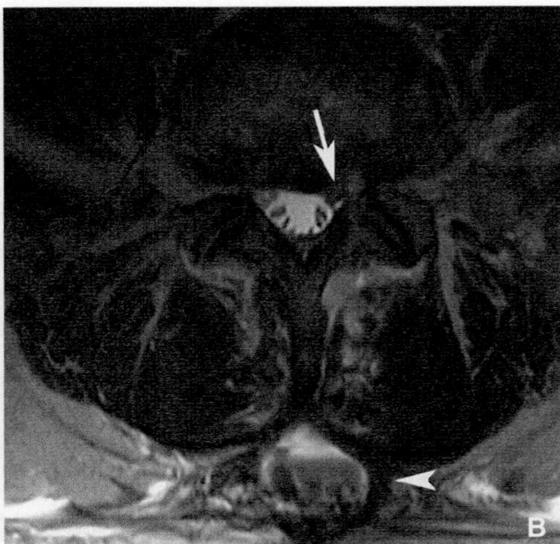

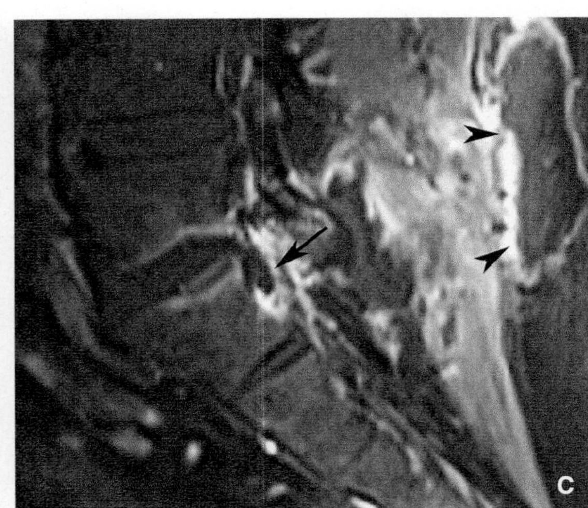

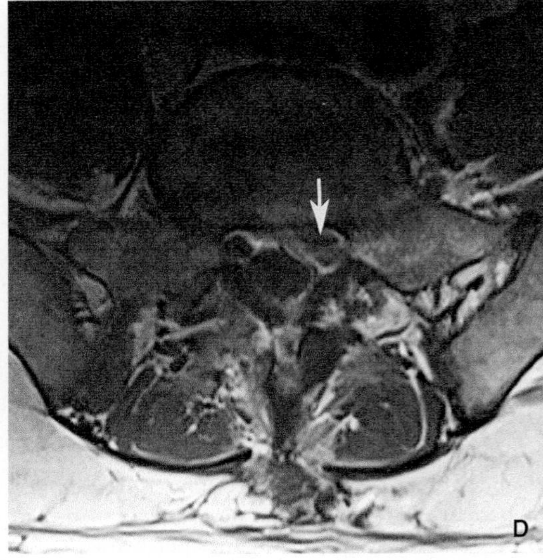

FIGURE 11.109 **MRI of recurrent disk herniation following diskectomy.** Young adult presented with recurrent left radiculopathy after L5-S1 hemilaminectomy and diskectomy. **(A)** Left parasagittal T2-weighted image and **(B)** axial T2-weighted image show a low–signal intensity lesion located in the left lateral recess and extending caudally *(arrows)*. This could represent a recurrent disk herniation or scar tissue. Note a posterior subcutaneous posthemilaminectomy hematoma *(arrowhead)*. **(C)** Left parasagittal and **(D)** axial T1-weighted fat-saturated MR images obtained following intravenous injection of gadolinium demonstrate nonenhancing hypointense lesion *(arrows)* surrounded by enhancing granulation tissue in the left lateral recess. Note the peripherally enhancing postsurgical hematoma in the posterior subcutaneous tissues (*arrowheads* in **C**). (Courtesy of Oleg Opsha, MS, Brooklyn, New York.)

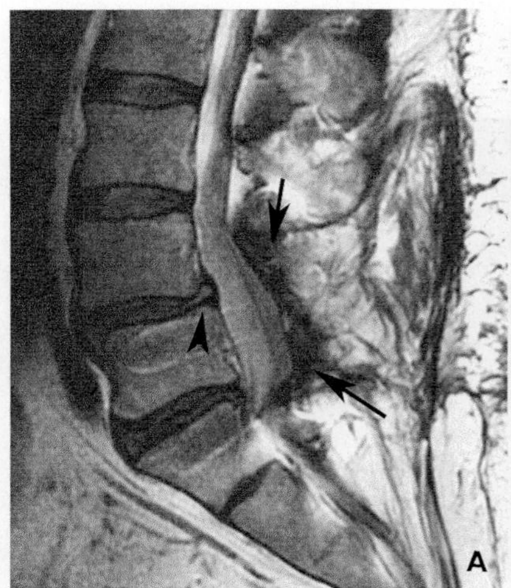

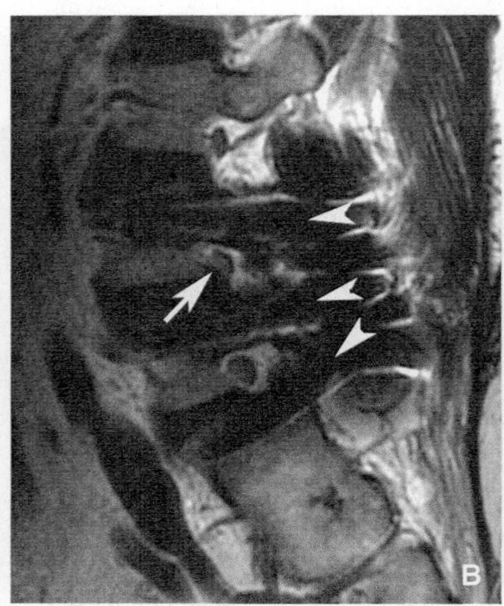

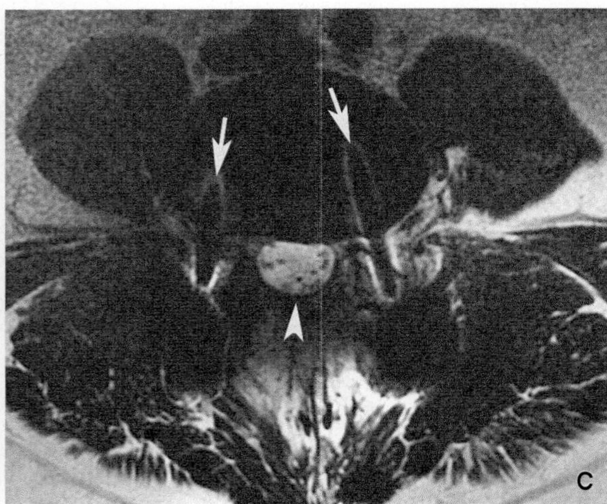

FIGURE 11.110 **MRI of postdecompressive laminectomy and posterior transpedicular screw fixation.** **(A)** Sagittal midline T2-weighted MR image demonstrates laminectomy at L4 and L5 *(arrows)*, with successful decompression of the spinal canal. Note the residual anterolisthesis of L4 on L5 *(arrowhead)*. **(B)** Right parasagittal T2-weighted MR image demonstrates the proper transpedicular position of the screws *(arrowheads)*. Note the residual impingement of the right exiting L4 nerve root *(arrow)*. **(C)** Axial T2-weighted MR image shows again the successful decompression of the spinal canal *(arrowhead)* and the proper position of the transpedicular screws *(arrows)*.

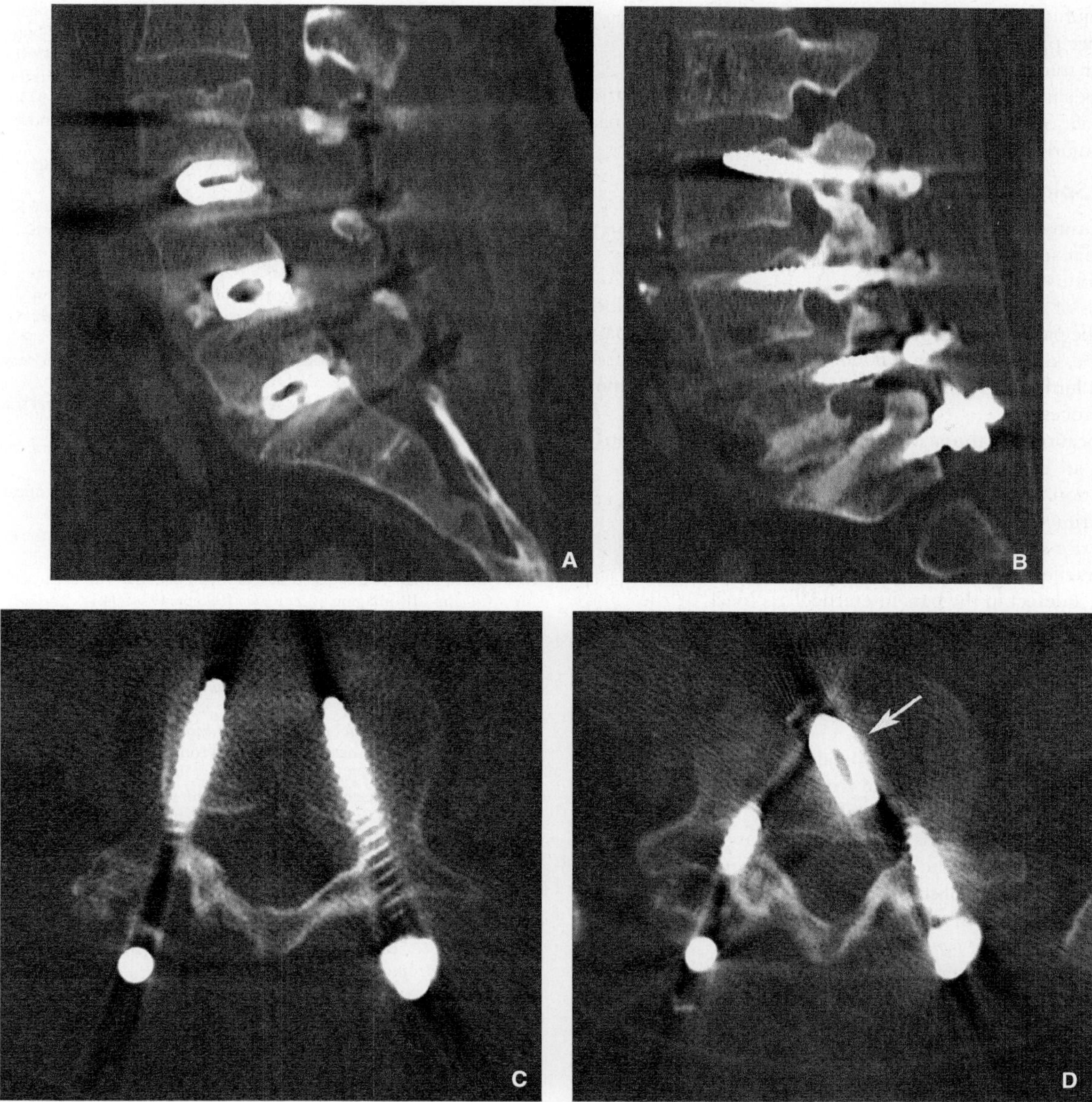

FIGURE 11.111 CT of posterior and anterior lumbar spine fusion. **(A)** Reformatted midline sagittal CT image demonstrates the properly placed interbody metallic spacers at L3-4, L4-5, and L5-S1. **(B)** Reformatted right parasagittal CT image demonstrates the proper position of the screws within the pedicles of L3, L4, L5, and S1. **(C)** Axial CT image through the L4 pedicles confirms the proper intrapedicular location of the screws. **(D)** Axial CT through the L4-5 disk space confirms the proper location of the metallic interbody spacer *(arrow)*.

PRACTICAL POINTS TO REMEMBER

Cervical Spine

1. The single most important projection in the radiographic examination of the cervical spine is the lateral view—either the erect or cross-table lateral.
2. In the evaluation of injury to the cervical spine, it is mandatory to visualize the C7 vertebra, the site of the most commonly missed fractures. If this cannot be accomplished on the lateral projection, the swimmer's view should be attempted.
3. CT examination and MRI are useful techniques for evaluating vertebral-column trauma and associated soft-tissue and spinal cord injuries.
4. Stability of a cervical spine fracture is the most important practical factor in the evaluation of injuries to this region.
5. Fractures of the occipital condyles are best demonstrated on CT with coronal reformation.
6. A classification system of three types of occipital condyle fractures devised by Anderson and Montesano is based on fracture morphology, pertinent anatomy, and biomechanics.
7. Occipitocervical dislocation is effectively demonstrated on the lateral radiographs supplemented with CT reformatted images.
8. Jefferson fracture—a symmetrical fracture of the anterior and posterior arches of C1—can be diagnosed on the anteroposterior open-mouth radiograph by the lateral displacement of the lateral masses.
9. In the evaluation of fractures of the odontoid process (dens), note that:
   - type I (an oblique fracture cephalad to the base) and type III (a fracture through the base extending into the body) are stable
   - type II (a transverse fracture through the base) is unstable.
10. Teardrop fracture, a flexion injury representing a variant of a burst fracture, is the most severe and unstable of cervical spine fractures; it is frequently associated with spinal cord damage.
11. Extension teardrop fracture, which usually occurs at the level of C2 or C3, is a stable injury without the potentially dangerous complications of the flexion teardrop fracture.
12. Clay shoveler's fracture, involving the spinous processes of C6 or C7, can be recognized on the anteroposterior projection of the cervical spine by the ghost sign produced by caudal displacement of the fractured spinous process.

13. In the radiographic evaluation of locked facets, a bow-tie or bat-wing appearance of the dislocated articular pillars on the lateral projection is characteristic.
14. MRI is the modality of choice to demonstrate extraosseous posttraumatic abnormalities such as ligamentous tears, epidural hematomas, cervical cord injuries, and similar conditions.

Thoracolumbar Spine

1. The three-column spine classification of acute injuries to the thoracic and lumbar segments is a practical approach to defining the stability of various fractures.
2. Subtle fractures of the thoracic vertebrae can be recognized by a localized bulge in the paraspinal line secondary to edema and hemorrhage.
3. Chance fracture, known also as a *seat-belt fracture*, is a horizontal fracture through a lumbar vertebral body with extension into the lamina and spinous process.
4. Fracture–dislocations of thoracic and lumbar spine, which are unstable injuries, are classified into four types:
   - flexion-rotation injury
   - posteroanterior shear injury
   - anteroposterior shear injury
   - flexion-distraction injury.
5. Spondylolysis, a defect in the pars interarticularis (neck of the "Scotty dog"), leads to ventral slipping of one vertebra on the vertebra beneath it—spondylolisthesis.
6. Spondylolisthesis:
   - may be associated with a defect in the pars interarticularis, so-called *true spondylolisthesis*
   - or exist without an isthmic defect, so-called *pseudospondylolisthesis* or *degenerative spondylolisthesis* (associated with degenerative changes in the intervertebral disk and apophyseal joints).
7. A simple test on the radiographs to distinguish between the two types of spondylolisthesis is the spinous-process sign.
8. A severe degree of spondylolisthesis at the L5-S1 level can be recognized on the anteroposterior radiograph by the phenomenon known as the *inverted Napoleon's hat sign*.
9. An intervertebral disk can herniate anteriorly or anterolaterally as well as posteriorly or posterolaterally. Intraosseous herniation into a vertebral body may occur caudad or ventrocaudad, cephalad, or ventrocephalad.
10. Intravertebral ventrocaudad or ventrocephalad herniation results in the separation of a small, triangular segment of a vertebra. This limbus vertebra should not be mistaken for a fracture.
11. Posterior disk herniation can be documented by:
    - CT
    - myelography
    - diskography
    - MRI
    - or a combination of these.
12. As a rule, diskography is performed if the results of CT, myelography, and MRI are equivocal.
13. Provocative diskography serves as an important diagnostic clue to the orthopaedic surgeon regarding the level of intervertebral disk to be operated on.

SUGGESTED READINGS

Anderson LD, D'Alonzo RT. Fractures of the odontoid process of the axis. *J Bone Joint Surg Am* 1974;56(8):1668–1674.

Anderson PA, Montesano PX. Morphology and treatment of occipital condyle fractures. *Spine (Phila Pa 1976)* 1988;13:731–736.

Anderson PA, Montesano PX. Treatment of sacral fractures and lumbosacral injuries. In: Chapman MW, ed. *Operative orthopaedics*, vol. 4, 2nd ed. Philadelphia: JB Lippincott; 1993:2699–2710.

Bertolotti M. Contributo alla conoscenza dei vizi differenziazione regionale del rachide con speciale riguardo all assimilazione sacrale della V. lombare. *Radiol Med* 1917;4:113–144.

Bierry G, Venkatasamy A, Kremer S, et al. Dual-energy CT in vertebral compression fractures: performance of visual and quantitative analysis for bone marrow edema demonstration with comparison to MRI. *Skeletal Radiol* 2014;43:485–492.

Brown RC, Evans ET. What causes the "eye in the Scotty dog" in the oblique projection of the lumbar spine? *Am J Roentgenol Radium Ther Nucl Med* 1973;118:435–437.

Bryk D, Rosenkranz W. True spondylolisthesis and pseudospondylolisthesis—the spinous process sign. *J Can Assoc Radiol* 1969;20:53–56.

Cancelmo JJ Jr. Clay shoveler's fracture. A helpful diagnostic sign. *Am J Roentgenol Radium Ther Nucl Med* 1972;115:540–543.

Chance GQ. Note on a type of flexion fracture of the spine. *Br J Radiol* 1948;21:452.

Daffner RH. Helical CT of the cervical spine for trauma patients: a time study. *AJR Am J Roentgenol* 2001;177:677–679.

Daffner RH. *Imaging of vertebral trauma*, 2nd ed. Philadelphia: Lippincott-Raven; 1996.

Daffner RH. Injuries of the thoracolumbar vertebral column. In: Dalinka MK, Kaye JJ, eds. *Radiology in emergency room medicine*. New York: Churchill Livingstone; 1984:317–341.

Daffner RH, Brown RR, Goldberg AL. A new classification for cervical vertebral injuries: influence of CT. *Skeletal Radiol* 2000;29:125–132.

Daffner RH, Deeb ZL, Rothfus WE. "Fingerprints" of vertebral trauma—a unifying concept based on mechanisms. *Skeletal Radiol* 1986;15:518–525.

Denis F. Spinal instability as defined by the three-column spine concept in acute spinal trauma. *Clin Orthop Relat Res* 1984;189:65–76.

Denis F. The three column spine and its significance in the classification of acute thoracolumbar spinal injuries. *Spine (Phila Pa 1976)* 1983;8:817–831.

Dietz GW, Christensen EE. Normal "Cupid's bow" contour of the lower lumbar vertebrae. *Radiology* 1976;121:577–579.

Dullerud R, Johansen JG. CT-diskography in patients with sciatica. Comparison with plain CT and MR imaging. *Acta Radiol* 1995;36:497–504.

Firooznia H, Benjamin V, Kricheff II, et al. CT of lumbar spine disk herniation: correlation with surgical findings. *AJR Am J Roentgenol* 1984;142:587–592.

Freyschmidt J, Brossmann J, Wiens J, et al. *Freyschmidt's "Koehler/Zimmer" borderlands of normal and early pathological findings in skeletal radiography*, 5th ed. Stuttgart, Germany: Thieme; 2003:671–730.

Fuchs AW. Cervical vertebrae (part I). *Radiogr Clin Photogr* 1940;16:2–17.

Gerlock AJ Jr, Mirfakhraee M. Computed tomography and hangman's fractures. *South Med J* 1983;76:727–728.

Greenspan A. CT-discography vs. MRI in intervertebral disk herniation. *Appl Radiol* 1993;22:34–40.

Greenspan A, Amparo EG, Gorczyca D, et al. Is there a role for diskography in the era of magnetic resonance imaging? Prospective correlation and quantitative analysis of computed tomography-diskography, magnetic resonance imaging, and surgical findings. *J Spinal Disord* 1992;5:26–31.

Greenspan A, Beltran J, Ledermann E. Radiologic imaging of the spine. In: Chapman MW, James MA, eds. *Chapman's comprehensive orthopaedic surgery*, 4th ed. New Delhi, India: Jaypee Brothers Medical; 2019.

Hayes CW, Conway WF, Walsh JW, et al. Seat belt injuries: radiologic findings and clinical correlation. *Radiographics* 1991;11:23–36.

Holdsworth F. Fractures, dislocations and fracture-dislocations of the spine. *J Bone Joint Surg Am* 1970;52(8):1534–1551.

Hyman RA, Gorey MT. Imaging strategies for MR of the spine. *Radiol Clin North Am* 1988;26:505–533.

Jancucska JB, Spivak JM, Bendo JA. A review of symptomatic lumbosacral transitional vertebrae: Bertolotti's syndrome. *Int J Spine Surg* 2015;9:42.

Jefferson G. Fractures of the atlas vertebra. Report of four cases, and a review of those previously recorded. *Br J Surg* 1920;7:407–422.

Kathol MH. Cervical spine trauma. What is new? *Radiol Clin North Am* 1997;35:507–532.

Leone A, Cianfoni A, Cerase A, et al. Lumbar spondylolysis: a review. *Skeletal Radiol* 2011;40:683–700.

Montesano PX, Benson DR. The thoracocolumbar spine. In: Rockwood CA, Green DP, Bucholz RW, eds. *Rockwood and Green's fractures in adults*, 3rd ed. Philadelphia: JB Lippincott; 1991:1359–1397.

Montesano PX, Benson DR. Thoracolumbar spine fractures. In: Chapman MW, ed. *Operative orthopaedics*, vol. 4, 2nd ed. Philadelphia: JB Lippincott; 1993:2665–2697.

Munter FM, Wasserman BA, Wu H-M, et al. Serial MR imaging of annular tears in lumbar intervertebral disks. *AJNR Am J Neuroradiol* 2002;23:1105–1109.

Myerding HW. Spondylolisthesis. *Surg Gynecol Obstet* 1932;34:371–377.

Ranawat CS, O'Leary P, Pellicci P, et al. Cervical spine fusion in rheumatoid arthritis. *J Bone Joint Surg Am* 1979;61:1003–1010.

Slone RM, MacMillan M, Montgomery WJ. Spinal fixation. Part 1. Principles, basic hardware, and fixation techniques for the cervical spine. *Radiographics* 1993;13:341–356.

Slone RM, MacMillan M, Montgomery WJ, et al. Spinal fixation. Part 2. Fixation techniques and hardware for the thoracic and lumbosacral spine. *Radiographics* 1993;13:521–543.

Traynelis VC, Marano GD, Dunker RO, et al. Traumatic atlanto-occipital dislocation. Case report. *J Neurosurg* 1986;65:863–870.

Wiltse LL. Spondylolisthesis: classification and etiology. In: *AAOS Symposium on the Spine. American Academy of Orthopedic Surgeons*. St. Louis, MO: Mosby; 1969:143–167.

Wood-Jones F. The ideal lesion produced by judicial hanging. *Lancet* 1913;1:53–55.

Yu S, Sether JA, Ho PS, et al. Tears of the annulus fibrosus: correlation between MR and pathologic findings in cadavers. *AJNR Am J Neuroradiol* 1988;9:367–370.

Zanca P, Lodmell EA. Fracture of spinous processes; a new sign for the recognition of fractures of cervical and upper dorsal spinous processes. *Radiology* 1951;56:427–429.

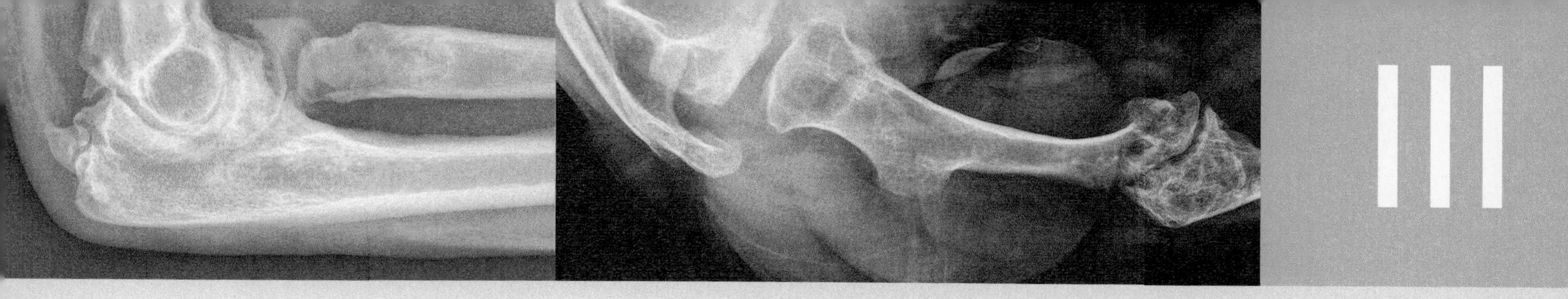

III

ARTHRITIDES

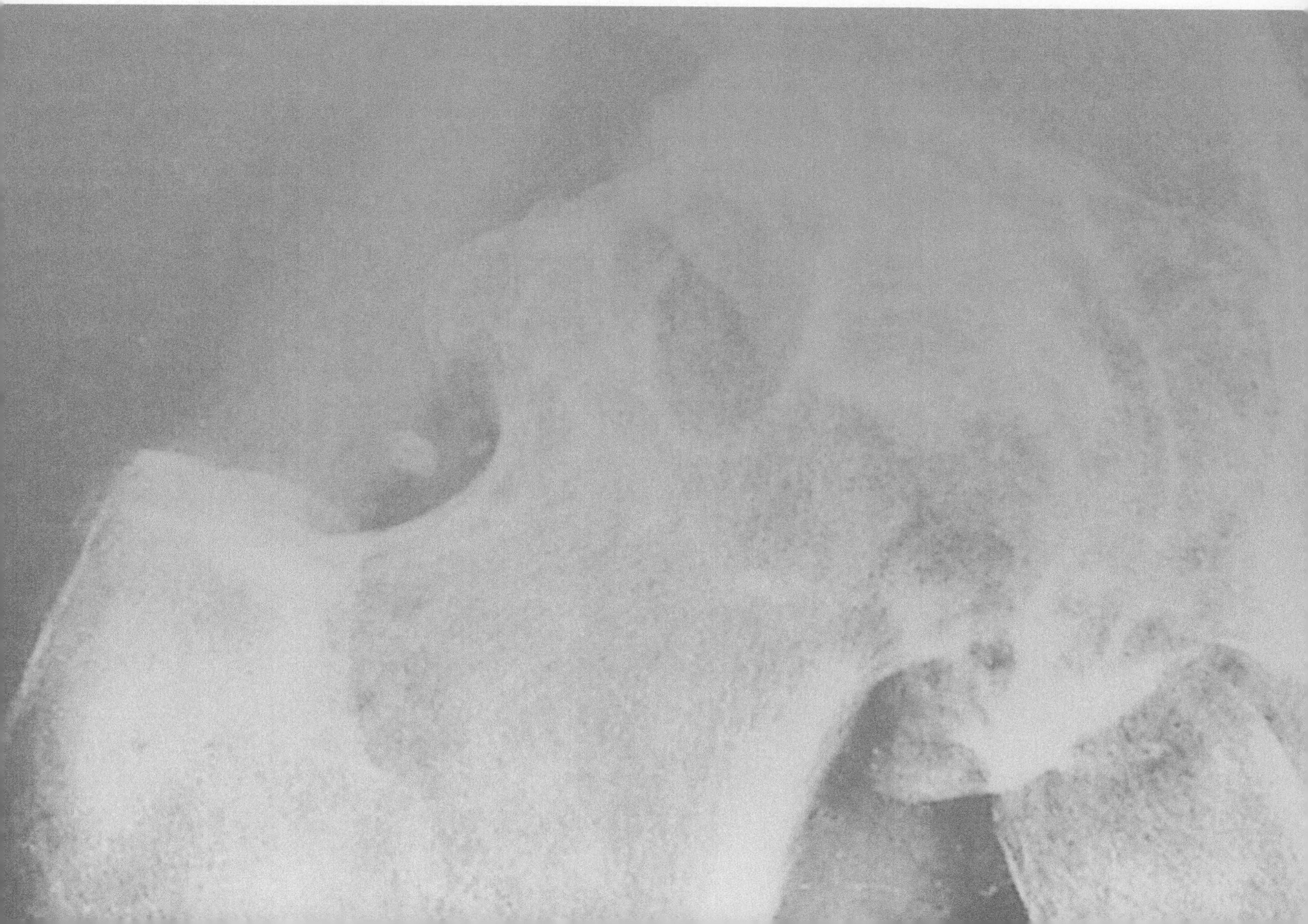

12

Clinical, Imaging, and Pathologic Evaluation of the Arthritides and Arthropathies

In its general meaning, the term *arthritis* indicates an abnormality of the joint as the result of a degenerative, inflammatory, or infectious process. Arthritis is distinguished from *arthralgia*, which implies aches and pains in the joint. In addition to arthritis and arthralgia, there is also a term known as *arthropathy*, a generic term applied to more than 100 different genetic, autoimmune, metabolic, connective tissue, and other acquired diseases that produce pathologic processes of the joint or joints (Fig. 12.1). Distinguishing these different processes is key to proper imaging and treatment and plays a major role in the critical element of patient's care.

Radiologic Imaging Modalities

Conventional Radiography

The radiologic modalities used to evaluate arthritis are very similar to those used in traumatic conditions involving the bones and joints (see Chapter 4), although there are some modifications. The most important modality for the evaluation of arthritis is conventional radiography. As in the radiographic examination of traumatic conditions, standard radiographs of the involved joint should be obtained in at least two projections at 90 degrees to each other (Fig. 12.2; see also Fig. 4.1). A weight-bearing view may be of value, particularly for a dynamic evaluation of any decrement in the joint space under the weight of the body (Fig. 12.3). Special projections may at times be required to demonstrate destructive changes in the joint to better advantages. The radial head–capitellum view (see Chapter 6), by eliminating overlap of the radial head and coronoid process and by more clearly demonstrating the humeroradial and humeroulnar joints, shows the inflammatory changes in the elbow joint to better advantage (Fig. 12.4). The semisupinated oblique view of the hand and wrist (the so-called *ball-catcher's view*), introduced by Norgaard in 1965, effectively demonstrates the radial aspects of the metacarpal heads and of the base of the proximal phalanges in the hand and the triquetrum and pisiform in the wrist (Fig. 12.5). Because the earliest erosive changes of some inflammatory arthritides begin in these areas, the Norgaard view may provide important information at the early stages of arthritides (Fig. 12.6). It may also demonstrate subtle subluxations in metacarpophalangeal joints frequently seen in systemic lupus erythematosus (SLE).

Magnification Radiography

This technique was used in the past to diagnose the very early articular changes of arthritis, which were not well appreciated on standard projections. The method involved a special screen-film system and geometric enlargement that yielded magnified images of the bones and joints with greater sharpness and bony detail. Magnification radiography is now completely replaced by digital radiography and cutting-edge technology of picture archiving and communication system (PACS) for radiology images, allowing filmless high-resolution image display format with advanced radiology reading workstations.

Tomography and Computed Tomography

Among the ancillary imaging techniques, conventional tomography was used in the past—its major purpose being demonstration to better advantage the degree of joint destruction. Currently, it has been replaced by computed tomography (CT), which is effective in evaluating degenerative and inflammatory changes of various joints (Fig. 12.7A–C) and in the spine to document spinal stenosis (Fig. 12.7D). In the assessment of spinal stenosis secondary to degenerative changes, CT examination may also be performed after myelography (Fig. 12.8), although myelography alone is often sufficient (Fig. 12.9). Recently, dual-energy CT gained a wide acceptance as a modality used for detection or exclusion of tophaceous gout (Figs. 12.10 and 12.11; see also Figs. 2.15, 15.37, and 15.38). In addition, in patients with known tophaceous gout, this technique may be used for serial volumetric quantification of subclinical tophus to evaluate response to treatment.

Scintigraphy

Radionuclide bone scan is much more commonly used than those other techniques, mainly for evaluating the distribution of arthritis in different joints (see Chapter 2). The radiopharmaceuticals currently in use in bone scan include organic diphosphonates—ethylene diphosphonate (EHDP) and methylene diphosphonate (MDP)—labeled with technetium-99m (^{99m}Tc), a gamma emitter with a 6-hour half-life; MDP is more commonly used, typically in a dose that provides 15 mCi (555 MBq) of ^{99m}Tc. After intravenous injection of the radiopharmaceutical, approximately 50% of the dose localizes in bone, with the remainder circulating freely in the

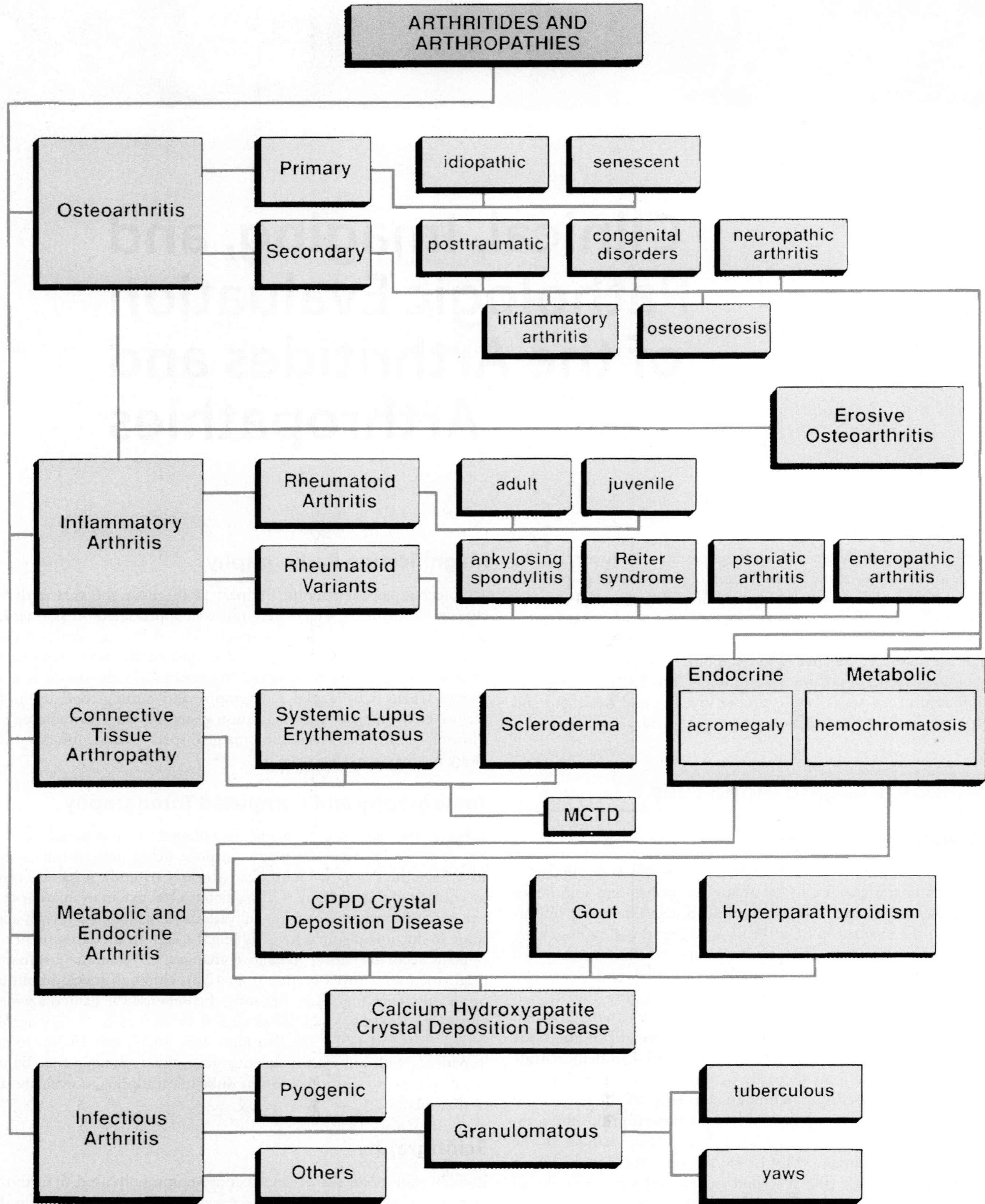

FIGURE 12.1 Classification of the arthritides. *MCTD*, mixed connective tissue disease; *CPPD*, calcium pyrophosphate dihydrate.

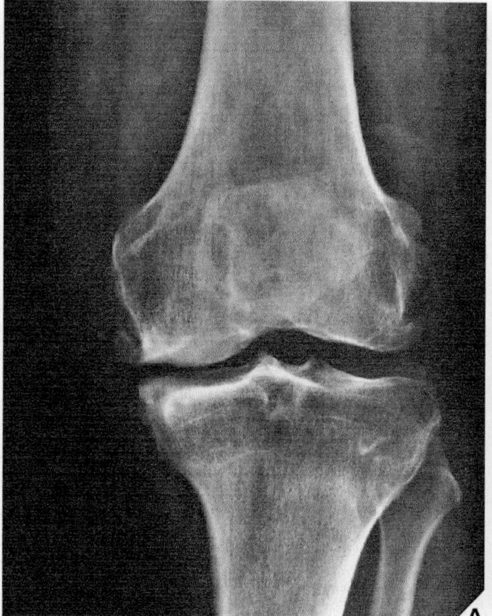

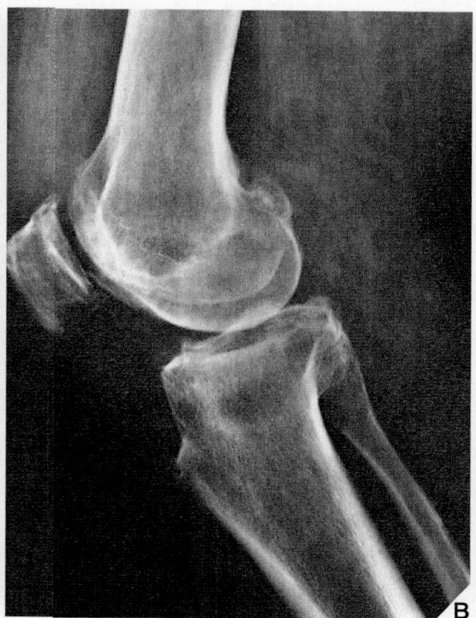

FIGURE 12.2 **Osteoarthritis.** A 58-year-old woman presented with a history of pain in the left knee. **(A)** Anteroposterior radiograph of the knee demonstrates narrowing of the medial femorotibial joint compartment and marginal osteophytes arising from both the medial and lateral femoral condyles—findings typical of OA (degenerative joint disease). **(B)** Lateral radiograph demonstrates, in addition, osteophytes at the anterior and posterior aspects of the articular end of the tibia, which are not appreciated on the anteroposterior projection. Involvement of the femoropatellar joint compartment and the presence of synovitis, represented by suprapatellar joint effusion, are also well demonstrated.

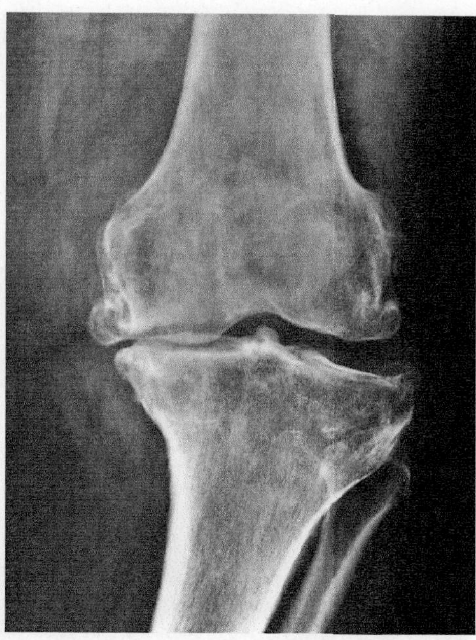

FIGURE 12.3 **Osteoarthritis.** Weight-bearing anteroposterior radiograph of the left knee of the same patient shown in Figure 12.2 demonstrates collapse of the medial femorotibial compartment under the weight of the body, with a resulting varus configuration of the knee.

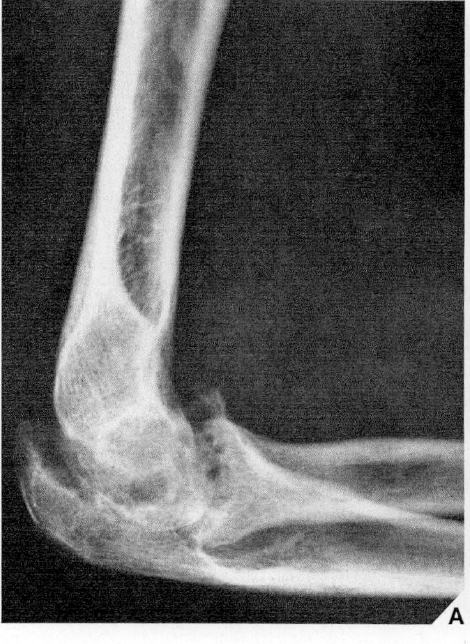

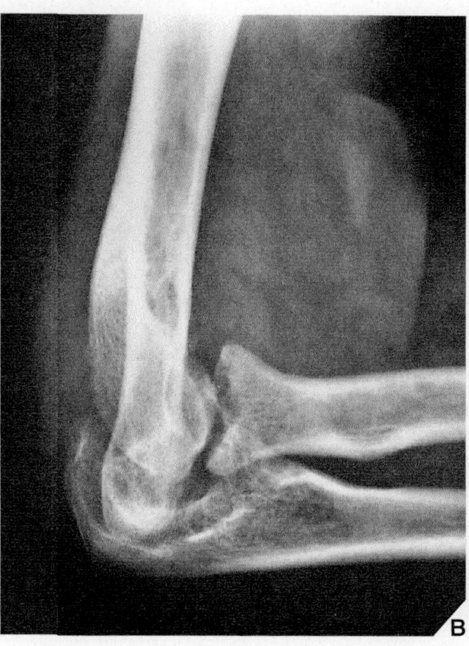

FIGURE 12.4 **Rheumatoid arthritis.** **(A)** Standard lateral radiograph of the elbow of a 48-year-old woman with known RA of several years' duration shows destructive changes typical of inflammatory arthritis. **(B)** A special projection known as the *radial head–capitellum view* (see also Fig. 6.14) demonstrates to better advantage the details of the arthritic process involving the humeroradial and humeroulnar joints. (Reprinted from Greenspan A, Norman A. Radial head-capitellum view in elbow trauma [Letter]. *Am J Roentgenol* 1983;140:1273–1275. Copyright © 1983 American Roentgen Ray Society.)

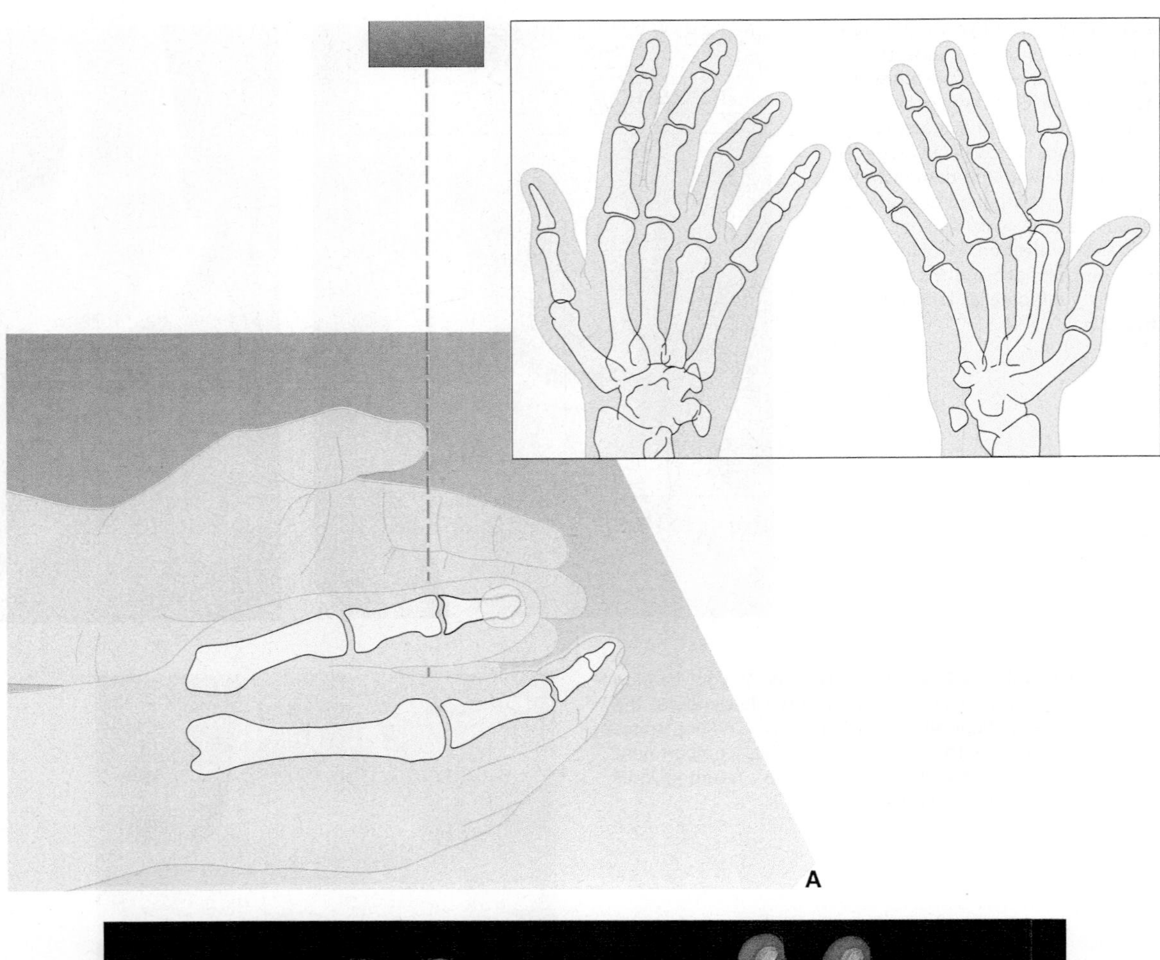

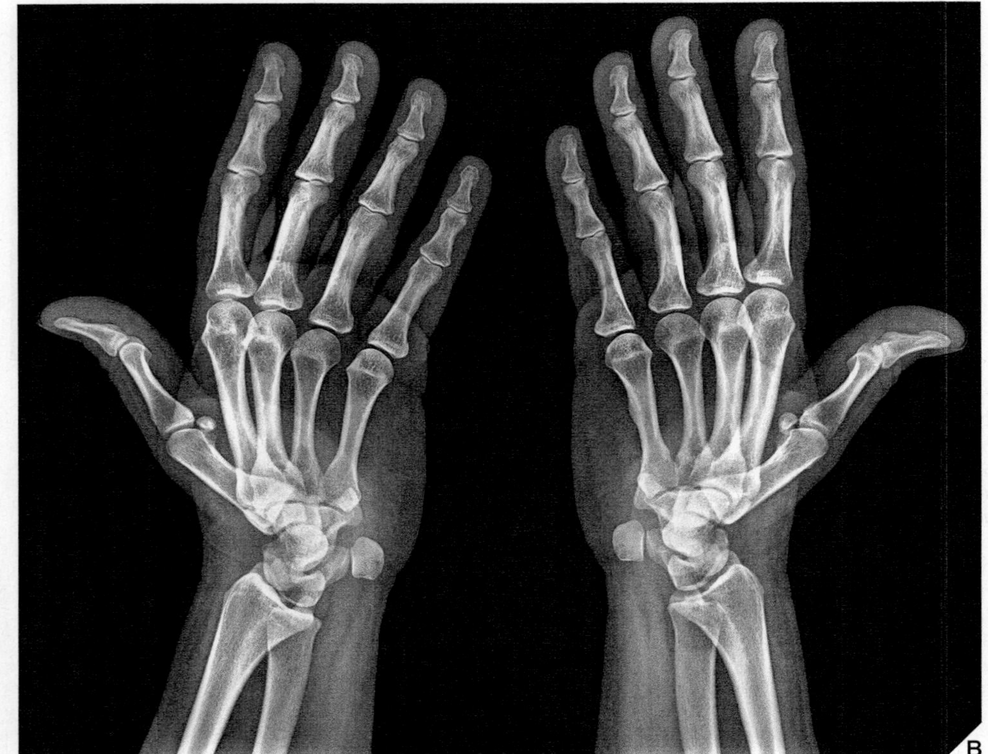

FIGURE 12.5 Ball-catcher's view. **(A)** For the Norgaard view of the hands and wrists, the patient's arm is fully extended and resting on its ulnar side. Fingers are extended. The hands are in slight pronation, as when catching a ball. The central beam is directed toward the metacarpal heads. **(B)** On the radiograph in this projection, the radial aspects of the base of the proximal phalanges, the triquetrum, and pisiform bones as well as triquetropisiform joint are well demonstrated.

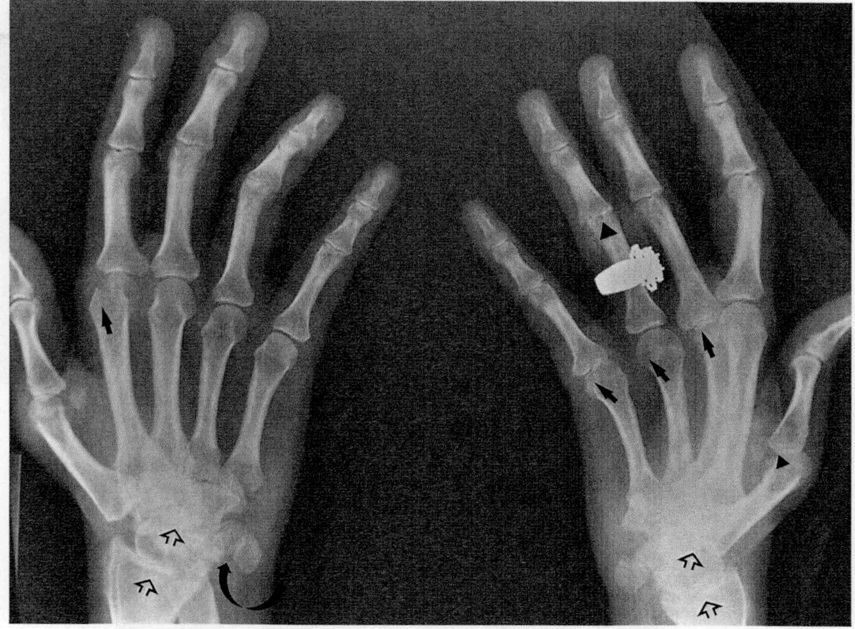

FIGURE 12.6 Rheumatoid arthritis. The Norgaard view of the hands and the wrists of this 62-year-old woman with RA demonstrates erosions in the radiocarpal and intercarpal articulations as well as the carpometacarpal joint, bilaterally *(open arrows)*. Note, in addition, subtle erosions of the head of the first, third, fourth, and fifth metacarpals of the left hand and of the head of the second metacarpal of the right hand *(arrows)*. A small erosion at the base of the middle phalanx of the ring finger of the left hand *(arrowheads)* and the erosion in the right triquetropisiform joint *(curved arrow)* are also well seen.

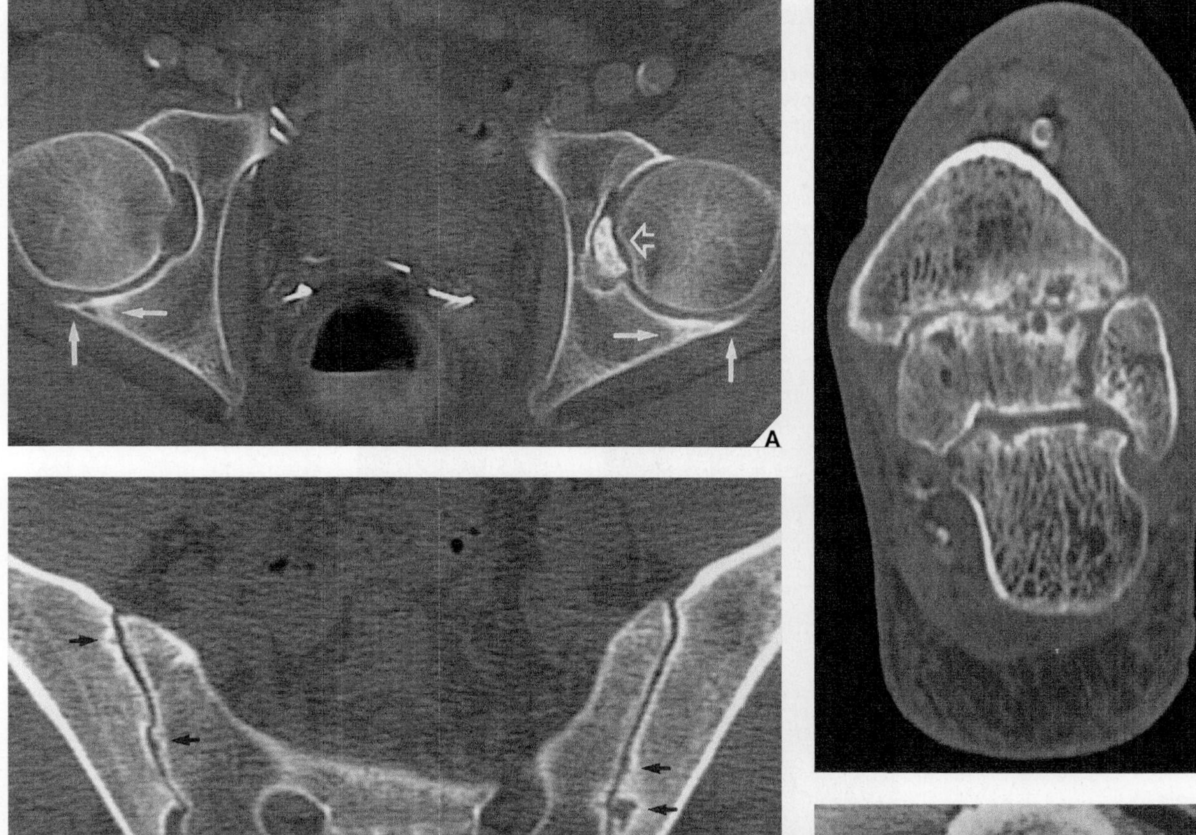

FIGURE 12.7 Evaluation of arthritides with CT. **(A)** Axial CT section through the hip joints of a 55-year-old man with hip OA shows narrowing of the joint spaces, subchondral sclerosis, and osteophytes *(arrows)*. The intraarticular osteochondral body *(open arrow)* was not clearly demonstrated on conventional radiographs. **(B)** Axial CT section through the sacroiliac joints of a 49-year-old man with psoriatic arthritis shows diffuse narrowing of the joints and articular erosions *(arrows)*. **(C)** Coronal CT section through the ankle and foot of a 52-year-old woman with RA shows erosions of the tibiotalar and subtalar joints. **(D)** CT scan of the lumbar spine in a 66-year-old patient with advanced OA of the facet joints shows marked narrowing of the spinal canal secondary to degenerative changes. At 8 mm, the transverse diameter is well below normal.

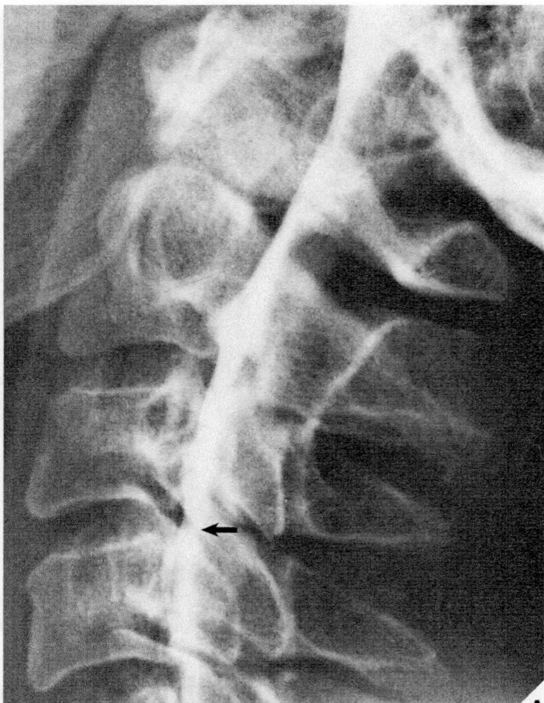

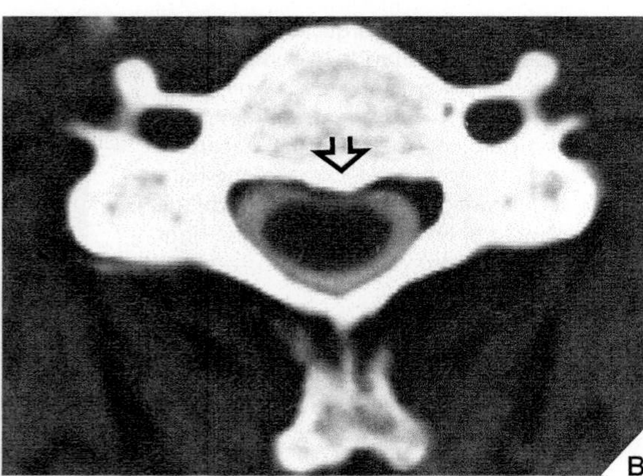

FIGURE 12.8 **CT myelography of impingement of the thecal sac.** A 56-year-old man reported constant pain in the neck radiating to the left arm; there was also associated weakness and numbness in the left hand. **(A)** Cervical myelogram in the lateral projection shows a small extradural defect on the ventral aspect of the thecal sac at C3-4 *(arrow)*. **(B)** CT section obtained after myelography shows impingement of a posterior osteophyte on the thecal sac at the corresponding level *(open arrow)*.

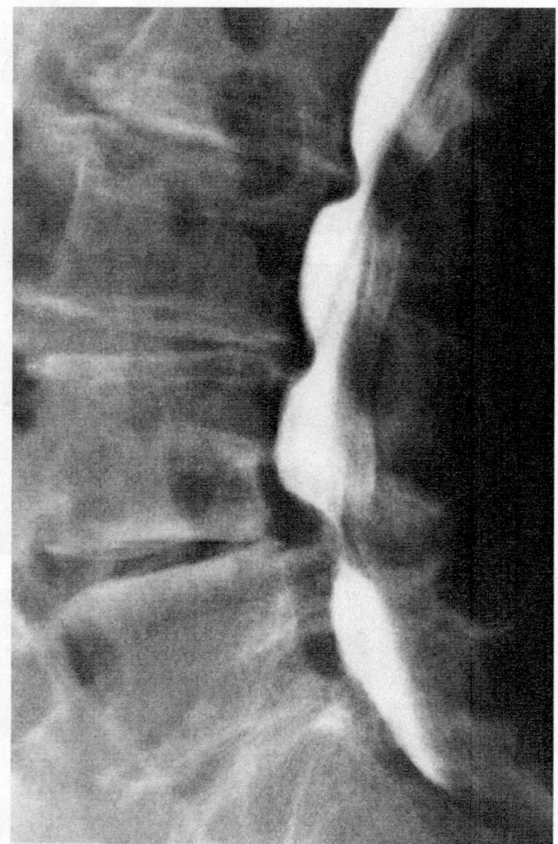

FIGURE 12.9 **Myelography of spinal stenosis.** Lateral radiograph of the lumbosacral spine obtained after injection of metrizamide into the subarachnoid space shows an "hourglass" configuration of the contrast agent in the thecal sac, a feature characteristic of spinal stenosis. This appearance results from concomitant hypertrophy of the facet joints and posterior bulging of the intervertebral disks.

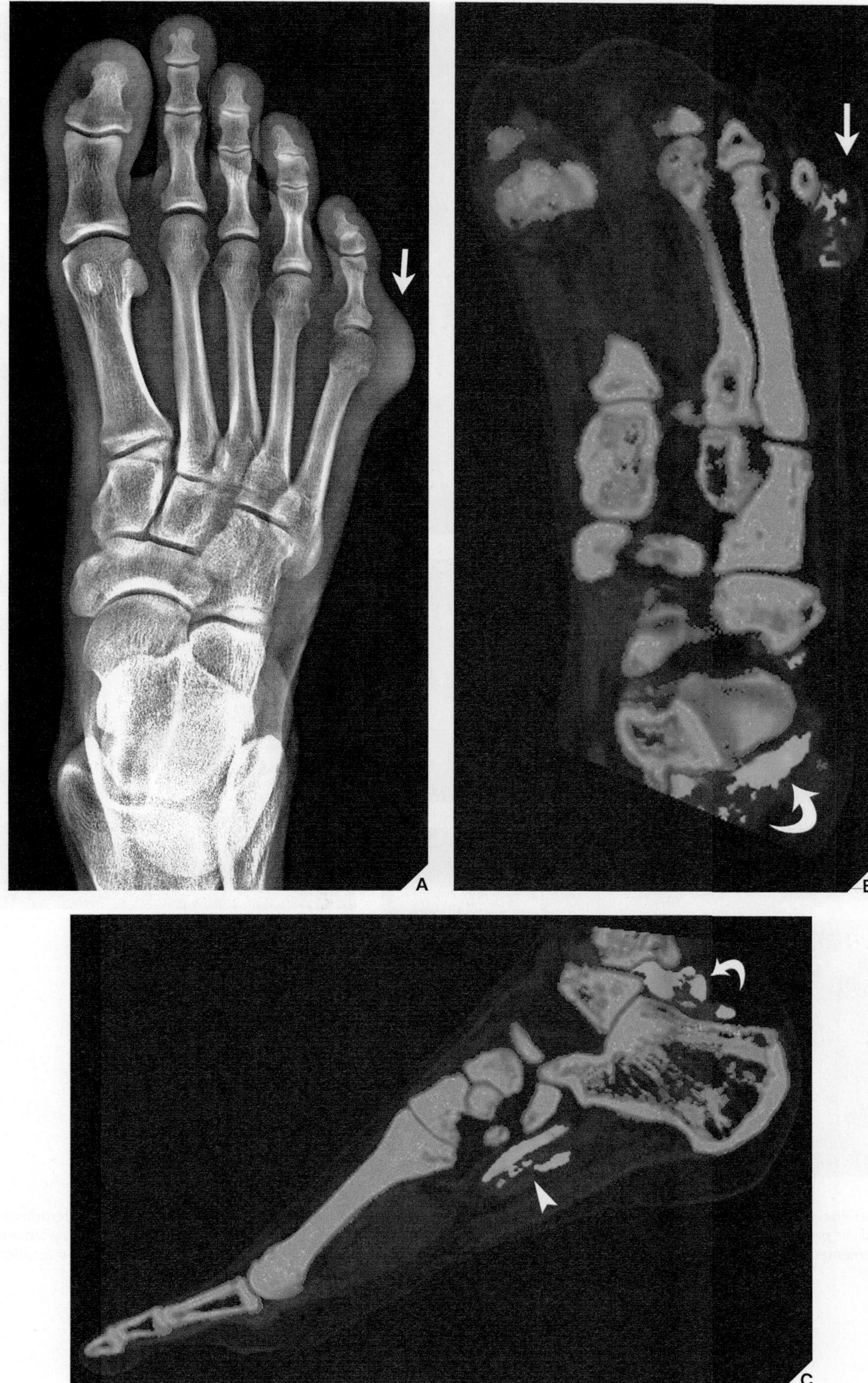

FIGURE 12.10 Dual-energy CT of tophaceous gout. A 45-year-old man presented with a painful mass of the small toe of the left foot for past 4 months. **(A)** Anteroposterior radiograph shows a soft-tissue mass at the lateral aspect of the fifth metatarsophalangeal joint *(arrow)*. The osseous structures are intact, and there is no evidence of erosions. Dual-energy coronal **(B)** and sagittal **(C)** reformatted color-coded CT images, in addition to the mass at the small toe *(arrow)*, reveal unsuspected masses *(green areas)* in the plantar *(arrowhead)* and posterior aspects *(curved arrows)* of the hindfoot, consistent with uric acid crystals deposition within the gouty tophi in clinically occult sites.

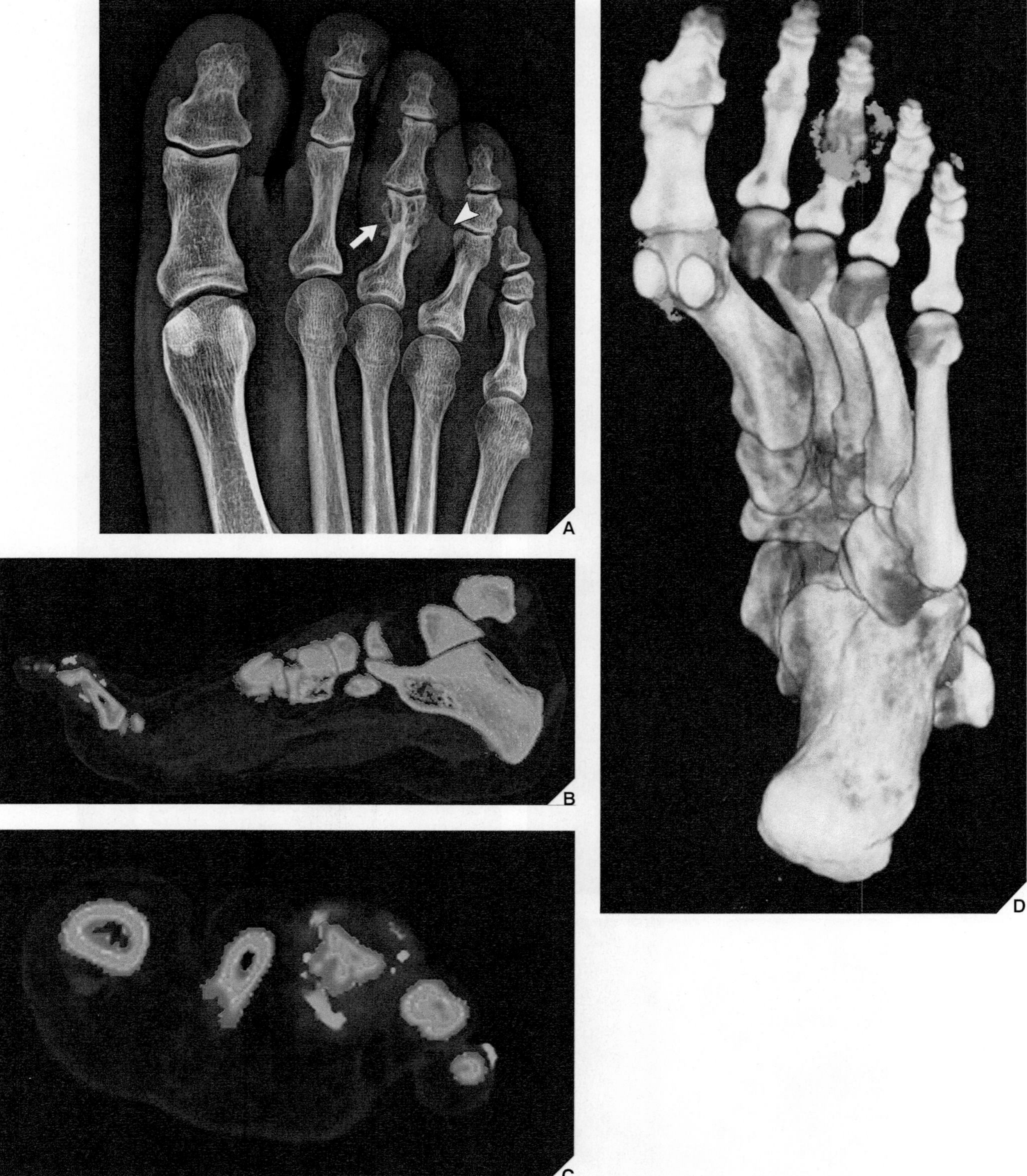

FIGURE 12.11 **Dual-energy CT of tophaceous gout.** A 50-year-old man presented with painful swollen third toe of the left foot. **(A)** Anteroposterior radiograph shows a paraarticular erosion of the proximal phalanx of the third toe *(arrow)*, associated with a fusiform mass *(arrowhead)*. Dual-energy **(B)** sagittal reformatted and **(C)** axial color-coded CT images supplemented with **(D)** 3D reconstructed CT image viewed from the plantar aspect were diagnostic of gouty tophi in several locations *(green areas)*.

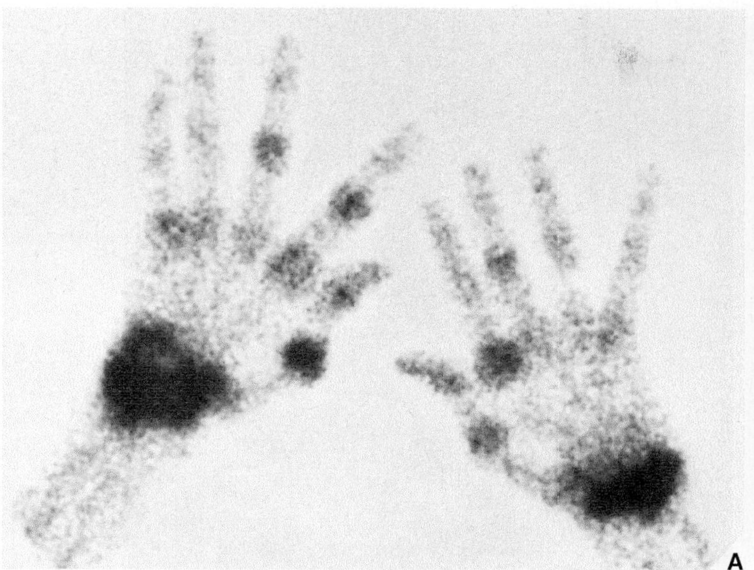

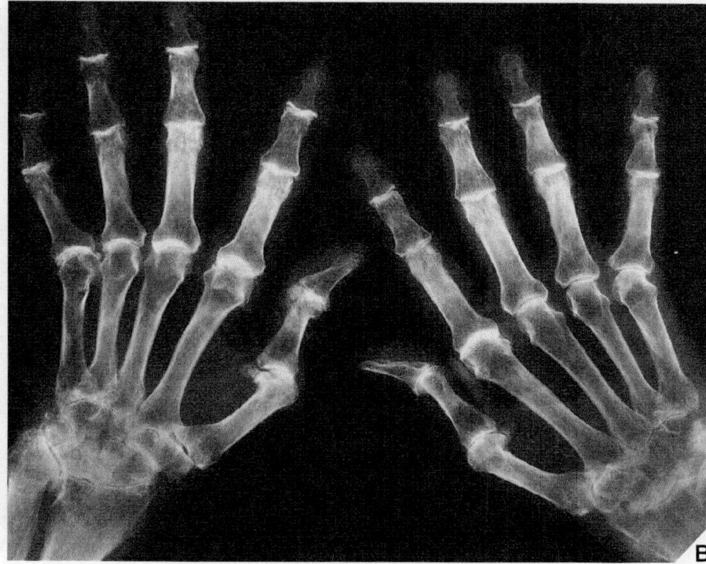

FIGURE 12.12 **Scintigraphy of psoriatic arthritis.** Radionuclide bone scan **(A)** obtained 2 hours after the intravenous injection of 15 mCi (555 MBq) of ^{99m}Tc-labeled MDP shows an increased uptake of radiopharmaceutical in several joints of the hand and wrist. A conventional radiograph **(B)** of the same patient shows advanced psoriatic arthritis.

body and eventually excreted by the kidneys. A gamma camera can then be used in a procedure known as a *three-phase radionuclide bone scan*. Scintigraphy can determine the distribution of arthritic changes in large and small joints (Fig. 12.12). It can also distinguish an infected joint from infected periarticular soft tissues (see Fig. 24.10). To distinguish infectious arthritis from other forms of arthritides, Indium-111 (^{111}In)-labeled leukocytes and gallium-57 (^{57}Ga) scans are employed (see Chapter 2, "Scintigraphy [Radionuclide Bone Scan]" section). Serial examinations with bone scintigraphy have also been helpful in evaluating the activity of given arthritis at a particular point in time. Such examinations may differentiate active disease from arthritis in remission. High-resolution single-photon emission CT (SPECT) trials have been attempted to detect osseous alterations in early stages of rheumatoid arthritis (RA) and erosive osteoarthritis (EOA) with promising results.

Ultrasound

Ultrasound (US) is frequently used in the evaluation of joint abnormalities. This technique helps to differentiate popliteal fossa masses in patients with RA, in whom complications of an arthritic process (such as popliteal cyst or hypertrophied synovium) may be distinguished from conditions not related to arthritis (such as popliteal artery aneurysm) (see Figs. 2.22 and 2.24). It also effectively diagnose deep vein thrombosis, occasionally seen in patients with RA (see Fig. 2.23). US has also been used to demonstrate osseous erosions. Doppler US is useful to demonstrate inflammatory pannus and rheumatoid synovitis. US-guided needle aspiration of synovial fluid in the joints and tendons with injection of steroids is a commonly used interventional technique.

Magnetic Resonance Imaging

Magnetic resonance imaging (MRI) of the joints provides excellent contrast between soft tissues and bone. Articular cartilage, fibrocartilage, cortex, and spongy bone can be distinguished from each other by their specific signal intensities. It is an excellent modality for demonstrating the rheumatoid nodules and synovial abnormalities in patients with RA. MRI's ability to contrast the synovium-covered joint from other soft-tissue structures allows for noninvasive delineation of the degree of synovial hypertrophy that accompanies synovitis, previously demonstrable only by means of arthrography or arthroscopy. Because synovitis is often accompanied by joint effusion, this too can be effectively demonstrated by MRI (Fig. 12.13). In particular, when this technique is combined with intravenous administration of gadolinium diethylenetriamine pentaacetic acid (Gd-DTPA), it is highly effective in differentiation between fluid-filled joints and tendon sheaths from synovitis. Both fluid and intraarticular synovial tissues exhibit an intermediate signal intensity on T1-weighted images and a high signal on T2 weighting. However, gadolinium-enhanced T1-weighted images will show high-intensity signal of inflammatory pannus/synovial tissue, whereas fluid will not enhance (Figs. 12.14 and 12.15). MRI is also helpful in diagnosing Baker cyst (Fig. 12.16). Although MRI is sensitive in detecting joint effusion, it cannot yet distinguish between inflammatory fluid and noninflammatory fluid. Occasionally, MRI may provide some additional information on osteoarthritis (OA) (Figs. 12.17 and 12.18) and hemophilic arthropathy (Figs. 12.19 and 12.20). With the development of more sophisticated orthopaedic methods for cartilage repair in OA, such as new articular cartilage replacement techniques, including chondrocyte transplantation, osteochondral transplantation, and cartilage growth-stimulating factors, optimized MRI of these interventions for diagnosis and treatment planning in OA is essential (see discussion in Chapter 9). Recent investigations of the value of contrast-enhanced MRI with subtraction technique proved to be useful for early detection of active sacroiliitis.

MRI plays an important role in the evaluation of the spine. MR images in the sagittal plane are useful for demonstrating hypertrophy of the ligamentum flavum or the vertebral facets, grading the degree of foramina stenosis, and measuring the sagittal diameter of the spinal canal and the spinal cord. MR images in the axial plane facilitate detailed analysis of the facet joints and more accurate measurement of the thickness of the ligamentum flavum and the diameter of the spinal canal. The quality of evaluation of spinal cord abnormalities by MRI in the cervical area in patients with RA and of spinal stenosis in patients with advanced degenerative changes of the spine surpasses that obtained with other modalities. MRI is particularly useful in the examination of patients with pain related to disk disease because it can differentiate normal, degenerated, and herniated disks noninvasively (see Chapter 11). In fact, the changes of disk degeneration can be identified by MRI long before they can be detected by conventional radiography or CT.

The Arthritides

Diagnosis

Clinical Information

The accurate diagnosis of specific arthritis depends on many factors; however, the most important is to understand the patterns of symptoms and the mechanism of disease.

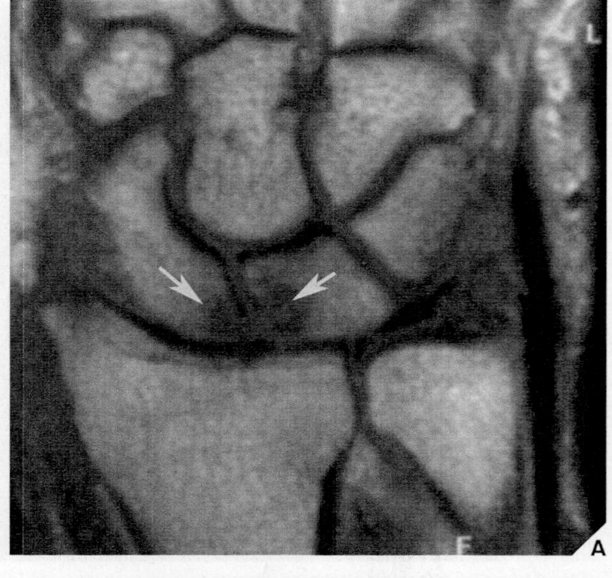

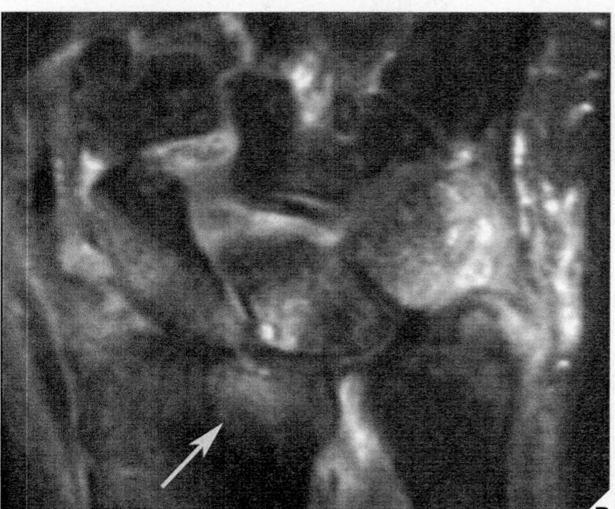

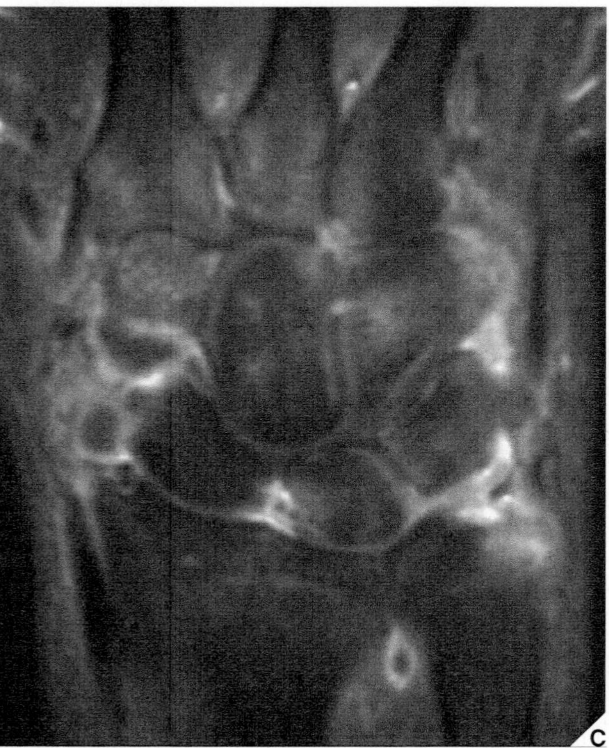

FIGURE 12.13 MRI of RA. Conventional radiographs (not shown here) showed questionable erosions in the scaphoid and lunate bones. **(A)** Coronal T1-weighted MRI confirms the presence of scaphoid and lunate erosions *(arrows)*. **(B)** Coronal short time inversion recovery (STIR) MRI demonstrates additionally extensive bone marrow edema of the entire proximal carpal row, ulnar styloid process, and distal radius *(arrow)* (pre-erosive edema). **(C)** Coronal T1-weighted fat-saturated MRI obtained after intravenous injection of gadolinium demonstrates strong enhancement of the synovium and multiple areas within the carpal bones, proximal metacarpals, and ulnar styloid, the hallmarks of severity and extension of the inflammation. (Courtesy of Luis Cerezal, MD, Santander, Spain.)

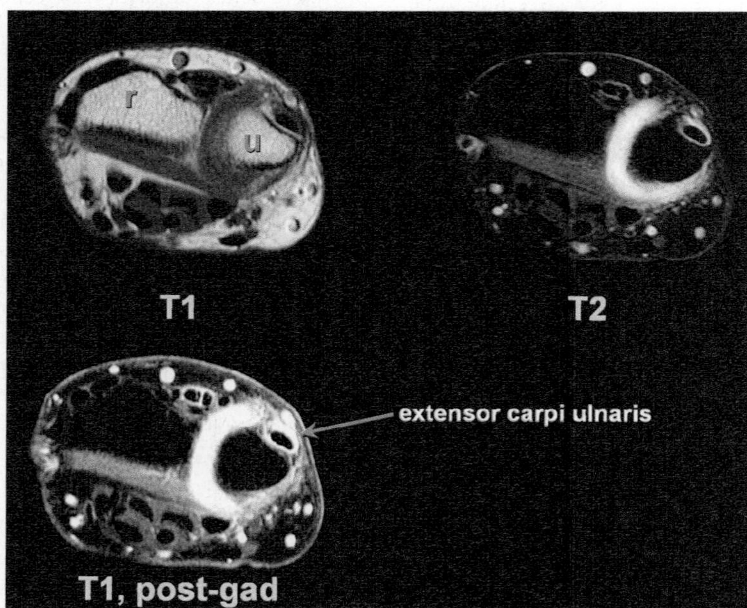

FIGURE 12.14 Magnetic resonance arthrography of RA. Axial T1-weighted, T2-weighted, and contrast-enhanced T1-weighted MR images of the wrist of the 28-year-old woman with clinical diagnosis of RA show advantage of postgadolinium study for diagnosis of synovitis of the distal radioulnar joint and extensor carpi ulnaris tendon. Although the high signal on T2 weighting may indicate either fluid or inflammatory pannus, the marked enhancement on postgadolinium sequences confirms the presence of the latter because fluid would not enhance. *r*, radius; *u*, ulna.

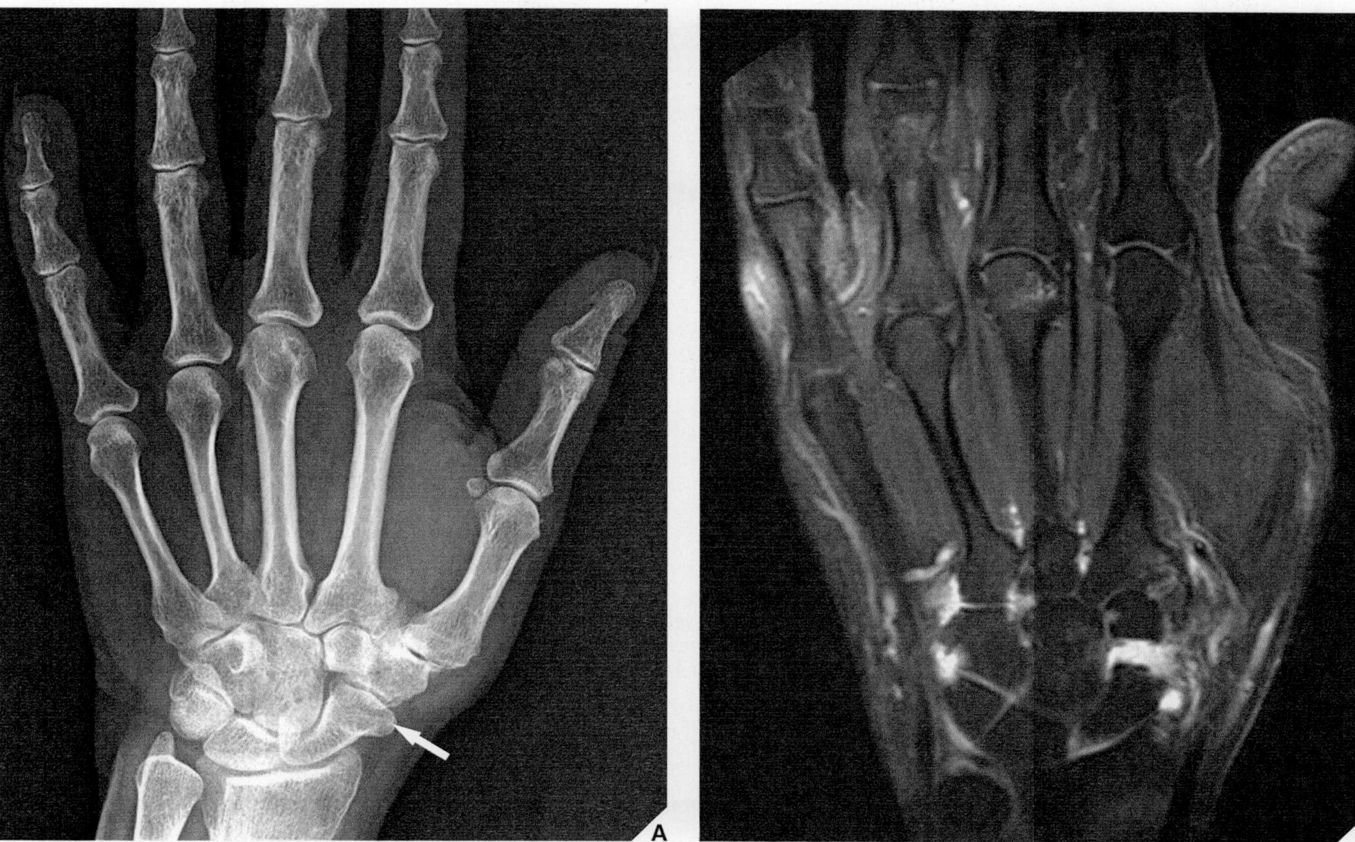

FIGURE 12.15 **Magnetic resonance arthrography of psoriatic arthritis.** A 42-year-old man with skin lesions clinically diagnosed as psoriasis, presented with 4-month history of pain in the right wrist. **(A)** Dorsovolar radiograph shows small cyst-like lesion in the distal scaphoid *(arrow)* but no erosions or other radiographic features of inflammatory arthritis. **(B)** Coronal T1-weighted fat-suppressed MRI obtained after intravenous administration of gadolinium shows erosions of the head of the third metacarpal, scaphoid, triquetrum, and hamate bones, and extensive synovitis in the intercarpal articulations, consistent with inflammatory arthritis.

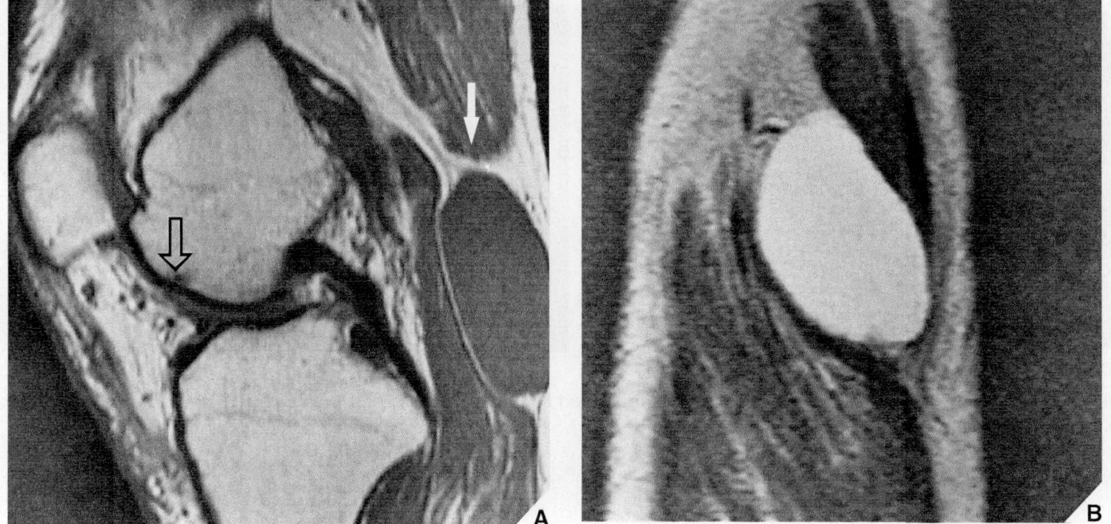

FIGURE 12.16 **MRI of the Baker cyst.** A 68-year-old woman with RA reported pain in the region of the popliteal fossa. The presumptive diagnosis of thrombophlebitis was made. **(A)** Sagittal MRI (spin echo [SE]; recovery time [TR] 900/echo time [TE] 20 msec) demonstrates an oval structure in the popliteal fossa displaying intermediate signal intensity *(arrow)*. Also note a small subchondral erosion of the anterior aspect of the medial femoral condyle *(open arrow)*. **(B)** Coronal MRI (SE; TR 1800/TE 80 msec) at the level of the popliteal fossa demonstrates a large Baker cyst that displays a high signal intensity caused by fluid content.

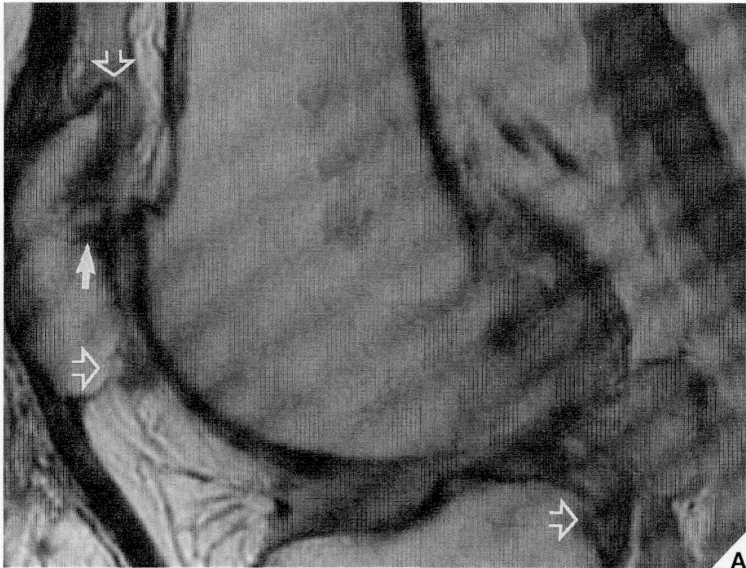

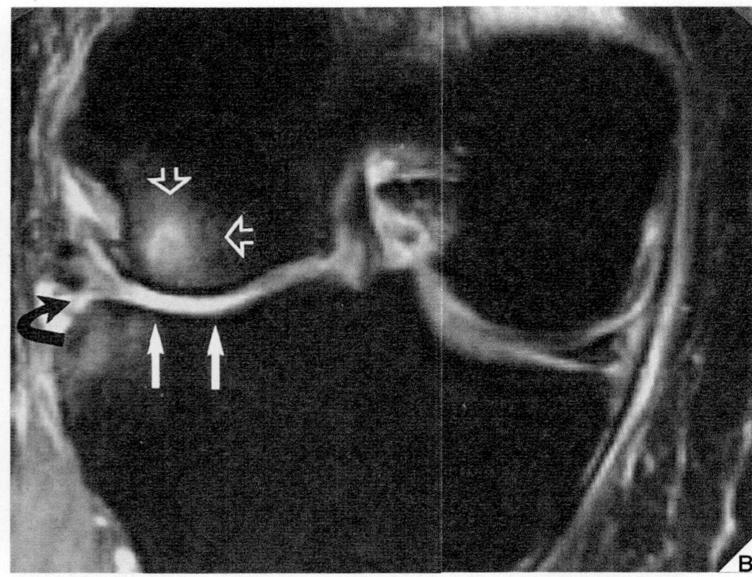

FIGURE 12.17 MRI of OA. **(A)** Sagittal proton density–weighted MRI of a 62-year-old woman with OA of the right knee shows involvement of the femoropatellar compartment. Note joint space narrowing, subchondral cyst *(arrow)*, and osteophytes *(open arrows)*. **(B)** Coronal T2-weighted fat-suppressed MR image shows complete destruction of articular cartilage of the lateral joint compartment *(arrows)*, subchondral edema *(open arrows)*, and degenerative tear of the lateral meniscus *(curved arrow)*.

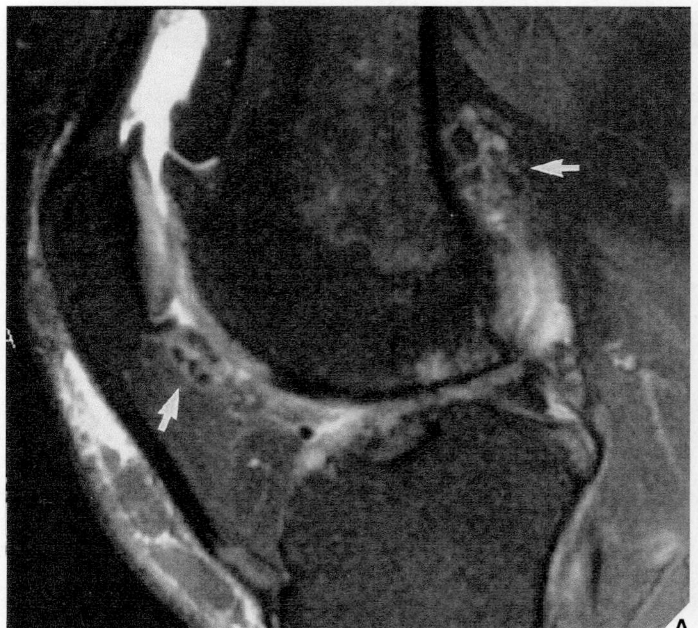

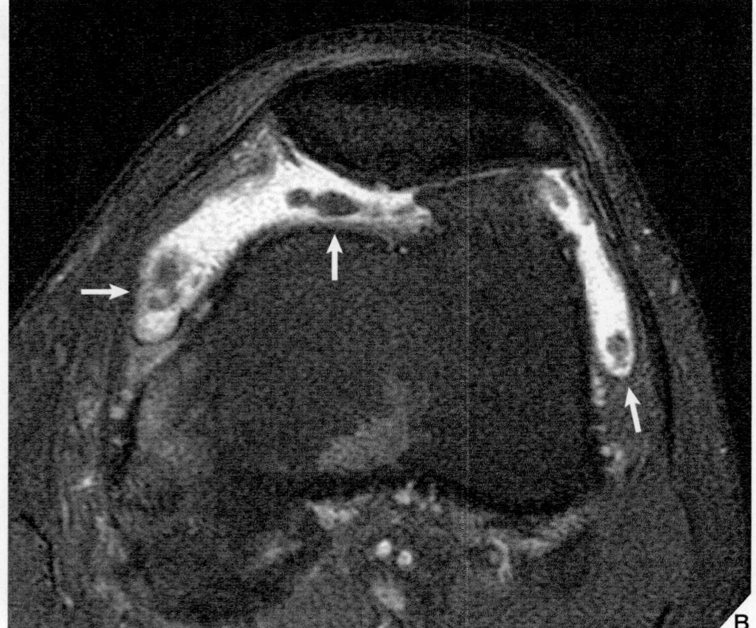

FIGURE 12.18 MRI of OA. **(A)** Sagittal and **(B)** axial T2-weighted fat-suppressed MR images of the knee of a 60-year-old man show OA complicated by multiple osteochondral bodies *(arrows)*.

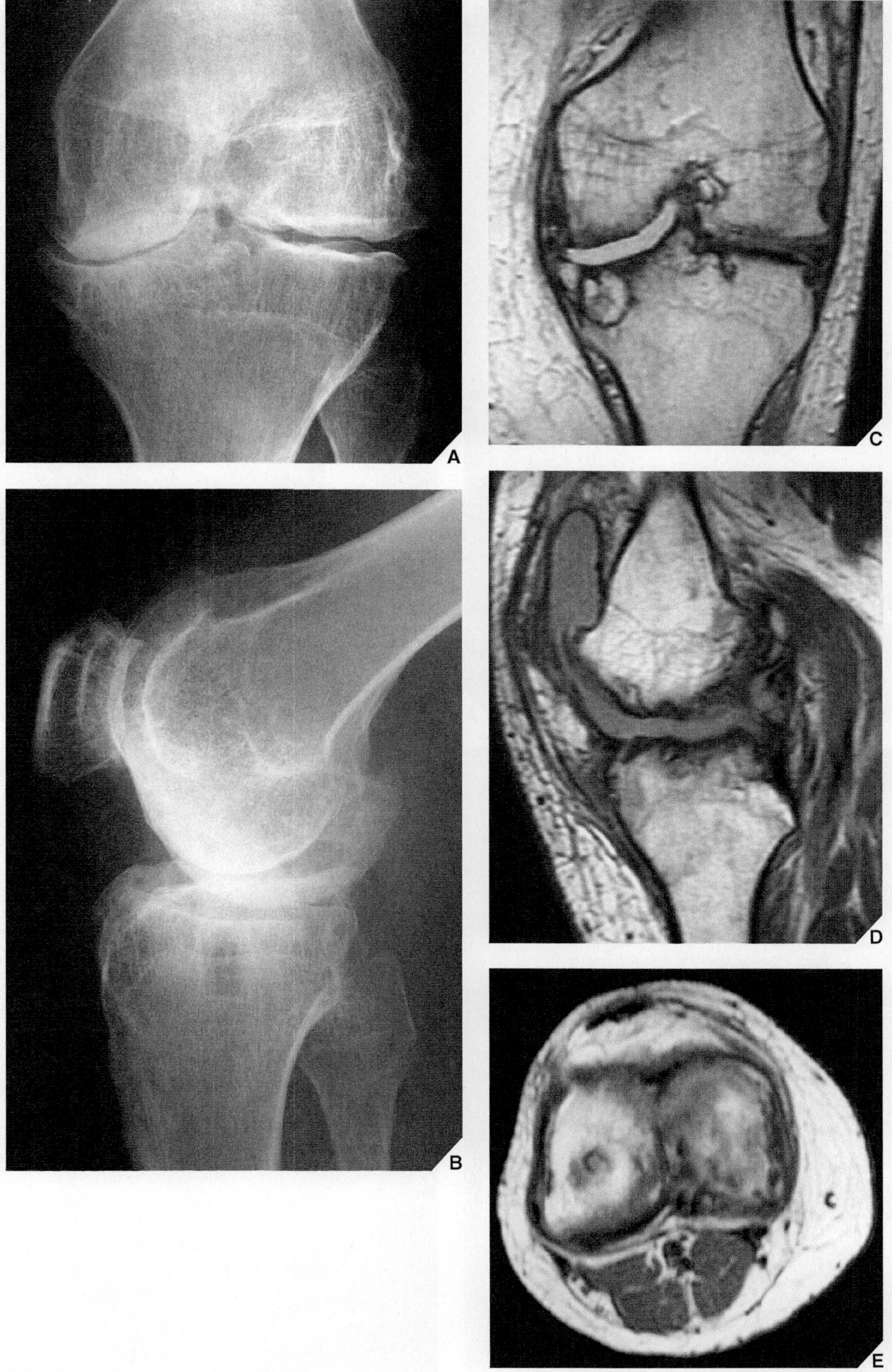

FIGURE 12.19 MRI of hemophilic arthropathy. A 29-year-old man with hemophilia presented with history of multiple episodes of intraarticular bleeding. **(A)** Anteroposterior and **(B)** lateral radiographs of the left knee demonstrate an advanced stage of hemophilic arthropathy. Abnormalities include periarticular osteoporosis, irregularity of subchondral bone at the tibial plateau and femoral condyles, narrowing of the radiographic joint space, and erosion of the subchondral bone. **(C)** Coronal MRI (spin echo [SE]; recovery time [TR] 1900/echo time [TE] 20 msec) demonstrates, in addition, complete destruction of articular cartilage at the medial joint compartment and a large, subchondral cyst in the proximal tibia, not well appreciated on the radiographic films. **(D)** Sagittal MRI (SE; TR 800/TE 20 msec) demonstrates to better advantage the intraarticular blood, and blood in suprapatellar recess and infrapatellar bursa, displaying intermediate signal intensity. **(E)** Axial MRI (TR 400/TE 20 msec) shows erosive changes of the articular cartilage of the femoral condyles.

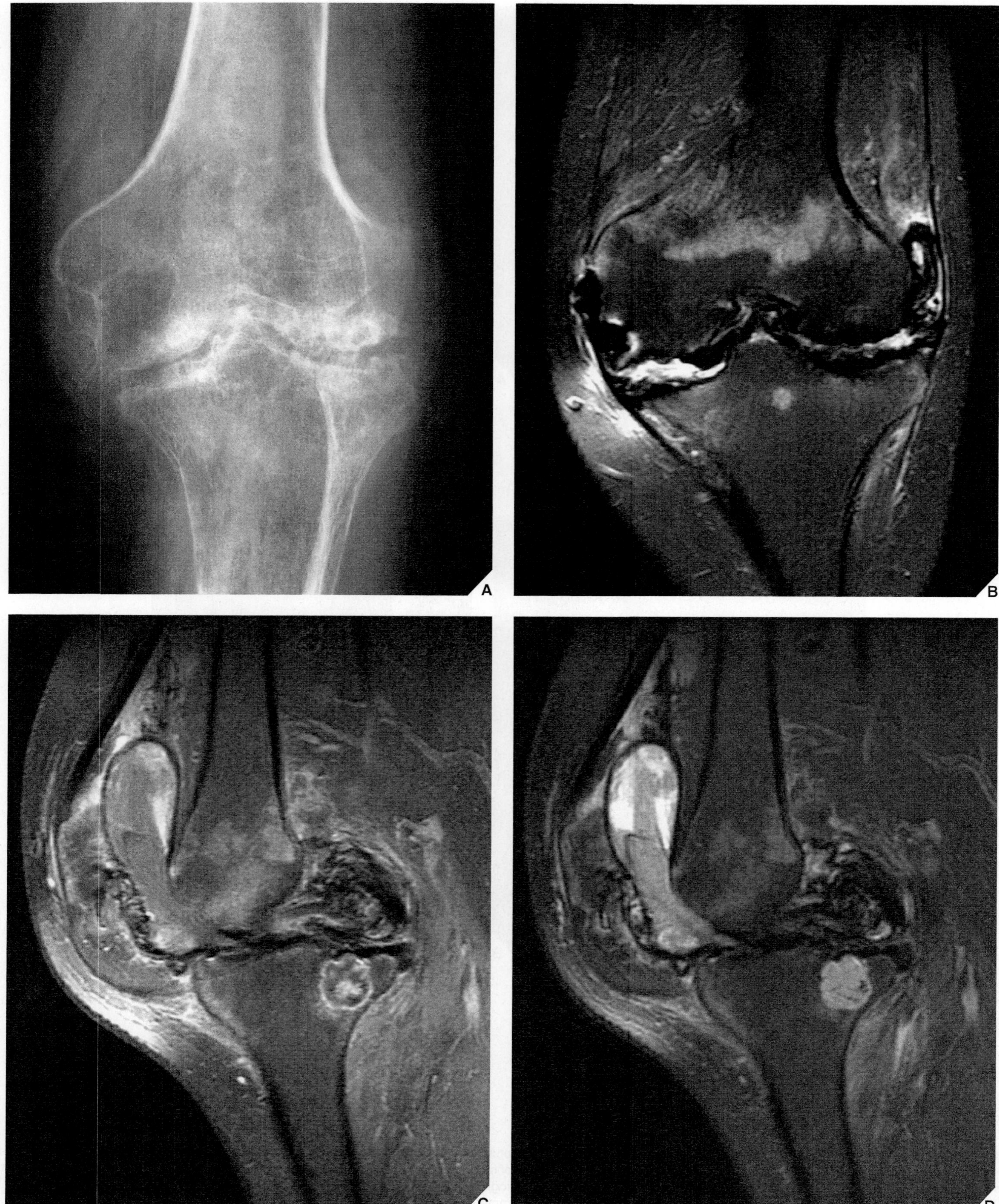

FIGURE 12.20 **MRI of hemophilic arthropathy.** **(A)** Anteroposterior radiograph of the left knee, **(B)** coronal proton density–weighted fat-suppressed, **(C)** sagittal T1-weighted contrast-enhanced fat-suppressed, and **(D)** sagittal proton density–weighted fat-suppressed MR images of a 34-year-old man show destructive changes of all three joint compartments. Note heterogeneous appearance of bloody effusion in the joint and suprapatellar recess.

The clinical manifestations and laboratory data, in conjunction with the imaging findings, are of significant help in making the diagnosis of a specific arthritic process. The most critical component of an examination in clinical practice is the determination of whether inflammation is present in the joint—that is, is it an inflammatory or noninflammatory process? The presence of inflammatory process is much more serious and, in some cases such as infection, creates rheumatology emergency. It should be clarified that the cardinal features of inflammation include the presence of pain (*dolor*), swelling (*tumor*), erythema (*rubor*), and warmth (*calor*), which are typically detected on physical examination, at least with respect to the peripheral joints. In addition, the elevation of white blood cell (WBC) count in the synovial fluid (>2,000 per μL), elevated erythrocyte sedimentation rate (ESR), and a high C-reactive protein (CRP) level are also the reliable factors.

A large number of standardized objective parameters that are useful to determine whether inflammation is or is not present are now available for the clinician. The most important is a quality physical examination looking for the four key components of inflammation described earlier. In addition, there are blood tests available that include the measurements of ESR and CRP. ESR is a valuable but nonspecific test that measures the rate at which red blood cells sediment in standardized Westergren tube in a period of 1 hour. The CRP is a protein produced by the liver, induced and generated by cytokine interleukin-6 (IL-6) in response to infection or other cause of inflammation. An elevation of ESR or CRP is a clear indicator of the presence of an inflammatory systemic process and strongly implicates the need for further evaluation of the patient that must incorporate a thorough physical examination as well as synovial fluid analysis, including quantification of cells, the presence or absence of crystals, a Gram stain, and culture for microorganisms. These tests, in conjunction with careful clinical evaluation, provide the cornerstone for the diagnosis and management of patient with joint abnormalities.

The fundamentals of physical examination remain the cornerstone of rheumatology, and the examination technique is universally recognized as a sensitive detector of crucial abnormalities. The GALS (gait, arms, legs, spine) locomotor system was devised to rapidly screen the patient for musculoskeletal disorders. The physical examination should be focused among others on the following features: type of gait, joint swelling, deformities and contractures, joint movements (active and passive), skin changes including redness and rashes, and wasting of muscles. Each joint should be individually and systematically examined. Particular attention should be directed to the appearance of the hand because distinctive patterns of hand involvement and several characteristic abnormalities can point to the specific diagnosis. Swelling of the joints and deformity of the digits resulting from loss of alignment may be consequence of destructive arthritis such as rheumatoid (Fig. 12.21). Swan-neck and boutonnière deformities have characteristic clinical appearance suggesting inflammatory arthritis (Fig. 12.22); the presence of Heberden or Bouchard nodes may point to the diagnosis of interphalangeal OA (Fig. 12.23); swelling of the proximal and distal interphalangeal joints (Fig. 12.24A) and nail changes such as onycholysis (separation of the nail plate from the nail bed) (Fig. 12.24B), pitting of the nails (Fig. 12.24C), leukonychia (white nails, milk spots) (Fig. 12.24D), splinting hemorrhages (Fig. 12.24E), subungual hyperkeratosis (Fig. 12.24F), and swelling of the entire finger (dactylitis or "sausage digit") (Fig. 12.24G) are commonly seen in psoriasis; flexible, easy-reducible joint contractures combined with redness and telangiectasia of the nail fold capillaries may be indicative of SLE; tapering of the ends of digits and sclerodactyly is characteristic of scleroderma. In the foot, the redness and swelling of the big toe, as well as the presence of soft-tissue masses representing chronic tophi, may indicate the presence of gout (Fig. 12.25). Systemic symptoms should also be evaluated, such as urethritis, conjunctivitis, and mucocutaneous lesions that are typically present in patients with reactive arthritis.

In making a specific diagnosis, it has to be taken in consideration that the various arthritides have different frequencies of occurrence between the genders. RA is much more common in females, and EOA is seen almost exclusively in middle-aged women. Psoriatic arthritis, reactive arthritis, and gouty arthritis, however, are more common in males.

Laboratory data are also essential. Gouty arthritis, for instance, is associated with elevated serum uric acid concentrations, and a synovial fluid examination reveals monosodium urate crystals in leukocytes in the fluid. The synovial fluid of patients with pseudogout, however, contains calcium pyrophosphate crystals. The detection of autoantibodies is another important aid in the diagnostic workup. Rheumatoid factor (RF) is a typical finding in RA. RF is an antibody against the Fc portion of immunoglobulin G (IgG) produced by the immune system. It is detectable in the blood of approximately 80% of adults with RA. The presence of RF in serum, however, can also indicate the occurrence of autoimmune activity unrelated to RA, such as present in many other autoimmune diseases, chronic infections, sarcoidosis, and some malignancies as well as associated with tissue or organ rejection. The most common methods of detecting RF are latex fixation, using latex beads coated with human IgG, and nephelometry, using human IgG as the target antigen. For nearly 50 years, RF was felt to be a highly specific immunoassay for the detection of RA. It is, however, not nearly as specific as antibodies to anti–cyclic citrullinated peptide (CCP). Nevertheless, patients with high RF titer are more likely to have more severe disease and to suffer from extraarticular features of RA including Felty syndrome, rheumatoid disease of the lung, and lymphoma. Patients lacking the specific antibodies represented by RF are said to have "seronegative" arthritis.

Patients with lupus arthritis have a positive antinuclear antibody (ANA). ANAs are a heterogeneous group of antibodies directed against components normally present in all nucleated cells. They bind to contents

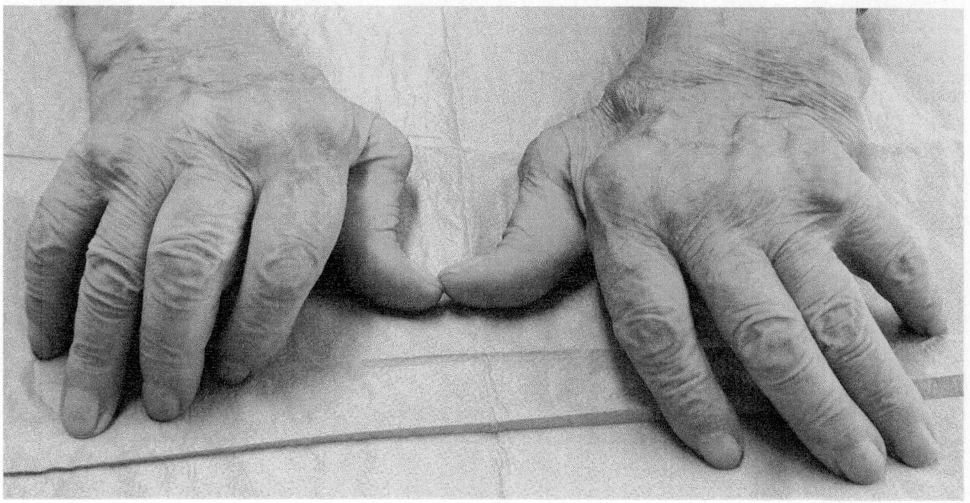

FIGURE 12.21 Rheumatoid arthritis. Clinical photograph of both hands of a patient with advanced RA shows ulnar deviation in the swollen metacarpophalangeal joints and hyperextension of the thumbs ("hitchhiker's thumbs"). (Reprinted with permission from Greenspan A, Gershwin ME. *Imaging in rheumatology: a clinical approach*, 1st ed. Philadelphia: Wolters Kluwer; 2018:5.)

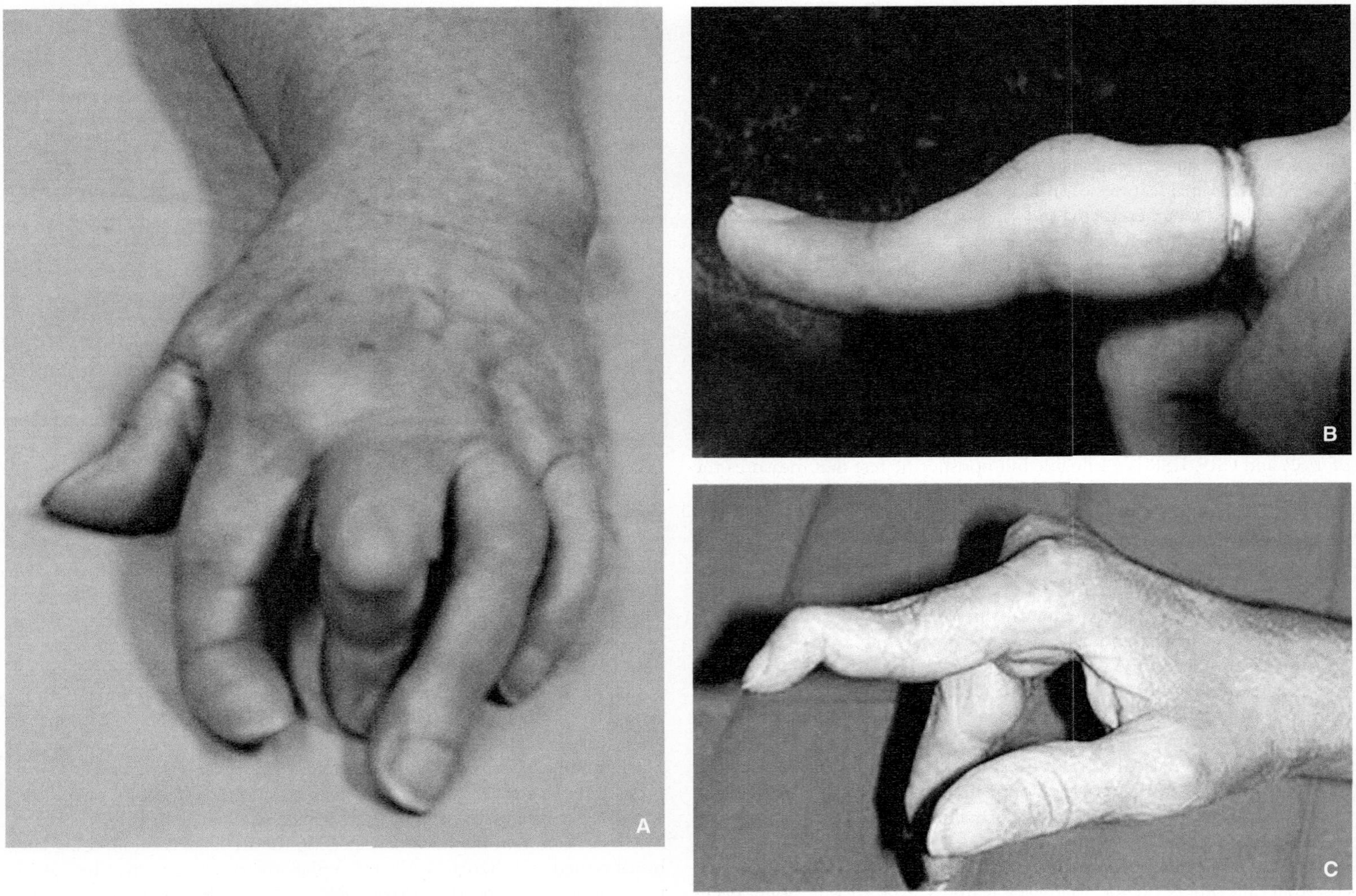

A

B

C

FIGURE 12.22 Rheumatoid arthritis. **(A)** Clinical photograph of the hand of a patient with advanced RA shows flexion in the proximal interphalangeal joints and extension in the distal interphalangeal joints of the index and middle fingers that resulted in boutonnière deformity. **(B)** In another patient, a clinical photograph of the index finger shows characteristic boutonnière deformity. **(C)** Extension in the proximal and flexion in the distal interphalangeal joint is known as a *swan-neck deformity*. (Reprinted with permission from Greenspan A, Gershwin ME. *Imaging in rheumatology: a clinical approach*, 1st ed. Philadelphia: Wolters Kluwer; 2018:5.)

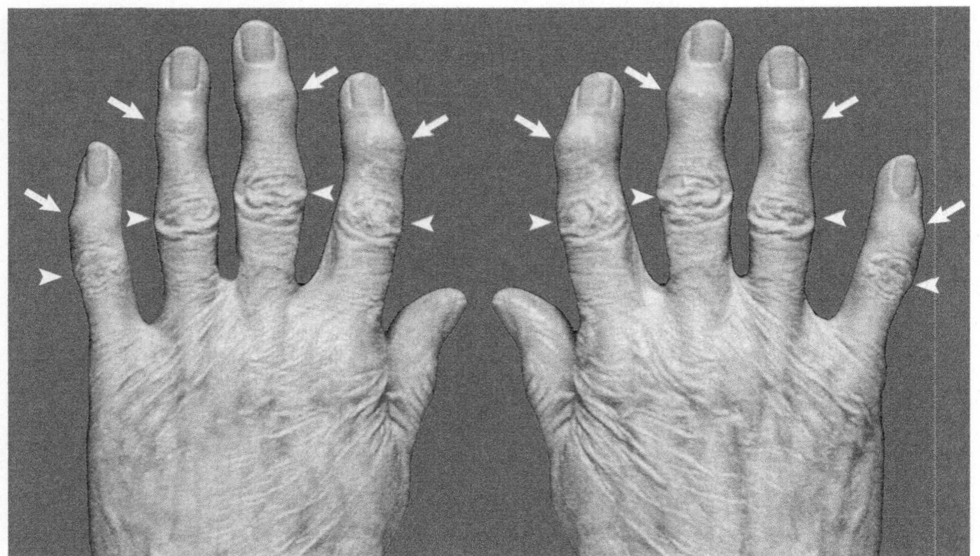

FIGURE 12.23 Interphalangeal OA. Clinical photograph of the hands of a 62-year-old woman shows prominence of the proximal interphalangeal joints known as *Bouchard nodes (arrowheads)* and distal interphalangeal joints known as *Heberden nodes (arrows)*. (Reprinted with permission from Greenspan A, Gershwin ME. *Imaging in rheumatology: a clinical approach*, 1st ed. Philadelphia: Wolters Kluwer; 2018:173.)

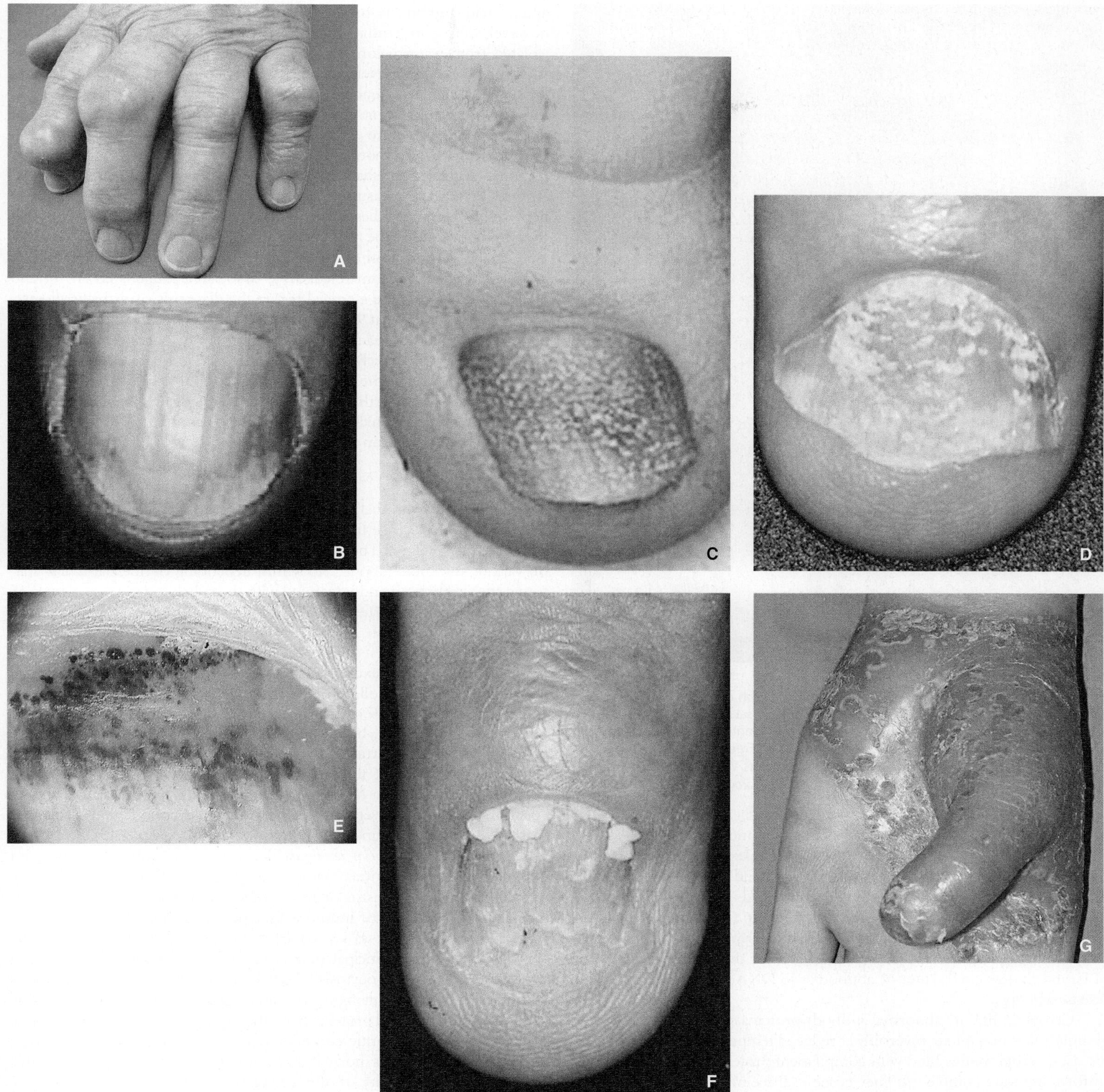

FIGURE 12.24 Psoriatic arthritis. **(A)** Note swelling of the proximal and distal interphalangeal joints and skin changes on the index, middle, and small fingers. **(B)** Detachment of the nail from the underlying nail bed is termed *onycholysis*. **(C)** The surface of the nail develops small pits that look like a surface of a thimble (nail pitting). The number of the pits can vary from a few to dozens. **(D)** White spots on the nail are termed *leukonychia*. **(E)** Reddish-brown lines and spots, termed *splinter hemorrhage*, represent tiny blood clots that run vertically under the nail because of damage of small capillaries. **(F)** Typical appearance of hyperkeratosis, a chalky substance that accumulates under the nail. **(G)** Diffusely swollen thumb (sausage digit) represents a dactylitis. Note also typical for psoriasis skin changes. (Reprinted with permission from Greenspan A, Gershwin ME. *Imaging in rheumatology: a clinical approach*, 1st ed. Philadelphia: Wolters Kluwer; 2018:6.)

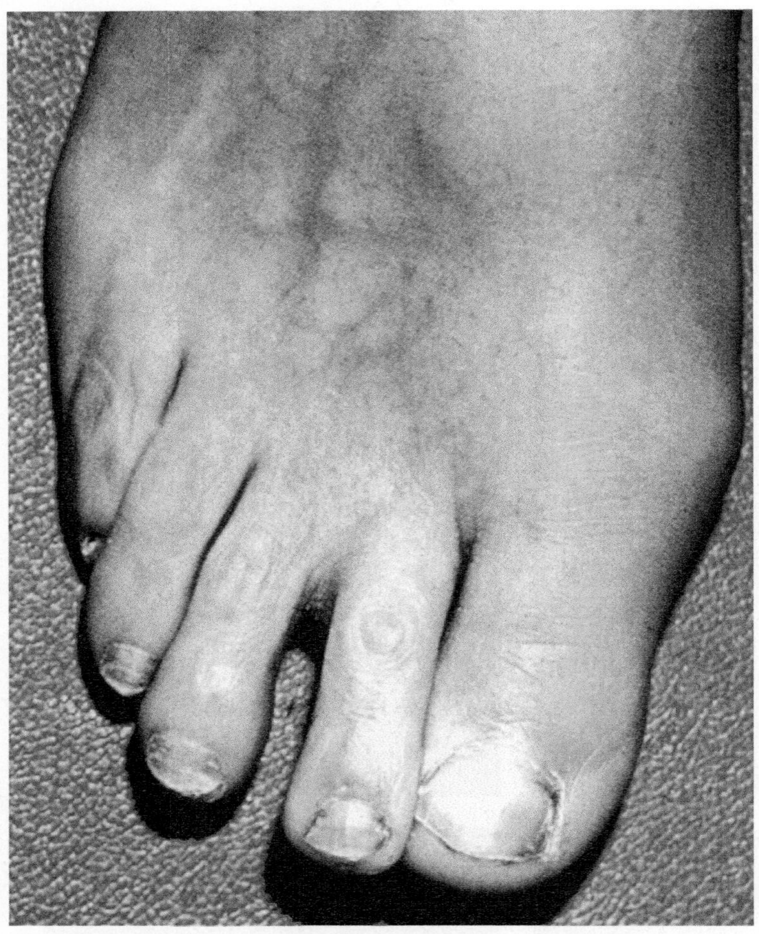

FIGURE 12.25 **Gouty arthritis.** Clinical photograph of the foot of the patient with gouty arthritis. Observe the big toe swelling and dorsal mass at the site of the first metatarsophalangeal joint representing a tophus. (Reprinted with permission from American Registry of Pathology, from Klein MJ, Bonar SF, Freemont T, et al. *Atlas of nontumor pathology. Non-neoplastic diseases of bones and joints.* Washington, DC: American Registry of Pathology and Armed Forces Institute of Pathology; 2011, Fig. 8.206.)

of the cell nucleus and are directed against histones, single- and double-stranded DNA, ribonucleoprotein (RNP) complexes, and other nuclear components. The common tests used to detect and to quantify ANAs are indirect immunofluorescence and enzyme-linked immunosorbent assay (ELISA). ANAs are found not only in SLE but also in other disorders such as RA, Sjögren syndrome, scleroderma, dermatomyositis, polymyositis, and multiple sclerosis. They are useful in the differential diagnosis of SLE, and changes in the titer of antibodies to DNA are useful in following disease activity.

Cryoglobulins are abnormal antibody proteins consisting of immunoglobulins that precipitate reversibly at reduced temperatures. In a variety of diseases, cryoglobulins bind with complement proteins and other peptides to form immune complexes. They come in three main types according to Brouet classification: type I (monoclonal immunoglobulins, commonly of the IgM isotype, directed against the Fc region of IgG), most common type II (a mixture of polyclonal IgG and monoclonal IgM), and type III (a combination of polyclonal IgG and polyclonal IgM molecules). Types II and III have RF activity and bind to polyclonal immunoglobulins. Cryoglobulins are not specific for any particular disorder; however, type I is linked to lymphoproliferative diseases and some malignancies; type II may be associated with chronic hepatitis C infection; and type III is associated with vasculitis, hepatitis C, subacute bacterial endocarditis, and autoimmune disorders such as SLE and RA.

Anti–cyclic citrullinated peptide antibodies (anti-CCP Abs) are the autoantibodies produced by the patient's immune system and directed against three unique proteins: α-enolase, fibrinogen, and vimentin. They are found in patients with seropositive RA and are actually directed at a modification of these three proteins. Under normal circumstances, the amino acid arginine is present in α-enolase, fibrinogen, and vimentin; however, during inflammation, an α-amino acid called *citrulline* (originally isolated from watermelon) replaces the arginine. The switch of arginine to citrulline occurs in everyone's body and is accelerated by smoking, but in RA, this change is enough to elicit a loss of immune tolerance and thus the production of autoantibodies. These antibodies are useful for the diagnosis of RA and are even detectable many years before clinical onset of disease. They are more specific than RF, and unlike RF, the immune response to these proteins is integrally related to the pathogenesis of RA. Anti-CCP Abs are measured by the ELISA using synthetic citrullinated peptides. These antibodies are frequently detectable in early RA, although they are not useful in the monitoring disease activity.

Lastly, identification of the antigens of the major histocompatibility complex, particularly human leukocyte–associated antigens HLA-B27 and HLA-DR4, has become a crucial test in the diagnosis of arthritic disease. It has been reported that 95% of patients with ankylosing spondylitis (AS), 86% of patients with reactive arthritis, and 60% of patients with psoriatic arthropathy test positively for antigen HLA-B27, whereas a majority of those with RA exhibit the HLA-DR4 antigen. This is helpful in differentiating certain types of arthritides as well as distinguishing psoriatic arthritis from RA in cases in which the radiographic presentation of these conditions may be very similar.

Pathology

The synovial (diarthrodial) joint consists of two bone ends cupped by the articular cartilage: dense fibrous capsule lined by the synovium, and synovial fluid (Fig. 12.26A). The articular cartilage consists of a hyaline cartilage of various thickness (about 2 to 4 mm depending of the particular anatomic site), resting on and integrated with the subchondral plate, a layer of bone resembling the cortex (Fig. 12.26B). In young people, hyaline cartilage is translucent and bluish white, whereas in older individuals, it is opaque and slightly yellowish (see Fig. 3.14). On microscopic examination, it is composed of a dense extracellular matrix containing sparsely distributed chondrocytes, type II collagen, and hydrophilic sulfated proteoglycans including aggrecan (which contains highly negatively charged glycosaminoglycan chains), decorin, biglycan, and fibromodulin. The distribution of proteoglycans in the cartilage matrix varies from joint to joint, but generally the surface layers of the cartilage contain much less proteoglycan than do the deeper layers. In histologic sections stained with hematoxylin and eosin, the junction between calcified cartilage and noncalcified cartilage is marked by a basophilic line known as the *tidemark* (see Fig. 3.19). Synovium, also referred to as *synovial membrane*, lines the inner surface of the joint capsule and all other intraarticular structures, with the exception of the articular cartilage. It consists of fibrous tissue and fat covered by an incomplete layer of two types of intimal cells: type A synoviocytes (deriving from macrophages) and type B synoviocytes (deriving from fibroblasts). The synovium has three principal functions: secretion of synovial fluid hyaluronate by B cells; phagocytosis of waste material derived from the various components of the joints by A cells; and regulation of the movements of solutes, electrolytes, and proteins from the capillaries into the synovial fluid.

In any of the arthritic conditions, there is anatomic and physiologic alteration of the joint's normal structure and function. In general, this includes loss of capacity of the articulating surfaces to move over one another and loss of joint stability. Regardless of the cause, joint injury is characterized by certain basic cellular and tissue responses. Usually, there is macroscopic and microscopic evidence of both degeneration and repair. The morphologic abnormalities of the articular cartilage and synovial membrane are depending on the specific arthritic process. *OA* is characterized by damage and loss of articular cartilage, subchondral bone sclerosis, degenerative cysts, and osteophytosis (Fig. 12.27A,B). The initial changes in articular cartilage are localized; however, the gradual damage and destruction of the cartilage eventually results in complete loss of articular cartilage exposing the underlying bone (Fig. 12.27C).

Microscopic findings include hypertrophy and hyperplasia of synoviocytes and synovial hypervascularity. The early changes within the cartilage include loss of proteoglycan, followed by flaking and cracking of the cartilaginous surface with formation of the fissures. In areas of residual cartilage, there is often irregularity, duplication, and reduplication of

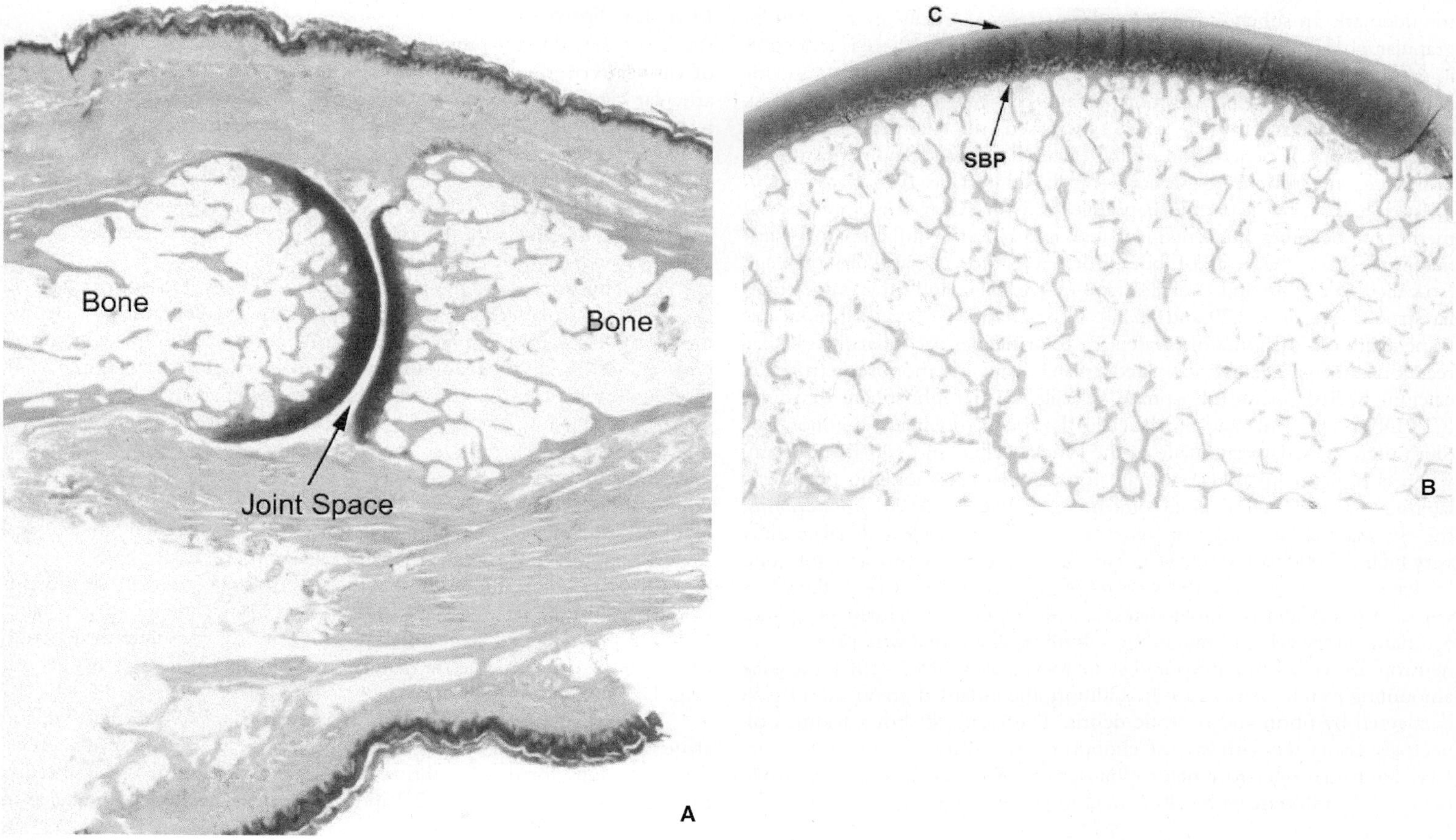

FIGURE 12.26 Normal diarthrodial (synovial) joint. **(A)** Longitudinal section through the interphalangeal joint demonstrates closely apposed convex and concave articular cartilage surfaces separated by a narrow fluid-filled cavity (joint space). **(B)** The cartilage *(C)* forms a thin layer on the surface of bone, beneath which is attached the subchondral bone plate *(SBP)*. (Reprinted with permission from American Registry of Pathology, from Klein MJ, Bonar SF, Freemont T, et al. *Atlas of nontumor pathology. Non-neoplastic diseases of bones and joints*. Washington, DC: American Registry of Pathology and Armed Forces Institute of Pathology; 2011:547, Figs. 7.5 and 7.9.)

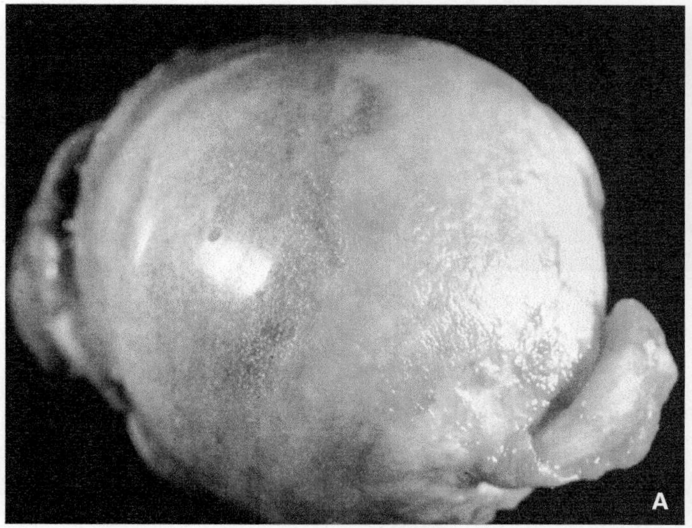

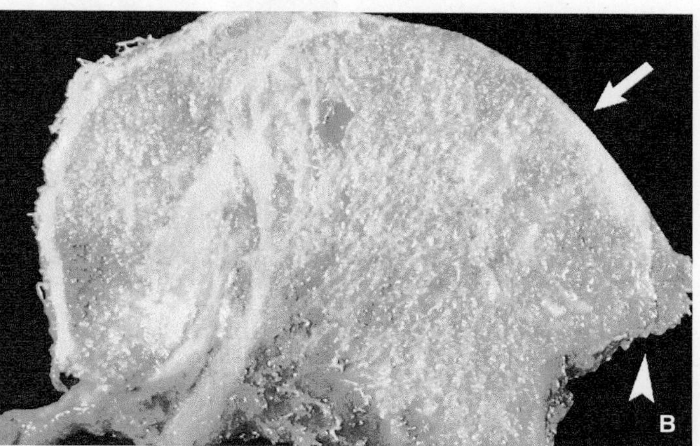

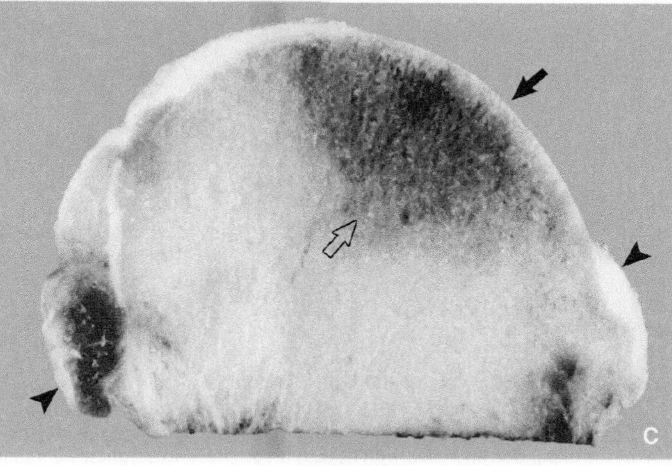

FIGURE 12.27 Pathology of OA. **(A)** Photograph of the gross specimen of the femoral head shows absence of the articular cartilage on the superior and lateral aspects and "polished" appearance of the exposed subchondral bone (eburnation). The remaining cartilage exhibits yellowish color and roughened surface. **(B)** Coronal section of resected femoral head shows marked thinning of the articular cartilage medially *(arrow)* and a large osteophyte *(arrowhead)*. (Reprinted from Bullough P. *Orthopaedic pathology*, 5th ed. Maryland Heights, MO: Mosby; 2009, with permission from Elsevier.) **(C)** Coronal section through the femoral head shows marked thinning of articular cartilage *(arrow)*, an area of eburnation *(open arrow)*, and osteophytes *(arrowheads)*. (Reprinted with permission from American Registry of Pathology, from Klein MJ, Bonar SF, Freemont T, et al. *Atlas of nontumor pathology. Non-neoplastic diseases of bones and joints*. Washington, DC: American Registry of Pathology and Armed Forces Institute of Pathology; 2011:604, Fig. 8.51.)

the tidemark. In subchondral bone, the marrow elements are replaced by granular, eosinophilic material lacking cellular elements. There is reduction in number of osteocytic lacunae, which in addition may become empty or may contain cellular debris. In more advanced stages, there is complete loss of the articular cartilage (Fig. 12.28); increased endochondral ossification; increased vascular penetration of the calcified cartilage; and deposition if immature, woven bone at the bone–cartilage interface. *Inflammatory arthritis*, such as RA, has a particular predilection for synovium. The synovial membrane becomes thickened, swollen, and red. The inflammatory pannus erodes first the parts of bone not covered by the articular cartilage (so-called *bare areas*) and later destroys the cartilage and other intraarticular structures (Figs. 12.29 and 12.30). *Crystal-induced arthropathies* represent a spectrum of inflammatory articular abnormalities secondary to cellular reaction directed against deposited crystals (such as monosodium urate, calcium hydroxyapatite phosphate, or calcium pyrophosphate dihydrate [CPPD]) in the joints and periarticular tissues. For instance, the monosodium urate crystals accumulate in the synovial fluid and soft-tissue tophi, whereas pyrophosphate crystals are found most commonly in fibrocartilaginous tissues, such as knee joint menisci (Fig. 12.31). In *septic arthritis*, the synovial fluid is opaque or frankly purulent. The nucleated cell count is very high (20,000 to 100,000 cells/mm^3), and there is progressive infiltrate in synovium, associated with vascular congestion, and increase in the number of types A and B synoviocytes. The synovium is inflamed, and there is inflammatory cell infiltrate in the subintima associated with presence of neutrophils within subintima and synoviocyte layer, often with aggregates amounting to microabscesses. In addition, the inflamed granulation tissue is covered by fibrin and necrotic debris. The cartilage shows features of necrosis associated with loss of chondrocytes and irregularity of the surface due to damage from neutrophil-derived enzymes. There is extensive neutrophilic infiltrate with cells containing coarse ragocyte granules.

Imaging Features

As already stated in the previous text, the true or diarthrodial joint consists of cartilage covering the articular ends of the bones forming the joint; the articular capsule, which is reinforced by ligamentous structures; and the joint space, which is lined with synovial membrane and filled with synovial fluid (Fig. 12.32; see also Fig. 12.26A). Because of its physicochemical constitution, articular cartilage absorbs only a minimal amount of x-rays, thus appearing radiolucent on a radiographic film. The radiolucent articular cartilage, together with the joint cavity filled with synovial fluid, creates the so-called *radiographic joint space*.

The abnormality of the joint in arthritis usually consists of destruction of the articular cartilage, which appears on a radiograph as a narrowing of the radiographic joint space, usually accompanied by subchondral erosion; narrowing of the joint is the cardinal sign of arthritis (Fig. 12.33). It should be kept in mind, however, that in some arthritic processes, the joint space may not become narrow, appearing instead slightly expanded. This happens, for example, in the early stages of some arthritides, when joint effusion and ligamentous laxity cause distention of the joint with fluid, but the articular cartilage has not yet been destroyed. It may also be seen in rare instances when granulation pannus erodes the subchondral bone without destroying the articular cartilage (Fig. 12.34).

Other radiographic signs specific to different types of arthritis include periarticular soft-tissue swelling, periarticular osteoporosis, and, in the more advanced stages of some arthritides, complete destruction of the joint with subluxation or dislocation and ankylosis (joint fusion) (Fig. 12.35).

The radiographic presentation of arthritis depends on the type and stage of the disease as well as the site of the original insult characteristic for the various forms of arthritis (Fig. 12.36), whether it is the articular cartilage, as in OA (see Figs. 12.2 and 12.40); the synovial membrane, as in

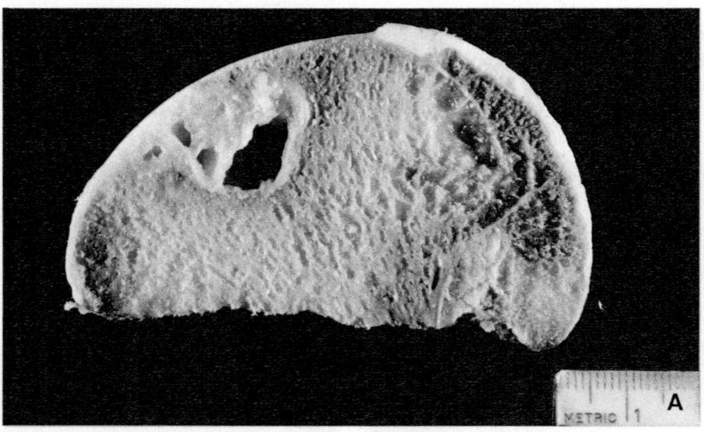

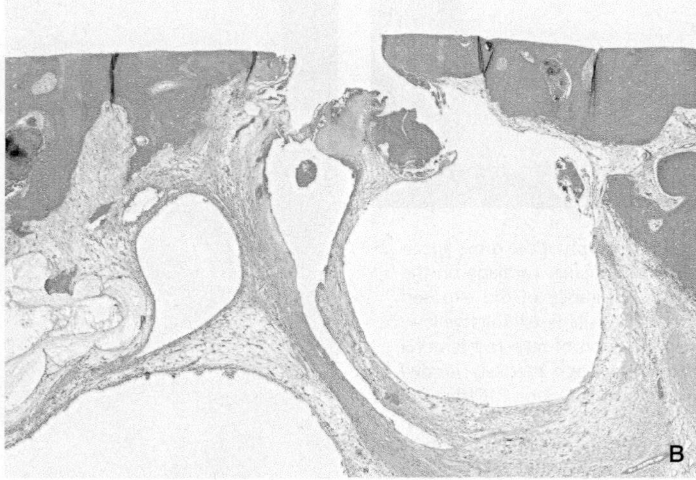

FIGURE 12.28 Pathology of OA. **(A)** Photograph of coronal section of the femoral head resected from the patient with advanced osteoarthritis of the hip joint shows complete absence of the articular cartilage *(left)* with focal subarticular sclerosis and secondary cysts formation. Observe a large peripheral osteophyte containing dark-red hematopoietic marrow *(right)*. **(B)** Photomicrograph demonstrates complete erosion of the articular cartilage associated with sclerosis and interruption of the subarticular plate. The intertrabecular spaces are expanded and filled with fibrous tissue showing secondary encystification (H&E, original magnification ×25). (Courtesy of Michael J. Klein, MD, New York.)

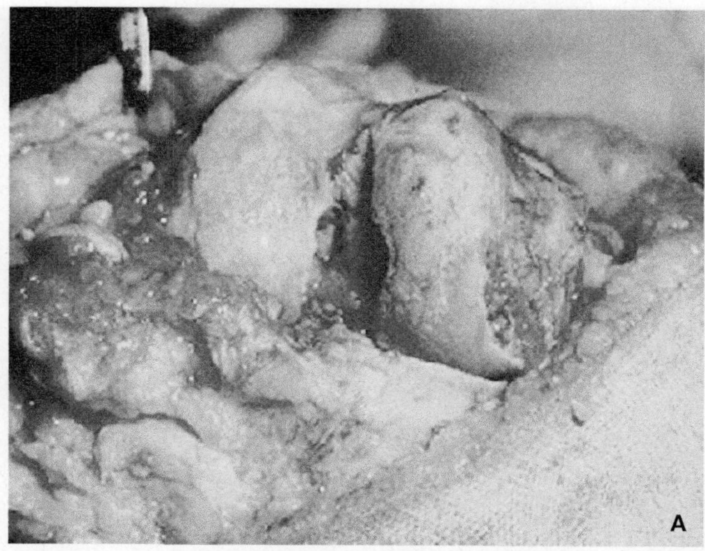

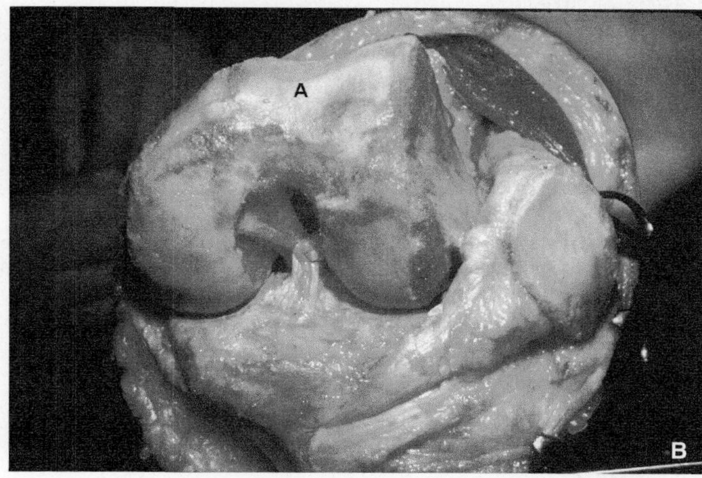

FIGURE 12.29 Pathology of RA. **(A)** Intraoperative photograph of the distal end of the femur shows inflammatory pannus and peripheral erosions of the articular cartilage of the femoral condyles. **(B)** In another patient, observe erosion of the articular cartilage *(A)* by pannus invading the articular surface from periphery. (Reprinted with permission from American Registry of Pathology, from Klein MJ, Bonar SF, Freemont T, et al. *Atlas of nontumor pathology. Non-neoplastic diseases of bones and joints*. Washington, DC: American Registry of Pathology and Armed Forces Institute of Pathology; 2011:605, 692, Figs. 8.52 and 8.171.)

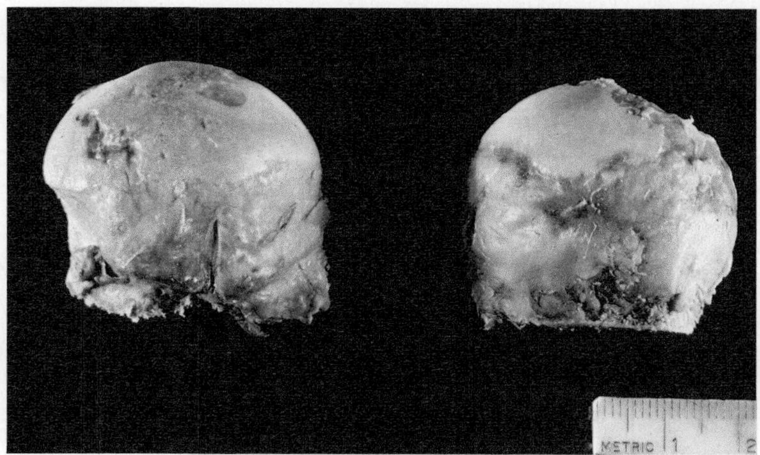

FIGURE 12.30 Pathology of RA. Photograph of the specimen of the resected femoral head shows erosions of the articular cartilage by inflammatory pannus growing over the articular surface from its periphery, and replacement by fibrovascular tissue. (Courtesy of Michael J. Klein, MD, New York.)

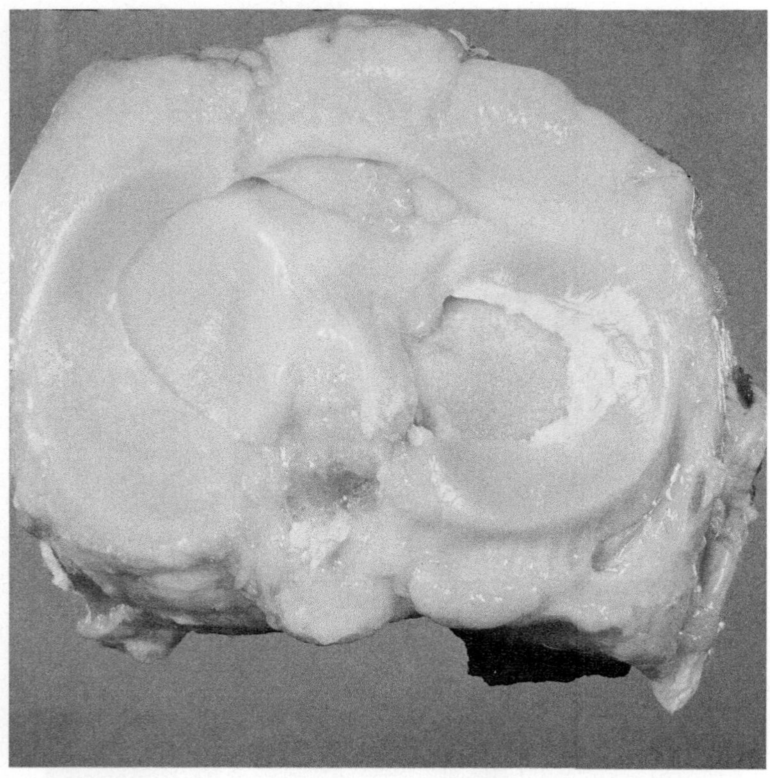

FIGURE 12.31 Pathology of calcium pyrophosphate crystal deposition disease. Gross specimen of the knee shows deposit of the CPPD within the lateral semilunar cartilage (meniscus). (Reprinted with permission from American Registry of Pathology, from Klein MJ, Bonar SF, Freemont T, et al. *Atlas of nontumor pathology. Non-neoplastic diseases of bones and joints*. Washington, DC: American Registry of Pathology and Armed Forces Institute of Pathology; 2011.)

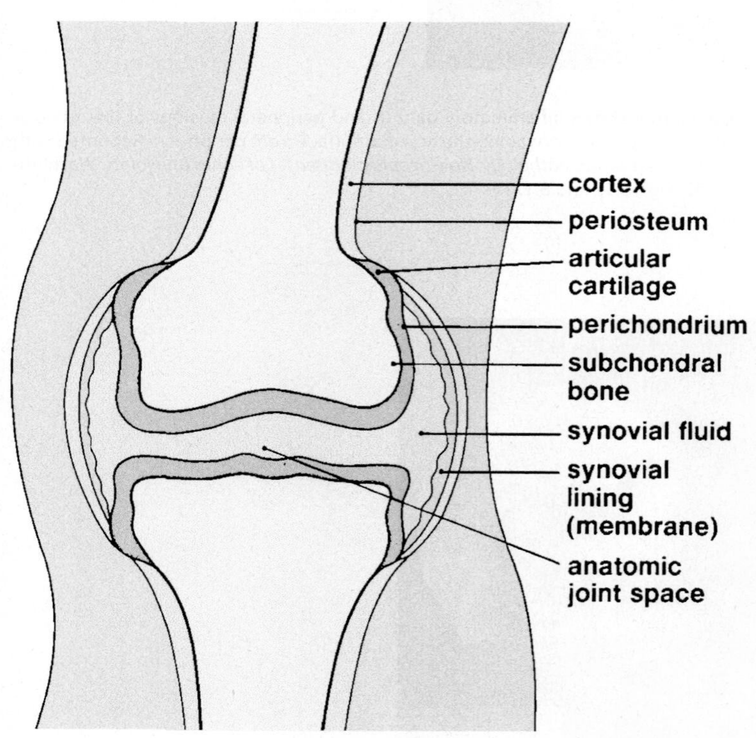

FIGURE 12.32 The constituent structures of a true or diarthrodial joint.

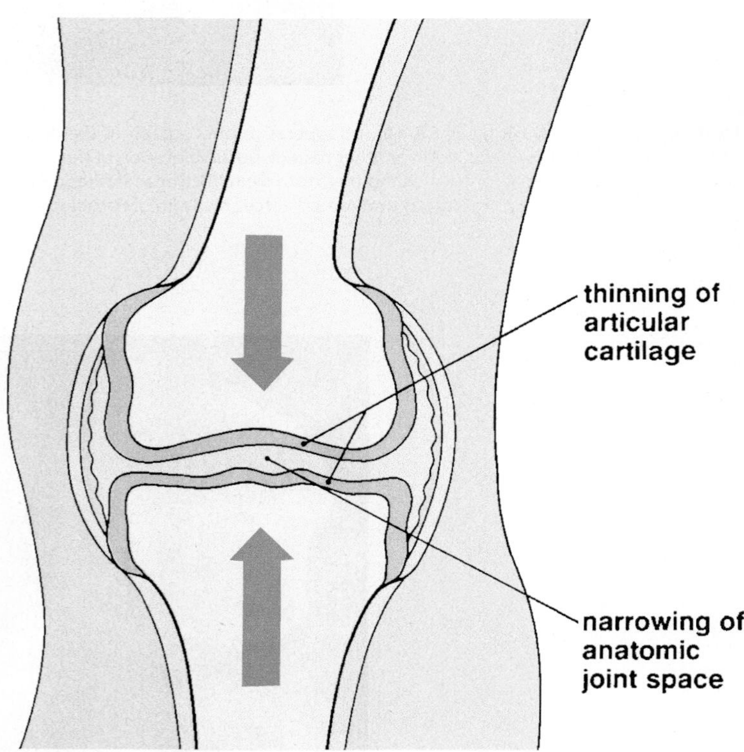

FIGURE 12.33 Narrowing of the joint space. The cardinal sign of an arthritic process is narrowing of the radiographic joint space. Thinning of the articular cartilage reduces the space mechanically.

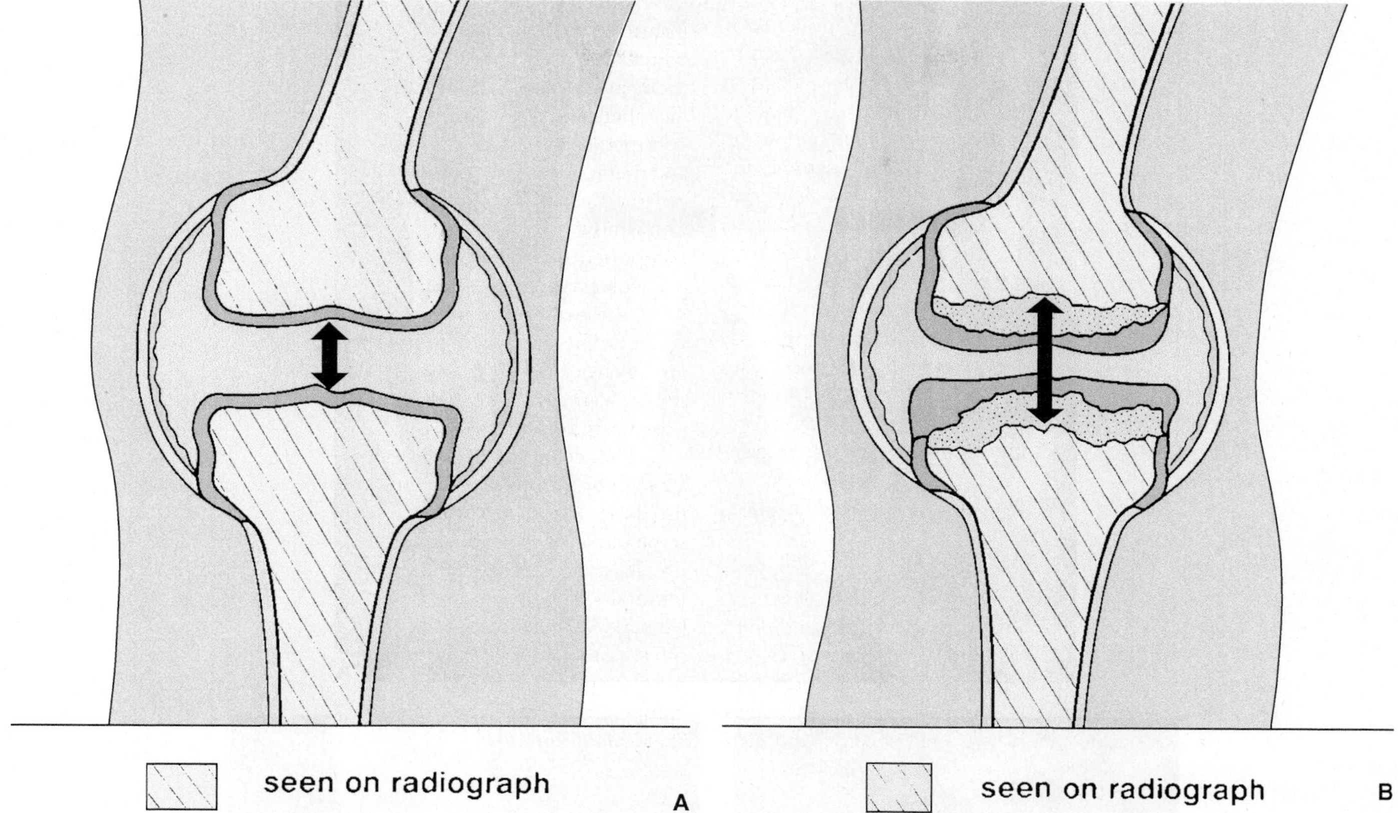

FIGURE 12.34 Variations in the width of the joint space. In the early stage of some arthritides, widening rather than narrowing of the joint space may be seen radiographically. This may be caused by distention of the joint with fluid **(A)** or erosion of the subchondral bone by granulation pannus with some preservation of the articular cartilage **(B)**.

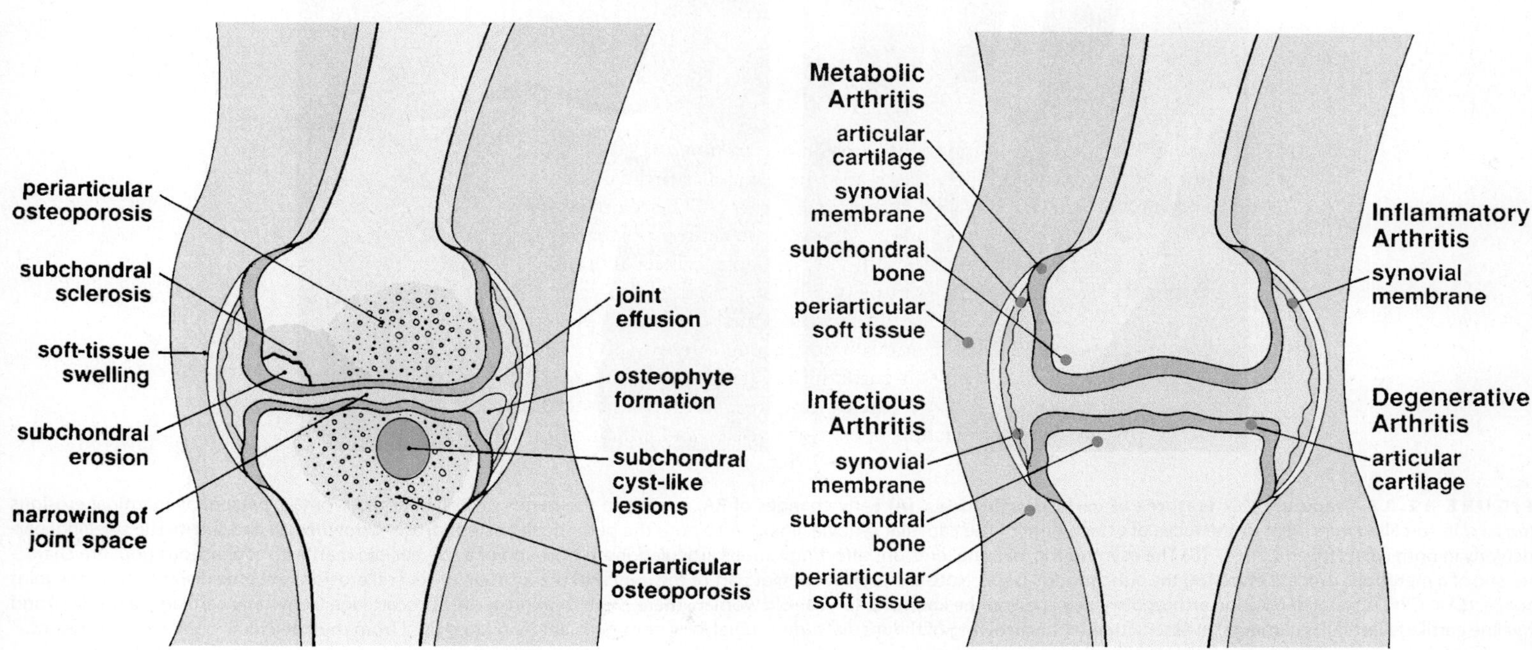

FIGURE 12.35 Radiographic features of arthritides. Summary representation of radiographic features seen in the arthritides. Not all of these features are seen in every type of arthritis.

FIGURE 12.36 Target sites of various arthritides in a joint.

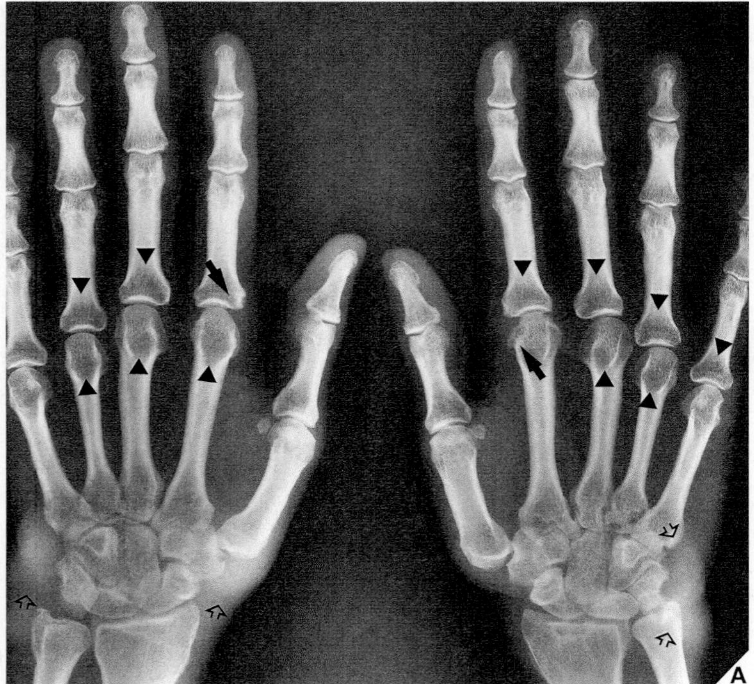

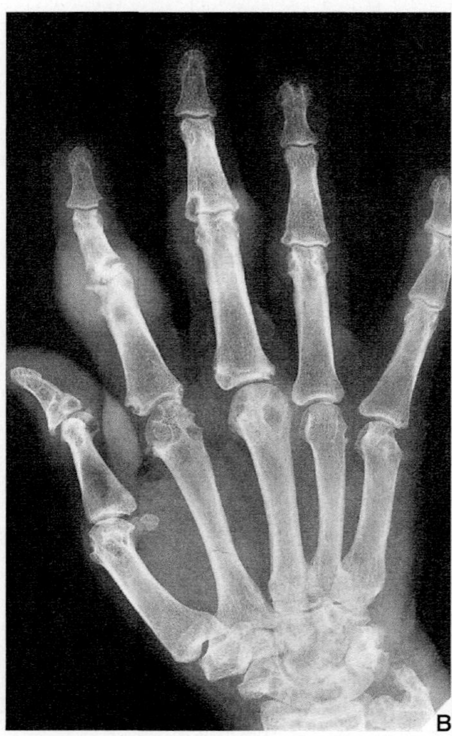

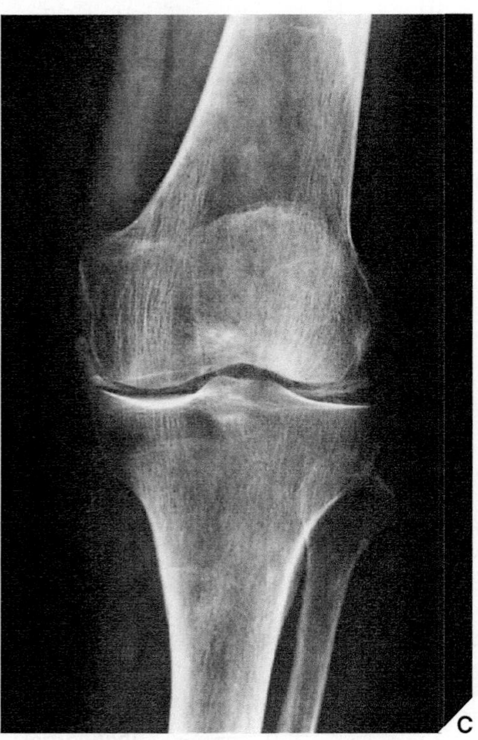

FIGURE 12.37 Radiographic features of various arthritides. (A) Early changes of RA, as seen in the hands of a 40-year-old woman, present as marginal erosions *(arrows)* in so-called *bare areas* at the locus of attachment of the capsular synovial lining. Also note the periarticular osteoporosis *(arrowheads)* and soft-tissue swelling, particularly in both wrists *(open arrows)*. **(B)** The asymmetric marginal erosions affecting various articulations in the hand of a 38-year-old man with tophaceous gout are characteristic of a metabolic process involving the subchondral bone. Note the preservation of part of the joint and the location of several erosions at some distance from the joint space. **(C)** In CPPD crystal deposition arthropathy, seen here in the knee of a 45-year-old woman, there is calcification of the fibrocartilage (semilunar cartilage or menisci) and hyaline cartilage (articular cartilage) in association with narrowing of the medial femorotibial joint compartment. Aspirated fluid from the knee joint yielded CPPD crystals.

inflammatory arthritis (Fig. 12.37A); the synovial membrane, subchondral bone, and periarticular soft tissues, as in infectious arthritis (see Fig. 25.23); or the synovial membrane, articular cartilage, subchondral bone, and periarticular soft tissues, as in some metabolic arthropathies (Fig. 12.37B,C).

The radiographic diagnosis of arthritis, as Resnick observed, is based on the evaluation of two fundamental parameters: the *morphology* of the articular lesion and its *distribution* in the skeleton. If these findings are combined with the history, physical examination, and relevant laboratory data in a given case, then the accuracy of the diagnosis is markedly improved.

Morphology of the Articular Lesion

The various arthritides exhibit morphologically distinct features, as observed radiographically in the large (Fig. 12.38) and small (Fig. 12.39) joints. In the degenerative form of the disease known as *osteoarthritis* (osteoarthrosis), thinning of the articular cartilage results in localized narrowing of the joint space; there is also subchondral sclerosis and osteophyte and cyst formation, but generally osteoporosis is absent (Fig. 12.40). *EOA* is characterized by central articular erosions and marginal proliferation of bone assuming the so-called *gull-wing deformity*

RADIOGRAPHIC MORPHOLOGY OF ARTHRITIDES IN A LARGE JOINT

Osteoarthritis

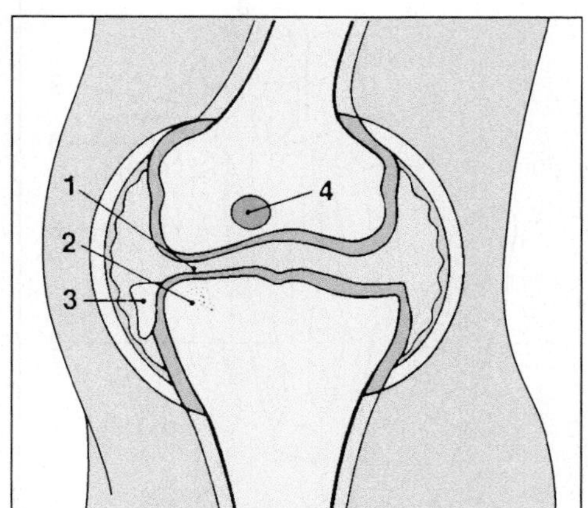

1 localized joint-space narrowing
2 subchondral sclerosis
3 osteophytes
4 cyst or pseudocyst

Inflammatory Arthritis (Rheumatoid Arthritis)

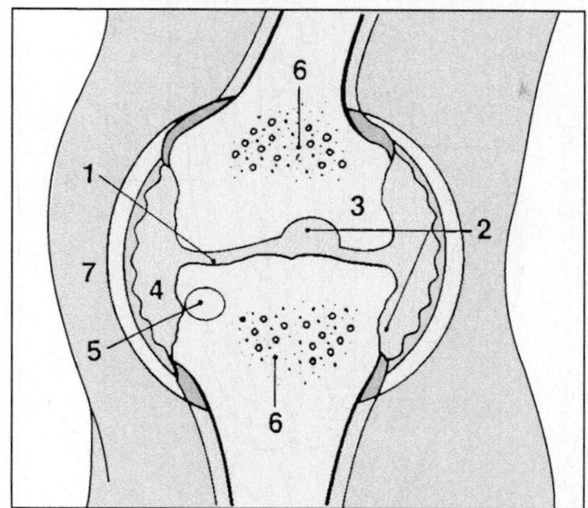

1 diffuse joint-space narrowing
2 marginal or central erosions
3 absent or minimal subchondral sclerosis
4 lack of osteophytes
5 cystic lesions
6 osteoporosis
7 periarticular soft-tissue swelling (symmetric, usually fusiform)

Metabolic Arthritis (Gout)

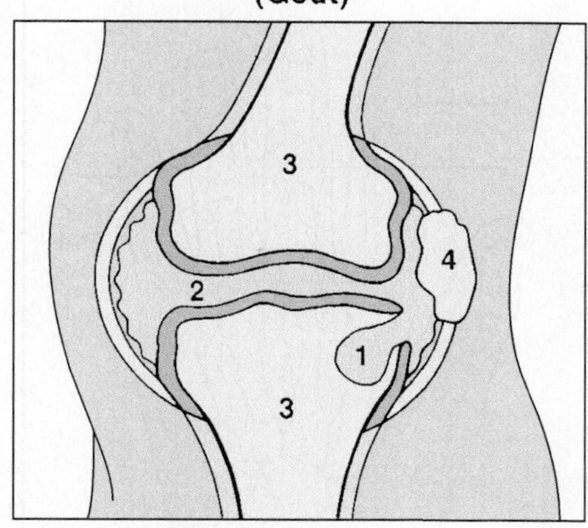

1 marginal erosion with overhanging edge
2 partial preservation of joint space
3 lack of osteoporosis
4 lobulated, asymmetric soft tissue mass

Infectious Arthritis

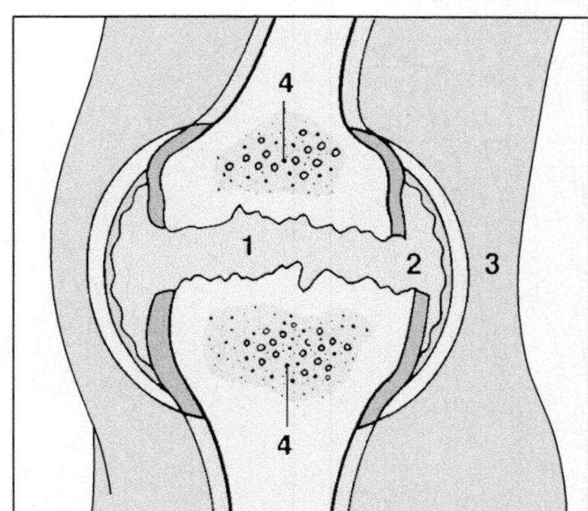

1 destruction of joint space
2 joint effusion
3 soft-tissue swelling
4 osteoporosis

Neuropathic Joint

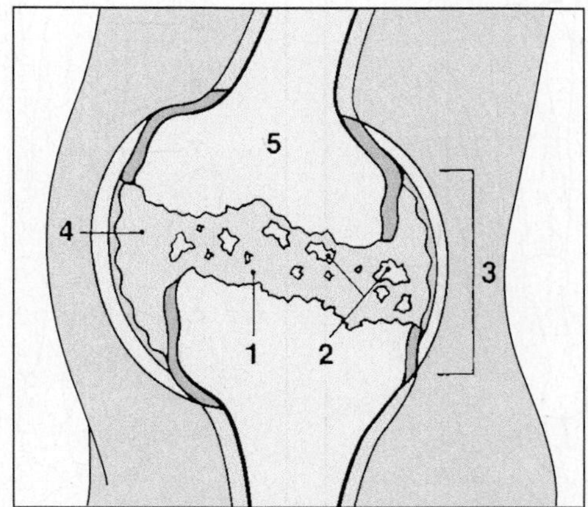

1 destruction of joint with gross disorganization
2 bony debris
3 joint instability
4 joint effusion
5 (usual) lack of osteoporosis

FIGURE 12.38 Morphologic features distinguishing the various arthritides in a large joint.

RADIOGRAPHIC MORPHOLOGY OF ARTHRITIDES IN THE HAND

Osteoarthritis

1 Heberden nodes
2 Bouchard nodes
3 joint space narrowing
4 subchondral sclerosis

Erosive Osteoarthritis

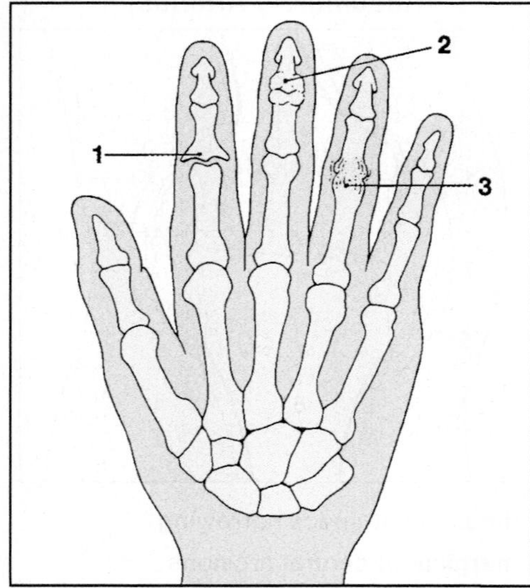

1 gull-wing erosion
2 Heberden nodes (occasionally)
3 interphalangeal ankylosis

Rheumatoid Arthritis

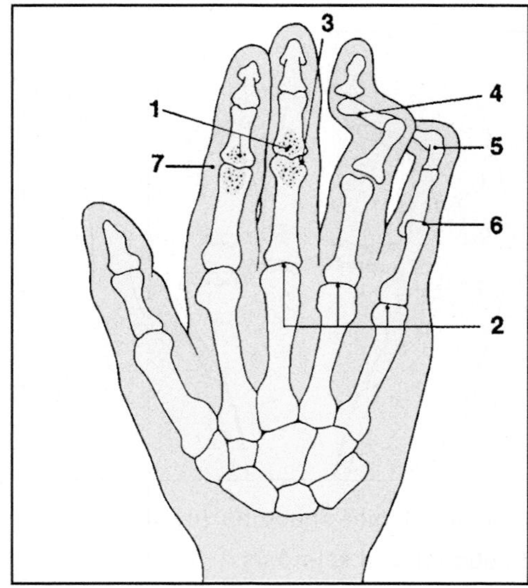

1 periarticular osteoporosis
2 joint space narrowing
3 marginal erosions
4 boutonniére deformity
5 swan-neck deformity
6 subluxations and dislocations
7 soft-tissue swelling (symmetric, fusiform)

Gouty Arthritis

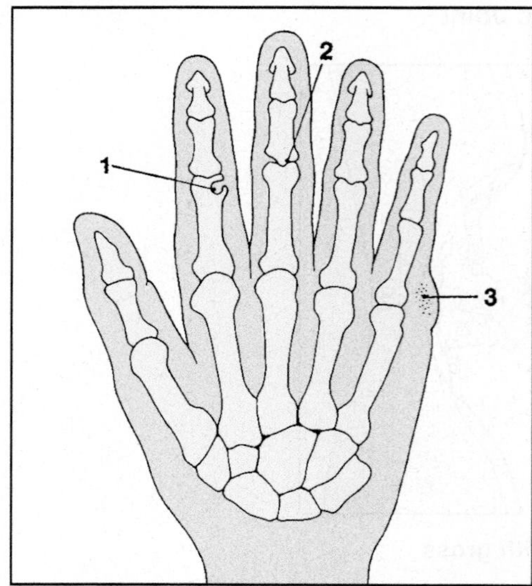

1 asymmetric erosion with overhanging edge
2 partial preservation of joint space
3 asymmetric soft-tissue swelling with or without calcifications (tophus) (usually at dorsal aspect)

Psoriatic Arthritis

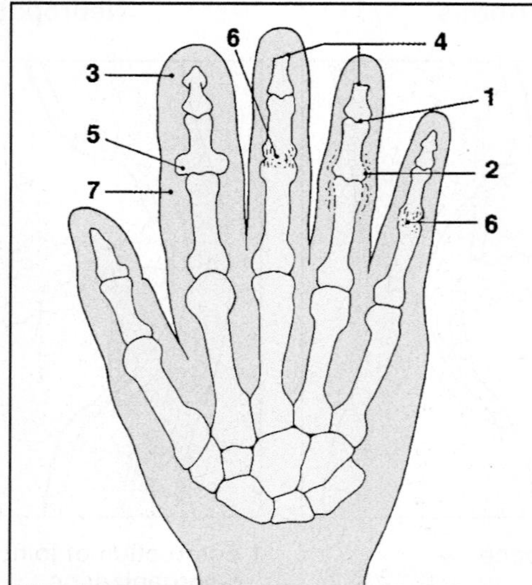

1 joint space narrowing
2 fluffy periostitis
3 "sausage digit" (soft tissue swelling of single digit)
4 erosion of terminal tufts
5 "mouse-ear" type of articular erosion
6 interphalangeal ankylosis
7 soft-tissue swelling

Lupus Arthritis

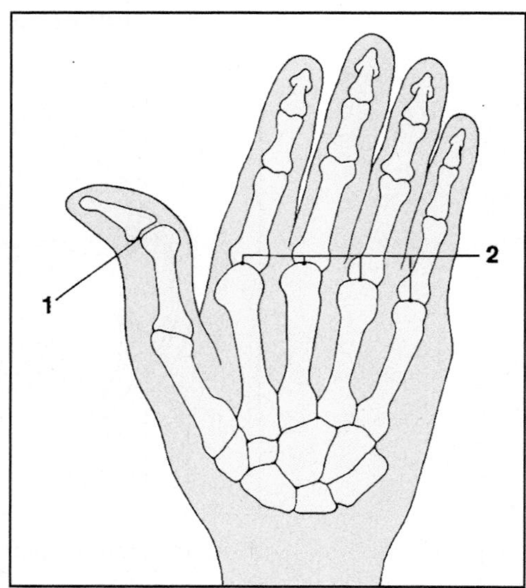

1 hitchhiker's thumb deformity
2 flexible deformities (subluxations)

FIGURE 12.39 Morphologic features distinguishing the various arthritides in the small joints of the hand.

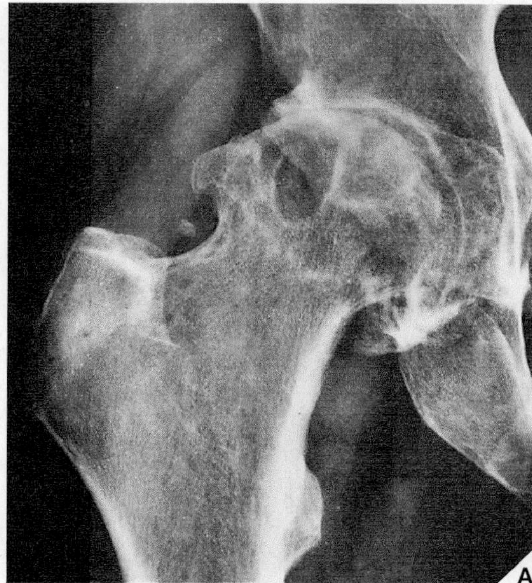

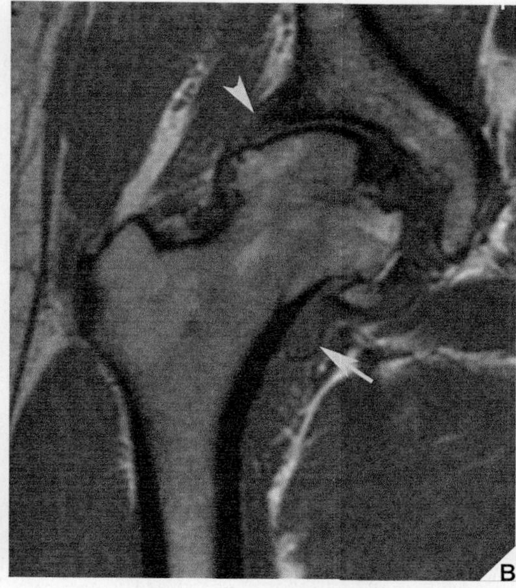

FIGURE 12.40 Osteoarthritis. **(A)** Conventional radiograph of the hip demonstrates the typical morphologic changes seen in degenerative joint disease (OA): focal narrowing of the joint space (here at the weight-bearing segment), subchondral sclerosis, cyst-like lesions, and marginal osteophytes. Note the lack of osteoporosis. **(B)** Coronal T1-weighted MRI demonstrates superior joint space narrowing secondary to the loss of articular cartilage, marginal osteophytes at the femoral head/neck junction and around the fovea capitis, joint effusion *(arrow)*, and degeneration and tearing of the superior acetabular labrum *(arrowhead)*.

(Fig. 12.41). *Inflammatory arthritides*, such as RA, are characterized by a diffuse, usually multicompartmental narrowing of the joint space associated with marginal or central erosions, periarticular osteoporosis, and symmetric periarticular soft-tissue swelling; subchondral sclerosis is minimal or absent, and formation of osteophytes is lacking (Fig. 12.42). In a *metabolic arthropathies* such as gout, well-defined osseous erosions displaying a so-called *overhanging edge* are usually associated with preservation of part of the joint space and a localized, asymmetric soft-tissue nodules; osteophyte formation and osteoporosis are absent (Fig. 12.43). *Infectious arthritis* is characterized by the complete destruction of both articular ends of the bones forming the joint; all communicating joint compartments are invariably involved, with diffuse osteoporosis, joint effusion, and periarticular soft-tissue swelling (Fig. 12.44; see also Fig. 25.24A). *Neuropathic arthritis* is marked by destruction of the articular surfaces, which leaves bony debris, and a substantial joint effusion; osteoporosis is usually lacking. Depending on the amount of destruction, varying degrees of joint instability are present (Fig. 12.45).

Analysis of the morphologic features of an arthritic lesion at certain sites other than the diarthrodial joints may be of further assistance in differentiating the various arthritides and reaching a correct diagnosis. Two such sites that are frequently affected are the heel and the spine. In the heel (Fig. 12.46), degenerative changes are usually manifested by a traction osteophyte at the posterior and plantar aspects of the calcaneus (Fig. 12.47A). RA produces erosive changes in the area of the retrocalcaneal bursa secondary to inflammatory rheumatoid bursitis (Fig. 12.47B). Psoriatic arthritis (Fig. 12.47C), reactive arthritis (Fig. 12.47D), and AS all produce a characteristic "fluffy" periostitis that results in a broad-based osteophyte at the site of attachment of the fascia plantaris on the plantar aspect of the calcaneus, associated with erosions of the plantar surface and the posterior aspect of this bone.

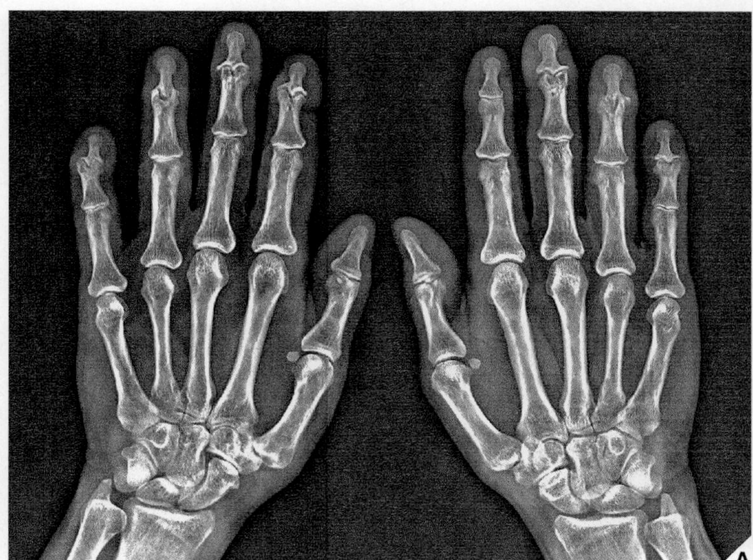

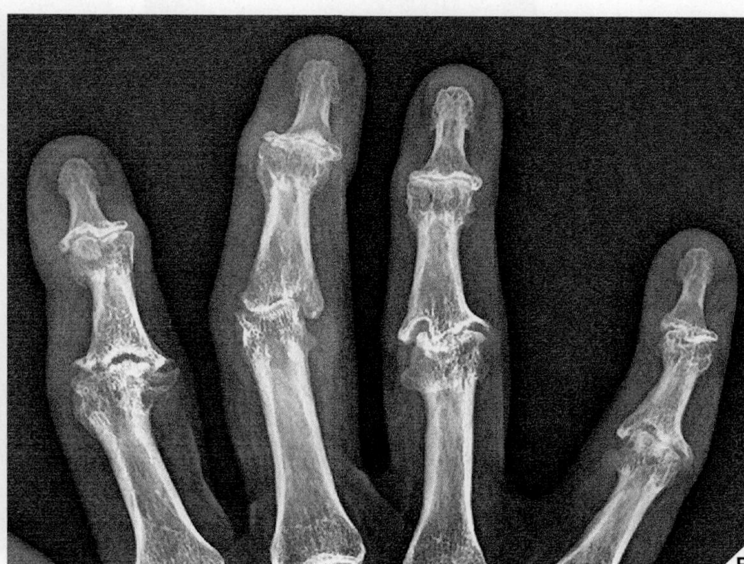

FIGURE 12.41 Erosive OA. **(A)** Dorsovolar radiograph of both hands of a 59-year-old woman who presented with long history of joint pains shows erosions of the distal interphalangeal joints with typical "gull-wing" configuration due to central erosions and peripheral osseous proliferation. **(B)** In another patient, a 63-year-old woman, the characteristic gull-wing erosions are present in the proximal and distal interphalangeal joints.

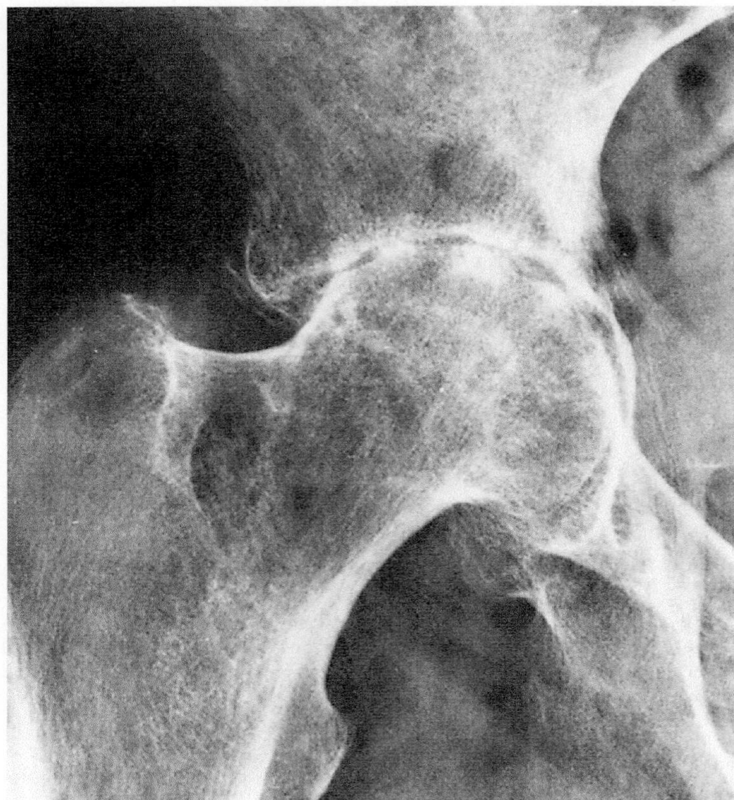

FIGURE 12.42 Rheumatoid arthritis. Inflammatory arthritis, seen here in the hip, is marked by diffuse, uniform narrowing of the joint space, axial migration of the femoral head, marginal and central subchondral erosions, and severe periarticular osteoporosis. Note the almost total absence of reactive subchondral sclerosis and the lack of osteophyte formation.

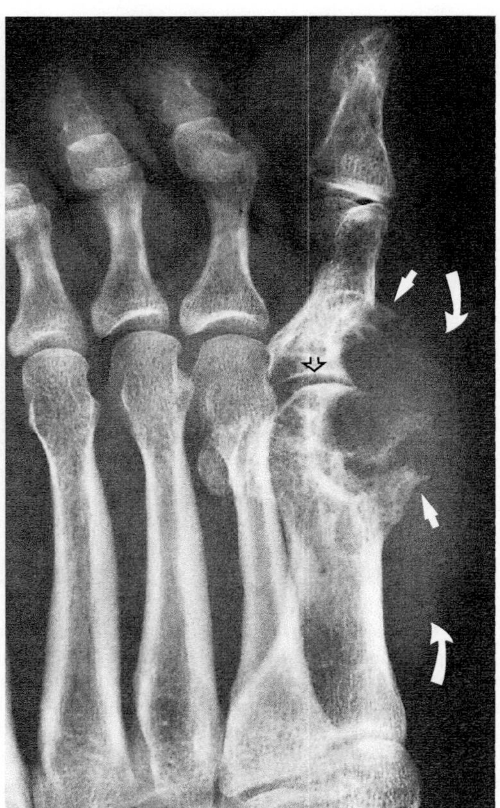

FIGURE 12.43 Gouty arthritis. Asymmetric periarticular erosions that spare part of the joint are typical of gouty arthritis, seen here involving the first metatarsophalangeal joint of the right foot. Note the characteristic overhanging edge at the site of erosion *(arrows)* and the soft-tissue mass representing a tophus *(curved arrows)*; osteophytes and osteoporosis are absent, and the joint is partially preserved *(open arrow)*.

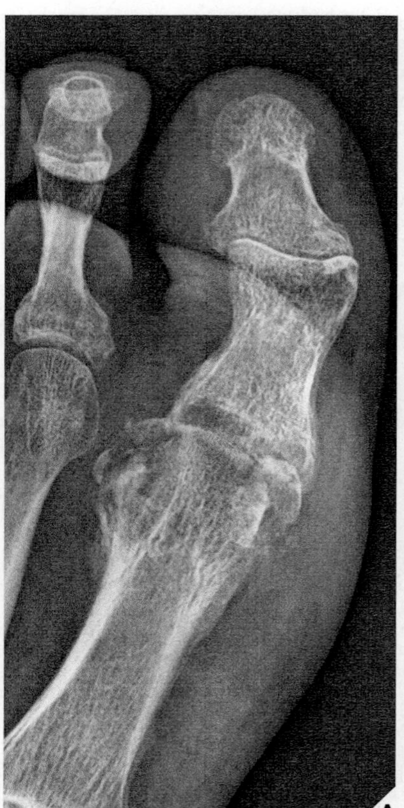

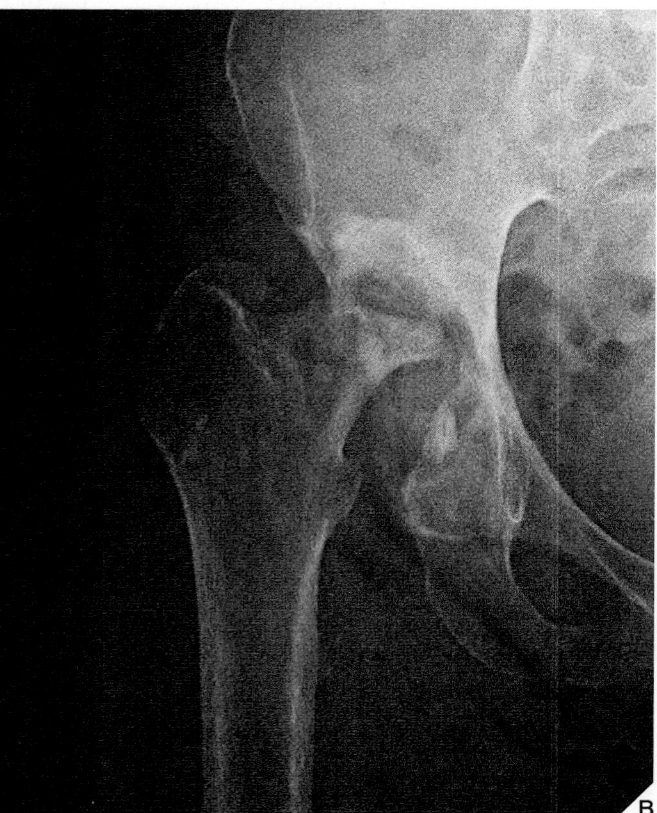

FIGURE 12.44 Infectious arthritis. **(A)** A 48-year-old diabetic man presented with pain and soft-tissue swelling of the right big toe for the past 3 months. Anteroposterior radiograph shows destruction of the first metatarsophalangeal joint associated with soft-tissue swelling and edema typical for septic arthritis. **(B)** In another patient, a 45-year-old human immunodeficiency virus (HIV)-positive man, who presented with a history of right hip joint pain for several months, anteroposterior radiograph shows extensive destruction of the right femoral head and neck and right acetabulum consistent with septic arthritis. Hip joint aspiration and culture revealed methicillin-resistant *Staphylococcus aureus* (MRSA) infection.

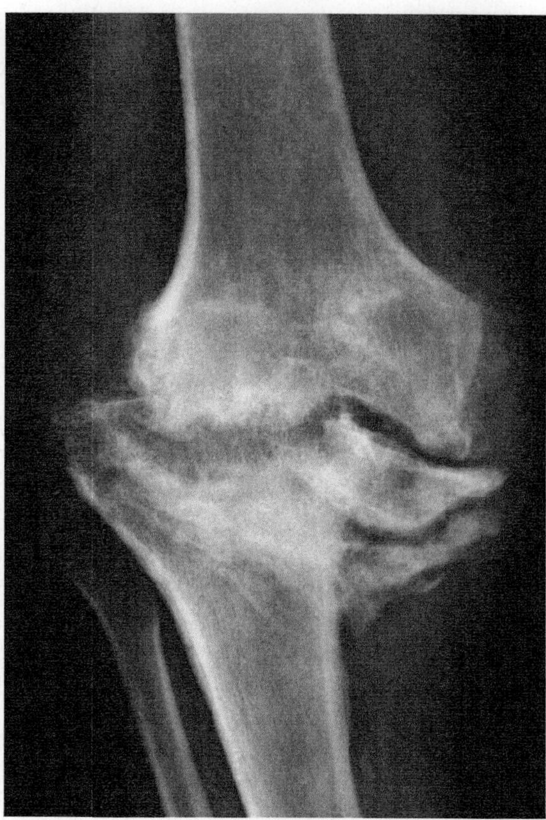

FIGURE 12.45 Neuropathic joint. The neuropathic joint is morphologically identified by gross articular disorganization, multiple bony debris, and joint effusion, as seen here in the knee. Note the lack of osteoporosis. The amount of destruction evident in this case results in severe joint instability.

RADIOGRAPHIC MORPHOLOGY OF ARTHRITIDES IN THE HEEL

Degenerative Arthritis

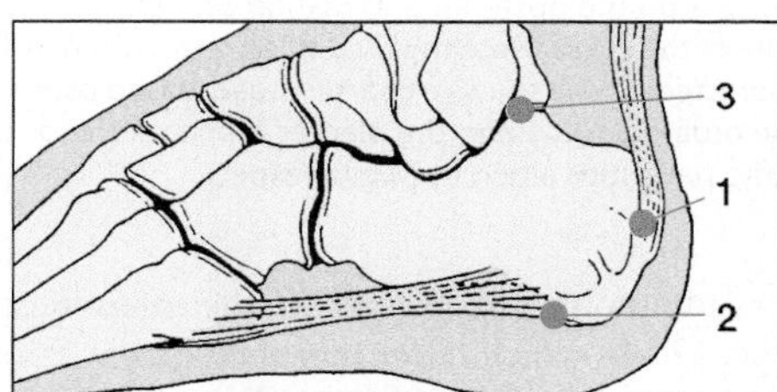

traction osteophytes at
1 posterior aspect of os calcis (insertion of Achilles tendon) and
2 plantar aspect of os calcis (insertion of fascia plantaris)
3 osteophytes at the posterior facet of subtalar joint

Rheumatoid Arthritis

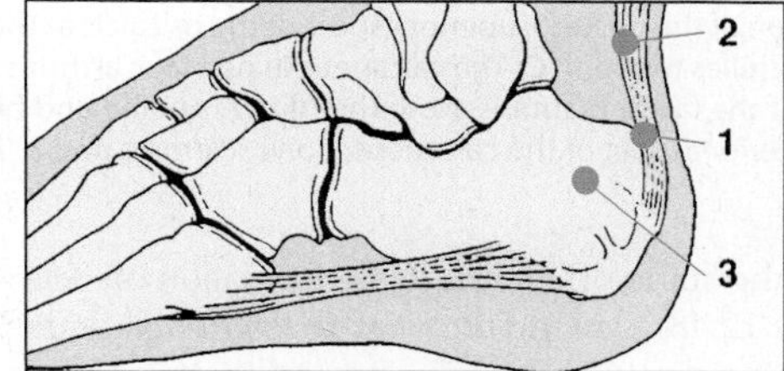

1 erosion at posterosuperior aspect of os calcis (secondary to retrocalcaneal bursitis)
2 thickening of Achilles tendon
3 focal osteoporosis

Psoriatic Arthritis, Ankylosing Spondylitis, and Reactive Arthritis

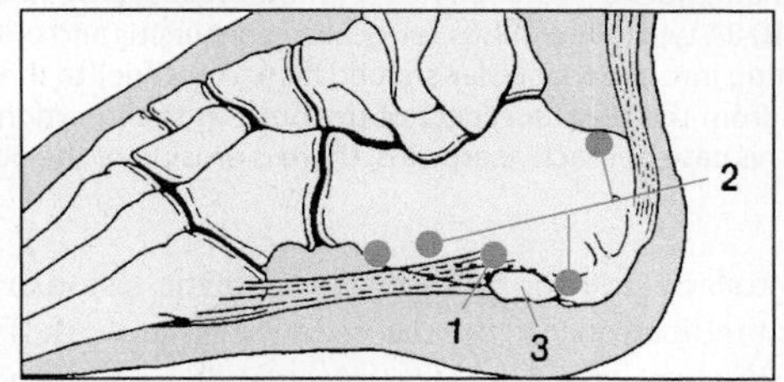

1 fluffy periostitis
2 erosions at posterior aspect of os calcis above attachment of Achilles tendon, at attachment of plantar fascia, and at plantar surface of os calcis anterior to aponeurotic attachment
3 broad-based osteophyte

FIGURE 12.46 Arthritic changes in the heel. Morphologic features distinguishing the various arthritides as manifest in arthritic lesions at the heel.

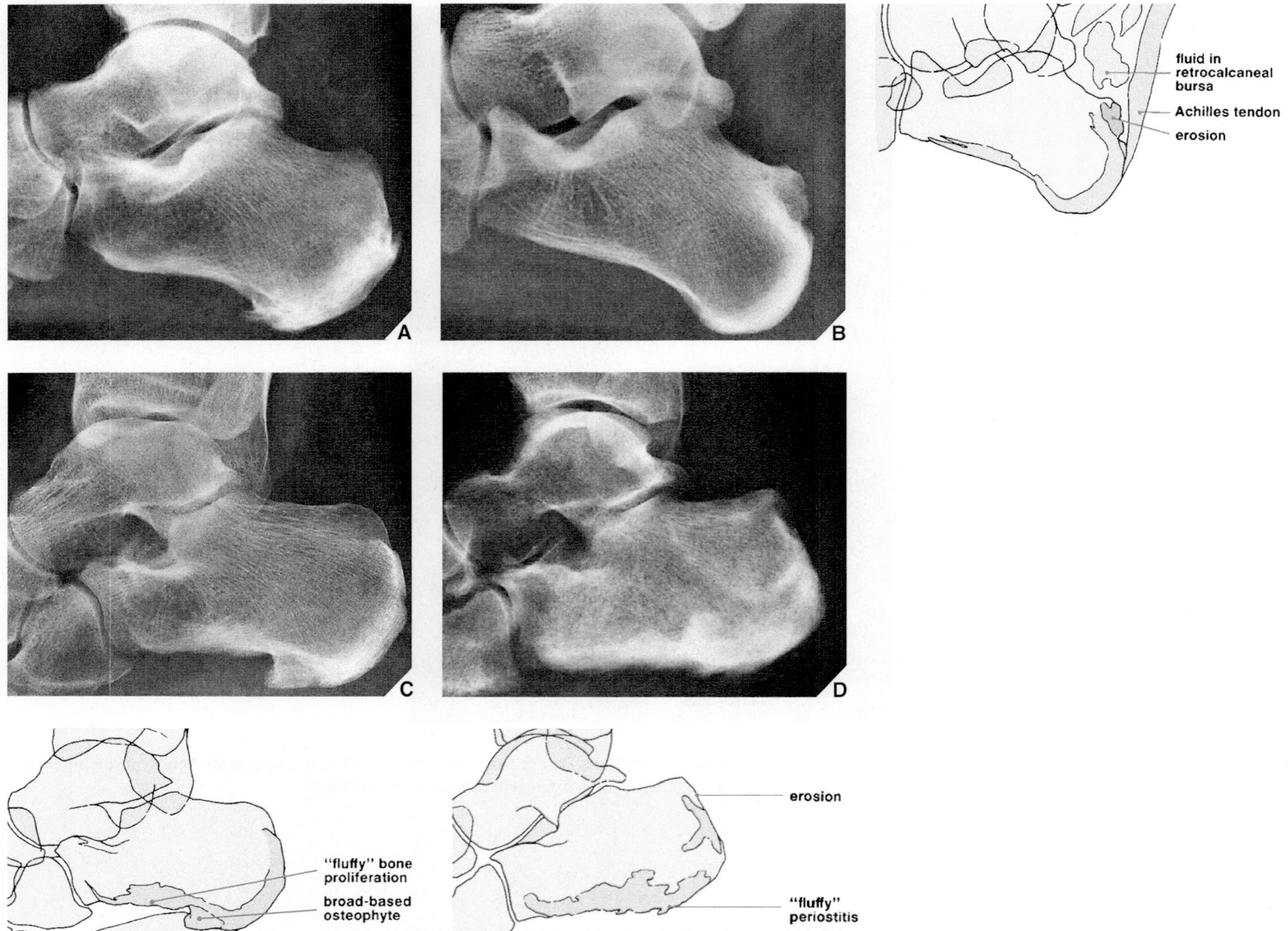

FIGURE 12.47 **Arthritic changes in the heel.** The morphology of arthritic lesions in the heel can be helpful in differentiating the various arthritides. **(A)** In the degenerative variant, traction osteophytes (enthesophytes) are evident at the insertions of the Achilles tendon and fascia plantaris on the posterior and plantar aspects of the calcaneus. **(B)** RA typically exhibits retrocalcaneal bursitis and erosion of the posterosuperior aspect of the os calcis at the site of the bursa. Note the fluid-filled retrocalcaneal bursa projecting into the triangular-shaped fat pad anterior to the Achilles tendon. **(C)** The calcaneus in psoriatic arthritis characteristically shows a coarse, broad-based osteophyte arising from the plantar aspect of the bone at the insertion of the fascia plantaris. Note the "fluffy" outline and bone proliferation along the plantar aspect of the os calcis. **(D)** In this case of reactive arthritis, there is erosion of the posterior aspect of the calcaneus, bone sclerosis, and a "fluffy" periostitis along its plantar aspect.

Similarly, the morphology of arthritic lesions in the spine offers important indications of the disease process at work (Fig. 12.48). Among the inflammatory arthritides, for instance, RA causes a characteristic erosion of the odontoid process (Fig. 12.49). Moreover, as a result of inflammatory pannus and erosion of the transverse ligament between the anterior arch of the atlas and C2, there may be subluxation in the atlantoaxial joint. This is usually manifested by an increase to more than 3 mm in the distance between the arch of the atlas and the dens, as demonstrated on a lateral view of the cervical spine in flexion (Fig. 12.50). Erosion of the apophyseal joints of the cervical spine, sometimes leading to fusion, is frequently seen in juvenile idiopathic arthritis (JIA) (Fig. 12.51).

Arthritic lesions involving other segments of the spine also exhibit distinguishing features that help in differentiating the disease process. Degenerative changes may manifest in the cervical, thoracic, or lumbar (Fig. 12.52) spine by the appearance of marginal osteophytes, narrowing and sclerosis of the apophyseal joints and narrowing of the disk spaces. In AS, in the early stages of the disease, there is a characteristic "squaring" of the vertebral bodies associated with sclerotic changes at the anterior aspect at the site of anterior longitudinal ligament due to osteitis (anterior spondylitis) and secondary reactive bone formation, as well as small erosions at the corners of the vertebral bodies, at the site of attachment of the annulus fibrosus to the vertebral end plate, surrounded by reactive sclerosis and osseous proliferation, so-called *shiny corners* or *Romanus lesion* (Fig. 12.53). This follows the formation of delicate syndesmophytes arising from the anterior aspects of the vertebral bodies (Fig. 12.54), which differ morphologically from degenerative osteophytes. In the later stages of this condition, inflammation and fusion of the apophyseal joints lead to the appearance of what has been called *bamboo spine*; the sacroiliac joints are also invariably affected (Fig. 12.55). In psoriasis and reactive arthritis, one can occasionally see a single, coarse osteophyte/syndesmophyte in the lumbar spine, frequently bridging adjacent vertebral bodies as well as paravertebral ossifications; there are also associated inflammatory changes in the sacroiliac joints (Fig. 12.56).

Distribution of the Articular Lesion

OA tends to have a characteristic distribution in the skeletal system. Typically, the large joints such as the hip and knee and the small joints of the hand and wrist are involved, whereas the shoulder, elbow, and ankle are spared (Fig. 12.57). Inflammatory arthritides, however, have different sites of predilection in the skeleton, depending on the specific variant of the disease. RA, for example, involves most of the large joints such as the hip, knee, elbows, and shoulders. In the hand, the metacarpophalangeal and proximal interphalangeal joints are commonly affected. In the cervical spine the C1-2 articulation and the apophyseal joints are frequently affected. JIA has a similar pattern of distribution, except that the distal interphalangeal joints of the hand may also be affected. Psoriatic arthritis, in contrast to RA, has a predilection for the distal interphalangeal joints, as well as the

RADIOGRAPHIC MORPHOLOGY OF ARTHRITIDES IN THE SPINE

Rheumatoid Arthritis

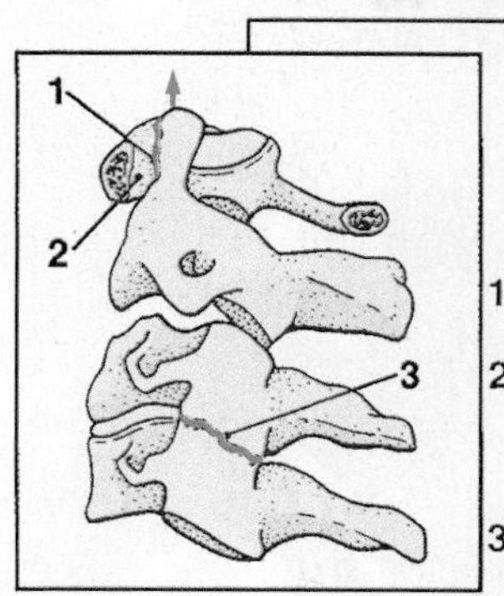

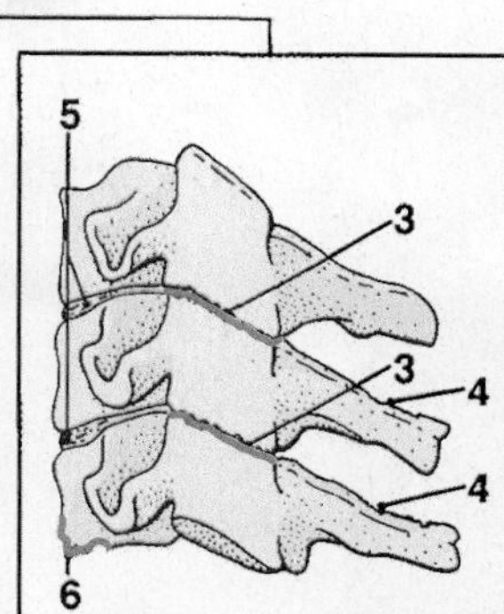

Degenerative Spine Disease

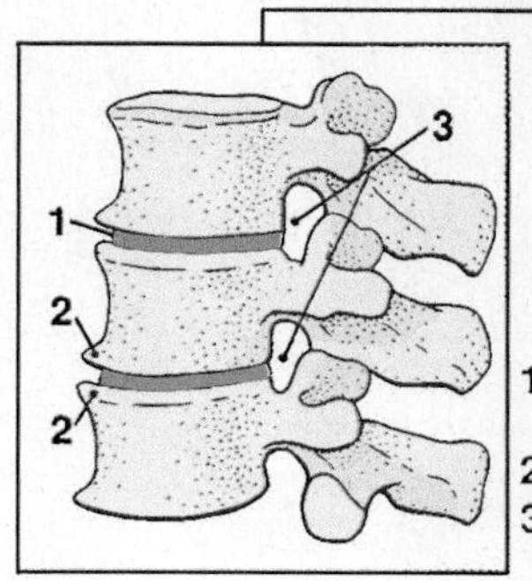

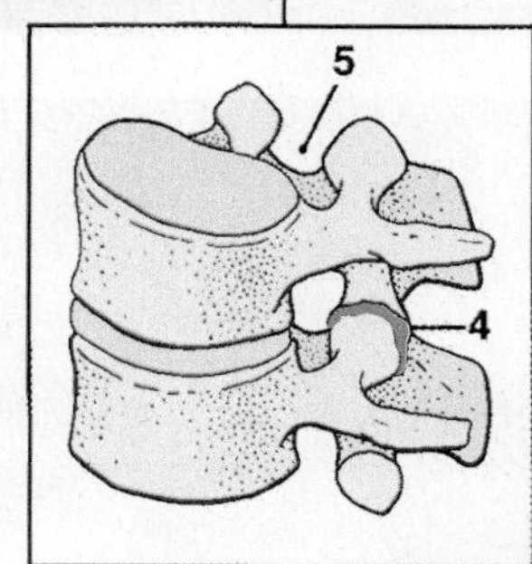

Ankylosing Spondylitis

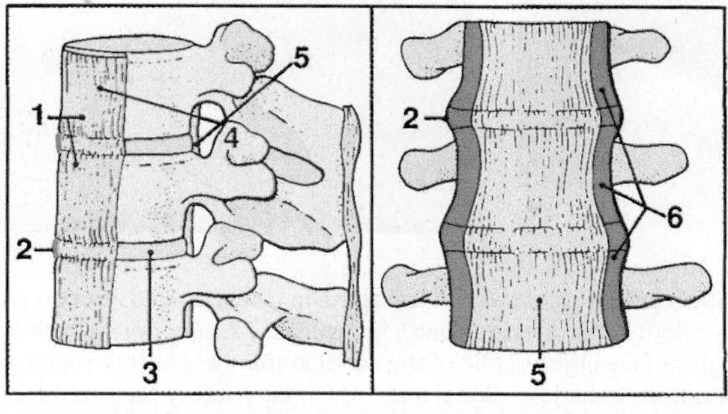

Psoriatic Arthritis and Reactive Arthritis

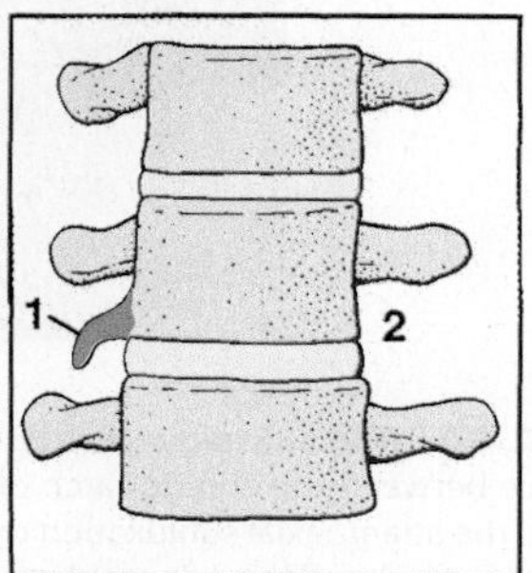

FIGURE 12.48 **Arthritides of the spine.** Morphologic features distinguishing the various arthritides as manifested in the spine.

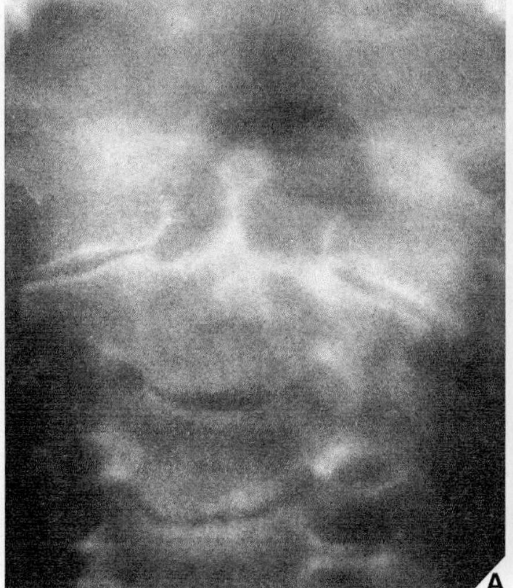

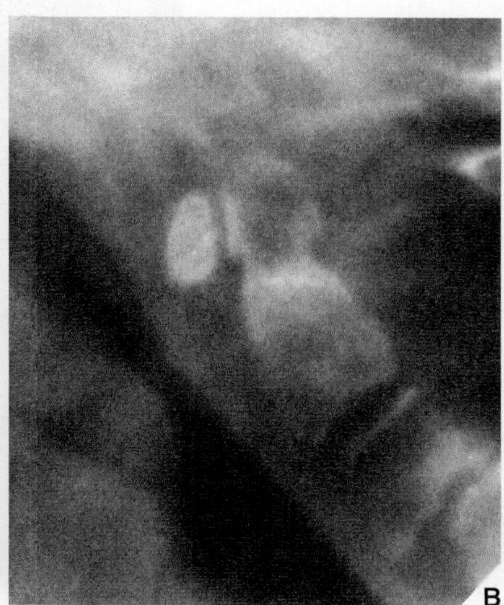

FIGURE 12.49 **Rheumatoid arthritis.** **(A)** Anteroposterior and **(B)** lateral trispiral tomograms of the cervical spine in a 55-year-old woman with a 15-year history of RA show erosion of the odontoid process typical for this condition.

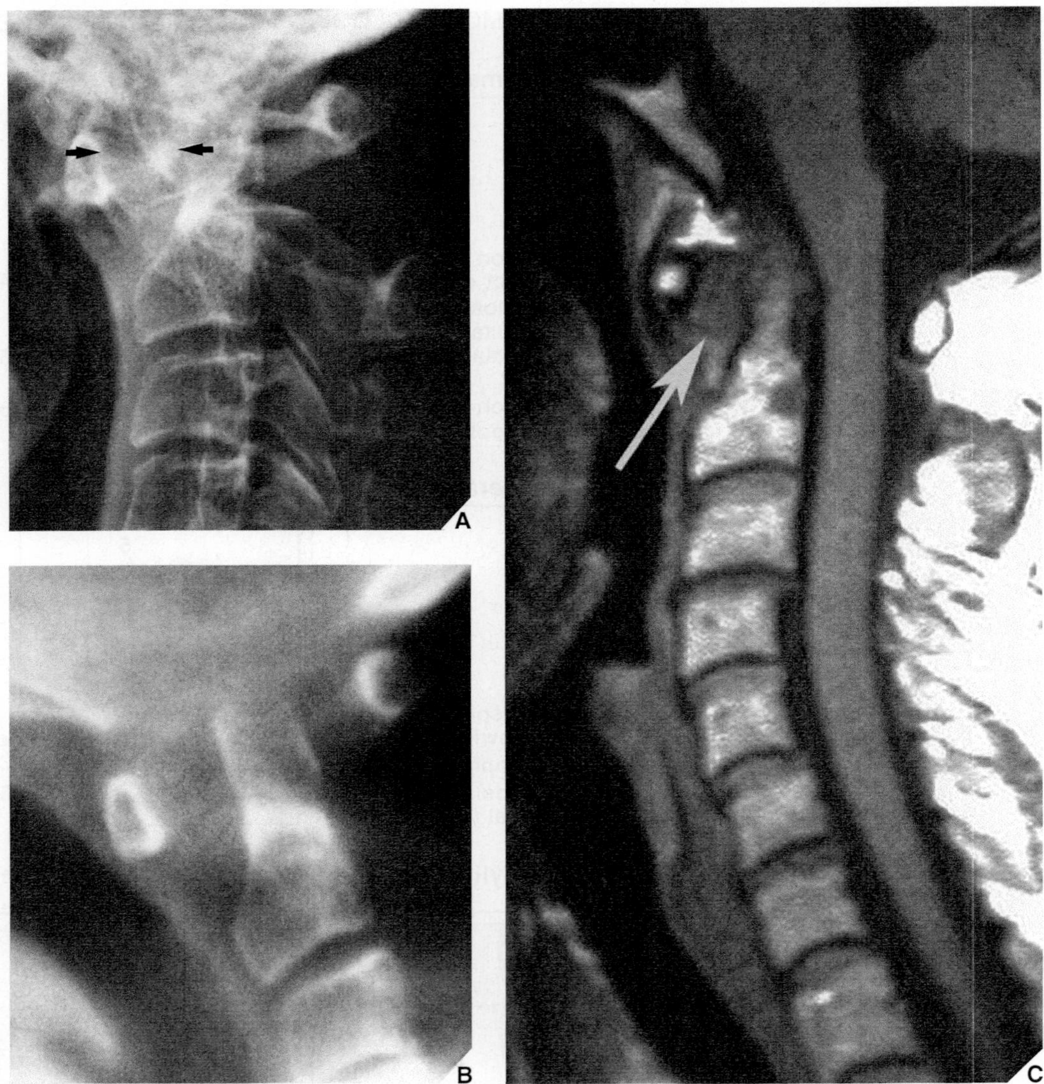

FIGURE 12.50 Rheumatoid arthritis. (A) Lateral radiograph in flexion of the cervical spine in a 68-year-old woman with a long history of RA shows a marked increase in the distance between the anterior arch of the atlas and the odontoid process *(arrows)*, measuring 12 mm; normally, it should not exceed 3 mm. **(B)** Trispiral tomogram demonstrates the atlantoaxial subluxation more clearly. **(C)** Sagittal T1-weighted MRI of the cervical spine in another patient with RA demonstrates increased space between the anterior arch of C1 and the odontoid process, which is eroded. Note the low-signal intensity inflammatory pannus *(arrow)*.

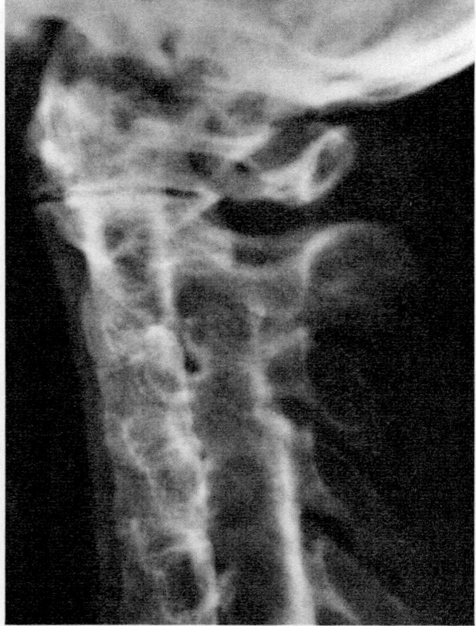

FIGURE 12.51 Juvenile idiopathic arthritis. Lateral radiograph of the cervical spine in a 34-year-old woman with JIA since age 20 shows the typical involvement of the apophyseal joints. In this case, there is complete fusion of these joints.

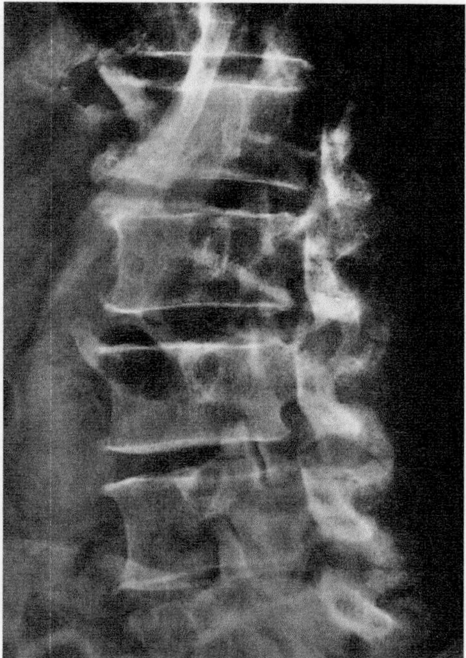

FIGURE 12.52 **Degenerative spine disease.** Oblique radiograph of the lumbar spine of a 72-year-old woman shows narrowing and eburnation of the articular margins of the facet joints, osteophytosis, and narrowing of the intervertebral disk spaces—a combination of the effects of true facet joint arthritis, spondylosis deformans, and degenerative disk disease.

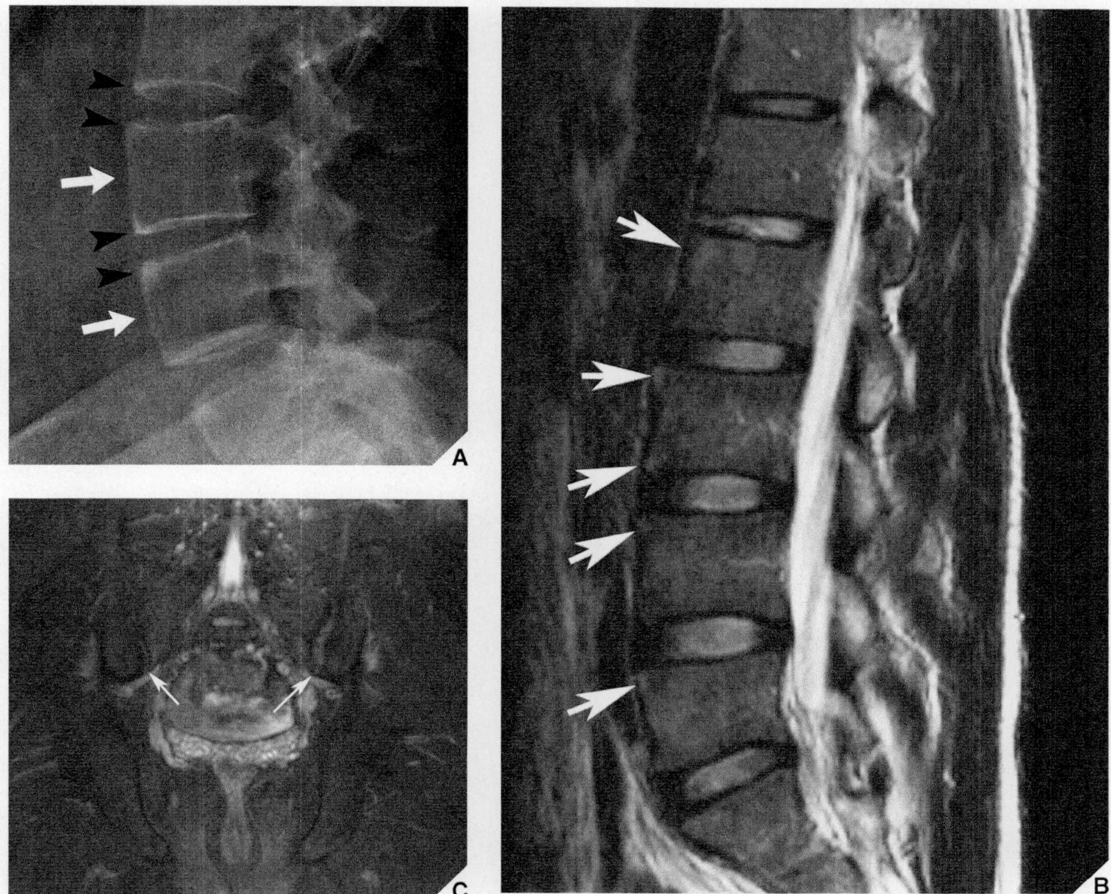

FIGURE 12.53 **AS—early changes.** **(A)** A lateral radiograph of the lower lumbar spine of a 33-year-old man shows early inflammatory changes manifesting by so-called *shiny corners* (Romanus lesion) *(arrowheads)* and squaring of the vertebral bodies *(arrows)*. **(B)** T2-weighted MRI in a 26-year-old man shows early signs of AS of the lumbar spine, the shiny corners *(arrows)*. **(C)** T2-weighted MRI of the sacroiliac joints in the same patient demonstrates bone marrow edema adjacent to the sacroiliac joints and erosive changes bilaterally, more prominent on the left *(arrows)*. (Courtesy of Luis Beltran, MD, Boston.)

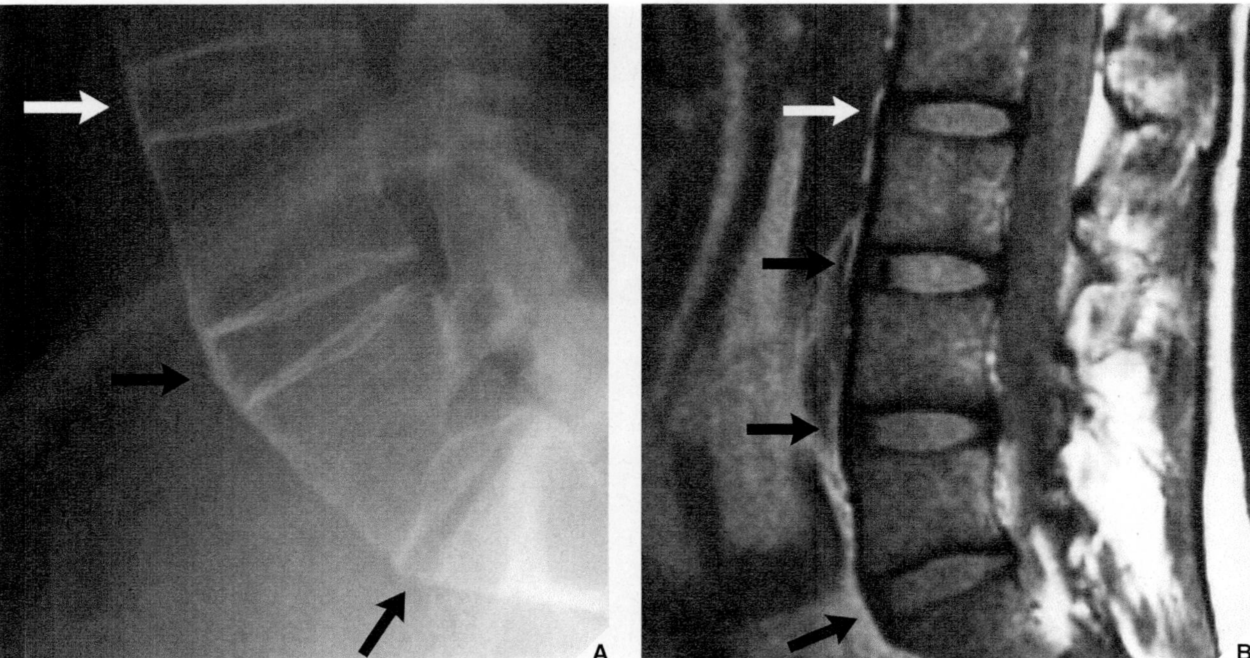

FIGURE 12.54 AS—syndesmophytes. **(A)** Lateral radiograph and **(B)** sagittal T1-weighted MR image of the lumbar spine show characteristic delicate, vertically oriented syndesmophytes *(arrows)*. Compare this inflammatory feature with degenerative coarse osteophytes in Figure 12.52.

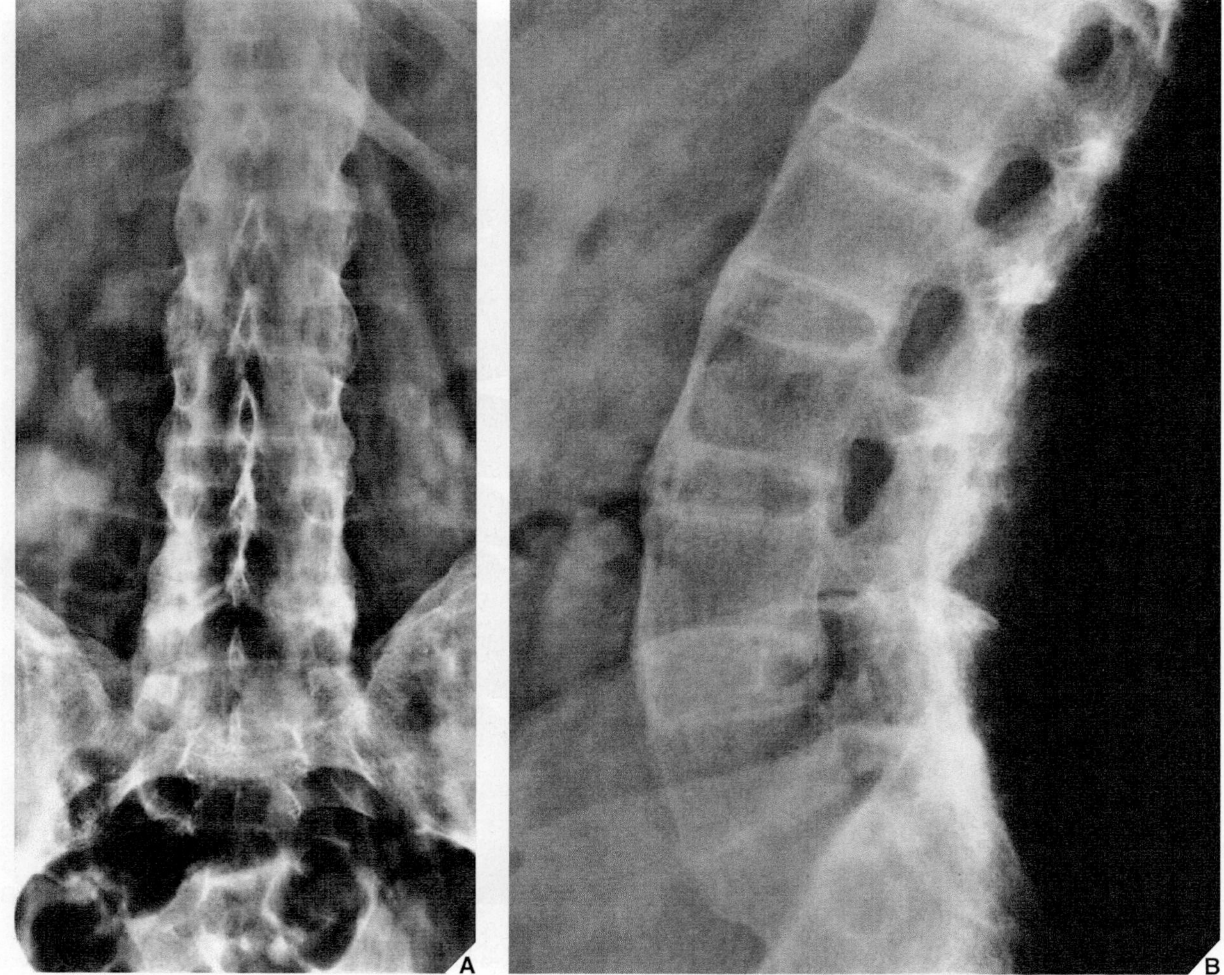

FIGURE 12.55 AS—advanced changes. **(A)** Anteroposterior and **(B)** lateral radiographs of the lumbar spine in a 31-year-old man with advanced AS demonstrate the typical appearance of "bamboo spine" secondary to inflammation, ossification, and fusion of the apophyseal joints associated with ossification of the anterior and posterior longitudinal ligaments as well as the supraspinous and interspinous ligaments. Note also the fusion of the sacroiliac joints.

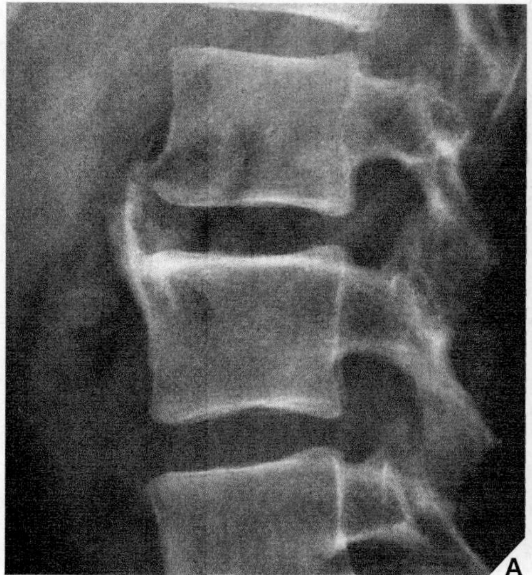

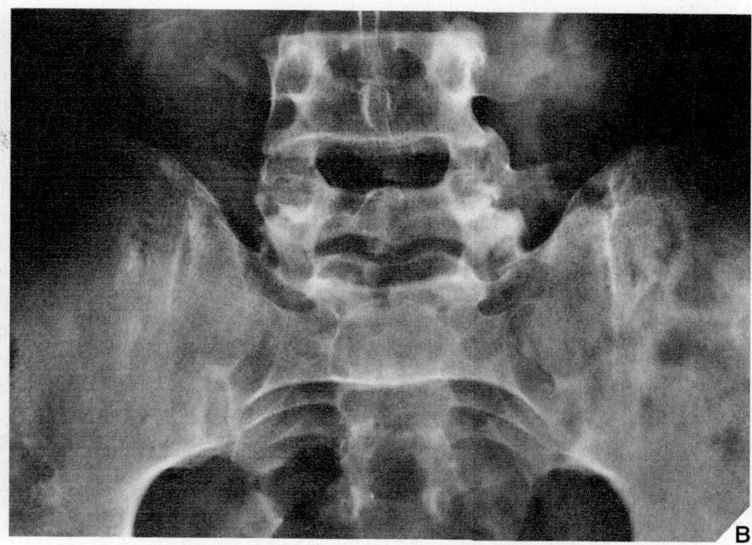

FIGURE 12.56 Reactive arthritis (Reiter syndrome). **(A)** Lateral radiograph of the lumbar spine in a 27-year-old man shows a single, coarse osteophyte/syndesmophyte bridging the bodies of L1 and L2. **(B)** Anteroposterior radiograph of the lumbosacral segment shows the effects of the inflammatory process on the sacroiliac joints (sacroiliitis).

FIGURE 12.57 Distribution of arthritic lesions in the skeleton in various arthritides.

DISTRIBUTION OF LESIONS IN VARIOUS ARTHRITIDES

Osteoarthritis

Rheumatoid Arthritis

adult

juvenile

Psoriatic Arthritis

Reactive Arthritis

asymmetric

symmetric

asymmetric

sacroiliac joints, resembling reactive arthritis in this respect (see Fig. 12.56). EOA, which some investigators consider a variant of OA, others a variant of RA, and still others a distinct form of arthritis, has a tendency to affect the proximal and distal interphalangeal joints of the hand (see Fig. 12.41).

Management

Medical Treatment

The treatment of rheumatologic diseases has undergone a revolution in the past decade. In the past, the standard model for the management of inflammatory arthritides such as RA, psoriatic arthritis, and AS was to treat with nonsteroidal antiinflammatory drugs (NSAIDs), followed by increasing use of more potent medication; this was often called a *pyramid scheme*. The current approach is to treat patients early and aggressively with disease-modifying drugs and, in particular, to include the use of the biologic drugs such as agents that inhibit tumor necrosis factor (TNF), IL-6, or CD20-bearing B cells. Discussion of these therapies is beyond the scope of this textbook, but it is important to note that the biologic drugs have a significant potential to modify disease, reduce the systemic manifestations, and slow the progression of destructive changes in the joints. They do, however, carry significant side effects and must be monitored on a regular basis. Interestingly, this is likewise the case for patients with gout. In the past, treatment consisted of antiinflammatory drugs and often the use of allopurinol. However, a whole variety of new drugs have been introduced that modulate different levels of uric acid metabolism. Treatment for CPPD crystal deposition disease associated with pseudogout syndrome is essentially the same as for gout, including oral administration of colchicine. Unfortunately, the treatment model has not significantly changed for SLE, in which there have been no significant improvements in drugs or drug protocols for more than a decade. Although there are agents that block B-cell activation and have been approved for SLE, they are, for the most part, disappointing. The treatment of first choice for reactive arthritis consists of NSAIDs, such as ibuprofen. Systemic glucocorticoids or intraarticular injections of steroids can also be beneficial. Because reactive arthritis is associated with infection caused by *Shigella*, *Salmonella*, *Campylobacter*, *Yersinia*, or *Chlamydia trachomatis*, appropriate antibiotic treatment should be administered if infection is active.

Finally, we note that despite intensive efforts at understanding cartilage repair and new bone formation, the treatment of OA has remained unchanged. The major handicap is a late diagnosis of the disease because majority of the patients present to the medical facilities with the already advanced, nondiagnosed OA lasted for years. There are already pathologic changes in cartilage water content and an age-related influence of normal tissue repair. These factors are superimposed, among others, on influence of obesity, prior injury, and poor conditioning. Most patients with OA can be managed through nonpharmacologic and pharmacologic therapy. The former includes education, weight management, bracing, and appropriate exercise with goal to delay the progression of the disease, alleviate symptoms, and improve function. Nutritional supplements such as glucosamine and chondroitin sulfate may be beneficial for some patients. Occasionally, therapeutic US and pulsed electromagnetic field therapy proved to be helpful. The pharmacologic therapy includes nonnarcotic analgesics such as acetaminophen and NSAIDs. The use of opiates is strongly discouraged. Some patients benefit from intraarticular injections of corticosteroids or hyaluronan, particularly for OA of the knee. The latter drug produces symptomatic relief through one or more of a large number of mechanisms. It decreases the sensitivity of pain fibers, enhances proteoglycan synthesis by chondrocytes, reduces quantities and activity of proinflammatory mediators and matrix metalloproteinases, and alters the behavior of immune system cells.

The most recent trials using platelet-rich plasma intraarticular injections proved to be very promising in the treatment of OA of the knee and hip joints.

Radiotherapy

Radiotherapy was used in the past in several rheumatologic disorders in an attempt to relieve symptoms of inflammation. In particular, radiotherapy for AS was used extensively in the 1950s. With the recognition of significant long-term complications from high doses of radiation, including the development of pulmonary fibrosis, leukemias, lymphomas, osteosarcomas, and other malignant tumors, this approach has generally been abandoned. More recently, radiosynovectomy that involves an intraarticular injection of small radioactive particles became a well-established therapy for arthritic disorders to treat synovitis. Intraarticular radiotherapy using yttrium-90 (^{90}Y) was attempted in patients with RA. Some investigators reported promising results after radiation synovectomy for inflamed small joints of the hands injecting under fluoroscopic or sonographic guidance erbium-169 (^{169}Er) citrate colloid. The other radiopharmaceutical used for this purpose included rhenium-186 (^{186}Re) sulfur colloid, lutetium-177 (^{177}Lu)-labeled hydroxyapatite particles, colloidal chromium phosphate (^{32}P), and radioactive colloid gold (^{198}Au). In selected patients with SLE and with RA, the use of the total lymphoid irradiation (TLI) as a localized means of immune suppression has been studied. In Europe, teleradiotherapy of inflamed joints in the patients with RA has been tried, using a 20 MeV linear accelerator delivering a total dose of 20 Gy, without, however, significant results.

Orthopaedic Treatment

Similar modalities as for diagnosis are also used for monitoring the results of orthopaedic treatment of arthritis. Because the most effective treatment, particularly when large joints are involved, entails corrective and reconstructive procedures such as femoral or tibial osteotomy or total joint replacement of the hip, knee, or shoulder, the surgeon follows the postsurgical progress of the patient with sequential radiographic examinations. In OA of the hip, the corrective procedures most often performed are varus or valgus osteotomies of the proximal femur to improve the congruence of the articular surfaces and redistribute the stress forces over different areas of the joint. Similarly, a high tibial osteotomy is performed to correct severe varus or valgus deformities in OA of the knee, particularly in cases of unicompartmental involvement (Fig. 12.58). The radiographic techniques used in monitoring the outcome of these procedures, which in fact represent iatrogenic surgical fractures, are similar to those used in evaluating traumatic fractures. As in traumatic fractures, the radiologist also pays attention to similar features, such as bone union, nonunion, or delayed union (see Chapter 4). In patients in whom ***total hip arthroplasties*** are performed, radiographic scrutiny is also essential. At present, two basic types of hip arthroplasty are used in orthopaedic practice: bipolar hip hemiarthroplasty and total hip arthroplasty. The first type is used mainly for patients with fracture of the femoral head and neck and those with advanced femoral head osteonecrosis. Bipolar prosthesis has a metallic cup the size of the resected femoral head filled with polyethylene, providing an articular cavity to accommodate the metallic femoral head attached to the stem (Fig. 12.59). The principle of this type of construction is that the motion between the metallic femoral head and the inner polyethylene insert reduces the wear of the native acetabulum. Total hip arthroplasty is commonly used in patients with advanced arthritis of the hip joint. The modern systems are modular, meaning that the femoral stem, head, acetabular shell, and liner consist of separate pieces. The prosthetic components, commonly composed of cobalt-chrome alloy or titanium (femoral stem) and metal or ceramic (femoral head), are usually cemented to the bone with polymethylmethacrylate (PMMA) (Fig. 12.60), although cementless fixation is now gaining popularity. After total hip replacement using cemented components, it is important to evaluate the position of the prosthesis, with particular reference to the degree of inclination of the acetabular component, the position of the stem of the prosthesis (whether it is in valgus, varus, or the neutral position), and the status of the separated and rejoined greater trochanter, among other features. Equally important is the evaluation of cement–bone interface to detect the radiolucent area suggestive of prosthesis loosening (see Figs. 12.60 and 12.82).

The technique of noncemented hip prosthesis is based on the use of a rough or porous surface on the prosthetic parts that enables ingrowth of the bone. A bioactive coating (i.e., hydroxyapatite) can also be used for the same purpose. Acetabular components, which contain a polyethylene liner, usually have a porous coating over the entire surface of the cup, whereas femoral components can be either partially or fully coated (Fig. 12.61A). Cementless acetabular components are sometimes reinforced with the rim screws or spikes (Figs. 12.61B and 12.62). Occasionally, so-called *hybrid arthroplasties* are performed with cementless acetabular and cemented femoral components (Fig. 12.63). In order to assess quantitatively the extent of mechanical loosening of a hip prosthesis, the areas of the interface between the

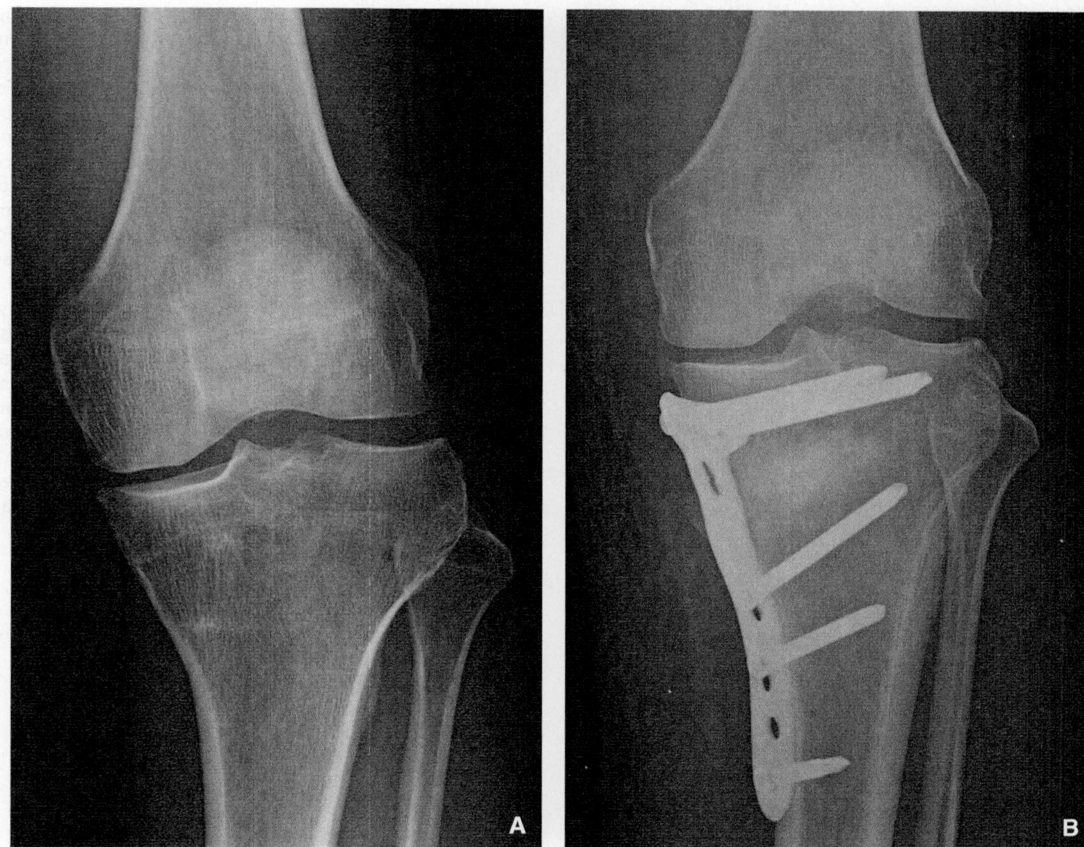

FIGURE 12.58 **Corrective high tibial valgus osteotomy.** **(A)** A 37-year-old man presented with OA affecting the medial joint compartment of the left knee, which resulted in varus deformity. **(B)** To alleviate the symptoms and to correct the deformity, a proximal tibia wedge valgus osteotomy combined with reamed intramedullary autograft was performed. Observe correction of varus deformity after surgery.

FIGURE 12.59 **Hemiarthroplasty of the hip joint.** Anteroposterior radiograph of the left hip of a 61-year-old woman, who was diagnosed with advanced osteonecrosis of the femoral head, shows status post hemiarthroplasty using bipolar type of the prosthesis. The cemented stem of the prosthesis is in a neutral position within the femoral shaft.

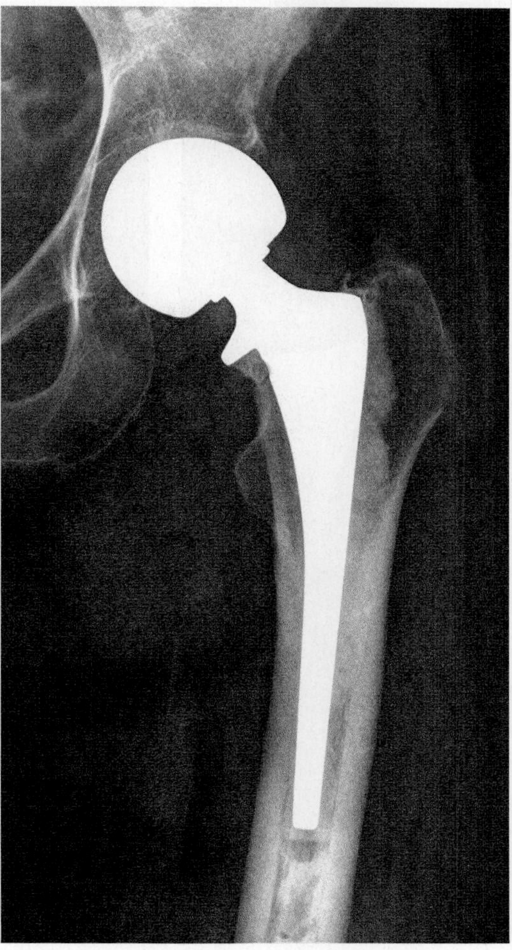

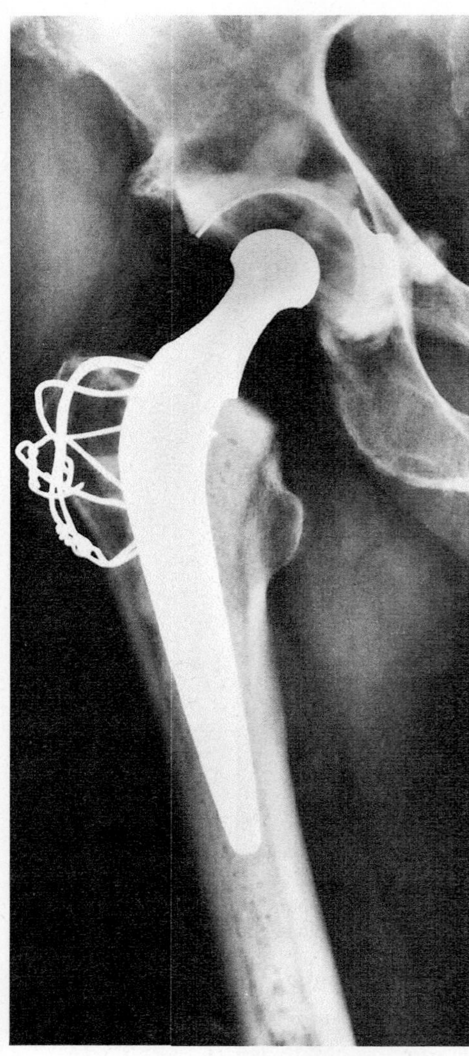

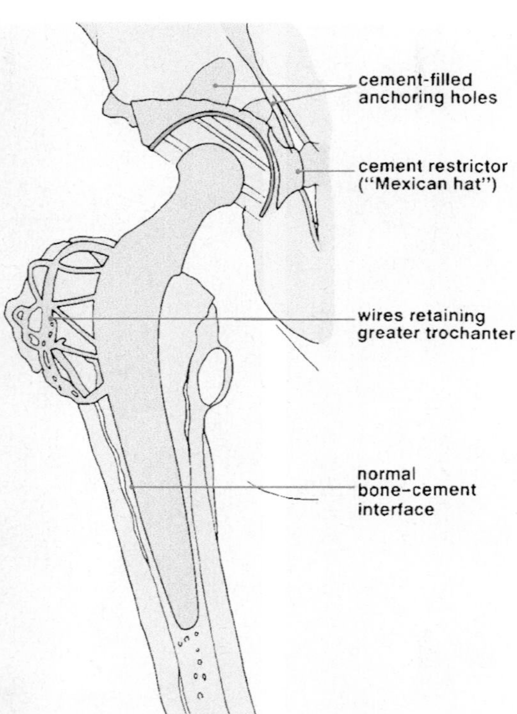

FIGURE 12.60 Cemented total hip arthroplasty. A 69-year-old man underwent total hip replacement because of advanced degenerative joint disease; a Charnley low-friction arthroplasty was performed. On the anteroposterior radiograph of the right hip, one can evaluate all the parts of the prosthesis. Note that the acetabular component is oriented approximately 45 degrees to the horizontal plane and is cemented to the bone with methylmethacrylate previously impregnated with barium sulfate to make it visible radiographically. A wire-mesh cement restrictor ("Mexican hat") prevents significant leakage of methylmethacrylate into the pelvis. The stem of the prosthesis is in the neutral position in the medullary canal of the femur. Note the extent of cement below the distal end of the prosthesis, for secure anchoring. The greater trochanter, which was osteotomized to facilitate exposure of the joint, has been reattached by metallic wires slightly distal and lateral for improved stability. Note the normal appearance of the bone–cement interface.

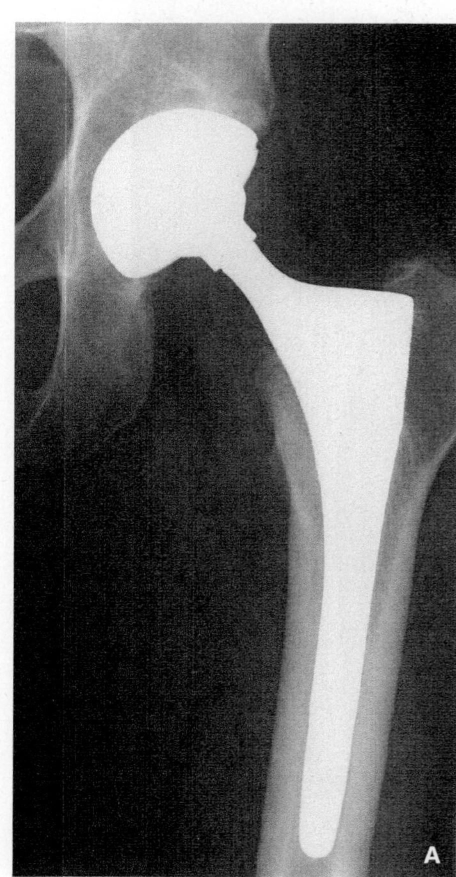

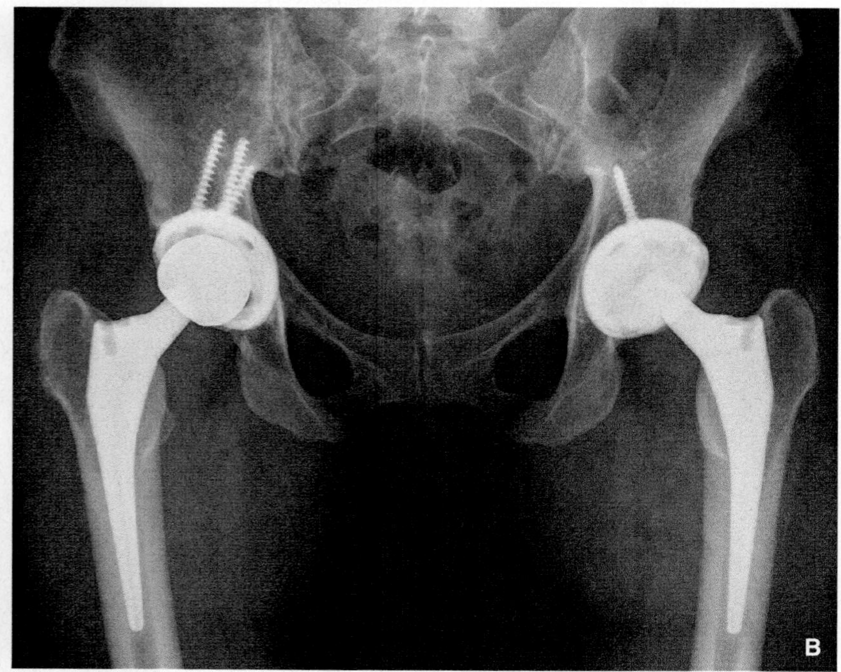

FIGURE 12.61 Cementless total hip arthroplasty. (A) A 48-year-old woman underwent total hip arthroplasty because of advanced OA. Note porous-coated acetabular component and partially coated femoral stem. The prosthetic components are in anatomic alignment, the femoral stem is in neutral position, the endocortex is intact, and there are no signs of loosening. **(B)** Anteroposterior radiograph of the pelvis of a 64-year-old woman shows status post bilateral total noncemented hip arthroplasties. The right acetabular component was reinforced with three rim screws, whereas the left one with a single rim screw.

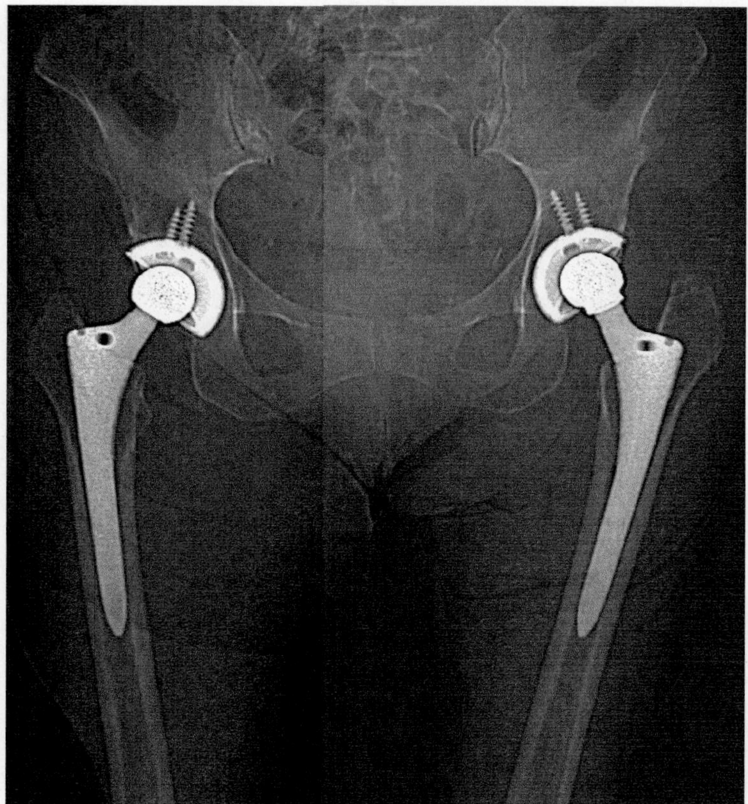

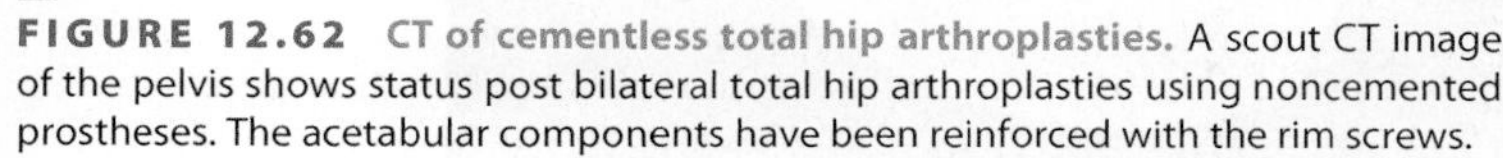

FIGURE 12.62 **CT of cementless total hip arthroplasties.** A scout CT image of the pelvis shows status post bilateral total hip arthroplasties using noncemented prostheses. The acetabular components have been reinforced with the rim screws.

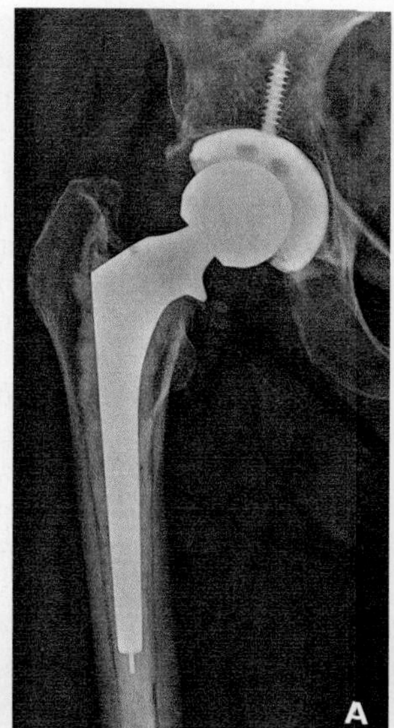

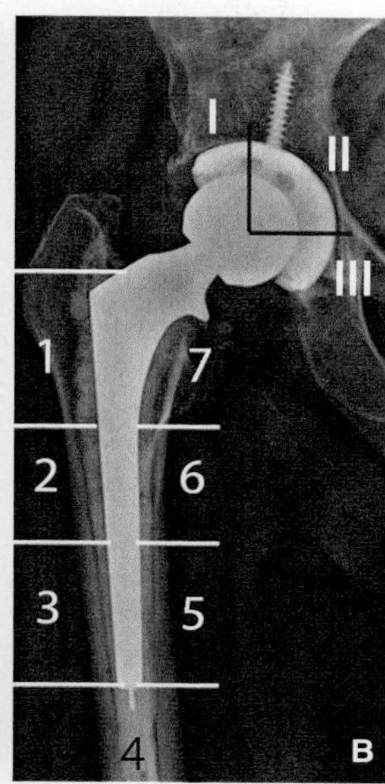

FIGURE 12.63 **Hybrid total hip arthroplasty and Gruen zones. (A)** Anteroposterior radiograph of the right hip of a 66-year-old woman shows a hybrid type of total hip prosthesis. Note that the femoral stem of the prosthesis has been cemented in a neutral position within the femoral shaft, and the noncemented acetabular component has been reinforced with a single rim screw. **(B)** The Gruen zones are labeled 1 through 7 in the femoral component of the prosthesis and I through III (in roman numbers) in the acetabular component of the prosthesis. These regions are used as references to quantify the extent of mechanical loosening.

device and the adjacent bone has been divided in the so-called *Gruen zones* (Fig. 12.63B). Alternative to conventional total hip arthroplasty, especially in younger patients, metal-on-metal hip resurfacing arthroplasty (HRA) has been advocated (Fig. 12.64). There are different types of this prosthesis, but most of them are made from high carbon cobalt-chromium alloys and consist of a femoral component, which can be cemented or noncemented, and an uncemented acetabular component that achieves primary fixation through press-fit and circumferential fins. The acetabular components are coated using various methods and material providing a bone ingrowth surface at the implant–bone interface to achieve maximum stability. The advantages of this type of arthroplasty include the durability of the prosthetic components, low volumetric wear rate, an increased level of inherent stability using large heads with reduced rate of dislocation, preservation of metaphyseal and diaphyseal bone stock, optimization of stress transfer to the proximal femur, optimal range of movement, and improved biomechanics of the hip joint. The disadvantage of this type of hip arthroplasty is shedding metal particles leading to periprosthetic osteolysis and metallosis with formation of pseudotumors (see in the following text).

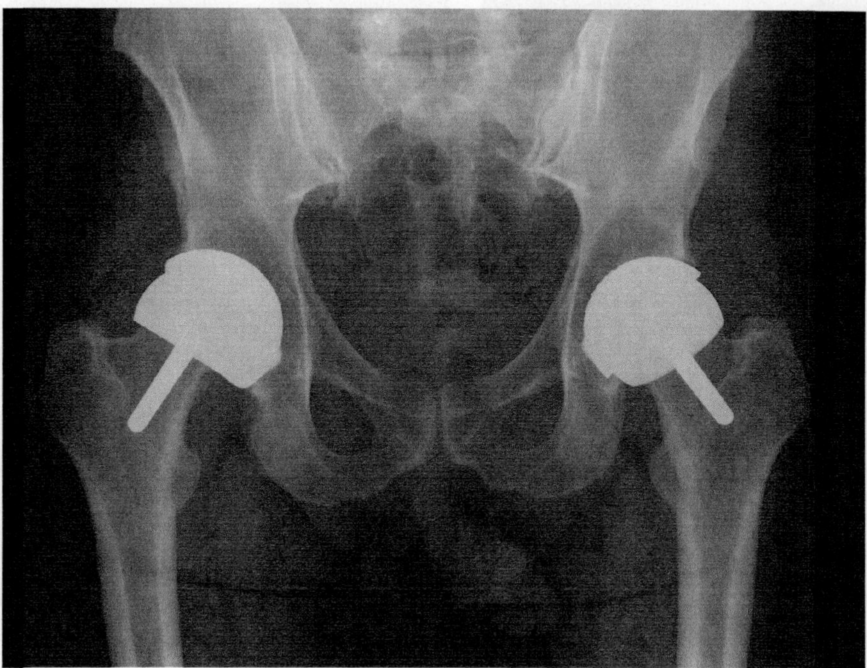

FIGURE 12.64 **Total hip metal-on-metal resurfacing arthroplasty.** A 42-year-old man with OA of both hip joints underwent metal-on-metal total resurfacing hip arthroplasties.

After total hip arthroplasty using noncemented components, imaging evaluation should focus on the interface between the prosthesis and the bone to detect areas of bone resorption (focal osteolysis) that may indicate loosening of the prosthesis. Additional abnormalities to look for are progressive subsidence, migration, or tilt of the components. With HRA, there is well-documented risk of femoral neck fracture. Groin pain may occur secondary to impingement of the femoral neck on the acetabular component resulting in femoral neck scalloping. Because the implant consists of a metal-on-metal articulation made from cast cobalt-chromium alloys, the incidents of production of wear particles and hence the occurrence of metallosis, pseudotumors, and inflammatory reaction known as *aseptic lymphocyte-dominated vasculitis associated lesion (ALVAL)* are increased (see in the following text).

Although two-compartmental and unicompartmental knee arthroplasties are occasionally performed, the most common type is a *total knee arthroplasty*. This procedure combines resurfacing the femoral, tibial, and patellar articular surfaces by using metal and polyethylene-bearing surfaces. The major prosthesis categories include posterior cruciate ligament-retaining, posterior cruciate ligament-substituting or stabilized, unlinked constrained or varus-valgus constrained, and rotating-hinge knee implants. Femoral and tibial components can be either cemented, noncemented, or anchored with the screws. A patellar component invariably consists of high-density polyethylene, which can be metal backed. Modern three-part (three-compartmental) condylar cemented nonconstrained arthroplasty is performed using metal femoral component, which resurfaces both condyles and the trochlear notch, and a tibial component, that consists of a metal-backed polyethylene tray that articulates with the femoral component (Fig. 12.65). Some tibial components may contain a locking-mechanism clip that locks the tibial polyethylene tray into the tibial base plate. Occasionally, femoral and tibial components can include varying lengths

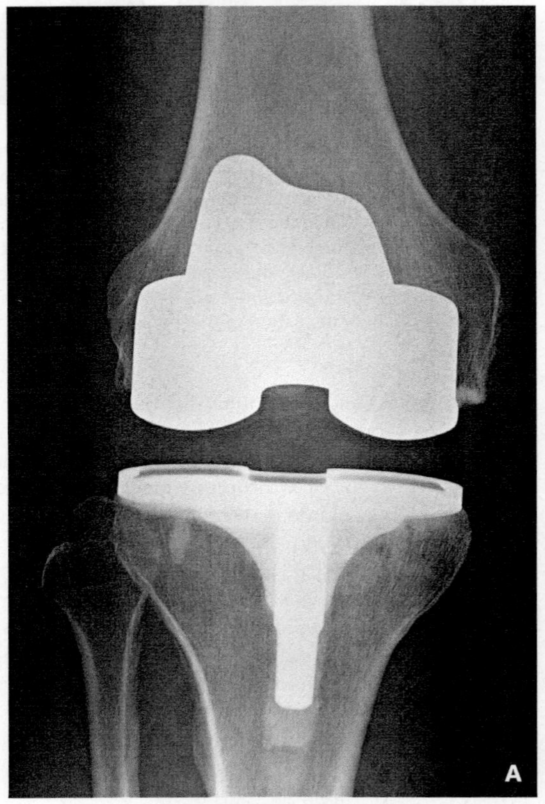

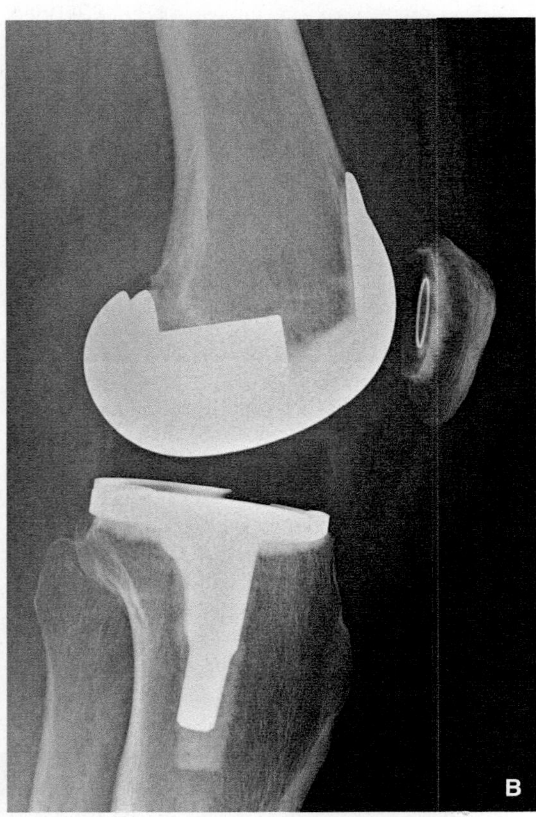

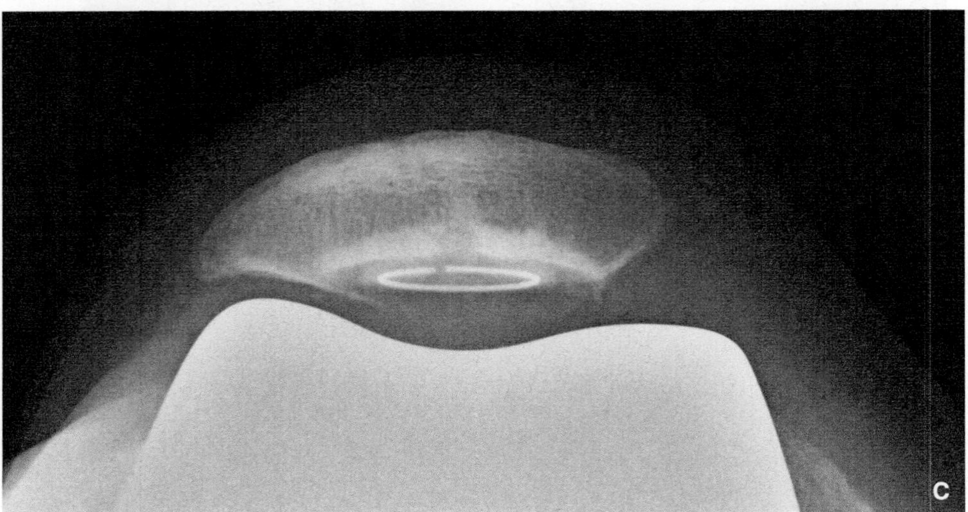

FIGURE 12.65 Cemented total knee arthroplasty. A 62-year-old woman underwent total knee arthroplasty using a nonconstrained three-part cemented posterior cruciate ligament-substituting condylar prosthesis. **(A)** Anteroposterior radiograph demonstrates that the tibial component is aligned with the surface of the bone, forming a 90-degree angle with the long axis of the tibia. There is no evidence of a radiolucent line at the cement–bone interface. The slight valgus configuration at the knee (approximately 7 degrees) is acceptable. **(B)** On the lateral knee radiograph, note the tight adherence of the anterior and posterior brackets of the femoral component of the prosthesis to the bone. **(C)** The Merchant projection shows anatomic alignment of the patella within the anterior femoral bracket of the prosthesis.

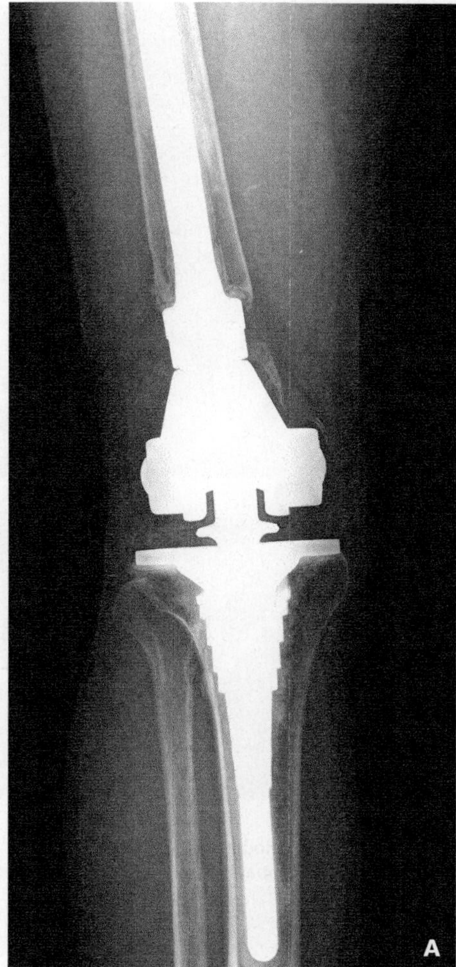

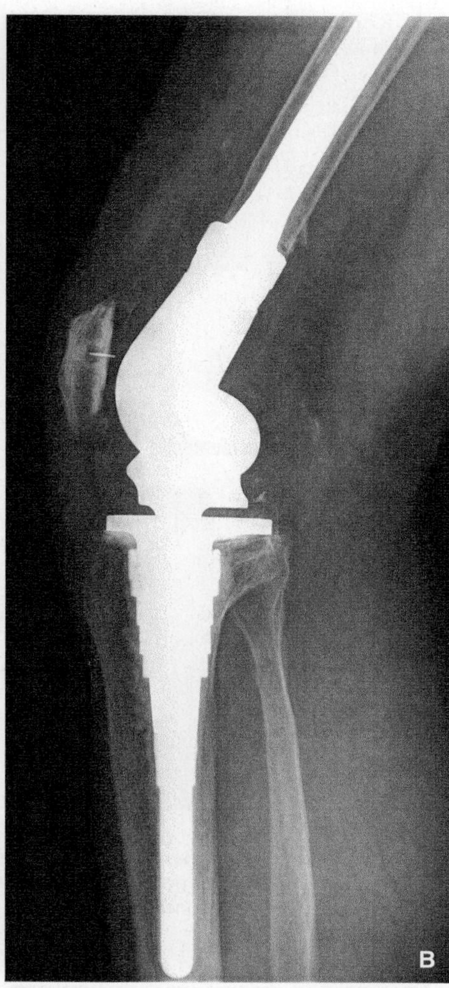

FIGURE 12.66 Total hinged knee arthroplasty. A 74-year-old man presented with two failed total nonconstrained knee arthroplasties performed for advanced OA. In the third attempt, the three-part constrained hinge prosthesis was implanted, as seen here on **(A)** anteroposterior and **(B)** lateral radiographs of the right knee.

stems that supplement prosthesis fixation, and tibial component may be augmented with prominent pegs for additional stability. Fully constrained rotating-hinge total knee arthroplasty is usually performed for revision of failed nonconstrained knee arthroplasty and in patients with ligament deficiency, severe bone loss, or severe knee joint instability (Fig. 12.66). This type of implant allows the flexion-extension movement combined with rotation of the femur on the tibial component, or with rotation of the tibial polyethylene liner on the metal tibial tray, thus allowing a more physiologic range of motion and reducing the stress transfer to the bone–prosthesis interface compared with the old fixed-hinge models.

After a total knee arthroplasty with a condylar type of prothesis, it is important to evaluate the position of the tibial component relative to the tibial shaft as well as the axial alignment and the status of the methylmethacrylate fixation of the components (see Fig. 12.65). The tibial component should be aligned perpendicular to the long axis of the tibia on the anteroposterior view of the knee and perpendicular or in slight (up to 6 degrees) flexion on the lateral view. The anterior bracket (flange) of the femoral component should be flushed with the anterior femoral cortex.

Unicompartmental arthroplasty is performed for isolated unicompartmental OA, usually in the medial or lateral compartment (Fig. 12.67), although femoropatellar unicompartmental arthroplasty is also occasionally performed (Fig. 12.68).

Total ankle arthroplasty devices incorporate two basic designs: three-component (mobile bearing) and two-component (fixed bearing) types. Three-component types are characterized by separate tibial and talar components separated by a fully conforming mobile polyethylene spacer. Two-component types have only a single partially conforming articulation between the tibial and talar components, with the polyethylene spacer fixed to the tibial component. Recently, third-generation ankle implants became increasingly favored over first- and second-generation prostheses, which were cemented and constrained, hence leading to a higher failure rate. The most popular among the third-generation implants is the INBONE prosthesis, a fixed-bearing design with a modular system for both the tibial and talar components (Fig. 12.69A,B). Another popular implant is a Zimmer third-generation trabecular metal prosthesis (Fig. 12.69C,D). After total ankle arthroplasty, in addition to assessing the position and alignment of the prosthetic parts, attention should be paid to the possible subsidence of the talar component, which should not exceed 5 mm, best evaluated on the lateral radiograph of the ankle. Furthermore, syndesmotic fusion (if performed) and status of adjacent osseous structures should be evaluated.

After a *total shoulder arthroplasty*, whether conventional (Fig. 12.70) or the one using reverse (Delta or Aequalis) shoulder prosthesis (Fig. 12.71), alignment of the prosthetic components and metal–cement and cement–bone interface must be evaluated. Reverse shoulder arthroplasty makes use of a semiconstrained prosthesis that comprises a humeral component, lateralized polyethylene insert, glenosphere, and metaglene, consisting of a base plate that is secured by locking and nonlocking screws to the native glenoid. The humeral component consists of a metal stem that is monoblock or modular and a cup-shaped proximal portion. All humeral components are cemented. With the latter arthroplasty, imaging evaluation will include, in addition to the position of the anchoring screws within the scapula, relationship of the humeral component to the scapula and status of supporting bone. In particular, the inferior border of the glenoid should be examined for erosions and heterotopic ossifications and one should look for unique for this prosthesis complication such as notching of the inferior scapula by the humeral component and acromial stress fractures.

There are three basic types of *total elbow arthroplasty*: nonconstrained or resurfacing elbow arthroplasty, semiconstrained elbow arthroplasty, and constrained elbow arthroplasty (Fig. 12.72). In the first type,

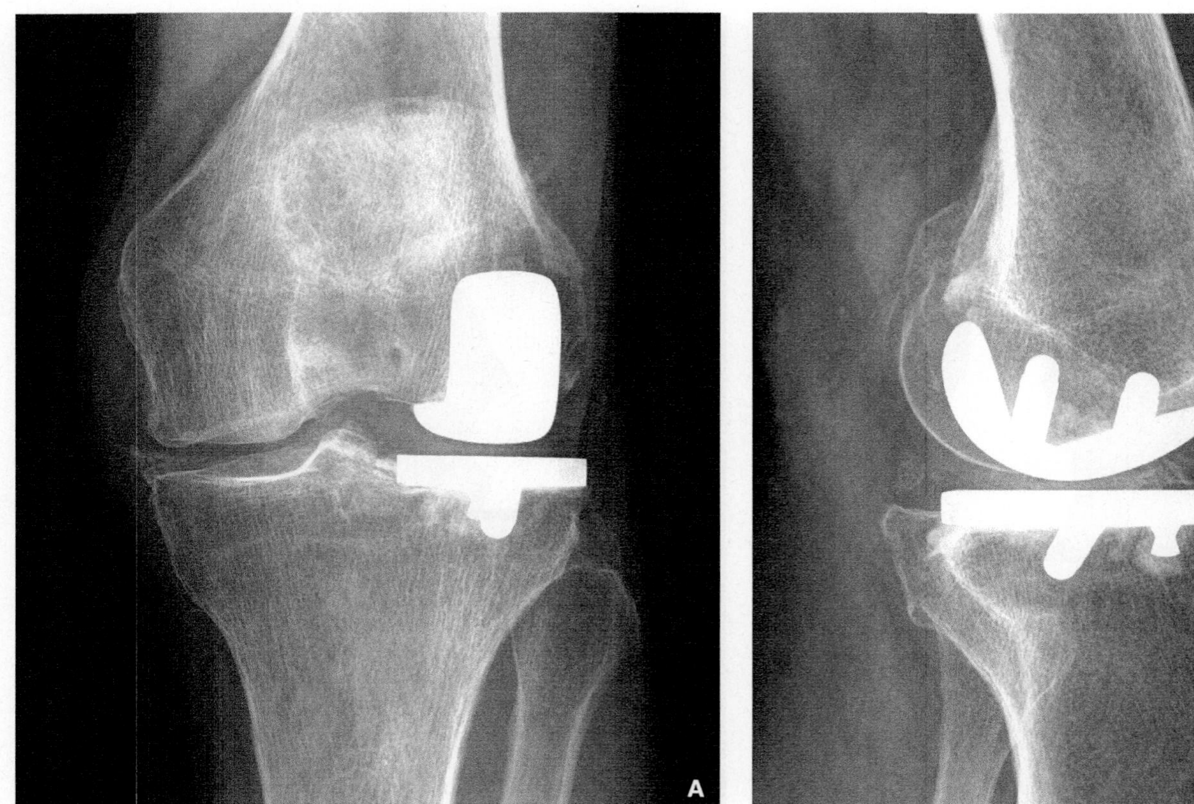

FIGURE 12.67 Unicompartmental lateral knee arthroplasty. **(A)** Anteroposterior and **(B)** lateral radiographs of the left knee of a 73-year-old man, who, because of advanced OA of the lateral joint compartment but relatively good preservation of the medial and femoropatellar compartments, underwent a unicompartmental knee arthroplasty, show anatomic alignment of the prosthetic components.

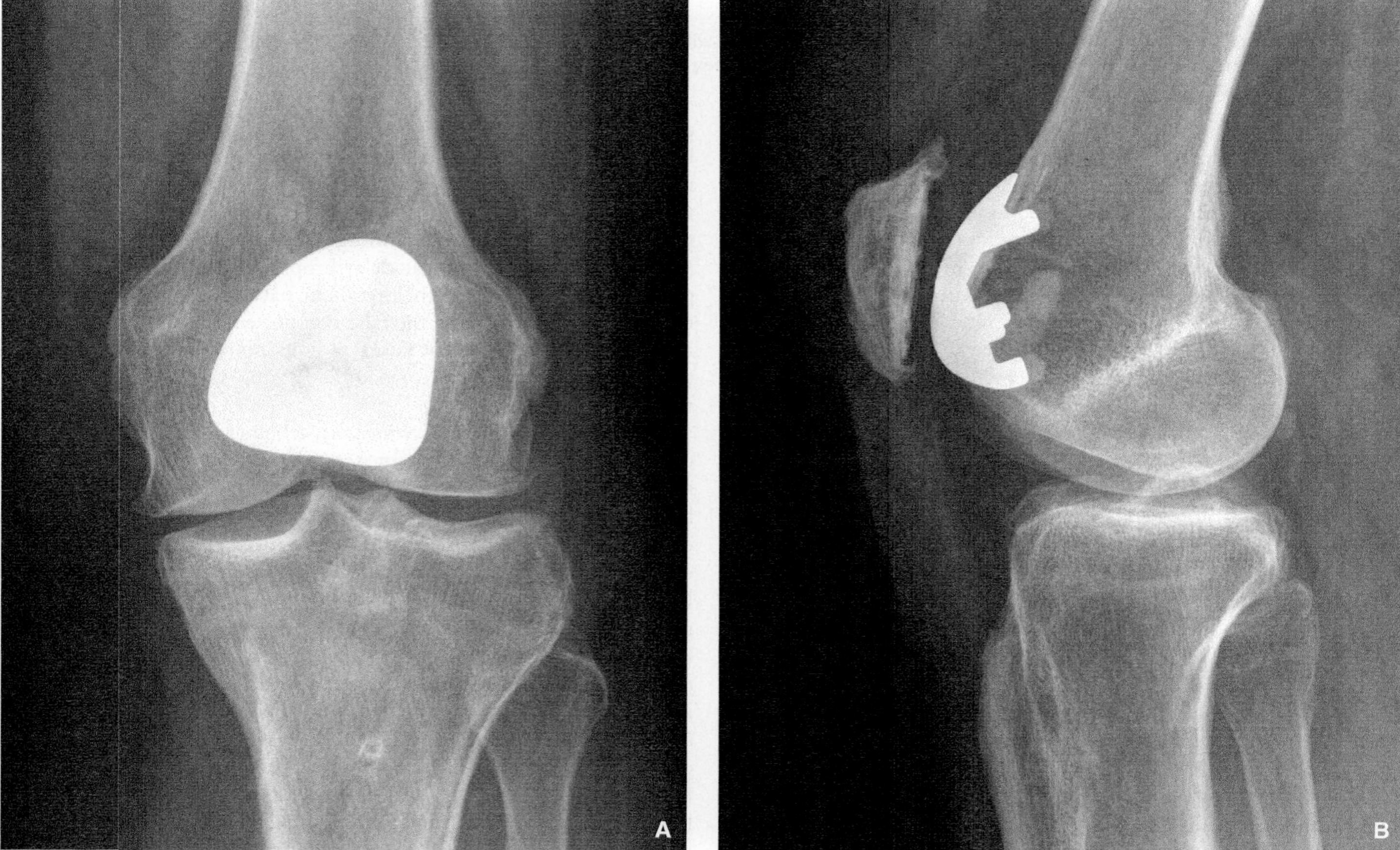

FIGURE 12.68 Unicompartmental knee arthroplasty. **(A)** Anteroposterior and **(B)** lateral radiographs of the left knee of a 68-year-old woman show femoropatellar unicompartmental arthroplasty.

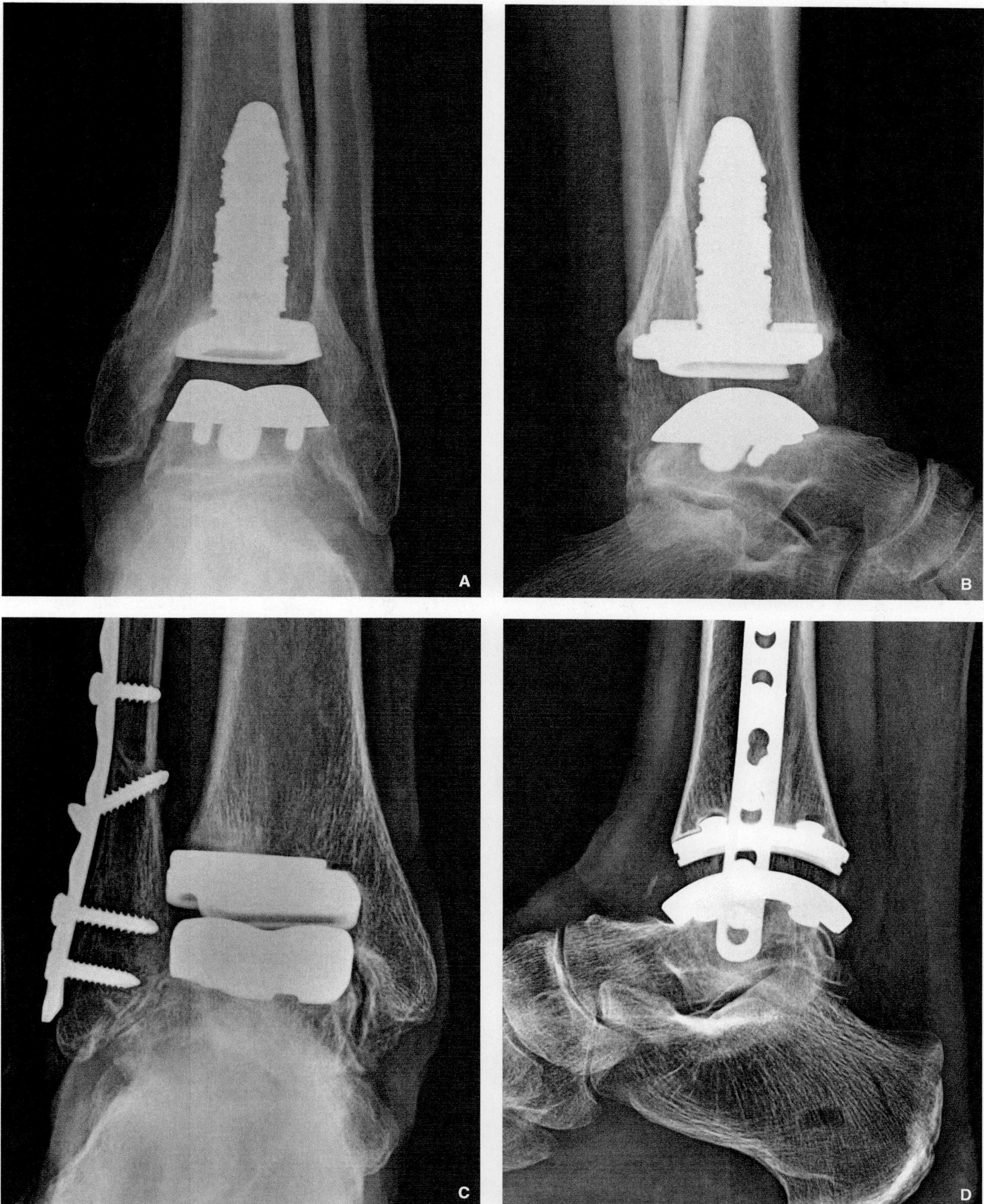

FIGURE 12.69 Total ankle arthroplasty. **(A)** Anteroposterior and **(B)** lateral radiographs of the left ankle show intramedullary fixation of total INBONE ankle prosthesis. The noncemented prosthetic components made from a titanium alloy and incorporating a cobalt-chrome polyethylene articulation are porous coated for bone ingrowth. **(C)** Anteroposterior and **(D)** lateral radiographs of the right ankle of another patient show a third-generation Zimmer trabecular metal total ankle prosthesis. Note status post fibular osteotomy with a side plate cortical screws fixation.

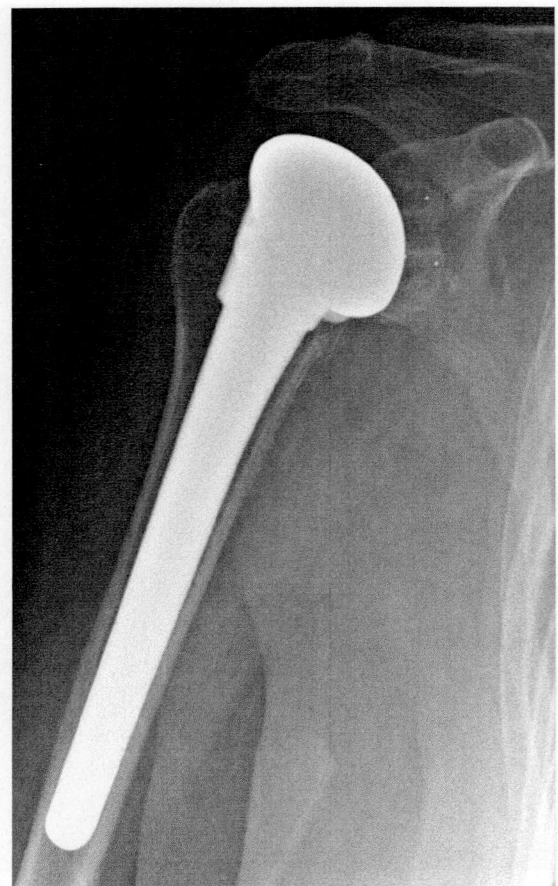

FIGURE 12.70 Total shoulder prosthesis. Anteroposterior radiograph of the right shoulder shows status post total shoulder arthroplasty with a conventional prosthesis in anatomic alignment.

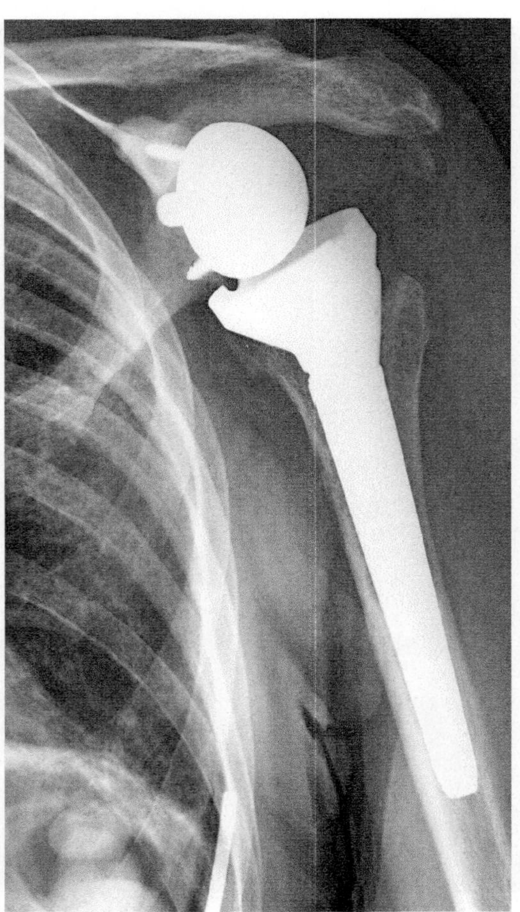

FIGURE 12.71 Total reverse shoulder prosthesis. Anteroposterior radiograph of the left shoulder shows status post total shoulder arthroplasty with a Delta reverse shoulder system in anatomic alignment.

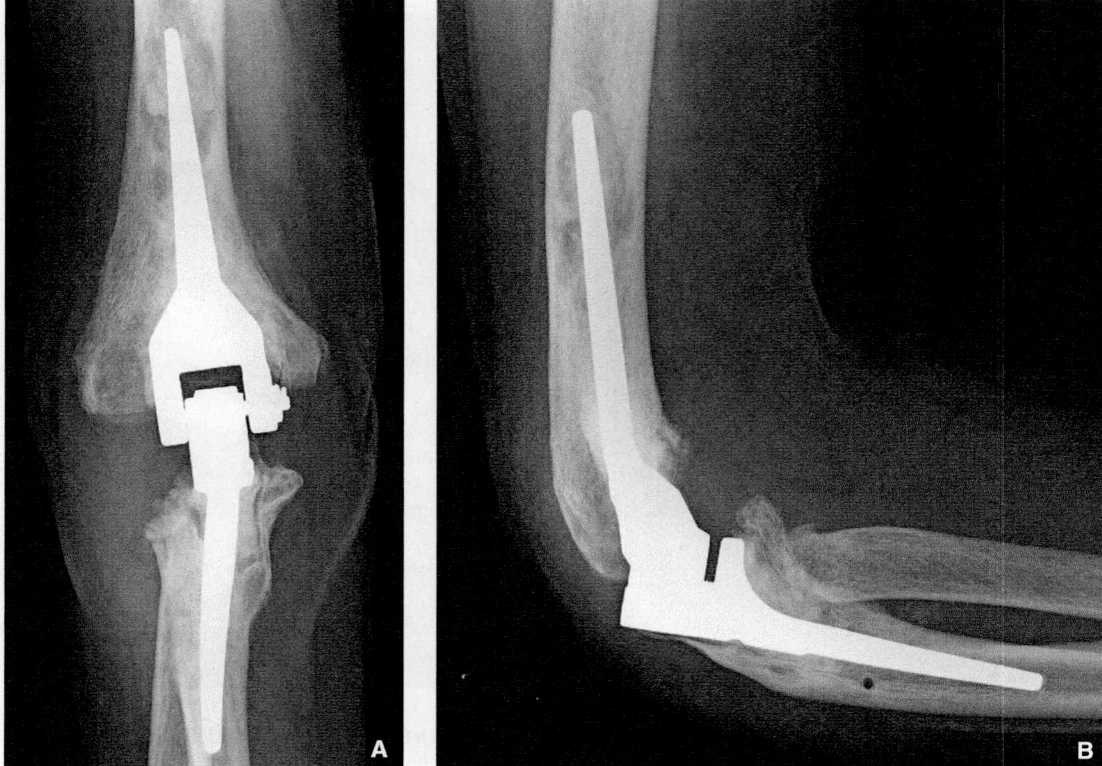

FIGURE 12.72 Total elbow arthroplasty. **(A)** Anteroposterior and **(B)** lateral radiographs of the right elbow of a 72-year-old woman with RA show total hinged elbow prosthesis. Note that radial head has been resected.

the prosthesis consists of two separate metal components, humeral and ulnar, which articulate by a high-density polyethylene component. The major complication with this implant is subluxation and dislocation. The semiconstrained prosthesis consists of titanium or cobalt-chromium ulnar and humeral stems that are linked by a pin and bushing, which consists of a polyethylene ring in between the metal components to reduce friction. Constrained elbow prosthesis consists of rigid hinges, constructed with either metal-on-metal or metal and high-density polyethylene parts connected through either a bushing or a separate polyethylene piece that links the humeral and ulnar components. The radial head is commonly resected proximally to the annular ligament. Imaging evaluation focuses on emerging complications, such as heterotopic ossifications, perihardware lucency indicative of loosening (the humeral component is more prone to this complication), periprosthetic fracture, subluxation or dislocation of the prosthesis, wear and breakdown of bushing, and hardware fracture.

In the *hands and feet*, occasionally, either *hemiarthroplasties* or *total joint arthroplasties* are performed for OA and RA using either metal (Figs. 12.73 and 12.74) or silastic (elastomer–rubber or silicone-polymer) type of prostheses (Figs. 12.75 and 12.76). These implants provide instant stability with excellent pain relief, leading to improve range of motion and function. The complications of silastic prostheses are discussed in the following text.

Complications of Surgical Treatment

As important as evaluating the outcome of the surgical treatment of arthritic disease is monitoring the complications that may arise from such treatment, especially those after osteotomies and joint-replacement procedures. These complications include among others thrombophlebitis, hematomas, heterotopic bone formation, the intrapelvic leakage of acrylic cement, infection, loosening, subluxation or dislocation of a prosthesis, fracture of a prosthesis, prosthetic component wear, particle disease (giant cell granulomatosis), inflammatory reaction and formation of pseudotumors, and periprosthetic fracture.

Venous Thrombosis and Thrombophlebitis

A rather frequent complication in the immediate postoperative period, particularly in patients with previous circulatory problems, thrombophlebitis is related to venous stasis and the lack of movement of the surgically treated extremity; sudden pain and swelling of the leg are common clinical findings. The venous soleal plexus in the calf is the most common site of thrombus formation. Radiologically, this complication can be detected by venography (Fig. 12.77), radionuclide scanning, or US. On radionuclide scan, an increased gamma count rate in an area of the lower extremities following intravenous administration of ^{125}I-labeled fibrinogen suggests adherence of the tracer to a developing clot. US can detect venous thrombosis using compression technique. Lack of compressibility of a vein is

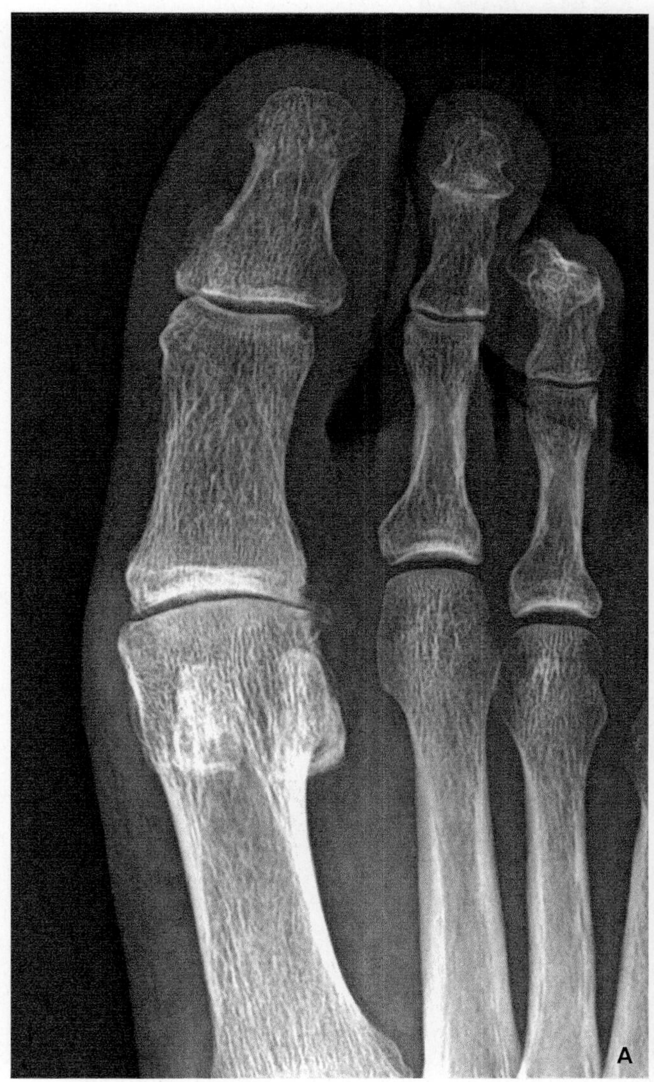

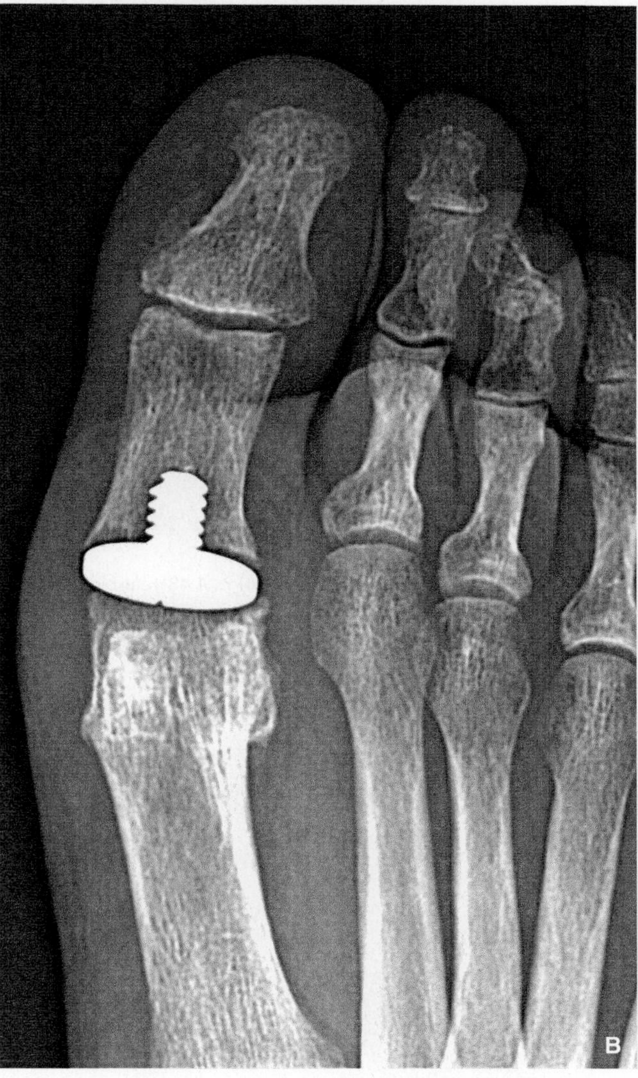

FIGURE 12.73 Metallic hemiarthroplasty of a small joint. A 62-year-old woman presented with chronic pain in her left great toe. **(A)** Dorsoplantar radiograph shows narrowing of the first metatarsophalangeal joint associated with formation of marginal osteophytes, consistent with OA. **(B)** Hemiarthroplasty was performed using metallic prosthesis implanted into the proximal phalanx.

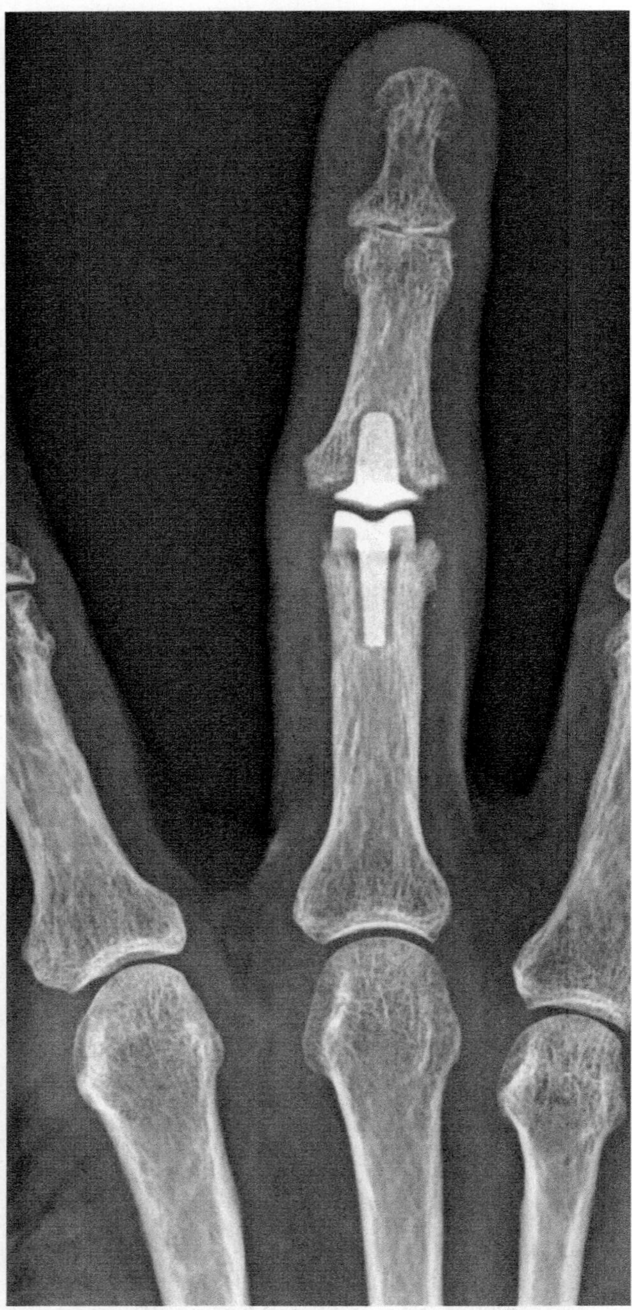

FIGURE 12.74 Metallic arthroplasty of a small joint. A 48-year-old man underwent noncemented metallic arthroplasty of the proximal interphalangeal joint of the middle finger for posttraumatic arthritis.

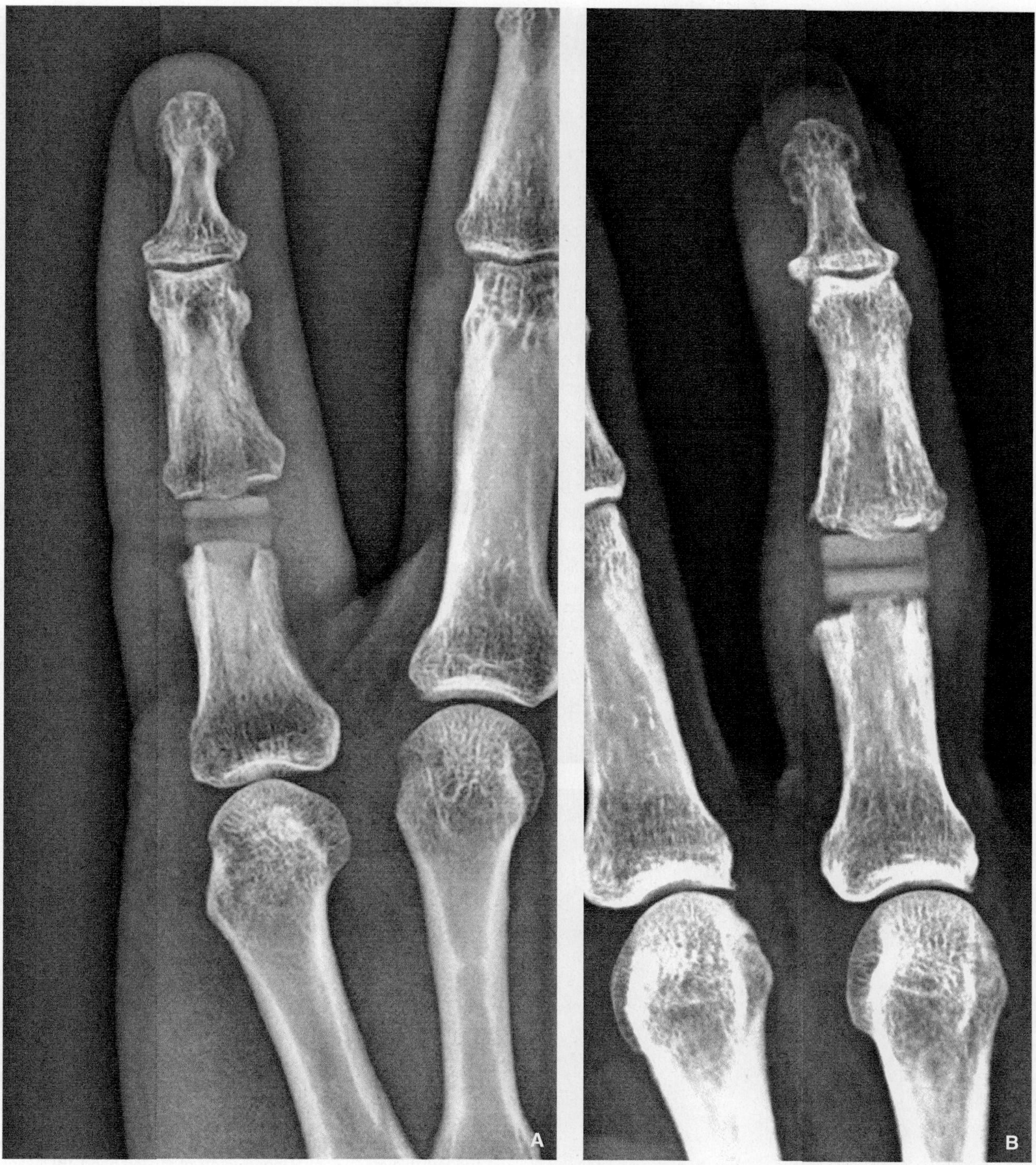

FIGURE 12.75 Silastic arthroplasty of a small joint. **(A)** Swanson silastic prosthesis was implanted in the proximal interphalangeal joint of the small finger of this 39-year-old woman with posttraumatic arthritis. **(B)** Dorsovolar radiograph of the index finger of another patient shows status post silastic arthroplasty of proximal interphalangeal joint.

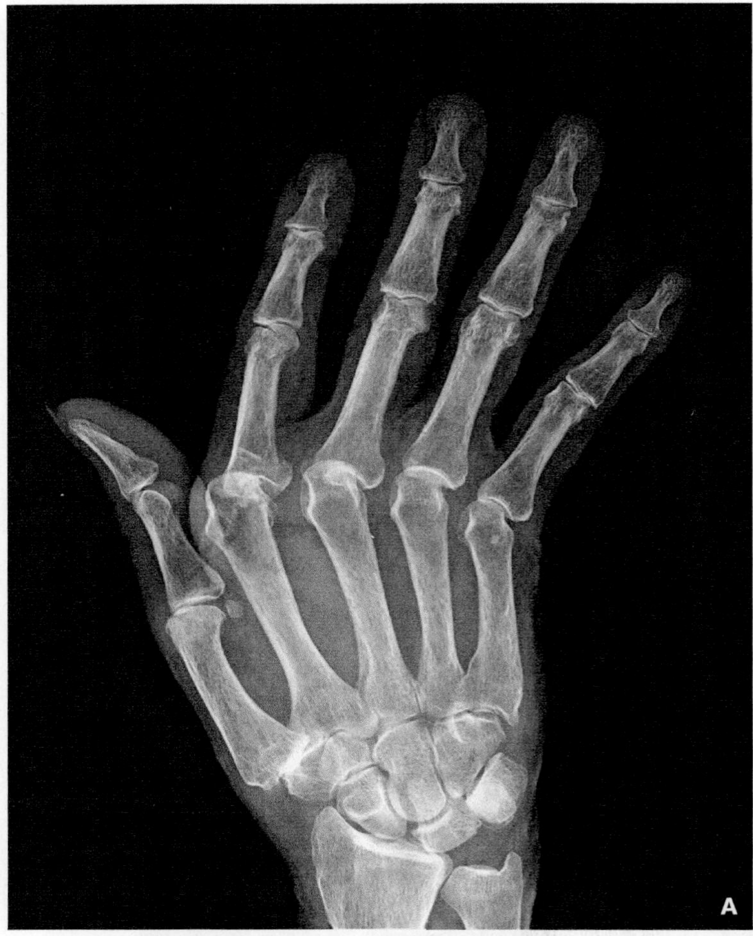

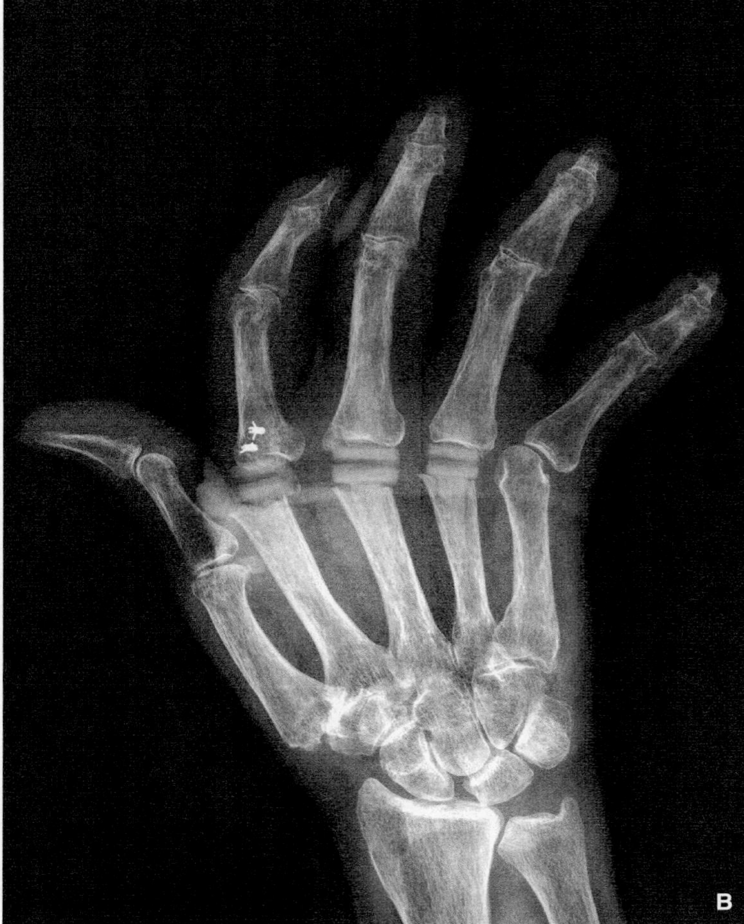

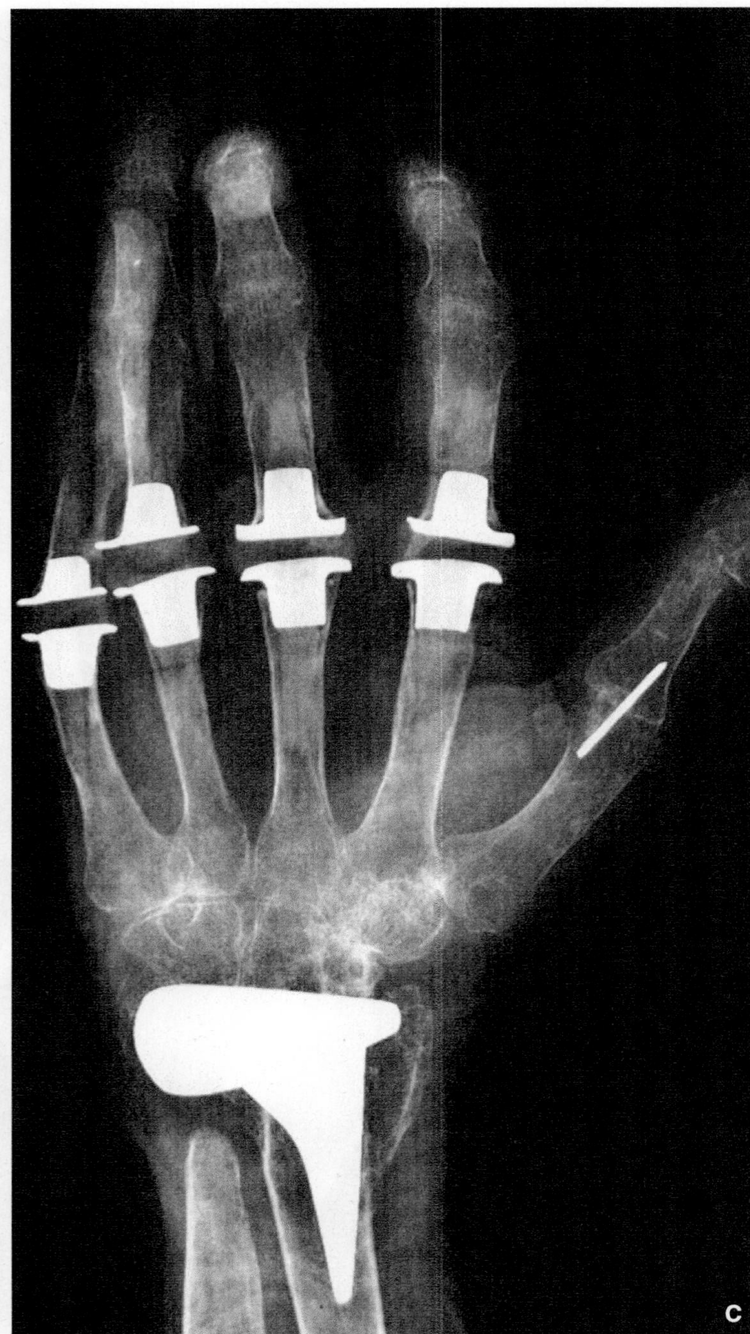

FIGURE 12.76 **Silastic arthroplasties of the small joints.** **(A)** A 68-year-old man was diagnosed with CPPD crystal deposition disease affecting second, third, and fourth metacarpophalangeal joints of the left hand. **(B)** Swanson silicone implants were used to replace the affected joints. **(C)** In another patient, a woman with advanced JIA, silastic flexible hinge (two-stem) prostheses with circumferential titanium grommets were implanted in the second to fifth metacarpophalangeal joints. In addition, note the radiocarpal metallic prosthesis and fusion of the first metacarpophalangeal joint.

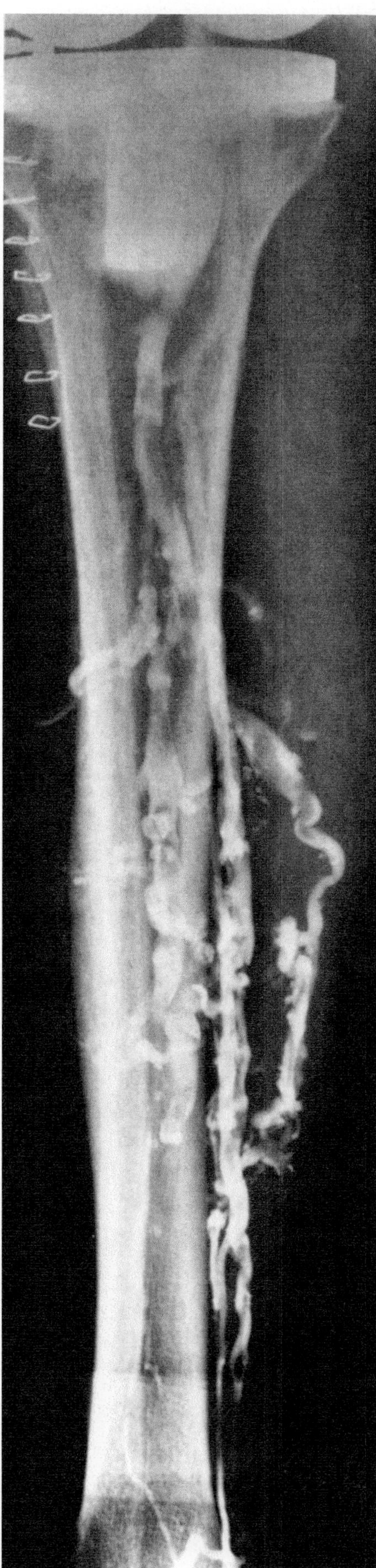

FIGURE 12.77 Venography of venous thrombosis. A 67-year-old woman with RA, who recently underwent total knee arthroplasty, presented with pain and swelling of the left leg. A venogram shows multiple thrombi in the soleal venous plexus of the lower extremity.

thought to be the single most reliable finding in differentiating between thrombosed and normal veins. Other criteria useful in detection of vein thrombosis are the presence of echogenic intraluminal material and enlargement of the vein.

Hematoma

The formation of a hematoma is a common complication of surgery for arthritic disease. However, it usually subsides within a short time, unless it is associated with infection. This complication can be easily detected with MRI.

Leakage of Acrylic Cement

Intrapelvic leakage of methylmethacrylate may lead to vascular and neurologic damage, visceral necrosis, and urinary tract disorders, as a result of the heat of polymerization of the acrylic cement (Fig. 12.78). To prevent an accidental leak, a wire mesh restrictor ("Mexican hat") is applied around the acetabular anchoring holes of the prosthesis (see Fig. 12.60).

Heterotopic Bone Formation

This is a relatively frequent complication of surgery for arthritic disease in the hip. The amount of new bone that forms in the adjacent soft tissues varies: If extensive, it may interfere with function of the hip joint. Conventional radiography (Fig. 12.79) and occasionally CT are sufficient to evaluate this complication.

Infection

Although infection may occur at any time postoperatively, it is usually observed shortly after the joint-replacement procedure. Clinically, it is manifested by pain, elevation of temperature, and discharge from the wound. The imaging findings in cases of infection include soft-tissue swelling, rarefaction of bone, and, occasionally, a periosteal reaction. Scintigraphy using either ^{99m}Tc-labeled MDP (Fig. 12.80) or ^{111}In-oxine–labeled WBCs (Fig. 12.81) has been reported to be very useful in these circumstances. More recently, SPECT/CT imaging also effectively demonstrated this complication (see Fig. 2.34).

Loosening of a Prosthesis

Infection after a joint-replacement procedure may result in loosening of a prosthesis, but loosening may also be seen as a late complication resulting from mechanical factors. The standard radiographic projections are usually sufficient to reveal this development (Figs. 12.82 to 12.85). In cemented prosthesis, the circumferential radiolucent gap at the cement–bone interface 2 mm or wider suggests loosening of the implant. In the past, arthrography with subtraction technique used to be performed to demonstrate the cardinal sign of loosening—the extension of contrast agent into the gap that develops at the interface of the bone and acrylic cement (Fig. 12.86).

A radionuclide bone scan may occasionally be helpful in differentiating mechanical loosening from infectious loosening (Fig. 12.87; see also Fig. 12.80). Foci of increased activity, representing accumulation of radiopharmaceutical agent, are consistent with mechanical loosening, whereas diffuse increased activity indicates infection. SPECT/CT is also effective in demonstration of failure of arthroplasty (see Fig. 2.33).

Subluxation and Dislocation of a Prosthesis

These complications are easily diagnosed on the conventional radiography: on the anteroposterior view of the hip (Fig. 12.88A,B), lateral view of the knee (Fig. 12.88C,D), or anteroposterior view of the shoulder (Fig. 12.88E). CT examination is equally effective in this respect (Fig. 12.89).

Fracture of Prosthesis

Similarly to the subluxations and dislocations, this rare complication is also effectively demonstrated on conventional radiography (Fig. 12.90).

Prosthetic Component Wear

Most commonly, this complication is related to the wear of a polyethylene lining of the acetabular cup of the hip prosthesis on the superolateral side. It is recognized on the radiography by asymmetric position of the prosthetic head within the acetabular component (Fig. 12.91).

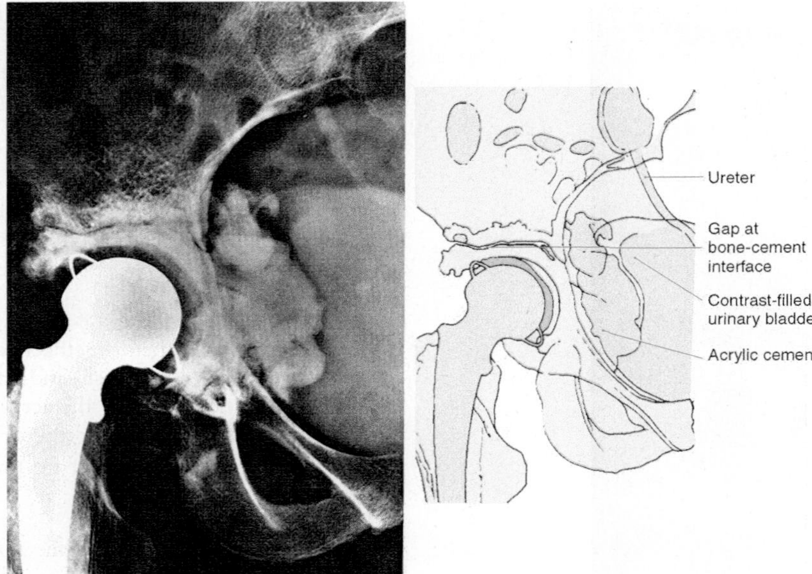

FIGURE 12.78 **Intrapelvic leakage of the cement.** A 46-year-old woman, who underwent total cemented right hip arthroplasty, presented with right hip pain, and intermittent symptoms related to the urinary tract. An intravenous urogram shows a large mass of acrylic cement extruded into the pelvis compressing the right wall of the urinary bladder. (Reprinted with permission from Greenspan A, Gershwin ME. *Imaging in rheumatology: a clinical approach*, 1st ed. Philadelphia: Wolters Kluwer; 2018:126.)

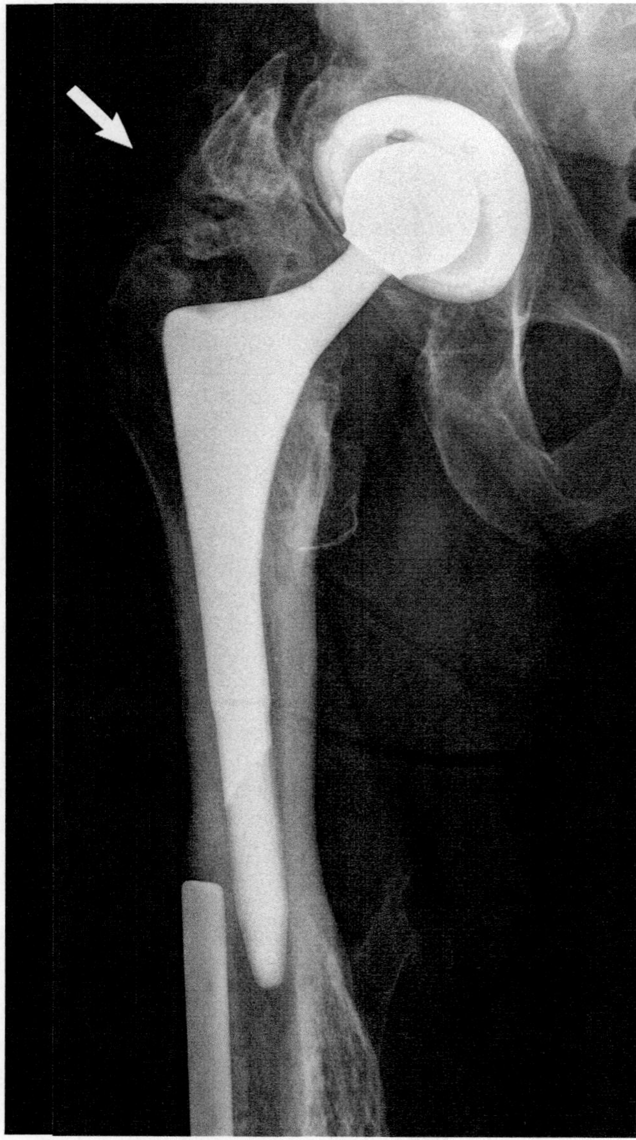

FIGURE 12.79 **Heterotopic bone formation.** Anteroposterior radiograph of the right hip of a 58-year-old man who underwent a total hip arthroplasty for OA shows one of the common complications of this procedure—heterotopic bone formation *(arrow)*.

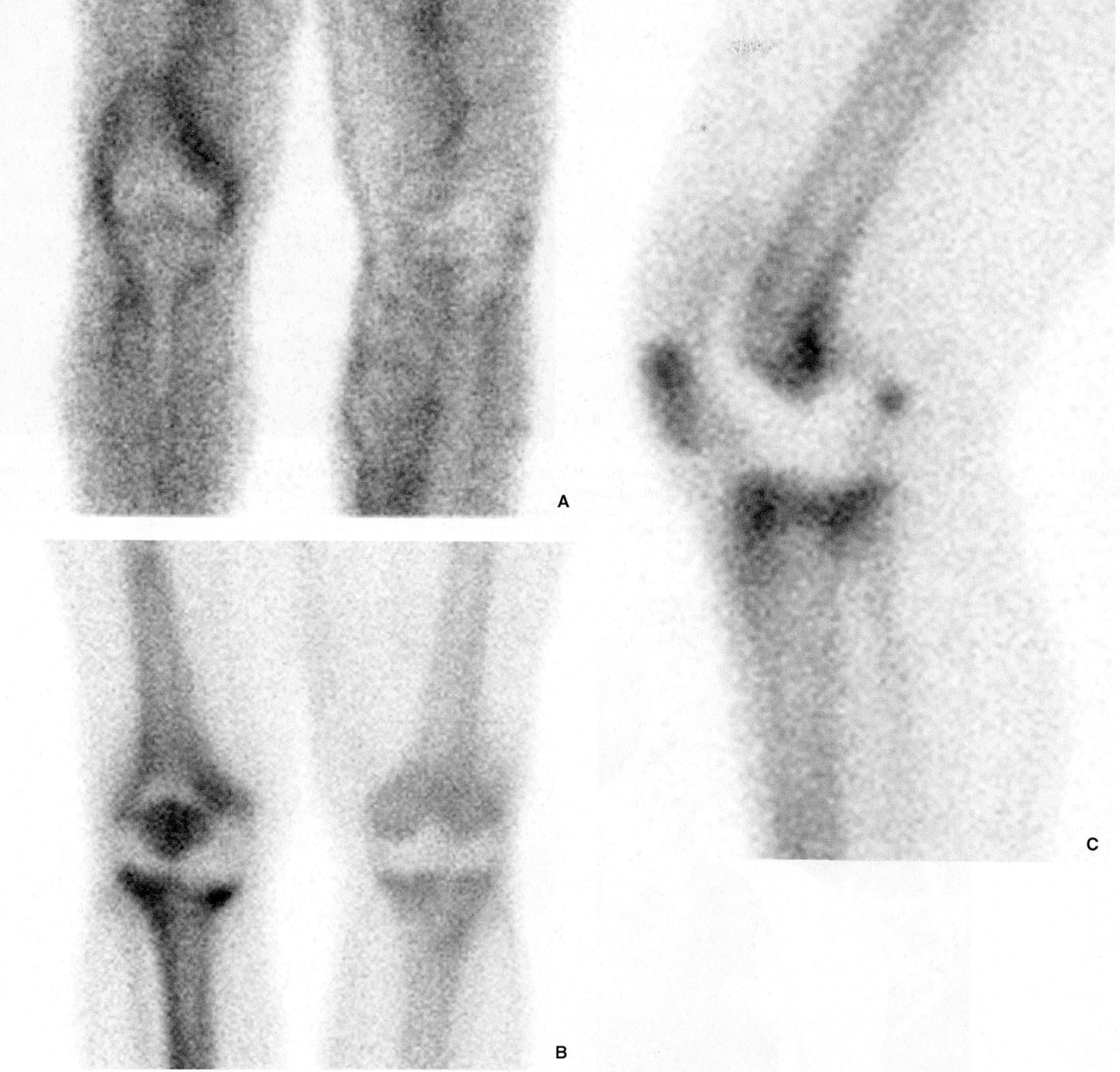

FIGURE 12.80 **Scintigraphy (technetium) of infected prosthesis.** A 63-year-old woman underwent bilateral total knee arthroplasty. A radionuclide bone scan using 25.0 mCi of ^{99m}Tc-labeled MDP was performed to evaluate possible infection. **(A)** Anterior blood pool image of both knees shows increased activity around the right knee prosthesis. The activity around the left knee prosthesis is normal. **(B)** The anterior planar delayed image of both knee and **(C)** lateral image of the right knee show increased uptake of the radiopharmaceutical tracer localized to all three components of the right knee prosthesis. The left knee prosthesis shows no abnormalities. The infection was confirmed by knee joint aspiration followed by fluid analysis and culture.

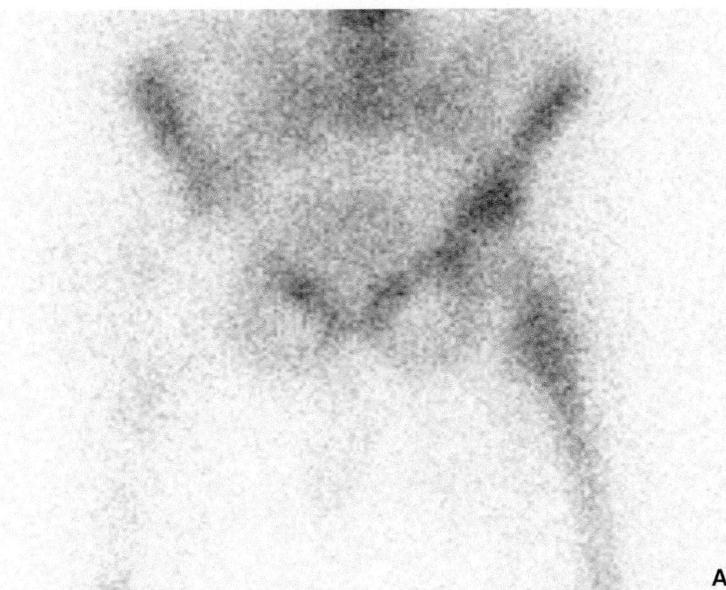

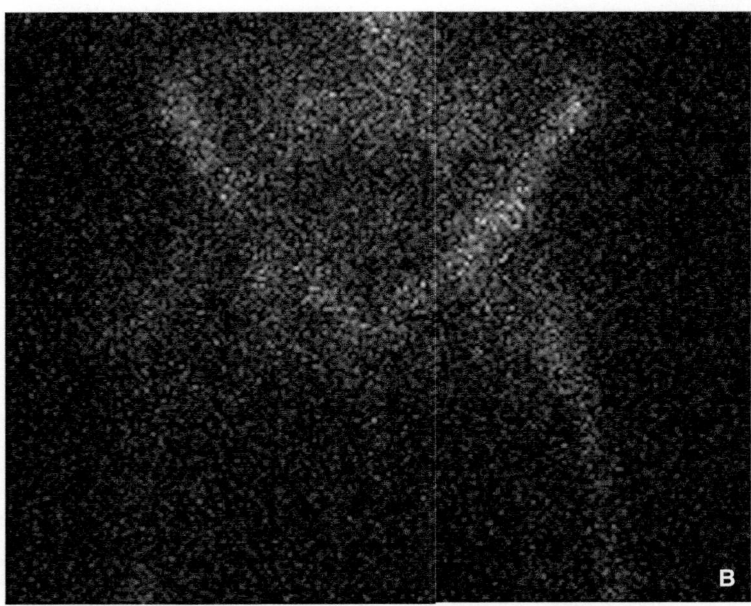

FIGURE 12.81 Scintigraphy (technetium and indium) of infected prosthesis. A 59-year-old man had bilateral total hip arthroplasties for advanced OA. He presented with fever and severe pain in the left hip. **(A)** Delayed image of the planar radionuclide technetium bone scan shows increased uptake of the radiopharmaceutical tracer in the region of the left hip prosthesis. Observe normal uptake at the site of the right hip prosthesis. **(B)** Indium bone scan using ^{111}In oxine-labeled WBCs shows increased uptake around the left hip prosthesis. The diagnosis of infection was confirmed by fluid aspiration and microbiologic examination that revealed methicillin-resistant strain of *Staphylococcus aureus* (MRSA).

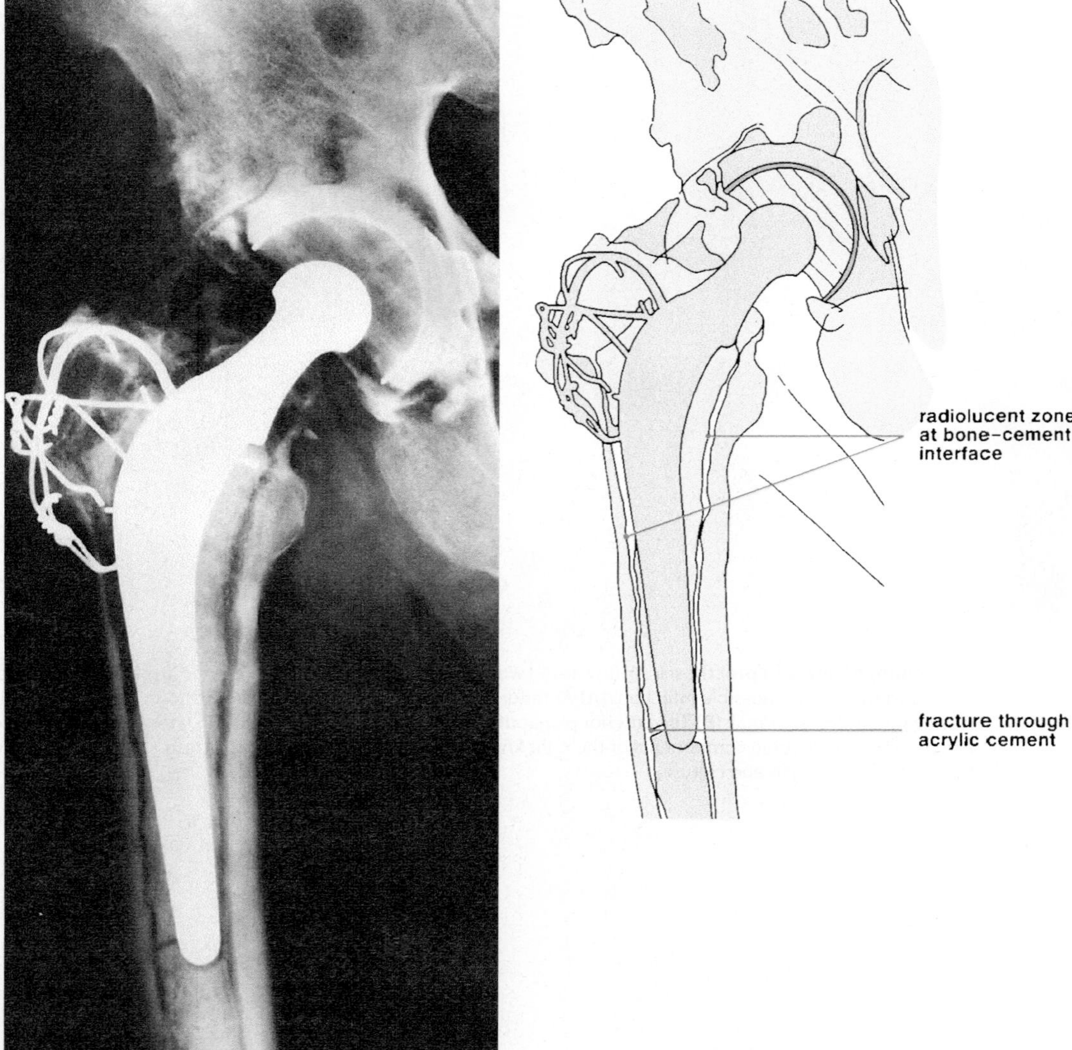

FIGURE 12.82 Failure of cemented total hip arthroplasty. Anteroposterior radiograph of the right hip of a 69-year-old woman shows a wide radiolucent zone at the bone–cement interface characteristic of loosening of a Charnley prosthesis. Note the fracture through the acrylic cement at the distal segment of the prosthetic stem.

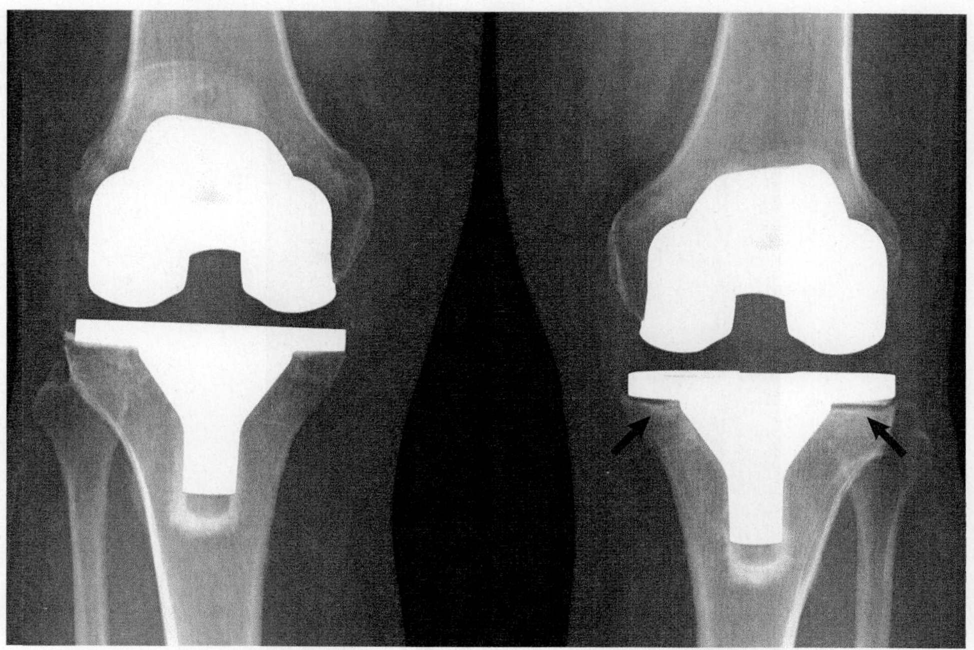

FIGURE 12.83 Failure of total knee arthroplasty. Anteroposterior radiograph of both knees of a 67-year-old man who underwent bilateral total knee arthroplasties for OA shows loosening of the tibial component of the left prosthesis *(arrows)*.

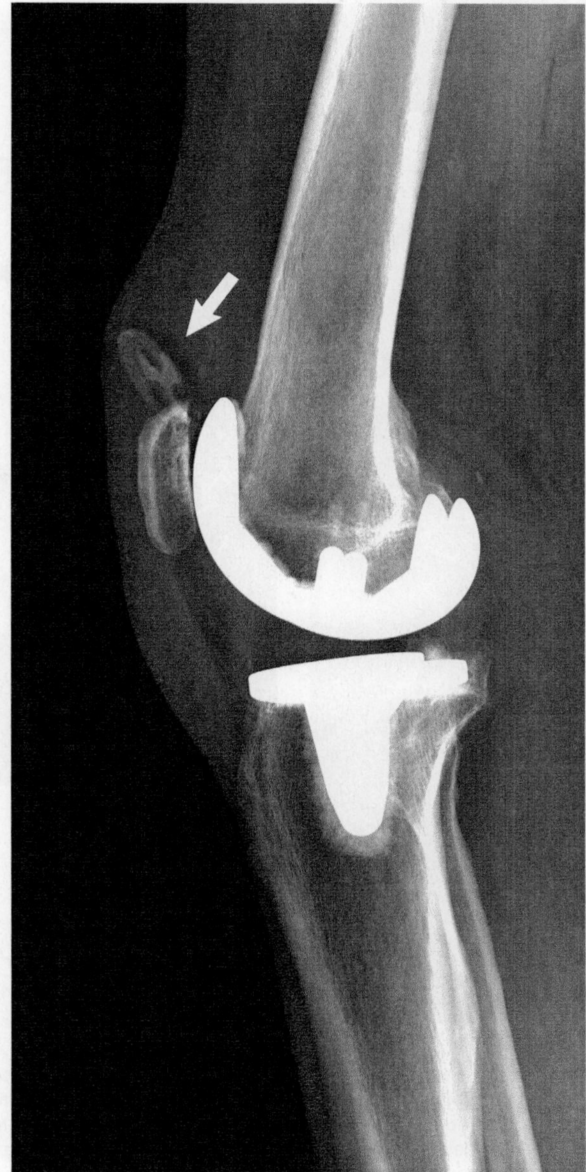

FIGURE 12.84 Failure of total knee arthroplasty. A lateral knee radiograph shows dislodgement of the patellar component of the prosthesis *(arrow)*.

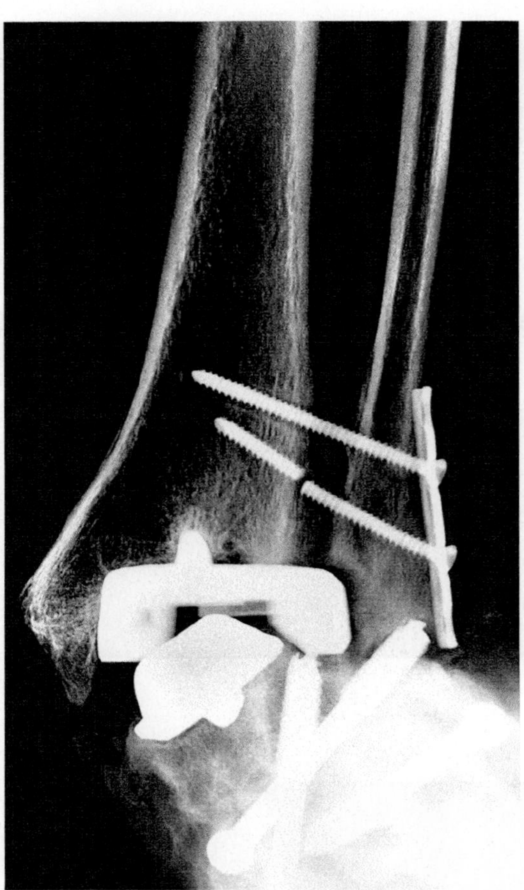

◀ **FIGURE 12.85 Failure of total ankle arthroplasty.** Oblique radiograph of the left ankle shows a failure of total ankle arthroplasty after placement of Agility prosthesis. Note malalignment of the tibial and talar parts of the prosthesis and a break of the distal syndesmotic screw.

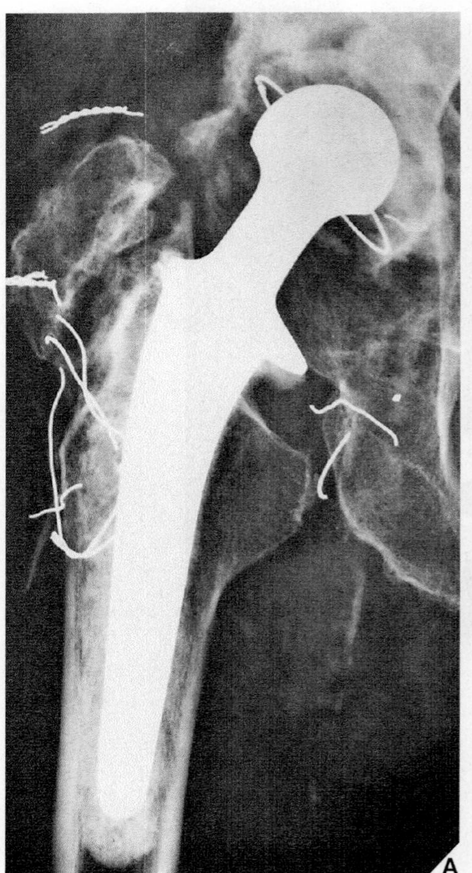

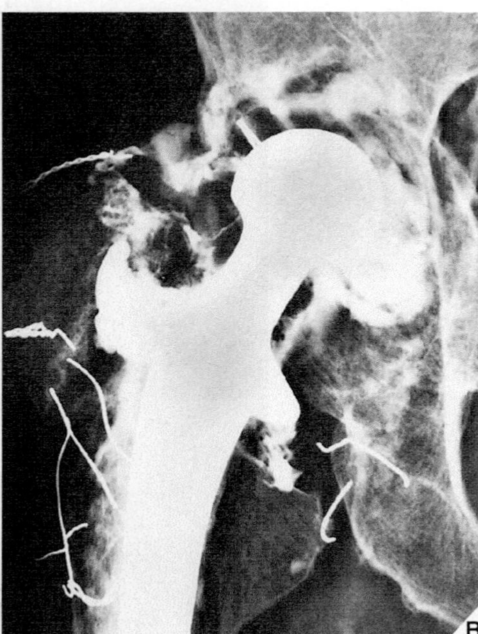

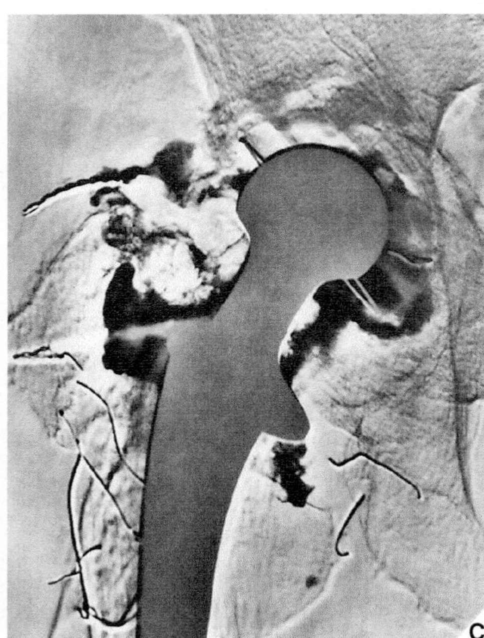

▲ **FIGURE 12.86 Failure of cemented total hip arthroplasty—value of subtraction arthrography.** An 80-year-old man had his right hip replaced 8 years before this radiographic examination. **(A)** Anteroposterior radiograph shows nonunion of the greater trochanter, broken wire sutures, and the suggestion of a radiolucent zone at the interface of the acrylic cement and bone in the acetabular component of the Charnley-Müller prosthesis. **(B)** On a subsequent arthrogram and **(C)** a subtraction-enhanced film, loosening of the prosthesis is clearly evident from the contrast agent seen entering the bone–cement gap and leaking medial and lateral to the neck of the prosthesis; the gap between the femur and separated greater trochanter is also opacified.

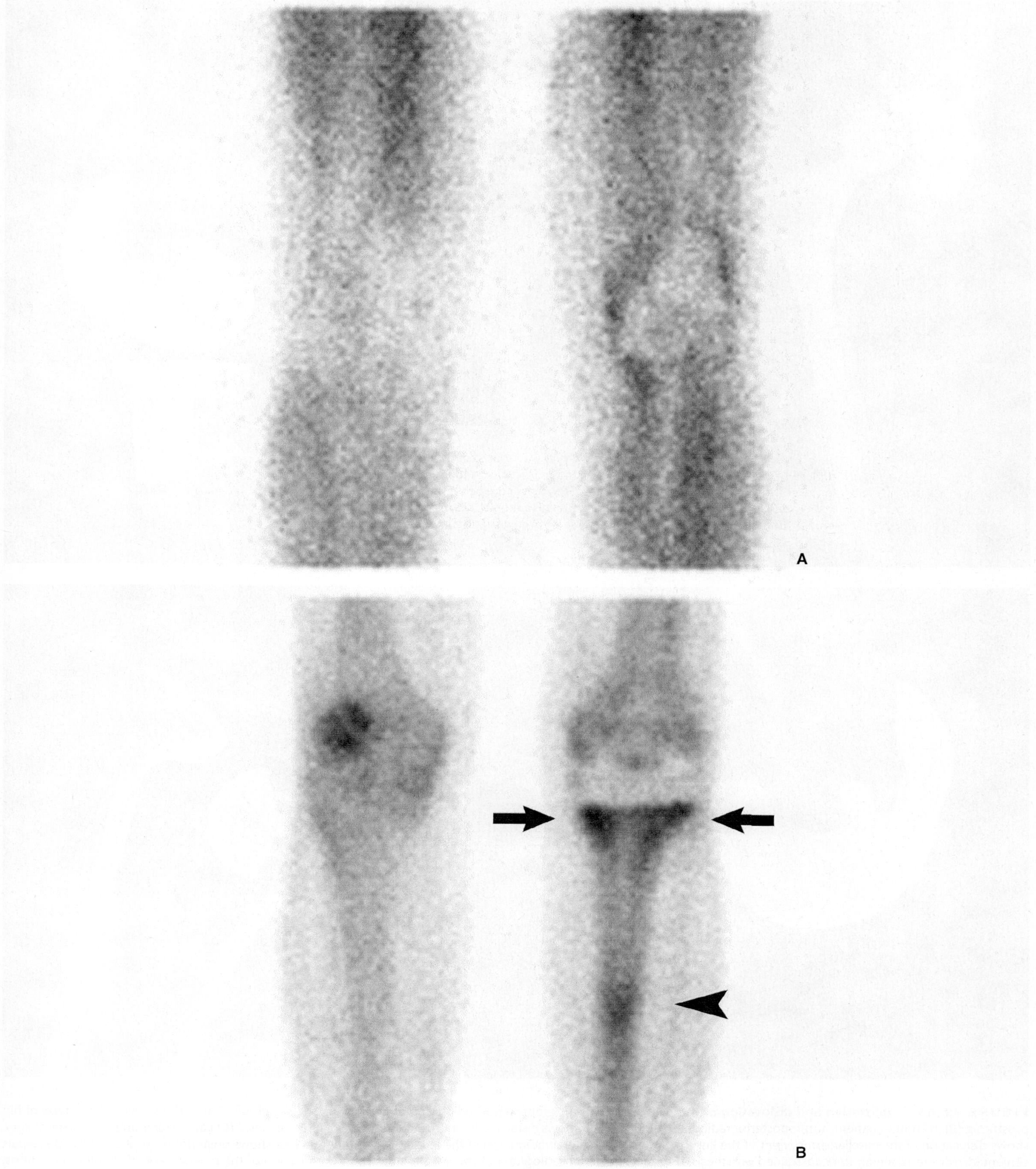

FIGURE 12.87 Scintigraphy of mechanical loosening of the prosthesis. Twenty-four months after undergoing left total knee arthroplasty, a 58-year-old man presented with discomfort and occasional pain at the site of the knee replacement. The radiographs (not shown here) demonstrated no obvious abnormalities. Radionuclide bone scan was performed next. **(A)** The blood pool image obtained after intravenous administration of 22.2 mCi of ^{99m}Tc-labeled MDP shows increased activity of the radiopharmaceutical tracer mostly at the site of the tibial component of the prosthesis. **(B)** The planar delayed image shows increased activity of the radiopharmaceutical tracer mostly at the site of the tibial plateau *(arrows)* and at the distal end of the tibial stem *(arrowhead)*. The focal increased uptake in the right patella is due to the prior fracture. (Reprinted with permission from Greenspan A, Gershwin ME. *Imaging in rheumatology: a clinical approach*. Philadelphia: Wolters Kluwer; 2018:60, Fig. 2.59; Courtesy of PZWL Wydawnictwo Lekarskie, Warsaw, Poland.)

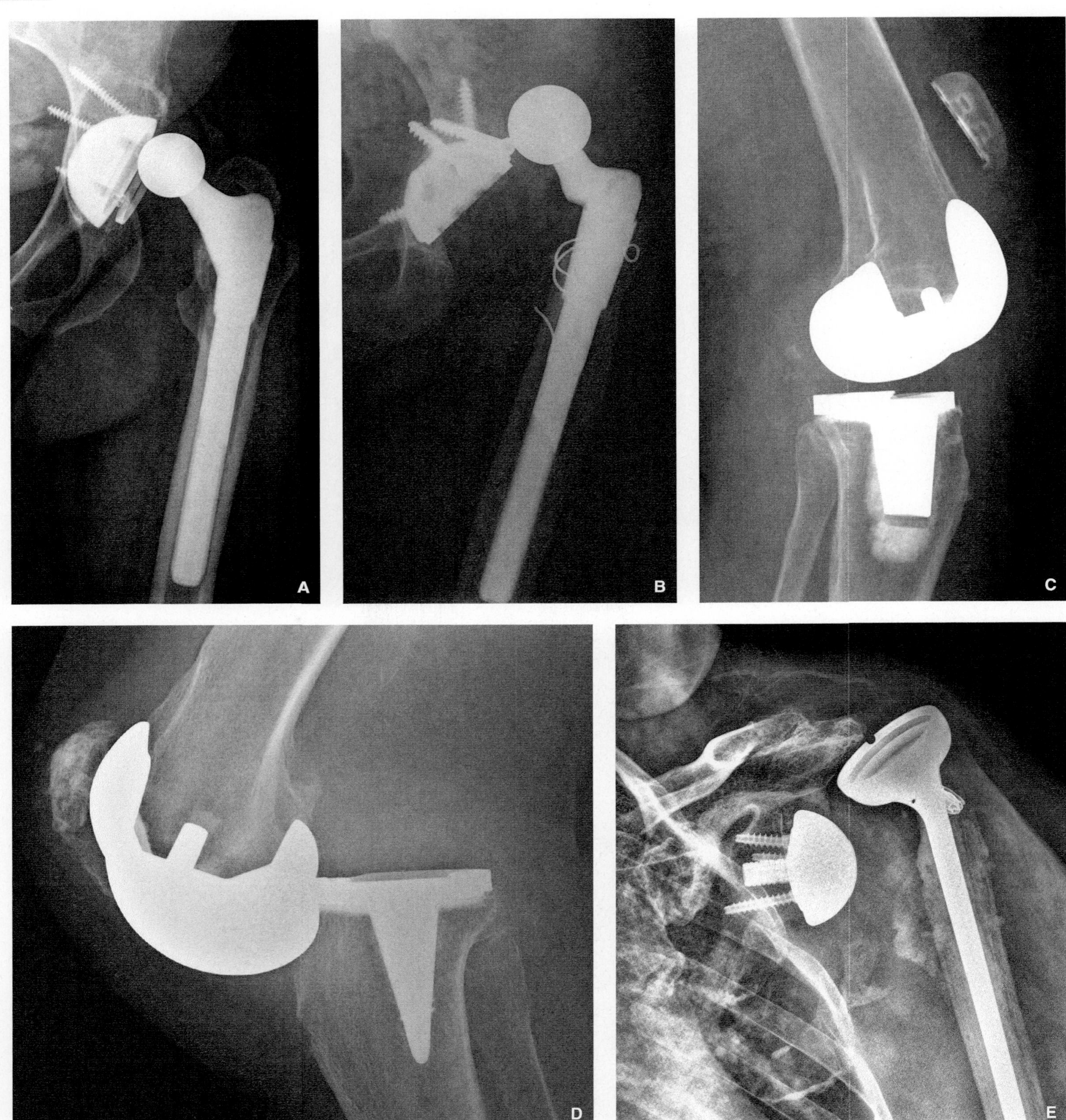

FIGURE 12.88 Subluxation and dislocation of the prosthesis. (A) Anteroposterior radiograph of the left hip shows subluxation of the noncemented type of hip prosthesis. **(B)** In another patient, anteroposterior radiograph of the left hip shows dislocation of noncemented type of hip prosthesis. **(C)** Lateral radiograph of the right knee shows dislocation of the patellar component of the knee prosthesis. **(D)** Lateral radiograph of the left knee of another patient shows posterior dislocation of the three-part cemented cruciate-retaining nonconstrained prosthesis. **(E)** Anteroposterior radiograph of the left shoulder shows dislocation of the reverse type of shoulder prosthesis. (Reprinted with permission from Greenspan A, Gerswhin ME. *Imaging in rheumatology*. Philadelphia: Wolters Kluwer; 2018:131, Fig. 4.28E.)

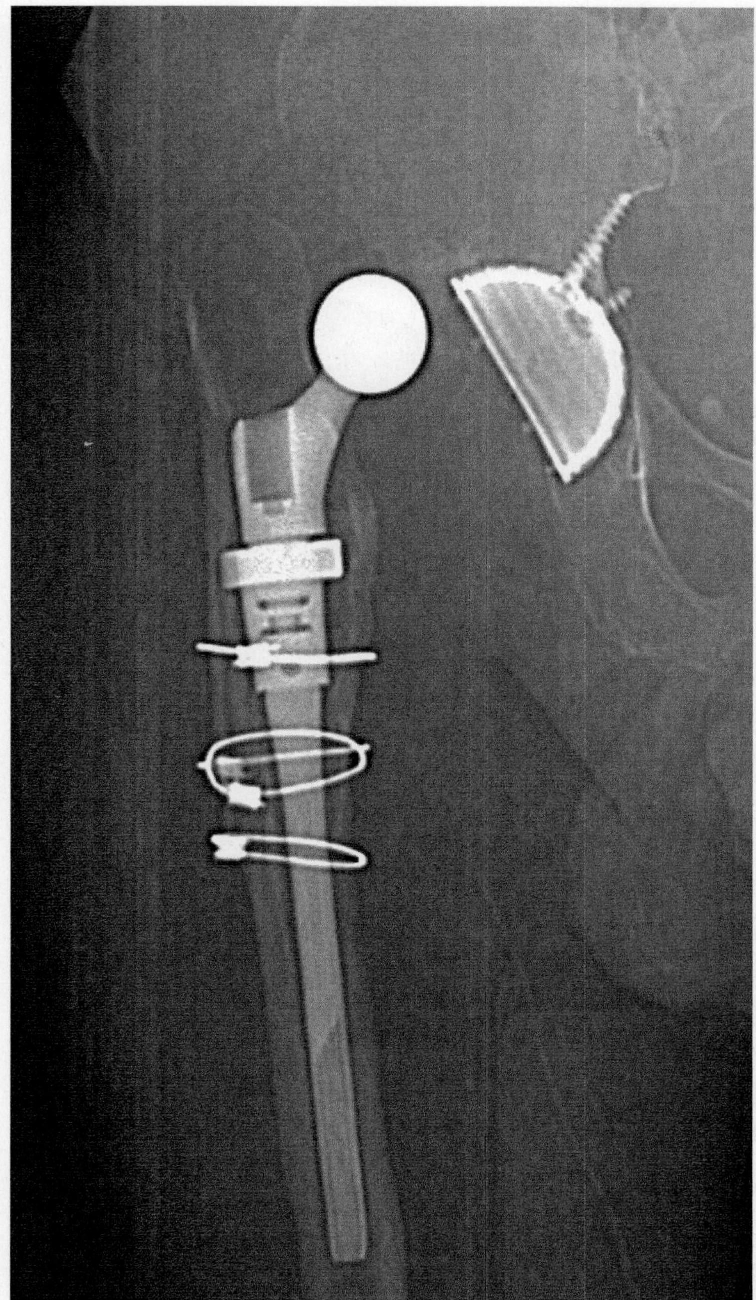

FIGURE 12.89 CT of prosthesis dislocation. Scout CT image shows superolateral dislocation of the femoral component of the total right hip prosthesis.

After total knee arthroplasty, similar complication may occur. The smallest polyethylene-wear particles induce a cytokine-mediated, intraarticular inflammatory reaction, referred to as *particle disease* (see in the following text), which may result in polyethylene wear-induced synovitis. This complication shows on MRI synovial thickening associated with dense synovial proliferation and debris with low-to-intermediate signal intensity (similar to that of skeletal muscle) and variable amounts of interspersed fluid and joint distention.

Particle Disease (Metallosis)

This complication, also known as *particle inclusion disease*, *giant cell granulomatosis*, or *aggressive granulomatosis*, is the result of inflammation and osteolysis secondary to shedding of micron- and submicron-size portions of the prosthesis. It commonly occurs from 1 to 5 years after implantation of cementless prosthesis. It has been reported in the setting of total hip, total shoulder, total knee, and unicompartmental knee arthroplasties. It may occur secondary to wear in metal-on-metal arthroplasties or in arthroplasties with a polyethylene component due to abnormal contact between metal surfaces following erosion or displacement of the polyethylene. The rate of metallosis complication depends on the material used—titanium components are more likely to cause this complication than cobalt-chromium components.

The patient may be asymptomatic until substantial loss of bone, at which time he or she may experience pain and limitation of motion. Radiography is usually diagnostic, demonstrating fluffy increased densities in the periprosthetic soft tissues ("cloud sign"), radiolucency at the metal–bone interface, endosteal scalloping without reactive sclerosis, or large focal defects. At times, metallic particles are seen in the vicinity of the prosthesis (Figs. 12.92 and 12.93).

Inflammatory Reaction and Pseudotumors

Approximately 35% of second-generation metal-on-metal hip prosthesis develop an inflammatory reaction called ALVAL, which can evolve into formation of pseudotumors around the hip prosthesis. This complication is probably related to the release of metal ions from the prosthesis producing a hypersensitivity response in the local soft tissues (Fig. 12.94).

Loosening of Silicon Prosthesis, Silicone Synovitis, and Infection

Mechanical loosening of the silicon prosthesis is best evaluated by CT (Fig. 12.95). Silicone synovitis, which represents the tissue response to the shedding of silicone particles from the implants that are damaged by shear and compressive forces, is more serious complication. The radiographic findings include nodular soft-tissue swelling and well-defined subchondral lytic defects and osseous erosions as well as deformity or fracture of the prosthesis (Figs. 12.96 and 12.97). Infection of silastic implant is best evaluated with MRI. In addition to multiple small hypointense particles in the vicinity of the implants, this modality shows intermediate-to-mild hyperintensity osseous lesions on proton- and T2-weighted sequences. These signal intensities characteristics are consistent with the presence of inflammatory and fibrous tissue (Fig. 12.98).

Arthrofibrosis

This is a complication following knee arthroplasty characterized by chronic pain, global capsular contraction, and progressive loss of range of motion, and may lead to complete joint stiffness. Arthrofibrosis is caused by the formation of dense fibrous tissue along the synovial lining of the entire joint due to excessive fibroplasia with resulting adhesions and impairment of the extensor mechanism of the knee.

Patellar Clunk Syndrome

This is a complication of total knee arthroplasty at the site of patellofemoral prosthetic components that manifests by a locking sensation or impaired motion during flexion and extension of the knee prosthesis. At physical examination, an audible clunking noise occurs during knee extension. This syndrome is caused by formation of focal fibrous tissue at the junction of the superior pole of the patella and quadriceps tendon, occurring usually about a year after joint replacement. One of the mechanisms of this complication is the entrance of the fibrous tissue into the intercondylar notch with knee flexion and its displacement with knee extension, resulting in audible clunk.

Periprosthetic Fracture

Periprosthetic fracture occurs as a result of the direct traumatic insult to the limb (low-energy trauma) or because the bone is weakened due to osteoporosis, periprosthetic osseous resorption, particle disease, or infection (osteomyelitis), leading to a form of pathologic fracture. The femur is most commonly affected after hip or knee arthroplasties (Figs. 12.99 to 12.101), following by the tibia and the humerus (Fig. 12.102). On rare occasion, the periprosthetic fracture may involve the acetabulum (Fig. 12.103).

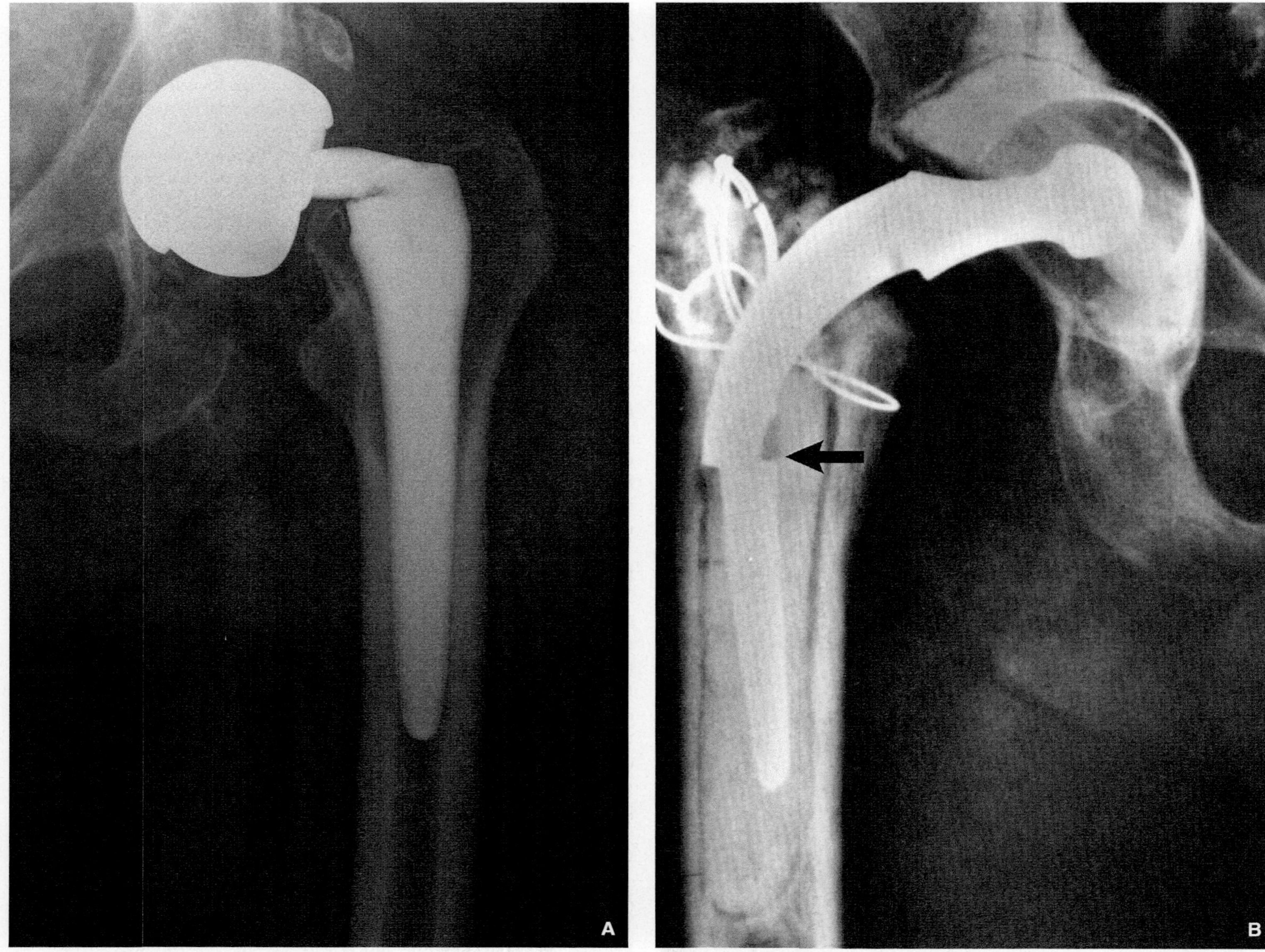

FIGURE 12.90 **Fracture of the prosthesis.** **(A)** Anteroposterior radiograph of the left hip shows a fracture of the femoral component of hip prosthesis. **(B)** Anteroposterior radiograph of the right hip of another patient shows a fracture of the stem of the femoral component of the cemented total hip prosthesis *(arrow)*. In addition, observe the break of the wires retaining the previously osteotomized greater trochanter and a radiolucent gap at the cement–bone interface of the femoral and acetabular components, diagnostic of loosening of the prosthesis.

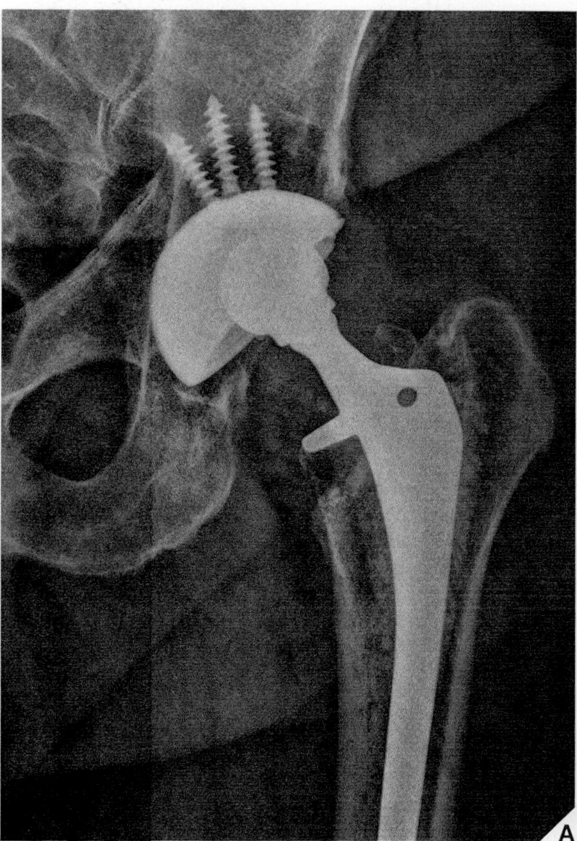

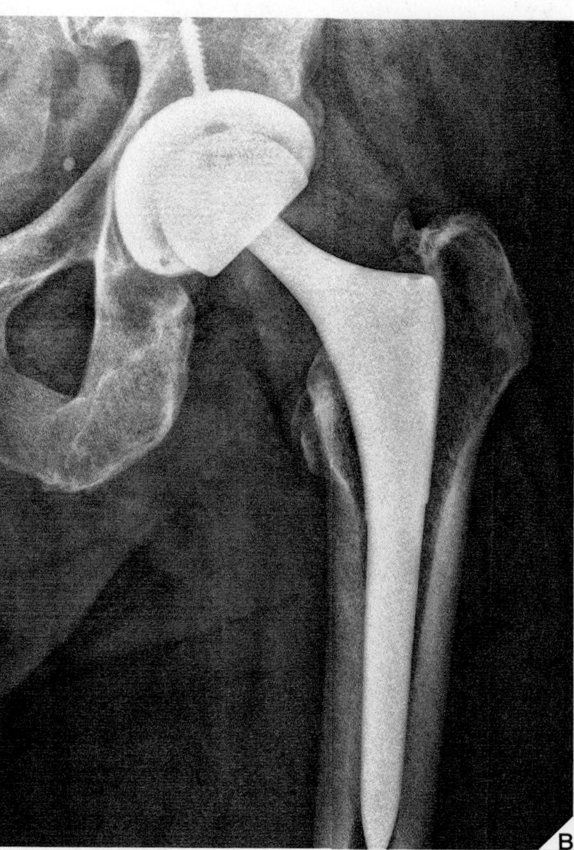

FIGURE 12.91 **Complication of total hip arthroplasty—polyethylene wear.** A 72-year-old man presented with hip pain after left total hip arthroplasty performed 4 years prior to the current admission. **(A)** Anteroposterior radiograph of the hip shows eccentric position of the prosthetic femoral head within the acetabular cup secondary to the wear of polyethylene lining. Note in addition the bone resorption at the site of the acetabular rim screws. **(B)** Normal symmetric position of the prosthetic femoral head within the acetabular cup and proper alignment is shown for comparison.

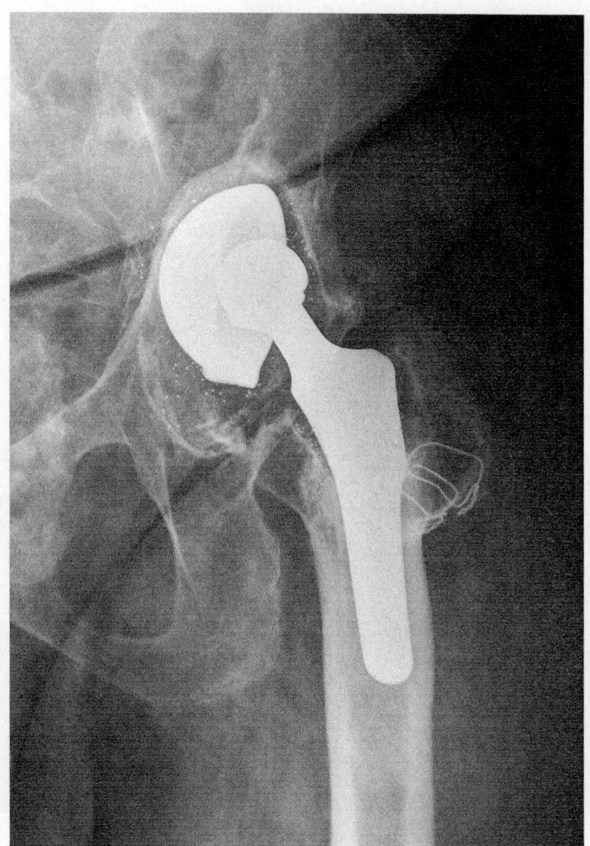

FIGURE 12.92 **Particle disease (metallosis).** A 60-year-old man had total noncemented hip arthroplasty performed 5 years prior to this examination. There is extensive bone destruction surrounding the acetabular component of the prosthesis which represents giant cell granulomatosis. Note also numerous metallic particles in the vicinity of the prosthesis.

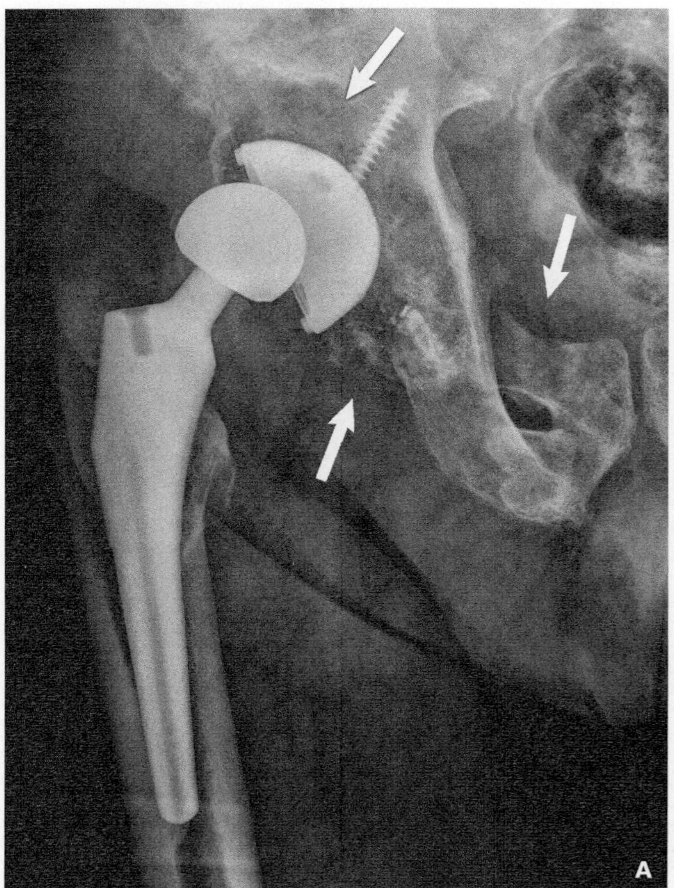

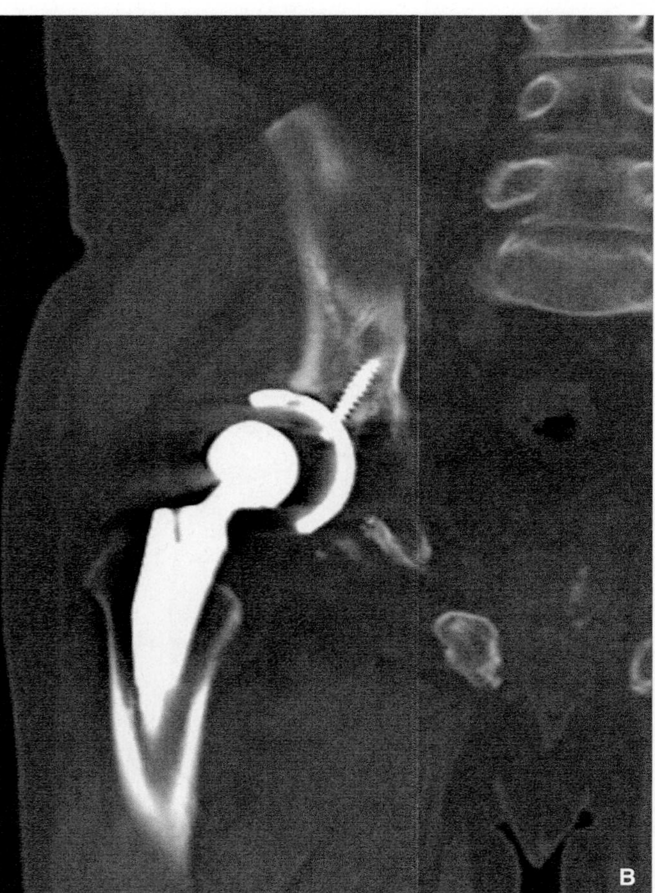

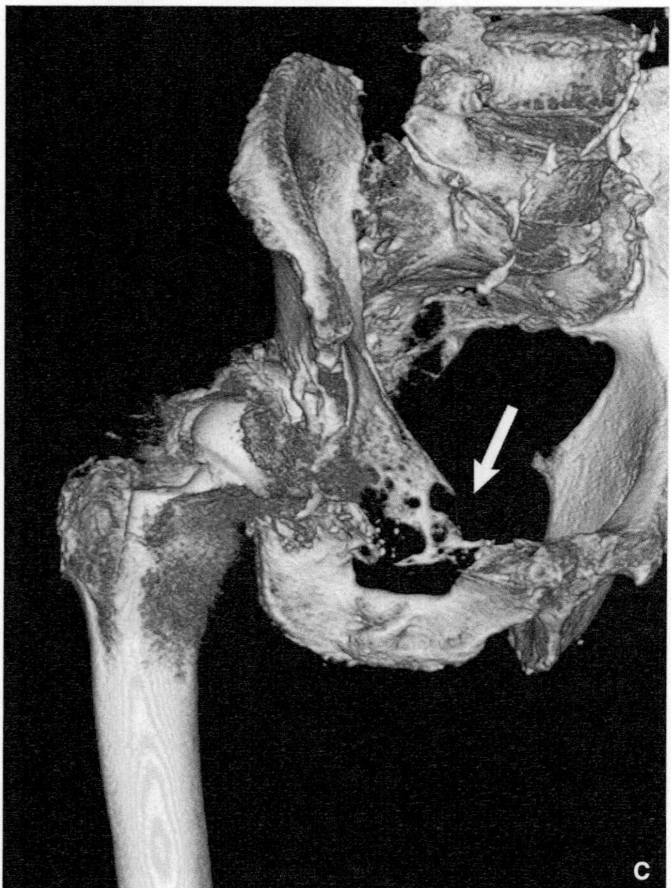

FIGURE 12.93 CT and 3D CT of particle disease (metallosis). A 61-year-old woman presented with severe pain at the site of right total hip arthroplasty. **(A)** Anteroposterior radiograph of the right hip shows subluxation of noncemented hip prosthesis. In addition, note destructive changes of the bone at the site of acetabular component and in the pubic and ischial bones *(arrows)*. **(B)** Coronal reformatted and **(C)** 3D reconstructed CT images demonstrate the bone destruction more accurately. Particularly, the destruction of the pubic bone is well depicted *(arrow)*. (Reprinted with permission from Greenspan A, Gershwin ME. *Imaging in rheumatology: a clinical approach*, 1st ed. Philadelphia: Wolters Kluwer; 2018:134.)

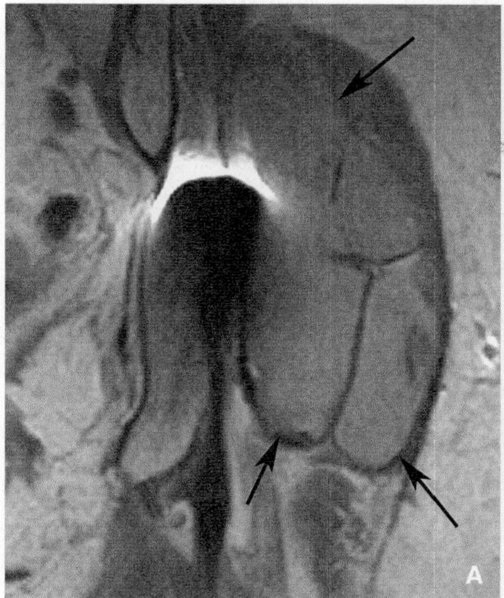

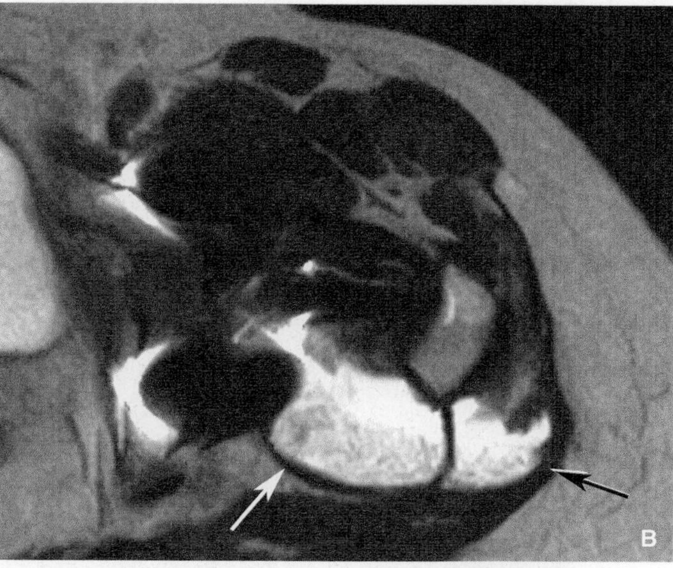

FIGURE 12.94 **Aseptic lymphocyte-dominated vasculitis associate lesion.** **(A)** Coronal proton density–weighted and **(B)** axial T2-weighted MR pulse sequences of the left hip obtained in a patient, who presented with pain after undergoing metal-on-metal total hip arthroplasty, demonstrate a fluid collection adjacent to the metallic prosthesis and extending inferiorly and posteriorly *(arrows)*. Pathologic examination of the aspirated material revealed abundant lymphocytes and vasculitis, consistent with ALVAL.

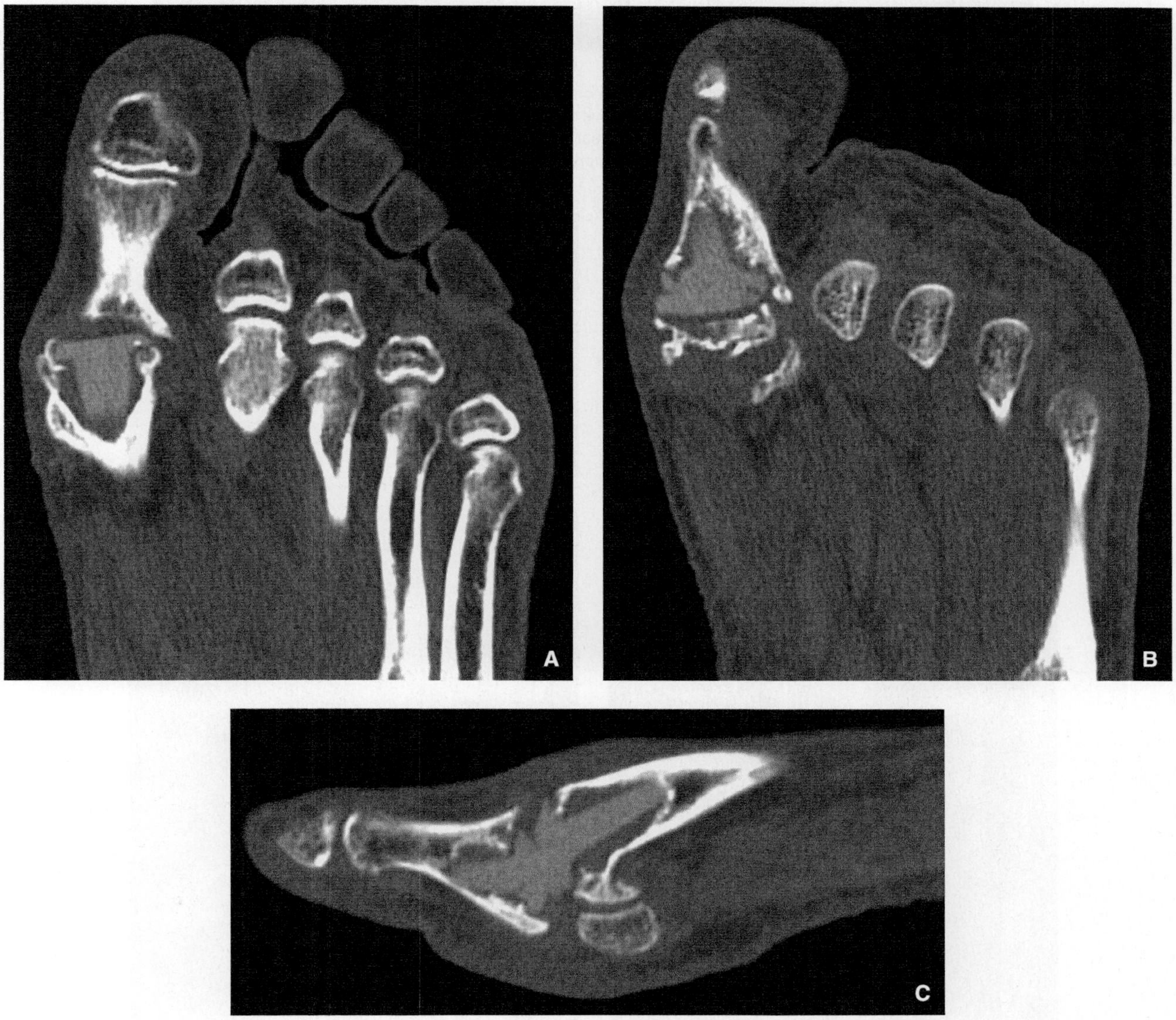

FIGURE 12.95 **Failure of silastic prosthesis.** Two coronal reformatted CT images of the left foot of a patient who underwent silastic arthroplasty of the first metatarsophalangeal joint demonstrate a wide gap separating **(A)** the metatarsal and **(B)** the phalangeal part of the prosthesis from bone. **(C)** Sagittal reformatted CT image of the great toe shows loosening of the prosthesis more clearly. (Reprinted with permission from Greenspan A, Gershwin ME. *Imaging in rheumatology: a clinical approach*, 1st ed. Philadelphia: Wolters Kluwer; 2018:135.)

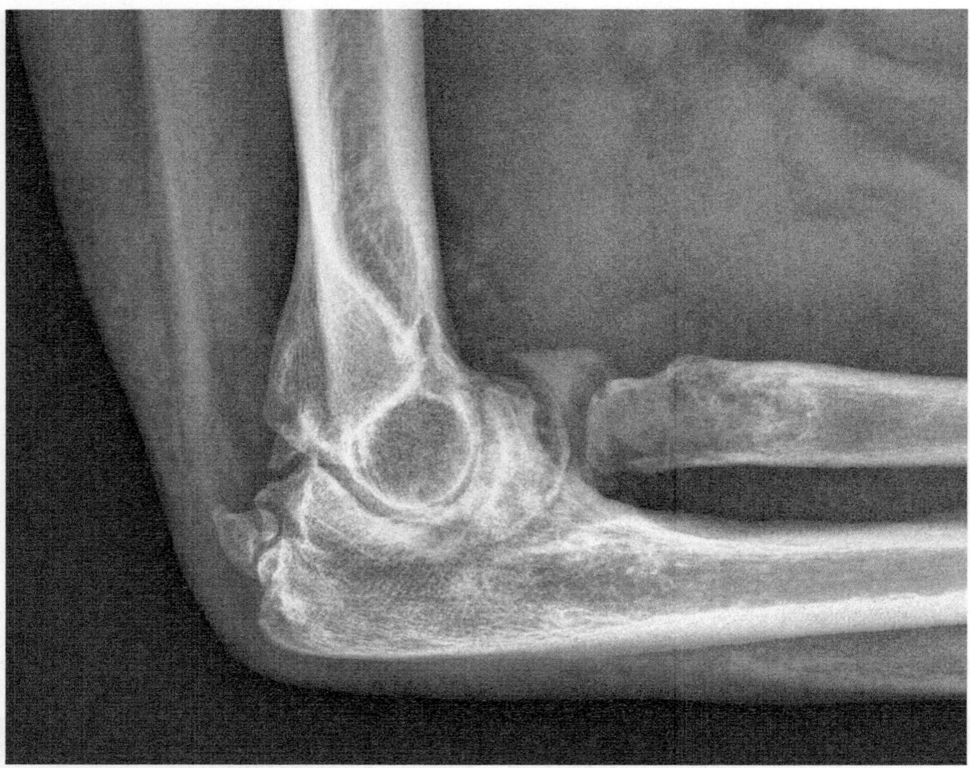

FIGURE 12.96 Silicone synovitis. A 67-year-old woman with posttraumatic OA of the right elbow had resection of the radial head and replacement with silastic radial head prosthesis. A lateral radiograph of the elbow shows fracture of the implant, erosive changes in the proximal radius and capitellum, and elbow joint effusion with silicone debris, all features consistent with silicone synovitis. Note also OA of the ulna–trochlear joint compartment and heterotopic ossifications around the olecranon. (Reprinted with permission from Greenspan A, Gershwin ME. *Imaging in rheumatology: a clinical approach*, 1st ed. Philadelphia: Wolters Kluwer; 2018:135.)

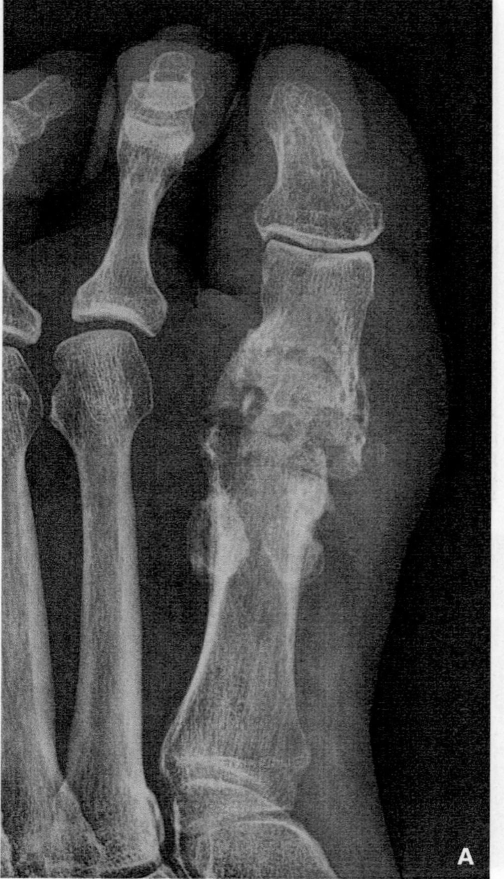

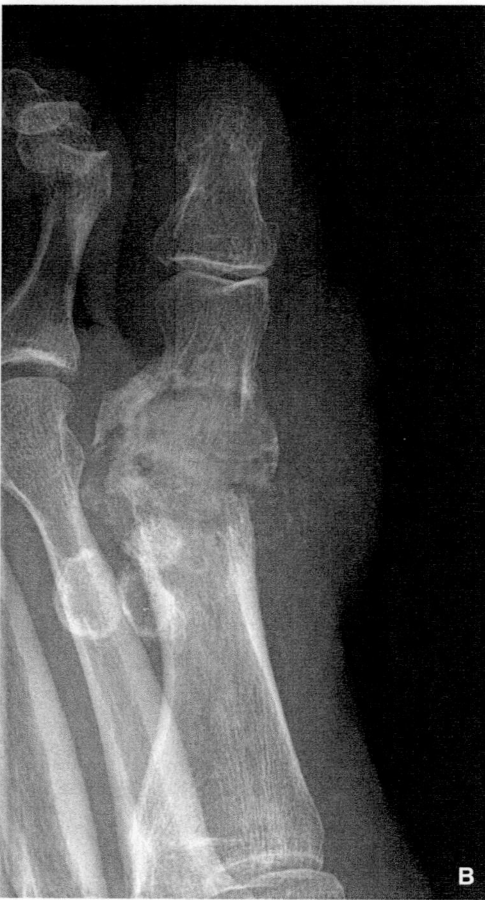

FIGURE 12.97 Silicone synovitis. A 72-year-old woman who underwent first metatarsophalangeal joint arthroplasty for OA presented with pain and swelling of the great toe. **(A)** Anteroposterior and **(B)** oblique radiographs of the great toe show fragmentation of the prosthesis, silastic debris, osseous erosions, and a large soft-tissue swelling, typical findings of silicone synovitis.

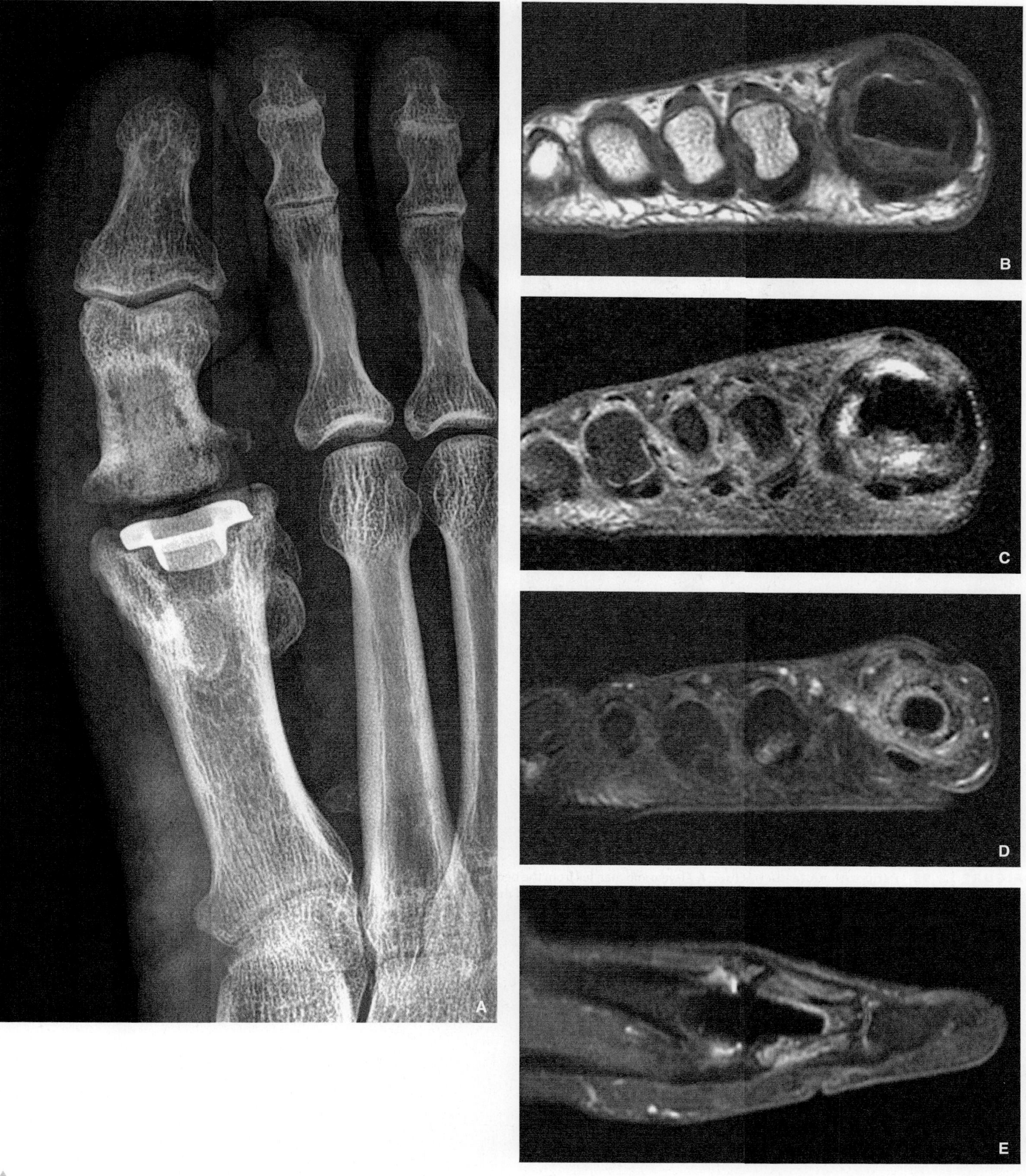

FIGURE 12.98 **MRI of infection of silastic prosthesis.** **(A)** Anteroposterior radiograph of the great toe of the left foot shows status post first metatarsophalangeal arthroplasty using Swanson silicone device with circumferential titanium grommet. There is soft-tissue swelling surrounding the prosthesis. In addition, there is radiolucent zone surrounding the prosthetic stems. **(B)** Axial (short axis) T1-weighted MR image through the metatarsal heads shows low-intensity implant in place. **(C)** Axial STIR MR image shows high-signal edema surrounding the implant. **(D)** Axial and **(E)** sagittal T1-weighted fat-suppressed MR images obtained after intravenous administration of gadolinium show enhancement of the bone and soft tissue surrounding the distal portion of the prosthesis. (Reprinted with permission from Greenspan A, Gershwin ME. *Imaging in rheumatology: a clinical approach*, 1st ed. Philadelphia: Wolters Kluwer; 2018:137.)

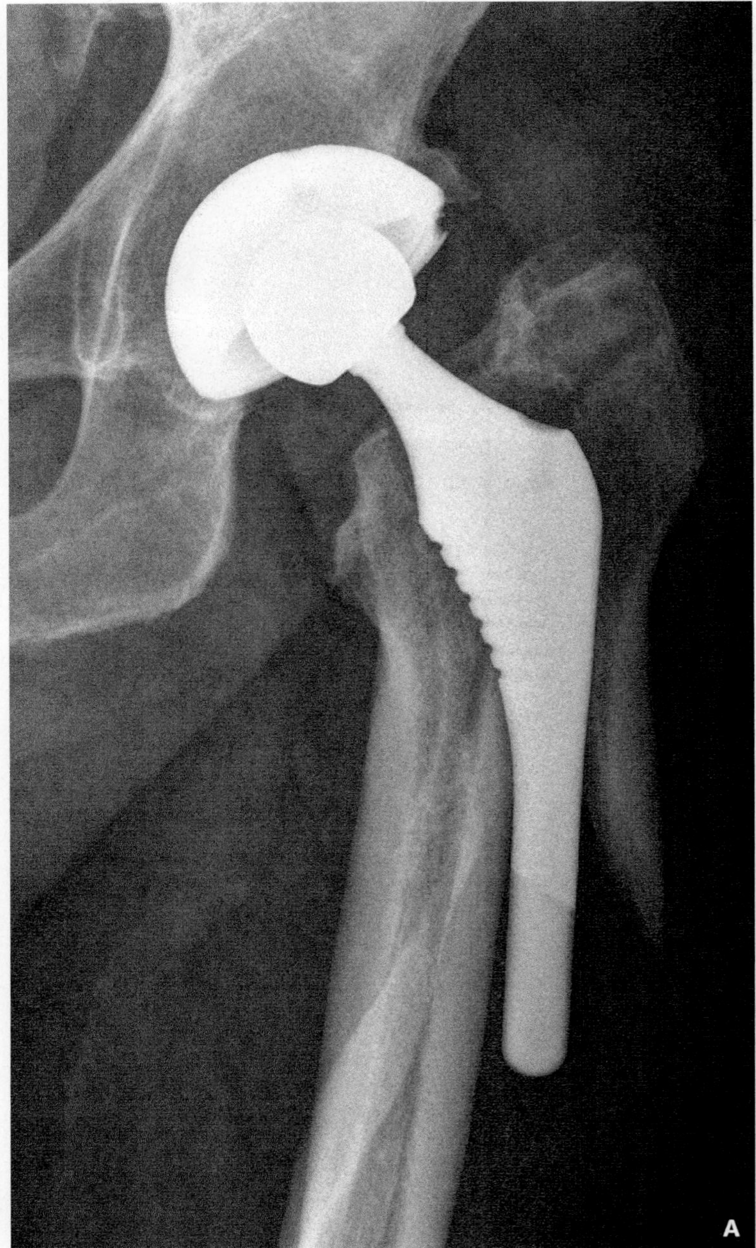

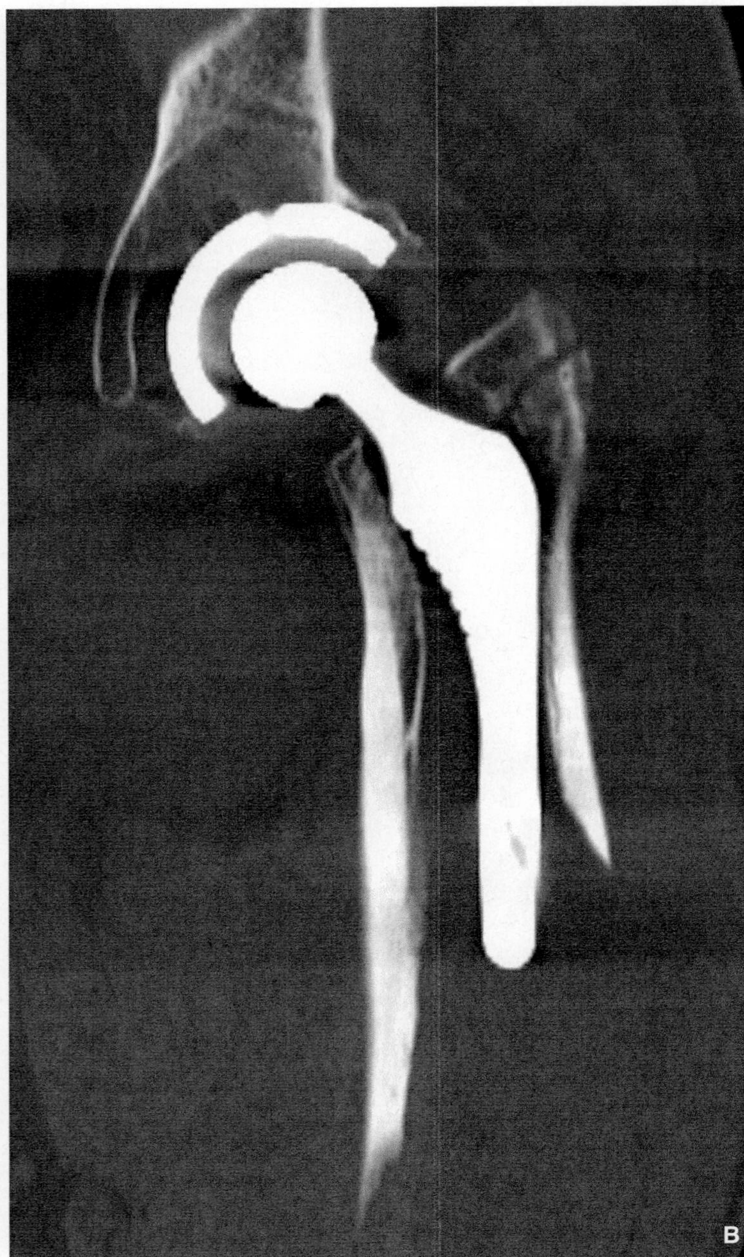

FIGURE 12.99 **Periprosthetic femur fracture.** A 71-year-old man fell from the bed. **(A)** Anteroposterior radiograph of the left hip and **(B)** coronal reformatted CT image show status post noncemented total hip arthroplasty. Note periprosthetic fracture of the femoral shaft at the site of the femoral component of the prosthesis.

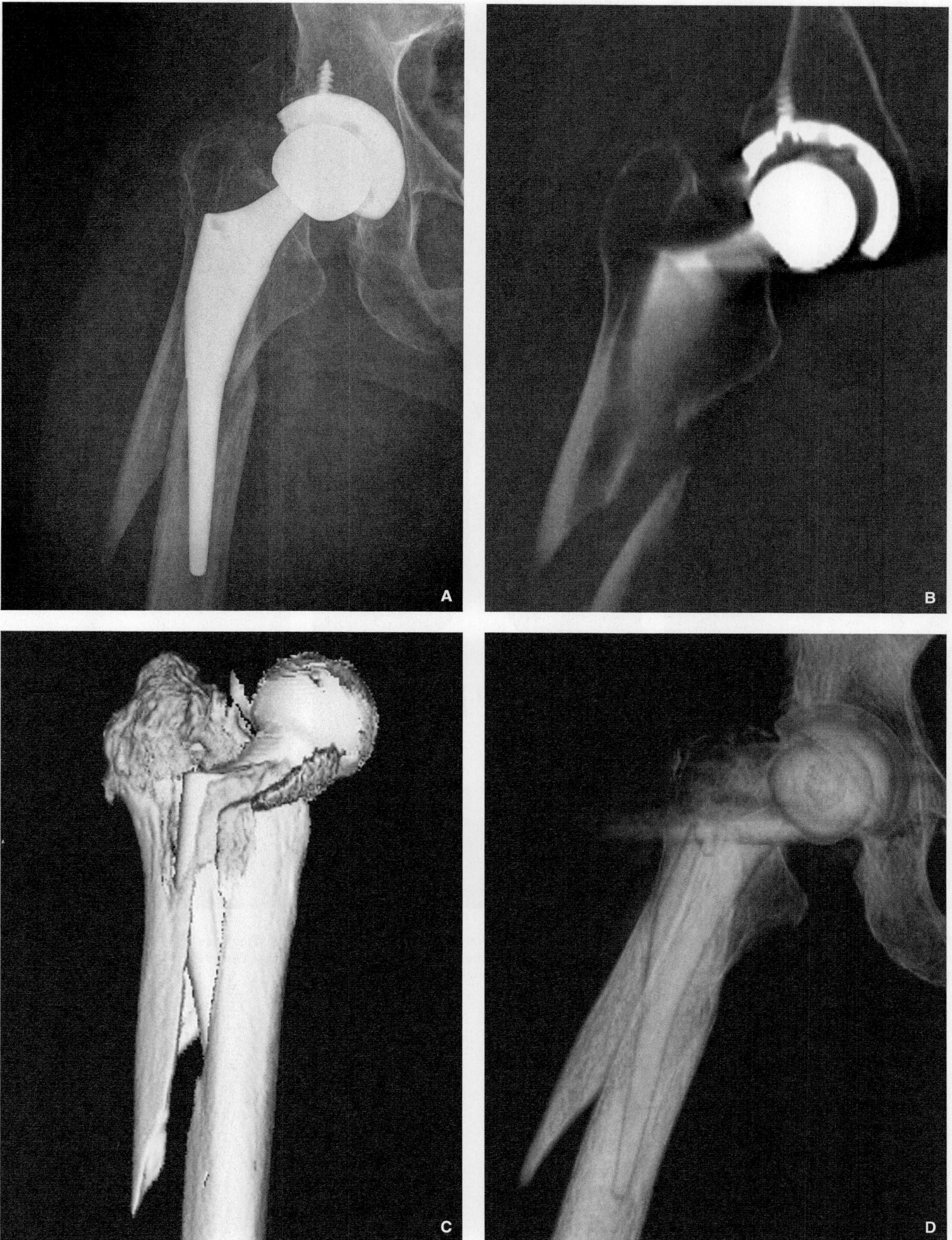

FIGURE 12.100 **Periprosthetic femur fracture.** A 77-year-old man fell from the bike. **(A)** Anteroposterior radiograph of the right hip, **(B)** coronal reformatted CT image, **(C)** 3D reconstructed CT image, and **(D)** 3D reconstructed volume-rendered CT image with metal-enhancing algorithm show status post total noncemented hip arthroplasty complicated by a periprosthetic fracture of the femoral shaft at the site of the femoral component of the prosthesis.

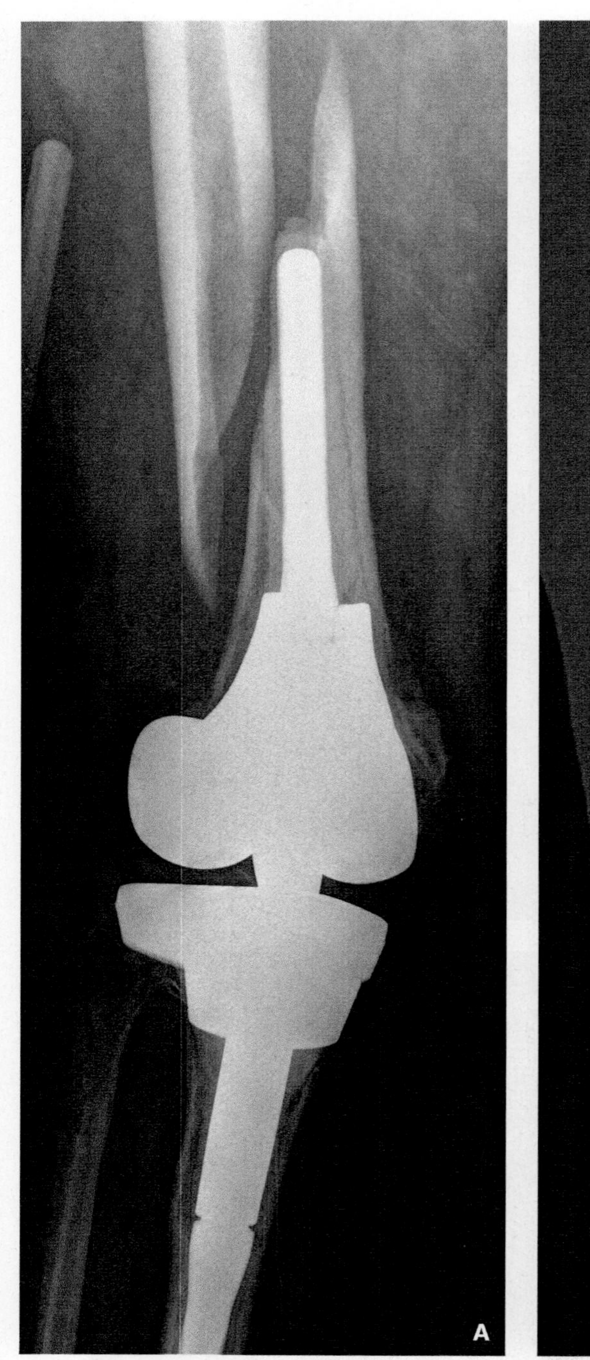

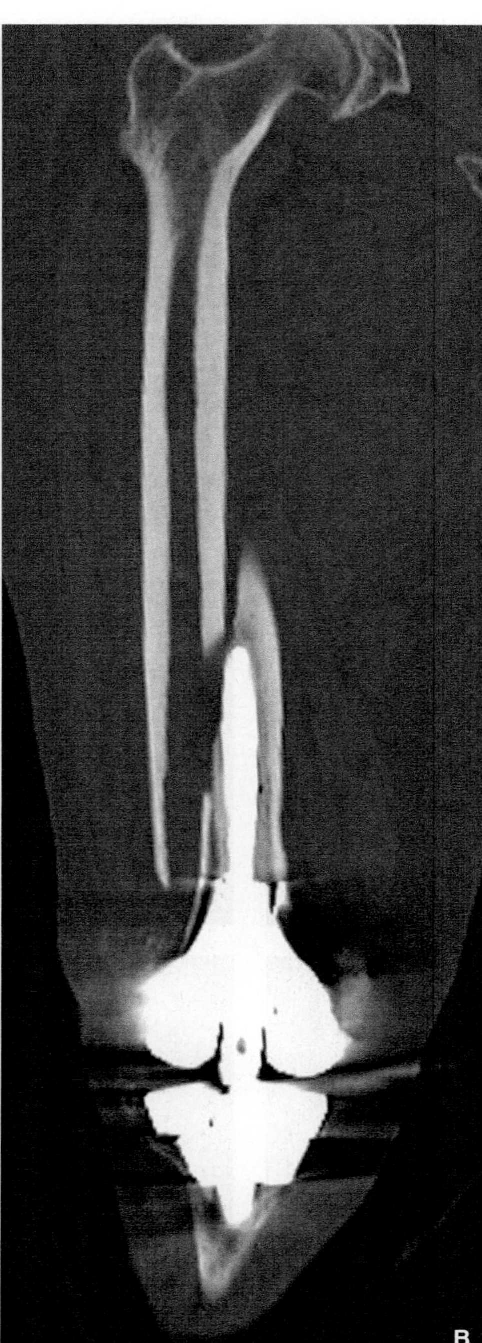

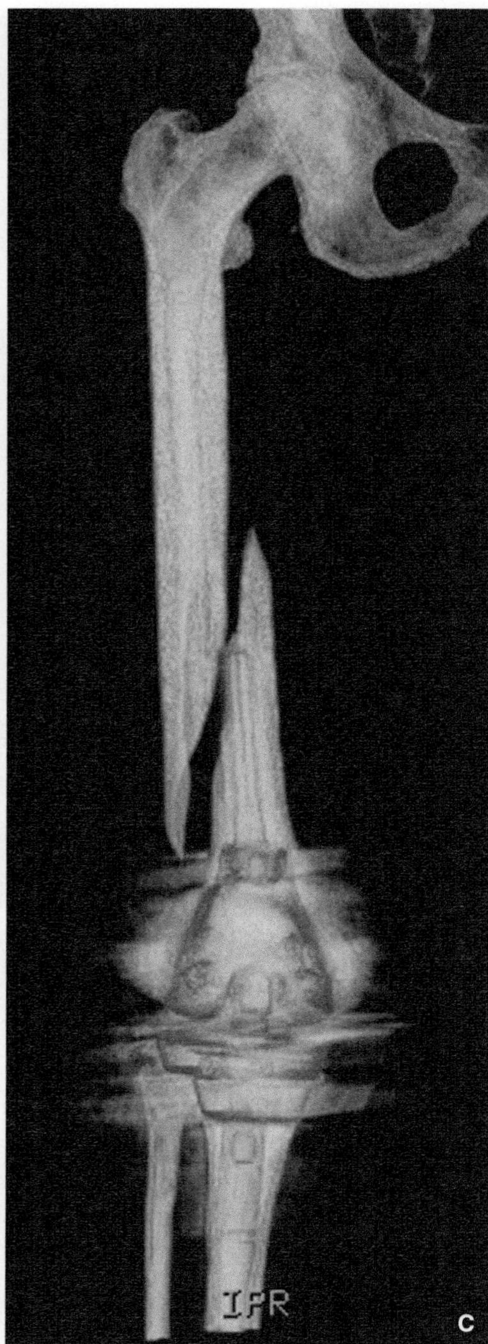

FIGURE 12.101 **Periprosthetic femur fracture.** A 71-year-old man, who recently underwent total constrained hinged knee arthroplasty for advanced OA, tripped over a step and twisted his knee in a fall. **(A)** Anteroposterior radiograph of the right knee, **(B)** coronal reformatted CT image of the femur, and **(C)** 3D reconstructed volume-rendered CT image with metal-enhancing algorithm show periprosthetic fracture of the distal part of the femoral shaft.

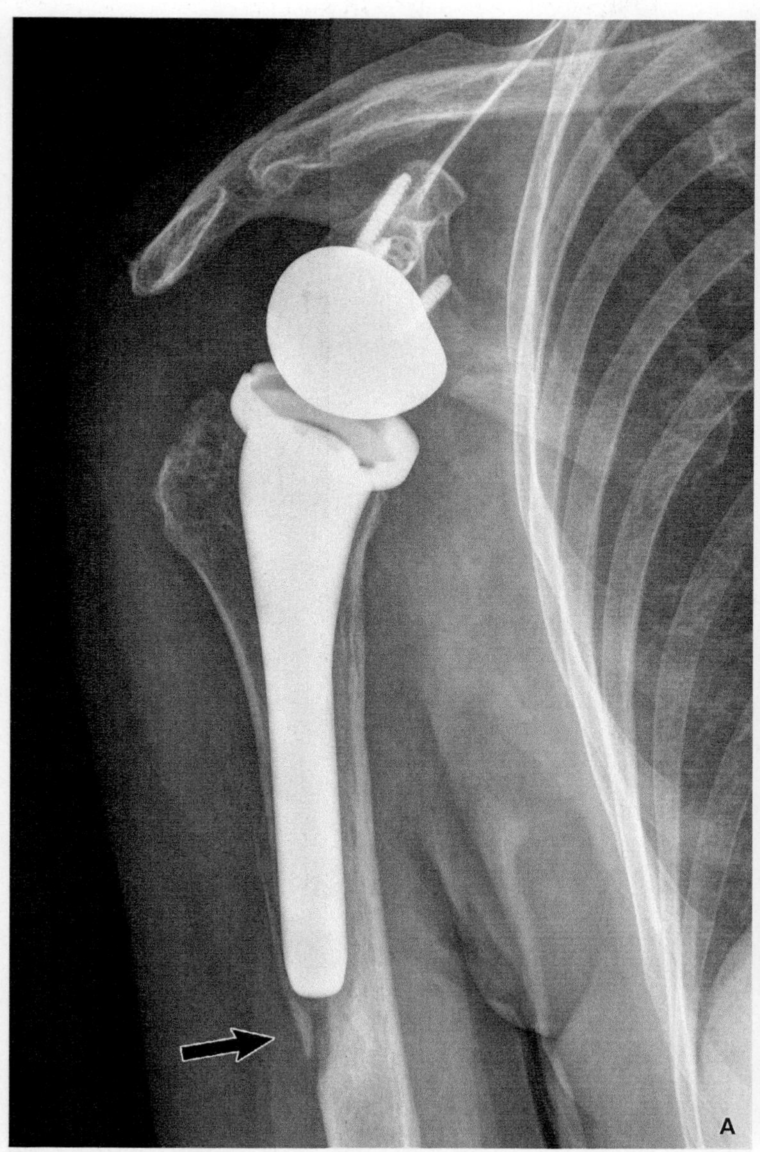

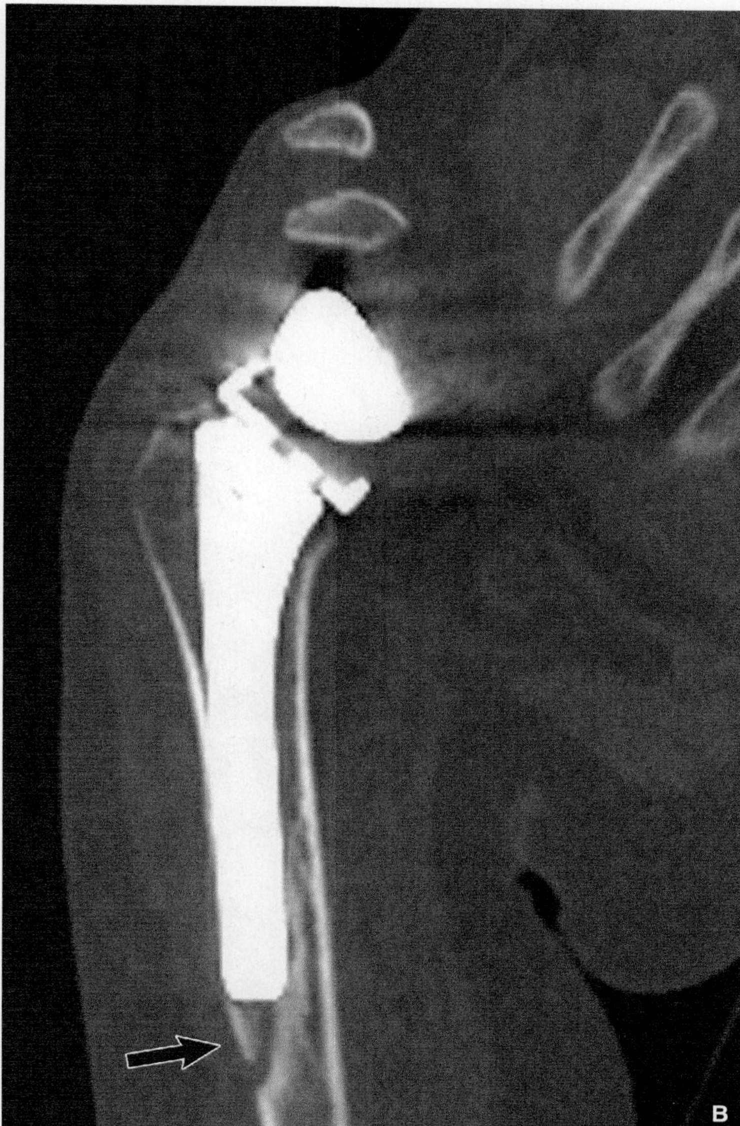

FIGURE 12.102 **Periprosthetic humerus fracture.** **(A)** Anteroposterior radiograph of the right shoulder and **(B)** coronal reformatted CT image show status post total reverse shoulder arthroplasty. Observe periprosthetic fracture of the humeral shaft at the distal end of the humeral prosthetic component *(arrows)*.

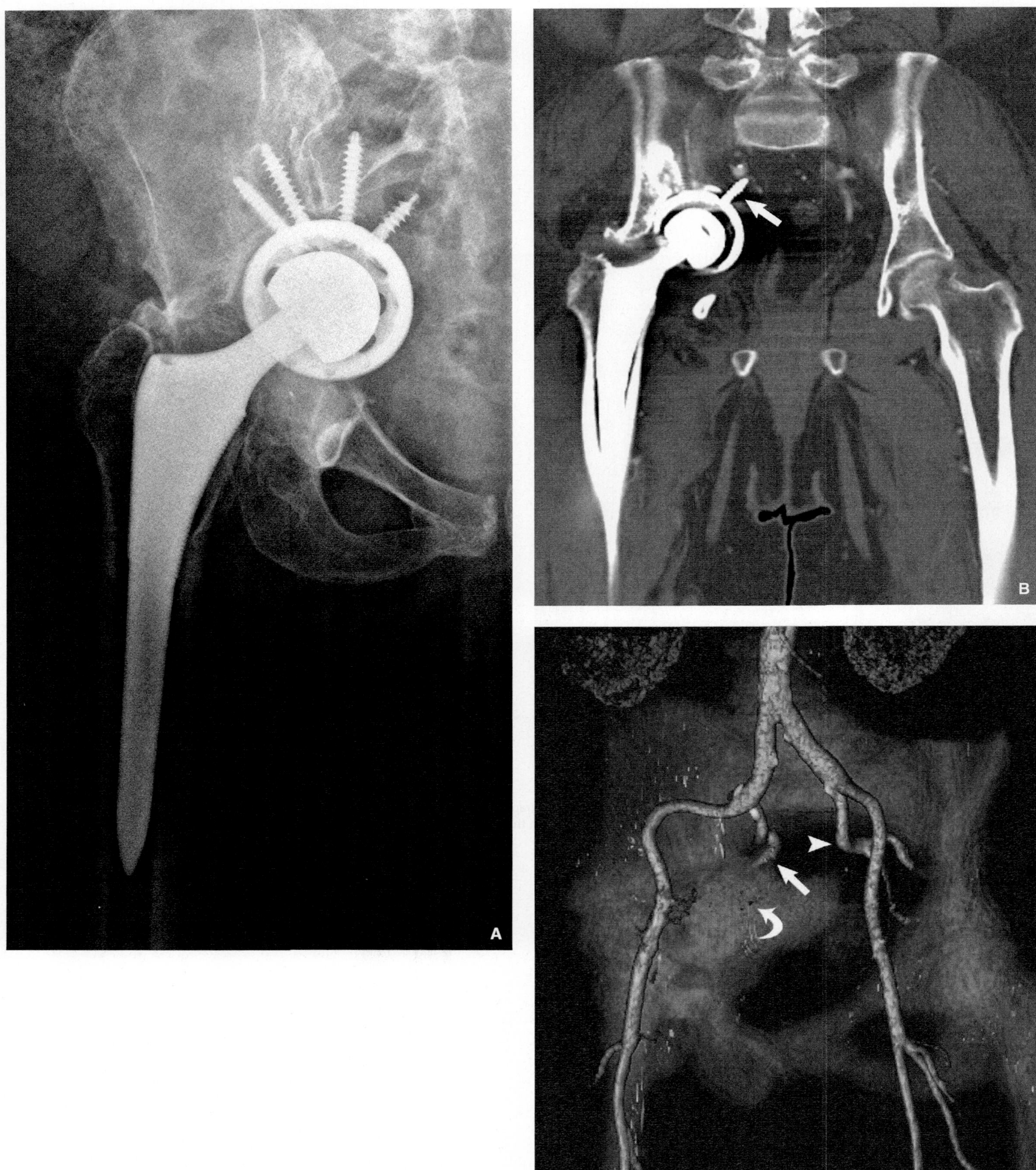

FIGURE 12.103 Periprosthetic acetabular fracture. A 65-year-old woman was injured in a car accident. **(A)** Anteroposterior radiograph of the right hip shows status post noncemented total hip arthroplasty. The acetabular component has been reinforced with four rim screws. Observe the fracture of the acetabulum and axial migration of the retroverted acetabular cup into the pelvic cavity. **(B)** Coronal reformatted CT image of the pelvis shows the most medial rim screw being in the vicinity of the right iliac artery *(arrow)*. **(C)** 3D reconstructed volume-rendered CT-angiogram obtained after administration of 125 mL of Omnipaque 350 shows the most medial acetabular rim screw penetrating the right internal iliac artery *(arrow)*. Note the normal left internal iliac artery *(arrowhead)*. The *curved arrow* points to the location of acetabular component of the prosthesis.

PRACTICAL POINTS TO REMEMBER

1. The term *arthritis* indicates an abnormality of the joint as a result of a degenerative, inflammatory, or infectious process. The term *arthralgia* implies aches and pains in the joint. The term *arthropathy* applies to numerous different genetic, autoimmune, metabolic, connective tissue, and other acquired diseases that produce pathologic process of the joint.
2. The radiographic hallmarks of an arthritic process regardless of cause are:
   - narrowing of the joint space
   - bony erosion of various forms depending on the specific type of arthritis.
3. The most effective radiologic imaging modality for evaluating arthritis is conventional radiography. Ancillary techniques, in order of their frequency of use, include:
   - radionuclide bone scan
   - MRI
   - CT and three-dimensional (3D) CT.
4. Radionuclide imaging is an effective technique for:
   - determining the skeletal distribution of arthritic changes
   - differentiating arthritis from periarticular soft-tissue infection
   - narrowing the differential diagnosis between infectious arthritis and other arthritides
   - monitoring the various complications of joint-replacement surgery.
5. CT is effective in demonstrating complications of degenerative spine disease, such as spinal stenosis.
6. MRI is effective in demonstrating abnormalities of the articular cartilage, synovial abnormalities, inflammatory pannus, joint effusion, rheumatoid nodules, early subchondral erosions, and bone marrow edema.
7. The radiographic diagnosis of arthritis is based on:
   - the morphology of an articular lesion
   - its distribution in the skeleton.
8. The morphologic changes characteristic of different arthritides can be effectively analyzed in several important anatomic sites, including the hand, heel, and spine. These changes, together with the characteristic distribution of lesions in the skeleton and the clinical and laboratory data in a given case, facilitate a specific diagnosis.
9. In the hand, the various arthritides have predilections for specific sites:
   - in OA and EOA—the proximal and distal interphalangeal joints
   - in psoriatic arthritis—the distal interphalangeal joints
   - in RA—the metacarpophalangeal and proximal interphalangeal joints
   - in multicentric reticulohistiocytosis—distal and proximal interphalangeal joints
   - in gouty arthritis—metacarpophalangeal and interphalangeal joints
   - in hyperparathyroid arthropathy—distal and proximal interphalangeal joints and metacarpophalangeal joints
   - in CPPD crystal deposition disease—metacarpophalangeal joints
   - in scleroderma—distal interphalangeal joints.
10. Patterns of migration of the femoral head within the acetabulum may suggest the etiology of hip arthritis:
    - OA: superior, superolateral, superomedial, and medial migrations
    - inflammatory arthritides: axial migration.
11. In the spine, the various arthritides exhibit characteristic morphologic features in:
    - degenerative disease—marginal osteophytes and narrowing of the apophyseal joints and intervertebral disk spaces
    - RA—atlantoaxial subluxation and erosion of the odontoid process
    - JIA—fusion of the apophyseal joints of the cervical spine
    - psoriatic arthritis and reactive arthritis—coarse, asymmetric paraspinal ossifications
    - AS—delicate syndesmophytes.
12. Certain arthritides generally show lack of periarticular osteoporosis–OA, gouty arthritis, CPPD crystal deposition disease, and multicentric reticulohistiocytosis.
13. Sacroiliitis is commonly seen in AS (in which it is bilateral and symmetrical) and in psoriatic arthritis and reactive arthritis (in which it is either unilateral or bilateral but asymmetric in terms of degree of involvement).
14. Monitoring the results of treatment of the arthritides involves detecting possible complications of various osteotomies and joint-replacement procedures. These complications include:
    - thrombophlebitis
    - intrapelvic leakage of methylmethacrylate cement
    - heterotopic bone formation
    - infection
    - loosening, dislocation, and fracture of a prosthesis
    - wear of the polyethylene lining of the prosthetic components
    - particle disease (metallosis)
    - ALVAL
    - patellar clunk syndrome
    - periprosthetic fracture.
15. Scintigraphy and SPECT/CT are useful in detecting loosening of a prosthesis.

SUGGESTED READINGS

Alazraki NP, Fierer J, Resnick D. The role of gallium and bone scanning in monitoring response to therapy in chronic osteomyelitis. *J Nucl Med* 1978;19:696–697.

Aletaha D, Neogi T, Silman AJ, et al. 2010 Rheumatoid arthritis classification criteria: an American College of Rheumatology/European League Against Rheumatism collaborative initiative. *Arthritis Rheum* 2010;62:2569–2581.

Algin O, Gokalp G, Baran B, et al. Evaluation of sacroiliitis: contrast-enhanced MRI with subtraction technique. *Skeletal Radiol* 2009;38:983–988.

Allen AM, Ward WG, Pope TL Jr. Imaging of the total knee arthroplasty. *Radiol Clin North Am* 1995;33:289–303.

Archer CW, Morrison H, Pitsillides AA. Cellular aspects of the development of diarthrodial joints and articular cartilage. *J Anat* 1994;184:447–456.

Ash Z, Marzo-Ortega H. Ankylosing spondylitis—the changing role of imaging. *Skeletal Radiol* 2012;41:1031–1034.

Aufdermaur M. Pathogenesis of square bodies in ankylosing spondylitis. *Ann Rheum Dis* 1989;48:628–631.

Bayliss MT, Dudhia J. Articular cartilage: structure, function and physiology. In: Fitzgerald RH, Kaufer H, Malkani AL, eds. *Orthopaedics*. St. Louis, MO: Mosby; 2002:160–167.

Bianchi S, Martinoli C, Abdelwahab IF. High-frequency ultrasound examination of the wrist and hand. *Skeletal Radiol* 1999;28:121–129.

Boileau P. Complications and revision of reverse total shoulder arthroplasty. *Orthop Traumatol Surg Res* 2016;102:S33–S43.

Boutry N, Morel M, Flipo R-M, et al. Early rheumatoid arthritis: a review of MRI and sonographic findings. *AJR Am J Roentgenol* 2007;189:1502–1509.

Brigden M. The erythrocyte sedimentation rate. Still a helpful test when used judiciously. *Postgrad Med* 1998;103:257–262.

Brower AC, Flemming DJ. *Arthritis in black and white*, 2nd ed. Philadelphia: WB Saunders; 1997.

Bruhlmann P, Michel BA. History and clinical examination in rheumatology—key to diagnosis and prognosis. *Ther Umsch* 2006;63:485–490.

Bullough PG. *Atlas of orthopedic pathology: with clinical and radiologic correlation*, 2nd ed. New York: Gower Medical; 1992.

Capone A, Congia S, Civinini R, et al. Periprosthetic fractures: epidemiology and current treatment. *Clin Cases Miner Bone Metabol* 2017;14:189–196.

Castrejón I, McCollum L, Tanriover MD, et al. Importance of patient history and physical examination in rheumatoid arthritis compared to other chronic diseases: results of a physician survey. *Arthritis Care Res (Hoboken)* 2012;64:1250–1255.

Chen LX, Clayburne G, Schumacher HR. Update on identification of pathogenic crystals in joint fluid. *Curr Rheumatol Rep* 2004;6:217–220.

Datz FL, Morton KA. New radiopharmaceuticals for detecting infection. *Invest Radiol* 1993;28:356–365.

Desai MA, Peterson JJ, Garner HW, et al. Clinical utility of dual-energy CT for evaluation of tophaceous gout. *Radiographics* 2011;31:1365–1375.

Doherty M, Dacre J, Dieppe P, et al. The 'GALS' locomotor screen. *Ann Rheum Dis* 1992;51:1165–1169.

Eustace S, DiMasi M, Adams J, et al. In vitro and in vivo spin echo diffusion imaging characteristics of synovial fluid: potential non-invasive differentiation of inflammatory and degenerative arthritis. *Skeletal Radiol* 2000;29:320–323.

Farrant JM, Grainger AJ, O'Connor PJ. Advanced imaging in rheumatoid arthritis. Part 2: erosions. *Skeletal Radiol* 2007;36:381–389.

Farrant JM, O'Connor PJ, Grainger AJ. Advanced imaging in rheumatoid arthritis. Part 1: synovitis. *Skeletal Radiol* 2007;36:269–279.

Fernandes JC, Martel-Pelletier J, Pelletier JP. The role of cytokines in osteoarthritis pathophysiology. *Biorheology* 2002;39:237–246.

Ferri C, Zignego AL, Pileri SA. Cryoglobulins. *J Clin Pathol* 2002;55:4–13.

Forrester DM. Imaging of the sacroiliac joints. *Radiol Clin North Am* 1990;28:1055–1072.

Fremont AJ. The pathophysiology of cartilage and synovium. *Br J Rheumatol* 1996;35 (suppl 3):10–13.

Fritz J, Lurie B, Potter HG. MR imaging of knee arthroplasty implants. *Radiographics* 2015;35:1483–1501.

Gallo J, Kaminek P, Ticha V, et al. Particle disease. A comprehensive theory of periprosthetic osteolysis: a review. *Biomed Papers* 2002;146:21–28.

Gee R, Munk PL, Keogh C, et al. Radiography of the PROSTALAC (prosthesis with antibiotic-loaded acrylic cement) orthopedic implant. *AJR Am J Roentgenol* 2003;180:1701–1706.

Gonzalez S, Martina-Barra J, Lopez-Larrea C. Immunogenetics. HLA-B27 and spondyloarthropathies. *Curr Opin Rheumatol* 1999;11:257–264.

Grammont PM, Baulot E. Delta shoulder prosthesis for rotator cuff rupture. *Orthopedics* 1993;16:65–68.

Greenspan A. Back to the future—conventional radiography in rheumatology. *J Ultrason* 2016;16:225–228.

Greenspan A, Beltran J. *Orthopedic imaging: a practical approach*, 6th ed. Philadelphia: Wolters Kluwer; 2015:527–535.

Greenspan A, Gershwin ME. *Imaging in rheumatology: a clinical approach*. Philadelphia: Wolters Kluwer; 2018:3–22, 93–113, 114–139.

Greenspan A, Grainger AJ. Articular abnormalities that may mimic arthritis. *J Ultrason* 2018;18:126–137.

Greenspan A, Norman A. Gross hematuria: a complication of intrapelvic cement intrusion in total hip replacement. *AJR Am J Roentgenol* 1978;130:327–329.

Greenspan A, Norman A. Radial head-capitellum view: an expanded imaging approach to elbow injury. *Radiology* 1987;164:272–274.

Gruen TA, McNeice GM, Amstutz HC. "Modes of failure" of cemented stem-type femoral components: a radiographic analysis of loosening. *Clin Orthop Relat Res* 1979;141: 17–27.

Harris WH. Osteolysis and particle disease in hip replacement. A review. *Acta Orthop Scand* 1994;65:113–123.

Imboden JB. Approach to the patient with arthritis. In: Imboden JB, Hellmann DB, Stone JH, eds. *Current diagnosis & treatment: rheumatology*, 3rd ed. New York: McGraw-Hill; 2013:1–6.

Ingegnoli F, Castelli R, Gualtierotti R. Rheumatoid factors: clinical application. *Dis Markers* 2013;35:727–734.

Iwanaga T, Shikichi M, Kitamura H, et al. Morphology and functional roles of synoviocytes in the joint. *Arch Histol Cytol* 2000;63:17–31.

Kamishima T, Tanimura K, Henmi M, et al. Power Doppler ultrasound of rheumatoid synovitis: quantification of vascular signal and analysis of intraobserver variability. *Skeletal Radiol* 2009;38:467–472.

Kim NR, Choi J-Y, Hong SH, et al. "MR corner sign": value for predicting presence of ankylosing spondylitis. *AJR Am J Roentgenol* 2008;191:124–128.

Kim S-H, Chung S-K, Bahk Y-W, et al. Whole-body and pinhole bone scintigraphic manifestations of Reiter's syndrome: distribution patterns and early and characteristic signs. *Eur J Nucl Med* 1999;26:163–170.

Klein MJ. Radiographic correlation in orthopedic pathology. *Adv Anat Pathol* 2005;12:155–179.

Klein MJ, Bonar SF, Freemont T, et al. *Atlas of nontumor pathology. Non-neoplastic diseases of bones and joints*. Washington, DC: American Registry of Pathology and Armed Forces Institute of Pathology; 2011:1–53, 545–575, 577–767.

Klein-Nulend J, Nijweide PJ, Burger EH. Osteocyte and bone structure. *Curr Osteoporos Rep* 2003;1:5–10.

Lajeunesse D, Reboul P. Subchondral bone in osteoarthritis: a biologic link with articular cartilage leading to abnormal remodeling. *Curr Opin Rheumatol* 2003;15:628–633.

Lawrence C, Williams GR, Namdari S. Influence of glenosphere design on outcome and complications of reverse arthroplasty: a systemic review. *Clin Orthop Surg* 2016;8: 288–297.

Lumbreras B, Pascual E, Frasquet J, et al. Analysis of the crystals in synovial fluid: training of the analysts results in high consistency. *Ann Rheum Dis* 2005;64:612–615.

Lund PJ, Heikal A, Maricic MJ, et al. Ultrasonographic imaging of the hand and wrist in rheumatoid arthritis. *Skeletal Radiol* 1995;24:591–596.

Lyon R, Narain S, Nichols C, et al. Effective use of autoantibody tests in the diagnosis of systemic autoimmune disease. *Ann N Y Acad Sci* 2005;1050:217–228.

Manaster BJ. Total hip arthroplasty: radiographic evaluation. *Radiographics* 1996;16:645–660.

Marsland D, Mears SC. A review of periprosthetic femoral fractures associated with total hip arthroplasty. *Geriatr Orthop Surg Rehabil* 2012;3:107–120.

Mauri C, Ehrenstein MR. Cells of the synovium in rheumatoid arthritis. B cells. *Arthritis Res Ther* 2007;9:205.

McFarland EG, Sanguanjit P, Tasaki A, et al. The reverse shoulder prosthesis: a review of imaging features and complications. *Skeletal Radiol* 2006;35:488–496.

McGonagle D. The history of erosions in rheumatoid arthritis: are erosions history? *Arthritis Rheum* 2010;62:312–315.

Mills JA. Physical examination of the musculoskeletal system. In: Imboden JB, Hellmann DB, Stone JH, eds. *Current diagnosis & treatment: rheumatology*, 3rd ed. New York: McGraw-Hill; 2013:1–6.

Nakamura MC, Imboden JB. Laboratory diagnosis. In: Imboden JB, Hellmann DB, Stone JH, eds. *Current diagnosis & treatment: rheumatology*, 3rd ed. New York: McGraw-Hill; 2013:15–25.

Nalbant S, Martinez JA, Kitumnuaypong T, et al. Synovial fluid features and their relations to osteoarthritis severity: new findings from sequential studies. *Osteoarthr Cartil* 2003;11:50–54.

Niewold TB, Harrison MJ, Paget SA. Anti-CCP antibody testing as a diagnostic and prognostic tool in rheumatoid arthritis. *QJM* 2007;100:193–201.

Nikac V, Blazar P, Earp B, et al. Radiographic and surgical considerations in arthritis surgery of the hand. *Skeletal Radiol* 2017;46:591–604.

Norgaard F. Earliest roentgenological changes in polyarthritis of the rheumatoid type: rheumatoid arthritis. *Radiology* 1965;85:325–329.

Ostendorf B, Mattes-György K, Reichelt DC, et al. Early detection of bony alterations in rheumatoid and erosive arthritis of finger joints with high-resolution single photon emission computed tomography, and differentiation between them. *Skeletal Radiol* 2010;39:55–61.

Østergaard M, Ejbjerg B, Szkudlarek M. Imaging in early rheumatoid arthritis: roles of magnetic resonance imaging, ultrasonography, conventional radiography and computed tomography. *Best Pract Res Clin Rheumatol* 2005;19:91–116.

Pasqual E, Jovani V. Synovial fluid analysis. *Best Pract Res Clin Rheumatol* 2005;19:371–386.

Peterfy CG, Genant HK. Emerging applications of magnetic resonance imaging in the evaluation of articular cartilage. *Radiol Clin North Am* 1996;34:195–213.

Peterfy CG, Majumdar S, Lang P, et al. MR imaging of the arthritic knee: improved discrimination of cartilage, synovia, and effusion with pulsed saturation transfer and fat-suppressed T1-weighted sequences. *Radiology* 1994;191:413–419.

Petri M. Review of classification criteria for systemic lupus erythematosus. *Rheum Dis Clin North Am* 2005;31:245–254.

Punzi L, Oliviero F, Plebani M. New biochemical insight into the pathogenesis of osteoarthritis and the role of laboratory investigations in clinical assessment. *Crit Rev Clin Lab Sci* 2005;42:279–309.

Puszczewicz M, Iwaszkiewicz C. Role of anti-citrullinated protein antibodies in diagnosis and prognosis of rheumatoid arthritis. *Arch Med Sci* 2011;7:189–194.

Rastogi AK, Davis KW, Ross A, et al. Fundamentals of joint injection. *AJR Am J Roentgenol* 2016;207:484–494.

Recht MP, Resnick D. MR imaging of articular cartilage: current status and future directions. *AJR Am J Roentgenol* 1994;163:283–290.

Resnick D. Common disorders of synovium-lined joints: pathogenesis, imaging abnormalities, and complications. *AJR Am J Roentgenol* 1988;151:1079–1088.

Reynolds PPM, Heron C, Pilcher J, et al. Prediction of erosion progression using ultrasound in established rheumatoid arthritis: a 2-year follow-up study. *Skeletal Radiol* 2009;38:473–478.

Roberts CC, Ekelund AL, Renfree KJ, et al. Radiologic assessment of reverse shoulder arthroplasty. *Radiographics* 2007;27:223–235.

Robinson DB, El-Gabalawy HS. Evaluation of the patient. A. History and physical examination. In: Klippel JH, Stone JH, Crofford LJ, et al., eds. *Primer of the rheumatic diseases*, 13th ed. New York: Springer; 2008:6–41.

Russo R, Rotonda GD, Ciccarelli M, et al. Analysis of complications of reverse shoulder arthroplasty. *Joints* 2015;3:62–66.

Samitier G, Alentorn-Geli E, Torrens C, et al. Reverse shoulder arthroplasty. Part 1: systemic review of clinical and functional outcomes. *Int J Shoulder Surg* 2015;9:24–31.

Sebes JI, Nasrallah NS, Rabinowitz JG, et al. The relationship between HLA-B27 positive peripheral arthritis and sacroiliitis. *Radiology* 1978;126:299–302.

Sigurdson LA. The structure and function of articular synovial membranes. *J Bone Joint Surg* 1930;12:603–639.

Singhal O, Kaur V, Kalhan S, et al. Arthroscopic synovial biopsy in definitive diagnosis of joint diseases: an evaluation of efficacy and precision. *Int J Appl Basic Med Res* 2012;2:102–106.

Swan A, Amer H, Dieppe P. The value of synovial fluid assays in the diagnosis of joint disease: a literature survey. *Ann Rheum Dis* 2002;61:493–498.

Talbot BS, Weinberg E. MR imaging with metal-suppression sequences for evaluation of total joint arthroplasty. *Radiographics* 2016;36:209–225.

Taljanovic MS, Jones MD, Hunter TB, et al. Joint arthroplasties and prostheses. *Radiographics* 2003;23:1295–1310.

Taylor P, Gartemann J, Hsieh J, et al. A systematic review of serum biomarkers anti-cyclic citrullinated peptide and rheumatoid factor as tests for rheumatoid arthritis. *Autoimmune Dis* 2011;259:414–420.

Tehranzadeh J, Ashikyan O, Anavim A, et al. Enhanced MR imaging of tenosynovitis of hand and wrist in inflammatory arthritis. *Skeletal Radiol* 2006;35:814–822.

Tehranzadeh J, Ashikyan O, Dascalos J. Advanced imaging of early rheumatoid arthritis. *Radiol Clin North Am* 2004;42:89–107.

Vervoordeldonk MJ, Tak PP. Cytokines in rheumatoid arthritis. *Curr Rheumatol Rep* 2002;4:208–217.

Watters TS, Cardona DM, Menon KS, et al. Aseptic lymphocyte-dominated vasculitis-associated lesion: a clinicopathologic review of an underrecognized cause of prosthetic failure. *Am J Clin Pathol* 2010;134:886–893.

Weber U, Østergaard M, Lambert RGW, et al. The impact of MRI on the clinical management of inflammatory arthritides. *Skeletal Radiol* 2011;40:1153–1173.

Weissman BN. Spondyloarthropathies. *Radiol Clin North Am* 1987;25:1235–1262.

Woolf AD, Akesson K. Primer: history and examination in the assessment of musculoskeletal problems. *Nat Clin Pract Rheumatol* 2008;4:26–33.

Zendman AJW, van Venroij WJ, Pruijn GJM. Use and significance of anti-CCP autoantibodies in rheumatoid arthritis. *Rheumatology* 2006;45:20–25.

13

Degenerative Joint Disease

Osteoarthritis

Degenerative joint disease (osteoarthritis [OA], osteoarthrosis) is the most common form of arthritis and represents a heterogeneous group of joint abnormalities with similar clinical, pathologic, and imaging features. Symptomatic OA is defined by the American College of Rheumatology as a group of conditions that lead to joint symptoms and signs, which are associated with the defective integrity of articular cartilage, in addition to related changes in the underlying bone at the joint margins. In 1994, at a meeting of the World Health Organization (WHO) and the American Academy of Orthopedic Surgery, a definition of OA was proposed as follows: "OA is the result of both mechanical and biologic events that destabilize the normal coupling of degradation and synthesis of articular cartilage and subchondral bone. Although it may be initiated by multiple factors including genetic, developmental, metabolic and traumatic, OA involves all of the tissues of the diarthrodial joint. Ultimately, OA is manifested by morphologic, biochemical, molecular, and biomechanical changes in both cells and matrix, which leads to softening, fibrillation, ulceration and loss of articular cartilage, sclerosis and eburnation of subchondral bone, osteophytes, and subchondral cysts. When clinically evident, OA is characterized by joint pain, tenderness, limitation of movement, crepitus, occasional effusion, and variable degrees of local inflammation." In its primary (idiopathic) form, OA affects individuals aged 50 years and older; in its secondary form, however, OA may be seen in a much younger age group. Patients in the latter group have clearly defined underlying conditions leading to the development of degenerative joint disease (see Fig. 12.1).

Some authorities postulate that there are two types of primary degenerative joint disease. The first form is apparently closely related to the aging process ("wear and tear") and represents not a true arthritis but a senescent process of the joint. It characteristically shows limited destruction of the cartilage, slow progression, lack of significant joint deformity, and no restriction of joint function. This process is not affected by gender or race. The second type, a true OA, is unrelated to the aging process, although it shows an increased prevalence with age. Genetic factors have been found to be strong determination of this form of OA. The nature of the genetic influence, however, is partially speculative and may involve either a structural defect (i.e., collagen), alterations in cartilage or bone metabolism, or alternatively a genetic influence on a known environmental risk factors such as obesity, sports, and trauma. Several studies have implicated linkages to OA on chromosomes 2q, 9q, 11q, and 16p, among others. Implicated genes include VDR; AGC1; IGF-1; ER alpha; TGF beta; cartilage matrix protein (CRTM); cartilage link protein (CRTL); and collagen II, IX, and XI. Most recent studies also suggested that mutations in the gene *GDF5*, also known as *cartilage-derived morphogenetic protein 1*, can be linked with etiology of OA of the hip and knee. Some investigators suggested that OA in some families may be caused by the mutations in the type II collagen gene *COL2A1*, which encodes a protein expressed almost exclusively in cartilage. Marked by progressive destruction of the articular cartilage and reparative processes such as osteophyte formation and subchondral sclerosis, true OA progresses rapidly, leading to significant joint deformity. This form may be related to genetic factors as well as to gender, race, and obesity. It has been shown that OA tends to affect women more commonly than men, particularly in the proximal and distal interphalangeal joints and the first carpometacarpal joints. In the population older than 65 years, OA affects Caucasians more commonly than African Americans. Obesity is associated with a higher incidence of OA in the knees, which may be related to an excessive weight-bearing load on these joints.

Generally, in OA, the large diarthrodial joints such as the hip or knee and the small joints such as the interphalangeal joints of the hand are most often affected; the spine, however, is just as frequently involved in the degenerative process (Fig. 13.1). The shoulder, elbow, wrist, and ankle are unusual sites for primary OA, and if degenerative changes are encountered in these locations, secondary OA should be considered. It should be kept in mind, however, that evidence exists for an association between degenerative arthritis in unusual sites and certain occupations. Even primary osteoarthritic changes may develop more rapidly, for example, in the lumbar spine, knees, and elbows of coal miners and in the wrists, elbows, and shoulders of pneumatic drill operators. Degenerative changes are also commonly seen in the ankles and feet of ballet dancers and in the femoropatellar joints of bicyclists.

Ordinarily, OA manifests clinically by two cardinal symptoms: joint pain exacerbated by activity and usually short-lasting joints stiffness. Some other symptoms include focal swelling of the joints, cracking of the joints, locking of the joints, and difficulty with daily activities.

An overview of the clinical and radiographic hallmarks of degenerative joint disease is presented in Table 13.1.

Osteoarthritis of the Large Joints

The hip and knee joints are the most common sites of OA. The severity of imaging changes does not always correlate with the clinical symptoms, which may vary from stiffness and pain to severe deformities and limitation of joint function.

Osteoarthritis of the Hip

Clinical Features

Commonly, the patient presents with a history of gradual onset of slowly worsening hip pain, localized primarily in the groin, aggravated by movement in the joint and by weight bearing. This is accompanied by decreasing range of motion. The patient is limping and has difficulty to walk normally, particularly going up and down the stairs. Not infrequently, the patient may experience pain in the knee. This phenomenon occurs because branches of the obturator nerve innervate both the knee and the hip joints.

Pathology

Some of the pathologic features of OA were already outlined in Chapter 12. Generally, the disease is described as occurring in two stages: loss of articular cartilage, followed by reparative process in adjacent bone and cartilage in an attempt to remodel the joint.

HIGHLIGHTS OF PRIMARY OSTEOARTHRITIS

Morphology

Large Joints

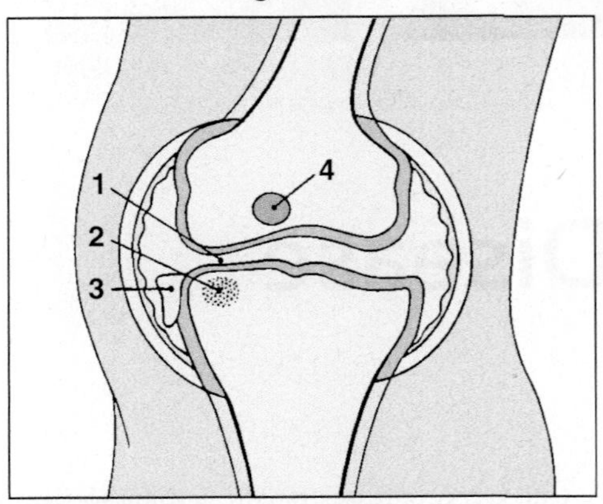

1 localized joint-space narrowing
2 subchondral sclerosis
3 osteophytes
4 cyst or pseudocyst

Small Joints

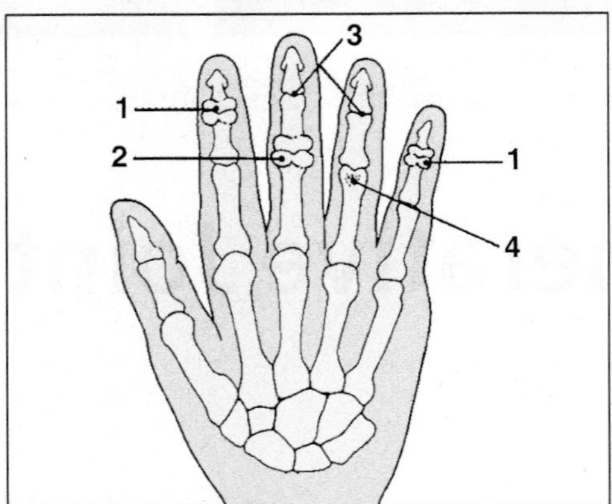

1 Heberden nodes
2 Bouchard nodes
3 joint-space narrowing
4 subchondral sclerosis

Spine

1 facet narrowing and eburnation
2 foraminal stenosis
3 stenosis of spinal canal

Distribution

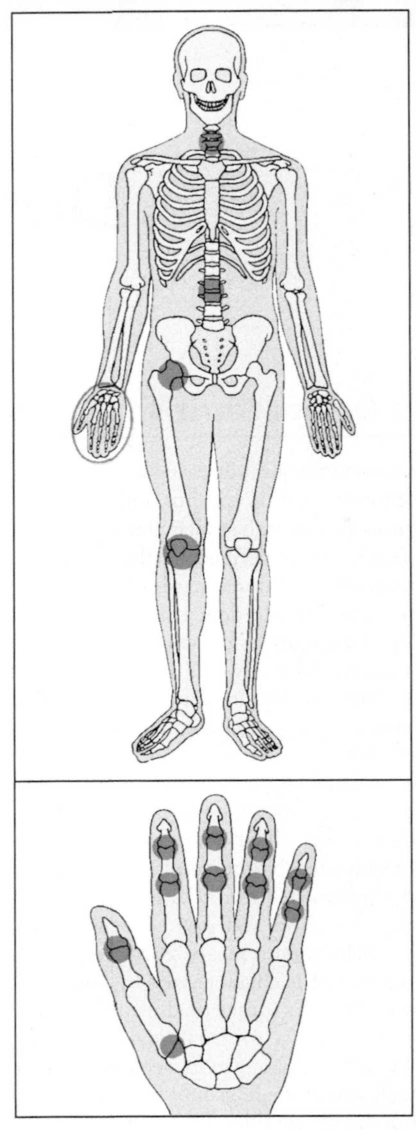

FIGURE 13.1 Highlights of the morphology and distribution of arthritic lesions in primary OA.

Gross specimens of resected osteoarthritic femoral head show alterations in the shape of the articular surface and damaged cartilage. In the weight-bearing areas, the cartilage may be entirely absent, and the subchondral bone has a dense, polished, marble-like appearance, termed *eburnation* (see Figs. 12.27A,C). Cystic-like defects, known as *geodes*, may be found, filled either with thick fluid or with loose fibromyxoid tissue (see Fig. 12.28). In the non–weight-bearing areas and around its margins, osteophytes develop (Fig. 13.2; see also Fig. 12.27B). As the articular cartilage is progressively destroyed, the underlying subchondral bone is subjected to increasingly localized overload, leading to pressure necrosis (Fig. 13.3). This superficial necrosis is, however, different from primary avascular necrosis (osteonecrosis) that has distinct etiology and pathogenesis.

Histopathology shows hypertrophy and hyperplasia of the synoviocytes. Also present are areas of fibrillation, and increase in the ratio of water to the proteoglycan in the cartilage matrix leads to cartilage softening (chondromalacia), followed by formation of the fissures on the cartilaginous surface. Extension of the hyperplastic synovium (pannus) into the articular surface of the hip joint is a common finding. In deeper sections, at the cartilage-subchondral bone junction, there is often present marked irregularity and duplication of the tidemark. In the more advanced stages, subchondral sclerosis predominates due to accelerated bone turnover and apposition of small strips of new bone through the process of increased endochondral ossification and osteoblastic deposition (see Fig. 12.28B,C).

Imaging Features

There are four cardinal imaging features of degenerative joint disease in the hip:

1. Narrowing of the joint space as a result of thinning of the articular cartilage
2. Subchondral sclerosis (eburnation) caused by reparative processes (remodeling)
3. Osteophyte formation (osteophytosis) as a result of reparative processes in sites not subjected to stress (so-called *low-stress areas*), which are usually marginal (peripheral) in distribution
4. Cyst or pseudocyst formation resulting from bone contusions that lead to microfractures and intrusion of synovial fluid into the altered spongy bone; in the acetabulum, these subchondral cyst-like lesions are referred to as *Eggers cysts*.

TABLE 13.1 Clinical and Radiographic Hallmarks of Degenerative Joint Disease

Type of Arthritis	Site	Crucial Abnormalities	Technique[a]/Projection
Primary osteoarthritis (F > M; >50 y)	Hand	Degenerative changes in Proximal interphalangeal joints (Bouchard nodes) Distal interphalangeal joints (Heberden nodes)	Dorsovolar view
	Hip	Narrowing of joint space Subchondral sclerosis Marginal osteophytes Cysts and pseudocysts Superolateral subluxation	Anteroposterior view
	Knee	Same changes as in hip Varus or valgus deformity Degenerative changes in Femoropatellar compartment Patella (tooth sign)	Anteroposterior view Weight-bearing anteroposterior view Lateral view Axial view of patella
	Spine	Degenerative disk disease Narrowing of disk space Degenerative spondylolisthesis Osteophytosis Spondylosis deformans Degenerative changes in apophyseal joints Foraminal stenosis Spinal stenosis	 Lateral view Lateral flexion/extension views Anteroposterior and lateral views Anteroposterior and lateral views Oblique views (cervical, lumbar) CT, myelogram, MRI
Secondary osteoarthritis Posttraumatic	Hip Knee Shoulder, elbow, wrist, ankle (unusual sites)	Similar changes to those in primary osteoarthritis History of previous trauma Younger age	Standard views
FAI syndrome	Hips	Bone formation at the head/neck junction Acetabular crossover sign	MRI/MRa
Slipped capital femoral epiphysis	Hips	Herndon hump Narrowing of joint space Osteophytosis	Anteroposterior and frog-lateral views
Congenital hip dislocation (F > M)	Hips	Signs of acetabular hypoplasia	Anteroposterior and frog-lateral views
Perthes disease (M > F)	Hip	Unilateral or bilateral Osteonecrosis of femoral head Coxa magna Lateral subluxation	Anteroposterior and frog-lateral views
Inflammatory arthritis	Hip Knee	Medial and axial migration of femoral head Periarticular osteoporosis Limited osteophytosis	Standard views
Osteonecrosis	Hip Shoulder	Increased bone density Joint space usually preserved or only slightly narrowed Crescent sign	Anteroposterior views (hip, shoulder) Grashey view (shoulder) Frog-lateral view (hip)
Paget disease (>40 y)	Hips, knees, shoulders	Coarse trabeculations Thickening of cortex	Standard views of affected joints Radionuclide bone scan
Multiple epiphyseal dysplasia	Epiphyses of long bones	Dysplastic changes Narrowing of joint space Osteophytes	Standard views of affected joints
Hemochromatosis	Hands	Degenerative changes in second and third metacarpophalangeal joints with beak-like osteophytes Chondrocalcinosis	Dorsovolar view
Acromegaly	Large joints Hands	Joint spaces widened or only slightly narrowed Enlargement of terminal tufts Beak-like osteophytes in heads of metacarpals	Standard views of affected joint Dorsovolar view

[a]Radionuclide bone scan is used to determine the distribution of arthritic lesions in the skeleton.

F, female; M, male; CT, computed tomography; MRI, magnetic resonance imaging; FAI, femoroacetabular impingement; MRa, magnetic resonance arthrography.

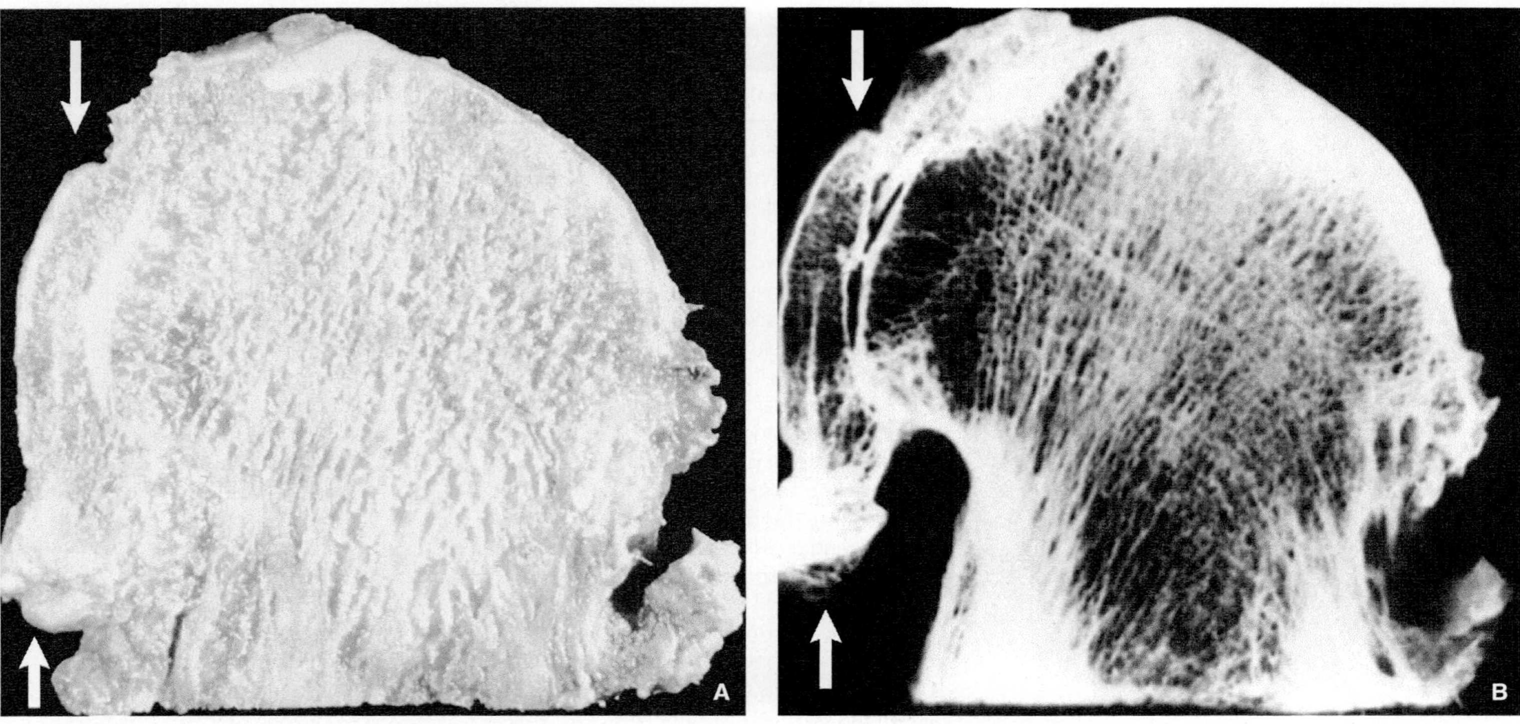

FIGURE 13.2 **Pathology of OA of hip joint.** **(A)** Coronal section of the resected femoral head and **(B)** radiograph of the gross specimen show a large flat osteophyte extending from the medial aspect to the region of fovea *(arrows)*. (Reprinted from Bullough P. *Orthopaedic pathology*, 5th ed. Maryland Heights, MO: Mosby; 2009, with permission from Elsevier.)

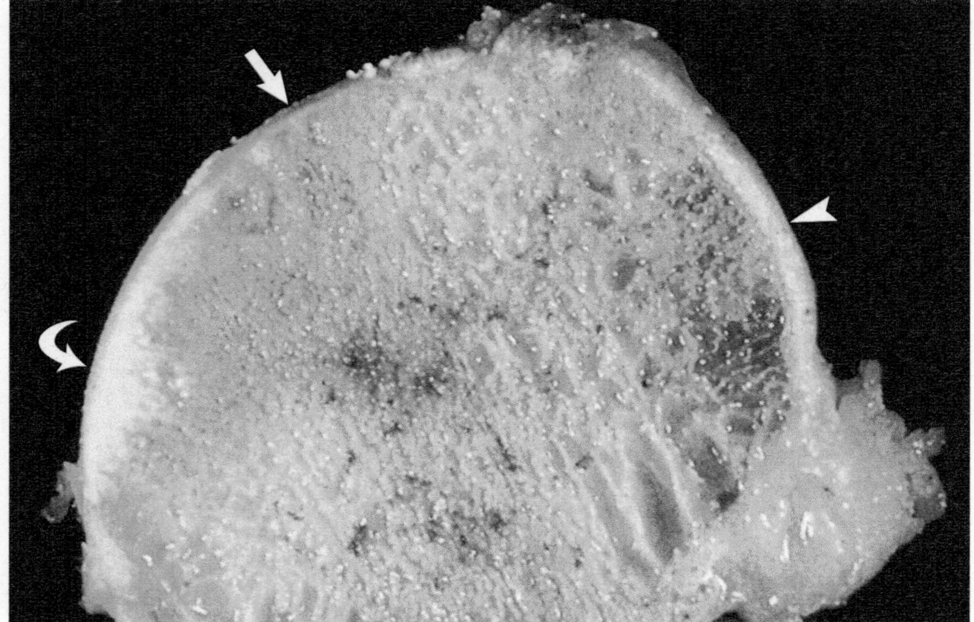

FIGURE 13.3 **Pathology of OA of hip joint.** Coronal section of the osteoarthritic femoral head shows subchondral bone partially denuded of articular cartilage *(arrow)*. Some articular cartilage remains intact *(arrowhead)*. Observe in the exposed subchondral bone focal bone marrow necrosis *(yellow area)* due to localized overloading *(curved arrow)*. (Reprinted from Bullough P. *Orthopaedic pathology*, 5th ed. Maryland Heights, MO: Mosby; 2009, with permission from Elsevier.)

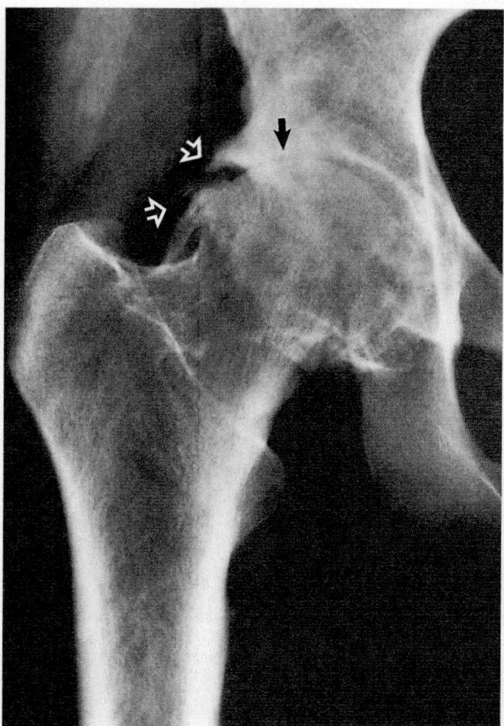

FIGURE 13.4 **OA of the hip joint.** A 51-year-old woman presented with a history of right hip pain for the past 10 years and no previous history suggesting predisposing factors for OA. Anteroposterior radiograph of the hip demonstrates the radiographic hallmarks of OA: narrowing of the joint space, particularly at the weight-bearing segment *(arrow)*; formation of marginal osteophytes *(open arrows)*; and subchondral sclerosis. Note the lack of osteoporosis.

These hallmarks of degenerative joint disease can be readily demonstrated on the standard radiographs of the hip (Figs. 13.4 to 13.6). Computed tomography (CT) (Figs. 13.7 to 13.9 and 13.10B) and magnetic resonance imaging (MRI) (Figs. 13.10C and 13.11) may further delineate the characteristic features of OA.

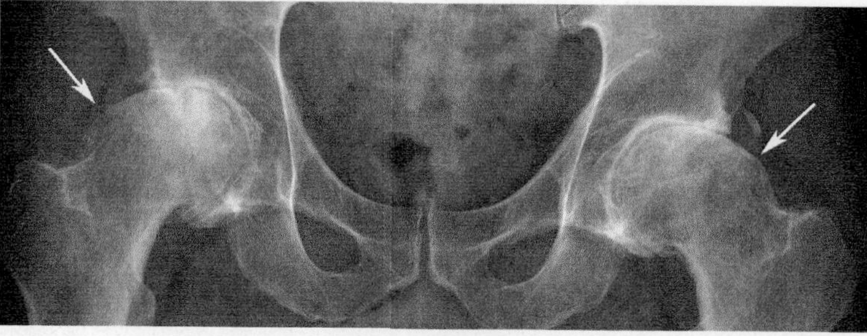

FIGURE 13.6 **OA of both hip joints.** Anteroposterior radiograph shows advanced OA of both hip joints in this 70-year-old man. There are features of bilateral cam-type femoroacetabular impingement (FAI) with loss of the normal concavity of the superolateral aspect of the femoral head-neck junction (*arrows*). See discussion of FAI in the text that follows.

As articular cartilage is destroyed and reparative changes develop, evidence emerges of a change in the relation of the femoral head with respect to the acetabulum, known as *migration*. Generally, three patterns of femoral head migration can be observed: superior, which may be either superolateral or superomedial; medial; and axial (Fig. 13.12). The most common pattern is superolateral migration; the medial pattern is less common, whereas axial migration is only exceptionally seen. It should be kept in mind, however, that in inflammatory arthritis of the hip, such as rheumatoid arthritis (RA), in which a previous axial migration of the femoral head is commonly associated with acetabular protrusio, degenerative changes might develop as a complication of the inflammatory process. Thus, one may see secondary OA with axial migration (Fig. 13.13).

The OA of the hip joint is typically characterized by the presence of osteophytes, which are commonly the most prominent imaging feature of the disease and represent the reparative response to joint destruction. Osteophytes are of two types: peripheral, which arise at the osseous-chondral junction of the femoral neck and head at the sites of capsular attachments, formed through the process of intramembranous ossification; and surface, central osteophytes, occasionally referred to as *surface bumps* because they produce a lumpy and irregular contour to the femoral head, which develop at low-pressure areas at the perimeter of the pressure zones, formed by the

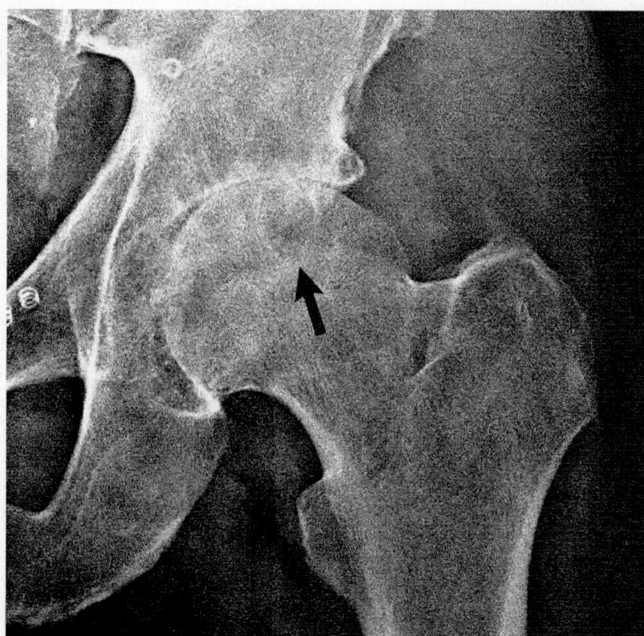

FIGURE 13.5 **OA of the hip joint.** Anteroposterior radiograph of the left hip of a 76-year-old man shows narrowing of the joint space mainly at the weight-bearing segment, subchondral sclerosis, and geode within the femoral head *(arrow)*.

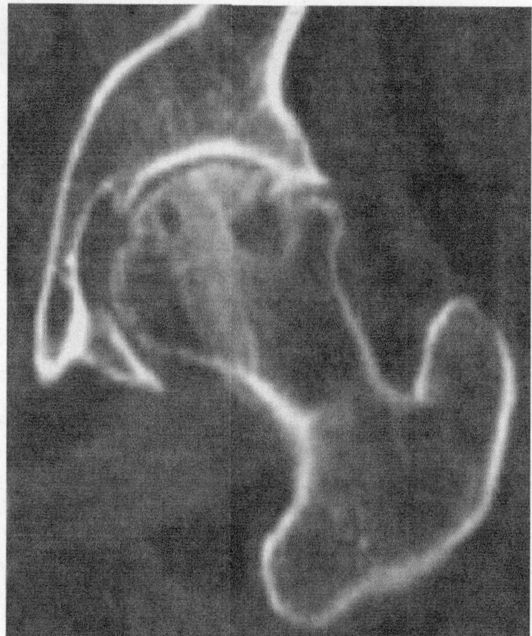

FIGURE 13.7 **CT of OA of the hip joint.** Coronal reformatted image shows diminution of the joint space, osteophytes, and subchondral cysts in the femoral head.

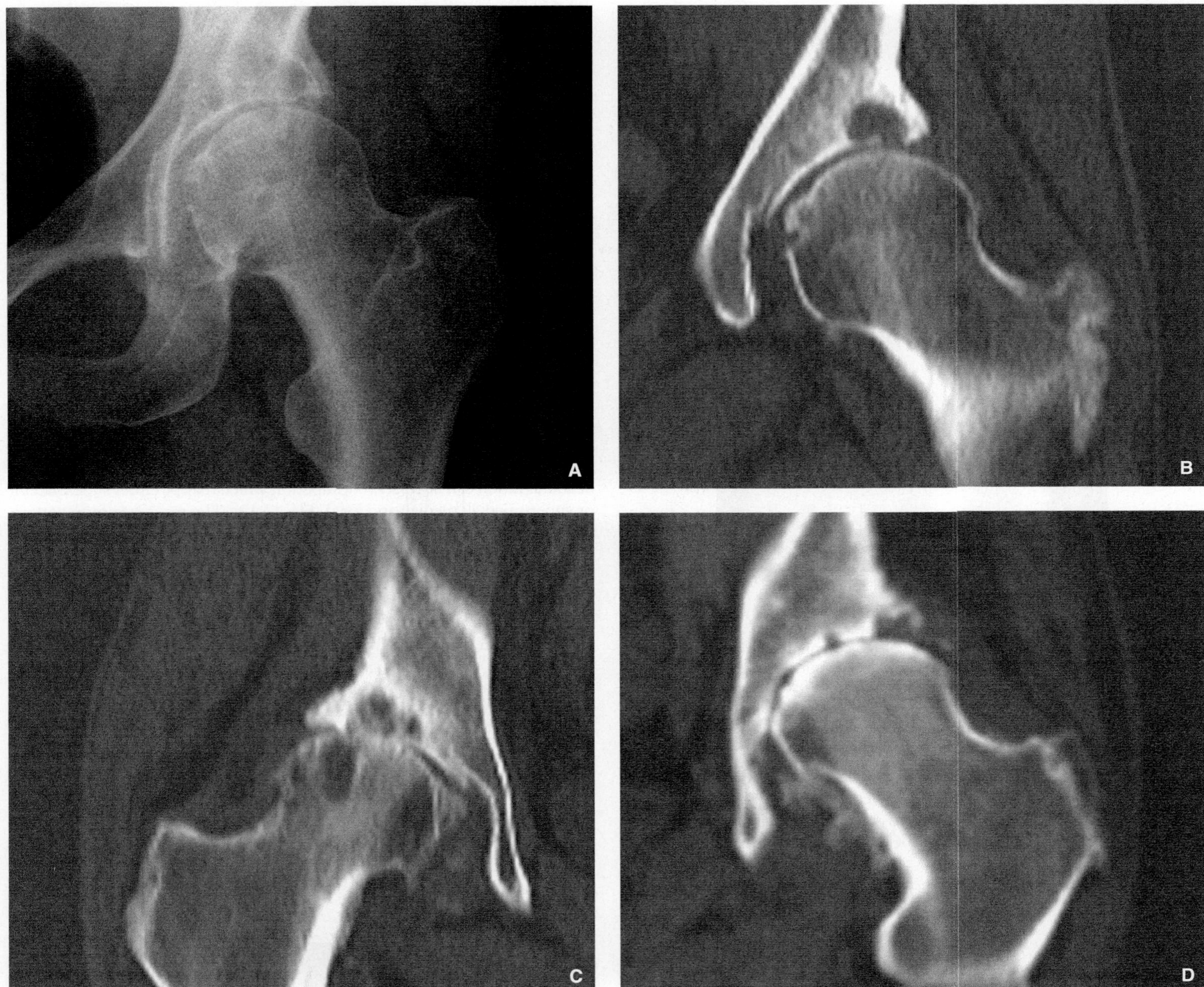

FIGURE 13.8 CT of OA of the hip joint. **(A)** Anteroposterior radiograph of the left hip of a 66-year-old woman shows narrowing of the joint space, subchondral sclerosis, and cystic-like lesion in the acetabulum, better demonstrated on **(B)** the coronal reformatted CT image. **(C)** In another patient, a 71-year-old woman, coronal reformatted CT image of the right hip joint shows geodes in the femoral head and acetabulum. **(D)** Coronal reformatted CT image of the left hip joint of a 55-year-old woman shows narrowing of the joint space, subchondral sclerosis, and osteophytosis.

process of endochondral bone formation. Similar hypertrophic changes occur on the inferior-posterior wall of the acetabulum. Osteophytes do not develop in the weight-bearing areas because these segments are subjected to constant mechanical abrasions.

Degenerative "cysts" are one of the imaging hallmarks of OA, although only some of these structures on histopathologic examination exhibit character of a true cystic lesion. More often, these are solid foci of fibrous or cartilaginous metaplasia; therefore, the term *pseudocysts*, *cyst-like lesions*, or *geodes* is probably more accurate. They are usually small, circular, or piriform in shape and confined to subarticular area of sclerotic bone within the segment of high pressure. Larger lesion may also develop deeper in the femoral head and acetabulum. In some cases, a communication channel from the neck of the lesion into the joint cavity can be identified.

Occasionally, the degenerative process in the hip may run a more rapid course. In a matter of months and sometimes weeks, a traditionally slowly progressive OA of the hip is converted into the rapidly progressive, aggressively destructive disease that completely destroys the hip joint. In some of the patients, the major portion of the femoral head may completely disappear. The acetabulum became concentrically enlarged (Figs. 13.14 and 13.15). The pain in the hip is typically disabling and unrelenting. This destructive arthrosis of the hip joint is known as *Postel coxarthropathy*, a condition characterized by rapid chondrolysis that may quickly lead to complete destruction of the hip joint. Originally described by Lequesne and also by Postel and Kerboull in 1970, this unique hip disorder occurs predominantly in women, with age of onset at 60 to 70 years. In all cases, a rapid clinical course of hip pain is the consistent common symptom. The histologic findings are those of conventional OA with severe degenerative changes in the articular cartilage. However, osteophyte formation is absent or minimal. Hypervascularity in the subchondral bone is a common finding. The bone trabeculae are either abnormally thickened or abnormally thinned. Occasionally, one can observe foci of fibrosis, interstitial edema and hemorrhage in the marrow spaces, focal marrow fat fibrosis, and focal

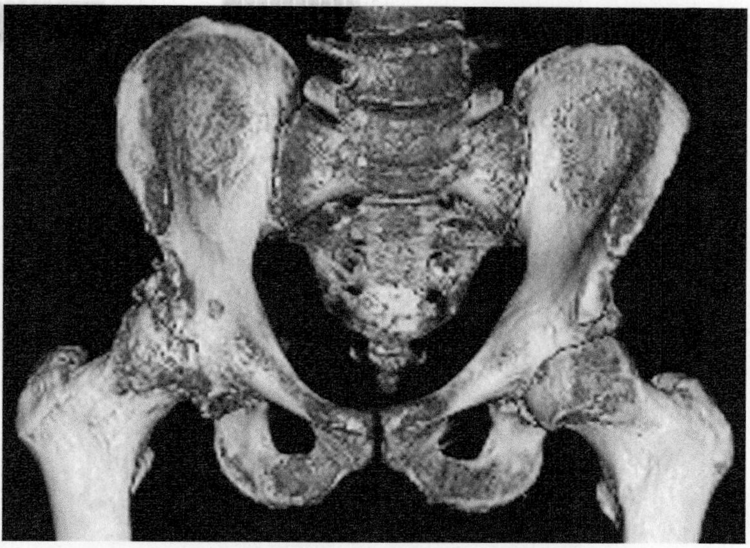

FIGURE 13.9 **3D CT of OA of the hip joints.** 3D reconstructed CT image of the pelvis shows advanced OA of the right hip joint and moderate OA of the left hip joint in a 69-year-old man.

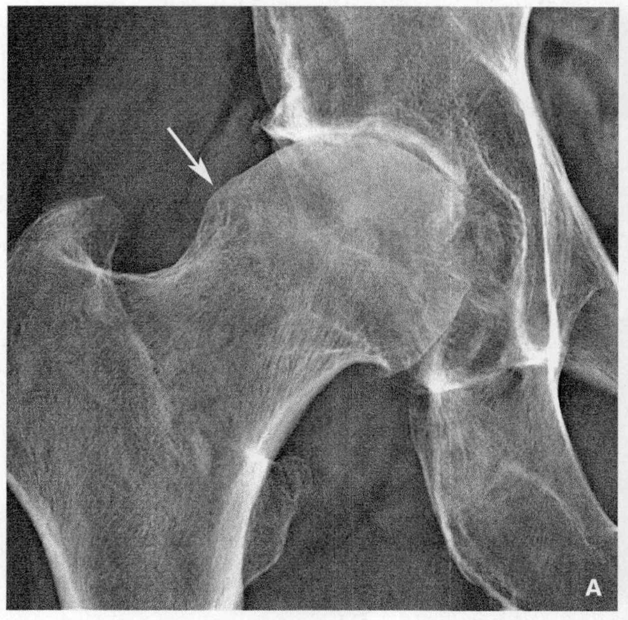

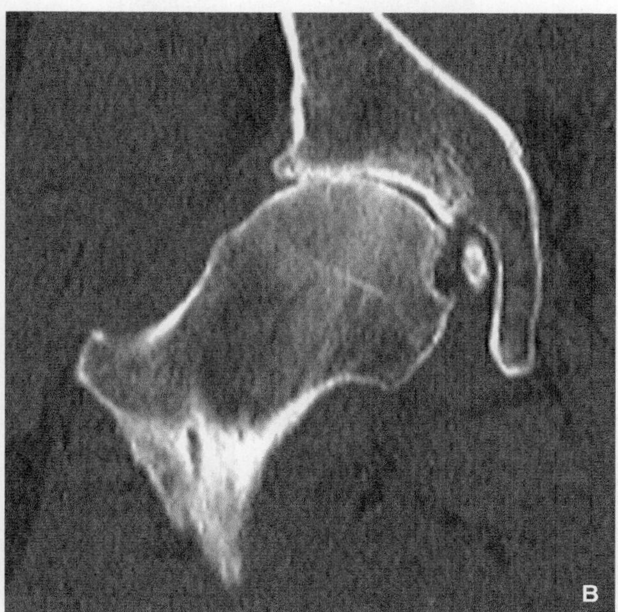

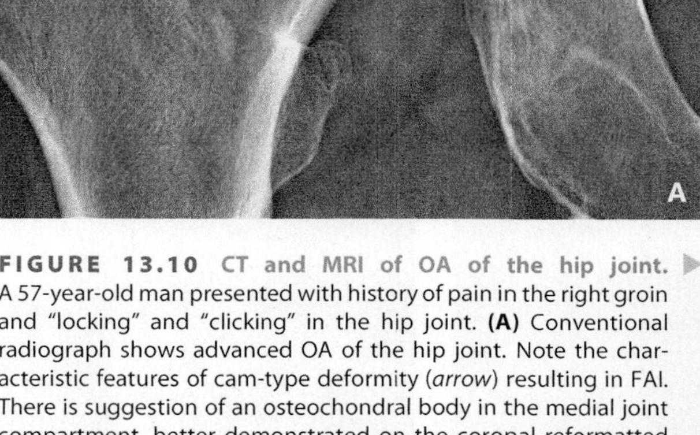

FIGURE 13.10 **CT and MRI of OA of the hip joint.** A 57-year-old man presented with history of pain in the right groin and "locking" and "clicking" in the hip joint. **(A)** Conventional radiograph shows advanced OA of the hip joint. Note the characteristic features of cam-type deformity (*arrow*) resulting in FAI. There is suggestion of an osteochondral body in the medial joint compartment, better demonstrated on the coronal reformatted CT image **(B)**. **(C)** Coronal T2-weighted fat-suppressed MR image shows in addition a large joint effusion.

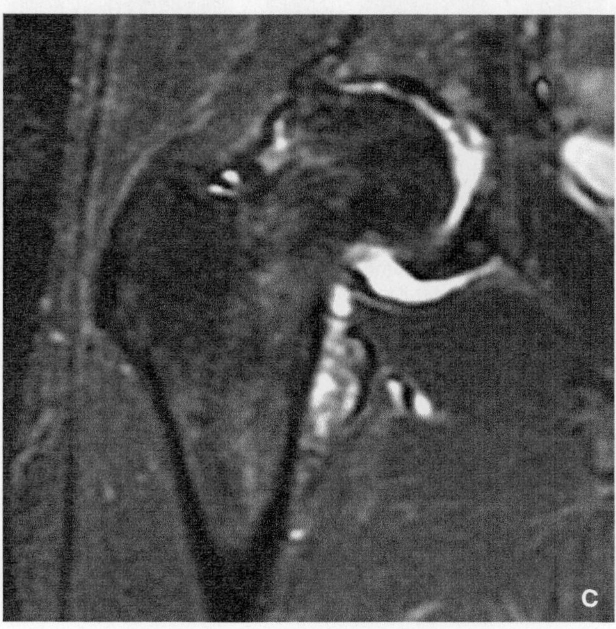

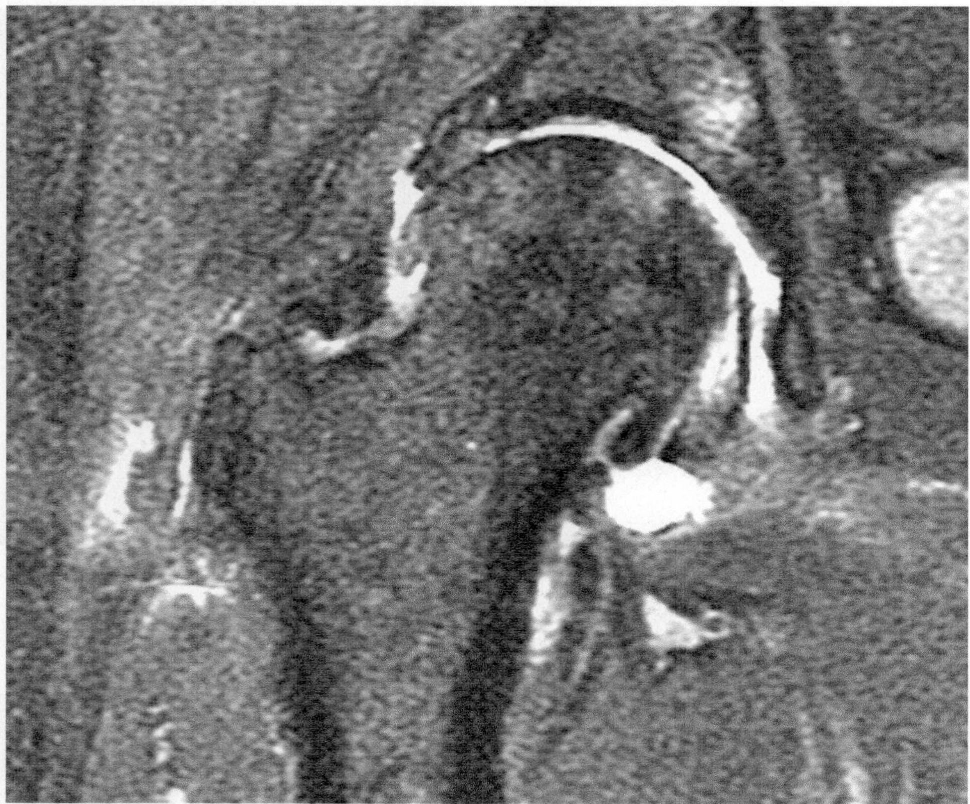

FIGURE 13.11 **MRI of OA of the hip joint.** Coronal proton density–weighted fat-suppressed MR image of the right hip of a 68-year-old woman shows joint space narrowing, subchondral sclerosis and bone marrow edema, osteophytes arising from the femoral head and acetabulum, and joint effusion.

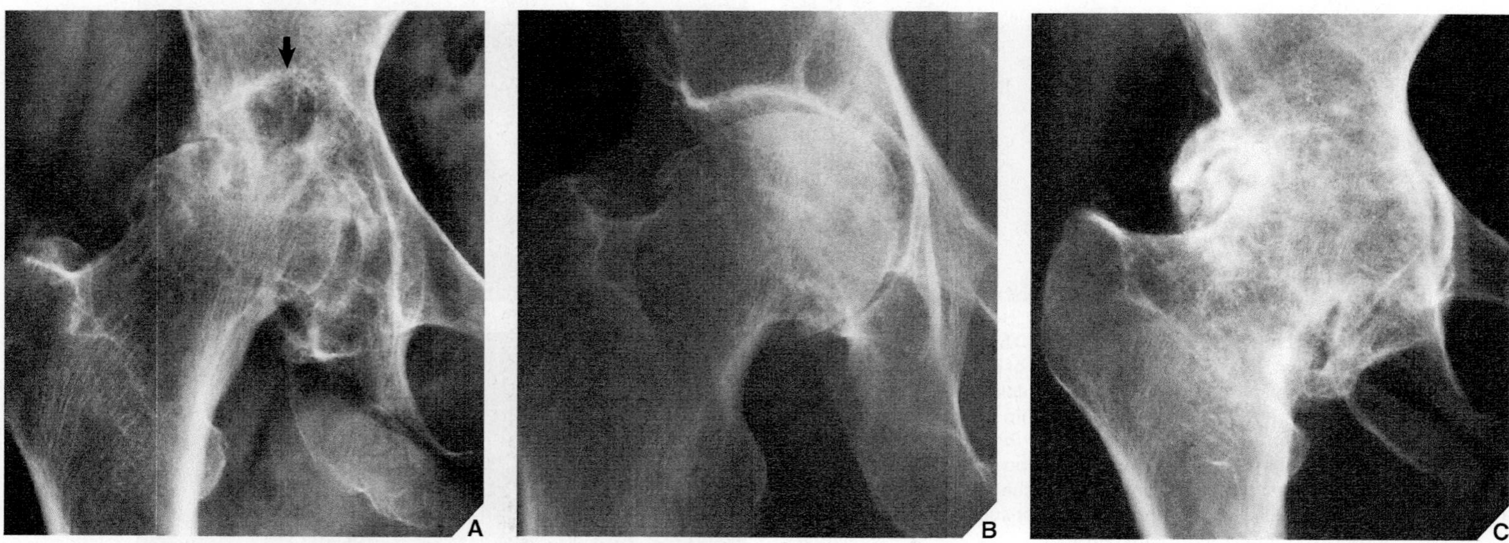

FIGURE 13.12 **Migration of the femoral head.** **(A)** Anteroposterior radiograph of the right hip of a 65-year-old woman with long-standing degenerative joint disease in both hips demonstrates superolateral migration of the femoral head, the most common pattern seen in OA of the hip joint. Note the typical Eggers cyst in the acetabulum *(arrow)*. **(B)** Medial migration of the femoral head is apparent in this 48-year-old woman with OA of the right hip. **(C)** Axial migration of the femoral head is evident in this 57-year-old woman who was suspected of having inflammatory arthritis. Clinical and laboratory investigations, however, led to a diagnosis of idiopathic OA, which was confirmed on histopathologic examination after total hip replacement.

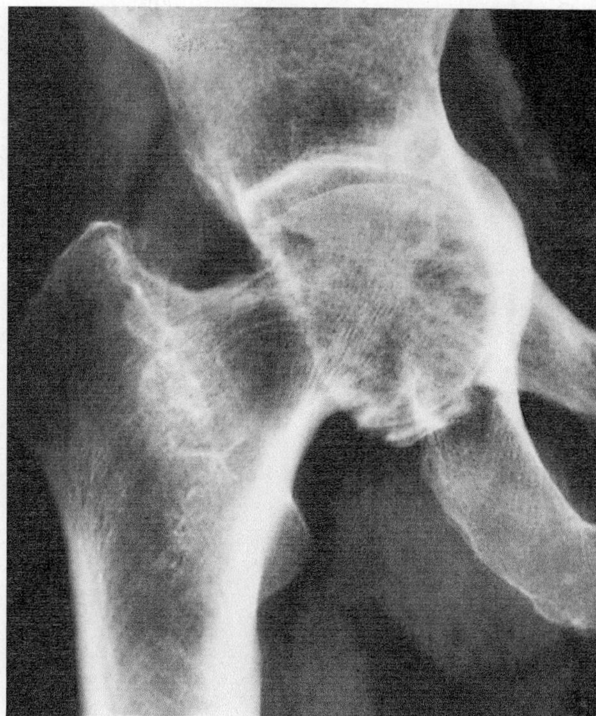

FIGURE 13.13 RA with superimposed OA. Anteroposterior radiograph of the right hip of a 42-year-old woman with a known history of long-standing RA shows the typical changes of inflammatory arthritis, including axial migration of the femoral head and acetabular protrusio. Superimposition of secondary OA is evident in subchondral sclerosis and marginal osteophytes.

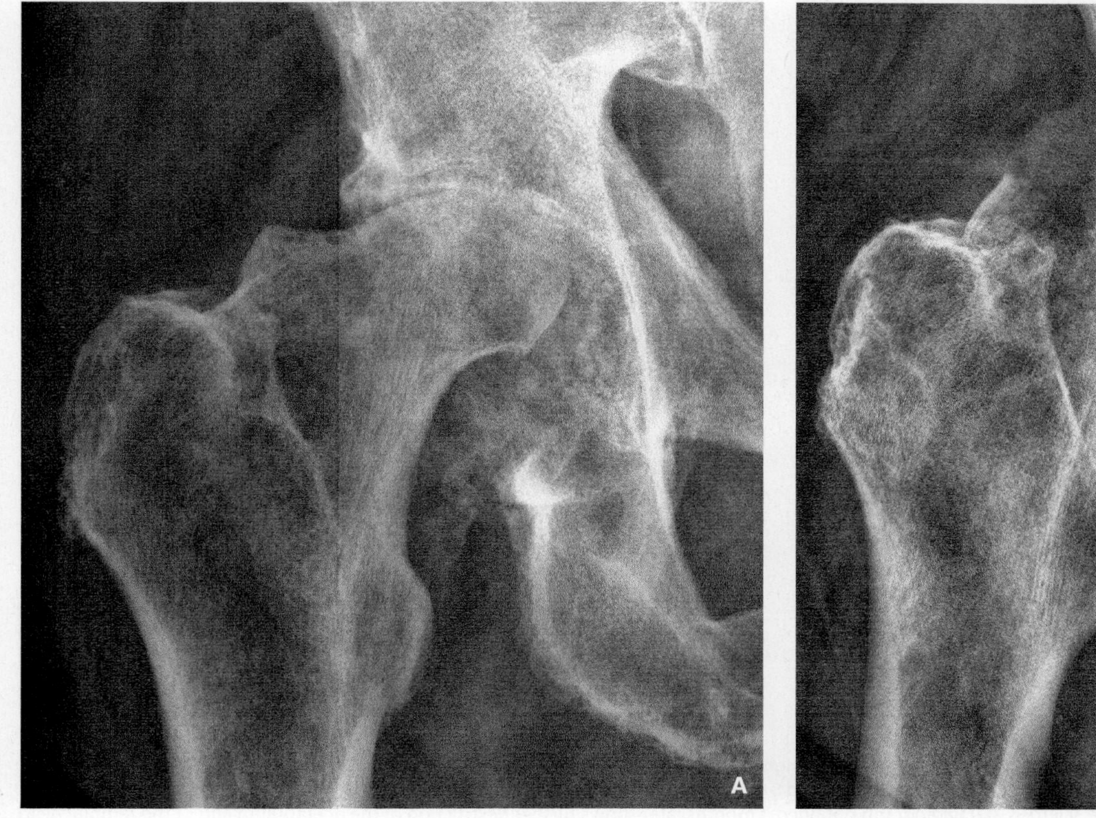

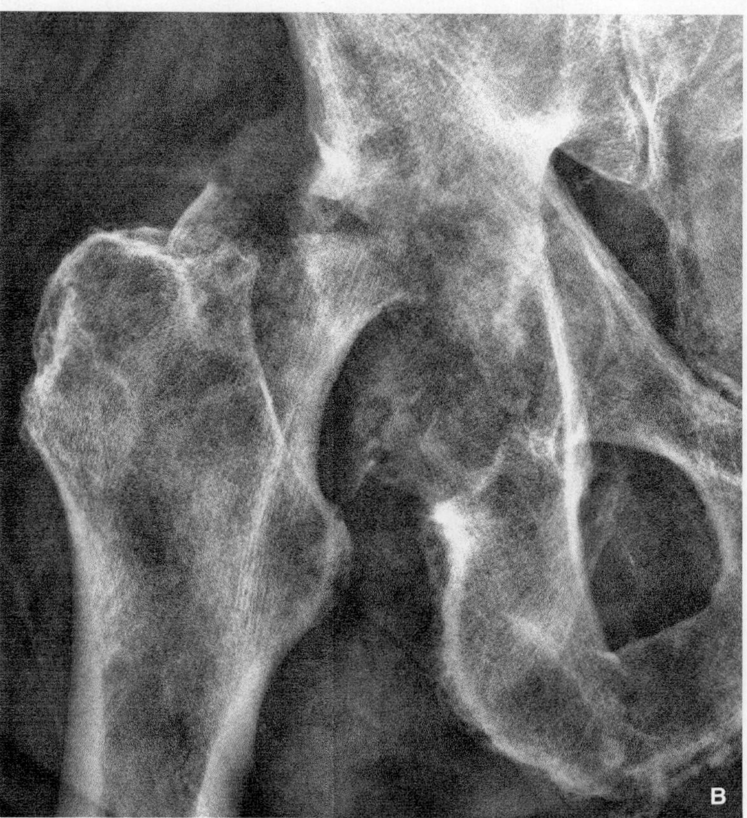

FIGURE 13.14 Postel coxarthropathy. **(A)** OA of the right hip joint in this 61-year-old woman markedly progressed in a very short time as seen here on the radiograph obtained 5 months later **(B)**.

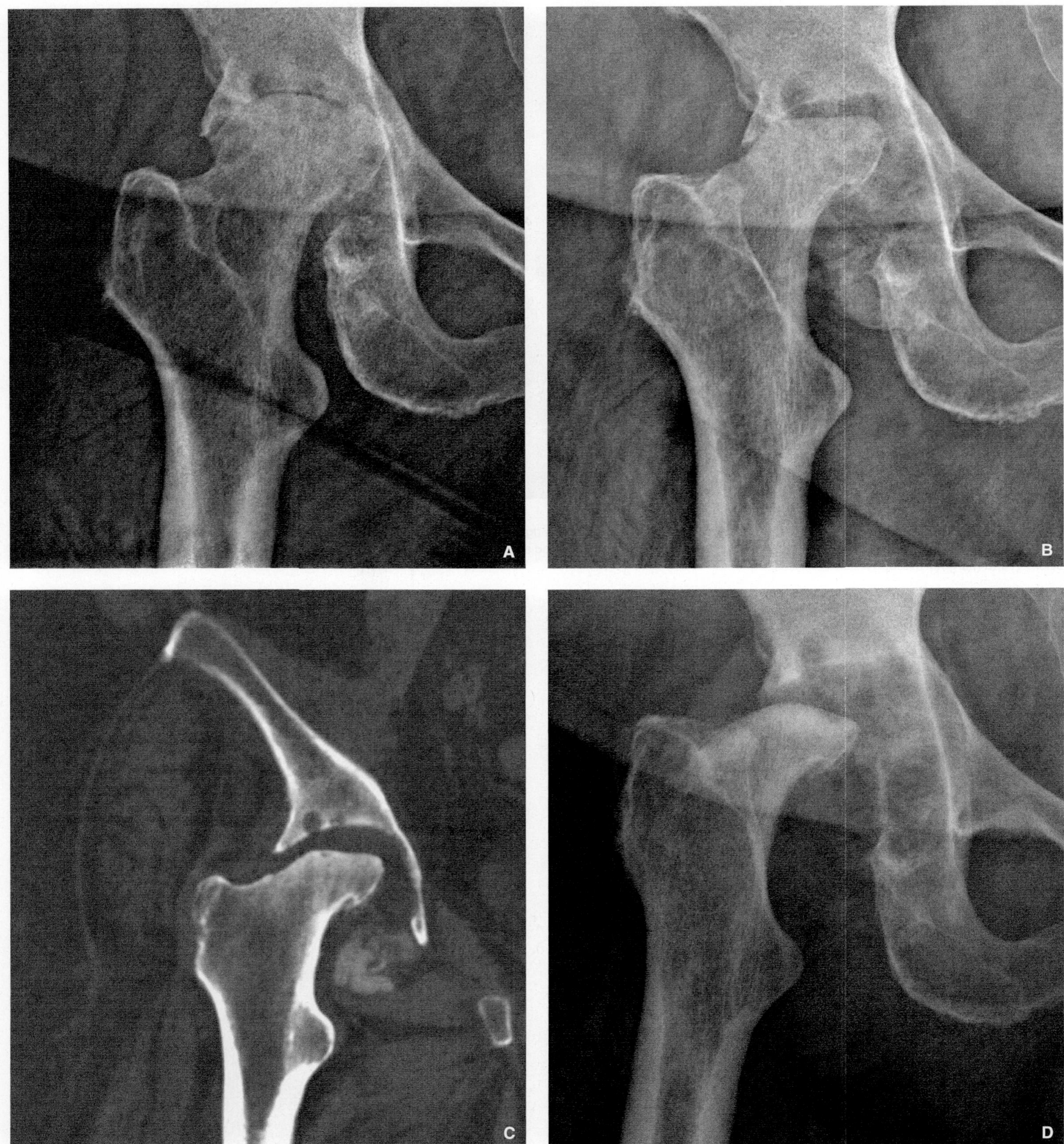

FIGURE 13.15 Postel coxarthropathy. **(A)** Anteroposterior radiograph of the right hip of a 53-year-old woman shows narrowing of the joint and superior migration of the femoral head. **(B)** The radiograph and **(C)** coronal reformatted CT image obtained 8 months later show destruction of the acetabulum and femoral head. Observe almost complete lack of osteophytes and minimal reactive sclerosis. **(D)** Radiograph obtained 3 months later shows further destruction of the acetabulum and of the femoral head with progression of superolateral migration.

areas of bone resorption. The precise pathogenesis of this condition remains unclear, although direct drug toxicity and the analgesic effects of nonsteroidal antiinflammatory drugs have been implicated. Some investigators have suggested that intraarticular deposition of hydroxyapatite crystals might lead to joint destruction. Others have proposed subchondral insufficiency fracture of the femoral head as a cause of this arthritis. Some investigators demonstrated elevated levels of interleukin-6 (IL-6) and interleukin-1β (IL-1β) in the joint fluid as well as elevated secretion of matrix metalloproteinases by fibroblasts from the synovium and subchondral cysts.

Because of the rapidity of the process, the radiographic presentation of this condition is marked by very little, if any, reparative changes, mimicking infectious or neuropathic arthritis (Charcot joint) (Fig. 13.16). Boutry and colleagues reported MRI findings of this form of OA. These included joint effusion, a bone marrow edema-like pattern in the femoral head, neck, and acetabulum; femoral head flattening; and cyst-like subchondral defects (Fig. 13.17).

Secondary Osteoarthritis of the Hip

Secondary OA is often seen in the hip joint in patients with predisposing conditions such as previous trauma (Figs. 13.18 and 13.19), slipped capital femoral epiphysis (Fig. 13.20), congenital hip dysplasia/dislocation (Fig. 13.21), osteonecrosis (Fig. 13.22), Paget disease (see Fig. 29.25), infectious arthritis (Fig. 13.23), inflammatory arthritis (Figs. 13.24 and 13.25), Perthes disease, and femoroacetabular impingement (FAI) syndrome (see text and figures in the following section). The imaging findings

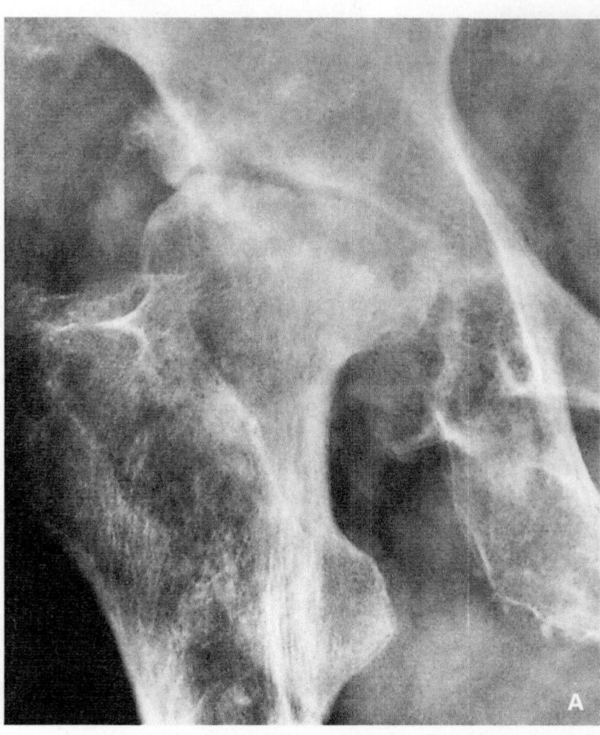

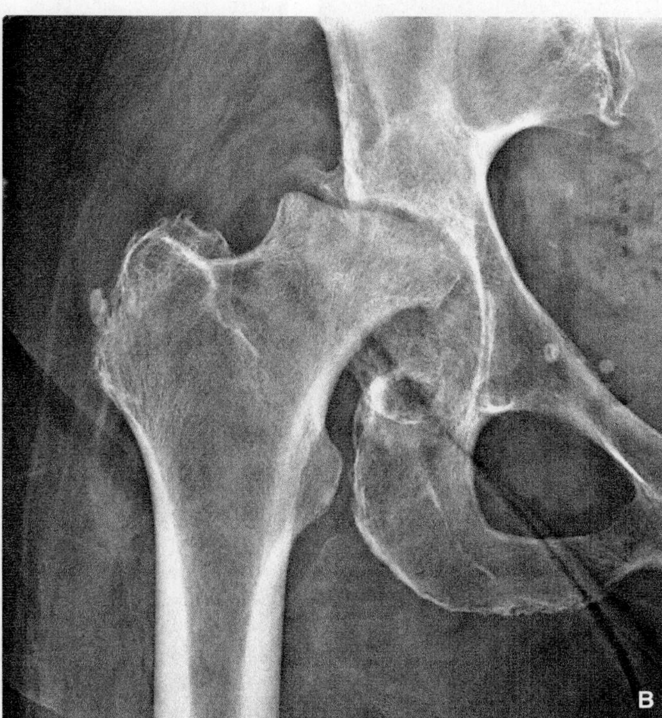

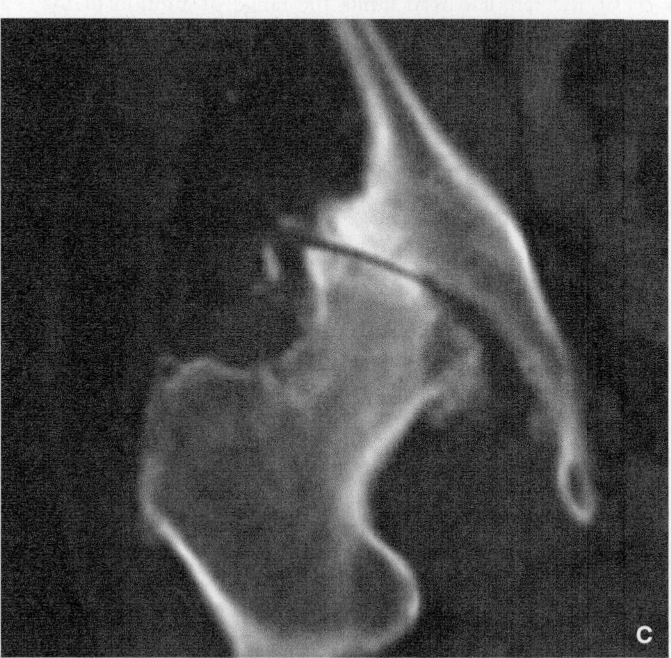

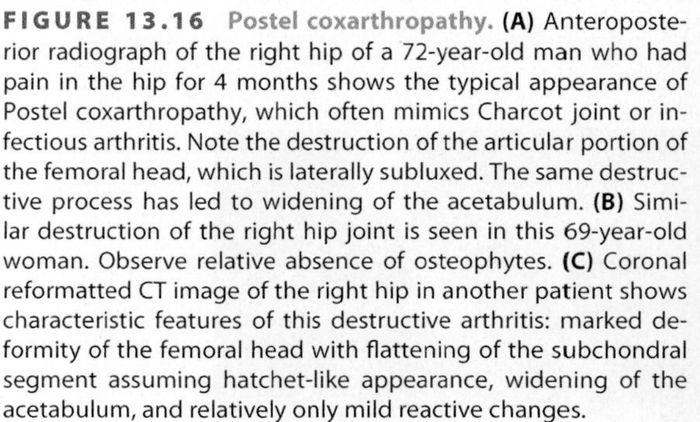
FIGURE 13.16 Postel coxarthropathy. (A) Anteroposterior radiograph of the right hip of a 72-year-old man who had pain in the hip for 4 months shows the typical appearance of Postel coxarthropathy, which often mimics Charcot joint or infectious arthritis. Note the destruction of the articular portion of the femoral head, which is laterally subluxed. The same destructive process has led to widening of the acetabulum. **(B)** Similar destruction of the right hip joint is seen in this 69-year-old woman. Observe relative absence of osteophytes. **(C)** Coronal reformatted CT image of the right hip in another patient shows characteristic features of this destructive arthritis: marked deformity of the femoral head with flattening of the subchondral segment assuming hatchet-like appearance, widening of the acetabulum, and relatively only mild reactive changes.

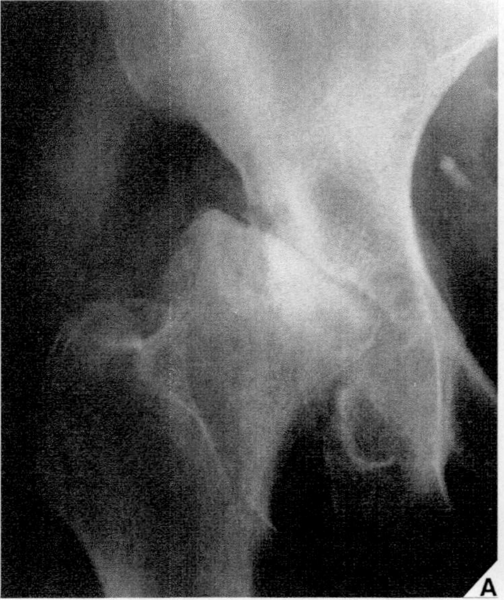

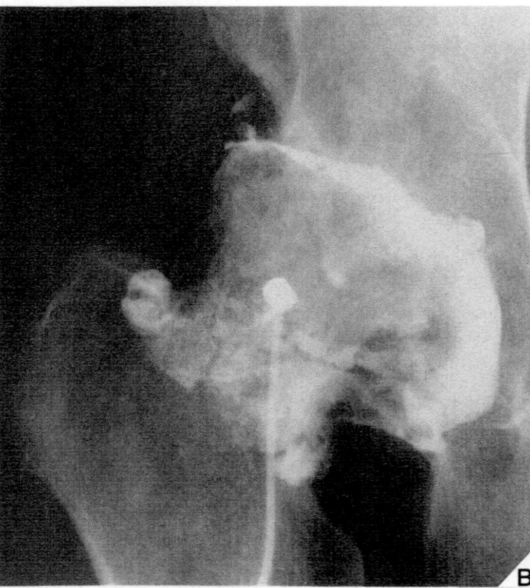

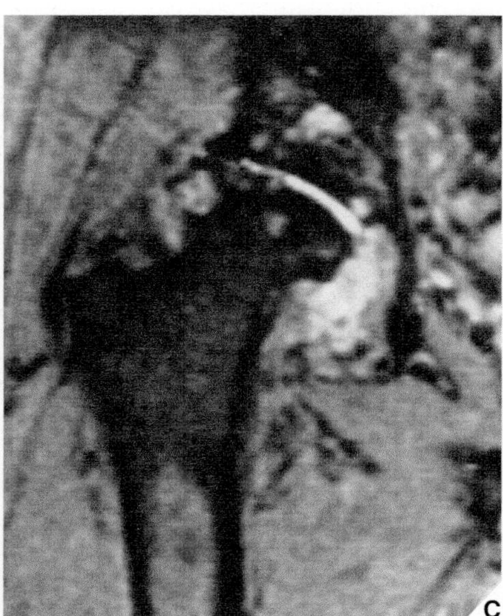

FIGURE 13.17 Arthrography and MRI of Postel coxarthropathy. **(A)** Anteroposterior radiograph of the right hip of a 44-year-old man shows destructive changes of the femoral head and acetabulum. **(B)** Aspiration arthrogram, which was performed to rule out infection, shows hypertrophic synovitis. **(C)** Gradient-echo T2*-weighted MRI shows joint effusion, hypertrophied synovium, and subchondral cysts in the acetabulum and femoral head.

of the secondary OA are the same as those described for primary OA, but the features of the underlying process also can often be detected. Although the standard radiographic views are usually sufficient for demonstrating these changes, CT, arthrography, or MRI may at times be needed for a more accurate assessment of the status of the articular cartilage.

Femoroacetabular Impingement Syndrome

FAI results from incongruity of the femoral head and acetabulum and is one of the leading causes of precocious OA of the hip joint. Two types of FAI have been described based on the predominance of anatomic abnormalities affecting either femoral head or acetabulum. In *cam type*, the nonspherical shape of the femoral head secondary to excessive bone formation at the junction of head and neck results in abutment against the acetabular rim. In *pincer type*, because of deep acetabulum (coxa profunda), acetabular protrusio, or acetabular retroversion, acetabular "overcoverage" of the femoral head limits the range of motion in the hip joint and leads to abnormal stresses on acetabular rim. In both types of FAI, the abnormal mechanism results in damage of the acetabular labrum, thus promoting secondary OA. The diagnosis of FAI is based on (a) the patient's clinical history of chronic pain; (b) physical examination revealing reduced range of motion in the hip joint, particularly flexion and internal rotation; and (c) imaging findings on conventional radiography, CT, and MRI. In cam type, conventional radiography demonstrates excessive bone formation at the femoral head/neck junction with loss of normal anatomic "waist" at this site (Fig. 13.26A, see also Figs. 13.6 and 13.10), occasionally resembling the smooth hand grip of some pistols ("pistol grip deformity" or a "cam effect") (Fig. 13.26B); an os acetabulum, which more likely represents an osseous metaplasia of the cartilaginous labrum or a fragment of damaged acetabular rim; and a radiolucent lesion at the head/neck junction, formerly called *synovial herniation pit*, and now designated as fibroosseous lesion. CT shows these abnormalities even better (Fig. 13.27). Magnetic resonance arthrography

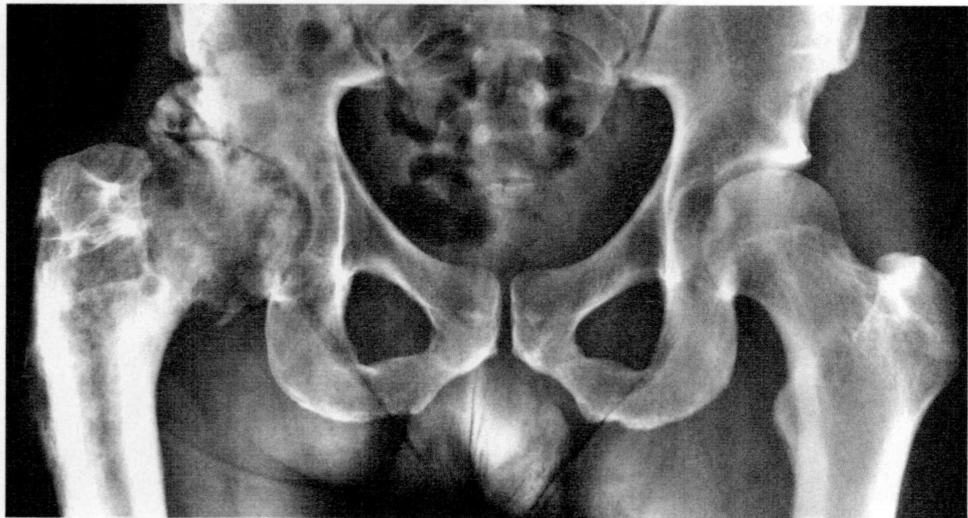

FIGURE 13.18 Posttraumatic OA. Anteroposterior radiograph of the pelvis of a 40-year-old man, who, 7 years prior to this examination, sustained a complex fracture of the right proximal femur and acetabulum, shows a deformity of the femoral head and neck associated with narrowing of the hip joint space, subchondral sclerosis, and osteophyte formation. Note the completely normal left hip joint.

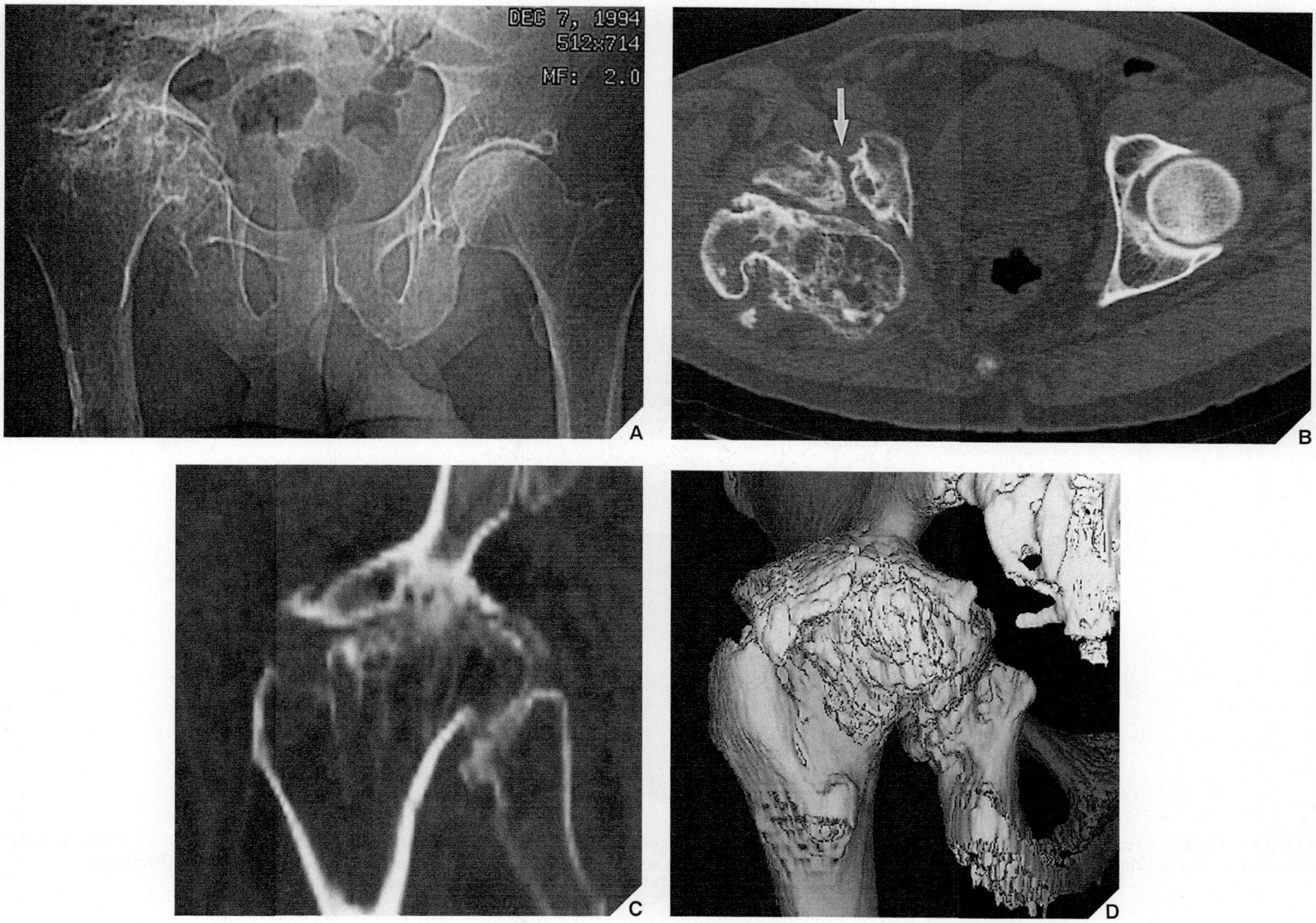

FIGURE 13.19 CT and 3D CT of posttraumatic OA. A 64-year-old man, who in the past sustained complex right acetabular and femoral fractures, developed secondary OA. **(A)** Preliminary scout CT image shows posttraumatic deformity of the acetabulum and femoral head associated with acetabular protrusio. **(B)** Axial CT section through both hips shows osteoarthritic changes of the right femoral head and ununited fracture of the anterior column *(arrow)*. **(C)** Coronal reformatted image demonstrates significant narrowing of the joint space, deformity of the femoral head, and periarticular sclerosis. **(D)** 3D CT reconstructed image shows almost complete obliteration of the hip joint, acetabular protrusio, and osteophyte formation. All CT findings are consistent with posttraumatic OA.

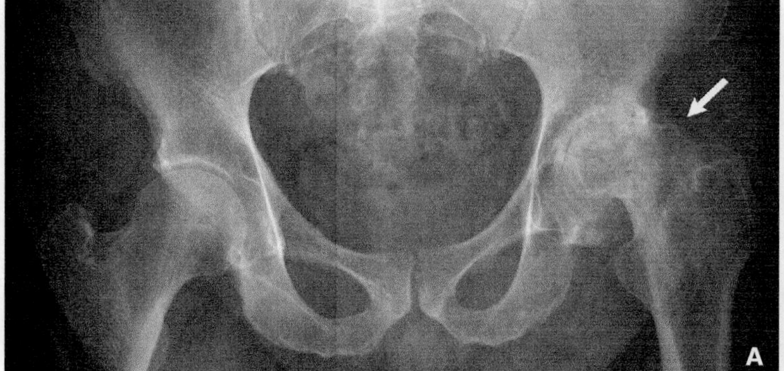

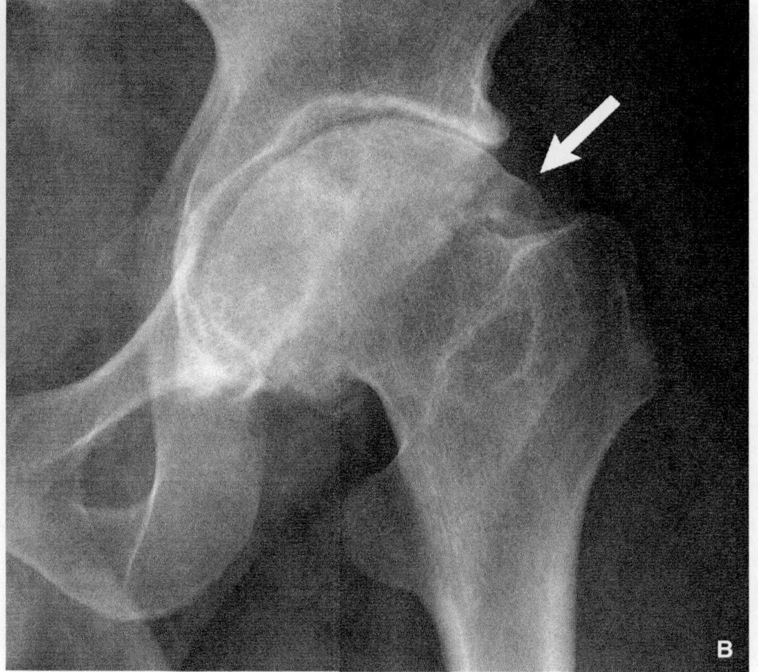

FIGURE 13.20 Secondary OA due to slipped capital femoral epiphysis (SCFE). **(A)** Anteroposterior radiograph of the pelvis of a 40-year-old man with history of SCFE shows osteoarthritic changes of the left hip joint. Note osseous remodeling at the junction of the femoral head and neck, a hallmark of this condition, known as a *Herndon hump (arrow)*. **(B)** In another patient, a 24-year-old woman with OA of the left hip joint, observe a characteristic Herndon hump *(arrow)* pointing to SCFE as the underlying cause of arthritis.

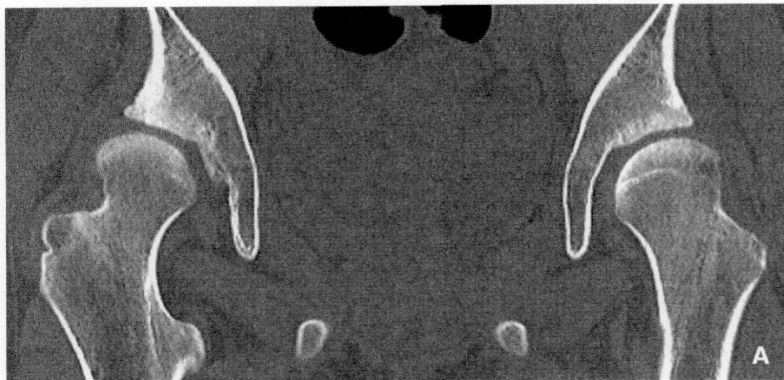

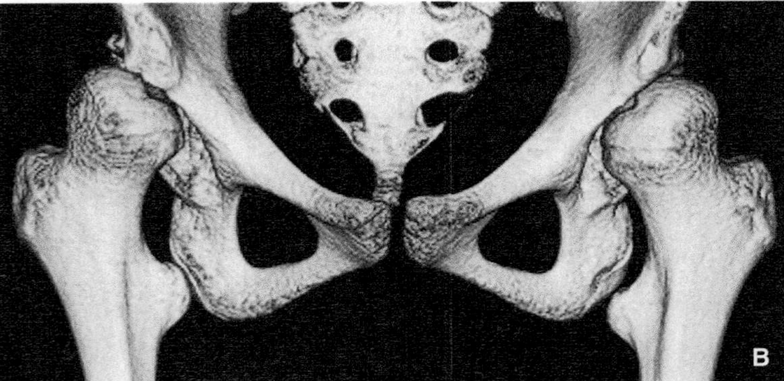

FIGURE 13.21 **Secondary OA due to developmental dysplasia of the hips (DDH).** **(A)** Coronal reformatted and **(B)** 3D reconstructed with surface-rendering algorithm CT images of the hips of a 30-year-old woman with history of bilateral congenital hip dislocation show dysplastic changes of both hip joints. There is evidence of secondary OA manifested by narrowing of the joint spaces, subchondral sclerosis at the site of femoral heads and acetabula, and formation of small marginal osteophytes at the periphery of both acetabula.

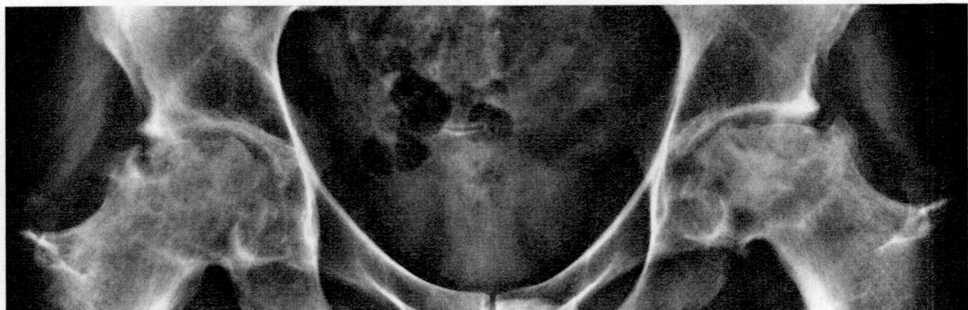

FIGURE 13.22 **Secondary OA due to osteonecrosis.** A 48-year-old man, a chronic alcoholic, developed osteonecrosis of both femoral heads, marked by increased bone density and subchondral collapse. Secondary OA is distinguished by narrowing of the joint space, marginal osteophytosis, and subchondral cyst formation.

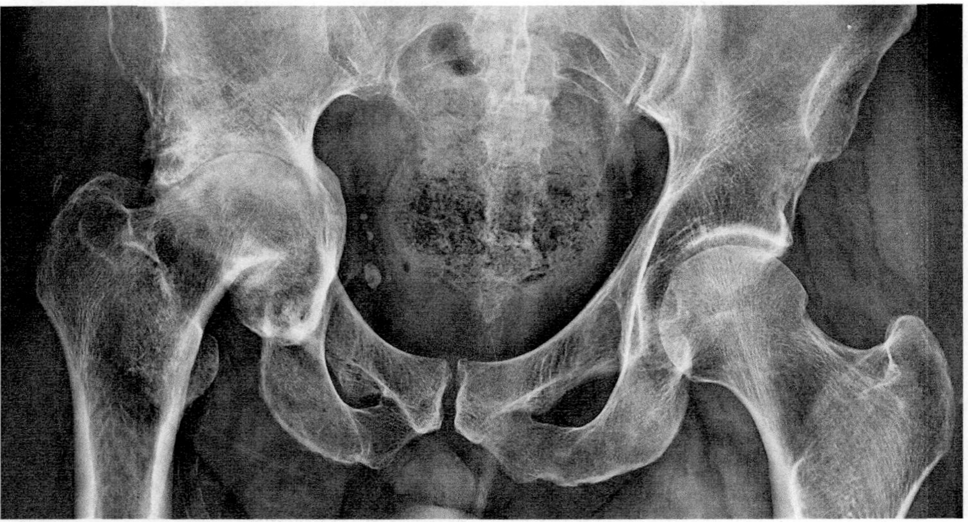

FIGURE 13.23 **Secondary OA due to joint infection.** Anteroposterior radiograph of the pelvis of a 49-year-old man with history of septic arthritis of the right hip joint and acetabular osteomyelitis shows deformity of the acetabulum, subchondral sclerosis, and significant narrowing of the joint space. Note unremarkable left hip joint. (Reprinted with permission from Greenspan A, Gershwin ME. *Imaging in rheumatology: a clinical approach*, 1st ed. Philadelphia: Wolters Kluwer; 2018:156.)

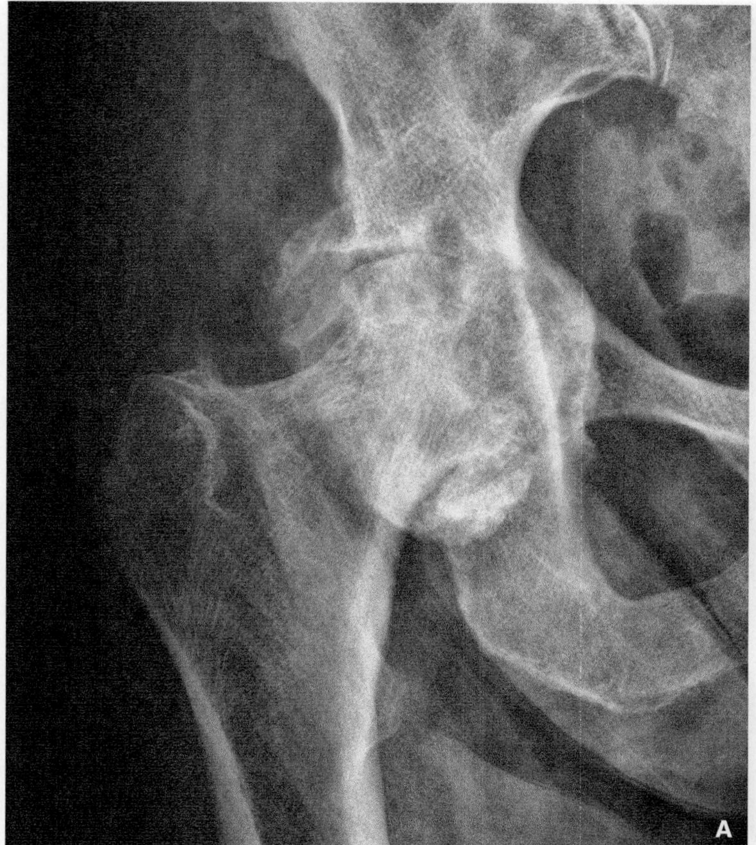

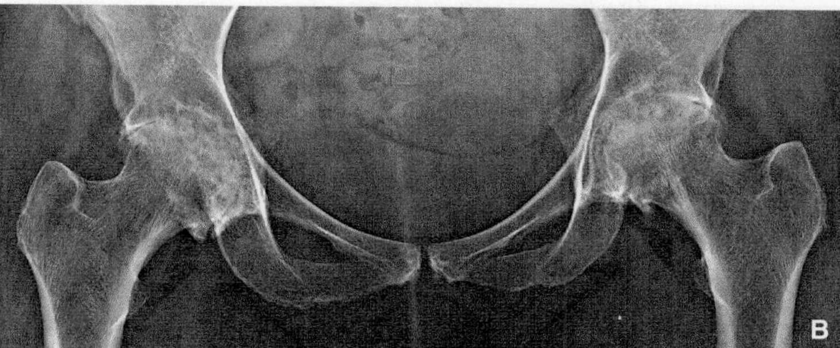

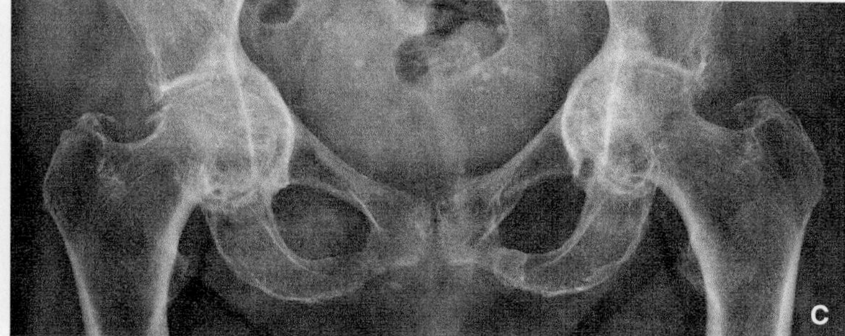

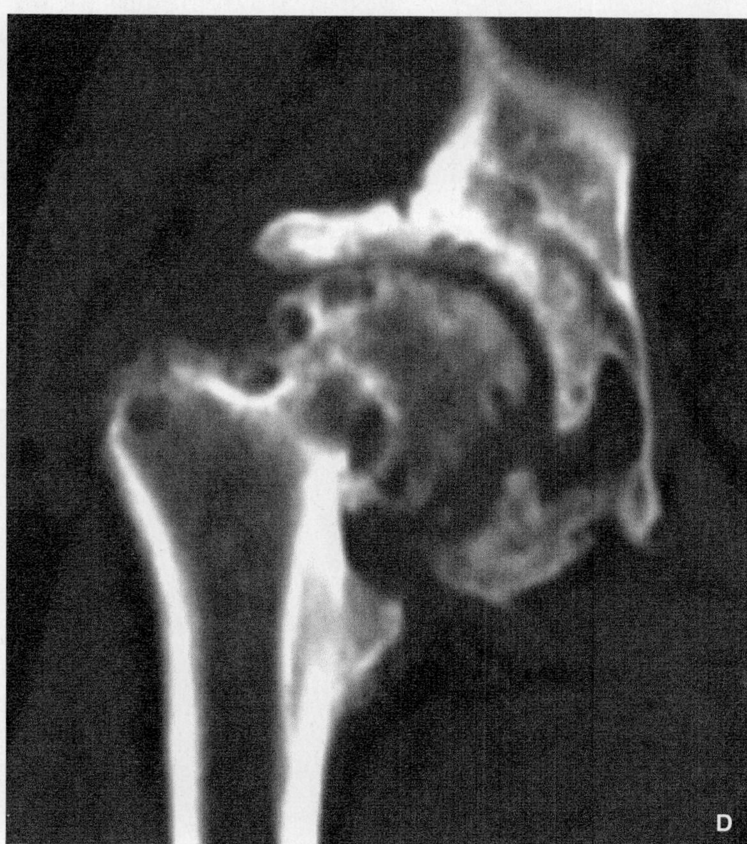

FIGURE 13.24 Secondary OA due to inflammatory arthritis (RA). **(A)** Radiograph of the right hip of a 60-year-old woman shows concentric narrowing of the joint space and acetabular protrusio, features of inflammatory arthritis. Superimposed are features of OA comprising sclerotic changes of the femoral head and acetabulum and osteophytosis. **(B)** In another patient, a 38-year-old woman with bilateral hip RA, observe typical features of inflammatory arthritis and secondary osteoarthritic changes manifesting mainly by formation of prominent osteophytes. **(C)** Similar example of secondary OA superimposed on RA affecting both hip joints is seen in an 81-year-old woman. **(D)** Coronal reformatted CT image of the right hip of a 40-year-old woman with RA shows subchondral and osseous erosions of the femoral head and acetabulum and superimposed secondary osteoarthritic changes in form of subchondral sclerosis of the acetabulum and osteophyte formation.

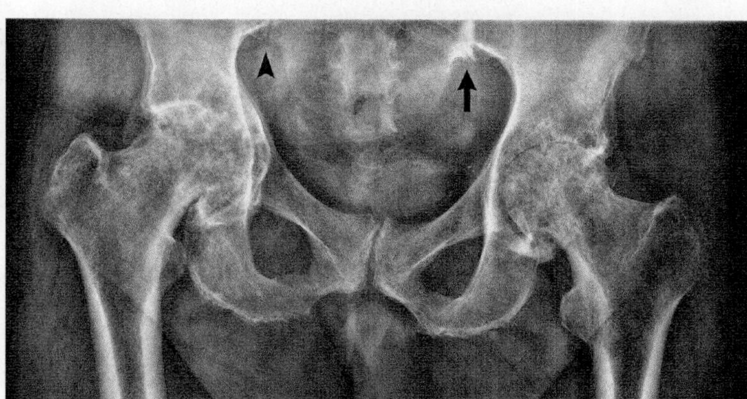

FIGURE 13.25 Secondary OA due to inflammatory arthritis (psoriasis). Radiograph of the pelvis of a 64-year-old man with clinically documented psoriasis shows characteristic for inflammatory arthritis concentric narrowing of the hip joints and axial migration of the femoral heads. In addition, note the changes of superimposed secondary OA marked by subchondral sclerosis, osteophytosis, and cyst formation in the left acetabulum and in the right femoral head. The patient also developed left-sided sacroiliitis *(arrow)*. The *arrowhead* points to unaffected right sacroiliac joint.

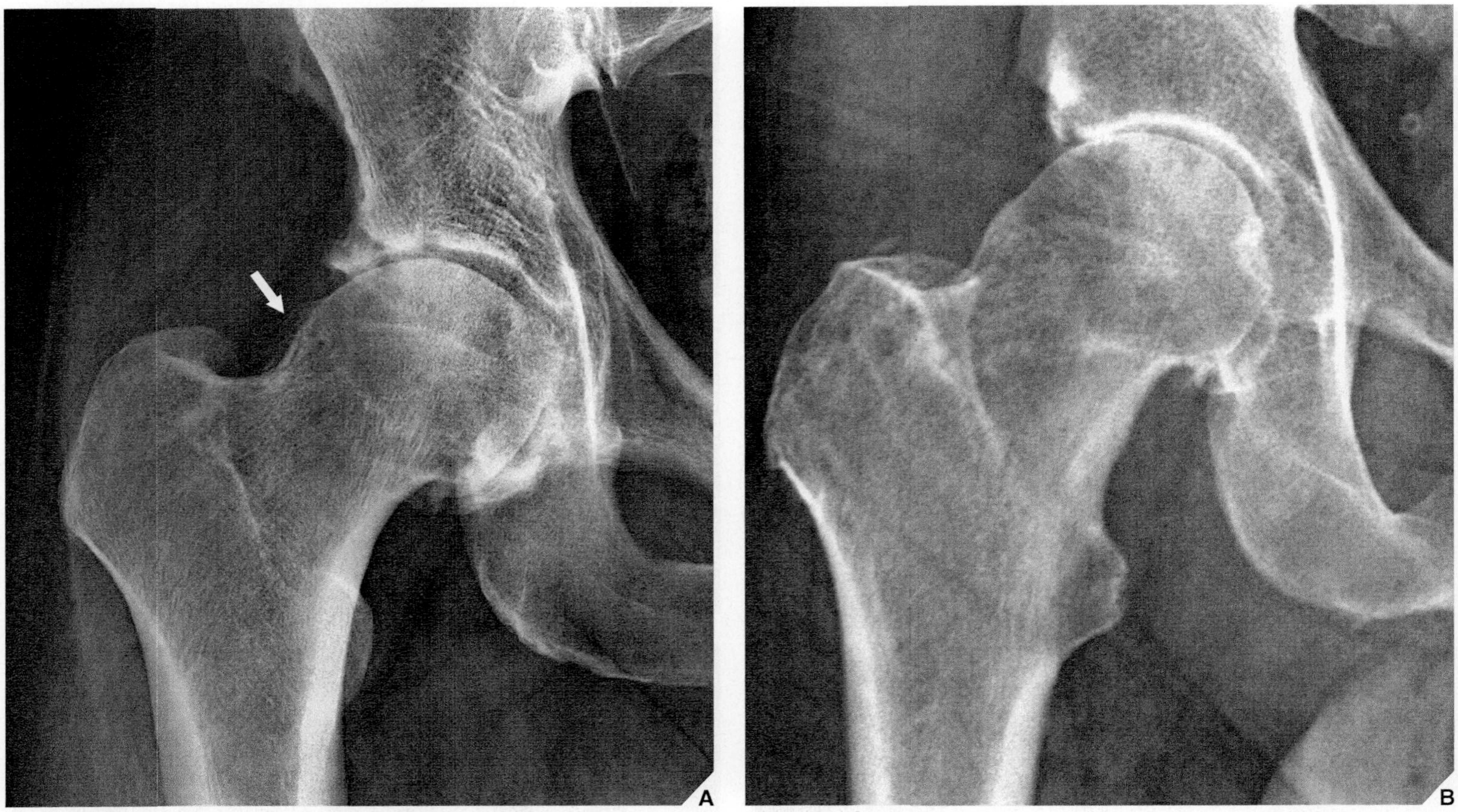

FIGURE 13.26 Cam type of FAI. **(A)** Anteroposterior radiograph of the right hip of a 39-year-old woman shows excessive bone buildup at the femoral head/neck junction *(arrow)*. Note secondary OA of the hip joint. **(B)** In another patient, a 41-year-old man, tubular appearance of the proximal right femur and the osseous prominence at the femoral head/neck junction assumed a "pistol grip" deformity. Also evident is OA of the hip joint.

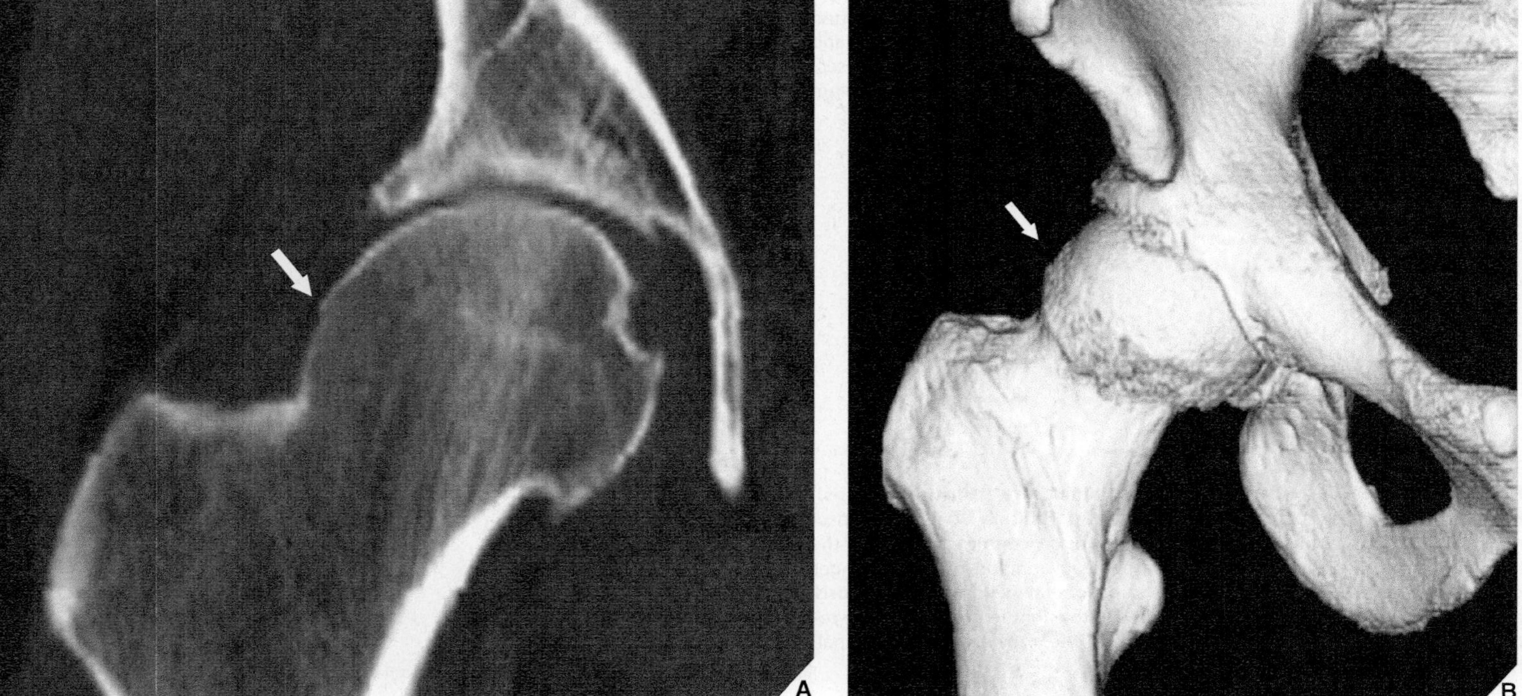

FIGURE 13.27 CT and 3D CT of cam type FAI. **(A)** Coronal reformatted CT image and **(B)** 3D reconstructed CT image in shaded surface display in a 34-year-old man show bone accretion at the femoral head/neck junction *(arrows)*.

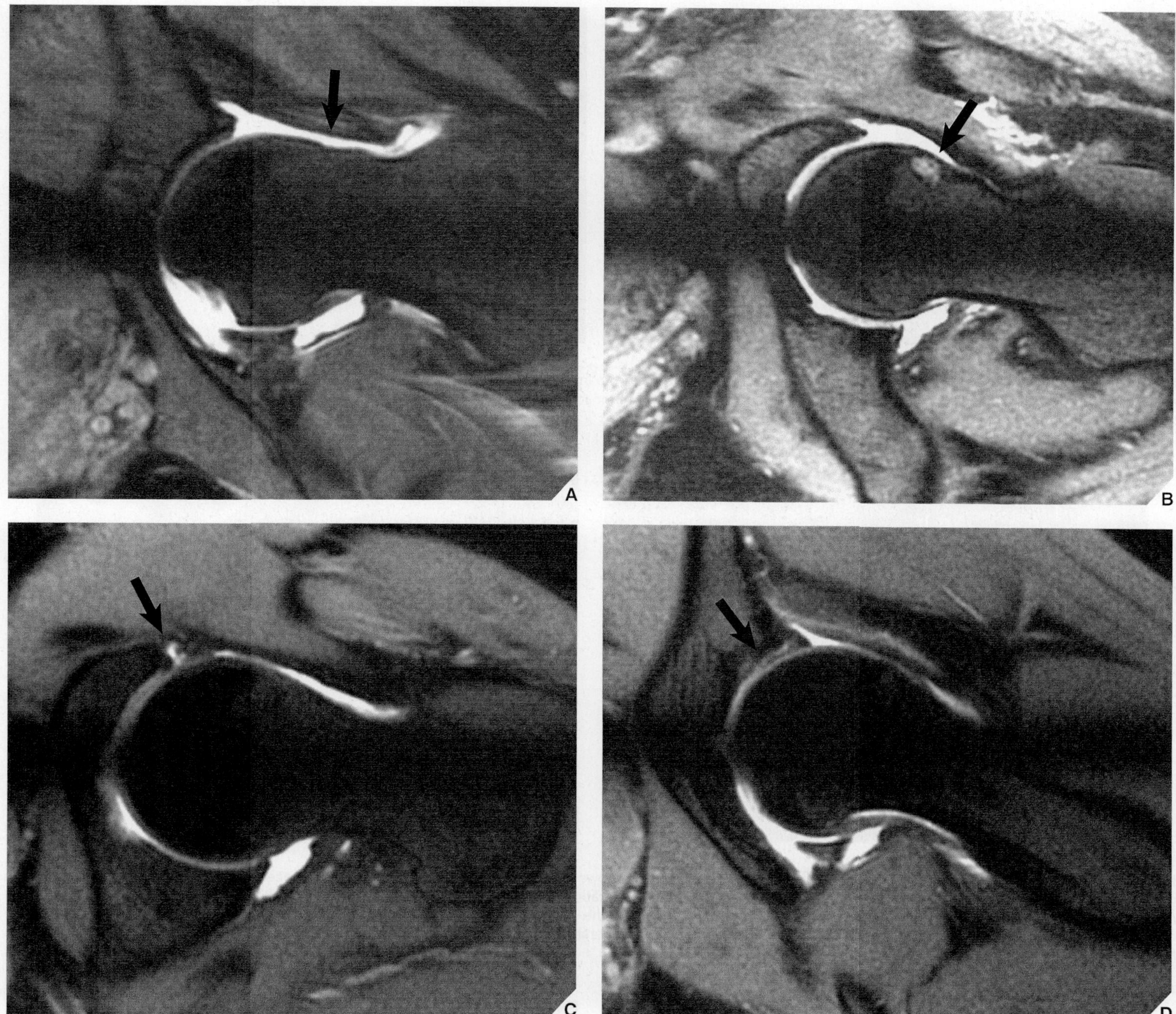

FIGURE 13.28 MRa of cam type FAI. Radial reconstructed MRa images of the hip joint show various characteristic features of this abnormality. **(A)** In a 34-year-old woman—a decreased femoral head/neck offset associated with hypertrophic ossification *(arrow)*. **(B)** In a 32-year-old woman—a fibroosseous lesion at the anterosuperior aspect of the femoral head/neck junction *(arrow)*. **(C)** In a 38-year-old man—a tear of the superior anterior cartilaginous labrum *(arrow)*. **(D)** In a 30-year-old woman—a delamination injury to the acetabular labrum *(arrow)*.

(MRa), particularly the radial reformatted images, in addition to the findings listed previously, clearly demonstrates abnormalities of the fibrocartilaginous labrum at the anterosuperior portion of the acetabulum (Fig. 13.28; see also Fig. 2.58). In pincer type, particularly in case of acetabular retroversion, conventional radiograph shows "crossover" sign, when more lateral projection of anterior acetabulum, which normally should project medially to the posterior acetabulum, "crosses" the posterior acetabular outline (Fig. 13.29). MRI demonstrates acetabular version and depth of the femoral head coverage (Fig. 13.30). To determine the sphericity of the femoral head and the prominence of the anterior femoral head/neck junction, the alpha angle is calculated on the oblique axial CT or oblique axial magnetic resonance (MR) images (Fig. 13.31). Radial reformatted MR images are of particular value in this respect because they allow optimal visualization of the anterosuperior region of the femoral head/neck junction, where the most significant changes in the alpha angle occur (see Fig. 13.31B). The normal alpha angle should not exceed 50 degrees. The larger the alpha angle, the more pronounced is nonspherical shape of the femoral head, and the greater is predisposition for anterior FAI.

Treatment

In very early stages of OA of the hip, particularly in the patients with FAI, open or arthroscopic trimming of acetabular rim and/or femoral head may be attempted. In younger patients, labral and acetabular repair

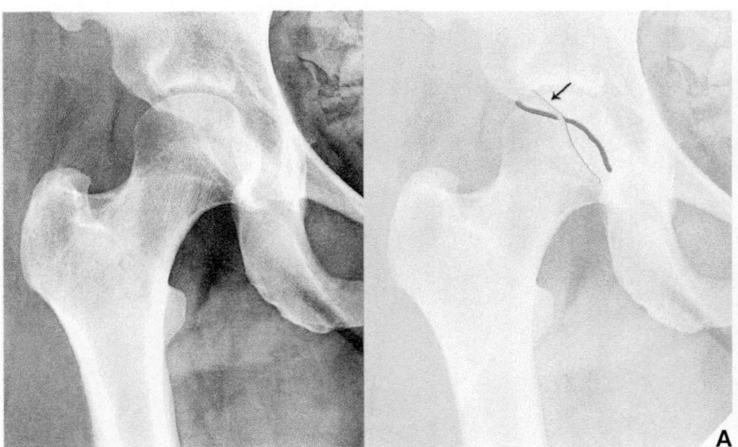

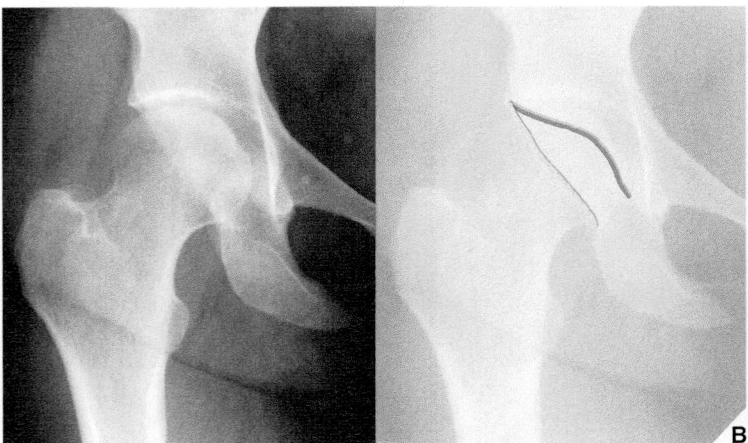

FIGURE 13.29 Pincer type FAI. **(A)** Anteroposterior radiograph of the left hip in a 29-year-old woman shows an acetabular crossover sign. Note that the posterior acetabular rim outline *(yellow line)* projects medially *(arrow)* in relation to the anterior acetabular rim *(red line)*, indicative of acetabular retroversion. **(B)** In a normal hip joint, the posterior acetabular rim outline projects laterally to the posterior acetabular rim.

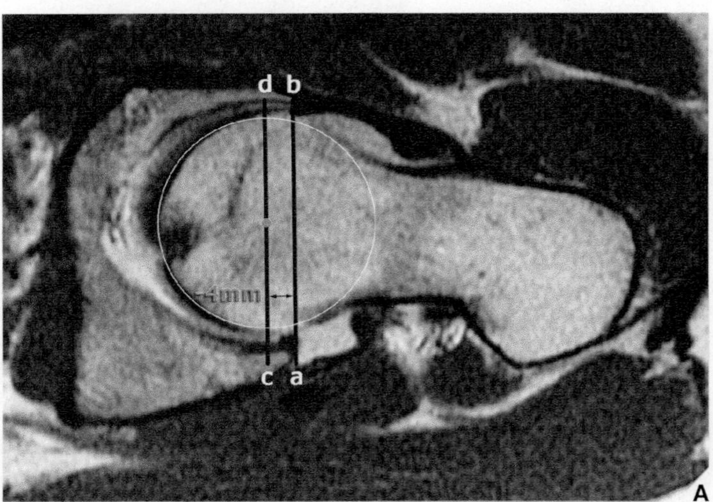

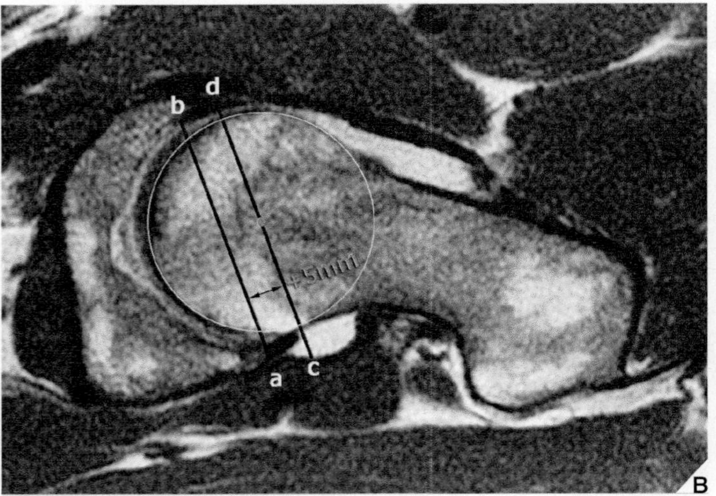

FIGURE 13.30 MRI of pincer FAI. **(A)** Axial oblique T1-weighted MR image shows deeply seated femoral head secondary to acetabular retroversion. Acetabular depth can be quantified by drawing a line *(ab)* connecting the posterior and anterior acetabular rims and a parallel line *(cd)* that passes through the center of the femoral head *(red dot)*. The distance between these two lines defines the acetabular depth, with the value being positive (+) if the center of the femoral head projects lateral to the line connecting the acetabular rims. Negative values (−) indicate deep seating of the femoral head within the acetabulum. **(B)** Axial oblique MR image of normal hip joint is shown for comparison.

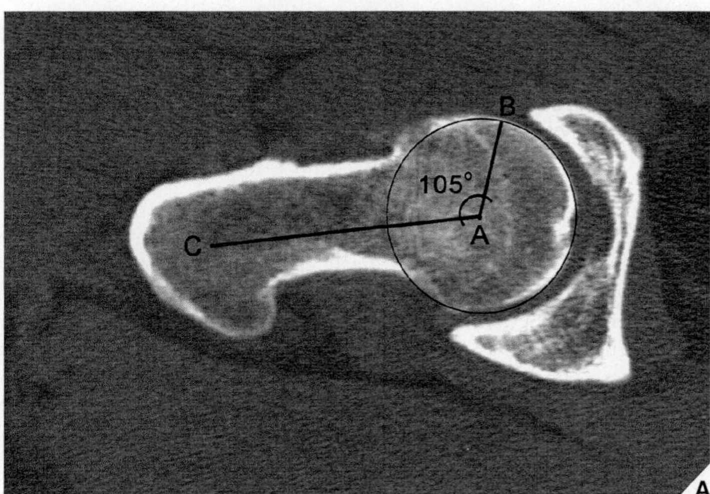

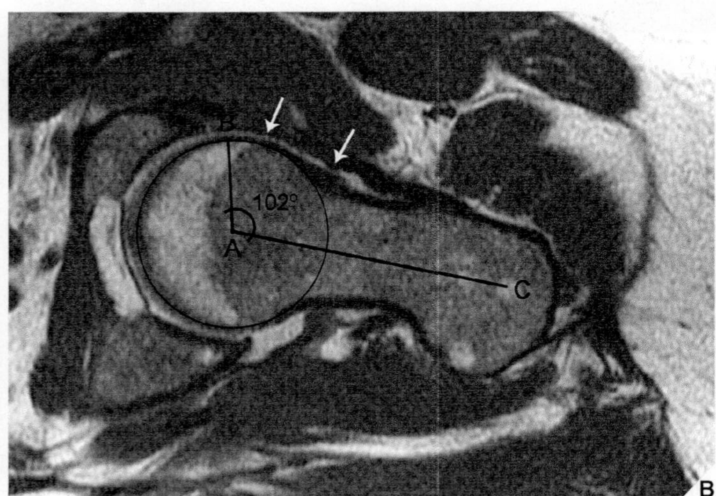

FIGURE 13.31 FAI—calculation of alpha angle. The alpha angle is formed by the intersection of two lines: line *AB*, drawn from the center of the femoral head *(A)* to the point where peripheral osseous contour of the anterior femoral head intersects the extrapolated circle of the femoral head *(B)*, and the second line *AC*, drawn from the center of the femoral head *(A)* through the longitudinal axis of the femoral neck *(C)*. Normal alpha angle should not exceed 50 degrees. **(A)** Alpha angle calculated on the oblique axial CT image of the right hip in a patient with cam FAI. **(B)** Alpha angle calculated on the oblique axial MR image of the left hip in a patient with cam FAI. The *arrows* point to excessive bone formation at the anterosuperior aspect of the femoral head/neck junction.

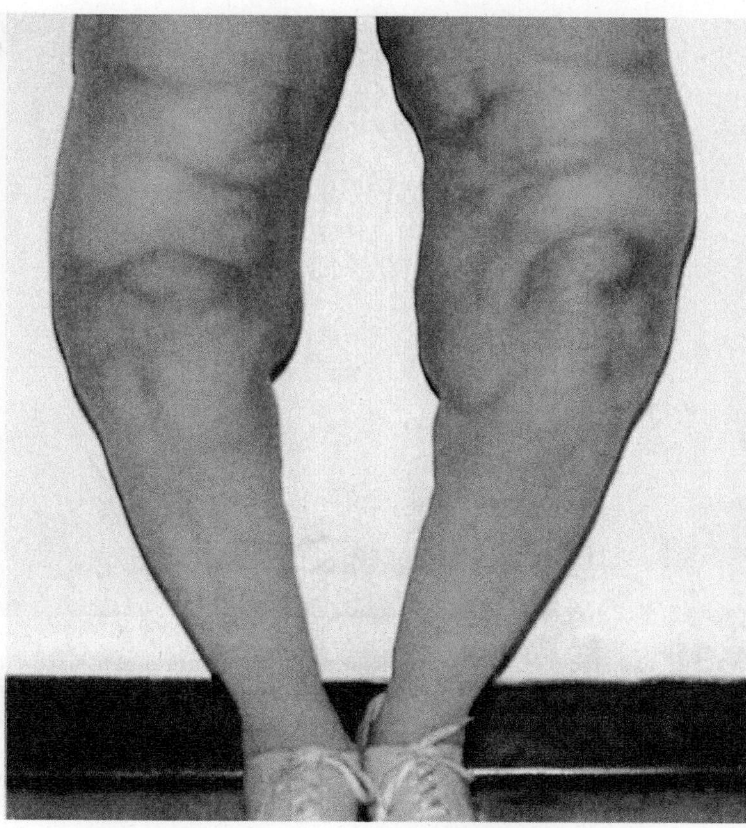

FIGURE 13.32 Knee deformities in OA. Clinical photograph of the knees of a patient with advanced OA of both knee joints affecting predominantly the medial compartments, which resulted in varus deformities. (Reprinted with permission from Greenspan A, Gershwin ME. *Imaging in rheumatology: a clinical approach,* 1st ed. Philadelphia: Wolters Kluwer; 2018:161.)

and/or osteoplasty with reshaping of femoral head/neck junction contributed to satisfactory results. Occasionally, intertrochanteric flexion-valgus osteotomy may also relieve the clinical symptoms. Periacetabular osteotomy is an effective way to reorient the acetabulum in young adults with symptomatic FAI due to acetabular retroversion. Advanced OA, whether primary or secondary, is usually treated surgically by total hip arthroplasty using, among the various types available, either a cemented or a noncemented prosthesis. The reader is referred to Chapter 12 for further discussion of management.

Osteoarthritis of the Knee

Clinical Features

The symptoms are similar to those experienced by the patients with hip OA: swelling around the knee joint, crepitus and joint locking, restricted range of motion, short-lasting morning stiffness, and pain that increases with activity and is relieved by rest. Some patients may experience sleep-disrupting pain at night. As the arthritis is progressing, gross deformities of the knees are become obvious, such as valgus or varus configuration (Fig. 13.32).

Pathology

The pathologic findings are also very similar to those described for OA of the hip. In the early stages, focal abnormalities are seen in the articular cartilage. Starting in the superficial layers, there is loss of proteoglycan, associated with flaking and surface cracking followed by formation of fissures and focal necrosis. In the later stages, the exposed subchondral bone exhibits characteristic eburnation (Fig. 13.33). Separated fragments of intraarticular osteophytes and fragments of fibrocartilage and hyaline cartilage remain free in the joint cavity as loose intraarticular bodies. Proliferation of cartilaginous cells may occur on the surface of these loose bodies, and consequently they grow larger. Sometimes, these chondral bodies may reattach to the synovial membrane in which case they are invaded by blood vessels, and through the process of endochondral ossification they become osteochondral bodies (Fig. 13.34).

Imaging Features

The knee is a complex joint comprising three major compartments—the medial femorotibial, the lateral femorotibial, and the femoropatellar—and each of which may be affected by degenerative changes. One of the hallmarks of OA of the knee is narrowing of the joint space. Narrowing can be expressed in both quantitative and semiquantitative terms. Ahlbäck proposed that narrowing, as a sign of cartilage loss, should be considered if the minimum joint space width is less than 3 mm, measured on the anteroposterior weight-bearing radiographs with the knee extended, and with the x-ray beam parallel to the tibial condyles. Most investigators have accepted this limit. Less frequently used are the semiquantitative parts of the Ahlbäck's definition, stating that joint space is narrowed when (a) it is narrower than half the width of the articular space in the same articulation of the other knee and (b) it is decreased in weight bearing as compared with non–weight-bearing position.

In 1957, J. H. Kellgren and J. S. Lawrence proposed a scoring system to assess the severity of knee OA on the conventional radiographs, which was in 1961 accepted by WHO. Based on this classification, *grade 0* was assigned if there were no radiographic features of OA; *grade 1*—if there was minimal joint space narrowing present on the anteroposterior weight-bearing radiographs and osteophyte formation; *grade 2*—if there was definite osteophyte formation with possible joint space narrowing; *grade 3*—if there were multiple osteophytes present associated with definite joint space narrowing, subchondral sclerosis, and possible bone deformity; and *grade 4*—if there were large osteophytes, marked joint narrowing, severe subchondral sclerosis, and definite bone deformity. More recently, P. R. Kornaat and associates have developed a Knee Osteoarthritis Scoring System (KOSS) based on the presence or absence of the following features on MRI: cartilaginous lesions, osteophytes, subchondral cysts, bone marrow edema, joint effusion, synovitis, Baker cyst, and meniscal abnormalities.

As Bennett and associates reported, the pathogenesis of OA in the knee joint begins on the surface of the articular cartilage. A loss of articular cartilage accounts for the narrowing of the joint space. If weight

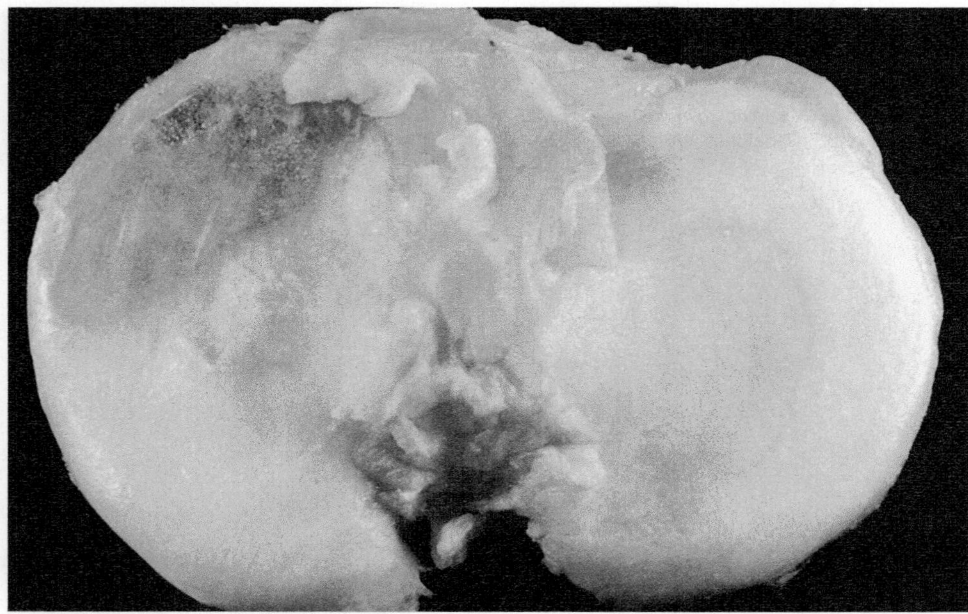

FIGURE 13.33 Pathology of OA of the knee joint. Specimen of the tibial plateau shows cartilage erosion with exposed subchondral bone. (Reprinted with permission from Greenspan A, Gershwin ME. *Imaging in rheumatology: a clinical approach*, 1st ed. Philadelphia: Wolters Kluwer; 2018:161.)

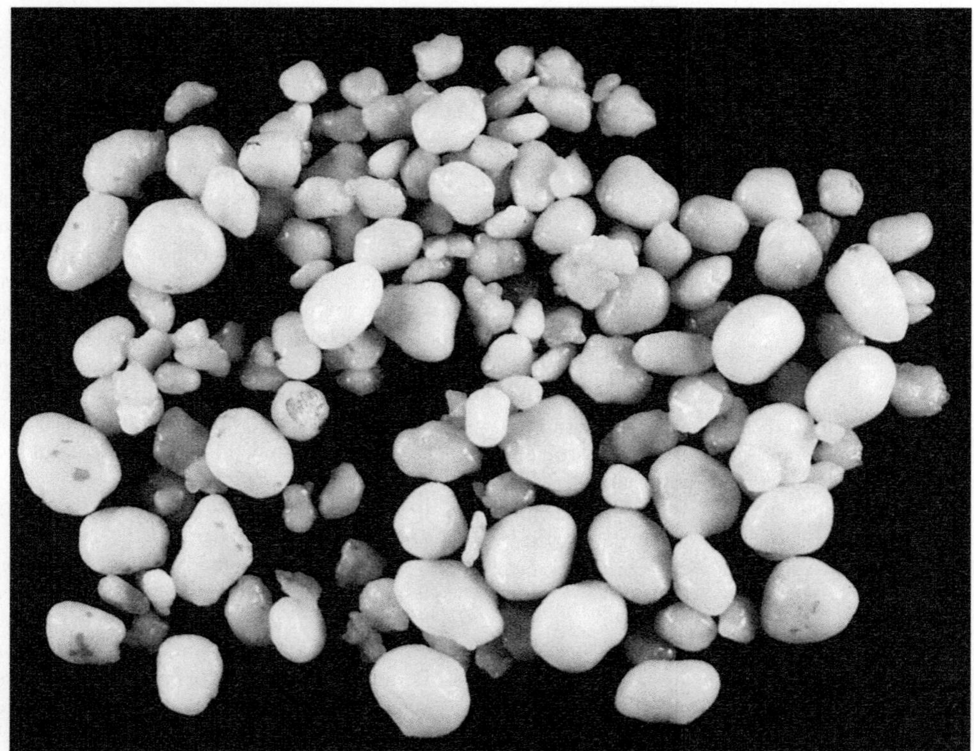

FIGURE 13.34 Osteochondral bodies. Photograph of multiple osteochondral bodies removed from the osteoarthritic joint. In contrast to the intraarticular bodies of primary synovial (osteo)chondromatosis, they are different in sizes. (Reprinted with permission from Bullough PG. *Atlas of orthopedic pathology: with clinical and radiologic correlations*, 2nd ed. New York: Gower Medical Publishing; 1992:9.16, Fig. 9.40.)

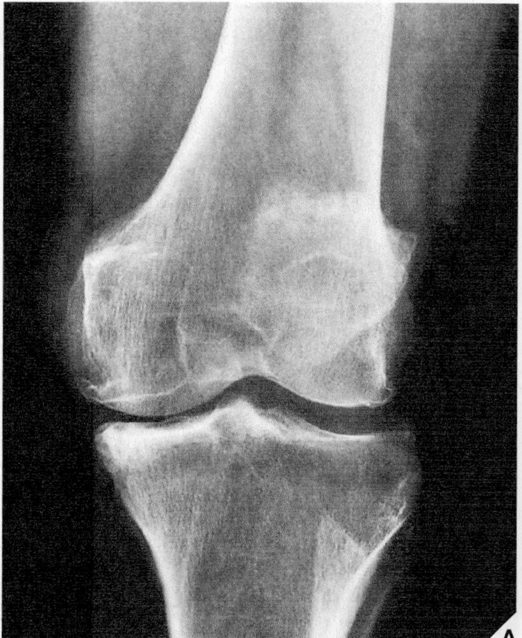

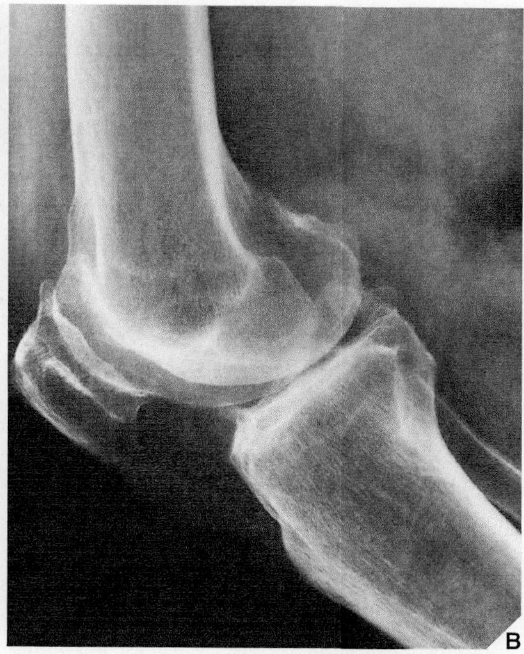

FIGURE 13.35 OA of the knee. **(A)** Anteroposterior and **(B)** lateral radiographs of the knee of a 57-year-old woman demonstrate narrowing of the medial femorotibial and femoropatellar compartments, subchondral sclerosis, and osteophytosis, which are the typical features of OA. Note that osteophytes that were not obvious on the frontal projection are much better demonstrated on the lateral radiograph.

bearing continues in an impaired joint, abnormalities develop not only in the cartilage but also in the subchondral bone, menisci, and synovium. Detritic fragments loosen from the joint surface and are discharge to the joint cavity. Shards of bone and cartilage are embedded in the synovial membrane, resulting in so-called *detritic synovitis*. Attrition of the menisci parallels the deterioration of the articular cartilage. The free edge of the meniscus becomes frayed and wavy, and meniscus may calcify. The imaging features of these changes are similar to those seen in OA of the hip, including narrowing of the joint space (usually one or two compartments), subchondral sclerosis, osteophytosis, and subchondral cyst (or pseudocyst) formation. These detritic cyst-like lesions, however, are not as common as in the hip joint, and when they do occur, they may be small and often obscured by subchondral sclerosis. Osteophytes are always marginal to the segment of weight bearing and are more pronounced when joint narrowing is advanced. The tibial spines became prominent, broadened, and small osteophytes may form on them as well ("peaking" of the tibial spines). In advanced OA, a "vacuum sign" may be seen within the joint space.

The standard weight-bearing anteroposterior and lateral projections of the knee are sufficient to demonstrate these processes (Fig. 13.35). If the medial joint compartment is affected, the knee may assume a varus configuration, which is best demonstrated on the weight-bearing anteroposterior view (Fig. 13.36A); involvement of the lateral compartment may lead to a valgus configuration (Fig. 13.36B). The femoropatellar joint compartment is also commonly involved in primary OA. The lateral radiograph of the knee and axial view of the patella are the most effective means of visualizing degenerative changes of the femoropatellar compartment (Fig. 13.37). Scintigraphy invariably shows increased uptake of radiopharmaceutical tracer localized to the involved compartment or compartments (Fig. 13.38).

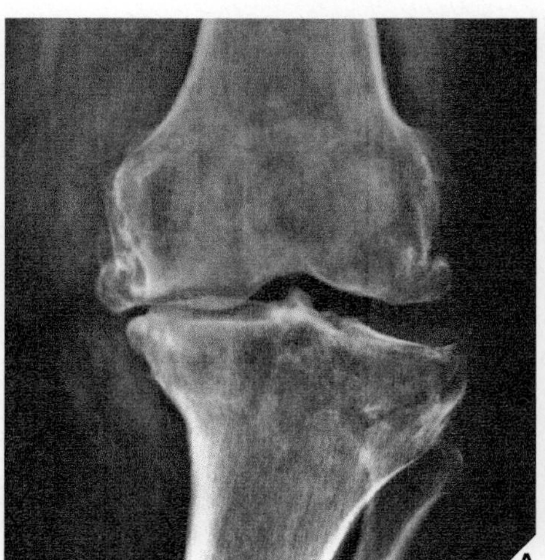

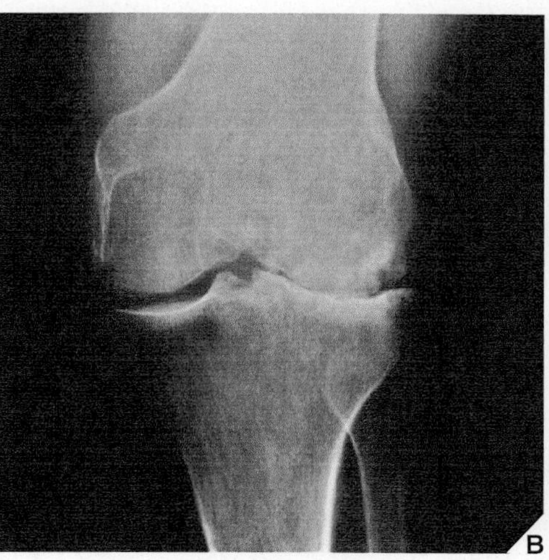

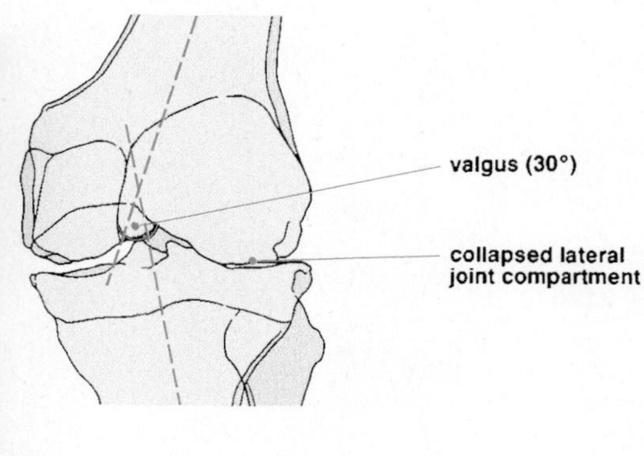

FIGURE 13.36 OA of the knee. **(A)** Weight-bearing anteroposterior radiograph of the knee of a 58-year-old woman demonstrates advanced OA of the medial femorotibial joint compartment, which has led to a varus configuration of the joint. **(B)** Involvement of the lateral femorotibial joint compartment in advanced OA as seen on this weight-bearing anteroposterior radiograph of another patient has resulted in a valgus configuration.

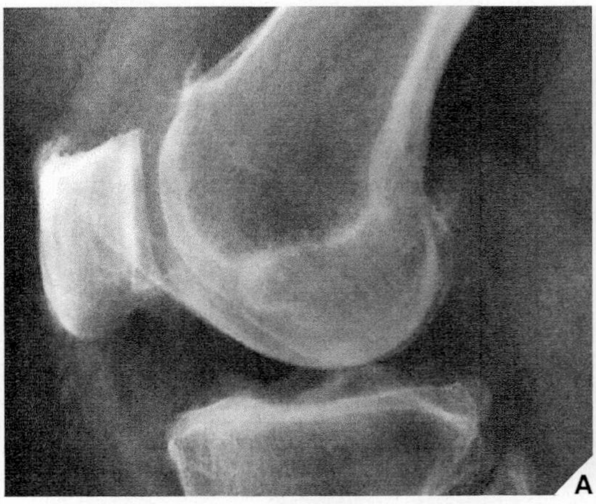

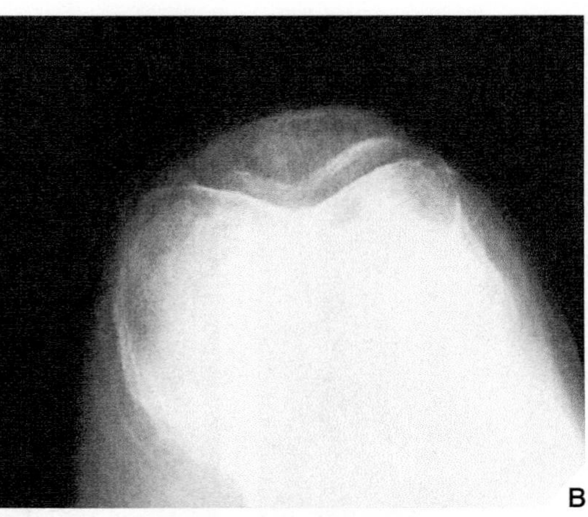

FIGURE 13.37 Femoropatellar OA. **(A)** Lateral radiograph of the knee and **(B)** axial radiograph of the patella of a 72-year-old woman demonstrate narrowing of the femoropatellar joint compartment and osteophytes formation.

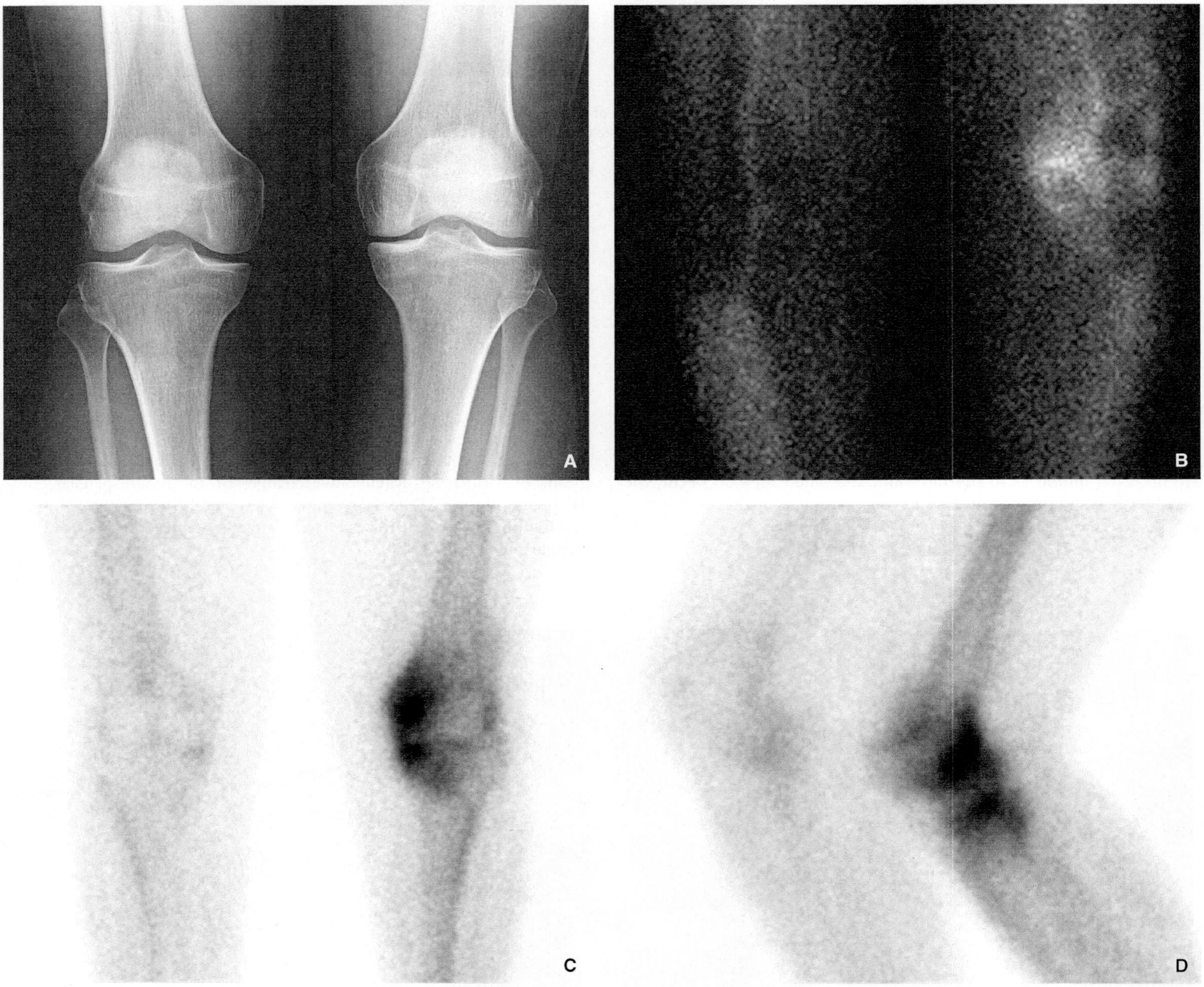

FIGURE 13.38 Scintigraphy of OA of the knee joint. **(A)** Anteroposterior radiograph of both knees shows narrowing of the medial joint compartment of the left knee, consistent with OA. **(B)** Technetium blood pool image shows increased activity in the region of the left knee. Delayed planar images in **(C)** frontal and **(D)** lateral projections show increased uptake of the radiopharmaceutical tracer localized to the medial joint compartment of the left knee. The right knee demonstrates normal activity.

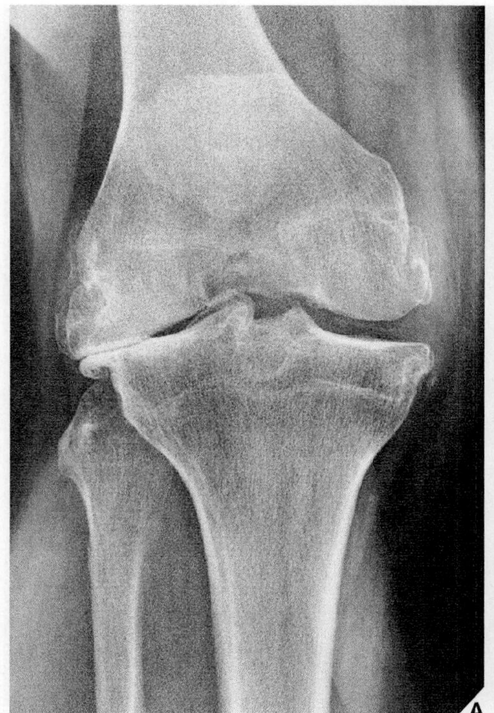
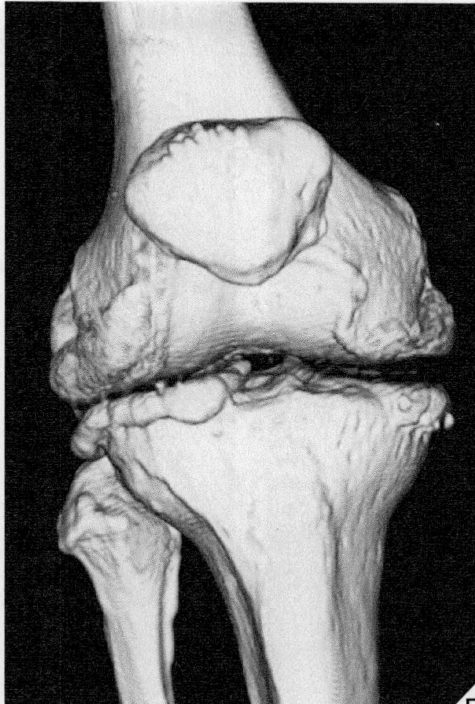
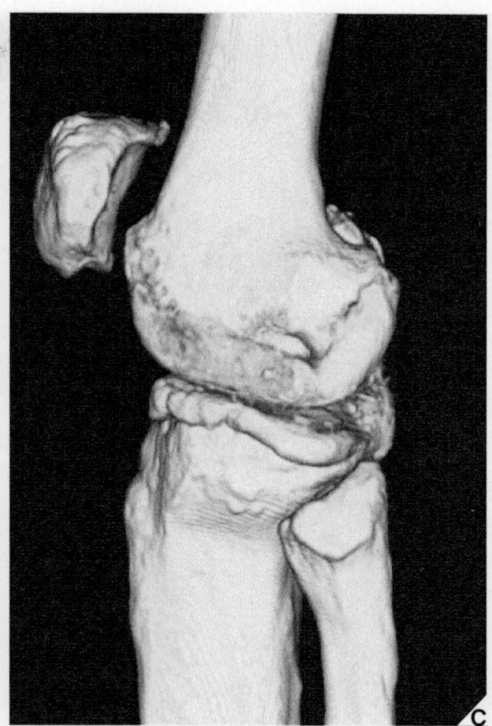

FIGURE 13.39 3D CT of OA. **(A)** Radiograph of the right knee of a 58-year-old man shows advanced OA. **(B,C)** 3D reconstructed CT images in shaded surface display demonstrate advanced three-compartmental OA.

CT and three-dimensional (3D) reconstructed CT images (Fig. 13.39) and MRI (Fig. 13.40) may provide additional information as to the status of osteoarthritic process. MRI is also very effective in demonstrating the very early degenerative changes affecting the cartilage such as chondromalacia and cartilage fibrillation and fissuring before they become apparent on other imaging modalities (Fig. 13.41).

A frequent complication of OA of the knee is the formation of osteochondral bodies, which can be demonstrated on the standard projections of the knee (Figs. 13.42 and 13.43); however, MRI may also be effective in this respect (Figs. 13.44 to 13.46).

Often, particularly in individuals past their fifth decade of life, degenerative changes unrelated to femoropatellar OA are seen at the insertion of the quadriceps tendon into the base of the patella. These changes are manifest as vertical ridges resembling teeth on an axial view of the patella and have been designated by Greenspan and colleagues as the "tooth" sign (Fig. 13.47A). The dentate structures represent an enthesopathy probably related to stress at the attachment of the quadriceps apparatus, and their nature is clearly demonstrated on the lateral projection (Fig. 13.47B). At times, they can be recognized on the anteroposterior radiograph of the knee as well (Fig. 13.47C). MRI also effectively demonstrates these changes (Fig. 13.48).

As in the hip joint, one may encounter secondary OA in the knee. One of the most common predisposing factors is previous trauma or surgery.

Osteoarthritis of Other Large Joints

Other large joints such as the shoulder (Figs. 13.49 and 13.50), elbow (Fig. 13.51), and ankle can be affected by OA, but involvement of these sites in the idiopathic form of the disease is much less common than involvement of the hip or knee. In fact, with evidence of degenerative changes in such sites (Figs. 13.52 and 13.53), one must consider the possibility of secondary rather than idiopathic OA (see Table 13.1).

Osteoarthritis of the Small Joints

Primary Osteoarthritis of the Hand

The most commonly affected small joints are those of the hand, particularly the proximal and distal interphalangeal and the first carpometacarpal articulations (see Figs. 12.39 and 13.1). In the distal interphalangeal joints, if hypertrophic phenomena supervene and osteophytes are prominent, degenerative changes are accompanied by *Heberden nodes.* Similar deformities in the proximal interphalangeal joints are called *Bouchard nodes* (Fig. 13.54). If the degenerative changes involve the first carpometacarpal joint (Fig. 13.55), they may result in an odd deformation of the thumb (Fig. 13.56). The midcarpal articulations may also be affected, particularly the scaphotrapeziotrapezoid (STT) joint (Fig. 13.57).

Secondary Osteoarthritis of the Hand

Acromegaly

The most characteristic secondary osteoarthritic changes in the small joints may be observed in acromegaly. Although the degenerative process in acromegaly also affects large joints such as the hip, knee, shoulder, and the spine, the hand displays the most typical features of this condition. These include soft-tissue prominence and enlargement of the terminal tufts and the bases of the terminal phalanges; there may also be widening of some articular spaces and narrowing of others; beak-like osteophytes at the heads of the metacarpals are a prominent feature (Fig. 13.58). Degenerative changes in acromegaly are the result of hypertrophy of articular cartilage, which is not properly nourished by synovial fluid because of its abnormal thickness. (The reader is also referred to the discussion of acromegaly in Chapters 15 and 30.)

Hemochromatosis

Commonly associated with the development of secondary OA in the small joints, hemochromatosis (iron storage disease) is a rare disorder characterized by iron deposition in internal organs, articular cartilage, and synovium.

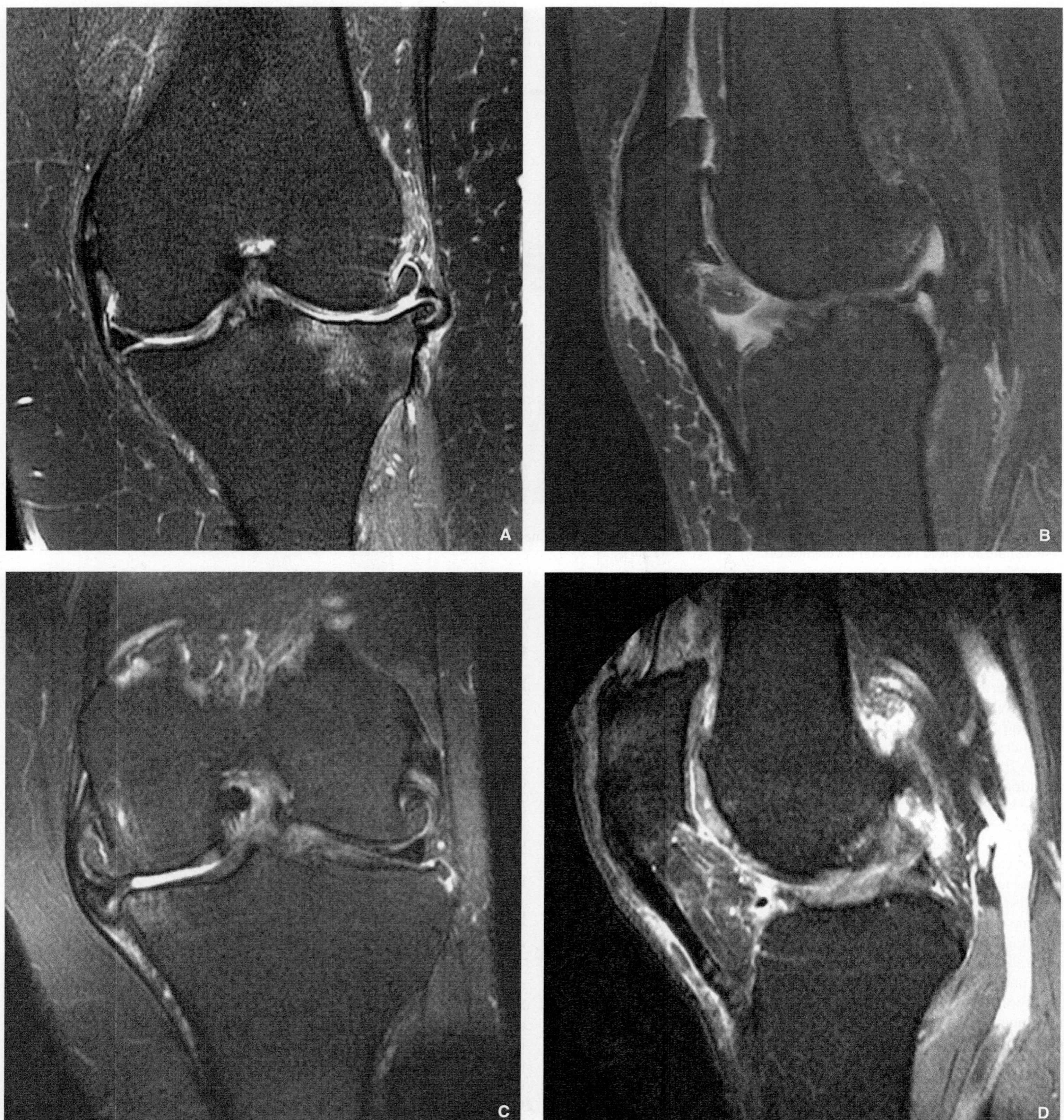

FIGURE 13.40 MRI of OA of the knee joint. **(A)** Coronal and **(B)** sagittal proton density–weighted fat-suppressed MR images of the left knee of a 74-year-old woman show prominent osteophytes at the lateral joint compartment as well as at the inferior pole of the patella. There is a marked thinning of the articular cartilage of the lateral femoral condyle, with a focal full-thickness cartilage defect, and complete loss of articular cartilage of the lateral tibial plateau associated with subchondral bone marrow edema. In addition, there is a degenerative tear of the lateral meniscus. **(C)** Coronal proton density–weighted fat-suppressed and **(D)** sagittal fast spin echo (FSE) proton density–weighted fat-suppressed MR images of the left knee of a 51-year-old woman show complete loss of articular cartilage of the medial femoral condyle and medial tibial plateau associated with subchondral bone marrow edema. There is degenerative tear of the medial meniscus, which is also medially extruded. The anterior cruciate ligament demonstrates degenerative tear, and there is diffuse nodular synovial thickening.

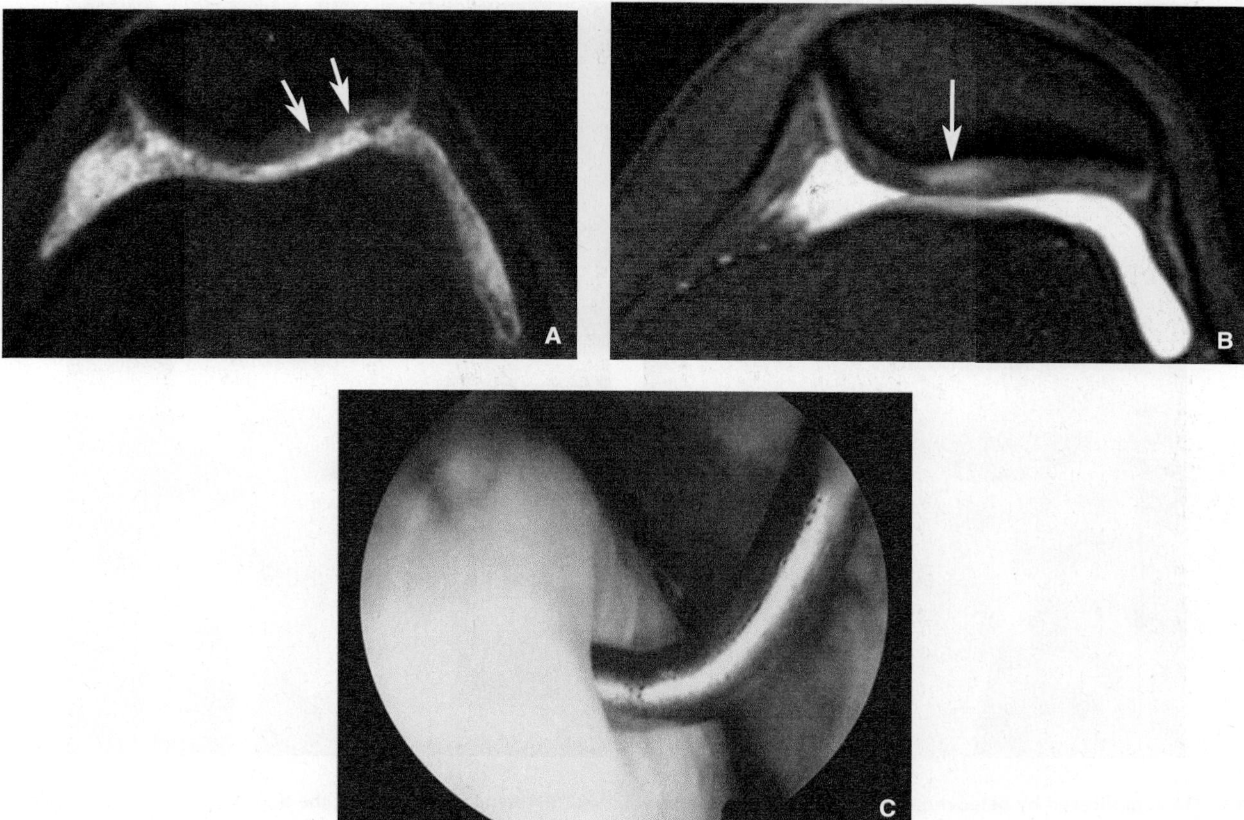

FIGURE 13.41 MRI and arthroscopy of chondral fibrillation and chondromalacia. **(A)** Axial T2-weighted fat-saturated MR image of the patella demonstrates surface chondral fibrillation in the lateral facet *(arrows)*. **(B)** Axial T2-weighted fat-saturated MR image of the patella of another patient shows a focal area of increased signal intensity within the articular cartilage of the lateral facet of the patella *(arrow)* reflecting focal increase water or "blister." **(C)** Arthroscopic image shows softening of the articular cartilage, as it is compressed with an instrument, with an otherwise normal-appearing chondral surface.

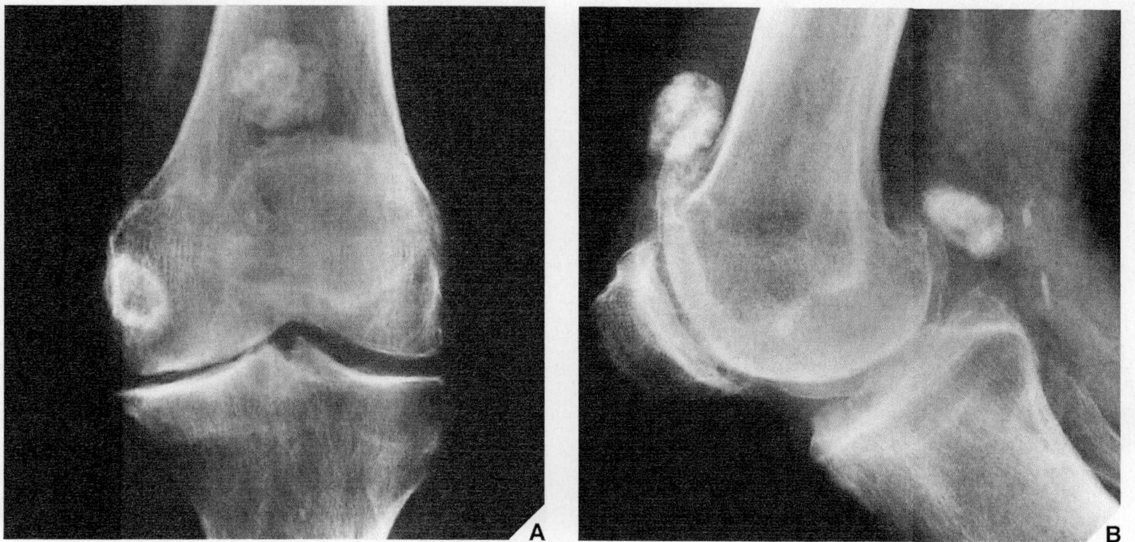

FIGURE 13.42 OA complicated by osteochondral bodies. **(A)** Anteroposterior and **(B)** lateral radiographs of the knee of a 66-year-old man with advanced OA demonstrate predominant involvement of the medial femorotibial and femoropatellar joint compartments, with formation of two large osteochondral bodies.

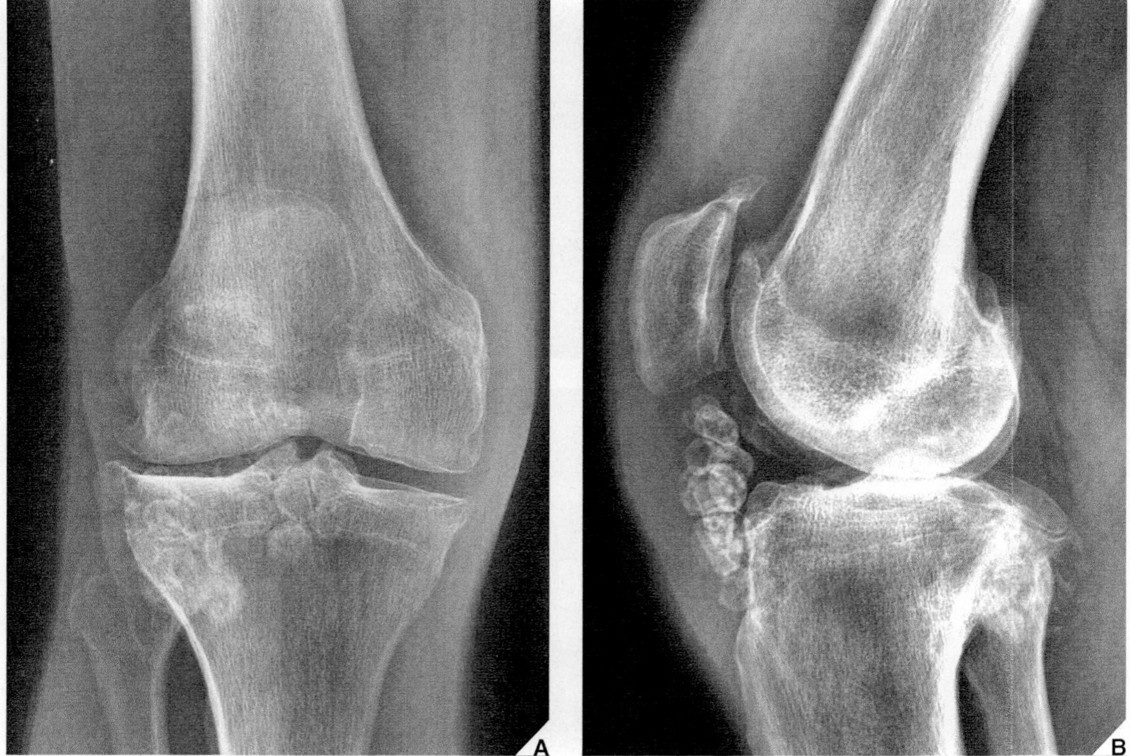

FIGURE 13.43 OA complicated by osteochondral bodies. **(A)** Anteroposterior and **(B)** lateral radiographs of the right knee show OA complicated by numerous osteochondral bodies.

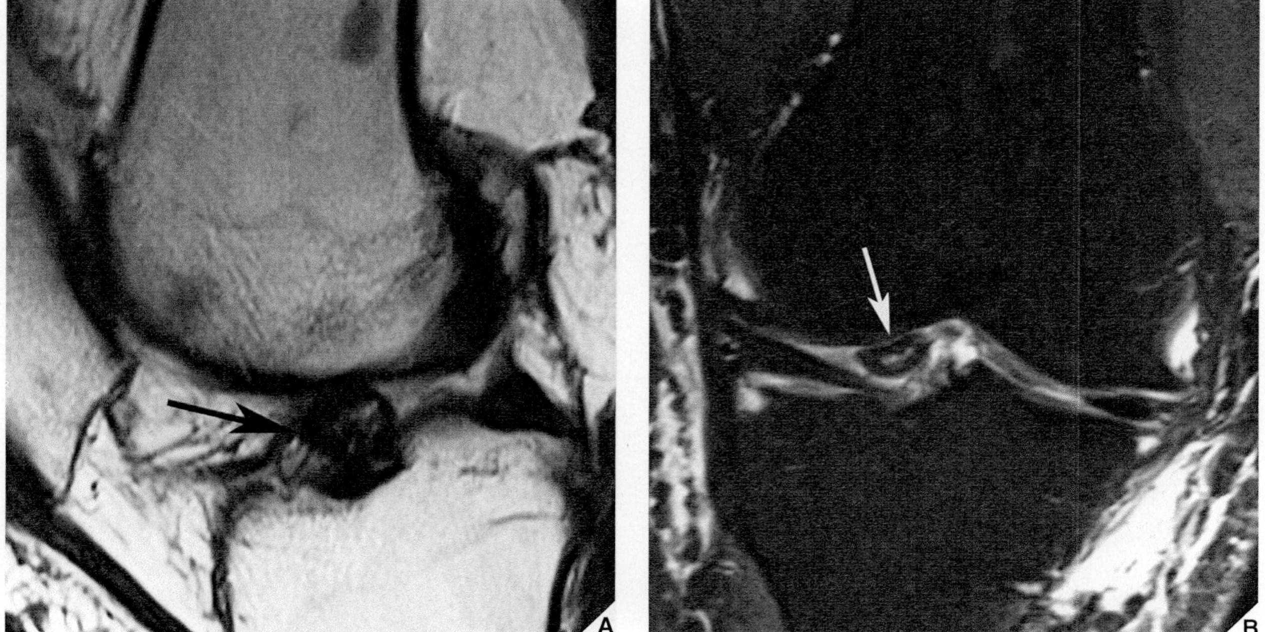

FIGURE 13.44 MRI of osteochondral body. A low–signal intensity osteocartilaginous loose body in the anterior joint space is revealed on T1-weighted **(A)** and T2-weighted **(B)** sagittal MR images of the knee *(arrows)*.

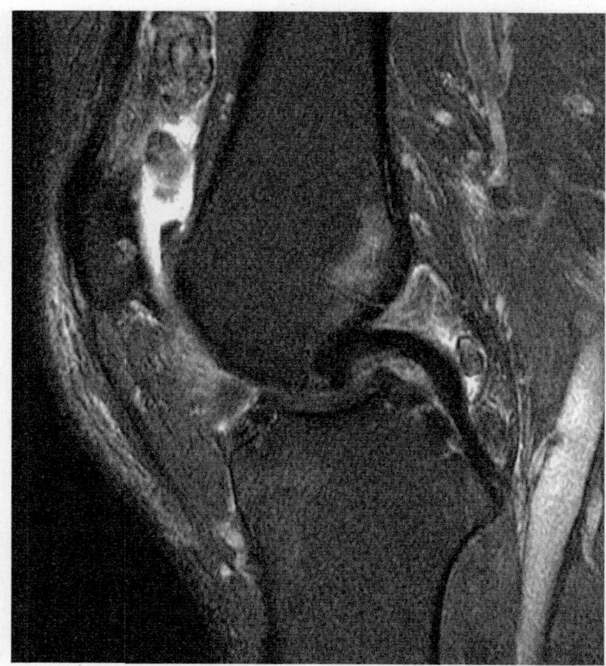

FIGURE 13.45 **MRI of osteochondral bodies.** Sagittal T2-weighted fat-suppressed MR image of the knee shows several intraarticular osteochondral bodies in this 67-year-old woman with OA.

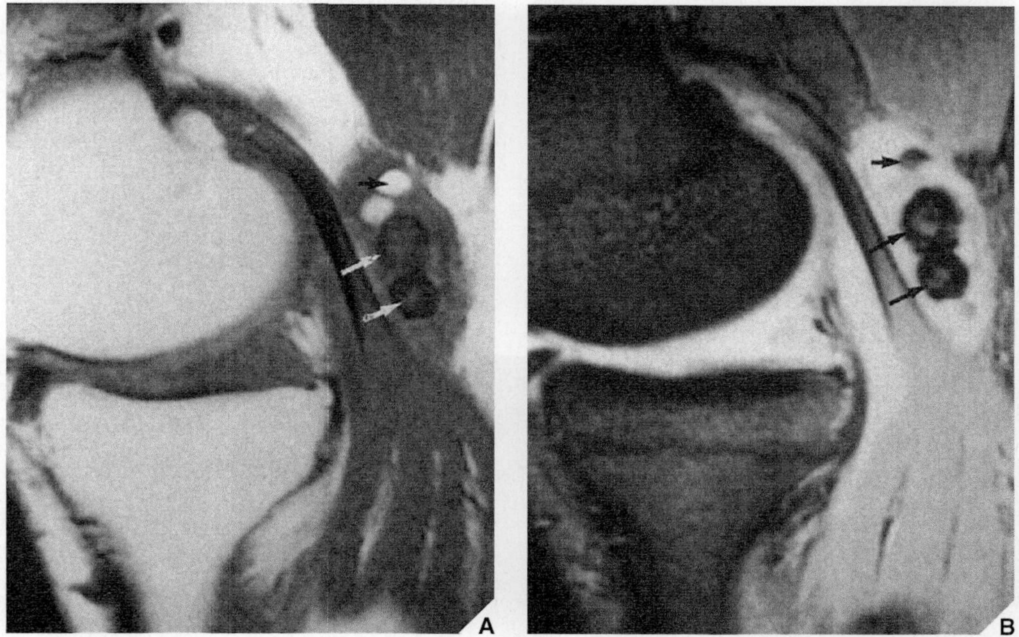

FIGURE 13.46 **Baker cyst with osteochondral bodies.** **(A)** Sagittal T1-weighted and **(B)** T2*-weighted MR images show multiple osteochondral loose bodies *(arrows)* in a popliteal (Baker) cyst adjacent to the medial head of gastrocnemius muscle. (Reprinted with permission from Stoller DW. *MRI in orthopaedics and sports medicine.* Philadelphia: JB Lippincott; 1993.)

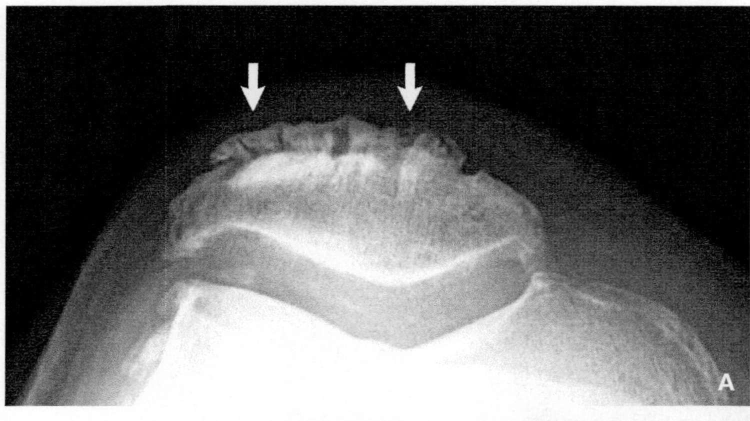

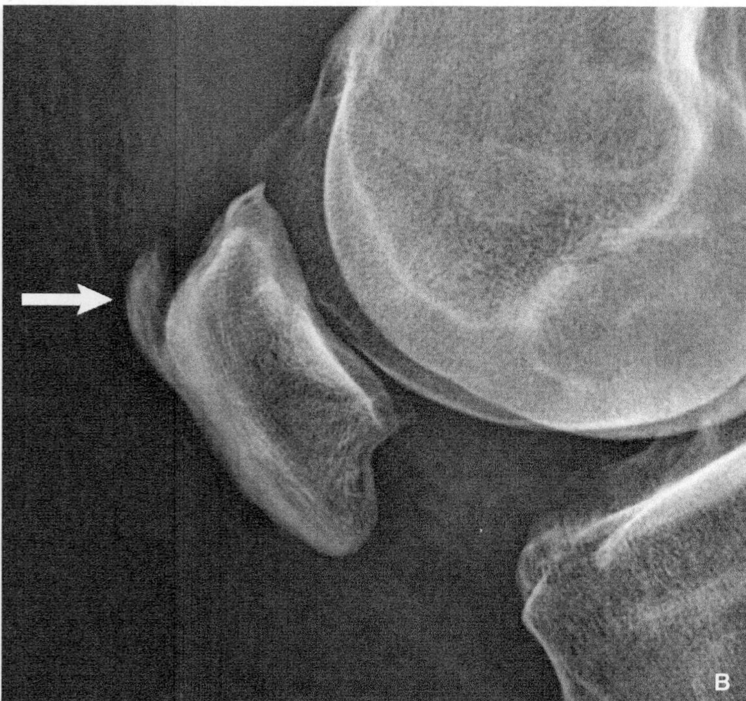

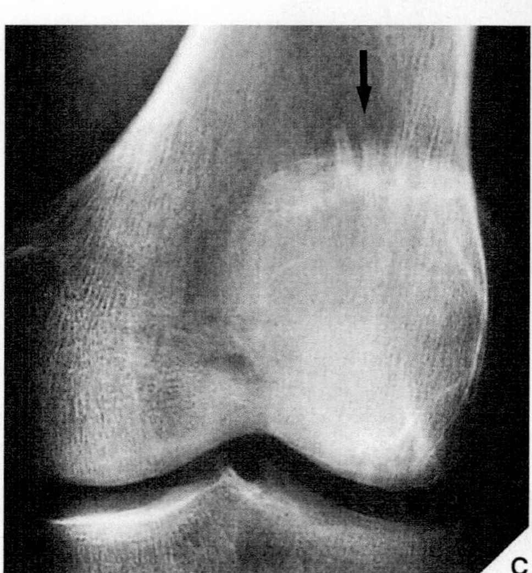

FIGURE 13.47 **Patellar enthesopathy.** **(A)** Axial view of the patella demonstrates dentate structures *(arrows)*—the tooth sign, which represent degenerative ossifications (enthesopathy) at the insertion of the quadriceps tendon into the base of patella *(arrow)*, as seen on the lateral view **(B)** in this 55-year-old man. **(C)** Occasionally, the tooth sign can also be demonstrated on the anteroposterior projection of the knee *(arrow)*, seen here in a 54-year-old woman.

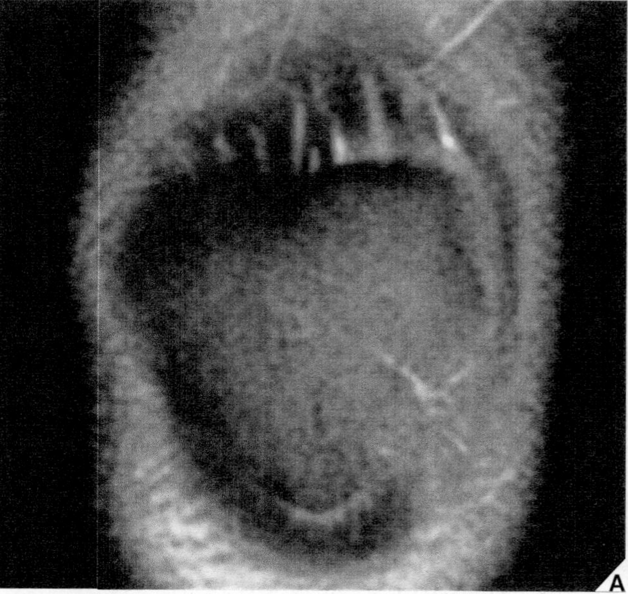

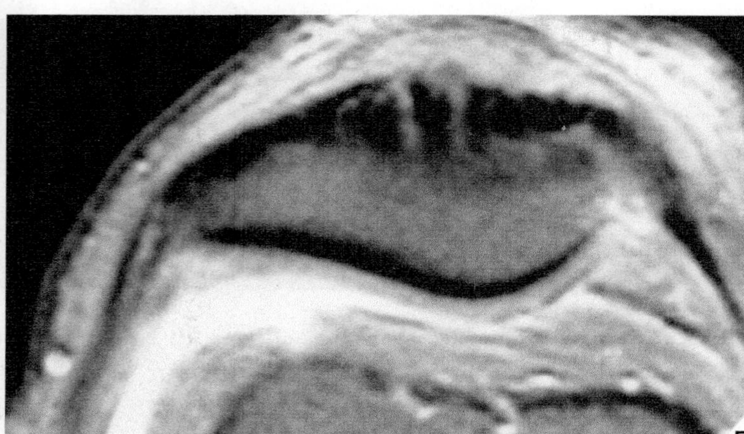

FIGURE 13.48 **MRI of patellar enthesopathy.** **(A)** Coronal T1-weighted and **(B)** axial T2-weighted MR images show tooth sign of the patella.

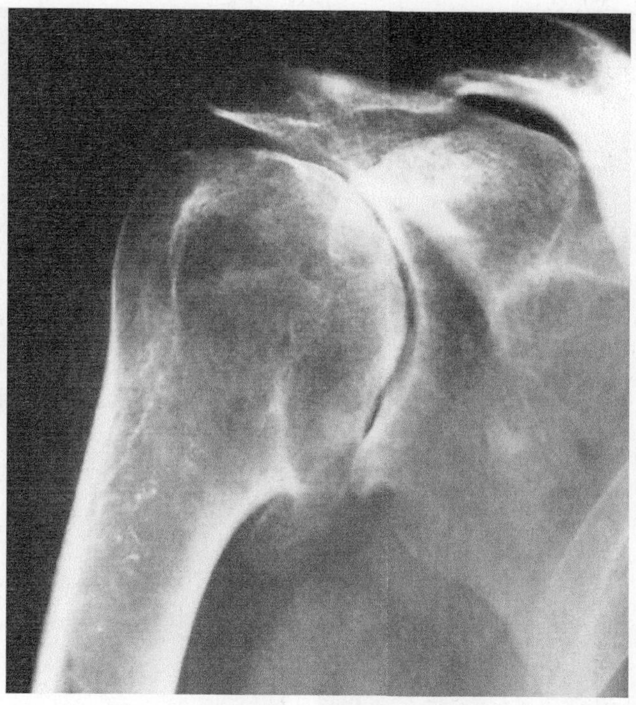

FIGURE 13.49 OA of the shoulder joint. Anteroposterior radiograph of the right shoulder of a 58-year-old man shows the typical features of OA; both shoulders were affected. The patient had no history of trauma or other underlying condition to suggest the possibility of secondary arthritis.

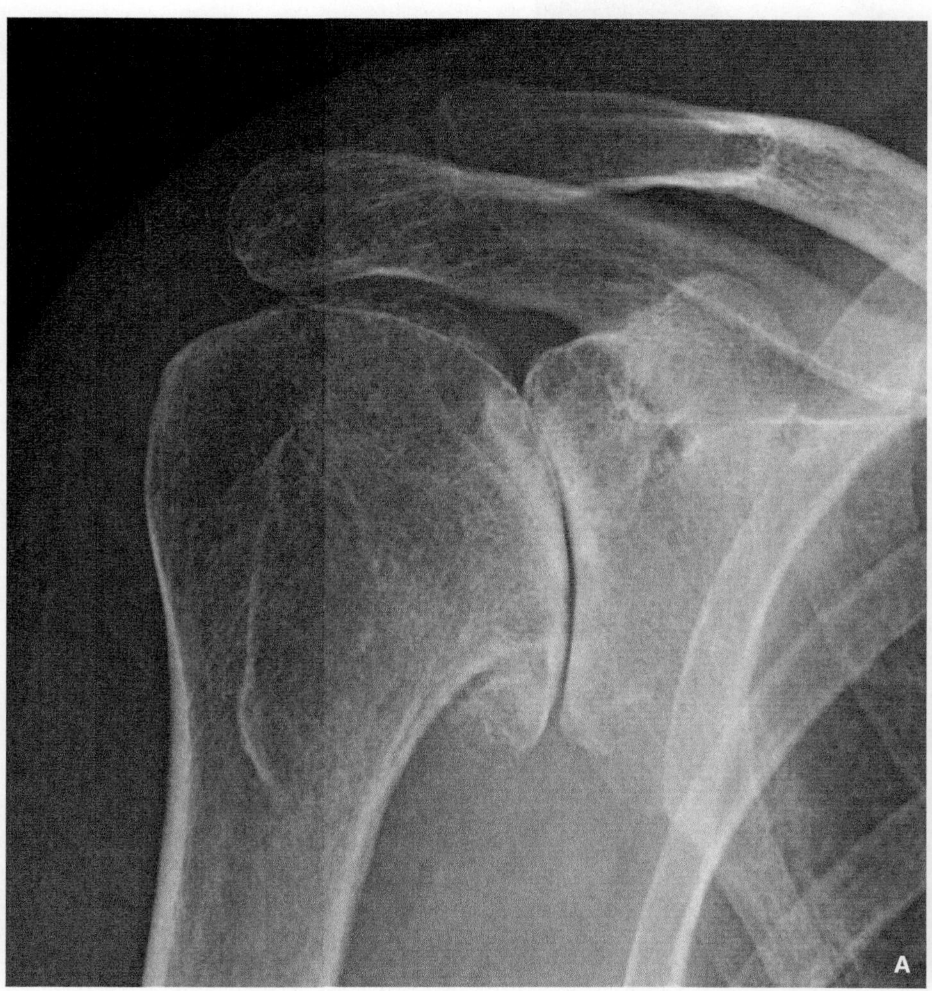

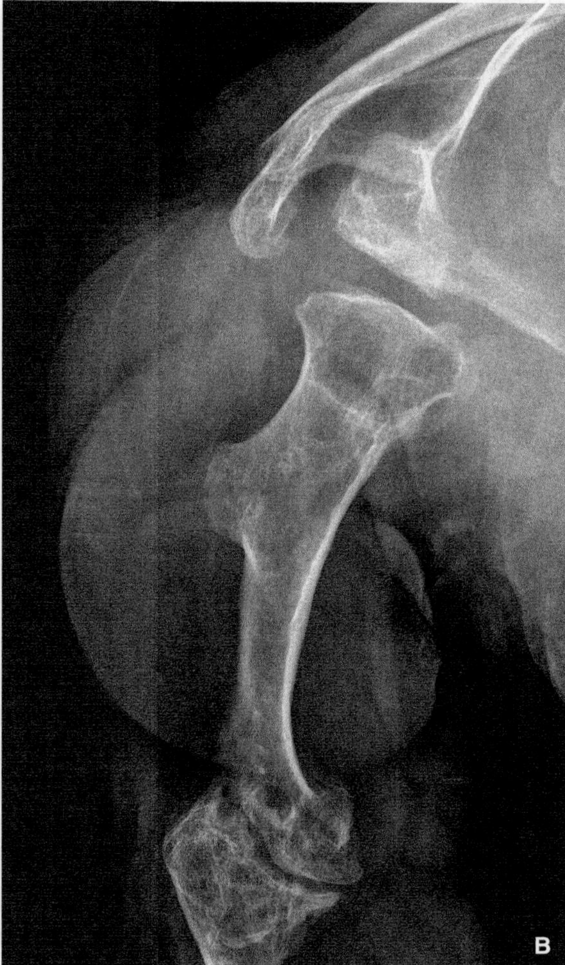

FIGURE 13.50 Secondary OA of the shoulder joint. **(A)** This 70-year-old woman presented with history of several dislocations in the right shoulder. Note advanced OA of the glenohumeral joint. **(B)** Radiograph of the right arm of a 30-year-old woman diagnosed with Morquio-Brailsford disease, a form of mucopolysaccharidosis, in addition to osteoporosis, hypoplasia, and deformities of the bones, demonstrates also OA of the shoulder and elbow joints. (Reprinted with permission from Greenspan A, Gershwin ME. *Imaging in rheumatology: a clinical approach*, 1st ed. Philadelphia: Wolters Kluwer; 2018:171.)

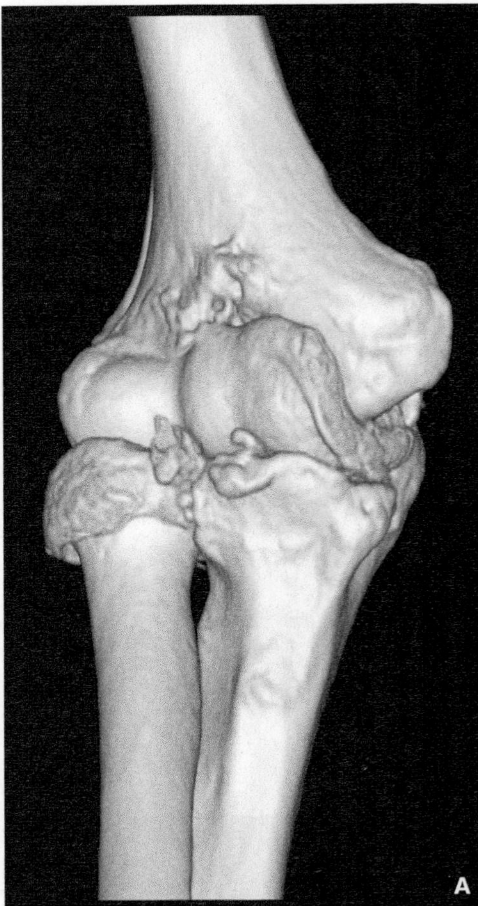

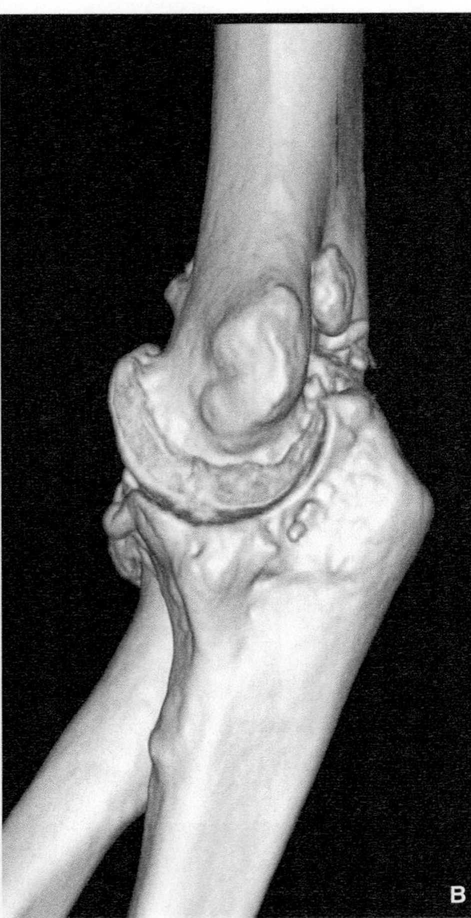

FIGURE 13.51 3D CT of OA of the elbow. **(A,B)** 3D CT reconstructed images of the elbow in shaded surface display of a 66-year-old woman, without past history of any significant trauma to this joint, show advanced OA. (Reprinted with permission from Greenspan A, Gershwin ME. *Imaging in rheumatology: a clinical approach*, 1st ed. Philadelphia: Wolters Kluwer; 2018:39.)

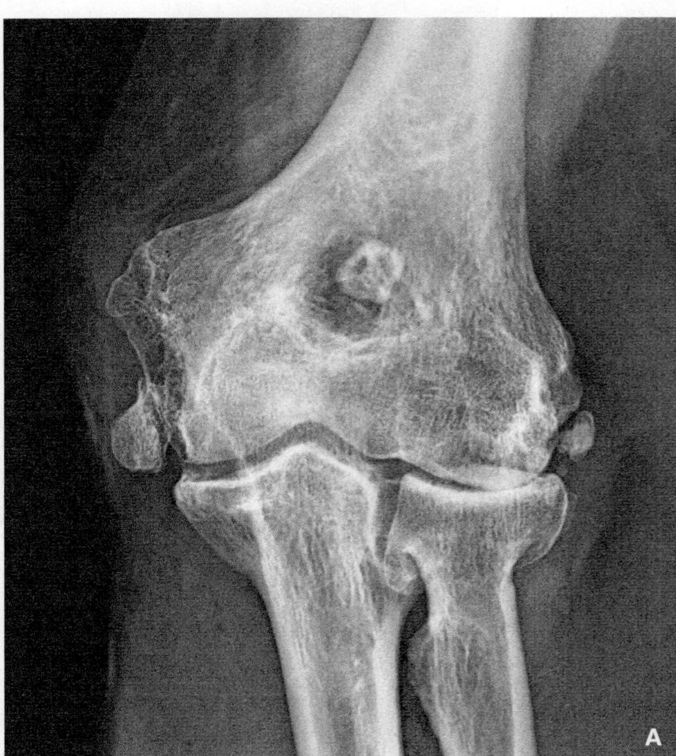

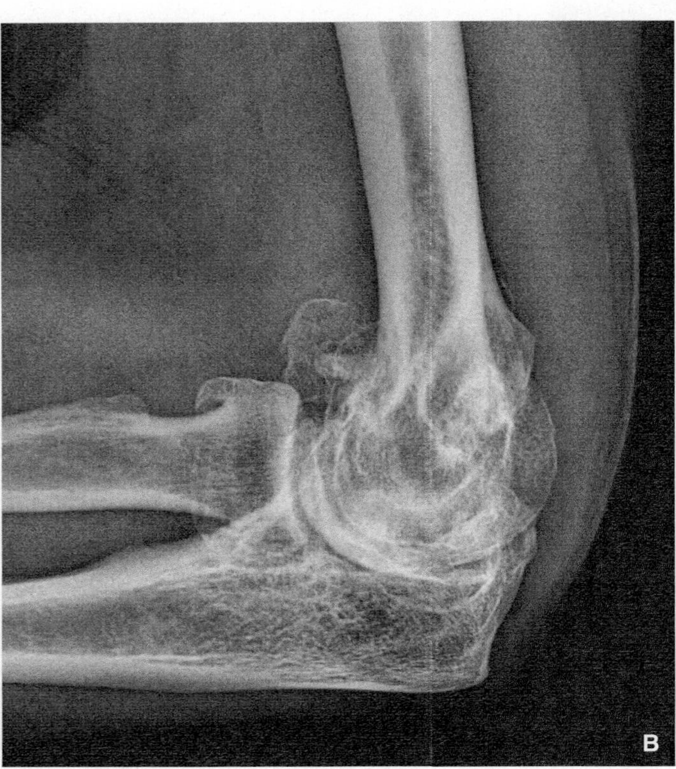

FIGURE 13.52 CT and 3D CT of secondary OA of the elbow joint. **(A)** Anteroposterior and **(B)** lateral radiographs of the elbow joint, supplemented with **(C)** coronal, **(D)** sagittal reformatted, and **(E)** 3D reconstructed CT images of a 57-year-old man, with history of several prior elbow joint dislocations, demonstrate OA complicated by the presence of numerous osteochondral bodies. An *arrow* points to the largest osteochondral body. (Reprinted with permission from Greenspan A, Gershwin ME. *Imaging in rheumatology: a clinical approach*, 1st ed. Philadelphia: Wolters Kluwer; 2018:172.) *(Continued)*

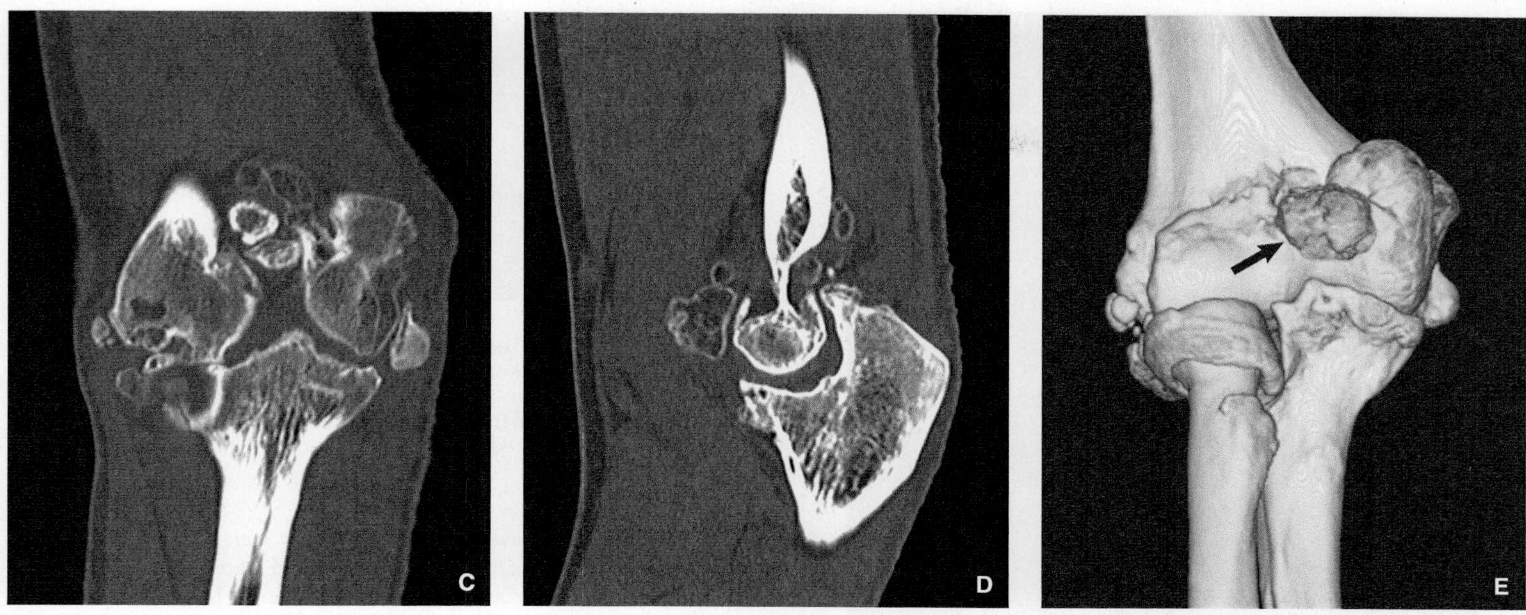

FIGURE 13.52 CT and 3D CT of secondary OA of the elbow joint. ***(Continued)***

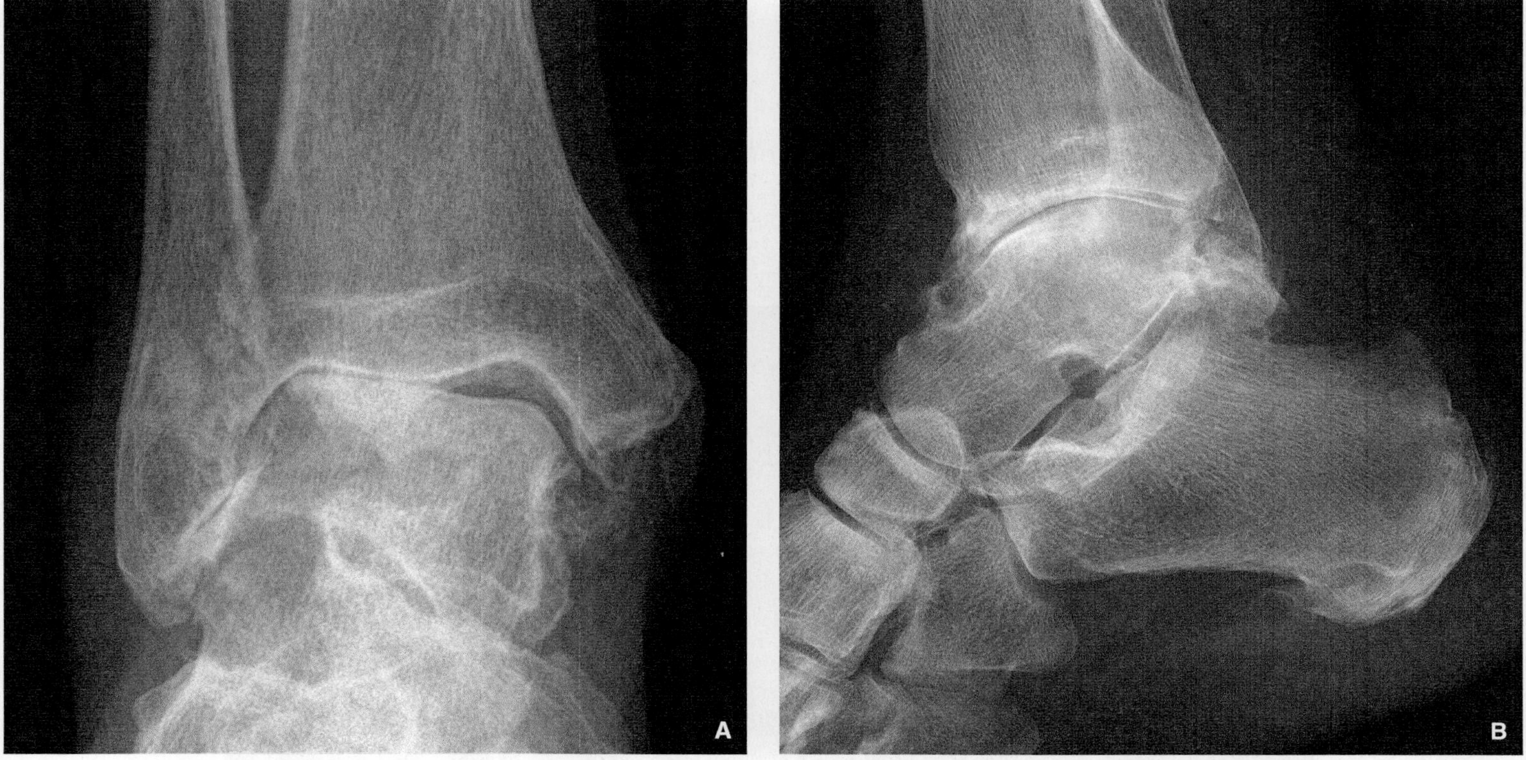

FIGURE 13.53 Secondary OA of the ankle. **(A)** Anteroposterior and **(B)** lateral radiographs of the ankle joint of a 55-year-old man show posttraumatic OA of tibiotalar articulation. (Reprinted with permission from Greenspan A, Gershwin ME. *Imaging in rheumatology: a clinical approach*, 1st ed. Philadelphia: Wolters Kluwer; 2018:172.)

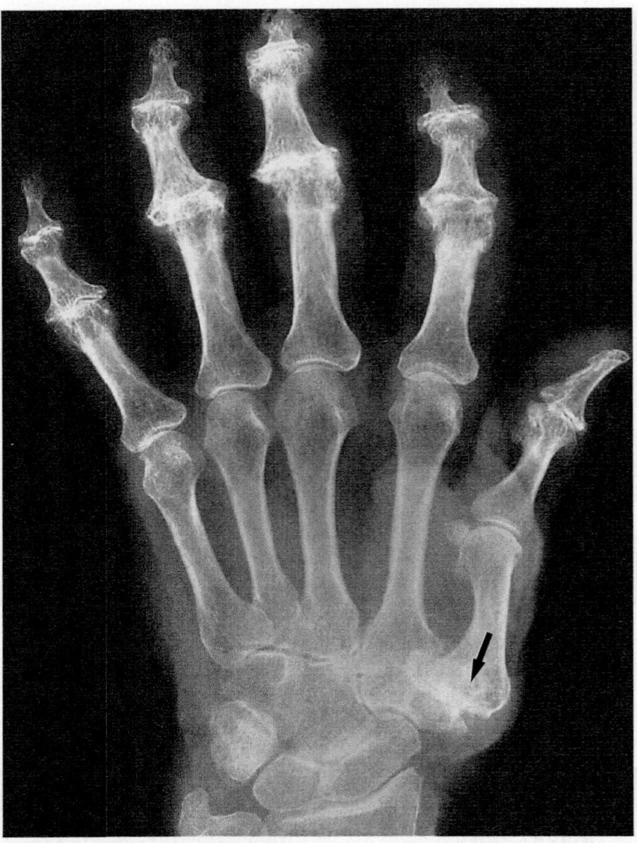

FIGURE 13.54 Interphalangeal OA. Dorsovolar radiograph of right hand of a 74-year-old woman shows degenerative changes in the distal interphalangeal joints, manifested by Heberden nodes, and in the proximal interphalangeal joints, manifested by Bouchard nodes. Note also degenerative changes in the first carpometacarpal joint *(arrow)*.

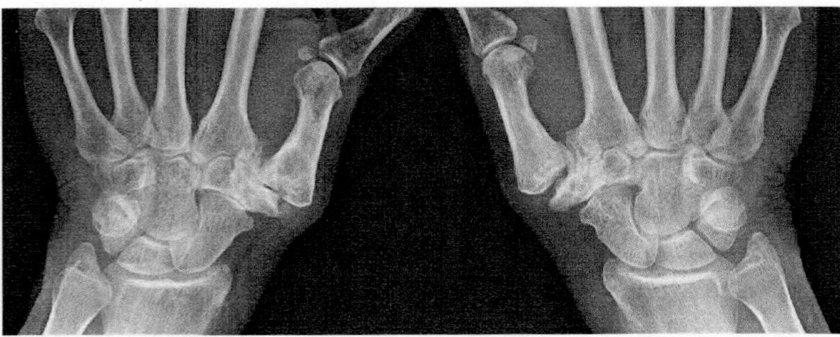

FIGURE 13.55 OA of the first carpometacarpal joints. Dorsovolar radiograph of both wrists of a 55-year-old woman shows joint space narrowing, subchondral sclerosis, subchondral cysts, and osteophytes at both first carpometacarpal joints. (Reprinted with permission from Greenspan A, Gershwin ME. *Imaging in rheumatology: a clinical approach*, 1st ed. Philadelphia: Wolters Kluwer; 2018:173.)

Some investigators believe that the arthropathy seen in this condition differs from typical degenerative joint disease and warrants classification in the group of metabolic arthropathies (see Chapter 15). In the hand, the second and third metacarpophalangeal joints are characteristically affected (Fig. 13.59), although other small joints such as the interphalangeal and carpal articulations may be involved. The changes may occasionally mimic those seen in calcium pyrophosphate dihydrate (CPPD) deposition disease and RA. Degenerative changes may also be seen at the shoulders, knees, hips, and ankles. Loss of the articular space, eburnation, subchondral cyst formation, and osteophytosis are the most prominent radiographic features of hemochromatosis.

Osteoarthritis of the Foot

In the foot, the most commonly affected articulation is the metatarsophalangeal joint of the great toe. This condition is known as *hallux rigidus* or *hallux limitus* (Figs. 13.60 and 13.61). Occasionally, osteoarthritic changes affecting other foot joints can be encountered (Fig. 13.62).

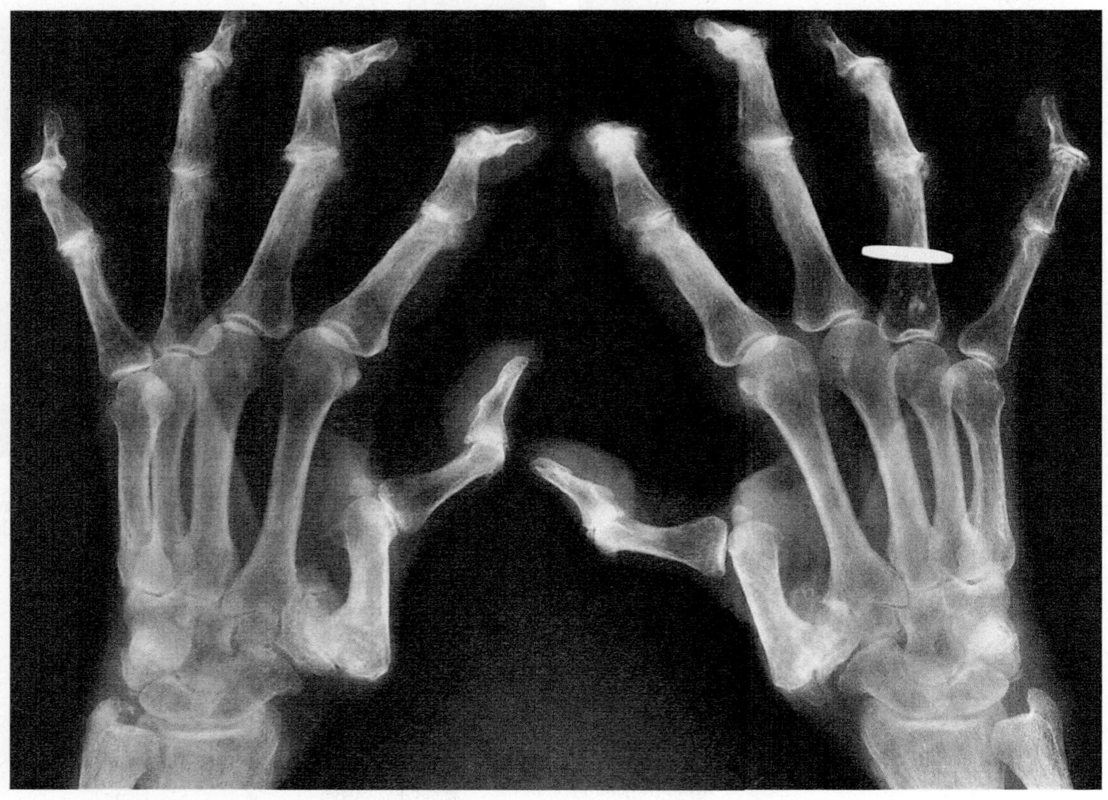

FIGURE 13.56 Interphalangeal and carpometacarpal OA. Dorsovolar radiograph of both hands of a 52-year-old woman in addition to the typical Heberden and Bouchard nodes shows deformative changes at the first carpometacarpal articulations, resulting in an odd configuration of both thumbs.

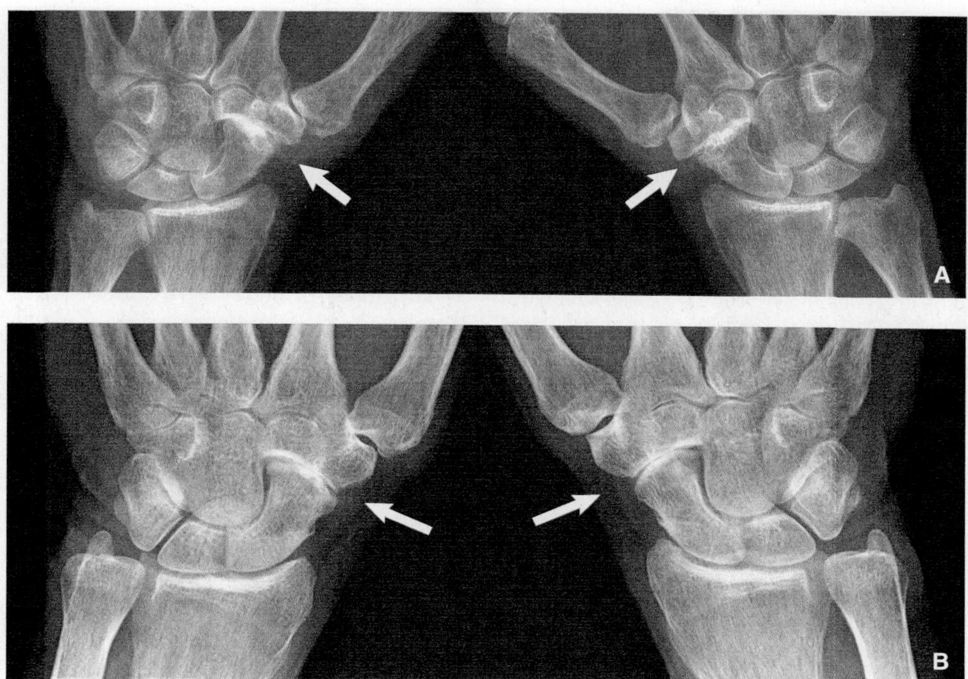

FIGURE 13.57 OA of STT joints. **(A)** Dorsovolar radiograph of both wrists of a 48-year-old woman shows narrowing and subchondral sclerosis of the STT joints *(arrows)*. **(B)** Dorsovolar radiograph of both wrists of a 63-year-old woman shows narrowing and sclerosis of the right and left STT joints *(arrows)*.

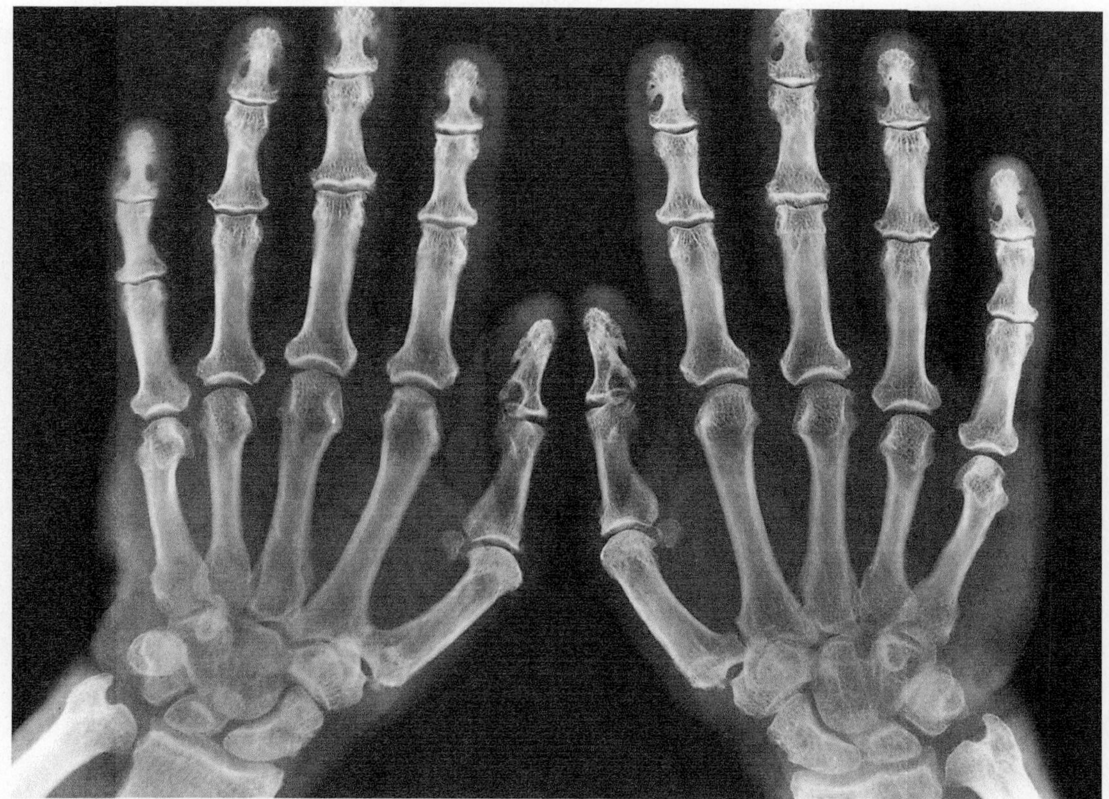

FIGURE 13.58 Acromegalic OA. Dorsovolar radiograph of both hands of a 42-year-old man shows widening of some and narrowing of other joint spaces, enlargement of the distal tufts and the bases of terminal phalanges, and beak-like osteophytes affecting particularly the heads of the metacarpals. Note the soft-tissue prominence and the large sesamoid bones at the first metacarpophalangeal joints. The sesamoid index (derived by multiplying the vertical and horizontal diameters of the sesamoid bone) is 48 in this patient; normally, it should not exceed 20 to 25.

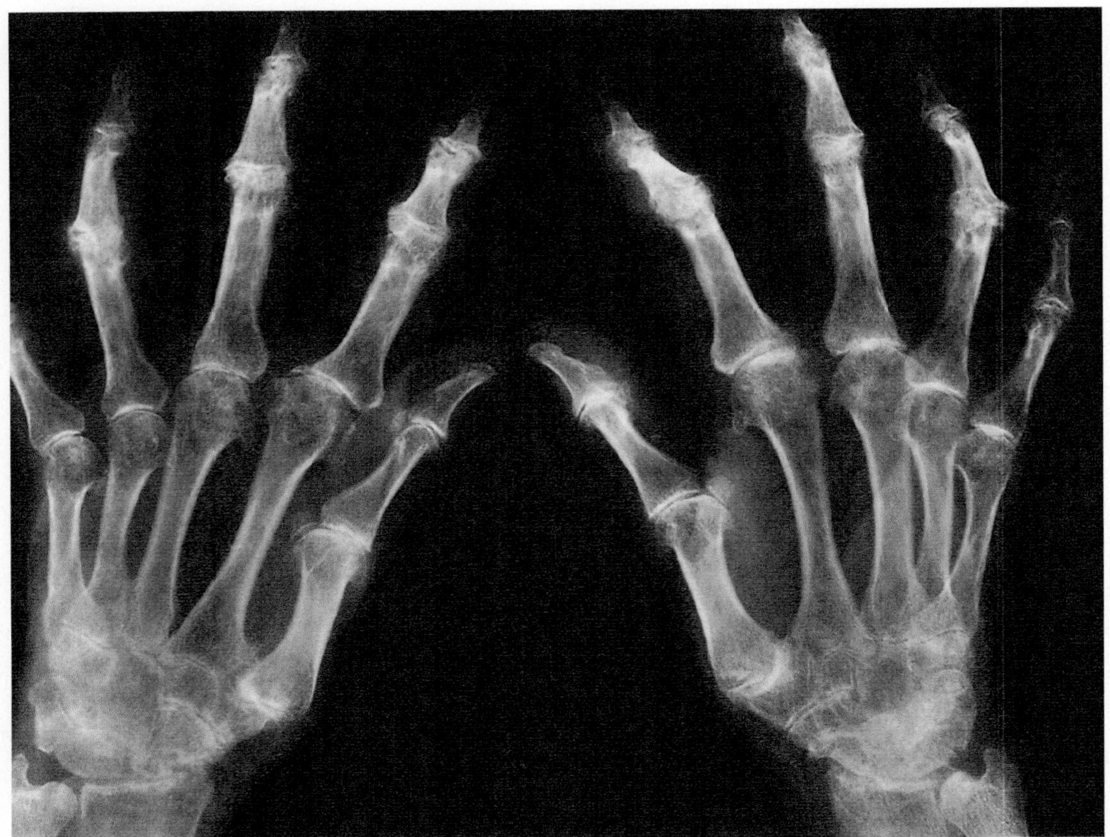

FIGURE 13.59 Hemochromatosis arthropathy. Oblique radiographs of both hands of a 53-year-old woman show beak-like osteophytes arising from the heads of the second and third metacarpals on the radial aspect of both hands. The interphalangeal, metacarpophalangeal, and carpal articulations are also affected.

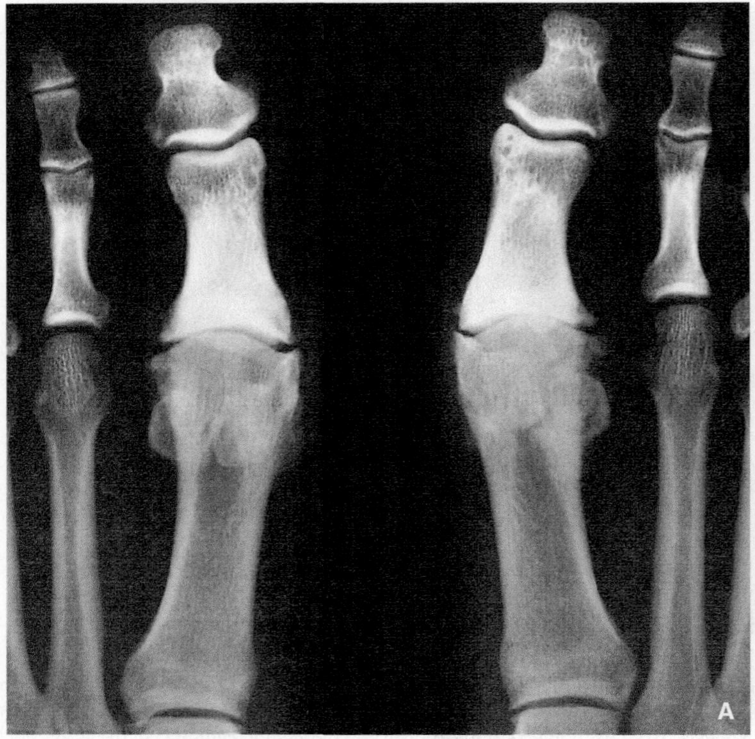

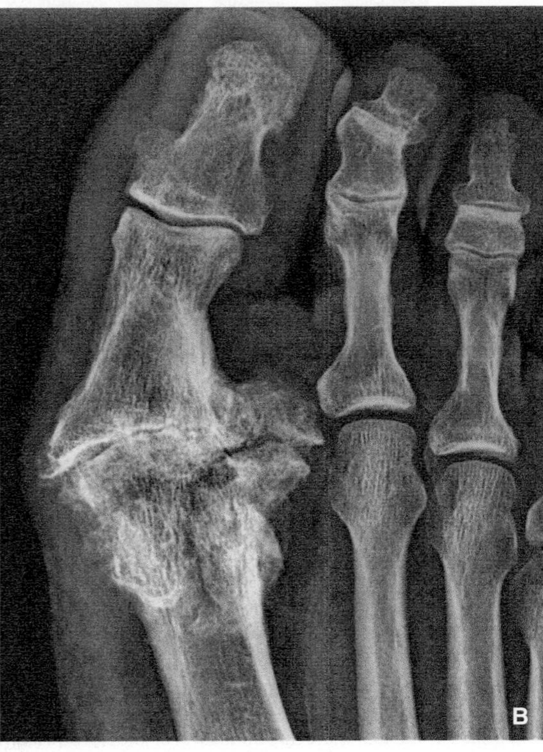

FIGURE 13.60 Hallux rigidus (hallux limitus). **(A)** Dorsoplantar radiograph of the great and second toes of the feet of a 33-year-old man shows OA of the first metatarsophalangeal joints, which are known as *hallux rigidus* (*hallux limitus*). Note the narrowing of the joint space, subchondral sclerosis, and marginal osteophytes. **(B)** More advanced OA of the first metatarsophalangeal joint is seen in this 72-year-old woman.

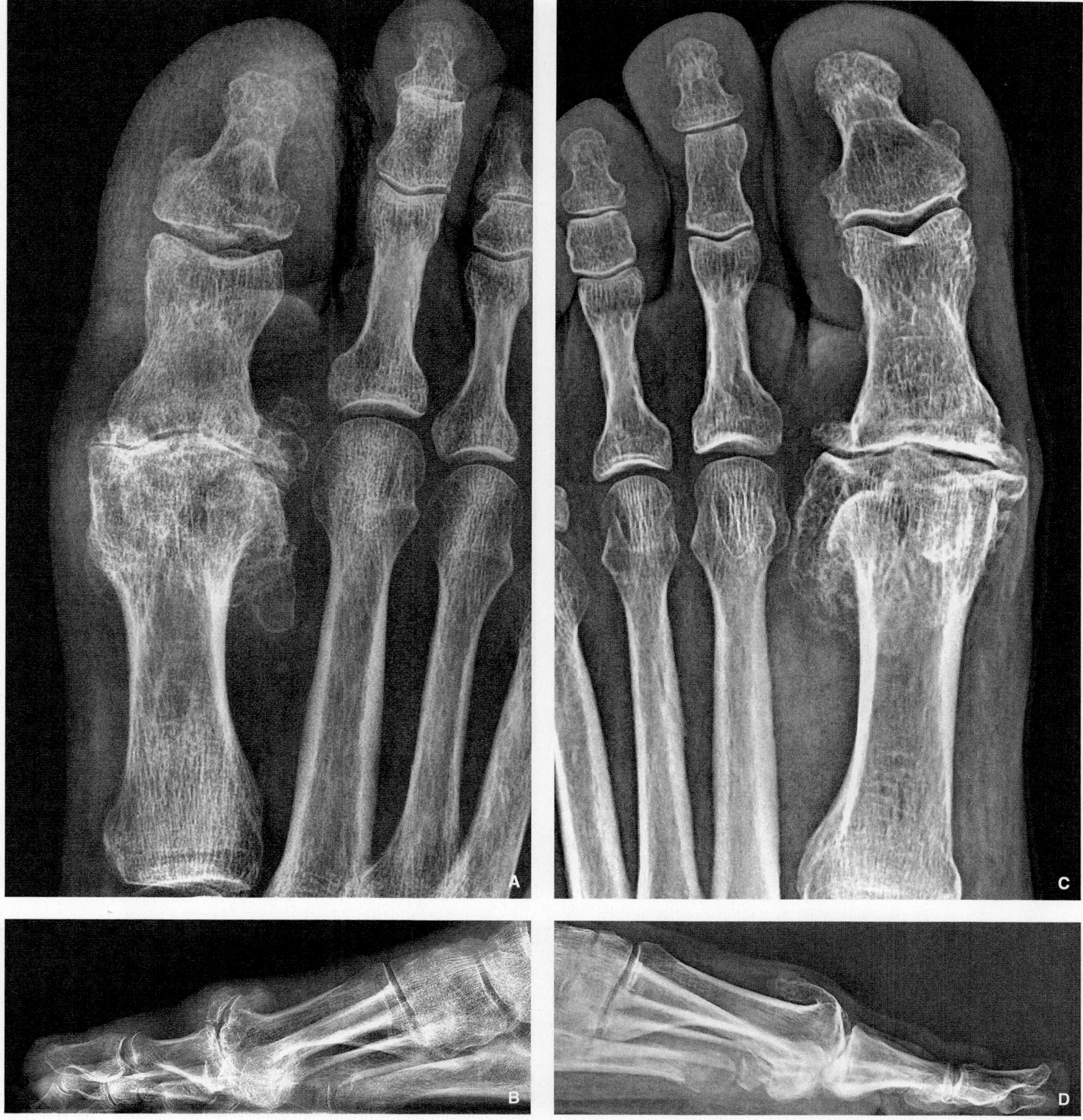

FIGURE 13.61 Hallux rigidus. **(A)** Anteroposterior and **(B)** lateral radiographs of the right great toe of an 80-year-old man show severe narrowing of the first metatarsophalangeal joint associated with subchondral sclerosis and formation of prominent osteophytes. **(C)** Anteroposterior and **(D)** lateral radiographs of the left great toe of a 69-year-old man demonstrate advanced OA of the first metatarsophalangeal joint. Observe on the lateral radiograph a very prominent dorsal osteophyte.

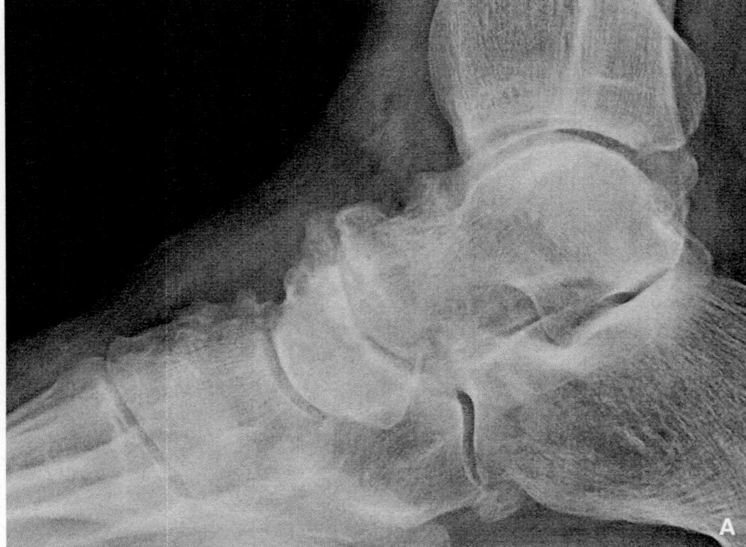

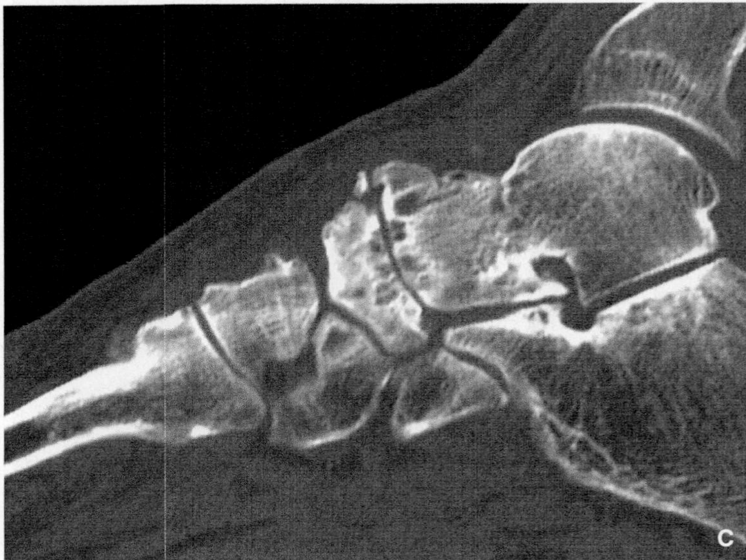

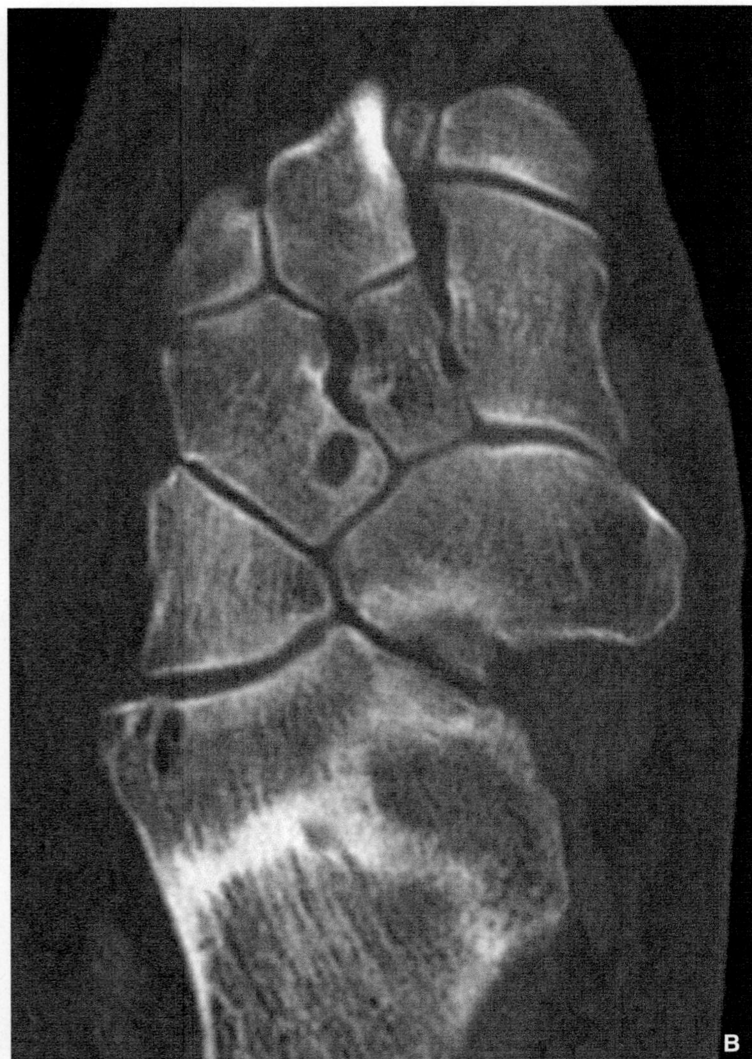

FIGURE 13.62 CT of OA of the foot joints. **(A)** Lateral radiograph of the right foot of a 60-year-old man shows narrowing of the talonavicular joint and formation of dorsal osteophytes. **(B)** Coronal and **(C)** sagittal reformatted CT images show in addition subchondral sclerosis and cyst-like lesions at the talonavicular, calcaneocuboid, naviculocuneiform, and subtalar joints.

Degenerative Diseases of the Spine

Degenerative changes may involve the spine at the following sites:

1. The synovial joints—atlantoaxial, apophyseal, costovertebral, and sacroiliac—leading to *OA* of these structures
2. The intervertebral disks, leading to the condition known as *degenerative disk disease*
3. The vertebral bodies and annulus fibrosus, leading to the condition known as *spondylosis deformans*
4. The fibrous articulations, ligaments, or sites of ligament attachment to the bone (entheses), leading to the condition known as *diffuse idiopathic skeletal hyperostosis* (DISH).

Frequently, all four conditions coexist in the same patient.

Clinical Features

Patients with *cervical facet joints OA* may complain of neck stiffness and pain, usually more severe during head and neck movements. In patients with *lumbar facet joints OA*, the pain may radiate to the posterior thigh and could be exacerbated by bending. Those patients with *degenerative disk disease* experience pain related to activity while twisting, bending, or lifting heavy objects. The symptoms may flare up at time and then return to a low-grade pain level. Some patients become symptomatic when sitting for a long time. Occasionally, back pain may be associated with leg weakness, numbness, or tingling. Assuming reclining position may alleviate the symptoms. The causes of back pain are not completely understood but include the following: ingrowths of nociceptive nerves into the intervertebral disk, nerve root compression by protruding disk tissue and osteophytes, sensitization of the nerve roots by tumor necrosis factor-α produced by protruding intervertebral disk tissue, and local nerve root ischemia. *Intervertebral disk herniation* is associated with radiculopathy and pain in the buttocks, legs, and feet. Commonly, the patients will experience sciatic pain. Patients with *DISH syndrome* are usually either asymptomatic or the pain is minimal, although generalized stiffness is a common complaint and there may be moderate limitation of spine motion. Posture is generally unaffected, although occasionally some patients may develop kyphosis. If the cervical spine is severely affected, the patient may complain of dysphagia. The complications of degenerative spine disease, such as spinal stenosis or spondylolisthesis bring more severe symptoms. The clinical hallmark of *spinal stenosis* is pseudoclaudication (so-called *neurogenic claudication*). Patient complain of pain and discomfort associated with weakness and paresthesias in the buttocks, thighs, and legs. The gait may become unsteady. Standing or walking induces the symptoms that are relieved by sitting, squatting, or flexing forward. Minimal *spondylolisthesis* may be asymptomatic; however, greater degree of vertebral displacement may result in low back pain with or without radiation into the leg, associated with signs of nerve root impingement, or even cauda equina syndrome.

Pathology

Facet joint arthritis results from the excessive load (combination of applied compression and torsion forces) on these anatomic structures. The morphologic features are identical to those seen in OA of other diarthrodial joints, namely, capsular laxity, synovitis, cartilage fibrillation followed by cartilage loss and eburnation of the exposed bone, and formation of marginal osteophytes.

In *degenerative disk disease*, the pathologic changes occur as a result of the disruption of the vertebral end plates. Evidence of degeneration of these structures is seen as microfractures at the bone–cartilage interface, advancing of calcification into the cartilage from the bone surface, and invasion of blood vessels from the subchondral bone into the cartilaginous end plate, with subsequent endochondral ossification. With disruption of the end plate, the disk components show a rapid progress of degeneration manifested by focal necrosis, fissuring, calcification, and tearing of annulus fibrosus. The fibrous tissue is replacing normal disk tissue, including the nucleus pulposus. Large horizontal clefts develop in the central part of the disk containing nitrogen gas, which is seen on the radiography as radiolucent areas termed *vacuum phenomenon*. As disk degeneration progresses, there is subsequent narrowing of the disk space, followed by new bone formation at the junction of the annulus fibrosus and the vertebral body. Ossification of the cartilaginous end plate also contributes to disk space narrowing (Fig. 13.63). Histopathologic features are characterized by variety of alternations in the nucleus pulposus, annulus fibrosus, and the vertebral end plate. In nucleus pulposus, there is loss of metachromasia due to reduced amounts of aggrecan and a reduction in the heavily sulfated glycosaminoglycan side chains. Mucoid material is replaced by fibrous tissue. Slits propagate from the nucleus pulposus into the annulus fibrosus. In the annulus fibrosus, blood vessels grow inward from the vasculature of the outer part of annulus. Microscopic tears appear, followed by fibrocartilaginous metaplasia. In the vertebral end plates, noted are microfractures and fracture repair. In general, the changes in the end plates are very similar to those occurring in the articular cartilage of diarthrodial joints in OA.

Tears in the periphery of the annulus fibrosus where the collagen bundles attach to the vertebral bodies by Sharpey fibers initiate the pathologic process of *spondylosis deformans*. This is followed by anterior and anterolateral protrusio/herniation of disk tissue. Once displacement has occurred, dissection of the anterior longitudinal ligament from its osseous attachment by the displaced disk permits extension of the disk tissue along the anterior aspect of vertebral body. Continuous tearing in these areas stimulates the development of bony outgrowths, termed *osteophytes*, along the anterior and lateral aspects of the vertebral body (Fig. 13.64).

DISH, also known as *ankylosing hyperostosis*, occurs as a result of ligamentous ossification without significant disk disease or facet arthropathy, leading to ankylosis of the vertebral column. Pathologic features include ligamentous calcification and ossification with periosteal new bone formation at the anterior vertebral surface, linked to "armor plating" (Fig. 13.65).

Osteoarthritis of the Synovial Joints

Degenerative changes of the vertebral facet joints are very common, particularly in the mid and lower cervical and the lower lumbar segments. As in the other synovial joints, the characteristic radiographic features include

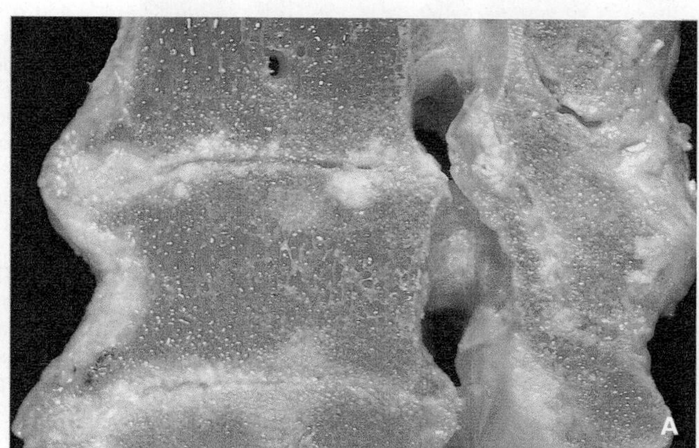

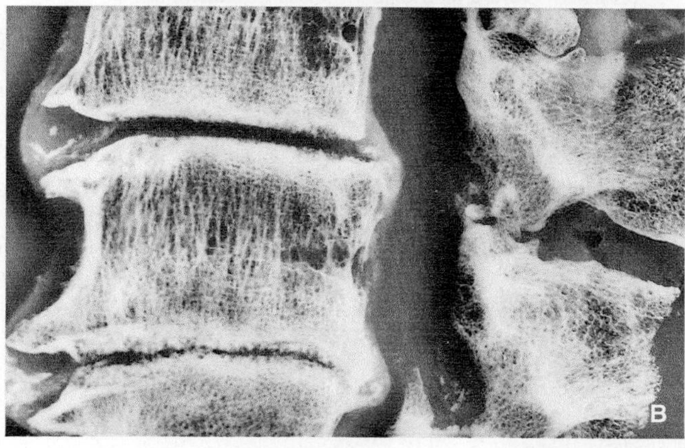

FIGURE 13.63 Pathology of the degenerative disk disease. (A) Photograph of sagittal section of the vertebrae of the mid-thoracic spine and **(B)** specimen radiograph show two degenerative disks. Note narrowing of the disk spaces, end plate sclerosis, and formation of anterior and posterior osteophytes. (Reprinted with permission from Vigorita JV, Ghelmsan B, Mintz D. *Orthopaedic pathology*, 3rd ed. Philadelphia: Wolters Kluwer; 2016:727.)

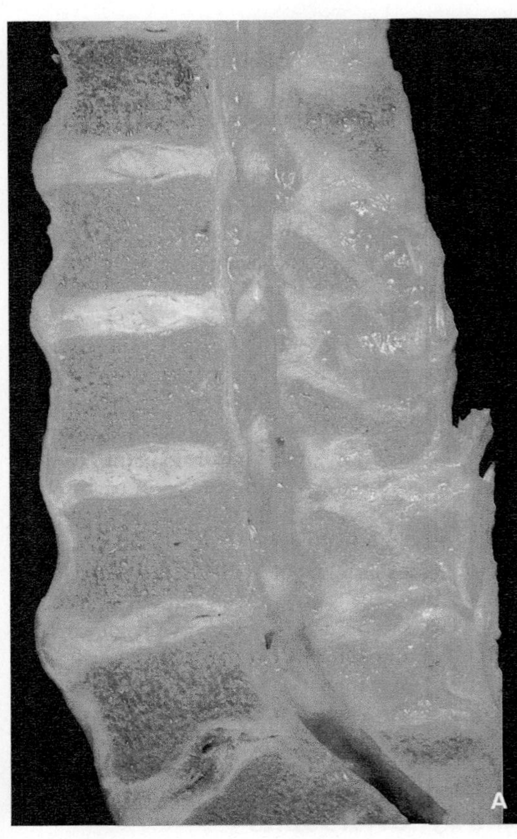

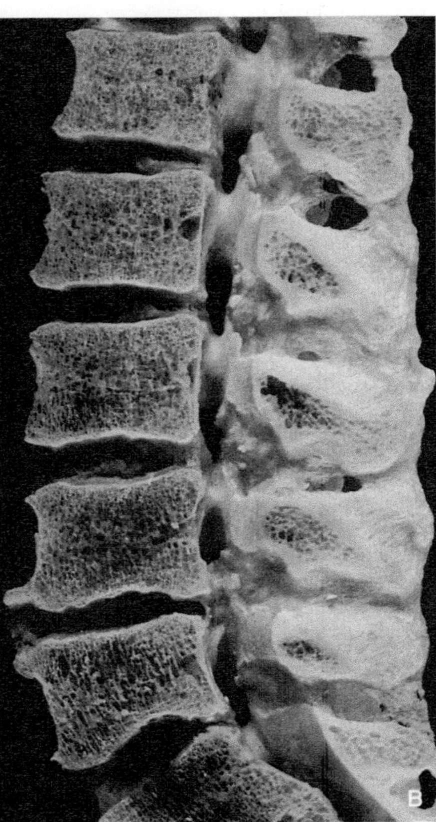

FIGURE 13.64 Pathology of spondylosis deformans. **(A)** Sagittal section of the lumbar spine and **(B)** macerated specimen show anterior protrusio of several intervertebral disks causing bulging of the annulus fibrosus and anterior longitudinal ligament. There is narrowing of the disk space L4-5 associated with formation of anterior osteophytes, but remaining disk spaces are relatively normal. (Reprinted from Bullough P. *Orthopaedic pathology*, 5th ed. Maryland Heights, MO: Mosby; 2009, with permission from Elsevier.)

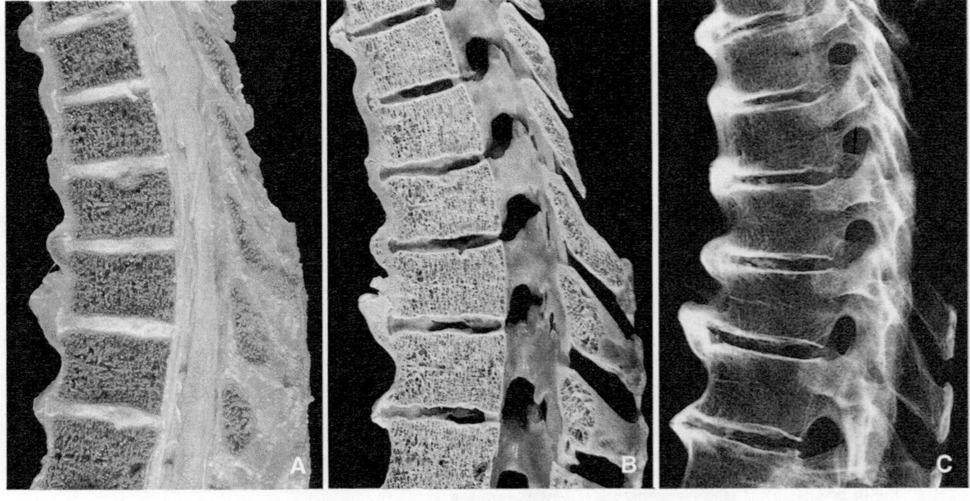

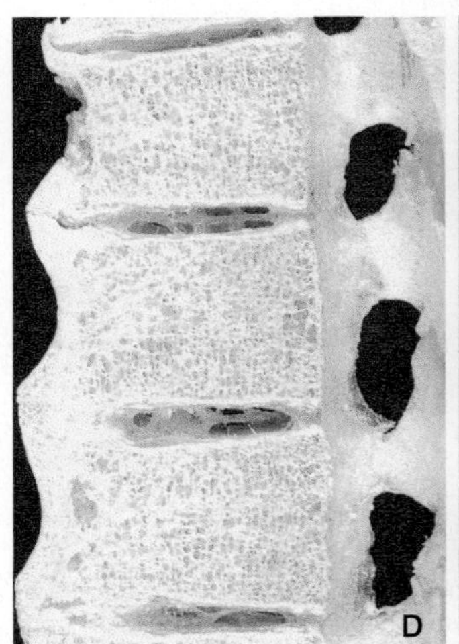

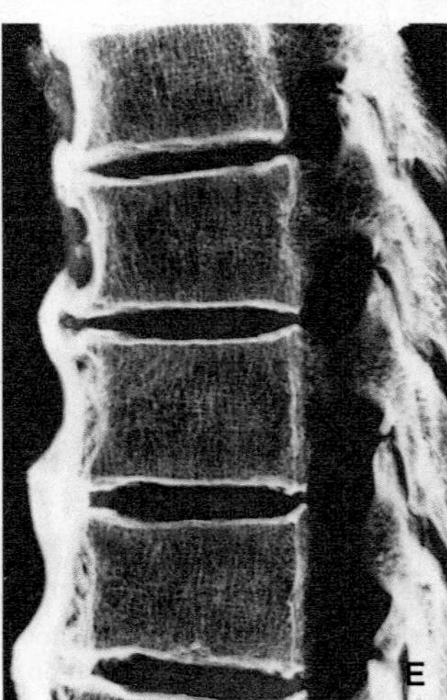

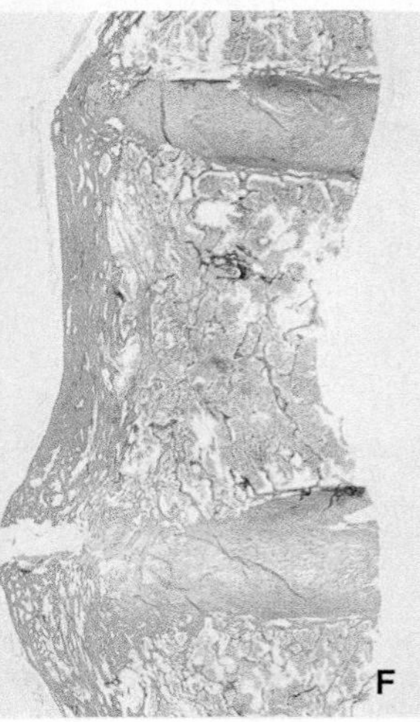

FIGURE 13.65 Pathology of DISH. **(A)** Sagittal section of the thoracic spine, **(B)** macerated specimen, and **(C)** radiograph of the macerated specimen show characteristic features of this condition, namely, flowing anterior hyperostosis bridging several vertebral bodies, relatively well-preserved disk spaces, and intact vertebral end plates. (Reprinted from Bullough P. *Orthopaedic pathology*, 5th ed. Maryland Heights, MO: Mosby; 2009, with permission from Elsevier.) **(D)** Lateral radiograph of another specimen of the thoracic spine shows anterior osseous ankylosis and thickening of the anterior surface of the vertebral bodies, creating "armor plate" appearance. The disk spaces are preserved. **(E)** On the sagittal section of the specimen, observe ossifications confined to the anterior longitudinal ligament. **(F)** A photomicrograph shows the details of anterior flowing hyperostosis. (Reprinted from Bullough PG, Boachie-Adjei O. *Atlas of spinal diseases*. Philadelphia: JB Lippincott; 1988:114, Fig. 9.33.)

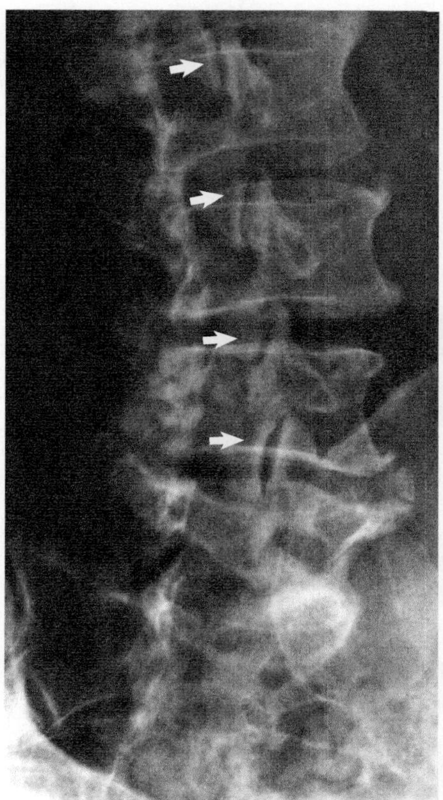

FIGURE 13.66 OA of the facet joints. Oblique radiograph of the lumbar spine in a 68-year-old man demonstrates advanced OA of the facet joints. Narrowing of the joint spaces, eburnation of the articular margins, and small osteophytes *(arrows)* are similar to the changes seen in OA of the large synovial joints.

diminution of the joint space, eburnation of subchondral bone, and osteophyte formation, all of which are most easily demonstrated on the oblique projection of the spine (Fig. 13.66). In the cervical spine, osteophytes on the posterior aspect of a vertebral body may encroach on the neural foramina or the thecal sac, causing various neurologic symptoms. In addition to the standard oblique views (Fig. 13.67), conventional tomography (in the past) or CT (at the present time) may demonstrate these changes (Fig. 13.68). Anterior osteophytes, however, are as a rule asymptomatic unless they are unusually prominent. Involvement of the apophyseal joints may exhibit a "vacuum phenomenon" (Fig. 13.69), which in fact represents gas in the joint. This finding is almost pathognomonic for a degenerative process.

As in other diarthrodial joints, degenerative changes of the sacroiliac joints are manifested by narrowing of the joint space, subchondral sclerosis, and osteophytosis (Fig. 13.70). It is important to note in the evaluation of the sacroiliac joints that only the lower half of the radiographic sacroiliac joint space is lined by synovium; the upper portion is a syndesmotic joint (Fig. 13.71).

Degenerative Disk Disease

In degenerative disk disease, the vacuum phenomenon in the disk space is common. These radiolucent collections of gas, principally nitrogen, are related to the negative pressure created by abnormally altered joint or disk spaces.

Other radiographic findings of degenerative disk disease include disk space narrowing and osteophytosis at the marginal borders of the adjacent vertebral bodies (Fig. 13.72). Degenerative disk disease, in combination with degenerative changes in the apophyseal joints, may lead to degenerative spondylolisthesis (see Fig. 13.72; see also Figs. 11.79 and 11.81B).

A destructive diskovertebral degenerative disease of the lumbar spine has been reported, similar to rapidly progressing coxarthropathy

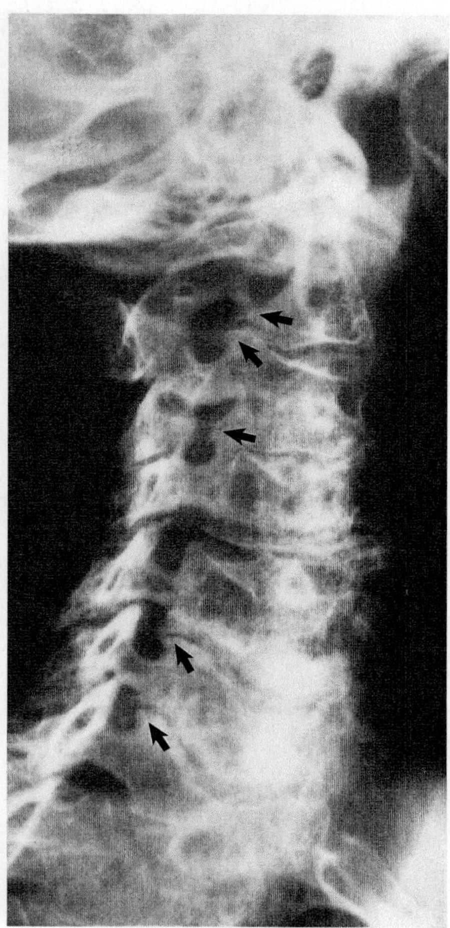

FIGURE 13.67 Encroachment of the neural foramina. Oblique radiograph of the cervical spine in a 72-year-old woman who reported neck pain radiating to both shoulders reveals multiple posterior osteophytes encroaching on numerous neural foramina *(arrows)*.

(see previous text), characterized by vertebral malalignment, severe disk resorption, intervertebral vacuum phenomenon, and "bone sand" formation secondary to vertebral fragmentation.

MRI is highly effective in demonstrating changes of disk degeneration. Decrease in the water content results in a decreased signal intensity of the nucleus pulposus on T2-weighted images (Fig. 13.73). Frequently, additional characteristic alterations are seen in the end plates of the vertebral bodies adjacent to the degenerative disk. These abnormalities consist of a focal decreased signal intensity of the marrow on T1-weighted images and increased signal on T2- or T2*-weighted images (Fig. 13.74). According to Modic, these alterations represent subchondral vascularized fibrous tissue associated with end plate fissuring and disruption (type I). These changes may progress to fatty marrow end plate conversion (type II) (Fig. 13.75) and later to sclerosis (type III).

Spondylosis Deformans

Spondylosis deformans is a degenerative condition marked by the formation of anterior and lateral osteophytes as a result of anterior and anterolateral disk herniation (see Fig. 11.90). As Schmorl and Junghanns and other investigators have pointed out, the initiating factors in the development of this condition are abnormalities in the peripheral fibers of the annulus fibrosus that result in weakening of the anchorage of the intervertebral disk to the vertebral body at the site where Sharpey fibers attach to the vertebral rim. Unlike degenerative disk disease, the intervertebral spaces in spondylosis deformans are relatively well preserved, with the primary radiographic feature being extensive osteophytosis (Fig. 13.76). These osteophytes must be differentiated from the delicate

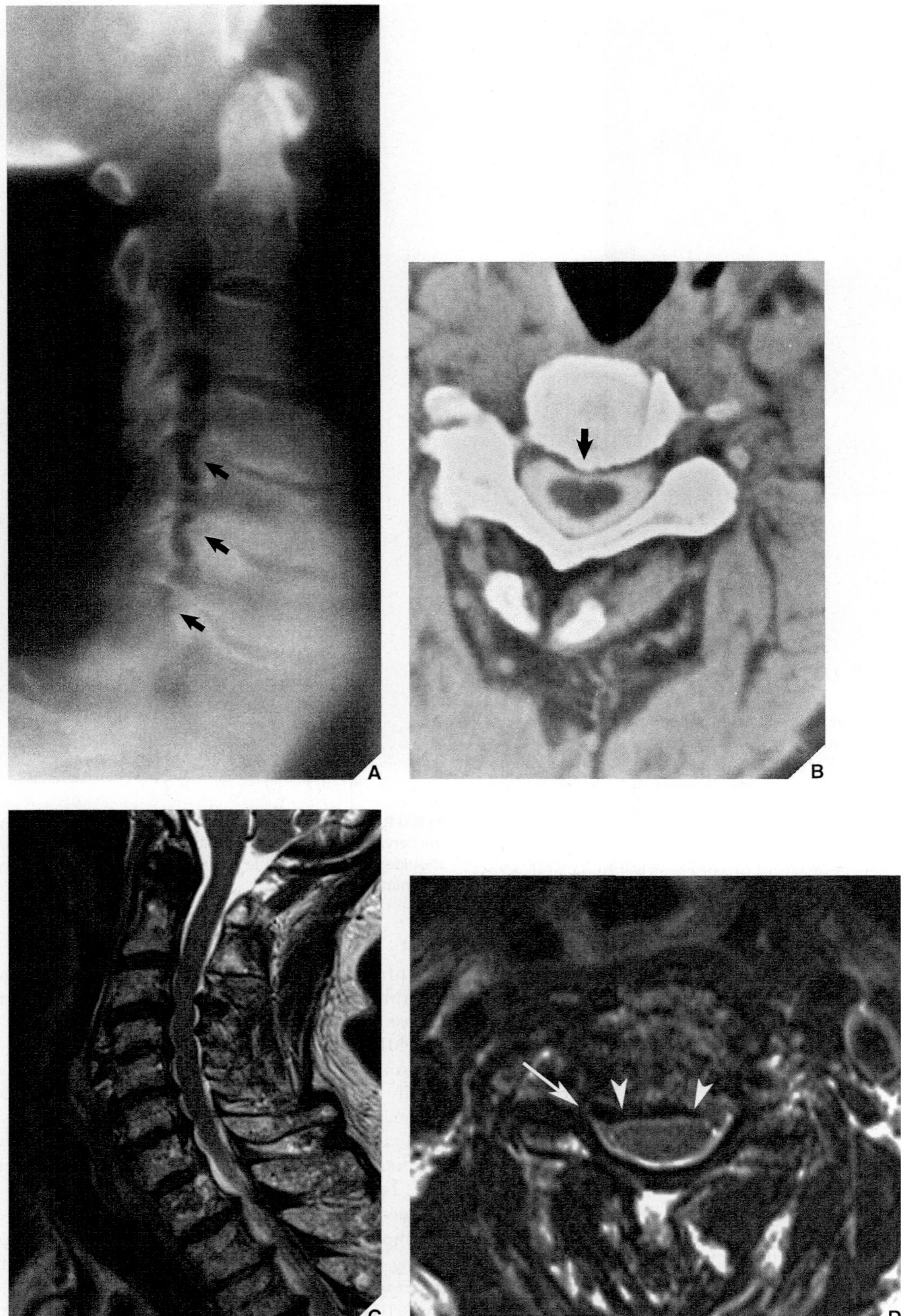

FIGURE 13.68 Encroachment of the neural foramina and the thecal sac. **(A)** Conventional lateral tomogram of the cervical spine in a 56-year-old man demonstrates encroachment of the neural foramina by posterior osteophytes *(arrows)*. **(B)** CT section at the level of C3 obtained during myelography demonstrates a large posterior osteophyte impinging on the thecal sac and compressing the subarachnoid space filled with contrast agent *(arrow)*. **(C)** Sagittal T2-weighted MRI in 73-year-old man demonstrates multilevel degenerative disk disease with anterior and posterior osteophytes impinging on the thecal sac. Note the deformity of the ventral aspect of the cord at C3-4, C4-5, and C6-7. **(D)** Axial T2-weighted MRI at C4-5 level demonstrates the posterior osteophytes deforming the ventral aspect of the cord *(arrowheads)* and the narrowing of the right neural foramen *(arrow)*.

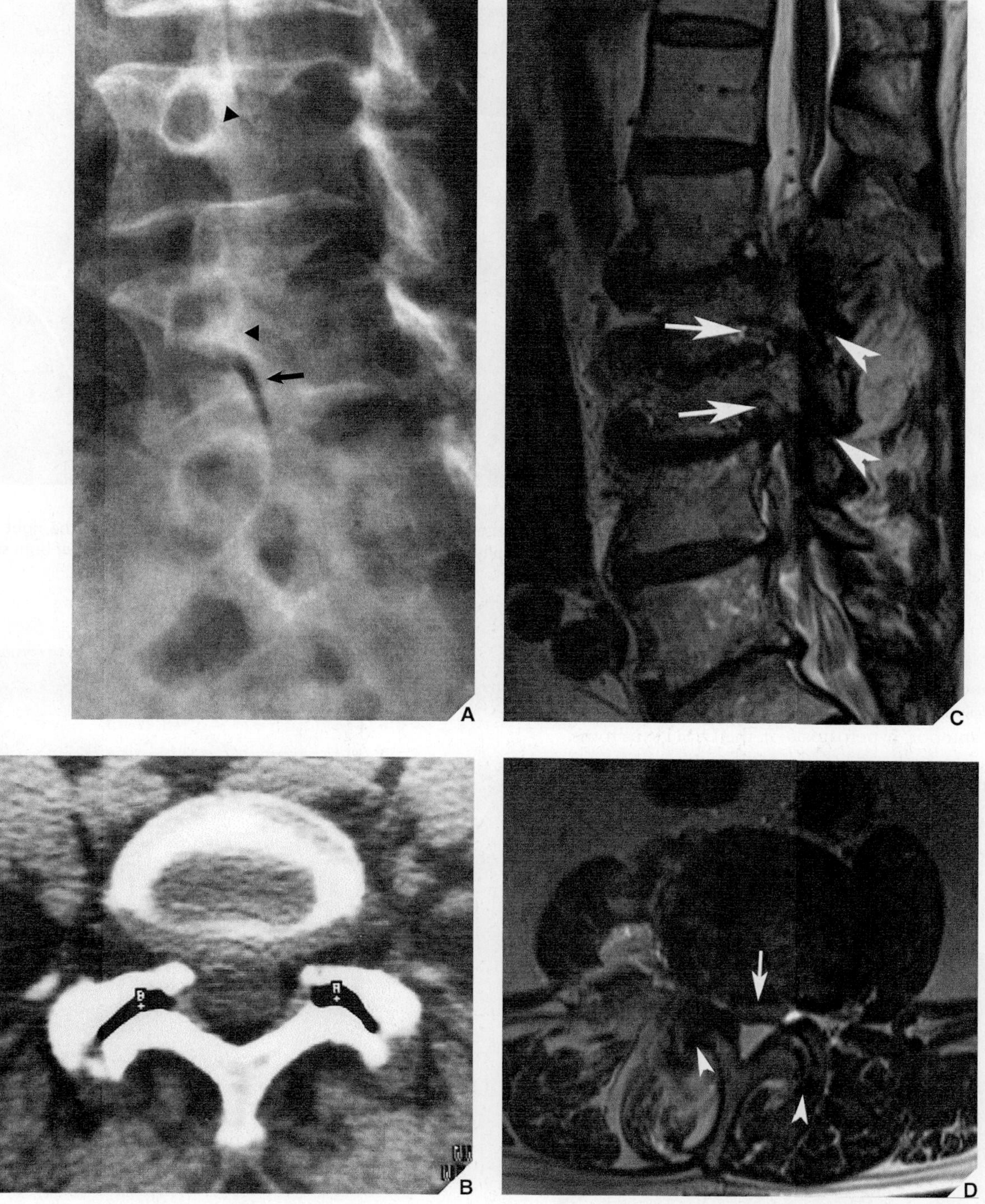

FIGURE 13.69 OA of the apophyseal joints. **(A)** Oblique radiograph of the lumbosacral spine in a 56-year-old man demonstrates a vacuum phenomenon of the facet joint L5-S1 *(arrow)* and eburnation of the subarticular bone *(arrowheads)*. **(B)** CT section through both facets clearly demonstrates the presence of gas, as confirmed by the Hounsfield values. These units are related to the attenuation coefficient for various tissues in the body and represent absorption values directly related to tissue density. Note also the hypertrophic spur arising from the right facet and encroaching on the spinal canal. **(C)** Sagittal T2-weighted MRI in an 84-year-old woman with scoliosis demonstrates advanced degenerative disk disease with severe facet arthrosis *(arrowheads)* associated with stenosis of the neural foramen and impingement of the exiting nerve roots *(arrows)*. **(D)** Axial T2-weighted MR image demonstrates an annular bulge with bilateral facet arthrosis *(arrowheads)*, severe stenosis of the thecal sac associated with clumping of the nerve roots *(arrow)*, and bilateral foraminal stenosis, more prominent on the right.

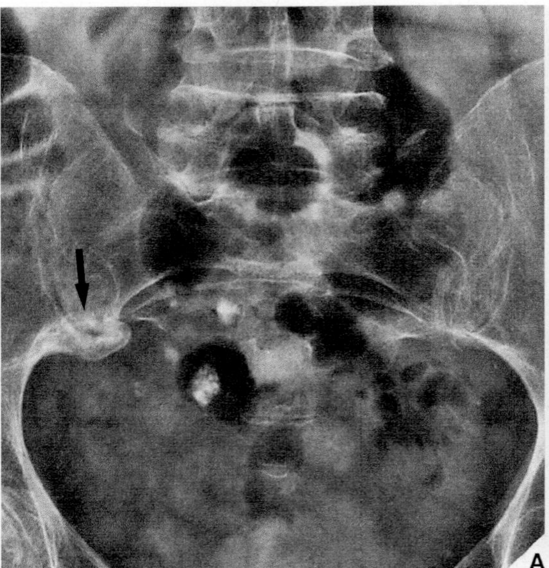

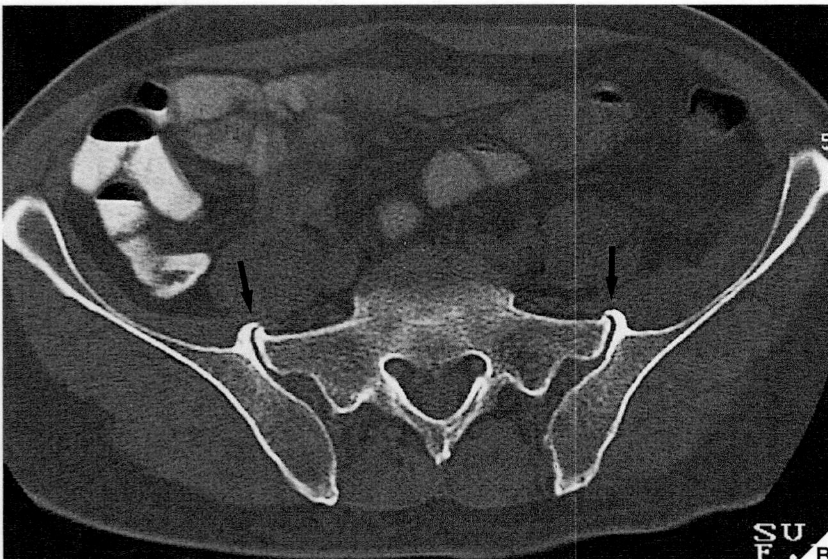

FIGURE 13.70 OA of the sacroiliac joints. **(A)** Degenerative changes in the sacroiliac joints, seen here affecting predominantly the right sacroiliac joint *(arrow)* in an 82-year-old woman, are manifested by narrowing of the joint space and osteophytosis. **(B)** In another patient, a 68-year-old man, OA of both sacroiliac joints *(arrows)* is demonstrated on axial CT image.

syndesmophytes of ankylosing spondylitis; from the large characteristically asymmetric bone excrescences that are seen in psoriatic arthritis and reactive arthritis involving the lateral aspect of vertebral bodies; and from the flowing, usually anterior, hyperostosis of the DISH syndrome.

Diffuse Idiopathic Skeletal Hyperostosis

DISH, a noninflammatory spondyloarthropathy, originally described by Forestier and popularized by Resnick, is characterized by flowing ossification along the anterior aspect of the vertebral bodies extending across the

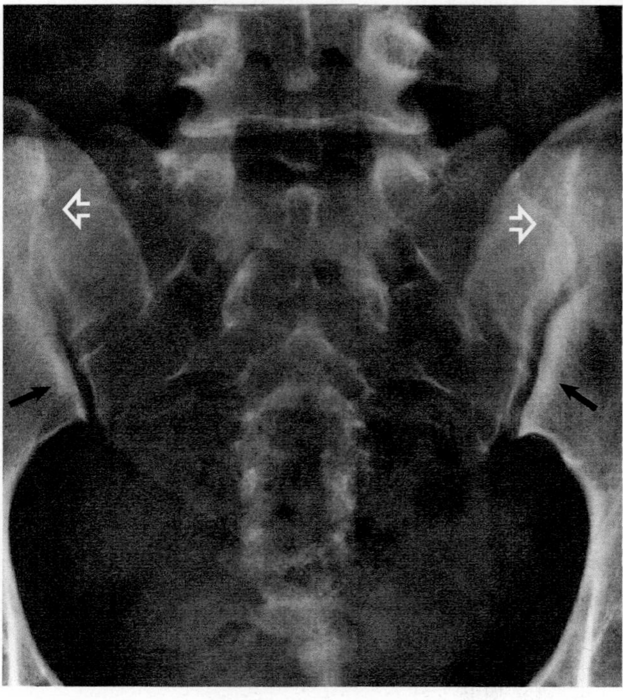

FIGURE 13.71 Sacroiliac joints. The true diarthrodial portion of the sacroiliac joint comprises only approximately 50% of the radiographic joint space *(arrows)*. The upper part is a syndesmotic joint *(open arrows)*.

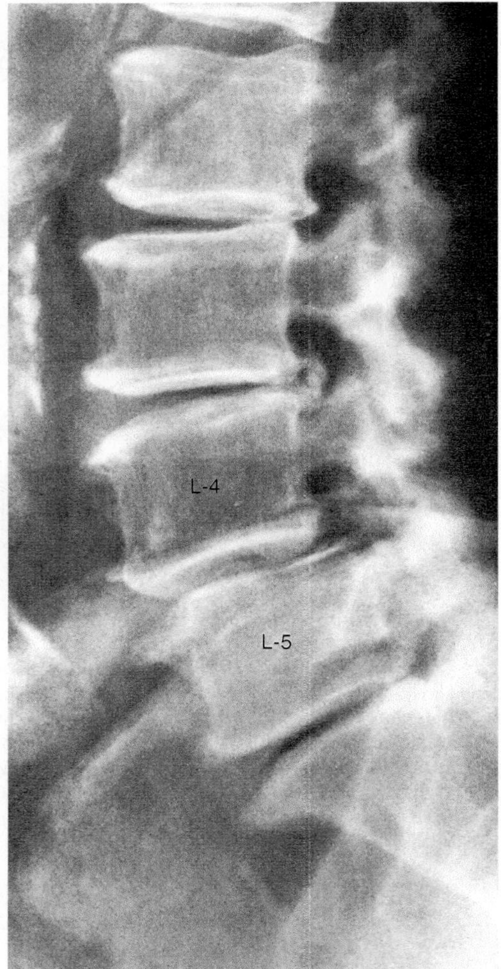

FIGURE 13.72 Degenerative disk disease. Lateral radiograph of the lumbosacral spine in a 66-year-old woman demonstrates advanced degenerative disk disease at multiple levels. Note the radiolucent collections of gas in several disks (the vacuum phenomenon) as well as the narrowing of the disk spaces and marginal osteophytes. Grade 1 degenerative spondylolisthesis is seen at the L4-5 level.

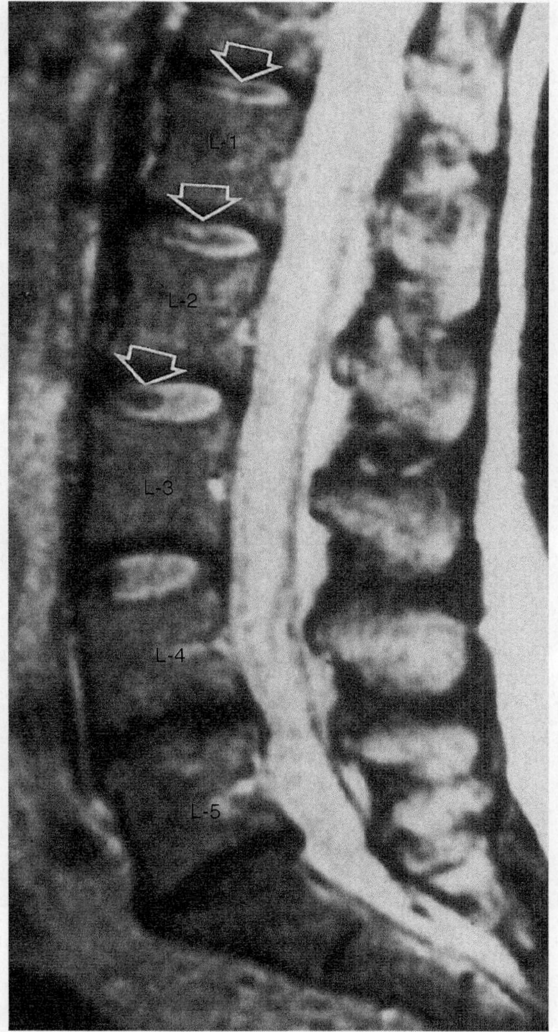

FIGURE 13.73 MRI of degenerative disk disease. Sagittal T2-weighted MR image shows early degenerative changes in the T12-L1, L1-2, and L2-3 intervertebral disks *(open arrows)*, more advanced process in the L3-4 disk, and severe degenerative disk disease at L4-5 and L5-S1. At the latter levels, markedly decreased intervertebral spaces and low signal intensity of degenerated disks are seen. (Reprinted with permission from Bloem JL, Sartoris DJ, eds. *MRI and CT of the musculoskeletal system. A text-atlas*. Baltimore: Williams Wilkins; 1992.)

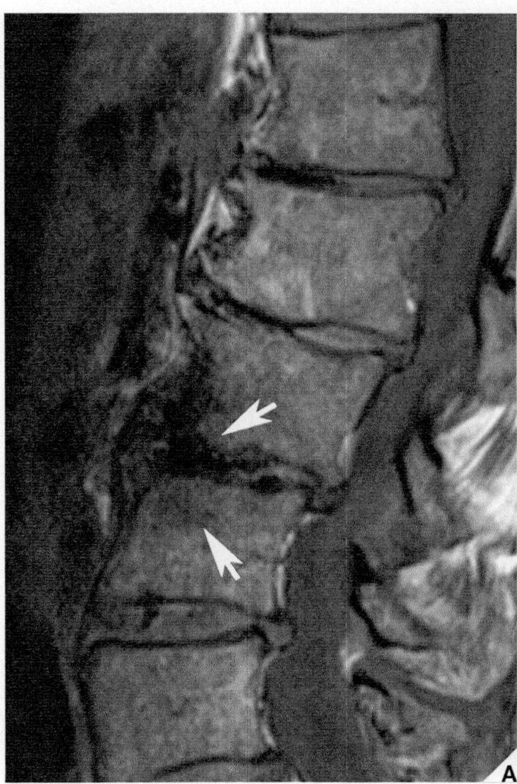

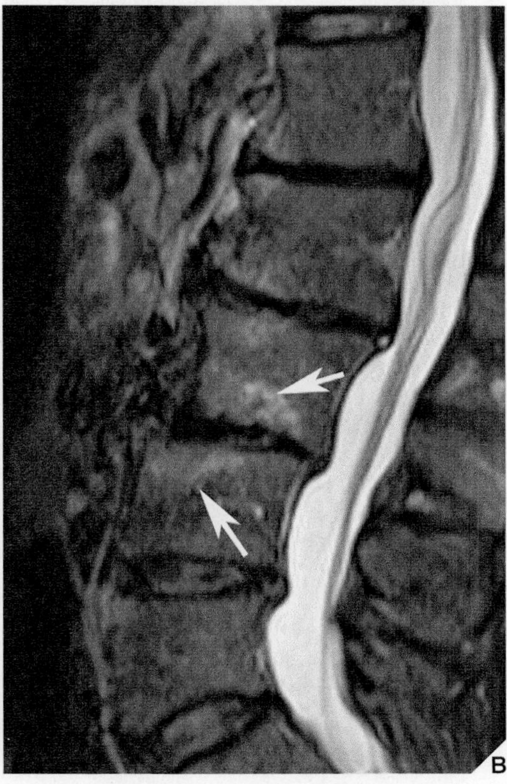

FIGURE 13.74 MRI of degenerative disk disease. Modic type I vertebral end plate change *(arrows)* demonstrates a focus of low signal intensity in subchondral marrow on a T1-weighted sagittal MRI **(A)** and a high signal intensity on short time inversion recovery (STIR) imaging **(B)**.

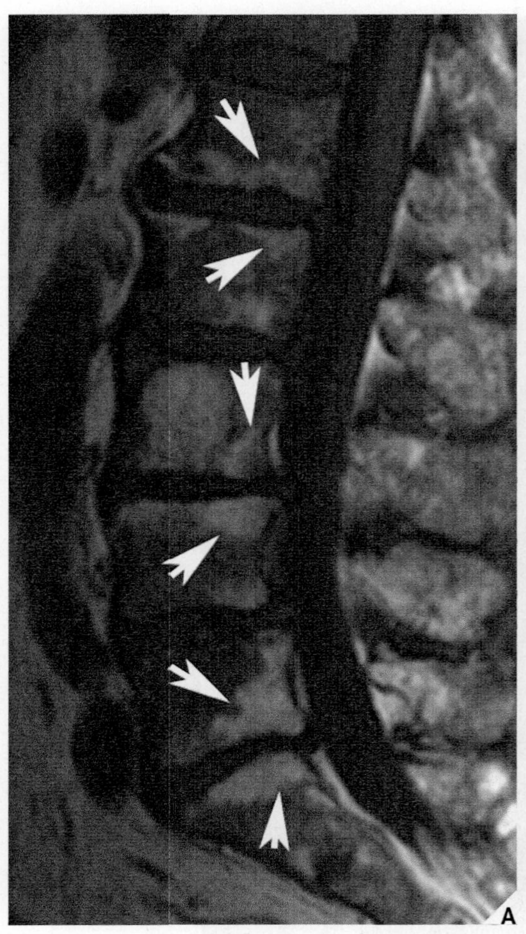

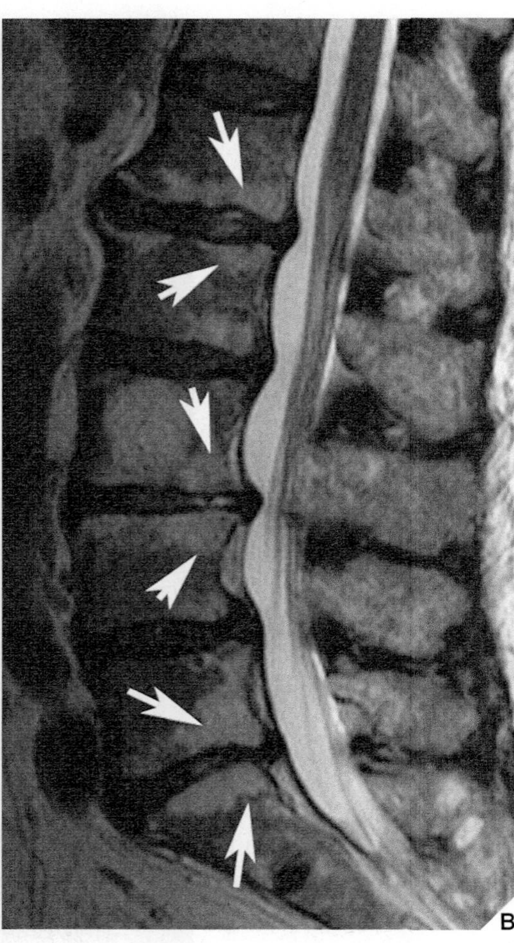

FIGURE 13.75 MRI of degenerative disk disease. Modic type II end plate changes in degenerative disk disease consisting of focal areas of yellow marrow conversion *(arrows)* are seen on a sagittal T1-weighted **(A)** and sagittal T2-weighted MR images **(B)**.

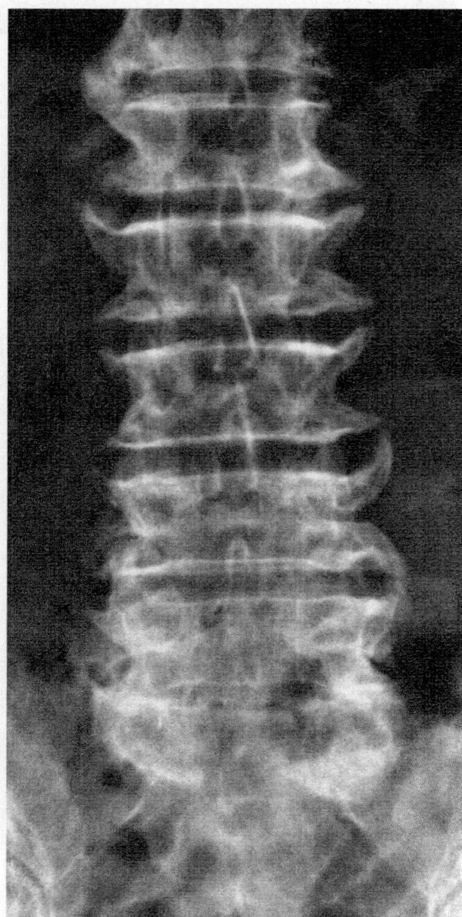

FIGURE 13.76 Spondylosis deformans. Anteroposterior radiograph of the lumbosacral spine in a 68-year-old woman exhibits the typical changes of spondylosis deformans. Note the extensive osteophytosis and relatively well-preserved intervertebral disk spaces.

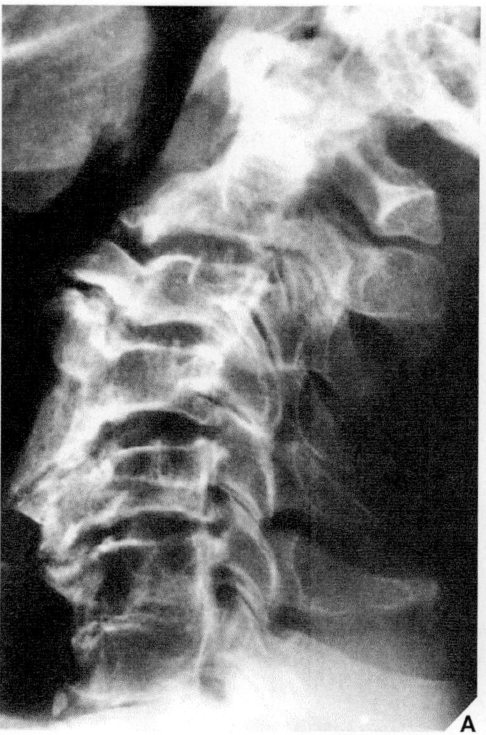

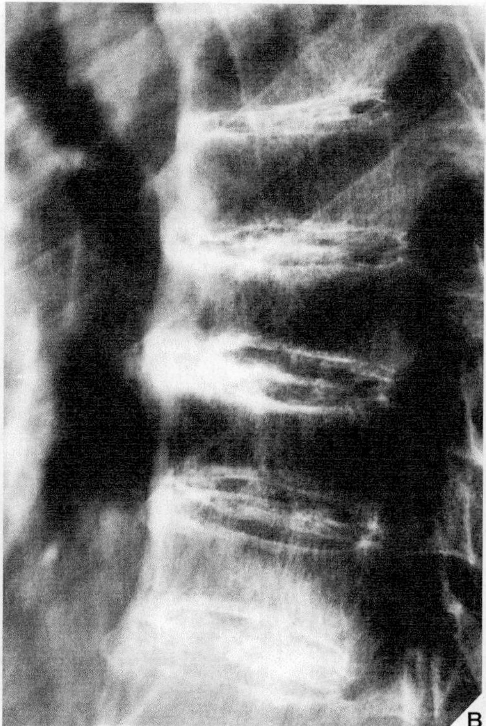

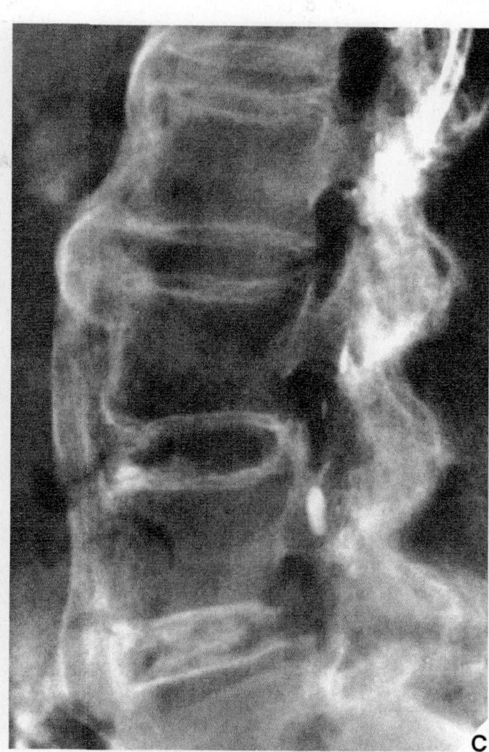

FIGURE 13.77 **Diffuse idiopathic skeletal hyperostosis.** Lateral radiographs of **(A)** the cervical, **(B)** thoracic, and **(C)** lumbar spine in a 72-year-old man with Forestier disease (DISH) show the characteristic flowing hyperostosis extending across the vertebral disk spaces, which are relatively well preserved.

disk spaces. Grossly, the appearance is that of a candle wax dripping down the anterior aspect of the spine, similar to melorheostosis. It is also associated with hyperostosis at the sites of tendon and ligament attachments to the bone, ligament ossification, and osteophytosis involving the axial and appendicular skeleton. A lateral radiograph of the spine best demonstrates these changes. As in spondylosis deformans, the disk spaces and facet joints are usually well preserved (Fig. 13.77). It is important to distinguish this condition from the apparently similar "bamboo spine" seen in ankylosing spondylitis (see Fig. 14.74).

Complications of Degenerative Disease of the Spine

Degenerative Spondylolisthesis

One of the most common complications of degenerative disease of the spine, degenerative spondylolisthesis results from degenerative changes in the disk and apophyseal joints. In this condition, there is anterior displacement of a vertebra onto the one below, which usually is easily recognized on the lateral view of the spine by the spinous-process sign (Fig. 13.78; see also Fig. 11.80). However, on occasion, the displacement may not be

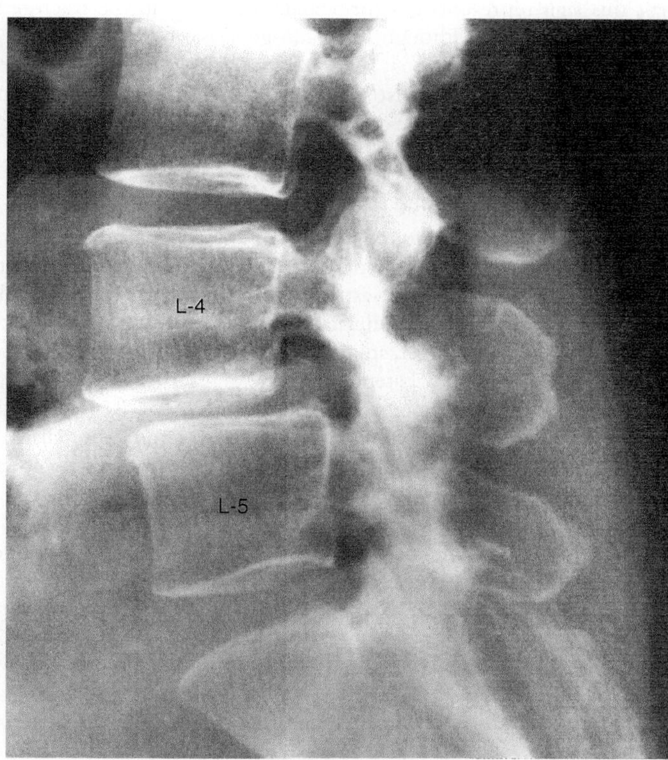

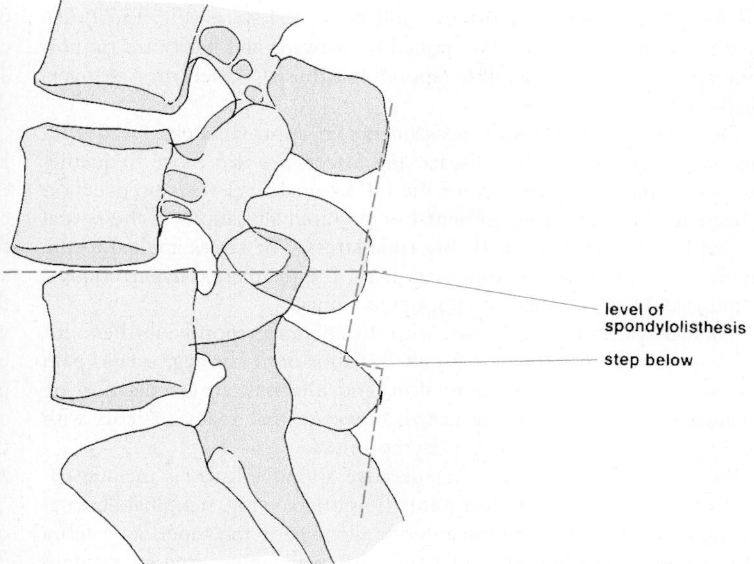

FIGURE 13.78 **Degenerative spondylolisthesis.** A 55-year-old woman with degenerative disk disease at L4-5 and degenerative facet arthritis developed spondylolisthesis, a common complication of this condition. Lateral radiograph of the lumbosacral spine is sufficient to differentiate this condition from spondylolisthesis associated with spondylolysis by the appearance of a step-off of the spinous process at the vertebra below the involved intervertebral space (see Fig. 11.90).

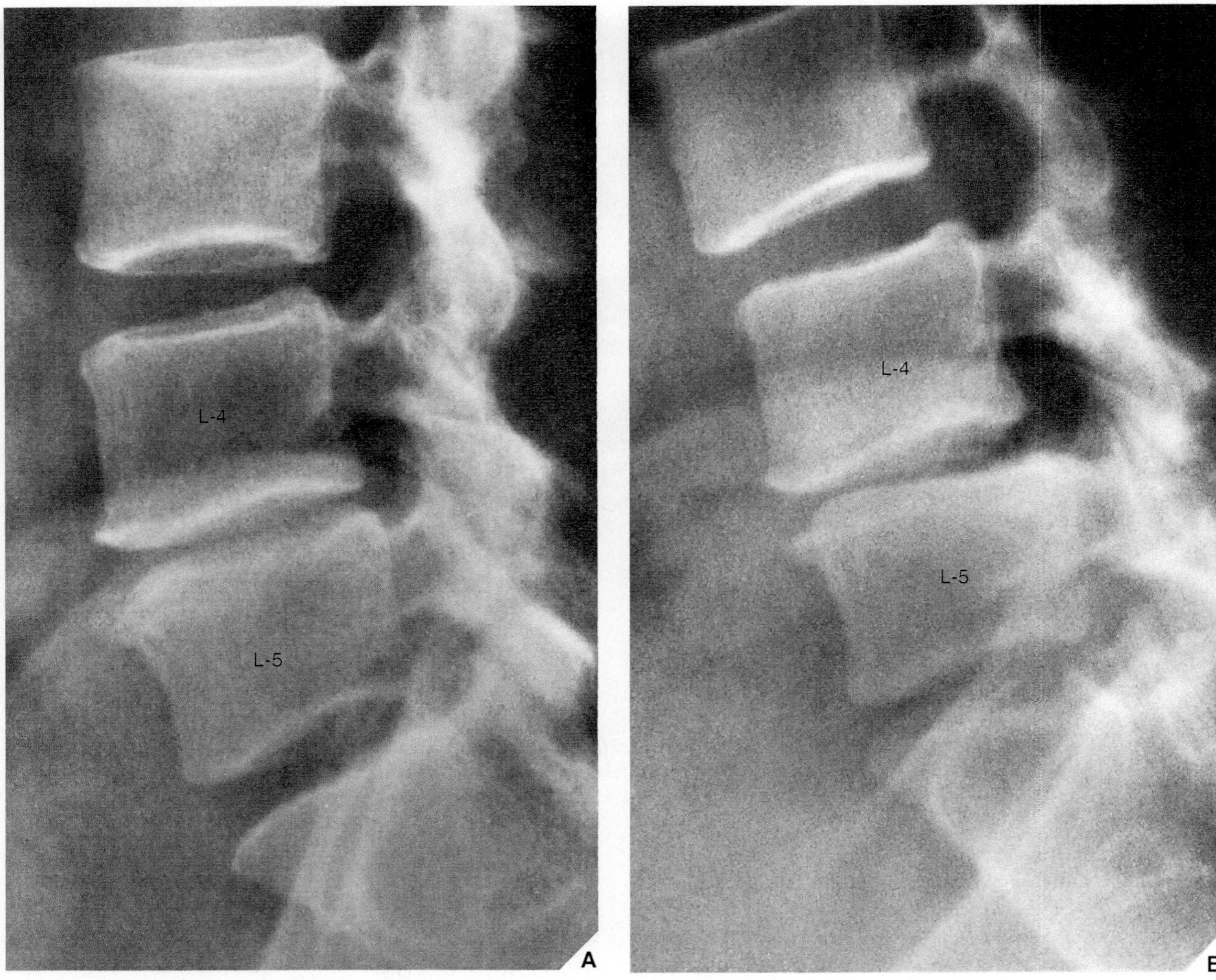

FIGURE 13.79 Degenerative spondylolisthesis. A 50-year-old man presented with chronic low back pain. **(A)** Standard lateral radiograph of the lumbosacral spine in the neutral position shows narrowing of the L4-5 disk space, indicating degenerative disk disease. There is no evidence of vertebral list. **(B)** Lateral radiograph in flexion, however, demonstrates grade 1 spondylolisthesis at L4-5.

obvious on the standard lateral film, and radiographs must be obtained while the patient maximally extends and flexes the spine (Fig. 13.79). As Milgram pointed out, the stress applied by forward and backward motion of the spine discloses instability (spondylolisthesis), which may be overlooked on other projections.

Degenerative spondylolisthesis occurs in approximately 4% of patients with degenerative disk disease and affects women more frequently than men. It has a predilection for the L4-5 spinal level. This predilection has been attributed to developmental or acquired alterations in the neural arch that lead to instability and abnormal stress. The stress applied to the vertebra may result in decompensation of the ligaments, hypermobility, instability, and OA of adjacent apophyseal joints.

Clinical symptoms associated with degenerative spondylolisthesis include low back pain with or without radiation into the leg, sciatic pain with signs of nerve root compression, and intermittent claudication of the cauda equina. It should be noted, however, that many patients with degenerative spondylolisthesis are asymptomatic.

Radiographic findings of degenerative spondylolisthesis include osteoarthritic changes of the facet joints (joint narrowing, marginal eburnation, and osteophyte formation), anterior slippage of the superior vertebra on the inferior vertebra, and, in many instances, intervertebral vacuum phenomenon (see Fig. 13.72). Invariably, the affected intervertebral disk space is narrowed. CT may also effectively demonstrate this complication.

The intervertebral vacuum phenomenon associated with degenerative disk disease should not be confused with the intravertebral vacuum cleft sign. This sign appears on radiographs as a transverse, linear, or semilunar radiolucency located within the vertebral body. According to recent reports, this sign represents gas (principally nitrogen) in the fracture line of the vertebral body. Although the pathogenesis of this process is not completely clear, the sign is most suggestive of ischemic necrosis of bone. This phenomenon has been also reported in association with Kümmell disease, a delayed posttraumatic collapse of the vertebral body (Fig. 13.80).

Spinal Stenosis

Spinal stenosis is a much more severe complication of degenerative disease of the spine. In its acquired form, it results from hypertrophy of the structures surrounding the spinal canal, such as the pedicles, laminae, articular processes, and posterior aspect of the vertebral bodies as well as the ligamentum flavum. These alternations usually are apparent on conventional radiography; however, spinal stenosis can be better demonstrated by ancillary techniques. Spinal stenosis can be demonstrated by myelography, which can show the impingement of the thecal sac by hypertrophic changes of the posterior parts of the vertebral body and bulging disks, but CT best delineates its details (Fig. 13.81). MRI is also an effective modality in this respect (Figs. 13.82 and 13.83).

Spinal stenosis in the lumbar segment can be divided into three groups on the basis of its anatomic location: stenosis of the spinal canal, stenosis of the subarticular or lateral recesses, and stenosis of the neural foramina.

The causes of stenosis of the central canal are related to hypertrophic changes of OA of the apophyseal joints, thickening of the ligamentum flavum, and osteophytes arising from the vertebral bodies. Bone hypertrophy at the site of the facet joints is a major cause of stenosis of the subarticular or lateral recesses, leading to encroachment on the neural elements in this region. Clinical manifestations of lateral recess syndrome include unilateral or

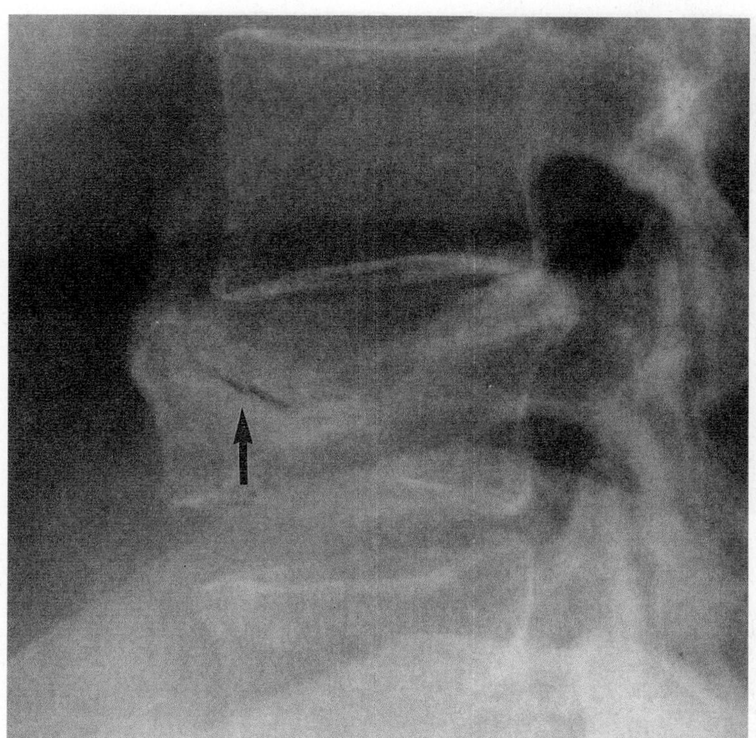

FIGURE 13.80 Kümmell disease. Lateral radiograph of the lumbar spine shows posttraumatic collapse of the vertebral body of L4 associated with intravertebral vacuum cleft sign *(arrow)*.

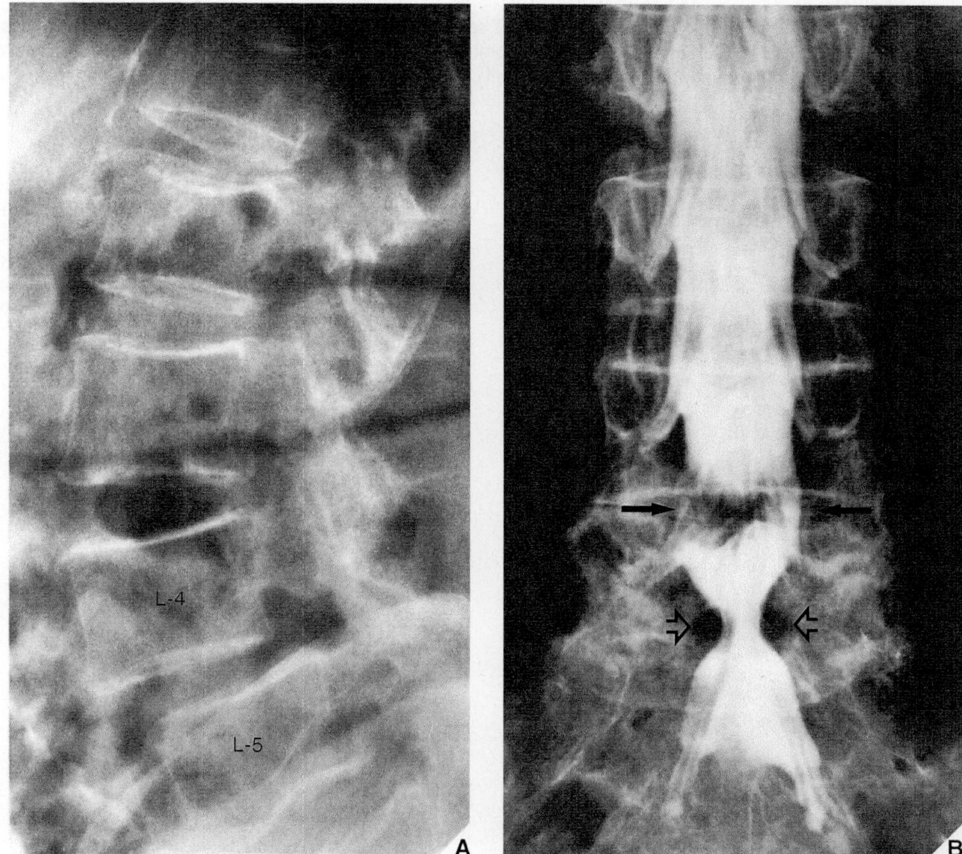

FIGURE 13.81 Myelography and CT of spinal stenosis. A 71-year-old woman was evaluated for severe low back pain. **(A)** Standard lateral radiograph of the lumbar spine shows degenerative spondylolisthesis at the L4-5 interspace. Note the short appearance of the pedicles. **(B)** Myelogram in the anteroposterior projection also discloses segmental narrowing of the thecal sac; the upper defect is related to spondylolisthesis *(arrows)*, the lower to spinal stenosis *(open arrows)*. *(Continued)*

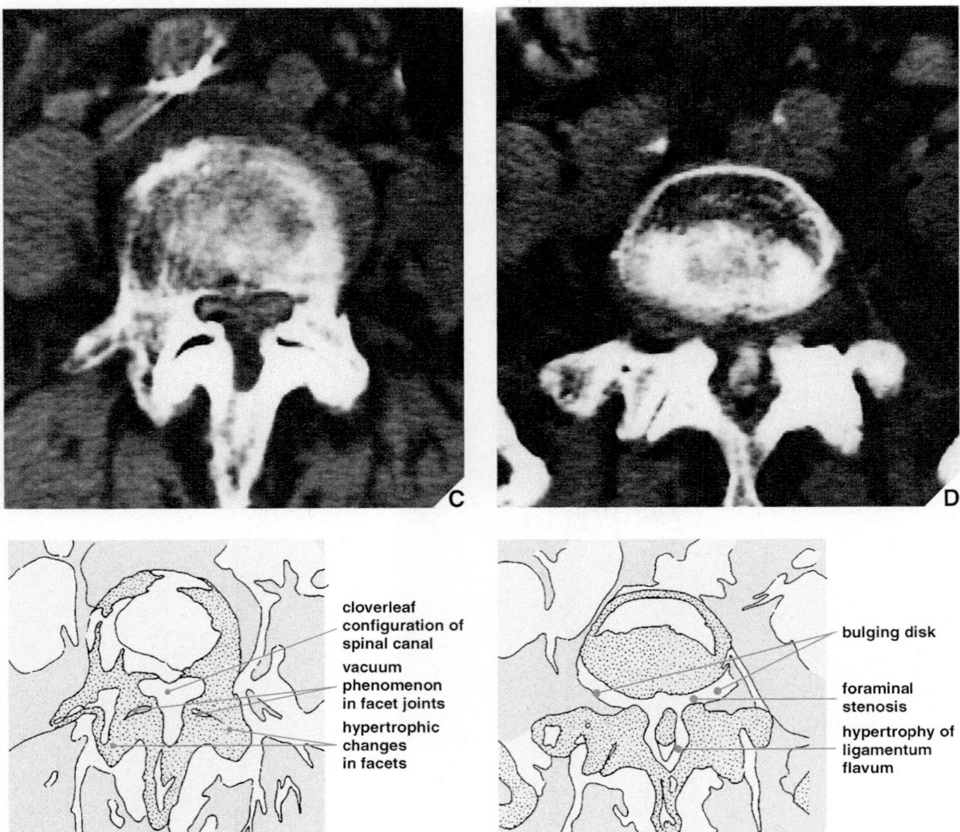

FIGURE 13.81 Myelography and CT of spinal stenosis. ***(Continued)*** **(C,D)** CT sections demonstrate the details of the abnormalities—severe spinal and foraminal stenosis, hypertrophy of the ligamenta flava, and posterior bulging of the intervertebral disk. Note the cloverleaf configuration of the spinal canal secondary to marked hypertrophy of the facet joints. The vacuum phenomenon in the apophyseal joints is well demonstrated.

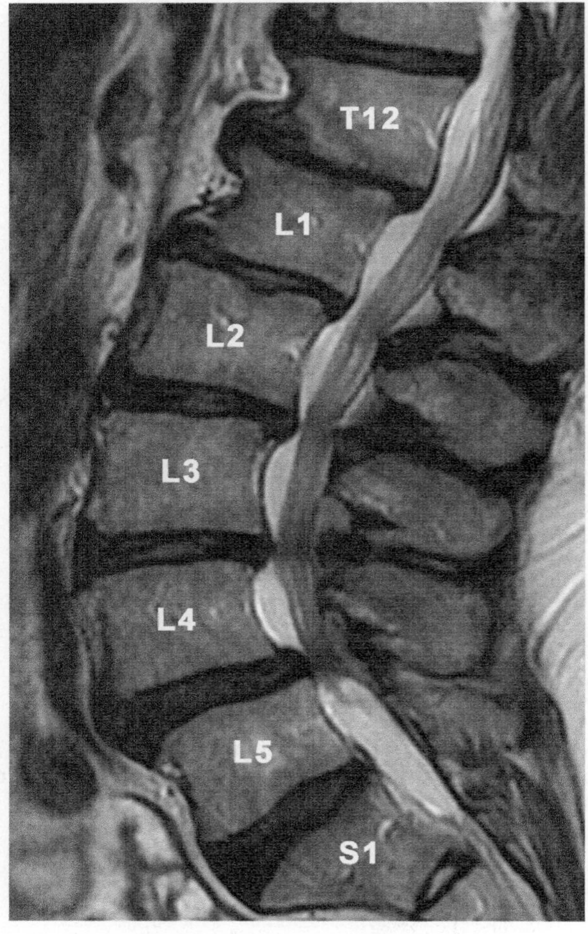

FIGURE 13.82 MRI of spinal stenosis. A 67-year-old man presented with low back pain and right-sided radiculopathy. Sagittal T2-weighted MR image shows exaggerated lumbar lordosis, degenerative disk disease at multiple levels associated with posterior bulging, retrospondylolisthesis at T12-L1, L1-2, L2-3, and L3-4 levels, anterolisthesis at L4-5 level, narrowing of the spinal canal, and compression of the cauda equina nerve roots.

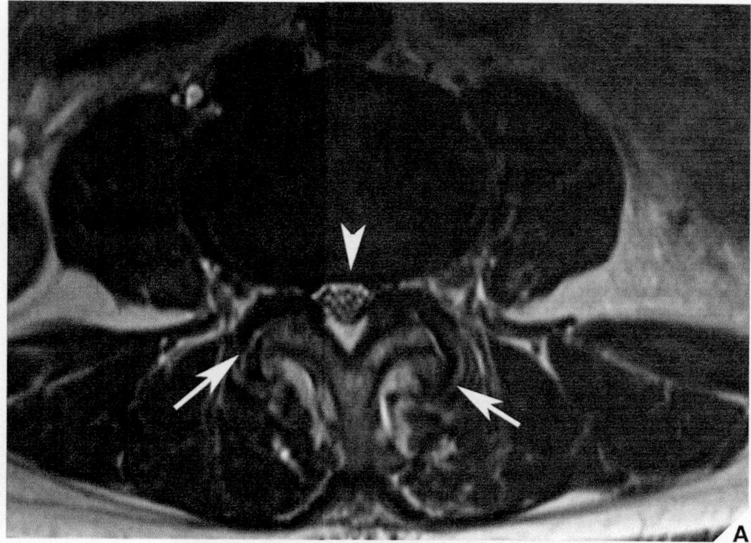

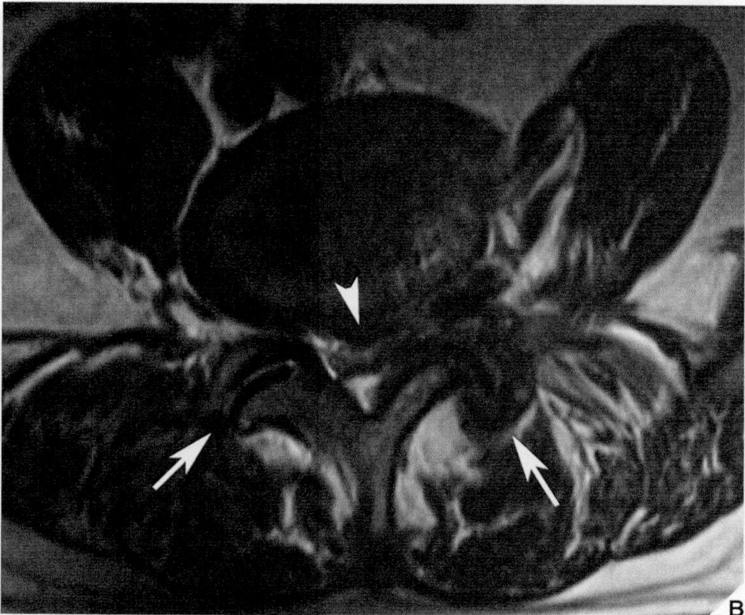

FIGURE 13.83 MRI of spinal stenosis. **(A)** Moderate spinal canal and thecal sac stenosis in a 45-year-old man. Degenerative changes of the facet joints *(arrows)* and disk bulging *(arrowhead)* contributed to central canal stenosis at the L4-5 disk level, as demonstrated here on T2-weighted axial MR image. Note the clumping of the nerve roots within the thecal sac. **(B)** Severe spinal canal stenosis in an 86-year-old woman. Axial T2-weighted MRI demonstrates almost complete collapse of the thecal sac at L4-5 level due to a combination of annular bulge with a central disk herniation *(arrowhead)* and severe facet arthrosis *(arrows)*.

bilateral leg pain, which is initiated or aggravated by long periods of standing or walking. These symptoms are usually relieved entirely by sitting or squatting. The stenosis of the neural foramina is caused by hypertrophic changes and osteophytosis involving the vertebral body and articular process. Moreover, degenerative spondylolisthesis may be associated with distortion of the intervertebral foramen and may lead to compromise of the exiting nerve.

Neuropathic Arthropathy

This acute or chronic destructive arthritis, also known as *Charcot joint*, is grouped with other degenerative joint diseases because it exhibits manifestations similar to those seen in other forms of OA—destruction of articular cartilage, subchondral sclerosis, and marginal osteophytosis—but in the most severe form. Neuropathic arthropathy comprises a spectrum of destructive processes in the joint associated with neurosensory deficit. Pathognomonic for neuropathic joints are fragmentation of the bone and cartilage, which are discharged as debris into the joint; chronic synovitis with accumulation of varying amounts of fluid in the joint; and joint instability manifested by subluxation and dislocation (Fig. 13.84). Underlying conditions leading to neuropathic joint include, among others, diabetes mellitus, syphilis, leprosy, syringomyelia, congenital indifference to pain, and spina bifida with meningomyelocele (Table 13.2). In diabetic patients, the condition has a greater predilection for the joints of the foot and ankle (Fig. 13.85); in patients with syringomyelia, joints of the upper extremities are more commonly affected (Fig. 13.86). The eponym *Charcot joint* was originally reserved for neuropathic joint in syphilitic patients with tabes dorsalis (Fig. 13.87). Currently, this term applies to any joint displaying features of neuropathic arthropathy, regardless of the causative factor. MRI is an effective modality to demonstrate the imaging details of this condition (Fig. 13.88).

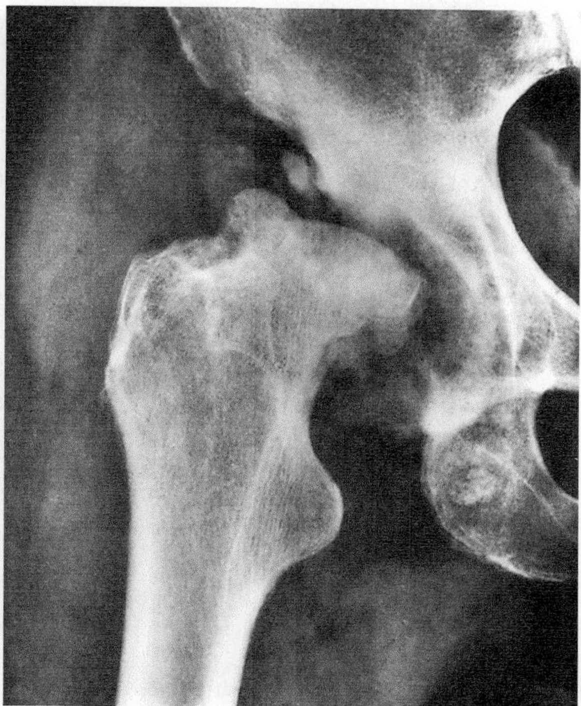

FIGURE 13.84 Neuropathic joint. Anteroposterior radiograph of the right hip of a 57-year-old woman with neurosyphilis (tabes dorsalis) shows the typical features of neuropathic (Charcot) joint. There is complete disorganization of the joint, fragmentation, and subluxation. The absence of osteoporosis is a characteristic feature of the neuropathic joint. This condition represents the most severe manifestation of degenerative joint disease.

TABLE 13.2 Causes of Neuropathic Arthropathy
Alcoholism
Amyloidosis
Charcot-Marie-Tooth disease
Congenital indifference to pain
Diabetes mellitus
Extrinsic compression of the spinal cord
Familial dysautonomia (Riley-Day syndrome)
Meningomyelocele
Multiple sclerosis
Peripheral nerve tumors
Pernicious anemia
Poliomyelitis
Spinal cord tumors
Steroids (systemic or intraarticular)
Syringomyelia
Tabes dorsalis (syphilis)
Uremia

Modified from Jones EA, Manaster BJ, May DA, et al. Neuropathic osteoarthropathy: diagnostic dilemmas and differential diagnosis. *Radiographics* 2000;20:S279–S293.

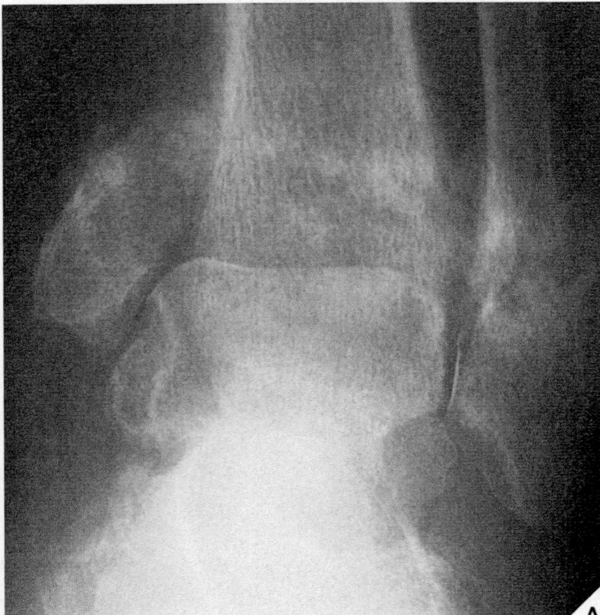

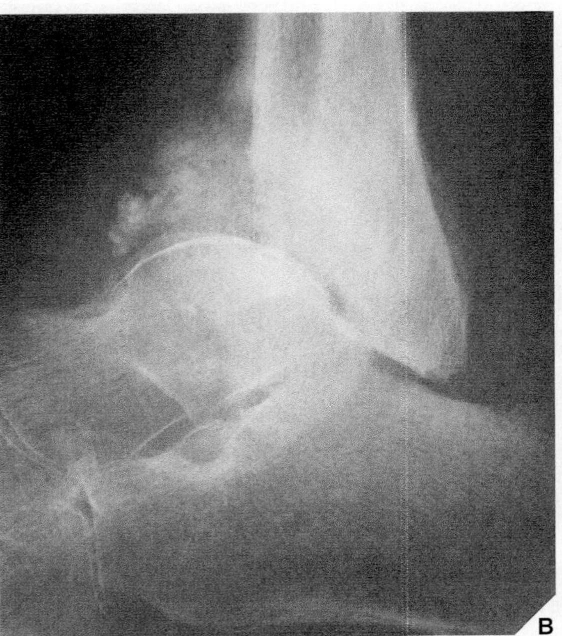

FIGURE 13.85 **Neuropathic joint.** A 59-year-old woman with long-standing diabetes mellitus presented with neuropathic changes of left ankle joint, demonstrated here on the anteroposterior **(A)** and lateral **(B)** radiographs.

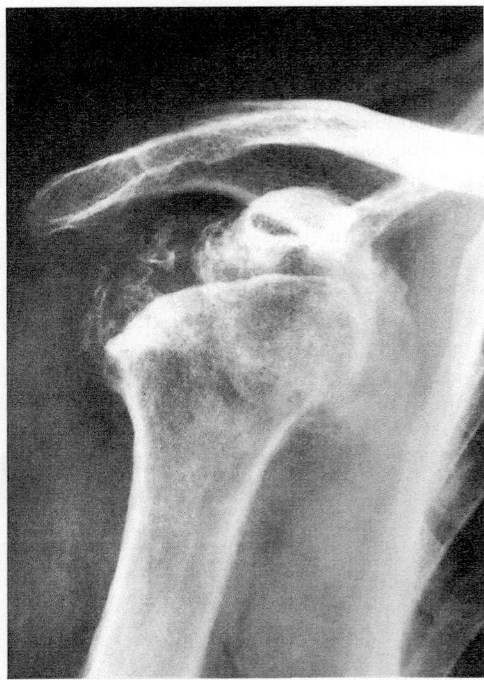

FIGURE 13.86 **Neuropathic joint.** A 59-year-old woman with syringomyelia developed a neuropathic shoulder joint. Anteroposterior radiograph shows destruction of the joint, bony debris, and subluxation of the humeral head.

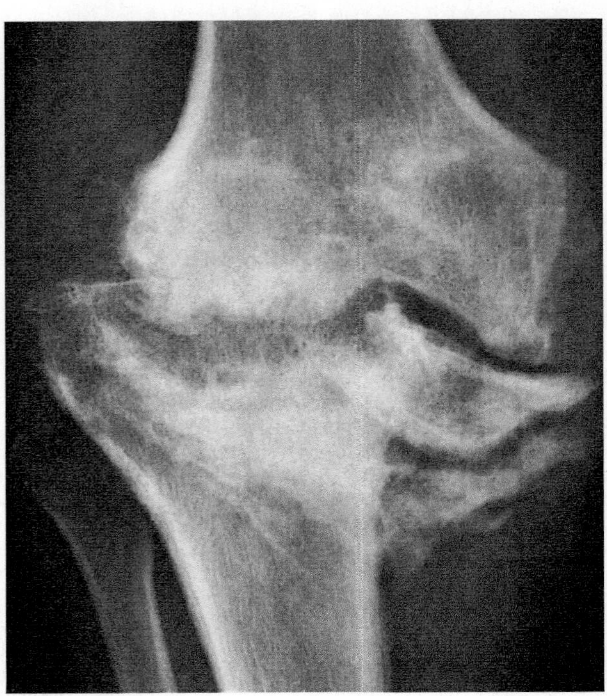

FIGURE 13.87 **Neuropathic joint.** A 62-year-old man with syphilis presented with a typical neuropathic (Charcot) knee joint.

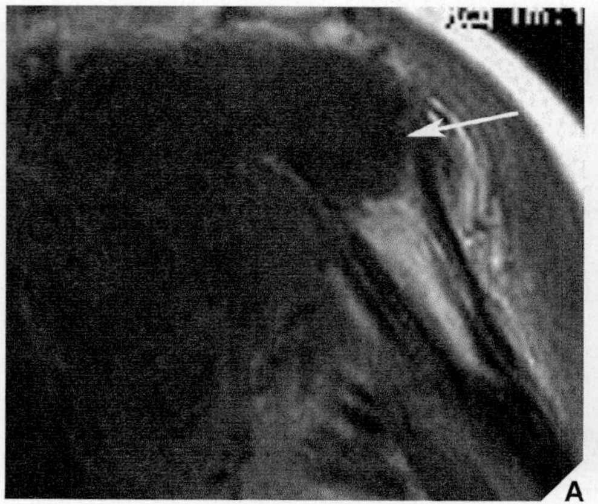

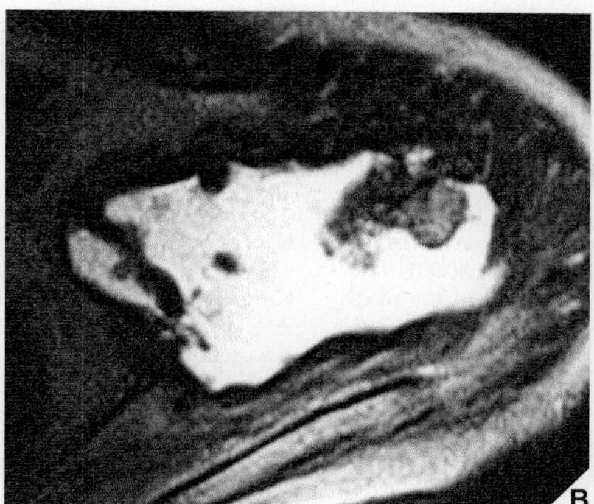

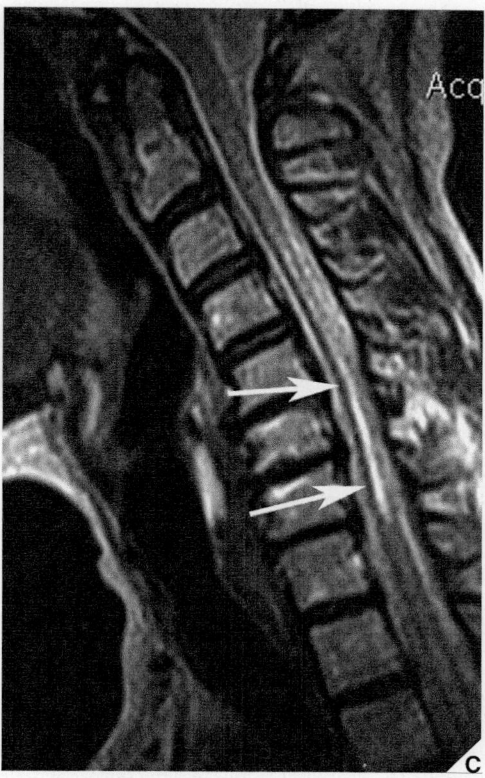

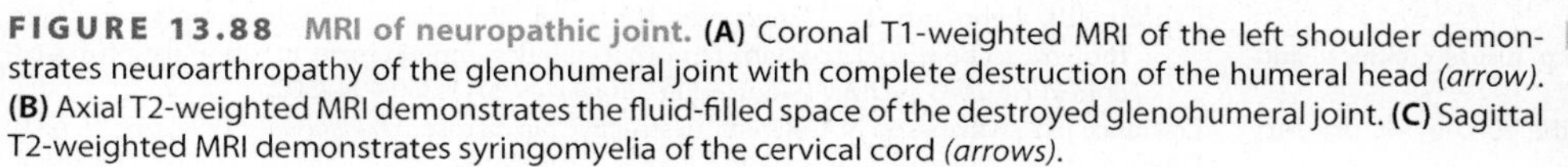

FIGURE 13.88 MRI of neuropathic joint. **(A)** Coronal T1-weighted MRI of the left shoulder demonstrates neuroarthropathy of the glenohumeral joint with complete destruction of the humeral head *(arrow)*. **(B)** Axial T2-weighted MRI demonstrates the fluid-filled space of the destroyed glenohumeral joint. **(C)** Sagittal T2-weighted MRI demonstrates syringomyelia of the cervical cord *(arrows)*.

PRACTICAL POINTS TO REMEMBER

Osteoarthritis

1. Degenerative joint disease (OA, osteoarthrosis, degenerative arthritis) is classified as primary (idiopathic) or secondary; in the latter, there is an underlying predisposing disorder.
2. The radiographic hallmarks of OA are:
   - diminution (narrowing) of the joint space
   - subchondral sclerosis
   - osteophytosis
   - cyst or pseudocyst formation
   - lack of pronounced osteoporosis.

Osteoarthritis of the Large Joints

1. In the hip joint, the degenerative process results in migration of the femoral head, most commonly in a superolateral direction.
2. One of the most common causes of precocious secondary OA of the hip joint is FAI syndrome. Two types have been recognized: cam, where abnormality is at the femoral head/neck junction; and pincer, commonly resulting from acetabular retroversion.
3. Postel coxarthropathy is a rapidly destructive arthrosis of the hip joint, which radiographically can mimic infection or neuropathic joint.
4. The medial femorotibial and femoropatellar compartments of the knee joint are commonly involved in OA. Weight-bearing examination may reveal a varus configuration of the knee.
5. The tooth sign of the patella, recognized on an axial view by vertical ridges at the insertion of the quadriceps tendon into the base of the patella, represents a type of degenerative change (enthesopathy) unrelated to femoropatellar OA. It is commonly seen after the fifth decade of life.
6. If the shoulder, elbow, or ankle joints are affected by degenerative joint disease, a diagnosis of secondary rather than primary OA should be considered.

Osteoarthritis of the Small Joints

1. In the hand, the hallmarks of primary degenerative joint disease are:
   - Heberden nodes affecting the distal interphalangeal joints
   - Bouchard nodes affecting the proximal interphalangeal joints.
2. The first carpometacarpal articulation is frequently involved in primary degenerative joint disease.

Degenerative Disease of the Spine

1. In the spine, degenerative changes may be present in four major forms:
   - as OA of the synovial joints, including the atlantoaxial, apophyseal, costovertebral, and sacroiliac
   - as spondylosis deformans, a condition manifested by formation of anterior and lateral marginal osteophytes with preservation of the disk spaces (at least in the early stages)
   - as degenerative disk disease, a condition primarily involving the intervertebral disks and manifested by the destruction of these structures, the vacuum phenomenon, and narrowing of the disk spaces
   - as DISH syndrome or Forestier disease, characterized by flowing ossifications along the anterior aspects of vertebral bodies extending across the disk spaces, relative preservation of the intervertebral disks, and hyperostosis at the sites of tendon and ligament attachment to the bone (enthesopathy).
2. Two common conditions can complicate degenerative spine disease:
   - degenerative spondylolisthesis
   - spinal stenosis.
3. Degenerative spondylolisthesis is marked by anterior (ventral) displacement of a vertebra onto the one below and recognized on the lateral view of the spine by the spinous-process sign.
4. Spinal stenosis can readily be diagnosed using CT or MRI.

Neuropathic Arthropathy

1. Neuropathic (Charcot) joint manifests with the same degenerative changes as OA but seen in the most severe form. This condition is also marked by:
   - fragmentation of the bone and cartilage, filling the joint with debris
   - chronic synovitis with joint effusion
   - joint instability with subluxation or dislocation.
2. The underlying conditions leading to neuropathic joint include diabetes mellitus, syphilis, leprosy, syringomyelia, and congenital indifference to pain.

SUGGESTED READINGS

Ahlbäck S. Osteoarthritis of the knee. A radiographic investigation. *Acta Radiol Diagn (Stockh)* 1968;(suppl 277):7–72.

Ali M, Mohamed A, Ahmed HE, et al. The use of ultrasound-guided platelet-rich plasma injections in the treatment of hip osteoarthritis: a systematic review of the literature. *J Ultrason* 2018;18:332–337.

Audenaert EA, Baelde N, Huysse W, et al. Development of three-dimensional detection method of cam deformities in femoroacetabular impingement. *Skeletal Radiol* 2011;40:921–927.

Bennett GL, Leeson MC, Michael A. Extensive hemosiderin deposition in the medial meniscus of a knee. Its possible relationship to degenerative joint disease. *Clin Orthop Relat Res* 1988;230:182–185.

Bhalla S, Reinus WR. The linear intravertebral vacuum: a sign of benign vertebral collapse. *AJR Am J Roentgenol* 1998;170:1563–1569.

Bittersohl B, Hosalkar HS, Apprich S, et al. Comparison of pre-operative dGEMRIC imaging with intra-operative findings in femoroacetabular impingement: preliminary findings. *Skeletal Radiol* 2011;40:553–561.

Blackburn WD Jr, Chivers S, Bernreuter W. Cartilage imaging in osteoarthritis. *Semin Arthritis Rheum* 1996;25:273–281.

Bock GW, Garcia A, Weisman MH, et al. Rapidly destructive hip disease: clinical and imaging abnormalities. *Radiology* 1993;186:461–466.

Bora FW Jr, Miller G. Joint physiology, cartilage metabolism, and the etiology of osteoarthritis. *Hand Clin* 1987;3:325–336.

Boutry N, Paul C, Leroy X, et al. Rapidly destructive osteoarthritis of the hip: MR imaging findings. *AJR Am J Roentgenol* 2002;179:657–663.

Broderick LS, Turner DA, Renfrew DL, et al. Severity of articular cartilage abnormality in patients with osteoarthritis: evaluation with fast spin-echo MR vs arthroscopy. *AJR Am J Roentgenol* 1994;162:99–103.

Brower AC, Downey EF. Kümmell disease: report of a case with serial radiographs. *Radiology* 1981;141:363–364.

Buckwalter JA, Mankin HG. Articular cartilage. II. Degeneration and osteoarthritis, repair, regeneration, and transplantation. *J Bone Joint Surg Am* 1997;79A:612–632.

Buckwalter JA, Mow VC. Cartilage repair in osteoarthritis. In: Moskowitz RW, Howell DS, Goldberg VM, et al, eds. *Osteoarthritis*, 2nd ed. Philadelphia: WB Saunders; 1992:71–107.

Bullough PG. The pathology of osteoarthritis. In: Moskowitz RW, Howell DS, Goldberg VM, et al, eds. *Osteoarthritis*, 2nd ed. Philadelphia: WB Saunders; 1992:39–69.

Bullough PG, Bansal M. The differential diagnosis of geodes. *Radiol Clin North Am* 1988;26:1165–1184.

Chan WP, Lang P, Stevens MP, et al. Osteoarthritis of the knee: comparison of radiography, CT, and MR imaging to assess extent and severity. *AJR Am J Roentgenol* 1991;157:799–806.

Charcot JM. Sur quelques arthropathies qui paraissent dépendre d'une lesion du cervean ou de la moëlle épindère. *Arch Physiol Norm Pathol* 1868;1:161–178.

Charran AK, Tony G, Lalam R, et al. Destructive discovertebral degenerative disease of the lumbar spine. *Skeletal Radiol* 2012;41:1213–1221.

Chen L, Boonthathip M, Cardoso F, et al. Acetabulum protrusio and center edge angle: new MR-imaging measurement criteria—a correlative study with measurement derived from conventional radiography. *Skeletal Radiol* 2009;38:123–129.

Chou L, Knight R. Idiopathic avascular necrosis of a vertebral body. Case report and literature review. *Spine (Phila Pa 1976)* 1997;22:1928–1932.

Cicuttini FM, Spector TD. Genetics of osteoarthritis. *Ann Rheum Dis* 1996;55:665–667.

Cohn EL, Maurer EJ, Keats TE, et al. Plain film evaluation of degenerative disk disease at the lumbosacral junction. *Skeletal Radiol* 1997;26:161–166.

Dandachli W, Najefi A, Iranpour F, et al. Quantifying the contribution of pincer deformity to femoro-acetabular impingement using 3D computerised tomography. *Skeletal Radiol* 2012;41:1295–1300.

Dieppe P, Cushnaghan J. The natural course and prognosis of osteoarthritis. In: Moskowitz RW, Howell DS, Goldberg VM, et al, eds. *Osteoarthritis*, 2nd ed. Philadelphia: WB Saunders; 1992:399–412.

Ellermann J, Ziegler C, Nissi MJ, et al. Acetabular cartilage assessment in patients with femoroacetabular impingement by using T2* mapping with arthroscopic verification. *Radiology* 2014;271:512–523.

Felson DT. The course of osteoarthritis and factors that affect it. *Rheum Dis Clin North Am* 1993;19:607–615.

Filardo G, Kon E, Buda R, et al. Platelet-rich plasma intra-articular knee injections for treatment of degenerative cartilage lesions and osteoarthritis. *Knee Surg Sports Traumatol Arthrosc* 2011;19:528–535.

Forestier J, Rotes-Querol J. Senile ankylosing hyperostosis of the spine. *Ann Rheum Dis* 1950;9:321–330.

Ganz R, Parvizi J, Beck M, et al. Femoroacetabular impingement: a cause for osteoarthritis of the hip. *Clin Orthop Relat Res* 2003;417:112–120.

Giori NJ, Trousdale RT. Acetabular retroversion is associated with osteoarthritis of the hip. *Clin Orthop Relat Res* 2003;417:263–269.

Golimbu C, Firooznia H, Rafii M. The intravertebral vacuum sign. *Spine (Phila Pa 1976)* 1986;11:1040–1043.

Greenspan A, Norman A, Tchang FKM. "Tooth" sign in patellar degenerative disease. *J Bone Joint Surg Am* 1977;59A:483–485.

Gross A, Ma CB. Approach to the patient with knee pain. In: Imboden JB, Hellmann DB, Stone JH, eds. *Current diagnosis & treatment in rheumatology*, 3rd ed. New York: McGraw-Hill; 2013:110–123.

Hashemi SA, Dehghani J, Vosoughi AR. Can the crossover sign be a reliable marker of global retroversion of the acetabulum? *Skeletal Radiol* 2017;46:17–21.

Hayward I, Björkengren AG, Pathria MN, et al. Patterns of femoral head migration in osteoarthritis of the hip: a reappraisal with CT and pathologic correlation. *Radiology* 1988;166:857–860.

Hill CL, Gale DG, Chaisson CE, et al. Knee effusions, popliteal cysts, and synovial thickening: association with knee pain in osteoarthritis. *J Rheumatol* 2001;28:1330–1337.

Jacobson JA, Girish G, Jiang Y, et al. Radiographic evaluation of arthritis: degenerative joint disease and variations. *Radiology* 2008;248:737–747.

Jones EA, Manaster BJ, May DA, et al. Neuropathic osteoarthropathy: diagnostic dilemmas and differential diagnosis. *Radiographics* 2000;20:S279–S293.

Jungmann PM, Liu F, Link TM. What has imaging contributed to the epidemiological understanding of osteoarthritis? *Skeletal Radiol* 2014;43:271–275.

Kassarjian A, Yoon LS, Belzile E, et al. Triad of MR arthrographic findings in patients with cam-type femoroacetabular impingement. *Radiology* 2005;236:588–592.

Kellgren JH, Lawrence JS. Radiological assessment of osteo-arthrosis. *Ann Rheum Dis* 1957;16:494–502.

Kellgren JH, Moore R. Generalized osteoarthritis and Heberden's nodes. *Br Med J* 1952;1:181–187.

Kim JA, Park JS, Jin W, et al. Herniation pits in the femoral neck: a radiographic indicator of femoroacetabular impingement? *Skeletal Radiol* 2011;40:167–172.

Kornaat PR, Ceulemans RY, Kroon HM, et al. MRI assessment of knee osteoarthritis: Knee Osteoarthritis Scoring System (KOSS)—inter-observer and intra-observer reproducibility of a compartment-based scoring system. *Skeletal Radiol* 2005;34:95–102.

Laborie LB, Lehmann TG, Engesæter IØ, et al. Prevalence of radiographic findings thought to be associated with femoroacetabular impingement in a population-based cohort of 2081 healthy young adults. *Radiology* 2011;260:494–502.

Lawrance JAL, Athanasou NA. Rapidly destructive hip disease. *Skeletal Radiol* 1995;24:639–641.

Leone A, Cassar-Pullicino VN, Semprini A, et al. Neuropathic osteoarthropathy with and without superimposed osteomyelitis in patients with a diabetic foot. *Skeletal Radiol* 2016;45:735–754.

Lequesne MG. La coxarthrose destructrice rapide. *Rhumatologie* 1970;22:51–63.

Lequesne MG, Laredo J-D. The faux profil (oblique view) of the hip in the standing position. Contribution to the evaluation of osteoarthritis of the adult hip. *Ann Rheum Dis* 1998;57:676–681.

Mankin HJ, Brandt KD. Biochemistry and metabolism of articular cartilage in osteoarthritis. In: Moskowitz RW, Howell DS, Goldberg VM, et al, eds. *Osteoarthritis*, 2nd ed. Philadelphia: WB Saunders; 1992:109–154.

Melville DM, Taljanovic MS, Scalcione LR, et al. Imaging and management of thumb carpometacarpal joint osteoarthritis. *Skeletal Radiol* 2015;44:165–177.

Milgram JE. Recurrent articular spondylolisthesis: common cause of vertebral instabilities, root pain, sciatica, and ultimately spinal stenosis. Early detection and blocking of specific dislocations. *Bull Hosp Jt Dis Orthop Inst* 1986;46:47–51.

Modic MT, Masaryk TJ, Ross JS, et al. Imaging of degenerative disk disease. *Radiology* 1988;168:177–186.

Modic MT, Steinberg PM, Ross JS, et al. Degenerative disk disease: assessment of changes in vertebral body marrow with MR imaging. *Radiology* 1988;166:193–199.

Nötzli HP, Wyss TF, Stoecklin CH, et al. The contour of the femoral head-neck junction as a predictor for the risk of anterior impingement. *J Bone Joint Surg Br* 2002;84:556–560.

Pfirrmann CWA, Mengiardi B, Dora C, et al. Cam and pincer femoroacetabular impingement: characteristic MR arthrographic findings in 50 patients. *Radiology* 2006;240:778–785.

Pollard TCB. A perspective on femoroacetabular impingement. *Skeletal Radiol* 2011;40:815–818.

Postel M, Kerboull M. Total prosthetic replacement in rapidly destructive arthrosis of the hip joint. *Clin Orthop Relat Res* 1970;72:138–144.

Ranawat AS, Schulz B, Baumbach SF, et al. Radiographic predictors of hip pain in femoroacetabular impingement. *HSS J* 2011;7:115–119.

Reichenbach S, Jüni P, Werlen S, et al. Prevalence of cam-type deformity on hip magnetic resonance imaging in young males: a cross-sectional study. *Arthritis Care Res (Hoboken)* 2010;62:1319–1327.

Resnick D. Patterns of migration of the femoral head in osteoarthritis of the hip. Roentgenographic-pathologic correlation and comparison with rheumatoid arthritis. *Am J Roentgenol Radium Ther Nucl Med* 1975;124:62–74.

Resnick D, Niwayama G. Diffuse idiopathic skeletal hyperostosis (DISH): ankylosing hyperostosis of Forestier and Rotes-Querol. In: Resnick D, ed. *Diagnosis of bone and joint disorders*, 3rd ed. Philadelphia: WB Saunders; 1995:1463–1495.

Resnick D, Shaul SR, Robins JM. Diffuse idiopathic skeletal hyperostosis (DISH). Forestier's disease with extraspinal manifestations. *Radiology* 1975;115:513–524.

Rosenberg ZS, Shankman S, Steiner GC, et al. Rapid destructive osteoarthritis: clinical, radiographic, and pathologic features. *Radiology* 1992;182:213–216.

Sánchez M, Guadilla J, Fiz N, et al. Ultrasound-guided platelet-rich plasma injections for the treatment of osteoarthritis of the hip. *Rheumatology (Oxford)* 2012;51:144–150.

Sandell LJ. Etiology of osteoarthritis: genetics and synovial joint involvement. *Nat Rev Rheumatol* 2012;8:77–89.

Schiebler ML, Grenier N, Fallon M, et al. Normal and degenerated intervertebral disk: in vivo and in vitro MR imaging with histopathologic correlation. *AJR Am J Roentgenol* 1991;157:93–97.

Schmorl G, Junghanns H. *The human spine in health and disease*, 2nd ed. New York: Grune & Stratton; 1971.

Schumacher HR. Articular cartilage in the degenerative arthropathy of hemochromatosis. *Arthritis Rheum* 1982;25:1460–1468.

Sienbenrock KA, Schoeniger R, Ganz R. Anterior femoroacetabular impingement due to acetabular retroversion: treatment with periacetabular osteotomy. *J Bone Joint Surg Am* 2003;85:278–286.

Watt I. Osteoarthritis revisited—again! *Skeletal Radiol* 2009;38:419–423.

Watt I, Dieppe P. Osteoarthritis revisited. *Skeletal Radiol* 1990;19:1–3.

Werner CML, Copeland CE, Stromberg J, et al. Correlation of the cross-over ratio of the cross-over sign on conventional pelvic radiographs with computed tomography retroversion measurements. *Skeletal Radiol* 2010;39:655–660.

Xu L, Hayashi D, Guermazi A, et al. The diagnostic performance of radiography for detection of osteoarthritis-associated features compared with MRI in hip joints with chronic pain. *Skeletal Radiol* 2013;42:1421–1428.

14

Inflammatory Arthritides

The inflammatory arthritides comprise a group of diverse monoarticular and systemic disorders (see Fig. 12.1) that have in common one important feature: inflammatory pannus eroding articular cartilage and bone (Fig. 14.1). An overview of the clinical and radiographic hallmarks of the various inflammatory arthritides is shown in Table 14.1.

Erosive Osteoarthritis

Erosive osteoarthritis (EOA) was first described by Kellgren and Moore in 1952 and reintroduced in 1961 by Crain, who called it *interphalangeal osteoarthritis* (OA). He defined this disorder as a localized variant of OA involving the finger joints, characterized by degenerative changes with intermittent inflammatory episodes leading to deformities and ankylosis. In 1966, Peter and Pearson coined the term *erosive osteoarthritis*, and Ehrlich in 1972 described it as inflammatory OA, based on the clinical symptoms of swelling, tenderness, erythema, and warmth. EOA can be defined as a progressive disorder of the interphalangeal joints with severe synovitis, superimposed on the changes of degenerative joint disease. Although the cause is still unclear, several investigators have suggested hormonal influences, metabolic background, autoimmunity, and heredity as being involved.

Clinical Features

EOA is a progressive inflammatory arthritis seen predominantly in middle-aged women. Only rarely are men affected, with an estimated female-to-male ratio of 12:1. Patients' ages range from 36 to 83 years, and mean age of onset is 50.5 years. This condition combines certain clinical manifestations of rheumatoid arthritis (RA) with certain imaging features of degenerative joint disease. Involvement is limited to the hands, with the proximal and distal interphalangeal joints being the most frequently affected. Large joints, such as the hip or shoulder, are only rarely involved. The arthritis usually begins abruptly and is characterized by pain, swelling, and tenderness of the small joints of the hands. Also described are throbbing paresthesias of the fingertips and morning stiffness.

Pathology

Proliferative synovitis is the most common histopathologic feature of EOA and cannot be distinguished from that of seen in RA. Moreover, Peter et al. described findings in some patients consisting of degenerative cartilage with prominent subchondral granulation tissue, lymphocyte aggregates, plasma cell infiltration, and subsynovial fibrosis. Loose fibrin-like material was noted interstitially as well as villous hypertrophy, hyperemia and thickening of the blood vessel walls, and organizing amorphous exudates that overlaid the synovium. Generally speaking, the pathologic synovium of EOA exhibits features that are consistent with both RA and OA.

Imaging Features

In the early stage of the disease, the main feature is symmetric synovitis of the interphalangeal joints. Later, this is followed by articular erosions, which exhibit a characteristic radiographic feature named the *gull-wing deformity* by Martel. This configuration is seen as a result of central erosion and marginal proliferation of bone (Figs. 14.2 and 14.3); Heberden nodes may also be present. Periosteal reaction taking the form of linear or fluffy bone apposition over the cortex near the affected joints is occasionally observed. Swelling of soft tissue, usually fusiform, may be present around involved articulations (see Fig. 14.2C); however, periarticular osteoporosis is rarely present. Later in the disease process, bone ankylosis of the phalanges may develop (see Figs. 14.3E and 14.4B). Approximately 15% of patients with EOA may have clinical, laboratory, and radiographic manifestations of RA (Fig. 14.4). The exact relationship between these two conditions is still unclear. Some investigators believe that EOA is actually RA originating in unusual sites but subsequently progressing to the articulations that are more typically involved. Others suggest that each is a distinct entity, citing as evidence the fact that the synovial fluid of patients with RA does not resemble that of patients with EOA, that the immunologic abnormalities commonly seen in RA are absent in the latter condition, and that the serologic test for rheumatoid factor is negative.

Because imaging presentation of erosive and non-EOA may be similar, the investigators were looking into the other means to distinguish these two conditions. The recent studies of serum biomarkers were very promising in this respect. They demonstrated elevation of myeloperoxidase, C-reactive protein, and serum levels of nitrated form of a marker of type II collagen denaturation (Coll2-1NO2) in patients with EOA.

Differential Diagnosis

The conditions to be considered in differential diagnosis of EOA include primarily classic interphalangeal OA, RA, and psoriatic arthritis (PsA). In interphalangeal OA, certain features, including osteophytosis, subchondral sclerosis, narrowing of the joint spaces, and Heberden and Bouchard nodes, are similar to those of EOA. However, joint erosions and interphalangeal ankylosis are absent. The relationship of EOA to OA and RA still remains a matter of controversy. Some investigators regard EOA as an entirely separate entity, whereas others believe that it represents the end spectrum of OA or perhaps an interface between OA and RA (see Fig. 14.4). Ehrlich noted the superimposition of clinical, laboratory, and imaging features of RA in 62 of 170 patients (15%) whose initial diagnosis was EOA. He was first to suggest a relationship between EOA and RA. Conversely, Martel and associates hypothesize that erosions in EOA reflect the intensity and duration of inflammation, favoring the OA spectrum of the disease rather than separate disease entities. The distribution of affected joints in OA and EOA in the hand is identical, with a distinct propensity for distal interphalangeal and proximal interphalangeal joints as well as occasional involvement of the first carpometacarpal and

TABLE 14.1 Clinical and Imaging Hallmarks of Inflammatory Arthritides

Type of Arthritis	Site	Crucial Abnormalities	Technique[a]/Projection
Erosive osteoarthritis (F; middle age)	Hands	Involvement of	Dorsovolar view
		Proximal interphalangeal joints	
		Distal interphalangeal joints	
		Gull-wing deformities associated with erosions	
		Heberden nodes	
		Joint ankylosis	
Rheumatoid arthritis (F > M; presence of rheumatoid factor and DRW4)	Hands and wrists	Involvement of	Dorsovolar view
		Metacarpophalangeal joints	
		Proximal interphalangeal joints	
		Central and marginal erosions	Dorsovolar and Norgaard views, MRI
		Periarticular osteoporosis	Dorsovolar view
		Joint deformities: swan-neck, boutonnière, *main-en-lorgnette*, hitchhiker's thumb	Dorsovolar view
		Synovitis	Postcontrast MRI
		Pre-erosive edema	MRI
	Hip	Narrowing of joint space	Anteroposterior and lateral views
		Erosions	Anteroposterior and lateral views
		Acetabular protrusio	MRI
			Anteroposterior view
	Knee	Narrowing of joint space	Anteroposterior and lateral views
		Erosions	
		Synovial cysts	MRI
	Ankle and foot	Involvement of subtalar joint	Lateral view
		Erosions of calcaneus	Lateral and Broden views
			Lateral view (heel)
Juvenile idiopathic arthritis (JIA)	Hands	Joint ankylosis	Dorsovolar view (wrist and hand)
		Periosteal reaction	
		Growth abnormalities	
	Knees	Growth abnormalities	Anteroposterior and lateral views
	Cervical spine	Fusion of apophyseal joints	Anteroposterior, lateral, and oblique views
Rheumatoid variants		C1-2 subluxation	Lateral view in flexion
Ankylosing spondylitis (M > F; young adult; 95% positive for HLA-B27)	Spine	Squaring of vertebral bodies	Anteroposterior and lateral views
		Syndesmophytes	
		Bamboo spine	
		Paravertebral ossifications	
		Shiny corners	Lateral view
	Sacroiliac joints	Inflammatory changes	Posteroanterior and Ferguson views
		Fusion	
	Pelvis	Whiskering of iliac crests and ischial tuberosity	Anteroposterior view
Reactive arthritis (M > F)	Foot	Involvement of great toe articulations	Anteroposterior and lateral views
		Erosions of calcaneus	
	Spine	Single, coarse syndesmophyte	Anteroposterior and lateral views
	Sacroiliac joints	Unilateral or bilateral but asymmetric involvement	Posteroanterior and Ferguson views
			Computed tomography
			Postcontrast MRI
Psoriatic arthritis (M ≥ F; skin changes HLA-B27 positive)	Hands	Involvement of distal interphalangeal joints	Dorsovolar view
		Erosion of terminal tufts	
		Mouse-ear erosions	
		Pencil-in-cup deformities	
		Sausage digit	
		Joint ankylosis	
		Fluffy periosteal reaction	
	Foot	Involvement of distal interphalangeal joints	Anteroposterior and lateral views (ankle and foot)
		Erosions of terminal tufts and calcaneus	
	Spine	Single, coarse syndesmophyte	Anteroposterior and lateral views
	Sacroiliac joints	Unilateral or bilateral but asymmetric involvement	Posteroanterior and Ferguson views
			Postcontrast MRI
Enteropathic arthropathies	Sacroiliac joints	Symmetric involvement	Posteroanterior and Ferguson views
			CT (coronal and sagittal reformatted images)
SAPHO syndrome	Sternoclavicular, manubriosternal, and costosternal joints	Osteosclerosis, hyperostosis, cortical thickening, narrowing of the medullary canal	Postcontrast MRI
			Coronal CT

[a]Radionuclide bone scan is used to determine the distribution of arthritic lesions in the skeleton.

F, female; M, male; CT, computed tomography; MRI, magnetic resonance imaging.

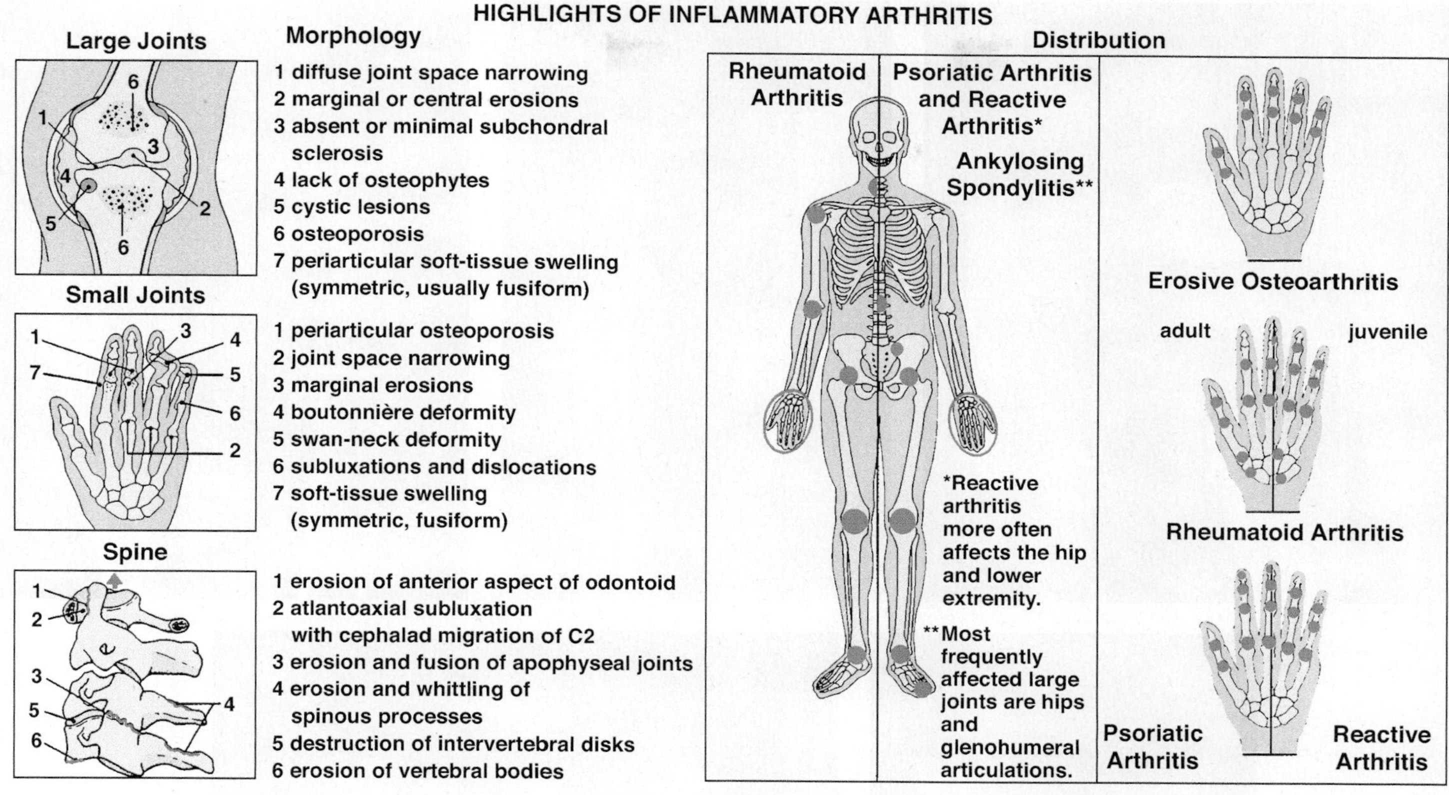

FIGURE 14.1 Inflammatory arthritides. Highlights of the morphology and distribution of arthritic lesions in the inflammatory arthritides.

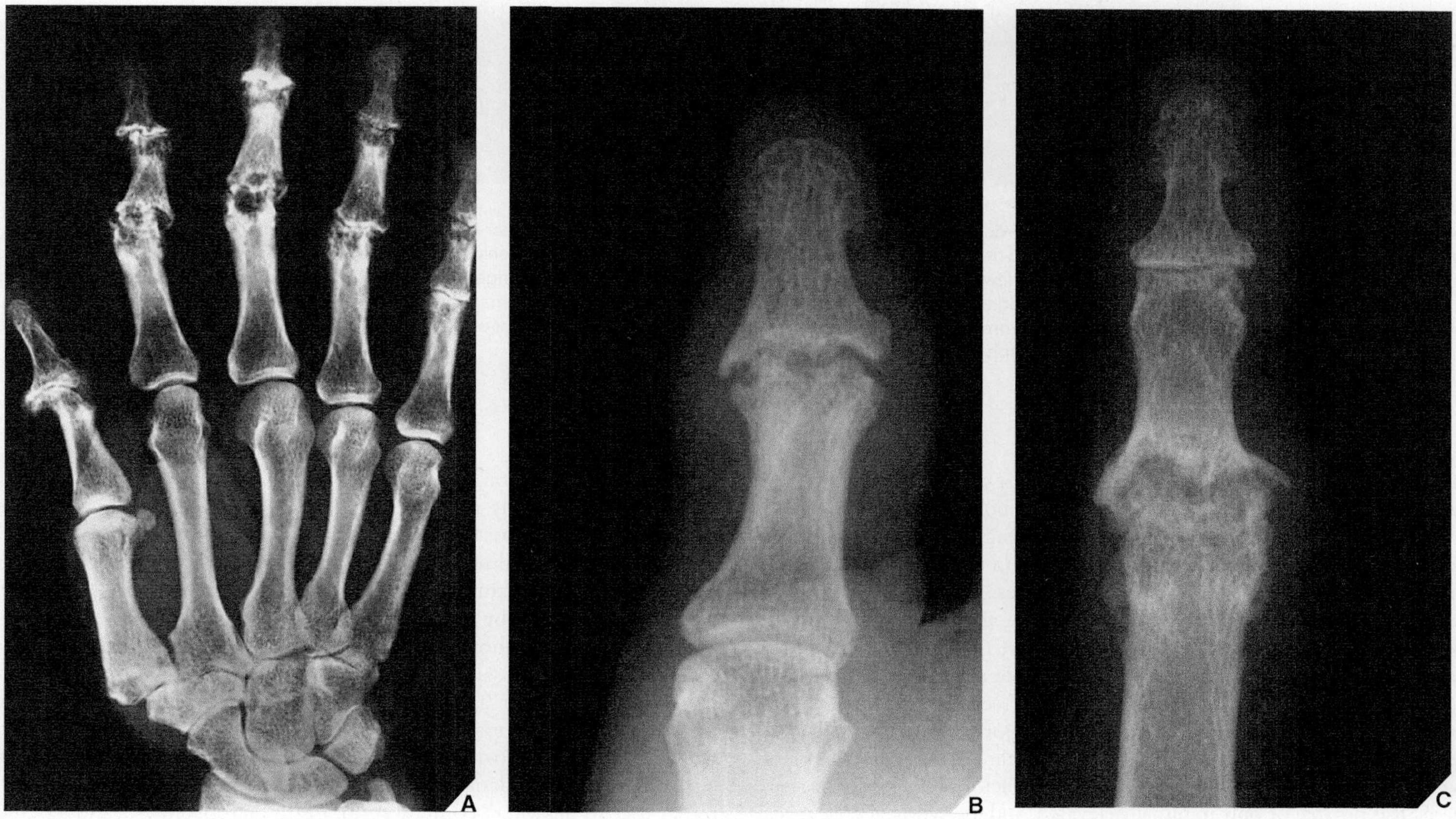

FIGURE 14.2 Erosive osteoarthritis. **(A)** Dorsovolar radiograph of the left hand of a 48-year-old woman with EOA shows the typical involvement of the proximal and distal interphalangeal joints. Note the "gull-wing" pattern of articular erosion, a configuration resulting from peripheral bone erosion in the distal side of the joint and central erosion in the proximal side of the joint associated with marginal bone proliferation. **(B)** Dorsovolar radiograph of the left thumb of a 51-year-old woman shows characteristic gull-wing erosion of the interphalangeal joint. Note adjacent fusiform soft-tissue swelling and lack of periarticular osteoporosis. **(C)** In another patient, a 50-year-old woman, gull-wing erosion is accompanied by periosteal reaction and fusiform soft-tissue swelling, very similar to PsA.

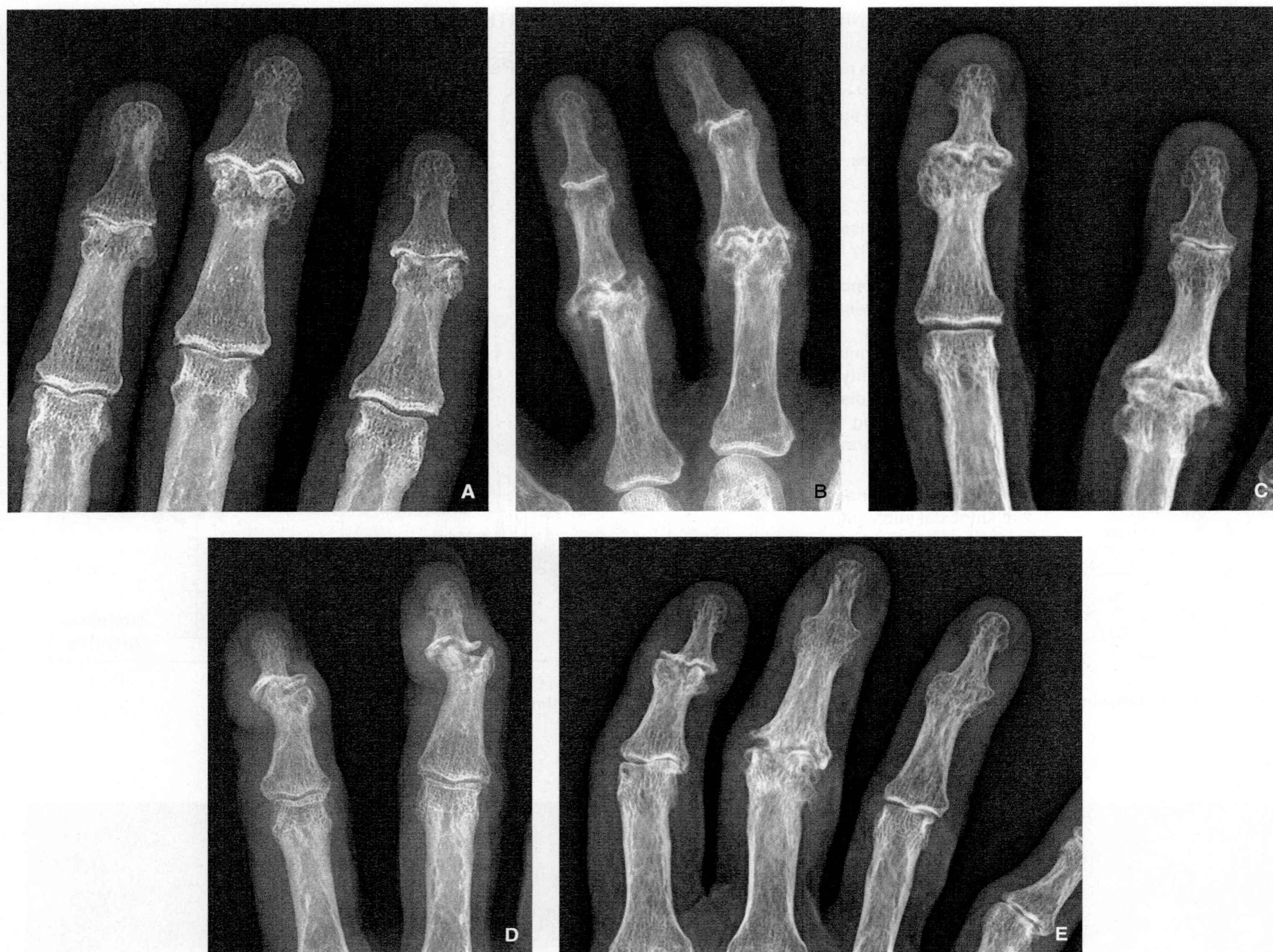

FIGURE 14.3 Erosive osteoarthritis. **(A)** Coned-down view of the index, middle, and ring fingers of a 70-year-old man shows gull-wing erosions of the distal interphalangeal joints. **(B)** Coned-down view of the middle and ring fingers of a 66-year-old woman shows advanced erosions of the proximal interphalangeal joints and early erosions of the distal interphalangeal joints. **(C)** Coned-down view shows characteristic erosion of the proximal interphalangeal joint of the ring finger and distal interphalangeal joint of the index finger of a 53-year-old woman. **(D)** Radiograph of the index and middle fingers of a 50-year-old woman shows gull-wing erosions of the distal interphalangeal joints. **(E)** In this patient, a 69-year-old woman, apart from the typical erosions of the proximal interphalangeal joint of the middle finger and distal interphalangeal joint of the index finger, observe also the fusion of the distal interphalangeal joints of the middle and ring fingers.

metacarpophalangeal articulations. However, in classic OA affecting the hand, the articular erosions are absent. In addition, Smith and coworkers in their research study of OA and EOA observed that patients with EOA exhibited more severe imaging features of OA in those joints with erosive changes than in the joints without such changes. It is worthwhile to indicate that in adult onset of RA, unlike in EOA, the distal interphalangeal joints are commonly spared, and the erosions are marginal rather than central. In juvenile-onset of RA (juvenile idiopathic arthritis [JIA]), however, the distal interphalangeal joints may also be affected. Both forms of RA are characterized by notable periarticular osteoporosis, which usually is absent in EOA. There are also differences in the clinical and laboratory findings. Latex agglutination tests for rheumatoid factor are typically negative, the ESR is normal or only minimally elevated, and the synovial fluid reveals no significant inflammatory changes. Moreover, patients do not experience prolonged morning stiffness. Subcutaneous nodules, a common clinical feature of RA, are absent, and no subluxation or dislocation is observed in the interphalangeal joints.

Another condition to be distinguished from EOA is PsA. Both arthritides preferentially affect the distal interphalangeal joints, but the erosions of PsA are usually marginally located, similar to those of RA. Unlike EOA, which almost invariably has a symmetric distribution, most patients with PsA exhibit asymmetrical joint involvement. Moreover, PsA is characterized by other abnormalities not seen in EOA, including skin lesions, nails abnormalities, involvement of sacroiliac joints (sacroiliitis), paraspinal ossifications, and formation of broad-based osteophytes at the plantar aspect of the calcaneus, accompanied by fluffy periostitis. Fluffy periostitis is also seen in the short tubular bones, unlike linear bone apposition observed in EOA. The articular erosions at the distal interphalangeal joints are also different, with "mouse-ear" rather than "gull-wing" configuration. Lastly, acroosteolysis and tapered erosions with pencil-like deformities, leading to the so-called *arthritis mutilans* typical for PsA, are absent in EOA. Although osteophytosis is a consistent phenomenon in EOA, it is almost never seen in RA or PsA. When osteophytes accompany the latter conditions, it is secondary

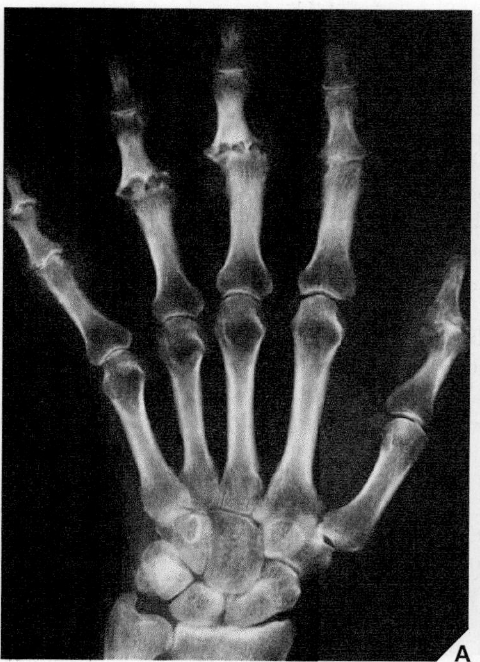

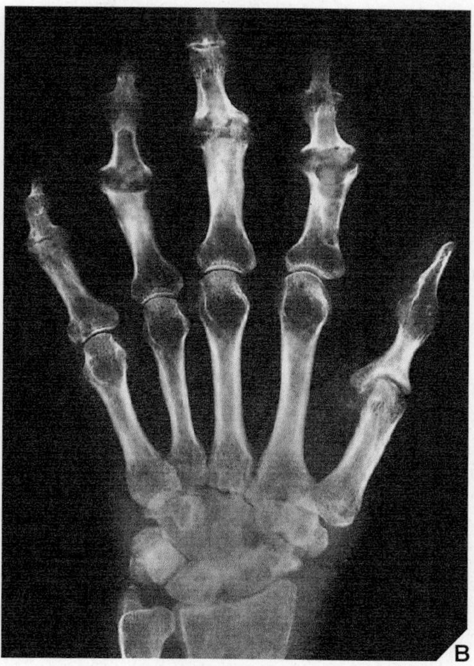

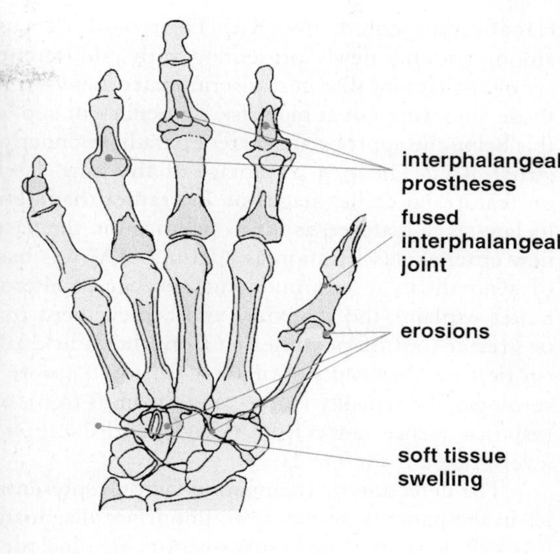

FIGURE 14.4 Progression of EOA into RA. **(A)** Dorsovolar radiograph of the hand of a 58-year-old woman demonstrates the gull-wing configuration of erosive changes in the proximal interphalangeal joints and the distal interphalangeal joint of the small finger. Because of protracted pain and lack of response to conservative treatment, she underwent joint resection followed by implantation of silicone–rubber prostheses in the proximal interphalangeal joints of the index, middle, and ring fingers, together with fusion of the interphalangeal joint of the thumb and the distal interphalangeal joint of the small finger. Five years after surgery, the classic radiographic features of RA developed, involving the wrists **(B)**, elbows, shoulders, hips, and cervical spine. Note the surgical fusion of interphalangeal joints of the thumb and fifth finger as well as the spontaneous fusion of the distal interphalangeal joints of the index and ring fingers.

phenomenon due to superimposed degenerative changes rather than a primary feature.

Rarely, erosive changes in the interphalangeal joints seen in hyperparathyroidism arthropathy can simulate those present in EOA. However, differential features include osteopenia, invariably accompanying the changes of hyperparathyroidism, and frequent occurrence of acroosteolysis, a hallmark of former condition. Moreover, the erosions seen in hyperparathyroidism arthropathy are not as sharply demarcated as in EOA, being the result of periosteal, chondral, and subchondral resorption. Other features of hyperparathyroidism, including cortical "tunneling," "brown" tumors, soft-tissue calcifications, and involvement of ligaments and tendons leading to joint laxity and instability, are additional differentiating features.

Occasionally, a variant of EOA may be seen as one of the features of Cronkhite-Canada syndrome. This rare systemic disorder also manifests with generalized gastrointestinal polyposis, hyperpigmentation of the skin, and nail atrophy.

Treatment

The main objective of therapy in patients with inflammatory EOA is relief of pain and restoration of joint function. Nonpharmacologic therapy includes physical and occupational therapy. Range-of-motion exercises and moist heat, in the form of a paraffin bath, are helpful. Pharmacologic methods include analgesics, nonsteroidal antiinflammatory drugs (NSAIDs), and corticosteroids. Selected cases have also been treated with methotrexate and oral gold salts. Recently, promising results have been achieved with administration of hydroxychloroquine in patients who did not respond to NSAIDs. Also, good results have been reported after subcutaneous injections of adalimumab and intraarticular injections of infliximab. Surgical intervention is often necessary for the relief of persistent pain and the correction of severe deformities. One of the most effective procedures is joint replacement by means of silicone–rubber arthroplasties (see Fig. 14.4). The indications for this type of surgery are loss of the joint space, synovial proliferation with joint destruction, loss of normal alignment, and uncontrollable pain.

Rheumatoid Arthritis

Adult Rheumatoid Arthritis

RA is a progressive, chronic, systemic inflammatory disease affecting primarily the synovial joints; women are affected 3 times more often than men. The course of the disease varies from patient to patient, and there is a striking tendency toward spontaneous remissions and exacerbations. Currently, RA is considered to be a heterogeneous autoimmune disorder, with genetic factors playing an important role in the disease expression.

Multiple genome-wide association studies have been conducted, but the results have generally been disappointing. The genetics is complex, multifactorial, and varies between ethnic populations. The best association is with the major histocompatibility complex (MHC), but the data have yielded no practical clues that can be translated to the bedside.

Although the association with the susceptibility loci of HLA-DRB1 and PTPN22 genes is best understood, several non-HLA loci have been linked to this arthritis, including the 18q21 chromosome region of the TNFRSR11A gene, which encodes the receptor activator of nuclear factor κB. In addition, a common genetic variant at the TRAF1-C5 locus on chromosome 9 is associated with an increased risk of anti-citrullinated protein (CCP)–positive RA. Allelic variants of HLA-DRB1 associated with risk for RA encode a similar sequence, namely amino acids 70–74, known as the *shared epitope*. The detection of antibodies to CCP, representing specific autoantibodies in the patient's serum, is an important diagnostic finding.

In 2010, the American College of Rheumatology in collaboration with European League Against Rheumatism established new classification criteria for RA. Their work "focused on identifying, among patients newly presenting with undifferentiated inflammatory synovitis, factors that best discriminated between those who were and those who were not at high risk for persistent and/or erosive disease—this being the appropriate current paradigm underlying the disease construct 'RA'." The main advantage of this new classification is focusing on features at earlier stages of RA rather than defining the disease by its late-stage features, as it was practiced in the past. In the established new criteria, classification as "definite RA" was based on the presence of synovitis in at least one joint, absence of alternative diagnosis that better explains the synovitis, and achievement of a total score of 6 or greater (out of possible 10) from the individual scores in four categories: number and site of involved joints (score range from 0 to 5), serologic abnormality (score range from 0 to 3), elevated acute-phase response (score range from 0 to 1), and duration of symptoms (two levels; range from 0 to 1).

The detection of rheumatoid factor, representing specific antibodies in the patient's serum, is an important diagnostic finding. Although it is still debatable, some investigators also include under this rubric a condition called *seronegative RA* (see later), in which patients present without rheumatoid factor but with the clinical and radiographic picture of RA.

Rheumatoid Factors

Rheumatoid factors, so widely used by clinicians, are antigamma-globulin antibodies that are elaborated in part by rheumatoid synovium. They are generally immunoglobulin M (IgM) and combine with their antigens (immunoglobulin G [IgG]) to form immune complexes. Because rheumatoid factors can be found in the serum and in joint fluids of patients with nonrheumatoid disorders, their presence alone is not diagnostic of RA. They have been studied for decades and were once thought to be the only critical serologic marker of RA; this, however, is not the case, because rheumatoid factors can be found in the joint fluid of patients with nonrheumatoid disorders. Although the rheumatoid factor is still widely used, it has lost much of the luster of the past. Nevertheless, finding high titers of these factors in a joint effusion strongly suggests the diagnosis of RA. Early in the course of disease, rheumatoid factors may be demonstrated in the synovial fluid before they are positive in the serum, allowing early diagnosis.

Rheumatoid factors do participate in the pathogenesis of RA through the formation of local and circulating antigen–antibody complexes. In synovial fluid, IgM and IgG rheumatoid factors can combine to form immune complexes. The complement system is activated, resulting in the attraction of polymorphonuclear leukocytes into the joint space. Discharge of their hydrolytic enzymes causes the destruction of joint tissues. The process initiating these events is as yet unknown. Patients with RA with subcutaneous nodules almost always will have positive rheumatoid factors, generally in high titer. Interesting, however, is the fact that frequency and severity of rheumatoid nodules has greatly decreased in population and the disease is strikingly different in this respect from two generations ago.

However, finding high titers of these factors in a joint effusion strongly suggests the diagnosis of RA. Early in the course of disease, rheumatoid factors may be demonstrated in the synovial fluid before they are positive in the serum, allowing early diagnosis.

As already discussed in the text earlier, autoantibodies against the group of *CCPs* are more pathognomonic for RA than rheumatoid factors. The second-generation enzyme-linked immunosorbent assay (ELISA) tests for anti-cyclic citrullinated peptide-2 (anti-CCP2) antibodies have specificity for RA as high as 97%. These antibodies are directed at one or all of the following proteins: α enolase, fibrinogen, and vimentin. In all cases, the arginine in these proteins has been replaced by the plant amino acid citrulline. In people with a genetic predisposition to loss of tolerance, autoantibodies to these CCPs appear and may be detected many years before the clinical onset of RA. There are several factors known to accelerate this loss of tolerance, including smoking and infections, particularly proteus infections of the gums.

Clinical Features

Articular and periarticular manifestations include joint swelling and tenderness to palpation, with morning stiffness and severe motion impairment in the affected joints. The clinical presentation varies between the patients, but an insidious onset of pain with symmetrical swelling of the joints of the hands is the most common finding. Some patients may present with palindromic onset; monoarticular presentation; extraarticular synovitis (such as tenosynovitis and bursitis); and general symptoms such as malaise, fatigue, anorexia, weight loss, and low-grade fever.

Imaging Features

RA is characterized by a diffuse, usually multicompartmental, symmetric narrowing of the joint space associated with marginal or central erosions, periarticular osteoporosis, and periarticular soft-tissue swelling; subchondral sclerosis is minimal or absent; and formation of osteophytes is lacking.

Large Joint Involvement

Any of the large weight-bearing and non–weight-bearing joints can be affected by RA. Regardless of the size of the joint and the site of involvement, certain imaging features can be identified that are characteristic of this inflammatory process.

Osteoporosis. In RA, unlike OA, osteoporosis is a striking feature. In the early stage of the disease, osteoporosis is localized to periarticular areas, but with progression of the condition, a generalized osteoporosis can be observed.

Joint Space Narrowing. This is usually a symmetric process with concentric narrowing of the joint. In the knee, all three joint compartments are involved (Figs. 14.5 and 14.6). Concentric narrowing in the hip joint leads to axial migration of the femoral head, which in more advanced stages may result in acetabular protrusio (Fig. 14.7). Similar concentric narrowing is observed in the shoulder joint (Fig. 14.8). Cephalad migration of the humeral head may also be seen secondary to destructive changes in the shoulder joint and rupture of the rotator cuff (Fig. 14.9); resorption of the distal end of the clavicle, which assumes a pencil-like appearance, may also be observed. Tear of the rotator cuff in this condition (Fig. 14.10) must be differentiated from the chronic traumatic form of this abnormality (see Fig. 5.67). When ankle joint is affected, uniform narrowing of the joint is also observed (Fig.14.11).

Articular Erosions. Erosive destruction of a joint may be central or peripheral in location. As a rule, reparative processes are absent or very minimal; thus, there is no evidence of subchondral sclerosis or osteophytosis (Figs. 14.12 and 14.13), which may be present only if secondary degenerative changes are superimposed on the underlying inflammatory process (see Fig. 13.13). Magnetic resonance imaging (MRI) effectively shows articular erosions (Figs. 14.14 to 14.16).

Extraarticular Osseous Erosions. Loss of the normal radiolucent triangle between the posterosuperior margin of the calcaneus and the adjacent Achilles tendon is consistent with the presence of inflammatory fluid within the retrocalcaneal bursa, commonly associated with erosion of the calcaneus (Fig. 14.17). Osseous erosions may also be seen in other parts of the foot (Fig. 14.18) and hand and wrist (Figs. 14.19 to 14.22).

Synovial Cysts and Pseudocysts. These radiolucent defects are usually seen in close proximity to the joint (Fig. 14.23). They may or may not communicate with the joint space.

Popliteal (Baker) Cyst. Baker cyst, named after the surgeon William Morrant Baker, who first described it, arises in the popliteal fossa between the medial head of the gastrocnemius tendon and the semimembranosus tendon, and is a common finding, seen in approximately 48% of patients with RA. It can be detected with ultrasound (US) (Fig. 14.24), with computed tomography (CT) (see Fig. 14.57A,B), or with MRI (Fig. 14.25; see also Fig. 14.57C–E). It extends posteriorly and may be directed inferiorly or superiorly in the soft tissues in the posterior aspect of the knee joint. Rupture of the popliteal cyst (Fig. 14.26) leads to extravasation of the inflammatory content into the soft tissues of calf, producing pain and swelling that may be mistaken for thrombophlebitis (see also the following text).

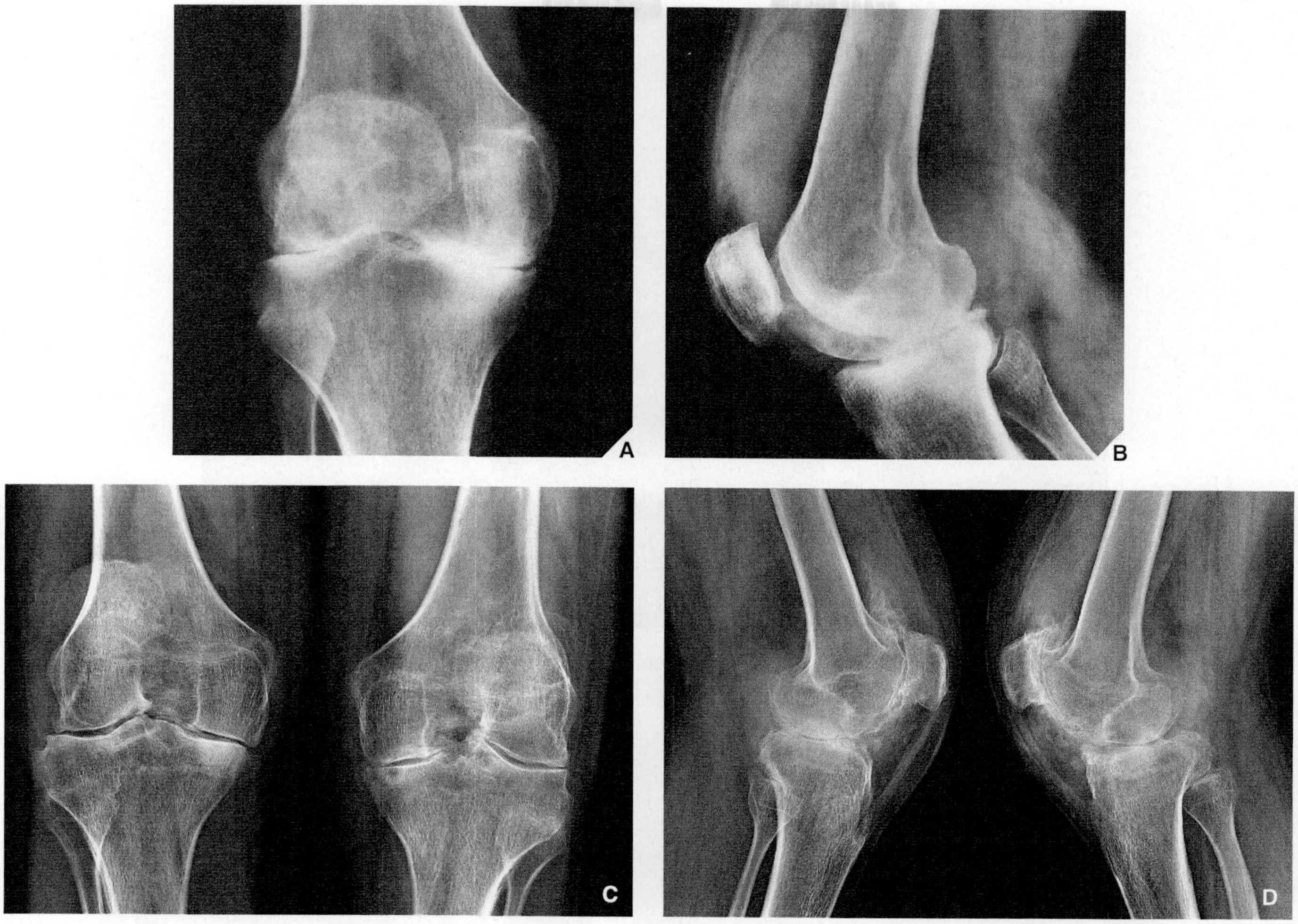

FIGURE 14.5 RA of the knee joints. **(A)** Anteroposterior and **(B)** lateral radiographs of the knee of a 52-year-old woman with RA affecting several joints show tricompartmental involvement. Note the periarticular osteoporosis, joint effusion, and lack of osteophytosis. **(C)** Anteroposterior and **(D)** lateral radiographs of both knees of a 50-year-old man show uniform narrowing of the medial, lateral, and femoropatellar joint compartments associated with joint effusions.

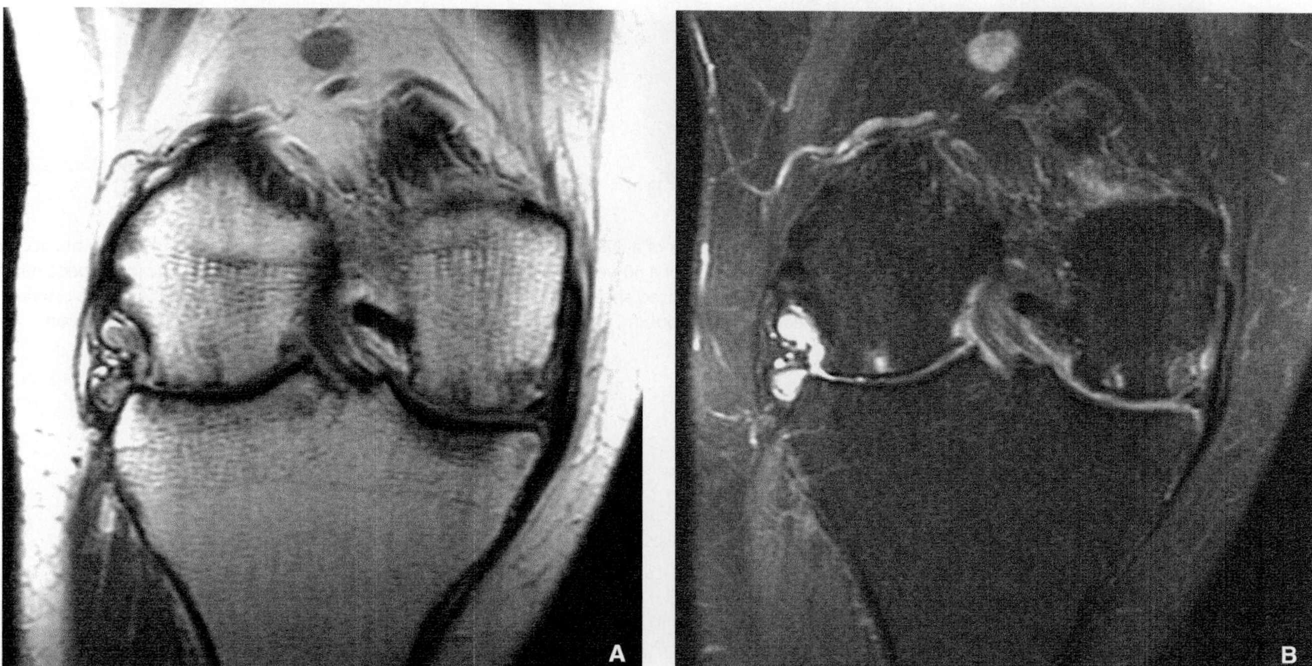

FIGURE 14.6 MRI of RA of the knee joint. **(A)** Coronal T1-weighted and **(B)** coronal proton density–weighted fat-suppressed MR images of the left knee of a 50-year-old woman show uniform joint space narrowing of the lateral and medial compartments, destruction of the articular cartilage, subchondral bone erosions, and tear of the lateral and medial menisci. Note the absence of bone proliferation/osteophytes formation despite severe chondral loss. (Reprinted with permission from Greenspan A, Gershwin ME. *Imaging in rheumatology: a clinical approach*, 1st ed. Philadelphia: Wolters Kluwer; 2018:213.)

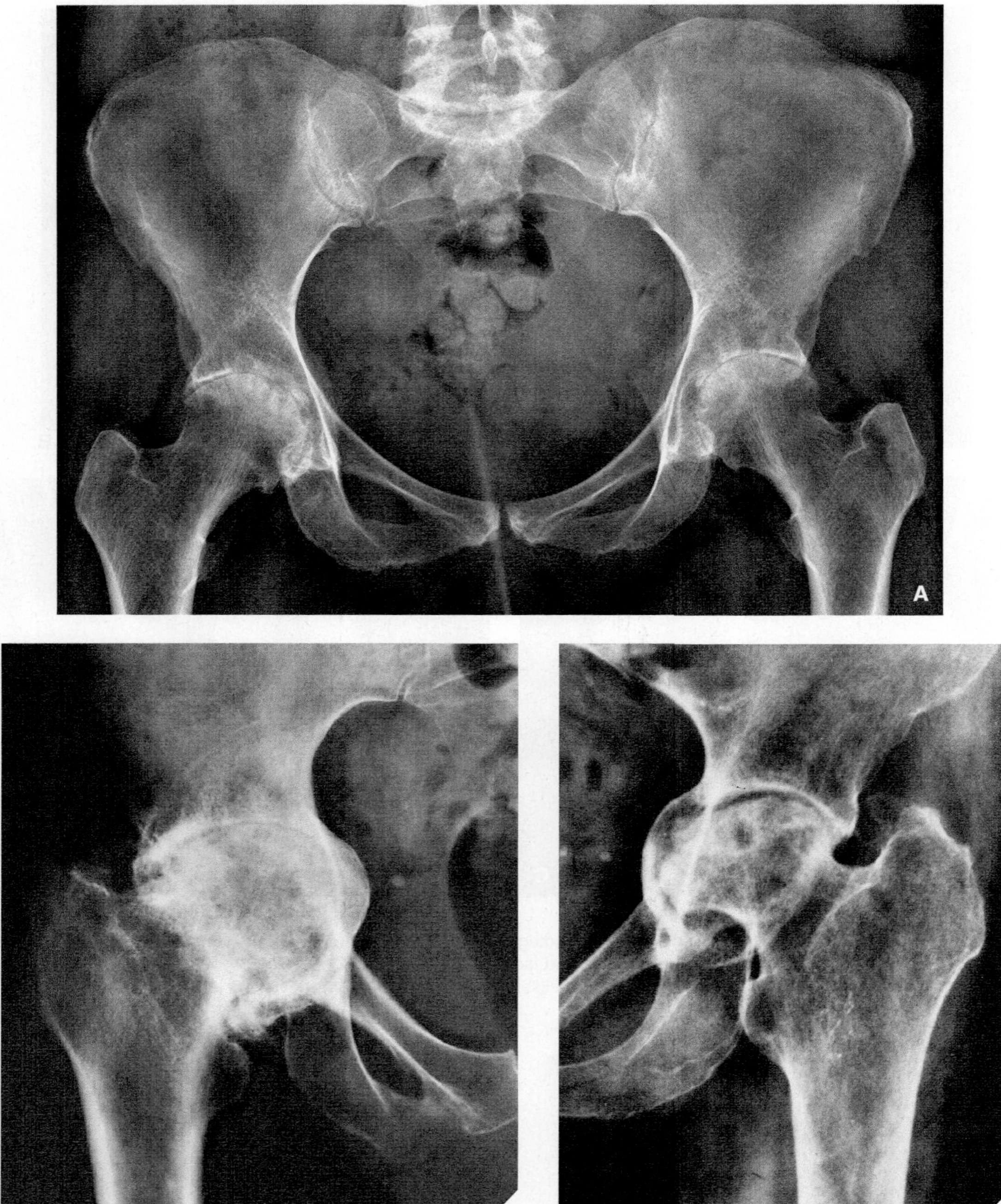

FIGURE 14.7 RA of the hip joints. **(A)** Anteroposterior radiograph of the pelvis of a 47-year-old woman shows uniform narrowing of both hip joints accompanied by axial migration of the femoral heads. **(B)** Anteroposterior radiograph of the right hip of a 60-year-old woman with advanced RA shows concentric joint space narrowing, with axial migration of the femoral head leading to acetabular protrusio. Some superimposed secondary osteoarthritic changes are also present. **(C)** Anteroposterior radiograph of the left hip of a 64-year-old woman shows erosions of the femoral head and acetabulum, concentric narrowing of the hip joint, and acetabular protrusion.

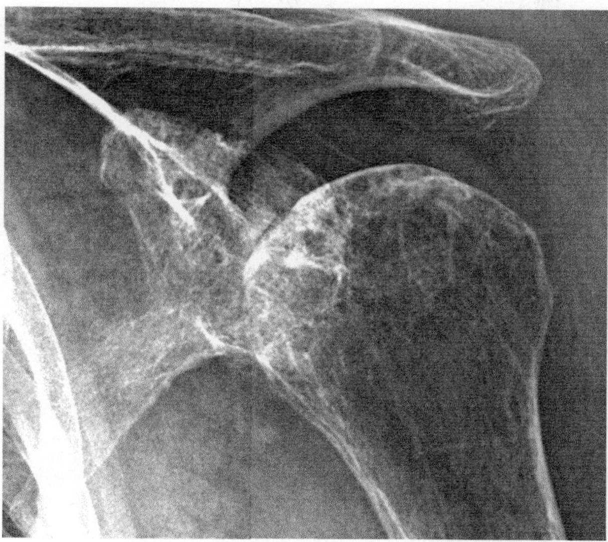

FIGURE 14.8 RA of the shoulder joint. Anteroposterior radiograph of the left shoulder of a 70-year-old woman shows periarticular osteoporosis and concentric narrowing of the glenohumeral joint. Also present are erosions of the glenoid and humeral head.

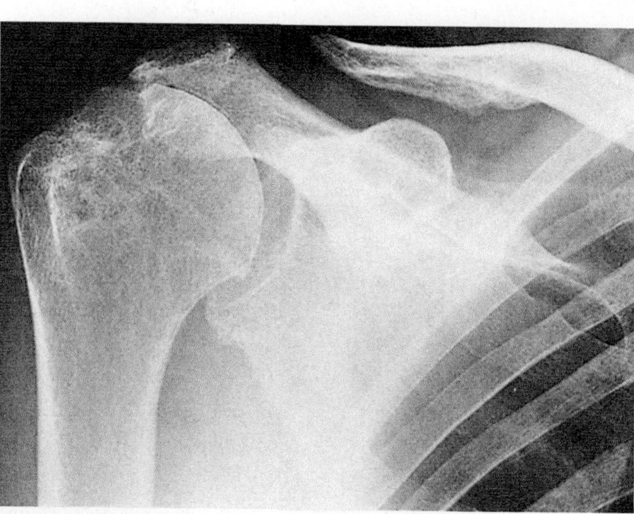

FIGURE 14.9 RA of the shoulder joint. Anteroposterior radiograph of the right shoulder of a 72-year-old man with advanced RA shows upward migration of the humeral head secondary to rotator cuff tear, a common complication of rheumatoid changes in the shoulder joint. Note the characteristic tapered erosion of the distal end of the clavicle, erosions of the humeral head, and the substantial degree of periarticular osteoporosis.

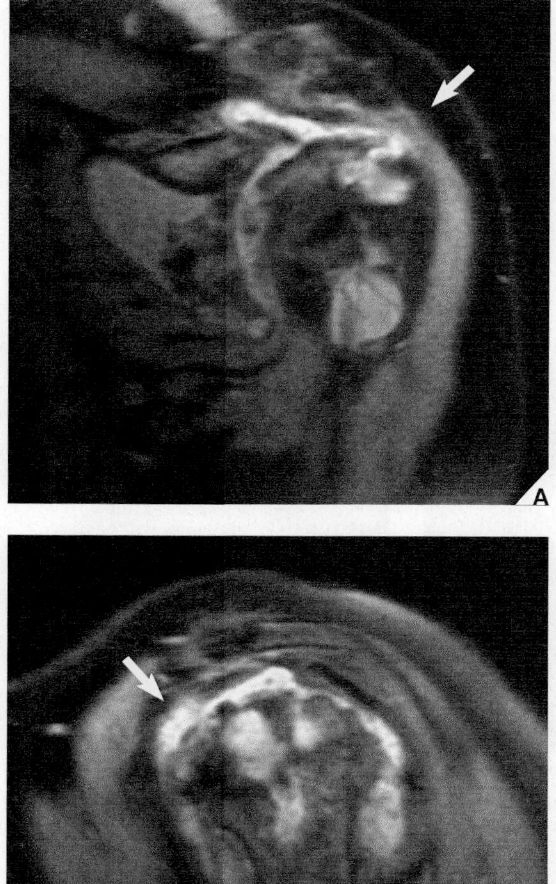

FIGURE 14.10 MRI of RA of the shoulder joint. **(A)** Oblique coronal and **(B)** sagittal proton density–weighted fat-suppressed MR images of the left shoulder of a 64-year-old woman show large articular and periarticular erosions, joint space narrowing, joint effusion, and a tear of the supraspinatus tendon *(arrows)*, all features of advanced RA.

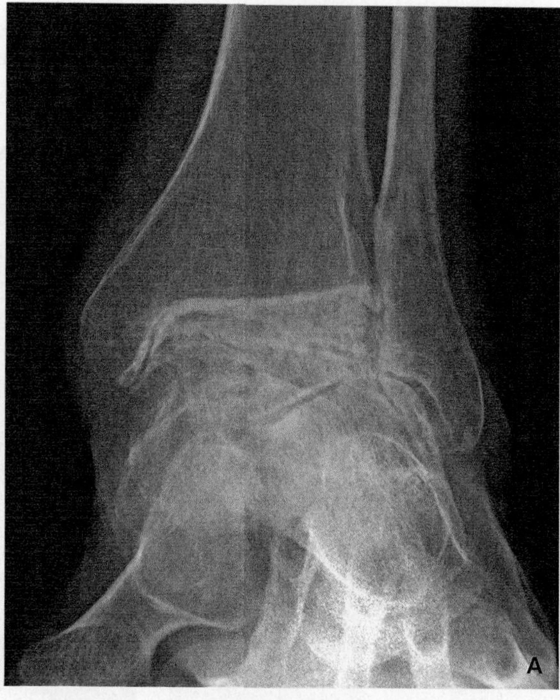

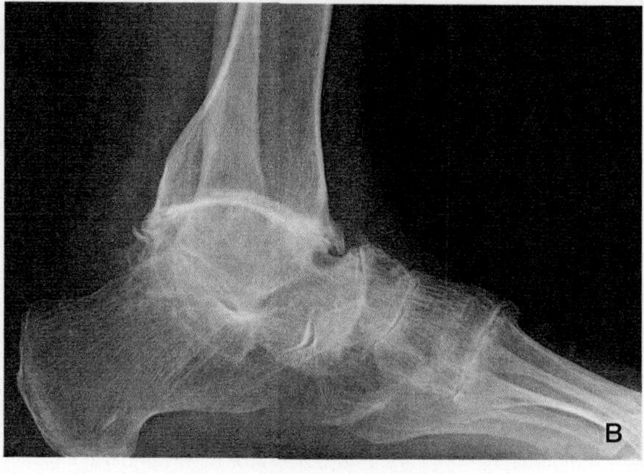

FIGURE 14.11 RA of the ankle. **(A)** Anteroposterior and **(B)** lateral radiographs of the left ankle show uniform joint space narrowing of the tibiotalar, subtalar, Chopart, and Lisfranc joints.

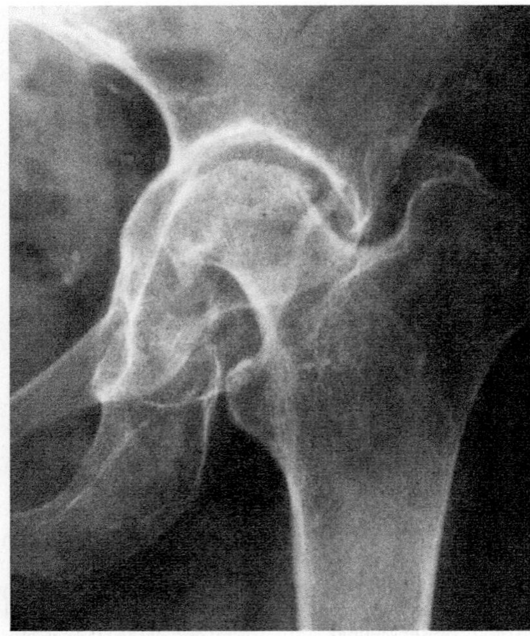

FIGURE 14.12 RA of the hip. Anteroposterior radiograph of the left hip of a 59-year-old woman with advanced rheumatoid polyarthritis demonstrates the typical erosions of the femoral head and acetabulum. Note the lack of osteophytosis and the only very minimal reactive sclerosis.

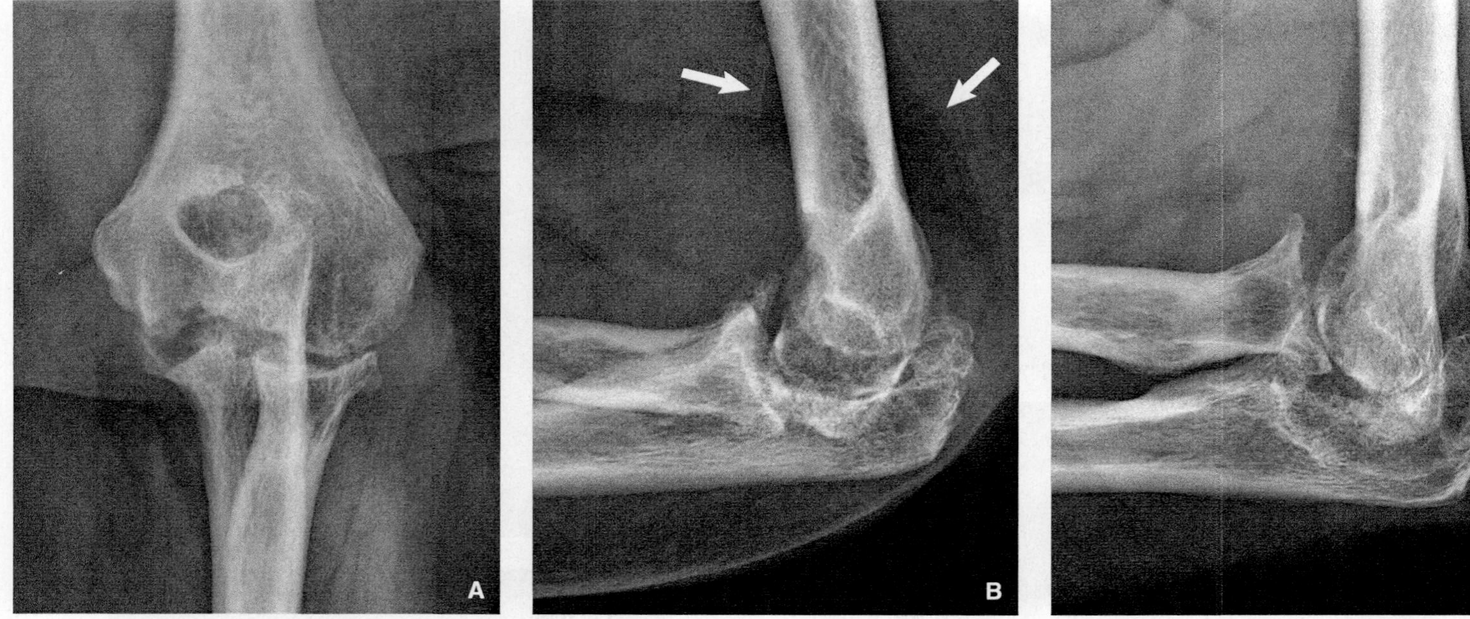

FIGURE 14.13 RA of the elbow joint. **(A)** Anteroposterior, **(B)** lateral, and **(C)** radial head–capitellum views of the left elbow of a 61-year-old woman show narrowing of the joint spaces, erosions of the subchondral bone of the capitellum, radial head, and trochlea, and joint effusion manifested by the positive anterior and posterior fat-pad sign *(arrows)*.

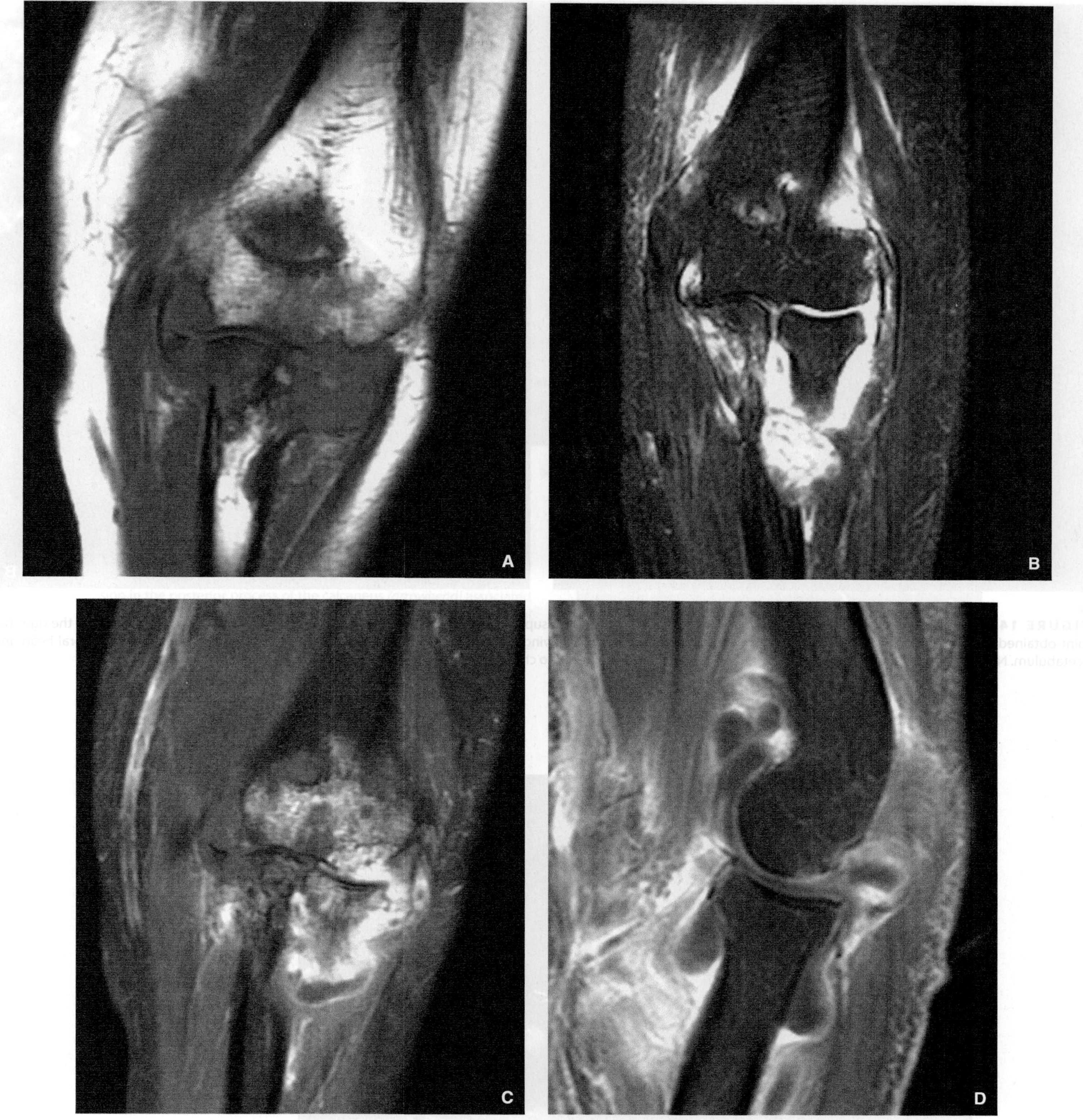

FIGURE 14.14 MRI of RA of the elbow. **(A)** Coronal T1-weighted, **(B)** coronal inversion recovery (IR), and **(C)** coronal and **(D)** sagittal T1-weighted fat-suppressed MR images of the elbow joint obtained after intravenous administration of gadolinium show extensive synovitis, joint effusion, and articular erosions in a 52-year-old woman. Note the enhancing pericapsular edema following gadolinium injection.

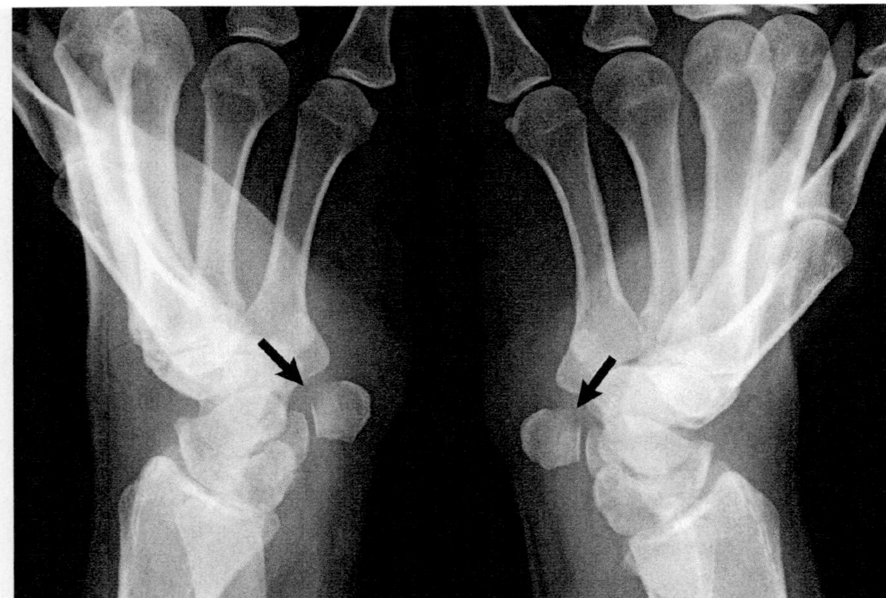

FIGURE 14.19 RA: osseous erosions. Norgaard view of both hands of a 33-year-old woman shows early erosions of both pisiform bones *(arrows)*.

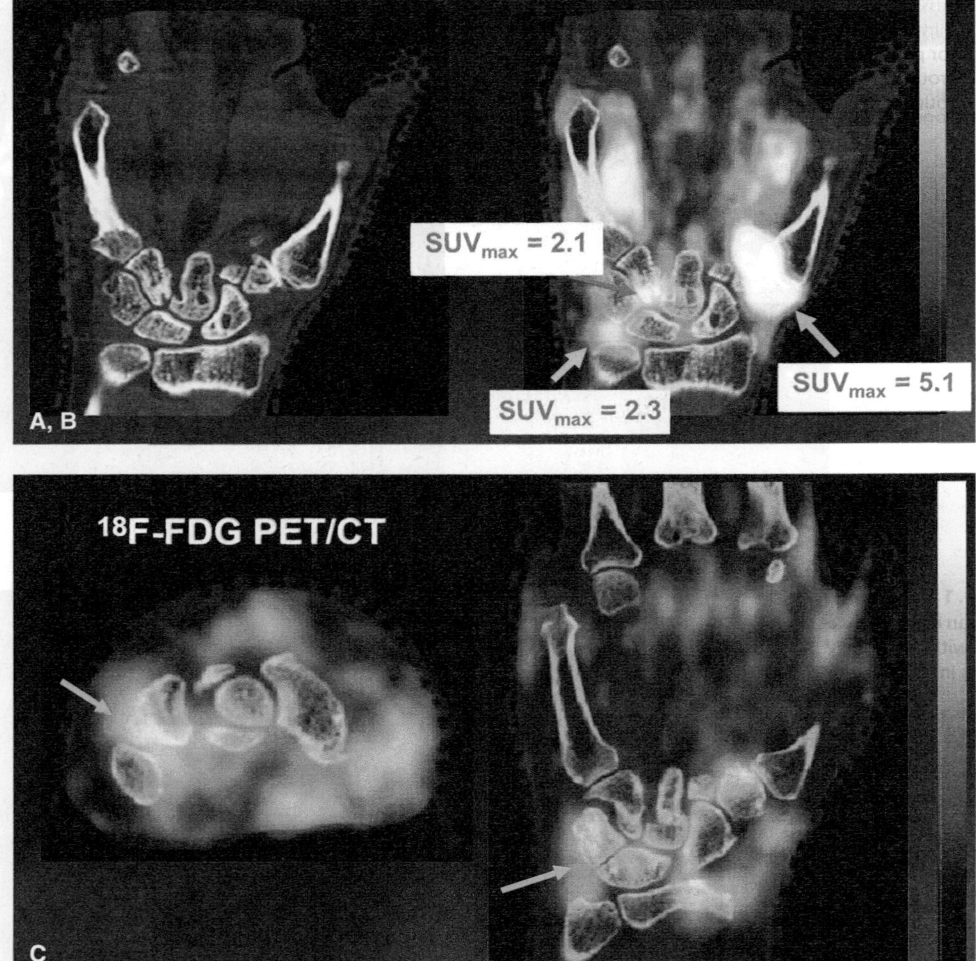

FIGURE 14.20 CT and ^{18}F-FDG PET/CT of osseous erosion. **(A)** Coronal reformatted CT image of the right wrist of a 49-year-old woman with clinically documented RA shows erosions of several carpal bones, including the hamate, triquetrum, capitate, and scaphoid. In addition, there is narrowing, subchondral sclerosis, and osteophyte formation of the first carpometacarpal joint typical of OA. **(B)** Coronal fused PET/CT image shows increased accumulation of the FDG radiotracer (increased metabolic activity) at the sites of active inflammatory synovitis and erosions *(blue and turquoise arrows)*, and at the site of OA *(green arrow)*. SUV$_{max}$, standarized uptake value. **(C)** Axial and coronal reformatted fused ^{18}F-FDG PET/CT images of the right wrist of a 59-year-old woman with RA show high glucose uptake in the pisiform-triquetral compartment and erosion of the triquetral bone *(arrows)*. (Courtesy of Abhijit J. Chaudhari, MD, Sacramento, California.)

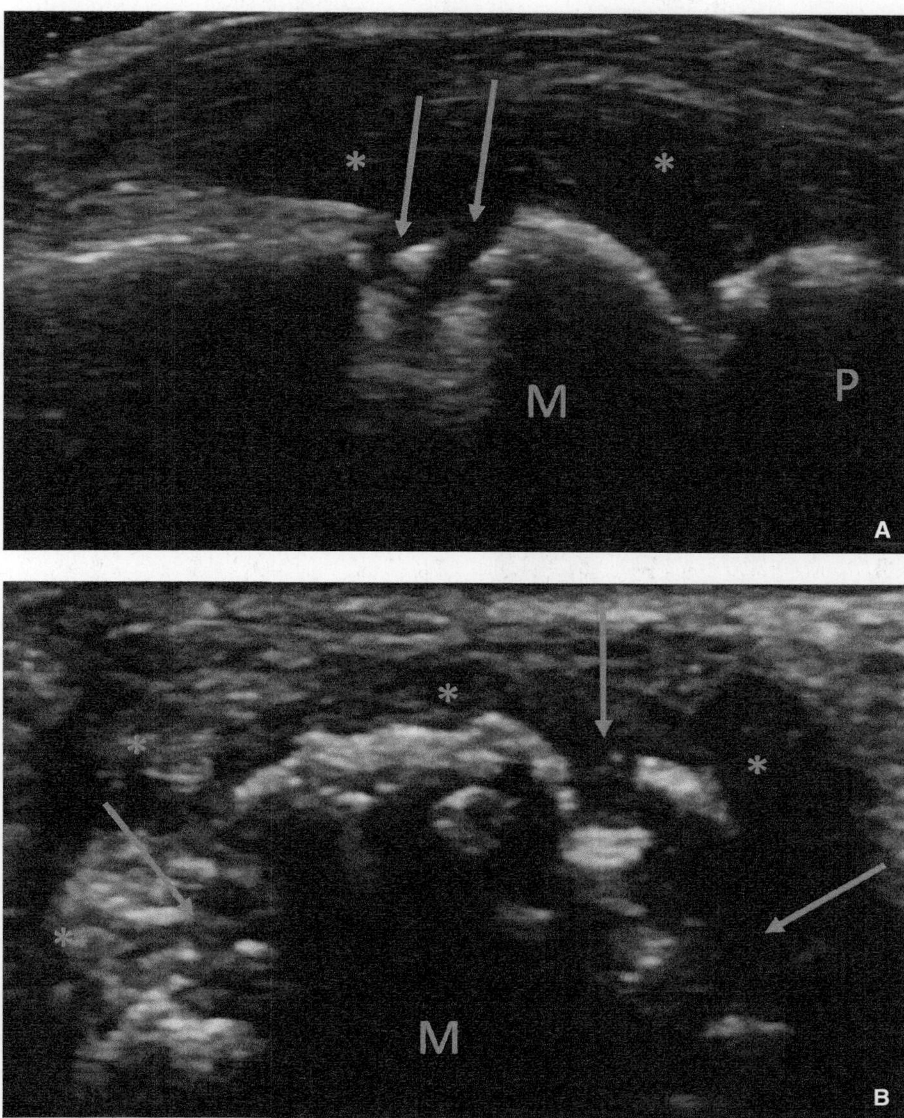

FIGURE 14.21 US of osseous erosion. **(A)** US image in the longitudinal plane of the hand in a patient with RA shows erosion in the dorsal aspect of the second metacarpal head *(arrows)*. *M*, metacarpal head; *P*, proximal phalanx of the index finger; *asterisks*, synovitis and effusion. **(B)** Image in the transverse plane of the wrist in another patient with RA shows large erosions at the base of the third metacarpal bone *(arrows)* associated with synovitis *(asterisks)*. *M*, third metacarpal bone. (Courtesy of Prof. Andrew J. Grainger, Cambridge, United Kingdom.)

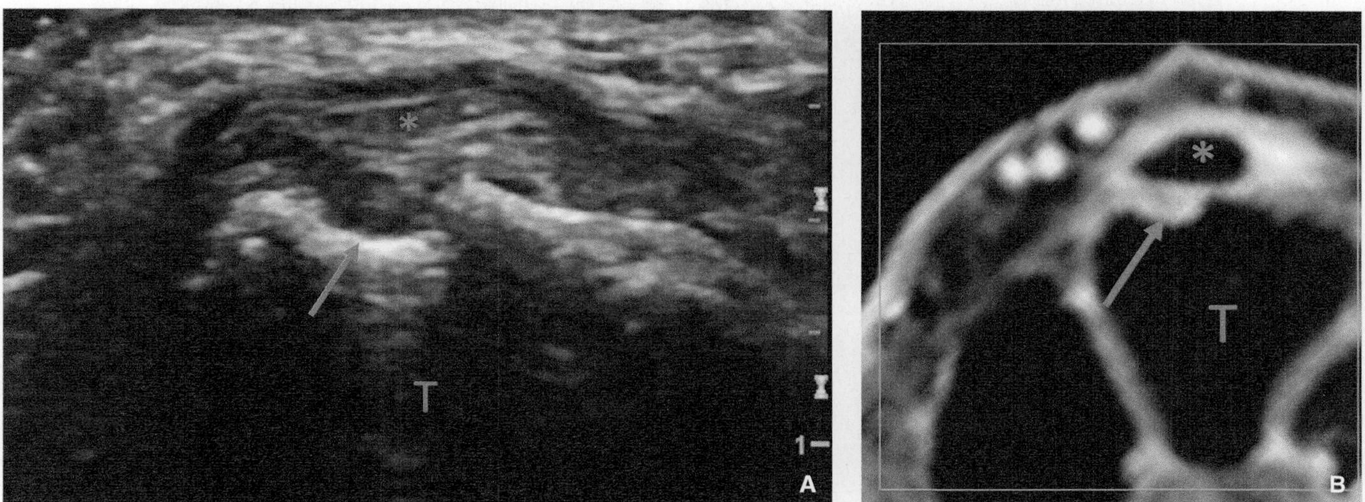

FIGURE 14.22 US and MRI of osseous erosion. **(A)** US image and **(B)** water excitation spoiled gradient-echo (SPGR) MR image of the wrist of a patient with RA show erosion *(arrow)* in the dorsal aspect of the triquetral bone *(T)*. The extensor carpi ulnaris tendon *(asterisks)* overlies the erosion. (Courtesy of Prof. Andrew J. Grainger, Cambridge, United Kingdom.)

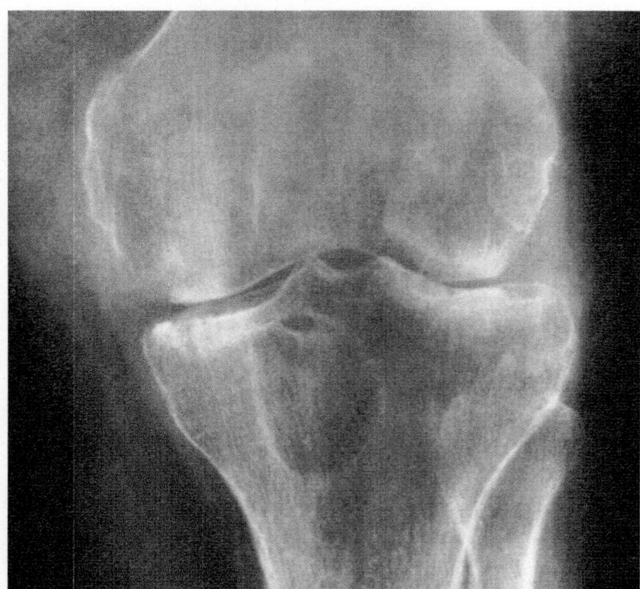

FIGURE 14.23 **Rheumatoid cyst.** Anteroposterior radiograph of the left knee of a 35-year-old woman with RA shows a large synovial cyst in the proximal tibia. Note also articular erosions and periarticular osteoporosis.

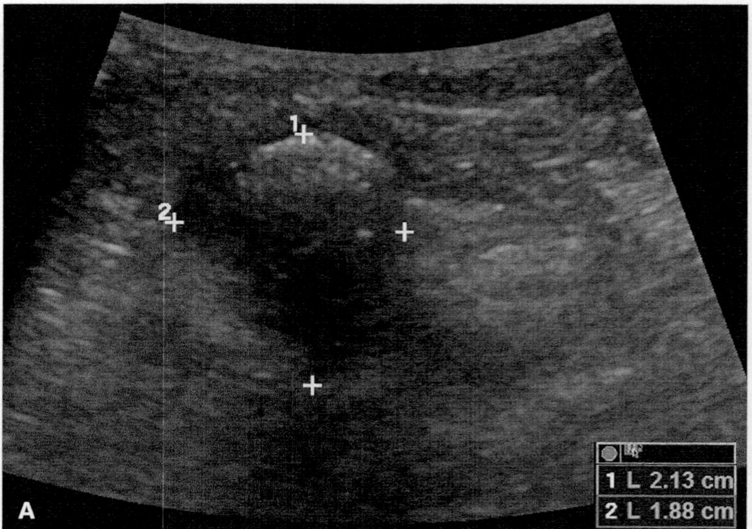

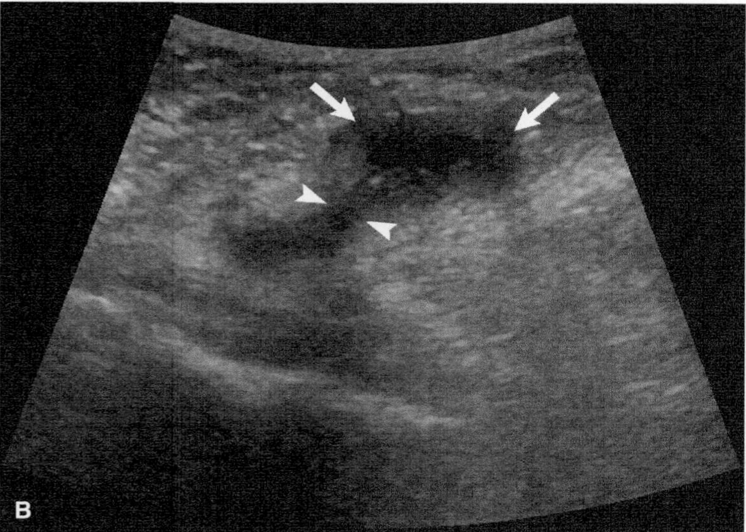

FIGURE 14.24 **US of the Baker cyst.** **(A)** US of the popliteal fossa performed in a 51-year-old woman with RA shows a Baker cyst (marked with +). **(B)** Transverse US image of the knee of a 42-year-old woman with RA shows an oval in shape hypoechoic area *(arrows)* that communicates with the knee joint *(arrowheads)*.

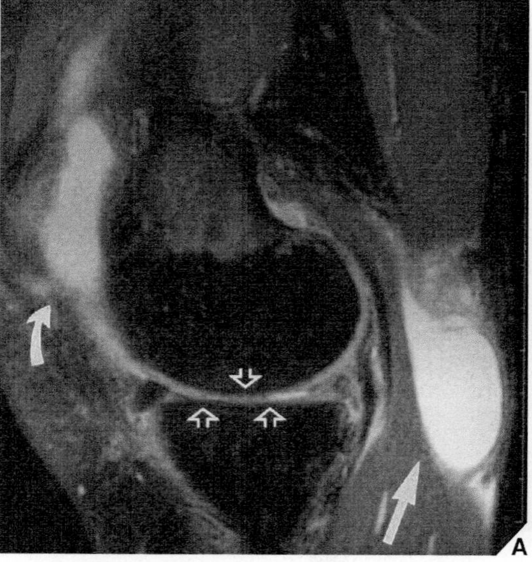

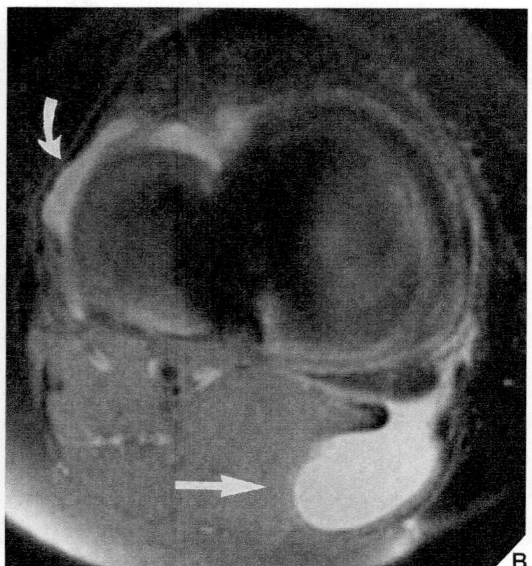

FIGURE 14.25 **MRI of the Baker cyst.** **(A)** Sagittal and **(B)** axial T2-weighted fat-suppressed MR images of a 60-year-old woman with RA demonstrate a large popliteal cyst *(arrows)*. *Open arrows* point to erosive changes of the articular cartilage and subchondral bone; *curved arrows* indicate joint effusion.

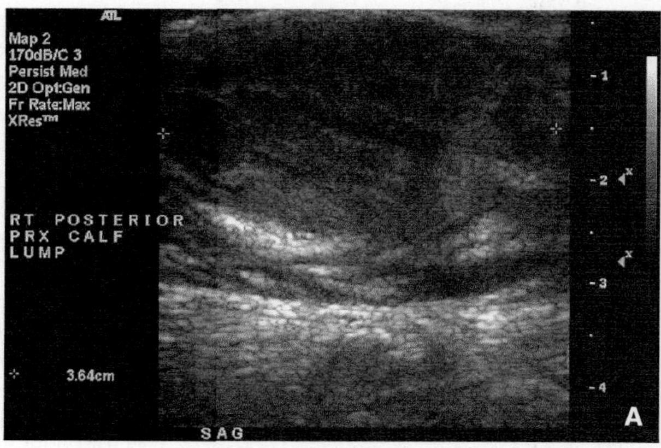

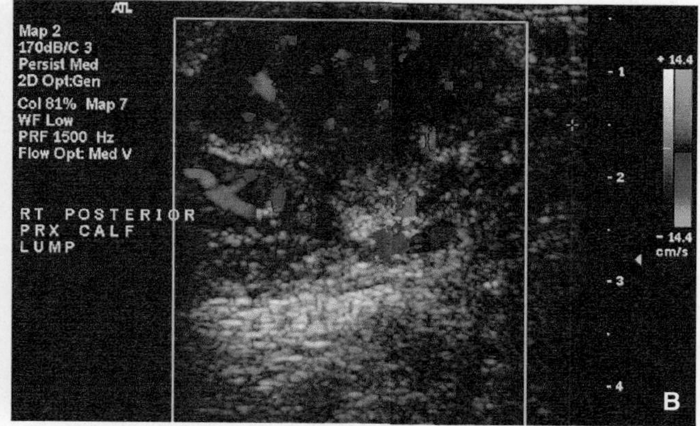

FIGURE 14.26 US of ruptured Baker cyst. A 41-year-old woman presented with a painful mass in the popliteal region. **(A)** Color-flow US shows a portion of the intact Baker cyst with hyperechoic heterogenous fluid collection. **(B)** This image shows the site of chronic rupture of the cyst associated with internal debris, secondary inflammatory changes, and hypervascularity. (Reprinted with permission from Greenspan A, Gershwin ME. *Imaging in rheumatology: a clinical approach*. Philadelphia: Wolters Kluwer; 2018:71, Fig. 2.77.)

Joint Effusion. Fluid can be best demonstrated in the knee joint on the lateral projection (see Fig. 14.5B,D), or by MRI (see Fig. 14.25). The latter modality is also effective in demonstrating fluid in the other large joints such as the shoulder (see Fig. 14.10), elbow (see Fig. 14.14), and hip (see Fig. 14.15B).

Rice Bodies. Bearing macroscopic similarity to grains of polished white rice, these small, usually uniform in size intraarticular or intrabursal loose bodies are commonly associated with RA and are thought to represent a complication of chronic inflammatory process. Occasionally, they also may be seen in seronegative inflammatory arthritis and even in tuberculous arthritis. These particles contain collagen, fibrinogen, fibrin, reticulin, elastin, mononuclear cells, blood cells, and some amorphous material. On radiography (Fig. 14.27), this condition occasionally can be mistaken for synovial chondromatosis (see Chapter 23). On MR T1-weighted images, rice bodies exhibit intermediate signal intensity, whereas on T2 weighting, they are only slightly hyperintense relative to muscle (Figs. 14.28 and 14.29).

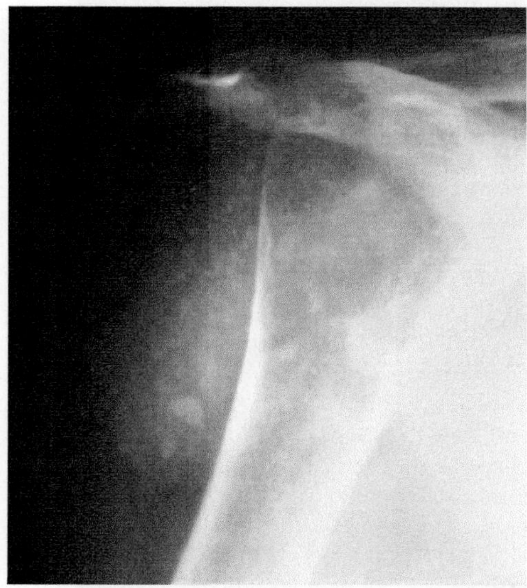

FIGURE 14.27 Rice bodies. Anteroposterior radiograph of the right shoulder of a 60-year-old woman with advanced RA demonstrates multiple rice bodies within subacromial–subdeltoid bursae complex.

Rheumatoid Nodules. Rheumatoid nodules are relatively common, with a reported frequency of about 25%. They usually develop over pressure areas such as elbow (Fig. 14.30), heel, or ischial tuberosities.

Small Joint Involvement

RA characteristically affects the small joints of the wrist as well as the metacarpophalangeal and proximal interphalangeal joints of the hands and feet (Figs. 14.31 and 14.32). As a rule, the distal interphalangeal joints in the hand are spared, although in advanced stages of the disease, even these may be affected. This latter point, however, is controversial because some investigators believe that if the distal interphalangeal joints are involved, the condition may represent JIA or another form of polyarthritis, not classic RA.

In addition to the characteristic changes exhibited in large joint involvement, the small joints may also show radiographic features specific for these sites.

Soft-Tissue Swelling. This earliest sign of RA usually has a fusiform, symmetric shape. It is periarticular in location and represents a combination of joint effusion, edema, and tenosynovitis. Although it can be seen on the radiographs (see Fig. 14.40A,B), the MRI provides a more effective way of demonstration of this critical feature of preerosive RA (see Fig. 14.32). MRI is also a modality of choice to show early changes of tenosynovitis (Fig. 14.33), although US may also effectively demonstrate soft-tissue abnormalities around the joints (Figs. 14.34 and 14.35) as well as tenosynovitis in the hands (Figs. 14.36 and 14.37) and feet (see Fig. 14.34).

Loss of Articular Cortex. This is another early radiographic sign of inflammatory arthritis, when the so-called *articular (or subchondral) cortex* becomes indistinct or completely lost (Fig. 14.38).

Marginal Erosions. Other early imaging signs of articular abnormalities manifest as marginal erosions at so-called *bare areas*. These are the sites within the small joints that are not covered by articular cartilage (Fig. 14.39). The most common locations for these erosions are the radial aspects of the second and third metacarpal heads and the radial and ulnar aspects of the bases of the proximal phalanges (Fig. 14.40). Synovial inflammation in the prestyloid recess, a diverticulum of the radiocarpal joint that is intimate with the styloid process of ulna, as Resnick pointed out, produces marginal erosion of the styloid tip.

Articular Erosions. In more advanced stages of RA, articular erosions are commonly seen. In the hand, the metacarpophalangeal and proximal interphalangeal joints are usually affected (Fig. 14.41), and in the foot, the metatarsophalangeal and proximal interphalangeal joints (Figs. 14.42 and 14.43). The subtalar joint may be affected as well (Fig. 14.44).

Joint Deformities. Although not pathognomonic for RA, certain deformations such as the swan-neck deformity and the boutonnière deformity are more often seen in this form of arthritis than in other inflammatory arthritides. The first of these represents hyperextension in the proximal interphalangeal joint and flexion in the distal interphalangeal joint, a configuration resembling a swan's neck (Fig. 14.45). In the boutonnière deformity, the configuration is just the opposite, with flexion in the proximal joint and extension in the distal interphalangeal joint (Fig. 14.46). The word *boutonnière* is French for "buttonhole," the term for this deformity deriving from the configuration of the finger while securing a flower to a lapel. A similar deformation of the thumb is called *hitchhiker's thumb*.

Moreover, subluxations and dislocations with malalignment of the fingers are common findings in advanced stages of RA. Particularly, characteristic are ulnar deviation of the fingers in the metacarpophalangeal joints and radial deviation of the wrist in the radiocarpal articulation (Fig. 14.47). In far-advanced stages of RA, shortening of several phalanges may be encountered secondary to destructive changes in the joints associated with dislocations in the metacarpophalangeal joints. This deformity appears as a "telescoping" of the fingers, hence, its name, *main-en-lorgnette*, from the French name for the telescoping type of opera glass (Fig. 14.48). An abnormally wide space between the lunate and the scaphoid may also be encountered in advanced stages of the disease secondary to erosion and rupture of the scapholunate ligament (Fig. 14.49); this phenomenon resembles the Terry-Thomas sign seen secondary to trauma (see Figs. 7.94 and 7.95). Joint deformities are also often seen in the foot; the subtalar joint is frequently affected, and subluxation in the metatarsophalangeal joints often leads to deformities such as hallux valgus and hammertoes (Fig. 14.50).

Joint Ankylosis. A rare finding that may be observed in advanced stages of RA is joint ankylosis, which is most commonly encountered in the midcarpal articulations (see Figs. 14.47 and 14.48). Ankylotic changes in the wrist are more common in patients with JIA and with so-called *seronegative RA*.

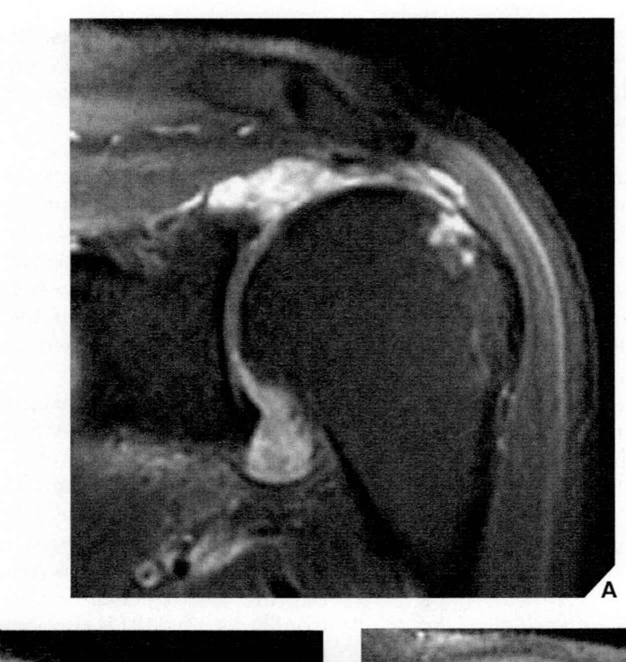

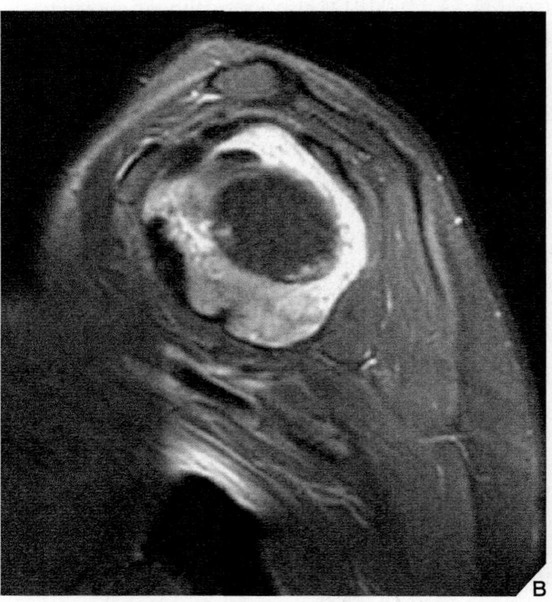

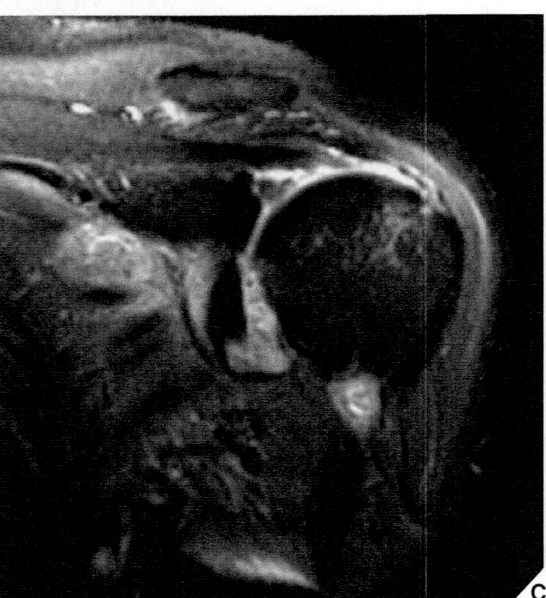

FIGURE 14.28 MRI of rice bodies. **(A)** Oblique coronal proton density–weighted, **(B)** sagittal proton density–weighted, and **(C)** oblique coronal T2-weighted fat-suppressed MR images of the left shoulder of a 66-year-old woman with RA show numerous rice bodies within the shoulder joint.

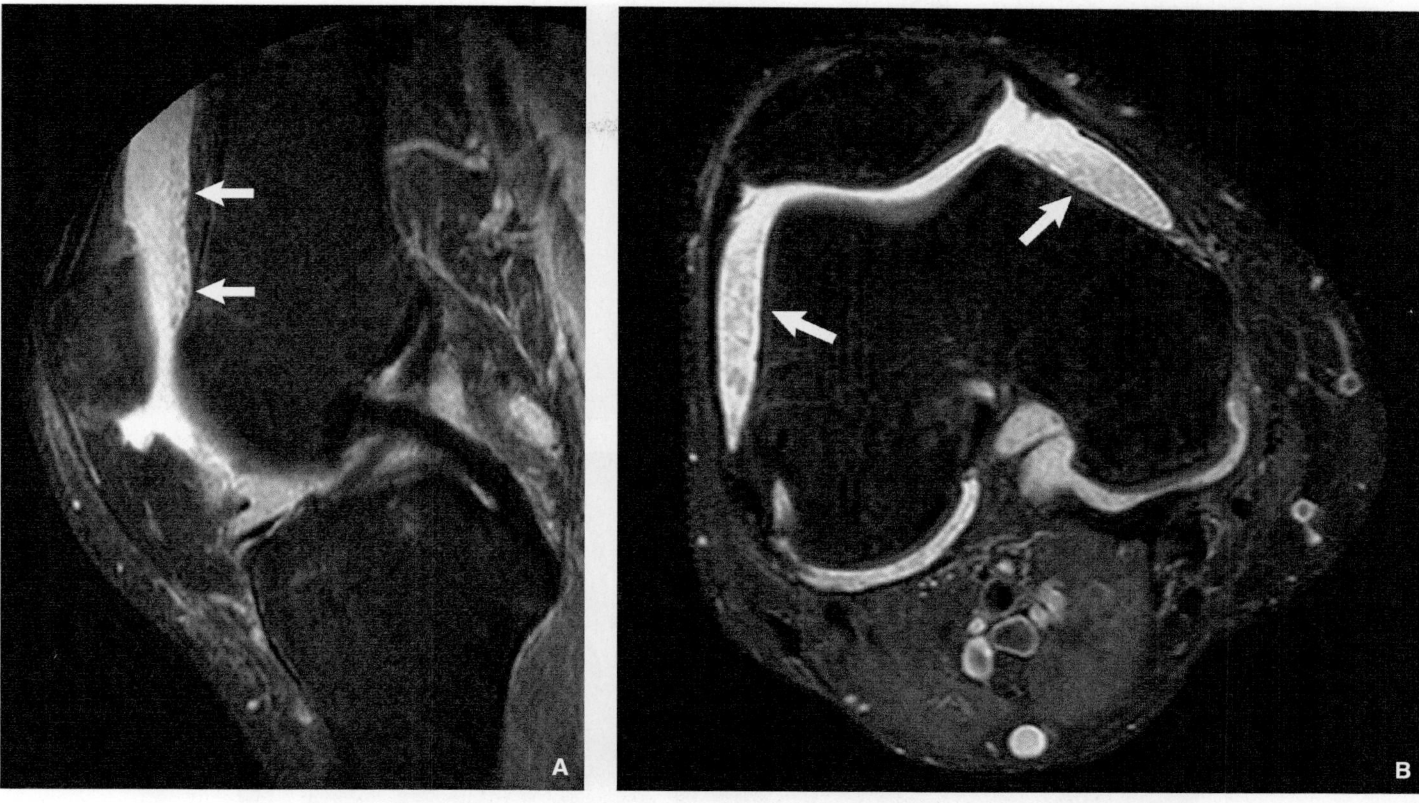

FIGURE 14.29 MRI of rice bodies. **(A)** Sagittal and **(B)** axial fast spin-echo (FSE) proton density–weighted fat-suppressed MR images of the right knee of a 68-year-old woman with RA show numerous rice bodies within the joint fluid *(arrows)*.

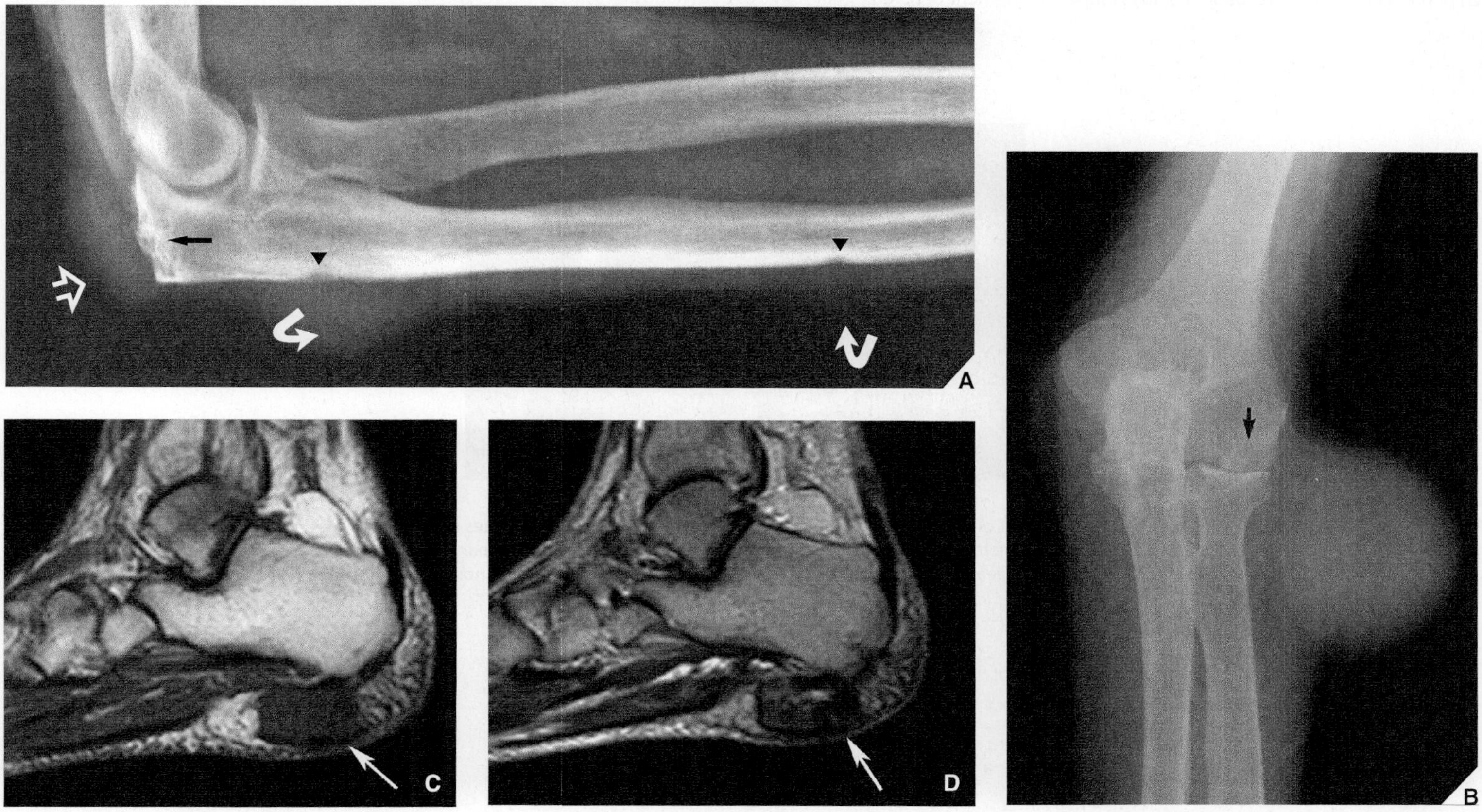

FIGURE 14.30 Rheumatoid nodules. **(A)** Lateral radiograph of the right elbow of a 39-year-old man with RA demonstrates erosions of the olecranon process *(arrow)*, olecranon bursitis *(open arrow)*, and rheumatoid nodules on the dorsal aspect of the forearm *(curved arrows)*. Note the characteristic pit-like cortical erosions at the site of the rheumatoid nodules *(arrowheads)*. This presentation of RA should not be mistaken for rheumatoid nodulosis. **(B)** A 68-year-old woman with RA had a large rheumatoid nodule at the lateral side of the elbow joint. Note erosions at the radiocapitellar joint *(arrow)*. **(C)** Sagittal T1-weighted and **(D)** sagittal T2-weighted MR images of the ankle in another patient with RA demonstrate a hypointense rheumatoid nodule in the plantar aspect of the heel *(arrows)*.

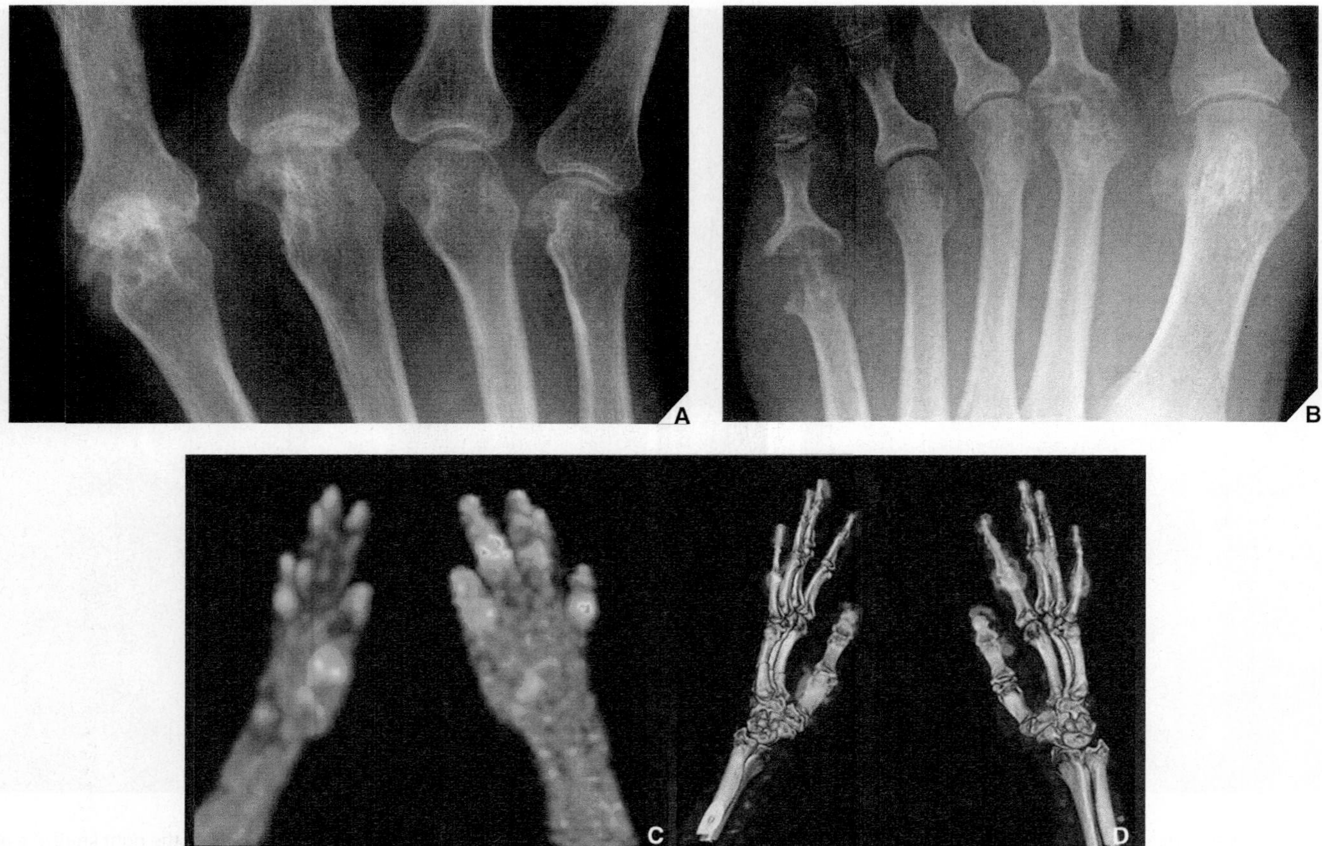

FIGURE 14.31 RA of the small joints. Radiographs of the hand **(A)** and foot **(B)** of a 51-year-old woman show typical erosions of the small joints. Technetium-99m (^{99m}Tc)-labeled methylene diphosphonate (MDP) single-photon emission computed tomography (SPECT) **(C)** and SPECT/CT three-dimensional (3D) reconstructed image **(D)** of the hands of another patient with RA show involvement of several small joints of both hands.

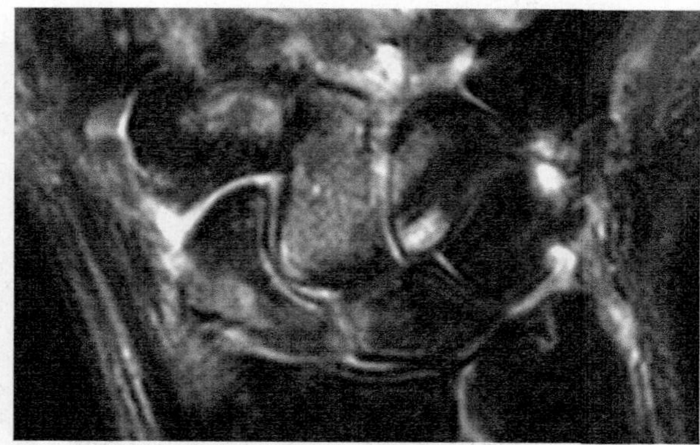

FIGURE 14.32 MRI of very early changes of RA. Coronal short time inversion recovery (STIR) MRI demonstrates bone marrow edema involving the carpal bones and radial styloid process, without discrete bone erosions. There are small joint effusions and pericapsular edema. Bone marrow edema may be seen on MRI before the bone erosions are seen on radiographs (pre-erosive edema). This feature makes MRI a good tool for establishing an early diagnosis thus leading to early therapy of RA.

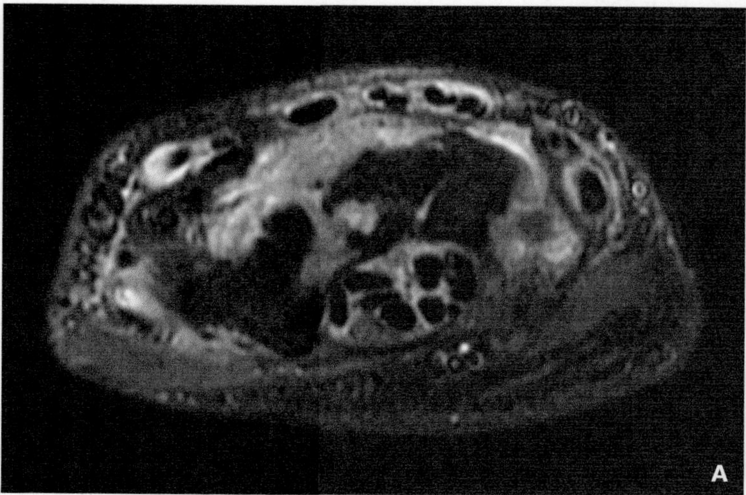

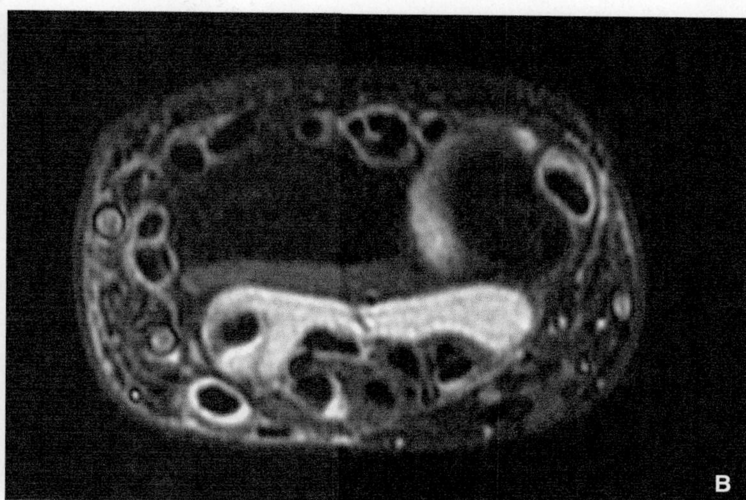

FIGURE 14.33 MRI of tenosynovitis. **(A,B)** Two axial short time inversion recovery (STIR) and **(C)** axial T1-weighted fat-suppressed MR post contrast image in a 67-year-old woman with RA show enhancing synovial thickening of the extensor tendons and enhancing tenosynovitis of the flexor tendons. (Courtesy of Prof. Andrew J. Grainger, Cambridge, United Kingdom.)

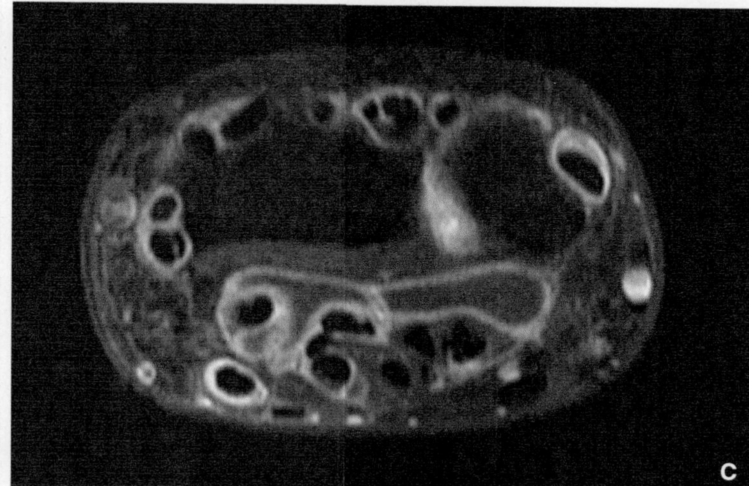

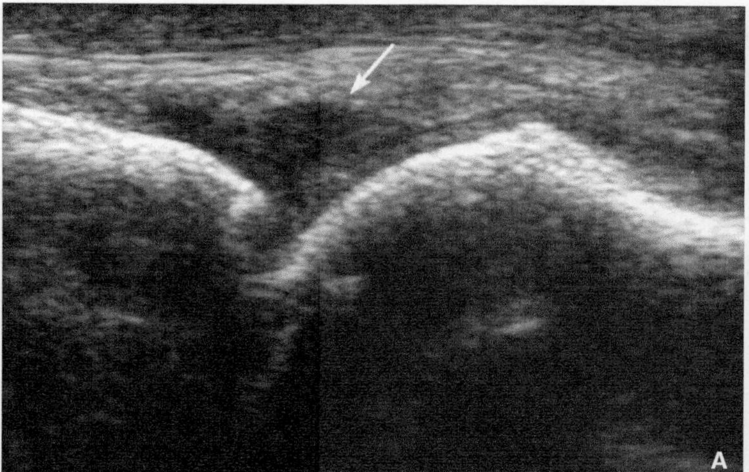

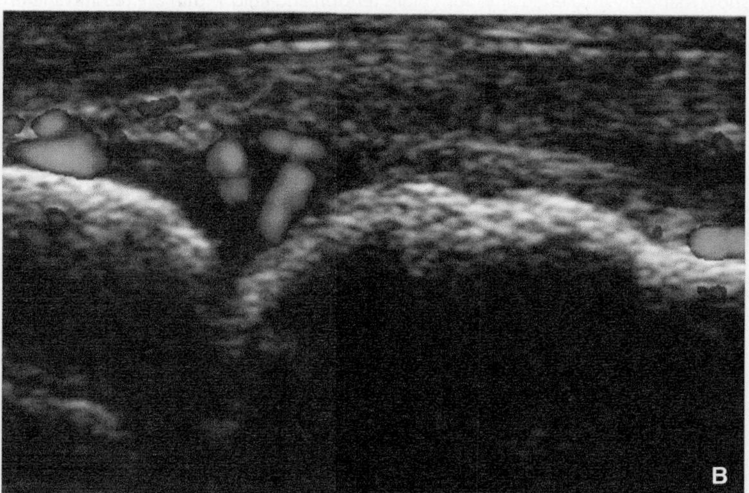

FIGURE 14.34 US of small joint synovitis. **(A)** Longitudinal US image of the left second metacarpophalangeal joint of a 60-year-old man with RA shows hypoechoic triangular area at the site of distended joint capsule *(arrow)*, representing joint effusion and synovial thickening. **(B)** Power Doppler color scale of the same area shows increased vascularity consistent with synovial hyperemia from active inflammation. (Reprinted with permission from American Registry of Pathology, from Klein MJ, Bonar SF, Freemont T, et al, eds. *Atlas of nontumor pathology. Non-neoplastic diseases of bones and joints*. Washington, DC: American Registry of Pathology and Armed Forces Institute of Pathology; 2011:68, Fig. 2.17.)

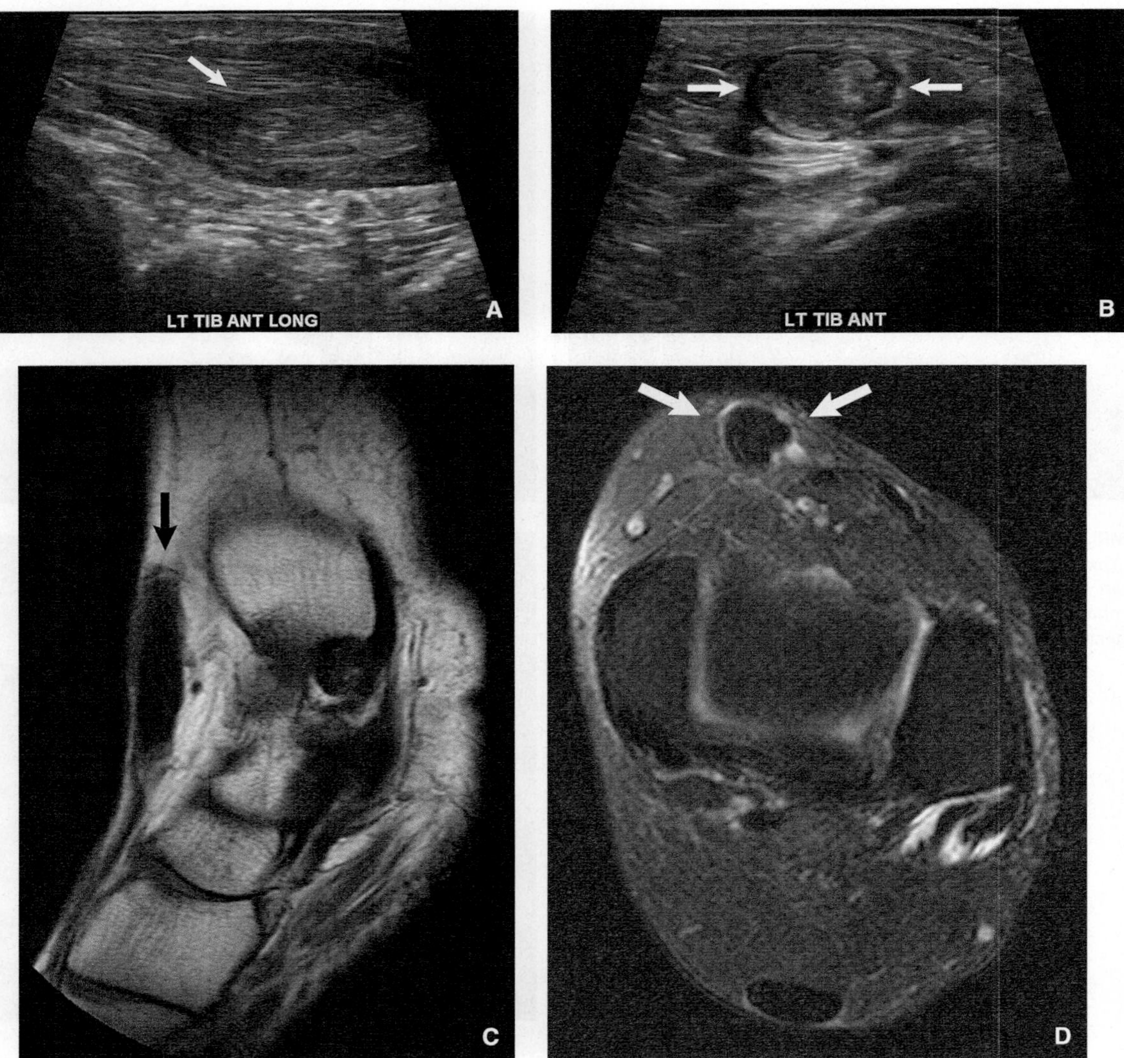

FIGURE 14.35 US and MRI of tenosynovitis. **(A)** Longitudinal and **(B)** transverse US images of the anterior aspect of the left ankle of a 65-year-old woman with RA show markedly thickened anterior tibialis tendon and fluid within the tendon sheath *(arrows)*. **(C)** Sagittal T1-weighted MR image confirms the thickening of the anterior tibialis tendon. **(D)** Axial proton density–weighted fat-suppressed MR image shows in addition fluid within the anterior tibialis tendon sheath *(arrows)* and tenosynovitis of the peroneus longus and brevis tendons *(arrowheads)*. (Courtesy of Cyrus Bateni, MD, Sacramento, California.)

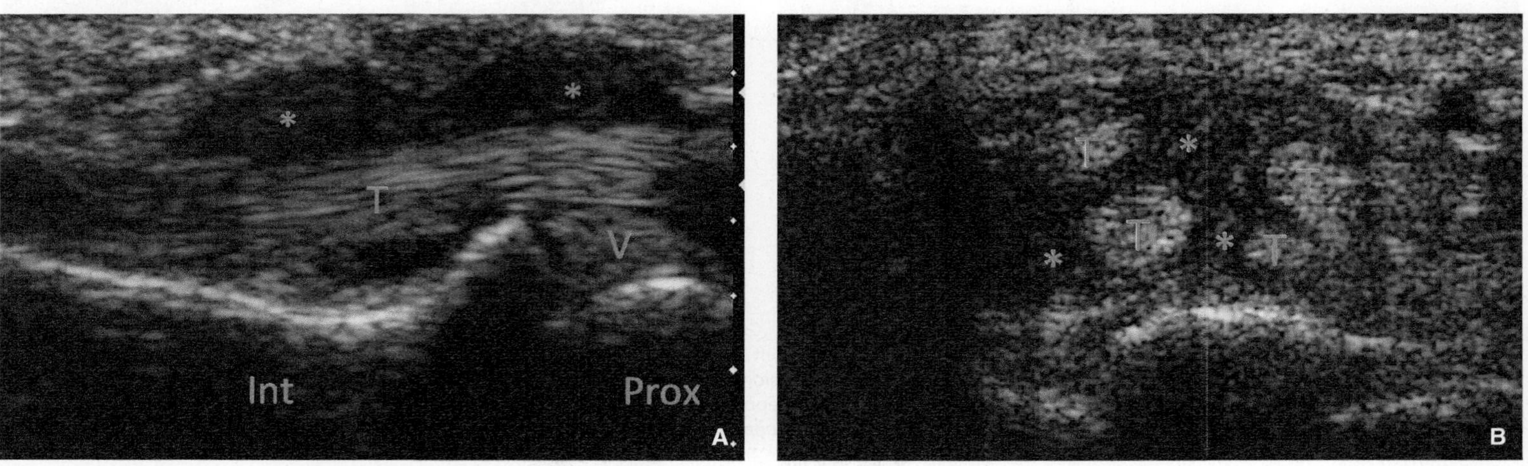

FIGURE 14.36 US of tenosynovitis. **(A)** Image in the longitudinal plane at the level of the proximal interphalangeal joint of the index finger of a woman with RA shows low reflective synovitis *(asterisks)* surrounding the flexor digitorum profunda tendon *(T)*. *Int*, intermediate phalanx; *Prox*, proximal phalangeal head; *V*, volar plate. **(B)** In another patient with RA, the synovitis *(asterisks)* surrounding the flexor tendons within the carpal tunnel is seen as low reflective change around the tendons. *T*, flexor tendons. (Courtesy of Prof. Andrew J. Grainger, Cambridge, United Kingdom.)

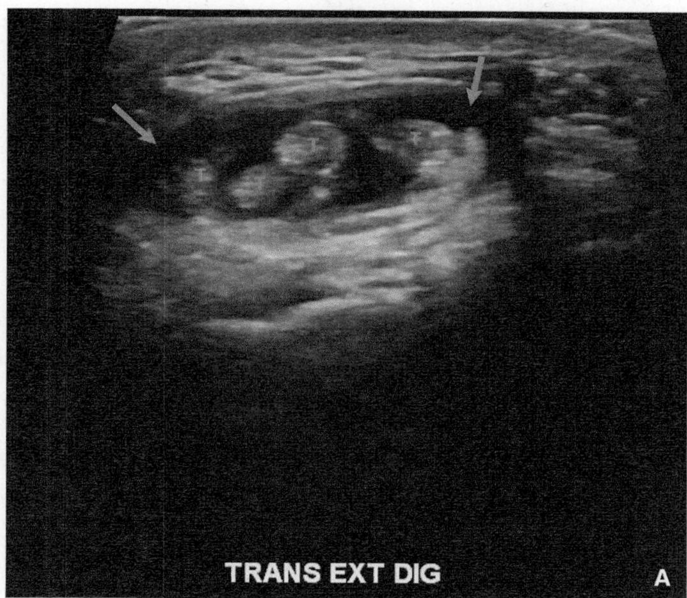

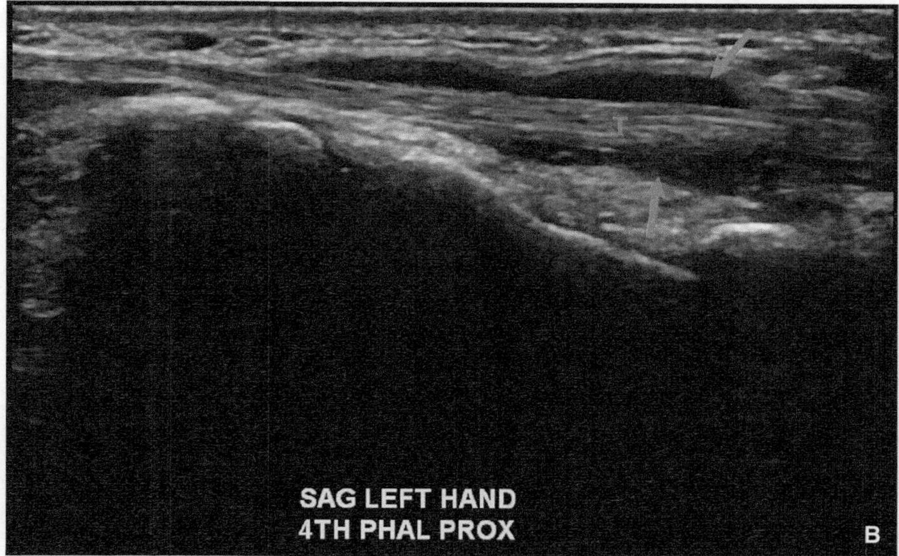

FIGURE 14.37 US of tenosynovitis. **(A)** Image in the transverse plane of the left wrist shows fluid *(arrows)* surrounding the thickened extensor tendons *(T)*. **(B)** Image in the sagittal plane shows lobulated fluid *(arrows)* tracking along the thickened extensor digitorum tendon of the ring finger *(T)*. (Courtesy of Cyrus Bateni, MD, Sacramento, California.)

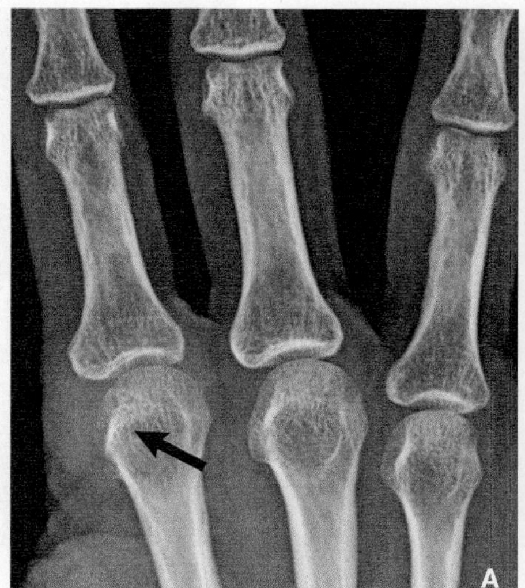

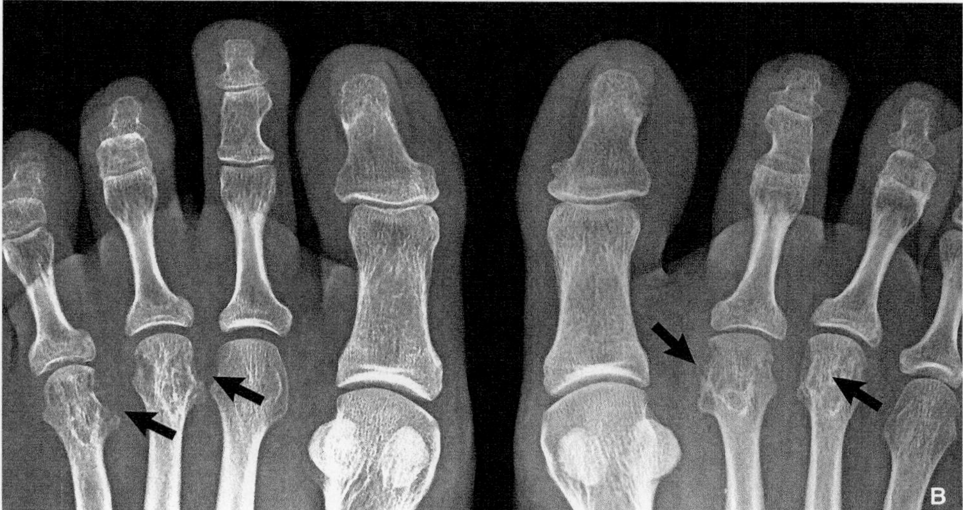

FIGURE 14.38 RA—loss of articular cortex. **(A)** Very early radiographic feature is the loss of so-called *articular cortex* of the second metacarpal head on the radial aspect *(arrow)*. Compare with the intact outline of the normal third and fourth metacarpal heads. **(B)** In another patient, the metatarsal heads are affected in similar manner *(arrows)*.

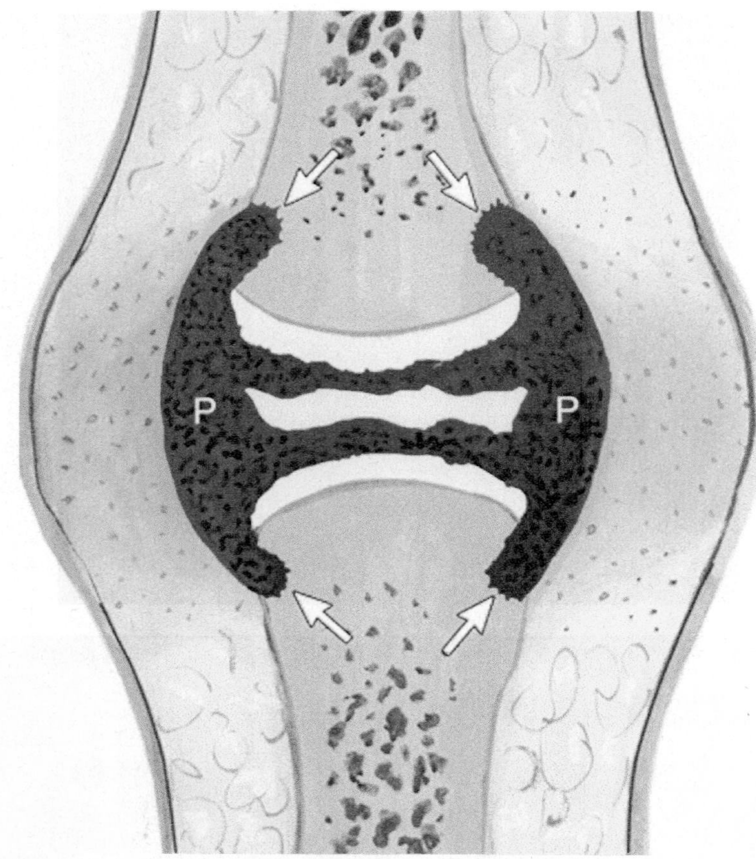

FIGURE 14.39 RA—erosions in bare areas. Invasion of inflammatory pannus *(P)* into the articular areas not covered by the articular cartilage (so-called *bare areas*) causes marginal erosions *(arrows)*.

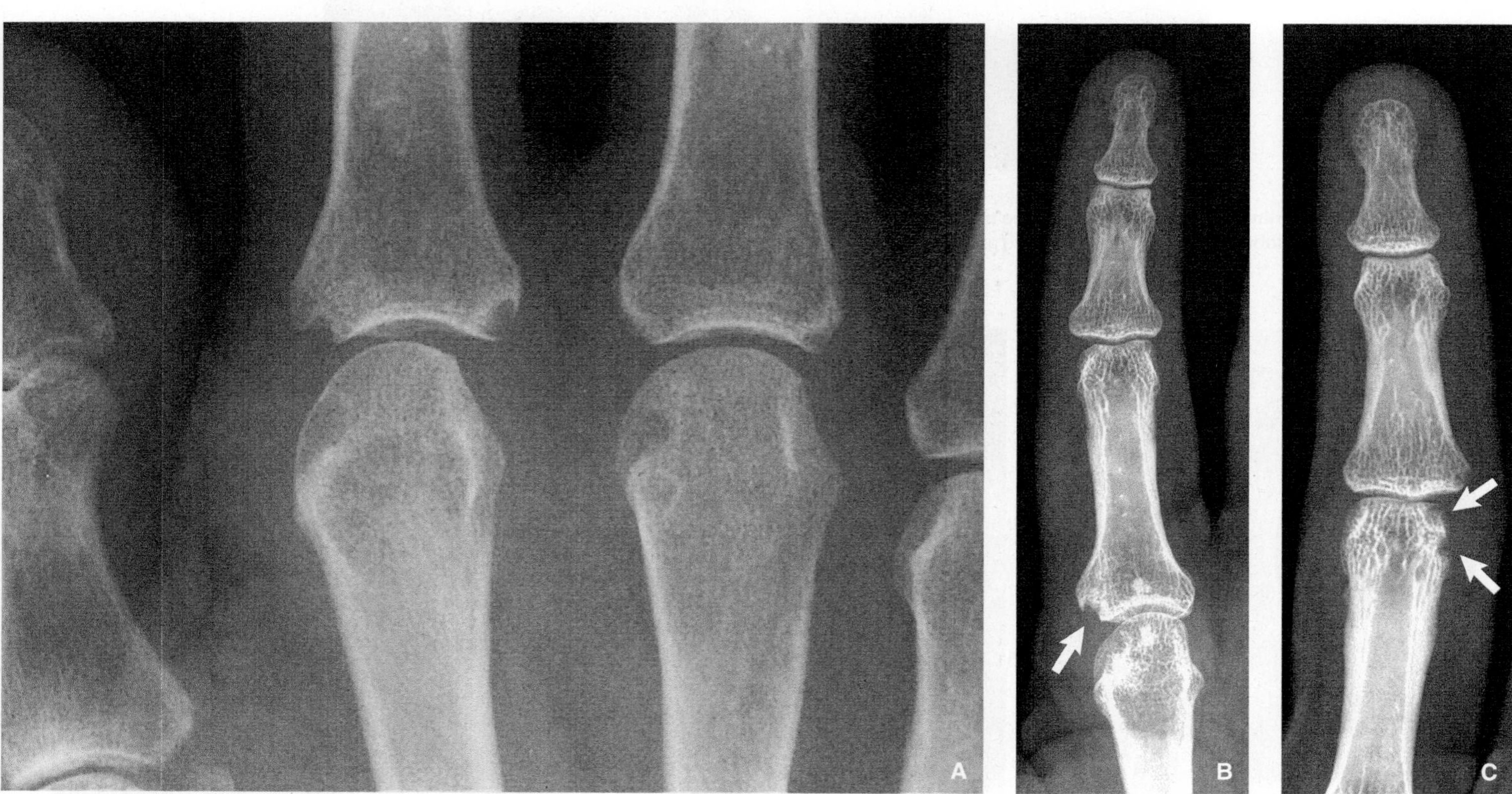

FIGURE 14.40 RA—erosions in bare areas. **(A)** Typical erosions in the bare areas are seen in this 55-year-old woman with RA. Note also periarticular osteoporosis and soft-tissue swelling. **(B)** Radiograph of the index finger shows erosion in the bare area at the base of the proximal phalanx *(arrow)* associated with soft-tissue swelling. **(C)** Radiograph of the middle finger of another patient shows erosions in the bare areas at the distal end of the proximal phalanx *(arrows)*. **B** and **C**, Reprinted with permission from Greenspan A, Gershwin ME. *Imaging in rheumatology: a clinical approach*. Philadelphia: Wolters Kluwer; 2018:225, Fig. 6.34B,C.)

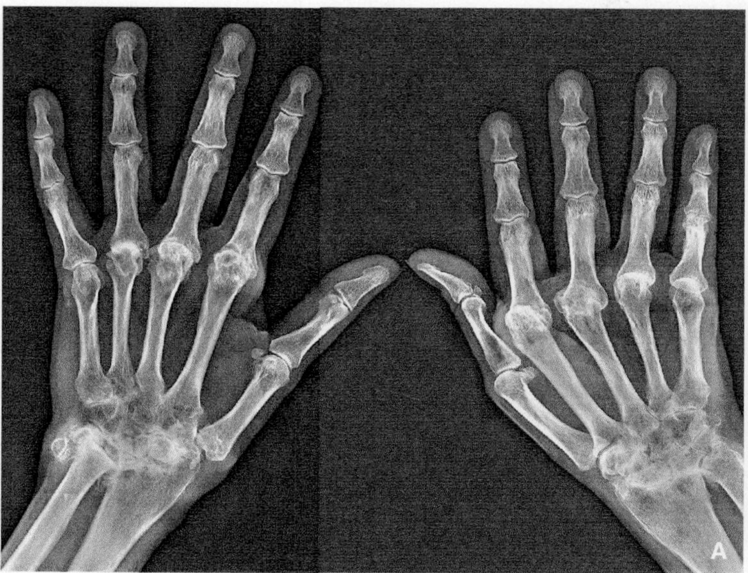

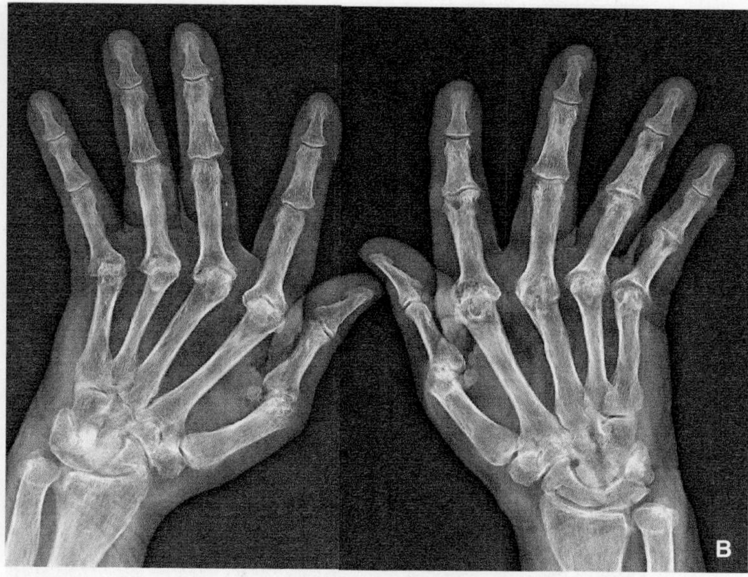

FIGURE 14.41 RA of the hands. **(A)** Dorsovolar radiograph of both hands of a 63-year-old woman shows typical for this disease loss of articular cartilage and subchondral erosions affecting predominantly metacarpophalangeal, radiocarpal, and intercarpal joints. Observe that the distal interphalangeal joints are spared. **(B)** Dorsovolar radiograph of both hands of a 72-year-old woman shows articular erosions affecting metacarpophalangeal joints of both hands. The proximal interphalangeal joints of the left hand are also affected. The distal interphalangeal joints are normal.

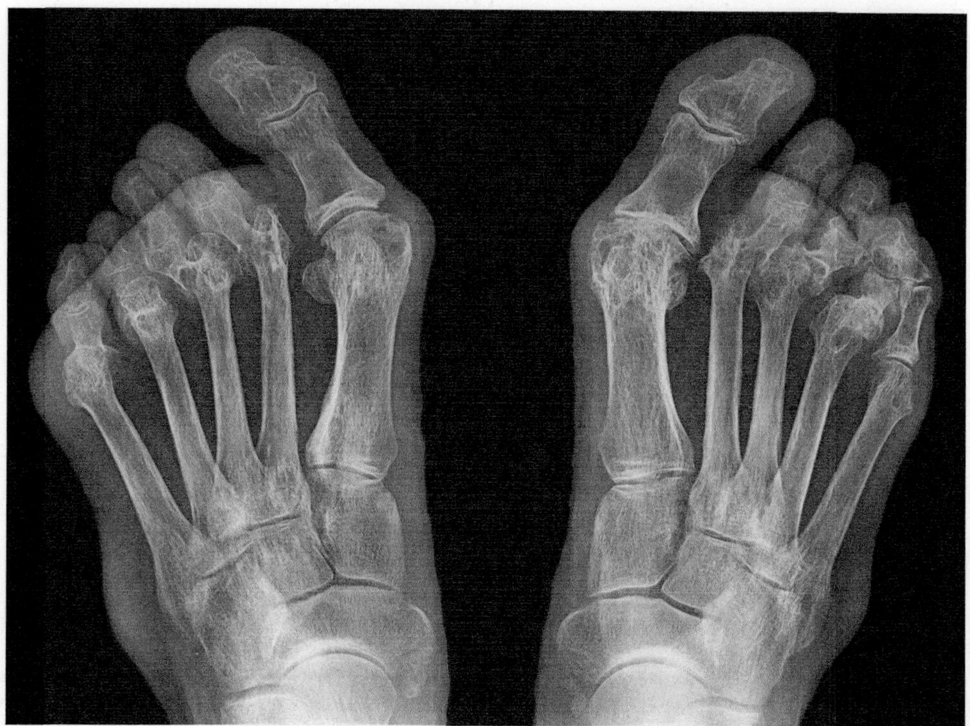

FIGURE 14.42 RA of the feet. Dorsoplantar radiograph of both feet of a 55-year-old woman shows erosions and subluxations of metatarsophalangeal joints.

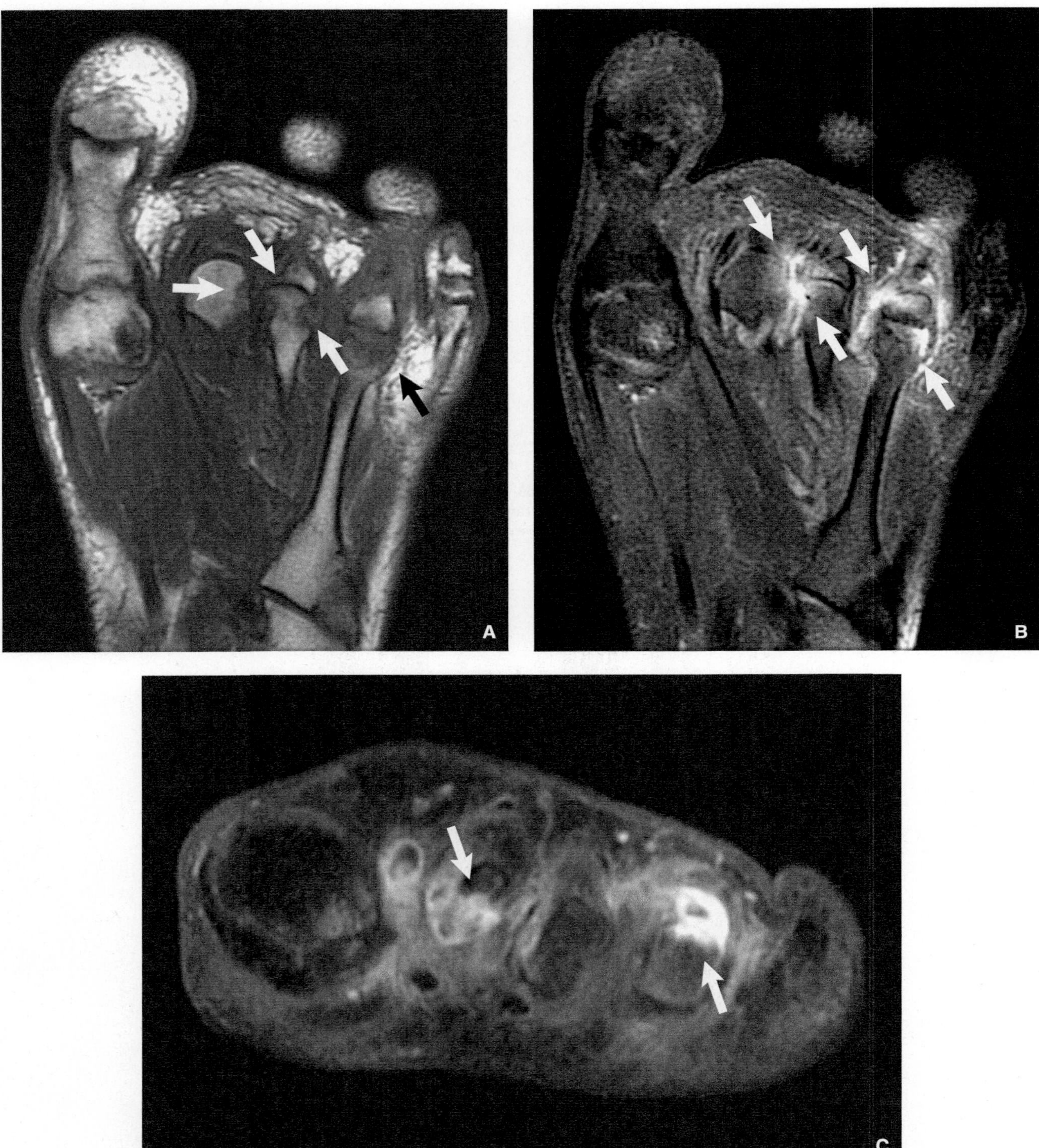

FIGURE 14.43 MRI of RA of the foot. **(A)** Long axis T1-weighted, **(B)** long axis proton density–weighted fat-suppressed, and **(C)** short axis T1-weighted fat-suppressed postcontrast MR images of the left foot of a 64-year-old woman show erosions of the second, third, and fourth metatarsophalangeal joints *(arrows)* accompanied by synovitis. (Reprinted with permission from Greenspan A, Gershwin ME. *Imaging in rheumatology: a clinical approach*, 1st ed. Philadelphia: Wolters Kluwer; 2018:227.)

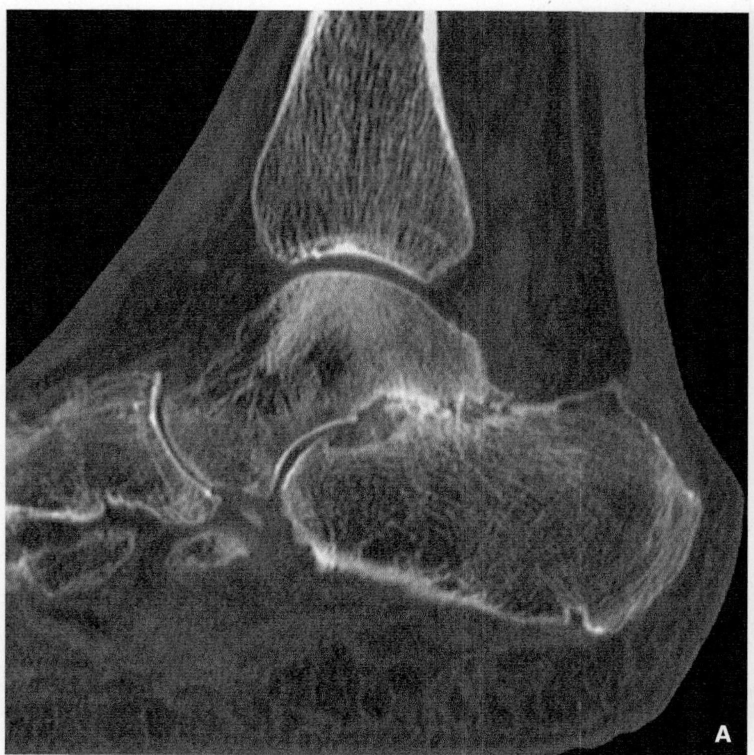

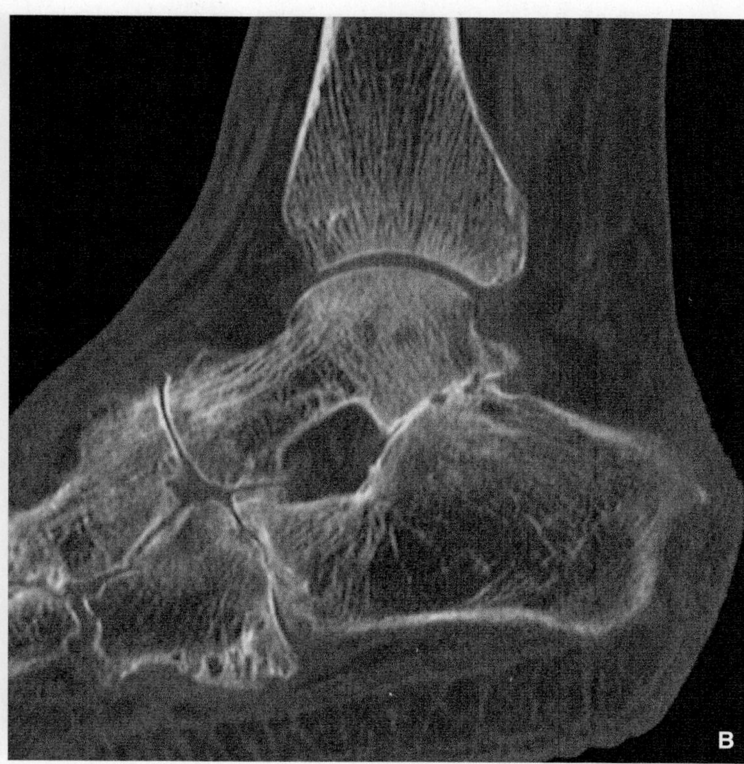

FIGURE 14.44 CT of RA of the foot. **(A,B)** Two sagittal reformatted CT images of the hindfoot of a 52-year-old man show erosions of the subtalar and calcaneocuboid joints.

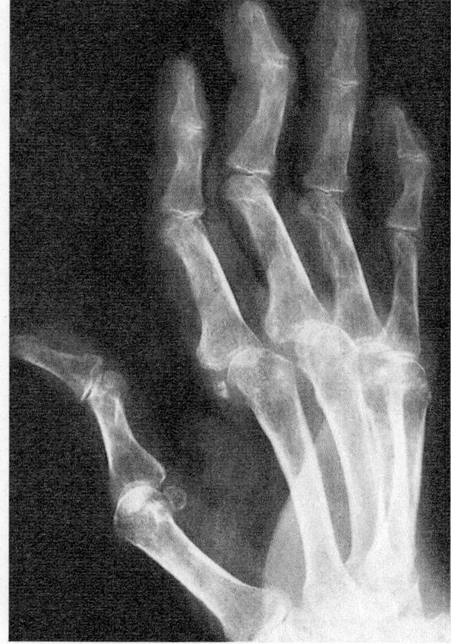

FIGURE 14.45 Rheumatoid arthritis. Oblique radiograph of the hand of a 59-year-old woman shows the swan-neck deformity of the second through fifth fingers. Note the flexion in the distal interphalangeal joints and the extension in the proximal interphalangeal joints, the hallmarks of this abnormality.

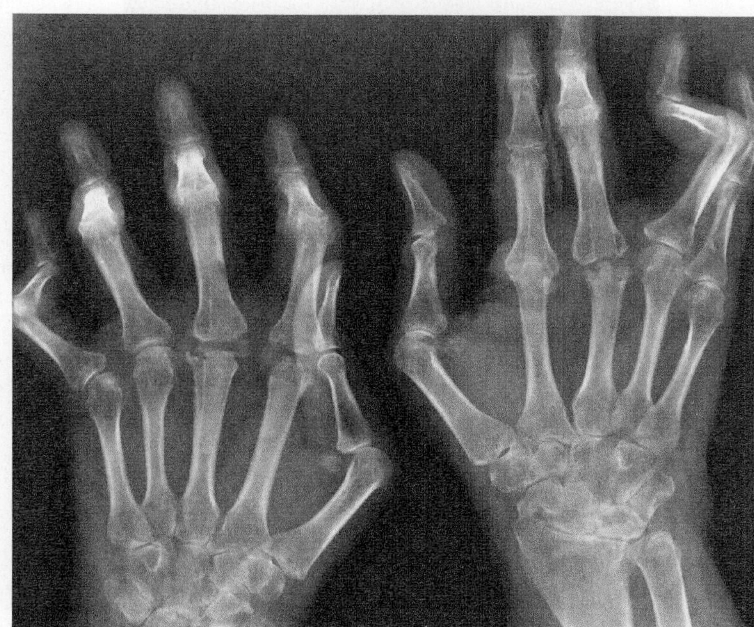

FIGURE 14.46 Rheumatoid arthritis. Dorsovolar radiograph of the hands of a 48-year-old woman demonstrates the boutonnière deformity in the small and ring fingers of the right hand and in the ring finger of the left hand.

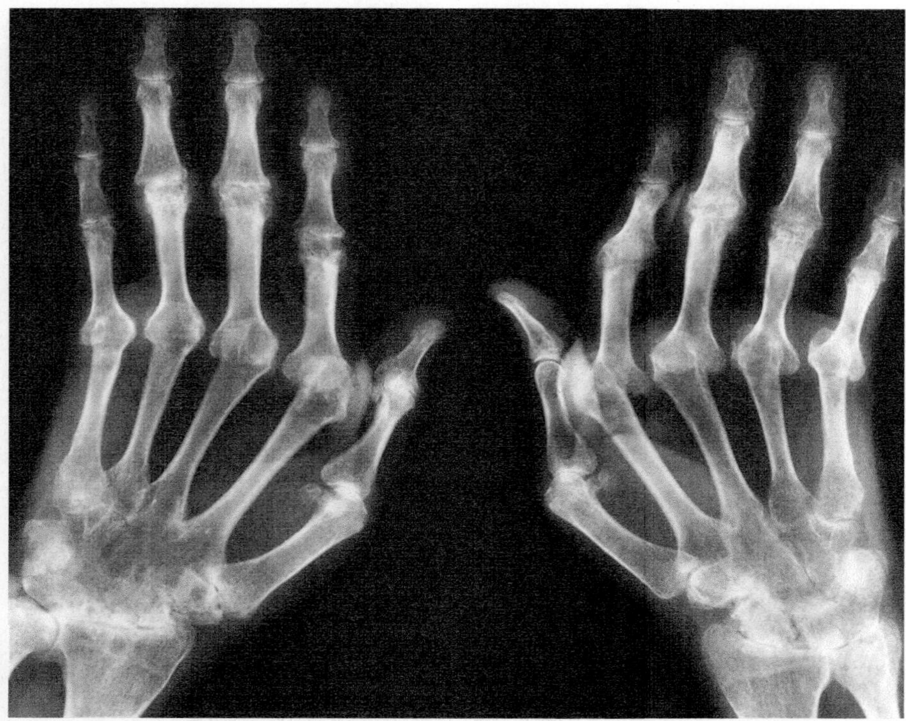

FIGURE 14.47 Rheumatoid arthritis. Dorsovolar radiographs of both hands of a 51-year-old woman shows subluxation in the metacarpophalangeal joints resulting in ulnar deviation of the fingers and radial deviation in the radiocarpal articulations. Note also ankylosis of the midcarpal articulations of the right hand.

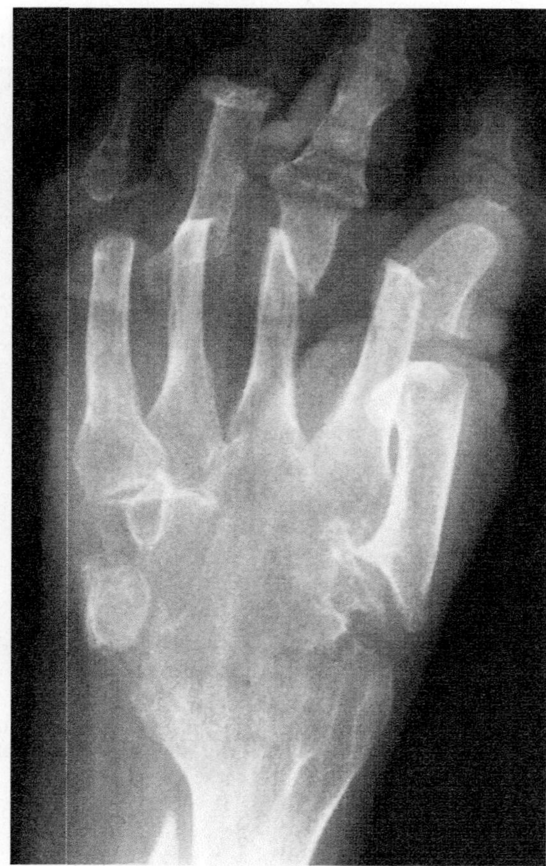

FIGURE 14.48 Rheumatoid arthritis. Dorsovolar view of the right hand of a 54-year-old woman with long-standing advanced RA demonstrates the *main-en-lorgnette* deformity. Note the telescoping of the fingers secondary to destructive joint changes and dislocations in the metacarpophalangeal joints. There is also ankylosis of the radiocarpal and intercarpal articulations and "penciling" of the distal ulna.

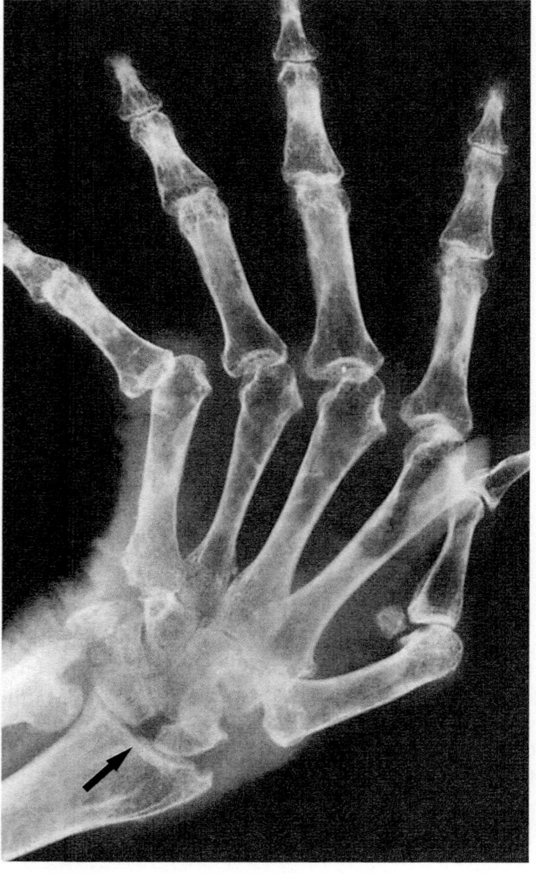

FIGURE 14.49 Rheumatoid arthritis. Dorsovolar view of the hand of a 60-year-old woman shows a gap between the scaphoid and lunate *(arrow)*, indicating destruction of the scapholunate ligament. Note also the subluxation in the metacarpophalangeal joints resulting in ulnar deviation of the fingers.

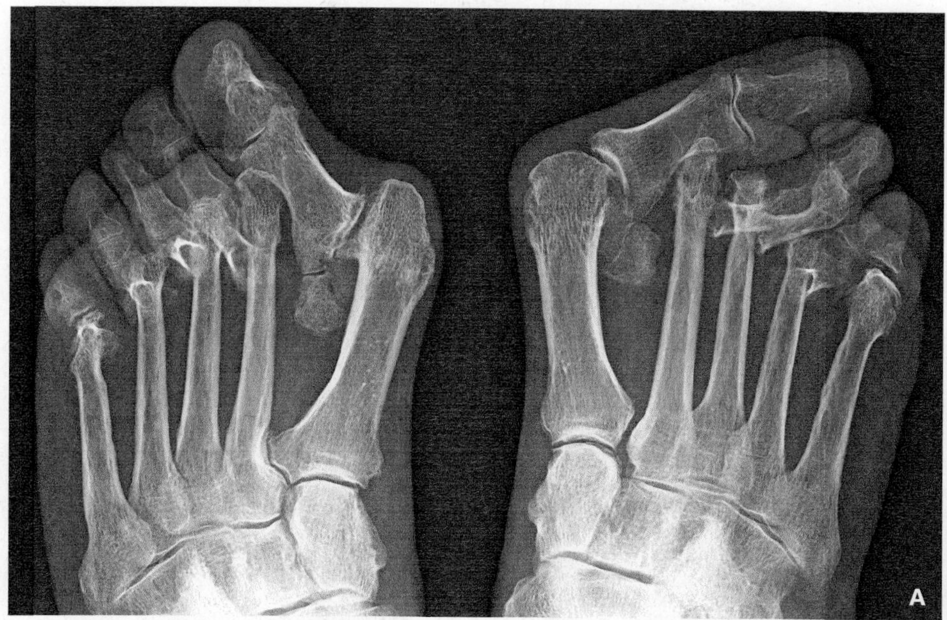

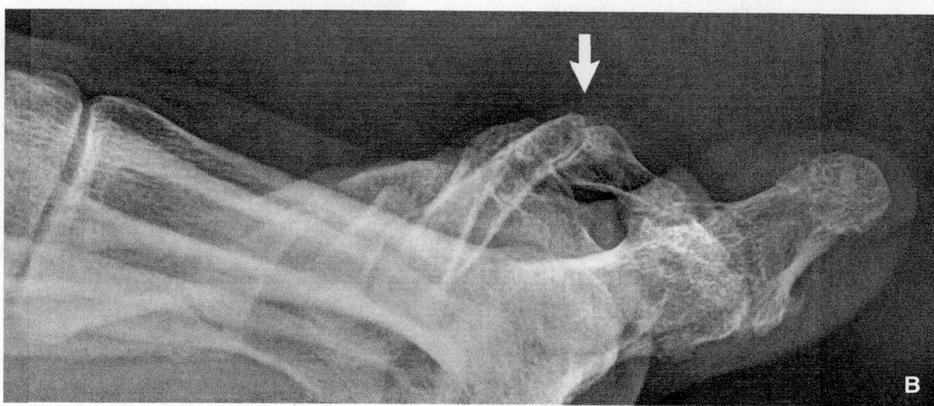

FIGURE 14.50 Rheumatoid arthritis. **(A)** Dorsoplantar radiograph of both feet and **(B)** lateral radiograph of the toes of the left foot of a 71-year-old woman show erosions of the metatarsophalangeal joints associated with subluxations and dislocations, severe hallux valgus deformity, and hammertoes *(arrow)*.

Involvement of the Spine

The thoracic and lumbar segments are affected in RA only on rare occasions. The cervical spine, however, is involved in approximately 50% of individuals with this condition (Table 14.2). The most characteristic radiographic features of RA in the cervical spine can be observed in the odontoid process, the atlantoaxial joints, and the apophyseal joints.

TABLE 14.2 Abnormalities of the Cervical Spine in Rheumatoid Arthritis

Osteoporosis
Erosion of the odontoid process
Atlantoaxial (C1-2) subluxation
Vertical translation of the odontoid (cranial settling)
Erosions of the apophyseal joints
Fusion of the apophyseal joints
Erosions of the Luschka joints
Disk space narrowing
Erosions and sclerosis of the vertebral body margins
Erosions (whittling) of the spinous processes
Subluxations of the vertebral bodies ("stepladder" or "doorstep" appearance on lateral radiographs)

Modified from Resnick D, Niwayama G. Rheumatoid arthritis and the seronegative spondyloarthropathies: radiographic and pathologic concepts. In: Resnick D, ed. *Diagnosis of bone and joint disorders*, 3rd ed. Philadelphia: WB Saunders; 1995:807–865. Copyright © 1995 Elsevier. With permission.

Erosive changes may be encountered in the odontoid process and apophyseal joints (Figs. 14.51 and 14.52; see also Fig. 12.49), whereas subluxation is a common finding in the atlantoaxial joint (see Fig. 12.50), frequently accompanied by vertical translocation of the odontoid process (also known as *cranial settling* or *atlantoaxial impaction*) (Figs. 14.53 and 14.54). The most common abnormality is laxity of the transverse ligament connecting the odontoid to the atlas. This laxity becomes apparent on the radiograph obtained in the lateral view of the flexed cervical spine, is expressed by subluxation in the atlantoaxial joint (Fig. 14.55), and is frequently accompanied by cephalad migration of the odontoid process. This complication often requires surgical intervention, and the most common procedure to correct this is posterior fusion.

Severe involvement of the apophyseal joints leads to subluxations. In extremely rare cases, in a manner similar to that in JIA, the apophyseal joints may ankylose. The other structures occasionally affected by rheumatoid process are the intervertebral disks and adjacent vertebral bodies, which become involved as a result of synovitis extending from the joints of Luschka. Only a small percentage of patients with cervical disease may have cervical myelopathy. MRI is an ideal modality to evaluate spinal cord involvement in these patients (see Fig. 14.54).

Complications of Rheumatoid Arthritis

The complications of RA are related not only to the inflammatory process itself but also to the sequelae of treatment (see the discussion on the "Complications of Surgical Treatment" in Chapter 12). The large doses of steroids that are commonly prescribed in therapy often lead to the development of generalized osteoporosis. Severe osteoporosis and large

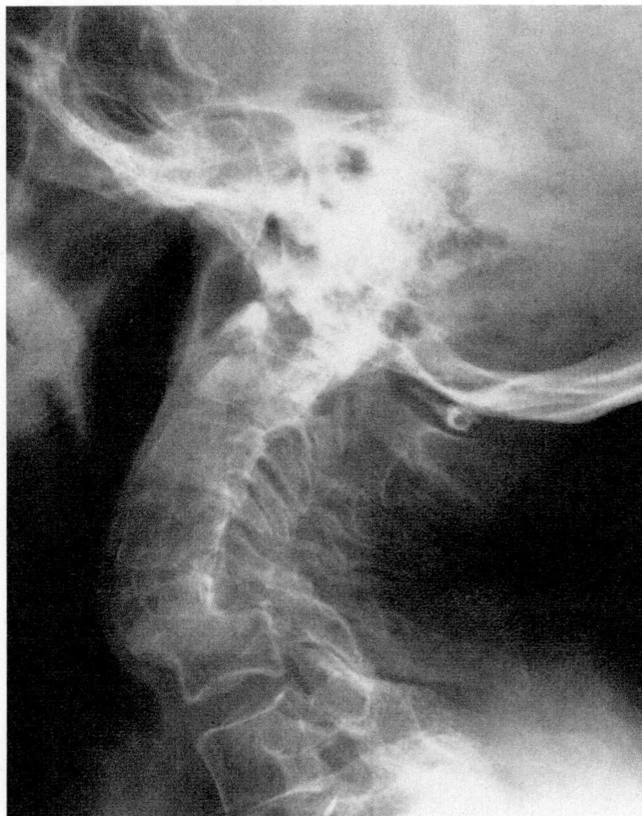

FIGURE 14.51 Rheumatoid arthritis of the cervical spine. Lateral radiograph of the cervical spine of a 52-year-old woman with advanced RA shows erosive changes of the apophyseal joints. In addition, note osteoporosis, erosion of the odontoid, erosions at the diskovertebral junctions, and whittling of the spinous processes.

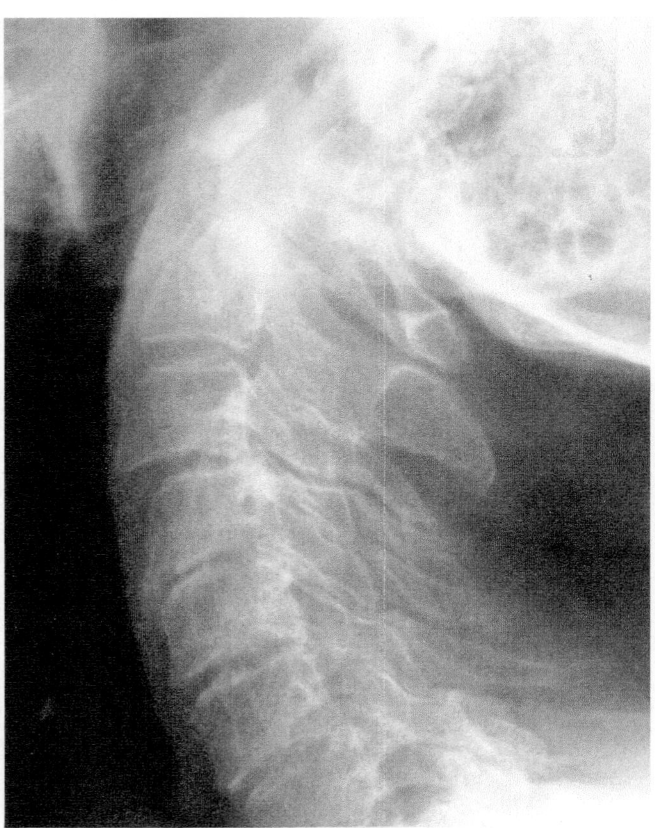

FIGURE 14.53 RA of the cervical spine. Lateral radiograph of the cervical spine of a 41-year-old woman shows a vertical translocation of the odontoid process (cranial settling). Note also erosive changes at the diskovertebral junctions, erosions of the apophyseal joints, and whittling of the spinous processes.

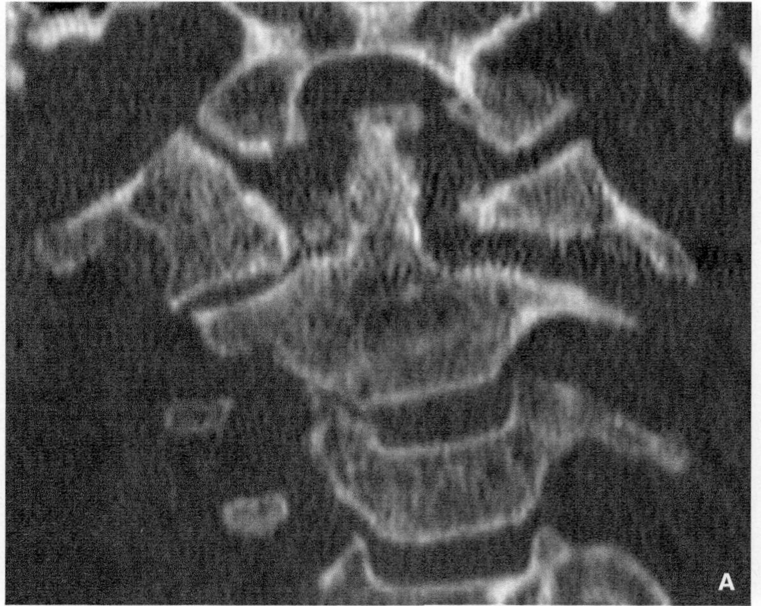

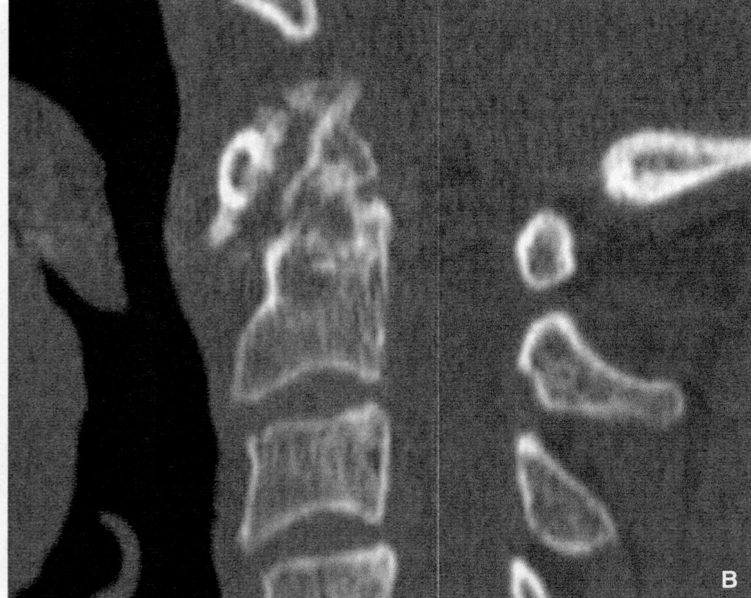

FIGURE 14.52 CT of RA of the cervical spine. **(A)** Coronal and **(B)** sagittal reformatted CT images of the upper cervical spine of a 47-year-old woman show erosions of the odontoid process.

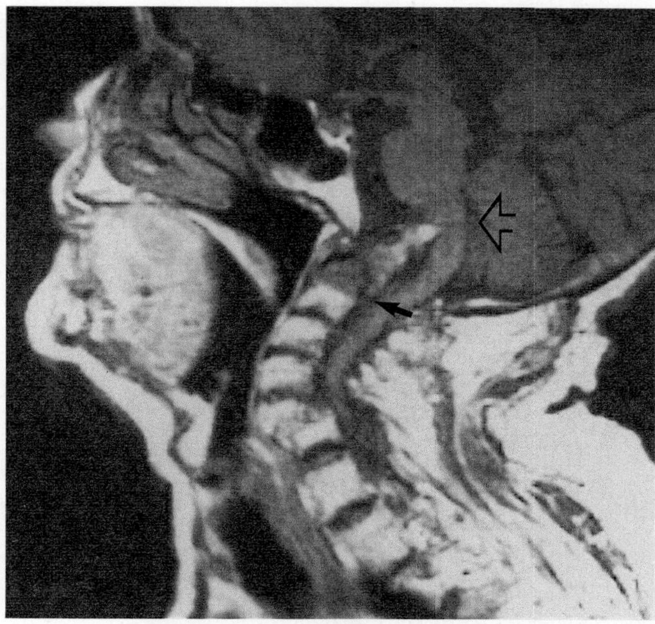

FIGURE 14.54 MRI of RA of the cervical spine. A 52-year-old woman with advanced RA presented with chronic neck pain, weakness of the upper limbs, numbness in both hands, and occasional dyspnea and cardiac arrhythmia. A sagittal spin echo T1-weighted MR image shows inflammatory pannus eroding odontoid *(arrow)* and cranial settling with cephalad migration of C2 impinging on the medulla oblongata *(open arrow)*.

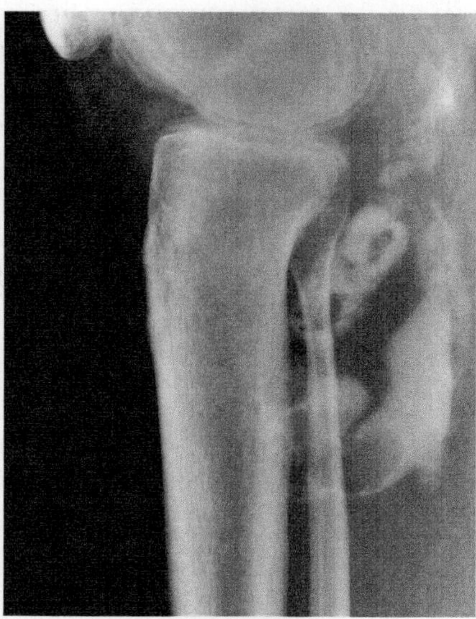

FIGURE 14.56 RA complicated with a ruptured popliteal cyst. A 31-year-old woman with a 2-year history of seropositive RA developed swelling of the upper calf and tenderness in the popliteal fossa. A presumptive diagnosis of thrombophlebitis was made, but a venogram failed to corroborate this. This lateral view of a knee arthrogram shows a large ruptured popliteal cyst (Baker) dissecting into the medial aspect of the calf. This condition is a well-documented complication in patients with RA. (Reprinted with permission from NYU Grossman School of Medicine, from Greenspan A, Baker ND, Norman A. Rheumatoid arthritis simulating other lesions. *Bull Hosp Joint Dis Orthop Inst* 1983;43:70–77.)

bony erosions may in turn precipitate pathologic fracture, a frequent complication. Tear of the rotator cuff may also occur because of erosion by inflammatory pannus in the shoulder joint (see Fig. 14.9). In the knee, a large popliteal (Baker) cyst may complicate RA changes (Figs. 14.56 and 14.57; see also Figs. 14.24 and 14.25); this condition may be misdiagnosed as thrombophlebitis (see Fig. 2.22).

Rheumatoid Nodulosis

A variant of RA is rheumatoid nodulosis, which occurs predominantly in men. It is a nonsystemic disorder characterized by the presence of multiple subcutaneous nodules (Fig. 14.58) and a very high rheumatoid factor titer; as a rule, there are no joint abnormalities. Occasionally, small cystic lesions may be present in various bones. Nodules are usually different in size and consistency, and distribution is over the elbows, extensor surfaces of hands and feet, and other pressure points. The most striking feature is the lack of systemic manifestations of RA.

On histologic examination, the nodules show typical rheumatoid changes, including central necrosis surrounded by palisading histiocytes and fibroblasts, with an outer layer of connective tissue and chronic inflammatory cells. Only occasionally will the histologic appearance be atypical. In these cases, the nodule may contain abundant cholesterol clefts and lipid-loaded macrophages, suggestive of xanthoma or even multicentric reticulohistiocytosis.

Therapy is usually limited to the occasional use of NSAIDs. Nodules that cause local pain because of nerve compression can be surgically removed. Some investigators have reported a decrease in nodule size after the use of penicillamine. These reports are controversial, however, because the regression and even disappearance of rheumatoid nodules may occur without any treatment at all.

In classic RA, small-vessel vasculitis is a primary factor in nodule development, and circulating immune complexes used by rheumatoid synovium are responsible for such extraarticular manifestations as

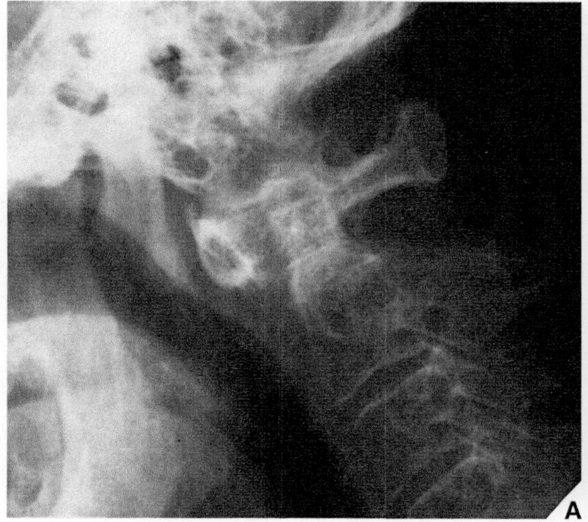

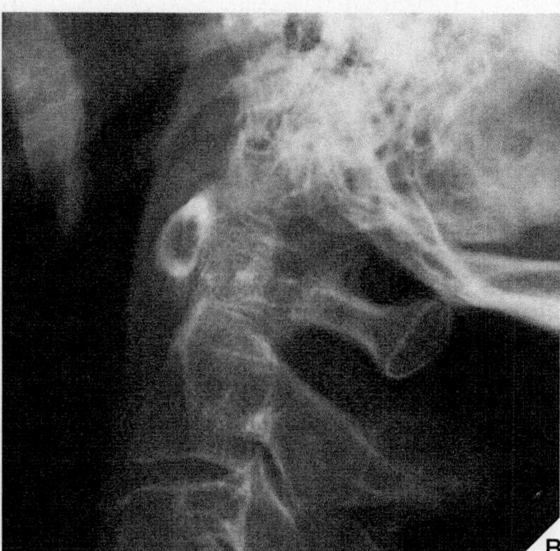

FIGURE 14.55 RA: C1-2 instability. **(A)** Flexion and **(B)** extension lateral radiographs demonstrate C1-2 subluxation in a 66-year-old woman with RA.

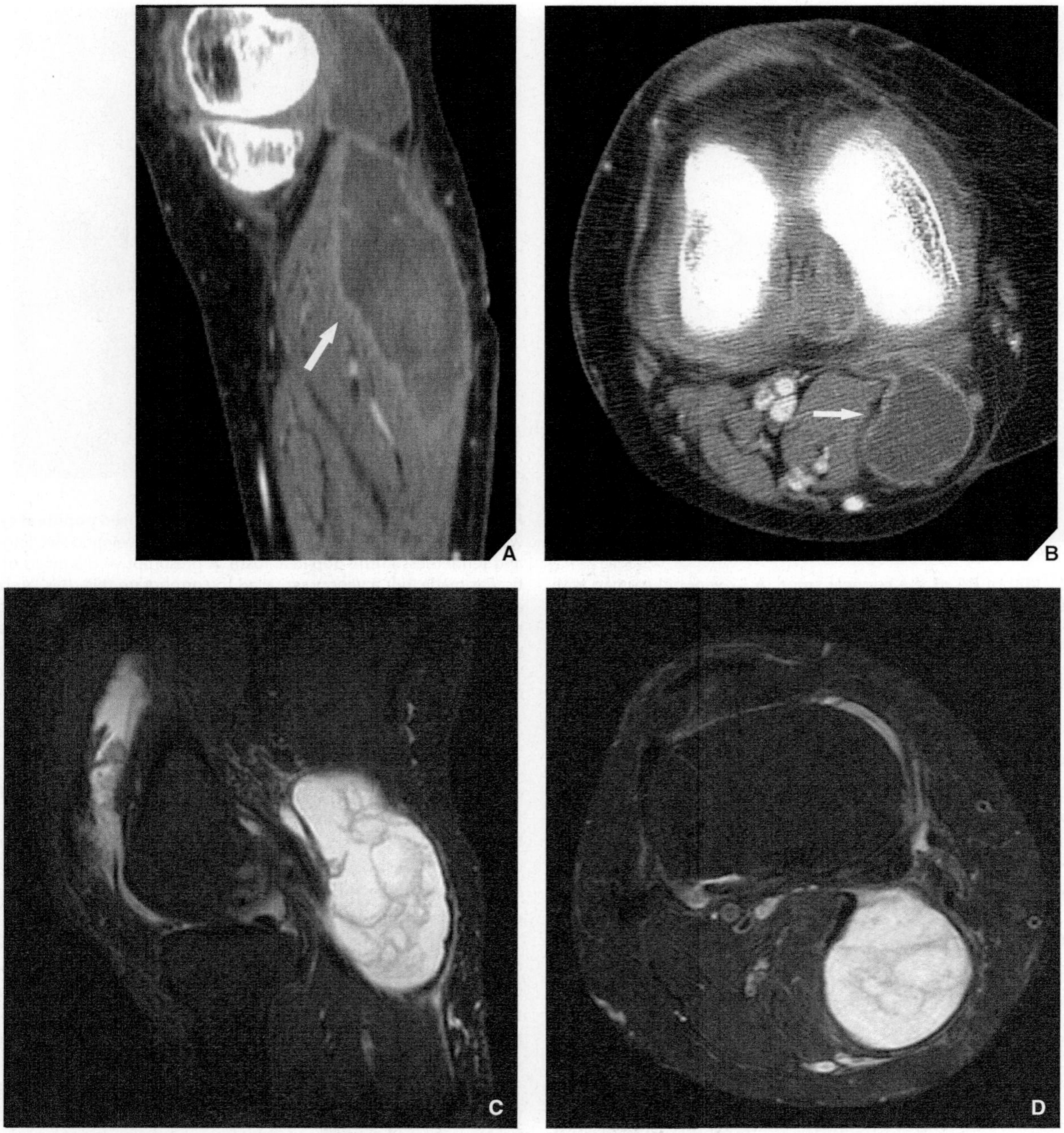

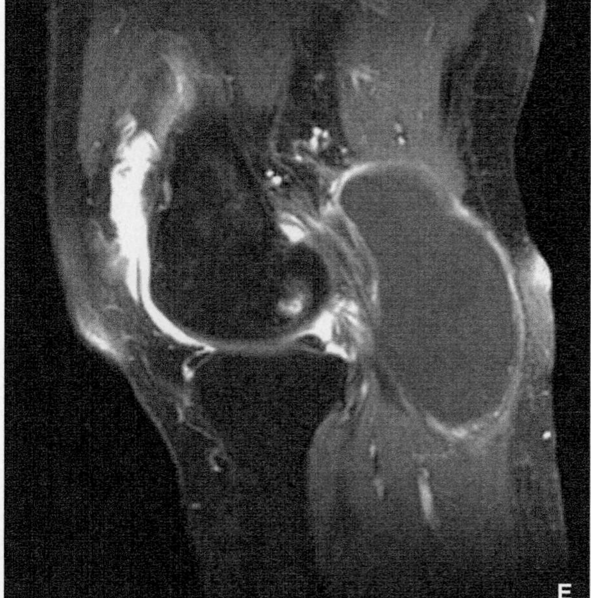

FIGURE 14.57 CT and MRI of the Baker cyst and the ruptured Baker cyst. **(A)** Sagittal reformatted and **(B)** axial CT images, obtained after intravenous administration of contrast agent, show a large Baker cyst *(arrows)* in a patient diagnosed with RA. **(C)** Sagittal inversion recovery (IR), **(D)** axial T2-weighted, and **(E)** sagittal T1-weighted fat-suppressed post-contrast MR images of another patient with RA show a large Baker cyst. *(Continued)*

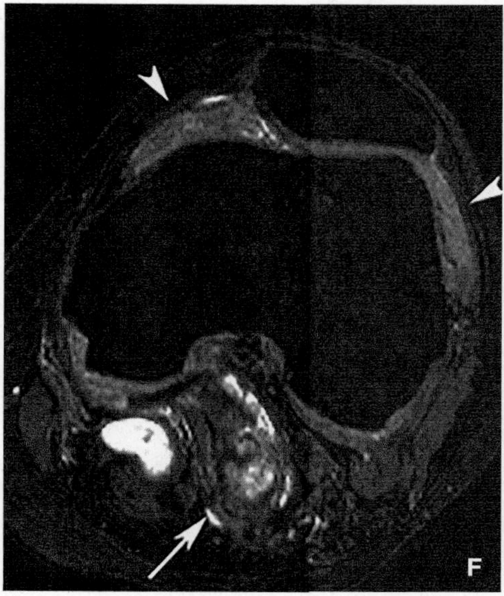

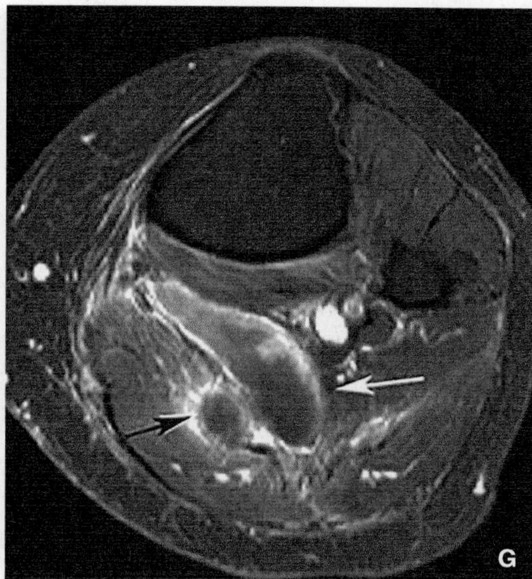

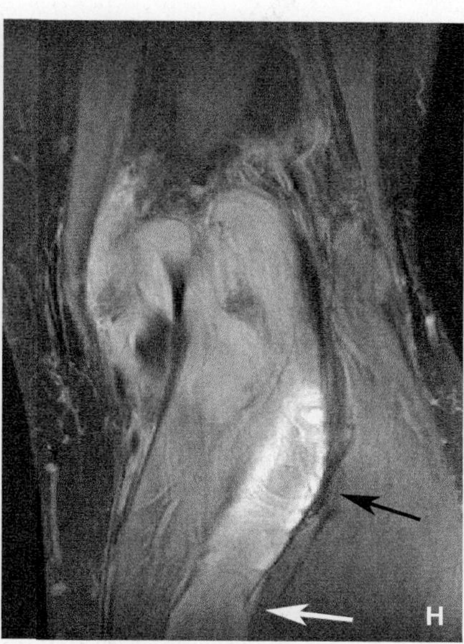

FIGURE 14.57 CT and MRI of the Baker cyst and the ruptured Baker cyst. ***(Continued)*** In another patient, **(F)** axial gradient-echo MR image demonstrates pannus formation in the knee *(arrowheads)* and within the popliteal cyst *(arrow)*. **(G)** T1-weighted fat-saturated MR image obtained after intravenous injection of gadolinium shows the distal extension of the popliteal cyst in the posterior compartment of the leg with peripheral enhancement *(arrows)*. **(H)** Coronal T1-weighted fat-saturated MR image obtained after intravenous injection of gadolinium shows the distal extension of the popliteal cyst in the leg with areas of contrast enhancement *(arrows)*, indicative of rupture.

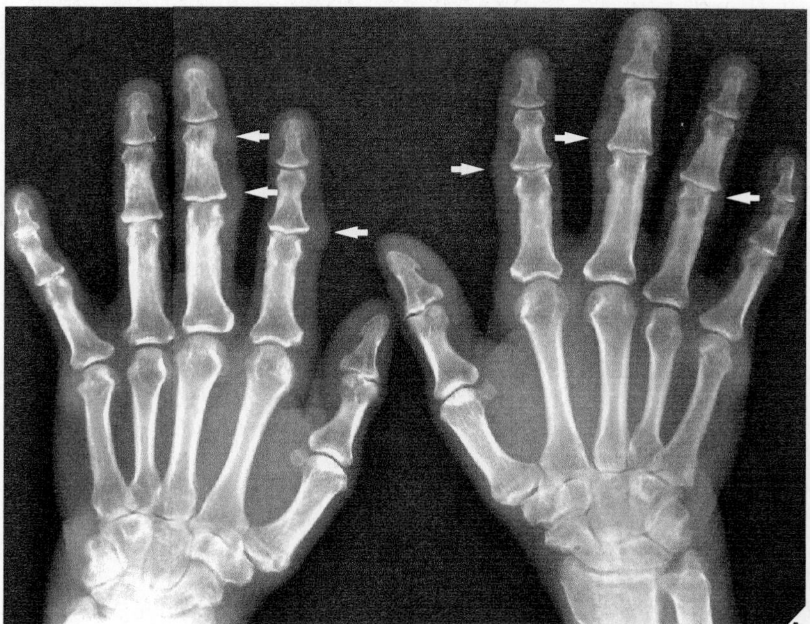

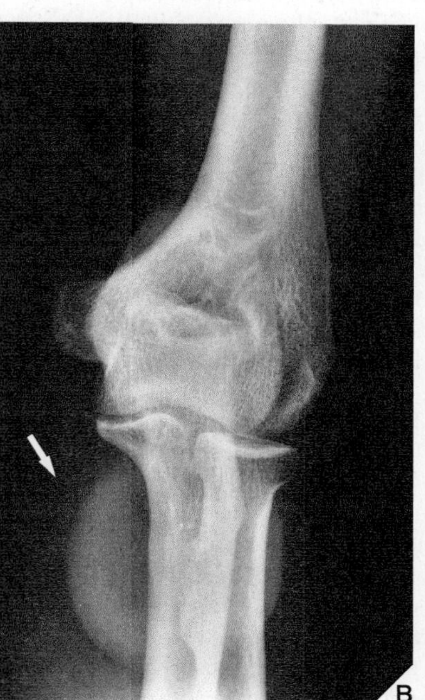

FIGURE 14.58 Rheumatoid nodulosis. A 52-year-old man with a 15-year history of polyarthritis presented with large, fluctuant nodules on the dorsal aspect of the hands and elbows. A high titer of rheumatoid factor (1:1,280) was identified in his serum. **(A)** Dorsovolar radiographs of both hands show several soft-tissue nodules adjacent to joints *(arrows)*. Note the lack of joint abnormalities. **(B)** Anteroposterior and **(C)** lateral radiographs of the left elbow demonstrate similar soft-tissue masses at the dorsal aspect of the proximal forearm *(arrows)*. The elbow joint is intact. (Reprinted with permission from NYU Grossman School of Medicine, from Greenspan A, Baker ND, Norman A. Rheumatoid arthritis simulating other lesions. *Bull Hosp Joint Dis Orthop Inst* 1983;43:70–77.)

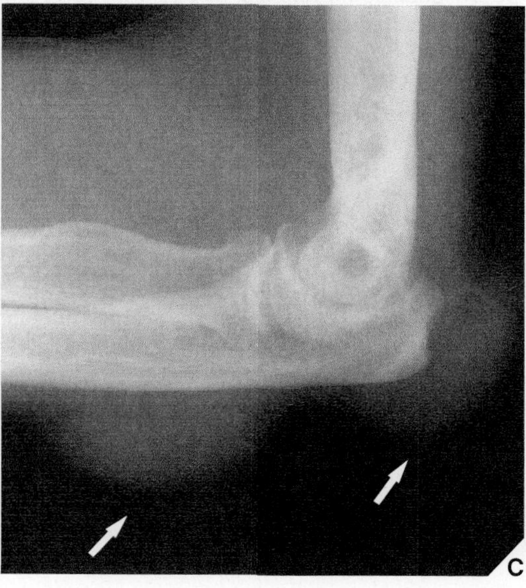

vasculitis, polyserositis, and nodules. In rheumatoid nodulosis, however, nodules develop in the absence of active joint disease. Thus, the pathogenesis of rheumatoid nodulosis remains unclear.

A positive family history of RA in some patients with rheumatoid nodulosis and the occurrence of familial nodulosis suggest the involvement of hereditary factors. Investigations into tissue typing, particularly the search for DW4/DRW4 antigens, may illustrate the pathogenesis of this rheumatoid variant. The strong male preponderance suggests that androgens may modify disease expression in genetically predisposed individuals. Rheumatoid nodulosis is often misdiagnosed as gout or xanthomatosis. Moreover, it should be kept in mind when evaluating this condition that approximately 20% of patients with classic RA have rheumatoid nodules, which are usually located at sites of pressure or stress such as the dorsal aspect of the hands and forearms (see Fig. 14.30). Articular involvement in nodular RA distinguishes it from rheumatoid nodulosis, which consequently has a better prognosis.

Juvenile Idiopathic Arthritis

JIA, formerly termed *juvenile rheumatoid arthritis*, is a heterogenous group of at least three chronic inflammatory synovial diseases that affect children; girls are more frequently affected than boys. The term *JIA* was introduced by the International League of Associations for Rheumatology (ILAR) to replace two other terms: juvenile RA and juvenile chronic arthritis. JIA is classified on the basis of the number of joints affected, variety of symptoms, family history, and serologic findings.

The three defined subtypes are Still disease, polyarticular arthritis, and pauciarticular (oligoarticular) arthritis. Some investigators include under this rubric also enthesitis-related arthritis (ERA) and juvenile PsA. Each of these subgroups has distinct clinical and laboratory findings and different natural histories. There is no pathognomonic laboratory test for any of them, and the diagnosis is based on the clinical spectrum exhibited by a given patient. The etiology is unknown, and the genetic component is complex, making clear distinction between the various subtypes sometimes difficult. The involvement of tumor necrosis factor (TNF) protein and its receptors in the pathology of JIA has been suggested by multiple studies. Studies of non-HLA genes with the MHC, cytokine, and T cell–related genes have been all positively associated with this arthritis, and most recently, link between MHC-encoded LMP7 gene and early-onset pauciarticular JIA and between the gene encoding Tapasin and systemic-onset JIA has been established.

Still Disease

Still disease, included by some authorities into the group of polyarticular JIA, is well known for sudden onset of spiking fever, lymphadenopathy, and an evanescent salmon-colored skin rash. Patients may exhibit hepatosplenomegaly, pleuritis, pericarditis, fatigue, anorexia, and weight loss. The majority of patients have chronic and recurrent arthralgias. A significant number of patients, depending on the series, may also subsequently have chronic polyarthritis. A poorly understood Still-like disease with fever and arthralgias may develop in some adult patients, recently designated as macrophage activation syndrome (MAS) (see in the following text). In all cases, etiology can be related to immunologic storm, namely, uncontrolled activation of macrophages and secretion of variety of proinflammatory cytokines.

Polyarticular Juvenile Idiopathic Arthritis

Polyarticular JIA consists of inflammation of five or more joints within 6 months of onset, with associated findings of anorexia, weight loss, fatigue, and adenopathy. Growth retardation is common. This disorder also results in the following abnormalities: undergrowth of the mandible; early closure of the growth plates resulting in shortening of metacarpals and metatarsals; and overgrowths of the epiphyses at the knees, hips, and shoulders. A worse prognosis occurs in patients with positive rheumatoid factors.

Juvenile Idiopathic Arthritis with Pauciarticular Onset (Oligoarthritis)

The third subtype of JIA has pauciarticular onset, with four or fewer joints involved within 6 months of onset. Approximately 40% of patients with JIA exhibit involvement of fewer than four joints in the first 6 months of the disease. Some of these patients may even present with negative rheumatoid factor, whereas others may have positive antigen HLA-B27. Pediatric rheumatologists have attempted to define other subgroups within this pauciarticular subgroup, but, with the exception of HLA-B27–positive children with sacroiliitis, such definitions are broad and clinically dependent on unique systemic features such as iridocyclitis. However, involvement of the sacroiliac joints is not a feature of JIA as was thought in the past; rather, it represents juvenile onset of ankylosing spondylitis (AS). Similarly, some investigators believe that patients with pauciarticular arthritis, particularly those with positive histocompatibility antigen HLA-B27, may in fact have atypical AS syndrome or spondyloarthropathy; both these conditions are different from RA.

Arthritis with Enthesitis

This type of arthritis that constitutes about 5% to 10% of all JIA cases, predominantly affects boys over 6 years of age and is typify by enthesopathy (enthesitis) at the site of attachment of Achilles tendon and fascia plantaris, associated with asymmetric arthritis affecting articulations of the lower extremities and hip joint. Sacroiliac joints are usually affected. Most patients present with positive HLA-B27 antigen.

Juvenile Psoriatic Arthritis

This form of arthritis, first described by Ansell and Bywaters in 1962, is defined as a seronegative inflammatory arthritis presenting before the age of 16 years with either typical for psoriasis features, or at least three of the four minor criteria: dactylitis, nail pitting, psoriasis-like skin changes, and family history of psoriasis. Girls are affected more commonly than boys. Clinically, the patients may present with joint pain and swelling, reddish scaly skin rash, nail changes, and ocular involvement. Early imaging findings can be demonstrated by MRI, including synovial abnormalities (thickening and enhancement), joint effusion, bone marrow edema, tendon abnormalities (thickening, edema, tenosynovitis), and joint abnormalities (joint space narrowing and articular erosions). Some patients may present with acroosteolysis.

Imaging Features of JIA

JIA exhibits many of the features of adult RA, although the destructive joint changes are much more striking (Fig. 14.59). However, some additional features that are almost pathognomonic for this condition have been identified.

Periosteal Reaction

This feature is usually seen along the shafts of the proximal phalanges and metacarpals (Fig. 14.60).

Joint Ankylosis

Ankylosis has been reported to occur within 3 to 5 years after onset of the disease. It may occur not only in the wrist (Figs. 14.61 and 14.62) but also in the interphalangeal articulations (Fig. 14.63). Fusion in the apophyseal joints of the cervical spine is also a characteristic finding (Figs. 14.64 and 14.65).

Growth Abnormalities

Because the onset of JIA frequently occurs before completion of skeletal maturation, alterations in growth of the bones is a common finding. The involvement of epiphyseal sites often leads to fusion of the growth plate, with resultant retardation of bone growth (Fig. 14.66); it may also precipitate acceleration of growth caused by stimulation of the growth plates by hyperemia. Enlargement of the epiphysis of the distal femur leads to characteristic overgrowth of the condyles in the knee associated with widening of the intercondylar notch and squaring of the patella (Fig. 14.67).

Sacroiliitis

This feature is seen in approximately 30% of children with the ERA subtype of JIA. Imaging identification of this abnormality is crucial because, despite the inflammatory changes of sacroiliac joints, the clinical symptoms (pain) may be a relative late development in the pediatric population.

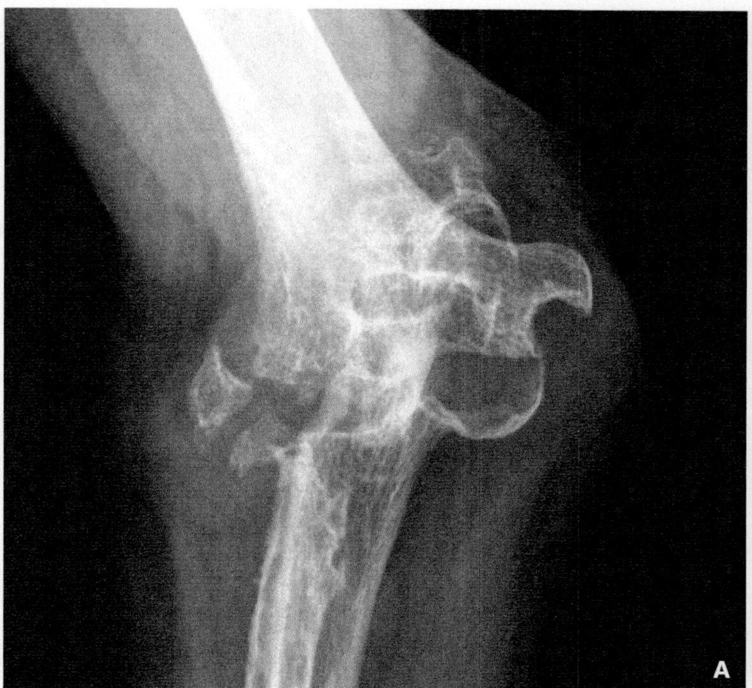

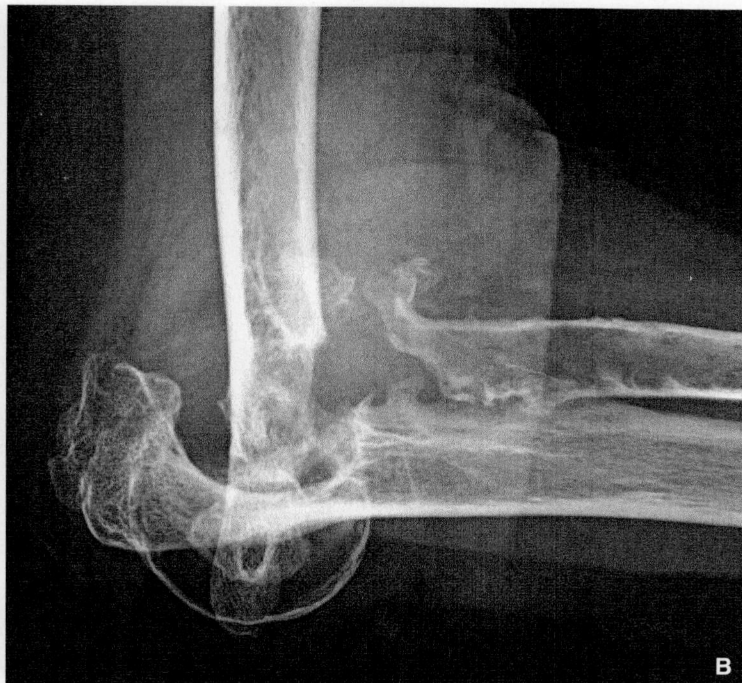

FIGURE 14.59 **Juvenile idiopathic arthritis.** **(A)** Anteroposterior and **(B)** lateral radiographs of the elbow of a 35-year-old woman show severe destruction and subluxation of the elbow joint associated with joint effusion.

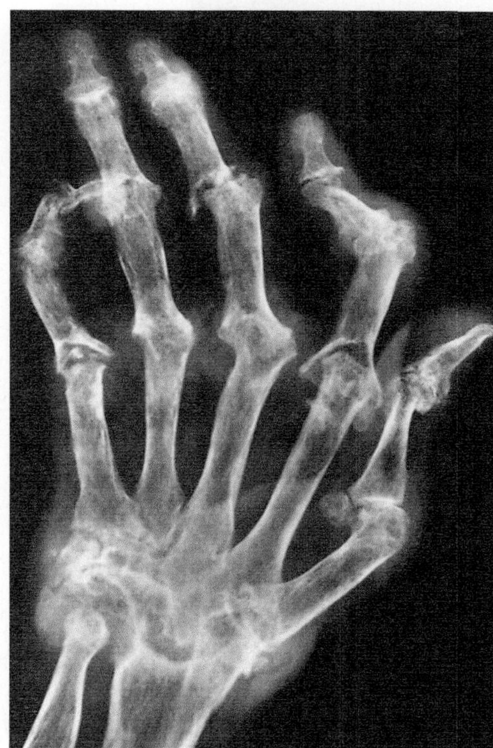

FIGURE 14.60 **Juvenile idiopathic arthritis.** Dorsovolar radiograph of the wrist and hand of a 26-year-old woman with a 14-year history of arthritis shows severe destructive changes in the wrist and in the metacarpophalangeal and proximal interphalangeal articulations. Note ankylosis of the third and fourth metacarpophalangeal joints and periostitis involving the proximal phalanges and metacarpals.

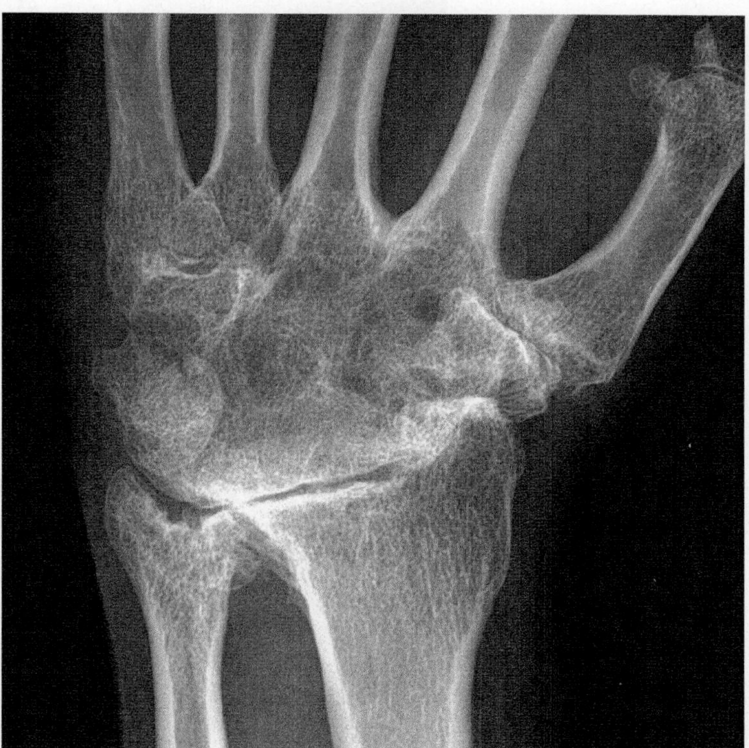

FIGURE 14.61 **Juvenile idiopathic arthritis.** A dorsovolar radiograph of the right wrist of a 28-year-old man shows fusion of the several carpal and carpometacarpal joints.

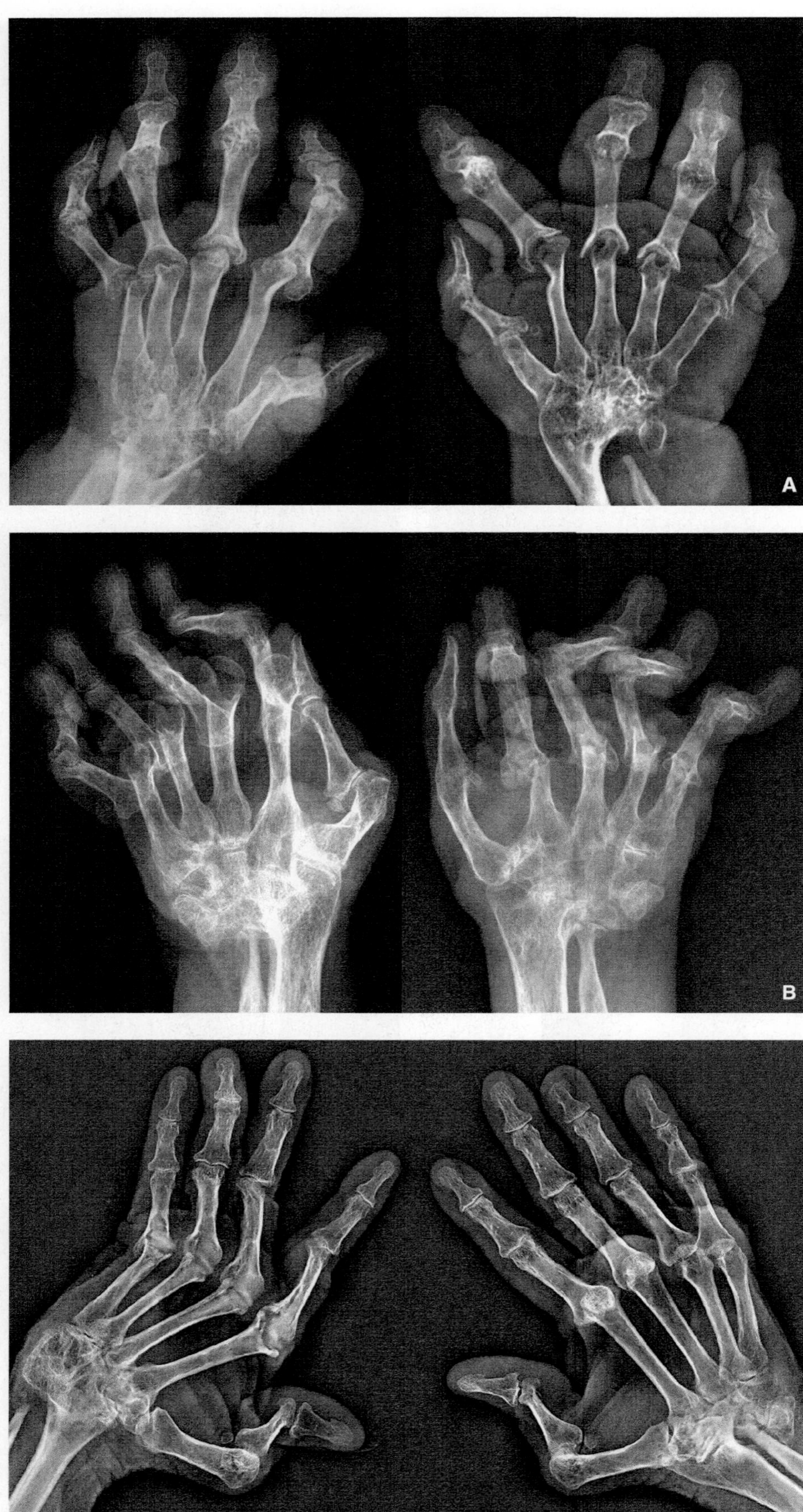

FIGURE 14.62 **Juvenile idiopathic arthritis.** **(A)** Dorsovolar radiograph of both hands of a 42-year-old woman with a history of 27-year polyarthritis shows destructive changes in the metacarpophalangeal and interphalangeal joints. Note also joints ankylosis in both wrists. **(B)** In another patient, a 51-year-old woman, observe erosions, subluxations, and dislocations in several metacarpophalangeal joints of both hands, and striking deformities of the fingers. In addition, there is fusion of the radiocarpal and midcarpal joints as well as of the first metacarpophalangeal and interphalangeal joints of the left thumb. **(C)** Radiograph of both hands of a 62-year-old woman demonstrates erosions and subluxations of the radiocarpal, midcarpal, and metacarpophalangeal joints of the left hand. The radiocarpal and midcarpal joints of the right wrist are fused. The metacarpophalangeal joints of the right hand show status post silastic arthroplasties.

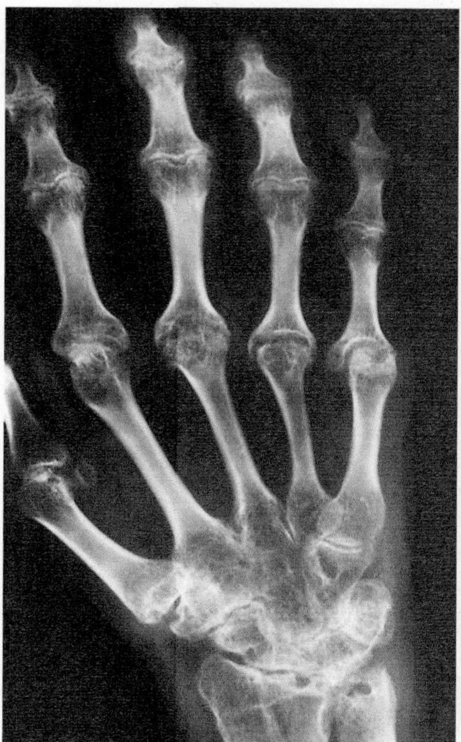

FIGURE 14.63 Juvenile idiopathic arthritis. Dorsovolar radiograph of the hand of a 25-year-old woman with a 10-year history of JIA shows advanced destructive changes in multiple joints of the hand and wrist. Joint ankylosis is evident in several articulations.

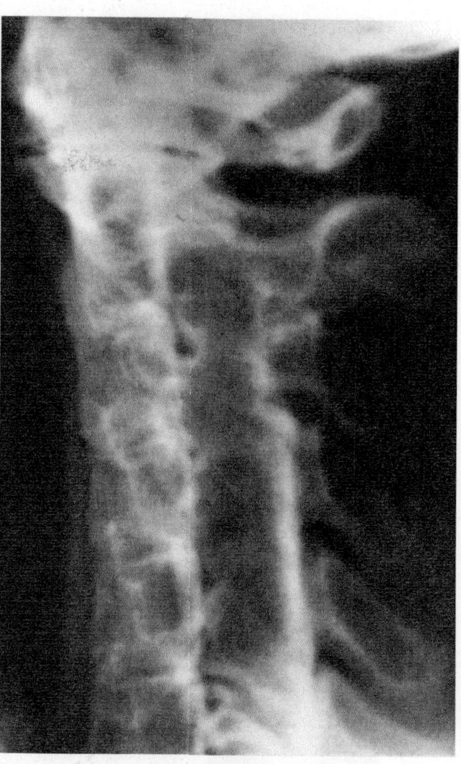

FIGURE 14.64 Juvenile idiopathic arthritis. Lateral radiograph of the cervical spine in a 25-year-old woman with a 15-year history of polyarthritis shows fusion of the apophyseal joints, a common finding in JIA.

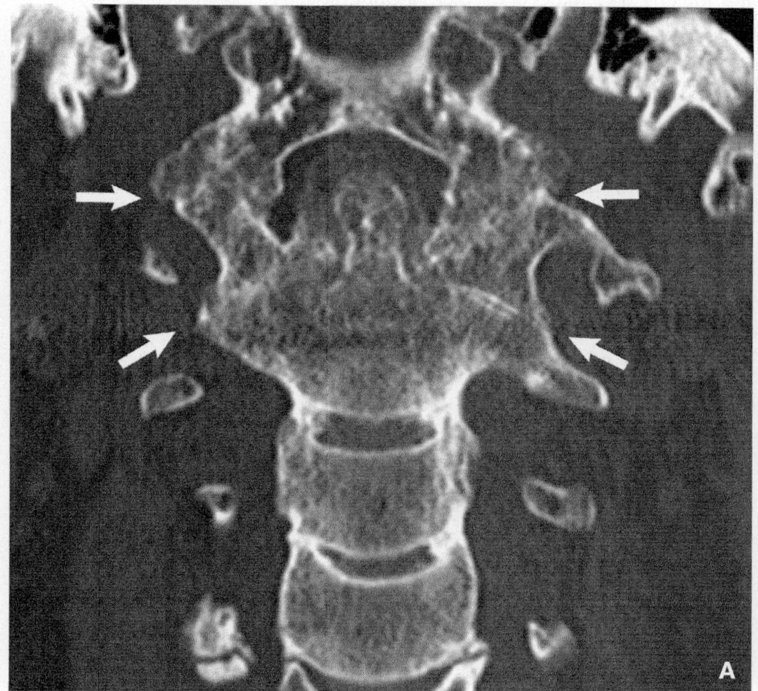

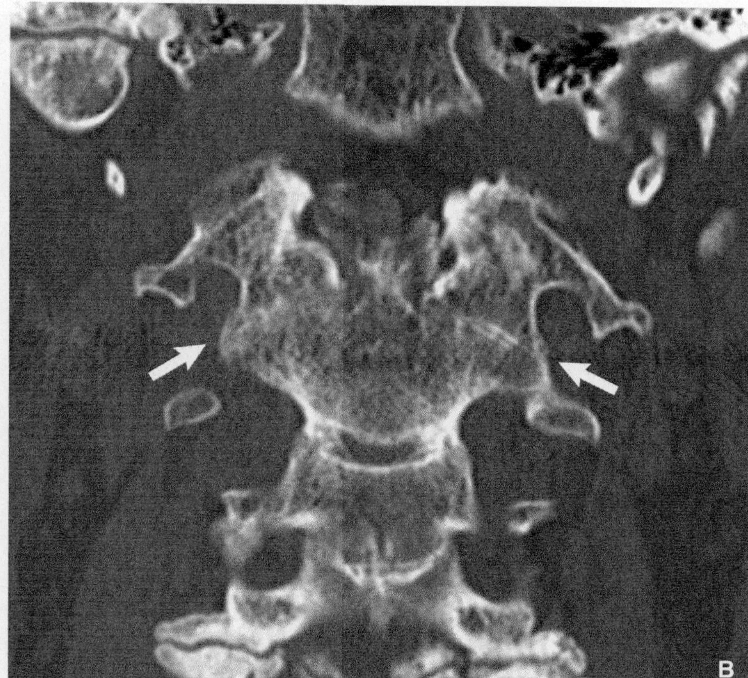

FIGURE 14.65 CT of JIA. **(A,B)** Two coronal reformatted CT sections of the upper cervical spine of a 56-year-old man show atlantoaxial fusion *(arrows)*.

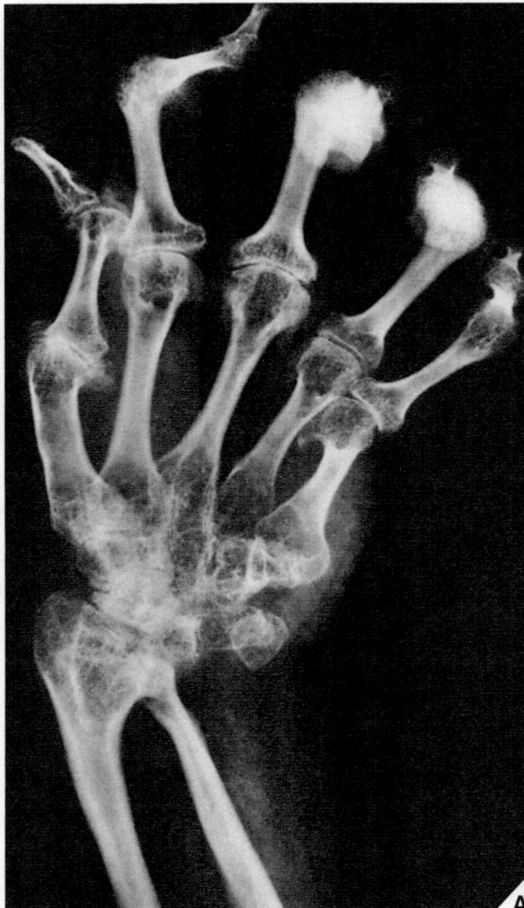

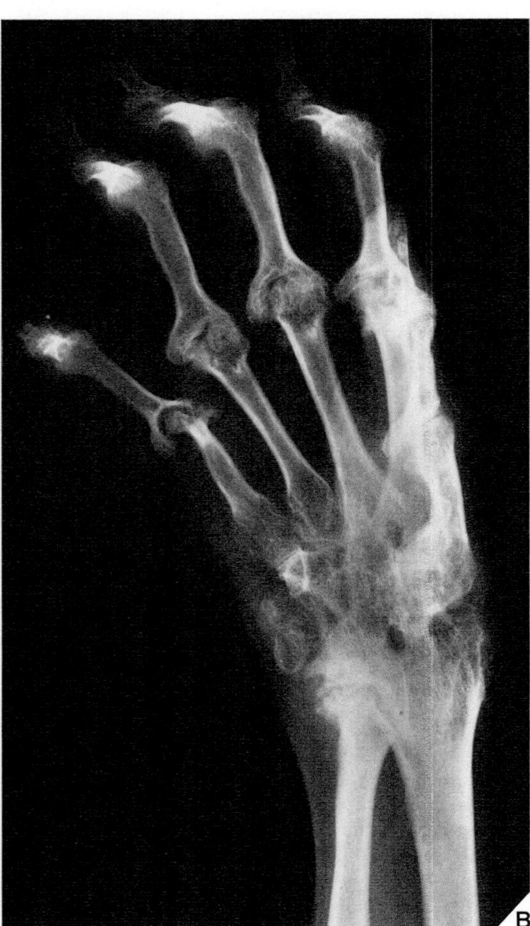

FIGURE 14.66 **Juvenile idiopathic arthritis.** **(A,B)** Dorsovolar radiograph of the hands of a 24-year-old woman with advanced JIA, which was diagnosed when she was 7 years old, shows retarded growth of the bones caused by early fusion of the growth plates. Multiple deformities of the digits include hitchhiker's thumb and a boutonnière configuration of the fingers.

Macrophage Activation Syndrome

MAS refers to a clinicopathologic entity caused by excessive uncontrolled activation and expansion of T lymphocytes and macrophagic histiocytes that exhibit hemophagocytic activity. The expansion of these cells leads to a massive systemic inflammatory response associated with pancytopenia, liver and spleen dysfunction, hypertriglyceridemia, hyperferritinemia, and coagulopathy resembling disseminated intravascular coagulation. Because expansion of tissue macrophages and histiocytes is often triggered by infections or modifications in the drug therapy, some investigators prefer the term *reactive hemophagocytic lymphohistiocytosis* for this condition. MAS is severe and potentially life-threatening complication of several chronic rheumatologic disorders of childhood. It occurs most commonly with systemic JIA and adult-onset Still disease.

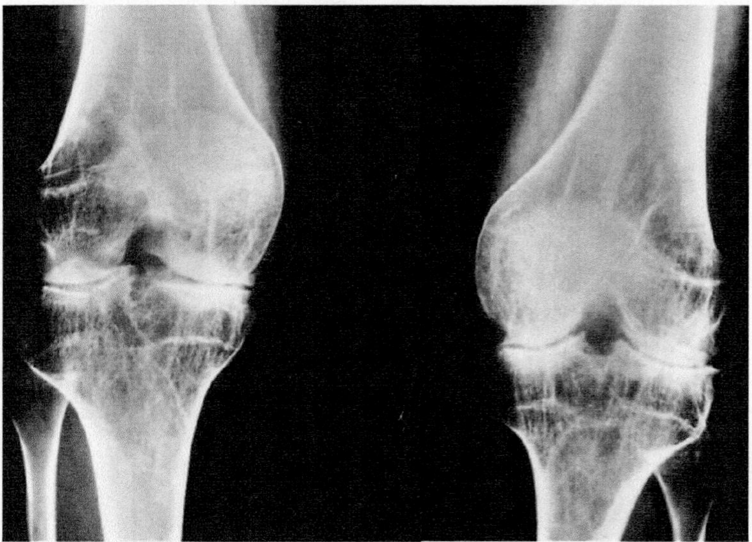

FIGURE 14.67 **Juvenile idiopathic arthritis.** Anteroposterior radiograph of both knees of a 20-year-old woman shows overgrowth of the medial condyles, one of the characteristic features of this disorder.

Treatment of Rheumatoid Arthritis

Medical

Over the past several years, there has been significant change in treatment of RA that contributed to major improvement in clinical outcome of patients with this debilitating disease. These encouraging results were mainly achieved through the introduction of the newer biologic agents that have revolutionized the treatment of RA and should be offered and discussed with each and every patient with this disease. Historically, treatment included methotrexate, sulfasalazine, leflunomide, hydroxychloroquine, azathioprine, cyclosporine, etanercept, minocycline, and gold salts. However, now, all patients receive methotrexate with or without biologic agents. They comprise TNF-blocking agents (so-called *anti-TNF agents*—infliximab, etanercept, and adalimumab), rituximab (monoclonal antibody against the protein CD 20), abatacept (CTLA4-Ig fusion protein), and tocilizumab (interleukin-6 receptor–inhibiting monoclonal antibodies). In clinical trials, cyclosporine alone or in combination with methotrexate also has been shown to reduce the arthritic symptoms, and even to delay the development of articular erosions, but is rarely used. Similarly, low doses of glucocorticoids (such as prednisone) can provide rapid improvement of articular symptoms.

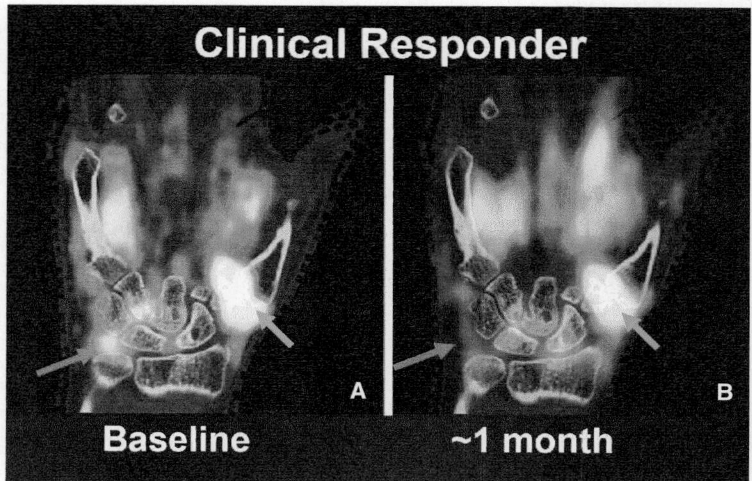

FIGURE 14.68 ^{18}F-FDG PET/CT evaluation of response of RA to treatment. **(A)** Coronal fused PET/CT image of the wrist of a 49-year-old woman with RA shows increased accumulation of the ^{18}F-FDG radiotracer at sites of multiple osseous erosions including triquetro-pisiform joint *(red arrow)*. There is also increased metabolic activity in the first carpometacarpal joint due to OA *(green arrow)*. **(B)** Coronal PET/CT fused image of the wrist obtained after 1 month of treatment with TNF-α inhibitor (etanercept) shows significant reduction in signal at the sites of inflammatory arthritis *(red arrow)*, suggesting reduced inflammation in the synovium. Note lack of improvement at the site of OA *(green arrow)*. (Courtesy of Abhijit Chaudhari, MD, Sacramento, California.)

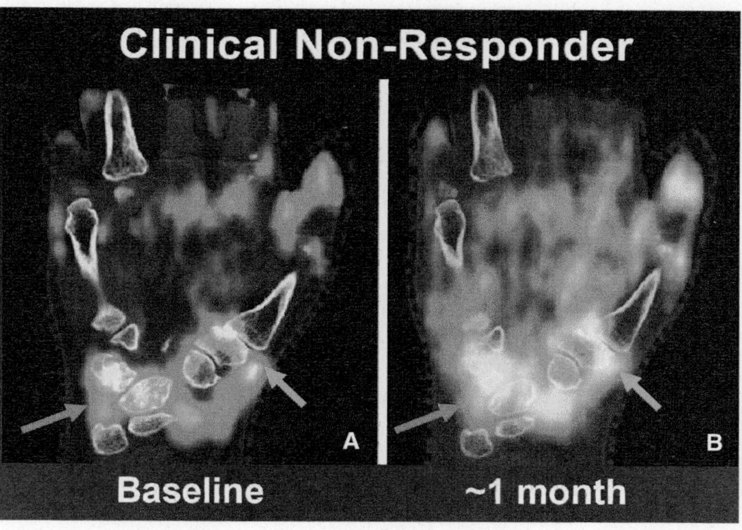

FIGURE 14.69 ^{18}F-FDG PET/CT evaluation of response of RA to treatment. **(A)** Coronal fused PET/CT image of the wrist of 63-year-old woman with RA shows high metabolic activity at the sites of synovitis in the carpal joints *(red and green arrows)*. **(B)** Same image obtained after 1 month of treatment with TNF-α inhibitor shows further increase in metabolic activity *(red and green arrows)*, indicating lack of response to therapy. (Courtesy of Abhijit Chaudhari, MD, Sacramento, California.)

If indicated, intraarticular injections of steroids can suppress joint inflammation. Positron emission tomography (PET)/CT may occasionally be used to monitor and evaluate response to treatment (Fig. 14.68 and 14.69).

NSAIDs play only a minor role in the treatment, and their use is mainly reserve to symptomatic relief.

Surgical

Surgical treatment includes mainly total joint arthroplasties performed not only on the large joints like hip, knee, shoulder, and elbow but also replacement of small joints of the hands and feet (see Chapter 12).

Seronegative Spondyloarthropathies

Ankylosing Spondylitis

Clinical Features

AS, known in the European literature as *Bechterew disease* or *Marie-Strümpell disease*, belongs to a heterogeneous group of inflammatory arthritides known collectively as the *seronegative spondyloarthropathies*. It is a chronic, progressive, inflammatory arthritis principally affecting the synovial joints of the spine and adjacent soft tissues as well as the sacroiliac joints; however, the peripheral joints such as the hips, shoulders, and knees may also be involved. Historically, AS was thought to be a disease almost exclusively affecting young men. More recent studies suggest a male-to-female ratio from 3:1 to 7:1 depending on geographical and ethnic factors. Low back pain and neck pain are the most typical presenting symptoms, although patients with AS frequently exhibit extraarticular features of disease including iritis (uveitis), pulmonary fibrosis, cardiac conduction defects, aortic incompetence, spinal cord compression, and amyloidosis. Patients may also have low-grade fever, anorexia, fatigue, and weight loss. Early mortality has been reported, associated mainly with an increased risk of cardiovascular morbidity.

Rheumatoid factor is negative in patients with AS, which is the prototype of the spondyloarthropathies. A high percentage of patients (up to 95%), however, possess histocompatibility antigen HLA-B27. A positive family history can be found in 15% to 20% of cases.

Pathology

Pathologically, AS is a diffuse proliferative synovitis of the diarthrodial joints exhibiting features similar to those seen in RA. In addition, there is inflammatory enthesopathy at the anterior and posterior aspects of the vertebral bodies, followed by a secondary process of progressive calcification and ossification, initially limited to the spinal ligaments and annulus fibrosus, and gradually spreading throughout the spine resulting in partial or total spine fusion (Fig. 14.70).

Imaging Features

Squaring of the anterior border of the lower thoracic and lumbar vertebrae and so-called *shiny corners* are one of the earliest radiographic features of AS, best demonstrated on the lateral radiograph of the spine (Fig. 14.71; see also Fig. 12.53). As the condition progresses, syndesmophytes form, bridging the vertebral bodies (Fig. 14.72; see also Fig. 12.54). The delicate appearance of these excrescences and their vertical rather than horizontal orientation distinguish them from the osteophytes of degenerative spine disease (Fig. 14.73). Paravertebral ossifications are common. When the apophyseal joints and vertebral bodies fuse late in the course of the disease, a radiographic hallmark of this condition, the "bamboo" spine, can be observed (Fig. 14.74; see also Fig. 12.55). On the anteroposterior radiographs of the lumbar spine, a single radiodense central line (so-called a *dagger sign*) may be identified, representing ossification of the supraspinous and interspinous ligaments (Fig. 14.75). Sites of ankylosis are prone to "banana stick" fractures and subsequent pseudoarthrosis formation. The sacroiliac joints are also invariably affected in this process (Fig. 14.76).

Among conditions affecting vertebral column that should not be mistaken for AS is progressive noninfectious anterior vertebral fusion, so-called *Copenhagen syndrome*. The disease usually presents in early childhood and adolescent age and is characterized by disk-spaces obliteration and anterior osseous ankylosis with fusion of the vertebral bodies (Fig. 14.77).

In the peripheral joints, inflammatory changes of AS may be indistinguishable from those seen in RA (see Fig. 14.41). In the foot, erosions characteristically occur at certain tendinous insertions, particularly in the calcaneus (see Figs. 12.46 and 12.47). Involvement of the ischial tuberosities and iliac crests exhibits a lace-like formation of new bone called *whiskering*.

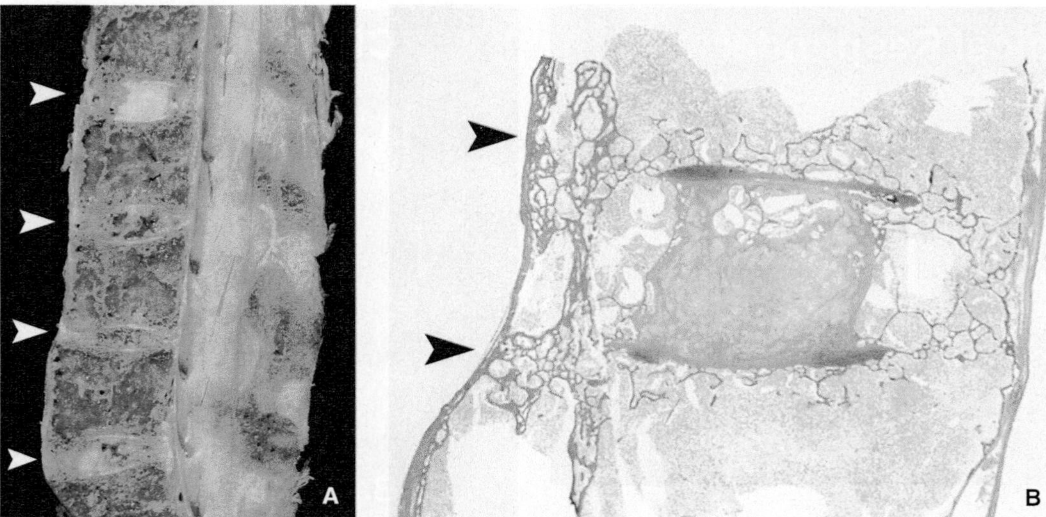

FIGURE 14.70 Pathology of AS. **(A)** Photograph of the sagittal section of the lumbar spine shows anterior syndesmophytes *(arrowheads)* fusing the intervertebral disk spaces, which are not significantly narrowed. **(B)** Photomicrograph shows marginal syndesmophytes *(arrowheads)* at the site of annulus fibrosus. (Reprinted from Bullough P. *Orthopaedic pathology*, 5th ed. Maryland Heights, MO: Mosby; 2009, with permission from Elsevier.)

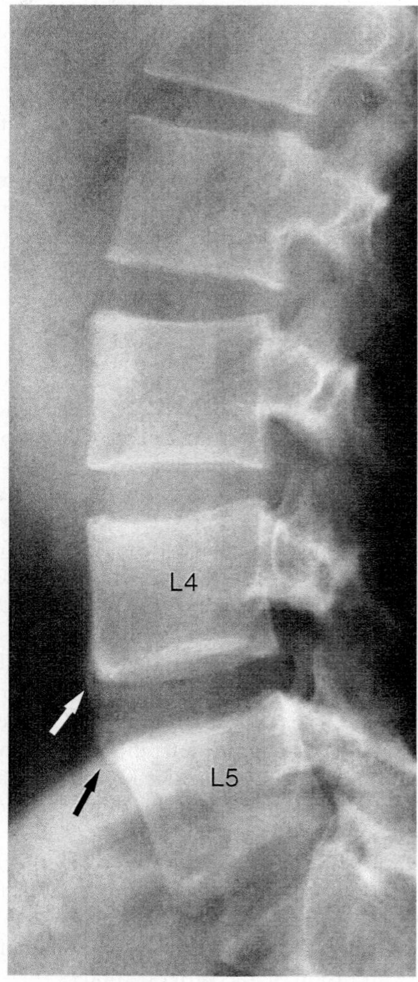

FIGURE 14.71 Ankylosing spondylitis. Lateral radiograph of the lumbar spine in a 28-year-old man demonstrates squaring of the vertebral bodies secondary to small osseous erosions at the corners. This finding is an early radiographic feature of AS. Note also the formation of syndesmophytes at the L4-5 disk space *(arrows)*.

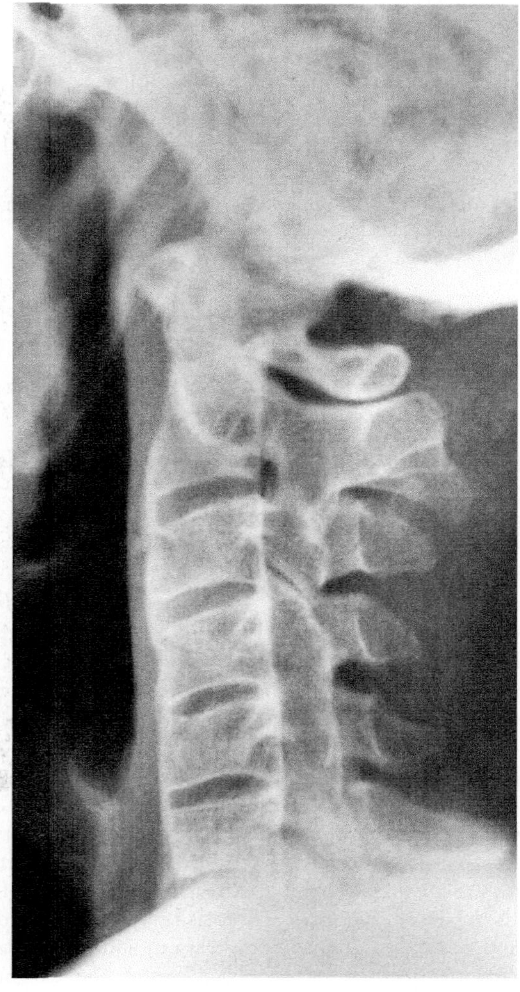

FIGURE 14.72 Ankylosing spondylitis. Lateral radiograph of the cervical spine in a 31-year-old man demonstrates delicate syndesmophytes bridging the vertebral bodies, a common feature of AS. Note the fusion of several apophyseal joints.

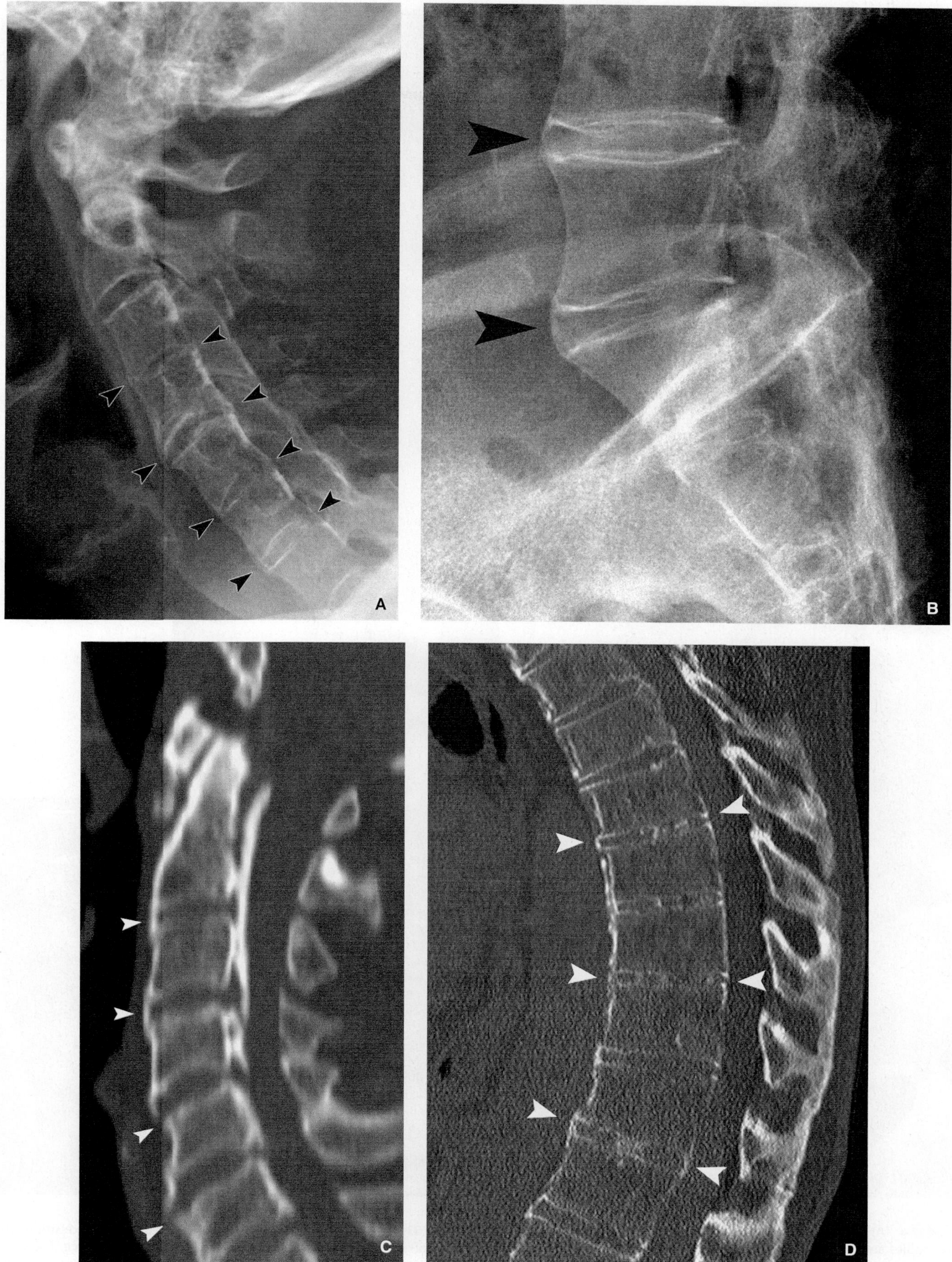

FIGURE 14.73 CT of AS. **(A)** Lateral radiograph of the cervical spine of a 32-year-old man shows delicate vertically oriented anterior and posterior syndesmophytes *(arrowheads)*. **(B)** Lateral coned-down radiograph of the lumbosacral segment of a 29-year-old man shows delicate vertically oriented anterior syndesmophytes *(arrowheads)*. **(C)** Sagittal reformatted CT image of the cervical spine and **(D)** sagittal reformatted image of the thoracic spine of another patient demonstrate delicate vertically oriented anterior and posterior syndesmophytes *(arrowheads)*.

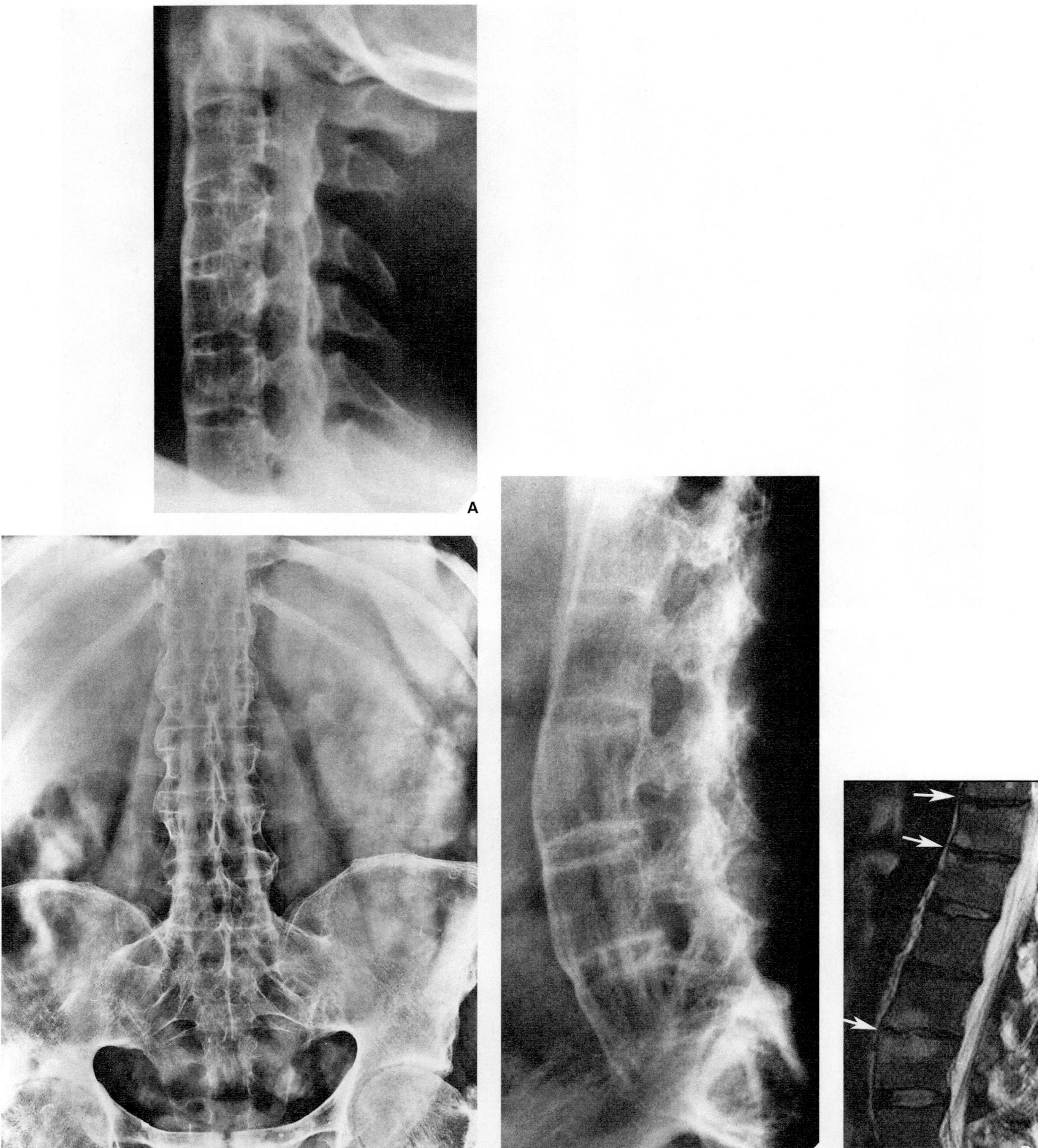

FIGURE 14.74 Ankylosing spondylitis. (A) Lateral radiograph of the cervical spine in a 53-year-old man with advanced AS shows anterior syndesmophytes bridging the vertebral bodies and posterior fusion of the apophyseal joints, together with paravertebral ossifications, producing a "bamboo-spine" appearance. The same phenomenon is seen on the anteroposterior **(B)** and lateral **(C)** radiographs of the lumbosacral spine. Note on the anteroposterior radiograph the fusion of the sacroiliac joints and the involvement of both hip joints, which show axial migration of the femoral heads similar to that seen in RA. In another patient, a 36-year-old man, **(D)** sagittal T2-weighted MR image demonstrates squaring of the vertebral bodies and high–signal intensity areas in the anterior end plates at different levels ("shiny corner sign") *(arrows)*.

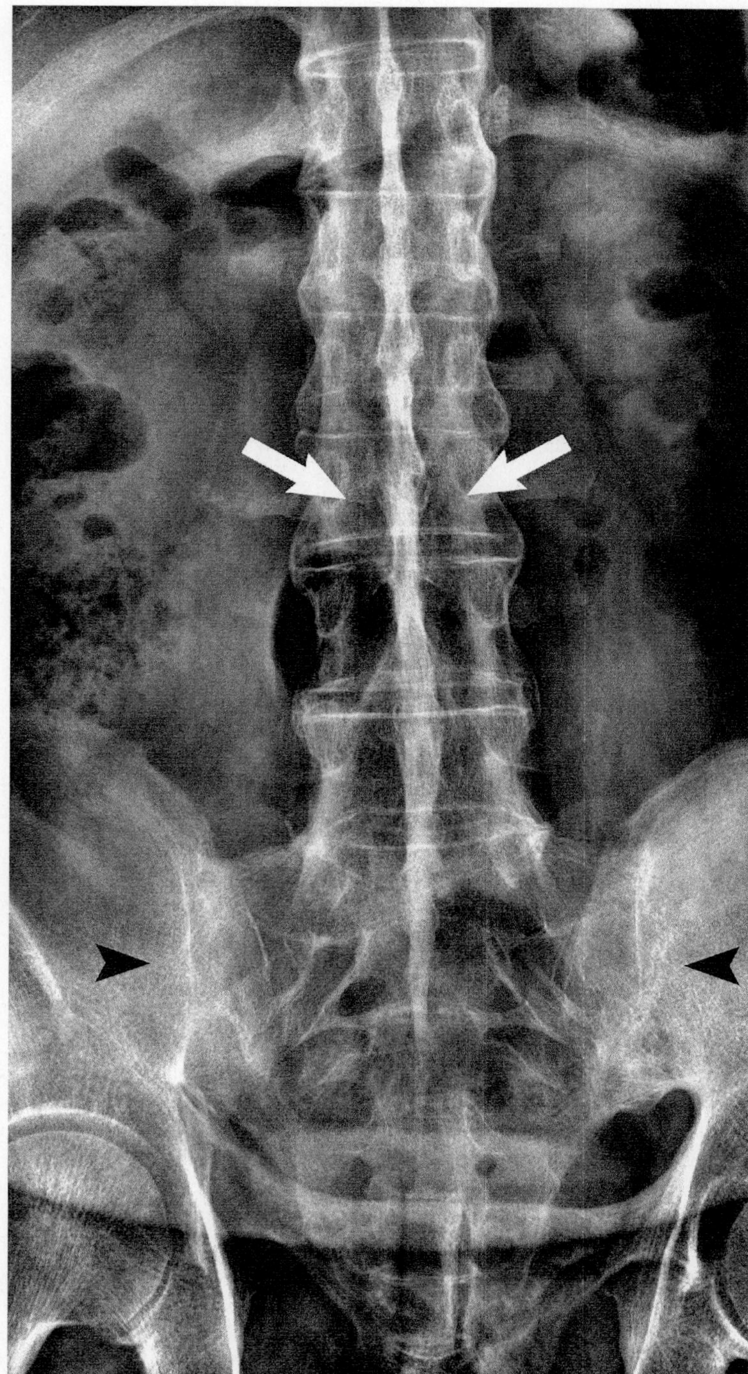

FIGURE 14.75 **Ankylosing spondylitis.** Anteroposterior radiograph of the lumbar spine of a 42-year-old man shows ossifications of the supraspinous and interspinous ligaments, producing a "dagger sign" *(arrows)*. Note symmetrical bilateral fusion of the sacroiliac joints *(arrowheads)*.

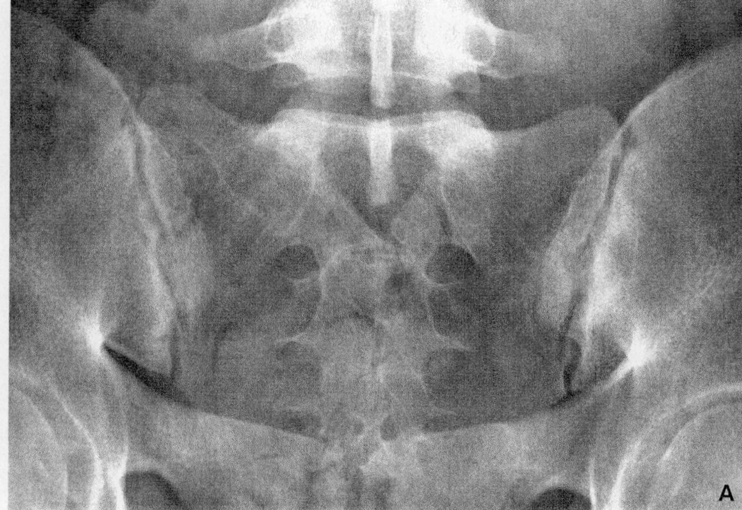

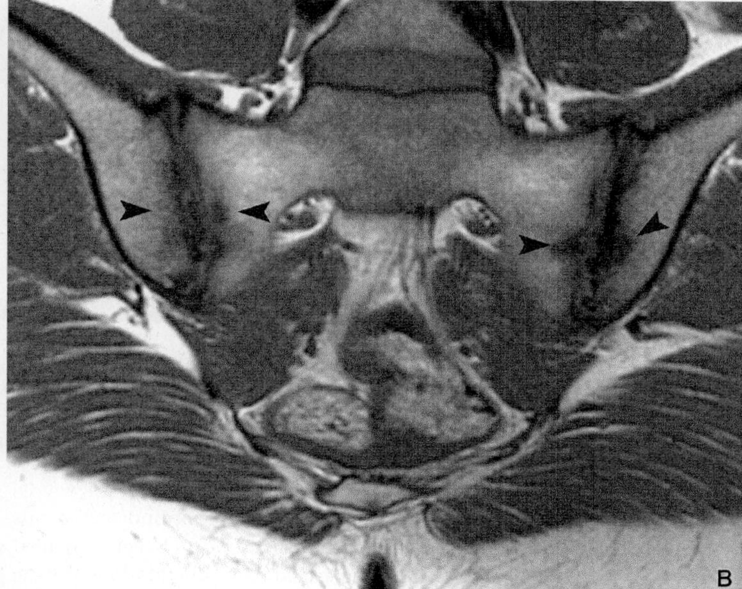

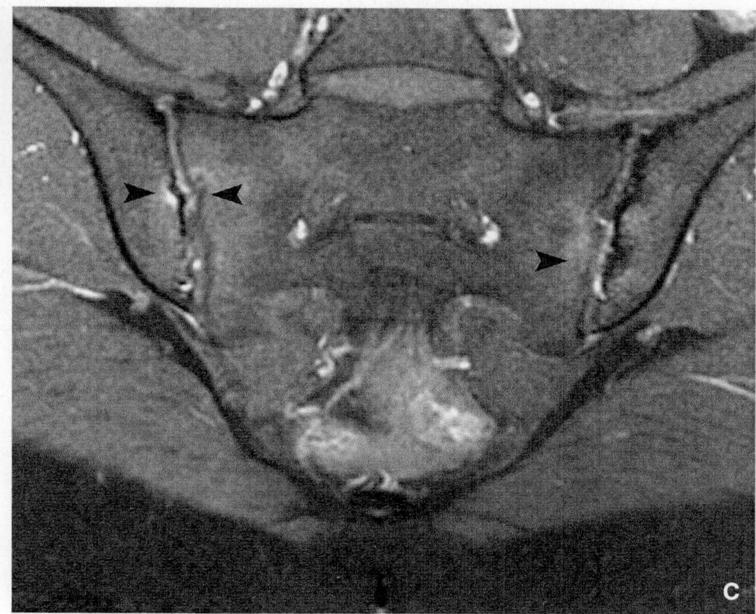

FIGURE 14.76 **MRI of AS.** **(A)** Fergusson view of the pelvis of a 25-year-old man shows bilateral symmetric sacroiliitis, confirmed on **(B)** coronal T1-weighted and **(C)** coronal T1-weighted fat-suppressed postcontrast MR images *(arrowheads)*.

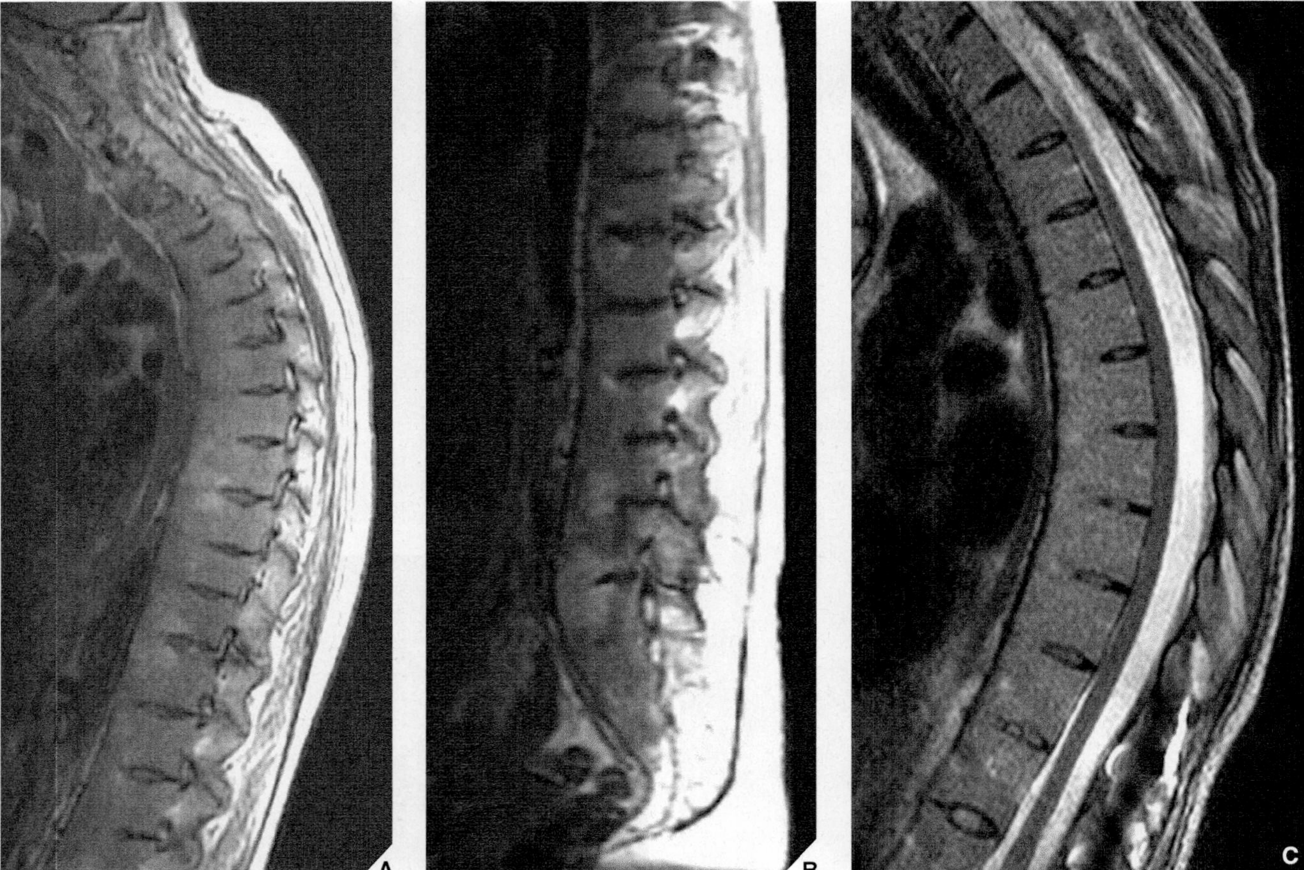

FIGURE 14.77 Copenhagen syndrome. Sagittal T1-weighted MR images of the **(A)** thoracic and **(B)** lumbar spine and **(C)** T2-weighted MRI of the thoracic spine of a 16-year-old girl show fusion of the anterior aspects of the vertebral bodies. Unlike in AS, the apophyseal joints are normal.

Treatment

The International Assessment in AS (Assessment of SpondyloArthritis international Society [ASAS]) Group and the European League Against Rheumatism recently developed evidence-based recommendations for the management of AS. These recommendations emphasize that the optimal management of patients with AS "requires a combination of nonpharmacologic and pharmacologic treatment" and stress the importance of patient education, regular exercise and/or physical therapy, and possibly social support groups. Physical therapy is important to prevent spinal deformity and loss of motion in the joints. NSAIDs are used as first-line medical treatment to relieve the pain. Disease-modifying antirheumatic drugs (DMARDs) proved to be not very effective, although they can alleviate the symptoms from coexisting peripheral arthritis. Clinical trials showed that symptoms in some patients had improved after treatment with TNF inhibitors. Surgery is usually limited to stabilization of spinal fractures, one of the complications of AS.

Reactive Arthritis (Reiter Syndrome)

Clinical Features

Reactive arthritis, formerly known as a *Reiter syndrome*, an autoimmune condition that develops in response to an infection in another part of the body, affects 5 times more males than females and is characterized by arthritis, conjunctivitis, and urethritis. It was first reported in 1916 by the German military physician Hans Conrad Julius Reiter (who later was prosecuted in Nuremberg as a war criminal for his involvement in forced human experimentation in the Buchenwald concentration camp), and in the same year, it was described by the French physicians Fiessinger and LeRoy. Reactive arthritis is also well-known for the presence of mucocutaneous rash, keratoderma blenorrhagica. Like in AS, eye involvement is common and can include conjunctivitis, iritis, uveitis, and episcleritis. About 20% to 40% of the men develop penile lesions called *balanitis circinata*. Approximately 60% to 80% of patients are positive for HLA-B27 gene on chromosome 6. This frequency varies according to the ethnic origin of the patient. Unlike AS, reactive arthritis may exhibit unilateral sacroiliac diseases.

Two types of this syndrome have been identified. First, the sporadic or endemic type, which is common in the United States, is associated with nongonococcal urethritis, prostatitis, or hemorrhagic cystitis, although recently genital infections with *Chlamydia trachomatis* and *Neisseria gonorrhoeae* have been reported. It occurs almost exclusively in males. In Europe, a second type has been identified, which is an epidemic form associated with bacillary (Shigella) dysentery. It may be seen in women as well. There has been considerable research on the putative role of *Yersinia enterocolitica* in inducing disease, particularly in Scandinavia, where such infections are more prevalent than in North America. The frequency in the general population is estimated to be 3.5 to 5 cases per 100,000, but in the era before effective therapy for HIV, it was as high as 75% incidence in HIV-positive males expressing positive HLA-B27.

Imaging Features

Radiographically, reactive arthritis is marked by peripheral and usually asymmetric arthritis, with a predilection for the joints of the lower limb (Fig. 14.78). The foot is the most common site of involvement, particularly the metatarsophalangeal joints and the heels (Fig. 14.78B; see also Fig. 12.47C). Periosteal new bone formation is not uncommon. Involvement of the sacroiliac joints, which is frequently encountered, may be either asymmetric unilateral (Fig. 14.79), asymmetric bilateral (Fig. 14.80), or symmetric bilateral (Fig. 14.81). In the thoracic and lumbar spine, coarse syndesmophytes or paraspinal ossifications may be present, characteristically bridging adjacent vertebrae (Fig. 14.82).

Treatment

NSAIDs remain the treatment of choice for the articular manifestations, and in most cases, provided adequate control of acute synovitis and enthesitis. DMARDs may be considered in patients not responding to

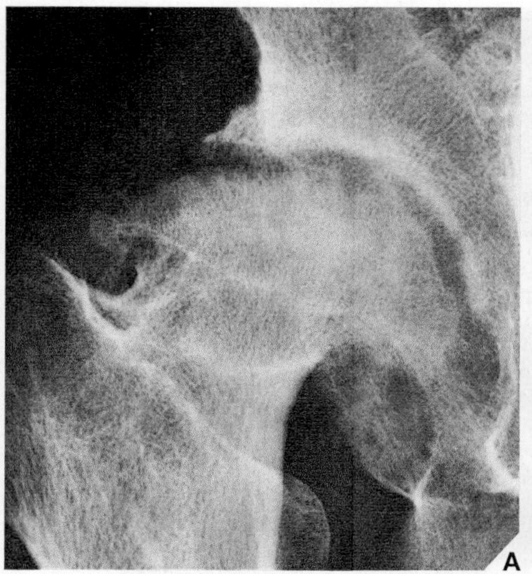

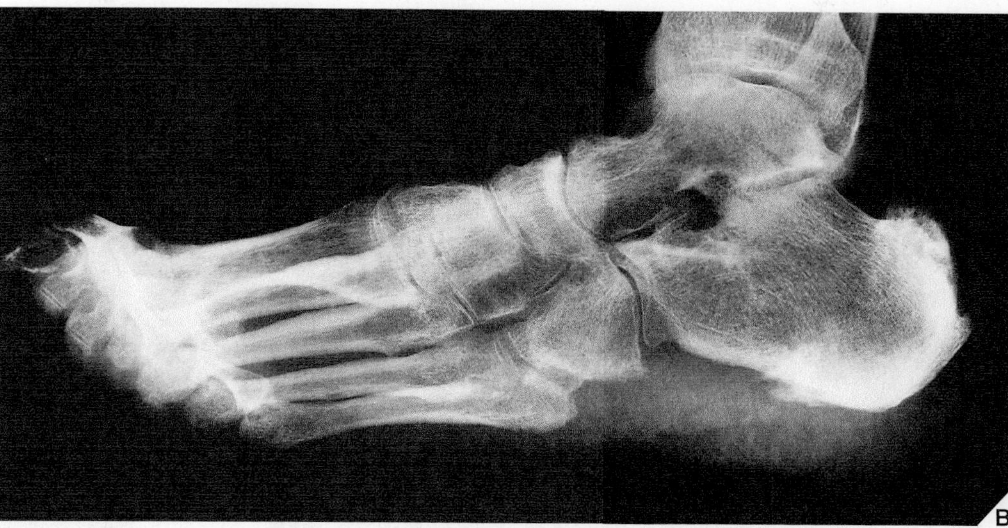

FIGURE 14.78 Reactive arthritis. **(A)** Anteroposterior radiograph of right hip joint of a 39-year-old man shows characteristic changes of inflammatory arthritis. **(B)** Lateral radiograph of the foot of a 28-year-old man demonstrates the "fluffy" periostitis of the calcaneus and inflammatory changes of the metatarsophalangeal joints typical of this condition.

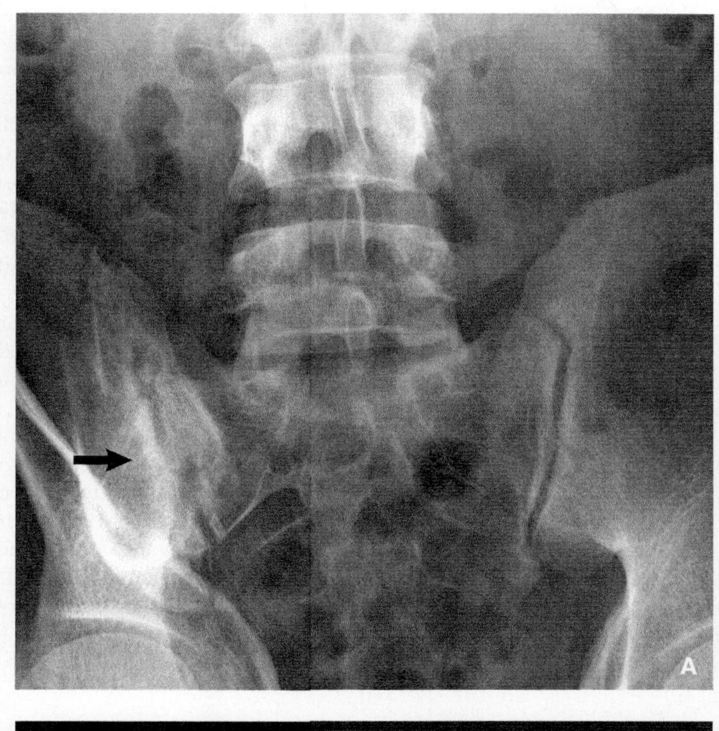

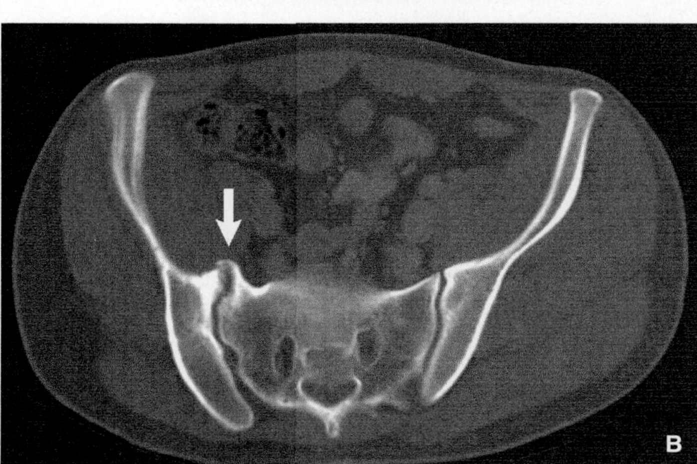

FIGURE 14.79 CT of reactive arthritis. **(A)** Fergusson view of the sacroiliac joints and **(B)** axial CT image of the pelvis of a 38-year-old man show unilateral right-sided sacroiliitis *(arrows)*.

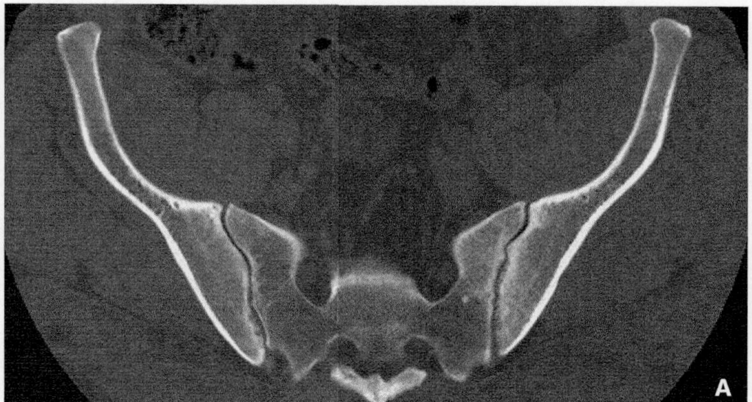

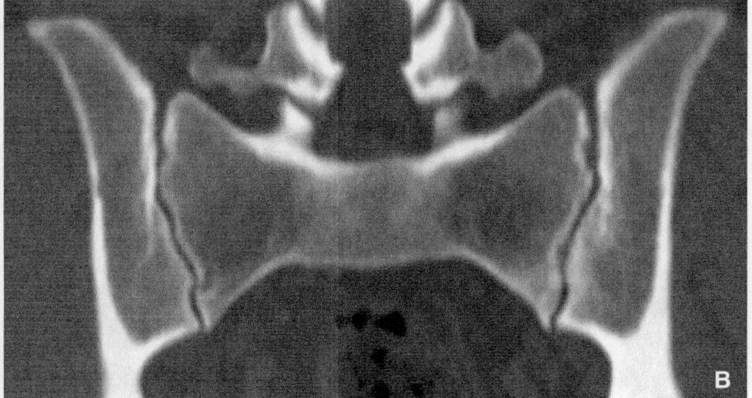

FIGURE 14.80 CT of reactive arthritis. **(A)** Axial and **(B)** coronal reformatted CT images of the pelvis of a 41-year-old man show bilateral but asymmetric (more advanced on the left side) sacroiliitis.

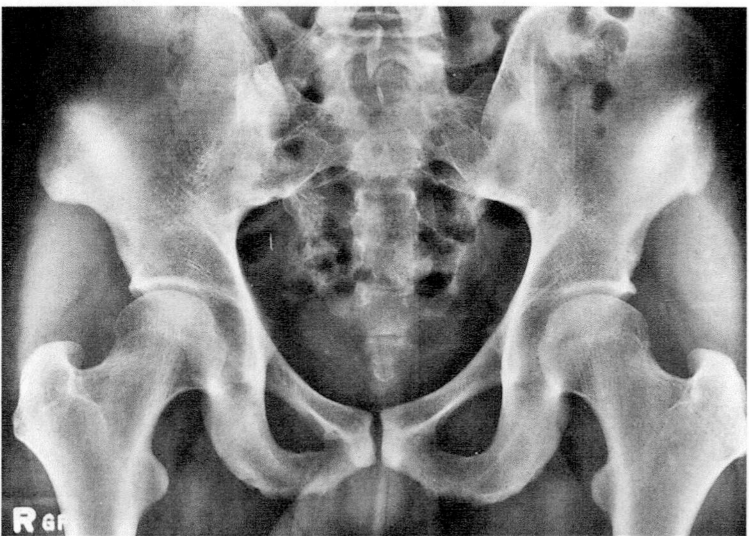

FIGURE 14.81 Reactive arthritis. Anteroposterior radiograph of the pelvis of the patient shown in Figure 14.78B demonstrates symmetric bilateral involvement of the sacroiliac joints.

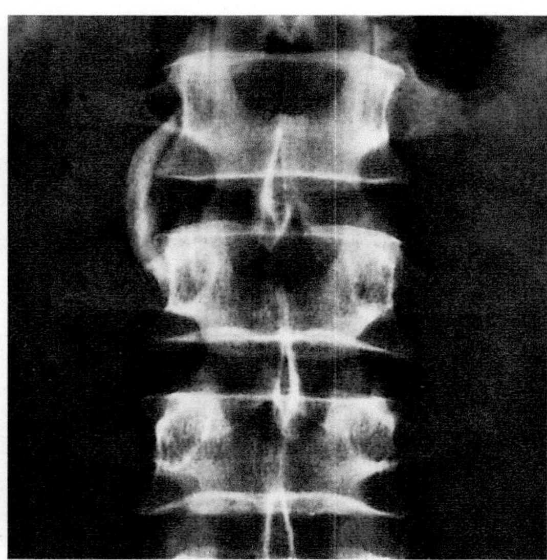

FIGURE 14.82 Reactive arthritis. Anteroposterior radiograph of the lumbar spine of a 23-year-old man with reactive arthritis demonstrates a paraspinal ossification bridging the L2 and L3 vertebrae.

treatment with NSAIDs and glucocorticoids. Appropriate short-term antibiotic therapy should be administered if the infection remains active.

Psoriatic Arthritis

Clinical Features

Psoriasis is a dermatologic disorder that affects approximately 1% to 2% of the population. The macular and papular skin lesions of psoriasis display characteristic focal plaques covered with silvery white scales and are commonly located over extensor surfaces of the extremities. Nail abnormalities, including discoloration, fragmentation, pitting, and onycholysis, may provide an early diagnostic clue (see Fig. 12.24). Approximately 10% to 15% of patients with psoriasis develop inflammatory arthritis, which usually predates the onset of cutaneous abnormalities by about 10 years. Articular disease is more common in patients with moderate or severe skin abnormalities, and according to Wright, severe and mutilating arthropathy is often associated with extensive exfoliative skin abnormalities. The entheses are an important site of inflammation and subsequent pathology in this disorder. These are locations where tendons, ligaments, and fascia insert into bone. Histopathology is characterized by chronic inflammatory infiltrates similar to that present in RA.

The cause of PsA is unknown, and its relationship to RA and spondyloarthropathies is still unsettled. It has been postulated that some mutations in the genes CARD14, HLA-B, HLA-C, HLA-DRB1, IL12B, IL13, IL23R, and TRAF3IP2 are associated with this arthritis. Regarding HLA, a haplotype epidemiologic association involves the expression of both class I and class II HLA alleles, including HLA-B13, HLA-B17, HLA-B27, HLA-B38, HLA-B39, HLA-Cw6, HLA-DR4, and HLA-DR7. It is worthwhile to notice that HLA-B27 is present in 60% of patients with disease, as compared with 8% of the general population.

The arthritis predominantly affects the distal interphalangeal joints of the hands and feet, although other sites of involvement—the proximal interphalangeal joints as well as the hips, knees, ankles, shoulders, and spine—may also be encountered.

According to the original classification of PsA by Moll and Wright, five specific subgroups of arthritic syndromes have been described in PsA.

Subgroup 1, or classic PsA, includes nail pathology with frequent erosion of the terminal tufts termed *acroosteolysis* (Fig. 14.83). It is important, however, to remember that other conditions may also exhibit acroosteolysis (Table 14.3). The involvement of the distal and occasionally proximal interphalangeal joints of the hand and foot is also a common finding (Figs. 14.84 and 14.85).

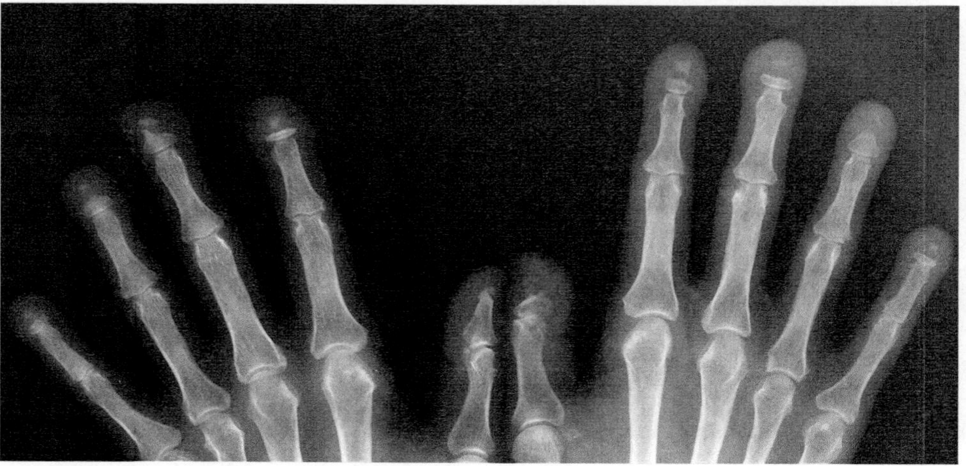

FIGURE 14.83 Psoriatic arthritis. A 57-year-old woman with long-standing psoriasis developed resorption of the tufts of the distal phalanges (acroosteolysis) of both hands, typical of this condition.

TABLE 14.3 Most Common Causes of Acroosteolysis

Trauma	Hyperparathyroidism (primary, secondary)	Sarcoidosis
Diabetic gangrene	Frostbite	Sjögren syndrome
Psoriasis	Burn (thermal, electrical)	Polyvinyl chloride
Scleroderma	Congenital (Hajdu-Cheney syndrome)	Pachydermoperiostosis
Dermatomyositis	Leprosy	Thromboangiitis obliterans
Rheumatoid arthritis	Gout	Syringomyelia
Raynaud disease	Pyknodysostosis	

Data from Reeder MM, Felson B. *Gamuts in radiology*. Cincinnati, OH: Audiovisual Radiology of Cincinnati, Inc.; 1975:D87–D89.

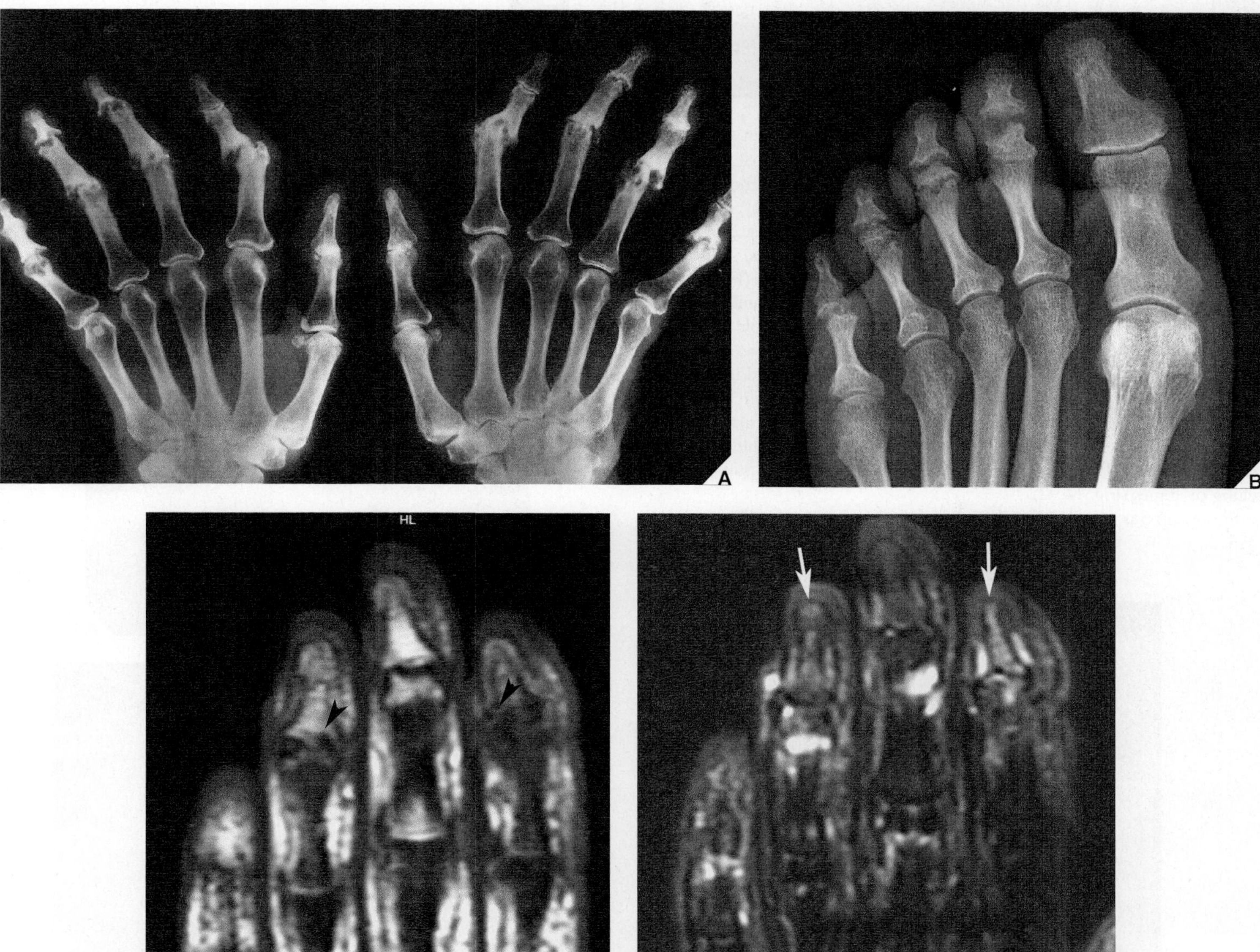

FIGURE 14.84 MRI of PsA. **(A)** Dorsovolar radiograph of both hands of a 55-year-old woman who presented with skin changes typical of psoriasis shows destructive changes in the proximal and distal interphalangeal joints. **(B)** Anteroposterior radiograph of the right foot shows similar erosions of the interphalangeal joints of her toes. **(C)** Coronal T1-weighted MR image of the fingers in another patient shows erosive changes in the distal interphalangeal joints of the second and fourth digits *(arrowheads)*. **(D)** Coronal T2-weighted fat-saturated MR image shows bone marrow edema of the distal phalanges of the second and fourth digits *(arrows)* with small joint effusions and pericapsular edema.

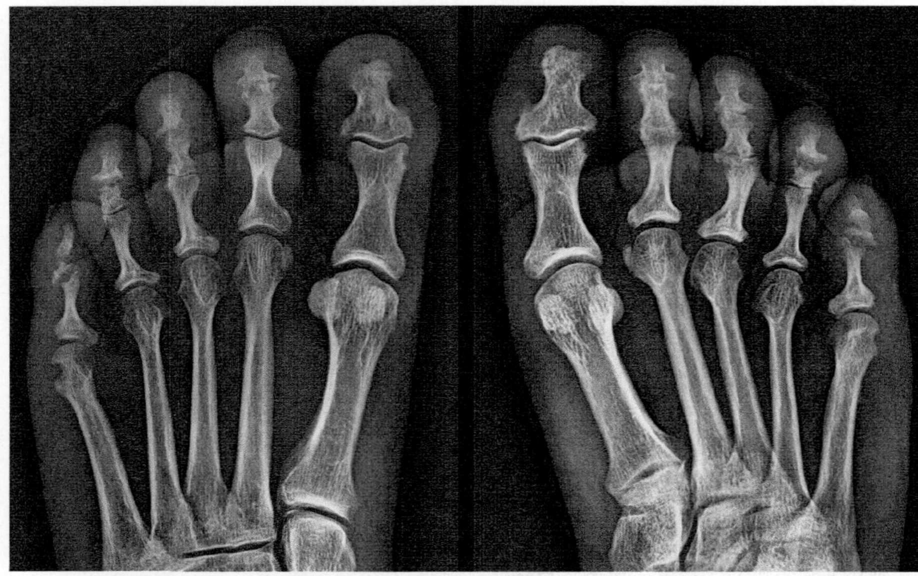

FIGURE 14.85 Psoriatic arthritis. Anteroposterior radiograph of both feet of a 46-year-old woman shows characteristic erosions of several distal interphalangeal joints and erosion of the right fifth metatarsal head. Note also fusion of the proximal interphalangeal joint of the second left toe.

Subgroup 2, well known for the "opera glass" deformity of the hand, is termed *arthritis mutilans* because of the extensive destruction of the phalanges and metacarpal joints, including the "pencil-in-cup" deformity (Fig. 14.86). Other joints such as hip or elbow (Fig. 14.87) are also frequently affected. Patients with arthritis mutilans often will have sacroiliitis.

Subgroup 3 is characterized by symmetric polyarthritis (Figs. 14.88 and 14.89) and may result in ankylosis of the proximal and distal interphalangeal joints. In this form, PsA is frequently indistinguishable from RA (Fig. 14.90).

Subgroup 4 is characterized by oligoarticular arthritis, and in contrast to subgroup 3, the joint involvement is asymmetric, generally including the proximal and distal interphalangeal and metacarpophalangeal articulations (Fig. 14.91). Patients with this oligoarticular arthritis form the most frequent subgroup of PsA and are known for the appearance of sausage-like swelling of digits (Fig. 14.92).

Subgroup 5 is a spondyloarthropathy that has features similar to those of AS.

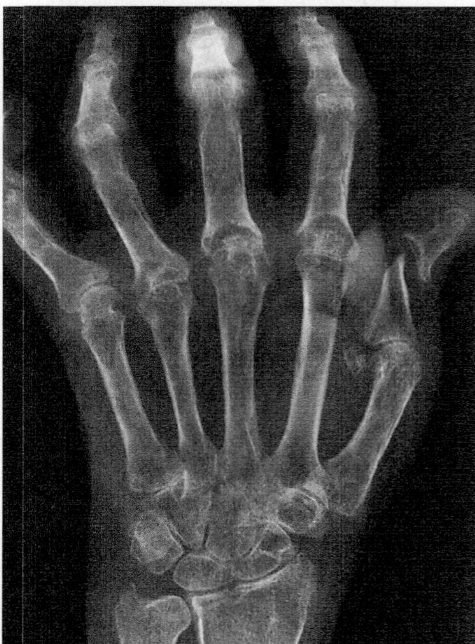

FIGURE 14.86 Psoriatic arthritis. Dorsovolar radiograph of the hand of a 57-year-old woman shows the typical presentation of psoriatic polyarthritis. The "pencil-in-cup" deformity in the interphalangeal joint of the thumb is characteristic of this form of psoriasis.

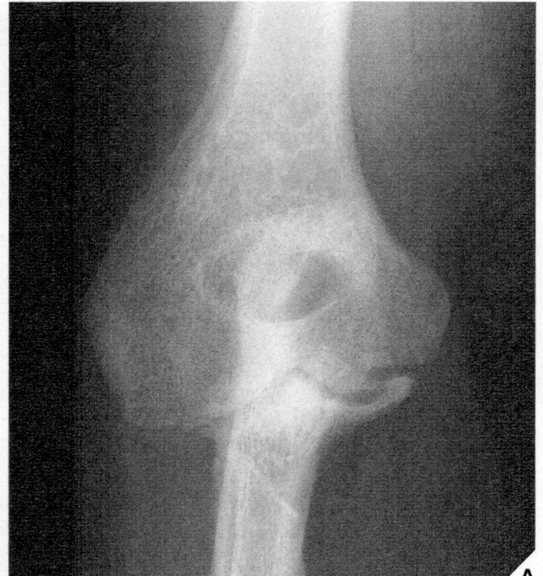

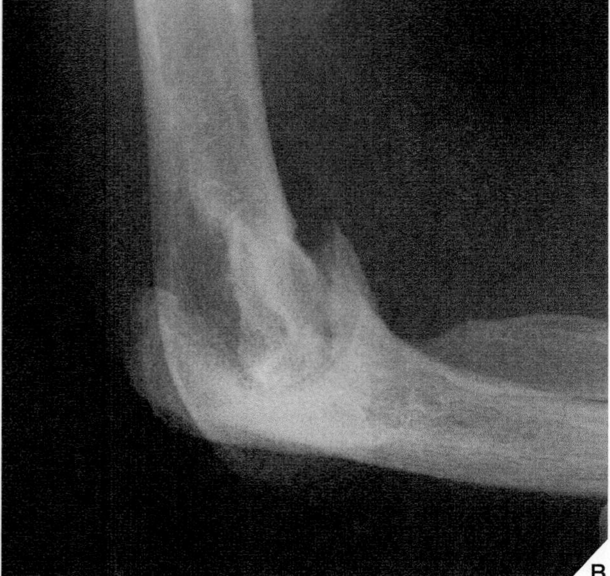

FIGURE 14.87 Psoriatic arthritis. A 49-year-old man presented with PsA mutilans. **(A)** Anteroposterior and **(B)** lateral radiographs of the right elbow show extensive articular erosions. Elevated anterior fat pad indicates a joint effusion.

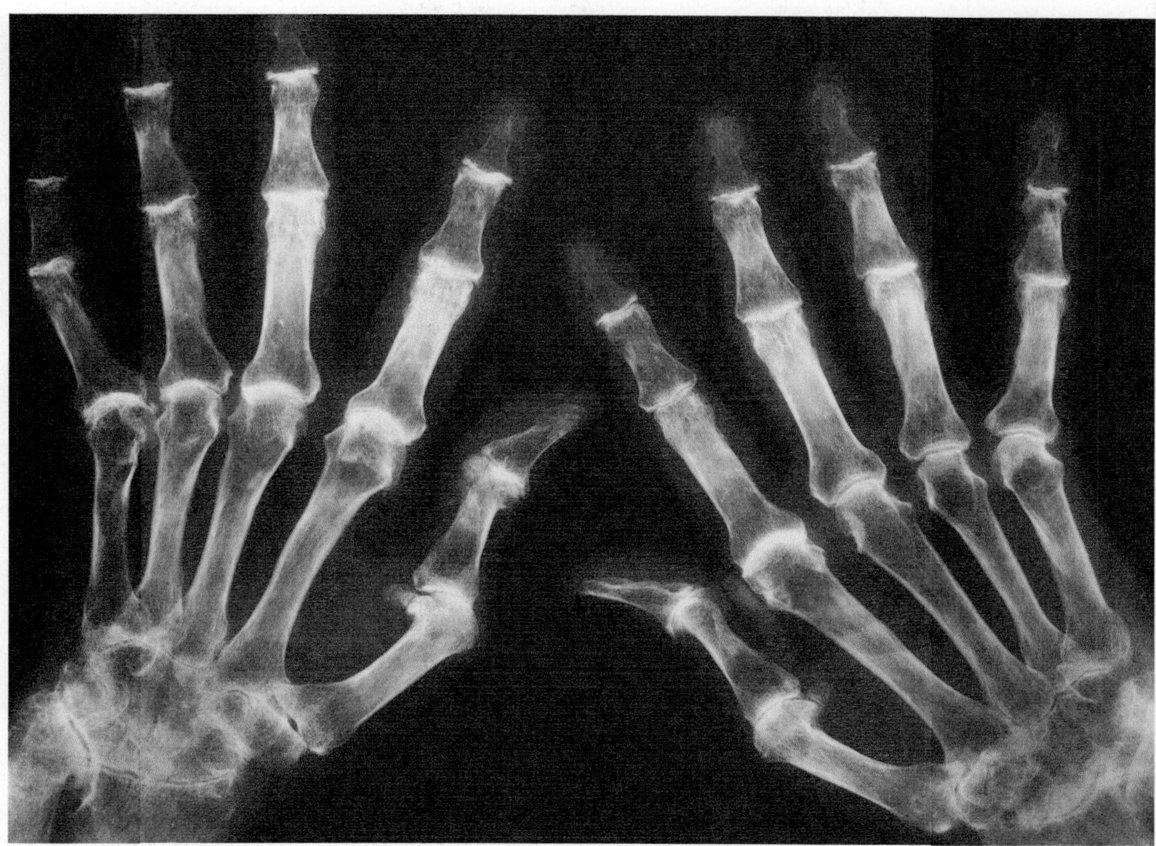

FIGURE 14.88 Psoriatic arthritis. A 75-year-old woman presented with symmetric psoriatic polyarthritis affecting all joints of the hands and wrists. Unlike in adult-onset type of RA, the distal interphalangeal joints are also involved.

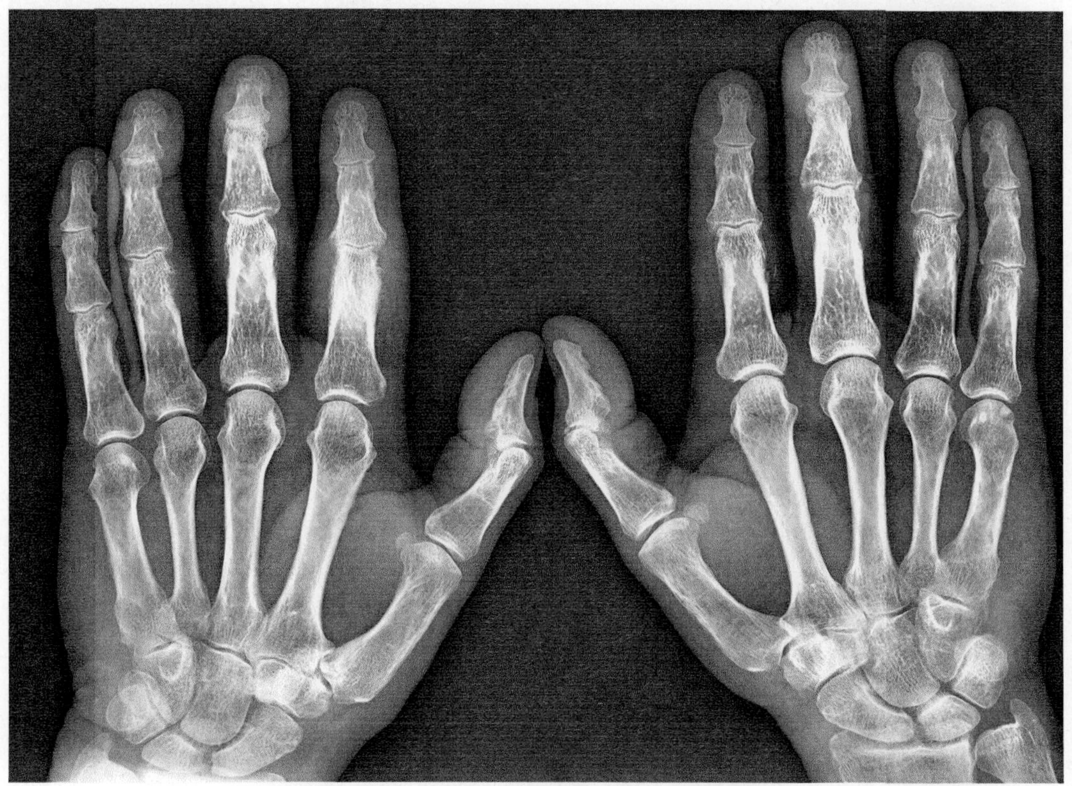

FIGURE 14.89 Psoriatic arthritis. A 65-year-old man presented with PsA affecting symmetrically both hands. Note soft-tissue swelling, articular erosions, and periostitis.

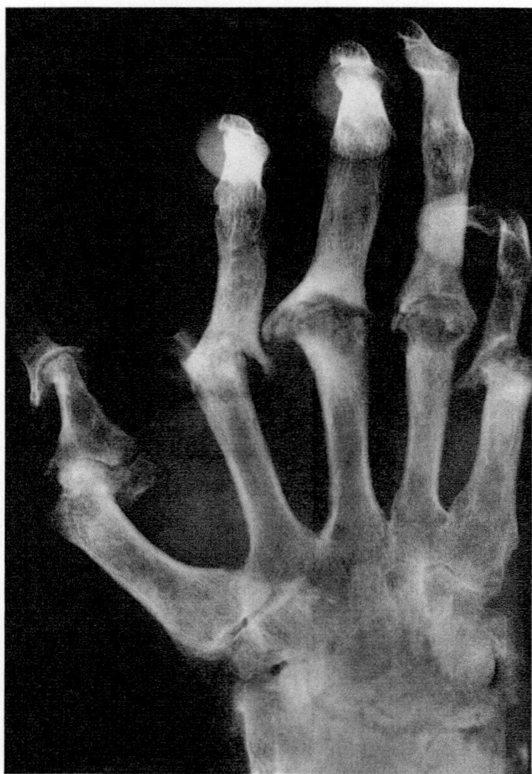

FIGURE 14.90 Psoriatic arthritis. Dorsovolar radiograph of the left hand of a 67-year-old man with the polyarthritic form of PsA demonstrates erosions and fusion of multiple joints. The swan-neck deformity of the small finger is similar to that seen in patients with RA.

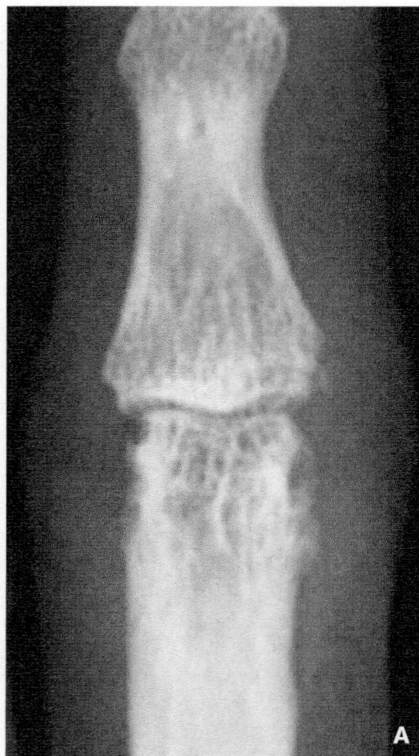

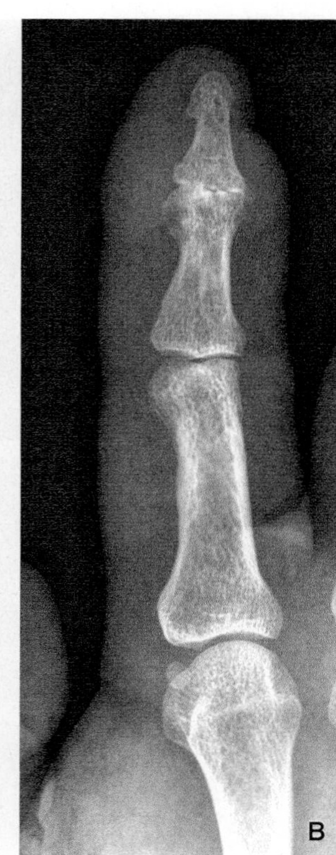

FIGURE 14.91 Psoriatic arthritis. **(A)** A 39-year-old man with psoriasis presented with a painful and swollen middle finger of his right hand. Note subtle periarticular erosions, fluffy periosteal reaction, and soft-tissue swelling, features characteristic of oligoarticular PsA. **(B)** A 42-year-old man presented with swollen index finger. The radiograph shows erosive changes of the distal interphalangeal joint and diffuse swelling of the entire finger, typical for "sausage digit."

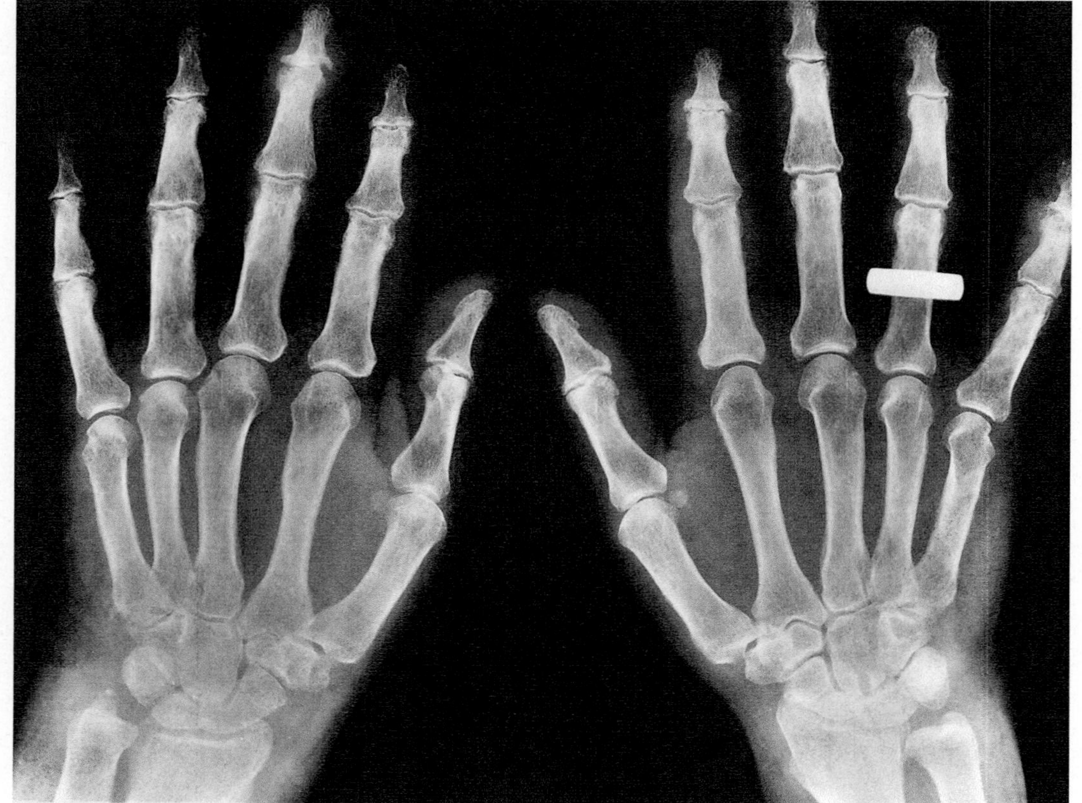

FIGURE 14.92 Psoriatic arthritis. Dorsovolar radiograph of the hands of a 33-year-old man with psoriasis and oligoarticular involvement shows destructive changes in the distal interphalangeal joints of the right middle finger and the left index and small fingers. The right middle and left index fingers presented as "sausage digits."

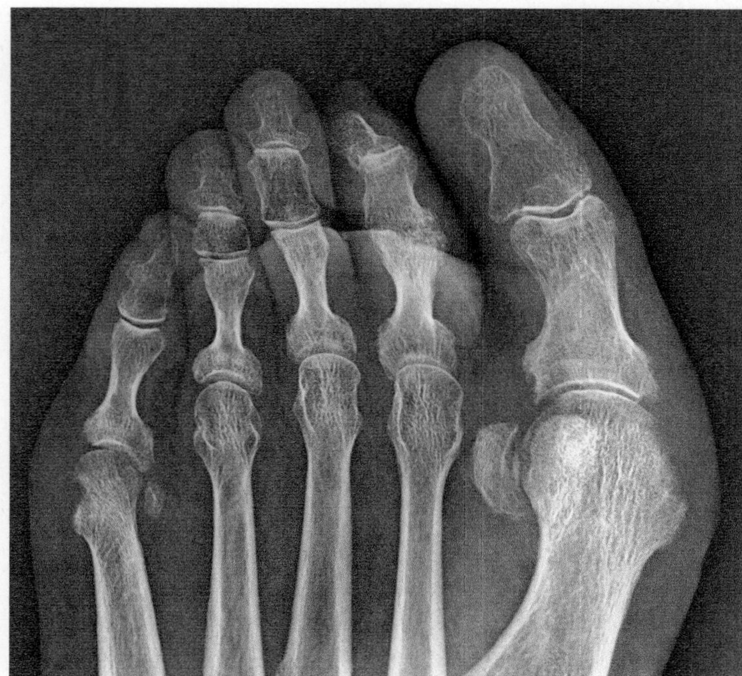

FIGURE 14.93 Psoriatic arthritis. Periarticular erosions at the first metatarsophalangeal joint and proximal interphalangeal joint of the second toe are accompanied by fluffy periostitis.

More recently, The Classification of Psoriatic Arthritis (CASPAR) Study Group criteria were introduced in 2006 as a new classification for this disorder. To the contrary to the original classification, CASPAR Study Group provided the diagnosis of PsA in patients without skin lesions. To increase the sensitivity, additional features were included, such as dactylitis ("sausage digit"), nail changes, and family history.

Imaging Features

In general, there are few characteristic radiographic features of PsA that help to make a correct diagnosis. In the phalanges of the hand or foot, a periosteal reaction in the form of a "fluffy" new bone apposition may often be noted (Fig. 14.93; see also Fig. 14.91). If this new bone is periarticular in location and associated with erosions of the interphalangeal joints, it exhibits a "mouse-ear" appearance (Fig. 14.94). Some investigators have reported that psoriatic hand arthropathy can cause significant enlargement of the thumb sesamoids, similar to one described in acromegaly (see Chapter 30). In the advanced arthritis mutilans stage of PsA, severe deformities such as the "pencil-in-cup" configuration (see Fig. 14.86) and interphalangeal ankylosis may be observed. In the heel, late-stage changes may be seen in the formation of broad-based osteophytes and in the presence of erosions and a fluffy periostitis (see Fig. 12.47D). Very early inflammatory changes, not so obvious on other imaging modalities, can be demonstrated by ^{18}F-labeled 2-fluoro-2 deoxyglucose (^{18}FDG). PET and PET/CT techniques (Fig. 14.95). Isolated tenosynovitis, especially of the flexor tendon sheaths, with additional synovitis and soft-tissue edema results in dactylitis (sausage digit), which is a hallmark of PsA. Less commonly, the extensor tenosynovitis is observed. MRI, in addition to articular erosions, may also detect proliferative synovitis, subarticular bone marrow edema, enthesitis, and tenosynovitis.

PsA of the spine is associated with a particularly high incidence of sacroiliitis, which may be bilateral and symmetric (Fig. 14.96), bilateral and asymmetric, or unilateral (Fig. 14.97). As in reactive arthritis, coarse asymmetric syndesmophytes and paraspinal ossifications may form (Figs. 14.98 and 14.99) and, as Resnick pointed out, this may represent an early manifestation of the disease.

The diagnosis of PsA at times may be challenging, particularly when skin manifestations are subtle, or the arthritis antedates the skin lesions. The lack of clearly defined diagnostic criteria and the possibility of overlap syndromes of other rheumatologic disorders further add to the complexity of diagnosis. The differential diagnosis of PsA includes other forms of inflammatory arthritides, such as other seronegative spondyloarthropathies, in particular those associated with sacroiliitis and enthesitis, as well as RA. The appearance of periostitis and joint ankylosis in PsA usually leads to the correct diagnosis. Because on conventional radiography the appearance of articular erosions may be very similar in both diseases, some investigators suggested using dynamic contrast-enhanced MRI to discriminate these two entities. Schwenzer and collaborators found significant correlations between inflammatory parameters and dynamic contrast-enhanced findings in patients with RA but not in those with PsA. Specifically, they found a statistically significant difference in synovial enhancement 15 minutes after intravenous administration of gadolinium in patients with RA.

Treatment

Patients with PsA are treated with biologic agents as first-line therapy, and this approach has dramatically improved the outcome of the disease.

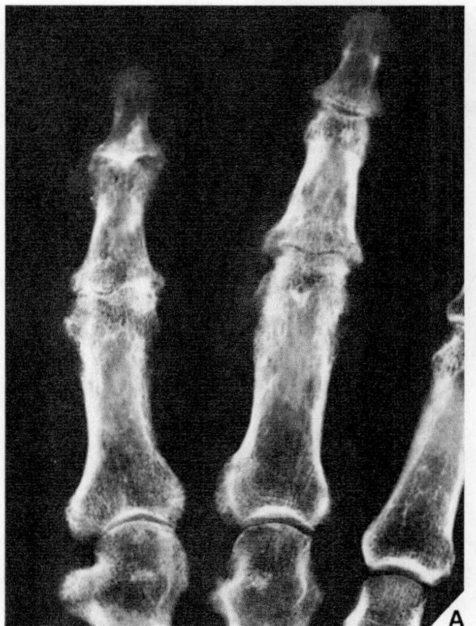

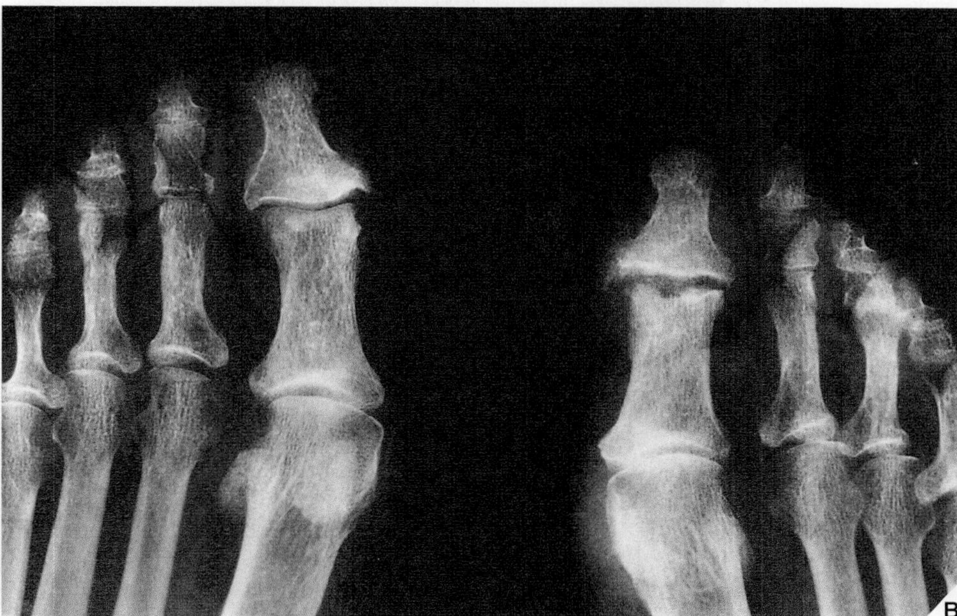

FIGURE 14.94 Psoriatic arthritis. **(A)** Dorsovolar radiograph of the ring and small fingers of a 48-year-old man who presented with clinically documented psoriasis shows marginal erosions and new bone apposition in the proximal and distal interphalangeal joints, resembling mouse ears. Note the fluffy periostitis in the juxtaarticular areas of the phalanges and distal metacarpals. **(B)** In the feet, the same process has led to a "mouse-ear" appearance at the interphalangeal joints of the great toes.

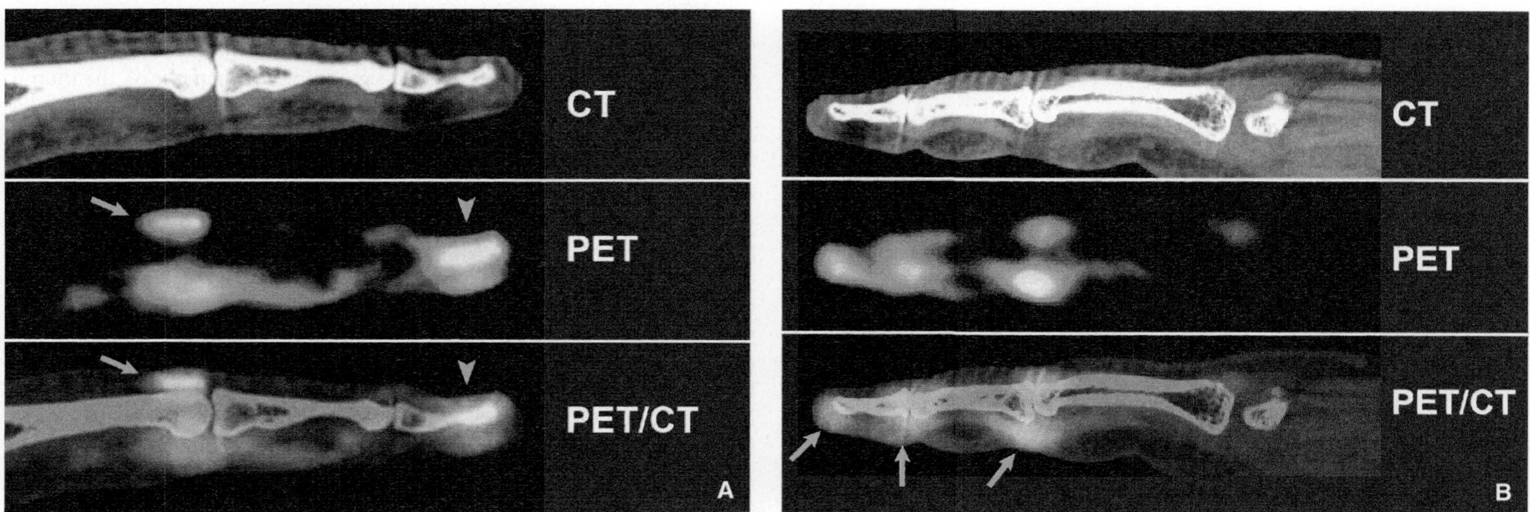

FIGURE 14.95 CT, ^{18}F-FDG PET, and PET/CT of PsA. **(A)** Along the extensor tendon *(arrows)* and its insertion into the nail bed *(arrowheads)* of the middle finger of a 53-year-old man, the inflammatory changes are well demonstrated by increased metabolic activity. **(B)** In another patient, a 50-year-old man, note the inflammatory changes at the flexor tendon of the index finger *(arrows)*. (Courtesy of Abhijit J. Chaudhari, MD, Sacramento, California.)

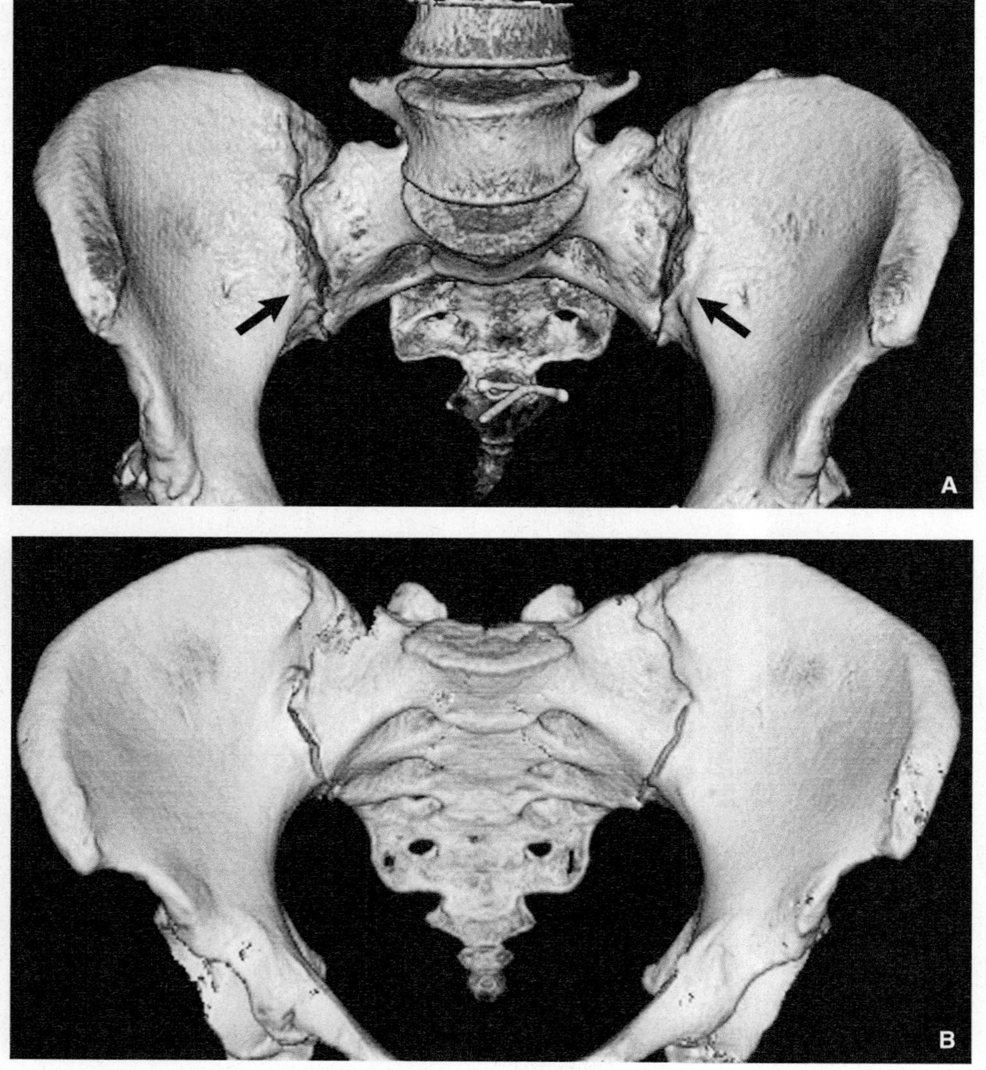

FIGURE 14.96 Three-dimensional (3D) CT of sacroiliitis in PsA. **(A)** 3D reconstructed CT image of the pelvis of a 38-year-old woman shows early subtle erosions of synovial portion of both sacroiliac joints *(arrows)*. **(B)** 3D reconstructed CT image of normal sacroiliac joints is shown for comparison.

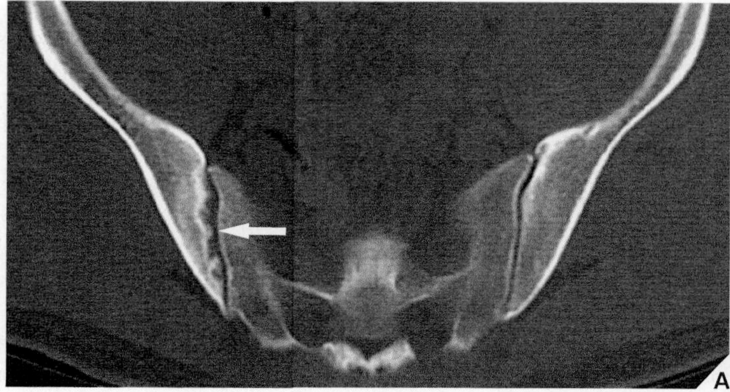

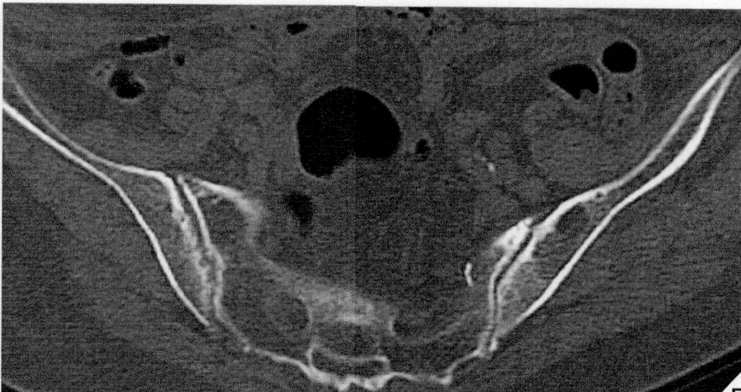

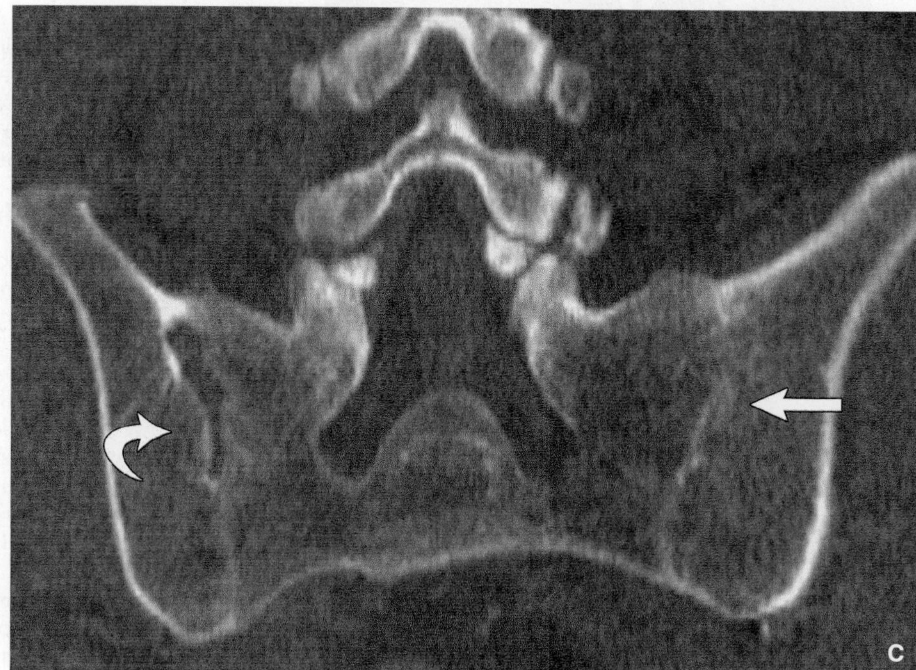

FIGURE 14.97 **Sacroiliitis in PsA.** **(A)** Axial CT section through the sacroiliac joints of a 28-year-old man with clinical diagnosis of psoriasis shows unilateral involvement of the right sacroiliac joint *(arrow)*. **(B)** Axial CT image of sacroiliac joints of a 61-year-old woman with PsA and bilateral sacroiliitis demonstrates asymmetric involvement. **(C)** Coronal reformatted CT image of sacroiliac joints of a 70-year-old man shows complete fusion of the left *(arrow)* and incomplete fusion of the right *(curved arrow)* sacroiliac joint.

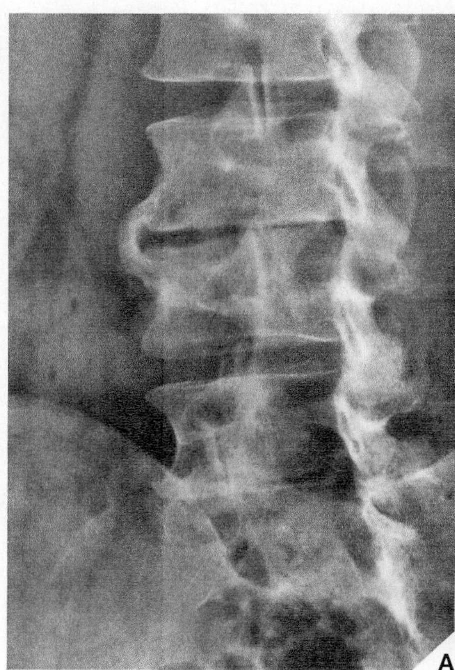

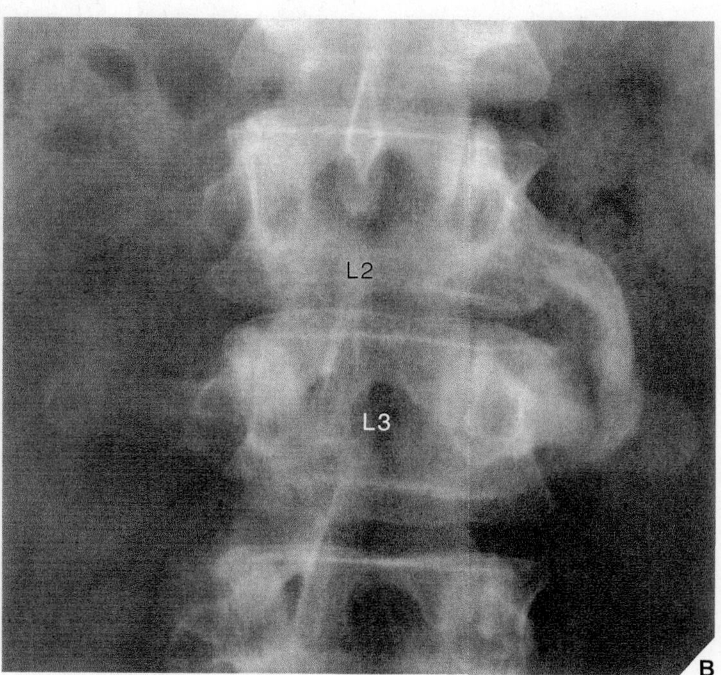

FIGURE 14.98 **Spinal abnormalities in PsA.** **(A)** Oblique radiograph of the lumbar spine in a 30-year-old man with psoriasis shows a characteristic single coarse syndesmophyte bridging the bodies of L3 and L4. The right sacroiliac joint is also affected. **(B)** Anteroposterior radiograph of the lumbar spine in a 45-year-old man with psoriasis reveals paraspinal ossification at the level of L2-3.

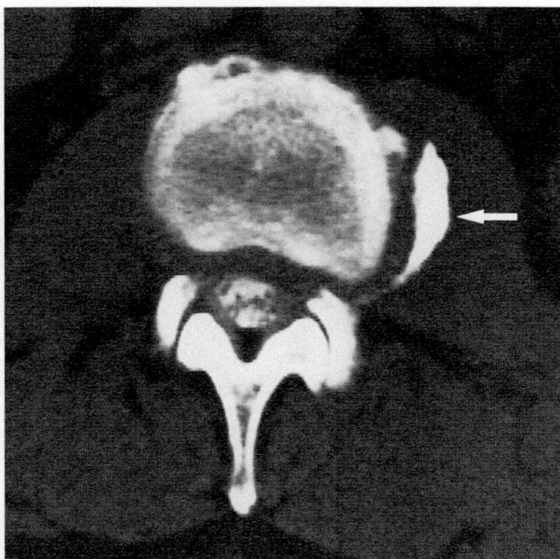

FIGURE 14.99 **Spinal abnormalities in PsA.** A postmyelographic CT scan through the lumbar spine shows a paraspinal ossification *(arrow)* in a 48-year-old man with psoriasis.

Biologic inhibitors of TNF including etanercept, adalimumab, certolizumab, infliximab, and golimumab decrease the symptoms of articular and skin manifestations of psoriasis. However, there are many other new drugs introduced to treat both psoriasis and PsA; therefore, the reader is referred to recent reviews in the literature on this important subject.

Enteropathic Arthropathies

This group comprises arthritides associated with inflammatory intestinal diseases such as ulcerative colitis, regional enteritis (Crohn disease), and intestinal lipodystrophy (Whipple disease), the last of which predominantly affects men in their fourth and fifth decades. The histocompatibility antigen HLA-B27 is present in most patients with enteropathic abnormalities. In all three conditions, the spine and the sacroiliac and peripheral joints may be affected. In the spine, squaring of the vertebral bodies and the formation of syndesmophytes are common features. Sacroiliitis, which is usually bilateral and symmetric, is radiographically indistinguishable from AS (Fig. 14.100). In addition, patients may also exhibit a peripheral arthritis, the activity of which generally approximates the activity of the bowel disease.

Finally, it should be noted that arthritis may follow intestinal bypass procedures. The synovitis is polyarticular and symmetric, but radiographically, the lesions are nonerosive.

Undifferentiated Spondyloarthritis

The term *undifferentiated spondyloarthritis* is applied to patients exhibiting increased HLA-B27 positivity and who also have peripheral arthritis, sacroiliitis, and/or enthesitis but who lack of clinical or imaging features allowing further subclassification. A subset of patients with this designation may progress to AS or PsA, but it is not clear which clinical or laboratory features may be predictive of such progression. According to Taurog et al., the concept of undifferentiated spondyloarthritis is becoming gradually subsumed under the general rubric of axial and peripheral spondyloarthropathy.

SAPHO Syndrome

In 1987, Chomot and collaborators coined the acronym SAPHO (**s**ynovitis, **a**cne, **p**ustulosis, **h**yperostosis, **o**steitis) for a group of patients with pustular acne (palmoplantar pustulosis) and hyperostotic inflammation of bone. Some investigators link SAPHO syndrome with seronegative spondyloarthropathies because significant number of patients with this condition fulfill the accepted criteria for spondyloarthropathy. However, not all of the individuals affected with this disorder have the genetic predisposition found in the patients with the other seronegative spondyloarthropthies discussed earlier. Specifically, only some patients with this syndrome tested positive for human leukocyte antigen HLA-B27. SAPHO, whose etiology is still not known, affects patients in any age, more commonly women than men. The most common site of involvement is the sternoclavicular, manubriosternal, and costosternal joints. Imaging findings include osteosclerosis, hyperostosis, cortical thickening, narrowing of the medullary canal, with external surface

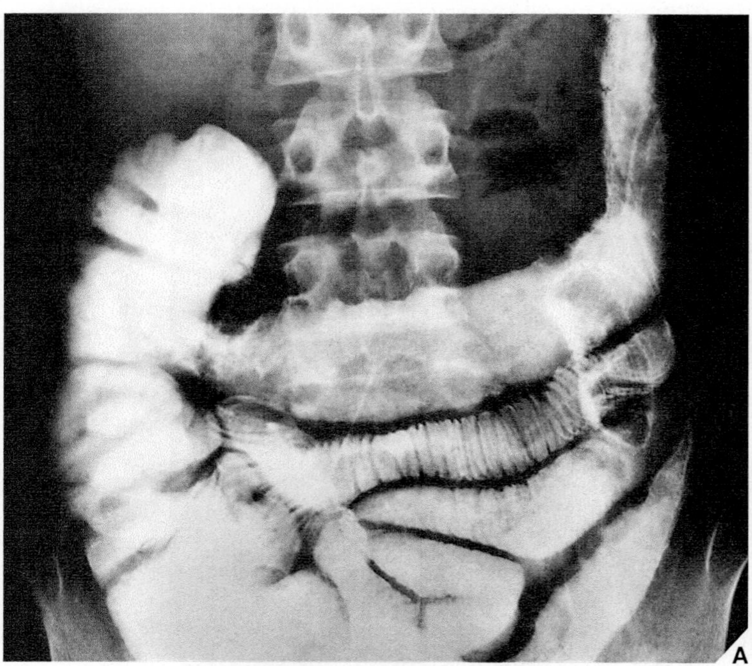

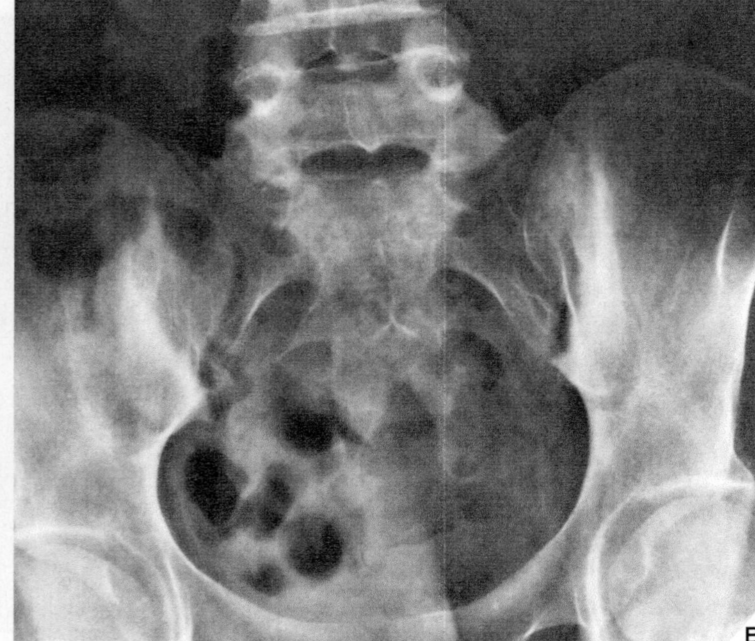

FIGURE 14.100 **Ulcerative colitis complicated by sacroiliitis.** A 20-year-old woman with known ulcerative colitis developed severe low back pain localized to the sacroiliac joints. **(A)** Barium enema study shows extensive involvement of the transverse and descending colon, consistent with ulcerative colitis. **(B)** Posteroanterior radiograph of the pelvis shows symmetric, bilateral sacroiliitis similar to that seen in AS.

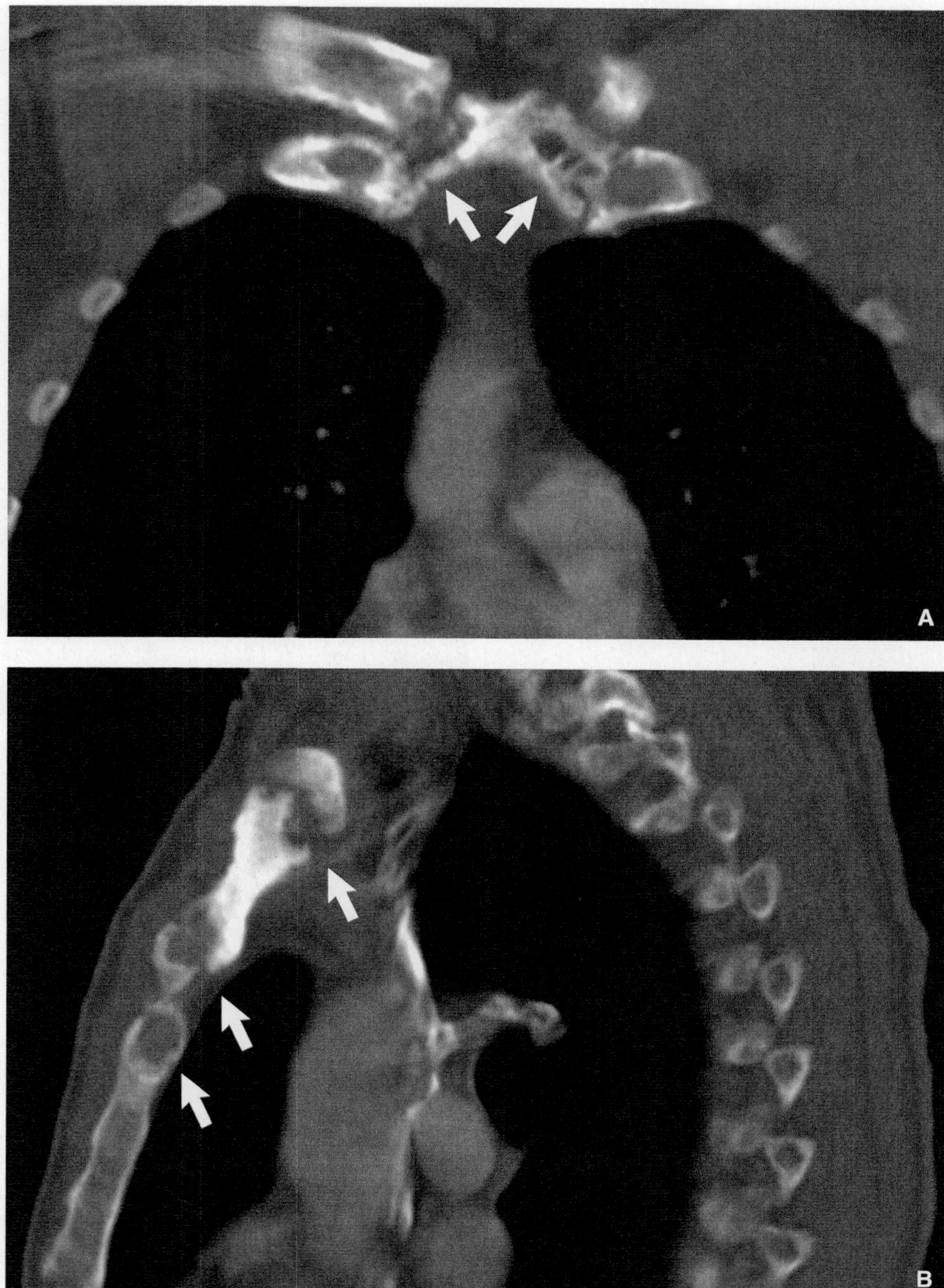

FIGURE 14.101 SAPHO syndrome. A 49-year-old man presented with pustulosis on his palms and soles and anterior chest wall pain. **(A)** Coronal reformatted CT image of the sternum shows sclerotic changes and erosions of the sternoclavicular and costosternal joints *(arrows)*. **(B)** Sagittal reformatted CT image in addition shows osteolytic foci in the sternum *(arrows)*.

of bone appearing sometimes expanded, indistinct, or irregular, better depicted with CT (Figs. 14.101 and 14.102). Articular manifestations become apparent sometime after the onset of skin lesions. Cutaneous manifestations include palmoplantar pustulosis, severe forms of acne (acne fulminans or conglobata, hidradenitis suppurativa), and various forms of psoriatic-like skin lesions. The treatment with antibiotics (clindamycin) and NSAIDs (lornoxicam) proved to be very effective in rapid symptoms resolution. Recent clinical trials suggested that pamidronate might be an effective drug for this condition.

Some researchers combine SAPHO together with chronic recurrent multifocal osteomyelitis (CRMO), an acute inflammatory multifocal process affecting more than one bone, occurring mostly in children and adolescents, with clinical and imaging manifestations similar to osteomyelitis (Fig. 14.103) but without infection and lack of known pathogen. Giedion et al. described this entity in 1972, and some authors contended that CRMO is in fact the pediatric presentation of SAPHO. Yet, there are also many investigators who believe that these are two separate entities with the different localization of inflammation: in pediatric CRMO, the extremities are more often affected, whereas in SAPHO, the axial skeleton, and particularly costosternoclavicular region is the focus of abnormalities. Moreover, CRMO is now considered to be an inherited autoinflammatory disease caused by immune dysregulation, without autoantibodies or antigen-specific T cells. Some investigators suggested a link between CRMO and a rare allele of marker D18S60, resulting in a haplotype relative risk (HRR) of chromosome 18 (18q21.3-18q22).

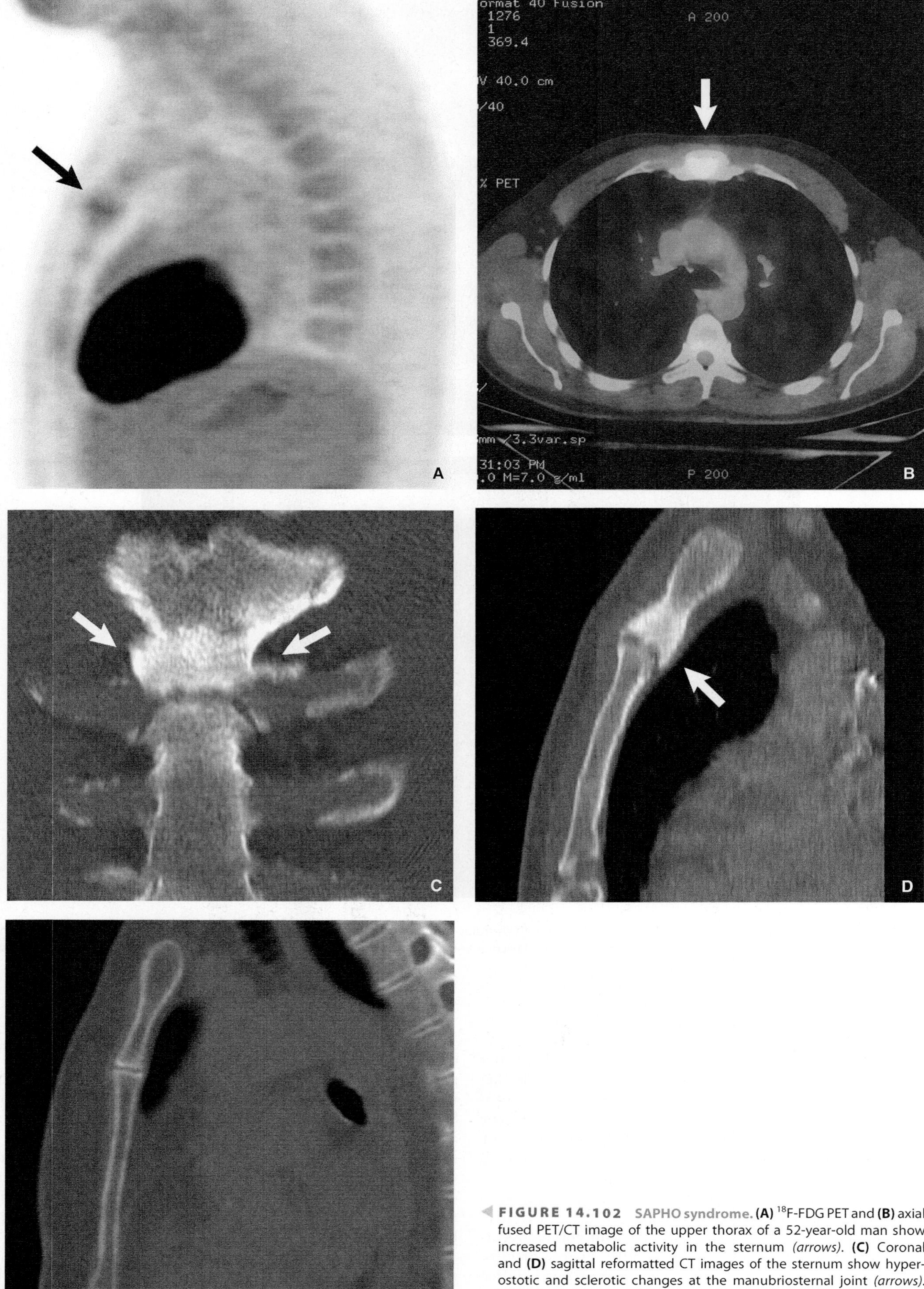

FIGURE 14.102 SAPHO syndrome. **(A)** ^{18}F-FDG PET and **(B)** axial fused PET/CT image of the upper thorax of a 52-year-old man show increased metabolic activity in the sternum *(arrows)*. **(C)** Coronal and **(D)** sagittal reformatted CT images of the sternum show hyperostotic and sclerotic changes at the manubriosternal joint *(arrows)*. **(E)** Sagittal reformatted CT image of a normal manubriosternal joint is shown for comparison.

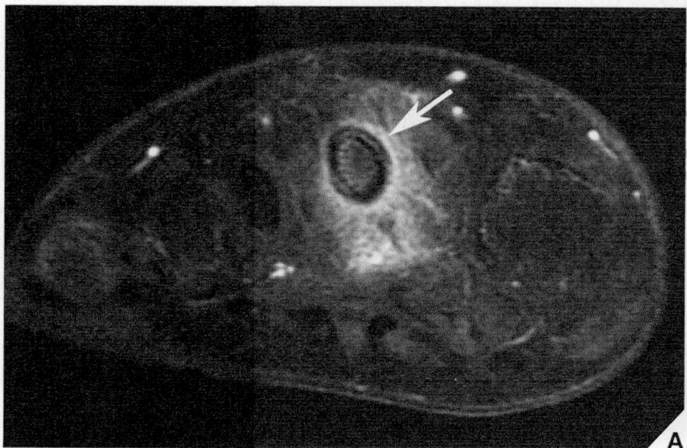

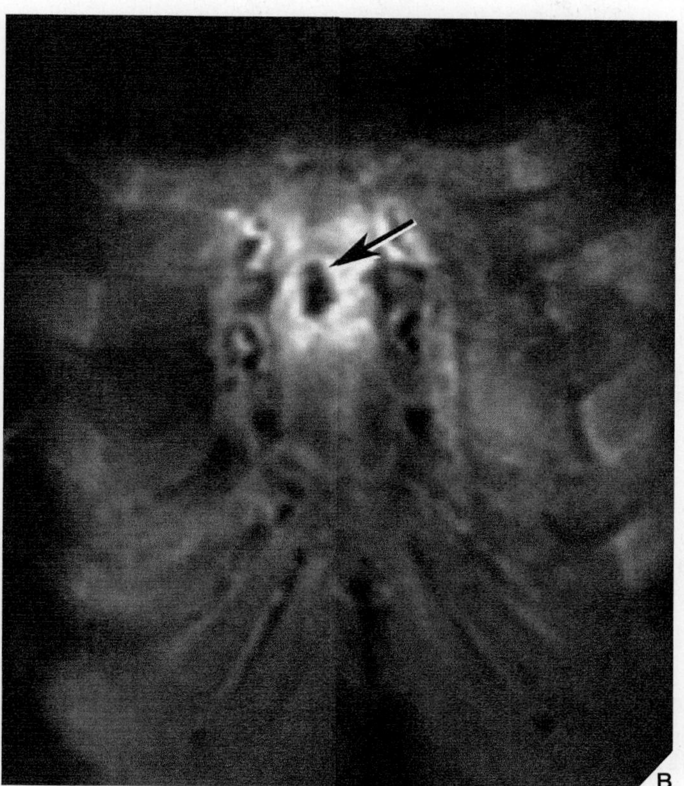

FIGURE 14.103 MRI of chronic recurrent multifocal osteomyelitis (CRMO). A 12-year-old girl presented with history of chronic foot pain and anterior chest wall pain. **(A)** Short-axis T2-weighted fat-suppressed MR image of the forefoot shows signal alteration of the second metatarsal bone associated with periosteal reaction *(arrow)* and surrounding soft-tissue edema. **(B)** Coronal T1-weighted fat-suppressed MR image of the sternum obtained after intravenous administration of gadolinium shows a focal area of low signal intensity in the body of the sternum *(arrow)* surrounded by enhancing edema.

PRACTICAL POINTS TO REMEMBER

Erosive Osteoarthritis

1. EOA, a condition seen predominantly in middle-aged women, combines the clinical manifestations of RA with the radiographic features of OA.
2. EOA can be recognized by:
   - involvement of the proximal and distal interphalangeal joints
   - a characteristic "gull-wing" configuration of articular erosions. Spontaneous fusion (ankylosis) in the interphalangeal joints may develop.

Rheumatoid Arthritis

1. RA has a predilection for:
   - the large joints (knees and hips)
   - the small joints in the hand (metacarpophalangeal and proximal interphalangeal)
   - the carpal articulations.

   The distal interphalangeal and sacroiliac joints are usually spared.
2. The radiographic hallmarks of RA include:
   - diffuse, symmetric narrowing of the joint space
   - periarticular osteoporosis
   - fusiform soft-tissue swelling
   - rheumatoid nodules
   - marginal and central articular erosions
   - periarticular synovial cysts
   - subluxations and other joint deformities—swan-neck, boutonnière, hitchhiker's thumb.
3. In the cervical spine, RA is characterized by:
   - erosion of the odontoid process associated with subluxation in the atlantoaxial joints and, frequently, cephalad translocation of C2 (cranial settling)
   - involvement of the apophyseal joints
   - erosions of vertebral bodies
   - destruction of intervertebral disks
   - erosions (whittling) of the spinous processes.
4. In RA:
   - axial or, less frequently, medial migration of the femoral head and acetabular protrusio are characteristic in the hip joint
   - rotator cuff tear is a frequent complication in the shoulder joint
   - the subtalar joint is most often affected in the foot, and a hallux valgus deformity is observed.
5. MRI provides an effective way to demonstrate critical features of preerosive RA: joint effusion, edema, inflammatory pannus, and tenosynovitis.
6. Rheumatoid nodulosis, a condition occurring predominantly in men, is a variant of RA. It exhibits:
   - a characteristic lack of joint abnormalities
   - multiple subcutaneous nodules
   - a high titer of rheumatoid factor.
7. JIA (juvenile RA) displays several characteristic features that are either rare or not present in adult-onset disease:
   - a periosteal reaction
   - joint ankylosis, particularly affecting the apophyseal joints of the cervical spine
   - growth abnormalities secondary to involvement of epiphyseal sites.
8. MAS is severe and potentially life-threatening complication of several chronic rheumatologic disorders of childhood. It occurs most commonly with systemic JIA and adult-onset Still disease.

Other Inflammatory Arthritides

1. Spondyloarthropathies comprise four distinctive entities: AS, PsA, reactive arthritis (Reiter syndrome), and arthritides associated with inflammatory bowel disease.
2. AS (Bechterew or Marie-Strümpell disease), a condition seen predominantly in young men, characteristically affects the spine and sacroiliac joints. Histocompatibility antigen HLA-B27 is invariably present in 95% of patients. The radiographic hallmarks of this condition include:
   - squaring of the vertebral bodies
   - "shiny corners"

- the development of delicate syndesmophytes
- in a later stage of disease, complete fusion of the apophyseal joints and vertebrae, leading to "bamboo" spine.

3. Reactive arthritis, formerly known as *Reiter syndrome*, consists of inflammatory arthritis, urethritis, conjunctivitis, and mucocutaneous rash. Its radiographic features include:
   - a peripheral, usually asymmetric arthritis that shows a predilection for the lower limb joints, particularly in the foot
   - coarse syndesmophytes and paraspinal ossifications bridging vertebral bodies
   - sacroiliitis, which usually is asymmetric.
4. PsA has a predilection for the distal interphalangeal joints. Oligoarticular involvement may yield a phenomenon known as *sausage digit*. Radiographically, PsA is marked by:
   - fluffy periostitis
   - "pencil-in-cup" deformity of the joints (arthritis mutilans)
   - coarse syndesmophytes and paraspinal ossifications that are indistinguishable from those seen in reactive arthritis
   - involvement of the sacroiliac joints.
5. Enteropathic arthropathies are associated with:
   - ulcerative colitis
   - regional enteritis (Crohn disease)
   - intestinal lipodystrophy (Whipple disease)
   - intestinal bypass procedures.

   Characteristically, there is symmetric involvement of the sacroiliac joints.
6. Undifferentiated spondyloarthritis is characterized by increased HLA-B27 positivity, peripheral arthritis, sacroiliitis, and enthesitis. Some patients with this designation may progress to AS or PsA.
7. SAPHO syndrome is characterized by synovitis, acne, pustulosis, hyperostosis, and osteitis in addition to palmoplantar pustulosis and hyperostotic inflammation of bones. It is closely related to CRMO.
8. CRMO is an acute, inflammatory multifocal process affecting many bones, and occuring mostly in children and adolescents. It is considered to be an inherited autoinflammatory disease caused by immune dysregulation.

SUGGESTED READINGS

Adam G, Dammer M, Bohndorf K, et al. Rheumatoid arthritis of the knee: value of gadopentetate dimeglumine-enhanced MR imaging. *AJR Am J Roentgenol* 1991;156:125–129.

Agten CA, Zubler V, Rosskopf AB, et al. Enthesitis of lumbar spine ligaments in clinically suspected spondyloarthritis: value of gadolinium-enhanced MR images in comparison to STIR. *Skeletal Radiol* 2016;45:187–195.

Aletaha D, Neogi T, Silman AJ, et al. 2010 Rheumatoid arthritis classification criteria: an American College of Rheumatology/European League Against Rheumatism Collaborative Initiative. *Arthritis Rheum* 2010;62:2569–2581.

Algin O, Gokalp G, Baran B, et al. Evaluation of sacroiliitis: contrast-enhanced MRI with subtraction technique. *Skeletal Radiol* 2009;38:983–988.

Ansell BM. Juvenile psoriatic arthritis. *Baillieres Clin Rheumatol* 1994;8:317–332.

Ansell BM, Bywaters EGL. Diagnosis of "probable" Still's disease and its outcome. *Ann Rheum Dis* 1962;21:253.

Ansell BM, Wigley RA. Arthritic manifestations in regional enteritis. *Ann Rheum Dis* 1964;23:64–72.

Arnett FC, Edworthy SM, Bloch DA, et al. The American Rheumatism Association 1987 revised criteria for the classification of rheumatoid arthritis. *Arthritis Rheum* 1988;31:315–324.

Ash Z, Marzo-Ortega H. Ankylosing spondylitis—the changing role of imaging. *Skeletal Radiol* 2012;41:1031–1034.

Azouz EM, Duffy CM. Juvenile spondyloarthropathies: clinical manifestations and medical imaging. *Skeletal Radiol* 1995;24:399–408.

Belhorn LR, Hess EV. Erosive osteoarthritis. *Semin Arthritis Rheum* 1993;22:298–306.

Boden SD, Dodge LD, Bohlman HH, et al. Rheumatoid arthritis of the cervical spine. A long-term analysis with predictors of paralysis and recovery. *J Bone Joint Surg Am* 1993;75:1282–1297.

Bollow M, Braun J, Biedermann T, et al. Use of contrast-enhanced MR imaging to detect sacroiliitis in children. *Skeletal Radiol* 1998;27:606–616.

Boutin RD, Resnick D. The SAPHO syndrome: an evolving concept for unifying several idiopathic disorders of bone and skin. *AJR Am J Roentgenol* 1998;170:585–591.

Breton S, Jousse-Joulin S, Cangemi C, et al. Comparison of clinical and ultrasonographic evaluation for peripheral synovitis in juvenile idiopathic arthritis. *Semin Arthritis Rheum* 2011;41:272–278.

Burgos-Vargas R, Vázquez-Mellado J. The early clinical recognition of juvenile-onset ankylosing spondylitis and its differentiation from juvenile rheumatoid arthritis. *Arthritis Rheum* 1995;38:835–844.

Canella C, Schau B, Ribeiro E, et al. MRI in seronegative spondyloarthritis: imaging features and differential diagnosis in the spine and sacroiliac joints. *AJR Am J Roentgenol* 2013;200:149–157.

Carmona R, Harish S, Linda DD, et al. MR imaging of the spine and sacroiliac joints for spondyloarthritis: influence on clinical diagnostic confidence and patient management. *Radiology* 2013;269:208–215.

Chamot AM, Benhamou CL, Kahn MF, et al. Acne-postulosis-hyperostosis-osteitis syndrome. Result of a national survey. 85 cases. *Rev Rhum Mal Osteoartic* 1987;54:187–196.

Chung C, Coley BD, Martin LC. Rice bodies in juvenile rheumatoid arthritis. *AJR Am J Roentgenol* 1998;170:698–700.

Clark RL, Muhletaler CA, Margulies SI. Colitic arthritis: clinical and radiographic manifestations. *Radiology* 1971;101:585–594.

Coates LC, Hodgson R, Conaghan PG, et al. MRI and ultrasonography for diagnosis and monitoring of psoriatic arthritis. *Best Pract Res Clin Rheumatol* 2012;26:805–822.

Cobby M, Cushnaghan J, Creamer P, et al. Erosive osteoarthritis: is it a separate disease entity? *Clin Radiol* 1990;42:258–263.

Crain DC. Interphalangeal osteoarthritis. *JAMA* 1961;175:1049–1053.

Ehrlich GE. Erosive osteoarthritis: presentation, clinical pearls, and therapy. *Curr Rheumatol Rep* 2001;3:484–488.

Ehrlich GE. Inflammatory osteoarthritis. II. The superimposition of rheumatoid arthritis. *J Chronic Dis* 1972;25:635–643.

el-Noueam KI, Giuliano V, Schweitzer ME, et al. Rheumatoid nodules: MR/pathological correlation. *J Comput Assist Tomogr* 1997;21:796–799.

Forrester DM. Imaging of the sacroiliac joints. *Radiol Clin North Am* 1990;28:1055–1072.

Gálvez J, Sola J, Ortuño G, et al. Microscopic rice bodies in rheumatoid synovial fluid sediments. *J Rheumatol* 1992;19:1851–1858.

Garg N, van den Bosch F, Deodhar F. The concept of spondyloarthritis: where are we now? *Best Pract Res Clin Rheumatol* 2014;28:663–672.

Giedion A, Holthusen K-H, Eriksson B, et al. Chronic recurrent multifocal osteomyelitis and pustulosis palmoplantaris. *J Pediatr* 1978;93:227–231.

Ginsberg MH, Genant HK, Yü TF, et al. Rheumatoid nodulosis: an unusual variant of rheumatoid disease. *Arthritis Rheum* 1975;18:49–58.

Golla A, Jansson A, Ramser J, et al. Chronic recurrent multifocal osteomyelitis (CRMO): evidence for a susceptibility gene located on chromosome 18q21.3-18q22. *Eur J Hum Genet* 2002;10:217–221.

Greenspan A. Erosive osteoarthritis. *Semin Musculoskel Radiol* 2003;7:155–159.

Greenspan A, Baker ND, Norman A. Rheumatoid arthritis simulating other lesions. *Bull Hosp Jt Dis Orthop Inst* 1983;43:70–77.

Handly B, Moore M, Creutzberg G, et al. Bisphosphonate therapy for chronic recurrent multifocal osteomyelitis. *Skeletal Radiol* 2013;42:1777–1778.

Hazlewood GS, Barnabe C, Tomlison G, et al. Methotrexate monotherapy and methotrexate combination therapy with traditional and biologic disease modifying anti-rheumatic drugs for rheumatoid arthritis: a network meta-analysis. *Cochrane Database Syst Rev* 2016;(8):CD010227. doi:10.1002/14651858.

Helliwell PS, Wright V. Clinical features of psoriatic arthritis. In: Klippel JH, Dieppe PA, eds. *Practical rheumatology*. London, United Kingdom: Mosby; 1995:235–242.

Hermann K-GA, Bollow M. Magnetic resonance imaging of sacroiliitis in patients with spondyloarthritis: correlation with anatomy and histology. *Rofo* 2014;186:230–237.

Herregods N, Jaremko JL, Baraliakos X, et al. Limited role of gadolinium to detect active sacroiliitis on MRI in juvenile spondyloarthritis. *Skeletal Radiol* 2015;44:1637–1646.

Hughes RJ, Saifuddin A. Progressive non-infectious anterior vertebral fusion (Copenhagen syndrome) in three children: features on radiographs and MR imaging. *Skeletal Radiol* 2006;35:397–401.

Kahn MF. Why the "SAPHO" syndrome? *J Rheumatol* 1995;22:2017–2019.

Kamishima T, Tanimura K, Shimizu M, et al. Monitoring anti-interleukin 6 receptor antibody treatment for rheumatoid arthritis by quantitative magnetic resonance imaging of the hand and power Doppler ultrasonography of the finger. *Skeletal Radiol* 2011;40:745–755.

Kellgren JH, Moore R. Generalized osteoarthritis and Heberden's nodes. *Br Med J* 1952;1:181–187.

Kettering JM, Towers JD, Rubin DA. The seronegative spondyloarthropathies. *Semin Roentgenol* 1996;31:220–228.

Kim NR, Choi J-Y, Hong SH, et al. "MR corner sign": value for predicting presence of ankylosing spondylitis. *AJR Am J Roentgenol* 2008;191:124–128.

Klecker R, Weissman BN. Imaging features of psoriatic arthritis and Reiter's syndrome. *Semin Musculoskelet Radiol* 2003;7:115–126.

Larbi A, Viala P, Molinari N, et al. Assessment of MRI abnormalities of the sacroiliac joints and their ability to predict axial spondyloarthritis: a retrospective pilot study on 110 patients. *Skeletal Radiol* 2014;43:351–358.

Mak W, Hunter JC. MRI of early diagnosis of inflammatory arthritis. *J Musculoskeletal Med* 2009;26:478–486.

Maksymowych WP, Crowther SM, Dhillon SS, et al. Systemic assessment of inflammation by magnetic resonance imaging in the posterior elements of the spine in ankylosing spondylitis. *Arthritis Care Res (Hoboken)* 2010;62:4–10.

Mansour M, Cheema G, Naguwa S, et al. Ankylosing spondylitis: a contemporary perspective on diagnosis and treatment. *Semin Arthritis Rheum* 2007;36:210–223.

Marsal L, Winblad S, Wollheim FA. *Yersinia enterocolitica* arthritis in southern Sweden: a four-year follow-up study. *Br Med J (Clin Res Ed)* 1981;283:101–103.

Martel W, Snarr JW, Horn JR. The metacarpophalangeal joints in interphalangeal osteoarthritis. *Radiology* 1973;108:1–7.

Martel W, Stuck KJ, Dworin AM, et al. Erosive osteoarthritis and psoriatic arthritis: a radiologic comparison in the hand, wrist, and foot. *AJR Am J Roentgenol* 1980;134:125–135.

Martini A. It is time to rethink juvenile idiopathic arthritis classification and nomenclature. *Ann Rheum Dis* 2012;71:1437–1439.

Martini A, Lovell DJ. Juvenile idiopathic arthritis: state of the art and future perspectives. *Ann Rheum Dis* 2010;69:1260–1263.

McGonagle D. The history of erosions in rheumatoid arthritis: are erosions history? *Arthritis Rheum* 2010;62:312–315.

Moll JMH, Wright V. Psoriatic arthritis. *Semin Arthritis Rheum* 1973;3:55–78.

Mutlu H, Silit E, Pekkafali Z, et al. Multiple rice body formation in the subacromial-subdeltoid bursa and knee joint. *Skeletal Radiol* 2004;33:531–533.

Nakayamada S, Kubo S, Iwata S, et al. Recent progress in JAK inhibitors for the treatment of rheumatoid arthritis. *BioDrugs* 2016;30:407–419.

Navalho M, Resende C, Rodrigues AM, et al. Bilateral MR imaging of the hand and wrist in early and very early inflammatory arthritis: tenosynovitis is associated with progression to rheumatoid arthritis. *Radiology* 2012;264:823–833.

Navallas M, Ares J, Beltrán B, et al. Sacroiliitis associated with axial spondyloarthropathy: new concepts and latest trends. *Radiographics* 2013;33:933–956.

Navallas M, Inarejos EJ, Iglesias E, et al. MR imaging of the temporomandibular joint in juvenile idiopathic arthritis: technique and findings. *Radiographics* 2017;37:595–612.

Oloff-Solomon J, Oloff LM, Jacobs AM. Rheumatoid nodulosis in the foot: a variant of rheumatoid disease. *J Foot Surg* 1984;23:382–385.

Ostendorf B, Mattes-György K, Reichelt DC, et al. Early detection of bony alterations in rheumatoid and erosive arthritis of finger joints with high-resolution single photon emission computed tomography, and differentiation between them. *Skeletal Radiol* 2010;39:55–61.

Ostensen H, Pettersson H, Davies AM, eds. *The WHO manual of diagnostic imaging.* Geneva, Switzerland: World Health Organization; 2002:129–142.

Paparo F, Ravelli M, Semprini A, et al. Seronegative spondyloarthropathies: what radiologists should know. *Radiol Med* 2014;119:156–163.

Peter JB, Pearson CM, Marmor L. Erosive osteoarthritis of the hands. *Arthritis Rheum* 1966;9:365–388.

Petty RE, Southwood TR, Baum J, et al. Revision of the proposed classification criteria for juvenile idiopathic arthritis: Durban, 1997. *J Rheumatol* 1998;25:1991–1994.

Plenge RM, Seielstad M, Padyukov L, et al. TRAF1-C5 as a risk locus for rheumatoid arthritis—a genomewide study. *N Engl J Med* 2007;357:1199–1209.

Polster JM, Winalski CS, Sundaram M, et al. Rheumatoid arthritis: evaluation with contrast-enhanced CT with digital bone masking. *Radiology* 2009;252:225–231.

Porter-Young FM, Offiah AC, Broadley P, et al. Inter- and intra-observer reliability of contrast-enhanced magnetic resonance imaging parameters in children with suspected juvenile idiopathic arthritis of the hip. *Pediatr Radiol* 2018;48:1891–1900.

Punzi L, Ramonda R, Deberg M, et al. Coll2-1, Coll2-1NO2, and myeloperoxidase serum levels in erosive and non-erosive osteoarthritis of the hands. *Osteoarthritis Cartilage* 2012;20:557–561.

Qubti MA, Flynn JA. Ankylosing spondylitis & the arthritis of inflammatory bowel disease. In: Imboden JB, Hellmann DB, Stone JH, eds. *Current diagnosis & treatment: rheumatology*, 3rd ed. New York: McGraw-Hill; 2007:159–166.

Raychaudhuri SB, Deodhar A. The classification and diagnostic criteria of ankylosing spondylitis. *J Autoimmun* 2014;48–49:128–133.

Reiter H. Ueber eine bisher unerkannte Spirochaeteninfektion (Spirochaetosis arthritica). *Dtsch Med Wochenschr* 1916;42:1535–1536.

Resnick D, Niwayama G. Rheumatoid arthritis and the seronegative spondyloarthropathies: radiographic and pathologic concepts. In: Resnick D, ed. *Diagnosis of bone and joint disorders*, 3rd ed. Philadelphia: WB Saunders; 1995:807–865.

Roderick MR, Ramanan AV. Chronic recurrent multifocal osteomyelitis. *Adv Exp Med Biol* 2013;764:99–107.

Rosendahl K. Juvenile idiopathic arthritis: recent advances. *Pediatr Radiol* 2011;41(suppl 1):110–112.

Rukavina I. SAPHO syndrome: a review. *J Child Orthop* 2015;9:19–27.

Sanders KM, Resnik CS, Owen DS. Erosive arthritis in Cronkhite-Canada syndrome. *Radiology* 1985;156:309–310.

Sankowski AJ, Lebkowska UM, Cwikła J, et al. Psoriatic arthritis. *Pol J Radiol* 2013; 78:1–17.

Schueller-Weidekamm C, Lodemann K-P, Grisar J, et al. Contrast-enhanced MR imaging of hand and finger joints in patients with early rheumatoid arthritis: do we really need a full dose of gadobenate dimeglumine for assessing synovial enhancement at 3T? *Radiology* 2013;268:161–169.

Schwenzer NF, Kötter I, Henes JC, et al. The role of dynamic contrast-enhanced MRI in the differential diagnosis of psoriatic and rheumatoid arthritis. *AJR Am J Roentgenol* 2010;194:715–720.

Sheybani EF, Khanna G, White AJ, et al. Imaging of juvenile idiopathic arthritis: a multimodality approach. *Radiographics* 2013;33:1253–1273.

Smith D, Braunstein EM, Brandt KD, et al. A radiographic comparison of erosive osteoarthritis and idiopathic nodal osteoarthritis. *Ann Rheum Dis* 2011;70:326–330.

Soldatos T, Pezeshk P, Ezzani F, et al. Cross-sectional imaging of adult crystal and inflammatory arthropathies. *Skeletal Radiol* 2016;45:1173–1191.

Stiskal MA, Neuhold A, Szolar DH, et al. Rheumatoid arthritis of the craniocervical region by MR imaging: detection and characterization. *AJR Am J Roentgenol* 1995;165:585–592.

Sudoł-Szopińska I, Grochowska E, Gietka P, et al. Imaging of juvenile idiopathic arthritis. Part II: ultrasonography and MRI. *J Ultrason* 2016;16:237–251.

Sudoł-Szopińska I, Jans L, Teh J. Rheumatoid arthritis: what do MRI and ultrasound show. *J Ultrason* 2017;17:5–16.

Sudoł-Szopińska I, Jurik AG, Eshed I, et al. Recommendations of the ESSR Arthritis Subcommittee for the use of magnetic resonance imaging in musculoskeletal rheumatic diseases. *Semin Musculoskeletal Radiol* 2015;19:396–411.

Sudoł-Szopińska I, Kwiatkowska B, Prochorec-Sobieszek M, et al. Enthesopathies and enthesitis. Part 2: imaging studies. *J Ultrason* 2015;15:196–207.

Sudoł-Szopińska I, Matuszewska G, Gietka P, et al. Imaging of juvenile idiopathic arthritis. Part I: clinical classifications and radiographs. *J Ultrason* 2016;16:225–236.

Sudoł-Szopińska I, Matuszewska G, Kwiatkowska B, et al. Diagnostic imaging of psoriatic arthritis. Part I: etiopathogenesis, classification and radiographic features. *J Ultrason* 2016;16:65–77.

Sudoł-Szopińska I, Pracoń G. Diagnostic imaging of psoriatic arthritis. Part II: magnetic resonance imaging and ultrasonography. *J Ultrason* 2016;16:163–174.

Swett HA, Jaffe RB, McIff EB. Popliteal cysts: presentation as thrombophlebitis. *Radiology* 1975;115:613–615.

Taurog JD, Chhabra A, Colbert RA. Ankylosing spondylitis and axial spondyloarthritis. *N Engl J Med* 2016;374:2563–2574.

Tehranzadeh J, Ashikyan O, Dascalos J. Magnetic resonance imaging in early detection of rheumatoid arthritis. *Semin Musculoskel Radiol* 2003;7:79–94.

Thompson W, Donn R. Juvenile idiopathic arthritis genetics—what's new? What's next? *Arthritis Res* 2002;4:302–306.

Turesson C, Matteson EL. Genetics of rheumatoid arthritis. *Mayo Clin Proc* 2006;81:94–101.

van der Kooij SM, Allaart CF, Dijkmans BA, et al. Innovative treatment strategies for patients with rheumatoid arthritis. *Curr Opin Rheumatol* 2008;20:287–294.

van der Woude D, Rantapää-Dahlqvist S, Ioan-Fascinay A, et al. Epitope spreading of the anti-citrullinated protein antibody response occurs before disease onset and is associated with the disease course of early arthritis. *Ann Rheum Dis* 2010;69:54–60.

Villeneuve E, Emery P. Rheumatoid arthritis: what has changed? *Skeletal Radiol* 2009;38:109–112.

Weber U, Østergaard M, Lambert RGW, et al. The impact of MRI on the clinical management of inflammatory arthritides. *Skeletal Radiol* 2011;40:1153–1173.

Whitehouse RW, Aslam R, Bukhari M, et al. The sesamoid index in psoriatic arthropathy. *Skeletal Radiol* 2005;34:217–220.

Wisnieski JJ, Askari AD. Rheumatoid nodulosis. A relatively benign rheumatoid variant. *Arch Intern Med* 1981;141:615–619.

Wright V. Seronegative polyarthritis: a unified concept. *Arthritis Rheum* 1978;21:619–633.

Zochling J, van der Heijde D, Burgos-Vargas R, et al. ASAS/EULAR recommendations for the management of ankylosing spondylitis. *Ann Rheum Dis* 2006;65:442–452.

15

Miscellaneous Arthritides and Arthropathies

Connective Tissue Arthropathies

An overview of the clinical and radiographic hallmarks of the forms of arthritides and arthropathies associated with connective tissue disorders is presented in Table 15.1.

Systemic Lupus Erythematosus

Systemic lupus erythematosus (SLE) is a chronic, inflammatory, connective tissue disorder of unknown cause characterized by significant immunologic abnormalities and involvement of multiple organs. Although the etiology of this disorder still remains unsettled, genetic, hormonal, and environmental influence play a role in disease pathogenesis. SLE is characterized by activation of polyclonal B cells to a variety of antigens and may be associated with hypergammaglobulinemia. Abnormalities of cytokines have been also reported including interleukin (IL)-1, IL-2, IL-6, and IL-10. There is increasing evidence that interferon α (IFN α) plays an important role in the pathogenesis of SLE. Various investigations have shown that plasmacytoid dendritic cells are responsible for release of IFN α factor stimulation with immune complexes containing nucleic acid. The risk of acquiring SLE is in part genetic, but it is a complex genetic disorder with no clear Mendelian pattern of inheritance, although it occurs in families.

The first described genetic link to SLE was the major histocompatibility complex (MHC) on chromosome 6, which contains the human leukocyte antigens (HLA)-DR. The other genes implicated included those that encode components of the complement pathway, Fcg receptors, protein tyrosine phosphatase nonreceptor type 22 (PTPN22), and cytotoxic T-lymphocyte–associated antigen 4 (CTLA4). Eight of the best-supported SLE susceptibility loci are 1q23, 1q25-31, 1q41-42, 2q35-37, 4p16-15.2, 6p11-21, 12p24, and 16q12. More recent investigations concluded that *PDCD1* (programmed cell death 1) gene is responsible for the linkage at chromosome 2q34 or 2q37 and is associated with lupus nephritis. Women, particularly adolescents and young adults, are affected 9 times as frequently as men, and this prevalence may be linked to *TLR7* gene. In men with Klinefelter syndrome (47, XXY), the risk of SLE is 14-fold higher than in healthy male controls. Smoking is a risk factor as well and has been associated with anti-dsDNA production. SLE is more common in blacks in the United States, but it is rare among blacks in Africa. Cumulative results have shown that hereditary deficiencies of complement component C4A (an MHC class III gene) confer risk for SLE in almost all ethnic group studied.

Clinical Features

The clinical manifestations of SLE vary according to the distribution and extent of systemic alterations. The most common symptoms are malaise, weakness, fever, anorexia, and weight loss. Women are affected 9 times as often as men. Consistent and characteristic features of this disease are serologic abnormalities, including a variety of serum autoantibodies to nuclear antigens, which have been historically associated with the presence of lupus erythematosus cells and neutrophilic leukocytes filled with cytoplasmic inclusion bodies.

Antinuclear antibodies (ANAs) are useful in the differential diagnosis of SLE, and changes in the titer of antibodies to DNA are useful in following disease activity. ANAs are a heterogeneous group of antibodies directed against a number of discrete nuclear macromolecular proteins. They represent what has classically been referred to as *autoantibodies* because they are directed against components normally present in all nucleated cells. They generally lack tissue or species specificity; therefore, they will cross-react with nuclei from different sources. The primary sources for study of these antibodies are patients with SLE and related systemic rheumatic diseases. Many studies have centered on defining the specificity of these antibodies and have contributed extensively to our understanding of their immunopathologic role in connective tissue disorders. It is worthwhile to state that 100% patients with SLE are ANA positive; the concept of ANA-negative lupus is no longer valid. Furthermore, autoantibodies against small nuclear ribonucleoprotein (snRNP), also known as *anti-Smith antibodies*, were found to be highly specific for SLE, although they are present in only 15% to 30% of SLE patients. They are present more frequently (about 60%) in young black women with SLE. The immunobiology of lupus is well-beyond the scope of this text, but we have to emphasize that despite exhaustive studies of tolerance and the existence of mouse model of lupus, there have not been any clinically significant advances in the specific treatment of SLE in nearly two decades.

Pathology

Pathology reveals widespread vasculitis affecting capillaries, arterioles, and venules. There is villous hypertrophy of the synovium covered by fibrin. In addition, a low-grade lymphoplasmacytic inflammatory cell infiltrate in the subintima may be encountered. The synovial fluid is characterized by an inflammatory pattern in which lymphocytes often predominate, and lupus erythematosus cells are commonly seen.

Imaging Features

The musculoskeletal system is a common site of involvement in SLE, and joint abnormalities, exhibited by 90% of patients during the course of the disease, represent a significant part of the clinical and radiologic picture. Arthritic involvement is symmetric, and articular deformities without fixed contractures are a hallmark of this disorder. The hands are the predominant site of involvement. Typically, the conventional radiography discloses malalignments, most commonly at the metacarpophalangeal and proximal interphalangeal joints of the fingers and the first carpometacarpal, metacarpophalangeal, and the interphalangeal joints of the thumb (Fig. 15.1).

TABLE 15.1 Clinical and Imaging Hallmarks of Connective Tissue Arthritides and Arthropathies

Type of Arthritis	Site	Crucial Abnormalities	Technique/Projection
Systemic lupus erythematosus (SLE) (F > M; young adults; blacks > whites; skin changes: rash)	Hands	Flexible joint contractures	Lateral view
	Hips, ankles, shoulders	Osteonecrosis	Standard views of affected joints Scintigraphy Magnetic resonance imaging (MRI)
Scleroderma (F > M; skin changes: edema, thickening)	Hands	Soft-tissue calcifications Acroosteolysis Tapering of distal phalanges Interphalangeal destructive changes	Dorsovolar and lateral views
	Gastrointestinal tract	Dilatation of esophagus	Esophagram
		Decreased peristalsis	Esophagram (cine or video study)
		Dilatation of duodenum and small bowel	Upper gastrointestinal and small bowel series
		Pseudodiverticulosis of colon	Barium enema
Polymyositis/dermatomyositis	Upper and lower extremities (proximal parts)	Soft-tissue calcifications Periarticular osteoporosis	Xeroradiography; digital radiography
	Hands	Erosions and destructive changes in distal interphalangeal articulations	Dorsovolar and lateral views
Mixed connective tissue disease (MCTD) (overlap of clinical features of SLE, scleroderma, dermatomyositis, and rheumatoid arthritis)	Hands, wrists	Erosions and destructive changes in proximal interphalangeal, metacarpophalangeal, radiocarpal, and midcarpal articulations, associated with joint space narrowing	Dorsovolar and lateral views
		Symmetric soft-tissue swelling	MRI
		Soft-tissue atrophy and calcifications	Posteroanterior and lateral views
	Chest	Pleural and pericardial effusions	Ultrasound

F, female; M, male.

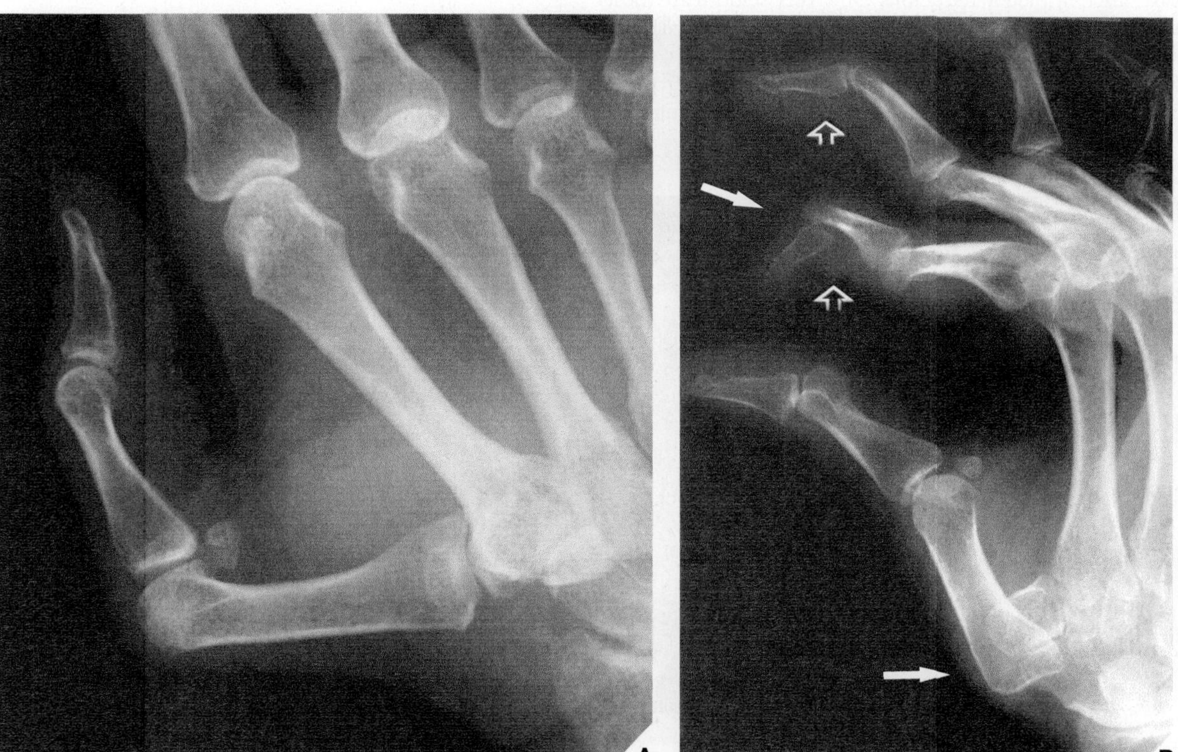

FIGURE 15.1 Systemic lupus erythematosus. (A) Typical appearance of the thumb in a 43-year-old woman with SLE. Note subluxations in the first carpometacarpal and metacarpophalangeal joints without articular erosions. **(B)** In another patient, a 32-year-old woman, the oblique radiograph of her left hand shows dislocations at the first carpometacarpal joint and distal interphalangeal joint of the index finger *(arrows)*, and subluxations in the metacarpophalangeal joints of the index and middle fingers associated with swan-neck deformities *(open arrows)*.

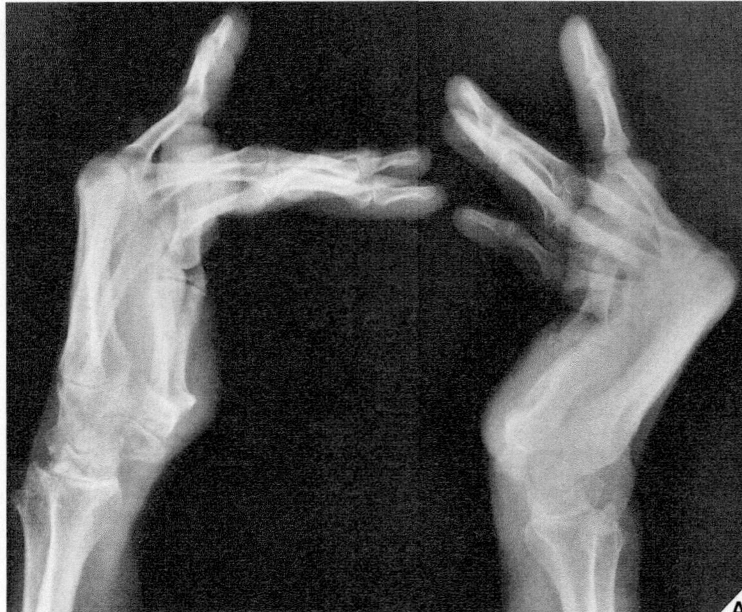

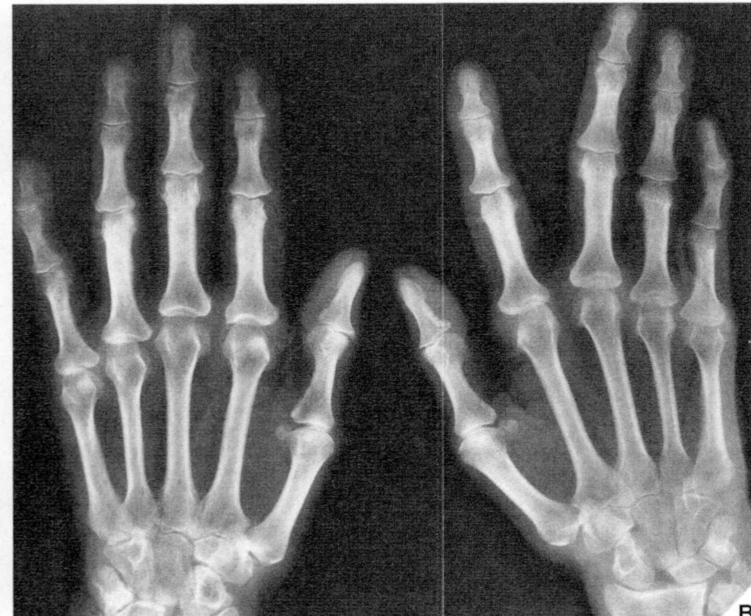

FIGURE 15.2 Systemic lupus erythematosus. **(A)** Lateral radiograph of both hands of a 42-year-old woman with documented SLE for the past 4 years demonstrates flexion deformities in the metacarpophalangeal joints. On the dorsovolar projection **(B)**, the flexion deformities have been corrected by the pressure of the hands against the radiographic cassette.

These abnormalities may not be apparent on a dorsovolar radiograph because the malalignments are flexible and are corrected by the pressure of the hand against the radiographic cassette (Fig. 15.2). These pathognomonic deformities usually occur secondary to a loss of support from the ligamentous and capsular structures about the joint and, at least in the early stage of disease, are completely reducible. Only very seldom are these abnormalities fixed and/or accompanied by articular erosions (Fig. 15.3).

Some patients present with sclerosis of the distal phalanges (acral sclerosis) (Fig. 15.4) or with resorption of the terminal tufts (acroosteolysis). Osteonecrosis, which is frequently seen, has been attributed to complications of treatment with corticosteroids (Fig. 15.5A–D). However, current investigations suggest the vital role of the inflammatory process (vasculitis) in the development of this complication. Nonspecific joint effusions with synovial proliferation may be seen on magnetic resonance imaging (MRI) (Fig. 15.5E).

Treatment

The treatment of SLE consists of using antimalarial drugs (such as hydroxychloroquine), corticosteroids (such as prednisone), and especially immunosuppressants (such as cyclophosphamide, azathioprine, mycophenolate,

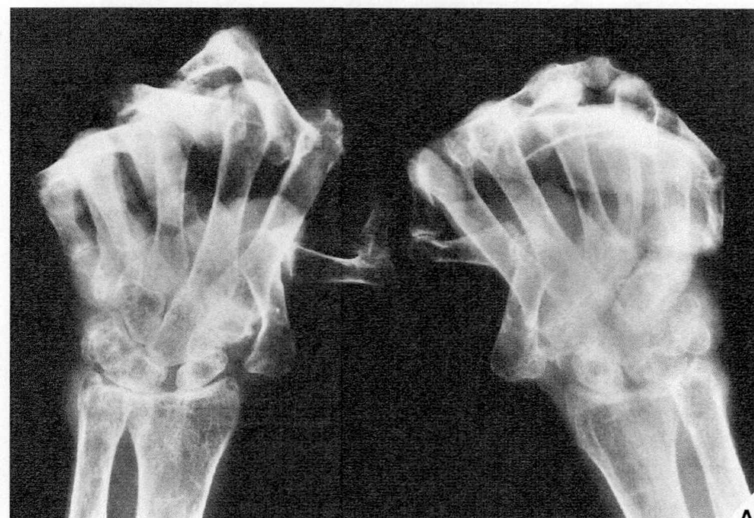

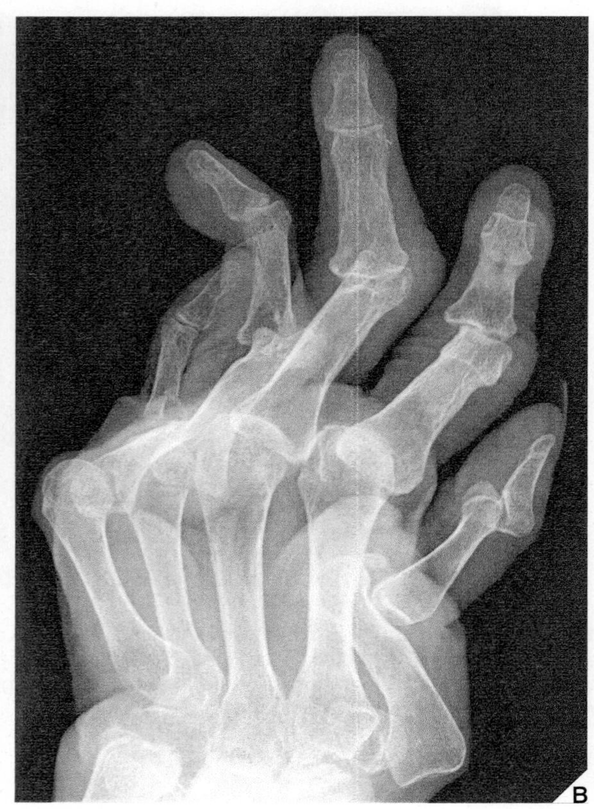

FIGURE 15.3 Systemic lupus erythematosus. **(A)** A 62-year-old woman presented with a 15-year history of SLE. Dorsovolar radiograph of both hands shows severe deformities, subluxations, and articular erosions. Note the advanced osteoporosis secondary to disuse of the extremities and treatment with corticosteroids. **(B)** In another patient, a 51-year-old woman, note flexion contractions, subluxations, and dislocations in the several joints of the right hand.

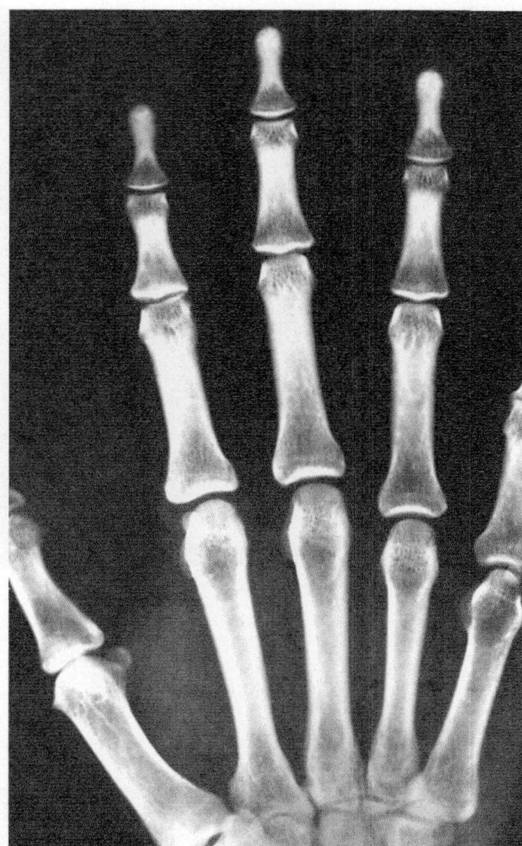

FIGURE 15.4 **Systemic lupus erythematosus.** Dorsovolar radiograph of the hand of a 29-year-old woman with SLE demonstrates sclerosis of the distal phalanges (acral sclerosis). Similar sclerotic changes are also occasionally seen in rheumatoid arthritis and scleroderma.

and methotrexate). Rituximab, a humanized monoclonal antibody against B cells, plasmapheresis, and intravenous administration of immunoglobulin (IVIG) are also used under special circumstances. The details of the therapy, which is frequently individualized, are beyond the scope of this chapter; however, it is worthwhile to mention that SLE may become one of the first rheumatic diseases with a personalized therapeutic approach.

Scleroderma

Clinical Features

Scleroderma (progressive systemic sclerosis) is a generalized disorder of unknown cause. It is seen predominantly in young women, usually becoming apparent in their third and fourth decades. Primarily, a connective tissue disorder characterized by deposition of collagen and other components of extracellular matrix in the skin and internal organs, it is distinguished by thickening and fibrosis of the skin and subcutaneous tissues, with frequent involvement of the musculoskeletal system. Scleroderma has an autoimmune basis with disease-specific ANAs, most commonly antitopoisomerase-1 and anticentromere. Recently, researchers have identified a new genetic link to systemic form of scleroderma, a susceptibility locus involving the genome *CD247* (that encodes the T-cell receptor zeta subunit modulating T-cell activation), in addition to previously known genes *MHC*, *IRF5*, and *STAT4* (that encodes a regulatory protein important to immune system). Clinically, many patients develop joint involvement, which is manifesting as arthralgia and arthritis leading to flexion contractions of the fingers. Most patients have the so-called *CREST syndrome*, which refers to the coexistence of **c**alcinosis, **R**aynaud phenomenon (episodes of intermittent pallor of the fingers and toes on exposure to cold, secondary to vasoconstriction of the small blood vessels), **e**sophageal abnormalities (dilatation and hypoperistalsis), **s**clerodactyly, and **t**elangiectasia; 30% to 40% of patients have a positive serologic test for rheumatoid factor and a positive ANA test.

Pathology

Pathology shows symmetrical intimal thickening of affected arteries associated with endothelial necrosis and telangiectasia of capillaries. In the dermis, there is excessive deposition of fibrous tissue.

Imaging Features

Radiographically, scleroderma presents with characteristic abnormalities of the bone and soft tissues. The hands usually exhibit atrophy of the soft tissues at the tips of the fingers (Fig. 15.6), resorption of the distal phalanges (acroosteolysis), osteopenia, subcutaneous and periarticular calcifications (Figs. 15.7 and 15.8A), and destructive changes of the small articulations, usually the interphalangeal joints (Fig. 15.9). Soft-tissue calcifications within the upper limbs can occasionally be quite prominent (see Fig. 15.8B). Corroborative findings are seen in the gastrointestinal tract, where dilatation of the esophagus and small bowel, together with a pseudoobstruction pattern, is characteristic (Fig. 15.10). Pseudodiverticula in the colon are also commonly seen.

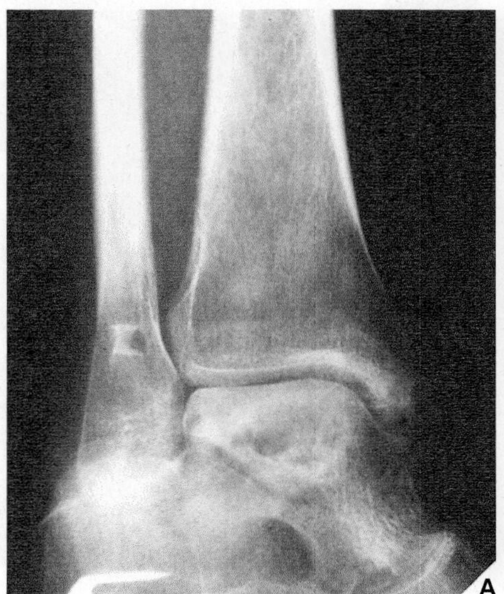

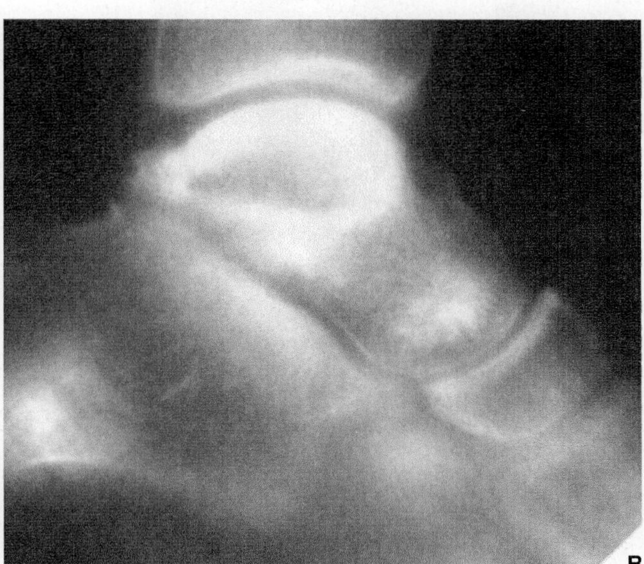

FIGURE 15.5 **SLE complicated by osteonecrosis and synovial proliferation.** **(A)** Oblique radiograph and **(B)** lateral tomogram of the ankle demonstrate osteonecrosis of the talus in a 26-year-old woman with lupus who was treated with massive doses of steroids. *(Continued)*

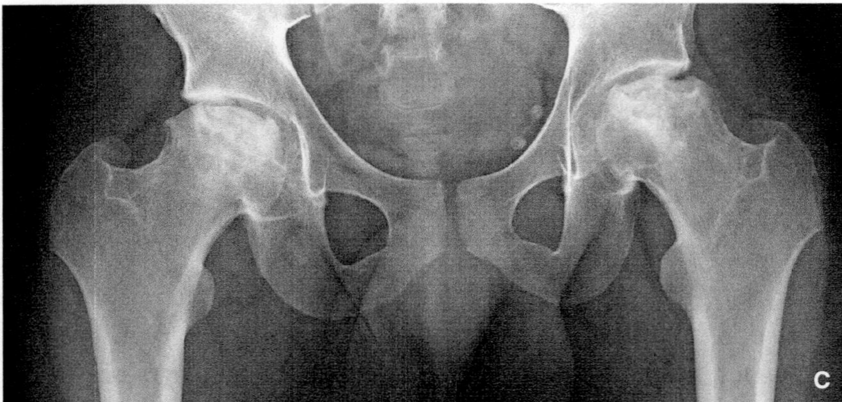

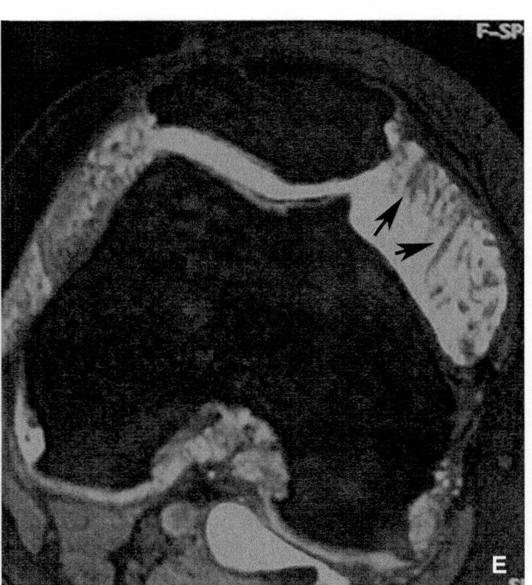

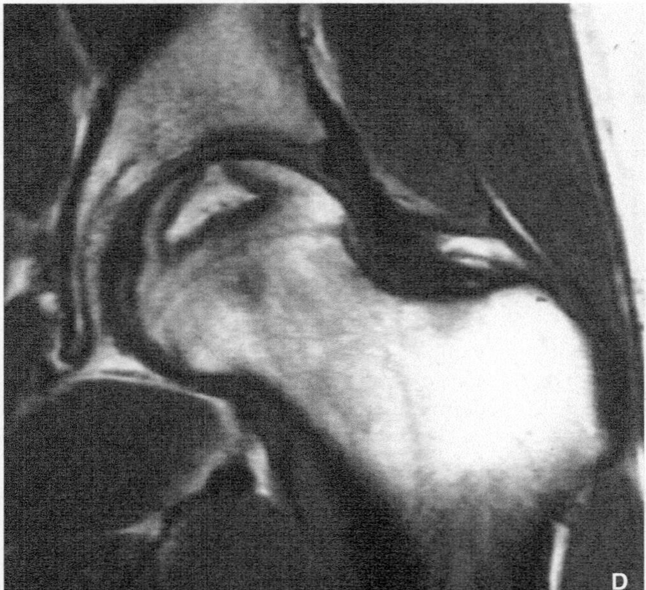

FIGURE 15.5 SLE complicated by osteonecrosis and synovial proliferation. *(Continued)* **(C)** Anteroposterior radiograph of the pelvis of a 27-year-old man treated with corticosteroids shows advanced osteonecrosis of both femoral heads. **(D)** Coronal T2-weighted MRI in an 18-year-old woman with SLE demonstrates a focal area of osteonecrosis of the femoral head. **(E)** Axial gradient recalled echo (GRE) MR image of the knee of a 35-year-old woman shows large joint effusion with frond-like synovial proliferation *(arrows)*.

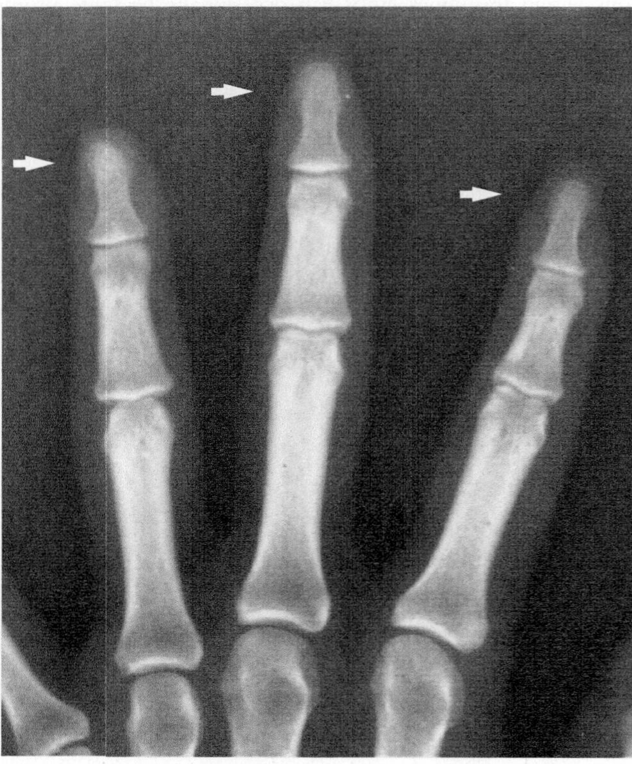

FIGURE 15.6 Scleroderma. A 24-year-old woman presented with atrophy of the soft tissues at the distal phalanges of the index, middle, and ring fingers *(arrows)*.

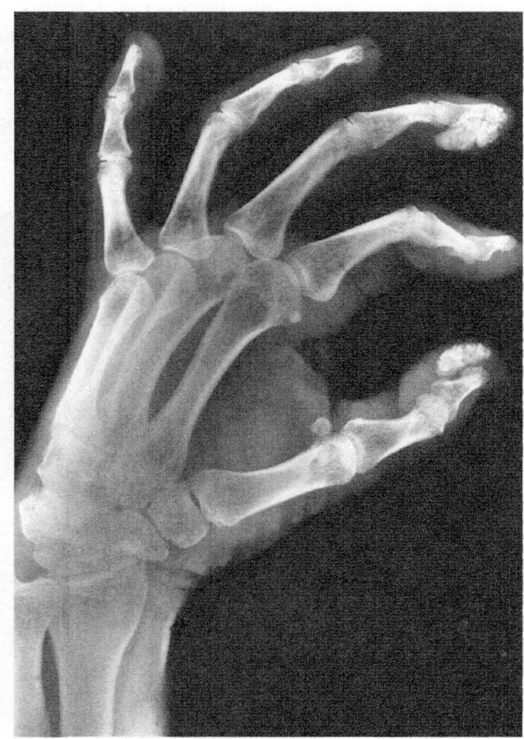

FIGURE 15.7 Scleroderma. A 32-year-old woman with progressive systemic sclerosis exhibits soft-tissue calcifications in the distal phalanges of the right hand *(arrows)*, a typical feature of this disorder.

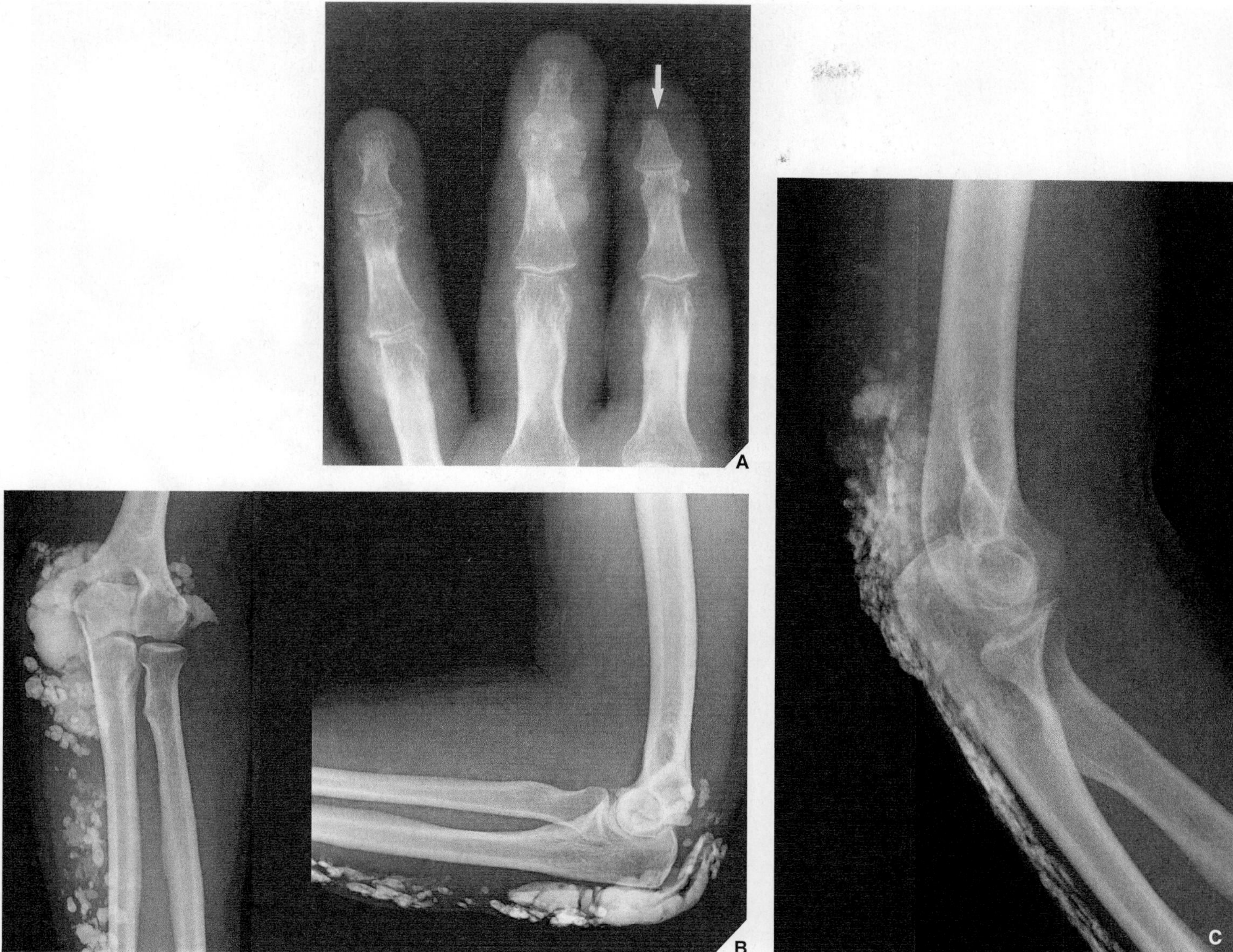

FIGURE 15.8 Scleroderma. **(A)** Dorsovolar radiograph of the fingers of a 44-year-old woman reveals acroosteolysis *(arrow)*, soft-tissue calcifications, and destructive changes of the distal interphalangeal joint of the middle finger. **(B)** In another patient, a 46-year-old woman, extensive soft-tissue calcifications are present around the elbow and the forearm. **(C)** Calcifications are present in the soft tissues of the posterior aspect of the distal arm and proximal forearm in this 37-year-old woman.

Treatment

The treatment of scleroderma is elusive and there are no specific guidelines. Therapy includes the use of antiinflammatory drugs such as nonsteroidal antiinflammatory drugs (NSAIDs), corticosteroids such as prednisone, immunosuppressive therapy, that is, cyclophosphamide, antiinterferon agents such as sifalimumab, anti–B-cell agents such as rituximab, and anticytokine therapy (anti-IL6R). Recent trials using autologous bone marrow transplantation yielded promising results but are not practical for most patients. Patients with pulmonary hypertension, a complication of scleroderma, are treated with prostaglandin inhibitors to reduce wedge pressure.

Polymyositis and Dermatomyositis

Clinical Features

Polymyositis and dermatomyositis belong to the rare heterogeneous group of autoimmune myopathies. They represent disorders of striated muscle and skin and are characterized by diffuse, nonsuppurative inflammation as well as degeneration. In adults, they can occur at any age, but the peak is seen between 45 and 60 years of age. Most patients have both skin and muscle involvement. Early diagnosis and subsequent management of patients with any type of myopathy, including polymyositis and dermatomyositis, can be facilitated by the use of appropriate laboratory tests. The four tests most helpful in evaluating muscle disorders include (a) serum enzymes, (b) urinary creatine and creatinine excretion, (c) electromyogram, and (d) muscle biopsy.

Different serum enzyme determinations have been advocated, but the most valuable tests include serum creatine phosphokinase (CPK), serum aldolase (ALD), serum lactate dehydrogenase (LDH), serum glutamic oxalacetic transaminase (SGOT), and serum glutamic pyruvic transaminase (SGPT). Furthermore, the determination of serum enzyme levels and urinary creatine excretion is helpful for the clinical management of polymyositis and dermatomyositis because the two tests provide a broader perspective than either test alone.

Polymyositis is characterized by a cytotoxic T-cell response targeting as yet unidentified muscle antigens presented by MHC class I molecules and can occur in isolation or more often as a part of multisystem overlap syndrome. Over the past decade, myositis-specific autoantibodies (MSAs) have been better characterized, including those directed against the aminoacyl-tRNA synthetase enzymes, the signal-recognition particle and the Mi-2 protein. In addition, clinically significant novel autoantibodies—anti-CADM-140, anti-SAE (small ubiquitin-like modifier activating enzyme), anti-p155/140, and anti-p140, have been described. MSAs are

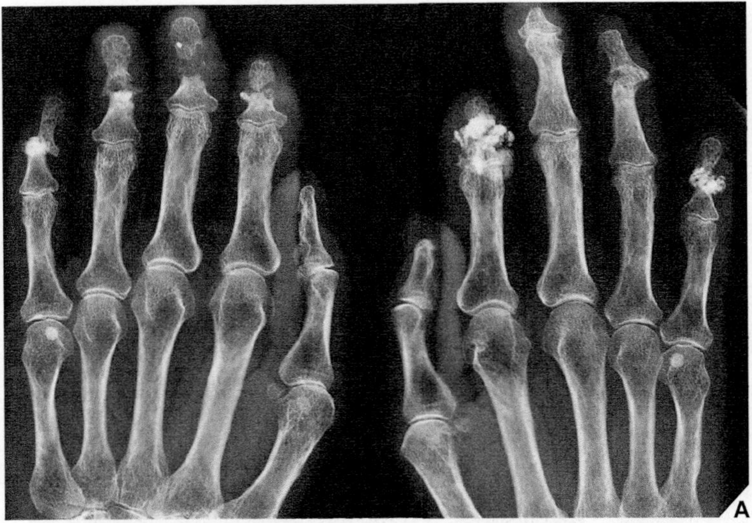

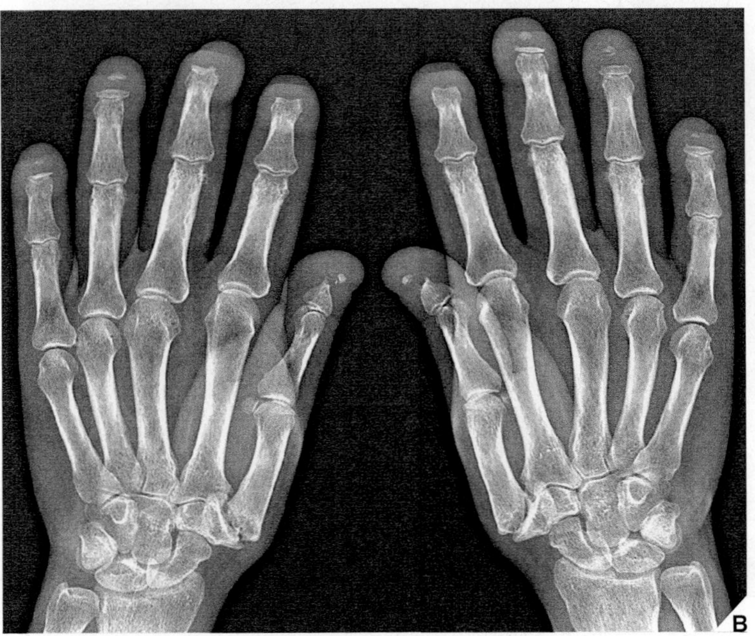

FIGURE 15.9 Scleroderma. **(A)** Dorsovolar radiograph of the hands of a 50-year-old man with documented systemic sclerosis shows destructive changes in the distal interphalangeal joints as well as soft-tissue calcifications and resorption of the tip of the distal phalanx of the left middle finger. **(B)** Dorsovolar radiograph of the hands of a 53-year-old woman with long-standing systemic sclerosis shows acroosteolysis of all distal phalanges. Note also erosions of the first carpometacarpal joints.

directed against cytoplasmic or nuclear components involved in key regulatory intracellular processes including protein synthesis, translocations, and gene transcriptions. A number of different autoantibodies are found exclusively in dermatomyositis. Antibodies directed against the chromatin-remodeling enzyme Mi-2 are found in about 20% of patients. The anti-MDA5 antibodies have been reported in patients with amyopathic dermatomyositis, particularly in those with interstitial lung disease. In some patients, anti–small ubiquitin-like modifier 1 (anti–SUMO-1) antibodies have been identified. ANAs were found in about 50% of patients with polymyositis and dermatomyositis and were found to be associated with the presence of antibodies directed against a nuclear protein Mi-2. A positive biopsy may not only demonstrate that the disease process is myopathic, thus enabling the physician to rule out a neurogenic lower motor neuron lesion but may also identify those patients whose muscle disease is more severe pathologically than was suspected on clinical grounds. This is important with respect to prognosis. With the aid of histochemical and electron microscopic techniques, muscle biopsy will occasionally enable the pathologist to diagnose one of the rare forms of myopathy that can clinically mimic polymyositis. Such diseases include sarcoid myopathy, central core disease, and muscle diseases associated with abnormal mitochondria.

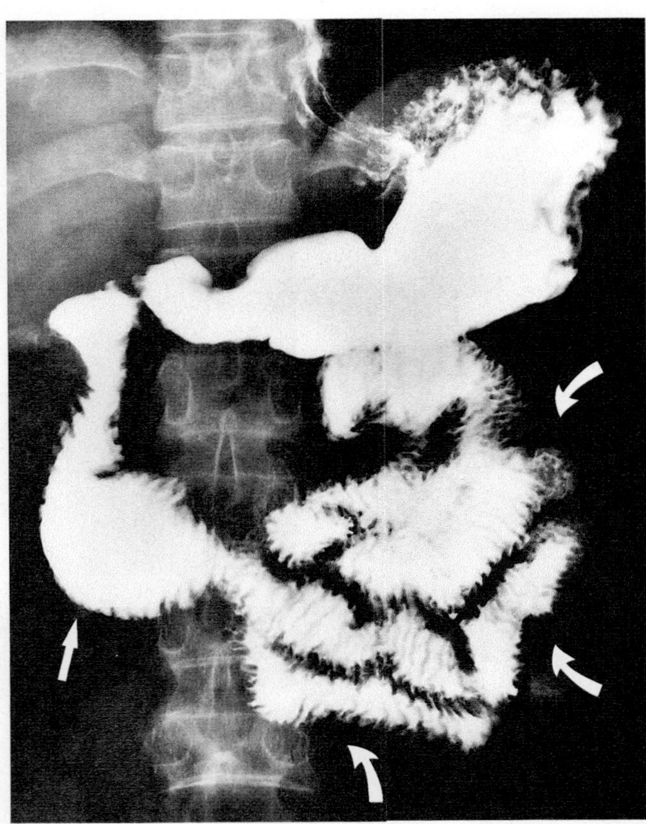

FIGURE 15.10 Scleroderma. Upper gastrointestinal series and small bowel study in the patient shown in Figure 15.9A demonstrate dilatation of the second and third portions of the duodenum *(straight arrow)* and jejunum *(curved arrows)*, with a pseudoobstruction pattern.

Clinical symptoms consist of symmetric muscle weakness, especially in the proximal parts of the extremities. Additional symptoms include arthralgias, myalgias, and severe fatigue; Raynaud phenomenon may also be encountered. Dyspnea may reflect diaphragmatic weakness. Patients with dermatomyositis may present with cutaneous manifestations, including Gottron papules (raised violaceous lesions on the extensor surfaces of the elbows, knees, and the hands—particularly at the site of metacarpophalangeal and interphalangeal joints), and heliotrope rash (red or purple discoloration of the eyelids). Less common, erythematous or poikilodermatous rash across the posterior neck and shoulders (the shawl sign), and on the anterior neck and chest (the V-sign) may be observed. Some patients exhibit hyperkeratotic skin thickening, often associated with painful cracking either on the radial surfaces of the fingers (so-called *mechanic's hands*) or toes (*mechanic's feet*). Periungual telangiectasias and nailfold capillary changes identical to those seen in scleroderma also have been reported.

Pathology

The pathologic changes found on muscle biopsy in polymyositis have been well described. The degree of pathologic change may vary widely; one patient may show only negligible pathologic changes in muscle fibers on biopsy results, whereas another patient presenting similar clinical features may show extensive necrosis and fiber replacement. This variability in histologic findings is probably responsible for the frequent normal muscle biopsy results from patients with otherwise classic polymyositis. The overall rate of positive findings from muscle biopsy in several studies of polymyositis was in the range of 55% to 80%. The most common finding is lymphocytic infiltration. Areas of myonecrosis may be encountered.

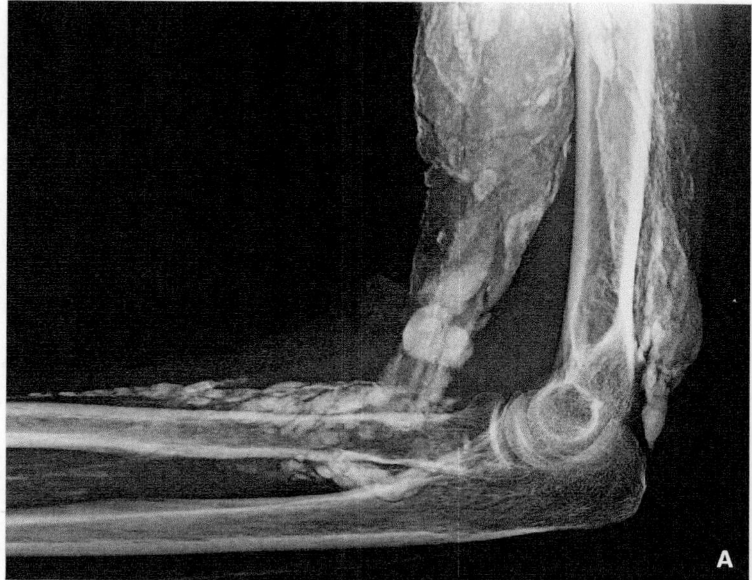

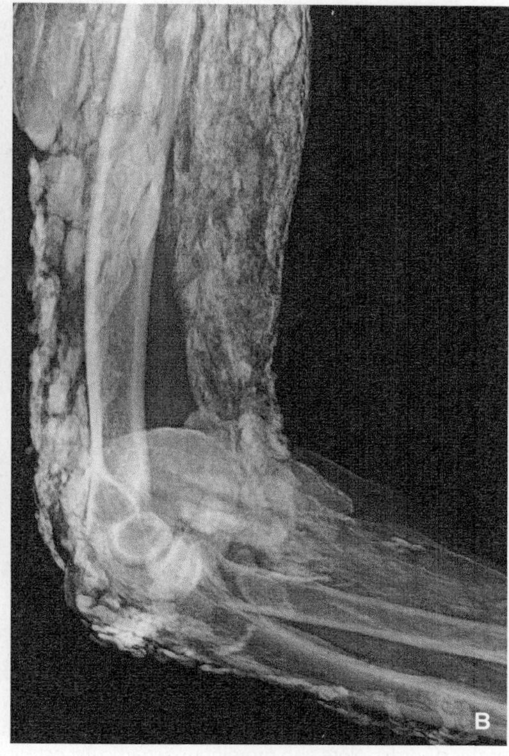

FIGURE 15.11 Dermatomyositis. Lateral radiographs of the **(A)** left and **(B)** right elbow of a 50-year-old woman show extensive calcifications of the muscles of the arm and forearm.

Imaging Features

Imaging abnormalities in polymyositis and dermatomyositis are divided into two types: those involving soft tissues and those involving joints. The most characteristic soft-tissue abnormality in both conditions is soft-tissue calcifications. The favorite sites of intermuscular calcification are the large muscles in the proximal parts of upper and lower extremities (Figs. 15.11 and 15.12). In addition, subcutaneous calcifications similar to those of scleroderma are seen (Figs. 15.12B, 15.13, and 15.14). MRI offers the best evaluation of abnormalities of the soft tissues including muscles. Muscle edema is an indicator of active inflammation (Figs. 15.15 and 15.16), and fatty infiltration is an indicator of chronic process (Fig. 15.17). MRI is also effective modality to determine the site for muscle biopsy. It is also important technique in monitoring the disease progression and response to therapy.

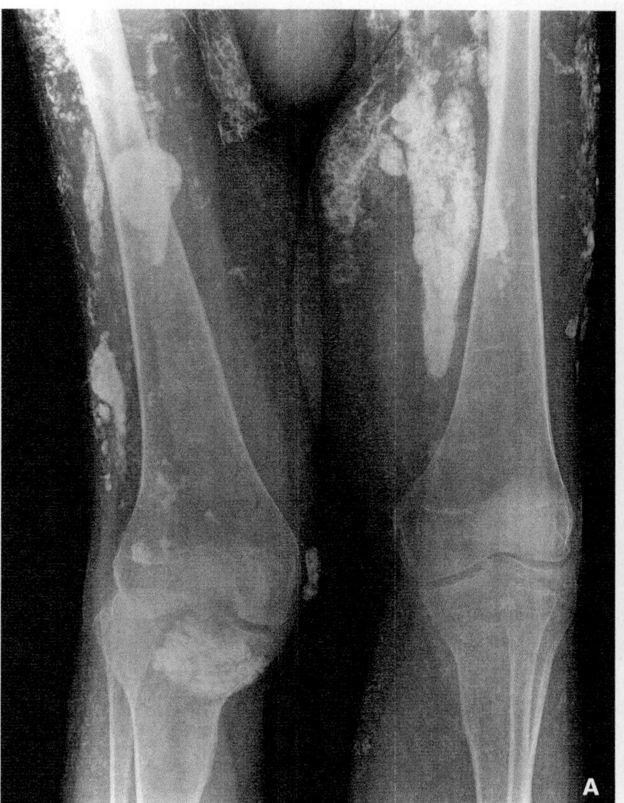

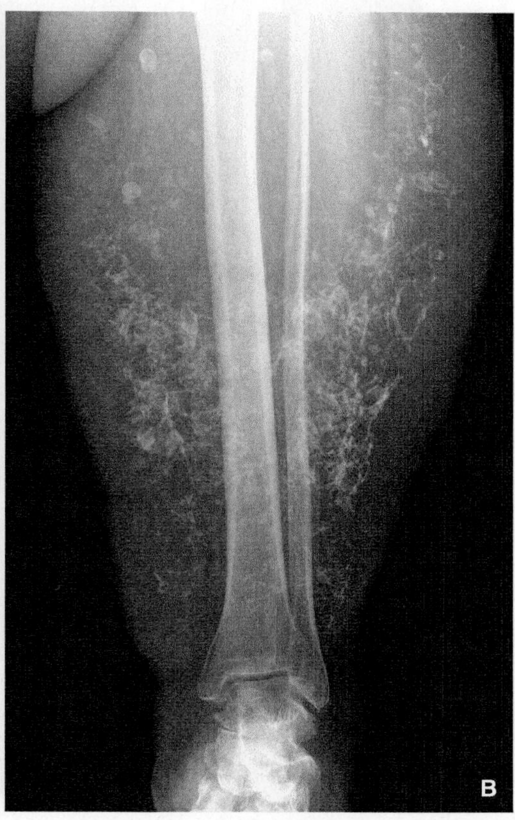

FIGURE 15.12 Dermatomyositis. **(A)** Anteroposterior radiograph of both knees shows extensive calcifications within the muscles. Observe also subcutaneous calcifications. The bones are markedly osteoporotic. **(B)** Anteroposterior radiograph of the left leg of a 66-year-old woman shows subcutaneous and muscle calcifications.

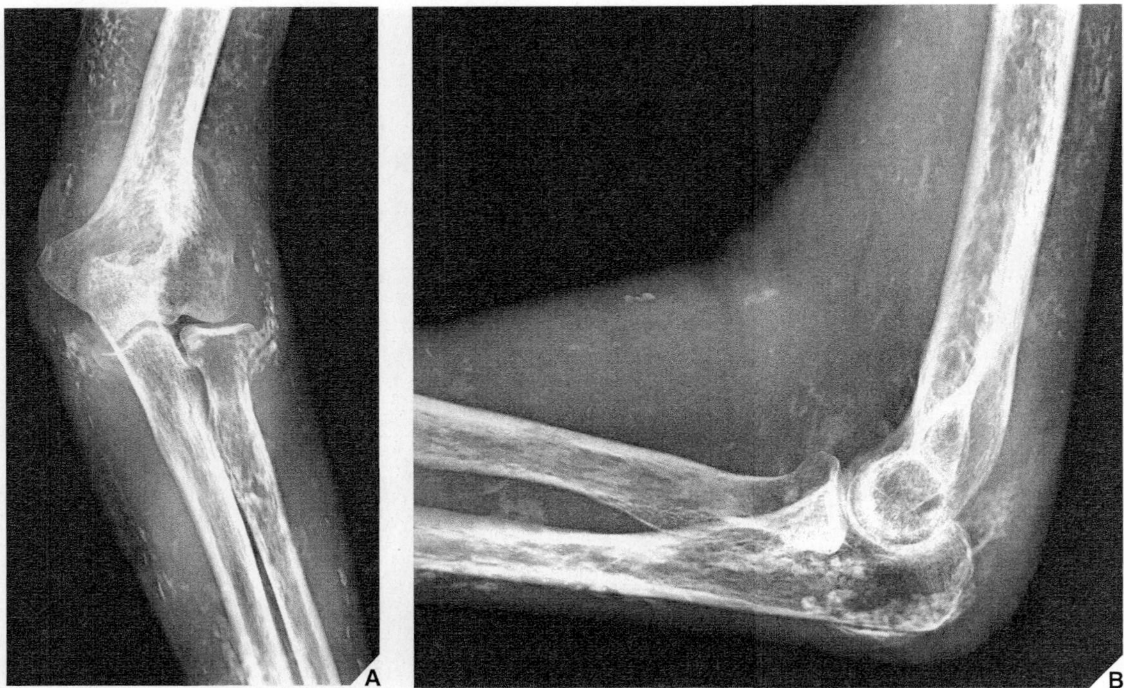

FIGURE 15.13 Dermatomyositis. **(A)** External oblique and **(B)** lateral radiographs of the left elbow of a 64-year-old woman show extensive soft-tissue calcifications, characteristic for this disorder. Note also prominent periarticular osteoporosis.

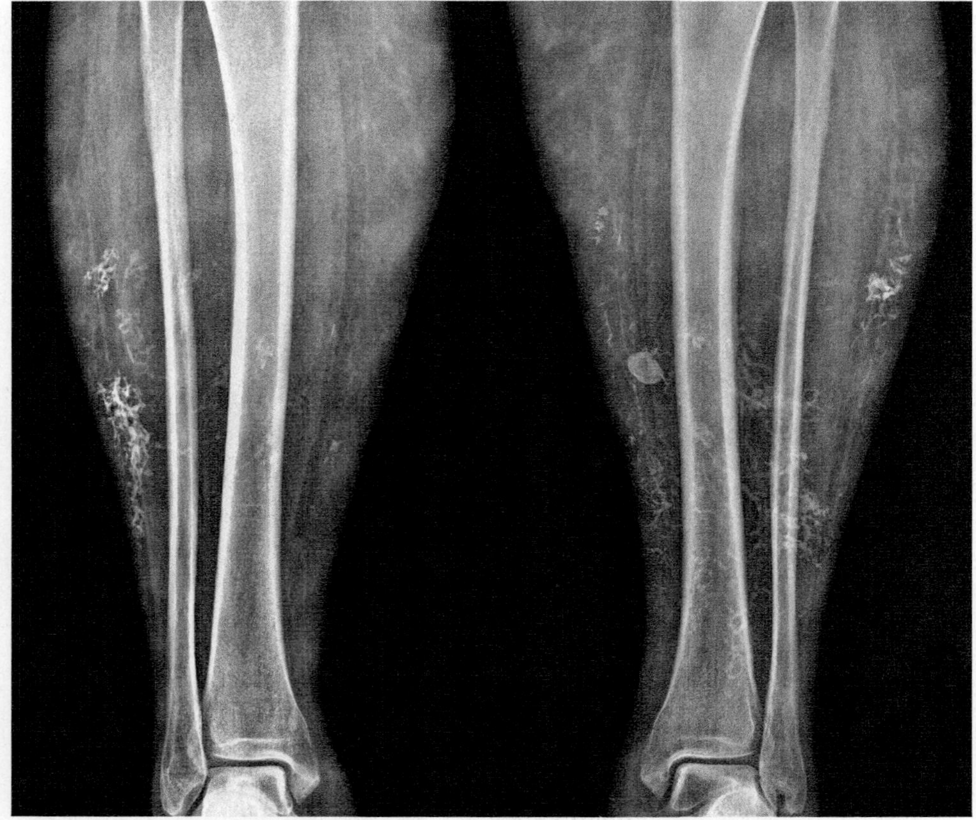

FIGURE 15.14 Dermatomyositis. Anteroposterior radiograph of both legs of a 55-year-old woman shows predominantly cutaneous and subcutaneous calcifications.

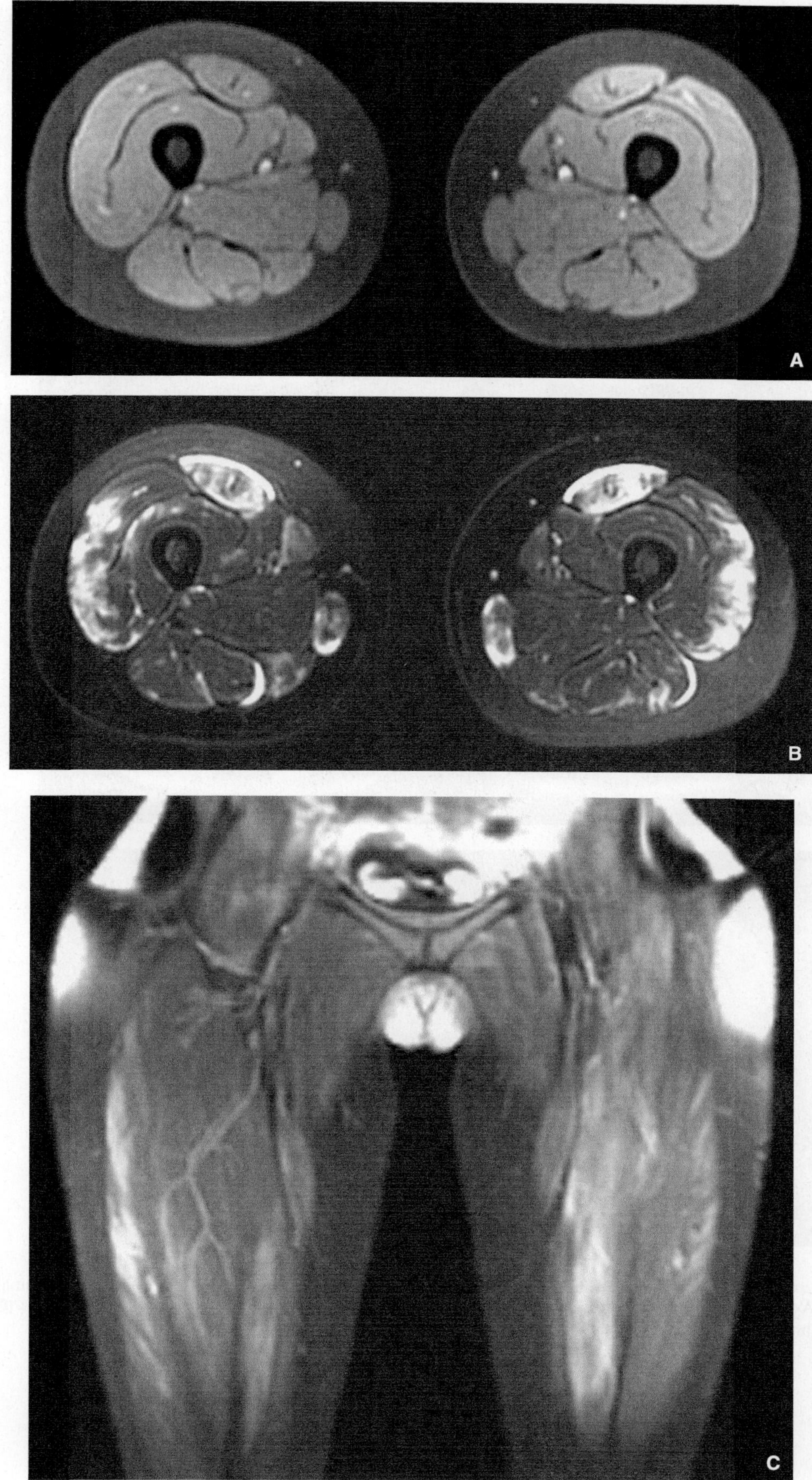

FIGURE 15.15 MRI of polymyositis. **(A)** Axial T1-weighted and **(B)** axial and **(C)** coronal T1-weighted fat-suppressed MR images obtained after intravenous administration of gadolinium, show enhancement of several group of muscles of the thighs of a 23-year-old woman, including abductors, rectus femoris, vastus lateralis, vastus intermedius, sartorius, gracilis, semimembranosus, and semitendinosus.

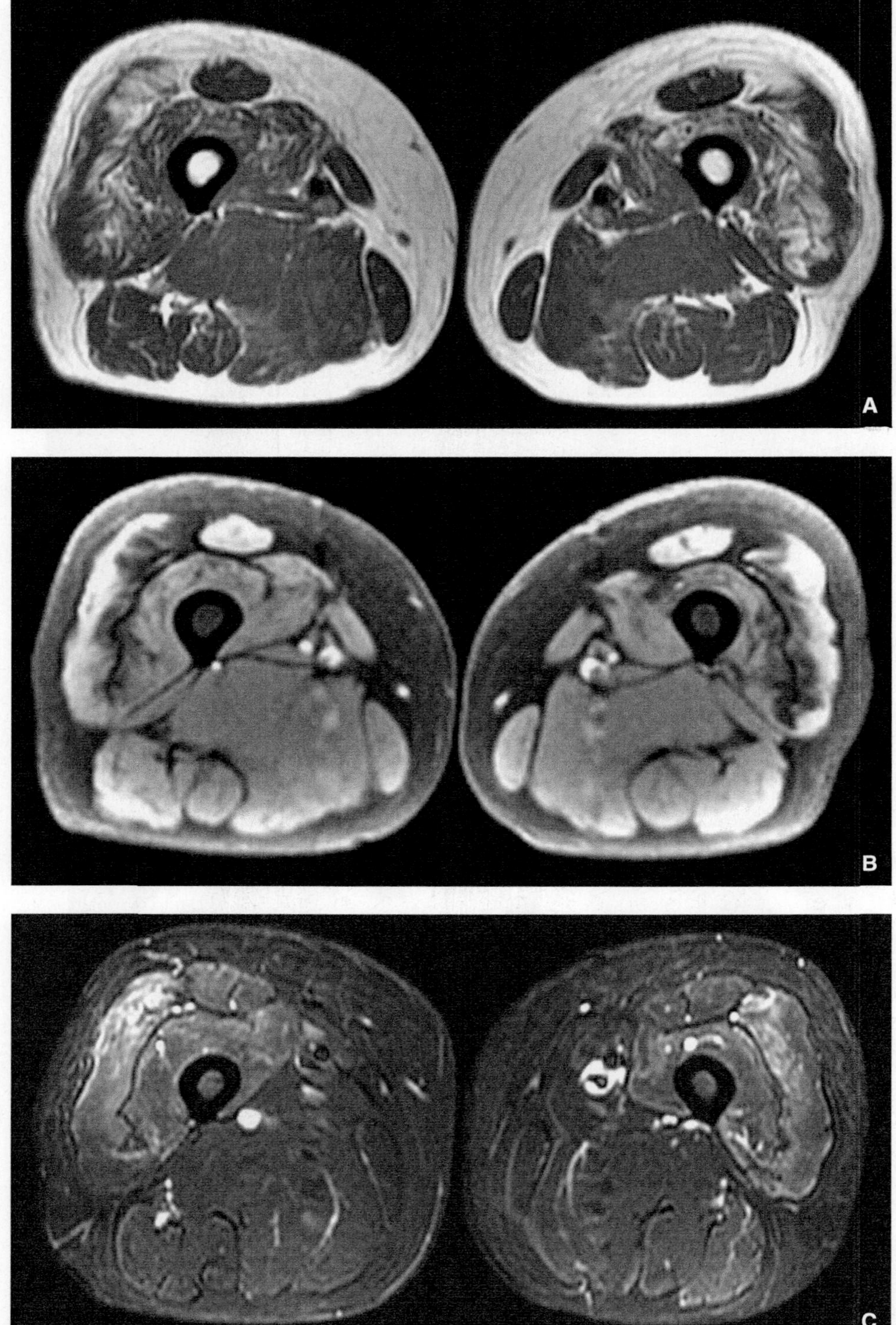

FIGURE 15.16 MRI of polymyositis. **(A)** Axial T1-weighted MR image of both thighs of a 65-year-old woman shows fatty atrophy predominantly affecting vastus lateralis and rectus femoris muscles. **(B)** Axial T1-weighted fat-suppressed image shows areas of high signal intensities within the muscle structures. **(C)** Axial short time inversion recovery (STIR) image shows high signal within the vastus lateralis muscles representing edema. *(Continued)*

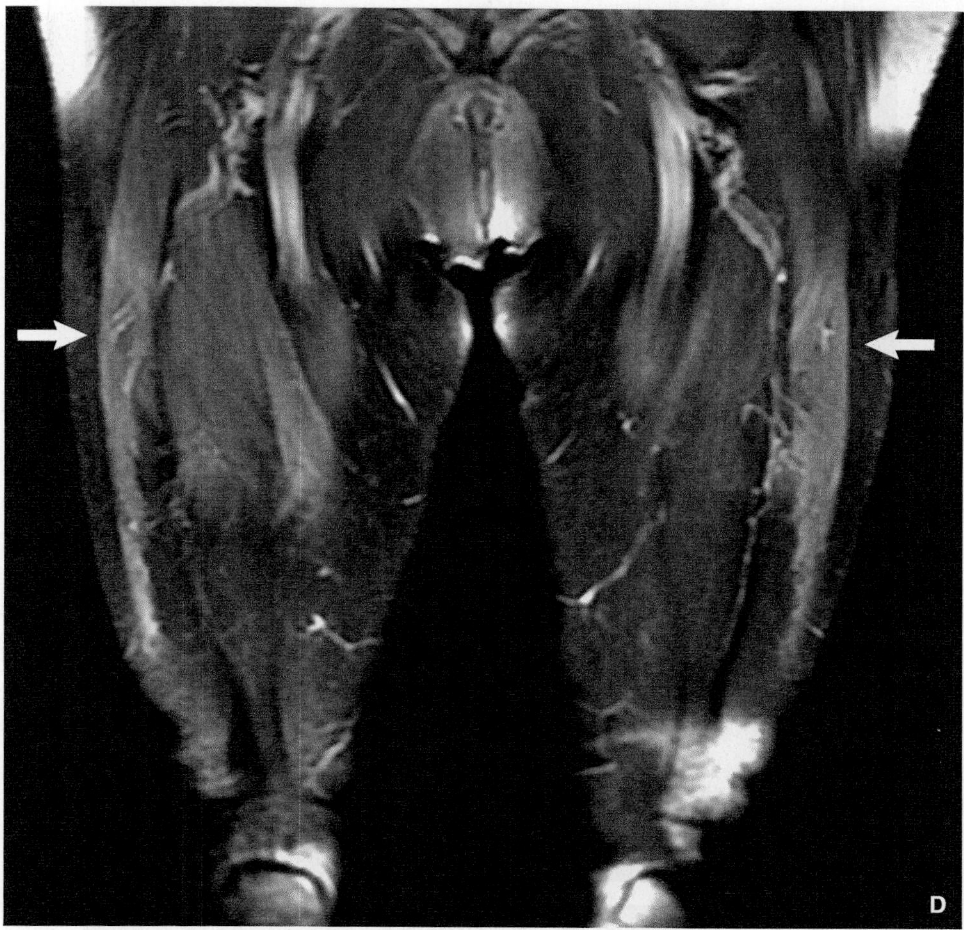

FIGURE 15.16 MRI of polymyositis. ***(Continued)*** **(D)** Coronal T1-weighted fat-suppressed image obtained after intravenous administration of gadolinium shows subtle symmetrical enhancement of vastus lateralis *(arrows)*.

Articular abnormalities are rare. The most frequently reported, however, is periarticular osteoporosis. Destructive joint changes have been reported only occasionally and primarily in the distal interphalangeal articulations of the hands.

Treatment

The therapy is directed to control inflammation through corticosteroids drugs. Immunosuppressive agents, including methotrexate, azathioprine, cyclophosphamide, cyclosporine A, and chlorambucil, may be used for patients who do not respond to corticosteroids. Rituximab and mycophenolate mofetil have shown some benefit in patients who have been resistant to other therapies. Combination therapy such as azathioprine plus methotrexate and methotrexate plus cyclosporine A also have been tried. Intravenous administration of gamma globulins has been tried with mixed results.

Mixed Connective Tissue Disease

Mixed connective tissue disease (MCTD) was first reported as a distinctive syndrome by Sharp and associates in 1972. This syndrome is characterized by clinical abnormalities that combine the features of SLE, scleroderma, dermatomyositis, and rheumatoid arthritis. The one feature that distinguishes MCTD as a separate entity is a positive serologic test for antibody to the ribonucleoprotein (RNP) component of extractable nuclear antigen (ENA). Furthermore, anti-RNP antibodies, particularly those directed against ribonuclear protein U1-RNP were found to be associated with MCTD. Detection of anti-RNP antibodies, in the absence of other antibodies, strongly suggests the diagnosis of MCTD.

The typical clinical pattern consists of Raynaud phenomenon, polyarthralgia, swelling of the hands, esophageal hypomotility, inflammatory myopathy, and pulmonary disease. Women constitute approximately 80% of affected patients. Patients with MCTD have prominent joint abnormalities, with typical involvement of the small articulations of the hand, wrist, and foot; large joints such as the knee, elbow, and shoulder may also be affected. The joint deformities mimic those seen in rheumatoid arthritis, but occasionally, joint subluxation may be nonerosive, as in SLE. Soft-tissue abnormalities are identical to those encountered in scleroderma (Figs. 15.18 to 15.20).

Vasculitis

There is a diverse clinical spectrum of the vasculitides that includes systemic necrotizing vasculitis, hypersensitivity vasculitis, Wegener granulomatosis, lymphomatoid granulomatosis, giant cell arteritis (Takayasu arteritis), and a variety of miscellaneous syndromes (e.g., Kawasaki disease, Behçet disease, Churg-Strauss syndrome, and others). A discussion of these diverse but often overlapping diseases is far beyond the scope of this volume, but the reader is referred to several key references at the end of this chapter. The demonstration of vasculitis by angiograms can often be documented by the presence of aneurysmal dilatation in affected vessels. Generally, an angiogram is performed when the diagnosis cannot be established by tissue biopsy. Most recently, more advanced imaging modalities are applied for diagnosis of the earlier-referenced condition, including CT-angiography (Figs. 15.21 and 15.22), magnetic resonance angiography (Fig. 15.23), and 18F-fluorodeoxyglucose (^{18}F-FDG) positron emission tomography (PET) and PET/CT (Fig. 15.24).

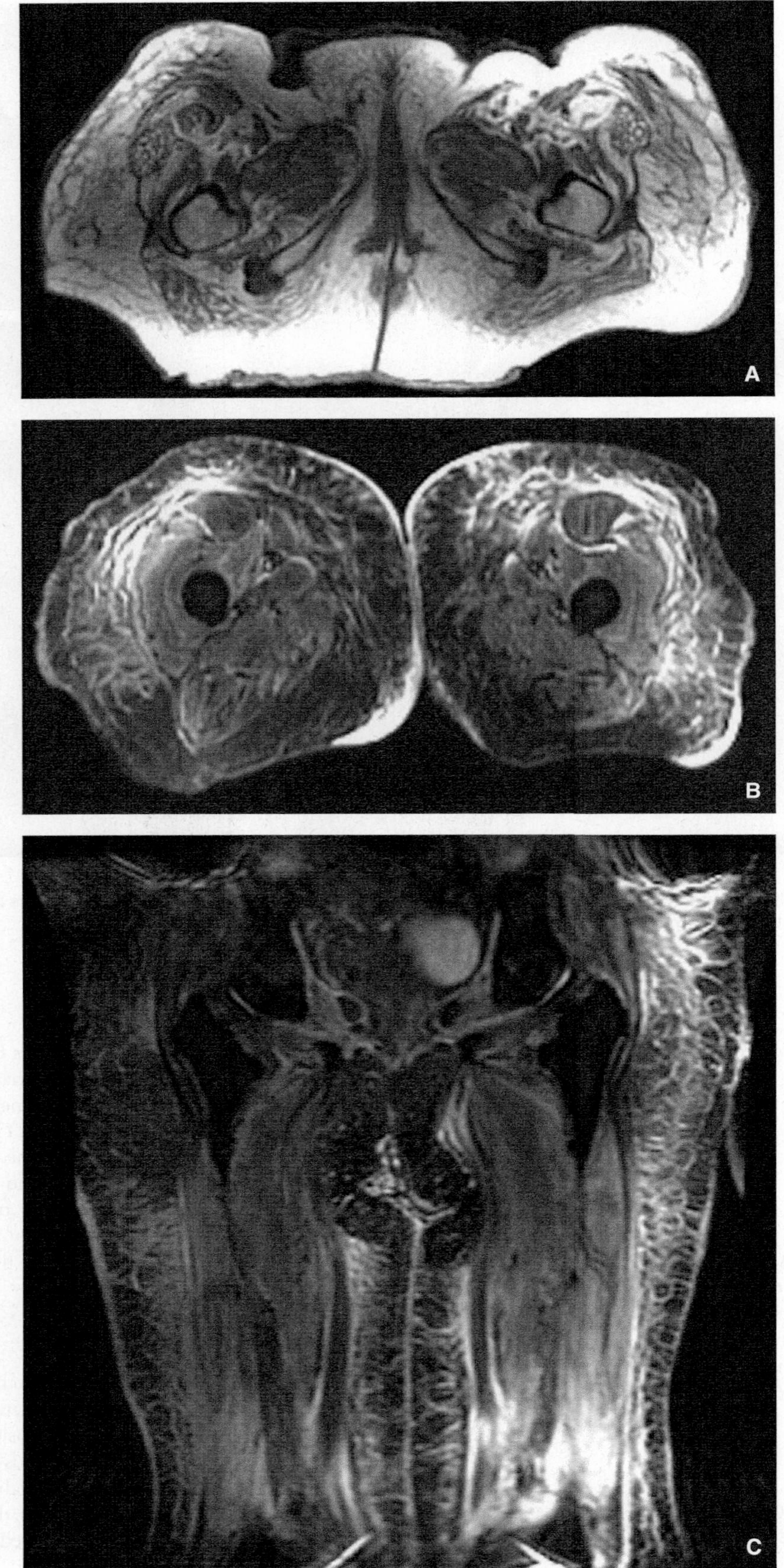

FIGURE 15.17 MRI of polymyositis. **(A)** Axial T1-weighted MR image of the proximal thighs of a 57-year-old woman shows fatty atrophies of all groups of muscles. **(B)** Axial and **(C)** coronal inversion recovery (IR) MR images demonstrate extensive subcutaneous fat and muscle edema.

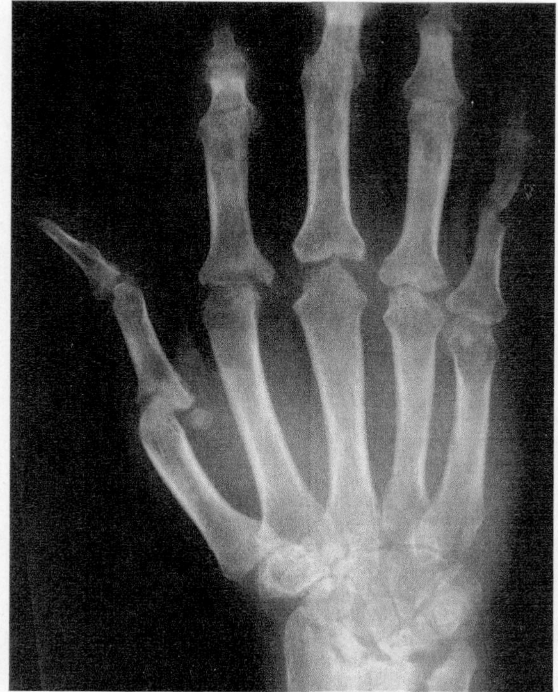

FIGURE 15.18 Mixed connective tissue disease. A 44-year-old woman presented with clinical and imaging features of rheumatoid arthritis. In addition, she had clinically documented dermatomyositis. A dorsovolar radiograph of her left hand shows extensive articular erosions at radiocarpal, metacarpophalangeal, and proximal interphalangeal joints, typical for rheumatoid arthritis. The muscle biopsy result was consistent with polymyositis.

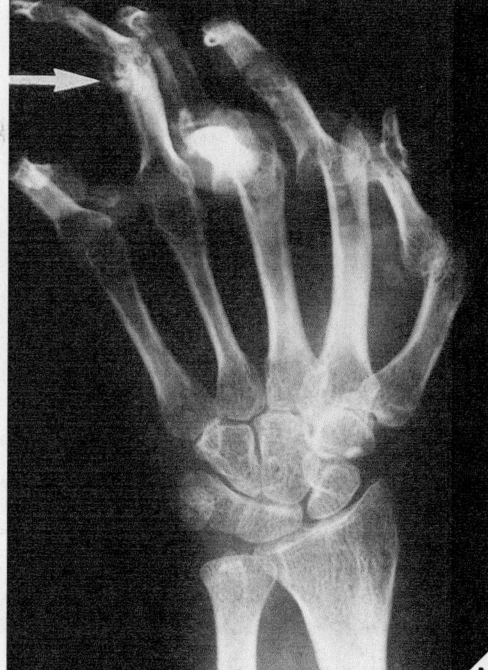

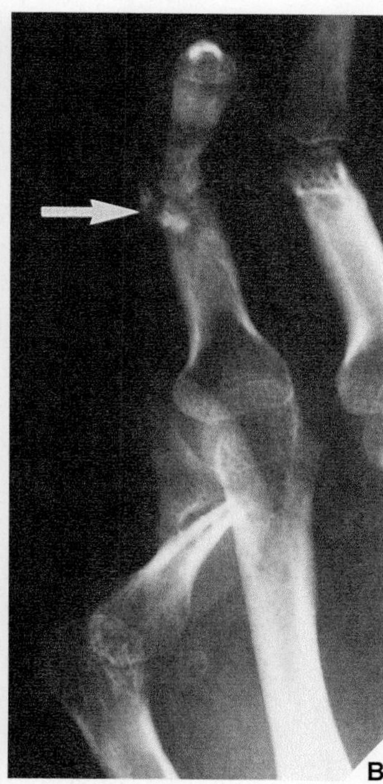

FIGURE 15.19 Mixed connective tissue disease. A 26-year-old woman presented with swelling of both hands, polyarthralgia, and Raynaud phenomenon. She tested positively for the rheumatoid factors and ANAs, and her clinical findings were characteristic for SLE and scleroderma. **(A)** Oblique radiograph of the right hand and **(B)** coned-down view of the thumb and index finger of the left hand show flexion deformities and subluxations in the multiple joints. Deformities of both thumbs are characteristic for SLE, whereas soft-tissue calcifications *(arrows)* are typical for scleroderma. The clinical diagnosis was MCTD.

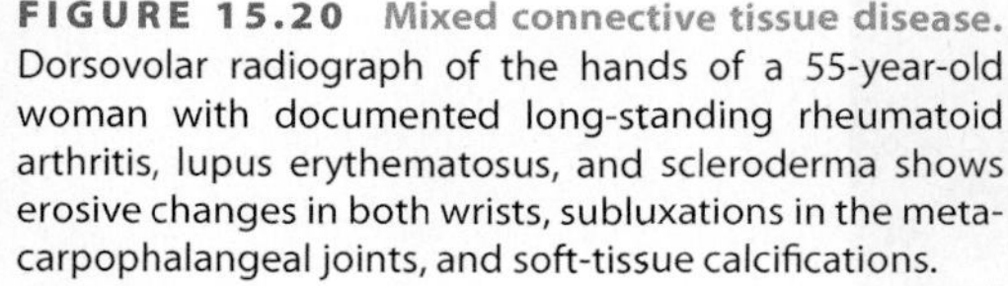

FIGURE 15.20 Mixed connective tissue disease. Dorsovolar radiograph of the hands of a 55-year-old woman with documented long-standing rheumatoid arthritis, lupus erythematosus, and scleroderma shows erosive changes in both wrists, subluxations in the metacarpophalangeal joints, and soft-tissue calcifications.

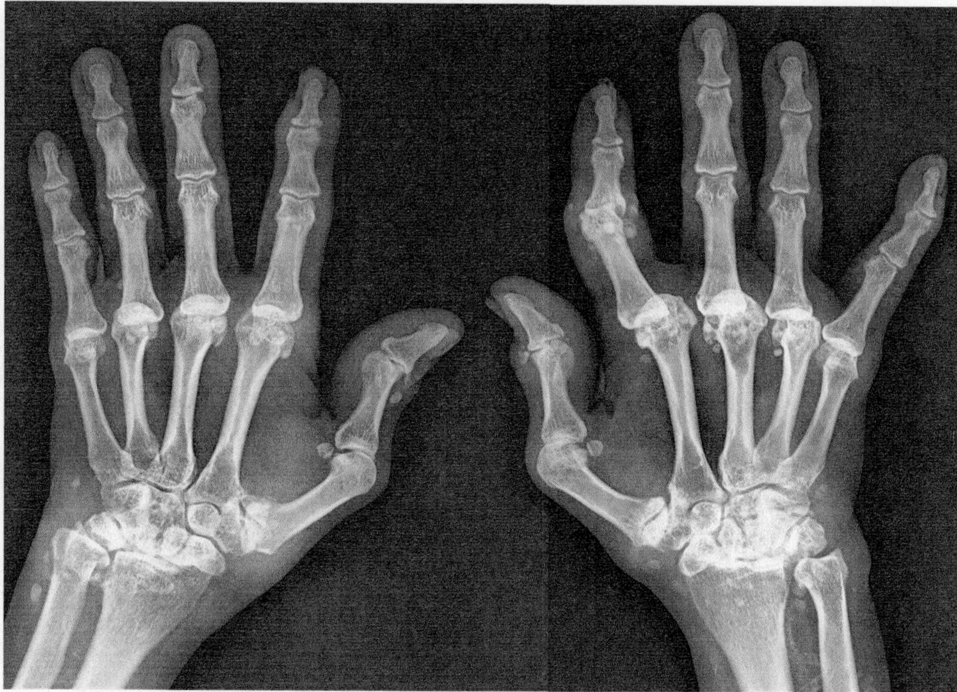

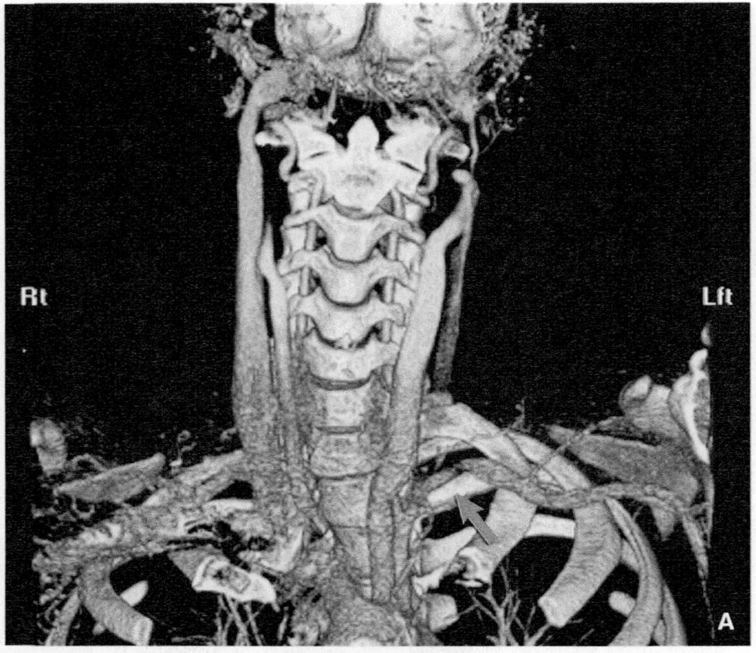

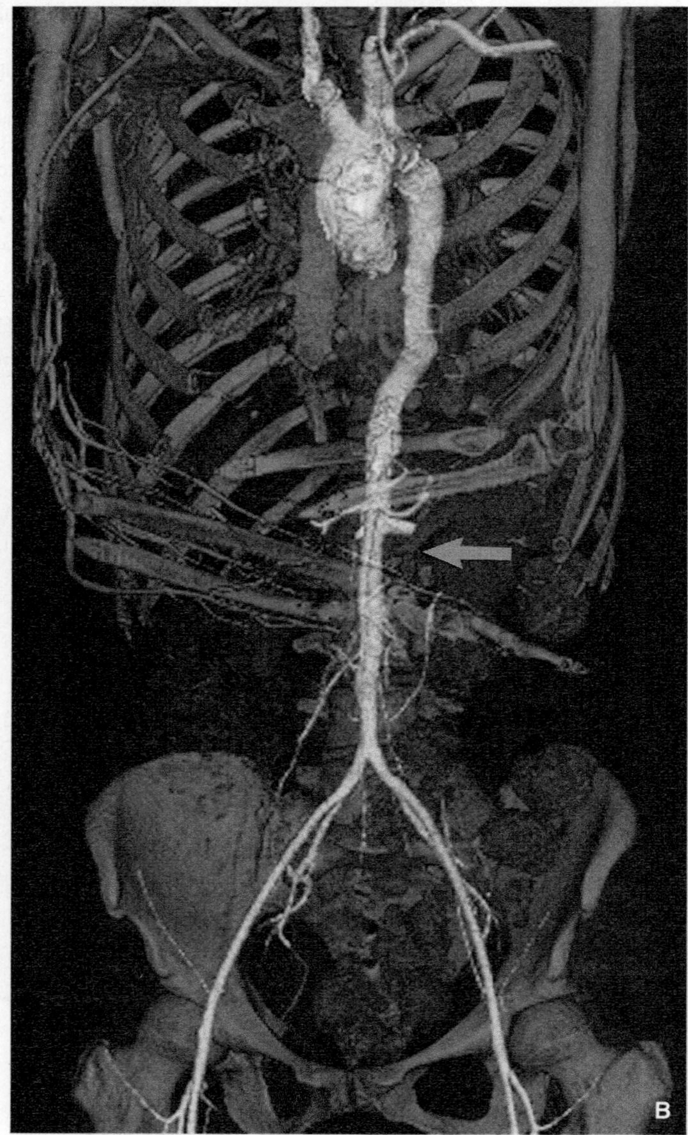

FIGURE 15.21 CT-angiography of Takayasu arteritis. **(A)** Three-dimensional (3D) reconstructed volume-rendering image of the neck of a 37-year-old woman obtained after intravenous administration of 125 mL of Omnipaque 350 shows narrowing of the left subclavian artery distal to the origin of the carotid artery *(arrow)*. **(B)** 3D CT reconstructed volume-rendering image of the thoracic and abdominal aorta shows diffuse narrowing of the abdominal aorta *(arrow)*, calcified plaque art the diaphragmatic hiatus, stenosis at the origin of the celiac axis, and occlusion of the right main renal artery.

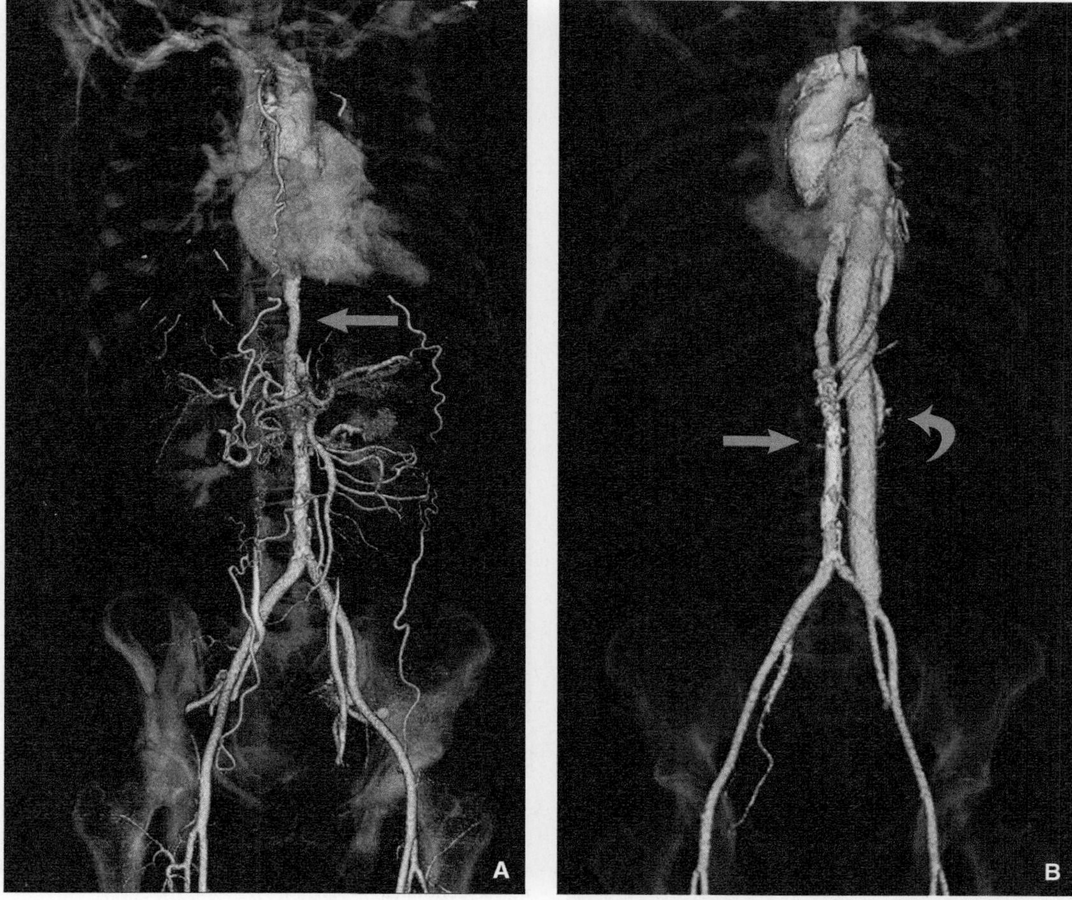

FIGURE 15.22 CT-angiography of Takayasu arteritis. A 56-year-old woman, who was diagnosed with Takayasu arteritis 3 years before, presented with high blood pressure, pain in the abdomen and lower extremities, dizziness, and headache. **(A)** After intravenous administration of 100 mL of Omnipaque 350, three-dimensional (3D) CT reconstructed volume-rendering image shows significant narrowing of the lower thoracic and abdominal aortic segments, most pronounced at the diaphragmatic hiatus *(arrow)*. There is also mild dilatation of proximal renal and mesenteric arteries. **(B)** After surgery, which consisted of placement of abdominal aorta graft, 3D CT reconstructed volume-rendering image obtained after intravenous administration of 125 mL of Omnipaque 350 injected at a rate of 4.0 mL/sec demonstrates the abdominal aorta graft *(curved arrow)* that extends from the thoracic aorta to the bifurcation. The native abdominal aorta is diffusely narrowed *(arrow)* and shows sclerotic plaques. Visualized branches of the bypass graft include the left renal artery, celiac artery, and superior mesenteric artery, all of which are patent.

FIGURE 15.23 MR angiography of Takayasu arteritis. After intravenous administration of 20 mL of gadodiamide (a gadolinium-based contrast agent), 3D MR angiography of the chest and neck was performed in a 64-year-old man diagnosed with myelodysplastic syndrome and large vessel arteritis. In the arterial phase, note the narrowing of the left subclavian *(arrow)* and left carotid *(arrowheads)* arteries. In addition, the venous phase (not shown here) demonstrated occlusion of the left subclavian, left internal jugular, and left brachiocephalic veins.

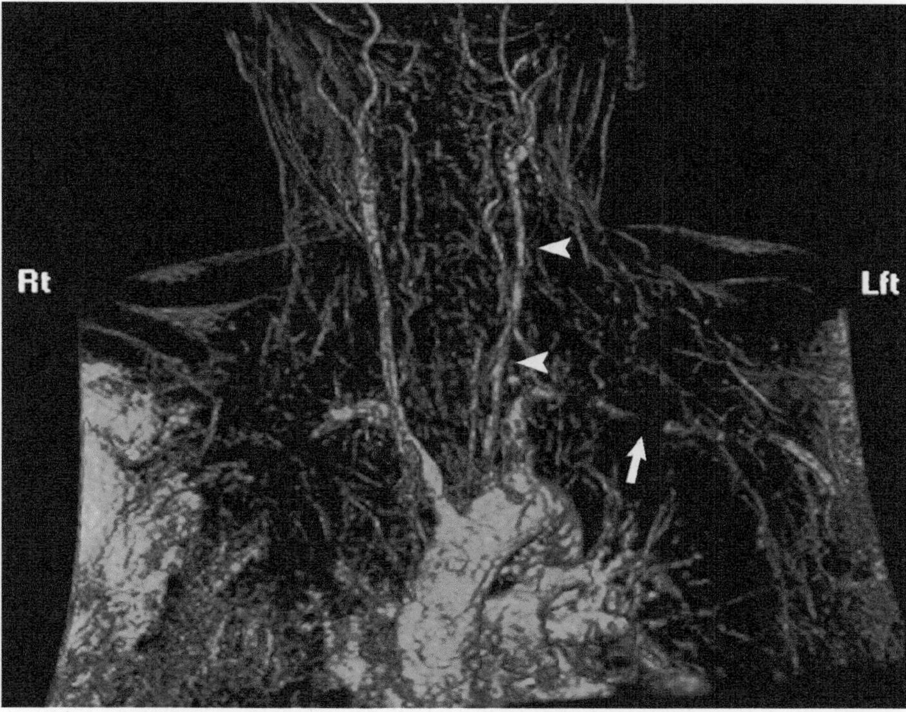

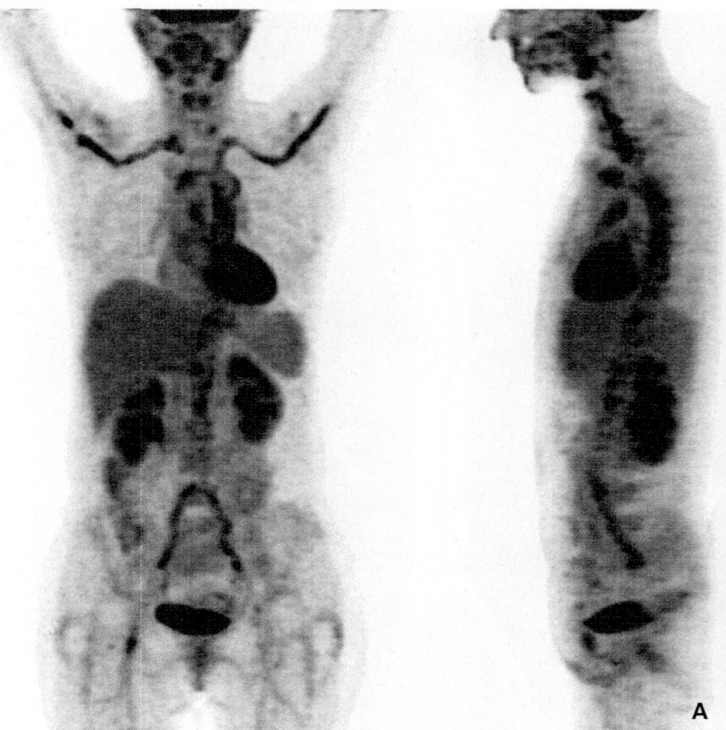

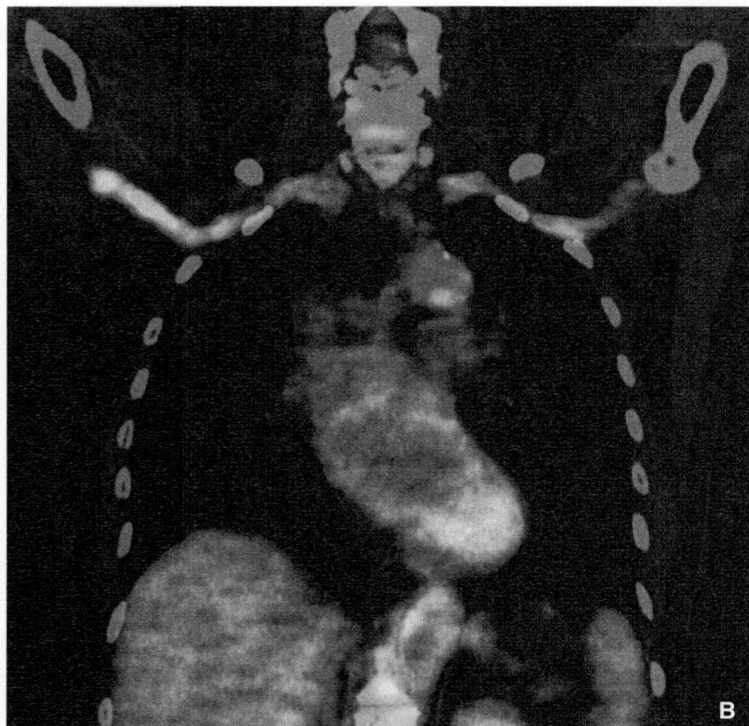

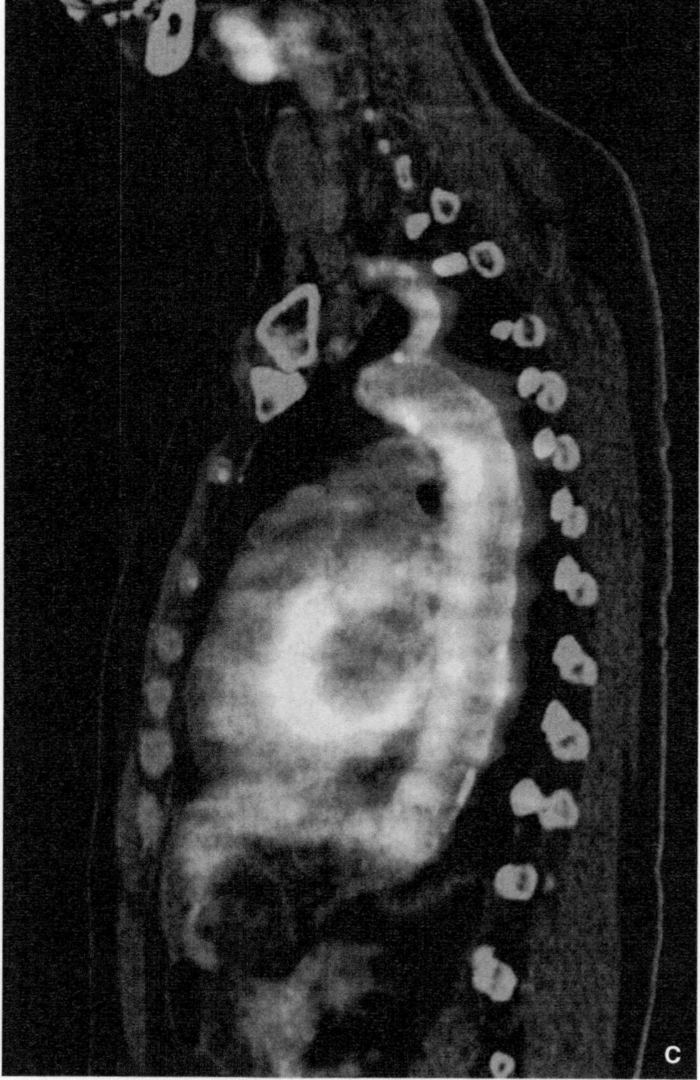

FIGURE 15.24 ^{18}F-FDG PET and PET/CT of Takayasu arteritis. **(A)** Frontal and lateral whole-body ^{18}F-FDG PET performed in a 58-year-old woman shows increased metabolic activity in the aorta, both subclavian arteries, and common iliac arteries. **(B)** Fused PET/CT image demonstrates increased metabolic activity in both subclavian arteries. **(C)** Lateral projection shows increased metabolic activity in thoracic aorta. *(Continued)*

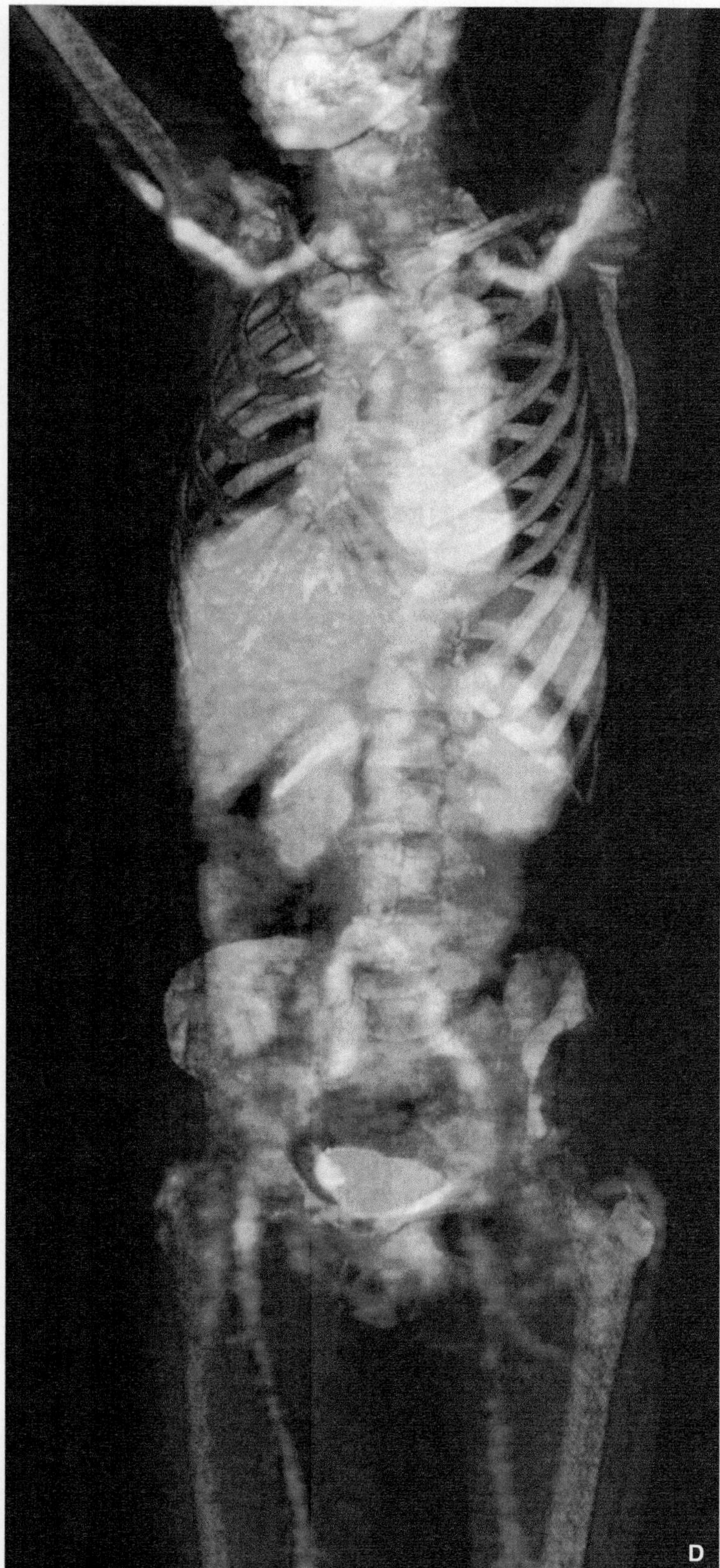

FIGURE 15.24 ^{18}F-FDG PET and PET/CT of Takayasu arteritis. ***(Continued)*** **(D)** Fused reconstructed PET/CT image in volume rendering technique more effectively demonstrates the abnormalities depicted in parts A–C. (Courtesy of PZWL Wydawnictwo Lekarskie, Warsaw, Poland.)

Metabolic, Endocrine, and Crystal Deposition Arthropathies and Arthritides

An overview of the clinical and radiographic hallmarks of the arthropathies and arthritides associated with metabolic, endocrine, and crystal deposition abnormalities is shown in Table 15.2.

Gout

Clinical Features

Gout is a metabolic disorder of purine metabolism characterized by recurrent episodes of arthritis associated with the presence of monosodium urate monohydrate crystals in the synovial fluid leukocytes and, in many cases, gross deposits of sodium urate (tophi) in periarticular soft tissues.

Tophi, a pathognomonic feature of gout, typically form on pressure points in and around the inflamed joints. Serum uric acid concentrations are elevated; however, hyperuricemia does not necessarily lead to gout, and patients with gout may occasionally present with normal serum uric acid levels. Crystal deposits cause acute inflammation of the articular and periarticular soft tissues, whereas recurrent acute intermittent flares can result in chronic gouty arthritis leading to cartilage and bone destruction.

Gouty arthritis accounts for approximately 5% of all arthritides. Four stages of the disease have been recognized: asymptomatic hyperuricemia, acute gouty arthritis, intercritical gout, and chronic tophaceous gout. Articular manifestations occur in the different stages of the disease. Ninety percent of the first gout attacks are monoarticular. The great toe is the most common site of involvement in gouty arthritis; the condition known as *podagra*, which involves the first metatarsophalangeal joint, occurs in approximately 75% of patients. Other frequently affected sites include the ankle, knee, elbow, and wrist. Most patients are men, but gouty arthritis is seen in postmenopausal women as well. Recent data from genome-wide association studies (GWAS) shows that genetic variants of SLC2A9/GLUT9 were associated with lower serum uric acid levels and the values were higher among women, and, conversely, genetic variants of protein ABCG2 were associated with higher serum uric acid levels, and the values were higher among men. These studies point to GLUT9 and ABCG2 as being important modulators of uric acid levels and playing important role in the risk of gout.

Hyperuricemia

An increased miscible pool of uric acid with resulting hyperuricemia can occur in two principal ways. First, urate is produced in such large quantities that, even though excretion routes are of normal capacity, they are inadequate to handle the excessive load. Second, the capacity for uric acid excretion is critically reduced so that even a normal quantity of uric acid cannot be eliminated.

In 25% to 30% of gouty patients, a primary defect in the rate of purine synthesis causes excessive uric acid formation, as reflected in excessive urinary uric acid excretion (more than 600 mg/day) measured while the patient is maintained on a standard purine-free diet. Increased production can also be seen in gout secondary to myeloproliferative disorders associated with increased destruction of cells and result in increased breakdown of nucleic acids. Decreased excretion occurs in primary gout in patients with a dysfunction in the renal tubular capacity to excrete urate and in patients with chronic renal disease. In most patients, however, there is evidence of both uric acid overproduction and diminished renal excretion of uric acid.

The chance of development of gouty arthritis in hyperuricemic individuals should increase in proportion to the duration and, even more, to the degree of hyperuricemia. Monosodium urate, however, has a marked tendency to form relatively stable supersaturated solutions; therefore, the proportion of hyperuricemic patients in whom gouty arthritis actually develops is relatively low. The clinical development of gouty arthritis in the hyperuricemic subject is also substantially influenced by other factors, such

TABLE 15.2 Clinical and Imaging Hallmarks of Metabolic, Endocrine, and Miscellaneous Arthritides

Type of Arthritis	Site	Crucial Abnormalities	Technique/Projection
Gout (M > F)	Great toe Large joints (knee, elbow) Hand	Articular erosion with preservation of part of joint Overhanging edge of erosion Lack of osteoporosis Periarticular swelling	Standard views of affected joints
		Tophi	Dual-energy color-coded computed tomography (CT)
Calcium pyrophosphate dihydrate (CPPD) crystal deposition disease (M = F)	Variable joints	Chondrocalcinosis (calcification of articular cartilage and menisci) Calcifications of tendons, ligaments, and capsule	Standard views of affected joints
	Femoropatellar joint	Joint space narrowing Subchondral sclerosis Osteophytes	Lateral (knee) and axial (patella) views
	Wrists, elbows, shoulders, ankles	Degenerative changes with chondrocalcinosis	Standard views of affected joints
Calcium hydroxyapatite (CHA) crystal deposition disease (F > M)	Variable joints but predilection for shoulder joint (supraspinatus tendon)	Pericapsular calcifications Calcifications of tendons	Standard views of affected joints
Hemochromatosis (M > F)	Hands	Involvement of second and third metacarpophalangeal joints with beak-like osteophytes	Dorsovolar view
	Large joints	Chondrocalcinosis	Standard views of affected joints
Alkaptonuria (ochronosis) (M = F)	Intervertebral disks, sacroiliac joints, symphysis pubis, large joints (knees, hips)	Calcification and ossification of intervertebral disks, narrowing of disks, osteoporosis, joint space narrowing, periarticular sclerosis	Anteroposterior and lateral views of spine; standard views of affected joints
Hyperparathyroidism (F > M)	Hands	Destructive changes in interphalangeal joints	Dorsovolar view
		Subperiosteal resorption	Dorsovolar and oblique views
	Multiple bones	Bone cysts (brown tumors)	Standard views specific for locations
	Skull	Salt-and-pepper appearance	Lateral view
	Spine	Rugger-jersey appearance	Lateral view
Acromegaly (M > F)	Hands	Widened joint spaces Large sesamoid Degenerative changes (beak-like osteophytes)	Dorsovolar view
	Skull	Large sinuses	Lateral view
	Facial bones	Large mandible (prognathism)	Lateral view
	Heel	Thick heel pad (>25 mm)	Lateral view
	Spine	Thoracic kyphosis	Lateral view (thoracic spine)
Amyloidosis (M > F)	Large joints (hips, knees, shoulders, elbows)	Articular and periarticular erosions, osteoporosis (periarticular), joint subluxations, pathologic fractures	Standard views of affected joints Radionuclide bone scan (scintigraphy)
Multicentric reticulohistiocytosis (F > M)	Hands (distal and proximal interphalangeal joints) Feet	Soft-tissue swelling, articular erosions, lack of osteoporosis	Dorsovolar view Norgaard (ball-catcher's) view Dorsoplantar view Oblique view
Hemophilia (M > F)	Large joints (hips, knees, shoulders) Elbows, ankles	Joint effusion, osteoporosis, symmetrical and concentric joint space narrowing, articular erosions, widening of intercondylar notch, squaring of patella; very similar to changes of juvenile rheumatoid arthritis	Standard views of affected joints Magnetic resonance imaging (MRI)

M, male; F, female.

as binding of urate to plasma proteins or the presence of promoters or inhibitors of crystallization.

Examination of Synovial Fluid

A wet preparation of fresh synovial fluid is best for the examination of crystals. Although crystals may often be seen by ordinary light microscopy, reliable identification requires polarization equipment. To differentiate between urate and pyrophosphate crystals—characteristics of gout and pseudogout, respectively—a compensated, polarized light microscope is advisable. Because both types of crystals are birefringent, they refract the polarized light that passes through them. The birefringence phenomenon is caused by the refractive index for light, which vibrates either parallel or perpendicular to the axis of the crystal being viewed. Color is the key to negative or positive birefringence. Urates are strongly birefringent; therefore, they are brightly colored in polarized light, with a red compensator. They are usually seen as needles. During an acute gouty attack, many intraleukocytic crystals are present. Monosodium urate crystals are negatively birefringent, that is, they appear yellow when the longitudinal axis of the crystal is parallel to the axis of slow vibrations of the red compensator on the polarizing system, and they appear blue when perpendicular.

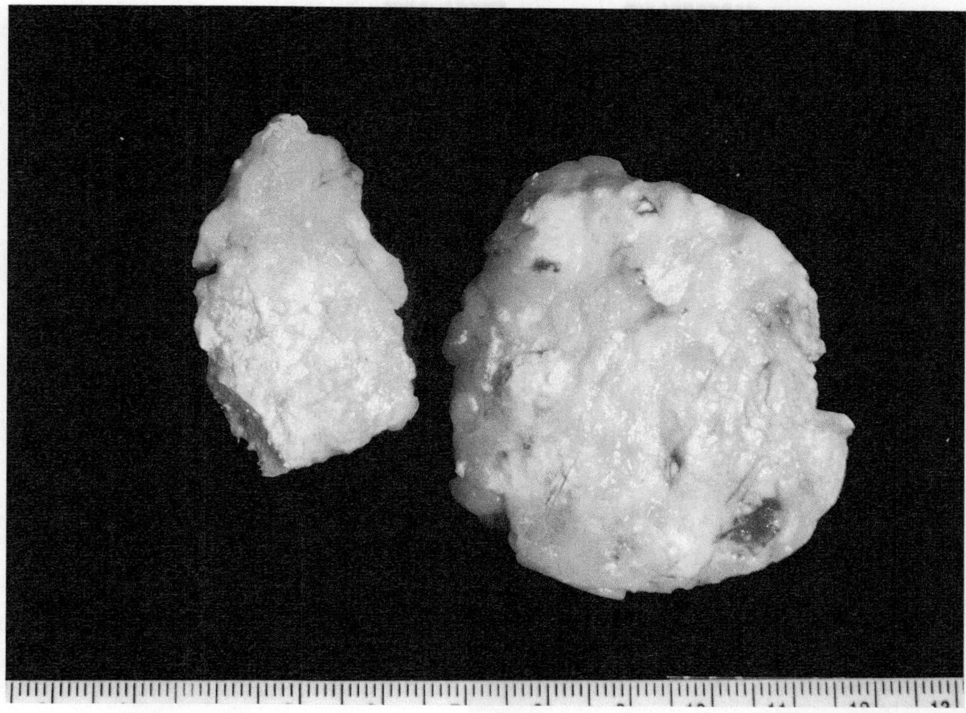

FIGURE 15.25 Pathology of gouty tophus. Photograph of gross specimen of the gouty tophus shows nodular, pasty tan-white material deposited in fibroadipose tissue. (Courtesy of Michael J. Klein, MD, New York.)

Conversely, calcium pyrophosphate dihydrate (CPPD) crystals are usually rhomboidal and exhibit weakly positive birefringence, appearing blue and less bright than urate crystals when their long axis is aligned with the line on the compensating filter.

Monosodium urate crystals, the pathogens of gouty arthritis, range in length from 2 to 10 μm and are found within synovial leukocytes or extracellularly in virtually every case of acute gout, although the likelihood of finding such crystals varies inversely with the amount of time elapsed from the onset of symptoms to the time of examination. Crystals from tophi may be larger.

Pathology

Prolonged hyperuricemia leads to the accumulation of monosodium urate crystals in the joints and soft tissues, which usually results in the formation of nodular masses known as *tophi* (Fig. 15.25). The accumulation of the crystals within bone marrow and articular cartilage induces a chronic inflammatory reaction with consequent bone resorption and erosions. The chalky tophi consist of large deposits of crystal surrounded by highly vascularized inflammatory tissue rich in mononuclear histiocytes, fibroblasts, and giant cells. The synovium of a joint affected by acute gout shows villous hyperplasia and synoviocyte hypertrophy and hyperplasia. The subintima and synoviocyte layer are heavily infiltrated by large number of polymorphonuclear leukocytes and fewer macrophages and lymphocytes.

Imaging Features

Gouty arthritis has several characteristic imaging features. Erosions, which are usually sharply marginated, are initially periarticular in location and are later seen to extend into the joint (Fig. 15.26); an "overhanging edge" of erosion is a frequent identifying feature (Figs. 15.27 and 15.28). Occasionally, intraosseous defects are present secondary to the formation of intraosseous tophi (Figs. 15.29 and 15.30). Usually, there is a striking lack of osteoporosis, which helps differentiate this condition from rheumatoid arthritis. The reason for the absence of osteoporosis is that the duration of an acute gouty attack is too short to allow the development of the disuse osteoporosis so often seen in patients with rheumatoid arthritis. If erosion involves the articular end of the bone and extends into the joint, part of the joint is usually preserved (Fig. 15.31; see also Fig. 15.27). Unlike rheumatoid arthritis, periarticular and articular erosions are asymmetric in distribution (Fig. 15.32). In chronic tophaceous gout, sodium urate deposits in and around the joint are seen, creating a dense mass in the soft tissues called a *tophus*, which frequently exhibits calcifications (Figs. 15.33 to 15.35; see also Figs. 15.26 and 15.27). Characteristically, tophi are randomly distributed and are usually asymmetric; if they occur in the hands or feet, they are more often seen on the dorsal aspect (Fig. 15.36). Currently, dual-energy color-coded CT images can accurately depict gouty tophi (Figs. 15.37 to 15.39; see also Figs. 12.10, and 12.11). Reported sensitivity of this technique varies between 78% and 100% and specifically between 89% and 100%. MRI is also effective way to detect articular and soft-tissue abnormalities of gouty arthritis. Tophaceous gouty deposits exhibit a wide spectrum of signal intensities characteristics, which reflects their variable composition and relative proportion of protein, fibrous tissue, crystals, and hemosiderin. Most lesions are isointense relative to muscle on T1-weighted images, and low-to-intermediate heterogeneous signal intensity on proton density–weighted and water-sensitive (IR, T2) sequences (see Figs. 15.35C,D and 15.39B,C). There is strong enhancement following intravenous injection of gadolinium, although contrast enhancement of the tophus is variable and depends on the vascularity of the affected synovium and surrounding granulation tissue (see Fig. 15.30). Concomitant enhancement of adjacent tendon sheaths, ligaments, muscles, and bone marrow may also be present, reflecting intense inflammatory reaction. PET and PET/CT may also accurately localize the joint affected by gout (Fig. 15.40).

Differential Diagnosis

Although imaging findings of gouty arthritis are generally very characteristic and most of the time even pathognomonic, clinical presentation of acute gouty arthritis may be sometimes mistaken for septic arthritis. The two conditions may present with similar symptoms including joint pain, swelling, tenderness, and occasionally similar laboratory findings such as elevated white blood cell count and sedimentation rate. Soft-tissue tophi may at times mimic rheumatoid nodules. Intraosseous tophi may have aggressive appearance and thus may simulate malignant bone tumor. On radiography, articular gouty erosions, particularly affecting the proximal and distal interphalangeal joints, may sometimes mimic erosive osteoarthritis. Amyloid infiltrate of the articular structures may cause soft-tissue masses accompanied by cystic and erosive lesions indistinguishable from those of gout. Finally, it has to be pointed out that gout may coexist with other arthropathic conditions such as rheumatoid arthritis, osteoarthritis, and infectious arthritis.

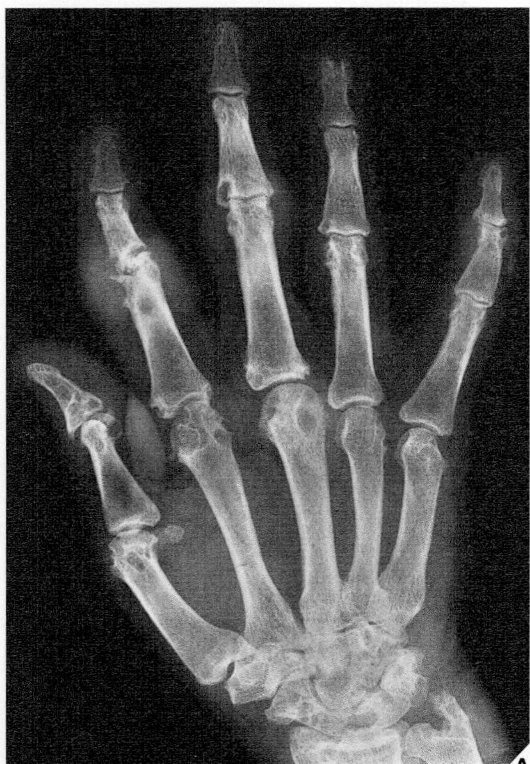

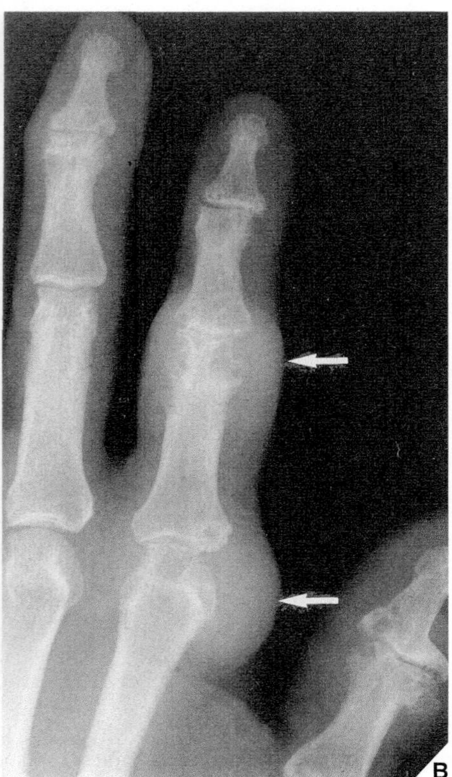

FIGURE 15.26 Gouty arthritis. **(A)** Dorsovolar radiograph of the left hand of a 43-year-old man with tophaceous gout shows multiple sharply marginated articular and periarticular erosions and soft-tissue masses at the proximal interphalangeal joints of the index and middle fingers, representing tophi. Observe also erosions at the second and third metacarpophalangeal joints, and erosions of the radiocarpal and midcarpal joints. **(B)** Dorsovolar radiograph of the fingers of a 70-year-old man with gouty arthritis shows multiple articular and periarticular erosions associated with large tophi *(arrows)*.

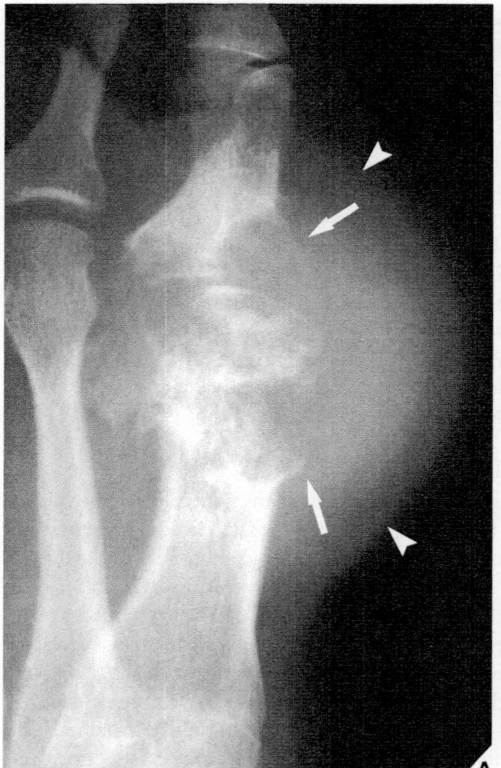

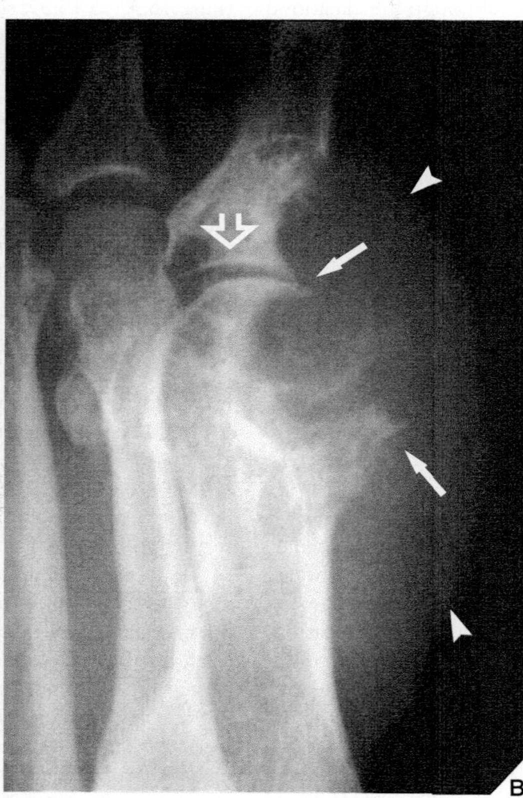

FIGURE 15.27 Gouty arthritis. **(A)** Anteroposterior and **(B)** oblique radiographs of the right great toe of a 58-year-old man with a 3-month history of gout shows the typical involvement of the first metatarsophalangeal joint. Note the characteristic overhanging edge of the erosive changes *(arrows)*, preservation of the lateral portion of the joint *(open arrow)*, and a large tophus *(arrowheads)*.

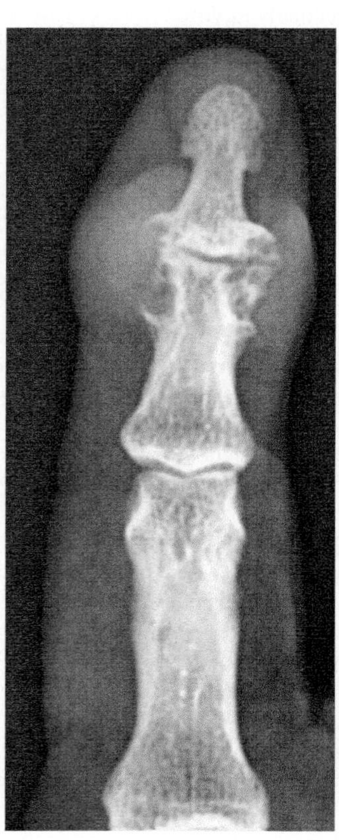

FIGURE 15.28 Gouty arthritis. Typical paraarticular erosions in the distal interphalangeal joint of the index finger exhibiting an overhanging edge are associated with a large tophus.

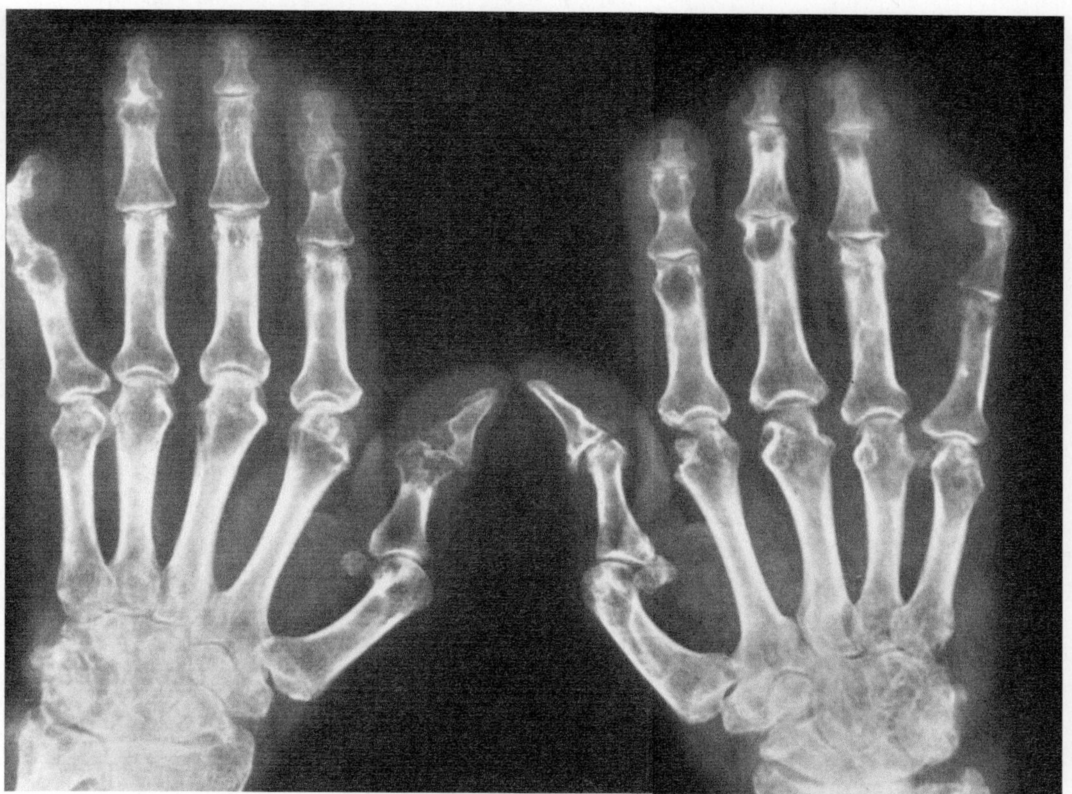

FIGURE 15.29 Gouty arthritis. Dorsovolar radiograph of both hands of a 60-year-old man shows articular and paraarticular erosions of several joints. In addition, note the presence of intraosseous defects in the phalanges consistent with intraosseous tophi.

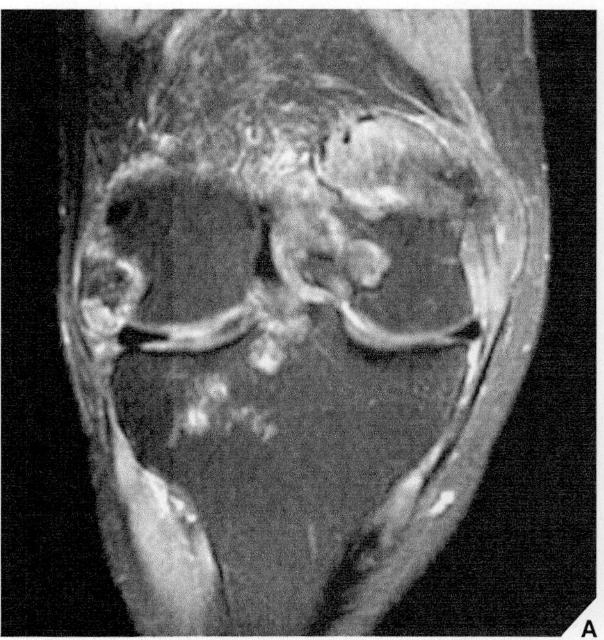

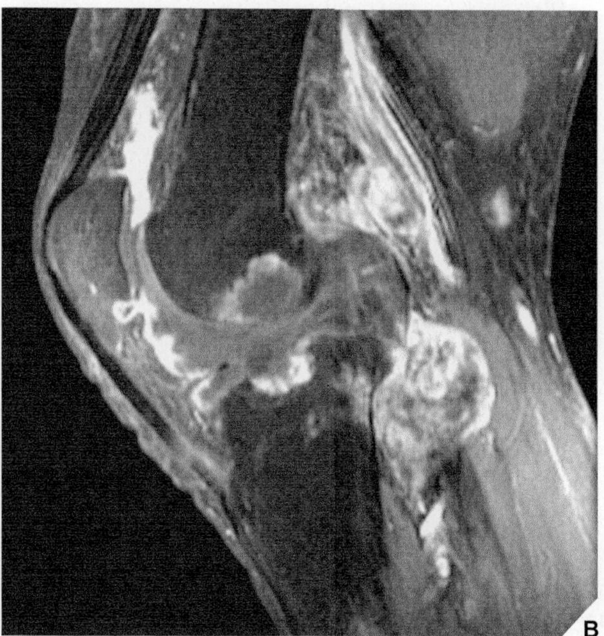

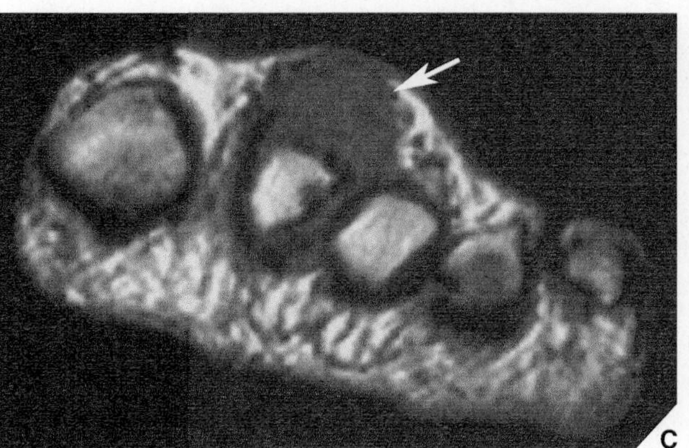

FIGURE 15.30 MRI of gouty arthritis. **(A)** Coronal proton density–weighted fat-suppressed and **(B)** sagittal T1-weighted fat-suppressed contrast-enhanced MR images of the right knee of a 53-year-old man show multiple articular and paraarticular erosions associated with intraosseous as well as soft-tissue tophi. **(C)** Short axis T1-weighted MRI of the foot in another patient with gouty arthritis demonstrates a low–signal intensity tophaceous deposit in the dorsal aspect of the second metatarsal *(arrow)*. *(Continued)*

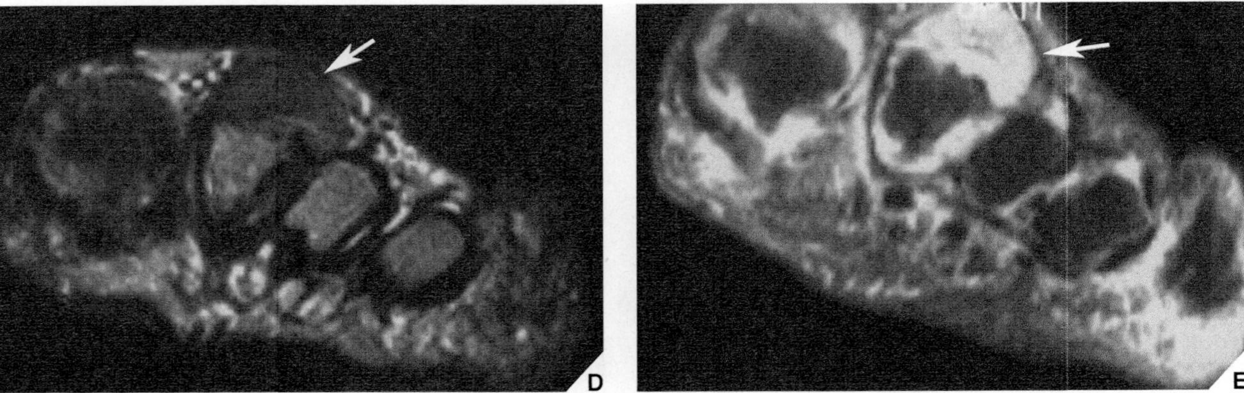

FIGURE 15.30 MRI of gouty arthritis. ***(Continued)*** **(D)** Short-axis T2-weighted MRI of the same patient shows the low–signal intensity tophaceous deposit *(arrow)*. **(E)** Short-axis postcontrast T1-weighted fat-saturated MRI demonstrates strong enhancement of the tophaceous deposit *(arrow)*.

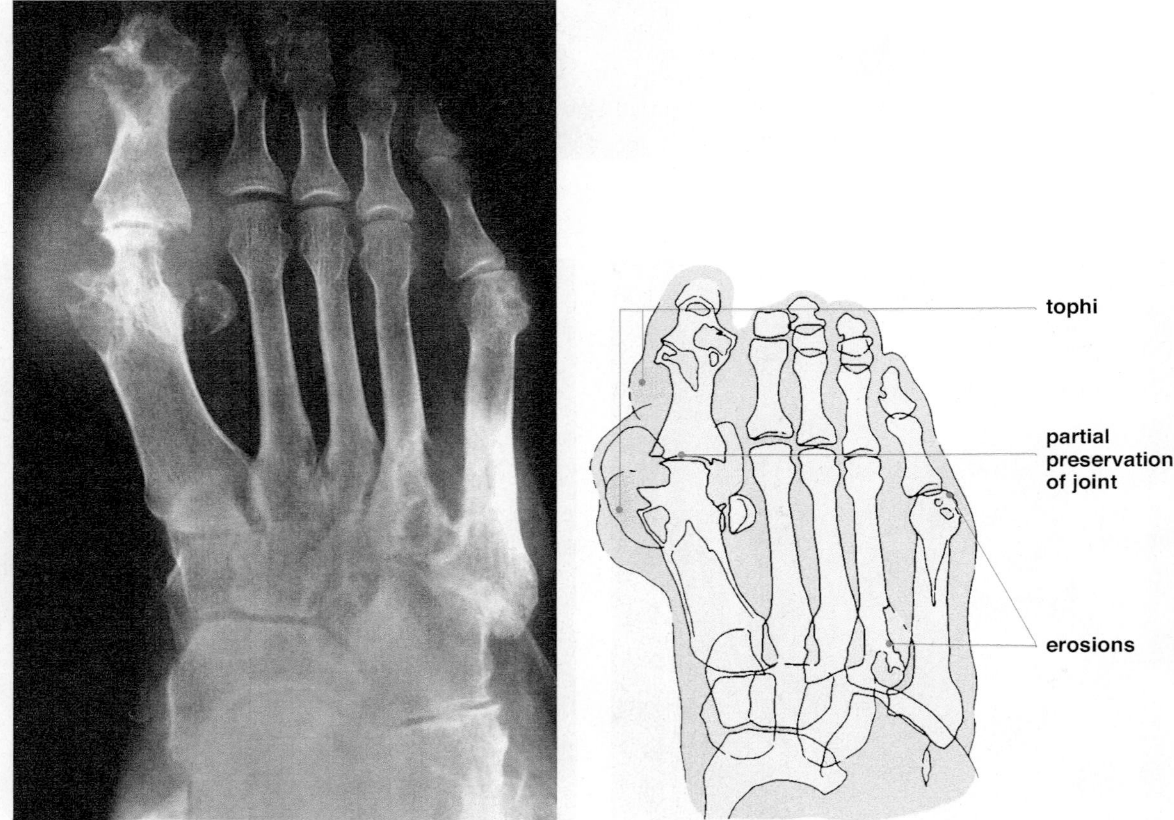

FIGURE 15.31 Gouty arthritis. Dorsoplantar radiograph of the left foot of a 62-year-old man with a long history of tophaceous gout shows multiple erosions involving the big and small toes and the base of the fourth and fifth metatarsals. The first metatarsophalangeal joint is partially preserved, a characteristic feature of gouty arthritis. A large soft-tissue mass of the great toe represents a tophus.

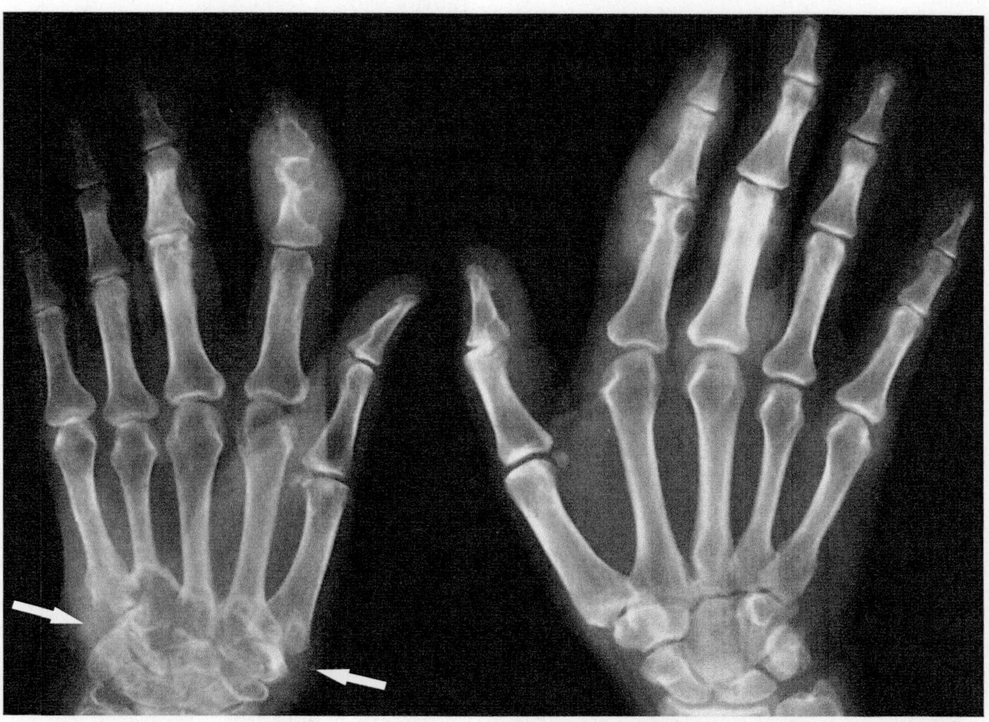

FIGURE 15.32 Gouty arthritis. Dorsovolar radiograph of the hands of a 64-year-old woman shows the typical asymmetric distribution of periarticular and articular erosions. Note involvement of the carpometacarpal joints of the right hand *(arrows)*, a typical site for gout.

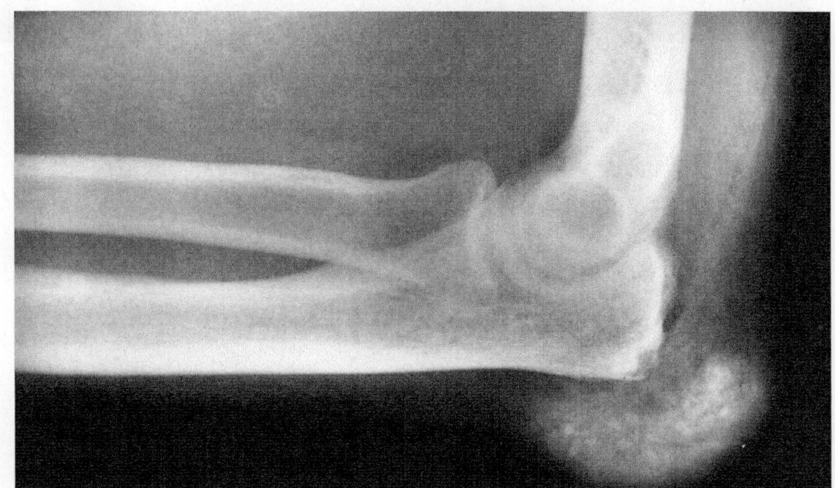

FIGURE 15.33 Gouty tophus. Lateral radiograph of the elbow of a 73-year-old man with a 30-year history of gout shows a tophus with dense calcifications adjacent to the olecranon process, which exhibits a small erosion.

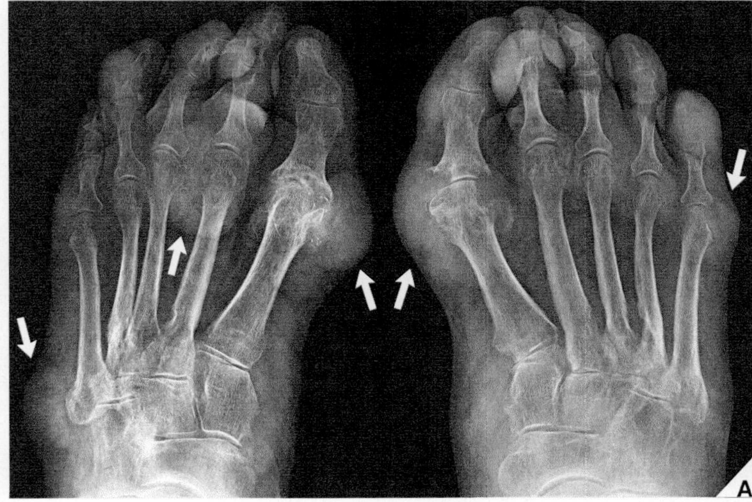

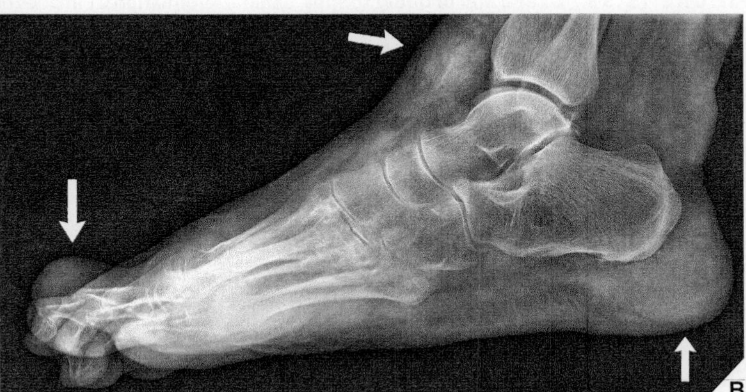

FIGURE 15.34 Tophaceous gout. **(A)** Anteroposterior radiograph of both feet and **(B)** lateral radiograph of the left foot of a 69-year-old man show numerous gouty tophi *(arrows)*. Note also a characteristic for this arthritis erosion of the first metatarsophalangeal joint of the left foot.

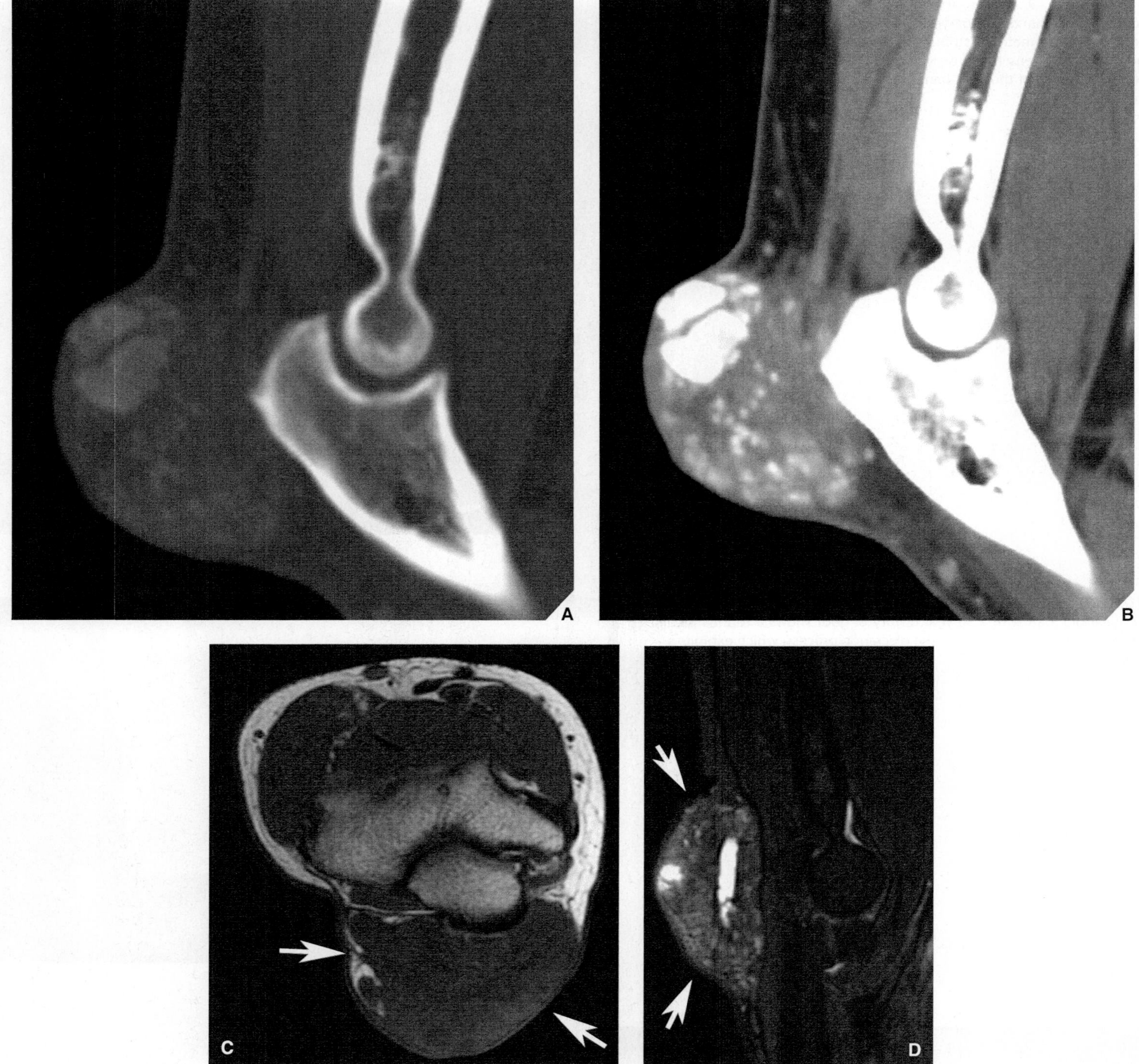

FIGURE 15.35 CT and MRI of gouty tophus. Sagittal reformatted CT images of the elbow viewed in **(A)** bone and **(B)** soft-tissue window show a large soft-tissue mass with numerous calcifications adjacent to the olecranon process of ulna. **(C)** Axial T1-weighted and **(D)** sagittal T2-weighted fat-saturated MR images demonstrate heterogeneous but mostly hypointense large gouty tophi within the olecranon bursa *(arrows)*.

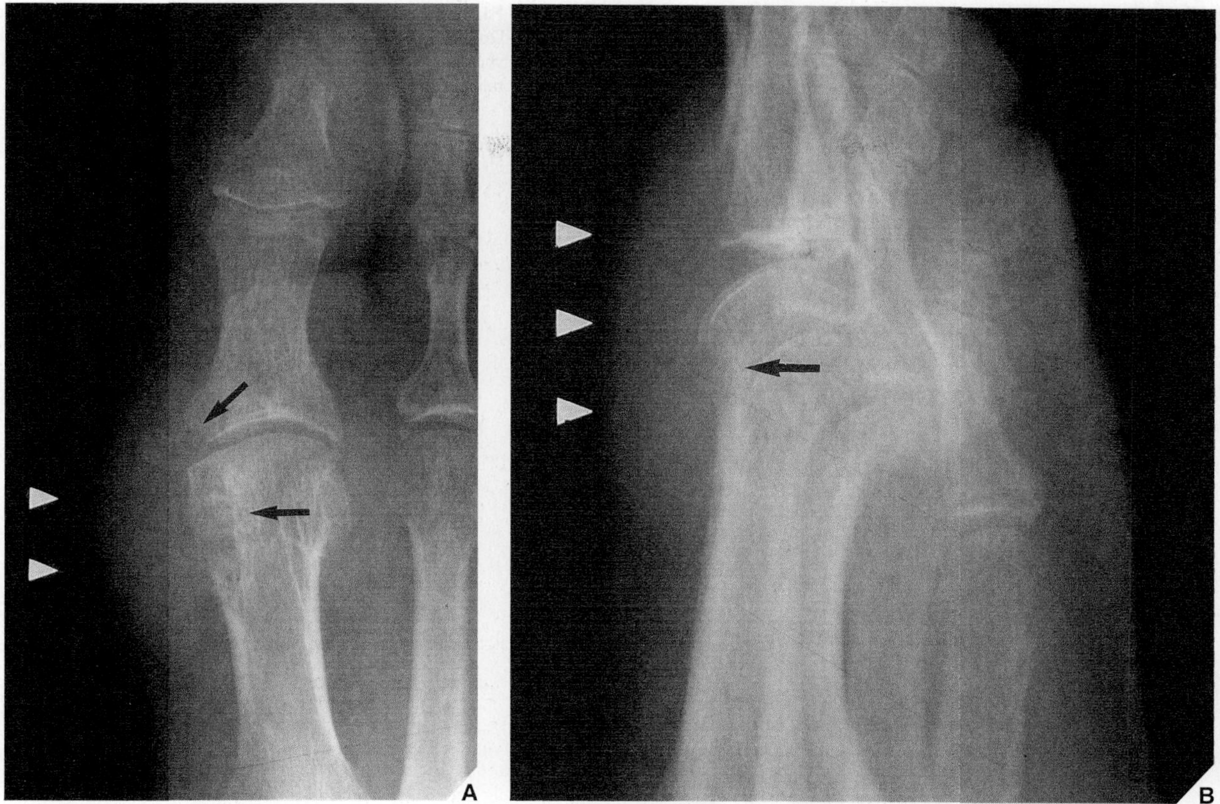

FIGURE 15.36 Gouty tophus. **(A)** Dorsoplantar and **(B)** lateral radiographs of the great toe show articular and periarticular erosions *(arrows)* associated with a large tophus on the dorsal aspect of the first metatarsophalangeal joint *(arrowheads)*.

FIGURE 15.37 Dual-energy CT of tophaceous gout. **(A)** Anteroposterior radiograph of the right foot of a 48-year-old man shows nonspecific erosion at the third tarsometatarsal joint *(arrow)*, confirmed on **(B)** the coronal reformatted CT image. *(Continued)*

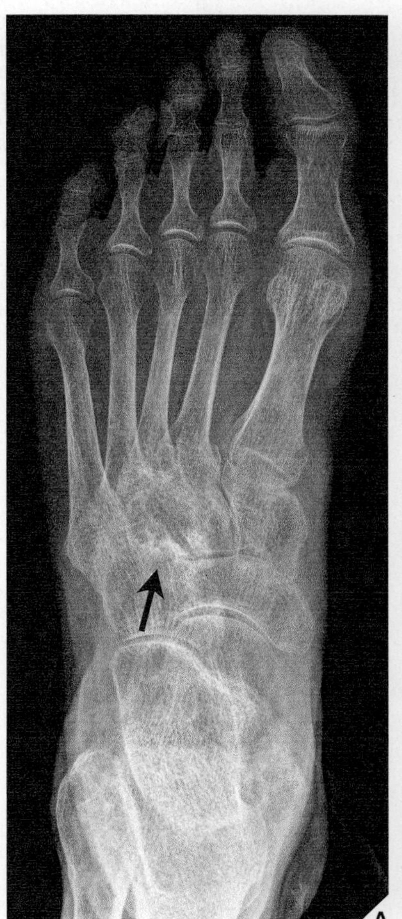

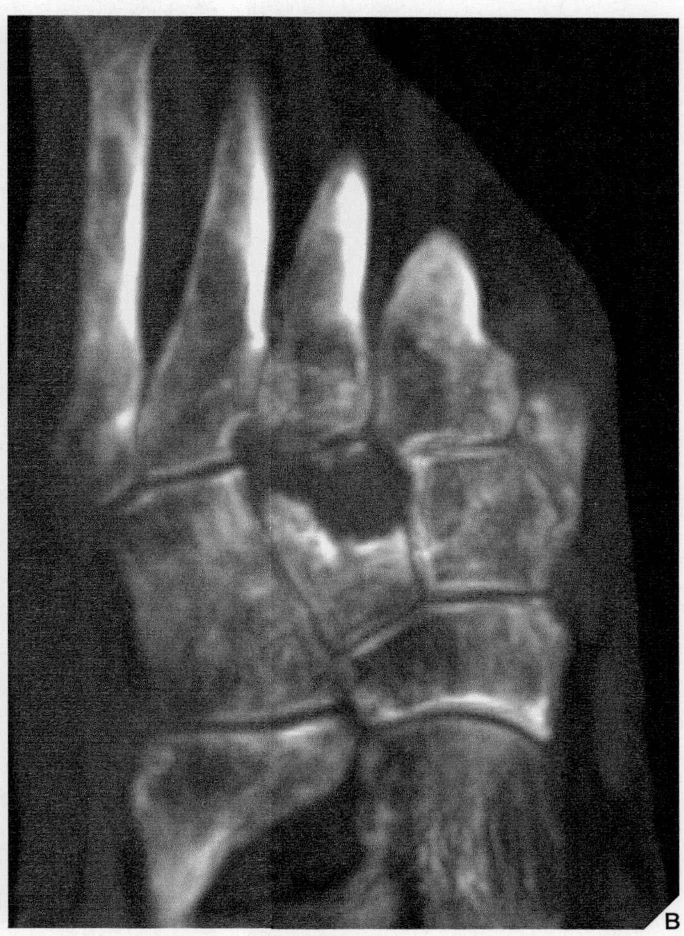

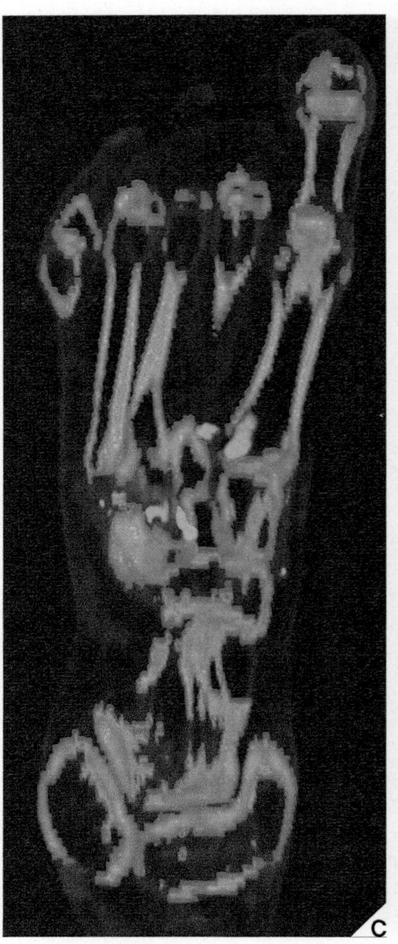

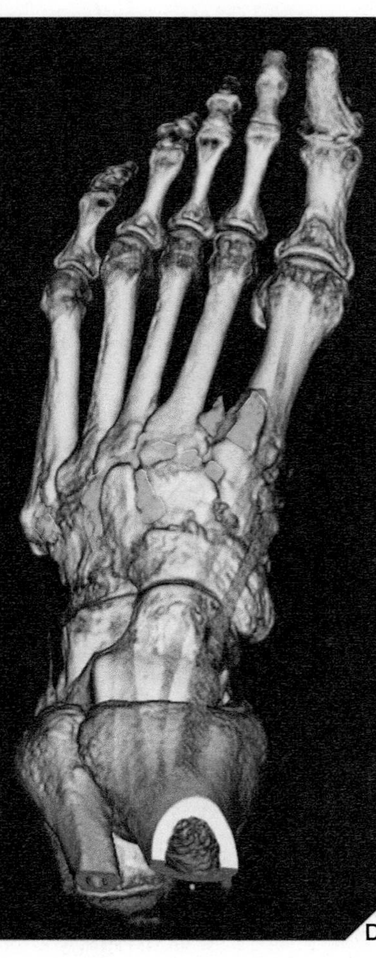

FIGURE 15.37 Dual-energy CT of tophaceous gout. ***(Continued)*** Dual-energy **(C)** coronal and **(D)** 3D reconstructed color-coded CT images show in addition several masses *(green areas)* representing uric acid crystals within the gouty tophi.

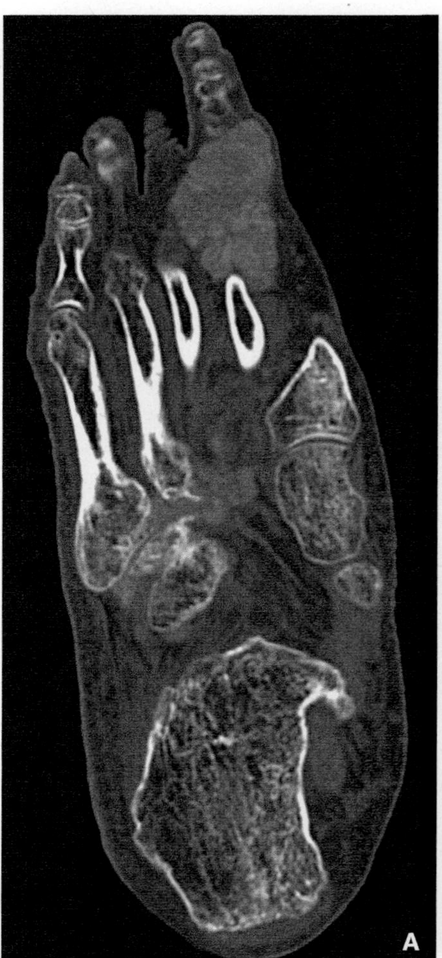

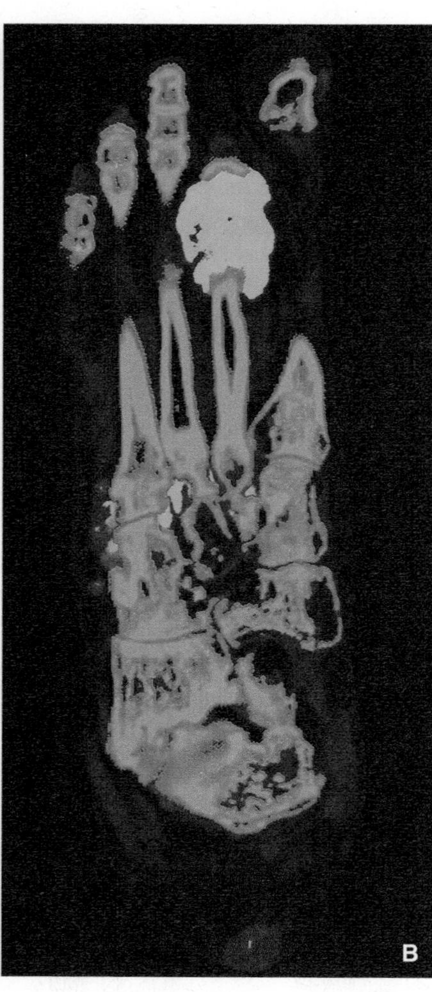

FIGURE 15.38 Dual-energy CT of tophaceous gout. **(A)** Long axis CT image of the right foot of a 71-year-old man shows a nonspecific low-attenuation mass in the region of the second toe. **(B)** Long axis and **(C)** sagittal reformatted dual-energy color-coded CT images identify the mass as being a large tophus containing monosodium urate crystals *(green area)*. *(Continued)*

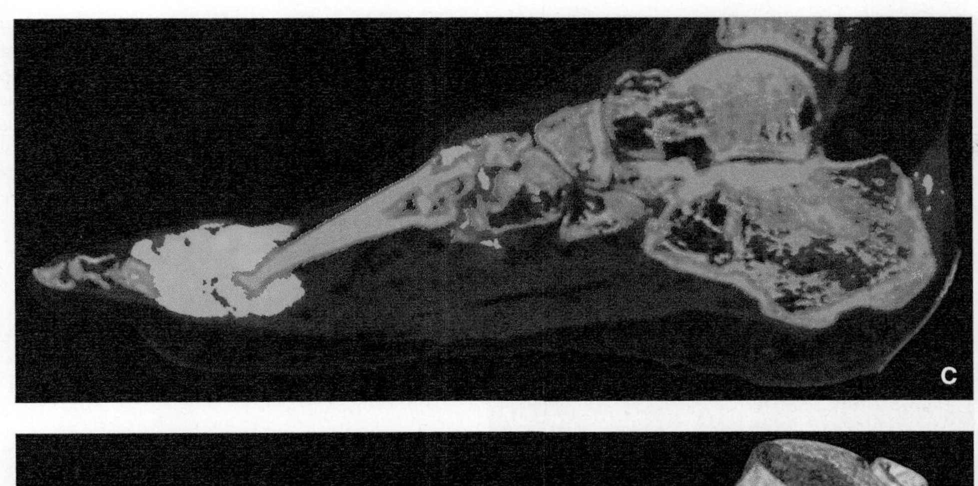

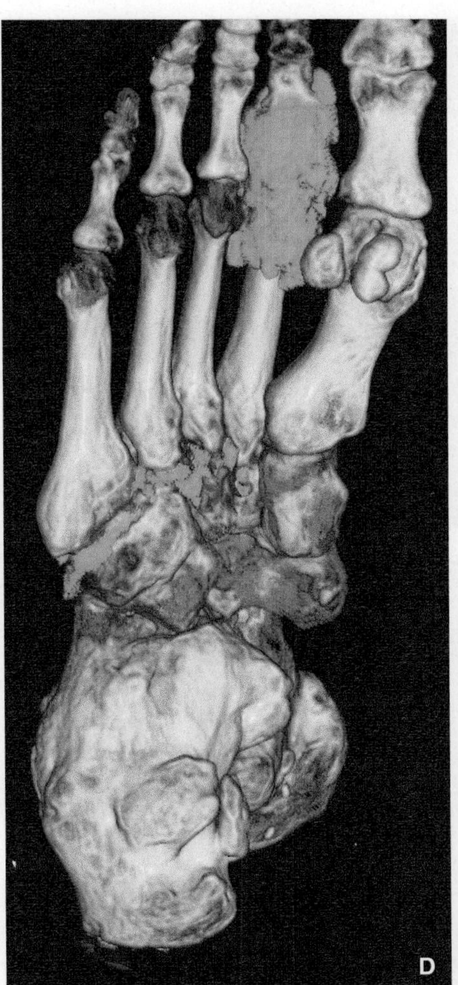

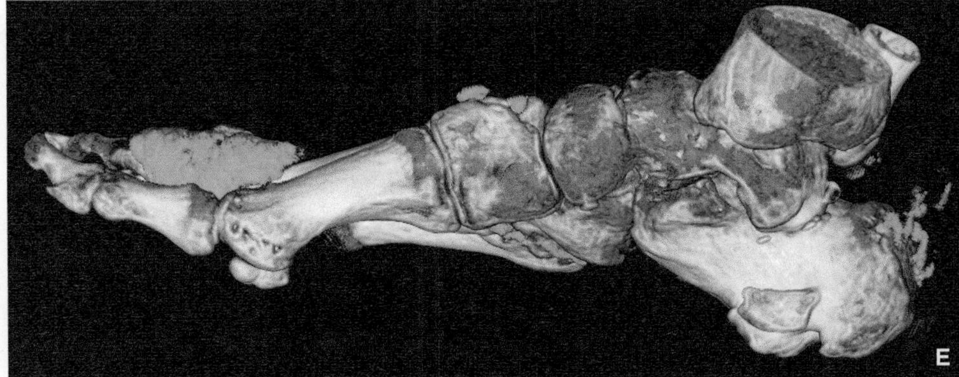

FIGURE 15.38 Dual-energy CT of tophaceous gout. ***(Continued)*** In addition, several smaller tophi are identified at the site of Lisfranc joint and at the site of Achilles tendon attachment to the calcaneus. Three-dimensional reconstructed dual-energy CT color-coded images viewed from the plantar **(D)** and medial **(E)** aspects of the foot better demonstrate the spatial distribution of the urate tophi. (Reprinted with permission from Greenspan A, Gershwin ME. *Imaging in rheumatology*, 1st ed. Philadelphia: Wolters Kluwer; 2018:282, Fig. 7-20A–E.)

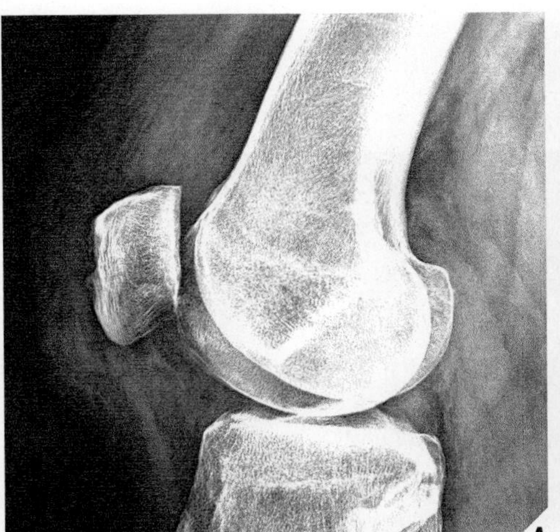

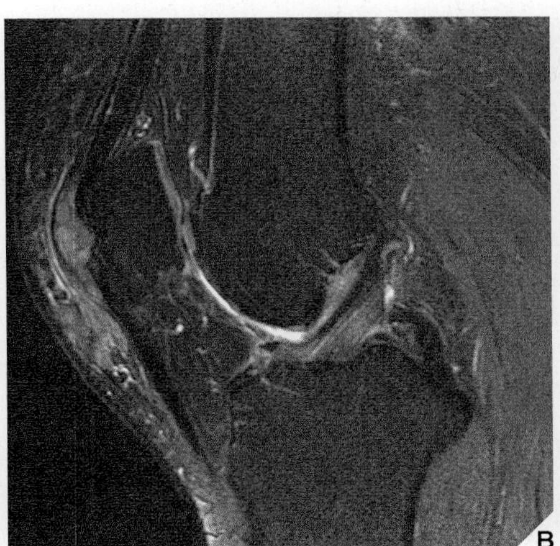

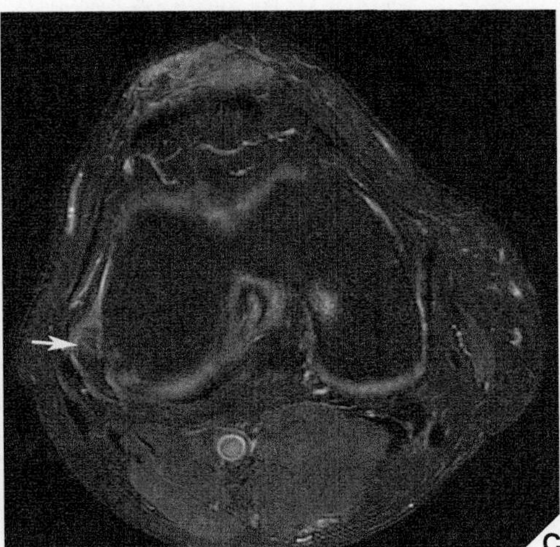

FIGURE 15.39 MRI and dual-energy CT of tophaceous gout. **(A)** Lateral radiograph of the knee of a 65-year-old man, who presented with right knee pain, shows prepatellar soft-tissue mass eroding the anterior cortex of the patella. **(B)** Sagittal and **(C)** axial proton density–weighted fat-suppressed MR images demonstrate heterogeneous mass adjacent to the patella and smaller mass eroding the lateral femoral condyle *(arrow)*. *(Continued)*

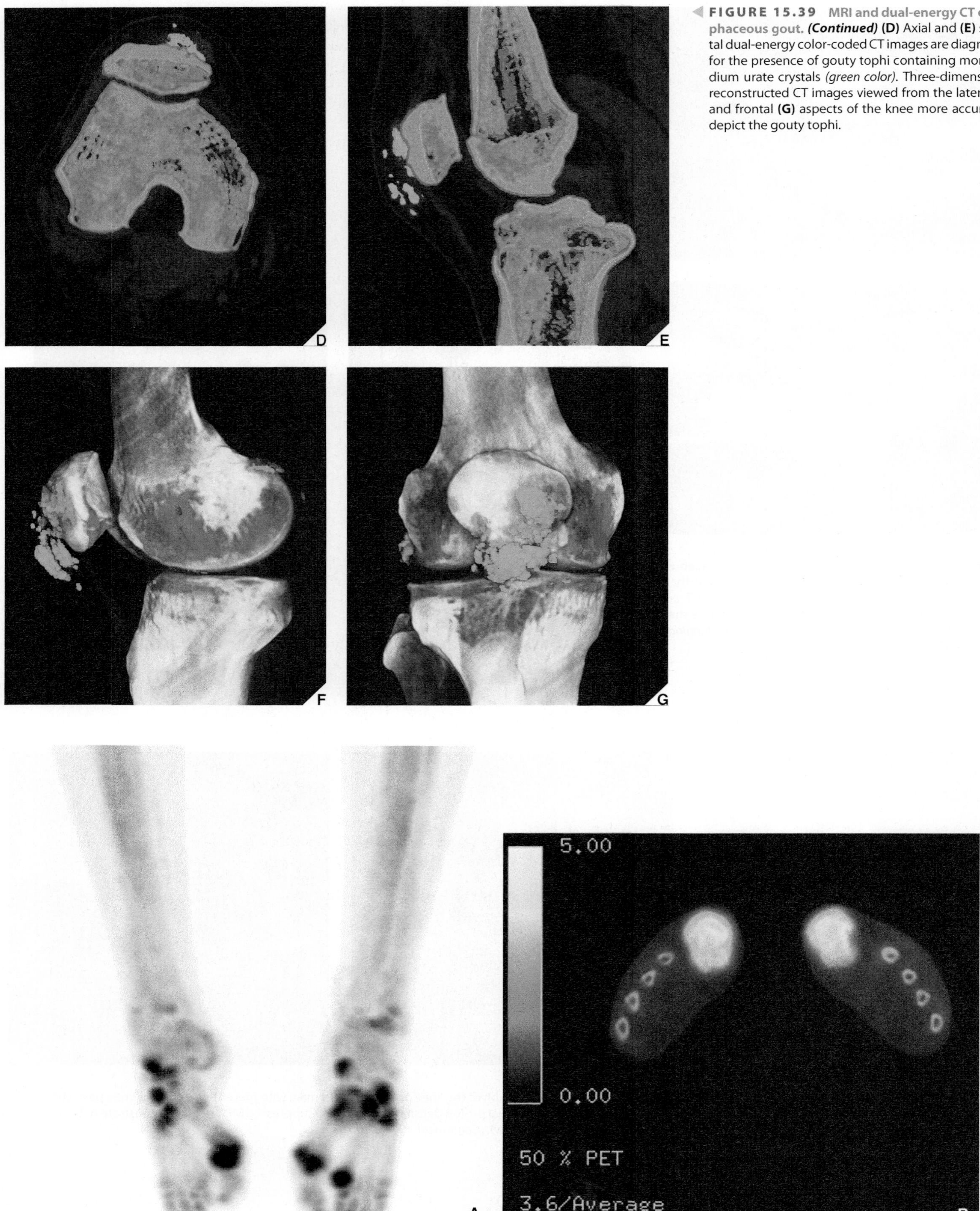

FIGURE 15.39 MRI and dual-energy CT of tophaceous gout. ***(Continued)*** **(D)** Axial and **(E)** sagittal dual-energy color-coded CT images are diagnostic for the presence of gouty tophi containing monosodium urate crystals *(green color)*. Three-dimensional reconstructed CT images viewed from the lateral **(F)** and frontal **(G)** aspects of the knee more accurately depict the gouty tophi.

FIGURE 15.40 ^{18}F-FDG PET and PET/CT of gout. **(A)** Image of both feet shows several foci of increased metabolic activity at the site of tophaceous gouty arthritis in a 61-year-old man. **(B)** Fused PET/CT axial (short axis) image of both feet of a 49-year-old man shows increased metabolic activity in both first metatarsophalangeal joints.

Treatment

The treatment of gout depends on the stages of the disease. Recently, the American College of Physicians (ACP) developed guidelines and clinical recommendations on the management of gout. The acute gouty attacks respond well to colchicine, as well as to NSAIDs such as ibuprofen, naproxen, or indomethacin. In chronic stages, corticosteroids control inflammation and pain. In addition, the drugs that block uric acid production, such as xanthine oxidase inhibitors (allopurinol or febuxostat), and medications that improve removal of uric acid from the body (probenecid), are used to prevent complications of gout. Most recently, rheumatologists reported that urate-lowering therapy using pegloticase, a pegylated mammalian (porcine-like) recombinant uricase, resulted in reduction of the gouty tophus size both at subcutaneous sites and within the joints. However, ACP recommends that clinicians should discuss benefits, harms, costs, and individual preferences with patients before initiating urate-lowering therapy in patients with recurrent gout attacks. This includes the risk of Stevens-Johnson syndrome in patients receiving allopurinol.

Calcium Pyrophosphate Dihydrate Crystal Deposition Disease

Clinical Features

CPPD crystal deposition disease is a metabolic disorder, which is characterized by the accumulation of CPPD crystals in intraarticular and periarticular tissues, most commonly within fibrocartilage and hyaline cartilage. In addition, synovial, bursal, ligamentous, and tendinous calcifications are encountered. It rarely presents as a soft-tissue mass in extraarticular location, which is known as *tumoral* or *tophaceous pseudogout*. The condition may occur as a hereditary or sporadic disorder. Some investigators suggested that a putative pyrophosphate transporter, the progressive ankylosis protein homolog, a protein encoded by *ANKH* gene, might be responsible for this disease. *ANKH* may also play a role in modulating the enzymes involved in mineralization, such as alkaline phosphatase, thus potentially contributing to the disease process. The men and women are equally affected; most commonly, patients are middle-aged and older. The disease may be asymptomatic, in which case the only imaging finding may be *chondrocalcinosis* (see in the following text). When symptomatic, it is called *pseudogout*. There is, however, a great deal of confusion about these terms, and they are often misused.

In an effort to explain the relationship between chondrocalcinosis, calcium pyrophosphate arthropathy, and the pseudogout syndrome, Resnick has proposed an integration of these terms under the rubric CPPD crystal deposition disease. *Chondrocalcinosis*, a condition in which calcification of the hyaline (articular) cartilage or fibrocartilage (menisci) occurs, may be seen in other disorders as well, such as gout, hyperparathyroidism, hemochromatosis, hepatolenticular degeneration (Wilson disease), and degenerative joint disease (Table 15.3). *Calcium pyrophosphate arthropathy* refers to CPPD crystal deposition disease affecting the joints and producing structural damage to the articular cartilage. It displays distinctive radiographic abnormalities such as narrowing of the joint space, subchondral sclerosis, and osteophytosis, similar to osteoarthritis. The *pseudogout syndrome* represents a condition in which symptoms such as acute pain is similar to those seen in gouty arthritis; however, it does not respond to the usual treatment (colchicine) for the latter disease.

Pathology

Calcium pyrophosphate crystals, the pathogens in pseudogout, range up to 10 μm in length. As in gout, many intracellular crystals are seen during an acute episode. The colors are usually but not always much less intense than urates; that is, they are weakly birefringent. Pyrophosphate crystals are generally chunkier and often show a line down the middle. The most common form of calcium pyrophosphate crystal is a rhomboid. Pyrophosphate crystals are positively birefringent in that they are blue when the longitudinal axis of the crystal is parallel to the slow vibrations axis of the red compensator and yellow when it is perpendicular. Pathologic findings consist of punctate or linear calcium deposits, usually in the hyaline cartilage paralleling the subchondral bone end plate, also referred to as a *subchondral* or *articular cortex* (Fig. 15.41). Pyrophosphate crystals also commonly are found in fibrocartilaginous tissue, such as knee joint menisci (see Fig. 12.31). Punctate calcifications may also be seen in synovial tissue. On microscopic examination, the chalky-white deposits appear either crystalline or amorphous. In the vascularized tissue, there is associated inflammatory infiltrate that includes monophages and phagocytic polykaryons. In nonvascularized tissue, no inflammatory reaction is present. The pyrophosphate crystals are distinguished from urate crystals by their rhomboid shape and by their weakly positive birefringence (see prior text).

TABLE 15.3 Most Common Causes of Chondrocalcinosis

Senescent (aging process)
Osteoarthritis
Posttraumatic
Calcium pyrophosphate arthropathy (CPPD crystal deposition disease)
Gout
Hemochromatosis
Hyperparathyroidism
Hypophosphatasia
Ochronosis
Oxalosis
Wilson disease
Acromegaly
Idiopathic

Data from Reeder MM, Felson B. *Gamuts in radiology*. Cincinnati, OH: Audiovisual Radiology of Cincinnati; 1975:D142–D143.

Imaging Features

The radiographic appearance of asymptomatic CPPD crystal deposition disease is merely marked by chondrocalcinosis (Fig. 15.42). The arthritic changes encountered in this condition are similar to those seen in osteoarthritis. Any joint in the body may be affected, including spine (see Fig. 15.50). The most common sites, however, are the knee (Figs. 15.43 to 15.45) and the wrist/hand (particularly the second and third metacarpophalangeal joints) (Figs. 15.46 and 15.47), but other joints, such as the elbow (Figs. 15.48 and 15.49), shoulder (see Fig. 15.42A), ankle, and hip, may also be affected. MRI demonstrates the calcium deposits in the articular cartilage because of the contrast between the high signal intensity of the cartilage and the low signal intensity of the calcium deposits (see Fig. 15.45A). The presence of large subchondral cysts associated degenerative changes in a non–weight-bearing joint should raise the suspicion of calcium pyrophosphate arthropathy (see Fig. 15.45B).

One of the complications of the wrist involvement is development of scapholunate advanced collapse (SLAC) deformity (see Fig. 15.46B). In the knee joint, typically, the femoropatellar joint compartment is affected to significantly greater degree than medial or lateral joint compartments (see Figs. 15.43B, 15.44B, and 15.45B). As mentioned in the prior text, CPPD crystal deposition disease is characterized by calcification of the articular cartilage and fibrocartilage; the tendons, ligaments, and joint capsule may exhibit calcifications as well (see Fig. 15.44).

Deposits of CPPD crystals in the spine are relatively rare. Clinically, patients complain of nonspecific back pain. The disease can manifest itself as calcium deposits in the periarticular capsular and ligamentous soft tissues of the apophyseal joints, retro-odontoid mass-like calcium deposits (crowned dens syndrome), and diskitis-like changes simulating septic diskitis (Fig. 15.50).

Differential Diagnosis

Differential diagnosis of CPPD crystal deposition disease arthropathy should include osteoarthritis and neuropathic arthropathy, and if the second and third metacarpophalangeal joints are affected, hemochromatosis and acromegalic arthropathy should be additional considerations.

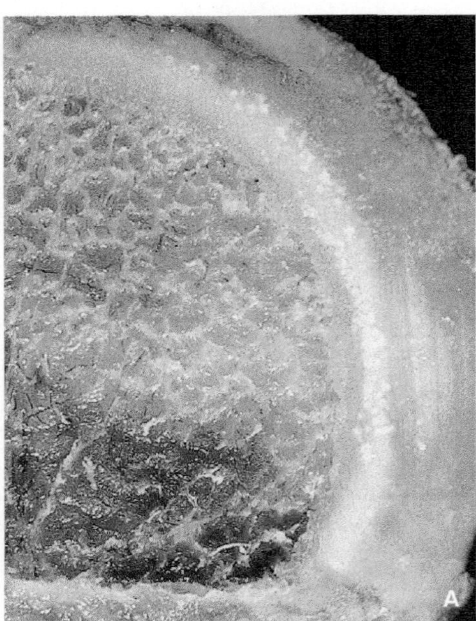
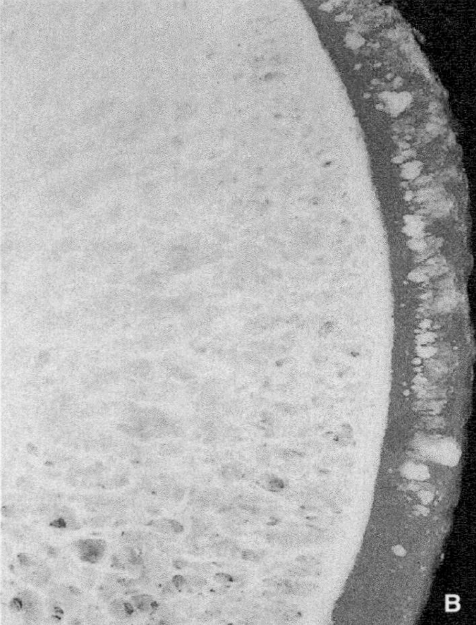
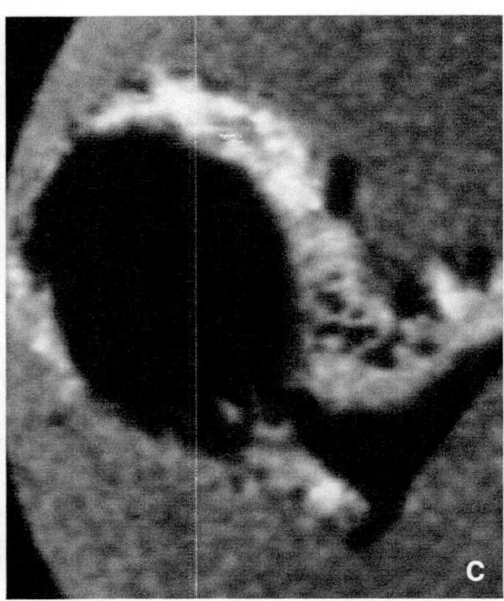

FIGURE 15.41 Pathology of CPPD crystal deposition disease. **(A)** Sagittal section of the femoral head shows chalky-white deposits of CPPD within the articular cartilage. **(B)** Radiograph of the specimen clearly demonstrates the calcific nature of the deposit. (Reprinted with permission from Vigorita VJ. *Orthopaedic pathology*. Philadelphia: Wolters Kluwer Health; 2015, Figure 15.22D). **(C)** Gradient recalled echo (GRE) MR image of the knee specimen shows multiple punctate low–signal intensity calcium deposits within the articular cartilage.

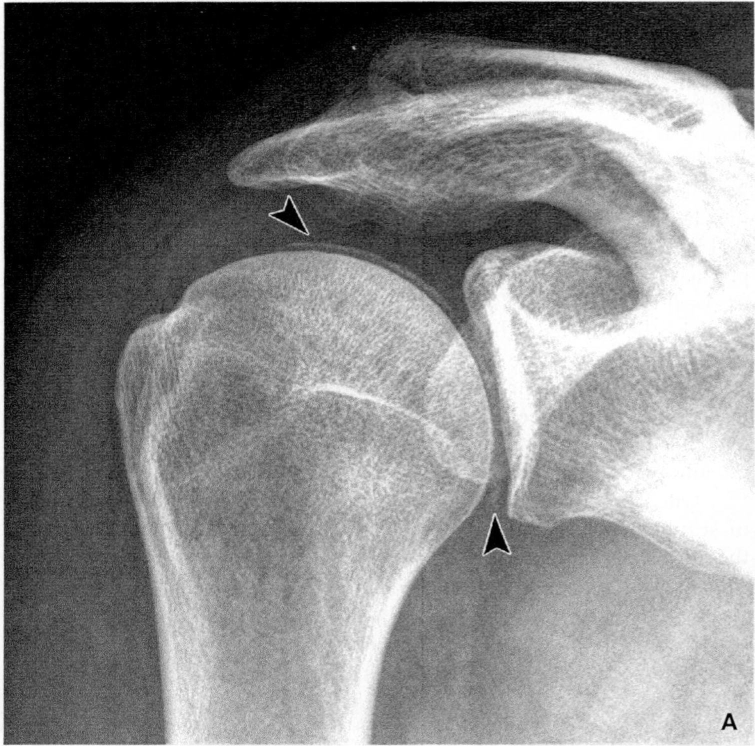
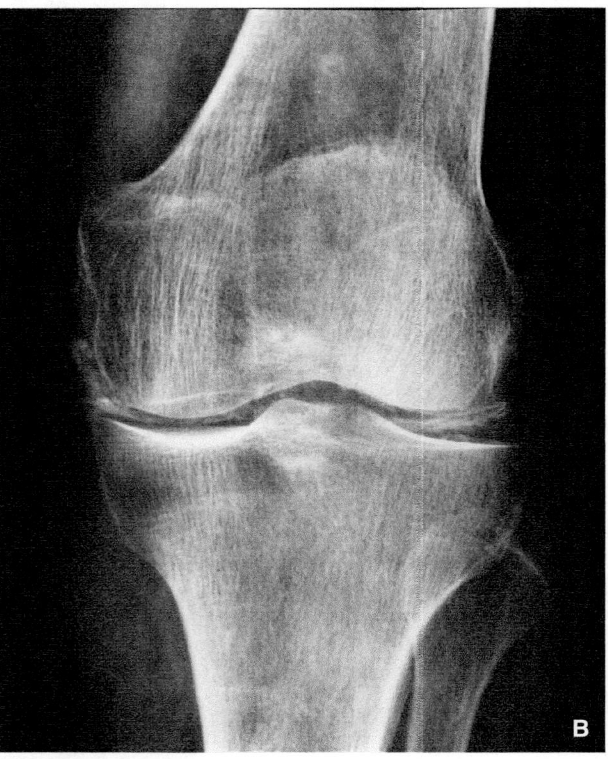
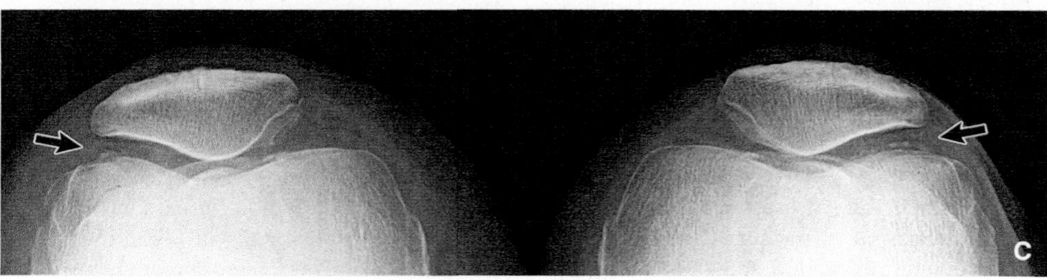

FIGURE 15.42 CPPD crystal deposition disease. One of the hallmarks of this condition is chondrocalcinosis as shown on this **(A)** Grashey view of the right shoulder of a 32-year-old within the hyaline cartilage of the humeral head *(arrowheads)*, **(B)** anteroposterior radiograph of the left knee of a 51-year-old man within the medial and lateral menisci, and **(C)** Merchant view of the knees of a 40-year-old woman, within the hyaline cartilage of the patellae *(arrowheads)*.

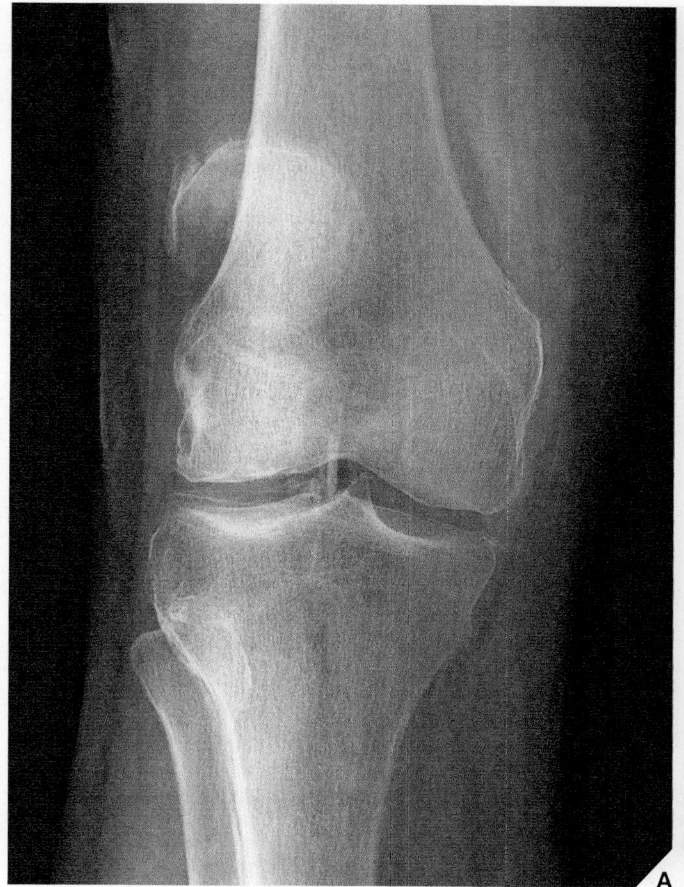

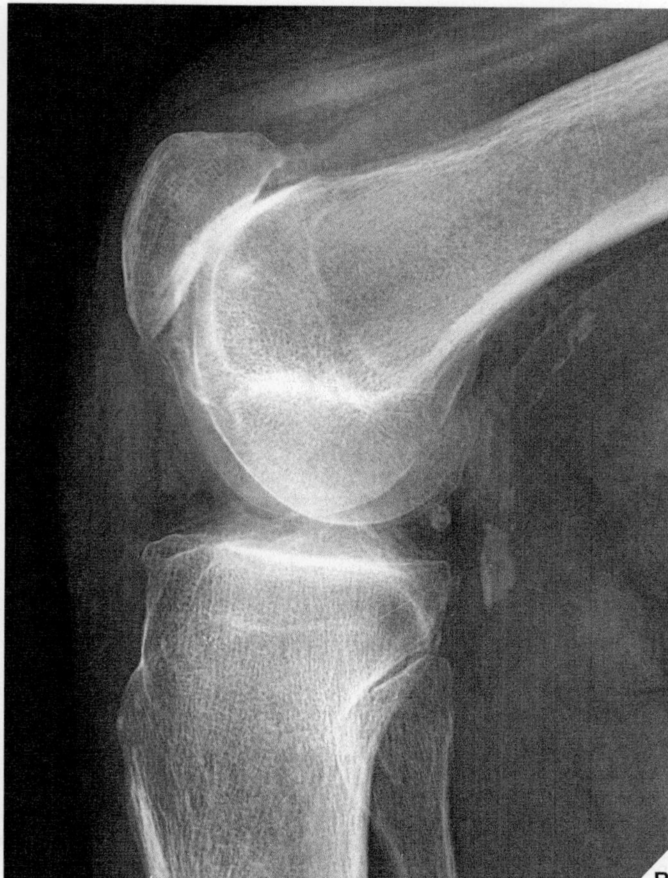

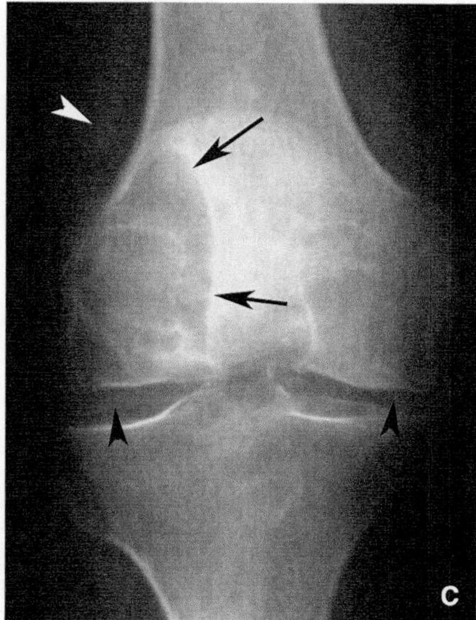

FIGURE 15.43 CPPD crystal deposition disease. **(A)** Anteroposterior and **(B)** lateral radiographs of the right knee of a 58-year-old woman, whose knee joint aspiration revealed calcium pyrophosphate crystals, show chondrocalcinosis and marked narrowing of the femoropatellar joint. **(C)** Anteroposterior radiograph of the right knee in another patient with intermittent knee pain and swelling demonstrates chondrocalcinosis of the menisci, articular cartilage, and joint capsule *(arrowheads)*, with a large subchondral cyst in the lateral femoral condyle *(arrows)*.

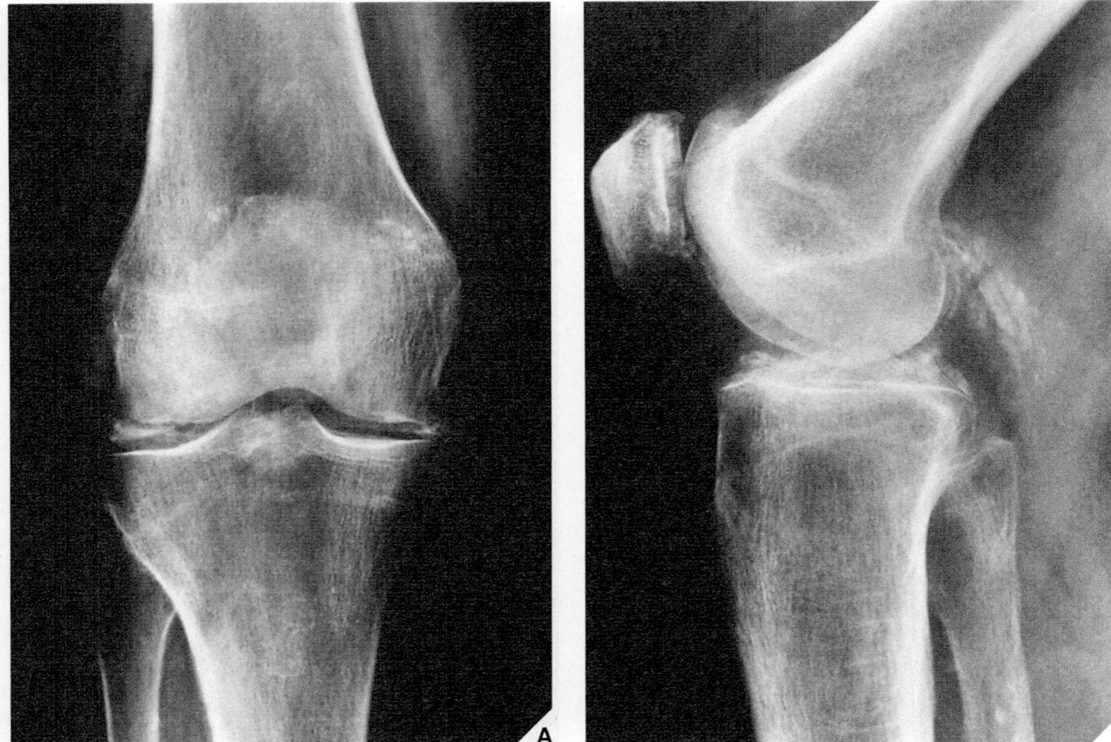

FIGURE 15.44 CPPD crystal deposition disease. A 70-year-old woman presented with acute onset of pain in her right knee and was treated with colchicine for acute gouty arthritis without relief of her pain. Synovial fluid yielded calcium pyrophosphate crystals. **(A)** Anteroposterior and **(B)** lateral radiographs of the knee demonstrate calcification of the hyaline and fibrocartilage. Capsular calcifications are also apparent, as well as narrowing of the femoropatellar joint compartment, a characteristic feature of CPPD crystal deposition disease.

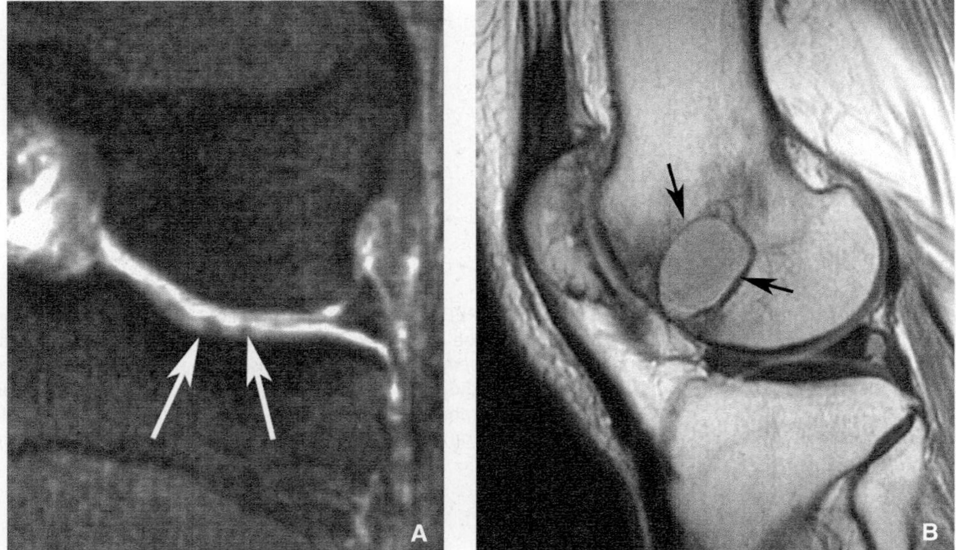

FIGURE 15.45 MRI of CPPD crystal deposition disease. **(A)** Coronal gradient recalled echo (GRE) MR image of the knee shows areas of low signal intensity *(arrows)* within the hyperintense articular cartilage, representing chondrocalcinosis. **(B)** Sagittal proton density–weighted MRI in another patient with symptoms of pseudogout demonstrates a large subchondral cyst in the lateral femoral condyle *(arrows)* and severe arthrosis of the femoropatellar joint.

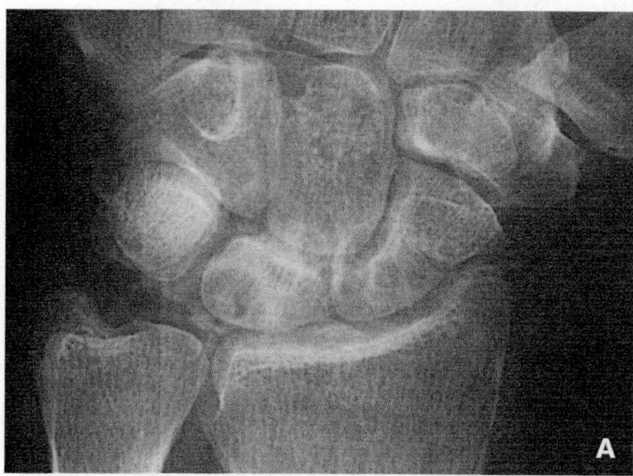

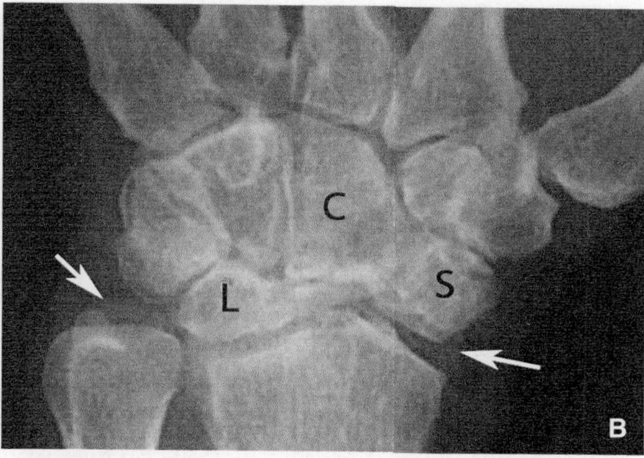

FIGURE 15.46 CPPD crystal deposition disease. **(A)** A 63-year-old man presented with an acute onset of pain in the wrist. A dorsovolar radiograph shows chondrocalcinosis of the triangular fibrocartilage, cystic changes in the scaphoid and lunate, and narrowing of the radiocarpal joint. **(B)** Dorsovolar radiograph of the right wrist in another patient with long-term history of intermittent pain and swelling demonstrates SLAC with the proximal migration of the capitate bone *(C)* wedged between the lunate *(L)* and scaphoid *(S)*. Note the presence of chondrocalcinosis in the triangular fibrocartilage complex and articular cartilage *(arrows)*.

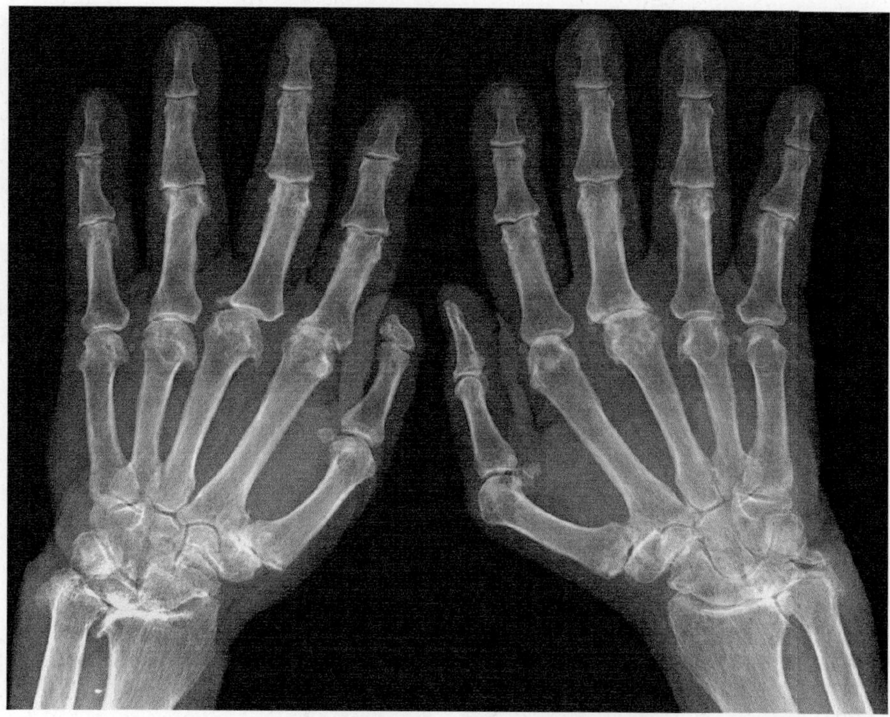

FIGURE 15.47 CPPD crystal deposition disease. Dorsovolar radiograph of both hands of a 60-year-old man shows typical for this condition arthropathy of the radiocarpal, metacarpophalangeal, and proximal interphalangeal joints.

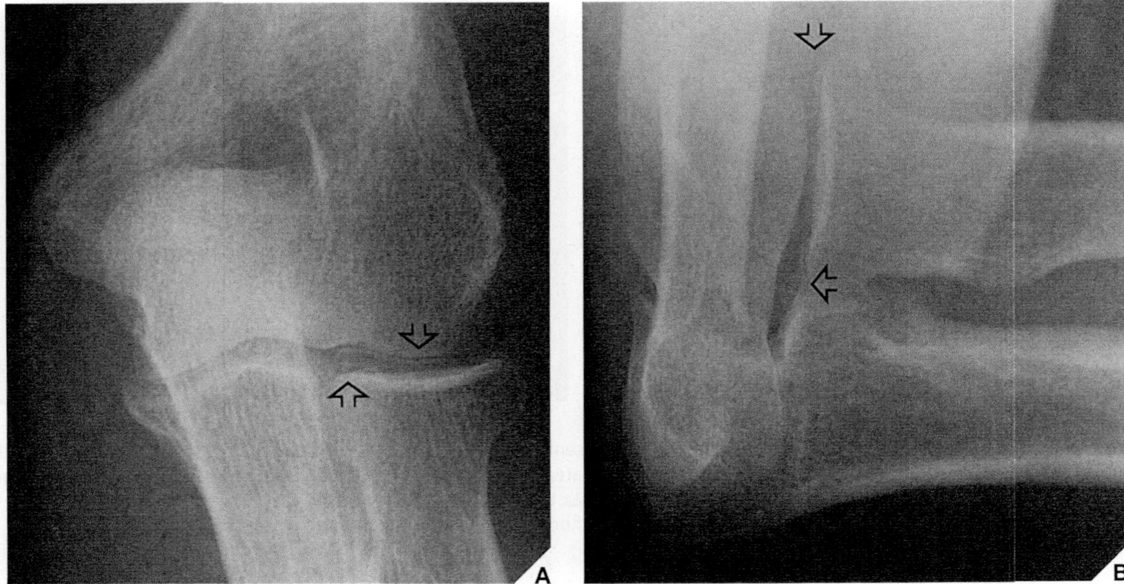

FIGURE 15.48 CPPD crystal deposition disease. **(A)** Anteroposterior and **(B)** radial head–capitellum views of the right elbow of a 52-year-old woman with pseudogout syndrome demonstrate chondrocalcinosis *(open arrows)* but no other alterations of the joint space.

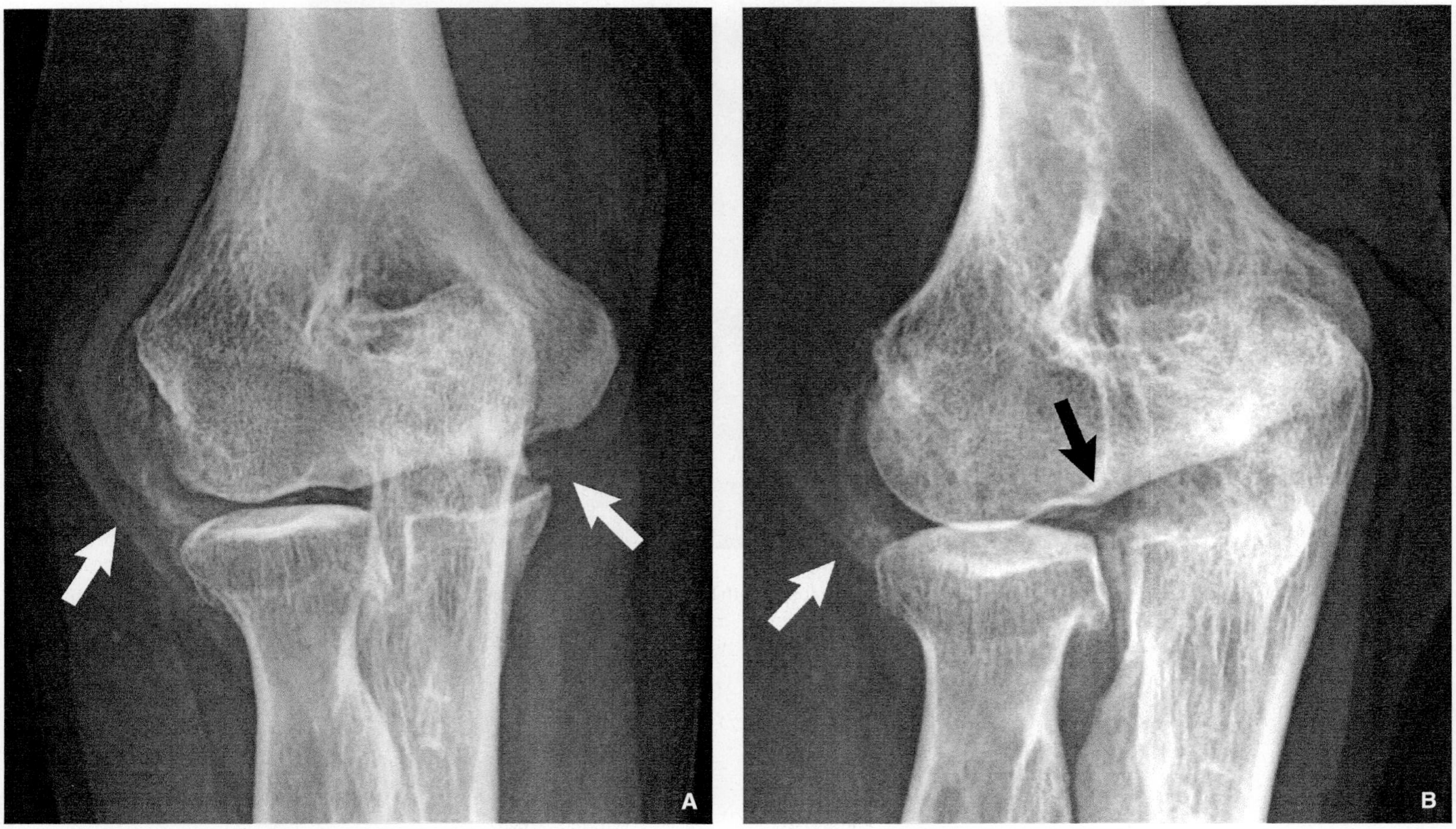

FIGURE 15.49 CPPD crystal deposition disease. **(A)** Anteroposterior and **(B)** external oblique radiographs of the right elbow of a 57-year-old man, in addition to extensive chondrocalcinosis *(arrows)* demonstrate also early osteoarthritic-like changes of the radiocapitellar joint.

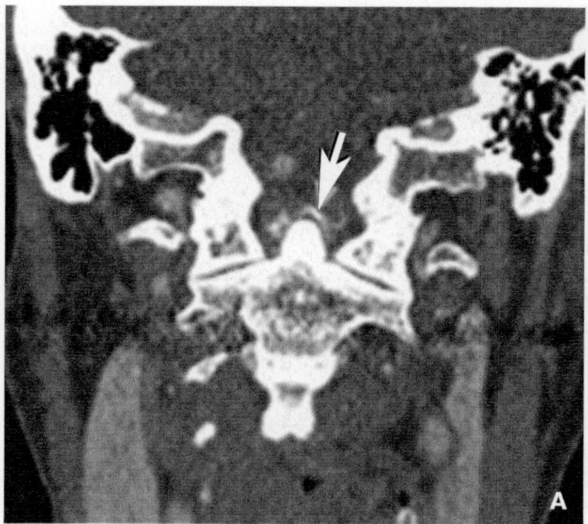

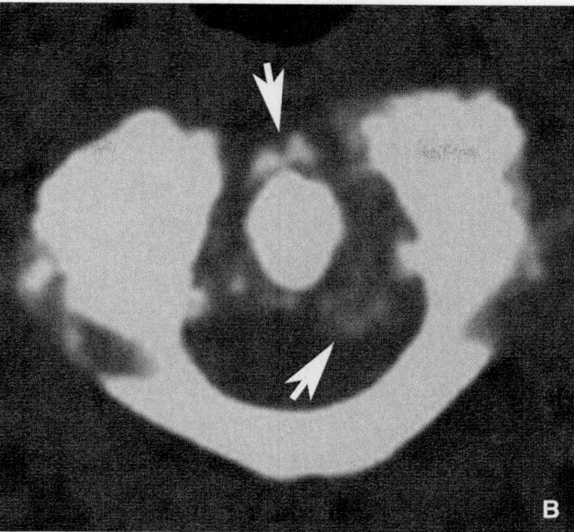

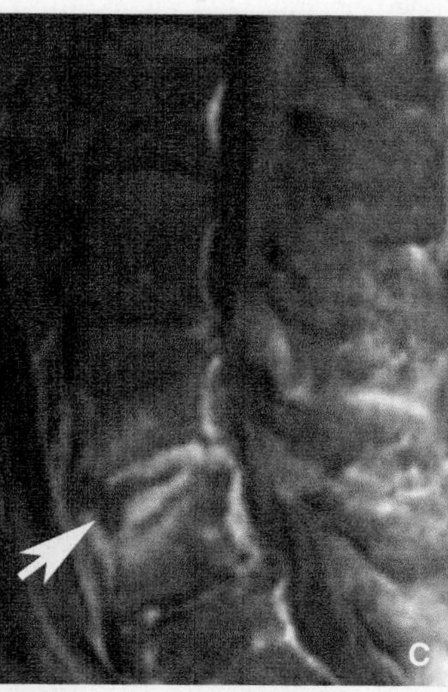

FIGURE 15.50 CPPD crystal deposition disease of the spine. (A) Coronal reformatted CT image demonstrates CPPD adjacent to the tip of the odontoid process (crowned dens) *(arrow)*. **(B)** Axial CT image shows mass-like retro-odontoid and preodontoid pyrophosphate crystal deposits *(arrows)*. **(C)** Sagittal T1-weighted fat-saturated MR image of the lumbar spine obtained after intravenous injection of gadolinium demonstrates erosion of the superior end plate of L4 and enhancing edematous changes in the corresponding end plates and margins of the intervertebral disk simulating infectious diskitis *(arrow)*.

Rarely, CPPD deposits can assume the form of bulky tumor-like masses located in the joint and paraarticular soft tissues (Fig. 15.51). In these instances, it may mimic a malignant tumor; hence, this form of CPPD deposition was termed by Sissons and associates, *tumoral calcium pyrophosphate deposition disease.* The mineral deposits are associated with a tissue reaction characterized by the presence of histiocytes and multinucleated giant cells, sometimes with bone and cartilage formation. The differential diagnosis should include tumoral calcinosis, a disorder characterized by the presence of single or multiple lobulated cystic masses in the soft tissues, usually near the major joints, containing chalky material consisting of calcium phosphate, calcium carbonate, or hydroxyapatite. The calcified deposits fail to show a crystalline appearance when examined by polarization microscopy. In this condition, the masses are painless and usually occur in children and adolescents, a majority of whom are black.

Fragmentation and bone resorption in the absence of peripheral neuropathy simulating Charcot neuroarthropathy is an unusual manifestation of pyrophosphate arthropathy and thus called *pseudoneuroarthropathy* (Fig. 15.52).

Calcium Hydroxyapatite Crystal Deposition Disease

Clinical Features

Resulting from abnormal deposition of calcium hydroxyapatite (CHA) crystals in and around the joints, CHA crystal deposition disease is more common in women and may at times simulate gout or pseudogout syndrome. Acute symptoms include pain, tenderness on palpation, and local swelling and edema. The syndrome may be associated with other disorders, such as scleroderma, dermatomyositis, MCTD, and chronic renal disease, particularly one treated by hemodialysis. Recent investigations suggested a genetic predisposition for this condition. Amor and associates raised the possibility of an inherited defect that might be responsible for the development of CHA crystal deposition disease by demonstrating an increased prevalence of the histocompatibility antigen of HLA-A2 and HLA-BW35 in patients affected by this disorder.

CHA crystals are most frequently deposited in periarticular locations, usually in and around tendons, joint capsule, or bursae. This is the feature that distinguishes the syndrome from CPPD crystal deposition disease, which affects primarily hyaline cartilage and fibrocartilage.

Although laboratory findings are usually normal, CHA crystal deposition disease may occasionally cause fever, elevated concentration of C-reactive protein, and elevated erythrocyte sedimentation rate (ESR).

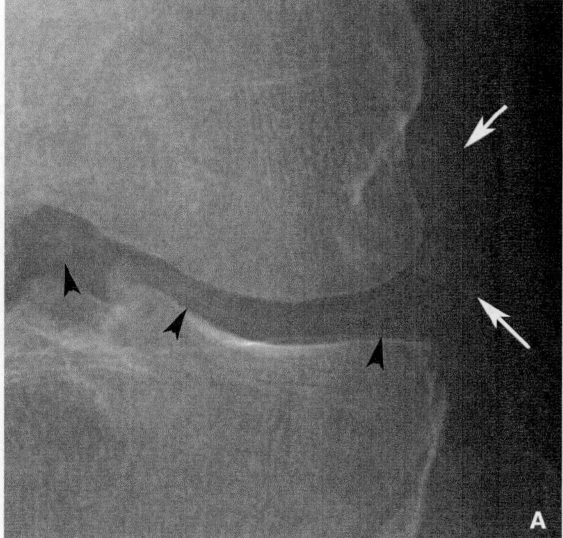

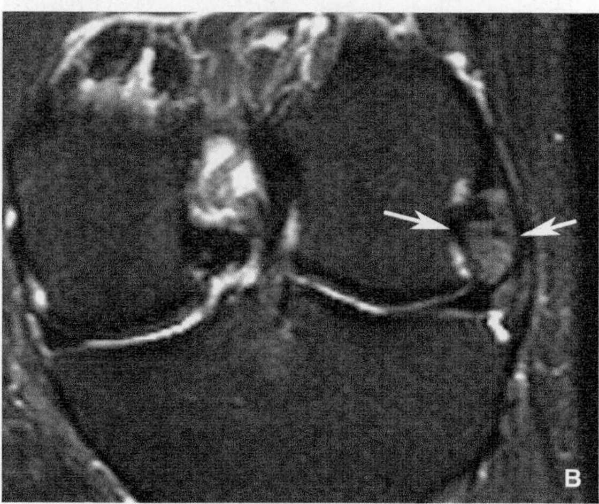

FIGURE 15.51 Tumoral CPPD crystal deposition disease. (A) Anteroposterior radiograph of the left knee demonstrates classic chondrocalcinosis *(arrowheads)* and a calcified mass in the lateral aspect of the joint *(arrows)*. **(B)** Coronal T2-weighted fat-saturated MR image shows the lateral mass to be hypointense *(arrows)*, consistent with the tumoral form of CPPD crystal deposition disease.

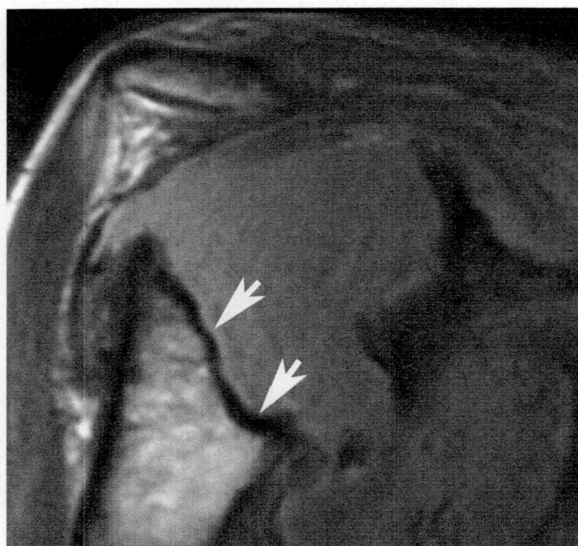

FIGURE 15.52 Pseudoneuroarthropathy of CPPD crystal deposition disease. Coronal proton density–weighted MR image in a patient with chronic intermittent right shoulder pain demonstrates complete bone resorption of the humeral head and glenoid *(arrows)* with fluid filling the large glenohumeral joint space. Joint aspiration revealed pyrophosphate crystals. In the absence of neuropathy, these findings are consistent with pseudoneuroarthropathy.

Imaging Features

Radiographic features depend on the site of involvement, but usually cloud-like or dense homogeneous calcific deposits are seen around the joint and tendons. The most common location is around the shoulder joint at the site of the supraspinatus tendon (Fig. 15.53). At this location, it is commonly referred to as *calcific peritendinitis or tendinitis* (tendinosis or tendinopathy). The MRI manifestations of calcific peritendinitis include low–signal intensity deposits adjacent to the tendon with marked inflammatory reaction (Fig. 15.54A,B). Calcific deposits can migrate into the adjacent bone, into the adjacent bursa, or into the tendon extending along the myotendinous plane (Fig. 15.54C,D).

Treatment

Treatment of this condition includes application of shockwave therapy (using sound waves), acetic acid iontophoresis, and drugs such as corticosteroids and cimetidine. Occasionally, arthroscopic or open shoulder surgery is required to remove the calcific deposits.

Hemochromatosis

Clinical Features

Hemochromatosis is a rare autosomal recessive disorder of iron metabolism, characterized by increased intestinal absorption of iron from a normal diet and presenting with iron deposition in various organs, particularly the liver, skin, and pancreas. It may be primary (endogenous or idiopathic), caused by an error in metabolizing iron, or secondary, caused by iron overload. Idiopathic hemochromatosis, with a prevalence of about 4 cases per 1,000 in Europe and North America, may be familial and has been linked with histocompatibility antigens HLA-A3 (placing the gene on the short arm of chromosome 6), HLA-B7, and HLA-B14. The newest studies using a positional cloning technique discovered a novel MHC class 1–type gene, originally called *HLA-H*, and now termed *HFE*, containing two missense mutations C282Y and H63D.

In the classical form of the disease, cysteine in substituted by tyrosine at amino acid 282 in both alleles. The so-called *compound heterozygote* is less common (representing about 10% of cases) but is also compatible with hereditary hemochromatosis. In this form, histidine is substituted by aspartic acid at amino acid 63 in one allele and cysteine by tyrosine at amino acid 282 in the other (C282Y/H63D). More recently, additional mutations in other molecules involved in iron metabolism, including hepcidin, hemojuvelin, and ferroportin, have been identified.

The secondary form of hemochromatosis is related to iron overload (such as transfusions or dietary intake) and may be associated with alcohol abuse. Hemochromatosis affects men 10 times more frequently than women. It is generally diagnosed between the ages of 40 and 60 years on the basis of markedly elevated serum iron levels. For confirmation, biopsy of the liver or synovium may be performed. Fifty percent of patients with hemochromatosis will have a slowly progressing arthritis, starting in the small joints of the hands, but eventually, the large joints and intervertebral disks in the cervical and lumbar region may become affected. Some investigators believe that the arthropathy seen in this condition differs from

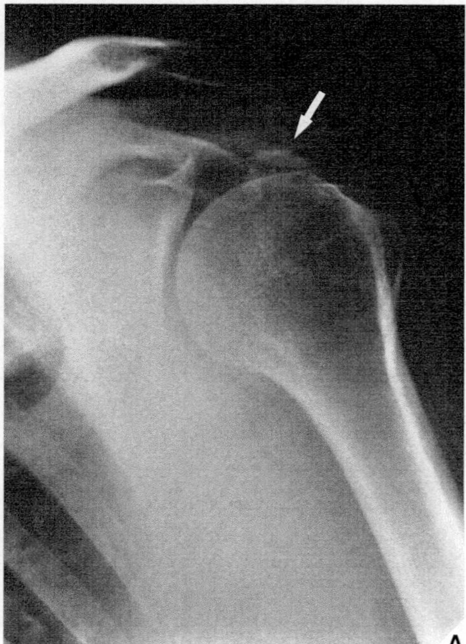

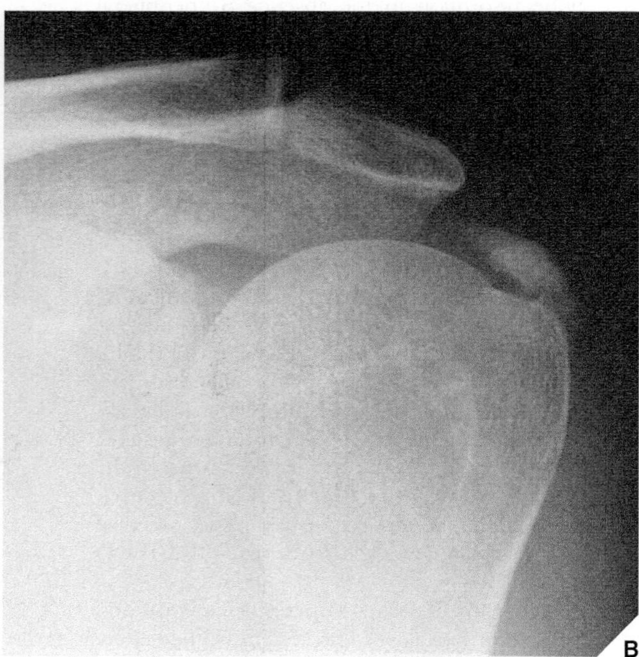

FIGURE 15.53 CHA crystal deposition disease. **(A)** Anteroposterior radiograph of the left shoulder of a 50-year-old woman who had been experiencing pain in this region for several months demonstrates an amorphous, homogenous calcific deposit in the soft tissues at the site of supraspinatus tendon *(arrow)*. This finding is typical of CHA crystal deposition disease. **(B)** In another patient, a 38-year-old woman who presented with left shoulder pain, a similar calcific deposit is seen at the site of insertion of the supraspinatus tendon to the greater tuberosity of the humerus.

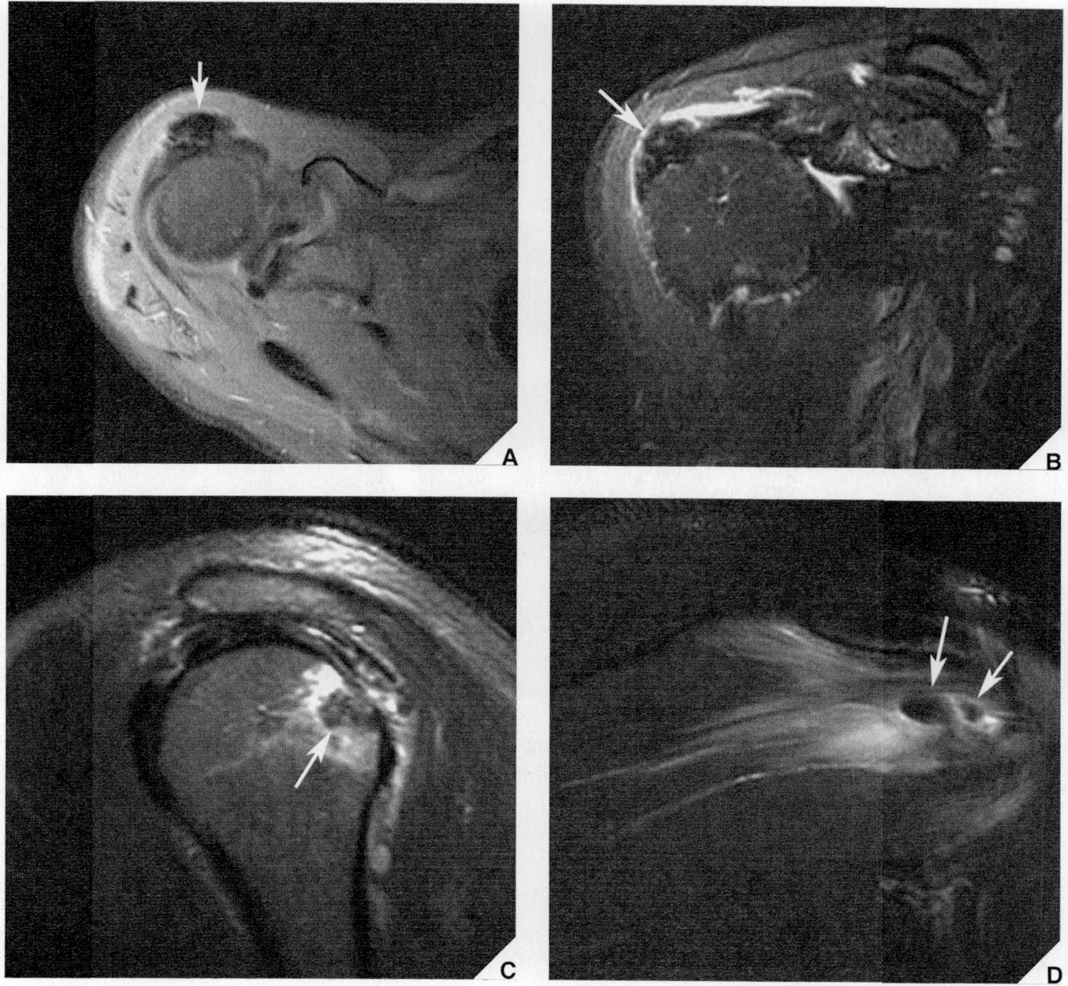

FIGURE 15.54 **MRI of CHA crystal deposition disease. (A)** Axial proton density–weighted fat-saturated MRI of the shoulder demonstrates low-signal intensity calcium deposit adjacent to the supraspinatus tendon *(arrow)*. **(B)** Coronal oblique T2-weighted MRI of the same patient shows the hypointense calcific deposit *(arrow)* with surrounding inflammatory changes and subacromial–subdeltoid bursitis. **(C)** Sagittal oblique T2-weighted MRI of the shoulder in another patient demonstrates intraosseous migration of the calcific deposits *(arrow)*. **(D)** Oblique coronal T2-weighted MRI of the shoulder in the same patient shows intramuscular migration of the calcific deposits *(arrows)*. Note the severe muscular inflammatory reaction.

typical degenerative joint disease and warrants classification in the group of metabolic arthritides.

Pathology

Pathologic findings include hemosiderin granules accumulation either in the synovioblasts or in the perivascular histiocytes. Occasionally, synovial villous hypertrophy may be present. Calcification may be seen within the fibrocartilage and hyaline cartilage (chondrocalcinosis). The explanation of the mechanism of this abnormality is based on the fact that ferric salts promote the formation and deposition of intraarticular calcium pyrophosphate crystals by inhibiting the activity of synovial pyrophosphates and decreasing the clearance of intraarticular immune complexes by inhibiting the activity of synovial reticuloendothelial cells.

Imaging Features

In the hand, the second and third metacarpophalangeal joints are characteristically affected (Figs. 15.55 and 15.56; see also Fig. 13.59), although other small joints such as the interphalangeal and carpal articulations may also be involved. Degenerative changes may also be seen in the shoulders, knees, hips (Fig. 15.57), and ankles. Loss of the articular space, eburnation, subchondral cyst formation, and osteophytosis are the most prominent radiographic features of hemochromatosis. The changes may occasionally mimic those seen in CPPD crystal deposition disease and rheumatoid arthritis. MRI has been used for detection and quantification of iron overload in the liver, spleen, and pancreas, as the strong paramagnetic properties of the stored iron cause a significant decrease in T2 relaxation times of the affected tissues. However, accumulation of iron in the synovium or in articular cartilage is less pronounced, unless gradient-echo sequences, which are more susceptible to the paramagnetic properties of iron, are used (Fig. 15.58). Nevertheless, magnetic resonance (MR) imaging may demonstrate abnormalities of the menisci and articular cartilage including erosive changes and cyst formation.

Treatment

The treatment of hemochromatosis consists of phlebotomy on a regular basis.

Early diagnosis is essential to positive results. Unfortunately, one survey of 2,851 patients with hemochromatosis showed that patients had consulted a physician after an average 2 years of symptoms, and on average, it took additional 10 years before the diagnosis was made.

Wilson Disease

Clinical Features

Known also as *hepatolenticular degeneration*, Wilson disease is a rare autosomal recessive inherited genetic disorder of copper metabolism. A defective *ATP7B* gene and related mutations has been mapped to chromosome 13 (13q14.3). The gene encodes intracellular copper-transporting P-type ATPase that transports copper into bile and incorporates it into ceruloplasmin, a 132-kDa protein produced by the liver. The condition is

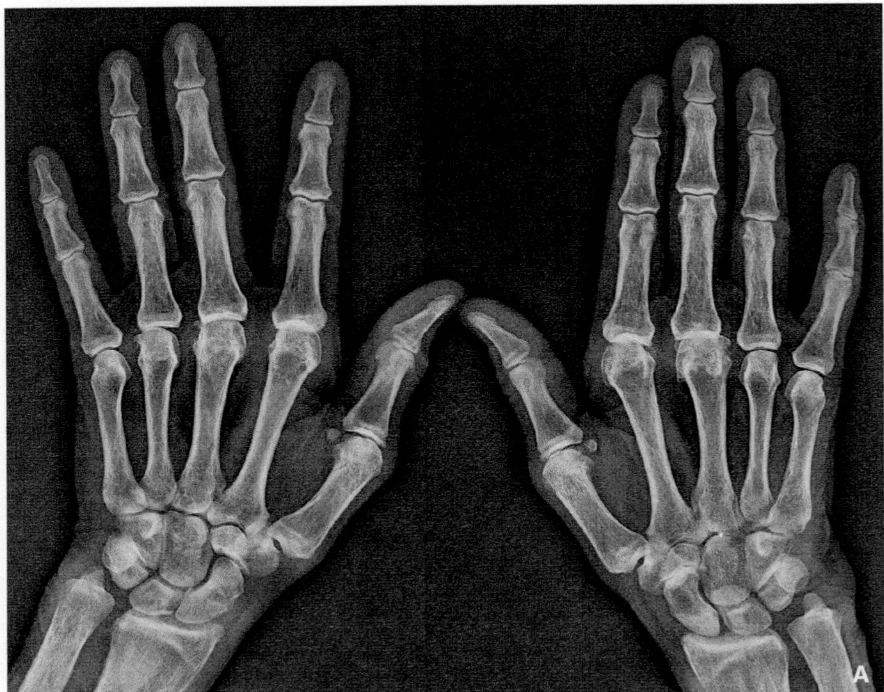

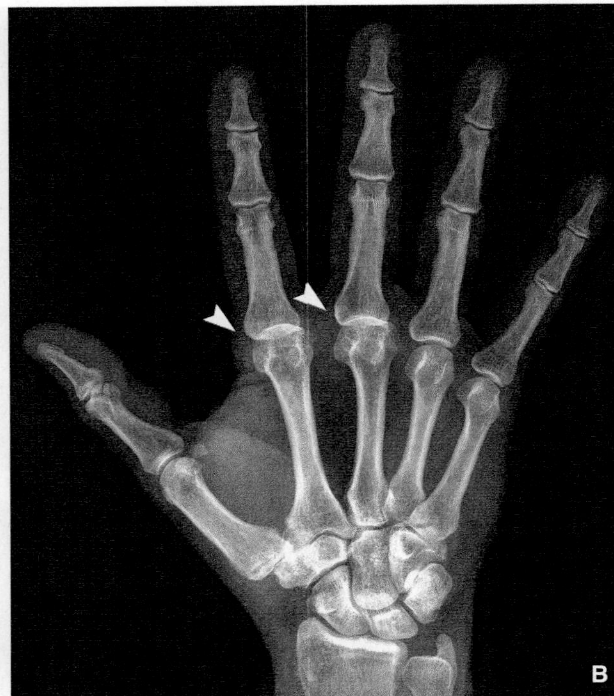

FIGURE 15.55 **Hemochromatosis arthropathy.** **(A)** Dorsovolar radiograph of the hands of a 50-year-old man shows characteristic involvement of the second and third metacarpophalangeal joints. **(B)** In another patient, a 41-year-old man, observe arthropathy of the second and third metacarpophalangeal joints of the left hand *(arrowheads)*.

more common in men than in women. It is characterized by degenerative changes in the brain (basal ganglia), cirrhosis of the liver, and pathognomonic Kayser-Fleischer rings of greenish-brown pigment deposited in the Descemet membrane in the limbus of the cornea. The clinical symptoms result from accumulation of copper in the body, particularly in the liver and brain. Increased amount of copper within the liver overwhelms the proteins that normally bind it, causing oxidative damage through the process known as *Fenton chemistry* (or *Fenton reaction*). This damage eventually leads to chronic hepatitis, fibrosis, and liver cirrhosis. Lenticular degeneration leads to neurologic symptoms, including tremor, rigidity, dysarthria, and dyscoordination. Articular abnormalities may be present in about 50% of affected adults. The affected joints include those of the hand, wrist, elbow, shoulder, hip, and knee. Light and electron microscopy failed to detect crystal-containing calcium neither in synovial fluid nor in synovial biopsies. Synovial biopsies showed hyperplasia of synovial lining cells with mild inflammatory response. In the serum, levels of copper and copper-binding protein ceruloplasmin are decreased, and urinary copper excretion is increased. Electron microscopic detection of copper-containing hepatocytic lysosomes, in addition to the quantification of hepatic copper by atomic absorption spectrophotometry, is helpful in the diagnosis of the early stages of Wilson disease.

Imaging Features

Subchondral bone fragmentation, cyst formation, cortical irregularities and sclerosis, and joint narrowing have been described in the literature. The imaging findings resemble those present in CPPD crystal deposition

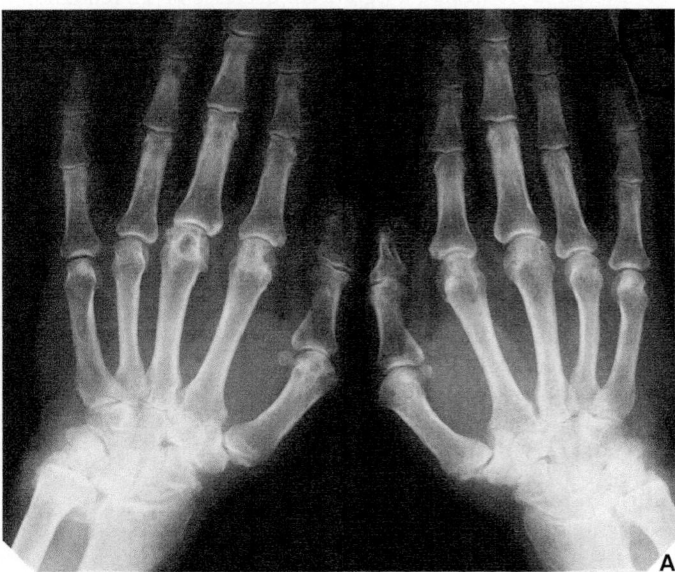

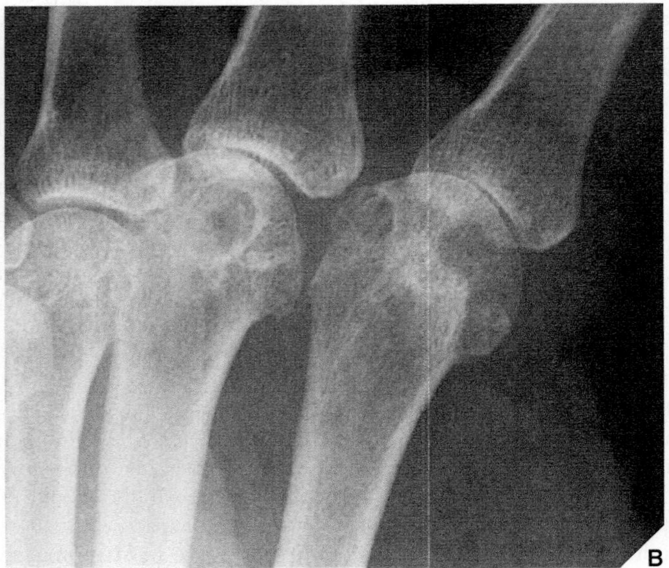

FIGURE 15.56 **Hemochromatosis arthropathy.** **(A)** Dorsovolar radiograph of both hands of a 45-year-old man shows typical abnormalities of hemochromatosis predominantly affecting wrists and metacarpophalangeal joints. **(B)** Coned-down magnified radiograph of the second and third metacarpophalangeal joints of the right hand demonstrates characteristic involvement of the metacarpal heads.

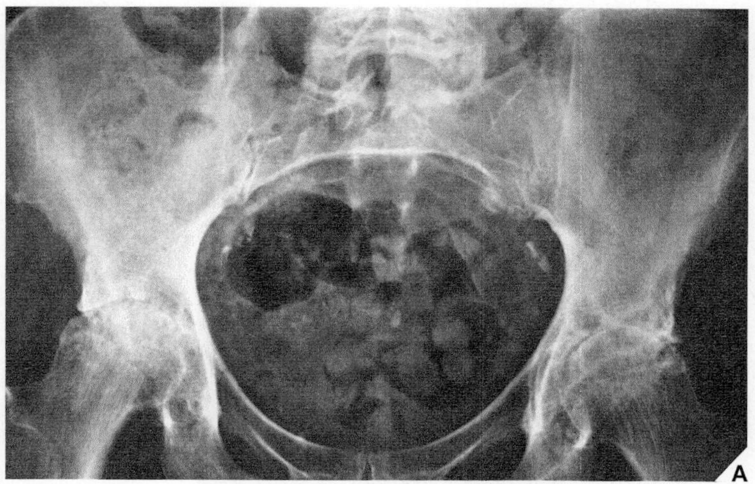

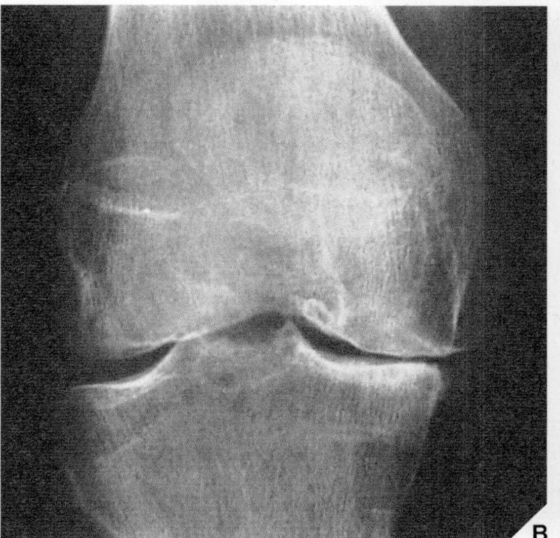

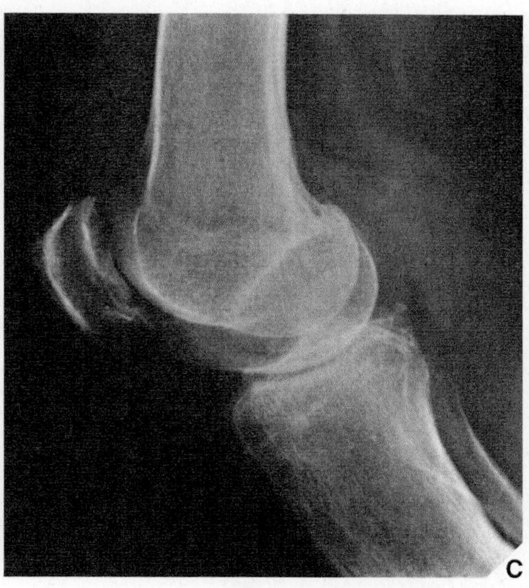

FIGURE 15.57 Hemochromatosis arthropathy. A 67-year-old woman was diagnosed with hemochromatosis arthropathy. **(A)** Anteroposterior radiograph of the pelvis shows advanced arthritis of both hip joints. Severe concentric narrowing of joint space, subchondral sclerosis, and periarticular cysts are typical of hemochromatosis. **(B)** Anteroposterior and **(C)** lateral radiographs of the right knee demonstrate predilection for medial and femoropatellar compartments. Joint space narrowing and marked subarticular sclerosis with small osteophyte formation are characteristic. (Reprinted with permission from Baker ND. Hemochromatosis. In: Taveras JM, Ferrucci JT, eds. *Radiology—diagnosis, imaging, intervention*. Philadelphia: JB Lippincott; 1986:1–6.)

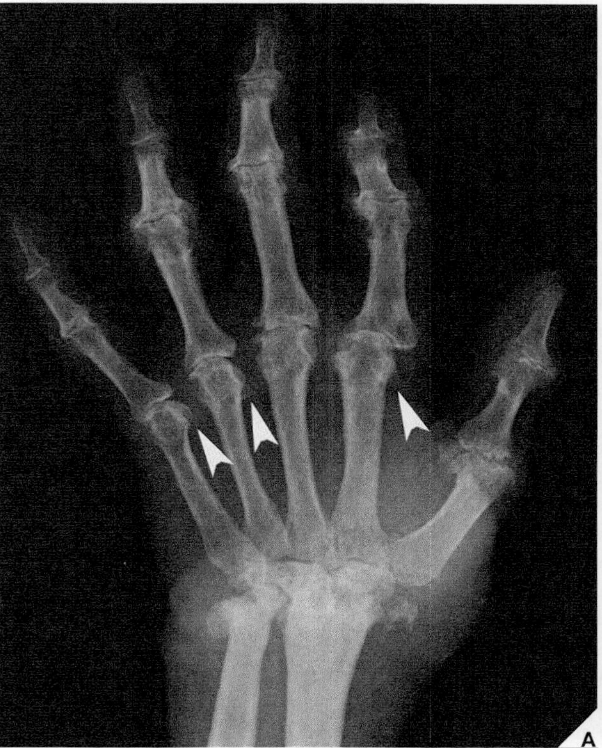

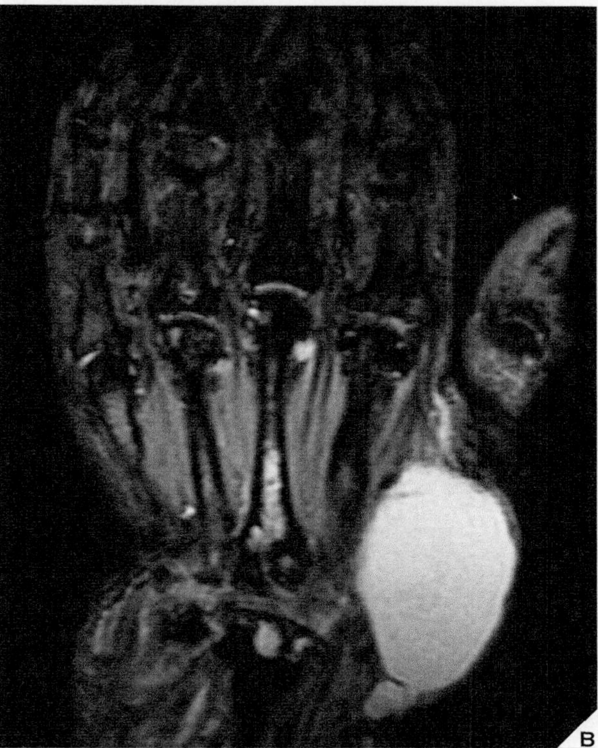

FIGURE 15.58 MRI of hemochromatosis arthropathy. (A) Dorsovolar radiograph of the hand of a patient with advanced arthropathy due to hemochromatosis shows the characteristic "hooks" of the heads of the metacarpals *(arrowheads)*. **(B)** Coronal gradient recalled echo (GRE) MRI demonstrates the multiple erosions of the distal radius, metacarpals and phalanges, and the secondary severe degenerative arthropathy. The patient also had a large ganglion cyst in the radial aspect of the wrist.

disease and hemochromatosis. Articular cartilage calcifications may occur, but generally are rare.

Treatment

Copper-chelating agents such as trientine, zinc salt, and D-penicillamine along with dietary copper restriction are the treatment of choice. A diet low in copper-containing foods is recommended with avoidance of mushrooms, nuts, chocolate, dried fruit, liver, and shellfish.

Alkaptonuria (Ochronosis)

Clinical Features

Alkaptonuria is a rare autosomal recessive inherited disease characterized by the presence of homogentisic acid in the urine that turns black when oxidized (Fig. 15.59). This metabolic abnormality results from the absence of the enzyme homogentisic acid oxidase, which plays a part in the normal degradation process of the aromatic amino acids tyrosine and phenylalanine. As a consequence, there is significant accumulation of homogentisic acid in various organs, with predilection for connective tissues. The genetic defect is mapped to the *HGO* gene located on the arm of chromosome 3q1. The deposition of an abnormal brown-black pigment, a polymer of homogentisic acid, within the intervertebral disks and in the articular cartilage is termed *ochronosis* (Fig. 15.60). This deposition leads to spondylosis and peripheral arthropathy. As a rule, ochronotic arthropathy is a manifestation of long-standing alkaptonuria. The condition affects men and women equally and is more common in certain areas in Slovakia, Dominican Republic, Jordan, and India. In general, the affected individuals are asymptomatic until adult life, at which time ochronotic arthropathy may develop in the joints of the axial and appendicular skeleton. The clinical signs consist of mild pain and a decreased range of motion in various joints. When the spine is involved, back pain and stiffness are the usual symptoms. Nonarticular features of ochronosis include bluish discoloration and calcification of the ear pinnae, triangular pigmentation of the sclera, and pigmentation over the nose, axillae, and groins.

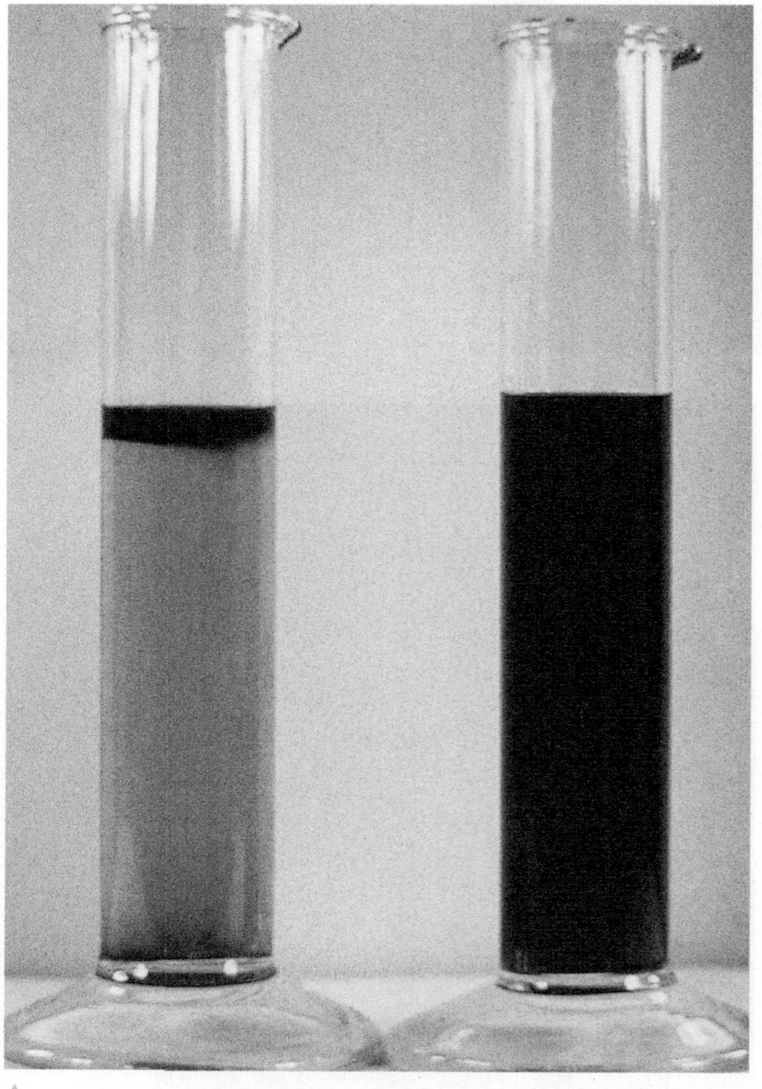

FIGURE 15.59 Alkaptonuria. Two flasks contain urine from a patient with ochronosis. In the flask on the left-hand side, the urine has been left to stand for 15 minutes. Some darkening is apparent on the surface due to oxidation of homogentisic acid. In the flask on the right, after 2 hours, the urine has become entirely black. (Reprinted with permission from Vigorita VJ. *Orthopaedic pathology*. Philadelphia: Wolters Kluwer Health; 2015, Figure 16.51A.)

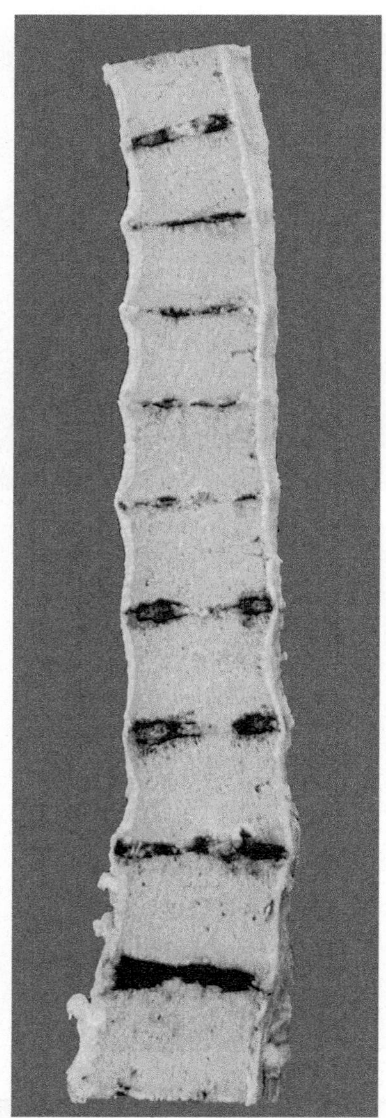

FIGURE 15.60 Pathology of ochronosis. Sagittally sectioned spine specimen shows black pigmentation within the narrowed intervertebral disks. (From Bullough PG, Boachie-Adjei O. *Atlas of spinal diseases*. New York: Gower Medical; 1988:75, Fig. 6.15.)

Imaging Features

The radiographic presentation includes dystrophic calcifications, most commonly in the intervertebral disks and the articular cartilage, tendons, and ligaments (Fig. 15.61). Osteoporosis is usually present. Disk spaces are narrowed, with occasional vacuum phenomena. The extraspinal abnormalities are limited to involvement of the sacroiliac joints, the symphysis pubis, and the large peripheral joints, which are likewise narrowed and show periarticular sclerosis with occasional small osteophytes. Tendinous calcifications and ossifications may occur, at times leading to tendon rupture.

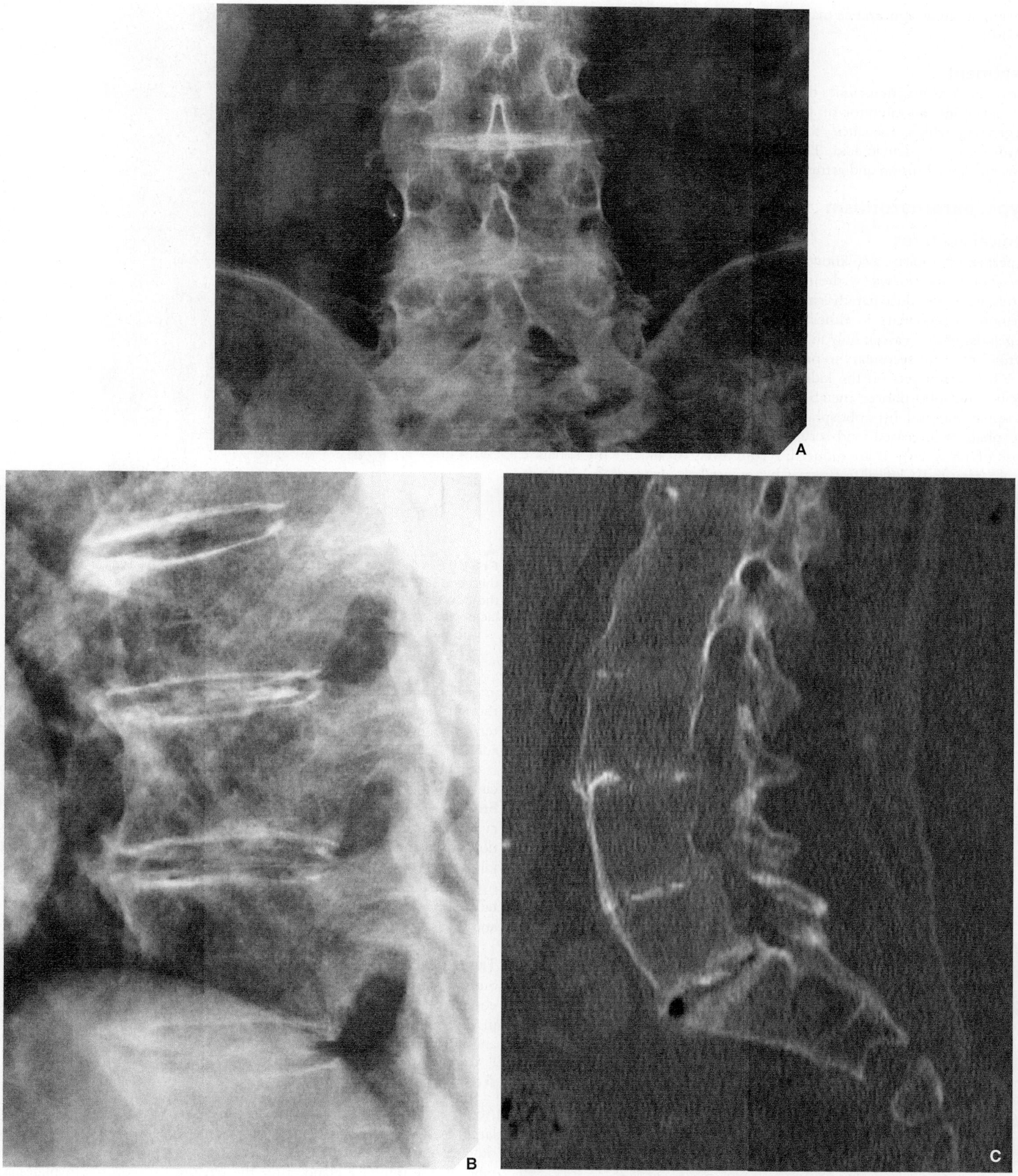

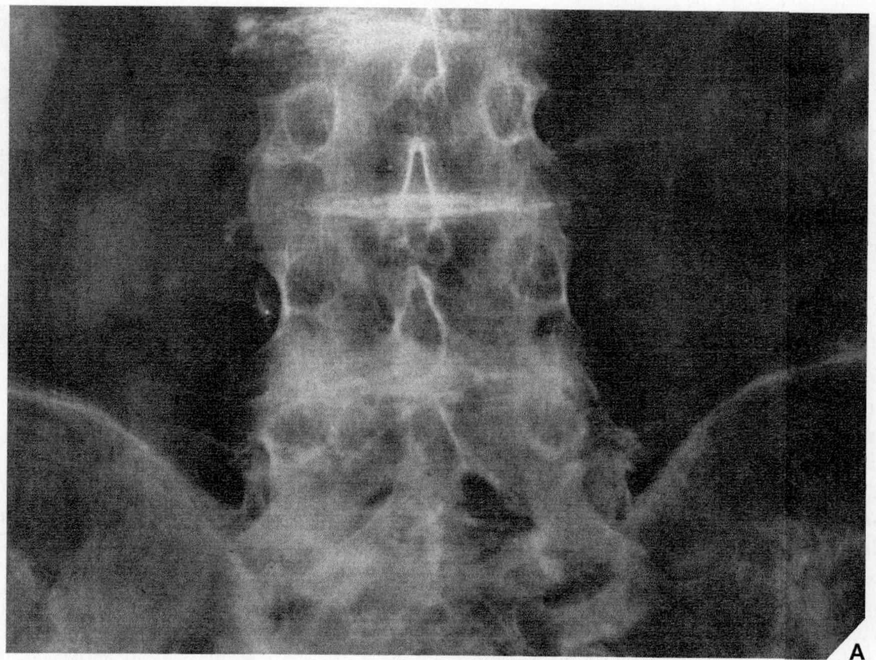

FIGURE 15.61 Ochronosis. **(A)** Anteroposterior radiograph of the lumbar spine and **(B)** lateral radiograph of the thoracic spine of a 64-year-old woman with a clinical diagnosis of alkaptonuria demonstrate narrowing of several intervertebral disk spaces associated with marginal anterior osteophytes and moderate osteoporosis. Characteristic calcifications of multiple intervertebral disks are a hallmark of ochronosis. (Courtesy of J. Tehranzadeh, MD, Orange, California.) **(C)** In another patient, a sagittal reformatted CT image shows disks calcification in the lower lumbar spine.

The radiographic appearance may mimic that of degenerative joint disease or CPPD.

Treatment

The medical treatment includes the high doses of ascorbic acid (vitamin C) and nitisinone, an inhibitor of the enzyme 4-hydroxyphenylpyruvate dioxygenase, which mediates formation of homogentisic acid from 4-hydroxyphenulpyruvic acid. The surgical intervention includes diskectomy and spinal fusion and arthroplasties of the affected joints.

Hyperparathyroidism

Clinical Features

Hyperparathyroidism, also known as *generalized osteitis fibrosa cystica* or *Recklinghausen disease of bone*, is the result of overactivity of the parathyroid glands, which produce parathormone (PTH). Increased production of this hormone is secondary to either adenoma (90% of cases) or hyperplasia of glands (9% of cases); only in very rare instances (1%) does hyperparathyroidism occur secondary to parathyroid carcinoma. Excessive secretion of PTH, which acts on the kidneys and bones, leads to disturbances in calcium and phosphorus metabolism, resulting in hypercalcemia, hyperphosphaturia, and hypophosphatemia. Renal excretion of calcium and phosphate is increased, and serum levels of calcium are elevated while those of phosphorous are reduced; serum levels of alkaline phosphatase are also elevated. Clinical features of hyperparathyroidism are usually fairly characteristic. Classic medical textbooks have described hyperparathyroidism as a disease of "stones and bones", in reference to nephrolithiasis and bone abnormalities encountered in this condition. Patient may present with kidney stones and bone pain, and occasionally with a pathologic fracture due to osteopenia (see also text in Chapter 28).

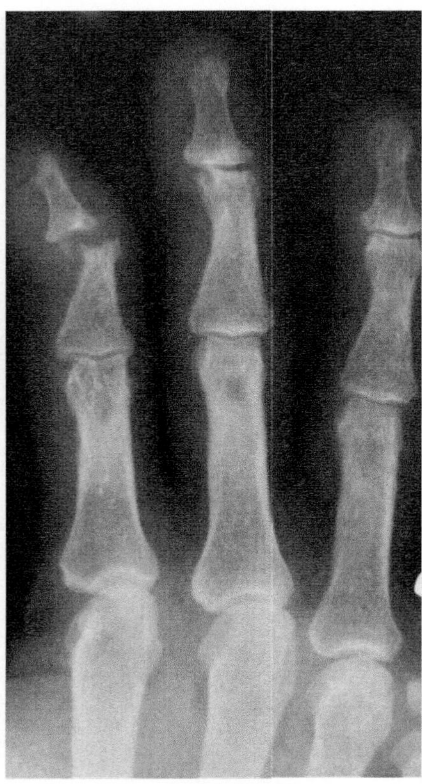

FIGURE 15.63 Hyperparathyroidism arthropathy. Typical abnormalities of this condition are manifested in this patient at the distal interphalangeal joints of the index and middle fingers. Note also beginning of the resorption of the distal tufts (acroosteolysis).

Pathology

Pathologic findings consist of ragging and scalloping of bone trabeculae and increased number of osteoclasts on the bone surfaces resulting in characteristic "tunneling" or "dissecting resorption" of trabeculae. In addition, noted is fibrovascular proliferation that displaces the bone marrow in a paratrabecular distribution. Other findings include increased amounts of woven bone, and marrow fibrosis, particularly abutting trabecular surfaces.

Imaging Features

One of the most characteristic features of hyperparathyroidism is subperiosteal and subchondral bone resorption that appears at the margins of certain joints, thus accounting for articular manifestation or "arthropathy" of hyperparathyroidism. This is frequently noted at the acromioclavicular joint, at the sternoclavicular and sacroiliac articulations (Fig. 15.62), at the symphysis pubis, and sometimes at the metacarpophalangeal and interphalangeal joints. The erosions can mimic rheumatoid arthritis, although they are usually asymptomatic, involve more commonly distal interphalangeal joints (Fig. 15.63), and almost invariably are associated with subperiosteal bone resorption, typical for hyperparathyroidism.

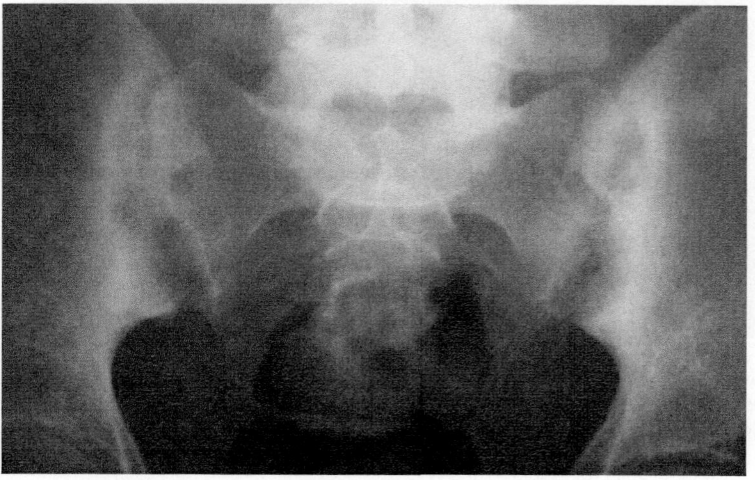

FIGURE 15.62 Hyperparathyroidism arthropathy. Subchondral resorption resulted in widening of the sacroiliac joints in this patient with hyperparathyroidism arthropathy.

The other feature of hyperparathyroidism arthropathy is chondrocalcinosis, which involves calcium deposition in the articular cartilage and fibrocartilage. This finding may mimic degenerative joint disease and CPPD crystal deposition arthropathy. It may be distinguished from the calcification of degenerative joint disease by the absence of arthritic changes in the joint and from CPPD crystal deposition arthropathy by the presence of osteopenia and other typical features of hyperparathyroidism. A more detailed description of hyperparathyroidism is provided in Part VI: Metabolic and Endocrine Disorders.

Treatment

Surgery, consisting of removal of the parathyroid gland/glands, is the most common treatment for primary hyperparathyroidism and provides a cure in about 95% of all cases. Medical treatment includes calcimimetic drugs and hormone replacement therapy.

Acromegaly

Acromegaly (from Greek *akros*—extreme or extremities, and *megalos*—large) is a syndrome resulting from the overproduction of growth hormone (somatotropin or HGH—human growth hormone) by the anterior lobe of the pituitary gland, after the closure of the growth plates. Degenerative joint changes in this condition are the result of hypertrophy of articular cartilage, which is not adequately nourished by synovial fluid because of its abnormal thickness.

After initial overgrowth of cartilage, as reflected by widening of the radiographic joint spaces in the hand, particularly at the metacarpophalangeal joints (Fig. 15.64), a later manifestation of this disorder is thinning of the joint cartilages with osteophyte formation caused by secondary osteoarthritis. Arthritis-like symptoms including pain and stiffness are

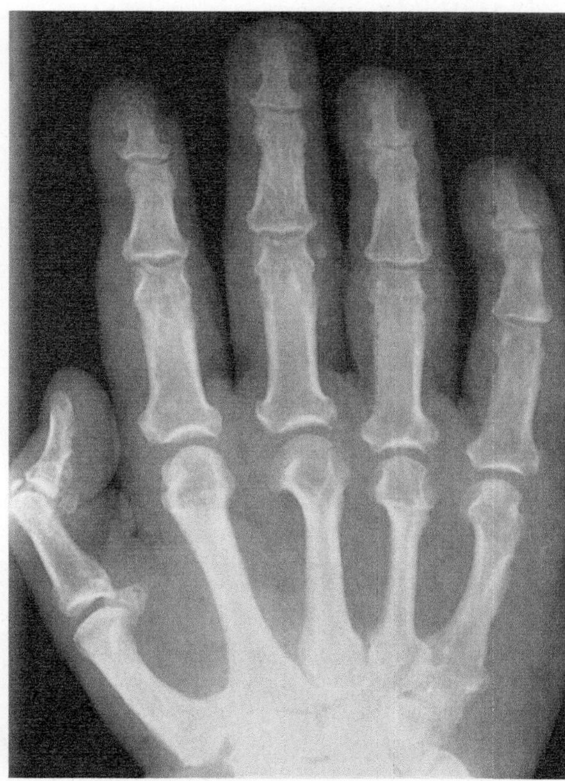

FIGURE 15.64 Acromegalic arthropathy. Characteristic abnormalities in acromegalic hand include prominence of the soft tissue, enlargement of the tufts and bases of the distal phalanges, widening of the metacarpophalangeal joints, and beak-like osteophytes at the radial aspect of the metacarpal heads. Note also markedly enlarged sesamoid bone at the first metacarpophalangeal joint.

common, and limitation of joint motion becomes apparent. Besides articulations of the hands, large joints such as the hip, knee, and even shoulder or elbow may be affected. In particular, beak-like osteophytes on the inferior aspect of the humeral head, the lateral aspect of the acetabulum, the superior margin of the symphysis pubis, and radial aspects of the heads of metacarpals are characteristic (see Fig. 13.58). Additional information is provided in Chapter 30.

Miscellaneous Conditions

Amyloidosis

Amyloidosis is a systematic disorder characterized by the infiltration of various organs by a homogeneous eosinophilic material consisting of protein fibers in a ground substance of mucopolysaccharides. There are three major types of systemic amyloidosis: (a) *primary amyloidosis*, the most common form, in which bone marrow produces too much of certain fragments of antibody protein, which builds up in the bloodstream and deposits in the body tissues; (b) *familial (hereditary) amyloidosis*, which is a genetic form, due to mutations in the gene *TTR*, inherited in autosomal dominant manner; and (c) *secondary amyloidosis*, which develops secondary to certain chronic conditions such as tuberculosis or rheumatoid arthritis. Amyloid arthropathy is a sign of acquired idiopathic systemic amyloidosis and is a condition that results in noninflammatory arthropathy.

Clinical Features

Clinically, amyloidosis bears a striking resemblance to rheumatoid arthritis because the joints are stiff and painful and the arthropathy is bilateral and symmetric. There is a predilection for large joints such as the hips, knees, shoulders, and elbows. Subcutaneous nodules are noted over the extensor surfaces of the forearm and dorsum of the hand, often mimicking the rheumatoid nodules. Another characteristic feature is the massive involvement of the soft tissues, giving the patient an almost pathognomonic appearance known as *shoulder-pad sign* or *football player shoulders*. Carpal tunnel syndrome is frequently an associated abnormality.

The bone abnormalities and arthropathy associated with deposition of B_2-microglobulin (B_2-MG) amyloid are well-recognized complications of long-term hemodialysis and chronic renal failure. B_2-MG, a low-molecular-weight serum protein, is not filtered by standard dialysis membranes. It therefore accumulates in the bones, joints, and soft tissues. Clinically, characteristic pain and decreased joint mobility occur in the shoulders, hips, and knees.

Pathology

All forms of amyloidosis are characterized pathologically by extracellular deposition of insoluble non–branching β-pleated protein fibrils formed as a result of abnormal protein synthesis. Amyloid is seen within the synovium and bone marrow as extensive extracellular deposits of brightly eosinophilic/hyaline amorphous material. Histopathologic sections stained with Congo red have a characteristic apple-green birefringence when examined under polarized light.

Imaging Features

Regardless of cause, imaging studies show massive accumulation of amyloid around the joints, and there is invasion of the periarticular tissue, capsule, and joint. Also, deposits can be seen in the synovium. The articular ends of the bone can be destroyed, and both subluxations and pathologic fractures are frequently encountered. In addition, focal osteolytic lesions, particularly in the bones of the upper extremities and in the proximal ends of the femora, can be seen (Fig. 15.65A,B). The MRI manifestations of amyloidosis include intermediate–signal intensity to low–signal intensity deposits of amyloid material in the synovium, ligaments, and tendons with or without erosive changes (Fig. 15.65C,D).

Treatment

Although there is no cure for amyloidosis, therapy is directed toward relieving the symptoms and limitation of further production of amyloid protein. Treatment includes chemotherapy agents such as melphalan or cyclophosphamide, and corticosteroids such as dexamethasone. Recently, other drugs such as bortezomib, thalidomide, and lenalidomide, which is a thalidomide derivative, have been tried with some promising results. In most severe cases, autologous peripheral blood stem cell transplantation using high-dose chemotherapy and transfusion of stem cells has been advocated. Surgical treatment consists of removal of affected organs followed by organ transplantation.

Multicentric Reticulohistiocytosis

Clinical Features

Multicentric reticulohistiocytosis is a rare systemic granulomatous disorder of unknown cause seen in adulthood and is characterized by the proliferation of the histiocytes (macrophages) in the skin, the mucosa, the subcutaneous tissue, and the synovium. It was first described in 1937 as a nondiabetic cutaneous xanthomatosis. The disorder has been also called *lipoid dermatoarthritis*, *reticulohistiocytoma*, *lipid rheumatism*, *giant cell reticulohistiocytosis*, *giant cell histiocytoma*, and *giant cell histiocytosis*. Goltz and Laymon proposed the name of this condition in 1954 because of the multifocal origin and systemic nature of the disease. It usually begins during the fourth decade of life, and women are more commonly affected than men, with ratio of 3:1. In approximately 60% to 70% of patients, polyarthralgia is the first manifestation of the disease. Clinical findings, like those of rheumatoid arthritis, consist of soft-tissue swelling, stiffness, and tenderness, particularly of hands (Fig. 15.66).

Imaging Features

Like the clinical features, imaging findings of multicentric reticulohistiocytosis are also similar in appearance to rheumatoid arthritis. Unlike rheumatoid arthritis, however, the distal interphalangeal joints are most frequently affected. Less commonly affected are the proximal interphalangeal, metacarpophalangeal, shoulder, and elbow joints. Occasionally, the articular lesions may be marked by severe destruction similar to arthritis mutilans of

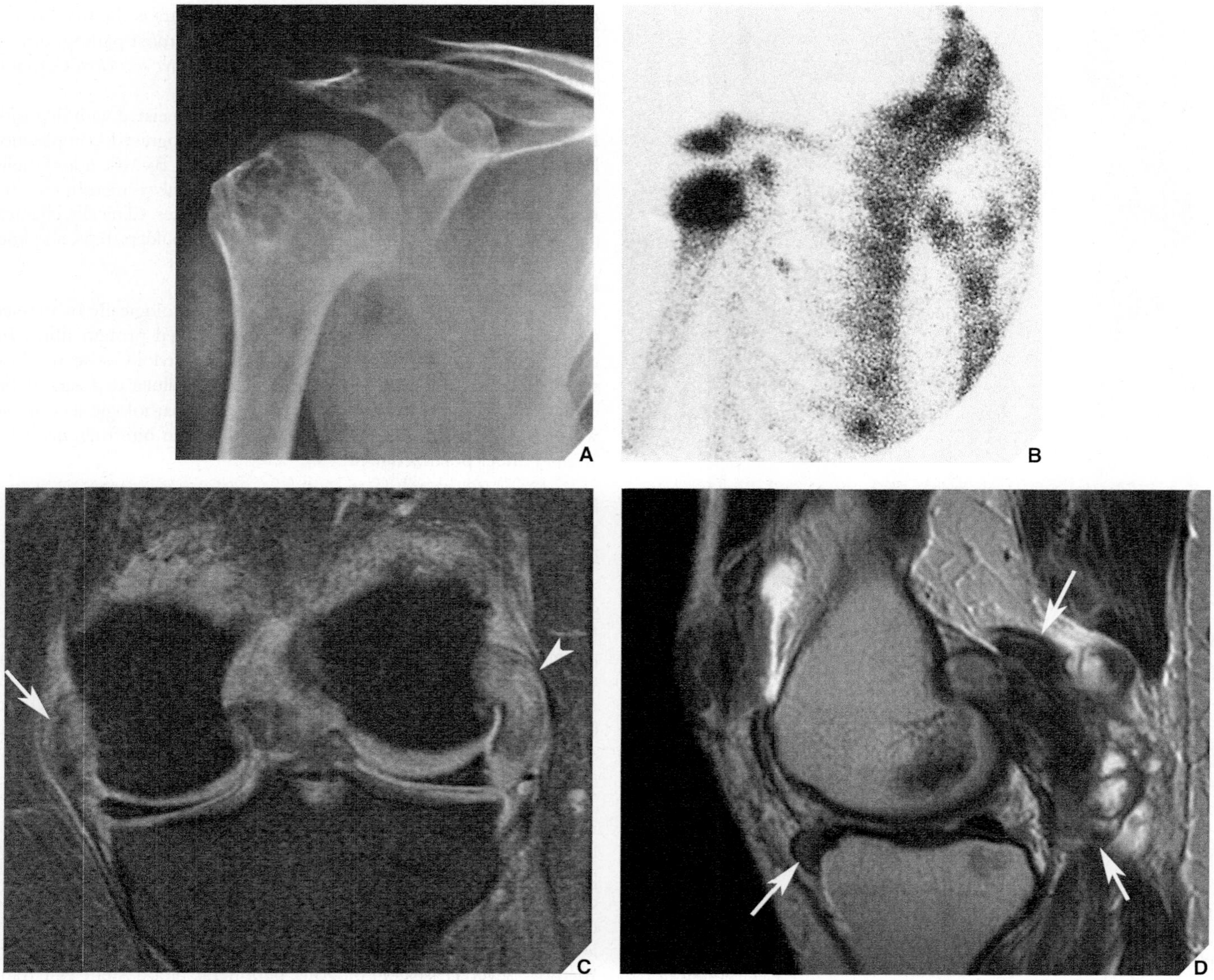

FIGURE 15.65 **Amyloidosis.** **(A)** Anteroposterior radiograph of the right shoulder of an 80-year-old man demonstrates a moderate degree of juxtaarticular osteoporosis, soft-tissue swelling, and a large osteolytic lesion in the humeral head. The glenohumeral joint space is relatively well preserved. **(B)** Radionuclide bone scan shows an increased uptake of technetium-labeled methylene diphosphonate (MDP) around the shoulder. **(C)** Coronal T2-weighted fat-saturated MRI of the knee in another patient with primary amyloidosis demonstrates thickening of the popliteus tendon *(arrowhead)* and the proximal superficial fibers of the medial collateral ligament *(arrow)* due to extensive deposits of intermediate–signal intensity amyloid tissue. Note also amyloid deposition in the intercondylar notch. **(D)** Sagittal T2-weighted MRI of the knee in the same patient shows the hypointense synovial deposits of amyloid tissue *(arrows)*.

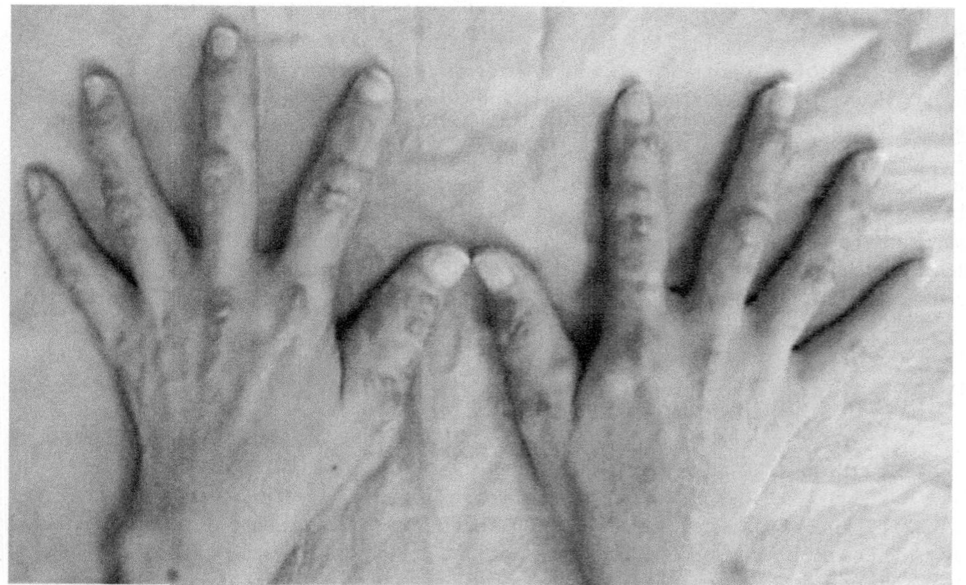

FIGURE 15.66 **Multicentric reticulohistiocytosis.** Clinical photograph of the hands of the patient with multicentric reticulohistiocytosis shows characteristic erythematous nodules on the dorsal aspect of the metacarpophalangeal and interphalangeal joints. (Reprinted with permission from Greenspan A, Gershwin ME. *Imaging in rheumatology: a clinical approach*. Philadelphia: Wolters Kluwer; 2018:363, Fig. 10.4.)

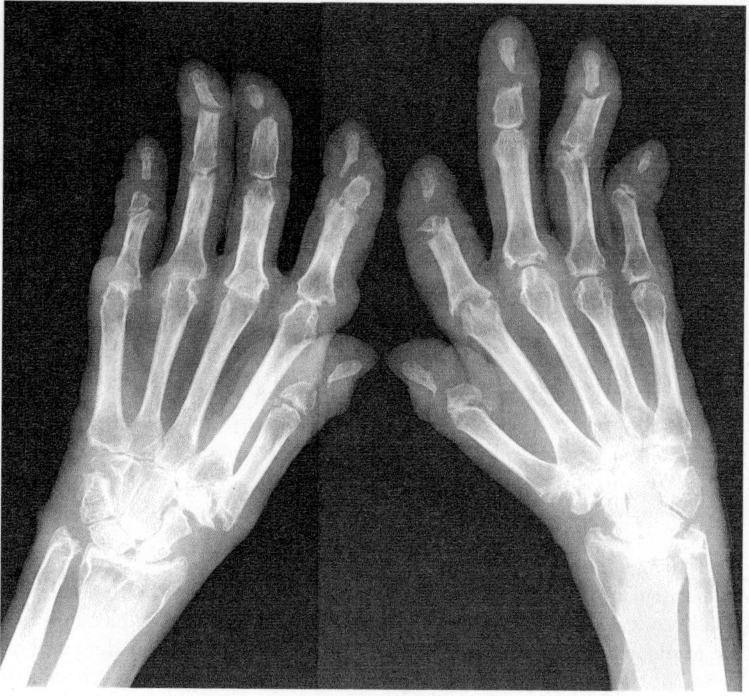

FIGURE 15.67 **Multicentric reticulohistiocytosis.** Dorsovolar radiograph of both hands of a 57-year-old woman with long-standing polyarthralgia, soft-tissue swelling, and deformities of the fingers demonstrates severe destruction of multiple carpometacarpal, metacarpophalangeals, and interphalangeals joints similar to those seen in rheumatoid or psoriatic arthritis.

rheumatoid arthritis or psoriatic arthritis (Figs. 15.67 and 15.68). The characteristic absence of significant periarticular osteoporosis distinguishes this disorder from the inflammatory arthritides, and there is also no periosteal new bone formation, which distinguishes it from psoriatic arthritis or juvenile idiopathic arthritis. Lack of osteophytes and interphalangeal ankylosis, and the presence of soft-tissue nodules and atlantoaxial abnormalities including subluxation and erosion of the odontoid process distinguish this arthropathy from erosive osteoarthritis. At times, the pattern of bone

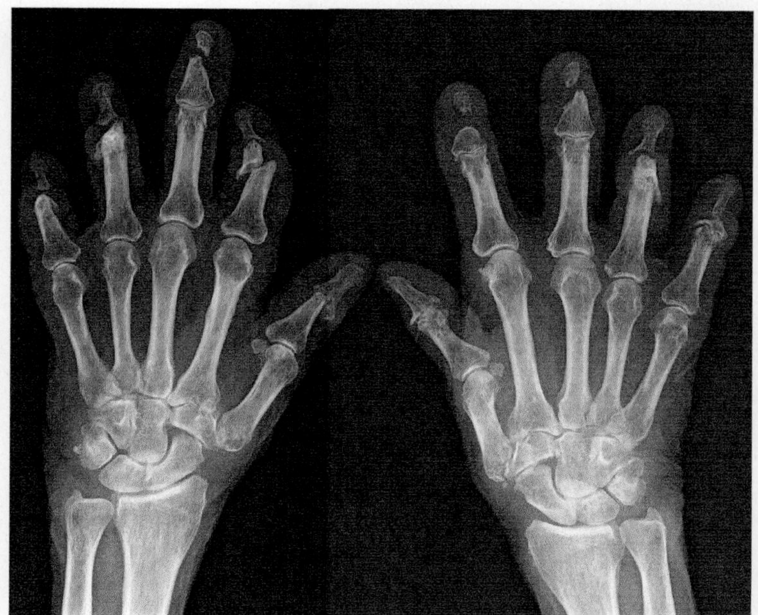

FIGURE 15.68 **Multicentric reticulohistiocytosis.** Dorsovolar radiograph of both hands of a 63-year-old man shows arthritis mutilans affecting mainly distal interphalangeal joints.

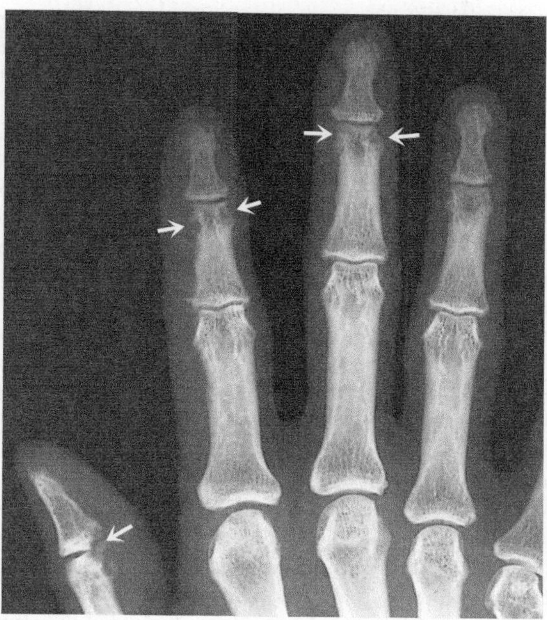

FIGURE 15.69 **Multicentric reticulohistiocytosis.** A 46-year-old woman presented with distal interphalangeal joints pain and soft-tissue swelling. Note sharply marginated erosions at the distal interphalangeal joints *(arrows)* resembling gout.

erosions with sclerotic margins and overhanging edges may mimic those of gout (Fig. 15.69). Unlike gout, however, there is symmetrical distribution of the lesions in the hands and feet and lack of calcification within soft-tissue nodules.

Pathology

On histopathology, dermal infiltration of multinucleated giant cells with eosinophilic ground-glass cytoplasm is characteristic. Immunohistologically, there is expressed positivity for tartrate-resistant acid phosphatase (TRAP), CD68, lysosome, and human alveolar macrophage-56 (HAM-56); however, there is conspicuous negativity for S-100 protein, CD1a, and factor XIIIa.

Treatment

Treatment consists of systemic steroids, cytotoxic drugs such as cyclophosphamide, chlorambucil, methotrexate, and infliximab. Bisphosphonates such as alendronate and zoledronate have been reported to improve skin lesions and arthritis.

Sarcoidosis

Clinical Features

Sarcoidosis is a systemic inflammatory disorder predominantly affecting young adults, characterized by the presence of noncaseating granulomas in affected organs. The disease has a worldwide distribution, with the greatest incidence in Sweden. Although the etiology still remains unsettled, the evidence that sarcoidosis most commonly involves the lungs, eyes, and skin, focused the search for environmental causes such as exposures to airborne antigens. In fact, some of the earliest studies have reported association of sarcoidosis with exposures irritants found in rural settings, such as emissions from wood-burning stoves and tree pollen. More recently, association of sarcoidosis with exposure to inorganic particles, insecticides, and moldy environments have been suggested. Currently, the investigators found compelling evidence to support the hypothesis implying certain environmental foreign nonparticulates, as a plausible cause of this condition in individuals with a genetically based immune dysregulational predisposition. Some researchers suggested that a predisposition to acute sarcoid arthritis is carried by the HLA DQ2-DR3 haplotype that appears to be transmitted as a dominant genetic trait. Many genetic associations have been linked sarcoidosis with genes within the MHC locus. Most recent studies suggested the novel gene BTNL2 (butyrophilin-like) has been associated with sarcoidosis of Caucasian patients. The active granulomatous inflammation is associated with a dominant expression of T-helper (Th) 1 cytokines (interferon γ [IFN-γ]), IL-12 and IL-18, and tumor necrosis factor (TNF).

Clinical presentation varies depending on organs involved. Systemic symptoms such as fatigue, weight loss, and night sweats are common. Dyspnea, cough, and wheezing occur when respiratory system is affected. Soft-tissue swelling and cutaneous lesions of the hands and feet can be associated with osseous changes. Maculae, papules, and plaques are common manifestation of skin involvement. The joints are rarely affected and may be present in about 10% to 35% of patients with sarcoidosis. Arthralgia tends to occur in patients with acute presentation of disease, that includes a triad of arthritis, erythema nodosum, and bilateral hilar adenopathy (Löfgren syndrome); however, more often the inflammation is present in the periarticular region (periarthritis).

Pathology

On histopathologic examination sarcoid granulomas consist of compact aggregates of epithelioid histiocytes with rare foreign body-type giant cells, encompassed by an outer zone of fibrosis with lymphocytes and plasma cells. Characteristic but not pathognomonic findings include the presence of intracytoplasmic inclusions of two types: laminated concretions composed of calcium and proteins (so-called *Schaumann bodies*), and stellate inclusions with a central core of degenerating organelles encompassed by multiple rays of collagen filaments (so-called *asteroid bodies*).

Laboratory findings include anemia, leucopenia, eosinophilia, decrease in serum albumins, elevation of serum globulins, and hypercalcemia.

Imaging Features

When the skeletal system is affected, cystic, punch-out lesions, lacy reticulations, and honeycomb pattern of destruction are commonly observed in the short tubular bones of the hands and feet (Fig. 15.70). Less frequently, nodular opacities in the medullary portion of these bones and osteosclerosis of the terminal tufts can be seen. Occasionally, generalized osteosclerosis may be present. Involvement of the spinal column is rare, and if present, it is usually limited to the cervical segment (Fig. 15.71).

Treatment

Corticosteroids, including prednisone, are considered the first line of treatment of sarcoidosis. The antimalarial drug hydroxychloroquine is effective in patients with dermatologic involvement, joint arthropathy, and hypercalcemia. Some patients benefit from receiving methotrexate, azathioprine, mycophenolate mofetil, leflunomide, and cyclophosphamide.

Hemophilia

Hemophilia A is an inherited bleeding disorder characterized by an anomaly of blood coagulation caused by functional deficiency of antihemophilic factor (AHF) VIII. It is inherited as an X-linked recessive trait and essentially occurs only in males, although female carriers transmit the abnormal gene. In hemophilia B, also known as *Christmas disease*, there is a deficiency of plasma thromboplastin component, factor IX. This disorder may also affect females.

Imaging Features

The articular changes in hemophilia most often occur in the first and second decades of life and are secondary to chronic repetitive bleeding into the joints and bones. Repeated episodes of intraarticular bleeding and inflammatory tissue response cause proliferation of synovium and erosion of cartilage and subchondral bone. Usually, there is no problem in the clinical recognition of this disorder; however, the changes of hemophilic arthropathy may radiographically mimic those of rheumatoid arthritis, particularly juvenile idiopathic arthritis (Fig. 15.72). Cartilage destruction, joint space narrowing, and erosions of the articular surfaces are identical to those seen in rheumatoid arthritis (Fig. 15.73; see also Figs. 12.19 and 12.20). The knee, ankle, and elbow are the most frequently involved articulations, and this involvement is usually bilateral. In the knee, the radiographic features include periarticular osteoporosis, joint effusion (hemarthrosis), overgrowth of femoral condyles with widening of the intercondylar notch and squaring of the patella. Frequently, multiple subchondral cysts and articular

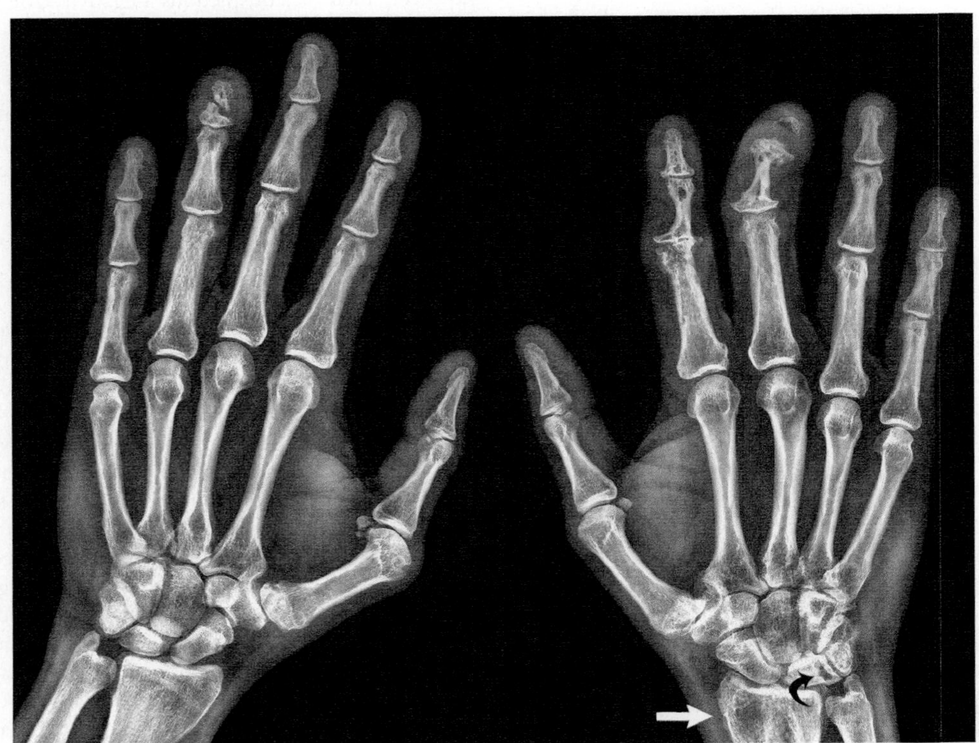

FIGURE 15.70 Sarcoidosis. Dorsovolar radiograph of the hands of a 55-year-old man shows destructive lesions of the distal phalanx of the ring finger of the right hand, and proximal and distal phalanges of the index and middle fingers of the left hand. Note also destructive lesion in the left lunate *(curved arrow)* and in the distal left radius *(arrow)*.

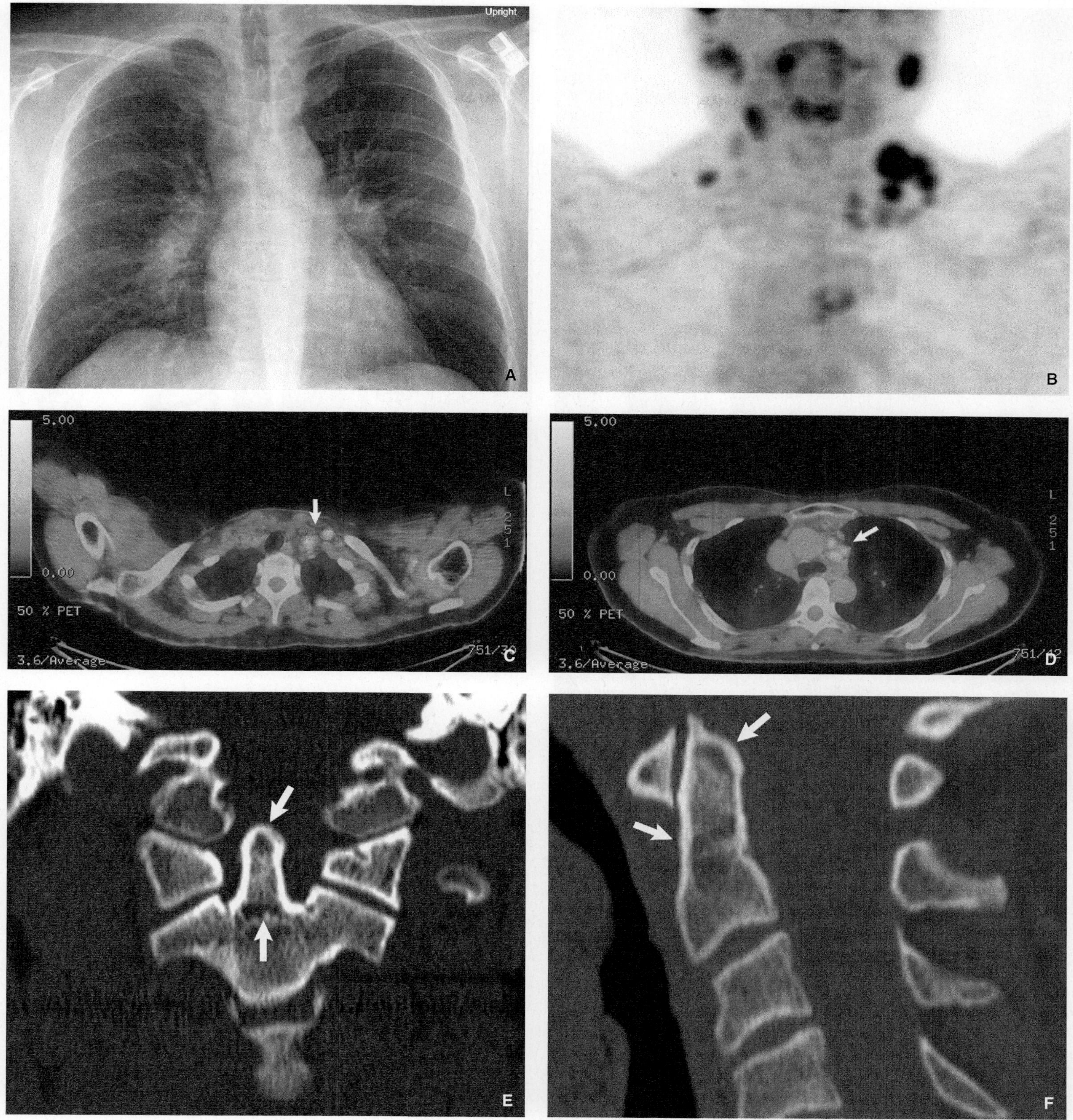

FIGURE 15.71 Sarcoidosis. A 38-year-old man with known pulmonary sarcoidosis presented with severe neck pain. **(A)** Posteroanterior radiograph of the chest shows perihilar and paratracheal adenopathy. **(B)** [18]FDG PET scan shows several hypermetabolic foci within neck, supraclavicular, and mediastinal lymph nodes. **(C,D)** Two axial fused PET/CT images of the upper chest show hypermetabolic activity within the affected lymph nodes. **(E)** Coronal and **(F)** sagittal reformatted CT images of the upper cervical spine show two osteolytic lesions in the odontoid process *(arrows)*. *(Continued)*

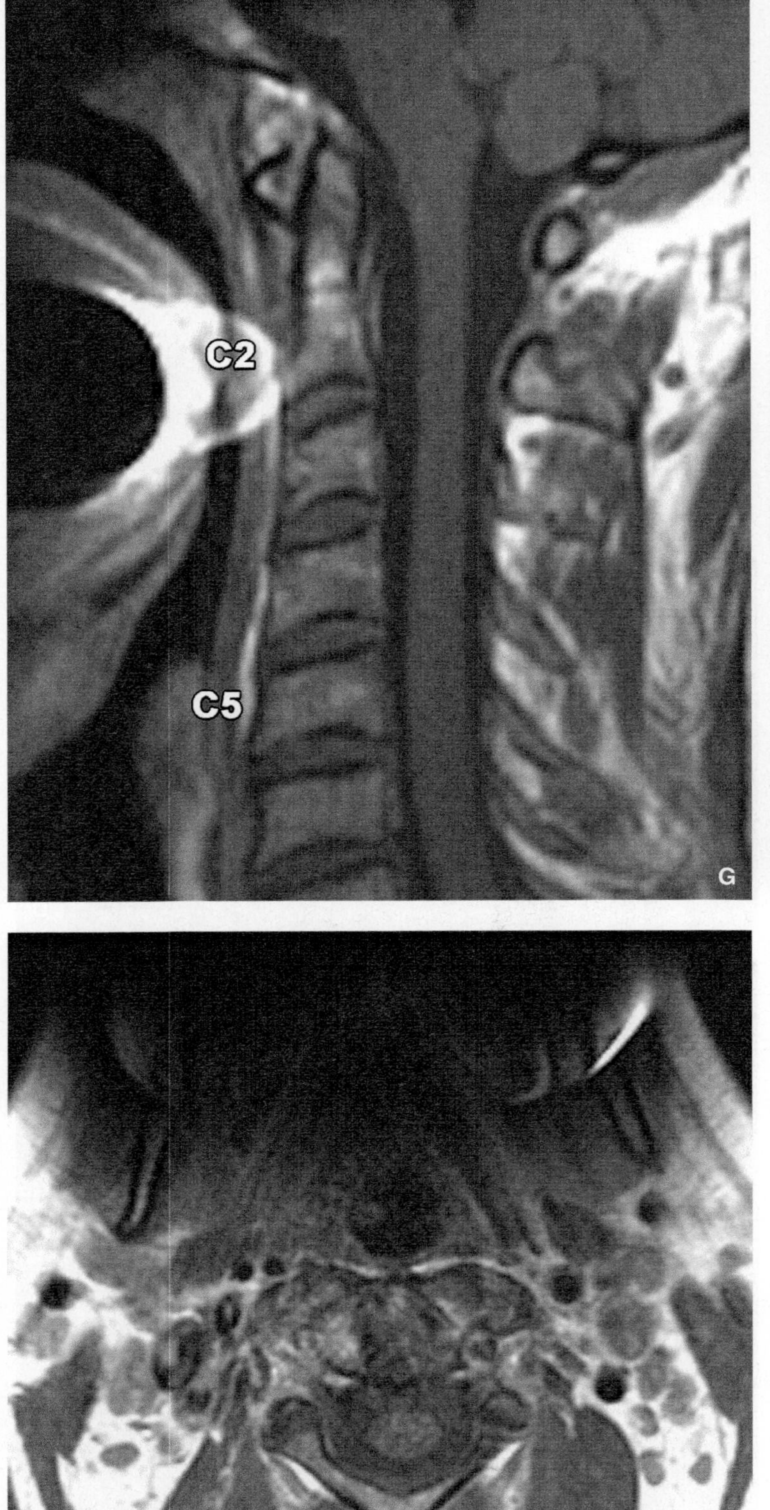

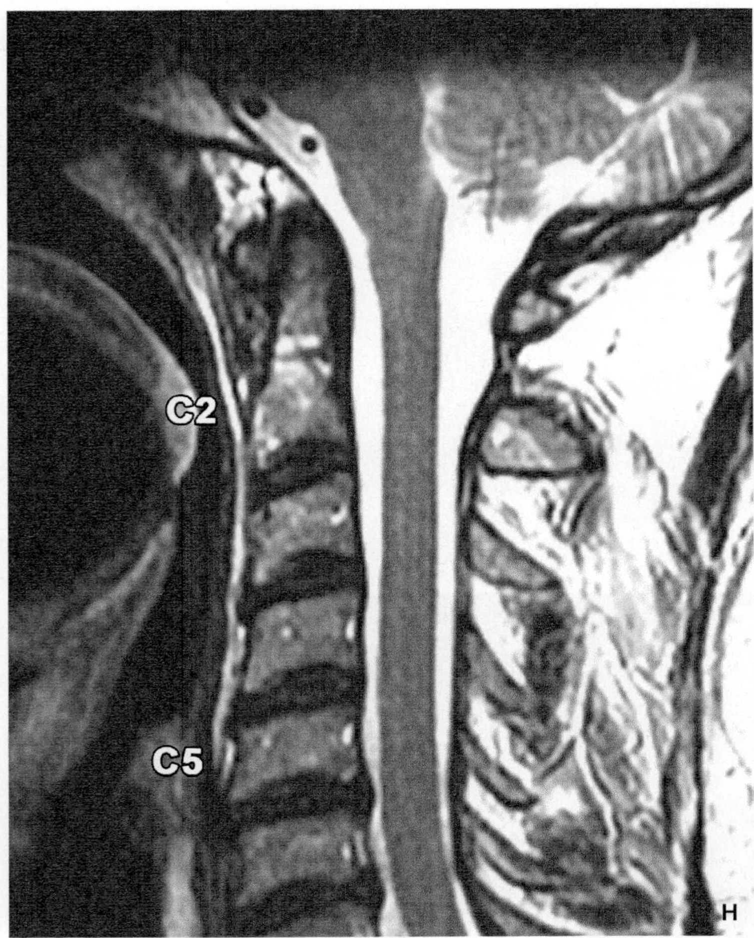

FIGURE 15.71 Sarcoidosis. ***(Continued)*** **(G)** Sagittal T2-weighted MR image of the cervical spine shows high–signal intensity lesions within the vertebral bodies of C2, C3, and C4. **(H)** Sagittal T1-weighted fat-suppressed MR image obtained after intravenous administration of gadolinium show mild enhancement of the vertebral lesions. **(I)** Axial T1-weighted postcontrast MRI shows enhancement of the lesion of the posterior arch of C2 *(arrows)*.

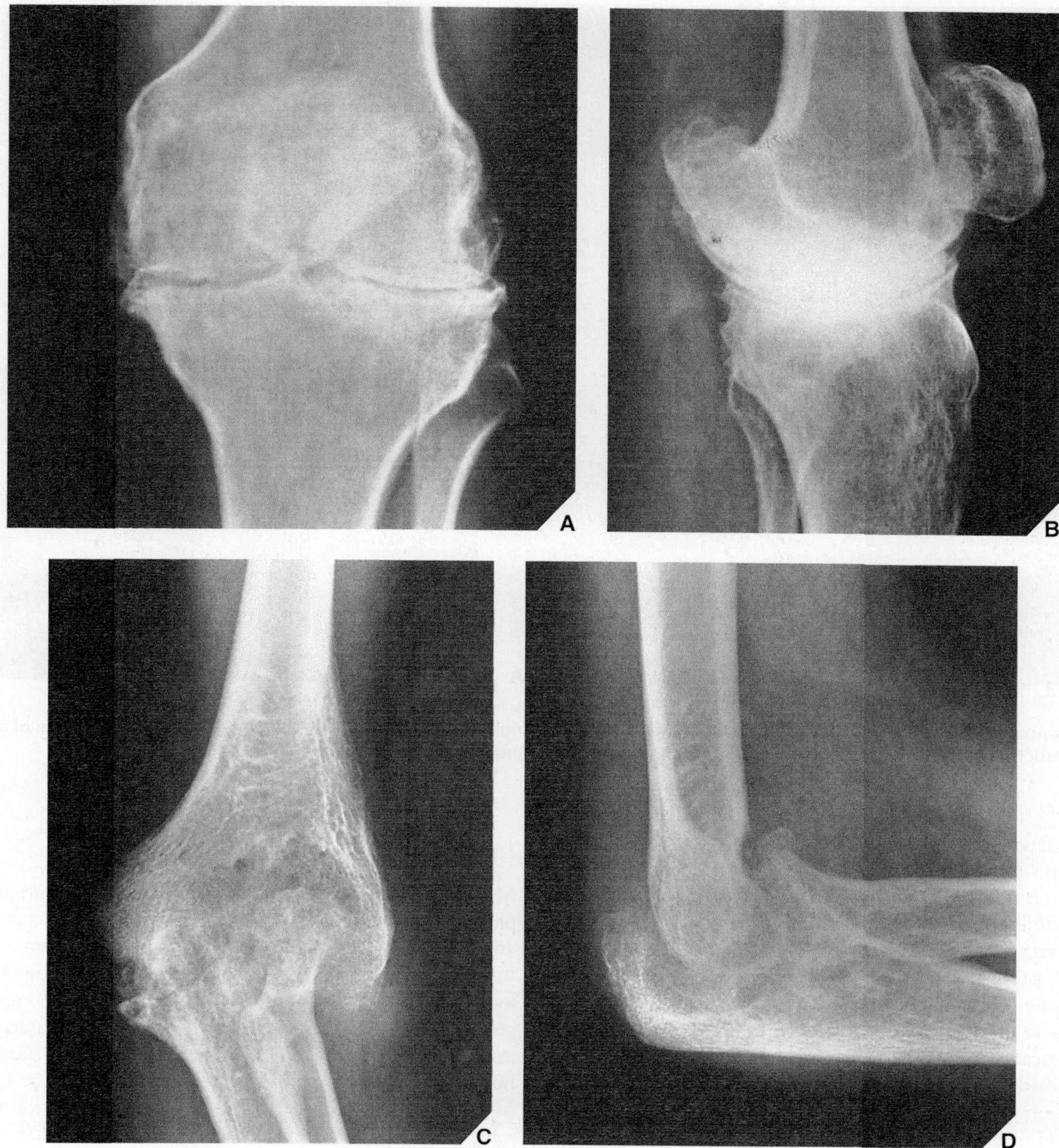

FIGURE 15.72 **Hemophilic arthropathy.** A 42-year-old man had several intraarticular bleeding episodes in his life. **(A)** Anteroposterior and **(B)** lateral radiographs of his left knee demonstrate advanced hemophilic arthropathy. Note the involvement of all three joint compartments. Similar destructive changes in the left elbow are demonstrated on **(C)** anteroposterior and **(D)** lateral radiographs of this joint.

erosions are evident. In the late stages of disease, the uniform narrowing of the joint space and secondary osteoarthritic changes may be observed. The differential diagnosis from juvenile idiopathic arthritis is based on evidence that there is no bony ankylosis, no evidence of growth inhibition, and frequent presence of pseudotumors. Recurrent episodes of hemarthrosis of the joint in patients with hemophilia lead to chronic synovitis and deposition of hemosiderin pigment in the synovium and joint capsule. These features are well depicted with MRI (Figs. 15.74 and 15.75).

Jaccoud Arthritis

Jaccoud arthritis is related to repeated attacks of rheumatic fever and migratory arthralgias. Usually, there is complete recovery, but residual stiffness in metacarpophalangeal joints may develop with subsequent attacks. The lesion appears to be periarticular rather than articular, and the changes are caused by mild flexion at the metacarpophalangeal joints with ulnar deviation, most notably in the fourth and fifth fingers, although any finger may be affected. The articular changes are not erosive, and patients can physically correct the deformity, particularly in the early course of the disease. The syndrome is rare and not well recognized in the United States.

Arthritis Associated with AIDS

AIDS results from infection with HIV, resulting in immunodeficiency state and pathologic disorders across multiple organ systems. Recently, an increased prevalence of rheumatologic disorders has been described in patients with HIV infection. Berman and colleagues stated that 71% of patients infected with HIV virus had rheumatic symptoms, including arthralgias, reactive arthritis, psoriatic arthritis, myositis, vasculitis, and undifferentiated spondyloarthropathy. Solomon and colleagues found that patients with HIV infection demonstrated a 144-fold increase in the prevalence of reactive arthritis and a 10-fold to 40-fold increase in the prevalence of psoriasis compared with the general population. It is interesting to note that arthritis was seen during various stages of HIV infection and often preceded clinical manifestations of the AIDS. The arthritis was more severe and was unresponsive to conventional treatment with NSAIDs. A few hypotheses have been suggested to explain the coexistence of inflammatory arthritis and HIV infection. One is that reactive arthritis entails an interaction between a genetic predisposition (e.g., HLA-B27 locus) and environmental factors, most often venereal infections. The immune system also plays a role in the pathogenesis of

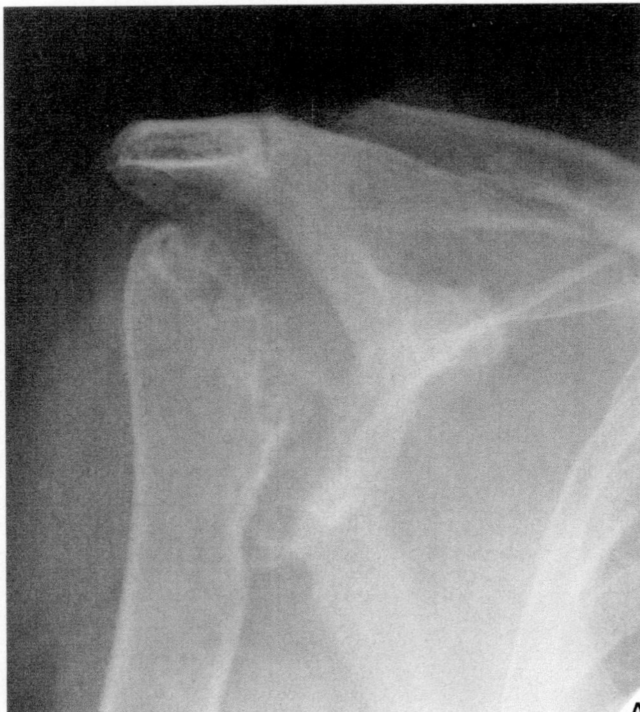

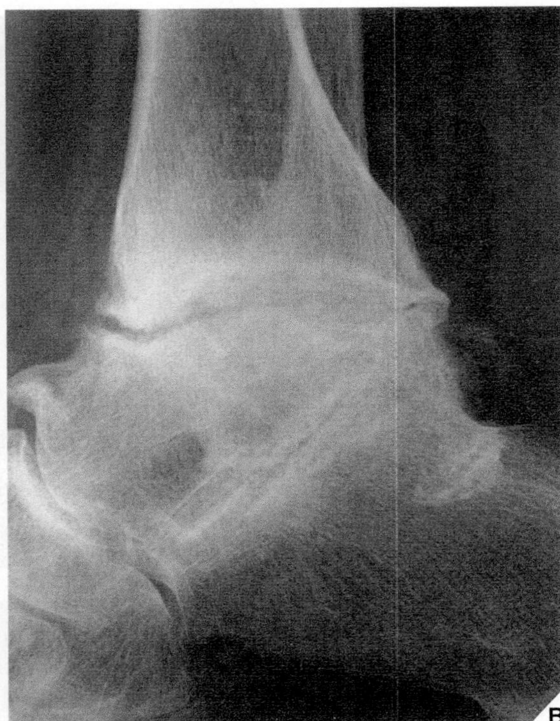

FIGURE 15.73 Hemophilic arthropathy. **(A)** Anteroposterior radiograph of the right shoulder and **(B)** lateral radiograph of the left ankle of a 49-year-old man with hemophilia A show destructive arthropathy of the glenohumeral, ankle, and subtalar joints.

reactive arthritis. Likewise, the pathogenesis of psoriatic arthritis may entail genetic predisposition (e.g., HLA-B27 or HLA-B38 loci). Because HIV infection is commonly followed by the development of immunodeficiency, it is possible that the altered immune mechanism noted in patients with AIDS triggered the onset of reactive arthritis or psoriatic arthritis in genetically predisposed patients. The second hypothesis is that HIV-related immunodeficiency causes susceptibility to infection with a variety of bacterial and viral organisms, which in turn trigger the onset of arthritis in a genetically predisposed patient. A third hypothesis is that there may be yet undiscovered causative factors that predispose an individual to arthritis when exposed to HIV. Finally, the arthritis may reflect the direct action of HIV infection on synovium. As Rosenberg and colleagues have pointed out, radiographic documentation of seronegative arthritis should raise the possibility of HIV-associated arthritis as part of the differential diagnosis, particularly in patients with known risk factors for HIV infection.

Infectious Arthritis

Most infectious arthritides demonstrate a positive radionuclide bone scan, particularly when using indium-labeled white cells as a tracer (see Chapter 2), and they also show a very similar radiographic picture, including joint effusion and destruction of cartilage and subchondral bone with consequent joint space narrowing (see Figs. 25.24A, 25.26A, and 25.27). However, certain clinical and radiographic features are characteristic of individual infectious processes as demonstrated at various target sites. In general, however, infectious arthritis is characterized by the complete destruction of both articular ends of the bones forming the joint; all communicating joint compartments are invariably involved, with diffuse osteoporosis, joint effusion, and periarticular soft-tissue swelling (see Fig. 12.44). A detailed description of pyogenic arthritis, tuberculous arthritis, fungal arthritis, and other infectious arthritides caused by viruses and spirochetes is provided in Part V: Infections.

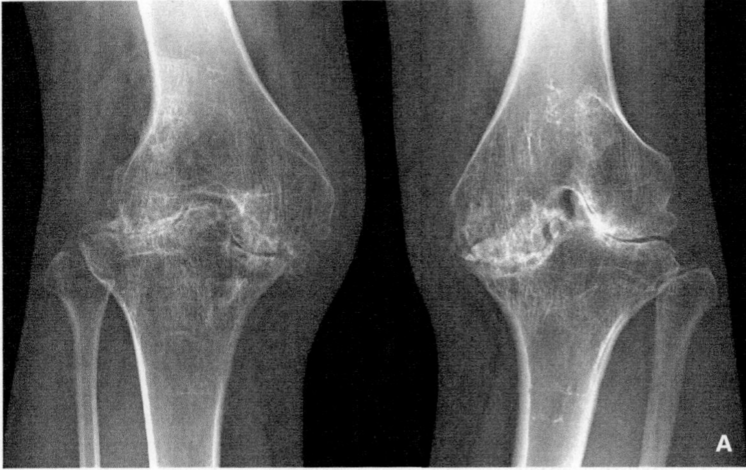

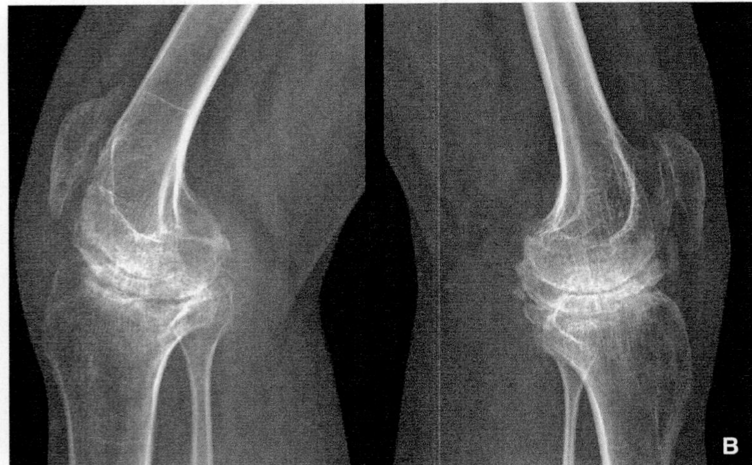

FIGURE 15.74 MRI of hemophilic arthropathy. **(A)** Anteroposterior and **(B)** lateral radiographs of the knees of a 33-year-old man show typical changes of this disorder, including periarticular osteoporosis and severe destruction of the articular cartilage associated with erosive changes of the subchondral bone. *(Continued)*

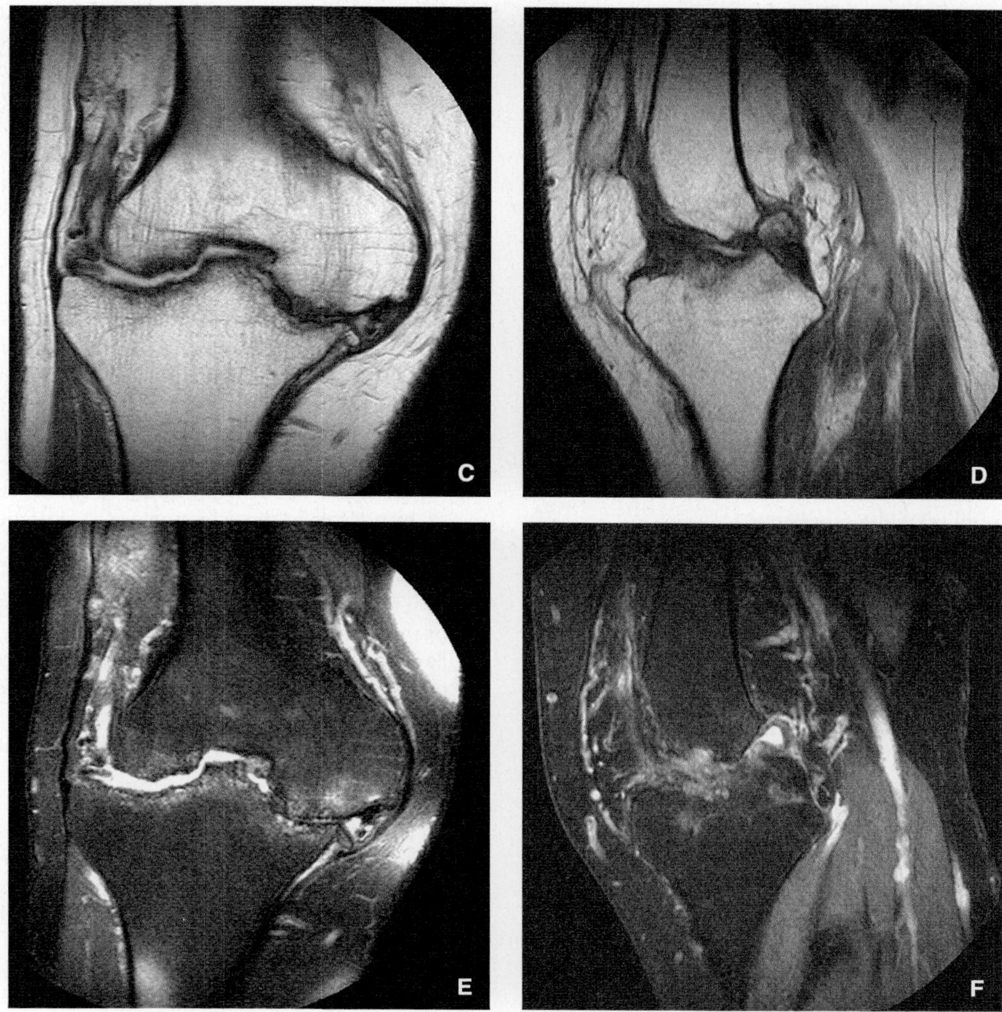

FIGURE 15.74 MRI of hemophilic arthropathy. ***(Continued)*** **(C)** Coronal and **(D)** sagittal T1-weighted, and **(E)** coronal and **(F)** sagittal T2-weighted MR images of the right knee demonstrate in addition the destruction of the lateral and medial menisci and chronic tears of the anterior and posterior cruciate ligaments. There is also small amount of joint fluid. Note also the overgrowth of the medial femoral condyle due to chronic hyperemia and the widening of the intercondylar notch.

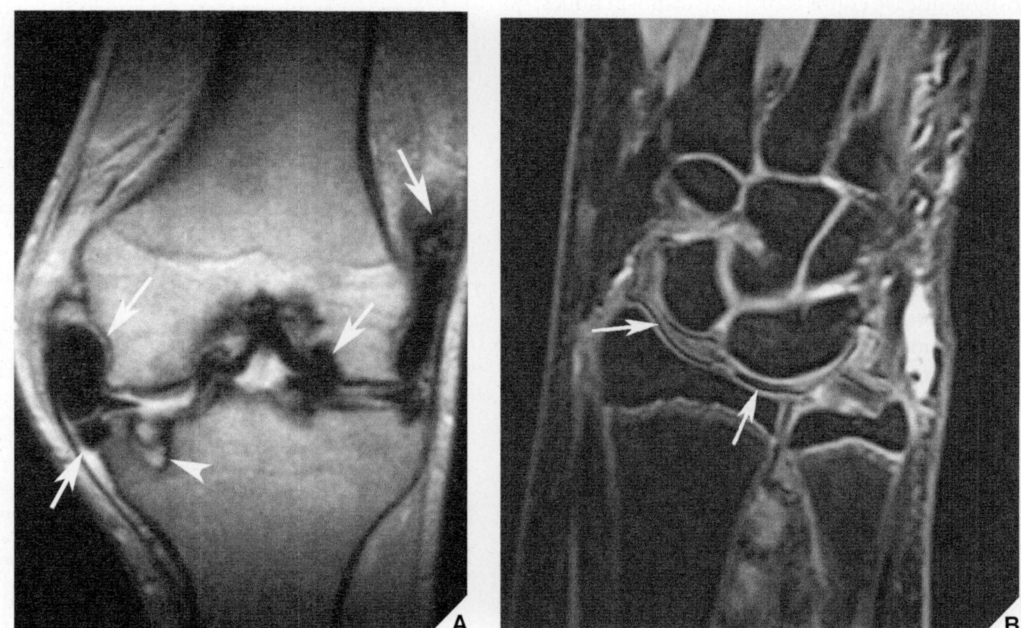

FIGURE 15.75 MRI of hemophilic arthropathy. **(A)** Coronal T2-weighted MRI of the knee in a young adult patient with hemophilia demonstrates hemosiderin deposition in the joint space related to repeated episodes of hemarthrosis *(arrows)*. Note the articular surface erosion in the medial tibial plateau *(arrowhead)* and the widening of the intercondylar notch. **(B)** Coronal T2-weighted fat-saturated MRI of a 10-year-old patient with early hemophilia shows low–signal intensity hemosiderin deposition outlining the synovium in the radiocarpal joint *(arrows)* and the absence of cartilage damage or bone erosions. (Courtesy of Francisco Aparisi, MD, Valencia, Spain.)

PRACTICAL POINTS TO REMEMBER

Connective Tissue Arthropathies

1. SLE is characterized by flexible joint contractures and malalignments of the metacarpophalangeal and proximal interphalangeal joints. These abnormalities are better demonstrated on the lateral radiographs because they can easily be reduced during positioning of the hand for the dorsovolar view.
2. Osteonecrosis is a frequent complication of SLE.
3. Radiographically, the musculoskeletal abnormalities associated with scleroderma are recognized by:
   - atrophy of the soft tissues, particularly the tips of fingers
   - resorption of the distal phalanges (acroosteolysis)
   - subcutaneous and periarticular calcifications
   - destructive changes in the interphalangeal joints.
4. In scleroderma, corroborative findings are seen in the gastrointestinal tract, where characteristically there is:
   - dilatation and hypomotility of the esophagus
   - dilatation of the duodenum and small bowel, with a pseudoobstruction pattern
   - pseudodiverticula of the colon.
5. MCTD is characterized by the clinical and radiologic features that combine the findings of SLE, scleroderma, dermatomyositis, and rheumatoid arthritis.

Metabolic, Endocrine, and Crystal Deposition Arthropathies and Arthritides

1. Gout is a metabolic disorder characterized by recurrent episodes of arthritis associated with the presence of monosodium urate monohydrate crystals in the synovial fluid.
2. Hyperuricemia may result from either increased uric acid production or decreased renal excretion.
3. Gouty arthritis can be recognized radiographically by:
   - sharply marginated periarticular and articular erosions, with an overhanging edge phenomenon
   - partial preservation of the joint space
   - asymmetric joint involvement
   - asymmetric distribution of tophi
   - the absence of osteoporosis.
4. Currently, dual-energy color-coded CT became a method of choice to identify the monosodium urate–containing gouty tophi.
5. CPPD crystal deposition disease consists of three distinct entities:
   - chondrocalcinosis
   - calcium pyrophosphate arthropathy
   - the pseudogout syndrome.
6. The presence of intraarticular crystals and calcifications of hyaline and fibrocartilage, occasionally associated with painful attacks similar to gout (pseudogout syndrome), are characteristic features of CPPD crystal deposition disease.
7. Chondrocalcinosis may also be seen in other conditions such as gout, hyperparathyroidism, hemochromatosis, ochronosis, oxalosis, Wilson disease, acromegaly, and degenerative joint disease.
8. CHA crystal deposition disease results from abnormal deposition of mineral crystals in and around the joints. The most common location is around the shoulder joint, at the site of supraspinatus tendon.
9. Hemochromatosis is a disorder resulting from an error of metabolism of iron or caused by iron overload. The arthropathy starts in the small joints of the hand with characteristic involvement of the heads of second and third metacarpals.
10. Alkaptonuria (ochronosis) is characterized by narrowing of the intervertebral disk spaces, disk calcification and ossification, involvement of sacroiliac joints and symphysis pubis, and joint space narrowing with periarticular osteosclerosis. The radiographic appearance may occasionally mimic degenerative joint disease or CPPD crystal deposition disease.
11. Wilson disease, known also as *hepatolenticular degeneration*, is an autosomal recessive inherited genetic disorder of copper metabolism. Imaging features include subchondral bone fragmentation, cyst formation, cortical irregularities and sclerosis, and joint space narrowing.
12. Hyperparathyroidism arthropathy results from subperiosteal and subchondral resorption at the site of small joints of the hand. This accounts for articular manifestation of this disorder.
13. Acromegaly arthropathy is the result of overgrowth of the articular cartilage and secondary degenerative changes (secondary osteoarthritis). The characteristic findings include:
    - beak-like osteophytes of the radial aspects of the metacarpal heads
    - beak-like osteophytes of the inferior aspects of the humeral heads
    - widening of the radiographic joint spaces.

Miscellaneous Arthropathies

1. Amyloid arthropathy is a noninflammatory symmetric polyarthritis. It may complicate long-term hemodialysis and chronic renal failure. The articular ends of the bone can be destroyed and subluxations and pathologic fractures occur. Focal osteolytic lesions, particularly of the bones of the upper extremities and in the proximal ends of the femora, can be seen.
2. Multicentric reticulohistiocytosis is characterized by proliferation of histiocytes in the skin, mucosa, subcutaneous tissue, and synovium. This may lead to severe articular destruction, but there is neither periarticular osteoporosis nor periosteal bone formation. The radiographic appearance may simulate gouty, rheumatoid, or psoriatic arthritis.
3. Sarcoidosis is a systemic inflammatory disorder characterized by the presence of noncaseating granulomas in affected organs. When the skeletal system is affected (most commonly short tubular bones of the hands and feet), the characteristic imaging features include:
   - cystic, punch-out lesions
   - lacy reticulations
   - honeycomb pattern of destruction.
4. The articular changes in hemophilia are due to repetitive bleeding into the joints and bone. The radiographic presentation is similar to that of juvenile rheumatoid arthritis. In the bones, pseudotumors are frequently encountered.
5. Jaccoud arthritis is a poorly defined entity resulting in periarticular stiffness in patients with repeated attacks of rheumatic fever. The articular changes are not erosive.
6. There is an increased prevalence of rheumatologic disorders in patients with AIDS, particularly reactive arthritis, psoriatic arthritis, and vasculitis.
7. Infectious arthritis is characterized by the complete destruction of both articular ends of the bones forming the joint. All communicating joint compartments are invariably involved, with diffuse osteoporosis, joint effusion, and periarticular soft-tissue swelling.

SUGGESTED READINGS

Adizie T, Moots RJ, Hodkinson B, et al. Inflammatory arthritis in HIV positive patients: a practical guide. *BMC Infect Dis* 2016;16:100–105.

Ali S, Huebner S. Multicentric reticulohistiocytosis. *Skeletal Radiol* 2013;42:1445, 1483–1484.

Amor B, Cherot A, Delbarre F, et al. Hydroxyapatite rheumatism and HLA markers. *J Rheumatol Suppl* 1977;3:101–104.

Arnett FC, Reveille JD, Duvic M. Psoriasis and psoriatic arthritis associated with human immunodeficiency virus infection. *Rheum Dis Clin North Am* 1991;17:59–78.

Assassi S, Radstake T, Mayes MD, et al. Genetics of scleroderma: implications for personalized medicine? *BMC Med* 2013;11:9.

Baker ND. Hemochromatosis. In: Taveras JM, Ferrucci JT, eds. *Radiology—diagnosis, imaging, intervention*. Philadelphia: JB Lippincott; 1986:1–6.

Beltran J, Marty-Delfaut E, Bencardino J, et al. Chondrocalcinosis of the hyaline cartilage of the knee: MRI manifestations. *Skeletal Radiol* 1998;27:369–374.

Benson MD. The hereditary amyloidoses. In: Picken M, Dogan A, Herrera G, eds. *Amyloid and related disorders: surgical pathology and clinical correlations*. New York: Springer; 2012:53.

Berman A, Espinoza LR, Diaz JD, et al. Rheumatic manifestations of human immunodeficiency virus infection. *Am J Med* 1988;85:59–64.

Berman MA, Sandborg CI, Calabia BS, et al. Interleukin 1 inhibitor masks high interleukin 1 production in acquired immunodeficiency syndrome (AIDS). *Clin Immunol Immunopathol* 1987;42:133–140.

Booth TC, Chhaya NC, Bell JRG, et al. Update on imaging of non-infectious musculoskeletal complications of HIV infection. *Skeletal Radiol* 2012;41:1349–1363.

Brandi ML, Falchetti A. Genetics of primary hyperparathyroidism. *Urol Int* 2004;72 (suppl 1):11–16.

Burke BJ, Escobedo EM, Wilson AJ, et al. Chondrocalcinosis mimicking a meniscal tear on MR imaging. *AJR Am J Roentgenol* 1998;170:69–70.

Bushara KO, Petermann G, Waclawik AJ, et al. Sarcoidosis of the spinal cord with extensive vertebral involvement: a case report. *Comput Med Imaging Graph* 1995;19:443–446.
Buxbaum JN, Tagoe CE. The genetics of the amyloidoses. *Annu Rev Med* 2000;51:543–569.
Calabrese LH. The rheumatic manifestations of infection with human immunodeficiency virus. *Semin Arthritis Rheum* 1989;18:225–239.
Chen C, Chandnani VP, Kang HS, et al. Scapholunate advanced collapse: a common wrist abnormality in calcium pyrophosphate dihydrate crystal deposition disease. *Radiology* 1990;177:459–461.
Chen CKH, Yeh LR, Pan H-B, et al. Intra-articular gouty tophi of the knee: CT and MR imaging in 12 patients. *Skeletal Radiol* 1999;28:75–80.
Choi HK, Burns LC, Shojania K, et al. Dual energy CT in gout: a prospective validation study. *Ann Rheum Dis* 2012;71:1466–1471.
Choi HK, Zhu Y, Mount DB. Genetics of gout. *Curr Opin Rheumatol* 2010;22:144–151.
Dalbeth N, Doyle AJ, McQueen FM, et al. Exploratory study of radiographic change in patients with tophaceous gout treated with intensive urate-lowering therapy. *Arthritis Care Res (Hoboken)* 2014;66:82–85.
Desai MA, Peterson JJ, Garner HW, et al. Clinical utility of dual-energy CT for evaluation of tophaceous gout. *Radiographics* 2011;31:1365–1377.
Dhanda S, Jagmohan P, Quek ST. A re-look at an old disease: a multimodality review on gout. *Clin Radiol* 2011;66:984–992.
Ebenbichler GR, Erdogmus CB, Resch KL, et al. Ultrasound therapy for calcific tendinitis of the shoulder. *N Engl J Med* 1999;340:1533–1538.
Elsaman AM, Radwan AR, Akmatov MK, et al. Amyloid arthropathy associated with multiple myeloma: a systematic analysis of 101 reported cases. *Semin Arthritis Rheum* 2013;43:405–412.
Escobedo EM, Hunter JC, Zink-Brody GC, et al. Magnetic resonance imaging of dialysis-related amyloidosis of the shoulder and hip. *Skeletal Radiol* 1996;25:41–48.
Fox C, Walker-Bone K. Evolving spectrum of HIV-associated rheumatic syndromes. *Best Pract Res Clin Rheumatol* 2015;29:244–258.
Girish G, Glazebrook KN, Jacobson JA. Advanced imaging in gout. *AJR Am J Roentgenol* 2013;201:515–525.
Glazebrook KN, Guimarães LS, Murthy NS, et al. Identification of intraarticular and periarticular uric acid crystals with dual-energy CT: initial evaluation. *Radiology* 2011;261:516–524.
Goltz RW, Laymon CW. Multicentric reticulohistiocytosis of the skin and synovia; reticulohistiocytoma or ganglioneuroma. *AMA Arch Derm Syphilol* 1954;69:717–731.
Govender P, Berman JS. The diagnosis of sarcoidosis. *Clin Chest Med* 2015;36:585–602.
Guerra SG, Vyse TJ, Cunninghame Graham DS. The genetics of lupus: a functional prospective. *Arthritis Res Ther* 2012;14:211.
Johansson M, Arlestig L, Moller B, et al. Association of a PDCD1 polymorphism with renal manifestations in systemic lupus erythematosus. *Arthritis Rheum* 2005;52:1665–1669.
Kandiah DA. Multicentric reticulohistiocytosis. *Mayo Clin Proc* 2014;89:e73.
Kelly D, Zhang QC, Soucie JM, et al. Prevalence of clinical hip abnormalities in haemophilia A and B: an analysis of the UDC database. *Haemophilia* 2013;19:424–431.
Kovach BT, Calamia KT, Walsh JS, et al. Treatment of multicentric reticulohistiocytosis with etanercept. *Arch Dermatol* 2004;140:919–921.
Laborde JM, Green DL, Ascari AD, et al. Arthritis in hemochromatosis: a case report. *J Bone Joint Surg Am* 1977;59:1103–1107.
La Montagna G, Sodano A, Capurro V, et al. The arthropathy of systemic sclerosis: a 12 month prospective clinical and imaging study. *Skeletal Radiol* 2005;34:35–41.
Lee DJ, Sartoris DJ. Musculoskeletal manifestations of human immunodeficiency virus infection: review of imaging characteristics. *Radiol Clin North Am* 1994;32:399–411.
Lima I, Ribeiro DS, Cesare A, et al. Typical Jaccoud's arthropathy in a patient with sarcoidosis. *Rheumatol Int* 2013;33:1615–1617.
Lomax A, Ferrero A, Cullen A, et al. Destructive pseudo-neuroarthropathy associated with calcium pyrophosphate deposition. *Foot Ankle Int* 2015;36:383–390.
Maclachlan J, Gough-Palmer A, Hargunani R, et al. Hemophilia imaging: a review. *Skeletal Radiol* 2009;38:949–957.
Major NM, Tehranzadeh J. Musculoskeletal manifestations of AIDS. *Radiol Clin North Am* 1997;35:1167–1189.
Mallinson PI, Reagan AC, Coupal T, et al. The distribution of urate deposition within the extremities in gout: a review of 148 dual-energy CT cases. *Skeletal Radiol* 2014;43: 277–281.
Mannoni A, Selvi E, Lorenzini S, et al. Alkaptonuria, ochronosis, and ochronotic arthropathy. *Semin Arthritis Rheum* 2004;33:239–248.
Martel W. The overhanging margin of bone: a roentgenologic manifestation of gout. *Radiology* 1968;91:755–756.
Martin J, Fonseca C. The genetics of scleroderma. *Curr Rheumatol Rep* 2011;13:13–20.
Martin JE, Bossini-Castillo L, et al. Unraveling the genetic component of systemic sclerosis. *Hum Genet* 2012;131:1023–1037.
Mikhael MM, Chioffe MA, Shapiro GS. Calcium pyrophosphate dihydrate crystal deposition disease (pseudogout) of lumbar spine mimicking osteomyelitis-discitis with epidural phlegmon. *Am J Orthop (Belle Mead NJ)* 2013;42:E64–E67.
Misra R, Darton K, Jewkes RF, et al. Arthritis in scleroderma. *Br J Rheumatol* 1995;34:831–837.
Moore SL, Teirstein AE. Musculoskeletal sarcoidosis: spectrum of appearances at MR imaging. *Radiographics* 2003;23:1389–1399.
Nicolaou S, Yong-Hing CJ, Galea-Soler S, et al. Dual-energy CT as a potential new diagnostic tool in the management of gout in the acute setting. *AJR Am J Roentgenol* 2010;194:1072–1078.
Oldenburg J, Zimmermann R, Katsarou O, et al. Controlled, cross-sectional MRI evaluation of joint status in severe haemophilia A patients treated with prophylaxis vs. on demand. *Haemophilia* 2015;21:171–179.
Pacheco-Tena C, Reyes-Cordero G, Ochoa-Albíztegui R, et al. Treatment of multicentric reticulohistiocytosis with tocilizumab. *J Clin Rheumatol* 2013;19:272–276.
Resnick D. Calcium hydroxyapatite crystal deposition disease. In: Resnick D, ed. *Diagnosis of bone and joint disorders*, 3rd ed. Philadelphia: WB Saunders; 1995:1615–1648.
Resnick D. Hemochromatosis and Wilson's disease. In: Resnick D, ed. *Diagnosis of bone and joint disorders*, 3rd ed. Philadelphia: WB Saunders; 1995:1649–1669.
Resnick D, Niwayama G. Calcium pyrophosphate dihydrate (CPPD) crystal deposition disease. In: Resnick D, ed. *Diagnosis of bone and joint disorders*, 3rd ed. Philadelphia: WB Saunders; 1995:1556–1614.
Resnick D, Niwayama G. Gouty arthritis. In: Resnick D, ed. *Diagnosis of bone and joint disorders*, 3rd ed. Philadelphia: WB Saunders; 1995:1511–1555.
Robledo G, Dávila-Fajardo CL, Márquez A, et al. Association between -174 interleukin-6 gene polymorphism and biological response to rituximab in several systemic autoimmune diseases. *DNA Cell Biol* 2012;31:1486–1491.
Rosenberg ZS, Norman A, Solomon G. Arthritis associated with HIV infection: radiographic manifestations. *Radiology* 1989;173:171–176.
Ross LV, Ross GJ, Mesgarzadeh M, et al. Hemodialysis-related amyloidomas of bone. *Radiology* 1991;178:263–265.
Sá Ribeiro D, Galvão V, Fernandes JL, et al. Magnetic resonance imaging of Jaccoud's arthropathy in systemic lupus erythematosus. *Joint Bone Spine* 2010;77:241–245.
Schanz S, Fierlbeck G, Ulmer A, et al. Localized scleroderma: MR findings and clinical features. *Radiology* 2011;260:817–824.
Scofield RH, Bruner GR, Namjou B, et al. Klinefelter's syndrome (47,XXY) in male systemic lupus erythematosus patients: support for the notion of a gene-dose effect from the X chromosome. *Arthritis Rheum* 2008;58:2511–2517.
Sekijima Y, Yoshida T, Ikeda S. CPPD crystal deposition disease of the cervical spine: a common cause of acute neck pain encountered in the neurology department. *J Neurol Sci* 2010;296:79–82.
Selmi C, Greenspan A, Huntley A, et al. Multicentric reticulohistiocytosis: a critical review. *Curr Rheumatol Rep* 2015;17:511.
Sestak AL, Nath SK, Sawalha AH, et al. Current status of lupus genetics. *Arthritis Res Ther* 2007;9:210.
Shah SP, Shah AM, Prajapati SM, et al. Multicentric reticulohistiocytosis. *Indian Dermatol Online J* 2011;2:85–87.
Sharp GC, Irwin WS, Tan EM, et al. Mixed connective tissue disease—an apparently distinct rheumatic disease syndrome associated with a specific antibody to an extractable nuclear antigen (ENA). *Am J Med* 1972;52:148–159.
Sissons HA, Steiner GC, Bonar F, et al. Tumoral calcium pyrophosphate deposition disease. *Skeletal Radiol* 1989;18:79–87.
Solomon G, Brancato L, Winchester R. An approach to the human immunodeficiency virus-positive patient with spondyloarthropathic disease. *Rheum Dis Clin North Am* 1991;17:43–55.
Sparks JA, McSparron JI, Shah N, et al. Osseous sarcoidosis: clinical characteristics, treatment, and outcomes—experience from a large, academic hospital. *Semin Arthritis Rheum* 2014;44:371–379.
Steinbach LS, Resnick D. Calcium pyrophosphate dihydrate crystal deposition disease revisited. *Radiology* 1996;200:1–9.
Steinbach LS, Tehranzadeh J, Fleckenstein J, et al. Human immunodeficiency virus infection: musculoskeletal manifestations. *Radiology* 1993;186:833–838.
Sweeney A, Hammer R, Evenski A, et al. Fulminant musculoskeletal and neurologic sarcoidosis: case report and literature update. *Skeletal Radiol* 2016;45:1571–1576.
Tehranzadeh J, Steinbach LS. *Musculoskeletal manifestations of AIDS*. St. Louis: Warren H. Green; 1994.
Udoff EJ, Genant HK, Kozin F, et al. Mixed connective tissue disease: the spectrum of radiographic manifestations. *Radiology* 1977;124:613–618.
Wilcox KA, Bharadwaj P, Sharma OP. Bone sarcoidosis. *Curr Opin Rheumatol* 2000;12: 321–330.
Yamada T, Kurohori YN, Kashiwazaki S, et al. MRI of multicentric reticulohistiocytosis. *J Comput Assist Tomogr* 1996;20:838–840.
Yang BY, Sartoris DJ, Djukic S, et al. Distribution of calcification in the triangular fibrocartilage region in 181 patients with calcium pyrophosphate dihydrate crystal deposition disease. *Radiology* 1995;196:547–550.
Yeter KC, Arkfeld DG. Treatment of multicentric reticulohistiocytosis with adalimumab, minocycline, methotrexate. *Int J Rheum Dis* 2013;16:105–106.
Yokoyama M, Aono H, Takeda A, et al. Cimetidine for chronic calcifying tendinitis of the shoulder. *Reg Anesth Pain Med* 2003;28:248–252.
Yu JS, Chung CB, Recht M, et al. MR imaging of tophaceous gout. *AJR Am J Roentgenol* 1997;168:523–527.
Zisman D, Schorr AF, Lynch JP III. Sarcoidosis involving the musculoskeletal system. *Semin Resp Crit Care Med* 2002;23:555–570.

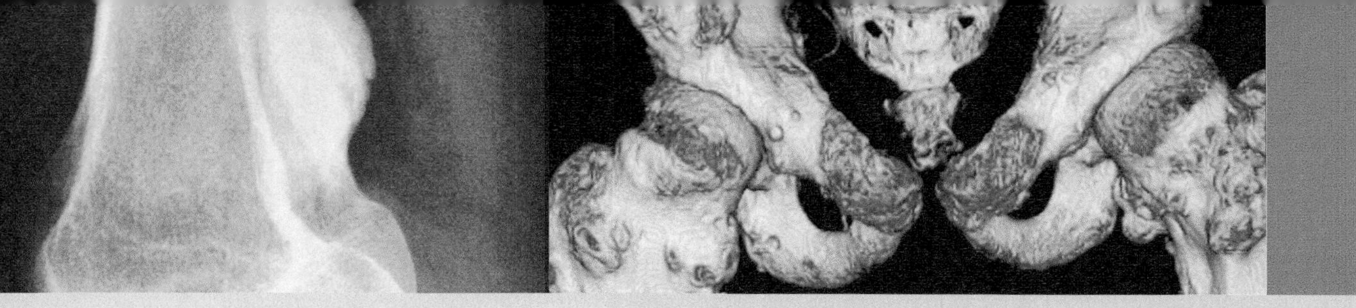

IV

TUMORS AND TUMOR-LIKE LESIONS

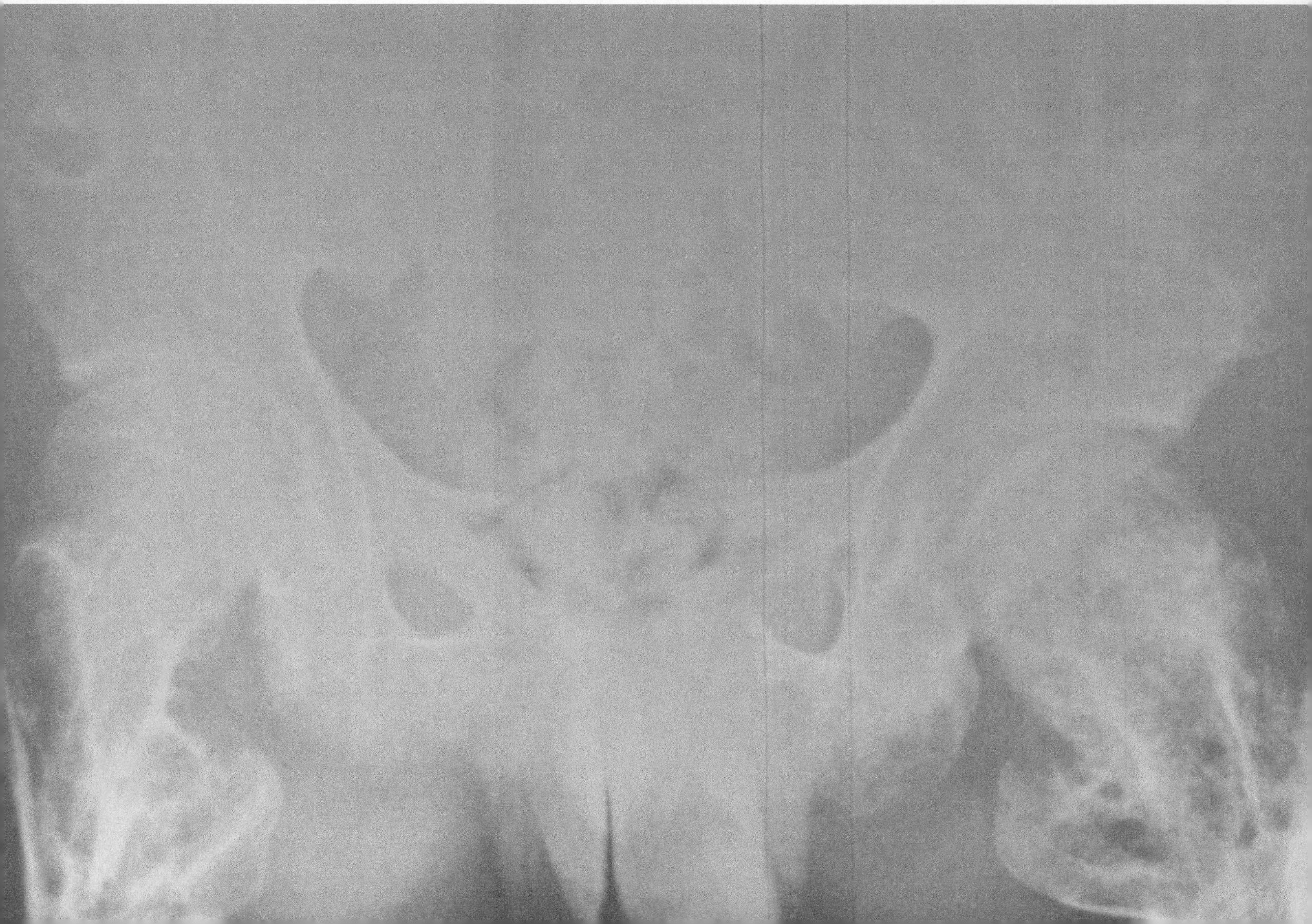

16

Imaging Evaluation of Tumors and Tumor-like Lesions

Classification of Tumors and Tumor-like Lesions

Tumors, including tumor-like lesions, can generally be divided into two groups: benign and malignant. The latter group can be further subclassified into primary malignant tumors, secondary malignant tumors (from the transformation of benign conditions), and metastatic tumors (Fig. 16.1). All of these lesions can be still further classified according to their tissue of origin (Table 16.1). Table 16.2 lists benign conditions that have the potential for malignant transformation.

To understand the terminology applied to tumors and tumor-like lesions of the bone, it is important to redefine certain terms pertinent to lesions and their location in the bone. The term *tumor* generally means *mass*; in common radiologic and orthopaedic parlance, however, it is the equivalent of the term *neoplasm*. By definition, a neoplasm, ruled by an uncontrolled process of aberrant cellular and morphologic mechanisms, demonstrates autonomous growth; if in addition it produces local or remote metastases, it is defined as a *malignant neoplasm* or *malignant tumor*. Beyond this (and not dealt within this chapter) are specific histopathologic criteria for defining a tumor as benign or malignant. It is nevertheless worth mentioning that certain giant cell tumors, despite a "benign" histopathology, may produce distant metastases and that certain cartilage tumors, despite adhering to a benign histopathologic pattern, can behave locally like malignant neoplasms, even though this is detectable only radiologically. Moreover, certain lesions discussed here and termed *tumor-like lesions* are not true neoplasms but rather have a developmental or inflammatory origin. They are included in this chapter because they display an imaging pattern that is almost indistinguishable from that of true neoplasms. Their cause is, in some cases, still being debated.

Equally important is the redefinition of certain terms pertinent to the location of a lesion in the bone. In the growing skeleton, one can clearly distinguish the epiphysis, growth plate (physis), metaphysis, and diaphysis (Fig. 16.2A), and when lesions are located at these sites, they are named accordingly. The greatest confusion is in the use of the term *metaphysis*. The metaphysis is a histologically very thin zone of active bone growth, adjacent to the growth plate. Consequently, for a lesion to be called *metaphyseal* in location, it must extend into and abut the growth plate. However, it is customary—however incorrect—to use the same term for locating a lesion after skeletal maturity has occurred. By the time of maturity, the growth plate is scarred, and neither the epiphysis nor metaphysis remains. More proper and less confusing would be a terminology such as *articular end of the bone* and *shaft* for locating lesions in the bone whose growth plate has been obliterated and whose metaphysis has ceased to exist (Fig. 16.2B). Some other terms used to describe the location of bone lesions are illustrated in Figure 16.3.

Imaging Modalities

In general, the imaging of musculoskeletal neoplasms can be considered from three standpoints: detection, diagnosis (and differential diagnosis), and staging (Fig. 16.4). The detection of a bone or a soft-tissue tumor does not always require the expertise of a radiologist. The clinical history and the physical examination are often sufficient to raise the suspicion of a tumor, although radiologic imaging is the most common means of revealing one. The radiologic modalities most often used in analyzing tumors and tumor-like lesions include (a) conventional radiography; (b) angiography (usually arteriography); (c) computed tomography (CT); (d) magnetic resonance imaging (MRI); (e) scintigraphy (radionuclide bone scan); (f) positron emission tomography (PET) and PET/CT; and (g) fluoroscopy-guided, ultrasound (US)-guided, or CT-guided percutaneous soft-tissue and bone biopsy.

Conventional Radiography

In most instances, the standard radiographic views specific for the anatomic site under investigation suffice to make a correct diagnosis (Fig. 16.5), which can subsequently be confirmed by biopsy and histopathologic examination. Conventional radiography yields the most useful information about the location and morphology of a lesion, particularly concerning the type of bone destruction, calcifications, ossifications, and periosteal reaction. Moreover, it is important to compare recent radiographic studies with earlier films. This point cannot be emphasized enough. The comparison can reveal not only the nature of a bone lesion (Fig. 16.6) but also its aggressiveness, a critical factor in a diagnostic workup. Chest radiography may also be required in cases of suspected metastasis, the most frequent complication of malignant lesions. This should be done before any treatment of a malignant primary bone tumor because most bone malignancies metastasize to the lung.

Computed Tomography

Although CT by itself is rarely helpful in making a specific diagnosis, it can provide a precise evaluation of the extent of a bone lesion and may demonstrate breakthrough of the cortex and involvement of surrounding

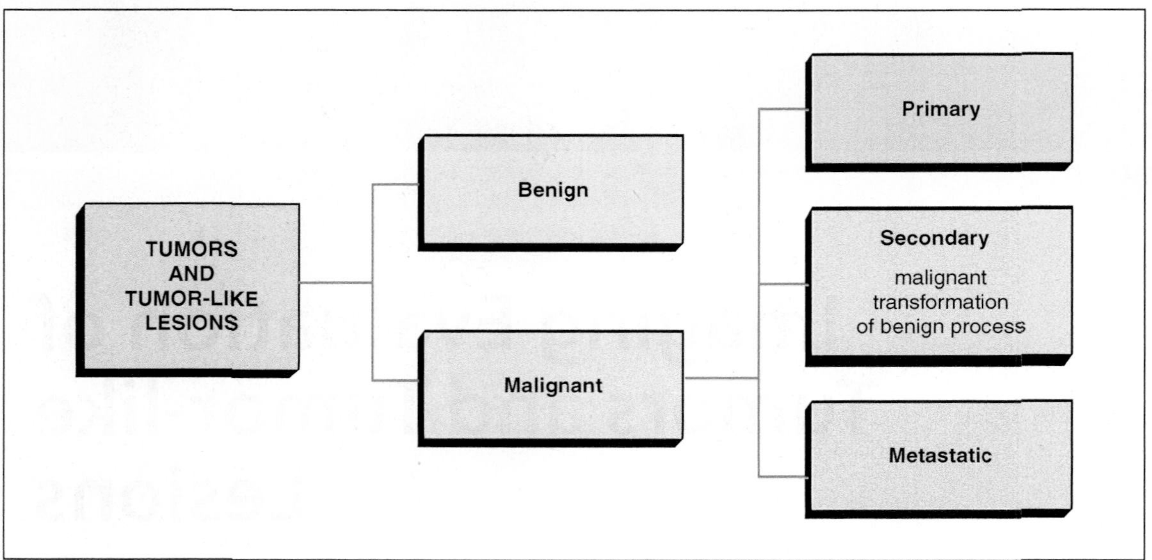

FIGURE 16.1 Classification of tumors and tumor-like lesions.

TABLE 16.1 Classification of Tumors and Tumor-like Lesions by Tissue of Origin

Tissue of Origin	Benign Lesion	Malignant Lesion
Bone forming (osteogenic)	Osteoma	Osteosarcoma (and variants)
	Osteoid osteoma	Juxtacortical osteosarcoma (and variants)
	Osteoblastoma	
Cartilage forming (chondrogenic)	Enchondroma (chondroma)	Chondrosarcoma (central)
	Periosteal (juxtacortical) chondroma	Conventional
	Enchondromatosis (Ollier disease)	Mesenchymal
	Osteochondroma (osteocartilaginous exostosis, solitary or multiple)	Clear cell
		Dedifferentiated
	Chondroblastoma	Chondrosarcoma (peripheral)
	Chondromyxoid fibroma	Periosteal (juxtacortical)
	Fibrocartilaginous mesenchymoma	
Fibrous, osteofibrous, and fibrohistiocytic (fibrogenic)	Fibrous cortical defect (metaphyseal fibrous defect)	Fibrosarcoma
	Nonossifying fibroma	Malignant fibrous histiocytoma
	Benign fibrous histiocytoma	
	Fibrous dysplasia (monostotic and polyostotic)	
	Fibrocartilaginous dysplasia	
	Focal fibrocartilaginous dysplasia of long bones	
	Periosteal desmoid	
	Desmoplastic fibroma	
	Osteofibrous dysplasia (Kempson-Campanacci lesion)	
	Ossifying fibroma (Sissons lesion)	
Vascular	Hemangioma	Angiosarcoma
	Glomus tumor	Hemangioendothelioma
	Cystic angiomatosis	Hemangiopericytoma
Hematopoietic, reticuloendothelial, and lymphatic	Giant cell tumor (osteoclastoma)	Malignant giant cell tumor
	Langerhans cell histiocytosis	Histiocytic lymphoma
	Lymphangioma	Hodgkin lymphoma
		Leukemia
		Myeloma (plasmacytoma)
		Ewing sarcoma
Neural (neurogenic)	Neurofibroma	Malignant schwannoma
	Neurilemoma	Neuroblastoma
	Morton neuroma	Primitive neuroectodermal tumor (PNET)
		Chordoma
Notochordal	Lipoma	Liposarcoma
Fat (lipogenic)	Simple bone cyst	
Unknown	Aneurysmal bone cyst	Adamantinoma
	Intraosseous ganglion	

TABLE 16.2 Benign Conditions with Potential for Malignant Transformation

Benign Lesion	Malignancy
Enchondroma (in the long or flat bones[a]; in the short, tubular bones almost always as a part of Ollier disease or Maffucci syndrome)	Chondrosarcoma
Osteochondroma	Peripheral chondrosarcoma
Synovial chondromatosis	Synovial chondrosarcoma
Fibrous dysplasia (usually polyostotic, or treated with radiation)	Fibrosarcoma Malignant fibrous histiocytoma Osteosarcoma
Osteofibrous dysplasia[b] (Kempson-Campanacci lesion)	Adamantinoma
Neurofibroma (in plexiform neuro-fibromatosis)	Malignant schwannoma Liposarcoma Malignant mesenchymoma
Medullary bone infarct	Fibrosarcoma Malignant fibrous histiocytoma
Osteomyelitis with chronic draining sinus tract (usually more than 15–20 years duration)	Squamous cell carcinoma Fibrosarcoma
Paget disease	Osteosarcoma Chondrosarcoma Fibrosarcoma Malignant fibrous histiocytoma

[a]Some authorities believe that at least in some "malignant transformations" of enchondroma to chondrosarcoma, there was in fact from the very beginning a malignant lesion masquerading as benign and not recognized as such.

[b]Some authorities believe that this is not a true malignant transformation but rather independent development of malignancy in the benign condition.

soft tissues (Fig. 16.7). CT is moreover very helpful in delineating a bone tumor within a complex anatomic structure. The scapula (Fig. 16.8), pelvis (Fig. 16.9), and sacrum, for example, may be difficult to image fully with conventional radiographic techniques. At times, three-dimensional (3D) CT reconstructed images are used to better and more comprehensively demonstrate the tumors. This technique can be useful, for example, in depicting surface lesions of bone, such as osteochondroma (Fig. 16.10), parosteal osteosarcoma, or juxtacortical chondrosarcoma. CT examination is crucial in determining the extent and spread of a tumor in the bone if limb salvage is contemplated so that a safe margin of resection can be planned (Fig. 16.11). It can effectively demonstrate the intraosseous extension of a tumor and its extraosseous involvement of soft tissues such as muscles and neurovascular bundles. CT is also useful for monitoring the results of treatment, evaluating for recurrence of a resected tumor, and demonstrating the effect of nonsurgical treatment such as radiation therapy or chemotherapy (Fig. 16.12). It is also helpful in evaluating soft-tissue tumors (Fig. 16.13), which on standard radiographs are indistinguishable from one another (with the exception of lipomas, which usually demonstrate low-density features), blending imperceptibly into the surrounding normal tissue.

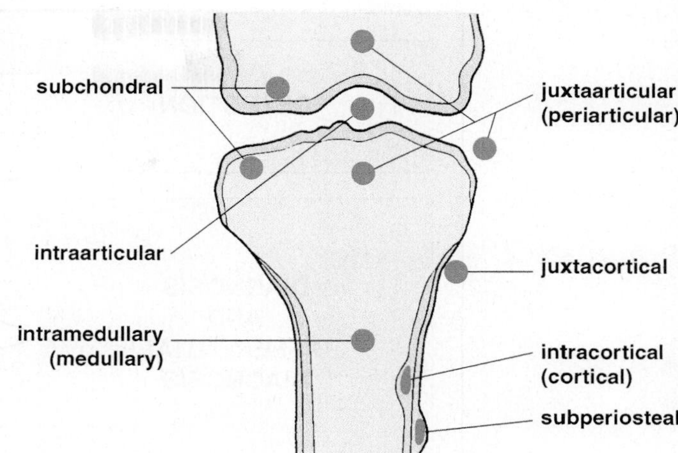

FIGURE 16.3 Terminology used to describe the location of lesions in the bone.

Contrast enhancement of CT images aids in the identification of major neurovascular structures and well-vascularized lesions. Evaluating the relationship between the tumor and the surrounding soft tissues and neurovascular structures is particularly important for planning limb-salvage surgery.

PET and PET/CT

Recently, 2-fluoro[fluorine-18]-2-deoxy-D-glucose (^{18}F-FDG) PET and PET/CT have emerged as very effective metabolic-anatomic imaging techniques for the assessment of variety of neoplastic conditions. The simultaneous detection and precise localization of metabolic and biochemical activities by PET combined with anatomic details obtained by CT

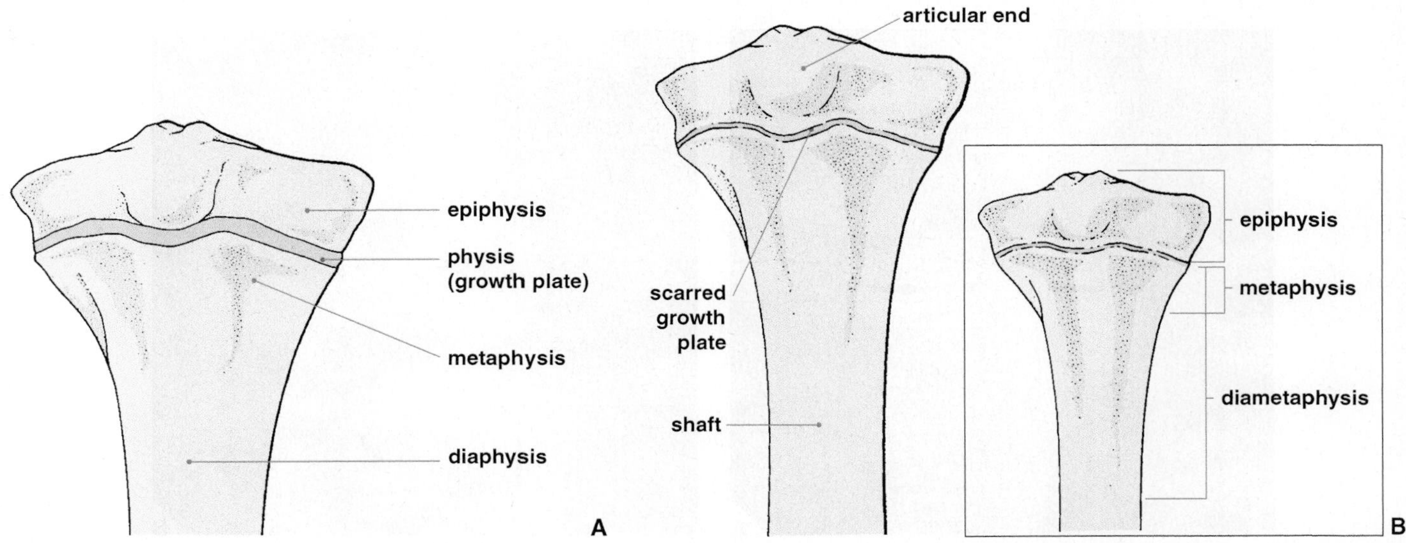

FIGURE 16.2 Parts of the bone. **(A)** In the maturing skeleton, the epiphysis, growth plate, metaphysis, and diaphysis are clearly recognizable areas. **(B)** With skeletal maturity, distinct epiphyseal and metaphyseal zones have ceased to exist. The terminology for describing the location of lesions should alter accordingly. The *inset* illustrates an alternate terminology.

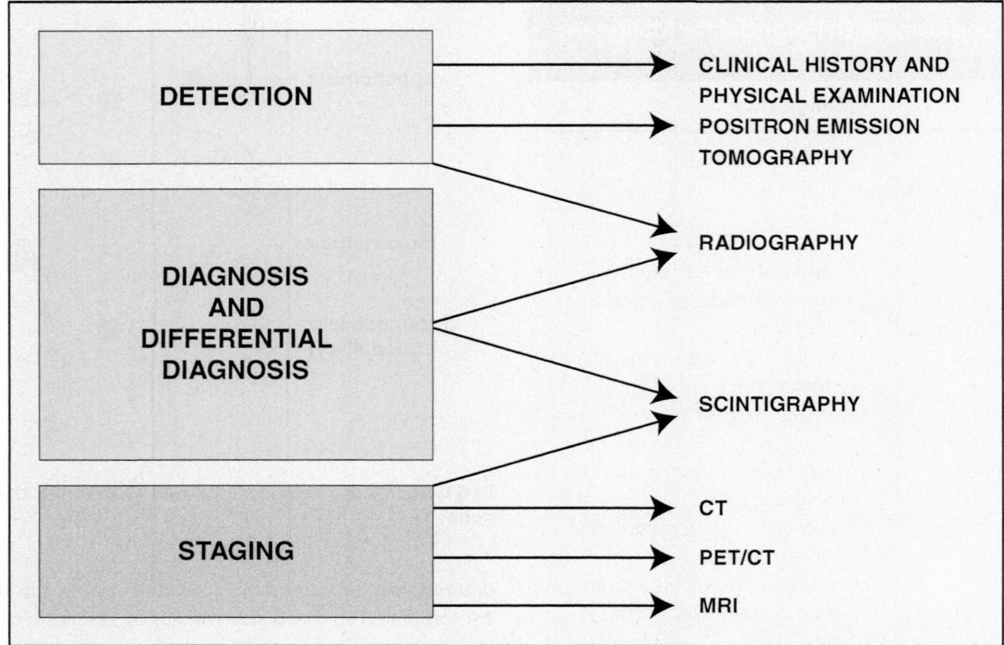

FIGURE 16.4 **Imaging of tumors.** Imaging of musculoskeletal neoplasms can be considered from three aspects: detection, diagnosis and differential diagnosis, and staging. CT, computed tomography ; PET/CT, positron emission tomography/computed tomography; MRI, magnetic resonance imaging. (Modified with permission from Greenspan A, Jundt G, Remagen W. *Differential diagnosis in orthopaedic oncology*, 2nd ed. Philadelphia: Lippincott Williams & Wilkins; 2007.)

into a single superimposed image provides the radiologist with a unique opportunity to make a distinction not only between the normal and pathologic processes but also frequently between the various pathologic disorders as well. Although the most common use of PET/CT is to improve the staging of musculoskeletal tumors and evaluate their response to therapy and emergence of recurrences, this technique is also a powerful tool for the detection and evaluation of metastatic disease (Fig. 16.14; see also Figs. 2.35B and 2.38) and some primary musculoskeletal tumors (Fig. 16.15; see also Figs. 2.36 and 2.37). In addition, recent trials using dual-time point ^{18}F-FDG PET to distinguish malignant tumors from benign conditions yielded promising results.

Arteriography

Arteriography is used mainly to map out bone lesions and to assess the extent of disease. It is also used to demonstrate the vascular supply of a tumor and to locate vessels suitable for preoperative intraarterial chemotherapy as well as to demonstrate the area suitable for open biopsy because the most vascular area of a tumor contains the most aggressive component. Occasionally, arteriography can be used to demonstrate abnormal tumor vessels, corroborating findings with conventional radiography (Fig. 16.16). Arteriography is often useful in planning for limb-salvage procedures because it demonstrates the regional vascular anatomy and thus permits a plan to be drawn up for the resection procedure. It is also sometimes used to outline the major vessels before resection of a benign tumor (Fig. 16.17), and it can be combined with an interventional procedure, such as embolization of hypervascular tumors, before further treatment (Fig. 16.18). In selected cases, arteriography may help make a differential diagnosis, such as of osteoid osteoma versus a bone abscess.

Myelography

Myelography may be helpful in dealing with tumors that invade the vertebral column and thecal sac (Fig. 16.19), although recently, this procedure has been almost completely replaced by MRI.

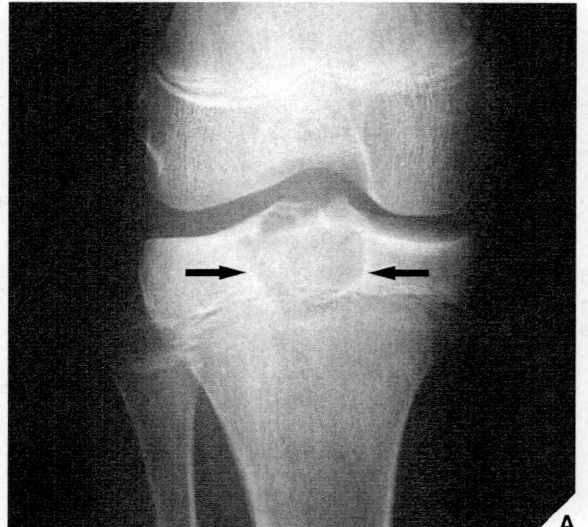

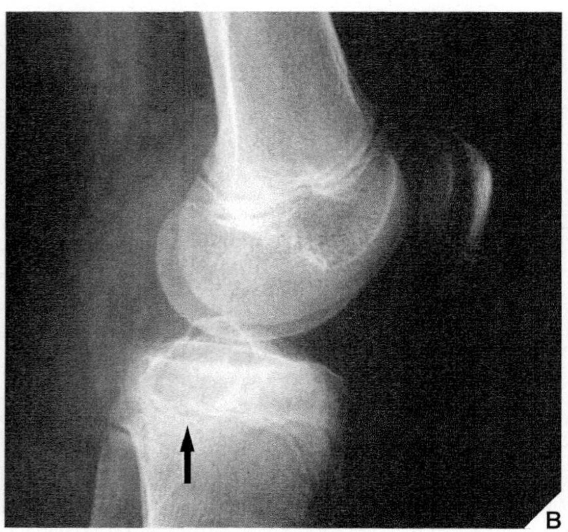

FIGURE 16.5 **Specific location of a tumor.** **(A)** Anteroposterior and **(B)** lateral radiographs of the right knee of a 13-year-old girl reveal a radiolucent lesion located eccentrically in the proximal epiphysis of the tibia, with sharply defined borders and a thin, sclerotic margin *(arrows)*. Here, the lesion's location and appearance on the standard radiographs led to the correct diagnosis of chondroblastoma.

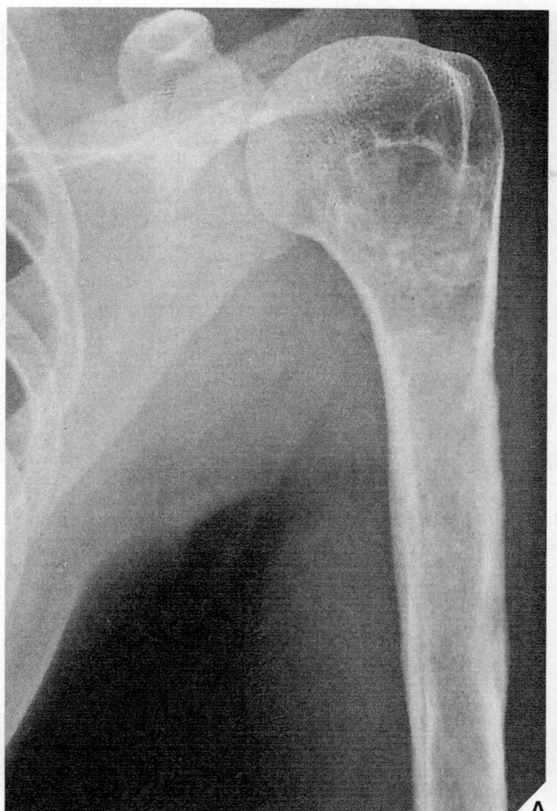

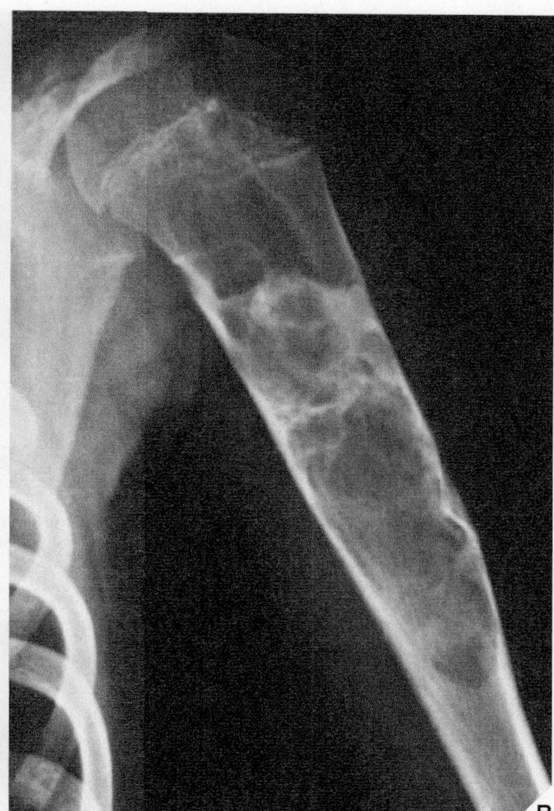

FIGURE 16.6 Comparison radiography: a simple bone cyst. (A) Anteroposterior radiograph of the left humerus in a 26-year-old woman with vague pain for 2 months shows an ill-defined lesion in the medullary region, with a periosteal reaction medially and laterally. There appear to be scattered calcifications in the proximal portion of the lesion. The possibility of a cartilage tumor such as chondrosarcoma was considered, but a radiograph taken 17 years earlier **(B)** shows an unquestionably benign lesion (a simple bone cyst) that had been treated by curettage and the application of bone chips. In view of this, the later findings were interpreted as representing a healed bone cyst. The patient's pain was found to be related to muscle strain.

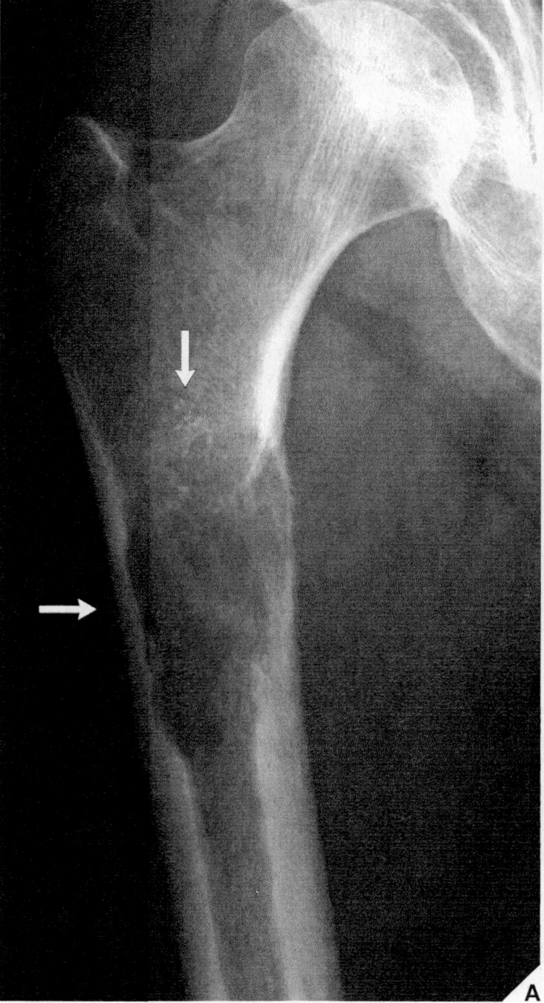

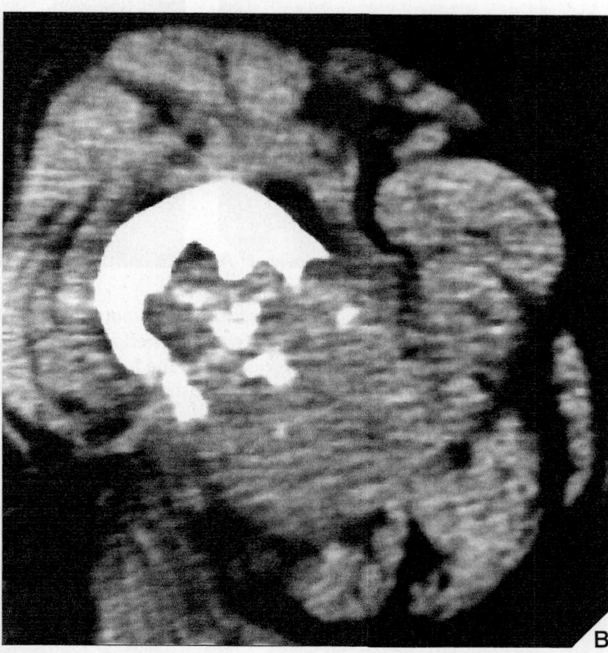

FIGURE 16.7 Soft-tissue extension of malignant tumor: effectiveness of CT. (A) Anteroposterior radiograph of the right proximal femur of a 70-year-old man shows a destructive lesion in the medullary portion of the bone *(arrows)* displaying focal chondroid calcifications. The soft-tissue extension of the tumor cannot be well evaluated. **(B)** Axial CT demonstrates a large soft-tissue mass, which on biopsy proved to be a chondrosarcoma.

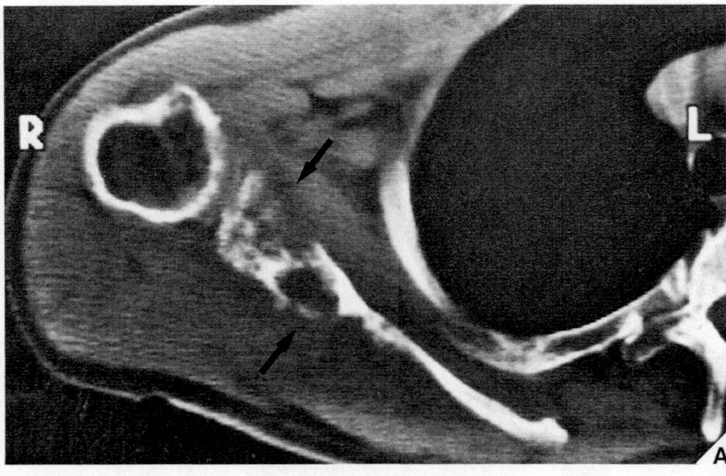

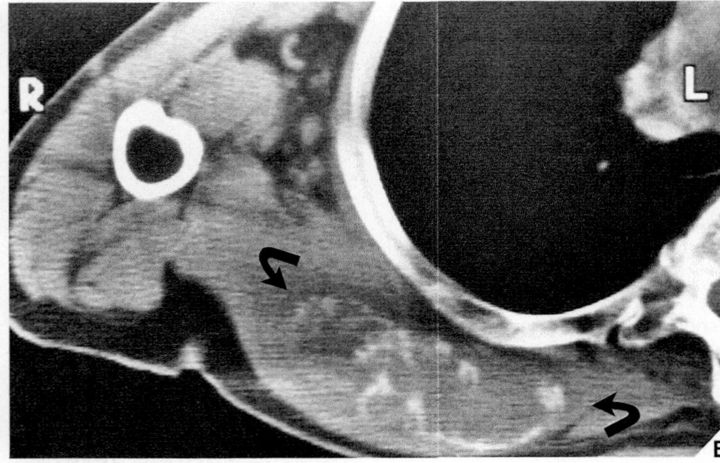

FIGURE 16.8 CT of chondrosarcoma. Standard radiographs were ambiguous in this 70-year-old man with a palpable mass over the right scapula. However, two axial CT sections demonstrate a destructive lesion of the glenoid portion and body of the scapula *(arrows)* **(A)**, with a large soft-tissue mass extending to the rib cage and containing calcifications *(curved arrows)* **(B)**.

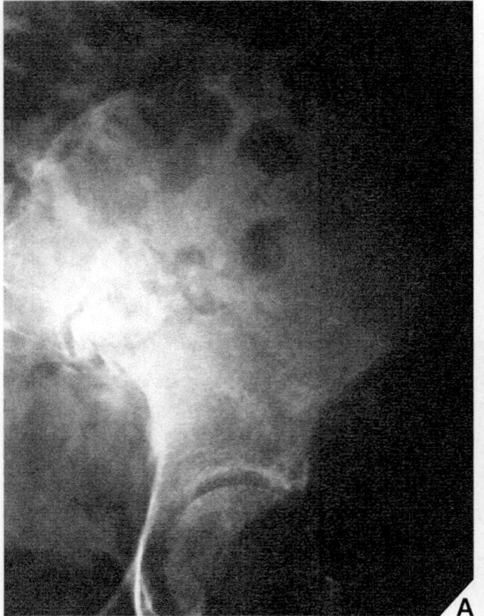

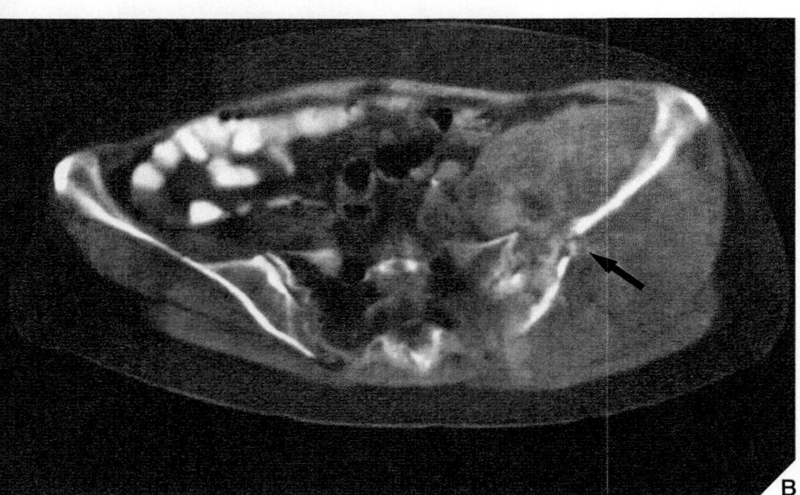

FIGURE 16.9 CT of osteosarcoma. **(A)** Standard anteroposterior radiograph of the pelvis was not sufficient to delineate the full extent of the destructive lesion of the iliac bone in this 66-year-old woman. **(B)** CT image, however, showed a pathologic fracture of the ilium *(arrow)* and the full extent of soft-tissue involvement. The high Hounsfield values of the multiple soft-tissue densities suggested bone formation. Enhancement of the CT images with contrast agent showed an increased vascularity of the lesion. Collectively, the CT findings suggested a diagnosis of osteosarcoma that, although unusual for a person of this age, was confirmed by open biopsy.

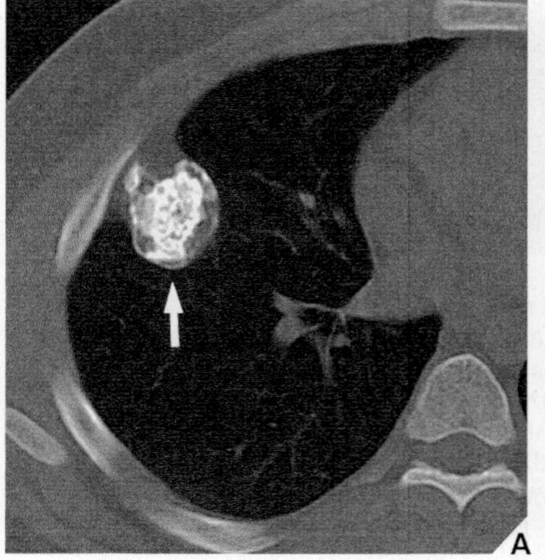

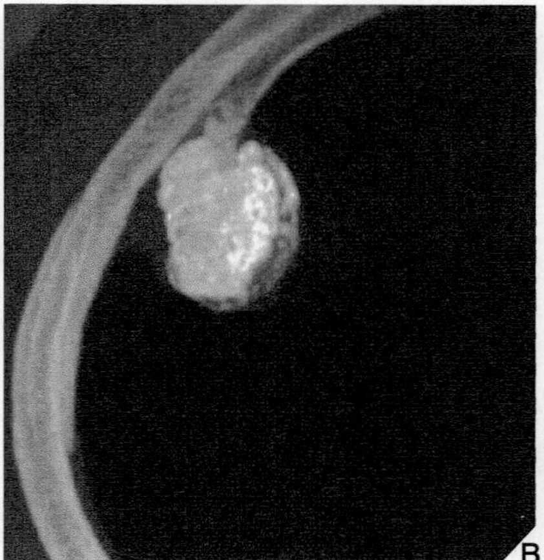

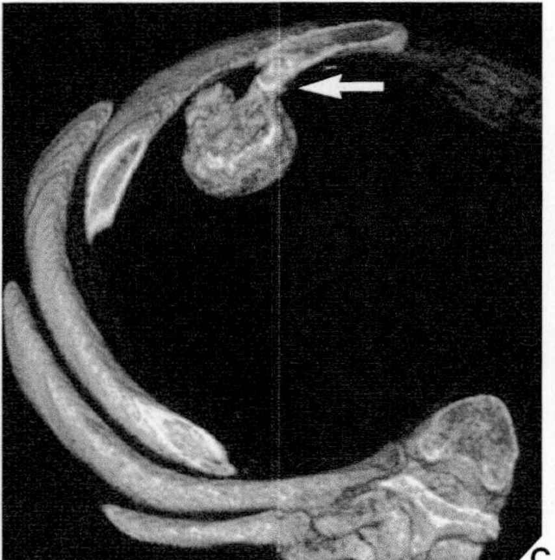

FIGURE 16.10 Osteochondroma: effectiveness of 3D CT. **(A)** Conventional CT section through the chest shows an osteochondroma at the site of the anteromedial portion of the right forth rib *(arrow)*. It is difficult to determine if the lesion is sessile or pedunculated. **(B)** 3D CT reconstructed image in maximum intensity projection (MIP) delivers a much more informative image of osteochondroma and allows one to characterize the internal architecture of the lesion; note typical chondroid matrix of the tumor. **(C)** 3D CT reconstructed image in shaded surface display (SSD) renders better conspicuity of the lesion; the pedicle of osteochondroma *(arrow)* is now clearly demonstrated. (Reprinted with permission from Greenspan A, Jundt G, Remagen W. *Differential diagnosis in orthopaedic oncology*, 2nd ed. Philadelphia: Lippincott Williams & Wilkins; 2007.)

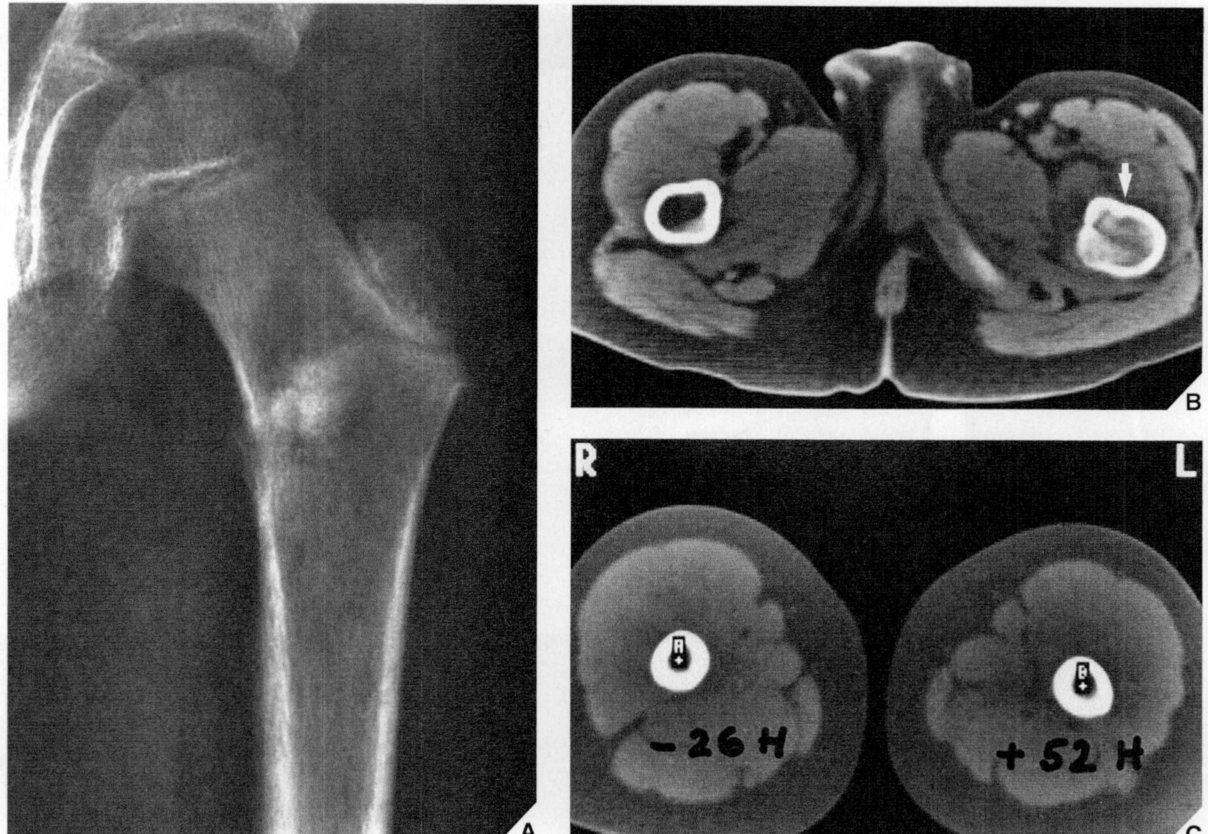

FIGURE 16.11 Osteosarcoma: effectiveness of CT. **(A)** Anteroposterior radiograph of the left proximal femur of a 12-year-old boy demonstrates an osteolytic lesion in the intertrochanteric region, with a poorly defined margin and amorphous densities in the center associated with a periosteal reaction medially—features suggesting osteosarcoma, which was confirmed on open biopsy. Because a limb-salvage procedure was contemplated, a CT scan was performed to determine the extent of marrow infiltration and the required level of bone resection. The most proximal section **(B)** shows obvious gross tumor involvement of the marrow cavity of the left femur *(arrow)*. A more distal section **(C)** shows no gross marrow abnormality, but a positive Hounsfield value of 52 units indicates tumor involvement of the marrow, which was not shown on the standard radiographs. By comparison, the section of the right femur shows a normal Hounsfield value of −26 for bone marrow.

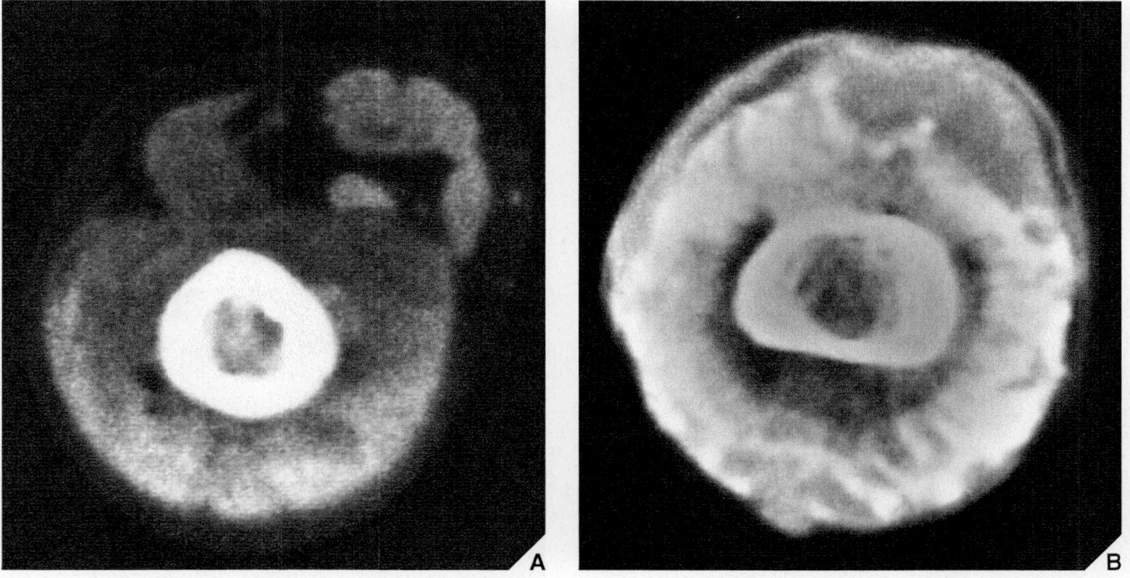

FIGURE 16.12 Osteosarcoma after chemotherapy: effectiveness of CT. Before surgery, this 14-year-old girl with an osteosarcoma of the left femur underwent a full course of chemotherapy. **(A)** CT section before the therapy was begun shows involvement of the bone and marrow cavity. Note the soft-tissue extension of the tumor, with heterogeneous, amorphous tumor bone formation. After combined treatment with doxorubicin hydrochloride, vincristine, methotrexate, and cisplatin, a repeat CT scan **(B)** shows calcifications and ossifications in the periphery of the lesion, which represents reactive rather than tumor bone and demonstrates the success of chemotherapy. Radical excision of the femur and a subsequent histopathologic examination showed almost complete eradication of malignant cells, confirming the CT findings.

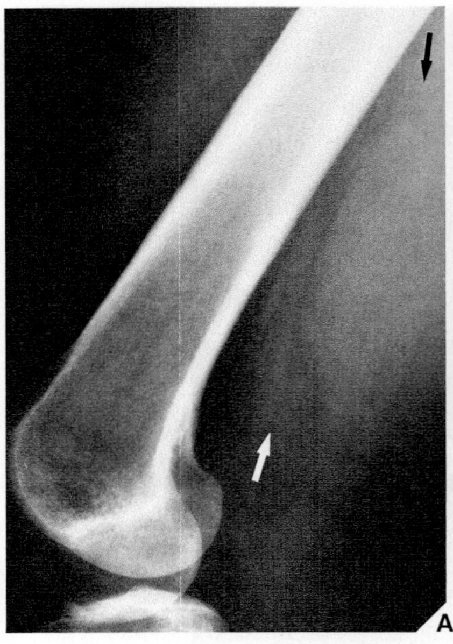

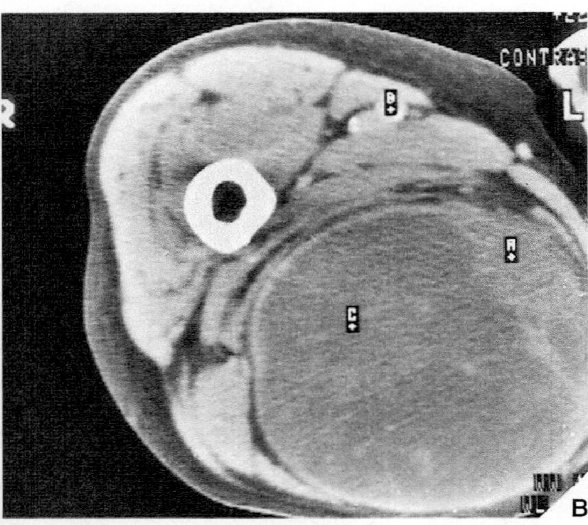

FIGURE 16.13 **CT of malignant fibrous histiocytoma (MFH) of the soft tissue.** A 56-year-old woman presented with a soft-tissue mass on the posteromedial aspect of the right thigh. **(A)** Lateral radiograph of the femur demonstrates only a soft-tissue prominence posteriorly *(arrows)*. **(B)** CT section shows an axial image of the mass, which is contained by a fibrotic capsule. The overlying skin is not infiltrated. Despite the benign appearance, the mass proved on biopsy to be an MFH.

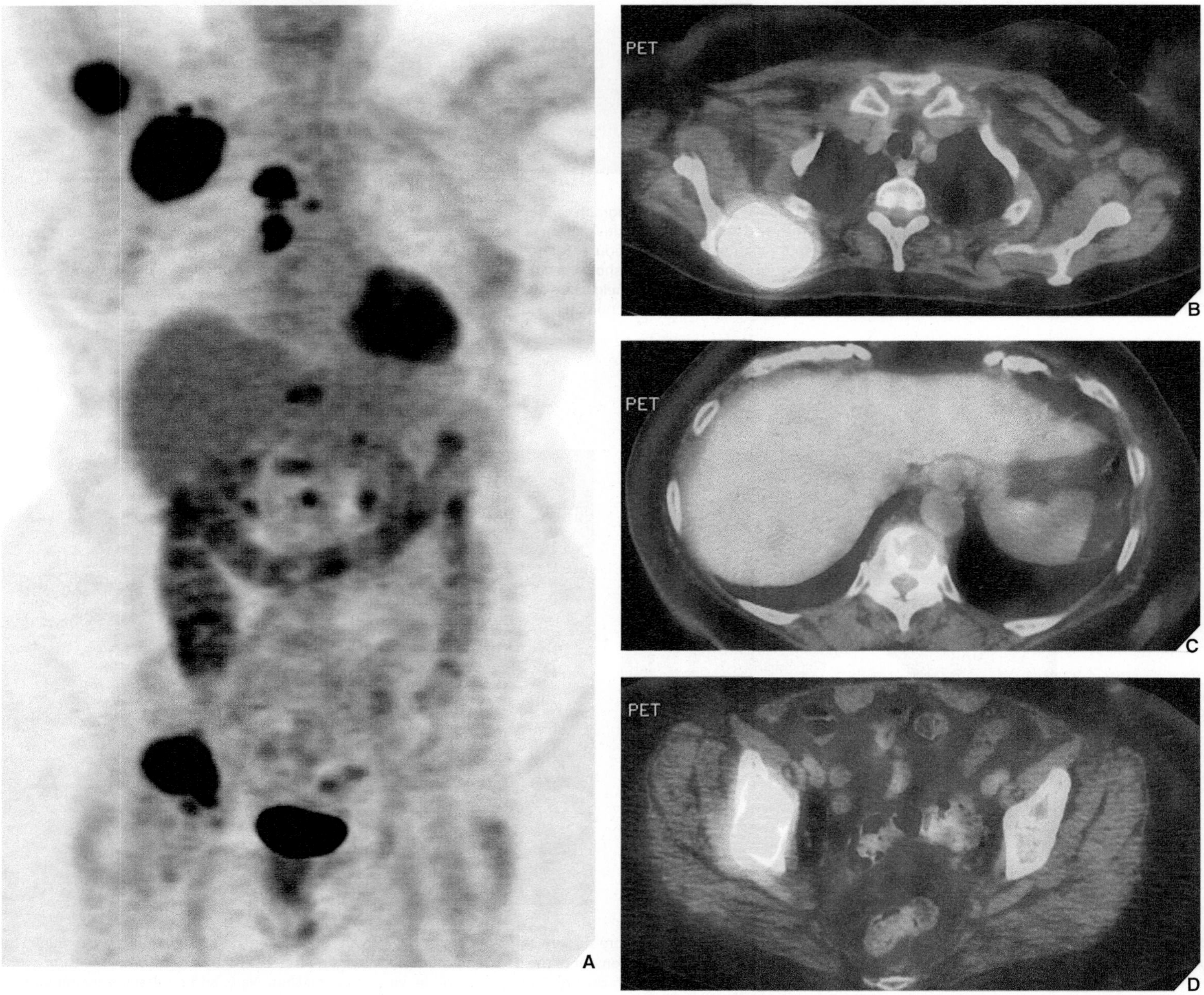

FIGURE 16.14 **PET and PET/CT of metastases.** A 61-year-old woman was diagnosed with lung carcinoma. **(A)** A whole-body PET scan shows several hypermetabolic foci in the internal organs, lymph nodes, and osseous structures, representing metastatic disease. The fused PET/CT images demonstrate metastatic lesions in the right scapula **(B)**, thoracic vertebral body **(C)**, and right ilium **(D)**.

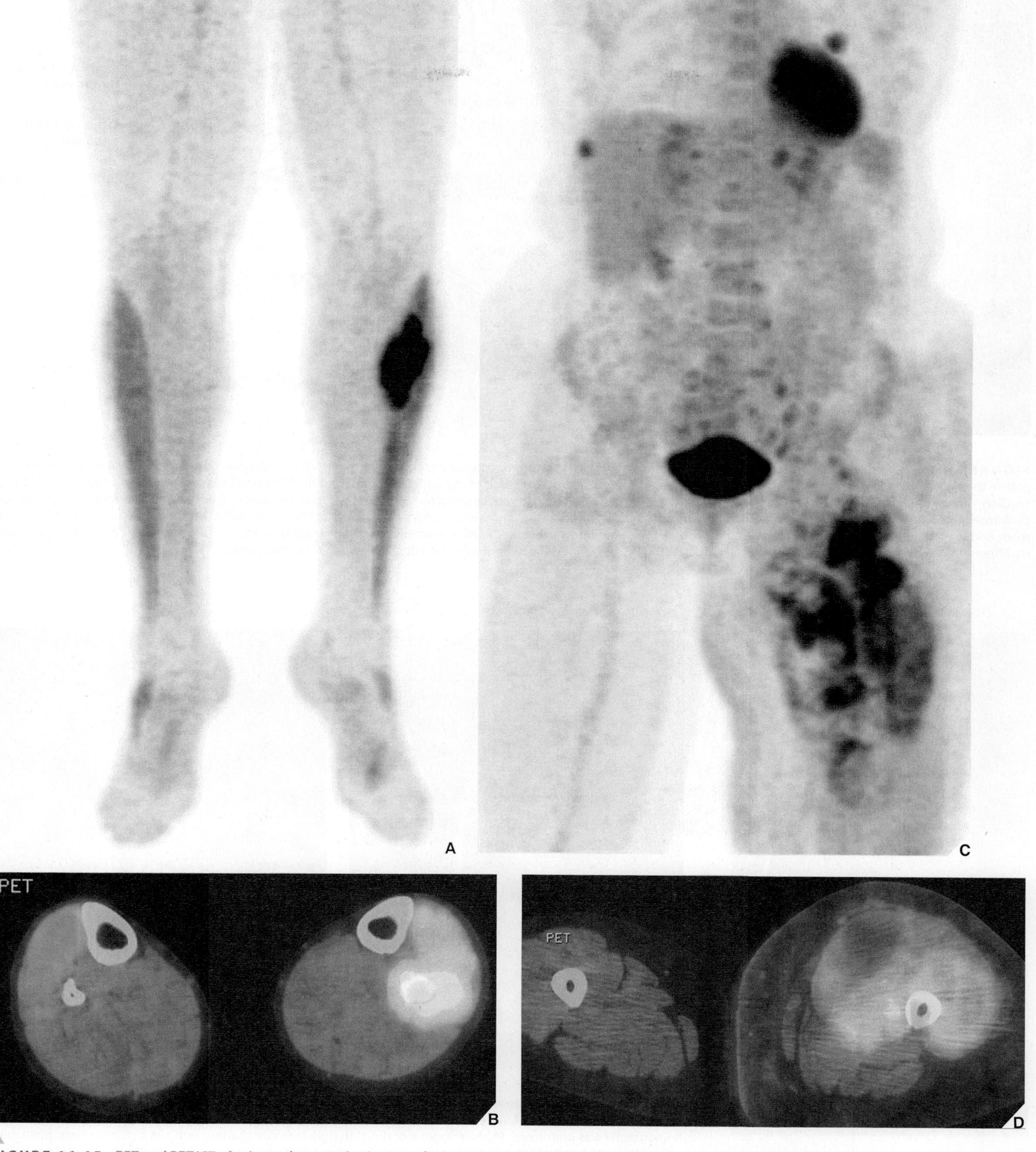

FIGURE 16.15 PET and PET/CT of primary bone and primary soft-tissue tumors. **(A,B)** Hypermetabolic focus in the proximal left fibula in a 23-year-old man proved to be an Ewing sarcoma. **(C,D)** Hypermetabolic lesion in the vastus lateralis and medialis in the proximal left thigh in a 58-year-old woman was diagnosed on histopathologic examination as malignant fibrous histiocytoma of the soft tissues.

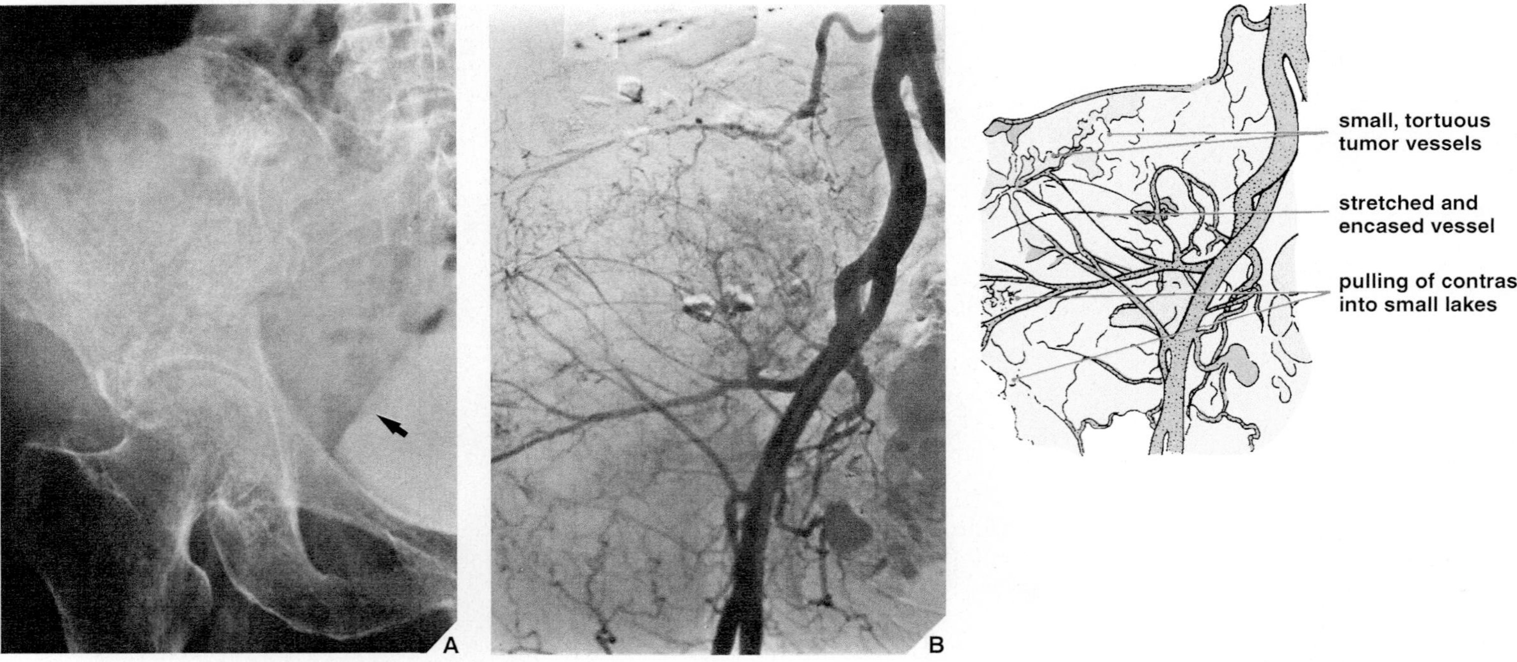

FIGURE 16.16 Arteriography of dedifferentiated chondrosarcoma. **(A)** Anteroposterior radiograph of the pelvis in a 79-year-old woman with an 8-month history of pain in the right buttock and weight loss demonstrates a poorly defined destructive lesion of the right iliac bone, with multiple small calcifications and a soft-tissue mass extending into the pelvic cavity. Note the effect of the mass on the urinary bladder filled with contrast *(arrow)*. A chondrosarcoma was suspected, and a femoral arteriogram was performed as part of the diagnostic workup. **(B)** Subtraction study of an arteriogram demonstrates hypervascularity of the tumor. Note the abnormal tumor vessels, encasement and stretching of some vessels, and "pulling" of contrast medium into small "lakes"—all characteristic signs of a malignant lesion. Biopsy revealed a highly malignant, dedifferentiated chondrosarcoma. In this case, the vascular study corroborated the radiographic findings of a malignant bone tumor.

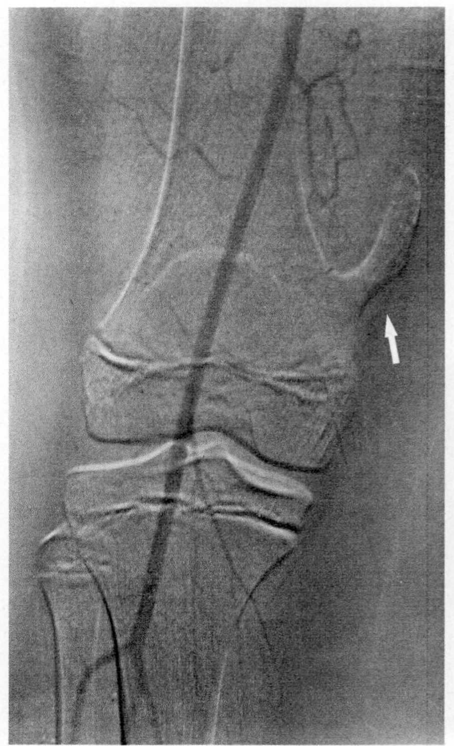

FIGURE 16.17 Arteriography of osteochondroma. A 12-year-old boy with osteochondroma of the distal femur *(arrow)* underwent arteriography to demonstrate the relationship of the distal superficial femoral artery to the lesion. This subtraction study shows no major vessels near the planned site of resection at the base of the lesion, important information for surgical planning.

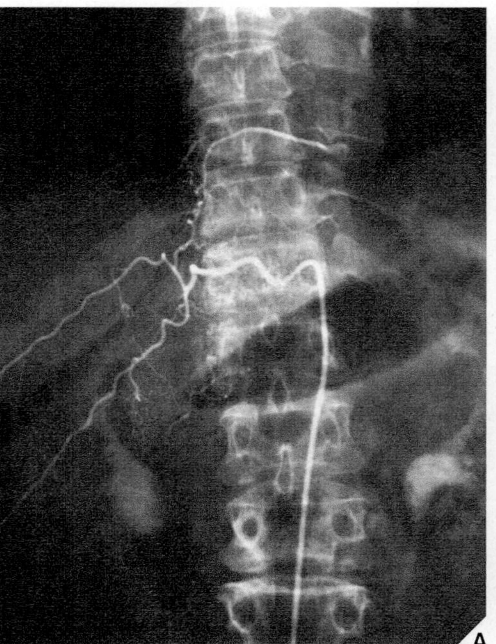

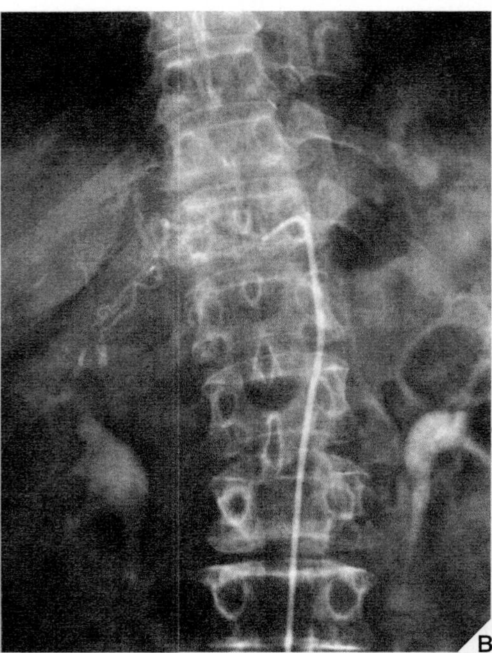

FIGURE 16.18 Vertebral arteriography and embolization of hemangioma. A 73-year-old woman presented with a collapsed T11 vertebra, which showed a corduroy-like pattern suggestive of hemangioma. Vertebral angiography was performed. **(A)** Arteriogram of the 11th right intercostal artery outlines a vascular paraspinal mass associated with hemangioma and indicating extension of the lesion into the soft tissues. **(B)** After embolization, the lesion shows a marked decrease in vascularity. Subsequently, the patient underwent decompression laminectomy and anterior fusion at T10-11 using a fibular strut graft.

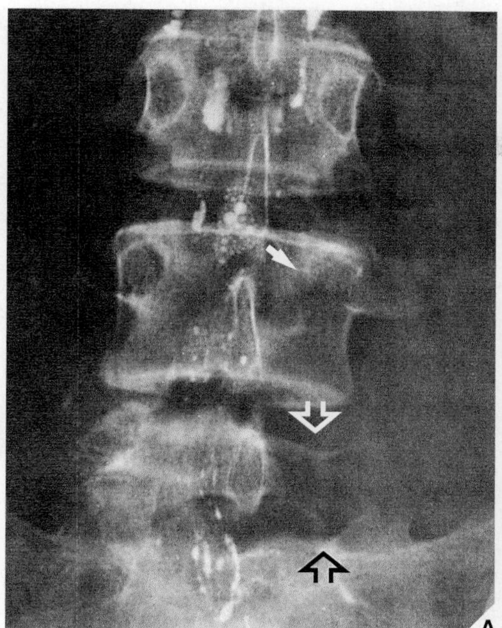

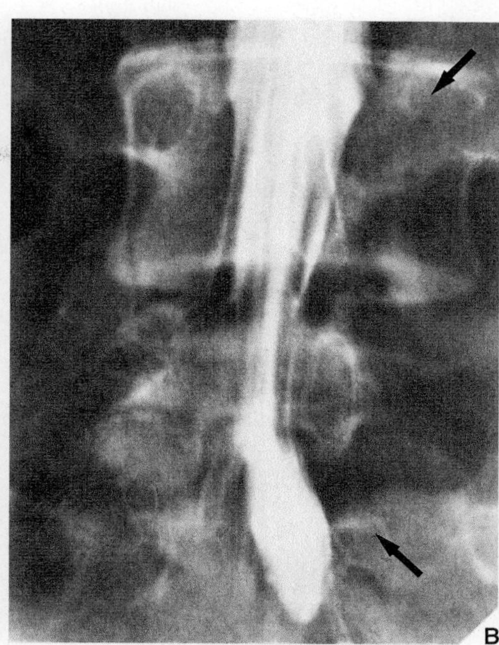

FIGURE 16.19 Myelography of aneurysmal bone cyst. Initial radiographic examination of the lumbar spine of this 14-year-old girl with an 18-month history of pain in the lower back and sciatica of the left leg did not disclose any abnormalities; myelography was performed because of suspected herniation of a lumbar disk, but it was inconclusive. A repeat study was requested when the symptoms became more severe after 3 months. **(A)** Posteroanterior radiograph of the lumbosacral spine shows destruction of the left pedicle of L4 *(arrow)* and the left part of the L5 body *(open arrows)*. Note the residual contrast in the subarachnoid space. A repeat myelogram using a water-soluble contrast (metrizamide) shows, on the posteroanterior view **(B)**, extradural compression of the thecal sac on the left side with displacement of the nerve roots *(arrows)*. Biopsy confirmed the radiographic diagnosis of an aneurysmal bone cyst.

Magnetic Resonance Imaging

MRI is indispensable in evaluating bone and soft-tissue tumors. Particularly with soft-tissue masses, MRI offers distinct advantages over CT. There is improved visualization of tissue planes surrounding the lesion, for example, and neurovascular involvement can be evaluated without the use of intravenous contrast.

In the evaluation of intraosseous and extraosseous extensions of a tumor, MRI is crucial because it can determine with high accuracy the presence or absence of soft-tissue invasion by a tumor (Fig. 16.20). MRI has often proved to be superior to CT in delineating the extraosseous and intramedullary extent of the tumor and its relationship to surrounding structures (Fig. 16.21). By showing sharper demarcation between normal and abnormal tissue than CT, MRI—particularly in evaluation of the extremities—reliably identifies the spatial boundaries of tumor masses (Fig. 16.22), the encasement and displacement of major neurovascular bundles, and the extent of joint involvement. Spin echo (SE) T1-weighted images enhance tumor contrast with bone, bone marrow, and fatty tissue, whereas SE T2-weighted images enhance tumor contrast with muscle

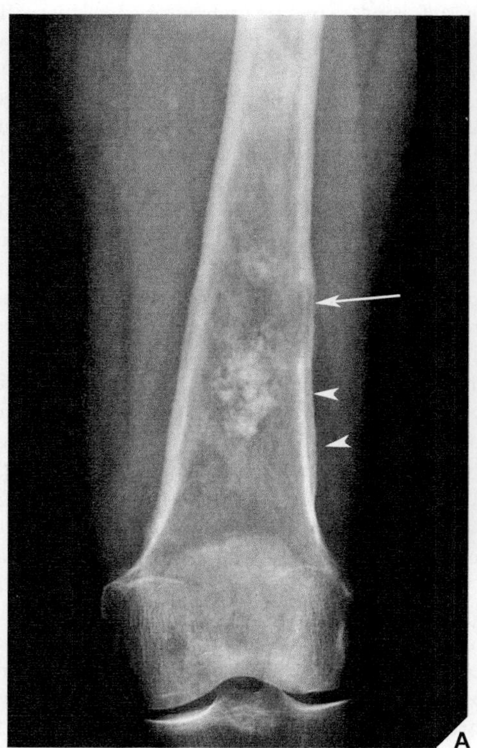

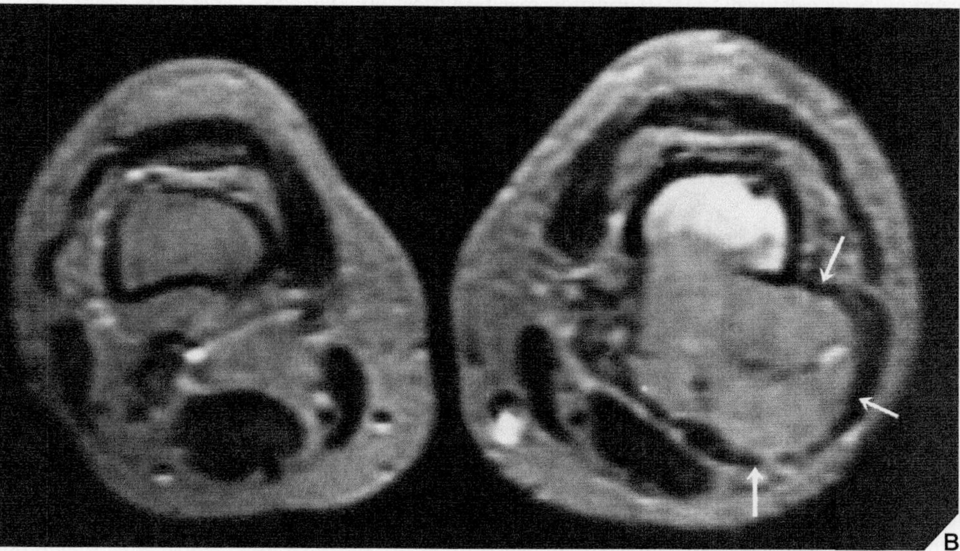

FIGURE 16.20 MRI of chondrosarcoma. (A) Conventional radiograph of the left femur in anteroposterior projection of a 67-year-old woman demonstrates a tumor in the distal shaft destroying the medullary portion of the bone and breaking through the cortex (*arrow*). Note the associated thick periosteal reaction (*arrowheads*). The soft-tissue extension cannot be precisely determined. **(B)** Axial T2-weighted MR image (SE; repetition time [TR] 2500/echo time [TE] 70 msec) demonstrates a tumor infiltrating bone marrow, destroying the posteromedial cortex, and breaking into the soft tissues with the formation of a large mass *(arrows)*. Compare with a normal contralateral extremity.

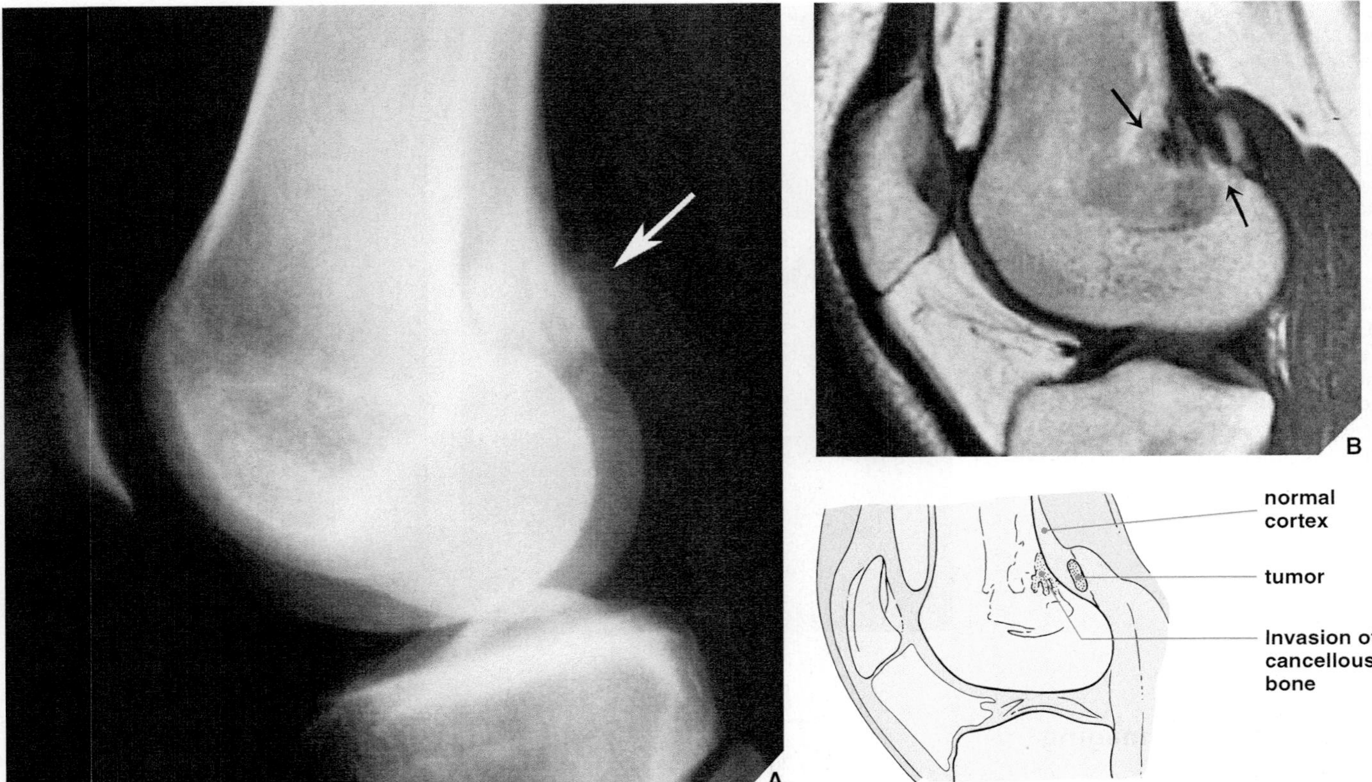

FIGURE 16.21 MRI of parosteal osteosarcoma. **(A)** From this lateral radiograph of the distal femur of a 22-year-old woman with parosteal osteosarcoma, it is difficult to evaluate if the tumor *(arrow)* is on the surface of the bone or already infiltrated through the cortex. **(B)** Sagittal T1-weighted MRI (SE; repetition time [TR] 500/echo time [TE] 20 msec) demonstrates invasion of the cancellous portion of the bone, as represented by an area of low signal intensity *(arrows)*.

and accentuate peritumoral edema. Axial and coronal images have been used in determining the extent of soft-tissue invasion in relation to important vascular structures. However, in comparison with CT, MR images do not clearly demonstrate calcification in the tumor matrix; in fact, large amounts of calcification or ossification may be almost undetectable. Moreover, MRI has been shown to be less satisfactory than CT in the demonstration of cortical destruction. It is important to realize that both MRI and CT have advantages and disadvantages, and circumstances exist in which either can be the preferential or complementary study. But it is even more important that the surgeon tell the radiologist who is performing and interpreting the study what information is needed.

Several investigators have stressed the superior contrast enhancement of MR images using intravenous injection of gadopentetate dimeglumine (gadolinium diethylenetriamine-penta-acetic acid [Gd-DTPA]). Enhancement was found to give better delineation of the tumor's richly vascularized parts and of the compressed tissue immediately surrounding the tumor. It was also found to assist in the differentiation of intraarticular tumor extension from joint effusion, and, as Erlemann et al. pointed out, improved the differentiation of necrotic tissue from viable areas in various malignant tumors.

MRI has an additional application in evaluating both the tumor's response to radiation and chemotherapy and any local recurrence. On gadolinium-enhanced T1-weighted images, signal intensity remains low in avascular, necrotic areas of tumor while it increases in viable tissue. Although static MRI was of little value for the assessment of response to the treatment, dynamic MRI using Gd-DTPA as a contrast enhancement, according to Erlemann et al., had the highest degree of accuracy (85.7%) and was superior to scintigraphy, particularly in patients who were receiving intraarterial chemotherapy. In general, drug-sensitive tumors display slower uptake of Gd-DTPA after preoperative chemotherapy than do nonresponsive lesions. The rapid uptake of Gd-DTPA by malignant tissues may be due to increased vascularity and more rapid perfusion of the contrast material through an expanded interstitial space.

It must be stressed, however, that most of the time MRI is not suitable for establishing the precise histologic nature of a bone tumor. In particular, too much faith has been placed in MRI as a method of distinguishing benign lesions from malignant ones. An overlap between the classic characteristics of benign and malignant tumors is often observed. Moreover, some malignant bone tumors can appear misleadingly benign on MR images and, conversely, some benign lesions may exhibit a misleadingly malignant appearance. Attempts to formulate precise criteria for correlating MRI findings with histologic diagnosis have been largely unsuccessful. Tissue characterization on the basis of MRI signal intensities is unreliable. Because of the wide spectrum of bone tumor composition and their differing histologic patterns, as well as in tumors of similar histologic diagnosis, signal intensities of histologically different tumors may overlap or there may be variability of signal intensity in histologically similar tumors.

Trials using combined hydrogen-1 MRI and phosphorus-31 (^{31}P) MR spectroscopy also failed to distinguish most benign lesions from malignant tumors. Despite the use of various criteria, the application of MRI to tissue diagnosis has rarely brought satisfactory results. This is because, in general, the small number of protons in calcified structures renders MRI less effective in diagnosing bone lesions, and hence, valuable evidence concerning the production of the tumor matrix can be missed. Moreover, as several investigations have shown, MRI is an imaging modality of low specificity. T1 and T2 measurements are generally of limited value for histologic characterization of musculoskeletal tumors. There are, however, some exceptions to this general rule. Some bone tumors demonstrate morphologic characteristic that allows a specific diagnosis, such as the typical "popcorn" appearance of chondroid matrix (Fig. 16.23) or "fluid–fluid" levels characteristic of aneurysmal bone cyst (see Fig. 20.23E,F) and telangiectatic osteosarcoma (Fig. 16.24). Quantitative determination of relaxation times has not proved to be clinically valuable in identifying various tumor types, although, as noted by Sundaram and McLeod, it has proved to be an important technique in the staging of osteosarcoma and chondrosarcoma. T2-weighted images in particular are a crucial factor in delineating extraosseous tumor extension and peritumoral edema as well as in assessing the involvement of major neurovascular bundles. Necrotic areas change from a low-intensity signal in the T1-weighted image to a very bright, intense signal in the T2-weighted image and can be differentiated from viable, solid tumor tissue. Although MRI cannot predict the histology of bone tumors,

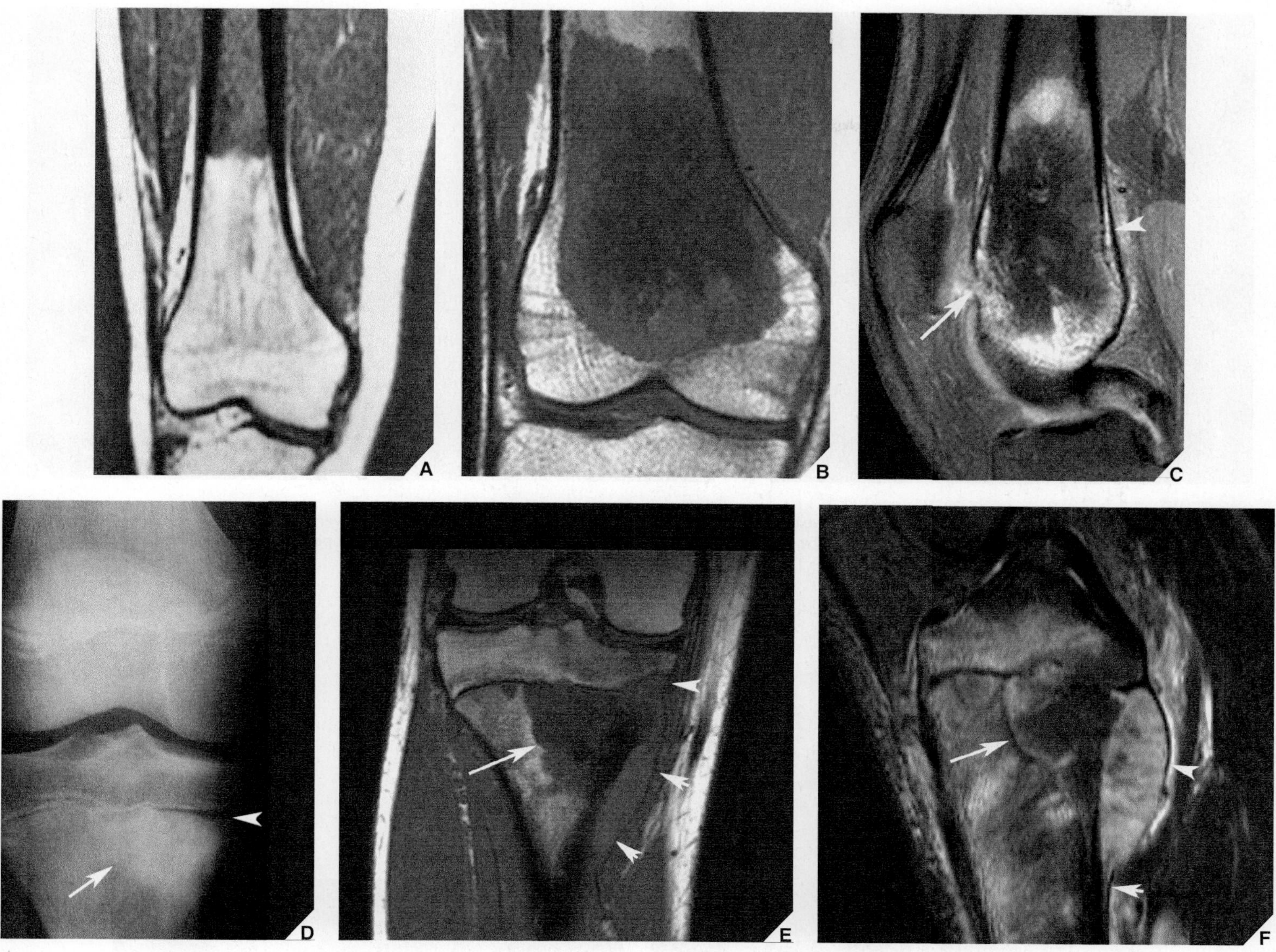

FIGURE 16.22 MRI of malignant fibrous histiocytoma (MFH) and osteosarcoma. **(A)** Coronal T1-weighted MRI (SE; repetition time [TR] 500/echo time [TE] 20 msec) demonstrates involvement of the medullary cavity of the right femur in this 16-year-old girl with MFH (the entire tumor is not imaged on this study). Note the excellent demonstration of the interface between normal bone displaying high signal intensity and a tumor displaying intermediate signal intensity. **(B)** Coronal T1-weighted MRI in another patient with osteosarcoma of the distal femur demonstrates the intramedullary extension of the tumor. Again, note demonstration of sharp interface between tumor and not affected bone. **(C)** Sagittal T2-weighted MRI shows a small focal area of cortical breakthrough in the anterior cortex of the distal femur *(arrow)* and posterior periosteal elevation *(arrowhead)*. **(D)** Anteroposterior radiograph of the knee of another patient shows a sclerotic lesion within the medullary cavity of the proximal tibia *(arrow)*. Note the subtle widening of the medial aspect of the physis *(arrowhead)*, suspicious for transphyseal extension of the tumor. **(E)** Coronal T1-weighted MRI of the proximal tibia outlines the intramedullary extent of osteosarcoma *(long arrow)*, the extraosseous mass *(short arrows)*, and confirms the extension of the tumor across the physis into the epiphysis *(arrowhead)*. **(F)** Sagittal T2-weighted MR image demonstrates the intramedullary *(long arrow)* and extraosseous *(arrowhead)* extension of the tumor. Note the typical Codman triangle in the inferior aspect of the lesion *(short arrow)* and the surrounding bone marrow and soft-tissue edema.

as Sundaram and McLeod pointed out, it is a useful tool for distinguishing round cell tumors and metastases from stress fractures or medullary infarcts in symptomatic patients with normal radiographs, and, it can occasionally differentiate benign from pathologic fracture.

Diffusion weighted imaging (DWI) is a method of signal contrast generation based on the differences in Brownian motion. This methodology allows evaluation of molecular function and microarchitecture of the human body, and it can be quantified by generation of apparent diffusion coefficient maps, which can be used to evaluate treatment response and disease progression. Diffusion tensor imaging (DTI) is a tool that allows detection and quantification of anisotropy of diffusion in highly organized fiber structure. These techniques are widely used in neuroimaging for brain ischemia, tumors, white matter disease, pediatric brain development, and aging and also in oncologic applications including head and neck malignancies, thoracic malignancies, breast cancer, hepatobiliary and pancreatic cancer, gastrointestinal and genitourinary disorders, peripheral nerve imaging, and in the musculoskeletal system. The use of DWI has been particularly useful in differentiating between acute osteoporotic fractures of the spine and malignant compression fractures.

Thanks to technical developments, whole-body MRI is increasingly being used for cancer assessment, including multichannel surface receive coils, parallel imaging, and continuously moving table acquisition mode, which allows high spatial resolution T1- and T2-weighted images with good contrast-to-noise ratio in a relatively short time. The addition DWI aids in detection of cellular disease. Using both techniques combined allows tumor staging, assessment of neoplastic activity, and response to treatment not only in the skeleton but also in the entire body. Oncologic applications of whole-body MRI include multiple myeloma, lymphoma, lung cancer, and ovarian cancer.

Skeletal Scintigraphy (Radionuclide Bone Scan)

The radionuclide bone scan is an indicator of mineral turnover, and because there is usually enhanced deposition of bone-seeking radiopharmaceuticals

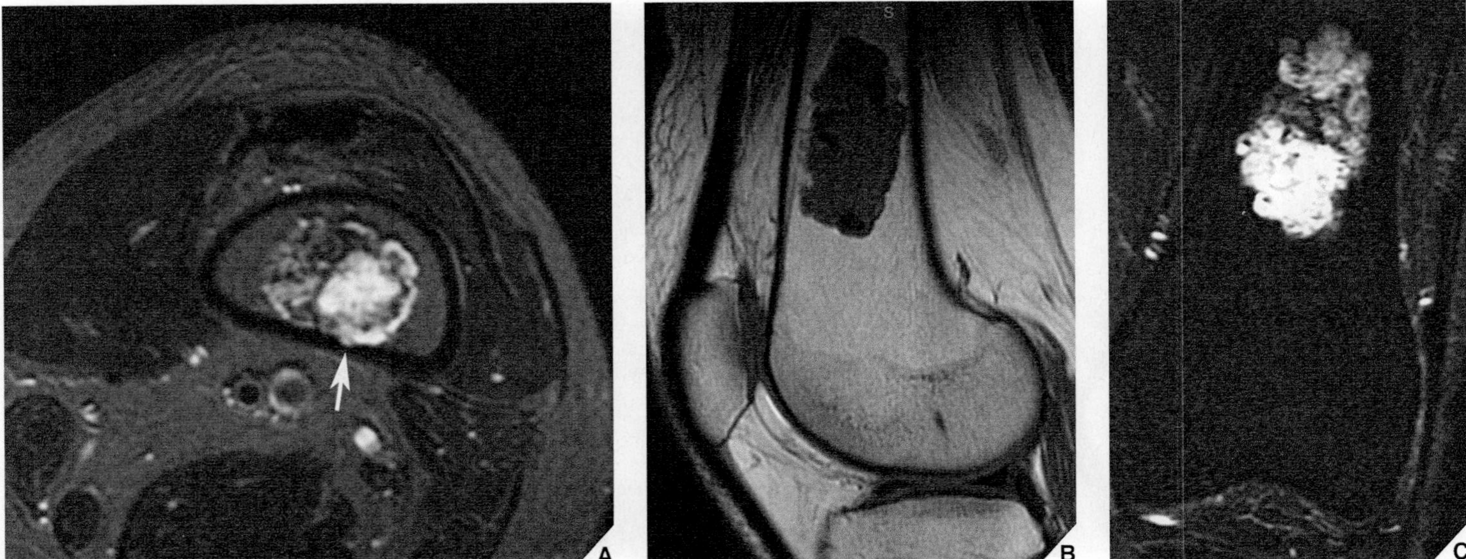

FIGURE 16.23 MRI of chondroid matrix. **(A)** Axial T2-weighted, **(B)** sagittal T1-weighted, and **(C)** coronal short time inversion recovery (STIR) images demonstrate a typical popcorn pattern of chondroid matrix in the bone marrow space of the distal femur. Note also the slight endosteal scalloping on the axial image *(arrow)*. The excision biopsy revealed the lesion to be an enchondroma.

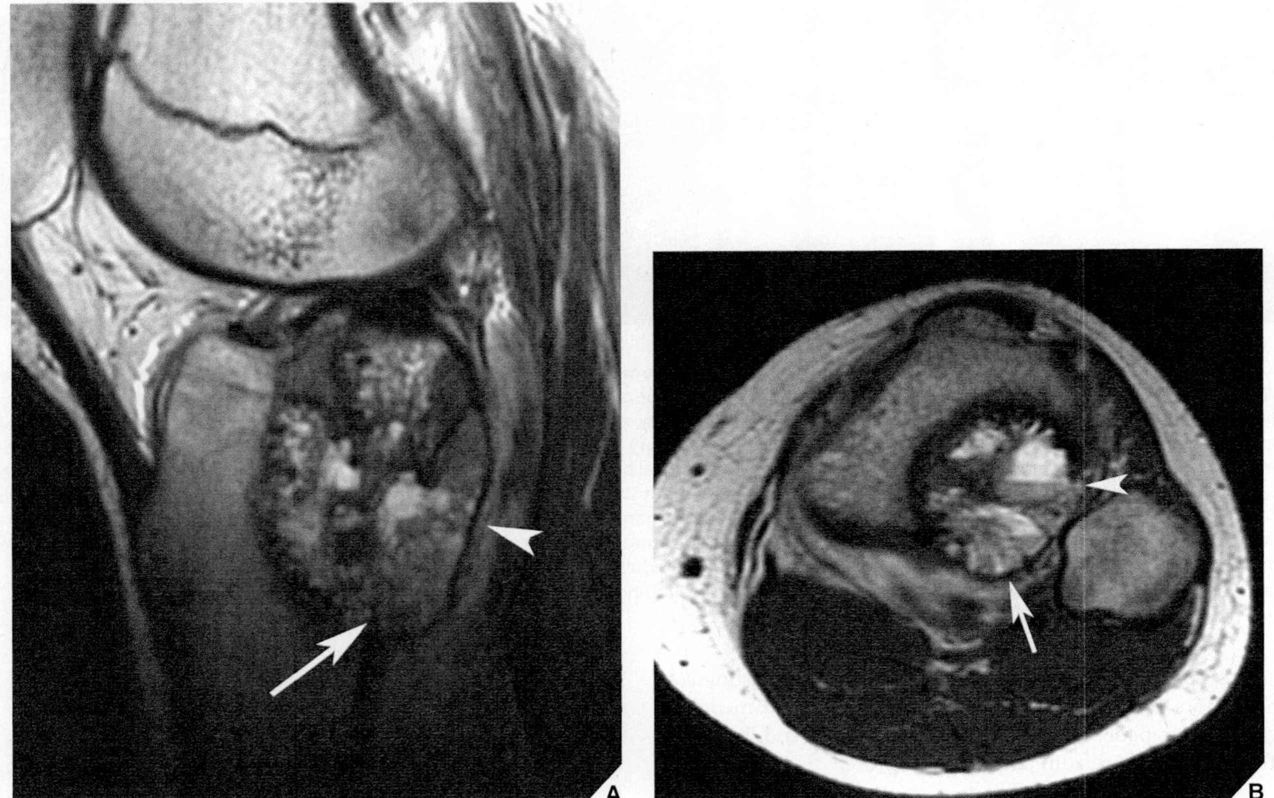

FIGURE 16.24 MRI of telangiectatic osteosarcoma. **(A)** Sagittal T2-weighted MRI shows the intramedullary extension of the tumor *(arrow)* and the invasion of the soft tissues posteriorly *(arrowhead)*. **(B)** Axial T2-weighted MR image shows posterior extension of the tumor *(arrow)* and the presence of characteristic fluid–fluid levels *(arrowhead)*.

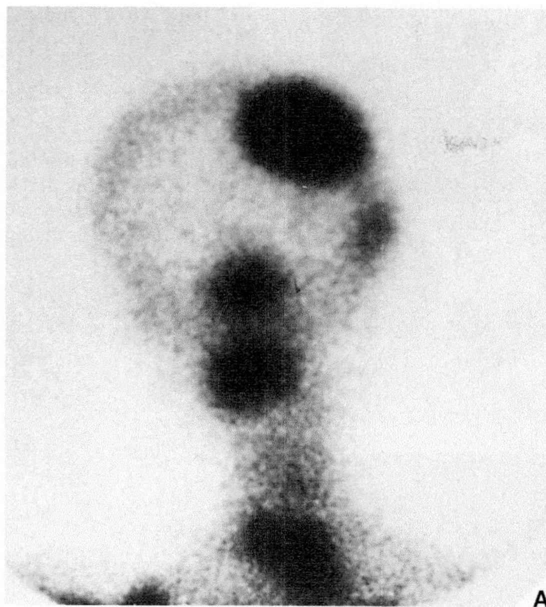

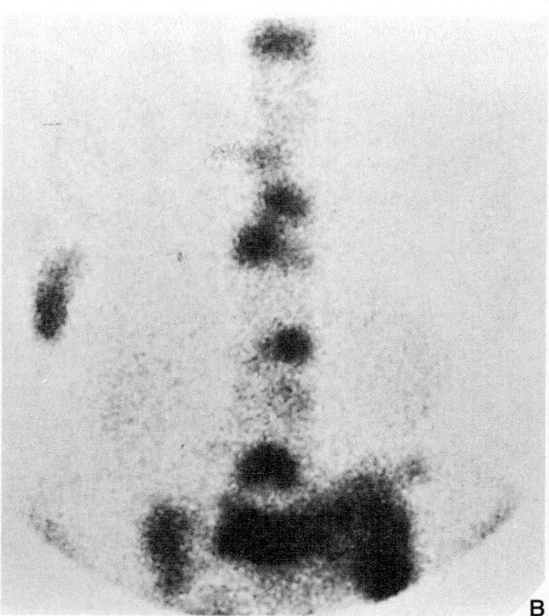

FIGURE 16.25 **Scintigraphy of the metastases.** A radionuclide bone scan was performed on a 68-year-old woman with metastatic breast carcinoma to determine the distribution of metastases. After an intravenous injection of 15 mCi (555 MBq) of ^{99m}Tc diphosphonate, an increased uptake of the radiopharmaceutical agent is seen in the skull and cervical spine **(A)** and lumbar spine and pelvis **(B)**, localizing the site of the multiple metastases.

in areas of bone undergoing change and repair, a bone scan is useful in localizing tumors and tumor-like lesions in the skeleton, particularly in such conditions as fibrous dysplasia, Langerhans cell histiocytosis, or metastatic cancer, in which more than one lesion is encountered (Fig. 16.25). It also plays an important role in localizing small lesions such as osteoid osteomas, which may not always be seen on conventional radiographs (see Fig. 17.12B). Although in most instances, a radionuclide bone scan cannot distinguish benign lesions from malignant tumors, because increased blood flow with increased isotope deposition and increased osteoblastic activity takes place in benign and malignant conditions, it is still occasionally capable of making such differentiation in benign lesions that do not absorb the radioactive isotope (Fig. 16.26). The radionuclide bone scan is sometimes also useful for differentiating multiple myeloma, which usually shows no significant uptake of the tracer, from metastatic cancer, which usually does.

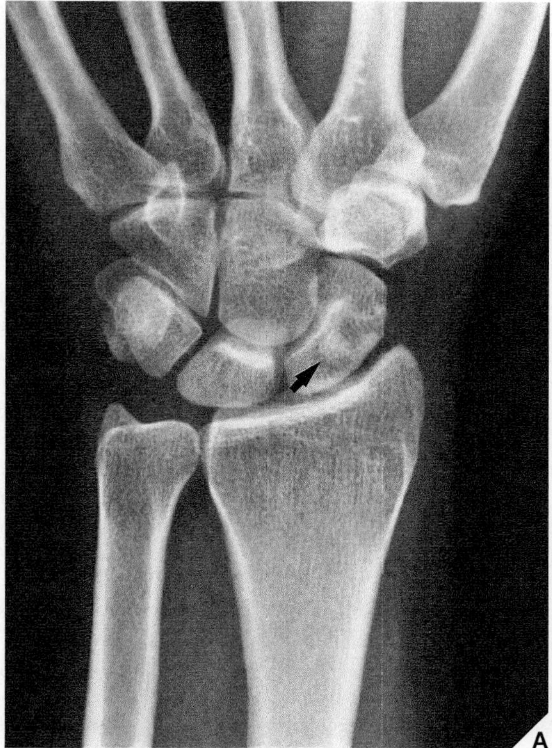

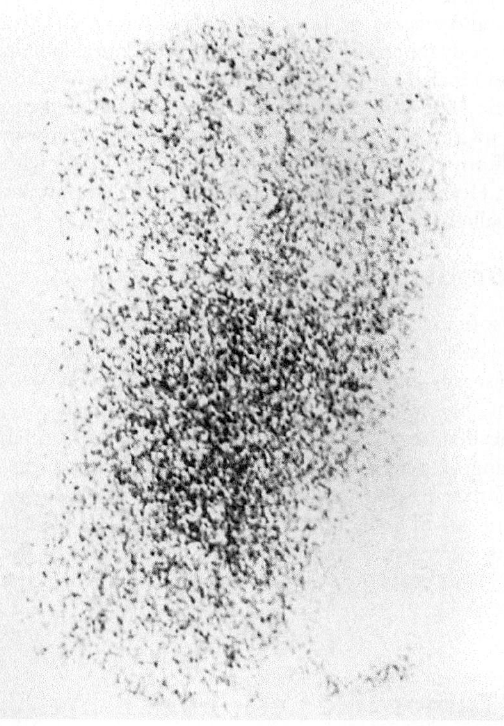

FIGURE 16.26 **Scintigraphy of enostosis.** A 32-year-old woman presented with pain localized in the wrist area. **(A)** Dorsovolar radiograph of the wrist demonstrates a sclerotic round lesion in the scaphoid *(arrow)*, and a diagnosis of osteoid osteoma was considered. **(B)** Radionuclide bone scan reveals normal isotope uptake, ruling out osteoid osteoma, which is invariably associated with an increased uptake of radiopharmaceutical. The lesion instead proved to be a bone island (enostosis), an asymptomatic developmental error of endochondral ossification without any consequence to the patient. The pain was unrelated to the island, coming instead from tenosynovitis; it disappeared after the patient was treated for the latter condition.

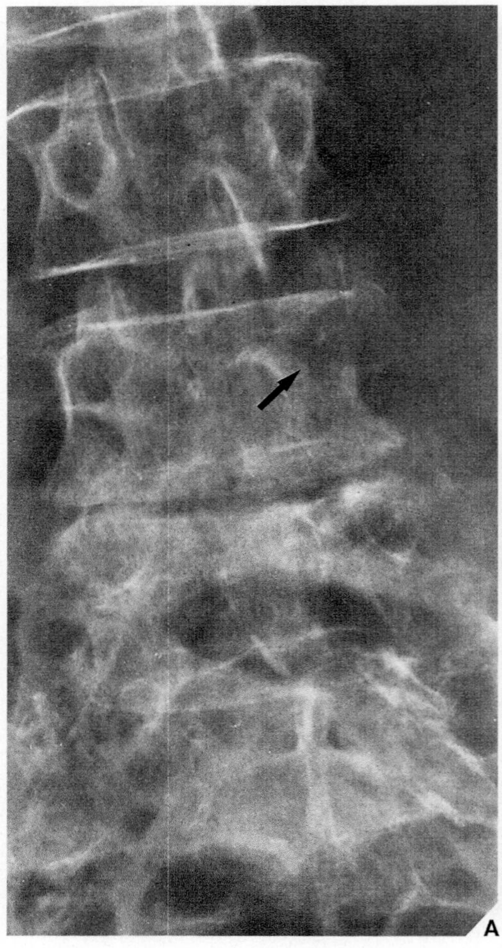
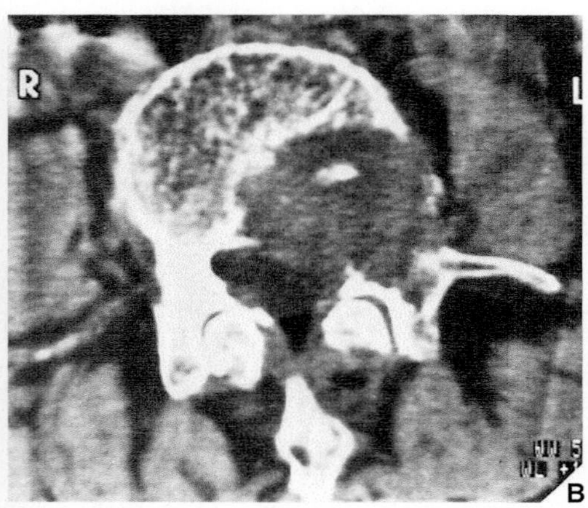
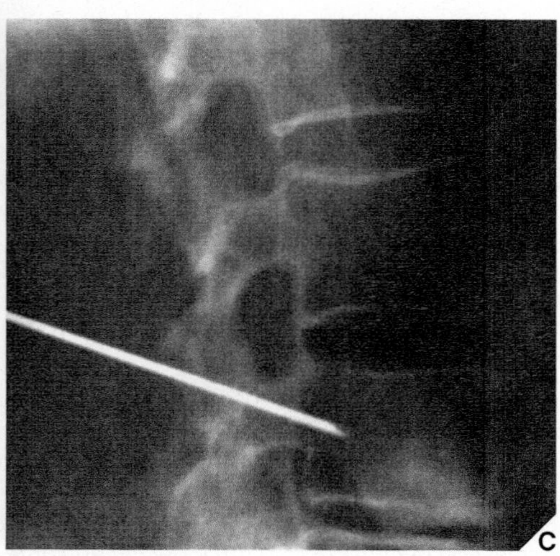

FIGURE 16.27 Percutaneous bone biopsy. **(A)** Anteroposterior radiograph of the lumbar spine in a 67-year-old woman with lower back pain for 4 months demonstrates destruction of the left pedicle of the L4 vertebra *(arrow)*. **(B)** CT section shows, in addition, involvement of the vertebral body by the tumor. **(C)** Percutaneous biopsy of the lesion, performed in the radiology suite for the purpose of rapid histopathologic diagnosis, revealed a metastatic adenocarcinoma from the colon.

Aside from routine radionuclide scans performed using technetium-99m (^{99m}Tc)-labeled phosphate compounds, occasionally, gallium-67 (^{67}Ga) is used for the detection and staging of bone and soft-tissue neoplasms. Gallium is handled by the body much like iron in that the protein transferrin carries it in the plasma, and it also competes for extravascular iron-binding proteins such as lactoferrin. The administered dose for adults ranges from 3 mCi (111 MBq) to 10 mCi (370 MBq) per study. The exact mechanism of tumor uptake of gallium remains unsettled, and its uptake varies with tumor type. In particular, Hodgkin lymphomas and histiocytic lymphomas are prone to significant gallium uptake.

Interventional Procedures

Percutaneous bone and soft-tissue biopsy performed in the radiology department has in recent years gained its place in the diagnostic workup for various neoplastic diseases, including bone tumors. In patients with primary bone neoplasms, it is a helpful diagnostic and evaluative tool, allowing rapid histologic diagnosis, which is now considered essential, particularly in the planning of a limb-salvage procedure. It also helps assess the effect of chemotherapy and radiation therapy and helps locate the site of the primary tumor in cases of metastatic disease (Fig. 16.27). In addition, percutaneous bone and soft-tissue biopsy performed in the radiology suite is simpler and costs less than a biopsy performed in the operating room.

Tumors and Tumor-like Lesions of Bone

Diagnosis

Clinical Information

Patient age and determination of whether a lesion is solitary or multiple are the starting approaches in the diagnosis of bone tumors (Fig. 16.28). The age of the patient is probably the single most important item of clinical data in radiographically establishing the diagnosis of a tumor (Fig. 16.29). Certain tumors have a predilection for specific age groups. Aneurysmal bone cysts, for example, rarely occur beyond age 20 years, and giant cell tumors as a rule are found only after the growth plate is closed. Other lesions may have different radiographic presentations or occur in different locations in patients of different ages. Simple bone cysts, which before skeletal maturity present almost exclusively in the long bones such as the proximal humerus and proximal femur, may appear in other locations (pelvis, scapula, calcaneus) and have unconventional radiographic presentations with progressing age (Fig. 16.30).

Also important for clinically differentiating lesions of similar radiographic presentation—such as Langerhans cell histiocytosis (formerly called *eosinophilic granuloma*), osteomyelitis, and Ewing sarcoma—is the duration of the patient's symptoms. In Langerhans cell histiocytosis, for example, the amount of bone destruction seen radiographically after 1 week of symptoms is usually the same as that seen after 4 to 6 weeks of symptoms in osteomyelitis and 3 to 4 months in Ewing sarcoma.

The growth rate of the tumor may be an additional factor in differentiating malignant tumors (usually rapid growing) from benign tumors (usually slow growing).

Laboratory data, such as an increased erythrocyte sedimentation rate or an elevated alkaline or acid phosphatase level in the serum, occasionally can be a corroborative factor in diagnosis.

Choice of Imaging Modality

With so many imaging techniques available to diagnose and characterize the bone tumor further, radiologists and clinicians are frequently at a loss as to how to proceed in a given case, what modality to use for this particular problem, in what order of preference to use the modalities, and when to stop. It is important to keep in mind that the choice of techniques for imaging the bone or soft-tissue tumor should be dictated not only by the clinical presentation and the technique's expected effectiveness but also by

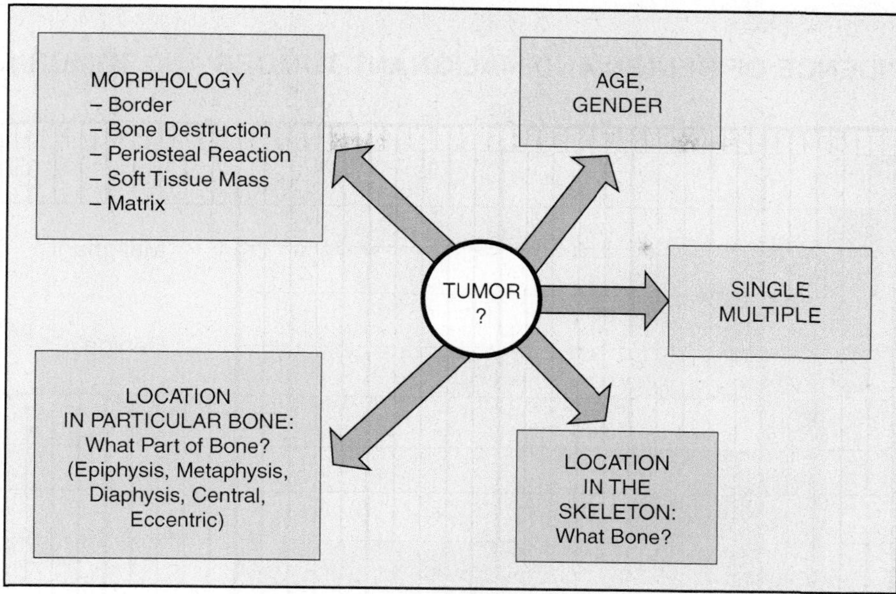

FIGURE 16.28 Diagnosis of bone lesion. Analytic approach to evaluation of the bone neoplasm must include patient age, multiplicity of a lesion, location in the skeleton and in the particular bone, and radiographic morphology. (Reprinted with permission from Greenspan A, Remagen W. *Differential diagnosis of tumors and tumor-like lesions*. Philadelphia: Lippincott-Raven; 1998.)

equipment availability, expertise, cost, and restrictions applicable to individual patients (e.g., allergy to ionic or nonionic iodinated contrast agents may preclude the use of arthrography, presence of a pacemaker may preclude the use of MRI, or physiologic states such as pregnancy warrant the use of US over the use of ionized radiation). Some of these problems were discussed in general in Chapters 1 and 2.

Here, we give a general guideline related to the most effective modality for diagnosing and evaluating bone and soft-tissue tumors. In the evaluation of bone tumors, conventional radiography is still the standard diagnostic procedure. No matter what ancillary technique is used, the conventional radiograph should always be available for comparison. Most of the time, the choice of imaging technique is dictated by the type of suspected tumor. For instance, if osteoid osteoma is suspected based on the clinical history (see Fig. 1.5), conventional radiography followed by scintigraphy should be performed first, and after the lesion is localized to the particular bone, CT should be used for more specific localization and for obtaining quantitative information (measurements). However, if a soft-tissue tumor is suspected, MRI is the best technique able to localize and characterize the lesion accurately. Likewise, if radiographs are suggestive of a malignant bone tumor, MRI or CT should be used next to evaluate both the intraosseous extent of the tumor and the extraosseous involvement of the soft tissues.

The use of CT versus MRI is based on the radiographs: If there is no definite evidence of soft-tissue extension, then CT is superior to MRI for detecting subtle cortical erosions and periosteal reaction while providing at the same time an accurate means of determining the intraosseous extension of the tumor; if, however, the radiographs suggest cortical destruction and soft-tissue mass, then MRI would be the preferred modality because it provides an excellent soft-tissue contrast and can determine the extraosseous extension of the tumor much better than CT.

In evaluating the results of malignant tumors treated by radiotherapy and chemotherapy, dynamic MRI using Gd-DTPA as a contrast enhancement is much superior to scintigraphy, CT, or even plain MRI.

Figure 16.31 depicts an algorithm for evaluating a bone lesion discovered on the standard radiographs. Note that the proper order of the various imaging modalities depends on two main factors: whether the radiographic findings are or are not diagnostic for any particular tumor and the lesion's uptake of a tracer on the radionuclide bone scan. Scintigraphy plays a crucial role here, dictating further steps in using the different techniques.

Radiographic Features of Bone Lesions

The radiographic features that help the radiologist diagnose a tumor or tumor-like bone lesion include (a) the site of the lesion (location in the skeleton and in the individual bone), (b) the borders of the lesion (the so-called *zone of transition*), (c) the type of matrix of the lesion (composition of the tumor tissue), (d) the type of bone destruction, (e) the type of periosteal response to the lesion (periosteal reaction), (f) the nature and extent of soft-tissue involvement, and (g) the single or multiple nature of the lesion (Fig. 16.32).

Site of the Lesion

The site of a bone lesion is an important feature because some tumors have a predilection for specific bones (Table 16.3 and Fig. 16.33) or specific sites in the bone (Table 16.4 and Fig. 16.34). The sites of some lesions are so characteristic that a diagnosis can be suggested on this basis alone, as in the case of parosteal osteosarcoma (Fig. 16.35), giant cell tumor (Fig. 16.36), or chondroblastoma (Fig. 16.37). Moreover, certain entities can be readily excluded from the differential diagnosis on the basis of the lesion's location. Thus, for example, the diagnosis of a giant cell tumor should not be made for a lesion that does not reach the articular end of the bone because very few of these tumors develop in sites remote from the joint.

The relation of tumor to the central axis of bone—especially a long tubular bone like humerus, radius, tibia, and femur—is an equally significant component in assessing the site of the lesion. Some lesions appear centrally located; these include simple bone cyst (Fig. 16.38A), a focus of fibrous dysplasia (Fig. 16.38B), or enchondroma (Fig. 16.38C). An eccentric location is more typical of aneurysmal bone cyst (Fig. 16.39A), nonossifying fibroma (Fig. 16.39B), or chondromyxoid fibroma (Fig. 16.39C).

Borders of the Lesion

Evaluation of the borders or margins of a lesion is crucial in determining whether it is slow growing or fast growing (aggressive) (Fig. 16.40). Three types of lesion margins have been described: (a) a margin with sharp demarcation by sclerosis between the peripheral aspect of the tumor and the adjacent host bone (1A margin), (b) a margin with sharp demarcation without sclerosis around the periphery of the lesion (1B margin), and (c) a margin with an ill-defined region (either the entire circumference or only a portion of it) at the interface between lesion and host bone (1C margin) (Fig. 16.41). Slow-growing lesions, which are usually benign, have sharply outlined sclerotic borders (a narrow zone of transition) (Fig. 16.42A), whereas malignant

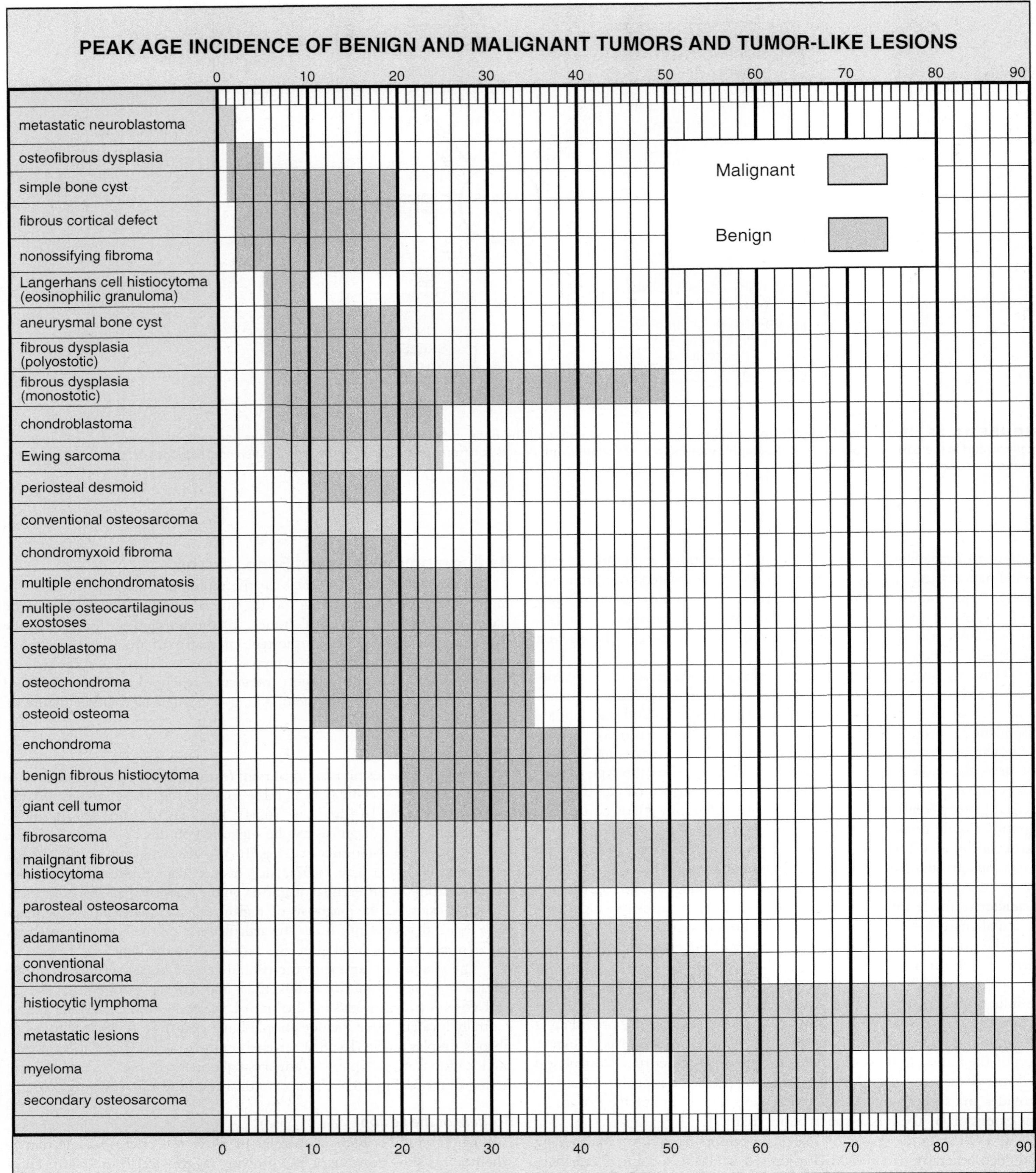

FIGURE 16.29 **Peak age incidence of benign and malignant tumors and tumor-like lesions.** (Data from Dahlin DC, Unni KK. *Bone tumors: general aspects and data on 8,542 cases*, 4th ed. Springfield, MO: Charles C. Thomas Publishers; 1986; Dorfman HD, Czerniak B. *Bone tumors*. St. Louis: Mosby; 1998:1–33; Fechner RE, Mills SE. *Tumors of the bones and joints*. Washington, DC: Armed Forces Institute of Pathology; 1993:1–16; Huvos AG, 1979; Jaffe HL, 1968; Mirra JM, 1989; Moser RP, 1990; Schajowicz F, 1994; Unni KK, 1988; Wilner D, 1982.)

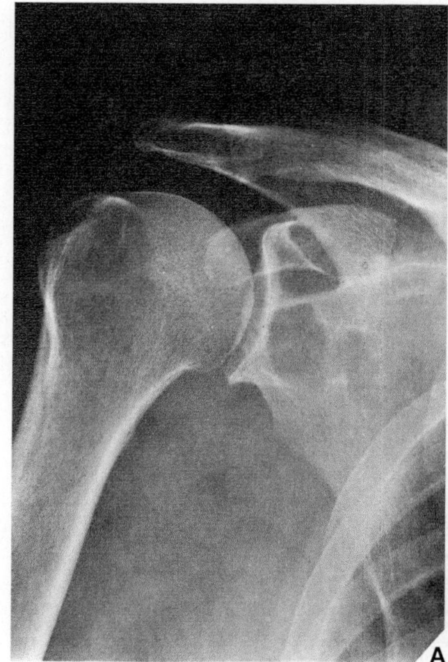

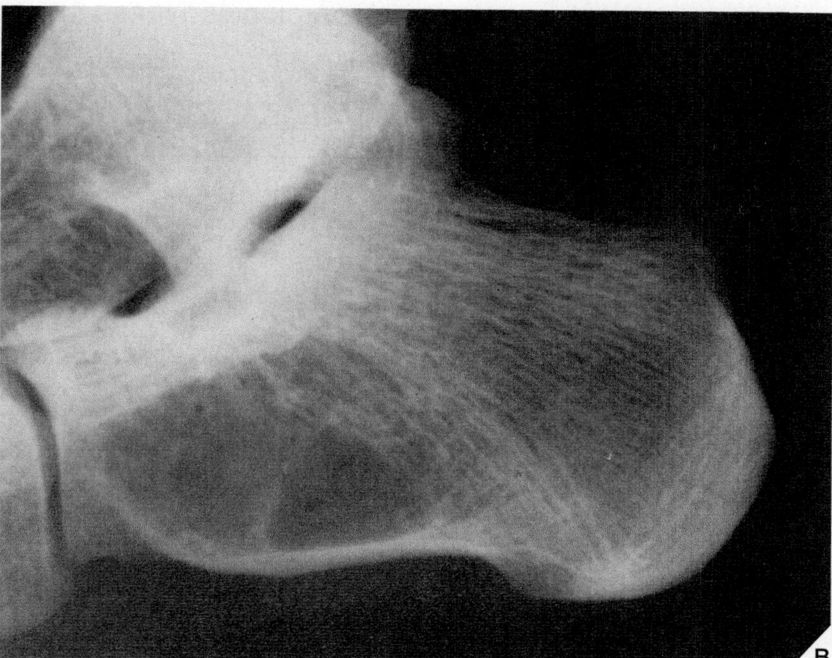

FIGURE 16.30 Simple bone cyst. **(A)** Anteroposterior radiograph of the right shoulder of a 69-year-old man with shoulder pain for 8 months demonstrates a well-defined radiolucent lesion with a sclerotic border in the glenoid portion of the scapula. Because the patient had a history of gout, the lesion was thought to represent an intraosseous tophus. In the differential diagnosis, an intraosseous ganglion and even a cartilage tumor were also considered. An excision biopsy, however, revealed a simple bone cyst, which is very unusual in the glenoid part of the scapula. **(B)** Lateral radiograph of the left hindfoot of a 50-year-old woman shows a radiolucent lesion in the calcaneus proven on the excision biopsy to be a simple bone cyst.

or aggressive lesions typically have indistinct borders (a wide zone of transition) with either minimal or no reactive sclerosis (Fig. 16.42B). Some lesions ordinarily lack a sclerotic border (Table 16.5), and some lesions commonly display a sclerotic border (Table 16.6). It must be emphasized that treatment can alter the appearance of malignant bone tumors; after radiation or chemotherapy, they may exhibit significant sclerosis as well as a narrow zone of transition (Fig. 16.43).

Type of Matrix

All bone tumors are composed of characteristic tissue components, the so-called *tumor matrix*. Only two of these—osteoblastic and cartilaginous tissue—can usually be clearly demonstrated radiographically. If one can identify bone or cartilage within a tumor, one can assume that it is osteoblastic or cartilaginous (Fig. 16.44). The identification of tumor bone within or adjacent to the area of destruction should alert the radiologist to the possibility of osteosarcoma. However, the deposition of new bone may also be the result of a reparative process secondary to bone destruction—so-called *reactive sclerosis*—rather than production of osteoid or bone by malignant cells. This new tumor bone is often radiographically indistinguishable from reactive bone; however, fluffy, cotton-like, or cloud-like densities within the medullary cavity and in the adjacent soft tissue should suggest the presence of tumorous bone and hence the diagnosis of osteosarcoma (Fig. 16.45; see also Figs. 16.11A and 16.22D).

Cartilage is identified by the presence of typically popcorn-like, punctate, annular, or comma-shaped calcifications (Fig. 16.46; see also Fig. 16.23). Because cartilage usually grows in lobules, a tumor of cartilaginous origin can often be suggested by lobulated growth. A completely radiolucent lesion may be either fibrous or cartilaginous in origin, although hollow structures produced by tumor-like lesions, such as simple bone cysts or intraosseous ganglia, can also present as radiolucent areas (Table 16.7). The list of tumors and pseudotumors that may present as radiodense lesions is provided in Table 16.8.

Type of Bone Destruction

The type of bone destruction caused by a tumor is primarily related to the tumor growth rate. Although not pathognomonic for any specific neoplasm, the type of destruction, which can be described as geographic, moth-eaten, or permeative (Fig. 16.47), may suggest not only a benign or malignant neoplastic process (Fig. 16.48A,B) but also, at times, the histologic type of a tumor, as in the permeative type of bone destruction characteristically produced by the so-called *round cell tumors*—Ewing sarcoma (Fig. 16.48D) and lymphoma.

Periosteal Response

The periosteal reaction to a neoplastic process in the bone is usually categorized as uninterrupted or interrupted (Fig. 16.49 and Table 16.9). The first type of reaction is marked by solid layers of periosteal density, indicating a long-standing benign process, such as that seen in osteoid osteoma (Fig. 16.50) or osteoblastoma (see Fig. 17.39). Uninterrupted reaction is also seen in nonneoplastic processes, such as Langerhans cell histiocytosis, osteomyelitis, bone abscess (Fig. 16.51), or pachydermoperiostosis, in fractures in the healing stage, or in hypertrophic pulmonary osteoarthropathy (Fig. 16.52). The interrupted type of periosteal reaction suggests malignancy or a highly aggressive nonmalignant process. It may present as a sunburst pattern, a lamellated (onion-skin) pattern, a velvet pattern, or a Codman triangle, and it is commonly seen in malignant primary tumors such as osteosarcoma or Ewing sarcoma (Fig. 16.53).

Soft-Tissue Extension

With few exceptions—such as giant cell tumors, aneurysmal bone cysts, osteoblastomas, or desmoplastic fibromas—benign tumors and tumor-like bone lesions usually do not exhibit soft-tissue extension; thus, almost invariably, a soft-tissue mass indicates an aggressive lesion and one that is in many instances malignant (Fig. 16.54). It should be kept in mind, however, that nonneoplastic conditions such as osteomyelitis also exhibit a soft-tissue component, but the involvement of the soft tissues is usually poorly defined, with obliteration of fatty tissue layers. In malignant processes, however, the tumor mass is sharply defined, extending through the destroyed cortex with preservation of the tissue planes (Fig. 16.55).

In the case of a bone lesion associated with a soft-tissue mass, it is always helpful to determine which condition arose first. Is the soft-tissue lesion, in other words, an extension of a primary bone tumor or is it itself a primary lesion that has invaded the bone? Although not always applicable, certain imaging criteria may help in deciding this issue (Fig. 16.56). In most instances, for example, a large soft-tissue mass and a smaller bone lesion indicate secondary skeletal involvement. Ewing sarcoma breaks this

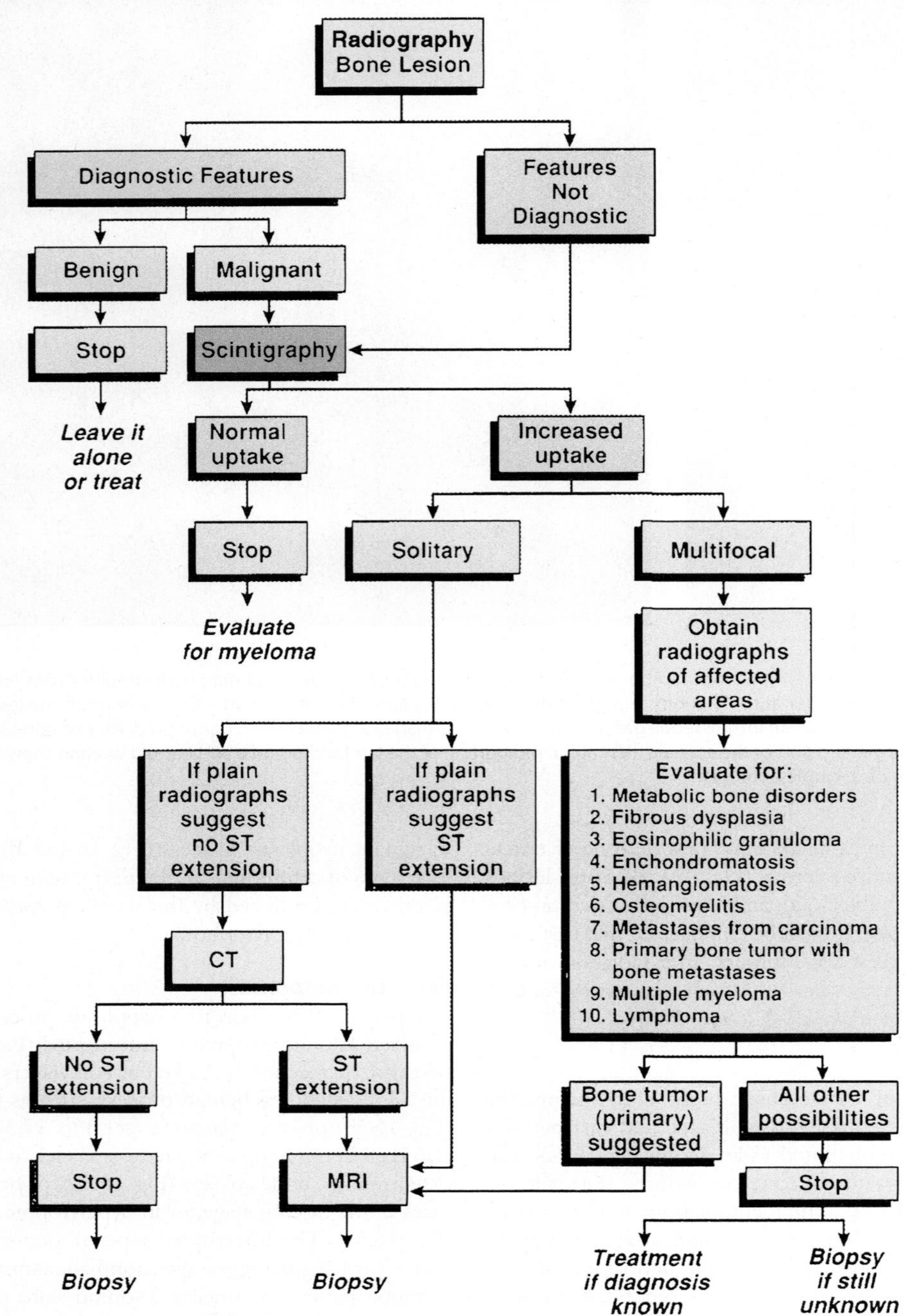

FIGURE 16.31 Algorithm to evaluate and manage a bone lesion discovered on standard radiographs.

rule, however. Its destructive primary bone lesion may be small and often accompanied by a large soft-tissue mass. A destructive lesion of bone lacking a periosteal reaction and adjacent to a soft-tissue mass may indicate secondary invasion by a primary soft-tissue tumor, which usually destroys the neighboring periosteum. This contrasts with primary bone lesions, which usually prompt a periosteal reaction when they break through the cortex and extend into adjacent soft tissues. Because these observations are not universally applicable, however, they should be taken only as indicators and not as pathognomonic features.

Multiplicity of Lesions

A multiplicity of malignant lesions usually indicates metastatic disease, multiple myeloma, or lymphoma (Fig. 16.57). Very rarely do primary malignant lesions, such as an osteosarcoma or Ewing sarcoma, present as multifocal disease. Benign lesions, however, tend to involve multiple sites, as in polyostotic fibrous dysplasia (Fig. 16.58), multiple osteochondromas (see Figs. 18.55 and 18.56A), enchondromatosis (see Figs. 18.27 and 18.29), Langerhans cell histiocytosis, hemangiomatosis, and fibromatosis.

Benign versus Malignant

Although it is sometimes very difficult to distinguish benign from malignant bone lesions on the basis of radiography alone, certain characteristic features favor one designation over the other (Fig. 16.59). Benign lesions usually present with well-defined, sclerotic borders, a geographic type of bone destruction; an uninterrupted, solid periosteal reaction; and no soft-tissue mass (see Figs. 16.42A,B, 16.48B, and 16.50). Conversely, malignant tumors tend to demonstrate poorly defined borders with a wide zone of transition, a moth-eaten or permeative pattern of bone destruction, an interrupted periosteal reaction of the sunburst or onion-skin type, and an adjacent soft-tissue mass (see Figs. 16.42C,D, 16.48C,D, 16.53, and 16.55A). It should be kept in mind, however, that some benign lesions may also exhibit aggressive features (Table 16.10).

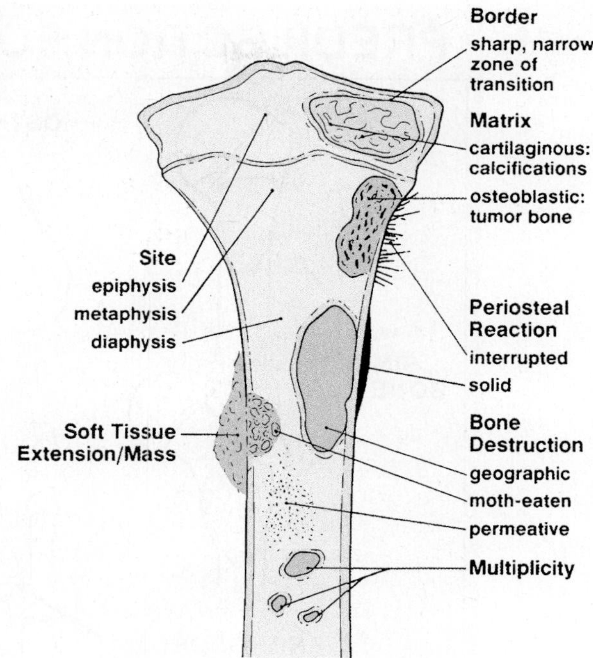

FIGURE 16.32 Radiographic features of tumors and tumor-like lesions of bone.

TABLE 16.3 Most Common Skeletal Location of Bone Tumors

Lesions	Most Common Skeletal Sites
Ewing sarcoma Multiple myeloma Leukemia/lymphoma Metastatic cancers	Hematopoietic marrow sites in the axial skeleton (vertebrae, ribs, sternum, pelvis, cranium) and proximal long bones (femur, humerus)
Nonossifying fibroma	Femur and distal tibia
Simple bone cyst	Proximal humerus (50%); proximal femur (25%)
Chordoma	Base of the skull, C2, and sacrum (90%)
Adamantinoma	Midshaft of the tibia (90%); jaw bones
Chondroblastoma	75% long bones (distal and proximal femur, proximal tibia, and proximal humerus)
Giant cell tumor	Ends of long bones, the distal femur, proximal tibia, distal radius, and proximal humerus
Enchondroma	Most common in short tubular bones of the hand (~40% of cases)
Chondrosarcoma (primary and less commonly secondary)	About 75% occurs in the trunk, femur, and humerus; 25%–30% occurring in the pelvic bones
Fibrous dysplasia	Craniofacial bones and the femur are the most common sites for monostotic and polyostotic forms. In monostotic fibrous dysplasia, most lesions are located in the femur, skull, and tibia.
Osteochondroma	Most common in metaphyseal region of the distal femur, upper humerus, proximal tibia, and fibula
Osteoblastoma	Posterior elements of the spine and sacrum (40%–55%)
Aneurysmal bone cyst	Can affect any bone but usually arises in the metaphysis of long bones: femur, tibia, and humerus
Chondromyxoid fibroma	Knee area (30%), pelvic bones, small bones of the feet
Hemangioma	Vertebral bodies are most common to be involved followed by craniofacial and long bones.

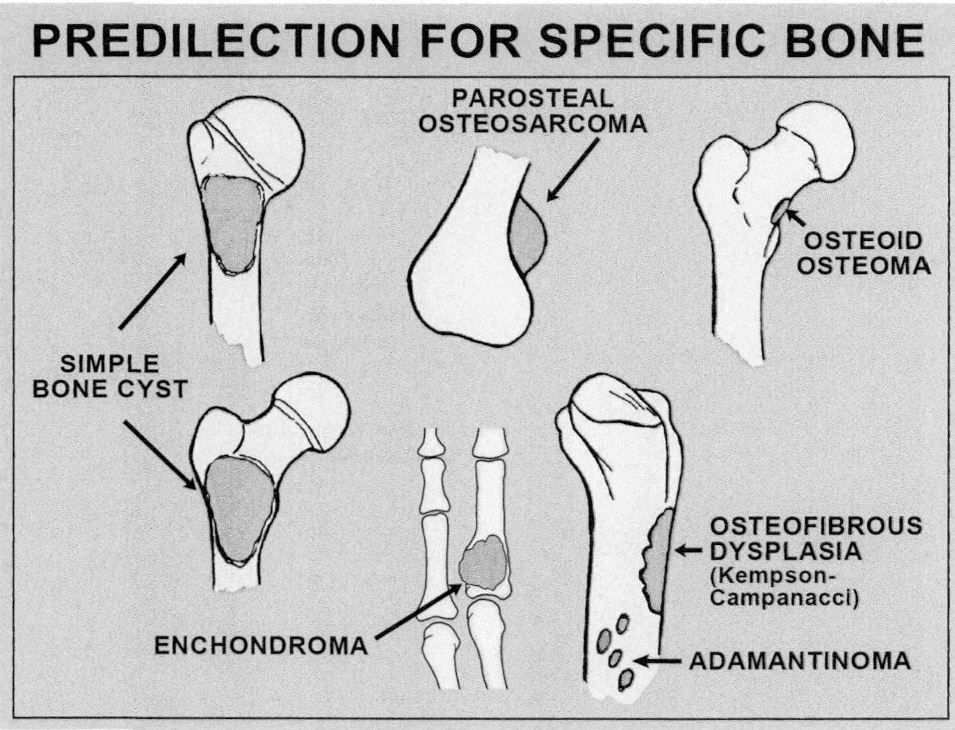

FIGURE 16.33 **Site of the lesion: predilection for specific bone.** Examples of typical preference of some tumors for specific bones.

TABLE 16.4 Predilection of Tumors for Specific Sites in the Skeleton

	Skeletal Predilection of Benign Osseous Neoplasms and Tumor-like Lesions	Skeletal Predilection of Malignant Osseous Neoplasms
Axial skeleton	*Skull and facial bones*: osteoma, osteoblastoma, Langerhans cell histiocytosis, fibrous dysplasia, solitary hemangioma, osteoporosis circumscripta (lytic phase of Paget disease)	*Skull and facial bones*: mesenchymal chondrosarcoma, multiple myeloma, metastatic neuroblastoma, metastatic carcinoma
	Jaw: giant cell reparative granuloma, myxoma, ossifying fibroma, desmoplastic fibroma	*Mandible*: osteosarcoma
	Spine: aneurysmal bone cyst, osteoblastoma, Langerhans cell histiocytosis, hemangioma	*Spine*: chordoma, myeloma, metastases
Appendicular skeleton	*Long tubular bones*: osteoid osteoma, simple bone cyst, aneurysmal bone cyst, osteochondroma, enchondroma, periosteal chondroma, chondroblastoma, chondromyxoid fibroma, nonossifying fibroma, giant cell tumor, osteofibrous dysplasia, desmoplastic fibroma, intraosseous ganglion	*Long tubular bones*: osteosarcoma (all variants), adamantinoma, malignant fibrous histiocytoma, primary lymphoma, chondrosarcoma, angiosarcoma, fibrosarcoma
	Hands and feet: giant cell reparative granuloma, florid reactive periostitis, enchondroma, glomus tumor, epidermoid cyst, subungual exostosis, bizarre parosteal osteochondromatous lesion	*Hands and feet*: none
Specific predilections	Simple bone cyst—proximal humerus, proximal femur Osteofibrous dysplasia—tibia, fibula (anterior cortex) Osteoid osteoma—femur, tibia Chondromyxoid fibroma—tibia, metaphyses Chondroblastoma—epiphyses Giant cell tumor—articular ends of femur, tibia, radius Liposclerosing myxofibrous tumor—intertrochanteric region of femur	Adamantinoma—tibia, fibula Parosteal osteosarcoma—distal femur (posterior cortex) Periosteal osteosarcoma—tibia Clear cell chondrosarcoma—proximal femur and humerus Chordoma—sacrum, clivus, C2 Multiple myeloma—pelvis, spine, skull

Data from Fechner RE, Mills SE. *Tumors of the bones and joints*. Washington, DC: Armed Forces Institute of Pathology; 1993:1–16.

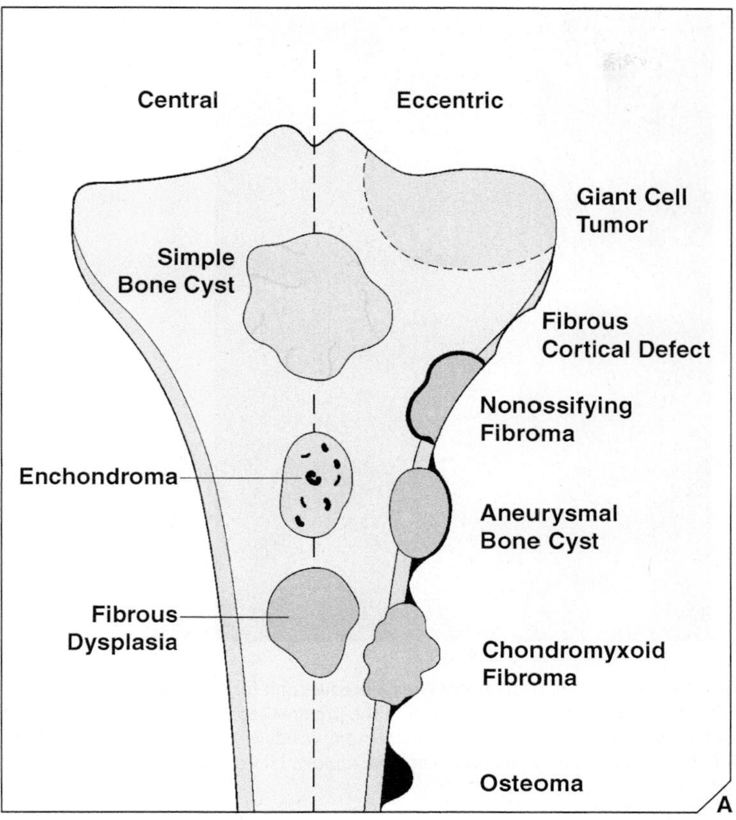

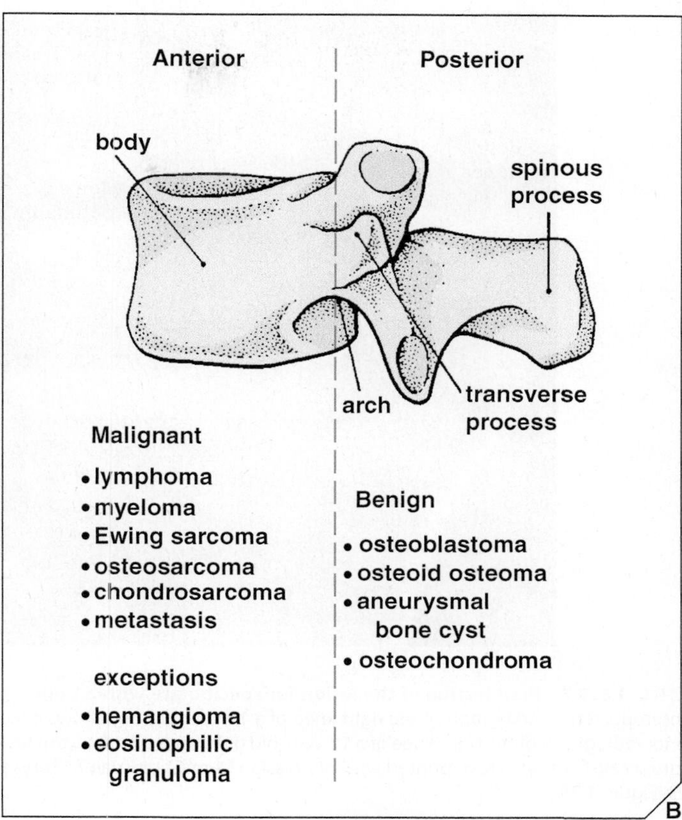

FIGURE 16.34 Site of the lesion. **(A)** Eccentric versus central location of the similar-appearing lesions is helpful in differential diagnosis. **(B)** Distribution of various tumors and tumor-like lesions in a vertebra. Malignant lesions are seen predominantly in its anterior part (body), whereas benign lesions predominate in its posterior elements (neural arch).

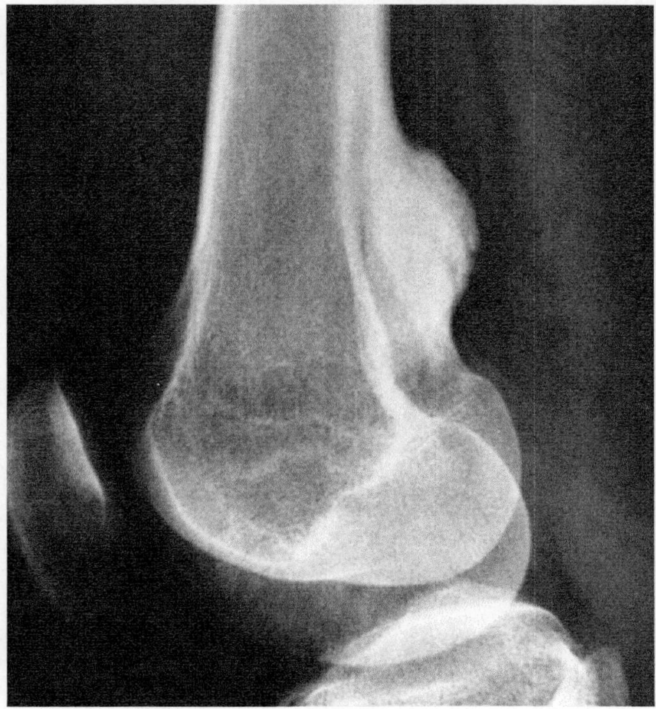

FIGURE 16.35 Predilection of the lesion for specific site within bone—parosteal osteosarcoma. This tumor has a predilection for the posterior aspect of the distal femur.

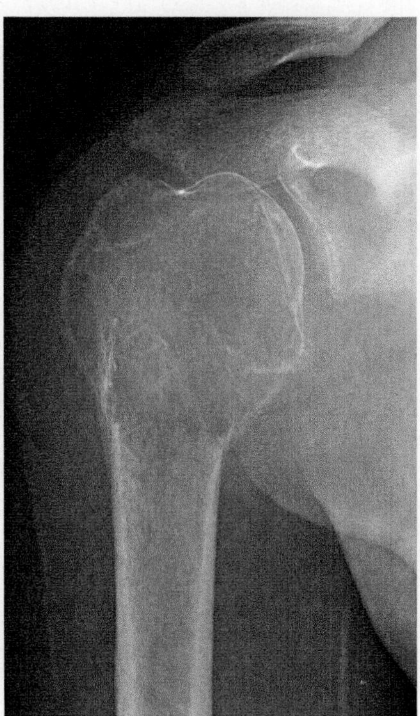

FIGURE 16.36 Predilection of the lesion for specific site within bone—giant cell tumor. One of the characteristic features of the giant cell tumor is its location in the articular end of a long bone, as seen here in a 35-year-old woman who has a slightly expansive purely lytic lesion affecting right proximal humerus.

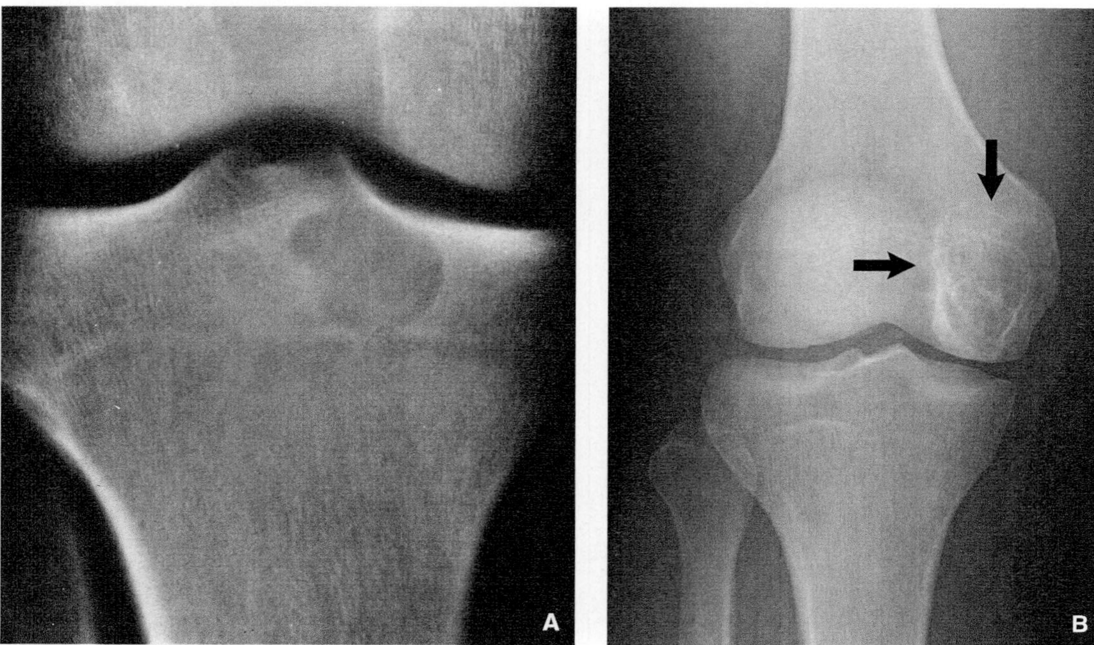

FIGURE 16.37 Predilection of the lesion for specific site within bone—chondroblastoma. Chondroblastoma has a predilection for the epiphysis of a long bone. **(A)** Anteroposterior radiograph of the right knee of a 14-year-old boy shows a radiolucent lesion with the sclerotic border in the proximal epiphysis of the tibia. **(B)** Anteroposterior radiograph of the right knee of a 17-year-old girl shows a radiolucent lesion with sclerotic border within the medial femoral condyle of the femur *(arrows)* exhibiting chondroid calcifications. (**A**, Reprinted with permission from Greenspan A, Borys D. *Radiology and pathology correlation of bone tumors*, 1st ed. Philadelphia: Wolters Kluwer; 2015:3, Figure 1.2A.

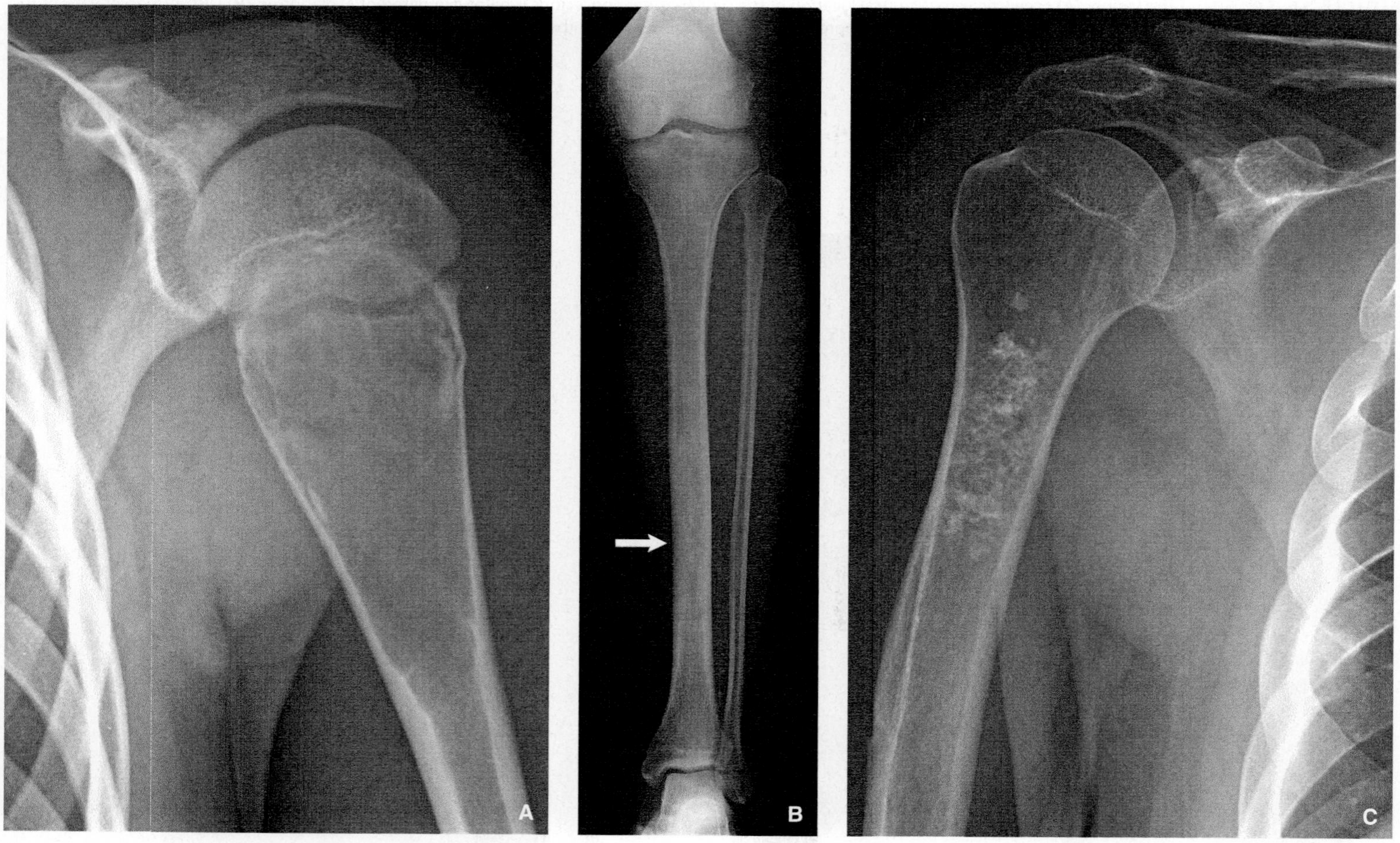

FIGURE 16.38 Central location of the lesion within bone. (A) Simple bone cyst is typically centrally located within the long bone, as seen here in 12-year-old boy who has a radiolucent lesion abutting the growth plate of the proximal left humerus. **(B)** Majority of fibrous dysplasias are centrally located, as in this 28-year-old man with a sclerotic lesion affecting medullary portion of the left tibia, exhibiting "ground-glass" appearance *(arrow)*. **(C)** Enchondroma is typically a central lesion, as demonstrated on this anteroposterior radiograph of the right humerus of a 52-year-old man.

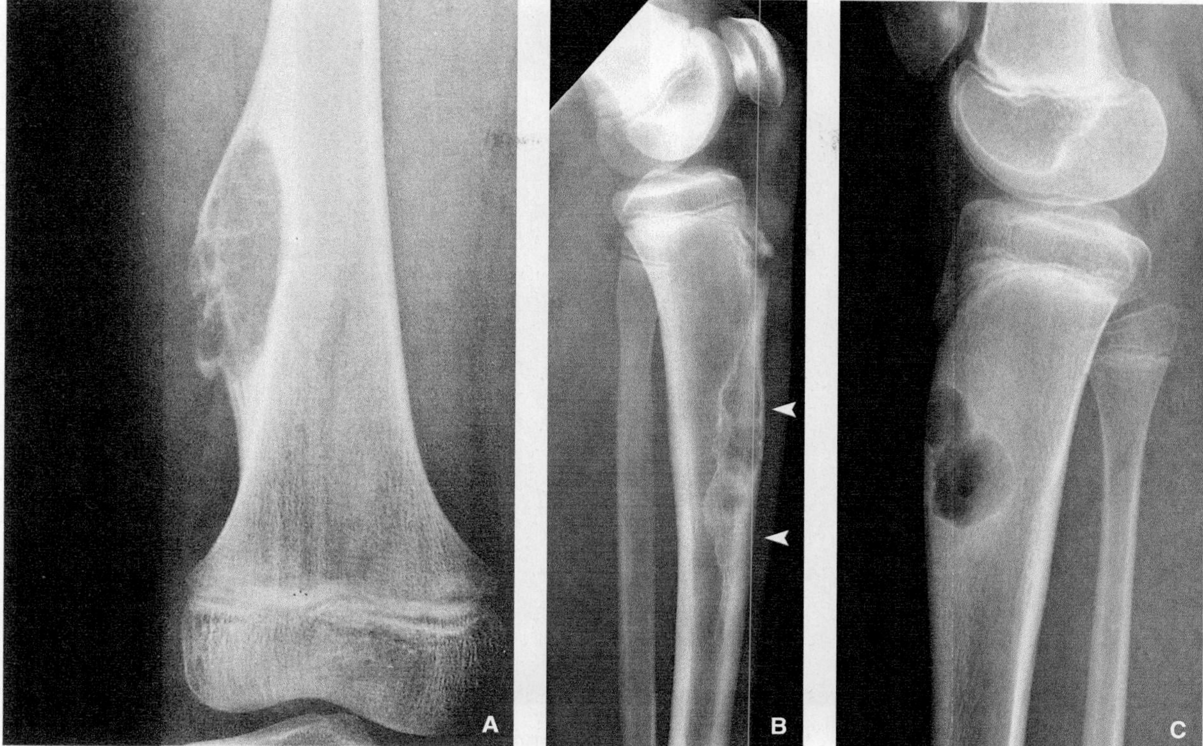

FIGURE 16.39 Eccentric location of the lesion within bone. **(A)** Aneurysmal bone cyst affecting the diaphysis of the right femur of an 8-year-old boy shows characteristic eccentric expansion of the cortex. **(B)** Nonossifying fibroma, seen here in the anterior aspect of the tibia of a 12-year-old girl, exhibits a lobulated posterior margin and eccentric location within the bone *(arrowheads)*. **(C)** Chondromyxoid fibroma, seen here in a 17-year-old girl, is affecting the anterior aspect of the tibial diaphysis. (**A**, Reprinted with permission from Greenspan A, Borys D. *Radiology and pathology correlation of bone tumors*, 1st ed. Philadelphia: Wolters Kluwer; 2015:5, Figure 1.7A.

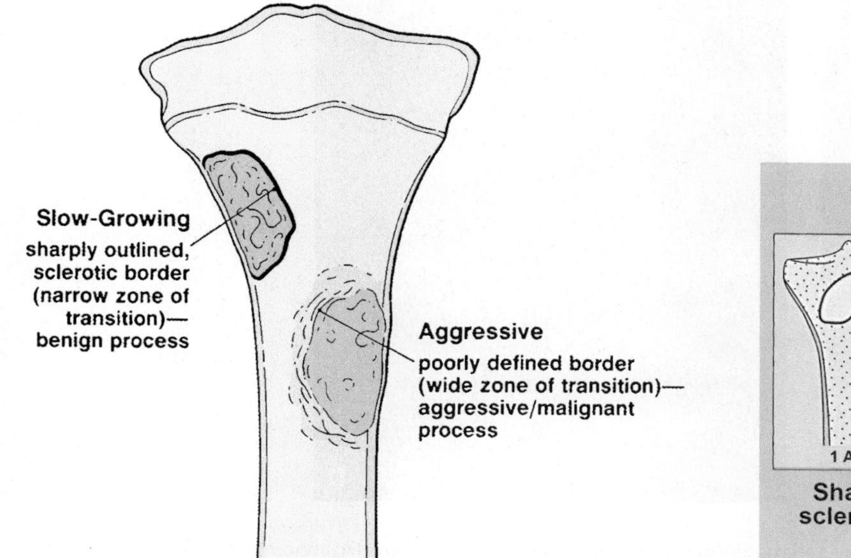

FIGURE 16.40 Borders of the lesion. The radiographic features of the borders of a lesion characterize it as either slow growing (and most likely benign) or aggressive (and most likely malignant).

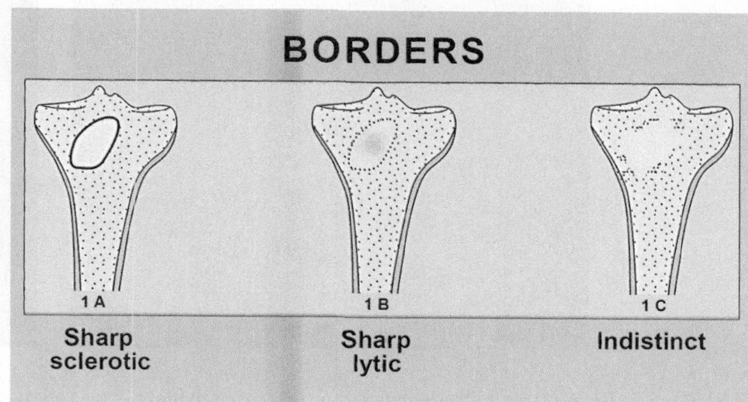

FIGURE 16.41 Borders of the lesion. Borders of the lesion determine its growth rate. (Modified from Madewell JE, Ragsdale BD, Sweet DE. Radiologic and pathologic analysis of solitary bone lesions. Part I: internal margins. *Radiol Clin North Am* 1981;19(4):715–748. Copyright © 1981 Elsevier. With permission.)

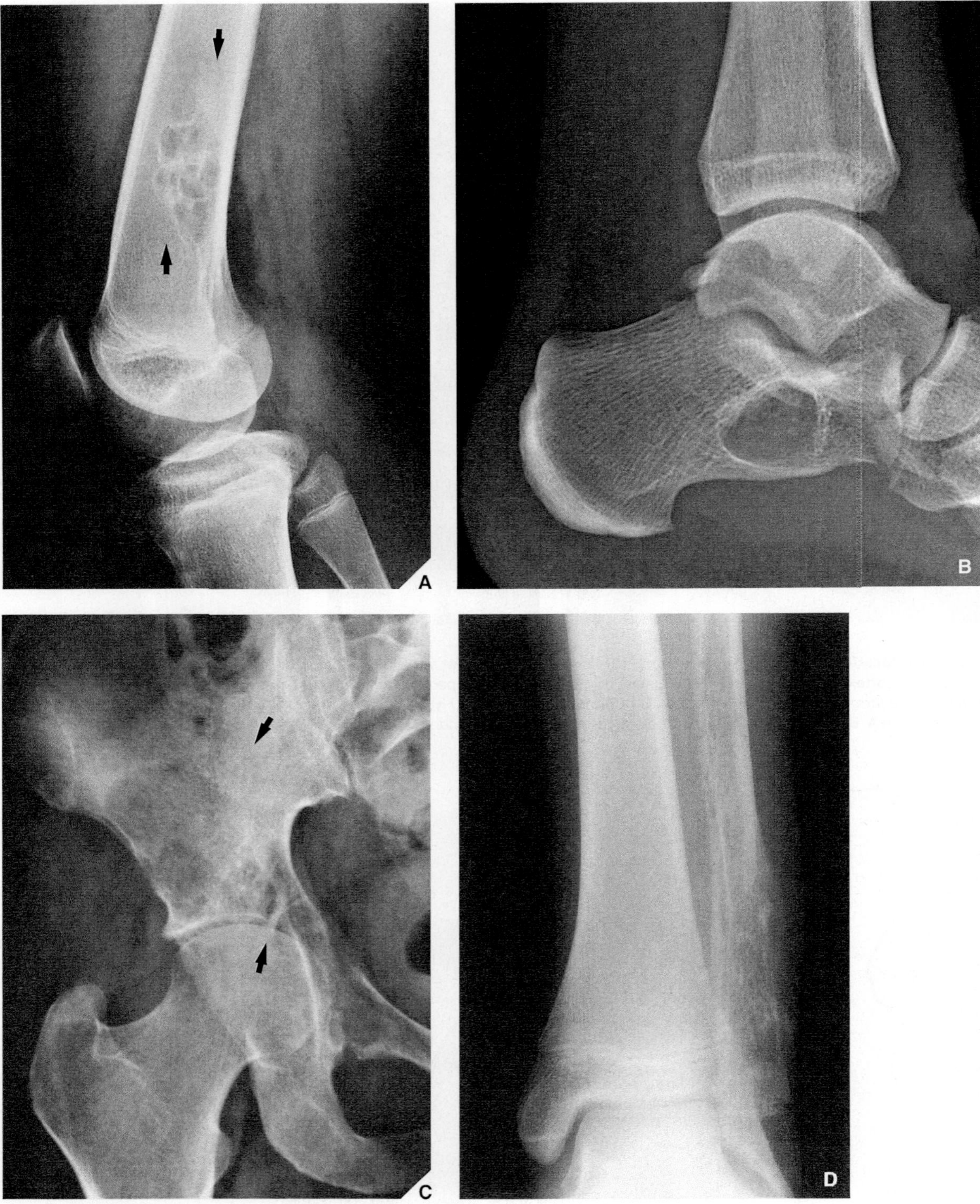

FIGURE 16.42 **Borders of the lesion: benign versus malignant.** A sclerotic border or narrow zone of transition from normal to abnormal bone typifies a benign lesion, as in this example of **(A)** nonossifying fibroma *(arrows)* and **(B)** simple bone cyst. A wide zone of transition typifies an aggressive/malignant lesion, in this case **(C)** solitary plasmacytoma involving the pubic bone and the supra-acetabular portion of the right ilium *(arrows)* and **(D)** Ewing sarcoma located in the distal fibula. (**B**, **D**, Reprinted with permission from Greenspan A, Borys D. *Radiology and pathology correlation of bone tumors: a quick reference and review*. Philadelphia: Wolters Kluwer; 2016:5, Fig. 1.8A–B.)

TABLE 16.5 Bone Lesions Usually Lacking a Sclerotic Border

Benign	Malignant
Acute osteomyelitis	Angiosarcoma
Brown tumor of hyperparathyroidism	Fibrosarcoma
Enchondroma in short tubular bone	Leiomyosarcoma of bone
Fibrocartilaginous mesenchymoma	Leukemia
Giant cell tumor	Lymphoma
Langerhans cell histiocytosis (sometimes)	Malignant fibrous histiocytoma
Osteolytic phase of Paget disease	Metastases from primary tumor in lung, gastrointestinal tract, kidney, breast, or thyroid
	Myeloma (plasmacytoma)
	Telangiectatic osteosarcoma

TABLE 16.6 Bone Lesions Commonly Displaying a Sclerotic Border

Benign	Malignant
Aneurysmal bone cyst	Chordoma
Benign fibrous histiocytoma	Clear-cell chondrosarcoma
Bone abscess	Conventional chondrosarcoma (sometimes)
Chondroblastoma	Low-grade central osteosarcoma
Chondromyxoid fibroma	Some malignant tumors after treatment with radiation or chemotherapy
Epidermoid inclusion cyst	
Fibrous cortical defect	
Fibrous dysplasia	
Giant cell reparative granuloma	
Intraosseous ganglion	
Intraosseous lipoma	
Medullary bone infarct	
Nonossifying fibroma	
Osteoblastoma	
Osteofibrous dysplasia	
Periosteal chondroma	
Simple bone cyst	

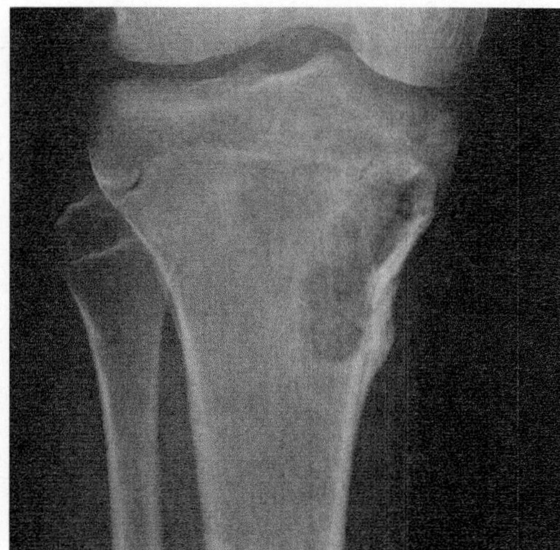

FIGURE 16.43 Osteosarcoma after chemotherapy. After 3 months of combined therapy with methotrexate, doxorubicin hydrochloride, and vincristine, the anteroposterior radiograph of the knee of this 16-year-old boy with a conventional osteosarcoma of the right tibia reveals reactive sclerosis at the borders of the tumor and a narrow zone of transition, features more often seen in benign lesions. The patient underwent a limb-salvage procedure.

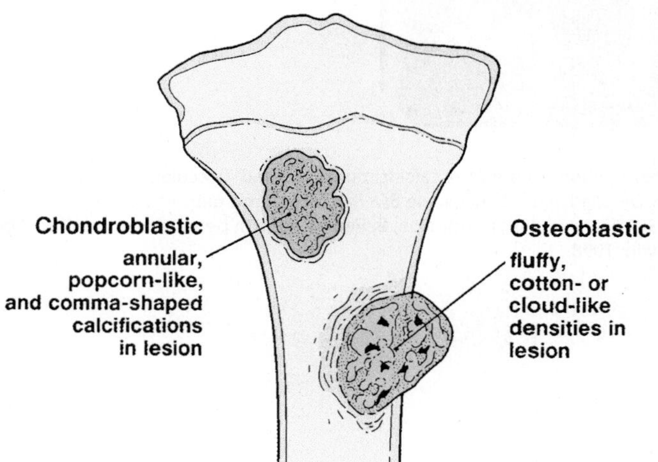

FIGURE 16.44 Tumor matrix. Radiographic features of the matrix of tumors and tumor-like lesions that characterize a lesion as cartilage forming or bone forming.

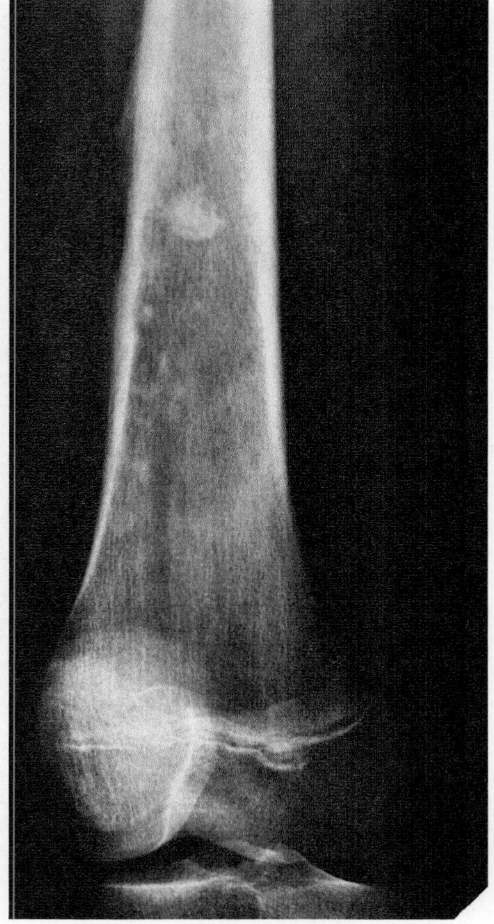

FIGURE 16.45 Osteoblastic matrix. The matrix of a typical osteoblastic lesion, in this case an osteosarcoma, is characterized by the presence of fluffy, cotton-like densities within the medullary cavity of the distal femur.

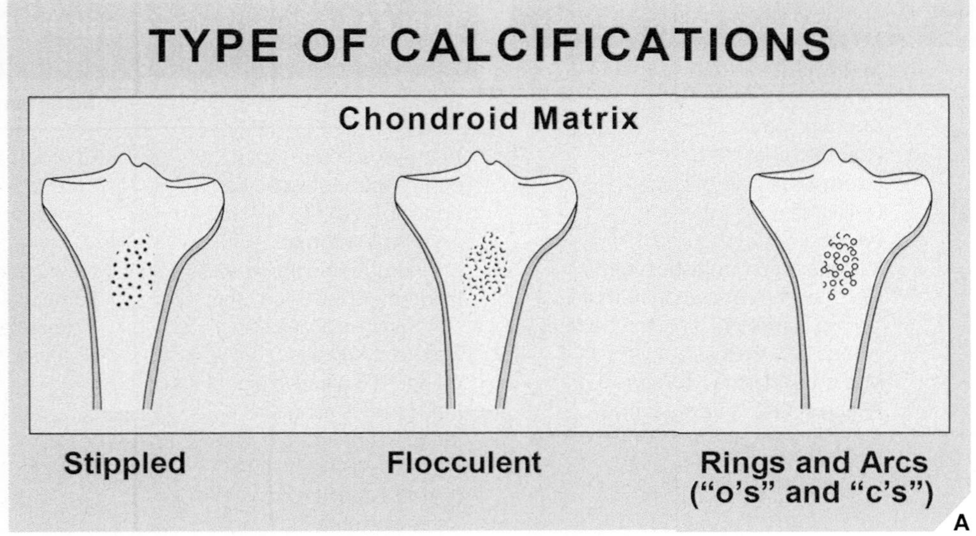

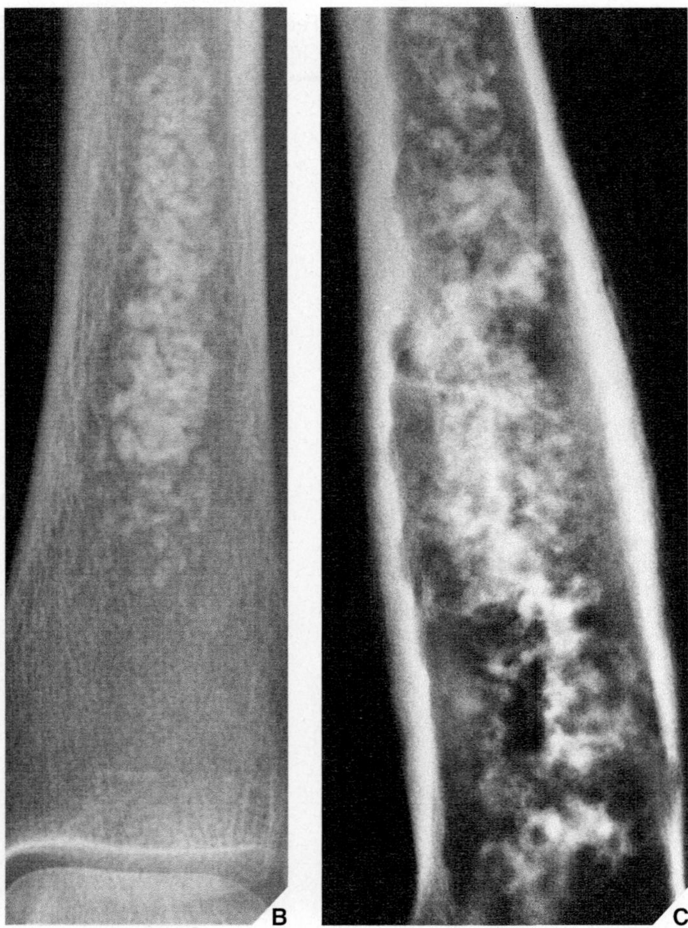

FIGURE 16.46 **Chondroid matrix.** **(A)** Schematic representation of various appearances of chondroid matrix calcifications: stippled, flocculent, and rings and arcs. **(B)** The matrix of enchondroma. **(C)** The matrix of chondrosarcoma. (**A**, Modified from Sweet DE, Madewell JE, Ragsdale BD. Radiologic and pathologic analysis of solitary bone lesions. Part III: matrix patterns. *Radiol Clin North Am* 1981;19(4):785–814. Copyright © 1981 Elsevier. With permission; **B**, Reprinted with permission from Greenspan A, Remagen W. *Differential diagnosis of tumors and tumor-like lesions.* Philadelphia: Lippincott-Raven; 1998.)

TABLE 16.7 Tumors and Pseudotumors That May Present as Radiolucent Lesions

Solid	Cystic
Cartilaginous (enchondroma, chondroblastoma, chondromyxoid fibroma, chondrosarcoma)	Aneurysmal bone cyst
Ewing sarcoma	Bone abscess
Fibrous and histiocytic (nonossifying fibroma, fibrous dysplasia, osteofibrous dysplasia, desmoplastic fibroma, fibrosarcoma, malignant fibrous histiocytoma)	Brown tumor of hyperparathyroidism
Giant cell reparative granuloma	Cystic angiomatosis
Giant cell tumor	Hemophilic pseudotumor
Langerhans cell histiocytosis	Hydatid cyst
Lymphoma	Intraosseous ganglion
Metastatic (from lung, breast, gastrointestinal tract, kidney, thyroid)	Intraosseous lipoma
Myeloma (plasmacytoma)	Simple bone cyst
Osteoblastic (osteoid osteoma, osteoblastoma, telangiectatic osteosarcoma)	Various bone cysts (synovial, degenerative)
Paget disease (osteolytic phase—osteoporosis circumscripta)	Vascular lesions

TABLE 16.8 Tumors and Pseudotumors That May Present as Radiodense Lesions

Benign	Malignant
Bone island	Adamantinoma
Caffey disease	Chondrosarcoma
Calcifying enchondroma	Ewing sarcoma (after chemotherapy)
Condensing osteitis	Lymphoma
Diskogenic vertebral sclerosis	Osteoblastic metastasis
Healed fibrous cortical defect	Osteosarcoma, conventional
Healed nonossifying fibroma	Parosteal osteosarcoma
Healing or healed fracture	
Liposclerosing myxofibrous tumor	
Mastocytosis	
Medullary bone infarct	
Melorheostosis	
Osteoblastoma	
Osteofibrous dysplasia	
Osteoid osteoma	
Osteoma	
Osteonecrosis	
Osteopoikilosis	
Sclerosing hemangioma	

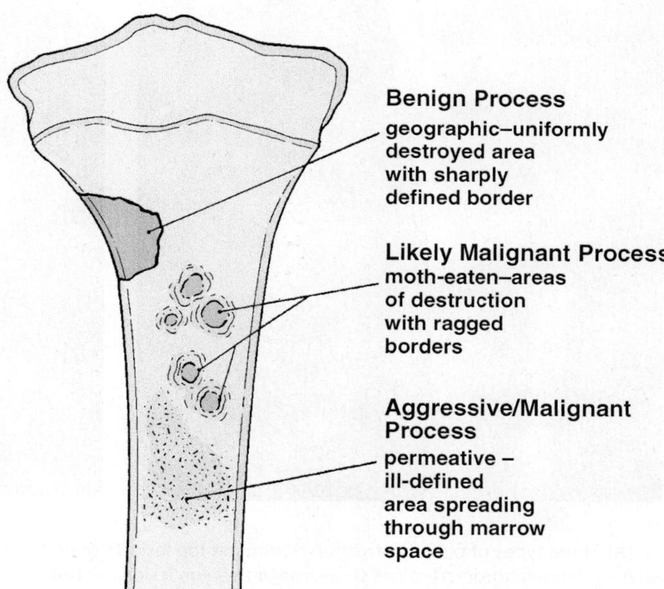

FIGURE 16.47 Pattern of bone destruction. The radiographic features of the type of bone destruction may suggest a benign or malignant neoplastic process.

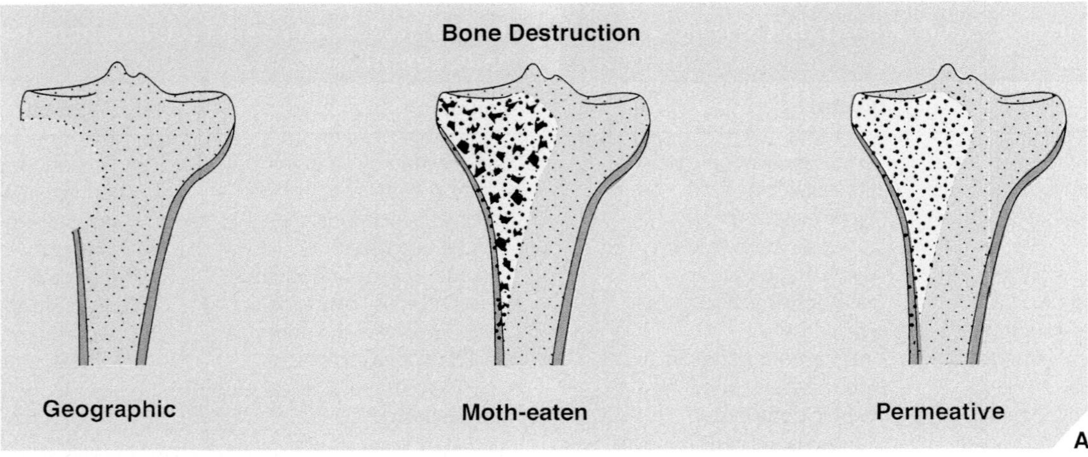

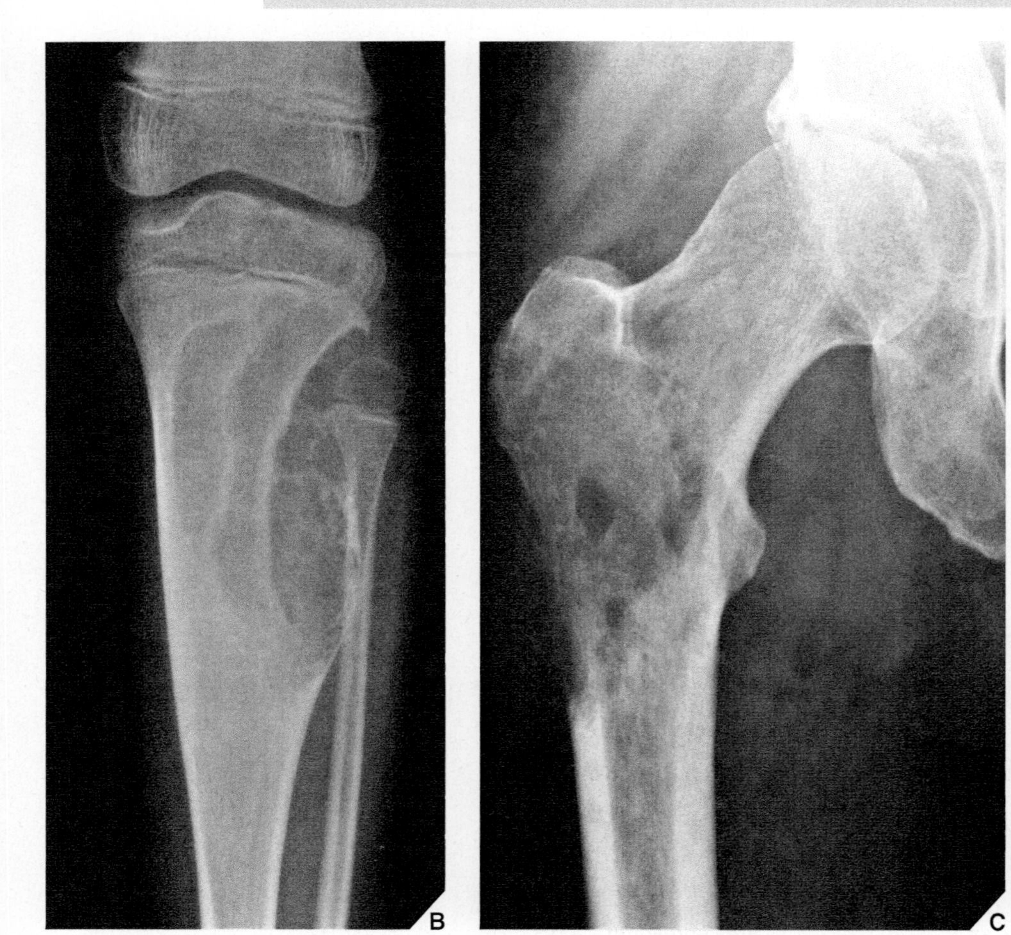

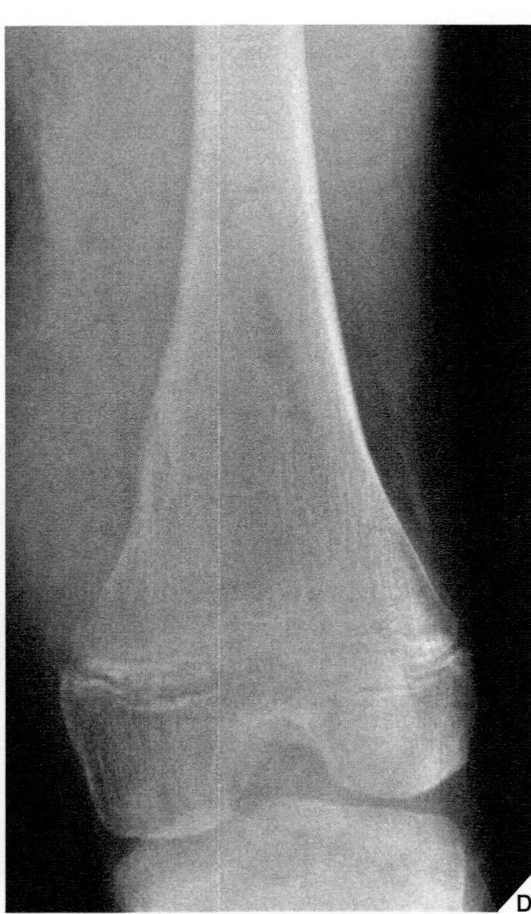

FIGURE 16.48 Pattern of bone destruction. **(A)** Three types of bone destruction determine the lesion's growth rate. **(B)** The geographic type of bone destruction, characterized by a uniformly affected area within sharply defined borders, typifies slow-growing benign lesions, in this case a chondromyxoid fibroma. **(C)** Moth-eaten bone destruction is characteristic of rapidly growing infiltrating lesions, in this case myeloma. **(D)** The permeative type of bone destruction is characteristic of round cell tumors, in this case Ewing sarcoma. Note the almost imperceptible destruction of the metaphysis of the femur by a tumor that has infiltrated the medullary cavity and cortex and extended into the surrounding soft tissues, forming a large mass. (**A**, Modified from Madewell JE, Ragsdale BD, Sweet DE. Radiologic and pathologic analysis of solitary bone lesions. Part I: internal margins. *Radiol Clin North Am* 1981;19(4):715–748. Copyright © 1981 Elsevier. With permission; **B**, Reproduced with permission of AAOS, from Lewis MM, Sissons HA, Norman A, Greenspan A. Benign and malignant cartilage tumors. In: Griffin PP, ed. *Instructional course lectures*. Chicago: American Academy of Orthopaedic Surgeons; 1987:87–114.)

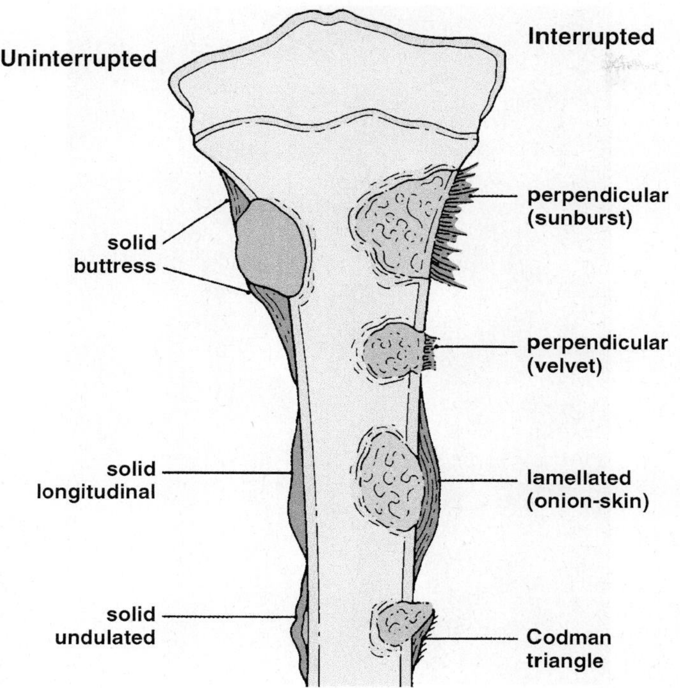

FIGURE 16.49 Types of periosteal reaction. Radiographic characteristics of uninterrupted and interrupted types of periosteal reaction. Uninterrupted periosteal reaction indicates a benign process, whereas interrupted reaction indicates a malignant or aggressive nonmalignant process.

Pathology

Stains

One of the principals and most widely used stains in histology is hematoxylin and eosin (H&E) stain. Special stains are used when the H&E stain cannot provide answers to diagnostic, pathogenetic, and etiologic questions. Van Gieson stain, which is more commonly used in Europe, helps to identify the presence and amount of collagen in bone and other connective tissues by staining it intensively red. Giemsa stain is occasionally used in the differentiation of small round cell tumors, particularly the lymphomas. Reticulin fibers are usually stained with Gomori stain or Novotny stain. Periodic acid-Schiff (PAS) stain coupled with diastase digestion is used to demonstrate intracytoplasmic glycogen. In bone tumor pathologic studies, PAS is often used to reveal glycogen in Ewing sarcoma and in clear cell chondrosarcoma. Mucin stain can demonstrate metastatic adenocarcinoma whenever the tumor cells do not form glandular structures. Trichrome stain can reveal extracellular substances such as collagen. The Congo red stain is used to highlight amyloid deposition. The von Kossa technique is used as a calcium stain, which proves useful in the histomorphometric assessment of metabolic bone disorders involving calcium. The Gram stain is used to classify bacterial organism as gram-positive or gram-negative. Grocott methenamine silver (GMS) stain identifies fungal organisms, and Warthin-Starry stain is used to detect spirochetes and rickettsiae.

Immunohistochemistry

The immunohistochemistry (IHC) method is based on binding a specific cell antigen with a specific antibody on the cell surface or inner structures. Techniques using IHC are very helpful in distinguishing between tumors with similar histology but different origin. For example, this technique is

TABLE 16.9 Examples of Nonneoplastic and Neoplastic Processes Categorized by Type of Periosteal Reaction

Uninterrupted Periosteal Reaction	
Benign Tumors and Tumor-like Lesions	*Nonneoplastic Conditions*
Osteoid osteoma	Osteomyelitis, bone abscess
Osteoblastoma	Langerhans cell histiocytosis
Aneurysmal bone cyst	Healing fracture
Chondromyxoid fibroma	Juxtacortical myositis ossificans
Periosteal chondroma	Hypertrophic pulmonary osteoarthropathy
Chondroblastoma	Hemophilia (subperiosteal bleeding)
	Varicose veins and peripheral vascular insufficiency
	Caffey disease
	Thyroid acropachy
	Treated scurvy
	Pachydermoperiostosis
	Gaucher disease
Malignant Tumors	
Chondrosarcoma (rare)	
Some malignant tumors after treatment with radiation or chemotherapy	
Interrupted Periosteal Reaction	
Malignant Tumors	*Nonneoplastic Conditions*
Osteosarcoma	Acute osteomyelitis
Ewing sarcoma	Langerhans cell histiocytosis (occasionally)
Chondrosarcoma	Subperiosteal hemorrhage (occasionally)
Lymphoma (rare)	Hemophilia (rare)
Fibrosarcoma (rare)	
Malignant fibrous histiocytoma (rare)	
Metastatic carcinoma	

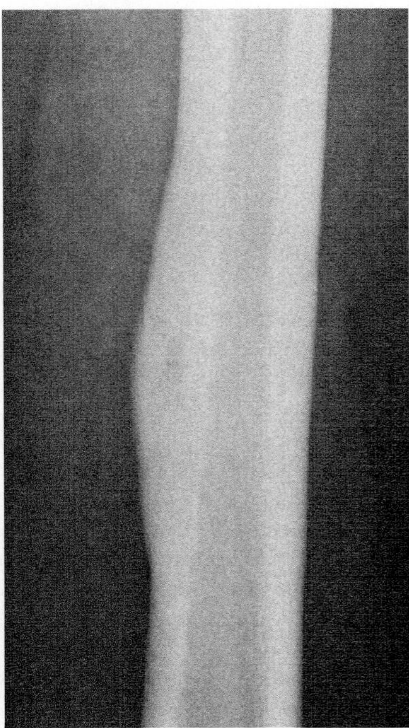

FIGURE 16.50 **Solid periosteal reaction: osteoid osteoma.** An uninterrupted solid periosteal reaction is characteristic of benign lesions, in this case a cortical osteoid osteoma.

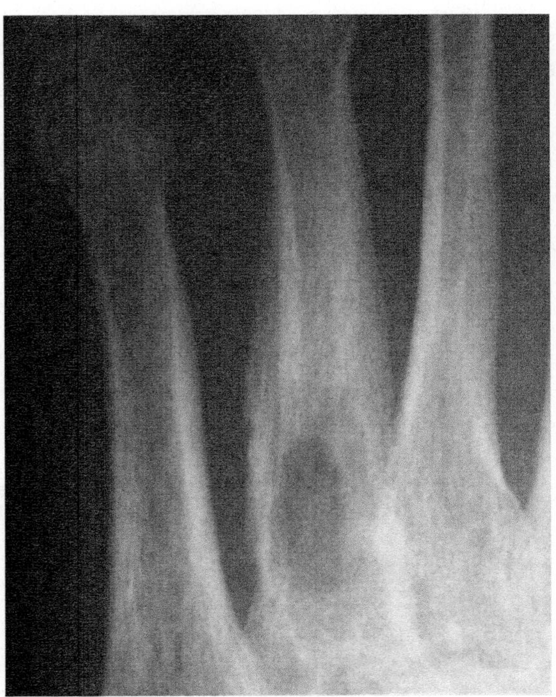

FIGURE 16.51 **Solid periosteal reaction: bone abscess.** A bone abscess located at the base of the fourth metatarsal bone elicits a solid type of periosteal reaction.

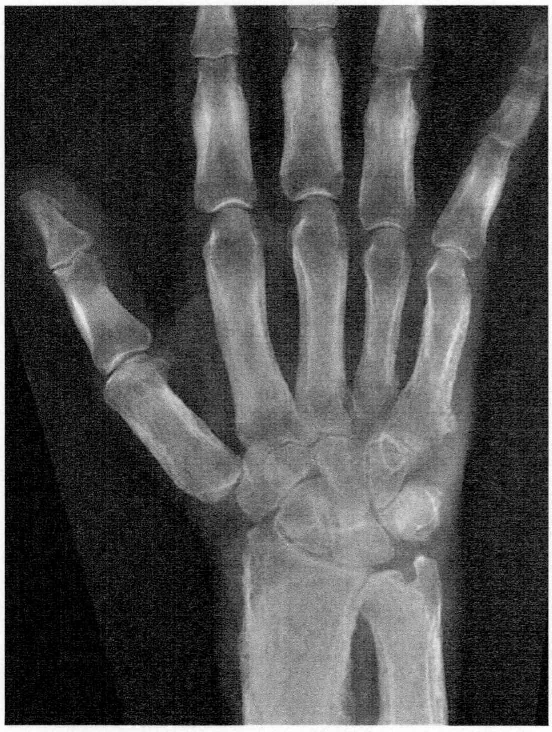

FIGURE 16.52 **Solid periosteal reaction: hypertrophic pulmonary osteoarthropathy.** An uninterrupted periosteal reaction typifies changes of hypertrophic pulmonary osteoarthropathy as seen here in the distal forearm and hand in a patient with carcinoma of the lung.

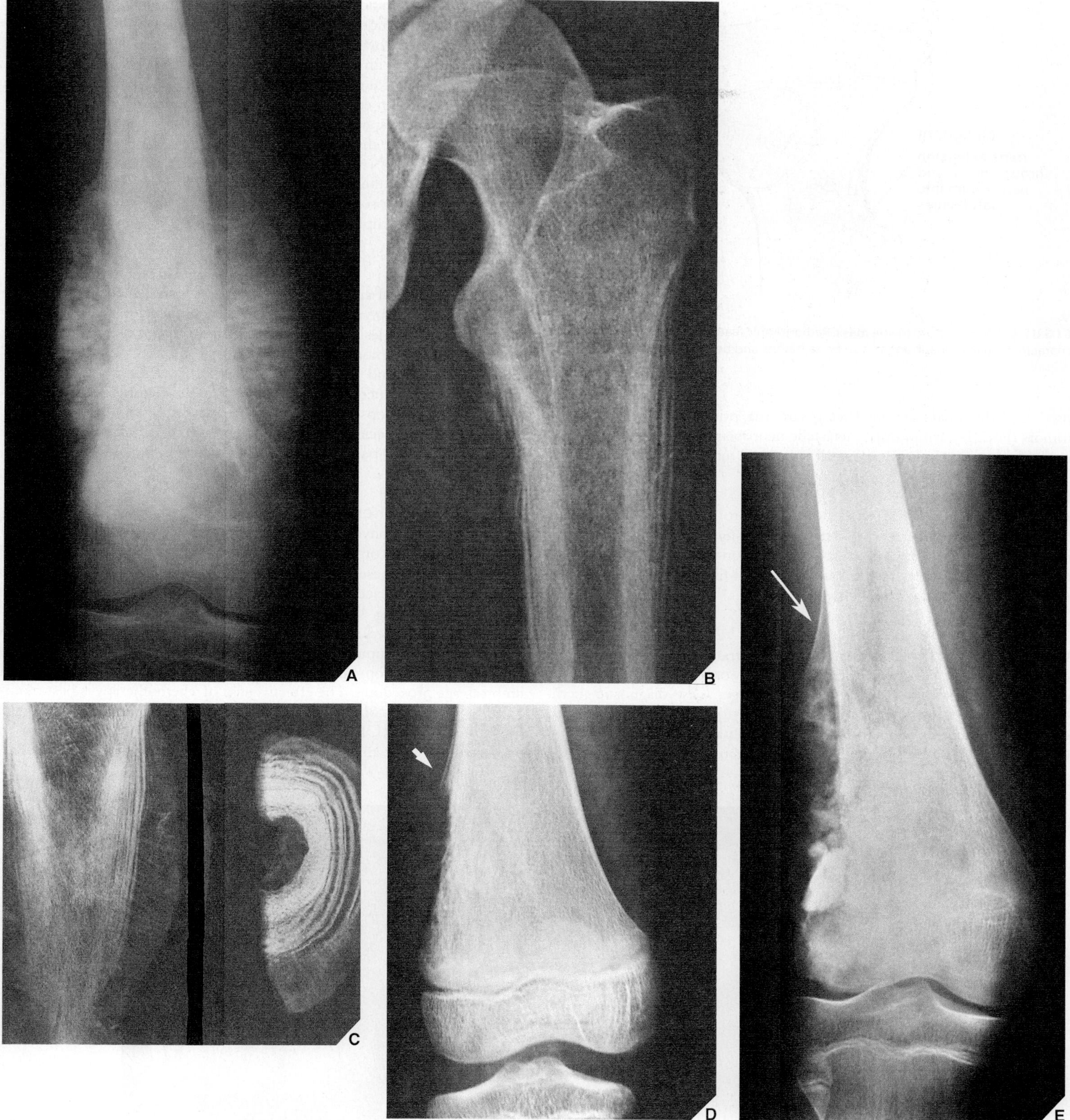

▲
FIGURE 16.53 Interrupted type of periosteal reaction. (A) Highly aggressive and malignant lesions may present radiographically with a sunburst pattern of periosteal reaction, as seen in this case of osteosarcoma. **(B)** Another pattern of interrupted periosteal reaction is the lamellated or onion-skin type, as seen here in Ewing sarcoma involving the proximal left femur. **(C)** Radiograph of the slab sections (coronal at left and transverse at right) of the resected specimen from Ewing sarcoma demonstrates lamellated type in more detail. **(D)** Codman triangle *(arrows)* also reflects an aggressive, usually malignant type of periosteal reaction, as seen here in a patient with Ewing sarcoma and **(E)** in a patient with osteosarcoma. (**C**, Reprinted with permission from Greenspan A, Remagen W. *Differential diagnosis of tumors and tumor-like lesions*. Philadelphia: Lippincott-Raven; 1998.)

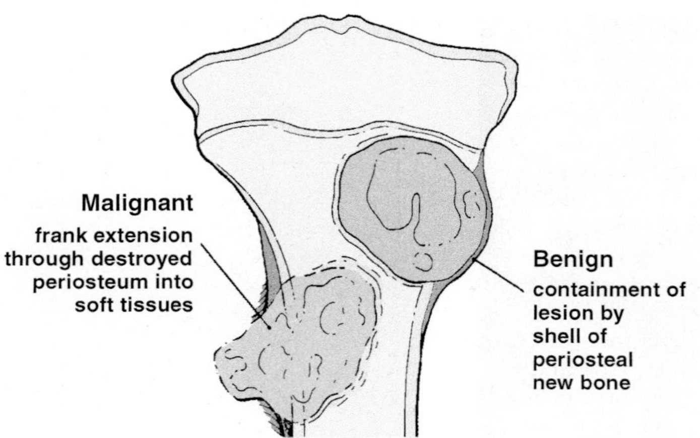

FIGURE 16.54 Soft-tissue mass. Radiographic features of soft-tissue extension characterizing malignant/aggressive bone lesions and benign neoplastic processes.

used to differentiate among Ewing sarcoma/primitive neuroectodermal tumors (PNETs), lymphoma, metastatic neuroblastoma, and Wilms tumor in the differential diagnosis of small round cell tumors.

Electron Microscopy

Electron microscopy (EM) does not have a prominent role in the study of bone tumor pathology. Ultrastructural investigations, however, are still of help in the evaluation of small cell neoplasms (e.g., PNET may show neurosecretory granules), or in Langerhans cell histiocytosis, demonstrating characteristic Birbeck granules.

Genetics of Bone Tumors

Genetic studies of bone tumors may demonstrate specific chromosomal changes in cancer cells, which may act as diagnostic, prognostic, and targeted therapy markers. To detect these changes, new diagnostic methods such as flow cytometry (FCM), digital cytogenetics, and molecular cytogenetics were developed. FCM is a quantitative automated method used to analyze the DNA content and proliferation rate of isolated cells. Cytogenetics is a branch of genetics that is concerned with studying the structure and function of the cell, especially chromosomes. Molecular cytogenetic is a branch of genetics that combines molecular biology and cytogenetics. With the development of fluorescent in situ hybridization (FISH), genetic analyses of interphase nuclei became possible, even in fixed and paraffin-embedded material, by application of differentially labeled centromere-specific and sequence-specific probes to nuclear material. The polymerase chain reaction (PCR) is a revolutionary method based on the ability of DNA polymerase to synthesize new strands of DNA complementary to the offered template strands. This method enables detection of chromosomal translocation t(11;22) in Ewing sarcoma from even a very small sample of biopsy tissue.

Management

When all the clinical and imaging information concerning a patient with a bone lesion has been analyzed, the most important diagnostic decision is whether the lesion is definitely benign and not to undergo biopsy but rather merely monitored or completely ignored—a "don't touch" lesion (Fig. 16.60 and Table 16.11)—or whether it has an aggressive or ambiguous appearance and should be further investigated via percutaneous or open biopsy (Fig. 16.61). The results of the histopathologic examination of a specimen determine whether the further management in a given case should be surgical, chemotherapeutic, radiotherapeutic, or a combination of these.

Monitoring the Results of Treatment

Five modalities—conventional radiography, CT, MRI, scintigraphy, and arteriography—are commonly used to monitor the results of treatment for bone tumors. Of these five, radiography is used mainly to document the results of surgical resection of benign lesions such as osteochondroma or osteoid osteoma (Fig. 16.62), or to follow up after curettage of benign tumors or tumor-like lesions and application of bone graft (Fig. 16.63). In the case of malignant tumors, radiographic films permit one to demonstrate the position of endoprostheses (Fig. 16.64) or bone grafts (Fig. 16.65) in limb-salvage procedures. The effectiveness of chemotherapy is best monitored by a combination of radiography, arteriography (Fig. 16.66), CT (see Fig. 16.12), and MRI. Recurrence or metastatic spread of a tumor can be effectively shown at an early stage on scintigraphy, CT, PET/CT, or MRI.

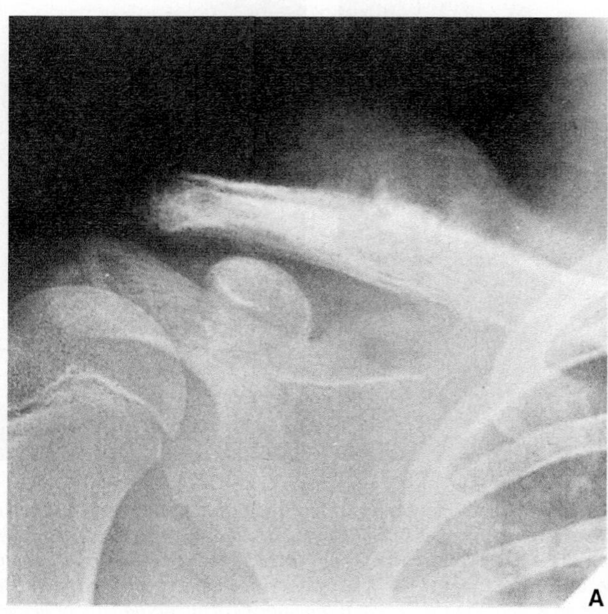

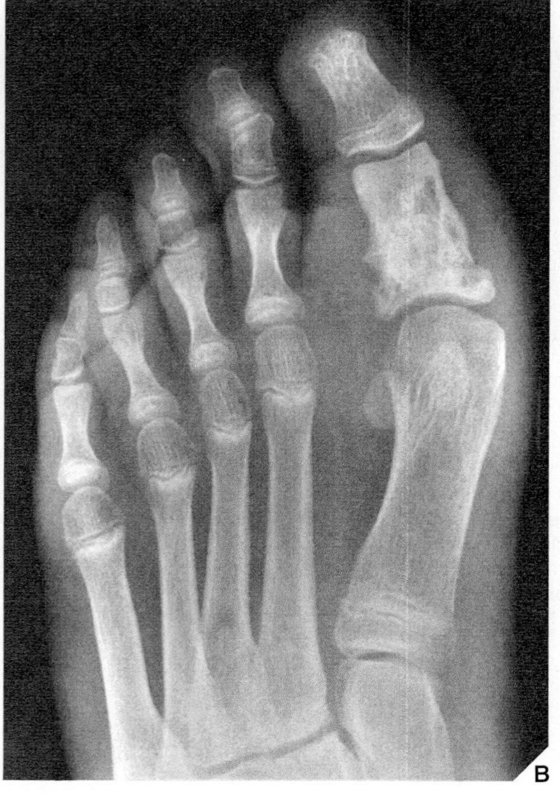

FIGURE 16.55 Soft-tissue mass. (A) A malignant tumor of the clavicle, in this case Ewing sarcoma, exhibits a distinct, sharply outlined soft-tissue mass. **(B)** In osteomyelitis, in this case affecting the proximal phalanx of the great toe, the tissue planes are obliterated, and the soft-tissue mass has an indistinct border.

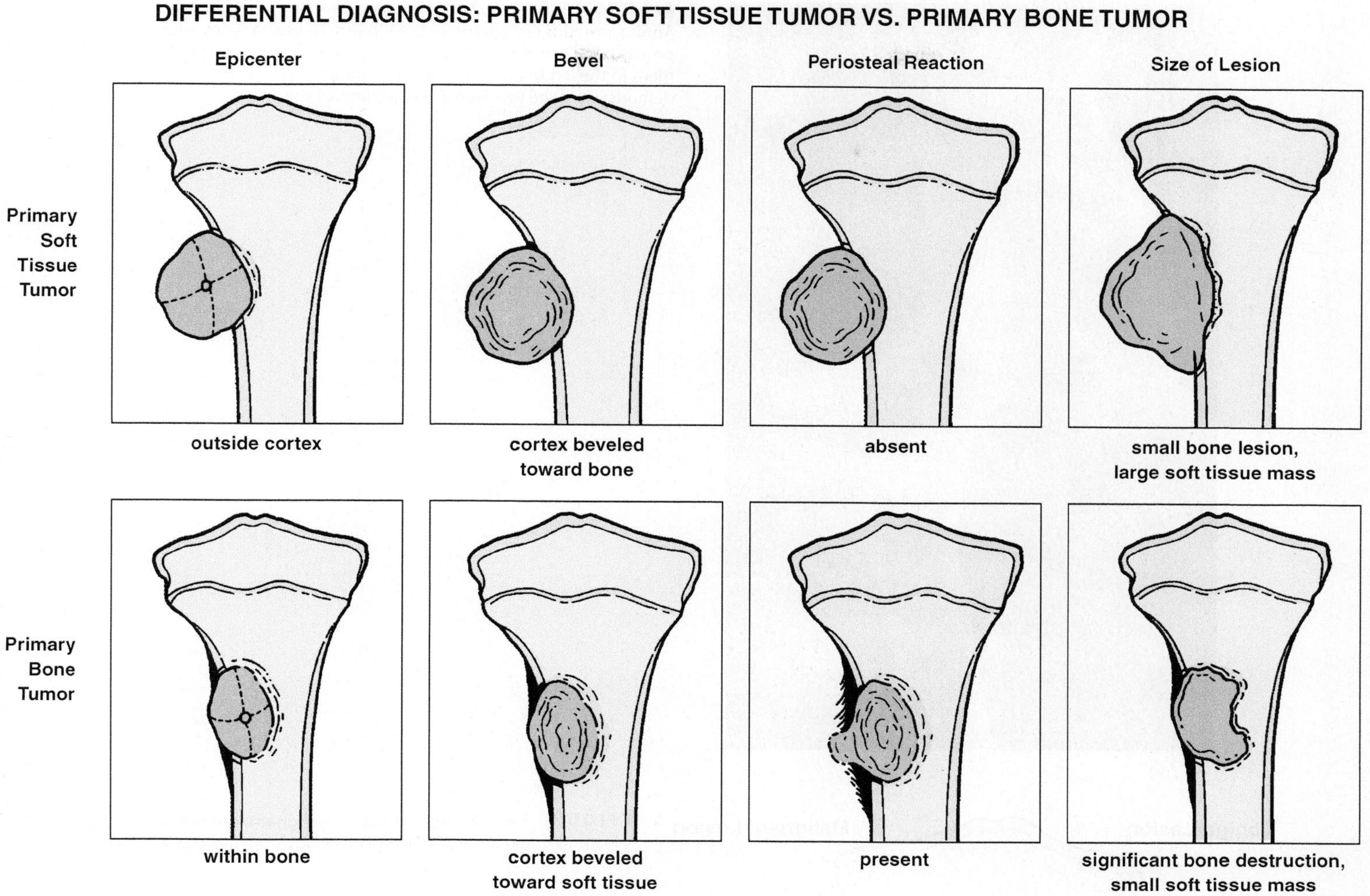

DIFFERENTIAL DIAGNOSIS: PRIMARY SOFT TISSUE TUMOR VS. PRIMARY BONE TUMOR

	Epicenter	Bevel	Periosteal Reaction	Size of Lesion
Primary Soft Tissue Tumor	outside cortex	cortex beveled toward bone	absent	small bone lesion, large soft tissue mass
Primary Bone Tumor	within bone	cortex beveled toward soft tissue	present	significant bone destruction, small soft tissue mass

FIGURE 16.56 Primary soft-tissue tumor versus primary bone tumor. Certain radiographic features of bone and soft-tissue lesions may help differentiate a primary soft-tissue tumor invading the bone from a primary bone tumor invading soft tissues.

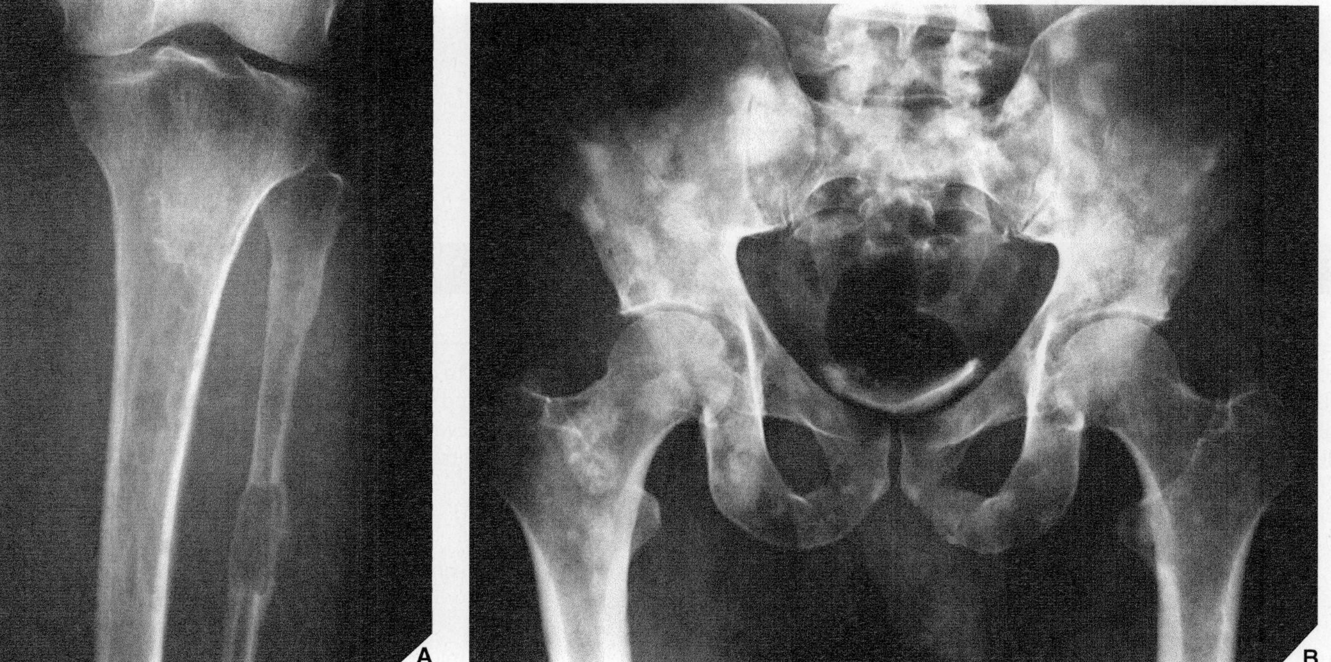

FIGURE 16.57 Multiplicity of lesion. **(A)** Multiple myeloma is characterized by numerous osteolytic lesions. **(B)** Metastatic disease may also present with multiple foci, as seen in this 66-year-old man with carcinoma of the prostate. Note several osteoblastic lesions scattered throughout the pelvis and both femora.

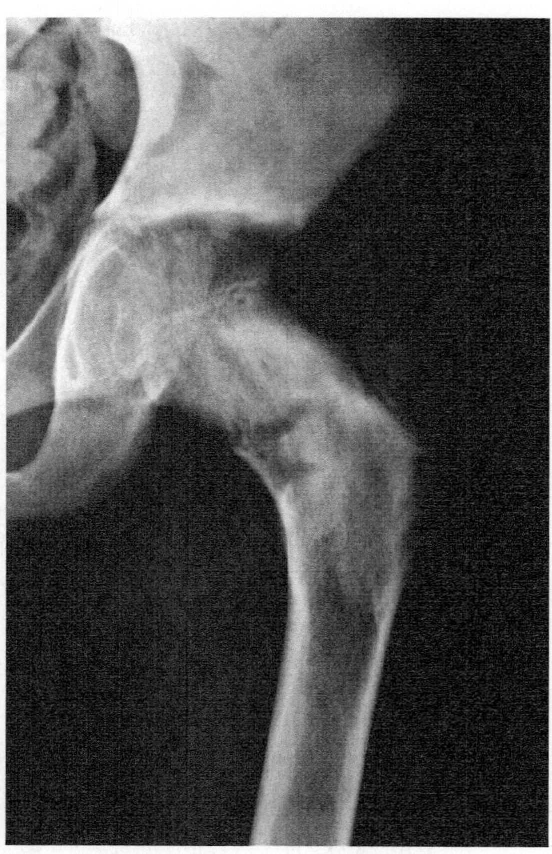

FIGURE 16.58 Multiplicity of lesion—fibrous dysplasia. Anteroposterior radiograph of the hip in a 10-year-old boy with polyostotic fibrous dysplasia shows numerous sites of involvement in the left femur and ilium. Scintigraphy (not shown here) demonstrated the involvement of additional sites.

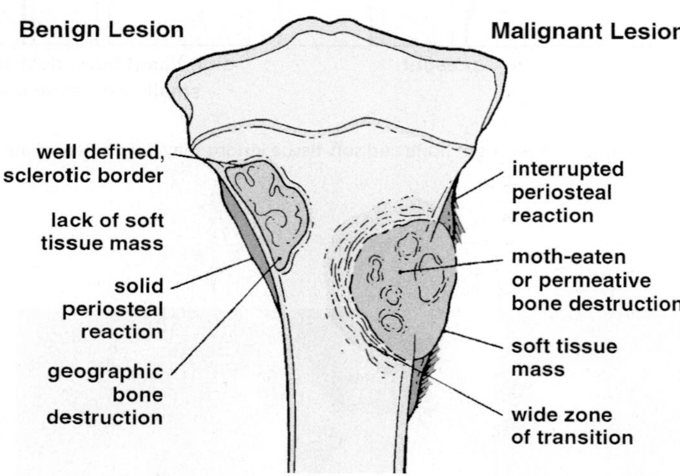

FIGURE 16.59 Benign versus malignant lesion. Radiographic features that may help differentiate benign from malignant lesions.

TABLE 16.10 Benign Lesions with Aggressive Features

Lesion	Radiographic Presentation
Osteoblastoma (aggressive)	Bone destruction and soft-tissue extension similar to osteosarcoma
Desmoplastic fibroma	Expansive destructive lesion, frequently trabeculated
Periosteal desmoid	Irregular cortical outline, mimics osteosarcoma or Ewing sarcoma
Giant cell tumor	Occasionally aggressive features such as osteolytic bone destruction, cortical penetration, and soft-tissue extension
Aneurysmal bone cyst	Soft-tissue extension, occasionally mimicking malignant tumor (i.e., telangiectatic osteosarcoma)
Osteomyelitis	Bone destruction, aggressive periosteal reaction Occasionally, features resembling osteosarcoma, Ewing sarcoma, or lymphoma
Langerhans cell histiocytosis	Bone destruction, aggressive periosteal reaction Occasionally, features resembling Ewing sarcoma
Pseudotumor of hemophilia	Bone destruction, periosteal reaction occasionally mimics malignant tumor
Myositis ossificans	Features of parosteal or periosteal osteosarcoma, soft-tissue osteosarcoma, or liposarcoma
Brown tumor of hyperparathyroidism	Lytic bone lesion, resembling malignant tumor

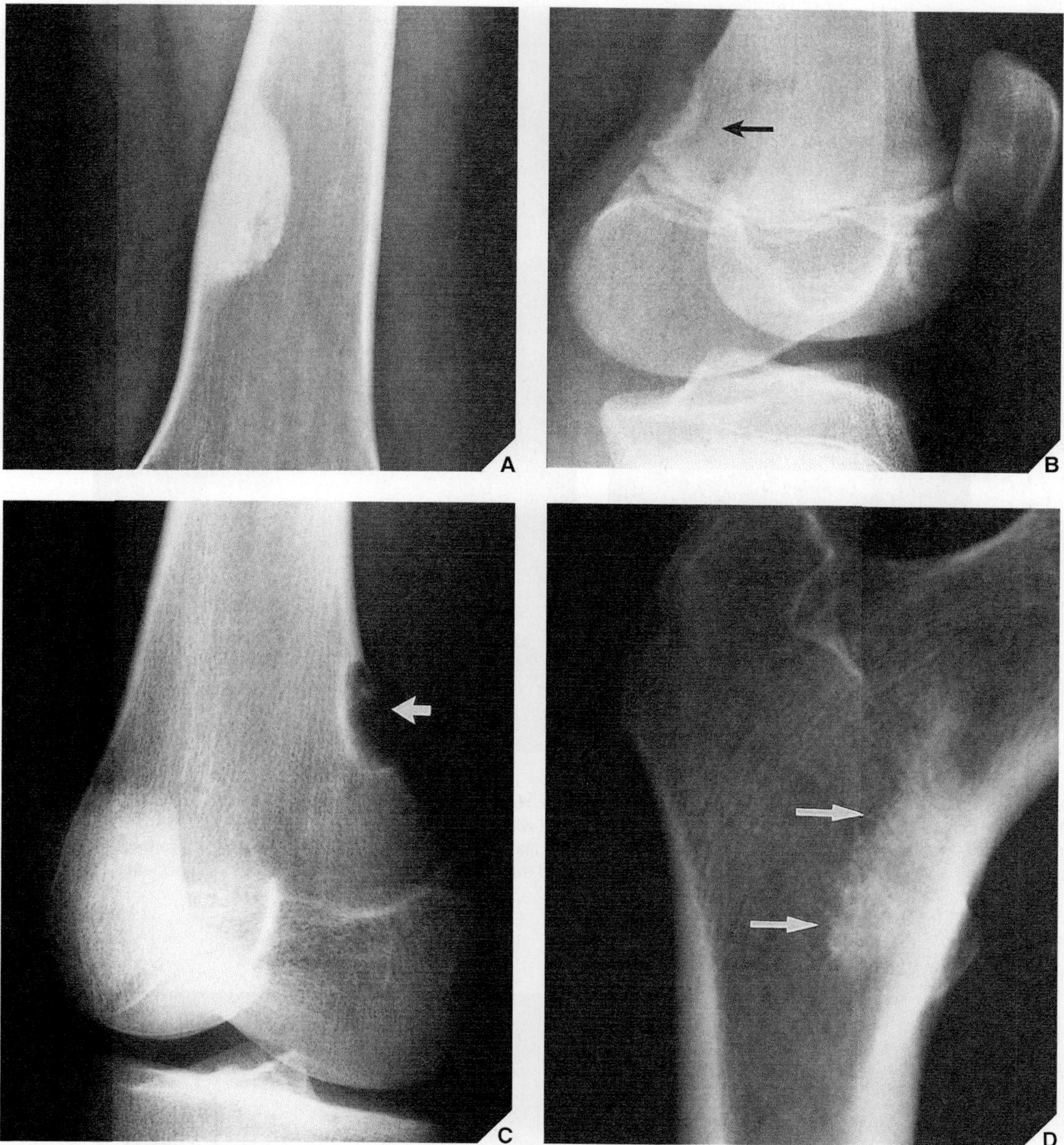

FIGURE 16.60 "Don't touch" lesions. **(A)** A typical benign "don't touch" lesion, in this case a nonossifying fibroma in healing phase, should not be mistaken for a malignant tumor of bone. **(B)** Another "don't touch" lesion, a periosteal (cortical) desmoid *(arrow)* in a typical location at the distal femoral metaphysis, medially. **(C)** A fibrous cortical defect *(arrow)* is an innocent fibrous lesion that never requires biopsy. **(D)** A bone island *(arrows)* should be recognized by a characteristic brush border and not to be mistaken for a sclerotic neoplasm.

TABLE 16.11 "Don't Touch" Lesions That Should Not Undergo Biopsy

Tumors and Tumor-like Lesions	Nonneoplastic Processes
Fibrous cortical defect	Stress fracture
Nonossifying fibroma (healing phase)	Avulsion fracture (healing stage)
Periosteal (cortical) desmoid	Bone infarct
Small, solitary focus of fibrous dysplasia	Bone island (enostosis)
Pseudotumor of hemophilia	Myositis ossificans
Intraosseous ganglion	Degenerative and posttraumatic cysts
Enchondroma in a short, tubular bone	Brown tumor of hyperparathyroidism
Intraosseous hemangioma	Diskogenic vertebral sclerosis

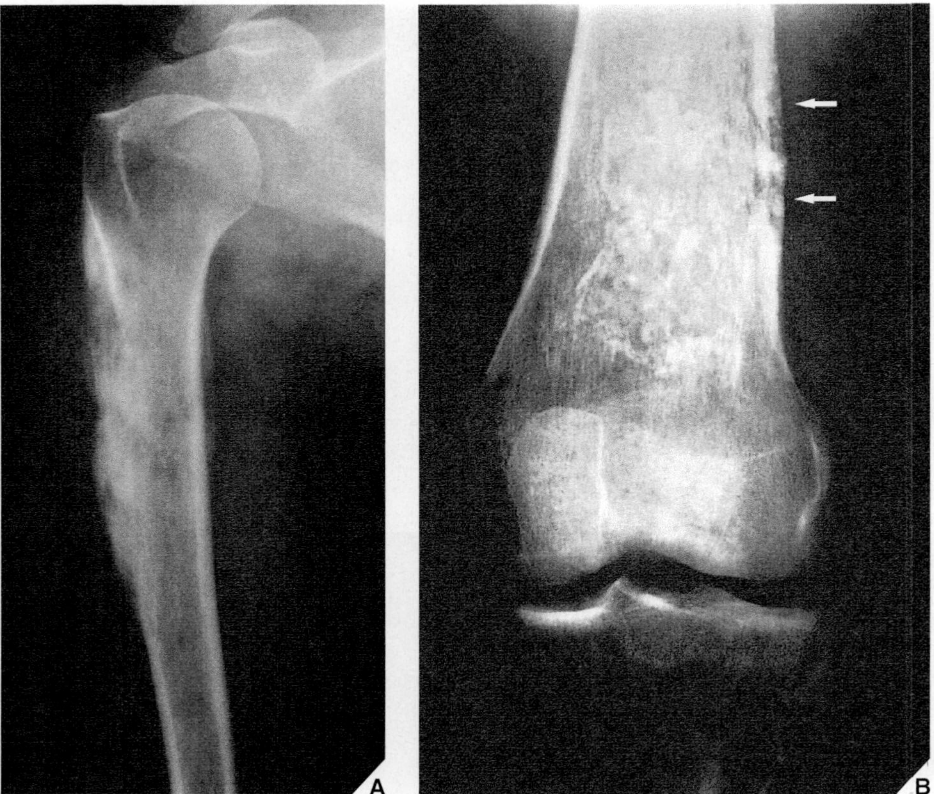

FIGURE 16.61 Ambiguous lesions: chronic osteomyelitis and bone infarction. **(A)** A typical "ambiguous" lesion exhibiting aggressive characteristics requires biopsy. The radiographic differential diagnosis in this case included osteosarcoma, Ewing sarcoma, lymphoma, and bone infection. Biopsy revealed chronic osteomyelitis. **(B)** Although the lesion in the distal femur exhibits all the characteristics of the medullary bone infarct, the lateral cortex shows some permeation and lamellated periosteal reaction *(arrows)*, features not ordinarily seen with benign condition. Biopsy revealed malignant fibrous histiocytoma arising in bone infarct.

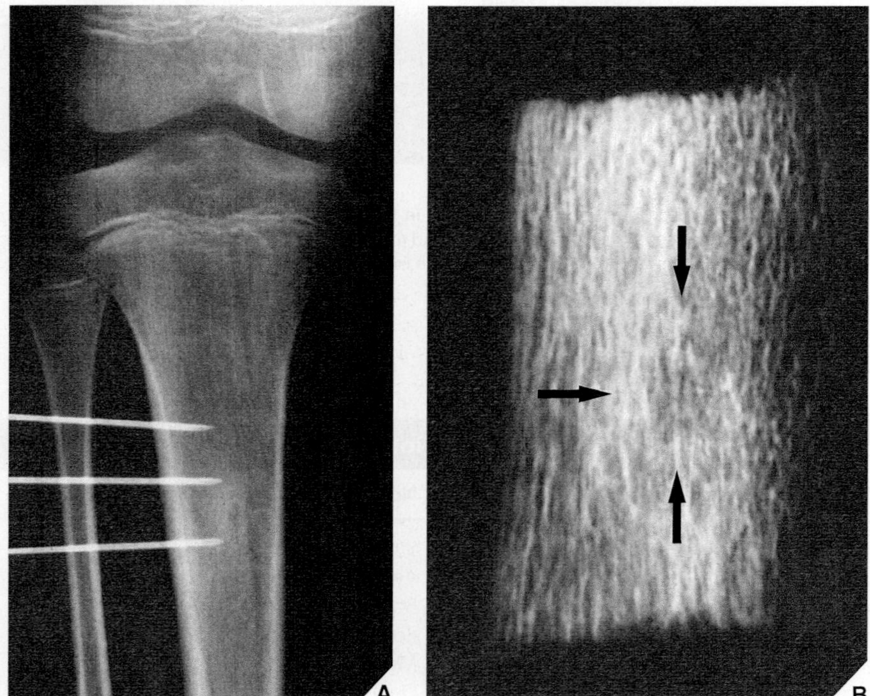

FIGURE 16.62 Osteoid osteoma. **(A)** During surgery for resection of a nidus of osteoid osteoma in the proximal diaphysis of the tibia of a 10-year-old boy, needles are taped into the skin to localize the nidus. **(B)** Radiograph of the resected specimen demonstrates complete excision of the lesion *(arrows)*.

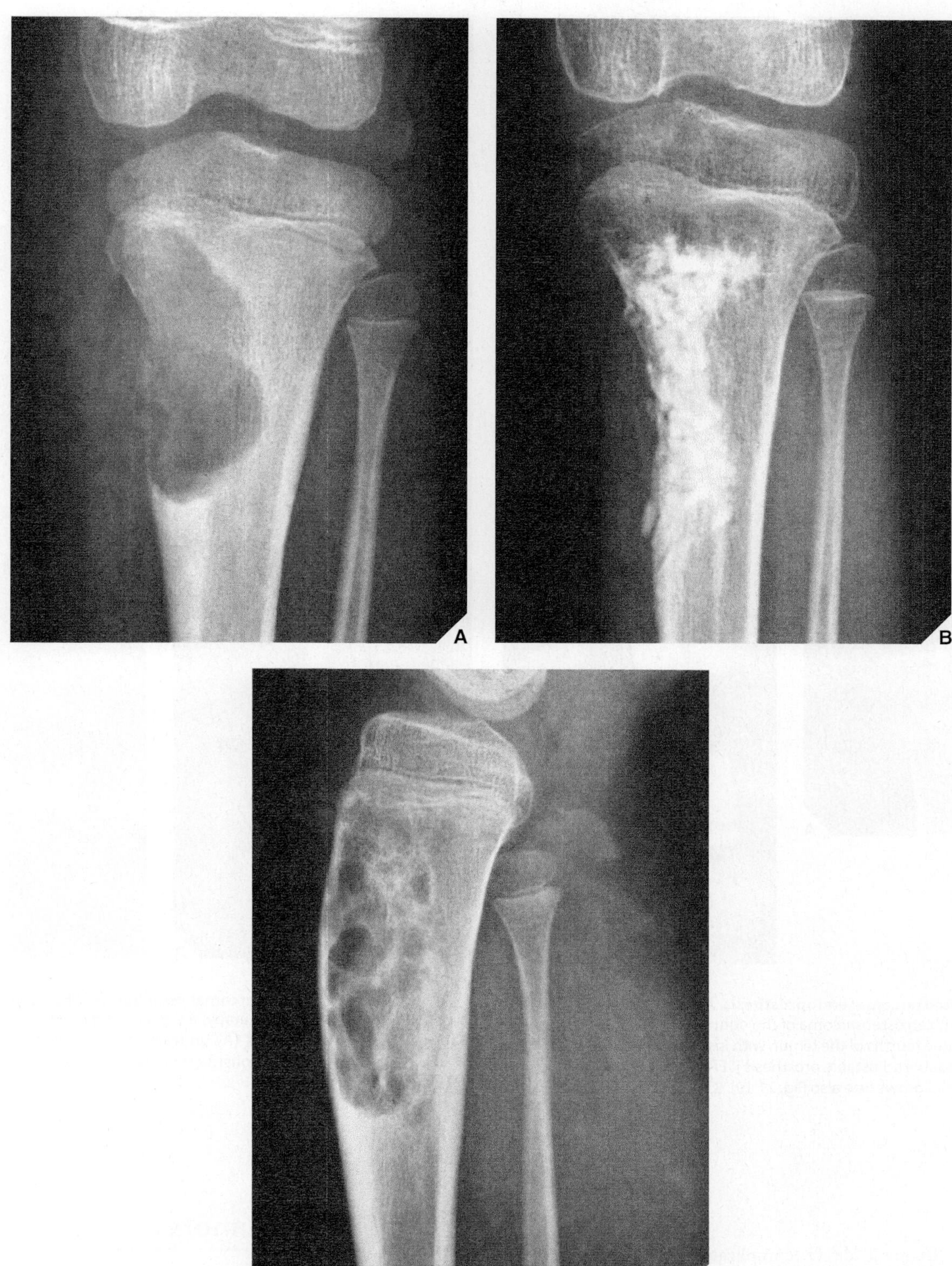

FIGURE 16.63 Chondromyxoid fibroma: recurrence. A 9-year-old boy was treated for a chondromyxoid fibroma, a benign cartilaginous lesion in the proximal left tibia. **(A)** Preoperative radiograph shows a lesion exhibiting a thin sclerotic border with endosteal scalloping, a geographic-type bone destruction, and a solid buttress of periosteal new bone formation at its distal part. **(B)** Postoperative film shows the lesion's cavity packed with bone chips after curettage. **(C)** Two years later, the tumor recurred.

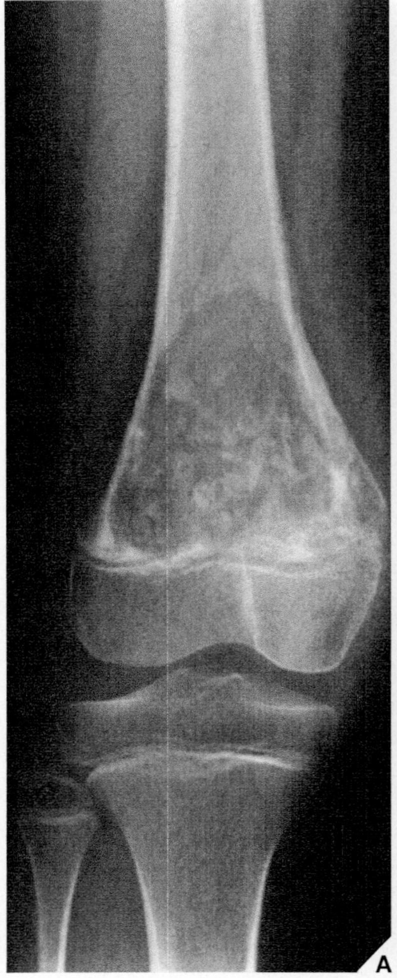

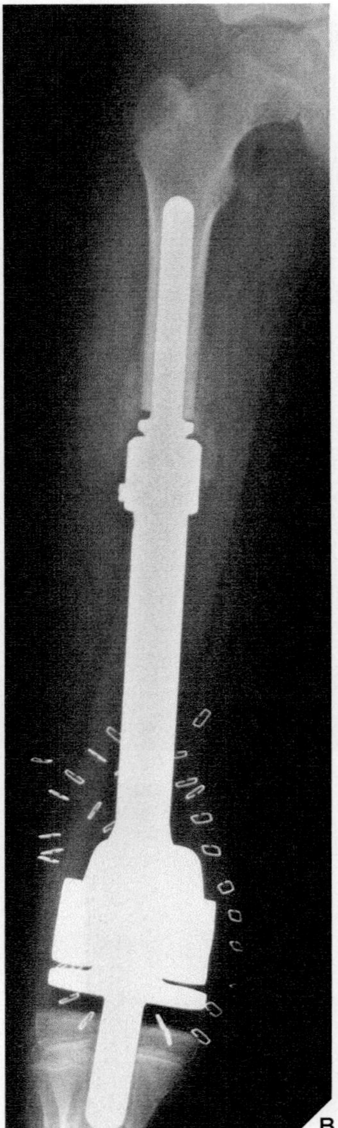

FIGURE 16.64 **Osteosarcoma: endoprosthesis.** After a course of chemotherapy, an 8-year-old girl with an osteosarcoma of the right femur **(A)** underwent radical resection of the distal three fourths of the femur, with insertion of an expandable and adjustable (Lewis expandable adjustable prosthesis [LEAP]) prosthesis **(B)**, which can be lengthened as the child grows (see also Fig. 21.19). (Courtesy of Michael M. Lewis, MD, Santa Barbara, CA.)

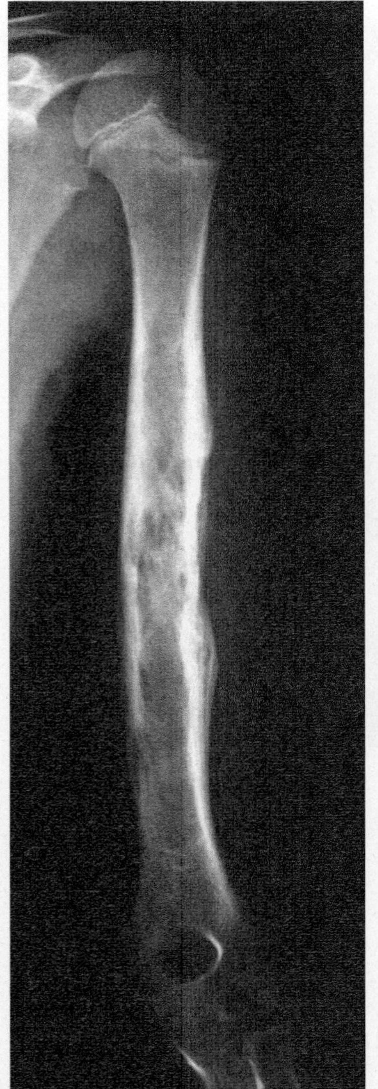

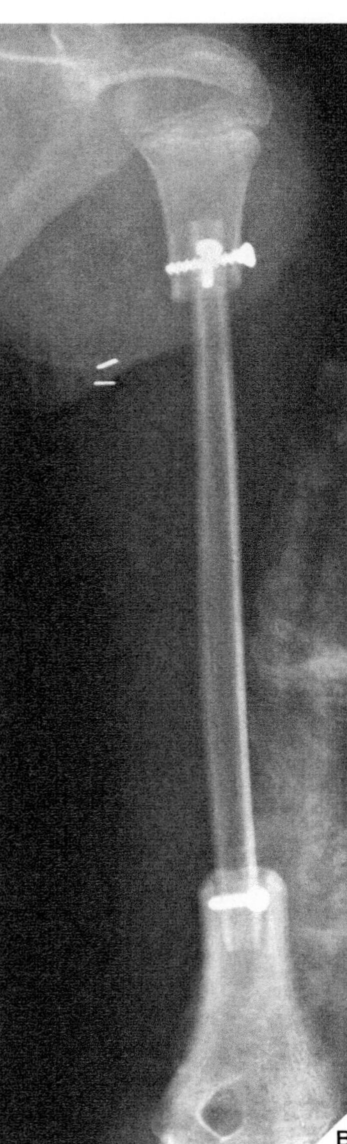

FIGURE 16.65 **Ewing sarcoma: resection and bone grafting.** After a course of radiotherapy and chemotherapy, a 9-year-old girl with an Ewing sarcoma in the diaphysis of the left humerus **(A)** underwent radical resection of the middle segment of the humerus. **(B)** Reconstruction was accomplished with the application of a fibular autograft.

Complications

Although the most frequent direct complication of malignant bone tumors is metastasis, particularly to the lung, the most serious complication of some benign lesions is their potential for malignant transformation (Fig. 16.67; see also Table 16.2). Moreover, some benign lesions, such as those seen in multiple cartilaginous exostoses (Fig. 16.68) or enchondromatosis (see Figs. 18.33B and 18.34C), may result in severe growth disturbance. The most common complication of tumors and tumor-like lesions in general, however, is pathologic fracture. Although not a diagnostic feature, this may complicate both benign and malignant lesions. Among lesions with a high potential for fracture are simple bone cysts, large nonossifying fibromas (Fig. 16.69), fibrous dysplasia, and enchondromas (see Figs. 18.7 and 18.8). Occasionally, pathologic fracture is the first sign of a neoplastic process. Other complications, such as pressure erosion of adjacent bone (Fig. 16.70) or compression of adjacent blood vessels or nerves (see Fig. 18.48B), may occur with growth of a lesion beyond the cortex.

Soft-Tissue Tumors

Unlike tumors and tumor-like lesions of bone, most soft-tissue tumors (Table 16.12) lack specific radiographic characteristics that might be helpful in their diagnosis. Some findings, however, may point to a particular kind of lesion. For instance, calcified phleboliths in a soft-tissue mass suggest a hemangioma or hemangiomatosis (Fig. 16.71); radiolucency within a mass suggests a lipoma (Fig. 16.72); mottled lucencies within a dense mass, in association with bone formation, suggest liposarcoma (Fig. 16.73); popcorn-like calcifications suggest soft-tissue chondroma or chondrosarcoma; similar calcifications in the vicinity of a joint, particularly when associated with bone destruction, suggest synovial sarcoma (see Figs. 23.31A and 23.32A,B); and ill-defined, nonhomogeneous, smudgy bone in a soft-tissue mass may indicate a soft-tissue osteosarcoma (Fig. 16.74). Several investigators implied the efficacy of MRI in the characterization and evaluation of soft-tissue masses; its superiority over CT stems from the lack of ionizing radiation, its capability of multidirectional and multiplanar imaging, and its excellent

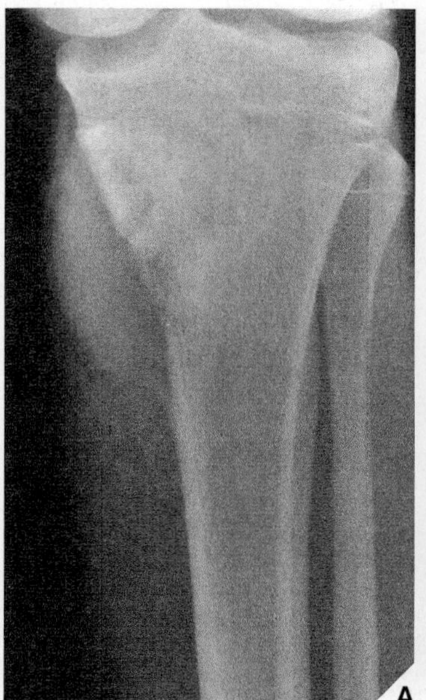

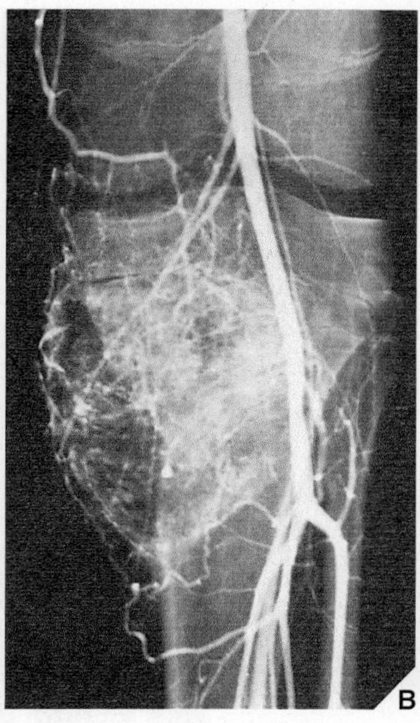

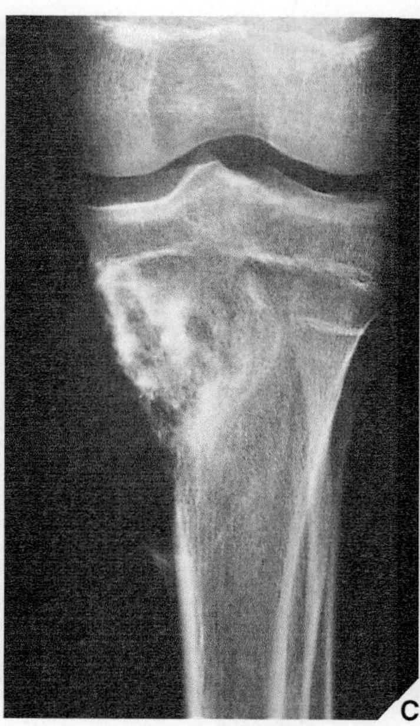

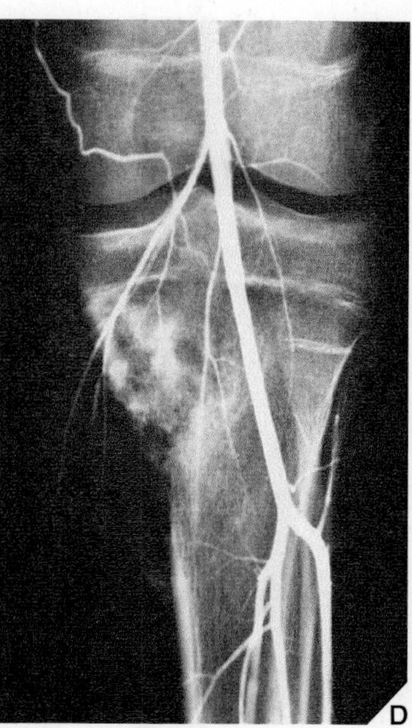

FIGURE 16.66 **Osteosarcoma after chemotherapy.** **(A)** Anteroposterior radiograph of the proximal left tibia of a 15-year-old boy demonstrates an osteosarcoma in the metaphysis associated with a large soft-tissue mass. **(B)** An arteriogram done prior to treatment shows the soft-tissue mass to be hypervascular. After combination chemotherapy with methotrexate, vincristine, doxorubicin hydrochloride, and cisplatin, a repeated radiograph **(C)** and an arteriogram **(D)** show marked reduction of the tumor mass. Subsequently, a wide resection of the proximal tibia was performed, and a metallic spacer similar to the one shown in Figure 16.64B was implanted.

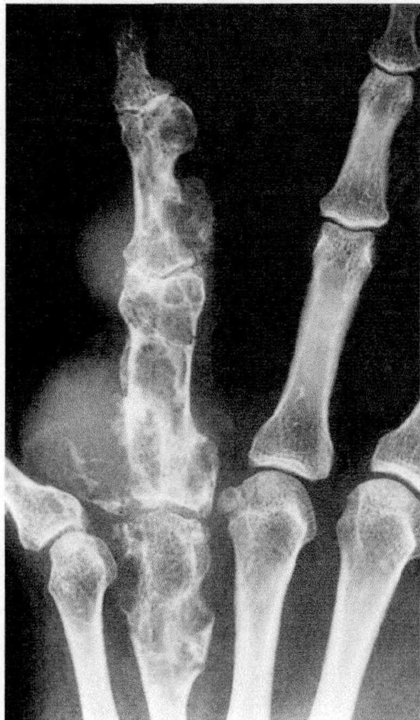

FIGURE 16.67 **Malignant transformation to chondrosarcoma.** An enchondroma at the base of the ring finger of this 32-year-old man with multiple enchondromatosis underwent sarcomatous transformation to a chondrosarcoma.

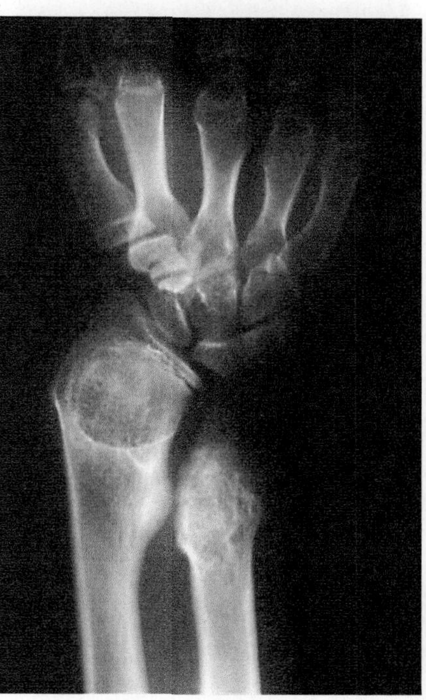

FIGURE 16.68 **Multiple cartilaginous exostoses: growth disturbance.** Anteroposterior radiograph of the wrist of a 14-year-old boy with multiple cartilaginous exostoses (osteochondromas) shows marked growth disturbance of the distal ends of the radius and ulna.

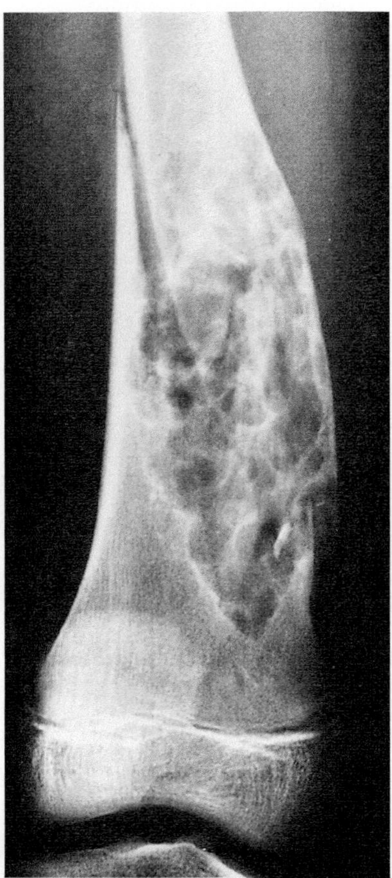

FIGURE 16.69 Nonossifying fibroma complicated by a pathologic fracture. A 9-year-old boy with a giant nonossifying fibroma of the distal diaphysis of the right femur developed a pathologic fracture, a common complication of this lesion.

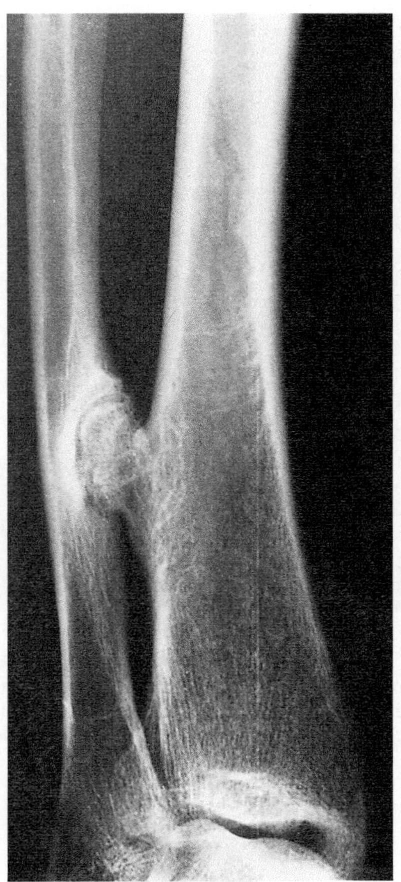

FIGURE 16.70 Osteochondroma eroding the adjacent bone. Extension of a lesion arising from the posterolateral aspect of the distal tibia in a 24-year-old man with an osteochondroma erodes the adjacent fibula.

contrast resolution and accurate anatomic definition of soft-tissue tumors. On T1-weighted pulsing sequences, the majority of soft-tissue masses display low-to-intermediate signal intensity, whereas on T2-weighted images, they display high signal intensity. There are, however, masses that show high signal intensity on T1 weighting because of blood or fat content, such as lipomas, hemangiomas, and chronic hematomas. One of the fatty tumors that do not show a high signal on T1 weighting is myxoid liposarcoma. At present, however, as Sundaram and McLeod contended based on MRI results, neither visual characteristics nor signal intensity values permit one to distinguish or predict the histology of soft-tissue masses. Nevertheless, certain criteria are

TABLE 16.12 Most Common Benign and Malignant Soft-Tissue Lesions

Benign	Malignant
Ganglion	Rhabdomyosarcoma
Lipoma	Leiomyosarcoma
Myoma, leiomyoma	Malignant fibrous histiocytoma
Fibroma	Fibrosarcoma
Fibromatosis	Myxofibrosarcoma
Myxoma	Malignant schwannoma
Hemangioma, hemangiomatosis	Spindle-cell sarcoma
Lymphangioma	Liposarcoma
Chondroma	Synovial sarcoma
Neurofibroma	Extraskeletal osteosarcoma
Desmoid	Extraskeletal chondrosarcoma
Giant cell tumor of tendon sheath	Hemangioendothelioma
Morton neuroma	Kaposi sarcoma
Hamartoma	Angiosarcoma

very helpful to predict the benign or malignant nature of the tumor; sharp margination and homogeneity of the mass favor benignity, whereas prominent peritumoral edema and necrosis suggest malignancy. Recently, the application of high-resolution US including color Doppler US, power Doppler US, and spectral wave analysis was advocated for the initial assessment and sonographic-guided core biopsy of ambiguous soft-tissue masses.

The main role of the radiologist is not to make a specific diagnosis but rather to demonstrate the extent of the lesion and decide whether the lesion is a tumor or pseudotumor (Table 16.13), and in case of malignancy, whether it is a primary soft-tissue tumor invading the bone or an extracortical extension of a primary bone tumor (see Fig. 16.55A). Most often, this is achieved by using arteriography (Fig. 16.75), CT (Fig. 16.76), and MRI (Fig. 16.77). After this, the radiologist's role may become more active, involving fluoroscopy-guided, US-guided, or CT-guided percutaneous biopsy of the lesion. In this respect, arteriography helps select the proper area for biopsy, with the specimen usually taken from the most vascular part of the lesion (Fig. 16.78).

Nevertheless, some soft-tissue tumors exhibit specific features that allow a preoperative diagnosis. Vascular tumors, such as capillary hemangiomas, show characteristic intramuscular striations (see Fig. 16.77C). Cavernous hemangiomas demonstrate prominent vascular spaces with fluid–fluid levels (Fig. 16.79). Benign lipomatous tumors demonstrate characteristic fat signal throughout the entire tumor with thin capsule and thin or lack of intratumoral septae (Fig. 16.80). Low-grade liposarcomas or atypical lipomas may show thick septae within the fatty component of the tumor exhibiting some enhancement following intravenous administration of gadolinium (Fig. 16.81). High-grade liposarcomas contain minimal fat with a predominant nonlipomatous component of the tumor. Myxoid liposarcomas show fluid-like signal intensity on the nonenhanced MRI and prominent enhancement after gadolinium injection (Fig. 16.82). Fibrolipomatous hamartoma presents typically as soft-tissue mass adjacent to a nerve (more commonly the median nerve in the carpal tunnel), with characteristic "spaghetti"-like or "coaxial cable" striations (Fig. 16.83). Tumors of neural origin often exhibit a

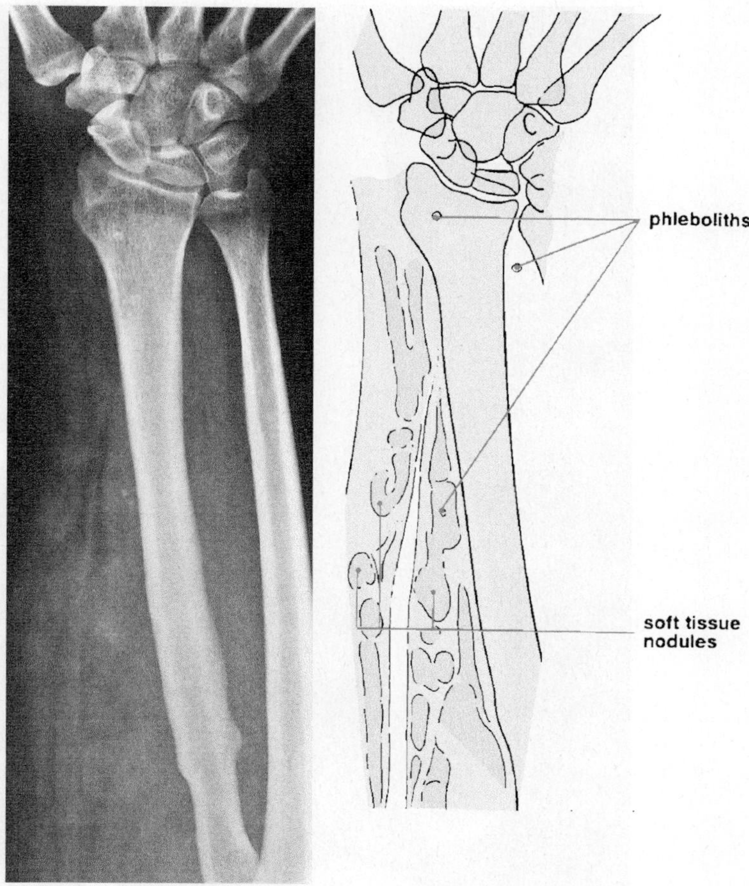

FIGURE 16.71 Soft-tissue hemangiomatosis. Conventional radiograph in a 39-year-old woman with a nodular swelling of the left forearm demonstrates multiple small calcified phleboliths, suggesting the diagnosis of hemangiomatosis.

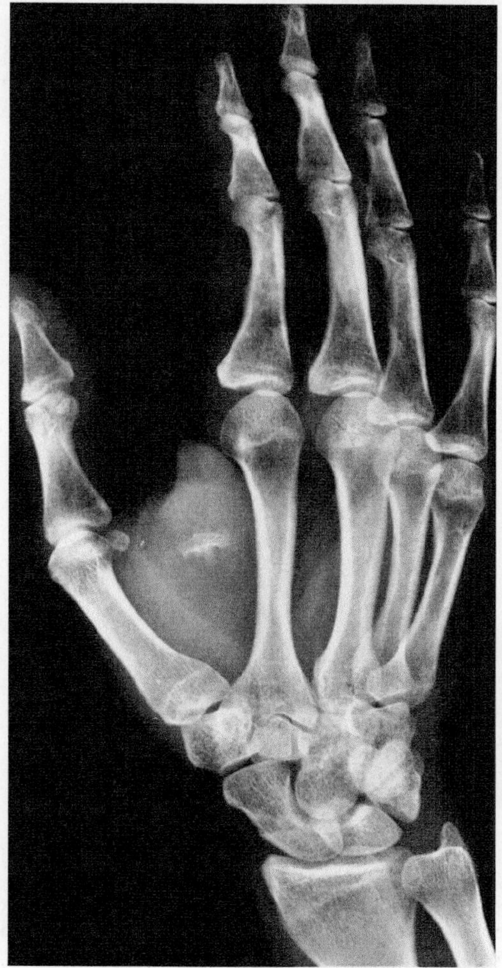

FIGURE 16.72 Soft-tissue lipoma. Oblique radiograph of the hand of a 27-year-old woman with a soft-tissue mass in the dorsal aspect shows a radiolucent lesion in the soft tissues adjacent to the radial aspect of the second metacarpal bone. Within the radiolucent area, there is evidence of bone formation.

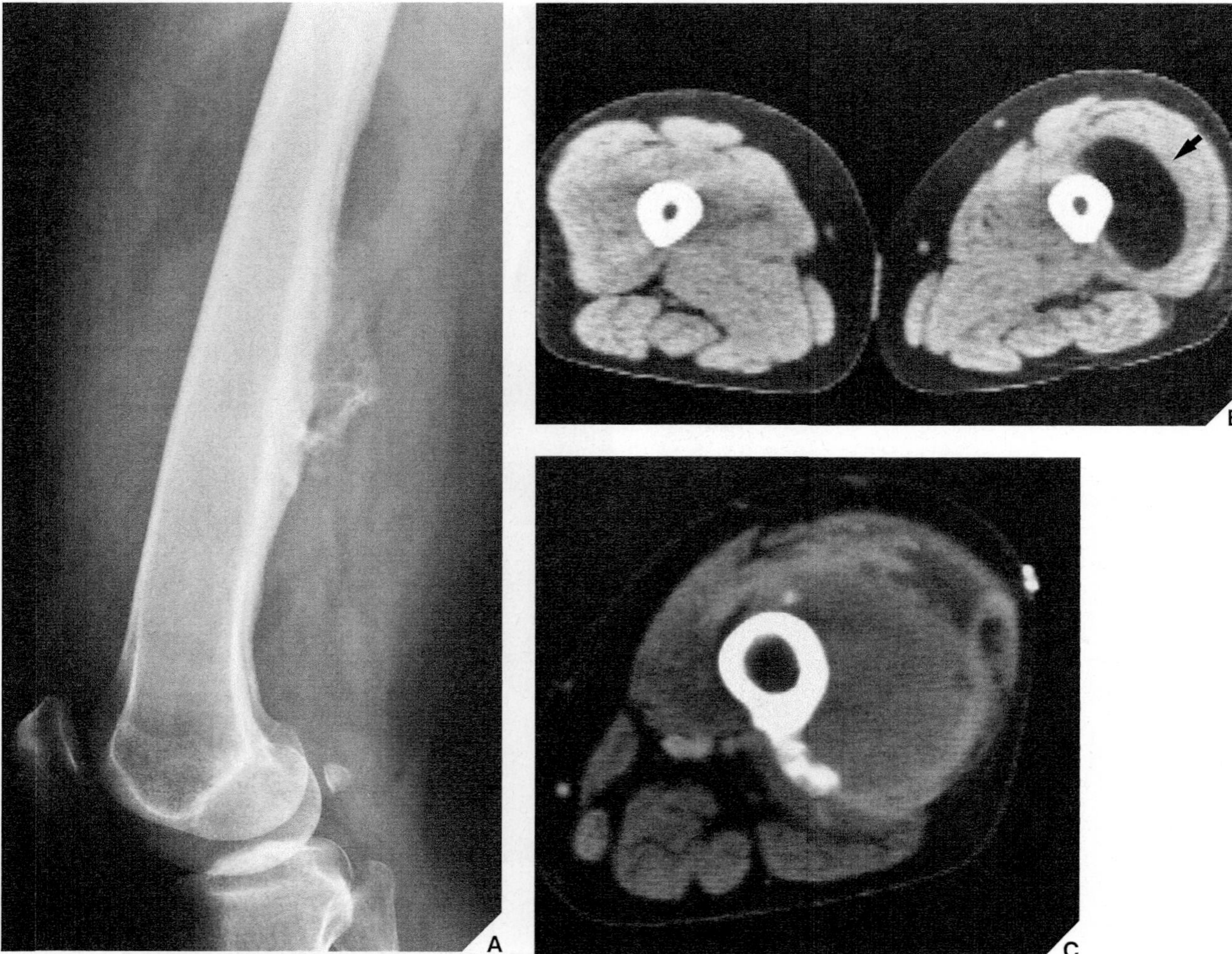

FIGURE 16.73 **Soft-tissue parosteal liposarcoma.** **(A)** Lateral radiograph in a 54-year-old man with a slowly enlarging mass on the posterior aspect of the thigh demonstrates a poorly defined soft-tissue mass with radiolucent areas and bone formation at the site of the posterior cortex of the femur. **(B)** CT section at the level of the radiolucency confirms the presence of fatty tissue *(arrow)*. **(C)** A CT section through the bone formation discloses a denser mass infiltrating surrounding muscular structures.

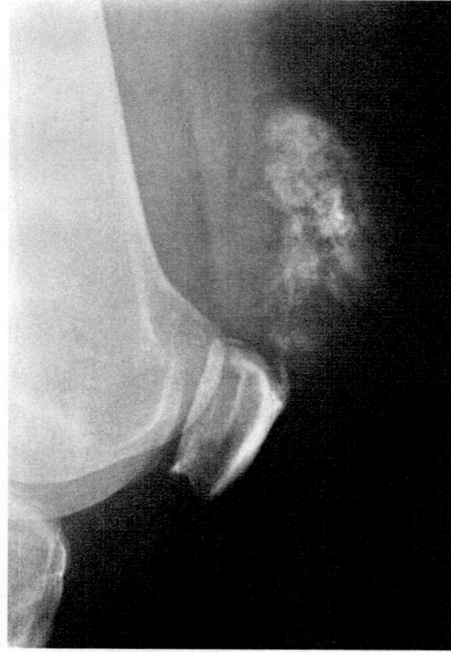

FIGURE 16.74 **Soft-tissue osteosarcoma.** A 51-year-old woman presented with a large suprapatellar soft-tissue mass. Lateral radiograph of the knee demonstrates a mass with ill-defined heterogeneous bone formation in the central part of the lesion. (Reprinted by permission from Springer: Greenspan A, Steiner G, Norman A, et al. Case report: osteosarcoma of the soft tissues of the distal end of the thigh. *Skeletal Radiol* 1987;16:489–492.)

continuation of the tumor with the nerve in a "tail-like" fashion (Fig. 16.84). Neurofibromas may demonstrate a "bull's-eye" pattern on MRI, with central areas of low signal intensity (Fig. 16.85). Most nerve-origin tumors also will demonstrate strong enhancement following intravenous gadolinium injection. Fibrous tumors often show poorly defined areas of low signal intensity (Fig. 16.86). Elastofibroma dorsi, another fibrous benign tumor, typically is found between the scapula and the chest wall (Fig. 16.87). Some tumors may demonstrate high signal intensity on T1- and T2-weighted pulse sequences. These include clear cell sarcoma, alveolar soft part sarcoma, and melanoma. Pigmented villonodular synovitis (PVNS) and giant cell tumors of the tendon sheaths show characteristic hypointense areas within the lesion due to deposits of hemosiderin (Fig. 16.88). However, most of the time, the MRI features of soft-tissue tumors are not characteristic, and only biopsy and histopathologic examination provides the final diagnosis (Fig. 16.89).

TABLE 16.13 Most Common Benign Soft-Tissue Masses That May Mimic Neoplasms

Abscess	Myositis ossificans
Amyloidoma	Nodular fasciitis
Calcific myonecrosis	Pigmented villonodular synovitis
Cyst	Pseudoaneurysm
Florid reactive periostitis	Reactive adenopathy
Foreign body granuloma	Rheumatoid nodule
Ganglion	Seroma
Gouty tophus	Synovial cyst
Hematoma	Tumoral calcinosis

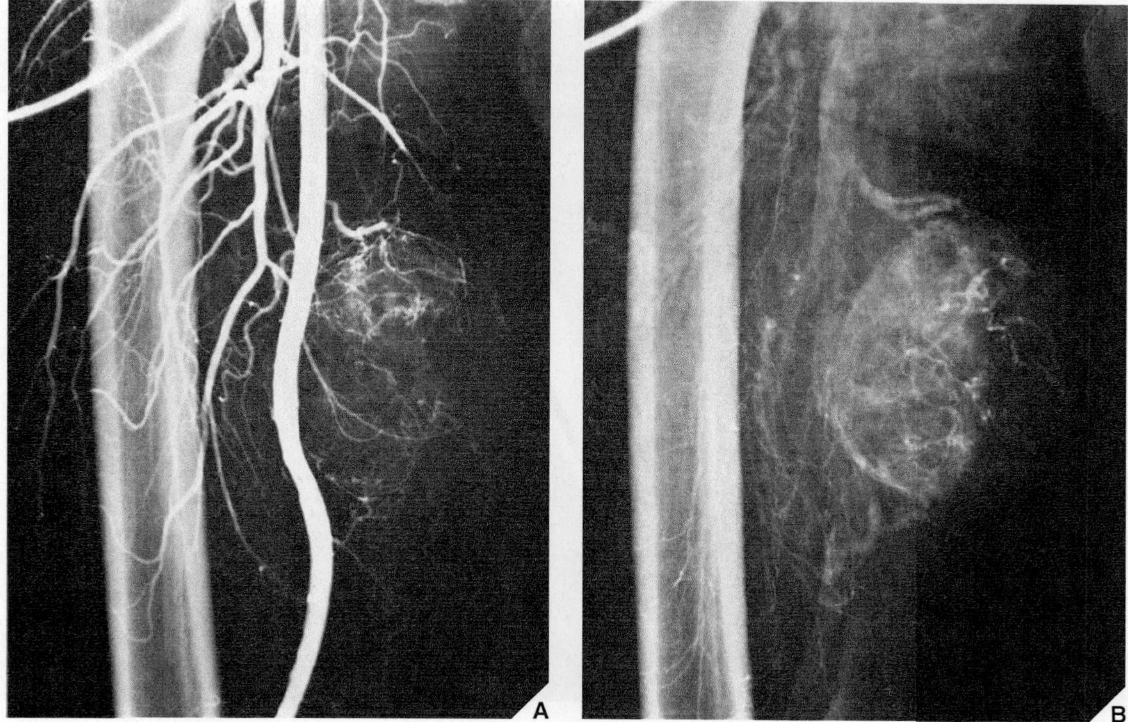

FIGURE 16.75 Soft-tissue malignant fibrous histiocytoma (MFH). Femoral arteriography was performed on a 56-year-old man with a tumor on the medial aspect of the right thigh, which proved to be an MFH of the soft tissues. **(A)** The arterial phase demonstrates the displacement of the superficial femoral artery by the tumor, the extent of the tumor and area of neovascularity, and the accumulation of contrast agent within the tumor. **(B)** The venous phase shows the accumulation of contrast in abnormal vessels and a tumor "stain" as well as the topography of venous structures.

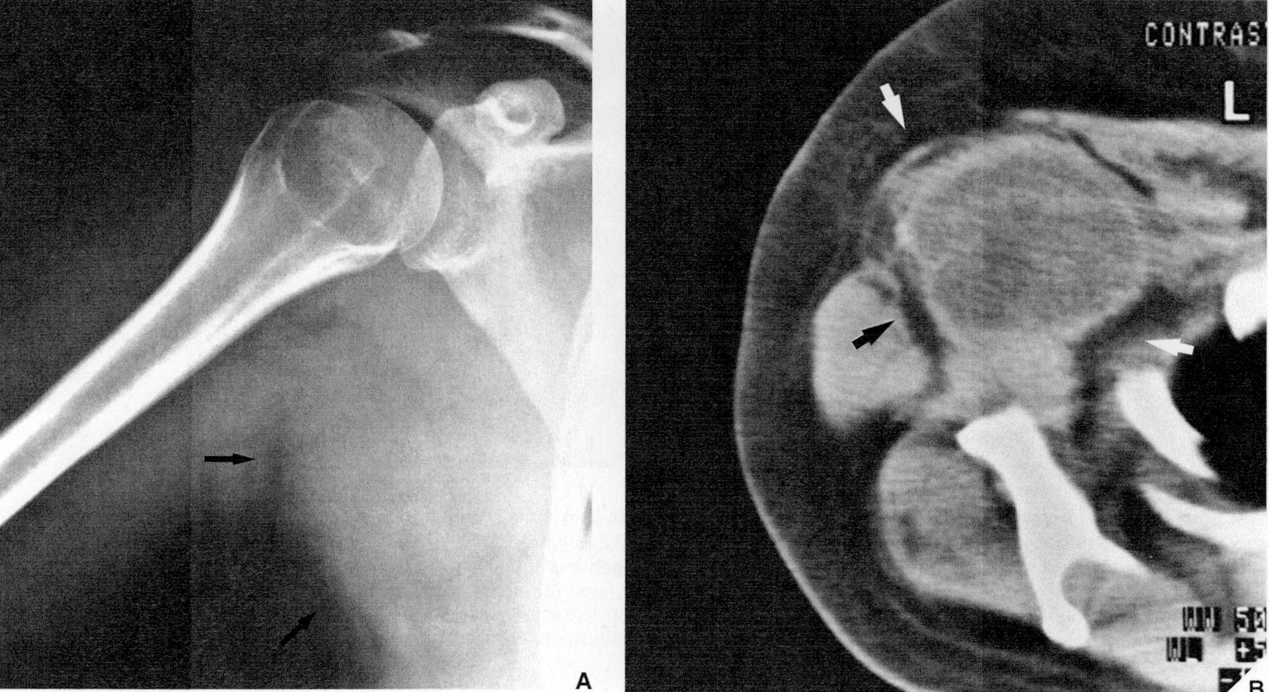

FIGURE 16.76 Soft-tissue fibrosarcoma. **(A)** Anteroposterior radiograph of the shoulder of a 40-year-old woman with a history of an enlarging mass in the right axilla shows an ill-defined mass *(arrows)* adjacent to the lateral border of the scapula. **(B)** CT section with contrast enhancement shows the extent of the mass *(arrows)* and the lack of bone involvement.

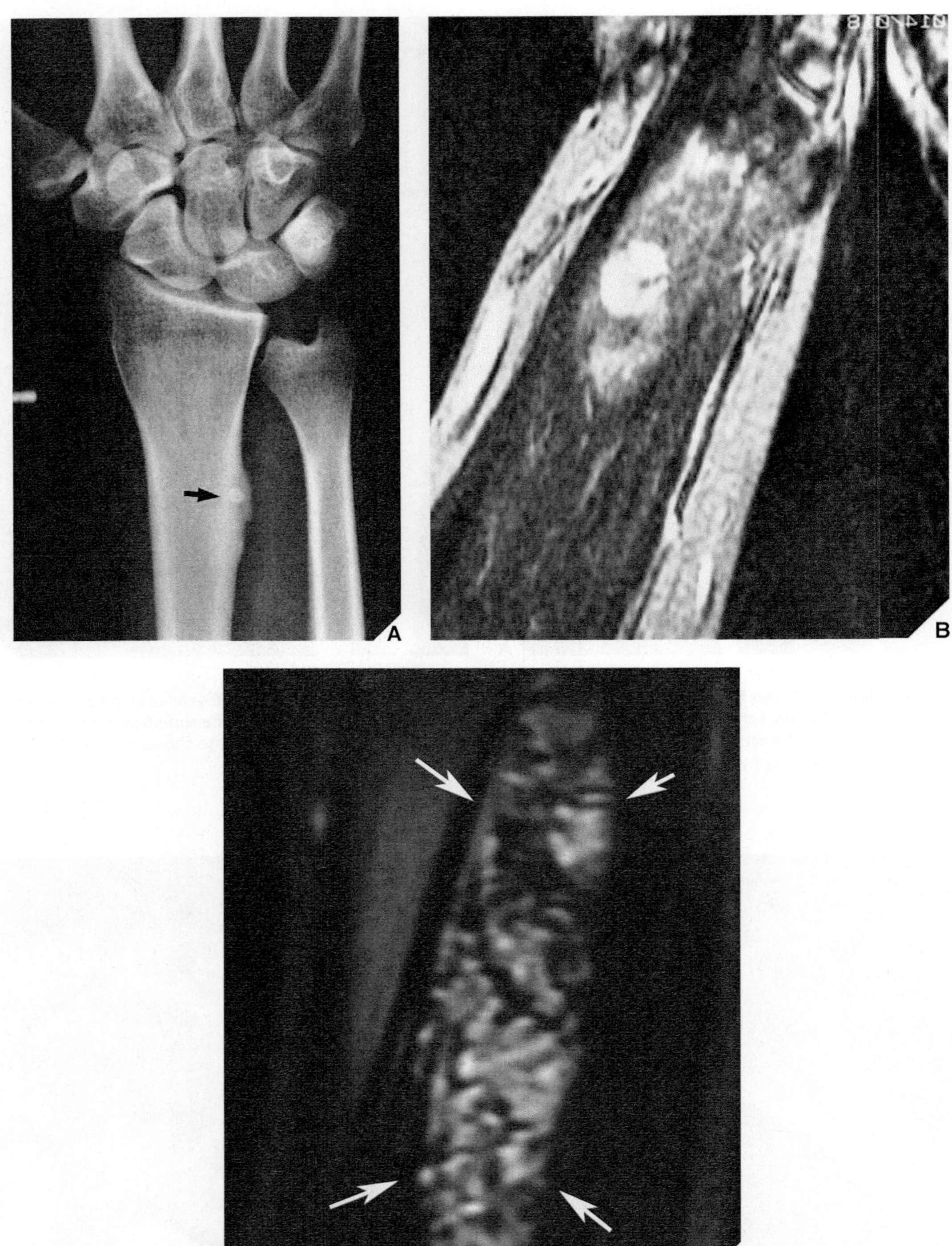

FIGURE 16.77 **Intramuscular hemangioma.** A 34-year-old woman presented with pain in the distal left forearm. **(A)** The radiograph demonstrates periosteal reaction at the ulnar border of the distal radius, associated with a phlebolith *(arrow)*. **(B)** Coronal T2-weighted MRI (SE; repetition time [TR] 2000/echo time [TE] 80 msec) shows a large mass situated in the pronator quadratus muscle of the distal forearm, displaying heterogeneous signal ranging from intermediate to high intensity. **(C)** Coronal T2-weighted MRI of the calf in another patient with an intramuscular capillary hemangioma *(arrows)* shows the striated pattern of the lesion. (**A,B**, Reprinted by permission from Springer: Greenspan A, McGahan JP, Vogelsang P, et al. Imaging strategies in the evaluation of soft-tissue hemangiomas of the extremities: correlation of the findings of plain radiography, angiography, CT, MRI, and ultrasonography in 12 histologically proven cases. *Skeletal Radiol* 1992;21:11–18.)

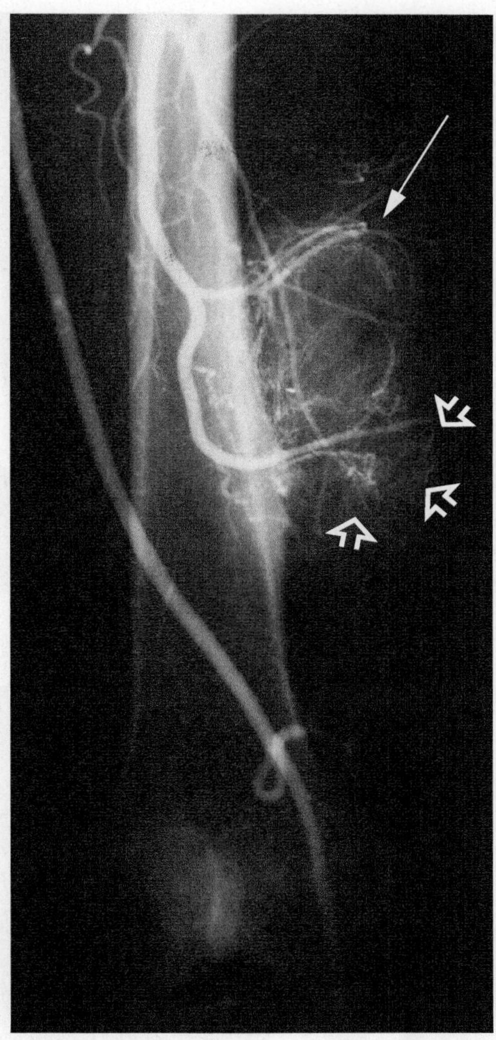

FIGURE 16.78 **Parosteal liposarcoma.** Vascular study of the patient shown in Figure 16.73 demonstrates that the lesion consists of two parts: The proximal part is more radiolucent and hypovascular *(arrow)*, whereas the distal part is denser and more hypervascular *(open arrows)*. The biopsy specimen on which the diagnosis of liposarcoma was made was obtained from the more vascular segment of the tumor. After radical resection and examination of the entire specimen, the more radiolucent hypovascular area revealed almost no malignant component. Had the biopsy been obtained only from that part of the tumor, the result probably would not have been consistent with the final diagnosis.

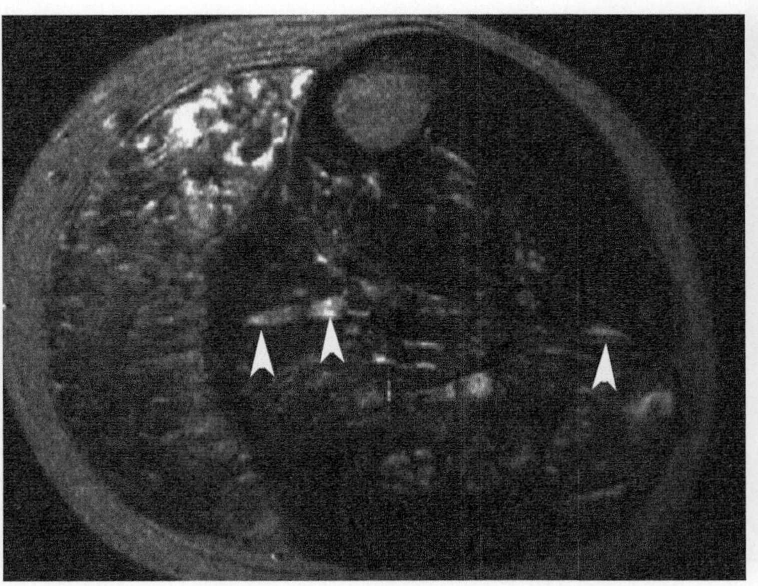

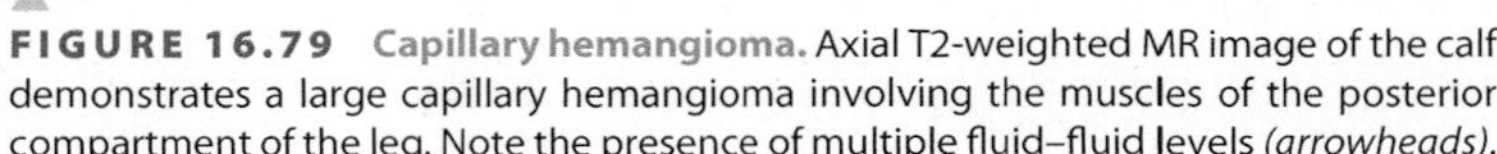

FIGURE 16.79 **Capillary hemangioma.** Axial T2-weighted MR image of the calf demonstrates a large capillary hemangioma involving the muscles of the posterior compartment of the leg. Note the presence of multiple fluid–fluid levels *(arrowheads)*.

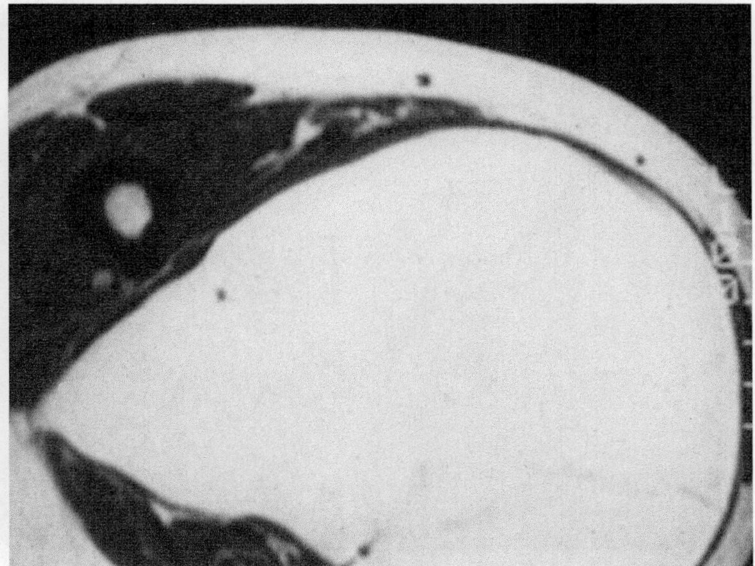

FIGURE 16.80 **Benign lipomatous tumor.** Axial T1-weighted MRI of the thigh demonstrates a large lipoma of the posterior compartment. Note the thin capsule and the absence of septae within the tumor.

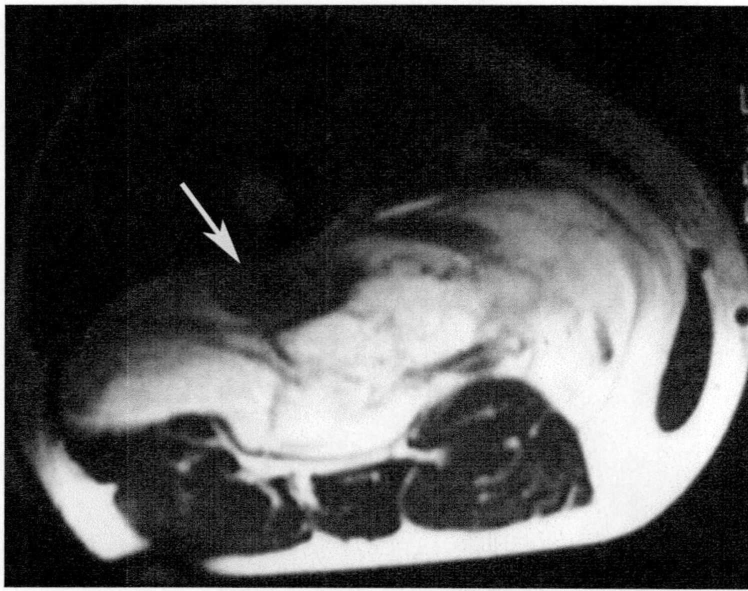

FIGURE 16.81 Atypical lipoma (low-grade liposarcoma). Axial T1-weighted MRI of the thigh demonstrates a lipomatous tumor of the posterior compartment. Note the presence of a solid nonfatty component within the tumor *(arrow)*.

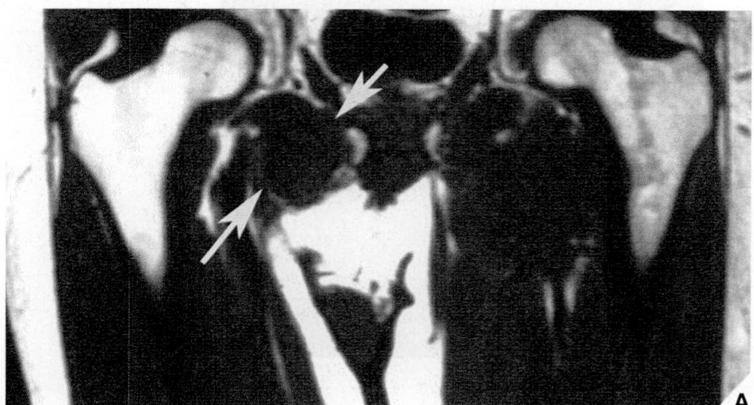

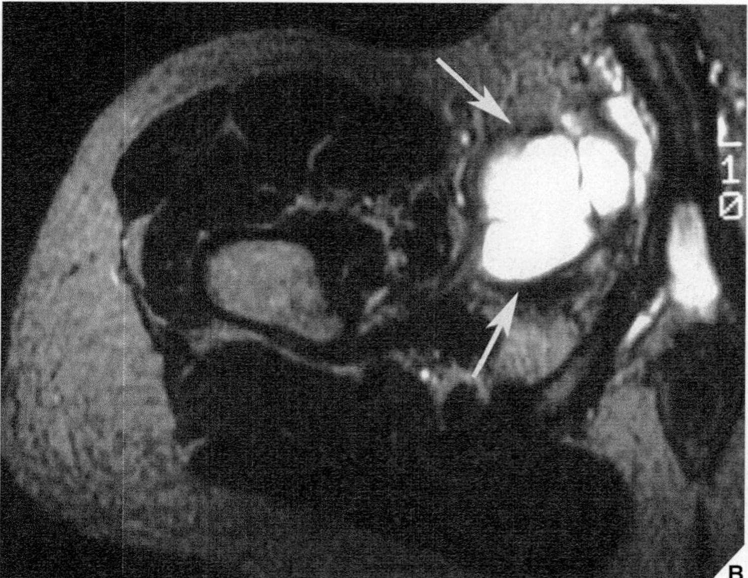

FIGURE 16.82 Myxoid liposarcoma. (A) Coronal T1-weighted MRI demonstrates a hypointense, fluid-like lesion in the right inguinal area *(arrows)*. **(B)** Axial T2-weighted MRI demonstrates a uniform hyperintense character of the lesion *(arrows)*. These findings could be easily misinterpreted as a fluid collection.

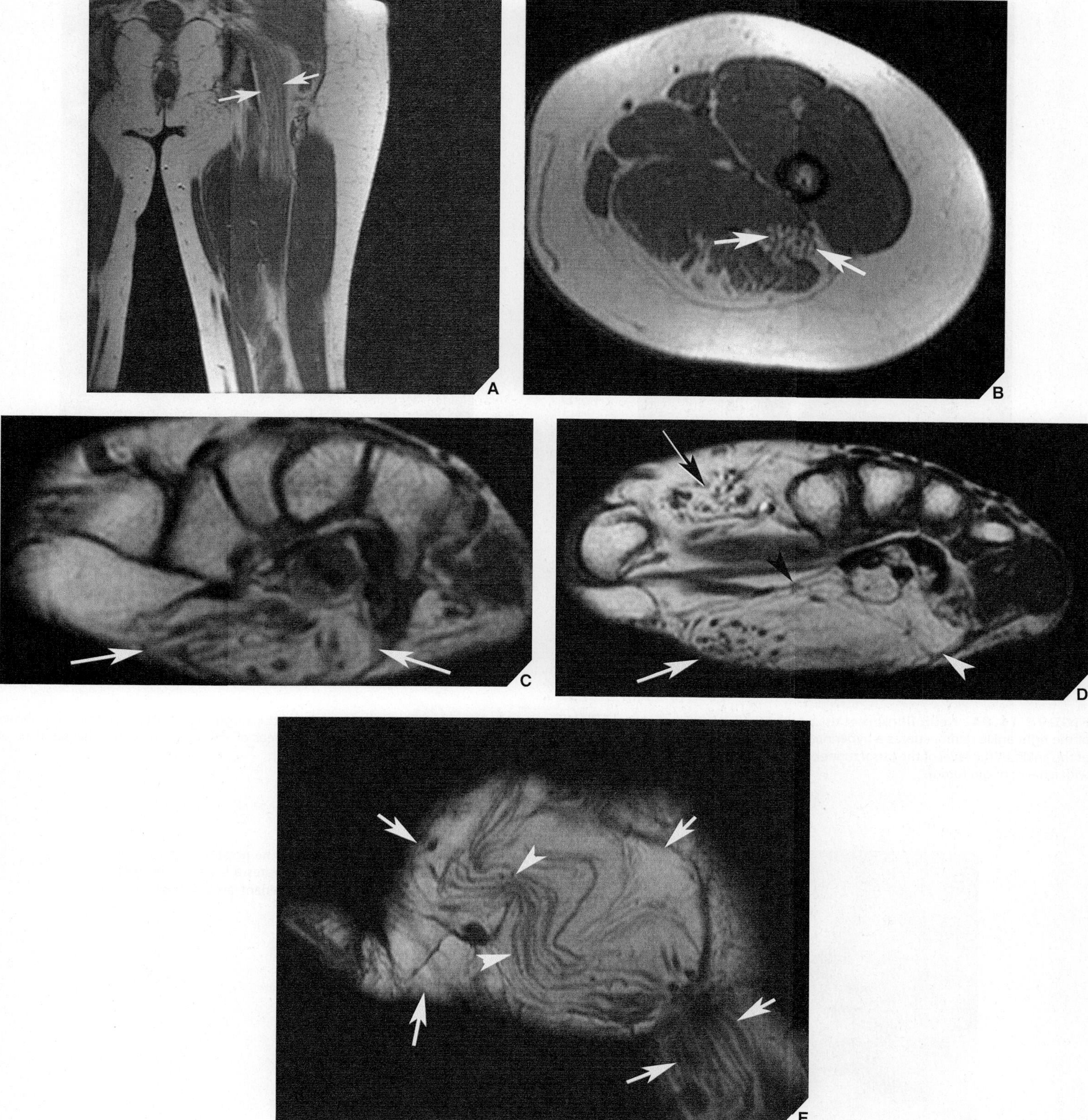

FIGURE 16.83 Fibrolipomatous hamartoma. **(A)** Coronal T1-weighted MRI demonstrates "spaghetti-like" appearance of the sciatic nerve *(arrows)*. **(B)** Axial T1-weighted MRI demonstrates a "coaxial cable" appearance of the sciatic nerve *(arrows)*. **(C)** Axial T1-weighted MRI of the wrist in another patient demonstrates a large fibrolipomatous tumor of the median nerve within the carpal tunnel *(arrows)*. **(D)** Axial T1-weighted MRI of the hand in the same patient demonstrates the extension of the fibrolipomatous hamartoma to the palm of the hand *(arrowheads)* and the first and second digits. Note the "coaxial cable" appearance of the nerve fibers *(arrows)*. **(E)** Coronal T1-weighted MRI of the same patient demonstrates the extension of the tumor from the region of the carpal tunnel to the hand *(arrows)*. Note the spaghetti-like configuration of the fibers of the median nerve and its digital branches *(arrowheads)*.

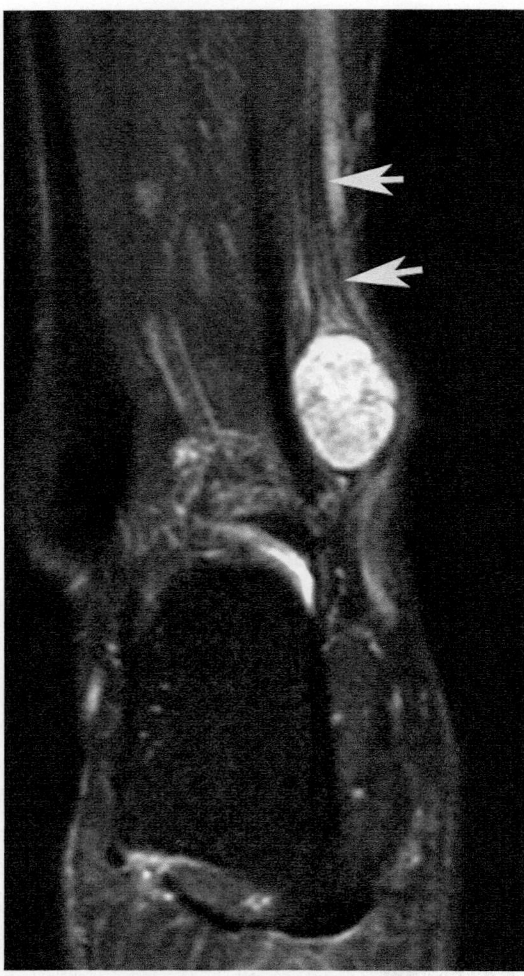

FIGURE 16.84 Neurofibroma of the posterior tibial nerve. Coronal STIR MRI of the right ankle demonstrates a hyperintense mass in the posterior medial aspect of the ankle, at the level of the tarsal tunnel, with a superior "tail" *(arrows)*, consistent with a nerve origin tumor.

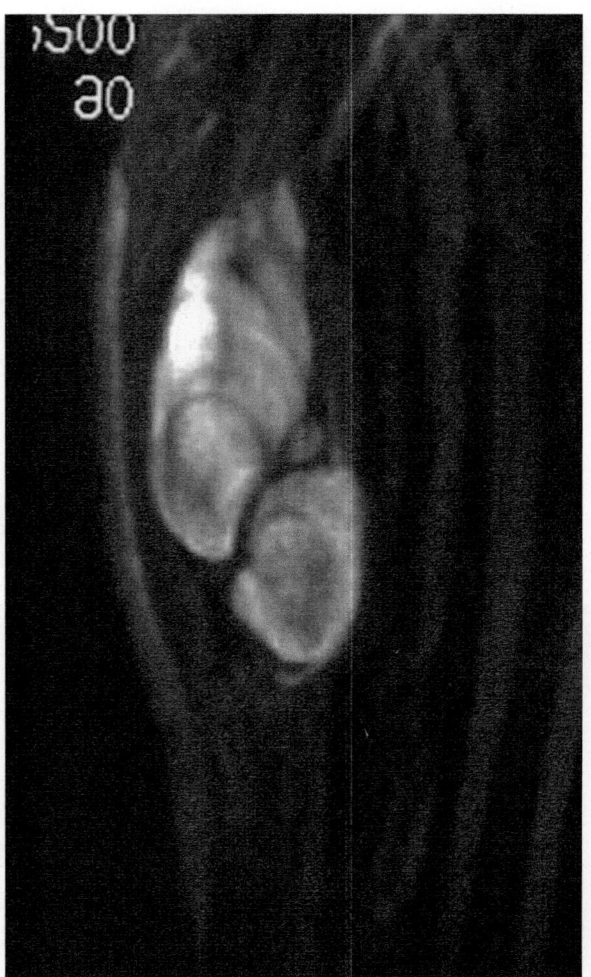

FIGURE 16.85 Neurofibroma of the thigh. Sagittal T2-weighted MRI shows a large mass in the thigh with central areas of low signal intensity, characteristic of neurofibroma.

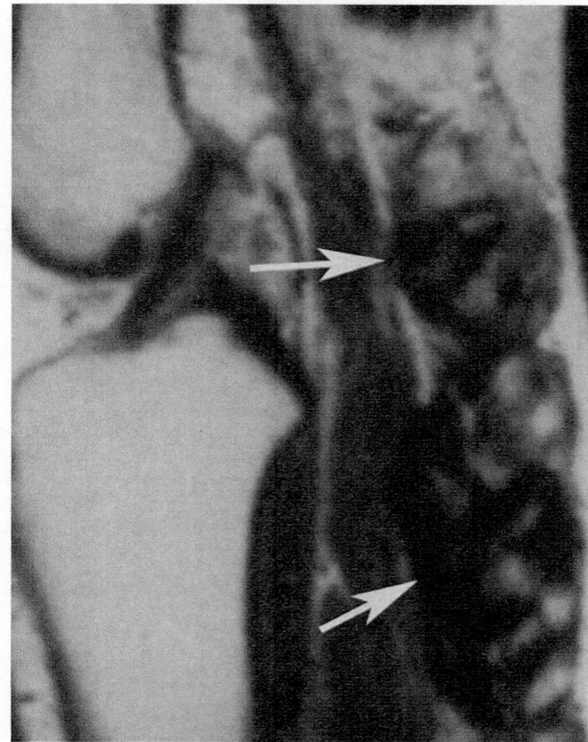

FIGURE 16.86 Fibromatosis in the popliteal space. Sagittal T1-weighted MR image demonstrates a large tumor in the popliteal space *(arrows)* with predominant areas of low signal intensity.

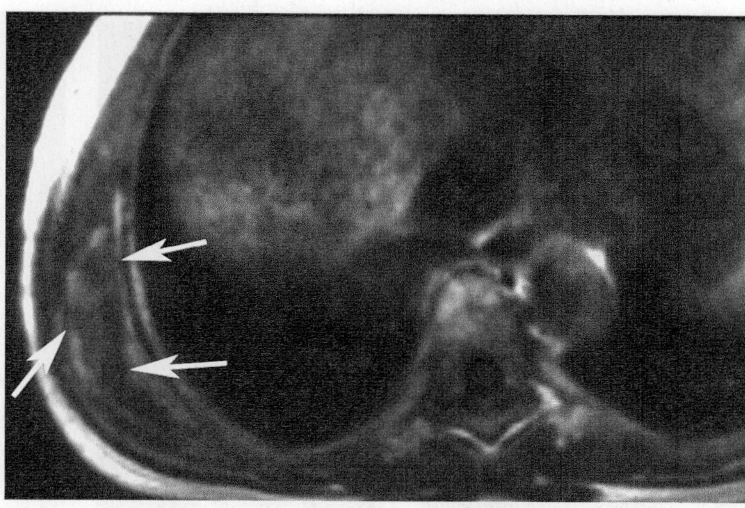

FIGURE 16.87 **Elastofibroma dorsi.** Axial T1-weighted MR image of the right chest wall demonstrates a hypointense tumor between the scapula and the thoracic wall *(arrows)*.

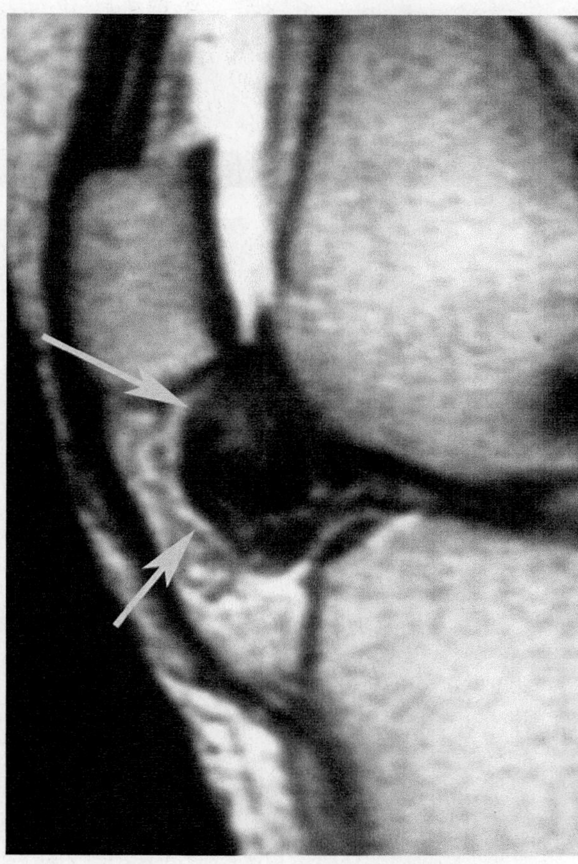

FIGURE 16.88 **Pigmented villonodular synovitis.** Sagittal T2-weighted MRI of the knee demonstrates a hypointense mass in the anterior aspect of the knee *(arrows)*, consistent with hemosiderin deposition in a focal nodule of PVNS (see Fig. 23.12).

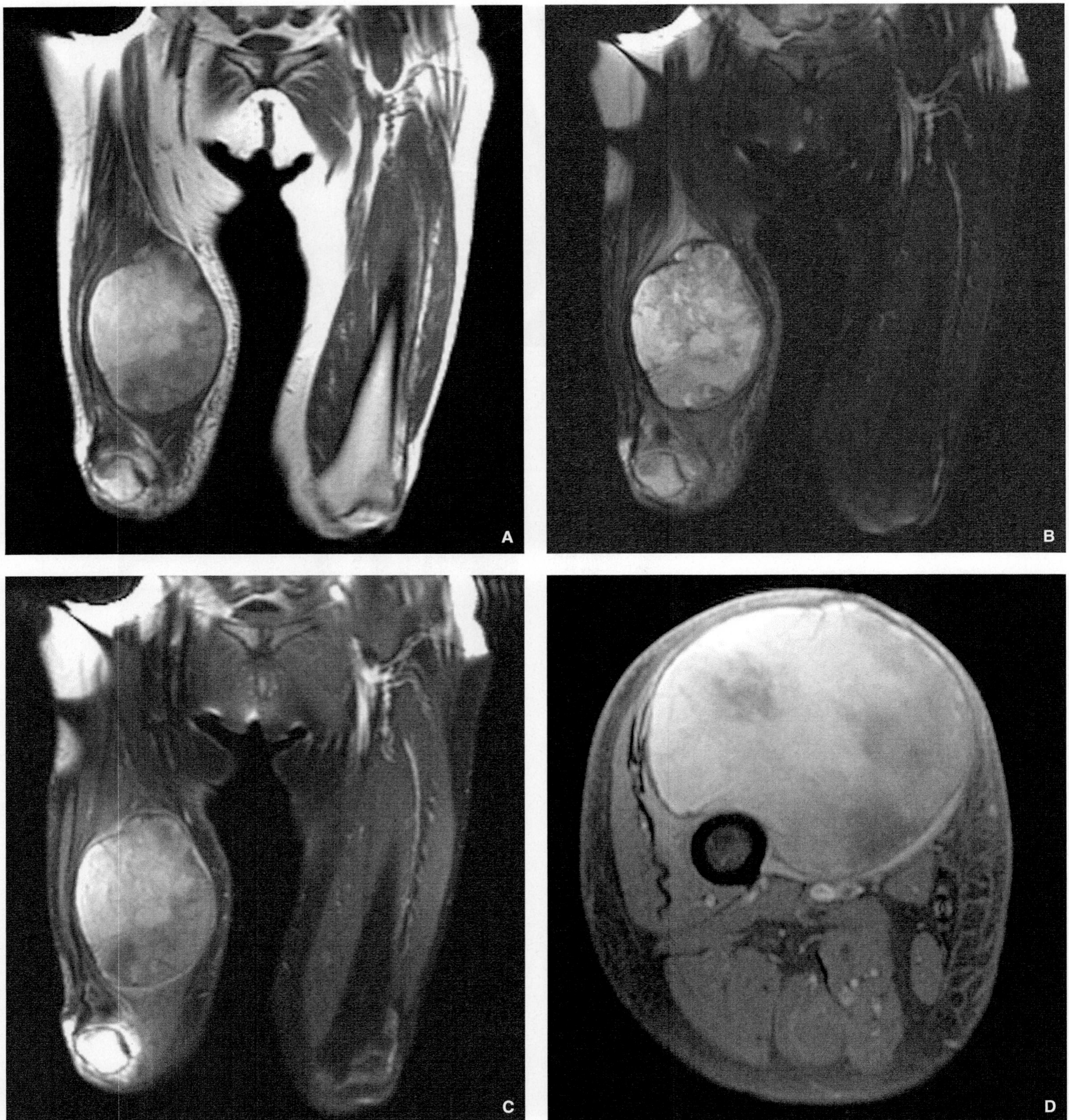

FIGURE 16.89 **MRI of pleomorphic undifferentiated soft-tissue sarcoma.** A 70-year-old woman presented with a large soft-tissue mass in her right thigh. **(A)** Coronal T1-weighted and **(B)** coronal T2-weighted fat-suppressed MR images show a well-circumscribed mass in the anterior compartment displaying heterogenous signal. **(C)** Coronal and **(D)** axial T1-weighted fat-suppressed MR images obtained after intravenous administration of gadolinium show moderate enhancement of the tumor. The diagnosis was established after excision biopsy and histopathologic examination.

PRACTICAL POINTS TO REMEMBER

1. The most helpful clinical data concerning patients presenting with suspected bone or soft-tissue lesions are:
   - the age of the patient
   - the duration of the symptoms
   - the growth rate of the tumor.
2. In the evaluation of tumors or tumor-like bone lesions, several key radiographic features should be sought, including:
   - the site of the lesion (the particular bone and site in the bone affected)
   - the nature of the border of the lesion (narrow or wide zone of transition)
   - the type of matrix (calcified, ossified, or hollow)
   - the type of bone destruction (geographic, moth-eaten, or permeative)
   - the periosteal reaction (solid or interrupted—sunburst, velvet, lamellated, Codman triangle)
   - the presence or absence of soft-tissue extension.
3. A lytic (radiolucent) lesion located in the epiphysis and showing a narrow zone of transition is most likely a chondroblastoma.
4. A lytic lesion lacking a sclerotic border and extending into the articular end of a bone after closure of the growth plate is most likely a giant cell tumor. The absence of extension into the articular end of the bone virtually excludes giant cell tumor.
5. A centrally located lesion having a sclerotic border and abutting the growth plate in the proximal humerus or proximal femur is most likely a simple bone cyst.
6. A radiolucent lesion located in the lateral aspect of the calcaneus is most likely a simple bone cyst.
7. An eccentrically located lesion ballooning out from the cortex and seen in a patient younger than 20 years of age is most likely an aneurysmal bone cyst or a chondromyxoid fibroma. If the patient is 30 or older, these possibilities are remote.
8. A radiolucent lesion in a short tubular bone is most likely an enchondroma.
9. A lesion with a sclerotic margin located in the anterior aspect of the tibia in a child is most likely an osteofibrous dysplasia (Kempson-Campanacci lesion). A similar lesion or multiple osteolytic lesions in the tibia in adults most likely represent adamantinoma.
10. A lesion in the medial aspect of distal femur lying close to the linea aspera and showing cortical irregularity is most likely a periosteal desmoid.
11. An intramedullary lesion in the posterior aspect of the distal femur having a scalloped, sclerotic margin is most likely a nonossifying fibroma.
12. A sclerotic, lobulated lesion on the surface of the posterior aspect of distal femur should be considered to represent a parosteal osteosarcoma.
13. An ill-defined lesion displaying calcifications and located on the anterior aspect of the tibia should raise the possibility of periosteal osteosarcoma.
14. A lesion in a vertebral body is most often a metastasis, myeloma, lymphoma, hemangioma, or Langerhans cell histiocytosis.
15. A lesion in the posterior vertebral arch is most likely an aneurysmal bone cyst, osteoblastoma, or osteoid osteoma.
16. A lesion most likely represents a benign tumor when it exhibits:
   - geographic bone destruction
   - a sclerotic margin
   - solid, uninterrupted periosteal reaction, or no periosteal response
   - no soft-tissue mass.
17. A lesion most likely represents a malignant tumor when it shows:
   - poorly defined margins (a wide zone of transition)
   - a moth-eaten or permeative type of bone destruction
   - an interrupted periosteal reaction
   - a soft-tissue mass.
18. A lesion most likely represents a cartilage tumor (e.g., enchondroma or chondrosarcoma) when it exhibits:
   - lobulation (endosteal scalloping)
   - punctate, annular, or comma-like calcifications in the matrix.
19. An eccentric lesion displaying a solid buttress of periosteal reaction is most likely an aneurysmal bone cyst, chondromyxoid fibroma, or juxtacortical chondroma.
20. A lesion exhibiting a moth-eaten or permeative type of bone destruction and associated with a large soft-tissue mass without ossifications or calcifications is most likely an Ewing sarcoma. If the patient is younger than age 5 years or is black, Ewing sarcoma is unlikely.
21. When a soft-tissue mass and a destructive bone lesion coexist, certain radiographic features of the lesion may help differentiate a primary soft-tissue tumor invading bone from a primary bone tumor invading soft tissue:
   - the epicenter of the lesion: if outside the bone, then it is probable that it is primary soft tissue; if within it, then it is probable that it is primary bone
   - the bevel of cortical destruction: if directed toward the bone, then it is probable that it is primary soft tissue; if toward the soft tissue, then it is probable that it is primary bone
   - the absence of periosteal reaction: probable primary soft tissue
   - a large soft-tissue mass and a small bone lesion: probable primary soft tissue (with the exception of Ewing sarcoma).
22. Benign lesions such as fibrous dysplasia, nonossifying fibroma, Langerhans cell histiocytosis, hemangioma, cartilaginous exostoses, and enchondroma tend to be multiple. Multiple malignant lesions, on the other hand, should raise the possibility of metastatic disease, multiple myeloma, and lymphoma.
23. In the evaluation of soft-tissue lesions, some imaging findings can help suggest a diagnosis. Among these are:
   - phleboliths (hemangioma)
   - radiolucent areas within the mass (lipoma)
   - dense areas dispersed with radiolucencies and ossifications (liposarcoma)
   - ill-defined ossifications within the dense mass (osteosarcoma)
   - mass near the joint with calcifications (synovial sarcoma)
   - popcorn-like calcifications within the mass (chondroma or chondrosarcoma).
24. MRI features suggesting a benign soft-tissue mass include sharp margination and homogeneity of the lesion, whereas prominent peritumoral edema and necrosis suggest malignant nature.
25. Some soft-tissue lesions exhibit specific MRI characteristics that allow a preoperative diagnosis:
   - prominent vascular spaces with fluid–fluid levels (cavernous hemangioma)
   - thick intratumoral septae within fatty component of tumor (low-grade liposarcoma)
   - minimal fat with predominant nonlipomatous component of tumor (high-grade liposarcoma)
   - fluid-like signal intensity on the nonenhanced images and prominent enhancement after gadolinium injection (myxoid liposarcoma)
   - tail-like extension from the tumor (tumors of neural origin)
   - high signal intensity on both T1- and T2-weighted pulse sequences (clear cell sarcoma, alveolar soft part sarcoma, melanoma).
26. DWI and DTI are imaging techniques used not only in general oncology but also in musculoskeletal system, for instance, to differentiate acute osteoporotic fractures of the spine from malignant compression fractures.
27. Whole-body MRI is effective in imaging multiple myeloma, lymphoma, lung cancer, and ovarian cancer.

SUGGESTED READINGS

Aoki J, Wanatabe H, Shinozaki T, et al. FDG PET of primary benign and malignant bone tumors: standardized uptake value in 52 lesions. *Radiology* 2001;219:774–777.

Baliyan V, Das CJ, Sharma R, et al. Diffusion weighted imaging: technique and applications. *World J Radiol* 2016;8:785–798.

Barnes G Jr, Gwinn J. Distal irregularities of the femur simulating malignancy. *Am J Roentgenol Radium Ther Nucl Med* 1974;122:180–185.

Berquist TH. Magnetic resonance imaging of primary skeletal neoplasms. *Radiol Clin North Am* 1993;31:411–424.

Bisseret D, Kaci R, Lafage-Proust M-H, et al. Periosteum: characteristic imaging findings with emphasis on radiologic-pathologic comparisons. *Skeletal Radiol* 2015;44:321–338.

Bloem JL. *Radiological staging of primary malignant musculoskeletal tumors. A correlative study of CT, MRI, ^{99m}Tc scintigraphy and angiography*. The Hague, Netherlands: A. Jongbloed; 1988.

Bloem JL, Reiser MF, Vanel D. Magnetic resonance contrast agents in the evaluation of the musculoskeletal system. *Magn Res Q* 1990;6:136–163.

Bodner G, Schocke MFH, Rachbauer F, et al. Differentiation of malignant and benign musculoskeletal tumors: combined color and power Doppler US and spectral wave analysis. *Radiology* 2002;223:410–416.

Calleja M, Dimigen M, Saifuddin A. MRI of superficial soft tissue masses: analysis of features useful in distinguishing between benign and malignant lesions. *Skeletal Radiol* 2012;41:1517–1524.

Conrad EU III, Enneking WF. Common soft tissue tumors. *Clin Symp* 1990;42:2–32.

Crim JR, Seeger LL, Yao L, et al. Diagnosis of soft-tissue masses with MR imaging: can benign masses be differentiated from malignant ones? *Radiology* 1992;185:581–586.

Dahlin DC, Unni KK. *Bone tumors: general aspects and data on 8,542 cases*, 4th ed. Springfield, MO: Charles C. Thomas Publishers; 1986.

Dinauer PA, Brixey CJ, Moncur JT, et al. Pathologic and MR imaging features of benign fibrous soft-tissue tumors in adults. *Radiographics* 2007;27:173–187.

Dorfman HD, Czerniak B. *Bone tumors*. St. Louis: Mosby; 1998:1–33.

Edeiken J, Hodes PJ, Caplan LH. New bone production and periosteal reaction. *Am J Roentgenol Radium Ther Nucl Med* 1966;97:708–718.

Elias DA, White LM, Simpson DJ, et al. Osseous invasion by soft-tissue sarcoma: assessment with MR imaging. *Radiology* 2003;229:145–152.

Enneking WF. Staging of musculoskeletal neoplasms. *Skeletal Radiol* 1985;13:183–194.

Enzinger FM, Weiss SW. *Soft tissue tumors*, 3rd ed. St. Louis: Mosby; 1995:3–56.

Erlemann R, Sciuk J, Bosse A, et al. Response of osteosarcoma and Ewing sarcoma to preoperative chemotherapy: assessment with dynamic and static MR imaging and skeletal scintigraphy. *Radiology* 1990;175:791–796.

Ewing J. A review and classification of bone sarcomas. *Arch Surg* 1922;4:485–533.

Fayad LM, Bluemke DA, Weber KL, et al. Characterization of pediatric skeletal tumors and tumor-like conditions: specific cross-sectional imaging signs. *Skeletal Radiol* 2006;35:259–268.

Fechner RE, Mills SE. *Tumors of the bones and joints*. Washington, DC: Armed Forces Institute of Pathology; 1993:1–16.

Fletcher CDM, Bridge JA, Hogendoorn P, et al. *WHO classification of tumors of soft tissue and bone*, vol. 5, 4th ed. Lyon, France; 2013.

Fletcher CDM, Unni KK, Mertens F, eds. *Pathology & genetics: tumors of soft tissue and bones*, vol. 5, 3rd ed. Lyon, France: IARC Press; 2013.

Frank JA, Ling A, Patronas NJ, et al. Detection of malignant bone tumors: MR imaging vs scintigraphy. *AJR Am J Roentgenol* 1990;155:1043–1048.

Gartner L, Pearce CJ, Saifuddin A. The role of the plain radiograph in the characterisation of soft tissue tumours. *Skeletal Radiol* 2009;38:549–558.

Gaskin CM, Helms CA. Lipomas, lipoma variants, and well-differentiated liposarcomas (atypical lipomas): results of MRI evaluations of 126 consecutive fatty masses. *AJR Am J Roentgenol* 2004;182:733–739.

Greenspan A. Bone island (enostosis): current concept—a review. *Skeletal Radiol* 1995; 24:111–115.

Greenspan A. Pragmatic approach to bone tumors. *Semin Orthop* 1991;6:125–133.

Greenspan A, Borys D. *Radiology and pathology correlation of bone tumors: a quick reference and review*. Philadelphia: Wolters Kluwer; 2016:1–31.

Greenspan A, Jundt G, Remagen W. *Differential diagnosis in orthopaedic oncology*, 2nd ed. Philadelphia: Lippincott Williams & Wilkins; 2007:1–35.

Greenspan A, Klein MJ. Radiology and pathology of bone tumors. In: Lewis MM, ed. *Musculoskeletal oncology: a multidisciplinary approach*. Philadelphia: WB Saunders; 1992:13–72.

Greenspan A, McGahan JP, Vogelsang P, et al. Imaging strategies in the evaluation of soft-tissue hemangiomas of the extremities: correlation of the findings of plain radiography, angiography, CT, MRI, and ultrasonography in 12 histologically proven cases. *Skeletal Radiol* 1992;21:11–18.

Greenspan A, Stadalnik RC. Bone island: scintigraphic findings and their clinical application. *Can Assoc Radiol J* 1995;46:368–379.

Greenspan A, Stadalnik RC. Central versus eccentric lesions of long tubular bones. *Semin Nucl Med* 1996;26:201–206.

Greenspan A, Steiner G, Norman A, et al. Case report 436: osteosarcoma of the soft tissues of the distal end of the thigh. *Skeletal Radiol* 1987;16:489–492.

Griffin N, Khan N, Thomas JM, et al. The radiological manifestations of intramuscular haemangiomas in adults: magnetic resonance imaging, computed tomography and ultrasound appearances. *Skeletal Radiol* 2007;36:1051–1059.

Hamada K, Ueda T, Tomita Y, et al. False positive 18F-FDG PET in an ischial chondroblastoma; an analysis of glucose transporter 1 and hexokinase II expression. *Skeletal Radiol* 2006;35:306–310.

Hanna SL, Fletcher BD, Parham DM, et al. Muscle edema in musculoskeletal tumors: MR imaging characteristics and clinical significance. *J Magn Reson Imaging* 1991;1:441–449.

Hayes CW, Conway WF, Sundaram M. Misleading aggressive MR imaging appearance of some benign musculoskeletal lesions. *Radiographics* 1992;12:1119–1134.

Helms CA. Skeletal "don't touch" lesions. In: Brant WE, Helms CA, eds. *Fundamentals of diagnostic radiology*. Baltimore: Williams & Wilkins; 1994:963–975.

Hermann G, Abdelwahab IF, Miller TT, et al. Tumor and tumor-like conditions of the soft tissue: magnetic resonance imaging features differentiating benign from malignant masses. *Br J Radiol* 1992;65:14–20.

Hong S-P, Lee SE, Choi Y-L, et al. Prognostic value of 18F-FDG PET/CT in patients with soft tissue sarcoma: comparisons between metabolic parameters. *Skeletal Radiol* 2014;43:641–648.

Hudson TM. *Radiologic-pathologic correlation of musculoskeletal lesions*. Baltimore: Williams & Wilkins; 1987.

Huvos AG. *Bone tumors: diagnosis, treatment and prognosis*. Philadelphia: WB Sanders; 1979.

Jaffe HL. *Tumors and tumorous conditions of the bones and joints*. Philadelphia: Lea & Febiger; 1968.

Jelinek JS, Murphey MD, Welker JA, et al. Diagnosis of primary bone tumors with image-guided percutaneous biopsy: experience with 110 tumors. *Radiology* 2002;223:731–737.

Khashper A, Zheng J, Nahal A, et al. Imaging characteristics of spindle cell lipoma and its variants. *Skeletal Radiol* 2014;43:591–597.

Kirwadi A, Abdul-Halim R, Fernando M, et al. MR imaging features of spindle cell lipoma. *Skeletal Radiol* 2014;43:191–196.

Kransdorf MJ. Magnetic resonance imaging of musculoskeletal tumors. *Orthopedics* 1994;17:1003–1016.

Kransdorf MJ. Malignant soft-tissue tumors in a large referral population: distribution of diagnoses by age, sex, and location. *AJR Am J Roentgenol* 1995;164:129–134.

Kransdorf MJ, Bancroft LW, Peterson JJ, et al. Imaging of fatty tumors: distinction of lipoma and well-differentiated liposarcoma. *Radiology* 2002;224:99–104.

Kransdorf MJ, Murphey MD, Sweet DE. Liposclerosing myxofibrous tumor: a radiologic-pathologic-distinct fibro-osseous lesion of bone with a marked predilection for the intertrochanteric region of the femur. *Radiology* 1999;212:693–698.

Lalam R, Bloem JL, Noebauer-Huhmann IM, et al. ESSR consensus document for detection, characterization, and referral pathway for tumors and tumorlike lesions of bone. *Semin Musculoskelet Radiol* 2017;21:630–647.

Lang P, Honda G, Roberts T, et al. Musculoskeletal neoplasm: perineoplastic edema versus tumor on dynamic postcontrast MR images with spatial mapping of instantaneous enhancement rates. *Radiology* 1995;197:831–839.

Lewis MM. The use of an expandable and adjustable prosthesis in the treatment of childhood malignant bone tumors of the extremity. *Cancer* 1986;57:499–502.

Lewis MM, Sissons HA, Norman A, et al. Benign and malignant cartilage tumors. In: Griffin PP, ed. *Instructional course lectures*. Chicago: American Academy of Orthopaedic Surgeons; 1987:87–114.

Lodwick GS. A systematic approach to the roentgen diagnosis of bone tumors. In: *M.D. Anderson Hospital and Tumor Institute—clinical conference on cancer: tumors of bone and soft tissue*. Chicago: Year Book; 1965:49–68.

Madewell JE, Ragsdale BD, Sweet DE. Radiologic and pathologic analysis of solitary bone lesions. Part I: internal margins. *Radiol Clin North Am* 1981;19:715–748.

Magid D. Two-dimensional and three-dimensional computed tomographic imaging in musculoskeletal tumors. *Radiol Clin North Am* 1993;31:425–447.

McCarthy EF. CT-guided needle biopsies of bone and soft tissue tumors: a pathologist's perspective. *Skeletal Radiol* 2007;36:181–182.

McCarthy EF. Histological grading of primary bone tumors. *Skeletal Radiol* 2009;38:947–948.

McCarville B. The role of positron emission tomography in pediatric musculoskeletal oncology. *Skeletal Radiol* 2006;35:553–554.

Miller TT. Bone tumors and tumorlike conditions: analysis with conventional radiography. *Radiology* 2008;246:662–674.

Mirra JM, Picci P, Gold RH. *Bone tumors: clinical, radiologic, and pathologic correlations*. Philadelphia: Lea & Febiger; 1989.

Morone M, Ball MA, Tunaru N, et al. Whole-body MRI: current applications in oncology. *AJR Am J Roentgenol* 2017;209:W336–W349.

Moser RP. Cartilaginous tumors of the skeleton. *AFIP Atlas of radiologic-pathologic correlations. Fascicle II*. St. Louis, MO: Mosby-Year Book; 1990.

Moulton JS, Blebea JS, Dunco DM, et al. MR imaging of soft-tissue masses: diagnostic efficacy and value of distinguishing between benign and malignant lesions. *AJR Am J Roentgenol* 1995;164:1191–1199.

Mulder JD, Kroon HM, Schutte HE, et al. *Radiologic atlas of bone tumors*. Amsterdam, Netherlands: Elsevier; 1993:9–46.

Mulligan ME, Badros AZ. PET/CT and MR imaging in myeloma. *Skeletal Radiol* 2007;36:5–16.

Munk PL, Lee MJ, Janzen DL, et al. Lipoma and liposarcoma: evaluation using CT and MR imaging. *Am J Roentgenol* 1997;169:589–594.

Norman A, Dorfman HD. Juxtacortical circumscribed myositis ossificans: evolution and radiographic features. *Radiology* 1970;96:301–306.

Olson P, Everson LI, Griffiths HJ. Staging of musculoskeletal tumors. *Radiol Clin North Am* 1994;32:151–162.

Peterson JJ, Kransdorf MJ, Bancroft LW, et al. Malignant fatty tumors: classification, clinical course, imaging appearance and treatment. *Skeletal Radiol* 2003;32:493–503.

Ragsdale BD, Madewell JE, Sweet DE. Radiologic and pathologic analysis of solitary bone lesions. Part II: periosteal reactions. *Radiol Clin North Am* 1981;19:749–783.

Reinus WR, Wilson AJ. Quantitative analysis of solitary lesions of bone. *Invest Radiol* 1995;30:427–432.

Schajowicz F. *Tumors and tumorlike lesions of bone. Pathology, radiology, and treatment*, 2nd ed. Berlin, Germany: Springer-Verlag; 1994:1–21.

Shin DS, Shon OJ, Han DS, et al. The clinical efficacy of (18)F-FDG-PET/CT in benign and malignant musculoskeletal tumors. *Ann Nucl Med* 2008;22:603–609.

Subhawong TK, Durand DJ, Thawait GK, et al. Characterization of soft tissue masses: can quantitative diffusion weighted imaging reliably distinguish cysts from solid masses? *Skeletal Radiol* 2013;42:1583–1592.

Sundaram M, McLeod R. MR imaging of tumor and tumorlike lesions of bone and soft tissue. *AJR Am J Roentgenol* 1990;155:817–824.

Sweet DE, Madewell JE, Ragsdale BD. Radiologic and pathologic analysis of solitary bone lesions. Part III: matrix patterns. *Radiol Clin North Am* 1981;19:785–814.

Tateishi U, Yamaguchi U, Seki K, et al. Bone and soft-tissue sarcoma: preoperative staging with fluorine 18 fluorodeoxyglucose PET/CT and conventional imaging. *Radiology* 2007;245:839–847.

Tian R, Su M, Tian Y, et al. Dual-time point PET/CT with F-18 FDG for the differentiation of malignant and benign bone lesions. *Skeletal Radiol* 2009;38:451–458.

Unni KK. *Bone tumors*. New York: Churchill Livingstone; 1988.

Widmann G, Riedl QA, Schoepf D, et al. State-of-the-art HR-US imaging findings of the most frequent musculoskeletal soft-tissue tumors. *Skeletal Radiol* 2009;38:637–649.

Wilner D. *Radiology of bone tumors and allied disorders*. Philadelphia: Lea & Febiger; 1982.

Zhao F, Ahlawat S, Farahani SJ, et al. Can MR imaging be used to predict tumor grade in soft-tissue sarcoma? *Radiology* 2014;272:192–201.

17

Benign Tumors and Tumor-like Lesions I

Bone-Forming Lesions

Benign Bone-Forming (Osteoblastic, Osteogenic) Lesions

Bone-forming neoplasms are characterized by the formation of osteoid or mature bone directly by the tumor cells. They include osteoma, osteoid osteoma, and osteoblastoma.

Osteoma

Clinical and Imaging Features

An osteoma is a slow-growing osteoblastic lesion commonly seen in the outer table of the calvarium and in the frontal and ethmoid sinuses. It is also occasionally encountered in long and short tubular bones, and at these sites, it is known as a *parosteal osteoma*. The lesion grows on the bone surface and has the radiographic appearance of a dense, ivory-like sclerotic mass attached to the cortex with sharply demarcated borders (Fig. 17.1). Osteomas have been reported in patients from ages 10 to 79 years, with most in the fourth and fifth decades. Men and women are equally affected (Fig. 17.2). An osteoma is an asymptomatic lesion that does not recur if excised surgically. Its importance lies in its similar radiographic presentation to the more aggressive parosteal osteosarcoma (see Figs. 16.35, 21.34, and 21.35A) and its common association with cutaneous and subcutaneous masses and intestinal polyps in the condition known as *Gardner syndrome* (Fig. 17.3). Intestinal adenomatous polyps, particularly in the colon, may undergo a malignant transformation to carcinoma. The syndrome is a familial, autosomal dominant disorder frequently seen in Mormons in Utah. The cause of this syndrome is linked to mutation in the *APC* gene located in chromosome 5q21.

Pathology

Histologically, osteoma is composed primarily of bone, with a mature lamellar architecture consisting of concentric rings as in compact bone or, more commonly, parallel plates as in cancellous bone.

Differential Diagnosis

The differential diagnosis of solitary parosteal osteoma should include parosteal osteosarcoma, sessile osteochondroma, juxtacortical myositis ossificans, periosteal osteoblastoma, ossified parosteal lipoma, and focus of melorheostosis (Fig. 17.4 and Table 17.1). Among these, parosteal osteosarcoma is the most important entity that needs to be excluded, which may be a difficult task radiographically because both lesions appear as ivory-like masses attached to the bone's surface. The keys to recognizing osteoma, however, are its usually exquisitely smooth borders and well-circumscribed, intensely homogeneous sclerotic appearance on conventional radiographs. Parosteal osteosarcoma, in contrast, usually appears less dense and homogeneous than osteoma and may show a zone of decreased density at the periphery.

Sessile osteochondroma can usually be identified by its characteristic radiographic features: The cortex of the lesion merges without interruption with the cortex of the host bone, and the cancellous portion is continuous with the host medullary cavity of the adjacent metaphysis or diaphysis (see Fig. 18.42).

A well-matured focus of myositis ossificans may occasionally mimic parosteal osteoma. The radiographic hallmark of myositis ossificans is the so-called *zonal phenomenon*, characterized by a radiolucent area in the center of the lesion that indicates immature bone formation and a dense zone of mature ossification at the periphery. Often, a thin radiolucent cleft separates the ossific mass from the adjacent cortex. At times, however, a mature lesion may adhere to and fuse with the cortex, thus mimicking a parosteal osteoma. In these instances, computed tomography (CT) may demonstrate the classic zonal phenomenon of the lesion (see Figs. 4.79 and 4.80).

Periosteal osteoblastoma and ossified parosteal lipoma rarely create a problem in terms of being mistaken for parosteal osteoma. Melorheostosis, a rare form of mixed sclerosing dysplasia, should be recognized on radiography by the characteristic appearance of segmental cortical thickening ("flowing hyperostosis"), often resembling wax dripping down one side of a candle. A typical focus of monostotic melorheostosis usually exhibits both parosteal and endosteal involvement, and the lesion commonly extends into the articular end of the bone, which are features that are almost never present in a parosteal osteoma (see Figs. 33.71 to 33.75).

Osteoid Osteoma

Clinical and Imaging Features

Osteoid osteoma is a benign osteoblastic lesion characterized by a nidus of osteoid tissue, which may be purely radiolucent or have a sclerotic center. The nidus has limited growth potential and usually measures less than 1 cm in diameter. It is often surrounded by a zone of reactive bone formation (Fig. 17.5). Very rarely, an osteoid osteoma may have more than one nidus, in which case it is called a *multicentric* or *multifocal osteoid osteoma* (Fig. 17.6). Depending on its location in the particular part of the bone, the lesion can be classified as cortical, medullary (cancellous), or subperiosteal. Osteoid osteomas can be further subclassified as extracapsular or intracapsular (intraarticular) (Fig. 17.7). These lesions occur in the young, usually

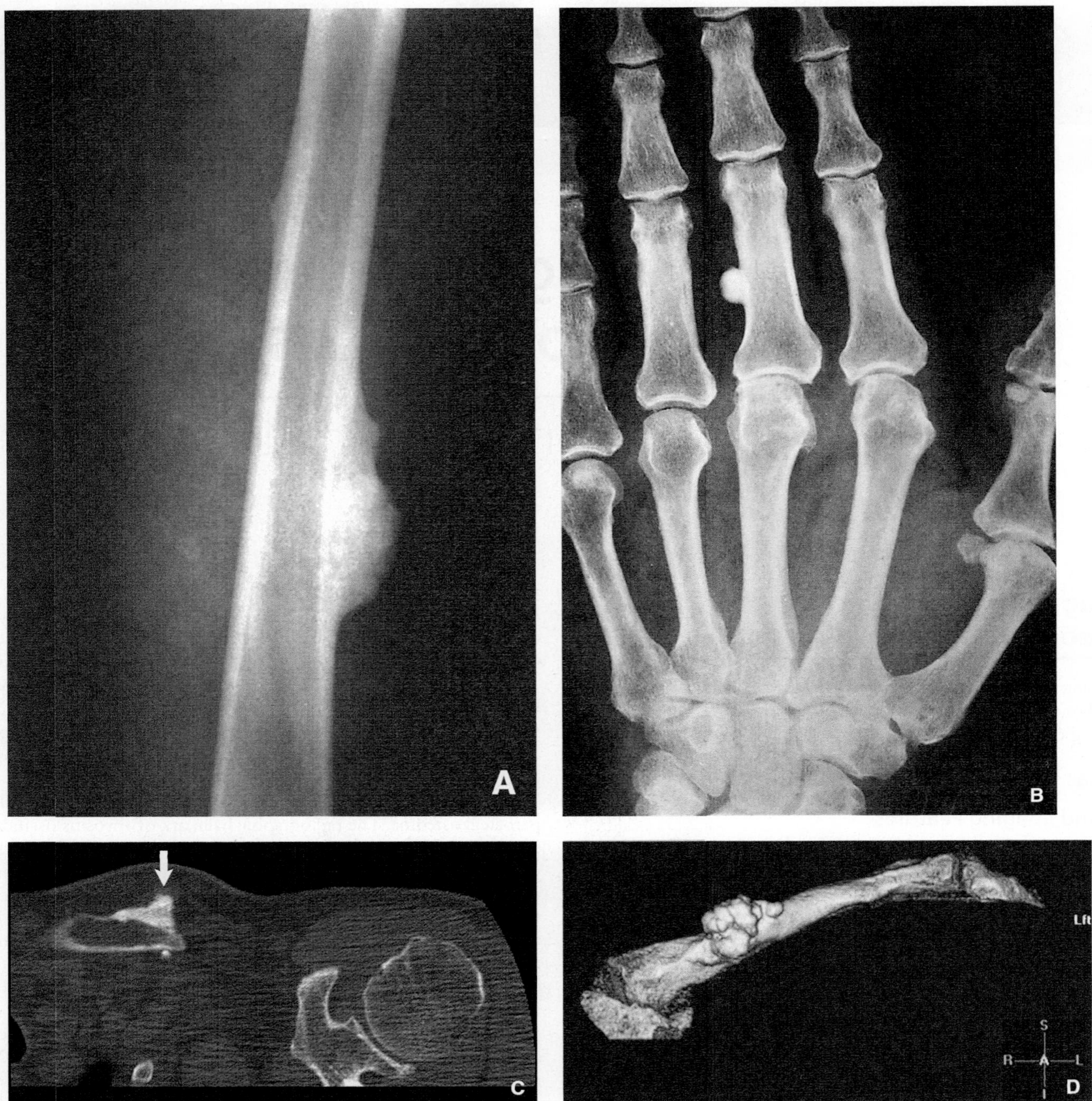

FIGURE 17.1 Parosteal osteoma. **(A)** Anteroposterior radiograph of the femur shows a sclerotic, ivory-like homogenous mass attached to the medial cortex. **(B)** Dorsovolar radiograph of the hand demonstrates a small homogenously sclerotic mass attached to the medial cortex of the proximal phalanx of the middle finger. **(C)** Coronal reformatted CT image of the left shoulder shows a sclerotic lesion attached to the clavicle *(arrow)*. Note lack of cortical invasion. **(D)** Three-dimensional (3D) CT reconstructed image of the clavicle shows slightly lobulated mass on the surface of the clavicle. (**A, C,** and **D,** Reprinted with permission from Greenspan A, Borys D. *Radiology and pathology correlation of bone tumors: a quick reference and review*. Philadelphia: Wolters Kluwer; 2016:33.)

between the ages of 10 and 35 years, and their sites of predilection are the long bones, particularly the femur and tibia (Fig. 17.8). Cytogenetic analysis performed in a few cases of this lesion reveled chromosomal alterations involving chromosome 22 [del(22)(q13.1)].

The most important clinical symptom of osteoid osteoma is pain that is more severe at night and is dramatically relieved by antiinflammatory medications such as salicylates, diclofenac, or ibuprofen within approximately 20 to 25 minutes. This typical history holds in more than 75% of cases and serves as an important clue to the diagnosis.

Standard radiographs may demonstrate the lesion, but CT (Figs. 17.9 and 17.10) is required to demonstrate the nidus and localize it precisely. CT has the added advantage of allowing exact measurement of the size of the nidus (Fig. 17.11A–C). Furthermore, a recent study indicated the high specificity of a new CT sign of osteoid osteoma, the so-called *vascular groove sign*. This sign reflects the vascular channels created by arterioles supplying the nidus of an osteoid osteoma (Fig. 17.11D). Frequently, when the lesion cannot be demonstrated radiographically, a radionuclide bone scan is helpful because osteoid osteoma invariably shows a marked increase in radiopharmaceutical tracer uptake (Fig. 17.12). This modality can be particularly helpful in cases for which the symptoms are atypical, and the initial radiographs appear normal. The use of a three-phase technique is recommended. Radionuclide tracer activity can be observed on both immediate and delayed images (Fig. 17.13). Not infrequently, the characteristic double density sign can be observed (Fig. 17.14). If the nidus is demonstrated

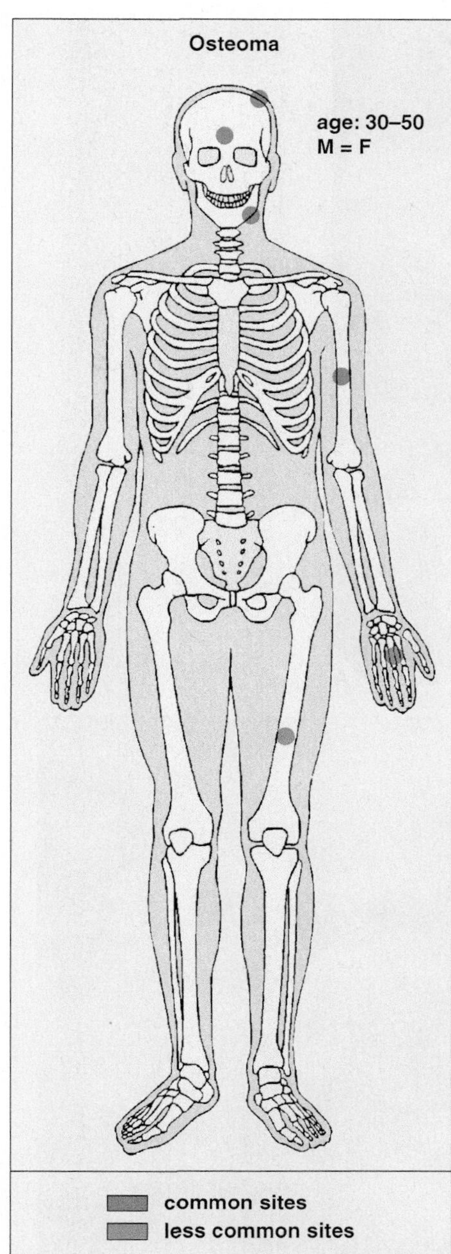

FIGURE 17.2 Osteoma: skeletal sites of predilection, peak age range, and male-to-female ratio.

radiographically, the diagnosis can usually be made with great assurance; only atypical presentations create diagnostic difficulty (Fig. 17.15).

The suitability of magnetic resonance imaging (MRI) for the detection of osteoid osteoma remains unclear, and published reports have shown mixed results. Goldman and associates reported on four cases of intracapsular osteoid osteoma of the femoral neck, in which the lesions were evaluated with bone scintigraphy, CT, and MRI. Although in all cases, abnormal findings were apparent in the MR images, the nidi could not be identified prospectively. On the basis of MRI findings of secondary bone marrow edema or synovitis, several incorrect diagnoses were made, which included Ewing sarcoma, osteonecrosis, stress fracture, and juvenile arthritis. In these cases, it is noteworthy that the correct diagnoses were made only after review of the radiographs and thin-section CT studies. Another report by Woods and associates involved three patients with a highly unusual association of osteoid osteoma with a reactive soft-tissue mass. In these cases, MRI studies might have led to confusion of osteoid osteoma with osteomyelitis or a malignant tumor. Moreover, in each case, the nidus displayed different signal characteristics. In one case, the intensity of signal was generally low on all pulse sequences, but mild enhancement was seen after administration of gadolinium. In another case, the signal was of intermediate intensity, and administration of gadolinium revealed in heterogeneous enhancement of the nidus. For the third case, in which radiographs showed the nidus to be intracortical, MRI could not identify the nidus distinctly.

However, some reports do suggest the effectiveness of MRI for demonstrating the nidus of osteoid osteoma (Figs. 17.16 and 17.17). Bell and colleagues clearly demonstrated an intracortical nidus on MRI that had not been seen on scintigraphy, angiography, or CT scans. In particular, imaging of osteoid osteoma with dynamic gadolinium-enhanced MR technique demonstrated greater conspicuity in detecting the lesion than with nonenhanced MRI (Fig.17.18).

Ebrahim and associates reported sonographic findings in patients with intraarticular osteoid osteoma. Ultrasound images revealed focal cortical irregularity and adjacent focal hypoechoic synovitis at the site of intraarticular lesions. The nidus was hypoechoic with posterior acoustic enhancement, and color Doppler imaging identified a vessel entering a focus of osteoid osteoma. It is noteworthy, however, that the authors concluded that the accuracy of sonography in the diagnosis of intraarticular osteoid osteoma cannot be certain because other intraarticular pathologic conditions, for example, inflammatory synovitis, may have a similar appearance. Therefore, one should seek corroborative features of this lesion using other imaging techniques, such as CT or MRI.

Pathology

Histologically, the nidus is composed of osteoid or even mineralized immature bone. It is a small, well-circumscribed, and self-limited lesion (Fig.17.19). Its microtrabeculae and irregular islets of osteoid matrix and bone are surrounded by a richly vascular fibrous stroma in which osteoblastic and osteoclastic activities are often prominent. The perilesional sclerosis is composed of dense bone displaying a variety of maturation patterns.

Differential Diagnosis

It must be emphasized that even when dealing with an apparent cortical osteoid osteoma of classic radiographic appearance, the differential diagnosis should include a stress fracture, a cortical abscess, and an osteosarcoma (Fig. 17.20). In a stress fracture, the radiolucency is usually more linear than in an osteoid osteoma, and it runs perpendicular or at an angle to the cortex rather than parallel to it (Fig. 17.21). A cortical bone abscess may have a similar radiographic appearance to that of osteoid osteoma, but it can usually be differentiated by a linear, serpentine tract that extends away from the abscess cavity (Fig. 17.22). An intracortical osteosarcoma is a rare bone-forming malignancy that arises solely within the cortex of bone and grossly involves neither the medullary cavity nor the soft tissues. On radiography, it appears as a radiolucent focus within the cortex (femur or tibia), surrounded by zone of sclerosis, and varying in size from 1.0 to 4.2 cm in reported cases. The cortex at the site of the lesion may bulge slightly or may be thickened. Periosteal reaction may or may not be present.

In intramedullary lesions, the differential diagnosis must consider a bone abscess (Brodie abscess), and in a lesion with calcified nidus, a bone island (enostosis). The larger lesions must be also differentiated from osteoblastoma (see Fig. 17.20B). A bone abscess may have a similar radiographic appearance, but one can usually detect a linear, serpentine tract extending from the abscess cavity toward the nearest growth plate (Fig. 17.23). A bone island is characterized on radiography by the lesion's brush borders, which blend with surrounding trabeculae in a pattern likened to "thorny radiation" or pseudopodia (Fig. 17.24). In addition, bone islands usually show no increased activity on radionuclide bone scan. Distinguishing osteoid osteoma from osteoblastoma can be very difficult, if not impossible. In general, osteoblastoma is larger than osteoid osteoma (usually more than 2 cm in diameter) and exhibits less reactive sclerosis, but the periosteal reaction may be more prominent.

For detailed features of the differential diagnosis of osteoid osteoma, see Table 17.2.

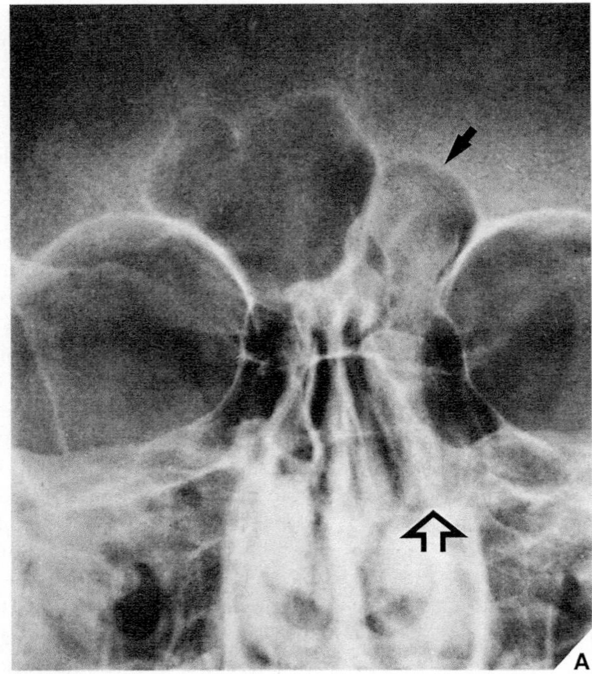

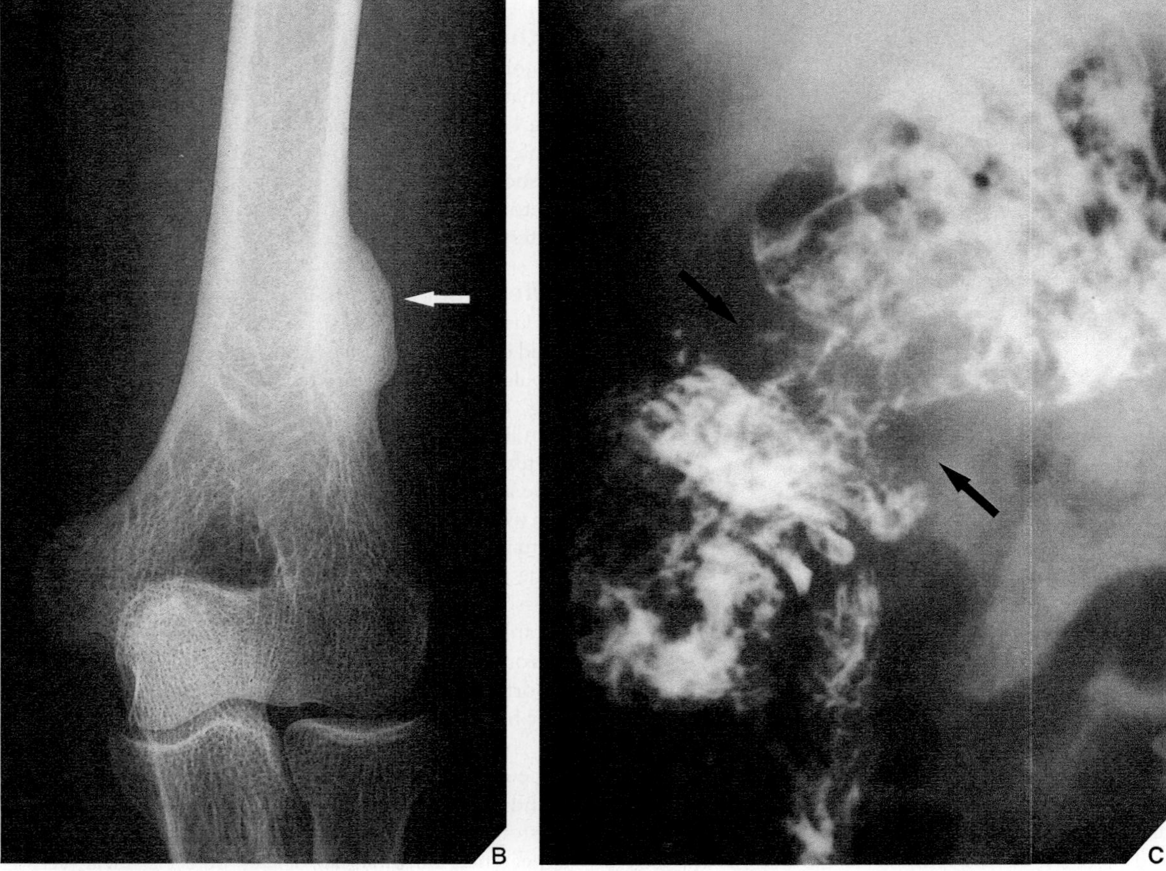

FIGURE 17.3 Gardner syndrome. (A) Frontal radiograph of the facial bones of a 36-year-old man shows the typical appearance of osteomas in the left frontal *(arrow)* and ethmoid *(open arrow)* sinuses. The dense, sclerotic masses are sharply demarcated from the surrounding structures by air. **(B)** This patient also had a parosteal osteoma of the distal left humerus *(arrow)*, multiple polyps in the colon, and subcutaneous masses, features of Gardner syndrome. **(C)** Barium enema shows several polyps in the cecum and an apple-core lesion *(arrows)*, proved by histologic examination to be adenocarcinoma.

RADIOLOGIC DIFFERENTIAL DIAGNOSIS OF OSTEOMA

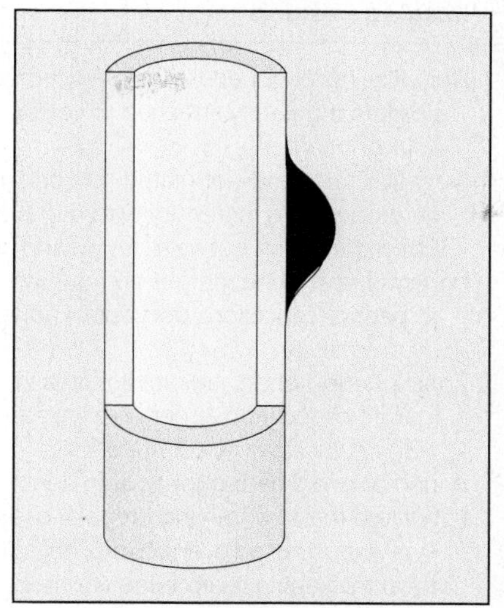
Osteoma

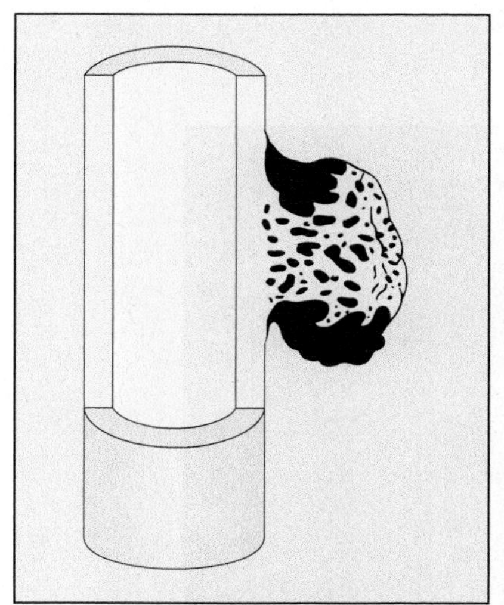
Parosteal Osteosarcoma

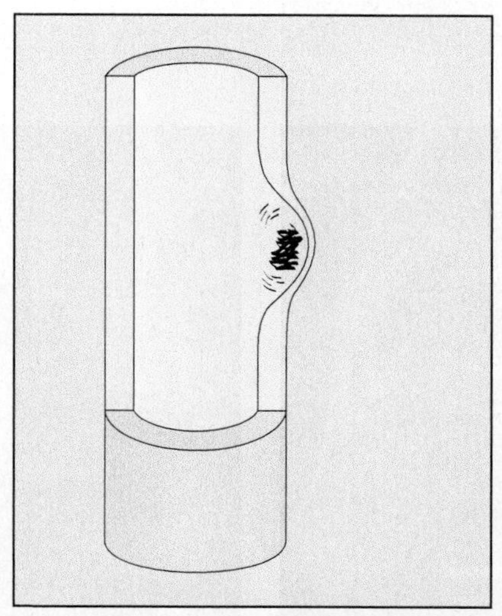
Sessile Osteochondroma

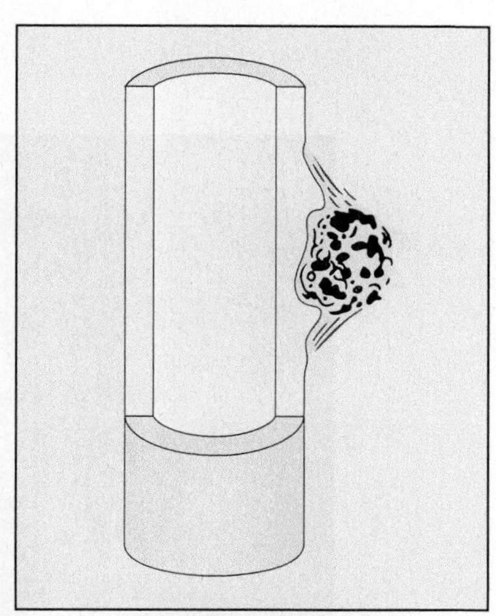
Periosteal Osteoblastoma

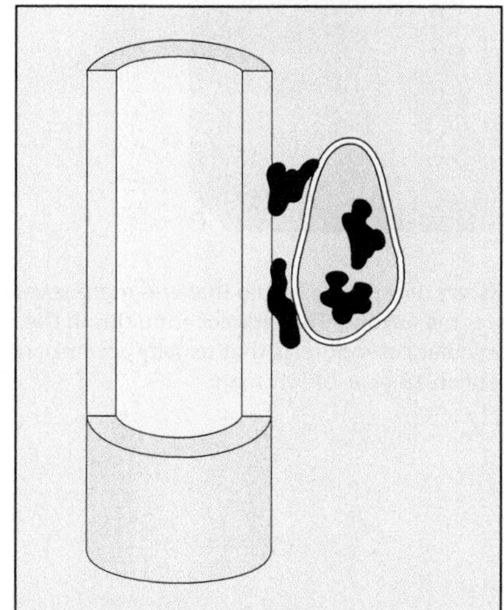
Ossified Parosteal Lipoma

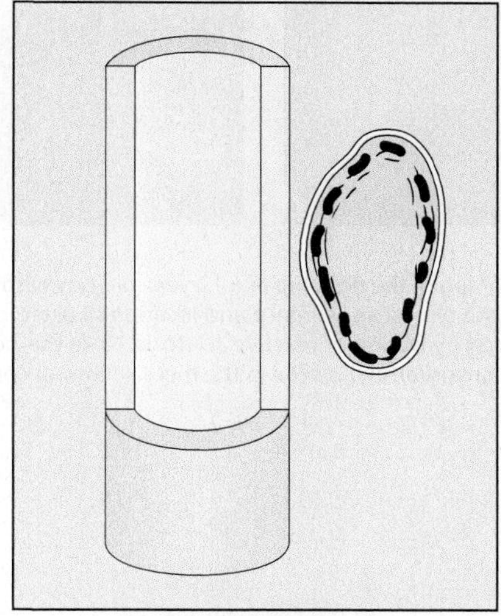
Myositis Ossificans

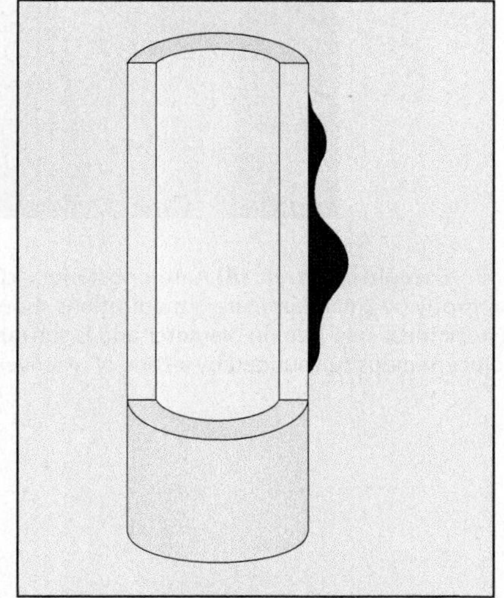
Melorheostosis

FIGURE 17.4 Differential diagnosis of parosteal osteoma. Schematic representation of various cortical and juxtacortical lesions having similar appearance to osteoma.

TABLE 17.1 Differential Diagnosis of Parosteal Osteoma

Condition (Lesion)	Imaging Features
Parosteal osteoma	Ivory-like, homogeneously dense sclerotic mass, with sharply demarcated borders, intimately attached to cortex; no cleft between lesion and adjacent cortex
Parosteal osteosarcoma	Ivory-like, frequently lobulated sclerotic mass, homogeneous or heterogeneous in density with more radiolucent areas at periphery; incomplete cleft between lesion and adjacent cortex occasionally present
Sessile osteochondroma	Cortex of host bone merges without interruption with cortex of lesion, and respective cancellous portions of adjacent bone and osteochondroma communicate
Juxtacortical myositis ossificans	Zonal phenomenon: radiolucent area in center of lesion and dense zone of mature ossification at periphery; frequently thin radiolucent cleft separates ossific mass from adjacent cortex
Periosteal osteoblastoma	Round or ovoid heterogeneous in density mass attached to cortex
Ossified parosteal (periosteal) lipoma	Lobulated mass containing irregular ossifications and radiolucent area of fat; hyperostosis of adjacent cortex occasionally present
Melorheostosis (monostotic)	Cortical thickening resembling wax dripping down on one side of a candle

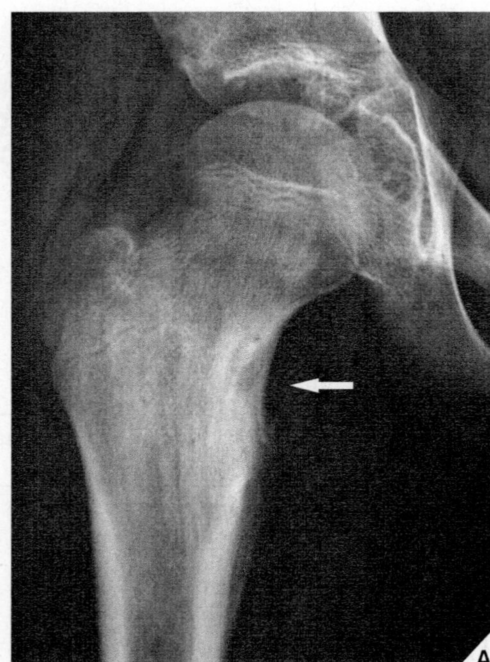

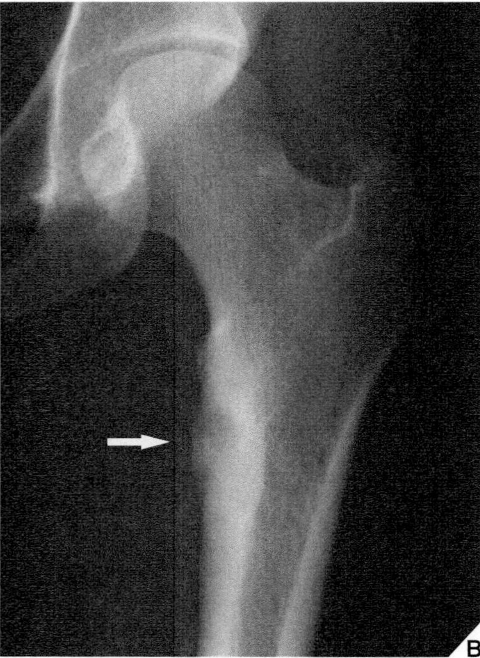

FIGURE 17.5 Osteoid osteoma. **(A)** Anteroposterior radiograph of the right hip of a 12-year-old boy with a history of right groin pain that was more severe at night and was relieved promptly by antiinflammatory medications shows the typical appearance and location of osteoid osteoma *(arrow)*. The radiolucent nidus in the medial aspect of the femoral neck measures 1 cm in diameter and is surrounded by a zone of reactive sclerosis. Note the periarticular osteoporosis that usually accompanies this lesion. **(B)** Purely radiolucent nidus surrounded by a zone of reactive sclerosis *(arrow)* is seen in the medial femoral cortex of an 18-year-old woman.

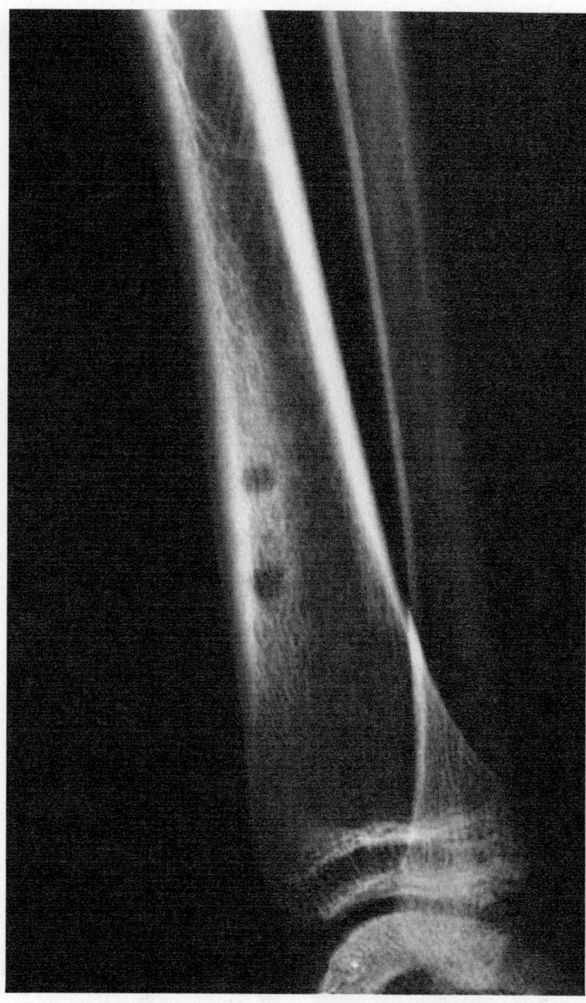

FIGURE 17.6 **Multifocal osteoid osteoma.** A 17-year-old boy presented with pain in the left lower leg for 3 months. It was promptly relieved by antiinflammatory medications. Lateral radiograph of the lower leg shows two well-defined radiolucencies within a sclerotic area in the anterior aspect of the distal tibia. A resected specimen showed three nidi of osteoid osteoma, the two most distal of which were fairly close to one another, creating a single radiolucency on the radiograph. (Reprinted from Greenspan A, Elguezabel A, Bryk D. Multifocal osteoid osteoma. A case report and review of the literature. *Am J Roentgenol Radium Ther Nucl Med* 1974;121:103–106. Copyright © 1974 American Roentgen Ray Society.)

Complications

Osteoid osteoma may be accompanied by a few complications. Accelerated bone growth may occur if the nidus is located near the growth plate, particularly in young children (Fig. 17.25). A vertebral lesion, particularly in the neural arch, may lead to painful scoliosis, with concavity of the curvature directed toward the side of the lesion (Fig. 17.26). An intracapsular lesion may result in arthritis of precocious onset (Fig. 17.27). As observed by Norman and associates, this latter complication may serve as an important diagnostic clue to an osteoid osteoma when a typical history of the condition is elicited from the patient, but the nidus is not recognizable radiographically (Fig. 17.28).

Treatment

The treatment of osteoid osteoma consists of complete *en bloc* resection of the nidus. The resected specimen and the involved bone should be radiographed promptly (Fig. 17.29) so as to exclude the possibility of incomplete resection, which can lead to recurrence (Fig. 17.30).

A variety of techniques other than *en bloc* excision have been tried, among them intralesional curettage, excision with trephines after surgical exposure, fluoroscopically guided or CT-guided percutaneous extraction, and percutaneous radiofrequency thermal ablation (RFTA). The latter technique, suggested by Rosenthal and colleagues, is an alternative to surgery in selected patients. It is performed through a small radiofrequency electrode that is introduced into the lesion through the biopsy track with CT guidance (Fig. 17.31) to produce thermal necrosis of an approximately 1-cm sphere of tissue. Several recent reports of successful RFTA of intramedullary osteoid osteoma confirmed the belief that this technique is an effective method of noninvasive treatment of these lesions.

Osteoblastoma

Clinical and Imaging Features

Osteoblastoma, which accounts for approximately 1% of all primary bone tumors and 3% of all benign bone tumors, is a lesion histologically similar to osteoid osteoma but characterized by a larger size (more than 1.5 cm in diameter and usually more than 2 cm). The age range of its occurrence is also similar to that of osteoid osteoma: The 75% of osteoblastomas are found in patients in their first, second, or third decade. Although the long bones are frequently involved, the lesion has a predilection for the vertebral column (Fig. 17.32). Its clinical presentation, however, is different from that of osteoid osteoma. Some patients are asymptomatic, but pain is not as readily relieved by salicylates. Their natural histories also differ. Whereas osteoid osteoma tends toward regression, osteoblastoma tends toward progression and even malignant transformation, although the possibility of the latter event remains controversial. Multifocal osteoblastomas have also been reported. Moreover, toxic osteoblastoma, a rare variant of this tumor, has been recognized. It is associated with systemic manifestations, including diffuse periostitis of multiple bones, fever, and weight loss.

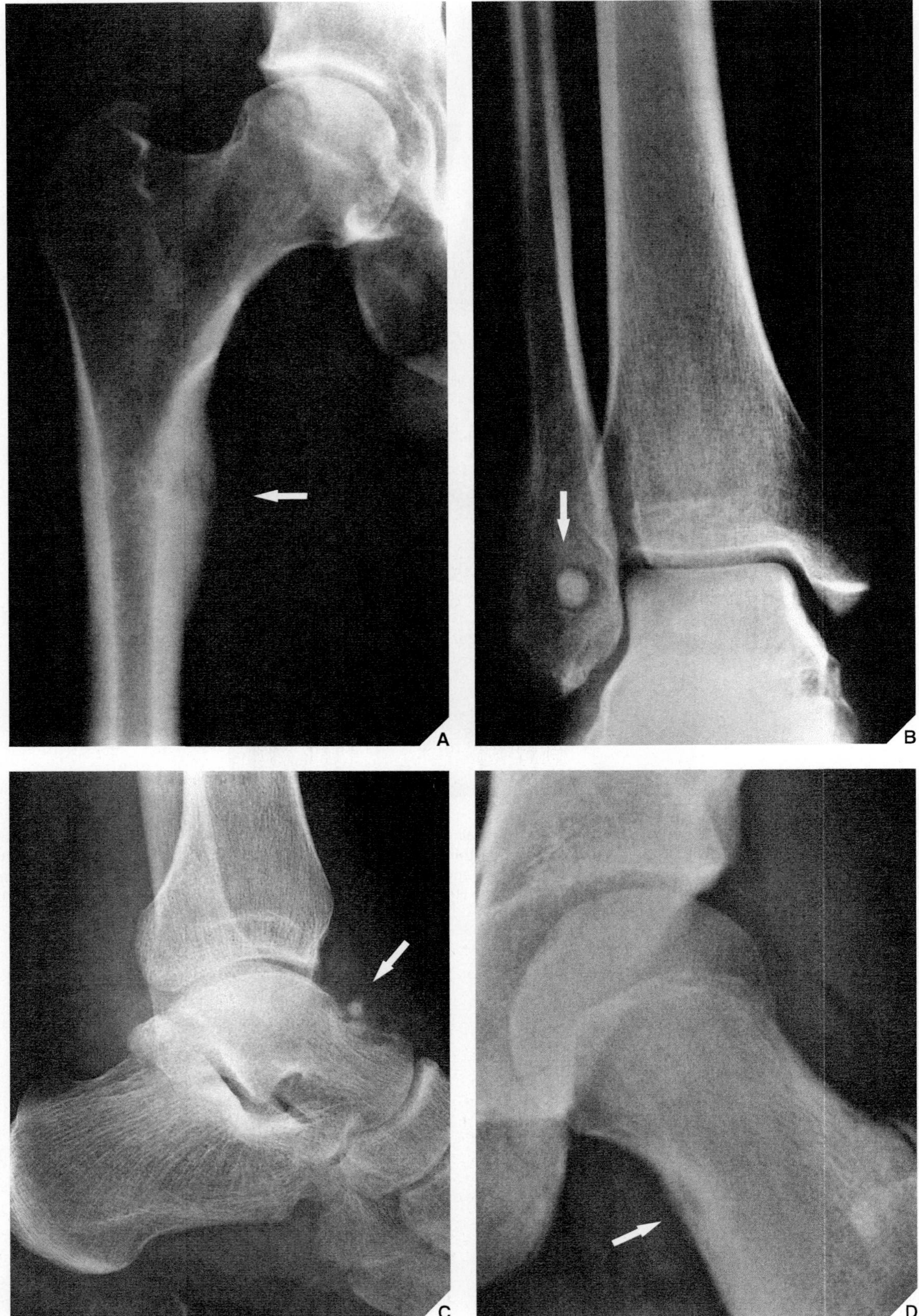

FIGURE 17.7 Types of osteoid osteoma. The radiographic presentation of osteoid osteoma differs according to its location in the bone. **(A)** In the cortical type, there is intense reactive sclerosis surrounding the nidus, as seen here in the medial cortex of the femur *(arrow)*. **(B)** The medullary variant, as seen here in the distal fibula, exhibits a dense, sclerotic nidus surrounded by a halo of radiolucent osteoid tissue *(arrow)*. Note the almost total lack of reactive sclerosis. **(C)** In subperiosteal osteoid osteoma, seen here on the surface of the talar bone *(arrow)*, periosteal response is minimal and reactive sclerosis is completely absent. **(D)** In the intracapsular osteoid osteoma, the radiolucent nidus seen here in the medial aspect of the proximal portion of the femoral neck *(arrow)* shows only minimal reactive sclerosis.

FIGURE 17.8 Skeletal sites of predilection, peak age range, and male-to-female ratio in osteoid osteoma.

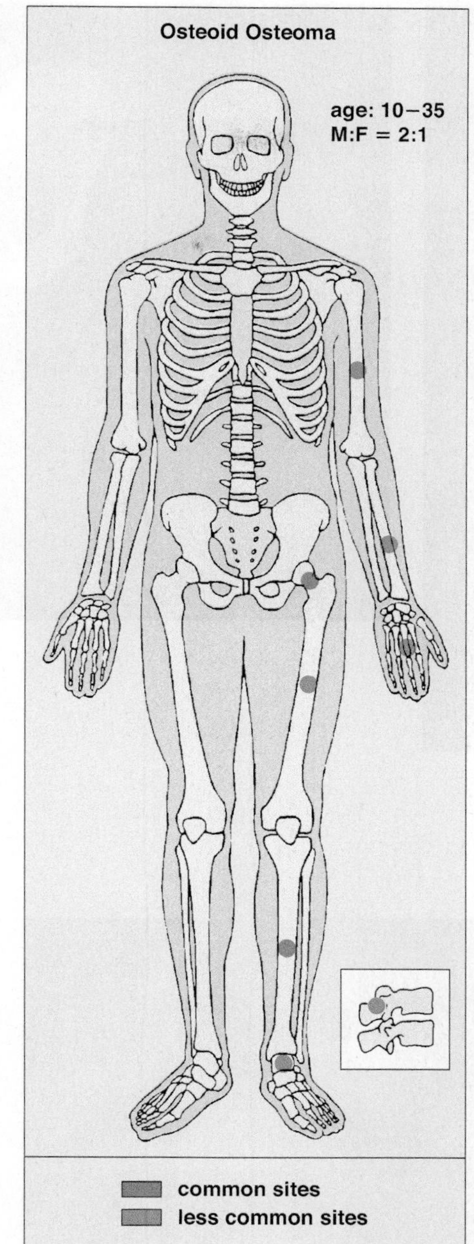

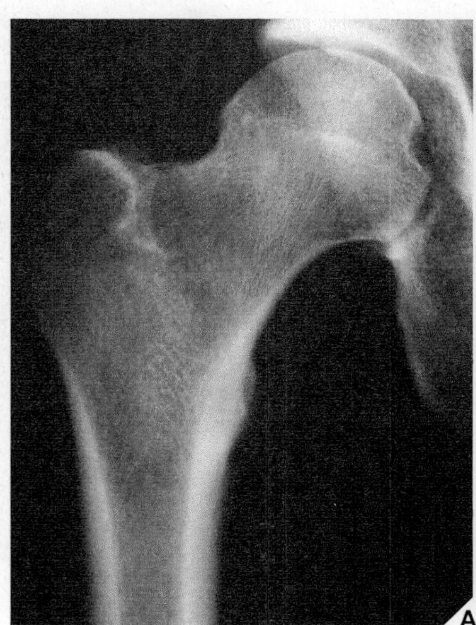

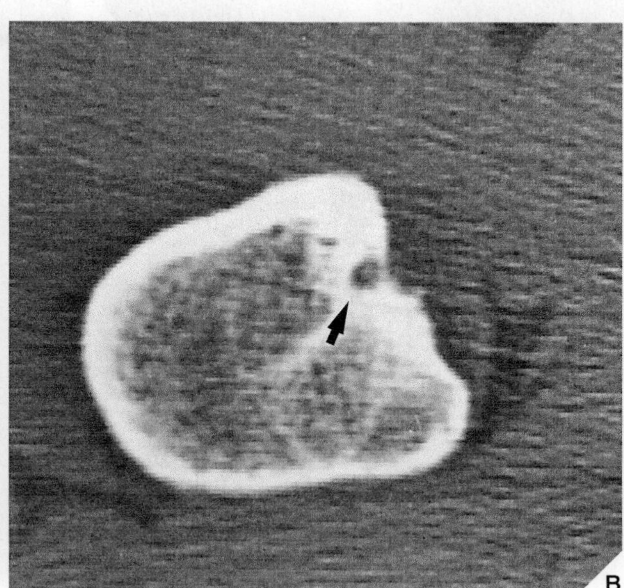

FIGURE 17.9 CT of osteoid osteoma. **(A)** Anteroposterior radiograph of the right hip of a 24-year-old man with pain in the upper thigh shows a lesion in the lesser trochanter, but a diagnosis of osteoid osteoma cannot be made unequivocally. **(B)** CT section, however, clearly demonstrates the nidus *(arrow)*.

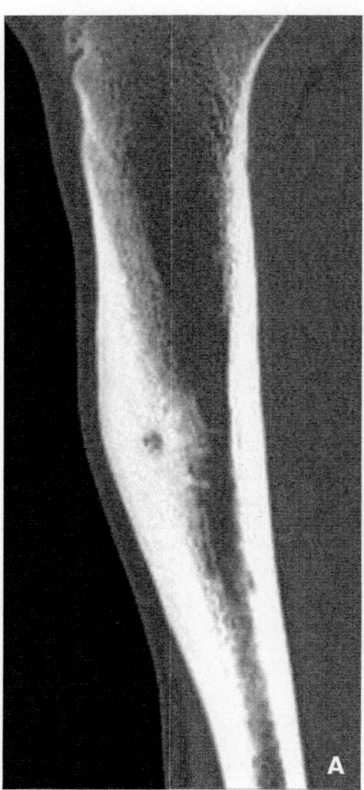

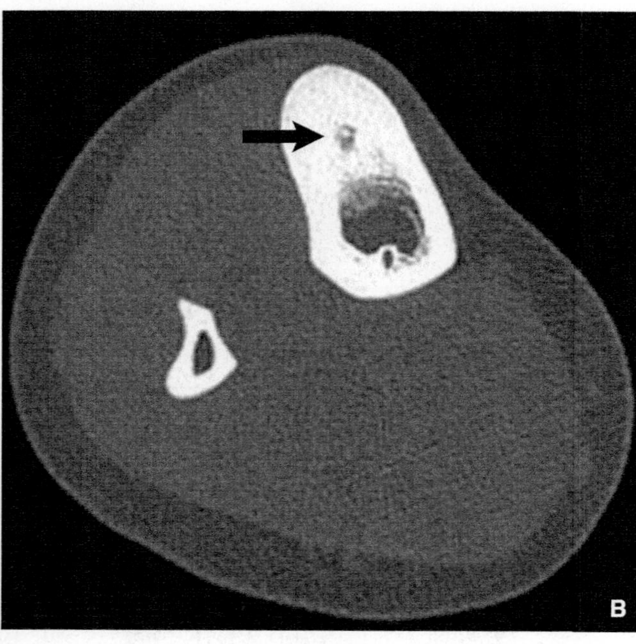

FIGURE 17.10 CT of osteoid osteoma. **(A)** Coronal reformatted CT image of the tibia and **(B)** axial CT section show a well-defined low-attenuation nidus with sclerotic center, located in the anterior cortex *(arrow)*. (Reprinted with permission from Greenspan A, Borys D. *Radiology and pathology correlation of bone tumors: a quick reference and review*. Philadelphia: Wolters Kluwer; 2016:38.)

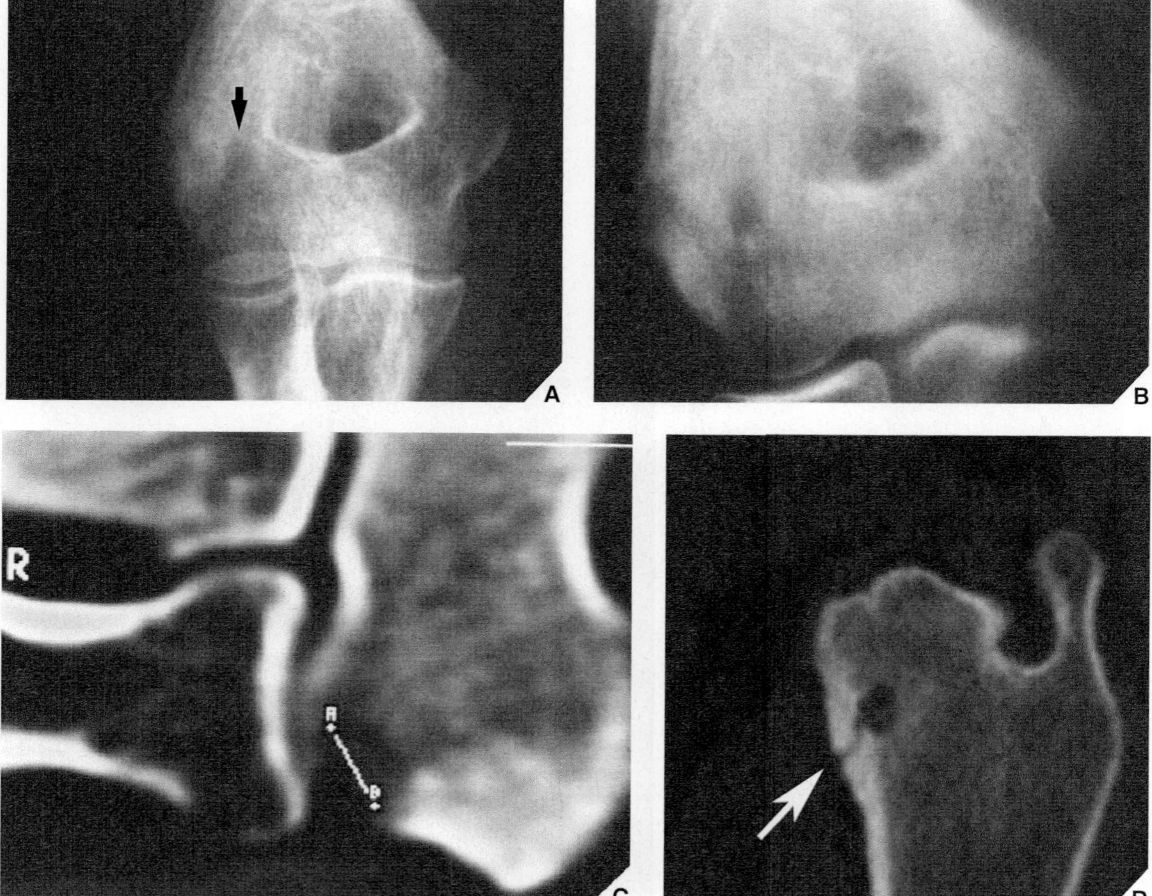

FIGURE 17.11 CT of osteoid osteoma. **(A)** Anteroposterior radiograph of the right elbow of a 31-year-old man with the typical clinical symptoms of osteoid osteoma demonstrates periarticular osteoporosis. There is the suggestion of a lesion in the capitellum *(arrow)*. **(B)** Conventional tomogram shows a radiolucent area surrounded by a zone of sclerotic reaction. **(C)** CT section unequivocally demonstrates a subarticular nidus, which measures 6.5 mm. **(D)** Sagittal reformatted CT image of the left femur in another patient with osteoid osteoma demonstrates the "vascular groove" sign *(arrow)*.

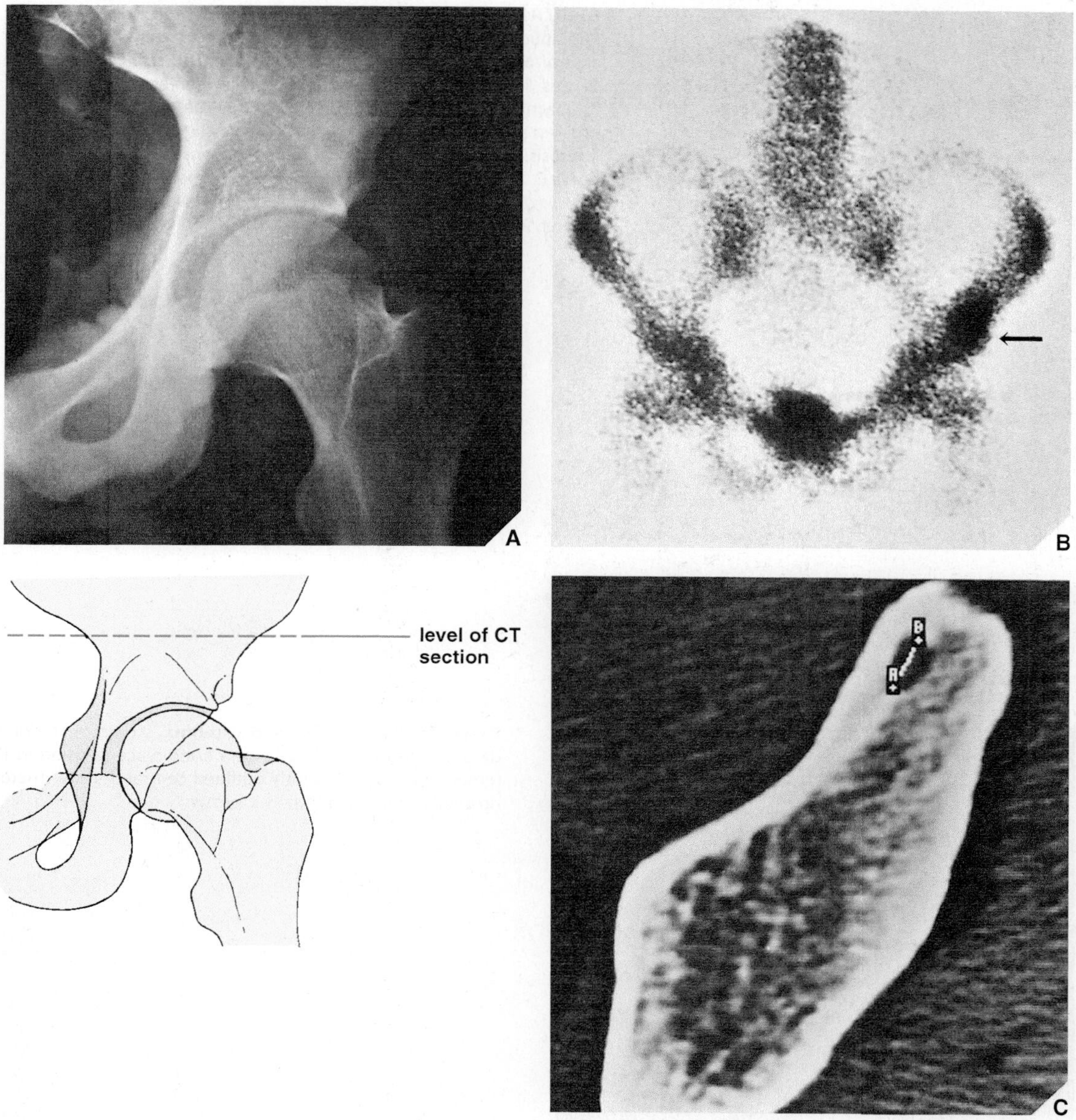

level of CT section

FIGURE 17.12 Scintigraphy and CT of osteoid osteoma. (A) Anteroposterior radiograph of the left hip of a 16-year-old boy with a typical history of osteoid osteoma is equivocal, although there is the suggestion of radiolucency in the supraacetabular portion of the ilium. **(B)** Radionuclide bone scan shows an increased uptake of radiopharmaceutical tracer in the supraacetabular portion of the left ilium *(arrow)*. **(C)** Subsequently performed CT scan not only demonstrated the lesion but also allowed its measurement (6.8 mm).

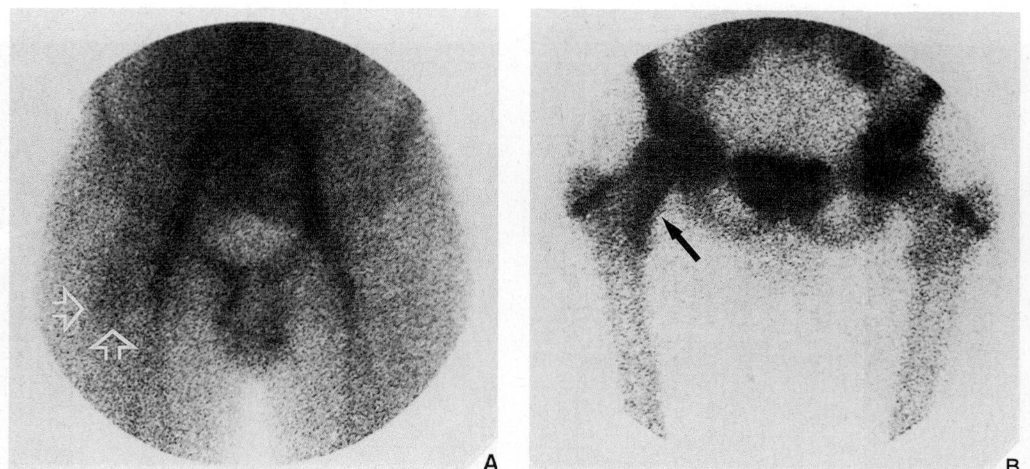

FIGURE 17.13 Scintigraphy of osteoid osteoma. (A) In the first phase of a three-phase radionuclide bone scan, 1 minute after intravenous injection of 15 mCi (555 MBq) technetium-99m (^{99m}Tc)-labeled methylene diphosphonate (MDP), there is increased activity in the iliac and femoral vessels. Discrete activity in the area of the medial femoral neck *(open arrows)* is related to the nidus of osteoid osteoma. **(B)** In the third phase, 2 hours after injection, there is accumulation of a bone-seeking tracer in the femoral neck lesion *(arrow)*. (Reprinted by permission from Springer: Greenspan A. Benign bone-forming lesions: osteoma, osteoid osteoma, and osteoblastoma. Clinical, imaging, pathologic, and differential considerations. *Skeletal Radiol* 1993;22:485–500.)

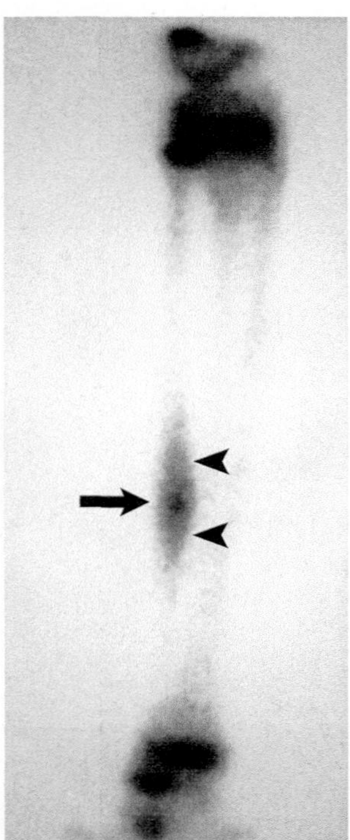

FIGURE 17.14 Scintigraphy of osteoid osteoma. Radionuclide bone scan shows a classic double density sign of osteoid osteoma located in the tibial diaphysis of this 14-year-old boy. Observe markedly increased radioactivity in the center *(arrow)* related to the nidus and less active areas *(arrowheads)* representing reactive sclerosis. (Reprinted with permission from Greenspan A, Borys D. *Radiology and pathology correlation of bone tumors: a quick reference and review*. Philadelphia: Wolters Kluwer; 2016:38.)

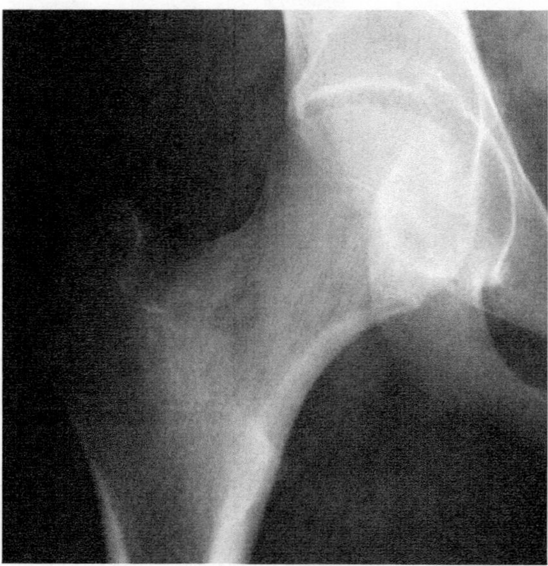

FIGURE 17.15 Osteoid osteoma. Anteroposterior radiograph of the right hip shows a radiolucent lesion in the femoral neck with a faintly outlined central density. There is no evidence of surrounding sclerosis.

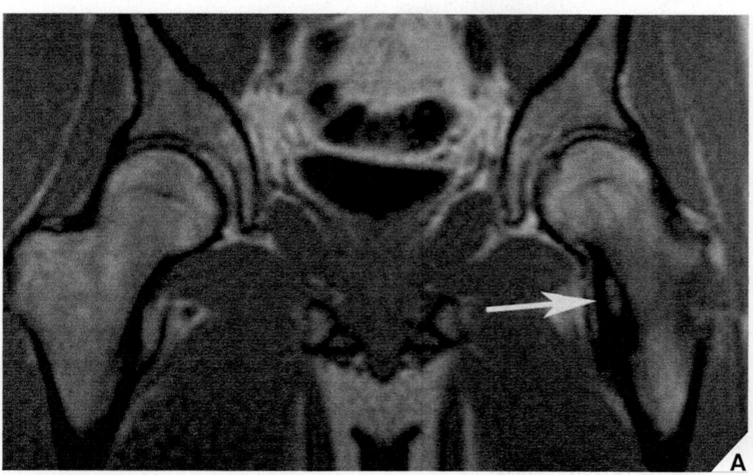

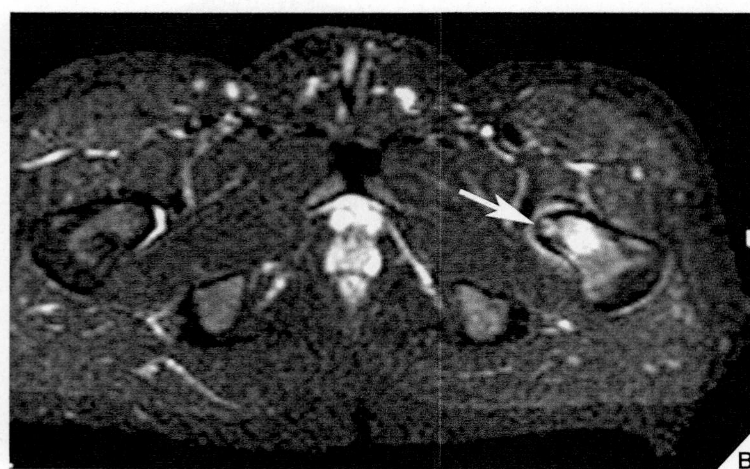

FIGURE 17.16 MRI of osteoid osteoma. (A) Coronal T1-weighted MRI demonstrates nidus of an osteoid osteoma in the medial aspect of the femoral neck *(arrow)* and cortical thickening. **(B)** Axial short time inversion recovery (STIR) MRI in the same patient demonstrates the nidus as a focal area of increased signal intensity in the femoral neck *(arrow)*, associated with cortical thickening and surrounding bone marrow and soft-tissue edema.

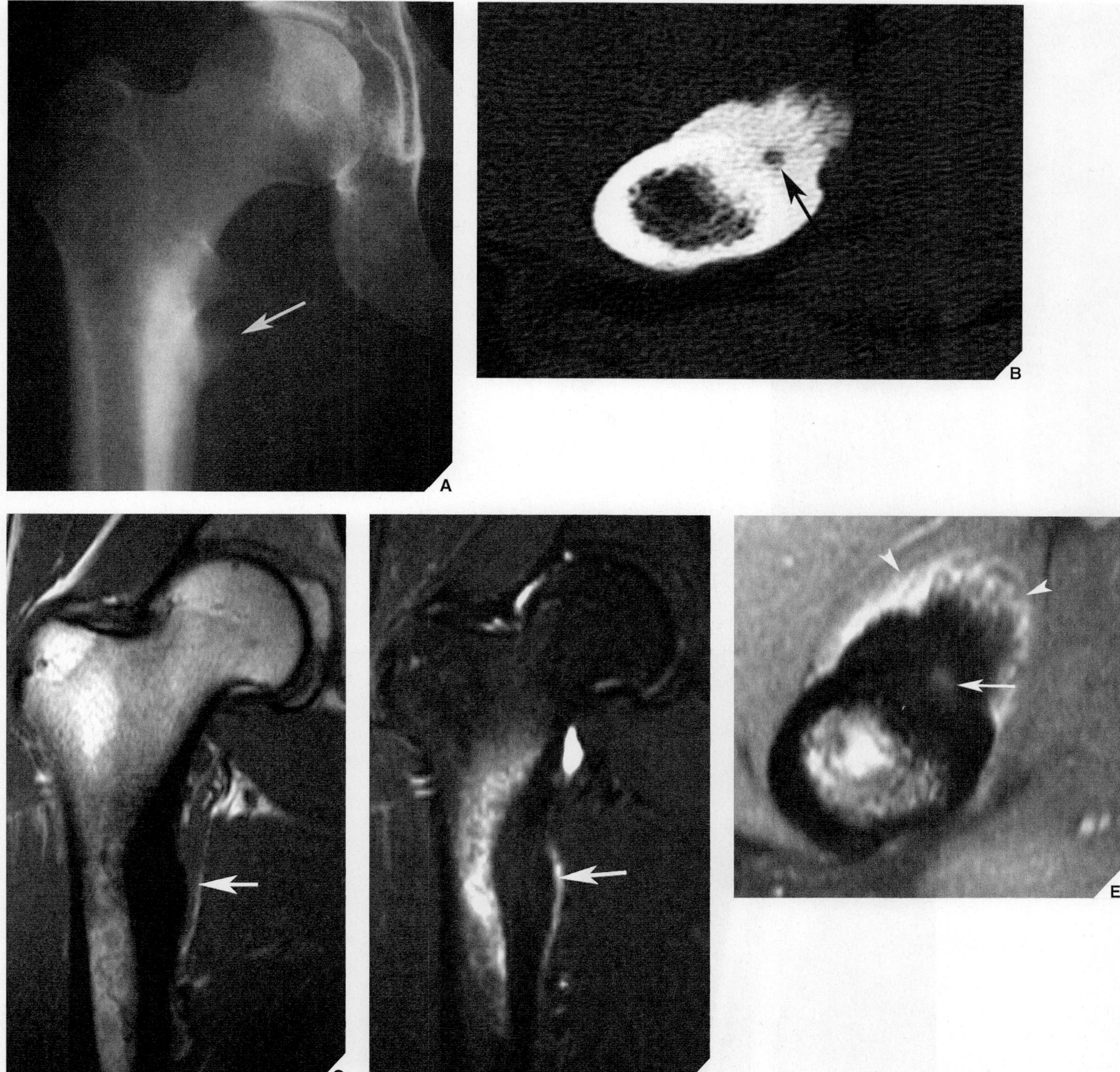

FIGURE 17.17 CT and MRI of osteoid osteoma. **(A)** Anteroposterior radiograph of the right femur shows marked cortical thickening of the medial aspect of the proximal femur with prominent focal periosteal reaction *(arrow)*. **(B)** Axial CT shows the nidus *(arrow)* associated with cortical thickening and periosteal reaction. **(C)** Coronal T1-weighted MRI demonstrates again the cortical thickening *(arrow)*, but the nidus is not identified. **(D)** Coronal T2-weighted MRI shows the cortical thickening *(arrow)*, extensive bone marrow edema, and mild soft-tissue edema, but the nidus is not visualized. **(E)** Axial T2-weighted MRI demonstrates the nidus clearly *(arrow)*, in addition to the cortical thickening with periosteal reaction *(arrowheads)* and the surrounding soft-tissue edema. (Courtesy of Steve Shankman, MD, Brooklyn, New York.)

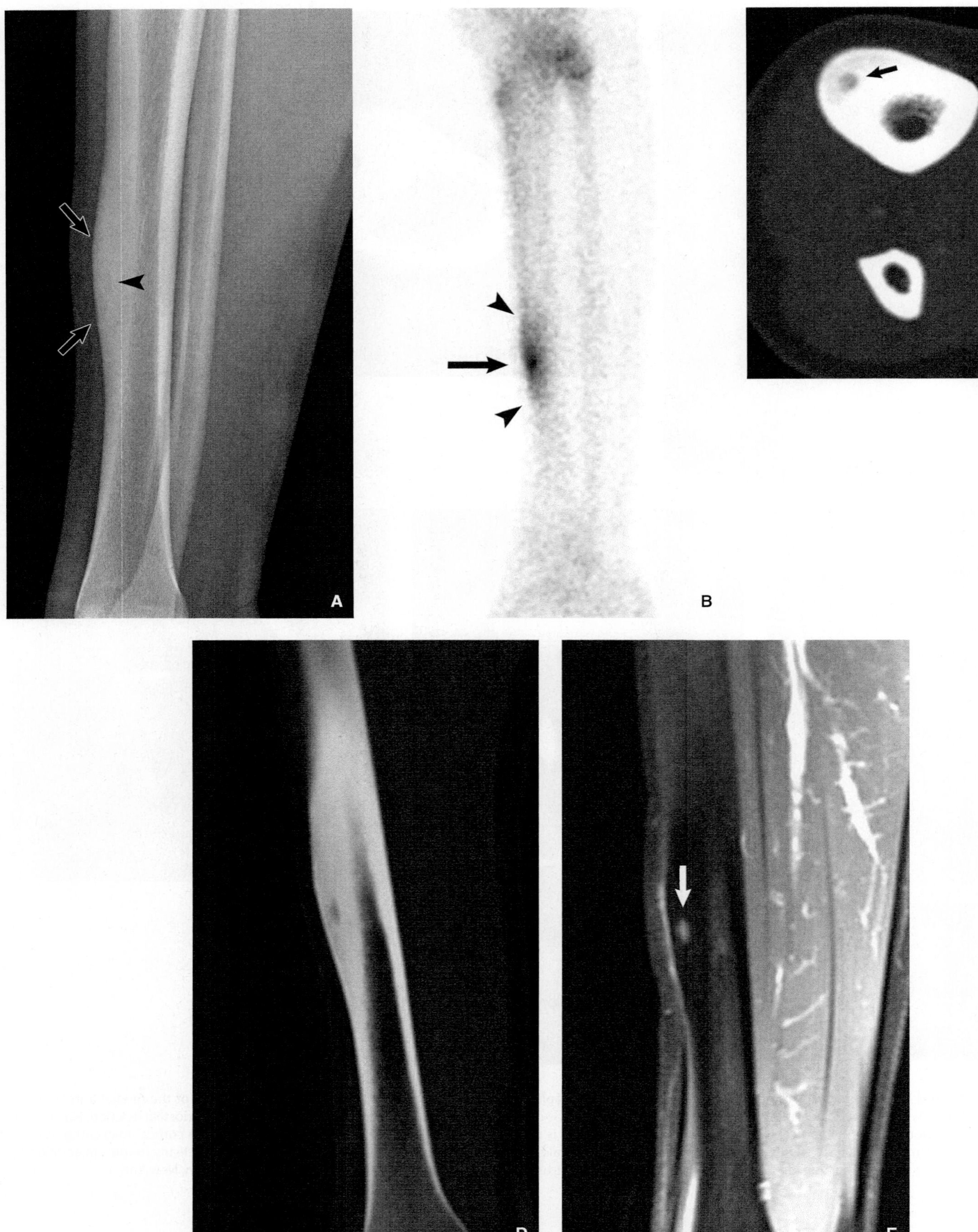

FIGURE 17.18 Scintigraphy, CT, and MRI of osteoid osteoma. A 20-year-old woman presented with nocturnal pain in her leg promptly relieved with antiinflammatory drugs. **(A)** Lateral radiograph shows a fusiform thickening of the anterior cortex of the tibia *(arrows)* associated with barely visible oval radiolucency *(arrowhead)*. **(B)** Radionuclide technetium bone scan shows typical for osteoid osteoma double density sign: markedly increased uptake of the radiopharmaceutical tracer in the center *(arrow)* corresponding to the nidus and only slightly increased uptake at the periphery of the lesion *(arrowheads)*, corresponding to reactive sclerosis. **(C)** Axial and **(D)** sagittal reformatted CT sections clearly demonstrate the nidus of osteoid osteoma in the anterior tibial cortex *(arrow)*. **(E)** Sagittal T1-weighted fat-suppressed MR image obtained after intravenous administration of gadolinium shows high–signal intensity nidus *(arrow)*.

FIGURE 17.19 **Pathology of osteoid osteoma.** Gross specimen shows well-circumscribed nidus *(arrow)* exhibiting a hypervascular zone with surrounding sclerotic rim *(arrowheads)*. (Reprinted with permission from Greenspan A, Borys D. *Radiology and pathology correlation of bone tumors: a quick reference and review*. Philadelphia: Wolters Kluwer; 2016:39.)

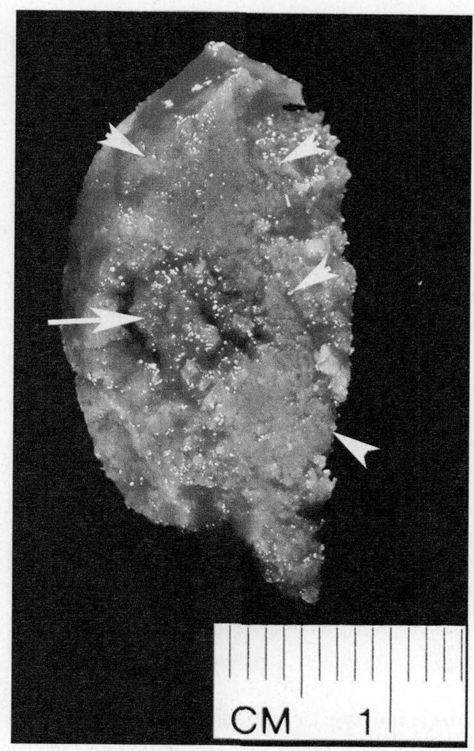

FIGURE 17.20 **Differential diagnosis of (A) cortical and (B) medullary osteoid osteoma.**

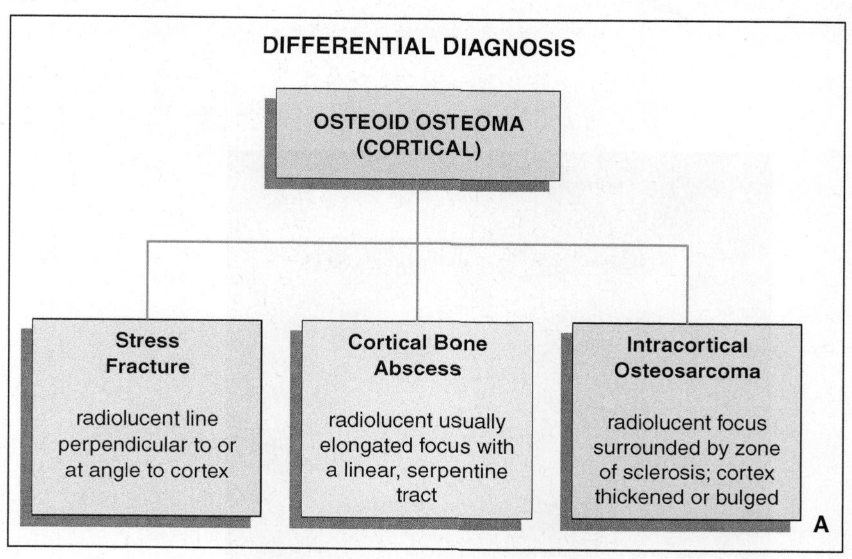

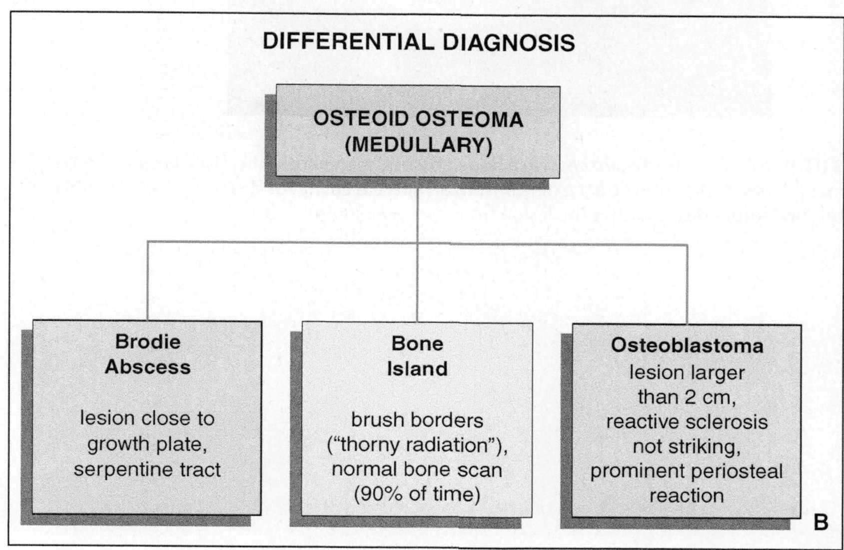

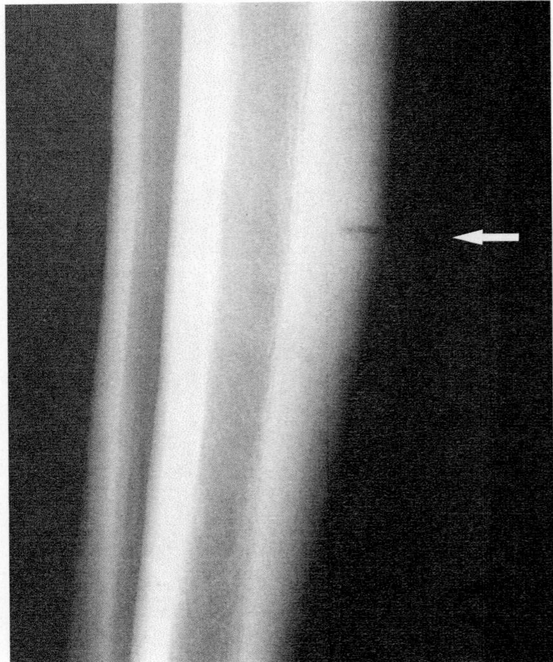

FIGURE 17.21 **Stress fracture.** Lateral radiograph demonstrates a stress fracture of the tibia *(arrow)*. Note the perpendicular direction of the radiolucency to the long axis of the tibial cortex. In osteoid osteoma, the radiolucent nidus is oriented parallel to the cortex.

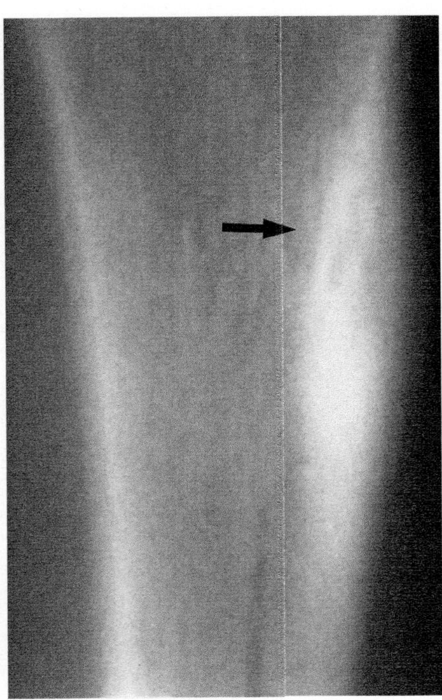

FIGURE 17.22 **Cortical abscess.** Lateral tomogram of the tibia shows a radiolucent, serpentine tract of a cortical bone abscess *(arrow)* that was originally misdiagnosed as osteoid osteoma. (Reprinted with permission from Greenspan A, Jundt G, Remagen W. *Differential diagnosis in orthopaedic oncology*, 2nd ed. Philadelphia: Lippincott Williams & Wilkins; 2007:70, Fig. 2.44.)

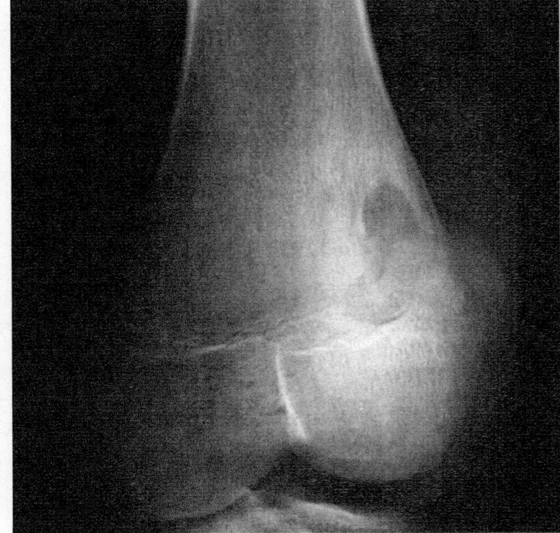

FIGURE 17.23 **Brodie abscess.** In a bone abscess, seen here in the distal femoral metaphysis, a serpentine tract extends from an abscess cavity toward the growth plate. This feature distinguishes the lesion from osteoid osteoma.

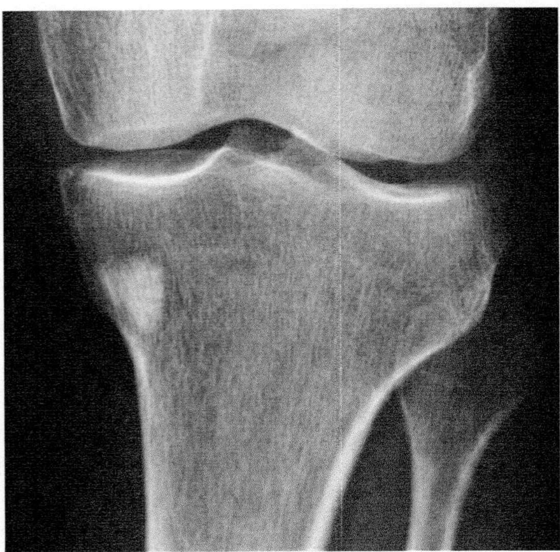

FIGURE 17.24 **Enostosis.** A bone island in the medial aspect of the proximal tibia exhibits the brush borders characteristic of this lesion.

TABLE 17.2 Differential Diagnosis of Osteoid Osteoma

Condition (Lesion)	Imaging Features
Cortical osteoid osteoma	Radiolucent nidus, round or elliptical, surrounded by radiodense reactive sclerosis; solid or laminated (but not interrupted) periosteal reaction; scintigraphy invariably shows increased uptake of radiotracer; "double-density" sign
Medullary osteoid osteoma	Radiolucent (or with central calcification) nidus, without or with only minimal perinidal sclerosis; usually no or only minimal periosteal reaction; scintigraphy—as above
Subperiosteal osteoid osteoma	Radiolucent or sclerotic nidus with or without reactive sclerosis; occasionally shaggy, crescent-like focus of periosteal reaction; scintigraphy—increased uptake of radiotracer
Intracapsular (periarticular) osteoid osteoma	Periarticular osteoporosis; premature onset of osteoarthritis; nidus may or may not be visualized; scintigraphy—as above
Osteoblastoma	Radiolucent lesion more than 2 cm, frequently with central opacities; perilesional sclerosis less intense than in osteoid osteoma; abundant periosteal reaction; scintigraphy—as above
Stress fracture (cortical)	Linear radiolucency runs perpendicular or at an angle to the cortex; scintigraphy—increased uptake of radiotracer
Bone abscess (Brodie)	Irregular in outline radiolucency, usually with a sclerotic rim, commonly associated with serpentine or linear tract; predilection for metaphysis and the ends of tubular bones; scintigraphy—increased uptake of radiotracer; MRI—on T1-weighted image a well-defined low-to-intermediate signal lesion outlined by a low-intensity rim; on T2-weighted image a very bright homogeneous signal, outlined by a low-signal rim
Bone island (enostosis)	Homogeneously dense, sclerotic focus in cancellous bone with distinctive radiating streaks (thorny radiation) that blend with the trabeculae of the host bone; scintigraphy—usually no increased uptake; MRI—low-intensity signal on T1- and T2-weighted images
Intracortical osteosarcoma	Intracortical radiolucent focus surrounded by zone of sclerosis; occasionally central "fluffy" densities; cortex thickened or bulged; scintigraphy—increased uptake of radiotracer

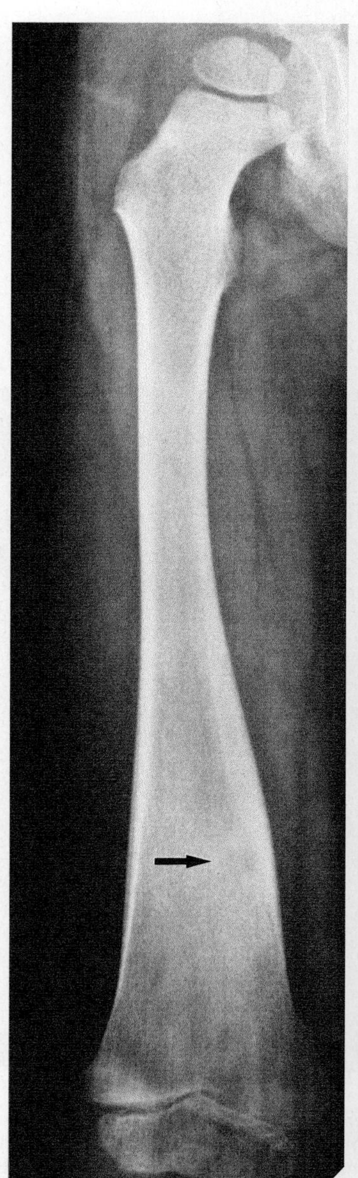

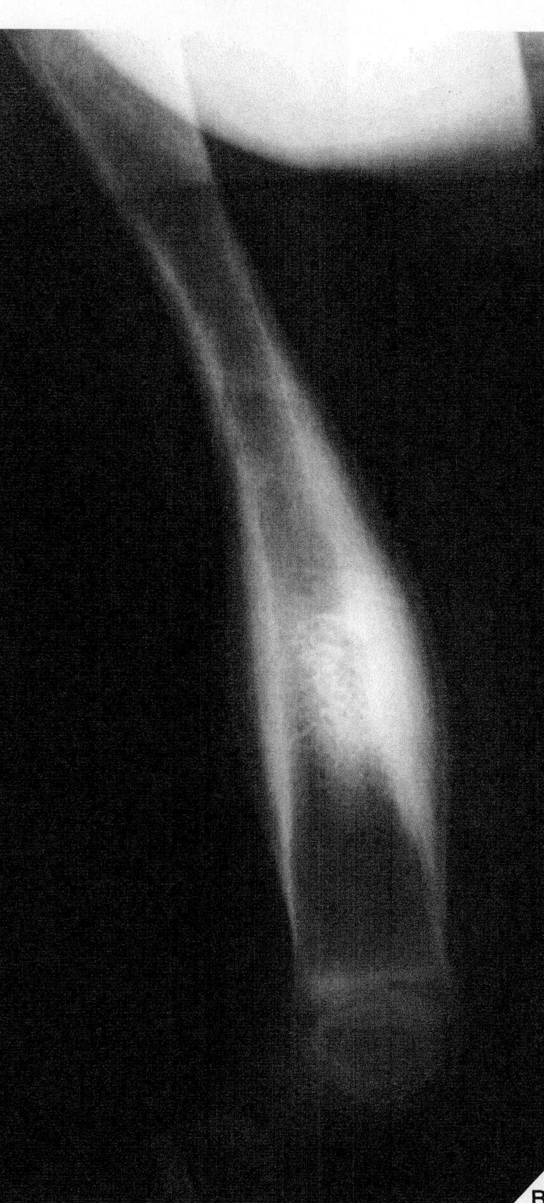

FIGURE 17.25 Complication of osteoid osteoma. **(A)** A 2-year-old boy has been diagnosed with an osteoid osteoma of the distal femoral diaphysis *(arrow)*. The proximity of the nidus to the growth plate caused accelerated growth of the bone, with marked widening of the distal femoral diaphysis. **(B)** In another patient, a 7-year-old girl with the lesion in the distal femur, note marked widening of the femoral diaphysis and hypertrophy of the anteromedial cortex.

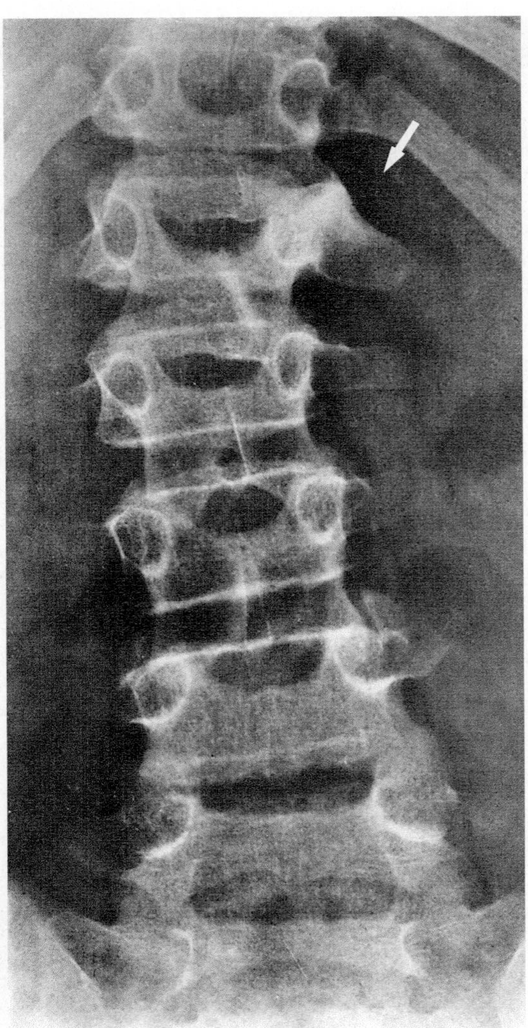

FIGURE 17.26 Complication of osteoid osteoma. Anteroposterior radiograph of the spine shows an osteoid osteoma in the left pedicle of L1 *(arrow)* in a 12-year-old boy. Note the shallow-curve scoliosis, with concavity directed toward the lesion.

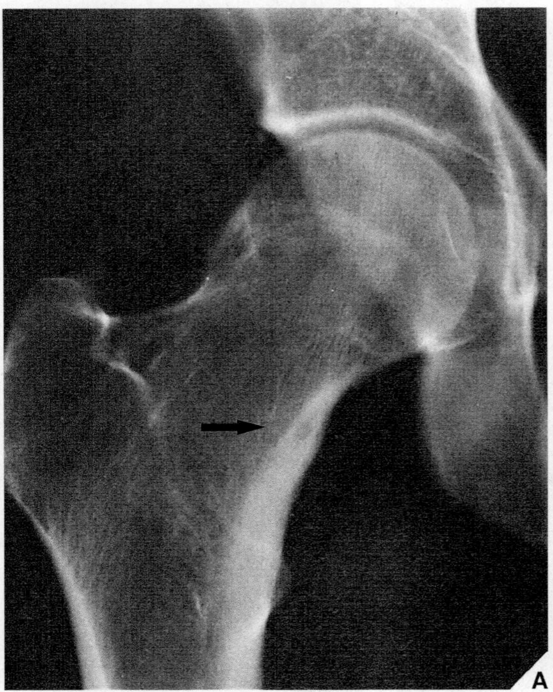

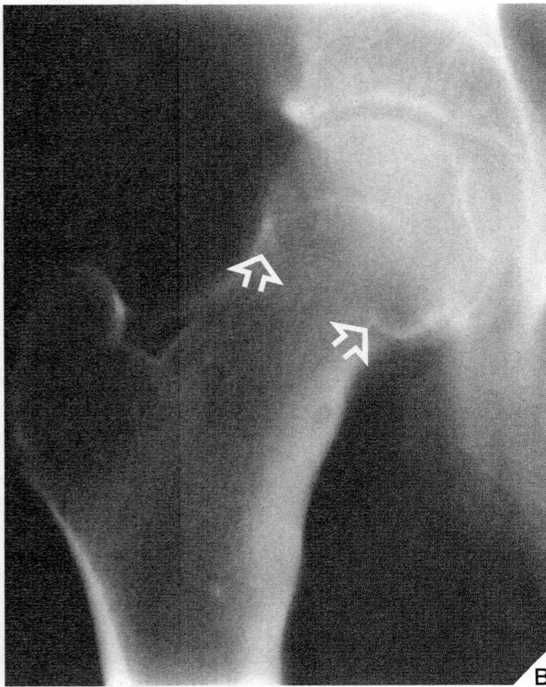

FIGURE 17.27 Complication of osteoid osteoma. **(A)** Anteroposterior radiograph of the right hip demonstrates an intracapsular osteoid osteoma located in the medial aspect of the neck of the right femur *(arrow)* in a 28-year-old man. **(B)** Tomographic cut shows the early changes of osteoarthritis. Note a collar osteophyte *(open arrows)* and slight narrowing of the weight-bearing segment of the hip joint. A radionuclide bone scan (not shown here) demonstrated an increased uptake not only at the site of the lesion but also at the site of the reactive bone formation resulting from the osteoarthritis.

FIGURE 17.28 **Complication of osteoid osteoma.** A 14-year-old boy presented with pain in the left hip for 8 months; it was more severe at night and was relieved by antiinflammatory medications within 15 to 20 minutes. Several previous radiographic examinations, including computed tomographic scans, had failed to demonstrate the nidus. A frog-lateral view shows evidence of periarticular osteoporosis and early degenerative changes *(arrows)*, both presumptive features of osteoid osteoma.

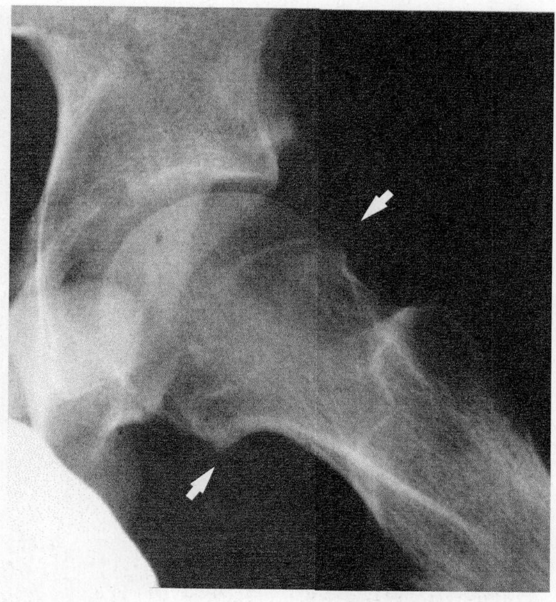

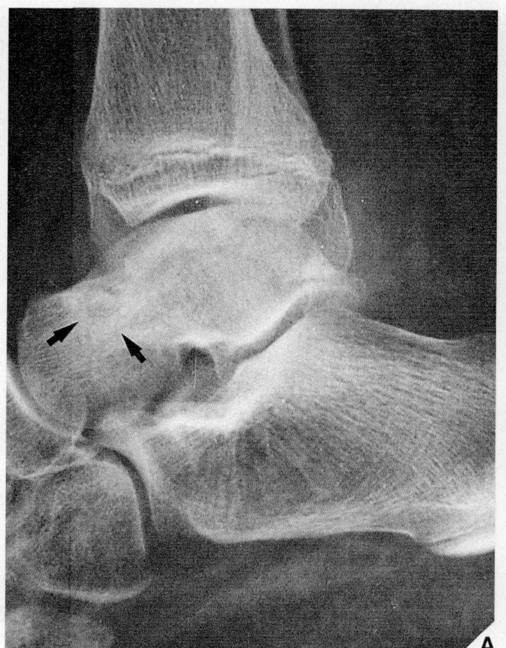

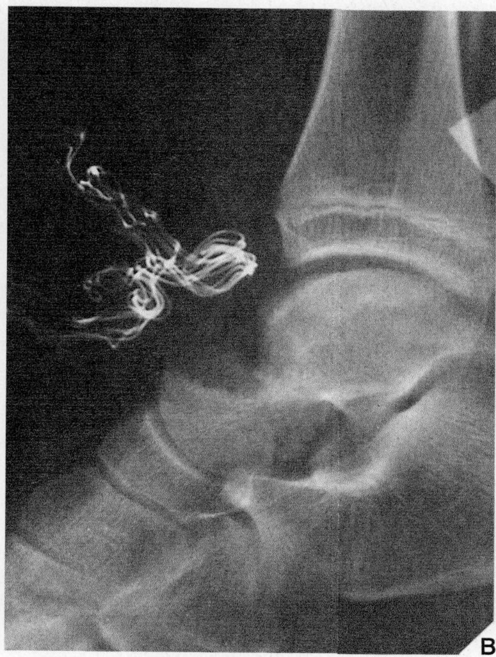

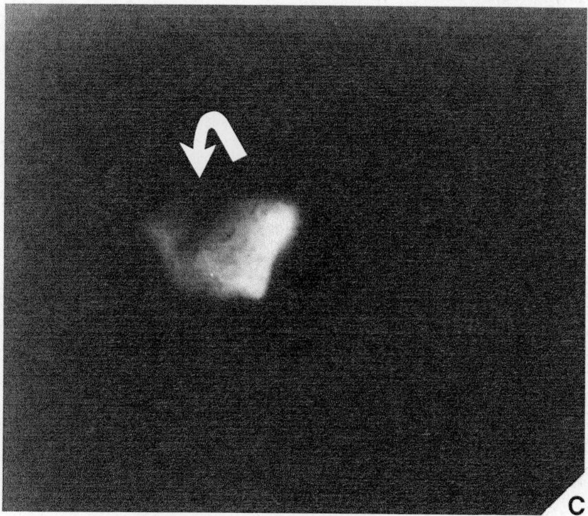

FIGURE 17.29 **Surgical treatment of osteoid osteoma.** **(A)** Preoperative lateral radiograph of the ankle of a 13-year-old boy demonstrates the nidus of osteoid osteoma in the talar bone *(arrows)*. Intraoperative films demonstrate the area of resection **(B)** and the resected specimen **(C)**, confirming that the lesion *(curved arrow)* was totally excised.

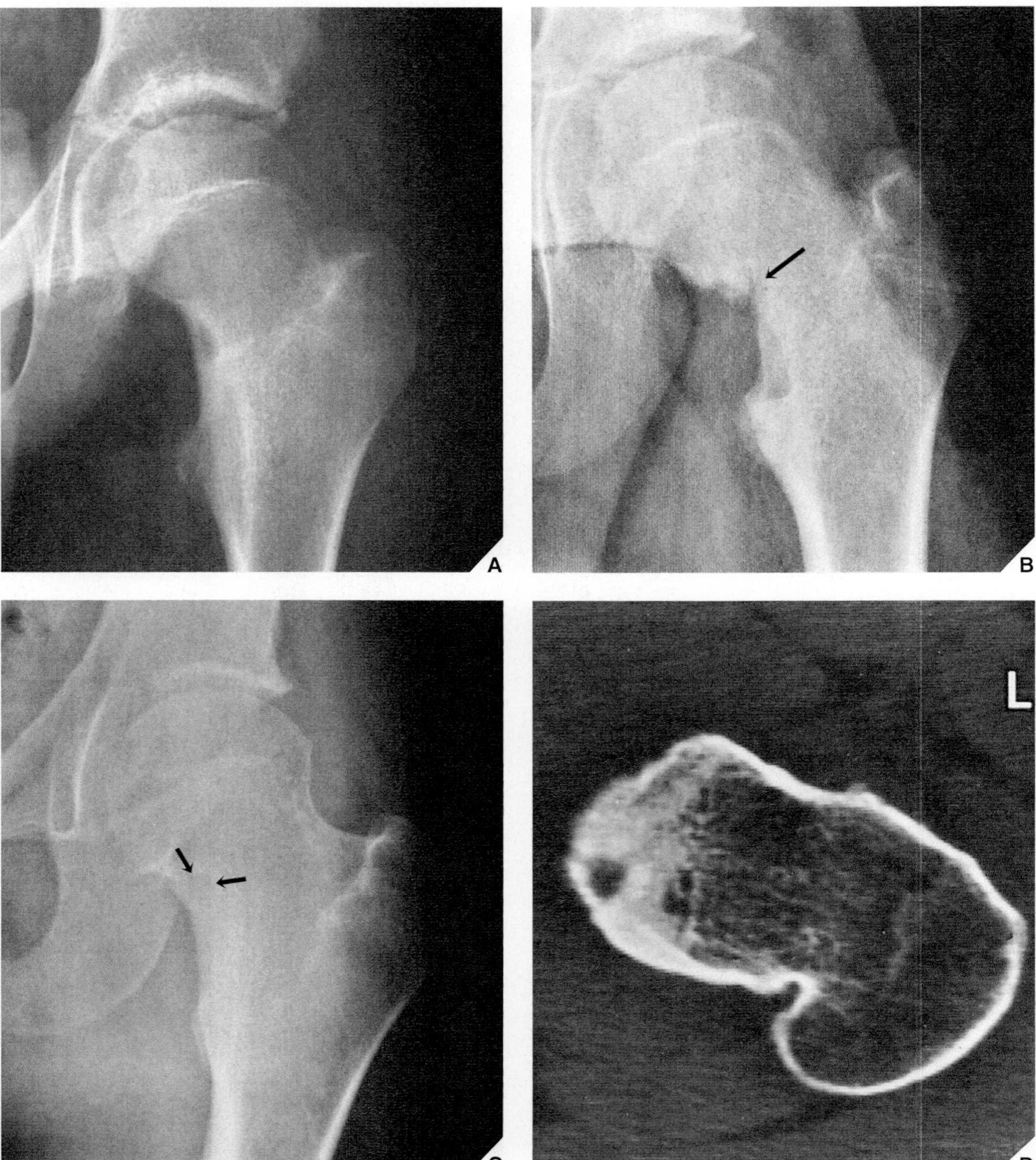

FIGURE 17.30 Recurrence of osteoid osteoma. **(A)** Anteroposterior radiograph of the left hip in a 17-year-old boy with pain in the left groin relieved promptly by salicylates demonstrates a nidus of osteoid osteoma in the medial cortex of the femoral neck. **(B)** The lesion was incompletely resected; note its remnants *(arrow)*. Two years later, the symptoms recurred. **(C)** Follow-up radiograph shows a radiolucent area in the medial femoral cortex *(arrows)*, and a CT section **(D)** demonstrates the nidus.

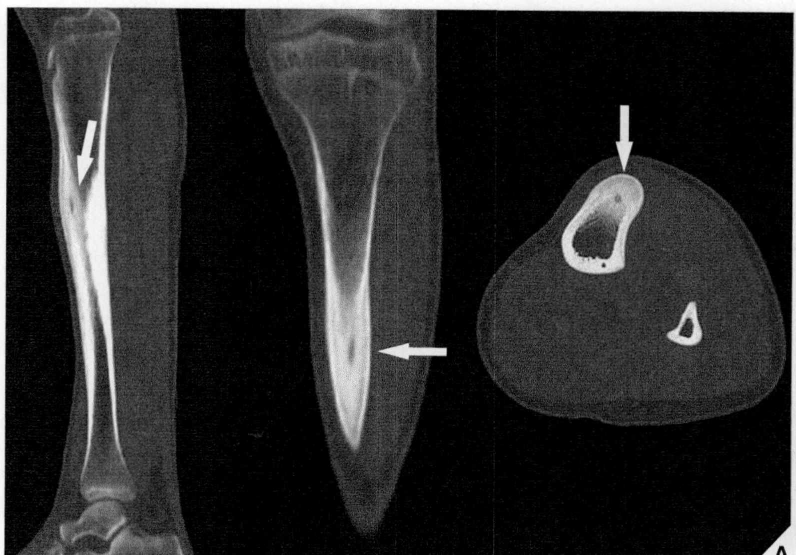

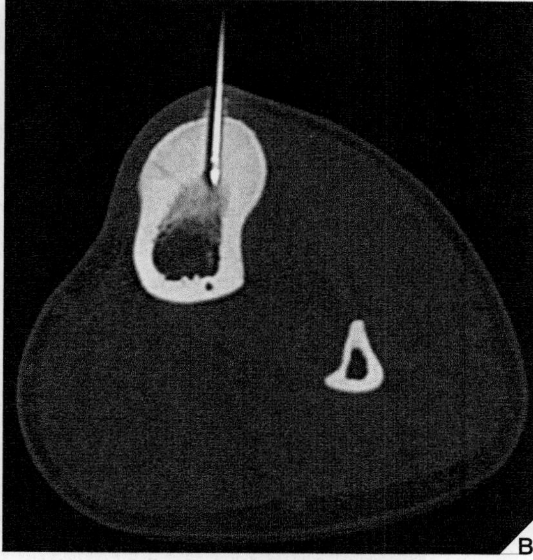

FIGURE 17.31 **CT-guided percutaneous radiofrequency ablation of osteoid osteoma.** **(A)** Sagittal, coronal, and axial CT images show a lesion in the anterior cortex of tibia *(arrows)*. **(B)** Axial CT image obtained during interventional procedure confirms the proper placement of the probe within the nidus of osteoid osteoma.

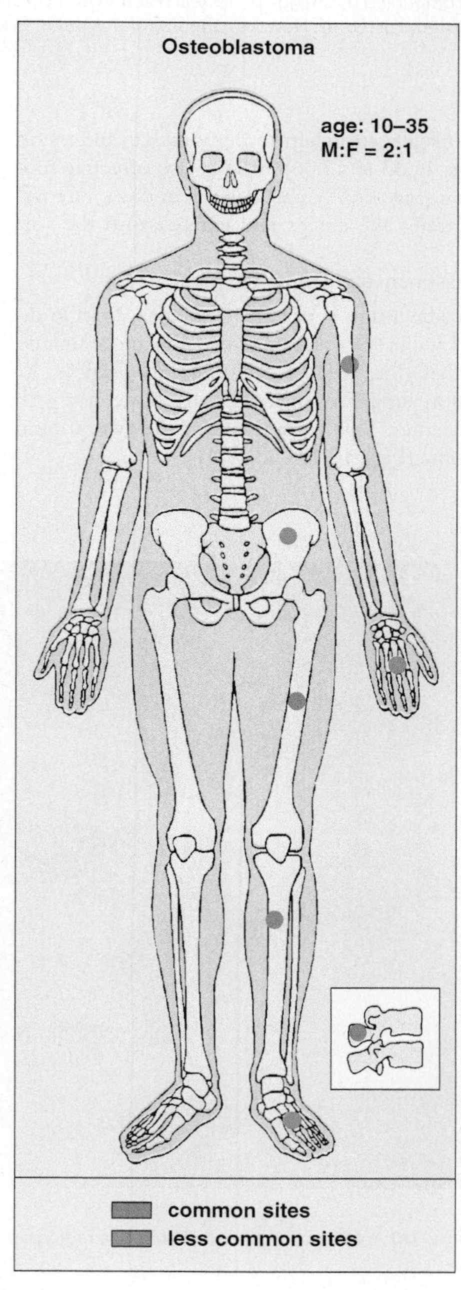

FIGURE 17.32 **Skeletal sites of predilection, peak age range, and male-to-female ratio in osteoblastoma.**

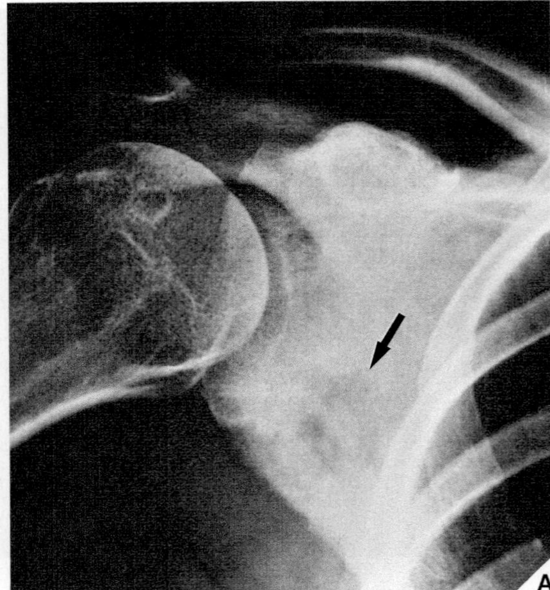
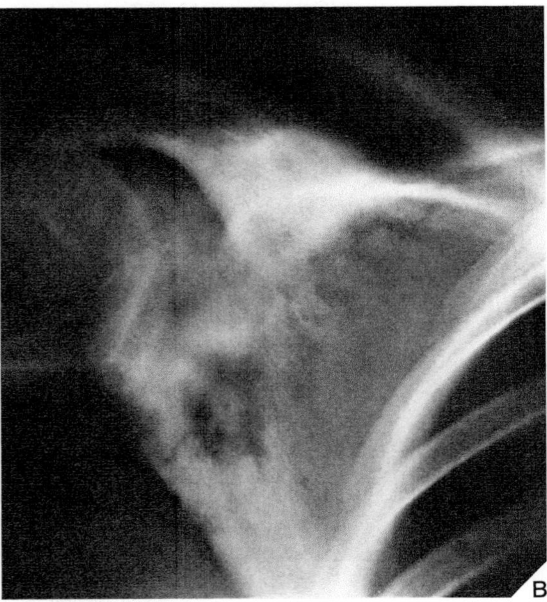

FIGURE 17.33 Osteoblastoma. **(A)** Anteroposterior radiograph of the right shoulder of a 28-year-old woman shows a faint radiolucent focus in the scapula *(arrow)* surrounded by a sclerotic area, accompanied by shaggy periosteal reaction at the axillary border. **(B)** Conventional tomogram clearly demonstrates a radiolucent nidus with a sclerotic border, resembling an osteoid osteoma. However, the size of this lesion (3 × 3 cm) marks it as an osteoblastoma, a diagnosis proved by excision biopsy.

Radiography and CT are usually sufficient to demonstrate the lesion and suggest the diagnosis (Figs. 17.33 to 17.36). MRI is also effective modality to demonstrate this lesion (Fig. 17.37), particularly on those rare occasions when the tumor penetrates the cortex and extends into the soft tissues (Fig. 17.38).

Osteoblastoma has four distinctive radiographic presentations:

1. A giant osteoid osteoma. The lesion is usually more than 2 cm in diameter and exhibits less reactive sclerosis and a possibly more prominent periosteal response than does osteoid osteoma (Fig. 17.39).
2. A blow-out expansive lesion similar to an aneurysmal bone cyst with small radiopacities in the center. This pattern is particularly common in lesions involving the spine (Figs. 17.40 and 17.41).
3. An aggressive lesion simulating a malignant tumor (Fig. 17.42)
4. Periosteal lesion that lacks perifocal bone sclerosis but exhibits a thin shell of newly formed periosteal bone (Figs. 17.43 and 17.44)

Pathology

Histopathologic differentiation between osteoid osteoma and osteoblastoma can be very difficult, and in a considerable number of patients, it can be impossible. Both are osteoid-producing lesions, but in the typical osteoblastoma, the bone trabeculae are broader and longer and seem less densely packed and less coherent than those in osteoid osteoma. Some authorities believe that because of its striking histologic similarity to osteoid osteoma, osteoblastoma represents a variant of clinical expression of the same pathologic process.

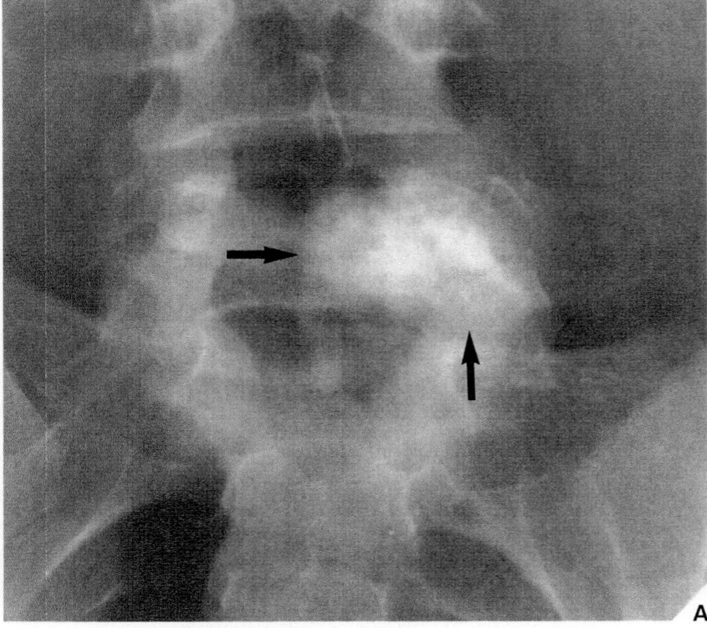
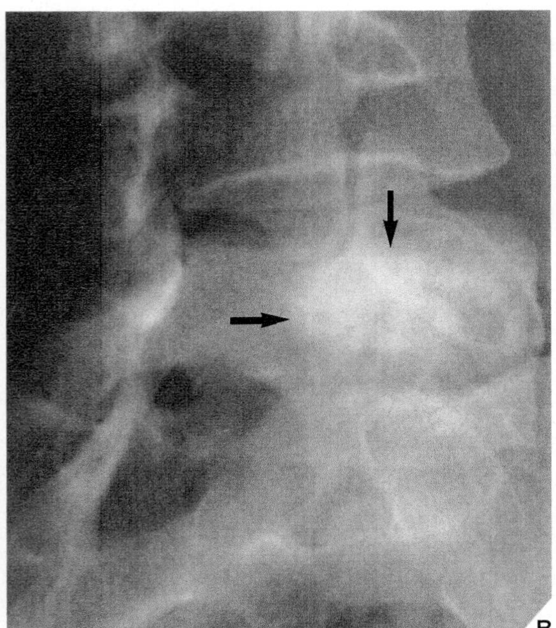

FIGURE 17.34 Osteoblastoma. **(A)** Anteroposterior and **(B)** oblique radiographs of the lumbosacral spine of an 18-year-old man show an expansive lesion in the left pedicle and lamina of L5 *(arrows)*.

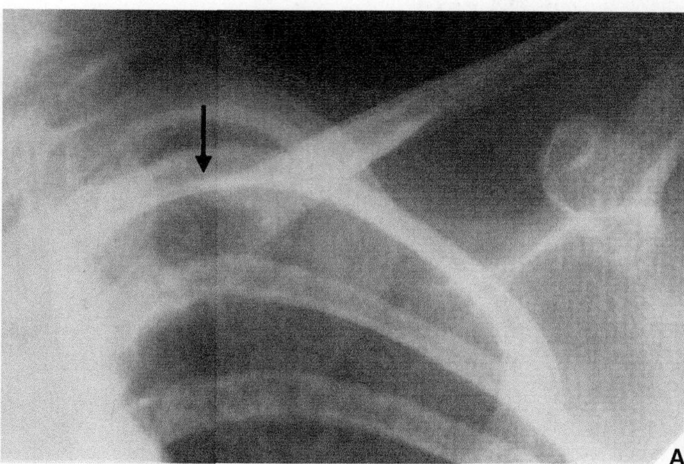

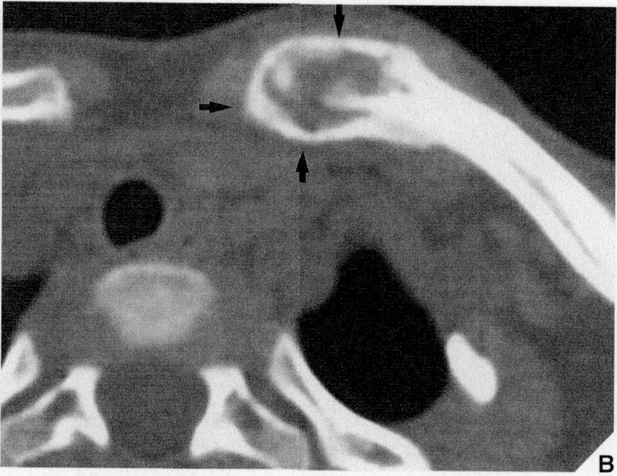

FIGURE 17.35 CT of osteoblastoma. **(A)** Conventional radiograph shows a radiolucent lesion in the sternal end of the left clavicle *(arrow)*. **(B)** Axial CT image demonstrates an expansive low-attenuation tumor *(arrows)* with high-attenuation foci of new bone formation. (Reprinted with permission from Greenspan A, Jundt G, Remagen W. *Differential diagnosis in orthopaedic oncology*, 2nd ed. Philadelphia: Lippincott Williams & Wilkins; 2007:59–74.)

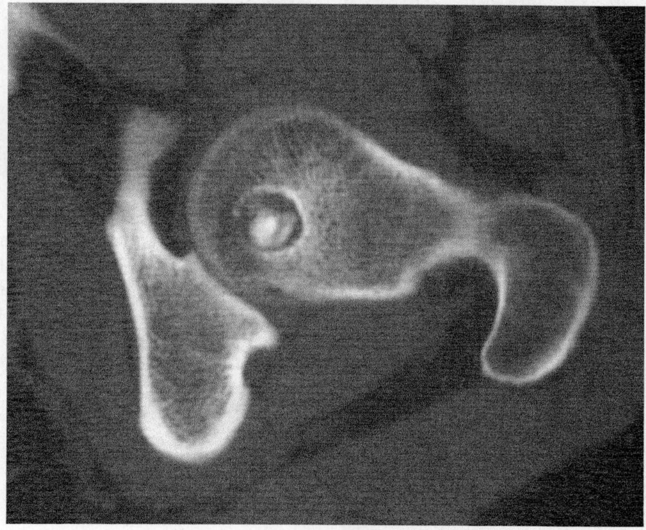

FIGURE 17.36 CT of osteoblastoma. Axial CT image of the left hip of a 20-year-old man shows a low-attenuated lesion with sclerotic center within the femoral head, measuring 2.75 cm. (Reprinted with permission from Greenspan A, Borys D. *Radiology and pathology correlation of bone tumors: a quick reference and review*. Philadelphia: Wolters Kluwer; 2016:44.)

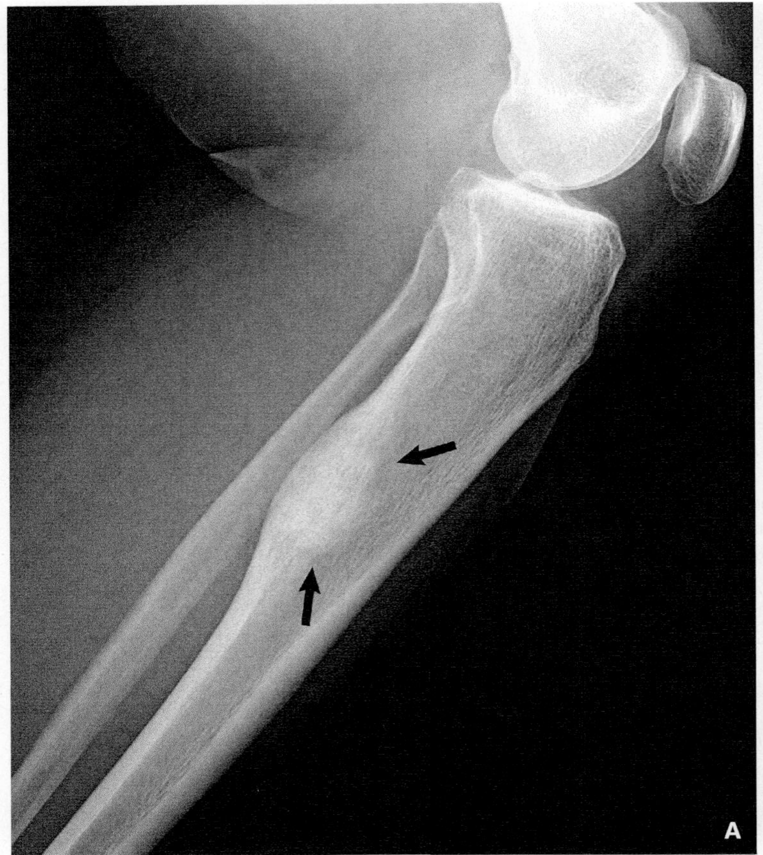

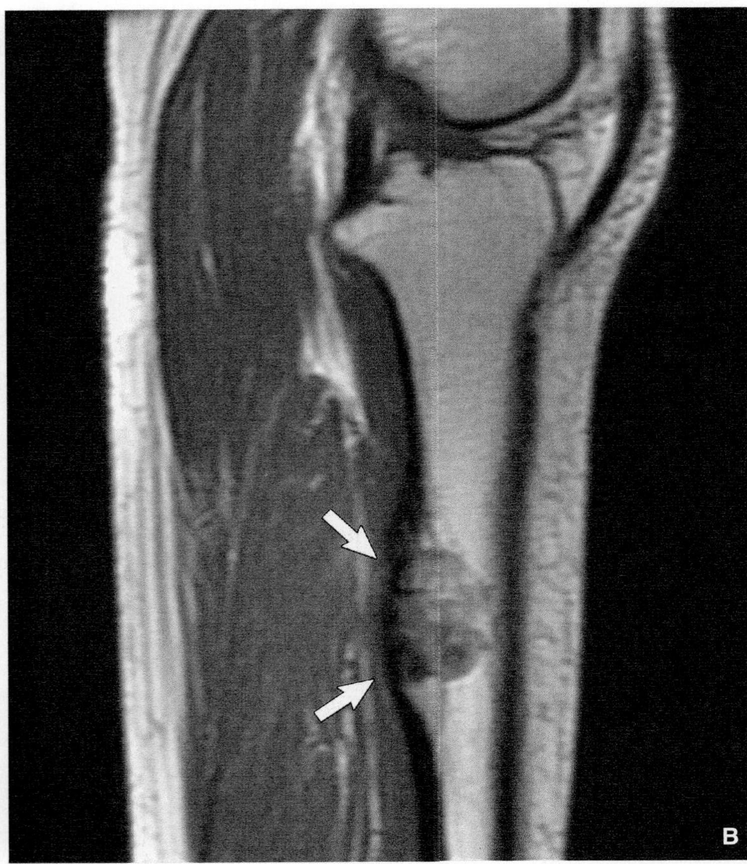

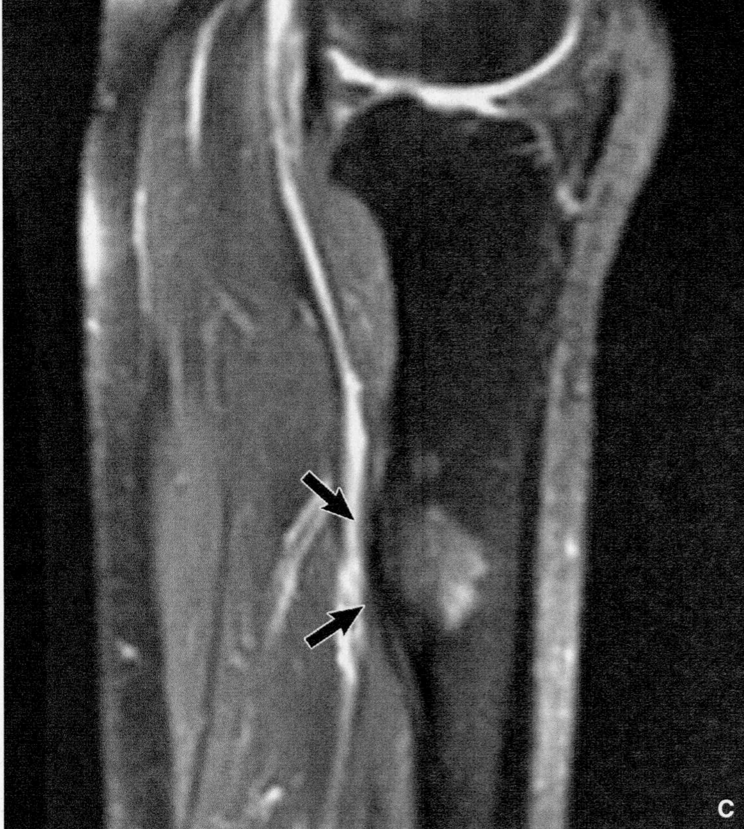

FIGURE 17.37 MRI of osteoblastoma. **(A)** Lateral radiograph of the leg of a 32-year-old woman shows a radiodense lesion with narrow zone of transition in the posterior aspect of proximal tibial shaft *(arrows)*. **(B)** Sagittal T1-weighted MR image demonstrates an intermediate– to low–signal intensity lesion with sharply defined borders, well demarcated from the normal bone *(arrows)*. **(C)** Sagittal T1-weighted fat-suppressed MR image obtained after intravenous administration of gadolinium shows prominent enhancement of the lesion *(arrows)*.

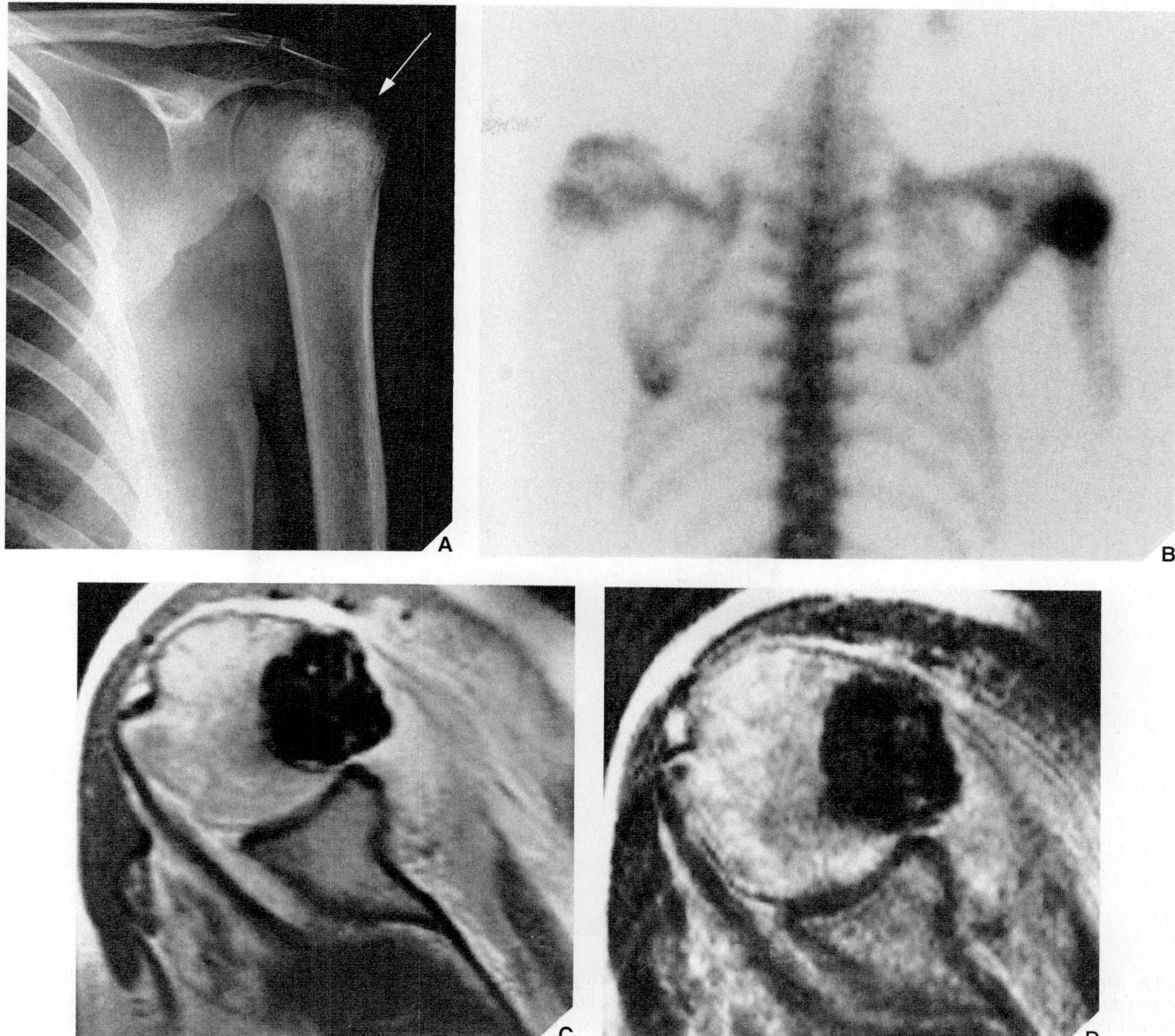

FIGURE 17.38 Scintigraphy and MRI of osteoblastoma. A 15-year-old girl presented with pain in her left shoulder. **(A)** Conventional radiograph demonstrates a sharply demarcated sclerotic lesion in the proximal metaphysis of the left humerus abutting the growth plate *(arrow)*. **(B)** Radionuclide bone scan obtained after injection of 15 mCi (555 MBq) of technetium-99m (^{99m}Tc)-labeled MDP shows an increased uptake of radiopharmaceutical tracer localized to the site of the lesion. **(C)** Axial spin echo T1-weighted MR image (repetition time [TR] 700/echo time [TE] 20 msec) demonstrates that the lesion is located posteromedially in the humeral head. The cortex is destroyed, and the tumor extends into the soft tissues. **(D)** Axial spin echo T2-weighted MR image (TR 2200/TE 60 msec) shows that the lesion remains of low signal intensity, indicating osseous matrix. The rim of high signal intensity adjacent to the posterolateral margin of the tumor reflects peritumoral edema.

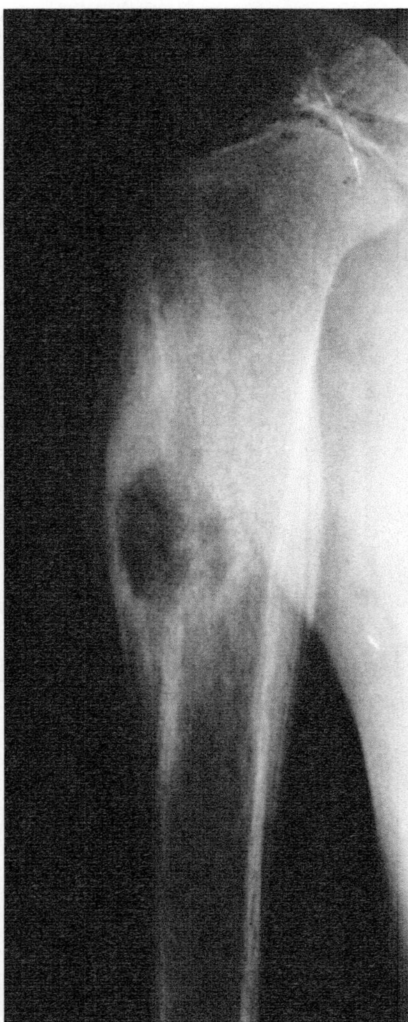

FIGURE 17.39 **Osteoblastoma.** Osteoblastoma in the proximal humerus of this 8-year-old boy is similar to the lesion of osteoid osteoma. This lesion, however, is larger (2.5 cm in its largest dimension), and there is a more pronounced periosteal response in the medial and lateral humeral cortices. Conversely, the extent of reactive bone surrounding the radiolucent nidus is less than that usually seen in osteoid osteoma. This type of osteoblastoma is frequently called a *giant osteoid osteoma*.

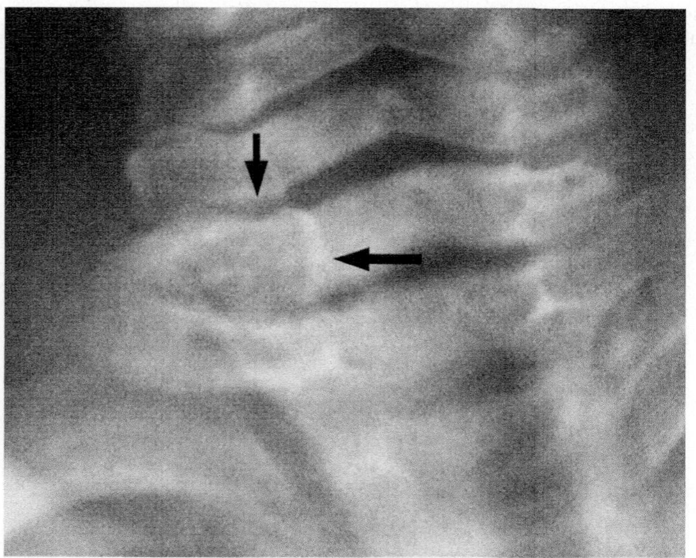

FIGURE 17.40 **Conventional tomography of osteoblastoma.** Tomographic section of the cervical spine shows an expanding, blow-out lesion of osteoblastoma, with several small central opacities, in the lamina of C6 *(arrows)*.

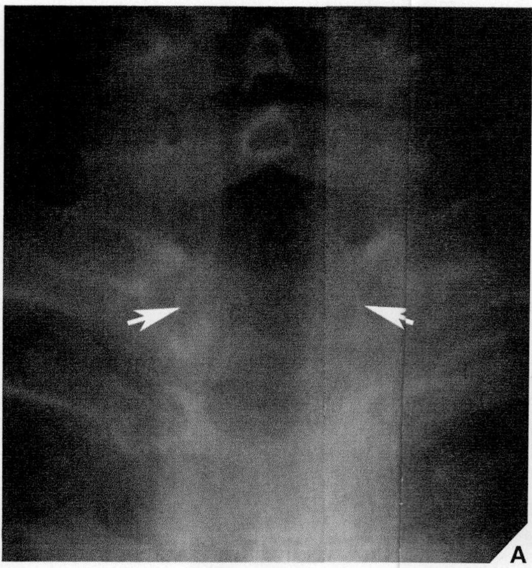

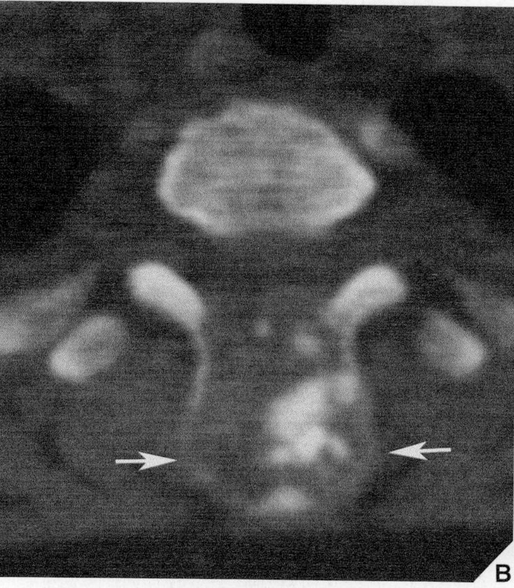

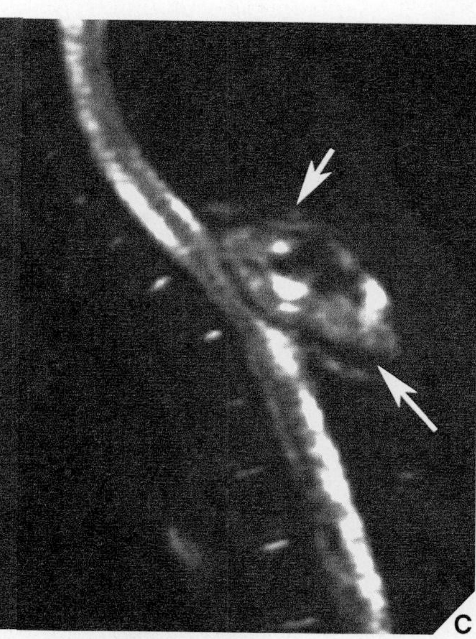

FIGURE 17.41 **MRI of osteoblastoma in the spine.** **(A)** Anteroposterior radiograph of the upper thoracic spine of a 19-year-old woman demonstrates expansion of the spinous process of T1 *(arrows)*. **(B)** Axial CT section confirms the expansion of the spinous process of T1 *(arrows)* and, in addition, shows matrix calcification within the tumor. **(C)** Sagittal T2-weighted MRI demonstrates the expanded spinous process *(arrows)* and the low signal areas within the tumor corresponding to the calcified matrix seen on CT section. Note the compression of the posterior aspect of the spinal cord by the tumor.

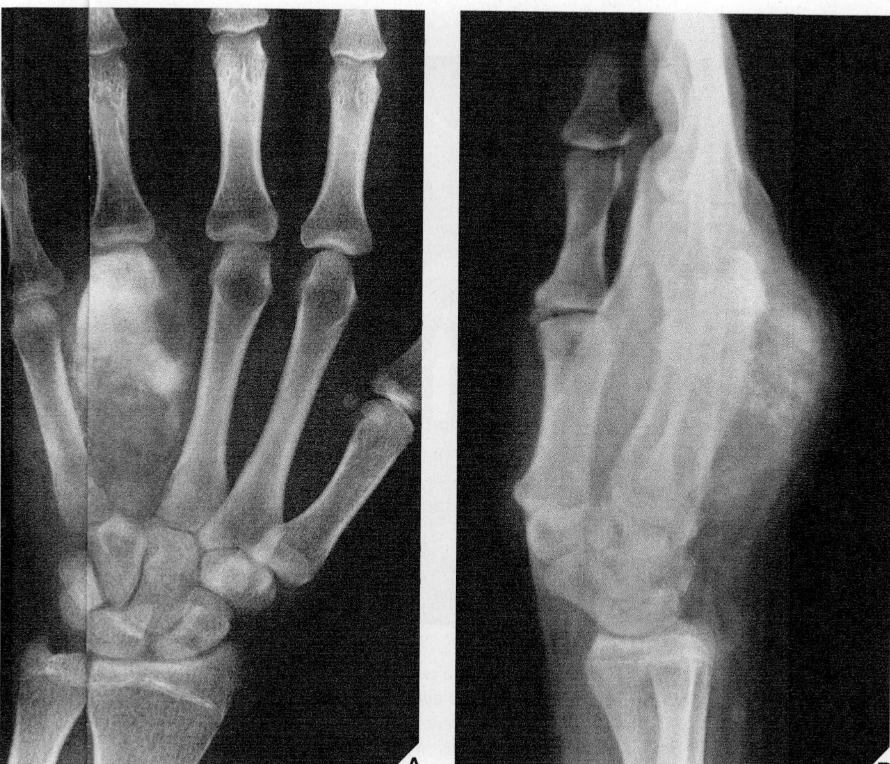

FIGURE 17.42 **Aggressive osteoblastoma.** **(A)** Dorsovolar and **(B)** lateral radiographs of the hand demonstrate an aggressive osteoblastoma. Note the destruction of the entire fourth metacarpal with massive bone formation, particularly in the distal portion. Although very similar in appearance to osteosarcoma, the lesion still appears to be contained by a shell of periosteal new bone formation.

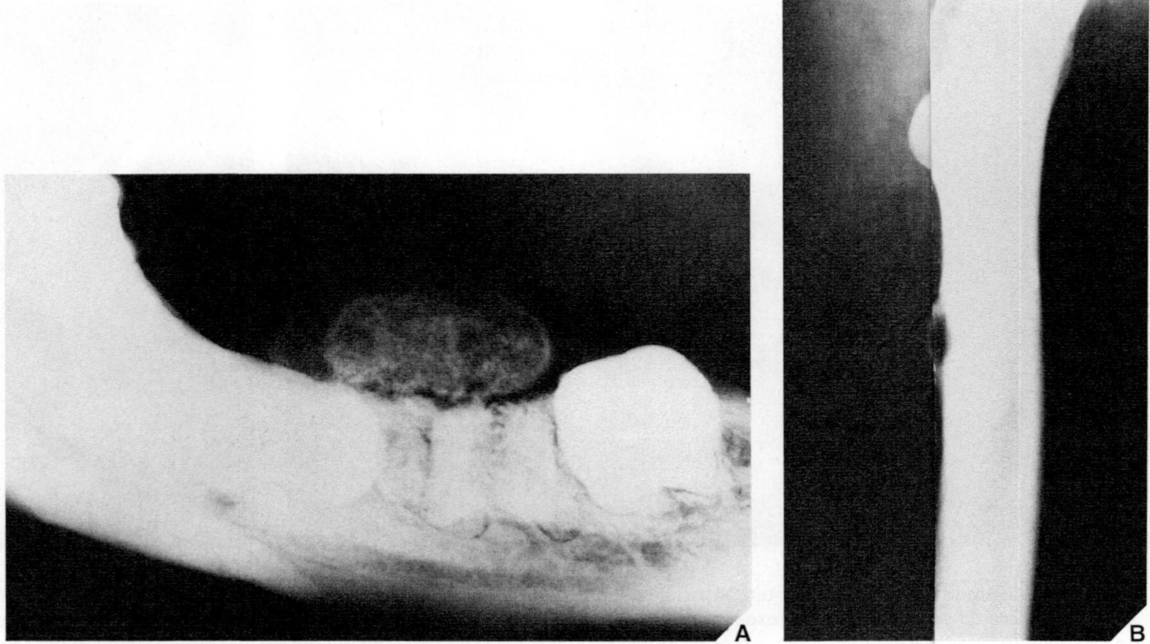

FIGURE 17.43 Periosteal osteoblastoma. **(A)** Periosteal osteoblastoma of the mandible and **(B)** periosteal osteoblastoma of the femur are covered by a thin shell of a new periosteal bone. (Courtesy of Prof. Wolfgang Remagen, Cologne, Germany.)

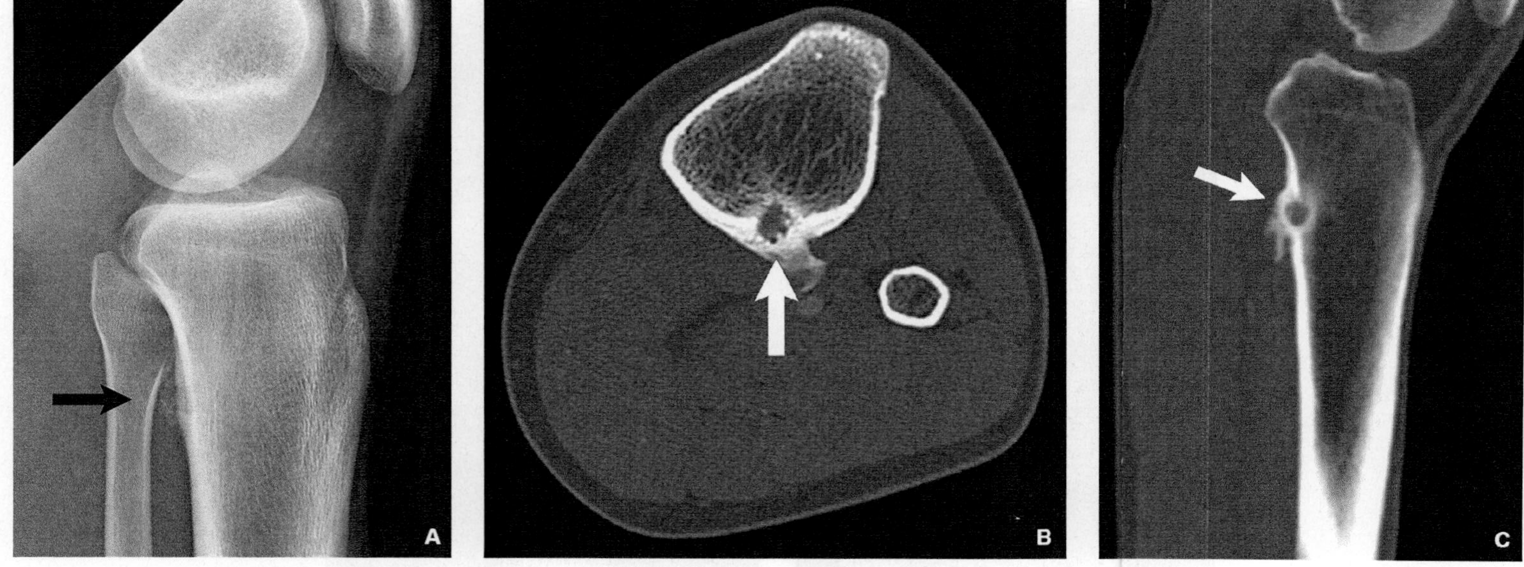

FIGURE 17.44 CT of periosteal osteoblastoma. **(A)** Lateral radiograph shows a periosteal lesion located in the posterior aspect of proximal tibia *(arrow)*. **(B)** Axial and **(C)** sagittal reformatted CT images show the lesion to invade the endocortex and to evoke the periosteal reaction *(arrows)*. (Reprinted with permission from Greenspan A, Borys D. *Radiology and pathology correlation of bone tumors: a quick reference and review*. Philadelphia: Wolters Kluwer; 2016:4-44.)

TABLE 17.3 Differential Diagnosis of Osteoblastoma

Condition (Lesion)	Imaging Features
Cortical and medullary osteoid osteoma–like osteoblastoma (giant osteoid osteoma)	Radiolucent lesion, spherical or oval, with well-defined margins; frequent perilesional sclerosis; abundant periosteal reaction; size of the nidus greater than 2 cm
Aneurysmal bone cyst-like expansive osteoblastoma	Blow-out lesion, similar to aneurysmal bone cyst, but with central opacities
Aggressive osteoblastoma (simulating malignant neoplasm)	Ill-defined borders, destruction of the cortex; aggressive-looking periosteal reaction; occasionally soft-tissue extension
Periosteal osteoblastoma	Round or ovoid heterogeneous in density mass attached to cortex, covered by shell of periosteal new bone
Osteoid osteoma	Radiolucent nidus ≤1.5 cm, occasionally with a sclerotic center
Aneurysmal bone cyst	Blow-out, expansive lesion; in long bone buttress of periosteal reaction; thin shell of reactive bone frequently covers the lesion but may be absent in rapidly growing lesions; soft-tissue extension may be present.
Enchondroma	Radiolucent lesion with or without sclerotic border, frequently displaying central calcifications in the form of dots, rings, and arcs
Osteosarcoma	Permeative or moth-eaten bone destruction; wide zone of transition; tumor-bone in form of cloud-like opacities; aggressive periosteal reaction; soft-tissue mass

Differential Diagnosis

The differential radiologic diagnosis of osteoblastoma should include an osteoid osteoma, a bone abscess, an aneurysmal bone cyst, an enchondroma, and an osteosarcoma (Table 17.3). A bone abscess is usually marked by a serpentine tract (see Figs. 17.22 and 17.23) or it is seen to cross the growth plate (Fig. 17.45), phenomena almost never seen in osteoblastoma. An aneurysmal bone cyst occasionally can assume a similar appearance to osteoblastoma but lacks central radiopacities. An enchondroma will usually display a calcified matrix assuming the form of dots, rings, and arcs. In addition, unless there has been a pathologic fracture, an enchondroma (see Figs. 18.7 to 18.9), unlike osteoblastoma (Fig. 17.46), does not elicit a periosteal reaction.

Aggressive osteoblastoma should be differentiated from osteosarcoma, for which CT may be helpful. CT may also help in the differential diagnosis of lesions located in complex anatomic regions such as the vertebrae (Fig. 17.47). If there is tumor extension into the thecal sac, MRI may be needed.

Treatment

The treatment for osteoblastoma is similar to that for osteoid osteoma; smaller lesions may be treated with percutaneous RFTA, whereas for larger lesions, *en bloc* resection should be performed. Larger lesions may also require additional bone grafting and internal fixation.

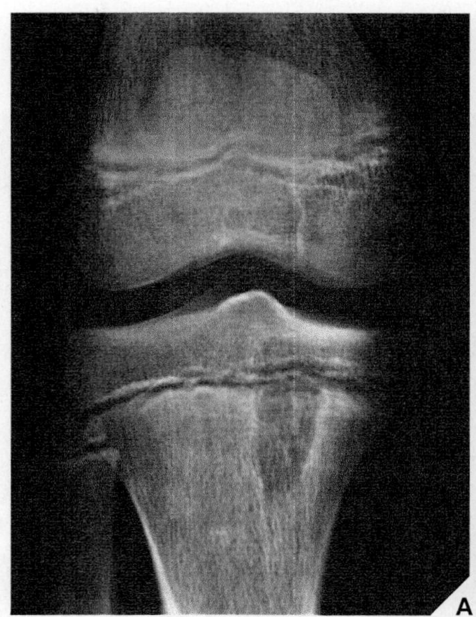

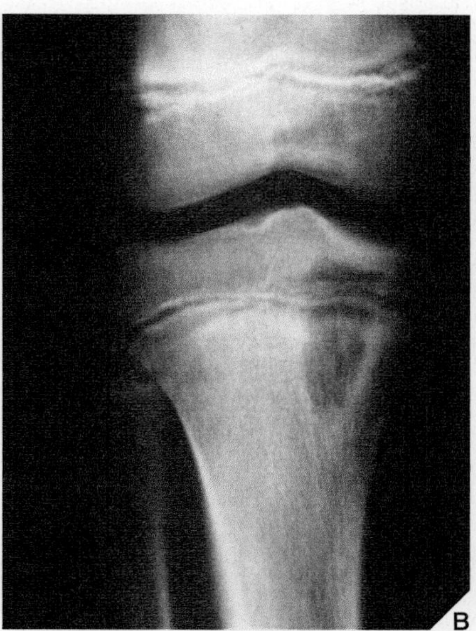

FIGURE 17.45 Brodie abscess. **(A)** Anteroposterior radiograph of the right knee of a 10-year-old boy demonstrates an oval radiolucent lesion abutting and crossing the growth plate of the proximal tibia. **(B)** Confirmation of extension of the lesion into the epiphysis is shown on an anteroposterior tomographic section. The lesion proved to be a bone abscess.

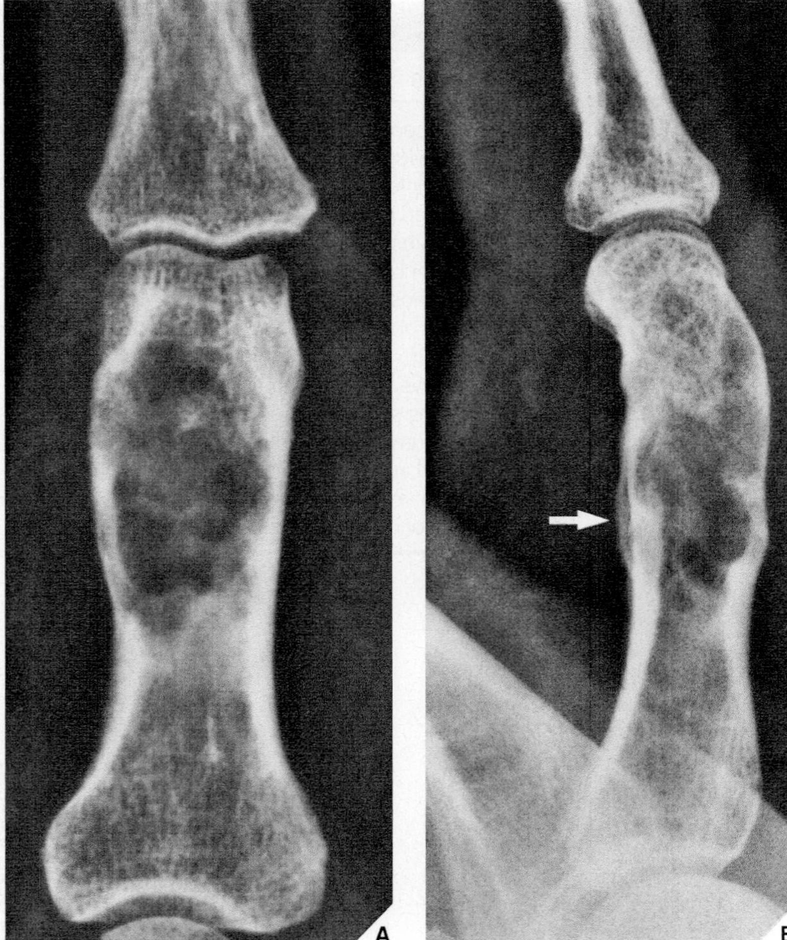

FIGURE 17.46 Osteoblastoma. Dorsovolar **(A)** and lateral **(B)** radiographs of the small finger show enchondroma-like osteoblastoma. Note the periosteal reaction *(arrow)* and lack of chondroid matrix, which are typical of enchondroma. Small radiopacities in the center of the lesion represent bone formation, a characteristic feature of osteoblastoma.

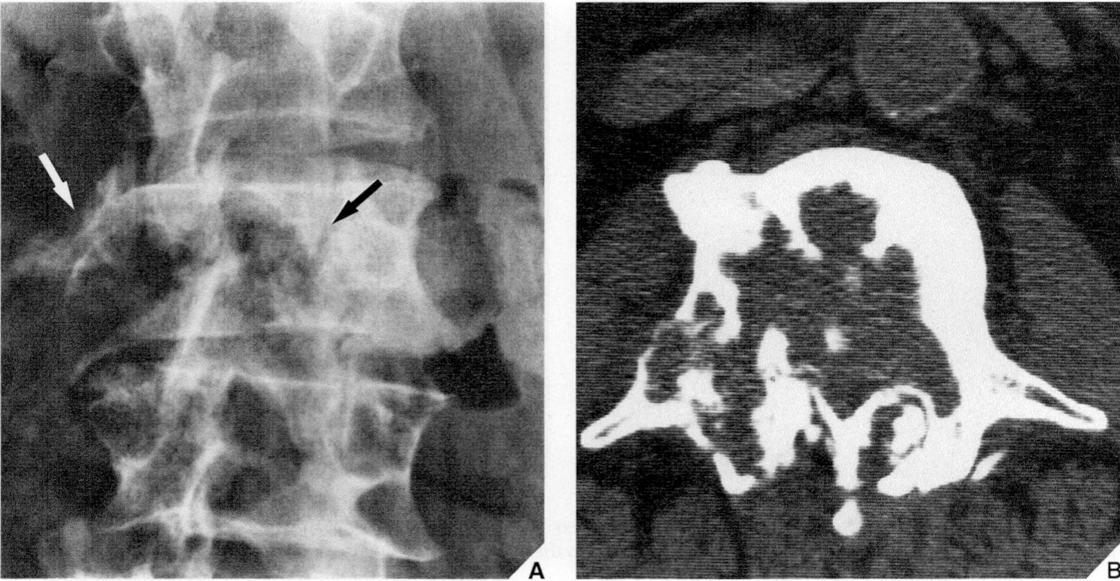

FIGURE 17.47 Aggressive osteoblastoma. **(A)** Anteroposterior radiograph of the lumbar spine shows a destructive lytic lesion affecting the right half of the vertebral body of L3 *(arrows)* in a 65-year-old man who presented with insidious onset of pain in the lower back radiating to the right lower extremity. **(B)** CT section demonstrates focal areas of bone formation within the lesion and invasion of the cortex. Subsequent biopsy revealed an aggressive osteoblastoma. (Courtesy of Ibrahim F. Abdelwahab, MD, New York.)

PRACTICAL POINTS TO REMEMBER

1. Parosteal osteoma, an asymptomatic bone-forming lesion, may be a part of the Gardner syndrome marked by sebaceous cysts, skin fibromas, desmoid tumors, and intestinal polyposis.
2. In the differential diagnosis of parosteal osteoma, the most important entity that needs to be excluded is parosteal osteosarcoma.
3. The most characteristic clinical symptom of osteoid osteoma is pain that is most severe at night and is promptly relieved by antiinflammatory medications.
4. In the radiographic evaluation of osteoid osteoma:
   - the lesion (nidus) consists of a small radiolucent area, sometimes with a sclerotic center; the dense zone surrounding the nidus represents reactive sclerosis, not a tumor
   - the imaging characteristics depend on the location of the lesion: intracortical, intramedullary, subperiosteal, or periarticular (intracapsular)
   - the differential diagnoses of osteoid osteoma should include osteoblastoma, stress fracture, bone abscess (Brodie abscess), bone island, and an intracortical osteosarcoma.
5. The complications of osteoid osteoma include:
   - recurrence of the lesion (if not completely resected)
   - accelerated growth (if the lesion is close to the growth plate)
   - scoliosis
   - arthritis of precocious onset (if nidus is intracapsular).
6. A well-prepared surgical approach to the treatment of osteoid osteoma requires:
   - imaging localization of the lesion (by scintigraphy, radiography, CT)
   - verification of total excision of the lesion in vivo (by examination of the host bone) and in vitro (by examination of the resected specimen).
7. A variety of techniques other than *en bloc* excision of osteoid osteoma are available, including intralesional curettage, excision with trephines after surgical exposure, percutaneous excision (usually CT-guided), and RFTA.
8. CT-guided RFTA of osteoid osteoma is a promising technique and alternative to surgery in selected patients. It is performed through a small radiofrequency electrode that is introduced into the lesion percutaneously to produce thermal necrosis of an approximately 1-cm sphere of tissue.
9. Osteoblastoma, histologically almost identical with osteoid osteoma, is nevertheless a distinct clinical entity. Its radiographic appearance is characterized by:
   - features similar to a giant osteoid osteoma
   - a blow-out type of expansive lesion with small radiopacities in the center, resembling aneurysmal bone cyst
   - a lesion exhibiting aggressive features resembling a malignant tumor (osteosarcoma).
10. The differential diagnosis of osteoblastoma includes osteoid osteoma, bone abscess, aneurysmal bone cyst, enchondroma, and osteosarcoma.
11. Unusual presentation of osteoblastoma includes lesion associated with diffuse periostitis and systemic manifestations (so-called *toxic osteoblastoma*) and lesion in multicentric location (so-called *multifocal osteoblastoma*).

SUGGESTED READINGS

Adler C-P. Multifocal osteoblastoma of the hand. *Skeletal Radiol* 2000;29:601–604.

Anderson RB, McAlister JA Jr, Wrenn RN. Case report 585. Intracortical osteosarcoma of tibia. *Skeletal Radiol* 1989;18:627–630.

Assoun J, Railhac JJ, Bonnevialle P, et al. Osteoid osteoma: percutaneous resection with CT guidance. *Radiology* 1993;188:541–547.

Assoun J, Richardi G, Railhac JJ, et al. Osteoid osteoma: MR imaging versus CT. *Radiology* 1994;191:217–223.

Atar D, Lehman WB, Grant AD. Tips of the trade. Computerized tomography—guided excision of osteoid osteoma. *Orthop Rev* 1992;21:1457–1458.

Baruffi MR, Volpon JB, Neto JB, et al. Osteoid osteomas with chromosome alterations involving 22q. *Cancer Genet Cytogenet* 2001;124:127–131.

Bauer TW, Zehr RJ, Belhobek GH, et al. Juxta-articular osteoid osteoma. *Am J Surg Pathol* 1991;15:381–387.

Bell RS, O'Connor GD, Waddell JP. Importance of magnetic resonance imaging in osteoid osteoma: a case report. *Can J Surg* 1989;32:276–278.

Bertoni F, Unni KK, Beabout JW, et al. Parosteal osteoma of bones other than of the skull and face. *Cancer* 1995;75:2466–2473.

Bertoni F, Unni KK, McLeod RA, et al. Osteosarcoma resembling osteoblastoma. *Cancer* 1985;55:416–426.

Bettelli G, Tigani D, Picci P. Recurring osteoblastoma initially presenting as a typical osteoid osteoma. Report of two cases. *Skeletal Radiol* 1991;20:1–4.

Biebuyck JC, Katz LD, McCauley T. Soft tissue edema in osteoid osteoma. *Skeletal Radiol* 1993;22:37–41.

Bullough PG. *Atlas of orthopedic pathology with clinical and radiologic correlations*, 2nd ed. New York: Gower Medical; 1992.

Campanacci M. *Bone and soft tissue tumors*. New York: Springer; 1990:355–373.

Carter TR. Osteoid osteoma of the hip: an alternate method of excision. *Orthop Rev* 1990;19:903–905.

Cassar-Pullicino VN, McCall IW, Wan S. Intra-articular osteoid osteoma. *Clin Radiol* 1992;45:153–160.

Chang CH, Piatt ED, Thomas KE, et al. Bone abnormalities in Gardner's syndrome. *Am J Roentgenol Radium Ther Nucl Med* 1968;103:645–652.

Crim JR, Mirra JM, Eckardt JJ, et al. Widespread inflammatory response to osteoblastoma: the flare phenomenon. *Radiology* 1990;177:835–836.

Dahlin DC. Osteoma. In: *Bone tumors. General aspects on 8,542 cases*, 4th ed. Springfield, IL: Charles C. Thomas; 1986:84–87, 308–321.

Dahlin DC, Johnson EW Jr. Giant osteoid osteoma. *J Bone Joint Surg Am* 1954;36-A:559–572.

Dahlin DC, Unni KK. *Bone tumors: general aspects and data on 8,542 cases*, 4th ed. Springfield, IL: Charles C. Thomas; 1987:88–101.

Dale S, Breidahl WH, Baker D, et al. Severe toxic osteoblastoma of the humerus associated with diffuse periostitis of multiple bones. *Skeletal Radiol* 2001;30:464–468.

Della Rocca C, Huvos AG. Osteoblastoma: varied histological presentations with a benign clinical course. 55 cases. *Am J Surg Pathol* 1996;20:841–850.

Denis F, Armstrong GW. Scoliogenic osteoblastoma of the posterior end of the rib. A case report. *Spine (Phila Pa 1976)* 1984;9:74–76.

Dolan K, Seibert J, Seibert R. Gardner's syndrome. A model for correlative radiology. *Am J Roentgenol Radium Ther Nucl Med* 1973;119:359–364.

Dorfman HD, Weiss SW. Borderline osteoblastic tumors: problems in the differential diagnosis of aggressive osteoblastoma and low-grade osteosarcoma. *Semin Diagn Pathol* 1984;1:215–234.

Ebrahim FS, Jacobson JA, Lin J, et al. Intraarticular osteoid osteoma: sonographic findings in three patients with radiographic, CT, and MR imaging correlation. *AJR Am J Roentgenol* 2001;177:1391–1395.

Ehara S, Rosenthal DI, Aoki J, et al. Peritumoral edema in osteoid osteoma on magnetic resonance imaging. *Skeletal Radiol* 1999;28:265–270.

Falappa P, Garganese MC, Crocoli A, et al. Particular imaging features and customized thermal ablation treatment for intramedullary osteoid osteoma in pediatric patients. *Skeletal Radiol* 2011;40:1523–1530.

Fechner RE, Mills SE. *Tumors of the bones and joints*. Washington, DC: Armed Forces Institute of Pathology; 1993:25–38.

Gardner EJ, Plenk HP. Hereditary pattern for multiple osteomas in a family group. *Am J Hum Genet* 1952;4:31–36.

Gardner EJ, Richards RC. Multiple cutaneous and subcutaneous lesions occurring simultaneously with hereditary polyposis and osteomatosis. *Am J Hum Genet* 1953;5:139–147.

Gil S, Marco SF, Arenas J, et al. Doppler duplex color localization of osteoid osteomas. *Skeletal Radiol* 1999;28:107–110.

Goldman AB, Schneider R, Pavlov H. Osteoid osteomas of the femoral neck: report of four cases evaluated with isotopic bone scanning, CT, and MR imaging. *Radiology* 1993;186:227–232.

Greenspan A. Benign bone-forming lesions: osteoma, osteoid osteoma, and osteoblastoma. Clinical, imaging, pathologic, and differential considerations. *Skeletal Radiol* 1993;22:485–500.

Greenspan A. Bone island (enostosis): current concept—a review. *Skeletal Radiol* 1995;24:111–115.

Greenspan A. Sclerosing bone dysplasias—a target-site approach. *Skeletal Radiol* 1991;20:561–583.

Greenspan A, Borys D. *Radiology and pathology correlation of bone tumors: a quick reference and review*. Philadelphia: Wolters Kluwer; 2016:32–89.

Greenspan A, Elguezabel A, Bryk D. Multifocal osteoid osteoma. A case report and review of the literature. *Am J Roentgenol Radium Ther Nucl Med* 1974;121:103–106.

Greenspan A, Jundt G, Remagen W. *Differential diagnosis in orthopaedic oncology*, 2nd ed. Philadelphia: Lippincott Williams & Wilkins; 2007:59–74.

Greenspan A, Stadalnik RC. Bone island: scintigraphic findings and their clinical application. *Can Assoc Radiol J* 1995;46:368–379.

Greenspan A, Steiner G, Knutzon R. Bone island (enostosis): clinical significance and radiologic and pathologic correlations. *Skeletal Radiol* 1991;20:85–90.

Griffith JF, Kumta SM, Chow LTC, et al. Intracortical osteosarcoma. *Skeletal Radiol* 1998;27:228–232.

Helms CA. Osteoid osteoma. The double density sign. *Clin Orthop Relat Res* 1987;222:167–173.

Jackson RP, Reckling FW, Mants FA. Osteoid osteoma and osteoblastoma. Similar histologic lesions with different natural histories. *Clin Orthop Relat Res* 1977;128:303–313.

Jaffe HL. Benign osteoblastoma. *Bull Hosp Joint Dis* 1956;17:141–151.

Jaffe HL. Osteoid osteoma: a benign osteoblastic tumor composed of osteoid and atypical bone. *Arch Surg* 1935;31:709–728.

Jaffe HL. Osteoid osteoma of bone. *Radiology* 1945;45:319–334.

Keim HA, Reina EG. Osteoid-osteoma as a cause of scoliosis. *J Bone Joint Surg Am* 1975;57:159–163.

Klein MH, Shankman S. Osteoid osteoma: radiologic and pathologic correlation. *Skeletal Radiol* 1992;21:23–31.

Kransdorf MJ, Stull MA, Gilkey FW, et al. Osteoid osteoma. *Radiographics* 1991;11:671–696.

Kricun ME. *Imaging of bone tumors*. Philadelphia: WB Saunders; 1993:114–116, 121–125.

Kroon HM, Schurmans J. Osteoblastoma: clinical and radiologic findings in 98 new cases. *Radiology* 1990;175:783–790.

Kyriakos M. Intracortical osteosarcoma. *Cancer* 1980;46:2525–2533.

Kyriakos M, El-Khoury GY, McDonald DJ, et al. Osteoblastomatosis of bone. A benign, multifocal osteoblastic lesion, distinct from osteoid osteoma and osteoblastoma, radiologically simulating a vascular tumor. *Skeletal Radiol* 2007;36:237–247.

Lawrie TR, Aterman K, Sinclair AM. Painless osteoid osteoma. A report of two cases. *J Bone Joint Surg Am* 1970;52:1357–1363.

Lee DH, Malawer MM. Staging and treatment of primary and persistent (recurrent) osteoid osteoma. Evaluation of intraoperative nuclear scanning, tetracycline fluorescence, and tomography. *Clin Orthop Relat Res* 1992;281:229–238.

Lichtenstein L. Benign osteoblastoma; a category of osteoid- and bone-forming tumors other than classical osteoid osteoma, which may be mistaken for giant-cell tumor or osteogenic sarcoma. *Cancer* 1956;9:1044–1052.

Liu PT, Chivers FS, Roberts CC, et al. Imaging of osteoid osteoma with dynamic gadolinium-enhanced MR imaging. *Radiology* 2003;227:691–700.

Liu TL, Kujak JL, Roberts CC, et al. The vascular groove sign: a new CT finding associated with osteoid osteomas. *AJR Am J Roentgenol* 2012;196:168–173.

Lucas DR, Unni KK, McLeod RA, et al. Osteoblastoma: clinicopathologic study of 306 cases. *Hum Pathol* 1994;25:117–134.

Marinelli A, Giacomini S, Bianchi G, et al. Osteoid osteoma simulating an osteocartilaginous exostosis. *Skeletal Radiol* 2004;33:181–185.

Mazoyer JF, Kohler R, Bossard D. Osteoid osteoma: CT-guided percutaneous treatment. *Radiology* 1991;181:269–271.

McLeod RA, Dahlin DC, Beabout JW. The spectrum of osteoblastoma. *AJR Am J Roentgenol* 1976;126:321–325.

Mirra JM, Picci P, Gold RH. *Bone tumors: clinical, pathologic, and radiologic correlations*. Philadelphia: Lea & Febiger; 1989:226–248.

Murphey MD, Andrews CL, Flemming DJ, et al. From the archives of the AFIP. Primary tumors of the spine: radiologic pathologic correlation. *Radiographics* 1996;16:1131–1158.

Mylona S, Patsoura S, Galani P, et al. Osteoid osteomas in common and in technically challenging locations treated with computed tomography-guided percutaneous radiofrequency ablation. *Skeletal Radiol* 2010;39:443–449.

Nogués P, Martí-Bonmatí L, Aparisi F, et al. MR imaging assessment of juxta cortical edema in osteoid osteoma in 28 patients. *Eur Radiol* 1998;8:236–238.

Norman A. Persistence or recurrence of pain: a sign of surgical failure in osteoid-osteoma. *Clin Orthop Relat Res* 1978;130:263–266.

Norman A, Abdelwahab IF, Buyon J, et al. Osteoid osteoma of the hip stimulating an early onset of osteoarthritis. *Radiology* 1986;158:417–420.

O'Connell JX, Rosenthal DI, Mankin HJ, et al. Solitary osteoma of a long bone. A case report. *J Bone Joint Surg Am* 1993;75:1830–1834.

Pettine KA, Klassen RA. Osteoid-osteoma and osteoblastoma of the spine. *J Bone Joint Surg Am* 1986;68:354–361.

Pinto CH, Taminiau AHM, Vanderschueren GM, et al. Technical considerations in CT-guided radiofrequency thermal ablation of osteoid osteoma: tricks of the trade. *AJR Am J Roentgenol* 2002;179:1633–1642.

Quílez-Caballero E, Martel-Villagran J, Bueno-Horcajadas ÁL, et al. Osteoblastomatosis: an unusual diagnosis and treatment. *Skeletal Radiol* 2018;47:1183–1189.

Resnick D, Kyriakos M, Greenway G. Tumors and tumor-like lesions of bone: imaging and pathology of specific lesions. In: Resnick D, ed. *Diagnosis of bone and joint disorders*, 3rd ed. Philadelphia: WB Saunders; 1995:3629–3647.

Roger B, Bellin M-F, Wioland M, et al. Osteoid osteoma: CT-guided percutaneous excision confirmed with immediate follow-up scintigraphy in 16 outpatients. *Radiology* 1996;201:239–242.

Rosenthal DI. Percutaneous radiofrequency treatment of osteoid osteomas. *Semin Musculoskelet Radiol* 1997;1:265–272.

Rosenthal DI, Hornicek FJ, Wolfe MW, et al. Percutaneous radiofrequency coagulation of osteoid osteoma compared with operative treatment. *J Bone Joint Surg Am* 1998;80:815–821.

Rosenthal DI, Springfield DS, Gebhardt MC, et al. Osteoid osteoma: percutaneous radiofrequency ablation. *Radiology* 1995;197:451–454.

Schai P, Friederich NB, Krüger A, et al. Discrete synchronous multifocal osteoid osteoma of the humerus. *Skeletal Radiol* 1996;25:667–670.

Schajowicz F. *Tumors and tumorlike lesions of bone: pathology, radiology and treatment*, 2nd ed. Berlin: Springer-Verlag; 1994:30–32, 48–56, 406–411.

Schajowicz F, Lemos C. Malignant osteoblastoma. *J Bone Joint Surg Br* 1976;58:202–211.

Schajowicz F, Lemos C. Osteoid osteoma and osteoblastoma. Closely related entities of osteoblastic derivation. *Acta Orthop Scand* 1970;41:272–291.

Shaikh MI, Saifuddin A, Pringle J, et al. Spinal osteoblastoma: CT and MR imaging with pathological correlation. *Skeletal Radiol* 1999;28:33–40.

Sherazi Z, Saifuddin A, Shaikh MI, et al. Unusual imaging findings in association with spinal osteoblastoma. *Clin Radiol* 1996;51:644–648.

Shukla S, Clarke AW, Saifuddin A. Imaging features of foot osteoid osteoma. *Skeletal Radiol* 2010;39:683–689.

Spjut HJ, Dorfman HD, Fechner RE, et al. Tumors of bone and cartilage. In: Firminger HI, ed. *Atlas of tumor pathology*, 2nd series, fascicle 5. Washington, DC: Armed Forces Institute of Pathology; 1971:117–119.

Sundaram M, Falbo S, McDonald D, et al. Surface osteomas of the appendicular skeleton. *AJR Am J Roentgenol* 1996;167:1529–1533.

Theologis T, Ostlere S, Gibbons CLMH, et al. Toxic osteoblastoma of the scapula. *Skeletal Radiol* 2007;36:253–257.

Thompson GH, Wong KM, Konsens RM, et al. Magnetic resonance imaging of an osteoid osteoma of the proximal femur: a potentially confusing appearance. *J Pediatr Orthop* 1990;10:800–804.

Towbin R, Kaye R, Meza MP, et al. Osteoid osteoma: percutaneous excision using a CT-guided coaxial technique. *AJR Am J Roentgenol* 1995;164:945–949.

Vanderschueren GM, Taminiau AHM, Obermann WR, et al. Osteoid osteoma: clinical results with thermocoagulation. *Radiology* 2002;224:82–86.

Verstraete KL, Van der Woude HJ, Hogendoorn PC, et al. Dynamic contrast-enhanced MR imaging of musculoskeletal tumors: basic principles and clinical applications. *J Magn Reson Imaging* 1996;6:311–321.

Wang B, Han S, Jiang L, et al. Percutaneous radiofrequency ablation for spinal osteoid osteoma and osteoblastoma. *Eur Spine J* 2017;26:1884–1892.

Weber M, Sprengel SD, Omlor GW, et al. Clinical long-term outcome, technical success, and cost analysis of radiofrequency ablation for the treatment of osteoblastomas and spinal osteoid osteomas in comparison to open surgical resection. *Skeletal Radiol* 2015;44:981–993.

Woods ER, Martel W, Mandell SH, et al. Reactive soft-tissue mass associated with osteoid osteoma: correlation of MR imaging features with pathologic findings. *Radiology* 1993;186:221–225.

Yalcinkaya U, Doganavsargil B, Sezak M, et al. Clinical and morphological characteristics of osteoid osteoma and osteoblastoma: a retrospective single-center analysis of 204 patients. *Ann Diagn Pathol* 2014;18:319–325.

Yaniv G, Shabshin N, Sharon M, et al. Osteoid osteoma—the CT vessel sign. *Skeletal Radiol* 2011;40:1311–1314.

Youssef BA, Haddad MC, Zahrani A, et al. Osteoid osteoma and osteoblastoma: MRI appearances and the significance of ring enhancement. *Eur Radiol* 1996;6:291–296.

18

Benign Tumors and Tumor-like Lesions II

Lesions of Cartilaginous Origin

Benign Chondroblastic Lesions

Diagnosis of a bone lesion as originating from cartilage is usually a simple task for the radiologist. The lesion's radiolucent matrix; scalloped margins; and annular, comma-shaped, or punctate calcifications usually suffice to establish its chondrogenic nature. However, whether a cartilage tumor is benign or malignant is sometimes extremely difficult for the radiologist to determine. It also may create a problem even to the experienced musculoskeletal pathologist. All cartilage tumors, regardless whether benign or malignant, exhibit a positive reaction for S100 protein, a helpful diagnostic hint.

Enchondroma (Chondroma)

Clinical and Imaging Features

Enchondroma is the second most common benign tumor of bone, constituting approximately 10% of all benign bone tumors and representing the most common tumor of the short tubular bones of the hand. When the lesion is located centrally in the bone, it is termed as an *enchondroma* (Fig. 18.1); if it is extracortical (periosteal) in location, it is called a *chondroma* (periosteal or juxtacortical) (see Figs. 18.16 and 18.17). Regardless of location, this benign lesion is characterized by the formation of mature hyaline cartilage. It has been widely postulated that enchondroma is formed as a consequence of displacement of embryonic rests of cartilage from the growth plate into the metaphysis. This contention, however, was recently challenged by some investigators whose work failed to confirm this theory. Douis and coworkers evaluated retrospectively 240 magnetic resonance imaging (MRI) studies of the knee performed in 209 children. They failed to identify any displacement of cartilage into the metaphysis. Furthermore, the study by Amary and colleagues identified somatic mutations in isocitrate dehydrogenase 1 and 2 (*IDH1* and *IDH2*) in many central, low-grade cartilaginous tumors, thus supporting the neoplastic origin of enchondromas. Moreover, most chondromas contain clonal chromosomal abnormalities involving chromosomes or chromosomal regions 4q, 5, 7, 11, 14q, 16q22-q24, 20, and particularly rearrangement of chromosome 6 and 12q12-q15. Although occurring throughout life, enchondromas are usually seen in patients in their second through fourth decades. There is no gender predilection. The short tubular bones of the hand (phalanges, particularly proximal and middle, and metacarpals) are the most common sites of occurrence (Fig. 18.2), although the lesions are also encountered in the long tubular bones, especially proximal humerus (Fig. 18.3) and proximal and distal femur (Figs. 18.4 and 18.5; see also Fig. 18.1). Sporadic cases have been reported in the rib, clavicle, sternum (Fig. 18.6), cuboid, and carpal bones. They are often asymptomatic; in the small bones of the hands and feet, they may present as palpable swelling with or without pain. A pathologic fracture through the tumor (Figs. 18.7 and 18.8) often calls attention to the lesion.

In most instances, radiography suffices to demonstrate the enchondroma. In the short bones, the lesion is often entirely radiolucent (Fig. 18.9), whereas in the long bones, it may display visible calcifications (see Figs. 18.1, 18.3, and 18.4). If the calcifications are extensive, enchondromas are called *calcifying* (Fig. 18.10). The lesions can also be recognized by shallow scalloping of the inner (endosteal) cortical margins because the cartilage in general grows in a lobular pattern (see Fig. 18.1).

Computed tomography (CT) and MRI may further delineate the tumor and more precisely localize it in the bone. On spin echo (SE) T1-weighted MR images, enchondromas demonstrate intermediate to low signal intensity, whereas on T2-weighted images, they exhibit high signal intensity. The calcifications within the tumor will image as low–signal intensity structures (Figs. 18.11 to 18.14). CT and MRI may provide additional morphological detail otherwise not well seen on radiographs, including cortical involvement, periosteal reaction, soft tissue extension, etc. that may help in differentiating benign from malignant lesions. Other MRI techniques such as diffusion imaging may provide further insights on the histological behavior of the lesions.

Skeletal scintigraphy usually reveals mild to moderate increased uptake of the tracer in uncomplicated enchondromas, whereas the presence of a pathologic fracture or malignant transformation is revealed by marked scintigraphic activity.

Intracortical chondroma is a very rare variant of conventional enchondroma. The lesion is located in cortical bone and is surrounded by sclerosis of the medullary bone and periosteal reaction. Some of these lesions may actually represent periosteal chondroma with an atypical radiographic appearance, as reported by Abdelwahab and associates. Intracortical chondroma can occasionally simulate an osteoid osteoma.

Enchondroma protuberans is a rare form of enchondroma, which arises in the medullary cavity, but exhibits an exophytic growth pattern extending beyond the cortical outline of bone (Fig. 18.15). The extraosseous mass may occasionally be partially encased by calcified rim. It is most commonly located in the phalanges and metacarpals but has also been reported in other sites. This lesion must be distinguished from osteochondroma or central chondrosarcoma that penetrates the cortex and extends to the surface of bone forming a juxtacortical mass.

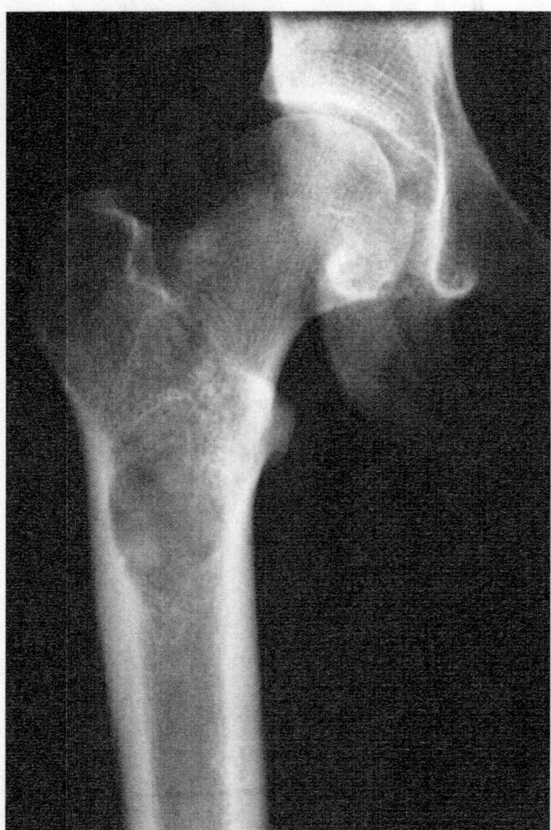

FIGURE 18.1 Enchondroma. A radiolucent lesion in the medullary portion of the proximal femur of a 22-year-old man is seen eroding the inner aspect of the lateral cortex. Note scalloped borders and matrix calcification.

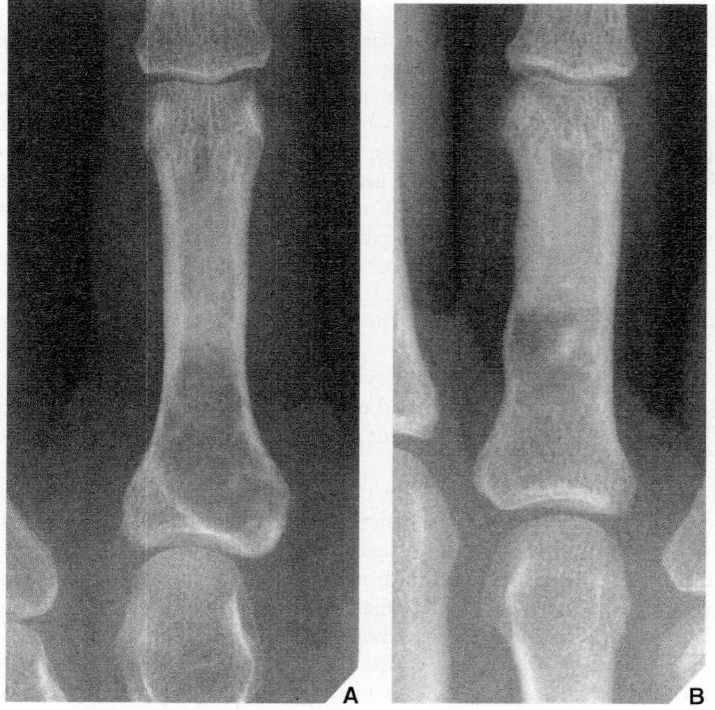

FIGURE 18.2 Enchondroma. **(A)** A radiolucent lesion in the proximal phalanx of the middle finger of a 40-year-old woman and **(B)** a similar lesion with central calcification in the proximal phalanx of the ring finger of a 42-year-old man are typical examples of enchondroma in the short tubular bones.

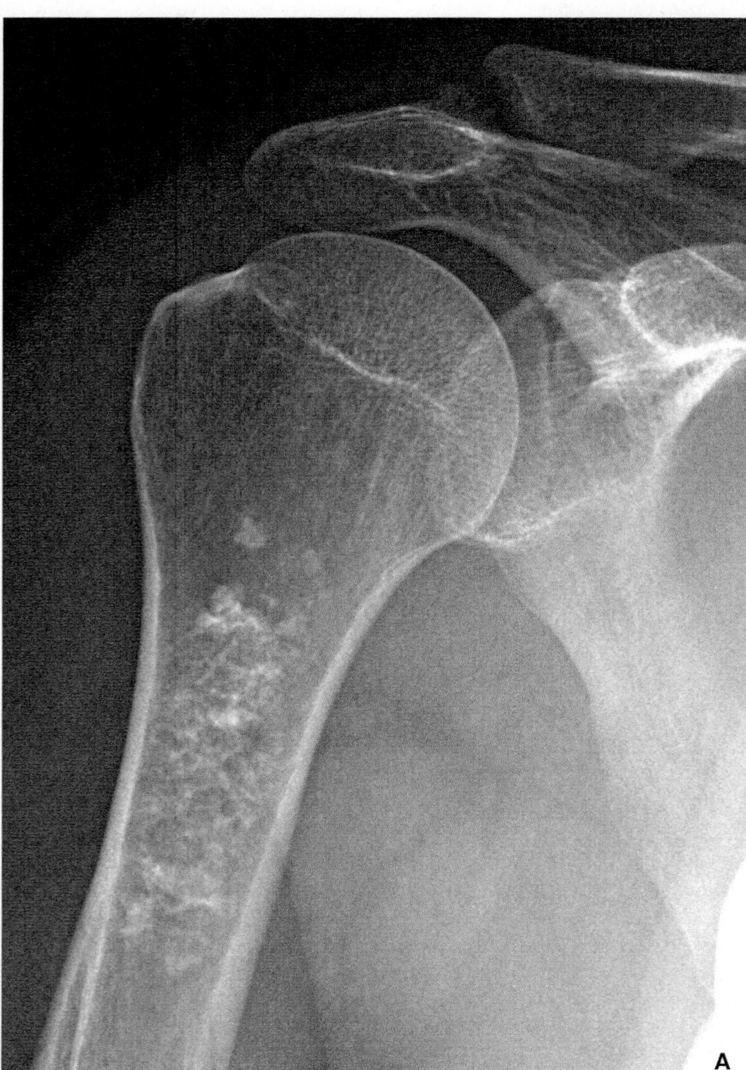

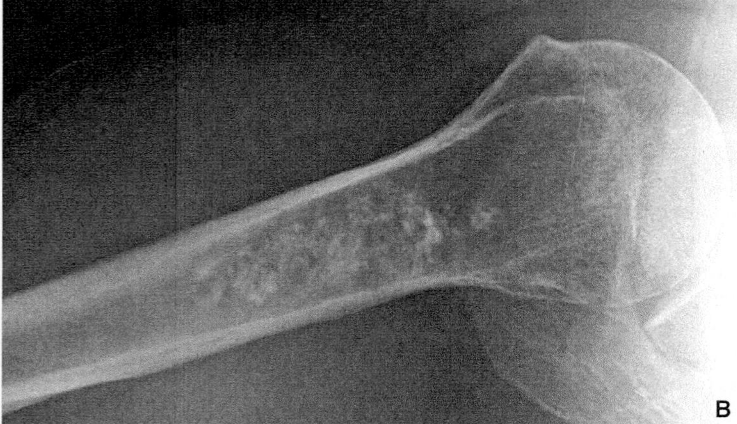

FIGURE 18.3 Enchondroma. **(A,B)** A radiolucent lesion containing "popcorn"-like calcifications occupies the proximal shaft of the left humerus. Observe that despite the size of the lesion, which extends from the lateral to medial cortex, there is no endosteal scalloping present and the cortex is not thickened.

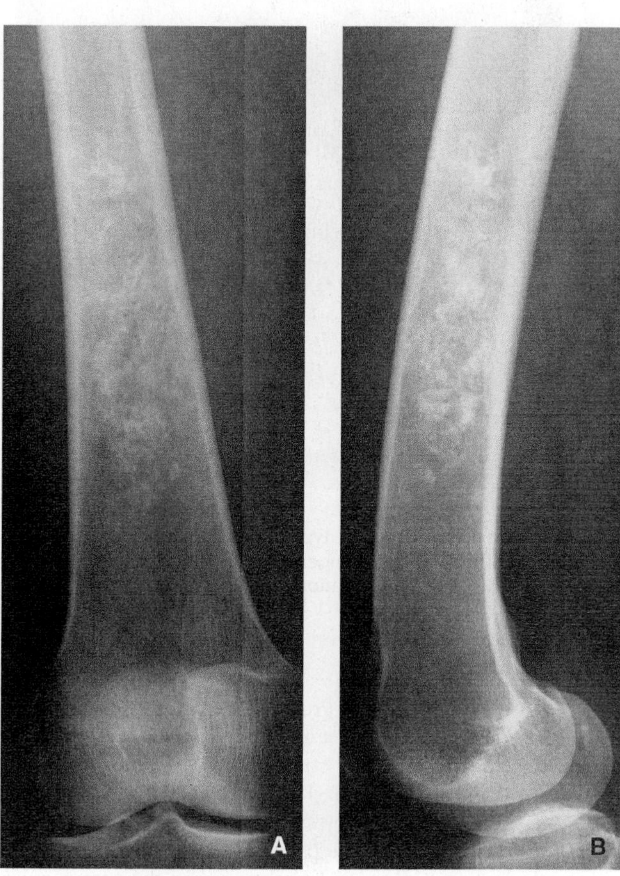

FIGURE 18.4 Enchondroma. **(A)** Anteroposterior and **(B)** lateral radiographs of the distal femur show a radiolucent lesion exhibiting typical chondroid calcifications. (Reprinted with permission from Greenspan A, Borys D. *Radiology and pathology correlation of bone tumors: a quick reference and review*. Philadelphia: Wolters Kluwer; 2016:92.)

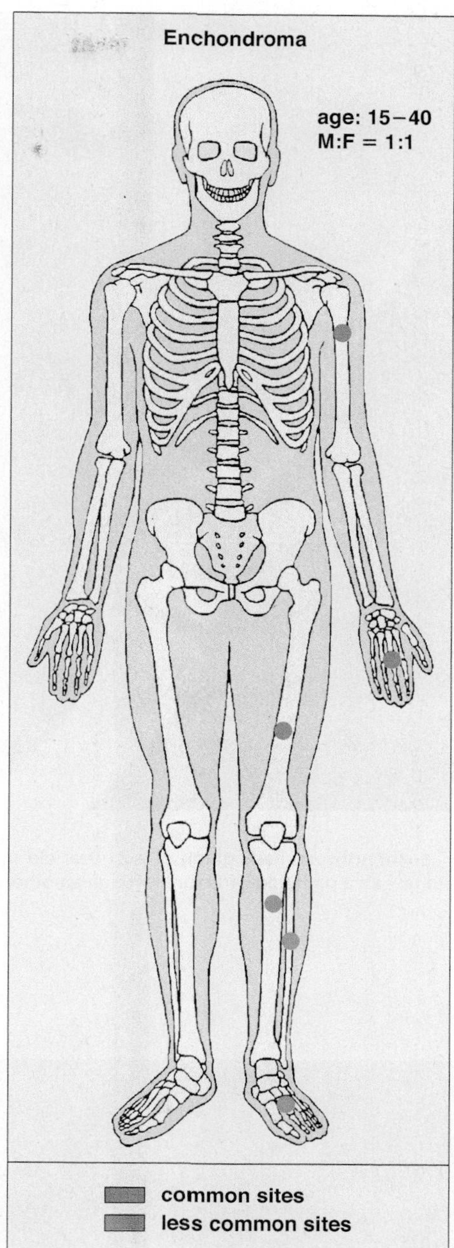

FIGURE 18.5 Skeletal sites of predilection, peak age range, and male-to-female ratio in enchondroma.

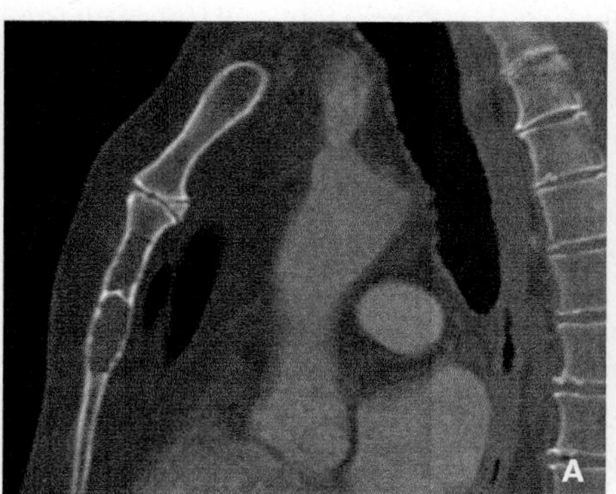

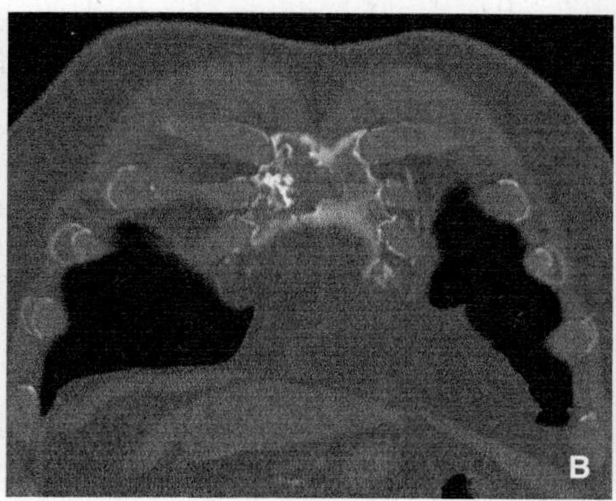

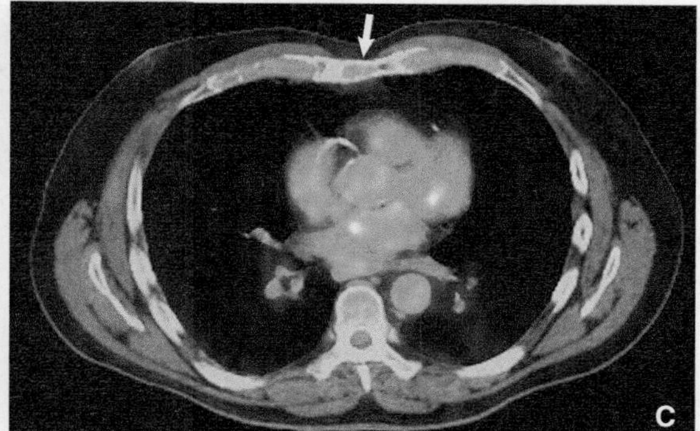

FIGURE 18.6 Enchondroma in the sternum. **(A)** Sagittal reformatted CT image of the upper chest of a 73-year-old man shows a low-attenuated lesion within the body of the sternum. Observe a shallow endosteal scalloping. **(B)** Coronal reformatted CT image shows chondroid calcifications within the large lobulated lesion. **(C)** Axial fused ^{18}F-FDG positron emission tomography (PET)/CT image shows that the lesion does not exhibit increased metabolic activity *(arrow)*.

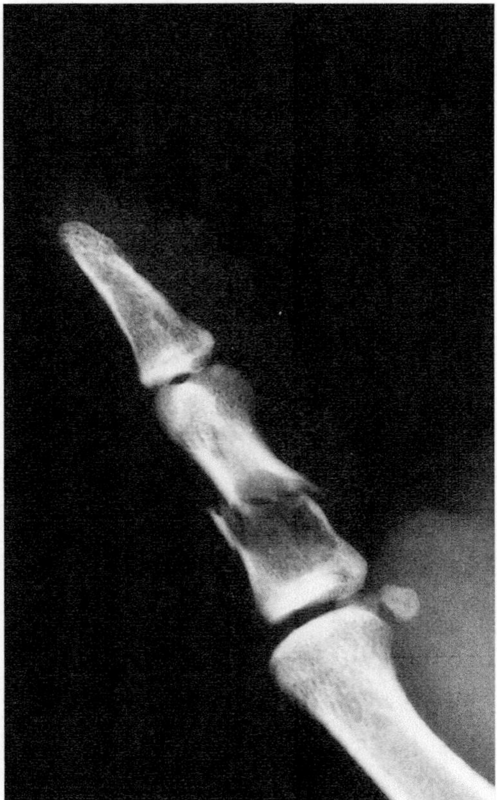

FIGURE 18.7 Enchondroma. Radiograph of a 31-year-old man who had injured his left thumb reveals a pathologic fracture through an otherwise asymptomatic lesion.

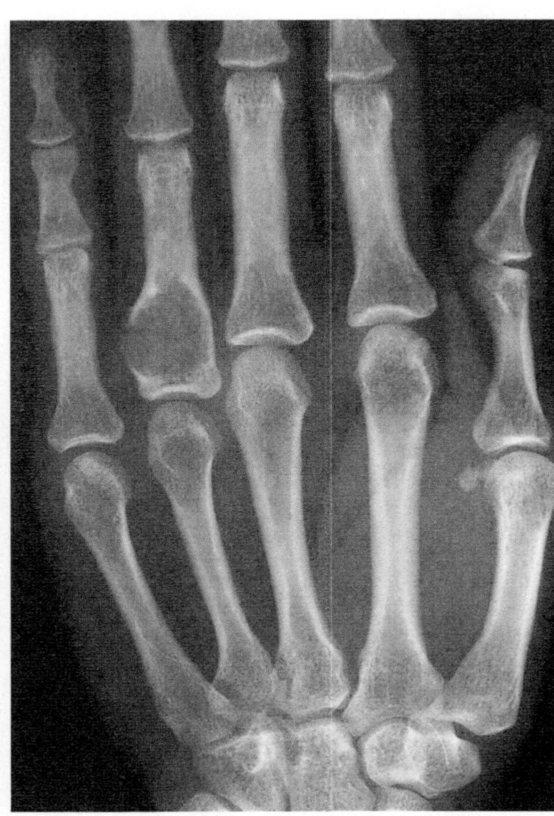

FIGURE 18.9 Enchondroma. A typical, purely radiolucent lesion at the base of the proximal phalanx of the ring finger of a 37-year-old woman represents an enchondroma. Note the marked attenuation of the ulnar side of the cortex.

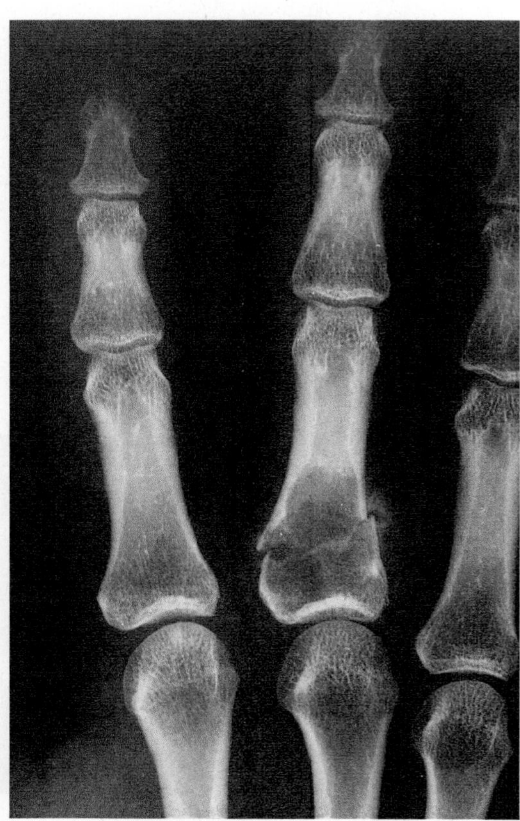

FIGURE 18.8 Enchondroma. Pathologic fracture through a large enchondroma is present in the proximal phalanx of the middle finger.

Periosteal chondroma is a slow-growing, benign cartilaginous lesion that arises on the surface of the cortex in or beneath the periosteum. It occurs in children as well as adults, most commonly in the third to fourth decades of life, with no sex predilection. There is usually a history of pain and tenderness, often accompanied by swelling at the site of the lesion, which is most commonly located in the proximal humerus. The other reported locations include femur, tibia, and phalanges. As the tumor enlarges, it is seen radiographically eroding the cortex in a saucer-like fashion, producing a solid buttress of periosteal new bone (Fig. 18.16). The lesion has a sharp sclerotic inner margin demarcating it from the buttress of periosteal new bone. Scattered calcifications are often seen within the lesion (Fig. 18.17).

CT may show to better advantage the scalloped cortex and matrix calcification (Figs. 18.18 and 18.19). It also may demonstrate the separation of a lesion from the medullary cavity, an important feature in differentiation from osteochondroma. MRI findings correspond to radiographic findings, depicting the cartilaginous soft-tissue component. If periosteal chondroma affects the medullary canal, MRI may be useful in depicting the extent of involvement (Fig. 18.20). Fat suppression or enhanced gradient-echo sequences may improve tumor–marrow contrast. The potential pitfall of MRI is marrow edema mimicking tumor invasion or vice versa. Unlike enchondroma and osteochondroma, periosteal chondroma may continue to grow after skeletal maturation. Some lesions may attain a large size (up to 6 cm) and may resemble osteochondromas (Figs. 18.21 and 18.22). Some lesions may mimic an aneurysmal bone cyst. Very rarely, the lesion may encase itself intracortically, thus mimicking other intracortical lesions (such as intracortical angioma, intracortical fibrous dysplasia, or intracortical bone abscess).

Pathology

Histologically, enchondroma consists of lobules of hyaline cartilage of varying cellularity and is recognized by the features of its intracellular matrix, which has a uniformly translucent appearance and contains relatively little collagen. It exhibits multinodular cartilaginous architecture well

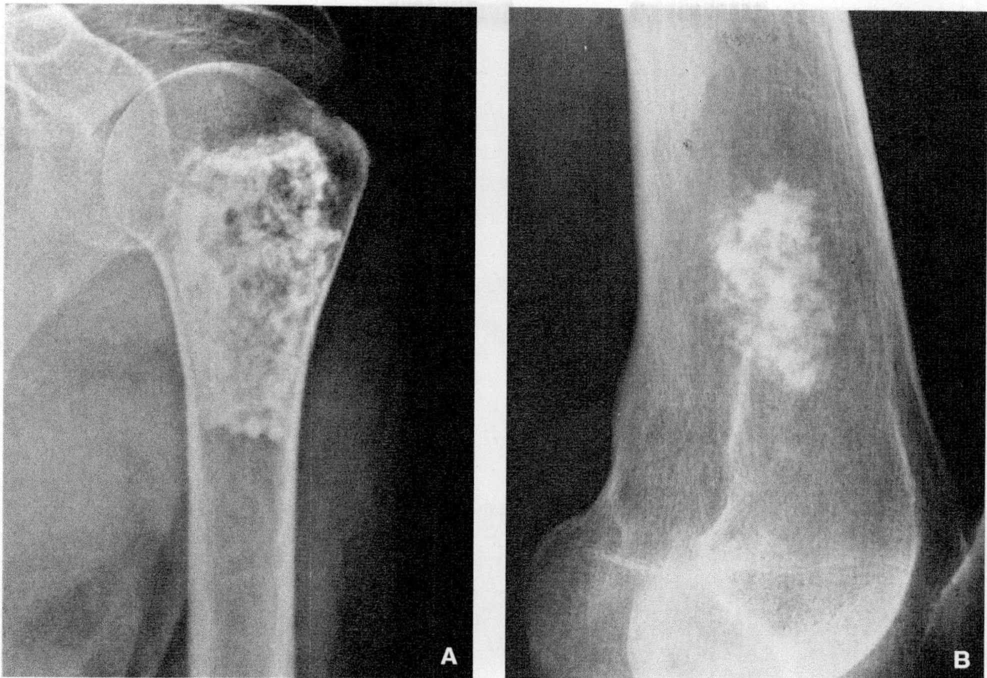

FIGURE 18.10 Calcifying enchondroma. **(A)** In this heavily calcified enchondroma of the proximal humerus of a 58-year-old woman, note the lobular appearance of the lesion and the minimal degree of scalloping of the lateral endocortex. **(B)** Similar heavy calcified lesion is present in the distal femur of a 30-year-old man. (Reprinted with permission from Greenspan A, Borys D. *Radiology and pathology correlation of bone tumors: a quick reference and review*. Philadelphia: Wolters Kluwer; 2016:92.)

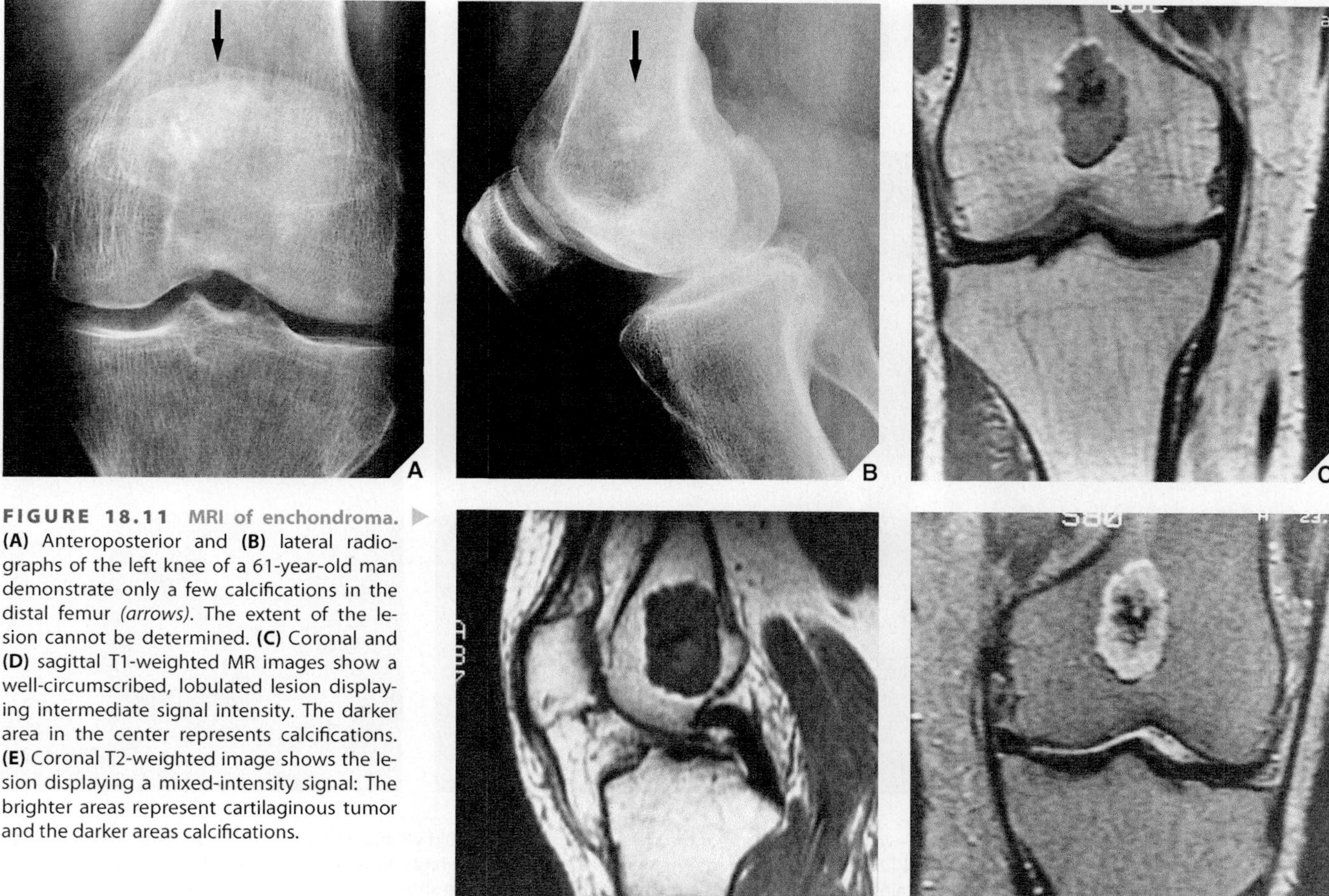

FIGURE 18.11 MRI of enchondroma. **(A)** Anteroposterior and **(B)** lateral radiographs of the left knee of a 61-year-old man demonstrate only a few calcifications in the distal femur *(arrows)*. The extent of the lesion cannot be determined. **(C)** Coronal and **(D)** sagittal T1-weighted MR images show a well-circumscribed, lobulated lesion displaying intermediate signal intensity. The darker area in the center represents calcifications. **(E)** Coronal T2-weighted image shows the lesion displaying a mixed-intensity signal: The brighter areas represent cartilaginous tumor and the darker areas calcifications.

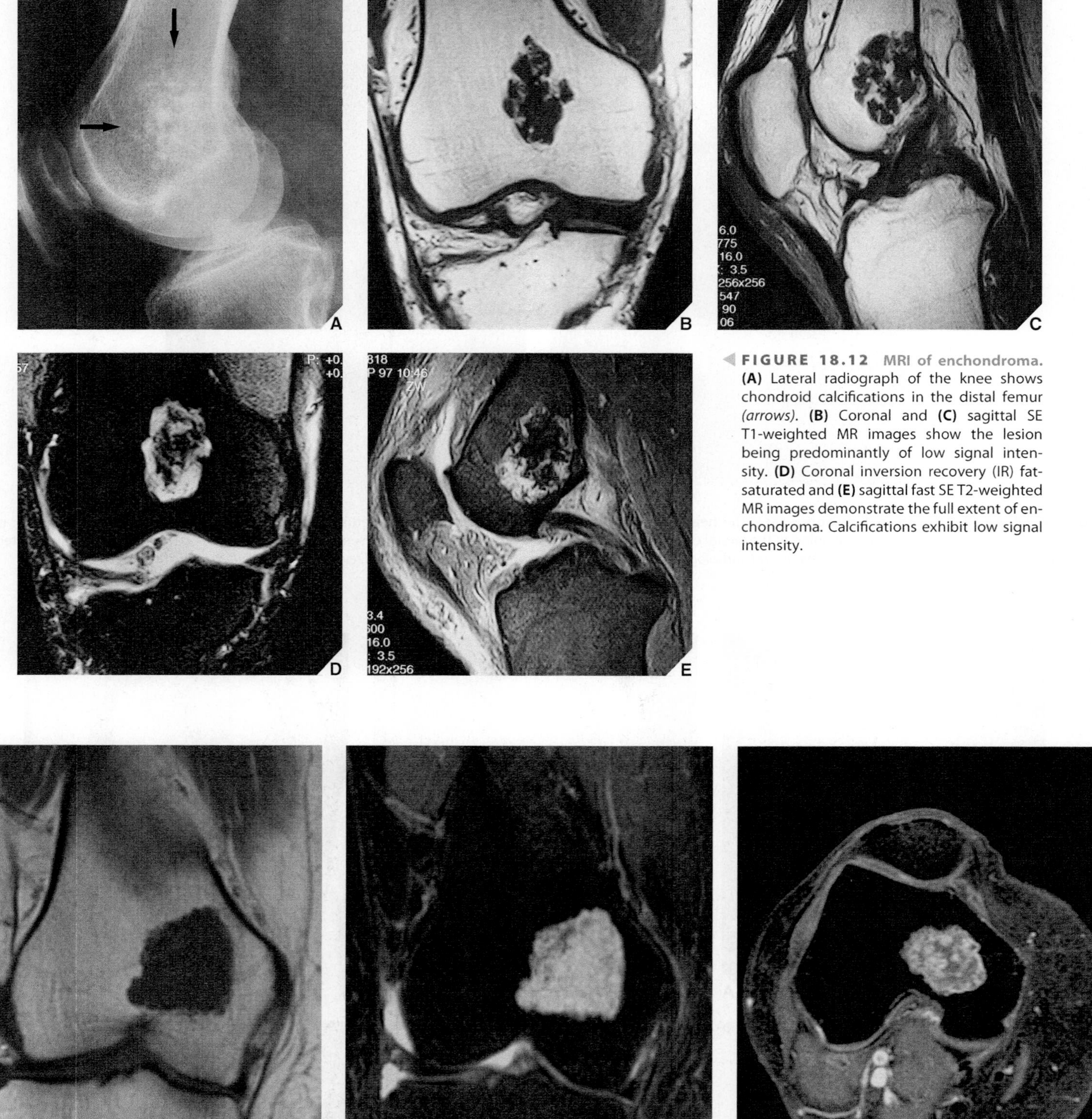

FIGURE 18.12 MRI of enchondroma. **(A)** Lateral radiograph of the knee shows chondroid calcifications in the distal femur *(arrows)*. **(B)** Coronal and **(C)** sagittal SE T1-weighted MR images show the lesion being predominantly of low signal intensity. **(D)** Coronal inversion recovery (IR) fat-saturated and **(E)** sagittal fast SE T2-weighted MR images demonstrate the full extent of enchondroma. Calcifications exhibit low signal intensity.

FIGURE 18.13 MRI of enchondroma. **(A)** Coronal T1-weighted MR image of the right knee of a 59-year-old woman shows a sharply demarcated lesion in the medial femoral condyle displaying low signal intensity. **(B)** Coronal T2-weighted MR image shows the lesion exhibiting high signal intensity with a few low signal foci, representing calcifications. **(C)** Axial T1-weighted fat-suppressed MRI obtained after intravenous administration of gadolinium shows significant enhancement of the tumor. Calcifications remain of low signal intensity.

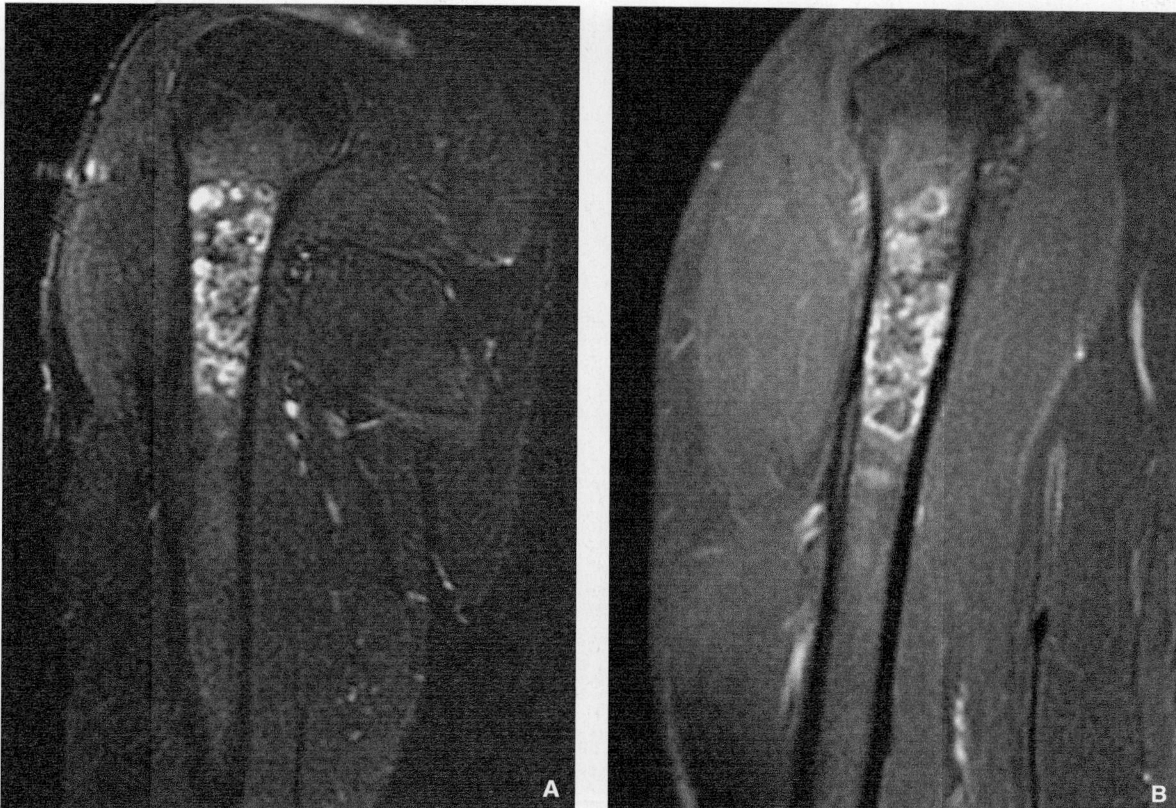

FIGURE 18.14 MRI of enchondroma. **(A)** Coronal inversion recovery (IR) and **(B)** sagittal T1-weighted fat-suppressed contrast-enhanced MR images show a long heterogeneous-appearing lesion within the medullary portion of the proximal humerus. Note that the cortex is intact, there is no periosteal reaction, and there is lack of soft-tissue extension.

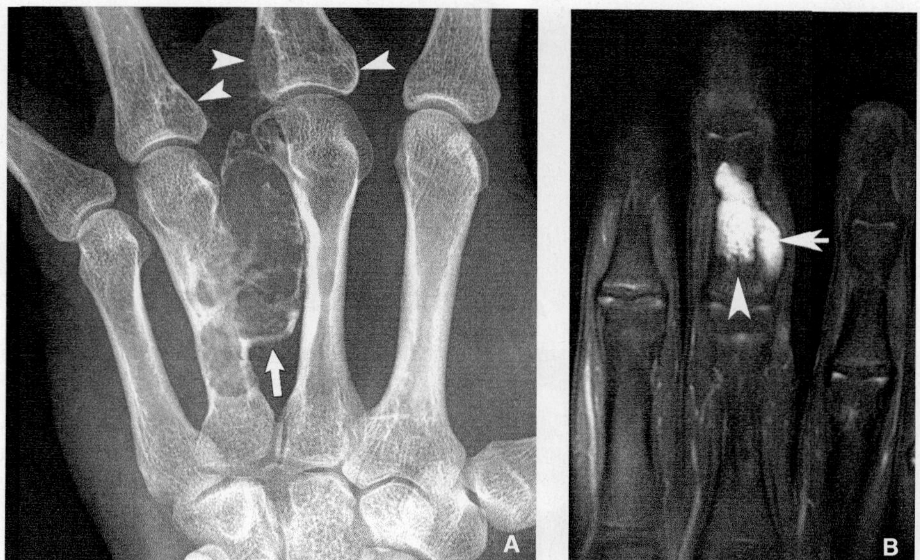

FIGURE 18.15 Enchondroma protuberans. **(A)** Coned-down dorsovolar radiograph of the right hand of a 27-year-old man diagnosed with enchondromatosis shows a typical appearance of enchondroma protuberans arising in the fourth metacarpal bone. Observe that intramedullary lesion extends out of the bone forming a large extraosseous mass contained by a thin sclerotic border *(arrow)*. Small intraosseous enchondromas are present within the bases of the proximal phalanges of the ring and middle fingers *(arrowheads)*. **(B)** Coronal T2-weighted MR image of the middle finger in another patient with a chronic palpable mass demonstrates an intramedullary lesion in the middle phalanx *(arrowhead)* extending to the surface of the bone *(arrow)*. Histopathologic examination revealed cartilage matrix.

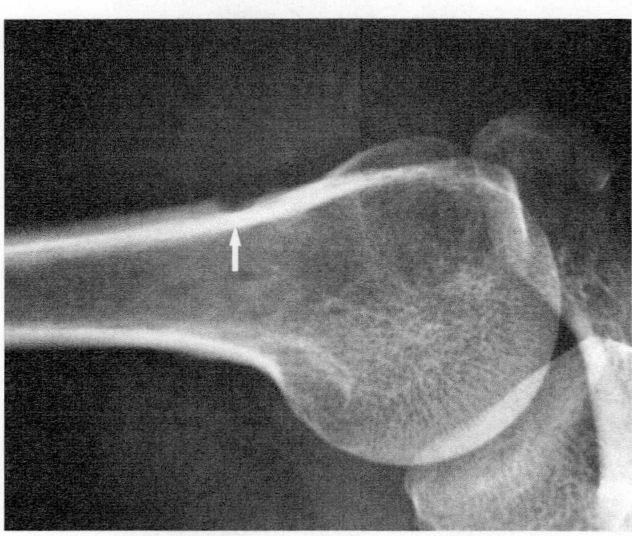

FIGURE 18.16 **Periosteal chondroma.** A radiolucent lesion *(arrow)* is eroding the external surface of the cortex of the proximal humerus of a 24-year-old man.

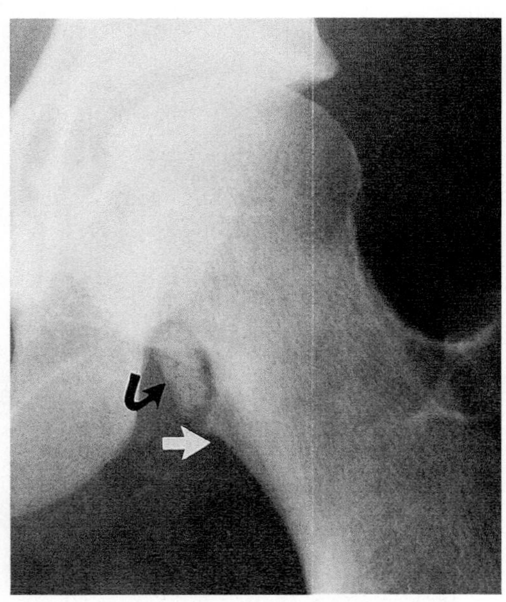

FIGURE 18.17 **Periosteal chondroma.** A periosteal chondroma at the medial aspect of the neck of the left femur eroded the cortex in a saucer-like fashion. The characteristic buttress of a periosteal reaction is seen at the inferior border of the lesion *(arrow)*. Note also cluster of calcification in the soft tissue *(curved arrow)*.

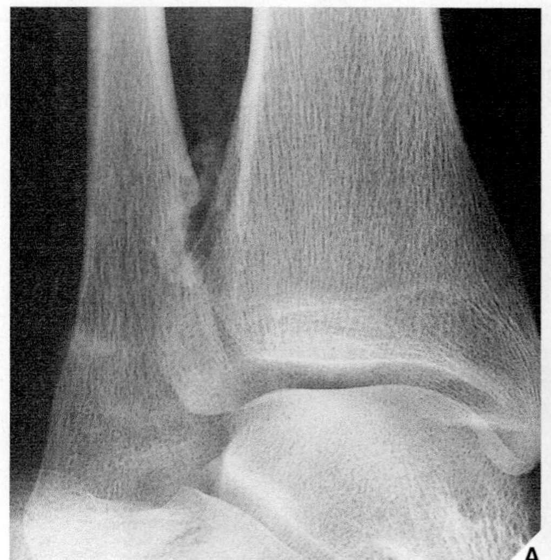

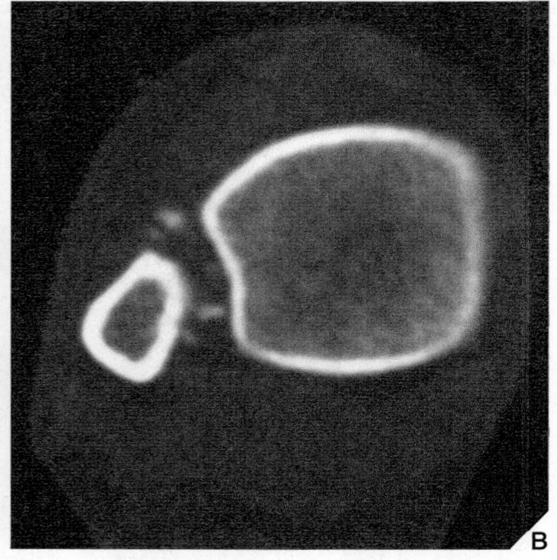

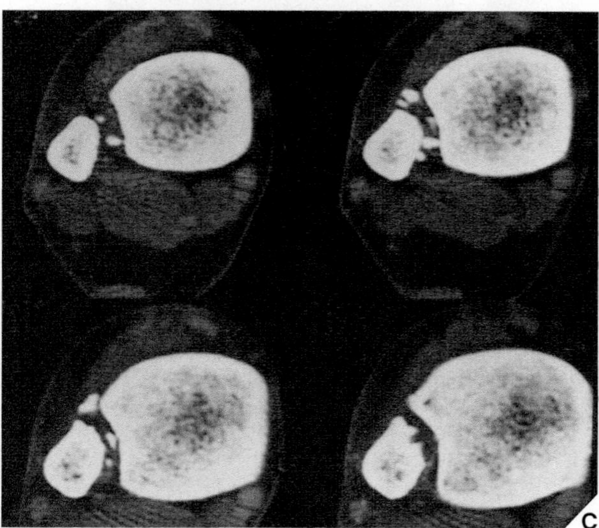

FIGURE 18.18 **CT of periosteal chondroma.** **(A)** Oblique radiograph of the right ankle shows a lesion containing calcifications eroding the medial cortex of the distal fibula. CT using a bone window **(B)** and a soft-tissue window **(C)** better demonstrates the extent of the lesion and the distribution of the calcifications.

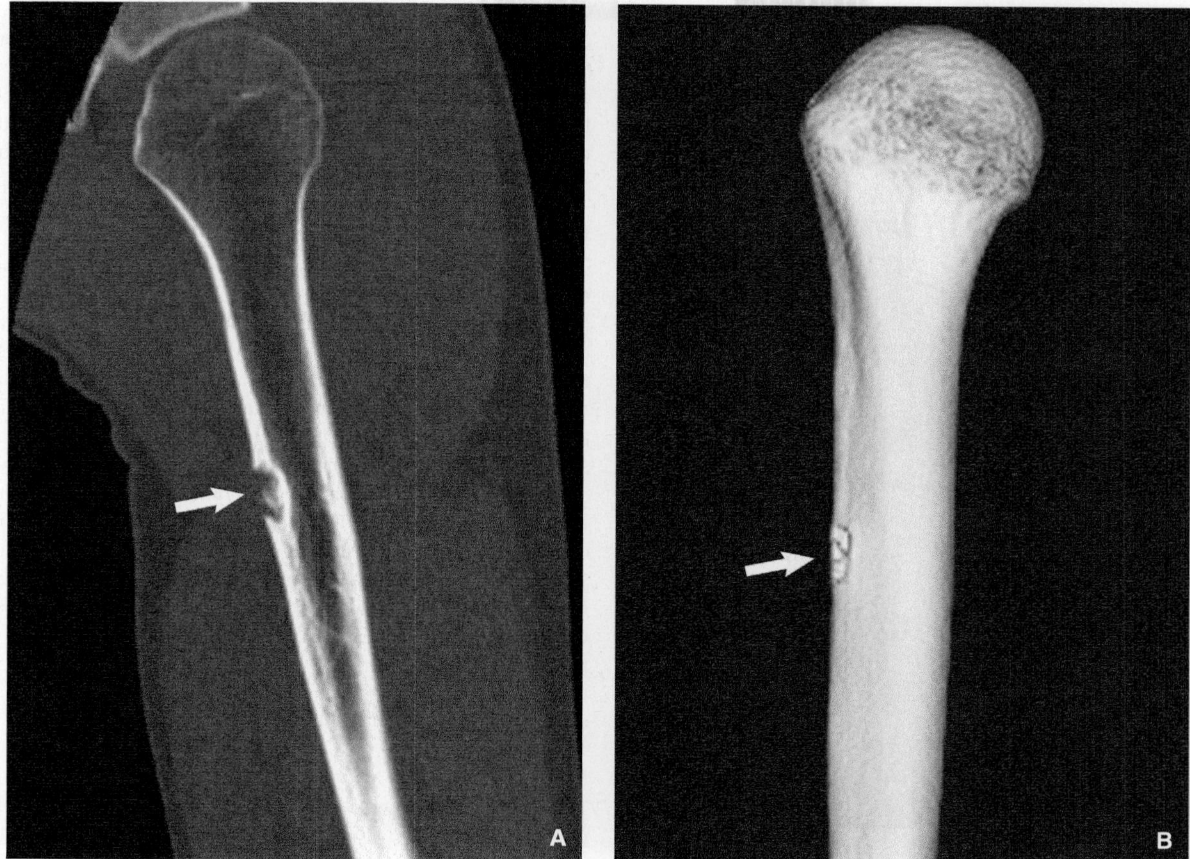

FIGURE 18.19 CT and 3D CT of periosteal chondroma. **(A)** Coronal reformatted and **(B)** 3D CT reconstructed images of the proximal left humerus of a 25-year-old man show juxtacortical lesion eroding the cortex and exhibiting chondroid calcifications *(arrows)*.

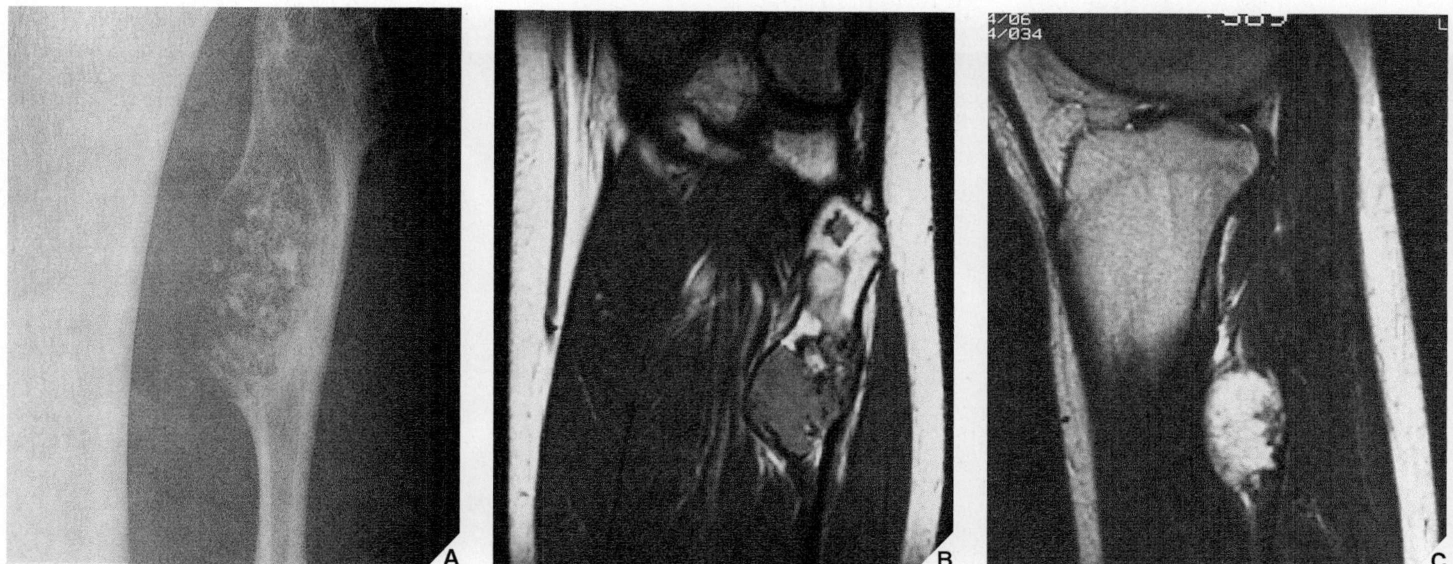

FIGURE 18.20 MRI of periosteal chondroma. **(A)** A large periosteal chondroma eroded the cortex of the proximal fibula and extended into the medullary cavity. **(B)** Coronal proton density–weighted (SE; repetition time [TR] 2000/echo time [TE] 19 msec) and **(C)** sagittal T2-weighted (SE; TR 2000/TE 70 msec) MR images show the lesion's extension into the bone marrow.

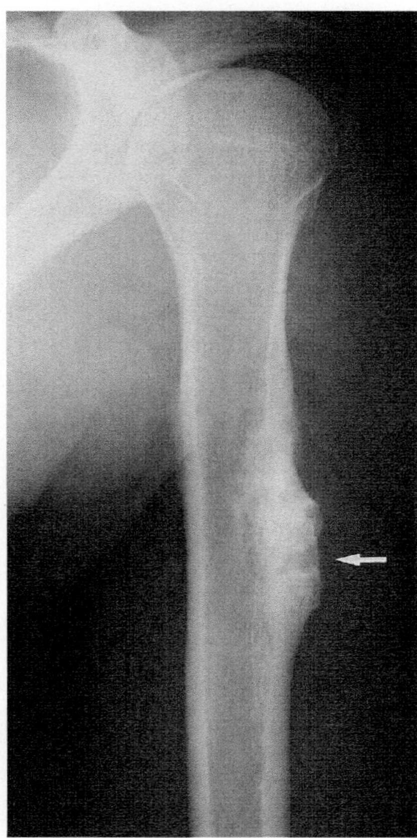

FIGURE 18.21 Periosteal chondroma resembling osteochondroma. A large periosteal chondroma *(arrow)* mimics an osteochondroma. Note, however, the periosteal reaction and separation of the tumor from the medullary cavity by a cortex, features that helped in the differentiation from osteochondroma. (Courtesy of K. K. Unni, MD, Rochester, MN.)

demarcated by surrounding bone marrow. The tissue is sparsely cellular, and the chondrocytes of variable size contain small and darkly staining hyperchromatic nuclei. The tumor cells are located in rounded spaces known as *lacunae*. Occasionally, scattered binucleated cells are present. Calcifications are commonly encountered. The histopathologic features of periosteal chondroma are identical to those of enchondroma, although the lesion sometimes exhibits higher cellularity, occasionally with atypical cells.

Differential Diagnosis

The main differential diagnosis of enchondroma, particularly in lesions of the long bones, is a medullary bone infarct (Fig. 18.23). At times, the two lesions may be difficult to distinguish from one another, particularly if the enchondroma is small, because both lesions present with similar calcifications. The radiographic features helpful in the differential diagnosis are the lobulation of the inner cortical margins in enchondroma; the annular, punctate, and comma-shaped calcifications in the matrix; and the lack of sclerotic rim that is usually seen in bone infarcts (Fig. 18.24).

The most difficult task for the radiologist is to distinguish a large solitary enchondroma from a slowly growing low-grade chondrosarcoma. One of the most significant findings pointing to a chondrosarcoma in the early stage of development is localized thickening of the cortex and deep endosteal scalloping (Fig. 18.25). The size of the lesion should also be taken into consideration. Lesions longer than 4 cm (or, according to some investigators, longer than 7 cm) are suggestive of malignancy. In more advanced tumors, destruction of the cortex and the presence of a soft-tissue mass are the hallmarks of malignancy.

Complications

The single most important complication of enchondroma, aside from pathologic fracture (see Figs. 18.7 and 18.8), is its malignant transformation to chondrosarcoma. With solitary enchondromas, this occurs almost exclusively in a long or flat bone and almost never in a short tubular bone. The radiographic signs of the transformation are thickening of the cortex, destruction of the cortex, and a soft-tissue mass. The development of pain in the absence of fracture at the site of the lesion is an important clinical sign.

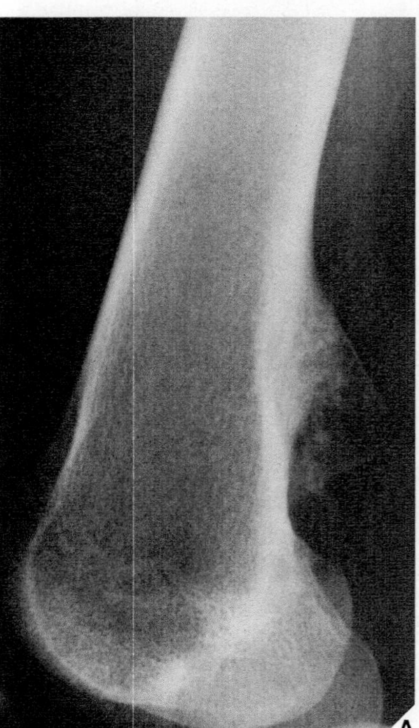

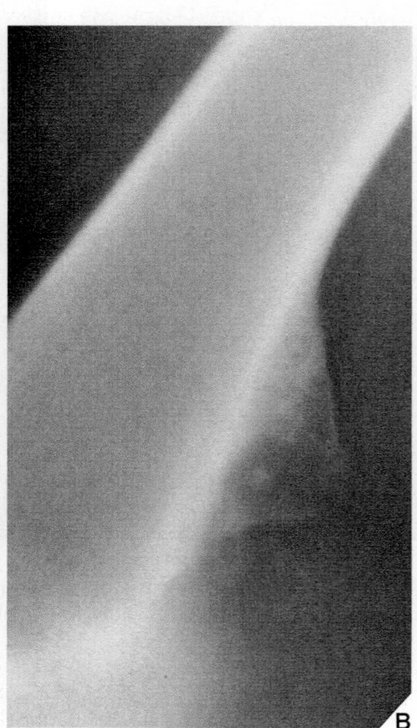

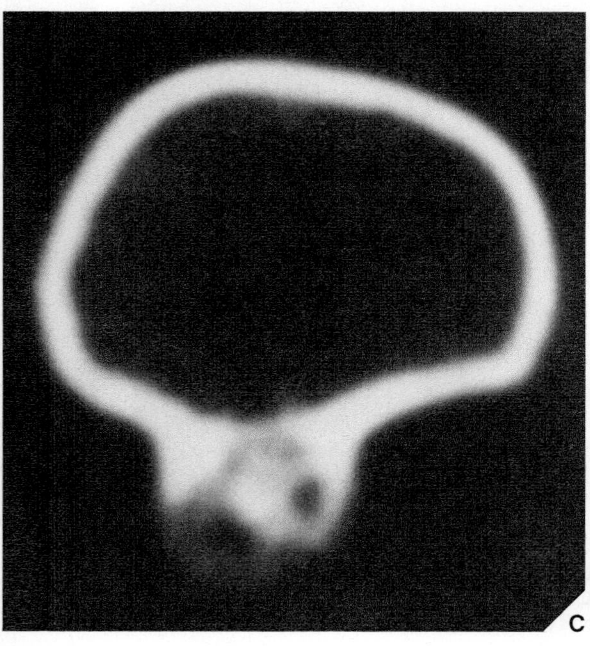

FIGURE 18.22 Periosteal chondroma resembling osteochondroma. **(A)** Lateral radiograph of the distal femur shows a lesion arising from the posterior cortex that resembles an osteochondroma. **(B)** Conventional tomography shows calcifications at the base of the lesion and continuity of the posterior cortex of the femur. **(C)** CT section demonstrates lack of communication between the medullary portion of the femur and the lesion, thus excluding the diagnosis of osteochondroma. (**A** and **C**, Reprinted from Greenspan A, Unni KK, Matthews J II. Periosteal chondroma masquerading as osteochondroma. *Can Assoc Radiol J* 1993;44(3):205–210. Copyright © 1993 Canadian Association of Radiologists. With permission.)

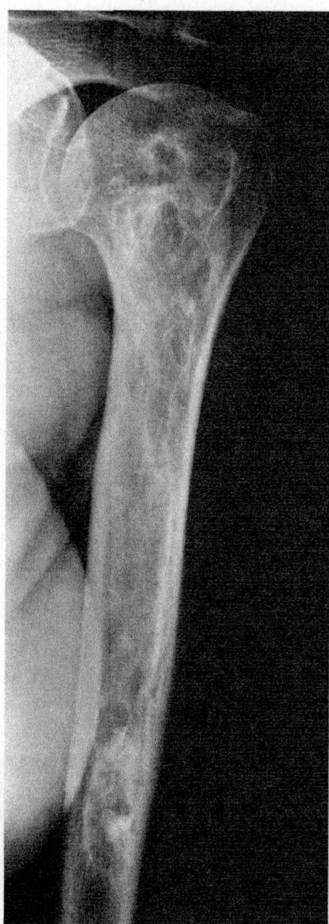

▲ **FIGURE 18.23** **Bone infarct.** In a medullary bone infarct, seen here in the proximal humerus of a 36-year-old man with sickle cell disease, there is no endosteal scalloping of the cortex, and the calcified area is surrounded by a thin, dense sclerotic rim, the hallmark of a bone infarct.

Treatment

Curettage of the lesion with the application of bone graft is the most common course of treatment.

Enchondromatosis, Ollier Disease, and Maffucci Syndrome

Clinical and Imaging Features

Enchondromatosis is a condition marked by multiple enchondromas, generally in the region of the metaphysis and diaphysis (Fig. 18.26). If the skeleton is extensively affected, with predominantly unilateral (monomelic) distribution, associated with bone growth disturbance, the term *Ollier disease* is applied. The clinical manifestations of multiple enchondromas, such as knobby swellings of the digits (Figs. 18.27 and 18.28) or gross disparity in the length of the forearms or legs, are frequently recognized in childhood and adolescence; the disease has a strong preference for one side of the body. The disorder has no hereditary or familial tendency. Some investigators claim that it is not a neoplastic lesion but rather a developmental bone dysplasia. Maffucci syndrome is a congenital, nonhereditary disorder, characterized by enchondromatosis and soft-tissue angiomatosis (hemangiomatosis). The hemangiomas may occur anywhere in the skin and subcutaneous tissue. They are usually cavernous in type and may form unilaterally or bilaterally. The enchondromas in Maffucci syndrome have predilection for the tubular bones and have the same distribution as in Ollier disease, with a strong predisposition for one side of the body, the metacarpals and the phalanges being the most common sites. The pathogenesis of Ollier disease and Maffucci syndrome is unknown. The recent investigations, however, suggested that these disorders represent two entities within continuum of enchondromatosis and that both conditions bear the risk of mesodermal and nonmesodermal malignancy, caused by somatic mosaic mutations of *IDH1* and *IDH2* genes.

Conventional radiography is usually sufficient to demonstrate the typical features of enchondromatosis/Ollier disease. Characteristically, interference of the lesion with the growth plate causes foreshortening of the limbs. Deformity of the bones is marked by radiolucent masses of

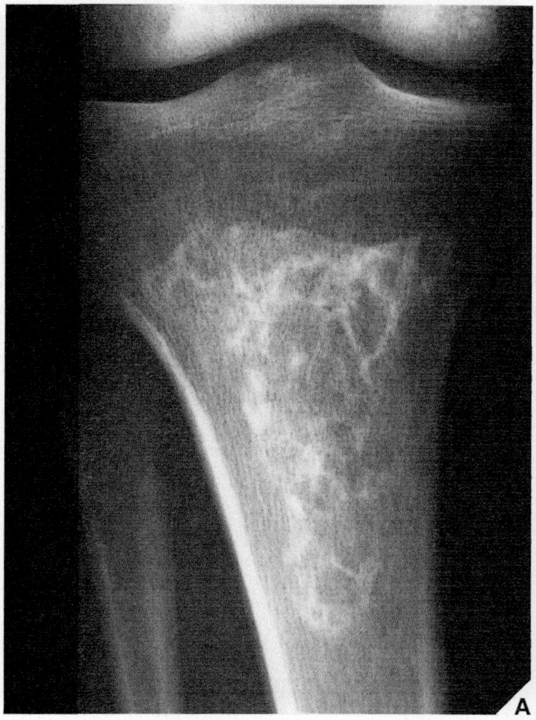

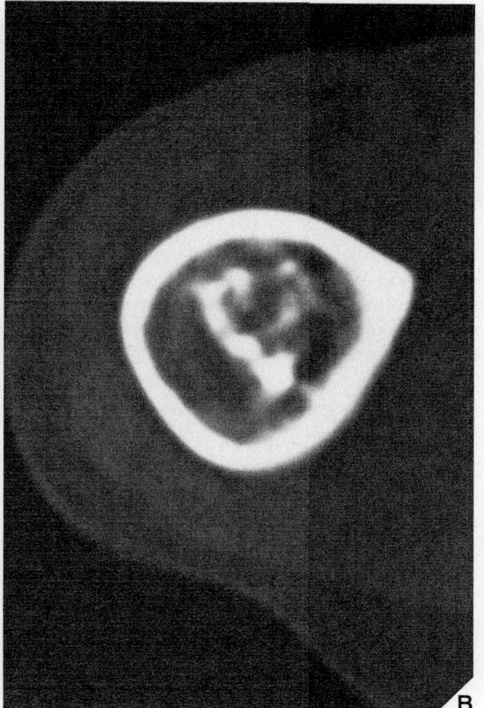

▲ **FIGURE 18.24** **Bone infarct.** **(A)** Conventional radiograph of the proximal tibia shows the typical coarse calcifications of medullary bone infarct. Note the sharply defined peripheral margin separating necrotic from viable bone and the lack of characteristics for chondroid tumor annular and comma-shaped calcifications. **(B)** In another patient with a bone infarct in the distal femur, a CT section reveals central coarse calcifications and lack of endosteal scalloping of the cortex.

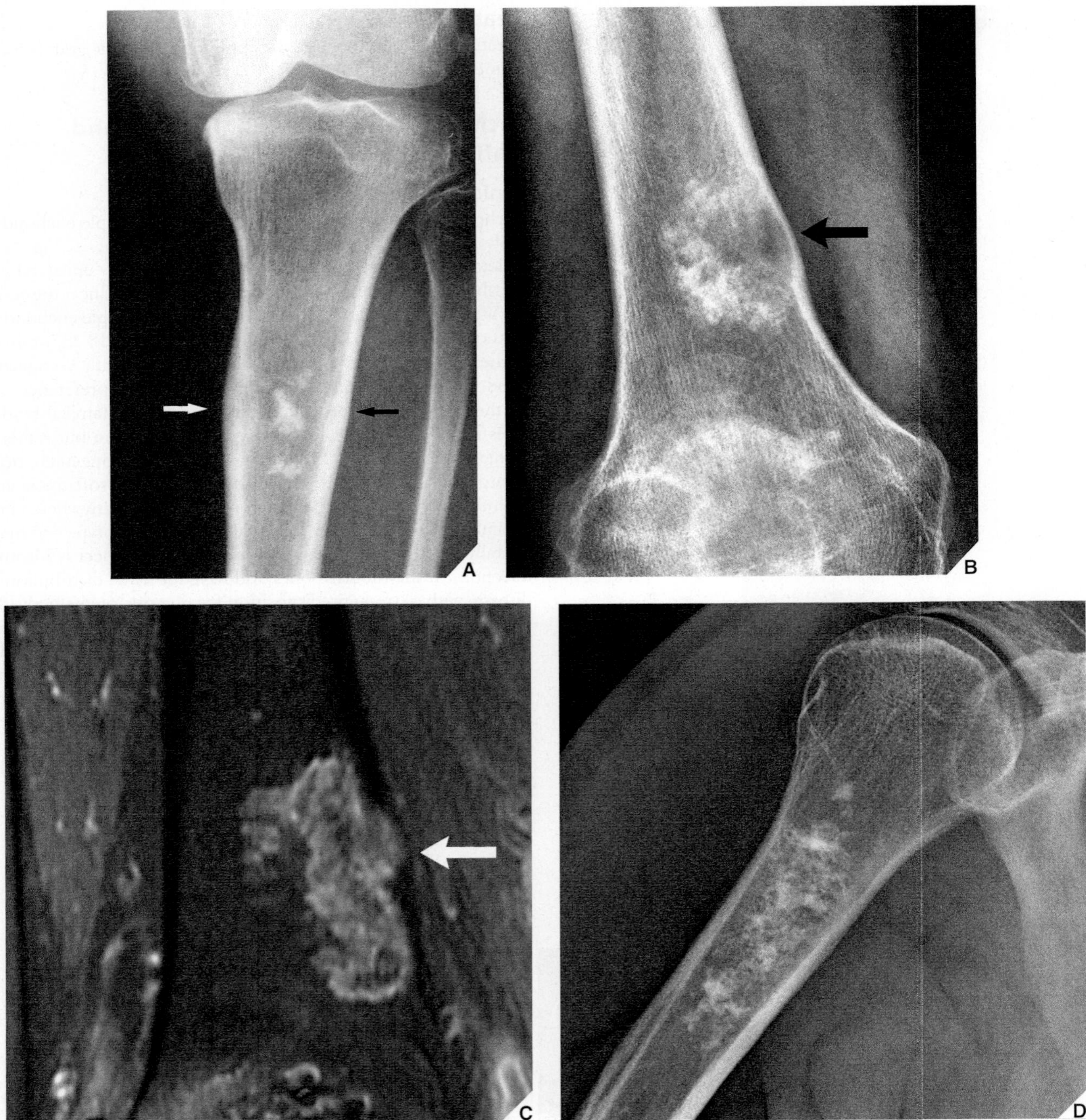

FIGURE 18.25 Low-grade chondrosarcoma. **(A)** A 48-year-old woman presented with pain in the upper leg. A radiograph shows a radiolucent lesion in the proximal tibia with a wide zone of transition and central calcifications. Note focal thickening of the cortex *(arrows)*, an important feature that distinguishes chondrosarcoma from similarly appearing enchondroma. In another patient, a 57-year-old woman, the radiograph of the distal femur **(B)** and coronal T1-weighted fat-suppressed MR image obtained after intravenous injection of gadolinium **(C)** show deep endosteal scalloping *(arrows)*. Excision biopsy revealed a low-grade chondrosarcoma. **(D)** Classic enchondroma is shown for comparison. Note that cortex is not thickened, and despite the size of the lesion that abuts the endocortex, there is lack of endosteal scalloping.

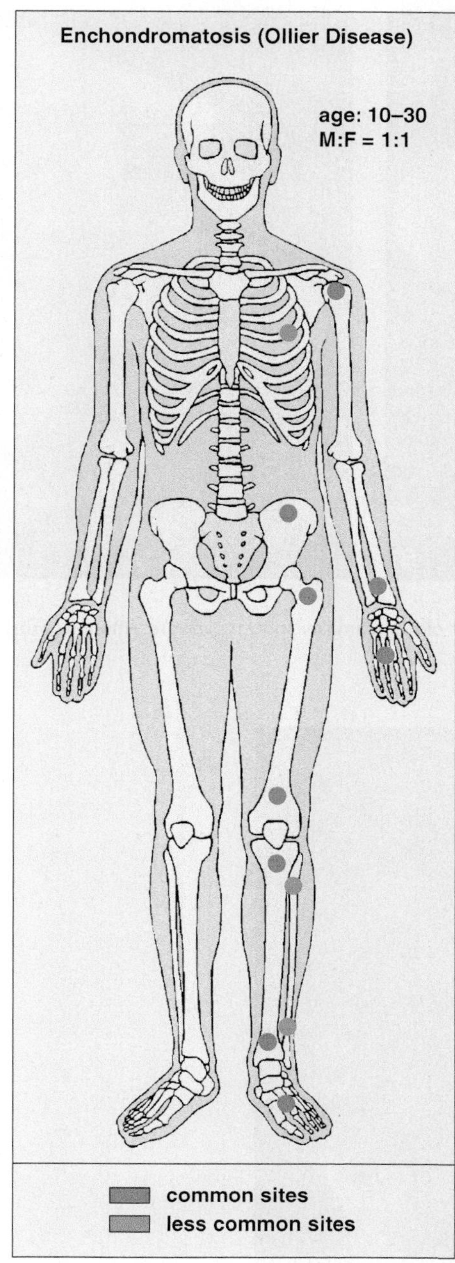

FIGURE 18.26 Skeletal sites of predilection, peak age range, and male-to-female ratio in enchondromatosis (Ollier disease).

cartilage, often in the hand and foot, with or without foci of calcification (Figs. 18.29 to 18.31). Enchondromas in this location may be intracortical and periosteal. They sometimes protrude from the shaft of the short or long tubular bone, thus resembling osteochondromas (Fig. 18.32). Linear columns of cartilage in the form of radiolucent streaks extend from the growth plate to the diaphysis, and a fan-like pattern is common in the iliac bones (Fig. 18.33). CT may better show the distribution of the lesions (Figs. 18.34 and 18.35). MRI demonstrates lobulated in contour masses exhibiting low-to-intermediate signal intensity on T1-weighted images and high signal on T2 weighting (Fig. 18.35C,D). After injection of gadolinium, there is various degree of enhancement (Fig. 18.36). The Maffucci syndrome, in addition to the typical osseous alterations of enchondromatosis, is recognized radiographically by the presence of multiple calcified phleboliths (Fig. 18.37).

Pathology

Histologically, the lesions of enchondromatosis, Ollier disease, and Maffucci syndrome are essentially indistinguishable from those of solitary enchondromas, although on occasion they tend to be more cellular, demonstrate cytologic atypia, and may contain myxoid stroma, which may suggest the diagnosis of chondrosarcoma.

Complications

The most frequent and severe complication of Ollier disease is malignant transformation to chondrosarcoma, reported in 25% to 30% of affected patients. In contrast to solitary enchondromas, even lesions in the short tubular bones may undergo sarcomatous change (Fig. 18.38). This is also true in patients with Maffucci syndrome (Fig. 18.39), with malignant transformation reported in more than 50% of the affected individuals.

Osteochondroma

Clinical and Imaging Features

Also known as *osteocartilaginous exostosis*, this lesion is characterized by a cartilage-capped bony projection on the external surface of a bone. It is the most common benign bone lesion, constituting approximately 20% to 50% of all benign bone tumors, and is usually diagnosed in patients before their third decade. It has been postulated that sporadic osteochondromas represent developmental abnormality; however, recent cytogenetic studies revealed mutations in the *EXT* gene encoding exostosin 1, suggesting their neoplastic nature. Apparently, these genetic mutations lead to abnormal processing and accumulation of heparan sulphate proteoglycans (HSPG) in the cytoplasm of the chondrocytes. This leads to a loss of polar organization of the growth plate allowing chondrocytes to grow in the wrong direction. Continued growth of these chondrocytes coupled with endochondral ossification result in the formation of outpouching of both medullary and cortical bone covered by the cartilaginous cap, thus forming

FIGURE 18.27 Enchondromatosis. Clinical photograph of hands of a 33-year-old man shows knobby masses affecting several fingers.

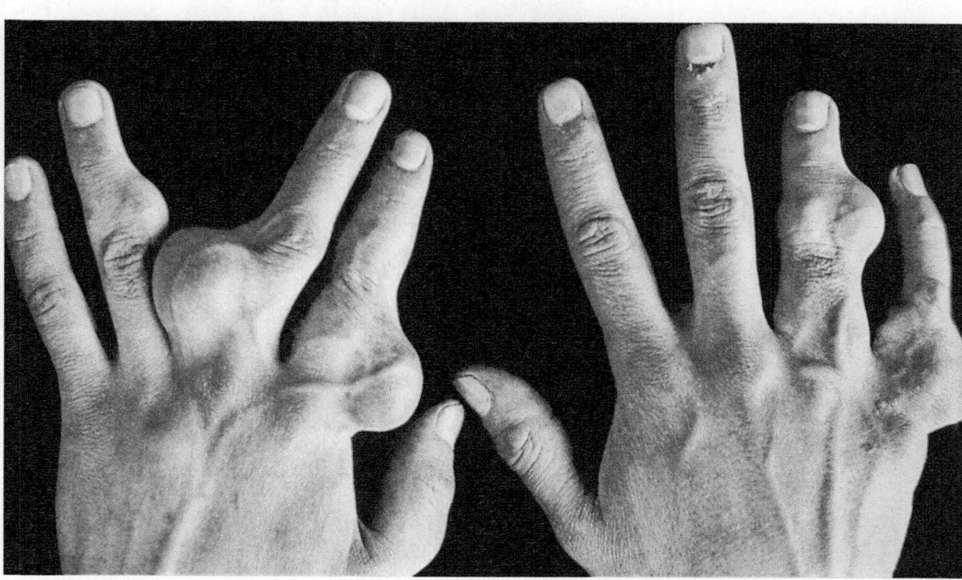

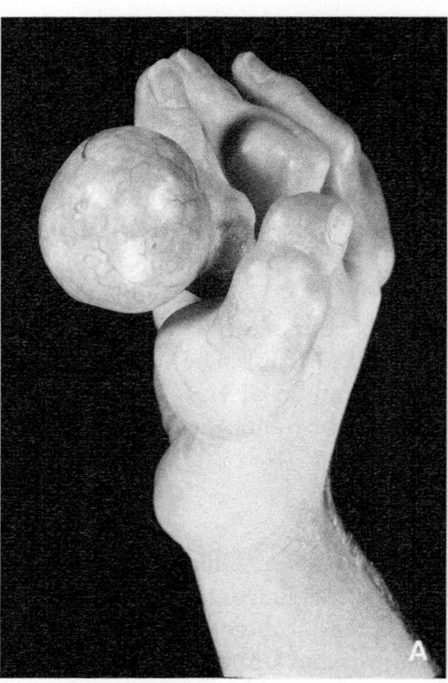

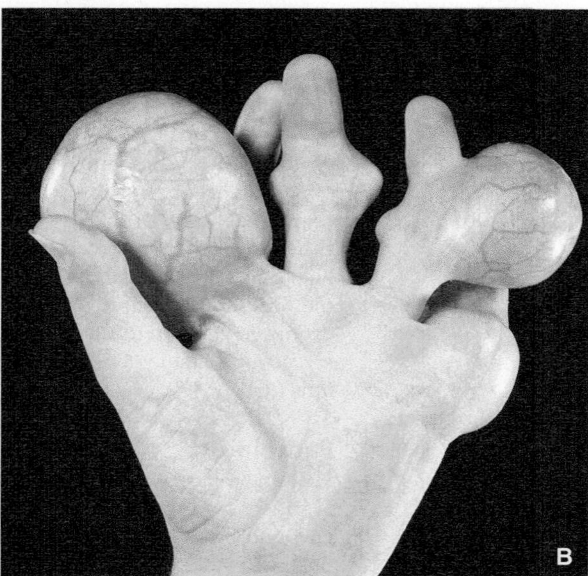

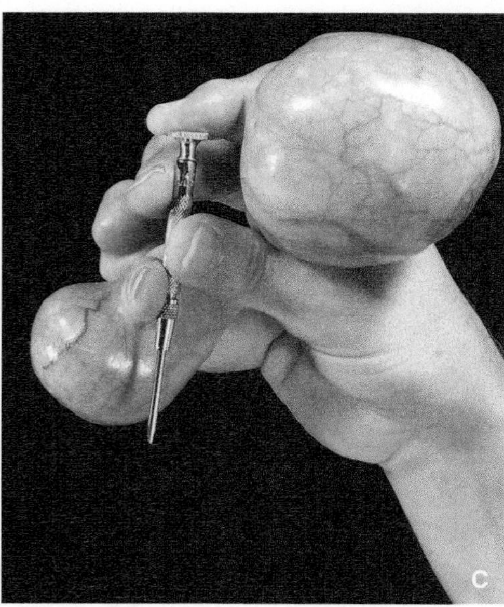

FIGURE 18.28 **Ollier disease.** Clinical photographs of **(A)** left hand and **(B,C)** right hand of a 41-year-old watchmaker show typical presentation of this condition.

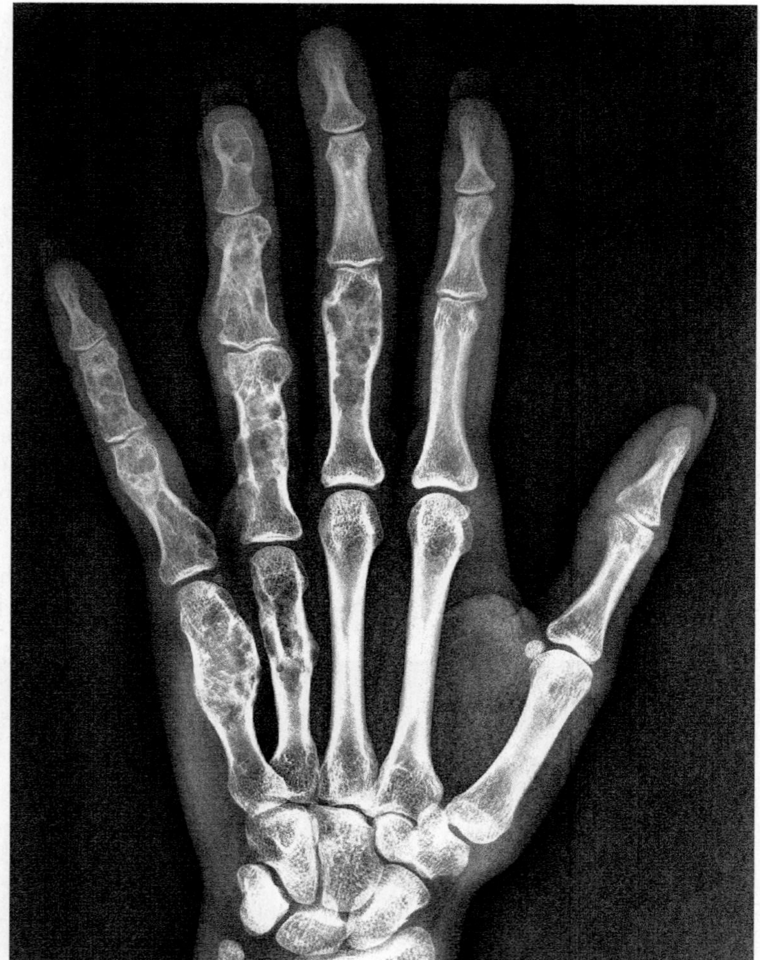

FIGURE 18.29 **Enchondromatosis.** Dorsovolar radiograph of the right hand of a 30-year-old woman shows several enchondromas affecting the fourth and fifth metacarpal bones as well as the phalanges of the middle, ring, and small fingers.

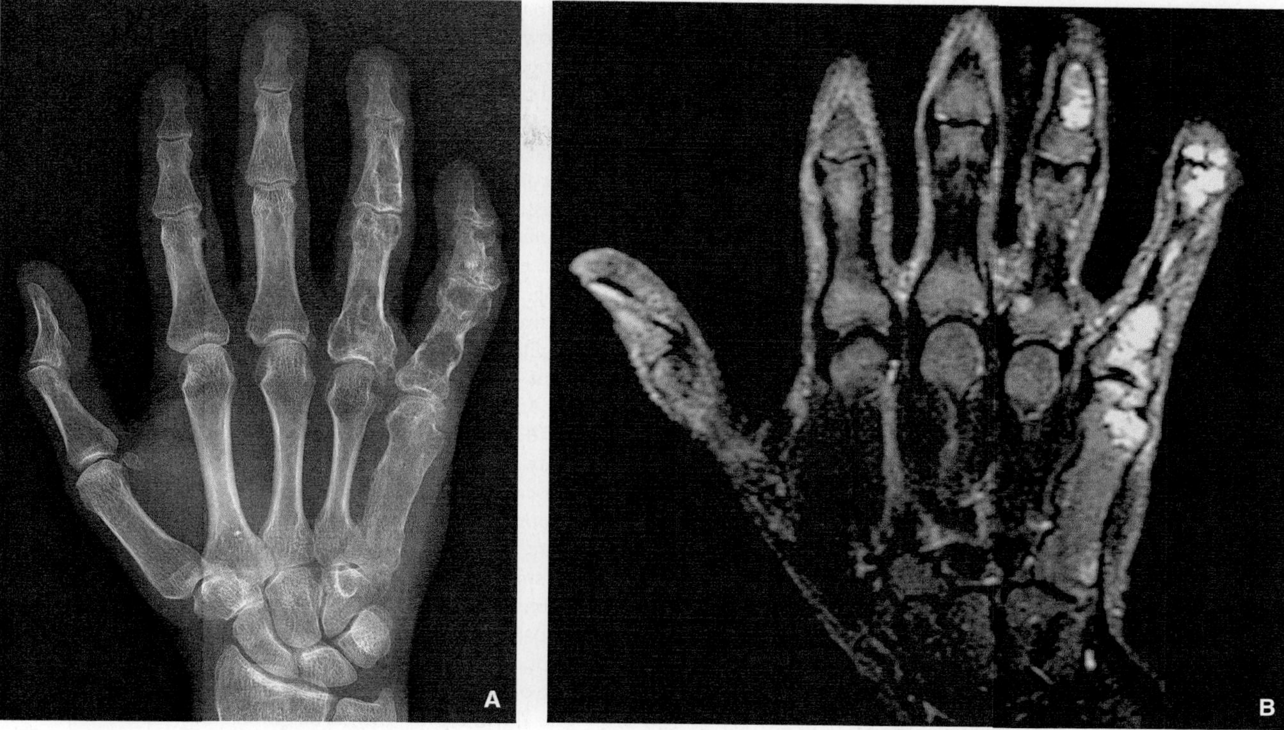

FIGURE 18.30 MRI of enchondromatosis. **(A)** Dorsovolar radiograph of the left hand of a 58-year-old man shows multiple enchondromas affecting the fifth metacarpal bone and phalanges of the ring and small fingers. **(B)** Coronal IR MR image shows that the lesions display high signal intensity.

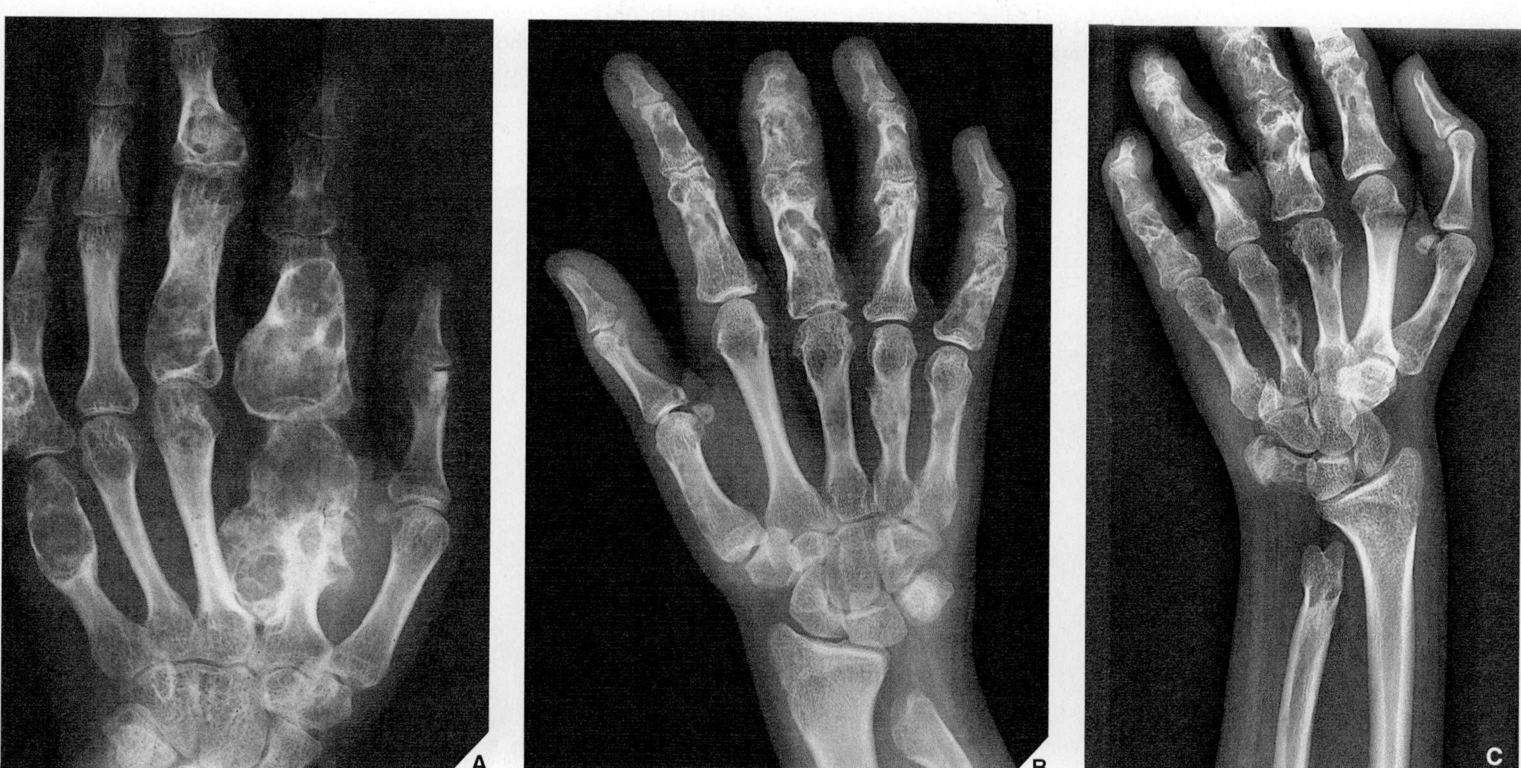

FIGURE 18.31 Ollier disease. **(A)** Large, lobulated cartilaginous masses markedly deform the bones of the hand in this 20-year-old man. **(B)** In another patient, a 29-year-old woman, multiple enchondromas are present within the phalanges and metacarpals. Note also growth stunting of the distal ulna. **(C)** Dorsovolar radiograph of the right hand of a 17-year-old girl shows extensive involvement of several metacarpals and phalanges by enchondromas. Note also involvement of the distal ulna, which in addition shows growth stunting, one of the features of this disorder.

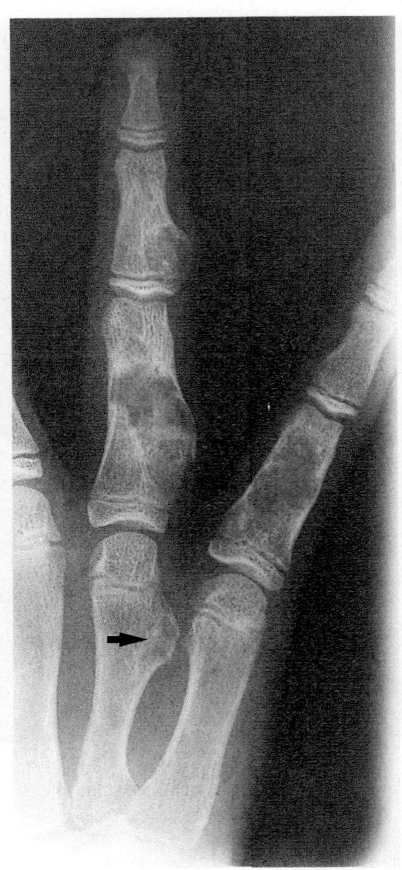

FIGURE 18.32 Enchondromatosis. In this 12-year-old boy, the intracortical lesion in the metaphysis of the fourth metacarpal protrudes from the bone *(arrow)*, thus resembling an osteochondroma.

an exostosis. Osteochondroma, which has its own growth plate, usually stops growing at skeletal maturity. The most common sites of involvement are the metaphyses of the long bones, particularly in the region around the knee and the proximal humerus (Fig. 18.40). Variants of osteochondroma include subungual exostosis (also known as *Dupuytren exostosis*), turret exostosis (also referred to as *acquired osteochondroma*), traction exostosis, bizarre parosteal osteochondromatous proliferation (BPOP), florid reactive periostitis, and dysplasia epiphysealis hemimelica (also called *intraarticular osteochondroma* or *Trevor-Fairbank disease*).

The radiographic presentation of osteochondroma is characteristic according to whether the lesion is pedunculated, with a slender pedicle usually directed away from the neighboring growth plate (Fig. 18.41), or sessile, with a broad base attached to the cortex (Fig. 18.42). The most important characteristic feature of either type of lesion is uninterrupted merging of the cortex of the host bone with the cortex of the osteochondroma; additionally, the medullary portion of the lesion and the medullary cavity of the adjacent bone communicate. CT scanning can establish unequivocally the lack of cortical interruption and the continuity of cancellous portions of the lesion and the host bone (Figs. 18.43 and 18.44). These are important features that distinguish this lesion from the occasionally similar looking bone masses of osteoma, periosteal chondroma, BPOP, juxtacortical osteosarcoma, soft-tissue osteosarcoma, and juxtacortical myositis ossificans (Fig. 18.45). The other characteristic feature of osteochondroma involves calcifications in the chondro-osseous portion of the stalk of the lesion (see Figs. 18.41B and 18.42A,B) and cartilaginous cap. The thickness of the cartilaginous cap ranges from 1 to 3 mm and rarely exceeds 1 cm. On MRI, the cartilaginous cap shows high signal intensity on T2-weighted and gradient-echo sequences. A narrow band of low signal intensity surrounding the cap represents the overlying perichondrium (Fig. 18.46).

Pathology

Pathology of osteochondroma reflects all characteristic features of the lesion seen on the imaging studies (Fig. 18.47). Histologically, the

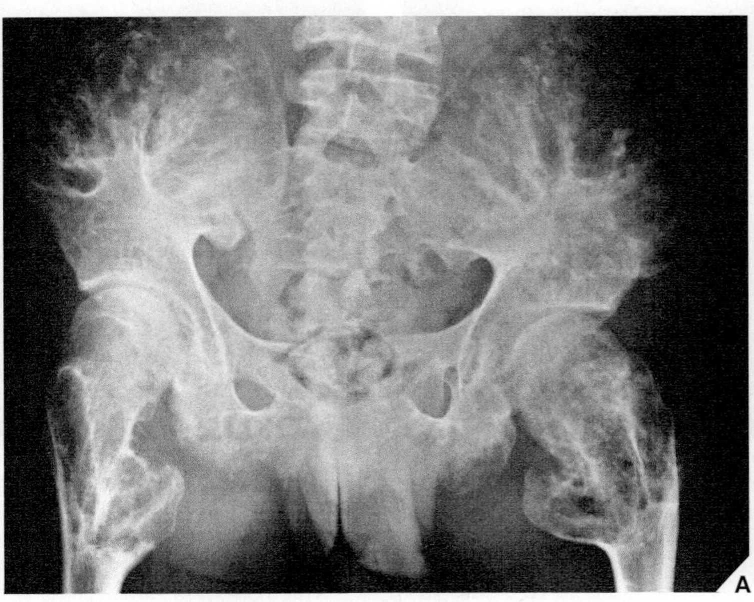

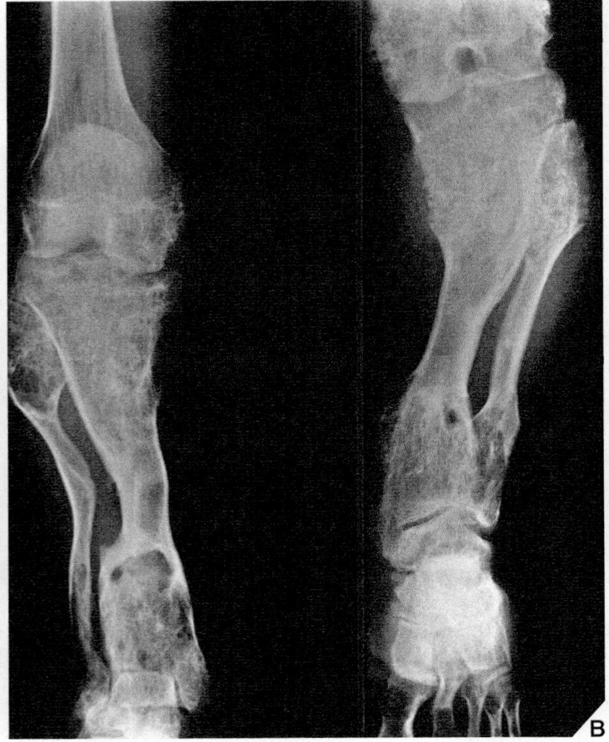

FIGURE 18.33 Ollier disease. The classic features of this disorder in a 17-year-old boy are exhibited in extensive involvement of multiple bones. **(A)** Anteroposterior radiograph of the pelvis demonstrates crescent-shaped and ring-like calcifications in tongues of cartilage extending from the iliac crests and proximal femora. **(B)** A radiograph of both legs shows growth stunting and deformities of the tibia and fibula. *(Continued)*

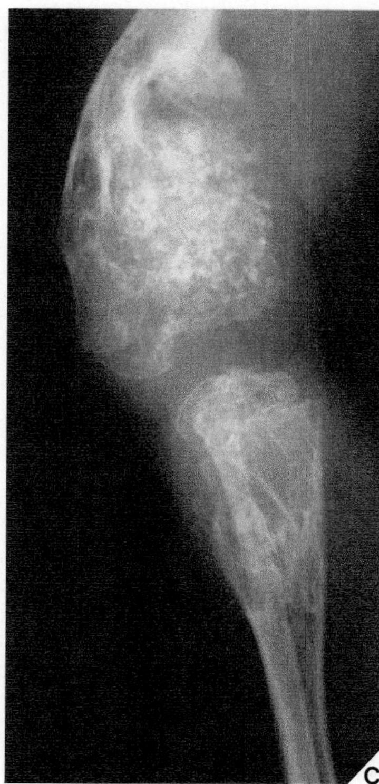

▲ **FIGURE 18.33** Ollier disease. ***(Continued)*** **(C)** In another patient, a 6-year-old boy, note extensive involvement of the proximal tibia and distal femur.

osteochondroma cap is composed of hyaline cartilage arranged similarly to that of a growth plate. A zone of calcification in the chondro-osseous portion of the stalk corresponds to the zone of provisional calcification in the physis. Beneath this zone, there is vascular invasion and replacement of the calcified cartilage by new bone formation, which undergoes maturation and merges with the cancellous bone of the host bone's medullary cavity.

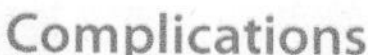

Complications

Osteochondroma may be complicated by a number of secondary abnormalities, including pressure on nerves or blood vessels (Fig. 18.48); pressure on the adjacent bone (Fig. 18.49; see also Fig. 16.70), with occasional fracture (Fig. 18.50); fracture through the lesion itself; and inflammatory changes of the bursa exostotica ("exostosis bursata") covering the cartilaginous cap (Fig. 18.51).

The least common complication of osteochondroma, seen in solitary lesions in less than 1% of cases, is malignant transformation to chondrosarcoma. Nevertheless, it is important to recognize this complication at an early stage. The chief clinical features suggesting malignant transformation are pain (in the absence of a fracture, bursitis, or pressure on nearby nerves) and a growth spurt or continued growth of the lesion beyond the age of skeletal maturity. Certain imaging features have also been identified that may help in the determination of malignancy (Table 18.1).

The most reliable imaging modalities for evaluating the possible malignant transformation of an osteochondroma are conventional radiography, CT, and MRI; the results of a radionuclide bone scan, which may show increased uptake of radiopharmaceutical at the site of the lesion, may not be reliable. The unreliability of radionuclide imaging is related to the fact that even benign exostoses exhibit an increased uptake of radiopharmaceutical tracer caused by endochondral ossification. Exostotic chondrosarcoma is also marked by isotope uptake, which is related to active ossification, osteoblastic activity, and hyperemia within the cartilage and bony stalk of the tumor. Thus, although the uptake is more intense in exostotic chondrosarcomas than in benign exostoses, various investigations show that this is not always a reliable feature distinguishing these lesions. The radiography usually demonstrates whether the calcifications in an osteochondroma are contained within the stalk of the lesion—a clear indication of benignity (see Figs. 18.41B and 18.42A,B). Similarly, CT can demonstrate both dispersed calcifications in the cartilaginous cap and increased thickness of the cap (greater than 2 cm), cardinal signs of malignant transformation of the lesion, as Norman and Sissons have pointed out (Fig. 18.52).

Treatment

Solitary lesions of osteochondroma usually can simply be monitored if they do not cause clinical problems. Surgical resection is indicated if the

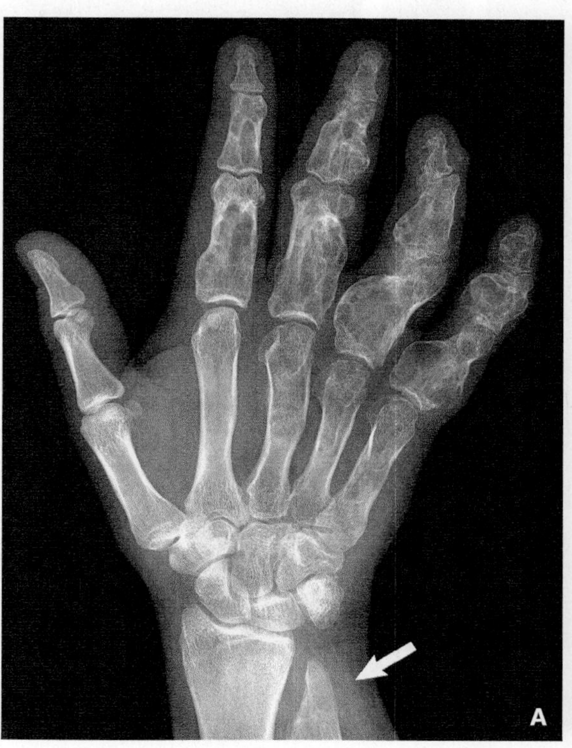

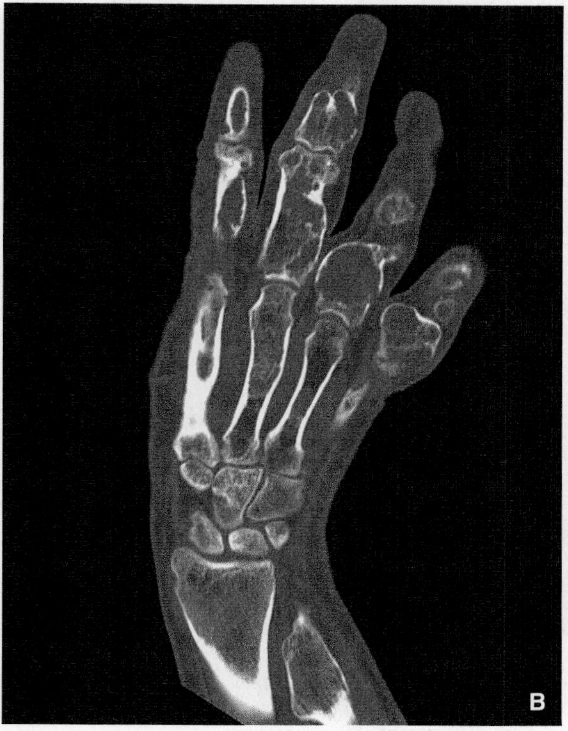

▲ **FIGURE 18.34** CT of Ollier disease. **(A)** Dorsovolar radiograph and **(B)** coronal reformatted CT image of the left hand of a 32-year-old man show numerous enchondromas affecting second to fifth metacarpals, and phalanges of all fingers except the thumb. Observe growth disturbance of the distal ulna *(arrow)*. *(Continued)*

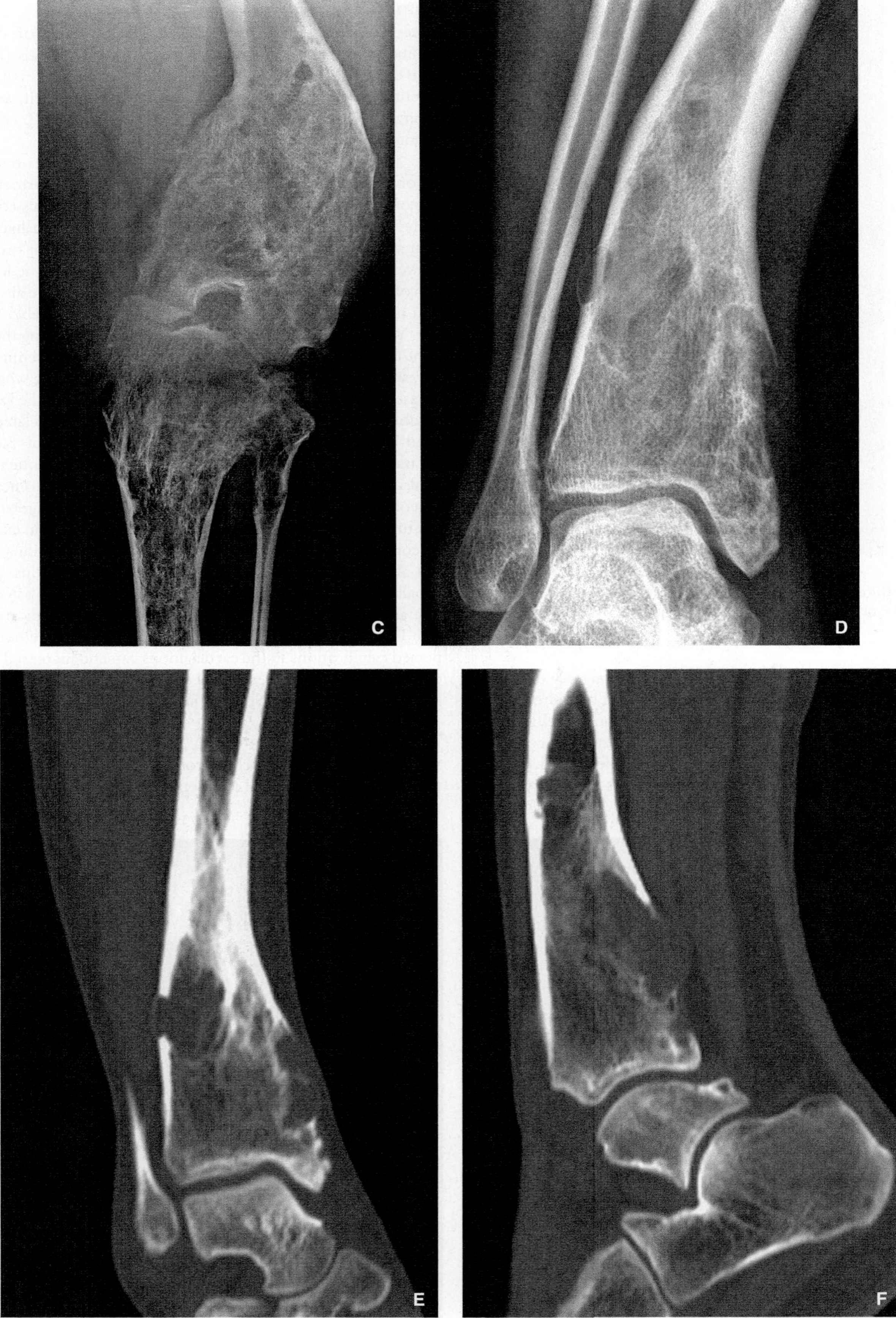

FIGURE 18.34 CT of Ollier disease. ***(Continued)*** In another patient, **(C)** anteroposterior radiograph of the right knee shows numerous enchondromas in the distal femur and proximal tibia and fibula associated with growth disturbance. **(D)** Anteroposterior radiograph of the right ankle of the same patient and **(E)** coronal and **(F)** sagittal reformatted CT images show involvement of the distal tibia.

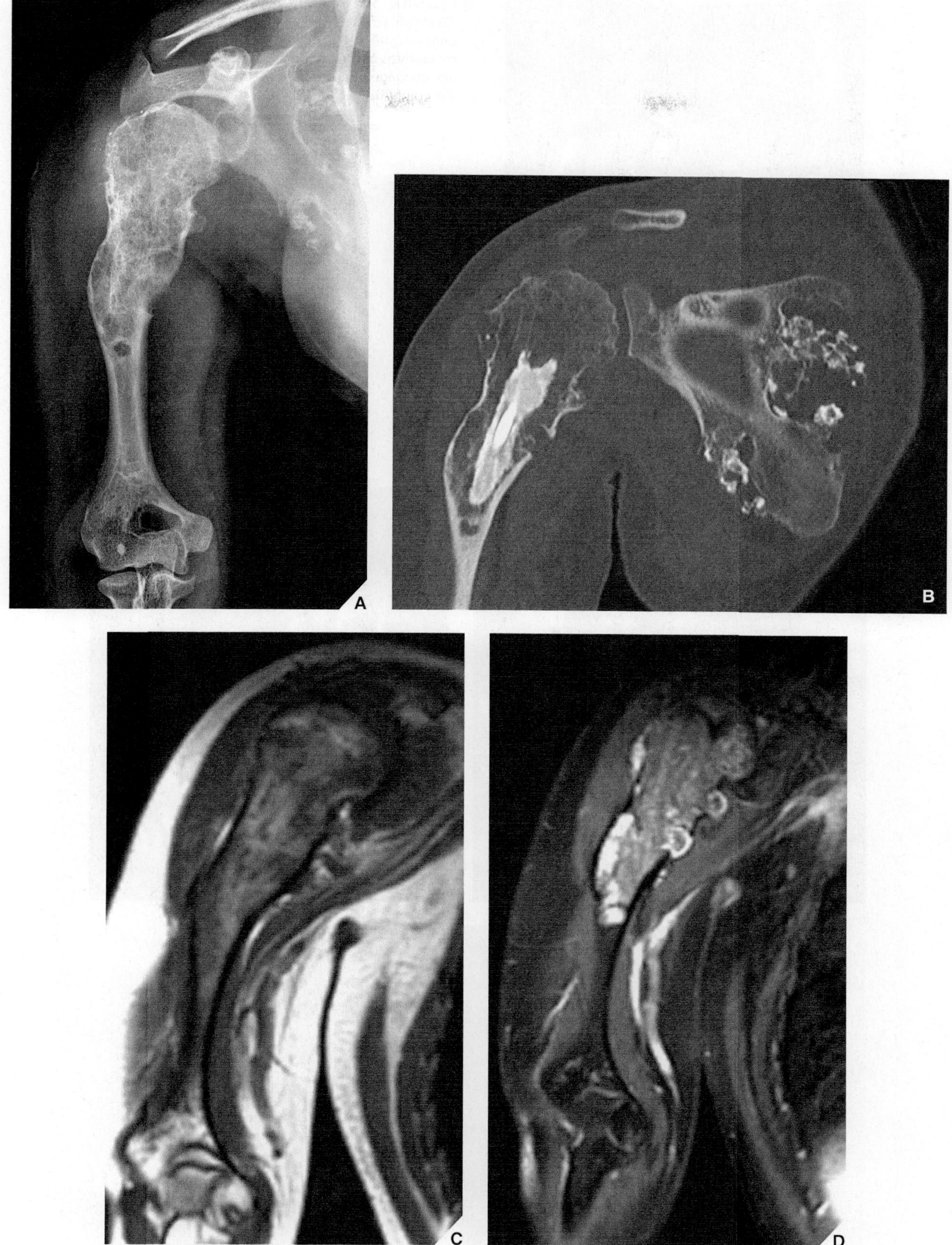

FIGURE 18.35 CT and MRI of Ollier disease. **(A)** Anteroposterior radiograph of the right humerus of a 23-year-old woman shows numerous enchondromas affecting proximal half of the bone. Observe also the lesions within the scapula. **(B)** Coronal reformatted CT image shows the distribution of numerous enchondromas within the proximal humerus and scapula to the better advantage. **(C)** Coronal T1-weighted MRI shows heterogenous signal intensity of the lesions. **(D)** Coronal T1-weighted fat-suppressed MR image obtained after intravenous administration of gadolinium demonstrates strong peripheral enhancement of the lesions.

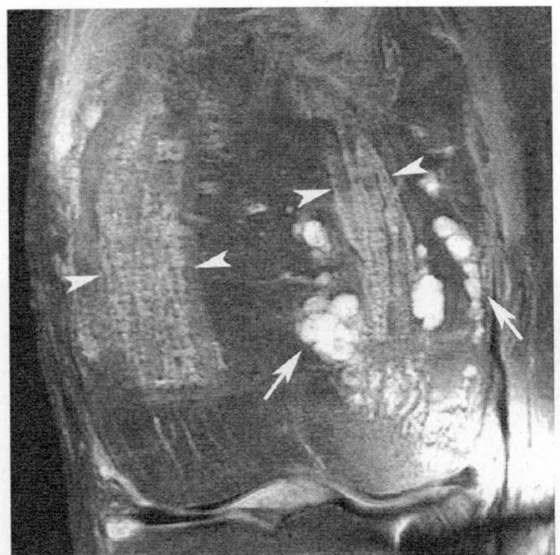

FIGURE 18.36 MRI of Ollier disease. Coronal T2-weighted fat-saturated MRI of the distal femur demonstrates linear columns of cartilage in the distal metaphysis of the femur *(arrowheads)* and more globular cartilage tumors *(arrows)*. Note the involvement of the epiphysis.

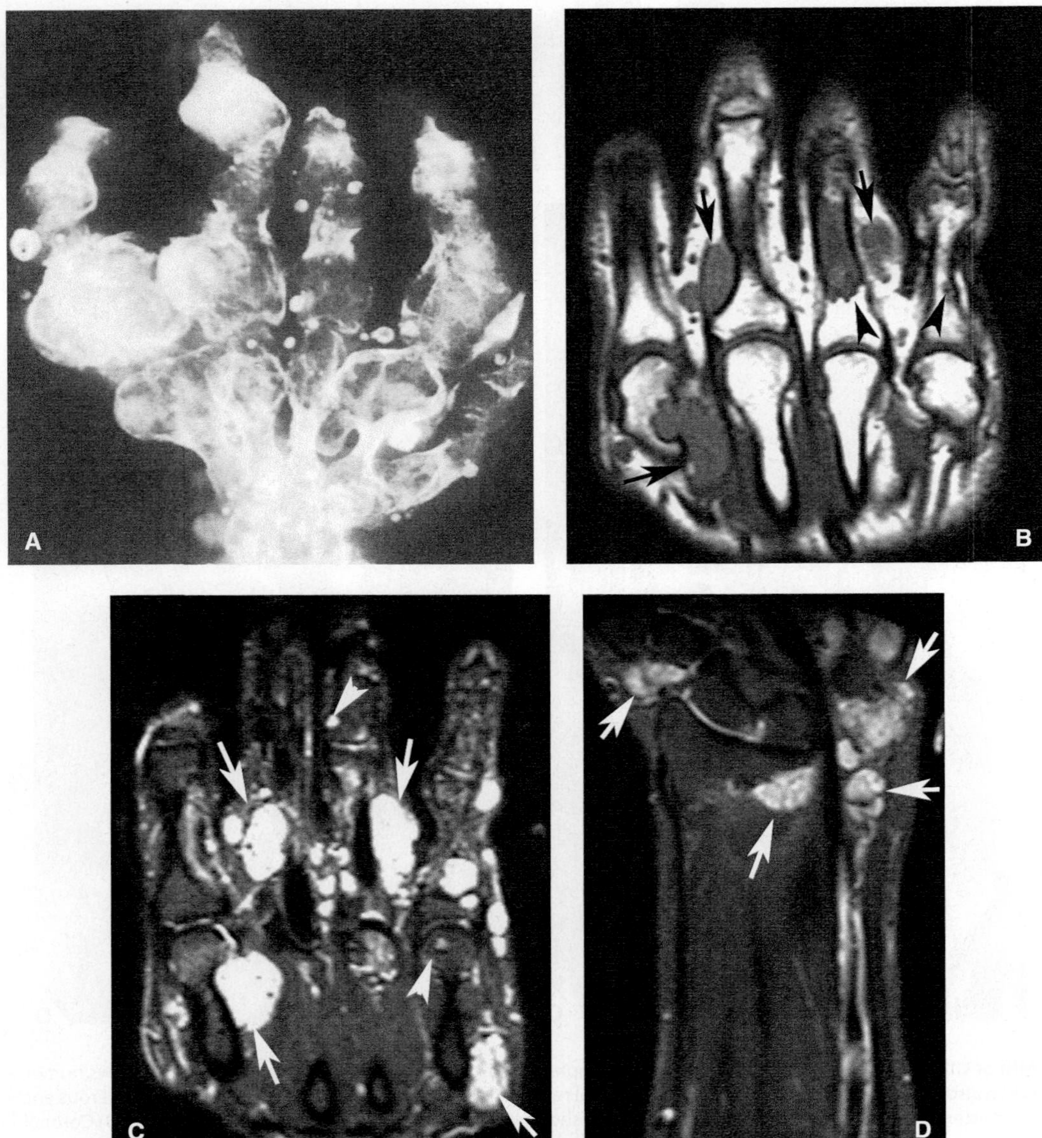

FIGURE 18.37 Maffucci syndrome. **(A)** Radiograph of the hand reveals typical changes of enchondromatosis, accompanied by calcified phleboliths in soft-tissue hemangiomas. (Reprinted from Bullough P. *Orthopaedic pathology*, 5th ed. Maryland Heights, MO: Mosby; 2009, with permission from Elsevier.) **(B)** Coronal T1-weighted and **(C)** coronal T2-weighted MR images of the hand of another patient with Maffucci syndrome supplemented with **(D)** coronal T2-weighted MR image of the forearm demonstrate multiple soft-tissue hemangiomas *(arrows)* and enchondromas *(arrowheads)*.

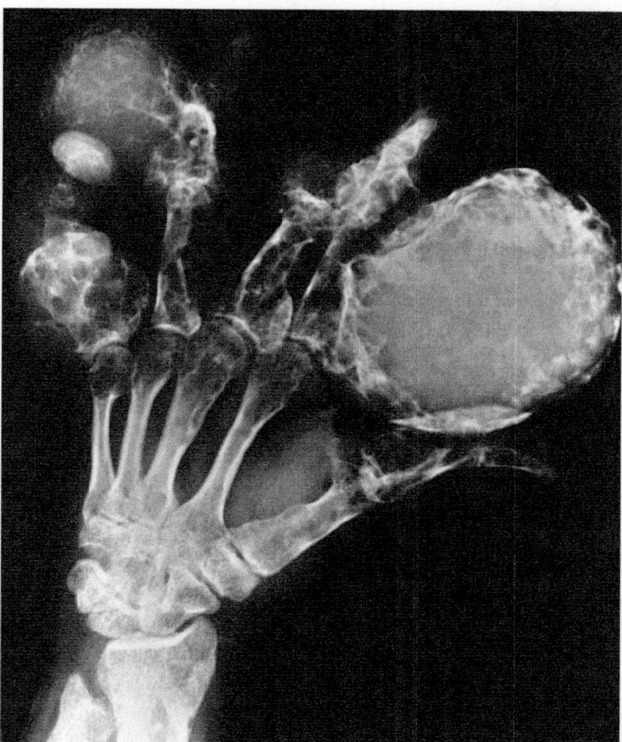

FIGURE 18.38 Chondrosarcoma in Ollier disease. In this case of sarcomatous transformation of enchondroma in the hand in a patient with Ollier disease, note the large, lobulated masses of cartilage in all fingers. The lesion of the middle phalanx of the ring finger shows destruction of the cortex and extension into the soft tissues (same patient as depicted in Fig. 18.28).

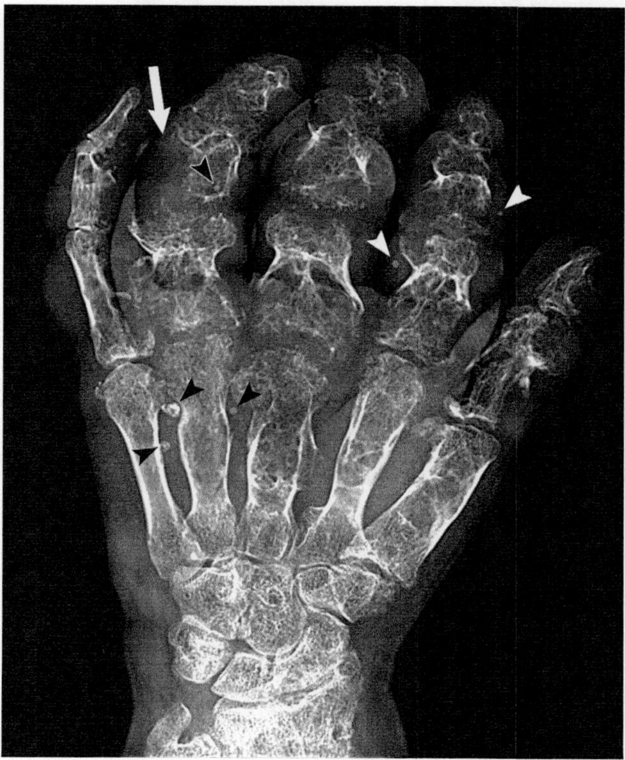

FIGURE 18.39 Chondrosarcoma in Maffucci syndrome. A 26-year-old woman, known to have Maffucci syndrome for several years, presented with slowly enlarging mass in the ring finger of her right hand. Dorsovolar radiograph shows numerous enchondromas affecting the carpal bones, metacarpals, and phalanges. Note several phleboliths within the soft tissues *(arrowheads)*. The lesion in the middle phalanx of the ring finger destroyed the cortex and extended into the soft tissues *(arrow)*. Excision biopsy revealed a chondrosarcoma.

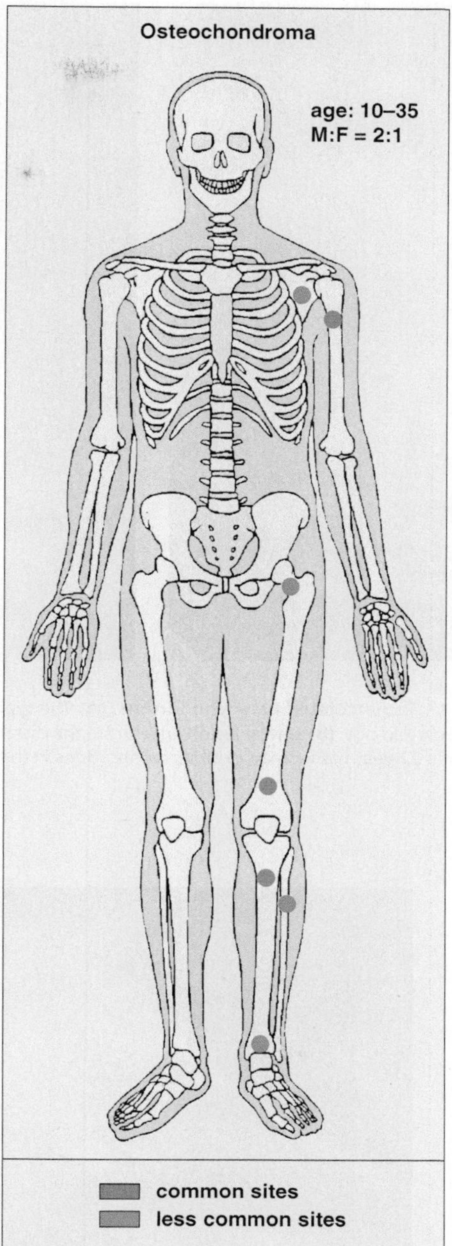

FIGURE 18.40 Skeletal sites of predilection, peak age range, and male-to-female ratio in osteochondroma (osteocartilaginous exostosis).

lesion becomes painful, if there is suspected encroachment on adjacent nerves or blood vessels, if pathologic fracture occurs, or if there is concern about the diagnosis.

Multiple Osteocartilaginous Exostoses

Clinical and Imaging Features

This condition, also known as *multiple hereditary osteochondromata*, *familial osteochondromatosis*, or *diaphyseal aclasis*, is classified by some authorities in the category of bone dysplasias. It is a hereditary, autosomal dominant disorder with incomplete penetrance in females. Approximately two thirds of affected individuals have a positive family history. The specific genetic defect has been recently identified, a novel mutation in genes *EXT1* that maps to chromosome 8q24.1, *EXT2* that maps to chromosome 11p13, and *EXT3* that maps to the short arm of chromosome 19. There is a decided 2:1 male predilection. The knees, ankles, and shoulders are the sites most frequently affected by the development of multiple osteochondromas (Fig. 18.53). The radiographic features are similar to those of single osteochondromas (see Figs. 18.41 and 18.42), but the lesions are more frequently of the sessile type (Figs. 18.54 and 18.55). MRI is effective to

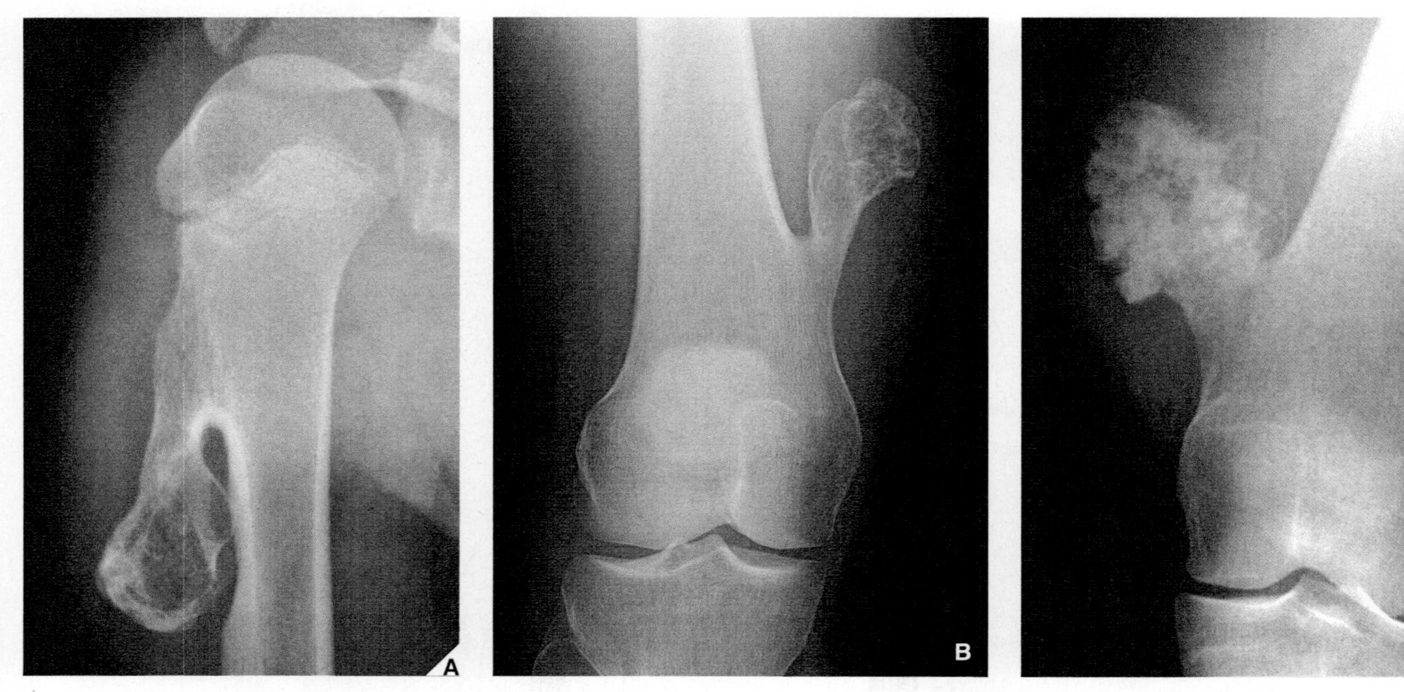

FIGURE 18.41 **Pedunculated osteochondroma.** **(A)** The typical pedunculated type of osteochondroma is seen arising near the proximal growth plate of the right humerus of a 13-year-old boy. **(B)** Similar lesion arises from the distal femur of a 21-year-old woman. **(C)** Pedunculated osteochondroma arising from the medial cortex of the distal left femur of a 22-year-old woman exhibits calcifications in the chondro-osseous zone of the stalk.

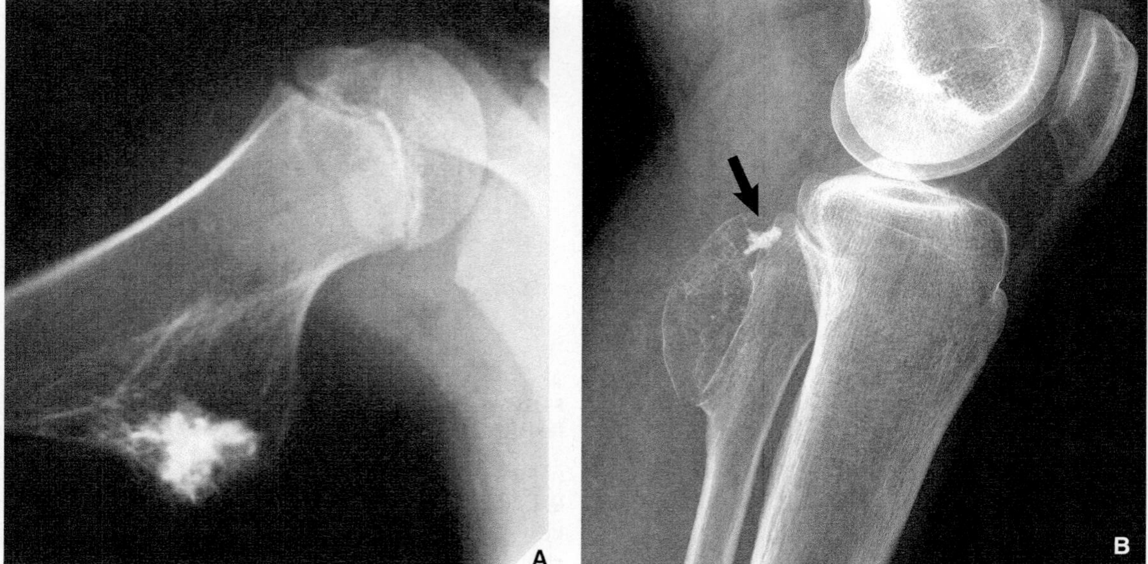

FIGURE 18.42 **Sessile osteochondroma.** **(A)** In the typical sessile or broad-based variant, seen here arising from the medial cortex of the proximal diaphysis of the right humerus in a 14-year-old boy, the cortex of the host bone merges without interruption with the cortex of the lesion. The cartilaginous cap is not visible on the conventional radiographs, but dense calcifications in the stalk can be seen. **(B)** In another patient, a 27-year-old woman, a sessile osteochondroma arising from the posterior aspect of the proximal fibula exhibits focal calcifications *(arrow)*. *(Continued)*

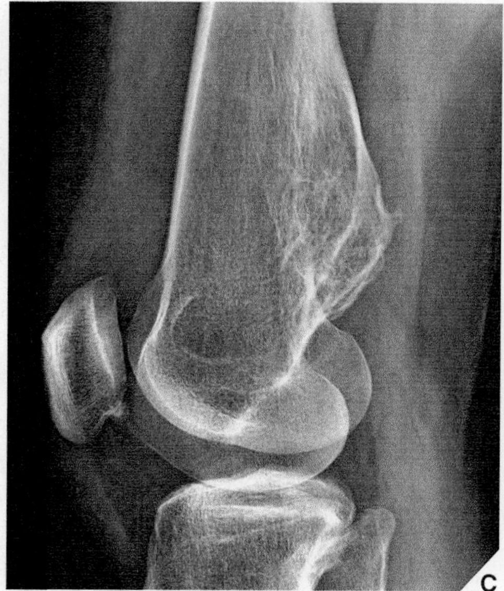

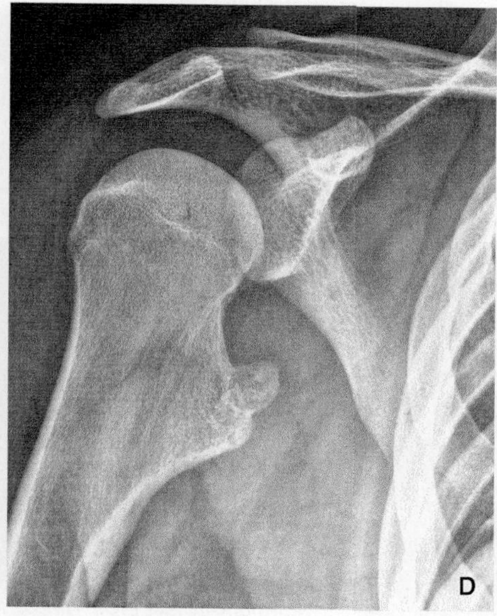

FIGURE 18.42 Sessile osteochondroma. ***(Continued)*** **(C)** In a 28-year-old man, a sessile osteochondroma of the distal femur exhibits no visible calcifications. **(D)** Anteroposterior radiograph of the right shoulder of a 15-year-old boy shows sessile osteochondroma without visible calcifications.

demonstrate continuity of the medullary portions of osteochondromas with the host bones (Figs. 18.56 and 18.57). CT and three-dimensional (3D) CT show spatial distribution of the lesions (Figs. 18.58 and 18.59). Occasionally, 3D CT angiogram is performed to confirm or rule out compression of the arteries by osteochondromas (Fig. 18.60).

The histopathologic features of multiple osteochondromas are the same as those of solitary lesions.

Two syndromes associated with multiple osteochondromas have been identified: *Langer-Giedion syndrome* and *Potocki-Shaffer syndrome*. The first one, also known as *trichorhinophalangeal syndrome type II* (TRPS2) or *Langer-Giedion chromosome region* (LGCR), is an autosomal dominant genetic disorder caused by deletion of gene *EXT2* and probably *ALX4*. Recent investigations points to loss of functional copies of the *trichorhinophalangeal syndrome type I* (TRPS1) gene encoding a zinc-finger protein, and *EXT1* gene at 8q23.2-q24.1 chromosome. Clinically, it characterizes by short stature, joint laxity, short fingers, microcephaly, craniofacial dysmorphism, mental retardation, and multiple osteochondromas. Potocki-Shaffer syndrome is caused by deletion of 11p11.2-p12 chromosome, and clinically, it manifests by enlarged parietal foramina, multiple osteochondromas, and sometimes craniofacial dysostosis and mental retardation.

Complications

There is a greater incidence of growth disturbance in multiple osteocartilaginous exostoses than in solitary osteochondroma. Growth abnormalities are primarily seen in the forearms (Fig. 18.61; see also Fig. 16.68) and legs (see Fig. 18.55). Malignant transformation to chondrosarcoma is also more common, seen in 5% to 15% of cases, with lesions at the shoulder girdle and around the pelvis at greater risk of undergoing transformation. The clinical and imaging signs of this complication are identical to those in the malignant transformation of a solitary osteochondroma (Fig. 18.62; see also Fig. 18.52 and Table 18.1).

Treatment

Multiple osteochondromas are treated individually. Like solitary lesions, they are likely to recur in younger children, and surgery may be deferred to a later date.

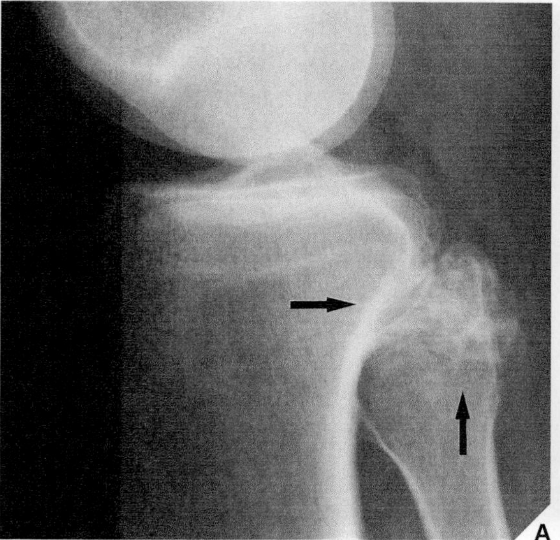

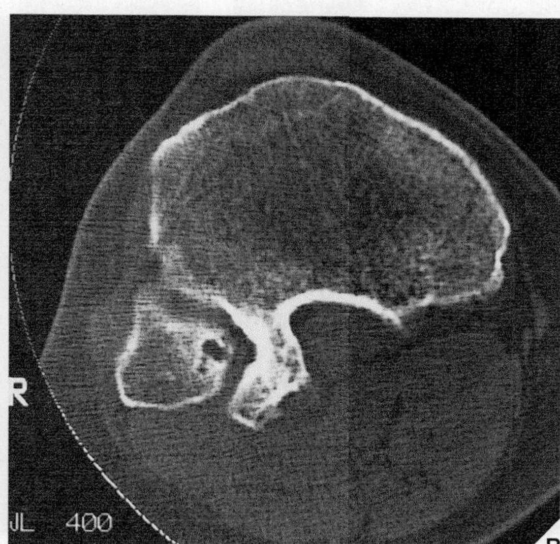

FIGURE 18.43 CT of osteochondroma. **(A)** Lateral radiograph of the knee shows a calcified lesion at the posterior aspect of the proximal tibia *(arrows)*. The exact nature of this lesion cannot be ascertained. **(B)** CT clearly establishes the continuity of the cortex, which extends without interruption from the osteochondroma into the tibia. Note also that the medullary portion of the lesion and the tibia communicate.

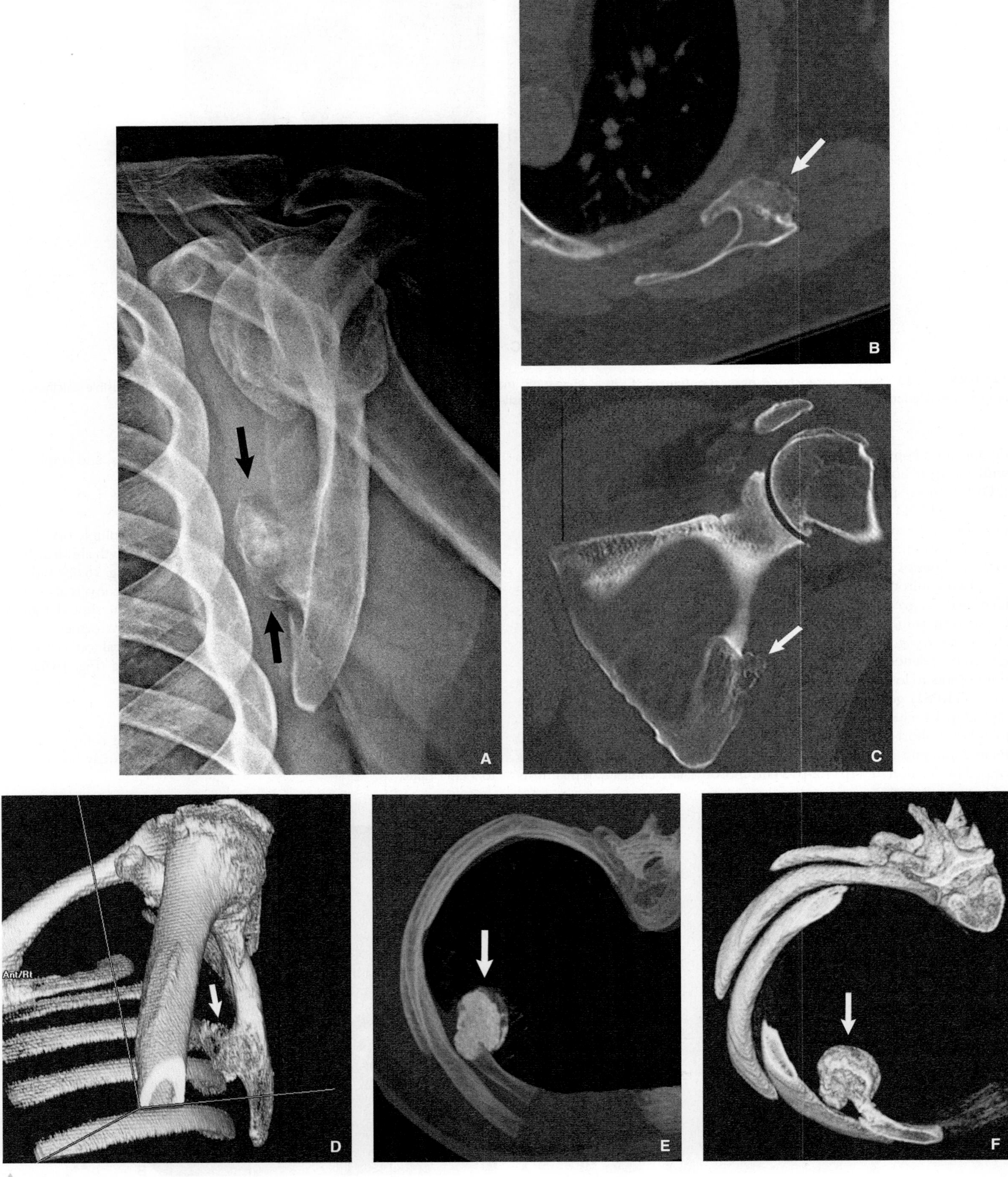

FIGURE 18.44 CT and 3D CT of osteochondroma. **(A)** "Y" view of the shoulder of a 62-year-old man shows an osteochondroma of the scapula *(arrows)*, better characterized on **(B)** axial *(arrow)*, **(C)** coronal reformatted *(arrow)*, and **(D)** 3D CT reconstructed images *(arrow)*. In another patient, a 34-year-old man, **(E)** 3D CT image of the right hemithorax reconstructed in maximum intensity projection (MIP) and **(F)** 3D CT image reconstructed in shaded surface display (SSD) show detailed features of the pedunculated osteochondroma arising from the rib *(arrows)*.

LESIONS OF SIMILAR APPEARANCE TO OSTEOCHONDROMA

Osteochondroma

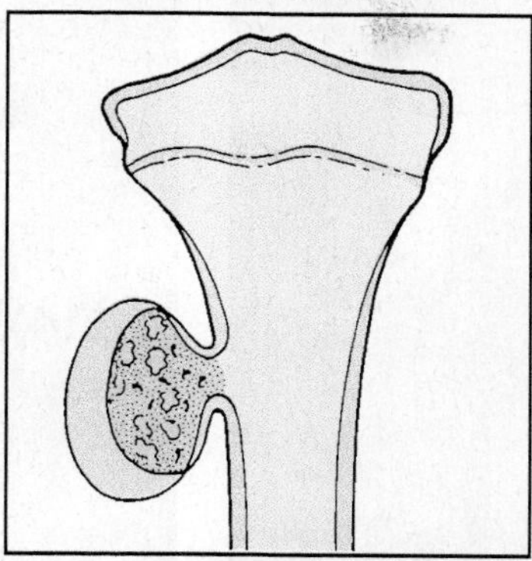

uninterrupted merging of cortex of host bone with cortex of lesion

Myositis Ossificans

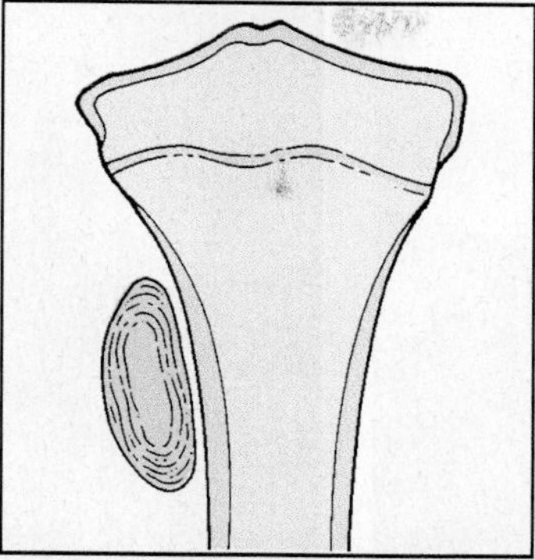

lesion with dense periphery and lucent center, cleft separating lesion from cortex

Juxtacortical Osteosarcoma

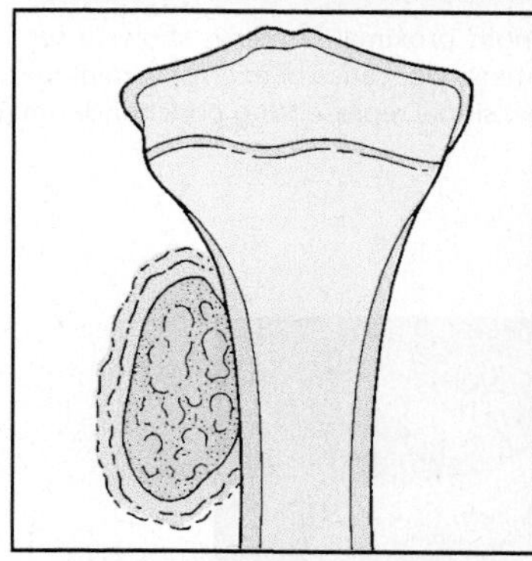

lesion with lucent periphery and dense center, no cleft

Soft Tissue Osteosarcoma

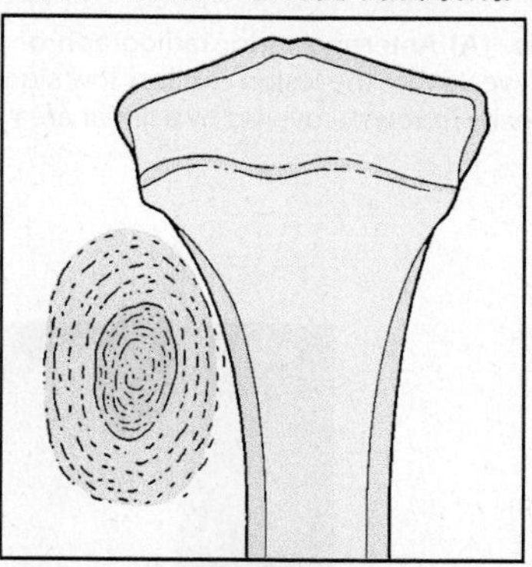

lesion with smudgy densities in center, more lucent at periphery

Juxtacortical Osteoma

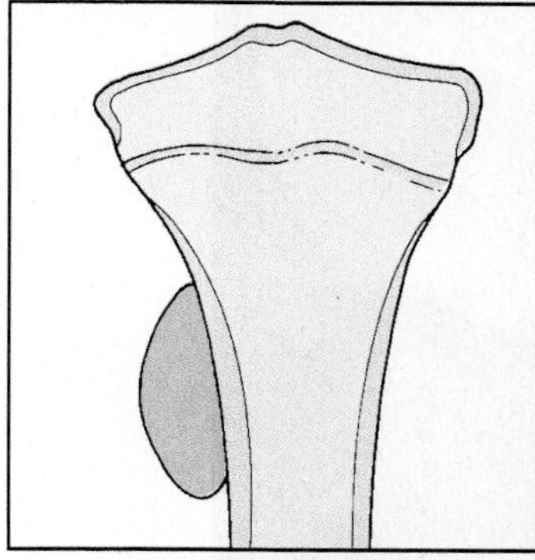

homogeneously dense (ivory) lesion, no cleft

Periosteal Chondroma

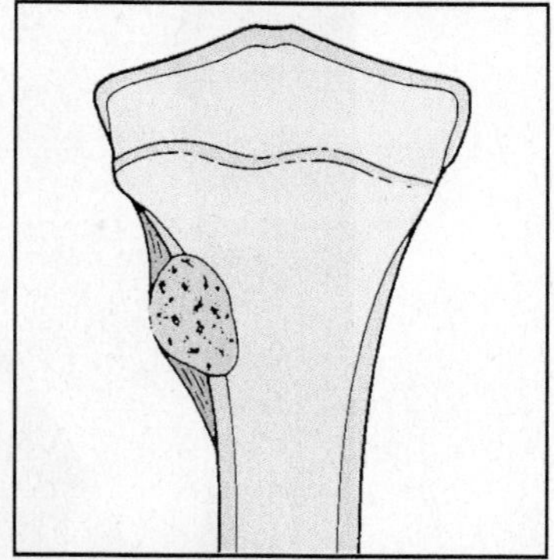

solid buttress of periosteal reaction, calcifications in center of lesion

FIGURE 18.45 Differential diagnosis of osteochondroma. Radiographic features characterizing lesions similar in appearance to osteochondroma.

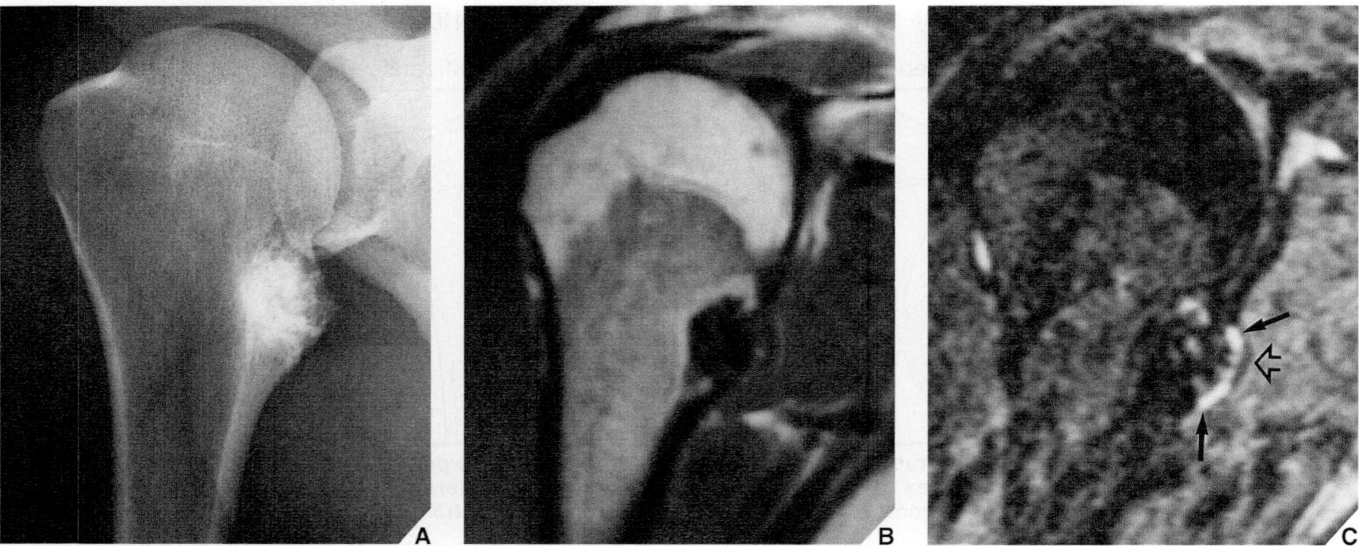

FIGURE 18.46 **MRI of osteochondroma.** **(A)** Anteroposterior radiograph of the right proximal humerus shows a sessile osteochondroma at the medial aspect of metadiaphysis. **(B)** T1-weighted coronal MRI reveals that the lesion exhibits low signal intensity because of extensive mineralization. **(C)** T2-weighted image shows the thin cartilaginous cap as a band of high signal intensity *(arrows)*, covered by a linear area of low signal representing perichondrium *(open arrow)*.

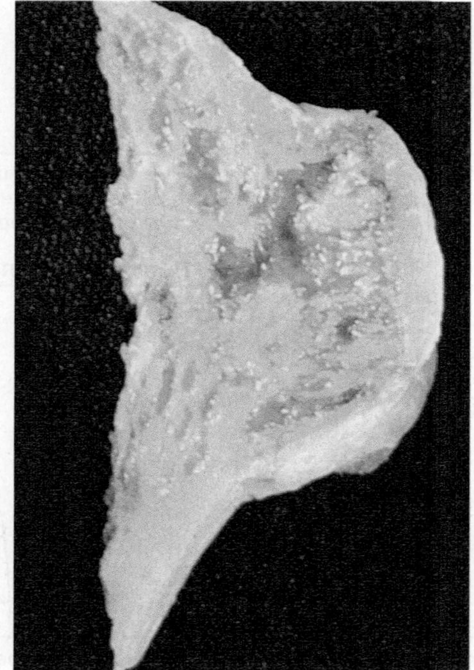

FIGURE 18.47 **Pathology of osteochondroma.** Gross specimen of sessile osteochondroma shows continuity of the medullary portion of the lesion and the host bone as well as continuity of the cortex of the host bone and the lesion. Observe a thin cartilaginous cap. (Reprinted with permission from Greenspan A, Borys D. *Radiology and pathology correlation of bone tumors: a quick reference and review*. Philadelphia: Wolters Kluwer; 2016:119.)

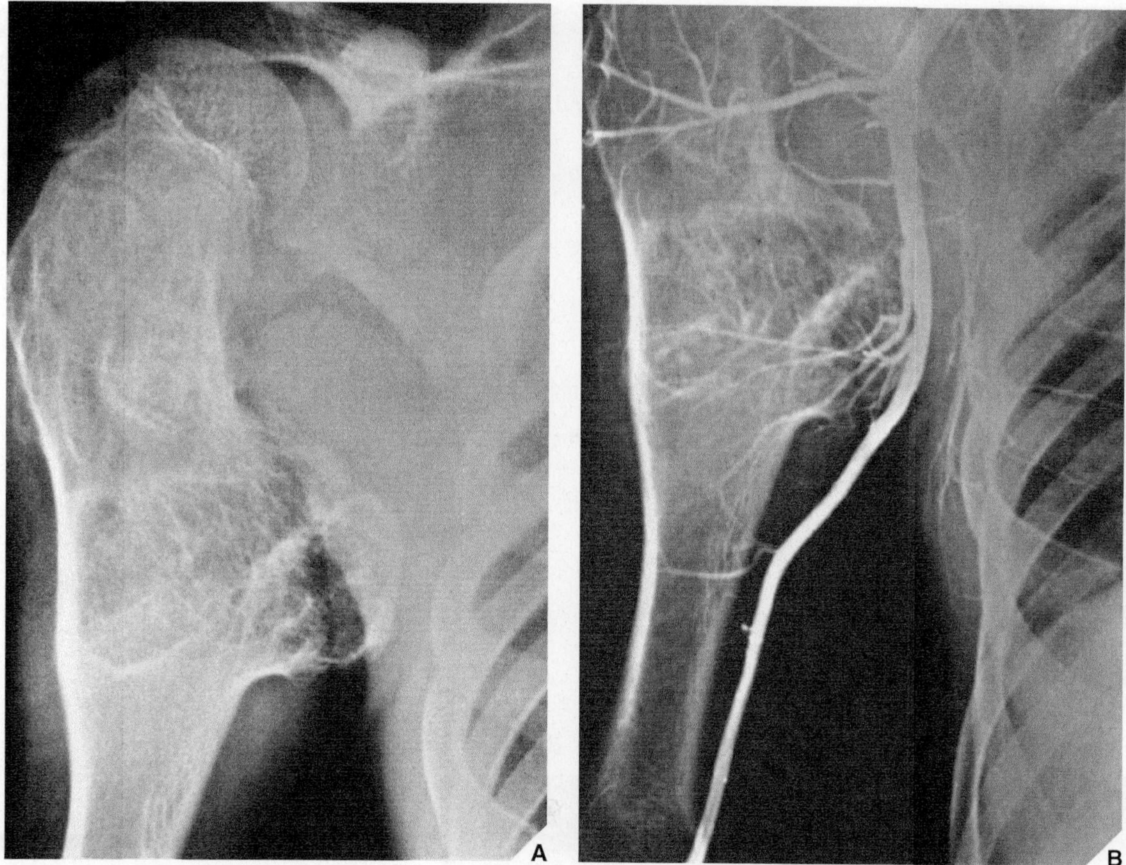

FIGURE 18.48 **Complication of osteochondroma.** A 14-year-old boy with a known osteochondroma of the right humerus complained of pain and numbness of the hand and fingers. **(A)** Radiograph of the right shoulder demonstrates a sessile-type osteochondroma arising from the medial aspect of the proximal diaphysis of the humerus. **(B)** Arteriography reveals compression and displacement of the brachial artery.

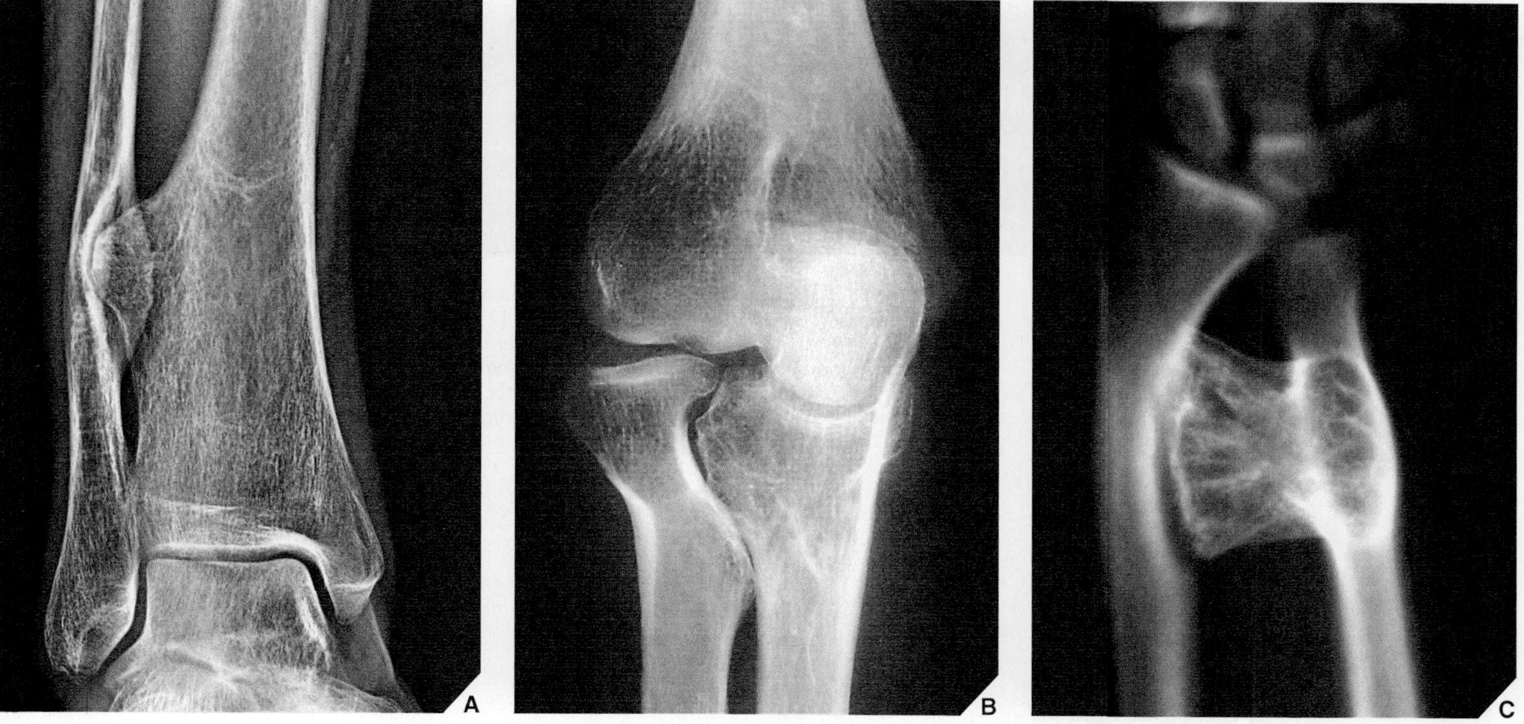

FIGURE 18.49 **Complication of osteochondroma.** **(A)** Sessile lesion of the distal tibia has caused erosion of the medial aspect of the fibula. **(B)** Continued growth of the sessile osteochondroma of the proximal ulna resulted in pressure erosion of the head and neck of the radius. **(C)** Pedunculated osteochondroma of the distal ulna has eroded medial aspect of the shaft of the radius.

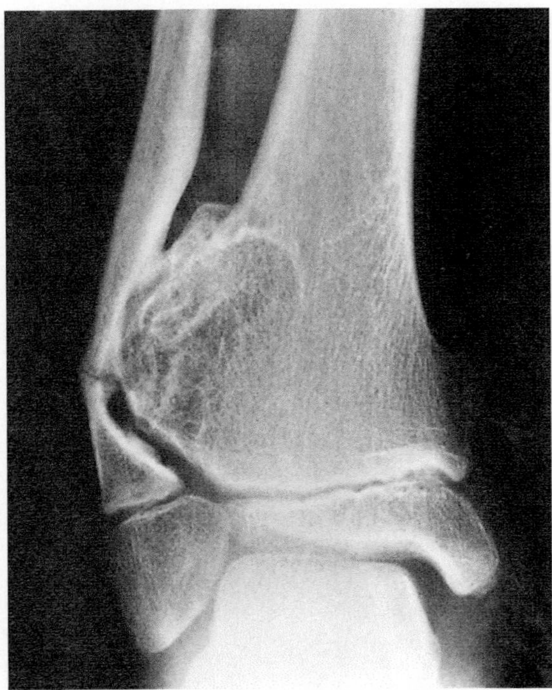

FIGURE 18.50 Complication of osteochondroma. A 9-year-old boy had a sessile osteochondroma of the distal tibia. The lesion produced pressure erosion and later bowing and attenuation of the fibula, with subsequent fracture of the bone.

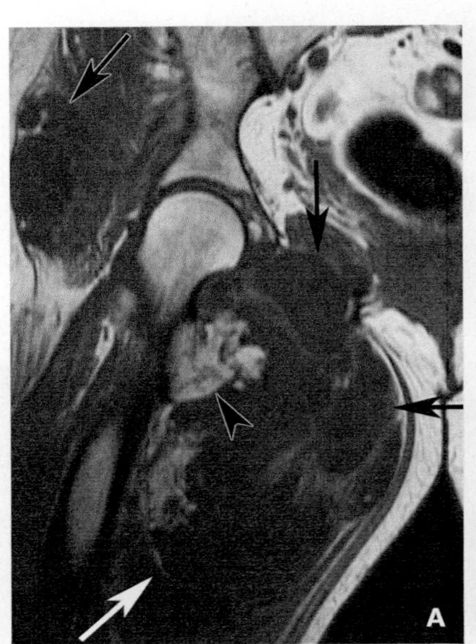

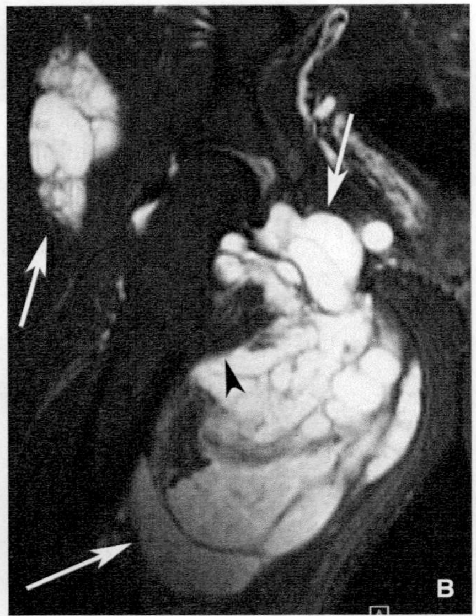

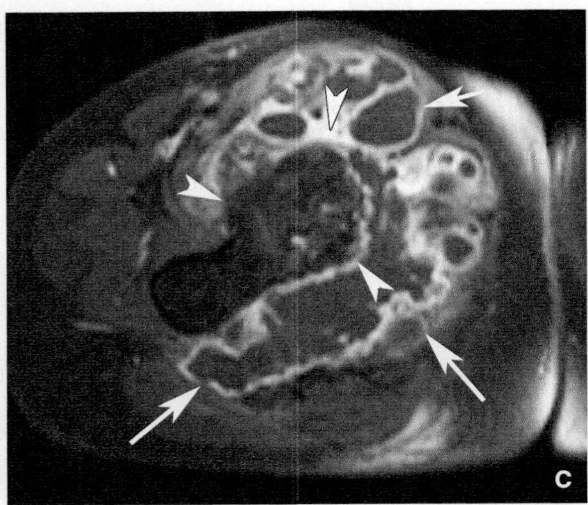

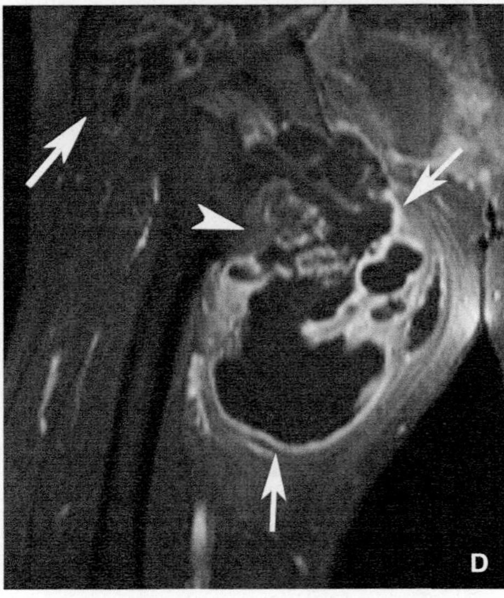

FIGURE 18.51 Bursa exostotica. A 58-year-old woman presented with a long history of right inguinal mass. **(A)** Coronal T1-weighted and **(B)** coronal T2-weighted MR images and **(C)** axial and **(D)** coronal T1-weighted fat-saturated MR images obtained after intravenous injection of gadolinium demonstrate a large osteochondroma in the proximal right femur *(arrowheads)*, surrounded by a large multilocular bursa filled with fluid, that extends into the thigh and buttocks *(arrows)*. Note the enhancement of the walls and septa of the bursa exostotica following contrast injection but lack of enhancement of the fluid.

TABLE 18.1 Clinical and Imaging Features Suggesting Malignant Transformation of Osteochondroma

Clinical Features	Imaging Features	Imaging Modality
Pain (in the absence of fracture, bursitis, or pressure on nearby nerves)	Enlargement of the lesion	Conventional radiography (comparison with earlier radiographs)
Growth spurt (after skeletal maturity)	Development of a bulky cartilaginous cap usually more than 2 cm thick	CT, MRI
	Dispersed calcifications in the cartilaginous cap	Radiography, CT, MRI
	Development of a soft-tissue mass with or without calcifications	
	Increased uptake of radiopharmaceutical tracer after closure of growth plate (not always reliable)	Scintigraphy

CT, computed tomography; MRI, magnetic resonance imaging.

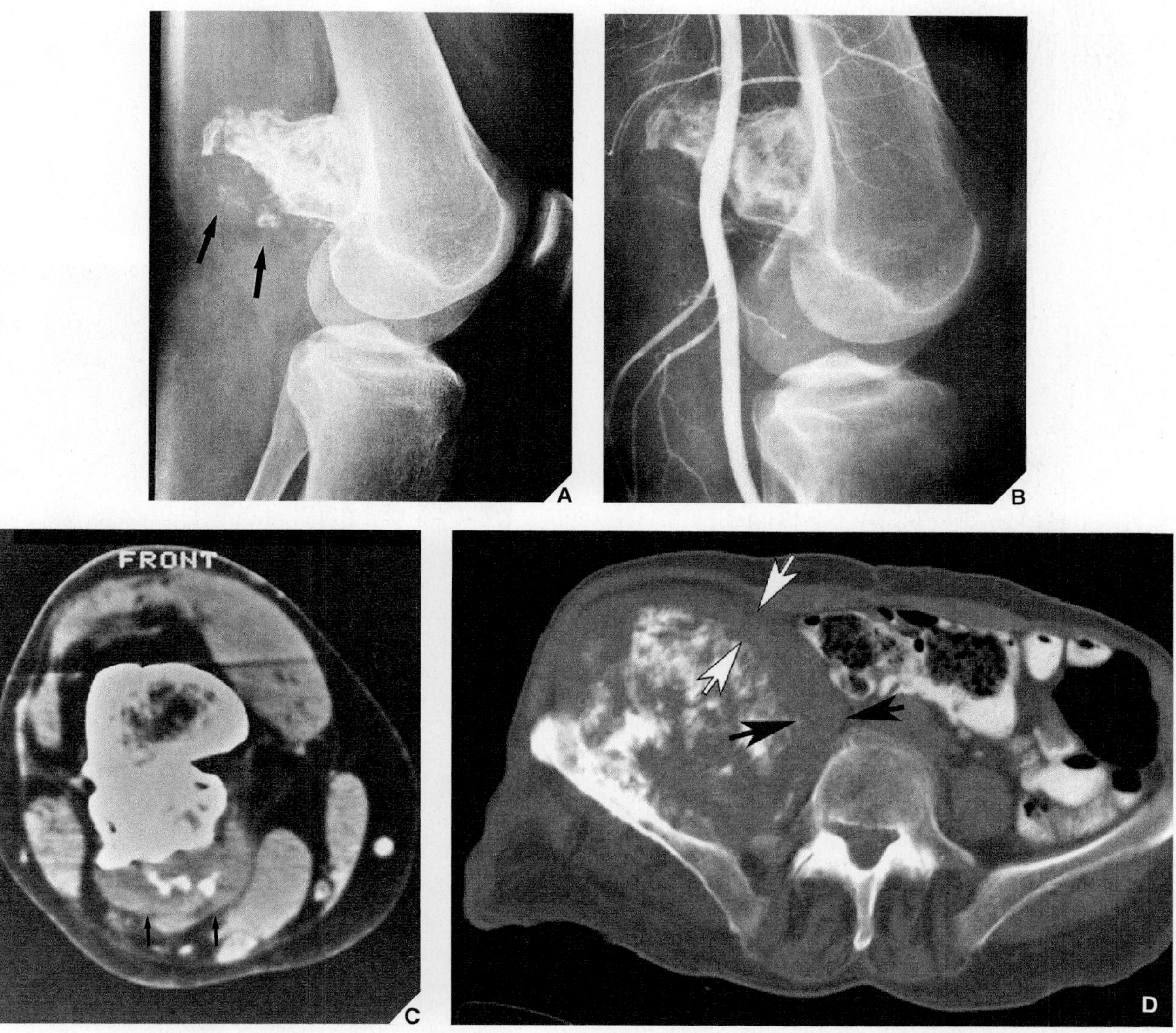

FIGURE 18.52 Transformation of osteochondroma to chondrosarcoma. A 28-year-old man had pain in the popliteal region and also noticed an increase in a mass he had been aware of for 15 years—important clinical information that warranted further investigation to rule out the malignant transformation of an osteochondroma. **(A)** Lateral radiograph of the knee demonstrates a sessile-type osteochondroma arising from the posterior cortex of the distal femur. Note that calcifications are present not only in the stalk of the lesion but also are dispersed in the cartilaginous cap *(arrows)*. **(B)** An arteriogram demonstrates displacement of the small vessels, which are draped over the invisible cartilaginous cap. **(C)** CT section confirms the increased thickness of the cartilaginous cap (2.5 cm) and dispersed calcifications within the cap *(arrows)*. These imaging features are consistent with a diagnosis of malignant transformation to chondrosarcoma, which was confirmed by excisional biopsy and histopathologic examination. **(D)** Axial CT image of the pelvis of another patient with a large solitary osteochondroma arising from the right iliac wing demonstrates marked thickening of the cartilaginous cap *(arrows)* containing scattered calcifications. Histopathologic examination revealed a low-grade chondrosarcoma.

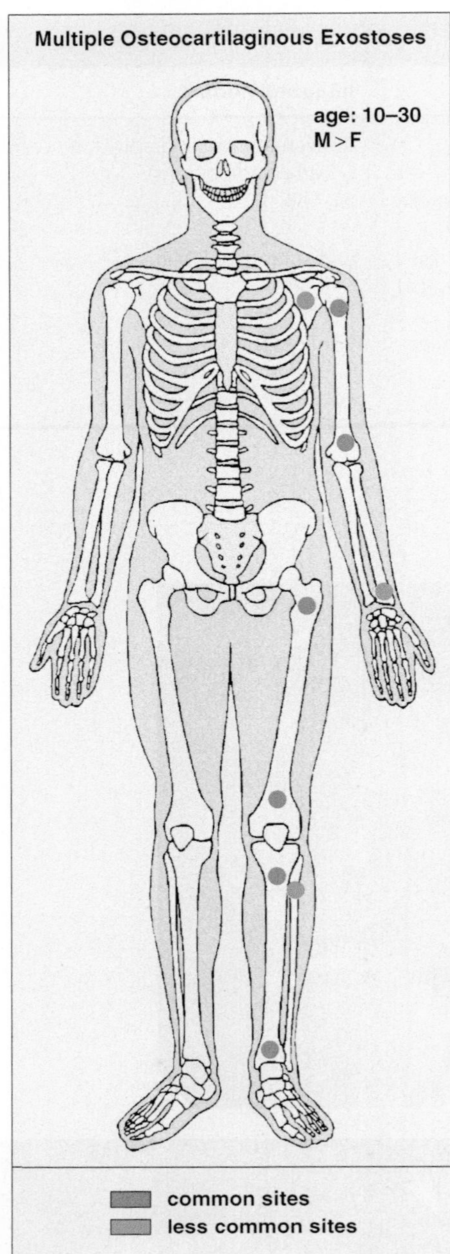

FIGURE 18.53 Skeletal sites of predilection, peak age range, and male-to-female ratio in multiple osteocartilaginous exostoses (multiple osteochondromata, diaphyseal aclasis).

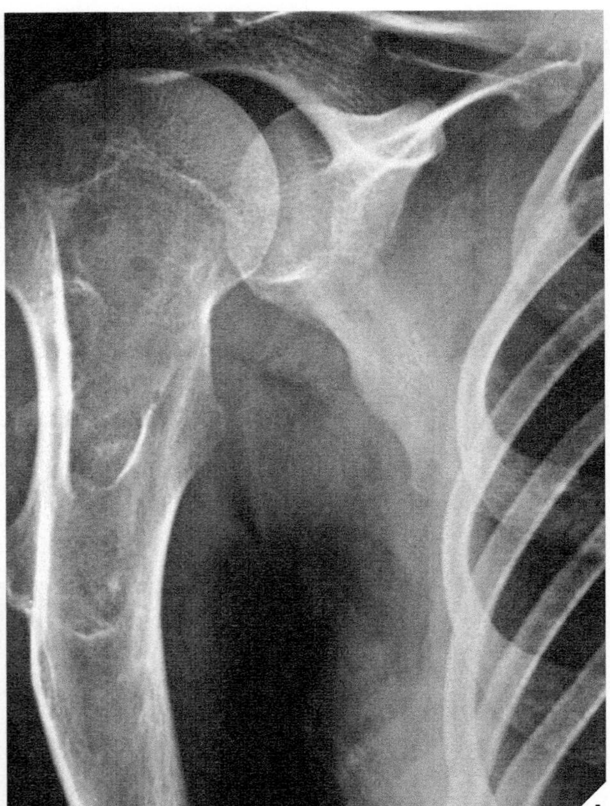

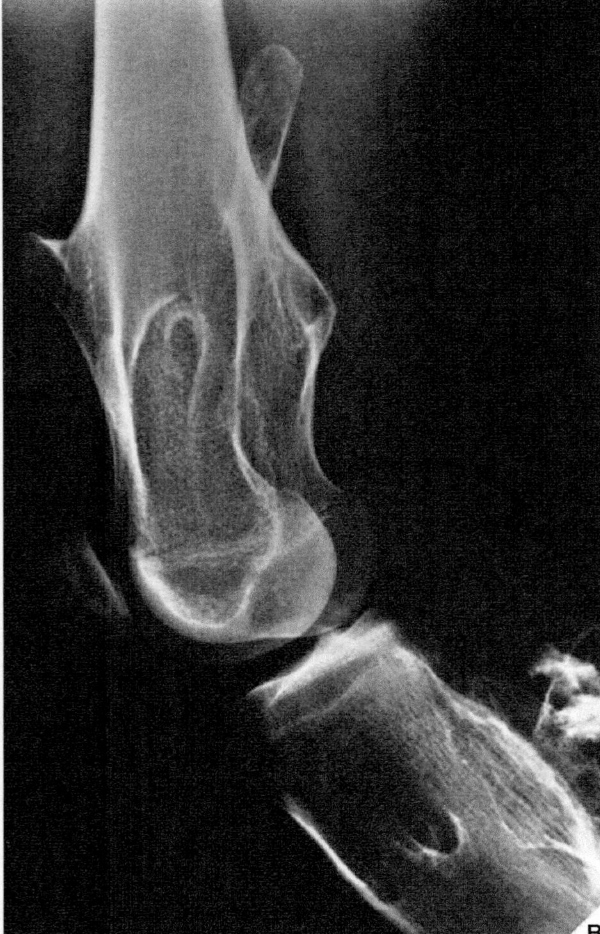

FIGURE 18.54 Hereditary multiple exostoses. **(A)** Anteroposterior radiograph of the shoulder of a 22-year-old man demonstrates multiple sessile lesions involving the proximal humerus, scapula, and ribs. **(B)** Involvement of the distal femur and proximal tibia is characteristic of this disorder.

Bizarre Parosteal Osteochondromatous Proliferation

Clinical and Imaging Features

Also known as *Nora lesion*, named for a pathologist F. E. Nora from Mayo Clinic, who first described this benign surface lesion in 1983, BPOP is part of a spectrum of reactive lesions, such as florid reactive periostitis or turret exostosis. It commonly affects the metacarpals and phalanges of the hand (proximal phalanges are more often affected than distal phalanges). The long bones are involved in about 25% of reported cases. The lesion is seen in the third and fourth decades, with men slightly more commonly affected than women. Patients typically present with a firm, slow-growing, nontender mass. The cause is unknown, but it may be related to trauma, although recently reported by Zambrano and associates, the cytogenetic changes put in question the lesion's nonneoplastic nature. Imaging studies commonly show a mushroom-like–shaped osseous or cartilaginous mass attached to the cortex (Figs. 18.63 and 18.64), although the imaging appearance of BPOP is dependent on the stage of evolution of the lesion. The contour of the mass is

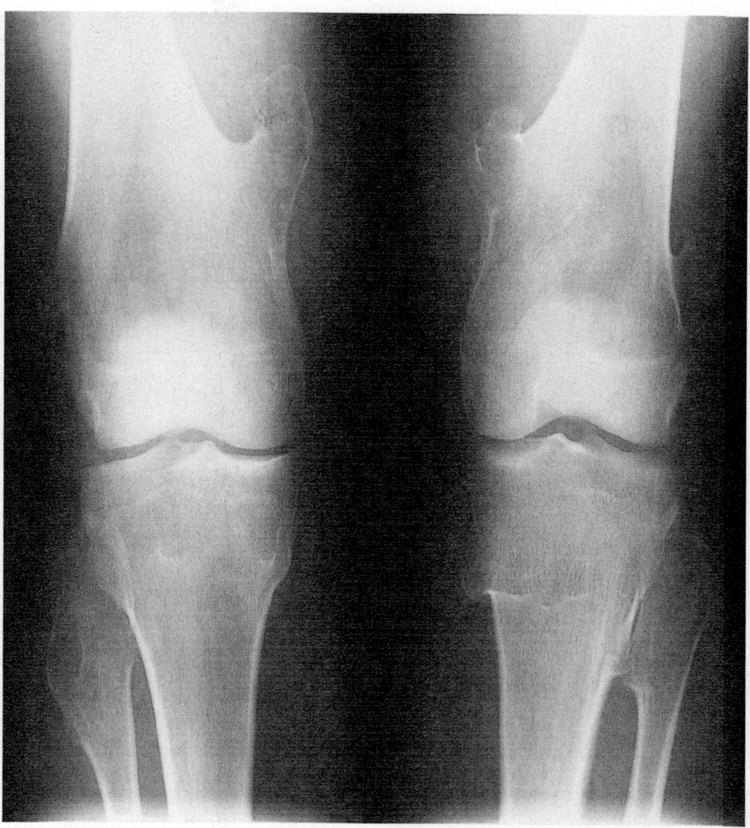

FIGURE 18.55 **Hereditary multiple exostoses.** An anteroposterior radiograph of both knees of a 17-year-old boy shows numerous sessile and pedunculated osteochondromas.

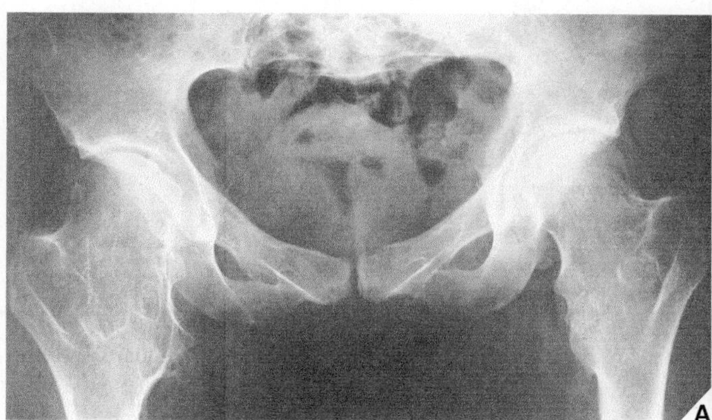

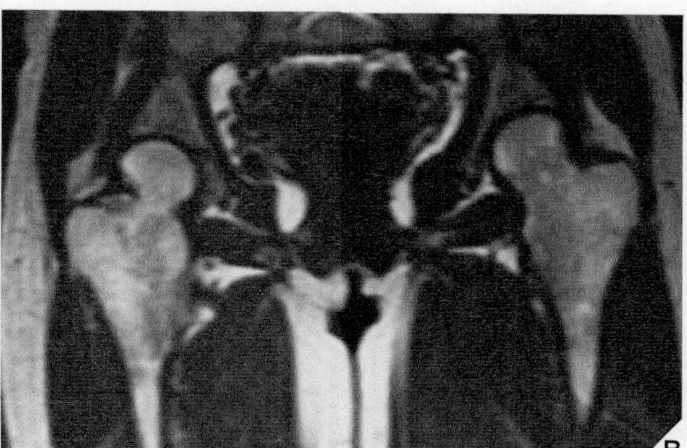

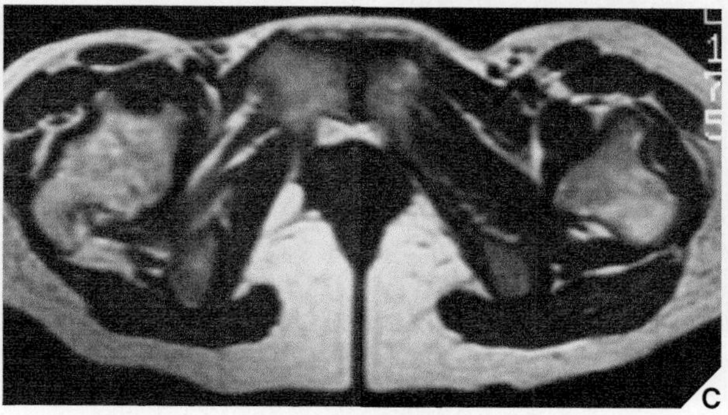

FIGURE 18.56 **MRI of hereditary multiple exostoses.** **(A)** Anteroposterior radiograph of the hips shows multiple sessile osteochondromas mainly affecting proximal femora. Some lesions are also present at the pubic bones. **(B)** Coronal and **(C)** axial T1-weighted (SE; repetition time [TR] 600/TE 20 msec) MR images demonstrate continuity of the lesions with the medullary portion of the femora. Note also dysplastic changes expressed by abnormal tubulation of the bones.

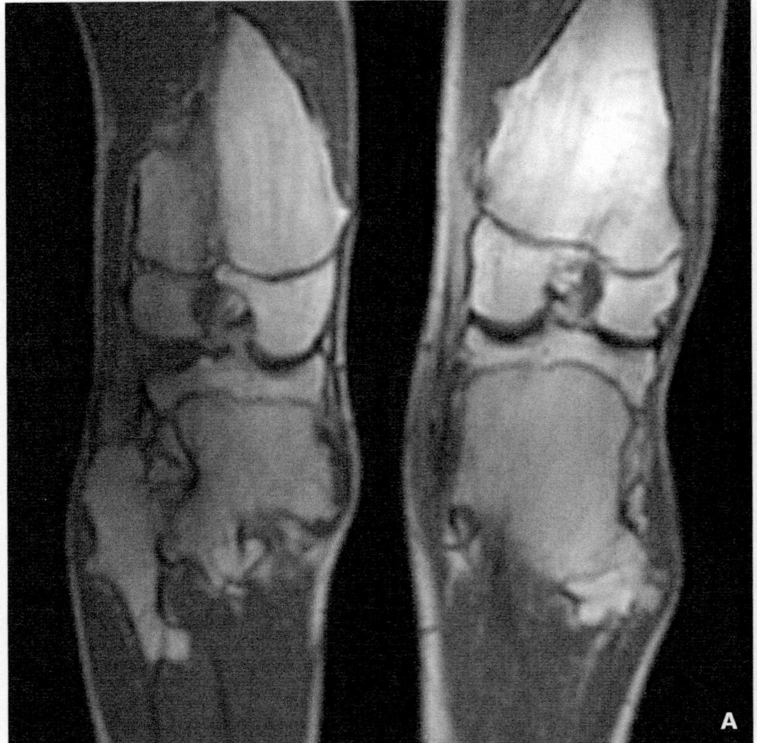

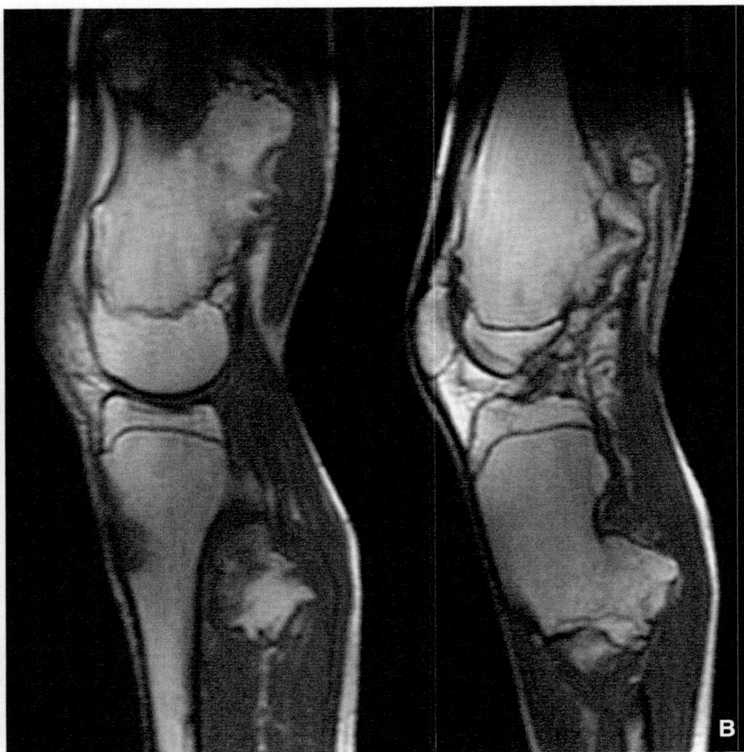

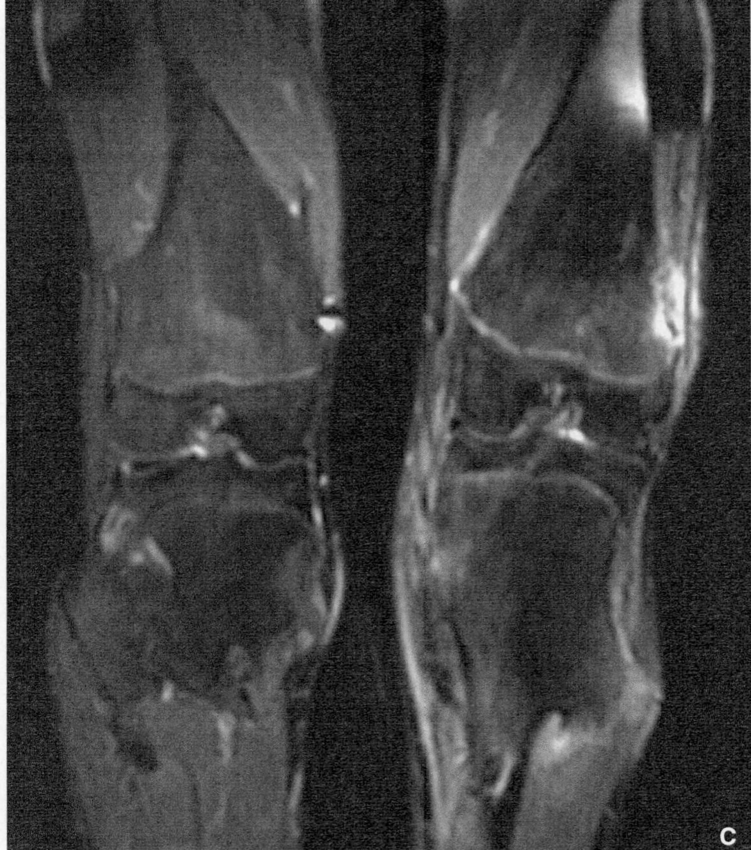

FIGURE 18.57 MRI of hereditary multiple exostoses. **(A)** Coronal T1-weighted, **(B)** two sagittal T1-weighted, and **(C)** coronal T2-weighted fat-suppressed MR images of the knees show multiple, predominantly sessile osteochondromas of the distal femora and proximal tibiae and fibulae. Observe that medullary portions of the host bones and the lesions communicate.

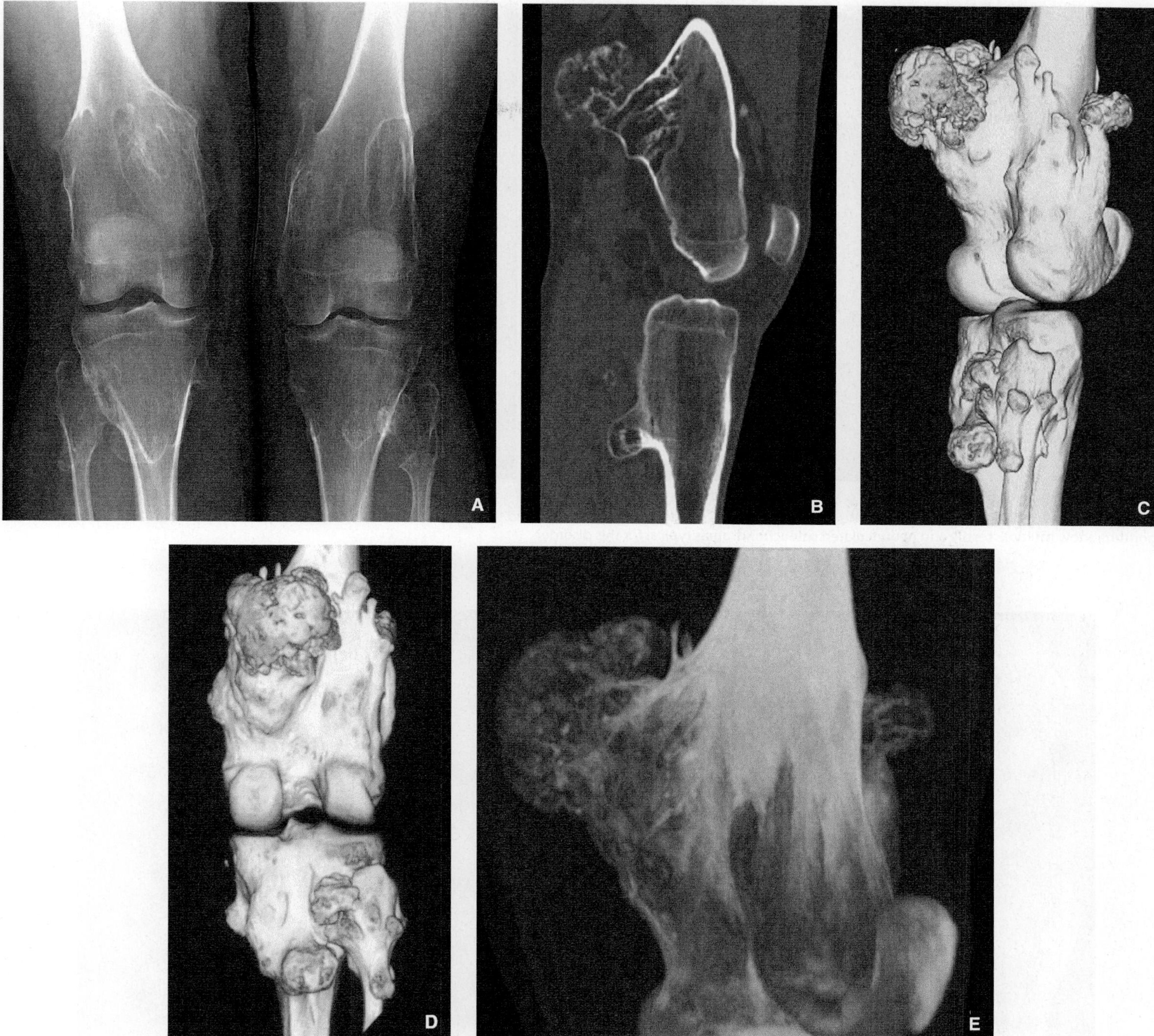

FIGURE 18.58 CT and 3D CT of hereditary multiple exostoses. **(A)** Anteroposterior radiograph of both knees of a 20-year-old man shows multiple osteochondromas arising from the distal femora and proximal tibiae and fibulae, associated with growth disturbance reflected by Erlenmeyer flask deformities of the femora. **(B)** Sagittal reformatted CT image shows osteochondromas arising from the posterior aspect of the distal femur and proximal tibia. 3D CT images reconstructed with surface-rendering algorithm viewed from the lateral **(C)** and posterior **(D)** aspects of the knee show spatial distribution of numerous osteochondromas. **(E)** 3D CT image of the distal femur reconstructed in maximum intensity projection (MIP) shows internal architecture of the sessile lesion. (**D**, Reprinted with permission from Greenspan A, Borys D. *Radiology and pathology correlation of bone tumors: a quick reference and review*. Philadelphia: Wolters Kluwer; 2016:126.)

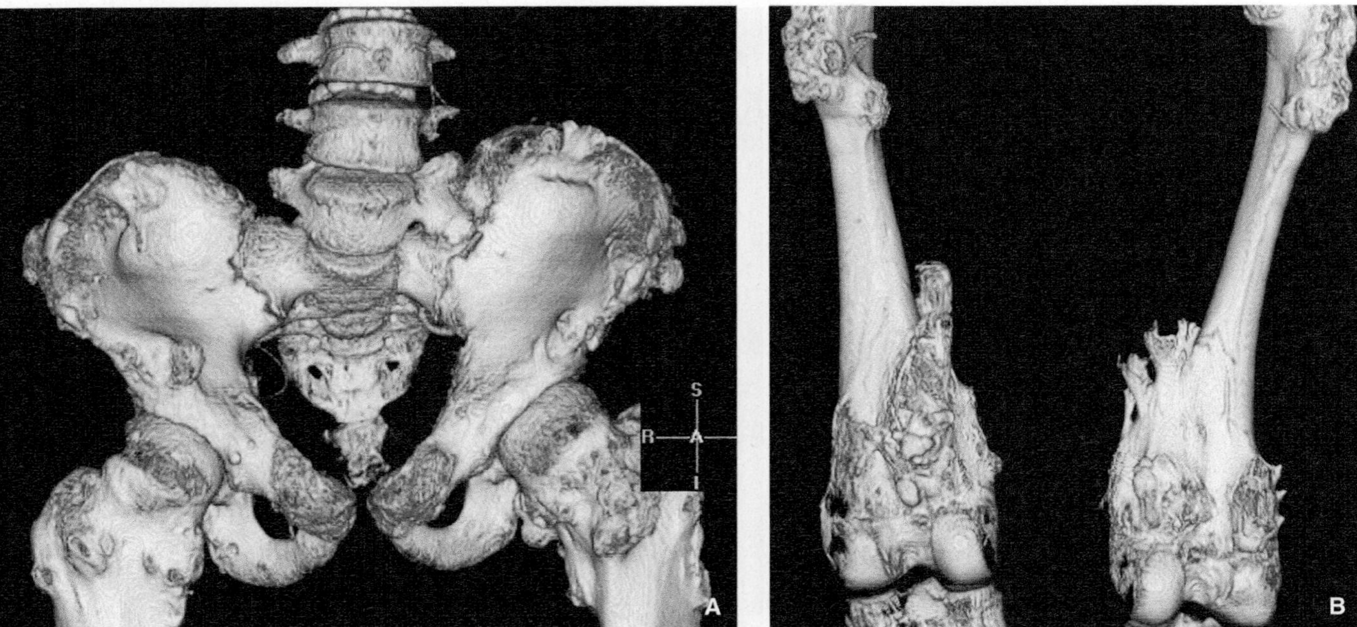

FIGURE 18.59 3D CT of hereditary multiple exostoses. 3D CT images of the pelvis **(A)** and the femora **(B)** of a 16-year-old boy, reconstructed with surface-rendering algorithm, show multiple sessile and pedunculated osteochondromas typical for this disorder.

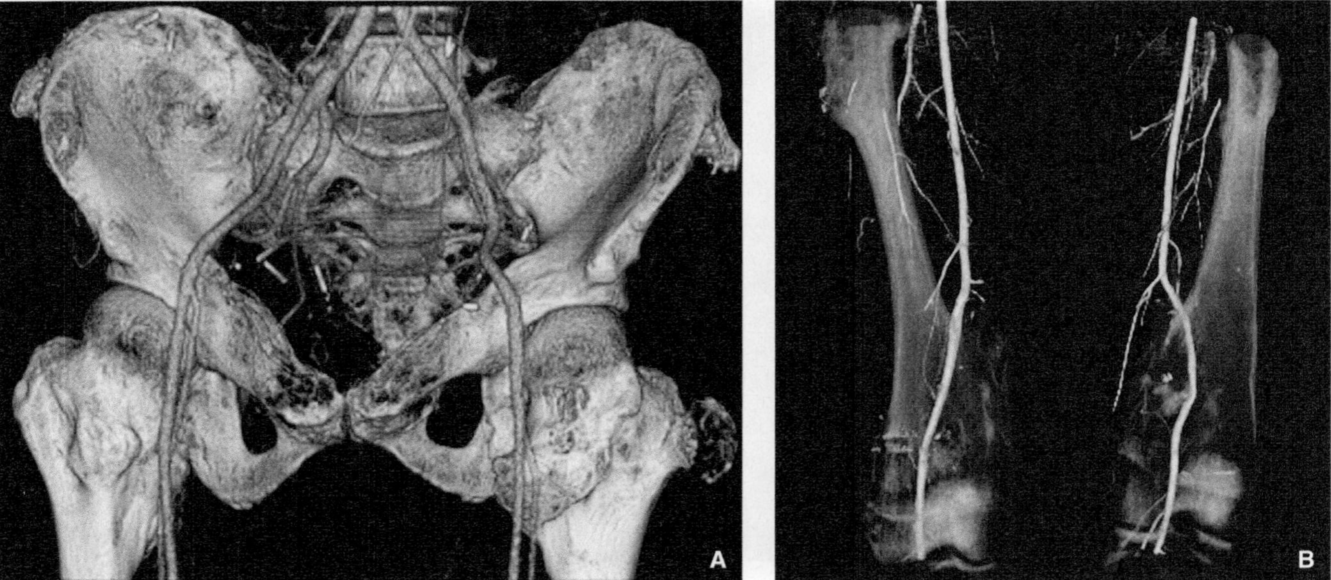

FIGURE 18.60 3D CT angiogram of hereditary multiple exostoses. **(A)** 3D CT angiogram of the pelvis of a 57-year-old woman reconstructed with surface-rendering algorithm shows multiple osteochondromas arising from the iliac wings, pubic bones, and proximal femora. The iliac and femoral arteries were not affected by the exostoses. **(B)** 3D CT angiogram of both lower extremities was performed in another patient to rule out compression of the arteries by osteochondromas. The femoral and popliteal arteries were not affected by the lesions.

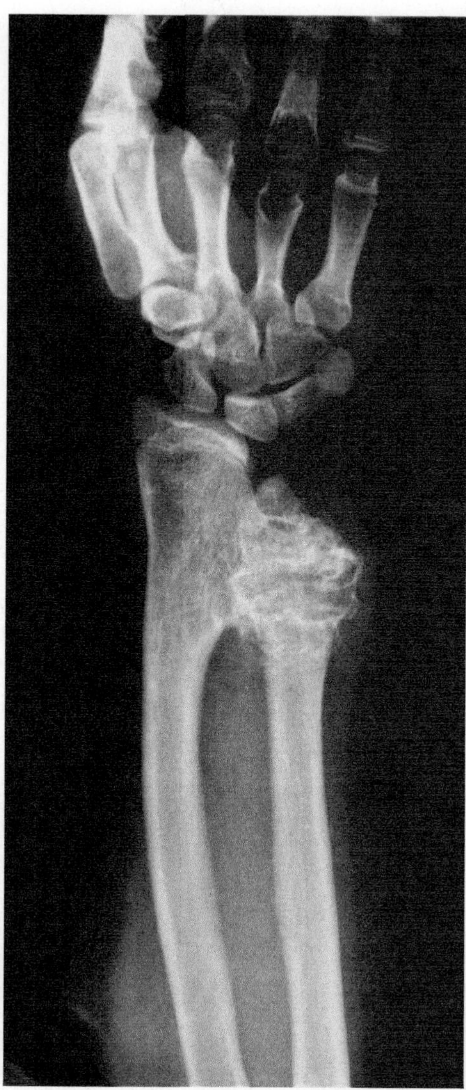

FIGURE 18.61 **Hereditary multiple exostoses: growth disturbance.** Posteroanterior radiograph of the forearm of an 8-year-old boy with multiple osteochondromas shows a growth disturbance in the distal radius and ulna, which is frequently seen as a complication in this disorder.

usually smooth but may be slightly lobulated. The absence of continuity between the lesion and medullary cavity of the adjacent bone differentiates this lesion from osteochondroma. The other similarly appearing lesions to consider in the differential diagnosis are juxtacortical myositis ossificans, periosteal chondroma, turret exostosis (Fig. 18.65), subungual exostosis (Fig. 18.66), florid reactive periostitis, and parosteal or periosteal osteosarcoma.

Pathology

The characteristic histologic feature of BPOP is the presence of irregular calcified matrix stained blue on hematoxylin and eosin staining referred to as *blue bone*. There is lack of cellular atypia of osteoblasts or fibrous tissue, and the bone is lamellar and well organized, features that distinguish this lesion from osteosarcoma.

Treatment

The treatment of BPOP is surgical excision; however, recurrence rate is high.

Chondroblastoma

Clinical and Imaging Features

Also known as a *Codman tumor*, chondroblastoma, representing fewer than 1% of all primary bone tumors, is a benign lesion occurring before skeletal maturity, characteristically presenting in the epiphyses of long bones such as the humerus, tibia, and femur (Fig. 18.67). Although secondary involvement of the metaphysis before or after skeletal maturity is recognized (see Figs. 18.71 and 18.72), a predominantly metaphyseal or diaphyseal location is exceedingly rare. Equally unusual is involvement of the vertebra or intracortical location in the long bones. Occasionally, the patella, which is considered equivalent to an epiphysis, is affected (see Fig. 18.70). Ten percent of chondroblastomas involve the small bones of the hands and feet, with the talus and calcaneus representing the most common sites. Although the lesion is usually seen in growing bones, some cases have been reported after obliteration of the growth plate (see Fig. 18.72). Chondroblastoma is usually located eccentrically, shows a sclerotic border, and often demonstrates scattered calcifications of the matrix (25% of cases) (Figs. 18.68 to 18.72). Brower and colleagues noticed a distinctively thick, solid periosteal reaction distal to the lesion in 57% of chondroblastomas in long bones (Figs. 18.73 and 18.74). This most likely represents an inflammatory reaction to the tumor. In most cases, radiography suffices to demonstrate the lesion but CT scan can help demonstrate the calcifications if they are not visible on the standard radiographs (see Fig. 18.72). MRI usually reveals a larger area of involvement than can be seen on radiography, including regional bone marrow and soft-tissue edema (Figs. 18.75 to 18.78).

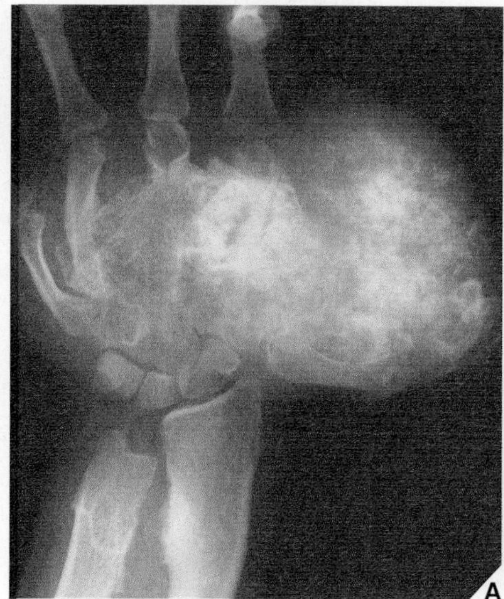

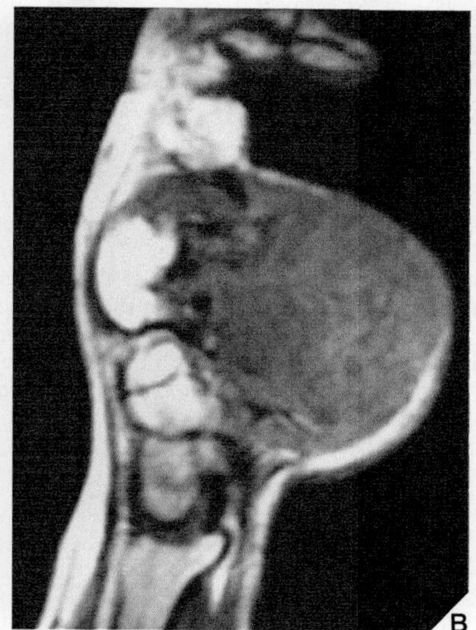

FIGURE 18.62 **Malignant transformation.** **(A)** Oblique radiograph of the right hand of a 22-year-old man shows multiple osteochondromas. A large soft-tissue mass situated between the index finger and thumb and containing chondroid calcifications indicates malignant transformation to chondrosarcoma. **(B)** Sagittal T1-weighted (SE; repetition time [TR] 600/TE 16 msec) MRI reveals volar extension of a large soft-tissue tumor. *(Continued)*

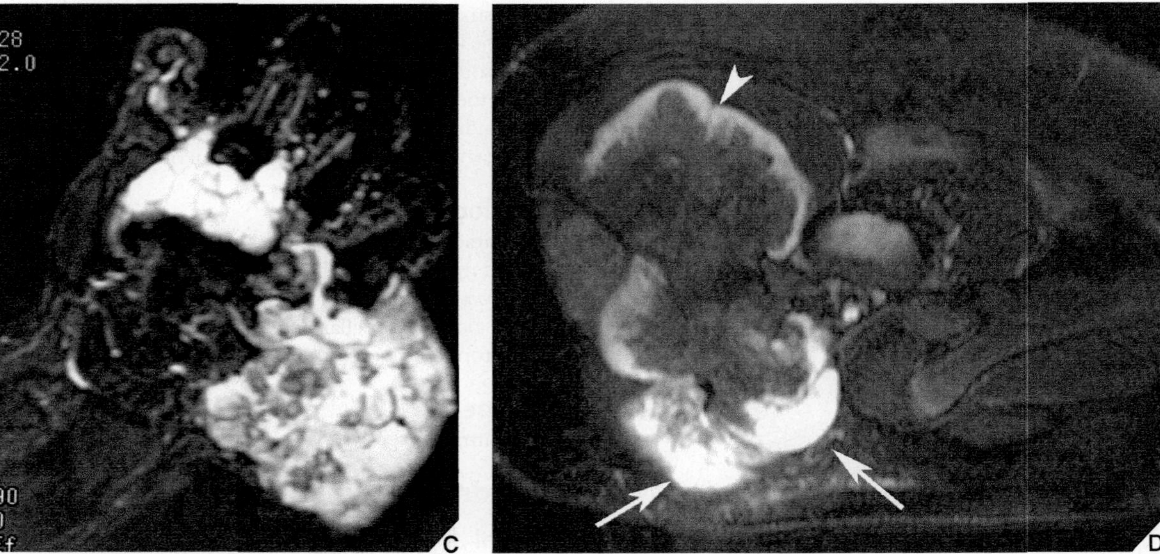

FIGURE 18.62 Malignant transformation. ***(Continued)*** **(C)** Coronal inversion recovery (fast multiplanar inversion recovery [FMPIR]/90; TR 4000/TE 64 msec/Ef) MR image shows malignant lobules of the cartilage invading the bones and soft tissues of the hand. **(D)** Axial T2-weighted fat-saturated MRI in another patient with a large osteochondroma of the pelvis that underwent malignant transformation. Observe the thin, hyperintense cartilage cap of the anterior aspect of the lesion *(arrowhead)*, in comparison to the thick cartilage cap of the posterior aspect undergoing malignant transformation to chondrosarcoma *(arrows)*. Biopsy of the posterior cartilage cap demonstrated malignant chondrocytes. (**A** and **B**, Courtesy of Robert Szabo, MD, Sacramento, CA; from Saunders C, Szabo RM, Mora S. Chondrosarcoma of the hand arising in a young patient with multiple hereditary exostoses. *J Hand Surg Br* 1997;22(2):237–242.)

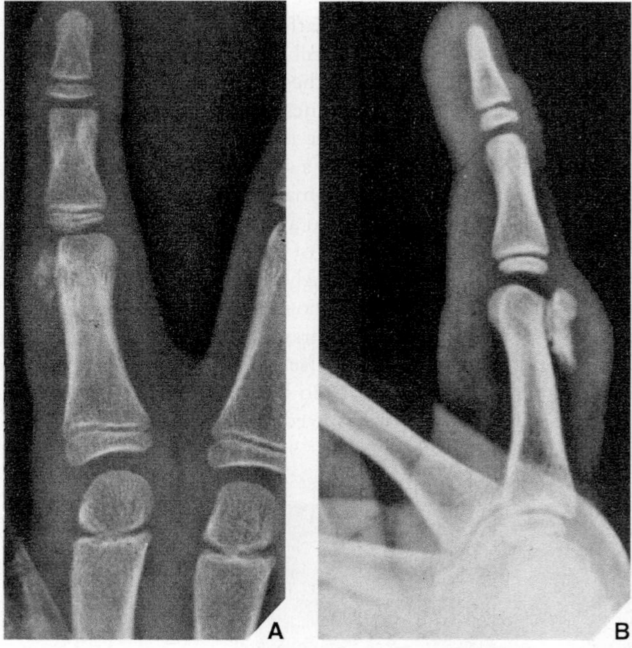

FIGURE 18.63 Bizarre parosteal osteochondromatous proliferation. **(A)** Anteroposterior and **(B)** lateral radiographs of the small finger of an 8-year-old boy show an ossific mass adjacent to the posteromedial cortex of the proximal phalanx. The lesion was excised, and histopathologic examination showed typical changes of Nora lesion, including bluish staining of the calcified cartilage matrix with hematoxylin and eosin, so-called *blue bone*. (Reprinted with permission from Greenspan A, Jundt G, Remagen W. *Differential diagnosis in orthopaedic pathology*, 2nd ed. Philadelphia: Lippincott Williams & Wilkins; 2007.)

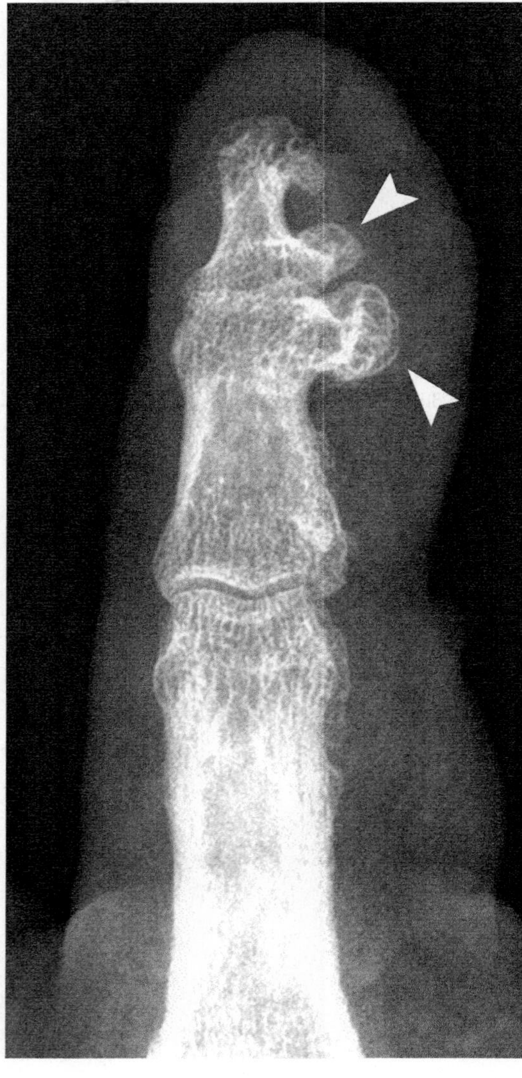

FIGURE 18.64 Bizarre parosteal osteochondromatous proliferation. Anteroposterior radiograph of the middle finger of a 63-year-old man shows mushroom-like osseous excrescences arising at the site of the distal interphalangeal joint *(arrowheads)*.

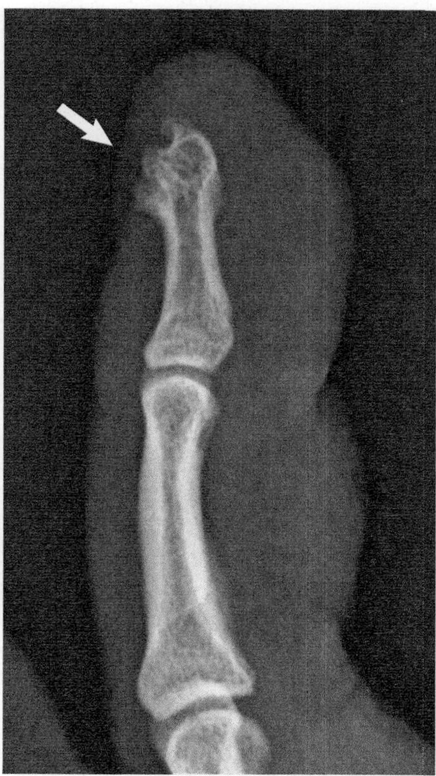

FIGURE 18.65 Turret exostosis. Lateral radiograph of the middle finger of a 30-year-old man shows a well-defined osseous mass fused to the underlying cortex of the distal phalanx *(arrow)*.

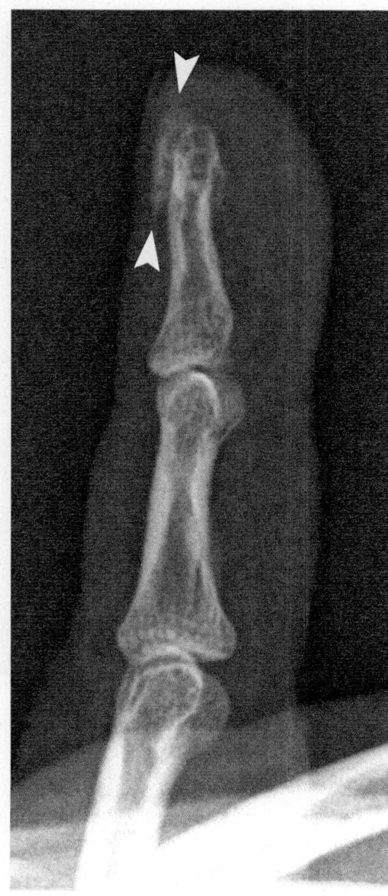

FIGURE 18.66 Subungual exostosis. Lateral radiograph of the small finger of a 55-year-old woman shows under her fingernail an osseous mass attached to the dorsal aspect of the distal tuft *(arrowheads)*.

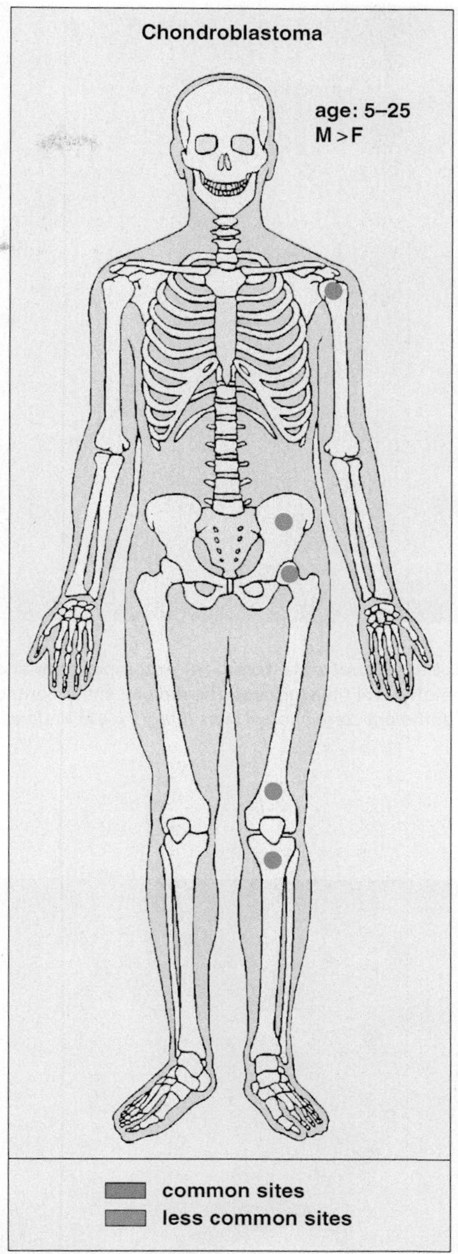

FIGURE 18.67 Skeletal sites of predilection, peak age incidence, and male-to-female ratio in chondroblastoma.

Clonal abnormalities in chondroblastoma have been reported, including recurrent structural alterations in chromosomes 5 and 8 with rearrangements of band 8q21 and recurrent breakpoints at 2q35, 3q21-q23, and 18q21.

Pathology

Histologically, chondroblastoma is composed of nodules of fairly mature cartilage matrix surrounded by a highly cellular tissue containing uniformly large round cells with ovoid nuclei and clear cytoplasm. Multinucleated osteoclast-like giant cells are a common finding. The matrix shows characteristic lattice-like fine calcifications surrounding apposing chondroblasts, having a spatial arrangement resembling the hexagonal configuration of chicken wire.

Treatment and Complications

Chondroblastoma is usually treated by curettage and bone grafting. Only few reported cases have been treated with percutaneous radiofrequency ablation.

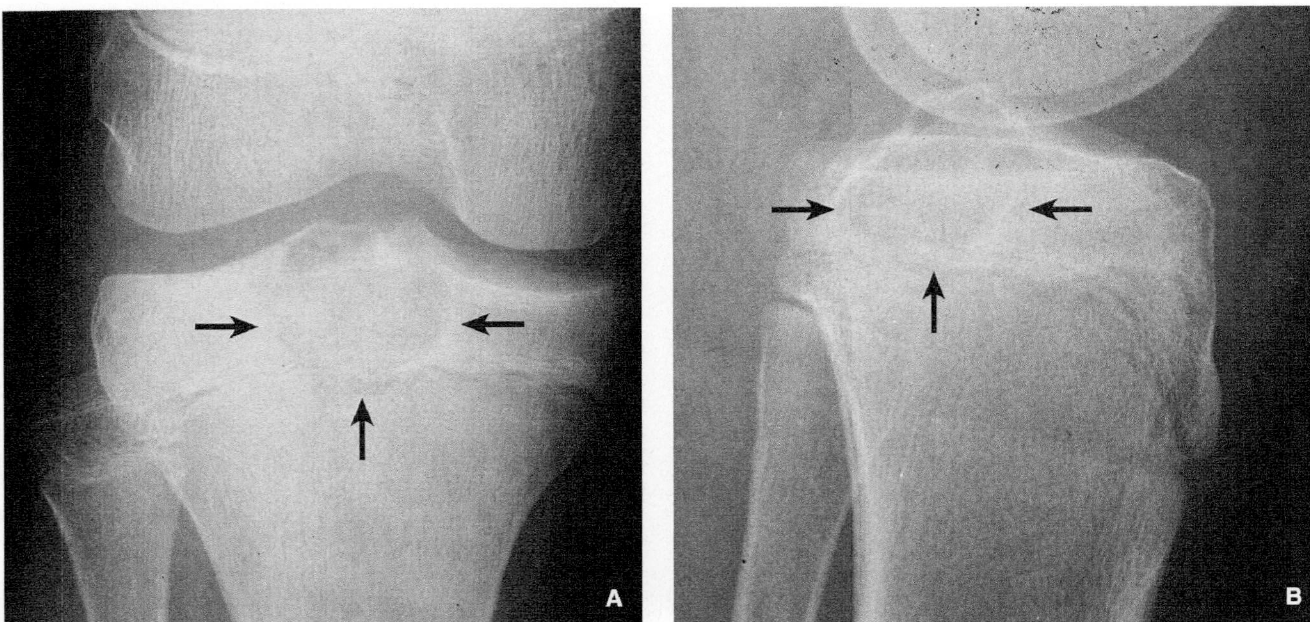

FIGURE 18.68 Chondroblastoma. **(A)** Anteroposterior and **(B)** lateral radiographs of the right knee of a 14-year-old boy show typical appearance of this tumor in the proximal epiphysis of tibia *(arrows)*. The radiolucent, eccentrically located lesion exhibits a thin sclerotic margin. (Reprinted with permission from Greenspan A, Borys D. *Radiology and pathology correlation of bone tumors: a quick reference and review*. Philadelphia: Wolters Kluwer; 2016:129.)

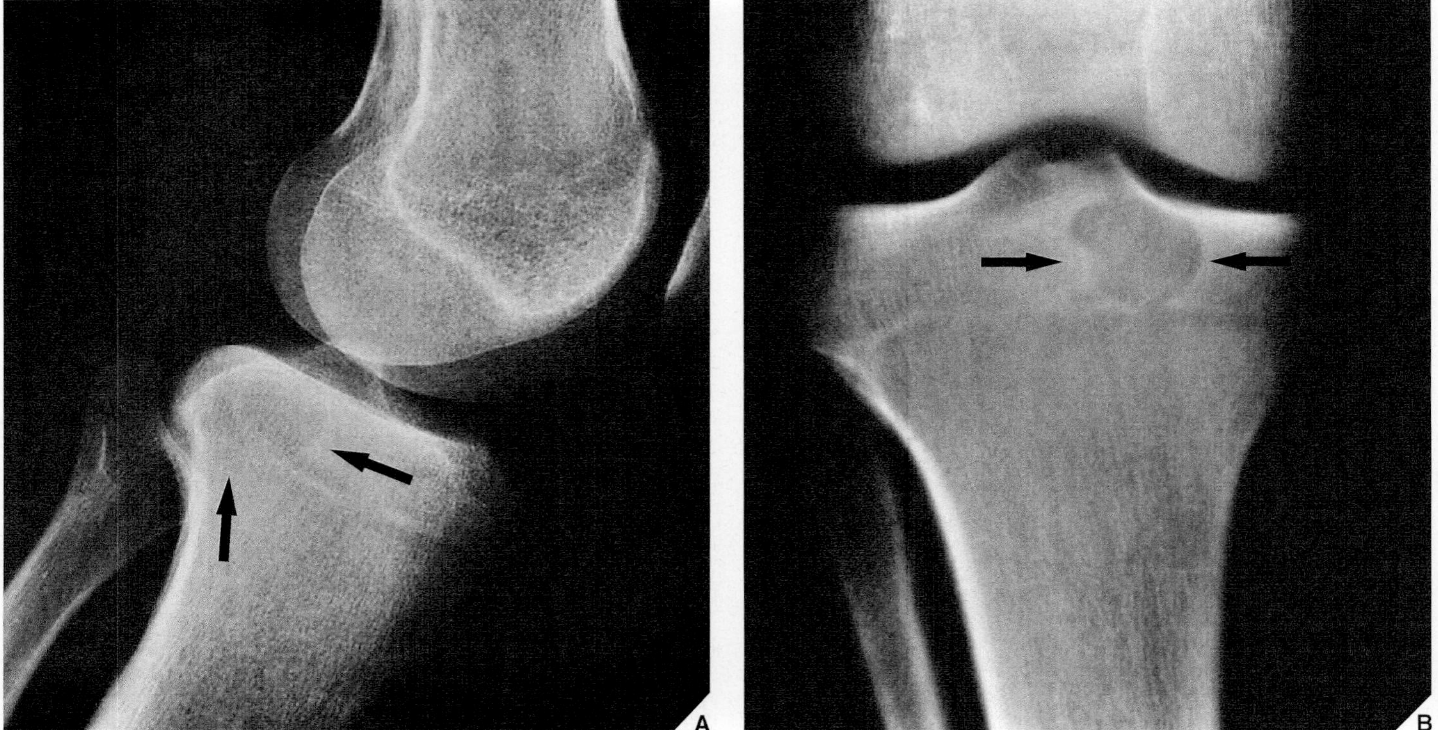

FIGURE 18.69 Chondroblastoma. **(A)** Anteroposterior and **(B)** lateral radiographs of the knee of a 16-year-old girl show the radiolucent, eccentrically located lesion with a thin, sclerotic margin *(arrows)*. There are small, scattered calcifications in the center of the lesion.

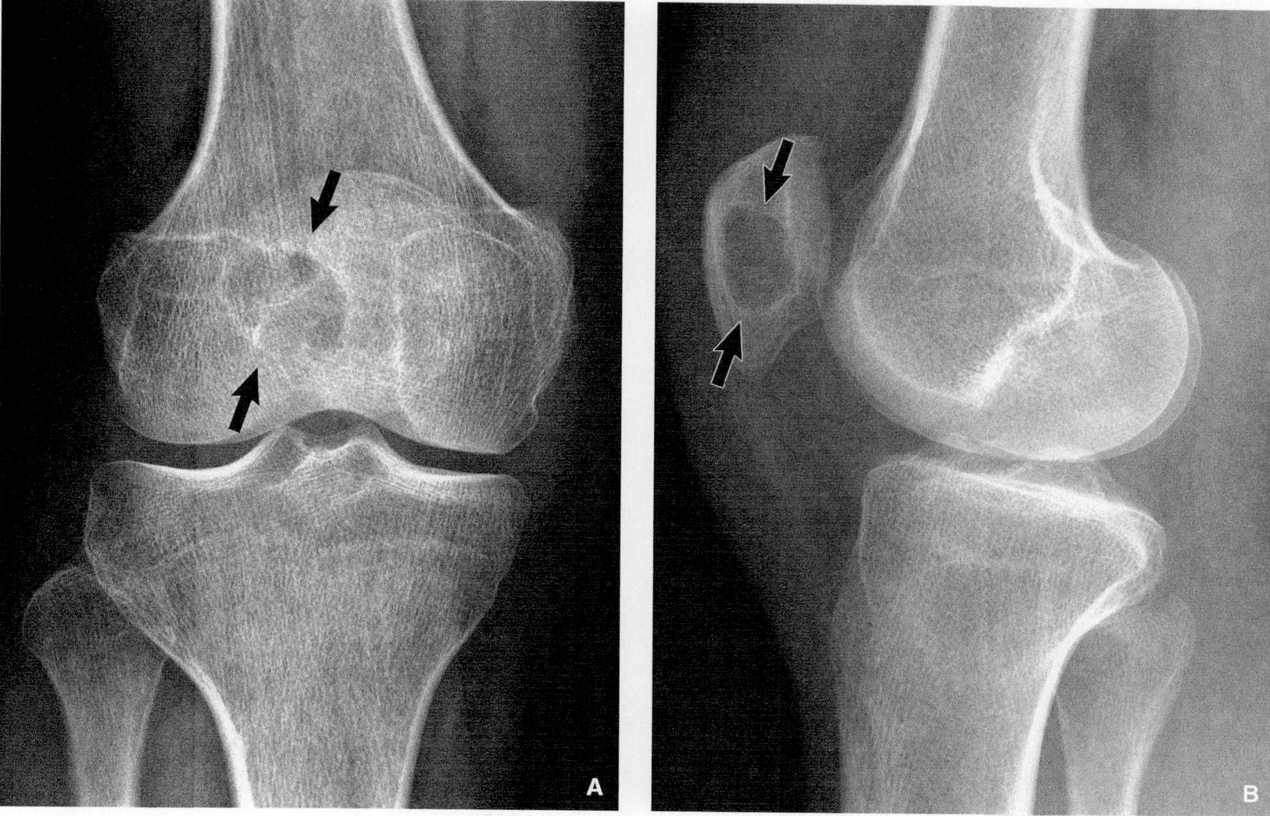

FIGURE 18.70 Chondroblastoma. **(A)** Anteroposterior and **(B)** lateral radiographs of the right knee of a 20-year-old man show well-circumscribed radiolucent lesion with thin sclerotic border within the patella *(arrows)*. There are no visible calcifications within the lesion.

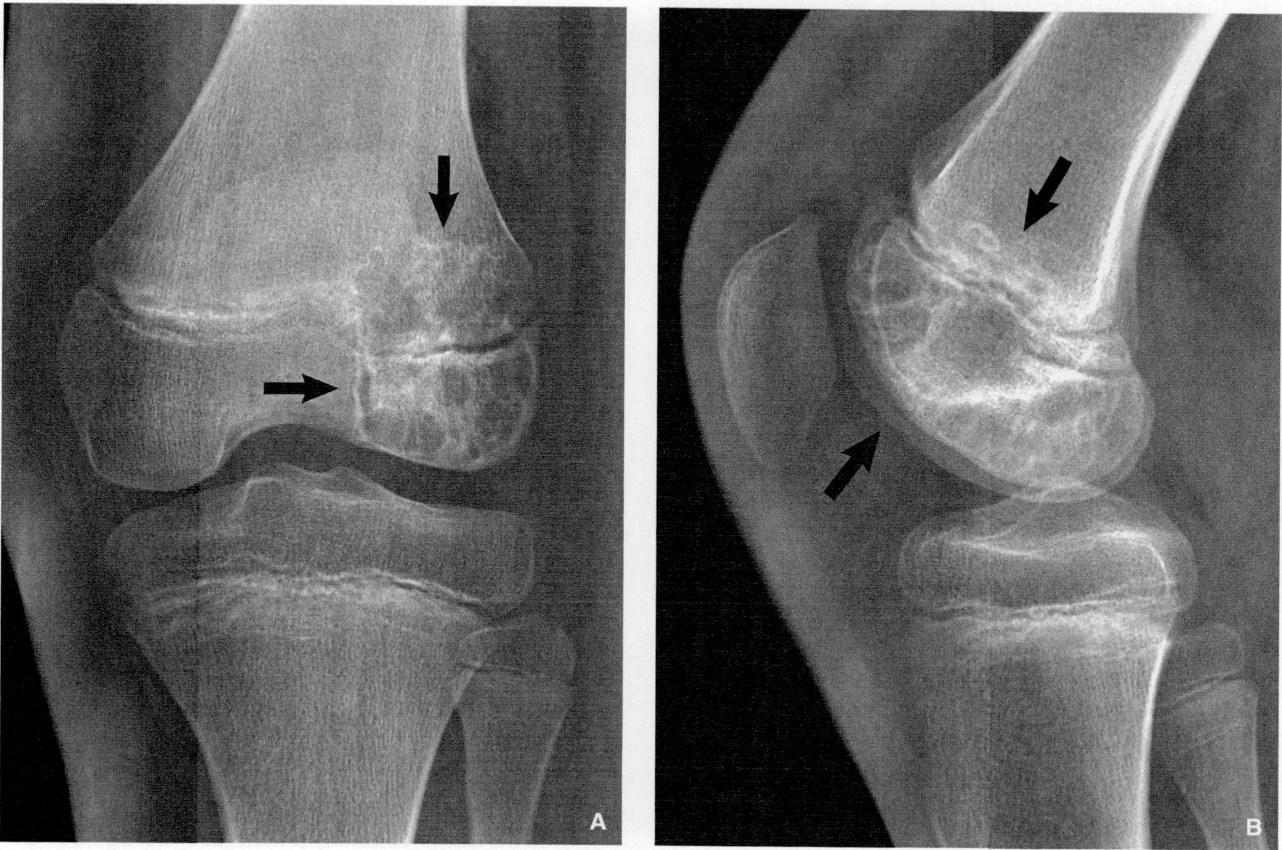

FIGURE 18.71 Chondroblastoma. **(A)** Anteroposterior and **(B)** lateral radiographs of the left knee of a 12-year-old boy show a radiolucent lesion with central mineralization within the lateral epiphysis of distal femur *(arrows)*. Observe that the lesion has crossed the growth plate and involves the metaphysis as well.

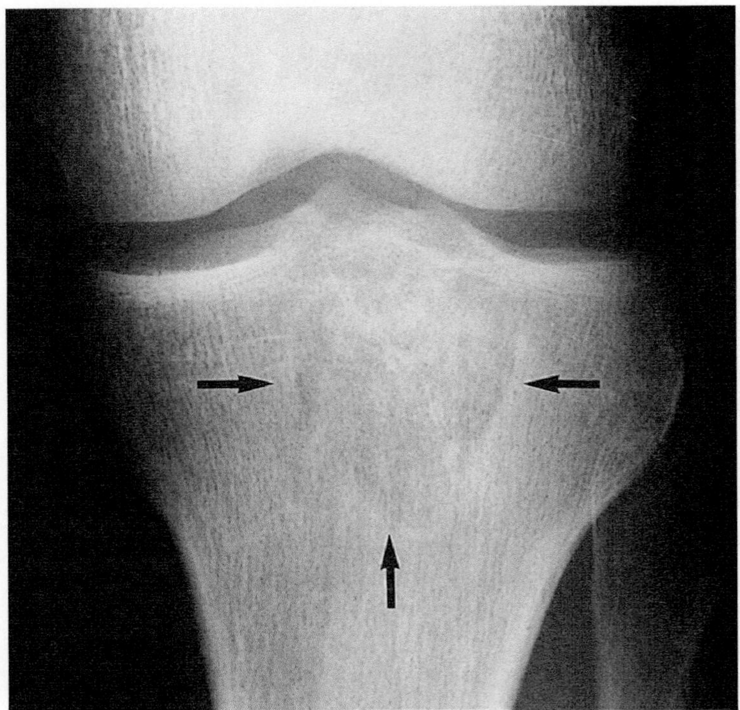

FIGURE 18.72 Chondroblastoma. Anteroposterior radiograph of a knee of a 20-year-old woman shows a radiolucent lesion in the proximal tibia, with a thin sclerotic border and central calcifications, crossing the scarred growth plate *(arrows)*.

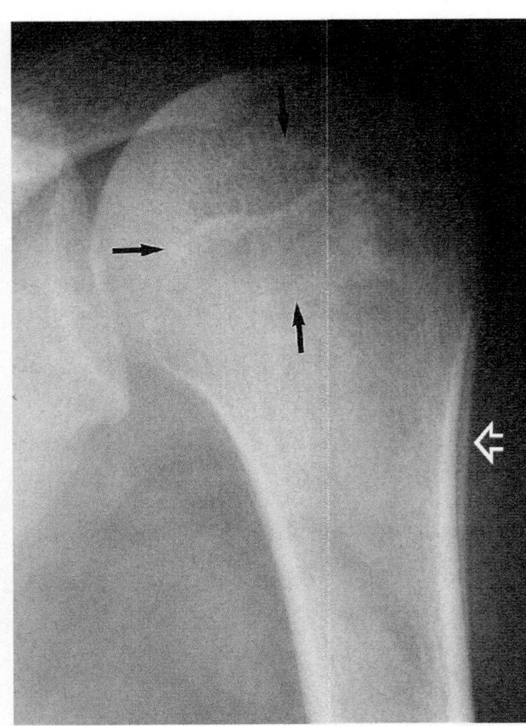

FIGURE 18.73 Chondroblastoma. A lesion in the proximal humerus *(arrows)* elicited periosteal reaction along the lateral cortex *(open arrow)*.

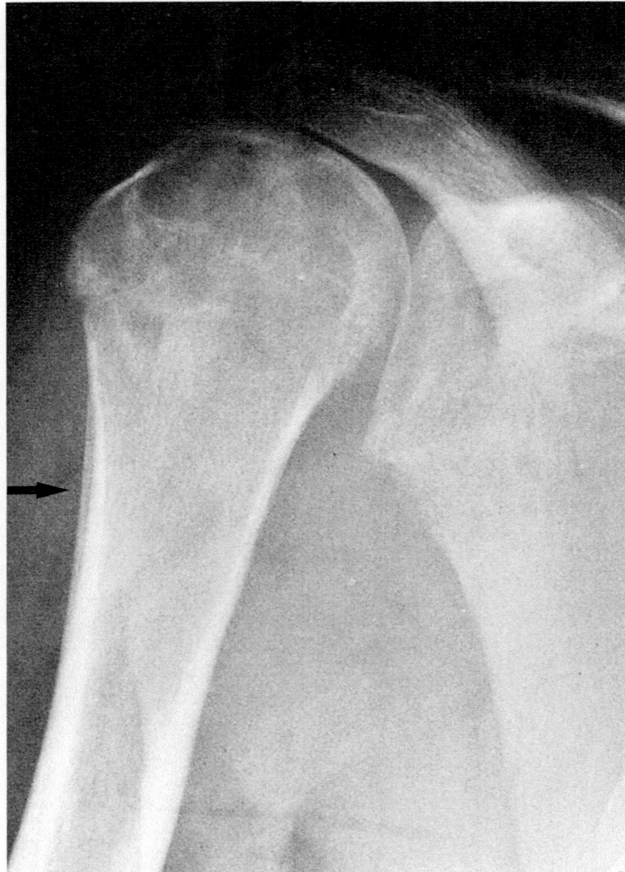

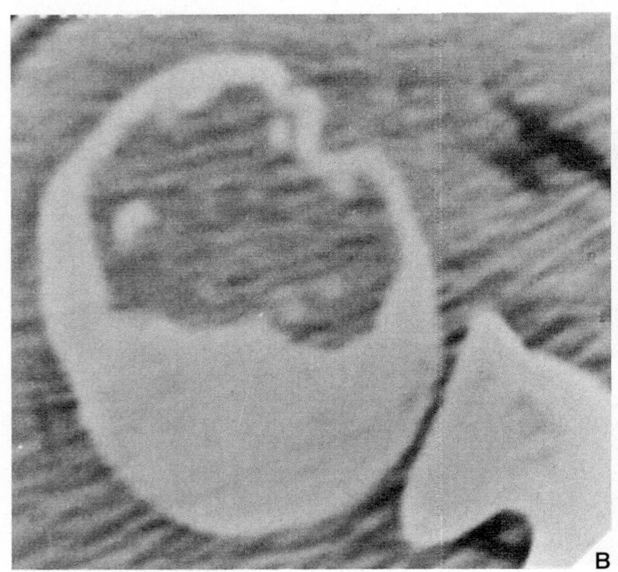

FIGURE 18.74 CT of chondroblastoma. **(A)** Anteroposterior radiograph of the right shoulder of a 16-year-old boy shows a lesion in the proximal humeral epiphysis, but calcifications are not well demonstrated. Note the well-organized layer of periosteal reaction at the lateral cortex *(arrow)*. **(B)** CT section shows the calcifications clearly.

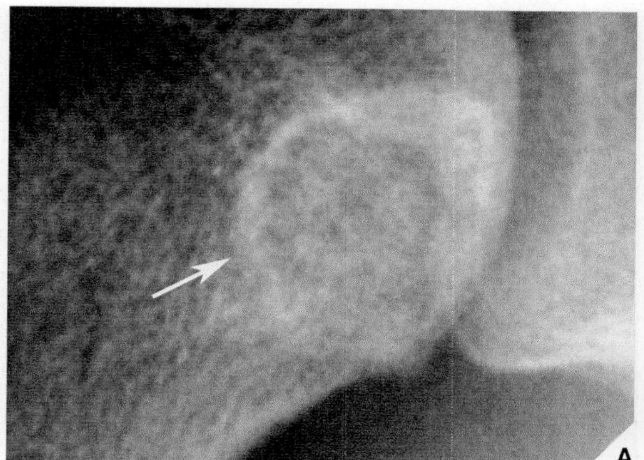

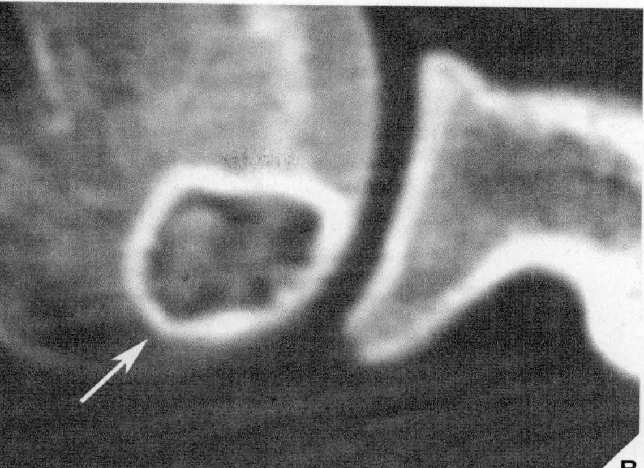

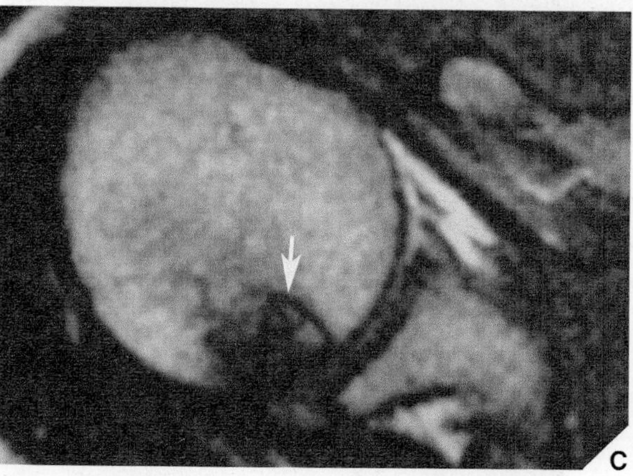

FIGURE 18.75 CT and MRI of chondroblastoma. **(A)** Anteroposterior radiograph of the shoulder demonstrates a well-demarcated lesion in the epiphysis of the humerus with a sclerotic rim *(arrow)* and internal calcifications. **(B)** Axial CT image shows the sclerotic rim *(arrow)* and chondral calcifications inside the lesion. **(C)** Axial T2-weighted MRI demonstrates the tumor *(arrow)* containing low–signal intensity calcified chondroid matrix.

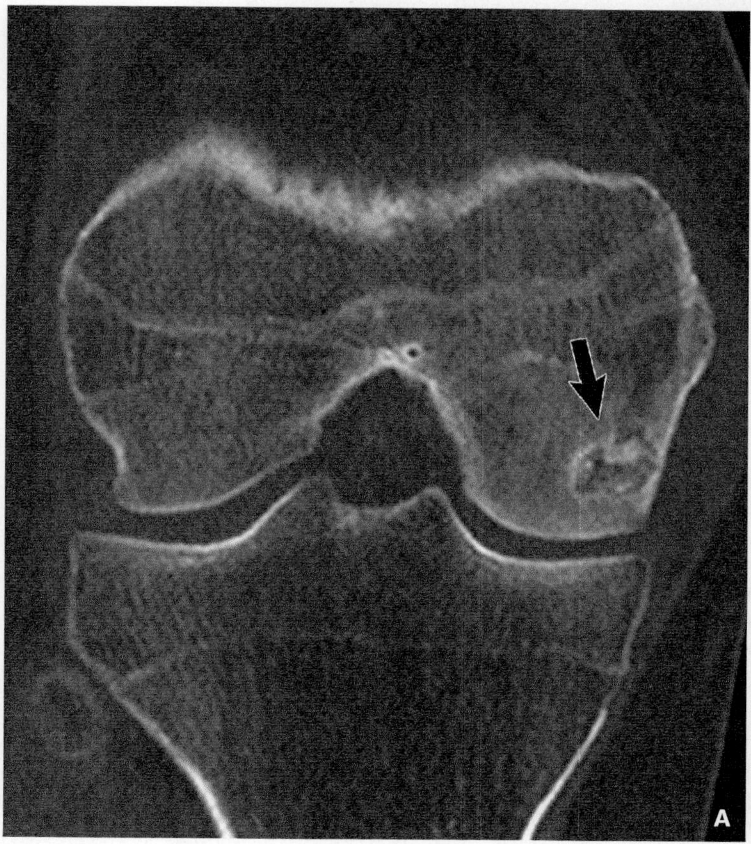

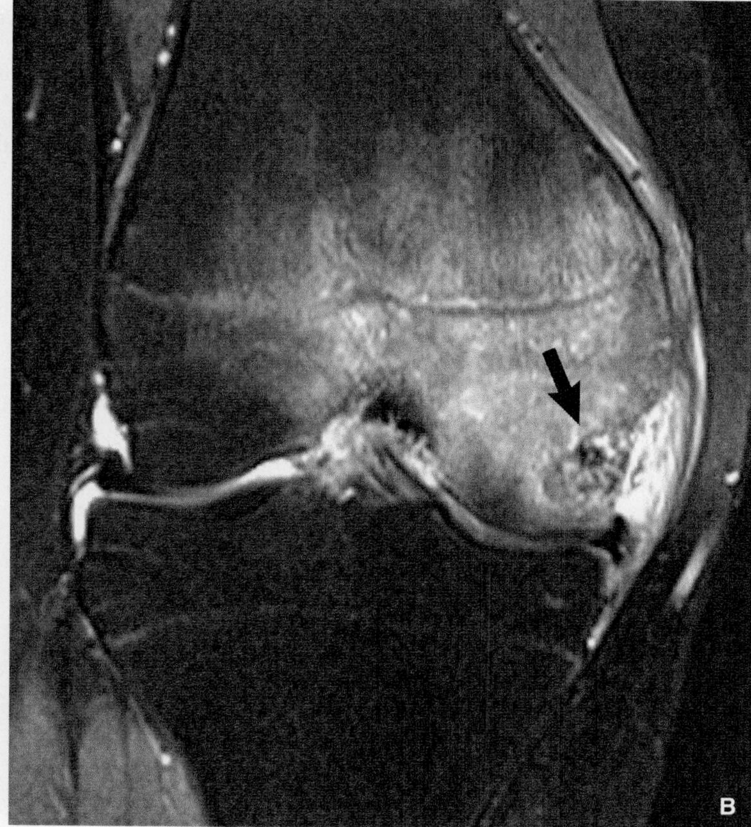

FIGURE 18.76 CT and MRI of chondroblastoma. **(A)** Coronal reformatted CT section and **(B)** coronal T2-weighted fat-suppressed MR image of the right knee of a 19-year-old woman show a small, eccentric in location lesion with sclerotic margin and central calcifications within the medial epiphysis of the distal femur *(arrows)*. Observe extensive peritumoral edema seen on MRI.

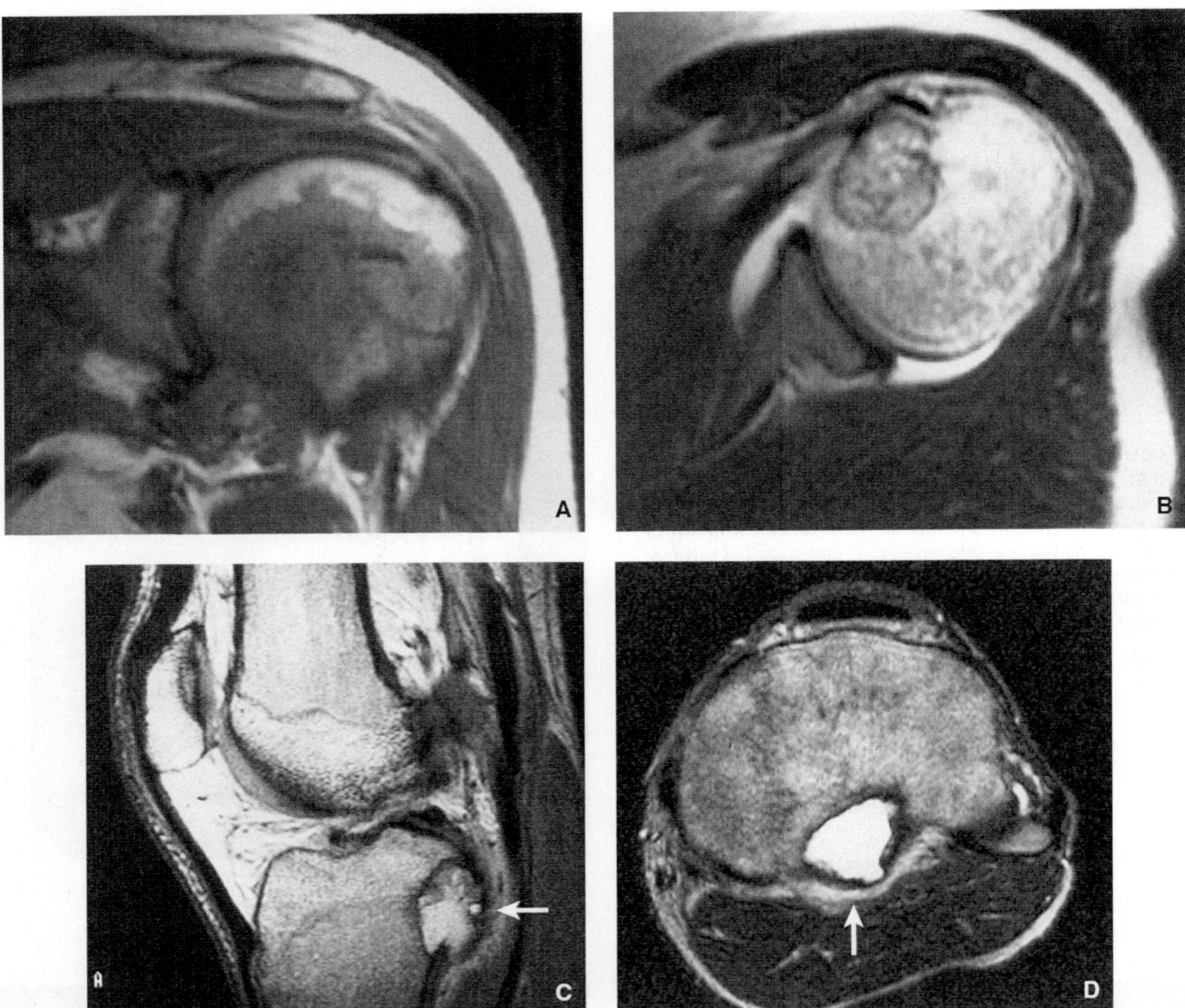

FIGURE 18.77 MRI of chondroblastoma. **(A)** Coronal T1-weighted MR image of the left shoulder shows a large lesion in the humeral head displaying intermediate-to-low signal intensity. **(B)** Axial T2-weighted MR image shows sharply demarcated lesion with low signal intensity border exhibiting a heterogenous but mostly high signal. **(C)** Sagittal proton density–weighted and **(D)** axial T2-weighted MR images of the knee of another patient show a lesion in the posterior aspect of the tibia displaying high signal intensity *(arrows)*. The sclerotic border is of low signal intensity. (Reprinted with permission from Greenspan A, Borys D. *Radiology and pathology correlation of bone tumors: a quick reference and review*. Philadelphia: Wolters Kluwer; 2016:131.)

In rare cases, pulmonary metastases develop in the absence of any histologic evidence of malignancy in either the primary bone tumor or the pulmonary lesions. Only in exceptional circumstances, pulmonary or widespread metastases led to patient death.

Chondromyxoid Fibroma

Clinical and Imaging Features

Chondromyxoid fibroma is a rare tumor of cartilaginous derivation, characterized by the production of chondroid, fibrous, and myxoid tissues in variable proportions, and accounts for 0.5% of all primary bone tumors and 2% of all benign bone tumors. It occurs predominantly in adolescents and young adults (males more than females), most commonly in the patient's second or third decade. It has a predilection for the bones of the lower extremities, with preferred sites in the proximal tibia (32%) and distal femur (17%) (Fig. 18.79). Exceedingly rare, the lesion may be located in the vertebra. Few cases of chondromyxoid fibroma have been reported in juxtacortical location.

Recently, a pericentric inversion of chromosome 6 [inv(6)(p25q13)] has been proposed as a specific genetic marker for chondromyxoid fibroma, and some other studies disclosed a breakpoint on a long arm (q25) of this chromosome. In addition, the clonal translocation t(1;5)(p13;p13) was suggested as a novel sole clone abnormality in this tumor.

Clinical symptoms of chondromyxoid fibroma include local swelling and pain, which are occasionally caused by pressure on adjacent neurovascular structures by a peripherally located mass.

Its characteristic radiographic picture is that of an eccentrically located radiolucent lesion in the bone, with an sclerotic scalloped margin often eroding or ballooning out the cortex (Figs. 18.80 and 18.81). The lesion may range from 1 to 10 cm in size, with an average of 3 to 4 cm. Calcifications are not apparent radiographically, but focal microscopic calcifications have been reported in as many as 27% of cases. Frequently, a buttress of periosteal new bone can be observed. MRI reveals characteristics of most cartilaginous tumors: intermediate-to-low signal intensity on T1-weighted and high signal on T2-weighted sequences (Fig. 18.82).

Pathology

Pathologically, the most important feature of the lesion is its lobular or pseudolobular arrangement into zones of varying cellularity. The center of the lobule is hypocellular. Within the matrix, loosely arranged spindle-shaped and stellate cells with elongated processes are present. The periphery of the lobule is densely cellular, containing a mixture of mononuclear spindle-shaped and polyhedral stromal cells with a variable number of multinucleated giant cells.

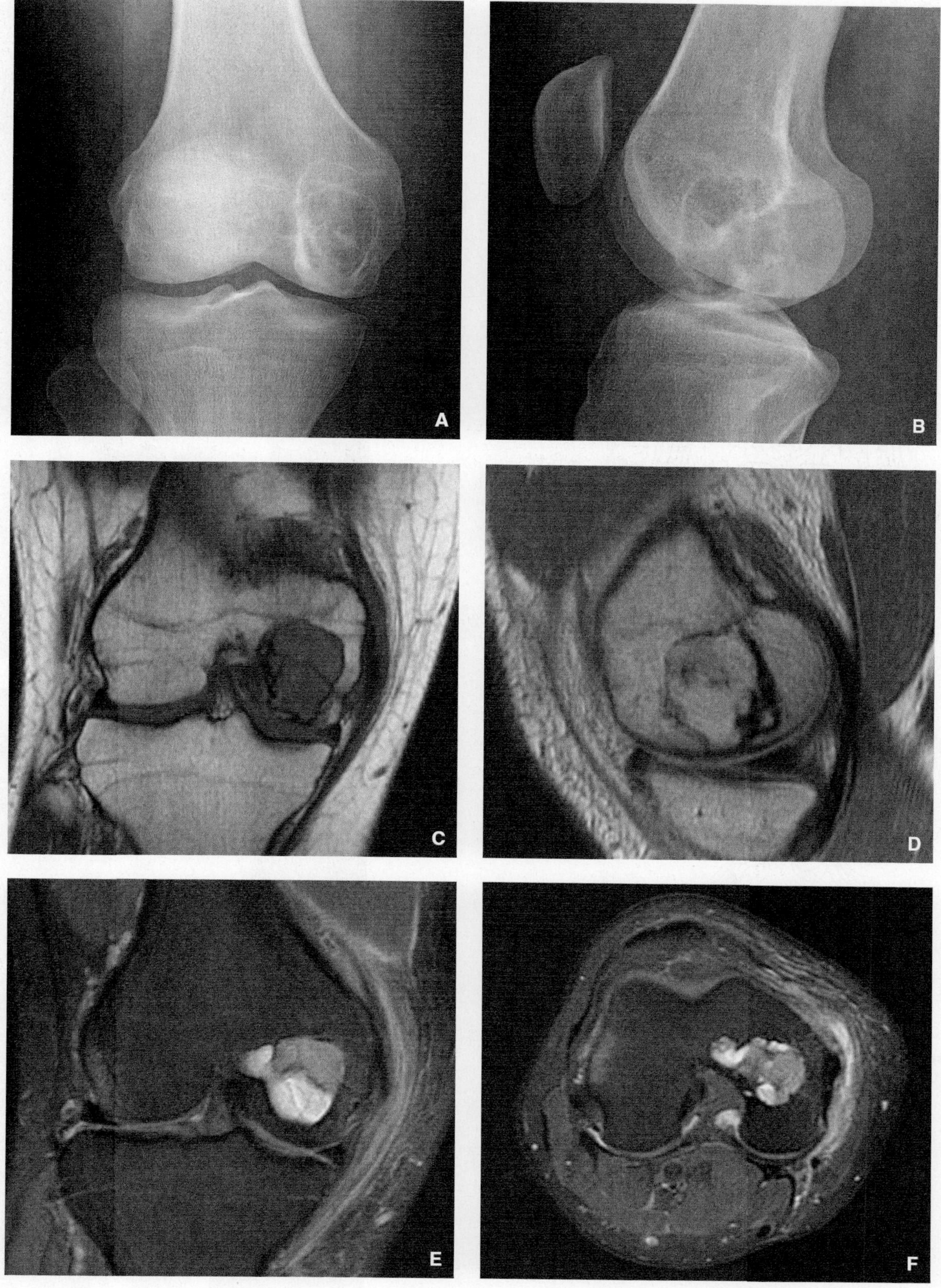

FIGURE 18.78 MRI of chondroblastoma. **(A)** Anteroposterior and **(B)** lateral radiographs of the right knee of a 22-year-old man show a radiolucent lesion with sclerotic border in the medial femoral condyle exhibiting chondroid calcifications. **(C)** Coronal and **(D)** sagittal T1-weighted MR images show the tumor displaying intermediate signal intensity. The sclerotic margin is of low signal intensity. **(E)** Coronal and **(F)** axial T2-weighted fat-suppressed MR images demonstrate heterogenous signal intensity of the lesion. (Reprinted with permission from Greenspan A, Borys D. *Radiology and pathology correlation of bone tumors: a quick reference and review*. Philadelphia: Wolters Kluwer; 2016:132.)

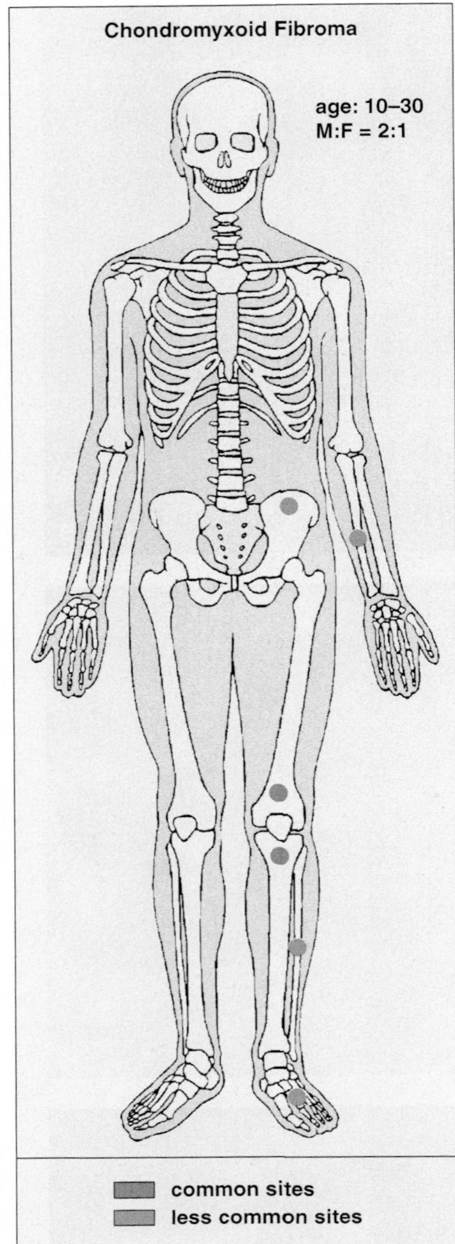

FIGURE 18.79 Skeletal sites of predilection, peak age range, and male-to-female ratio in chondromyxoid fibroma.

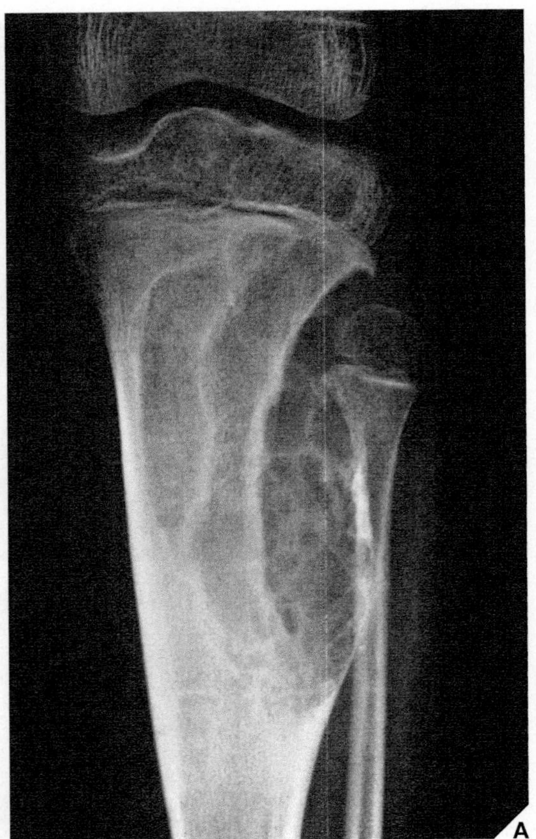

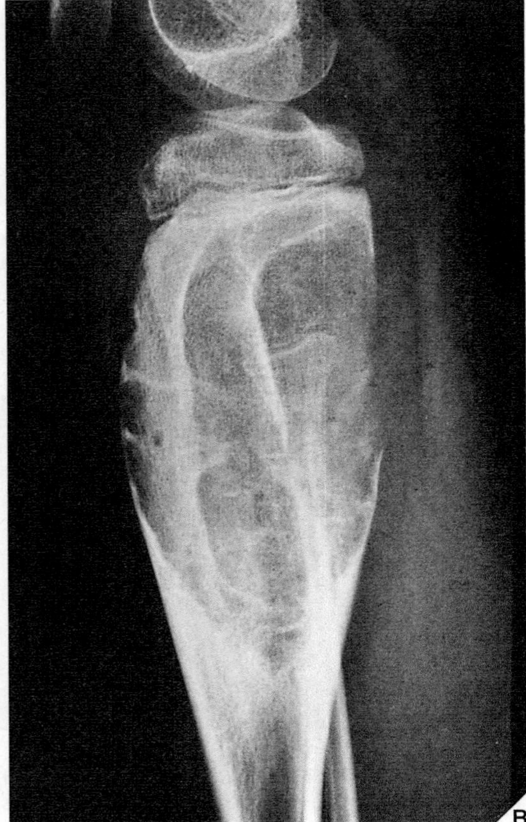

FIGURE 18.80 Chondromyxoid fibroma. **(A)** Anteroposterior and **(B)** lateral radiographs of the left leg of an 8-year-old girl demonstrate a radiolucent lesion extending from the metaphysis into the diaphysis of the tibia, with a geographic type of bone destruction and a sclerotic scalloped border.

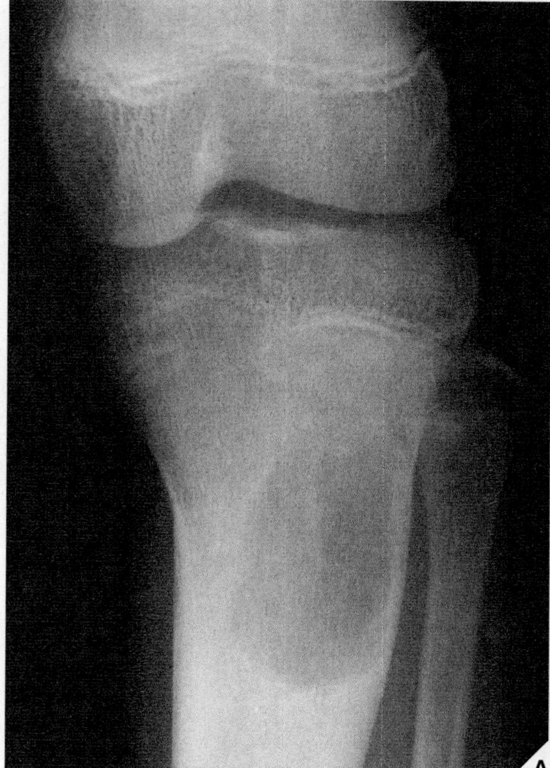
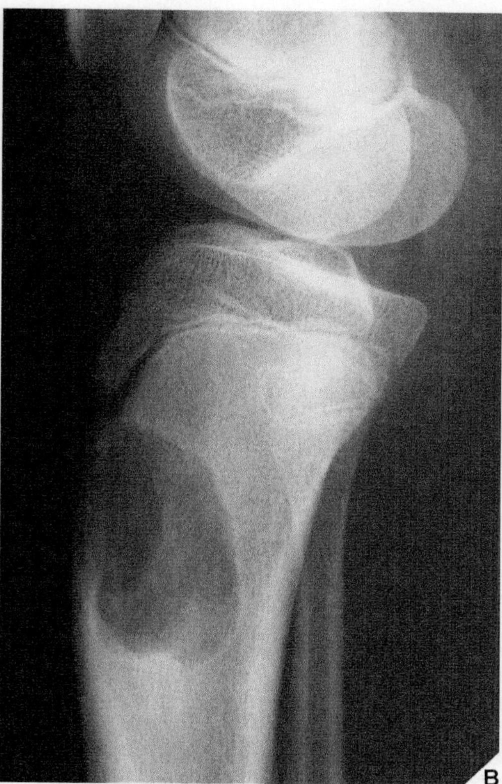

FIGURE 18.81 Chondromyxoid fibroma. **(A)** Anteroposterior and **(B)** lateral radiographs of the left knee of a 12-year-old girl show a radiolucent, slightly lobulated lesion with a thin sclerotic margin in the proximal tibial diaphysis. Note the lack of visible calcifications.

Differential Diagnosis

Commonly, one can observe a characteristic buttress of periosteal new bone formation (Fig. 18.83), in which case a chondromyxoid fibroma may be radiographically indistinguishable from an aneurysmal bone cyst. In unusual locations such as in short tubular or flat bones, it may mimic a giant cell tumor or desmoplastic fibroma.

Treatment

The treatment of this lesion usually consists of curettage and a bone graft. Recurrences are frequent, with the reported rate between 20% and 80% (see Fig. 16.63).

PRACTICAL POINTS TO REMEMBER

1. Enchondroma is characterized by the formation of mature hyaline cartilage and is seen:
   - most commonly in the short tubular bones of the hand, where the lesion is usually radiolucent
   - in the long bones, where scattered calcifications may be seen, resembling a medullary bone infarct.
2. The characteristic radiographic features of enchondroma include:
   - popcorn-like, annular, or punctate calcifications
   - a lobulated growth pattern with frequent shallow scalloping of the endosteal cortex.
3. Important clinical and radiographic features of the malignant transformation of an enchondroma include:
   - the development of pain, in the absence of a fracture, in a previously asymptomatic lesion
   - thickening or destruction of the cortex
   - development of a soft-tissue mass.
4. Enchondromatosis is a condition marked by multiple enchondromas, commonly in metaphysis and diaphysis. If skeleton is extensively affected and the lesions are distributed unilaterally, the term *Ollier disease* is applied.
5. Ollier disease and Maffucci syndrome (an association of Ollier disease with soft-tissue hemangiomatosis) both carry an increased risk for malignant transformation to chondrosarcoma.
6. In the radiographic evaluation of osteochondroma, the most common benign bone lesion, note that:
   - it can be seen as pedunculated or sessile (broad-based) variants
   - its two important radiographic features are uninterrupted merging of the lesion's cortex with the host bone cortex and continuity of the cancellous portion of the lesion with the medullary cavity of the host bone.
7. The most important differential diagnoses in suspected osteochondroma include:
   - juxtacortical osteoma
   - juxtacortical osteosarcoma
   - soft-tissue osteosarcoma
   - juxtacortical myositis ossificans.
8. Osteochondroma may be complicated by:
   - pressure on adjacent nerves or blood vessels
   - pressure on the adjacent bone, frequently leading to fracture
   - bursitis exostotica
   - malignant transformation to chondrosarcoma.
9. In the malignant transformation of osteochondroma, imaging signs include:
   - enlargement of the lesion
   - marked thickening of the cartilaginous cap of the lesion
   - dispersion of calcifications into the cartilaginous cap
   - development of a soft-tissue mass
   - increased isotope uptake by the lesion after skeletal maturity.
10. Variants of osteochondroma include subungual exostosis, turret exostosis, traction exostosis, BPOP, florid reactive periostitis, and dysplasia epiphysealis hemimelica (Trevor-Fairbank disease).

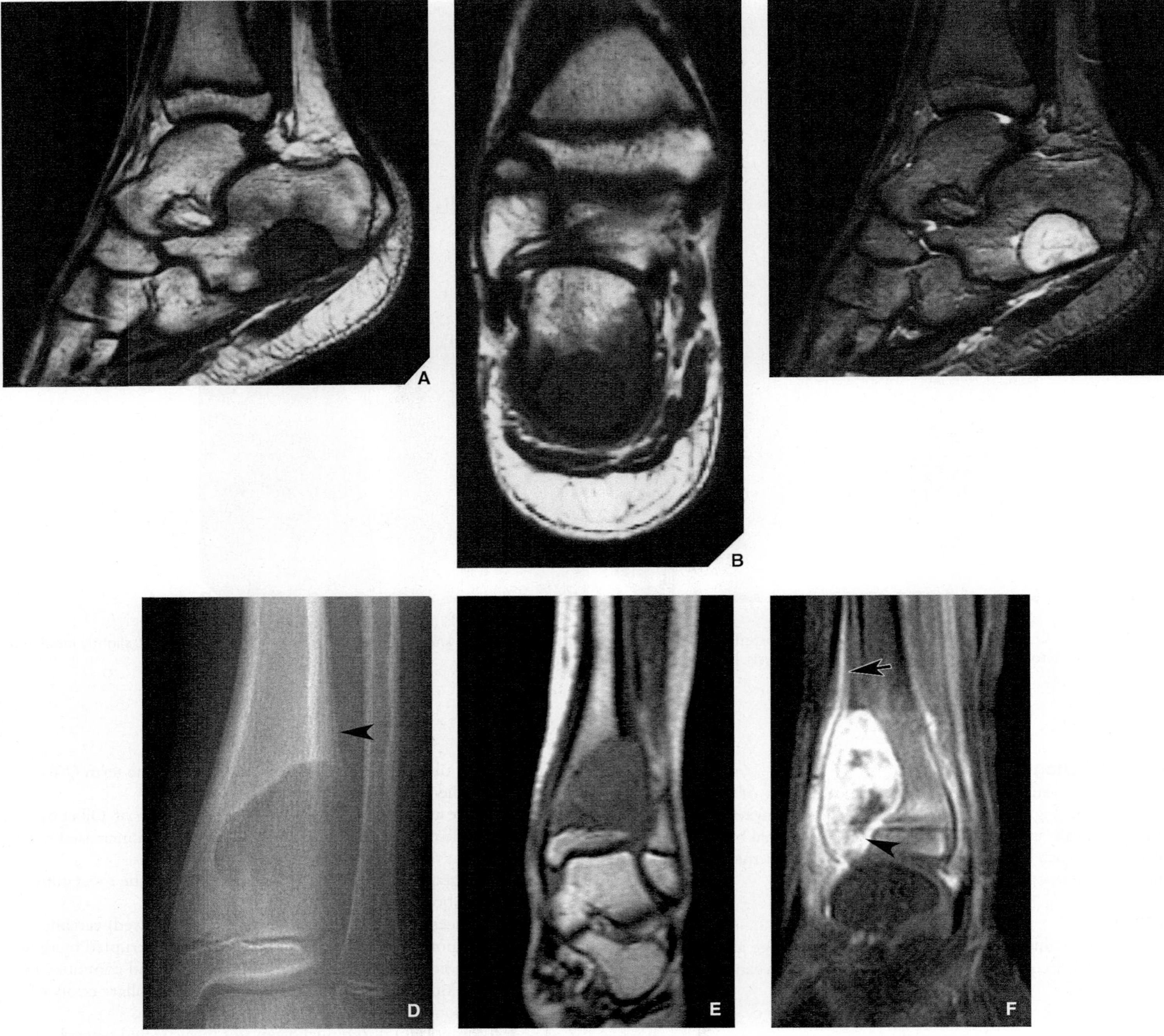

FIGURE 18.82 MRI of chondromyxoid fibroma. **(A)** Sagittal T1-weighted (SE; repetition time [TR] 600/TE 19 msec) MRI in a 10-year-old girl shows a well-demarcated lesion in the plantar aspect of the calcaneus, displaying low signal intensity. **(B)** Axial T1-weighted (SE; TR 600/TE 17 msec) MR image shows significant amount of peritumoral edema. **(C)** Sagittal T2-weighted (SE; TR 2000/TE 80 msec) MRI shows the lesion displaying high signal intensity. A sclerotic border is imaged as a rim of low signal intensity. **(D)** Anteroposterior radiograph of the left ankle of an 8-year-old girl who presented with sharp pain in this region, demonstrates a lytic lesion in the distal metaphysis of the tibia with narrow zone of transition, cortical destruction, and periosteal reaction *(arrowhead)*. **(E)** Coronal T1-weighted MR image and **(F)** sagittal T1-weighted fat-saturated MR image obtained after intravenous administration of gadolinium demonstrate more clearly the soft-tissue extension of the tumor and the invasion of the distal tibial epiphysis (*arrowhead* in **F**) not well demonstrated on the radiograph. Note the strong enhancement of the tumor following gadolinium injection and edema of the bone marrow and surrounding soft tissues as well as the periosteal reaction (*arrow* in **F**).

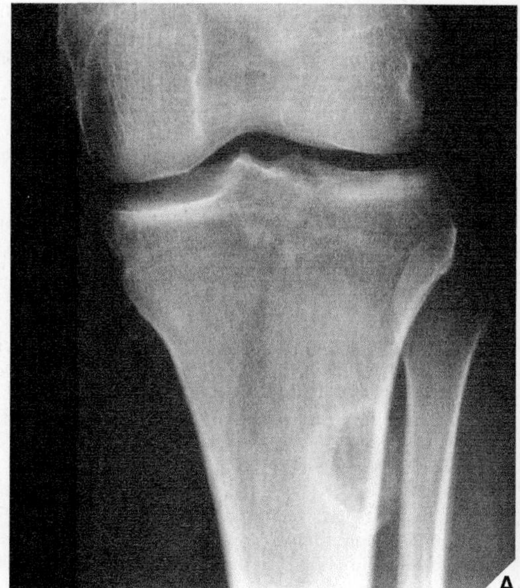

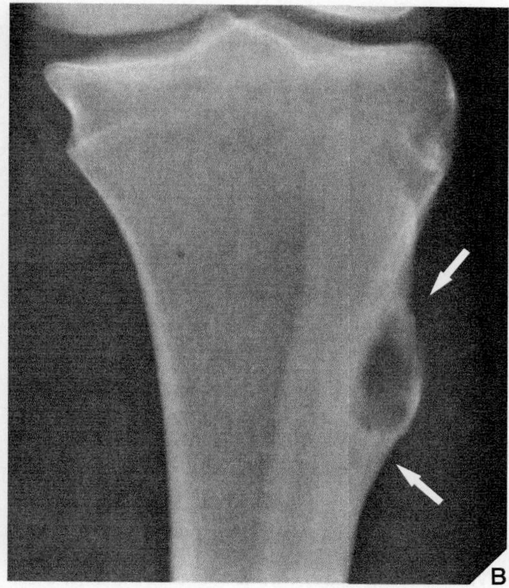

FIGURE 18.83 Chondromyxoid fibroma resembling an aneurysmal bone cyst. (A) Anteroposterior radiograph of the knee of an 18-year-old woman shows a lesion in the lateral aspect of the proximal tibia. The tumor balloons out from the cortex and is supported by a solid periosteal buttress resembling that seen in an aneurysmal bone cyst. The periosteal buttress *(arrows)* is better appreciated on a tomographic cut **(B)**.

11. Multiple osteocartilaginous exostoses, a familial hereditary condition, carry the increased risk of malignant transformation of an osteochondroma to a chondrosarcoma, particularly in the shoulder girdle and pelvis.
12. Chondroblastoma is characterized radiographically by:
    - its eccentric epiphyseal location
    - sclerotic margin
    - scattered calcifications
    - periosteal reaction (>50% cases).
13. Chondromyxoid fibroma is characterized radiographically by:
    - its location close to the growth plate
    - its scalloped, sclerotic border
    - a buttress of periosteal new bone
    - lack of visible calcifications.

    It may mimic an aneurysmal bone cyst.

SUGGESTED READINGS

Abdelwahab IF, Hermann G, Lewis MM, et al. Case report 588: intracortical chondroma of the left femur. *Skeletal Radiol* 1990;19:59–61.

Abdelwahab IF, Klein MJ. Surface chondromyxoid fibroma of the distal ulna: unusual tumor, site, and age. *Skeletal Radiol* 2014;43:243–246.

Amary MF, Bacsi K, Maggiani F, et al. IDH1 and IDH2 mutations are frequent events in central chondrosarcoma and central and periosteal chondromas but not in other mesenchymal tumours. *J Pathol* 2011;224:334–343.

Amary MF, Damato S, Halai D, et al. Ollier disease and Maffucci syndrome are caused by somatic mosaic mutations of IDH1 and IDH2. *Nature Genet* 2011;43:1262–1265.

Aoki JA, Sone S, Fujioka F, et al. MR of enchondroma and chondrosarcoma: rings and arcs of Gd-DTPA enhancement. *J Comput Assist Tomogr* 1991;15:1011–1016.

Armah HB, McGough RL, Goodman MA, et al. Chondromyxoid fibroma of rib with a novel chromosomal translocation: a report of four additional cases at unusual sites. *Diagn Pathol* 2007;2:44.

Azouz EM, Greenspan A, Marton D. CT evaluation of primary epiphyseal bone abscesses. *Skeletal Radiol* 1993;22:17–23.

Bandiera S, Bacchini P, Bertoni F. Bizarre parosteal osteochondromatous proliferation of bone. *Skeletal Radiol* 1998;27:154–156.

Bansal M, Goldman AB, DiCarlo EF, et al. Soft tissue chondromas: diagnosis and differential diagnosis. *Skeletal Radiol* 1993;22:309–315.

Bartsch O, Wuyts W, Van Hul W, et al. Delineation of a contiguous gene syndrome with multiple exostoses, enlarged parietal foramina, craniofacial dysostosis, and mental retardation, caused by deletions in the short arm of chromosome 11. *Am J Hum Genet* 1996;58:734–742.

Bernard SA, Murphey MD, Flemming DJ, et al. Improved differentiation of benign osteochondromas from secondary chondrosarcomas with standardized measurement of cartilage cap at CT and MR imaging. *Radiology* 2010;255:857–865.

Bierry G, Kerr DA, Nielsen GP, et al. Enchondromas in children: imaging appearance with pathological correlation. *Skeletal Radiol* 2012;41:1223–1229.

Bird JE, Wang W-L, Deavers MT, et al. Enchondroma with secondary aneurysmal bone cyst. *Skeletal Radiol* 2012;41:1475–1478.

Björnsson J, Unni KK, Dahlin DC, et al. Clear cell chondrosarcoma of bone. Observations in 47 cases. *Am J Surg Pathol* 1984;8:223–230.

Bloem JL, Mulder JD. Chondroblastoma: a clinical and radiological study of 104 cases. *Skeletal Radiol* 1985;14:1–9.

Borges AM, Huvos AG, Smith J. Bursa formation and synovial chondrometaplasia associated with osteochondromas. *Am J Clin Pathol* 1981;75:648–653.

Boriani S, Bacchini P, Bertoni F, et al. Periosteal chondroma. A review of twenty cases. *J Bone Joint Surg Am* 1983;65A:205–212.

Braunstein E, Martel W, Weatherbee L. Periosteal bone apposition in chondroblastoma. *Skeletal Radiol* 1979;4:34–36.

Brien EW, Mirra JM, Luck JV Jr. Benign and malignant cartilage tumors of bone and joint: their anatomic and theoretical basis with an emphasis on radiology, pathology and clinical biology. II. Juxtacortical cartilage tumors. *Skeletal Radiol* 1999;28:1–20.

Brower AC, Moser RP, Gilkey FW, et al. Chondroblastoma. In: Moser RP Jr, ed. *Cartilaginous tumors of the skeleton. AFIP atlas of radiologic-pathologic correlation, fascicle II.* Philadelphia: Hanley & Belfus; 1990:74–113.

Brower AC, Moser RP, Kransdorf MJ. The frequency and diagnostic significance of periostitis in chondroblastoma. *Am J Roentgenol* 1990;154:309–314.

Bruder E, Zanetti M, Boos N, et al. Chondromyxoid fibroma of two thoracic vertebrae. *Skeletal Radiol* 1999;28:286–289.

Buddingh EP, Naumann S, Nelson M, et al. Cytogenetic findings in benign cartilaginous neoplasms. *Cancer Genet Cytogenet* 2003;141:164–168.

Bui KL, Ilaslan H, Bauer TW, et al. Cortical scalloping and cortical penetration by small eccentric chondroid lesions in the long tubular bones: not a sign of malignancy? *Skeletal Radiol* 2009;38:791–796.

Bullough PG. *Atlas of orthopedic pathology*, 2nd ed. New York Medical: Gower; 1992:14.9.

Cannon CP, Nelson SD, Seeger L, et al. Clear cell chondrosarcoma mimicking chondroblastoma in a skeletally immature patient. *Skeletal Radiol* 2002;31:369–372.

Chung EB, Enzinger FM. Chondroma of soft parts. *Cancer* 1978;41:1414–1424.

Codman EA. Epiphyseal chondromatous giant cell tumors of the upper end of the humerus. *Surg Gynecol Obstet* 1931;52:543–548.

Cohen EK, Kressel HY, Frank TS, et al. Hyaline cartilage-origin bone and soft-tissue neoplasms: MR appearance and histologic correlation. *Radiology* 1988;167:477–481.

Collins PS, Han W, Williams LR, et al. Maffucci's syndrome (hemangiomatosis osteolytica): a report of four cases. *J Vasc Surg* 1992;16:364–371.

DaCambra MO, Gupta SK, Ferri-de-Barros F. Subungual exostosis of the toes: a systematic review. *Clin Orthop Relat Res* 2014;472:1251–1259.

Dahlin DC, Ivins JC. Benign chondroblastoma. A study of 125 cases. *Cancer* 1972;30:401–413.

Davids JR, Glancy GL, Eilert RE. Fracture through the stalk of pedunculated osteochondromas. A report of three cases. *Clin Orthop Relat Res* 1991;271:258–264.

De Beuckeleer LHL, De Schepper AMA, Ramon F. Magnetic resonance imaging of cartilaginous tumors: is it useful or necessary? *Skeletal Radiol* 1996;25:137–141.

De Beuckeleer LHL, De Schepper AMA, Ramon F, et al. Magnetic resonance imaging of cartilaginous tumors: a retrospective study of 79 patients. *Eur J Radiol* 1995;21:34–40.

deSantos LA, Spjut HJ. Periosteal chondroma: a radiographic spectrum. *Skeletal Radiol* 1981;6:15–20.

Devidayal A, Marwaha RK. Langer-Giedion syndrome. *Indian Pediatr* 2006;43:174–175.
Dharmshaktu GS, Pangtey T. Turret exostosis of proximal phalanx of thumb. *N Niger J Clin Res* 2016;5:64–65.
Dhondt E, Oudenhoven L, Khan S, et al. Nora's lesion, a distinct radiological entity? *Skeletal Radiol* 2006;35:497–502.
Douis H, Davies AM, James SL, et al. Can MR imaging challenge the commonly accepted theory of the pathogenesis of solitary enchondroma of long bone? *Skeletal Radiol* 2012;41:1537–1542.
Douis H, Saifuddin A. The imaging of cartilaginous bone tumours. I. Benign lesions. *Skeletal Radiol* 2012;41:1195–1212.
El-Khoury GY, Bassett GS. Symptomatic bursa formation with osteochondromas. *AJR Am J Roentgenol* 1979;133:895–898.
Erickson JK, Rosenthal DI, Zaleske DJ, et al. Primary treatment of chondroblastoma with percutaneous radio-frequency heat ablation: report of three cases. *Radiology* 2001;221:463–468.
Fairbank TJ. Dysplasia epiphysealis hemimelica (tarso-epiphyseal aclasis). *J Bone Joint Surg Br* 1956;38-B:237–257.
Flach HZ, Ginai AZ, Oosterhuis JW. Best cases from the AFIP. Maffucci syndrome: radiologic and pathologic findings. *Radiographics* 2001;21:1311–1316.
Garcia RA, Inwards CY, Unni KK. Benign bone tumors—recent developments. *Semin Diagn Pathol* 2011;28:73–85.
Garrison RC, Unni KK, McLeod RA, et al. Chondrosarcoma arising in osteochondroma. *Cancer* 1982;49:1890–1897.
Geirnaerdt MJA, Bloem JL, Eulderink F, et al. Cartilaginous tumors: correlation of gadolinium-enhanced MR imaging and histopathologic findings. *Radiology* 1993;186:813–817.
Goodman SB, Bell RS, Fornasier VS, et al. Ollier's disease with multiple sarcomatous transformations. *Hum Pathol* 1984;15:91–93.
Green P, Whittaker RP. Benign chondroblastoma. Case report with pulmonary metastasis. *J Bone Joint Surg Am* 1975;57:418–420.
Greenspan A. Tumors of cartilage origin. *Orthop Clin North Am* 1989;20:347–366.
Greenspan A, Borys D. Benign cartilage-forming lesions. In: *Radiology and pathology correlation of bone tumors: a quick reference and review*. Philadelphia: Wolters Kluwer; 2016:90–138.
Greenspan A, Jundt G, Remagen W. *Differential diagnosis in orthopaedic oncology*, 2nd ed. Philadelphia: Lippincott Williams & Wilkins; 2007.
Greenspan A, Klein MJ. Radiology and pathology of bone tumors. In: Lewis MM, ed. *Musculoskeletal oncology. A multidisciplinary approach*. Philadelphia: WB Saunders; 1992:13–72.
Greenspan A, Unni KK, Matthews J II. Periosteal chondroma masquerading as osteochondroma. *Can Assoc Radiol J* 1993;44:205–210.
Hameetman L, Szuhai K, Yavas A, et al. The role of EXT1 in nonhereditary osteochondroma: identification of homozygous deletions. *J Natl Cancer Inst* 2007;99:396–406.
Helliwell TR, O'Connor MA, Ritchie DA, et al. Bizarre parosteal osteochondromatous proliferation with cortical invasion. *Skeletal Radiol* 2001;30:282–285.
Hensinger RN, Cowell HR, Ramsey PL, et al. Familial dysplasia epiphysealis hemimelica, associated with chondromas and osteochondromas. Report of a kindred with variable presentations. *J Bone Joint Surg Am* 1974;56:1513–1516.
Hudson TM, Spriengfield DS, Spanier SS, et al. Benign exostoses and exostotic chondrosarcomas: evaluation of cartilage thickness by CT. *Radiology* 1984;152:595–599.
Huvos AG, Higinbotham NL, Marcove RC, et al. Aggressive chondroblastoma. Review of the literature on aggressive behavior and metastases with a report of one new case. *Clin Orthop Relat Res* 1977;(126):266–272.
Jaffe HL, Lichtenstein L. Benign chondroblastoma of bone: a reinterpretation of the so-called calcifying or chondromatous giant cell tumor. *Am J Pathol* 1942;18:969–991.
Jaffe HL, Lichtenstein L. Chondromyxoid fibroma of bone: a distinctive benign tumor likely to be mistaken especially for chondrosarcoma. *Arch Pathol (Chic)* 1948;45:541–551.
Janzen L, Logan PM, O'Connell JX, et al. Intramedullary chondroid tumors of bone: correlation of abnormal peritumoral marrow and soft-tissue MRI signal with tumor type. *Skeletal Radiol* 1997;26:100–106.
Kahn S, Taljanovic MS, Speer DP, et al. Kissing periosteal chondroma and osteochondroma. *Skeletal Radiol* 2002;31:235–239.
Kettelkamp DB, Campbell CJ, Bonfiglio M. Dysplasia epiphysealis hemimelica. A report of fifteen cases and a review of the literature. *J Bone Joint Surg Am* 1966;48:746–766.
Kontogeorgakos VA, Lykissas MG, Mavrodontidis AN, et al. Turret exostosis of the hallux. *J Foot Ankle Surg* 2007;46:130–132.
Lalam RK, Cribb GL, Tins BJ, et al. Image guided radiofrequency thermo-ablation therapy of chondroblastomas: should it replace surgery? *Skeletal Radiol* 2014;43:513–522.
Lang IM, Azouz EM. MRI appearances of dysplasia epiphysealis hemimelica of the knee. *Skeletal Radiol* 1997;26:226–229.
Lee KC, Davies AM, Cassar-Pullicino VN. Imaging the complications of osteochondromas. *Clin Radiol* 2002;57:18–28.
Lichtenstein L, Hall JE. Periosteal chondroma: a distinctive benign cartilage tumor. *J Bone Joint Surg Am* 1952;24 A:691–697.
Liu J, Hudkins PG, Swee RG, et al. Bone sarcomas associated with Ollier's disease. *Cancer* 1987;59:1376–1385.
Ly JQ, Beall DP. A rare case of infantile Ollier's disease demonstrating bilaterally symmetric extremity involvement. *Skeletal Radiol* 2003;32:227–230.
Maffucci A. Di un caso di encondroma el antioma multiplo. Contribuzone alla genesi embrionale dei tumori. *Movimento Med Chir Napoli* 1881;3:399–412.
Maheshwari AV, Jelinek JS, Song AJ, et al. Metaphyseal and diaphyseal chondroblastomas. *Skeletal Radiol* 2011;40:1563–1573.
McBrien J, Crolla JA, Huang S, et al. Further case of microdeletion of 8q24 with phenotype overlapping Langer-Giedion without TRPS1 deletion. *Am J Med Genet A* 2008;146A:1587–1592.
Mellon CD, Carter JE, Owen DB. Ollier's disease and Maffucci's syndrome: distinct entities or a continuum. Case report: enchondromatosis complicated by an intracranial glioma. *J Neurol* 1988;235:376–378.
Meneses MF, Unni KK, Swee RG. Bizarre parosteal osteochondromatous proliferation of bone (Nora's lesion). *Am J Surg Pathol* 1993;17:691–697.
Michelsen H, Abramovici L, Steiner G, et al. Bizarre parosteal osteochondromatous proliferation (Nora's lesion) in the hand. *J Hand Surg Am* 2004;29:520–525.
Moser RP Jr, Brockmole DM, Vinh TN, et al. Chondroblastoma of the patella. *Skeletal Radiol* 1988;17:413–419.
Murphey MD, Flemming DJ, Boyea SR, et al. Enchondroma versus chondrosarcoma in the appendicular skeleton: differentiating features. *Radiographics* 1998;18:1213–1237.
Nora FE, Dahlin DC, Beabout JW. Bizarre parosteal osteochondromatous proliferations of the hands and feet. *Am J Surg Pathol* 1983;7:245–250.
Norman A, Sissons HA. Radiographic hallmarks of peripheral chondrosarcoma. *Radiology* 1984;151:589–596.
Ollier L. De la dyschondroplasie. *Bull Soc Lyon Med* 1899;93:23–24.
Ozkoc G, Gonlusen G, Ozalay M, et al. Giant chondroblastoma of the scapula with pulmonary metastases. *Skeletal Radiol* 2006;35:42–48.
Pösl M, Werner M, Amling M, et al. Malignant transformation of chondroblastoma. *Histopathology* 1996;29:477–480.
Rappaport A, Moermans A, Delvaux S. Nora's lesion or bizarre parosteal osteochondromatous proliferation: a rare and relatively unknown entity. *JBR-BTR* 2014;97:100–102.
Safar A, Nelson M, Neff JR, et al. Recurrent anomalies of 6q25 in chondromyxoid fibroma. *Hum Pathol* 2000;31:306–311.
Schajowicz F, Sissons HA, Sobin LH. The World Health Organization's histologic classification of bone tumors. A commentary on the second edition. *Cancer* 1995;75:1208–1214.
Sjögren H, Orndal C, Tingby O, et al. Cytogenetic and spectral karyotype analyses of benign and malignant cartilage tumours. *Int J Oncol* 2004;24:1385–1391.
Stahl S, Schapira D, Nahir AM. Turret exostosis of the phalanges presenting as limited motion of the finger. *Eur J Plast Surg* 2000;23:82–84.
Sun TC, Swee RG, Shives TC, et al. Chondrosarcoma in Maffucci's syndrome. *J Bone Joint Surg Am* 1985;67A:1214–1219.
Unger EC, Kessler HB, Kowalyshyn MJ, et al. MR imaging of Maffucci syndrome. *Am J Roentgenol* 1988;150:351–353.
Unni KK, ed. Chondroma. In: *Dahlin's bone tumors. General aspect and data on 11,087 cases*, 5th ed. Philadelphia: Lippincott–Raven Publishers; 1996:25–45.
Viala P, Vanel D, Larbi A, et al. Bilateral ischiofemoral impingement in a patient with hereditary multiple exostoses. *Skeletal Radiol* 2012;41:1637–1640.
White PG, Saunders L, Orr W, et al. Chondromyxoid fibroma. *Skeletal Radiol* 1996;25:79–81.
Wuyts W, Van Hul W. Molecular basis of multiple exostoses: mutations in the EXT1 and EXT2 genes. *Hum Mutat* 2000;15:220–227.
Yamamura S, Sato K, Sugiura H, et al. Inflammatory reaction in chondroblastoma. *Skeletal Radiol* 1996;25:371–376.
Zambrano E, Nosé V, Perez-Atayde AR, et al. Distinct chromosomal rearrangements in subungual (Dupuytren) exostosis and bizarre parosteal osteochondromatous proliferation (Nora lesion). *Am J Surg Pathol* 2004;28:1033–1039.

19

Benign Tumors and Tumor-like Lesions III

Fibrous, Fibroosseous, and Fibrohistiocytic Lesions

Fibrous Cortical Defect and Nonossifying Fibroma

Clinical and Imaging Features

Fibrous cortical defects and nonossifying (nonosteogenic) fibromas are the most common fibrous lesions of bone and are predominantly seen in children and adolescents. More common in boys than in girls, they have a predilection for the long bones, particularly the femur and tibia (Fig. 19.1). Some authors prefer the term *fibroxanthoma* for both lesions, whereas Schajowicz prefers the term *histiocytic xanthogranuloma*. These lesions are not true neoplasms and are considered by many investigators developmental defects.

Fibrous cortical defect (metaphyseal fibrous defect) is a small asymptomatic lesion found in 30% of normal individuals in the first and second decades of life. The radiolucent lesion is elliptical and confined to the cortex of a long bone near the growth plate; it is demarcated by a thin margin of sclerosis (Figs. 19.2 and 19.3). Most of these lesions disappear spontaneously, but a few may continue to enlarge. When they encroach on the medullary region of a bone, they are designated *nonossifying fibromas* (Fig. 19.4). With continued growth, these lesions, which are typically located eccentrically in the bone, display a characteristic scalloped sclerotic border (Figs. 19.5 and 19.6).

Skeletal scintigraphy shows a minimal to mild increase in activity. During the healing phase, mild hyperemia may be seen on the blood pool image, and the positive delayed scan reflects the osteoblastic activity. Computed tomography (CT) may demonstrate to better advantage the cortical thinning and medullary involvement (Fig. 19.7) and may delineate early pathologic fracture more precisely. Hounsfield attenuation values for nonossifying fibroma are higher than for normal bone marrow. Magnetic resonance imaging (MRI), usually performed for another reason, shows intermediate-to-low signal intensity on T1-weighted and intermediate-to-high signal intensity on T2-weighted sequences (Fig. 19.8). Mineralization of the lesion during healing appears predominantly as low signal intensity on MR images. After intravenous injection of gadolinium diethylenetriamine pentaacetic acid (Gd-DTPA), both fibrous cortical defects and nonossifying fibromas invariably exhibit a hyperintense border and signal enhancement (Fig. 19.9).

Occasionally, nonossifying fibroma may involve several bones, in which case the condition is called *disseminated nonossifying fibromatosis*. Some of the patients with this presentation may exhibit on the skin café-au-lait spots with smooth ("coast of California") borders, similar to those seen in neurofibromatosis. Furthermore, they may develop neurofibromas affecting various nerves (see Chapter 33). This association is known as *Jaffe-Campanacci syndrome* (Fig. 19.10). Additional features of this syndrome include intellectual disability, kyphoscoliosis, hypogonadism or cryptorchidism, ocular malformations, cardiovascular malformations and giant cell granuloma of the jaw. Differential diagnosis includes polyostotic fibrous dysplasia and neurofibromatosis type 1.

Pathology

Gross pathologic specimen of nonossifying fibroma shows well-demarcated red-brownish lobulated lesion within the medullary portion of bone (Fig.19.11). Histologically identical, regardless of size, fibrous cortical defect and nonossifying fibroma are composed of spindle and histiocytic cells that have a clear, foamy cytoplasm. In addition, osteoclast-like multinucleated giant cells are present, and varying numbers of inflammatory cells (lymphocytes) and plasma cells are scattered in the background. The cells are often arranged in a storiform pattern, typifying fibrohistiocytic lesions. Some lesions contain an excessive amount of fat within the foam cells, and the term *xanthoma* or *fibroxanthoma* may be applied to such lesions.

Complications and Treatment

Most lesions undergo spontaneous involution (healing) by sclerosis or remodeling (Fig. 19.12). Some larger lesions may be complicated by pathologic fracture (Fig. 19.13). Therefore, if a lesion is large, extending across 50% or more of the medullary cavity, then curettage and bone grafting is the treatment of choice.

Benign Fibrous Histiocytoma

Clinical and Imaging Features

The term *benign fibrous histiocytoma*, although it may be controversial, is useful to subclassify lesions with histologic features similar to those of nonossifying fibroma but having an atypical clinical presentation and an atypical radiographic pattern. This lesion frequently has radiographic features very similar to those of nonossifying fibroma; it is radiolucent, with sharply defined and frequently sclerotic borders, without any mineralization of the matrix (Figs. 19.14 and 19.15). Its differentiation from nonossifying fibroma is made on purely clinical grounds because the histologic features

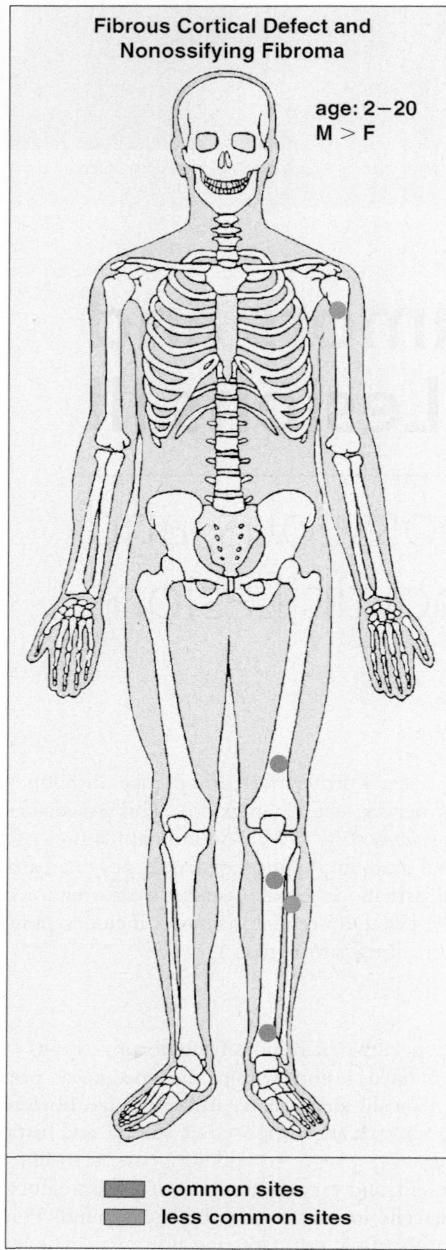

FIGURE 19.1 **Skeletal sites of predilection, peak age range, and male-to-female ratio in fibrous cortical defect and nonossifying fibroma.**

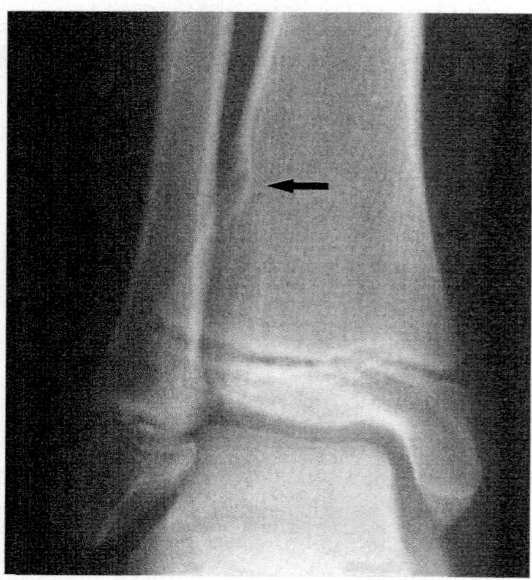

FIGURE 19.2 **Fibrous cortical defect.** Fibrous cortical defect, seen here in lateral cortex of the distal tibia *(arrow)* in a 13-year-old boy, typically presents as a radiolucent lesion demarcated by a thin zone of sclerosis.

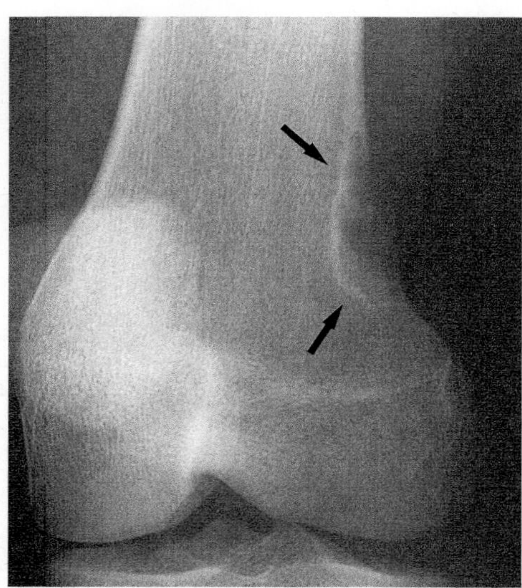

FIGURE 19.3 **Fibrous cortical defect.** Anteroposterior radiograph of the knee of a 21-year-old woman shows a lesion affecting medial cortex of the distal femur *(arrows)*.

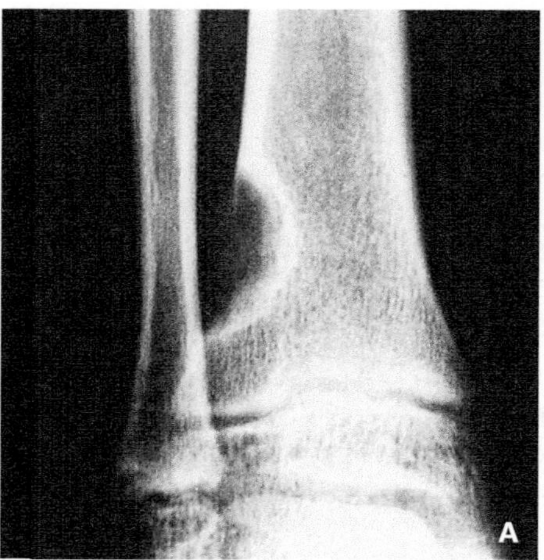

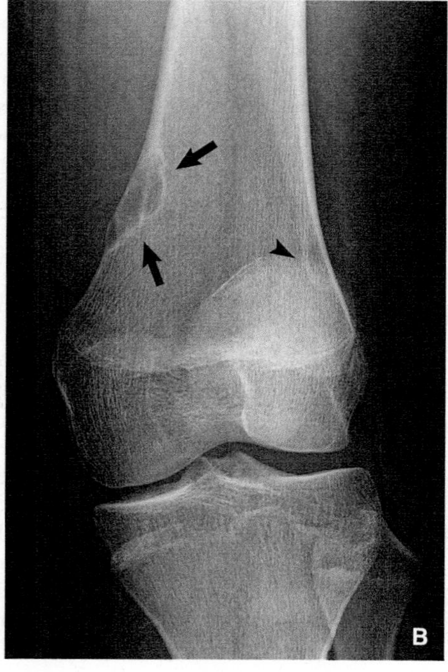

FIGURE 19.4 **Nonossifying fibroma.** **(A)** When a fibrous cortical defect encroaches on the medullary cavity, it is called a *nonossifying fibroma*. Note the similarity of the lesion to that in the previous figure. The only difference is that it is larger and extends beyond the cortex. **(B)** In another patient, a very small lesion with sclerotic lobulated border is encroaching on the medullary portion of the femur *(arrows)*. An incidental finding is a small fibrous cortical defect on the lateral aspect of bone *(arrowhead)*.

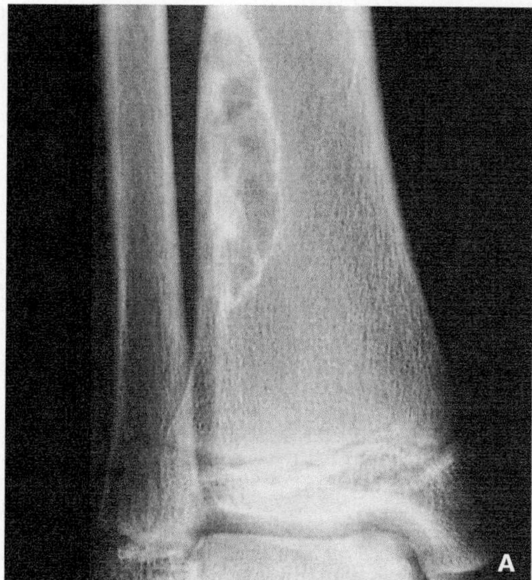

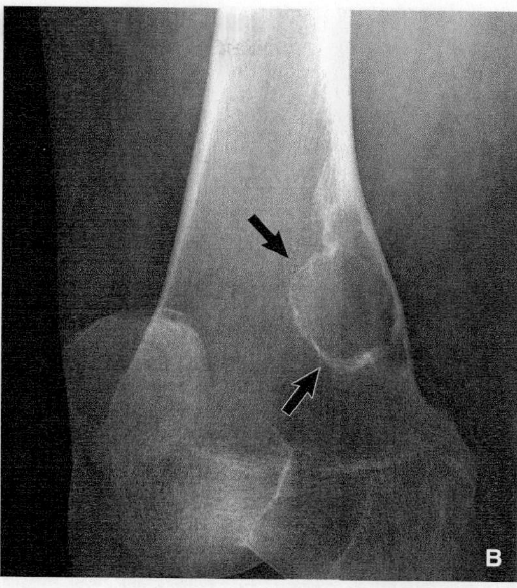

FIGURE 19.5 **Nonossifying fibroma.** **(A)** The lesion, seen here in the distal tibia in an asymptomatic 15-year-old boy, appears eccentrically located in the bone and has a scalloped sclerotic border. **(B)** Similar lesion with lobulated sclerotic border is abutting the medial cortex of the distal femur *(arrows)* in a 28-year-old man.

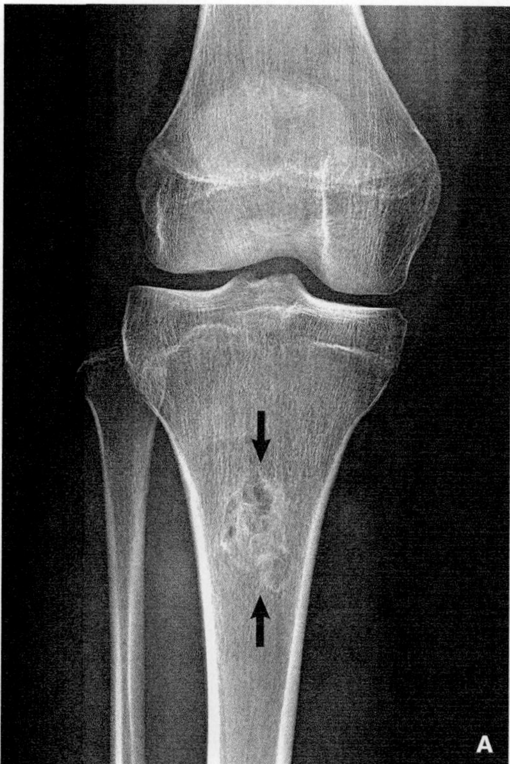

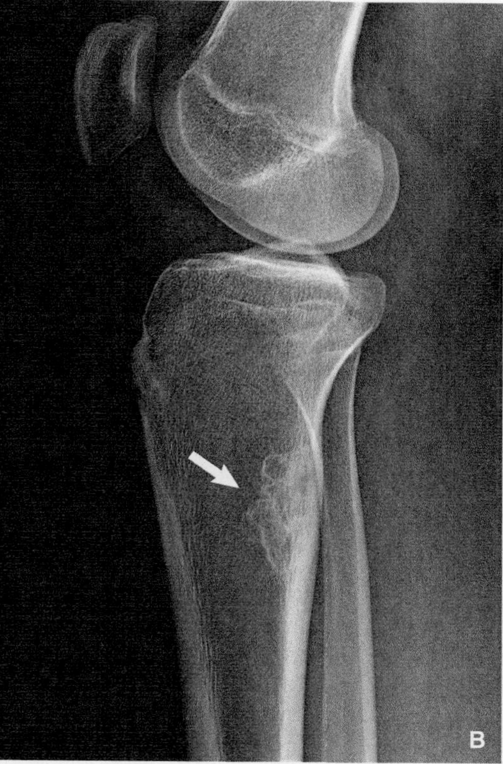

FIGURE 19.6 **Nonossifying fibroma.** **(A)** Anteroposterior and **(B)** lateral radiographs of the right knee of a 14-year-old girl show eccentric, radiolucent lesion with sclerotic border located in the proximal diaphysis of the tibia *(arrows)*.

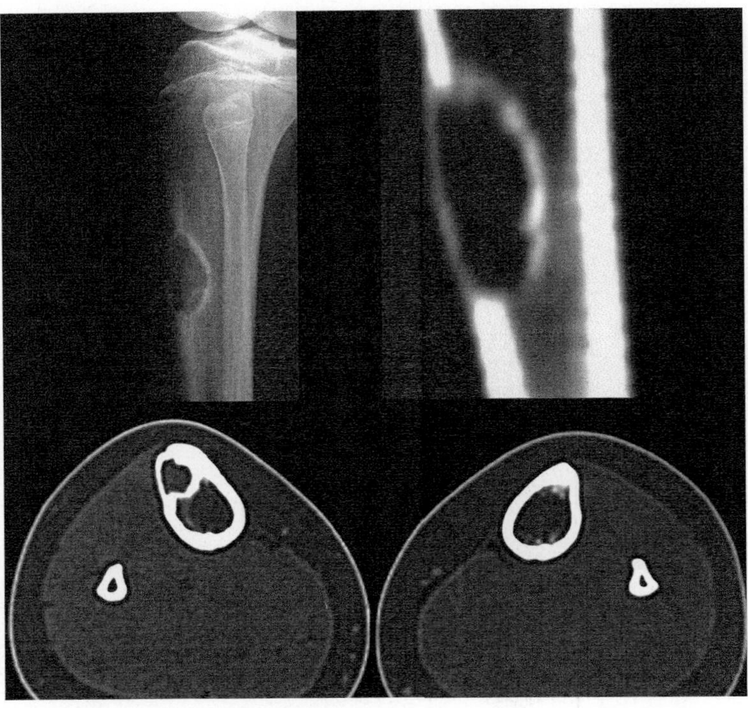

FIGURE 19.7 CT of nonossifying fibroma. Oblique radiograph of the right tibia of a 14-year-old girl shows an elliptical radiolucent lesion with sclerotic border. Axial and coronal reformatted CT images show low-attenuation lesion exhibiting a high-attenuation scalloped border and extending into the anterolateral cortex of tibia.

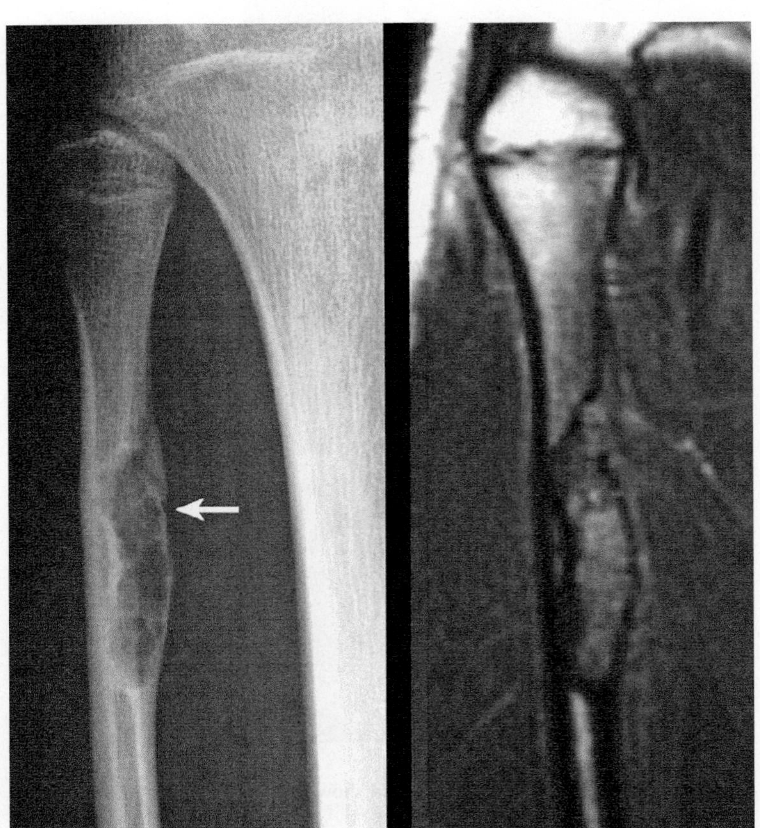

FIGURE 19.8 MRI of nonossifying fibroma. Anteroposterior radiograph of the right fibula of a 14-year-old girl shows an eccentric well-defined radiolucent lesion with sclerotic border. Note thinning of the medial cortex and a pathologic fracture *(arrow)*. Coronal T1-weighted MRI shows the lesion exhibiting intermediate signal intensity. (Reprinted with permission from Greenspan A, Jundt G, Remagen W. *Differential diagnosis in orthopaedic oncology*, 2nd ed. Philadelphia: Lippincott Williams & Wilkins; 2007.)

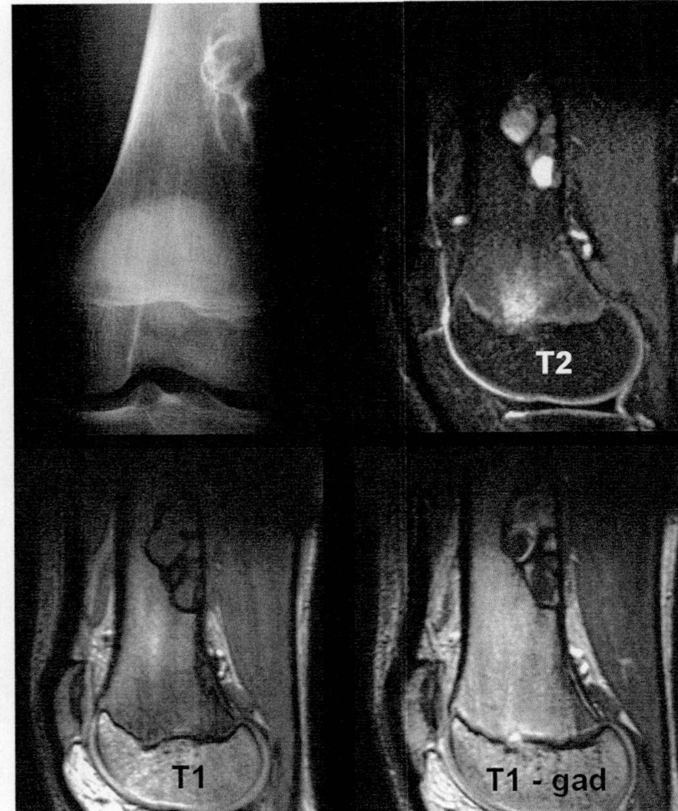

FIGURE 19.9 MRI of nonossifying fibroma. Anteroposterior radiograph shows a radiolucent lesion with sclerotic border abutting the posteromedial cortex of the right femur. Sagittal T1-weighted MR image shows predominantly intermediate signal intensity of the lesion. The sclerotic border exhibits low signal intensity. Sagittal T2-weighted image shows that the lesion exhibits heterogeneous but mostly high signal intensity. Sagittal T1-weighted MR images before and after intravenous injection of gadolinium shows slight heterogenous enhancement of nonossifying fibroma. (Reprinted with permission from Greenspan A, Jundt G, Remagen W. *Differential diagnosis in orthopaedic oncology*, 2nd ed. Philadelphia: Lippincott Williams & Wilkins; 2007.)

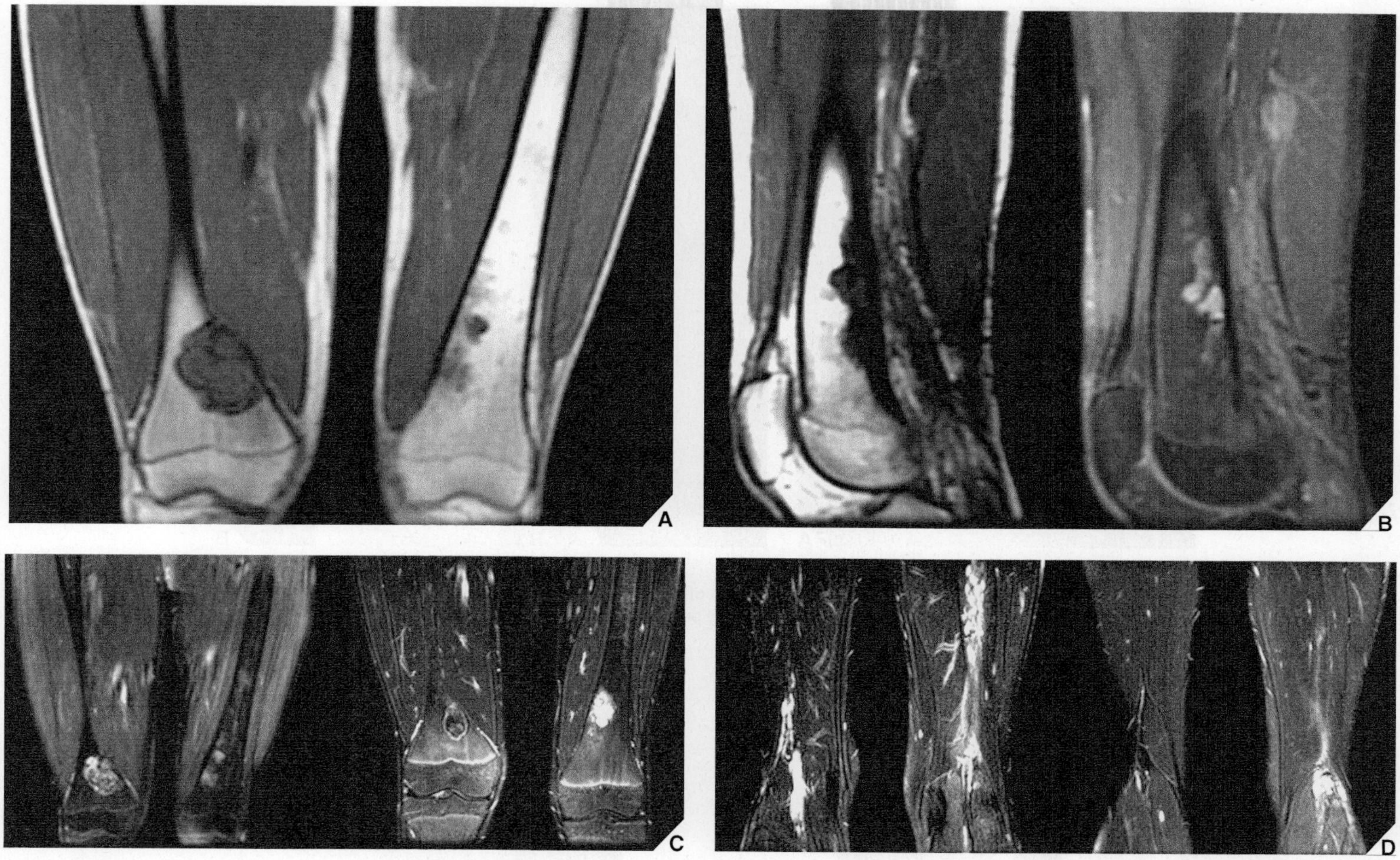

FIGURE 19.10 **MRI of Jaffe-Campanacci syndrome.** In a 15-year-old boy, **(A)** coronal T1-weighted MR image of both distal femora and **(B)** sagittal T1-weighted and proton density–weighted fat-suppressed MR images show multiple nonossifying fibromas. **(C)** Coronal inversion recovery MR image *(left part)* shows the lesions exhibiting high signal intensity and enhancement as seen on T1-weighted fat-suppressed image obtained after intravenous injection of gadolinium *(right part)*. **(D)** Coronal T2-weighted fat-suppressed MR images demonstrate multiple neurofibromas affecting popliteal, tibial, peroneal, and sciatic nerves.

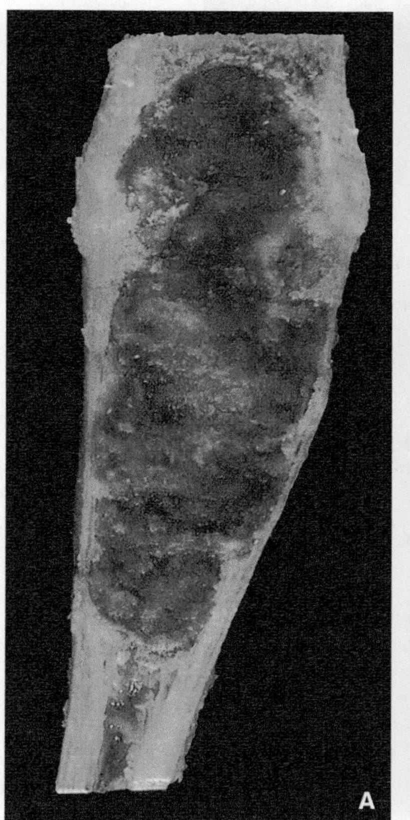

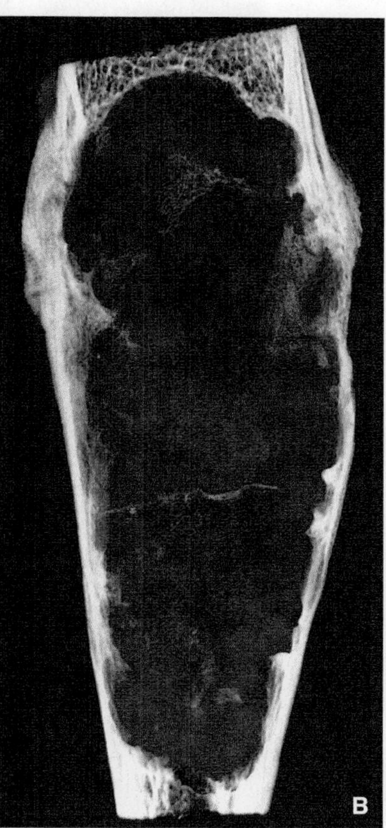

FIGURE 19.11 **Pathology of nonossifying fibroma.** **(A)** Section through the resected specimen of the proximal fibula shows red-brownish in color lesion with lobulated margins. **(B)** Radiograph of the specimen demonstrates endosteal scalloping and thinning of the cortex. (Reprinted from Bullough P. *Orthopaedic pathology*, 5th ed. Maryland Heights, MO: Mosby; 2009, with permission from Elsevier.)

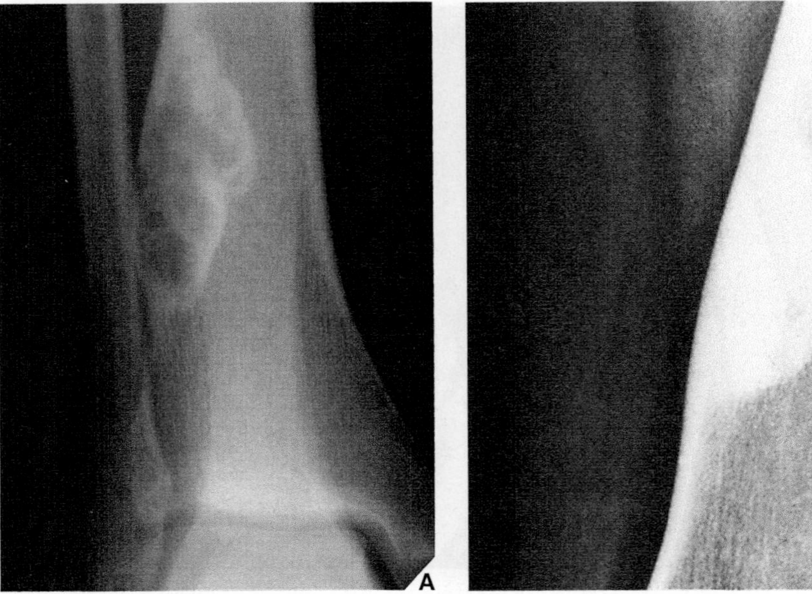

FIGURE 19.12 Healing of nonossifying fibroma. **(A)** Spontaneous involution of nonossifying fibroma in the distal tibia is characterized by progressive sclerosis of peripheral parts of the lesion. **(B)** A nonossifying fibroma that healed completely may persist as a sclerotic patch. Nonossifying fibromas in this sclerosing phase should not be mistaken for osteoblastic tumors or for sclerosing dysplasia.

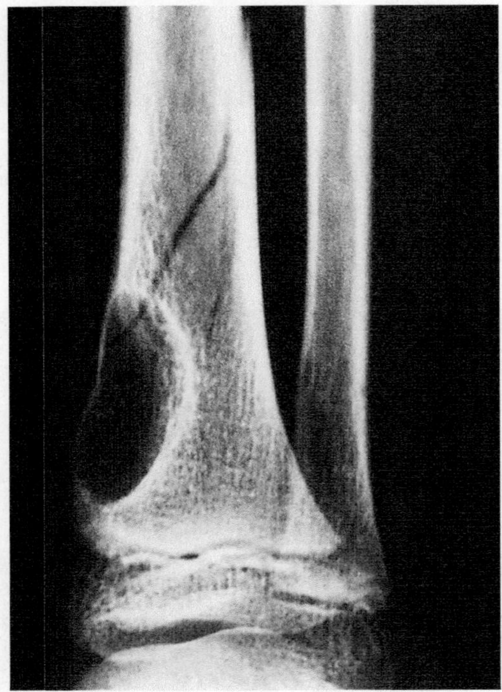

FIGURE 19.13 Complication of nonossifying fibroma. Pathologic fracture is a common complication of a large nonossifying fibroma, as seen here in the distal tibia of a 10-year-old boy.

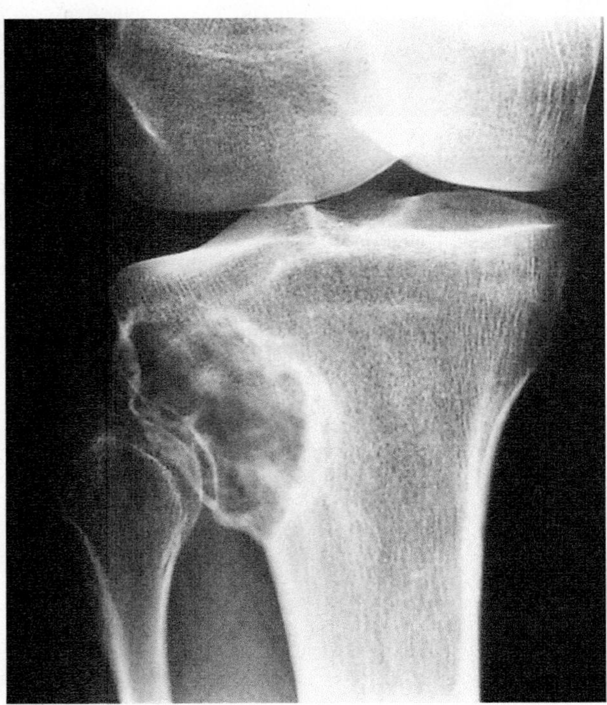

FIGURE 19.14 Benign fibrous histiocytoma. A 37-year-old man presented with occasional pain in the right knee. Oblique radiograph of the knee demonstrates a lobulated radiolucent lesion with a well-defined sclerotic border, located eccentrically in the proximal tibia. The diagnosis was confirmed by excision biopsy.

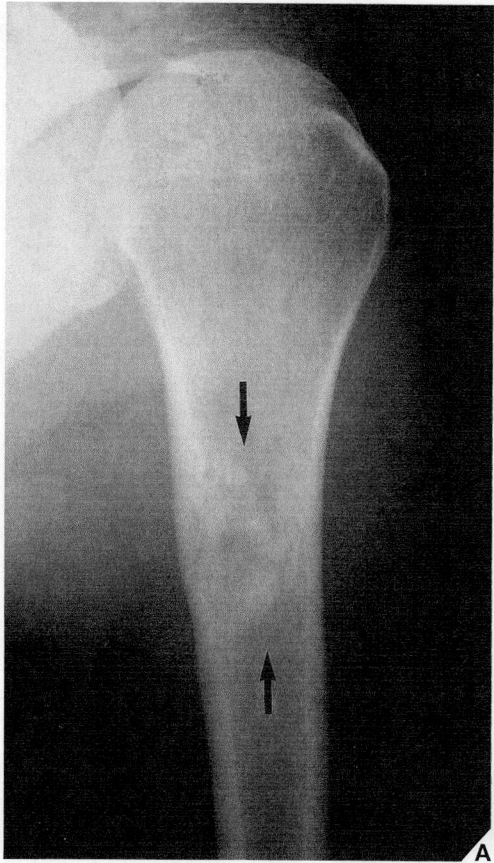
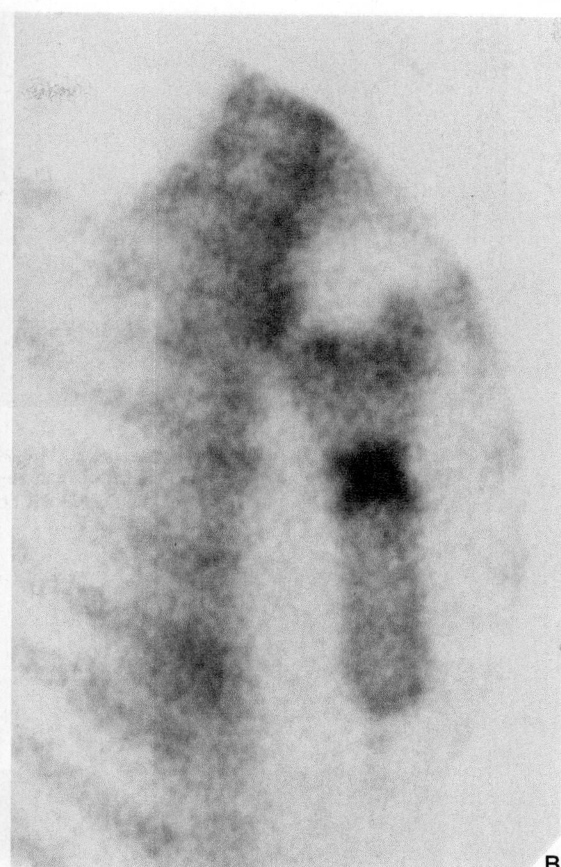

FIGURE 19.15 Benign fibrous histiocytoma. **(A)** Anteroposterior radiograph of the left proximal humerus in a 26-year-old woman with chronic arm pain shows eccentric, well-defined, partially sclerotic lesion *(arrows)*. **(B)** A radionuclide bone scan demonstrates a focal homogenous increased uptake of radiotracer. Excision biopsy was consistent with healing benign fibrous histiocytoma.

of both lesions are almost identical. Patients presenting with benign fibrous histiocytoma are older (usually older than 25 years) than those with nonossifying fibroma; unlike the latter lesion, benign fibrous histiocytomas may produce symptoms such as pain or discomfort in the involved bone. These lesions also seem to run a more aggressive clinical course and may recur after treatment, which consists of curettage and bone grafting.

Periosteal Desmoid

Clinical and Imaging Features

The periosteal desmoid is a tumor-like fibrous proliferation of the periosteum. It occurs in patients between the ages of 12 and 20 years and has a striking predilection for the posteromedial cortex of the medial femoral condyle. Many patients have a history of injury, although trauma is not necessarily a predisposing factor. The lesion simulates a fibrous cortical defect, except in the specificity of its location. Occasionally, it may simulate an aggressive and even malignant tumor. Radiographically, the hallmarks of a periosteal desmoid are its radiolucent saucer-shaped appearance, with sclerosis at the base eroding the cortex or producing cortical irregularity (Fig. 19.16). The radionuclide bone scan is usually normal but sometimes may show a focal increase in activity. CT shows a well-defined lesion, commonly with a sclerotic border (Fig. 19.17). On MRI, the lesion appears hypointense on T1-weighted and hyperintense on T2-weighted images, with a dark rim on both sequences at or near the sites of the bony attachment of the medial head of the gastrocnemius muscle (Fig. 19.18). Periosteal desmoid belongs to the "don't touch" lesions (see Table 16.10), so it should not undergo biopsy. Most lesions disappear spontaneously by the time the patient reaches age 20 years.

Pathology

The histologic appearance of the lesion demonstrates fibroblastic spindle cells that produce large amounts of collagen. Large areas of hyalinization and fibrocartilage and small fragments of bone may be scattered within the fibrous tissue.

Differential Diagnosis

Some authorities believe that periosteal desmoid should be differentiated from distal femoral cortical irregularity. This latter abnormality, which presents as cortical roughening just distal to the extension of the linea aspera, is a common finding in boys in the 10- to 15-year age group. Its cause is not settled. Although it was thought to represent an avulsion injury caused by traction of the adductor magnus aponeurosis, Brower and colleagues have shown that this lesion may exist in the area without any muscular or ligamentous attachment. Others consider periosteal desmoid and distal femoral cortical irregularity to be the same entity. Dahlin and Unni suggests that the

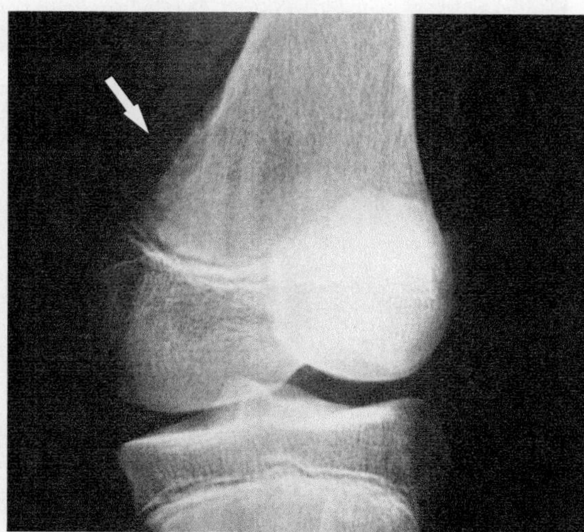

FIGURE 19.16 Periosteal desmoid. Oblique radiograph of the left knee of a 12-year-old boy shows the classic appearance of periosteal desmoid. Note the saucer-like radiolucency eroding the medial border of the distal femoral metaphysis at the linea aspera and producing cortical irregularity *(arrow)*. This lesion should not be mistaken for a malignant bone tumor.

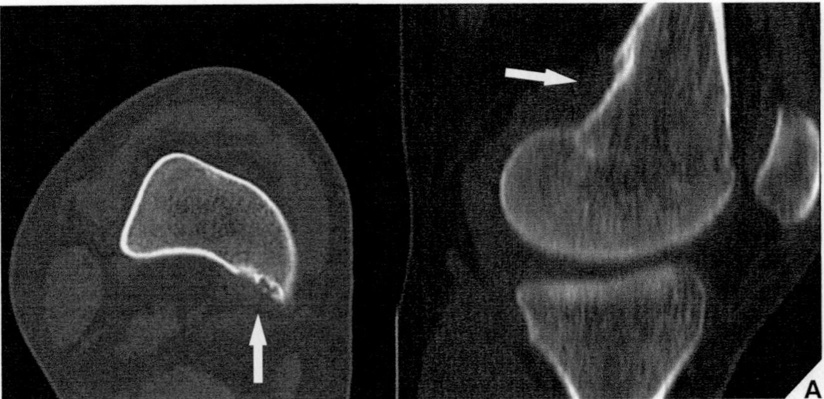

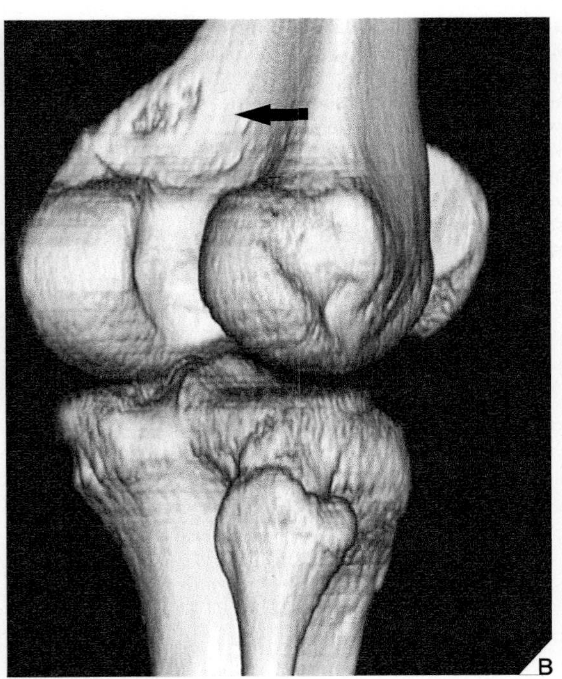

FIGURE 19.17 CT of periosteal desmoid. **(A)** Axial and sagittal reformatted CT images of the knee of a 17-year-old boy and **(B)** three-dimensional (3D) reconstructed CT image show well-marginated cortical defect in the posteromedial aspect of the distal femur *(arrows)*.

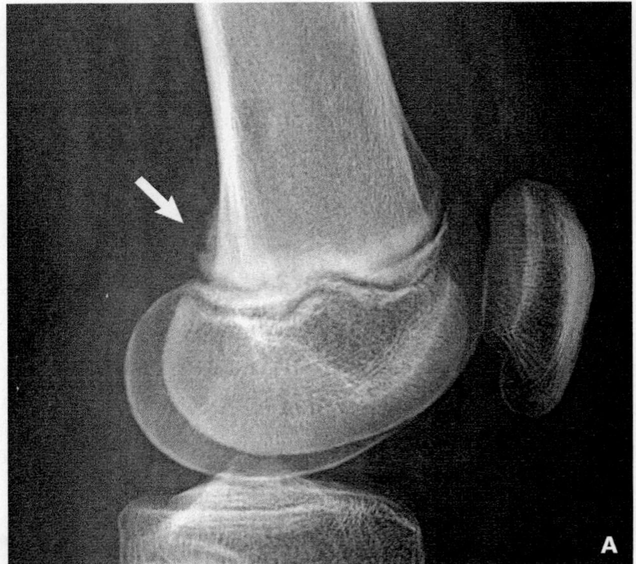

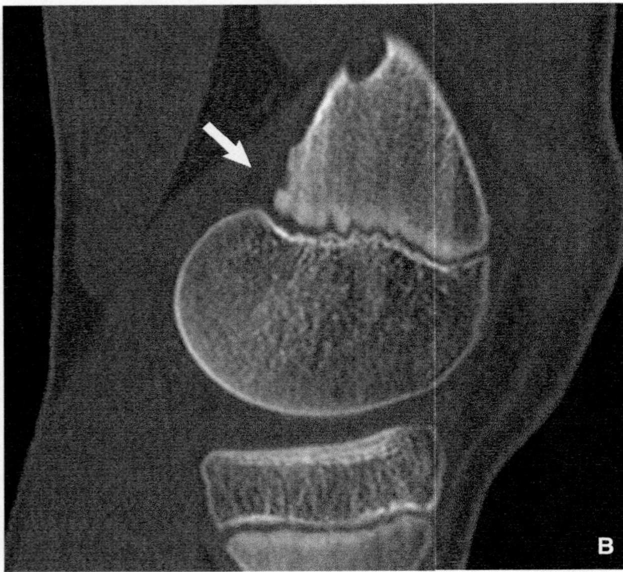

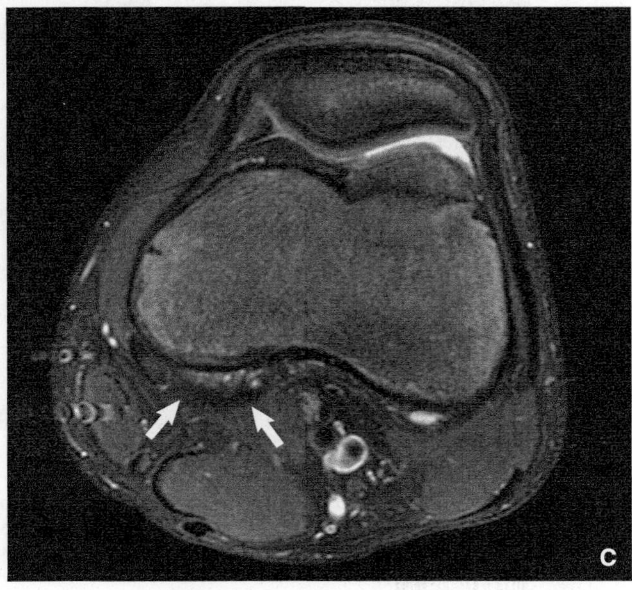

FIGURE 19.18 CT and MRI of periosteal desmoid. **(A)** Lateral radiograph of the left knee of a 15-year-old boy shows cortical irregularity and periosteal reaction at the site of the posteromedial metaphysis of the distal femur *(arrow)*. **(B)** Sagittal reformatted CT image shows small low-attenuated scalloped lesion and high-attenuation periosteal reaction in the same location *(arrow)*. **(C)** Axial T2-weighted fat-suppressed MR image shows a small high–signal intensity lesion at the posteromedial femoral condyle *(arrows)*.

periosteal desmoid is a hypocellular variant of nonossifying fibroma, and Schajowicz classifies it as a periosteal variant of desmoplastic fibroma. Other authors apply a broader definition to periosteal desmoid, considering it essentially a hypocellular variant of fibrous cortical defect. In any event, it is a self-limited benign lesion that requires no treatment, and its characteristic imaging appearance and location should serve as clues to the correct diagnosis.

Fibrous Dysplasia

Fibrous dysplasia, occasionally termed *fibrous osteodystrophy*, *osteodystrophia fibrosa*, or *osteitis fibrosa disseminata*, is a fibroosseous lesion that some authorities classify among the group of developmental dysplasias. The term *fibrous dysplasia* was coined in 1938 by L. Lichtenstein to describe the aberrant development of fibroosseous tissue replacing normal cancellous bone. At present time, this condition is considered to be a genetically based sporadic disorder due to mutation in the *GNAS1* gene, the defect that prevents osteoblasts to form a normal lamellar bone. There are two common *GNAS1* mutations associated with fibrous dysplasia, both occurring at codon 201, with arginine being substituted for either cysteine or histidine, R201C and R201H, respectively. Most recently reported, the third *GNAS1* gene mutation (Q227L) represents only about 5% of the *GNAS1* mutation in this condition. Clonal chromosomal alterations have also been reported, with structural recurrent aberrations of chromosome 12 (12p13).

Fibrous dysplasia may affect one bone (monostotic form) or several bones (polyostotic form). It is characterized by the replacement of normal lamellar cancellous bone by an abnormal fibrous tissue that contains small, abnormally arranged trabeculae of immature woven bone formed by metaplasia of the fibrous stroma.

Monostotic Fibrous Dysplasia

Clinical and Imaging Features

Monostotic fibrous dysplasia most commonly affects the femur—particularly the femoral neck—as well as the tibia and ribs (Fig. 19.19). The lesion arises centrally in the bone, usually sparing the epiphysis in children, and it is very rarely seen in the articular end of the bone in adults (Fig. 19.20). As the lesion enlarges, it expands the medullary cavity. The radiographic appearance of monostotic fibrous dysplasia varies, depending on the proportion of osseous-to-fibrous content. Lesions with greater osseous content are denser and more sclerotic, whereas those with greater fibrous content are more radiolucent, with a characteristic ground-glass appearance (Figs. 19.21 and 19.22; see also Fig. 19.19B). One of the lesions that mimics monostotic fibrous dysplasia, particularly when located in the intertrochanteric region of the femur, is the so-called *liposclerosing myxofibrous tumor* (Fig. 19.23), a benign fibroosseous lesion characterized by a complex mixture of histologic elements that include lipoma, fibroxanthoma, myxoma, myxofibroma, fat necrosis, bone, and cartilage.

Scintigraphy is helpful in determining the activity of fibrous dysplasia (Fig. 19.24) and the potential multicentricity of the lesion. Machida and associates reported that although a high incidence of increased uptake of radiopharmaceutical tracer was seen in 59 patients with fibrous dysplasia, 10% of the lesions with a ground-glass appearance failed to show similarly increased uptake.

The CT findings parallel those of conventional radiography. CT sections show areas of high attenuation in more sclerotic lesions and a low-attenuation matrix with an amorphous ground-glass texture in lesions with greater fibrous content (Figs. 19.25 to 19.30). The lesion of fibrous dysplasia shows a variety of appearances on MRI caused by the histologic composition of these lesions. Some lesions show a decreased signal on T1 and T2 sequences, and some show intermediate or low signal on T1-weighted but either mixed or high signal on T2-weighted images (Fig. 19.31). The sclerotic rim (rind sign) is invariably imaged as a band of low signal intensity on T1 and T2 sequences.

Pathologic fracture of the structurally weakened bone is the most frequent complication of monostotic fibrous dysplasia.

Pathology

Pathology of fibrous dysplasia is quite characteristic. Gross specimen shows well-circumscribed white-yellowish tan lesion of gritty and leather-like consistency (Fig. 19.32). Histologically, fibrous dysplasia presents as an aggregate of moderately dense fibrous connective tissue containing bony trabeculae in haphazard distribution instead of the stress-oriented distribution expected in normal cancellous bone. The trabeculae are curved and

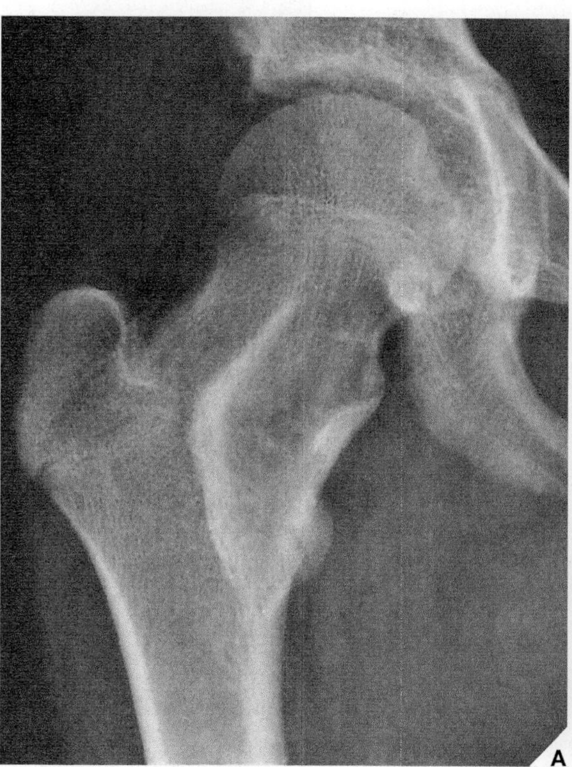

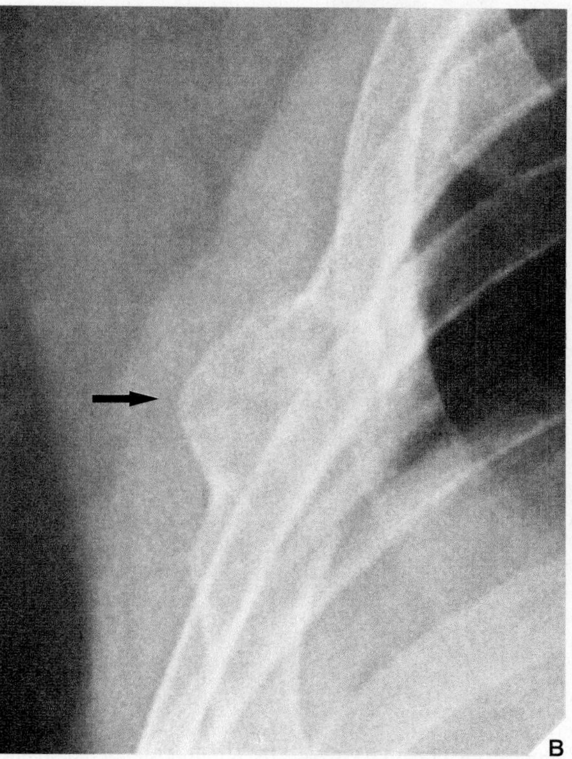

FIGURE 19.19 Monostotic fibrous dysplasia. **(A)** Typically, the focus of fibrous dysplasia is located in the femoral neck, as seen here in a 13-year-old girl. Note a characteristic sclerotic "rind" encapsulating the lesion. **(B)** The rib is a frequent site of fibrous dysplasia. Note the expansive lesion exhibiting a ground-glass appearance *(arrow)*.

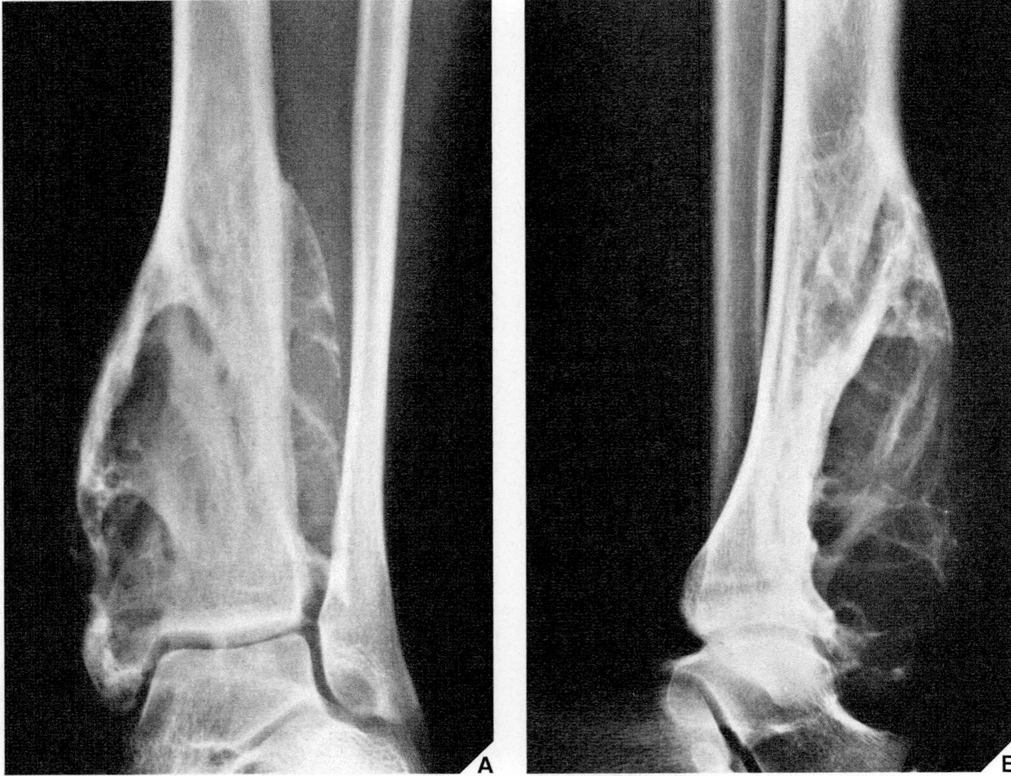

FIGURE 19.20 Monostotic fibrous dysplasia. **(A)** Oblique and **(B)** lateral radiographs of the left leg of a 32-year-old woman demonstrate a large, trabeculated radiolucent lesion in the distal tibia. Because of its aggressive features, it was thought to be a desmoplastic fibroma; however, biopsy proved it to be a fibrous dysplasia, a rare lesion at this site in adults.

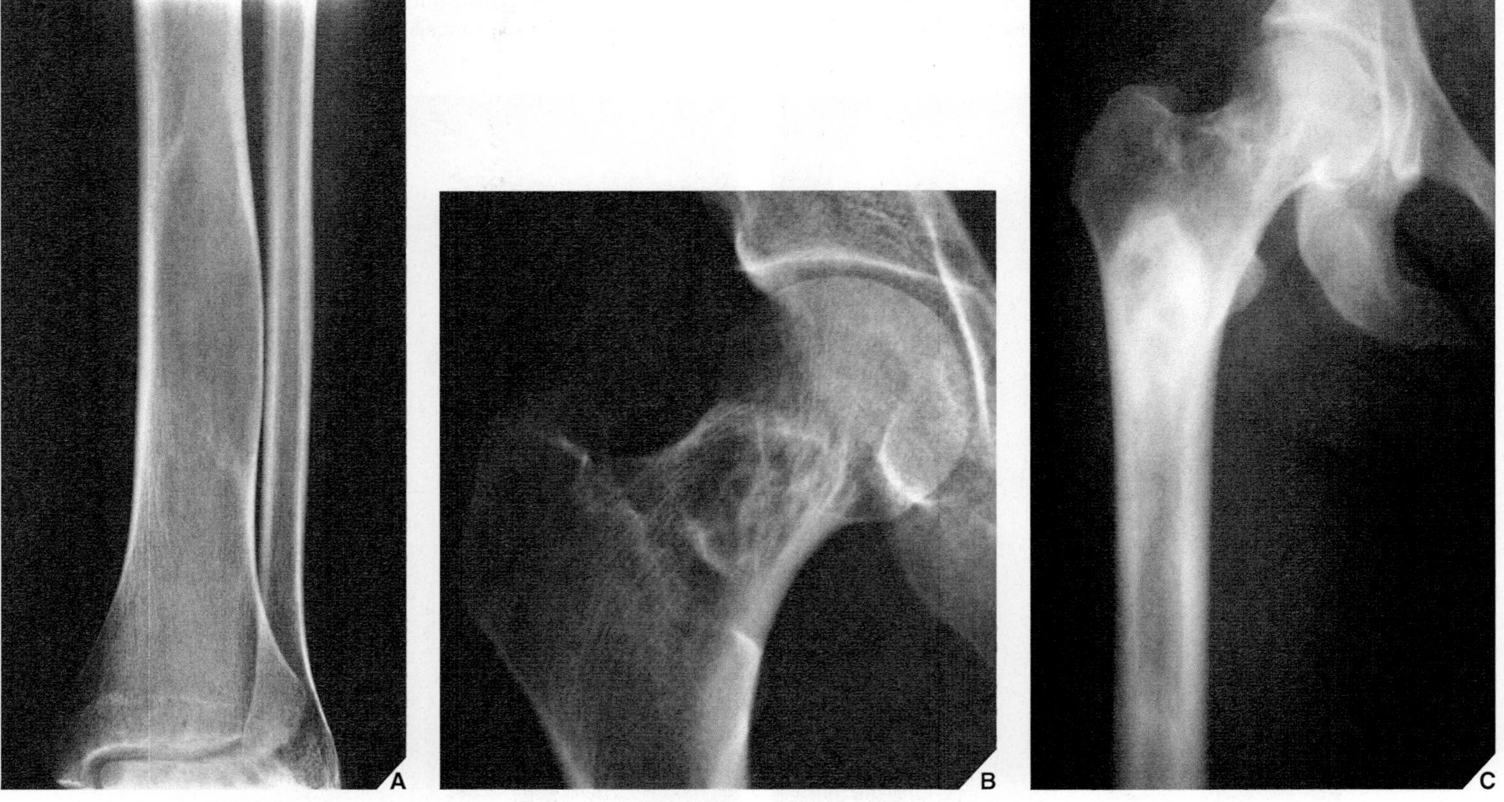

FIGURE 19.21 Monostotic fibrous dysplasia. **(A)** Anteroposterior radiograph of the distal leg of a 17-year-old girl shows a radiolucent lesion in the diaphysis of the tibia. Observe the slight expansion and thinning of the cortex and the partial loss of trabecular pattern in the cancellous bone, which gives the lesion a ground-glass or smoky appearance. **(B)** The focus of fibrous dysplasia in the femoral neck in this 25-year-old man exhibits a more sclerotic appearance than that seen in **A**. **(C)** Markedly sclerotic lesion of fibrous dysplasia in the proximal right femur of a 30-year-old woman.

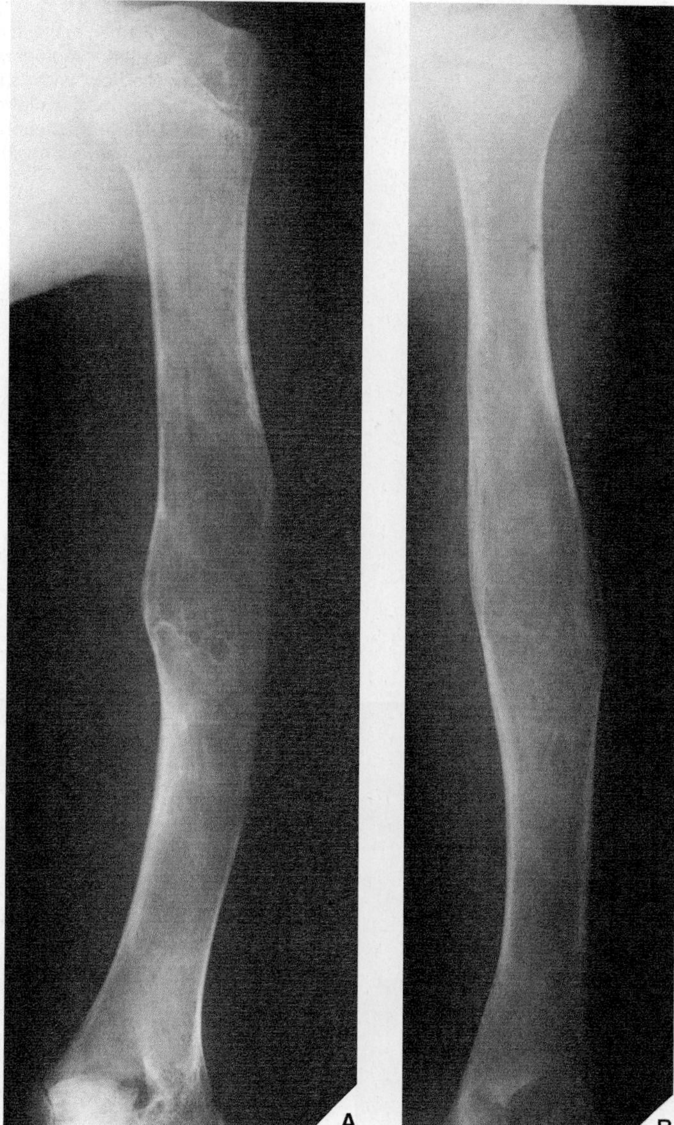

FIGURE 19.22 **Monostotic fibrous dysplasia.** Anteroposterior radiographs of the left humerus in neutral **(A)** and external rotation **(B)** projections of a 13-year-old boy show a radiolucent focus of fibrous dysplasia in the diaphysis of the bone.

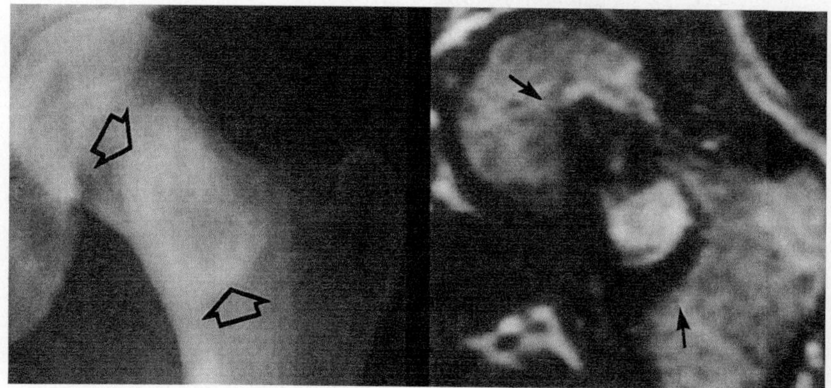

FIGURE 19.23 **Liposclerosing myxofibrous tumor.** Anteroposterior radiograph of the left hip of a 38-year-old woman presenting with vague hip pain shows a radiolucent lesion with well-defined thick sclerosing border in the intertrochanteric region of the femur *(open arrows)*. Coronal T2-weighted MR image shows the lesion *(arrows)* to exhibit heterogeneous signal intensity. Peripheral sclerotic "rind" displays signal void. (Reprinted from Kransdorf MJ, Murphey MD, Sweet DE. Liposclerosing myxofibrous tumor: a radiologic-pathologic-distinct fibroosseous lesion of bone with a marked predilection for the intertrochanteric region of the femur. *Radiology* 1999;212:693–698. Copyright © 1999 by The Radiological Society of North America, Inc.)

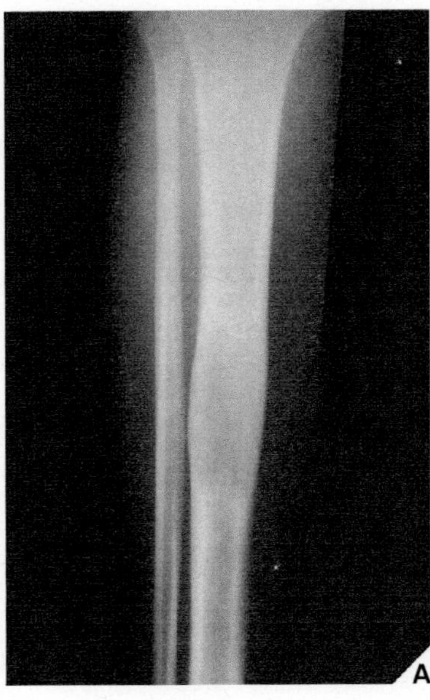

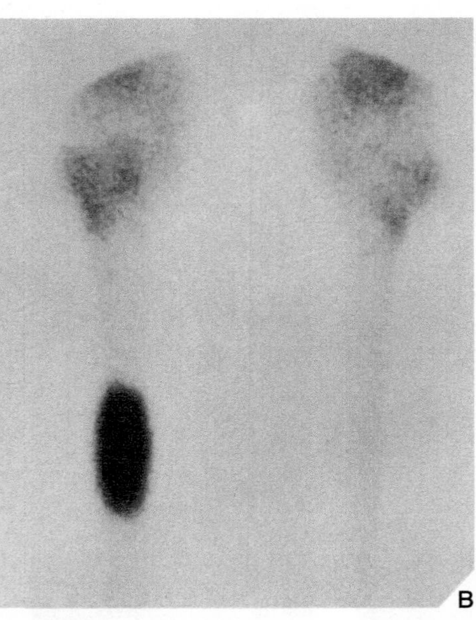

FIGURE 19.24 Scintigraphy of fibrous dysplasia. A 24-year-old woman presented with mild discomfort in the right leg. **(A)** Anteroposterior radiograph shows a radiolucent lesion in the midshaft of the tibia, with "smoky" appearance associated with thinning of the cortex and slight expansion, characteristic of fibrous dysplasia. **(B)** Radionuclide bone scan shows markedly increased uptake of the radiopharmaceutical tracer indicating an active lesion.

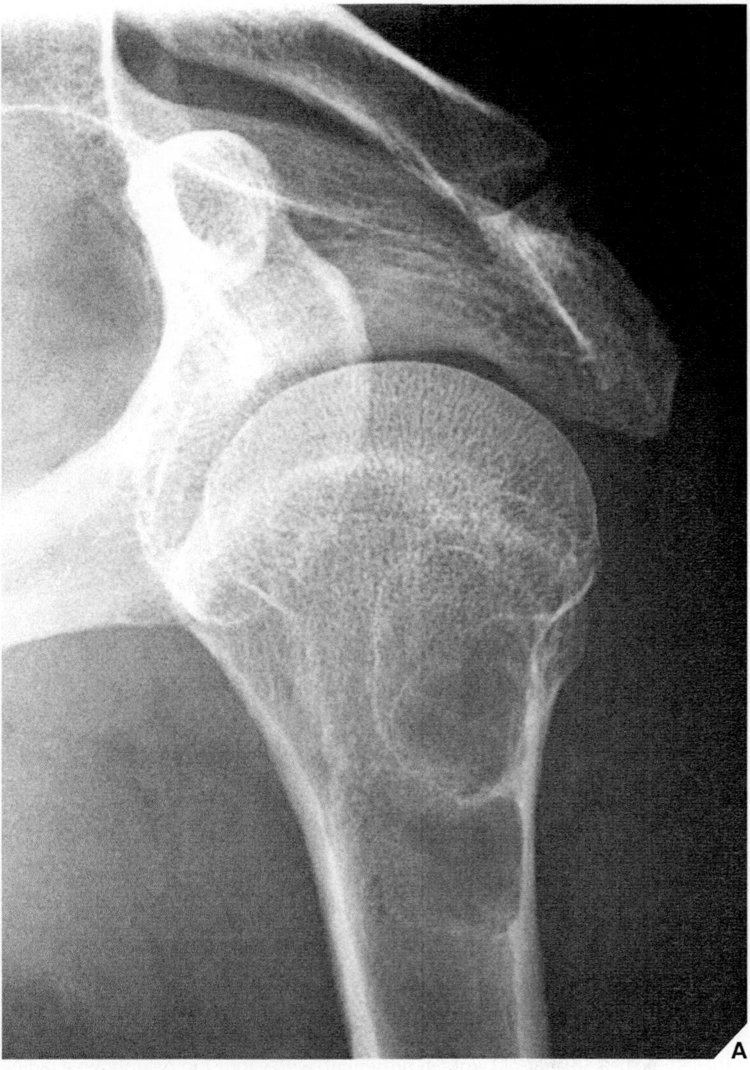

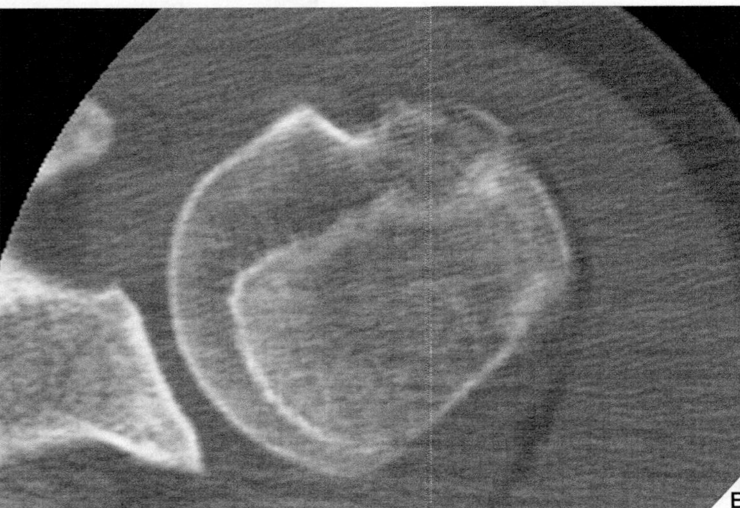

FIGURE 19.25 CT of monostotic fibrous dysplasia. **(A)** Conventional radiograph shows a monostotic focus in the neck and head of the left humerus. **(B)** CT section shows ground-glass appearance of the lesion and a sclerotic high-attenuation border.

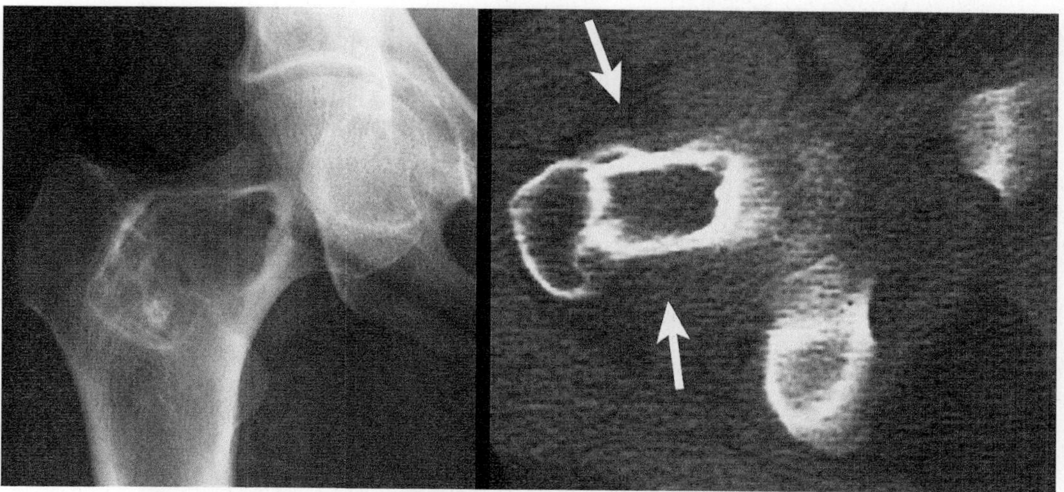

FIGURE 19.26 CT of monostotic fibrous dysplasia. Anteroposterior radiograph of the right hip and axial CT image shows a focus of fibrous dysplasia in the neck of the femur exhibiting a typical "rind sign"—thick sclerotic border surrounding a radiolucent/low-attenuation lesion *(arrows)*.

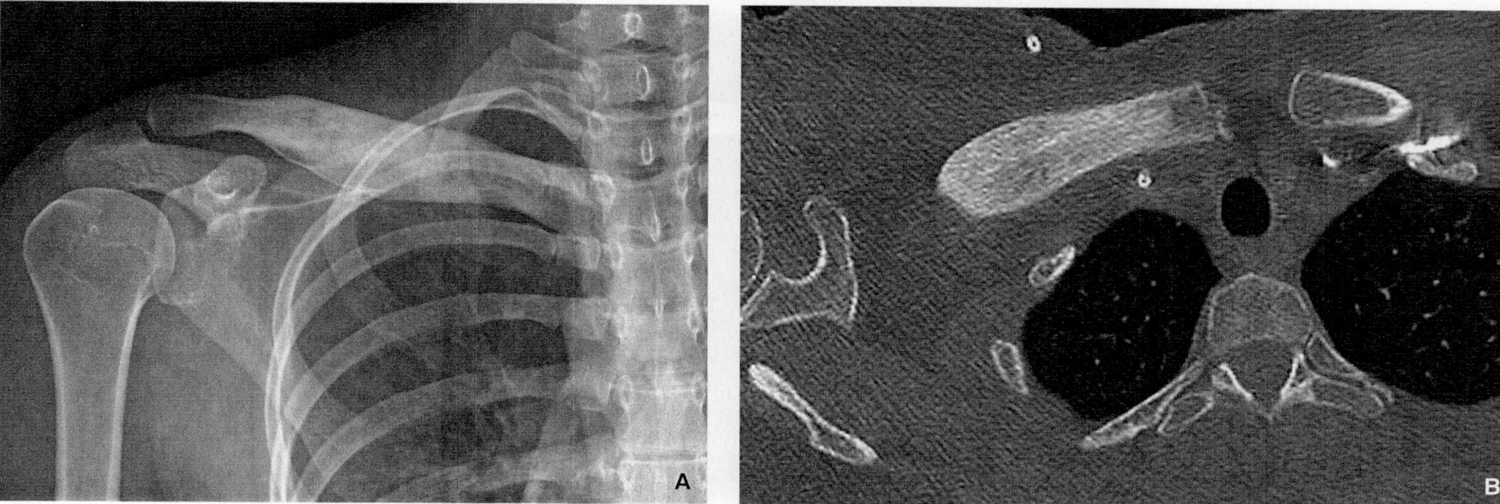

FIGURE 19.27 CT of monostotic fibrous dysplasia. **(A)** Anteroposterior radiograph of the right shoulder and **(B)** axial CT image of the upper thorax of a 28-year-old man show fibrous dysplasia affecting the right clavicle.

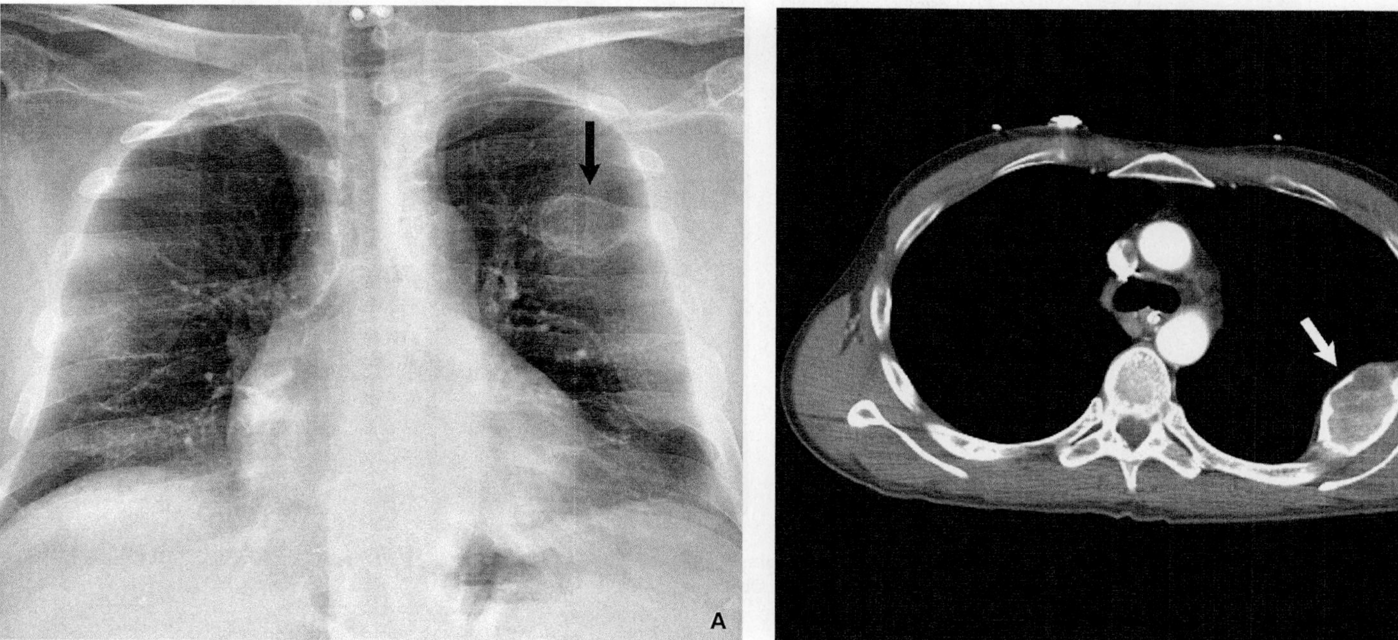

FIGURE 19.28 CT of monostotic fibrous dysplasia. **(A)** Posteroanterior radiograph and **(B)** axial CT image of the chest of a 56-year-old man show an expansive lesion affecting the fifth left posterior rib *(arrows)*.

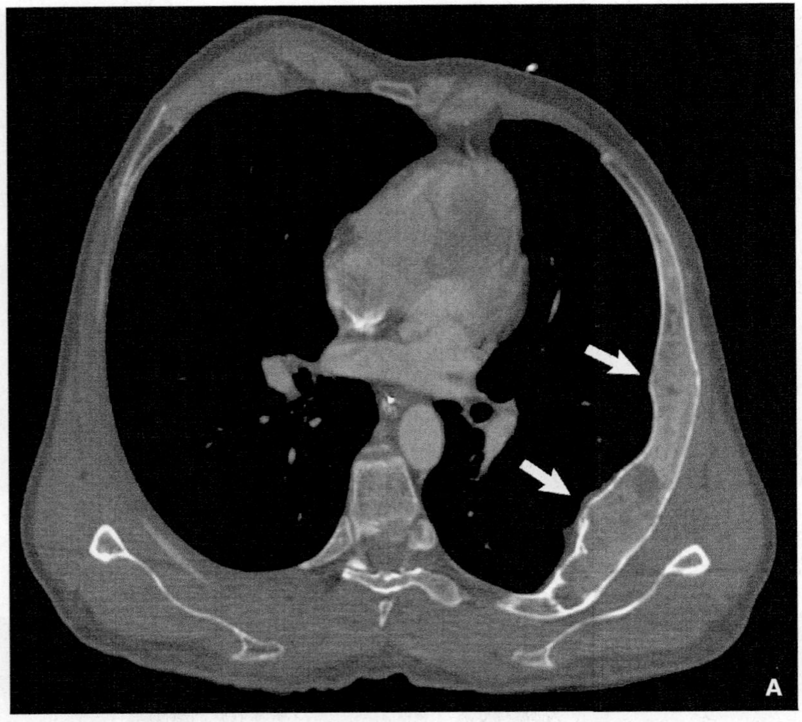

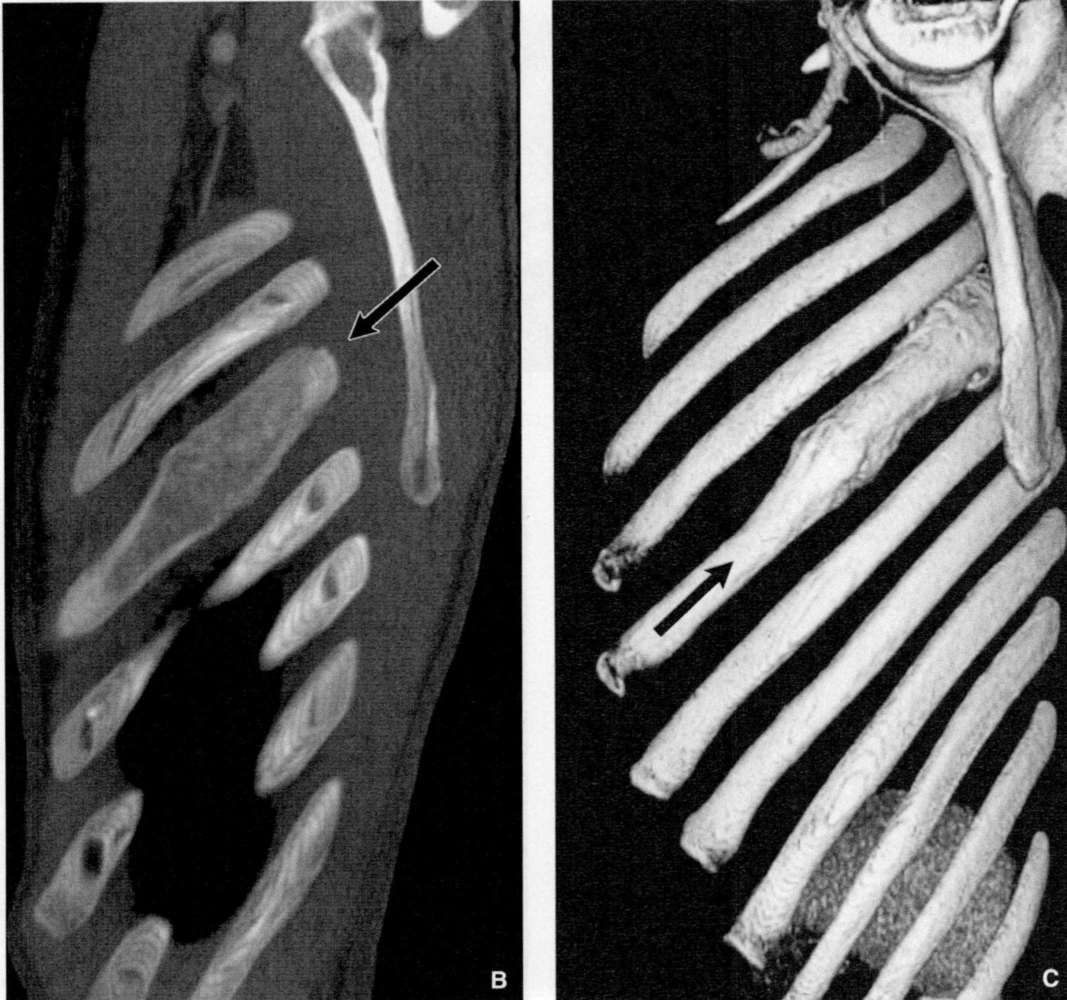

FIGURE 19.29 CT and three-dimensional (3D) CT of monostotic fibrous dysplasia. **(A)** Axial, **(B)** sagittal reformatted, and **(C)** and 3D reconstructed CT images show a lesion affecting posterior portion of the fourth left rib *(arrows)* of a 42-year-old man. Observe characteristic expansion of the bone and thinning of the cortex.

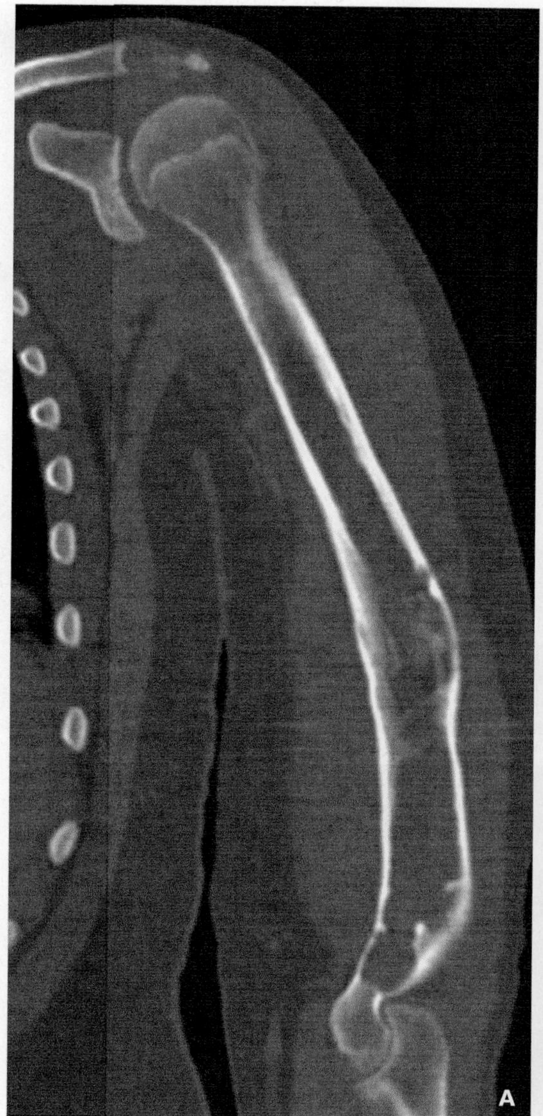

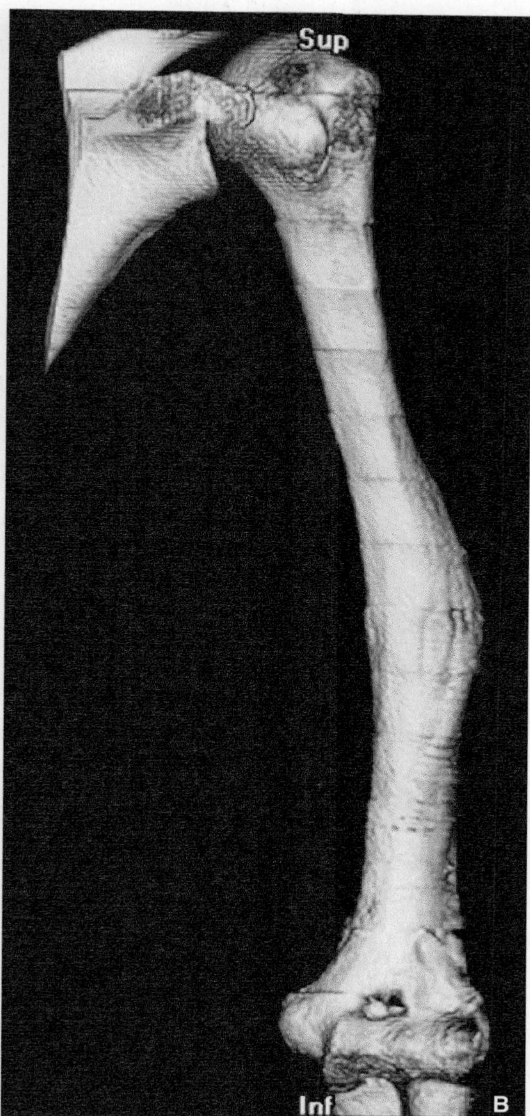

FIGURE 19.30 **CT and three-dimensional (3D) CT of monostotic fibrous dysplasia.** **(A)** Coronal reformatted and **(B)** 3D reconstructed in shaded surface display (SSD) CT images show solitary lesion affecting the diaphysis of the left humerus of a 13-year-old boy.

branching, with sparse interconnections. Low-power photomicrographs have been likened to "alphabet soup" or Chinese ideographs. They are composed of woven, immature bone and exhibit no evidence of osteoblastic activity ("naked trabeculae"). Occasionally, an area of cartilage formation may be present within the lesion.

Polyostotic Fibrous Dysplasia

Clinical and Imaging Features

Although radiographically similar to the monostotic form, polyostotic fibrous dysplasia is a more aggressive disorder. It also has a different distribution in the skeleton and a striking predilection for one side of the body (Fig. 19.33), a tendency that has been noted in more than 90% of cases. The pelvis is frequently affected, followed by the long bones, skull, and ribs; the proximal end of the femur is a common site of involvement (Fig. 19.34). The lesions generally progress in number and size until the end of skeletal maturation, at which time they become quiescent. In only 5% of cases do they continue to enlarge.

Radiographically, the changes typical of fibrous dysplasia may be recognized in a limited segment or a major portion of the long bones affected by the polyostotic form of the disease, but as in the monostotic form, the articular ends are usually spared. The cortex, which is generally left intact, is often thinned by the expansive component of the lesion, and the inner cortical margins may show scalloping. The lesion has a well-defined border. Occasionally, as in the monostotic form, the replacement of medullary bone by fibrous tissue leads to a loss of the trabecular pattern, giving the lesions a ground-glass, "milky," or "smoky" appearance (see Fig. 19.21A). More osseous lesions appear dense. The quickest means of determining the distribution of the lesion in the skeleton is radionuclide bone scan, which often discloses unsuspected sites of skeletal involvement (Fig. 19.35). Scintigraphy is also effective to determine the activity of fibrous dysplasia (Fig. 19.36).

CT can accurately delineate the extent of bone involvement (Figs. 19.37 and 19.38). Tissue attenuation values, as measured by Hounsfield units, are usually within the 70- to 400-HU range, apparently reflecting the presence of calcium and microscopic ossification throughout the abnormal tissue. As pointed out by Daffner and colleagues, CT is particularly useful to define the extent of craniofacial disease (Fig. 19.39), including impingement on orbital structures. On MRI, fibrous dysplasia exhibits homogeneous, intermediate or moderately low signal intensity on T1-weighted images, whereas on T2 weighting, the signal is bright or mixed. After intravenous injection of gadolinium, most lesions show central contrast enhancement and some peripheral rim enhancement (Figs. 19.40 and 19.41). In general, signal intensity on T1- and T2-weighted images and the degree of contrast enhancement on T1-weighted sequences depend on the amount and degree of bone trabeculae, collagen, and cystic and hemorrhagic changes in fibrous dysplasia.

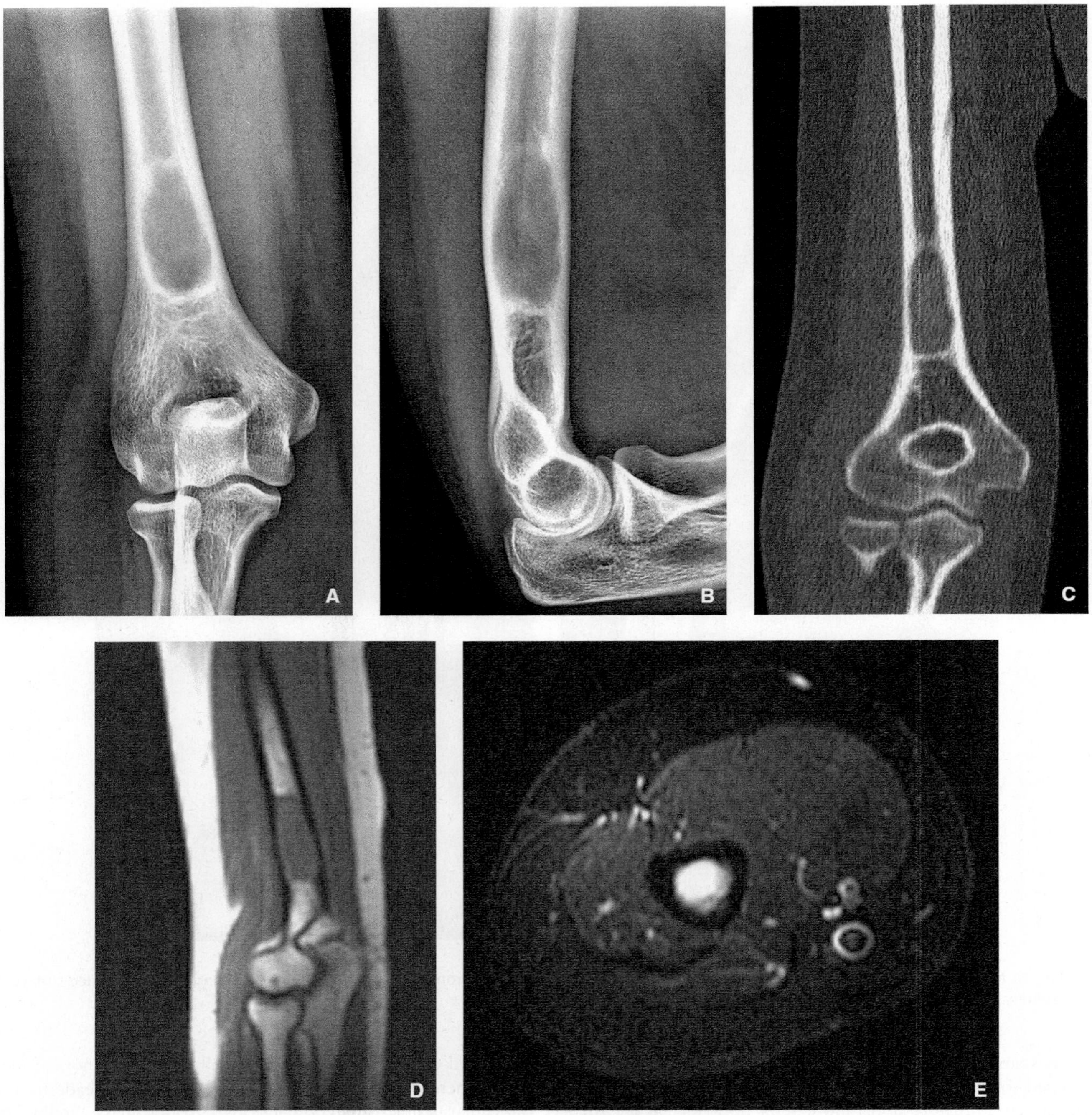

FIGURE 19.31 CT and MRI of monostotic fibrous dysplasia. **(A)** Anteroposterior and **(B)** lateral radiographs of the right elbow show a radiolucent lesion with sclerotic border in the distal humeral shaft of a 26-year-old woman. **(C)** Coronal reformatted CT image shows low-attenuation intramedullary lesion. Note thinning of the cortex. **(D)** Sagittal T1-weighted MR image shows the lesion to be of intermediate signal intensity, isointense with the surrounded skeletal muscles. **(E)** Axial IR MR image shows the lesion exhibiting high signal intensity. (Reprinted with permission from Greenspan A, Borys D. *Radiology and pathology correlation of bone tumors: a quick reference and review*. Philadelphia: Wolters Kluwer; 2016:202.)

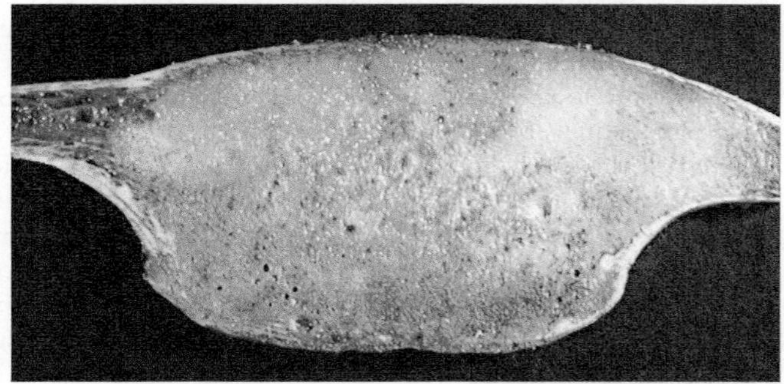

FIGURE 19.32 Pathology of monostotic fibrous dysplasia. Resected specimen of the rib shows yellow-reddish expansive lesion. Observe thinning of the cortex. (Reprinted from Bullough P. *Orthopaedic pathology*, 5th ed. Maryland Heights, MO: Mosby; 2009, with permission from Elsevier.)

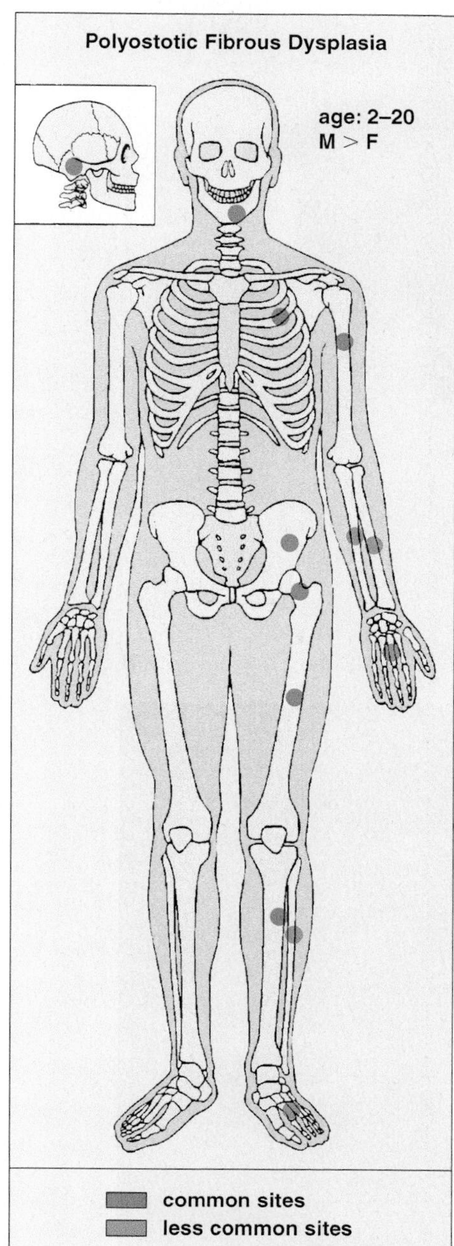

FIGURE 19.33 **Skeletal sites of predilection, peak age range, and male-to-female ratio in polyostotic fibrous dysplasia, which is usually seen in only one side of the skeleton.**

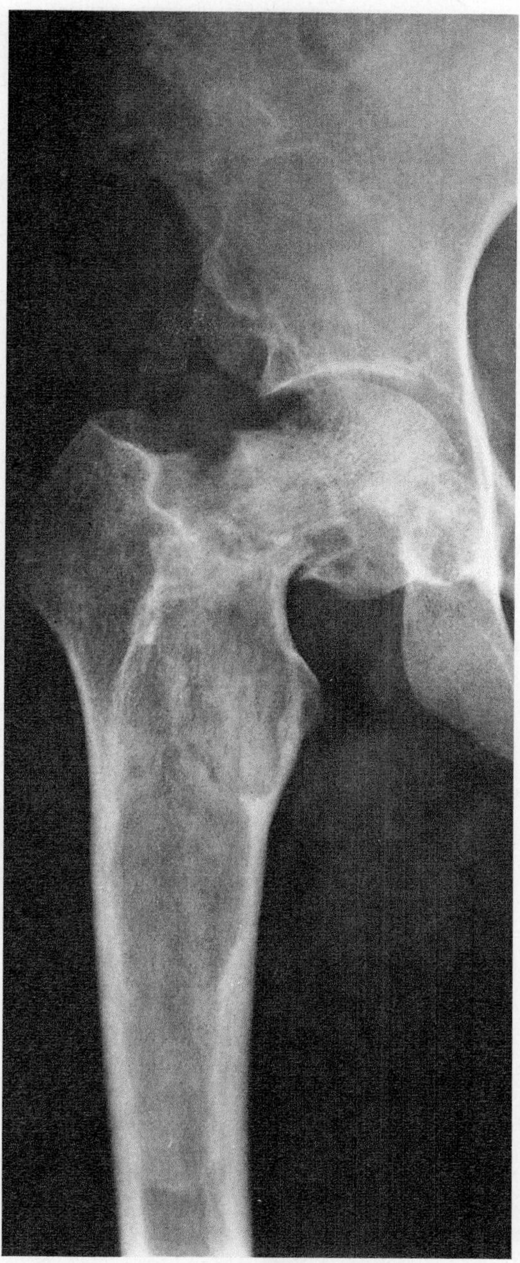

FIGURE 19.34 **Polyostotic fibrous dysplasia.** Anteroposterior radiograph of the right hip of an 18-year-old woman shows unilateral involvement of the ilium and femur. There is a pathologic fracture of the femoral neck with a varus deformity.

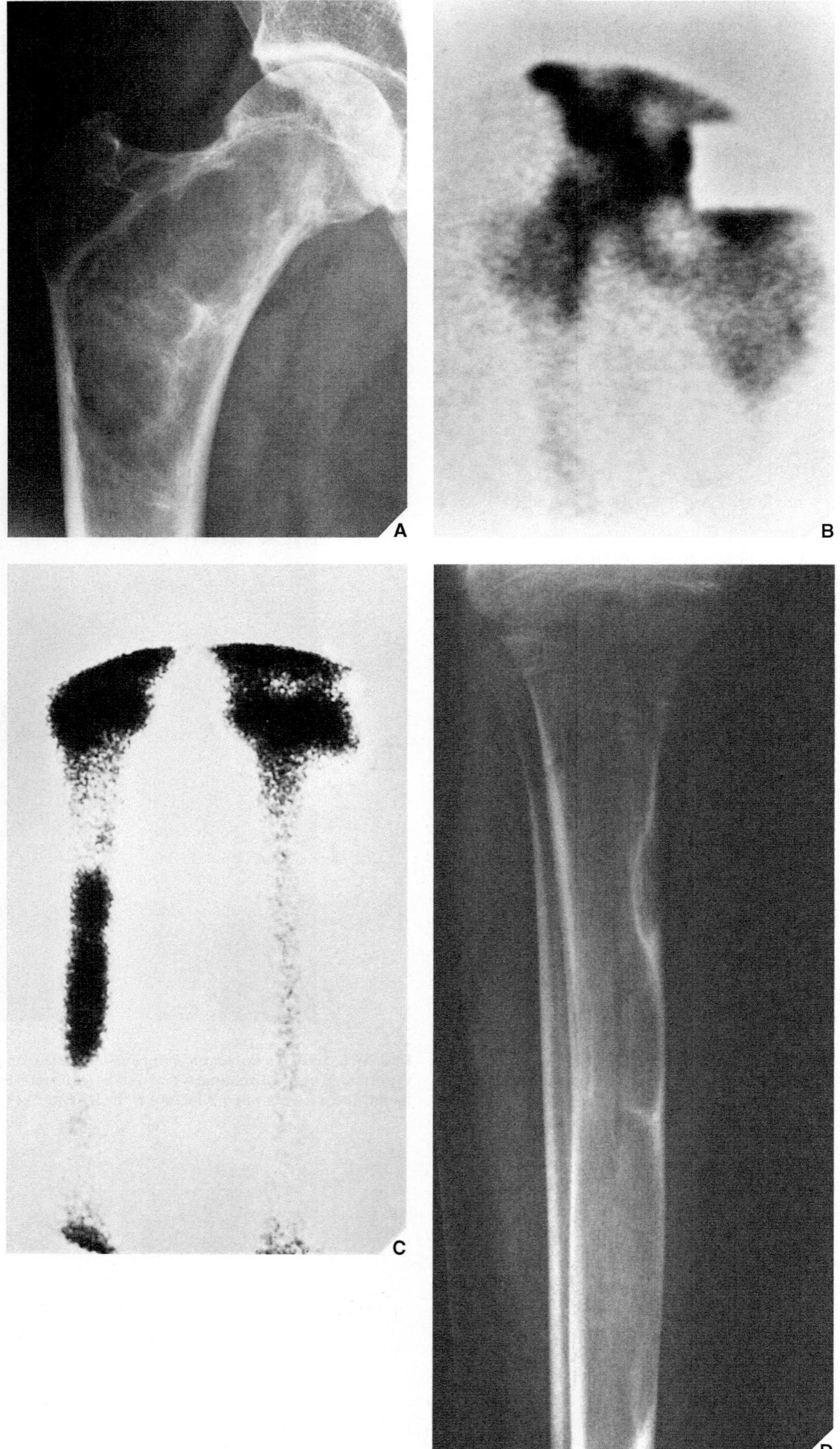

FIGURE 19.35 Scintigraphy of polyostotic fibrous dysplasia. A 13-year-old girl injured her right hip. **(A)** Anteroposterior radiograph of the hip, obtained to exclude a fracture, demonstrates a silent focus of fibrous dysplasia in the femoral neck. To determine other sites of involvement, a radionuclide bone scan was obtained. In addition to the focus in the femoral neck **(B)**, increased uptake of radiopharmaceutical tracer was demonstrated at various other sites but predominantly the right leg **(C)**. Subsequent radiograph of the right lower leg in the anteroposterior projection **(D)** confirms the presence of multiple foci of polyostotic fibrous dysplasia.

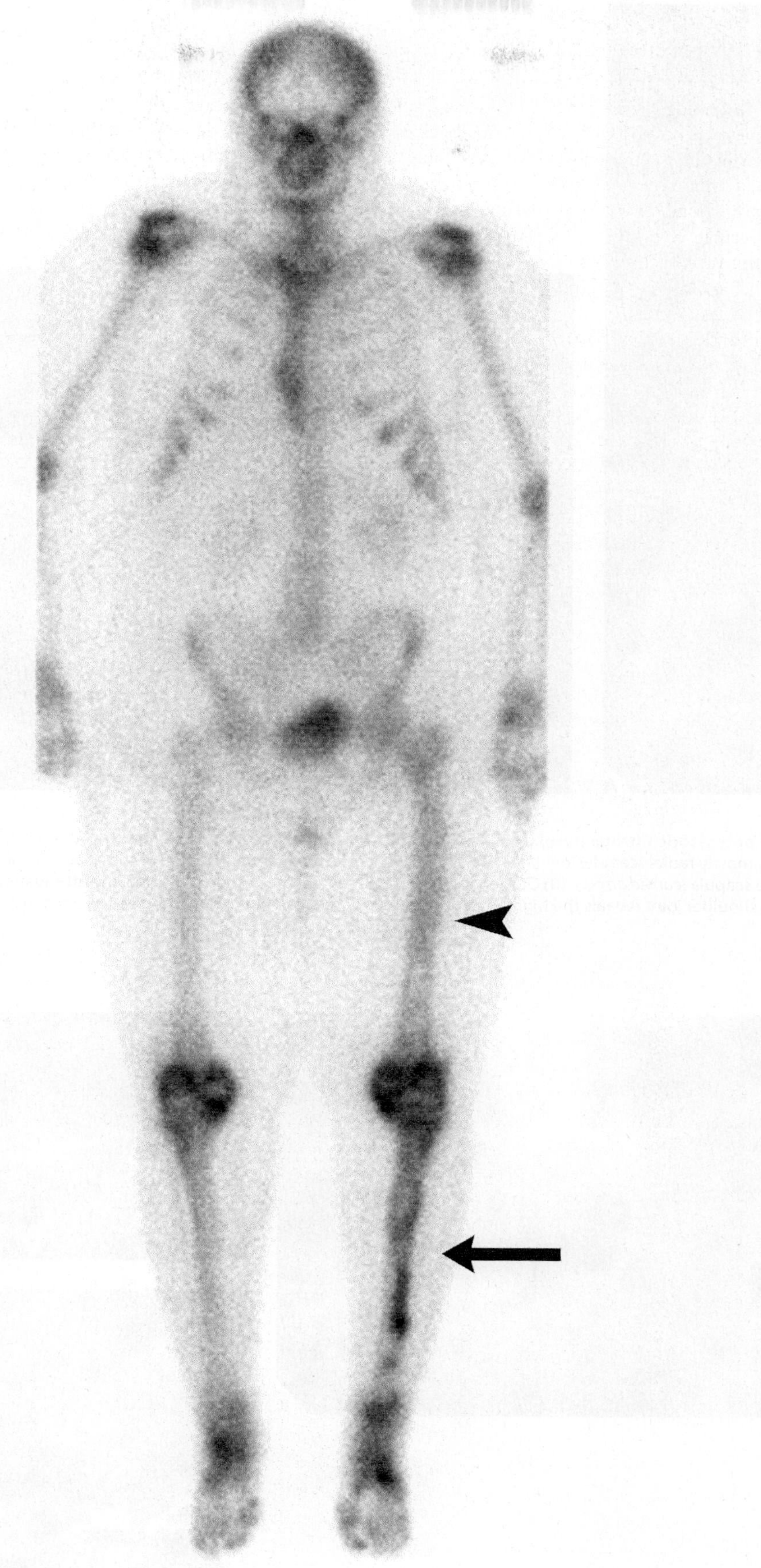

FIGURE 19.36 **Scintigraphy of polyostotic fibrous dysplasia.** Total body scan obtained in a 50-year-old woman after intravenous injection of 15mCi of technetium-99m (^{99m}Tc)-labeled methylene diphosphonate (MDP) shows markedly increased uptake of the radiotracer in the left tibia and fibula *(arrow)* and only slight activity in the left femur *(arrowhead)*.

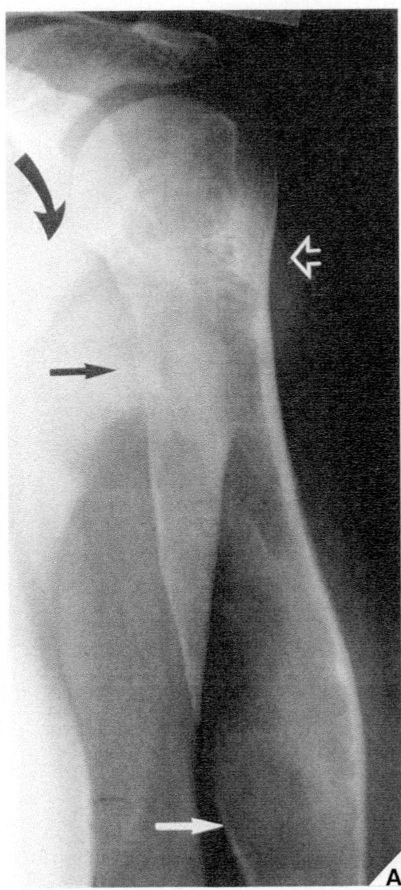

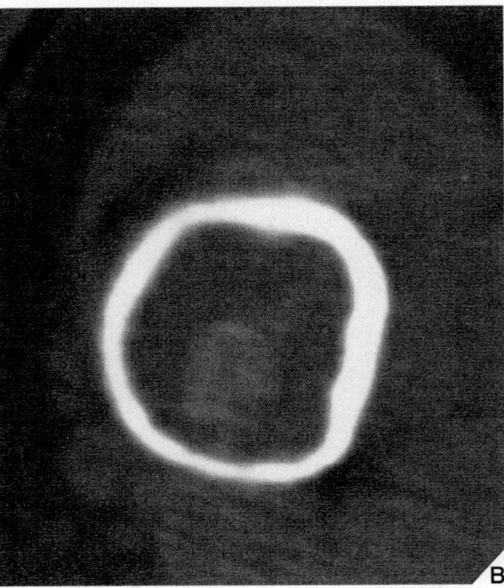

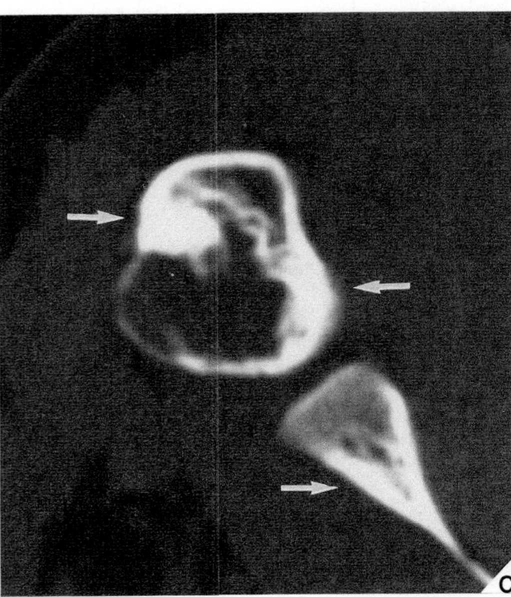

FIGURE 19.37 CT of polyostotic fibrous dysplasia. A 24-year-old woman presented with pain in the left arm. **(A)** Anteroposterior radiograph of the proximal left humerus shows expansive, mostly radiolucent lesion *(arrows)* with focal sclerotic areas at the junction of the head and neck *(open arrow)*. The cortex is thinned out. Another sclerotic focus is seen in the scapula *(curved arrow)*. **(B)** CT section through the shaft of the humerus shows a low-attenuation lesion with minimal scalloping of the endocortex. **(C)** CT section through the shoulder joint reveals the high-attenuation areas of sclerosis in the humeral head and scapula *(arrows)*.

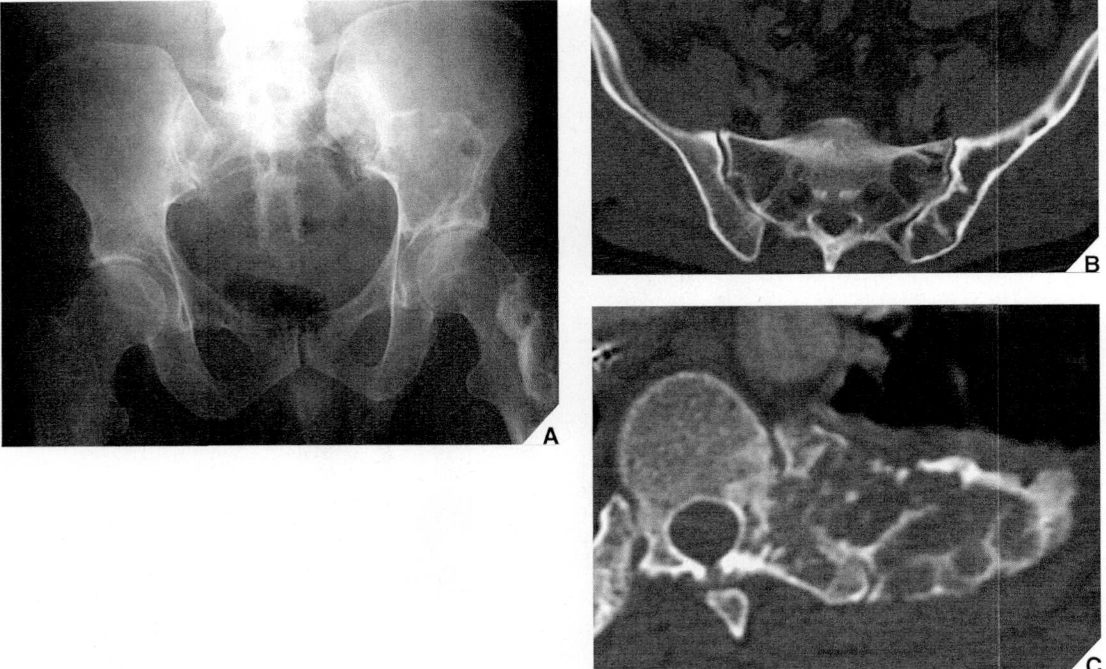

FIGURE 19.38 CT of polyostotic fibrous dysplasia. **(A)** Anteroposterior radiograph of the pelvis shows multiple lesions in the left ilium and proximal left femur. The involvement of the sacrum is not well demonstrated. **(B)** CT section of the pelvis precisely shows the extent of involvement of the ilium and sacrum. **(C)** Axial CT image of one of the thoracic vertebrae and ribs shows multiloculated appearance of the lesions, expansion of the bone, pseudosepta, thinning of the cortex, and a pathologic fracture. (Reprinted with permission from Greenspan A, Jundt G, Remagen W. *Differential diagnosis in orthopaedic oncology*, 2nd ed. Philadelphia: Lippincott Williams & Wilkins; 2007.)

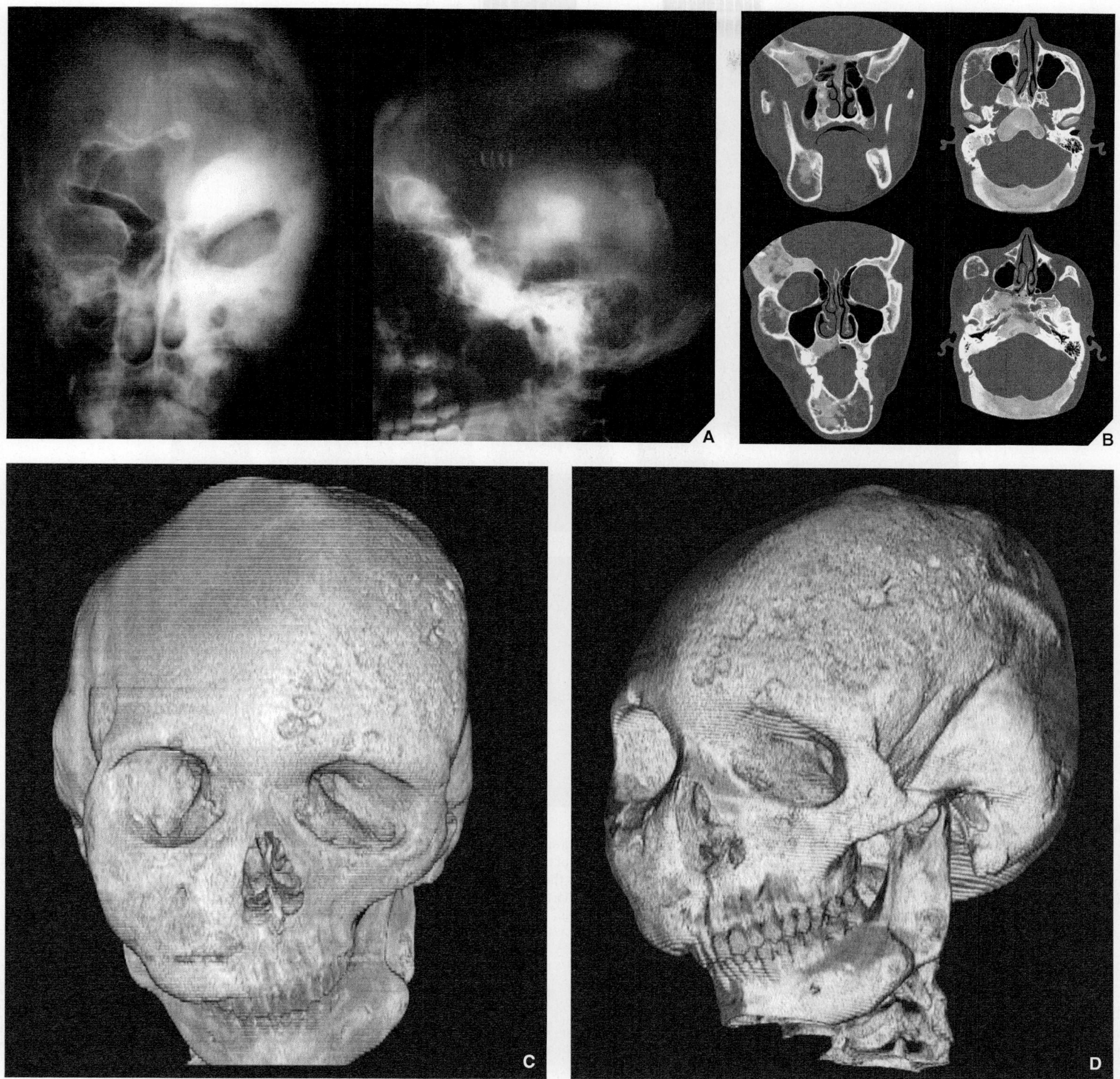

FIGURE 19.39 CT and three-dimensional (3D) CT of polyostotic fibrous dysplasia. **(A)** Anteroposterior and lateral radiographs of the skull of the 17-year-old boy show extensive involvement of the skull and the facial bones. **(B)** Several thin CT sections of the facial bones demonstrate the details and distribution of these lesions. 3D CT reconstructed images in SSD viewed from the **(C)** front and **(D)** side show extensive involvement and deformity of the facial bones and vault of the skull (calvaria) termed *leontiasis ossea*.

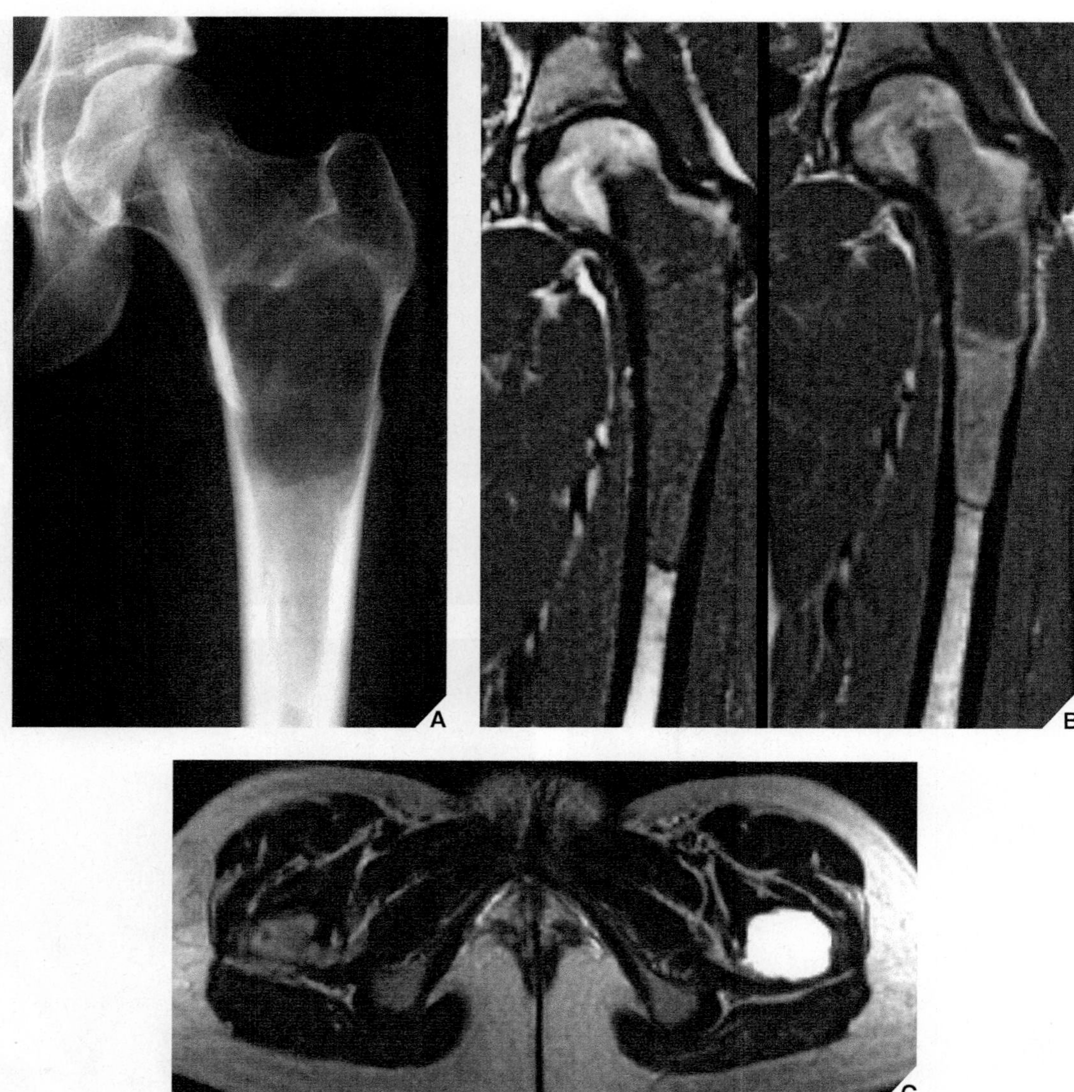

FIGURE 19.40 MRI of polyostotic fibrous dysplasia. **(A)** Anteroposterior radiograph of the proximal left femur of a 23-year-old woman shows a geographic radiolucent lesion in the subtrochanteric region of the bone. **(B)** Coronal MRI shows the full extent of the lesion, which is of intermediate signal intensity on T1-weighted image and exhibit mild enhancement on postcontrast sequence. **(C)** Axial T2-weighted MR image shows the lesion to be of high signal intensity. (Reprinted with permission from Greenspan A, Jundt G, Remagen W. *Differential diagnosis in orthopaedic oncology*, 2nd ed. Philadelphia: Lippincott Williams & Wilkins; 2007.)

Pathology

The histologic appearance of polyostotic fibrous dysplasia is identical to that of the monostotic form. The presence of small trabeculae of woven bone of various sizes and shapes, scattered within a fibrous tissue without the evidence of osteoblastic activity, is diagnostic for this disorder.

Complications

The most frequent complication of polyostotic fibrous dysplasia is pathologic fracture. If fracture occurs at the femoral neck, it commonly leads to a deformity called *shepherd's crook* (Fig. 19.42). Occasionally, accelerated growth of a bone or hypertrophy of a digit may be encountered (Fig. 19.43). The sarcomatous transformation of either form of fibrous dysplasia is extremely rare, but it may occur spontaneously (Fig. 19.44) or, more commonly, after radiation therapy (Fig. 19.45).

Fibrocartilaginous Dysplasia

Clinical, Pathologic, and Imaging Features

Massive cartilage hyperplasia (cartilaginous differentiation) may be seen in fibrous dysplasia resulting in the accumulation of cartilaginous masses in the medullary portion of the affected bone. This condition is commonly referred to as *fibrochondrodysplasia* or *fibrocartilaginous dysplasia*. Most common location is in the femur, humerus, and tibia. Imaging features are similar to fibrous dysplasia in addition to intralesional chondroid in type (stippled, comma-shaped, and ring-like) calcifications (Figs. 19.46 to 19.49). The lesion shows a variety of histopathologic features, ranging from purely dense fibrous tissue to benign fibrocartilaginous tissue. Moderate atypia of chondrocyte may be present.

Fibrocartilaginous dysplasia should not be confused with so-called *focal fibrocartilaginous dysplasia of long bones*. The latter occurs mainly in children and young adults. Characteristically, it affects the proximal tibia, although other long bones, such as the ulna and femur, may sometimes be involved.

Associated Disorders

McCune-Albright Syndrome

When polyostotic fibrous dysplasia is associated with endocrine disturbances (premature sexual development, hyperparathyroidism, and other endocrinopathies) and abnormal pigmentation marked by café-au-lait spots of the skin (Fig. 19.50), the disorder is called *McCune-Albright syndrome* (Fig. 19.51), described first in 1937 by Donovan James McCune and Fuller Albright. Overall, this condition almost exclusively affects girls who present with true sexual precocity secondary to acceleration of the normal process of gonadotropin release by the anterior lobe of the pituitary gland. The café-au-lait spots seen in McCune-Albright syndrome have

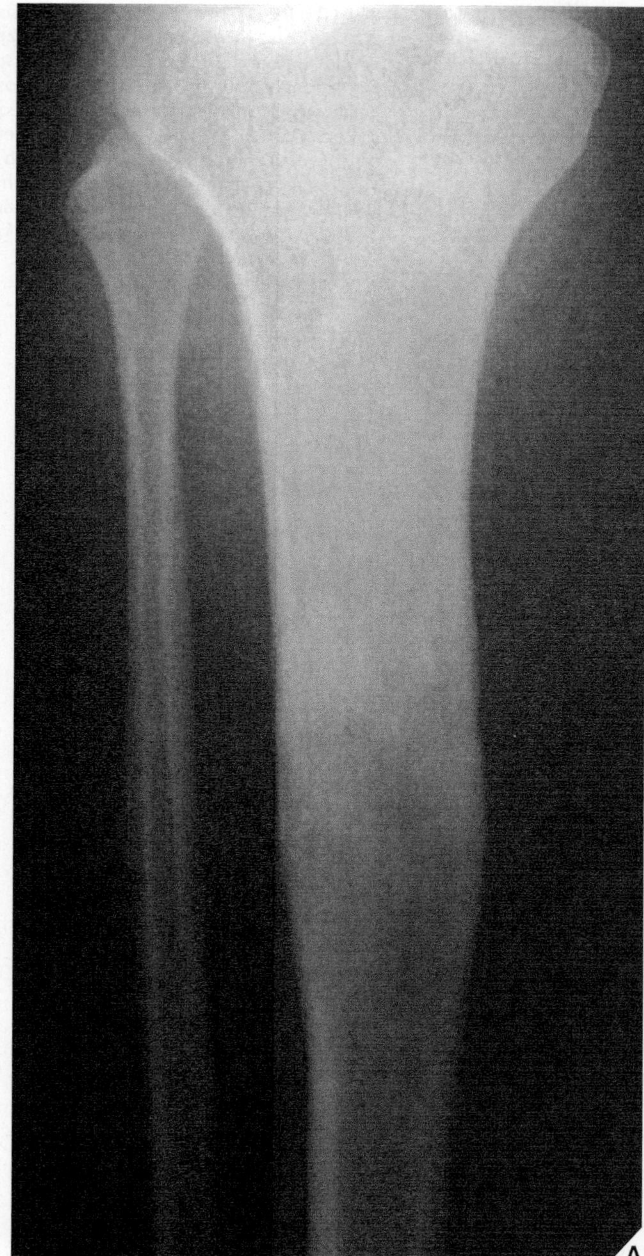

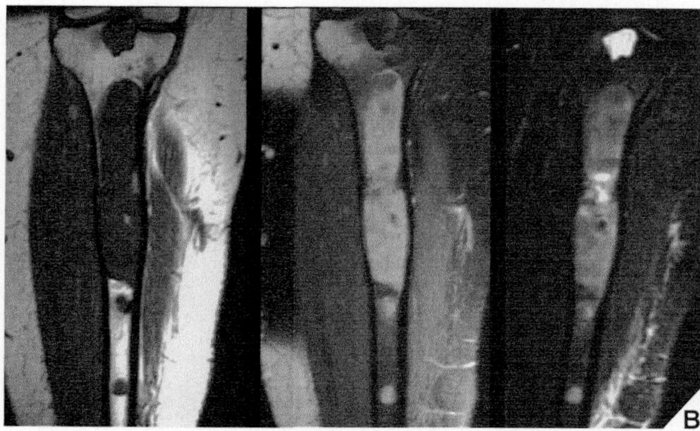

FIGURE 19.41 MRI of polyostotic fibrous dysplasia. **(A)** Anteroposterior radiograph of the proximal right leg of a 23-year-old woman shows a multifocal long lesion in the proximal tibia exhibiting a ground-glass appearance. The bone is mildly expanded; the cortex is thin. **(B)** Coronal T1-weighted, postcontrast fat-suppressed T1-weighted, and T2-weighted images show characteristic features of this lesion: intermediate signal intensity similar to that of the skeletal muscle on T1 weighting, heterogenous signal on T2 weighting, and slight enhancement after intravenous injection of gadolinium. (Reprinted with permission from Greenspan A, Jundt G, Remagen W. *Differential diagnosis in orthopaedic oncology*, 2nd ed. Philadelphia: Lippincott Williams & Wilkins; 2007.)

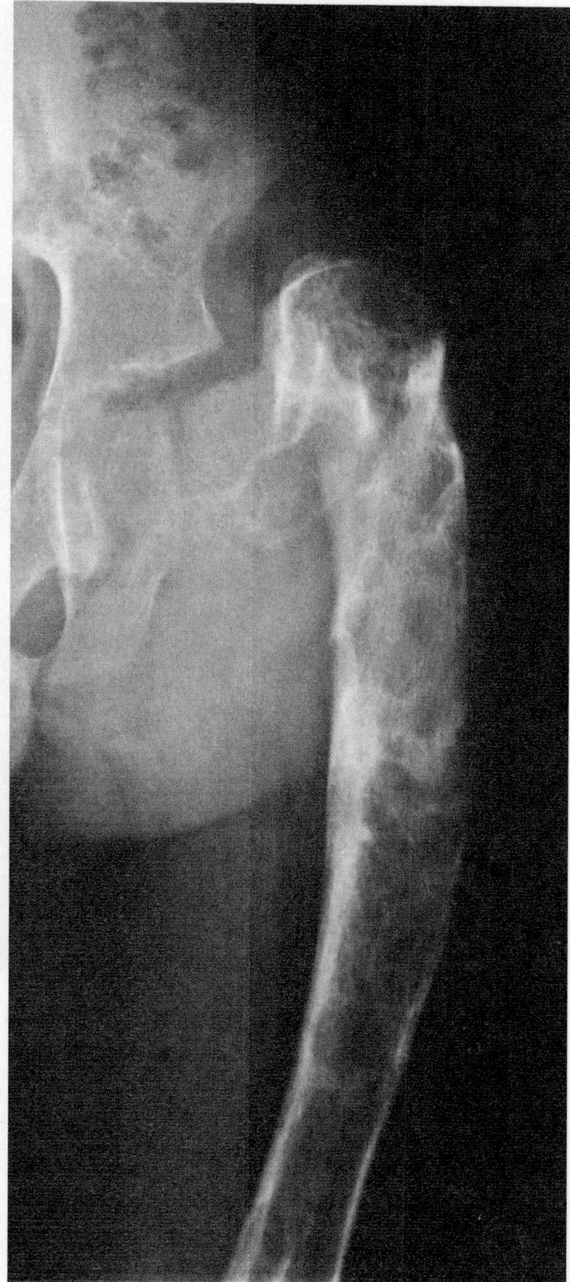

FIGURE 19.42 Polyostotic fibrous dysplasia. A "shepherd's crook" deformity, seen here in the proximal femur in a 12-year-old boy with polyostotic fibrous dysplasia, is often the result of multiple pathologic fractures.

characteristically irregular ragged borders (commonly called *coast of Maine borders*), as opposed to the smoothly marginated (*coast of California*) borders of the spots seen in neurofibromatosis. As fibrous dysplasia, also this syndrome is caused by gain-of-function random postzygomatic mutations in the *GNAS1* gene. The *GNAS1* regulates the process of formation of a guanine nucleotide-binding protein (G protein), responsible for activation of the enzyme adenylate cyclase, which in turn has influence on overproduction of several hormones.

Mazabraud Syndrome

This syndrome, which is characterized by an association of polyostotic fibrous dysplasia with soft-tissue myxomas (solitary or multiple), was first described by German pathologist F. Henschen in 1926 and later was reemphasized by French physician A. Mazabraud in 1967. Recently, Endo and associates reported a rare variant of Mazabraud syndrome—monostotic fibrous dysplasia coexisting with solitary intramuscular myxoma. The cause of Mazabraud syndrome remains unsettled. A variety of pathologic

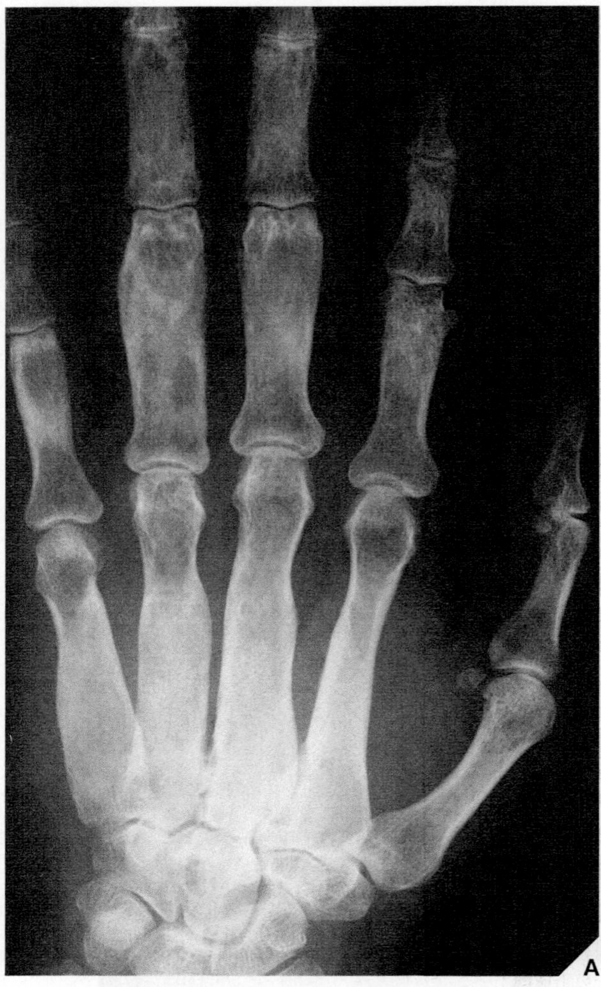

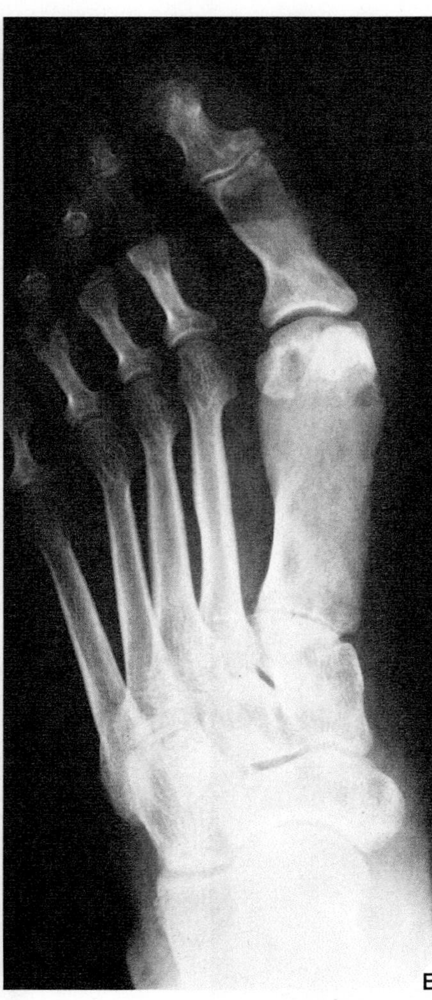

FIGURE 19.43 Complication of fibrous dysplasia. **(A)** Posteroanterior radiograph of the hand and **(B)** dorsoplantar radiograph of the foot of a 20-year-old man with polyostotic fibrous dysplasia demonstrate a frequent complication of this condition—accelerated growth of affected bones. In the hand, observe the enlargement of the third and fourth rays, including the metacarpals and phalanges, and in the foot, note the hypertrophy of the first metatarsal.

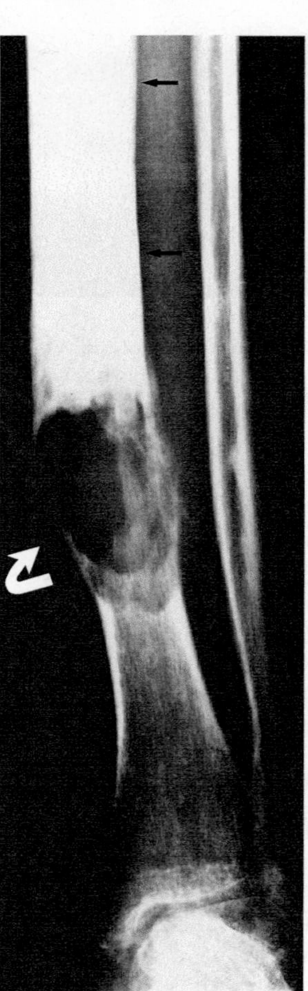

FIGURE 19.44 Complication of fibrous dysplasia. A 34-year-old man was noted to have a deformity of the left leg at age 5 years. Radiographic examination at that time showed typical involvement of the tibia by fibrous dysplasia, which subsequently was confirmed by biopsy. No treatment was given, and he was asymptomatic for 28 years until acute pain in his left leg developed. Conventional radiograph shows evidence of fibrous dysplasia affecting the proximal shaft of the tibia *(arrows)*. A large osteolytic destructive lesion in the distal third of the tibia is also seen encroaching on the dense segment of bone and affecting the medullary portion and the cortex *(curved arrow)*. There is a periosteal reaction and a soft-tissue mass. Biopsy revealed transformation of fibrous dysplasia to undifferentiated spindle-cell sarcoma.

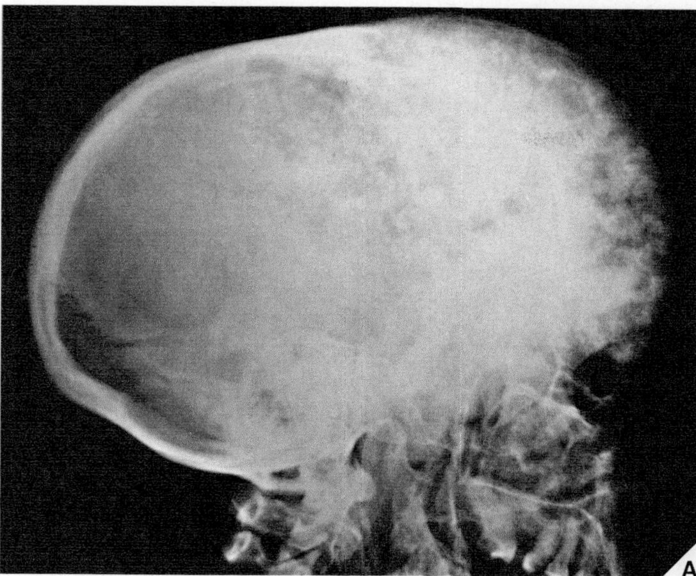

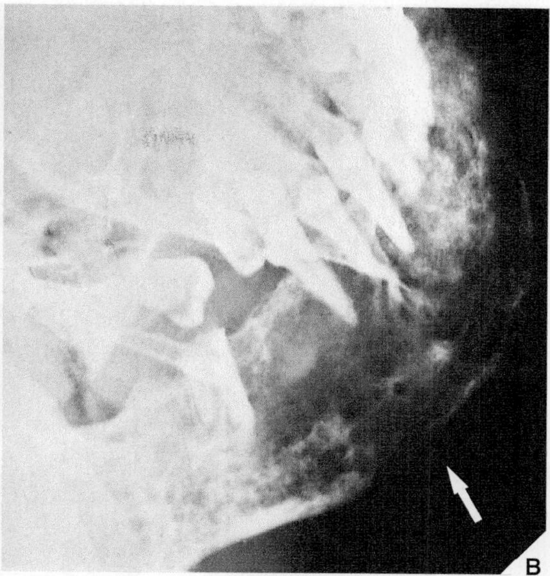

FIGURE 19.45 **Complication of fibrous dysplasia.** Eleven years before this examination, a 35-year-old woman with polyostotic fibrous dysplasia underwent radiation treatment of the mandible. **(A)** Lateral radiograph of the skull demonstrates predominant involvement of the frontal bones with a characteristic expansion of the outer table. The base of the skull, a frequent site of polyostotic fibrous dysplasia, is typically thickened, and the frontal and ethmoid sinuses are obliterated. The maxilla and mandible are also affected. This advanced stage of involvement of the skull and facial bones by polyostotic fibrous dysplasia is frequently termed *leontiasis ossea* (see also Fig. 19.39). **(B)** Oblique radiograph shows an expansive lytic lesion in the body of the left mandible, with partial destruction of the cortex *(arrow)*. Biopsy revealed an osteosarcoma.

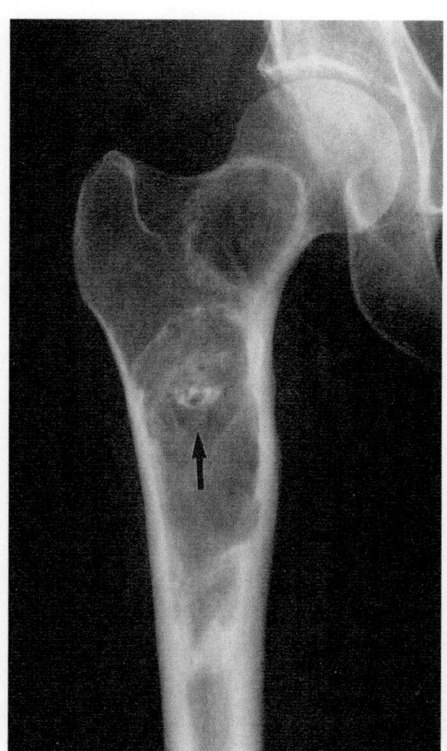

FIGURE 19.46 **Fibrocartilaginous dysplasia.** Anteroposterior radiograph of the right proximal femur in a 20-year-old man with polyostotic fibrous dysplasia shows foci of cartilage formation *(arrow)*, identifying this lesion as fibrocartilaginous dysplasia.

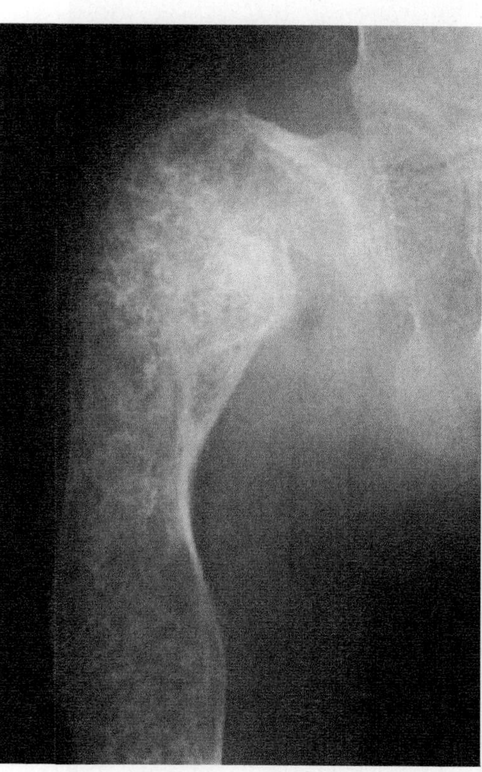

FIGURE 19.47 **Fibrocartilaginous dysplasia.** Anteroposterior radiograph of the proximal right femur of a 10-year-old boy with polyostotic fibrous dysplasia exhibits typical appearance of a massive formation of cartilage, known as *fibrocartilaginous dysplasia*.

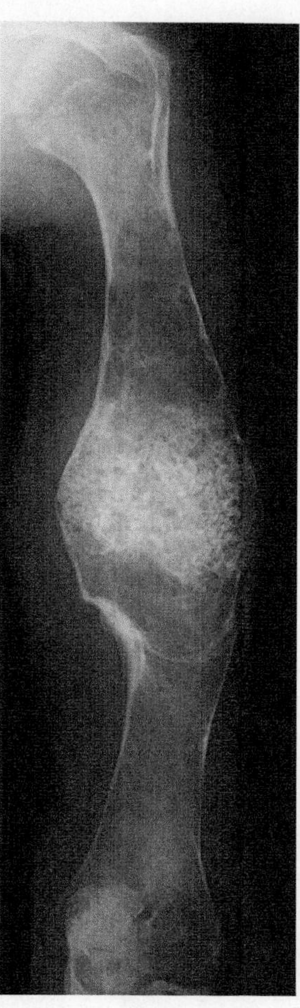

FIGURE 19.48 **Fibrocartilaginous dysplasia.** Anteroposterior radiograph of the left humerus in a 19-year-old man with polyostotic fibrous dysplasia shows an extensive involvement of almost the entire bone, with cartilage formation in the midportion of the diaphysis.

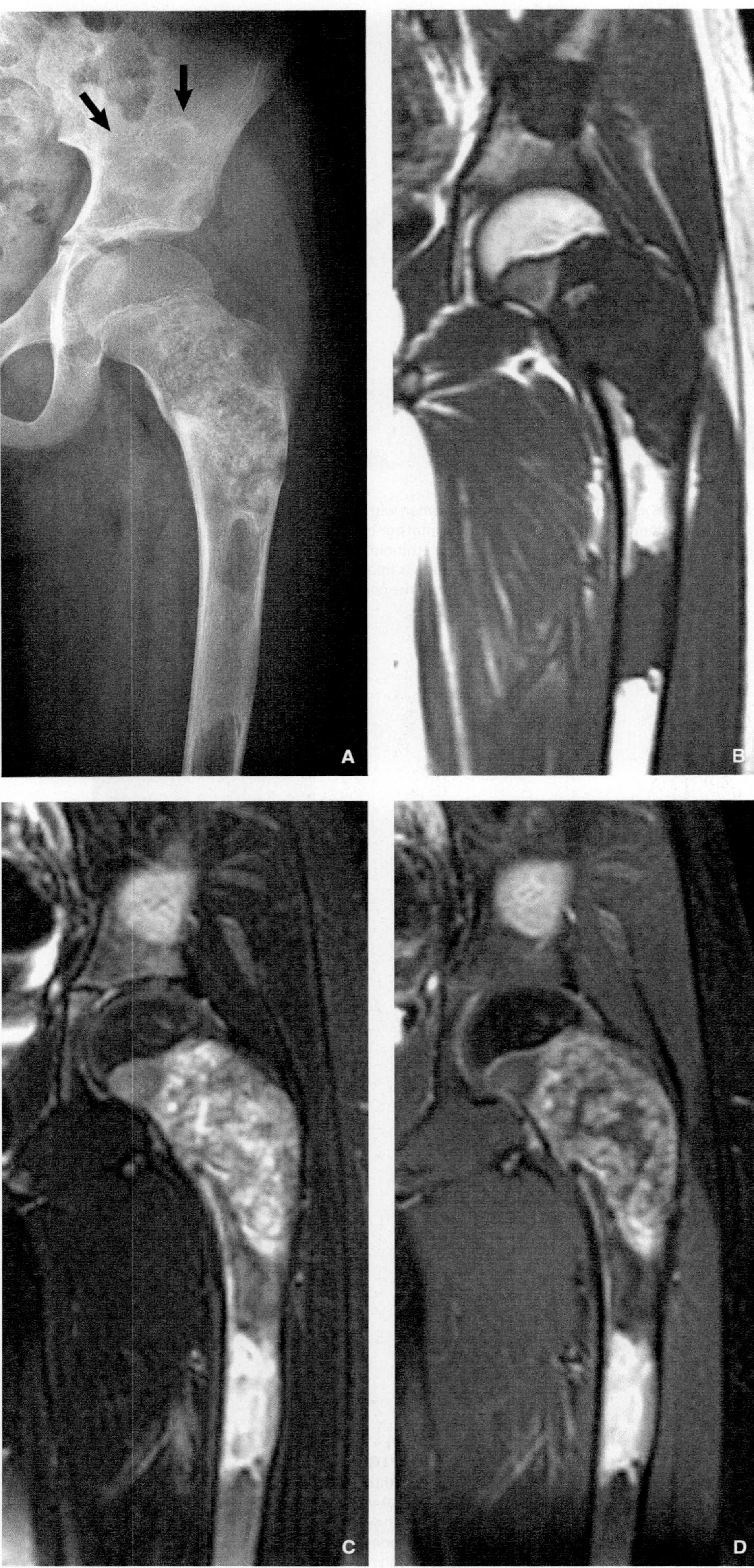

FIGURE 19.49 **MRI of fibrocartilaginous dysplasia.** **(A)** Anteroposterior radiograph of the left hip joint of an 11-year-old boy shows extensive involvement of proximal femur by fibrous dysplasia. Observe chondroid calcifications in the region of metaphysis and proximal diaphysis of the bone. There is also focus of fibrous dysplasia in the left ilium *(arrows)*. **(B)** Coronal T1-weighted MR image shows the lesions exhibit intermediate-to-low signal intensity. **(C)** Coronal T2-weighted fat-saturated MR image shows the lesions to become heterogenous but predominantly of high signal intensity with calcifications expressing low signal. **(D)** Coronal T1-weighted fat-suppressed MR image obtained after intravenous administration of gadolinium shows prominent enhancement of the lesions with calcifications remaining of low signal intensity.

FIGURE 19.50 McCune-Albright syndrome. **(A)** Clinical photograph of a 17-year-old girl with polyostotic fibrous dysplasia and history of precocious puberty shows typical "coast-of-Maine" café-au-lait spots over her neck. **(B)** Clinical photograph of the right leg of another patient, a 20-year-old woman affected by polyostotic fibrous dysplasia and history of precocious puberty shows café-au-lait spots over anterior aspect of the knee and the leg displaying rugged borders.

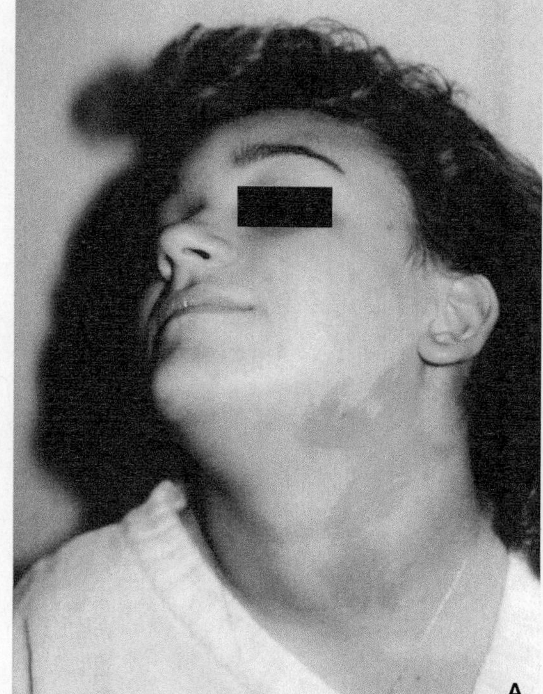

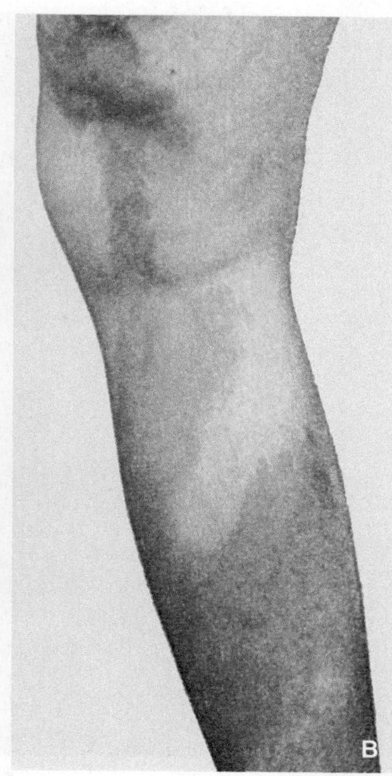

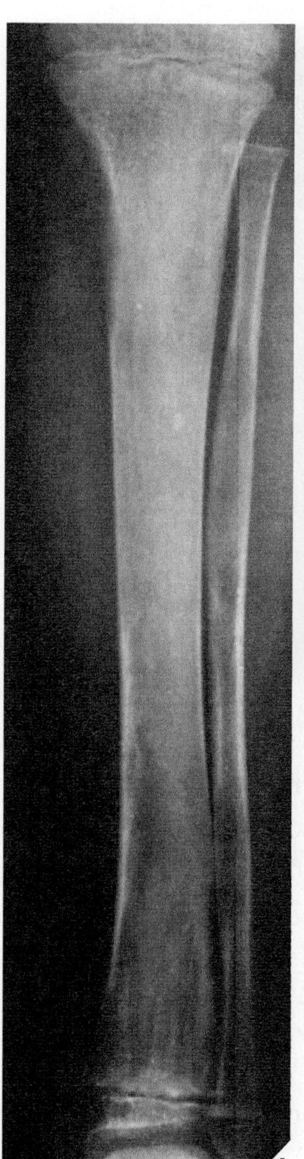

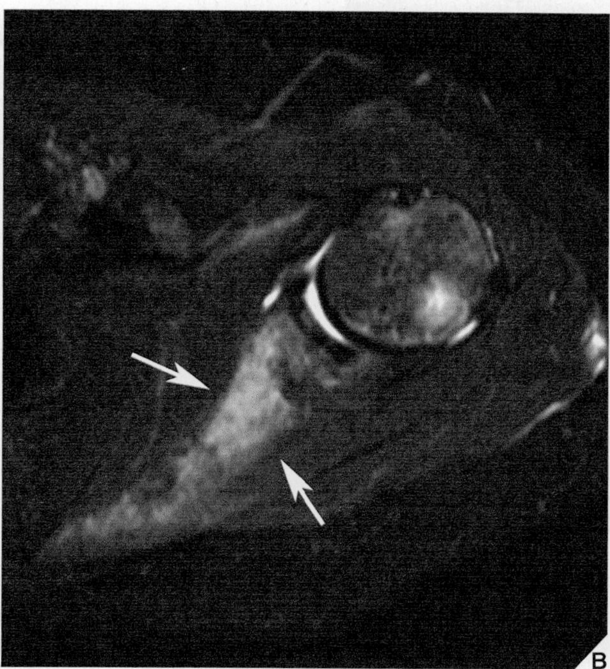

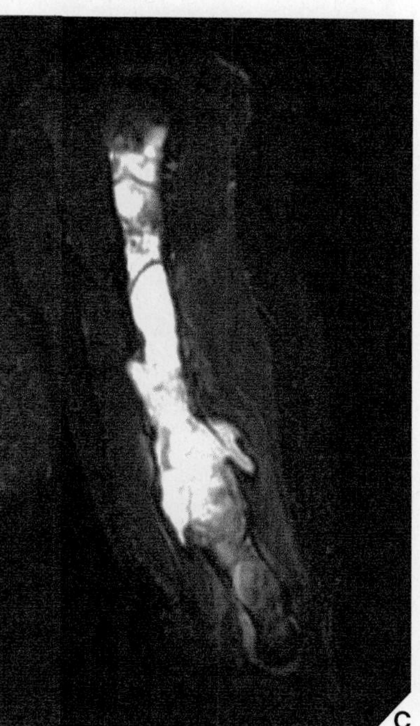

FIGURE 19.51 McCune-Albright syndrome. **(A)** Polyostotic fibrous dysplasia typically affects one side of the skeleton, as seen here in a 5-year-old girl with precocious puberty whose left upper and lower extremities were affected. Radiograph of the lower leg shows expansion of the tibia and fibula associated with thinning of the cortex. Note the ground-glass appearance of the medullary portion of these bones. **(B)** Axial T2-weighted MRI of the left shoulder of another patient with polyostotic fibrous dysplasia and McCune-Albright syndrome shows abnormal signal intensity and widening of the scapula *(arrows)* and abnormal signal intensity in the humeral head. **(C)** Short time inversion recovery (STIR) MRI of the left humerus demonstrates diffuse signal alteration of the humerus with marked deformity of the bone.

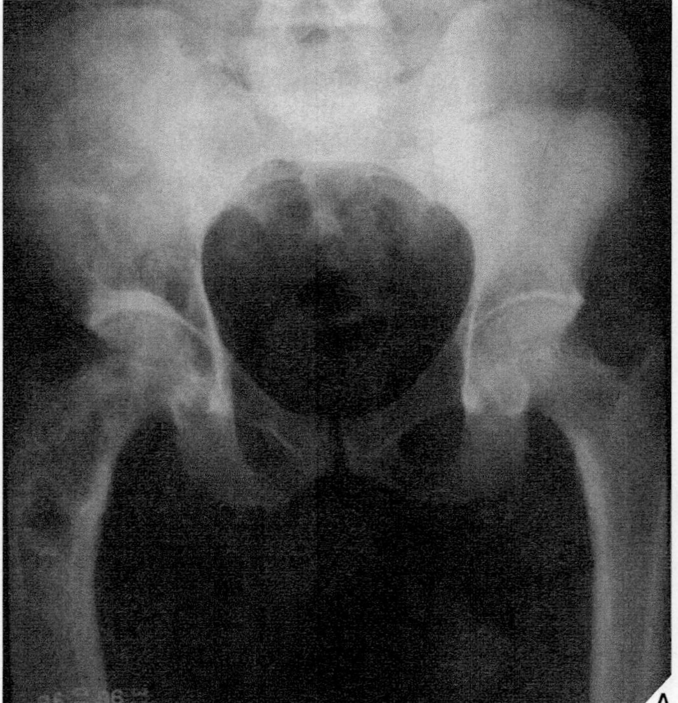

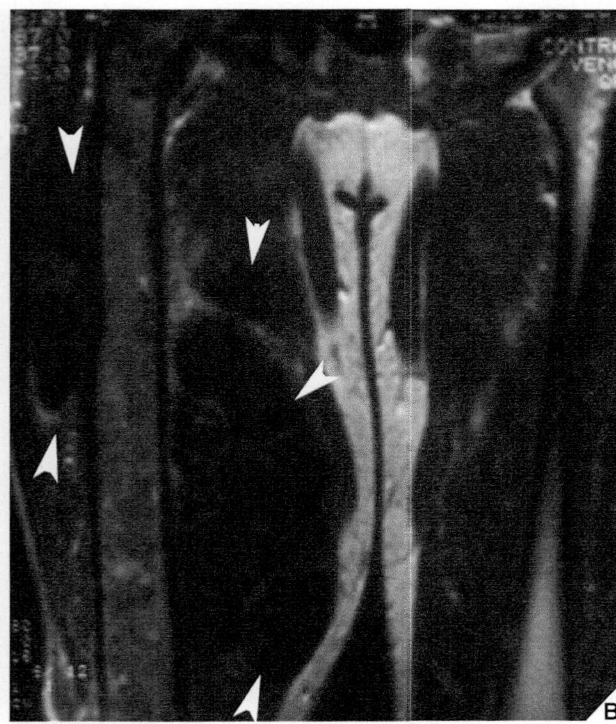

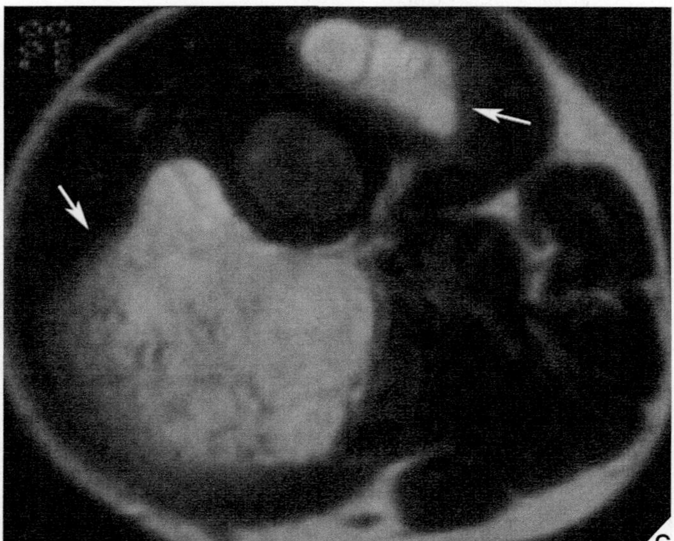

FIGURE 19.52 Mazabraud syndrome. **(A)** Frontal radiograph of the pelvis and hips demonstrates characteristic findings of fibrous dysplasia of the right femur and right iliac bone. **(B)** Coronal T1-weighted MRI of the right thigh demonstrates diffuse heterogenous signal alteration and dysplastic changes of the right femur, characteristic of fibrous dysplasia. Additionally, multiple hypointense intramuscular masses are noted *(arrowheads)*, representing multiple intramuscular myxomas. **(C)** Axial T2-weighted MRI of the right thigh demonstrates the multiple hyperintense intramuscular myxomas *(arrows)*.

mechanisms have been suggested to explain the link between fibrous dysplasia and soft-tissue myxomas. Some investigators have emphasized a common histiogenic origin or a shared abnormality in tissue metabolism. Others have suggested a collaborative developmental error, perhaps related to a genetic predisposition. In this syndrome, it is important to recognize the soft-tissue masses as benign myxomas and not to confuse them with malignant soft-tissue tumors that may develop *de novo* (e.g., malignant fibrous histiocytoma, malignant mesenchymoma, or liposarcoma) or those that may be present in cases of malignant transformation of fibrous dysplasia. MR imaging is very helpful because it reveals typical features of benign myxomas—that is, very sharply defined borders, homogeneous signal intensity before administration of contrast, and a heterogeneous pattern of enhancement after the intravenous injection of gadolinium. As pointed out by several investigators, the signal characteristics of myxoma on T1- and T2-weighted sequences are quite similar to those of fluid: low-to-intermediate signal intensity on T1-weighted and high signal intensity on T2-weighted images (Figs. 19.52 and 19.53).

Osteofibrous Dysplasia

Clinical, Imaging, and Histopathologic Features

Osteofibrous dysplasia (Kempson-Campanacci lesion), called *ossifying fibroma* in the past, is a rare, benign, fibroosseous lesion that occurs predominantly in children, although it may not be discovered until adolescence. Recently, familial occurrence has been reported. Cytogenetic studies revealed trisomies for chromosomes 7, 8, 12, and 22. Osteofibrous dysplasia has a decided preference for the tibia, being located with few exceptions in the proximal third or mid segment of the bone and often localized to its anterior cortex. In more than 80% of patients, there is some degree of anterior bowing. Larger lesions may destroy the cortex and invade the medullary cavity.

On radiography, the Kempson-Campanacci lesion exhibits a lobulated sclerotic margin and a striking resemblance to nonossifying fibroma and fibrous dysplasia (Figs. 19.54 to 19.56). CT and MRI features are also similar

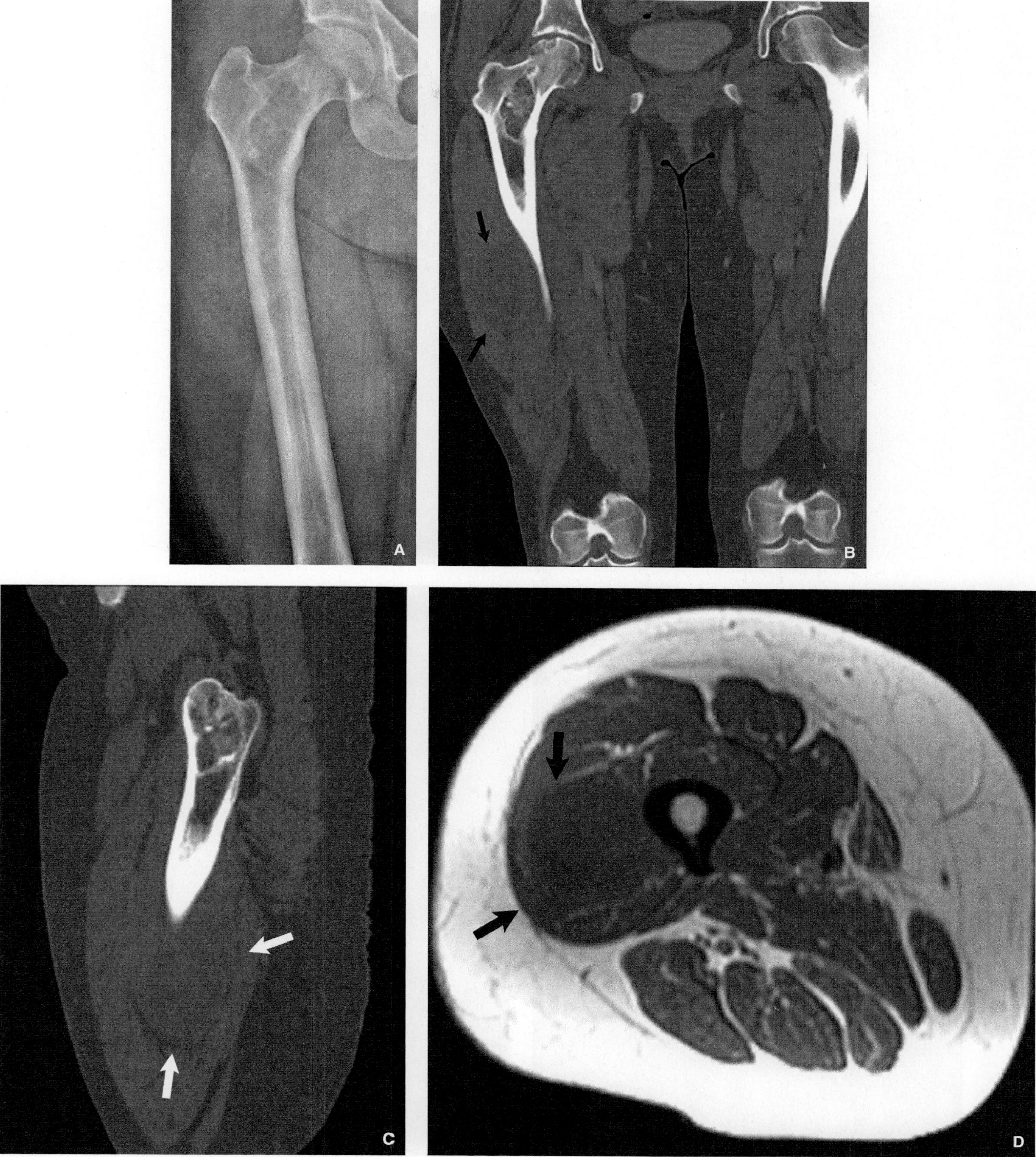

FIGURE 19.53 Mazabraud syndrome. **(A)** Anteroposterior radiograph of the right femur of a 49-year-old woman shows several radiolucent lesions in the proximal part of the bone. **(B)** Coronal and **(C)** sagittal reformatted CT images, in addition to osseous lesions, demonstrate a well-defined soft-tissue mass *(arrows)*. **(D)** Axial T1-weighted MR image shows a soft tissue mass, which exhibits intermediate signal intensity *(arrows)*, isointense with the skeletal muscles. *(Continued)*

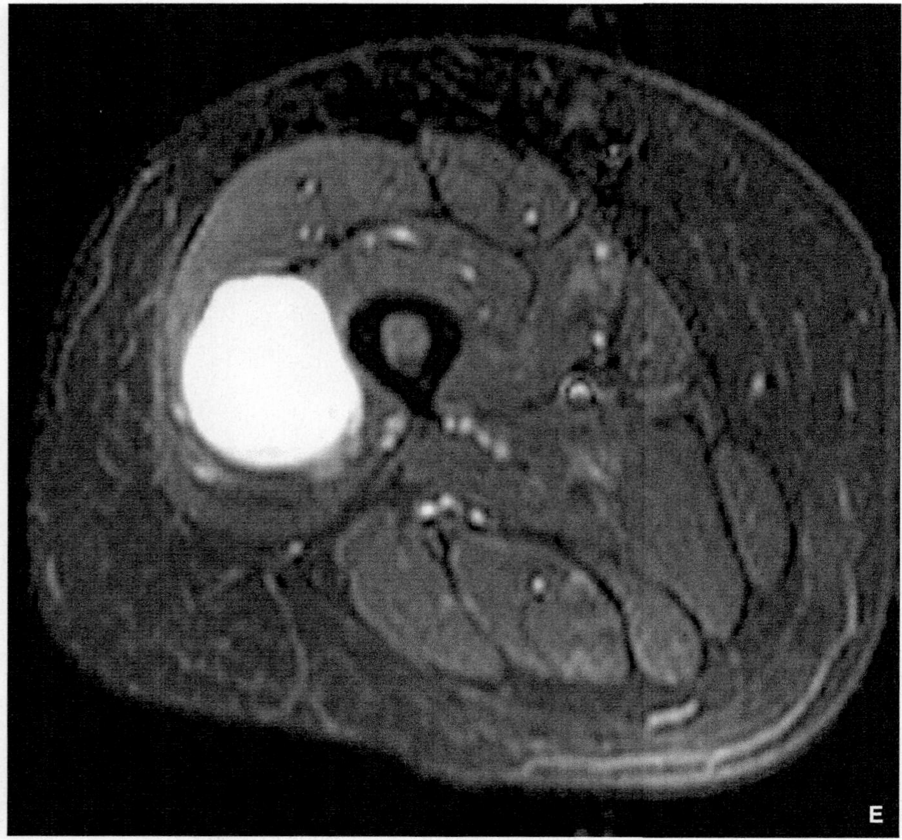

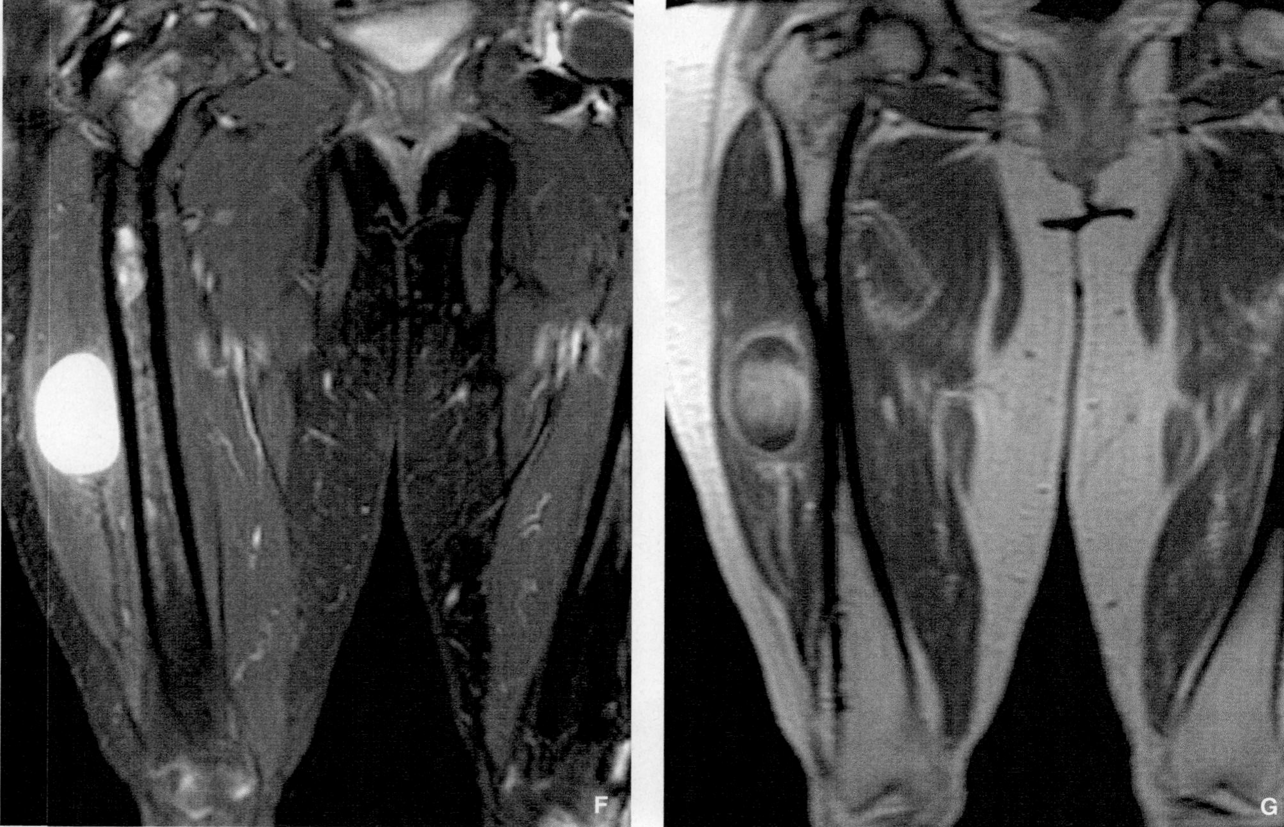

FIGURE 19.53 Mazabraud syndrome. ***(Continued)*** **(E)** Axial IR MR image shows the mass becoming bright. **(F)** Coronal T2-weighted fat-suppressed MR image shows the soft-tissue mass to be homogeneously of high signal intensity. **(G)** Coronal T1-weighted fat-suppressed MR image obtained after intravenous administration of gadolinium shows only minimal enhancement of the mass, proven on excision biopsy to represent a benign myxoma.

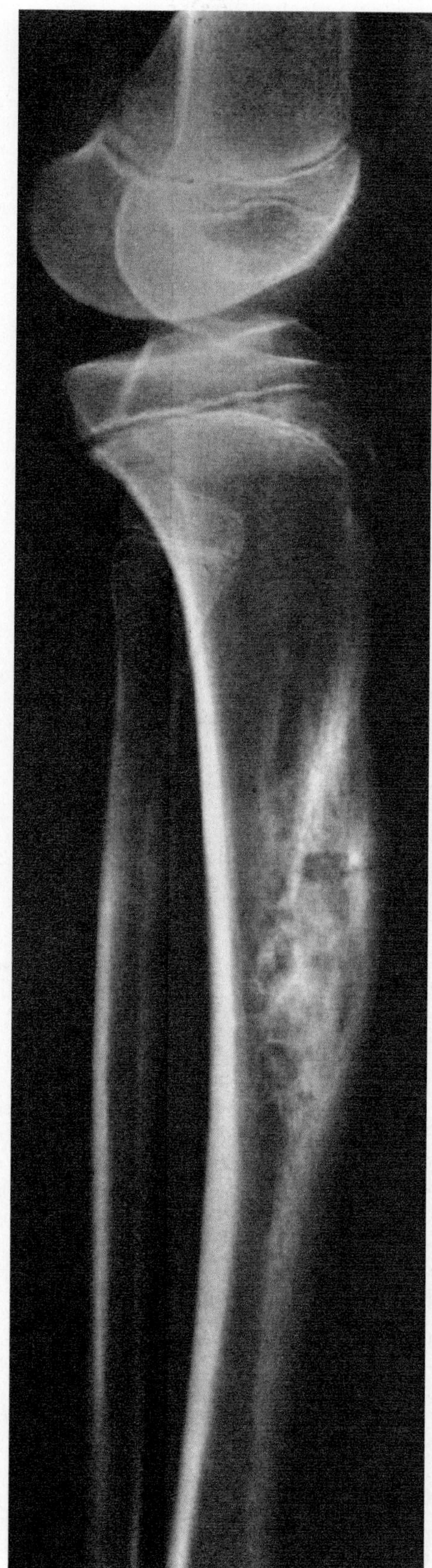

FIGURE 19.54 **Osteofibrous dysplasia.** This lesion in the anterior aspect of the right tibia of a 14-year-old girl was originally thought to be a nonossifying fibroma. Although it is similar to a nonossifying fibroma and fibrous dysplasia, its site is typical of osteofibrous dysplasia, which was confirmed by biopsy. Note the characteristic anterior bowing of the tibia.

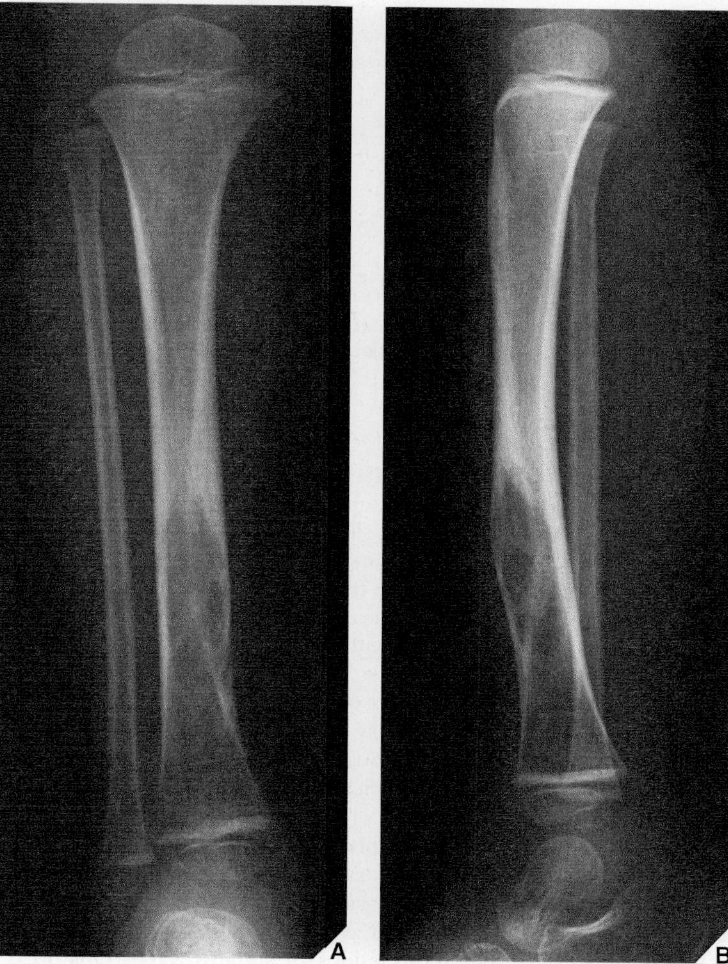

FIGURE 19.55 **Osteofibrous dysplasia.** **(A)** Anteroposterior and **(B)** lateral radiographs of the right leg in a 2-year-old boy show the lesion in the anterior aspect of the distal tibia.

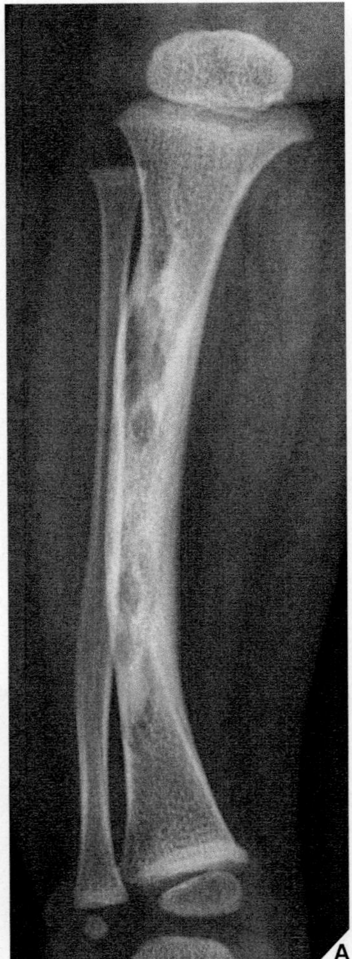

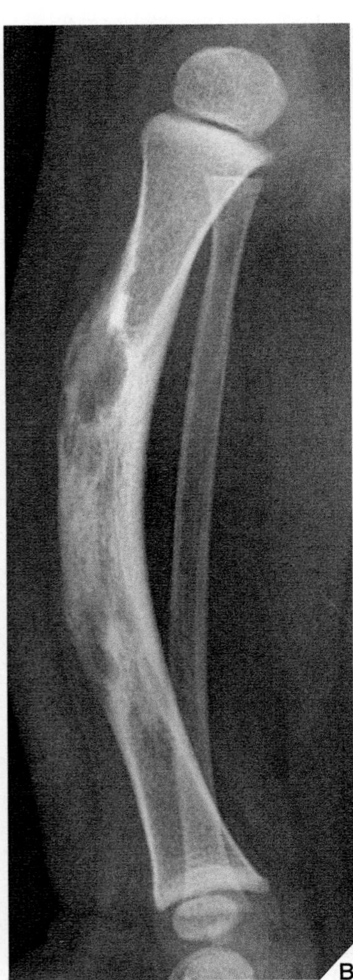

FIGURE 19.56 Osteofibrous dysplasia. **(A)** Anteroposterior and **(B)** lateral radiographs of the right leg of a 10-month-old girl show extensive involvement of the midtibial diaphysis. Note the characteristic anterior bowing of the tibia.

to those two lesions (Figs. 19.57 to 19.59). Furthermore, osteofibrous dysplasia and fibrous dysplasia, as the similarity in their names might suggest, display a remarkable histopathologic similarity. Like a lesion of fibrous dysplasia, osteofibrous dysplasia is composed of a fibrous background containing deformed trabeculae. These trabeculae, however, unlike those of fibrous dysplasia, display woven bone only in the center, being surrounded by an outer zone of lamellar bone with prominent appositional osteoblastic activity ("dressed trabeculae").

This lesion should not be confused with the lesion, also called *ossifying fibroma*, that is seen almost exclusively in the jaw (mandible) of women in their third and fourth decades, although it is still uncertain whether some of the latter lesions represent an atypical form of fibrous dysplasia. Sissons and colleagues reported two cases of fibroosseous lesions that differed histologically from osteofibrous dysplasia and fibrous dysplasia. They proposed the term ossifying fibroma for these, suggesting that the term osteofibrous dysplasia continue to be used for lesions of the tibia and fibula (Kempson-Campanacci lesions). To avoid confusion in terminology, the differential features of the various lesions are summarized in Table 19.1.

A relationship of osteofibrous dysplasia with fibrous dysplasia and adamantinoma has been suggested by some investigators. Although this remains a controversial matter, adamantinoma—a malignant tumor—may contain a fibroosseous component that on pathologic examination resembles both fibrous and osteofibrous dysplasia. Moreover, in recent years, patients have presented with lesions that contained foci of epithelial tissue corresponding to adamantinoma within areas of osteofibrous dysplasia. Czerniak and associates have termed such lesions *differentiated (regressing) adamantinomas*. According to these investigators, features characteristic of differentiated adamantinomas include onset during the first two decades of life, an exclusively intracortical location, uniform predominance of osteofibrous dysplasia, and scattered foci of epithelial elements that are identical to those observed in classic adamantinoma. This suggests that a single disease entity may exhibit a spectrum of manifestations with benign osteofibrous dysplasia at one end of the spectrum and malignant adamantinoma at the other end.

Complications and Treatment

Osteofibrous dysplasia is known to be an aggressive lesion that frequently recurs after local excision. According to some researchers, it may coexist with another very aggressive lesion, adamantinoma (see previous discussion).

Desmoplastic Fibroma

Clinical and Imaging Features

Desmoplastic fibroma (also called *intraosseous desmoid tumor*) is a rare, locally aggressive tumor that occurs in individuals younger than age 40 years, with 50% of all cases occurring in the patient's second decade. It was first described as a distinct entity in 1958 by H. Jaffe. Pain and local swelling are the most common symptoms, but some patients may be asymptomatic. The long bones (femur, tibia, fibula, humerus, and radius), the pelvis, and the mandible are frequent sites of involvement (Fig. 19.60). In the long bones, the lesion occurs in the diaphysis but often extends into the metaphysis. Although the epiphysis is spared, the lesion may extend into the articular end of the bone after closure of the growth plate.

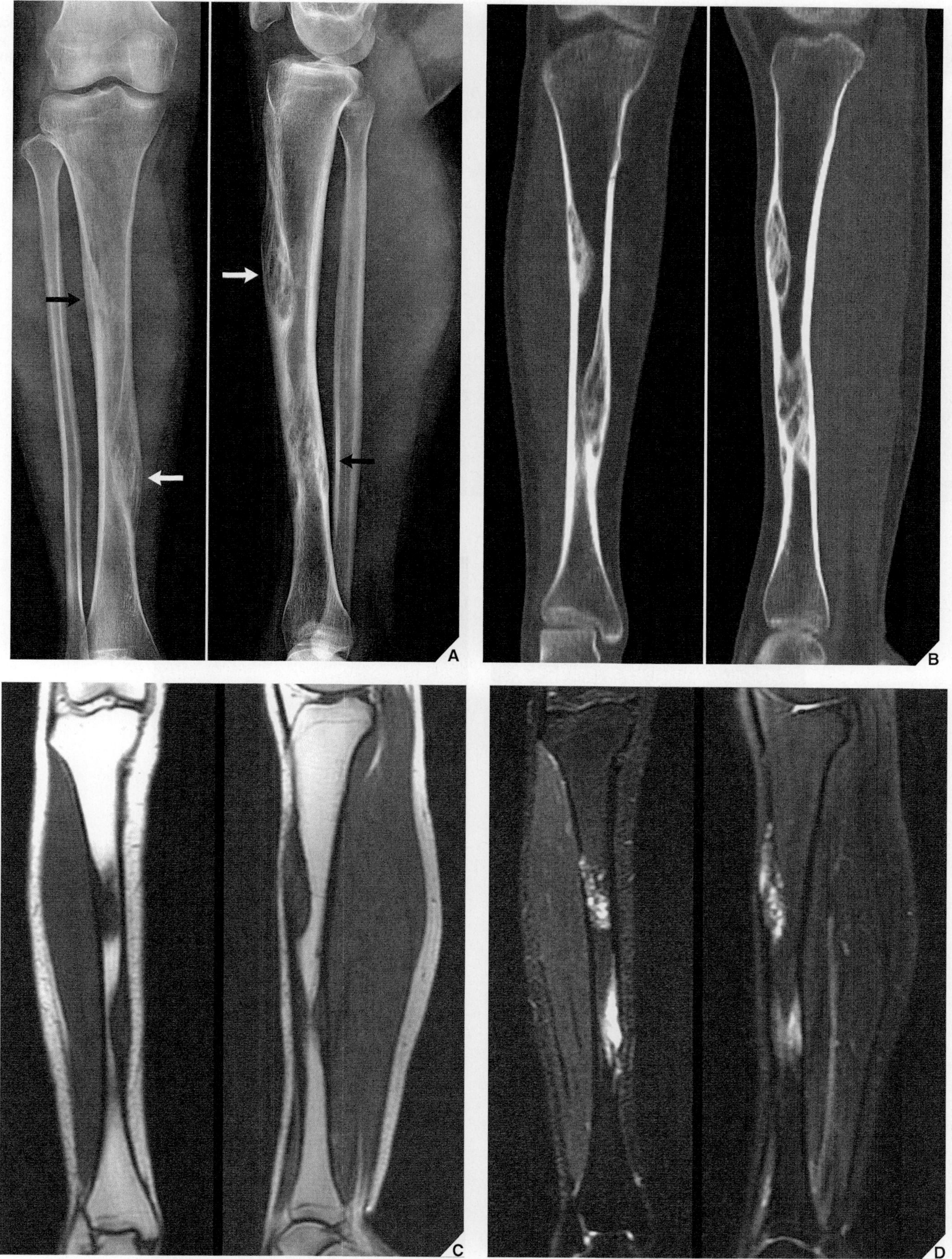

FIGURE 19.57 CT and MRI of osteofibrous dysplasia. **(A)** Anteroposterior and lateral radiographs of the right leg of a 14-year-old girl show fusiform in shape, trabeculated, predominantly cortical lesions affecting diaphysis of the tibia *(arrows)*. **(B)** Coronal and sagittal reformatted CT images demonstrate sharply demarcated mixed high- and low-attenuated lesions without evidence of periosteal reaction or soft-tissue mass. **(C)** Coronal and sagittal T1-weighted and **(D)** STIR MR images show the lesions exhibiting signal intensities similar to those of fibrous dysplasia.

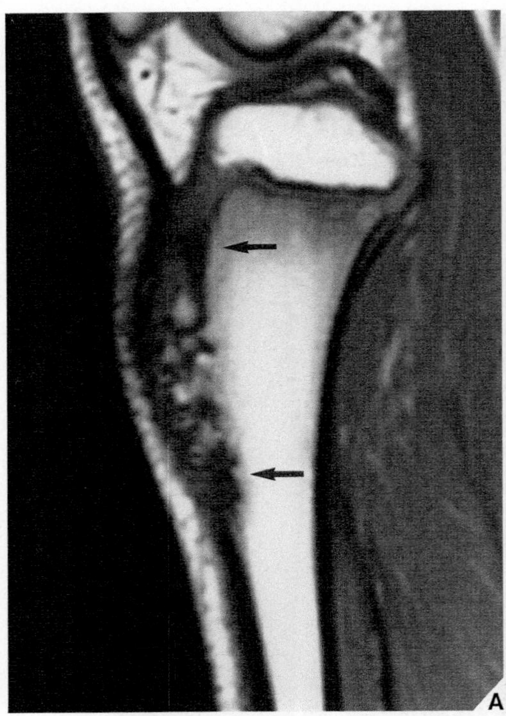
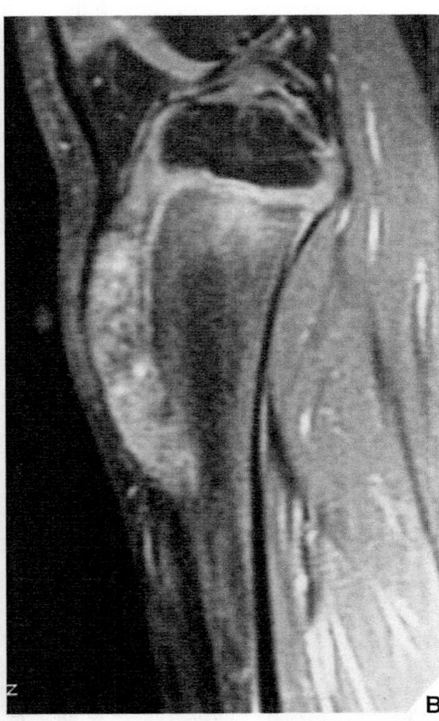

FIGURE 19.58 MRI of osteofibrous dysplasia. **(A)** Sagittal T1-weighted image shows an oblong lesion involving the anterior cortex of tibia, exhibiting heterogenous signal intensity *(arrows)*. **(B)** Sagittal T1-weighted fat-suppressed sequence obtained after intravenous injection of gadolinium shows significant enhancement of the lesion.

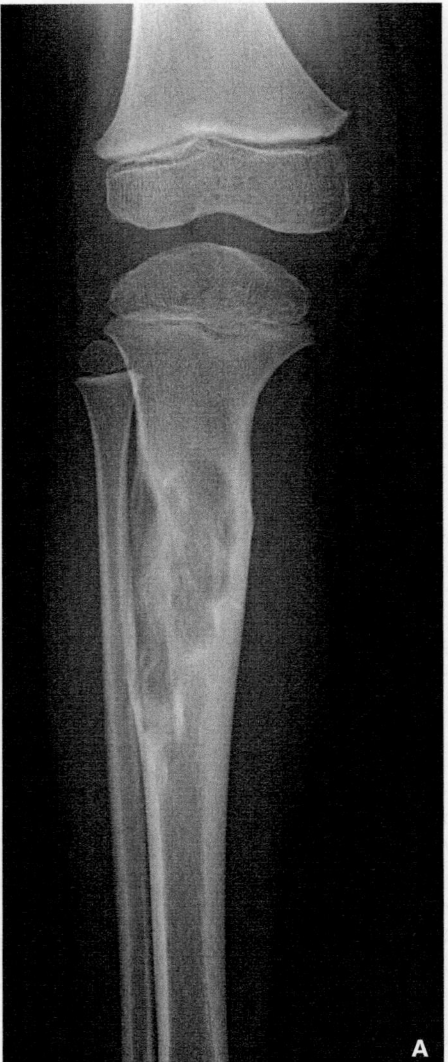
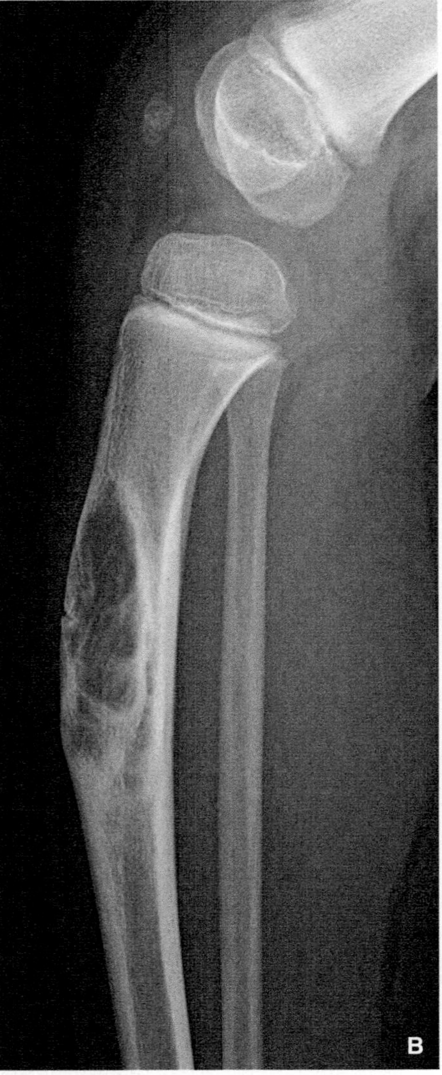

FIGURE 19.59 MRI of osteofibrous dysplasia. **(A)** Anteroposterior and **(B)** lateral radiographs of the right leg of a 6-year-old boy show a lobulated radiolucent lesion with sclerotic border in the anterior aspect of the tibial diaphysis. Observe characteristic anterior bowing of the tibia. *(Continued)*

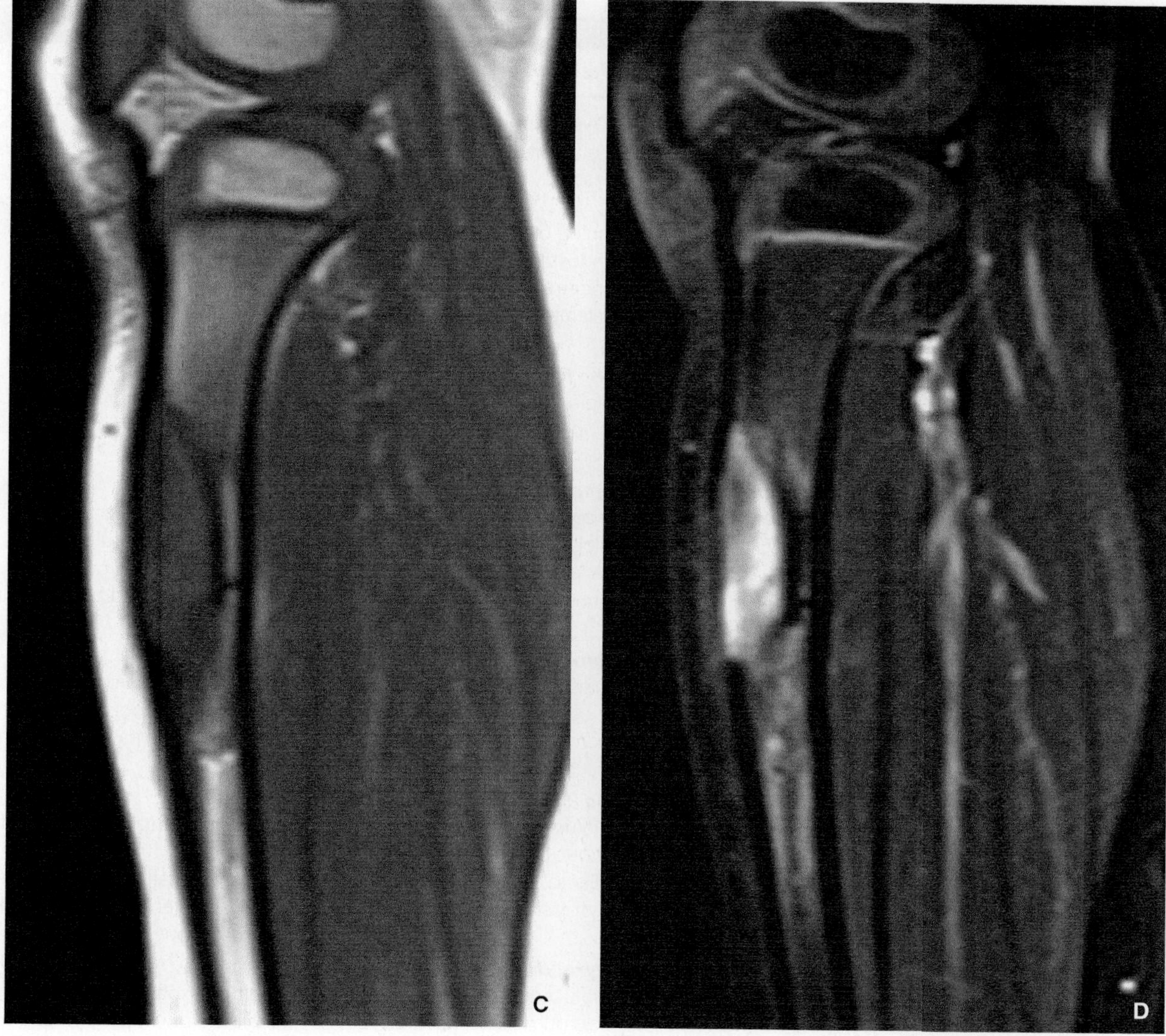

FIGURE 19.59 MRI of osteofibrous dysplasia. ***(Continued)*** **(C)** Sagittal T1-weighted MR image shows the lesion to be of intermediate signal intensity displaying a low–signal intensity sclerotic border. **(D)** Sagittal T1-weighted fat-saturated MR image obtained after intravenous administration of gadolinium shows significant enhancement of the lesion.

TABLE 19.1 Differential Features of Various Fibroosseous Lesions with Similar Radiographic Appearance

Sex	Age	Location	Radiographic Appearance	Histopathology
		Fibrous Dysplasia		
M/F	Any age (monostotic)	Femoral neck (frequent)	Radiolucent, ground-glass, or smoky lesion	Woven (nonlamellar) type of bone in loose to dense fibrous stroma; bony trabeculae lacking osteoblastic activity (naked trabeculae)
	First to third decades (polyostotic)	Long bones Pelvis Ends of bones usually spared Polyostotic: unilateral in skeleton	Thinning of cortex with endosteal scalloping Shepherd's crook deformity Accelerated growth	
		Nonossifying Fibroma		
M/F	First to third decades	Long bones (frequently posterior femur)	Radiolucent, eccentric lesion Scalloped, sclerotic border	Whorled pattern of fibrous tissue containing giant cells, hemosiderin, and lipid-filled histiocytes
		Osteofibrous Dysplasia (Kempson-Campanacci Lesion)		
M/F	First to second decades	Tibia (frequently anterior aspect) Fibula Intracortical (frequent)	Osteolytic, eccentric lesion Scalloped, sclerotic border Anterior bowing of long bone	Woven and mature (lamellar) type of bone surrounded by cellular fibrous spindle cell growth in whorled or matted pattern; bony trabeculae rimmed by osteoblasts (dressed trabeculae)
		Ossifying Fibroma of Jaw		
F	Third to fourth decades	Mandible (90%) Maxilla	Expansive radiolucent lesion Sclerotic, well-defined borders	Uniformly cellular fibrous spindle cell growth with varying amounts of lamellar bone formation and small, round cementum-like bodies
		Ossifying Fibroma (Sissons Lesion)		
M/F	Second decade	Tibia Humerus	Radiolucent lesion Sclerotic border Similar to osteofibrous dysplasia	Fibrous tissue containing rounded and spindle-shaped cells with scant intercellular collagen and small, partially calcified spherules resembling cementum-like bodies of ossifying fibroma of jaw
		Liposclerosing Myxofibrous Tumor		
M/F	Second to seventh decades	Intertrochanteric region of femur	Radiolucent or partially sclerotic lesion with well-defined sclerotic border, occasionally central matrix mineralization	Fibrous or myxofibrous areas with metaplastic curvilinear or circular woven bone ossicles and/or dystrophic mineralization in necrotic fat

M, male; F, female.

Recent cytogenetic and fluorescence in situ hybridization studies showed chromosome 11q13 breakpoint in desmoplastic fibroma of bone.

Desmoplastic fibroma has no characteristic radiographic features. The lesion is generally expansive and radiolucent, with sharply defined borders (Fig. 19.61); the cortex of the bone may be thickened or thinned, with no significant periosteal response. Usually, a geographic pattern of bone destruction is noted, with narrow zones of transition and nonsclerotic margins (76%). Internal pseudotrabeculation is present in 90% of cases (Figs. 19.62 and 19.63). Pathologic fractures through the tumor are rare (9%) (see Fig. 19.62B). Aggressive lesions of this type are marked by bone destruction and invasion of the soft tissues and may simulate malignant bone tumors (Fig. 19.64).

In addition to conventional radiography, radiologic evaluation of desmoplastic fibroma should include bone scintigraphy, CT, and MRI. Radionuclide bone scan shows an increase in the uptake of the radiopharmaceutical agent at the site of the lesion. CT is useful for evaluating cortical breakthrough and tumor extension into the soft tissues (see Fig.19.63C). MRI, also helpful in assessing intraosseous and extraosseous extension, can further characterize the tumor (Fig. 19.65; see also Fig. 19.63D). The lesion appears well defined on MR images, exhibiting an intermediate signal intensity on T1 weighting and a heterogeneous pattern on T2 weighting, marked by an area of increased signal intensity mixed with foci of intermediate and low signal intensity. The hypointensity of the signal reflects the dense connective tissue matrix and relative acellularity of the tumor. After intravenous administration of gadolinium contrast, a majority of the lesions demonstrate heterogenous enhancement, with peripheral areas enhancing more intensely than the central portions of the tumor.

Pathology

Histologically, the lesion is composed of spindle-shaped and occasionally stellate fibroblasts associated with a densely collagenized matrix. Cells are almost always in a smaller proportion to the matrix. The stroma usually contains large, thin-walled vessels similar to those seen in desmoid tumors of soft tissues. Desmoplastic fibroma may be difficult to distinguish from other fibrous tumors, particularly low-grade fibrosarcoma.

Treatment

Wide excision is the treatment of choice, although the recurrence rate is high even after complete excision of the tumor. Despite this aggressiveness, metastases have never been reported.

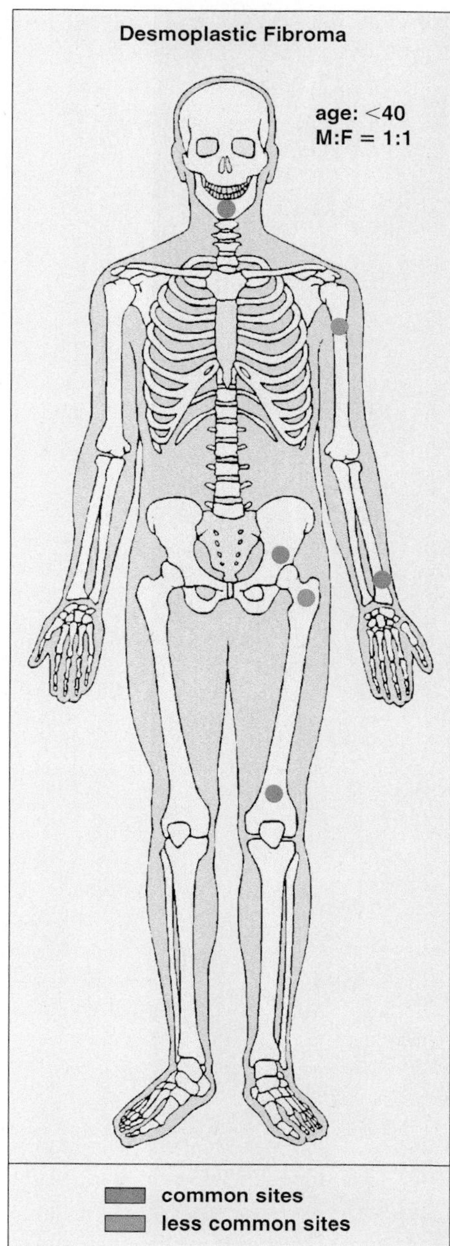

FIGURE 19.60 **Skeletal sites of predilection, peak age range, and male-to-female ratio in desmoplastic fibroma.**

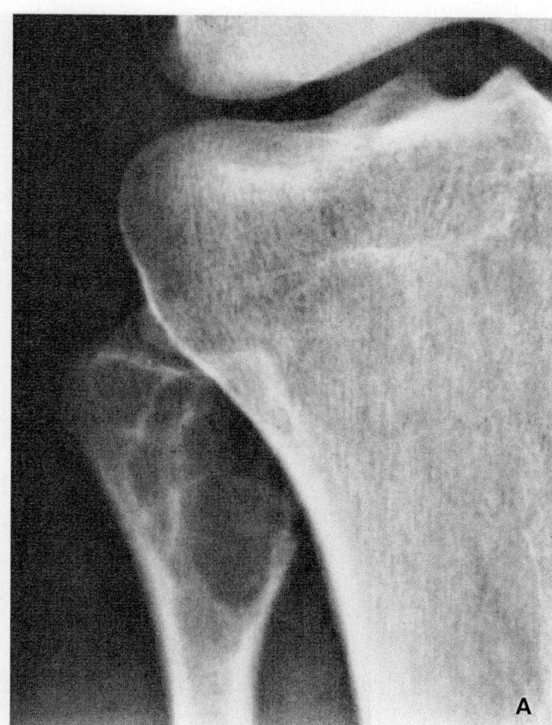

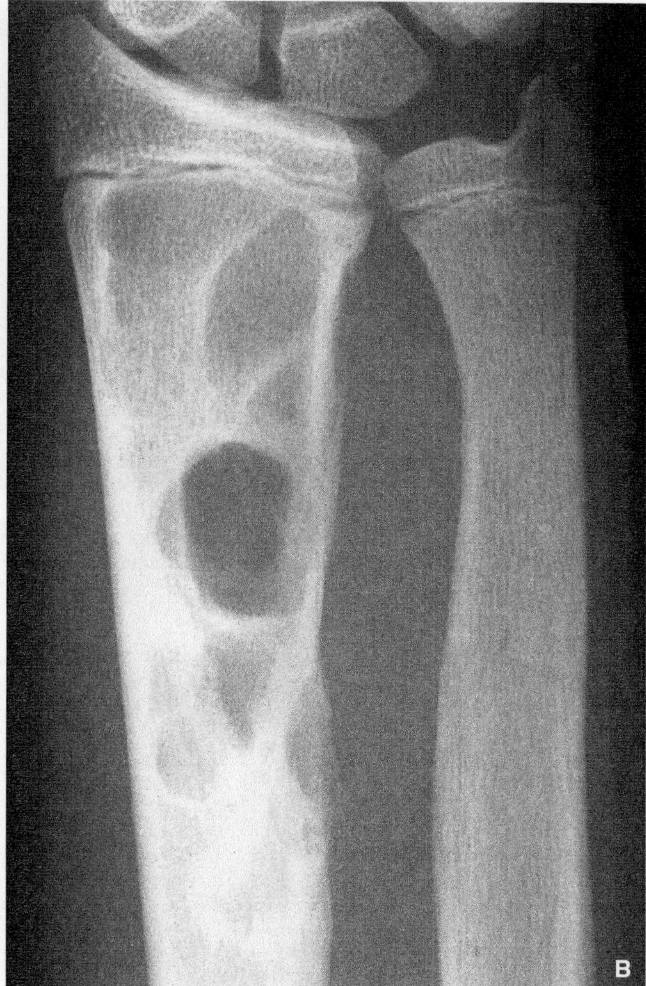

FIGURE 19.61 **Desmoplastic fibroma.** **(A)** Radiolucent, trabeculated, sharply marginated lesion occupies the proximal end of the right fibula in a 17-year-old girl. Note lack of periosteal reaction. **(B)** Radiolucent trabeculated lesion is present in the metadiaphyseal region of the distal radius of a 15-year-old boy. (**B**, Reprinted with permission from Greenspan A, Borys D. *Radiology and pathology correlation of bone tumors: a quick reference and review*. Philadelphia: Wolters Kluwer; 2016:215.)

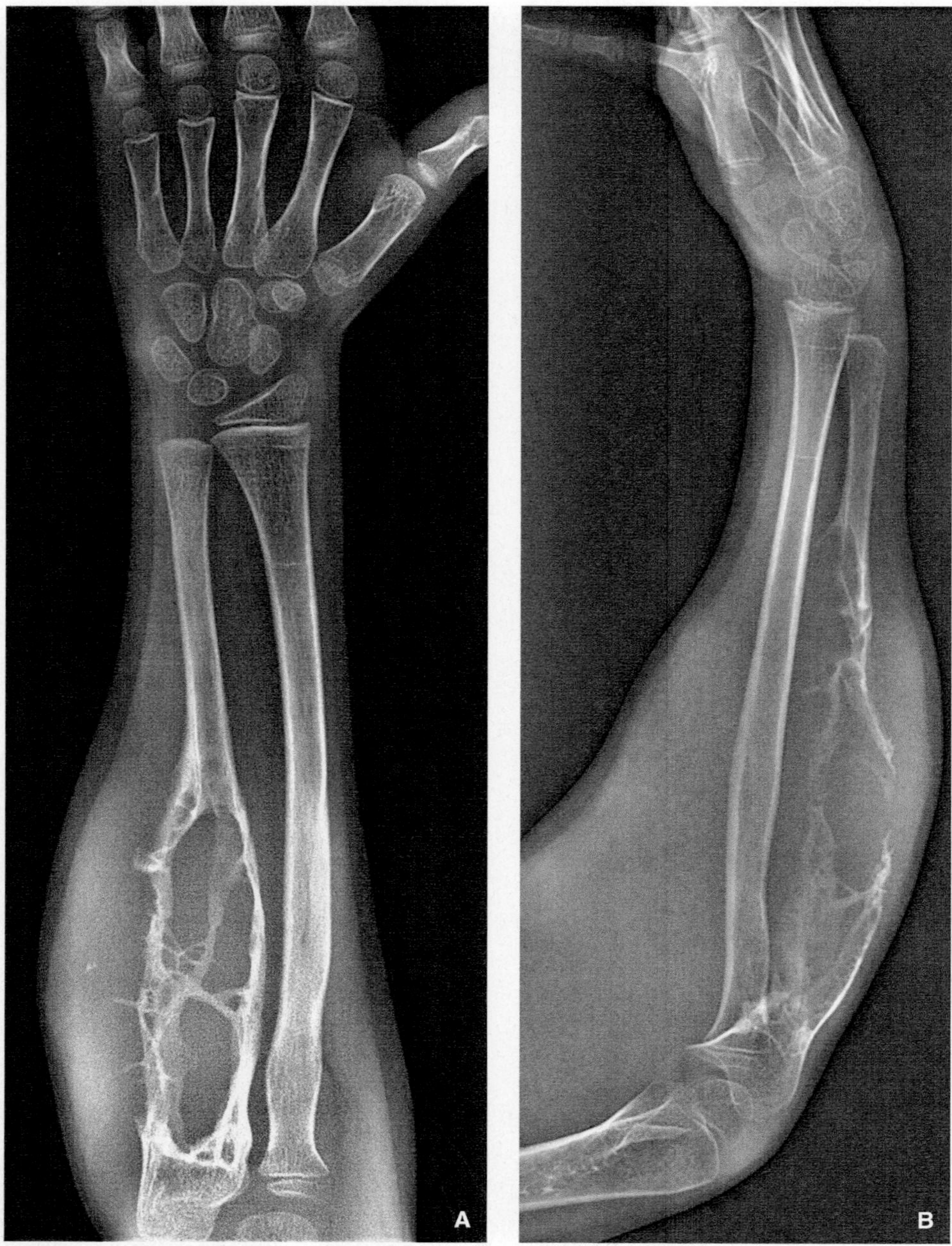

FIGURE 19.62 Desmoplastic fibroma. **(A)** Anteroposterior and **(B)** lateral radiographs of the left forearm of an 8-year-old boy show aggressive osteolytic, expansive, trabeculated lesion in the proximal ulna. Note a pathologic fracture of the posterior cortex and soft-tissue extension of the tumor.

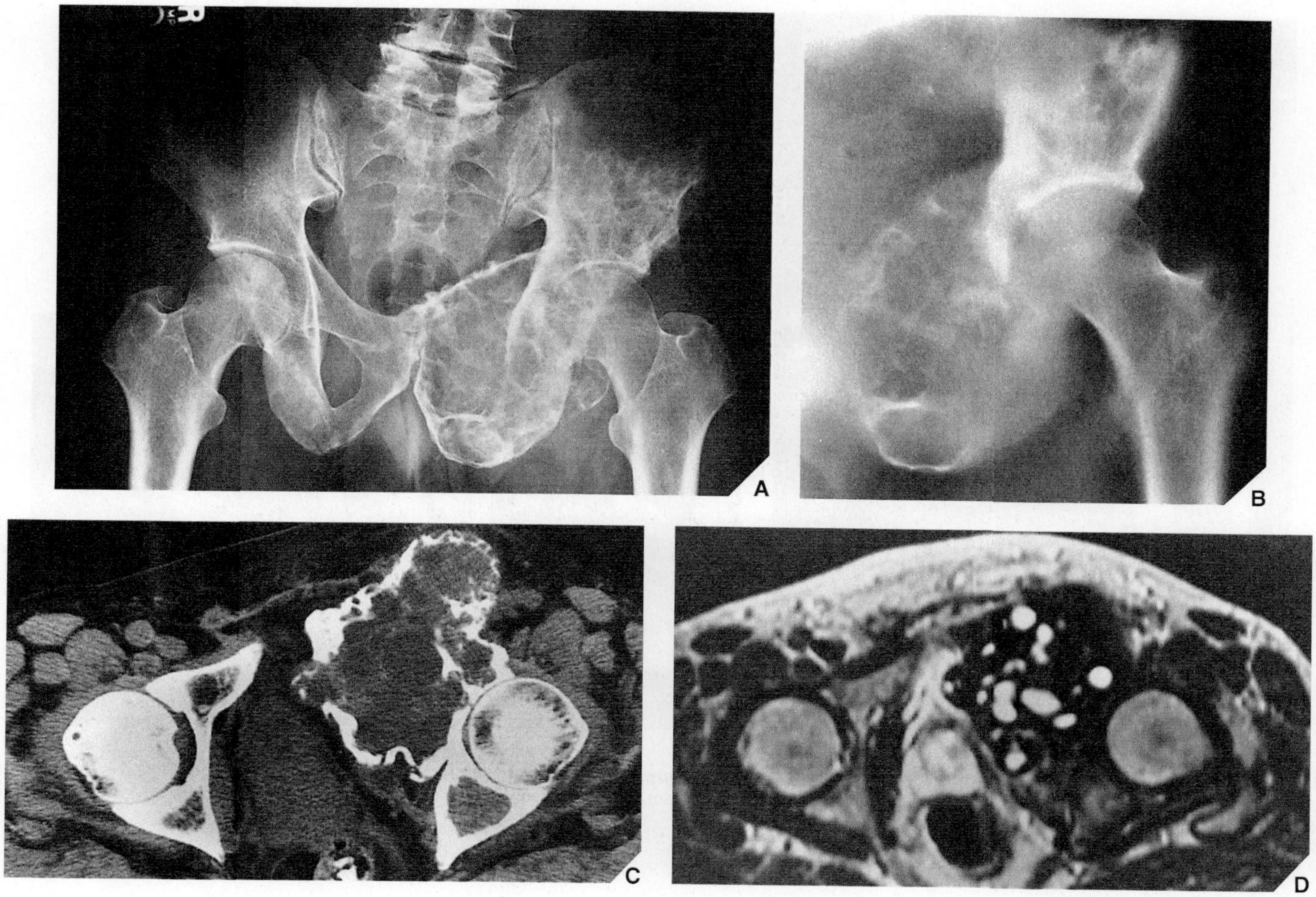

FIGURE 19.63 CT and MRI of desmoplastic fibroma. A 67-year-old man presented with a large pelvic mass. **(A)** Anteroposterior radiograph of the pelvis demonstrates an expansive trabeculated lytic lesion that involves ischium and pubis and extends into the supraacetabular portion of the ilium. **(B)** Conventional tomography confirms the lytic nature of the tumor and its expansive character. The involvement of ilium is better demonstrated. **(C)** CT section through the hip joint shows a lobulated appearance of the tumor and a thick, sclerotic margin. The lesion extends into the pelvic cavity, displacing the urinary bladder. **(D)** Axial spin echo T2-weighted MR image (repetition time [TR] 2000/echo time [TE] 80 msec) demonstrates heterogeneity of the signal from the tumor: The bulk of the lesion displays low-to-intermediate signal intensity with central areas of high signal intensity. An incision biopsy revealed desmoplastic fibroma. (Reprinted with permission from Greenspan A, Jundt G, Remagen W. *Differential diagnosis in orthopaedic oncology*, 2nd ed. Philadelphia: Lippincott Williams & Wilkins; 2007:299.)

FIGURE 19.64 Desmoplastic fibroma. **(A)** Anteroposterior and **(B)** lateral radiographs of the distal forearm in a 31-year-old woman show aggressive destructive lesions involving the radius and ulna, extending into the articular surfaces, complicated by pathologic fractures *(arrows)*. Excision biopsy followed by histopathologic examination confirmed the diagnosis.

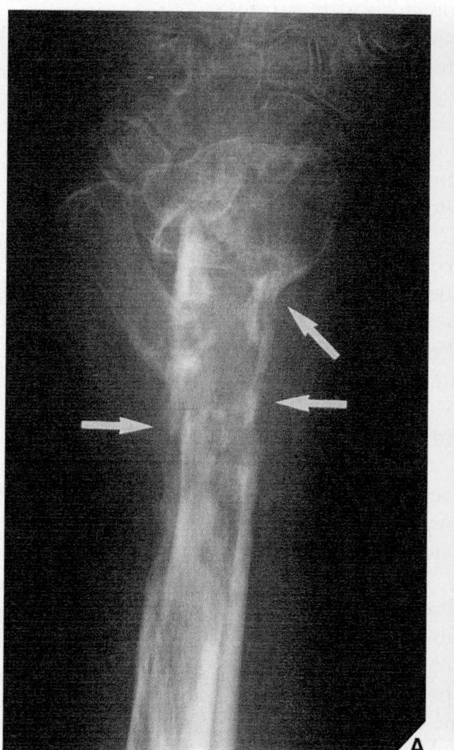

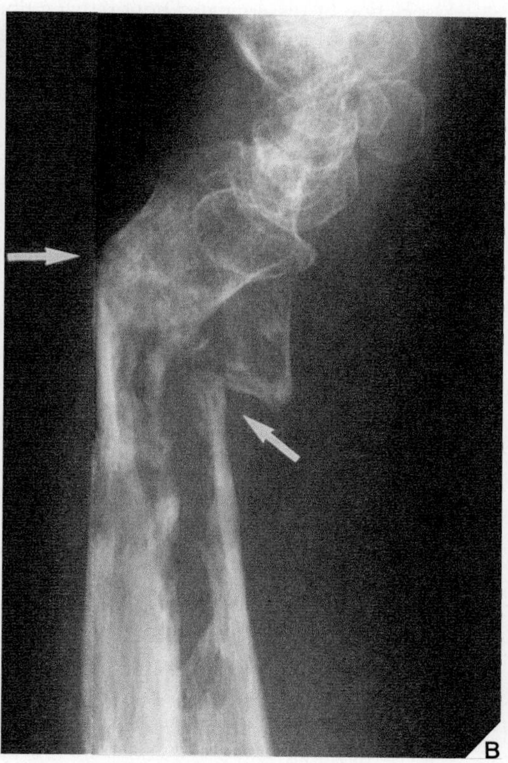

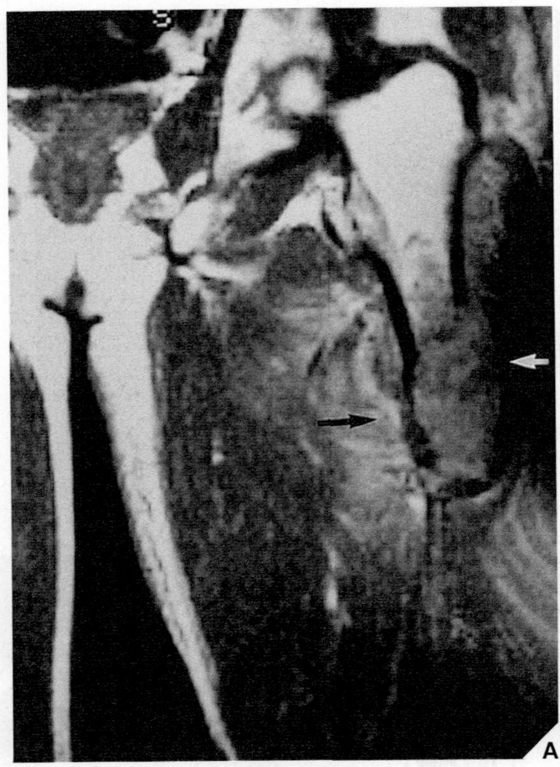

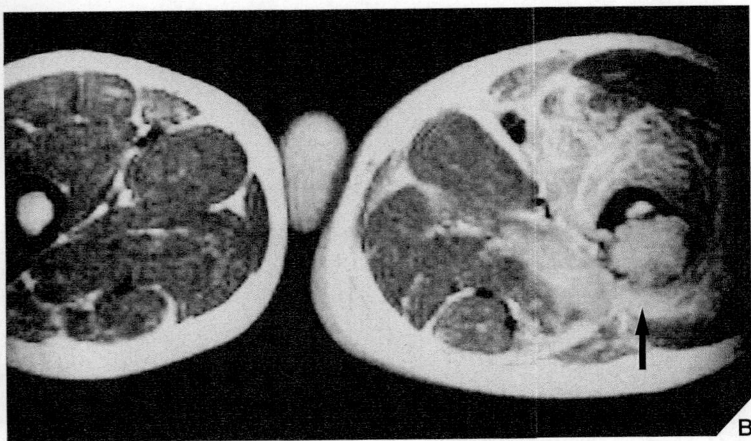

FIGURE 19.65 MRI of desmoplastic fibroma. **(A)** Coronal T1-weighted MRI shows the tumor in the left femoral shaft breaking through the cortex and extending into the soft tissues *(arrows)*. **(B)** Axial proton density MR image demonstrates replacement of the bone marrow by the tumor *(arrow)*, soft-tissue involvement, and peritumoral edema. (Courtesy of Prof. Wolfgang Remagen, Cologne, Germany.)

PRACTICAL POINTS TO REMEMBER

1. A fibrous cortical defect (metaphyseal fibrous defect) and nonossifying fibroma are closely related lesions of similar histopathologic structure. They differ radiologically only in their size.
2. Most of these lesions disappear spontaneously. With continued growth, they are eccentrically located and display a characteristic scalloped sclerotic border.
3. Association of disseminated nonossifying fibromatosis with café-au-lait spots is known as the *Jaffe-Campanacci syndrome*.
4. Benign fibrous histiocytoma has radiographic features similar to those of nonossifying fibroma; however, it affects older patients, may be symptomatic, and runs a more aggressive clinical course (may recur after surgical treatment).
5. Periosteal desmoid has a characteristic predilection for the posteromedial cortex of the medial femoral condyle. It should not be mistaken for a malignant bone tumor.
6. Fibrous dysplasia may be monostotic or polyostotic, with the latter having a decided preference for one side of the skeleton. The polyostotic form, if accompanied by precocious puberty and café-au-lait spots (with irregular, ragged, or "coast of Maine" borders), is called *McCune-Albright syndrome* and is seen predominantly in girls.
7. Association of polyostotic fibrous dysplasia with intramuscular myxomas is known as the *Mazabraud syndrome*.
8. Massive formation of cartilage may be observed in fibrous dysplasia, a condition known as *fibrocartilaginous dysplasia*. This variant can radiographically resemble a cartilaginous neoplasm, such as chondrosarcoma.
9. Fibrocartilaginous dysplasia (cartilaginous differentiation in fibrous dysplasia) should not be confused with focal fibrocartilaginous dysplasia of long bones, a condition seen predominantly in children and young adults that characteristically affects the proximal tibia.
10. The best radiologic technique for evaluating the distribution of fibrous dysplasia and its activity is radionuclide bone scan.
11. Osteofibrous dysplasia, a benign fibroosseous lesion seen in children and adolescents, has a decided predilection for the anterior aspect of the tibia. This lesion may be associated with adamantinoma.
12. Desmoplastic fibroma, a locally aggressive tumor, is frequently marked by bone destruction and invasion of the soft tissues, thus mimicking a malignant neoplasm.

SUGGESTED READINGS

Albright F, Butler AM, Hampton AO, et al. Syndrome characterized by osteitis fibrosa disseminata, areas of pigmentation and endocrine dysfunction with precocious puberty in females. *N Engl J Med* 1937;216:727–731.

Bahk W-J, Kang Y-K, Lee A-H, et al. Desmoid tumor of bone with enchondromatous nodules, mistaken for chondrosarcoma. *Skeletal Radiol* 2003;32:223–226.

Bancroft LW, Kransdorf MJ, Menke DM, et al. Intramuscular myxoma: characteristic MR imaging features. *AJR Am J Roentgenol* 2002;178:1255–1259.

Barnes GR Jr, Gwinn JL. Distal irregularities of the femur simulating malignancy. *Am J Roentgenol Radium Ther Nucl Med* 1974;122:180–185.

Bertoni F, Calderoni P, Bacchini P, et al. Benign fibrous histiocytoma of bone. *J Bone Joint Surg Am* 1986;68:1225–1230.

Bertoni F, Calderoni P, Bacchini P, et al. Desmoplastic fibroma of bone. A report of six cases. *J Bone Joint Surg Br* 1984;66:265–268.

Bridge JA, Dembinski A, DeBoer J, et al. Clonal chromosomal abnormalities in osteofibrous dysplasia. Implications for histopathogenesis and its relationship with adamantinoma. *Cancer* 1994;73:1746–1752.

Brower AC, Culver JE Jr, Keats TE. Histological nature of the cortical irregularity of the medial posterior distal femoral metaphysis in children. *Radiology* 1971;99:389–392.

Bufkin WJ. The avulsive cortical irregularity. *Am J Roentgenol Radium Ther Nucl Med* 1971;112:487–492.

Cabral CE, Guedes P, Fonseca T, et al. Polyostotic fibrous dysplasia associated with intramuscular myxomas: Mazabraud's syndrome. *Skeletal Radiol* 1998;27:278–282.

Camilleri AE. Craniofacial fibrous dysplasia. *J Laryngol Otol* 1991;105:662–666.

Campanacci M. Osteofibrous dysplasia of the long bones a new clinical entity. *Ital J Orthop Traumatol* 1976;2:221–237.

Campanacci M, Laus M, Boriani S. Multiple non-ossifying fibromata with extraskeletal anomalies: a new syndrome? *J Bone Joint Surg Br* 1983;65:627–632.

Choi IH, Kim CJ, Cho T-J, et al. Focal fibrocartilaginous dysplasia of long bones: report of eight additional cases and literature review. *J Pediatr Orthop* 2000;20:421–427.

Cohen DM, Dahlin DC, Pugh DG. Fibrous dysplasia associated with adamantinoma of the long bones. *Cancer* 1962;15:515–521.

Crim JR, Gold RH, Mirra JM, et al. Desmoplastic fibroma of bone: radiographic analysis. *Radiology* 1989;172:827–832.

Czerniak B, Rojas-Corona RR, Dorfman HD. Morphologic diversity of long bone adamantinoma. The concept of differentiated (regressing) adamantinoma and its relationship to osteofibrous dysplasia. *Cancer* 1989;64:2319–2334.

Daffner RH, Kirks DR, Gehweiler JA Jr, et al. Computed tomography of fibrous dysplasia. *AJR Am J Roentgenol* 1982;139:943–948.

Dahlin DC, Unni KK. *Bone tumors: general aspects and data on 8,542 cases*, 4th ed. Springfield, IL: Charles C. Thomas, 1986:141–148.

DiCaprio MR, Enneking WF. Fibrous dysplasia. Pathophysiology, evaluation, and treatment. *J Bone Joint Surg Am* 2005;87:1848–1864.

Dorfman HD, Ishida T, Tsuneyoshi M. Exophytic variant of fibrous dysplasia (fibrous dysplasia protuberans). *Hum Pathol* 1994;25:1234–1237.

Dreizin D, Glenn C, Jose J. Mazabraud syndrome. *Am J Orthop (Belle Mead NJ)* 2012;41: 332–335.

Endo M, Kawai A, Kobayashi E, et al. Solitary intramuscular myxoma with monostotic fibrous dysplasia as a rare variant of Mazabraud's syndrome. *Skeletal Radiol* 2007;36:523–529.

Flanagan AM, Delaney D, O'Donnell P. Benefits of molecular pathology in the diagnosis of musculoskeletal disease. Part II of a two-part review: bone tumors and metabolic disorders. *Skeletal Radiol* 2010;39:213–224.

Fletcher CDM, Unni KK, Mertens E, eds. *World Health Organization classification of tumours of soft tissues and bone*. Lyon, France: IARC Press; 2013:352–365.

Greenspan A, Borys D. *Radiology and pathology correlation of bone tumors: a quick reference and review*. Philadelphia: Wolters Kluwer; 2016:180–218.

Greenspan A, Jundt G, Remagen W. *Differential diagnosis in orthopaedic oncology*, 2nd ed. Philadelphia: Lippincott Williams & Wilkins; 2007.

Greenspan A, Unni KK. Case report 787: desmoplastic fibroma. *Skeletal Radiol* 1993;22:296–299.

Gross ML, Soberman N, Dorfman HD, et al. Case report 556: multiple non-ossifying fibromas of long bones in a patient with neurofibromatosis. *Skeletal Radiol* 1989;18: 389–391.

Hamada T, Ito H, Araki Y, et al. Benign fibrous histiocytoma of the femur: review of three cases. *Skeletal Radiol* 1996;25:25–29.

Henschen F. Fall von Osteitis fibrosa mit multiplen Tumoren in der umgebenden Muskulatur. *Verh Dtsch Ges Pathol* 1926;21:93–97.

Hermann G, Klein M, Abdelwahab IF, et al. Fibrocartilaginous dysplasia. *Skeletal Radiol* 1996;25:509–511.

Hoshi H, Futami S, Ohnishi T, et al. Gallium-67 uptake in fibrous dysplasia of the bone. *Ann Nucl Med* 1990;4:35–38.

Inamo Y, Hanawa Y, Kin H, et al. Findings on magnetic resonance imaging of the spine and femur in a case of McCune-Albright syndrome. *Pediatr Radiol* 1993;23:15–18.

Inwards CY, Unni KK, Beabout JW, et al. Desmoplastic fibroma of bone. *Cancer* 1991;68:1978–1983.

Ishida T, Dorfman HD. Massive chondroid differentiation in fibrous dysplasia of bone (fibrocartilaginous dysplasia). *Am J Surg Pathol* 1993;17:924–930.

Iwasko N, Steinbach LS, Disler D, et al. Imaging findings in Mazabraud's syndrome: seven new cases. *Skeletal Radiol* 2002;31:81–87.

Jaffe HL. Fibrous cortical defect and non-ossifying fibroma. In: *Tumors and tumorous conditions of the bones and joints*. Philadelphia: Lea & Febiger; 1958:76–91.

Jaffe HL, Lichtenstein L. Non-osteogenic fibroma of bone. *Am J Pathol* 1942;18:205–221.

Jee W-H, Choe B-Y, Kang H-S, et al. Nonossifying fibroma: characteristics at MR imaging with pathologic correlation. *Radiology* 1998;209:197–202.

Jee W-H, Choi K-H, Choe B-Y, et al. Fibrous dysplasia: MR imaging characteristics with radiopathologic correlation. *AJR Am J Roentgenol* 1996;167:1523–1527.

Kahn LB. Adamantinoma, osteofibrous dysplasia and differentiated adamantinoma. *Skeletal Radiol* 2003;32:245–258.

Kaushik S, Smoker WRK, Frable WJ. Malignant transformation of fibrous dysplasia into chondroblastic osteosarcoma. *Skeletal Radiol* 2002;31:103–106.

Kempson RL. Ossifying fibroma of the long bones. A light and electron microscopic study. *Arch Pathol* 1966;82:218–233.

Khanna M, Delaney D, Tirabosco R, et al. Osteofibrous dysplasia, osteofibrous dysplasia-like adamantinoma, and adamantinoma: correlation of radiological imaging features with surgical histology and assessment of the use of radiology in contributing to needle biopsy diagnosis. *Skeletal Radiol* 2008;37:1077–1084.

Kransdorf MJ, Murphey MD. Diagnosis please. Case 12: Mazabraud syndrome. *Radiology* 1999;212:129–132.

Kransdorf MJ, Murphey MD, Sweet DE. Liposclerosing myxofibrous tumor: a radiologic-pathologic-distinct fibro-osseous lesion of bone with a marked predilection for the intertrochanteric region of the femur. *Radiology* 1999;212:693–698.

Kumar R, Madewell JE, Lindell MM, et al. Fibrous lesions of bones. *Radiographics* 1990;10:237–256.

Kyriakos M, McDonald DJ, Sundaram M. Fibrous dysplasia with cartilaginous differentiation ("fibrocartilaginous dysplasia"): a review, with an illustrative case followed for 18 years. *Skeletal Radiol* 2004;33:51–62.

Lichtenstein L. Polyostotic fibrous dysplasia. *Arch Surg* 1938;36:874–898.

Lichtenstein L, Jaffe HL. Fibrous dysplasia of bone. *Arch Pathol* 1942;33:777–816.

Luna A, Martinez S, Bossen E. Magnetic resonance imaging of intramuscular myxoma with histological comparison and a review of the literature. *Skeletal Radiol* 2005;34:19–28.

Machida K, Makita K, Nishikawa J, et al. Scintigraphic manifestation of fibrous dysplasia. *Clin Nucl Med* 1986;11:426–429.

Matsuno T. Benign fibrous histiocytoma involving the ends of long bone. *Skeletal Radiol* 1990;19:561–566.

Mazabraud A, Semat P, Roze R. A propos de l'association de fibromyxomes des tissus mous à la dysplasie fibreuse des os. *Presse Med* 1967;75:2223–2228.

McCune DJ. Progress in pediatrics: osteodystrophia fibrosa. *Arch Pediatr Adolesc Med* 1937;54:806.

Mertens F, Romeo S, Bovée JV, et al. Reclassification and subtyping of so-called malignant fibrous histiocytoma of bone: comparison with cytogenetic features. *Clin Sarcoma Res* 2011;1:10.

Mirra JM, Gold RH. Fibrous dysplasia. In: Mirra JM, Picci P, Gold RH, eds. *Bone tumors*. Philadelphia: Lea & Febiger; 1989:191–226.

Mirra JM, Gold RH, Rand F. Disseminated nonossifying fibromas in association with café-au-lait spots (Jaffe-Campanacci syndrome). *Clin Orthop Relat Res* 1982;(168):192–205.

Mulder JD, Schütte HE, Kroon HM, et al. *Radiologic atlas of bone tumors*. Amsterdam, Netherlands: Elsevier; 1993:607–625.

Okubo T, Saito T, Takagi T, et al. Desmoplastic fibroma of the rib with cystic change: a case report and literature review. *Skeletal Radiol* 2014;43:703–708.

Park Y, Unni KK, McLeod RA, et al. Osteofibrous dysplasia: clinicopathologic study of 80 cases. *Hum Pathol* 1993;24:1339–1347.

Ragsdale BD. Polymorphic fibro-osseous lesions of bone: an almost site-specific diagnostic problem of the proximal femur. *Hum Pathol* 1993;24:505–512.

Riley GM, Greenspan A, Poirier VC. Fibrous dysplasia of a parietal bone. *J Comput Assist Tomogr* 1997;21:41–43.

Ruggieri P, Sim FH, Bond JA, et al. Malignancies in fibrous dysplasia. *Cancer* 1994;73: 1411–1424.

Schajowicz F. *Tumors and tumorlike lesions of bone. Pathology, radiology, and treatment*, 2nd ed. Berlin, Germany: Springer-Verlag; 1994.

Schajowicz F, Sissons HA, Sobin LH. The World Health Organization's histologic classification of bone tumors. A commentary on the second edition. *Cancer* 1995;75:1208–1214.

Singnurkar A, Phancao JP, Chatha DS, et al. The appearance of Mazabraud's syndrome on 18F-FDG PET/CT. *Skeletal Radiol* 2007;36:1085–1089.

Sissons HA, Kancherla PL, Lehman WB. Ossifying fibroma of bone. Report of two cases. *Bull Hosp Jt Dis Orthop Inst* 1983;43:1–14.

Springfield DS, Rosenberg AE, Mankin HJ, et al. Relationship between osteofibrous dysplasia and adamantinoma. *Clin Orthop Relat Res* 1994;309:234–244.

Stewart DR, Brems H, Gomes AG, et al. Jaffe-Campanacci syndrome, revisited: detailed clinical and molecular analyses determine whether patients have neurofibromatosis type 1, coincidental manifestations, or a distinct disorder. *Genet Med* 2014;16:448–459.

Sweet DE, Vinh TN, Devaney K. Cortical osteofibrous dysplasia of long bone and its relationship to adamantinoma. A clinicopathologic study of 30 cases. *Am J Surg Pathol* 1992;16:282–290.

Trombetta D, Macchia G, Mandahl N, et al. Molecular genetic characterization of the 11q13 breakpoint in a desmoplastic fibroma of bone. *Cancer Genet* 2012;205:410–413.

Ueda Y, Blasius S, Edel G, et al. Osteofibrous dysplasia of long bones—a reactive process to adamantinomatous tissue. *J Cancer Res Clin Oncol* 1992;118:152–156.

Yamazaki T, Maruoka S, Takahashi S, et al. MR findings of avulsive cortical irregularity of the distal femur. *Skeletal Radiol* 1995;24:43–46.

Zoccali C, Teori G, Erba F. Mazabraud's syndrome: a new case and review of the literature. *Int Orthop* 2009;33:605–610.

20

Benign Tumors and Tumor-like Lesions IV

Miscellaneous Lesions

Simple Bone Cyst

Clinical and Imaging Features

The simple bone cyst (SBC), also called a *unicameral bone cyst*, is a tumor-like lesion of unknown cause, representing approximately 3% of all primary bone lesions. It has been attributed to a local disturbance of bone growth. Although the pathogenesis is still unclear, SBC appears to be reactive or developmental rather than represent a true neoplasm. More common in males than in females, it is ordinarily seen during the first two decades of life. The majority of SBCs are located in the proximal diaphysis of the humerus and femur, especially in patients younger than age 17 years. In older patients, the incidence of bone cysts in atypical sites such as the calcaneus, talus, and ilium increases significantly (Fig. 20.1). The clinical symptoms include pain, swelling, or stiffness at the nearest joint. A pathologic fracture is often the first sign of the lesion. Radiographically, SBC appears as a radiolucent, centrally located, well-circumscribed lesion with sclerotic margins (Figs. 20.2 to 20.6). There is no periosteal reaction, a feature distinguishing an SBC from an aneurysmal bone cyst (ABC), which invariably shows some degree of periosteal response; however, in the presence of pathologic fracture, there is periosteal reaction. Conventional radiography usually suffices to make a diagnosis. Magnetic resonance imaging (MRI) of SBC shows the signal characteristics of fluid: a low-to-intermediate signal on T1-weighted images and a bright, homogeneous signal on T2 weighting (Figs. 20.7 and 20.8).

Pathology

Cadaveric specimens of SBC demonstrate well-demarcated cystic cavity with glistening membrane and occasionally thin grayish in color fragments (Fig. 20.9). Histologically, however, SBC is a diagnosis of exclusion. A surgical curettage yields almost no solid tissue, but the walls of the cavity may show remnants of fibrous tissue or a flattened single-cell lining. The fluid content of the cyst contains elevated levels of alkaline phosphatase.

Complications and Differential Diagnosis

The most common complication of SBC is pathologic fracture, which occurs in approximately 66% of cases. Occasionally, one can identify a piece of fractured cortex in the interior of the lesion—the "fallen fragment" sign (Fig. 20.10)—indicating that the lesion is either hollow or fluid filled, as most SBCs are. This sign permits the differentiation of a bone cyst, particularly in a slender bone, such as the fibula (Fig. 20.11), from other radiolucent, radiographically similar lesions containing solid fibrous or cartilaginous tissue, such as fibrous dysplasia, nonossifying fibroma (Fig. 20.12), or enchondroma. A bone abscess may occasionally mimic an SBC, particularly if located in the proximal humerus or proximal femur, the sites of predilection for SBCs. In such cases, the presence of a periosteal reaction and extension beyond the growth plate are important differentiating features favoring a bone abscess (Fig. 20.13). On rare occasions, an intraosseous ganglion may be mistaken for an SBC (Fig. 20.14).

Treatment

The treatment of SBCs is based on the premise that the induction of osteogenesis results in complete healing of the lesion. The simplest inducement for bone repair is fracture, but this alone is insufficient to obliterate the lesion completely, and SBCs usually do not disappear after spontaneous fracture. The most common treatment is curettage followed by grafting with small pieces of cancellous bone. With this procedure, however, there is a higher rate of recurrence in patients younger than age 10 years. Moreover, this approach may lead to damage to the growth plate because most solitary bone cysts occur about the physis. Some time ago, Scaglietti et al. reported treating bone cysts with simple injection of methylprednisolone acetate. In younger patients so treated, complete bone repair occurred more rapidly than in older patients, who sometimes had to be administered several injections.

Aneurysmal Bone Cyst

Clinical and Imaging Features

The term *ABC* was first used by Jaffe and Lichtenstein to describe two examples of blood-filled cyst in which tissue from the cyst wall contained conspicuous spaces, areas of hemosiderin deposition, giant cells, and occasional bone trabeculae. In a subsequent publication, Jaffe chose the designation *ABC* as a descriptive term for this lesion to emphasize the blown-out appearance. Although the cause of this lesion is unknown, alterations in local hemodynamics related to venous obstruction or arteriovenous fistula are believed to play an important role. Some investigators believe that the lesion is caused by a trauma. Dahlin and McLeod postulated that it may be similar to and related to other reactive nonneoplastic processes, such as giant cell reparative granuloma or traumatic reactions observed in periosteum and bone. ABC may arise *de novo* in bone, in which case no recognizable preexisting lesion can be demonstrated in the tissue, or it may

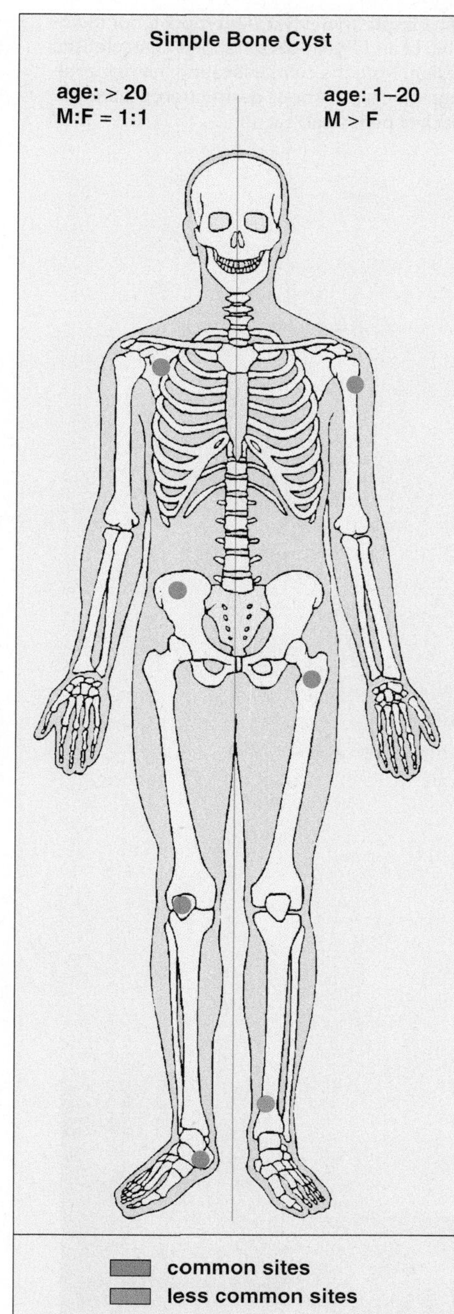

FIGURE 20.1 **Skeletal sites of predilection, peak age range, and male-to-female ratio in SBC.** The left half of the skeleton shows unusual sites of occurrence seen in an older patient population.

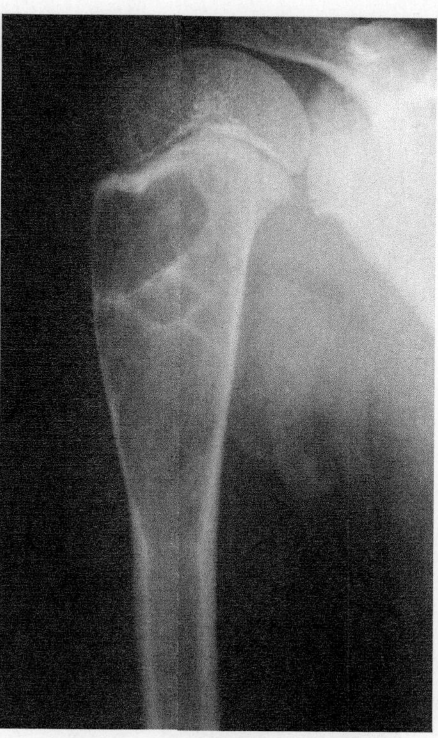

FIGURE 20.2 **Simple bone cyst.** Anteroposterior radiograph of the right proximal humerus demonstrates the typical appearance of an SBC in a 6-year-old boy. Its location in the metaphysis and the proximal diaphysis of the humerus is also characteristic. The radiolucent lesion is centrally located and shows pseudosepta. Note the slight thinning of the cortex and lack of periosteal reaction.

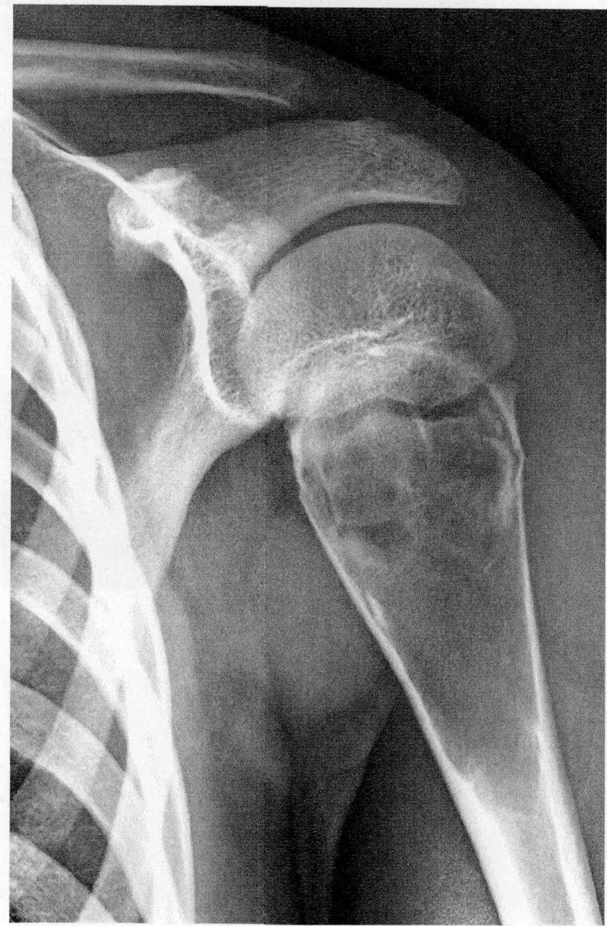

FIGURE 20.3 **Simple bone cyst.** Anteroposterior radiograph of the left shoulder of a 12-year-old boy shows a centrally located radiolucent lesion in the metadiaphysis of the humerus. The cortex is thin, and there is lack of periosteal reaction.

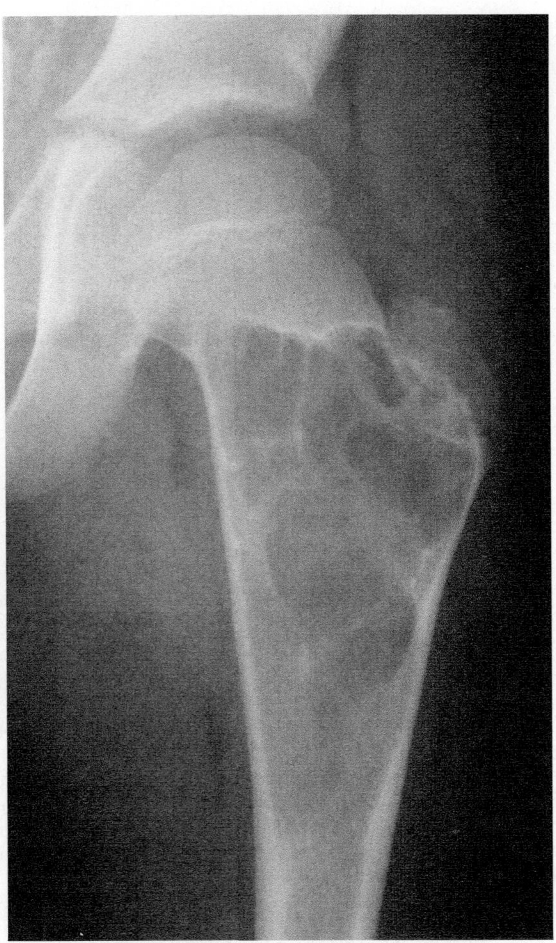

FIGURE 20.4 Simple bone cyst. Anteroposterior radiograph of the left hip of an 11-year-old girl shows characteristic features of this lesion. Note the central location, narrow zone of transition, geographic type of bone destruction, pseudotrabeculation, and lack of periosteal reaction.

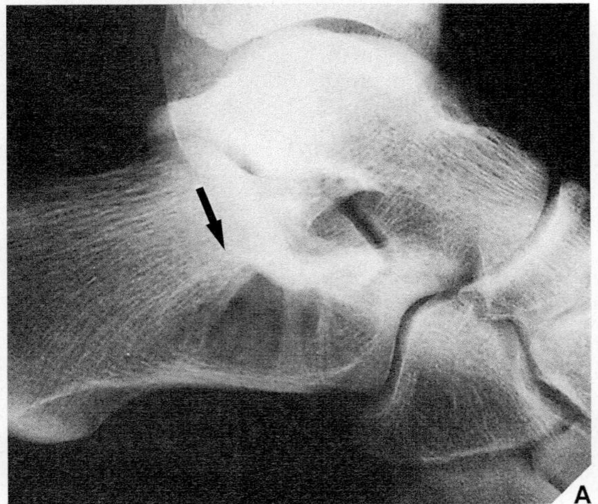

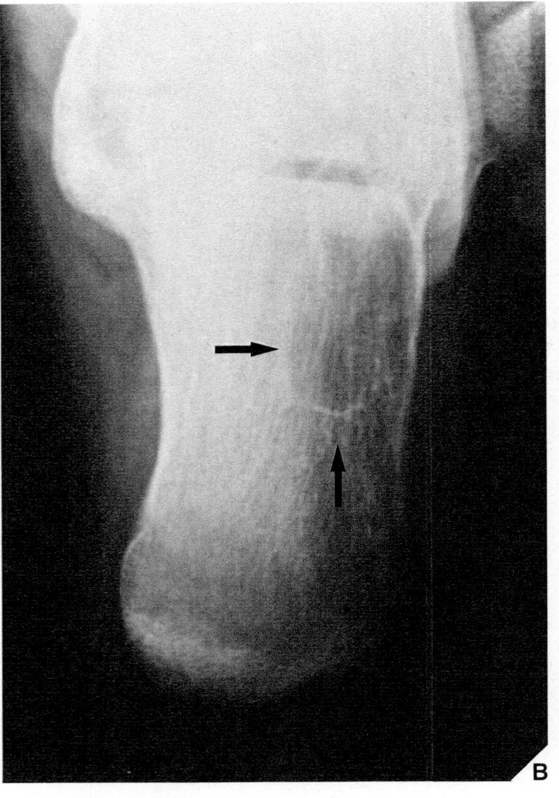

FIGURE 20.5 Simple bone cyst. **(A)** Lateral radiograph of the left hindfoot and **(B)** Harris-Beath view of the calcaneus of a 32-year-old man show an SBC in the os calcis *(arrows)*. Typically, bone cysts occurring at this site are located in the anterolateral aspect of the bone, as shown here.

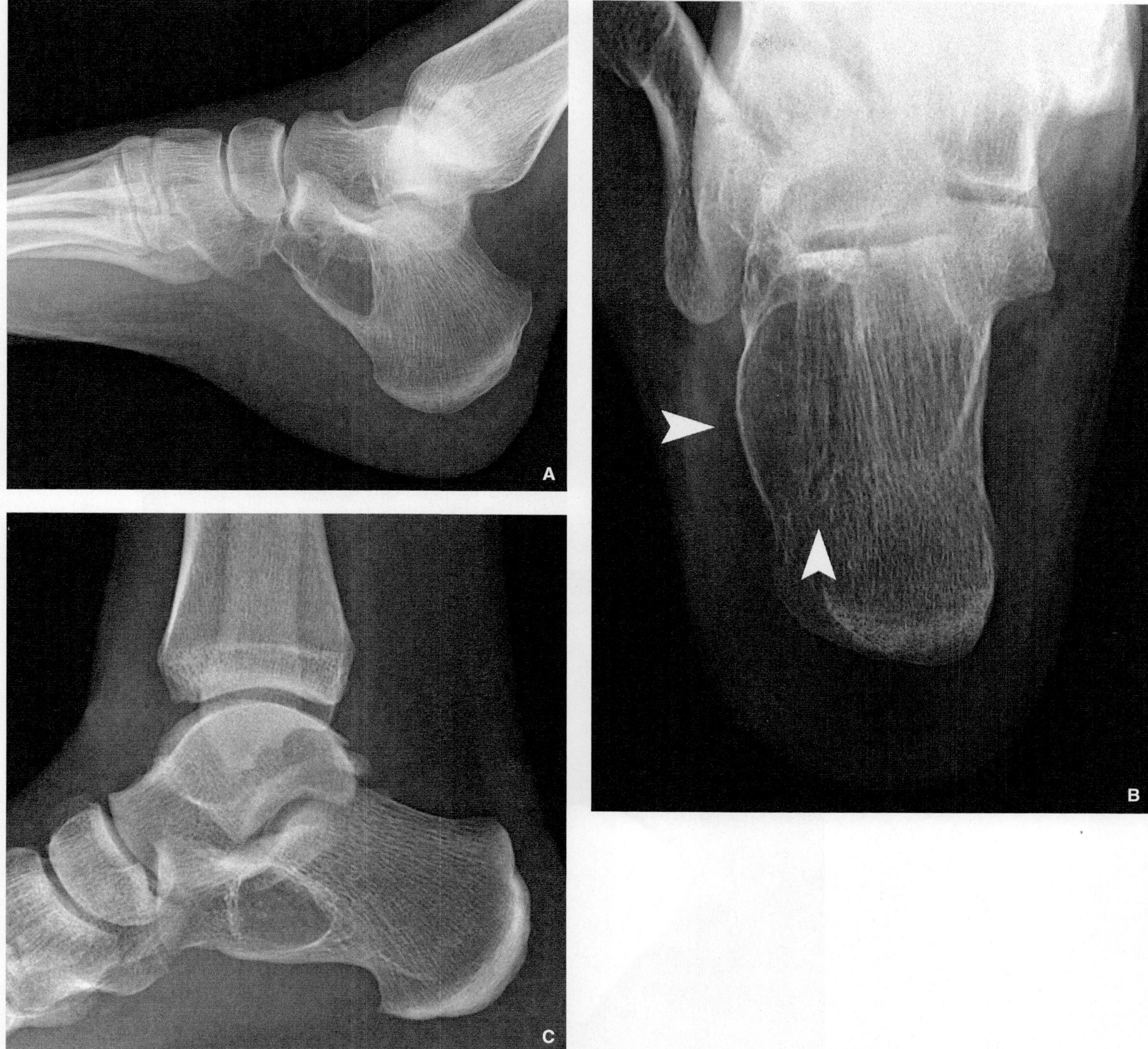

FIGURE 20.6 Simple bone cyst. **(A)** Lateral and **(B)** Harris-Beath views of the right hindfoot of a 35-year-old woman show a radiolucent lesion in the anterolateral aspect of the calcaneus *(arrowheads)*. **(C)** Lateral radiograph of the hindfoot of a 20-year-old man shows a similar radiolucent lesion in the anterior calcaneus exhibiting a narrow zone of transition and a thin sclerotic border.

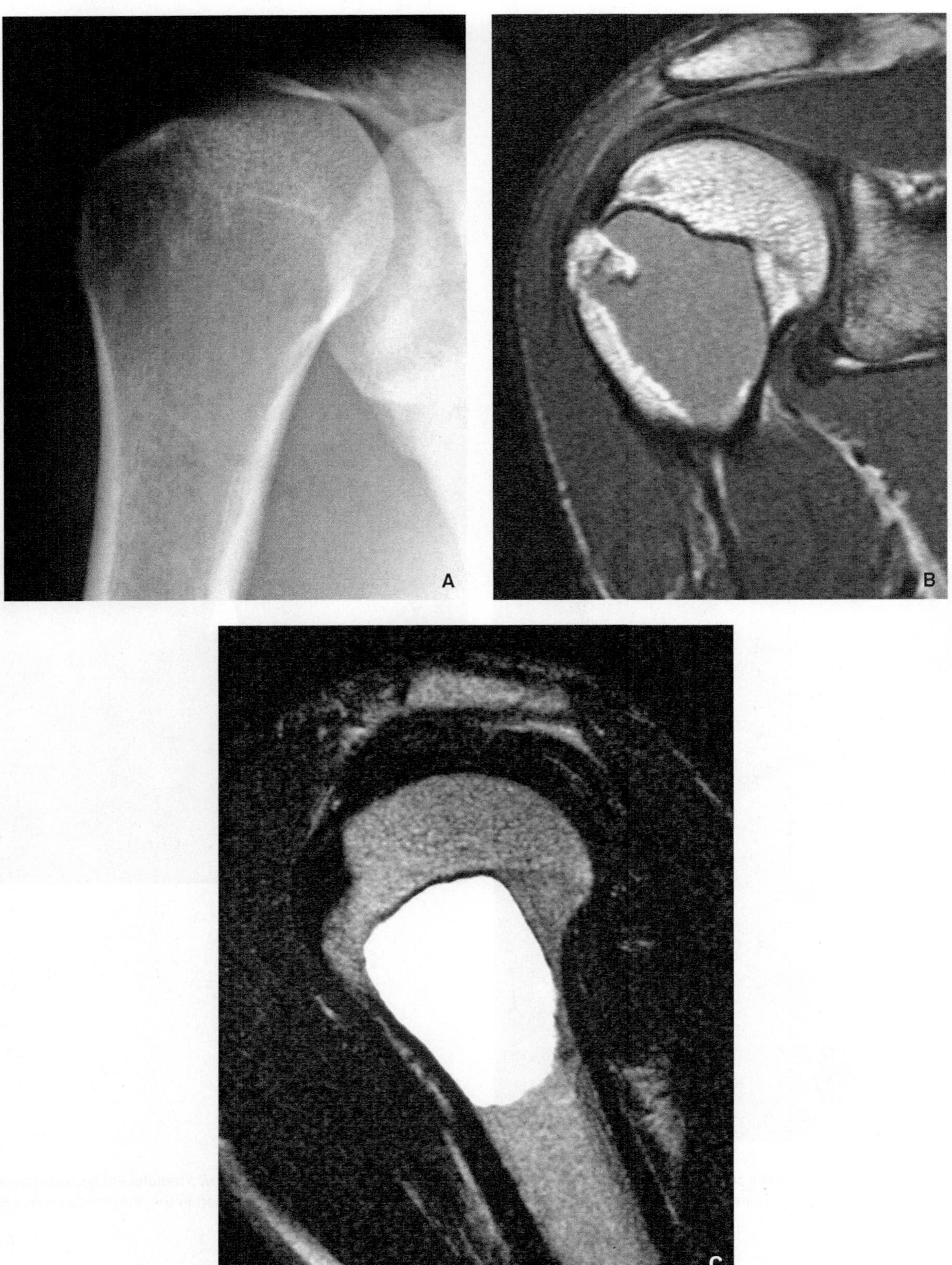

FIGURE 20.7 MRI of SBC. **(A)** Anteroposterior radiograph of the right shoulder of a 22-year-old man shows a radiolucent lesion with a narrow zone of transition in the proximal humeral shaft, abutting a scarred growth plate. **(B)** Coronal T1-weighted MR image shows the lesion to be of homogeneous intermediate signal intensity. **(C)** Sagittal T2-weighted MR image demonstrates homogeneous high signal intensity of the fluid-filled cyst. (Reprinted with permission from Greenspan A, Borys D. *Radiology and pathology correlation of bone tumors: a quick reference and review*. Philadelphia: Wolters Kluwer; 2016:313–314.)

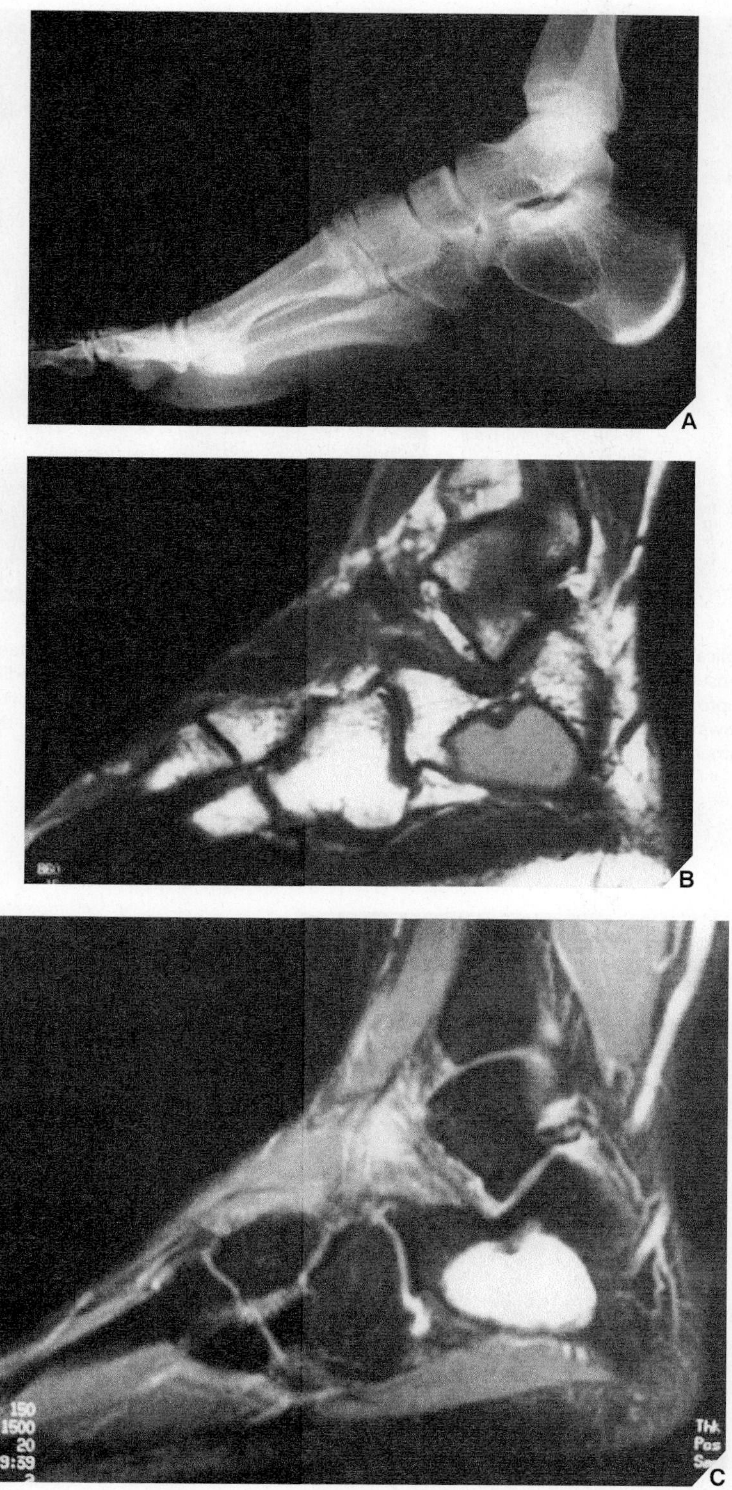

FIGURE 20.8 MRI of SBC. **(A)** Lateral radiograph of the foot of an 18-year-old man shows a radiolucent lesion in the calcaneus with a slightly sclerotic border. **(B)** Sagittal T1-weighted (spin echo [SE]; repetition time [TR] 850/echo time [TE] 15 msec) MR image demonstrates homogeneous intermediate signal intensity within the lesion, rimmed by low–signal intensity sclerotic margin. **(C)** Sagittal short time inversion recovery (STIR) MR image shows that the lesion now is of homogeneous high signal intensity. (Reprinted with permission from Greenfield GB, Arrington JA. *Imaging of bone tumors*. Philadelphia: JB Lippincott; 1995:217–218.)

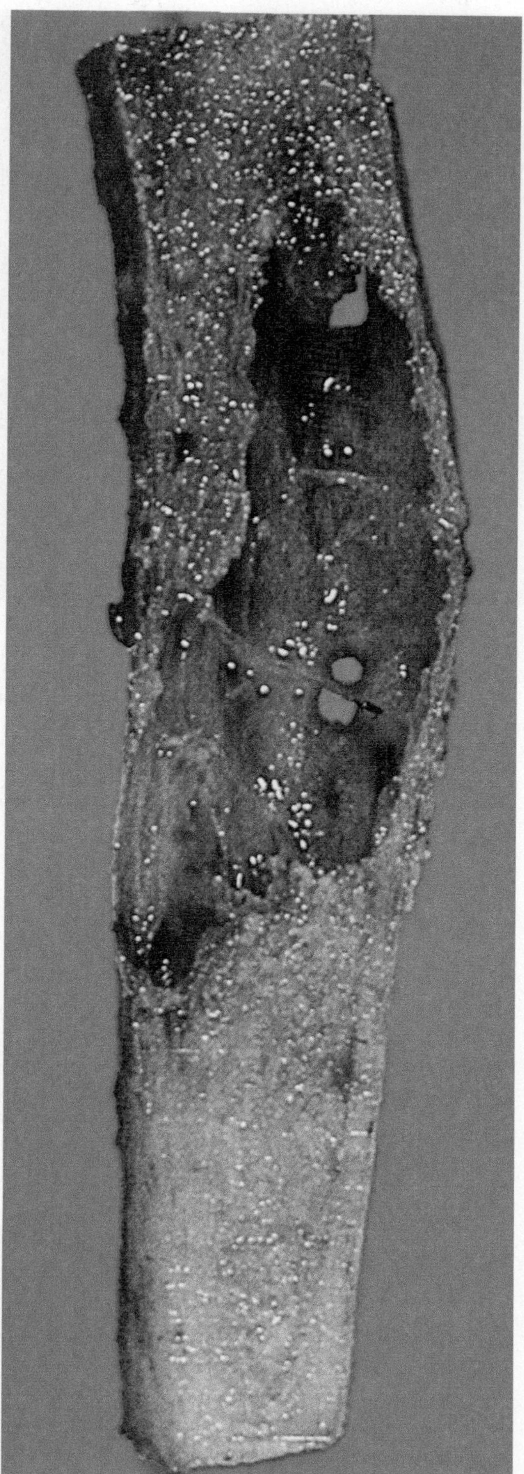

FIGURE 20.9 Pathology of SBC. Coronal section of gross specimen of the proximal humerus reveals a well-demarcated cystic cavity in the medullary portion of the bone. Observe cortical thinning and glistening lining of the cyst. (Reprinted from Bullough P. *Orthopaedic pathology*, 5th ed. Maryland Heights, MO: Mosby; 2009, with permission from Elsevier.)

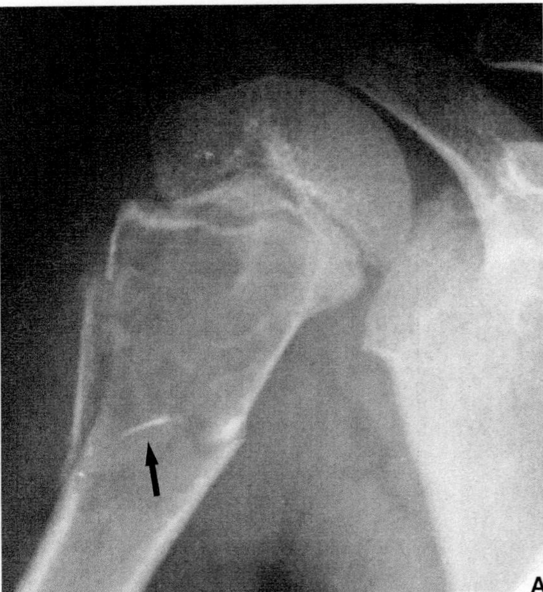

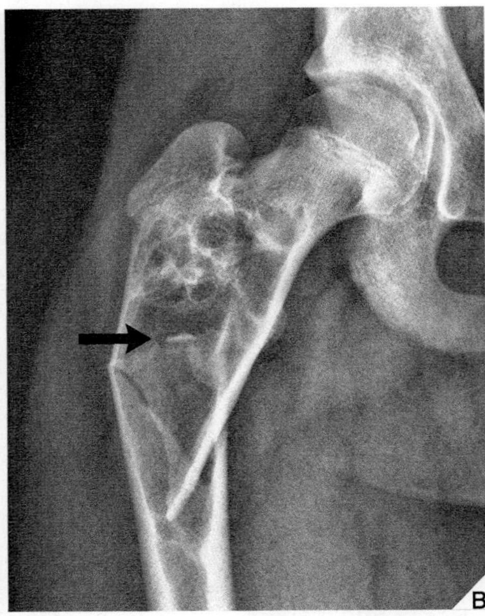

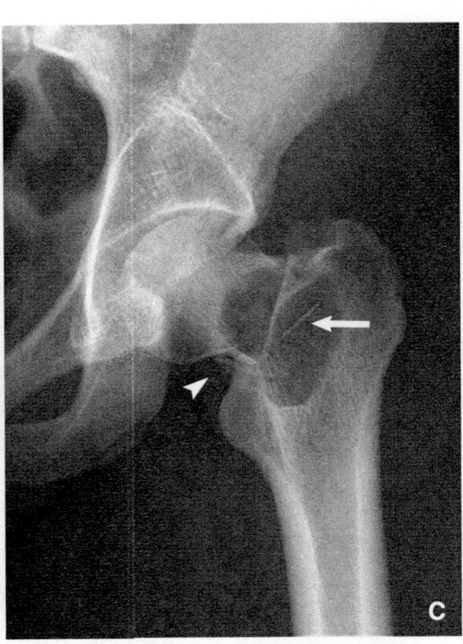

FIGURE 20.10 SBC with pathologic fracture. **(A)** One of the most common complications of SBC is pathologic fracture, as seen here in the proximal humeral metadiaphysis in a 6-year-old boy. The presence of the fallen fragment sign *(arrow)* is characteristic of this lesion. **(B)** In another patient, an 11-year-old girl, anteroposterior radiograph of the right hip shows sharply marginated radiolucent trabeculated lesion in the proximal femoral diaphysis with a pathologic fracture. An *arrow* points to the fallen fragment sign. **(C)** Anteroposterior radiograph of the left hip of a 20-year-old woman shows a radiolucent lesion in the intertrochanteric area of the femur extending into the femoral neck. The cyst had fractured *(arrowhead)*, and the *arrow* points to the fallen fragment sign.

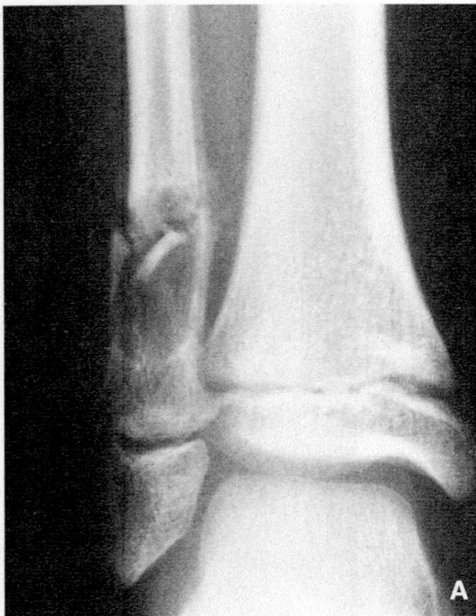

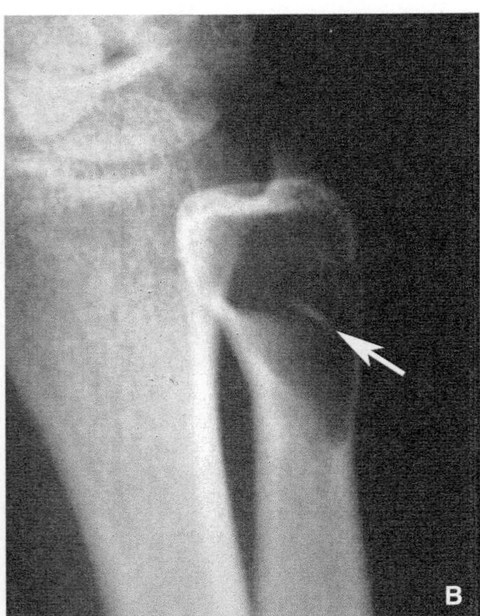

FIGURE 20.11 Fallen-fragment sign. **(A)** Anteroposterior radiograph demonstrates a radiolucent lesion in the distal diaphysis of the right fibula of a 5-year-old boy who sustained mild injury to the lower leg. Note the pathologic fracture through the lesion and the associated periosteal reaction. A radiodense cortical fragment in the center of the lesion represents the fallen fragment sign, identifying this lesion as an SBC. **(B)** Oblique radiograph of the wrist in another patient shows a radiolucent lesion in the distal ulna with a cortical fallen fragment inside the cystic lesion *(arrow)*.

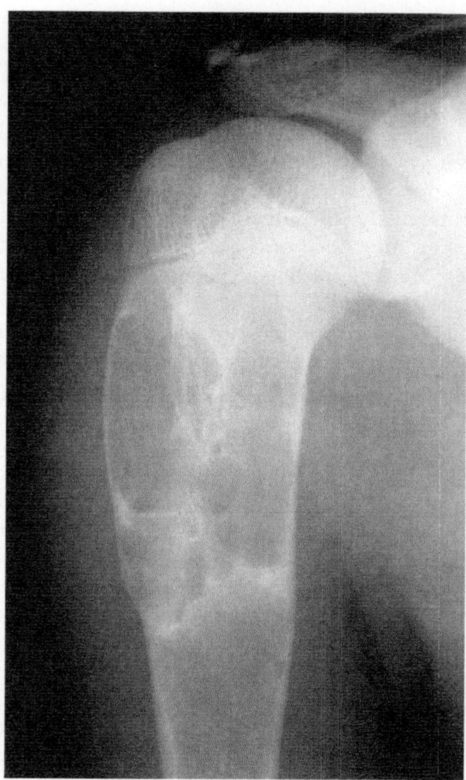

FIGURE 20.12 Nonossifying fibroma resembling an SBC. Anteroposterior radiograph of the right shoulder of a 10-year-old boy shows a radiolucent lesion in the metadiaphyseal region of the humerus, slightly eccentric in location, with a narrow zone of transition and a geographic type of bone destruction. The lateral cortex is significantly thinned and bulging. The lesion was believed to be an SBC; however, excision biopsy revealed a nonossifying fibroma.

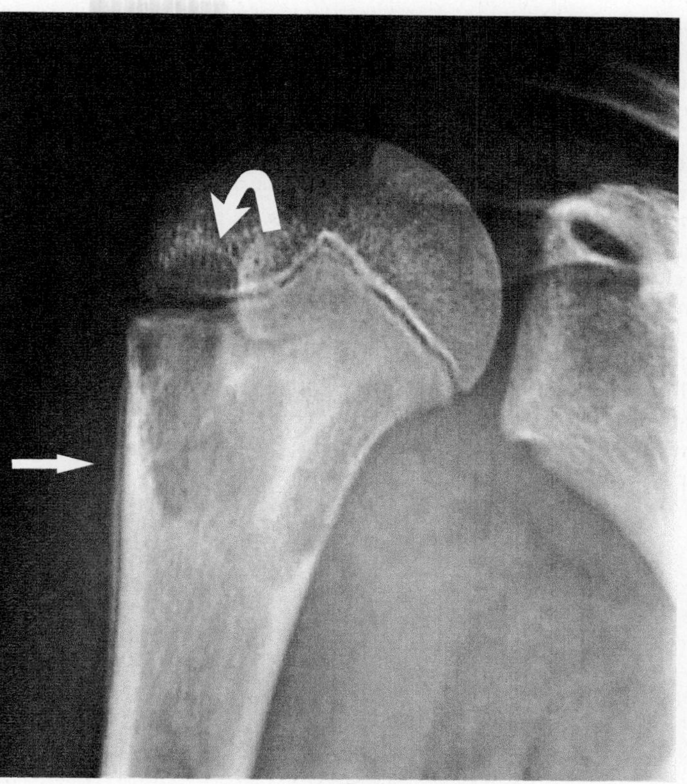

FIGURE 20.13 Bone abscess/osteomyelitis. A bone abscess may mimic an SBC, as seen here in the proximal humerus of a 12-year-old boy. The periosteal reaction *(arrow)* in the absence of pathologic fracture and the extension of the lesion into the epiphysis *(curved arrow)* favor the diagnosis of bone abscess/osteomyelitis.

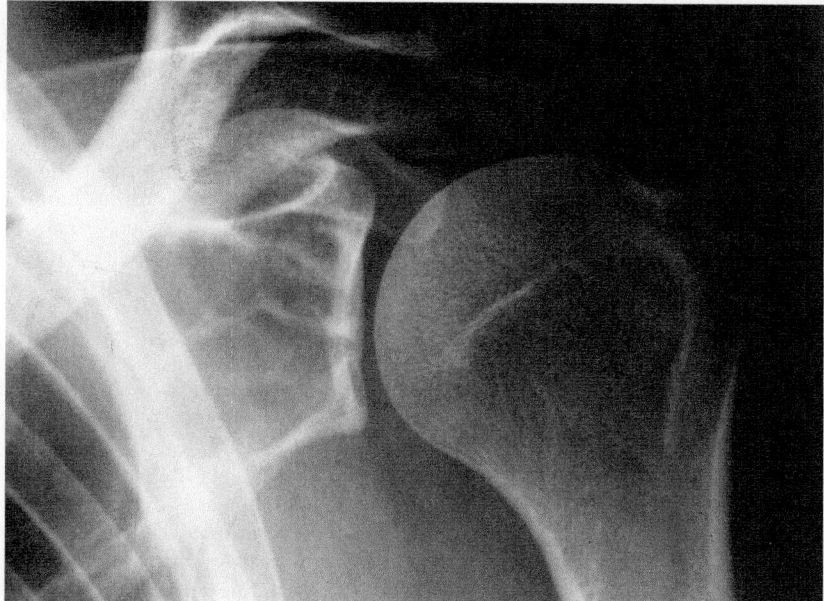

FIGURE 20.14 Intraosseous ganglion. An 18-year-old woman presented with left shoulder pain. Anteroposterior radiograph shows a radiolucent, trabeculated lesion in the glenoid, with the appearance of an SBC (compare with Fig. 16.30A). Excision biopsy was consistent with an intraosseous ganglion.

be associated with various benign (e.g., giant cell tumor [GCT], osteoblastoma, chondroblastoma, chondromyxoid fibroma, fibrous dysplasia) and malignant (e.g., osteosarcoma, fibrosarcoma, or chondrosarcoma) lesions. The concept of ABC as a secondary phenomenon occurring in a preexisting lesion has been validated by several researchers. Some investigators, however, regard ABC as a reparative process, probably the result of trauma or tumor-induced anomalous vascular process. Genetic and immunohistochemical studies suggest that primary ABC is a genetically predisposed bone lesion. Recent investigations demonstrated clonal rearrangements of chromosomal bands 16q22 and 17p13, namely, t(16,17)(q22;p13) and translocation of *TRE17/USP6* (ubiquitin-specific peptidase 8/Tre-2) gene at chromosome 17q13.

ABC constitutes approximately 6% of the primary lesions of bone and is seen predominantly in children; 90% of these lesions occur in patients younger than age 20 years. The metaphysis of long bones is a frequent site of predilection, although ABCs may sometimes be seen in the diaphysis of a long bone as well as in flat bones such as the scapula or pelvis and even in the vertebrae (Fig. 20.15). As already stated, these lesions can develop *de novo* or as a result of cystic changes in a preexisting lesion such as a chondroblastoma, osteoblastoma, GCT, or fibrous dysplasia (Fig. 20.16). The radiographic hallmark of an ABC is multicystic eccentric expansion (blow-out) of the bone, with a buttress or thin shell of periosteal response (Figs. 20.17 to 20.20). Although conventional radiographs usually suffice for evaluating the lesion, computed tomography (CT), MRI, and radionuclide bone scan can be of further assistance. CT is particularly helpful in determining the integrity of the cortex (Fig. 20.21). CT may also show internal ridges described on radiography as trabeculation or septation (Fig. 20.22). MRI is effective in demonstration of fluid–fluid levels (Fig. 20.23). These fluid levels are believed to represent the sedimentation of red blood cells and serum within the cystic cavities. To demonstrate this phenomenon, the patient must remain motionless for at least 10 minutes before scanning, and imaging must be performed in a plane perpendicular to the fluid levels.

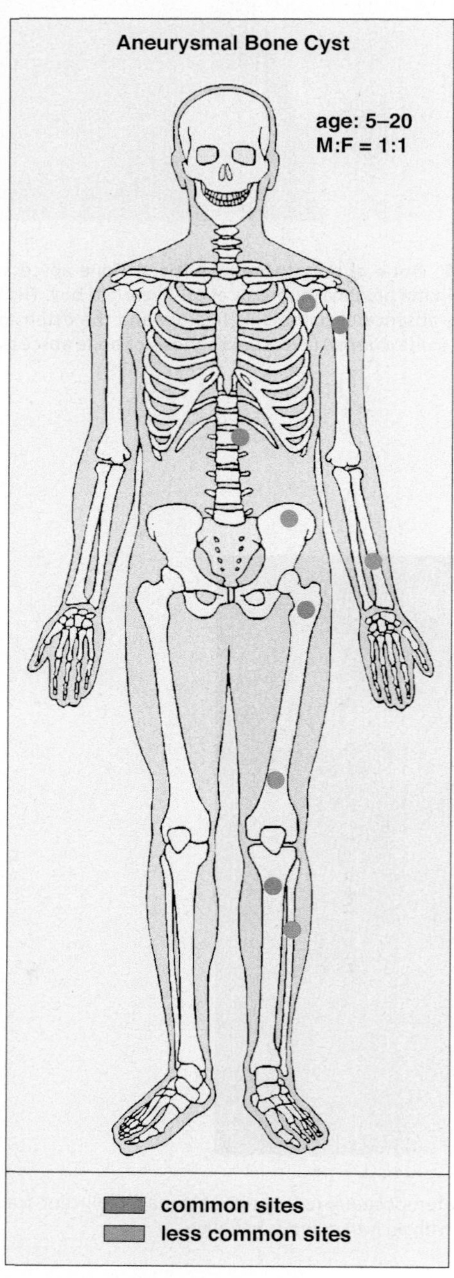

FIGURE 20.15 Skeletal sites of predilection, peak age range, and male-to-female ratio in ABC.

MRI findings are rather characteristic and usually allow a specific diagnosis of ABC. These include a well-defined lesion, often with lobulated contours, cystic cavities with fluid–fluid levels, multiple internal septations, and an intact rim of low-intensity signal surrounding the lesion (Figs. 20.24 to 20.28). This rim has been described as an indicator of a benign process. The wide range of signal intensities within the cyst on T1- and T2-weighted sequences is probably caused by settling of degraded blood products and reflects intracystic hemorrhages of different ages.

Skeletal scintigraphy (see Figs. 20.21C and 20.23B) may occasionally be helpful because it reflects the vascular nature of the lesion. Some investigators have reported an increased uptake of radiopharmaceutical tracer in a ring-like pattern around the periphery of ABC. Although this phenomenon is not specific for the lesion (it can also be observed in SBC and in bone infarct), the scintigraphic findings corroborate the radiographic presentation. Hudson, in his experience with 25 patients with ABC who underwent skeletal scintigraphy using technetium-99m methylene diphosphonate (^{99m}Tc-MDP) and ^{99m}Tc-pyrophosphate, found a correlation between the histopathologic features of the lesion, the amount and type of fluid contained within the cyst, and the scintigraphic pattern or intensity of uptake.

Pathology

Gross specimens of ABC show well-defined sponge-like mass composed of multiple blood-filled spaces separated by thin, tan-white septa; solid foci of various size may be present (Fig. 20.29). Histologically, the ABC consists of multiple blood-filled sinusoid spaces alternating with more solid areas. The solid tissue is richly vascular and composed of fibrous elements containing numerous multinucleated giant cells, usually in clusters, sometimes assuming arrangement of the cells "jumping into swimming pool" of cystic spaces. The sinusoids have fibrous walls, often containing reactive basophilic osteoid tissue or even mature bone, occasionally called the *blue bone*. Focal or diffuse collections of hemosiderin or reactive foam cells may be seen in the fibrous septa.

Complications and Differential Diagnosis

The most common complication of an ABC in a long bone is a pathologic fracture. Patients with spinal ABC may develop scoliosis and neurologic deficit.

The conditions that should always be included in the differential diagnosis at any age are SBC; chondromyxoid fibroma; and GCT, which occurs after skeletal maturity when the lesion extends into the articular end of bone. The most critical points in differentiation of ABC from SBC are that the former is an eccentric, expansive lesion, invariably associated with some degree of periosteal reaction (usually a solid layer or solid buttress). The latter is a centrally located lesion, showing little if any expansion and exhibiting periosteal reaction only when a pathologic fracture has occurred. In thin bones, such as the ulna, fibula, metacarpals, or metatarsals, the characteristic eccentricity of ABC may be lost and, conversely, SBC may demonstrate expansive features (Fig. 20.30). Because the former contains solid tissue, whereas SBC is a hollow structure filled with fluid, a fallen fragment

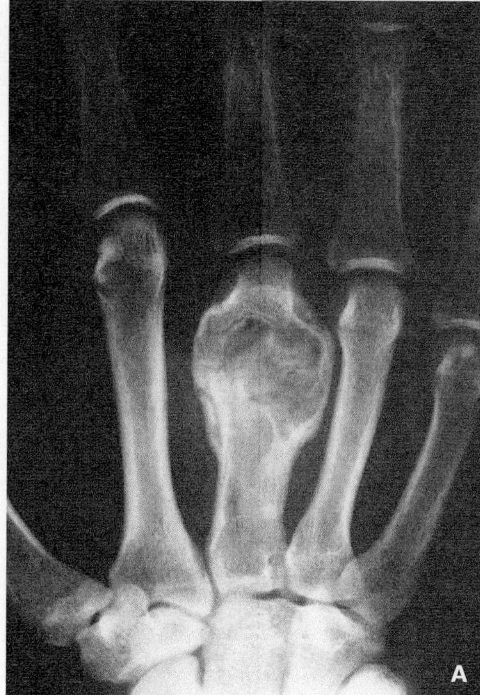

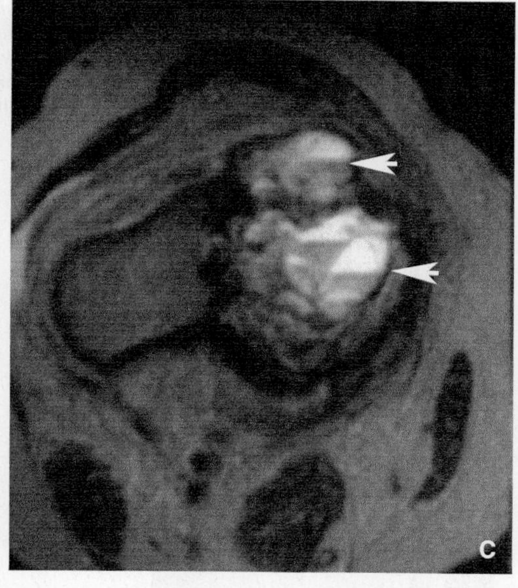

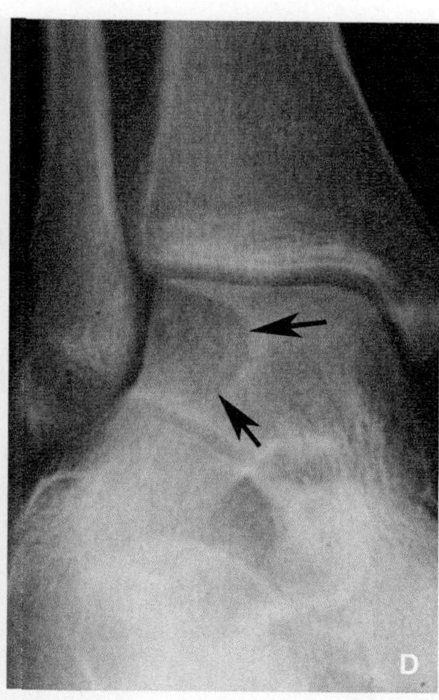

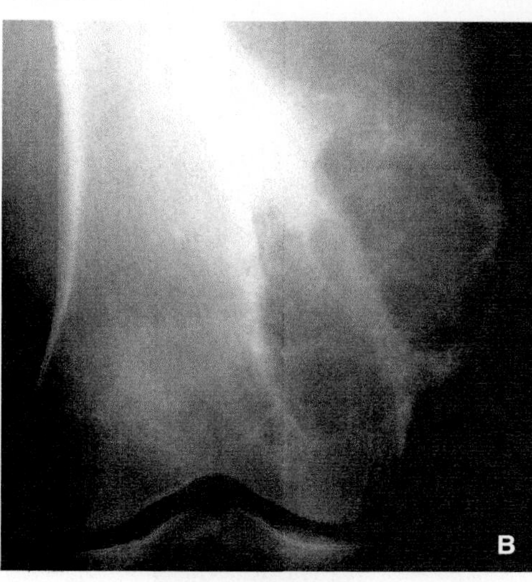

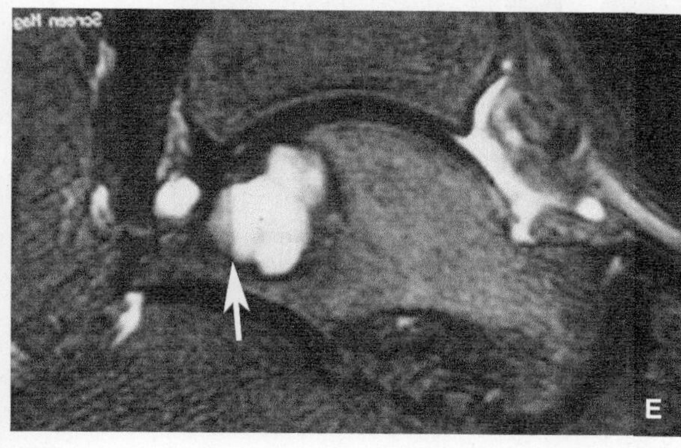

FIGURE 20.16 Secondary ABC. **(A)** A 14-year-old boy had a painless swelling on the dorsum of the left hand. Dorsovolar radiograph of the hand shows an expansive lesion in the distal segment of the third metacarpal. The lesion exhibits a well-organized periosteal reaction; the articular end of the bone is spared. Biopsy revealed an ABC engrafted on a monostotic focus of fibrous dysplasia. **(B)** Anteroposterior radiograph of the knee of another patient demonstrates an expansive lesion in the distal femur with thick cortex and internal septation. **(C)** Axial T2-weighted MRI shows multiple fluid–fluid levels within the lesion *(arrows)*. Histologic examination revealed a chondromyxoid fibroma with secondary ABC. **(D)** Anteroposterior radiograph of the right ankle of a young woman demonstrates a lytic lesion in the talus with a thick sclerotic rim *(arrows)*. **(E)** Sagittal T2-weighted MR image shows a fluid–fluid level within the lesion *(arrow)*. Histologic examinations demonstrated chondroblastoma with secondary ABC.

FIGURE 20.17 Aneurysmal bone cyst. **(A)** Anteroposterior and **(B)** lateral radiographs of the lower leg in an 8-year-old girl with a history of ankle pain demonstrate an expansive radiolucent lesion in the metaphysis of the distal tibia, extending into the diaphysis. Note its eccentric location in the bone and the buttress of periosteal response at the proximal aspect of the lesion *(arrows)*.

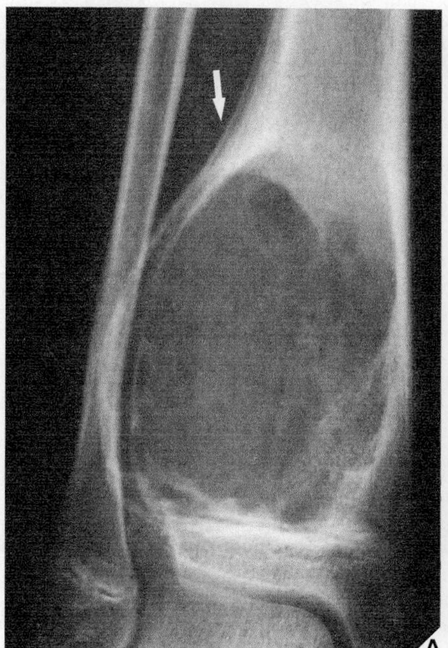

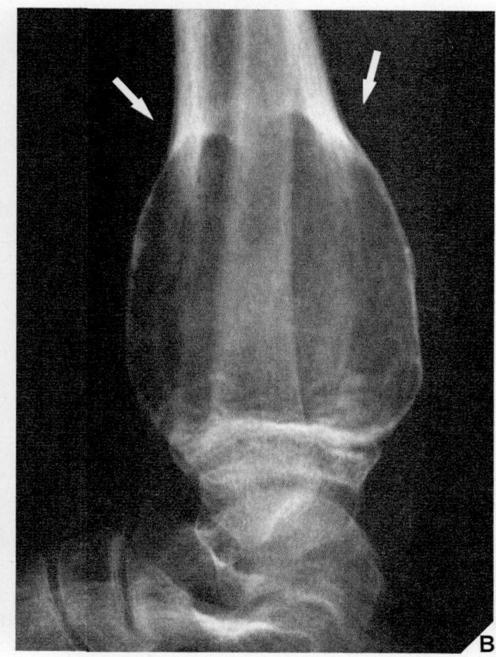

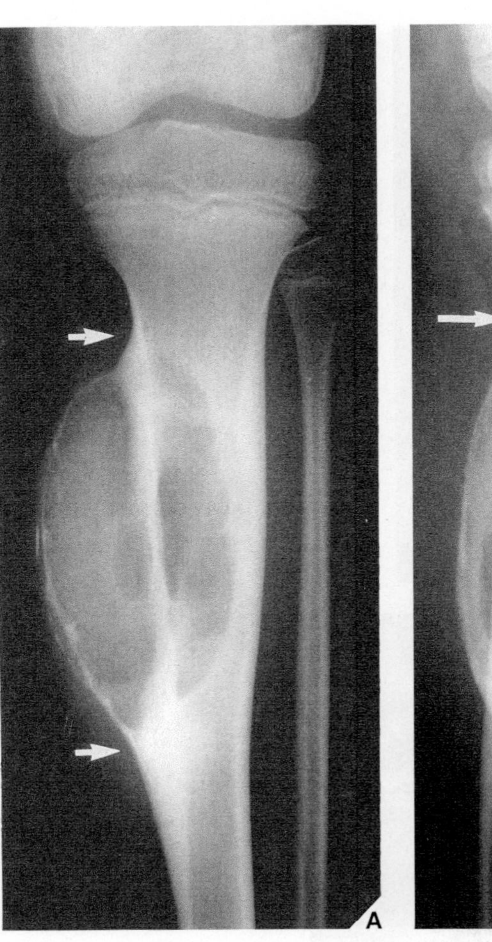

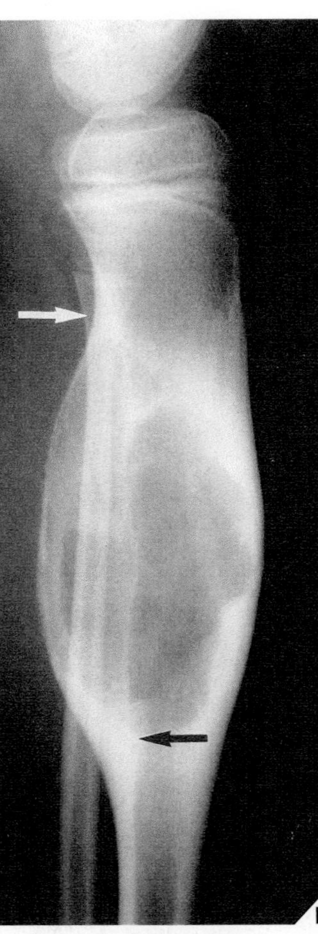

FIGURE 20.18 **Aneurysmal bone cyst.** **(A)** Anteroposterior and **(B)** lateral radiographs of the left proximal tibia of a 10-year-old girl show characteristic appearance of ABC, including eccentric location, expansive character, and a buttress of solid periosteal reaction proximally and distally *(arrows)*.

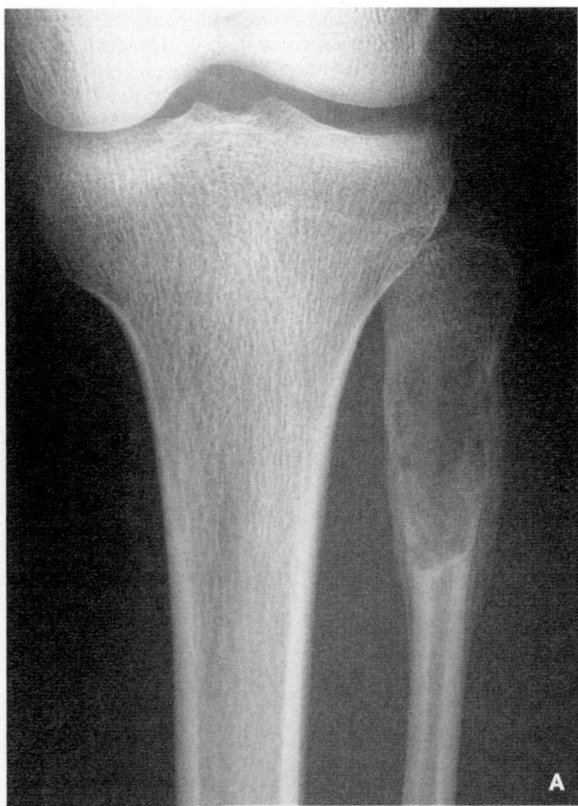

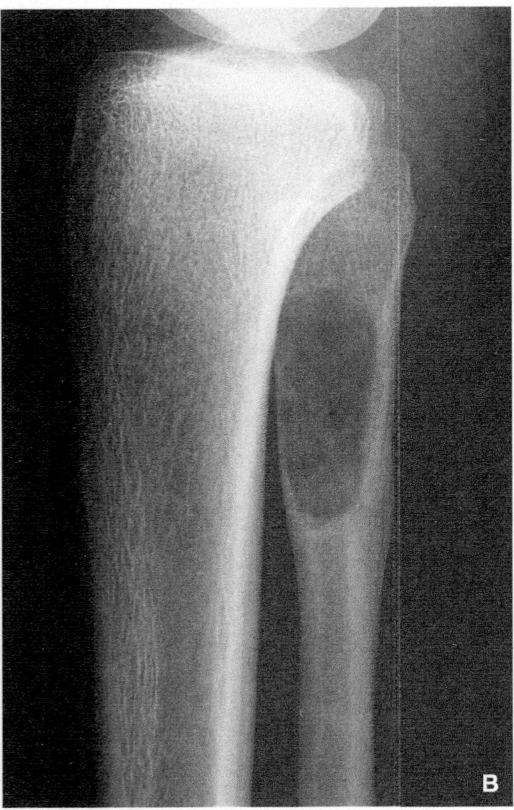

FIGURE 20.19 **Aneurysmal bone cyst.** **(A)** Anteroposterior and **(B)** lateral radiographs of the proximal leg of a 17-year-old girl show a radiolucent lesion in the fibula exhibiting a narrow zone of transition, a sclerotic border, and well-organized periosteal reaction. (Reprinted with permission from Greenspan A, Borys D. *Radiology and pathology correlation of bone tumors: a quick reference and review*. Philadelphia: Wolters Kluwer; 2016:317.)

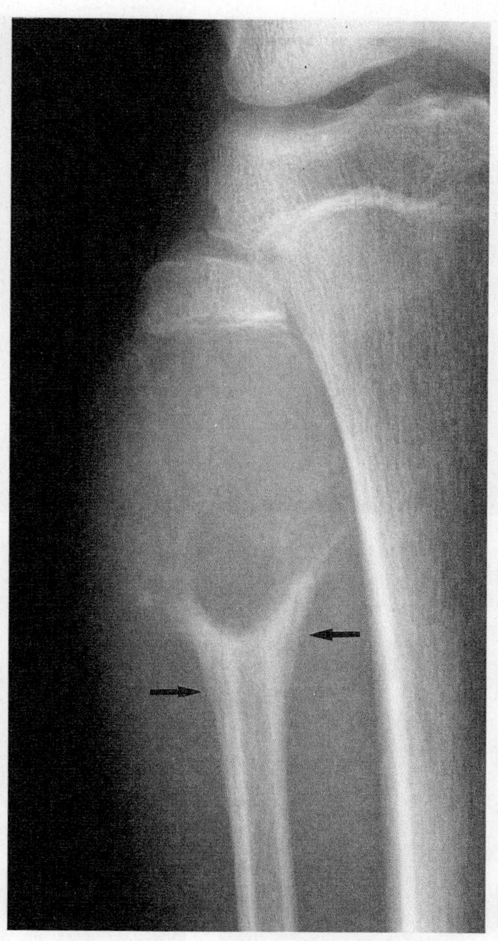

FIGURE 20.20 **Aneurysmal bone cyst.** A large, radiolucent expansive lesion in the proximal fibula of an 11-year-old girl reveals a buttress of periosteal reaction *(arrows)*.

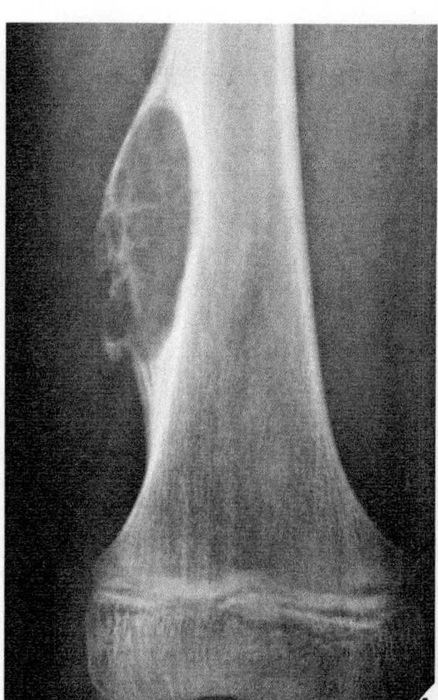

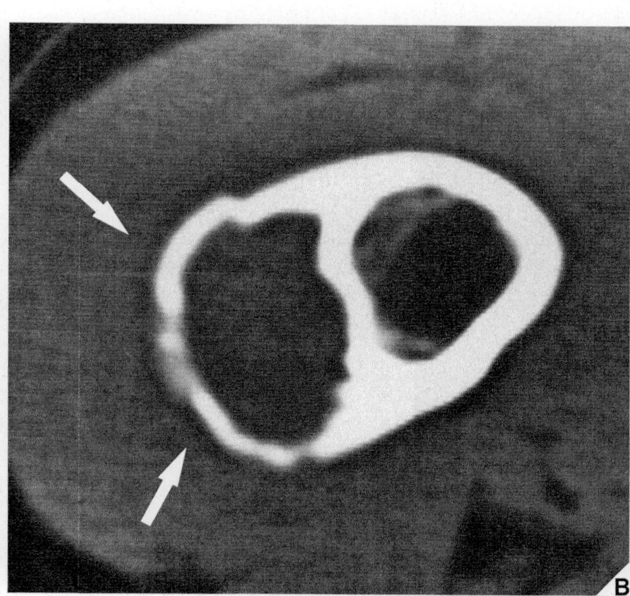

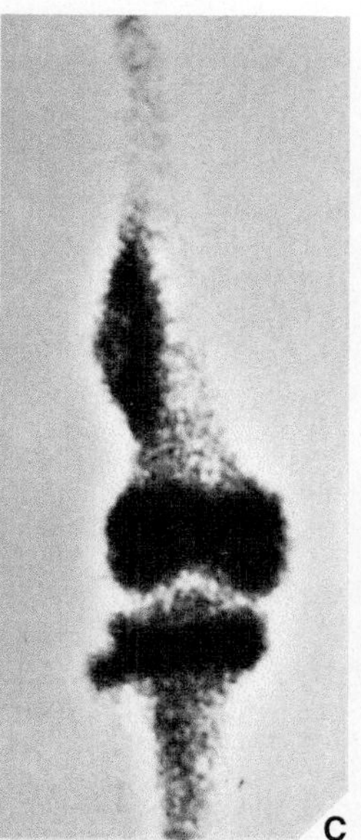

FIGURE 20.21 **CT and scintigraphy of ABC.** **(A)** Radiograph of the distal femur of an 8-year-old boy with a 6-month history of pain in the lower right thigh demonstrates a radiolucent expansive lesion located eccentrically in the femur and buttressed proximally and distally by a solid periosteal reaction, radiographic features consistent with an ABC. **(B)** CT section shows its intracortical location; the lesion balloons out from the lateral aspect of the femur but is contained within a thin uninterrupted shell of periosteal new bone *(arrows)*. **(C)** Radionuclide bone scan obtained after intravenous injection of 10 mCi (375 MBq) of ^{99m}Tc-labeled diphosphonate demonstrates increased uptake of radiopharmaceutical tracer by the lesion.

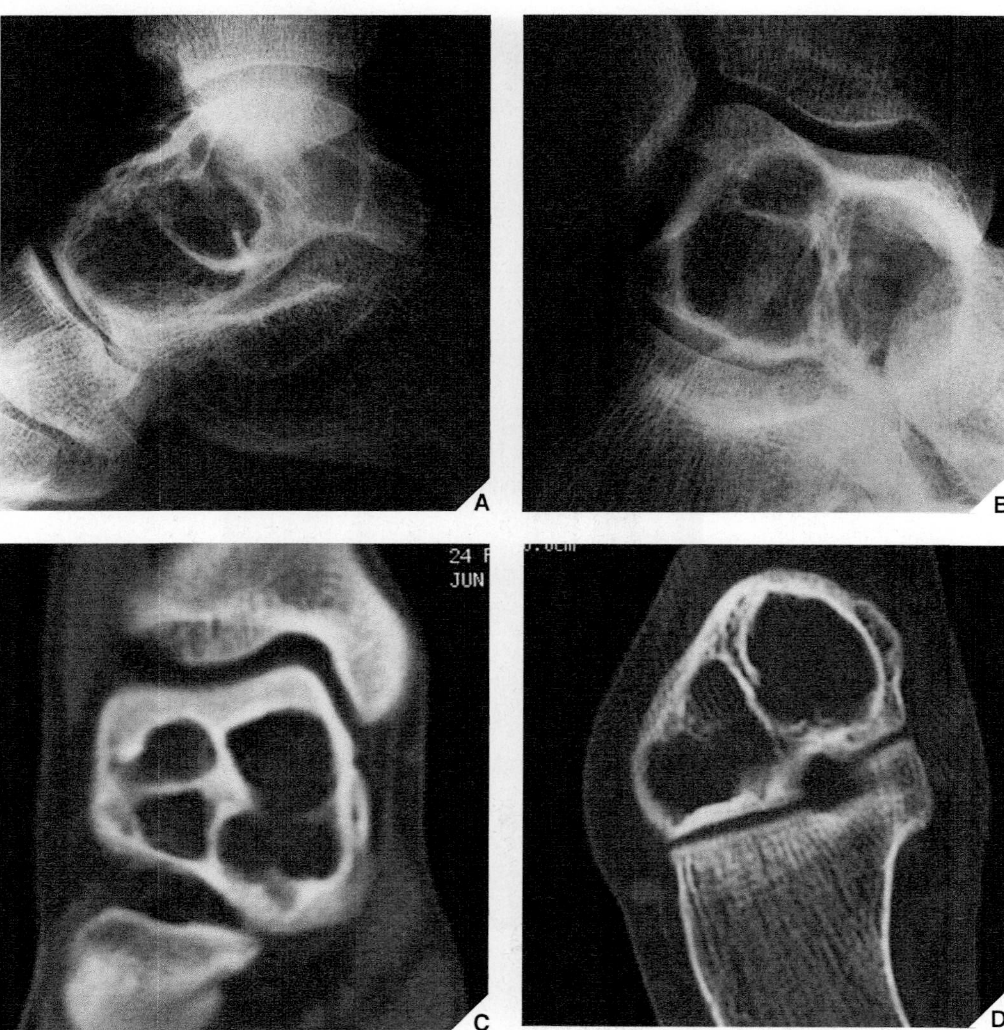

FIGURE 20.22 CT of ABC. **(A)** Lateral and **(B)** oblique radiographs of the right ankle of a 24-year-old woman show a radiolucent, trabeculated lesion in the talus. **(C)** Coronal anterior and **(D)** coronal posterior CT sections demonstrate the internal ridges of the lesion.

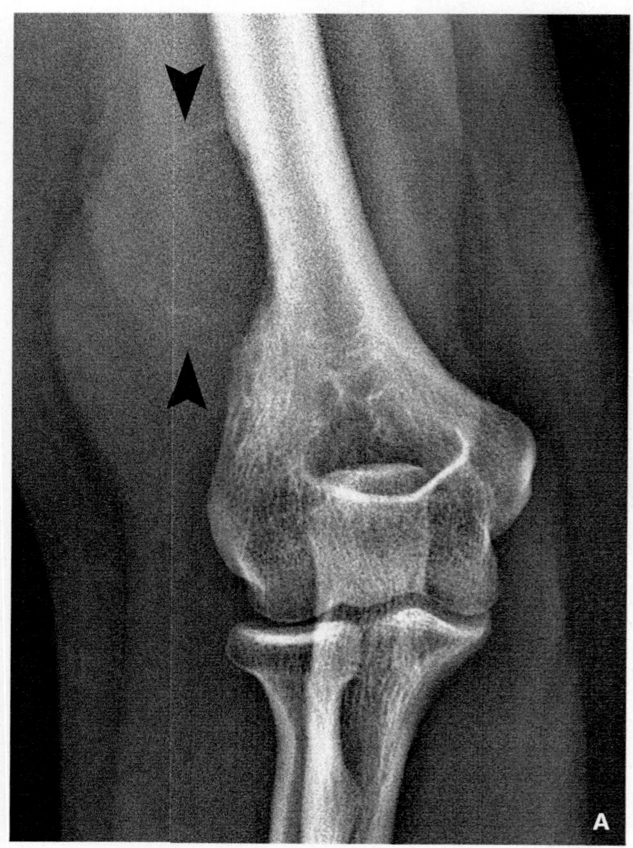

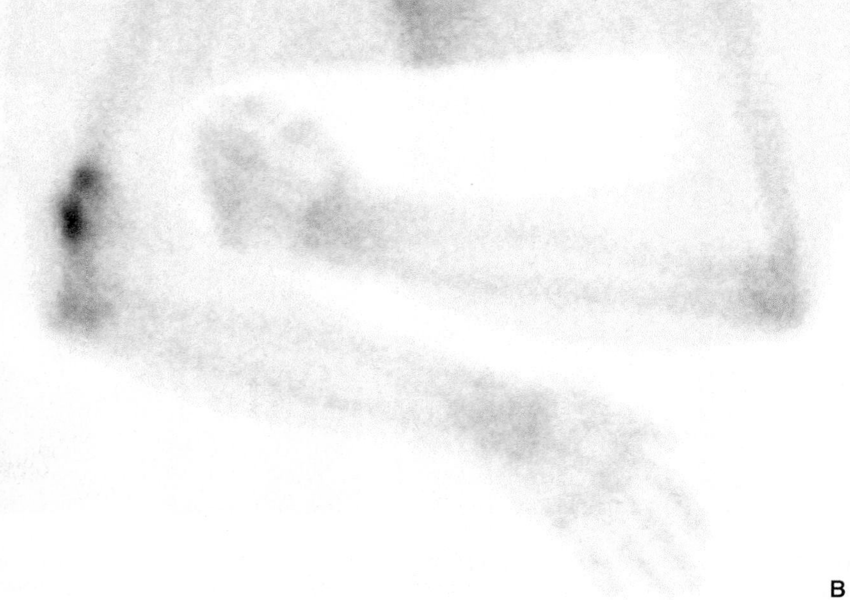

FIGURE 20.23 Scintigraphy, three-dimensional (3D) CT, and MRI of ABC. **(A)** Anteroposterior radiograph of the right elbow of a 21-year-old man shows an eccentric, expansive radiolucent lesion arising from the lateral cortex of the distal humerus. Observe the soft-tissue extension *(arrowheads)*. **(B)** Radionuclide bone scan shows increased uptake of the radiopharmaceutical tracer by the lesion. *(Continued)*

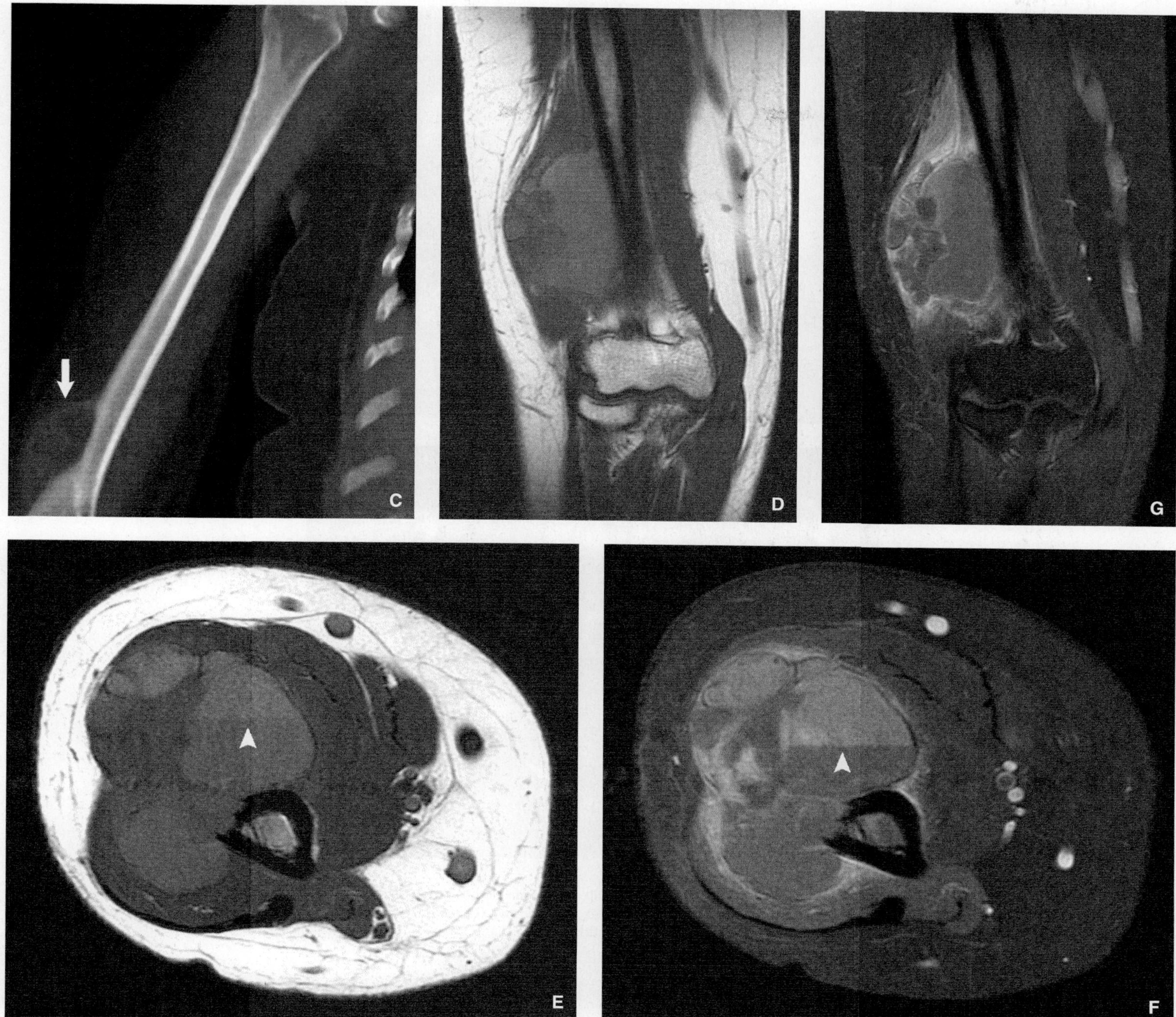

FIGURE 20.23 Scintigraphy, three-dimensional (3D) CT, and MRI of ABC. ***(Continued)*** **(C)** 3D CT image of the humerus reconstructed in maximum intensity projection (MIP) shows the soft-tissue mass contained by a thin shell of periosteal new bone *(arrow)*. **(D)** Coronal T1-weighted MR image shows heterogenous but predominantly intermediate signal intensity eccentric lesion extending into the soft tissues, compressing the high signal subcutaneous fat. **(E)** Axial T1-weighted and **(F)** axial T2-weighted MR images demonstrate fluid–fluid level within the lesion *(arrowheads)*. **(G)** Coronal T1-weighted fat-suppressed, contrast-enhanced MRI shows peripheral enhancement of the cyst.

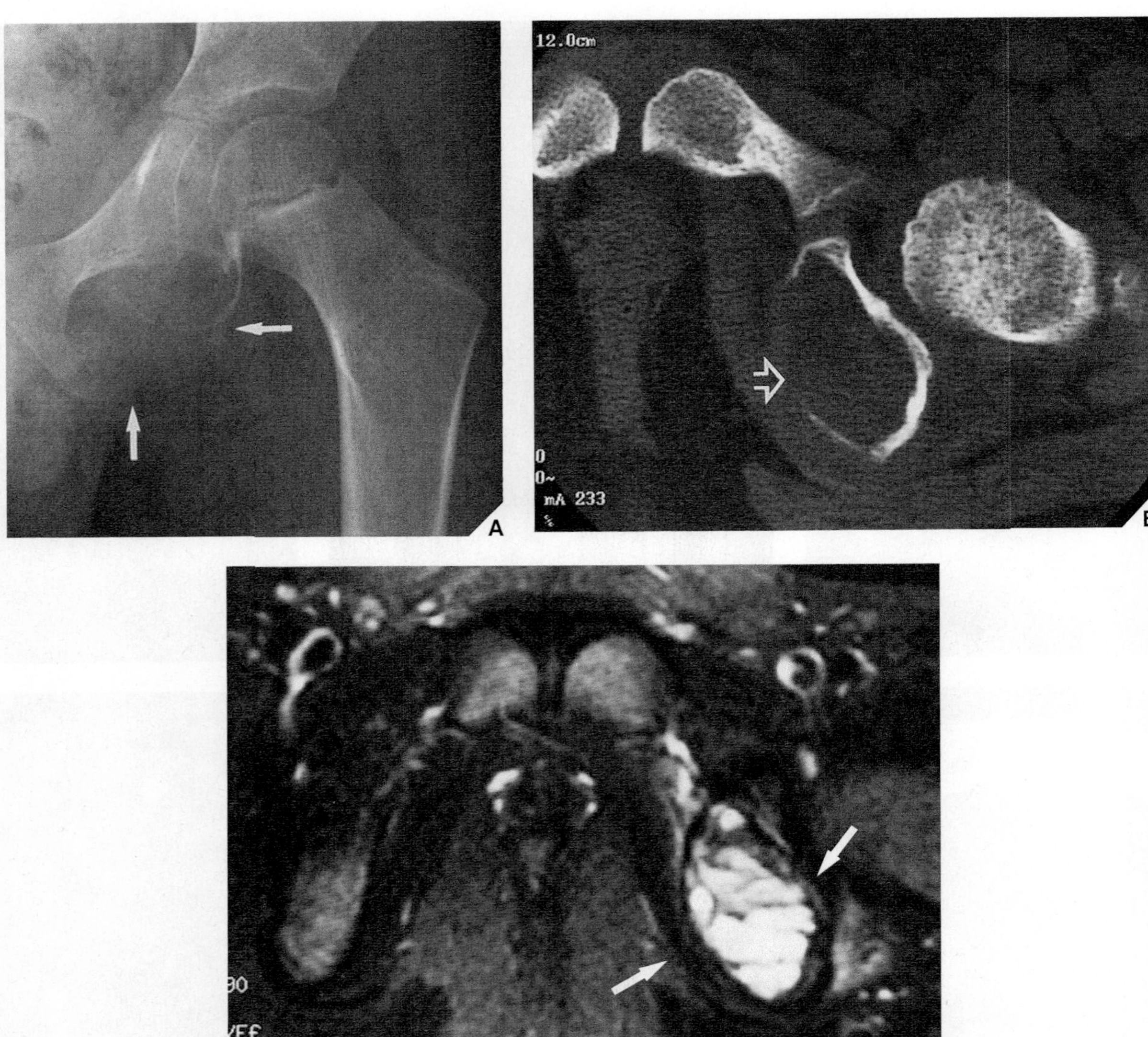

FIGURE 20.24 CT and MRI of ABC. **(A)** Anteroposterior radiograph of the left hip of a 4-year-old girl shows an expansive radiolucent lesion destroying the ischial bone *(arrows)*. **(B)** CT section demonstrates that the lesion broke through the medial cortex *(open arrow)*. **(C)** Axial T2-weighted MR image shows the lesion to be of high signal intensity *(arrows)*. Multiple fluid–fluid levels characteristic of an ABC are well demonstrated.

sign (if present) is a good differential feature, pointing to the latter diagnosis. Chondromyxoid fibroma may be indistinguishable from ABC (see Fig. 18.83) because both lesions are eccentric, expansive, and usually affect the metaphysis, exhibiting a reactive sclerotic rim and the aforementioned solid periosteal reaction (usually in the form of a buttress). CT and MRI are sometimes effective in making this distinction if they identify fluid–fluid levels, a phenomenon that points to the diagnosis of ABC because chondromyxoid fibroma is a solid lesion. However, occasionally chondromyxoid fibroma with secondary ABC have been reported (see Fig. 20.16B,C). As already mentioned in the previous text, secondary ABC has also been described in fibrous dysplasia, giant call tumor, chondroblastoma, and nonossifying fibroma (see Fig. 20.16D,E). In the mature skeleton, GCT may closely mimic ABC, although it usually is not associated with a periosteal reaction and rarely exhibits a zone of reactive sclerosis. Giant cell reparative granuloma (so-called *solid ABC*) may be indistinguishable from the conventional ABC. This lesion, however, unlike true ABC, usually involves the short tubular bones of the hands and feet. The cortex is thin but is characteristically intact. Extension into the surrounding soft tissues is distinctly uncommon, and the periosteal reaction is usually absent (see the following text). In thinner bones, such as the fibula, metacarpals, or metatarsals, ABC caused by expansive growth may destroy the cortex, mimicking an aggressive tumor such as telangiectatic osteosarcoma. Conversely, it is important to remember that at times, a telangiectatic osteosarcoma may masquerade as an ABC. Histopathologic differentiation is critical in these situations.

Treatment

The treatment for ABC consists of surgical removal of the entire lesion. At times, bone grafting to repair the resulting defect may be necessary (Fig. 20.31). The other methods of treatment include selective arterial embolization and use of adjuvant therapy such as liquid nitrogen, phenol, or polymethylmethacrylate (PMMA) to induce bone necrosis and microvascular damage to the wall of the cyst. Argon beam coagulation has also been used with mixed results. Percutaneous aspiration and injection of an aqueous solution of calcium sulphate have been tried in selected group of patients. Some investigators have advocated nonoperative treatment of recurrent spinal ABC by injection of ^{32}P chromic phosphate colloid into the cyst. Recently, percutaneous injections of Ethibloc, an alcoholic (ethanol) solution of corn protein which has thrombogenic and fibrogenic properties, have been advocated. Recurrence of the lesion, however, is frequent.

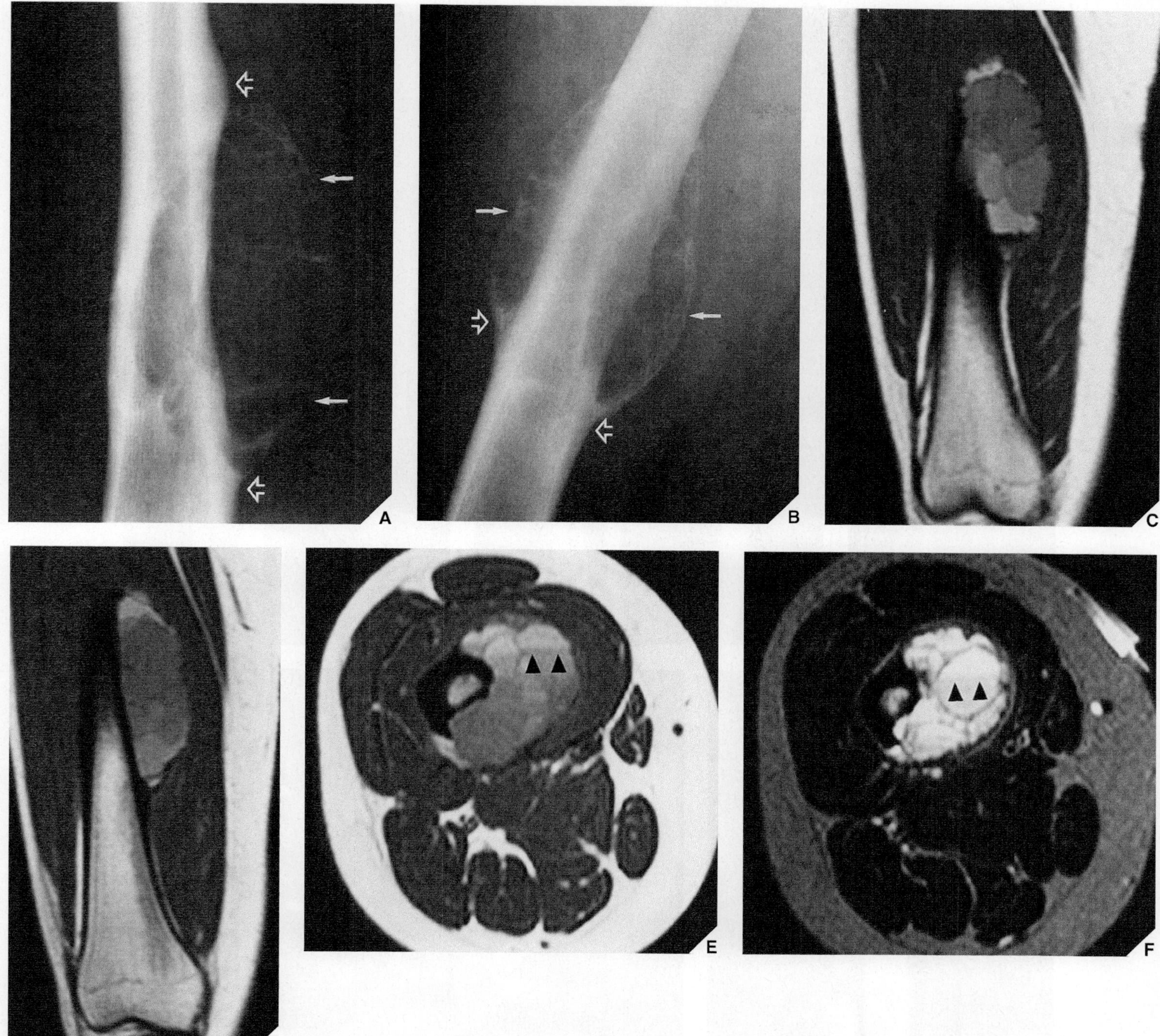

FIGURE 20.25 MRI of ABC. **(A)** Anteroposterior and **(B)** lateral radiographs of the midshaft of right femur of a 15-year-old girl show an expansive lesion arising eccentrically from the medial aspect of the bone. Note a thin shell of periosteal bone covering the lesion *(arrows)* and a buttress of periosteal reaction at its proximal and distal extent *(open arrows)*, characteristic for ABC. **(C,D)** Coronal T1-weighted (spin echo [SE]; repetition time [TR] 600/echo time [TE] 20 msec) MR images demonstrate heterogeneity of the lesion and internal septations. **(E)** Axial T1-weighted and **(F)** T2-weighted MR images show fluid–fluid levels *(arrowheads)*.

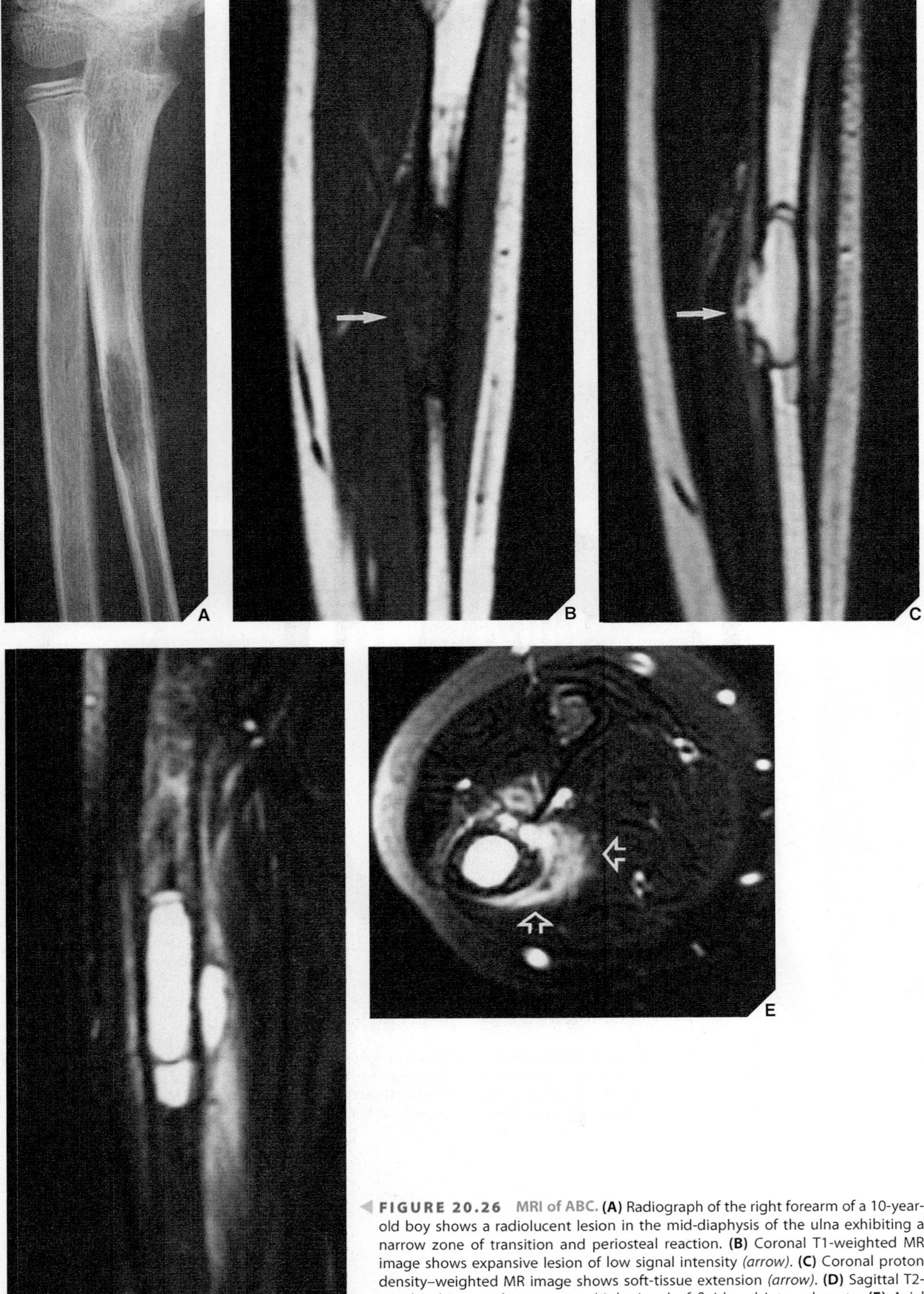

FIGURE 20.26 MRI of ABC. **(A)** Radiograph of the right forearm of a 10-year-old boy shows a radiolucent lesion in the mid-diaphysis of the ulna exhibiting a narrow zone of transition and periosteal reaction. **(B)** Coronal T1-weighted MR image shows expansive lesion of low signal intensity *(arrow)*. **(C)** Coronal proton density–weighted MR image shows soft-tissue extension *(arrow)*. **(D)** Sagittal T2-weighted image demonstrates high signal of fluid and internal septa. **(E)** Axial T2-weighted image shows cortical breakthrough and soft-tissue extension of the lesion and peritumoral edema *(open arrows)*.

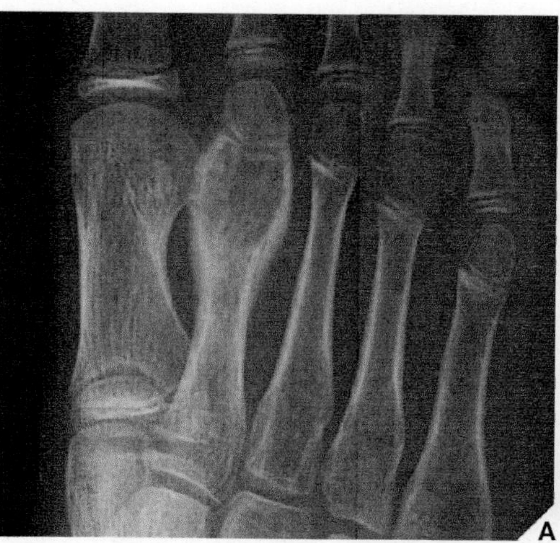

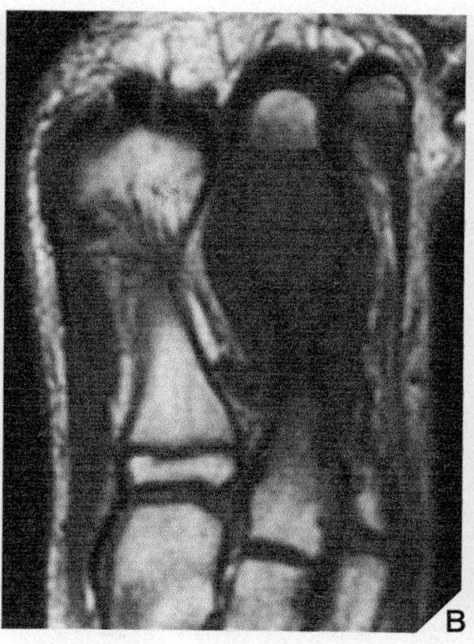

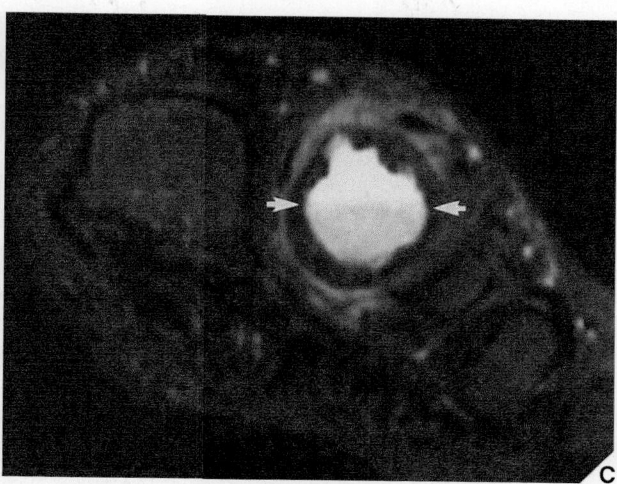

FIGURE 20.27 MRI of ABC. A 10-year-old boy presented with left foot pain for the previous 3 weeks. **(A)** Conventional radiograph shows an expansive lesion of the second metatarsal abutting the growth plate, associated with well-organized periosteal reaction. **(B)** Axial (long axis) T1-weighted (spin echo [SE]; repetition time [TR] 500/echo time [TE] 17 msec) MR image shows the lesion to exhibit an intermediate to low signal intensity. **(C)** Coronal (short axis) T2-weighted (fast spin echo [FSE]; TR 4500/TE 75 msec/Ef) image shows the lesion to become bright. Fluid–fluid level *(arrows)* is a typical finding in an ABC.

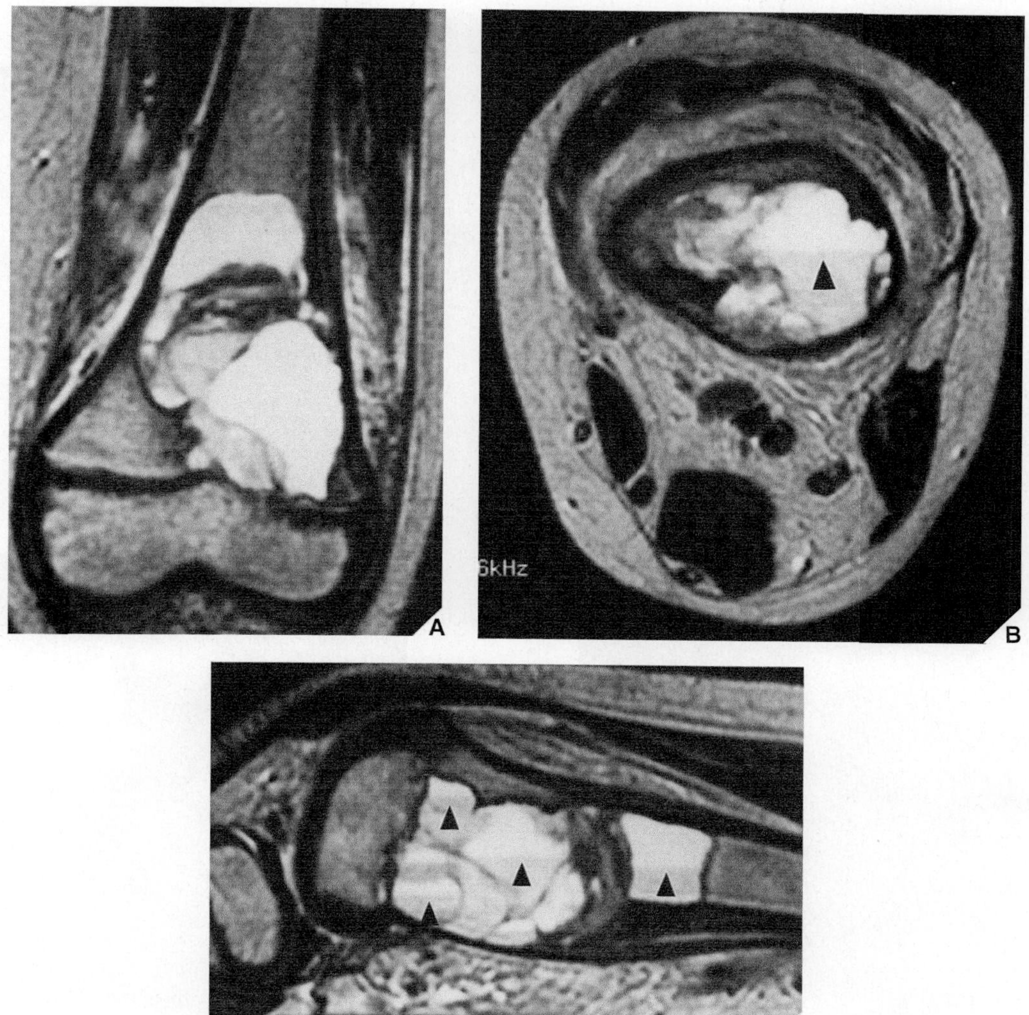

FIGURE 20.28 MRI of ABC. **(A)** Coronal T2-weighted (fast spin echo [FSE]; repetition time [TR] 2583/echo time [TE] 110 msec/Ef) MR image of a distal femur in a 5-year-old girl shows a heterogenous in appearance lesion extending into the growth plate. **(B)** Axial and **(C)** sagittal T2-weighted MR images demonstrate multiple fluid–fluid levels *(arrowheads)*.

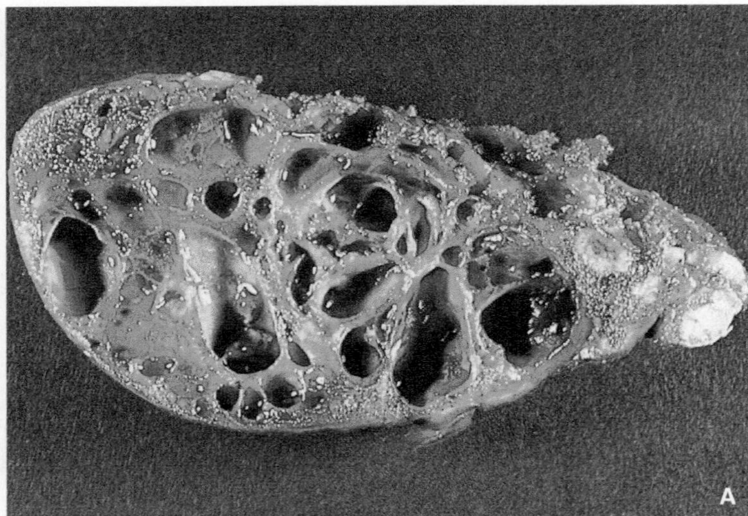

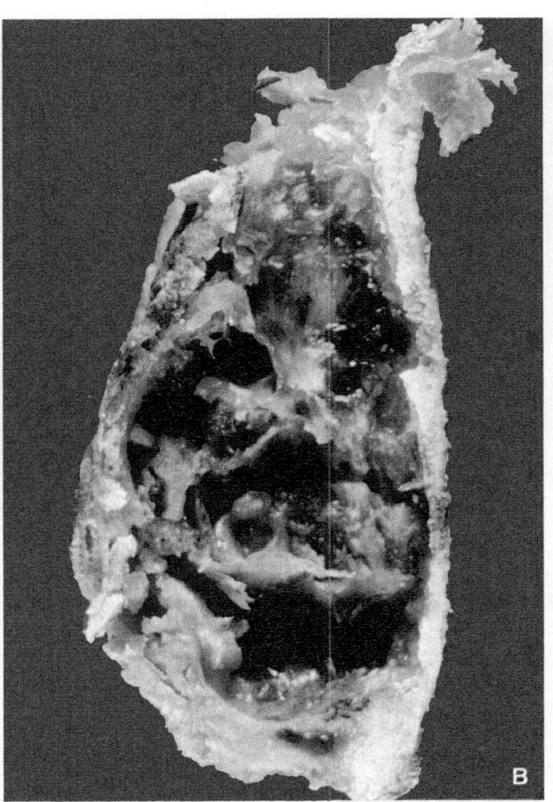

FIGURE 20.29 Pathology of ABC. **(A)** Gross specimen of ABC shows the tumor consisting of a red spongy, honeycomb mass with cystic spaces of various sizes filled with blood and osseous tissue within some of the septated walls. **(B)** Surgical specimen shows a gritty osseous tumor with multiple blood-filled cystic spaces separated by fibrous septa. (**A**, Modified from Bullough P. *Orthopaedic pathology*, 5th ed. Maryland Heights, MO: Mosby; 2009, with permission from Elsevier. **B**, Reprinted from Bullough P. *Orthopaedic pathology*, 5th ed. Maryland Heights, MO: Mosby; 2009, with permission from Elsevier.)

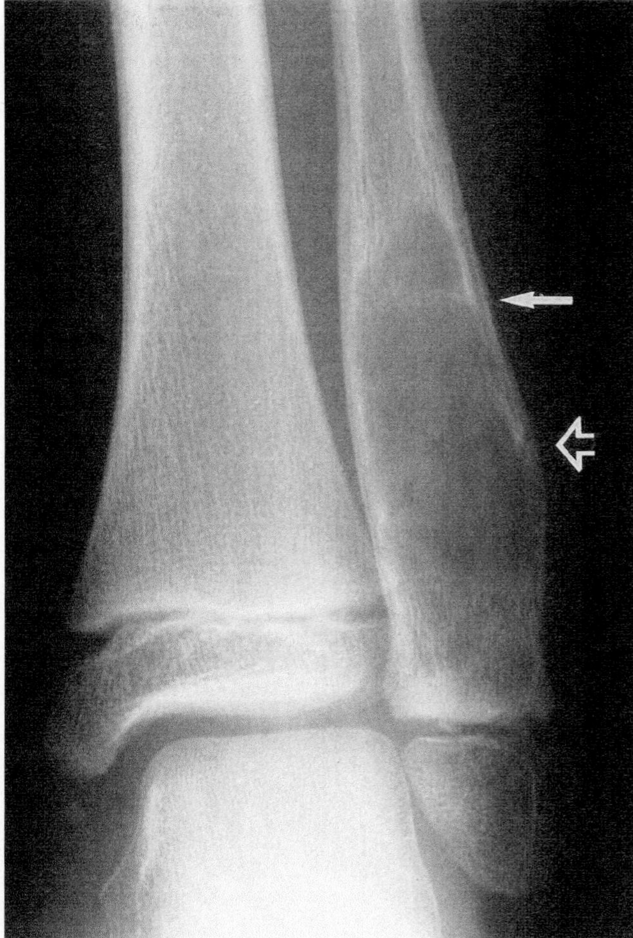

FIGURE 20.30 SBC mimicking ABC. A radiolucent expansive lesion in the distal fibula of an 8-year-old girl exhibits periosteal reaction *(arrow)* secondary to a healing pathologic fracture *(open arrow)*. Although diagnosis of an ABC was suggested, the excision biopsy was consistent with an SBC.

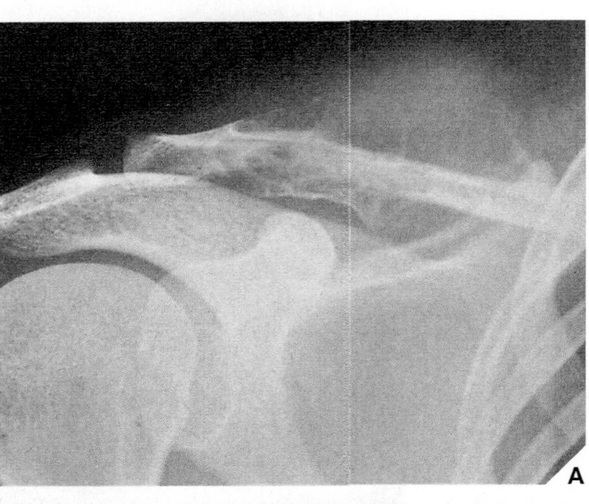

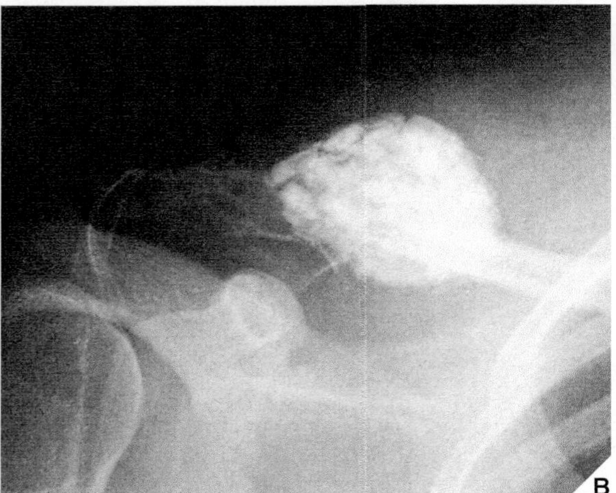

FIGURE 20.31 Treatment of ABC. **(A)** Anteroposterior radiograph of the shoulder of a 19-year-old woman shows an expansive lesion in the right clavicle. **(B)** The lesion was treated with curettage and the application of cancellous bone chips.

Solid Variant of Aneurysmal Bone Cyst

Clinical and Imaging Features

In 1983, Sanerkin and colleagues described a variant of ABC in which the predominant histology was that of the solid components of a conventional ABC. The histopathologic appearance of this lesion was very similar to that of another condition, reported originally by Jaffe in 1953 and later by Lorenzo and Dorfman in 1980, that represented a nonneoplastic hemorrhagic process in bones, termed *giant cell reparative granuloma*. The terms *solid ABC* and *giant cell reparative granuloma* are now being used interchangeably. These lesions are considered reactive and nonneoplastic, although they can lead to a mistaken diagnosis of malignancy. Although these lesions are seen primarily in craniofacial and short tubular bones of the hands and feet, they may also occur in the long bones, such as femur, tibia, and ulna. Multicentric presentation has been reported. Solid variant of ABC is seen most commonly in the second and third decades, with mean age of 18 years. Radiography reveals that most of these lesions are expansive and eccentric in location, commonly multiloculated with internal trabeculations, and with variably aggressive features. They may occasionally extend into the articular end of bone. At times, there is a thin shell of periosteal reaction indistinguishable from conventional ABC. MRI findings are variable, but most lesions show intermediate signal intensity on T1-weighted images, with heterogeneous but predominantly high signal intensity on T2 weighting (Fig. 20.32). The areas of low signal on T2-weighted sequences represent mineralization within the lesion.

Pathology

Histopathologic examination of these lesions reveals fibrous stroma, an admixture of spindle cells, and many multinucleated giant cells. Occasional formation of osteoid and even mature bone trabeculae can be noted. Vascular spaces and hemorrhagic areas are also present. Some of these lesions have a histologic appearance similar to that of the so-called *brown tumors of hyperparathyroidism*.

Treatment

Treatment of these lesions usually consists of curettage. The recurrence rate, as recently reported from the Rizzoli Institute in Bologna, Italy, is close to 24%, whereas the Mayo Clinic reports approximately 39%.

Giant Cell Tumor

Clinical and Imaging Features

Also known as *osteoclastoma*, a GCT of bone is an aggressive lesion characterized by richly vascularized tissue containing proliferating mononuclear stromal cells and numerous uniformly distributed giant cells of osteoclast type. It represents approximately 5% to 8.6% of all primary bone tumors and approximately 23% of benign bone tumors; it is the sixth most common primary osseous neoplasm. Sixty percent of these lesions occur in long bones, and almost all are localized to the articular end of the bone. Preferred sites include the proximal tibia, distal femur, distal radius, and proximal humerus (Fig. 20.33). GCTs are seen almost exclusively after skeletal maturity, when the growth plate is obliterated. Most patients are between ages 20 and 40 years, and there is a female predominance of 2:1.

Multifocal GCTs are rare, accounting for less than 1% of all cases of GCT of bone. They occur most commonly in patients with Paget disease. Multiple lesions can be discovered synchronously or metachronously. The preferential locations are skull and facial bones in Paget disease and small bones of the hands and feet in other patients.

Clinical symptoms in patients with solitary lesions are nonspecific. They include pain (usually reduced by rest), local swelling, and limitation of range of motion in the adjacent joint. When a lesion is located in the spine, neurologic symptoms may be present.

The imaging features of a GCT are characteristic. It is a purely osteolytic, radiolucent lesion with narrow zone of transition lacking sclerotic margins, revealing geographic bone destruction and usually no periosteal reaction (Figs. 20.34 to 20.38). Scintigraphy invariably shows increased uptake of radiopharmaceutical tracer by the tumor (see Fig. 20.41B). Occasionally, the bone scan may show more intense uptake of the tracer around the periphery of the lesion than within the lesion itself, which Hudson calls a "donut configuration," and is presumably caused by hyperemic changes in the bone surrounding the tumor. A soft-tissue mass may also be present, and CT or MRI is usually required for sufficient evaluation (Figs. 20.39 to 20.43). Approximately 5% of GCTs are malignant *de novo*. Having no characteristic imaging features, however, malignant lesions cannot be diagnosed radiologically (Figs. 20.44 to 20.46). It is also well known that benign GCT may evolve into a malignant lesion. Several authors have reported cases of malignant transformation of GCT of bone. In most cases,

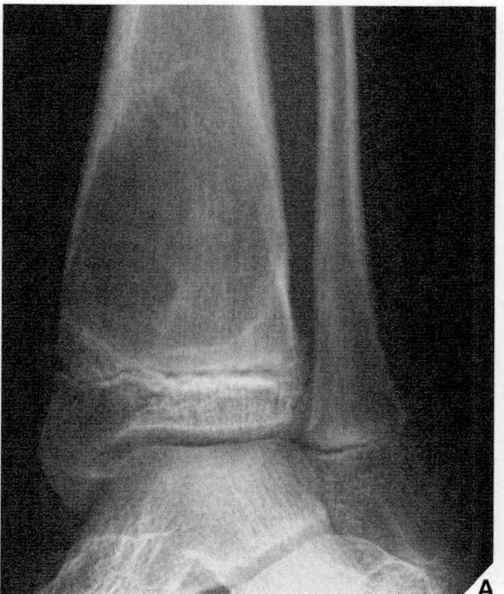

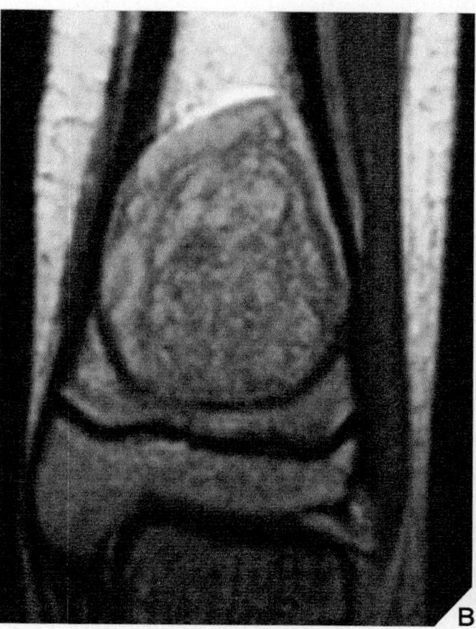

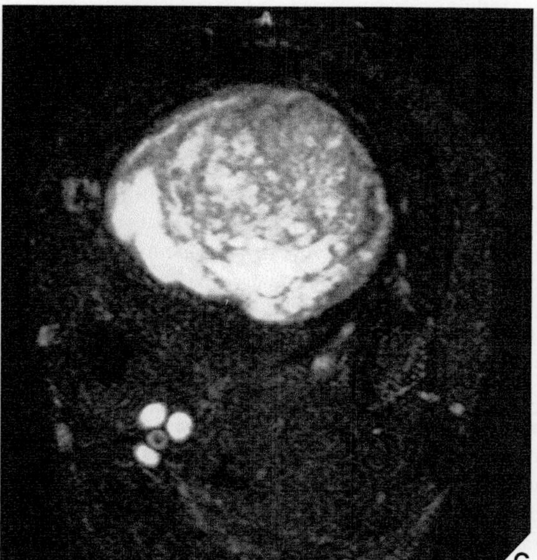

FIGURE 20.32 Solid variant of ABC. (A) Oblique radiograph of the left ankle of an 11-year-old girl shows a sharply marginated radiolucent lesion in the metadiaphysis of the tibia. **(B)** On coronal T1-weighted MR image, the lesion exhibits intermediate heterogeneous signal intensity. **(C)** On axial T2-weighted MRI, the lesion exhibits heterogeneous but predominantly high signal intensity. (Reprinted with permission from Greenspan A, Jundt G, Remagen W. *Differential diagnosis in orthopaedic oncology*, 2nd ed. Philadelphia: Lippincott Williams & Wilkins; 2007:387–431.)

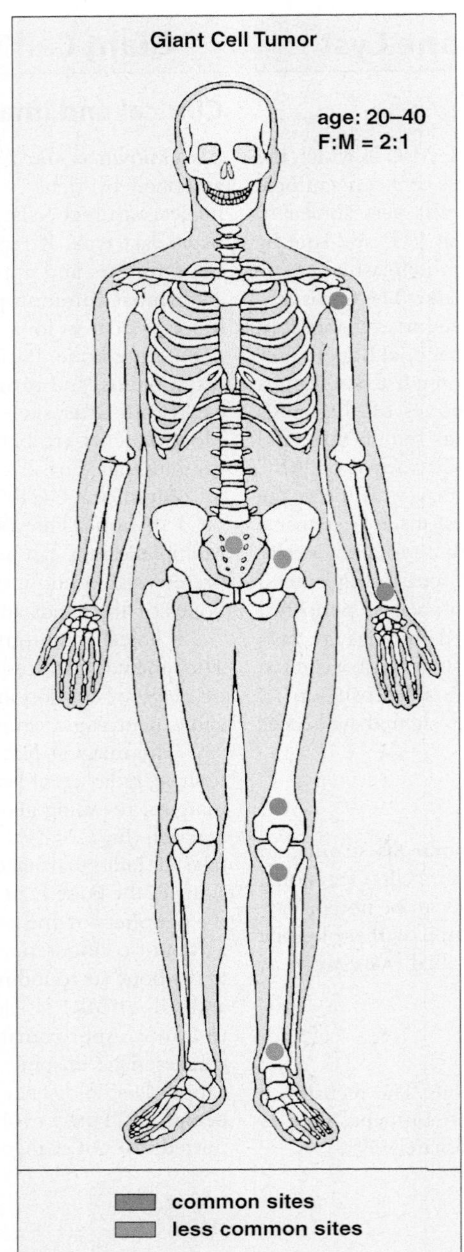

FIGURE 20.33 Skeletal sites of predilection, peak age range, and male-to-female ratio in GCT.

this transformation occurs after radiation therapy. Only a few cases have been reported of spontaneous malignant transformation after initial surgical therapy. Histologically, the secondary malignancies include malignant fibrous histiocytoma, fibrosarcoma, osteosarcoma, and undifferentiated sarcoma.

Historically, the imaging appearance and staging of GCTs have not accurately reflected the ultimate clinical outcome, but nevertheless several investigators, including Enneking, Campanacci, and Bertoni et al., have developed staging systems based on imaging and histologic appearance of this tumor. The stage 1 lesion has an indolent radiographic (well-marginated borders and intact cortex) and benign histologic appearance. The stage 2 lesion demonstrates a more aggressive radiographic appearance, with extensive remodeling of bone; thin cortex but without loss of continuity and intact periosteum; and still benign histologic pattern. Stage 3 GCT reveals aggressive growth with break through the cortex and extension into adjacent soft tissues but remains histologically benign, although distant metastases (predominantly to the lungs) may occur.

Pathology

On macroscopy, the tumor tissue is usually soft and reddish brown with occasional yellowish areas of xanthomatous change and firmer whitish areas representing fibrosis. Cystic and hemorrhagic spaces may be seen mimicking ABC (Fig. 20.47).

Histologically, a GCT is composed of a related dual population of mononuclear stromal cells and multinucleated giant cells. The tumor background contains varying amounts of collagen. Morphologically, the giant cells bear some resemblance to osteoclasts, and they display increased acid phosphatase activity. It is generally accepted that these cells are not neoplastic. The mononuclear cell, however, which arises from primitive mesenchymal stromal cells, represents the neoplastic component. These stromal cells, similar to osteoblasts, express factors necessary for osteoclast formation and differentiation (osteoclast differentiation factor or ODF). They exhibit the characteristics of osteoblast progenitors and express RANKL (receptor activator of nuclear factor kappa B [NF-κB] ligand), a growth factor that is essential for the recruitment of osteoclasts by osteoblasts

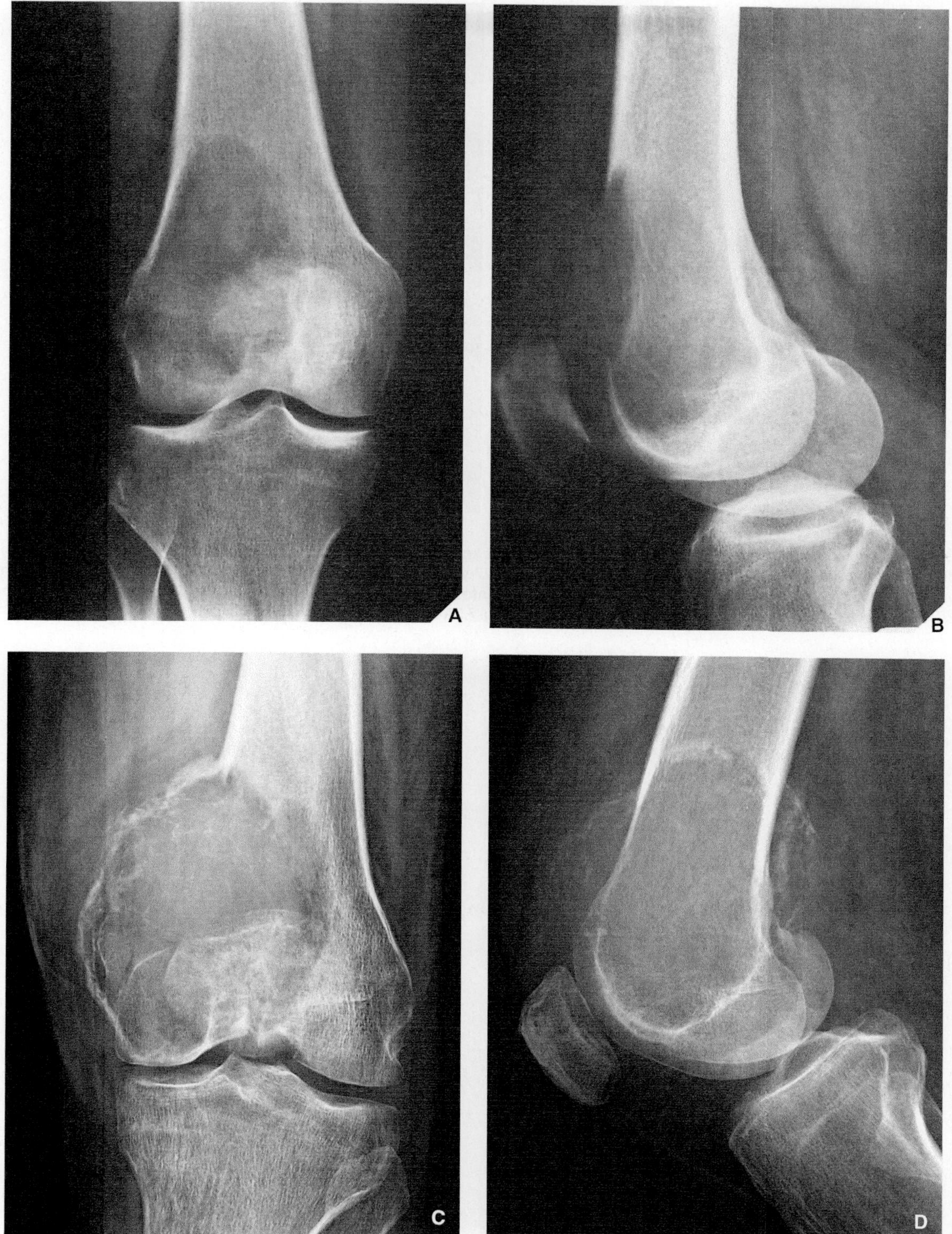

FIGURE 20.34 Giant cell tumor. **(A)** Anteroposterior and **(B)** lateral radiographs of the right knee of a 32-year-old man demonstrate a purely osteolytic lesion in the distal end of the femur. Note its eccentric location, the absence of reactive sclerosis, and the extension of the lesion into the articular end of the bone, all characteristic features of GCT. **(C)** Anteroposterior and **(D)** lateral radiographs of the left knee of a 58-year-old man show eccentric osteolytic expansive lesion in the medial femoral condyle.

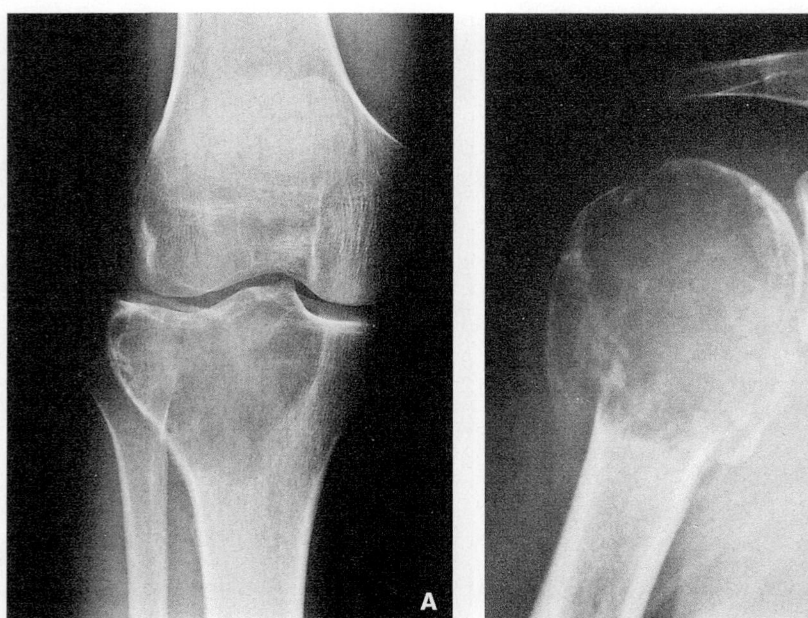

FIGURE 20.35 Giant cell tumor. **(A)** Anteroposterior radiograph of the right knee of a 30-year-old woman shows an osteolytic lesion eccentrically located in the proximal tibia, extending into the articular end of bone. **(B)** In another patient, a 27-year-old woman, a radiolucent lesion affects almost the entire proximal end of the right humerus. Observe a pathologic fracture at the distal extent of the tumor. (Reprinted with permission from Greenspan A, Borys D. *Radiology and pathology correlation of bone tumors: a quick reference and review*. Philadelphia: Wolters Kluwer; 2016: 300, Fig. 7.2A and C.)

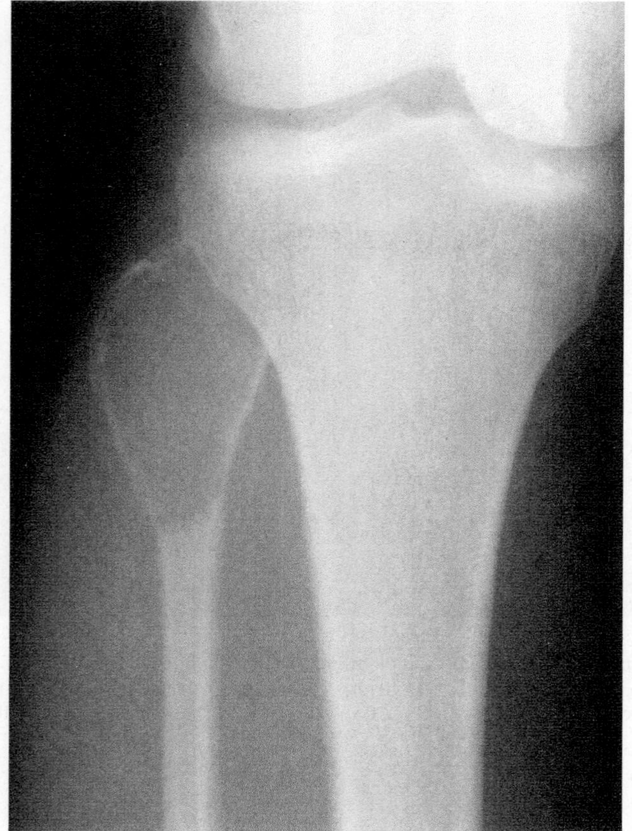

FIGURE 20.36 Giant cell tumor. Anteroposterior radiograph of the right knee in a 28-year-old woman shows an expansive radiolucent lesion in the head of the fibula.

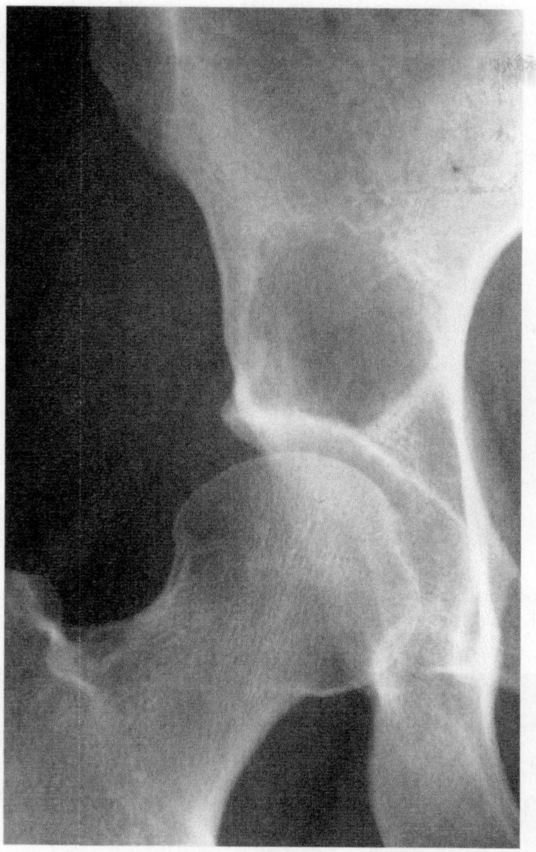

FIGURE 20.37 Giant cell tumor. Anteroposterior radiograph of the right hip in a 31-year-old woman shows a radiolucent lesion in the supraacetabular portion of the ilium, with a narrow zone of transition and a geographic type of bone destruction.

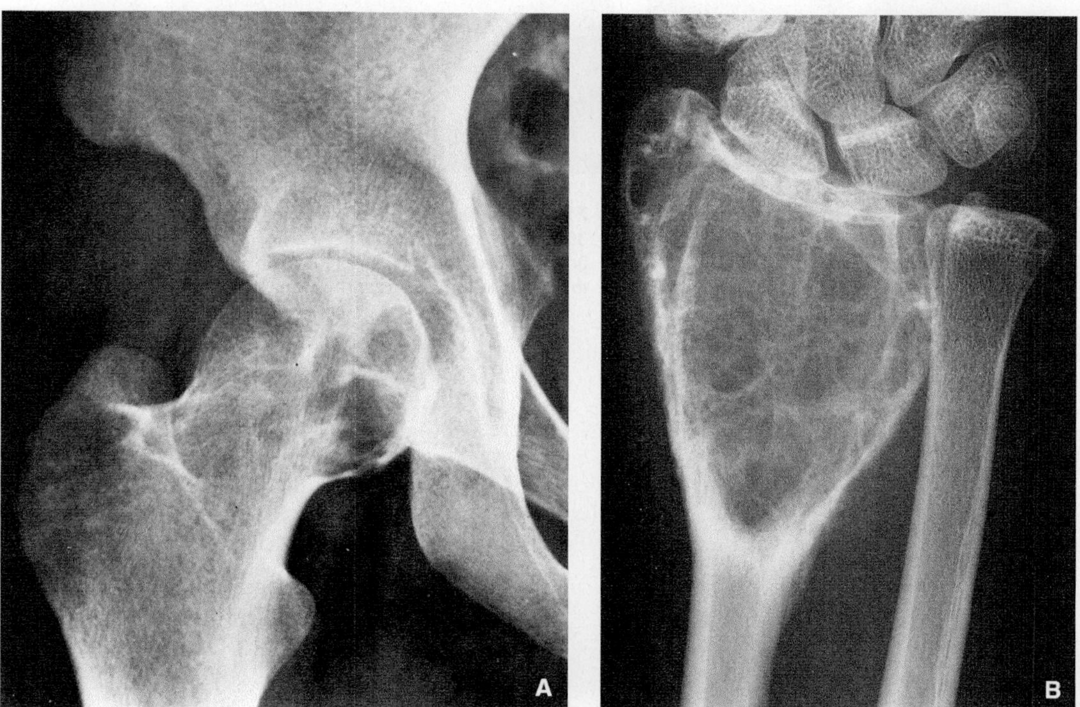

FIGURE 20.38 Giant cell tumor. **(A)** Anteroposterior radiograph of the right hip of a 27-year-old woman shows a radiolucent lesion with internal trabeculations in the femoral head. **(B)** Anteroposterior radiograph of the left wrist of a 36-year-old woman shows a trabeculated lesion in the distal radius. (Reprinted with permission from Greenspan A, Borys D. *Radiology and pathology correlation of bone tumors: a quick reference and review*. Philadelphia: Wolters Kluwer; 2016: 301, Fig. 7.3).

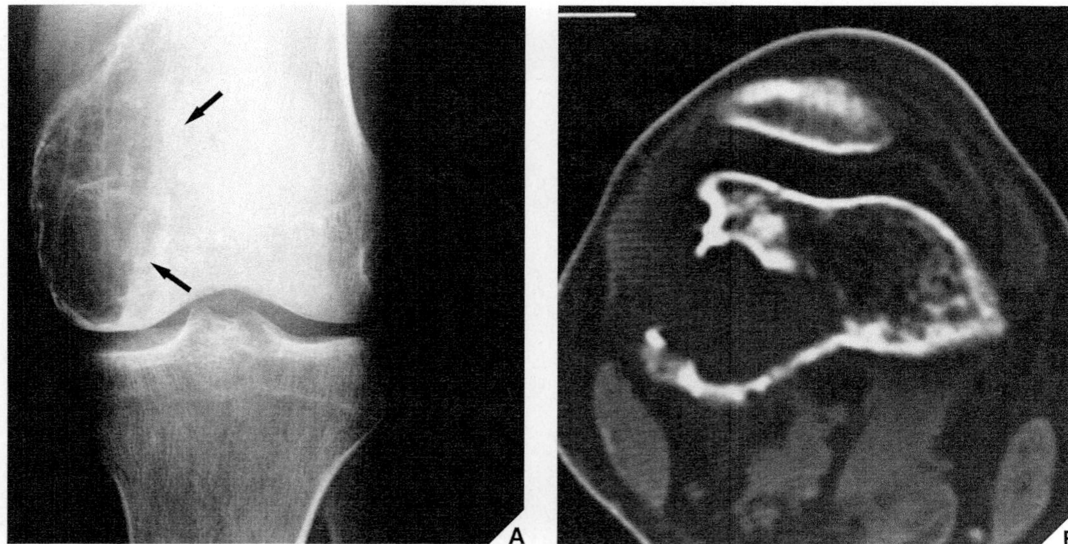

FIGURE 20.39 CT of giant cell tumor. **(A)** Anteroposterior radiograph of the knee of a 33-year-old woman shows a lytic lesion in the medial femoral condyle *(arrows)*. There is no definite evidence of a soft-tissue mass. **(B)** CT, however, demonstrates destruction of the cortex and the presence of a soft-tissue mass.

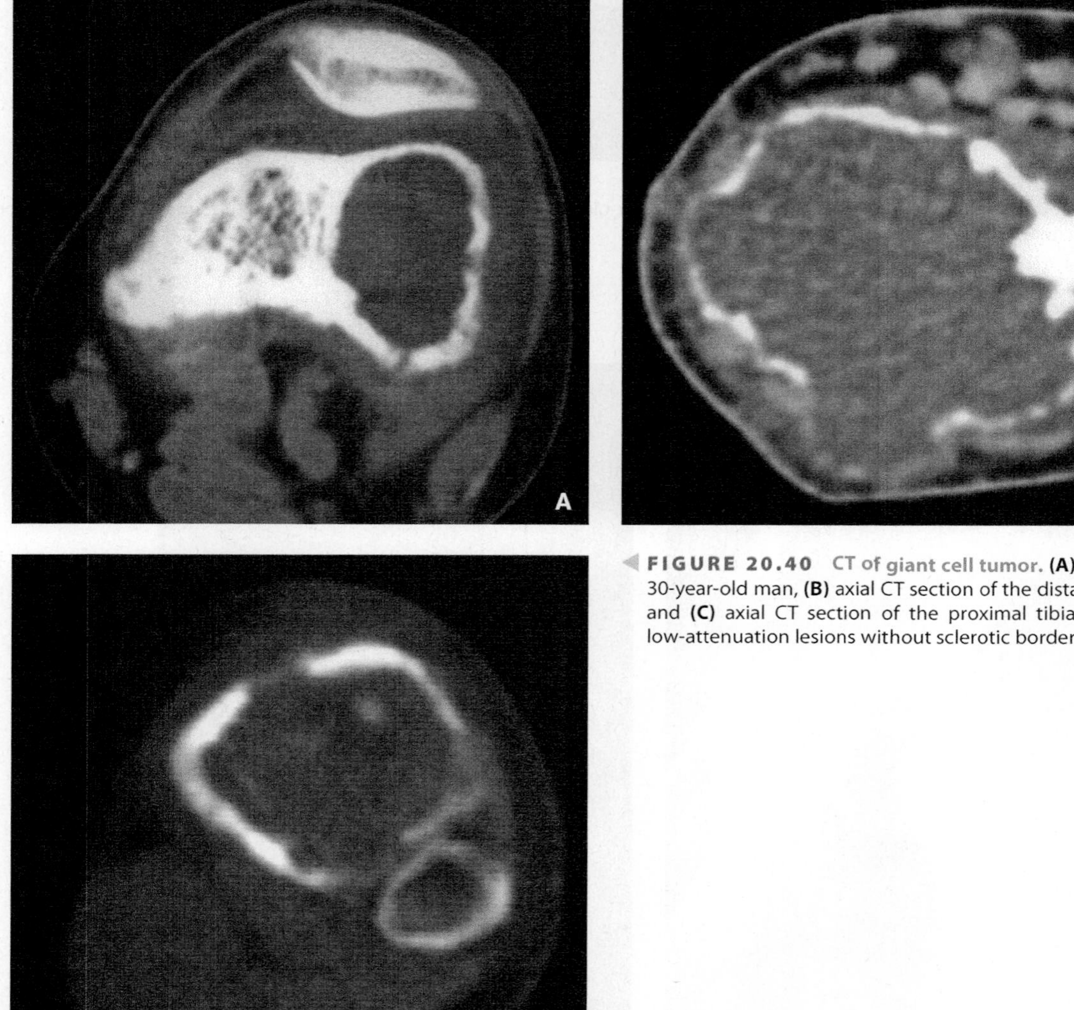

FIGURE 20.40 CT of giant cell tumor. **(A)** Axial CT section of the knee of a 30-year-old man, **(B)** axial CT section of the distal radius of a 35-year-old woman, and **(C)** axial CT section of the proximal tibia of a 22-year-old woman show low-attenuation lesions without sclerotic borders, typical of this tumor.

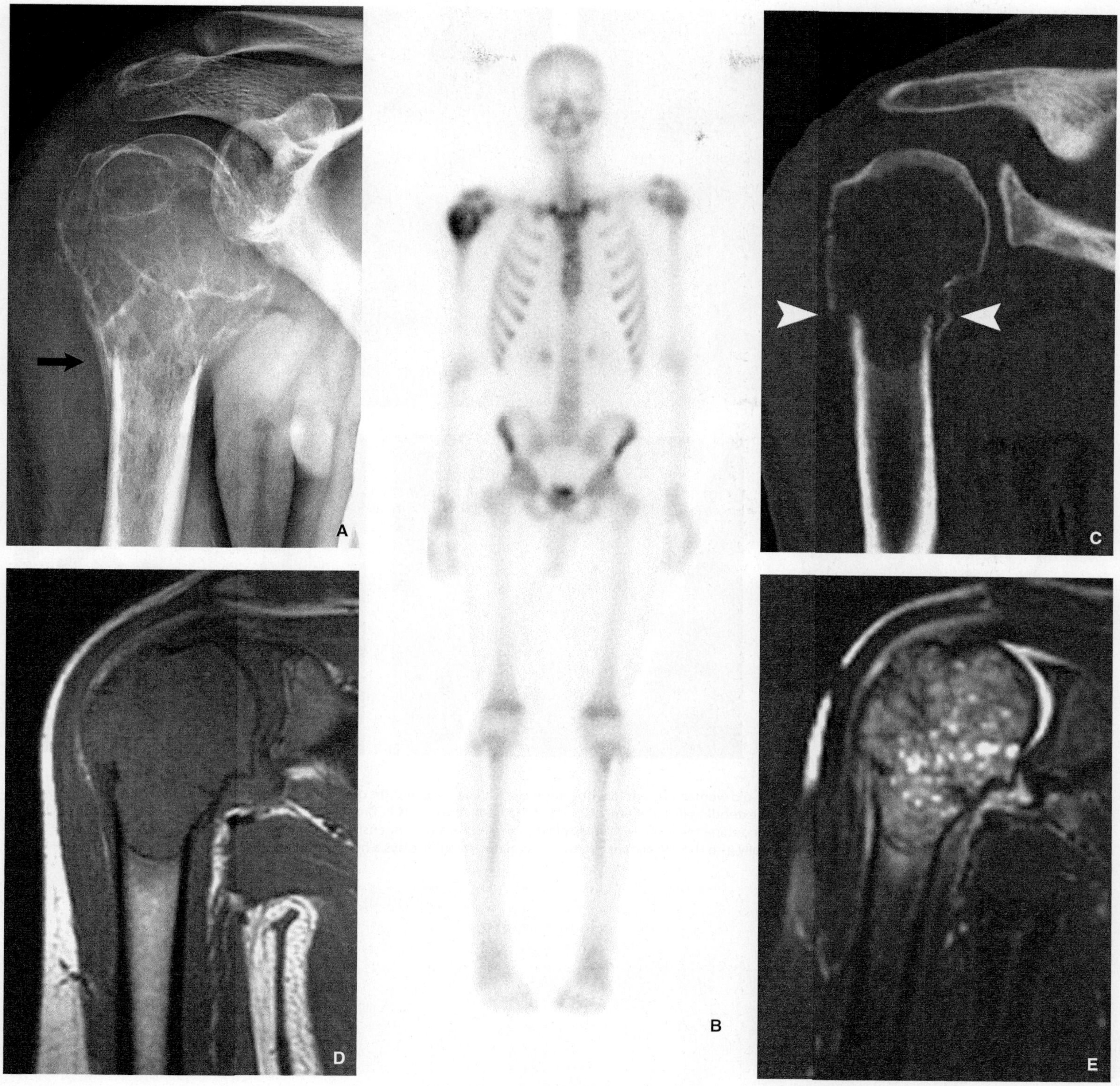

FIGURE 20.41 CT, scintigraphy, and MRI of giant cell tumor. **(A)** Anteroposterior radiograph of the right shoulder of a 19-year-old man shows an expansive osteolytic lesion in the proximal humerus with internal septations. Observe a pathologic fracture with early periosteal reaction *(arrow)*. **(B)** Total body radionuclide bone scan shows an increased uptake of the radiopharmaceutical tracer by the tumor. **(C)** Coronal reformatted CT image shows a pathologic fracture to the better advantage *(arrowheads)*. **(D)** Coronal T1-weighted MR image shows the lesion to be of homogeneous intermediate signal intensity. **(E)** Coronal T2-weighted fat-suppressed MR image shows heterogenous appearance of the tumor with foci of high signal intensity. Observe high-signal joint effusion. **(F)** Axial T1-weighted fat-suppressed MR image obtained after intravenous administration of gadolinium shows heterogenous enhancement of the tumor.

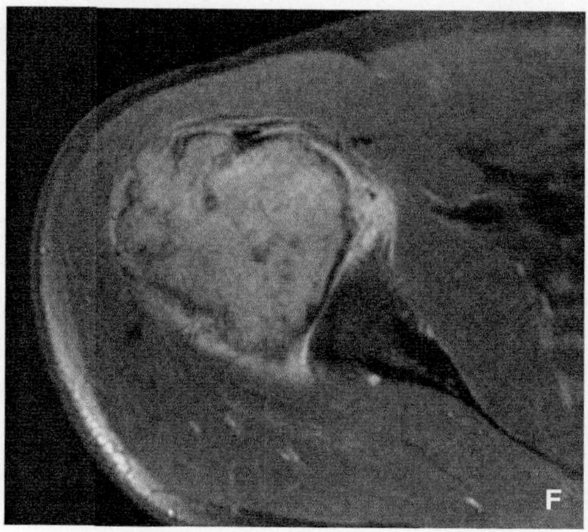

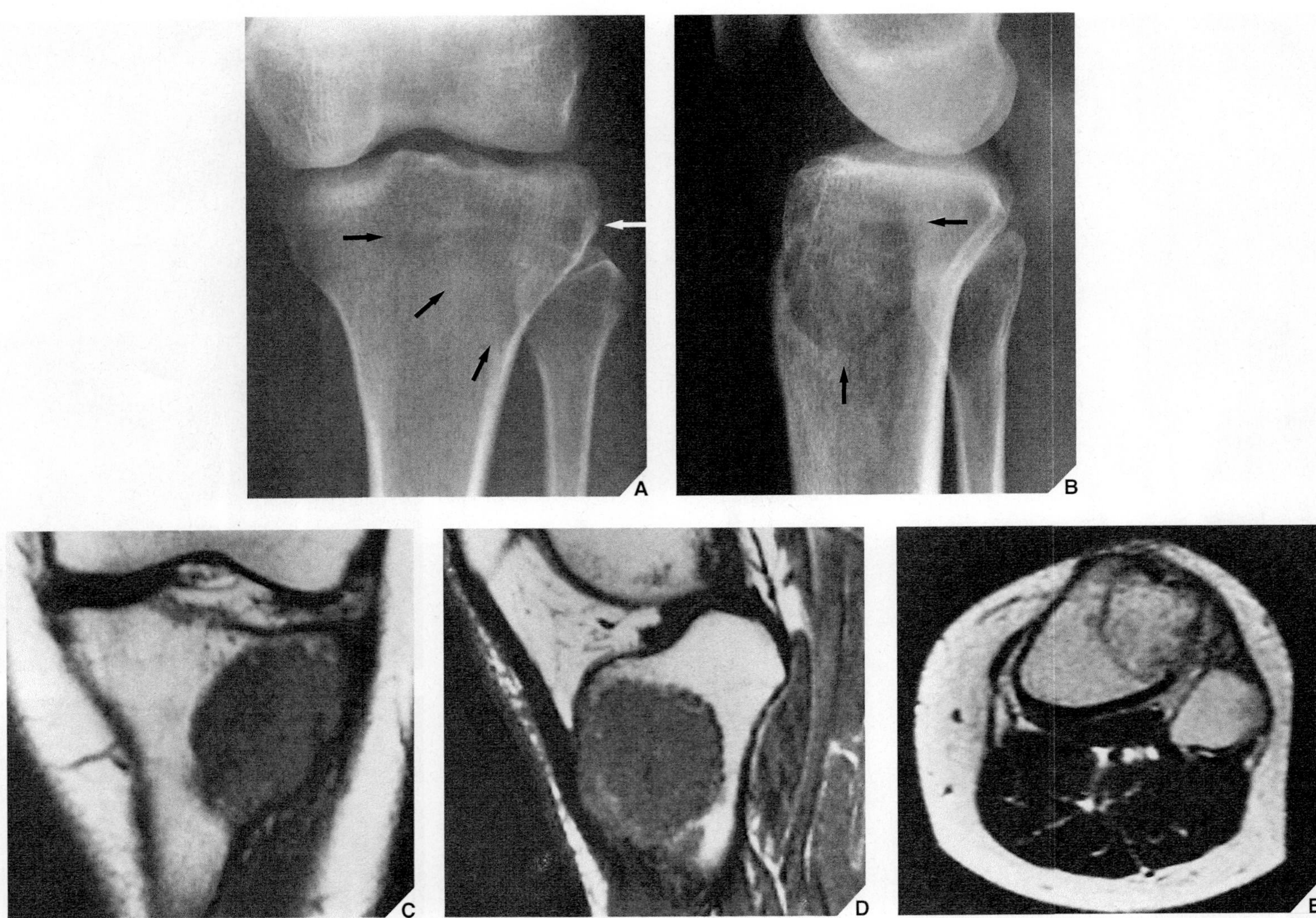

FIGURE 20.42 MRI of giant cell tumor. A 45-year-old woman presented with pain in the left knee of 6 months duration. **(A)** Anteroposterior and **(B)** lateral radiographs demonstrate a radiolucent lesion in the proximal tibia, extending into the articular end of the bone *(arrows)*. **(C)** Coronal and **(D)** sagittal spin echo T1-weighted MR images (repetition time [TR] 600/echo time [TE] 20 msec) better outline the lesion, which displays intermediate signal intensity. **(E)** Axial proton density-weighted MR image reveals that the lesion penetrates the cortex and extends laterally into the soft tissues. On this image, the lesion displays a heterogeneous signal varying from intermediate to high intensity.

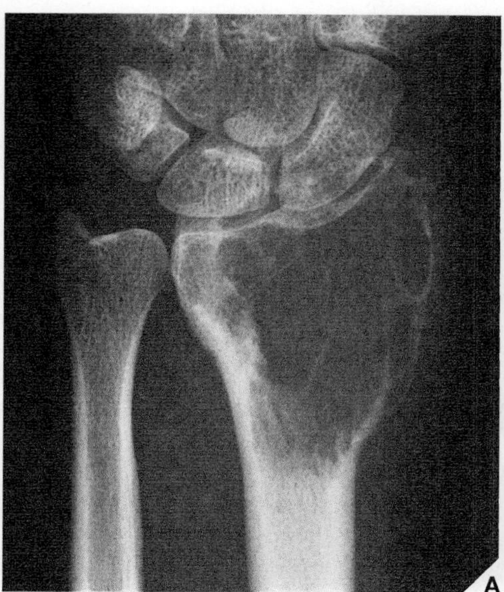

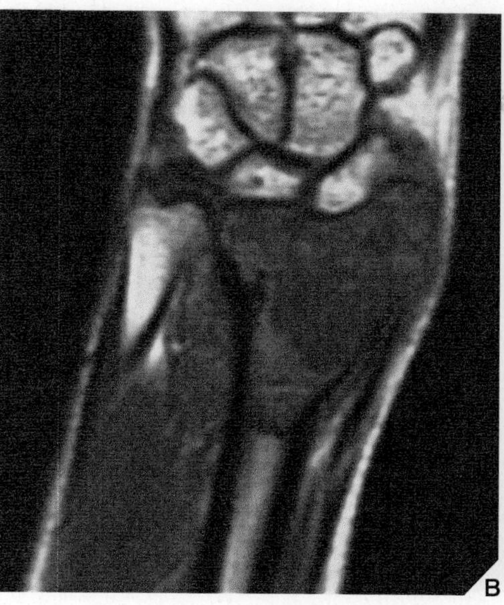

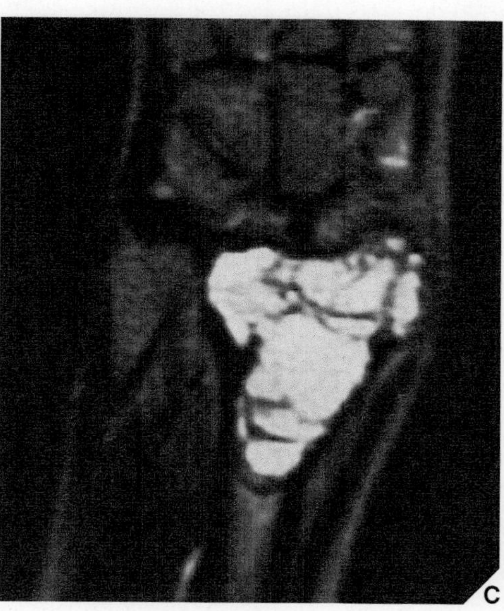

FIGURE 20.43 MRI of giant cell tumor. **(A)** Dorsovolar radiograph of the right wrist of a 36-year-old woman shows an osteolytic lesion in the distal radius. **(B)** Coronal T1-weighted (spin echo [SE]; repetition time [TR] 500/echo time [TE] 20 msec) MR image shows the tumor to be of intermediate-to-low signal intensity. **(C)** On coronal T2-weighted (SE; TR 2000/TE 80 msec) MRI, the lesion becomes bright, displaying low-signal septations.

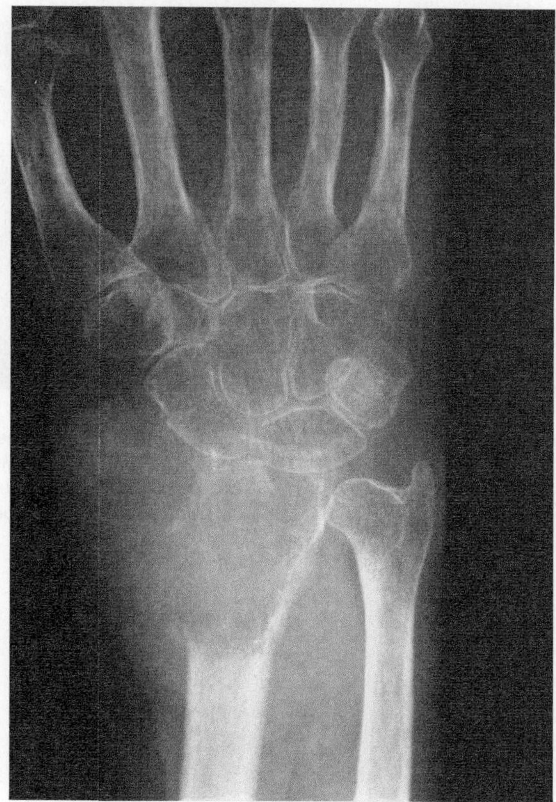

FIGURE 20.44 Giant cell tumor. Dorsovolar radiograph of the left wrist of a 56-year-old woman shows a lytic lesion of the distal radius that has destroyed the cortex and that extends into the soft tissues. Despite this aggressive radiographic presentation, on histopathologic examination, the tumor had a typically benign appearance, without malignant features. After wide resection, a 5-year follow-up showed no evidence of recurrence or of distant metastases.

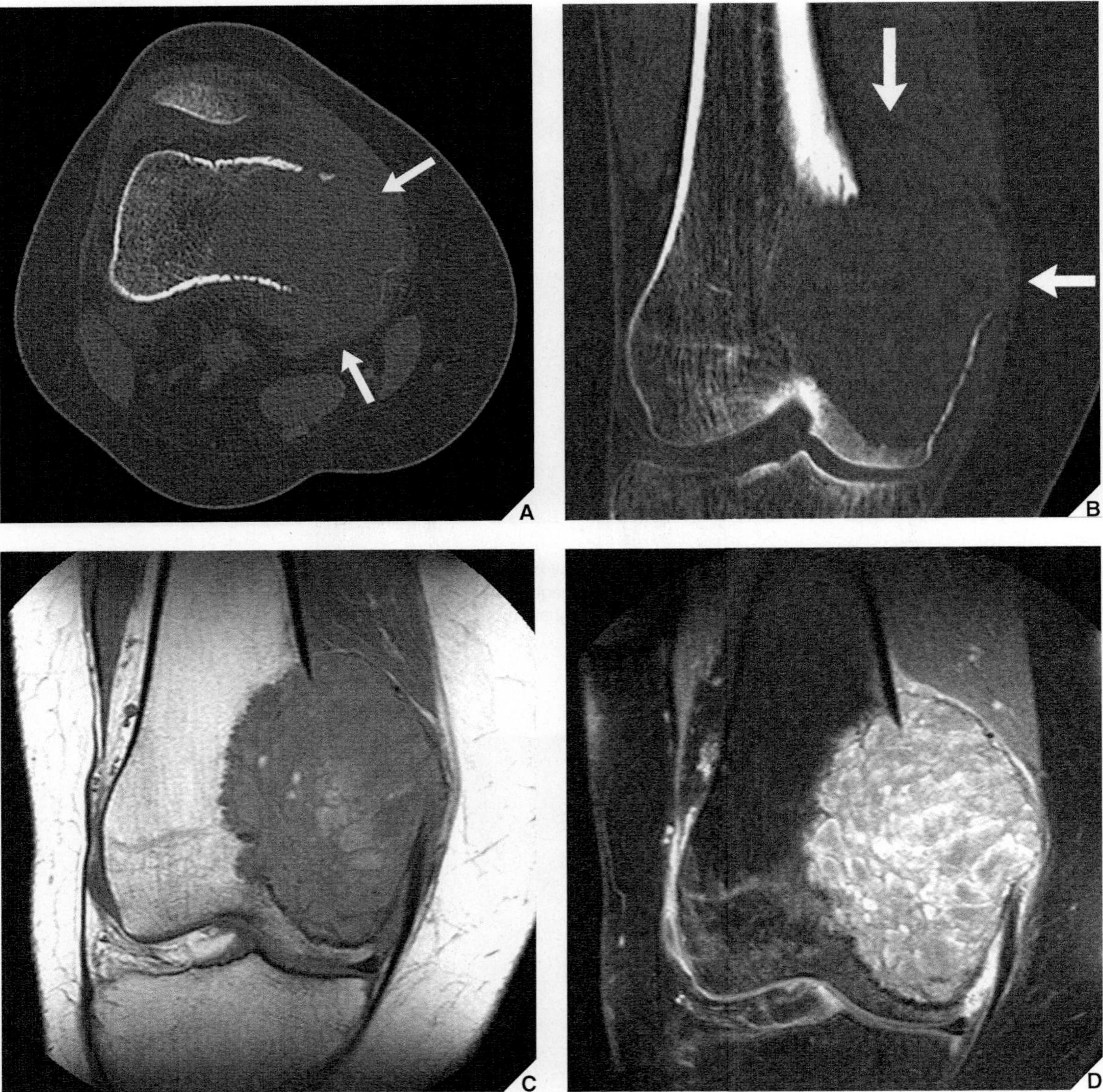

FIGURE 20.45 CT and MRI of giant cell tumor. **(A)** Axial and **(B)** coronal reformatted CT images of the right knee of a 31-year-old woman show a large tumor destroying the cortex of the medial femoral condyle and extending into the soft tissues *(arrows)*. **(C)** Coronal T1-weighted MRI demonstrates the tumor exhibiting an intermediate, slightly heterogenous signal due to the bleeding. **(D)** Coronal T1-weighted fat-suppressed MR image obtained after intravenous administration of gadolinium shows marked enhancement of the tumor. Histopathologic examination did not reveal any malignant features within the resected specimen.

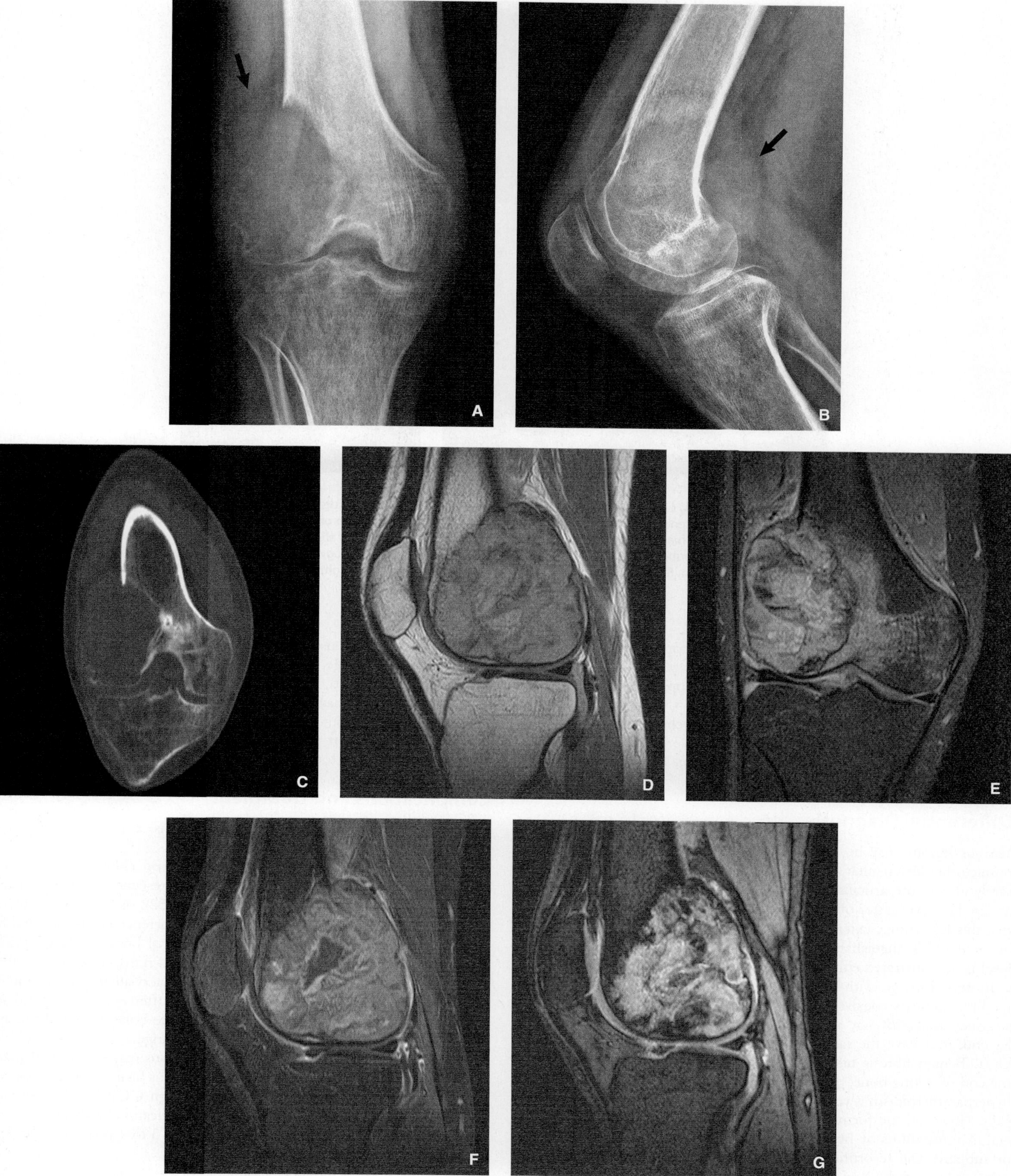

FIGURE 20.46 **CT and MRI of giant cell tumor.** **(A)** Anteroposterior and **(B)** lateral radiographs of the right knee of a 24-year-old man show an osteolytic lesion within the lateral femoral condyle. The tumor destroyed the lateral cortex and extended into the soft tissues forming a large mass *(arrows)*. Note a periarticular osteoporosis affecting the proximal tibia and fibula. **(C)** Coronal reformatted CT image of the knee shows better destruction of the cortex and a large soft-tissue mass. **(D)** Sagittal T1-weighted MR image shows heterogenous tumor but predominantly of intermediate signal intensity. **(E)** On coronal and **(F)** sagittal T2-weighted MR images, the tumor becomes bright with foci of low signal intensity. On coronal image, note high-signal peritumoral edema. **(G)** Sagittal T1-weighted fat-suppressed MR image obtained after intravenous administration of gadolinium shows prominent enhancement of the tumor. Despite aggressive features (stage 3), histopathologic examination of the resected specimen revealed no malignancy.

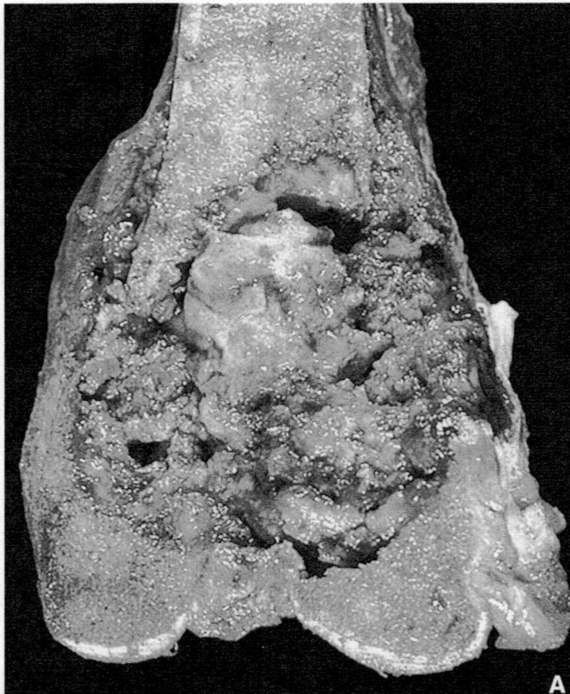

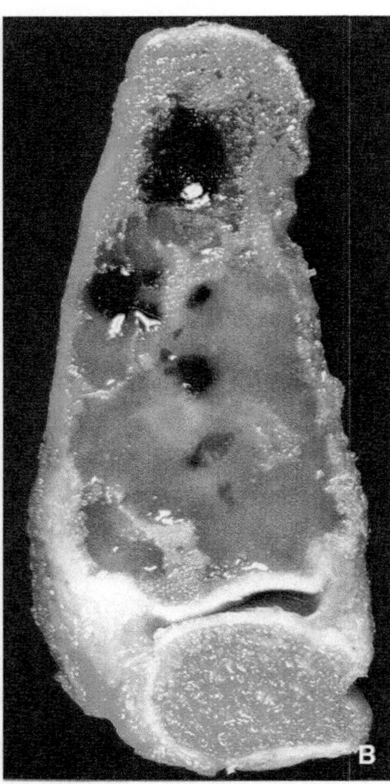

FIGURE 20.47 Pathology of giant cell tumor. **(A)** Coronal section of the resected surgical specimen of the distal femur shows a lobulated intramedullary tumor with hemorrhagic foci breaking through the cortex and extending into the articular end of bone. **(B)** Coronal section of the surgical specimen of the first metacarpal bone of another patient shows pinkish-tan soft intramedullary mass exhibiting foci of hemorrhage. Observe extension of the tumor to the proximal end of bone and preservation of the first carpometacarpal joint. (**A**, Reprinted with permission from Greenspan A, Borys D. *Radiology and pathology correlation of bone tumors: a quick reference and review*. Philadelphia: Wolters Kluwer; 2016:307; **B**, Modified from Bullough P. *Orthopaedic pathology*, 5th ed. Maryland Heights, MO: Mosby; 2009, with permission from Elsevier.)

and their maturation under normal physiologic conditions. *RANKL* gene is located at the chromosome 13q14 locus. In cytogenetic studies of GCTs, telomeric associations (end-to-end fusions of apparently intact chromosomes) involving chromosomes 11p, 13p, 14p, 15p, 19q, 20q, and 21p have been identified as the most commonly occurring chromosomal aberration. Some tumors show rearrangement of chromosomes 16q22 and 17p13. Loss of heterozygosity (LOH) of 1p, 3p, 5q, 9q, 10q, and 19q has been reported.

Differential Diagnosis

Various lesions may be mistaken for GCT and, conversely, GCT can mimic other lesions that affect the articular end of a bone. Primary ABC rarely affects the articular end of a bone and occurs in a younger age group. However, after obliteration of the growth plate at skeletal maturity, this lesion may extend into the subarticular region of a long bone, becoming indistinguishable from a GCT. Occasionally, if the fluid–fluid level is demonstrated either on CT or on MRI examination, this feature is more consistent with ABC. However, it should be noted that ABC might sometimes coexist with other lesions, among them the GCT. The so-called *solid ABC*, or a giant cell reparative granuloma at the articular end, may have the same radiologic characteristics as a conventional GCT. Benign fibrous histiocytoma, because of its frequent location at the end of a long bone, may appear identical to a GCT. Brown tumor of hyperparathyroidism is yet another lesion that can mimic GCT radiologically. However, the former lesion is usually accompanied by other skeletal manifestations of hyperparathyroidism, such as osteopenia, cortical or subperiosteal resorption, resorptive changes at the distal phalangeal tufts, or loss of the lamina dura of the teeth. Occasionally, an unusually large intraosseous ganglion may be mistaken for a GCT, although the former lesion invariably exhibits a sclerotic border. Some malignant lesions, such as chondrosarcoma, may extend into the articular end of bone and, particularly without radiographically identified calcifications, may closely mimic GCT. Myeloma and a lytic metastasis occupying subchondral segments of bone can usually be distinguished from GCT without much difficulty (the older age group in which the latter malignancies usually occur is a helpful hint), although at times the radiographic differences between the lesions may not be so obvious. Finally, on rare occasions, fibrosarcoma, malignant fibrous histiocytoma, or fibroblastic osteosarcoma (because of their purely lytic radiographic presentation) may exhibit some similarities to GCT.

Complications and Treatment

The most common complication of GCT is a pathologic fracture (Fig. 20.48; see also Figs. 20.35B and 20.41A).

The treatment of benign GCTs consists of either surgical curettage and bone grafting (Fig. 20.49) or wide resection with secondary implantation of an allograft (Figs. 20.50 to 20.52), or an endoprosthesis (see Fig. 20.54). Good healing and lack of recurrence are recognized by incorporation of the bone graft into the normal bone (see Fig. 20.52). Marcove recommended cryosurgery using liquid nitrogen, whereas other authorities recommended heat using methylmethacrylate to pack the tumor bed after intralesional excision. Recurrences are often encountered and are recognized radiographically by resorption of the bone graft and the appearance of radiolucent areas like those in the original tumor (Fig. 20.53). Especially after radiation therapy, recurrent lesions may exhibit malignant transformation to fibrosarcoma, malignant fibrous histiocytoma, or osteosarcoma. Occasionally, even histologically benign GCTs produce distant (to the lung) metastases (Fig. 20.54). This complication has been reported in 2% of the patients and is usually seen within 3 to 4 years after original diagnosis.

Recently, improved understanding of the molecular and cellular biology of this tumor, particularly identification of the osteoclast differentiation factor RANKL, a molecule that is critical to the pathogenesis of GCT, prompted trials of targeted treatment using a monoclonal antibody denosumab, directed against RANKL. This is a promising therapy in patients with either unresectable or recurrent GCT.

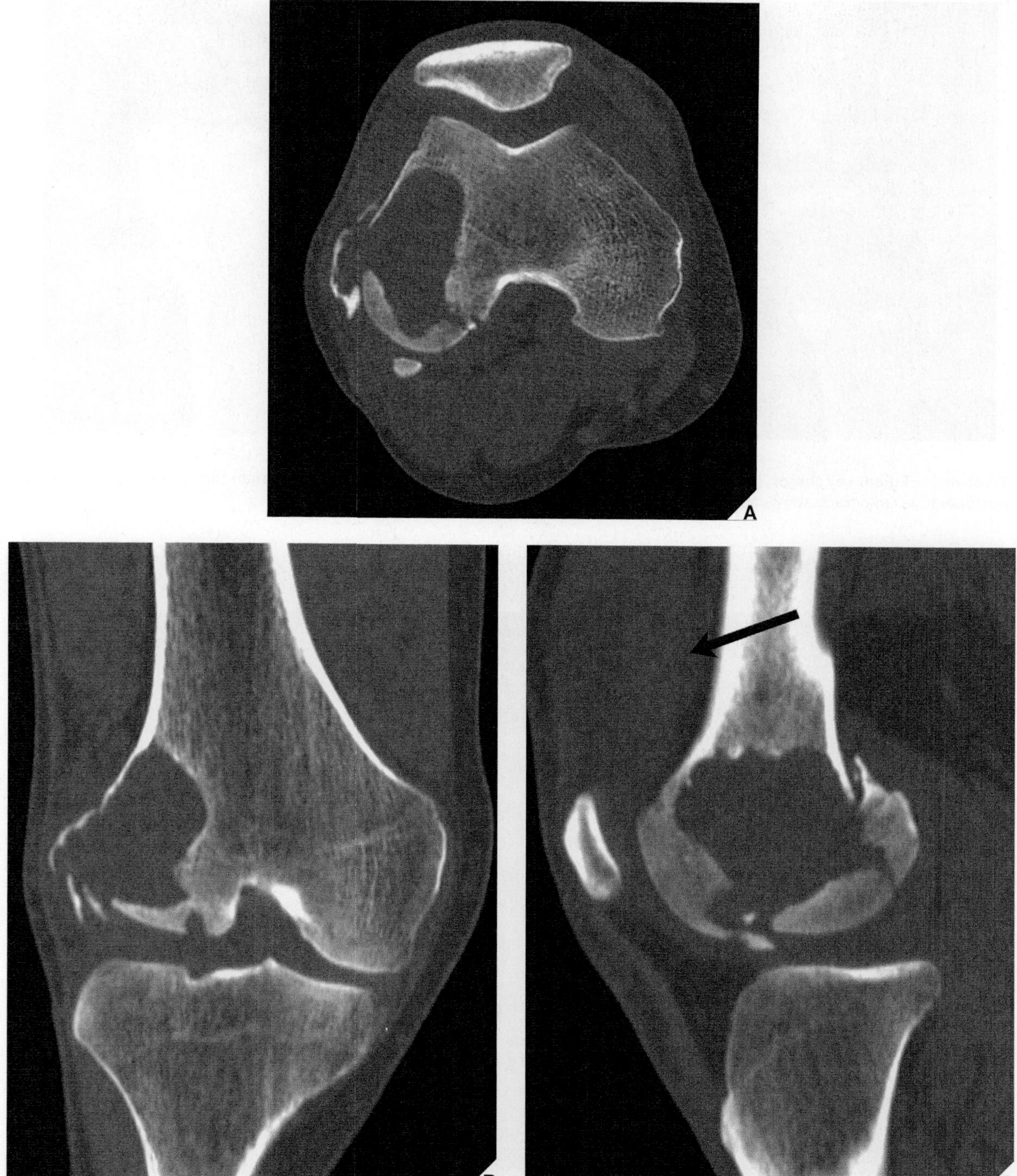

FIGURE 20.48 **Complication of giant cell tumor.** **(A)** Axial, **(B)** coronal reformatted, and **(C)** sagittal reformatted CT images of the right knee of a 40-year-old man show a comminuted pathologic fracture of a large GCT located in the lateral femoral condyle. Note opacification of the suprapatellar recess *(arrow)* due to a hemorrhage.

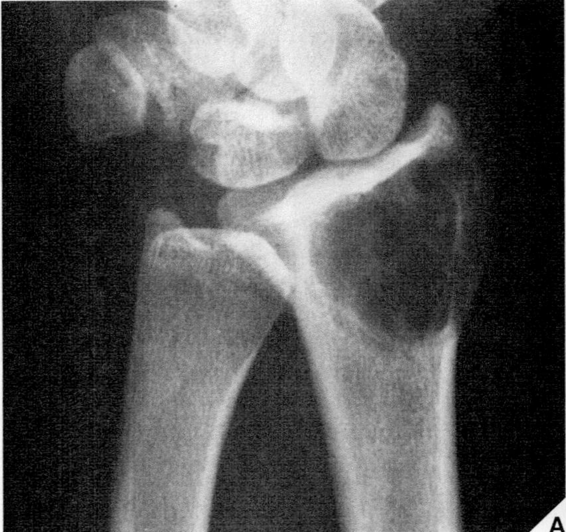

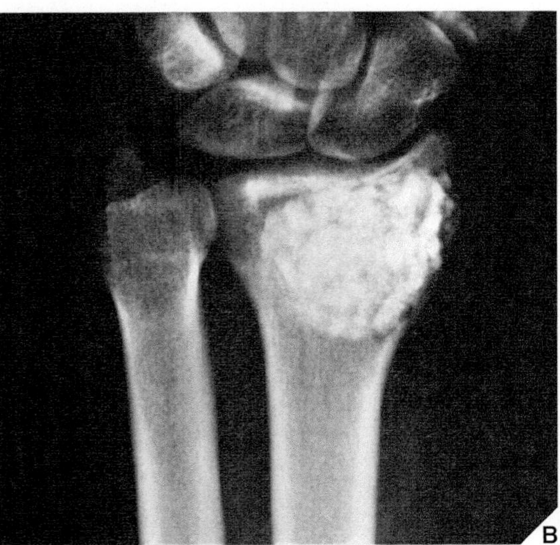

FIGURE 20.49 Treatment of giant cell tumor. (A) Conventional radiograph of the right wrist of a 32-year-old woman shows a lytic lesion in the distal radius. **(B)** After extensive curettage, postoperative radiograph shows application of bone chips.

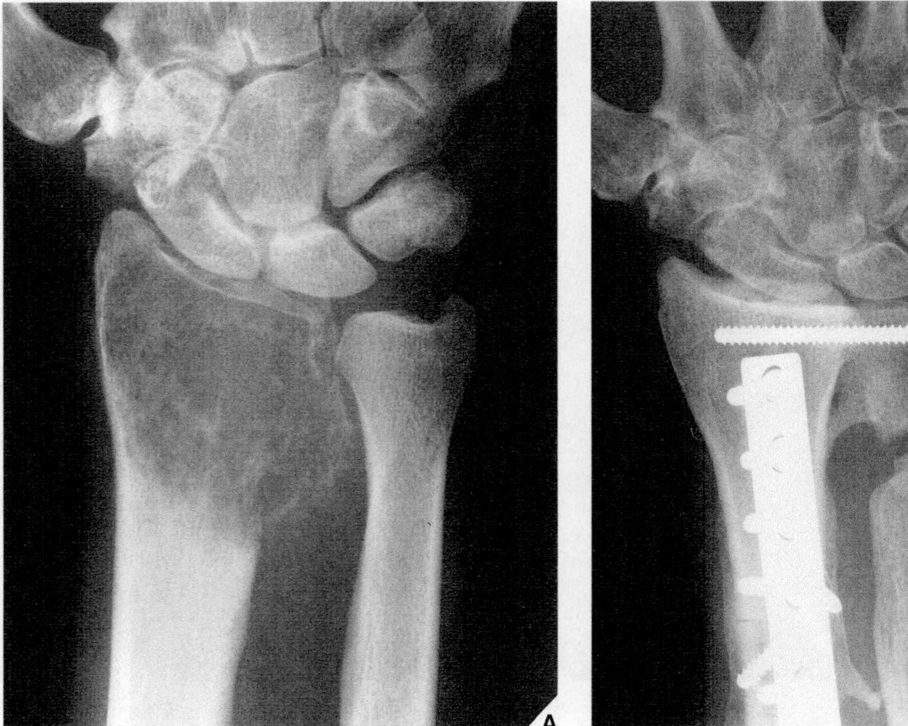

FIGURE 20.50 Treatment of giant cell tumor. (A) Dorsovolar radiograph of the left wrist of a 38-year-old woman shows the classic appearance of a GCT of the distal radius. **(B)** Treatment consisted of resection of the distal radius and application of an allograft. In addition, a Suavé-Kapandji procedure was performed, creating a pseudoarthrosis of the distal ulna and fusion of the distal radioulnar joint.

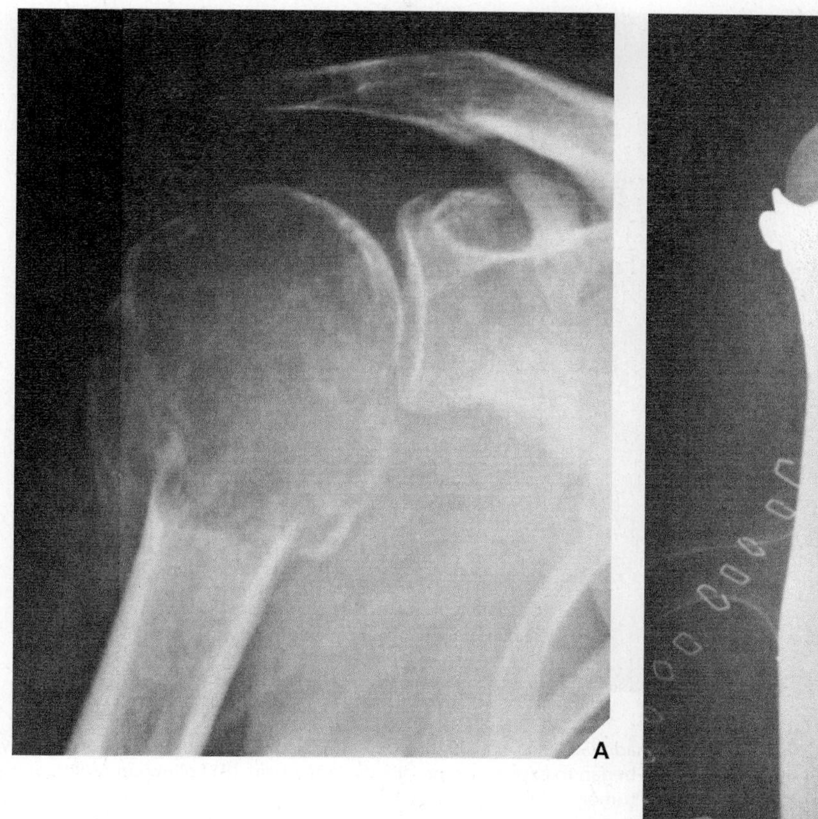

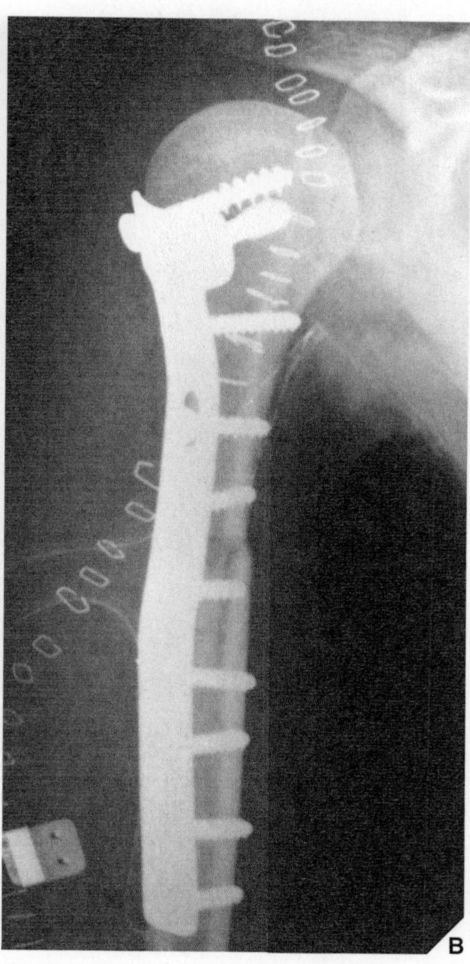

FIGURE 20.51 **Treatment of giant cell tumor.** **(A)** Anteroposterior radiograph of the right shoulder of a 27-year-old woman shows a GCT affecting almost the entire proximal end of the humerus (same patient as presented in Fig. 20.35B). **(B)** Wide resection was performed and the humerus was reconstructed by means of allograft.

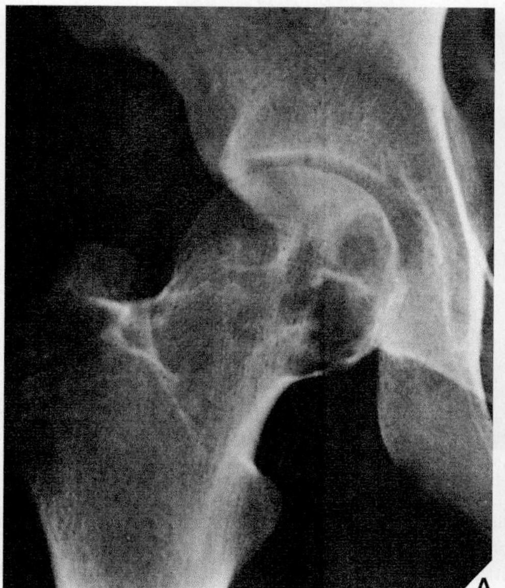

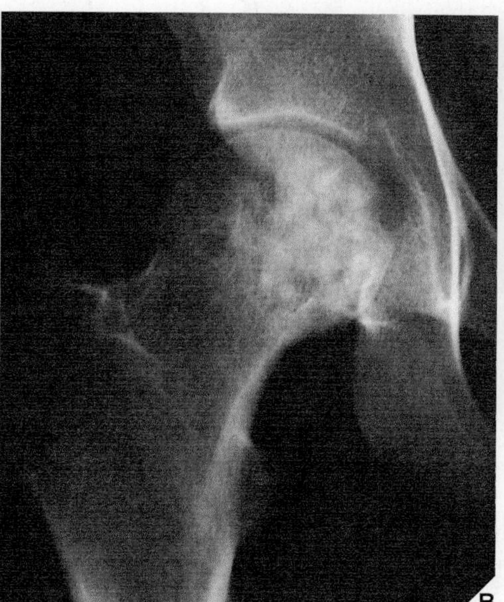

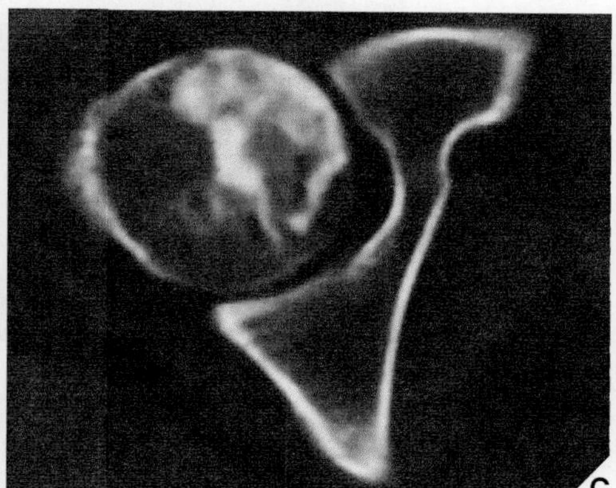

FIGURE 20.52 **Treatment of giant cell tumor.** **(A)** A 27-year-old woman was diagnosed with a GCT in the femoral head. **(B)** Two years after curettage and application of allograft, there was no recurrence of the lesion. **(C)** CT demonstrates good incorporation of the graft into the normal bone (compare with Fig. 20.53).

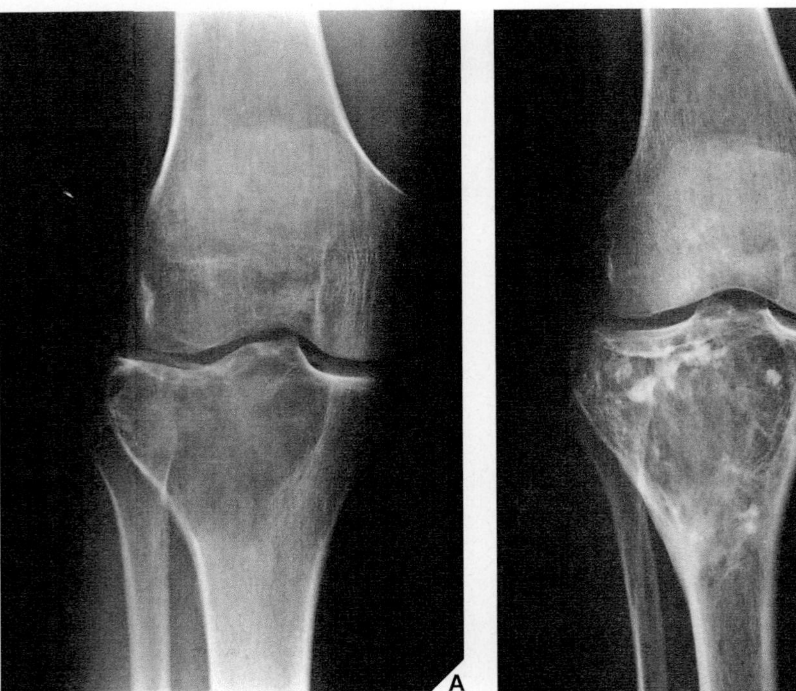

FIGURE 20.53 Recurrence of giant cell tumor. A 30-year-old woman had a GCT of the proximal end of the right tibia **(A)** and was subsequently treated with curettage and application of cancellous bone chips. Twenty months after surgery, she began to experience progressive knee pain. **(B)** Follow-up radiograph shows that most of the bone chips have been resorbed; the osteolytic foci indicate recurrence of the tumor.

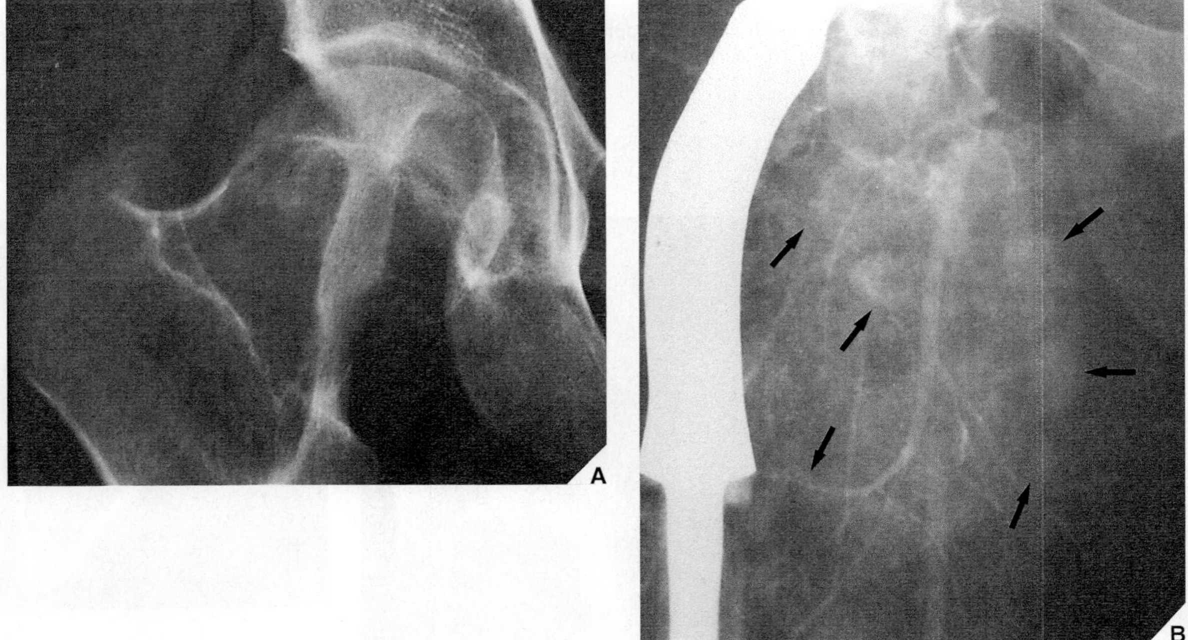

FIGURE 20.54 Complication of giant cell tumor. A 28-year-old man had a 4-month history of right hip pain. **(A)** Anteroposterior radiograph of the hip shows a destructive radiolucent lesion involving the medial aspect of the femoral head and extending into the femoral neck. Biopsy revealed an ABC. Five months after curettage and packing of the cavity with cancellous bone chips, the lesion recurred. This time the histopathologic examination revealed a benign GCT with an engrafted ABC. The proximal femur was resected and an endoprosthesis was implanted. Eight months after this procedure, the patient was readmitted to the hospital with increased pain and a significant increase in the circumference of the thigh. **(B)** A femoral arteriogram demonstrates multiple soft-tissue nodules *(arrows)*, which on biopsy proved to be metastases from the GCT. The patient also had pulmonary metastases.

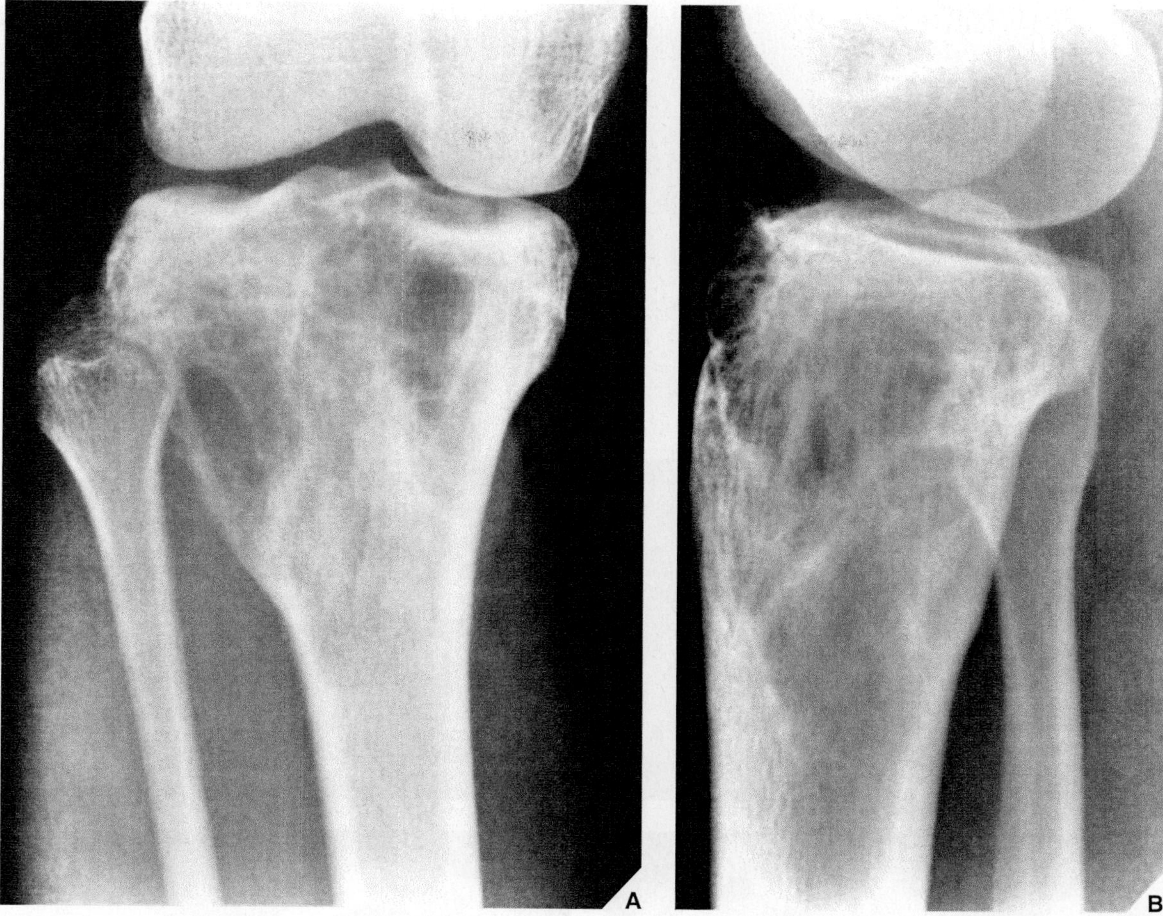

FIGURE 20.55 **Fibrocartilaginous mesenchymoma.** **(A)** Anteroposterior and **(B)** lateral radiographs of the right knee of a 23-year-old man show a radiolucent trabeculated lesion in the proximal tibia, bulging the anterolateral cortex and extending into the articular end of bone.

Fibrocartilaginous Mesenchymoma

Clinical and Imaging Features

Fibrocartilaginous mesenchymoma is an extremely rare tumor composed of two distinct tissues: one benign and cartilaginous, resembling an active growth plate, and the other resembling a low-grade fibrosarcoma. It was first described by Dahlin and colleagues in 1984 as a low-grade malignancy tumor. Mirra and associates classify this lesion as desmoid tumor with enchondroma-like nodules. The number of reported cases is probably less than 30, although several unpublished cases may exist. Fibrocartilaginous mesenchymoma has been reported in patients ranging from ages 1 to 25 years (mean age 13 years). Males were more frequently affected. The lesion is usually located in the epiphysis of a long bone, such as the fibula or humerus. The symptoms usually indicate a slow-growing tumor. They consist of slight discomfort and tenderness at the site of the lesion and occasionally a palpable mass.

On radiography, the lesion is radiolucent with scalloped borders, extending to or abutting the growth plate. After skeletal maturity, the lesion may extend into the articular end of bone (Fig. 20.55). Occasionally, the cortex is expanded and thinned. The cortex may be invaded, and in these cases, the lesion extends into the soft tissues (Fig. 20.56). This can be effectively demonstrated with CT and MRI. Although a periosteal reaction is usually absent, when present, it is sparse and of benign appearance. The tumor may contain visible calcifications typical of cartilaginous matrix.

Pathology

By microscopy, the lesion is composed of a tissue made of intersecting bundles of spindle cells and collagen fibers. The tissue is fairly cellular, the nuclei are plump, and there is evidence of pleomorphism and hyperchromatism, with occasional mitotic figures. Superimposed on this background are well-defined islands of obviously benign cartilage structured similarly to the growth plate. Characteristic feature is the presence of numerous curved cartilage particles surrounded by spindle-cell stroma, giving the tumor on H&E staining a "shrimp cocktail" appearance. In its first description, the tumor was named *fibrocartilaginous mesenchymoma with low-grade malignancy*. However, because metastases have never been observed thus far, the group at the Mayo Clinic later deleted that addition, simply calling it *fibrocartilaginous mesenchymoma*.

Hemangioma

Clinical and Imaging Features

A hemangioma is a benign bone lesion composed of newly formed blood vessels. It comprises approximately 2% of all benign and 0.8% of benign and malignant lesions of the skeletal system. Some investigators consider hemangiomas benign neoplasms; others put them into the category of congenital vascular malformations. They are classified, according to the type of vessels in the lesion, as capillary, cavernous, venous, or mixed.

Capillary hemangiomas are composed of small vessels that consist merely of a flat endothelium, surrounded only by a basal membrane. In bone, they most commonly occur in the vertebral body. *Cavernous hemangiomas* are composed of dilated, blood-filled spaces lined by the same flat endothelium with a basal membrane. Osseous cavernous hemangiomas most commonly involve the calvaria. *Venous hemangiomas* are composed of thick-walled vessels that possess a muscle layer. They frequently contain

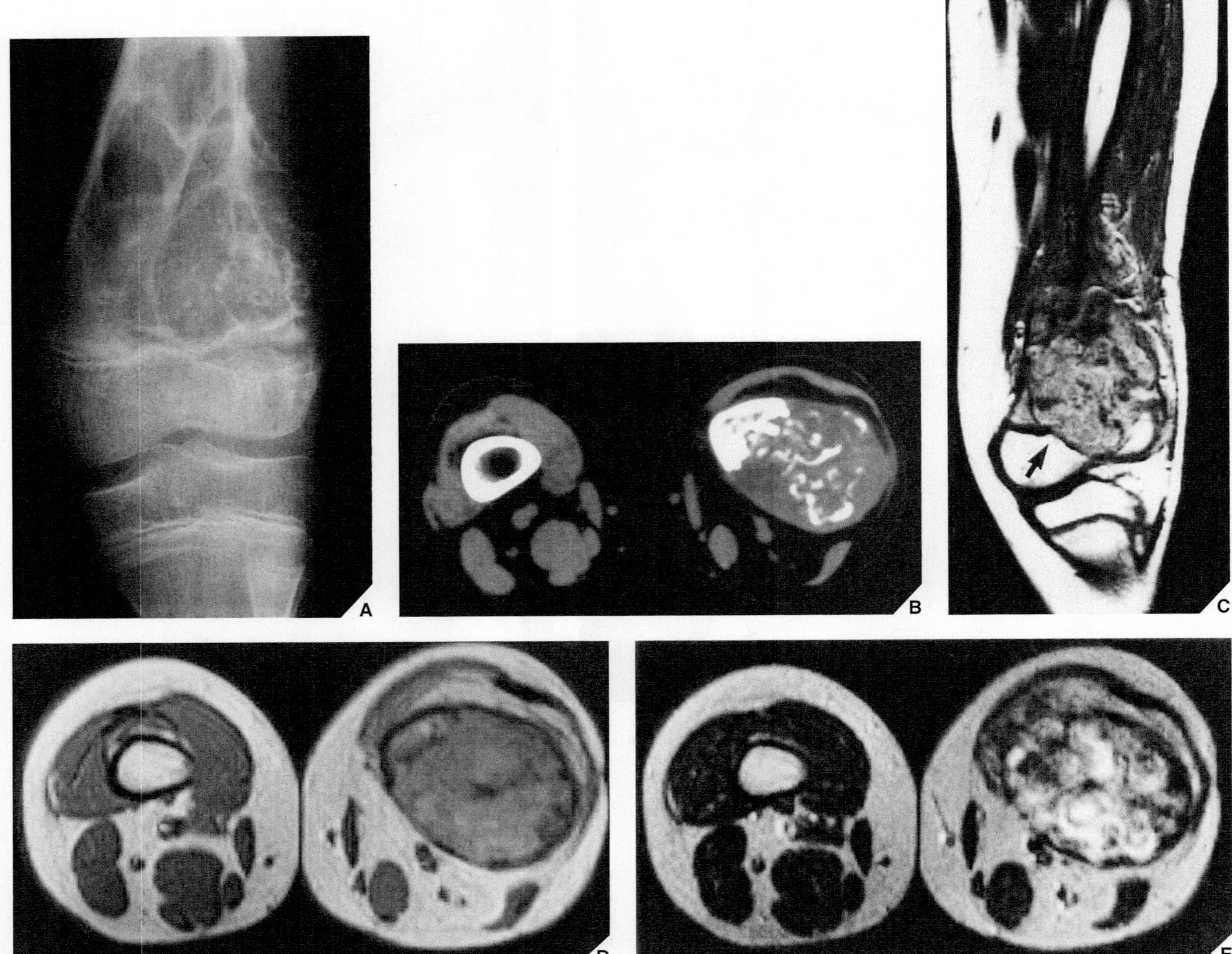

FIGURE 20.56 **MRI of fibrocartilaginous mesenchymoma.** **(A)** Oblique radiograph of the left knee of a 14-year-old boy shows an osteolytic trabeculated lesion in the distal femur abutting the growth plate. The lateral cortex is destroyed. **(B)** CT section through the tumor shows destruction of the posterolateral cortex and a large soft-tissue mass containing calcifications. **(C)** Coronal T1-weighted MRI shows heterogeneous signal of the tumor that violated the growth plate and extended into the distal femoral epiphysis *(arrow)*. **(D)** Axial T1-weighted MR image shows destruction of the cortex and a large soft-tissue mass of intermediate signal. Calcifications within the mass display low signal intensity. **(E)** On axial T2-weighted MR image, the tumor becomes for most part of high signal intensity. Pseudoseptation of the mass and its heterogeneous character are well demonstrated. (Courtesy Prof. Wolfgang Remagen, Cologne, Germany.)

phleboliths. *Arteriovenous hemangiomas* are characterized by abnormal communications between arteries and veins. These are extremely rare in bone and almost exclusively involve the soft tissues. The biologic classification of vascular anomalies have been reviewed by Mulliken and Glowacki, who advocate regarding hemangiomas as hamartomas rather than true neoplasms, this classification takes into consideration cellular turnover and histology as well as natural history and physical findings. It clearly separates hemangiomas of infancy, with their early proliferative and later involutional stages, from vascular malformations, which are congenital lesions and are characterized as arterial, venous, capillary, lymphatic, or combined. However, epithelioid hemangiomas have been observed that apparently are true tumors.

The incidence of hemangiomas seems to increase with age and is most frequent after middle age. Women are affected twice as often as men. The most common sites are the spine, particularly the thoracic segment, and the skull (Fig. 20.57). In the spine, the lesion typically involves a vertebral body, although it may extend into the pedicle or lamina and, rarely, to the spinous process. Occasionally, multiple vertebrae may be affected.

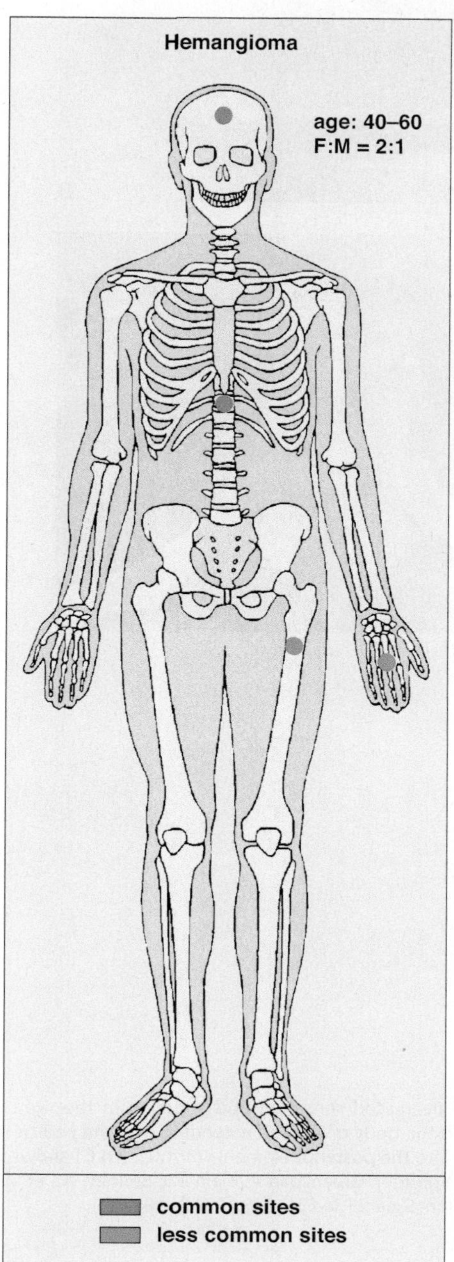

FIGURE 20.57 Skeletal sites of predilection, peak age range, and male-to-female ratio in hemangioma.

Most hemangiomas of the vertebral column are asymptomatic and discovered incidentally. Symptoms occur when the lesion in an affected vertebra compresses the nerve roots or spinal cord secondary to epidural extension. This neurologic complication is more commonly associated with lesions in the midthoracic spine (Fig. 20.58). Another mechanism considered responsible for compression of the cord, although seen less frequently, is fracture of the involved vertebral body with formation of an associated soft-tissue mass or hematoma.

On imaging studies, hemangioma is typified by the presence of multiloculated lytic foci (Fig. 20.59) or coarse vertical striations. In a vertebral body, this pattern is referred to as a *honeycomb* or *corduroy cloth pattern*, respectively (Fig. 20.60), and in the skull as a *spoke-wheel configuration.* When seen in the spine, this pattern is considered virtually pathognomonic for hemangioma. CT examination characteristically shows the pattern as multiple dots (often referred to as the *polka-dot appearance*), which represent a cross section of reinforced trabeculae (Fig. 20.61). On MRI, T1- and T2-weighted images usually reveal areas of a high-intensity signal that correspond to the vascular components (Fig. 20.62). Areas of trabecular thickening exhibit a low signal intensity regardless of the pulse sequence used. Both CT and MR images obtained after intravenous administration of gadolinium demonstrate lesion's enhancement. In the long and short tubular bones, hemangiomas are recognized by a typical lace-like pattern and honeycombing (Fig. 20.63A), but occasionally, they exhibit lytic, bubble-like expansive aggressively looking features (Fig. 20.63B). Not uncommonly, bone and adjacent soft tissue may be affected by hemangiomas (Figs. 20.64 and 20.65).

On scintigraphy, the appearance of osseous hemangiomas ranges from photopenia to a moderate increase in the uptake of radiopharmaceutical tracer. A recent study of planar images and single-photon emission CT (SPECT) of vertebral hemangiomas and their correlation with MRI showed that in most cases, hemangiomas exhibited normal uptake on planar images. SPECT images were also normal, particularly if the lesions were less than 3 cm in diameter. This study also showed a disparity between SPECT images and MRI: There was no correlation between MRI signal intensity changes and patterns of uptake on bone imaging. Arteriography of the hemangioma is rarely indicated.

Epithelioid hemangioma is a variant of conventional hemangioma. It has been previously described as *angiolymphoid hyperplasia with eosinophilia* and as *histiocytoid hemangioma* because of its morphologic features. Although it most commonly affects skin and subcutaneous tissue, epithelioid hemangioma may also involve bones, with a predilection for the vertebrae. Although majority of these lesions are solitary, there have been reports of multifocal affliction of the skeleton. The radiographic features of this lesion include expansive lytic areas with well-defined lobulated borders and marginal sclerosis. Rarely, the cortex is destroyed, causing formation of new periosteal bone. Histologically, as pointed out by Wenger and Wold, well-formed vessels with open lumina are observed, surrounded by multiple epithelioid endothelial cells with abundant eosinophilic cytoplasm. The vessels are usually of capillary size, and hemorrhage into the surrounding connective tissue may be present. The neighboring stroma may contain an inflammatory infiltrate. Occasionally, the histopathology of this lesion is similar to that of epithelioid hemangioendothelioma.

Diffuse involvement of bones by hemangiomatous lesions is defined as *hemangiomatosis* or *angiomatosis*. Occasionally, the soft tissues are also affected (Figs. 20.66 and 20.67). The imaging presentation of angiomatosis is that of lytic lesions, often with a honeycomb or latticework ("hole-within-hole") appearance. When bone is extensively involved, the term *cystic angiomatosis* is applied. Some other terms used for this condition include *diffuse skeletal hemangiomatosis*, *cystic lymphangiectasia*, and *hamartous hemolymphangiomatosis*. Schajowicz postulated that cystic hemangiomatosis should be distinguished from diffuse angiomatosis because of their different radiologic and macroscopic aspects. This is a rare bone disorder characterized by diffuse cystic lesions of bone, frequently (60% to 70% of cases) associated with visceral involvement. Patients with cystic angiomatosis usually present in the first three decades. There is 2:1 male-to-female predominance. The bones affected are most often those of the axial skeleton as well as the femur, humerus, tibia, radius, and fibula. The bone-related symptoms are usually secondary to pathologic

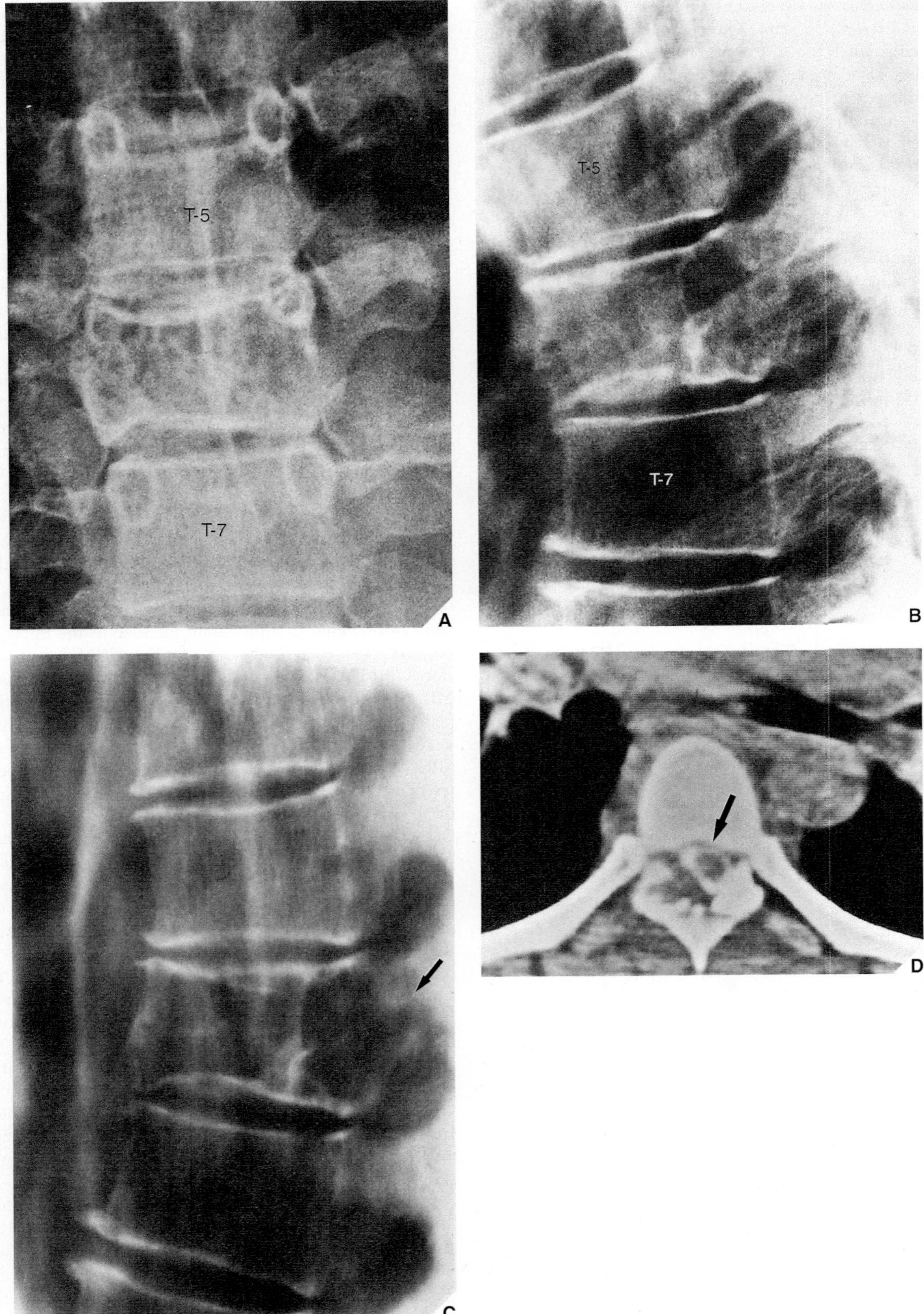

FIGURE 20.58 Vertebral hemangioma. A 39-year-old woman presented with back pain and decreased sensation and strength in the right upper extremity. **(A)** Anteroposterior and **(B)** lateral radiographs of the thoracic spine show a radiolucent lesion involving the body of T-6 and extending into the pedicle. **(C)** Lateral tomographic cut demonstrates ballooning of the posterior cortex of the vertebra and extension of the lesion into the posterior elements *(arrow)*. **(D)** CT shows a soft-tissue mass encroaching on the spinal canal and displacing the spinal cord *(arrow)*. (Reprinted by permission from Springer: Greenspan A, Klein MJ, Bennett AJ, et al. Case report 242. Hemangioma of the T6 vertebra with a compression fracture, extradural block and spinal cord compression. *Skeletal Radiol* 1978;10:183–188.)

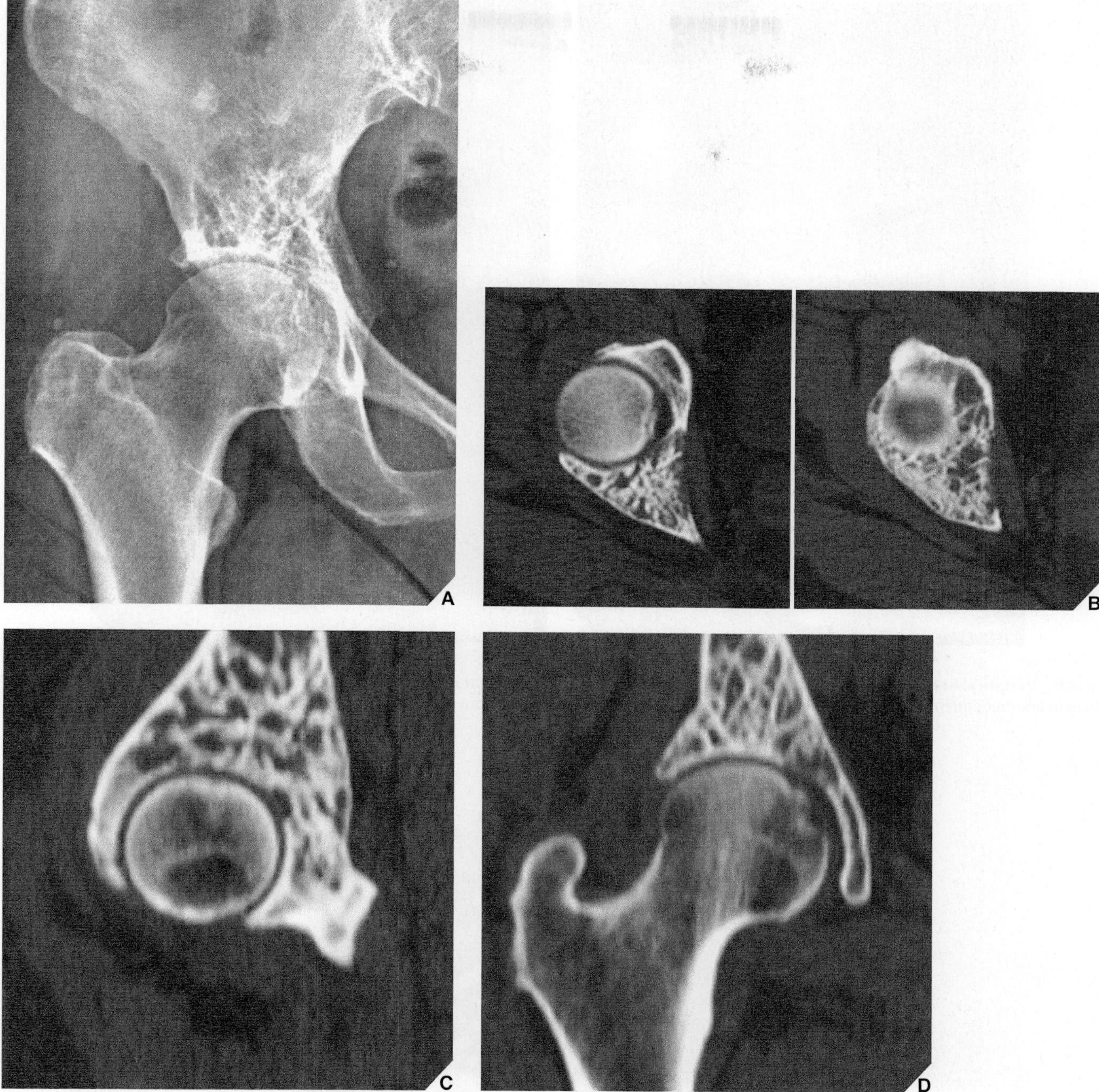

FIGURE 20.59 Hemangioma of the hip. A 58-year-old woman presented with right hip pain on and off for 1 year. **(A)** Anteroposterior radiograph of the right hip shows mixed radiolucent and sclerotic lesion in the ilium extending into the acetabulum. **(B)** Axial CT sections and **(C)** sagittal and **(D)** coronal reformatted CT images show a characteristic for hemangioma "honeycomb" pattern.

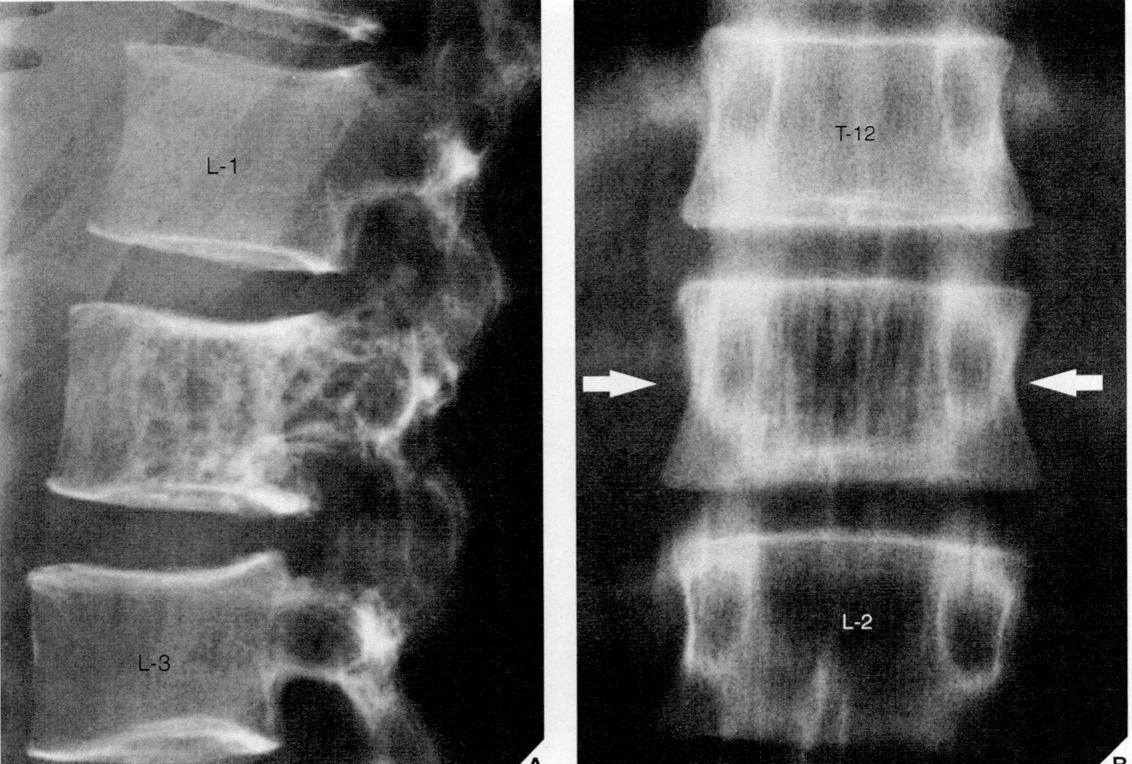

FIGURE 20.60 **Vertebral hemangioma.** **(A)** Lateral radiograph of the lumbar spine demonstrates a honeycomb pattern of hemangioma of L-2 vertebra. **(B)** Anteroposterior tomogram in another patient demonstrates vertical striations of hemangioma of L-1 vertebra *(arrows)*, referred to as a *corduroy cloth pattern*.

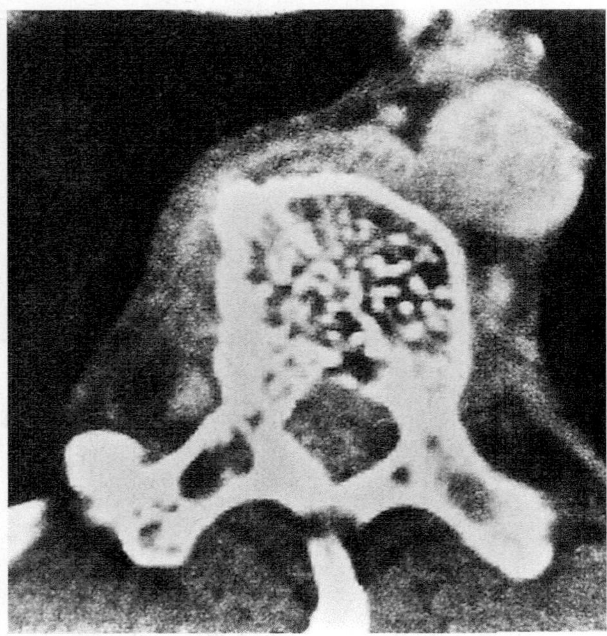

FIGURE 20.61 **CT of vertebral hemangioma.** CT section of a T-10 vertebra demonstrates coarse dots ("polka-dot" pattern) representing reinforced vertical trabeculae of the cancellous bone, characteristic of hemangioma.

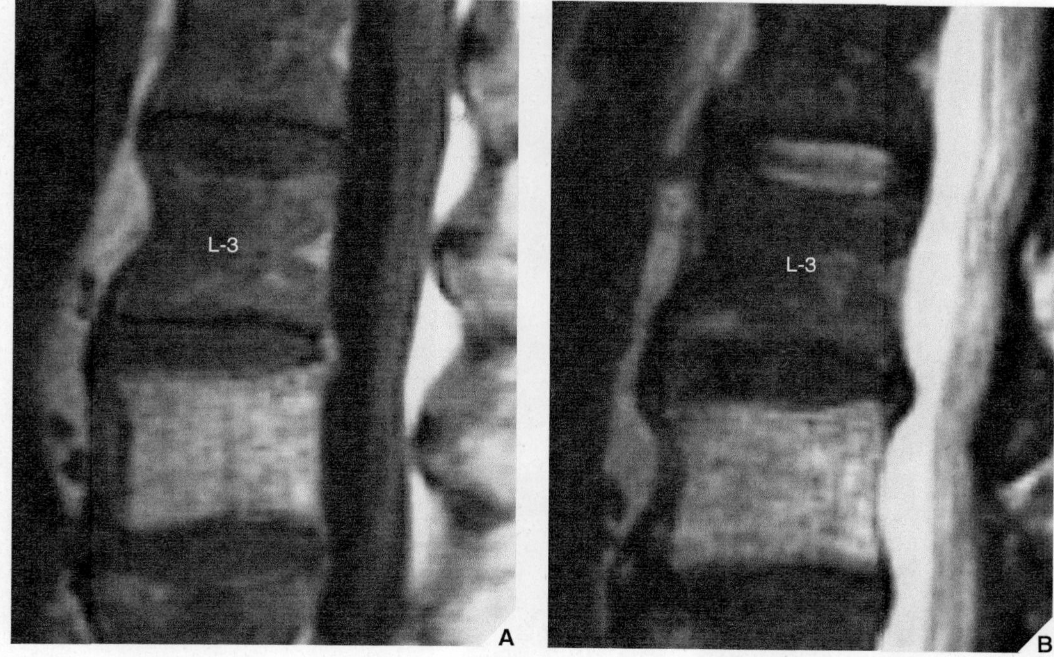

FIGURE 20.62 **MRI of vertebral hemangioma. (A)** Sagittal T1-weighted (spin echo [SE]; repetition time [TR] 517/echo time [TE] 12 msec) and **(B)** T2-weighted (SE; TR 2000/TE 80 msec) MR images show high signal intensity of hemangioma of L-4 vertebra.

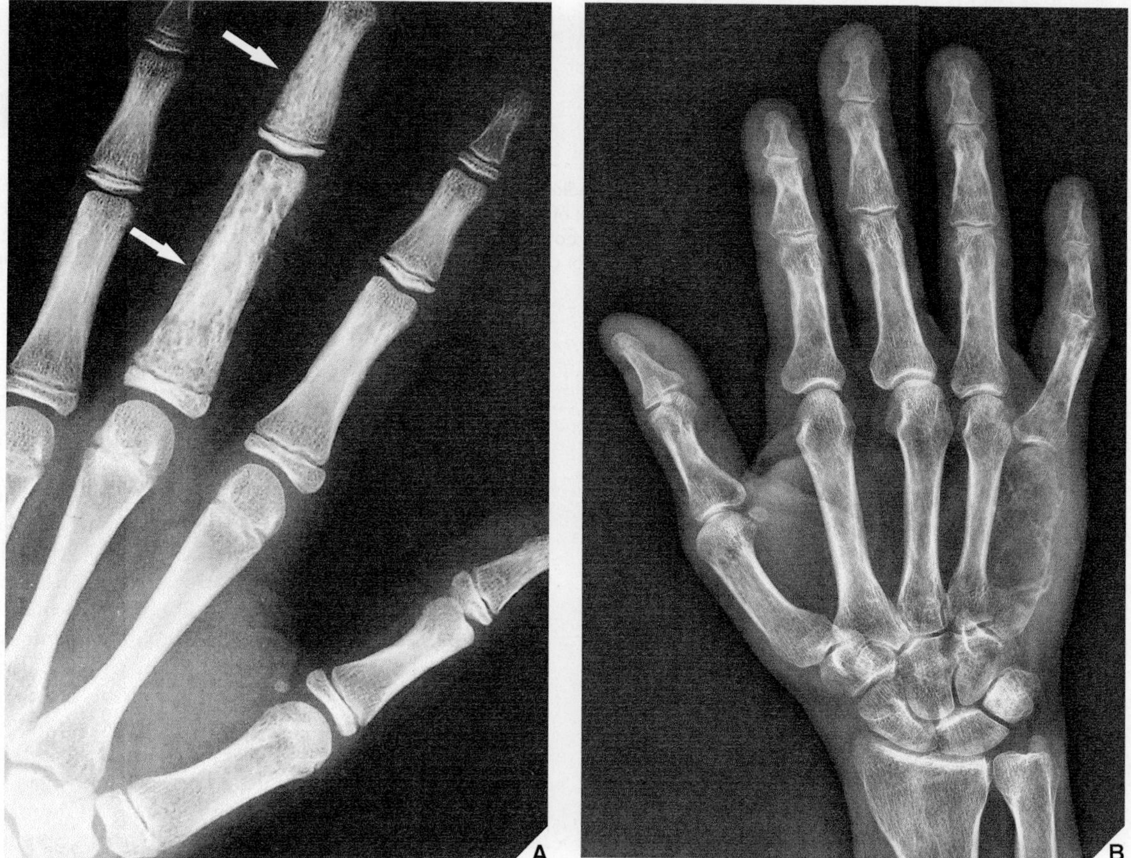

FIGURE 20.63 **Hemangioma of a short tubular bone. (A)** Dorsovolar radiograph of the hand of an 11-year-old girl shows the characteristic lace-like pattern and honeycombing of the middle finger's phalanges *(arrows)*. Overgrowth of the digit, as seen here, is a frequent complication of hemangioma. **(B)** In another patient, a 50-year-old man, observe the lytic, expansive, bubble-like lesion affecting the fifth metacarpal bone.

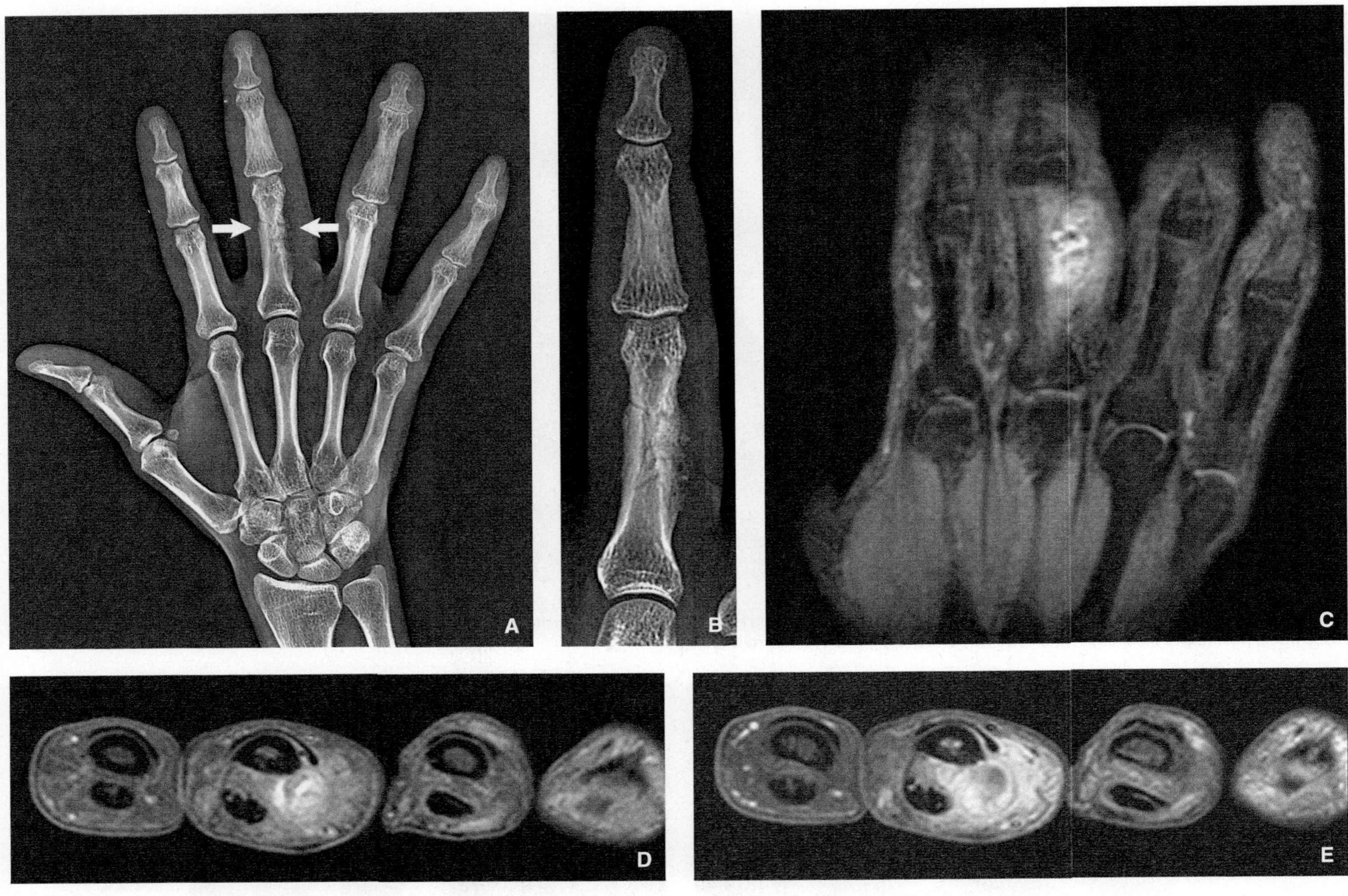

FIGURE 20.64 MRI of hemangioma of bone and soft tissue. **(A)** Dorsovolar radiograph of the left hand and **(B)** coned-down view of the middle finger of a 36-year-old woman show radiolucent channels traversing the medullary portion and the cortex of the proximal phalanx *(arrows)* associated with soft-tissue prominence. **(C)** Coronal T2-weighted fat-suppressed MR image shows high signal intensity lesion affecting both the bone and the soft tissue. **(D)** Axial T1-weighted fat-suppressed and **(E)** axial T1-weighted fat-suppressed MR images obtained after intravenous administration of gadolinium show significant enhancement of the lesion. (Courtesy of Robert Szabo, MD, Sacramento, CA.)

fractures through the cystic lesions. Most of the symptoms, however, are related to visceral involvement. On radiography, the osseous lesions are usually osteolytic (Fig. 20.68), occasionally with a honeycomb appearance (Fig. 20.69). They are well defined and surrounded by a rim of sclerosis, and they vary in size (Fig. 20.70). Although medullary involvement predominates, cortical invasion, osseous expansion, and periosteal reaction can occur. Rarely, sclerotic lesions may be present, and in these instances, the condition may mimic osteoblastic metastases. On MRI, the lesions usually show intermediate signal intensity on T1-weighted images, and T2-weighted images with fat saturation show a mixture of high, intermediate, and low signal intensities. On histologic examination, cystic angiomatosis is characterized by cavernous angiomatous spaces, indistinguishable from benign hemangioma of bone.

A condition that must be distinguished from angiomatosis is *Gorham disease* of bone, also known as *massive osteolysis*, *disappearing bone disease*, and *phantom bone disease*. It was originally described by Jackson in 1838 and subsequently properly defined by Gorham and Stout in a series of 24 patients in 1955. This entity is characterized by progressive, localized bone resorption, probably caused by multiple or diffuse cavernous hemangiomas or lymphangiomas of bone or by a combination of both. Gorham disease may develop in any site of the skeleton, but it commonly involves the shoulder girdle, the pelvic girdle, and the skull. Primary involvement of the long bones, short tubular bones, or the spine is rare. The radiographic presentation of Gorham disease consists of radiolucent areas in the cancellous bone or concentric destruction of the cortex, giving rise to a sucked-candy appearance (Fig. 20.71A). Eventually, the entire medullary cavity and the cortex are destroyed (Fig. 20.71B). MRI manifestation of Gorham disease include areas of bone resorption with low signal intensity on T1-weighted images and high signal intensity on T2-weighted images. Following intravenous injection of gadolinium, there is strong enhancement of the osseous lesions and the adjacent richly vascularized soft tissues (Fig. 20.72). On histologic examination, a marked increase is observed in intraosseous capillaries, which form an anastomosing network of endothelium-lined channels that are usually filled with erythrocytes or serum. Although some investigators claim that there is no evidence of osteoclasts in areas of bone resorption, studies by Spieth and coworkers suggest that osteoclastic activity plays a role in the pathogenesis of Gorham disease. Although multiple therapies have been attempted, only radiation therapy, complete excision of the bone defect, and cortical bone graft appear to halt the bone destruction.

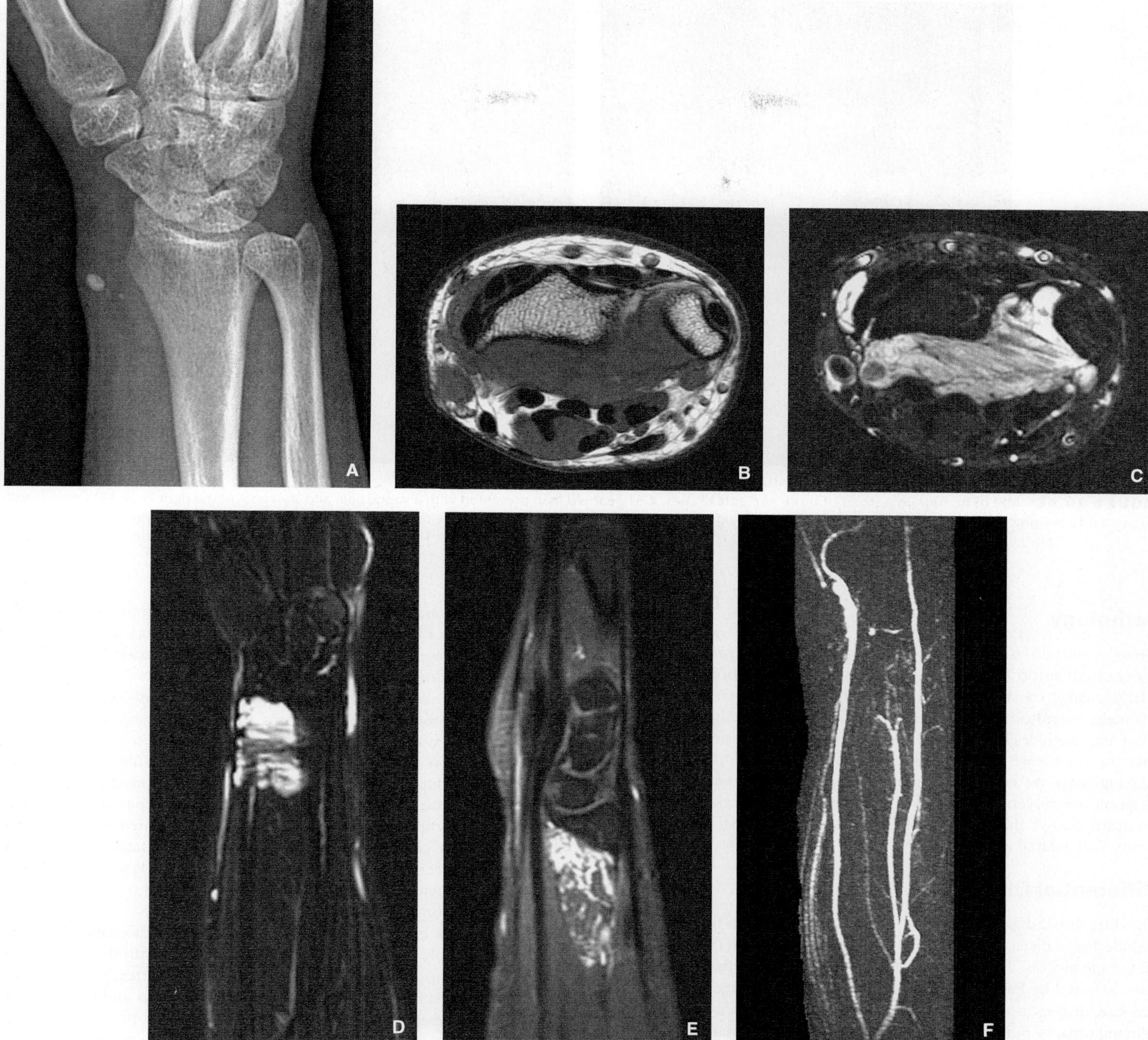

FIGURE 20.65 **MRI of hemangioma of bone and soft tissue.** **(A)** Oblique radiograph of the left wrist of a 21-year-old woman shows two phleboliths in the soft tissues adjacent to the distal radius. **(B)** Axial T1-weighted, **(C)** axial inversion recovery (IR), **(D)** coronal T2-weighted, and **(E)** sagittal T1-weighted fat-suppressed postcontrast MR images show a tubular lobulated soft-tissue mass within the quadratus pronator muscle that extends into the radiocarpal and distal radioulnar joints, with intraosseous involvement of the distal ulna and volar aspect of the distal radius. **(F)** Coronal MR angiogram shows puddling of the contrast in the region of the distal radial artery at the site of hemangioma. (Courtesy of Robert Szabo, MD, Sacramento, CA.)

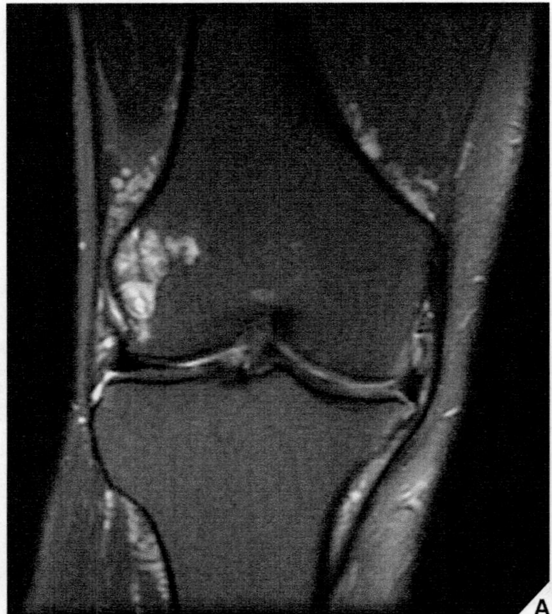

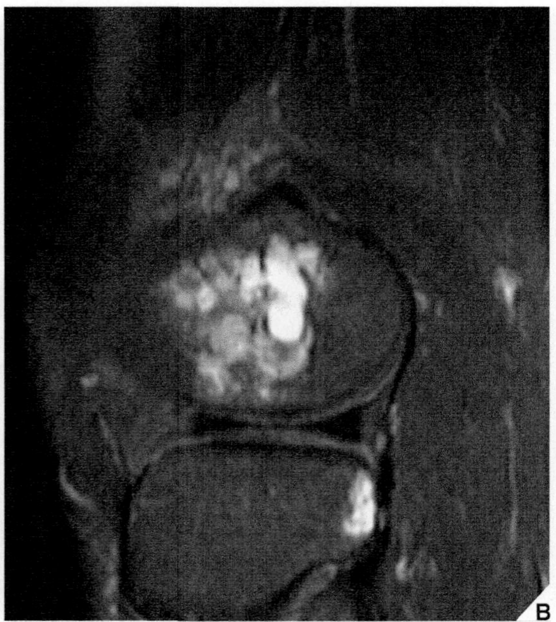

FIGURE 20.66 MRI of hemangiomatosis of bone and soft tissues. A 51-year-old man presented with a vague pain and "fullness" of the right knee. **(A)** Coronal and **(B)** sagittal T2-weighted fat-suppressed MR images show high–signal intensity multiple lesions affecting the osseous and soft-tissue structures of the knee.

Pathology

Gross specimen of hemangioma shows brown-red or dark-red well-demarcated lesion within the medullary portion of bone (Fig. 20.73). Histologically, most hemangiomas consist of simple endothelium-lined channels, morphologically identical with capillary endothelium. Some or all of the vascular channels may be enlarged and have a sinusoidal appearance, in which case the lesion is referred to as *cavernous type*. Occasionally, hemangiomas are composed of larger, thick-walled arteries or veins and resemble arteriovenous malformations of the soft tissues. Immunohistochemistry shows that endothelial cells are positive for CD31, CD34, and factor VIII-related antigen.

Differential Diagnosis

The differential diagnosis of hemangioma, particularly in the spine, should include Paget disease, Langerhans cell histiocytosis (LCH), myeloma, and metastatic lesions. The characteristic "picture frame" appearance of a vertebra affected by Paget disease (see Fig. 29.6) as well as its larger than normal size, distinguishes it from hemangioma. Myeloma in a vertebra, unlike hemangioma, is purely radiolucent—as are most metastatic lesions—and shows no vertical striations.

Treatment

Asymptomatic hemangiomas do not require treatment. Symptomatic lesions are usually treated with radiation therapy to ablate the venous channels forming the lesions. Embolization, laminectomy, spinal fusion, or a combination of these is also used in treatment.

Intraosseous Lipoma

Clinical and Imaging Features

Lipomas can be categorized according to their location in the bone as intraosseous, cortical, or parosteal lesions. Intraosseous lipoma is considered to be an extremely rare tumor (with an incidence of less than 1 in 1,000 primary bone tumors). In recent years, an increasing number of reports of intraosseous lipoma have appeared, particularly located in the intertrochanteric and subtrochanteric regions of the femur and in the calcaneus. The tumor has no gender predilection and occurs in a wide range of ages, from 5 to 75 years. It is usually an asymptomatic lesion, found on imaging examinations performed for other reasons. Some investigators report a higher incidence of symptomatic patients; however, even when a patient is symptomatic, the symptoms are not necessarily related to the lesion. In the large series of 61 intraosseous lipomas reported by Milgram, the most common sites were the intertrochanteric and subtrochanteric regions of the femur, followed by the calcaneus, ilium, proximal tibia, and sacrum. He classified intraosseous lipomas into three types, depending on the histologic composition. Type 1 is a sharply delineated, viable lipoma with uniform fat content. Type 2 is a predominantly fatty lesion with a central area of necrosis, calcification, and ossification. Type 3 is a heterogeneous lipoma with areas of necrosis, calcification, cyst formation, and reactive woven bone formation.

Intraosseous lipoma has a rather characteristic radiographic appearance. It is invariably a nonaggressive radiolucent lesion with sharply defined borders, associated with thinning and bulging of the cortex, particularly in thin bones such as fibula or rib. The central calcifications and ossifications are frequently present (Figs. 20.74 to 20.76). CT may be helpful in the diagnosis of these lesions because the Hounsfield units are consistent with fat (Fig. 20.77). MRI shows the lesion to have a signal similar to subcutaneous fat on T1- and T2-weighted images (Figs. 20.78 to 20.80). A thin circumferential rim of low signal intensity on T1- and T2-weighted images, consistent with reactive sclerosis, is commonly present demarcating the margin of the fatty lesion. After intravenous administration of gadolinium, there is no enhancement of the lesion. MRI is highly effective in demonstrating the exact intraosseous extension of the lesion.

Pathology

Gross specimen usually shows a well-defined, soft, yellow mass within the medullary portion of bone (Fig. 20.81). Histologically, intraosseous lipomas are composed of lobules of mature adipose tissue and are characterized by the presence of mature lipocytes, which are slightly larger than nonneoplastic fat cells, in a background of fibroblasts with occasional foci of fat necrosis. A capsule may occasionally encompass all or part of the tumor mass, and in most cases reported, atrophic bone trabeculae are found throughout the lesion. Immunohistochemistry shows that fat cells express positivity for vimentin and S-100 protein. As far as genetics is

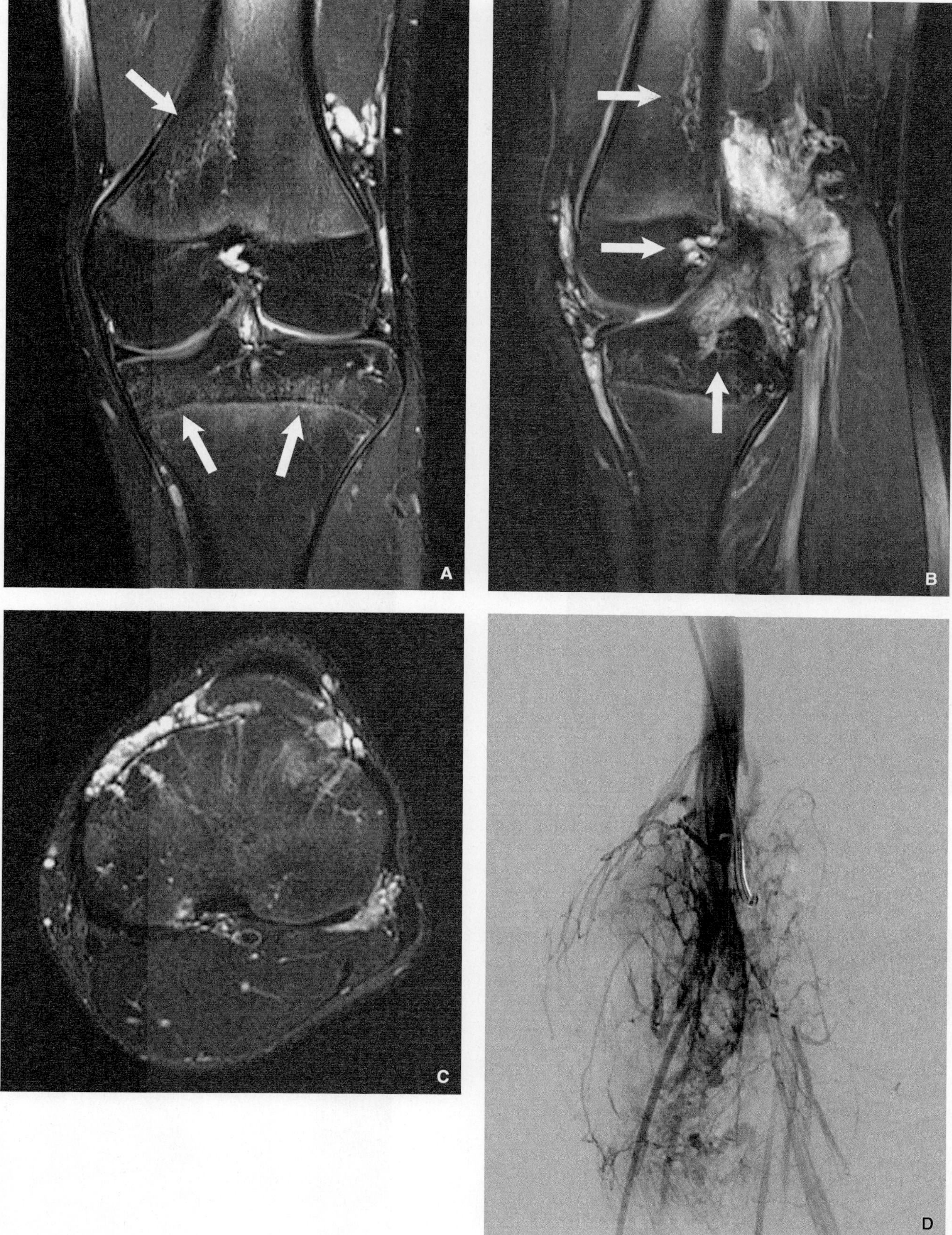

FIGURE 20.67 MRI of hemangiomatosis of bone and soft tissues. **(A)** Coronal and **(B)** sagittal T2-weighted fat-suppressed MR images of the knee of a 14-year-old boy show high-intensity lesions in the distal femur and proximal tibia *(arrows)*, associated with soft-tissue involvement. **(C)** Axial T2-weighted MRI shows involvement of the knee joint. **(D)** Angiogram shows a hypervascular lesion affecting both osseous structures and soft tissues.

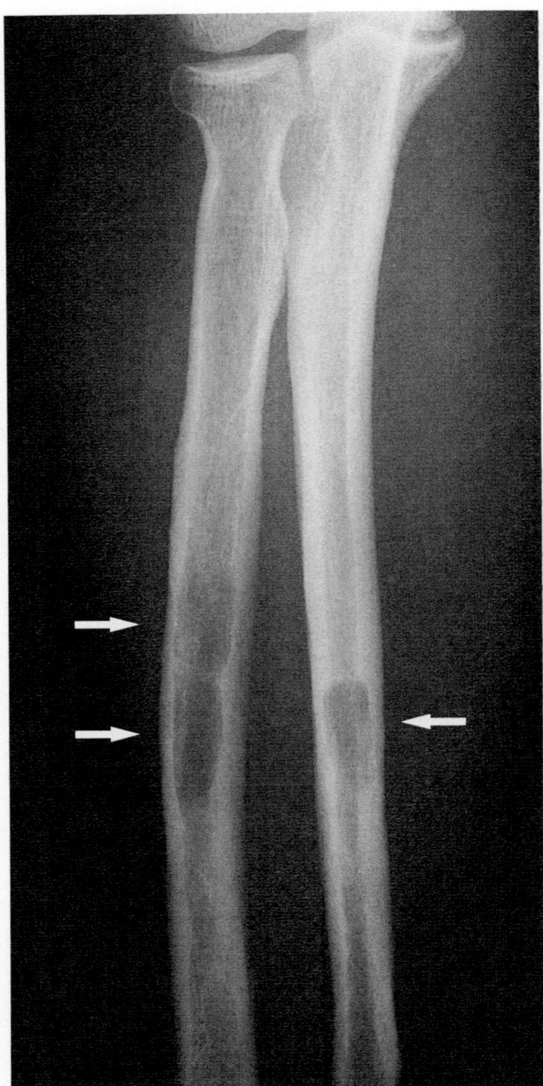

FIGURE 20.68 Cystic angiomatosis. Several osteolytic lesions *(arrows)* affect the shafts of the radius and ulna in this 25-year-old man.

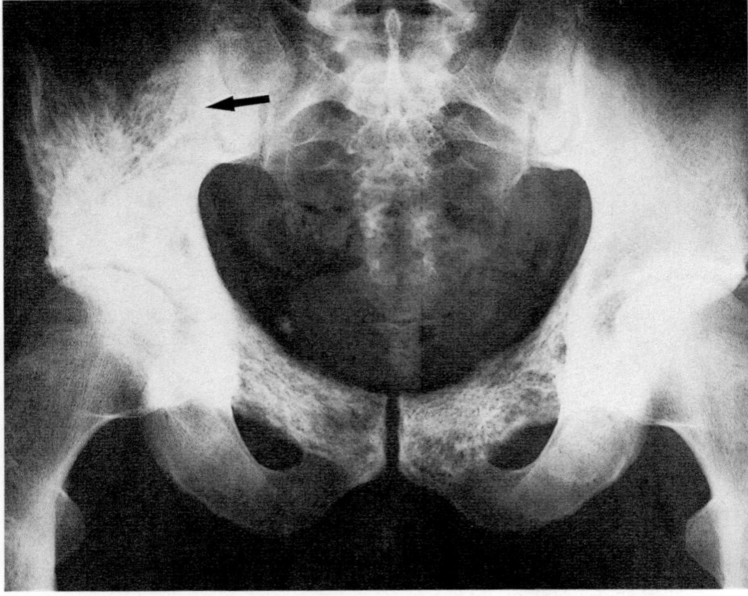

FIGURE 20.69 Cystic angiomatosis. A radiograph of the pelvis of a 28-year-old man shows a honeycomb pattern in the right ilium *(arrow)* and both pubic bones.

concerned, translocation t(3;12)(q28; q14) and its associated fusion transcript *HMGIC/LPP*, which is present in lipomas of the soft tissue, have been reported in parosteal tumors.

Nonneoplastic Lesions Simulating Tumors

Some nonneoplastic conditions that may mimic bone tumors include intraosseous ganglion, a "brown tumor" of hyperparathyroidism, LCH, Erdheim-Chester disease, encystified bone infarct, and myositis ossificans.

Intraosseous Ganglion

This lesion of unknown cause is frequently encountered in adults between ages 20 and 60 years. It has a predilection for the articular ends of the long bones, usually the non–weight-bearing segment. Radiographically, it exhibits the characteristic picture of a round or oval radiolucent area located eccentrically in the bone and rimmed by a sclerotic margin (Fig. 20.82). Its appearance is very similar to that of a degenerative cyst, but the adjacent joint does not show any degenerative changes; in most cases, the ganglion, in contrast to a degenerative cyst, does not communicate with the joint cavity. An intraosseous ganglion may also mimic chondroblastoma, osteoblastoma, enchondroma, pigmented villonodular synovitis, or bone abscess (Fig. 20.83).

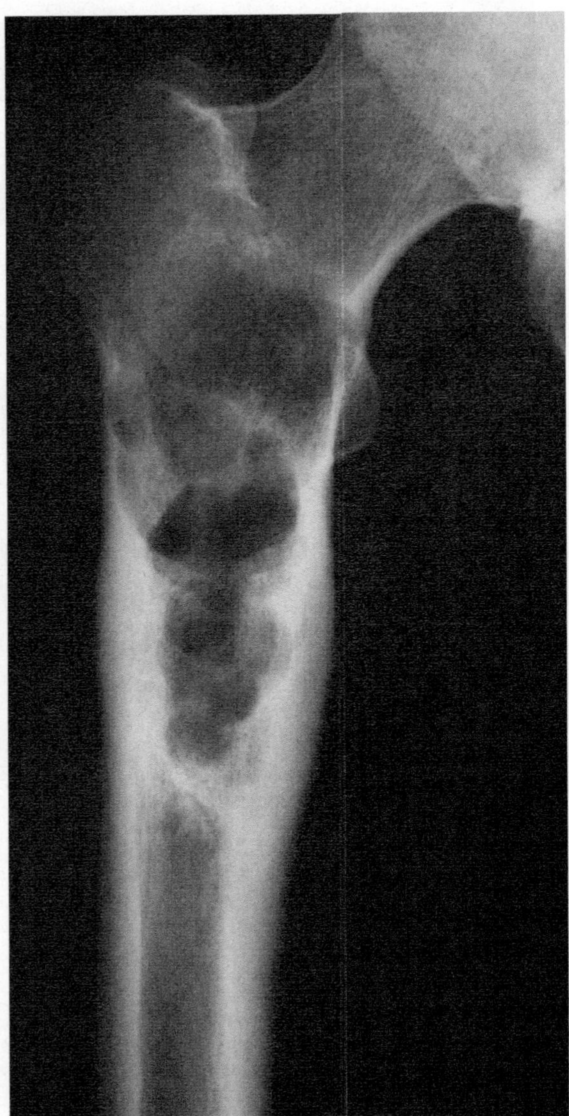

FIGURE 20.70 Cystic angiomatosis. Several confluent lesions with peripheral sclerosis and cortical thickening marked cystic angiomatosis in the right femur of a 20-year-old man.

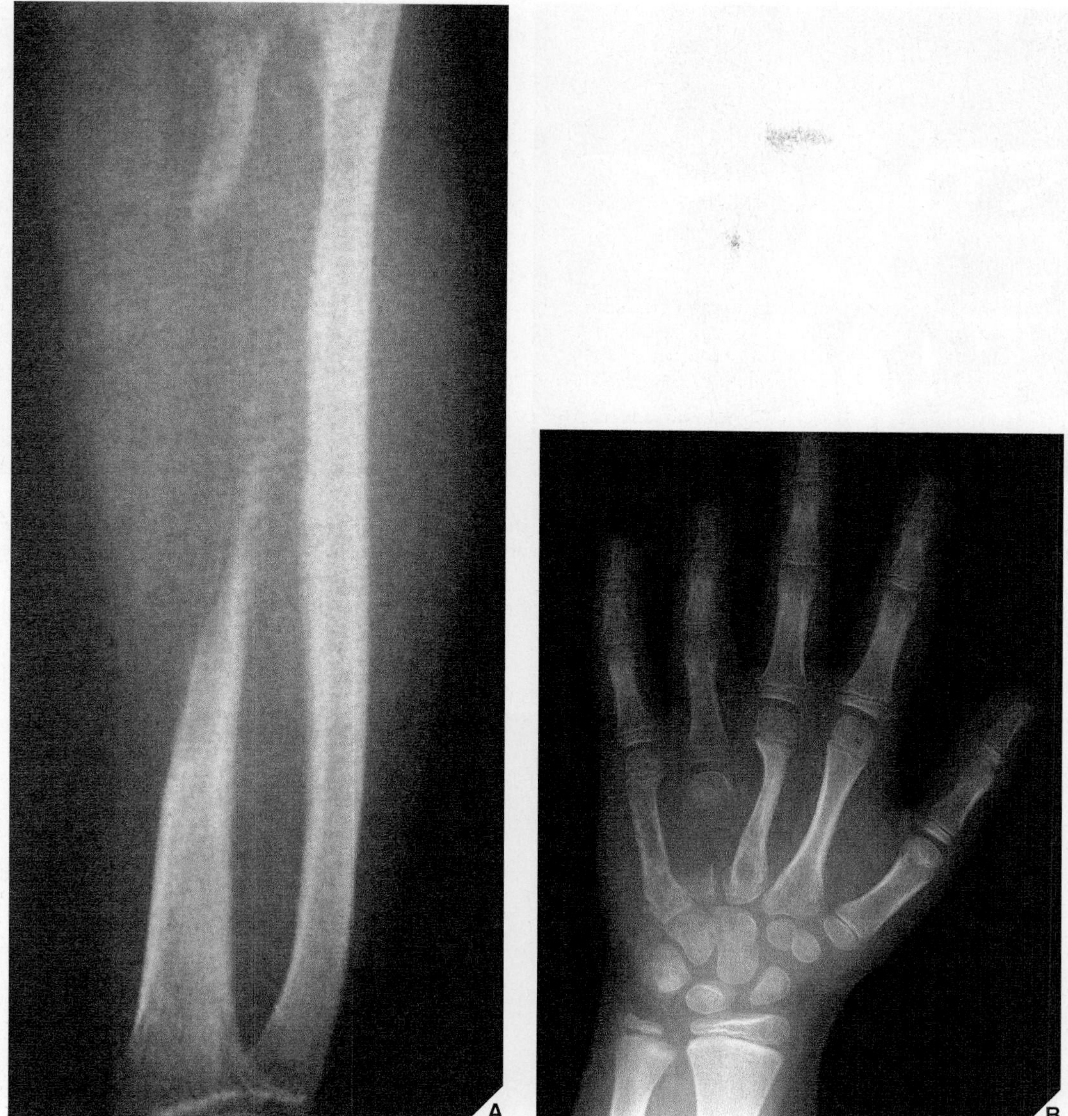

FIGURE 20.71 Gorham disease. **(A)** Anteroposterior radiograph of the right forearm of a 46-year-old woman shows osteolysis of the midportion of the radius. Observe characteristic tapering of the proximal end of the radius that assumed "sucked-candy" appearance. **(B)** Dorsovolar radiograph of the left hand of a 9-year-old boy shows complete resorption of the diaphysis of the fourth metacarpal bone and pressure-erosion of the ulnar aspect of the third metacarpal. (**B**, Courtesy of George Rab, MD, Sacramento, CA.)

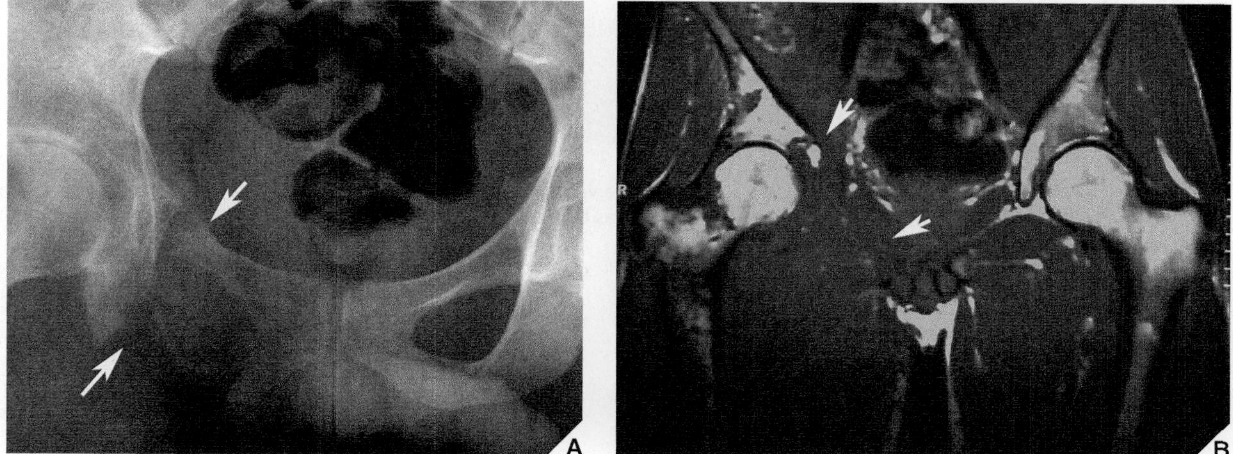

FIGURE 20.72 MRI of Gorham disease. **(A)** Anteroposterior radiograph of the pelvis of a young male demonstrates bone resorption of the right superior and inferior pubic rami *(arrows)*. **(B)** Coronal T1-weighted MRI shows bone destruction with a soft-tissue mass *(arrows)*. There are areas of signal alteration in the medullary space of the acetabulum and proximal right femur. *(Continued)*

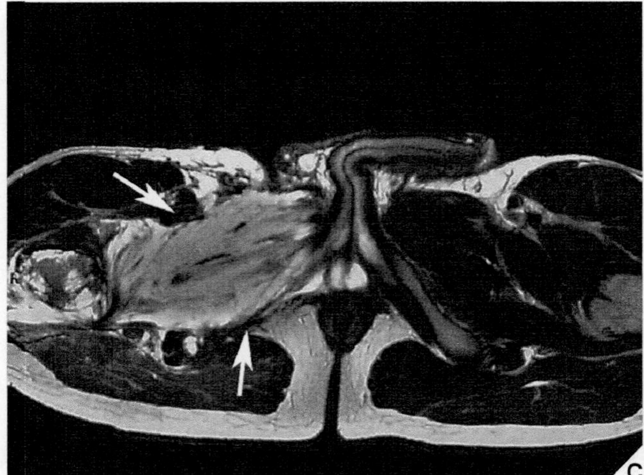

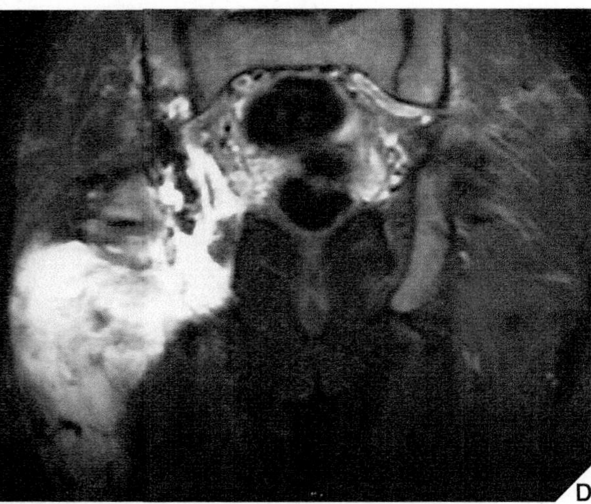

FIGURE 20.72 MRI of Gorham disease. ***(Continued)*** **(C)** Axial T2-weighted MRI shows the soft-tissue intramuscular mass *(arrows)* and the bone destruction of the inferior pubic ramus. **(D)** T1-weighted fat-saturated MRI following intravenous injection of gadolinium demonstrates extensive enhancement of the soft-tissue mass and the bone involvement.

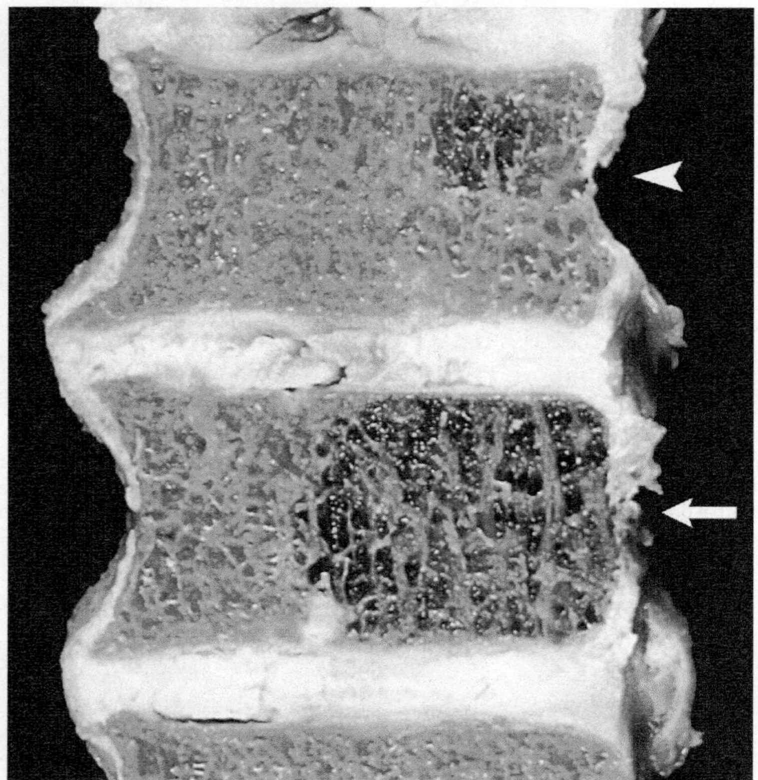

FIGURE 20.73 Pathology of intraosseous hemangioma. Gross specimen of the vertebrae shows two red-brown hemangiomas of the vertebral bodies, one small *(arrowhead)* and one large *(arrow)* that are well demarcated from the normal cancellous bone and exhibit coarse trabeculations. (Reprinted from Bullough P. *Orthopaedic pathology*, 5th ed. Maryland Heights, MO: Mosby; 2009, with permission from Elsevier.)

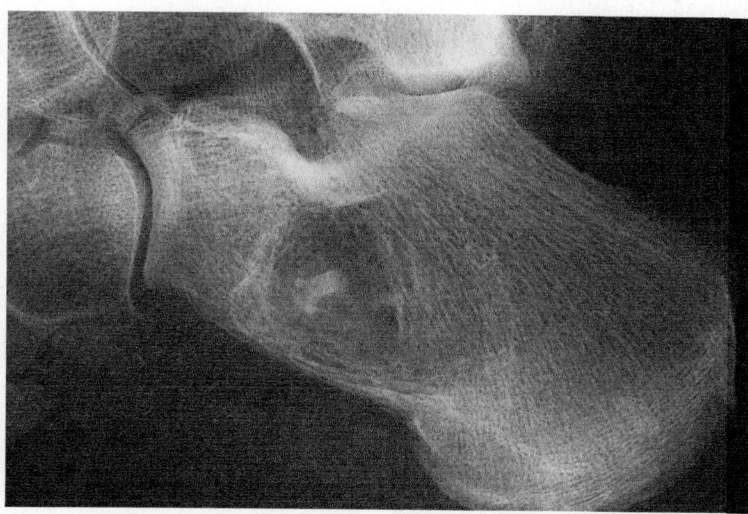

FIGURE 20.74 **Intraosseous lipoma.** Typical appearance of intraosseous lipoma in the calcaneus. Observe sharply marginated radiolucent lesion with central calcification.

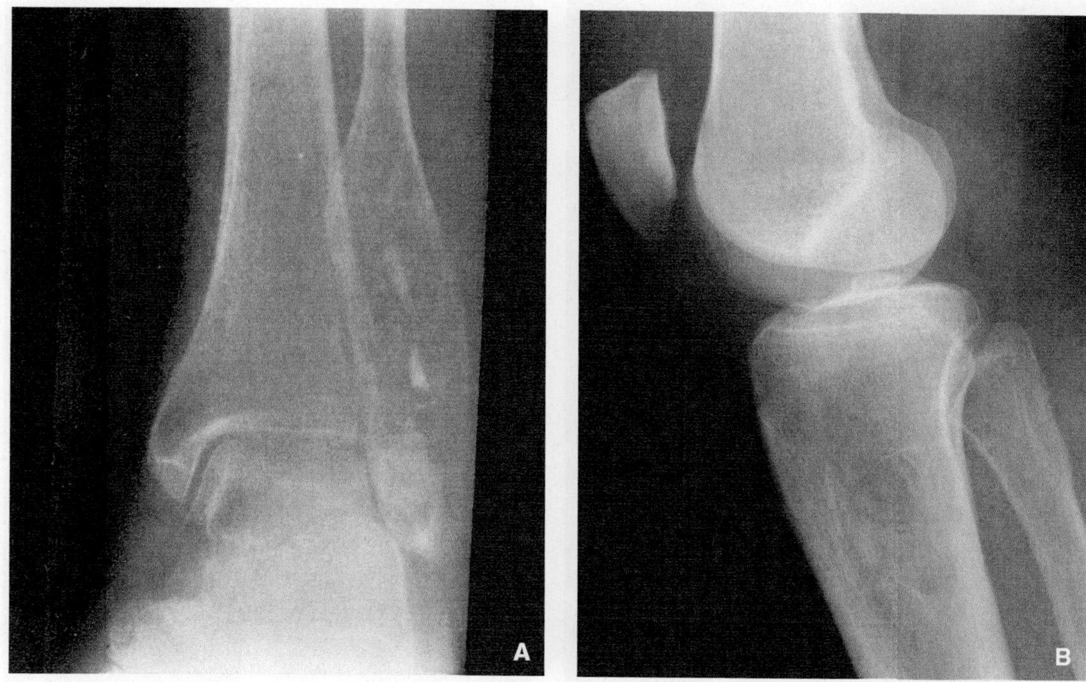

FIGURE 20.75 **Intraosseous lipoma.** **(A)** Anteroposterior radiograph of the left ankle shows a radiolucent lesion in the distal fibula exhibiting expansive features. Observe thinning of the cortex and central calcifications. **(B)** Lateral radiograph of the knee of another patient shows a radiolucent lesion with narrow zone of transition and central calcifications in the proximal tibia. (Reprinted with permission from Greenspan A, Borys D. *Radiology and pathology correlation of bone tumors: a quick reference and review*. Philadelphia: Wolters Kluwer; 2016: 331, Fig. 7.44.)

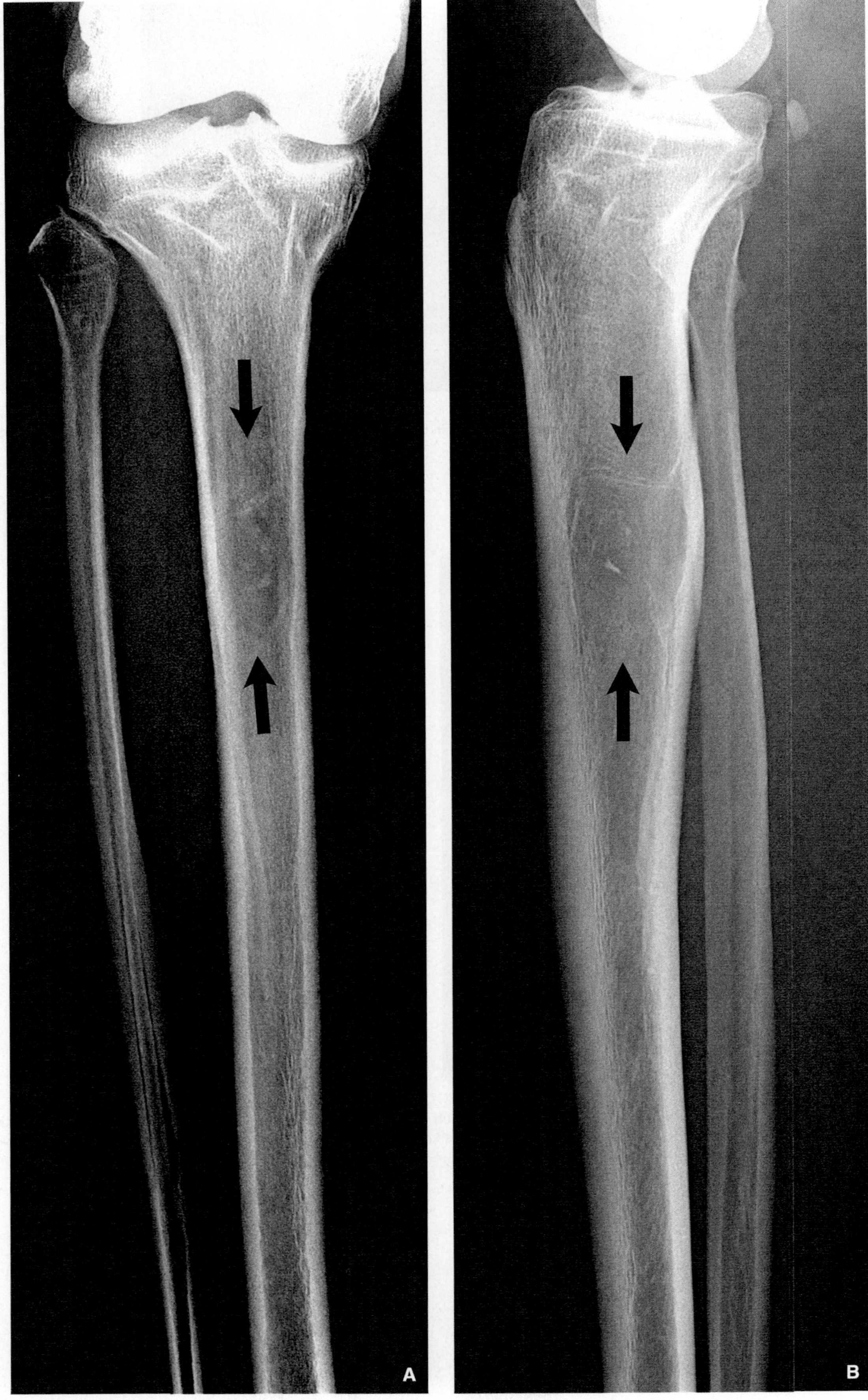

FIGURE 20.76 Intraosseous lipoma. **(A)** Anteroposterior and **(B)** lateral radiographs of the right leg of a 43-year-old man show a radiolucent lesion with narrow zone of transition within the proximal tibia *(arrows)*, with internal foci of calcifications.

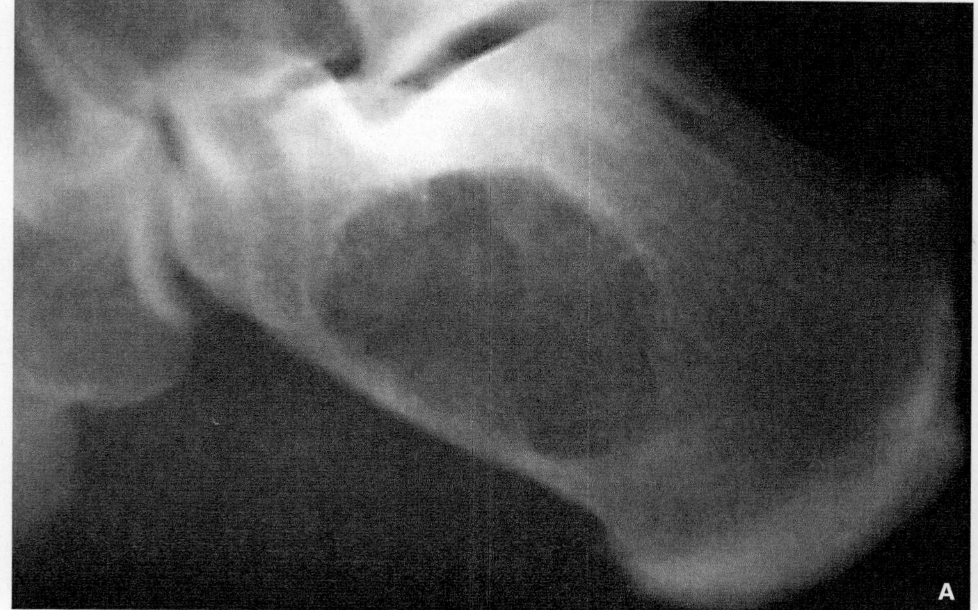

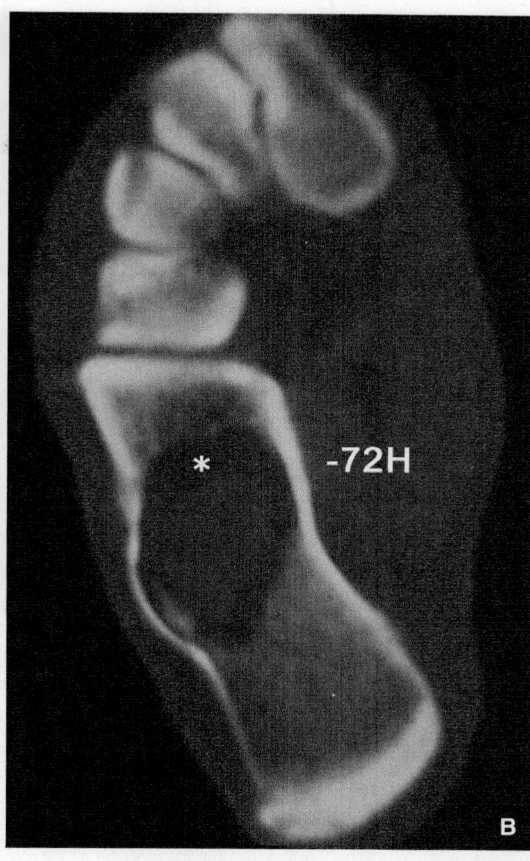

FIGURE 20.77 CT of intraosseous lipoma. **(A)** Lateral radiograph of the right hindfoot of a 40-year-old man shows a radiolucent lesion in the calcaneus. **(B)** CT image shows a lesion displaying low-attenuation values of −72 Hounsfield (H) units (*), consistent with fat.

Brown Tumor of Hyperparathyroidism

Hyperparathyroidism is a condition resulting from the excess secretion of parathormone by overactive parathyroid glands (see Chapter 28 for more detailed overview). Not infrequently, patients with this disorder present with solitary or multiple lytic lesions, most commonly in the long and short tubular bones; on radiographic examination, the lesions may resemble a tumor (Fig. 20.84). This lesion is called a *brown tumor* because, in addition to fibrous tissue, it contains decomposing blood, which gives specimens obtained for pathologic examination a brown coloration. The correct diagnosis can be made on radiography by observing associated abnormalities, including a decrease in bone density (osteopenia); subperiosteal bone resorption, which is best seen on the radial aspect of the proximal and middle phalanges of the second and third fingers; a granular "salt-and-pepper" appearance of the cranial vault; resorption of the acromial ends of the clavicles; and soft-tissue calcifications. Because of disturbed calcium and phosphorus metabolism, the serum calcium concentration is usually high (hypercalcemia) and the serum phosphorus concentration is low (hypophosphatemia), which are laboratory findings that usually confirm the diagnosis.

Langerhans Cell Histiocytosis (Eosinophilic Granuloma)

Clinical and Imaging Features

A nonneoplastic condition, eosinophilic granuloma, currently termed *LCH*, belongs to the group of disorders known as *reticuloendotheliosis* (or *histiocytosis X*, according to Lichtenstein's proposed name), which is a group that includes two other conditions, Hand-Schüller-Christian disease (xanthomatosis) and Letterer-Siwe disease (nonlipid reticulosis). The grouping has gained wide acceptance with the recognition that all three entities represent different clinical manifestations of a single pathologic disorder, characterized by granulomatous proliferation of the reticulum cell.

Although its causes and pathogenesis remain unsettled, LCH is now considered a disorder of immune regulation rather than neoplastic process. It belongs to a group of diseases now classified by the World Health Organization (WHO) as histiocytic and dendritic cell disorders. Molecular genetic studies using comparative genomic hybridization (CGH) and LOH experiments have revealed chromosomal alterations, with predominant losses affecting chromosomes 1p, 5p, 6q, 9, 16, 17, and 22q in CGH, and highest LOH frequencies on 1p and 17, leading to the hypothesis that loss of tumor suppressor genes located on chromosome 1p may be involved in development and progression of the disease. The term *Langerhans cell histiocytosis* has been accepted because it has been verified that the primary proliferative element in this disease is the Langerhans cell, a mononuclear cell of the dendritic type that is found in the epidermis but is derived from precursors in the bone marrow. The disorder exhibits a broad spectrum of clinical and imaging abnormalities. It is characterized by an abnormal proliferation of histiocytes in various parts of the reticuloendothelial system such as bone, lungs, central nervous system, skin, and lymph nodes.

LCH may manifest with solitary or with multiple lesions. It is usually seen in children, the common age of occurrence ranging from 1 to 15 years, with a peak incidence from 5 to 10 years. The most commonly affected sites are the skull, ribs, pelvis, spine, and long bones (Fig. 20.85). In the skull, the lytic lesions have a characteristic "punched-out" appearance, with sharply defined borders (Fig. 20.86). In the mandible or maxilla, the radiolucent lesions have the appearance of "floating teeth" (Fig. 20.87). In the spine, collapse of a vertebral body, the so-called *vertebra plana*, is a characteristic manifestation of the disease (Fig. 20.88). This finding was for a long time mistakenly interpreted as representing osteochondrosis of the vertebra and was called *Calve disease*.

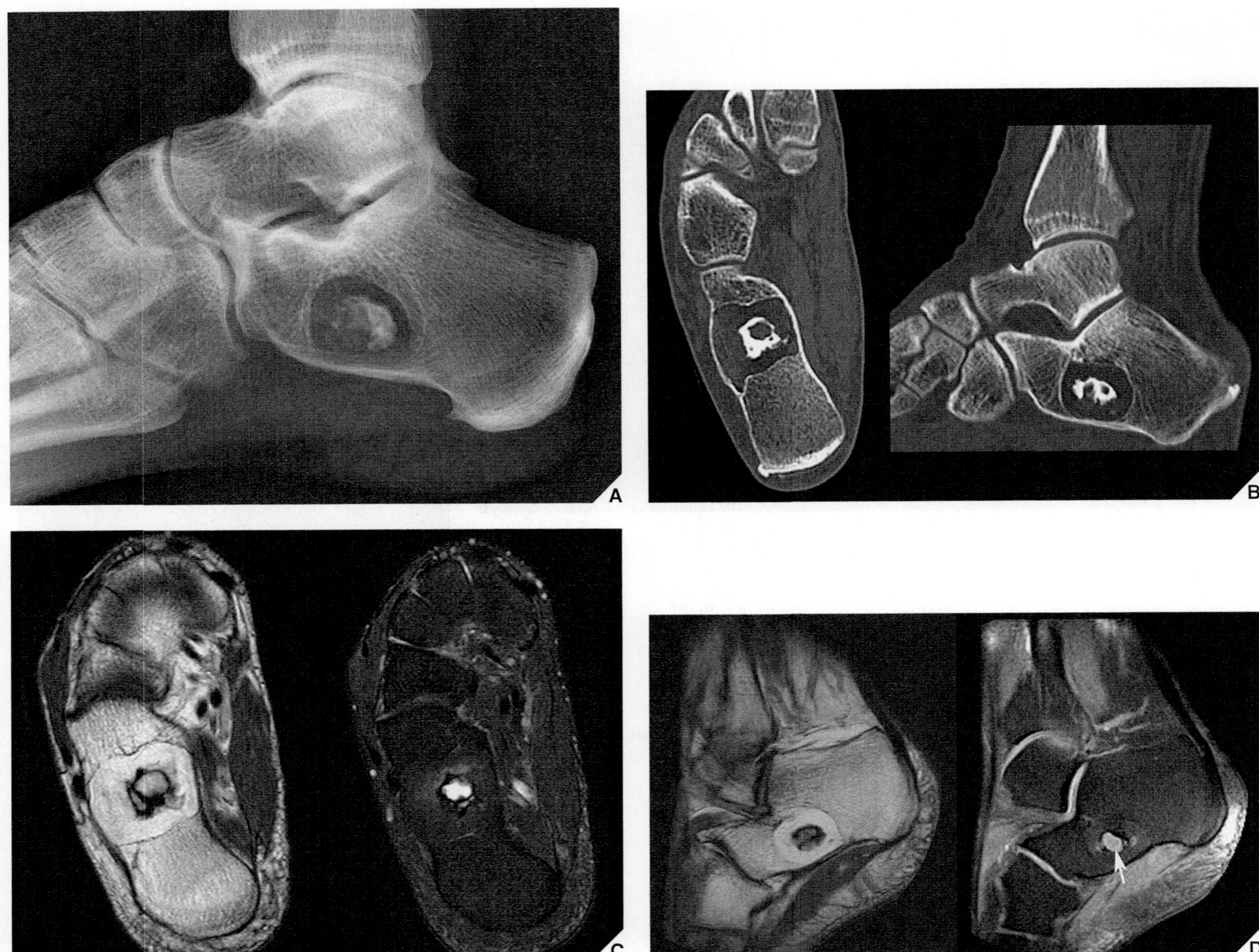

FIGURE 20.78 **CT and MRI of intraosseous lipoma. (A)** Lateral radiograph of the foot of a 54-year-old man shows a radiolucent lesion in the calcaneus with central ossification. **(B)** Short axial and sagittal reformatted CT images demonstrate low-attenuation lesion containing fat (Hounsfield values were −98 H) with central high-attenuation ossification. **(C)** Short axial T1-weighted and proton density–weighted fat-suppressed MR images show signal characteristics of a lesion similar to subcutaneous fat, confirming the diagnosis of intraosseous lipoma. **(D)** Sagittal T1-weighted and fast spin echo (FSE) fat-suppressed images demonstrate fat signal intensity surrounding the low signal intensity of the calcification noted on the radiographs and CT. Observe the central area of cyst formation within the calcified zone *(arrow)*. Areas of cyst formation within the intraosseous lipoma represent a type 3 lesion according to the Milgram classification.

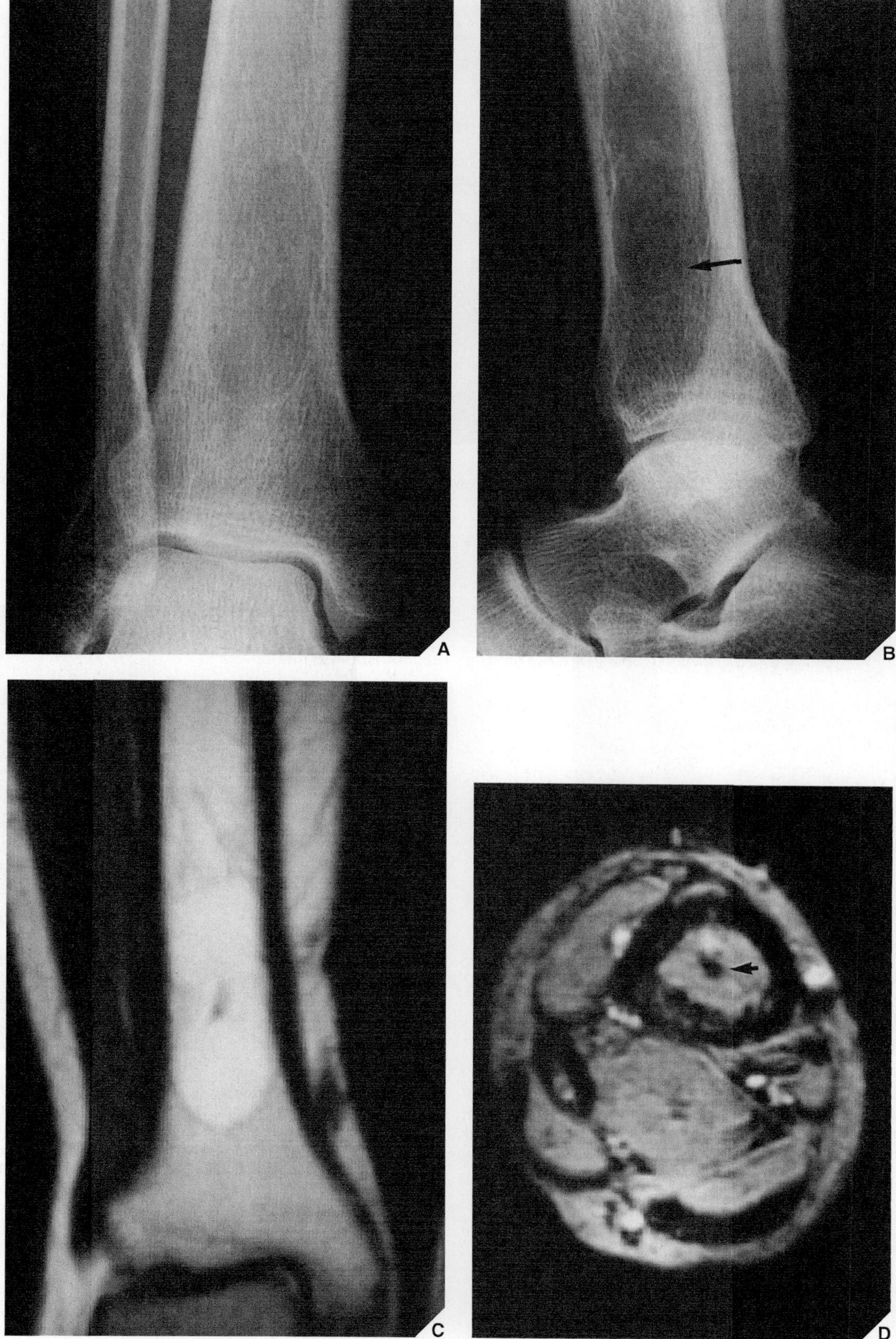

FIGURE 20.79 **MRI of intraosseous lipoma.** **(A)** Radiograph of the right lower leg in a 42-year-old man shows a radiolucent lesion in the distal tibia sharply delineated by a thin sclerotic margin. **(B)** On the lateral radiograph, there is a suggestion of a faint calcific body in the center of the lesion *(arrow)*. **(C)** Coronal T1-weighted (spin echo [SE]; repetition time [TR] 685/echo time [TE] 20 msec) MRI demonstrates the lesion to be of a high–signal intensity paralleling that of subcutaneous fat and thus consistent with intraosseous lipoma. A small focus of low signal is present within the lesion, corresponding to a calcific body seen on the conventional radiography. **(D)** Axial T2-weighted (SE; TR 2000/TE 70 msec) MR image shows that the lesion becomes of intermediate intensity, again paralleling the signal of subcutaneous fat. The central calcification exhibit signal void *(short arrow)*.

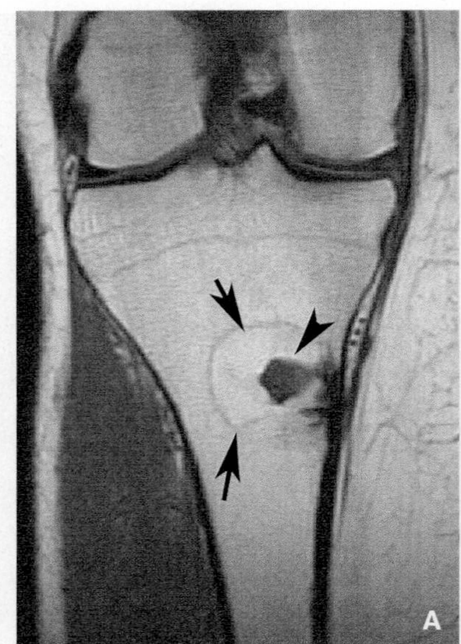

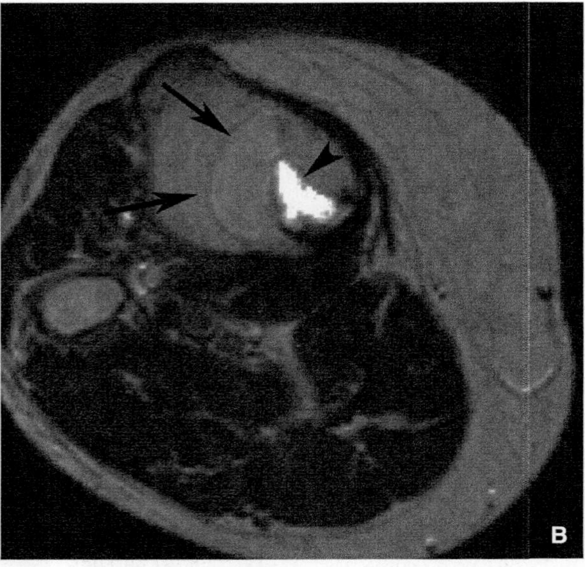

FIGURE 20.80 **MRI of intraosseous lipoma.** **(A)** Coronal T1-weighted and **(B)** axial T2-weighted MR images show a Milgram type 3 intraosseous lipoma in the proximal tibia *(arrows)* with an internal cystic component *(arrowheads)*.

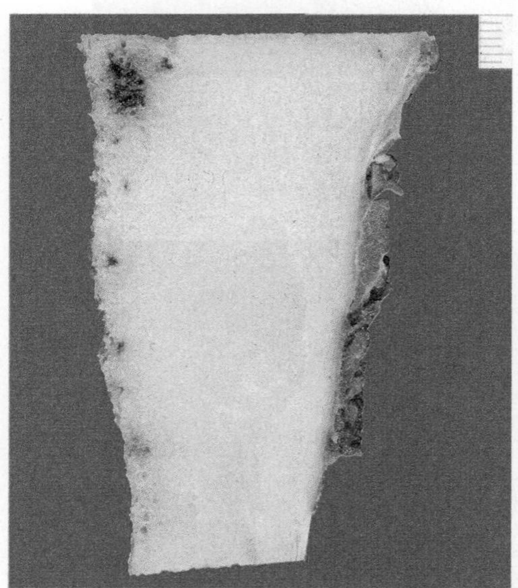

FIGURE 20.81 **Pathology of intraosseous lipoma.** Gross anatomic specimen of the proximal tibia shows oval, yellowish lesion surrounded by a thin fibrous capsule. (Reprinted with permission from Greenspan A, Borys D. *Radiology and pathology correlation of bone tumors: a quick reference and review*. Philadelphia: Wolters Kluwer; 2016:333.)

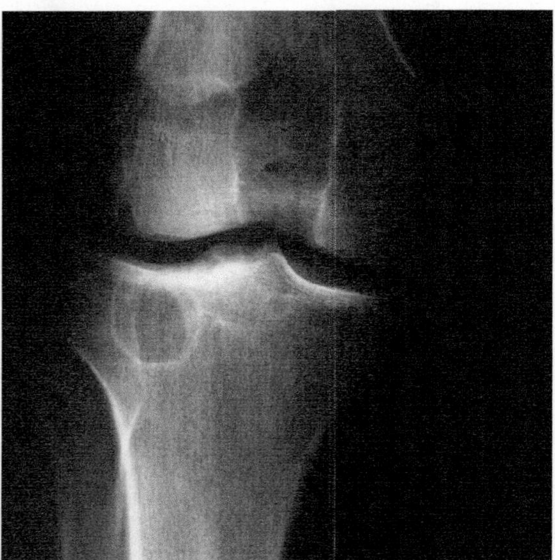

FIGURE 20.82 **Intraosseous ganglion.** A 28-year-old man sustained an injury to the right knee that tore the lateral meniscus. Anteroposterior radiograph of the knee discloses an eccentric radiolucent lesion in the articular end of the proximal tibia. During surgery to remove the meniscus, the lesion was biopsied and histopathologic examination revealed it to be an intraosseous ganglion.

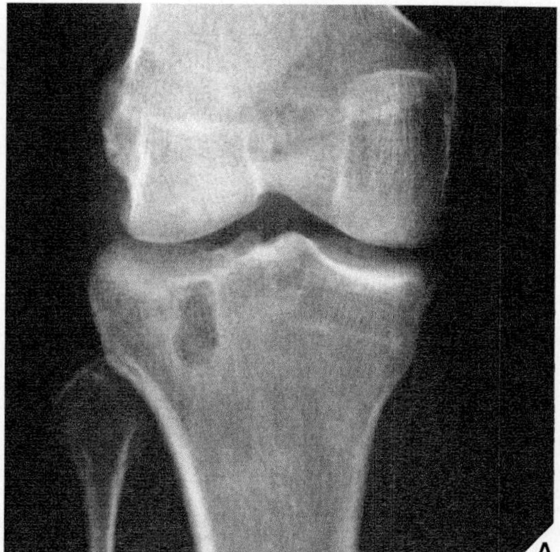

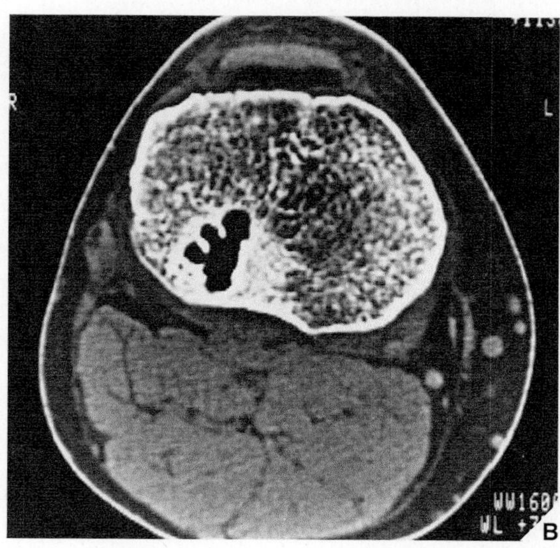

FIGURE 20.83 **CT of intraosseous ganglion.** A 24-year-old man presented with an 8-week history of pain in the knee. **(A)** Anteroposterior radiograph of the right knee and **(B)** CT section demonstrate an oval radiolucent lesion eccentrically located in the proximal tibia with ramifications, rimmed by a zone of reactive sclerosis. The differential diagnosis included a bone abscess, osteoblastoma, chondroblastoma, and an intraosseous ganglion. Biopsy confirmed an intraosseous ganglion.

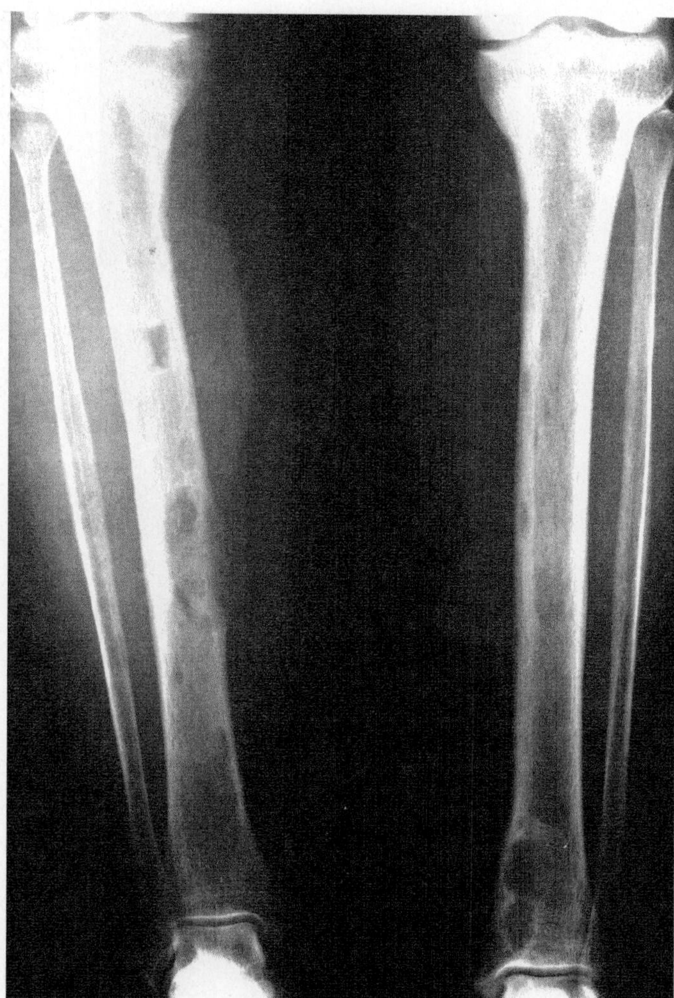

FIGURE 20.84 **Brown tumors of hyperparathyroidism.** Radiograph of the lower legs of a 28-year-old woman with clinically documented hyperparathyroidism shows multiple brown tumors involving both tibiae. This condition can easily be misdiagnosed as multiple myeloma or metastatic disease.

In the long bones, LCH presents as a destructive radiolucent lesion commonly associated with a lamellated periosteal reaction. It may mimic a malignant round cell tumor such as lymphoma or Ewing sarcoma (Fig. 20.89). In its later stages, the lesion becomes more sclerotic, with dispersed radiolucencies (Fig. 20.90). The distribution of the lesion and the detection of silent sites in the skeleton are best ascertained by a radionuclide bone scan; this may also be helpful in differentiating LCH from Ewing sarcoma, which rarely presents with multiple foci.

CT may be useful if conventional radiography inadequately defines the extent of the process, particularly in cases of spine and pelvic involvement. This modality effectively demonstrates periosteal reaction, beveled edges, and reactive sclerosis. There have been isolated reports of the usefulness of MRI in evaluating this condition. The MRI appearance varies and appears to correlate with the radiographic appearance. The MRI manifestations of LCH during the earlier stages are nonspecific and may simulate an aggressive lesion, such as osteomyelitis or Ewing sarcoma, and occasionally benign tumors, such as osteoid osteoma or chondroblastoma. After gadolinium diethylenetriamine pentaacetic acid (Gd-DTPA) injection, the lesions show variable degree of enhancement on T1-weighted images (Figs. 20.91 to 20.94). Occasionally, MRI can demonstrate early bone marrow involvement in the absence of radiographic or scintigraphic abnormalities. In some studies, on T1-weighted sequences, the lesions were isointense with adjacent structures. In the skull, lesions have been reported to show well-defined high–signal intensity areas of marrow replacement on T2-weighted sequences. The most recent investigations have shown that the most common MRI appearance of LCH is that of a focal lesion, surrounded by an extensive, ill-defined signal from bone marrow and by soft-tissue reaction with low signal intensity on T2-weighted images, considered to represent bone marrow and soft-tissue edema or the flare phenomenon.

The so-called *Langerhans cell sarcoma* represents an exceedingly rare but very aggressive form of LCH with multiorgan involvement. It can arise *de novo* or may progress from the conventional disorder.

Pathology

Histologically, LCH is composed of a variable admixture of two types of cells: eosinophilic leukocytes possessing bilobate nuclei and coarse eosinophilic cytoplasmic granules and histiocytes, identical with the Langerhans histiocytes seen in the skin. Proliferating Langerhans cells are arranged in aggregates, sheets, or individually within a loose fibrous stroma, exhibiting indistinct cytoplasmic borders and eosinophilic to clear cytoplasm. The nuclei are translucent, ovoid, coffee bean or kidney shaped with typical longitudinal grooves. Chromatin is either diffusely dispersed or condensed along the nuclear membranes. Special stains may reveal abundant droplets of sudanophilic fat peripherally or in the middle of the giant cell cytoplasm, so-called *Touton cells*. Langerhans cells are positive for CD1a, S-100 protein,

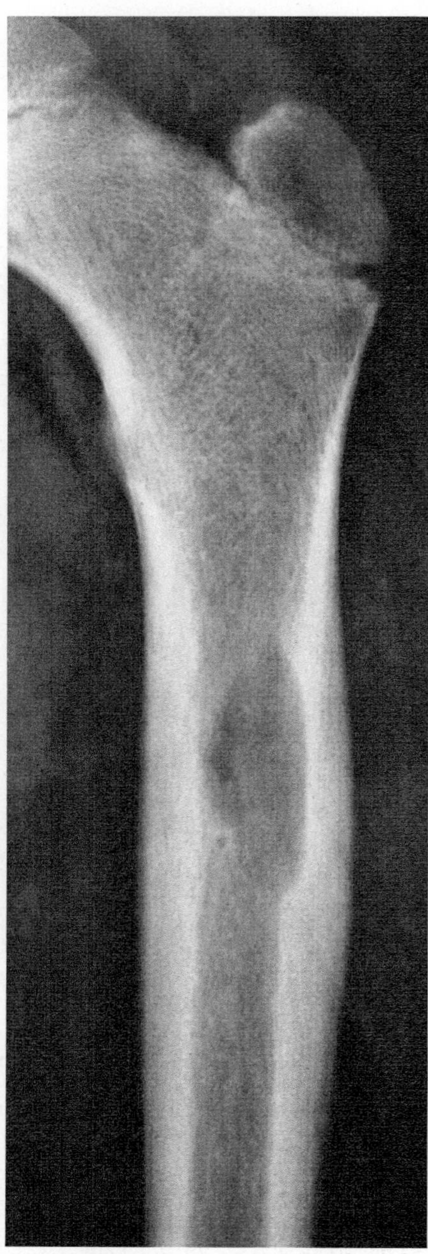

FIGURE 20.85 **Langerhans cell histiocytosis.** Radiograph of the proximal femur of a 3-year-old boy with a limp and tenderness localized to the upper thigh shows an osteolytic lesion in the medullary portion of the bone, without sclerotic changes. There is fusiform thickening of the cortex and a solid periosteal reaction. The patient's age, the location of the lesion, and its radiographic appearance are typical of LCH.

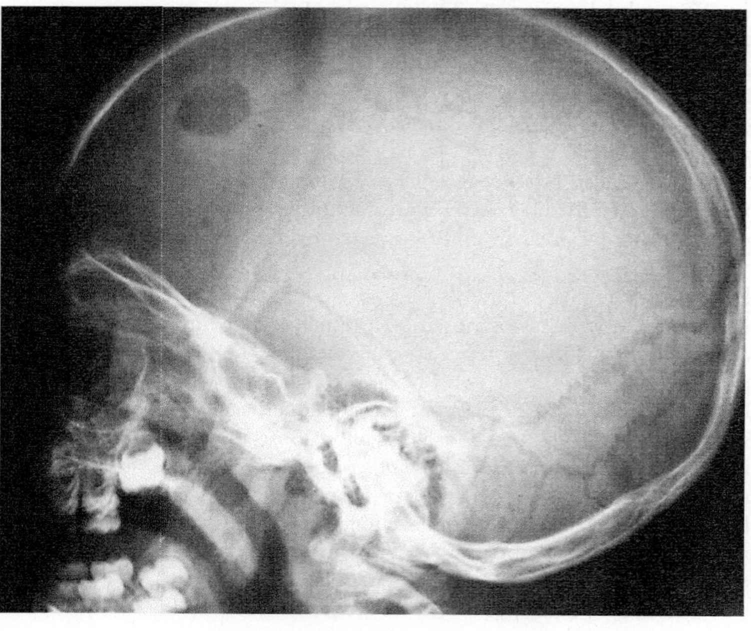

FIGURE 20.86 **Langerhans cell histiocytosis.** Lateral radiograph of the skull of a 2.5-year-old boy with disseminated disease shows an osteolytic lesion in the frontal bone with a sharply outlined margin, giving it a punched-out appearance. Uneven involvement of the inner and outer tables results in its beveled appearance.

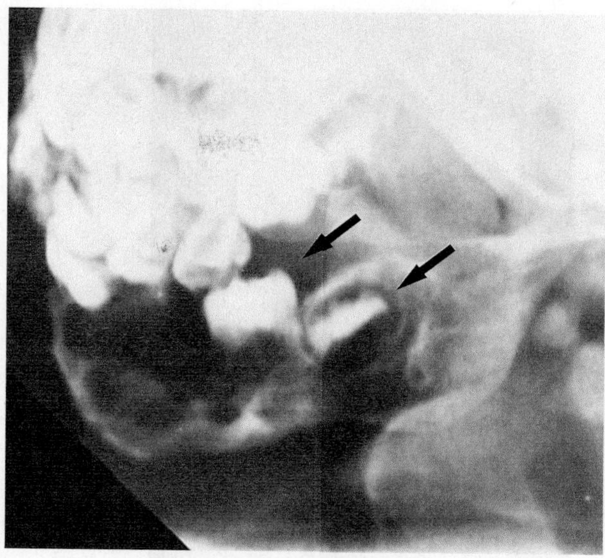

FIGURE 20.87 Langerhans cell histiocytosis. A 3-year-old girl with extensive skeletal involvement had in addition a large destructive lesion in the mandible. Note the characteristic appearance of the floating teeth *(arrows)*, which results from destruction of supportive alveolar bone.

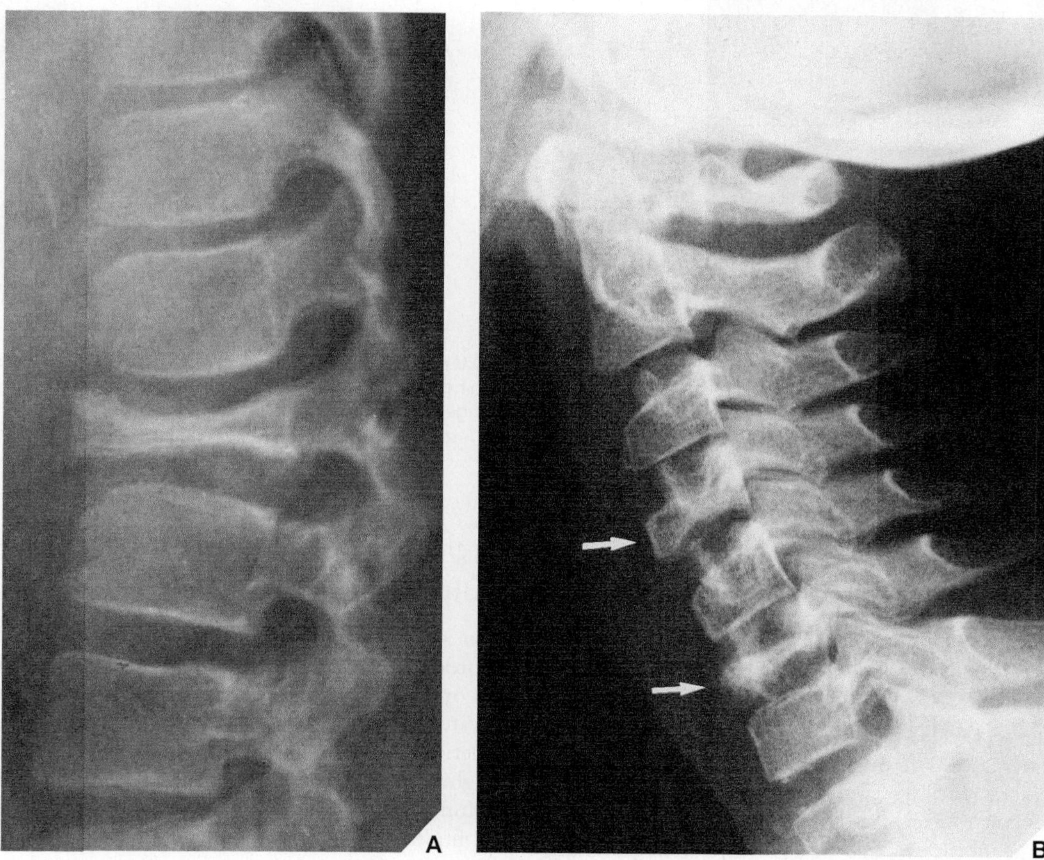

FIGURE 20.88 Langerhans cell histiocytosis. **(A)** Vertebra plana in LCH represents collapse of a vertebral body secondary to the destruction of bone by a granulomatous lesion. Note the preservation of the adjacent intervertebral disk spaces. **(B)** In another patient, observe compression fractures of the vertebral bodies C4 and C6 *(arrows)*.

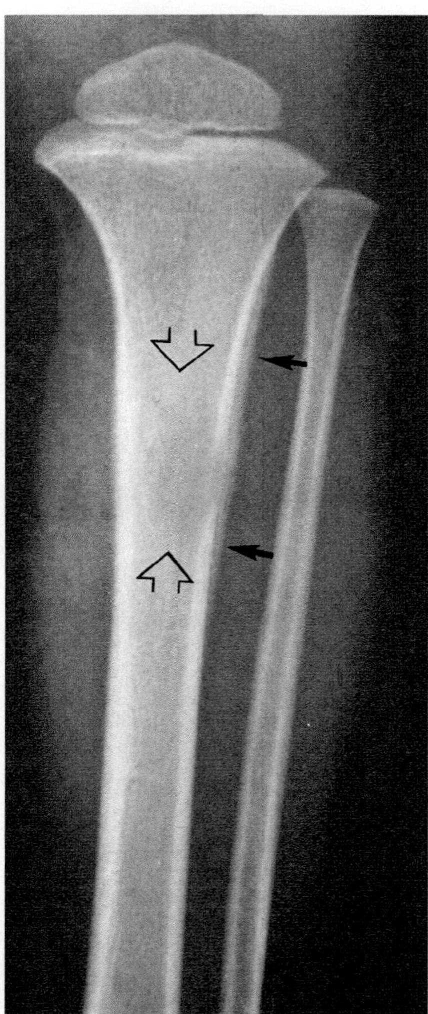

FIGURE 20.89 Langerhans cell histiocytosis. Radiograph of the left lower leg of a 4-year-old boy demonstrates a lesion in the diaphysis of the tibia exhibiting a permeative type of bone destruction *(open arrows)* and a lamellated (onion skin) type of periosteal response *(arrows)* not infrequently seen in osteomyelitis or Ewing sarcoma. The duration of the patient's symptoms (fever and pain for 10 days), however, favored LCH.

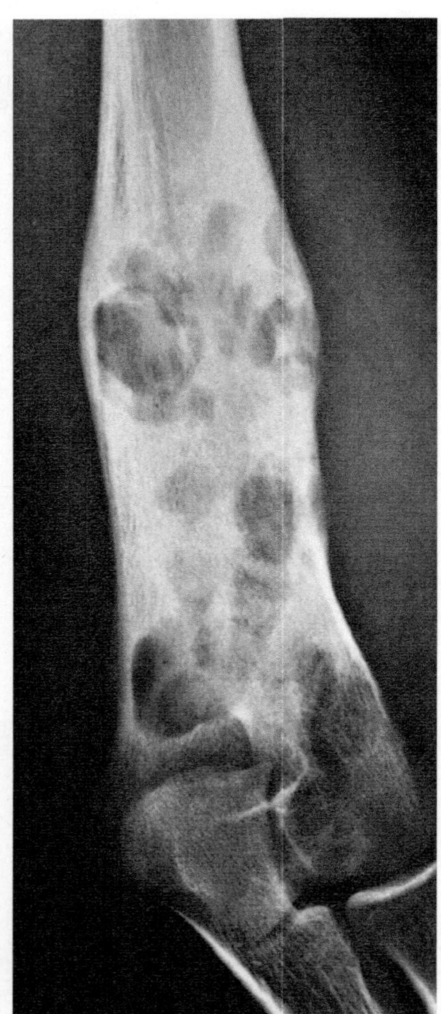

FIGURE 20.90 Langerhans cell histiocytosis. The healing stage of disease, seen here in the distal humerus of a 16-year-old girl, exhibits predominantly sclerotic changes with interspersed radiolucent foci, thickening of the cortex, and a well-organized periosteal reaction. In this stage, the lesion mimics chronic osteomyelitis.

and Langerhans/CD207, but negative for CD68 and CD45. Electron microscopy shows intracytoplasmic "tennis racquet"–shaped inclusion bodies (organelles) known as *Birbeck granules*, pathognomonic for this disorder.

Treatment and Prognosis

Treatment and prognosis of LCH depends on the site and size of the lesion, the age of the patient, and the presence or absence of multifocal disease. Monostotic disease is usually managed by curettage; however, lesions located in areas difficult to excise may be treated with low dose of radiation. Single- or multi-agent therapy may be administered in the setting of disseminated disease. Complete resolution may follow treatment or occasionally may occur spontaneously.

Infantile Myofibromatosis

Infantile myofibromatosis is a condition that can be mistaken for LCH. It is a nodular myofibroblastic lesion of unknown cause that occurs in either a solitary (more commonly) or a multicentric form. In addition to bones, the dermis, subcutis, muscle, and viscera (heart, lungs, gastrointestinal tract) may be affected. Infantile myofibromatosis usually affects children younger than age 2 years. On radiography, radiolucent areas with or without sclerotic border are identified in the long bones, facial bones, and calvaria. MRI shows the lesions to be of low signal intensity on T1-weighted sequences and high signal intensity on T2-weighted sequences.

Erdheim-Chester Disease (Lipogranulomatosis)

Also known as *Chester-Erdheim disease*, this rare disseminated histiocytic disorder of unknown cause affects the musculoskeletal system and various organs including heart, lungs, and skin. It was first described in the literature in 1930 by the Austrian pathologist Jakob Erdheim and the American pathologist William Chester. The clinical symptoms include weight loss, bone pain, abdominal pain, shortness of breath, neurologic dysfunction, exophthalmos, fever, and generalized weakness. The imaging findings are characteristic. Radiographs show extensive medullary sclerosis and cortical thickening affecting predominantly the long bones, with sparing of the articular ends (Fig. 20.95). The axial skeleton is usually not affected. MRI demonstrates decreased signal on T1-weighted images and increased signal on T2 weighting. The condition may mimic lymphoma and metastatic disease. Histologically, there is evidence of a dense infiltrate of lipid-laden foamy macrophages associated with cholesterol crystals, scattered giant cells, chronic inflammatory cells, and various amounts of fibrosis. Occasionally, Langerhans cells may be present, which raised the hypothesis of possible association of this disorder with LCH. Recently, the cytogenetic findings have been reported that included balanced chromosomal translocation t(12;15;20)(q11;q24;p13.3) among other numeric chromosomal abnormalities, such as BRAF V600E mutation. Furthermore, positivity for CD68 and negativity for CD1a and S-100 protein were described.

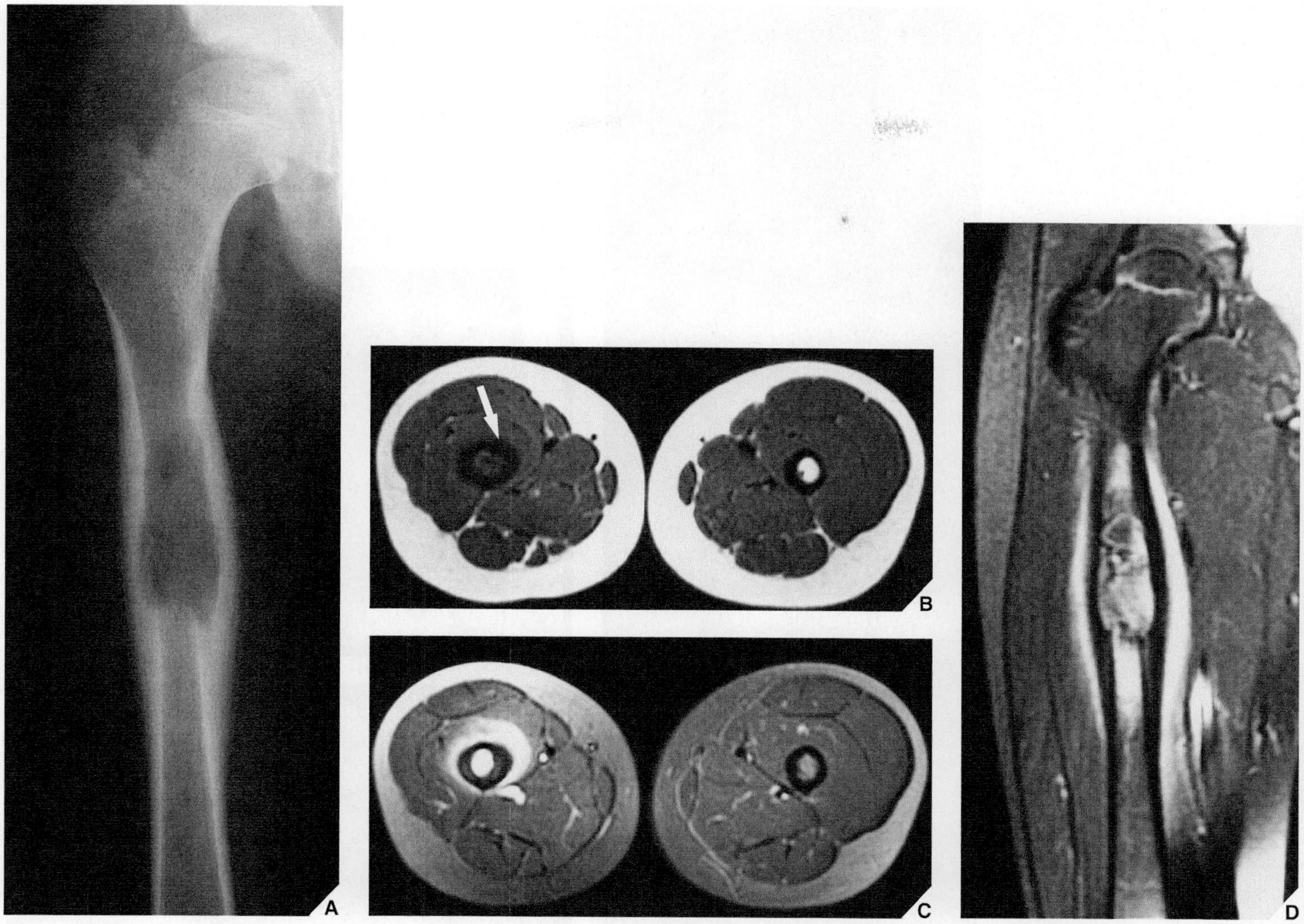

FIGURE 20.91 MRI of LCH. **(A)** Anteroposterior radiograph of the right femur of a 13-year-old boy shows a radiolucent lesion in the proximal femoral diaphysis associated with a lamellated periosteal reaction. **(B)** Axial T1-weighted (spin echo [SE]; repetition time [TR] 600/echo time [TE] 14 msec) MR image demonstrates the lesion to be of low signal intensity. The cortex is markedly thickened *(arrow)*. **(C)** Axial T2-weighted MR image shows high signal intensity of granuloma and perilesional edema. **(D)** Coronal fat-suppressed T1-weighted (SE; TR 500/TE 15 msec) MR image obtained after intravenous injection of gadolinium shows marked enhancement of the lesion and the soft tissues adjacent to the thickened femoral cortex.

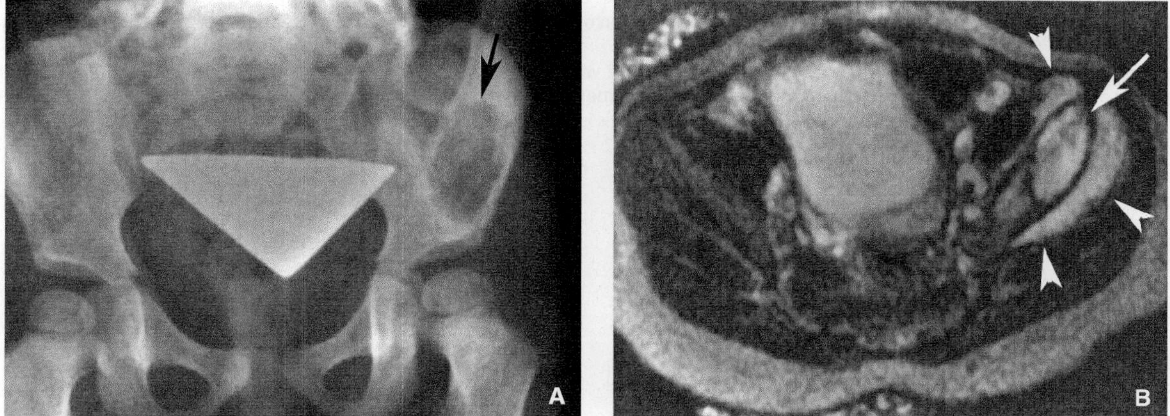

FIGURE 20.92 MRI of LCH. **(A)** Anteroposterior radiograph of the pelvis of a 4-year-old boy who presented with left-sided flank pain shows a well demarcated lytic lesion in the left iliac wing *(arrow)* with a rim of sclerosis. **(B)** Axial T2-weighted MR image demonstrates a lytic lesion in the left iliac wing *(arrow)* and surrounding mass-like soft-tissue edema *(arrowheads)*.

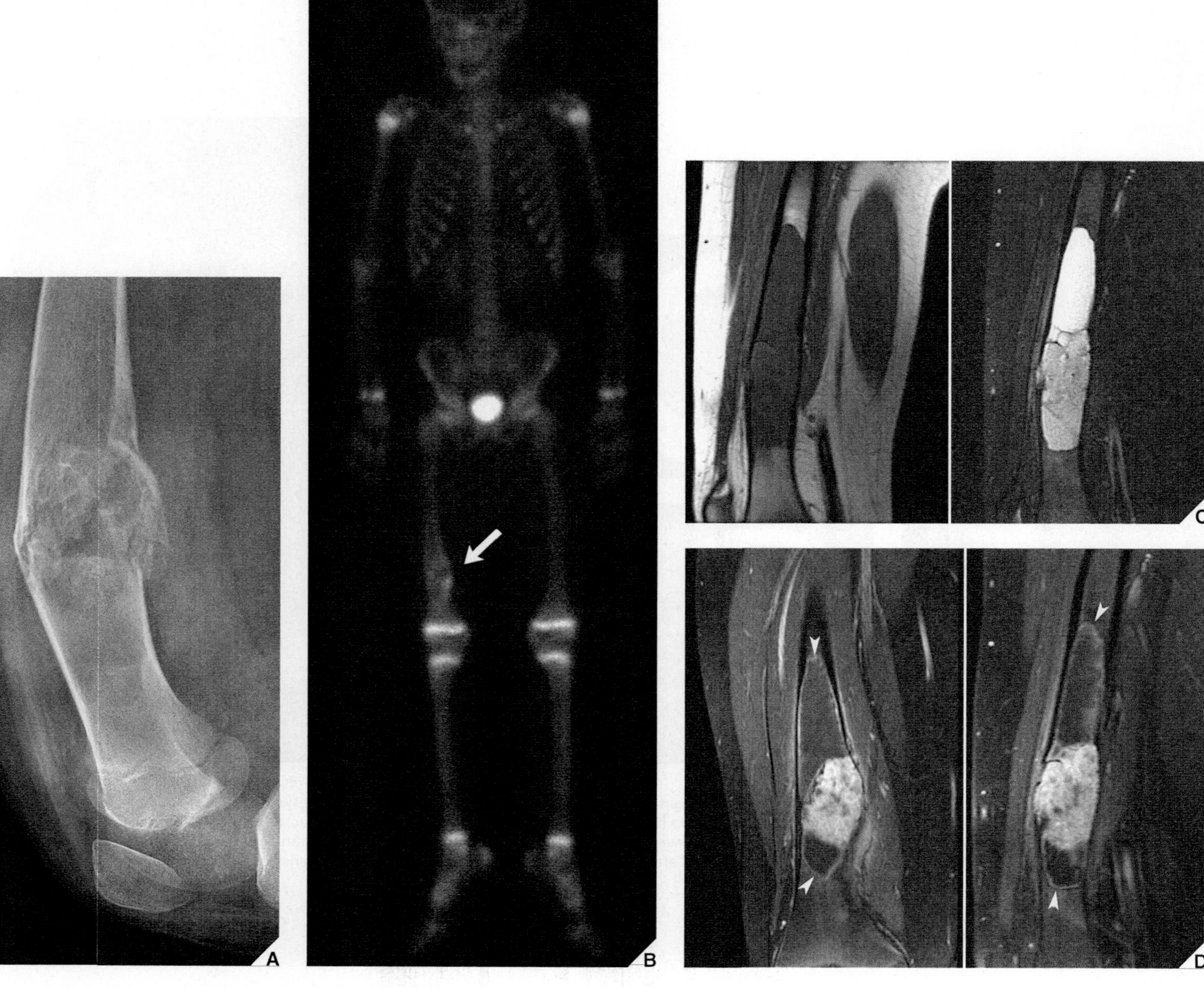

▲
FIGURE 20.93 MRI of LCH. **(A)** Lateral radiograph of the right knee of a 9-year-old boy shows an osteolytic lesion in the diaphysis of distal femur with a pathologic fracture. **(B)** Whole-body radionuclide bone scan obtained after intravenous injection of 15 mCi (555 MBq) of ^{99m}Tc-labeled MDP shows mildly increased uptake of the radiopharmaceutical agent at the site of the lesion *(arrow)*. There are no additional lesions present. **(C)** Sagittal T1-weighted MR image *(left part)* demonstrates sharply demarcated lesion exhibiting intermediate signal intensity, which changes to high signal with T2 weighting *(right part)*. **(D)** Sagittal and coronal T1-weighted fat-suppressed MR images obtained after intravenous administration of gadolinium show significant enhancement of the lesion. The solid, enhancing lesion is surrounded proximally and distally by intramedullary cyst formation with a thin enhancing peripheral rim *(arrowheads)*. This is a rare feature of LCH.

Medullary Bone Infarct

Radiographically, a medullary bone infarct presents with calcifications in the marrow cavity, usually surrounded by a well-defined hyalinized fibrotic or sclerotic border (see Figs. 18.23 and 18.24); occasionally, this presentation may be mistaken for a cartilage tumor such as an enchondroma. In the rare instances when a cyst develops in an infarcted segment of a long or flat bone, that is, an encystified bone infarct, it is visualized radiographically as an expanding radiolucent lesion associated with thinning of the surrounding cortex. Usually, the cyst cavity is sharply outlined, and the lesion is demarcated by a thin shell of reactive bone (Fig. 20.96). This encystification of a bone infarct can resemble an intraosseous lipoma or even a chondrosarcoma.

Myositis Ossificans

Myositis ossificans is a localized formation of heterotopic bone in the soft tissues that is initiated by trauma. Two types of these lesions have been identified. The first is a well-circumscribed lesion frequently seen adjacent to the cortex of a long tubular or flat bone, so-called *juxtacortical myositis ossificans circumscripta*; the other is a veil-like lesion that is less delineated. Radiographically, myositis ossificans circumscripta is characterized by a zonal phenomenon—dense, well-organized bone at the periphery of the lesion and less organized, immature bone at the center—and a radiolucent cleft that separates the lesion from the cortex of the adjacent bone (Fig. 20.97; see also Figs. 4.79, 4.80, and 21.38). The appearance of this lesion may mimic a malignant bone tumor such as parosteal or periosteal

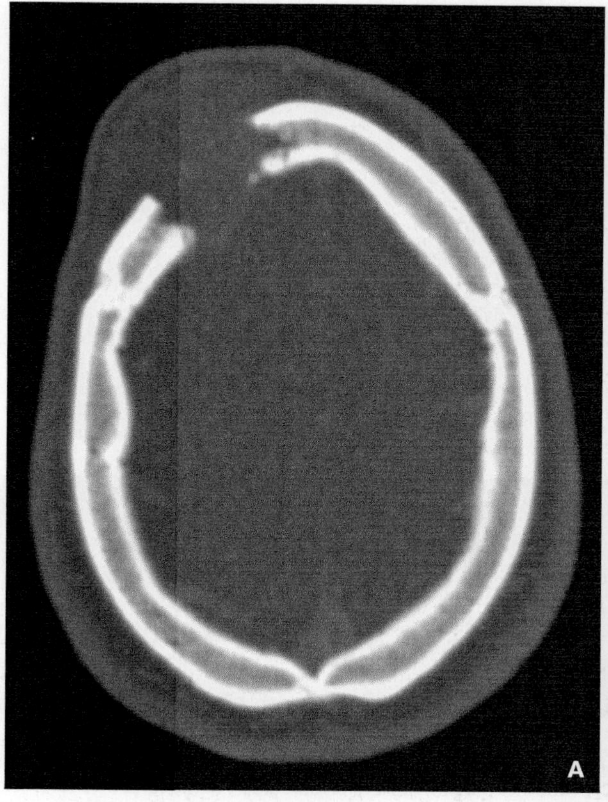

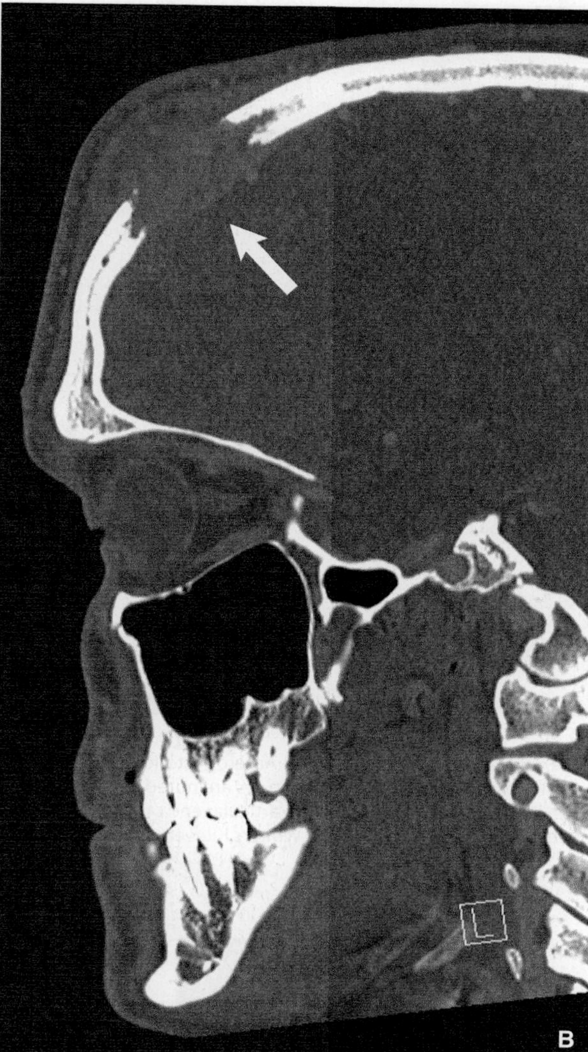

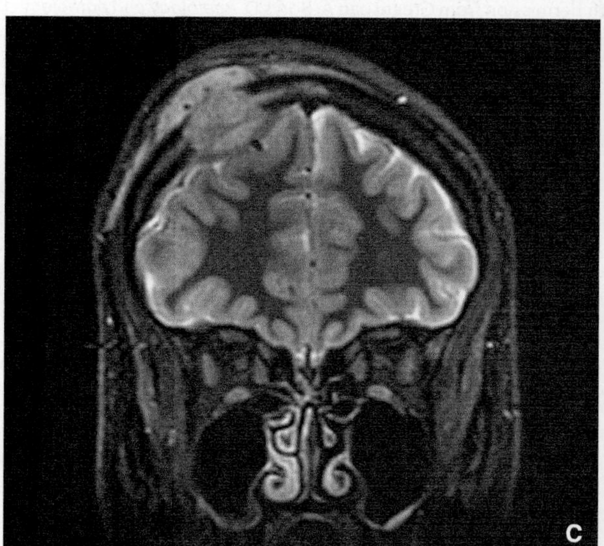

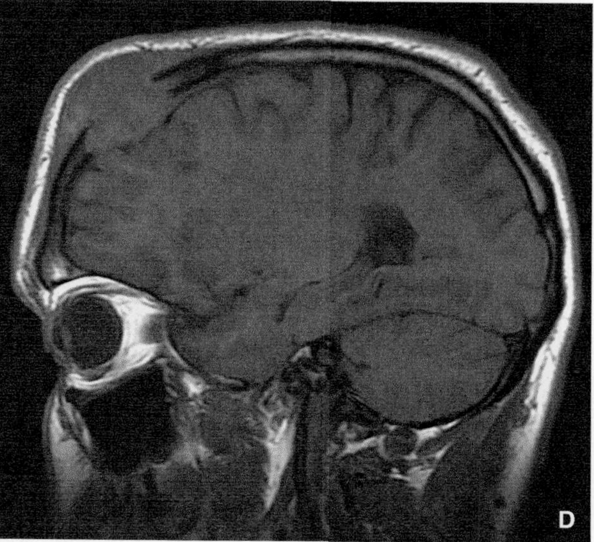

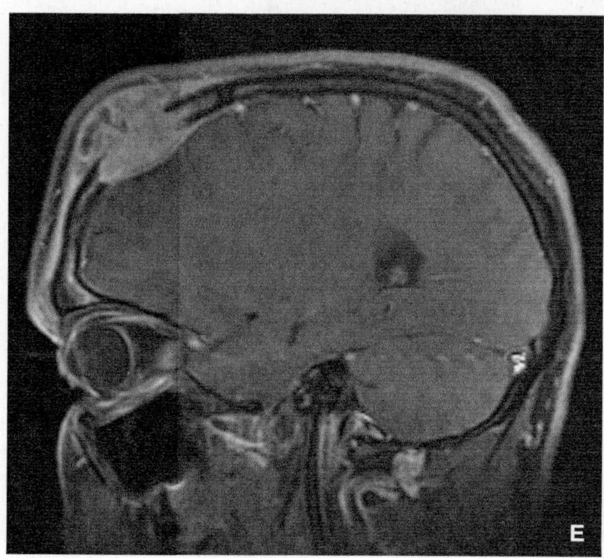

FIGURE 20.94 CT and MRI of LCH. **(A)** Axial and **(B)** sagittal reformatted CT images of the skull of a 19-year-old man show a destructive lesion in the right frontal bone associated with a soft-tissue mass *(arrow)*. **(C)** Coronal T2-weighted fat-suppressed MR image shows a soft-tissue mass to better advantage, displaying high signal intensity. The mass is compressing the right frontal lobe. Sagittal T1-weighted **(D)** and sagittal T1-weighted **(E)** fat-suppressed MR image obtained after intravenous administration of gadolinium show slight enhancement of both the intraosseous lesion and the soft-tissue mass.

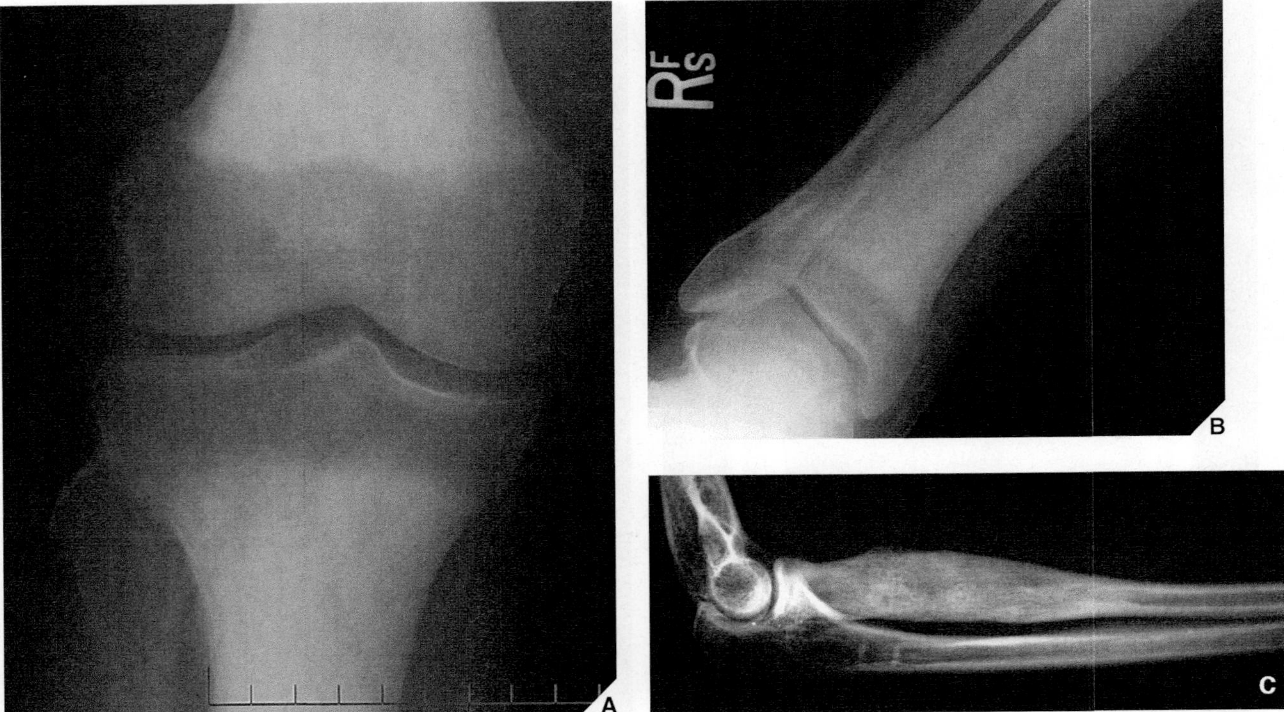

FIGURE 20.95 Erdheim-Chester disease. **(A)** Anteroposterior radiograph of the right knee shows the characteristic sclerosis of the long bones sparing the epiphysis of the distal femur and proximal tibia. **(B)** Similar features are noted in the distal tibia. **(C)** In another patient, the lateral radiograph of the forearm shows sclerotic changes in the shaft of the radius. Again, observe sparing of the articular end of bone. (Reprinted with permission from Greenspan A, Borys D. *Radiology and pathology correlation of bone tumors: a quick reference and review*. Philadelphia: Wolters Kluwer; 2016:242.)

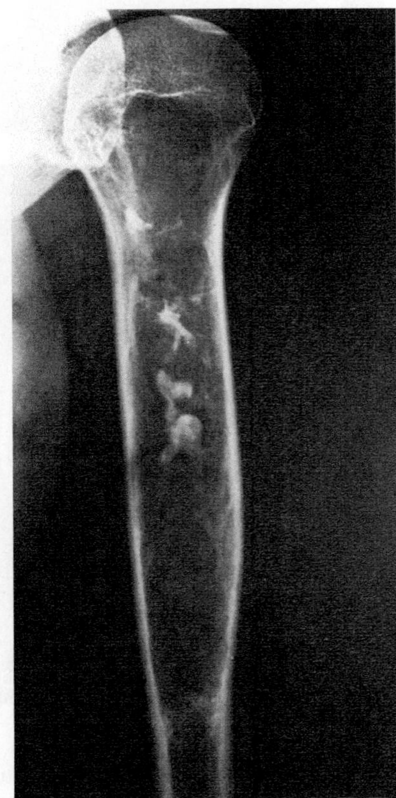

FIGURE 20.96 Encystified bone infarct. An expansive, radiolucent lesion in the proximal shaft of the left humerus was an incidental finding in a 31-year-old woman. The lesion exhibits the classic features of cyst formation within bone infarct: its location in the medullary portion of the bone with central coarse calcifications and a thin rim of reactive sclerosis. Note that although the cortex is thinned and expanded, there is no evidence of a periosteal reaction or soft-tissue mass. (Courtesy of Alex Norman, MD, New York.)

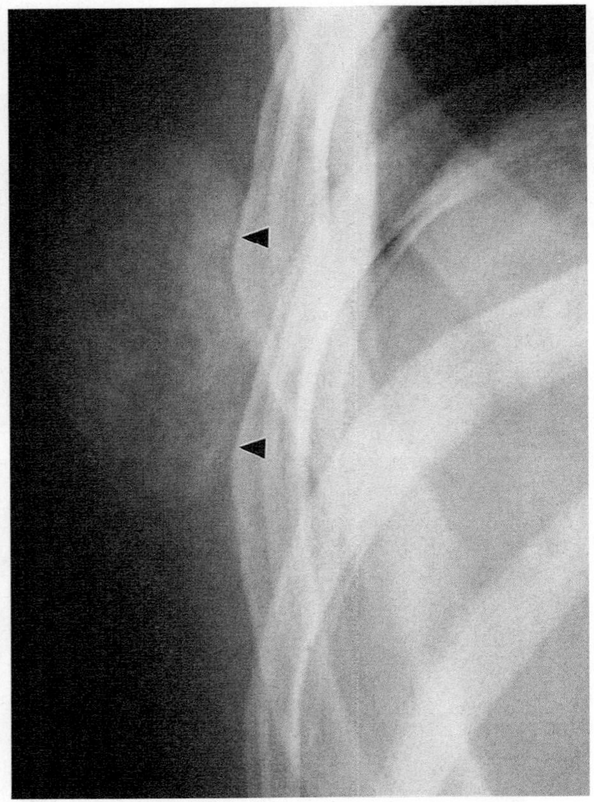

FIGURE 20.97 Myositis ossificans. Characteristic appearance of posttraumatic myositis ossificans circumscripta, adjacent to the right ribs. Note that periphery of the lesion is denser than the center. The *arrowheads* point to the narrow radiolucent cleft that separates the lesion from the cortex of the ribs.

osteosarcoma (see Figs. 21.33, 21.34, and 21.35A). Most errors in diagnosis occur when a biopsy of the lesion is performed too early in onset, when its histologic appearance may resemble sarcomatous tissue. (For more detailed information regarding myositis ossificans see Chapter 4).

PRACTICAL POINTS TO REMEMBER

1. SBCs have a predilection for:
   - the proximal diaphysis of the humerus and femur in children and adolescents
   - the pelvis and os calcis in adults.
2. SBC is characterized by:
   - its central location in a long bone
   - lack of periosteal reaction in the absence of fracture. It may be complicated by pathologic fracture, in which case the fallen fragment sign is often present and may help in the differential diagnosis.
3. ABC, seen almost exclusively in children and adolescents younger than age 20 years, is characterized by:
   - its eccentric location in a bone
   - a buttress of periosteal reaction
   - its usual containment by a thin shell of periosteum.
4. ABC can develop *de novo* or as a result of cystic changes in a preexisting benign (chondroblastoma, osteoblastoma, GCT, fibrous dysplasia) or malignant (osteosarcoma) tumors.
5. MRI of ABC usually shows rather characteristic fluid–fluid levels, which represent sedimentation of red blood cells and serum within cystic cavities.
6. Solid variant of ABC is commonly termed *giant cell reparative granuloma*. This lesion is seen primarily in craniofacial bones and short tubular bones of the hands and feet.
7. GCT, seen characteristically at the articular ends of long bones, most often presents as a purely radiolucent lesion without any sclerotic reaction at the periphery. It is impossible to determine radiologically whether a GCT is benign or malignant.
8. Multifocal GCTs are rare. Most commonly, they occur in patients with Paget disease.
9. Fibrocartilaginous mesenchymoma is a benign lesion composed of two distinct tissues: one cartilaginous, resembling an active growth plate, and one fibrous, resembling a low-grade fibrosarcoma.
10. Hemangiomas are commonly seen in a vertebral body. Although most frequently asymptomatic, they may produce symptoms if they expand into the spinal canal.
11. The characteristic MRI appearance of hemangioma includes high signal intensity on T1- and T2-weighted images.
12. Epithelioid hemangioma represents a variant of conventional hemangioma with predilection for the vertebrae.
13. Angiomatosis is defined as diffuse involvement of bones by hemangiomatous lesions. When bone is extensively involved, the term *cystic angiomatosis* is applied.
14. Gorham disease of bone, also known as *massive osteolysis* or *disappearing bone disease*, is characterized by progressive, localized bone resorption, giving rise to a "sucked-candy" appearance.
15. Intraosseous lipoma frequently presents with central calcification or ossification. The subtrochanteric region of the femur and the calcaneus are common sites for this lesion.
16. Nonneoplastic conditions frequently mistaken for tumors include:
   - intraosseous ganglion
   - brown tumor of hyperparathyroidism
   - LCH (eosinophilic granuloma)
   - Erdheim-Chester disease
   - encystified medullary bone infarct
   - posttraumatic myositis ossificans.
17. Intraosseous ganglion resembles a degenerative cyst and has a predilection for the non–weight-bearing segments of the articular end of the long bones.
18. Brown tumor of hyperparathyroidism appears on the radiographs as a lytic lesion, most commonly in the long and short tubular bones. The name derives from its pathologic appearance: The lesion contains decomposing blood, which gives specimens a brown coloration.
19. LCH is seen predominantly in children and may be mistaken for Ewing sarcoma.
20. Erdheim-Chester disease manifests on radiography by extensive medullary sclerosis and cortical thickening, mimicking lymphoma and osteoblastic metastases.
21. Myositis ossificans is characterized by a zonal phenomenon (well-organized, mature bone at the periphery of the lesion and immature bone at the center) and a radiolucent cleft that separates the lesion from the cortex of adjacent bone.

SUGGESTED READINGS

Abrahams TG, Bula W, Jones M. Epithelioid hemangioendothelioma of bone. A report of two cases and review of the literature. *Skeletal Radiol* 1992;21:509–513.

Adamsbaum C, Leclet H, Kalifa G. Intralesional Ethibloc injections in bone cysts. *Semin Musculoskelet Radiol* 1997;1:310–304.

Adamsbaum C, Mascard E, Guinebretière JM, et al. Intralesional Ethibloc injections in primary aneurysmal bone cysts: an efficient and safe treatment. *Skeletal Radiol* 2003;32(10):559–566.

Alles JU, Schulz A. Immunocytochemical markers (endothelial and histiocytic) and ultrastructure of primary aneurysmal bone cysts. *Hum Pathol* 1986;17:39–45.

Althof PA, Ohmori K, Zhou M, et al. Cytogenetic and molecular cytogenetic findings in 43 aneurysmal bone cysts: aberrations of 17p mapped to 17p13.2 by fluorescence in situ hybridization. *Mod Pathol* 2004;17:518–525.

Aoki J, Tanikawa H, Ishii K, et al. MR findings indicative of hemosiderin in giant-cell tumor of bone: frequency, cause, and diagnostic significance. *AJR Am J Roentgenol* 1996;166:145–148.

Aricò M, Danesino C. Langerhans' cell histiocytosis: is there a role for genetics? *Haematologica* 2001;86:1009–1014.

Assoun J, Richardi G, Railhac JJ, et al. CT and MRI of massive osteolysis of Gorham. *J Comput Assist Tomogr* 1994;18:981–984.

Athanasou NA, Bliss E, Gatter KC, et al. An immunohistological study of giant-cell tumour of bone: evidence for an osteoclast origin of the giant cells. *J Pathol* 1985;147:153–158.

Bacchini P, Bertoni F, Ruggieri P, et al. Multicentric giant cell tumor of skeleton. *Skeletal Radiol* 1995;24:371–374.

Bahk W-J, Kang Y-K, Lee A-H, et al. Desmoid tumor of bone with enchondromatous nodules, mistaken for chondrosarcoma. *Skeletal Radiol* 2003;32:223–226.

Baker ND, Klein MJ, Greenspan A, et al. Symptomatic vertebral hemangiomas: a report of four cases. *Skeletal Radiol* 1986;15:458–463.

Bancroft LW, Kransdorf MJ, Petersson JJ, et al. Benign fatty tumors: classification, clinical course, imaging appearance, and treatment. *Skeletal Radiol* 2006;35:719–733.

Baruffi MR, Neto JB, Barbieri CH, et al. Aneurysmal bone cyst with chromosomal changes involving 7q and 16p. *Cancer Genet Cytogenet* 2001;129:177–180.

Baudrez V, Galant C, Vande Berg BC. Benign vertebral hemangioma: MR-histological correlation. *Skeletal Radiol* 2001;30:442–446.

Beltran J, Aparisi F, Bonmati LM, et al. Eosinophilic granuloma: MRI manifestations. *Skeletal Radiol* 1993;22:157–161.

Beltran J, Simon DC, Levy M, et al. Aneurysmal bone cysts: MR imaging at 1.5 T. *Radiology* 1986;158:689–690.

Bergman AG, Rogero GW, Hellman B, et al. Case report 841. Skeletal cystic angiomatosis. *Skeletal Radiol* 1994;23:303–305.

Bertoni F, Bacchini P, Capanna R, et al. Solid variant of aneurysmal bone cyst. *Cancer* 1993;71:729–734.

Bertoni F, Bacchini P, Staals EL. Malignancy in giant cell tumor. *Skeletal Radiol* 2003;32:143–146.

Bertoni F, Present D, Sudanese A, et al. Giant-cell tumor of bone with pulmonary metastases. Six case reports and a review of the literature. *Clin Orthop Relat Res* 1988;(237):275–285.

Bhaduri A, Deshpande RB. Fibrocartilagenous mesenchymoma versus fibrocartilagenous dysplasia: are these a single entity? *Am J Surg Pathol* 1995;19:1447–1448.

Bindra J, Lam A, Lamba R, et al. Erdheim-Chester disease: an unusual presentation of an uncommon disease. *Skeletal Radiol* 2014;43:835–840.

Bisceglia M, Cammisa M, Suster S, et al. Erdheim-Chester disease: clinical and pathologic spectrum of four cases from the Arkadi M. Rywlin slide seminars. *Adv Anat Pathol* 2003;10:160–171.

Blacksin MF, Ende N, Benevenia J. Magnetic resonance imaging of intraosseous lipomas: a radiologic-pathologic correlation. *Skeletal Radiol* 1995;24:37–41.

Blombery P, Wong SQ, Lade S, et al. Erdheim-Chester disease harboring the BRAF V600E mutation. *J Clin Oncol* 2012;30:e331–e332.

Bonakdarpour A, Levy WM, Aegerter E. Primary and secondary aneurysmal bone cyst: a radiological study of 75 cases. *Radiology* 1978;126:75–83.

Bracko M, Cindro L, Golouh R. Familial occurrence of infantile myofibromatosis. *Cancer* 1992;69:1294–1299.

Bullough PG. *Atlas of orthopedic pathology: with clinical and radiologic correlations*, 2nd ed. New York: Gower Medical; 1992:15.12–15.14.

Bulychova IV, Unni KK, Bertoni F, et al. Fibrocartilagenous mesenchymoma of bone. *Am J Surg Pathol* 1993;17:830–836.

Bush CH, Drane WE. Treatment of an aneurysmal bone cyst of the spine by radionuclide ablation. *AJNR Am J Neuroradiol* 2000;21:592–594.

Campanacci M. *Bone and soft tissue tumors*. New York: Springer; 1986:345–348.

Campbell RSD, Grainger AJ, Mangham DC, et al. Intraosseous lipoma: report of 35 new cases and a review of the literature. *Skeletal Radiol* 2003;32:209–222.

Caudell JJ, Ballo MT, Zagars GK, et al. Radiotherapy in the management of giant cell tumor of bone. *Int J Radiat Oncol Biol Phys* 2003;57:158–165.

Chung EB, Enzinger FM. Infantile myofibromatosis. *Cancer* 1981;48:1807–1818.

Cohen J. Etiology of simple bone cyst. *J Bone Joint Surg Am* 1970;52:1493–1497.

Cohen MD, Rougraff B, Faught P. Cystic angiomatosis of bone: MR findings. *Pediatr Radiol* 1994;24:256–257.

Conway WF, Hayes CW. Miscellaneous lesions of bone. *Radiol Clin North Am* 1993;31:339–358.

da Costa CE, Annels NE, Faaij CM, et al. Presence of osteoclast-like multinucleated giant cells in the bone and nonostotic lesions of Langerhans cell histiocytosis. *J Exp Med* 2005;201:687–693.

Dahlin DC. Caldwell Lecture. Giant cell tumor of bone: highlights of 407 cases. *AJR Am J Roentgenol* 1985;144:955–960.

Dahlin DC, Bertoni F, Beabout JW, et al. Fibrocartilaginous mesenchymoma with low-grade malignancy. *Skeletal Radiol* 1984;12:263–269.

Dahlin DC. Giant-cell-bearing lesions of bone of the hands. *Hand Clin* 1987;3:291–297.

Dahlin DC, McLeod RA. Aneurysmal bone cyst and other nonneoplastic conditions. *Skeletal Radiol* 1982;8:243–250.

Dahlin DC, Unni KK. *Bone tumors: general aspects and data on 8,542 cases*, 4th ed. Springfield, MO: Charles C. Thomas Publishers; 1986:181–185.

Daoud A, Olivieri B, Feinberg D, et al. Soft tissue hemangioma with osseous extension: a case report and review of the literature. *Skeletal Radiol* 2015;44:597–603.

Drumond JMN. Efficacy of the Enneking staging system in relation to treating benign bone tumors and tumor-like bone lesions. *Rev Bras Ortop* 2010;45:46–52.

Dumford K, Moore TE, Walker CW, et al. Multifocal, metachronous, giant cell tumor of the lower limb. *Skeletal Radiol* 2003;32:147–150.

Duncan CP, Morton KS, Arthur JF. Giant cell tumour of bone: its aggressiveness and potential for malignant change. *Can J Surg* 1983;26:475–476.

Egan AJM, Boardman LA, Tazelaar HD, et al. Erdheim-Chester disease: clinical, radiologic, and histopathologic findings in five patients with interstitial lung disease. *Am J Surg Pathol* 1999;23:17–26.

Enneking WF. A system of staging musculoskeletal neoplasms. *Clin Orthop Relat Res* 1986;(204):9–24.

Errani C, Vanel D, Gambarotti M, et al. Vascular bone tumors: a proposal of a classification based on clinicopathological, radiographic and genetic features. *Skeletal Radiol* 2012;41:1495–1507.

Favara BE. Langerhans' cell histiocytosis pathobiology and pathogenesis. *Semin Oncol* 1991;18:3–7.

Fayad L, Hazirolan T, Bluemke D, et al. Vascular malformations in the extremities: emphasis on MR imaging features that guide treatment options. *Skeletal Radiol* 2006;35:127–137.

Fechner RE, Mills SE. *Atlas of tumor pathology: tumors of the bones and joints*. Washington, DC: Armed Forces Institute of Pathology; 1993:173–186, 203–209, 253–258.

Francis R, Lewis E. CT demonstration of giant cell tumor complicating Paget disease. *J Comput Assist Tomogr* 1983;7:917–918.

Freeby JA, Reinus WR, Wilson AJ. Quantitative analysis of the plain radiographic appearance of aneurysmal bone cysts. *Invest Radiol* 1995;30:433–439.

Friedman DP. Symptomatic vertebral hemangiomas: MR findings. *AJR Am J Roentgenol* 1996;167:359–364.

Garg NK, Carty H, Walsh HPJ, et al. Percutaneous Ethibloc injection in aneurysmal bone cysts. *Skeletal Radiol* 2000;29:211–216.

Ghert M, Simunovic N, Cowan RW, et al. Properties of the stromal cell in giant cell tumor of bone. *Clin Orthop Relat Res* 2007;459:8–13.

Glass TA, Mills SE, Fechner RE, et al. Giant-cell reparative granuloma of the hands and feet. *Radiology* 1983;149:65–68.

Gorham LW, Stout AP. Massive osteolysis (acute spontaneous absorption of bone, phantom bone, disappearing bone): its relation to hemangiomatosis. *J Bone Joint Surg Am* 1955;37-A:985–1004.

Gorham LW, Wright AW, Shultz HH, et al. Disappearing bones: a rare form of massive osteolysis. Report of two cases, one with autopsy findings. *Am J Med* 1954;17:674–682.

Greenspan A, Borys D, eds. Benign lesions. In: *Radiology and pathology correlation of bone tumors: a quick reference and review*. Philadelphia: Wolters Kluwer; 2016:298–334.

Greenspan A, Jundt G, Remagen W. *Differential diagnosis in orthopaedic oncology*, 2nd ed. Philadelphia: Lippincott Williams & Wilkins; 2007:387–431.

Greenspan A, Klein MJ, Bennett AJ, et al. Case report 242. Hemangioma of the T6 vertebra with a compression fracture, extradural block and spinal cord compression. *Skeletal Radiol* 1978;10:183–188.

Grote HJ, Braun M, Kalinski T, et al. Spontaneous malignant transformation of conventional giant cell tumor. *Skeletal Radiol* 2004;33:169–175.

Han BK, Ryu J-S, Moon DH, et al. Bone SPECT imaging of vertebral hemangioma correlation with MR imaging and symptoms. *Clin Nucl Med* 1995;20:916–921.

Haroche J, Charlotte F, Arnaud L, et al. High prevalence of BRAF V600E mutations in Erdheim-Chester disease but not in other non-Langerhans cell histiocytoses. *Blood* 2012;120:2700–2703.

Hoch B, Hermann G, Klein MJ, et al. Giant cell tumor complicating Paget disease of long bone. *Skeletal Radiol* 2007;36:973–978.

Hong WS, Sung MS, Kim J-H, et al. Giant cell tumor with secondary aneurysmal bone cyst: a unique presentation with an ossified extraosseous soft tissue mass. *Skeletal Radiol* 2013;42:1605–1610.

Hoover KB, Rosenthal DI, Mankin H. Langerhans cell histiocytosis. *Skeletal Radiol* 2007;36:95–104.

Hudson TM. Fluid levels in aneurysmal bone cysts: a CT feature. *AJR Am J Roentgenol* 1984;142:1001–1004.

Hudson TM, Hamlin DJ, Fitzsimmons JR. Magnetic resonance imaging of fluid levels in an aneurysmal bone cyst and in anticoagulated human blood. *Skeletal Radiol* 1985;13:267–270.

Ilaslan H, Sundaram M, Unni KK. Solid variant of aneurysmal bone cysts in long tubular bones: giant cell reparative granuloma. *AJR Am J Roentgenol* 2003;180:1681–1687.

Ishida T, Dorfman HD, Steiner GC, et al. Cystic angiomatosis of bone with sclerotic changes mimicking osteoblastic metastases. *Skeletal Radiol* 1994;23:247–252.

Jackson JBS. A boneless arm. *Boston Med Surg J* 1838;18:368–369.

Jaffe HL. Aneurysmal bone cyst. *Bull Hosp Joint Dis* 1950;11:3–13.

Jaffe HL. Giant-cell reparative granuloma, traumatic bone cyst, and fibrous (fibro-oseous) dysplasia of the jawbones. *Oral Surg Oral Med Oral Pathol* 1953;6:159–175.

Jaffe HL, Lichtenstein L. Solitary unicameral bone cyst with emphasis on the roentgen picture, the pathologic appearance and the pathogenesis. *Arch Surg* 1942;44:1004–1025.

Jaffe HL, Lichtenstein L, Perris RB. Giant cell tumor of bone. Its pathologic appearance, grading, supposed variants and treatment. *Arch Pathol* 1940;30:993–1031.

Jordanov MI. The "rising bubble" sign: a new aid in the diagnosis of unicameral bone cysts. *Skeletal Radiol* 2009;38:597–600.

Keats TE. *Atlas of normal roentgen variants that may simulate disease*, 5th ed. St. Louis: Mosby Year Book; 1992:637–648.

Kransdorf MJ, Sweet DE. Aneurysmal bone cyst: concept, controversy, clinical presentation, and imaging. *AJR Am J Roentgenol* 1995;164:573–580.

Kransdorf MJ, Sweet DE, Buetow PC, et al. Giant cell tumor in skeletally immature patients. *Radiology* 1992;184:233–237.

Kyriakos M, Hardy D. Malignant transformation of aneurysmal bone cyst, with an analysis of the literature. *Cancer* 1991;68:1770–1780.

Lateur L, Simoens CJ, Gryspeerdt S, et al. Skeletal cystic angiomatosis. *Skeletal Radiol* 1996;25:92–95.

Lichtenstein L. Aneurysmal bone cyst. Observations on fifty cases. *J Bone Joint Surg Am* 1957;39-A:873–882.

Lin J, Shulman SC, Steelman CK, et al. Fibrocartilaginous mesenchymoma, a unique osseous lesion: case report with review of the literature. *Skeletal Radiol* 2011;40:1495–1499.

Lomasney LM, Basu A, Demos TC, et al. Fibrous dysplasia complicated by aneurysmal bone cyst formation affecting multiple cervical vertebrae. *Skeletal Radiol* 2003;32:533–536.

Lorenzo JC, Dorfman HD. Giant-cell reparative granuloma of short tubular bones of the hands and feet. *Am J Surg Pathol* 1980;4:551–563.

Marcove RC, Weis LD, Vaghaiwalla MR, et al. Cryosurgery in the treatment of giant cell tumors of bone: a report of 52 consecutive cases. *Clin Orthop Relat Res* 1978;(134):275–289.

Martinez V, Sissons HA. Aneurysmal bone cyst. A review of 123 cases including primary lesions and those secondary to other bone pathology. *Cancer* 1988;61:2291–2304.

Marui T, Yamamoto T, Yoshihara H, et al. De novo malignant transformation of giant cell tumor of bone. *Skeletal Radiol* 2001;30:104–108.

McGlynn FJ, Mickelson MR, El-Khoury GY. The fallen fragment sign in unicameral bone cyst. *Clin Orthop* 1981;156:157–159.

Meyer JS, Hoffer FA, Barnes PD, et al. Biological classification of soft-tissue vascular anomalies: MR correlation. *AJR Am J Roentgenol* 1991;157:559–564.

Milgram JW. Intraosseous lipomas. A clinicopathologic study of 66 cases. *Clin Orthop Relat Res* 1988;(231):277–302.

Milgram JW. Intraosseous lipomas: radiologic and pathologic manifestations. *Radiology* 1988;167:155–160.

Moukaddam H, Pollak J, Haims AH. MRI characteristics and classification of peripheral vascular malformations and tumors. *Skeletal Radiol* 2009;38:535–547.

Mulliken JB, Glowacki J. Hemangiomas and vascular malformations in infants and children: a classification based on endothelial characteristics. *Plast Reconstr Surg* 1982;69:412–420.

Murphey MD, Nomikos GC, Flemming DJ, et al. From the archives of AFIP. Imaging of giant cell tumor and giant cell reparative granuloma of bone: radiologic-pathologic correlation. *Radiographics* 2001;21:1283–1309.

Norman A, Schiffman M. Simple bone cysts: factors of age dependency. *Radiology* 1977;124:779–782.

Norman A, Steiner GC. Radiographic and morphological features of cyst formation in idiopathic bone infarction. *Radiology* 1983;146:335–338.

O'Connell JX, Nielsen GP, Rosenberg AE. Epithelioid vascular tumors of bone: a review and proposal of a classification scheme. *Adv Anat Pathol* 2001;8:74–82.

Oliveira AM, Hsi BL, Weremowicz S, et al. USP6 (Tre2) fusion oncogenes in aneurysmal bone cyst. *Cancer Res* 2004;64:1920–1923.

Oliveira AM, Perez-Atayde AR, Dal Cin P, et al. Aneurysmal bone cyst variant translocations upregulate USP6 transcription by promoter swapping with the ZNF9, COL1A1, TRAP150, and OMD genes. *Oncogene* 2005;24:3419–3426.

Potter HG, Schneider R, Ghelman B, et al. Multiple giant cell tumors and Paget disease of bone: radiographic and clinical correlations. *Radiology* 1991;180:261–264.

Ratner V, Dorfman HD. Giant-cell reparative granuloma of the hand and foot bones. *Clin Orthop Relat Res* 1990;(260):251–258.

Remagen W. Pathologische Anatomie der Femurkopfnekrose. *Orthopäde* 1990;19:174–181.

Remagen W, Lampérth BE, Jundt G, et al. Das sogenannte osteolytische Dreieck de Calcaneus. Radiologische und pathoanatomische Befunde. *Osteologie* 1994;3:275–283.

Reynolds J. The "fallen fragment sign" in the diagnosis of unicameral bone cysts. *Radiology* 1969;92:949–953.

Rigopoulou A, Saifuddin A. Intraosseous hemangioma of the appendicular skeleton: imaging features of 15 cases, and a review of the literature. *Skeletal Radiol* 2012;41:1525–1536.

Ruggieri P, Montalti M, Angelini A, et al. Gorham-Stout disease: the experience of the Rizzoli Institute and review of the literature. *Skeletal Radiol* 2011;40:1391–1397.

Salerno M, Avnet S, Alberghini M, et al. Histogenetic characterization of giant cell tumor of bone. *Clin Orthop Relat Res* 2008;466:2081–2091.

Sanerkin NG, Mott MG, Roylance J. An unusual intraosseous lesion with fibroblastic, osteoclastic, osteoblastic, aneurysmal and fibromyxoid elements. "Solid" variant of aneurysmal bone cyst. *Cancer* 1983;51:2278–2286.

Scaglietti O, Marchetti PG, Bartolozzi P. The effects of methylprednisolone acetate in the treatment of bone cysts. Results of three years follow-up. *J Bone Joint Surg Br* 1979;61-B:200–204.

Schajowicz F, ed. Giant-cell tumor (osteoclastoma). In: *Tumors and tumorlike lesions of bone: pathology, radiology, and treatment*, 2nd ed. Berlin, Germany: Springer-Verlag; 1994:257–299.

Schajowicz F, Aiello CL, Francone MV, et al. Cystic angiomatosis (hamartous haemolymphangiomatosis) of bone. A clinicopathological study of three cases. *J Bone Joint Surg Br* 1978;60:100–106.

Schajowicz F, Slullitel I. Giant-cell tumor associated with Paget's disease of bone. A case report. *J Bone Joint Surg Am* 1966;48:1340–1349.

Schmidt H, Freyschmidt J, Holthusen W, et al, eds. *Kohler/Zimmer's borderlands of normal and early pathologic findings in skeletal radiography*, 13th ed. Stuttgart, Germany: Thieme Verlag; 1993:797–814.

Schoedel K, Shankman S, Desai P. Intracortical and subperiosteal aneurysmal bone cysts: a report of three cases. *Skeletal Radiol* 1996;25:455–459.

Shankman S, Greenspan A, Klein MJ, et al. Giant cell tumor of the ischium. A report of two cases and review of the literature. *Skeletal Radiol* 1988;17:46–51.

Skubitz KM, Cheng EY, Clohisy DR, et al. Gene expression in giant-cell tumors. *J Lab Clin Med* 2004;144:193–200.

Smith LT, Mayerson J, Nowak NJ, et al. 20q11.1 amplification in giant-cell tumor of bone: array CGH, FISH, and association with outcome. *Genes Chromosome Cancer* 2006;45:957–966.

Soper JR, De Silva M. Infantile myofibromatosis: a radiological review. *Pediatr Radial* 1993;23:189–194.

Spieth ME, Greenspan A, Forrester DM, et al. Gorham's disease of the radius: radiographic, scintigraphic, and MRI findings with pathologic correlation. A case report and review of the literature. *Skeletal Radiol* 1997;26:659–663.

Stacy GS, Peabody TD, Dixon LB. Pictorial essay. Mimics on radiography of giant cell tumor of bone. *AJR Am J Roentgenol* 2003;181:1583–1589.

Steiner GC, Ghosh L, Dorfman HD. Ultrastructure of giant cell tumor of bone. *Hum Pathol* 1972;3:569–586.

Struhl S, Edelson C, Pritzker H, et al. Solitary (unicameral) bone cyst. The fallen fragment sign revisited. *Skeletal Radiol* 1989;18:261–265.

Subach BR, Copay AG, Martin M, et al. An unusual occurrence of chondromyxoid fibroma with secondary aneurysmal bone cyst in the cervical spine. *Spine J* 2010;10:e5–e9.

Sung MS, Kim YS, Resnick D. Epithelioid hemangioma of bone. *Skeletal Radiol* 2000;29:530–534.

Tanaka H, Yasui N, Kuriskaki E, et al The Goltz syndrome associated with giant cell tumour of bone. A case report. *Int Orthop* 1990;14:179–181.

Thomas D, Henshaw R, Skubitz K, et al. Denosumab in patients with giant-cell tumour of bone: an open-label, phase 2 study. *Lancet Oncol* 2010;11:275–280.

Tsai JC, Dalinka MK, Fallon MD, et al. Fluid-fluid level: a nonspecific finding in tumors of bone and soft tissue. *Radiology* 1990;175:779–782.

Tubbs WS, Brown LR, Beabout JW, et al. Benign giant-cell tumor of bone with pulmonary metastases: clinical findings and radiologic appearance of metastases in 13 cases. *AJR Am J Roentgenol* 1992;158:331–334.

Vencio EF, Jenkins RB, Schiller JL, et al. Clonal cytogenetic abnormalities in Erdheim-Chester disease. *Am J Surg Pathol* 2007;31:319–321.

Vester H, Wegener B, Weiler C, et al. First report of a solid variant of aneurysmal bone cyst in the os sacrum. *Skeletal Radiol* 2010;39:73–77.

Vilanova JC, Barceló J, Smirniotopoulos JG, et al. Hemangioma from head to toe: MR imaging with pathologic correlation. *Radiographics* 2004;24:367–385.

Wenger DE, Wold LE. Benign vascular lesions of bone: radiologic and pathologic features. *Skeletal Radiol* 2000;29:63–74.

Wold LE, Swee RG, Sim FH. Vascular lesions of bone. *Pathol Annu* 1985;20(pt 2):101–137.

Wyatt-Ashmead J, Bao L, Eilert RE, et al. Primary aneurysmal bone cysts: 16q22 and/or 17p13 chromosome abnormalities. *Pediatr Dev Pathol* 2001;4:418–419.

Ye Y, Pringle LM, Lau AW, et al. TRE17/USP6 oncogene translocated in aneurysmal bone cyst induces matrix metalloproteinase production via activation of NF-kappaB. *Oncogene* 2010;29:3619–3629.

Zelger B. Position paper. Langerhans cell histiocytosis: a reactive or neoplastic disorder? *Med Pediatr Oncol* 2001;37:543–544.

Zenonos G, Jamil O, Governale LS, et al. Surgical treatment for primary spinal aneurysmal bone cysts: experience from Children's Hospital Boston. *J Neurosurg Pediatr* 2012;9:305–315.

21

Malignant Bone Tumors I

Osteosarcomas and Chondrosarcomas

Osteosarcomas

Osteosarcoma (osteogenic sarcoma) is one of the most common primary malignant bone tumors, comprising approximately 20% of all primary bone malignancies. There are several types of osteosarcoma (Fig. 21.1), each having distinctive clinical, imaging, and histologic characteristics. The common feature of all types is that the osteoid and bone matrix are formed by malignant cells of connective tissue.

The majority of osteosarcomas is of unknown cause and can therefore be referred to as *idiopathic*, or *primary*. A smaller number of tumors can be related to known factors predisposing to malignancy, such as Paget disease, fibrous dysplasia, external ionizing irradiation, or ingestion of radioactive substances. These lesions are referred to as *secondary osteosarcomas*. All types of osteosarcomas may be further subdivided by anatomic site into lesions of the appendicular skeleton and axial skeleton. Furthermore, they may be classified on the basis of their location in the bone as central (medullary), intracortical, and juxtacortical. A separate group consists of primary osteosarcoma originating in the soft tissues (so-called *extraskeletal* or *soft-tissue osteosarcomas*).

Histopathologically, osteosarcomas can be graded on the basis of their cellularity, nuclear pleomorphism, and degree of mitotic activity. According to Broder system, the numerical grade (1 to 4) indicates the degree of malignancy (grade 1 indicating the least undifferentiated tumor and grade 4 the most undifferentiated tumor) (Table 21.1). For example, well-differentiated central osteosarcomas and parosteal osteosarcomas are regarded as grade 1 or, rarely, grade 2 tumors; periosteal osteosarcomas and gnathic osteosarcomas as grade 2 or, rarely, grade 3; and conventional osteosarcoma as grade 3 or 4. Telangiectatic osteosarcomas, osteosarcomas developing in pagetic bone, postirradiation osteosarcomas, and multifocal osteosarcomas are usually grade 4 tumors. This grading has clinical, therapeutic, and prognostic importance. Generally speaking, central osteosarcomas are much more frequent than juxtacortical tumors, and they tend to have a higher histologic grade. Although pulmonary metastasis is the most common and most significant complication in high-grade osteosarcoma, it is rare in two subtypes: osteosarcoma of the jaw and multicentric osteosarcoma.

Almost all osteosarcomas harbor complex cytogenetic and molecular alterations; however, no specific findings have emerged that might be used as a molecular or cytogenetic marker for the diagnosis of this tumor. As extensively discussed by Sandberg and Bridge, conventional osteosarcomas reveal complex and unbalanced cytogenetic alterations, with pronounced variations in chromosome number and/or form, very often within the same tumor. Structural abnormalities are most often found in chromosomes 1p11-p13, 1q11-q12, 1q21-q22, 11p14-p15, 14p11-p13, 15p11-13, 17p, and 19q13. Losses of portions of chromosomes 3q, 6q, 9, 10, 13, 17p, and 18q and gains of portions of chromosomes 1p, 1q, 6p, 8q, and 17p are the most common abnormalities. Deregulation of *TP53* is also thought to be significant in the development of osteosarcoma and occurs due to mutations of the gene or gross changes to the gene locus at chromosome band 17p13.1. Aberrations of the gene *RECQL4* located at chromosome band 8q24.4 are also associated with development of this tumor. Amplification of the cyclin-dependent kinase gene (*CDK4*) located at chromosome band 12q13-14 has been detected in approximately 10% of the tumors. Deletion of 9p21 and the *CDKN2A* gene was reported in approximately 15% of the tumors. Loss of *CDKN2A* (p16) is associated with reduced survival. Amplification of the cyclin-dependent kinase gene (*CDK4*) located at chromosome band 12q13-14 has been detected in approximately 10% of the tumors. Deletion of 9p21 and the *CDKN2A* gene was reported in approximately 15% of the tumors. Loss of *CDKN2A* (p16) is associated with reduced survival. Amplification at 1q21-23 and 17p are frequent findings in conventional osteosarcoma.

Primary Osteosarcomas

Conventional Osteosarcoma

Clinical Features

Conventional osteosarcoma is the most common type, having its highest incidence in patients in their second decade and affecting males slightly more often than females. It has a predilection for the knee region (distal femur and proximal tibia), whereas the second most common site is the proximal humerus (Fig. 21.2). Patients usually present with bone pain, occasionally accompanied by a soft-tissue mass or swelling. At times, the first symptoms are related to pathologic fracture.

Imaging Features

The distinctive radiologic features of conventional osteosarcoma, as demonstrated by radiography, are medullary and cortical bone destruction, an aggressive periosteal reaction, a soft-tissue mass, and tumor bone either within the destructive lesion or at its periphery as well as within the soft-tissue mass (Fig. 21.3). In some instances, the type of bone destruction may not be obvious on the conventional studies, but patchy densities representing tumor bone and an aggressive periosteal reaction are clues to the diagnosis (Fig. 21.4).

The degree of radiopacity in the tumor reflects a combination of the amount of tumor bone production, calcified matrix, and osteoid. Tumors may present as purely sclerotic lesions or purely osteolytic lesions, but mostly a combination of both (Fig. 21.5). The borders are usually

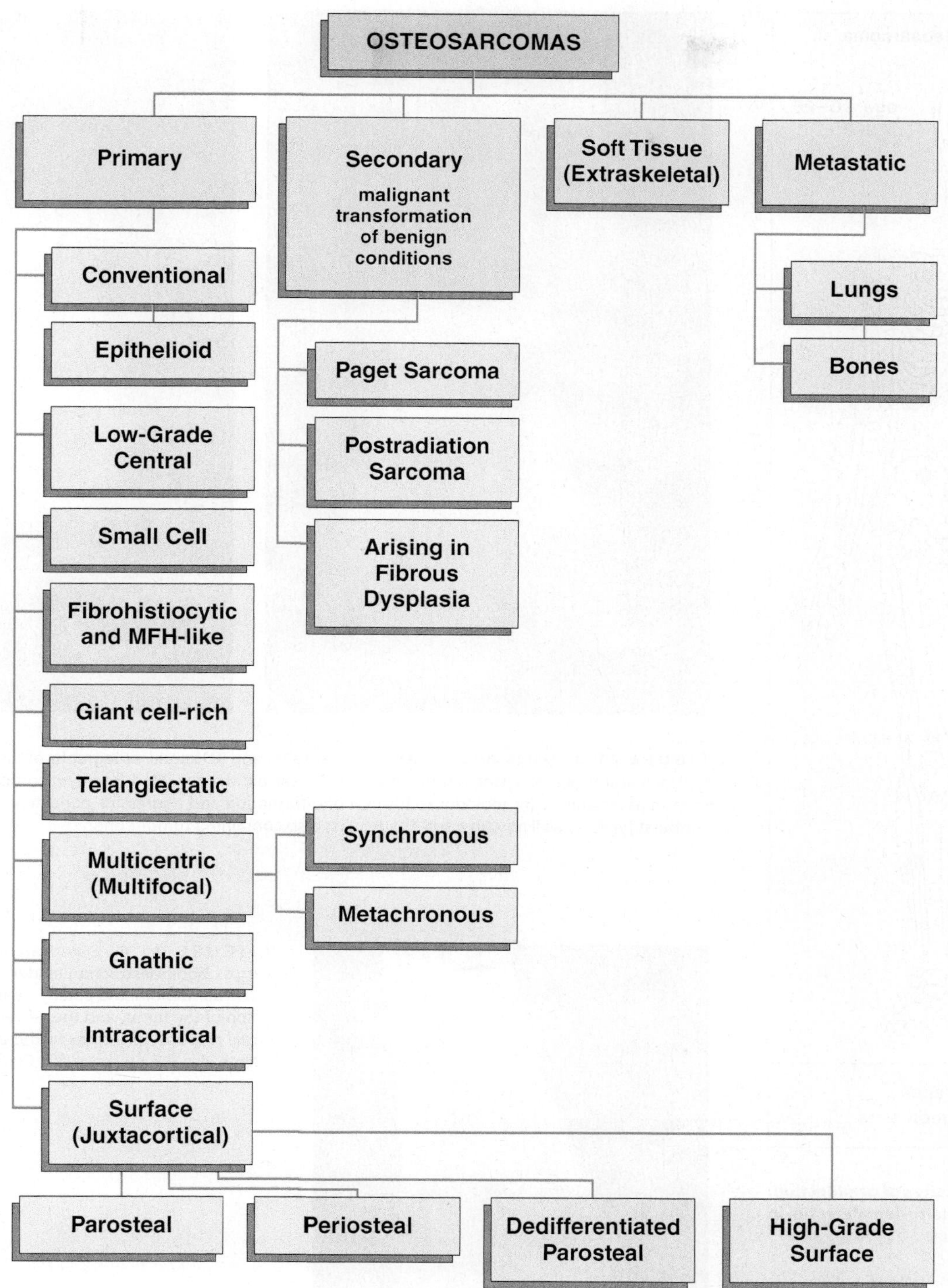

FIGURE 21.1 Classification of the types of osteosarcoma.

TABLE 21.1 Histologic Grading of Osteosarcoma

Grade	Histologic Features	Grade	Histologic Features
1	Cellularity: slightly increased Cytologic atypia: minimal to slight Mitotic activity: low Osteoid matrix: regular	3	Cellularity: increased Cytologic atypia: moderate to marked Mitotic activity: moderate to high Osteoid matrix: irregular
2	Cellularity: moderate Cytologic atypia: mild to moderate Mitotic activity: low to moderate Osteoid matrix: regular	4	Cellularity: markedly increased Cytologic atypia: markedly pleomorphic cells Mitotic activity: high Osteoid matrix: irregular, abundant

According to Unni KK, Dahlin DC. Grading of bone tumors. *Semin Diagn Pathol* 1984;1:165–172.

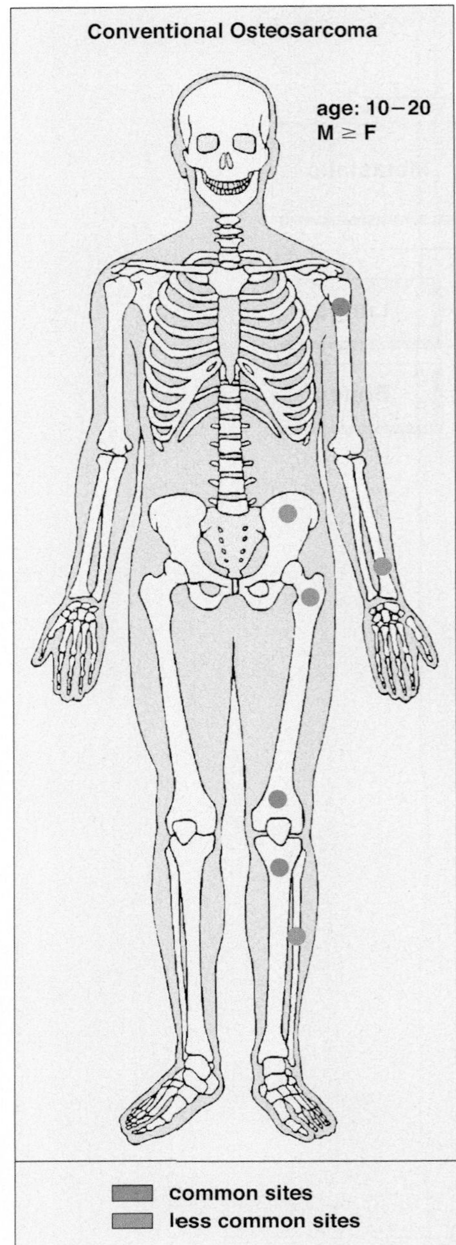

FIGURE 21.2 Skeletal sites of predilection, peak age range, and male-to-female ratio in conventional osteosarcoma.

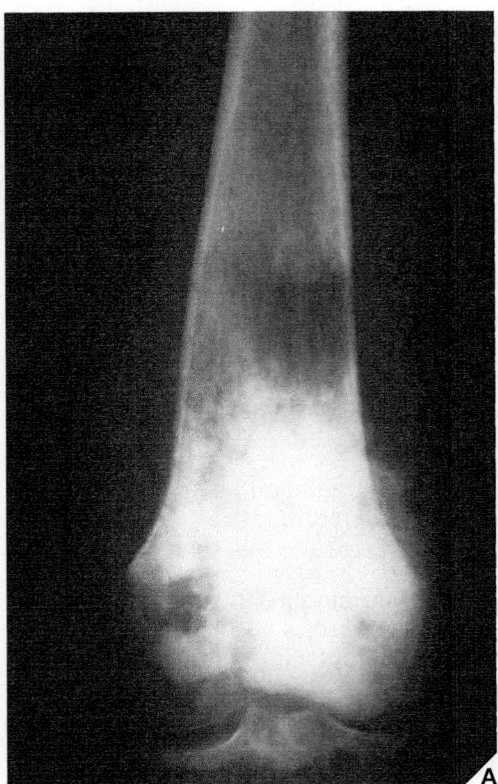

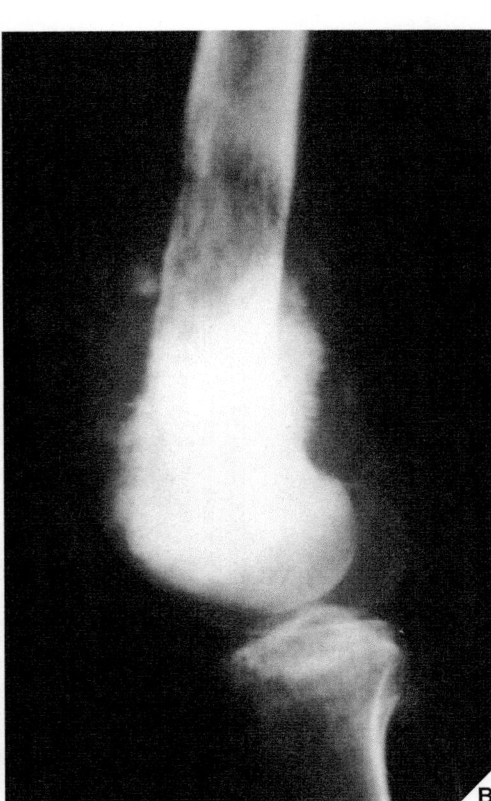

FIGURE 21.3 Osteosarcoma. **(A)** Anteroposterior and **(B)** lateral radiographs of the left knee demonstrate the typical features of this tumor in the femur of a 19-year-old woman. Medullary and cortical bone destruction can be seen in association with radiodense tumor-bone formation and aggressive periosteal response of the velvet and sunburst types as well as with a soft-tissue mass also containing tumor bone.

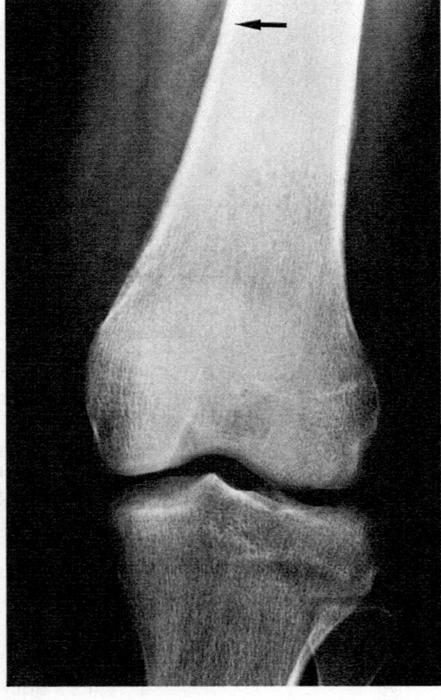

FIGURE 21.4 Osteosarcoma. Although there is no gross bone destruction evident in the distal femur of this 16-year-old girl, the patchy densities in the medullary portion of the femur and the velvet appearance of the periosteal response are clues to the diagnosis of osteosarcoma. Note also the presence of a Codman triangle *(arrow)*.

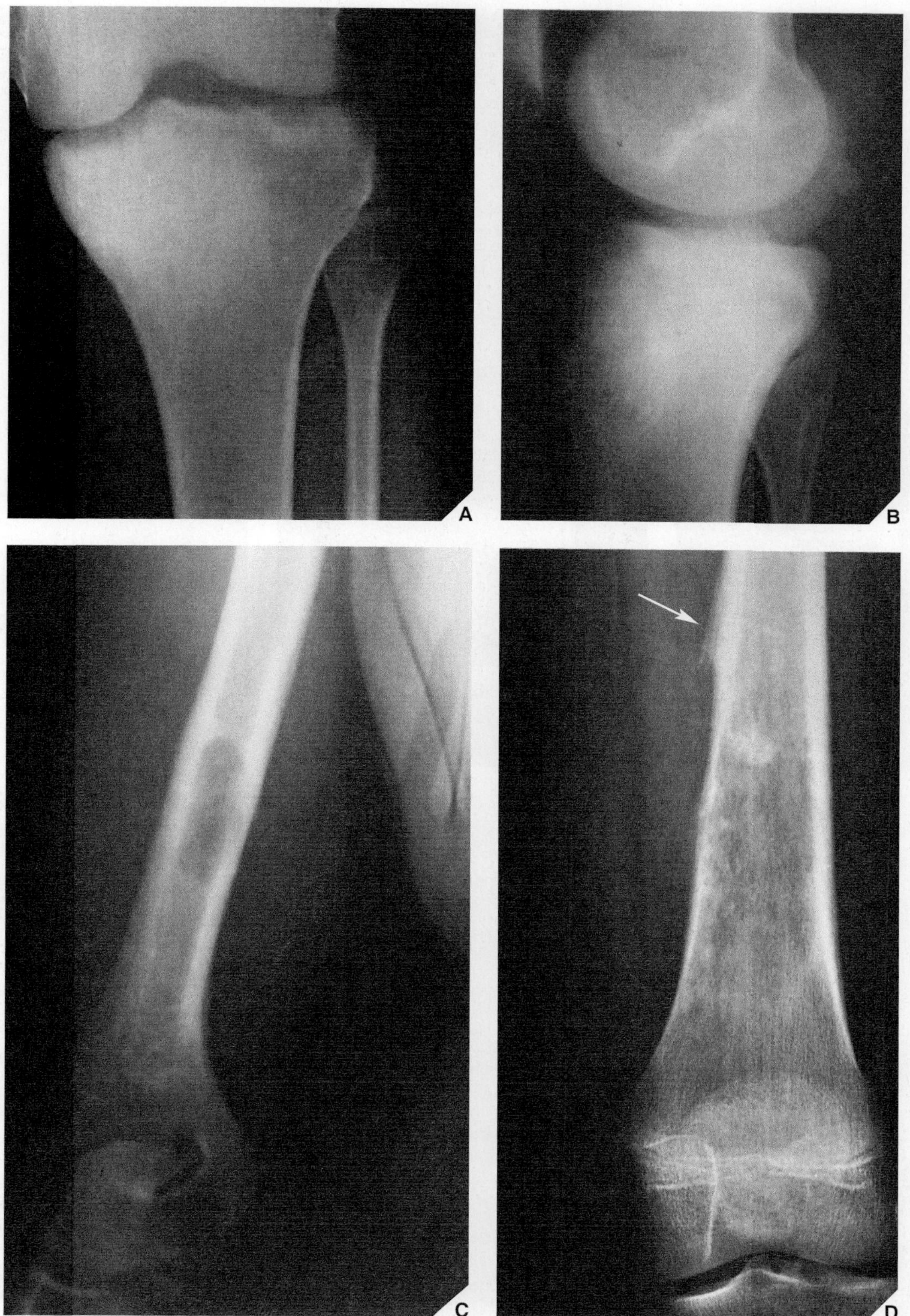

FIGURE 21.5 Various presentations of a conventional osteosarcoma. **(A)** Anteroposterior and **(B)** lateral radiographs of the left knee show sclerotic variant in the proximal tibia. **(C)** Anteroposterior radiograph shows a lytic variant in the distal humerus, which proved to be a fibroblastic osteosarcoma. **(D)** A radiograph of the distal femur shows a mixed variant: Areas of bone formation are present within a destructive lytic lesion. Note a Codman triangle in the upper part of the tumor *(arrow)*.

indistinct, with a wide zone of transition. The type of bone destruction is either moth-eaten or permeative and only rarely geographic.

The most common types of periosteal response encountered with osteosarcoma are the "sunburst" type and a Codman triangle; the lamellated (onionskin) type of reaction is less frequently seen (Fig. 21.6). Scintigraphy invariably shows increased uptake of the radiopharmaceutical tracer by the tumor (Fig. 21.7). It is also an effective modality to demonstrate the "skipped" lesions (Fig. 21.8). In the past, computed tomography (CT) was an indispensable technique for evaluating osteosarcomas (Figs. 21.9 and 21.10). This was particularly important if a limb-salvage procedure was contemplated because extension of the tumor into the medullary cavity is crucial information for effective surgical planning (see Fig. 16.11). Currently, magnetic resonance imaging (MRI) has become a modality of choice for evaluating these tumors, particularly for intraosseous tumor extension and soft-tissue involvement. On T1-weighted images, the solid nonmineralized parts of osteosarcoma generally present as areas of low-to-intermediate signal intensity. On T2-weighted images, the tumor demonstrates a high signal intensity. MRI can easily demonstrate transphyseal

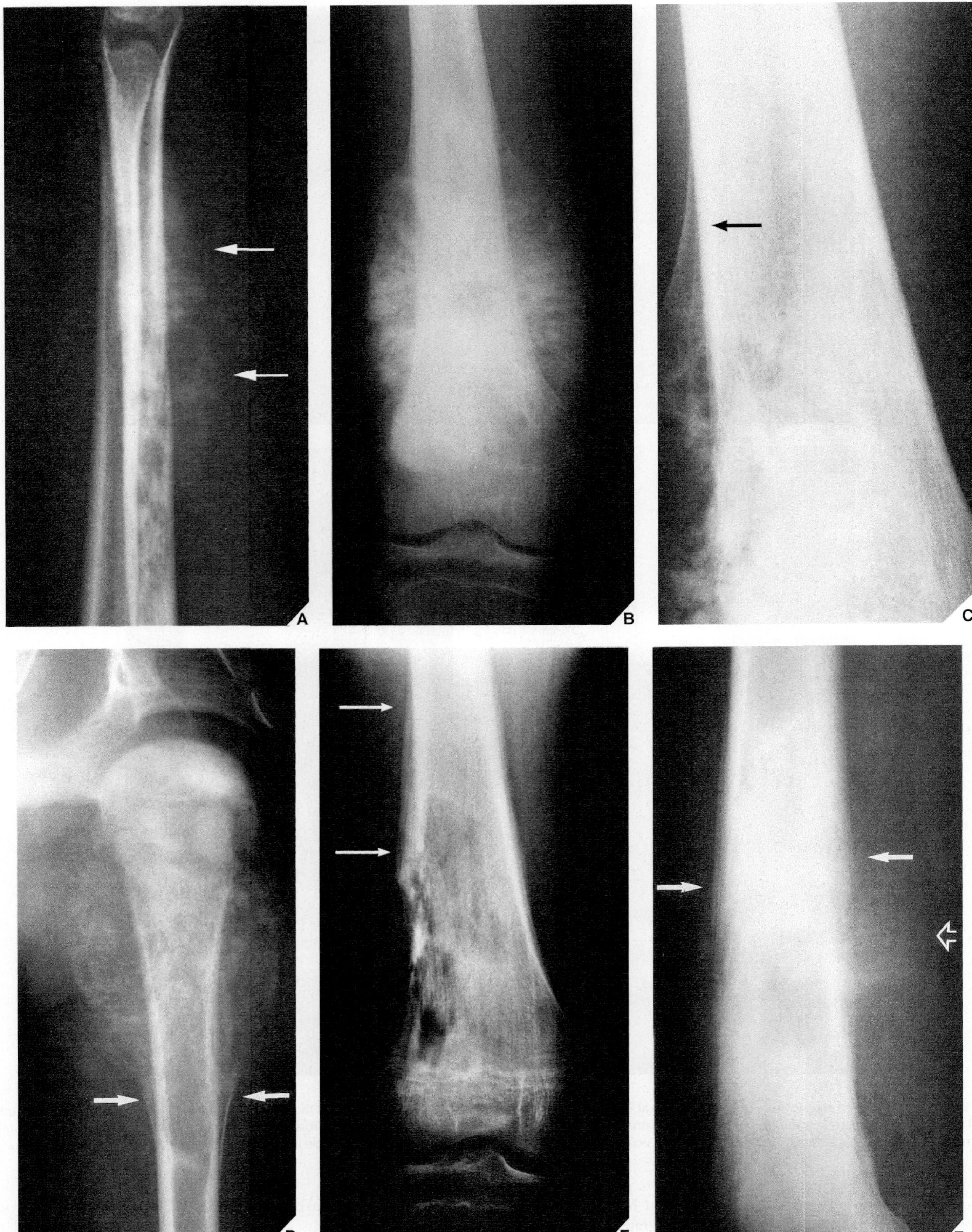

FIGURE 21.6 Periosteal reaction in osteosarcoma. Three types of periosteal reaction most commonly accompany osteosarcoma. **(A)** The sunburst or perpendicular type of periosteal reaction *(arrows)* is seen here on the lateral radiograph of the forearm in an 18-year-old woman with tumor in the radius and **(B)** on the anteroposterior radiograph of the distal femur in a 20-year-old man. **(C)** Codman triangle *(arrow)* may also be encountered, as seen here in a 15-year-old girl with tumor in the distal femur and **(D)** in an 11-year-old boy with tumor in the proximal humerus *(arrows)*. **(E)** The onion skin or lamellated type of periosteal response *(arrows)* is apparent in a 16-year-old girl with tumor in the distal femur. **(F)** Combination of lamellated *(arrows)* and sunburst *(open arrow)* periosteal reaction is present in a 16-year-old girl with osteosarcoma of the femur. (**B**, Reprinted with permission from Greenspan A, Remagen W. *Differential diagnosis of tumors and tumor-like lesions of bones and joints*. Philadelphia: Lippincott-Raven Publishers; 1998.)

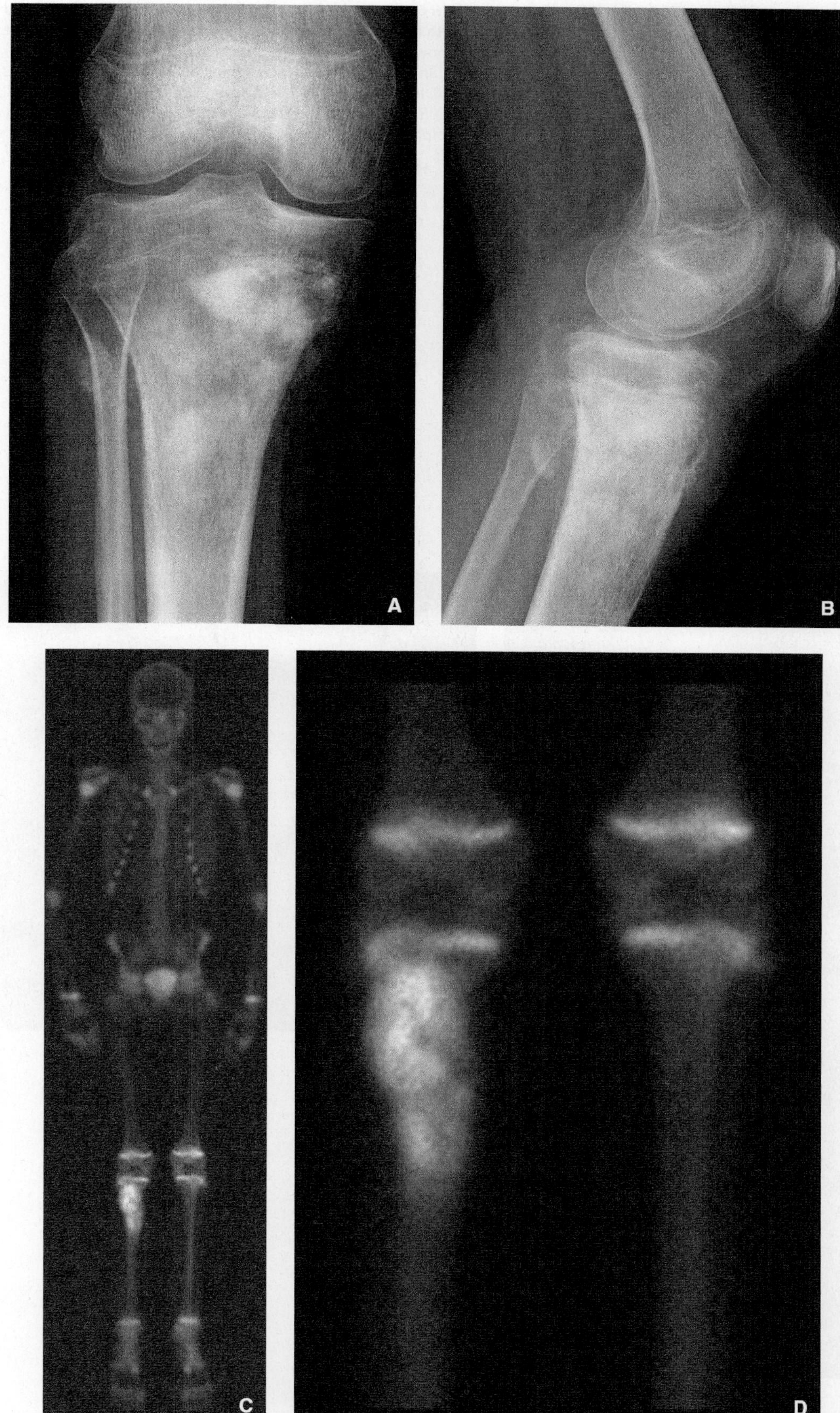

FIGURE 21.7 Scintigraphy of osteosarcoma. **(A)** Anteroposterior and **(B)** lateral radiographs of the right knee of a 13-year-old girl show a sclerotic tumor affecting the metaphysis and proximal diaphysis of the tibia. **(C)** A total-body technetium radionuclide bone scan and **(D)** coned-down scintigraphic images of the knees show significantly increased uptake of the radiopharmaceutical tracer by the tumor located in the right proximal tibia. (Reprinted with permission from Greenspan A, Borys D. *Radiology and pathology correlation of bone tumors,* 1st ed. Philadelphia: Wolters Kluwer, 2016:52–53.)

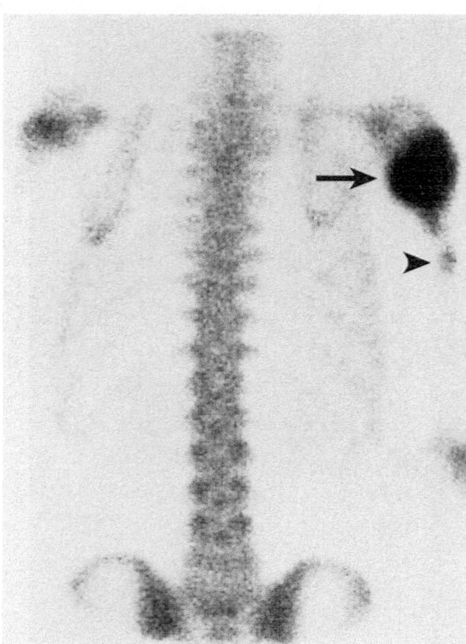

FIGURE 21.8 Scintigraphy of osteosarcoma. In a 7-year-old boy with a lesion in the proximal left humerus, radionuclide bone scan shows markedly increased uptake of the tracer by the tumor *(arrow)*. In addition, a small focus of activity *(arrowhead)* represents a "skip" lesion. (Reprinted with permission from Greenspan A, Borys D. *Radiology and pathology correlation of bone tumors,* 1st ed. Philadelphia: Wolters Kluwer, 2016:53.)

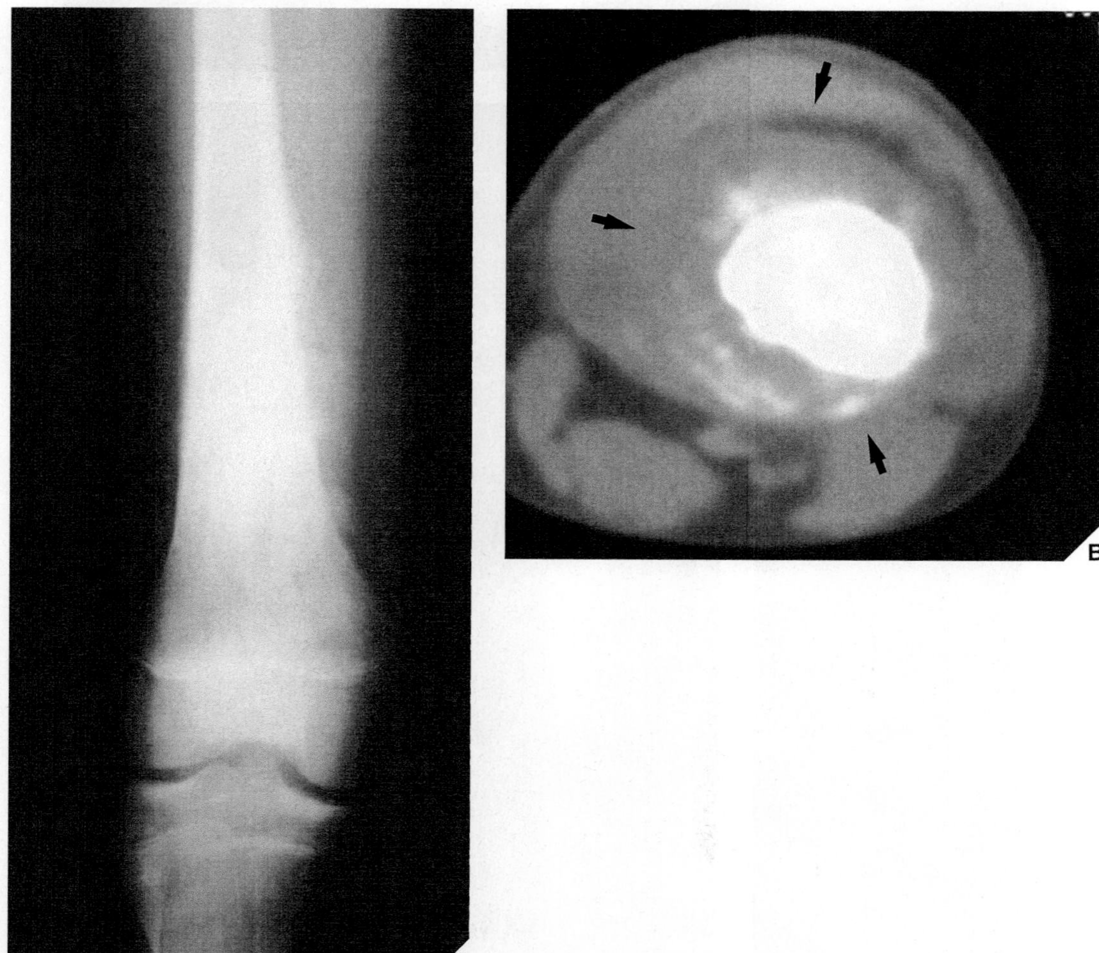

FIGURE 21.9 CT of osteosarcoma. **(A)** Conventional anteroposterior radiograph reveals a destructive lesion with poorly defined borders extending from the metaphysis of the femur into the diaphysis. Note the aggressive periosteal reaction and the formation of tumor bone. These features are sufficient for making a diagnosis of osteosarcoma in this 14-year-old boy. **(B)** Axial CT section demonstrates the extension of tumor into the soft tissues *(arrows)*. The tumor bone in the medullary portion of the bone and in the soft-tissue mass is seen to better advantage.

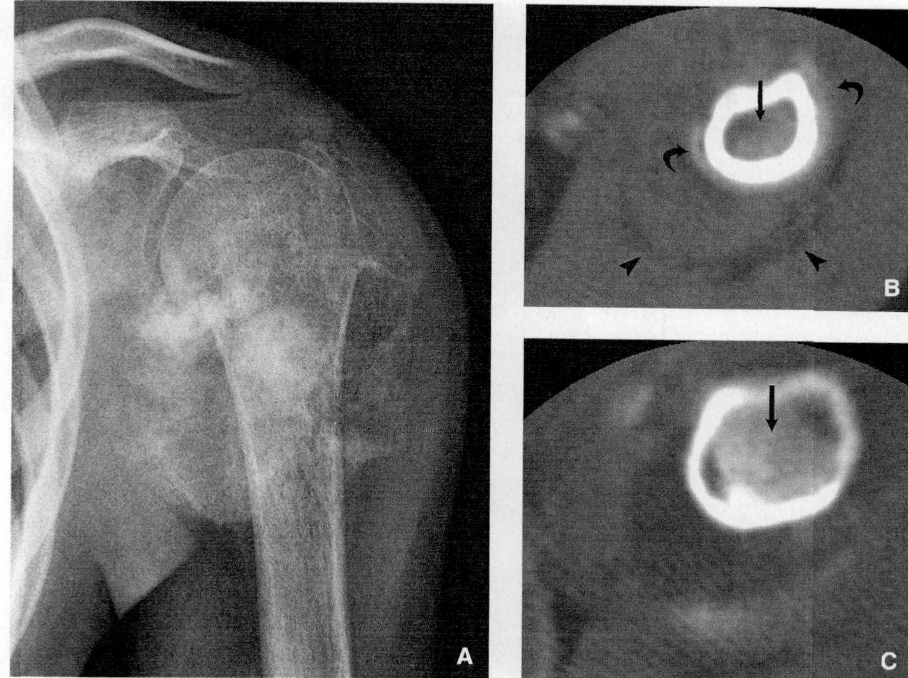

FIGURE 21.10 CT of osteosarcoma. **(A)** Anteroposterior radiograph of the left shoulder shows bone-forming tumor affecting the proximal humerus. Observe associated aggressive periosteal reaction and a soft-tissue mass. **(B,C)** Two CT axial sections show high-attenuation tumor replacing the bone marrow *(arrows)*, periosteal reaction *(curved arrows)*, and soft-tissue mass *(arrowheads)*. (Reprinted with permission from Greenspan A, Borys D. *Radiology and pathology correlation of bone tumors,* 1st ed. Philadelphia: Wolters Kluwer, 2016.)

and transarticular extension of the tumor. This is an important determination for surgical and radiotherapy planning. Osteosclerotic tumors demonstrate low signal intensity on all imaging sequences (Figs. 21.11 to 21.17). MRI may also effectively demonstrate peritumoral edema. This feature displays an intermediate intensity signal on T1-weighted and a high intensity on T2 weighting surrounding the tumor. CT and MRI are also essential in monitoring the results of treatment.

Pathology

Gross specimen shows heterogenous fleshy mass with ossified and nonossified components, and occasionally foci of cartilage (Fig. 21.18). Histopathology reveals tumor cells with prominent atypia and pleomorphism and most often eosinophilic cytoplasm producing osteoid or tumor bone. The cells may also produce varying amounts of cartilage and fibrous tissue. Based on the dominant histologic features, conventional osteosarcoma can be subdivided into three histologic subtypes: osteoblastic (50%), chondroblastic (25%), and fibroblastic (25%). In osteoblastic subtype, bone and/or osteoid is the predominant matrix. In chondroblastic subtype, chondroid matrix is predominant. The fibroblastic subtype, high-grade spindle-cell malignancy with sometimes minimal amount of osseous matrix with or without cartilage is present. The last subtype may occasionally mimic fibrosarcoma or malignant fibrous histiocytoma (MFH), which may be difficult to distinguish on small biopsy samples. At times, the tumor cells may be so undifferentiated that on a purely cytologic basis it is difficult to tell whether they are sarcomatous or epithelial. This variant of conventional osteosarcoma is sometimes referred to as *epithelioid osteosarcoma*. The diagnosis usually becomes evident from the patient's age, the production of obvious tumor matrix, and a radiographic appearance typical of osteosarcoma.

Complications and Treatment

The most frequent complications of conventional osteosarcoma are pathologic fracture and the development of pulmonary (most common) or intraosseous (less common) metastases.

If a limb-salvage procedure is feasible, a course of multidrug chemotherapy is used, followed by wide resection of the bone and insertion of an endoprosthesis (Fig. 21.19). Less frequently, amputation is performed, followed by chemotherapy. Currently, the 5-year survival rate after adequate therapy exceeds 50%.

Low-Grade Central Osteosarcoma

This rare form of osteosarcoma (1% of all osteosarcomas) usually occurs in patients older than those presenting with conventional osteosarcoma (the peak incidence is in the second to third decades of life), although the sites of predilection are similar. Radiographically, it may be indistinguishable from conventional osteosarcoma, but it grows more slowly and has a better prognosis. At times, its radiographic presentation clearly mimics fibrous dysplasia (Fig. 21.20) or another benign lesion (Fig. 21.21). Minor genetic alterations with gains at 13q13-14, 12p, and 6p21 have been reported, resulting in overexpression of *CDK4* and *MDM2* and amplification of *SAS* (*s*arcoma-*a*mplified *s*equence). Histologic examination typically reveals hypocellular-to-moderately cellular fibroblastic stroma with variable amounts of osteoid production. The spindle cells are prominent, but there is paucity of cellular atypia and mitotic figures. Small scattered foci of cartilage and multinucleated giant cells may occasionally be seen.

Telangiectatic Osteosarcoma

A very aggressive type of osteosarcoma, the telangiectatic variant, also called *hemorrhagic osteosarcoma* by Campanacci et al., is twice as common in males than in females and is seen predominantly in patients in their second and third decades of life. It is rare, comprising approximately 3% of all malignant bone tumors. It is characterized by a high degree of vascularity and large cystic spaces filled with blood, which account for its atypical imaging presentation. Most of these tumors arise in the femur and tibia. On radiography, telangiectatic osteosarcoma most commonly presents as an osteolytic destructive lesion with or without matrix mineralization, and with an almost complete absence of sclerotic changes; a soft-tissue mass may also be present (Figs. 21.22 to 21.24). An aggressive periosteal reaction (lamellar, sunburst, or Codman triangle) is present in most patients, reflecting the malignant nature of this tumor, and a pathologic fracture is not uncommon in the case of large lesions. On MRI, telangiectatic osteosarcoma often exhibits areas of high signal intensity on T1-weighted sequences, owing to the presence of methemoglobin. On T2 weighting, signal intensity is commonly heterogeneous (Fig. 21.25). Fluid–fluid levels can occasionally be seen (Fig. 21.26), similar to ones seen in aneurysmal bone cyst.

On gross pathologic examination, the tumor resembles a "bag of blood" and is characterized by blood-filled spaces, necrosis, and hemorrhage (Fig. 21.27). Histologically, it is composed of loculated blood-filled

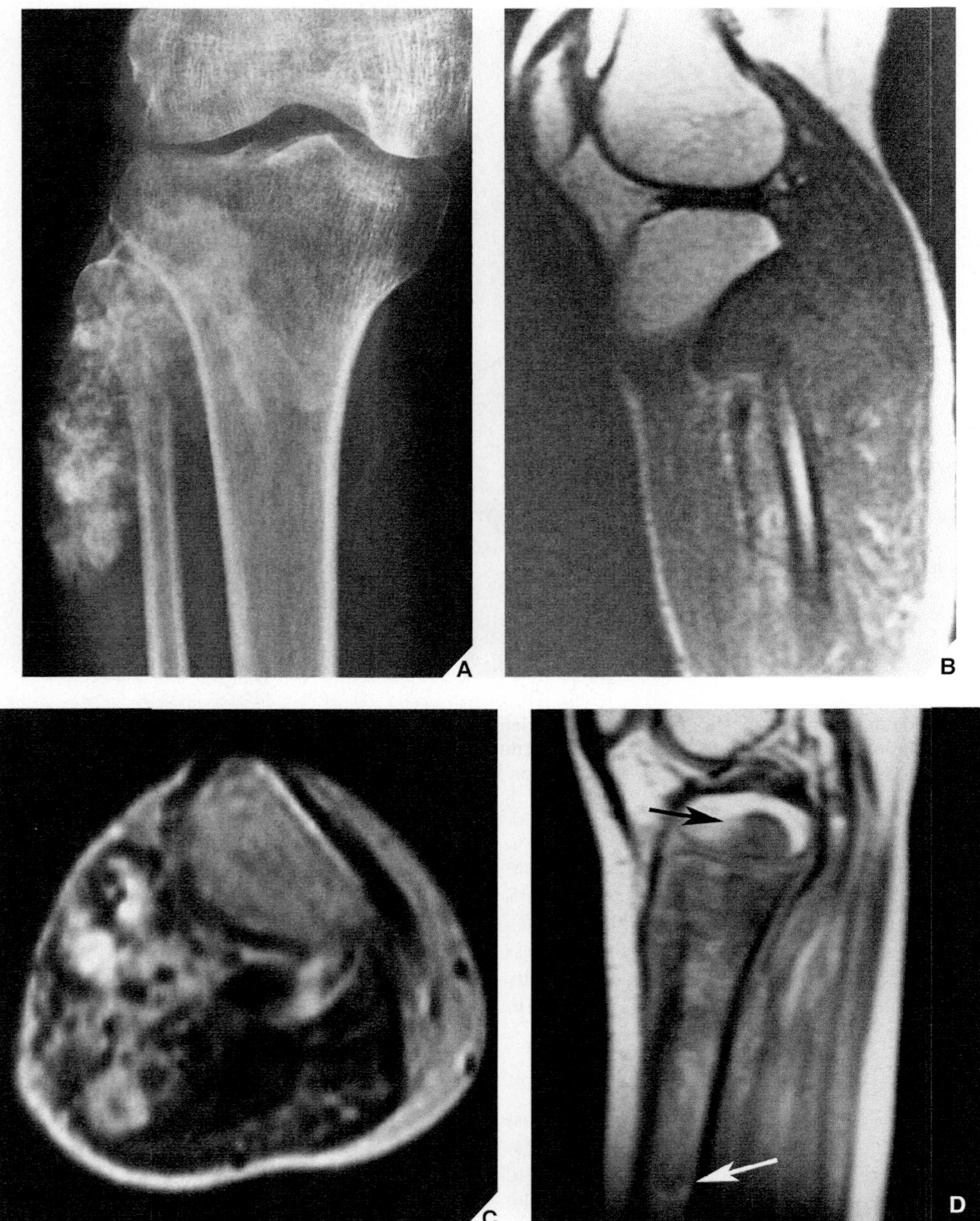

FIGURE 21.11 MRI of osteosarcoma. **(A)** Conventional radiograph demonstrates involvement of the head of the fibula and extensive soft-tissue infiltration with significant tumor-bone formation in a 20-year-old man. **(B)** Sagittal spin echo [SE] T1-weighted MR image shows that the tumor displays a predominantly intermediate signal, blending with the muscular structures. **(C)** On axial T2-weighted image, the tumor shows high signal intensity in both its intramedullary component and its soft-tissue extension. The foci of tumor-bone formation are imaged as areas of low signal intensity. **(D)** Sagittal T1-weighted image of the tibia in another patient with osteosarcoma shows the clear delineation of the distal intramedullary extension of the tumor *(white arrow)* and the proximal transphyseal extension of the tumor into the proximal tibial epiphysis *(black arrow)*.

spaces, separated by thin cellular septa partially lined by malignant cells producing sparse osteoid tissue. Tumor cells are hyperchromatic and pleomorphic with high mitotic activity, including atypical mitoses. It resembles an aneurysmal bone cyst, both radiologically and pathologically.

Giant Cell–Rich Osteosarcoma

This is a rare variant of osteosarcoma, which histologically appears as an undifferentiated sarcoma with an overabundance of giant cells (osteoclasts) and a paucity of tumor osteoid and tumor bone. It comprises approximately 3% of all osteosarcomas and histologically is related to telangiectatic osteosarcoma and MFH-like osteosarcoma. Many of the typical imaging features of conventional osteosarcoma are not present, periosteal reaction is either scant or absent, and the soft-tissue mass is small. This presentation may sometimes create the difficulties in differentiation of giant cell–rich osteosarcoma even from benign lesions. In most cases, however, on the radiographs, the lytic lesion exhibits poorly defined borders, and MRI characteristics confirm malignancy (Fig. 21.28). The common location of this tumor is the metaphysis or diaphysis of a long bone, usually the femur and tibia. Histologically, because of abundance of giant cells, and because tumor osteoid is usually scant and difficult to identify, giant cell–rich osteosarcoma bears striking resemblance to giant cell tumor.

Small Cell Osteosarcoma

Described by Sim and associates, small cell osteosarcoma with preferential sites of distal femur, proximal humerus, and proximal tibia, usually occurs as a radiolucent lesion with permeative borders and a large soft-tissue mass. Its radiographic appearance thus mimics that of a round cell bone sarcoma. These lesions usually exhibit small round cells in many histologic fields, much like Ewing sarcoma. Cytogenetic study for t(11,22) is the best diagnostic tool, which is negative in small cell osteosarcoma. In addition, the presence of spindled tumor cells, as well as the focal production of osteoid or bone, helps to make a histologic diagnosis of osteosarcoma.

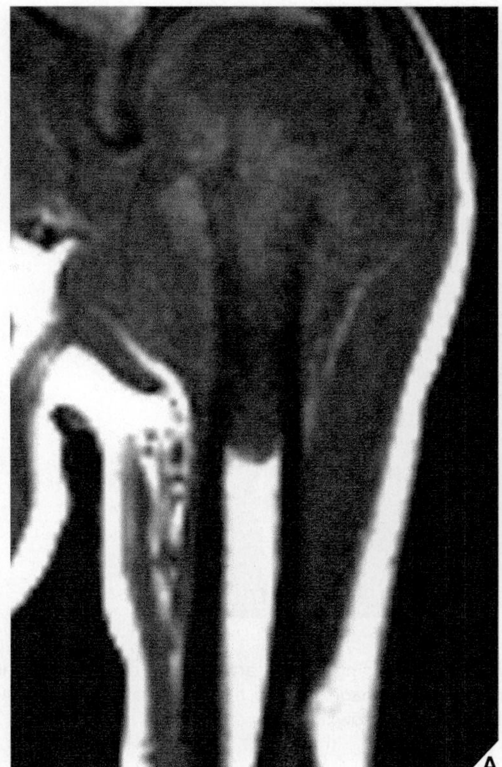

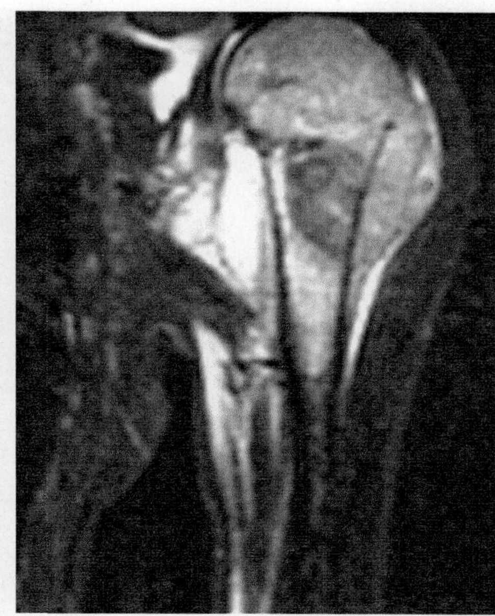

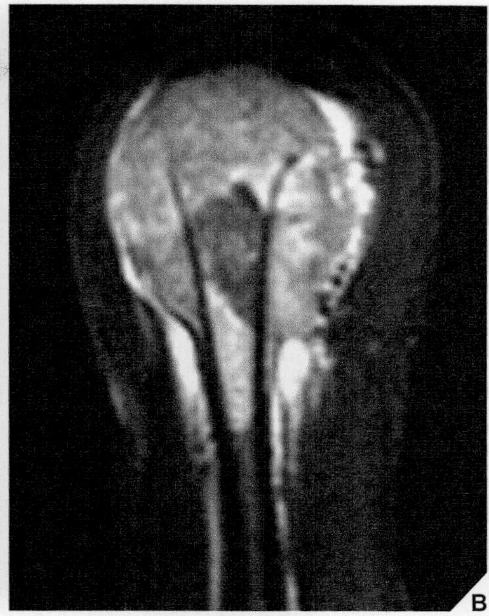

FIGURE 21.12 MRI of osteosarcoma. **(A)** Coronal T1-weighted MR image of the left proximal humerus of a 14-year-old boy shows an intermediate–signal to low–signal intensity tumor destroying the cortex and extending into the soft tissues. **(B)** Coronal and sagittal T2-weighted fat-suppressed MR images show that the tumor exhibits heterogeneous but mostly high signal. The areas of tumor-bone formation are of low signal intensity.

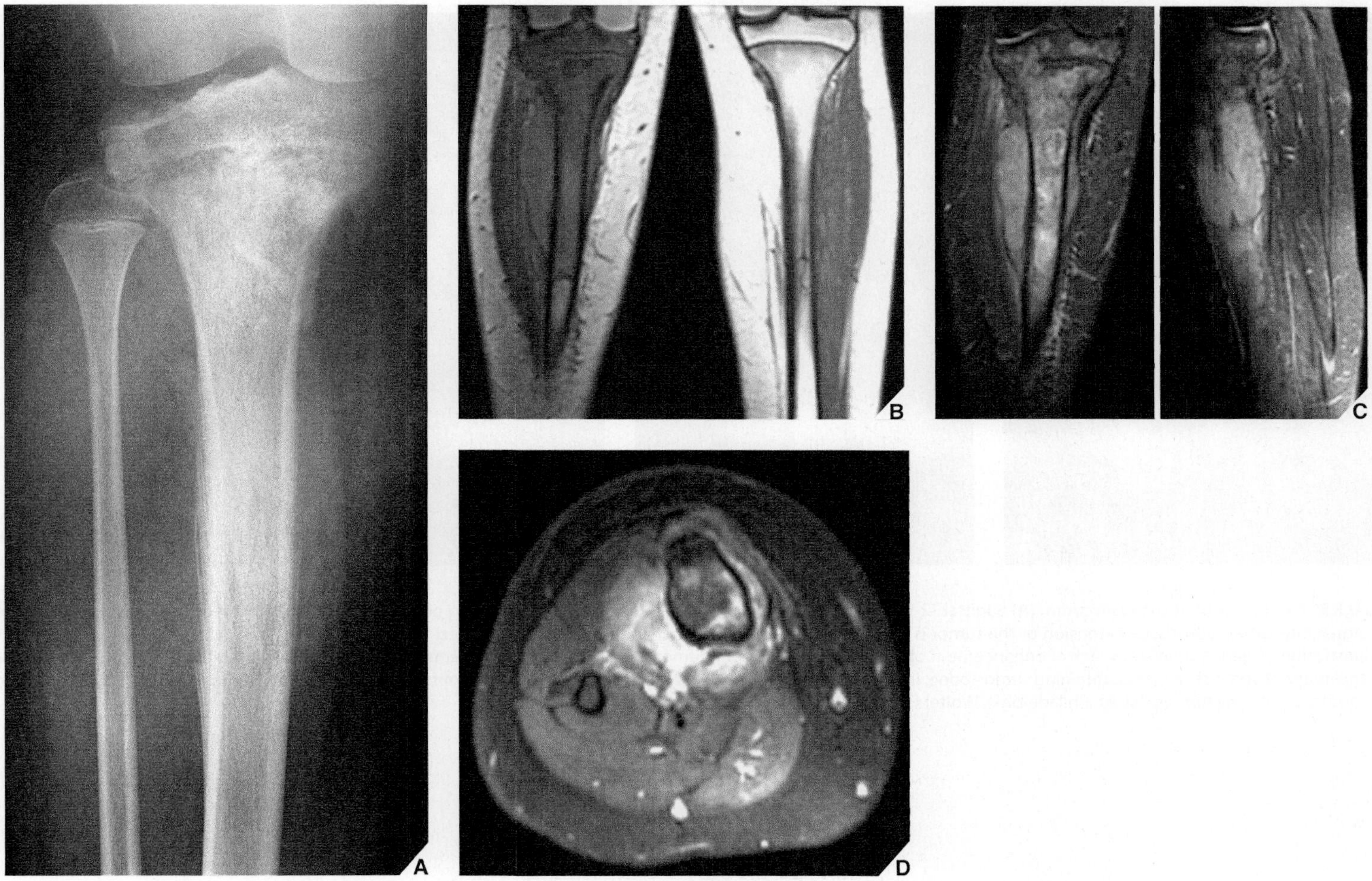

FIGURE 21.13 MRI of osteosarcoma. **(A)** Anteroposterior radiograph of the right leg of an 11-year-old girl shows an aggressive lesion in the tibial diaphysis and metaphysis, extending to the growth plate. Present is an interrupted periosteal reaction and a soft-tissue mass. **(B)** Coronal T1-weighted MR image shows both the osseous tumor and a soft-tissue mass to be of intermediate signal intensity. **(C)** Coronal and sagittal inversion recovery (IR) MR images show heterogeneous character of the tumor that exhibits foci of high signal. **(D)** Axial T1-weighted fat-suppressed MR image obtained after intravenous administration of gadolinium shows marked enhancement of the soft-tissue mass.

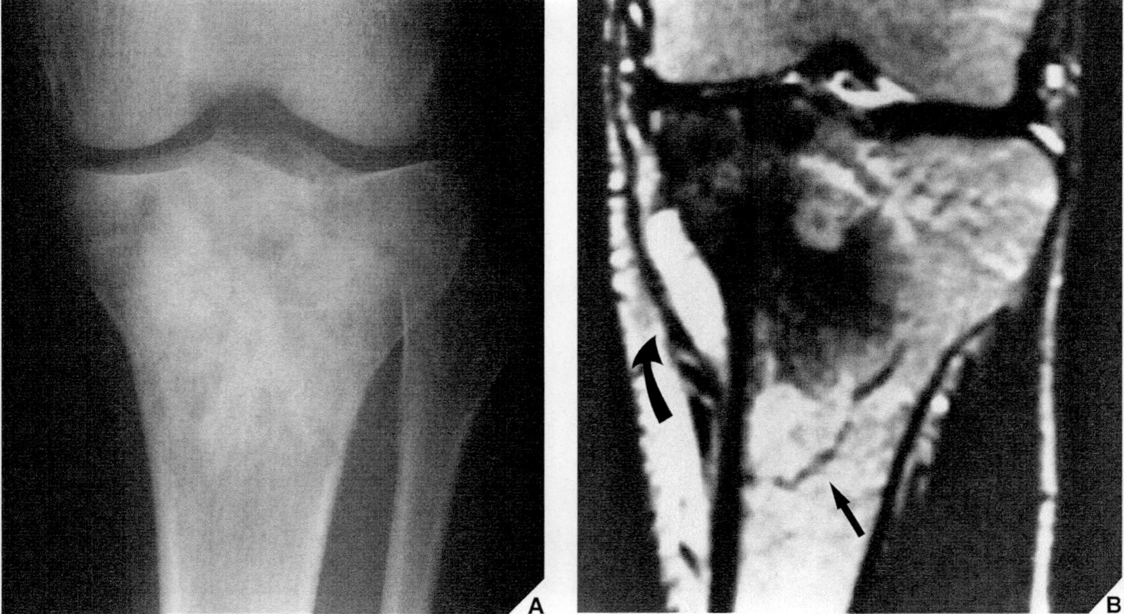

FIGURE 21.14 MRI of osteosarcoma. **(A)** Anteroposterior radiograph demonstrates a predominantly sclerotic tumor extending into the articular end of the left tibia in this 17-year-old boy. **(B)** The sclerotic parts of the lesion display low signal intensity on coronal spin echo (SE) T2-weighted MR image. Distally, a nonmineralized part of the tumor shows high signal intensity *(arrow)*. Likewise, the soft-tissue extension of the lesion displays high signal intensity *(curved arrow)*.

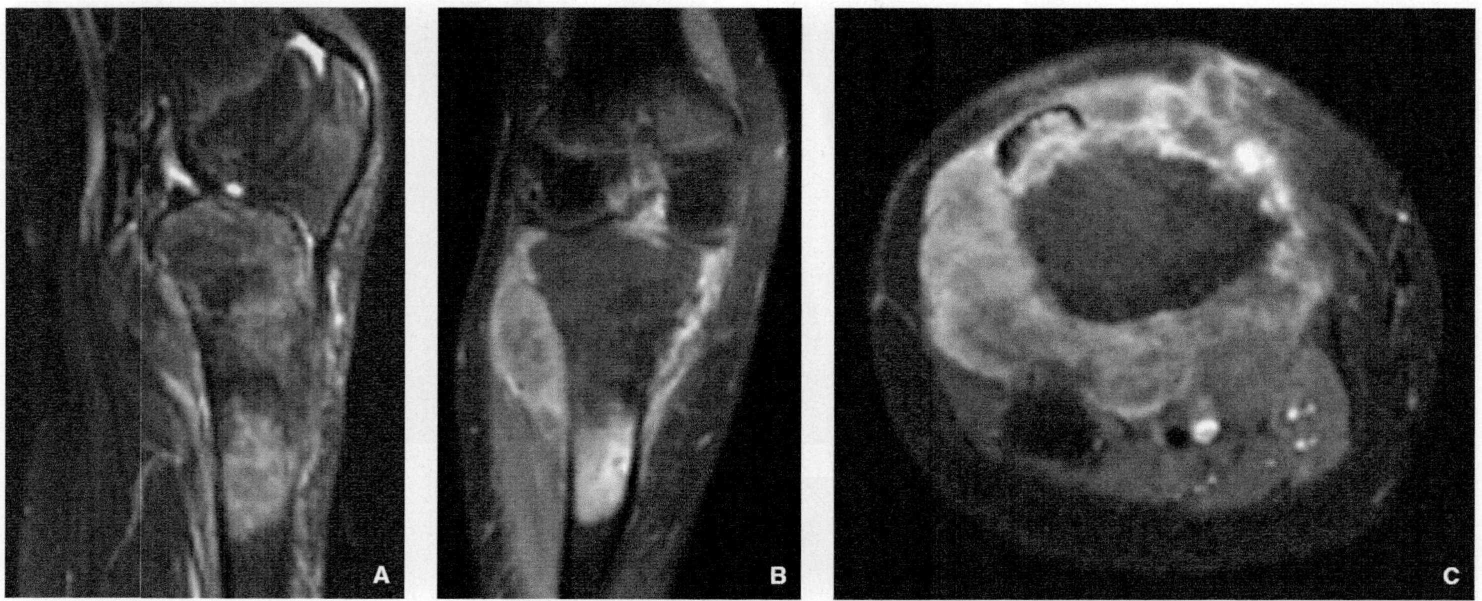

FIGURE 21.15 MRI of osteosarcoma. **(A)** Sagittal T2-weighted MR image of the knee shows a tumor affecting proximal tibia, exhibiting heterogenous mixed high and low signal intensities. Soft-tissue extension of the tumor is not well depicted. **(B)** Coronal and **(C)** axial T1-weighted fat-suppressed MR images obtained after intravenous administration of gadolinium show lack of enhancement of the sclerotic part of the tumor, but significant enhancement of the osteolytic distal part of the tumor. Note also enhancement of soft-tissue mass containing tumor-bone, imaged as low–signal intensity foci. (Reprinted with permission from Greenspan A, Borys D. *Radiology and pathology correlation of bone tumors,* 1st ed. Philadelphia: Wolters Kluwer, 2016:54.)

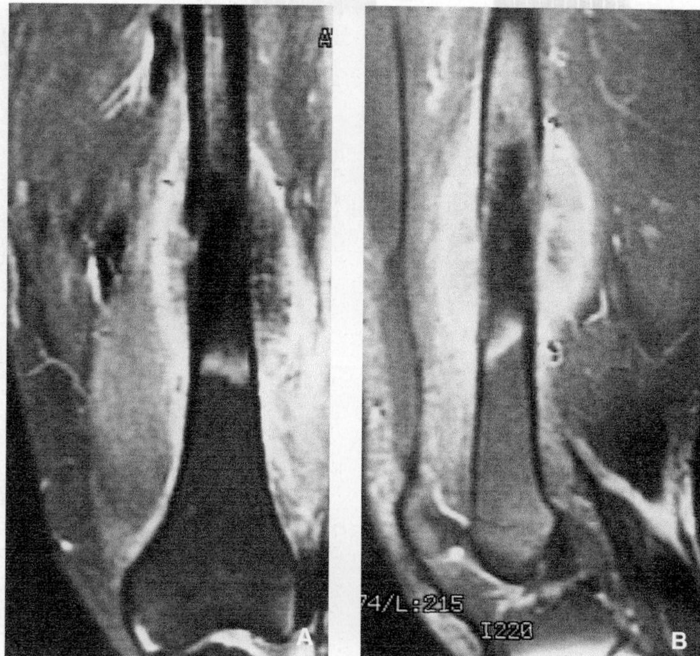

FIGURE 21.16 MRI of osteosarcoma. **(A)** Coronal and **(B)** sagittal T1-weighted fat-suppressed MR images of the distal femur of a 29-year-old man, obtained after intravenous administration of gadolinium, show tumor enhancement in the medullary portion of the femur and in the soft-tissue mass. Heavy mineralized portion of the tumor does not enhance and remains of low signal intensity. (Reprinted with permission from Greenspan A, Borys D. *Radiology and pathology correlation of bone tumors,* 1st ed. Philadelphia: Wolters Kluwer, 2016:55.)

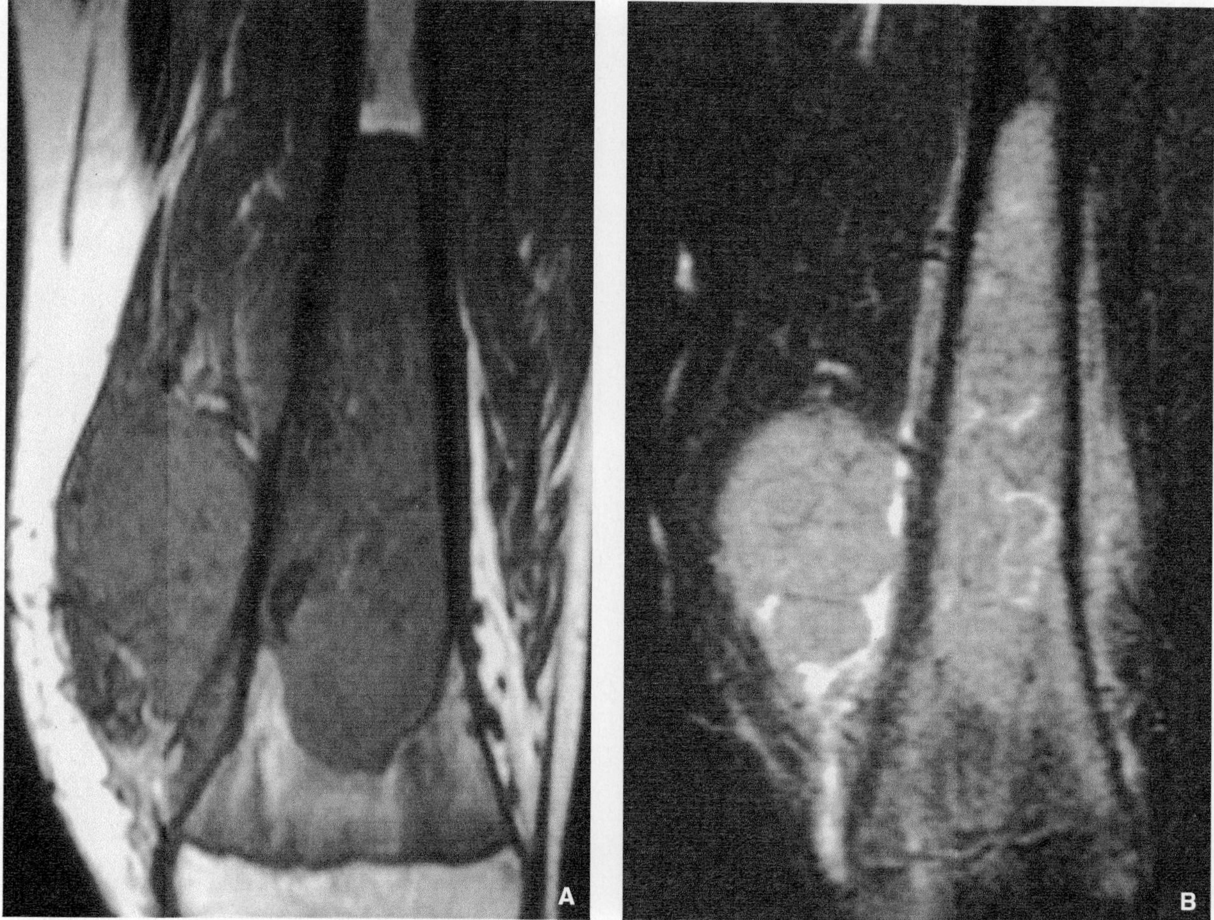

FIGURE 21.17 MRI of osteosarcoma. **(A)** Coronal T1-weighted MR image of the distal femur of a 14-year-old boy diagnosed with chondroblastic type of osteosarcoma shows a large intermediate–signal to low–signal intensity tumor in the bone marrow associated with a soft-tissue mass. **(B)** After intravenous administration of gadolinium, there is diffuse enhancement of both intramedullary tumor and soft-tissue mass. (Reprinted with permission from Greenspan A, Borys D. *Radiology and pathology correlation of bone tumors,* 1st ed. Philadelphia: Wolters Kluwer, 2016:55.)

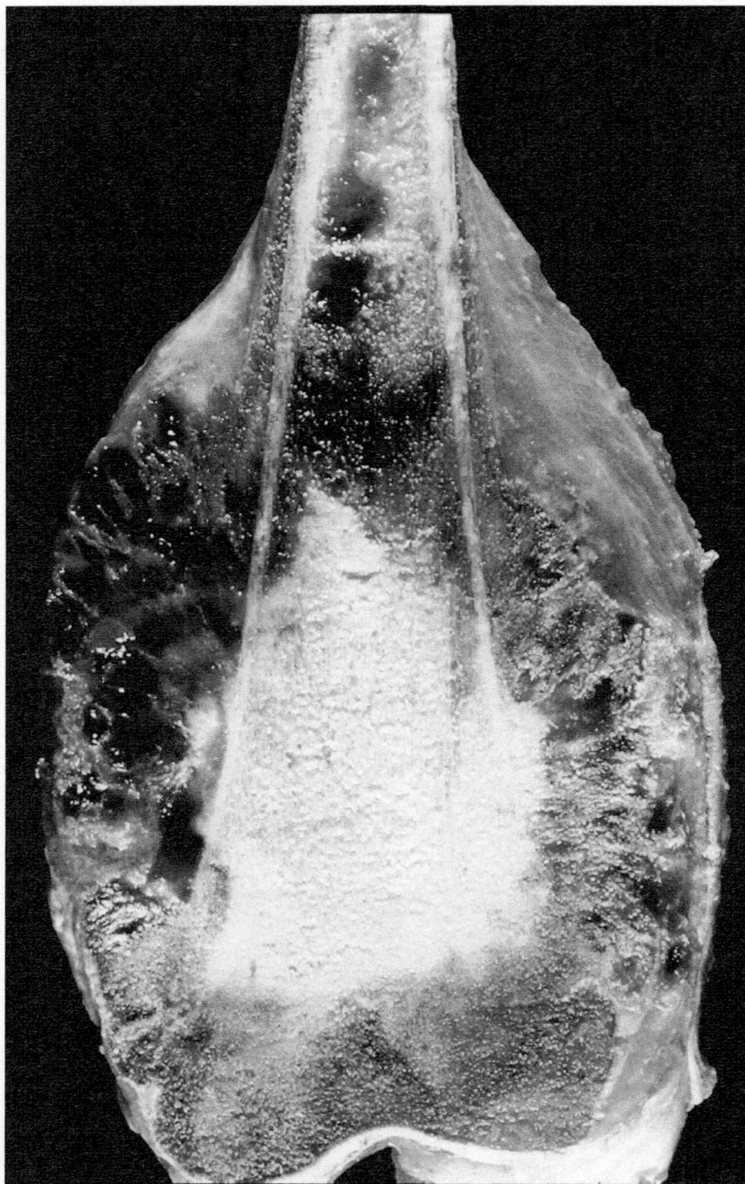

FIGURE 21.18 Pathology of conventional osteosarcoma. Gross specimen of resected distal femur shows predominantly osteoblastic intramedullary tumor breaking through the cortex and producing tumor-bone matrix in the soft-tissue mass. Areas of hemorrhage are present in the medullary cavity and in the soft-tissue mass.

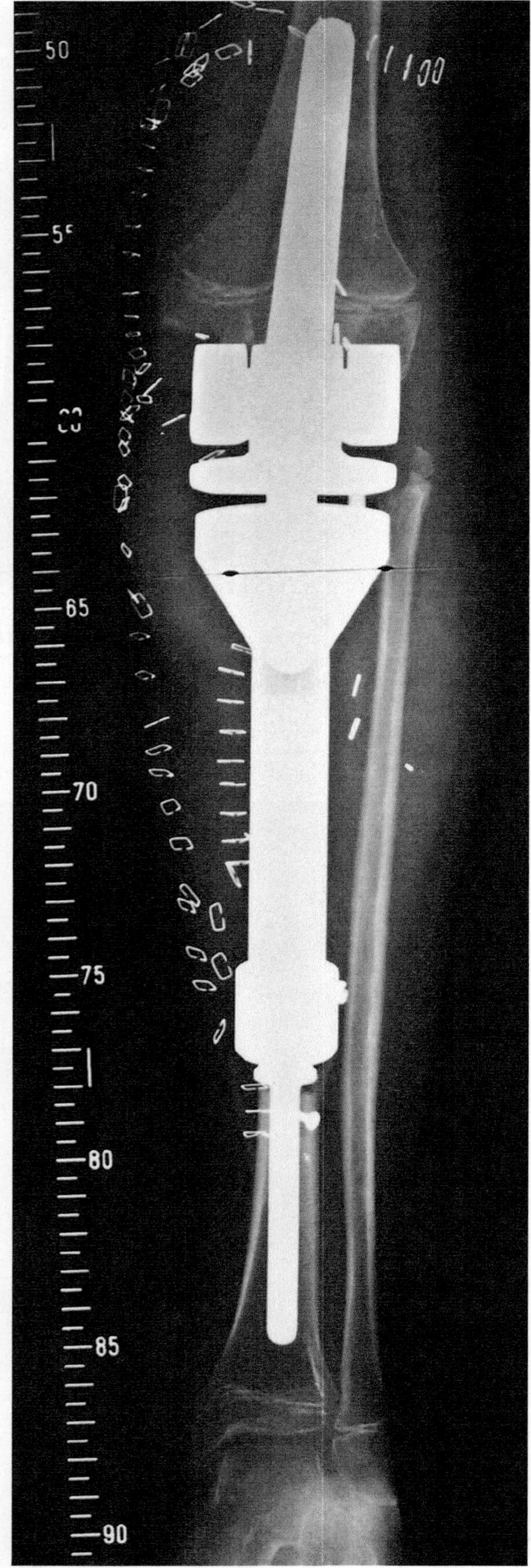

FIGURE 21.19 Treatment of osteosarcoma. An 8-year-old boy underwent a limb-salvage procedure for osteosarcoma in the left tibia. After a full course of chemotherapy, consisting of a combination of methotrexate, doxorubicin hydrochloride, and cisplatin, a wide resection of the proximal tibia was performed, and a LEAP metallic spacer inserted. This expandable prosthesis can be adjusted to maintain limb length with the normal contralateral limb as the child grows. (Courtesy of Michael M. Lewis, MD, Santa Barbara, California.)

Fibrohistiocytic Osteosarcoma

Fibrohistiocytic osteosarcoma, which resembles MFH, has recently been described in the literature. It can sometimes be confused with true MFH of bone because both of these tumors tend to arise at a greater age than conventional osteosarcoma, usually after the third decade. Both tend to involve the articular ends of long bones, and less periosteal reaction is typically present than in conventional osteosarcoma. Although on radiography both of these lesions tend to be radiolucent and thus do resemble giant cell tumor and fibrosarcoma, the MFH-like osteosarcoma usually exhibits areas of bone formation resembling cotton balls or cumulus clouds, whereas MFH does not. When such areas are identified on imaging studies, a diligent search should be made for tumor bone in the resected specimen. Histologically, MFH-like osteosarcoma is characterized by pleomorphic spindle cells and giant cells, many of which have bizarre nuclei. This lesion therefore resembles giant cell-rich osteosarcoma. An inflammatory background is not unusual, and the storiform or spiral nebular arrangement, characteristic of MFH, although sometimes a dominant feature, may be less prominent or may be replaced by areas of large pleomorphic

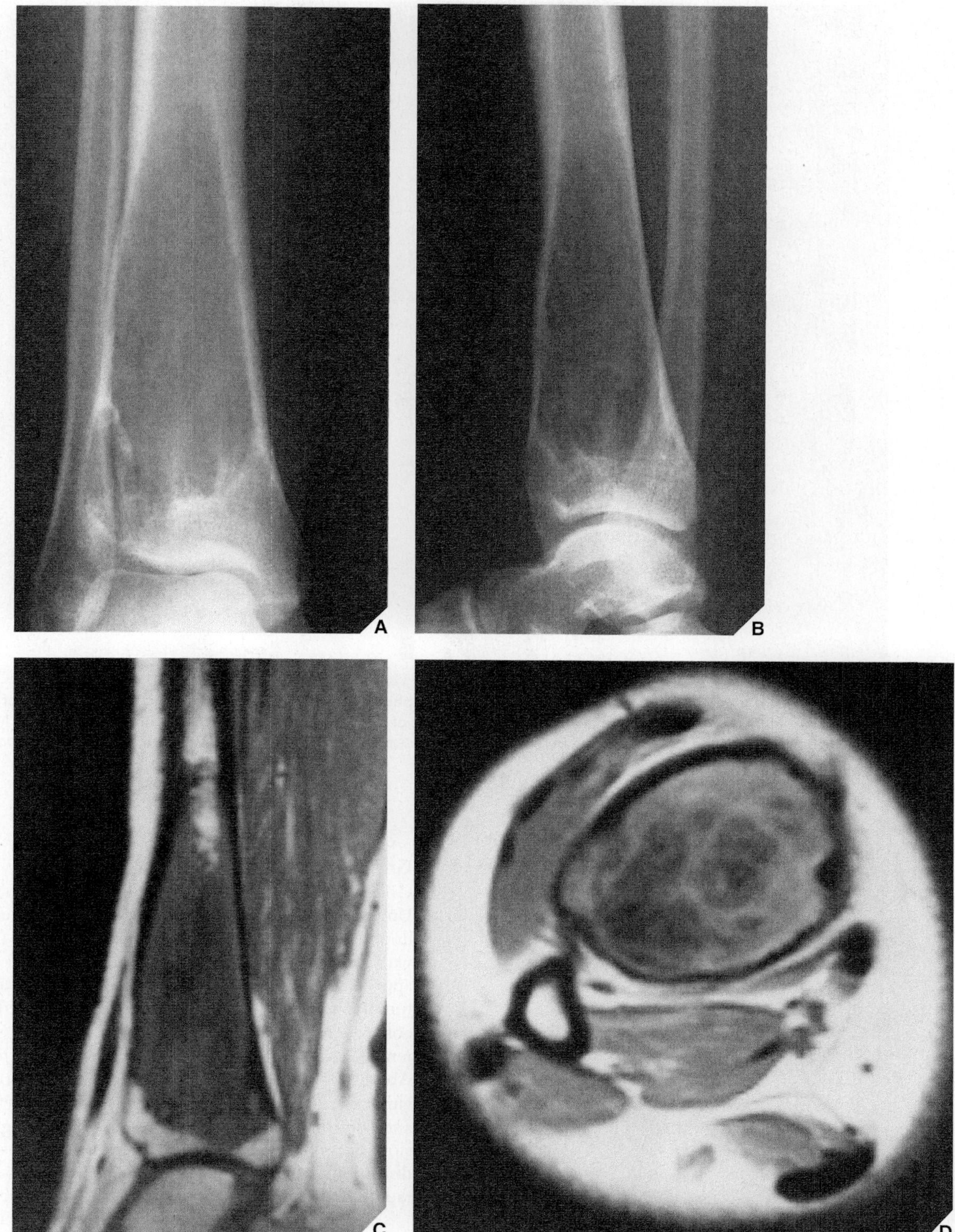

FIGURE 21.20 **Low-grade central osteosarcoma.** **(A)** Anteroposterior and **(B)** lateral radiographs of the distal leg in an 18-year-old woman were originally interpreted as showing fibrous dysplasia of the distal tibia. Note a benign-appearing radiolucent lesion exhibiting a geographic type of bone destruction with a narrow zone of transition and no evidence of periosteal reaction. **(C)** Sagittal and **(D)** axial T1-weighted (spin echo [SE]; repetition time [TR] 600/echo time [TE] 20 msec) MR images demonstrate intermediate to low signal intensity of the lesion and lack of a soft-tissue mass. Biopsy revealed a low-grade central osteosarcoma. (Courtesy of K. Krishnan Unni, MD, Rochester, Minnesota.)

cells arranged in diffuse sheets. As in all other subtypes of osteosarcoma, the distinction from other sarcomas depends on the demonstration of osteoid or bone formation by malignant cells in the very typical patterns seen in osteosarcomas.

Intracortical Osteosarcoma

Intracortical osteosarcoma is one of the rarest forms of osteosarcoma. Very few of these tumors have been reported, with an age range of 9 to 43 years (average 24 years) and a male predominance. The presenting symptom is pain, often associated with activity. In some patients, a history of previous trauma has been elicited. The tumor involves the cortex, without extension into the medullary portion of the bone or the soft tissues. The radiographic presentation is that of a radiolucent lesion with surrounding cortical sclerosis. The size of the lesion varies from 1.0 to 4.2 cm. In some instances, the lesion mimics osteoid osteoma or intracortical osteoblastoma.

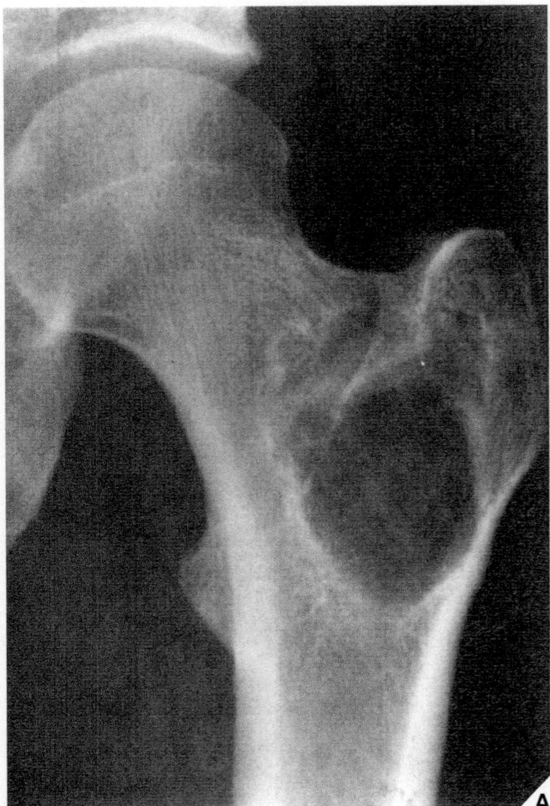

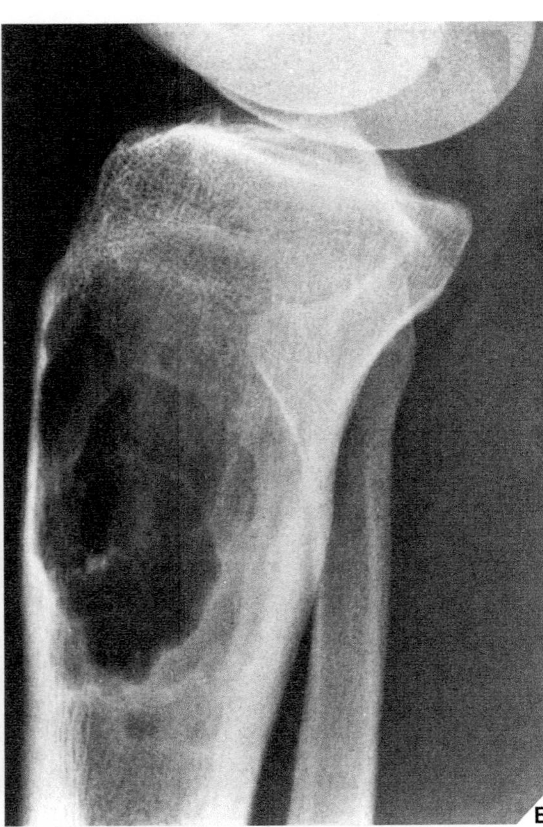

FIGURE 21.21 Low-grade central osteosarcoma. **(A)** A lytic lesion with geographic pattern of bone destruction and a narrow zone of transition is present in the intertrochanteric region of the left femur in a 24-year-old woman. **(B)** Lateral radiograph of the proximal tibia of a 30-year-old woman reveals a lytic lesion with well-defined borders and geographic type of bone destruction. (Reprinted with permission from Greenspan A, Jundt G, Remagen W. *Differential diagnosis in orthopaedic oncology*, 2nd ed. Philadelphia: Lippincott Williams & Wilkins; 2007:84–148, 212–249.)

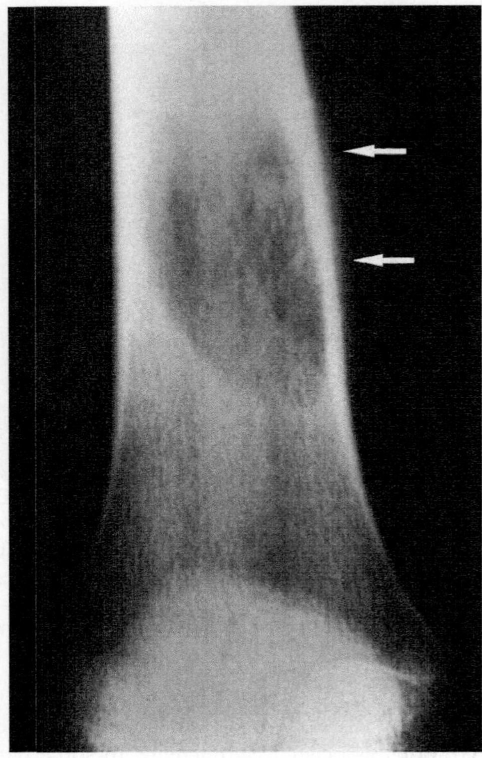

FIGURE 21.22 Telangiectatic osteosarcoma. A purely destructive lesion is present in the diaphysis of the femur of this 17-year-old girl. Note the velvet type of periosteal reaction *(arrows)*. The sclerotic changes usually seen in osteosarcomas are absent, and there is no radiographic evidence of tumor-bone. Biopsy revealed a telangiectatic osteosarcoma, one of the most aggressive types of this tumor. (Courtesy of Michael J. Klein, MD, New York.)

Gnathic Osteosarcoma

Gnathic osteosarcoma is osteosarcoma arising in the maxilla or mandible. Unlike osteosarcoma arising elsewhere in the skeleton, this tumor occurs in older patients with 60% male predominance (fourth to sixth decades, with a mean age of 35 years). This subtype of osteosarcoma represents approximately 6% of osteosarcomas. It is usually a well-differentiated tumor with a low mitotic rate, possessing a predominantly cartilaginous component in a high percentage of cases and with less malignant potential and a better prognosis than for other forms of osteosarcoma. About 60% of gnathic osteosarcomas are osteoblastic, and the rest are either fibroblastic or chondroblastic. Often they have aggressive appearance on imaging, including cortical breakthrough and soft-tissue extension. Secondary gnathic osteosarcomas are most often related to Paget disease, fibrous dysplasia, Ollier syndrome, or as a sequela of craniofacial radiotherapy.

Multicentric (Multifocal) Osteosarcoma

The simultaneous development of foci of osteosarcoma in multiple bones is a rare occurrence (Figs. 21.29 and 21.30). Whether this entity is truly separate or represents multiple bone metastases from a primary conventional osteosarcoma remains a controversy. This type of osteosarcoma is currently recognized as having two variants: synchronous and metachronous. Multifocal osteosarcoma must be differentiated from osteosarcoma metastasized to other bones.

Surface (Juxtacortical) Osteosarcomas

The term *juxtacortical* is a general designation for a group of osteosarcomas that arise on the bone surface (Fig. 21.31). Usually, these lesions are much rarer and occur a decade later than their intraosseous counterparts. The majority of juxtacortical osteosarcomas are low-grade tumors, although there are moderately and even highly malignant variants.

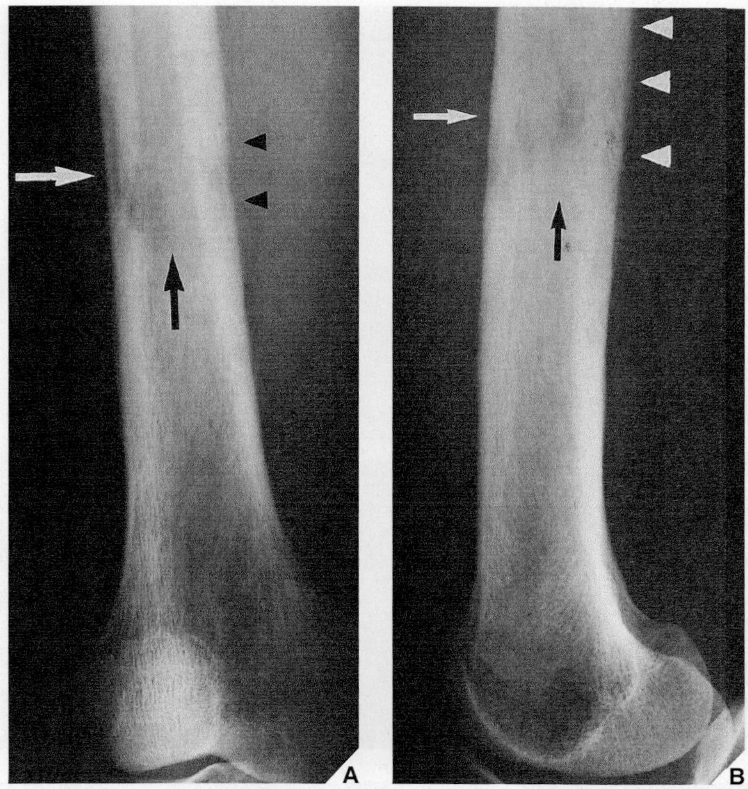

FIGURE 21.23 Telangiectatic osteosarcoma. **(A)** Anteroposterior and **(B)** lateral radiographs of the right femur of a 41-year-old man show an ill-defined lesion that exhibits a permeative type of bone destruction *(arrows)*. Note the velvet type of aggressive periosteal reaction *(arrowheads)*.

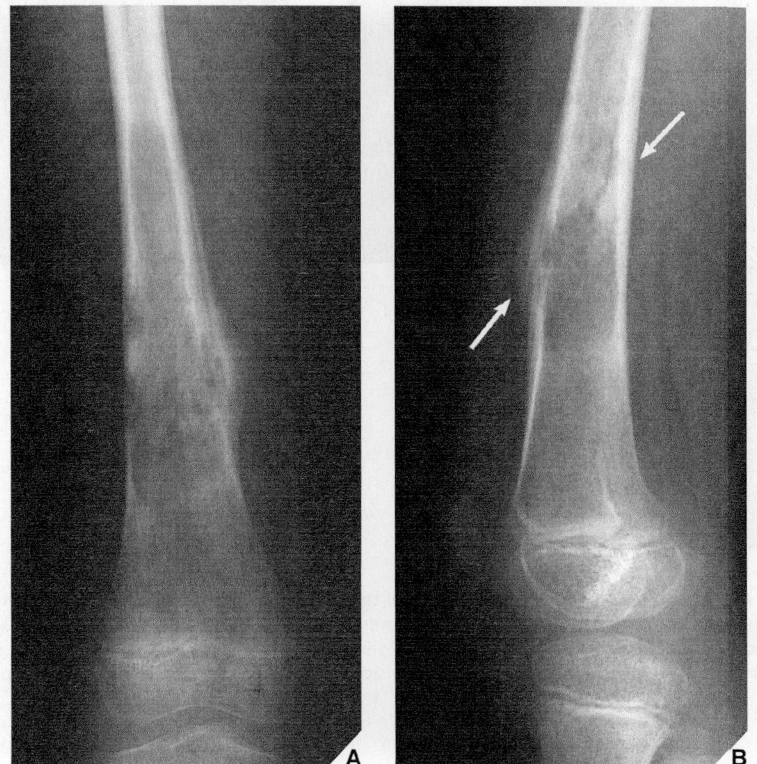

FIGURE 21.24 Telangiectatic osteosarcoma. **(A)** A predominantly lytic tumor associated with aggressive periosteal reaction is seen in the distal femoral diaphysis of this 6-year-old girl. **(B)** Lateral radiograph demonstrates an oblique pathologic fracture *(arrows)*. (Courtesy of K. Krishnan Unni, MD, Rochester, Minnesota.)

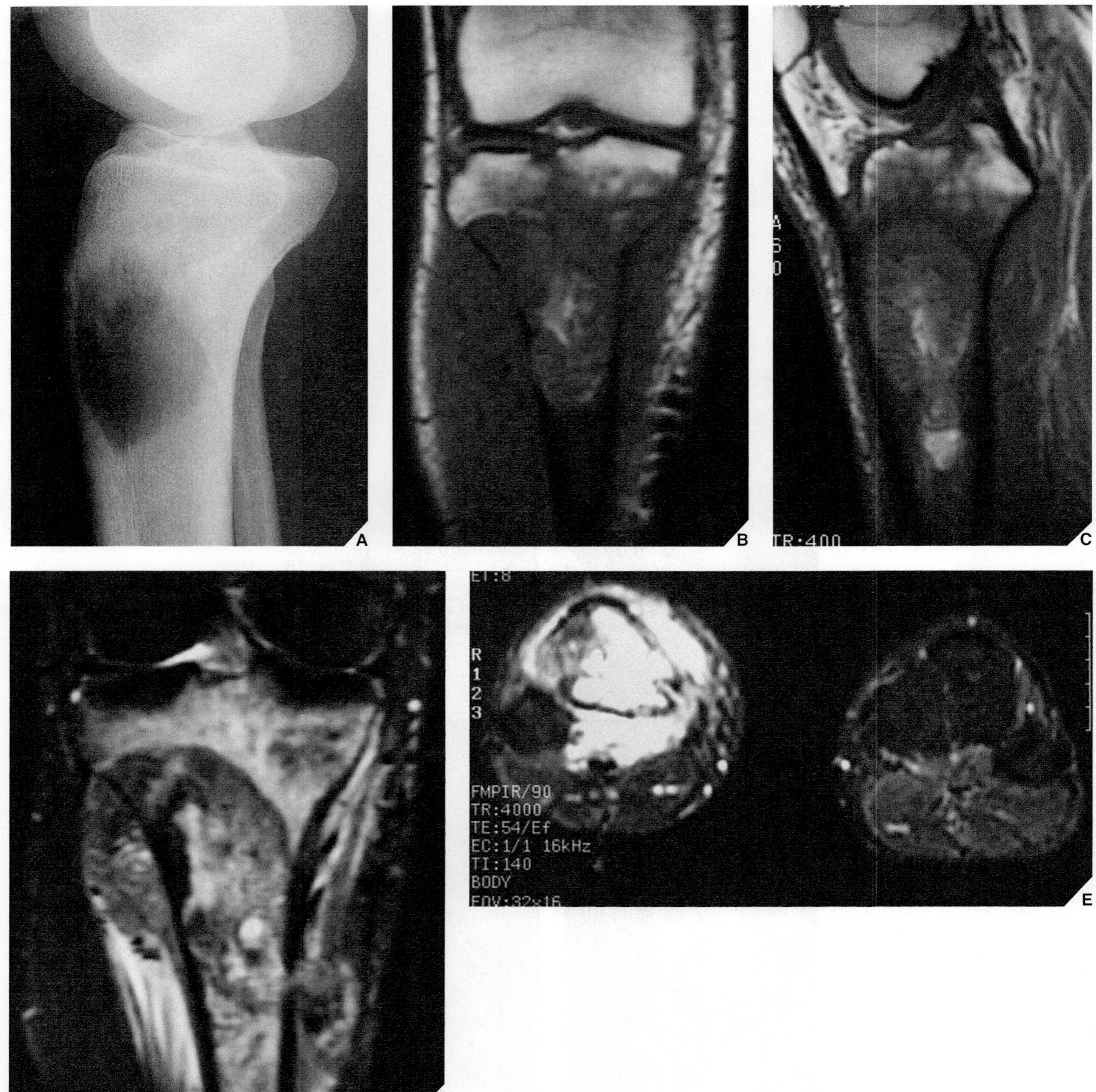

FIGURE 21.25 MRI of telangiectatic osteosarcoma. **(A)** Lateral radiograph of the proximal tibia of a 21-year-old man shows a lesion with relatively narrow zone of transition and no visible periosteal reaction. **(B)** Coronal and **(C)** sagittal T1-weighted (spin echo [SE]; repetition time [TR] 400/echo time [TE] 10 msec) MR images show the tumor to be predominantly of intermediate signal intensity with foci of high signal. **(D)** Coronal and **(E)** axial inversion recovery (fast multiplanar inversion recovery [FMPIR]/90 msec; TR 4000/TE 54/inversion time [TI] 140 msec) images show the extension of the tumor into the soft tissues and presence of peritumoral edema.

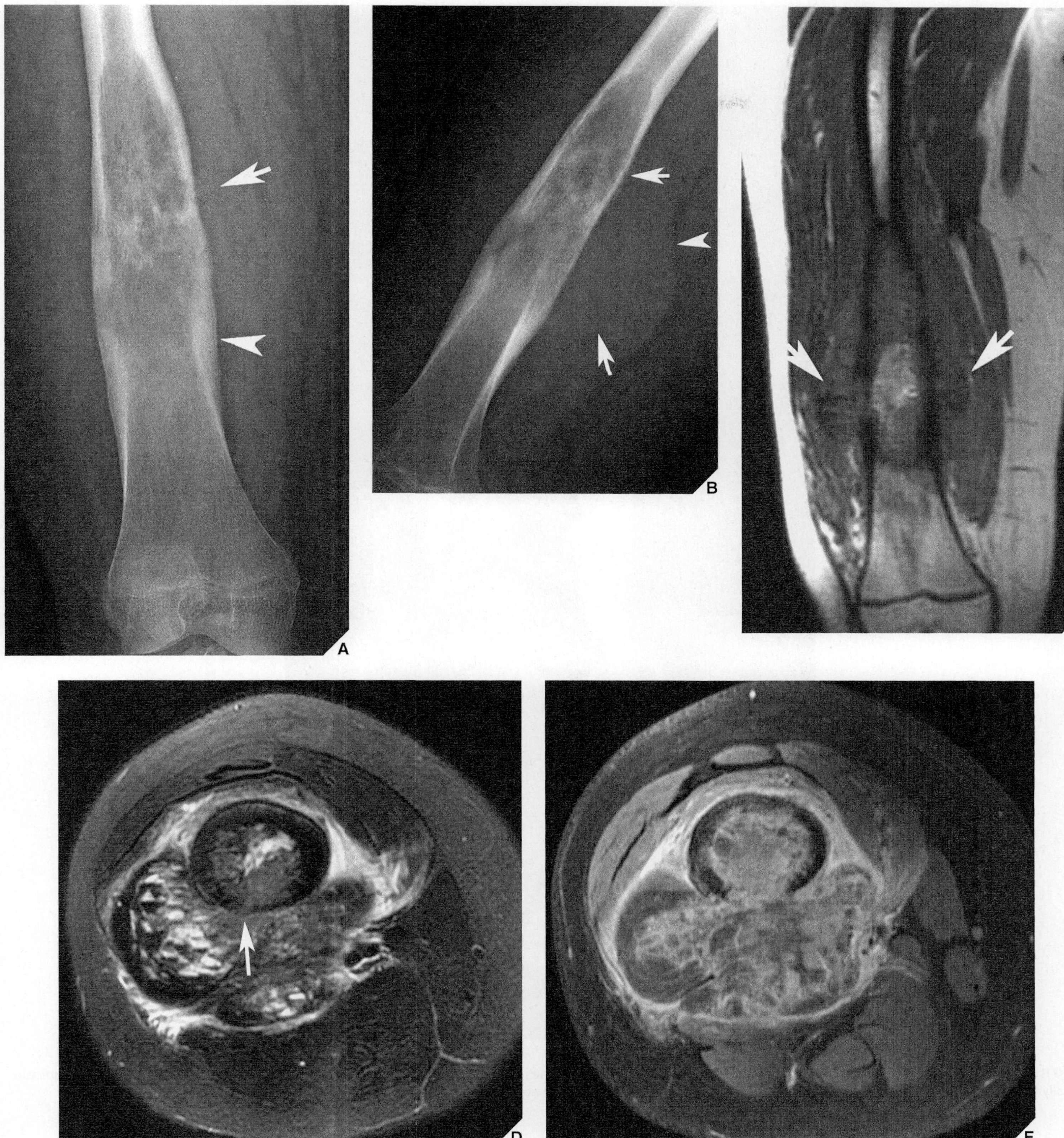

FIGURE 21.26 MRI of telangiectatic osteosarcoma. **(A)** Anteroposterior radiograph of the right femur of a 19-year-old man, who presented with history of pain for several months, shows an intramedullary lytic, expansive lesion of the midshaft of the femur, associated with periosteal reaction *(arrowhead)*. Note osteoid matrix calcification within the lesion and in the adjacent soft tissues *(arrow)*. **(B)** Lateral radiograph demonstrates periosteal reaction and tumor-bone formation *(arrows)* with a large posterior soft-tissue mass *(arrowhead)*. **(C)** Coronal T1-weighted MRI shows the intramedullary extension of the tumor and the soft-tissue extension *(arrows)*. **(D)** Axial T2-weighted MRI demonstrates cortical permeation of the tumor and an area of cortical breakthrough *(arrow)*. Note the large posterior soft-tissue mass with surrounding soft-tissue edema. The soft-tissue component of the tumor contains multiple short fluid–fluid levels, characteristic of telangiectatic osteosarcoma. **(E)** Axial T1-weighted fat-saturated MRI following intravenous injection of gadolinium reveals heterogeneous enhancement of the tumor due to the presence of vascular spaces in the central portion of the lesion. There is enhancement of the surrounding soft-tissue edema reflecting hyperemia.

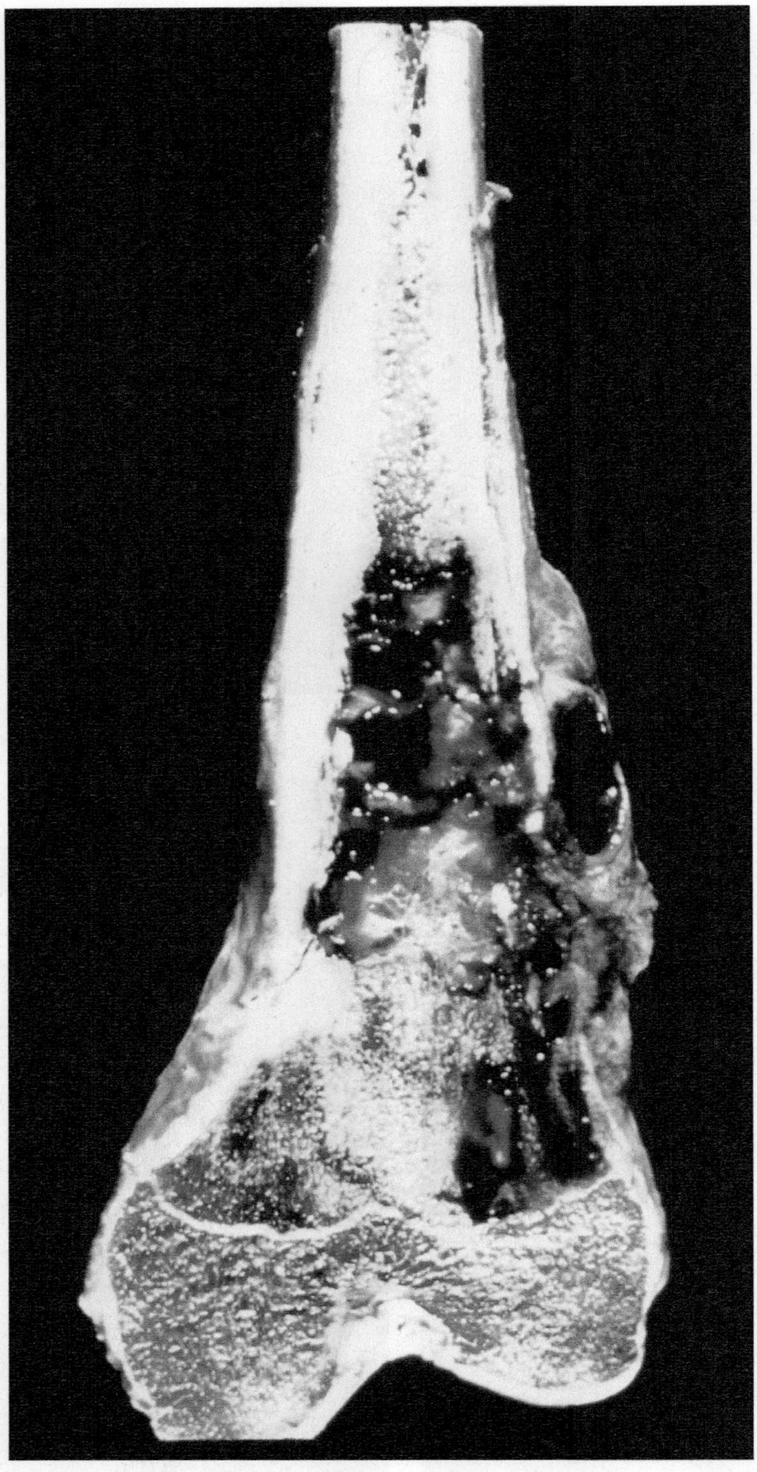

FIGURE 21.27 **Pathology of telangiectatic osteosarcoma.** Gross specimen of the resected distal femur shows areas of solid tumor and dominant cystic architecture partially filled with blood clots, characteristic for this type of neoplasm. Note that the tumor did not invade the growth plate.

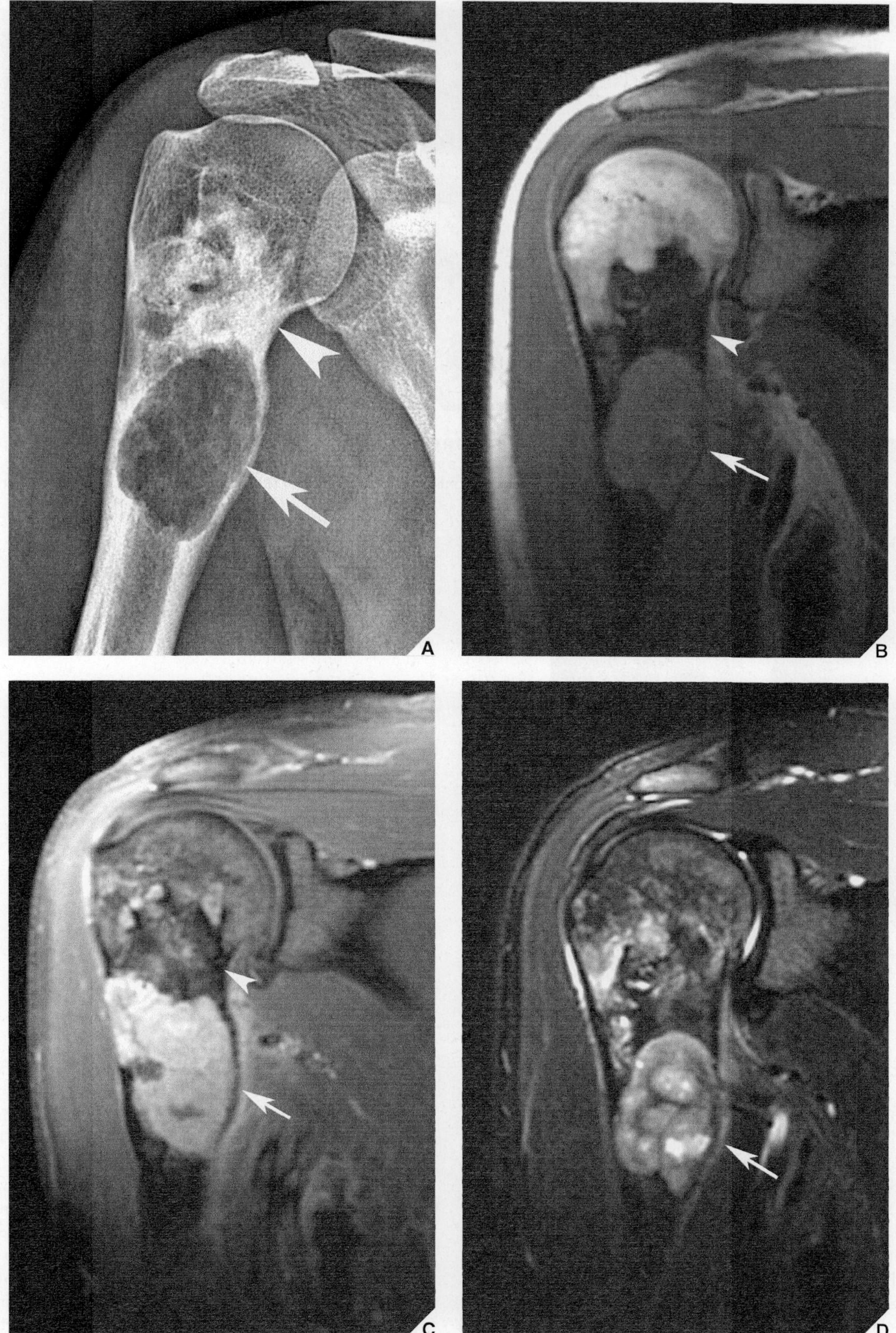

FIGURE 21.28 MRI of giant cell–rich osteosarcoma. **(A)** Anteroposterior radiograph of the right shoulder of a 22-year-old woman, who presented with a vague upper arm pain of 2-month duration, shows slightly expansive, mixed lytic *(arrow)* and sclerotic *(arrowhead)* lesion in the proximal humerus, exhibiting narrow zone of transition. **(B)** Coronal T1-weighted MR image shows the proximal sclerotic part of the tumor being of low signal intensity *(arrowhead)* and the distal lytic part of intermediate signal *(arrow)*. **(C)** Coronal T2-weighted MRI demonstrates that the proximal part is of mixed heterogeneous but predominantly of low signal *(arrowhead)*, whereas the distal part exhibits high signal intensity *(arrow)*. **(D)** Coronal T1-weighted fat-suppressed MRI obtained after intravenous administration of gadolinium shows various degree of enhancement of the entire tumor, more prominent in the distal part *(arrow)*. The cortex has not been violated and no soft-tissue mass is evident.

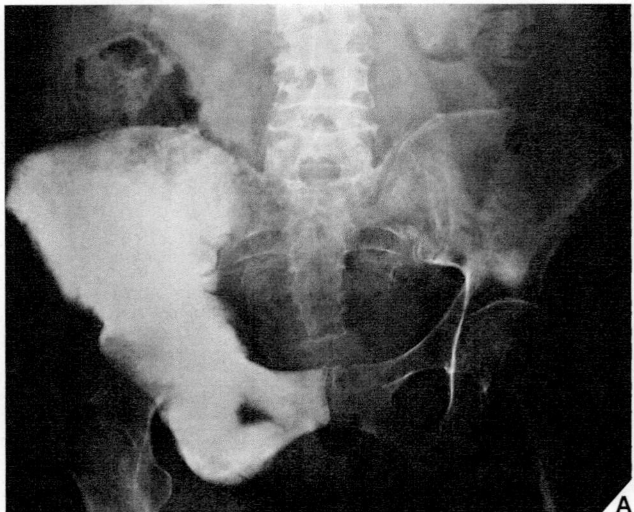

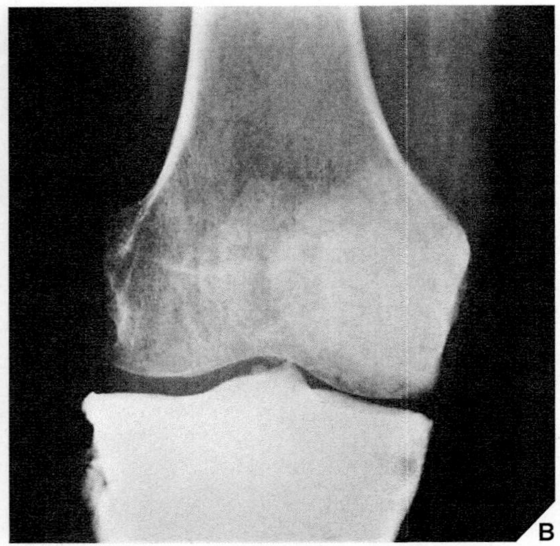

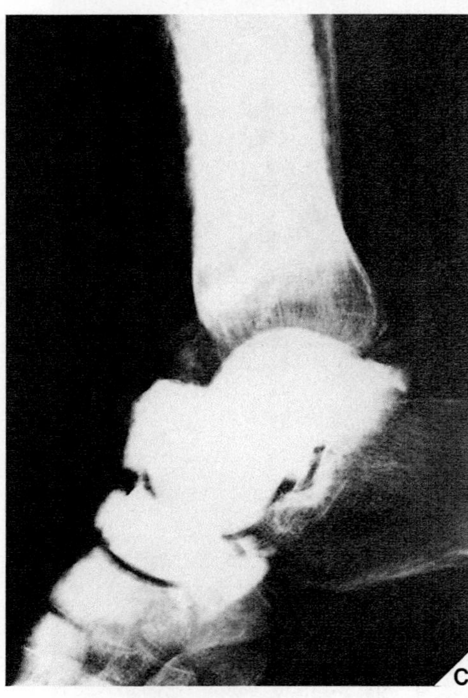

FIGURE 21.29 Multicentric osteosarcoma. Multicentric osteosarcoma, a very rare bone tumor, is demonstrated here in the right hemipelvis **(A)**, right tibia and distal femur **(B)**, and several bones of the right foot **(C)**.

Parosteal Osteosarcoma

Parosteal tumors are seen largely in patients in their third and fourth decades, with a characteristic site of predilection in the posterior aspect of the distal femur (Fig. 21.32).

Conventional radiography is usually adequate for making a diagnosis of parosteal osteosarcoma. The lesion presents as a dense oval or spherical mass attached to the cortical surface of the bone and sharply demarcated from the surrounding soft tissues (Figs. 21.33 to 21.36). CT (see Fig. 21.35B) or MRI (see Figs. 16.21B and 16.22E,F) is often necessary to determine whether the lesion has penetrated the cortex and invaded the medullary region of the bone.

Pathologic gross specimen shows a hard-lobulated mass attached to the underlying cortex and occasionally present osteochondroma-like incomplete cap-like cartilage covering the surface (Fig. 21.37). Histologically, the lesion consists of well-defined bone trabeculae in fibrous spindle-cell stroma, probably derived from the outer fibrous periosteal layer. Spindle cells show minimal atypia, osteoid formation, and rare mitotic figures. The osseous component is often trabeculated but is at least partially immature, particularly at the periphery of the tumor. This is an important point in differentiating it from the sometimes similar-appearing myositis ossificans, which, however, matures in a centripetal fashion, with its most mature portion outermost. Genetic abnormalities consisting of *SAS*, *CDK4*, and *MDM2* overexpression and coamplification were described in majority of cases.

Differential Diagnosis. Parosteal osteosarcoma must be differentiated from parosteal osteoma (see Figs. 17.3A and 17.4), myositis ossificans, soft-tissue osteosarcoma, parosteal liposarcoma with ossifications, and sessile osteochondroma. Differentiation from myositis ossificans and sessile osteochondroma is the most frequent source of confusion. Myositis ossificans is distinguished by a zonal phenomenon and by a cleft separating the ossific mass from the cortex (Fig. 21.38; see also Figs. 4.79 and 4.80). In sessile osteochondroma, however, the cortex of the lesion merges without interruption into the cortex of the host bone (see Fig. 18.42), a feature not seen in parosteal osteosarcoma. Because the lesion is relatively slow growing and most often involves only the surface of the bone, the prognosis for patients with parosteal osteosarcoma is much better than for those with other types of osteosarcoma. Simple wide resection of the lesion often constitutes sufficient treatment.

Dedifferentiated Parosteal Osteosarcoma

A rare and unusual bone tumor, dedifferentiated parosteal osteosarcoma, was identified by a group from the Mayo Clinic. Most cases reportedly originate as conventional parosteal osteosarcomas that, after resection and multiple local recurrences, have undergone transformation to histologically

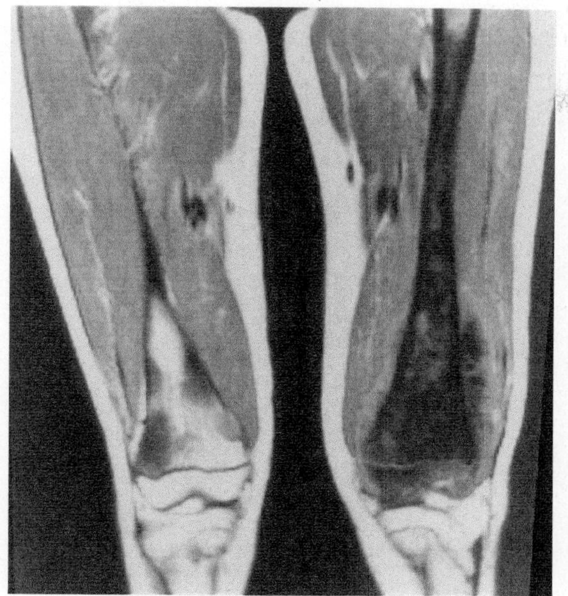

FIGURE 21.30 MRI of multicentric osteosarcoma. Coronal T1-weighted image shows multiple low-signal intensity lesions in both femora of a 12-year-old girl. (Reprinted with permission from Greenspan A, Jundt G, Remagen W. *Differential diagnosis in orthopaedic oncology*, 2nd ed. Philadelphia: Lippincott Williams & Wilkins; 2007:84–148, 212–249.)

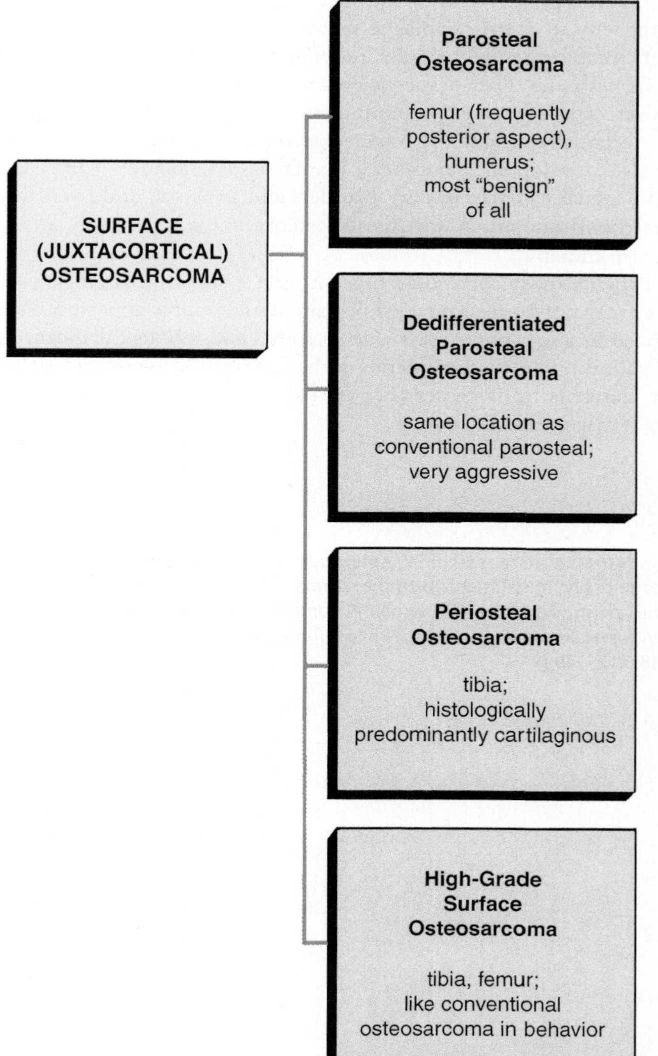

FIGURE 21.31 Variants of juxtacortical osteosarcoma.

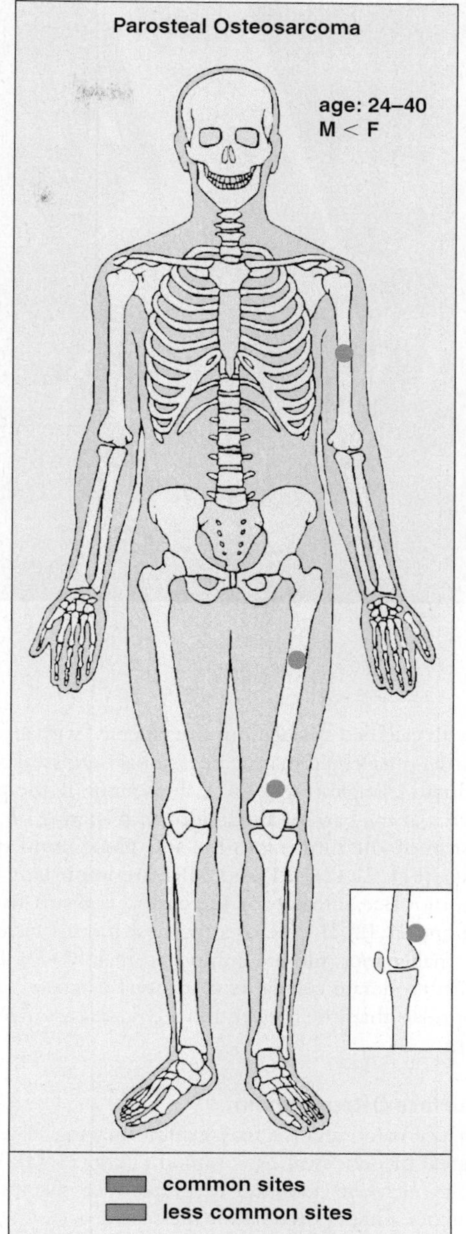

FIGURE 21.32 Skeletal sites of predilection, peak age range, and male-to-female ratio in parosteal osteosarcoma.

high-grade sarcomas. Some cases, however, have presented as primary tumors arising on the cortical surface of a bone *de novo*. Radiographically and histologically, dedifferentiated parosteal osteosarcoma mimics the features of conventional parosteal osteosarcoma. There are, however, some traits of a high-grade sarcoma, such as radiographically identifiable cortical destruction (Fig. 21.39) and histologically identifiable pleomorphic tumor cells with hyperchromatic nuclei and a high mitotic rate. Hence, the prognosis is much worse than that of parosteal osteosarcoma.

Periosteal Osteosarcoma

Most often occurring in adolescence, periosteal osteosarcoma is a very rare tumor (accounting for 1% to 2% of all osteosarcomas) that grows on the bone surface, usually at the midshaft of a long bone such as the tibia. The characteristic feature of this tumor, which radiographically may resemble myositis ossificans, is a predominance of cartilaginous tissue (Fig. 21.40). This may lead to an erroneous diagnosis of periosteal chondrosarcoma. The radiologic characteristics of periosteal osteosarcoma were defined by deSantos and colleagues. These include a heterogeneous

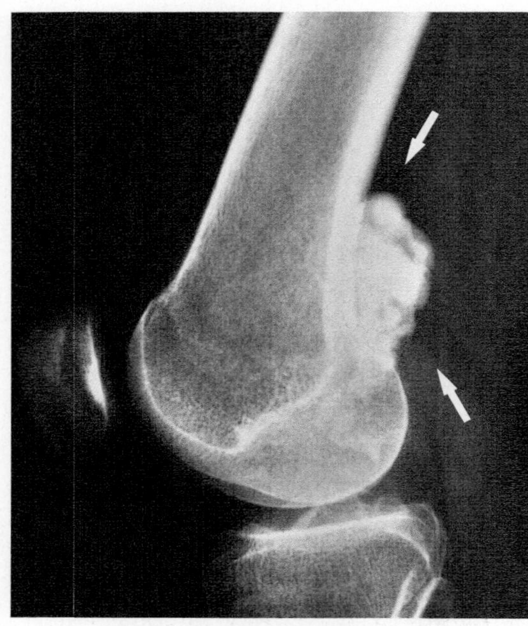

FIGURE 21.33 Parosteal osteosarcoma. Typical presentation of this tumor at the posterior aspect of the distal femur *(arrows)* in a 23-year-old woman.

tumor matrix with calcified spiculations interspersed with areas of radiolucency representing uncalcified matrix; occasional periosteal reaction in the form of a Codman triangle (Fig. 21.41); thickening of the periosteal surface of the cortex at the base of the lesion, with sparing of the endosteal surface; extension of the tumor into the soft tissues; and sparing of the medullary cavity (Fig. 21.42). CT and MRI are important techniques in evaluation of tumor size, integrity of the cortex, and soft-tissue extension (see Figs. 21.41 and 21.42). By microscopy, these tumors have low-grade to medium-grade malignancy and are composed mainly of lobulated chondroid tissue with moderate cellularity. Periosteal osteosarcoma is marked by a better prognosis than the conventional type but a worse one than the parosteal variant.

High-Grade Surface Osteosarcoma

High-grade surface osteosarcoma may exhibit imaging features similar to those of parosteal or periosteal osteosarcoma (Fig. 21.43). Histologically, this lesion shows elements identical to those of conventional osteosarcoma. It also carries a high potential for metastasis.

Soft-Tissue (Extraskeletal) Osteosarcoma

Osteosarcoma of the soft tissues (extraskeletal, extraosseous) is an uncommon malignant tumor of mesenchymal origin. This tumor possesses the capacity to form neoplastic osteoid, bone, and cartilage. It usually targets middle-aged and elderly individuals, with a mean age at presentation of 54 years. Soft-tissue osteosarcoma is much less common than osteosarcoma of bone, accounting for only 4% of all osteosarcomas. It preferentially affects the lower extremities and buttocks. This lesion may also develop in a number of soft tissues, including breast, lung, thyroid, renal capsule, urinary bladder, and prostate, and even the pelvic retroperitoneum. A soft-tissue osteosarcoma may rarely arise after radiation therapy.

Patients most commonly present with a slowly enlarging mass that may or may not be accompanied by pain. Radiographic appearance is characterized by a soft-tissue mass with scattered amorphous calcifications and ossifications. The tumor exhibits a disorganized arrangement of osteogenic elements in its center (Fig. 21.44). If the tumor develops close to bone, it may invade the cortex.

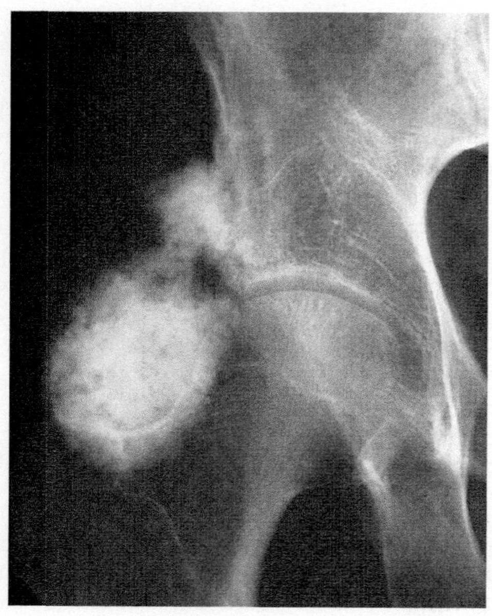

FIGURE 21.34 Parosteal osteosarcoma. Anteroposterior radiograph of the right hip shows a large ossific mass attached to the supraacetabular portion of the ilium. (Reprinted with permission from Greenspan A, Jundt G, Remagen W. *Differential diagnosis in orthopaedic oncology*, 2nd ed. Philadelphia: Lippincott Williams & Wilkins; 2007:84–148, 212–249.)

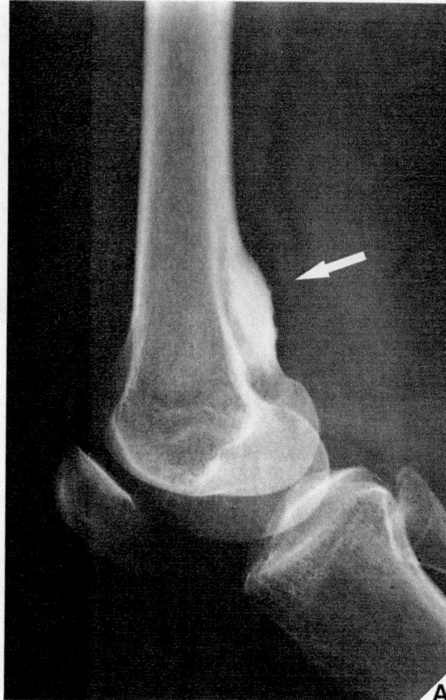

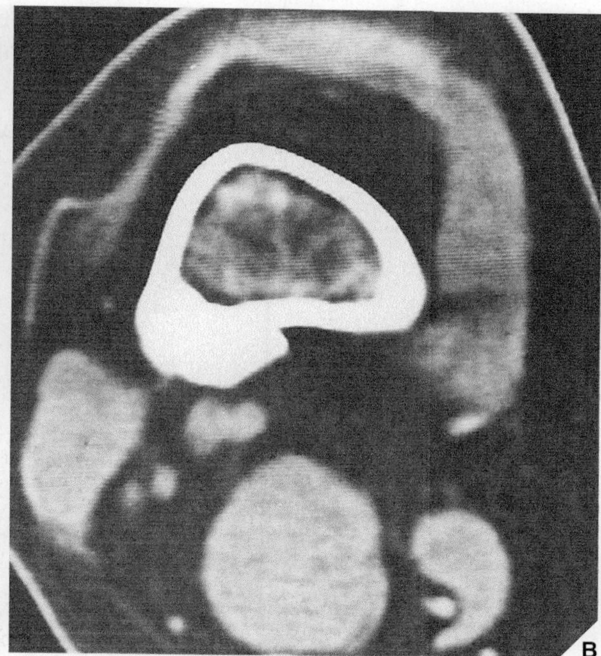

FIGURE 21.35 CT of parosteal osteosarcoma. **(A)** Lateral radiograph of the knee of a 37-year-old woman shows an ossific mass attached to the posterior cortex of the distal femur *(arrow)*. Its location and appearance are typical of parosteal osteosarcoma. **(B)** Contrast-enhanced axial CT section demonstrates that the medullary portion of the bone has not been invaded.

On CT, a heavily mineralized soft-tissue mass is usually seen, occasionally with necrotic areas. This technique is often better than radiography at revealing the pattern of central ossification, which is referred to as the *reverse zoning phenomenon*. CT also demonstrates a lack of attachment of the mass to the bone. On MRI, a mass with mixed low signal intensity on T1-weighted images and mixed but predominantly high signal intensity on T2-weighted and inversion recovery sequences is often seen. MRI may also reveal a pseudocapsule of tumor (Fig. 21.45).

Gross pathology of soft-tissue osteosarcoma shows fleshy mass with areas of bone and cartilage (Fig. 21.46). The histopathology of soft-tissue osteosarcoma is indistinguishable from that of a conventional osteosarcoma.

Differential Diagnosis

The differential diagnosis of extraskeletal osteosarcoma includes myositis ossificans, tumoral calcinosis, synovial sarcoma, extraskeletal chondrosarcoma, liposarcoma of soft tissues with ossification, and pseudomalignant osseous tumor of soft tissue.

Myositis ossificans is a benign, usually posttraumatic, lesion of the soft tissues that is observed predominantly in adolescents and young adults (see Fig. 21.38; see also Figs. 4.79 and 4.80). The zoning phenomenon reflects the maturation pattern of the lesion. The center of the lesion is undifferentiated and cellular, but increasingly mature ossification is observed toward the periphery constituting the histologic hallmark of this condition. Radiography reveals that the zoning phenomenon

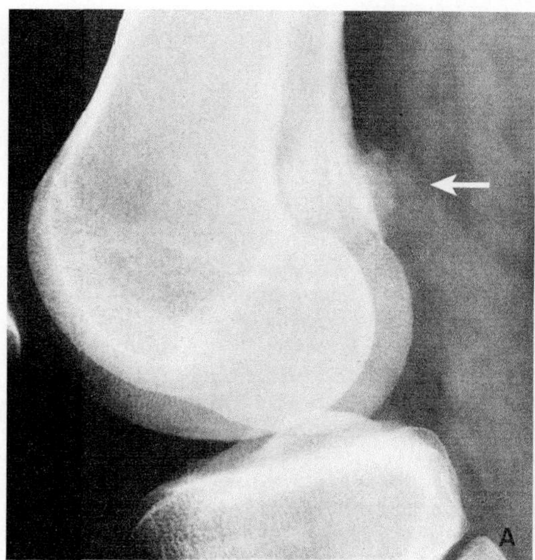

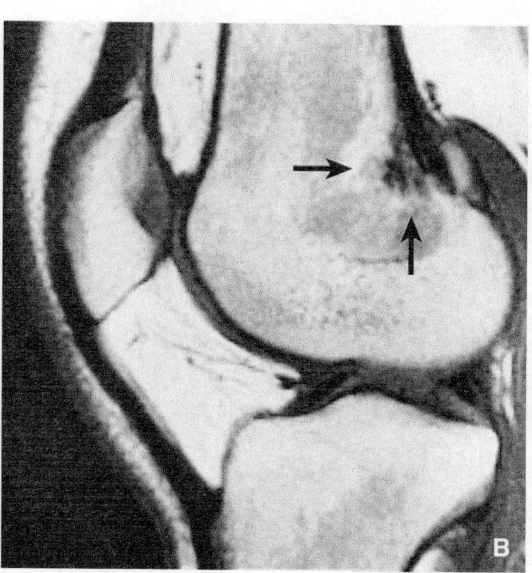

FIGURE 21.36 MRI of parosteal osteosarcoma. **(A)** Lateral radiograph of the knee of a 22-year-old woman shows a surface tumor involving the posterior aspect of the medial femoral condyle *(arrow)*. The invasion of the cortex cannot be determined. **(B)** Sagittal T1-weighted MR image demonstrates the invasion of medullary cavity *(arrows)*. (Reprinted with permission from Greenspan A, Borys D. *Radiology and pathology correlation of bone tumors,* 1st ed. Philadelphia: Wolters Kluwer, 2016:73.)

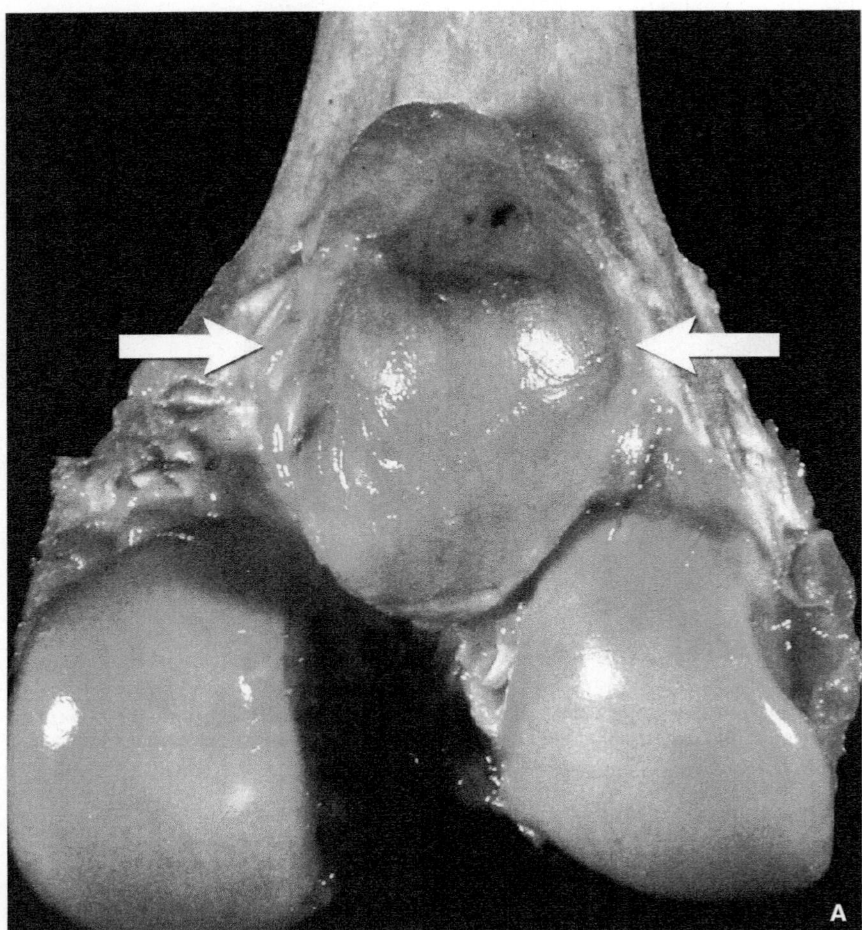

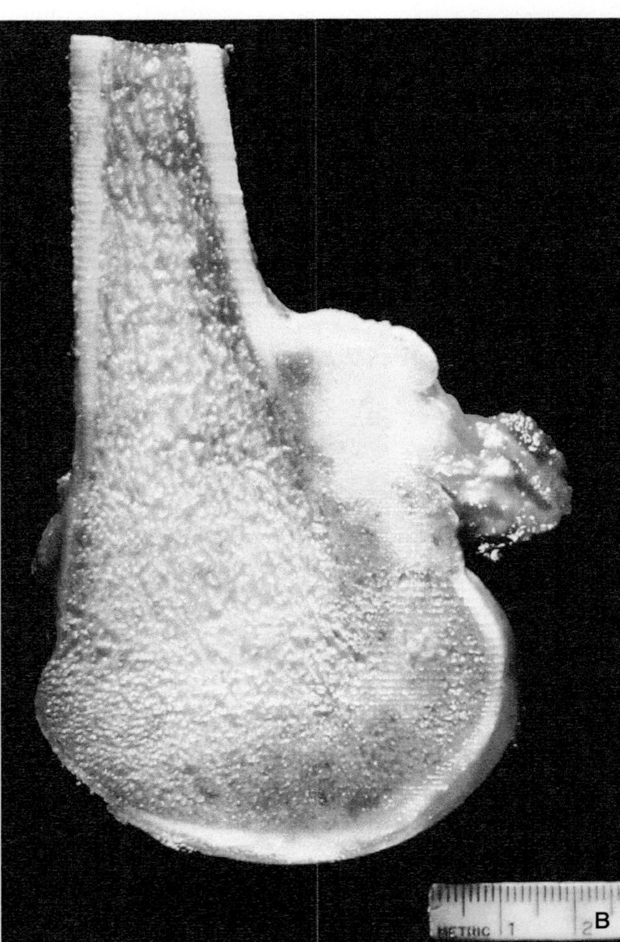

FIGURE 21.37 Pathology of parosteal osteosarcoma. **(A)** Gross specimen of the resected distal femur shows a large surface lesion in the posterior aspect of the bone exhibiting glistening cartilaginous-like cup *(arrows)*. **(B)** Sagittal section of gross specimen of the resected distal femur of another patient shows most of the tumor on the surface of the bone, but there is evidence of cortical invasion. (Reprinted with permission from Greenspan A, Borys D. *Radiology and pathology correlation of bone tumors: a quick reference and review*. Philadelphia: Wolters Kluwer, 2016:73, Figs 2.58 and 2.59.)

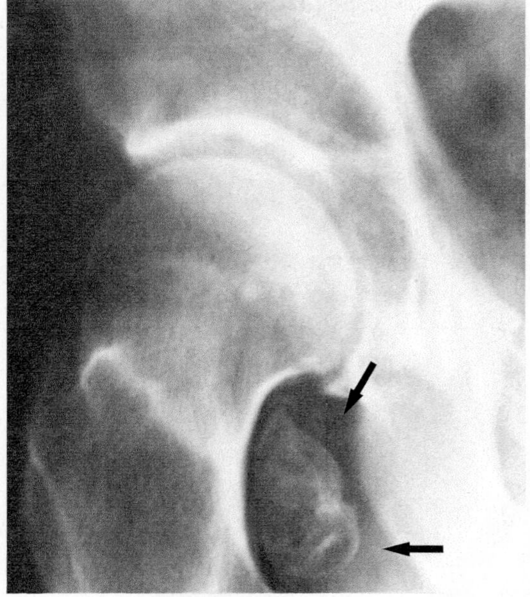

FIGURE 21.38 Myositis ossificans. Juxtacortical myositis ossificans, seen here near the medial cortex of the femoral neck *(arrows)*, typically presents as a more mature lesion at its periphery, with a center less dense than in parosteal osteosarcoma, and a clear zone representing complete separation of the lesion from the cortex.

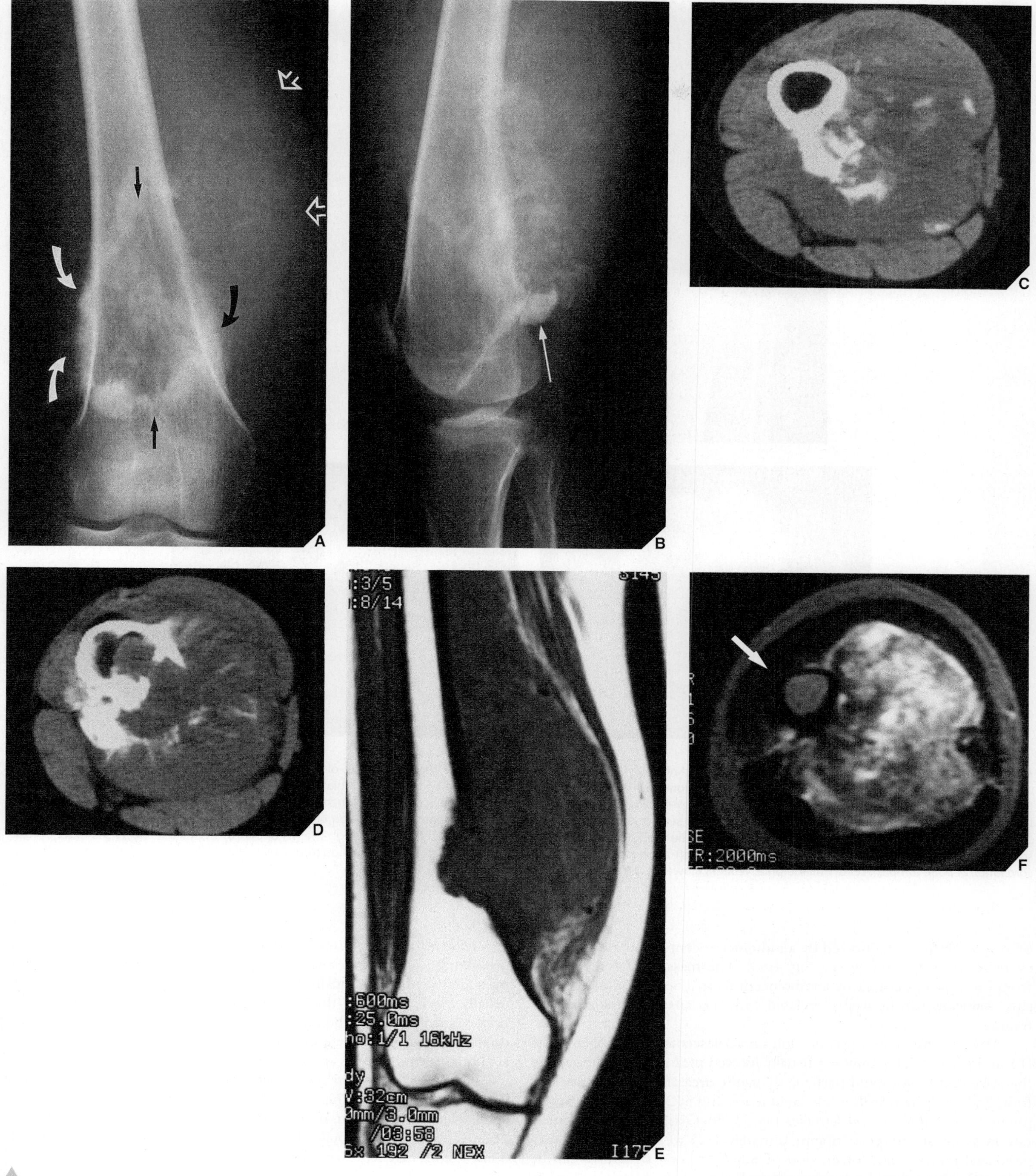

FIGURE 21.39 CT and MRI of dedifferentiated parosteal osteosarcoma. A 24-year-old woman presented with pain and palpable mass above the popliteal fossa of 2 months duration. Three years before the current symptoms, a parosteal osteosarcoma had been resected from her distal femur. **(A)** Anteroposterior radiograph of the distal femur shows a destructive lesion *(arrows)* associated with an aggressive type of periosteal reaction *(curved arrows)* and a large soft-tissue mass *(open arrows)* with foci of bone formation. **(B)** Lateral radiograph shows in addition the remnants of the previously resected parosteal osteosarcoma *(arrow)*. **(C)** The proximal CT section shows a surface tumor exhibiting bone formation and a large soft-tissue mass with foci of tumor-bone. At this level, the bone marrow is not invaded. **(D)** The more distal section reveals in addition the invasion of the medullary cavity, a feature not consistent with a conventional parosteal osteosarcoma. **(E)** Coronal T1-weighted (spin echo [SE]; repetition time [TR] 600/echo time [TE] 25 msec) MR image demonstrates the extent of both intramedullary invasion and a soft-tissue mass. **(F)** Axial T2-weighted (SE; TR 2000/TE 90 msec) MR image shows heterogeneous signal of a large soft-tissue mass. At the level of this section, the bone marrow is not infiltrated by a tumor *(arrow)*.

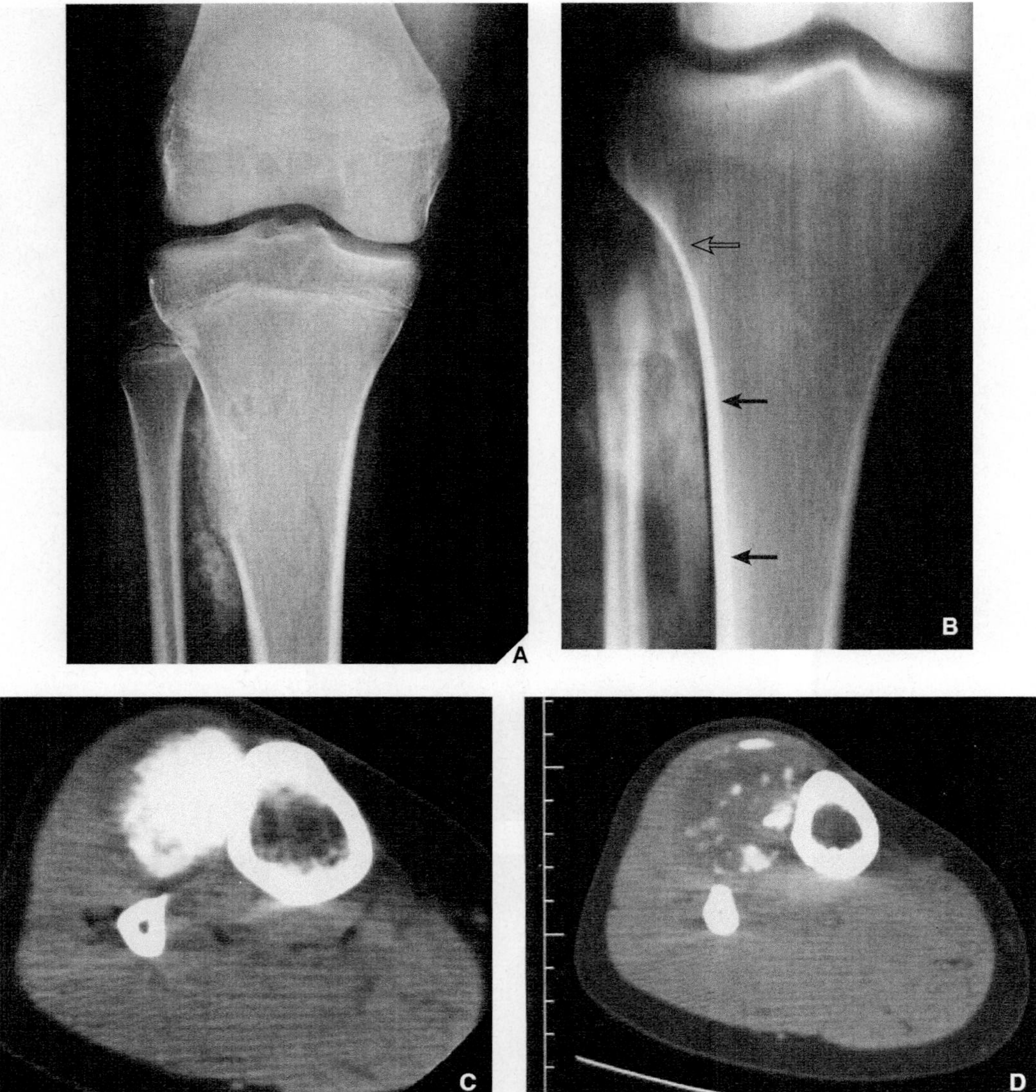

FIGURE 21.40 CT of periosteal osteosarcoma. **(A)** Anteroposterior radiograph of the right knee of a 12-year-old girl with "discomfort" in the upper leg for 2 months demonstrates poorly defined calcifications and ossifications in a mass attached to the surface of the lateral tibial cortex. There appears to be no bone destruction. **(B)** Anteroposterior conventional tomography shows the ossified mass. Although attached to the tibia proximally *(open arrow)*, it is partially separated from the lateral cortex by a narrow radiolucent cleft *(arrows)*, very similar to that seen in the juxtacortical myositis ossificans. **(C)** CT section obtained from the proximal part of the tumor clearly shows the attachment of the lesion to the tibial cortex. The medullary cavity is not affected. **(D)** CT section through the distal part of the tumor shows the extent of the soft-tissue mass. Note low attenuation of the mass and high-attenuation ossifications. (**B–D**, Reprinted with permission from Greenspan A, Borys D. *Radiology and pathology correlation of bone tumors,* 1st ed. Philadelphia: Wolters Kluwer, 2016.)

of this lesion is characterized by a radiolucent center and a denser and more sclerotic periphery (see Fig. 4.80). The mass is often separated from the adjacent cortex by a radiolucent cleft. The evolution of myositis ossificans can be well correlated with the lapse of time since the trauma.

Synovial sarcoma has a predilection for adolescents and younger adults (13 to 55 years). This tumor is usually located near a joint, especially in the lower extremities and particularly in the area around the knee and foot. Radiography reveals a lobulated mass, and in 25% of cases, amorphous calcifications are present (see Fig. 23.29). Ossification is extremely rare in synovial sarcoma. In approximately 15% to 20% of patients, a periosteal reaction and/or erosion of adjacent bone structures can be observed. There may be osteoporosis of the affected limb secondary to disuse.

Chondrosarcoma of soft tissue is a rare malignant tumor and is much less common than extraskeletal osteosarcoma. It appears as a soft-tissue mass with ring-like or punctate calcifications. Soft-tissue chondrosarcoma can be distinguished from soft-tissue osteosarcoma on imaging studies by the lack of bone formation.

Liposarcoma of soft tissues tends to affect older adults and has a male prevalence. This tumor may closely mimic soft-tissue osteosarcoma, particularly when ossification is present. However, the ossification is usually more organized than that in osteosarcoma of soft tissues, and fatty tissue can usually be identified. This lesion commonly affects the thigh, leg, and gluteal region. Growth of the tumor may proceed very slowly over many years, and erosion of adjacent bone is common.

Pseudomalignant osseous tumor of soft tissues was first described by Jaffe and later by Fine and Stout. These lesions are rare, are more common in females, and are located in the muscle and subcutaneous tissues. They are probably of infective origin, although this has not been unequivocally confirmed. Some lesions may represent unrecognized foci of myositis ossificans.

Osteosarcomas with Unusual Clinical Presentation

There are numerous genetic disorders, marked by chromosome instability, associated with the development of various tumors including osteosarcomas. Among these rare conditions are Rothmund-Thompson syndrome, Werner syndrome, Li-Fraumeni syndrome, retinoblastoma syndrome, and Bloom syndrome.

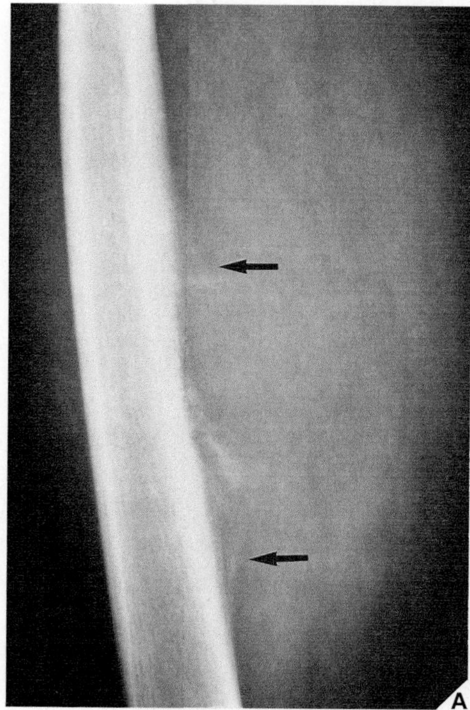

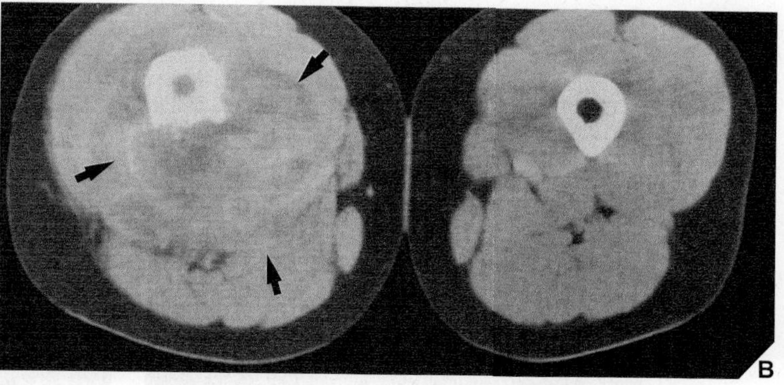

FIGURE 21.41 CT of periosteal osteosarcoma. **(A)** Anteroposterior radiograph of the right femur of a 16-year-old girl shows a surface lesion affecting the medial cortex, associated with a Codman triangle of periosteal reaction *(arrows)* and a large soft-tissue mass. **(B)** CT shows the soft-tissue component to better advantage *(arrows)*. The medullary cavity is not invaded by the tumor; however, an increase in attenuation value, compared with the contralateral marrow cavity, indicates bone marrow edema.

The *Rothmund-Thompson syndrome*, also known as *congenital poikiloderma*, is a hereditary disease with a male predominance of 2:1, appearing in the first year of life, and characterized by erythematous and maculopapular skin lesions with areas of hyperpigmentation. These lesions are associated with a variety of other abnormalities such as sensitivity to light, juvenile cataracts, short stature, growth retardation, premature baldness, hypogonadism, and development of skin malignancies (particularly basal cell and squamous cell carcinoma). Conventional osteosarcoma develops in about 30% of cases (particularly at a younger age), although the presence of multicentric osteosarcoma has also been reported. The syndrome, which is inherited in an autosomal recessive manner, has been attributed to mutations of *RECQL4* gene located at chromosome band 8q24.3 and coding for DNA helicase that unfolds double-stranded DNA into single-stranded DNA.

The *Werner syndrome*, also known as *adult progeria*, is a rare autosomal recessive genetic disorder caused by mutations in the *WRN* gene (*RECQL2*) that has been mapped at chromosome band 8p12-p11. This syndrome is characterized by the premature aging including graying of hair, alopecia, cataracts, scleroderma-like skin changes, osteoarthritis of peripheral joints, short stature, hypogonadism, osteoporosis, diabetes mellitus, and atherosclerotic cardiovascular disease. The patients with this syndrome are also at risk to develop epithelial neoplasms, melanoma, thyroid cancer, and osteosarcoma. Patients with osteosarcoma present at an older age and at atypical sites.

The *Li-Fraumeni syndrome* is a rare autosomal dominant inherited disorder associated with genetic heterozygous germ line R156H, R267Q, and R290H mutation in the *TP53* tumor suppressor gene. The disorder is characterized by multiple primary neoplasms in children and young adults, particularly soft-tissue sarcomas, osteosarcomas, breast cancer, brain tumors, and leukemias.

The *retinoblastoma syndrome* consists of the malignant tumor of the retina, originating from the embryonic neural retina. The following dysmorphic abnormalities are associated with this syndrome: microcephaly, broad and prominent nasal bridge, ptosis, protruding upper incisors, micrognathia, short neck, low-set ears, facial asymmetry, genital malformations, and mental retardation. Retinoblastoma is in 60% of patients nonhereditary and unilateral. However, 40% of the cases are inherited in an autosomal dominant manner with almost complete penetrance, and 25% of these patients present with bilateral tumors. The syndrome is caused by a genetic mutation found in the tumor suppressor gene *RB1* located on the long arm of chromosome 13 (13q14.1). Osteosarcoma is the most common secondary malignancy in patients with hereditary retinoblastoma. Furthermore, these mutations also increase the risk for developing an irradiation-induced secondary osteosarcoma.

The *Bloom syndrome*, also known as *Bloom-German syndrome*, is an autosomal recessive disorder characterized by congenital telangiectatic erythema of the face resembling lupus erythematosus, dolichocephaly with malar hypoplasia, sensitivity to sunlight, low birth weight and well-proportional dwarfism, immunoglobulin deficiency, limb abnormalities (including syndactyly, polydactyly, and clinodactyly), and propensity for development of malignant tumors, particularly osteosarcoma. This syndrome has been attributed to the functional alteration of DNA-helicase gene *BLM* of the RecQ-family (*RECQL3*), located on chromosome band 15q26.1.

Secondary Osteosarcomas

In contrast to primary osteosarcomas, secondary lesions occur in an older population. Many of these tumors are responsible for the complications of Paget disease (osteitis deformans) and, characteristically, develop in pagetic bone (Fig. 21.47). The typical radiographic changes in malignant transformation of Paget disease include a destructive lesion in the affected bone, the presence of tumor bone in the lesion, and an associated soft-tissue mass. Osteosarcoma in these patients must be differentiated from metastases to pagetic bone from primary carcinomas elsewhere in the body (most commonly the prostate, breast, and kidney (see Fig. 29.30). Secondary osteosarcoma may also develop spontaneously in fibrous dysplasia or after radiation therapy for benign bone lesions such as fibrous dysplasia and

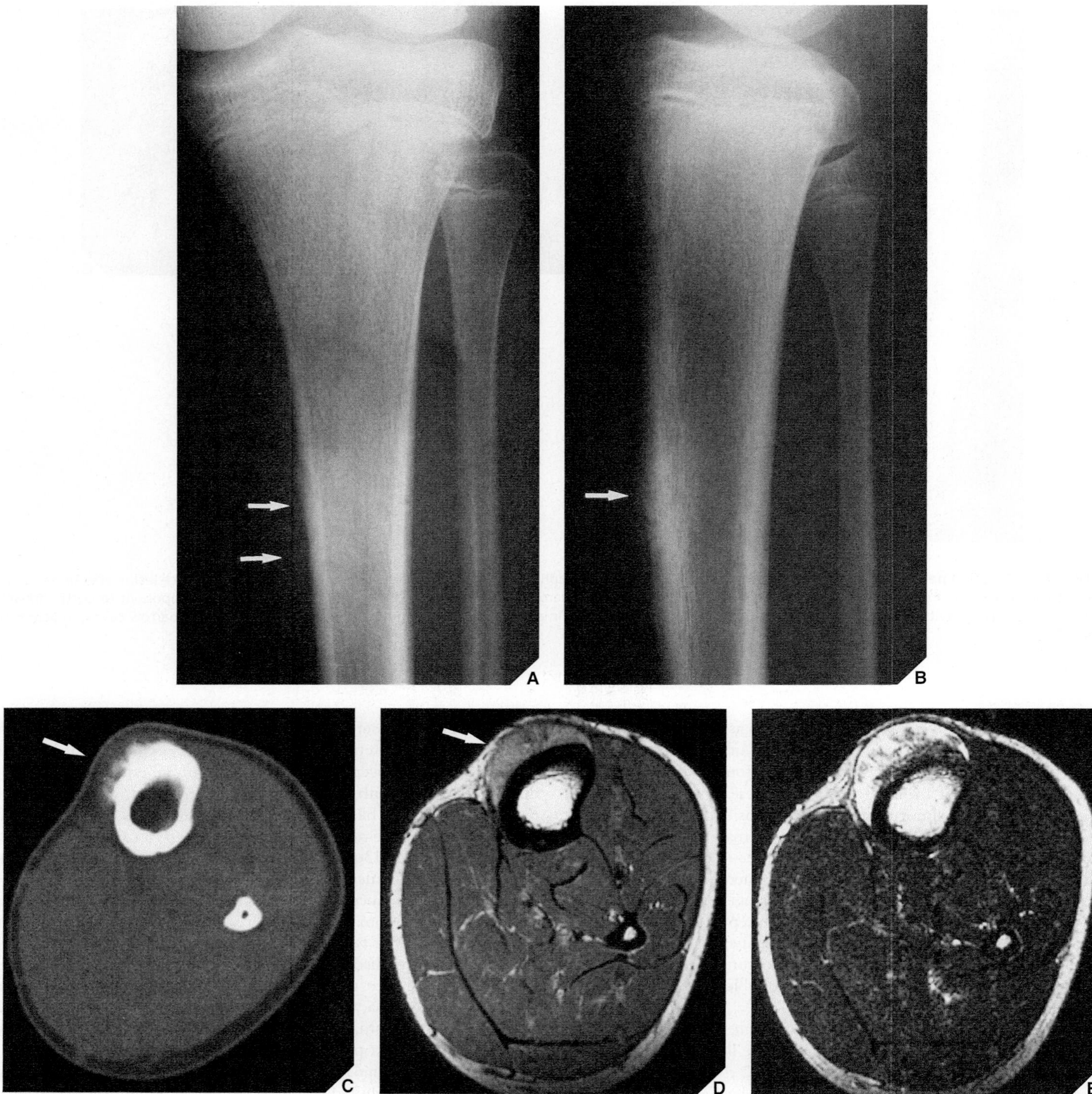

FIGURE 21.42 CT and MRI of periosteal osteosarcoma. **(A)** Anteroposterior and **(B)** lateral radiographs of the left leg of a 12-year-old boy show faint ossific densities on the anteromedial surface of the proximal tibia adjacent to the almost indistinct cortical destruction. An aggressive velvet type of periosteal reaction is evident *(arrows)*. **(C)** CT section through the tumor shows bone formation on the anterior surface of the tibia *(arrow)* and lack of invasion of the medullary cavity. **(D)** Axial spin echo (SE) T1-weighted MRI shows that tumor displays slightly higher signal than the muscles *(arrow)*. Note normal high signal of bone marrow. **(E)** On axial T2-weighted image (SE; repetition time [TR] 2000/echo time [TE] 80 msec), the mass becomes bright, except for the central areas at which bone formation displays low signal intensity.

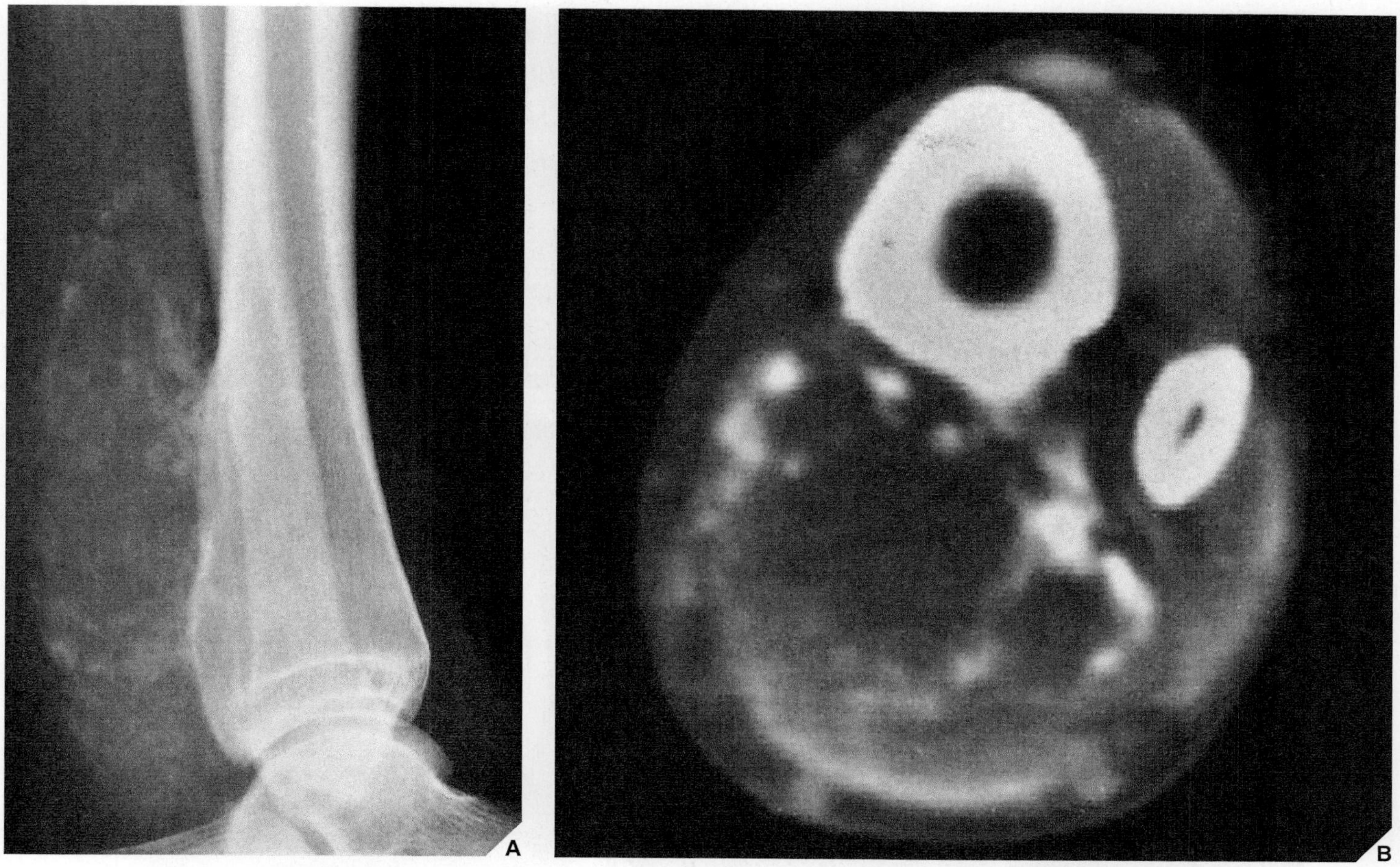

FIGURE 21.43 CT of high-grade surface osteosarcoma. **(A)** Lateral radiograph of the distal leg demonstrates a tumor attached to the posterior cortex of tibia in a 24-year-old man. Poorly defined ossific foci are seen within a large soft-tissue mass. Note the similarity of the tumor to periosteal osteosarcoma (see Figs. 21.29 and 21.30). **(B)** CT section demonstrates the extent of the lesion. Characteristically, the marrow cavity is not affected.

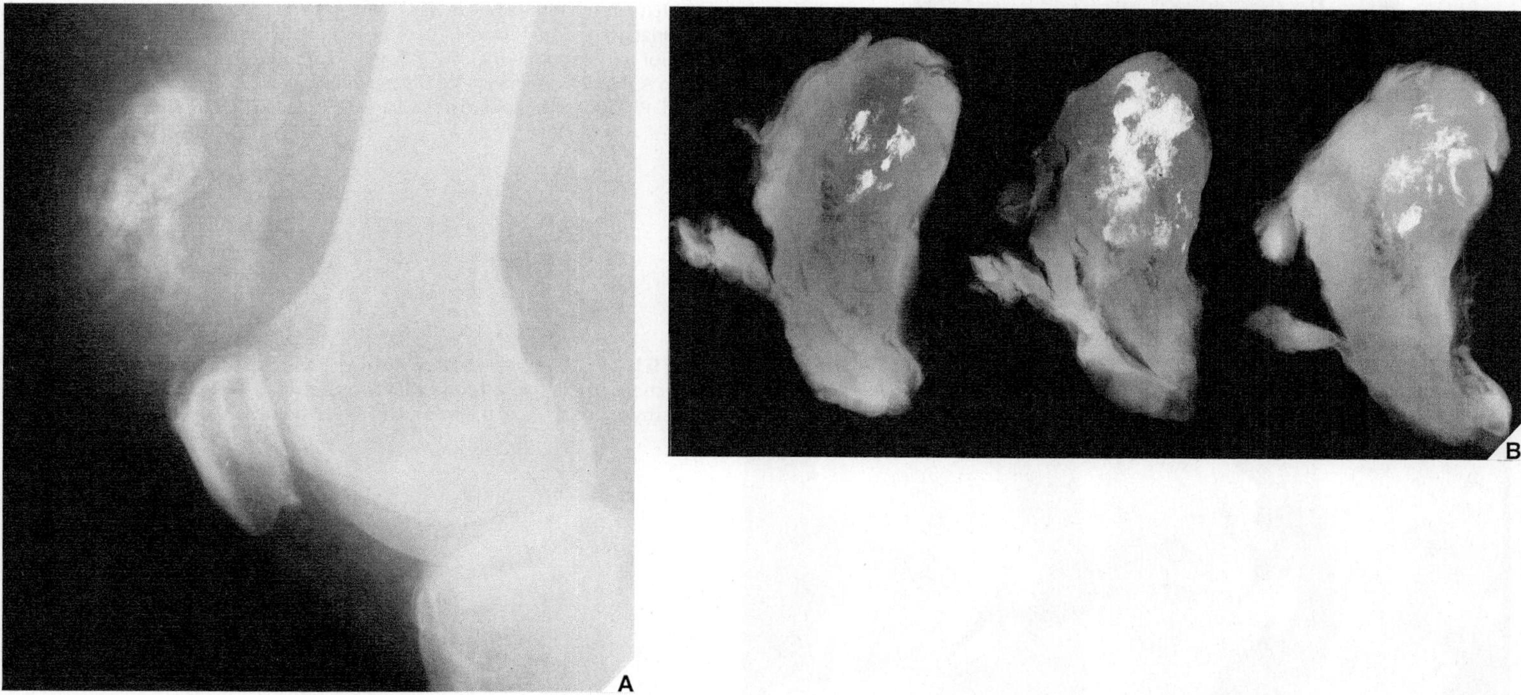

FIGURE 21.44 Soft-tissue osteosarcoma. **(A)** Lateral radiograph of the knee of a 51-year-old woman shows a poorly defined soft-tissue mass above the patella, merging with the quadriceps muscle. The center of the lesion exhibits amorphous calcifications and ossifications. **(B)** Radiograph of the resected specimen of the tumor reveals foci of ossifications in the center of the mass, surrounded by a radiolucent zone at the periphery (so-called *reverse zoning*). (Reprinted by permission from Springer: Greenspan A, Steiner G, Norman A, et al. Case report 436: osteosarcoma of the soft tissues of the distal end of the thigh. *Skeletal Radiol* 1987;16:489–492.)

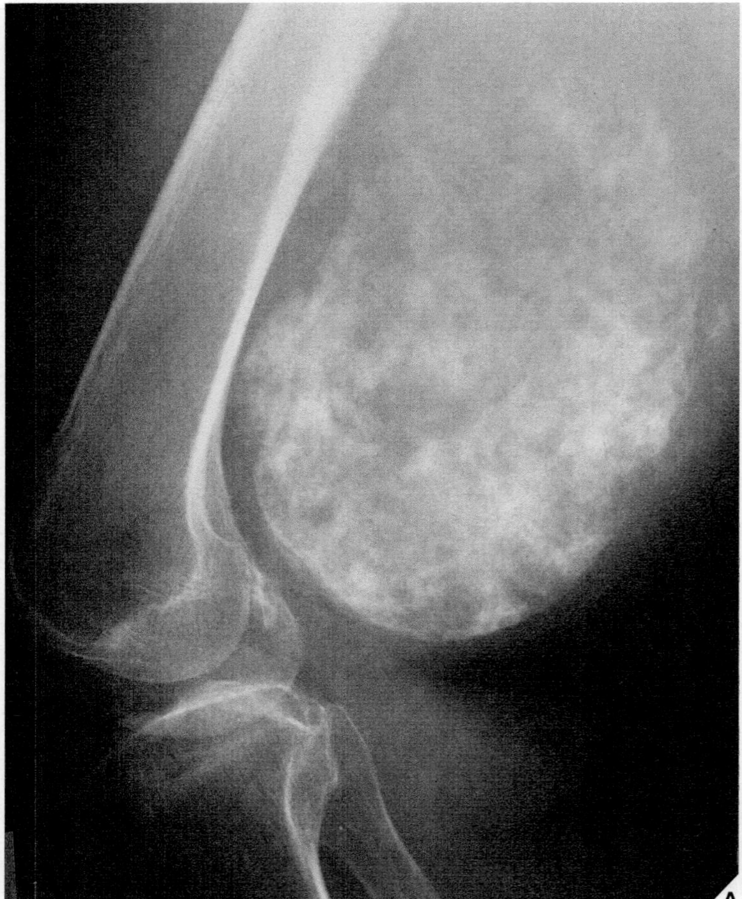

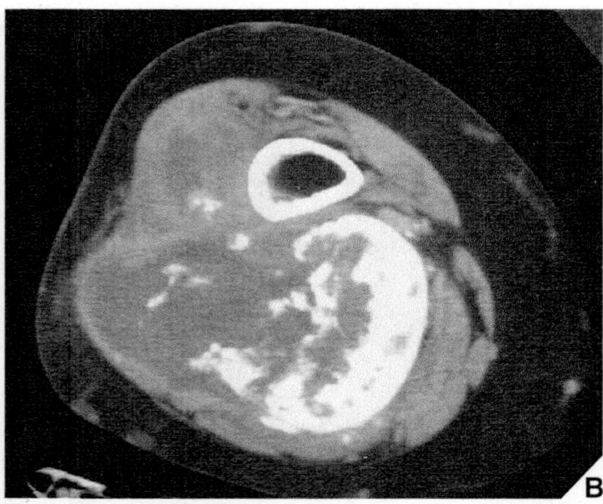

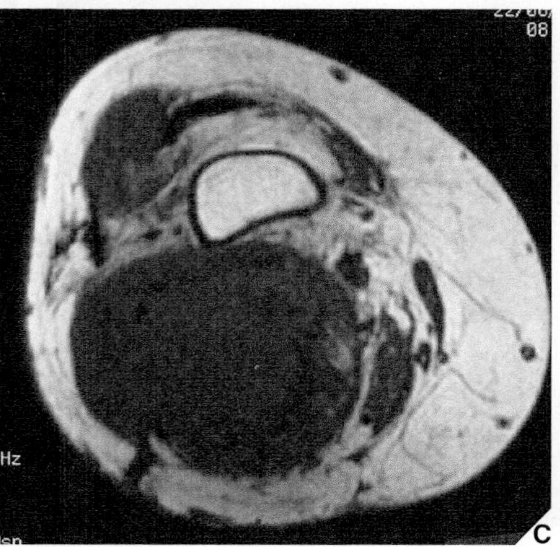

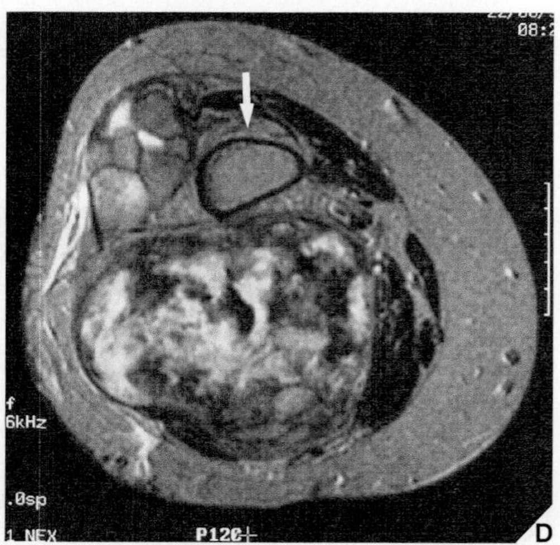

FIGURE 21.45 CT and MRI of soft-tissue osteosarcoma. A 68-year-old woman presented with a progressively enlarging soft-tissue mass in the popliteal region of the right knee. **(A)** Lateral radiograph shows a large soft-tissue mass, sharply outlined in its distal extent but poorly delineated at the proximal end. Calcifications and ossifications are present throughout the tumor. **(B)** Axial CT section reveals reverse zoning typical of soft-tissue osteosarcoma. **(C)** Axial T1-weighted MRI shows slightly heterogeneous mass exhibiting low signal intensity. **(D)** Axial T2-weighted MRI reveals marked heterogeneity of the tumor, displaying variation of signals from high to intermediate intensity. Note lack of involvement of femoral bone marrow *(arrow)*. (Reprinted with permission from Greenspan A, Jundt G, Remagen W. *Differential diagnosis in orthopaedic oncology*, 2nd ed. Philadelphia: Lippincott Williams & Wilkins; 2007:84–148, 212–249.)

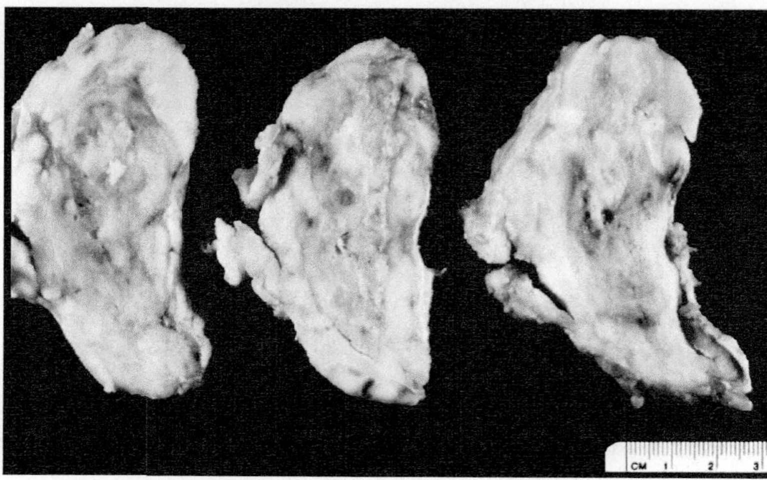

FIGURE 21.46 Pathology of soft-tissue osteosarcoma. Three slab sections of the tumor (same patient as depicted in Fig. 21.44) show gritty, fleshy appearance of the mass with foci of bone.

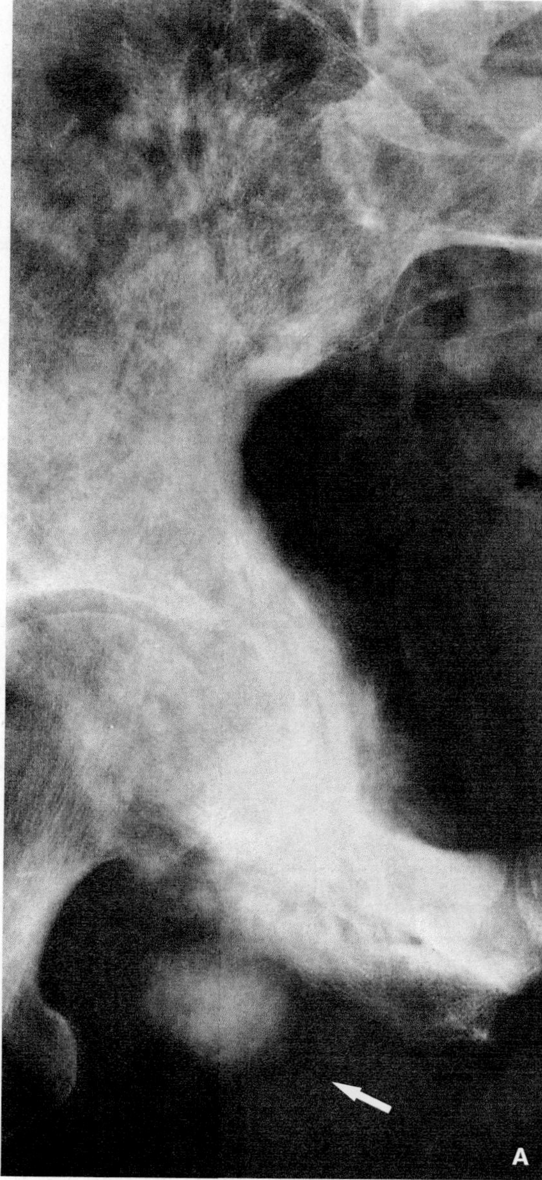

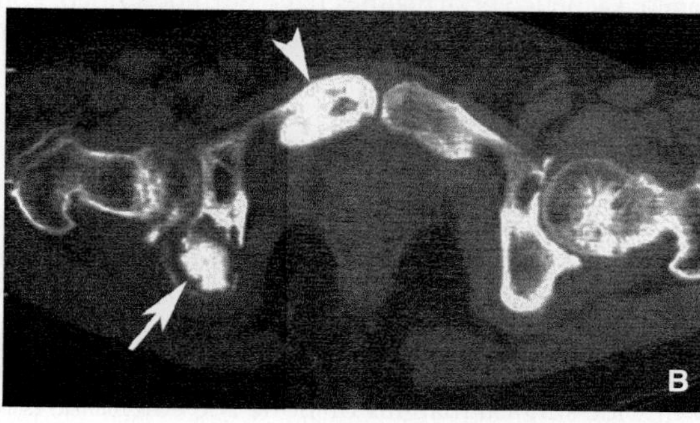

FIGURE 21.47 Secondary osteosarcoma. **(A)** Radiograph of a 66-year-old man who had extensive skeletal involvement by Paget disease and who had pain in the right hip shows the typical features of osteitis deformans in the right ilium and ischium. There is also destruction of the cortex associated with a soft-tissue mass containing tumor bone *(arrow)*—characteristic features of malignant transformation to osteosarcoma. **(B)** Secondary Paget osteosarcoma in the right ischial tuberosity in another patient. Axial CT image demonstrates a lytic lesion with osteoid matrix pubic ramus *(arrow)*. Note the cortical thickening and sclerosis on the inferior pubic ramus.

giant cell tumor as well as after irradiation of malignant processes in the soft tissues such as breast carcinoma and lymphoma. (For further discussion of malignant transformation, see the sections in Chapter 22 on Paget disease and radiation-induced sarcoma under the heading "Benign Conditions with Malignant Potential.")

Chondrosarcomas

Chondrosarcoma is a malignant bone tumor characterized by the formation of a cartilage matrix by tumor cells. As in osteosarcoma, there are several types of this tumor (Fig. 21.48), each with characteristic clinical, imaging, and pathologic features.

Primary Chondrosarcomas

Conventional Chondrosarcoma

Clinical and Imaging Features

Also known as *central* or *medullary chondrosarcoma,* this tumor is seen twice as frequently in males than in females and more commonly in adults, usually in those past their third decade. The most typical locations are the pelvis and long bones, particularly the femur and humerus (Fig. 21.49). Most conventional chondrosarcomas are slow-growing tumors, often discovered incidentally. Occasionally, local pain and tenderness may be present.

Radiographically, conventional chondrosarcoma appears as an expansive lesion in the medulla, with thickening of the cortex and characteristic deep endosteal scalloping; popcorn-like, annular or comma-shaped calcifications are seen in the medullary portion of the bone. A soft-tissue mass may sometimes be present (Figs. 21.50 and 21.51). In typical cases, conventional radiography is sufficient to make a diagnosis (Fig. 21.52). CT and MRI help delineate the extent of intraosseous and soft-tissue involvement (Figs. 21.53 to 21.59).

Pathology

Gross specimen shows translucent blue-gray or white in color mass, reflecting the presence of hyaline cartilage (Fig. 21.60). Lobular growth pattern is a consistent finding. There may be areas containing myxoid or mucoid material and cystic areas. Cortical thickening is almost always present. Erosion and destruction of the cortex with extension into the soft tissue may be present, especially in the pelvis, scapula, ribs, and sternum. The histopathologic hallmark is production of malignant cartilage by the tumor cells accompanied by infiltration of the marrow cavity and entrapment and permeation of preexisting bone trabeculae, and infiltration of Haversian systems. Present are varying in size and shape lobules of hyaline cartilage with areas of matrix mineralization in distinctive ring-and-arc–like pattern. The tissue is more cellular and pleomorphic in appearance than enchondroma and contains an appreciable number of plump cells, with large or double nuclei. Mitotic cells and necrosis can be present, particularly in high-grade tumors. Myxoid changes or chondroid matrix liquefaction is a common feature. The histologic distinction among low-grade, intermediate, and high-grade lesions is based on the cellularity of the tumor tissue, the degree of pleomorphism of the cells and nuclei, and the number of mitoses present. Some investigators (e.g., Unni) disregard the last feature in grading these tumors (Table 21.2).

Genetics of chondrosarcoma reveals that the most frequent numerical anomalies are loss of chromosomes 1, 6, 10, 13, 14, 15, and 22 and gain of chromosomes 2 and 20; also reported were rearrangements of chromosome bands 5q13, 1q21, 7p11, and 20q11.

Differential Diagnosis

In exceptional cases, particularly in the early stage of development, chondrosarcoma can be indistinguishable from an enchondroma. For this reason, all centrally located cartilage tumors in long bones, particularly in adult patients, should be regarded as malignant until proven otherwise. At the articular ends of the bone, chondrosarcomas frequently lack characteristic calcifications and may mimic a giant cell tumor.

Complications, Treatment, and Prognosis

Pathologic fractures through conventional chondrosarcomas are rare (Fig. 21.61). Moreover, conventional chondrosarcomas are slow-growing tumors, and only in rare cases do they metastasize to distant areas. Because they are not radiosensitive, surgical resection is the major means of

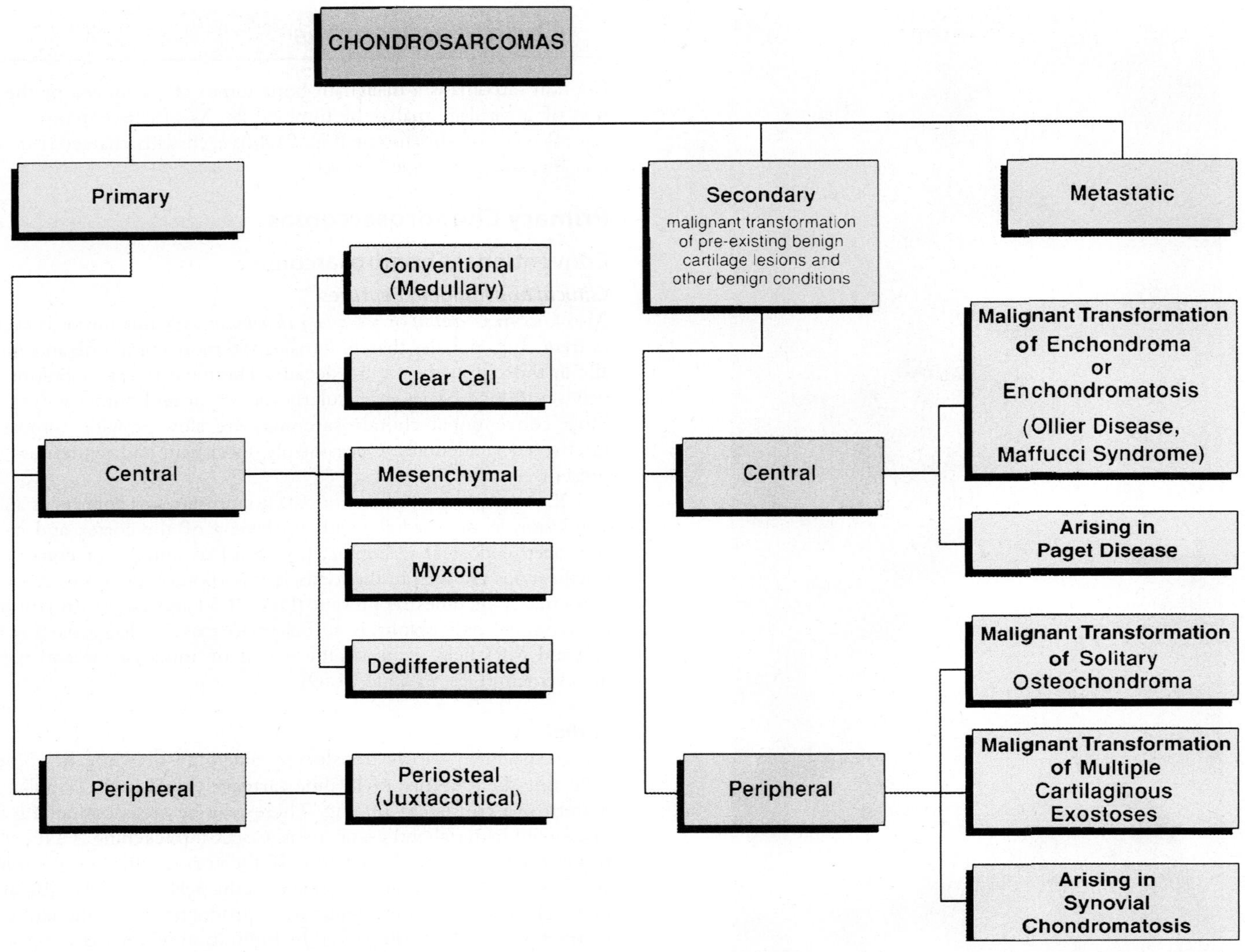

FIGURE 21.48 Classification of the types of chondrosarcoma.

therapy. Approximately 10% of tumors that recur have an increase in the degree of malignancy. Five-year survival is about 90% for patients with grade 1; the combined group of patients with grades 2 and 3 have a 5-year survival rate of 53%.

Clear Cell Chondrosarcoma

Clear cell chondrosarcoma is a rare (less than 4% of all chondrosarcomas in the Mayo Clinic series) variant of chondrosarcoma. First described by Unni and associates in 1976, it occurs twice as often in males than in females, usually in the third to fifth decades. It is predominantly a lytic lesion with a sclerotic border, which occasionally may contain calcifications. Many of these lesions resemble chondroblastomas or giant cell tumors, and many involve the proximal end of the humerus and femur (Figs. 21.62 and 21.63). Collins and colleagues reported MRI findings in 34 patients with pathologically documented cases of clear cell chondrosarcoma. The tumors revealed low signal intensity on T1-weighted sequences and moderately to significantly bright signal on T2 weighting. Heterogenic areas seen on T1- and T2-weighted images and on post-gadolinium T1-weighted images correlated pathologically to areas of mineralization, intralesional hemorrhage, and cystic changes within the tumor (Fig. 21.64).

Histologically, the clear cell variant exhibits larger and more rounded tumor cells than other chondrosarcomas with clear or vacuolated cytoplasm containing large amounts of glycogen. A chondroid matrix, trabeculae of reactive bone, and numerous osteoclast-like giant cells are distinctive features of this tumor. The tumor cells are positive for S-100 protein and type II collagen. Genetic abnormalities have been described, consisting of *CDKN2A*/p16 alterations, and loss or structural aberrations of chromosome 9 and gain of chromosome 20.

Treatment

Clear cell chondrosarcoma is considered a low-grade malignancy, although distant metastases have been reported. It has been managed in a variety of ways, from simple observation or curettage to wide resection and even amputation. Although it is a less aggressive tumor than conventional chondrosarcoma, inadequate treatment may lead to recurrence. Marginal excision or curettage results in high (about 86%) recurrence. Therefore, *en bloc* resection with wide surgical margins of bone and soft tissue is the current treatment of choice.

Mesenchymal Chondrosarcoma

Mesenchymal chondrosarcoma is very uncommon (less than 1% of all malignant bone tumors) and tends to occur in the patient's second or third decade. It presents radiographically with the permeative type of bone destruction seen in round cell tumors, and calcifications in the cartilaginous portion of the tumor (Fig. 21.65). It may be indistinguishable from conventional chondrosarcoma and is a highly malignant lesion with a strong capacity for metastases. Most common locations are craniofacial bones (mandible and maxilla), ribs, femur, fibula, ilium, and vertebrae. About 30% of cases develop in extraskeletal site. The tumor shows tendency toward local recurrence, and distant metastases were observed even after a delay of more than 20 years.

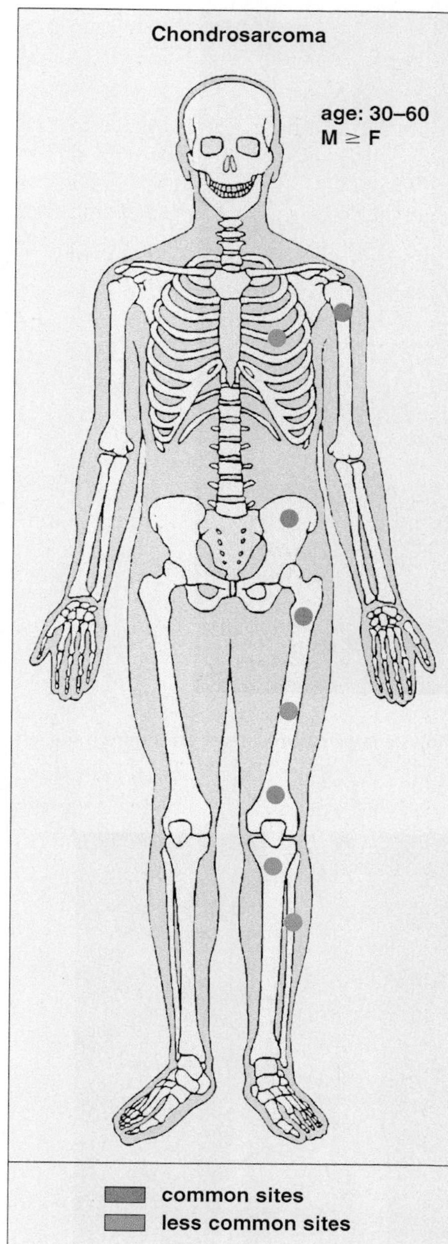

FIGURE 21.49 Skeletal sites of predilection, peak age range, and male-to-female ratio in conventional chondrosarcoma.

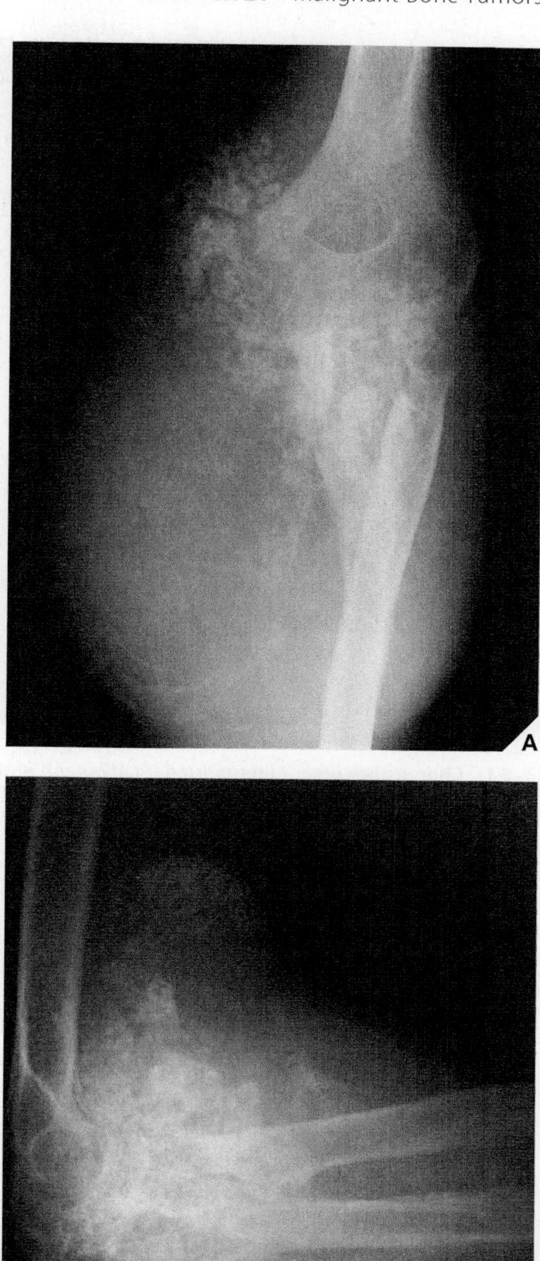

FIGURE 21.50 Chondrosarcoma. **(A)** Anteroposterior and **(B)** lateral radiographs of the right elbow in a 55-year-old man show a tumor arising from the proximal ulna. Note a huge soft-tissue mass containing chondroid calcifications.

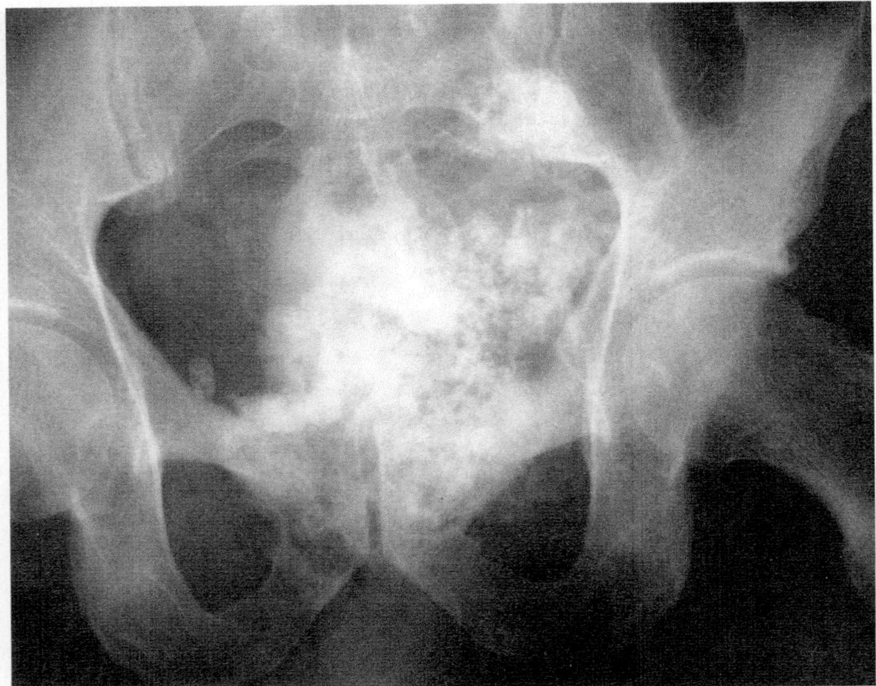

FIGURE 21.51 Chondrosarcoma. Anteroposterior radiograph of the pelvis in a 52-year-old man shows a large calcified mass arising from the left pubic bone and extending into the pelvic cavity.

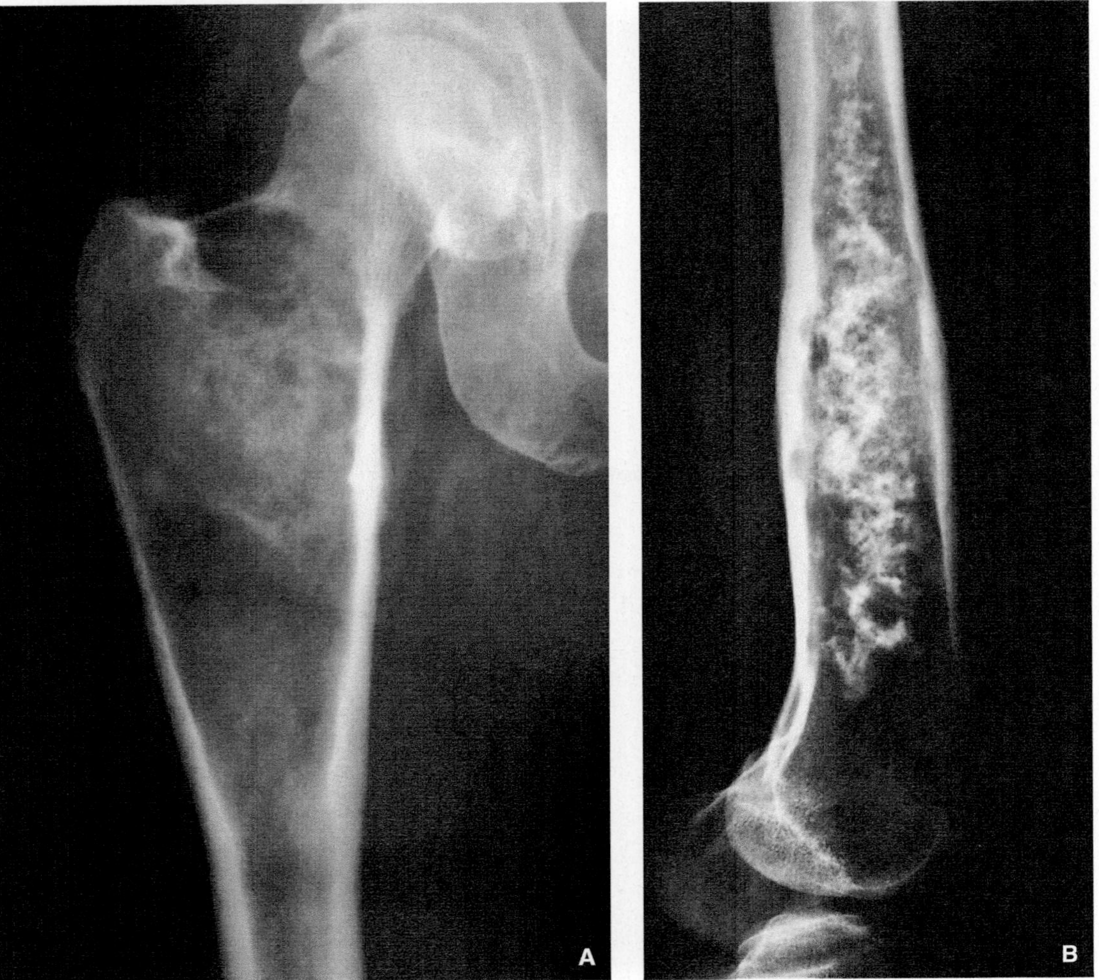

FIGURE 21.52 Chondrosarcoma. **(A)** Anteroposterior radiograph of the proximal right femur of a 66-year-old woman shows a radiolucent lesion containing chondroid calcifications. Although the tumor did not penetrate the cortex, the medial cortex is thickened. **(B)** Lateral radiograph of the distal femur of a 46-year-old man shows the characteristic features of a central chondrosarcoma. Within the destructive lesion in the medullary portion of the bone noted are annular and comma-shaped calcifications. The thickened cortex, which is caused by periosteal new bone formation in response to destruction of the cortex by the chondroblastic tumor, shows the typical deep endosteal scalloping.

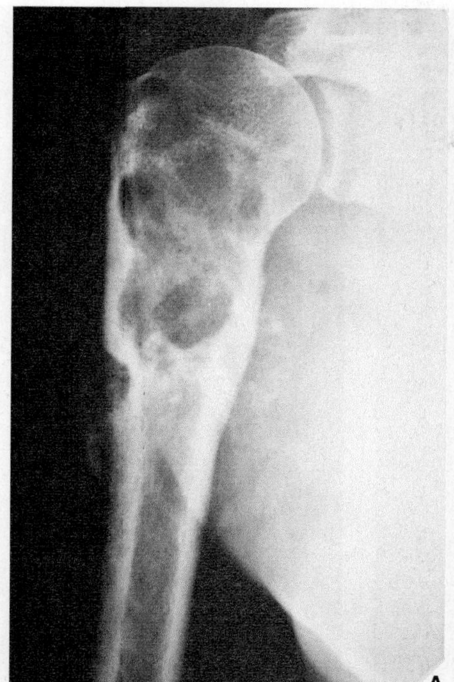

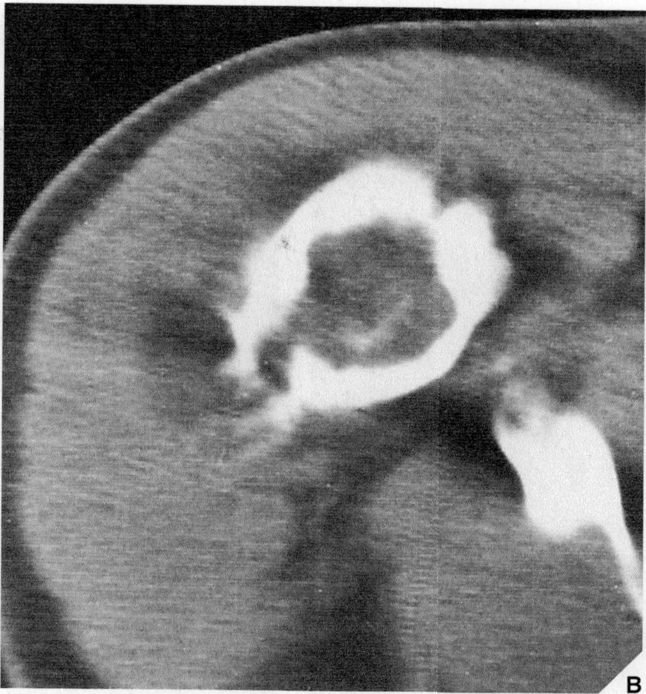

FIGURE 21.53 CT of chondrosarcoma. **(A)** Anteroposterior radiograph of the right shoulder of a 62-year-old man is not adequate for demonstrating the soft-tissue extension of the chondrosarcoma in the proximal humerus. **(B)** CT section through the lesion demonstrates cortical destruction and a large soft-tissue mass.

Histologically, the mesenchymal variant demonstrates a high degree of malignancy, typified by bimorphic pattern. The tumor is composed of more or less differentiated cartilage, together with highly vascular stroma of mesenchymal tissue containing spindle cells and round cells. Round cell component is positive for CD99, and cartilaginous component is positive for S-100 protein.

Genetic abnormalities were reported, in particular recurrent HEY1-NCOA2 fusion.

Myxoid Chondrosarcoma

Also known as *chordoid sarcoma*, it is a very rare (representing about 12% of all chondrosarcomas of bone) low-grade but locally aggressive malignant neoplasm showing chondroid differentiation. The age range of occurrence is wide, between 9 and 76 years, and males are predominantly affected. Clinically, it presents as a painful mass. Although the femur is most commonly affected (about 50% of reported cases), the tumor may involve the other bones (Fig. 21.66). Imaging shows a radiolucent, lobulated, sharply circumscribed lesion, commonly extending into the soft tissues (Fig. 21.67). Pathologic gross specimen shows a lobulated, frequently hemorrhagic mass braking from the bone into the soft tissues (Fig. 21.68). Histopathology shows lobulated cartilaginous nodules with round stellate cells, some with acidophilic cytoplasm, and abundant myxoid matrix. Occasionally, mitotic figures are present.

Dedifferentiated Chondrosarcoma

First described by Dahlin and Beabout in 1971, dedifferentiated chondrosarcoma is the most malignant of all chondrosarcomas and consequently carries a very poor prognosis; most patients die from the disease within 2 years of diagnosis. The patient typically has pain of long duration, followed by a more recent onset of rapid swelling and local tenderness. The prolonged pain probably reflects a slow-growing lesion, and the swelling and tenderness may be related to the development of a rapidly growing, more malignant component. The hallmark of this lesion is the appearance of an aggressive sarcoma engrafted on a benign chondral lesion or on a benign-appearing low-grade chondrosarcoma. Although it may radiographically resemble a conventional chondrosarcoma, its histologic composition differs. The dedifferentiated tissue may appear to be a fibrosarcoma, an MFH, or an osteosarcoma.

Radiographically, dedifferentiated chondrosarcomas exhibit calcific foci with aggressive bone destruction and are often accompanied by a large soft-tissue mass (Figs. 21.69 and 21.70). MRI findings of dedifferentiated chondrosarcoma, as reported by MacSweeney and associates, consist of three distinct patterns (Fig. 21.71). In one group of patients, clear demarcation was seen on T2-weighted images between the low-grade tumor that exhibited high signal intensity and the high-grade tumor that showed relatively reduced signal, a so-called *biphasic pattern*. In another group of patients, the only MRI evidence of an underlying chondroid lesion was the presence of several areas of signal void corresponding to matrix mineralization identified on the conventional radiography. The third MRI pattern consisted of relatively lower signal intensity of the tumor, accompanied by smaller areas revealing high signal and fluid–fluid levels on T2 weighting, presumably caused by tumor necrosis rather than chondroid tissue.

Gross pathologic specimen shows cartilaginous and noncartilaginous components in varying proportions (Figs. 21.72 to 21.75). Histologically, dedifferentiated chondrosarcoma often shows a cartilaginous component of low-grade malignancy combined with highly cellular sarcomatous tissue. MFH is the most frequent component of the high-grade sarcoma.

Genetic abnormalities reported in the literature consisted of structural and numerical aberrations of chromosomes 1 and 9. Heterozygous mutations of the isocitrate dehydrogenase 1 and 2 genes were found in both components in approximately 50% of these tumors.

Recently, the validity of the term *dedifferentiation* has been challenged. Studies using electron microscopy and immunohistochemistry indicate that sarcomatous dedifferentiation represents, in fact, the synchronous differentiation of separate clones of cells from a primitive spindle-cell sarcoma to various types of sarcoma.

Periosteal (Juxtacortical) Chondrosarcoma

This tumor originating in periosteal location accounts for about 4% of all malignant cartilage lesions. Adults in the third and fourth decade of life are most commonly affected, and there is slight male predilection. Long bones,

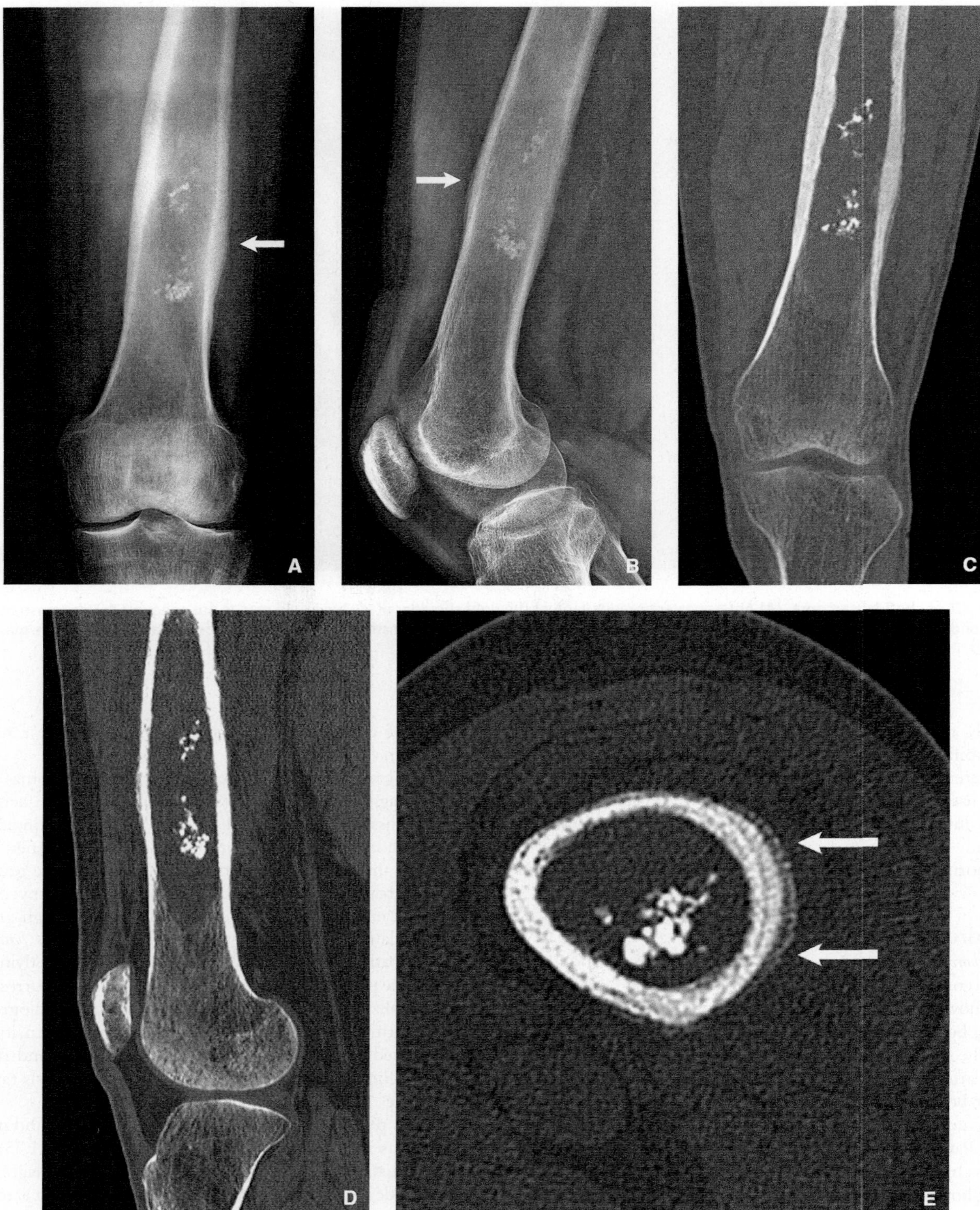

FIGURE 21.54 CT of chondrosarcoma. **(A)** Anteroposterior and **(B)** lateral radiographs of the left distal femur show a radiolucent lesion expanding the bone with chondroid calcifications, associated with cortical thickening and periosteal reaction *(arrows)*. **(C)** Coronal, **(D)** sagittal, and **(E)** axial CT images demonstrate cortical thickening and periosteal reaction *(arrows)* to better advantage. (Reprinted with permission from Greenspan A, Borys D. *Radiology and pathology correlation of bone tumors: a quick reference and review*. Philadelphia: Wolters Kluwer, 2016:144, Fig. 3.76.)

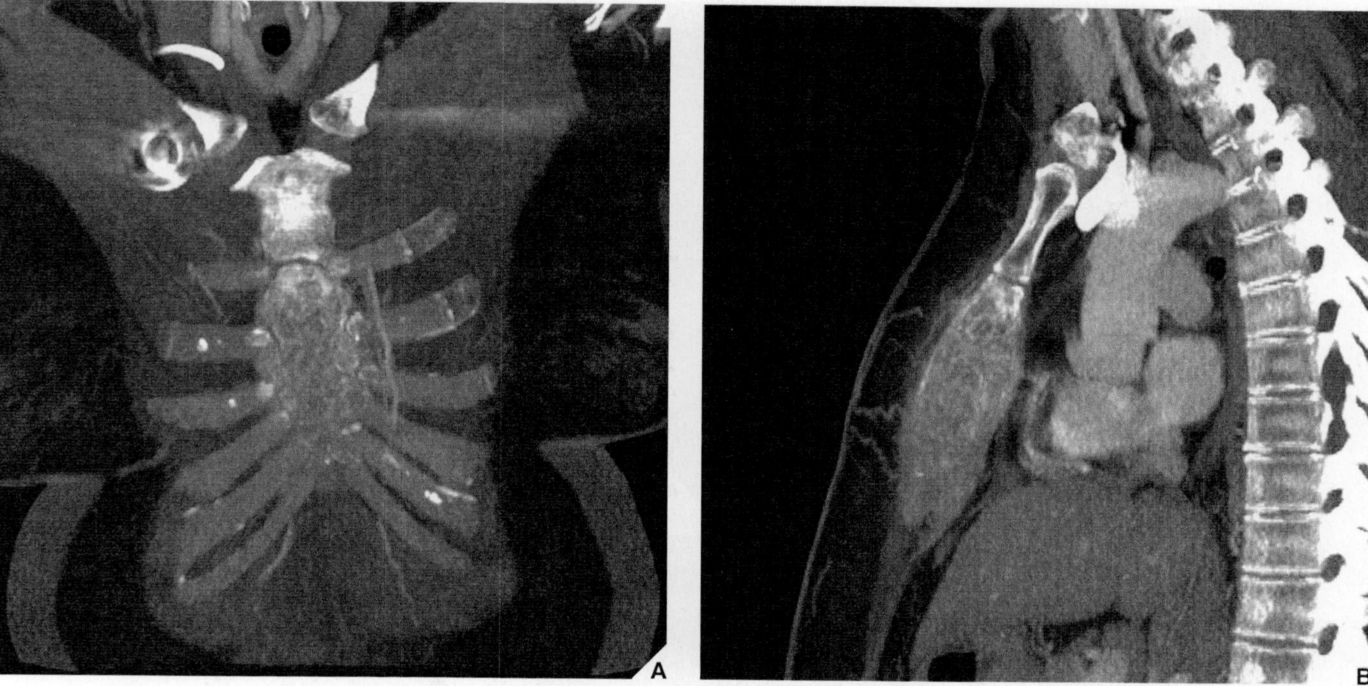

FIGURE 21.55 CT of chondrosarcoma. **(A)** Coronal and **(B)** sagittal reformatted CT images of the chest of a 50-year-old man show an expansive osteolytic lesion within the body of the sternum containing typical chondroid calcifications.

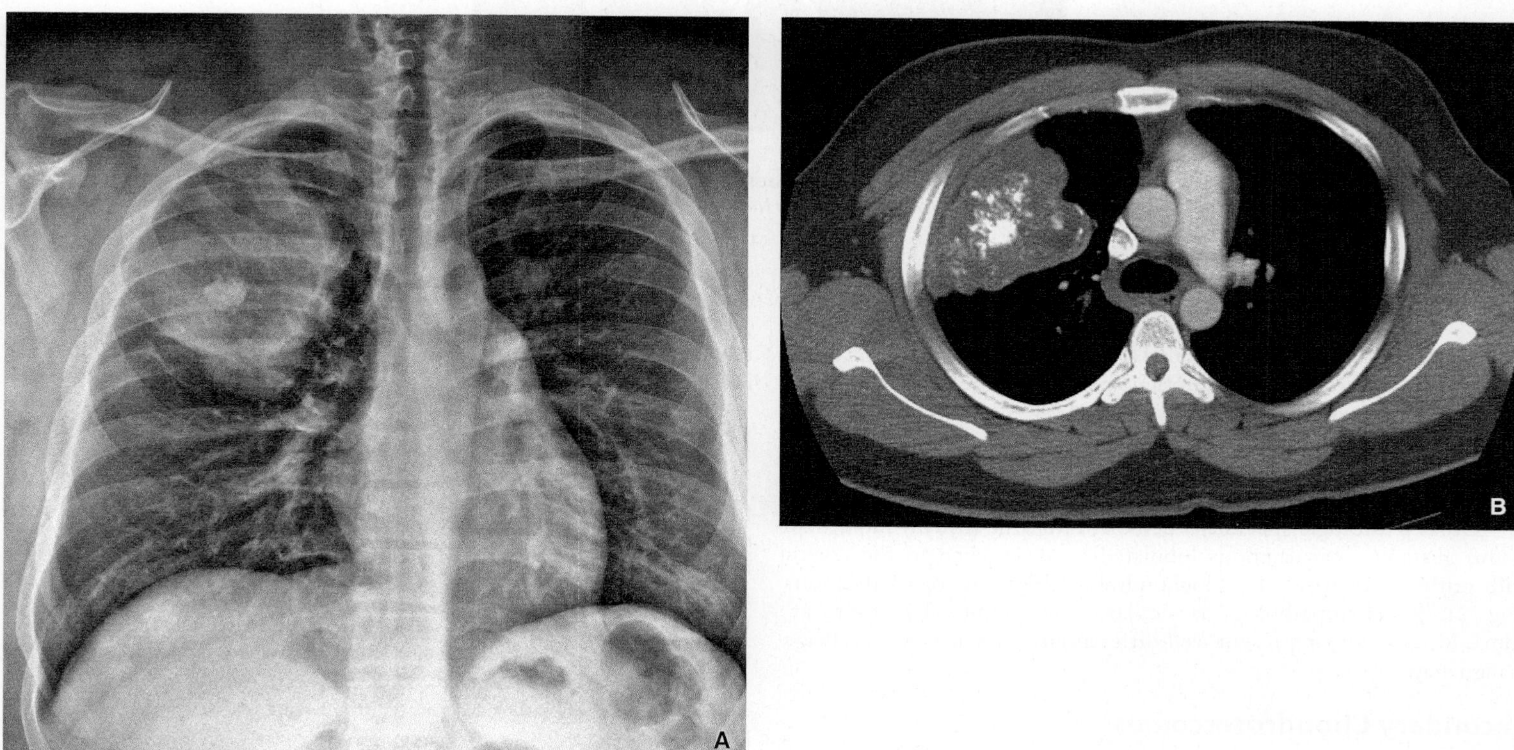

FIGURE 21.56 CT of chondrosarcoma. **(A)** Posteroanterior radiograph of the chest of a 20-year-old man shows a large mass with central chondroid calcifications overlying the right upper lobe. **(B)** Axial CT image shows a large lobulated mass containing chondroid calcifications, arising from and destroying the right third rib, and compressing the upper lobe of the right lung.

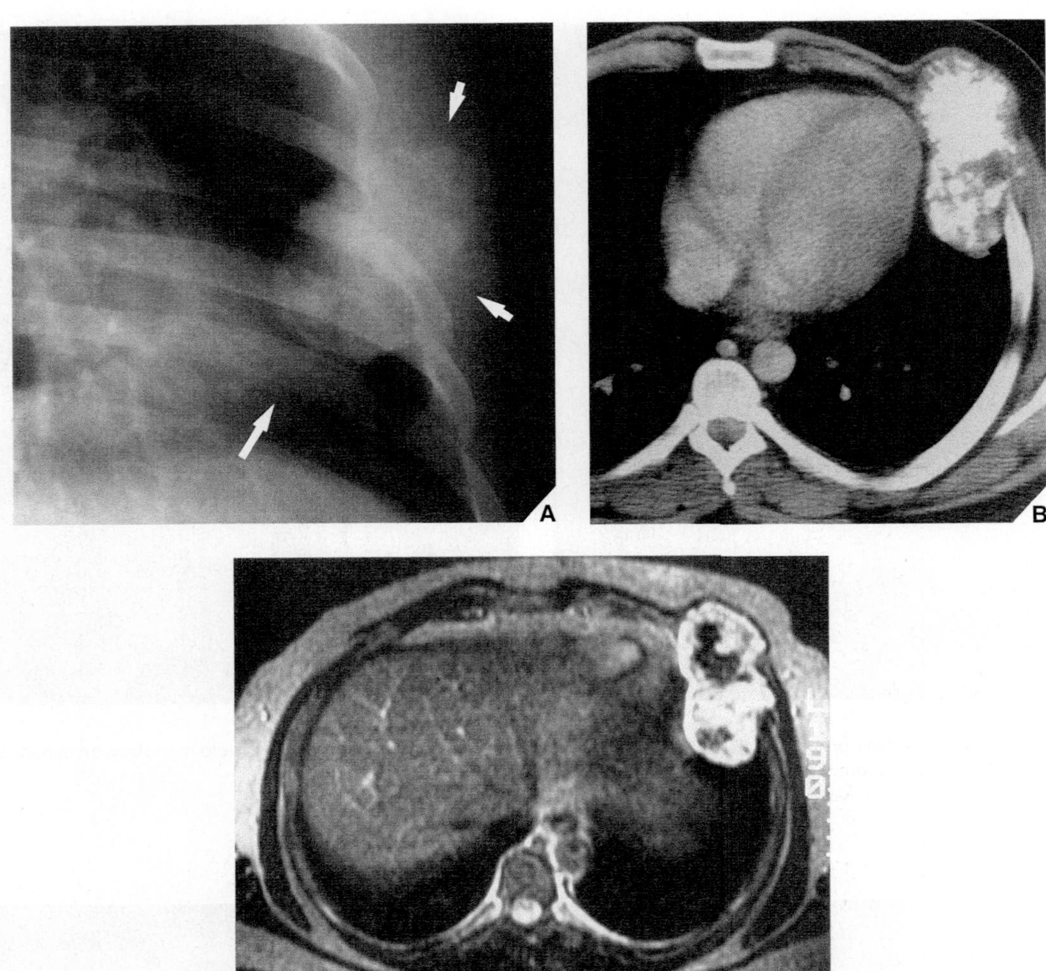

FIGURE 21.57 CT and MRI of chondrosarcoma. **(A)** A large calcified mass arises from the left anterior sixth rib *(arrows)*. **(B)** Axial CT section reveals destruction of the rib and intrathoracic and extrathoracic extension of tumor. **(C)** Axial T2-weighted MRI demonstrates heterogeneity of the tumor. Areas of low-intensity signal represent calcified portions of the mass.

particularly the distal femur, and spine are most common sites of involvement. Generally, periosteal chondrosarcoma has the same imaging features as central chondrosarcoma (Figs. 21.76 to 21.78). Because the lesion appears on the bone surface, it must be distinguished from periosteal osteosarcoma. The differentiation of this lesion may create problems for the radiologist and pathologist alike.

Gross pathologic specimens demonstrate large (usually more than 5 cm) glistening cartilaginous lobulated mass attached to the cortex with gritty white areas of endochondral calcifications or ossifications (Fig. 21.79). Histopathology is similar to conventional chondrosarcoma. Most lesions represent well-differentiated grade 1 or 2 cartilage malignancy.

Secondary Chondrosarcomas

The most common types of secondary chondrosarcomas are tumors developing in preexisting enchondromas or in multiple cartilaginous exostoses (see Figs. 18.52 and 18.62). Extremely rarely a solitary osteochondroma may undergo malignant transformation to chondrosarcoma (Fig. 21.80). These tumors develop in a slightly younger age group (age 20 to 40 years) than primary chondrosarcomas and have a more benign course. Because they are usually of low-grade malignancy, the prognosis is more favorable than in conventional chondrosarcoma. Total excision is the treatment of choice. (For further discussion of malignant transformation, see the sections under the heading “Benign Conditions with Malignant Potential” in Chapter 22.)

Soft-Tissue (Extraskeletal) Chondrosarcomas

These are very rare tumors, accounting for less than 3% of all soft-tissue sarcomas. They occur within deep soft tissues of the proximal extremities and limb girdles. Most common location is the thigh, followed by trunk, paraspinal region, foot, popliteal fossa, buttocks, and neck. Radiography shows soft-tissue mass with central chondroid calcifications, similar to conventional chondrosarcoma, in focal or uniform distribution (Fig. 21.81). Occasionally, soft-tissue mass may be present without prominent calcifications (Fig. 21.82). Scintigraphy shows increased uptake of radiopharmaceutical tracer. MRI shows the mass to be isointense with the muscles on T1-weighted sequences and of high signal intensity on T2 weighting and other water-sensitive sequences. On images obtained after intravenous administration of gadolinium, there is heterogenous enhancement of the tumor. Histopathology shows multinodular architecture with well-circumscribed pale-blue myxoid or chondromyxoid stroma separated by fibrous septa. Hyaline cartilage is rarely present. Undifferentiated mesenchymal tumor cells have uniform round to oval nuclei and fair amount of eosinophilic granular or vacuolated cytoplasm. The differential diagnosis should include myositis ossificans and soft-tissue osteosarcoma.

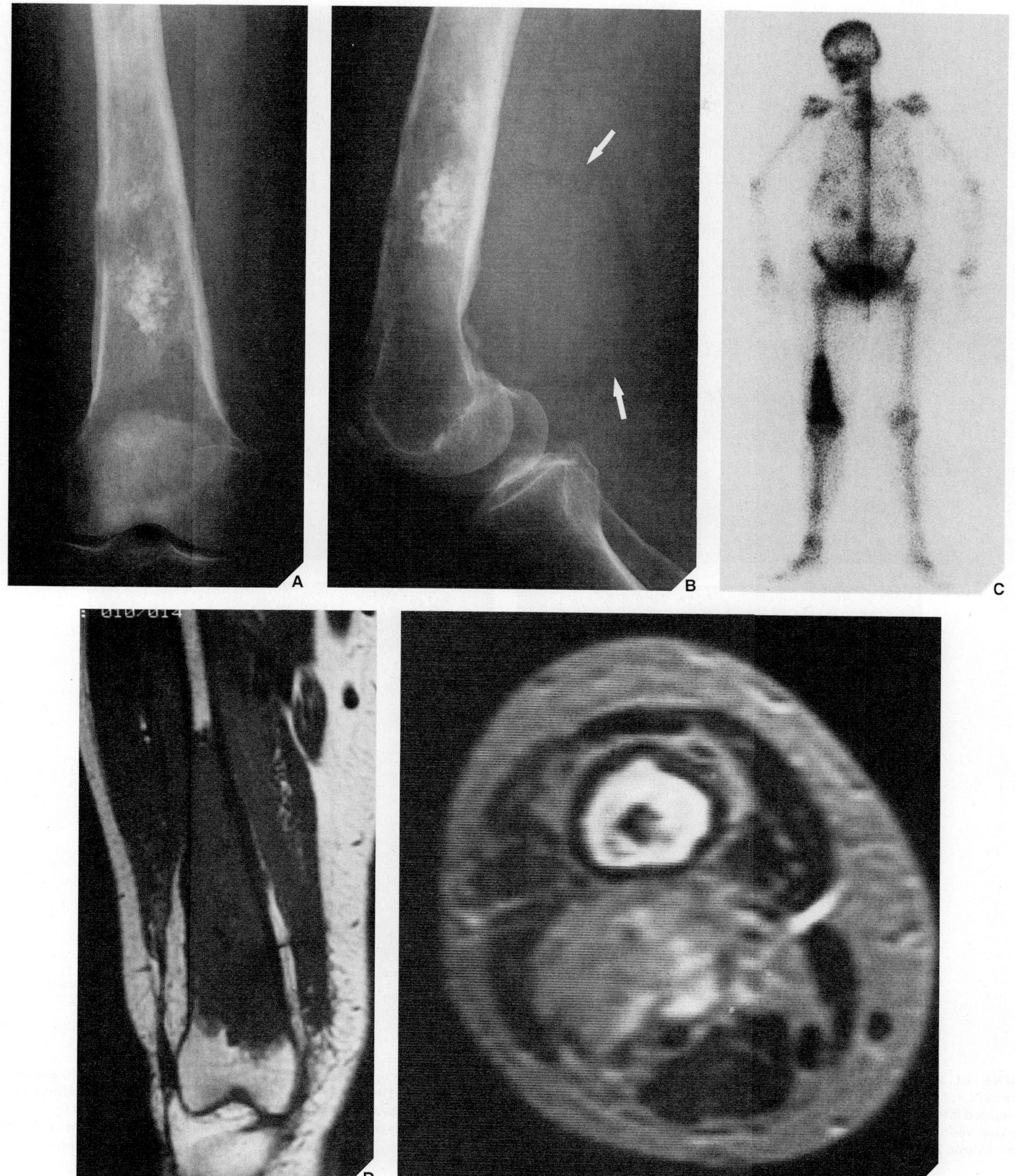

FIGURE 21.58 Scintigraphy and MRI of chondrosarcoma. **(A)** Anteroposterior and **(B)** lateral radiographs of the distal femur show typical appearance of central medullary chondrosarcoma. The cortex is destroyed, and there is a large soft-tissue mass projecting posteriorly *(arrows)*. **(C)** Radionuclide bone scan obtained after intravenous injection of 15 mCi (555 MBq) of technetium-99m (^{99m}Tc)-labeled methylene diphosphonate (MDP) shows increased uptake of tracer localized to the site of the tumor. **(D)** Coronal T1-weighted (spin echo [SE]; repetition time [TR] 700/TE 20 msec) MR image shows the tumor to be of intermediate-to-low signal intensity. The calcifications display signal void. **(E)** Axial T2-weighted (SE; TR 2000/TE 80 msec) image shows intramedullary tumor displaying a high signal intensity, whereas calcifications are of low signal. The soft-tissue mass shows heterogeneous signal.

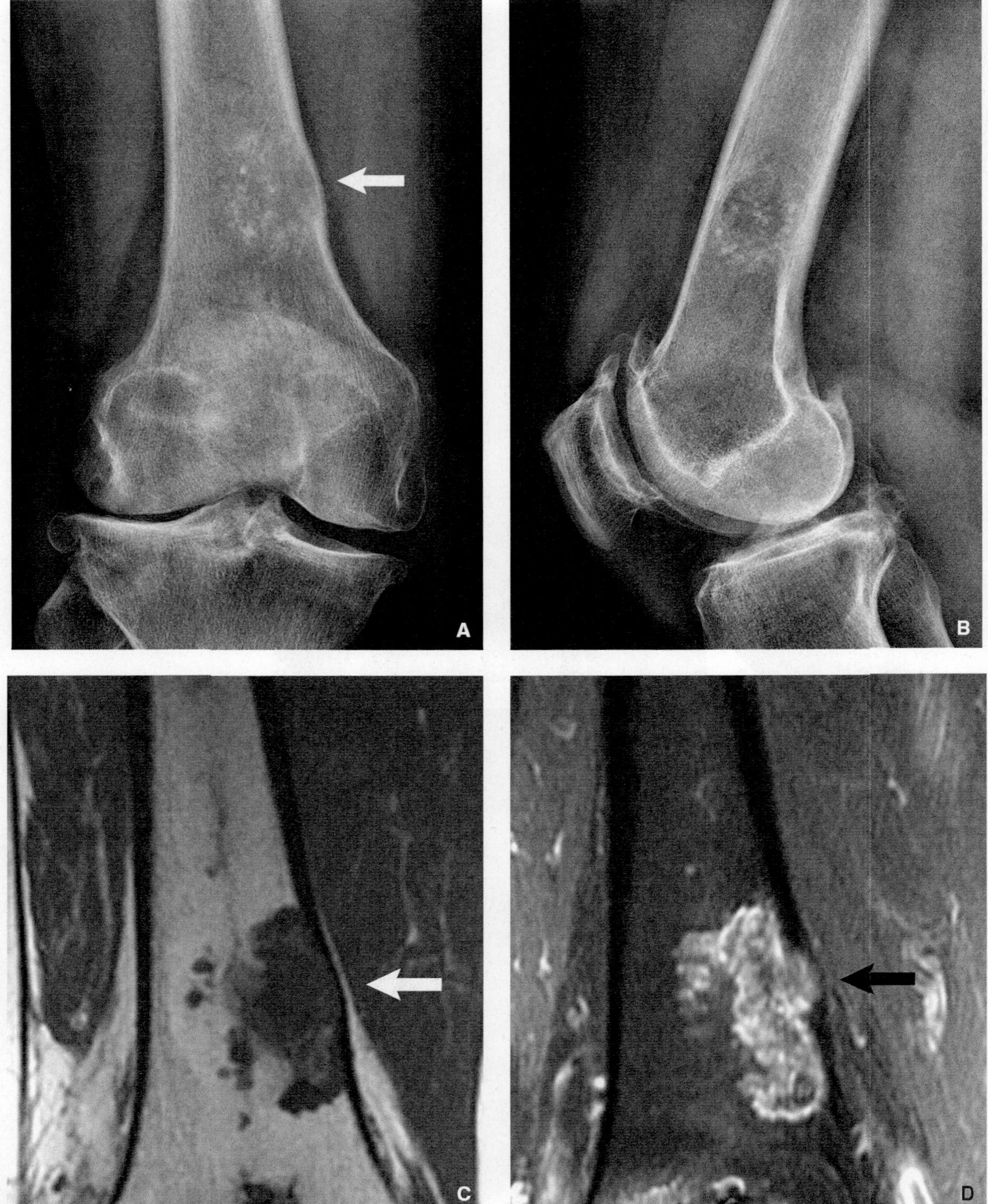

FIGURE 21.59 MRI of chondrosarcoma. **(A)** Anteroposterior and **(B)** lateral radiographs of the right knee of a 58-year-old woman show a radiolucent lesion with chondroid calcifications in the medullary portion of the distal femur. Note deep endosteal scalloping of the medial cortex *(arrow)*. **(C)** Coronal T1-weighted and **(D)** coronal T1-weighted fat-suppressed postcontrast MR images demonstrate the endosteal scalloping to better advantage *(arrows)*. Observe heterogenous signal of the tumor due to chondroid calcifications. (Reprinted with permission from Greenspan A, Borys D. *Radiology and pathology correlation of bone tumors: a quick reference and review*. Philadelphia: Wolters Kluwer; 2016:146, Fig. 3.79.)

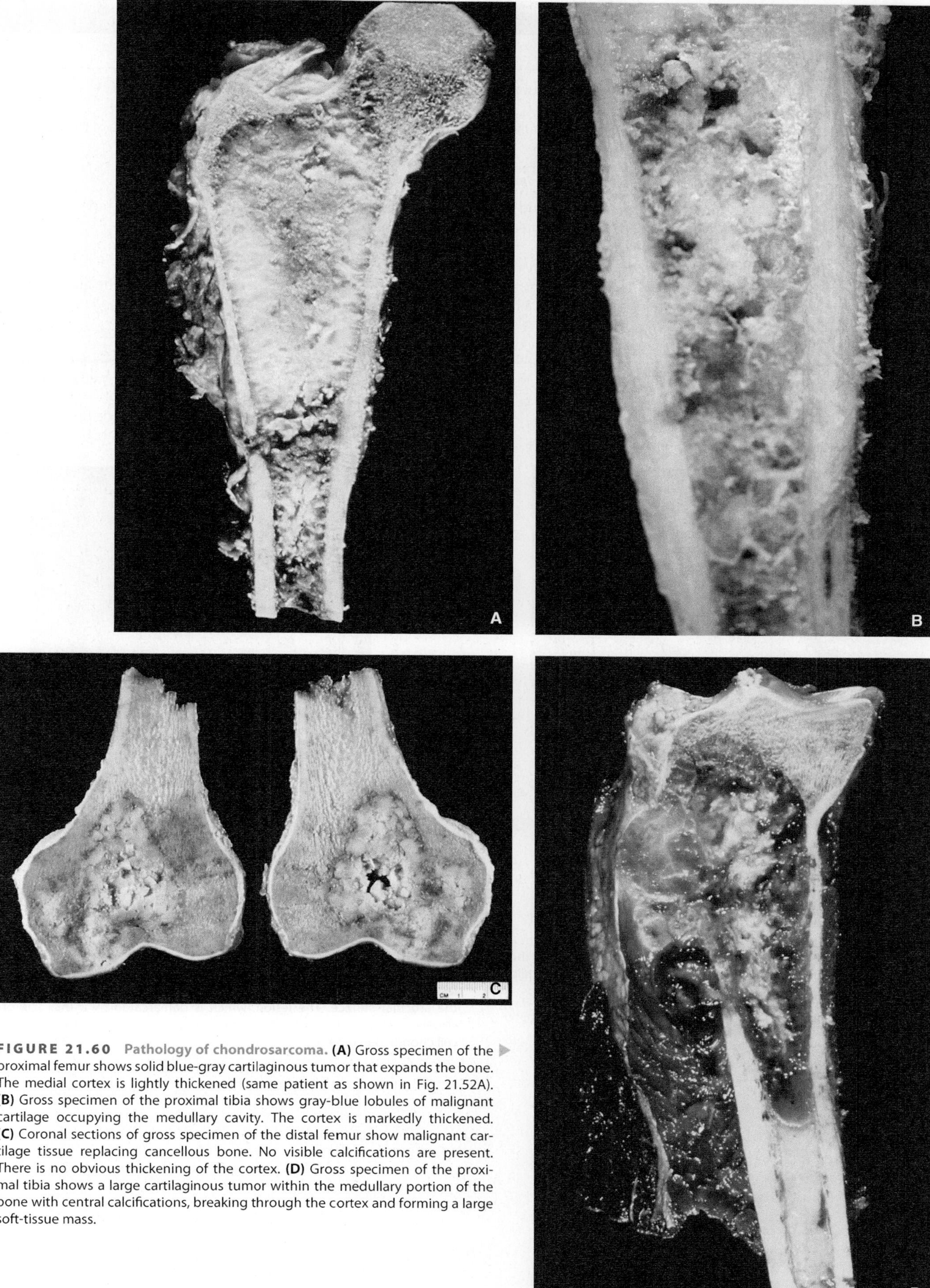

FIGURE 21.60 Pathology of chondrosarcoma. **(A)** Gross specimen of the proximal femur shows solid blue-gray cartilaginous tumor that expands the bone. The medial cortex is lightly thickened (same patient as shown in Fig. 21.52A). **(B)** Gross specimen of the proximal tibia shows gray-blue lobules of malignant cartilage occupying the medullary cavity. The cortex is markedly thickened. **(C)** Coronal sections of gross specimen of the distal femur show malignant cartilage tissue replacing cancellous bone. No visible calcifications are present. There is no obvious thickening of the cortex. **(D)** Gross specimen of the proximal tibia shows a large cartilaginous tumor within the medullary portion of the bone with central calcifications, breaking through the cortex and forming a large soft-tissue mass.

TABLE 21.2 Histologic Grading of Chondrosarcoma

Grade	Histologic Features
0.5 (borderline)	Histologic features similar to enchondroma, but imaging features more aggressive
1 (low grade)	Cellularity: slightly increased Cytologic atypia: slight increase in size and variation in shape of the nuclei; slightly increased hyperchromasia of the nuclei Binucleation: few binucleate cells are present Stromal myxoid change: may or may not be present
2 (intermediate)	Cellularity: moderately increased Cytologic atypia: moderate increase in size and variation in shape of the nuclei; moderately increased hyperchromasia of the nuclei Binucleation: large number of double-nucleated and trinucleated cells Stromal myxoid change: focally present
3 (high grade)	Cellularity: markedly increased Cytologic atypia: marked enlargement and irregularity of the nuclei; markedly increased hyperchromasia of the nuclei Binucleation: large number of double- and multinucleated cells Stromal myxoid change: commonly present Other: small foci of spindling at the periphery of the lobules of chondrocytes; foci of necrosis present

Modified from Dahlin DC. Grading of bone tumors. In: Unni KK, ed. *Bone tumors*. New York: Churchill Livingstone; 1988:35–45. Copyright © 1988 Elsevier. With permission.

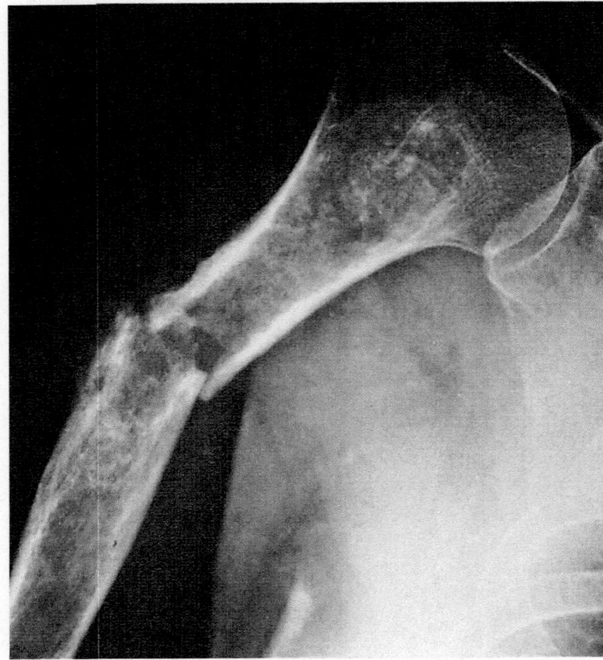

FIGURE 21.61 **Complication of chondrosarcoma.** Pathologic fracture through a tumor, as seen here in the right humerus in a 60-year-old man, is a rare complication of this lesion.

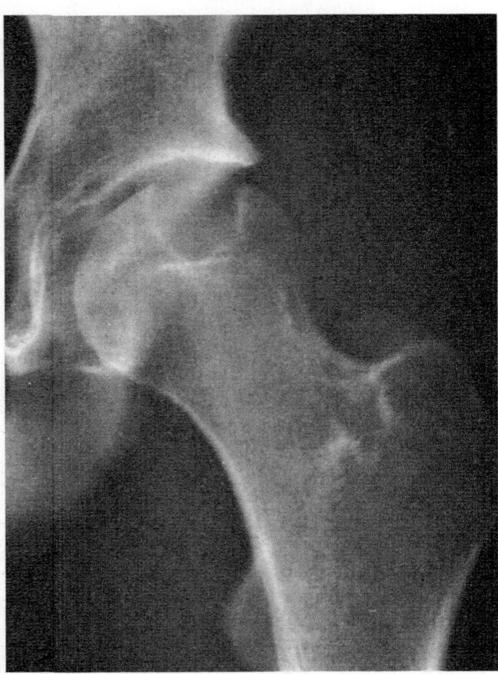

FIGURE 21.62 **Clear cell chondrosarcoma.** A 22-year-old man presented with left hip pain for 3 months. Anteroposterior radiograph demonstrates an osteolytic lesion located in the superolateral aspect of the femoral head and extending into the articular surface. The lesion, which is demarcated by a thin sclerotic border, closely resembles a chondroblastoma. On biopsy, however, it proved to be a clear cell chondrosarcoma.

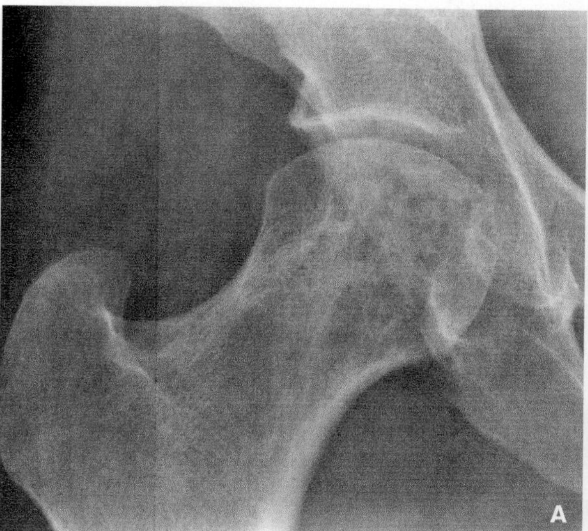

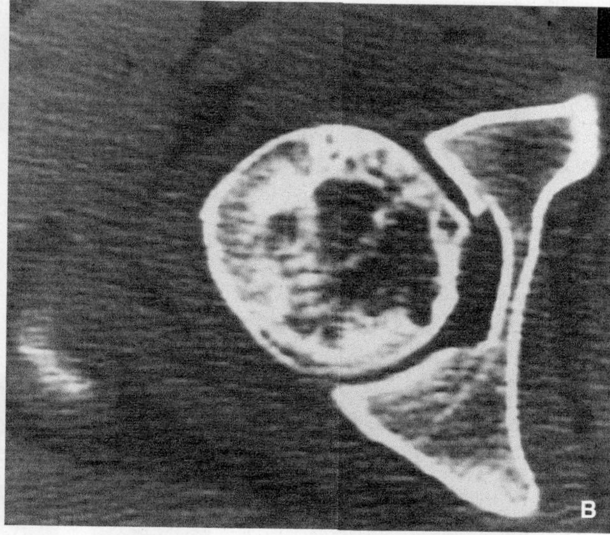

FIGURE 21.63 CT of clear cell chondrosarcoma. **(A)** Anteroposterior radiograph of the right hip shows a radiolucent lesion with chondroid calcifications within the femoral head. Note resemblance of this lesion to chondroblastoma. **(B)** Axial CT image shows the lytic character of the tumor and central calcifications to better advantage. (Reprinted with permission from Greenspan A, Borys D. *Radiology and pathology correlation of bone tumors,* 1st ed. Philadelphia: Wolters Kluwer, 2016:152.)

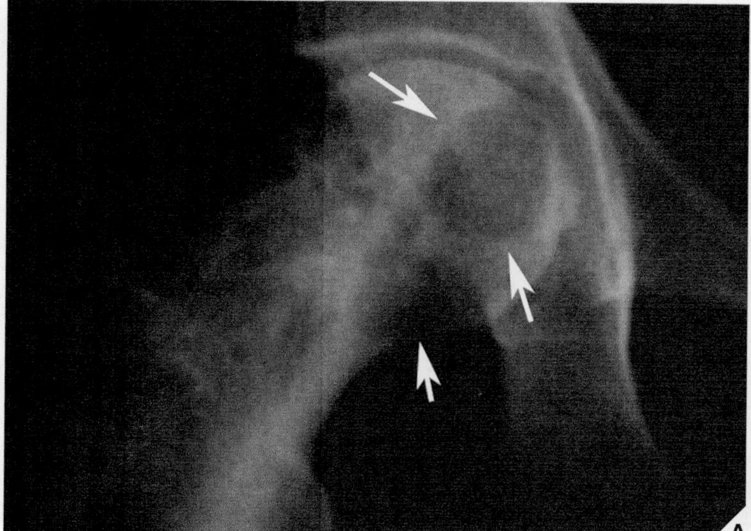

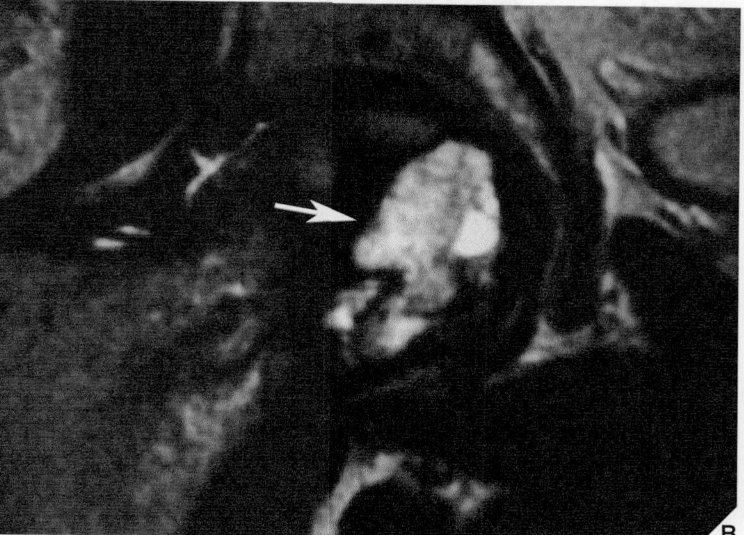

FIGURE 21.64 MRI of clear cell chondrosarcoma. **(A)** Anteroposterior radiograph of the right hip of a young male shows irregular lytic lesion with sclerotic rim in the femoral head extending to the neck *(arrows)*. **(B)** Coronal T2-weighted MRI demonstrates a hyperintense tumor in the femoral head extending to the neck *(arrow)*. The tumor is well demarcated exhibiting a narrow zone of transition and mild surrounding bone marrow edema in the femoral neck.

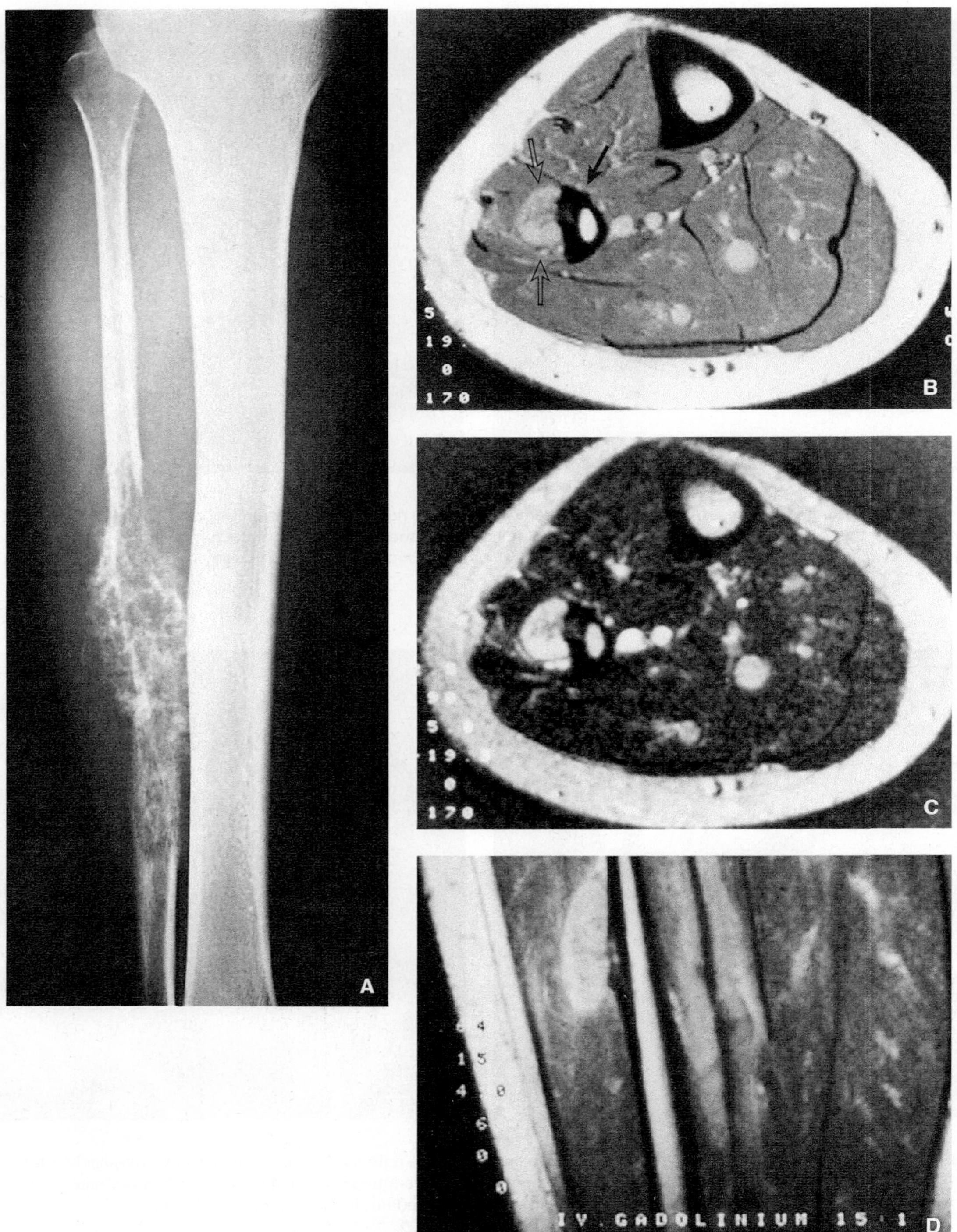

FIGURE 21.65 MRI of mesenchymal chondrosarcoma. **(A)** Anteroposterior radiograph of the right lower leg of a 43-year-old woman with a 6-month history of intermittent pain in the right calf shows a destructive lesion at the midportion of the fibula associated with a large soft-tissue mass. The central portion of the lesion exhibits annular and comma-shaped calcifications typical of a cartilage tumor, but its periphery shows a permeative type of bone destruction characteristic of round cell tumors. **(B)** Axial T1-weighted MR image shows a focus of intermediate signal intensity within the low signal intensity of the lateral cortex of fibula *(arrows)*. **(C)** Axial T2-weighted MR image shows the tumor displaying high signal intensity. Observe high signal intensity of the soft-tissue mass. **(D)** Coronal T1-weighted MR image obtained after intravenous administration of gadolinium shows marked enhancement of both, the intramedullary tumor and soft-tissue mass. (**B–D**, Reprinted with permission from Greenspan A, Borys D. *Radiology and pathology correlation of bone tumors*, 1st ed. Philadelphia: Wolters Kluwer, 2016:154–155.)

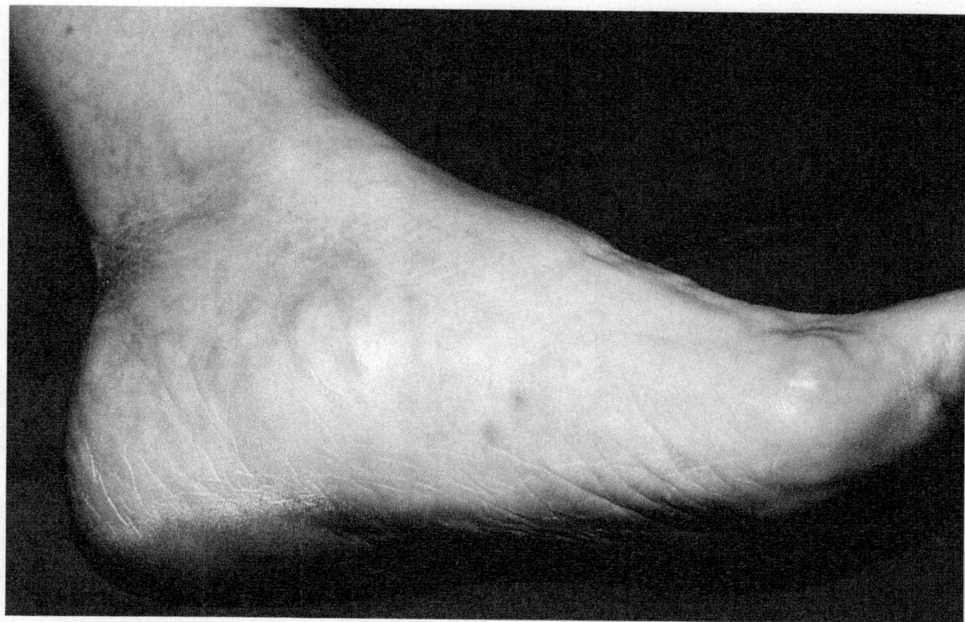

FIGURE 21.66 Myxoid chondrosarcoma. Clinical photograph of the foot of a 65-year-old woman who presented with rapidly growing painful mass on the medial aspect of her foot.

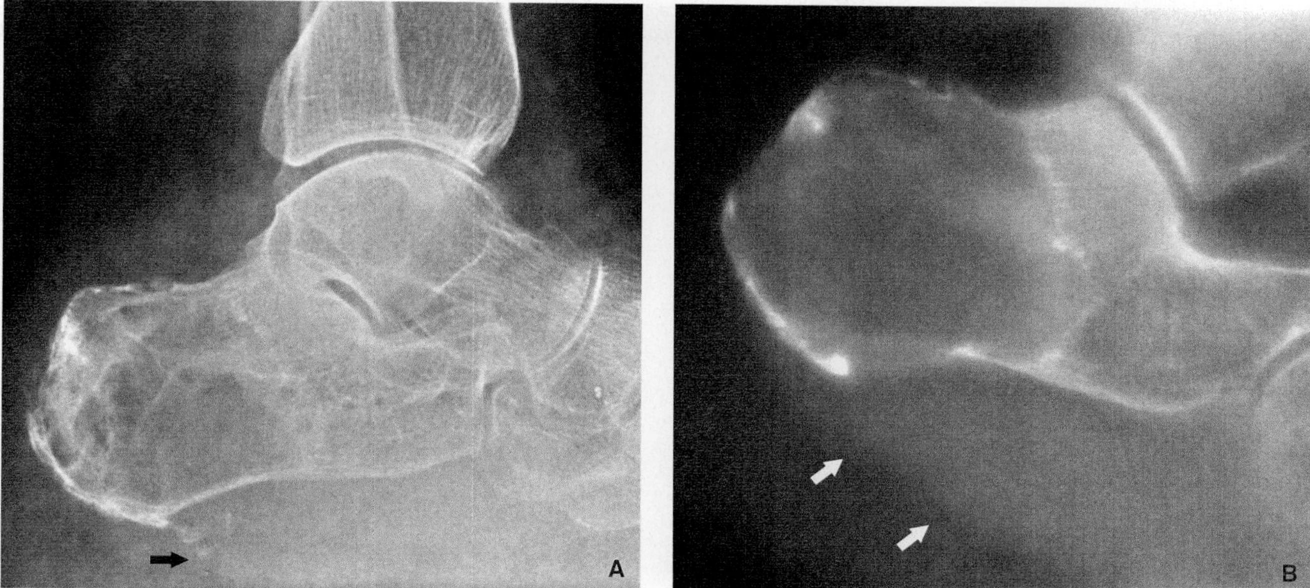

FIGURE 21.67 Myxoid chondrosarcoma. **(A)** Lateral radiograph of the hindfoot (same patient as depicted in Fig. 21.66) shows a large destructive lesion in the calcaneus. The tumor extends into the soft tissues *(arrow)*. **(B)** Lateral conventional tomogram demonstrates the soft-tissue mass more effectively *(arrows)*. (Reprinted with permission from Greenspan A, Borys D. *Radiology and pathology correlation of bone tumors: a quick reference and review*. Philadelphia: Wolters Kluwer; 2016:158, Fig. 3.98.)

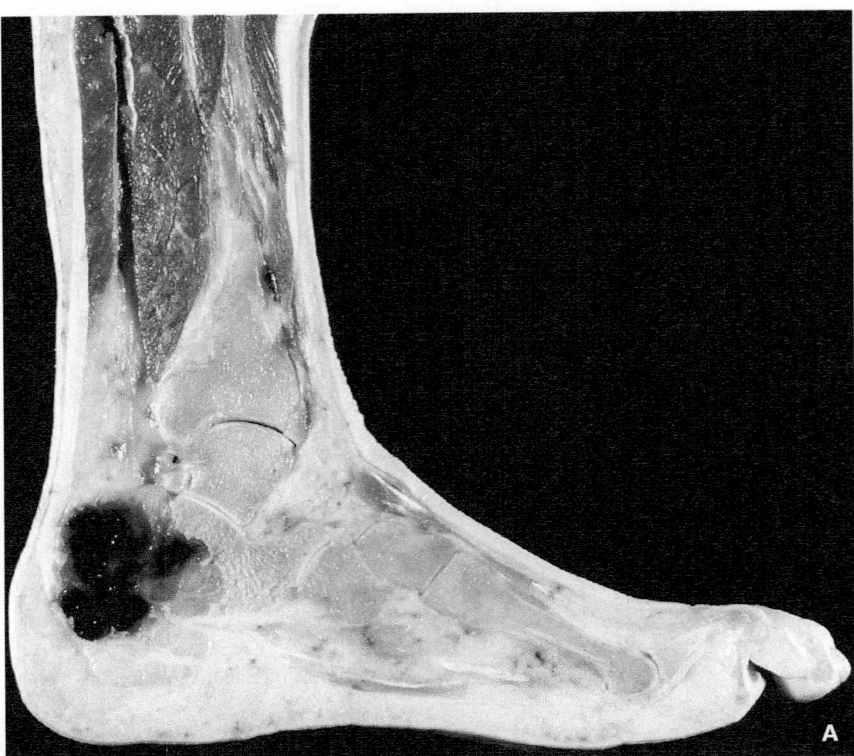

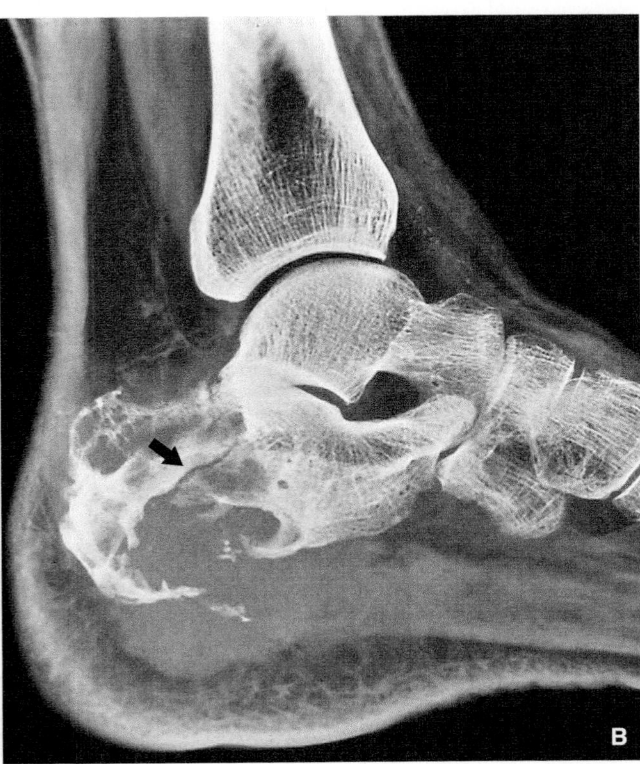

FIGURE 21.68 Pathology of myxoid chondrosarcoma. **(A)** Amputated specimen shows a hemorrhagic tumor within calcaneus, breaking through the cortex and extending into the soft tissues (same patient as presented in Figs. 21.66 and 21.67). Observe that the most plantar aspect of the tumor shows myxoid component. **(B)** Lateral radiograph of the amputated specimen shows a large osteolytic lesion in the posterior calcaneus with a pathologic fracture *(arrow)*. Soft-tissue extension of the tumor is clearly demonstrated. (Reprinted with permission from Greenspan A, Borys D. *Radiology and pathology correlation of bone tumors,* 1st ed. Philadelphia: Wolters Kluwer, 2016:158.)

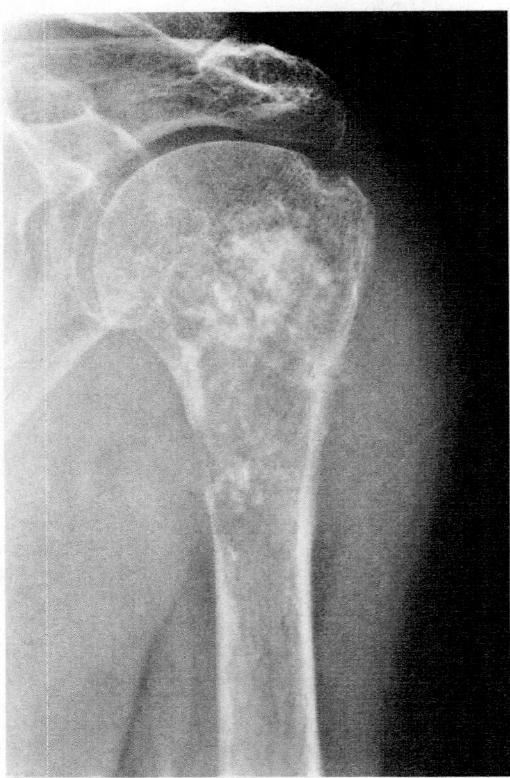

FIGURE 21.69 Dedifferentiated chondrosarcoma. A 70-year-old woman had a destructive lesion in the medullary cavity of the proximal shaft of the left humerus with calcifications typical of a cartilage tumor; there was also a soft-tissue mass. However, although the lesion seen on this radiograph exhibits features typical of medullary chondrosarcoma, biopsy revealed, in addition to typical chondrosarcomatous tissue, elements of a giant cell tumor and MFH, leading to a diagnosis of dedifferentiated chondrosarcoma—the most aggressive of all such tumors.

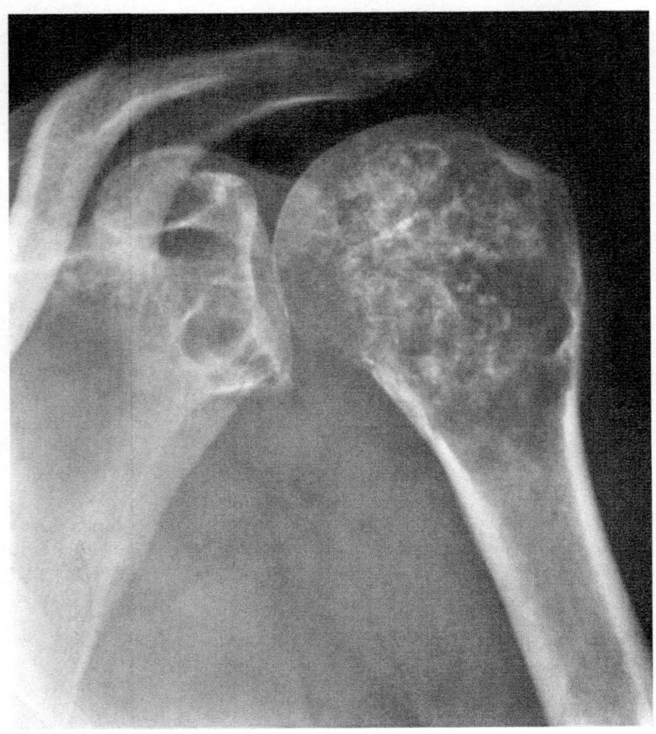

FIGURE 21.70 Dedifferentiated chondrosarcoma. Anteroposterior radiograph of the left shoulder of a 50-year-old man shows a lytic lesion in the humeral head, extending into the humeral neck, containing typical chondroid calcifications. The distal part of the tumor exhibits more destructive pattern. Observe deep endosteal scalloping. The incidentally discovered benign-appearing radiolucent, trabeculated lesion in the glenoid proved to be an intraosseous ganglion. (Reprinted with permission from Greenspan A, Borys D. *Radiology and pathology correlation of bone tumors: a quick reference and review*. Philadelphia: Wolters Kluwer; 2016:159, Fig. 3.100.)

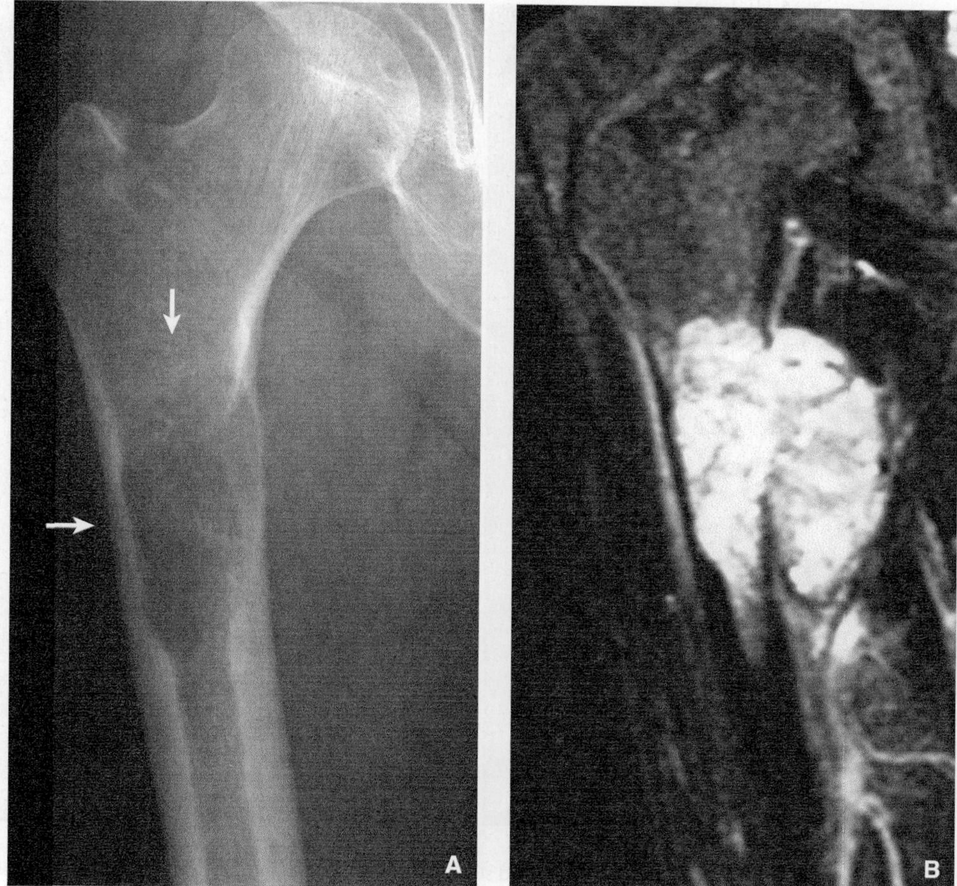

FIGURE 21.71 MRI of dedifferentiated chondrosarcoma. **(A)** Anteroposterior radiograph of the proximal femur of a 60-year-old man shows a predominantly osteolytic destructive lesion in the subtrochanteric region *(arrows)*. **(B)** Coronal short time inversion recovery (STIR) MR image shows the high–signal intensity tumor breaking through the medial cortex to form a large soft-tissue mass. (Reprinted with permission from Greenspan A, Borys D. *Radiology and pathology correlation of bone tumors: a quick reference and review*. Philadelphia: Wolters Kluwer; 2016:160, Fig. 3.102.)

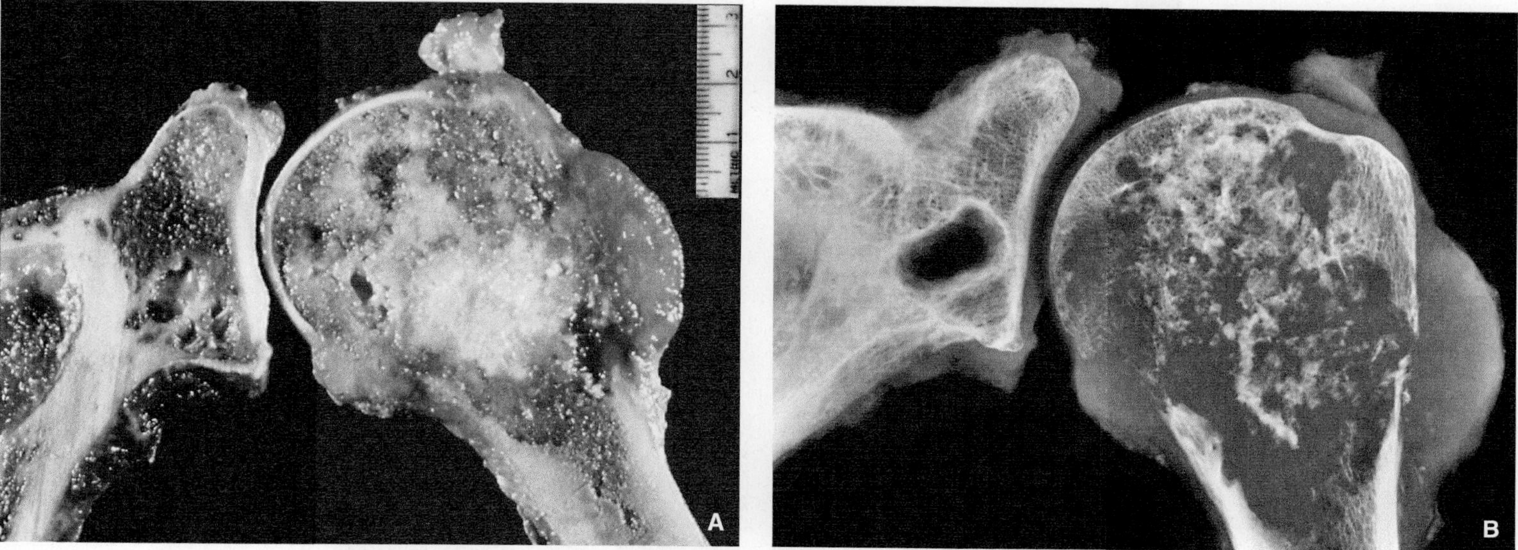

FIGURE 21.72 Pathology of dedifferentiated chondrosarcoma. **(A)** Gross specimen of the left shoulder (patient underwent three-quarter amputation) shows lobules of malignant cartilage invading humeral head and neck. Coarse calcifications are present proximally. **(B)** Radiograph of the resected specimen shows more aggressive destruction at the distal part of the tumor. Observe a benign lesion in the glenoid, proved to represent an intraosseous ganglion (same patient as depicted in Fig. 21.70). (Reprinted with permission from Greenspan A, Borys D. *Radiology and pathology correlation of bone tumors: a quick reference and review*. Philadelphia: Wolters Kluwer; 2016:160, Fig. 3.103.)

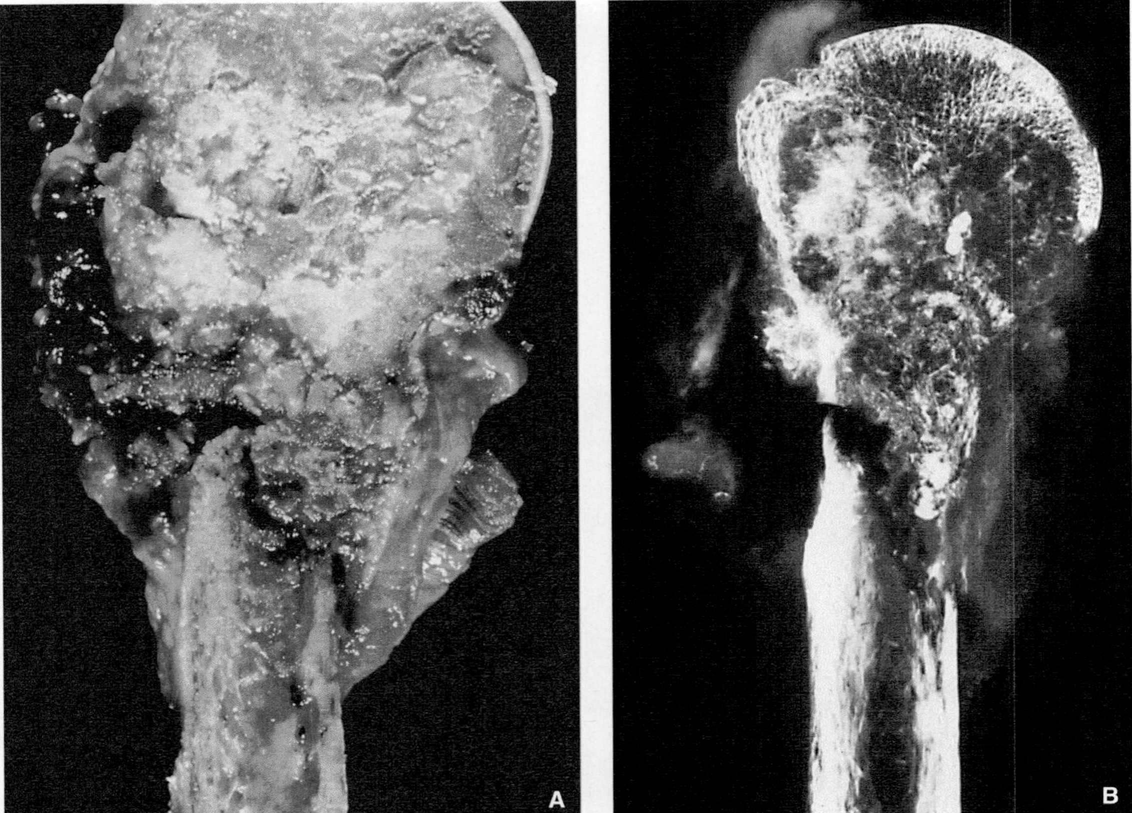

FIGURE 21.73 **Pathology of dedifferentiated chondrosarcoma.** **(A)** Resected surgical specimen of the proximal humerus and **(B)** radiograph of the specimen show biphasic appearance of cartilaginous tumor with a pathologic fracture through the more destructive portion of the lesion.

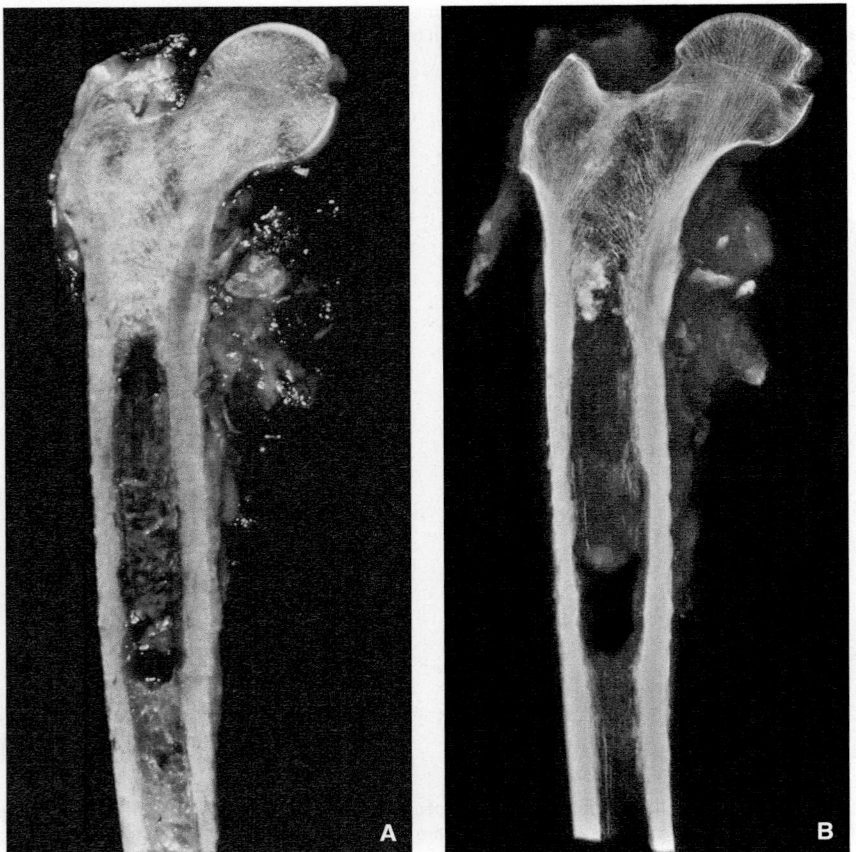

FIGURE 21.74 **Pathology of dedifferentiated chondrosarcoma.** **(A)** Resected surgical specimen of the right proximal femur and **(B)** radiograph of the specimen show biphasic appearance of cartilaginous tumor invading femoral shaft and femoral neck. The distal part of the tumor is lytic, the cortex is markedly thickened, and there are deep endosteal erosions. Large soft-tissue mass is present medially. The calcified portion of the tumor in the femoral neck showed histopathologic features of enchondroma; the tissue from the femoral shaft showed mixture of grade 3 chondrosarcoma and MFH.

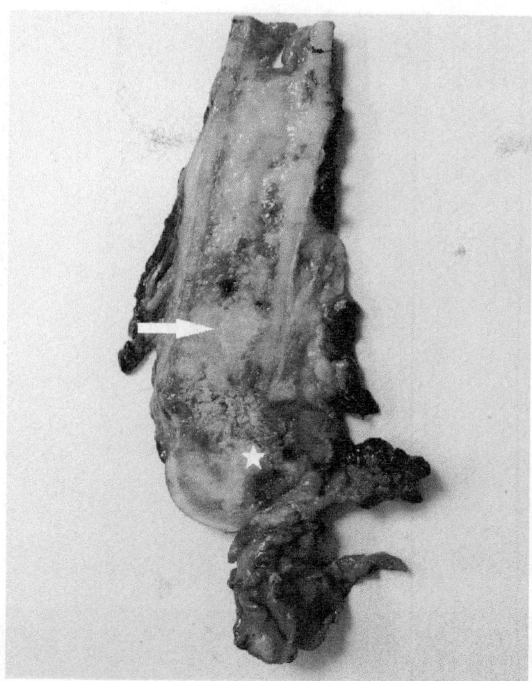

FIGURE 21.75 Pathology of dedifferentiated chondrosarcoma. In the resected surgical specimen of the distal femur, one can clearly distinguish two parts—gray-blue appearance of low-grade cartilaginous component *(arrow)* and yellow-tan to red-brown appearance of high-grade noncartilaginous sarcoma breaking through the cortex and extending into the soft tissues *(star)*. (Reprinted with permission from Greenspan A, Borys D. *Radiology and pathology correlation of bone tumors: a quick reference and review*. Philadelphia: Wolters Kluwer; 2016:161, Fig. 3.106.)

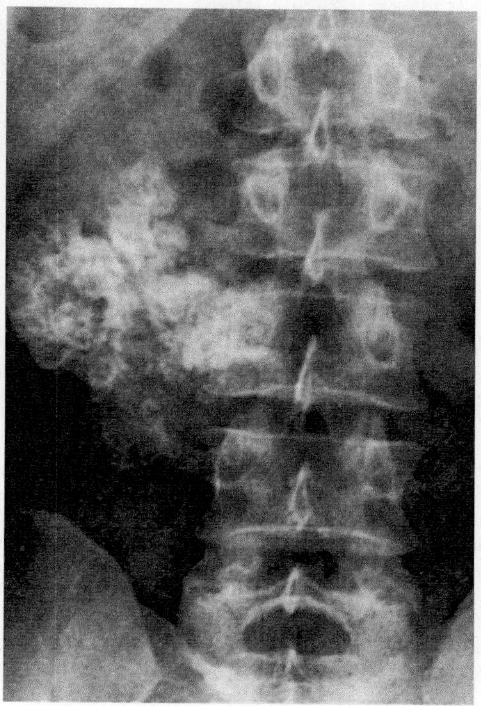

FIGURE 21.76 Periosteal chondrosarcoma. Anteroposterior radiograph of the lumbar spine shows a large calcified mass attached to the lateral aspect of the third lumbar vertebra. (Reprinted with permission from Greenspan A, Borys D. *Radiology and pathology correlation of bone tumors: a quick reference and review*. Philadelphia: Wolters Kluwer; 2016:165, Fig. 3.111.)

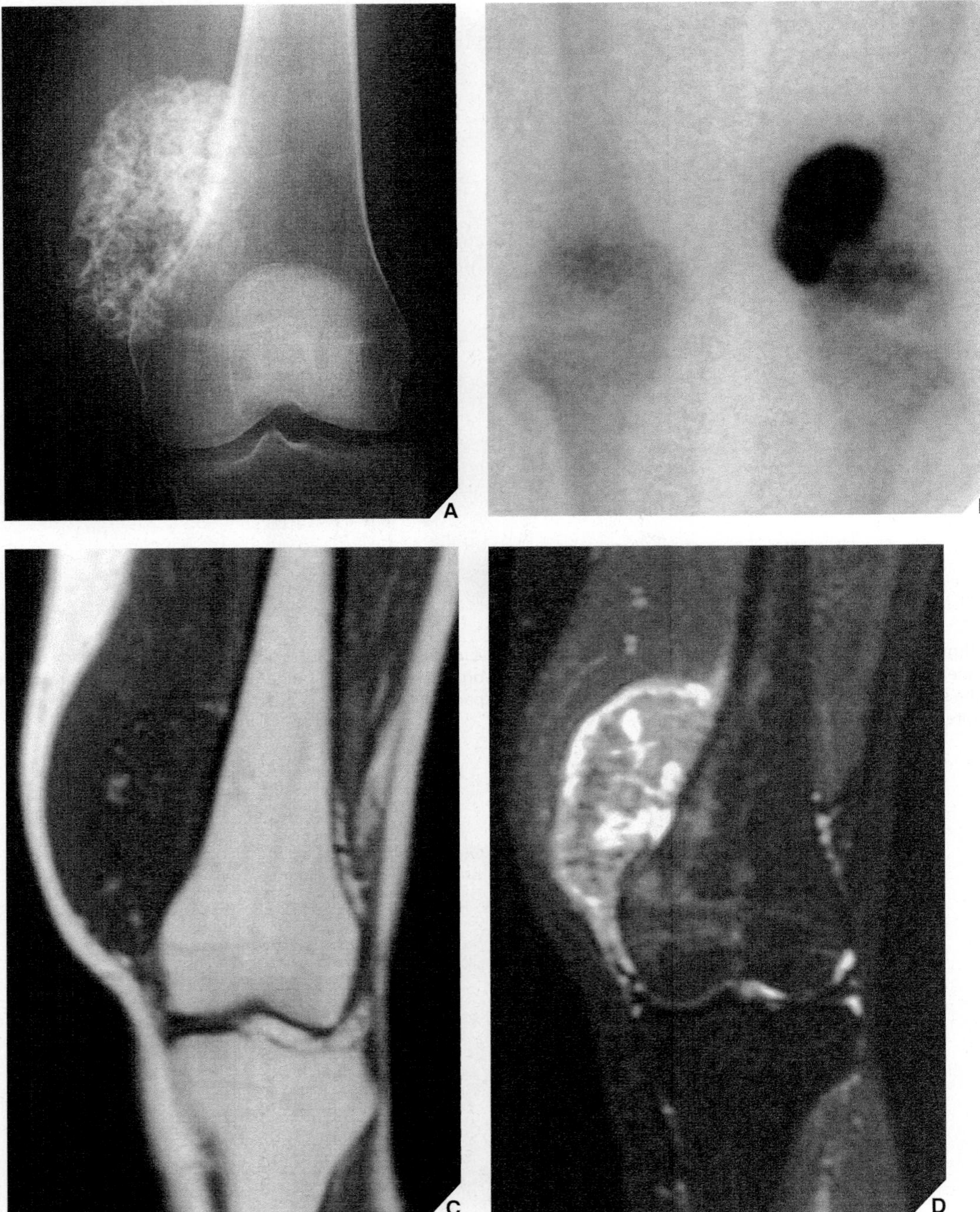

FIGURE 21.77 **Scintigraphy and MRI of periosteal chondrosarcoma.** **(A)** Anteroposterior radiograph of the left knee of a 30-year-old woman shows a parosteal calcified mass at the medial cortex of distal femur, exhibiting chondroid calcifications. **(B)** Radionuclide bone scan obtained after intravenous administration of 15 mCi (555 MBq) of technetium-99m (^{99m}Tc)-labeled methylene diphosphonate shows markedly increased uptake of radiotracer within the mass. **(C)** Coronal T1-weighted MR image shows the mass to be isointense with surrounding muscles displaying intermediate signal intensity. **(D)** On coronal T2-weighted MRI, the mass becomes bright, but the central calcifications exhibit low signal. (Reprinted with permission from Greenspan A, Jundt G, Remagen W. *Differential diagnosis in orthopaedic oncology*, 2nd ed. Philadelphia: Lippincott Williams & Wilkins; 2007:84–148, 212–249.)

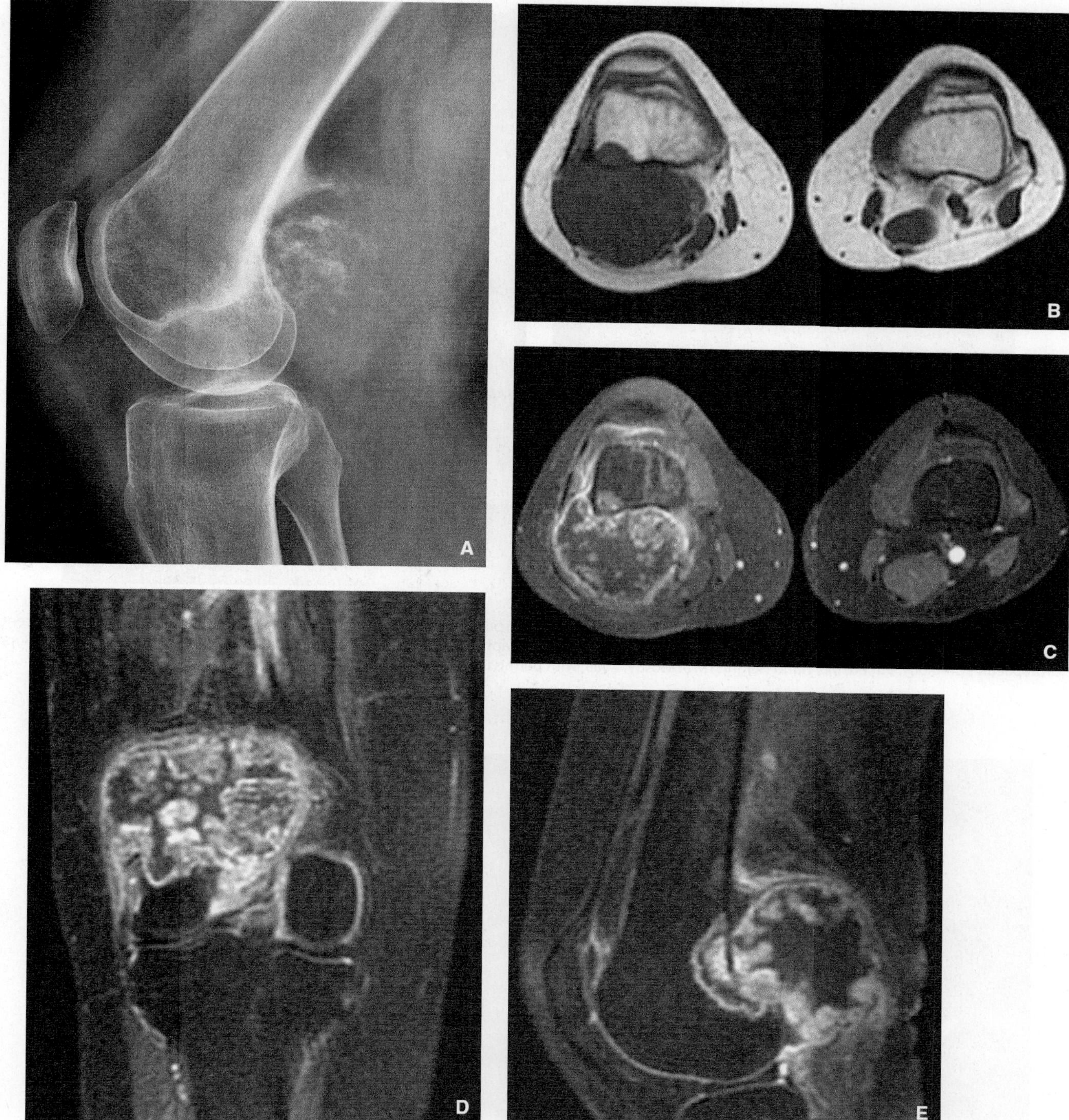

FIGURE 21.78 MRI of periosteal chondrosarcoma. **(A)** Lateral radiograph of the right knee of a 50-year-old woman shows a large soft-tissue mass abutting the posterior cortex of distal femur, containing chondroid calcifications. **(B)** Axial T1-weighted MR image and **(C)** axial T1-weighted fat-suppressed MRI obtained after intravenous administration of gadolinium show that the mass, exhibiting peripheral enhancement, is invading the lateral femoral condyle, better depicted on postcontrast coronal **(D)** and sagittal **(E)** fat-suppressed MR images. (Reprinted with permission from Greenspan A, Borys D. *Radiology and pathology correlation of bone tumors*, 1st ed. Philadelphia: Wolters Kluwer, 2016:166.)

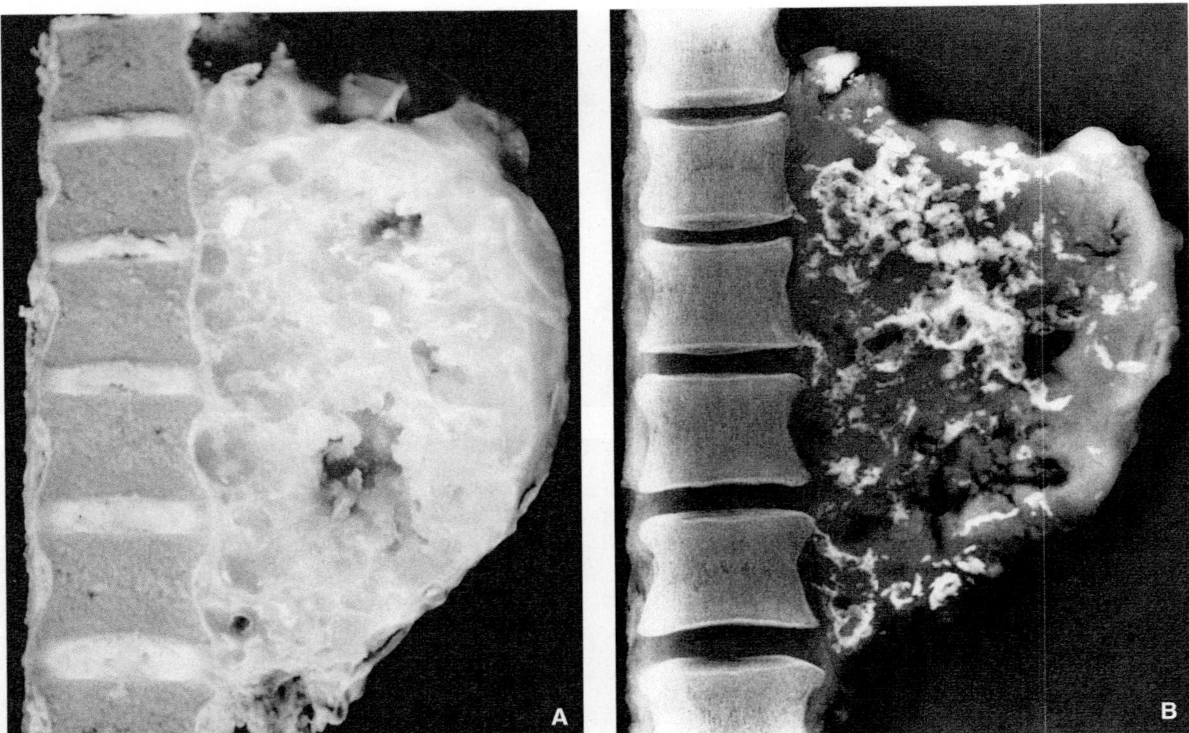

FIGURE 21.79 Pathology of periosteal chondrosarcoma. (A) Coronal section of a specimen of thoracolumbar spine junction shows a large mass adjacent to the five vertebral bodies. Note glistening cartilaginous matrix with foci of calcifications. **(B)** Radiograph of the specimen better demonstrates chondroid calcifications. (Reprinted from Bullough P. *Orthopaedic pathology*, 5th ed. Maryland Heights, MO: Mosby; 2009, with permission from Elsevier.)

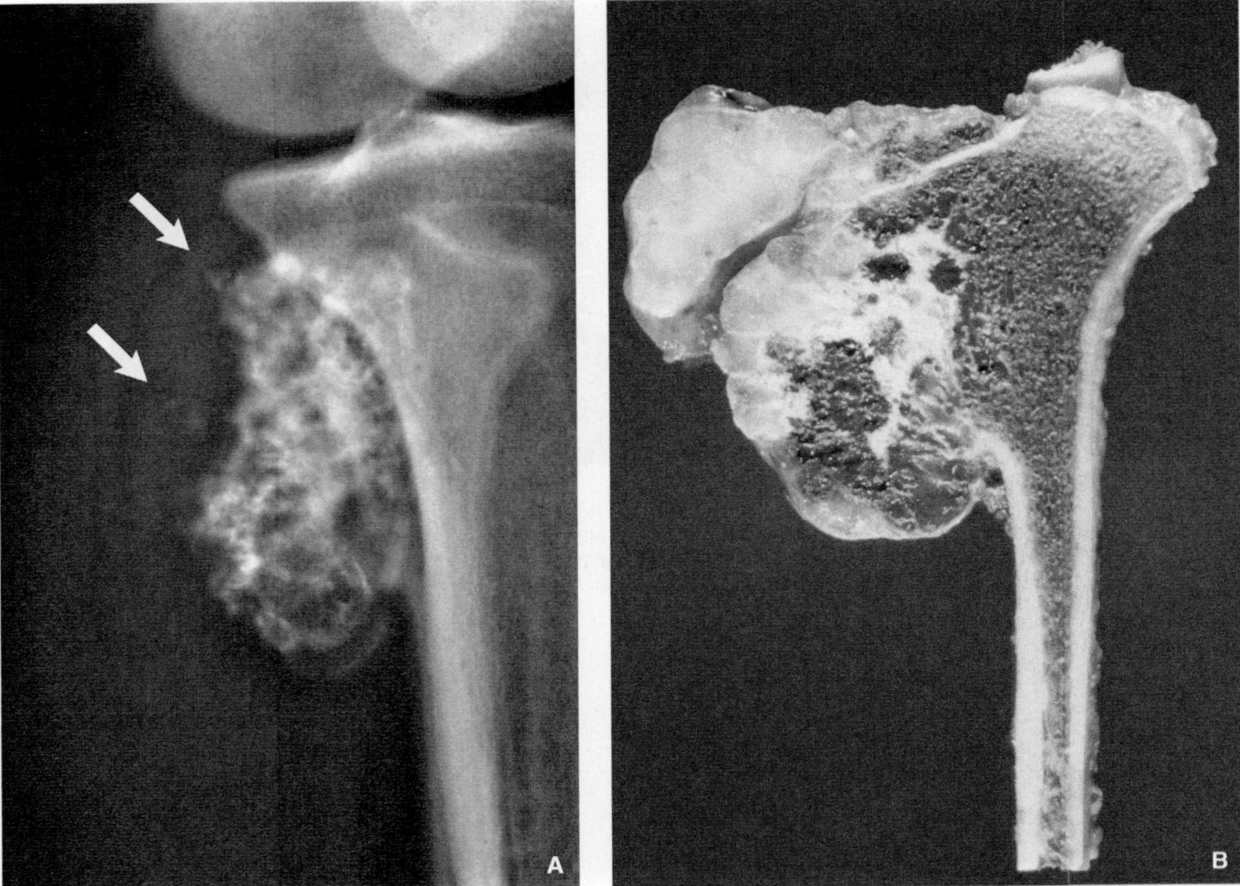

FIGURE 21.80 Malignant transformation of osteochondroma. (A) Large osteochondroma is seen arising from the proximal fibula of a 32-year-old woman. Note dispersed calcifications within the thick cartilaginous cap *(arrows)*. **(B)** Resected surgical specimen shows a large osseous tumor exhibiting a very thick cartilaginous cap. Note also flaring and destruction of the cortex. Histopathologic examination confirmed malignant transformation to chondrosarcoma.

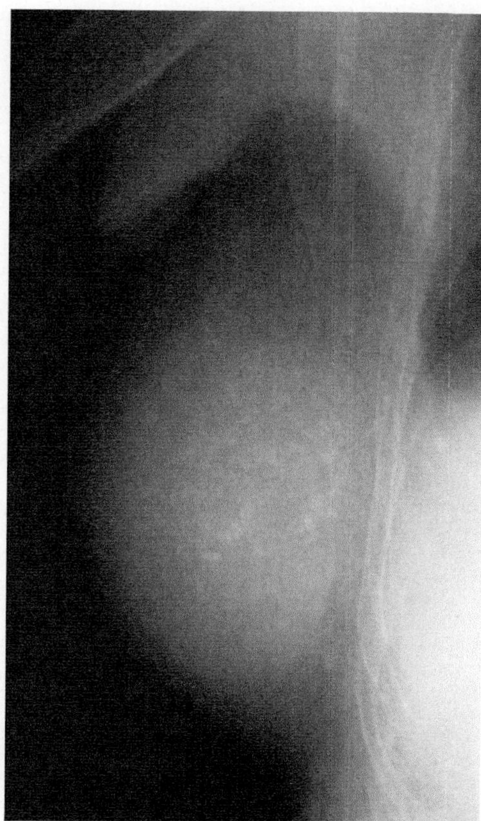

FIGURE 21.81 **Soft-tissue chondrosarcoma.** Conventional radiograph shows a large mineralized mass adjacent to the right lower ribs. Note the reverse zonal phenomenon that excludes the diagnosis of similarly appearing myositis ossificans, whereas extraskeletal osteosarcoma can be excluded because the tumor matrix exhibits typical chondroid calcifications in form of the dots, arcs, and rings. (Reprinted with permission from Greenspan A, Borys D. *Radiology and pathology correlation of bone tumors: a quick reference and review*. Philadelphia: Wolters Kluwer; 2016:170, Fig. 3.118.)

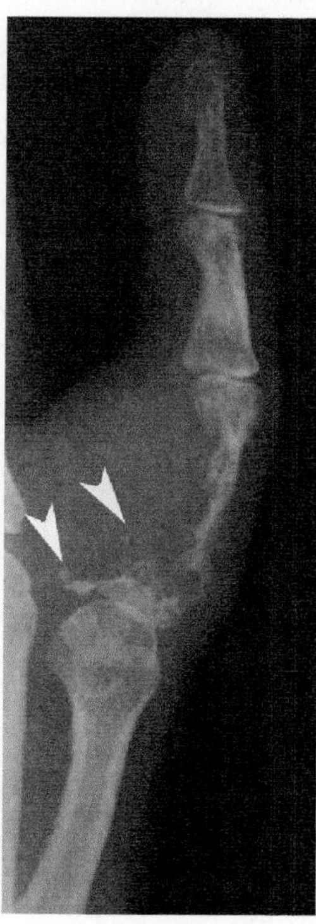

FIGURE 21.82 **Soft -tissue chondrosarcoma.** Oblique radiograph of the small finger of the left hand of a 47-year-old woman shows a soft-tissue mass invading and destroying the proximal phalanx. There are small calcifications within the soft tissue tumor (*arrowheads*). (Reprinted with permission from Greenspan A, Borys D. *Radiology and pathology correlation of bone tumors,* 1st ed. Philadelphia: Wolters Kluwer, 2016:170.)

PRACTICAL POINTS TO REMEMBER

Osteosarcoma

1. Osteosarcoma has the ability to produce osteoid tissue or bone. Its most characteristic radiographic features are:
   - the presence of tumor bone in the lesion—the hallmark of this malignancy
   - destruction of the medullary portion of the bone or cortex
   - an aggressive periosteal reaction—sunburst, lamellated, or Codman triangle
   - the presence of a soft-tissue mass.
2. In the radiologic evaluation of the different types of osteosarcoma—conventional, telangiectatic, multifocal, and juxtacortical:
   - conventional radiography is usually sufficient to identify the radiographic characteristics of each type and make a definitive diagnosis
   - CT and MRI are invaluable for defining the extent of the tumor in the bone and soft tissues and for monitoring the results of presurgical chemotherapy and radiation therapy.
3. Telangiectatic osteosarcoma, among the most aggressive of osteosarcomas, may present radiographically as a purely osteolytic lesion. It may resemble an aneurysmal bone cyst.
4. Parosteal osteosarcoma, the least malignant type of osteosarcoma:
   - has a predilection for the posterior aspect of the distal femur
   - is usually seen attached to the cortex, without invasion of the medullary cavity.
5. Periosteal osteosarcoma, like parosteal osteosarcoma, is a "surface" lesion. It is, however, more aggressive and contains an excessive amount of cartilaginous tissue. It may resemble periosteal chondrosarcoma and myositis ossificans.
6. Extraskeletal (soft-tissue) osteosarcoma is a rare malignant tumor of mesenchymal origin, most often affecting middle-aged and elderly individuals. The preferential sites for this neoplasm are lower extremities and buttocks. It may resemble myositis ossificans, tumoral calcinosis, and synovial sarcoma.
7. The most common form of secondary osteosarcoma is that complicating Paget disease. It is an extremely aggressive lesion; patients usually do not survive beyond 8 months after diagnosis.

Chondrosarcoma

1. Chondrosarcoma is a malignant bone tumor capable of forming cartilage. Its most characteristic radiographic features are:
   - an expansive, destructive lesion in the medullary portion of the bone
   - the presence of annular and comma-shaped calcifications within the tumor matrix
   - thickening of the cortex and deep endosteal scalloping
   - the presence of a soft-tissue mass.
2. Clear cell chondrosarcoma is characterized radiographically by lytic area occasionally containing calcifications and sclerotic border. It may resemble chondroblastoma.
3. Mesenchymal chondrosarcoma demonstrates radiographically two different appearances: side-by-side present are areas of permeative type of bone destruction similar to round cell tumors, and areas resembling typical cartilaginous tumor with calcifications.
4. Dedifferentiated chondrosarcoma, the most aggressive type of all cartilage tumors, carries a poor prognosis. In addition to chondrogenic tissue, it can contain elements of fibrosarcoma, MFH, or osteosarcoma.
5. Periosteal chondrosarcoma may be indistinguishable from periosteal osteosarcoma.
6. Secondary chondrosarcoma usually develops in a preexisting benign lesion such as an enchondromatosis or multiple cartilaginous exostoses. At risk are the patients with Ollier disease and Maffucci syndrome.
7. Soft-tissue chondrosarcoma should be differentiated from soft-tissue osteosarcoma and juxtacortical myositis ossificans.

SUGGESTED READINGS

Abe K, Kumagai K, Hayashi T, et al. High-grade surface osteosarcoma of the hand. *Skeletal Radiol* 2007;36:869–873.

Aisen AM, Martel W, Braunstein EM, et al. MRI and CT evaluation of primary bone and soft-tissue tumors. *AJR Am J Roentgenol* 1986;146:749–756.

Aizawa T, Okada K, Abe E, et al. Multicentric osteosarcoma with long-term survival. *Skeletal Radiol* 2004;33:41–45.

Alpert LI, Abaci IF, Werthamer S. Radiation-induced extraskeletal osteosarcoma. *Cancer* 1973;31:1359–1363.

Amary MF, Bacsi K, Maggiani F, et al. IDH1 and IDH2 mutations are frequent events in central chondrosarcoma and central and periosteal chondromas but not in other mesenchymal tumours. *J Pathol* 2011;224:334–343.

Aoki J, Sone S, Fujioka F, et al. MR of enchondroma and chondrosarcoma: rings and arcs of Gd-DTPA enhancement. *J Comput Assist Tomogr* 1991;15:1011–1016.

Azura M, Vanel D, Alberghini M, et al. Parosteal osteosarcoma dedifferentiating into telangiectatic osteosarcoma: importance of lytic changes and fluid cavities at imaging. *Skeletal Radiol* 2009;38:685–690.

Bagley L, Kneeland JB, Dalinka MK, et al. Unusual behavior of clear cell chondrosarcoma. *Skeletal Radiol* 1993;22:279–282.

Ballance WA Jr, Mendelsohn G, Carter JR, et al. Osteogenic sarcoma. Malignant fibrous histiocytoma subtype. *Cancer* 1988;62:763–771.

Bane BL, Evans HL, Ro JY, et al. Extra-skeletal osteosarcoma. A clinicopathologic study of 26 cases. *Cancer* 1990;65:2762–2770.

Bathurst N, Sanerkin N, Watt I. Osteoclast-rich osteosarcoma. *Br J Radiol* 1986;59: 667–673.

Berquist TH. Magnetic resonance imaging of primary skeletal neoplasms. *Radiol Clin North Am* 1993;31:411–424.

Bertoni F, Picci P, Bacchini P, et al. Mesenchymal chondrosarcoma of bone and soft tissues. *Cancer* 1983;52:533–541.

Bertoni F, Present DA, Enneking WF. Staging of bone tumors. In: Unni KK, ed. *Bone tumors*. New York: Churchill Livingstone; 1988:47–83.

Blasius S, Link TM, Hillmann A, et al. Intracortical low grade osteosarcoma. A unique case and review of the literature on intracortical osteosarcoma. *Gen Diagn Pathol* 1996;141:273–278.

Borys D, Cantor R. Mesenchymal chondrosarcoma of the chest wall. *Pathol Case Rev* 2012;17:10–13.

Brien EW, Mirra JM, Herr R. Benign and malignant cartilage tumors of bone and joints: their anatomic and theoretical basis with an emphasis on radiology, pathology, and clinical biology. I. The intramedullary cartilage tumors. *Skeletal Radiol* 1997;26:325–353.

Brien EW, Mirra JM, Luck JV Jr. Benign and malignant cartilage tumor of bone and joint: their anatomic and theoretical basis with an emphasis on radiology, pathology and clinical biology. II. Juxtacortical cartilage tumors. *Skeletal Radiol* 1999;28:1–20.

Broders AC. The microscopic grading of cancer. In: Pack CT, Ariel IM, eds. *Treatment of cancer and allied diseases*, vol. 1, 2nd ed. New York: Paul B. Hoeber; 1958:55–59.

Byun BH, Kong C-B, Lim I, et al. Comparison of (18)F-FDG PET/CT and (99m)Tc-MDP bone scintigraphy for detection of bone metastasis in osteosarcoma. *Skeletal Radiol* 2013;42:1673–1681.

Campanacci M, Cervellati G. Osteosarcoma: a review of 345 cases. *Ital J Orthop Traumatol* 1975;1:5–22.

Campanacci M, Pizzoferrato A. Osteosarcoma emorragico. *Chir Organi Mov* 1971;60: 409–421.

Cannon CP, Nelson SD, Seeger LL, et al. Clear cell chondrosarcoma mimicking chondroblastoma in a skeletally immature patient. *Skeletal Radiol* 2002;31:369–372.

Chung EB, Enzinger FM. Extraskeletal osteosarcoma. *Cancer* 1987;60:1132–1142.

Collins MS, Koyama T, Swee RG, et al. Clear cell chondrosarcoma: radiographic, computed tomographic, and magnetic resonance findings in 34 patients with pathologic correlation. *Skeletal Radiol* 2003;32:687–694.

Crim JR, Seeger LL. Diagnosis of low-grade chondrosarcoma. *Radiology* 1993;189:503–504.

Dahlin DC. Grading of bone tumors. In: Unni KK, ed. *Bone tumors*. New York: Churchill Livingstone; 1988:35–45.

Dahlin DC, Beabout JW. Dedifferentiation of low-grade chondrosarcomas. *Cancer* 1971;28:461–466.

Dahlin DC, Unni KK. *Bone tumors: general aspects and data on 8542 cases*, 4th ed. Springfield: Charles C. Thomas; 1986:227–259.

Dardick I, Schatz JE, Colgan TJ. Osteogenic sarcoma with epithelial differentiation. *Ultrastruct Pathol* 1992;16:463–474.

De Beuckeleer LHL, De Schepper AMA, Ramon F, et al. Magnetic resonance imaging of cartilaginous tumors: retrospective study of 79 patients. *Eur J Radiol* 1995;21:34–40.

deSantos LA, Murray JA, Finkelstein JB, et al. The radiographic spectrum of periosteal osteosarcoma. *Radiology* 1978;127:123–129.

DeSmet AA, Norris MA, Fisher DR. Magnetic resonance imaging of myositis ossificans: analysis of seven cases. *Skeletal Radiol* 1992;21:503–507.

Eustace S, Baker N, Lan H, et al. MR imaging of dedifferentiated chondrosarcoma. *Clin Imaging* 1997;21:170–174.

Farr GH, Huvos AG, Marcove RC, et al. Telangiectatic osteogenic sarcoma: a review of twenty-eight cases. *Cancer* 1974;34:1150–1158.

Fechner RE, Mills SE. Osseous lesions. In: Rosai J, Sobin L, eds. *Atlas of tumor pathology: tumors of the bones and joints*. Washington, DC: Armed Forces Institute of Pathology; 1993:25–77.

Fine G, Stout AP. Osteogenic sarcoma of the extraskeletal soft tissues. *Cancer* 1956;9: 1027–1043.

Frassica FJ, Unni KK, Beabout JW, et al. Dedifferentiated chondrosarcoma. A report of the clinicopathological features and treatment of seventy-eight cases. *J Bone Joint Surg Am* 1986;68A:1197–1205.

Geirnaerdt MJA, Bloem JL, Eulderink F, et al. Cartilaginous tumors: correlation of gadolinium-enhanced MR imaging and histopathologic findings. *Radiology* 1993;186: 813–817.

Geirnaerdt MJA, Bloem JL, van der Woude H-J, et al. Chondroblastic osteosarcoma: characterisation by gadolinium-enhanced MR imaging correlated with histopathology. *Skeletal Radiol* 1998;27:145–153.

Geirnaerdt MJA, Hogendoorn PCW, Bloem JL, et al. Cartilaginous tumors: fast contrast-enhanced MR imaging. *Radiology* 2000;214:539–546.

Gherlinzoni F, Antoci B, Canale V. Multicentric osteosarcomata (osteosarcomatosis). *Skeletal Radiol* 1983;10:281–285.

Goldman RL, Lichtenstein L. Synovial chondrosarcoma. *Cancer* 1964;17:1233–1240.

Greenspan A. Tumors of cartilage origin. *Orthop Clin North Am* 1989;20:347–366.

Greenspan A, Borys D. *Radiology and pathology correlations of bone tumors: a quick reference and review*. Philadelphia: Wolters Kluwer; 2016: 32–89; 90–179.

Greenspan A, Jundt G, Remagen W. *Differential diagnosis in orthopaedic oncology*, 2nd ed. Philadelphia: Lippincott Williams & Wilkins; 2007:84–148; 212–249.

Greenspan A, Klein MJ. Osteosarcoma: radiologic imaging, differential diagnosis, and pathological considerations. *Semin Orthop* 1991;6:156–166.

Greenspan A, Steiner G, Norman A, et al. Case report 436. Osteosarcoma of the soft tissues of the distal end of the thigh. *Skeletal Radiol* 1987;16:489–492.

Griffith JF, Kumta SM, Chow LTC, et al. Intracortical osteosarcoma. *Skeletal Radiol* 1998;27:228–232.

Hansen MF. Genetic and molecular aspects of osteosarcoma. *J Musculoskel Neuron Interact* 2002;2:554–560.

Hermann G, Abdelwahab IF, Kenan S, et al. Case report 795. High-grade surface osteosarcoma of the radius. *Skeletal Radiol* 1993;22:383–385.

Hermann G, Klein MJ, Springfield D, et al. Intracortical osteosarcoma; two-year delay in diagnosis. *Skeletal Radiol* 2002;31:592–596.

Hopper KD, Moser RP Jr, Haseman DB, et al. Osteosarcomatosis. *Radiology* 1990;175:233–239.

Hudson TM, Chew FS, Manaster BJ. Scintigraphy of benign exostoses and exostotic chondrosarcomas. *AJR Am J Roentgenol* 1983;140:581–586.

Hudson TM, Springfield DS, Spanier SS, et al. Benign exostoses and exostotic chondrosarcomas: evaluation of cartilage thickness by CT. *Radiology* 1984;152:595–599.

Ishida T, Dorfman HD, Habermann ET. Dedifferentiated chondrosarcoma of humerus with giant cell tumor-like features. *Skeletal Radiol* 1995;24:76–80.

Ishida T, Yamamoto M, Goto T, et al. Clear cell chondrosarcoma of the pelvis in a skeletally immature patient. *Skeletal Radiol* 1999;28:290–293.

Jaffe HL. *Tumors and tumorous conditions of the bones and joints*. Philadelphia: Lea & Febiger; 1968.

Jelinek JS, Murphey MD, Kransdorf MJ, et al. Parosteal osteosarcoma: value of MR imaging and CT in the prediction of histologic grade. *Radiology* 1996;201:837–842.

Jurik AG, Jørgensen PH, Mortensen MM. Whole-body MRI in assessing malignant transformation in multiple hereditary exostoses and enchondromatosis: audit results and literature review. *Skeletal Radiol* 2020;49:115–124.

Kaim AH, Hügli R, Bonél HM, et al. Chondroblastoma and clear cell chondrosarcoma: radiological and MRI characteristics with histopathological correlation. *Skeletal Radiol* 2002;31:88–95.

Kaufman RA, Towbin RB. Telangiectatic osteosarcoma simulating the appearance of an aneurysmal bone cyst. *Pediatr Radiol* 1981;11:102–104.

Kenan S, Ginat DT, Steiner GC. Dedifferentiated high-grade osteosarcoma originating from low-grade central osteosarcoma of the fibula. *Skeletal Radiol* 2007;36:347–351.

Klein MJ, Siegal GP. Osteosarcoma: anatomic and histologic variants. *Am J Clin Pathol* 2006;125:555–581.

Kramer K, Hicks D, Palis J, et al. Epithelioid osteosarcoma of bone. Immunocytochemical evidence suggesting divergent epithelial and mesenchymal differentiation in a primary osseous neoplasm. *Cancer* 1993;71:2977–2982.

Kransdorf MJ, Meis JM. Extraskeletal osseous and cartilaginous tumors of the extremities. *Radiographics* 1993;13:853–884.

Kyriakos M, Gilula LA, Besich MJ, et al. Intracortical small cell osteosarcoma. *Clin Orthop Relat Res* 1992;279:269–280.

Lichtenstein L, Jaffe HL. Chondrosarcoma of the bone. *Am J Pathol* 1943;19:553–589.

Lim C, Lee H, Schatz J, et al. Case report: periosteal osteosarcoma of the clavicle. *Skeletal Radiol* 2012;41:1011–1015.

Lopez BF, Rodriquez PJL, Gonzalez LJ, et al. Intracortical osteosarcoma. A case report. *Clin Orthop* 1991;278:218–222.

Lorigan JG, Lipshitz HI, Peuchot M. Radiation-induced sarcoma of bone: CT findings in 19 cases. *AJR Am J Roentgenol* 1989;153:791–794.

MacSweeney F, Darby A, Saifuddin A. Dedifferentiated chondrosarcoma of the appendicular skeleton: MRI-pathological correlation. *Skeletal Radiol* 2003;32:671–678.

Maheshwari AV, Jelinek JS, Seibel NL, et al. Bilateral synchronous tibial periosteal osteosarcoma with familial incidence. *Skeletal Radiol* 2012;41:1005–1009.

Mercuri M, Picci P, Campanacci M, et al. Dedifferentiated chondrosarcoma. *Skeletal Radiol* 1995;24:409–416.

Miller CW, Aslo A, Won A, et al. Alterations of the p53, Rb and MDM2 genes in osteosarcoma. *J Cancer Res Clin Oncol* 1996;122:559–565.

Moore TE, King AR, Kathol MH, et al. Sarcoma in Paget disease of bone: clinical, radiologic, and pathologic features in 22 cases. *AJR Am J Roentgenol* 1991;156:1199–1203.

Moser RP. *Cartilaginous tumors of the skeleton. AFIP atlas of radiologic-pathologic correlation*, vol 2. Philadelphia: Hanley & Belfus; 1990:190–197.

Mulder JD, Schütte HE, Kroon HM, et al. *Radiologic atlas of bone tumors*. Amsterdam, The Netherlands: Elsevier; 1993:51–76.

Murphey MD, Robbin MR, McRae GA, et al. The many faces of osteosarcoma. *Radiographics* 1997;17:1205–1231.

Murphey MD, Walker EA, Wilson AJ, et al. From the archives of the AFIP: imaging of primary chondrosarcoma: radiologic-pathologic correlation. *Radiographics* 2003;23:1245–1278.

Murphey MD, wan Joavisidha S, Temple HT, et al. Telangiectatic osteosarcoma: radiologic-pathologic comparison. *Radiology* 2003;229:545–553.

Norman A, Dorfman H. Juxtacortical circumscribed myositis ossificans: evolution and radiographic features. *Radiology* 1970;96:301–306.

Nuovo MA, Norman A, Chumas J, et al. Myositis ossificans with atypical clinical, radiographic, or pathologic findings: a review of 23 cases. *Skeletal Radiol* 1992;21:87–101.

Okada K, Kubota H, Ebina T, et al. High-grade surface osteosarcoma of the humerus. *Skeletal Radiol* 1995;24:531–534.

Okada K, Unni KK, Swee RG, et al. High grade surface osteosarcoma: a clinicopathologic study of 46 cases. *Cancer* 1999;85:1044–1054.

Onikul E, Fletcher BD, Parham DM, et al. Accuracy of MR imaging for estimating intraosseous extent of osteosarcoma. *AJR Am J Roentgenol* 1996;167:1211–1215.

Ontell F, Greenspan A. Chondrosarcoma complicating synovial chondromatosis: findings with magnetic resonance imaging. *Can Assoc Radiol J* 1994;45:318–323.

Park Y-K, Yang MH, Ryu KN, et al. Dedifferentiated chondrosarcoma arising in an osteochondroma. *Skeletal Radiol* 1995;24:617–619.

Partovi S, Logan PM, Janzen DL, et al. Low-grade parosteal osteosarcoma of the ulna with dedifferentiation into high-grade osteosarcoma. *Skeletal Radiol* 1996;25:497–500.

Pasic I, Shlien AD, Durbin AD, et al. Recurrent focal copy-number changes and loss of heterozygosity implicate two noncoding RNAs and one tumor suppressor gene at chromosome 3q13.31 in osteosarcoma. *Cancer Res* 2010;70:160–171.

Raymond AK, Ayala AG, Knuutila S. Conventional osteosarcoma. In: Fletcher CDM, Unni KK, Mertens F, eds. *Pathology and genetics of tumours of soft tissue and bone*. Lyon, France: IARC Press; 2002:264–270.

Saito T, Oda Y, Kawaguchi K, et al. Five-year evolution of a telangiectatic osteosarcoma initially managed as an aneurysmal bone cyst. *Skeletal Radiol* 2005;34:290–294.

Sandberg AA, Bridge JA. Updates on the cytogenetics and molecular genetics of bone and soft tissue tumors: osteosarcoma and related tumors. *Cancer Genet Cytogenet* 2003;145:1–30.

Saunders C, Szabo RM, Mora S. Chondrosarcoma of the hand arising in a young patient with multiple hereditary exostoses. *J Hand Surg Br* 1997;22(2):237–242.

Schajowicz F. *Tumors and tumorlike lesions of bone: pathology, radiology, and treatment*, 2nd ed. Berlin, Germany: Springer-Verlag; 1994:103–106.

Schajowicz F, Sissons HA, Sobin LH. The World Health Organization's histologic classification of bone tumors. A commentary on the second edition. *Cancer* 1995;75:1208–1214.

Sciot R, Samson I, Dal Cin P, et al. Giant cell rich parosteal osteosarcoma. *Histopathology* 1995;27:51–55.

Seeger LL, Farooki S, Yao L, et al. Custom endoprostheses for limb salvage: a historical perspective and image evaluation. *Am J Roentgenol* 1998;171:1525–1529.

Sheth DS, Yasko AW, Raymond AK, et al. Conventional and dedifferentiated parosteal osteosarcoma: diagnosis, treatment and outcome. *Cancer* 1996;78:2136–2145.

Shuhaibar H, Friedman L. Dedifferentiated parosteal osteosarcoma with high-grade osteoclast-rich osteogenic sarcoma at presentation. *Skeletal Radiol* 1998;27:574–577.

Sissons HA, Greenspan A. Paget's disease. In: Taveras JM, Ferrucci JT, eds. *Radiology: diagnosis, imaging, intervention*, vol. 5. Philadelphia: JB Lippincott; 1986:1–14.

Takeuchi K, Morii T, Yabe H, et al. Dedifferentiated parosteal osteosarcoma with well-differentiated metastases. *Skeletal Radiol* 2006;35:778–782.

Tateishi U, Hasegawa T, Nojima T, et al. MR features of extraskeletal myxoid chondrosarcoma. *Skeletal Radiol* 2006;35:27–33.

Torres FX, Kyriakos M. Bone infarct-associated osteosarcoma. *Cancer* 1992;70:2418–2430.

Unni KK. *Dahlin's bone tumors: general aspects and data on 11,087 cases*, 5th ed. Philadelphia: Lippincott-Raven; 1996:185–196.

Unni KK, Dahlin DC. Grading of bone tumors. *Semin Diagn Pathol* 1984;1:165–172.

Unni KK, Dahlin DC. Premalignant tumors and conditions of bone. *Am J Surg Pathol* 1979;3:47–60.

Unni KK, Dahlin DC, Beabout JW. Periosteal osteogenic sarcoma. *Cancer* 1976;37:2476–2485.

Unni KK, Dahlin DC, Beabout JW, et al. Parosteal osteogenic sarcoma. *Cancer* 1976;37:2644–2675.

Unni KK, Dahlin DC, Beabout JW, et al. Chondrosarcoma: clear-cell variant: a report of 16 cases. *J Bone Joint Surg Am* 1976;58A:676–683.

Vanel D, De Paolis M, Monti C, et al. Radiological features of 24 periosteal chondrosarcomas. *Skeletal Radiol* 2001;30:208–212.

Vanel D, Picci P, De Paolis M, et al. Radiological study of 12 high-grade surface osteosarcomas. *Skeletal Radiol* 2001;30:667–671.

West OC, Reinus WR, Wilson AJ. Quantitative analysis of the plain radiographic appearance of central chondrosarcoma of bone. *Invest Radiol* 1995;30:440–447.

Wootton-Georges SL. MR imaging of primary bone tumors and tumor-like conditions in children. *Magn Reson Imaging Clin N Am* 2009;17:469–487.

22

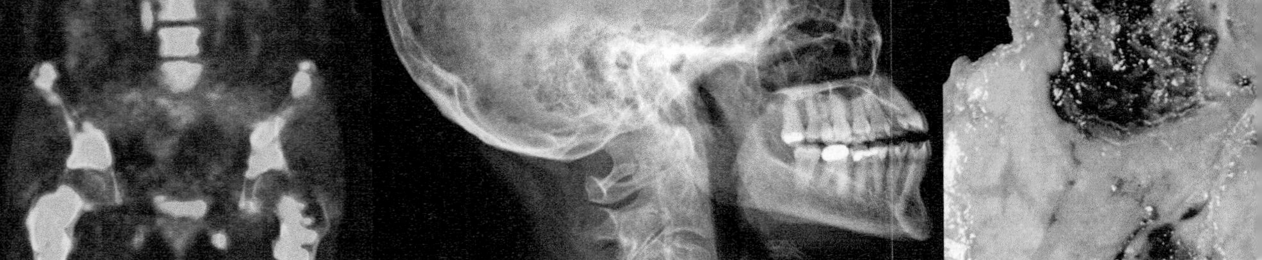

Malignant Bone Tumors II

Miscellaneous Tumors

Fibrosarcoma and Malignant Fibrous Histiocytoma

Clinical Features

Fibrosarcoma and malignant fibrous histiocytoma (MFH) are malignant fibrogenic tumors that have very similar imaging presentations and histologic patterns. Both typically occur in the third to sixth decades, and both have a predilection for the pelvis, femur, humerus, and tibia (Fig. 22.1).

Because there is no essential difference in the imaging features, clinical behavior, and survival data for these tumors, it is justified to regard them as a single group. Both fibrosarcoma and MFH can be either primary tumors or secondary to a preexisting benign condition, such as Paget disease, fibrous dysplasia, bone infarct, or chronic draining sinuses of osteomyelitis. These lesions may also arise in bones that were previously irradiated. Such lesions are termed *secondary fibrosarcomas* (or *secondary MFHs*). Rarely, fibrosarcoma can arise in a periosteal location (periosteal fibrosarcoma). Some investigators postulate, however, that in this location these lesions represent primary soft-tissue tumors abutting the bone and invading the underlying periosteum.

Imaging Features

Radiographically, fibrosarcoma and MFH are recognized by an osteolytic area of bone destruction and a wide zone of transition; the lesions are usually eccentrically located close to or in the articular end of the bone. They exhibit little or no reactive sclerosis and, in most cases, no periosteal reaction (Figs. 22.2 to 22.4); a soft-tissue mass, however, is commonly present.

On computed tomography (CT) examination, fibrosarcoma and MFH show a predominant density similar to that of normal muscle and exhibit the nonspecific tissue attenuation values of Hounsfield units encountered in most nonmineralized tissues. Hypodense areas reflect areas of necrosis within tumor. Magnetic resonance imaging (MRI) is useful to outline the intraosseous and extraosseous extension of these tumors, but there are no characteristic MRI findings for either one (Fig. 22.5). Several investigators found the signal characteristics comparable to those of other lytic bone tumors. Signal intensity is intermediate to low on T1-weighted images and high on T2 weighting, frequently heterogenous, and varying with the degree of necrosis and hemorrhage within the tumor.

Pathology

Gross specimens of fibrosarcoma and MFH are very similar, showing a solid tumor with trabeculated tan-to-white cut surface, occasionally with hemorrhagic and necrotic foci, commonly breaking the cortex and extending into the soft tissues (Fig. 22.6). Histologically, fibrosarcoma and MFH are characterized by tumor cells that produce collagen fibers. In fibrosarcoma, however, there is a herringbone pattern of fibrous growth with mild cellular pleomorphism, whereas histiocytic features of a characteristic storiform or pinwheel arrangement of fibrogenic tissue typify MFH. In addition, numerous large bizarre polyhedral cells (histiocytic component) are present. Mitotic activity may be present. Neither tumor is capable of producing osteoid matrix or bone, a factor distinguishing them from osteosarcoma.

It should be stressed, however, that the entity of MFH has recently fallen out of favor and into disrepute. One of the reasons was the fact that with advances of electron microscopy and increasing use of immunohistochemical and genetic investigations, it becomes obvious that some tumors, initially classified as MFH, have been reclassified as pleomorphic variants of other sarcomas such as leiomyosarcomas, liposarcomas, myxofibrosarcomas, and rhabdomyosarcomas. For example, in the new World Health Organization (WHO) classification of soft-tissue tumors, MFH is considered to represent a small group of undifferentiated pleomorphic sarcomas with no definable line of differentiation, and the term is used with reluctance, although MFH of bone still remains in this classification listed under the heading "fibrohistiocytic tumors." Recent genetic studies of MFH of bone disclosed loss of heterozygosity at chromosome 9p+g validated the hypothesis, that in the pathogenesis of these tumors, alterations of a putative tumor suppressor gene located at this chromosome may be involved. Mutation in *p53* gene was reported in secondary MFH associated with bone infarction.

More extensive genetic abnormalities were found in fibrosarcomas, such as gain of chromosomes 1q, 4q, 5p, 8q, 12p, 15q, 16q, 17q, 20q, 22q, and Xp, and loss at chromosomes 6q, 8p, 9p, 10, 13q, and 20p. In addition, gain of the *platelet-derived growth factor beta* (*PDGF-β*) gene, located at 22q12.3-q13.1, as well as homozygous deletion of *CDKN2A* and recurrent coamplification of KIT, PDGFRA, and KDR have also been reported.

Differential Diagnosis

Fibrosarcoma and MFH may resemble an aneurysmal bone cyst, giant cell tumor (Fig. 22.7), telangiectatic osteosarcoma (see Figs. 21.22 to 21.24), and plasmacytoma. They are also often mistaken for metastatic lesions (see Fig. 22.3). Some authorities believe that an almost pathognomonic sign of fibrosarcoma are small sequestrum-like fragments of cortical bone and spongy trabeculae, which may be demonstrated on conventional radiography or CT scan.

Immunohistochemical studies have been helpful in the diagnosis of MFH by demonstrating certain nonspecific markers of histiocytic enzymes such as lysozyme, α_1-antitrypsin, and α_1-antichymotrypsin in the tumor. Other antigens reported to variably stain MFH included vimentin, actin, desmin, and keratin.

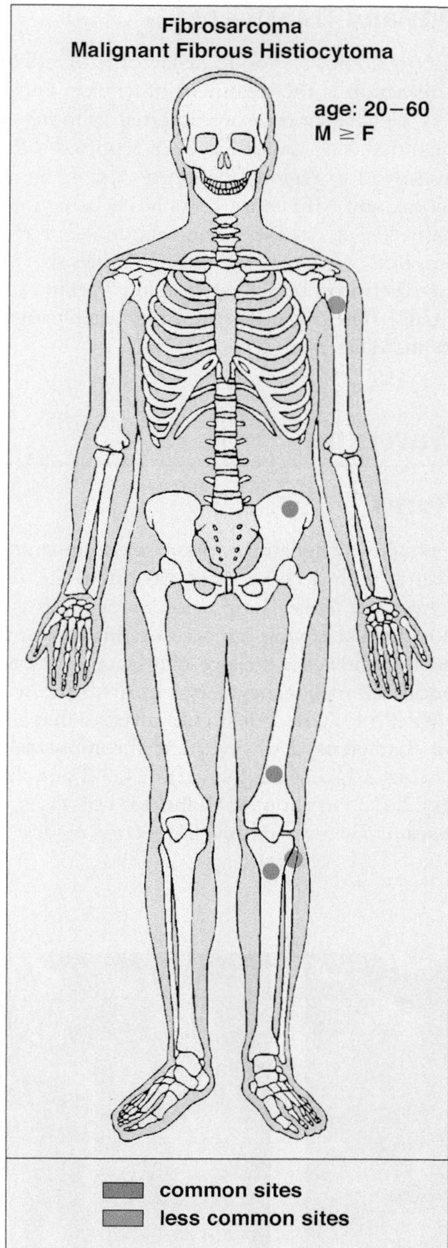

FIGURE 22.1 Skeletal sites of predilection, peak age range, and male-to-female ratio in fibrosarcoma and MFH.

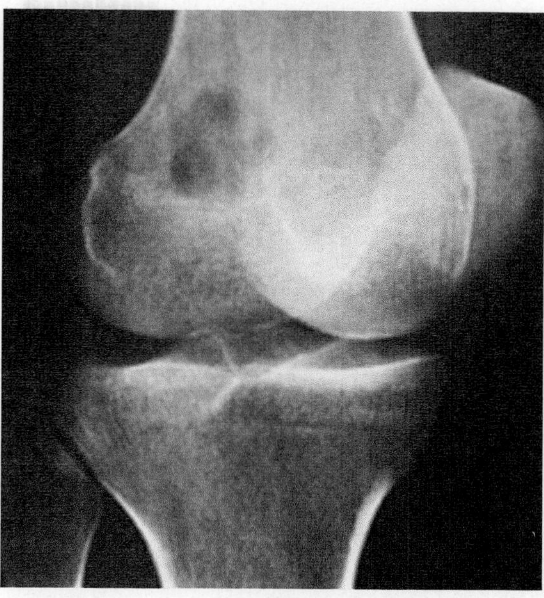

FIGURE 22.2 **Fibrosarcoma.** Oblique radiograph of the right knee of a 28-year-old woman shows a purely destructive osteolytic lesion in the intercondylar fossa of the distal femur. Note the absence of reactive sclerosis and periosteal response.

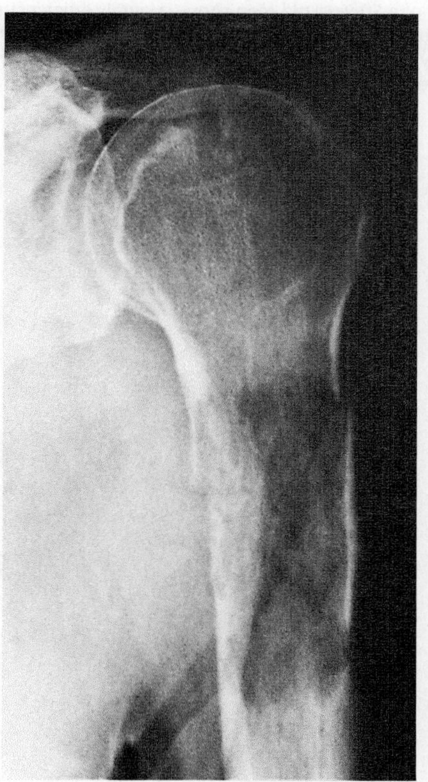

FIGURE 22.3 **Fibrosarcoma.** A 62-year-old man sustained a pathologic fracture through an osteolytic lesion in the proximal shaft of the left humerus. A metastatic lesion was suspected, but biopsy revealed a primary fibrosarcoma of the bone.

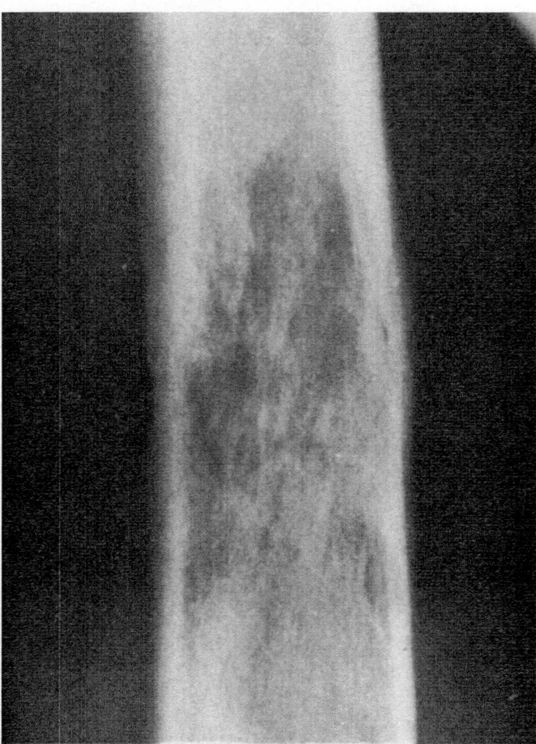

FIGURE 22.4 Malignant fibrous histiocytoma. A coned-down view of the shaft of the femur of a 50-year-old man shows a purely lytic destructive lesion with wide zone of transition and lack of reactive sclerosis. (Reprinted with permission from Greenspan A, Borys D. *Radiology and pathology correlation of bone tumors,* 1st ed. Philadelphia: Wolters Kluwer, 2016:221.)

Complications and Treatment

Because these tumors do not respond satisfactorily to radiation or chemotherapy, surgical resection is the treatment of choice. Pathologic fracture may occur, and as a palliative measure, internal splinting with a metallic implant may be justified. The tumor has been reported to recur after local excision and may spread to regional lymph nodes. As already stated previously, fibrosarcoma and MFH may complicate benign conditions such as fibrous dysplasia, Paget disease, bone infarction, or chronic draining sinuses of osteomyelitis. They may also arise in bones that were previously irradiated (see the discussion under the heading "Benign Conditions with Malignant Potential"). The 5-year survival rate after treatment varies according to different studies from 29% to 67%.

Ewing Sarcoma

Clinical Features

Ewing sarcoma, a highly malignant neoplasm predominantly affecting children and adolescents, with decisive male predominance, is representative of the so-called *round cell tumors*. Its precise histogenesis is unknown, but it is generally thought that Ewing sarcoma originates from bone marrow cells. Some authorities, however, believe that Ewing sarcoma is a neurally derived small round cell malignancy very similar to the so-called *primitive neuroectodermal tumor* (PNET). Recent studies revealed that all tumors of the Ewing family are characterized by recurrent chromosomal translocations involving chromosomes 11 and 22 [t(11;22)(q24;q12)] or chromosomes 21 and 22 [t(21;22)(q22;q12)] in about 85% and 15% of cases, respectively. In about 20% of cases of Ewing sarcoma, the second most common genetic

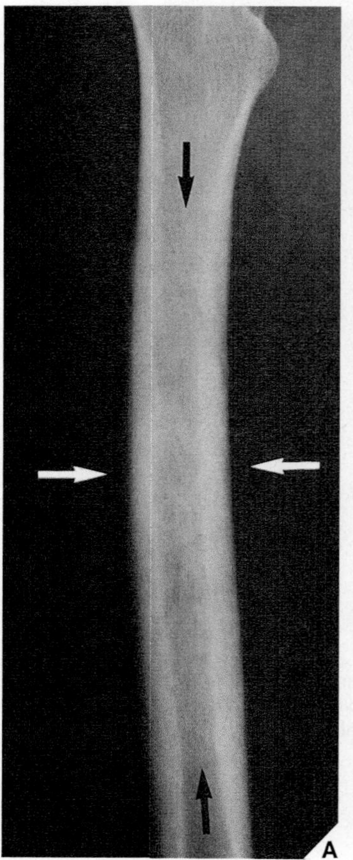

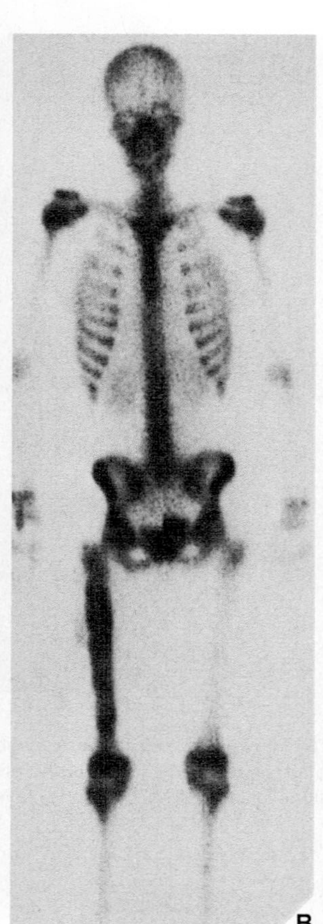

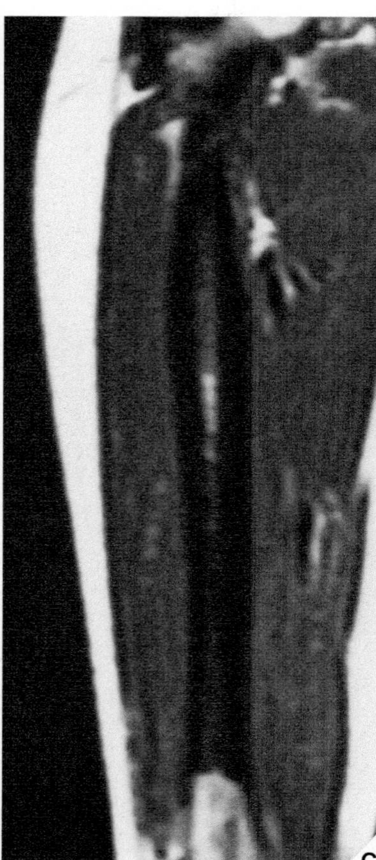

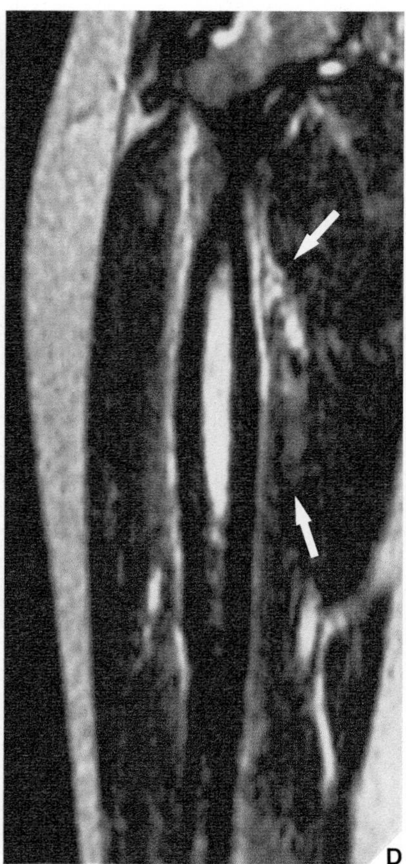

FIGURE 22.5 Scintigraphy and MRI of MFH. (A) Oblique radiograph of the right femur of a 16-year-old girl shows fusiform thickening of the cortex and permeative type of medullary bone destruction *(arrows)*. **(B)** Radionuclide bone scan (^{99m}Tc-MDP) shows increased uptake of the tracer in the right femur. **(C)** Coronal T1-weighted (spin echo [SE]; repetition time [TR] 500/echo time [TE] 20 msec) MR image demonstrates the extent of the tumor that involves about 75% of the length of the femur. **(D)** Coronal T2-weighted (SE; TR 2000/TE 80 msec) MR image shows that the tumor exhibits high signal intensity. The soft-tissue extension medially is also accurately depicted *(arrows)*.

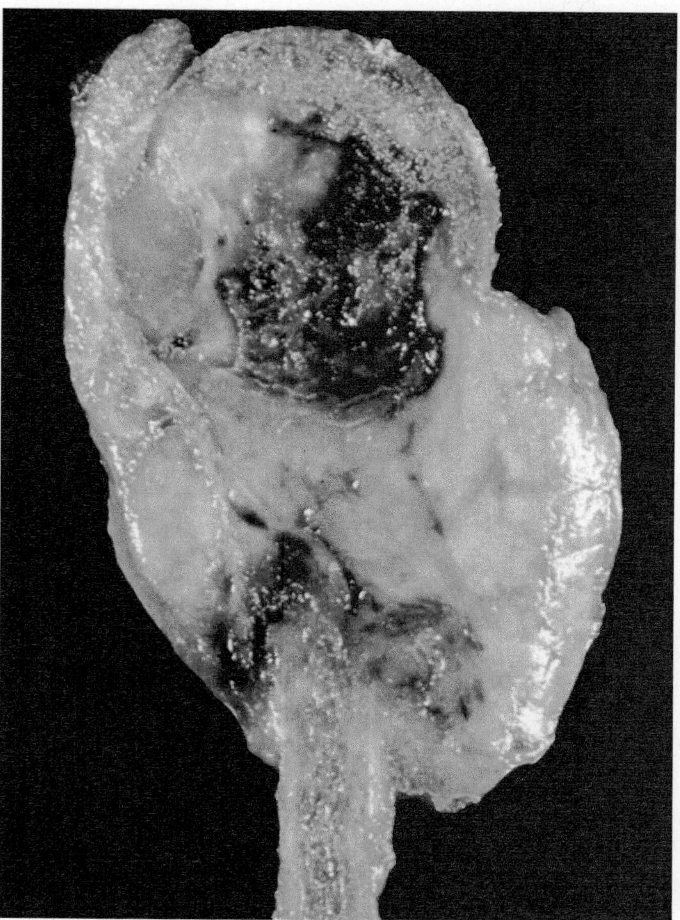

FIGURE 22.6 Pathology of fibrosarcoma. Resected specimen of the proximal humerus shows a solid tumor at the proximal end of bone breaking through the cortex and extending into the soft tissues. Observe focal areas of hemorrhage *(dark red)*. (Reprinted from Bullough P. *Orthopaedic pathology*, 5th ed. Maryland Heights, MO: Mosby; 2009, with permission from Elsevier.)

alteration is the inactivation of the gene *p16* or *INK4A*. In particular, *p16* deletions represent a significant negative predictive factor in Ewing tumor. Approximately 90% of Ewing sarcomas occur before age 25 years, and the disease is extremely rare in black persons. Ewing sarcoma has a predilection for the diaphysis of the long bones as well as the ribs and flat bones such as the scapula and pelvis (Fig. 22.8). Clinically, it may present as a localized painful mass or with systemic symptoms such as fever, malaise, weight loss, and an increased erythrocyte sedimentation rate. These systemic symptoms may lead to an erroneous diagnosis of osteomyelitis.

Imaging Features

The imaging presentation of this malignancy is usually rather characteristic; the lesion is poorly defined, marked by a permeative or moth-eaten type of bone destruction, and associated with an aggressive periosteal response that has an onion skin (or "onion peel") or, less commonly, a "sunburst" appearance, and a large soft-tissue mass (Figs. 22.9 and 22.10). Occasionally, the bone lesion itself is almost imperceptible, with the soft-tissue mass being the only prominent radiographic finding (Fig. 22.11).

On radionuclide bone scan, Ewing sarcoma shows an intense increase of technetium-99m methylene diphosphonate (^{99m}Tc-MDP) uptake. Gallium-67 (^{67}Ga) citrate more readily identifies soft-tissue tumor extension. Although scintigraphic findings are nonspecific, this technique provides reliable information concerning the presence of skeletal metastases. CT reveals the pattern of bone destruction, and attenuation values (Hounsfield units) provide information about the medullary extension. In addition, CT may help to delineate extraosseous involvement (see Fig. 22.11). MRI is essential for definite demonstration of the extent of intraosseous and extraosseous involvement by this tumor (Figs. 22.12 to 22.14). In particular, MRI may effectively reveal extension through the epiphyseal plate. T1-weighted images show intermediate to low signal intensity, which becomes bright on T2 weighting. Hypocellular regions and areas of necrosis are of lesser intensity. Imaging after injection of gadolinium diethylene triamine pentaacetic acid (Gd-DTPA) reveals signal enhancement of the tumor on T1-weighted sequences. Enhancement occurs only in the cellular areas, allowing differentiation of the tumor from the peritumoral edema. Fluorodeoxyglucose (FDG) positron emission tomography (PET) and PET/CT imaging invariably show hypermetabolic activity at the site of the tumor (Figs. 22.14 and 22.15).

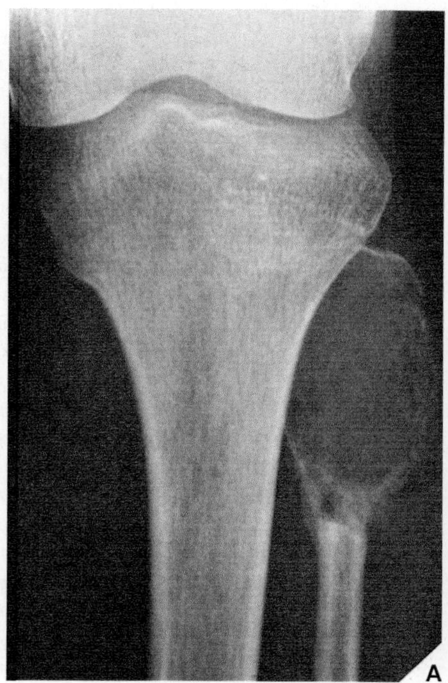

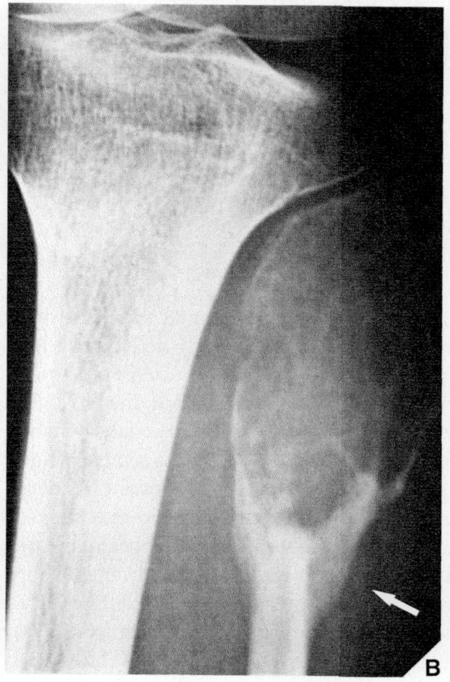

FIGURE 22.7 Malignant fibrous histiocytoma. **(A)** Anteroposterior radiograph of the left knee and **(B)** oblique projection demonstrate an expansive, lytic lesion in the proximal end of the fibula in a 13-year-old girl. The cortex has been partially destroyed, and there is a buttress of periosteal new bone formation *(arrow)* secondary to pathologic fracture. The differential diagnosis of this malignancy at this site should include giant cell tumor and aneurysmal bone cyst.

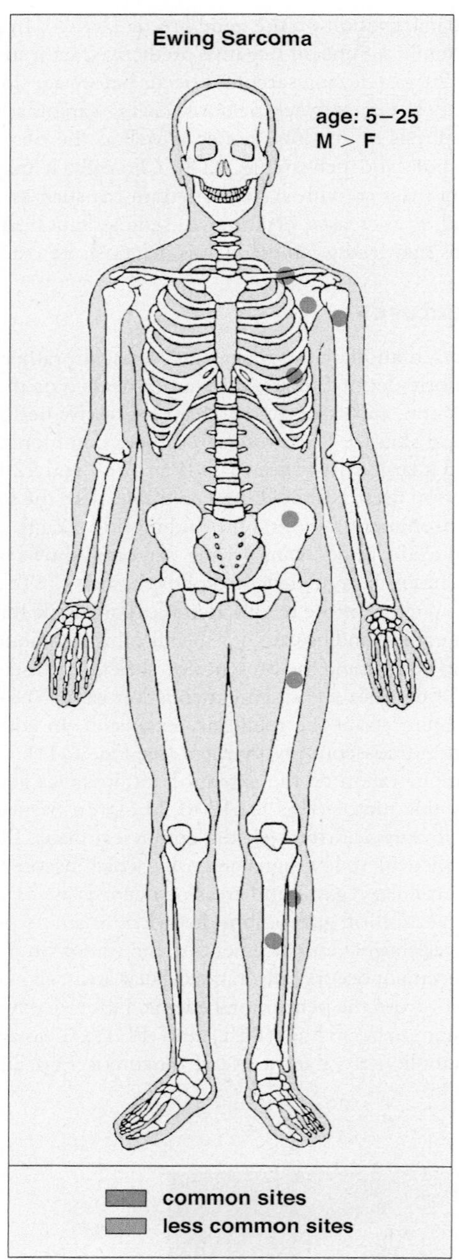

FIGURE 22.8 **Skeletal sites of predilection, peak age range, and male-to-female ratio in Ewing sarcoma.**

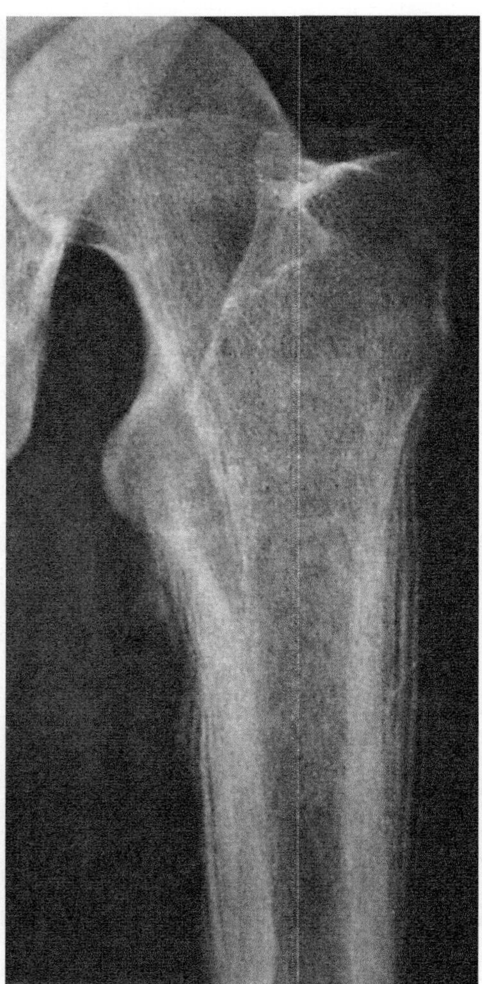

FIGURE 22.9 **Ewing sarcoma.** Anteroposterior radiograph of the right proximal femur of a 20-year-old woman shows permeative lesion associated with characteristic for this tumor onionskin periosteal reaction. (Reprinted with permission from Greenspan A, Borys D. *Radiology and pathology correlation of bone tumors,* 1st ed. Philadelphia: Wolters Kluwer, 2016:244.)

Pathology

Histologically, Ewing sarcoma consists of a uniform array of small cells with round hyperchromatic nuclei, scant cytoplasm, and poorly defined cell borders. The mitotic rate is high, and necrosis is frequently extensive. Usually, the cytoplasm contains a moderate amount of glycogen, demonstrable with the periodic acid–Schiff (PAS) stain. This PAS-positive material is washed away after digestion with diastase, confirming that, in fact, it represents glycogen. The demonstration of glycogen, which at one time was considered an absolutely distinctive marker for Ewing sarcoma, has fallen into disfavor because in some Ewing sarcomas, glycogen is not found. Moreover, malignant lymphoma and primitive neural tumors may at times contain glycogen. Since the advent of immunohistochemistry, lymphomas are usually differentiated from Ewing sarcomas by demonstrating leukocyte-common antigen, a pathognomic marker for lymphomas, and primitive neural tumors differ from Ewing sarcomas by the fact that they contain neural protein antibodies. Furthermore, immunohistochemistry reveals that almost all Ewing family tumors exhibit a positive membranous and cytoplasmic reaction for Fli-1, CD99, vimentin, and neuron-specific enolase (NSE), respectively. Conversely, there is negative reaction for S-100 protein, CD45, and muscular and vascular markers.

Differential Diagnosis

Ewing sarcoma may often mimic metastatic neuroblastoma or osteomyelitis (Fig. 22.16). At times, Ewing sarcoma exhibits a feature once thought to be almost pathognomonic, the "saucerization" of the cortex (Fig. 22.17), which may be related to destruction of the periosteal surface by the tumor combined with the effect of extrinsic pressure by the large soft-tissue mass. Although this sign has recently been reported in other tumors, and even in osteomyelitis, its presence in association with a permeative lesion and a soft-tissue mass favors the diagnosis of Ewing sarcoma. The radiographic distinction of Ewing sarcoma from metastatic neuroblastoma may occasionally be difficult; however, the latter usually occurs in the first 3 years, whereas Ewing sarcoma is uncommon in the first 5 years. Imaging features of solitary Langerhans cell histiocytosis may at times be very similar to those of Ewing sarcoma; however, the soft-tissue mass is usually smaller. In addition, slanting or beveling of the edges of the former lesion and "hole-in-hole" appearance is rather characteristic.

Occasionally, Ewing sarcoma may resemble an osteosarcoma, particularly when the former is accompanied by abundant periosteal new bone formation. Moreover, dystrophic calcifications in the soft-tissue mass may mimic tumor-bone formation in osteosarcoma (Fig. 22.18). Lymphoma must also be included in the differential diagnosis, although this lesion usually occurs in an older age group. The important radiologic difference is usually the absence of a soft-tissue mass in lymphoma, whereas in Ewing sarcoma a soft-tissue mass is almost invariably present, often being disproportionally large compared with the amount of bone destruction (see Figs. 22.8 and 22.9). The distinction between Ewing sarcoma and PNET cannot be made on the basis of imaging studies. Differentiation between these two tumors must rely entirely on immunohistochemistry, electron microscopy, and molecular genetic studies.

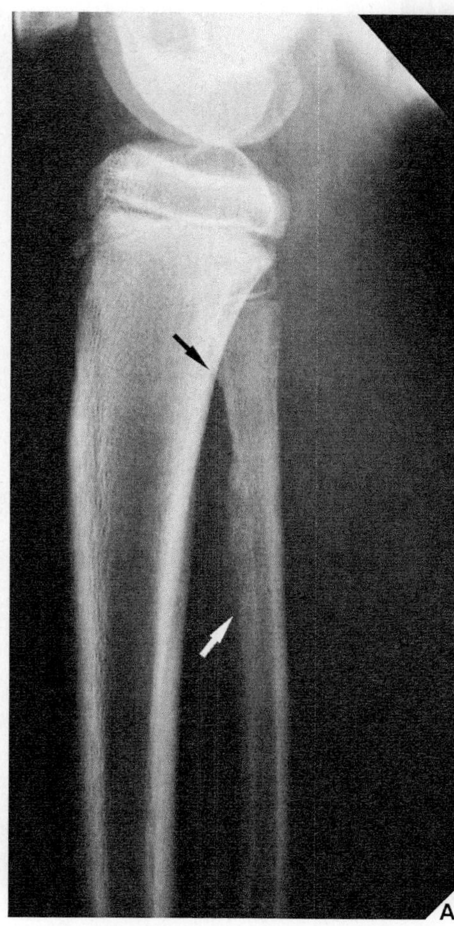

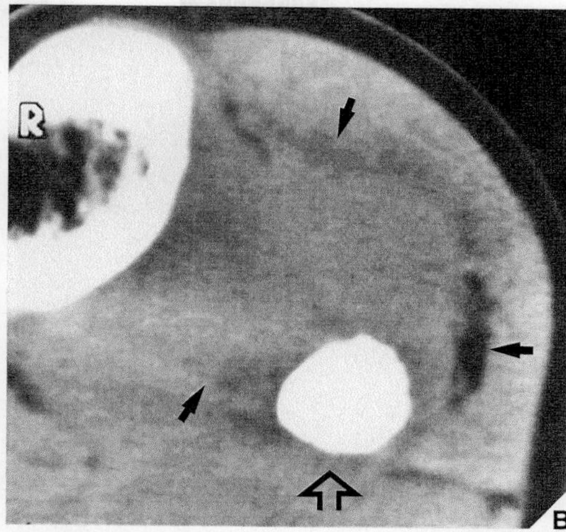

FIGURE 22.10 CT of Ewing sarcoma. **(A)** Lateral radiograph of a 12-year-old boy shows the typical appearance of this tumor in the fibula. The poorly defined lesion exhibits permeative bone destruction associated with an aggressive periosteal reaction *(arrows)*. **(B)** CT section through the lesion demonstrates a large soft-tissue mass *(arrows)*, which is not clear on the conventional study. Note the complete obliteration of the marrow cavity by tumor *(open arrow)*.

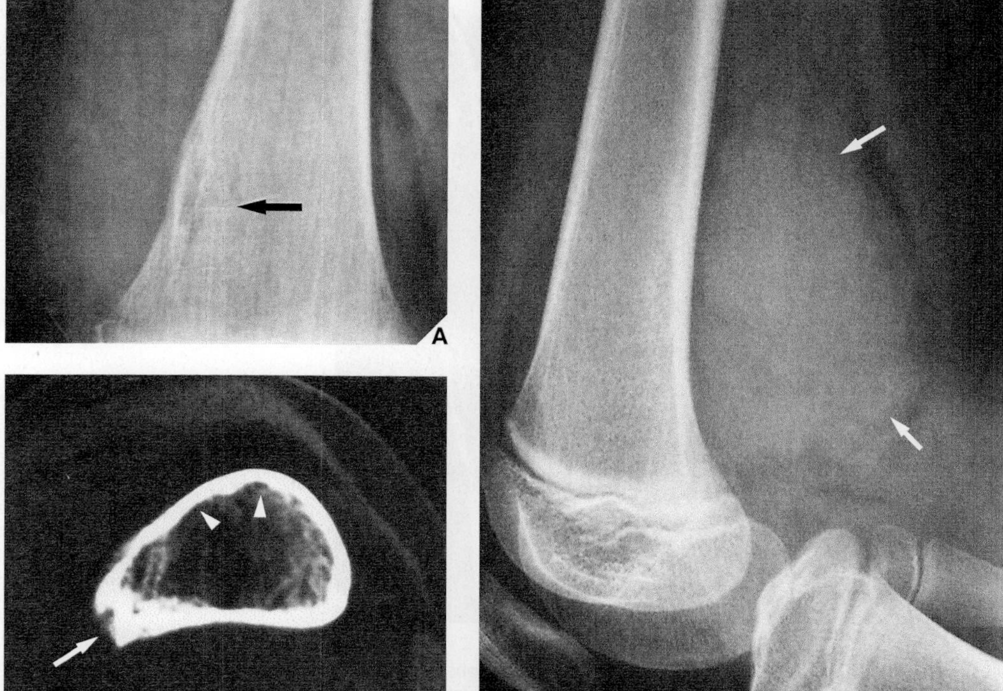

FIGURE 22.11 CT of Ewing sarcoma. **(A)** Bone destruction *(arrow)* is almost imperceptible on this radiograph of a 10-year-old girl with tumor in the distal femoral diaphysis. **(B)** Lateral radiograph of distal femur, however, shows a large soft-tissue mass *(arrows)*. **(C)** CT using bone "window" demonstrates destruction of the medullary portion of the bone, endosteal escalloping *(arrowheads)*, and invasion of the cortex *(arrow)*.

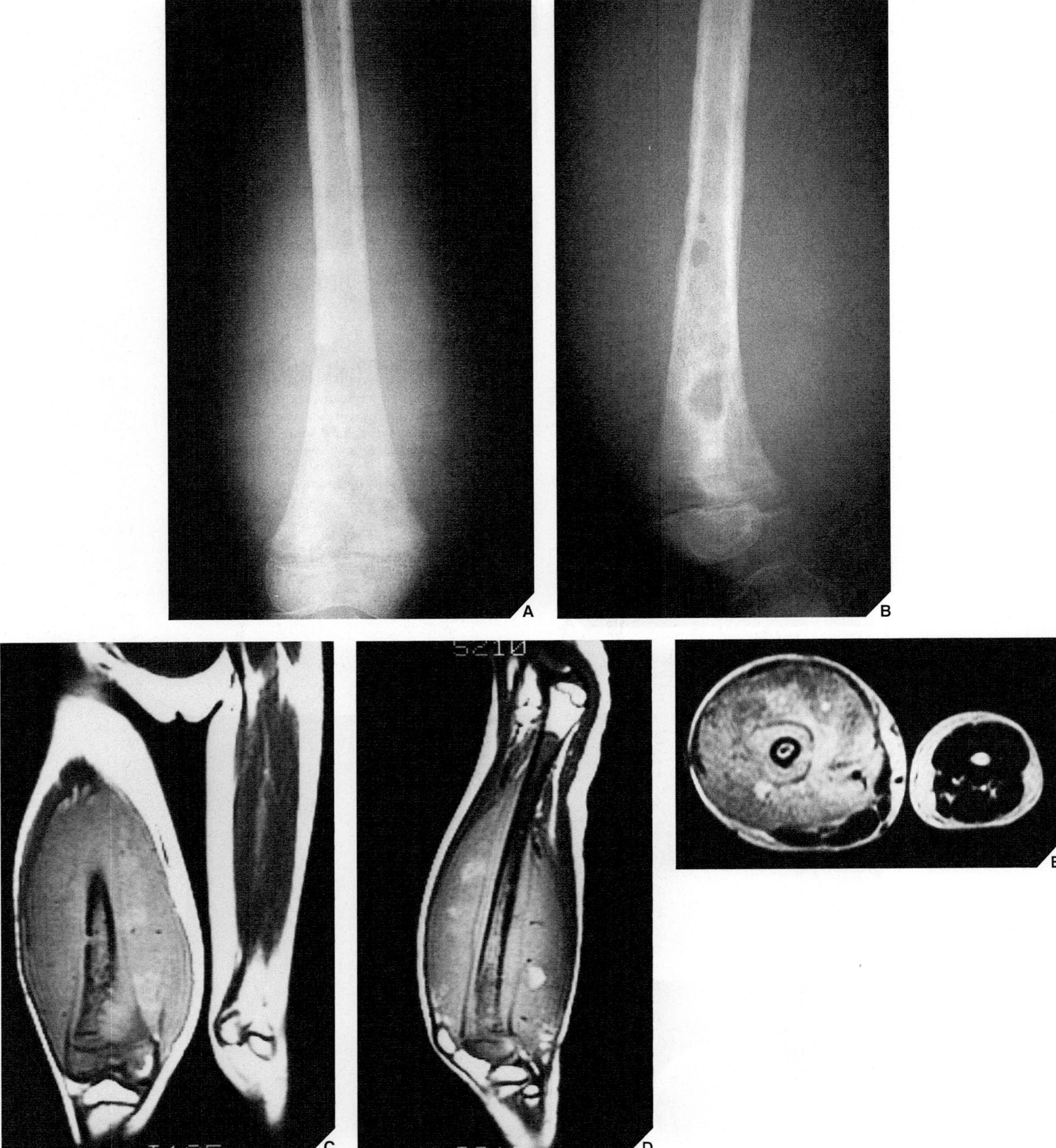

FIGURE 22.12 MRI of Ewing sarcoma. **(A)** Anteroposterior and **(B)** lateral radiographs of the right distal femur of a 7-year-old girl show permeative and moth-eaten types of bone destruction in the metaphysis and diaphysis associated with a large soft-tissue mass. **(C)** Coronal and **(D)** sagittal T1-weighted (spin echo [SE]; repetition time [TR] 750/echo time [TE] 20 msec) MR images demonstrate the intraosseous and extraosseous extent of the tumor. **(E)** Axial T2-weighted (SE; TR 2000/TE 80 msec) MR image shows heterogeneous but mostly high signal intensity of the soft-tissue mass. Note markedly enlarged circumference of the right thigh as compared to the contralateral normal thigh.

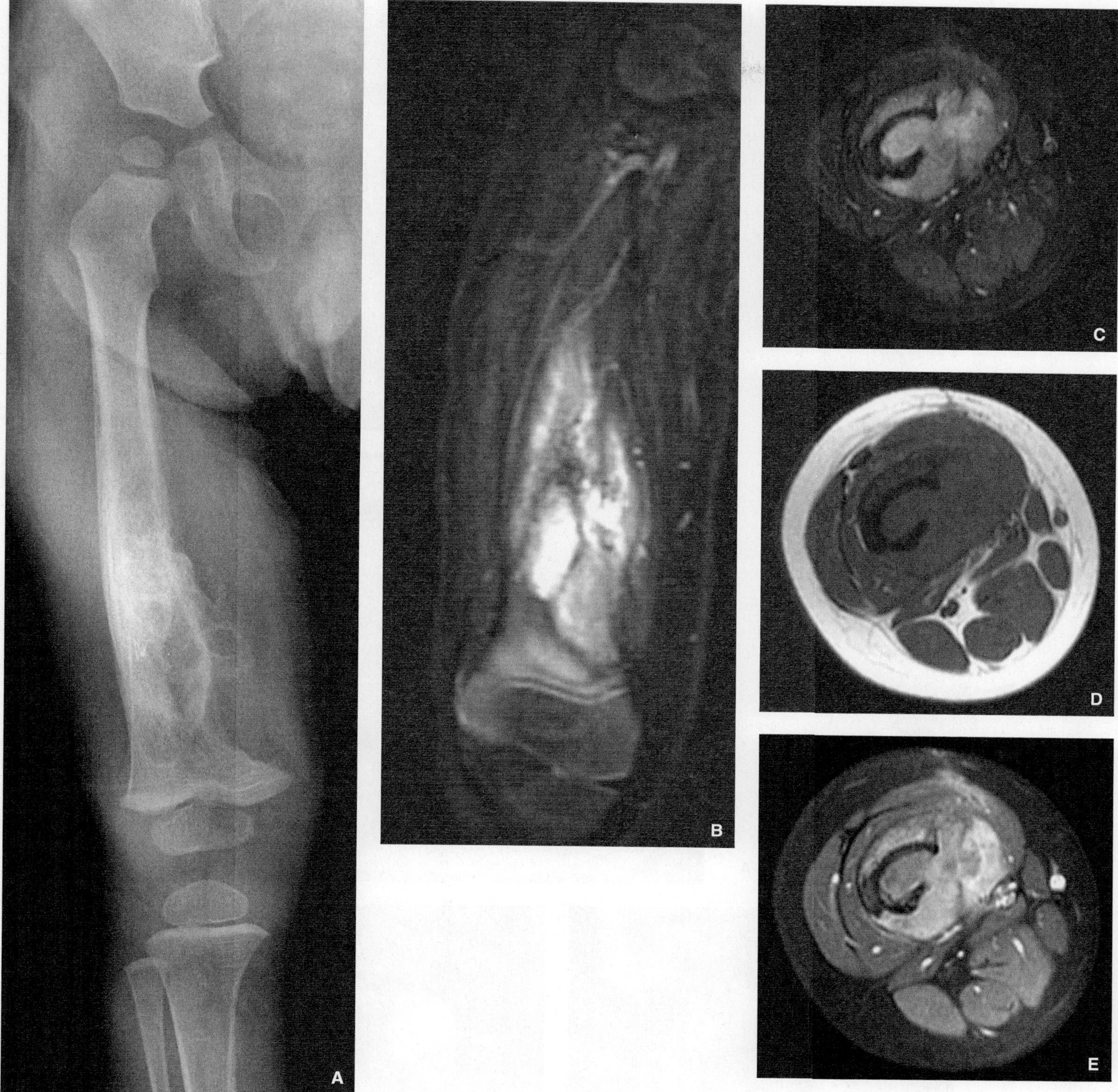

FIGURE 22.13 MRI of Ewing sarcoma. **(A)** Anteroposterior radiograph of the right femur of a 2-year-old boy shows a destructive lesion of the distal diaphysis associated with periosteal reaction and a soft-tissue mass. **(B)** Coronal and **(C)** axial short time inversion recovery (STIR) MR images show the tumor to exhibit heterogenous but predominantly high signal intensity. **(D)** Axial T1-weighted and **(E)** axial T1-weighted fat-suppressed MR images obtained after intravenous administration of gadolinium show significant enhancement of both intramedullary tumor and soft-tissue mass.

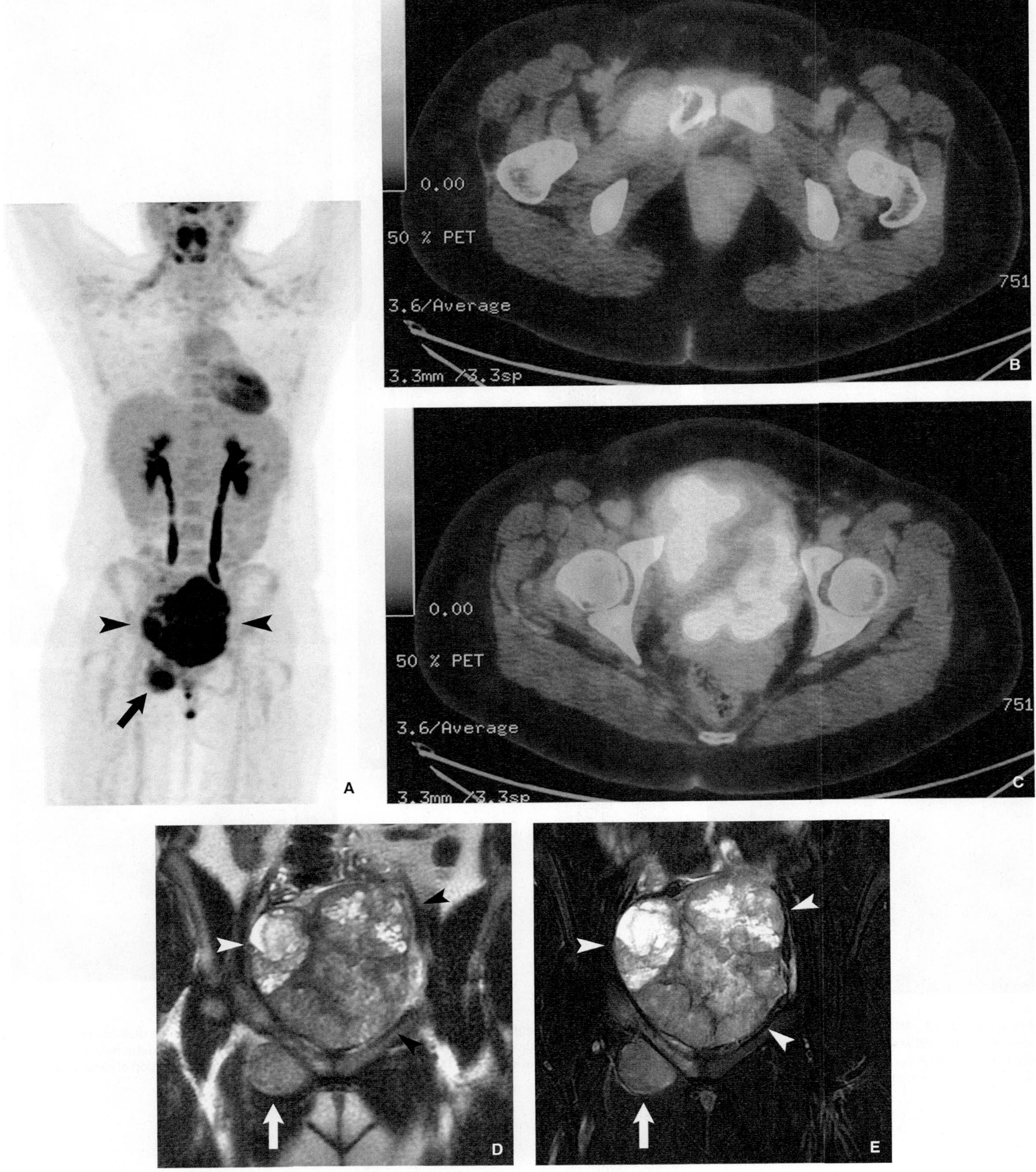

FIGURE 22.14 **FDG PET, PET/CT, and MRI of Ewing sarcoma.** **(A)** Total body ^{18}F-FDG PET scan of a 19-year-old woman shows small extrapelvic *(arrow)* and large intrapelvic *(arrowheads)* hypermetabolic foci. **(B)** Fused PET/CT image shows destructive lesion in the right pubic bone and extrapelvic mass. **(C)** Fused PET/CT image obtained more proximally through the hip joints demonstrate a large hypermetabolic intrapelvic mass. **(D)** Coronal T1-weighted and **(E)** T2-weighted MR images demonstrate the tumor within the right pubic bone, and the full extent of the extrapelvic *(arrow)* and intrapelvic *(arrowheads)* soft-tissue involvement.

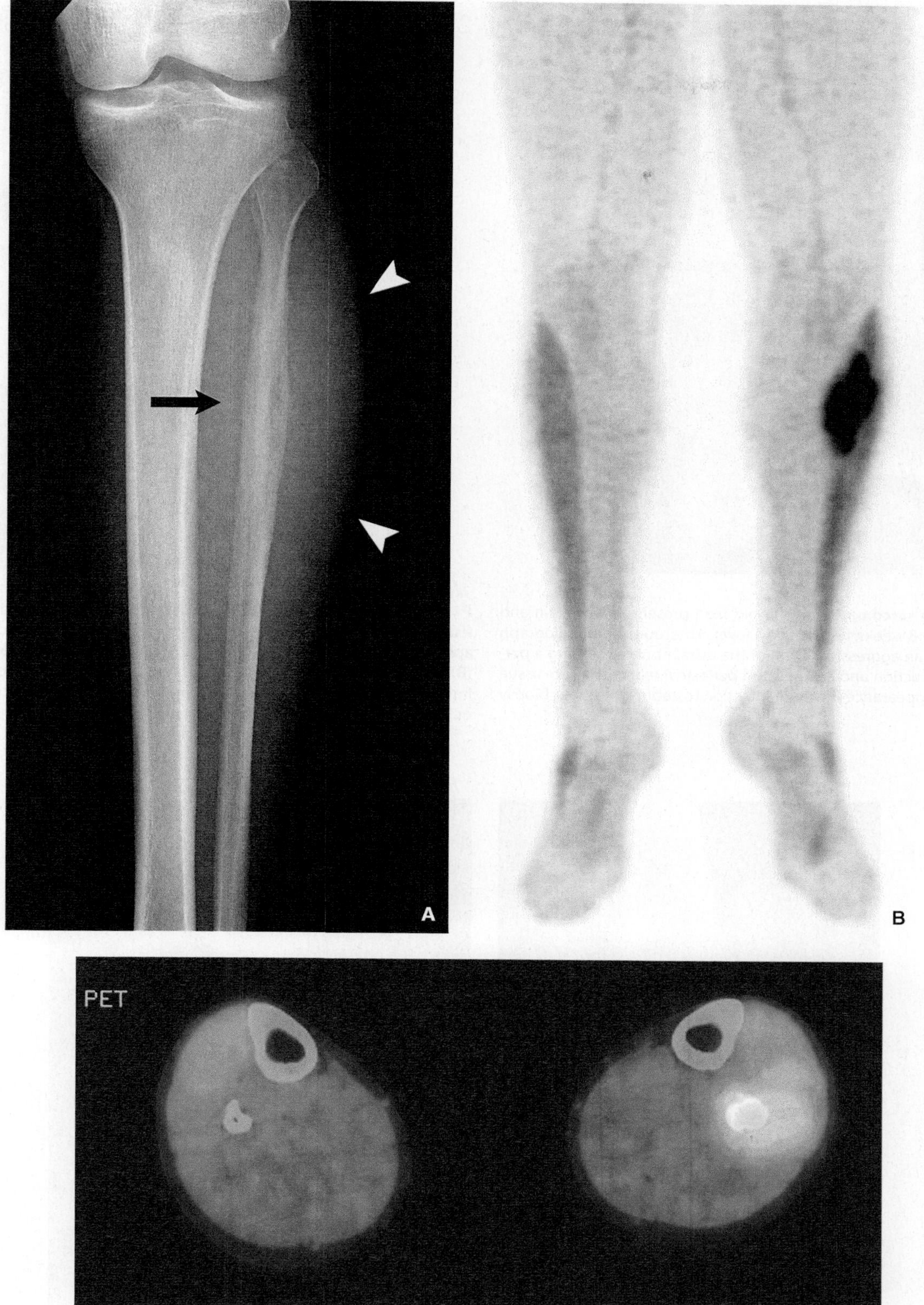

FIGURE 22.15 FDG PET and PET/CT of Ewing sarcoma. **(A)** Anteroposterior radiograph of the left leg of a 23-year-old man shows a slightly expansive lesion in the proximal fibula *(arrow)* associated with a soft-tissue mass *(arrowheads)*. **(B)** ^{18}F-FDG PET scan of the lower extremities and **(C)** fused PET/CT image show a hypermetabolic focus corresponding to the site of the tumor.

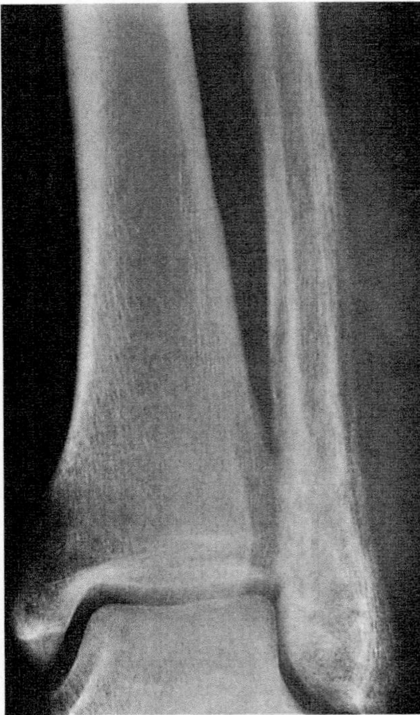

FIGURE 22.16 Ewing sarcoma. A 24-year-old man presented with pain and swelling of the left ankle for 8 weeks; he also had a fever. Anteroposterior radiograph of the ankle demonstrates an aggressive lesion of the distal fibula exhibiting a permeative type of bone destruction and a lamellated periosteal reaction; a soft-tissue mass is also evident. The appearance is that of infection (osteomyelitis), but biopsy confirmed malignancy.

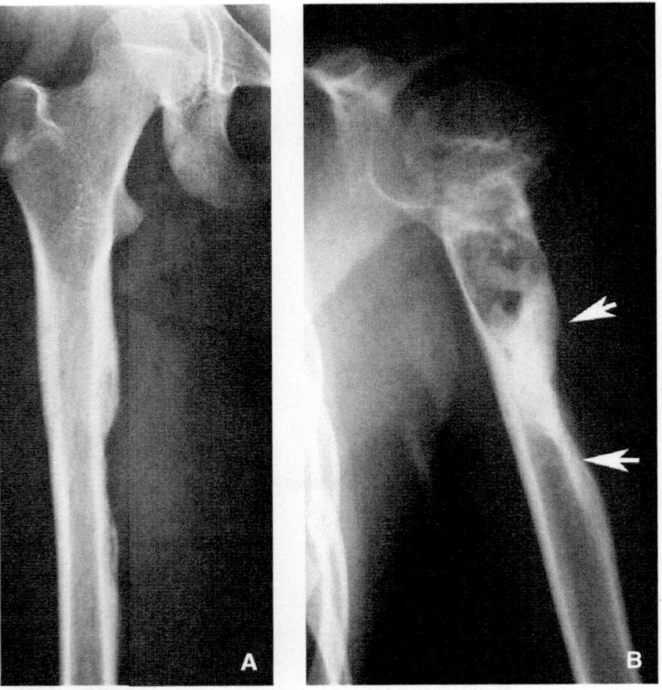

FIGURE 22.17 Ewing sarcoma. **(A)** Anteroposterior radiograph of the right femur of a 12-year-old girl shows "saucerization" of the medial cortex of the diaphysis, often seen in Ewing sarcoma; there is also an associated soft-tissue mass. **(B)** Anteroposterior radiograph of the humerus in another patient demonstrates the intramedullary involvement and the superficial erosion of the cortex of the humerus or "saucerization" *(arrows)*.

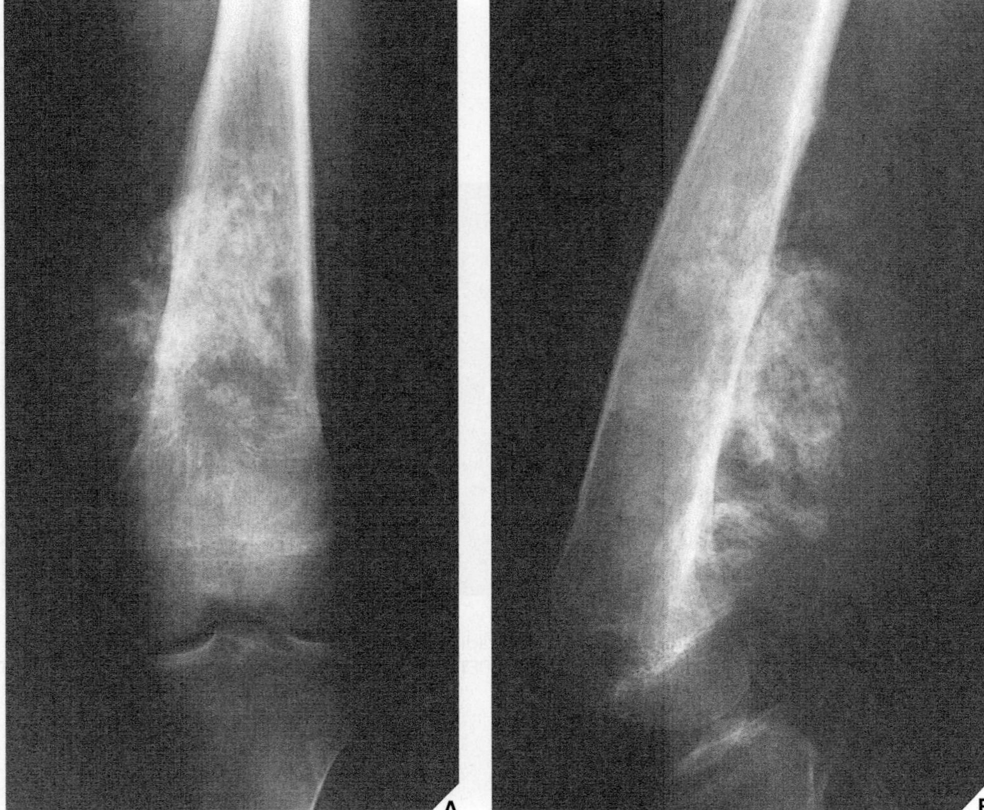

FIGURE 22.18 Ewing sarcoma. **(A)** Anteroposterior and **(B)** lateral radiographs of the left femur of a 17-year-old boy show a tumor displaying a significant degree of sclerosis and sunburst type of periosteal reaction that was originally misinterpreted as osteosarcoma.

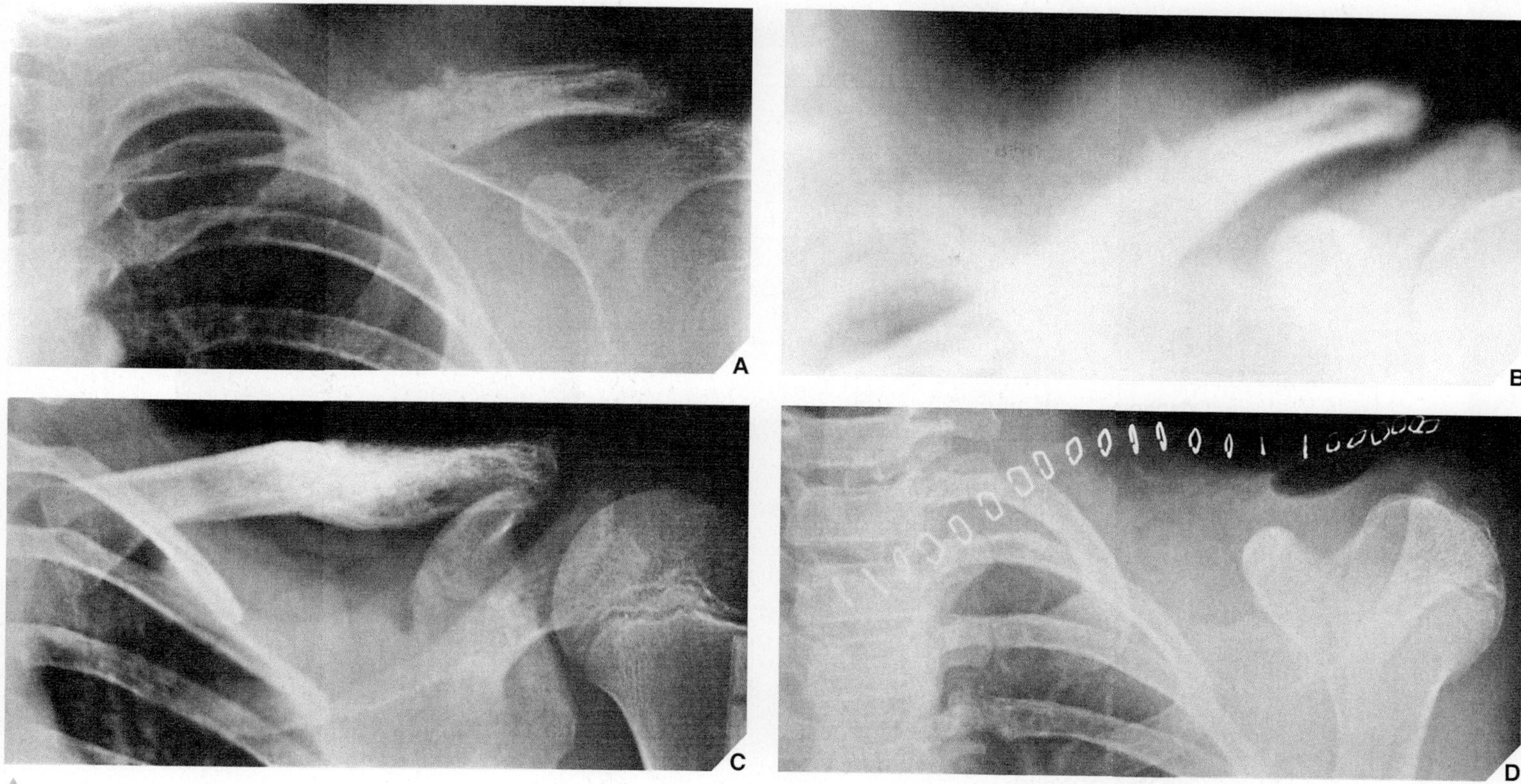

FIGURE 22.19 Treatment of Ewing sarcoma. **(A)** Radiograph of the shoulder of an 11-year-old boy shows the typical appearance of Ewing sarcoma involving the distal half of the left clavicle. The poorly defined destructive lesion is associated with an aggressive periosteal reaction and a large soft-tissue mass. **(B)** Tomographic cut gives a better picture of the soft-tissue mass. **(C)** After a 4-month course of chemotherapy, the lesion has become sclerotic, the periosteal reaction has disappeared, and the soft-tissue mass has shrunk substantially. **(D)** The clavicle was then removed en bloc.

Treatment and Prognosis

Ewing sarcoma is usually treated with a preoperative course of chemotherapy, either alone or combined with radiation therapy, to shrink the tumor, followed by wide resection (Fig. 22.19). Sometimes, the affected limb can be reconstructed with an endoprosthesis or an allograft. Prognosis has improved with adjuvant therapy. Important prognostic features include the stage, anatomic location, and size of the tumor. Patients with tumors that are already metastatic at the time of the diagnosis, particularly if they are large and arising in the pelvic bones, tend to do poorly.

Malignant Lymphoma

Clinical Features

The term *malignant lymphoma* refers to a group of neoplasms that are composed of lymphoid or histiocytic cells of different subtypes in various stages of maturation. Once called *reticulum cell sarcoma*, *non-Hodgkin lymphoma*, *lymphosarcoma*, or *osteolymphoma*, bone lymphoma is now known as *large cell* or *histiocytic lymphoma*. According to new WHO classification, malignant lymphomas of bone are subdivided into (a) those that affect one skeletal site with or without involvement of regional lymph nodes, (b) those that affect multiple bones without lymph nodes or visceral involvement, (c) those that present as a primary bone tumor but reveal nodal or visceral lesions, and (d) those occurring in the patients with known lymphoma elsewhere. Groups (a) and (b) are considered primary lymphoma of bone. Primary bone lymphoma is a rare tumor that accounts for less than 5% of all primary bone tumors. It occurs in the second to seventh decades, with a peak age of occurrence from 45 to 75 years; it has a slightly greater prevalence in males. The lesion develops in the long bones, vertebrae, pelvis, and ribs (Fig. 22.20). Patients may present with local symptoms, such as pain and swelling, or with systemic symptoms, such as fever and weight loss.

Imaging Features

Radiographically, histiocytic lymphoma produces a permeative or moth-eaten pattern of bone destruction or is a purely osteolytic lesion with or more commonly without a periosteal reaction (Fig. 22.21). The affected bone can also present with an "ivory" appearance, as is often the case in lesions of the vertebrae or flat bones (Figs. 22.22 and 22.23). Pathologic fractures are occasionally encountered (Figs. 22.24 and 22.25). Because lymphoma usually does not evoke significant periosteal new bone formation, this is an important feature in differentiating it from Ewing sarcoma. CT may better characterize the extent of osseous involvement (Figs. 22.26 to 22.28). Fluorine-18 (^{18}F)-FDG PET and MRI have been used for the diagnosis of lymphoma, but the sensitivity of MRI (whole-body MRI) is low compared to bone marrow biopsy. MRI and FDG PET are more sensitive in aggressive lymphoma than in indolent lymphoma (Figs. 22.29 and 22.30; see also Fig. 22.24). The MRI manifestations of lymphoma involving the bone marrow are relatively nonspecific. Areas of low signal intensity on T1-weighted images and high signal intensity on T2-weighted images, with enhancement following intravenous administration of gadolinium are the most common manifestations (see Figs. 22.24F, 22.29G, and 22.30). Soft-tissue masses and lymphadenopathy are often seen. Early manifestations of bone marrow involvement in lymphoma may be subtle (see Fig. 22.25A).

Recently, WHO adopted the Revised European-American Classification of Lymphoid Neoplasms (REAL) that originally was proposed by the International Lymphoma Study Group (Table 22.1).

Pathology

Histologically, lymphomas may be subdivided into non-Hodgkin lymphomas and Hodgkin lymphomas. Although secondary involvement of bones is relatively common in Hodgkin lymphoma, primary Hodgkin bone lymphoma is extremely rare. Non-Hodgkin bone lymphomas are considered primary only if a complete systemic workup reveals no evidence of extraosseous involvement. Histologically, the tumor consists of aggregates of malignant lymphoid cells replacing marrow spaces and osseous trabeculae. The cells contain irregular,

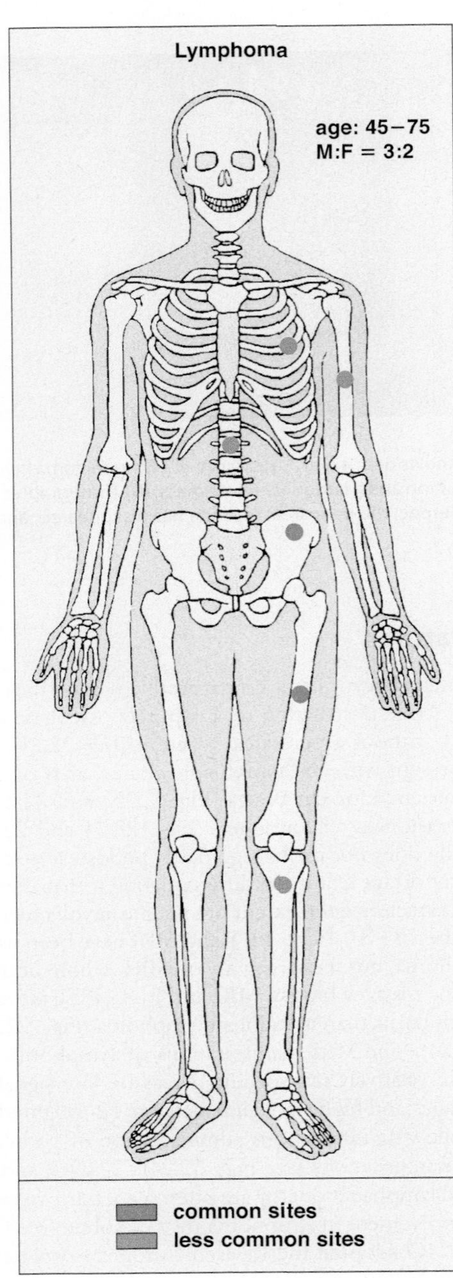

FIGURE 22.20 Skeletal sites of predilection, peak age range, and male-to-female ratio in primary bone lymphoma.

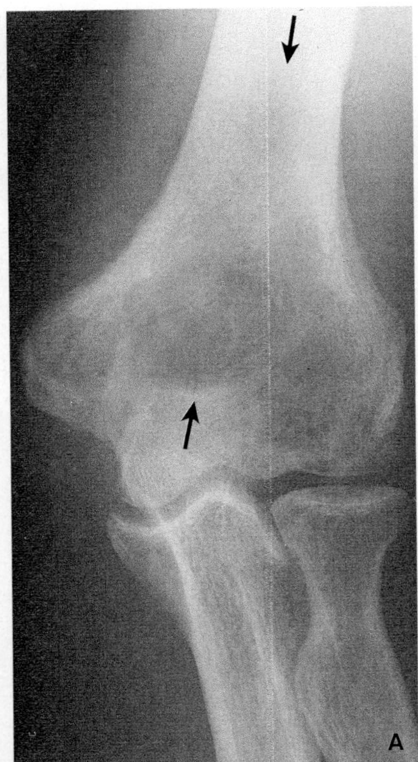

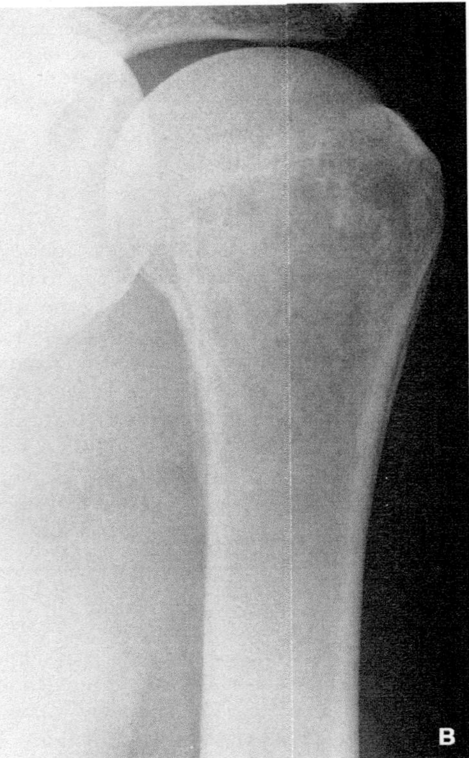

FIGURE 22.21 Lymphoma. **(A)** Anteroposterior radiograph of the left elbow of a 42-year-old man shows a large lytic lesion in the distal humerus *(arrows)*. **(B)** Anteroposterior radiograph of the left shoulder of a 30-year-old man shows a permeative pattern of bone destruction in the proximal humerus accompanied by a lamellated periosteal reaction. (Reprinted with permission from Greenspan A, Borys D. *Radiology and pathology correlation of bone tumors: a quick reference and review*. Philadelphia: Wolters Kluwer; 2016:255, Fig. 5.31.)

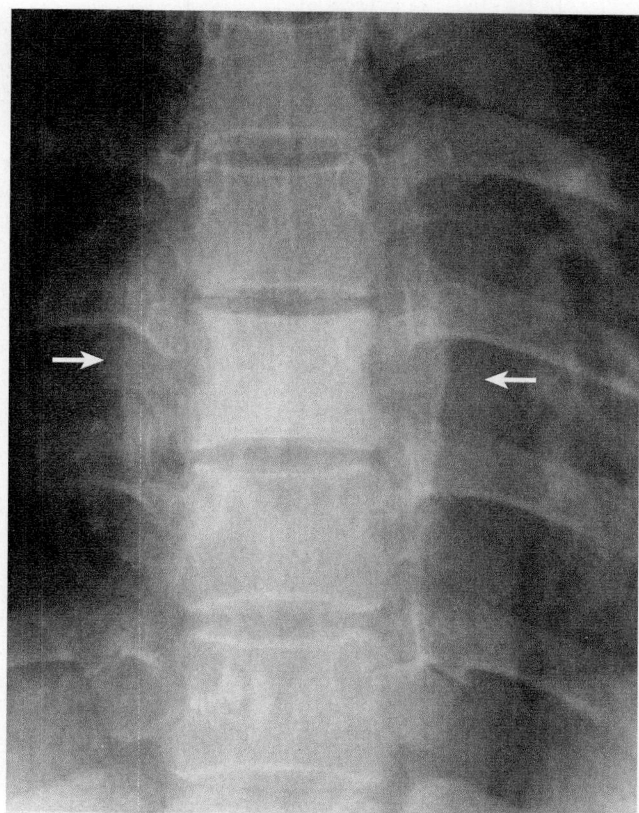

FIGURE 22.22 Lymphoma. Anteroposterior radiograph of the lower thoracic spine of a 32-year-old man shows sclerotic T7 vertebra. Note bulging of the paraspinal line *(arrows)*. (Reprinted with permission from Greenspan A, Borys D. *Radiology and pathology correlation of bone tumors: a quick reference and review*. Philadelphia: Wolters Kluwer; 2016:256, Fig. 5.32.)

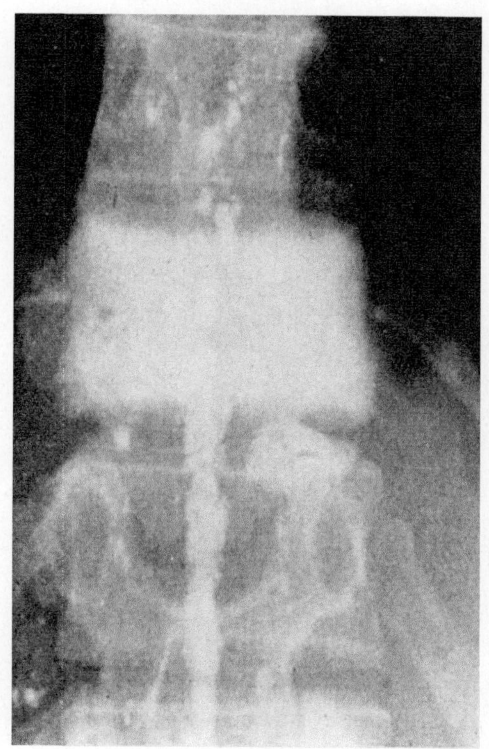

FIGURE 22.23 Hodgkin lymphoma. Anteroposterior radiograph of the lower thoracic spine of a 35-year-old man shows sclerotic T10 vertebra ("ivory vertebra"). (Reprinted from Bullough P. *Orthopaedic pathology*, 5th ed. Maryland Heights, MO: Mosby; 2009, with permission from Elsevier.)

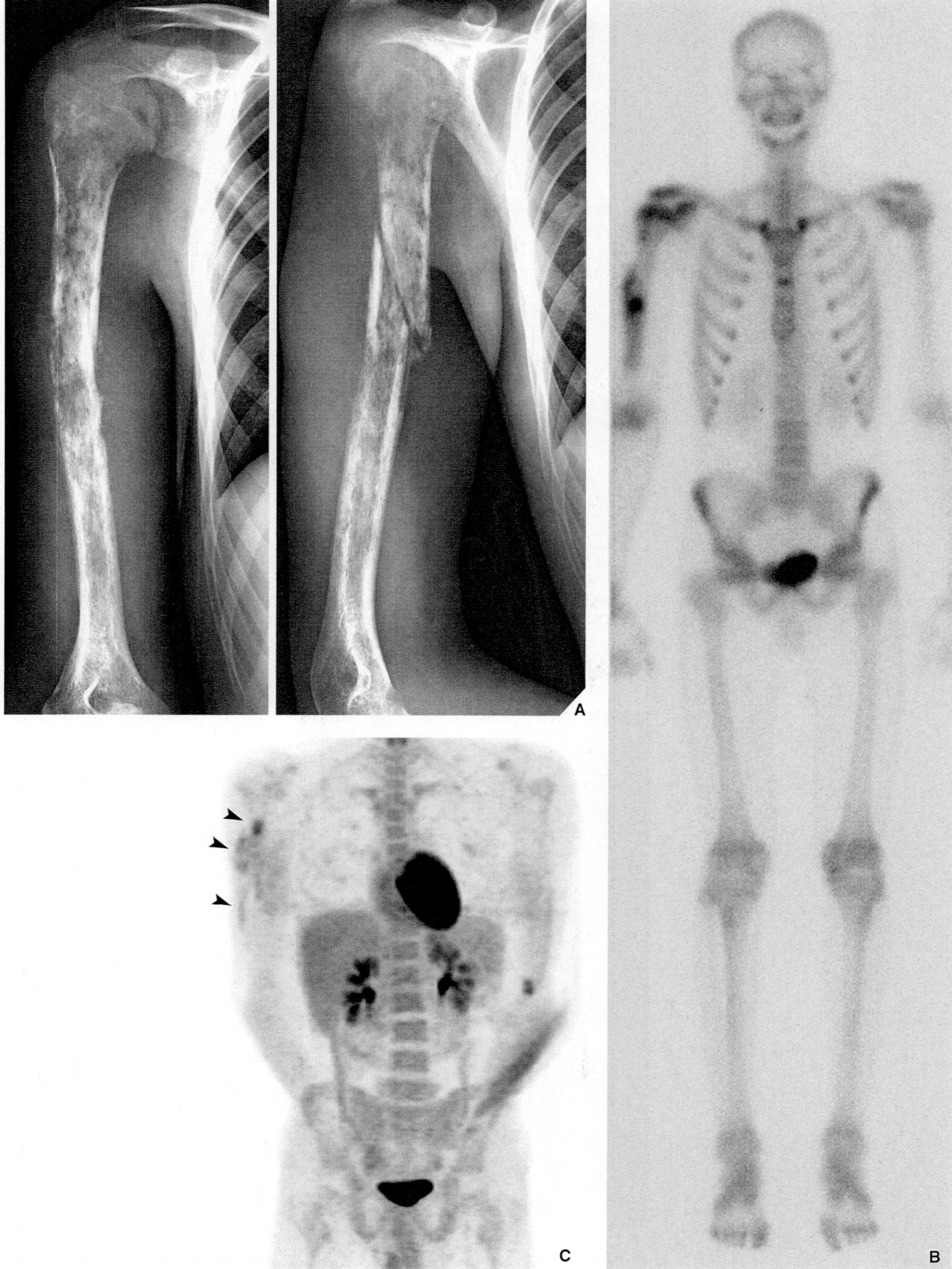

FIGURE 22.24 Scintigraphy, FDG PET, CT, and MRI of lymphoma. **(A)** Anteroposterior and oblique radiographs of the right humerus of a 20-year-old man show a long lesion exhibiting permeative and moth-eaten type of bone destruction. Periosteal reaction is secondary to the pathologic fracture. **(B)** Total body radionuclide bone scan shows increased uptake of radiopharmaceutical tracer at the site of the lesion, with most significant accumulation at the level of a pathologic fracture. **(C)** ^{18}F-FDG PET scan shows several hypermetabolic foci within the proximal humerus *(arrowheads)*. *(Continued)*

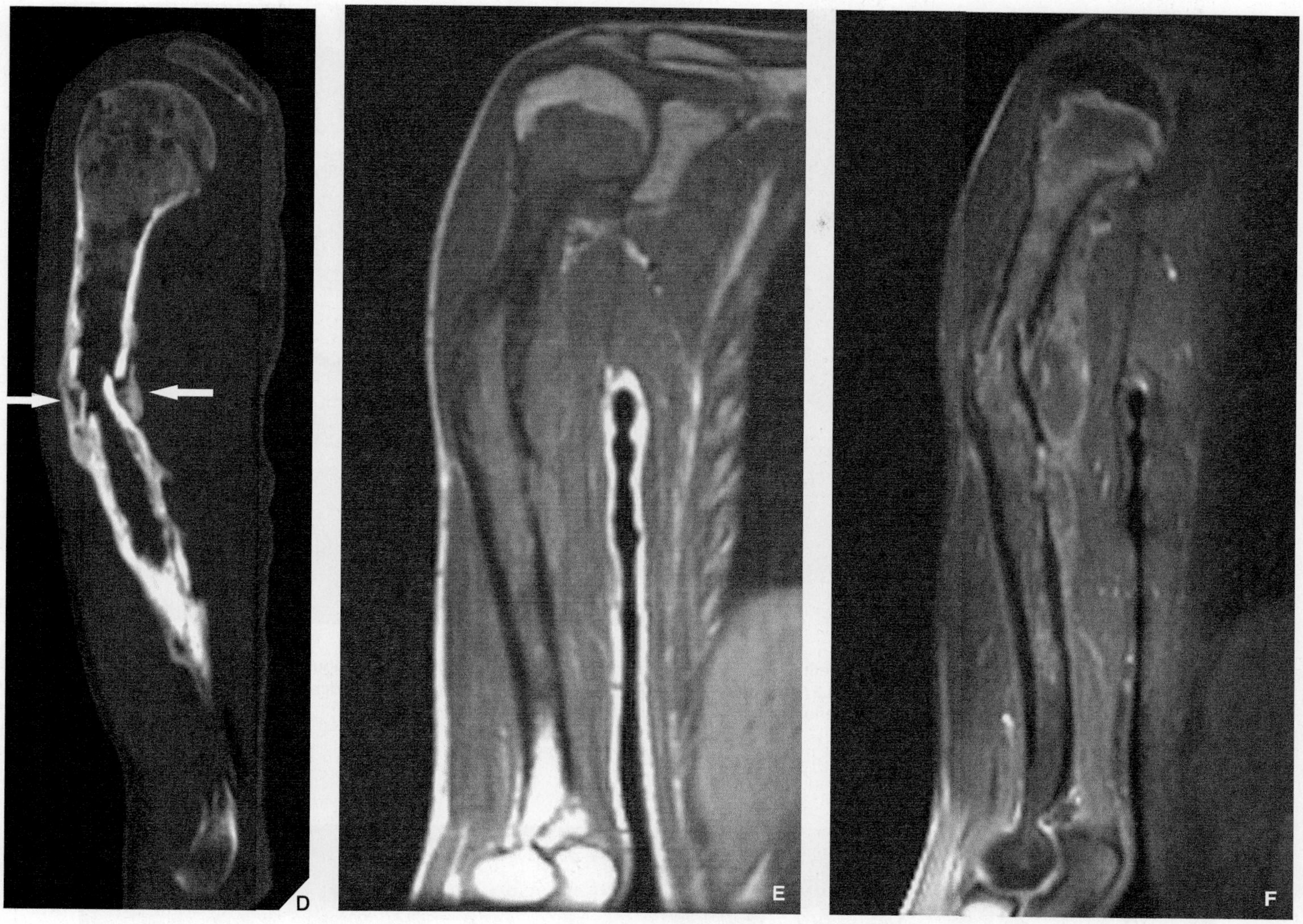

FIGURE 22.24 Scintigraphy, FDG PET, CT, and MRI of lymphoma. ***(Continued)*** **(D)** Sagittal reformatted CT image demonstrates endosteal scalloping and early callus formation at the site of a pathologic fracture *(arrows)*. **(E)** Coronal T1-weighted and **(F)** coronal T1-weighted fat-suppressed postcontrast MR image show enhancement of both, the intraosseous lesion and its extension into the soft tissues.

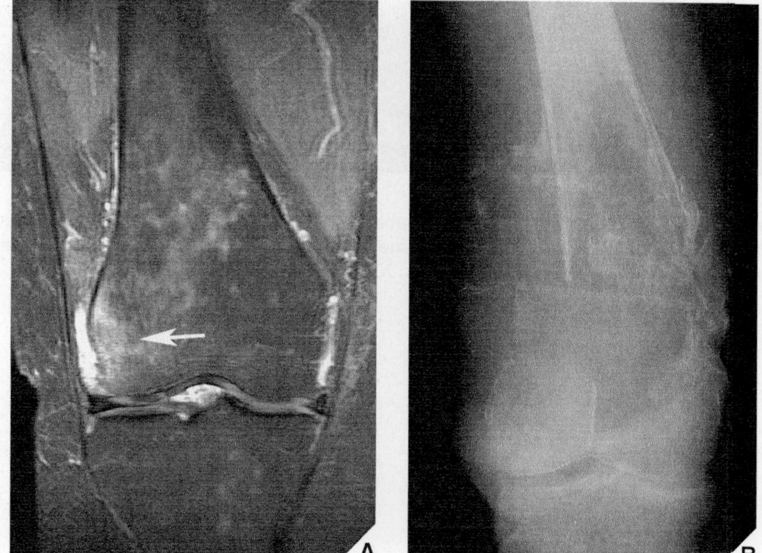

FIGURE 22.25 MRI of lymphoma. **(A)** Coronal proton density–weighted MRI of a patient with history of trauma shows an ill-defined area of increased signal intensity in the lateral femoral condyle *(arrow)*, originally interpreted as bone contusion. Multiple smaller areas of increased signal intensity noted in the distal femur were interpreted as red marrow islands. **(B)** Follow-up anteroposterior radiograph of the knee obtained a year later demonstrates a large lytic lesion of the distal femur with a pathologic fracture.

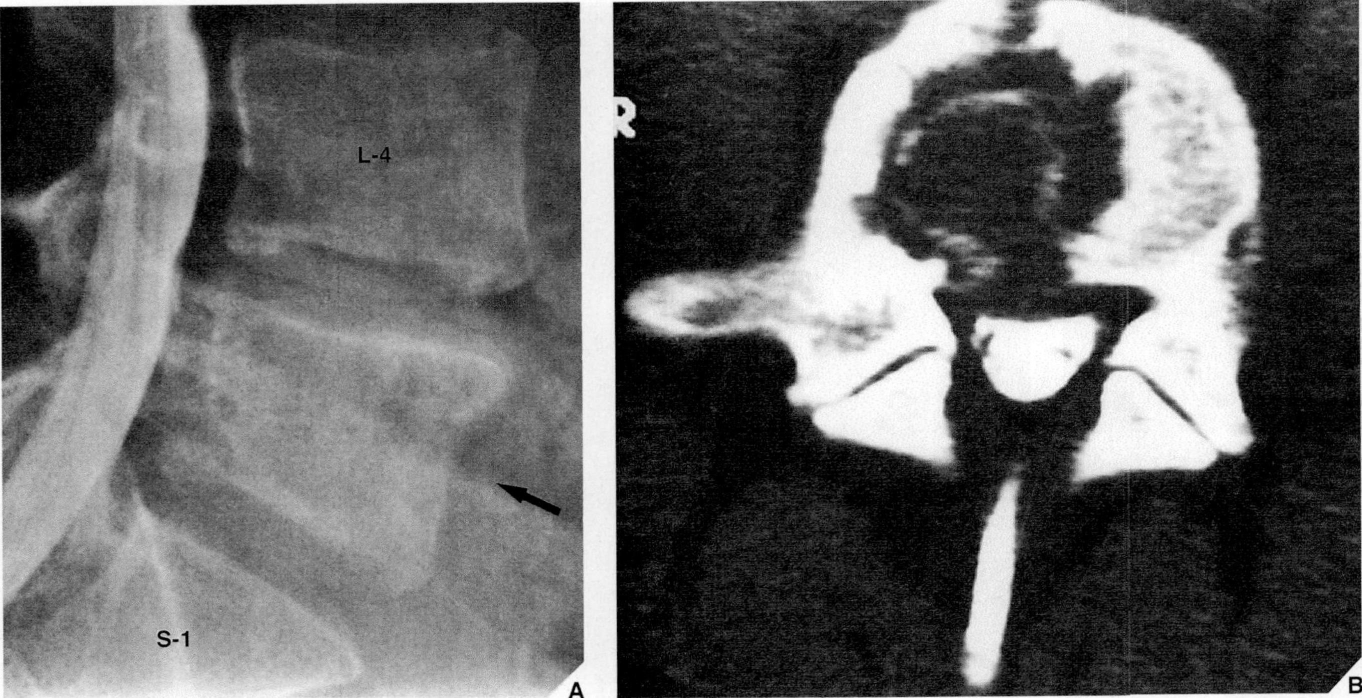

FIGURE 22.26 Lymphoma. An 18-year-old woman presented with low back pain for several months, which was attributed to herniation of an intervertebral disk. **(A)** Myelogram shows that the disk is normal, but the body of L5 *(arrow)* exhibits a mottled appearance and its posterior border is indistinct. **(B)** CT section demonstrates a large, osteolytic lesion extending from the anterior to the posterior margins of the vertebral body.

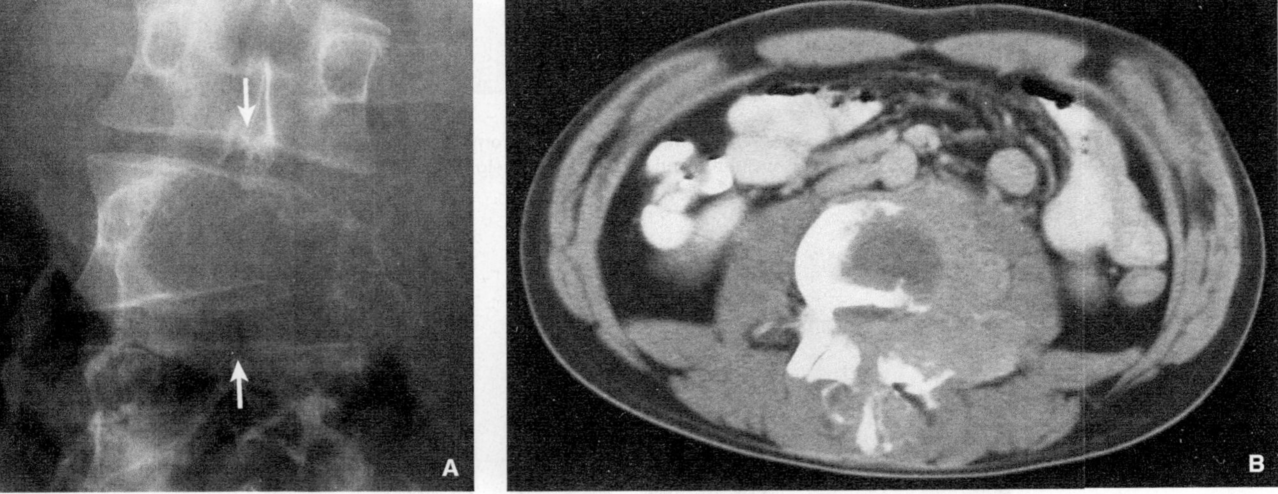

FIGURE 22.27 Lymphoma. **(A)** Anteroposterior radiograph of the upper lumbar spine of a 45-year-old man shows a destructive lesion of the L3 vertebra *(arrows)*. **(B)** Axial CT section shows the full extent of the lesion in the bone and a large soft-tissue mass. (Reprinted with permission from Greenspan A, Borys D. *Radiology and pathology correlation of bone tumors: a quick reference and review*. Philadelphia: Wolters Kluwer; 2016:256, Fig. 5.34.)

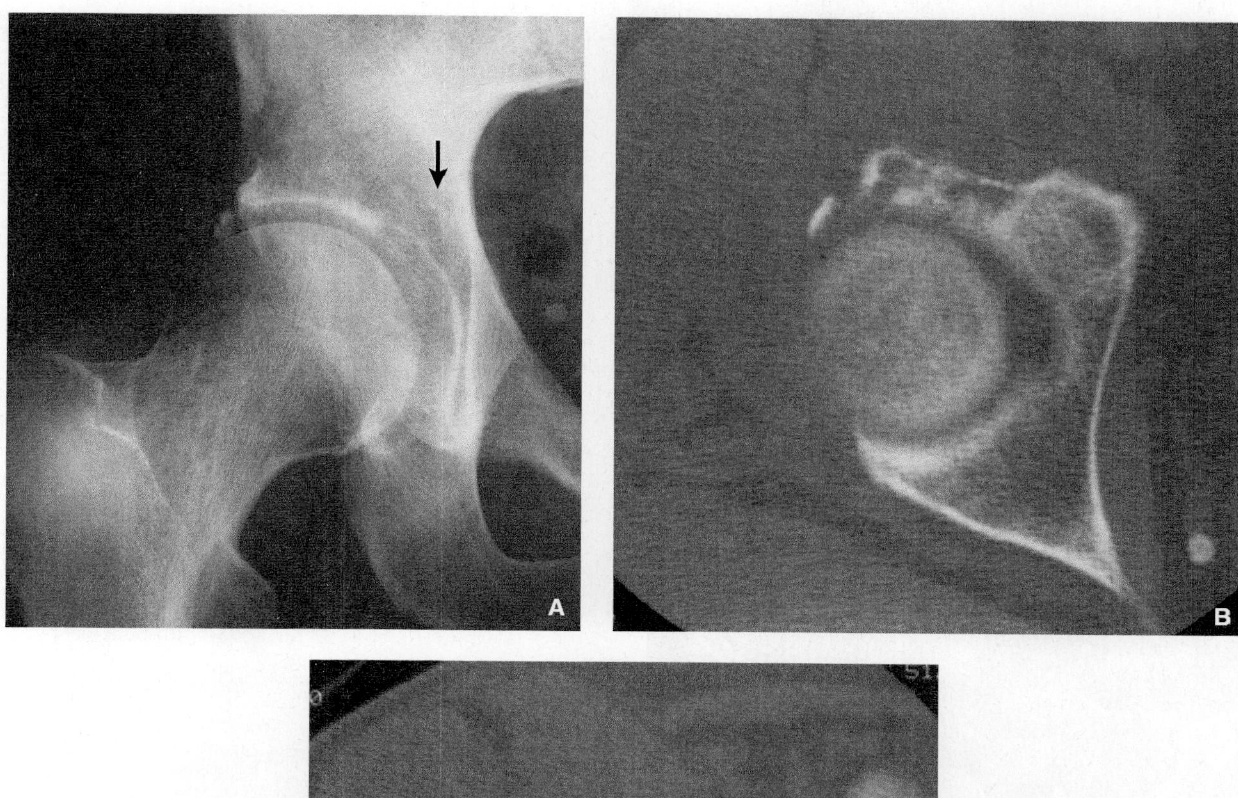

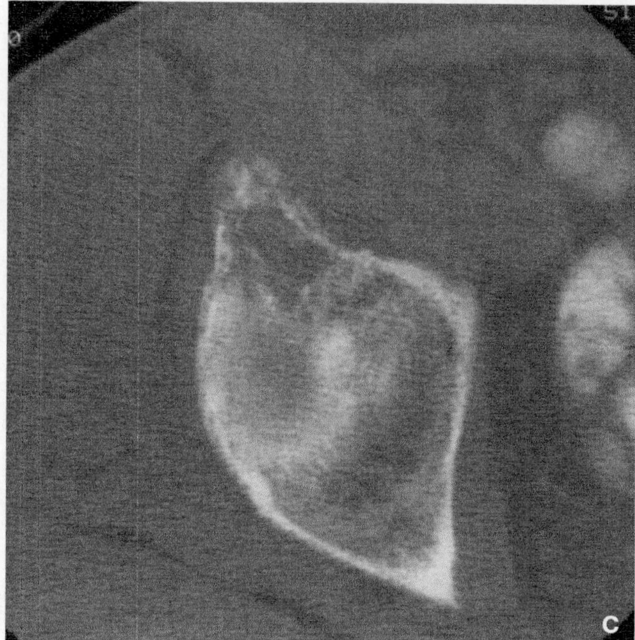

FIGURE 22.28 CT of lymphoma. **(A)** Anteroposterior radiograph of the right hip of a 36-year-old man shows a very subtle osteolytic lesion of the acetabulum *(arrow)*. **(B,C)** Two CT sections demonstrate more clearly the involvement of the anterior column and the roof of the acetabulum. (Reprinted with permission from Greenspan A, Borys D. *Radiology and pathology correlation of bone tumors: a quick reference and review*. Philadelphia: Wolters Kluwer; 2016:257, Fig. 5.35.)

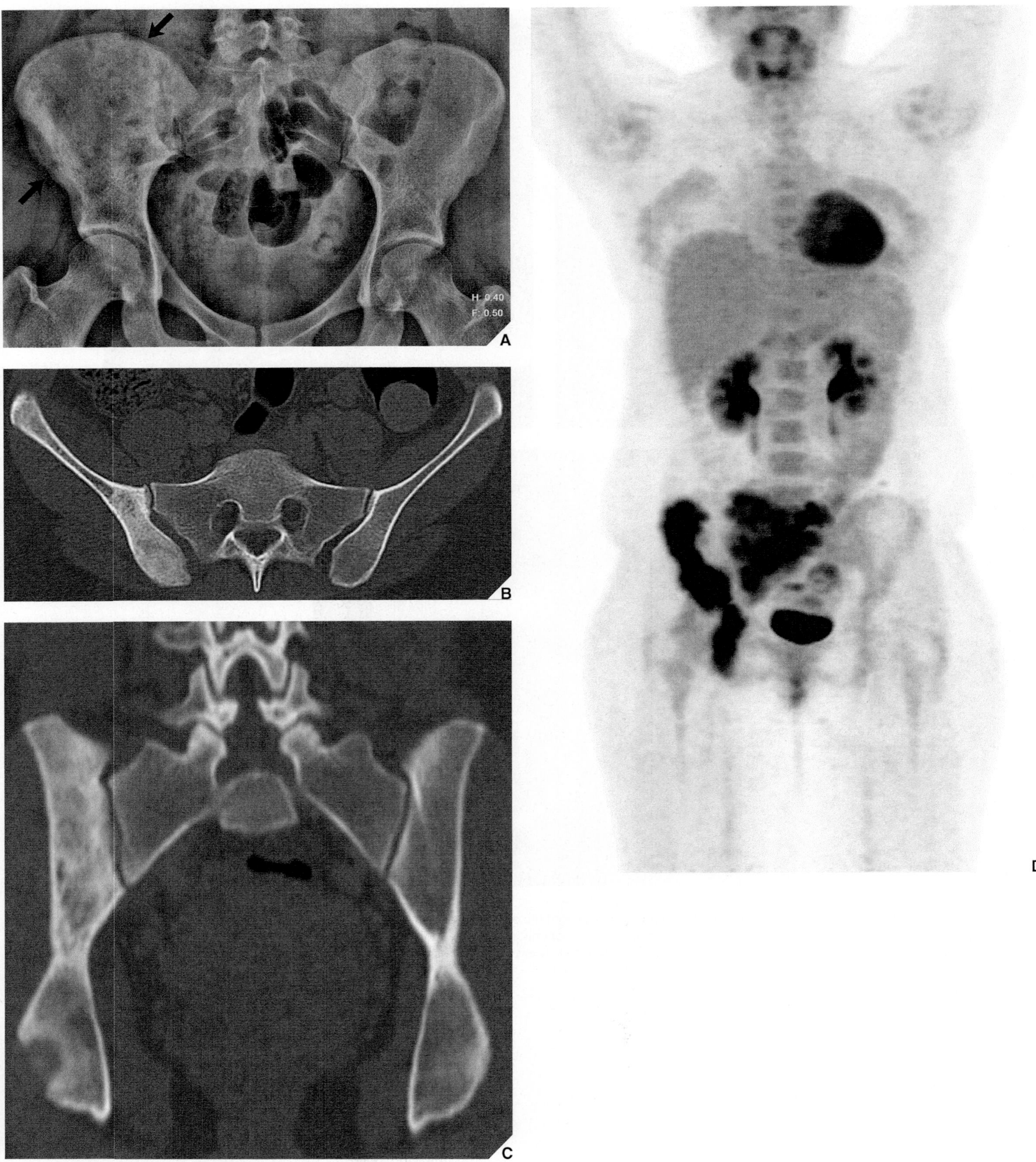

FIGURE 22.29 CT, FDG PET, PET/CT, and MRI of lymphoma. **(A)** Anteroposterior radiograph of the pelvis of a 19-year-old woman shows sclerosis of the right ilium *(arrows)*. **(B)** Axial and **(C)** coronal reformatted CT images confirm diffuse involvement of the ilium. **(D)** Total-body PET scan shows hypermetabolic tumor involving the right ilium, right ischium, and right-sided sacrum. *(Continued)*

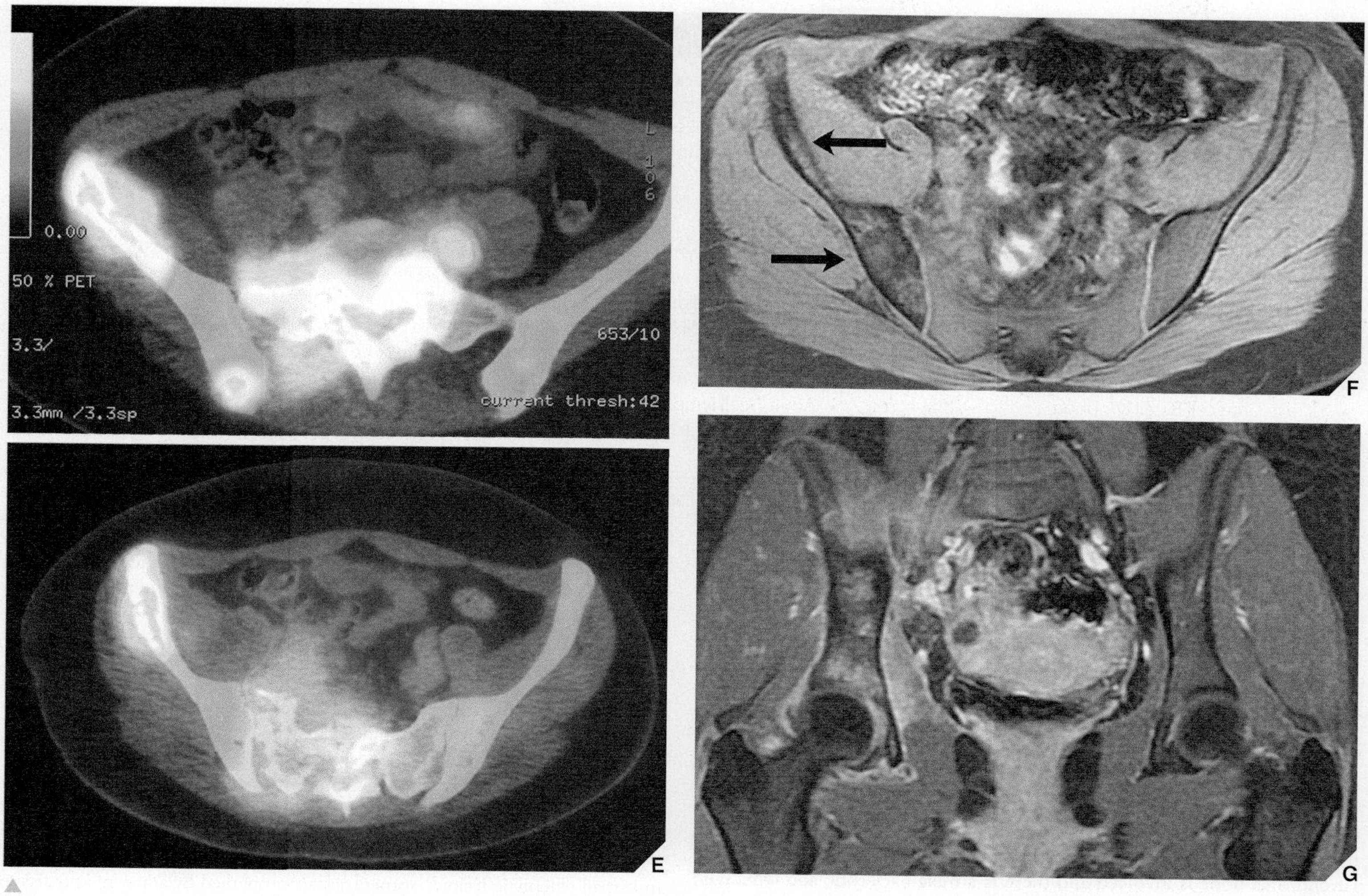

FIGURE 22.29 **CT, FDG PET, PET/CT, and MRI of lymphoma.** ***(Continued)*** **(E)** Two axial fused FDG PET/CT images confirm the location of the tumor in the ilium, ischium, and sacrum. **(F)** Axial T1-weighted MR image shows the tumor to be of low signal intensity *(arrows)*. **(G)** Coronal T1-weighted fat-saturated MR image obtained after intravenous administration of gadolinium demonstrates heterogenous enhancement of the tumor.

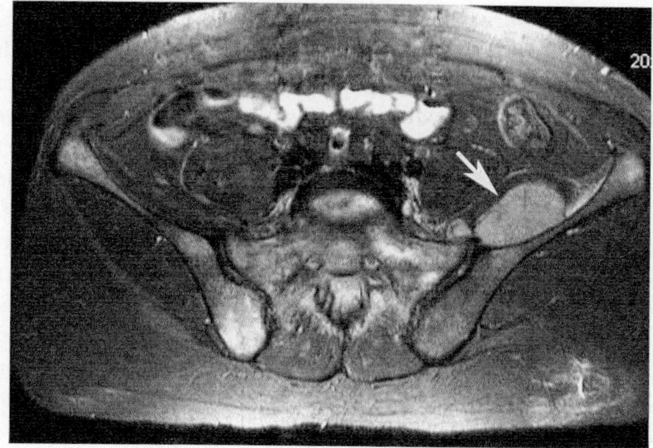

FIGURE 22.30 **MRI of lymphoma.** Axial T1-weighted fat-saturated MRI of the pelvis obtained after intravenous administration of gadolinium demonstrates multiple areas of diffuse enhancement in the bone marrow of the sacrum and pelvic bones and a soft-tissue mass *(arrow)*. (Courtesy of Maria Teresa Guedez, MD, Maracay, Venezuela.)

TABLE 22.1 Revised European American Lymphoma Classification

B-Cell Lymphomas	T-Cell and Natural Killer Cell Neoplasms	Hodgkin Disease
Precursor B-cell neoplasm • Precursor B-lymphoblastic leukemia or lymphoma Mature B-cell neoplasm • B-cell chronic lymphocytic leukemia, prolymphocytic leukemia, small lymphocytic leukemia • Lymphoplasmacytoid lymphoma • Mantle cell lymphoma • Follicle center lymphoma • Marginal zone B-cell lymphoma • Hairy cell lymphoma • Diffuse large cell B-cell lymphoma • Burkitt lymphoma • High-grade B-cell lymphoma	Precursor T-cell neoplasm • Precursor T-lymphoblastic lymphoma or leukemia Peripheral T-cell and natural killer cell neoplasm • T-cell chronic lymphocytic leukemia • Large granular lymphocyte leukemia • Mycosis fungoides, Sézary syndrome • Peripheral T-cell lymphoma • Angioimmunoblastic T-cell lymphoma • Angiocentric lymphoma • Adult T-cell lymphoma • Anaplastic large cell lymphoma	Nodular lymphocyte predominance (paragranuloma) Nodular sclerosis Mixed cellularity Lymphocyte depletion Lymphocyte-rich classic

Modified from Krishnan A, Shirkhoda A, Tehranzadeh J, et al. Primary bone lymphoma: radiographic-MR imaging correlation. *Radiographics* 2003;23:1371–1387. Copyright © 2003 by The Radiological Society of North America, Inc.

horseshoe-shaped or indented cleaved nuclei exhibiting scanty chromatin but prominent nucleoli. As mentioned in the section on Ewing sarcoma, the most important single procedure used to distinguish lymphoma from the other round cell tumors is the stain for leukocyte-common antigen because lymphoid cells are the only cells that stain positively with the immunoreaction for CD45, CD20, and CD3 (B-cell and T-cells markers). Hodgkin and Reed-Sternberg cells are positive for CD15 and CD30.

Differential Diagnosis

Histiocytic lymphoma must be distinguished from secondary involvement of the skeleton by systemic lymphoma. It may resemble Ewing sarcoma, particularly in younger patients (Fig. 22.31), or Paget disease if the articular end of a bone is involved and there is a mixed sclerotic and osteolytic pattern (Fig. 22.32).

Treatment and Prognosis

The treatment for primary bone lymphoma is controversial, and there is no consensus with regard to radiotherapy, although this tumor is radiosensitive. Some cases require chemotherapy as the mainstay (including rituximab, cyclophosphamide, doxorubicin, and vincristine) and additional adjuvant radiation therapy (dose of radiation greater than 4,000 cGy). The optimal treatment has not been determined and is still being debated. Prognosis of lymphoma depends on cell type and stage of disease. Patients older than 60 years have a worse overall survival and a worse progression-free period. Patients with immunoblastic subtype have a worse survival rate than those with the centroblastic mono/polymorphic subtype or the centroblastic multilobulated subtype.

Myeloma

Clinical Features

Myeloma, also known as *multiple myeloma* or *plasma cell myeloma*, is a tumor originating in the bone marrow and is the most common primary malignant bone tumor. It accounts for 10% of all hematologic malignancies and 1% of all cancers. It is usually seen between the fifth and seventh decades and is more frequent in men than in women. The axial skeleton (skull, spine, ribs, and pelvis) is the most commonly affected site, but no bone is exempt from involvement (Fig. 22.33). Rarely, the presentation can be that of a solitary lesion, in which case it is called a *solitary myeloma* or *plasmacytoma*; far more commonly, however, it presents with widespread involvement, in which case the name *multiple myeloma* is applied. Mild and transient pain exacerbated by heavy lifting or other activity is present in approximately 75% of cases and may be the initial symptom. Because of this, in its early course and before diagnosis, the disease may resemble sciatica or intercostal neuralgia. Rarely, a pathologic fracture through the lesion is the first sign of disease. The patient's urine in cases of myeloma contains Bence Jones protein; the serum albumin-to-globulin ratio is reversed and the total serum protein is elevated. Monoclonal γ-globulin is also present, with immunoglobulin G (IgG) and immunoglobulin A (IgA) peaks demonstrated on serum electrophoresis.

Imaging Features

Multiple myeloma may present in a variety of radiographic patterns (Fig. 22.34). Particularly in the spine, it may be seen only as diffuse osteoporosis with no clearly identifiable lesion; multiple compression fractures of the vertebral bodies may also be evident. More commonly, it exhibits multiple lytic lesions scattered throughout the skeleton. In the skull, characteristic "punched-out" areas of bone destruction, usually of uniform size, are noted (Fig. 22.35), whereas the ribs may contain lace-like areas of bone destruction and small osteolytic lesions, sometimes accompanied by adjacent soft-tissue masses. Areas of medullary bone destruction are noted in the flat and long bones, and if these appear about the cortex, they are accompanied by scalloping of the inner cortical margin (Figs. 22.36 and 22.37). Ordinarily, there is no evidence of sclerosis and no periosteal reaction. The radiographic characteristics in conjunction with the normal radionuclide bone scan are usually diagnostic for this condition, and CT is rarely performed (Fig. 22.38). In those rare instances when the solitary lesion is accompanied by a large soft-tissue mass (Fig. 22.39), the diagnosis may not be so obvious. On MRI, the lesions exhibit intermediate signal intensity on T1-weighted sequences, whereas on T2-weighted images the signal is usually high and homogenous. Post-contrast MR images show some degree of enhancement (Fig. 22.40).

Whereas in osteolytic myeloma, only 3% of patients have polyneuropathy, the incidence of polyneuropathy in the osteosclerotic variant has been reported as 30% to 50%. Compared with classic myeloma, this variant usually occurs in younger individuals and shows fewer plasma cells in the bone marrow, lower levels of monoclonal protein, and a better prognosis.

An interesting variant of sclerosing myeloma is the so-called *POEMS syndrome*, first described in 1968. It consists of polyneuropathy (P); organomegaly (O), particularly of the liver and the spleen; endocrine disturbances (E) such as amenorrhea and gynecomastia; monoclonal gammopathy (M); and skin changes (S) such as hyperpigmentation and hirsutism. Also known as *Crow-Fukase syndrome*, *Takatsuki syndrome*, and *PEP* (plasma cell dyscrasia, endocrinopathy, and polyneuropathy) *syndrome*, this condition represents a clinicopathologic complex of unknown etiology. On radiography and CT, the focal osseous lesions present as either a well-defined or fluffy sclerotic foci, or as a lytic areas with peripheral sclerosis. On MRI, the lesions exhibit decreased signal intensity on both T1- and T2-weighted sequences, and lack of enhancement on postcontrast (gadolinium) images.

A characteristic MRI appearance of solitary plasmacytoma involving the spine has been described as the "mini brain" sign. Expansion of the vertebral body with increased signal intensity areas separated by low–signal intensity linear struts, caused by compensatory hypertrophy of remaining trabecula, resemble the sulci of the brain (Fig. 22.41). ^{18}F-FDG PET and PET/CT images invariably show hypermetabolic activity of the tumor (Fig. 22.42).

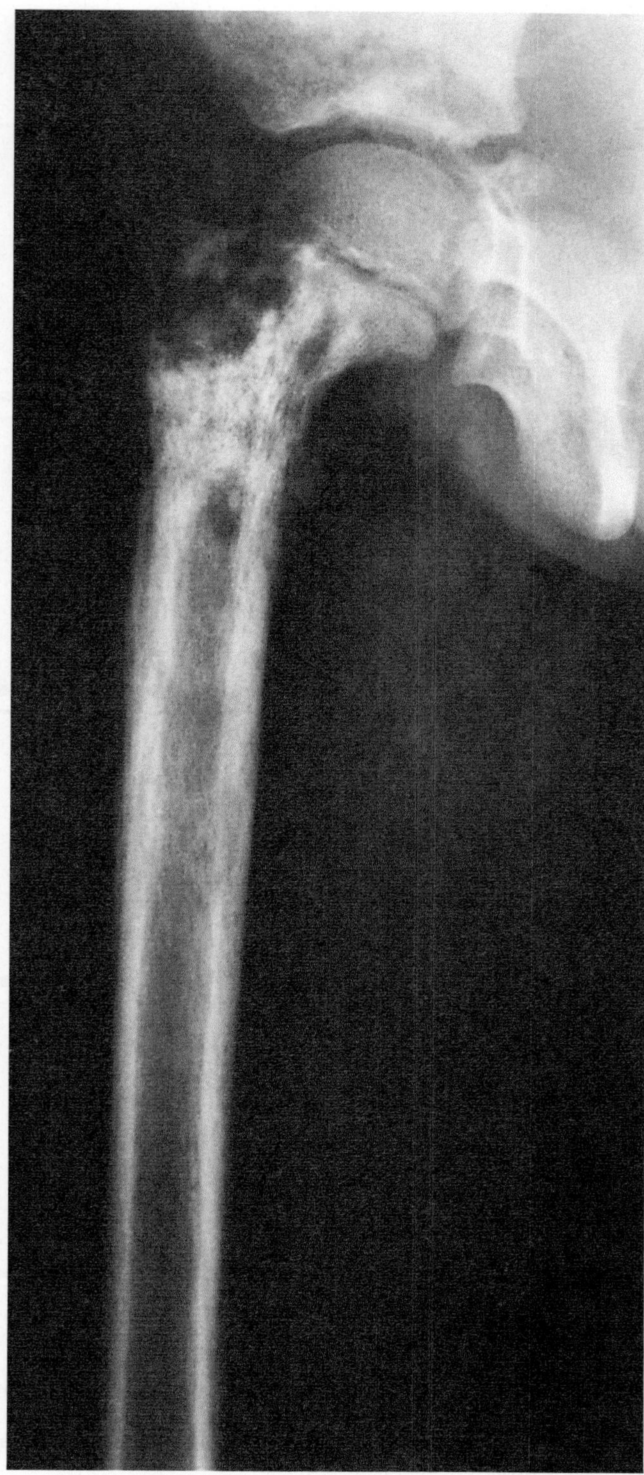

FIGURE 22.31 Lymphoma in a child. Conventional radiograph of the right femur of a 7-year-old girl with groin pain and a fever reveals a destructive lesion of the diaphysis extending to the growth plate; there is also a lamellated type of periosteal reaction. Because of the age of the patient, the primary differential diagnosis included Ewing sarcoma, osteomyelitis, and Langerhans cell histiocytosis, all three of which may have a similar radiographic presentation in a long bone. The main factor differentiating these lesions is the duration of the patient's symptoms. In this case, however, biopsy revealed a histiocytic lymphoma.

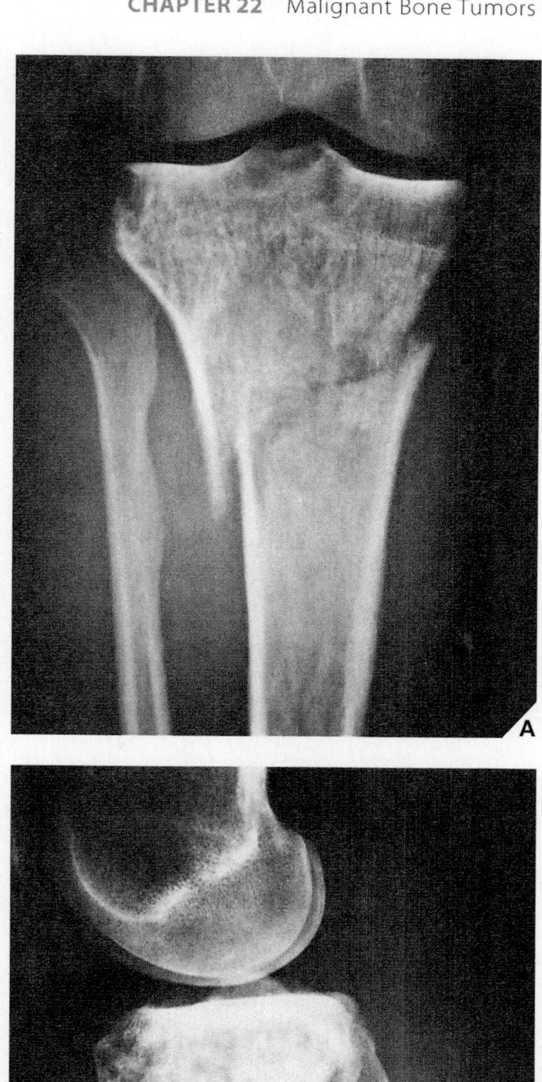

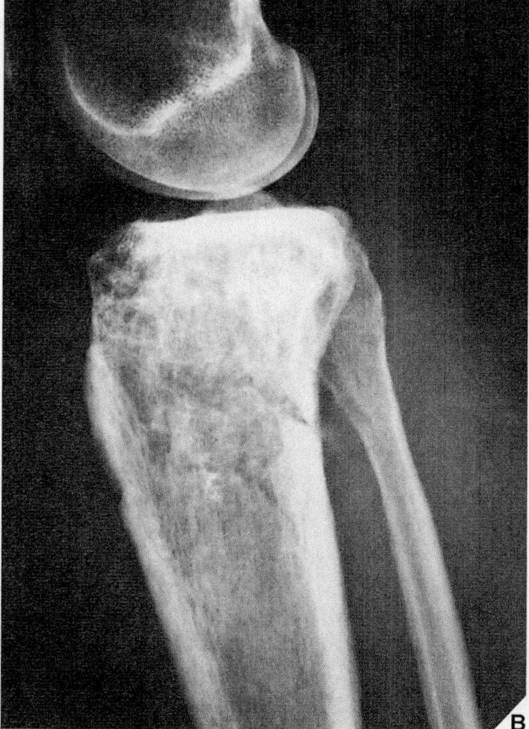

FIGURE 22.32 Lymphoma. **(A)** Anteroposterior and **(B)** lateral radiographs of the right knee of a 47-year-old woman, who had knee pain and initially was misdiagnosed with Paget disease, show a destructive lesion of the proximal tibia extending into the articular end of the bone. The mixed sclerotic and osteolytic character of this lesion may resemble the coarse trabecular pattern of Paget disease; however, there is a lack of cortical thickening. There is a pathologic fracture, but only a minimal periosteal response is evident.

Myeloma
age: ≥50
M > F
common sites
less common sites

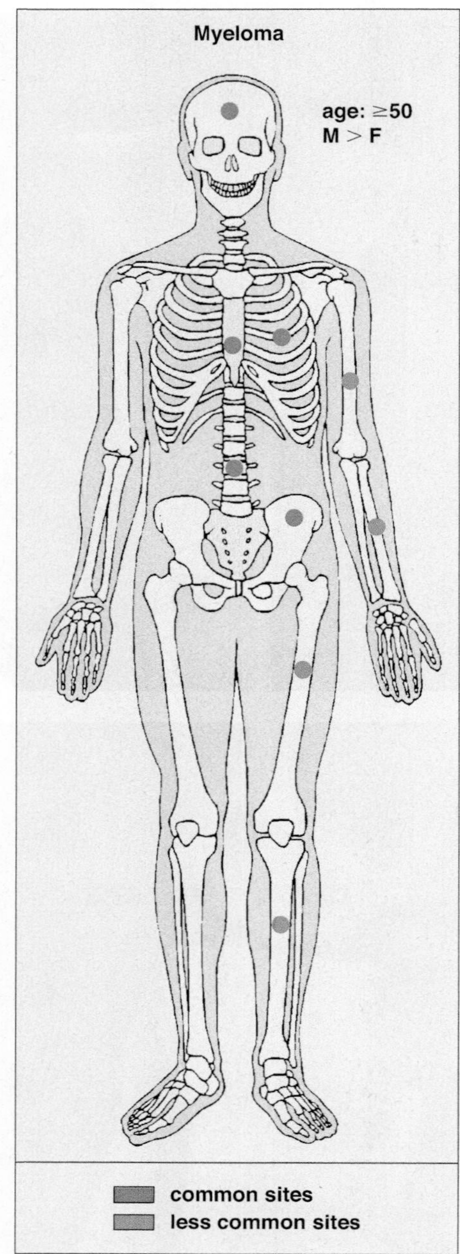

FIGURE 22.33 Skeletal sites of predilection, peak age range, and male-to-female ratio in myeloma.

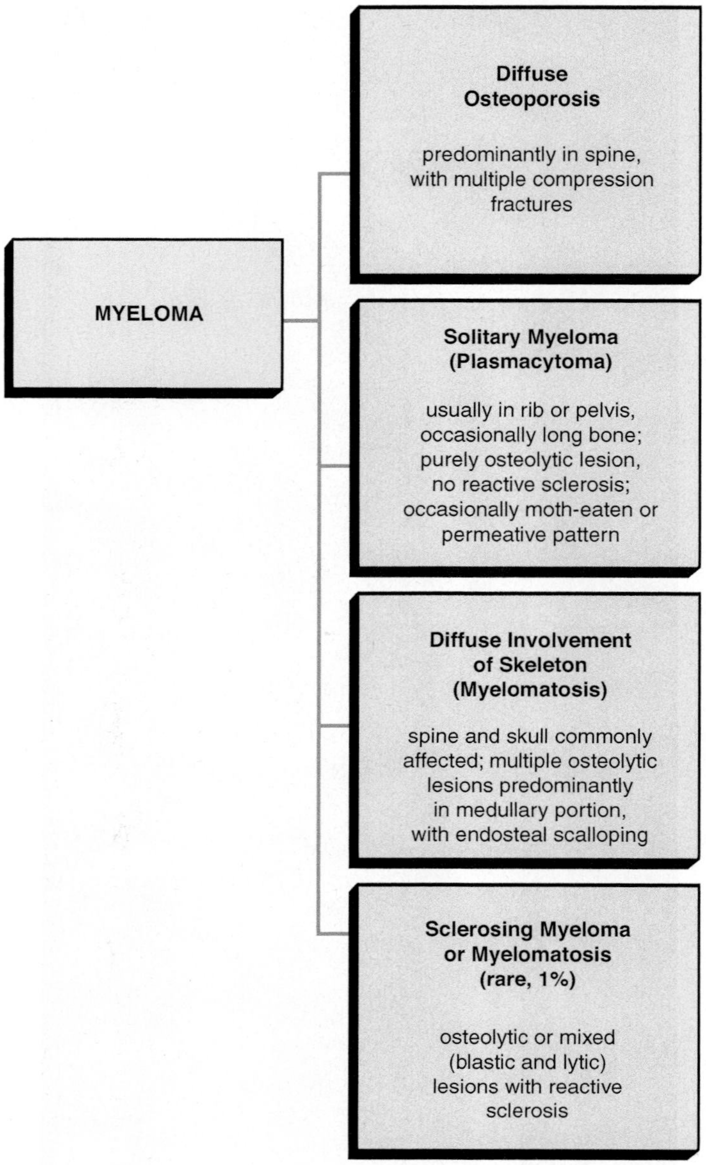

MYELOMA
Diffuse Osteoporosis
predominantly in spine, with multiple compression fractures
Solitary Myeloma (Plasmacytoma)
usually in rib or pelvis, occasionally long bone; purely osteolytic lesion, no reactive sclerosis; occasionally moth-eaten or permeative pattern
Diffuse Involvement of Skeleton (Myelomatosis)
spine and skull commonly affected; multiple osteolytic lesions predominantly in medullary portion, with endosteal scalloping
Sclerosing Myeloma or Myelomatosis (rare, 1%)
osteolytic or mixed (blastic and lytic) lesions with reactive sclerosis

FIGURE 22.34 Variants in the radiographic presentation of myeloma.

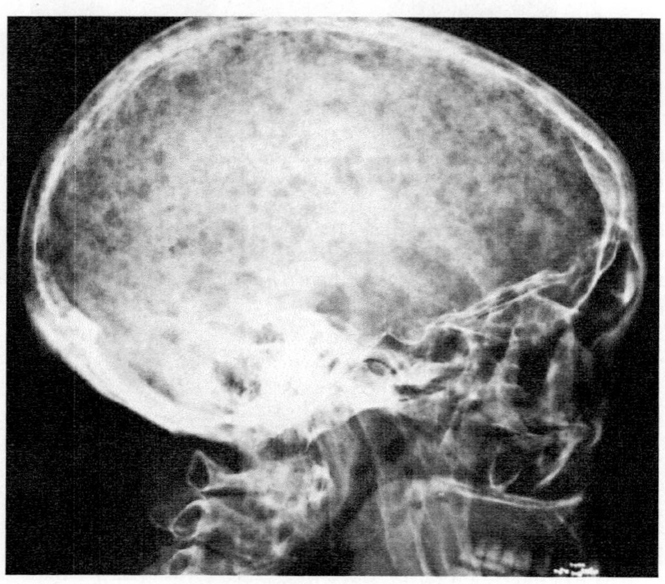

FIGURE 22.35 Multiple myeloma. Involvement of the skull is prominent in this 60-year-old woman. Note the characteristic punched-out, lytic lesions, most of which are uniform in size and lack sclerotic borders. Occasionally, this pattern may be seen in metastatic disease.

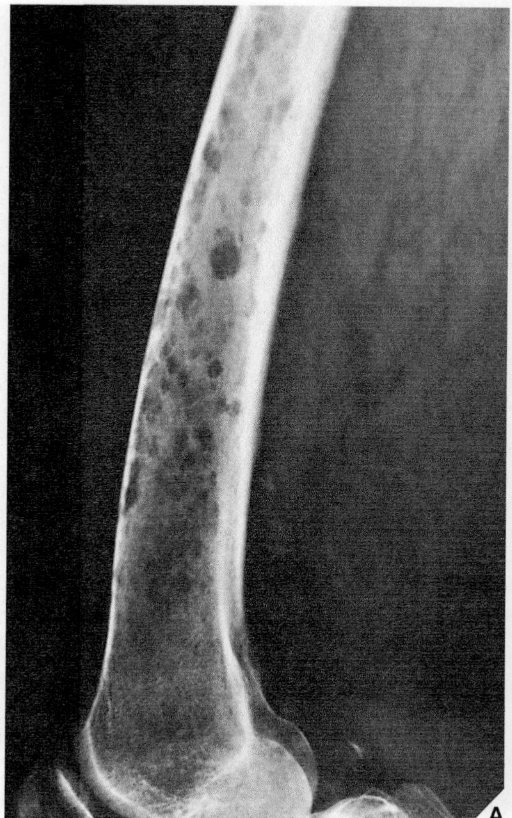

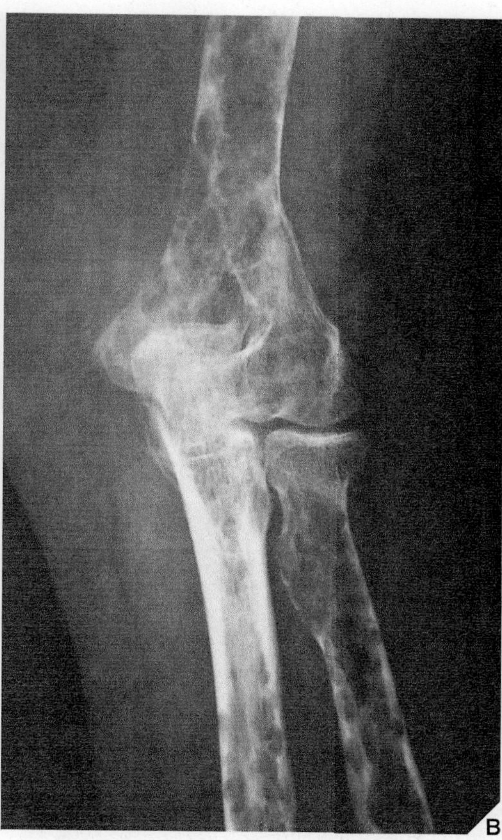

FIGURE 22.36 **Multiple myeloma.** **(A)** Lateral radiograph of the distal femur and **(B)** anteroposterior radiograph of the elbow in a 65-year-old woman show endosteal scalloping of the cortex typical of diffuse myelomatosis.

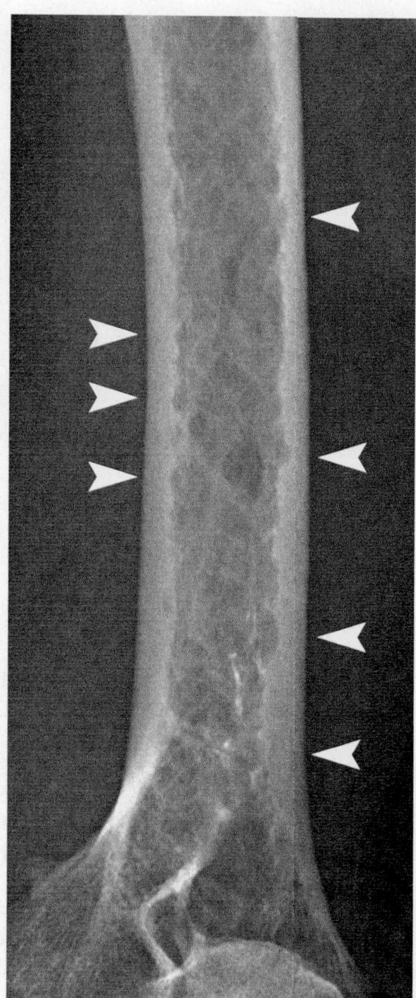

FIGURE 22.37 **Multiple myeloma.** Magnified radiograph of the distal humerus of a 72-year-old man shows characteristic for this malignancy endosteal scalloping *(arrowheads)*.

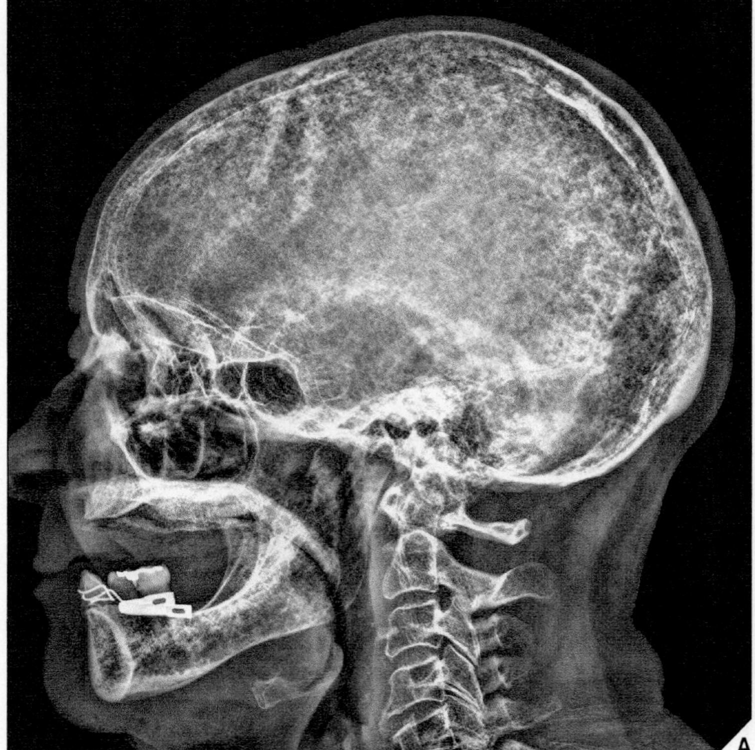

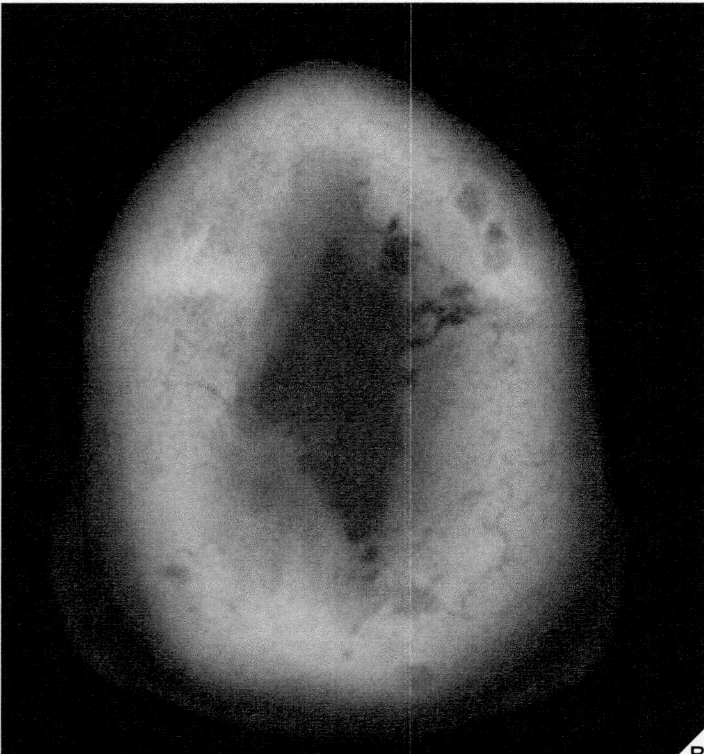

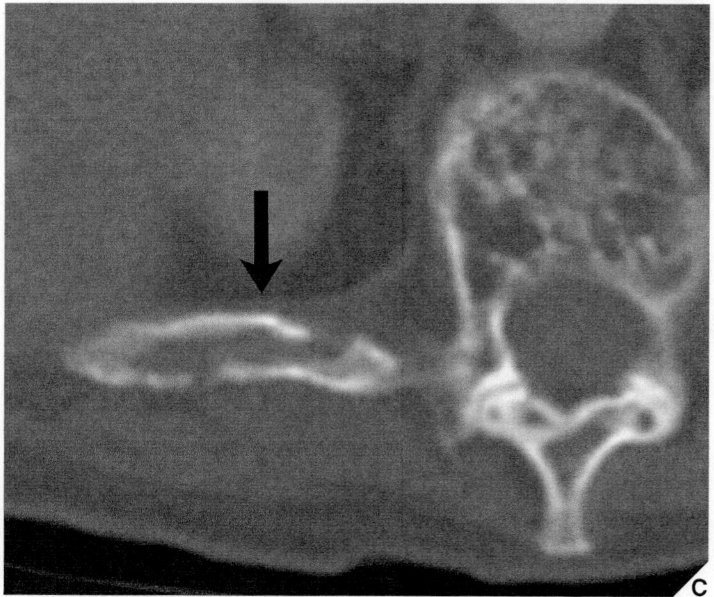

FIGURE 22.38 CT of multiple myeloma. **(A)** Lateral radiograph of the skull of a 76-year-old woman shows extensive involvement of the calvaria. Note also punched-out lesions in the mandible, not an unusual site of involvement. **(B)** CT image shows punched-out low-attenuated lesions in the occiput. **(C)** Axial CT section through the T10 vertebra shows involvement of the vertebral body and the adjacent right rib *(arrow)*.

Pathology

Histologically, the diagnosis is made by finding sheets of atypical plasmacytoid cells replacing the normal marrow spaces. The plasma cell is recognized by the presence of eccentrically situated nucleus within a large amount of cytoplasm that stains either light blue or pink. The neoplastic cells contain double or even multiple nuclei, usually hyperchromatic and enlarged, with prominent nucleoli. The tumor cells may accumulate immunoglobulins (Igs) in cytoplasm and show morular appearance or "Mott cells." Extracellular globules of polymerized globules called *Russell bodies* may be seen. Poorly differentiated tumors show atypical cells with brisk mitotic activity. Immunohistochemistry shows positivity for CD1 38, CD38, and MUM1 (multiple myeloma oncogene 1). Characteristic feature is expression of monotypic cytoplasmic Ig and lack of surface Ig. Monotypic expression of κ or λ Ig by the tumor cells establishes the diagnosis of malignancy. Majority of myelomas lack the pan-B antigen CD19 and CD20. Cyclin D1 protein may be expressed in 35% to 40% of cases and is associated with translocations t(11;14)(q13;32). The other genetic abnormalities include gains of chromosomes 1q, 3q, 9q, 11q, and 15q. Losses of chromosome13 at 13q14 was observed in 60% of cases. Deletion of gene *TP53* at 17q13 was reported in 25% of cases.

Differential Diagnosis

If the spine is involved, as is frequently the case, multiple myeloma must be differentiated from metastatic carcinoma. In this respect, the "vertebral pedicle" sign identified by Jacobson and colleagues may be helpful. They contended that in the early stages of myeloma, the pedicle (which does not contain as much red marrow as the vertebral body) is not involved, whereas even in an early stage of metastatic cancer the pedicle and vertebral body are both affected (Fig. 22.43). In the late stages of multiple myeloma, however, both the pedicle and vertebral body may be destroyed.

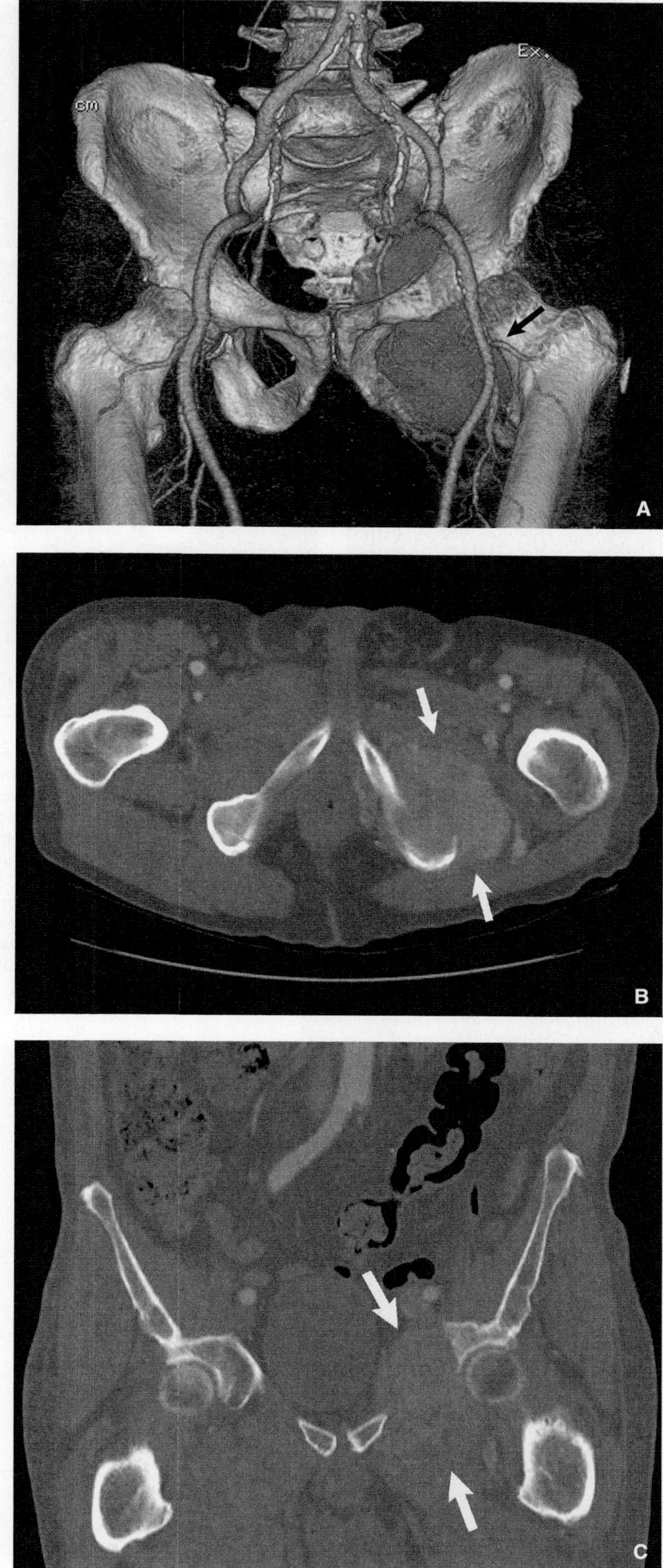

FIGURE 22.39 **Three-dimensional (3D) CT-angiogram and CT of solitary plasmacytoma.** **(A)** 3D CT-angiogram of the pelvis of a 79-year-old man shows destruction of the left ischial bone and a large soft-tissue mass occupying the obturator foramen and extending into the pelvic cavity. Observe narrowing of the left superficial femoral artery encased by the tumor *(arrow)*. **(B)** Axial and **(C)** coronal reformatted CT images of the pelvis show a low-attenuated tumor destroying the ischial bone and forming a large soft-tissue mass *(arrows)*.

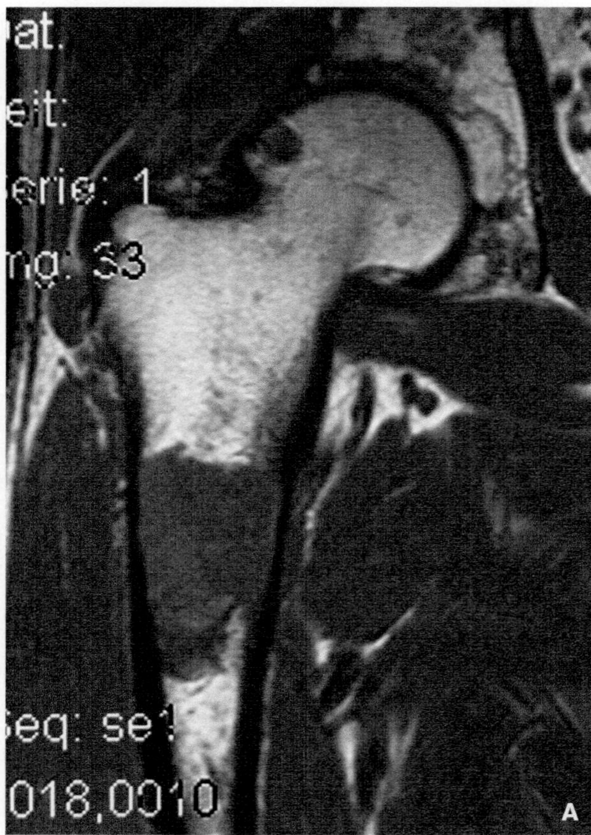

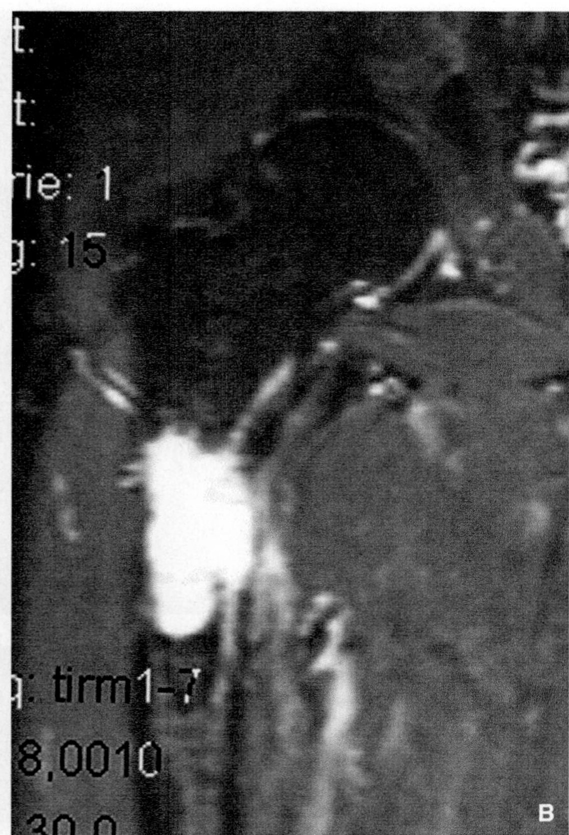

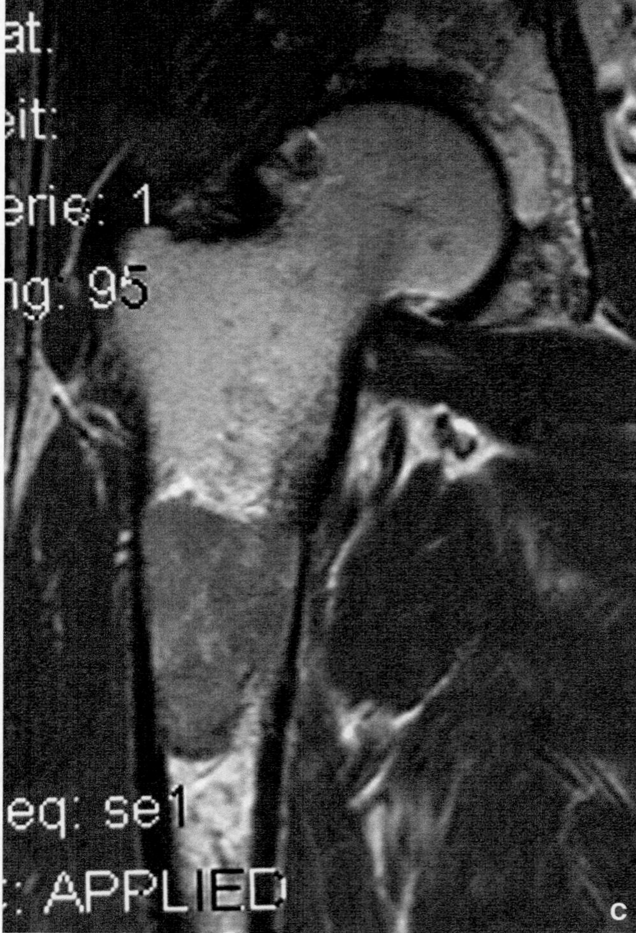

FIGURE 22.40 MRI of plasmacytoma. **(A)** Coronal T1-weighted MR image of the right hip of a 53-year-old man shows a lesion in the proximal femur exhibiting intermediate–signal intensity isointense with the skeletal muscles. **(B)** Coronal T2-weighted MR image shows the tumor to be of homogenous high signal intensity. **(C)** T1-weighted postcontrast MRI shows slight enhancement of the tumor. (Reprinted with permission from Greenspan A, Borys D. *Radiology and pathology correlation of bone tumors: a quick reference and review*. Philadelphia: Wolters Kluwer; 2016:266–267, Fig. 5.48.)

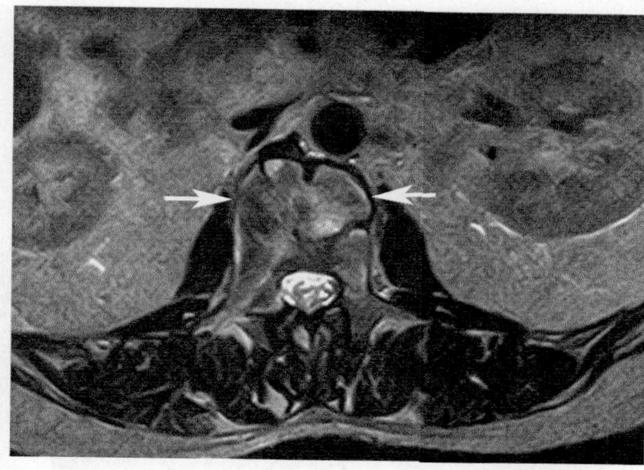

FIGURE 22.41 Multiple myeloma—mini brain sign. Axial T2-weighted MRI of the lumbar spine demonstrates expansion of the vertebral body *(arrows)* with anterior septa resembling the sulci of the brain. (Courtesy of Daniel Vanel, MD, Bologna, Italy.)

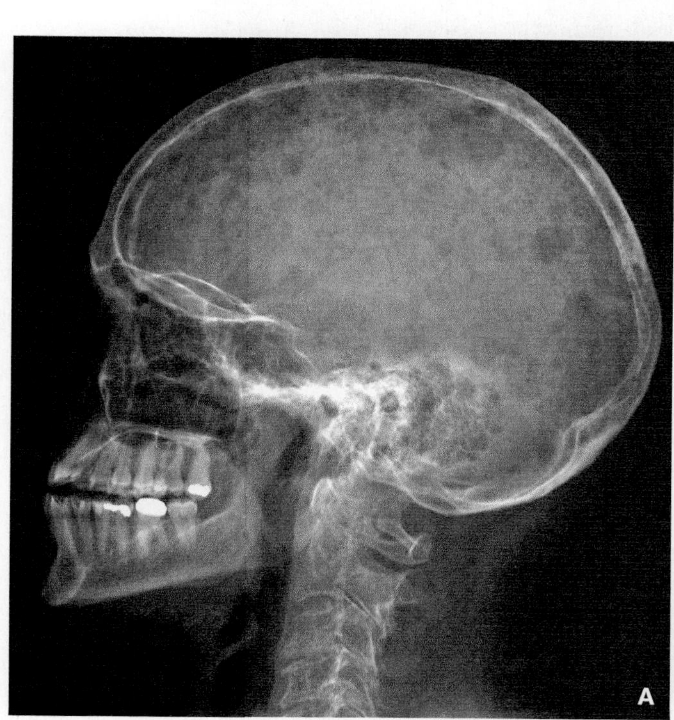

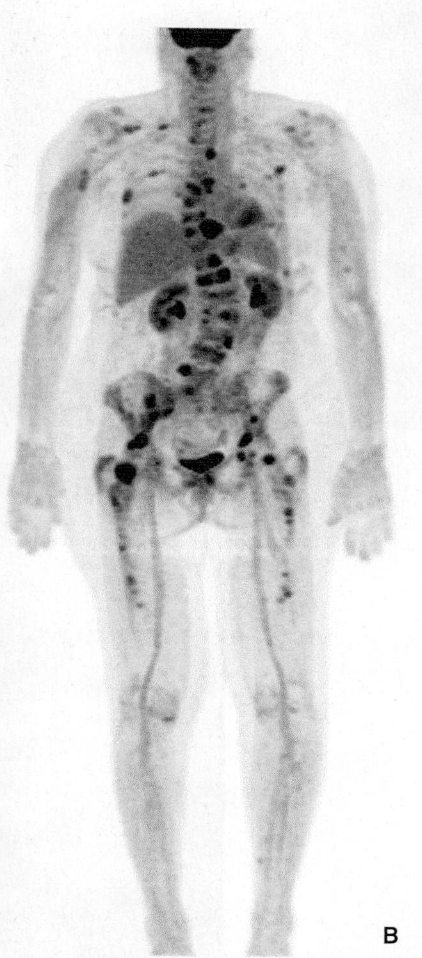

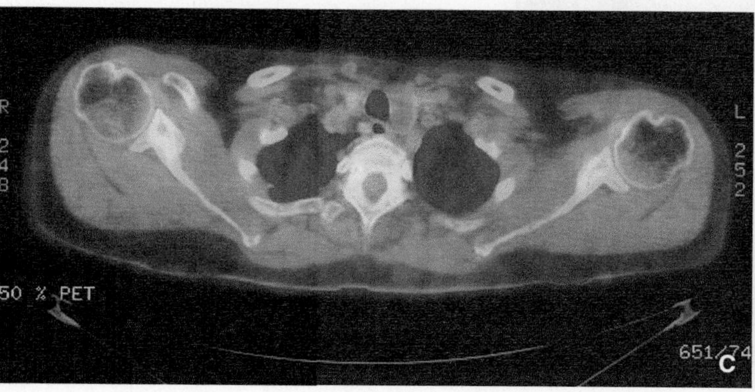

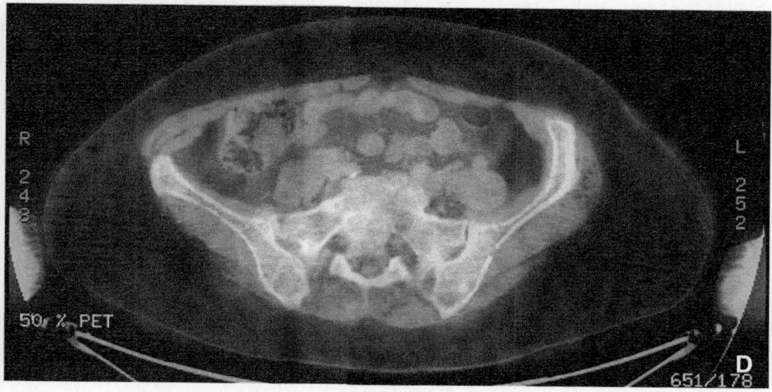

FIGURE 22.42 FDG PET and PET/CT of multiple myeloma. **(A)** Lateral radiograph of the skull of a 72-year woman shows numerous different in size lytic lesions. **(B)** Whole-body FDG PET scan shows multiple hypermetabolic foci within the spine, ribs, scapulae, pelvis, and proximal femora. **(C)** Fused axial PET/CT image obtained at the level of the shoulder girdles shows hypermetabolic foci within both scapulae and thoracic vertebra. **(D)** Fused axial PET/CT image obtained at the level of the pelvis shows hypermetabolic foci within the iliac bones and sacrum.

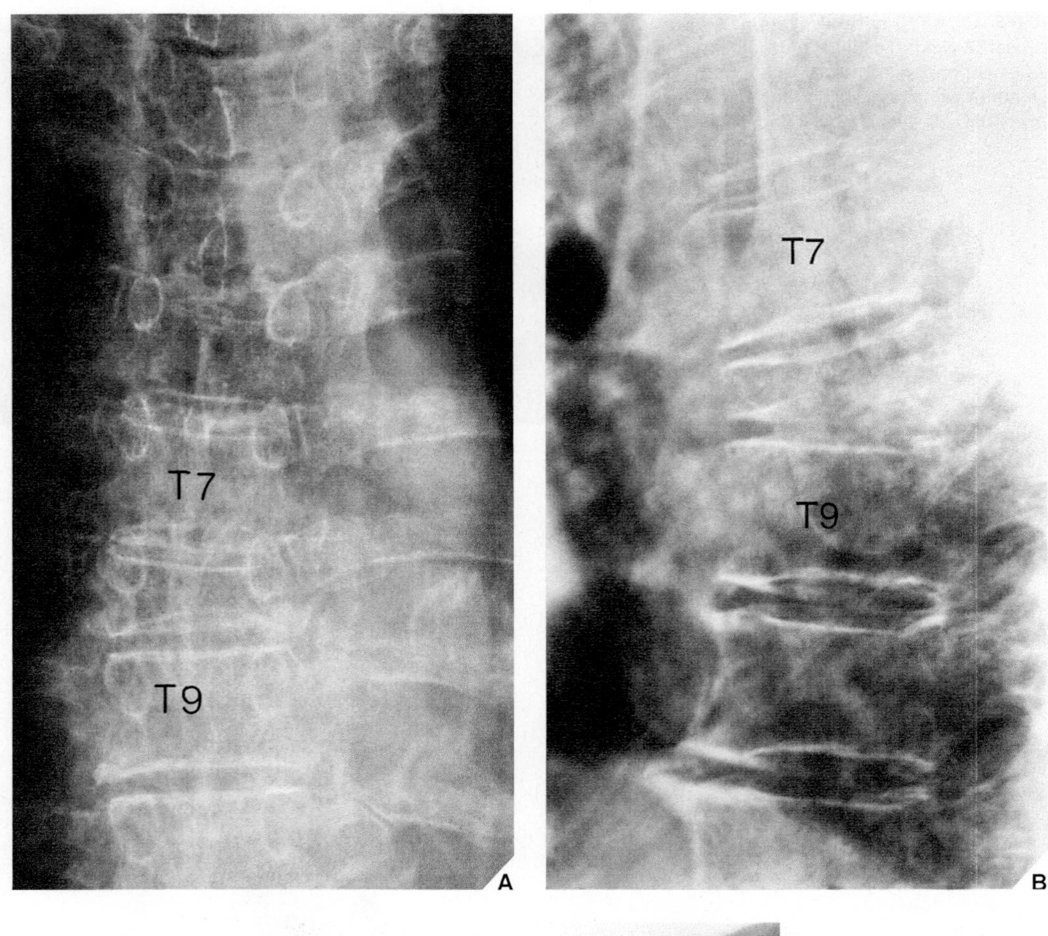

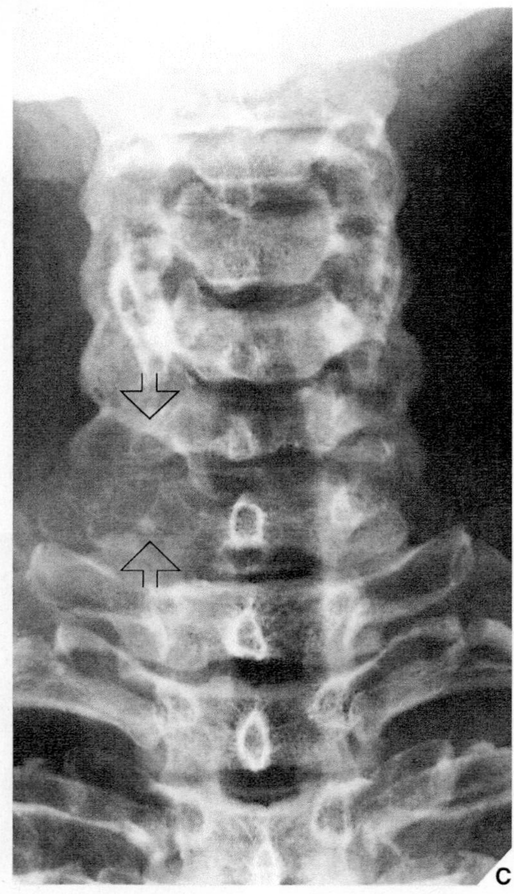

FIGURE 22.43 Multiple myeloma versus metastatic carcinoma. (A) Anteroposterior and lateral **(B)** radiographs of the spine in a 70-year-old man with multiple myeloma involving both the spine and appendicular skeleton show a compression fracture of the body of T8; several other vertebrae show only osteoporosis. The pedicles are preserved in contrast to metastatic disease of the spine, which usually also affects the pedicles, as seen on this anteroposterior radiograph of the cervical spine **(C)** in a 65-year-old man with colon carcinoma and multiple lytic metastases. Note the involvement of the right pedicle of C7 *(open arrows)*.

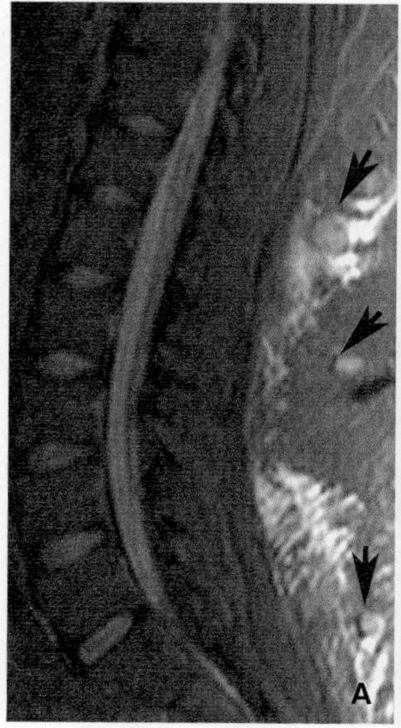

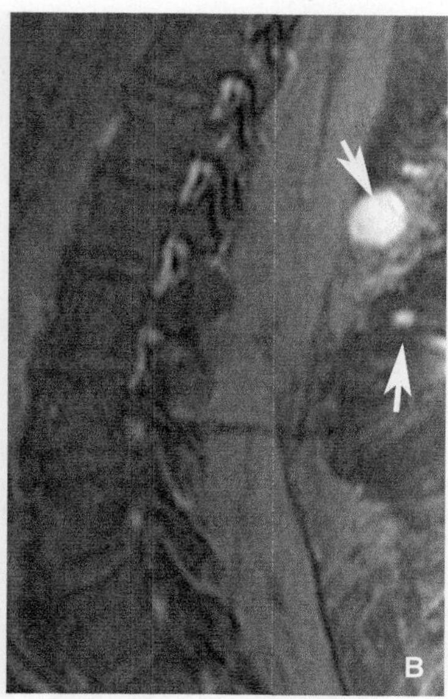

FIGURE 22.44 **MRI of soft tissue relapsing multiple myeloma.** **(A)** Sagittal short time inversion recovery (STIR) MR image of the spine and **(B)** sagittal T1-weighted fat-saturated MR image obtained after intravenous injection of gadolinium show multiple enhancing nodules in the posterior paraspinal subcutaneous soft tissues *(arrows)*. Note that the soft-tissue nodules are not contiguous with the osseous lesions. This feature indicates worst prognosis than in multiple myeloma with direct soft-tissue extension.

Radionuclide bone scan can more reliably distinguish these two malignancies at this stage. It is invariably positive in cases of metastatic carcinoma, whereas in most cases of multiple myeloma, there is no increased uptake of radiopharmaceutical tracer. This phenomenon appears to reflect the purely lytic nature of most myelomatous lesions and the absence of significant reactive new bone formation in response to the tumor.

A solitary myeloma/plasmacytoma may create even greater diagnostic difficulty. As a purely osteolytic lesion, it may mimic such other purely destructive processes as the brown tumor of hyperparathyroidism, giant cell tumor, fibrosarcoma, MFH, or a solitary metastatic focus of carcinoma from the kidney, thyroid, gastrointestinal tract, or lung (see Fig. 22.39).

Complications, Treatment, and Prognosis

A common complication of bone myelomas is pathologic fracture, especially in lesions of the long bones, ribs, sternum, and vertebrae. The development of amyloidosis has also been reported in approximately 15% of patients. Another reported complication of multiple myeloma is soft-tissue extramedullary involvement. This type of relapse has a significantly poorer prognosis than soft-tissue relapse related to adjacent bone involvement (Fig. 22.44).

Treatment consists of radiotherapy and systemic chemotherapy. Multiple myeloma is generally an incurable disease. Median survival is about 3 years, the 5-year survival rate is approximately 10%. Renal insufficiency, higher stage and degree of marrow replacement by tumor cells, increased proliferative activity, and certain karyotypic abnormalities are associated with shorter survival time. Chromosomal translocations t(4;14) and t(14;16) and deletion 17q13 (*TP53*) are associated with poorer prognosis.

Adamantinoma of Long Bones

Clinical and Imaging Features

Adamantinoma is a rare malignant tumor representing about 0.4% of all primary bone lesions, occurring equally in males and females between the second and fifth decades of life; 90% of cases involve the tibia. Clinical findings include localized swelling with or without pain. Physical examination reveals a firm, tender mass or swelling, usually firmly affixed to the underling bone. Radiographically, the tumor is marked by well-defined and elongated osteolytic defects of varying size, separated by areas of sclerotic bone, which occasionally give the lesion a "soap bubble" appearance; ordinarily, there is no periosteal reaction (Fig. 22.45). At times, adamantinoma may affect an entire bone with multiple satellite lesions (Fig. 22.46); "sawtooth" areas of cortical destruction in the tibia are quite distinctive of this tumor. Scintigraphy invariably demonstrates increased uptake of the radiopharmaceutical tracer (Fig. 22.47). MRI shows hypointense (compared to the normal bone marrow) signal on T1-weighted sequences and hyperintense signal on T2 weighting. Postcontrast images may or may not show enhancement of the tumor. Some investigators reported intense and homogeneous static enhancement but lack of uniform dynamic enhancement pattern.

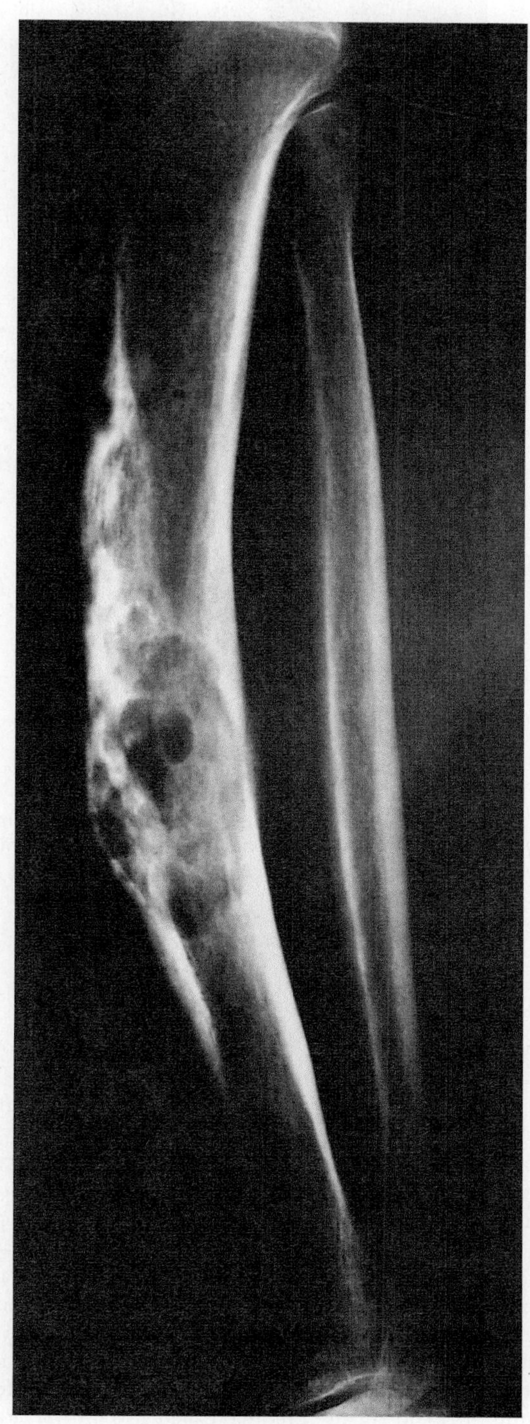

FIGURE 22.45 **Adamantinoma.** Lateral radiograph of a 64-year-old woman shows a lesion in the midshaft of the left tibia. The destructive lesion is multifocal and slightly expansive, with mixed osteolytic and sclerotic areas creating a soap bubble appearance resembling that of osteofibrous dysplasia (see Figs. 19.54 to 19.56, and 19.57A).

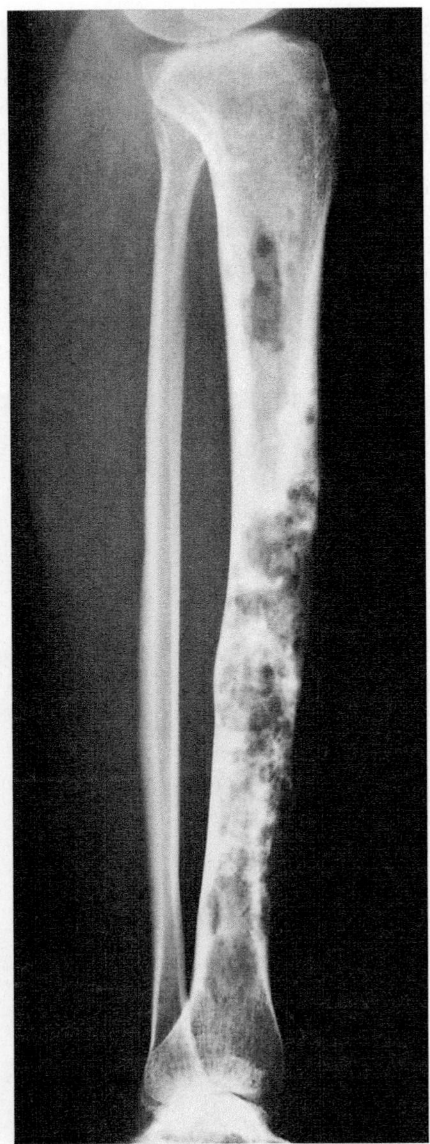

FIGURE 22.46 Adamantinoma. Lateral radiograph of the right leg of a 28-year-old woman shows multiple, confluent lytic lesions involving almost the entire tibia; only the articular ends are spared. The anterior cortex exhibits a predominantly sawtooth type of destruction.

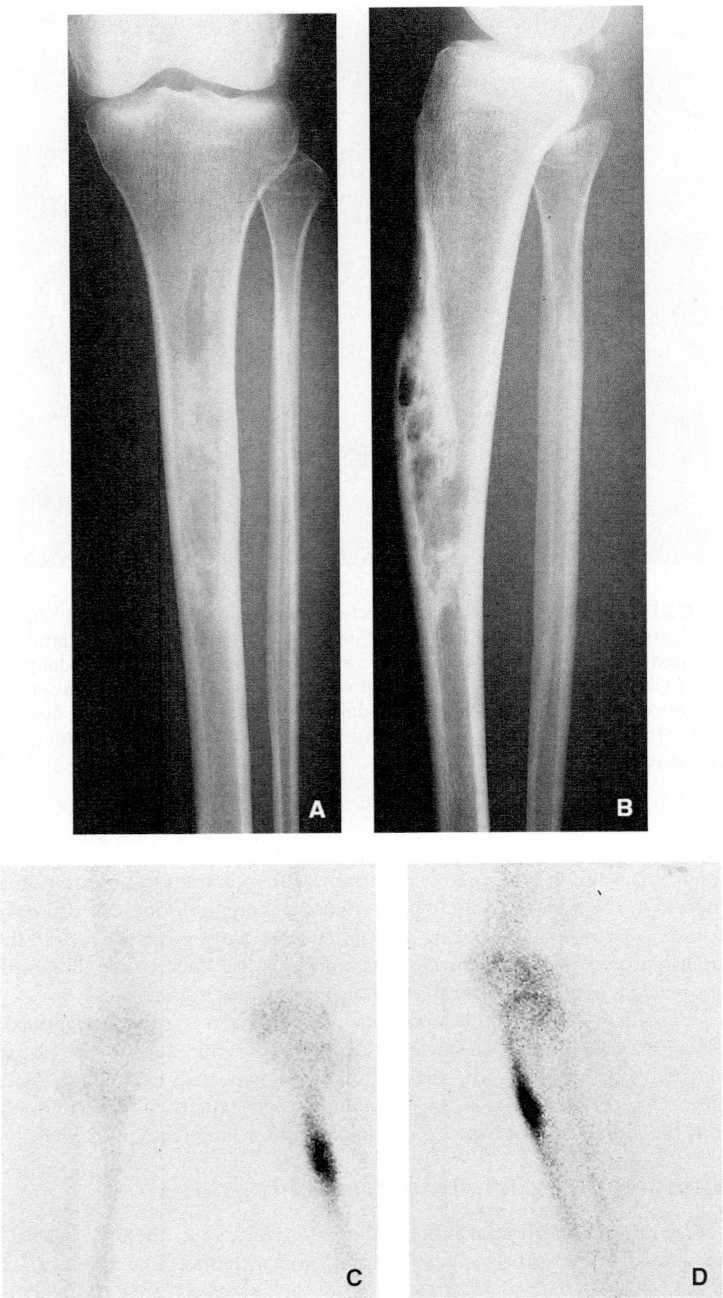

FIGURE 22.47 Scintigraphy of adamantinoma. **(A)** Anteroposterior radiograph of the left leg of a 46-year-old woman shows multiple radiolucent lesions in the midshaft of the tibia. The lateral cortex of the bone is slightly thickened. **(B)** Lateral radiograph shows a mixed sclerotic and lytic lesion predominantly affecting the anterior tibial cortex. **(C)** Frontal and **(D)** lateral radionuclide bone scan obtained after intravenous injection of 20 mCi (740 MBq) of ^{99m}Tc-labeled MDP show markedly increased uptake of radiopharmaceutical tracer by the tumor. (Reprinted with permission from Greenspan A, Borys D. *Radiology and pathology correlation of bone tumors: a quick reference and review*. Philadelphia: Wolters Kluwer; 2016:336, Fig. 7.50.)

Pathology

Gross specimen presents as a cortical, well-demarcated, yellowish-gray, lobulated firm consistency tumor with peripheral sclerosis. Although mostly a single lesion, occasionally may be multifocal with normal cortical bone between the lesions (Fig. 22.48).

Histologically, the tumor is biphasic and consists of an epithelial component intimately admixed in varying proportions with a fibrous component. Four main morphologic patterns may be present: basaloid, tubular, spindle cell, and squamous. Although it has been speculated that adamantinoma represents a form of vascular neoplasm, ultrastructural and immunohistochemical evidence points toward an epithelial derivation. Genetic abnormalities include gain of chromosomes 7, 8, 12, 19, and 21. *TP53* gene aberrations and DNA aneuploidy are limited to the epithelial component of tumor. Some cases that exhibited histopathologic features of both adamantinoma and Ewing sarcoma (called also *atypical adamantinoma* or *Ewing-like adamantinoma*) revealed translocations t(11;22), not present in classic adamantinoma.

A relationship of adamantinoma with osteofibrous dysplasia and fibrous dysplasia has been postulated and its coexistence with either of these lesions has been suggested. However, this is still controversial, with some investigators maintaining that the lesions of adamantinoma may contain a fibroosseous component that can resemble a Kempson-Campanacci lesion or fibrous dysplasia on histopathologic examination. (See also discussion in Chapter 19 in the section on "Osteofibrous Dysplasia.")

Treatment and Prognosis

Because adamantinoma is insensitive to radiotherapy, the treatment of choice is en bloc surgical resection with application of bone graft. Recurrence after limited (intralesional or marginal) surgical intervention is high (up to 90%). The tumor may spread to regional lymph nodes. Metastases (up to 29% of cases) have been recorded.

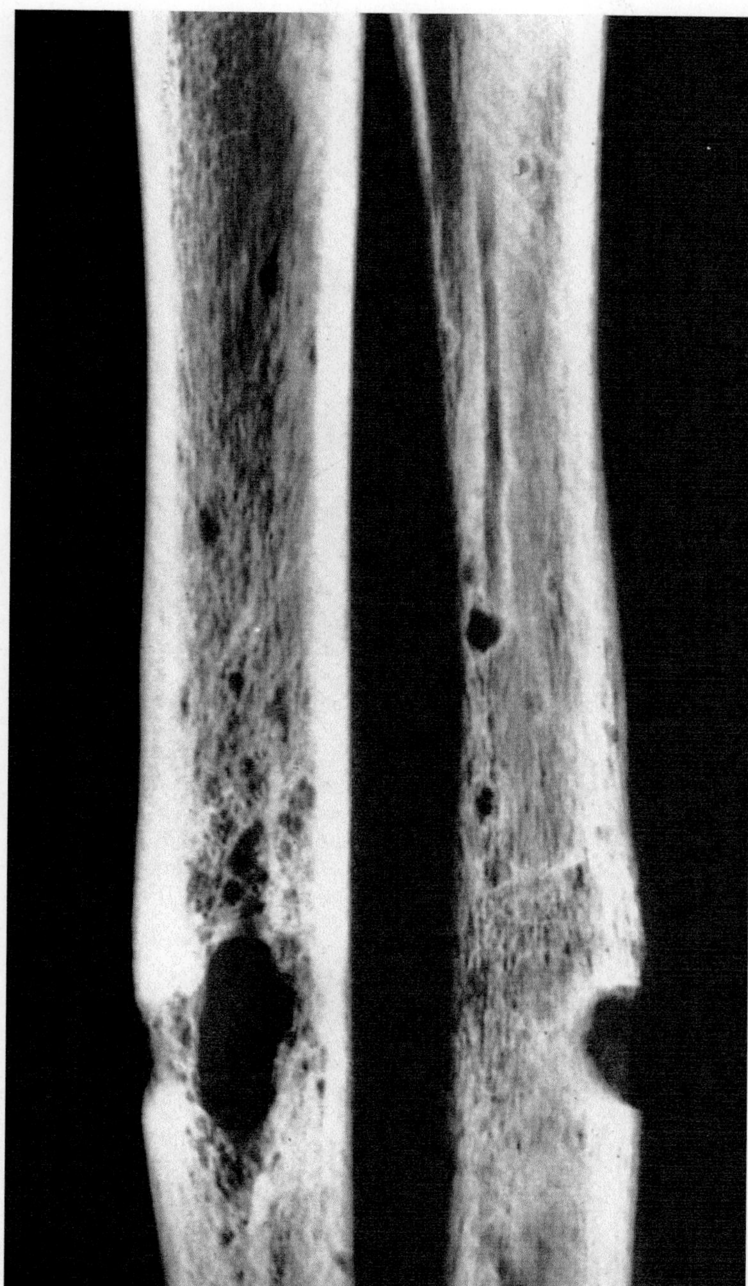

FIGURE 22.48 **Pathology of adamantinoma.** Anteroposterior *(left)* and lateral *(right)* radiographs of the resected specimen of the tibial diaphysis of a 9-year-old boy show several various in size osteolytic lesions affecting the cortex and the medullary cavity. (Reprinted from Bullough P. *Orthopaedic pathology*, 5th ed. Maryland Heights, MO: Mosby; 2009, with permission from Elsevier.)

Chordoma

Clinical Features

A chordoma is a malignant bone tumor arising from developmental remnants of the notochord. Consequently, these tumors occur almost exclusively in the midline of the axial skeleton. Chordomas represent from 1% to 4% of all primary malignant bone tumors. They arise between the fourth and seventh decades, with mean age of 56 years, and affect men slightly more often than women. The three most common sites for a chordoma are the sacrococcygeal area, the sphenooccipital area, and the C2 vertebra (Fig. 22.49). So-called *chondroid chordomas* occur exclusively at the base of the skull.

Imaging Features

The radiographic appearance is that of a highly destructive lesion with irregular scalloped borders; it is sometimes accompanied by calcifications in the matrix, probably as a result of extensive tumor necrosis (Fig. 22.50A). Bone sclerosis has been reported in 64% of cases. Soft-tissue masses are commonly associated with the lesion (Fig. 22.50B). Conventional radiography usually suffices to delineate the tumor (Fig. 22.51), but CT or MRI is required to demonstrate soft-tissue extension (Fig. 22.52) and invasion of the spinal canal. MRI shows the tumor to be of intermediate-to-low signal intensity on T1-weighted sequences and of high signal on T2-weighted and other water-sensitive sequences. Scintigraphy reveals an increased uptake of radiopharmaceutical tracer around the periphery of the tumor. Areas of abnormally decreased activity due to complete replacement of bone by the tumor may also be observed. Lack of uptake of the tracer within the tumor itself is probably secondary to the absence of vascularity and lack of new bone formation. Carbon-11 (^{11}C)-methionine (MET) PET shows high sensitivity (80%) for imaging of this tumor.

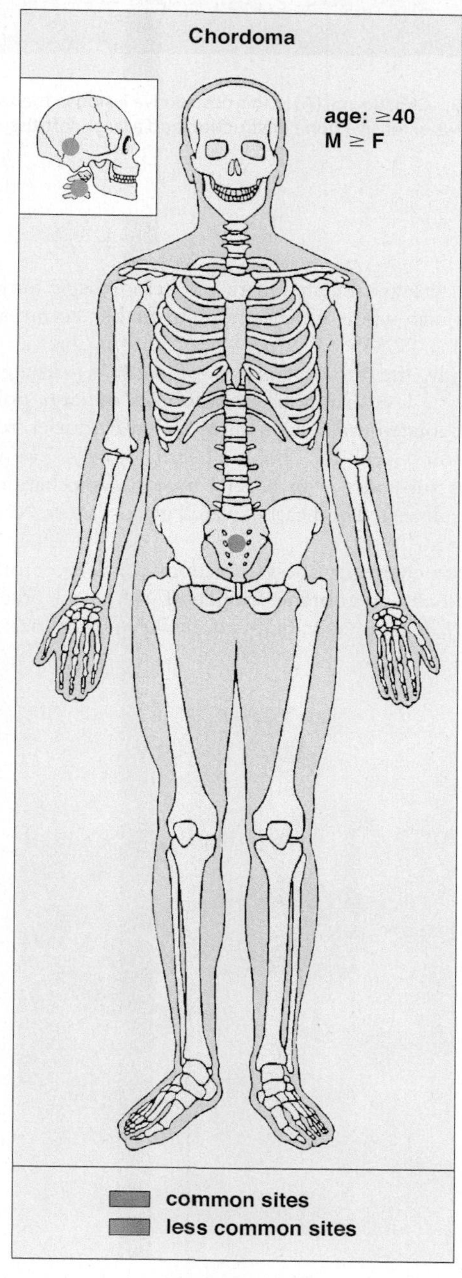

FIGURE 22.49 **Skeletal sites of predilection, peak age range, and male-to-female ratio in chordoma.**

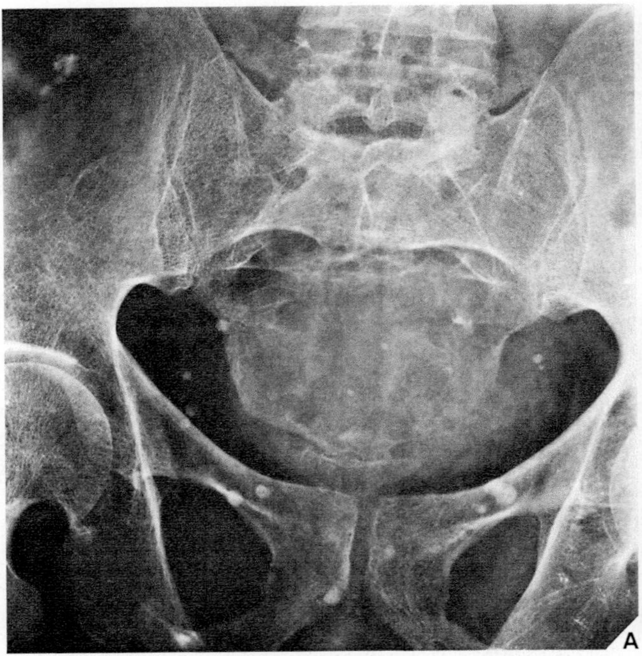

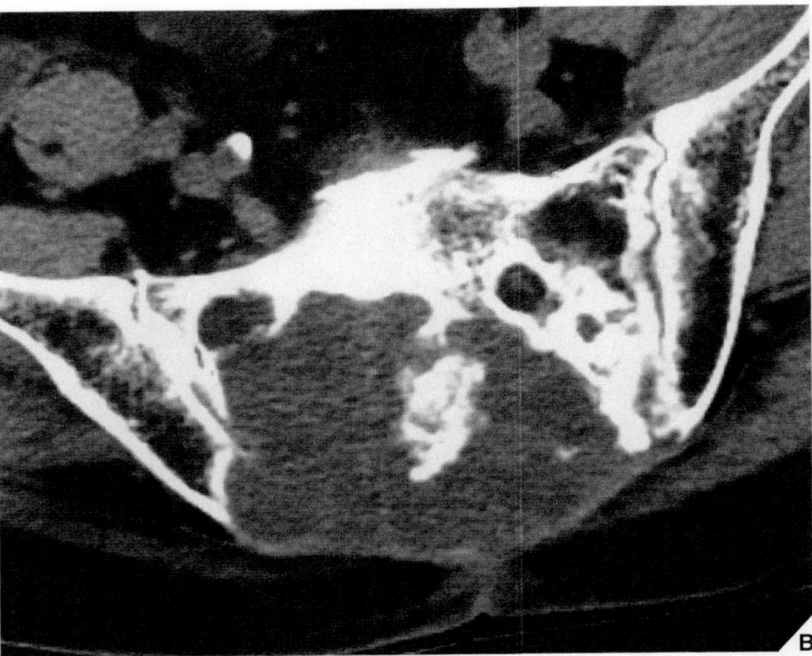

FIGURE 22.50 Chordoma. **(A)** In this destructive lesion in the sacrum of a 60-year-old woman, note its scalloped borders and the amorphous calcifications in the tumor matrix. **(B)** CT shows extensive bone destruction and a large soft-tissue mass.

Pathology

Gross specimen shows lobulated, dark-red hemorrhagic tumor, glistening, grayish tan-to-bluish white, mucilaginous to friable, commonly extending to soft tissues (Fig. 22.53).

Histologically, the tumor consists of loose aggregates of mucoid material separating cord-like arrays and lobules of large polyhedral cells, along with vacuolated cytoplasm and vesicular nuclei referred to as *physaliphorous* (from Greek for "bubble-bearing") cells. The vacuoles contain a mucinous substance with neutral mucopolysaccharides and a mixture of weakly sulfonated and carboxylated glycoprotein. Necrotic foci are commonly present.

Immunohistochemistry shows positivity for S-100 protein, cytokeratins (CKs), epithelial membrane antigen (EMA), and brachyury, a protein encoded by *T* gene (specificity about 90%). Genetics shows partial or complete *PTEN* gene deficiency and loss of chromosomes 3, 4, 10, and 13. Gain of chromosome arms 5q and 7q and chromosome 20 have been reported. Gain of brachyury 7q33 locus and the *EGFR7* (p12) locus is common.

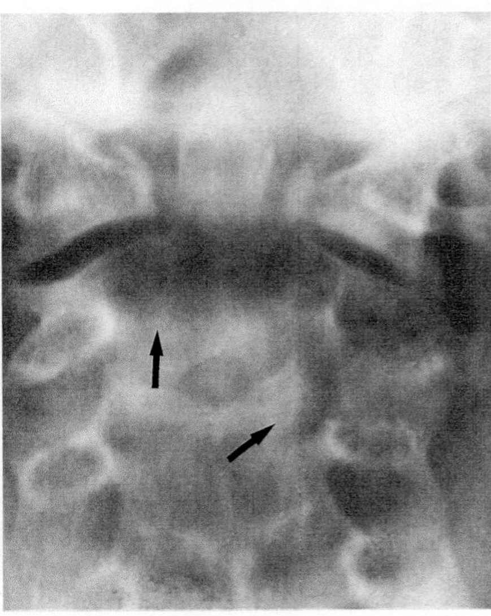

FIGURE 22.51 Chordoma. Open-mouth anteroposterior tomogram of the cervical spine of a 52-year-old man demonstrates an osteolytic lesion in the body of C2 *(arrows)*.

Complications, Treatment, and Prognosis

Invasion of the spinal canal by tumor may cause neurologic complications. Metastases are rare and usually late. The treatment for chordoma consists of complete resection, followed by radiation therapy. Cryosurgery with liquid nitrogen is occasionally used when complete tumor removal proves impossible. Overall median survival is 7 years, but it depends on the site and size of tumor. Dedifferentiated tumors have worse prognosis.

Primary Leiomyosarcoma of Bone

Clinical Features

Primary leiomyosarcomas of bone are very rare, with fewer than 150 cases reported in the world literature. More common are skeletal metastases from primary soft-tissue leiomyosarcoma. Therefore, an extraosseous primary tumor, mainly from the gastrointestinal tract or uterus, must be ruled out before a confident diagnosis of primary leiomyosarcoma of bone can be made. Leiomyosarcoma is a malignant, predominantly spindle cell, neoplasm that exhibits smooth muscle differentiation. Although the patients reported range from 9 to 80 years of age, occurrence before age 20 years is uncommon. Males are affected more often than females. The usual clinical presentation is pain of variable intensity and duration. A soft-tissue mass is occasionally observed. The most common sites are the distal femur, proximal tibia, proximal humerus, and iliac bone. Other bones occasionally may be affected, including the clavicle, ribs, and mandible.

Imaging Features

Although leiomyosarcoma exhibits no characteristic radiographic features, the tumor most often presents either as a lytic area of geographic bone destruction (Figs. 22.54A and 22.55A) or with aggressive-looking, ill-defined borders and a permeative or moth-eaten pattern. Approximately 50% of reported lesions exhibit fine periosteal reaction. CT is helpful in

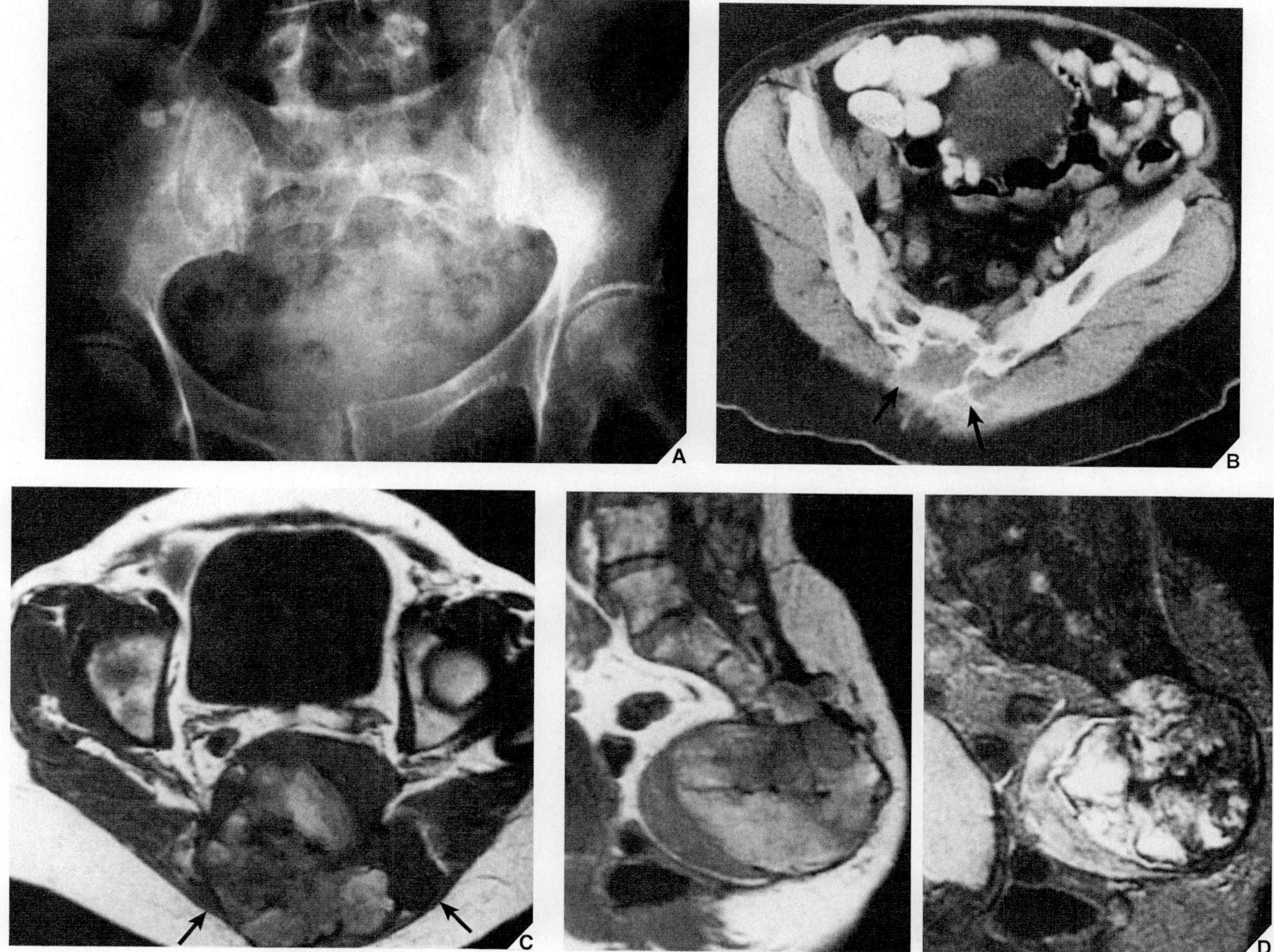

FIGURE 22.52 CT and MRI of chordoma. **(A)** Anteroposterior radiograph of the pelvis of a 68-year-old woman shows a destructive lesion in the lower part of the sacrum, associated with a soft-tissue mass. **(B)** Axial CT section demonstrates the low-attenuation tumor destroying the sacral bone *(arrows)*. **(C)** Axial T1-weighted MR image shows a large, heterogeneous tumor mass exhibiting predominantly intermediate signal intensity *(arrows)*. **(D)** Sagittal T1- and T2-weighted MR images show the lobulated tumor destroying distal part of the sacrum and coccyx and displaying a heterogeneous signal. (Reprinted with permission from Greenfield GB, Arrington JA. *Imaging of bone tumors. A multimodality approach*. Philadelphia: JB Lippincott; 1995.)

delineating the full intraosseous and extraosseous extent of the tumor (Figs. 22.54B and 22.55B). On MRI, the lesions are isointense to muscle on T1-weighted sequences, whereas on T2 weighting, they exhibit a heterogeneous but predominantly high signal (Fig. 22.55C,D).

Pathology

Microscopy reveals interlacing fascicles of spindle-shaped cells with eosinophilic (pyroninophilic) cytoplasm, which resemble leiomyosarcoma of soft tissue. The degree of cellularity, nuclear pleomorphism, and necrosis varies from case to case. The tumor cells have elongated, cigar-shaped nuclei with blunted (depressed) ends caused by a clear vacuole. Mitotic figures are common. Rarely, a storiform-like pattern, reminiscent of MFH, is seen. Immunohistochemical staining is positive for desmin, vimentin, and smooth muscle actin (SMA).

Genetics shows genomic losses and absence of phosphorylated Rb (retinoblastoma protein encoded by gene *RB1* located on 13q14-q14.2).

Differential Diagnosis

Because leiomyosarcoma of bone does not have a characteristic radiologic presentation, several possibilities should be considered in the differential diagnosis. The findings of aggressive bone destruction suggest that fibrosarcoma, MFH, and lymphoma should be considered. In younger patients, Ewing sarcoma is a possibility, as is a solitary metastasis in older patients.

Hemangioendothelioma and Angiosarcoma

Clinical Features

These tumors represent the most common malignant vascular lesions. The present nomenclature used to describe malignant vascular tumors is not uniform and is therefore rather confusing. Different terms, including *hemangiosarcoma* (*angiosarcoma*), *hemangioendothelioma*, and *hemangioendothelial sarcoma*, have been used as synonyms. The tumors have also been classified into different grades, from grade I hemangioendothelioma (well differentiated) to grade III hemangiosarcoma (poorly differentiated). Because of the prevailing confusion, the WHO classification system, although recently revised, continues to categorize these lesions as intermediate or indeterminate (including hemangioendothelioma and hemangiopericytoma) and

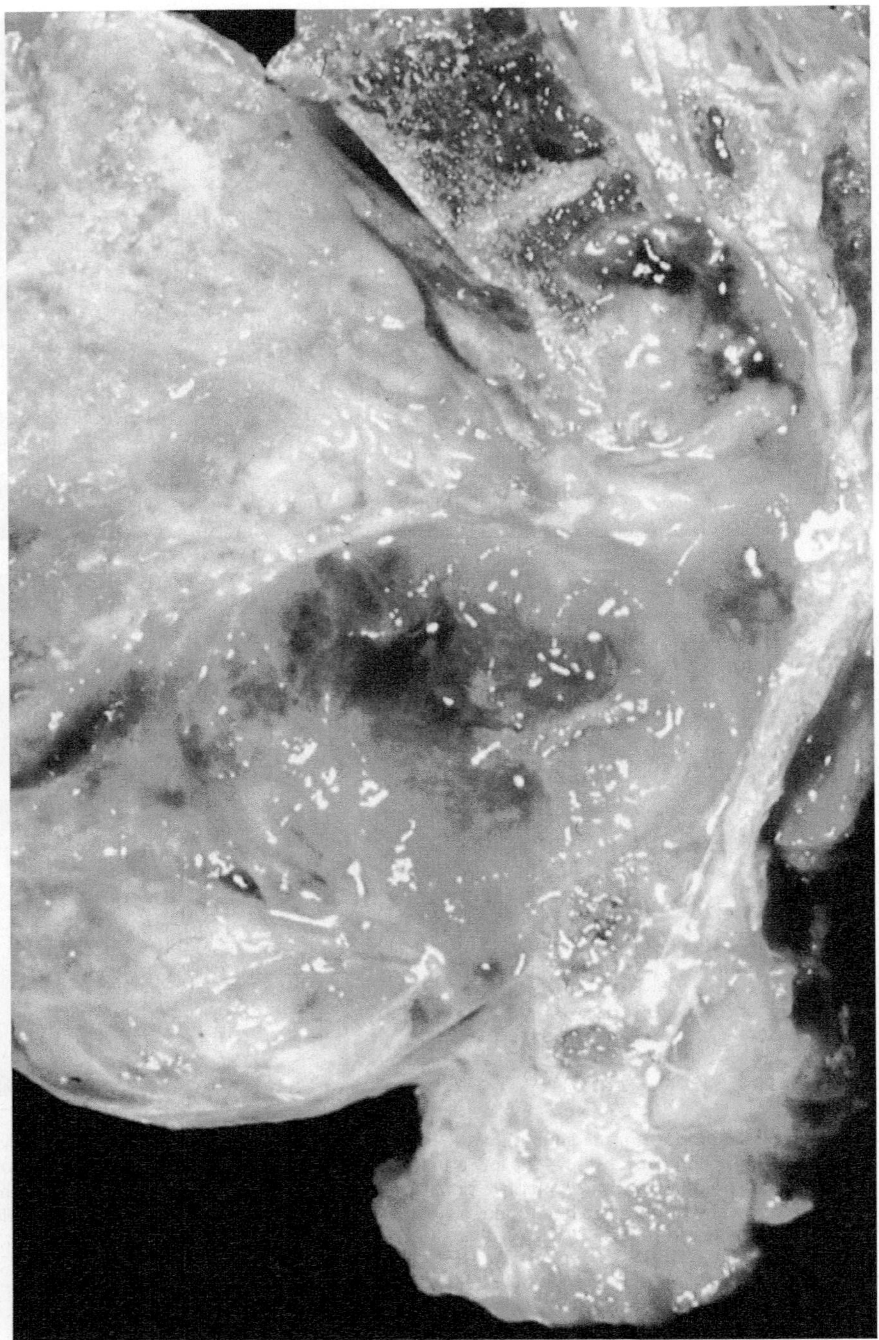

FIGURE 22.53 **Pathology of chordoma.** Sagittal section through the autopsy specimen of the lower lumbar vertebrae and sacrum shows a firm pink-gray-yellowish lobulated tumor destroying the sacral bone and L5 vertebra. A large fleshy soft-tissue mass is present anteriorly. Note prominent foci of hemorrhage *(dark red)*. (Reprinted from Bullough P. *Orthopaedic pathology*, 5th ed. Maryland Heights, MO: Mosby; 2009, with permission from Elsevier.)

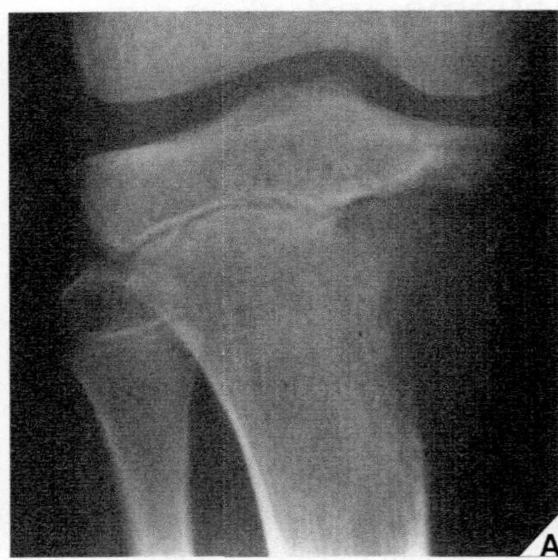

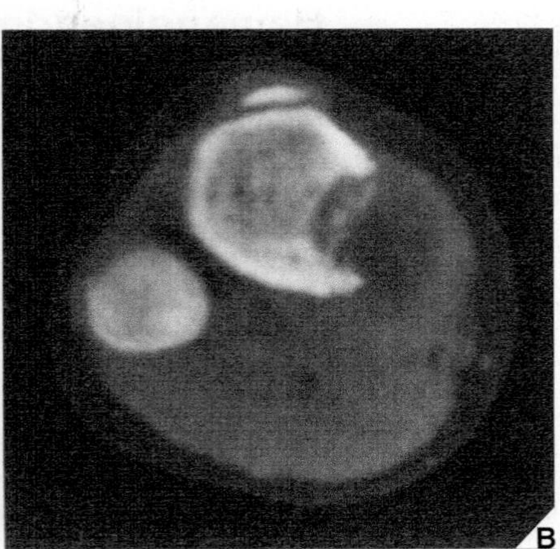

FIGURE 22.54 **Leiomyosarcoma of bone.** **(A)** Anteroposterior radiograph of the right knee of a 12-year-old boy reveals an osteolytic lesion in the proximal tibial metaphysis destroying the medial cortex and extending into the soft tissues. **(B)** Axial CT section shows destruction of the medial aspect of the tibia and an associated soft-tissue mass. (Reprinted with permission from Greenspan A, Remagen W. *Differential diagnosis of tumors and tumor-like lesions of bones and joints*. Philadelphia: Lippincott-Raven; 1998:369–371.)

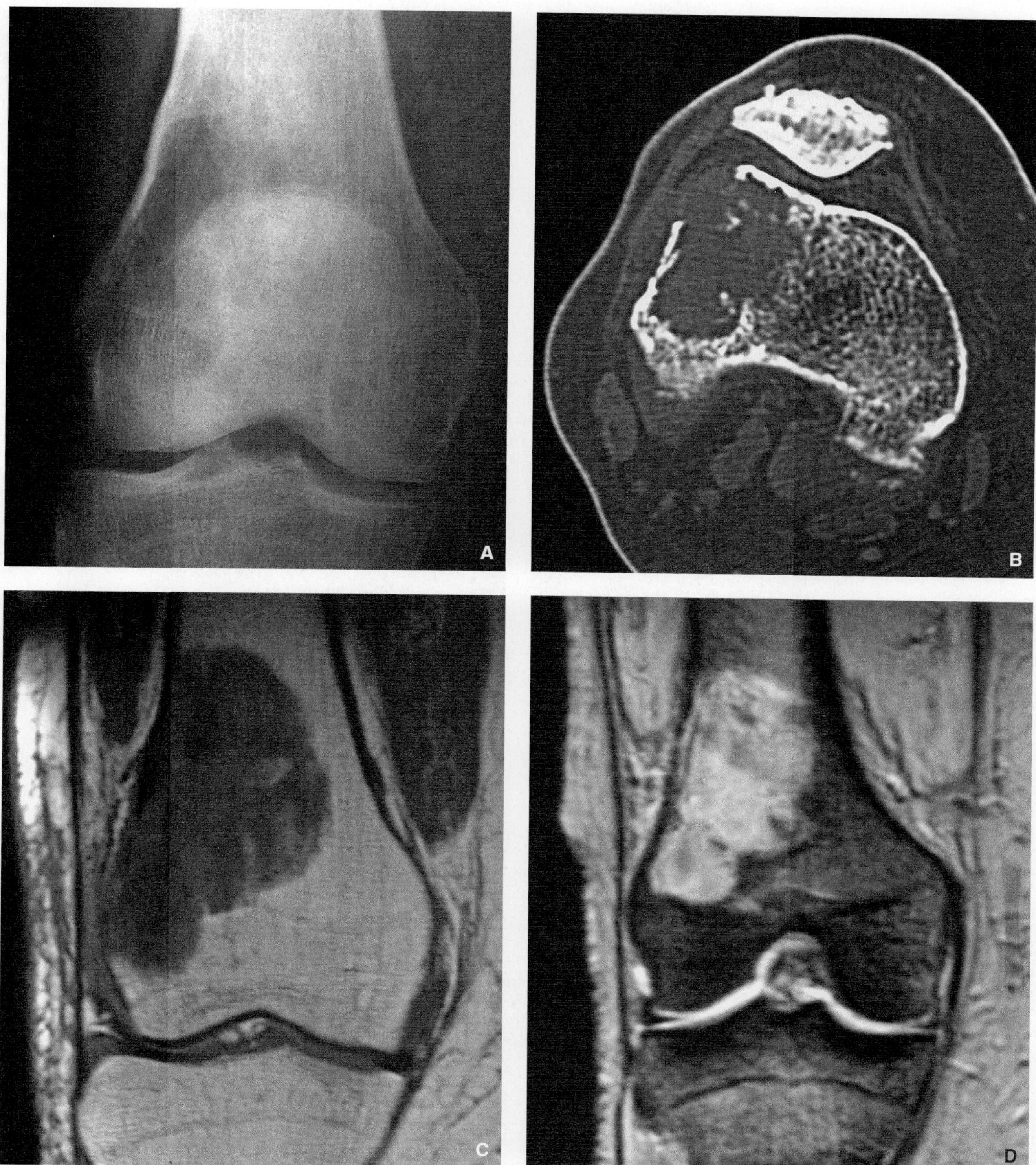

FIGURE 22.55 **CT and MRI of leiomyosarcoma of bone.** **(A)** Anteroposterior radiograph of the right knee of a 66-year-old woman shows a lytic eccentric lesion in the lateral aspect of the distal femur. **(B)** Axial CT section shows destruction of the cortex of the lateral femoral condyle and soft-tissue extension of the tumor. **(C)** Coronal T1-weighted MRI shows the lesion to be isointense with the skeletal muscles. **(D)** Coronal T2-weighted MR image shows that the tumor exhibits slightly heterogenous but predominantly high signal intensity. (Reprinted with permission from Greenspan A, Borys D. *Radiology and pathology correlation of bone tumors: a quick reference and review.* Philadelphia: Wolters Kluwer; 2016:345, Fig. 7.59.)

clearly malignant (angiosarcoma). Unequivocal distinction among these tumors is sometimes difficult.

Hemangioendothelioma and a recently identified lesion called *epithelioid hemangioendothelioma* are considered to represent true neoplasms because of their independent growth potential, the histopathologic demonstration of nuclear atypia accompanied by occasional mitotic activity, and because they commonly recur after inadequate local excision. Moreover, epithelioid hemangioendothelioma has been characterized by a specific chromosomal translocation [t(1;3)(p36.3:q25)] involving the *WWTR1-CAMTA1* genes fusion on chromosomes 1 and 3, a genetic hallmark that provides a diagnostic tool to distinguish this lesion from hemangioendothelioma. Both these tumors arise at any age within the range of 10 to 75 years, with a slight predilection for males. The lesion may be solitary or (usually epithelioid variant) multicentric. Patients with multifocal disease are usually 10 years younger than those with a solitary lesion. The most commonly affected sites are the calvaria, spine, and bones of the lower extremities. Clinical symptoms include dull local pain and tenderness. Some swelling and hemorrhagic joint effusion may sometimes be observed.

Angiosarcoma of bone represents the most malignant end of the spectrum of vascular tumors. This is an aggressive neoplasm, characterized by frequent local recurrence and distant metastases. The lesion occurs typically during the second to the seventh decade, with a peak in the fifth decade. Males are affected twice as frequently as females. Most common sites of occurrence are the long bones, particularly the tibia, femur, and humerus, and the most common symptoms are local pain and swelling. Metastases to the lungs and other internal organs occur in approximately 66% of cases.

Imaging Features

On radiography, hemangioendothelioma shows an osteolytic appearance, either well circumscribed or with a wide zone of transition (Fig. 22.56). Variable degrees of peripheral sclerosis may sharply demarcate the lesion. Some tumors may exhibit mixed lytic and sclerotic pattern. Occasionally, a soap-bubble appearance with expansion of bone is observed, with extension into the soft tissues. MRI reveals a mixed signal on T1-weighted sequences, with moderately increased signal intensity on T2 weighting (Fig. 22.57). On imaging studies, it is very difficult to differentiate hemangioendothelioma from other vascular lesions, either benign or malignant. A solitary osteolytic lesion may mimic a metastasis, fibrosarcoma, MFH, plasmacytoma, or lymphoma, and lesions that extend to the articular end of bone can be mistaken for giant cell tumor. Because the radiologic presentation of hemangioendothelioma is usually nonspecific, clinical information may be helpful in narrowing the differential diagnosis.

Angiosarcoma has imaging features similar to those of hemangioendothelioma, although more commonly it exhibits a wide zone of transition between the tumor and uninvolved bone (Fig. 22.58). Cortical permeation and associated soft-tissue masses are frequently observed.

Pathology

On histologic examination, hemangioendothelioma reveals markedly pleomorphic endothelial cells with abundant faintly eosinophilic or amphophilic cytoplasm and hyperchromatic nuclei with prominent nucleoli. The interanastomosing vascular channels, often arranged in an antler-like

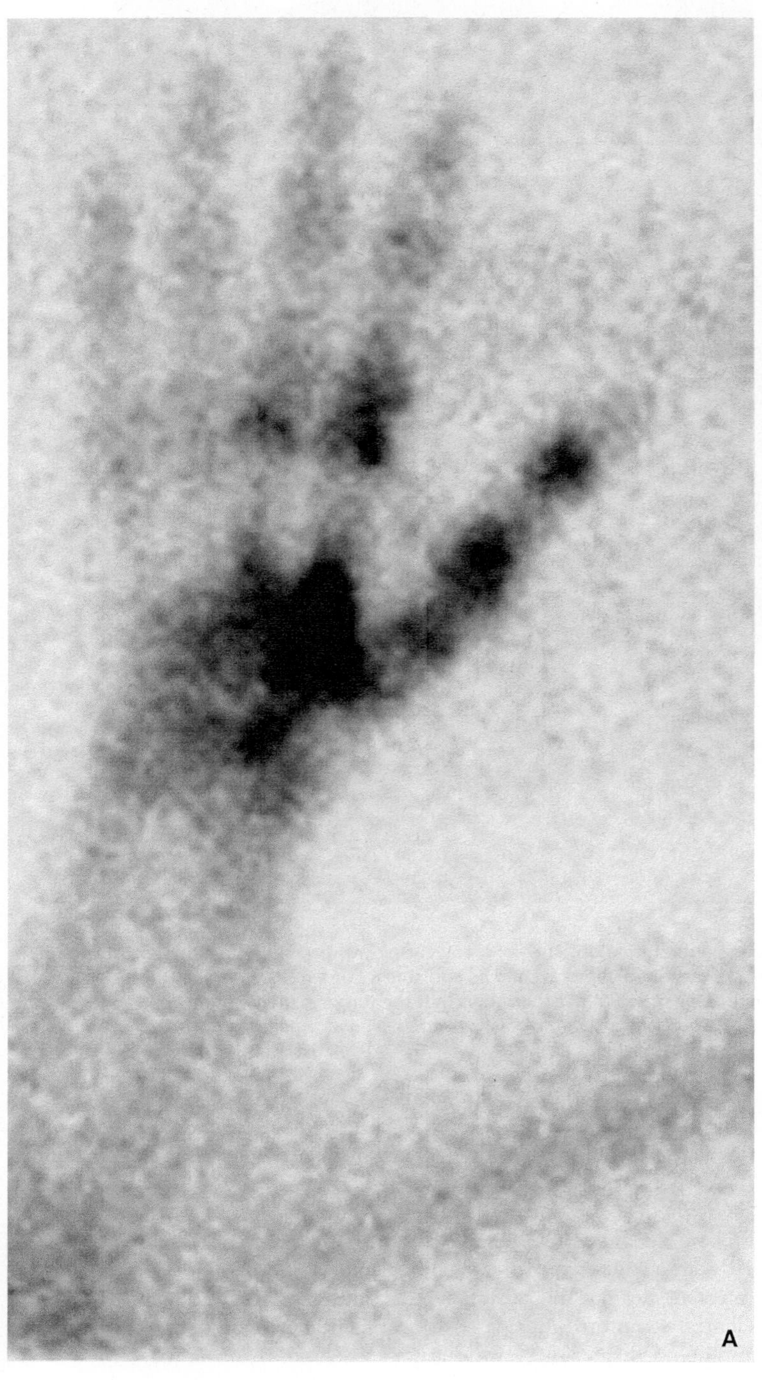

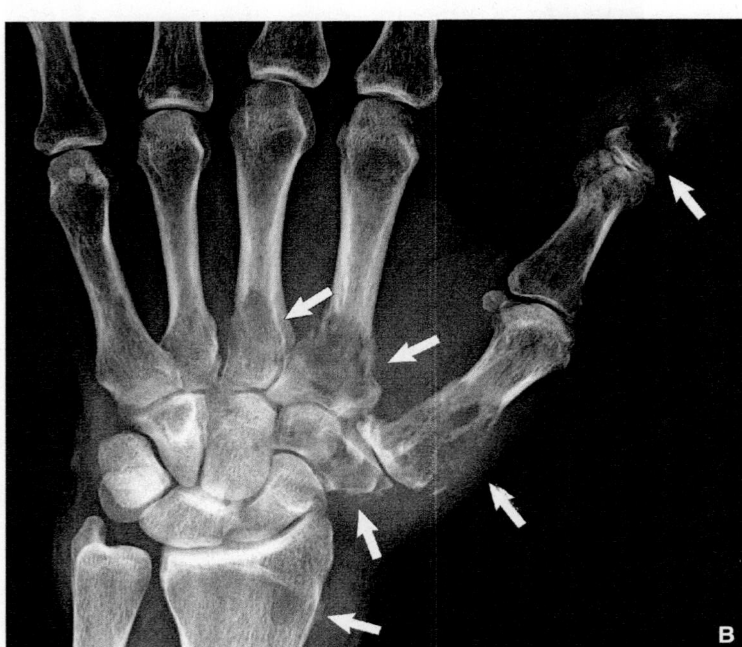

FIGURE 22.56 **Multifocal epithelioid hemangioendothelioma.** **(A)** Radionuclide bone scan of the right hand of a 66-year-old man shows several foci of increased activity of radiopharmaceutical tracer within the distal radius, carpal bones, metacarpals, and phalanges. **(B)** Dorsovolar radiograph of the right wrist shows destructive lytic lesions exhibiting wide zone of transition within the distal radius; trapezium; trapezoid; first, second, and third metacarpals; and proximal and distal phalanges of the thumb *(arrows)*.

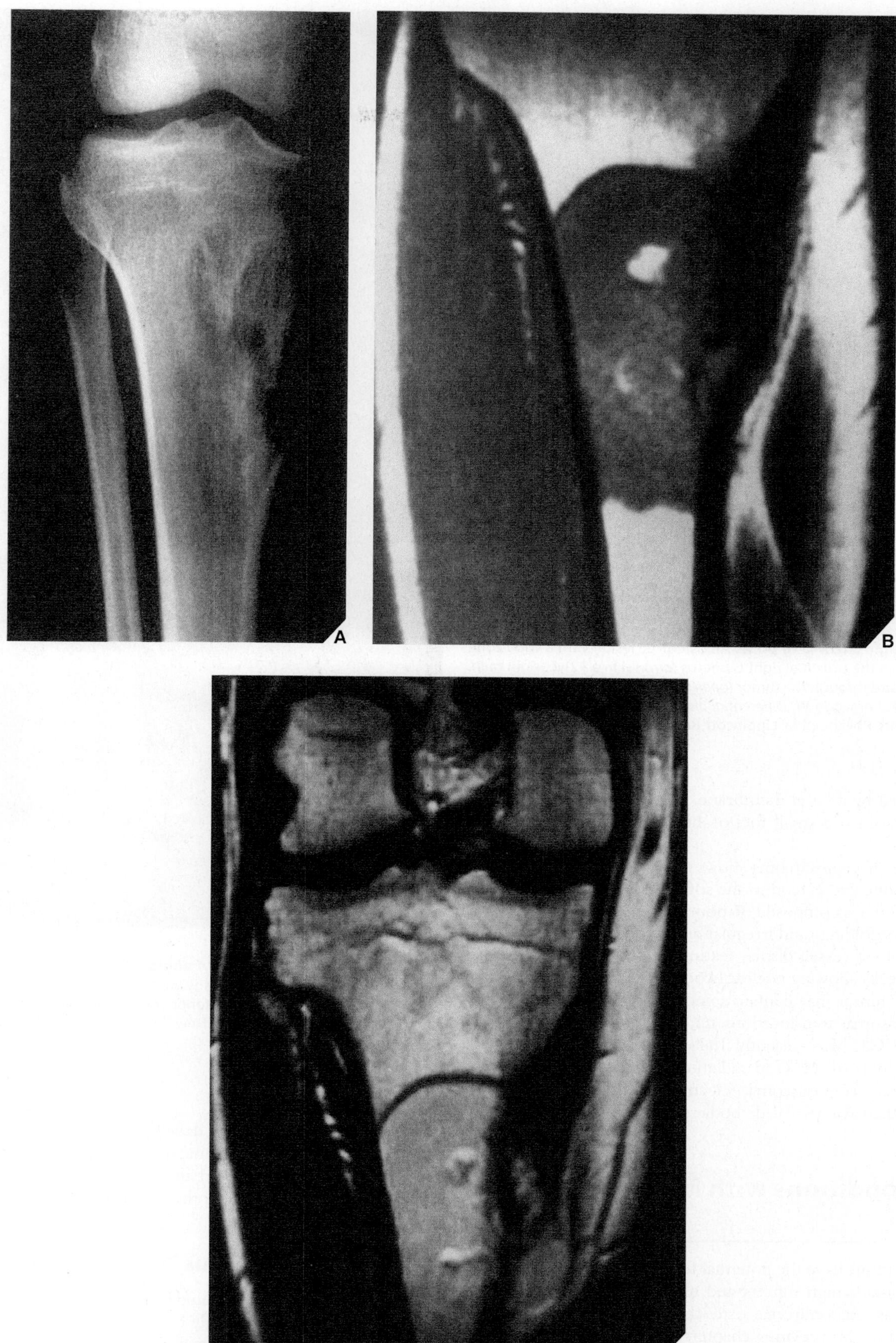

FIGURE 22.57 **MRI of hemangioendothelioma of bone.** **(A)** Anteroposterior radiograph of the right proximal tibia shows an osteolytic lesion destroying medial aspect of the bone. **(B)** Coronal T1-weighted MRI reveals a low–signal intensity tumor replacing bone marrow. **(C)** Coronal T2-weighted MRI shows an increase in the signal intensity of the tumor, which exhibits heterogeneous appearance. (Reprinted with permission from Greenfield GB, Arrington JA. *Imaging of bone tumors. A multimodality approach*. Philadelphia: JB Lippincott; 1995.)

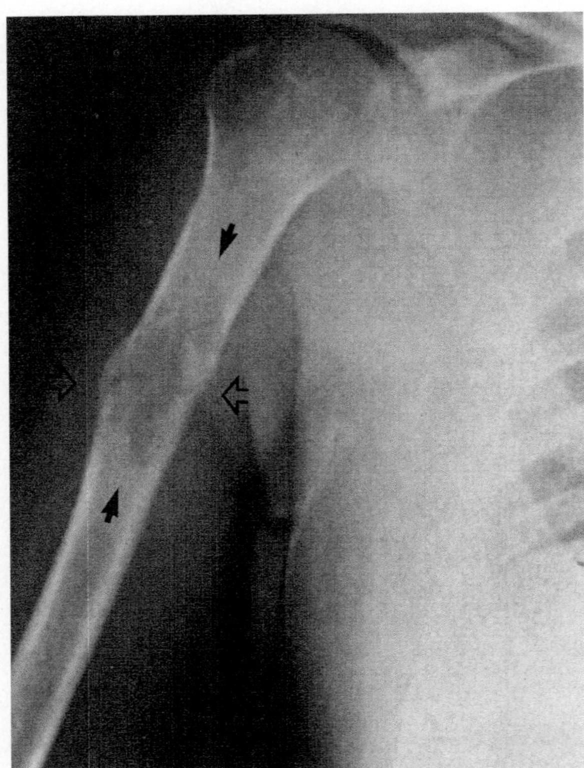

FIGURE 22.58 Angiosarcoma of bone. An osteolytic lesion with a wide zone of transition is present in the proximal right humerus *(arrows)* in a 42-year-old man. Note a pathologic fracture through the tumor *(open arrows)*. (Reprinted with permission from Greenspan A, Remagen W. *Differential diagnosis of tumors and tumor-like lesions of bones and joints*. Philadelphia: Lippincott-Raven; 1998:369–371.)

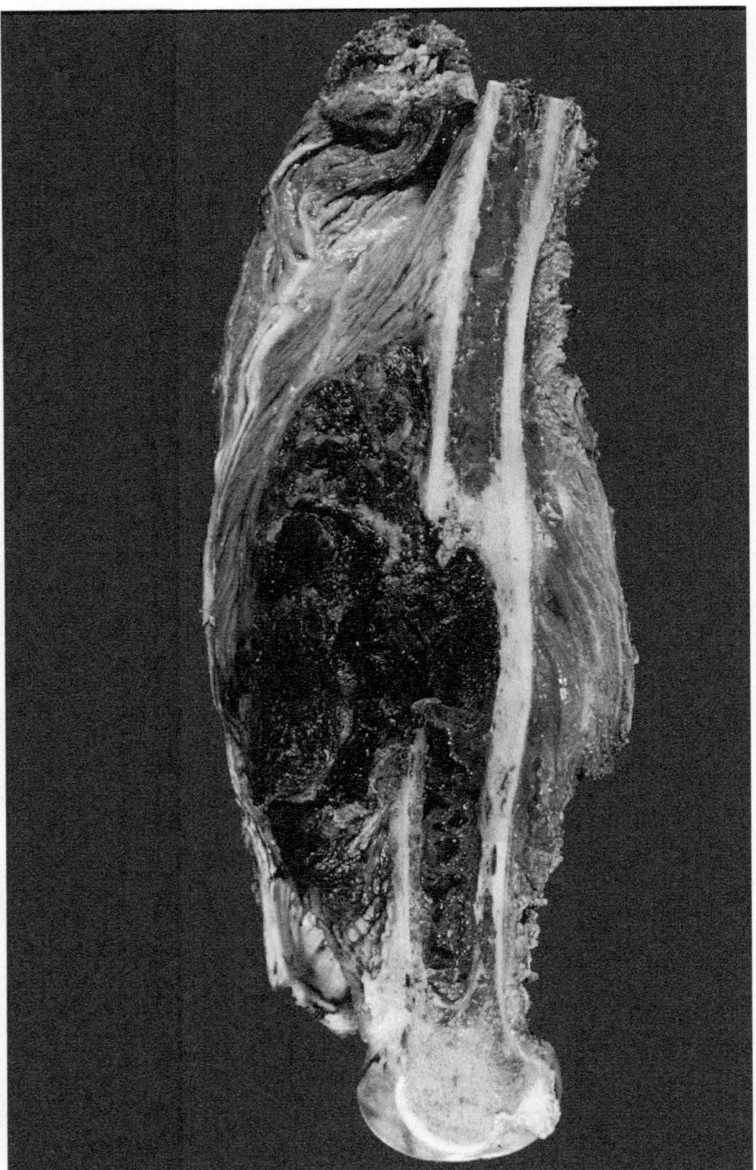

FIGURE 22.59 Pathology of angiosarcoma. Photograph of the sagittal section of the gross specimen of fleshy vascular tumor arising within the marrow cavity of the femur, invading the anterior cortex, and forming a large soft-tissue mass. (Courtesy of Michael J. Klein, MD, New York.)

pattern, are delimited by a basal membrane. The stroma typically varies from fibrous to myxoid and small foci of hemorrhage or necrosis may be observed.

Gross specimen of angiosarcoma shows firm, fleshy and bloody mass that can erode the bone and extend to the soft tissues (Fig. 22.59). Microscopically, angiosarcoma is composed of poorly formed blood vessels that exhibit complicated infoldings and irregular anastomoses. The endothelial cells that line these blood vessels display features of frank malignancy, with plump intraluminal cells showing nuclear hyperchromatin and atypical mitoses. Solid areas of tumor may contain spindle and epithelioid cells. Genetics show chromosomal translocations t(1;14)(p21;q24) and mutations of PTPRB and PLCG1. Most recently, Italiano and colleagues reported a genomic amplification of *MYC* in radiation-induced angiosarcoma as well as in the primary angiosarcoma. Electron microscopy shows that endothelial cells contain Weibel-Palade bodies.

Benign Conditions with Malignant Potential

Several benign conditions have the potential for malignant transformation (see Table 16.2). Some benign tumors and tumor-like lesions that are in this category, such as enchondroma, osteochondroma, and fibrous dysplasia, are discussed in the previous chapters (see Chapters 18 and 19). Several of the conditions discussed have also been touched on in Chapter 21. (See the sections on "Secondary Osteosarcomas" and "Secondary Chondrosarcomas.")

Medullary Bone Infarct

The development of a sarcoma in association with a medullary bone infarct is a rare event. The clinical sign that should alert the radiologist to this possibility is the development of bone pain in a previously asymptomatic patient. The imaging findings of bone destruction in the area of the medullary infarct in conjunction with a periosteal reaction and soft-tissue mass confirm the diagnosis of malignant transformation (Fig. 22.60).

Chronic Draining Sinus Tract of Osteomyelitis

Malignant transformation should be suspected when a long-standing sinus tract of osteomyelitis suddenly becomes painful and discharges purulent, foul material. In most patients with osteomyelitis, the history of the disease dates to childhood, and sinuses draining for more than 20 years are generally the precursors of malignant neoplasms. The development of squamous cell carcinoma is most commonly seen (Fig. 22.61), but fibrosarcoma and osteosarcoma may also be encountered. The incidence of neoplastic transformation, however, is low, ranging from 0.2% to 1.7%. The radiographic features of malignant transformation may occasionally be indistinguishable from those of chronic osteomyelitis, but an increase

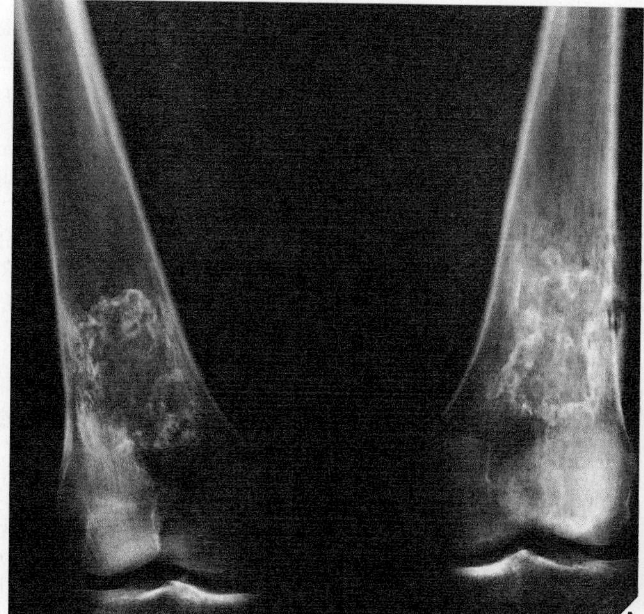

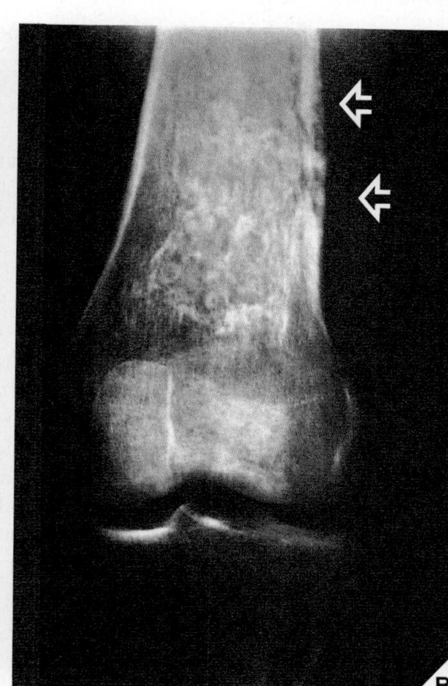

FIGURE 22.60 MFH arising in a bone infarct. A 39-year-old woman with known multiple idiopathic medullary bone infarcts had pain above the left knee. **(A)** Anteroposterior radiograph of both knees shows the typical appearance of medullary bone infarcts in the distal femora. In the left femur, there is evidence of a lamellated periosteal reaction along the lateral cortex. **(B)** Magnification study shows cortical destruction *(open arrows)*.

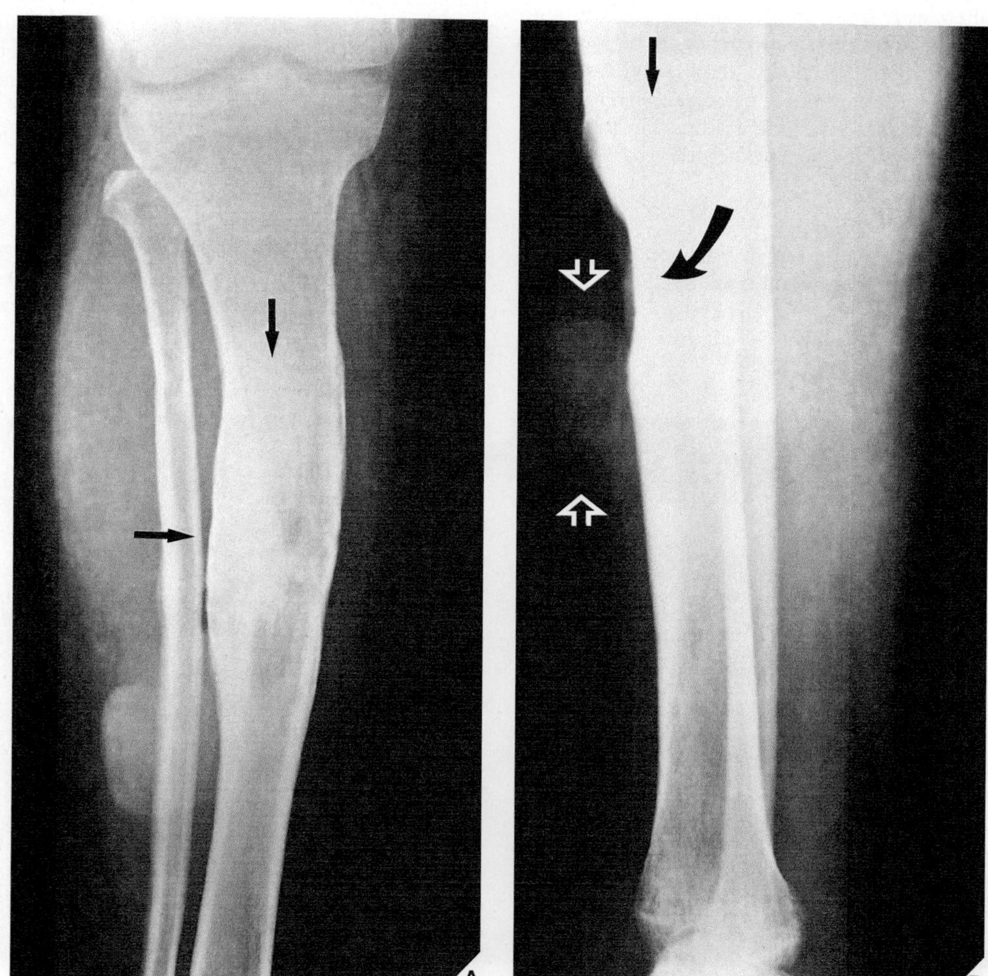

FIGURE 22.61 Squamous cell carcinoma arising in a chronic draining sinus of osteomyelitis. A 59-year-old man was admitted for treatment of an ulcer of the right leg that was present for 5 years. At age 13 years, he had an open fracture of the tibia that became infected, and he developed chronic osteomyelitis. **(A)** Anteroposterior and **(B)** lateral radiographs of the right leg show a large saucerized defect of the anterior cortex of the middle third of the tibia, with dense compact bone lining its base *(curved arrow)*. A large sharply circumscribed soft-tissue mass is also evident at this site *(open arrows)*. Above the defect, which is postsurgical, are medullary sclerosis and cortical thickening *(arrows)*, both characteristic of chronic osteomyelitis. (Reprinted by permission from Springer: Greenspan A, Norman A, Steiner G. Case Report 146. Squamous cell carcinoma arising in chronic, draining sinus tract secondary to osteomyelitis of right tibia. *Skeletal Radiol* 1981;6:149–151.)

in the extent of bone destruction usually indicates the onset of sarcoma or carcinoma.

Plexiform Neurofibromatosis

A spectrum of neoplastic disorders is associated with neurofibromatosis as the most serious complication of this disease. Sarcoma of the peripheral nerves and somatic soft tissues is well recognized in neurofibromatosis, with its incidence varying from 3% to 16%. Most such sarcomas are neural in origin, including neurosarcoma, neurofibrosarcoma, and malignant schwannoma; nonneurogenic sarcomas such as rhabdomyosarcoma and liposarcoma are less common. The precise origin of the sarcomas arising in neurofibromatosis is uncertain; in some instances, the mass clearly originates in a nerve trunk, whereas in others, there is no obvious relation to the nerve. The most common clinical features of malignant degeneration in a patient with neurofibromatosis are the development of pain, the rapid growth of a preexisting neurofibroma, and a new soft-tissue mass. Radiologically, the diagnosis of sarcomatous transformation is almost certain if abnormal tumor vessels (Fig. 22.62) or a "tumor stain" is demonstrated on arteriography.

Paget Disease

The development of a sarcoma in pagetic bone is a serious complication of Paget disease. Although Paget sarcoma is rare (less than 1%), individuals with Paget disease are 20 times more likely to have a malignant bone tumor develop than are other persons of comparable age. Radiographically, sarcomatous transformation is indicated by the development of a lytic lesion, often with evidence of cortical breakthrough and a soft-tissue mass (Fig. 22.63); a periosteal reaction is uncommon. The bones commonly affected include the pelvis, femur, and humerus. Histologically, the most common type of tumor is osteosarcoma, followed by MFH, fibrosarcoma, and chondrosarcoma, in that order. The prognosis for patients with Paget sarcoma is poor; few survive beyond 6 to 8 months.

Radiation-Induced Sarcoma

Radiation-induced sarcomas may arise in areas of normal bone exposed to radiation fields or may be caused by benign conditions treated by irradiation, such as fibrous dysplasia or giant cell tumor. Generally, a sarcoma can develop only if at least 3,000 rads are administered within a 4-week span, although cases have been reported after exposure to only 800 rads. The latency period for radiation-induced tumors varies from 4 to 40 years, with an average of 11 years. Their incidence is rather low, not exceeding 0.5%.

The criteria for diagnosis of postirradiation sarcoma are as follows:

1. The initial lesion and the postirradiation sarcoma must not be of the same histologic type.
2. The site of the new tumor must be within the field of irradiation.
3. At least 3 years must have elapsed since the previous radiation therapy.

Postirradiation osteosarcoma may also develop after the ingestion and intraosseous accumulation of radioisotopes, as has been described in painters of radium watch dials. Regardless of the source of radiation, the most common of such tumors is osteosarcoma, followed by fibrosarcoma and MFH (Fig. 22.64).

Skeletal Metastases

Clinical Features

Skeletal metastases are the most common malignant bone tumors and consequently should always be considered in the differential diagnosis of malignant lesions, particularly in older patients. Most metastatic lesions involve the axial skeleton—the skull, spine, and pelvis—as well as the proximal segments of the long bones; only very rarely is a metastasis seen distal to the elbows or knees (Fig. 22.65). These lesions result from the hematogenous spread of a malignancy, the usual mechanism by which a primary neoplasm erodes regional blood vessels, seeding malignant cells to the capillary beds of the lung and liver. Tumor emboli become lodged in the axial skeleton through communication with the vertebral venous plexus.

The incidence of metastases to bone varies with the type of primary neoplasm and the duration of disease. Some malignant tumors have a far greater propensity for osseous metastatic involvement than do others. Because of their frequency, cancers of the breast, lung, and prostate are responsible for the majority of bone metastases, although primary tumors of the kidney, small and large intestines, stomach, and thyroid may also metastasize to bone. Carcinoma of the prostate has been reported to underlie nearly 60% of all bone metastases in men, whereas in women, carcinoma of the breast is responsible for nearly 70% of all metastatic skeletal lesions.

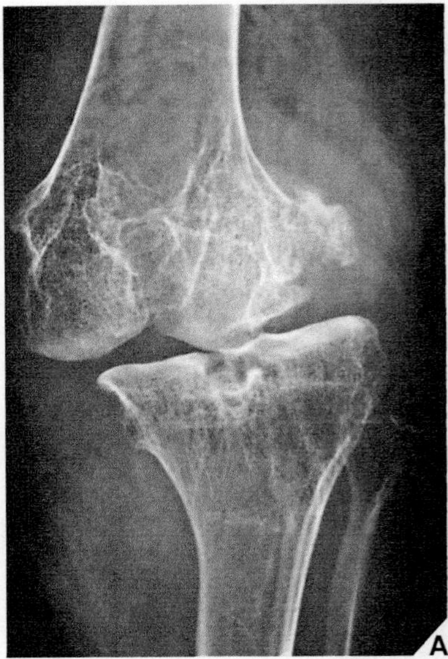

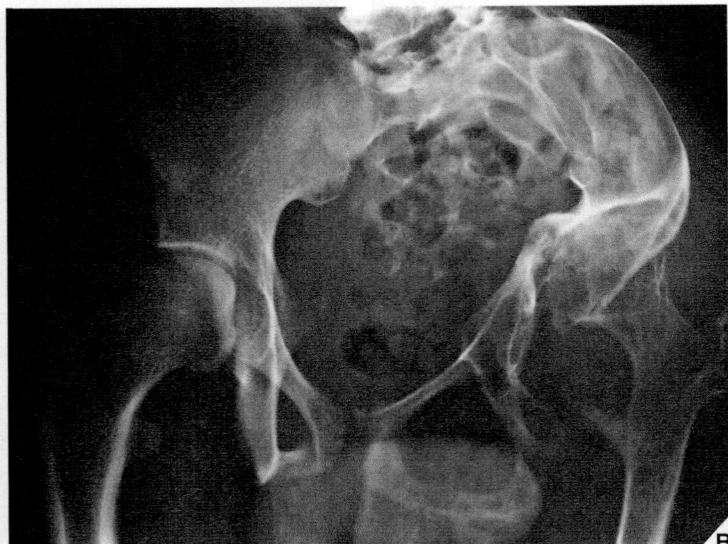

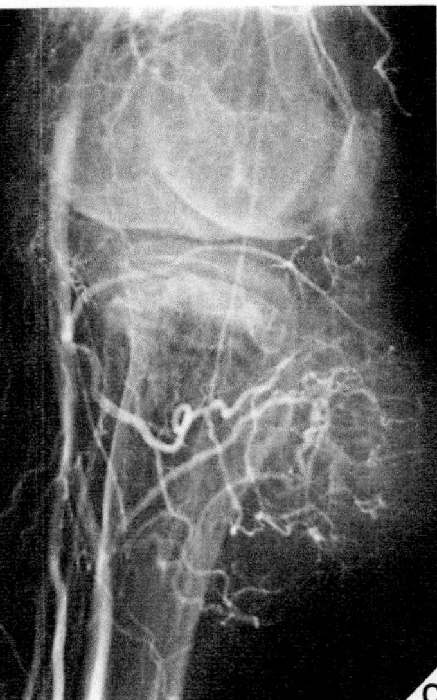

FIGURE 22.62 Liposarcoma arising in plexiform neurofibromatosis. An 18-year-old man with known neurofibromatosis since early childhood presented with an enlarging, painful pretibial mass of more than 10 months' duration. **(A)** Anteroposterior radiograph of the left knee shows instability with lateral subluxation. The medial cortex of the medial femoral condyle and the lateral cortex of the lateral femoral condyle are eroded at the site of a soft-tissue mass. **(B)** Anteroposterior radiograph of the pelvis shows asymmetry of the pelvis with a large deformed acetabulum, enlargement of the left obturator foramen, and superolateral subluxation of the left hip—all features typical of neurofibromatosis. **(C)** Femoral arteriogram shows the pretibial mass to be hypervascular, with numerous small tortuous tumor vessels. (Reprinted by permission from Springer: Baker ND, Greenspan A. Case Report 172: pleomorphic liposarcoma, grade IV, of the soft tissue, arising in generalized plexiform neurofibromatosis. *Skeletal Radiol* 1981;7:150–153.)

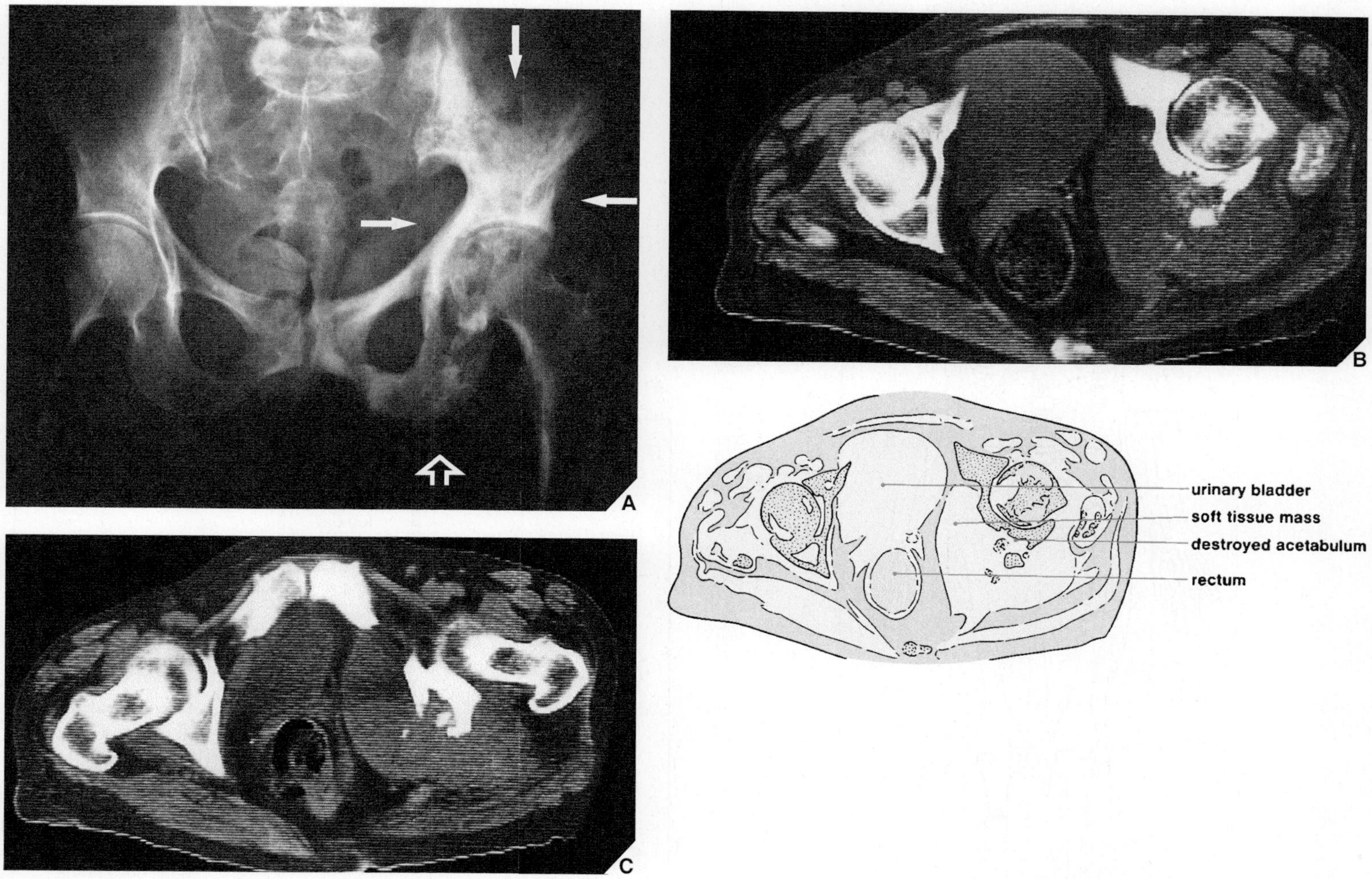

FIGURE 22.63 MFH arising in pagetic bone. A 66-year-old woman with known Paget disease had pain in the left hip joint radiating to the buttock. **(A)** Anteroposterior radiograph of the pelvis shows extensive involvement of the left hemipelvis by Paget disease *(arrows)*. There is also an osteolytic area of bone destruction in the left ischium *(open arrow)*. CT sections, one through the femoral heads and acetabula **(B)** and a second through the ischium and pubic symphysis **(C)**, demonstrate cortical destruction and a large soft-tissue mass—both signs of malignant transformation to sarcoma. Note the displacement of the rectum and urinary bladder.

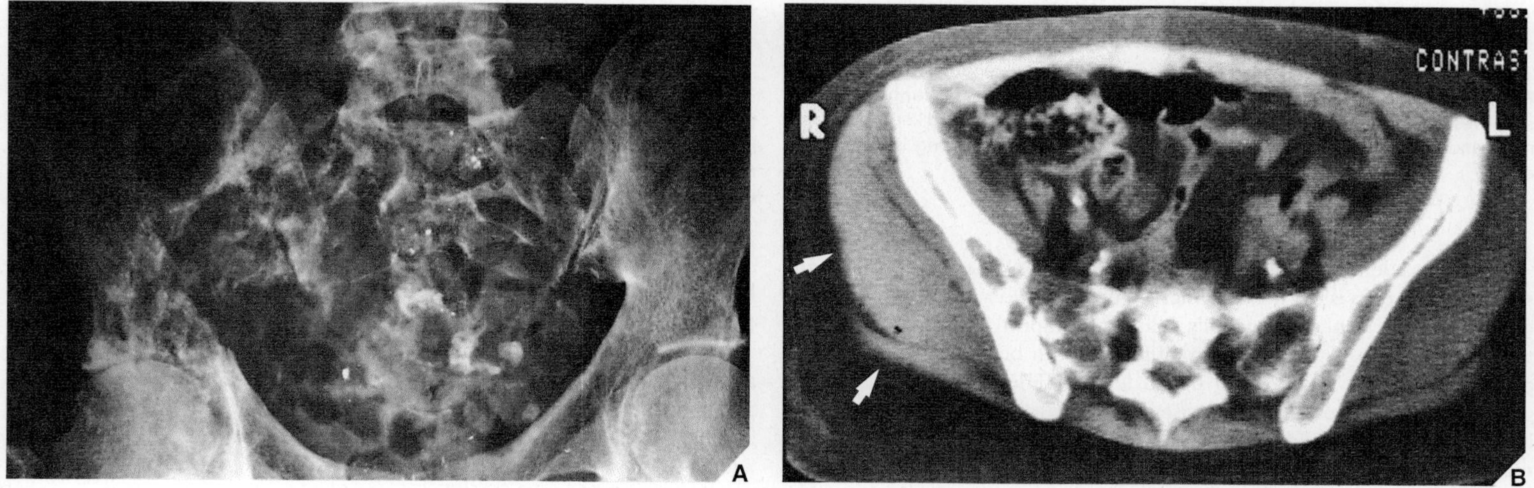

FIGURE 22.64 Radiation-induced MFH. A 63-year-old woman had been treated 15 years earlier with radium for carcinoma of the cervix. **(A)** Anteroposterior radiograph of the pelvis shows a large, destructive lesion involving the right ilium and extending into the supra-acetabular region, with destruction of the right wing of the sacral bone. **(B)** CT section, in addition to the changes seen on radiography, demonstrates a soft-tissue mass *(arrows)*. Biopsy revealed an MFH. The tumor developed in the ilium that had been exposed to radiation, extending into the soft tissue and invading the sacrum secondarily.

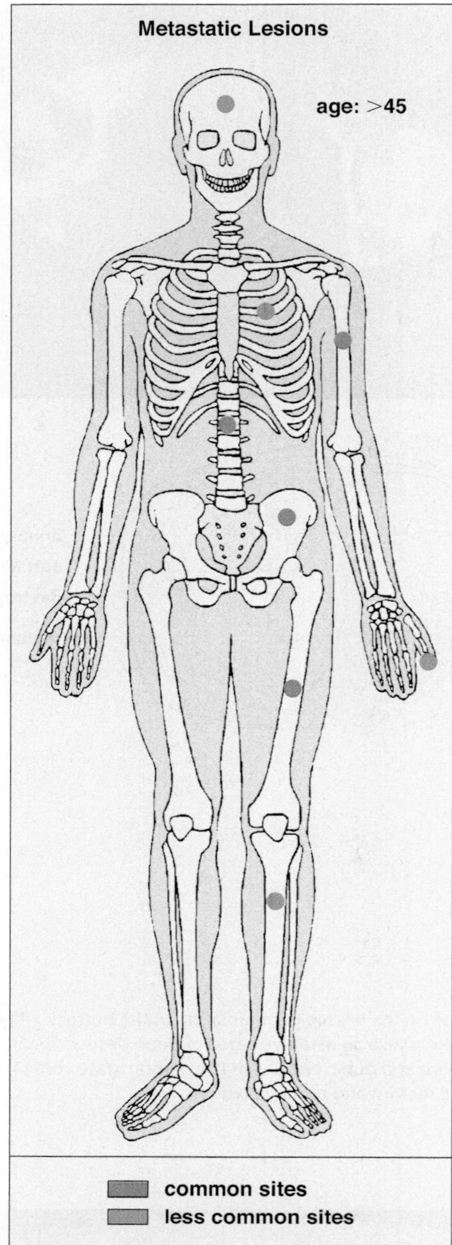

▲ **FIGURE 22.65 Skeletal sites of predilection and peak age range of metastatic lesions.** The occurrence of such lesions distal to the elbow and knee is uncommon, and in those sites, a primary malignancy of the breast or lung is usually the origin.

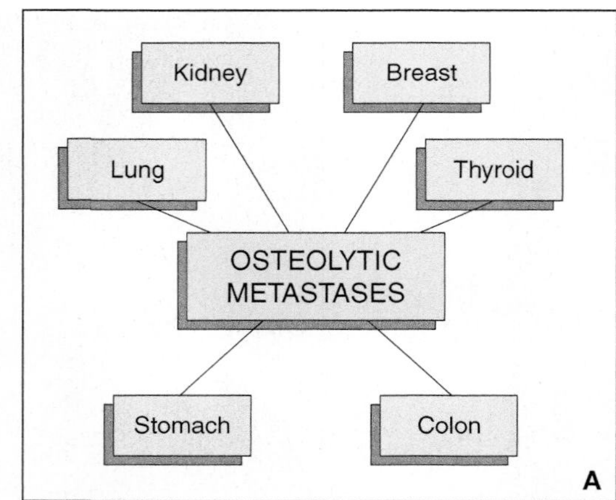

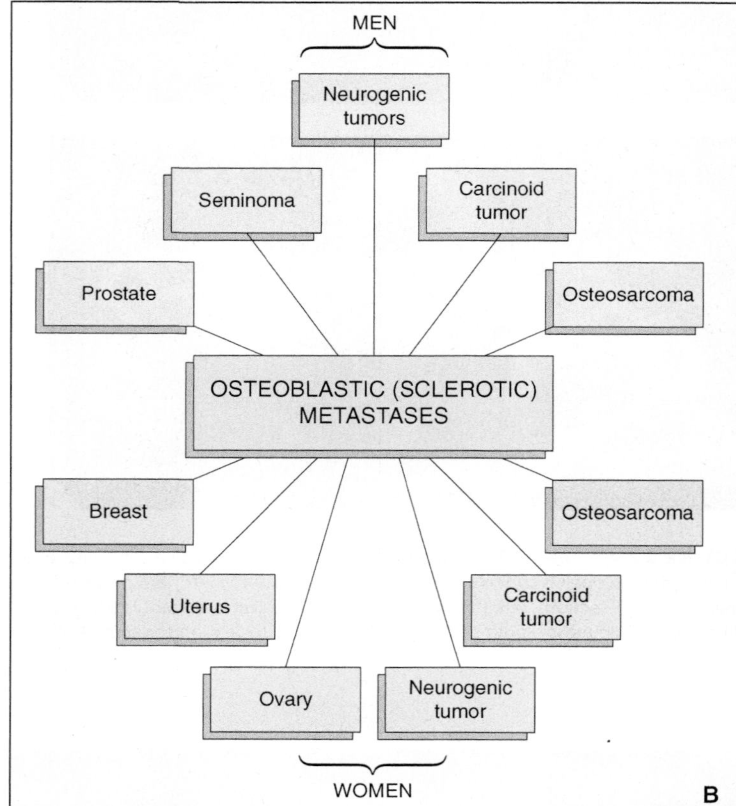

▲ **FIGURE 22.66 Skeletal metastases.** Origin of **(A)** osteolytic and **(B)** osteoblastic metastases. (Reprinted with permission from Greenspan A, Remagen W. *Differential diagnosis of tumors and tumor-like lesions of bones and joints*. Philadelphia: Lippincott-Raven; 1998:369–371.)

Most skeletal metastases are asymptomatic. When metastases are symptomatic, pain is the major clinical symptom, with a pathologic fracture through a lesion only occasionally calling attention to the disease. Metastasis to bone can be solitary or multiple and can be further divided into purely lytic, purely blastic, and mixed lesions. The primary tumors that give rise to purely osteolytic metastases are usually those of the kidney, lung, breast, thyroid, and gastrointestinal tract, although purely lytic lesions may become sclerotic after radiation therapy, chemotherapy, or hormonal therapy. Primary tumors responsible for purely osteoblastic metastases are generally those of the prostate gland, although other primary neoplasms may also be responsible (Fig. 22.66).

Imaging Features

The detection of skeletal metastases is not always possible on conventional radiographs because destruction of the bone may not be visible with this technique. Radionuclide bone scan is the best means of screening for early metastatic lesions whether they are lytic or blastic, although several investigators have pointed out the usefulness of MRI in detecting metastases, particularly in the spine (Fig. 22.67). The accuracy of MRI in identifying intramedullary lesions and assessing spinal cord and soft-tissue involvement has been demonstrated. Daldrup-Link and associates compared the diagnostic accuracy of whole-body MRI, skeletal scintigraphy, and FDG PET for the detection of bone metastases in children and young adults, suggest the superiority of FDG PET scan (Figs. 22.68 and 22.69; see also Figs. 2.36 and 2.38). The latter technique had 90% sensitivity compared with 82% for whole-body MRI and 71% for skeletal scintigraphy. CT scanning is effective in demonstrating the extent of bone destruction (Figs. 22.70 and 22.71).

In general terms, skeletal metastases may appear highly similar, irrespective of their primary source (Figs. 22.72 and 22.73). However, there are instances in which the morphologic appearance, location, and distribution of metastatic lesions may suggest their site of origin. Thus, for instance, 50% of skeletal metastases distal to the elbows and knees—rare

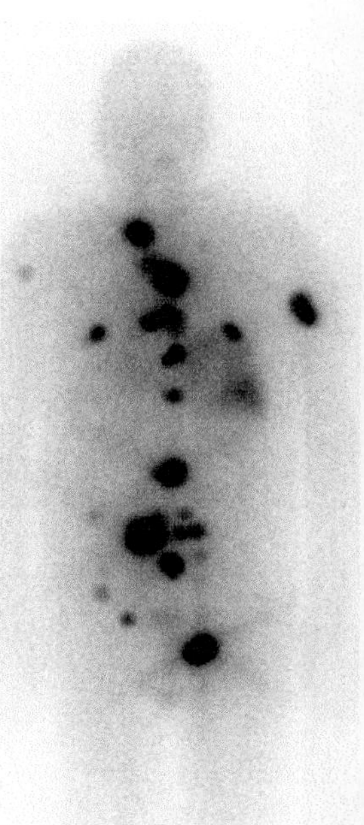

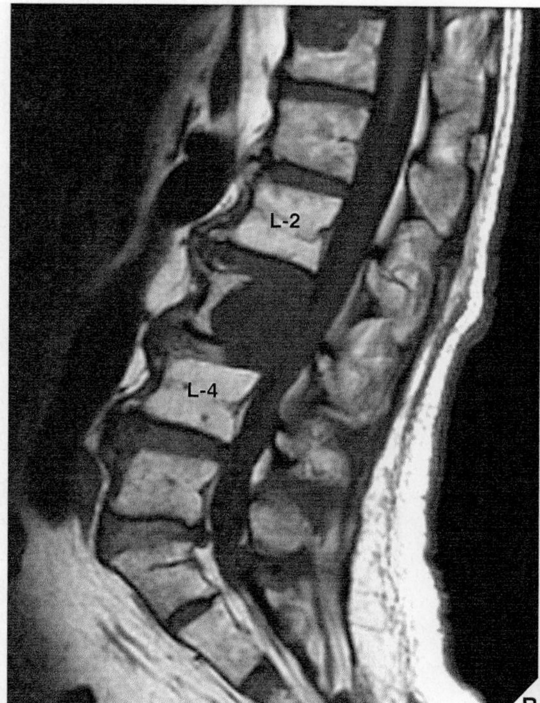

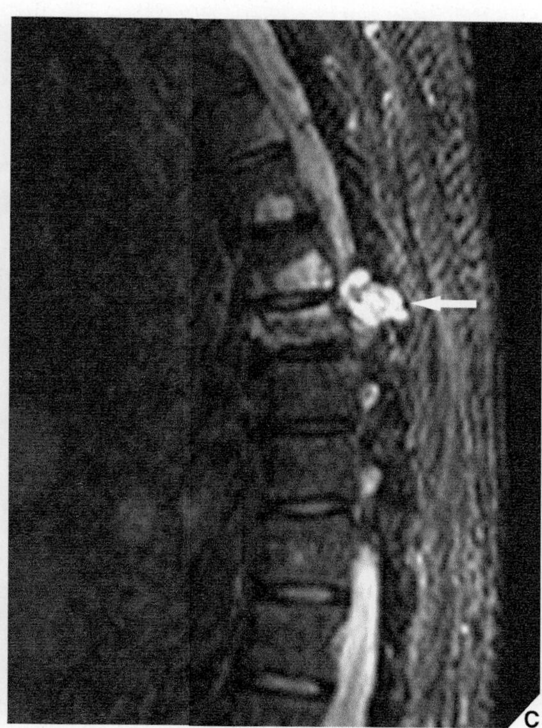

A

FIGURE 22.67 **Scintigraphy and MRI of metastases.** A 70-year-old man with known follicular thyroid carcinoma presented with severe back pain. **(A)** Total-body radionuclide bone scan performed after oral administration of 155 mCi iodine-131 (^{131}I) sodium iodide shows multiple skeletal metastases. **(B)** Sagittal T1-weighted MR image demonstrates the involvement of T12 and L3 vertebral bodies. **(C)** Sagittal short time inversion recovery (STIR) MR image shows extension of metastatic tumor affecting T12 vertebra into the spinal canal. Observe involvement of the spinal cord *(arrow)*.

sites for metastases—are secondary to breast or bronchogenic carcinomas (Fig. 22.74). Lesions that have an expansive, "blown-out" appearance on radiographs and are highly vascular on arteriography are characteristic of metastatic renal carcinoma (Fig. 22.75). Moreover, Choi and associates recently reported a flow-void sign on MRI, resulting from relatively rapid blood flow through dilated arteries that supply the hypervascular lesion and through dilated veins that drain the lesion, apparently characteristic for osseous metastases from renal cell carcinoma. Multiple round dense foci or diffuse bone density is often seen in metastatic carcinoma of the prostate (Figs. 22.76 and 22.77); in females, sclerotic metastases are usually from breast carcinoma.

Some time ago, characteristic cortical metastases have been described as originating from bronchogenic carcinoma; these metastases have been called by Resnick *cookie bite* or *cookie cutter* lesions of the cortices of the long bones (Figs. 22.78 and 22.79). Because the bulk of metastases that reach the skeleton via hematogenous spread lodge in the bone marrow and in spongy bone, the initial radiographic appearance of metastatic lesions in the skeleton is that of destruction of cancellous bone; only with further growth do such lesions affect the cortex. The anastomosing vascular systems of the cortex, originating in the overlying periosteum, probably serve as the pathway by which malignant cells from the lung reach the compact bone to produce destruction of the cortex. Occasionally, other primary tumors (e.g., breast and kidney) may also metastasize to the cortex.

Single metastatic lesions in a bone must be distinguished from primary malignant and benign bone tumors (Fig. 22.80). A few characteristic features of metastatic lesions may be helpful in making the distinction: (a) Metastatic lesions usually present without or with only a small adjacent soft-tissue mass and (b) they usually lack a periosteal reaction unless they have broken through the cortex. The latter feature, however, is not invariably reliable because in some series more than 30% of metastatic lesions—particularly metastases from carcinoma of the prostate—have been accompanied by a periosteal response. Metastatic lesions to the spine usually destroy the pedicle, a useful feature for distinguishing them from myeloma or neurofibroma invading the vertebra (Fig. 22.81; see also Fig. 22.43).

Pathology

Histologically, metastatic tumors are easier to diagnose than many primary tumors because of their essential epithelial pattern. Although biopsies of suspected metastases are useful for diagnosis in patients with unknown primary tumors, these procedures are seldom helpful in specifying an exact site of an unknown primary tumor. Occasionally, if gland formation is present, a specific diagnosis of metastatic adenocarcinoma can be made but rarely will a specific type of the tumor be detected. On occasion, a metastatic lesion may demonstrate a morphologic pattern that strongly suggests the site of a primary tumor, such as the clear cells of renal carcinoma or the pigment production of melanoma. The other studies may demonstrate nuclear transposition factors such as homeobox gene CDX2 (occurring in gastrointestinal cancers) or thyroid transcription termination factor I (TTFI, occurring in lung and thyroid cancers), or to analyze the pattern of CK filaments (e.g., presence of CK20 and absence of CK7 in gastrointestinal but not in lung cancers), supplemented by additional immunoreactions of CKs, classification determinant (CD) endothelial markers CD20, CD99, and NSE for the differentiation of small round blue cell tumors, all leading to identification of unknown primary tumor.

Complications

Although metastases are themselves complications of a primary malignant process, it must be emphasized that they can cause secondary complications such as pathologic fracture (Fig. 22.82) or, when occurring in the spine, compression of the thecal sac and spinal cord, thus producing neurologic symptoms (Fig. 22.83; see also Fig. 22.67).

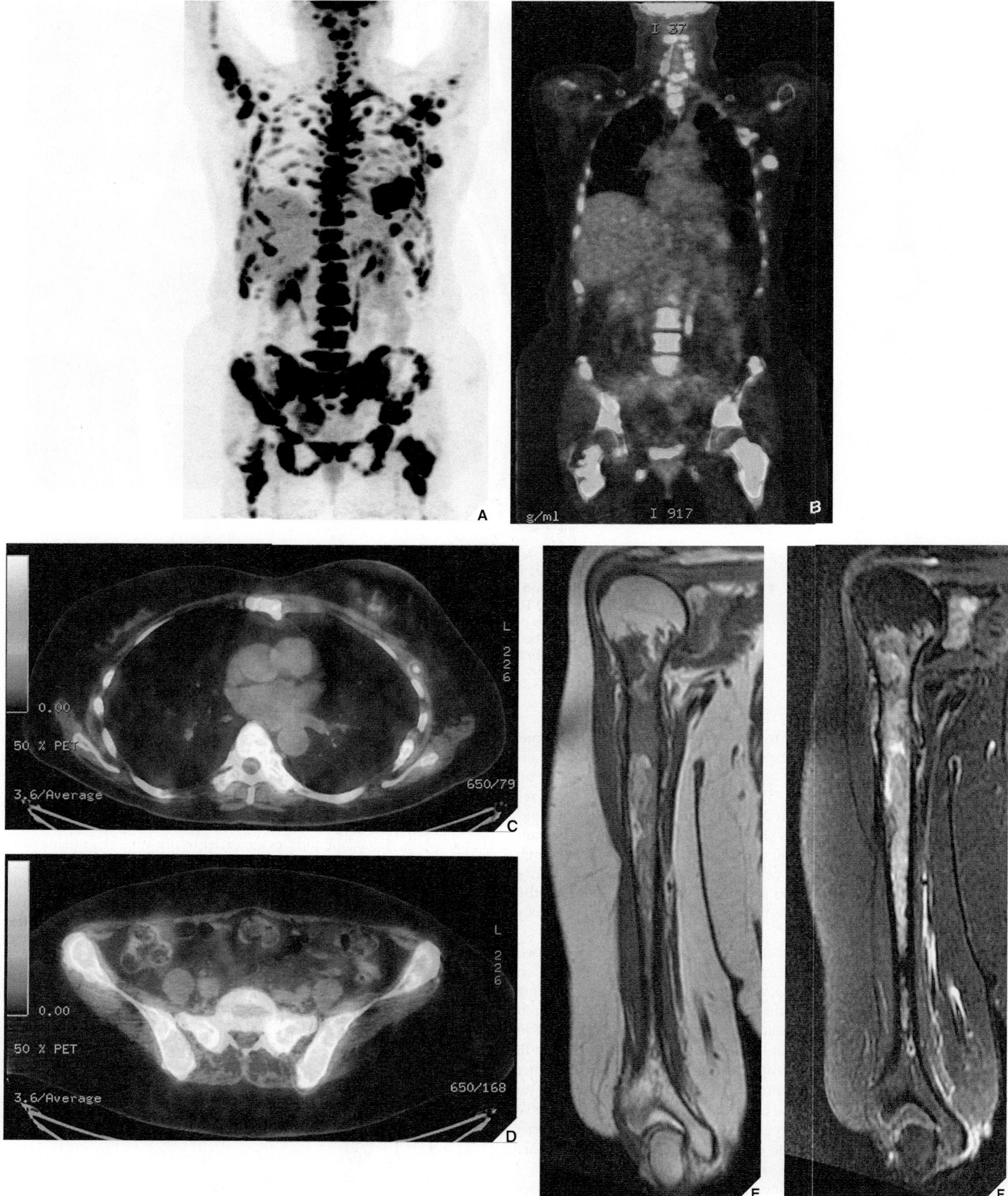

FIGURE 22.68 FDG PET, FDG PET/CT, and MRI of metastases. **(A)** Whole-body FDG PET scan and **(B)** coronal reformatted postcontrast PET/CT of 57-year-old woman with advanced adenocarcinoma of the breast shows numerous hypermetabolic foci in the bones, lymph nodes, and internal organs, representing diffuse metastatic disease. Axial fused PET/CT images obtained at the levels of the chest **(C)** and lower abdomen **(D)** demonstrate hypermetabolic metastases in the vertebrae, ribs, iliac bones, and sacrum. **(E)** Coronal T1-weighted and **(F)** coronal short time inversion recovery (STIR) MR images show diffuse involvement of the bone marrow of the right humerus. (Reprinted with permission from Greenspan A, Borys D. *Radiology and pathology correlation of bone tumors*. Philadelphia: Wolters Kluwer; 2016:391, Fig. 9.1B.)

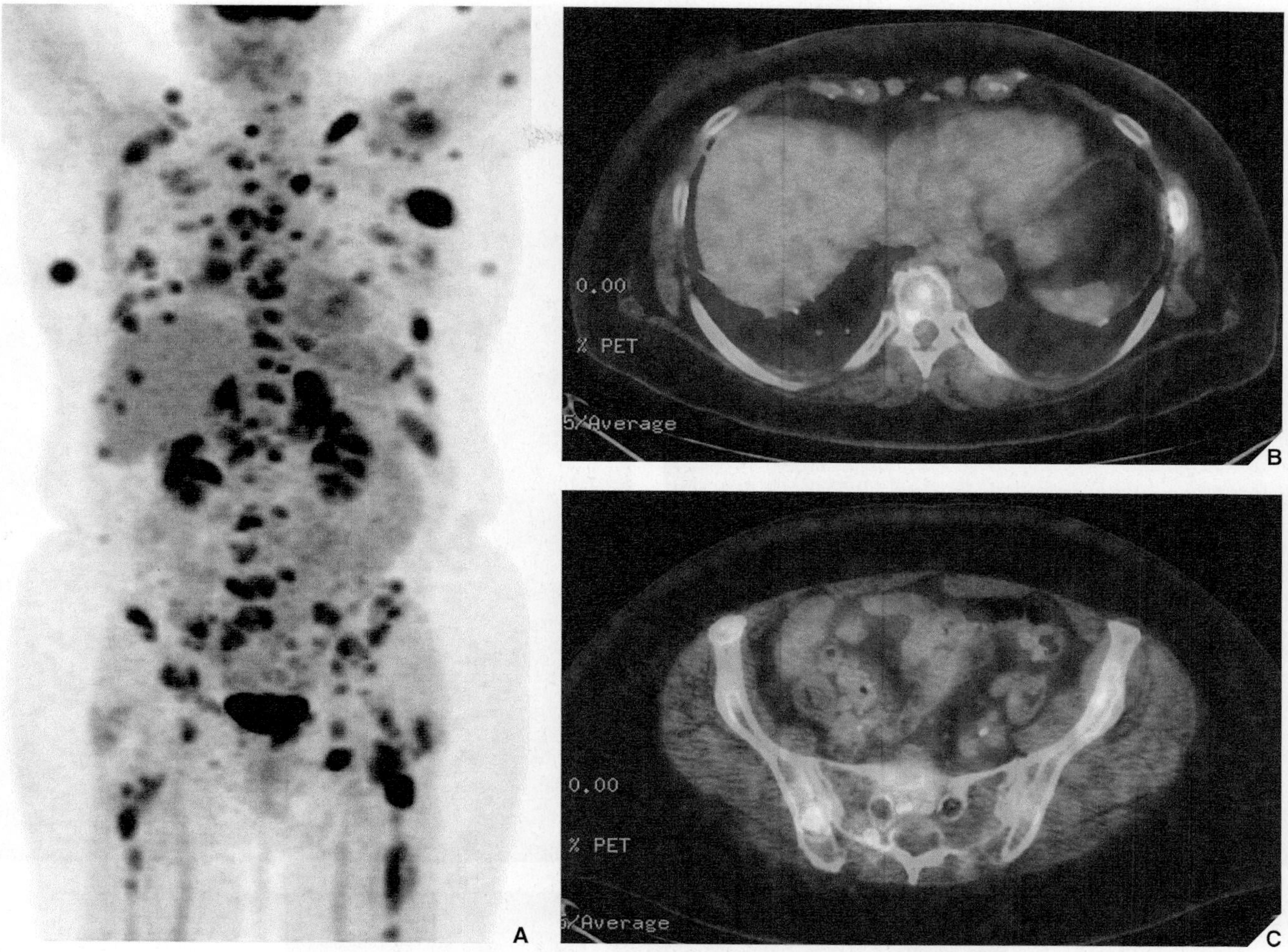

FIGURE 22.69 FDG PET and FDG PET/CT of metastases. **(A)** Whole-body FDG PET scan of a 60-year-old woman with adenocarcinoma of the breast shows several hypermetabolic foci within the osseous structures consistent with metastatic process. Axial fused PET/CT images obtained at the levels of the chest **(B)** and pelvis **(C)** demonstrate hypermetabolic lesions in the vertebra, ribs, sternum, pelvic bones, and sacrum.

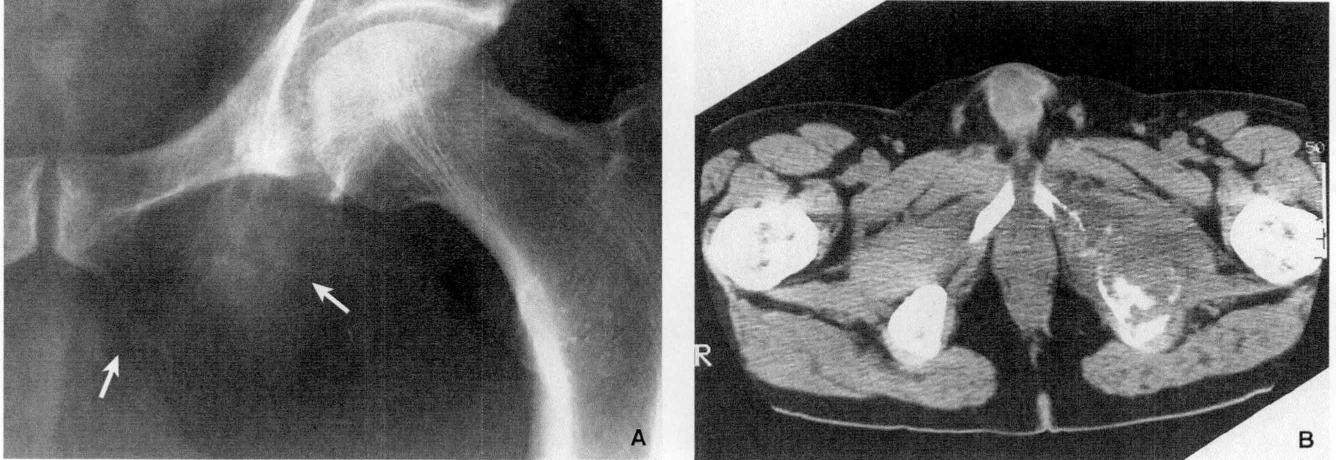

FIGURE 22.70 CT of osteolytic metastasis. **(A)** Anteroposterior radiograph of the left hip of a 50-year-old man diagnosed with renal cell carcinoma shows an osteolytic lesion almost completely destroying the ischium *(arrows)*. **(B)** Axial CT section demonstrates the extent of bone destruction and a soft-tissue extension. (Reprinted with permission from Greenspan A, Borys D. *Radiology and pathology correlation of bone tumors: a quick reference and review*. Philadelphia: Wolters Kluwer; 2016:384, Fig. 9.6.)

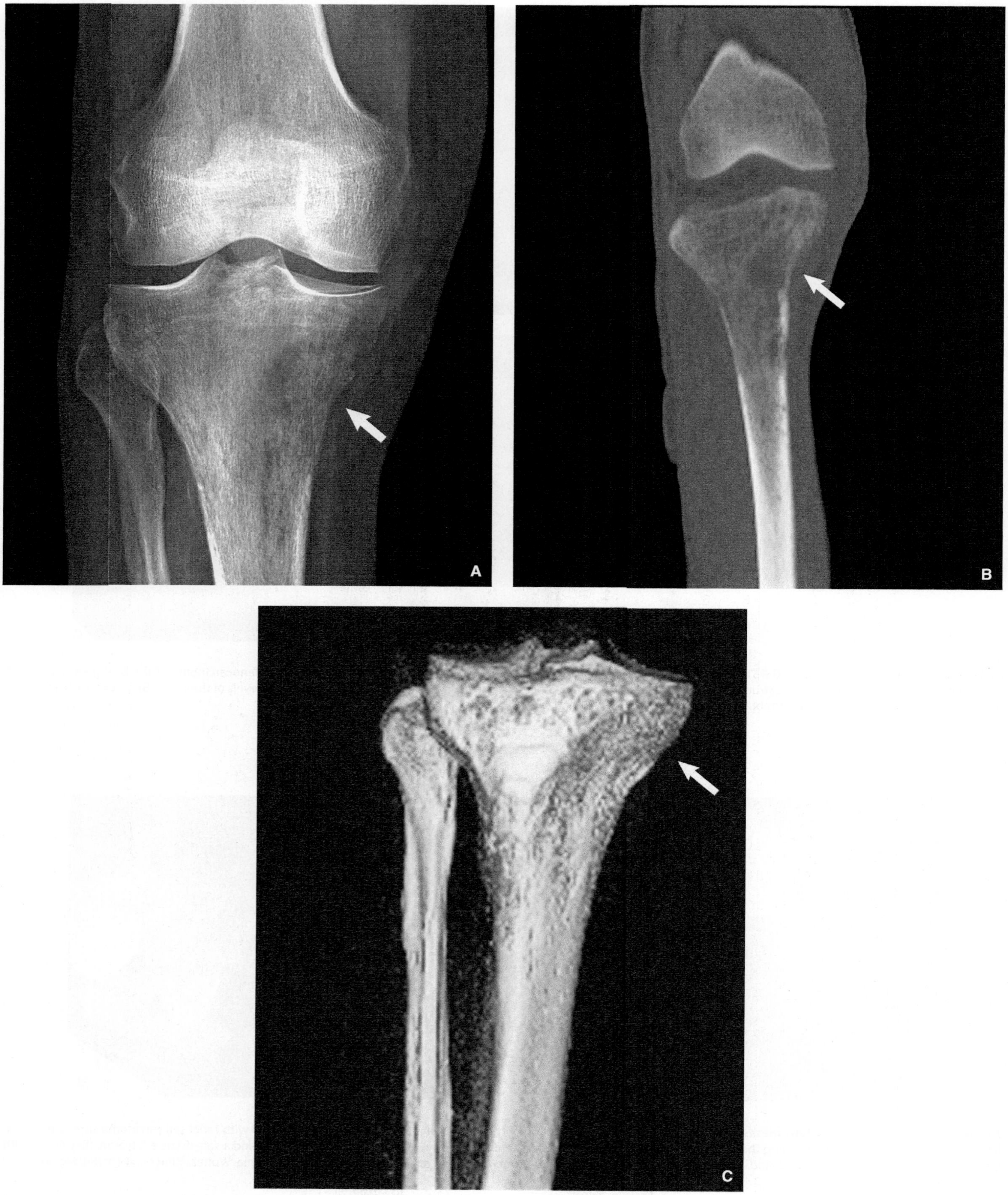

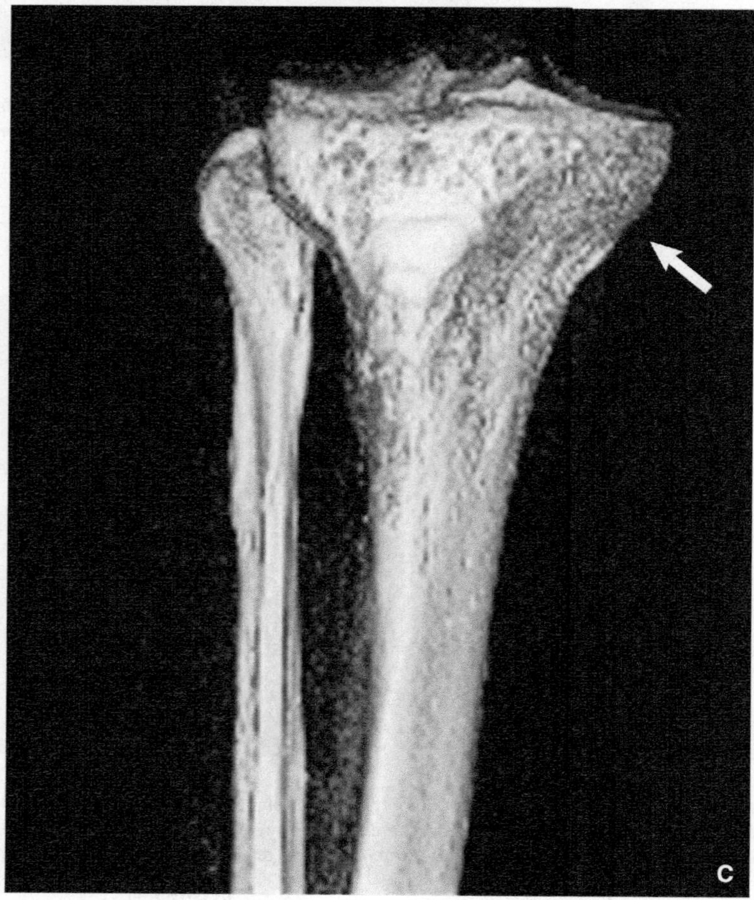

FIGURE 22.71 CT and three-dimensional (3D) CT of osteolytic metastasis. **(A)** Anteroposterior radiograph of the right knee of an 80-year-old man diagnosed with colon carcinoma shows a lytic lesion in the proximal tibia exhibiting a wide zone of transition *(arrow)*. **(B)** Coronal reformatted CT section and **(C)** 3D CT reconstruction image show full extent of bone destruction *(arrows)*.

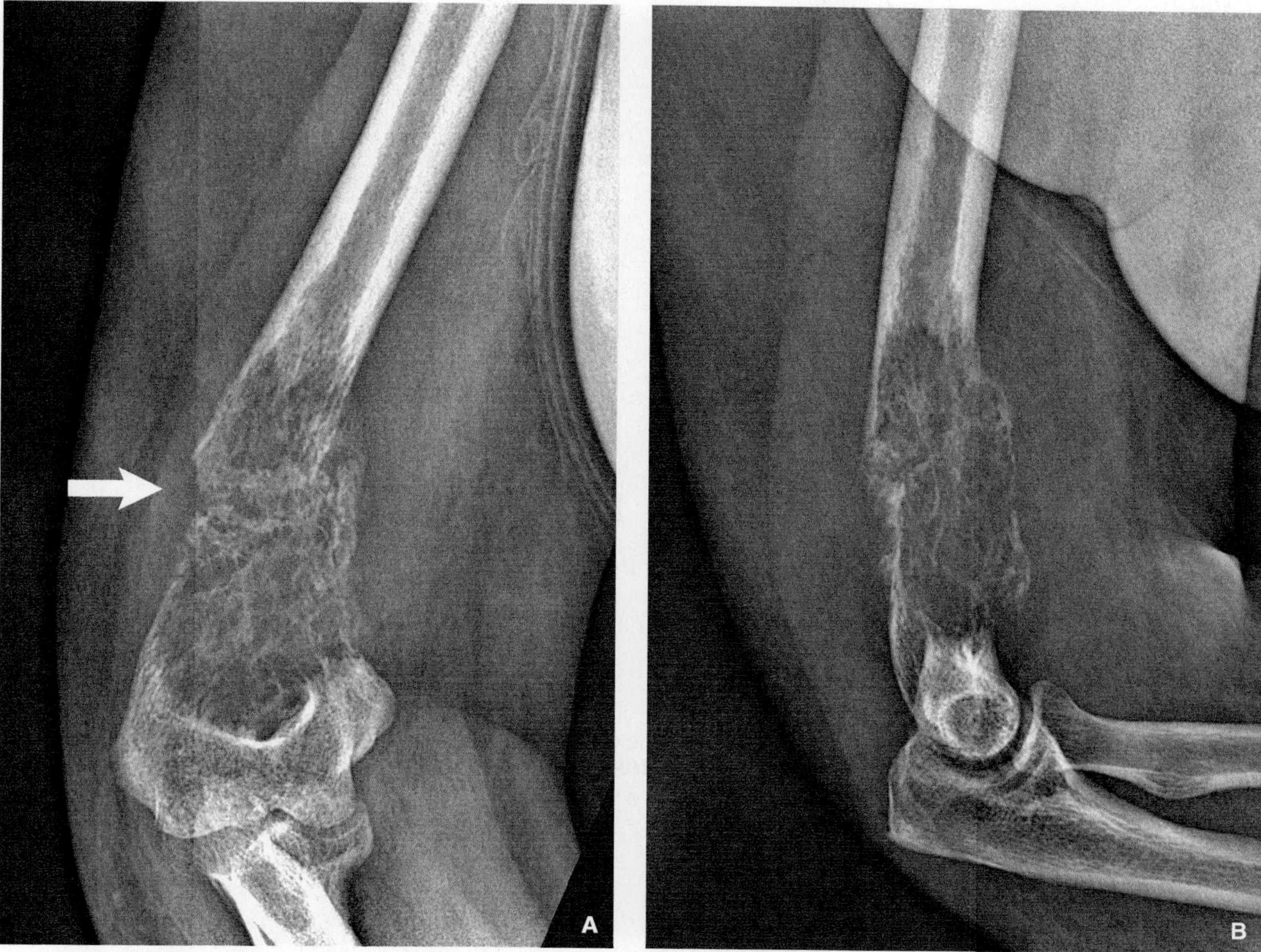

FIGURE 22.72 **Osteolytic metastasis.** **(A)** Anteroposterior and **(B)** lateral radiographs of the right elbow of a 44-year-old woman with soft-tissue leiomyosarcoma of the buttock show lytic metastasis to the distal humerus. Note associated pathologic fracture *(arrow)*.

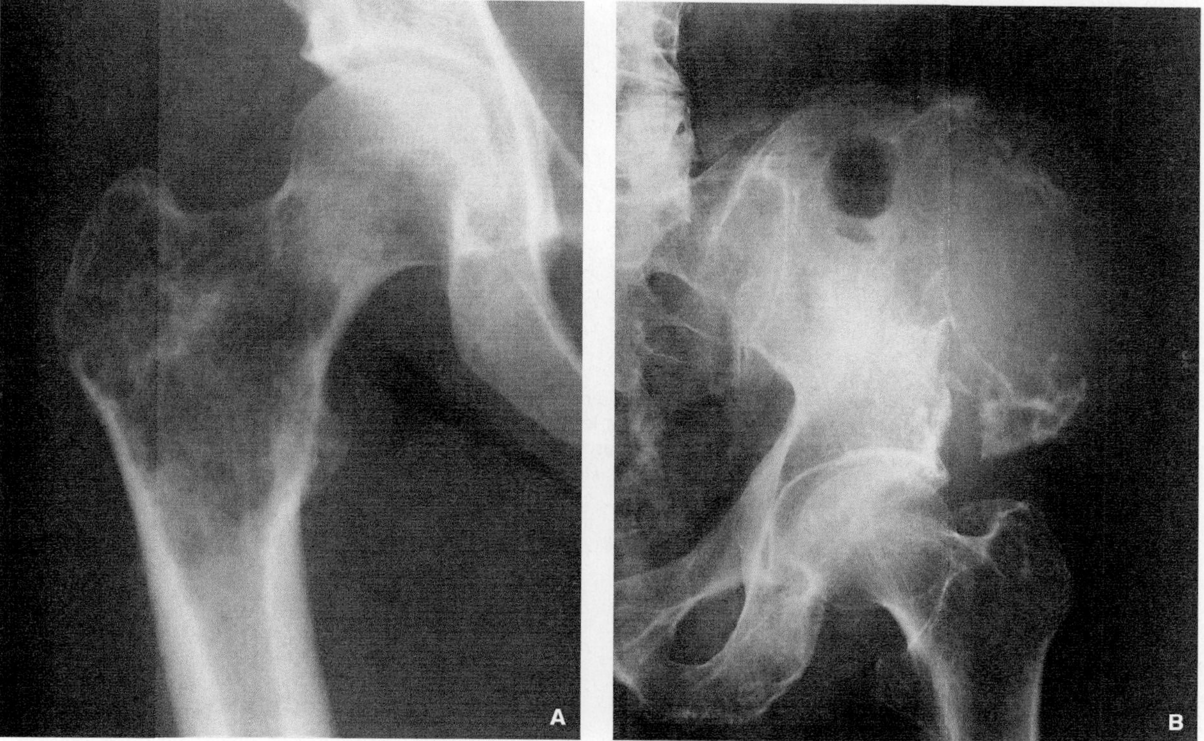

FIGURE 22.73 **Osteolytic metastasis.** **(A)** Anteroposterior radiograph of the right hip of a 52-year-old woman shows a large lytic lesion in the intertrochanteric region of the femur, proved to be a metastasis from carcinoma of the colon. **(B)** Anteroposterior radiograph of the left hemipelvis of an 83-year-old man shows an osteolytic lesion in the ilium, proved to be a metastasis from the thyroid carcinoma. (Reprinted with permission from Greenspan A, Borys D. *Radiology and pathology correlation of bone tumors: a quick reference and review*. Philadelphia: Wolters Kluwer; 2016:383, Fig. 9.4.)

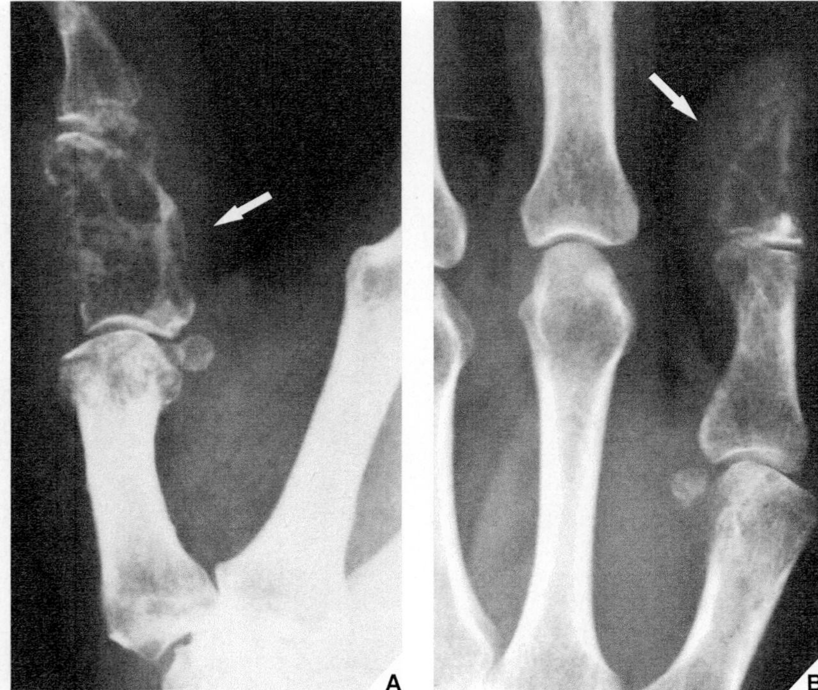

FIGURE 22.74 **Skeletal metastases.** **(A)** A 63-year-old man with bronchogenic carcinoma developed a single metastatic lesion in the proximal phalanx of the left thumb *(arrow)*. **(B)** A 50-year-old woman with breast carcinoma had a solitary metastatic lesion in the distal phalanx of the right thumb *(arrow)*.

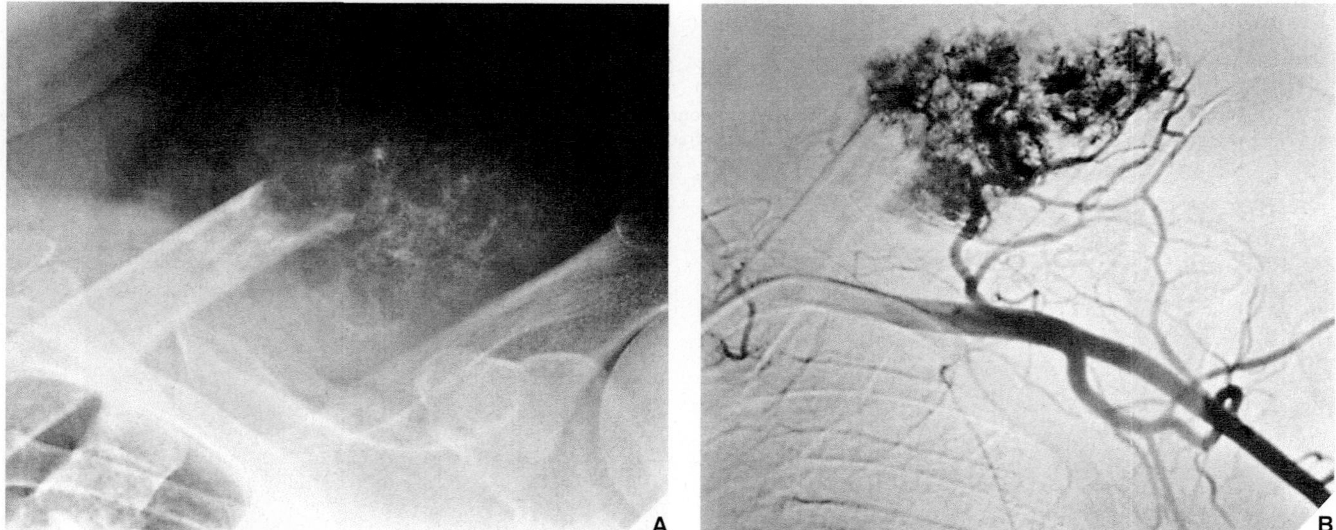

FIGURE 22.75 **Angiography of metastatic lesion.** A 52-year-old man with renal cell carcinoma (hypernephroma) presented with a solitary metastatic lesion in the acromial end of the left clavicle. **(A)** Radiograph shows an expansive blown-out lesion associated with a soft-tissue mass destroying the acromial end of the clavicle. **(B)** Subtraction study of a selective left subclavian arteriogram demonstrates hypervascularity of the tumor, a characteristic feature of metastatic hypernephroma.

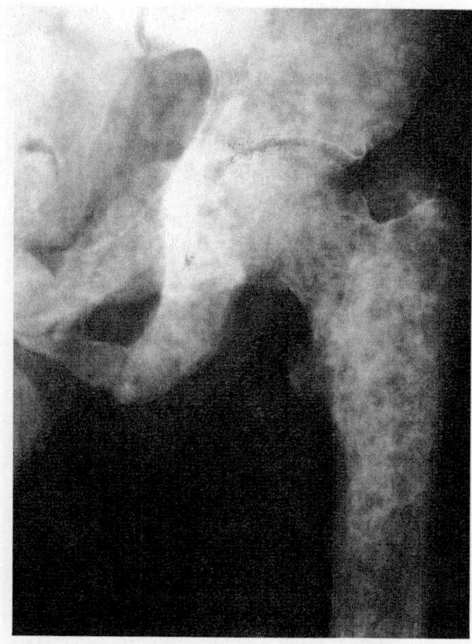

FIGURE 22.76 **Osteoblastic metastases.** Anteroposterior radiograph of the left hemipelvis and proximal femur of a 55-year-old man with carcinoma of the prostate shows extensive blastic skeletal metastases. Multiple sclerotic foci are scattered through the ilium, pubis, ischium, and femur.

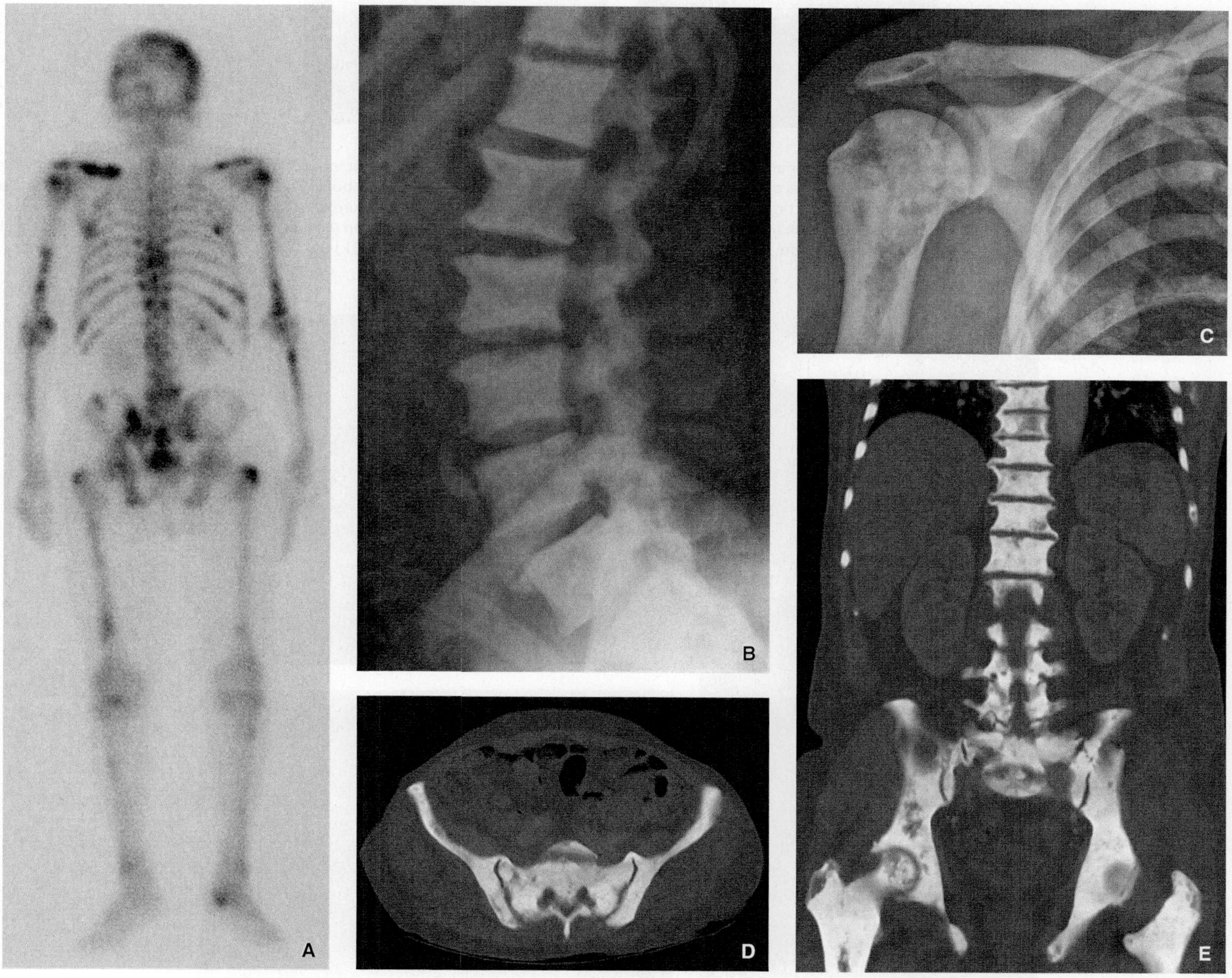

FIGURE 22.77 **Scintigraphy and CT of osteoblastic metastases.** **(A)** A whole-body radionuclide bone scan of a 68-year-old man diagnosed with prostate carcinoma shows widespread metastatic disease. **(B)** Lateral radiograph of the lumbar spine demonstrates sclerotic changes in all vertebrae. **(C)** Anteroposterior radiograph of the right shoulder shows sclerotic metastases in the proximal humerus, scapula, clavicle, and ribs. **(D)** Axial CT section and **(E)** coronal reformatted CT images of the pelvis and spine show extensive involvement of all visualized osseous structures.

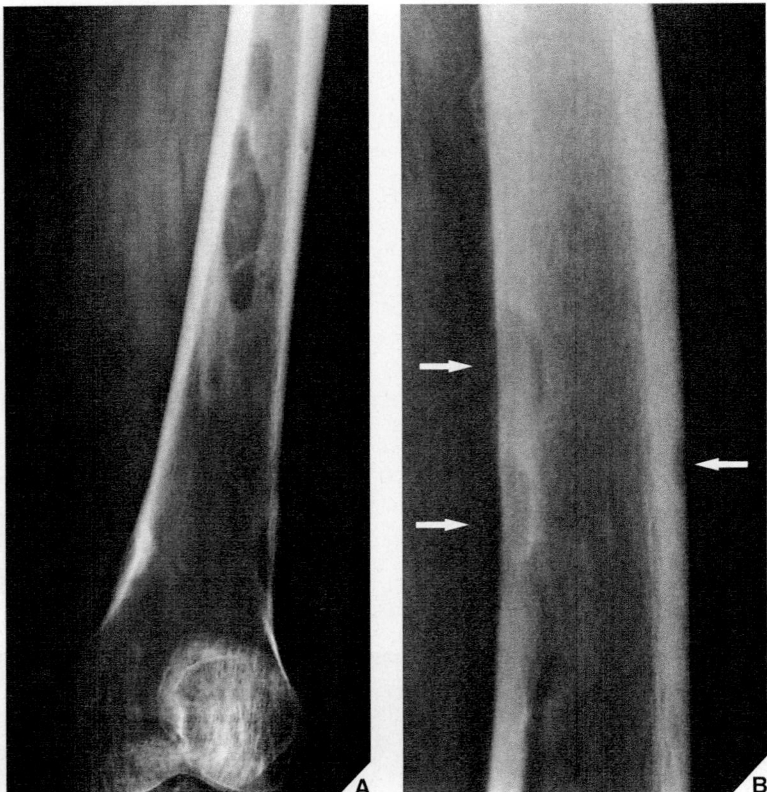

FIGURE 22.78 Cortical metastases. **(A)** Anteroposterior and **(B)** lateral magnification radiographs of the left femur in an 82-year-old man with progressive femoral pain demonstrate multiple sharply marginated osteolytic areas of bone destruction, predominantly affecting the cortical bone. There is no evidence of periosteal reaction. Note the characteristic "cookie-bite" appearance of the lesion on the lateral radiograph *(arrows)*. On the basis of this feature, attention was focused on the chest, where CT examination (not shown here) demonstrated bronchogenic carcinoma. (Reprinted by permission from Springer: Greenspan A, Klein MJ, Lewis MM. Case Report 272. Skeletal [predominately] cortical metastases in the left femur arising from bronchogenic carcinoma. *Skeletal Radiol* 1984;11:297–301.)

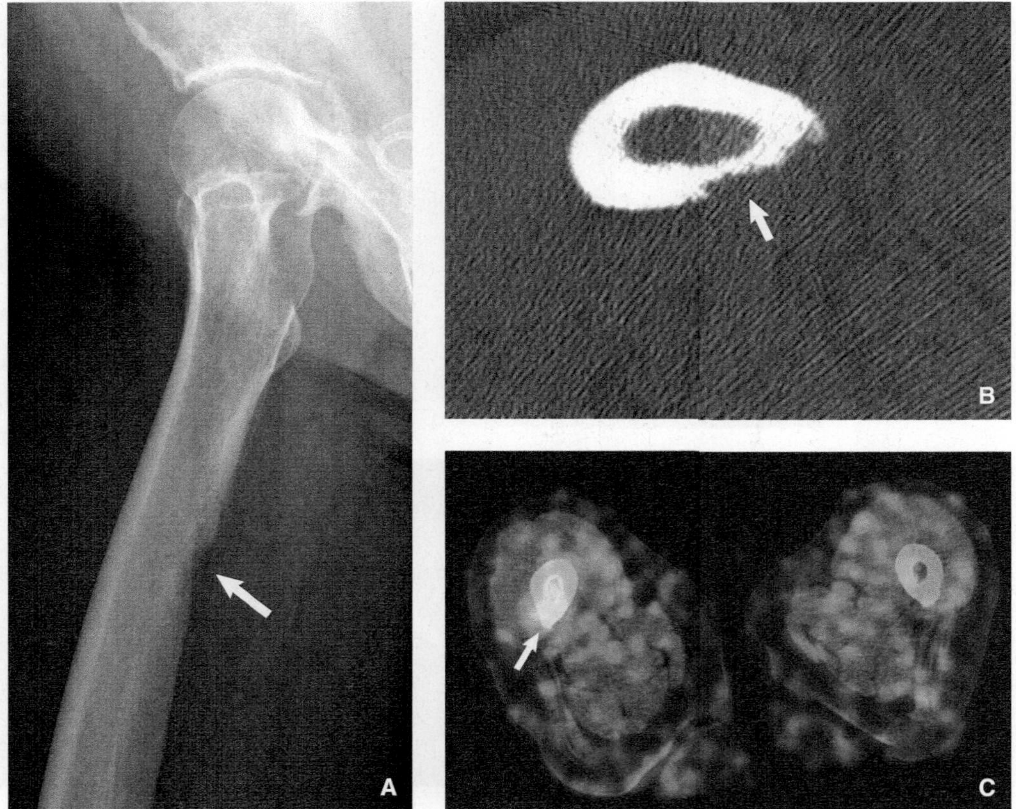

FIGURE 22.79 CT and FDG PET/CT of cortical metastasis. **(A)** Oblique radiograph of the proximal right femur of a 69-year-old woman diagnosed with bronchogenic carcinoma shows focal osteolytic destruction of the posteromedial cortex *(arrow)*. **(B)** Axial CT section shows "cookie-bite" type of a lesion *(arrow)*. **(C)** Fused FDG PET/CT image shows hypermetabolic focus within the femoral cortex *(arrow)*.

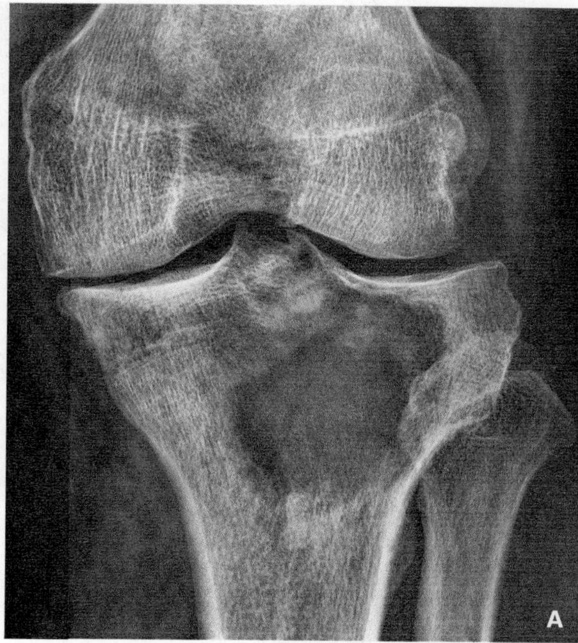

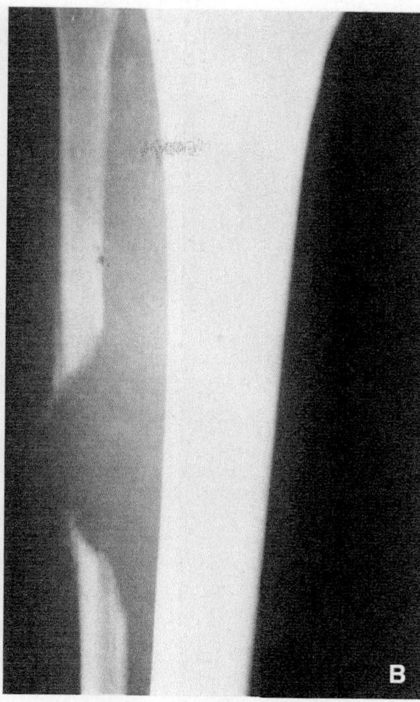

FIGURE 22.80 Osteolytic metastasis. **(A)** A 45-year-old man presented with a solitary osteolytic lesion in the left proximal tibia, originally misinterpreted as a giant cell tumor. An extensive clinical workup and excision biopsy lead to the diagnosis of metastasis from renal cell carcinoma. **(B)** Anteroposterior radiograph of the right leg of a 41-year-old woman shows a lytic lesion in the fibula, breaking through the cortex and extending into the soft tissues. At first, a diagnosis of a primary malignant bone tumor such as fibrosarcoma, MFH, or lymphoma was considered, but the clinical workup and excision biopsy established the diagnosis of metastasis from renal cell carcinoma. (**B**, Reprinted with permission from Greenspan A, Borys D. *Radiology and pathology correlation of bone tumors,* 1st ed. Philadelphia: Wolters Kluwer, 2016:384.)

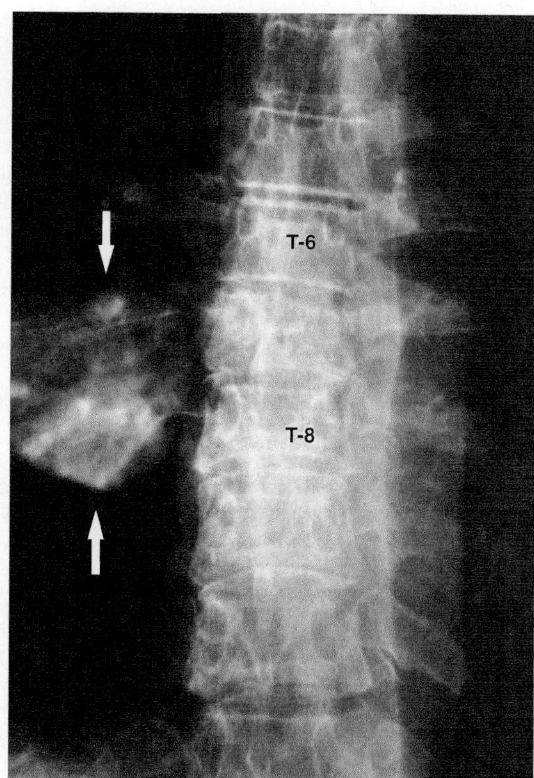

FIGURE 22.81 Vertebral metastasis. Anteroposterior radiograph of the thoracolumbar spine in a 59-year-old woman with bronchogenic carcinoma shows a metastatic lesion in the body of T7. Note the destroyed left pedicle and associated paraspinal mass, the features helpful in distinguishing this lesion from myeloma or neurofibroma. The lung tumor is obvious *(arrows).*

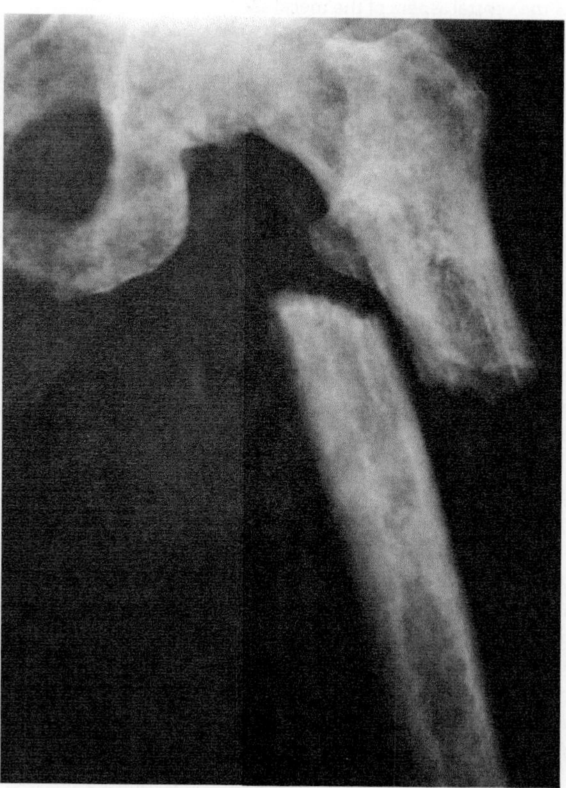

FIGURE 22.82 Skeletal metastases complicated by pathologic fracture. Pathologic fracture may complicate metastatic disease of the skeleton, as seen here in the proximal shaft of the left femur in a 74-year-old man with multiple skeletal metastases from a prostate carcinoma.

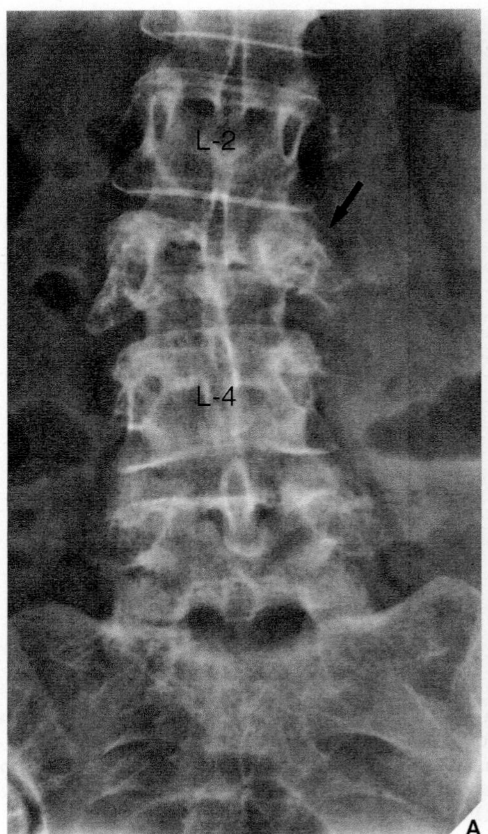

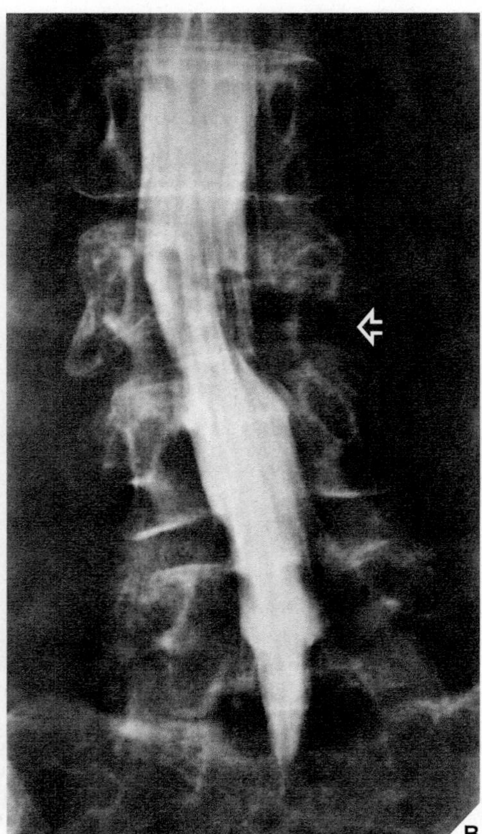

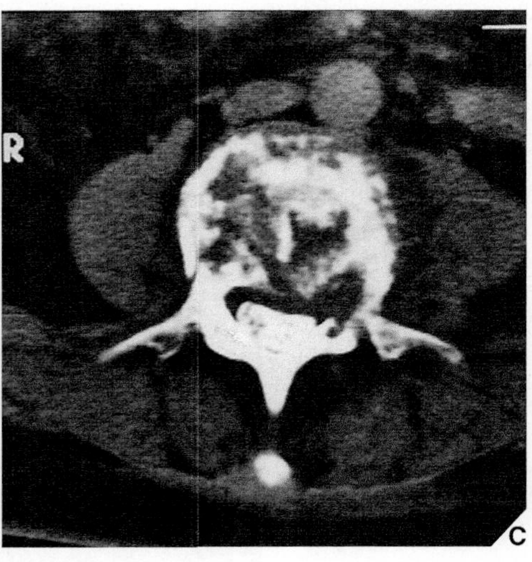

FIGURE 22.83 Neurologic complication of skeletal metastasis. **(A)** Anteroposterior radiograph of the lumbar spine in a 47-year-old woman with breast carcinoma shows destruction of the body of L3 with a pathologic fracture. Note the involvement of the left pedicle *(arrow)*. **(B)** A myelogram demonstrates compression of the thecal sac *(open arrow)*. **(C)** On CT section, compression fracture of the vertebral body and involvement of the left pedicle are evident; the tumor extends into the soft tissue and compresses the ventral aspect of the thecal sac.

PRACTICAL POINTS TO REMEMBER

1. Fibrosarcoma and MFH:
   - characteristically present as purely osteolytic lesions, frequently in the long bones
   - may resemble giant cell tumor, lymphoma, or telangiectatic osteosarcoma
   - may develop in certain benign conditions, such as fibrous dysplasia and bone infarct.
2. Ewing sarcoma, a round cell tumor, usually presents with characteristic radiographic features including:
   - a permeative type of bone destruction
   - cortical saucerization
   - an aggressive periosteal reaction, usually of onion-skin type
   - a soft-tissue mass.

   The diaphysis of long bones and the pelvis, ribs, and scapula are the most common sites of involvement.
3. In the differential diagnosis of Ewing sarcoma, osteomyelitis and Langerhans cell histiocytosis should always be considered, as well as metastatic neuroblastoma, particularly in patients in their first decade. The most important distinguishing feature is the duration of symptoms. The amount of bone destruction seen radiographically in patients with Ewing sarcoma reporting symptoms for 4 to 6 months is usually the same as that:
   - in patients with osteomyelitis reporting symptoms for 4 to 6 weeks
   - in patients with Langerhans cell histiocytosis reporting symptoms for 1 to 2 weeks.
4. Myeloma, the most common primary malignant bone tumor, has a predilection for the axial skeleton. Four distinctive forms of this lesion can be distinguished radiographically:
   - a solitary lesion (plasmacytoma), usually affecting the pelvis or ribs
   - diffuse myelomatosis
   - diffuse osteoporosis, usually seen in the vertebral column
   - sclerosing myeloma, the rarest manifestation of this tumor.
5. Primary myeloma of the spine can usually be distinguished from radiographically similar metastatic disease by the preservation of the pedicles (vertebral pedicle sign) in the early stages of the disease.
6. In myeloma, radionuclide bone scan usually shows no increase in uptake of radiopharmaceutical.
7. On MRI of solitary plasmacytoma affecting spine, so-called *mini brain sign* is characteristic.
8. Adamantinoma, a malignant tumor with a strong predilection for the tibia, is characterized radiographically by:
   - a soap bubble appearance of the lesion combining lytic and sclerotic areas
   - a sawtooth appearance of cortical destruction.
9. Chordoma, which arises from the remnants of the notochord, is located almost exclusively in the midline of the axial skeleton. It tends to arise in the sphenooccipital and sacrococcygeal areas and in the body of C2.
10. Primary leiomyosarcoma of bone, a rare bone malignancy, exhibits no characteristic radiographic features, although most often presents either as a lytic area of geographic bone destruction or with aggressive-looking, ill-defined borders and permeative or moth-eaten pattern.
11. Hemangioendothelioma of bone may be solitary or multicentric. The radiographic features include an osteolytic appearance, either well circumscribed or with a wide zone of transition, and occasionally a soap bubble character with extension into the soft tissues.
12. Angiosarcoma of bone represents the most malignant end of the spectrum of vascular tumors. The radiographic features include a wide zone of transition, cortical permeation, and soft-tissue mass.
13. Benign conditions with malignant potential include medullary bone infarct, the chronic draining sinus tract of osteomyelitis, plexiform

neurofibromatosis, Paget disease, normal tissue undergoing radiation, enchondroma, osteochondroma, synovial chondromatosis, and fibrous dysplasia.

14. Prostate carcinoma is the primary tumor most often responsible for blastic metastases to bone. The primary tumors most often responsible for osteolytic skeletal metastases are carcinomas of the kidney, lung, breast, thyroid, and gastrointestinal tract.
15. Bronchogenic carcinoma frequently produces cortical metastases ("cookie bite" lesions) and is responsible for metastases in sites distal to the elbow, including lesions of the phalanges.
16. Carcinoma of the kidney usually produces lytic, blown-out, hypervascular metastatic lesions.
17. The best technique for mapping metastatic lesions in the skeleton is radionuclide bone scan and FDG PET scan.

SUGGESTED READINGS

Abdelwahab IF, Hermann G, Kenan S, et al. Case Report 794. Primary leiomyosarcoma of the right femur (fig. 4). *Skeletal Radiol* 1993;22:379–381.

Abdelwahab IF, Kenan S, Hermann G, et al. Radiation-induced leiomyosarcoma. *Skeletal Radiol* 1995;24:81–83.

Abrahams TG, Bula W, Jones W. Epithelioid hemangioendothelioma of bone. A report of two cases and review of the literature. *Skeletal Radiol* 1992;21:509–513.

Adams HJA, Kwee TC, Vermoolen MA, et al. Whole-body MRI for the detection of bone marrow involvement in lymphoma: prospective study in 116 patients and comparison with FDG-PET. *Eur Radiol* 2013;23:2271–2278.

Adler C-P. Case Report 587: adamantinoma of the tibia mimicking osteofibrous dysplasia. *Skeletal Radiol* 1990;19:55–58.

Aggarwal S, Goulatia RK, Sood A, et al. POEMS syndrome: a rare variety of plasma cell dyscrasia. *AJR Am J Roentgenol* 1990;155:339–341.

Algra PR, Bloem JL, Tissing H, et al. Detection of vertebral metastases: comparison between MR imaging and bone scintigraphy. *Radiographics* 1991;11:219–232.

Algra PR, Heimans JJ, Valk J, et al. Do metastases in vertebrae begin in the body or the pedicles? Imaging study in 45 patients. *AJR Am J Roentgenol* 1992;158:1275–1279.

Aymoré IL, Meohas W, Brito de Almeida L, et al. Case report: periosteal Ewing's sarcoma: case report and literature review. *Clin Orthop Relat Res* 2005;434:265–272.

Bachman AS, Sproul EE. Correlation of radiographic and autopsy findings in suspected metastases in the spine. *Bull NY Acad Med* 1940;44:169–175.

Baker ND, Greenspan A. Case Report 172: pleomorphic liposarcoma, grade IV, of the soft tissue, arising in generalized plexiform neurofibromatosis. *Skeletal Radiol* 1981;7:150–153.

Baraga JJ, Amrami KK, Swee RG, et al. Radiographic features of Ewing's sarcoma of the bones of the hands and feet. *Skeletal Radiol* 2001;30:121–126.

Bardwick PA, Zvaifler NJ, Gill GN, et al. Plasma cell dyscrasia with polyneuropathy, organomegaly, endocrinopathy, M protein, and skin changes: the POEMS syndrome. Report on two cases and review of the literature. *Medicine (Baltimore)* 1980;59:311–322.

Berlin O, Angervall L, Kindblom LG, et al. Primary leiomyosarcoma of bone. A clinical, radiographic, pathologic-anatomic, and prognostic study of 16 cases. *Skeletal Radiol* 1987;16:364–376.

Bertoni F, Bacchini P, Ferruzzi A. Small round-cell malignancies of bone: Ewing's sarcoma, malignant lymphoma, and myeloma. *Semin Orthop* 1991;6:186–195.

Bessler W, Antonucci F, Stamm B, et al. Case Report 646. POEMS syndrome. *Skeletal Radiol* 1991;20:212–215.

Boutin RD, Speath HJ, Mangalic A, Sell JJ. Epithelioid hemangioendothelioma of bone. *Skeletal Radiol* 1996;25:391–395.

Brandon C, Martel W, Weatherbee L, et al. Case Report 572. Osteosclerotic myeloma (POEMS) syndrome. *Skeletal Radiol* 1989;18:542–546.

Breyer RJ III, Mulligan ME, Smith SE, et al. Comparison of imaging with FDG PET/CT with other imaging modalities in myeloma. *Skeletal Radiol* 2006;35:632–640.

Brown B, Laorr A, Greenspan A, et al. Negative bone scintigraphy with diffuse osteoblastic breast carcinoma metastases. *Clin Nucl Med* 1994;19:194–196.

Brown TS, Paterson CR. Osteosclerosis in myeloma. *J Bone Joint Surg Br* 1973;55:621–623.

Bullough PG. *Atlas of orthopedic pathology with clinical and radiologic correlations*, 2nd ed. New York: Gower Medical; 1992:17.1–17.29.

Bushnell DL, Kahn D, Huston B, et al. Utility of SPECT imaging for determination of vertebral metastases in patients with known primary tumors. *Skeletal Radiol* 1995;24:13–16.

Campanacci M. Osteofibrous dysplasia of long bones. A new clinical entity. *Ital J Orthop Traumatol* 1976;2:221–237.

Campanacci M, Laus M, Giunti A, et al. Adamantinoma of the long bones. The experience at the Istituto Ortopedico Rizzoli. *Am J Surg Pathol* 1981;5:533–542.

Choi J-A, Lee KH, Jun WS, et al. Osseous metastasis from renal cell carcinoma: "flow-void" sign at MR imaging. *Radiology* 2003;228:629–634.

Chong ST, Beasley HS, Daffner RH. POEMS syndrome: radiographic appearance with MRI correlation. *Skeletal Radiol* 2006;35:690–695.

Czerniak B, Rojas-Corona RR, Dorfman HD. Morphologic diversity of long bone adamantinoma. The concept of differentiated (regressing) adamantinoma and its relationship to osteofibrous dysplasia. *Cancer* 1989;64:2319–2334.

Dahlin DC. Grading of bone tumors. In: Unni KK, ed. *Bone tumors*. New York: Churchill Livingstone; 1988:35–45.

Dahlin DC, Unni KK, Matsuno T. Malignant (fibrous) histiocytoma of bone—fact or fancy? *Cancer* 1977;39:1508–1516.

Daldrup-Link HE, Franzius C, Link TM, et al. Whole-body MR imaging for detection of bone metastases in children and young adults: comparison with skeletal scintigraphy and FDG PET. *AJR Am J Roentgenol* 2001;177:229–236.

Dardick I, Schatz JE, Colgan TJ. Osteogenic sarcoma with epithelial differentiation. *Ultrastruct Pathol* 1992;16:463–474.

Deutsch A, Resnick D. Eccentric cortical metastases to the skeleton from bronchogenic carcinoma. *Radiology* 1980;137:49–52.

Deutsch A, Resnick D, Niwayama G. Case Report 145. Bilateral, almost symmetrical skeletal metastases (both femora) from bronchogenic carcinoma. *Skeletal Radiol* 1981;6:144–148.

Dorfman HD, Norman A, Wolff H. Fibrosarcoma complicating bone infarction in a caisson worker. A case report. *J Bone Joint Surg Am* 1966;48:528–532.

Enzinger FM, Weiss SW. Hemangioendothelioma: vascular tumors of intermediate malignancy. In: Enzinger FM, Weiss SW, eds. *Soft tissue tumors*, 3rd ed. St. Louis: Mosby; 1995.

Errani C, Vanel D, Gambarotti M, et al. Vascular bone tumors: a proposal of a classification based on clinicopathological, radiographic and genetic features. *Skeletal Radiol* 2012;41:1495–1507.

Errani C, Zhang L, Sung YS, et al. A novel WWTR1-CAMTA1 gene fusion is a consistent abnormality in epithelioid hemangioendothelioma of different anatomic sites. *Genes Chromosomes Cancer* 2011;50:644–653.

Fechner RE, Mills SE. Atlas of tumor pathology. *Tumors of the bones and joints*, 3rd series, fascicle 8. Washington, DC: Armed Forces Institute of Pathology; 1993:239–244.

Fletcher CDM. Pleomorphic malignant fibrous histiocytoma: fact or fiction? A critical reappraisal based on 159 tumors diagnosed as pleomorphic sarcoma. *Am J Surg Pathol* 1992;16:213–228.

Fletcher CDM, Unni KK, Mertens F, eds. *World Health Organization classification of tumors*. Pathology and genetics of tumours of soft tissue and bone. Lyon, France: IARC Press; 2002.

Fonseca R, Witzig TE, Gertz MA, et al. Multiple myeloma and the translocation t(11;14)(q13;32): a report on 13 cases. *Br J Haematol* 1998;101:296–301.

Fonesca R, Blood EA, Oken MM, et al. Myeloma and t(11;14)(q13;32); evidence for biologically defined unique subset of patients. *Blood* 2002;99:3735–3741.

Ford DR, Wilson D, Sothi S, et al. Primary bone lymphoma—treatment and outcome. *Clin Oncol (R Coll Radiol)* 2007;19:50–57.

Galasko CSB. The anatomy and pathways of skeletal metastases. In: Weiss L, Gilbert H, eds. *Bone metastasis*. Boston: GK Hall; 1981:49–63.

Galasko CSB. Mechanisms of lytic and blastic metastatic disease of bone. *Clin Orthop Relat Res* 1982;69:20–27.

Greenspan A, Gerscovich EO, Szabo RM, et al. Condensing osteitis of the clavicle: a rare but frequently misdiagnosed condition. *AJR Am J Roentgenol* 1991;156:1011–1015.

Greenspan A, Klein MJ, Lewis MM. Case Report 272. Skeletal (predominately) cortical metastases in the left femur arising from bronchogenic carcinoma. *Skeletal Radiol* 1984;11:297–301.

Greenspan A, Norman A. Osteolytic cortical destruction: an unusual pattern of skeletal metastases. *Skeletal Radiol* 1988;17:402–406.

Greenspan A, Norman A, Steiner G. Case Report 146. Squamous cell carcinoma arising in chronic, draining sinus tract secondary to osteomyelitis of right tibia. *Skeletal Radiol* 1981;6:149–151.

Greenspan A, Remagen W. *Differential diagnosis of tumors and tumor-like lesions of bones and joints*. Philadelphia: Lippincott-Raven; 1998:369–371.

Greenspan A, Stadalnik RC. Bone island: scintigraphic findings and their clinical application. *Can Assoc Radiol J* 1995;46:368–379.

Griffith B, Yadam S, Mayer T, et al. Angiosarcoma of the humerus presenting with fluid-fluid levels on MRI: a unique imaging presentation. *Skeletal Radiol* 2013;42:1611–1616.

Grover SB, Dhar A. Imaging spectrum in sclerotic myelomas: an experience of three cases. *Eur Radiol* 2000;10:1828–1831.

Gutzeit A, Doert A, Froehlich JM, et al. Comparison of diffusion-weighted whole body MRI and skeletal scintigraphy for the detection of bone metastases in patients with prostate or breast carcinoma. *Skeletal Radiol* 2010;39:333–343.

Healey JH, Turnbull AD, Miedema B, et al. Acrometastases. A study of twenty-nine patients with osseous involvement of the hands and feet. *J Bone Joint Surg Am* 1986;68:743–746.

Hendrix RW, Rogers LF, Davis TM Jr. Cortical bone metastases. *Radiology* 1991;181:409–413.

Heyning FH, Kroon HMJA, Hogendoorn PCW, et al. MR imaging characteristics in primary lymphoma of bone with emphasis on non-aggressive appearance. *Skeletal Radiol* 2007;36:937–944.

Hillemanns M, McLeod RA, Unni KK. Malignant lymphoma. *Skeletal Radiol* 1996;25:73–75.

Hudson TM. *Radiologic-pathologic correlation of musculoskeletal lesions*. Baltimore: Williams & Wilkins; 1987:287–303, 359–397, 421–440.

Huvos AG, Higinbotham NL, Miller TR. Bone sarcomas arising in fibrous dysplasia. *J Bone Joint Surg Am* 1972;54:1047–1056.

Huvos AG, Marcove RC. Adamantinoma of long bones. A clinicopathological study of fourteen cases with vascular origin suggested. *J Bone Joint Surg Am* 1975;57:148–154.

Ilievska Popovska B, Spirovski M, Trajkov D, et al. Neuron specific enolase—selective marker for small-cell lung cancer. *Radiol Oncol* 2004;38:21–26.

Ishida T, Iijima T, Kikuchi F, et al. A clinicopathological and immunohistochemical study of osteofibrous dysplasia, differentiated adamantinoma, and adamantinoma of long bones. *Skeletal Radiol* 1992;21:493–502.

Italiano A, Thomas R, Breen M, et al. The miR-17-92 cluster and its target THBS1 are differentially expressed in angiosarcomas dependent on MYC amplification. *Genes Chromosomes Cancer* 2012;51:569–578.

Jacobson HG, Poppel MH, Shapiro JH, et al. The vertebral pedicle sign: a roentgen finding to differentiate metastatic carcinoma from multiple myeloma. *Am J Roentgenol Radium Ther Nucl Med* 1958;80:817–821.

Jundt G, Moll C, Nidecker A, et al. Primary leiomyosarcoma of bone: report of eight cases. *Hum Pathol* 1994;25:1205–1212.

Jundt G, Remberger K, Roessner A, et al. Adamantinoma of long bones. A histopathological and immunohistochemical study of 23 cases. *Pathol Res Pract* 1995;191:112–120.

Kattapuram SV, Khurana JS, Scott JA, et al. Negative scintigraphy with positive magnetic resonance imaging in bone metastases. *Skeletal Radiol* 1990;19:113–116.

Keeney GL, Unni KK, Beabout JW, et al. Adamantinoma of long bones. A clinicopathologic study of 85 cases. *Cancer* 1989;64:730–737.

Kleer CG, Unni KK, McLeod RA. Epithelioid hemangioendothelioma of bone. *Am J Surg Pathol* 1996;20:1301–1311.

Klein MJ, Rudin BJ, Greenspan A, et al. Hodgkin disease presenting as a lesion in the wrist. A case report. *J Bone Joint Surg Am* 1987;69:1246–1249.

Koplas MC, Lefkowitz RA, Bauer TW, et al. Imaging findings, prevalence and outcome of de novo and secondary malignant fibrous histiocytoma of bone. *Skeletal Radiol* 2010;39:791–798.

Kramer K, Hicks D, Palis J, et al. Epithelioid osteosarcoma of bone. Immunocytochemical evidence suggesting divergent epithelial and mesenchymal differentiation in a primary osseous neoplasm. *Cancer* 1993;71:2977–2982.

Libshitz HI, Malthouse SR, Cunningham D, et al. Multiple myeloma: appearance at MR imaging. *Radiology* 1992;182:833–837.

Link TM, Haeussler MD, Poppek S, et al. Malignant fibrous histiocytoma of bone: conventional X-ray and MR imaging features. *Skeletal Radiol* 1998;27:552–558.

Llombart-Bosch A, Ortuño-Pacheco G. Ultrastructural findings supporting the angioblastic nature of the so-called adamantinoma of the tibia. *Histopathology* 1978;2:189–200.

Major N, Helms CA, Richardson WJ. The "mini brain": plasmacytoma in a vertebral body on MRI. *AJR Am J Roentgenol* 2000;175:261–263.

Markel SF. Ossifying fibroma of long bone: its distinction from fibrous dysplasia and its association with adamantinoma of long bone. *Am J Clin Pathol* 1978;69:91–97.

Mertens F, Romeo S, Bovée JV, et al. Reclassification and subtyping of so-called malignant fibrous histiocytoma of bone: comparison with cytogenetic features. *Clin Sarcoma Res* 2011;1:10.

Mirra JM, Gold RH, Marafiote R. Malignant (fibrous) histiocytoma arising in association with a bone infarct in sickle-cell disease: coincidence or cause-and-effect? *Cancer* 1977;39:186–194.

Mueller DL, Grant RM, Riding MD, et al. Cortical saucerization: an unusual imaging finding of Ewing sarcoma. *AJR Am J Roentgenol* 1994;163:401–403.

Mulder JD, Kroon HM, Schütte HE, et al. *Radiologic atlas of bone tumors.* Amsterdam, The Netherlands: Elsevier; 1993;267–274, 607–625.

Mulligan ME, Badros AZ. PET/CT and MR imaging in myeloma. *Skeletal Radiol* 2007;36:5–16.

Mulligan ME, Kransdorf MJ. Sequestra in primary lymphoma of bone: prevalence and radiologic features. *AJR Am J Roentgenol* 1993;160:1245–1248.

Murphey MD, Gross TM, Rosenthal HG. From the archives of the AFIP. Musculoskeletal malignant fibrous histiocytoma: radiologic-pathologic correlation. *Radiographics* 1994;14:807–828.

Myers JL, Arocho J, Bernreuter W, et al. Leiomyosarcoma of bone. A clinicopathologic, immunohistochemical, and ultrastructural study of five cases. *Cancer* 1991;67:1051–1056.

Ontell FK, Greenspan A. Blastic osseous metastases in ovarian carcinoma. *Can Assoc Radiol J* 1995;46:231–234.

Panchwagh Y, Puri A, Agarwal M, et al. Case report: metastatic adamantinoma of the tibia—an unusual presentation. *Skeletal Radiol* 2006;35:190–193.

Pour L, Sevcikova S, Gresilkova H, et al. Soft-tissue extramedullary multiple myeloma prognosis is significantly worse in comparison to bone-related extramedullary relapse. *Haematologica* 2014; 99:360–364.

Powell JM. Metastatic carcinoid of bone. Report of two cases and review of the literature. *Clin Orthop Relat Res* 1988;230:266–272.

Resnick D, Niwayama G. Skeletal metastases. In: Resnick D, ed. *Diagnosis of bone and joint disorders*, 3rd ed. Philadelphia: WB Saunders; 1995:3991–4065.

Romeo S, Bovee JV, Kroon HM, et al. Malignant fibrous histiocytoma and fibrosarcoma of bone: a re-assessment in the light of currently employed morphological, immunohistochemical and molecular approaches. *Virchows Arch* 2012;461:561–570.

Rosenberg AE. Malignant fibrous histiocytoma: past, present, and future. *Skeletal Radiol* 2003;32:613–618.

Rosenthal J, Cardona K, Sayyid SK, et al. Nodal metastases of soft tissue sarcomas: risk factors, imaging findings, and implications. *Skeletal Radiol* 2020;49:221–229.

Schajowicz F. *Tumors and tumorlike lesions of bone, pathology, radiology, and treatment*, 2nd ed. Berlin, Germany: Springer-Verlag; 1994:301–367, 468–481, 552–566.

Springfield DS, Rosenberg AE, Mankin HJ, et al. Relationship between osteofibrous dysplasia and adamantinoma. *Clin Orthop Relat Res* 1994;309:234–244.

Stäbler A, Baur A, Bartl R, et al. Contrast enhancement and quantitative signal analysis in MR imaging of multiple myeloma: assessment of focal and diffuse growth patterns in marrow correlated with biopsies and survival rates. *AJR Am J Roentgenol* 1996;167:1029–1036.

Steiner GC, Matano S, Present D. Ewing's sarcoma of humerus with epithelial differentiation. *Skeletal Radiol* 1995;24:379–382.

Sun T, Akalin A, Rodacker M, et al. CD20 positive T cell lymphoma: is it a real entity? *J Clin Pathol* 2004;57:442–444.

Sundaram M, Akduman I, White LM, et al. Primary leiomyosarcoma of bone. *AJR Am J Roentgenol* 1999;172:771–776.

Sung MS, Lee GK, Kang HS. Sacrococcygeal chordoma: MR imaging in 30 patients. *Skeletal Radiol* 2005;34:87–94.

Sweet DE, Vinh TN, Devaney K. Cortical osteofibrous dysplasia of long bone and its relationship to adamantinoma. A clinicopathologic study of 30 cases. *Am J Surg Pathol* 1992;16:282–290.

Tarkkanen M, Larramendy ML, Böhling T, et al. Malignant fibrous histiocytoma of bone: analysis of genomic imbalances by comparative genomic hybridisation and C-MYC expression by immunohistochemistry. *Eur J Cancer* 2006;42:1172–1180.

Treglia G, Salsano M, Stefanelli A, et al. Diagnostic accuracy of 18F-FDG-PET and PET/CT in patients with Ewing sarcoma family tumours: a systematic review and meta-analysis. *Skeletal Radiol* 2012;41:249–256.

Trias A, Fery A. Cortical circulation of long bones. *J Bone Joint Surg Am* 1979;61:1052–1059.

Ueda Y, Roessner A, Bosse A, et al. Juvenile intracortical adamantinoma of the tibia with predominant osteofibrous dysplasia-like features. *Pathol Res Pract* 1991;187:1039–1043.

Unni KK. Fibrous and fibrohistiocytic lesions of bone. *Semin Orthop* 1991;6:177–186.

Voss SD, Murphey MD, Hall FM. Solitary osteosclerotic plasmacytoma: association with demyelinating polyneuropathy and amyloid deposition. *Skeletal Radiol* 2001;30:527–529.

Wang J, Chen C, Lau S, et al. CD3-positive large B-cell lymphoma. *Am J Surg Pathol* 2009;33:505–512.

Weiss SW. Ultrastructure of the so-called "chordoid sarcoma." Evidence supporting cartilaginous differentiation. *Cancer* 1976;37:300–306.

Wenger DE, Wold LE. Malignant vascular lesions of bone: radiologic and pathologic features. *Skeletal Radiol* 2000;29:619–631.

Werling RW, Yaziji H, Bacchi CE, et al. CDX2, a highly sensitive and specific marker of adenocarcinomas of intestinal origin: an immunohistochemical survey of 476 primary and metastatic carcinomas. *Am J Surg Pathol* 2003;27:303–310.

Wong HH, Chu P. Immunohistochemical features of the gastrointestinal tract tumors. *J Gastrointest Oncol* 2012;3:262–284.

23

Tumors and Tumor-like Lesions of the Joints

Benign Lesions

Synovial (Osteo)Chondromatosis

Clinical Features

Synovial (osteo)chondromatosis (also known as *synovial chondromatosis* or *synovial chondrometaplasia*) is an uncommon benign disorder marked by the metaplastic proliferation of multiple cartilaginous nodules in the synovial membrane of the joints, bursae, or tendon sheaths. The cartilaginous nodules will frequently ossify at which point synovial chondromatosis becomes known as *synovial osteochondromatosis*. It is almost invariably monoarticular; rarely, multiple joints may be affected. The disorder is twice as common in men as in women and is usually discovered in the third to fifth decade. The knee is a preferential site of involvement, with the hip, shoulder, and elbow accounting for most of the remaining cases (Fig. 23.1). Patients usually report pain and swelling. Joint effusion, tenderness, limited motion in the joint, and a soft-tissue mass are common clinical findings.

Three phases of articular disease have been identified: an initial phase, characterized by metaplastic formation of cartilaginous nodules in the synovium; a transitional phase, characterized by detachment of those nodules and formation of free intraarticular bodies; and an inactive phase, in which synovial proliferation has resolved but loose bodies remain in the joint, usually with variable amounts of joint fluid.

Imaging Features

The imaging findings depend on the degree of calcification within the cartilaginous bodies, ranging from mere joint effusion to visualization of many radiopaque joint bodies, usually small and uniform in size (Figs. 23.2 to 23.4). The best proof that the bodies are indeed intraarticular is achieved by arthrography or computed tomography (CT) (Figs. 23.5 and 23.6). These modalities can visualize even noncalcified bodies. Ultrasound is hampered by its frequent inability to access all aspects of the joint. Nevertheless, it will readily identify both calcified and noncalcified bodies within the joint (Fig. 23.7). Magnetic resonance imaging (MRI) may also be helpful, although MRI appearance is variable and depends on the relative preponderance of synovial proliferation, loose bodies formation, and extent of calcification or ossification. Unmineralized hyperplastic synovial masses exhibit high signal intensity on T2-weighted images, whereas calcifications can be seen as signal void against the high–signal intensity fluid (Figs. 23.8 and 23.9). In addition to revealing loose bodies in the joint, CT and MRI may demonstrate bony erosion (see Fig. 23.6C).

Pathology

By microscopy, many cartilaginous nodules are observed as they form beneath the thin layer of cells that line the surface of the synovial membrane. These nodules covered by fibrous tissue are highly cellular, and the cells themselves may exhibit a moderate pleomorphism, with occasional plump and double nuclei. The cartilaginous nodules, which often are undergoing calcification and endochondral ossification, may detach and become loose bodies. The loose bodies continue to be viable and may increase in size as they receive nourishment from the synovial fluid.

Genetic abnormalities in most cases consist of near-diploid karyotypes with some cases exhibiting only numerical changes (−X, −Y, and +5, respectively). Recently, ERK and NOG (Noggin) gene association has been postulated.

Differential Diagnosis

Synovial (osteo)chondromatosis should be differentiated from the secondary osteochondromatosis caused by osteoarthritis, particularly in the knee and hip joints, and from synovial chondrosarcoma, either primary (arising *de novo* from the synovial membrane) or secondary (caused by malignant transformation). Distinguishing *primary* from *secondary osteochondromatosis* usually presents no problems. In the latter condition, there is invariably radiographic evidence of osteoarthritis with all of its typical features, such as narrowing of the radiographic joint space, subchondral sclerosis, and, occasionally, periarticular cysts or cyst-like lesions (Fig. 23.10). The loose bodies are fewer, larger, and invariably of different sizes. Conversely, in primary synovial (osteo)chondromatosis, the joint is not affected by any degenerative changes. In some cases, however, the bone may show erosions secondary to pressure of the calcified bodies on the outer aspects of the cortex (see Fig. 23.6C). The intraarticular bodies are numerous, small, and usually of uniform size (see Figs. 23.2 to 23.4).

It is more difficult to distinguish synovial chondromatosis from *synovial chondrosarcoma*. The clinical and radiographic features have not been useful in this differentiation and are equally ineffective in distinguishing a secondary malignant lesion arising in synovial (osteo)chondromatosis. In addition, both entities tend to have a protracted clinical course, and local recurrence is common after synovectomy for synovial chondromatosis or local resection of synovial chondrosarcoma. The presence of frank bone destruction rather than merely erosions, and the association of a soft-tissue mass, should always raise a concern for malignancy (see Fig. 23.35). Although extension beyond the joint capsule should heighten the suspicion of malignancy, some cases of synovial chondromatosis have been reported to have extraarticular extension.

The other conditions that can radiologically mimic synovial chondromatosis include pigmented villonodular synovitis (PVNS), synovial hemangioma, and lipoma arborescens. In PVNS (discussed in detail later in this chapter), the filling defects in the joint are more confluent and less distinct. MRI may show foci of decreased intensity of the synovium in all sequences because of the paramagnetic effects of deposition of hemosiderin (see Figs. 23.15 to 23.17). *Synovial hemangioma* usually presents as a single soft-tissue mass. On MRI, T1-weighted images show that the lesion is either isointense or slightly higher (brighter) in signal intensity

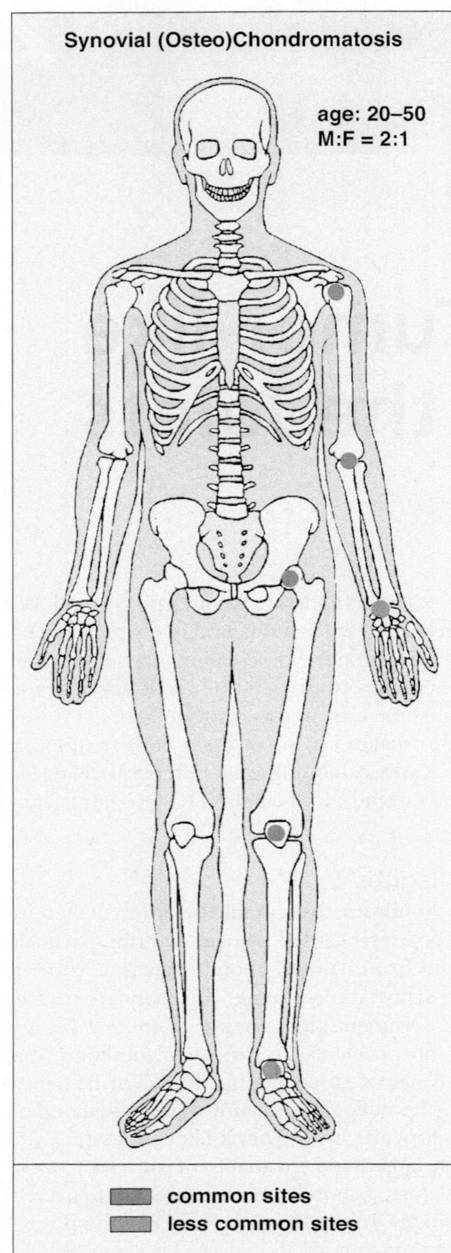

FIGURE 23.1 **Synovial (osteo)chondromatosis: skeletal sites of predilection, peak age range, and male-to-female ratio.** (Reprinted with permission from Greenspan A, Remagen W. *Differential diagnosis of tumors and tumor-like lesions of bones and joints.* Philadelphia: Lippincott-Raven; 1998.)

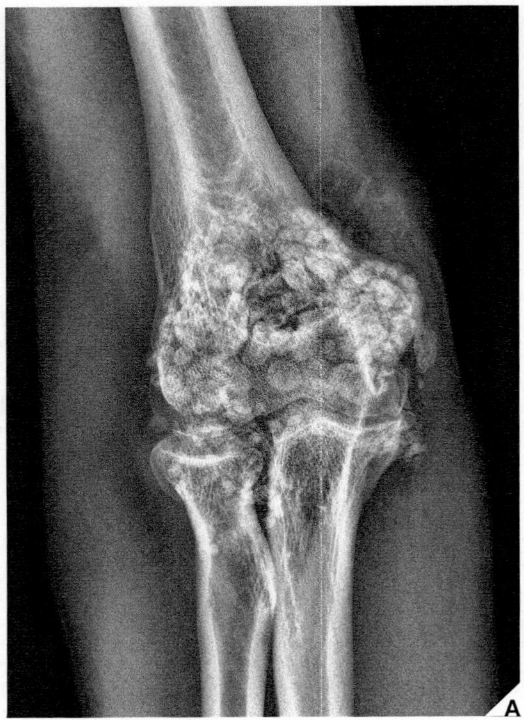

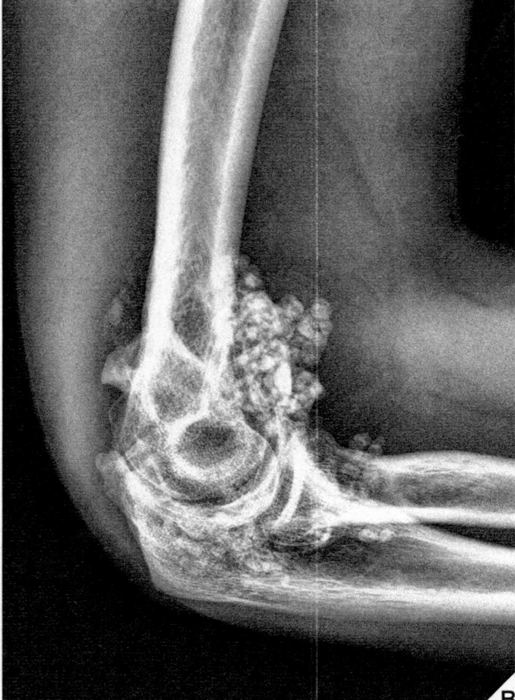

FIGURE 23.2 **Synovial (osteo)chondromatosis.** A 27-year-old man reported pain and occasional locking in the elbow joint; he had no history of trauma. **(A)** Anteroposterior and **(B)** lateral radiographs demonstrate multiple osteochondral bodies in the elbow joint, which are regularly shaped and uniform in size.

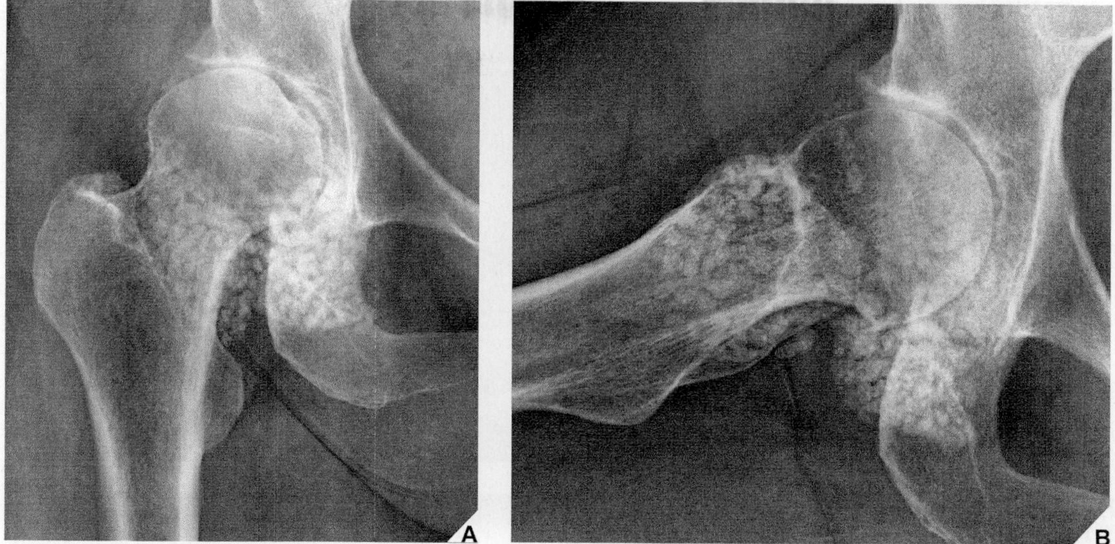

FIGURE 23.3 Synovial (osteo)chondromatosis. **(A)** Anteroposterior and **(B)** frog-lateral radiographs of the right hip of a 59-year-old woman show numerous, uniform in size, intraarticular osteochondral bodies.

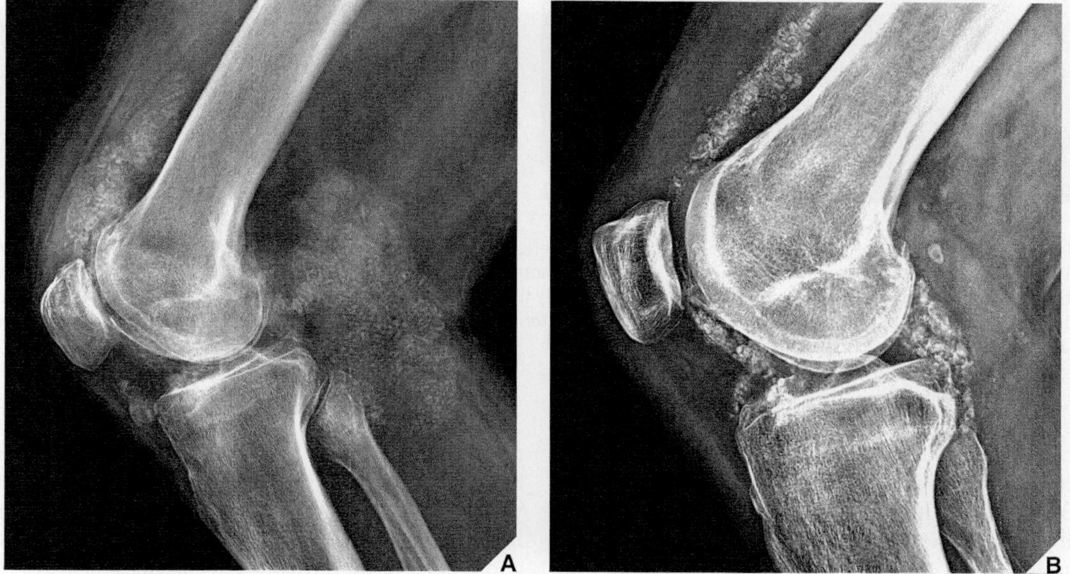

FIGURE 23.4 Synovial (osteo)chondromatosis. **(A)** Lateral radiograph of the knee of a 58-year-old man shows numerous small and uniform in size intraarticular osteochondral bodies. **(B)** Lateral radiograph of the knee of a 45-year-old woman shows typical appearance of synovial osteochondromatosis.

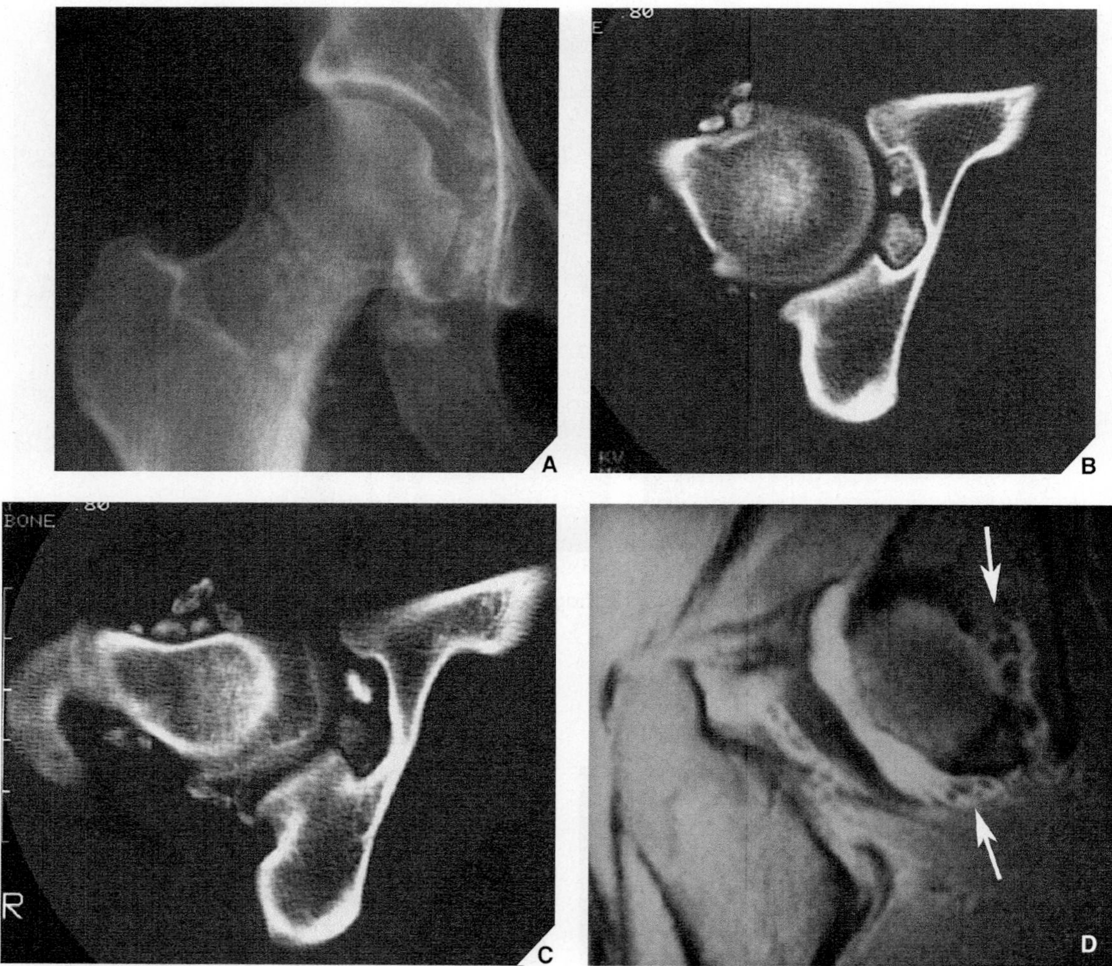

FIGURE 23.5 CT and MRI of synovial (osteo)chondromatosis. **(A)** Anteroposterior radiograph of the right hip of a 27-year-old woman shows multiple osteochondral bodies around the femoral head and neck. Note preservation of the joint space, a characteristic feature of synovial (osteo)chondromatosis. **(B,C)** Two CT sections, one through the femoral head and another through the femoral neck, demonstrate unquestionably the intraarticular location of multiple osteochondral bodies. **(D)** Coronal T2-weighted MR image of the right hip of another patient shows multiple small intraarticular osteochondral bodies lodged in the acetabular fossa and in the inferior capsular recess *(arrows)*. The osteochondral bodies were removed via arthroscopy.

than surrounding muscles but much lower in intensity than subcutaneous fat. On T2-weighted images, the mass is invariably much brighter than fat (see Figs. 23.23 and 23.24). Phleboliths and fibrofatty septa in the mass are common findings that show low-signal characteristics. *Lipoma arborescens* is a villous lipomatous proliferation of the synovial membrane. This rare condition usually affects the knee joint but has occasionally been reported in other joints, including the wrist and ankle. The disease has been variously reported to have a developmental, traumatic, inflammatory, or neoplastic origin, but its true cause is still unknown. The clinical findings include slowly increasing but painless synovial thickening as well as joint effusion with sporadic exacerbation. Imaging studies reveal a joint effusion occasionally accompanied by various degrees of osteoarthritis (see Figs 23.26 and 23.27). Histologic examination demonstrates complete replacement of the subsynovial tissue by mature fat cells and the formation of proliferative villous projections (see the following text).

Treatment and Prognosis

Treatment of synovial chondromatosis usually consists of removal of the intraarticular bodies and synovectomy, but local recurrence is not uncommon. Rare cases of chondrosarcoma arising in synovial chondromatosis have been described (see later text).

Pigmented Villonodular Synovitis

Clinical Features

PVNS is a locally destructive fibrohistiocytic proliferation, characterized by many villous and nodular synovial protrusions, which affects joints, bursae, and tendon sheaths. PVNS was first described by Jaffe, Lichtenstein, and Sutro in 1941, who used this name to identify the lesion because of its yellow-brown, villous, and nodular appearance. The yellow-brown pigmentation is caused by excessive deposits of lipid and hemosiderin. This condition can be diffuse or localized. When the entire synovium of the joint is affected, and when there is a major villous component, the condition is referred to as *diffuse PVNS*. When a discrete intraarticular mass is present, the condition is called *localized PVNS*. When the process affects the tendon sheaths, it is called *localized giant cell tumor of the tendon sheaths*. The diffuse form usually occurs in the knee, hip, elbow, or wrist and accounts for 23% of cases. The localized nodular form is often regarded as a separate entity. It consists of a single polypoid mass attached to the synovium. Nodular tenosynovitis is most often seen in the fingers and is the second most common soft-tissue tumor of the hand, exceeded only by the ganglion. In the new (2002) revised classification of soft-tissue tumors, the World Health Organization (WHO) classifies localized intraarticular and extraarticular lesions as *giant cell tumor of tendon sheath*, whereas diffuse intraarticular and extraarticular forms are categorized as *diffuse-type giant cell tumor* (keeping PVNS as a synonym).

Both the diffuse and the localized form of villonodular synovitis usually occur as a single lesion, mainly in young and middle-aged individuals of either sex. One of the most characteristic findings in PVNS is the ability of the hyperplastic synovium to invade the subchondral bone, producing cysts and erosions. Although the cause is unknown and is often controversial, some investigators have suggested an autoimmune pathogenesis. Trauma is also a suspected cause because similar effects

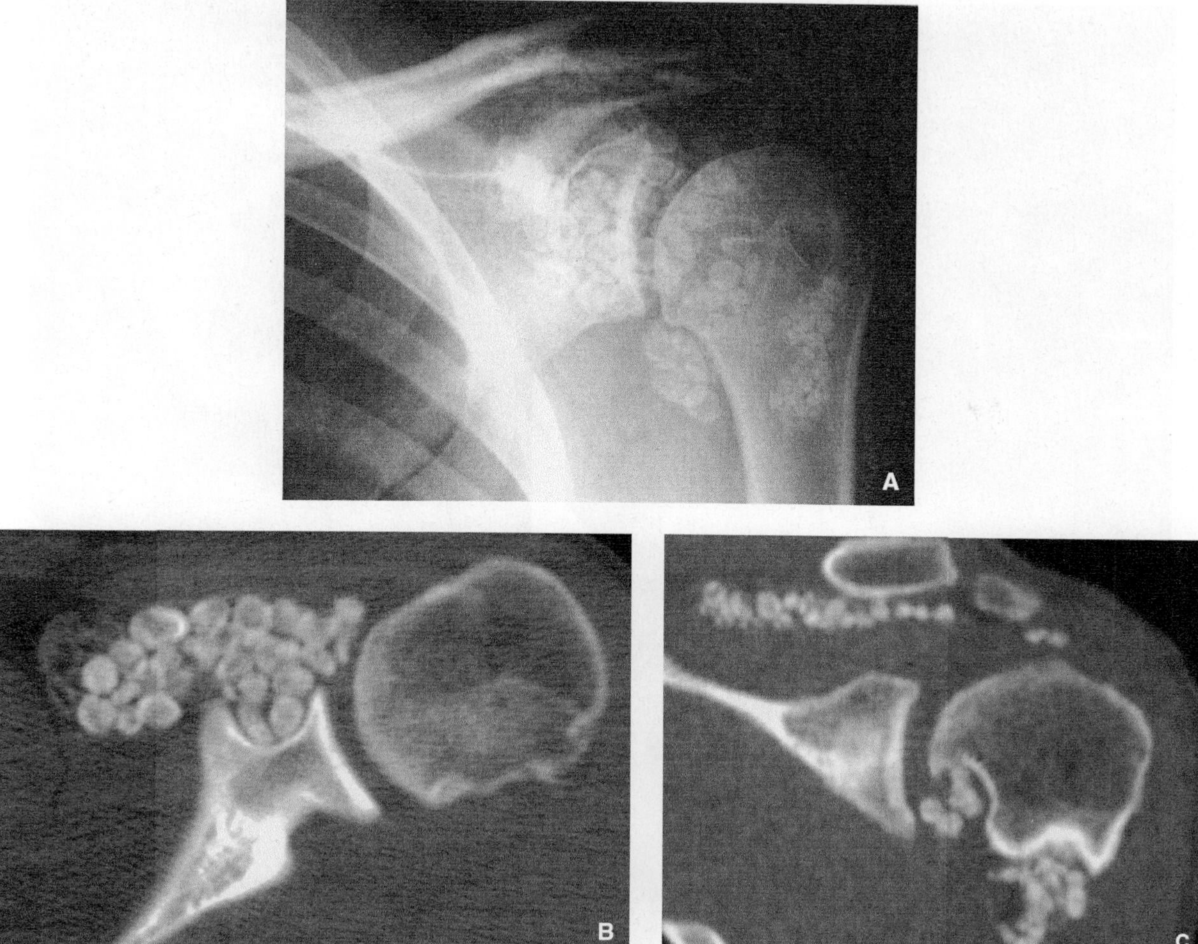

FIGURE 23.6 CT of synovial (osteo)chondromatosis. **(A)** Anteroposterior radiograph of the left shoulder of a 36-year-old man shows multiple osteochondral bodies around the glenohumeral joint. **(B)** Axial CT section confirms the intraarticular location of osteochondral bodies. **(C)** Coronal CT section effectively shows location of the uniform in size calcified bodies in the glenohumeral joint and subacromial bursa. Observe erosion of the humeral head. (Reprinted with permission from Greenspan A, Borys D. *Radiology and pathology correlation of bone tumors: a quick reference and review*. Philadelphia: Wolters Kluwer; 2016:111, Fig. 3.28.)

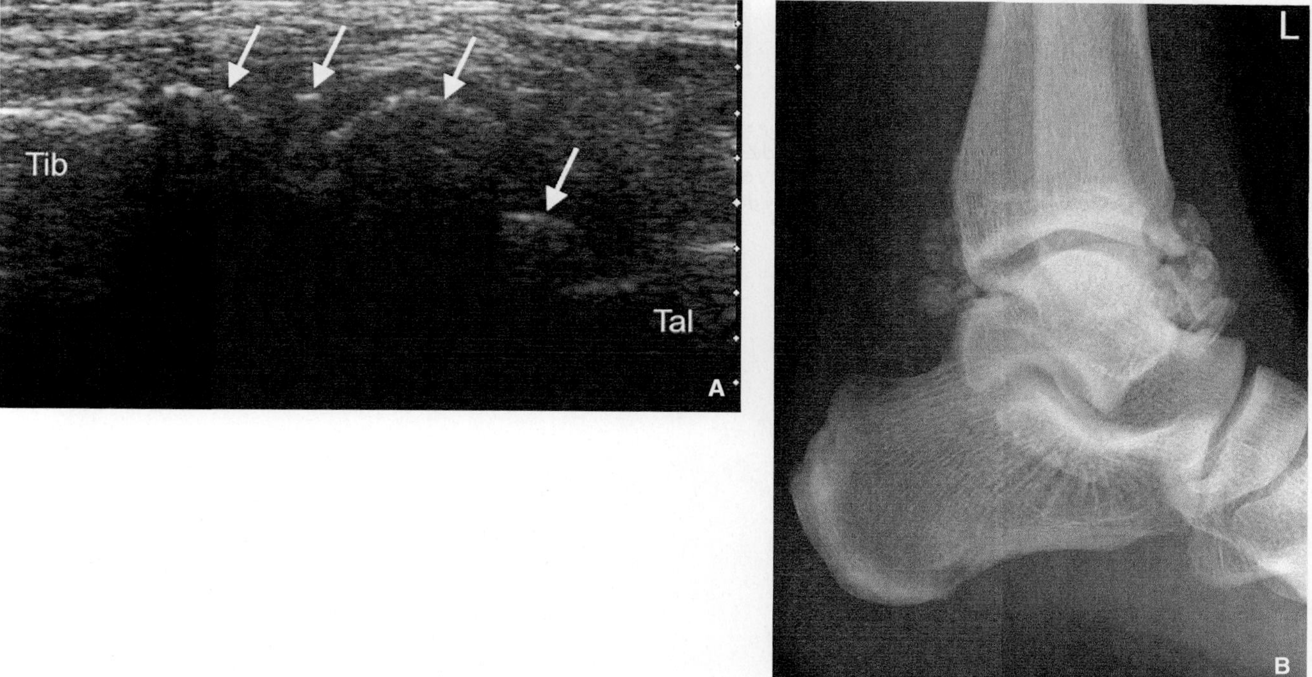

FIGURE 23.7 Ultrasound of synovial (osteo)chondromatosis. **(A)** Longitudinal ultrasound through the anterior aspect of the ankle joint of a 31-year-old man reveals multiple calcified loose bodies *(arrows)*, corresponding to ossified osteochondral bodies seen on the lateral radiograph of the ankle **(B)**. *Tib*, anterior tibia; *Tal*, dorsal talus. (Courtesy of Prof. Andrew J. Grainger, Cambridge, United Kingdom, from Greenspan A, Grainger AJ. Articular abnormalities that may mimic arthritis. *J Ultrason* 2018;18:212–223.)

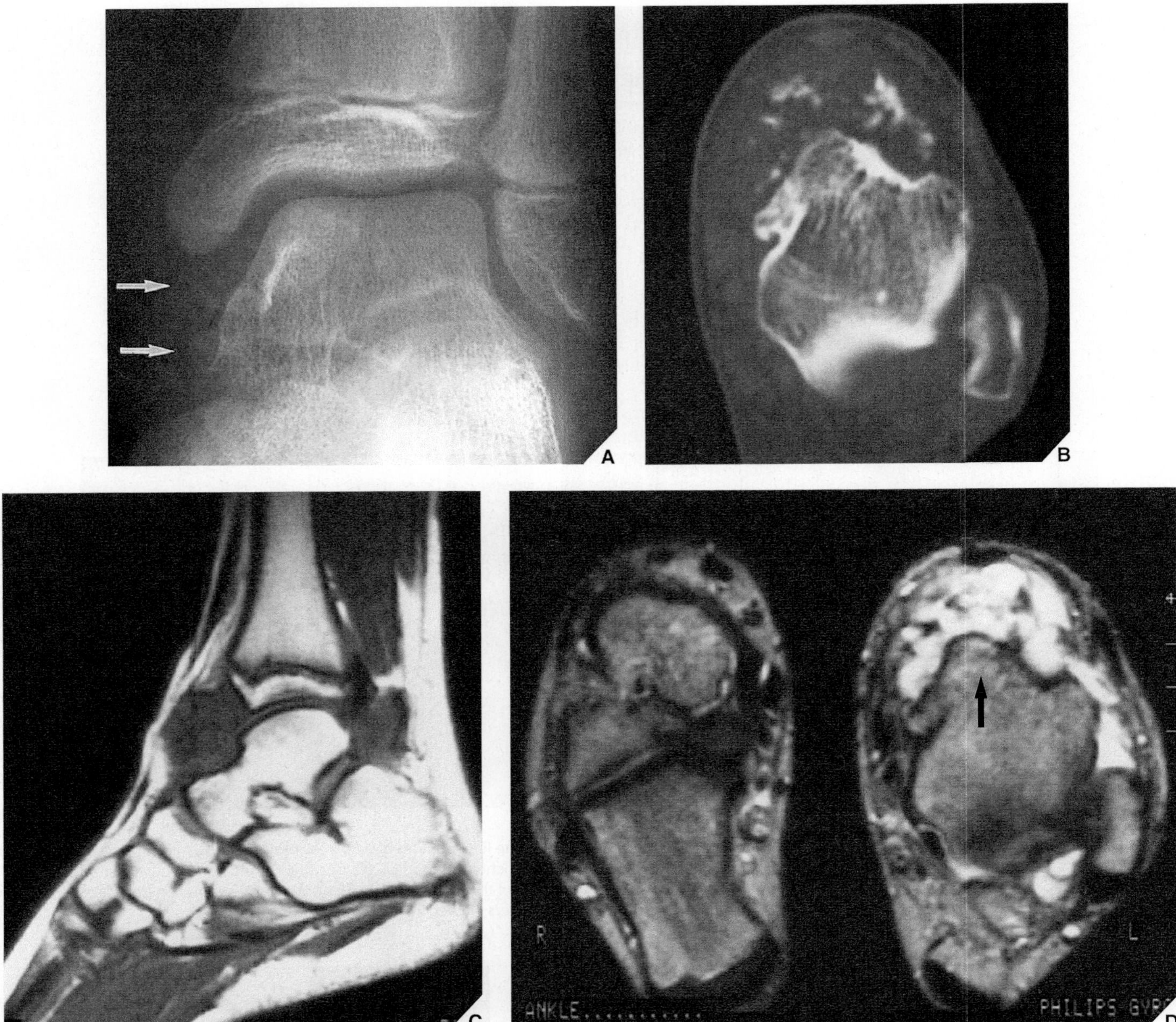

FIGURE 23.8 MRI of synovial (osteo)chondromatosis. **(A)** Oblique radiograph of the left ankle of a 14-year-old boy shows faint radiopaque foci projecting over the tibiotalar joint *(arrows)*. **(B)** CT section shows the location of calcified bodies in the anterior aspect of the joint. **(C)** Sagittal T1-weighted (spin echo [SE]; repetition time [TR] 640/echo time [TE] 20 msec) MR image shows intermediate signal intensity of the fluid in the ankle joint and dispersed low–signal intensity osteochondral bodies. **(D)** Coronal T2-weighted (SE; TR 2,000/TE 80 msec) MR image of the ankle joint clearly defines low–signal intensity osteochondral bodies within bright fluid *(arrow)*.

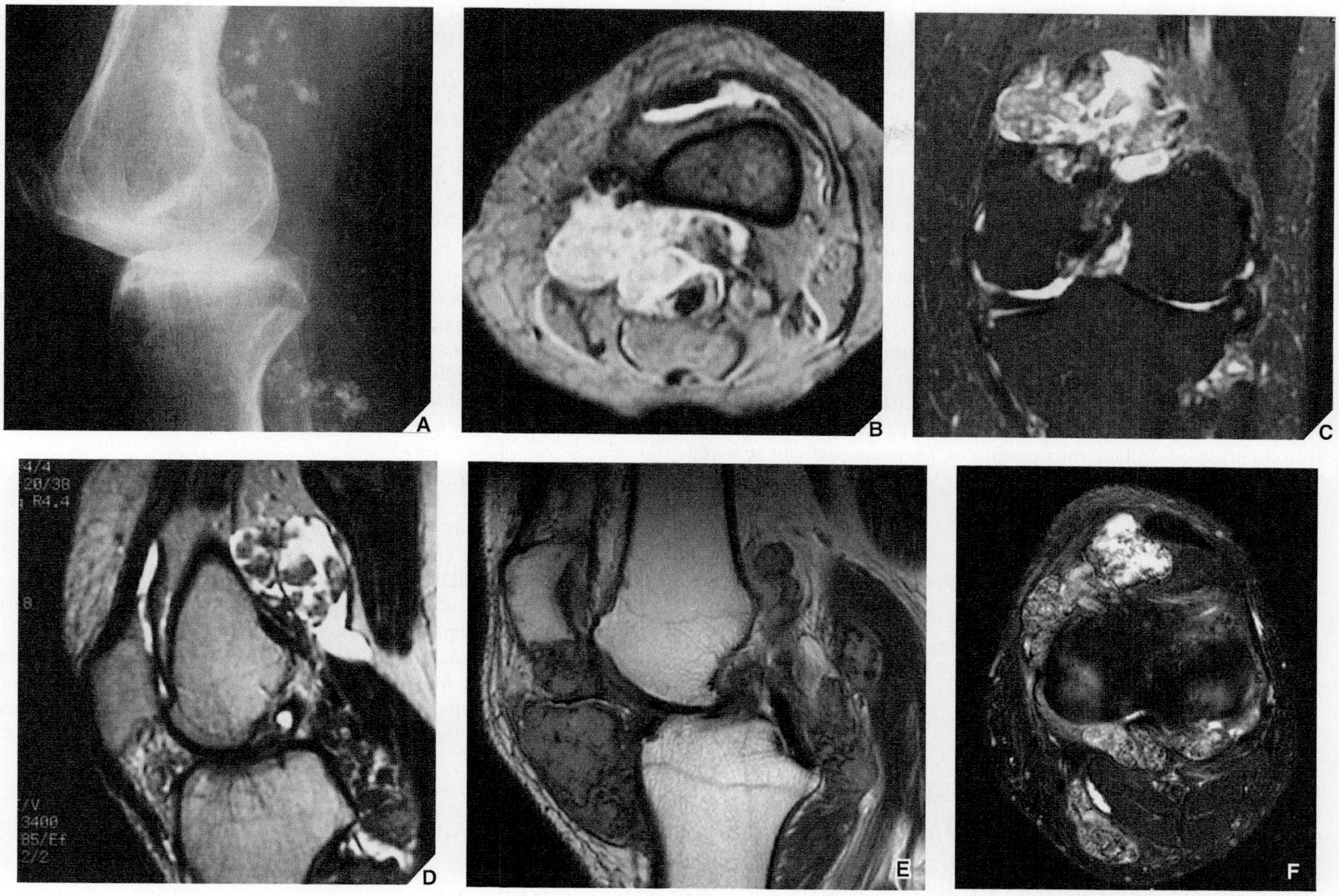

FIGURE 23.9 MRI of synovial (osteo)chondromatosis. **(A)** Lateral radiograph of the left knee of a 50-year-old man shows multiple osteochondral bodies in and around the joint. **(B)** Axial T2*-weighted (multiplanar gradient recalled [MPGR]; repetition time [TR] 500/echo time [TE] 20 msec, flip angle 30 degrees) MR image demonstrates high-signal joint effusion and multiple bodies of intermediate signal intensity, primarily located in a large popliteal cyst. **(C)** Coronal fast spin echo (SE) (TR 2,400/TE 85 Ef msec) and **(D)** sagittal fast SE (TR 3,400/TE 85 Ef msec) MR images show to better advantage the distribution of numerous osteochondral bodies. **(E)** Sagittal T1-weighted and **(F)** axial T2-weighted MR images of the knee of another patient demonstrate distension of the joint capsule and popliteal cyst by multiple intraarticular bodies with heterogeneous signal intensity representing areas of ossification and areas of cartilage.

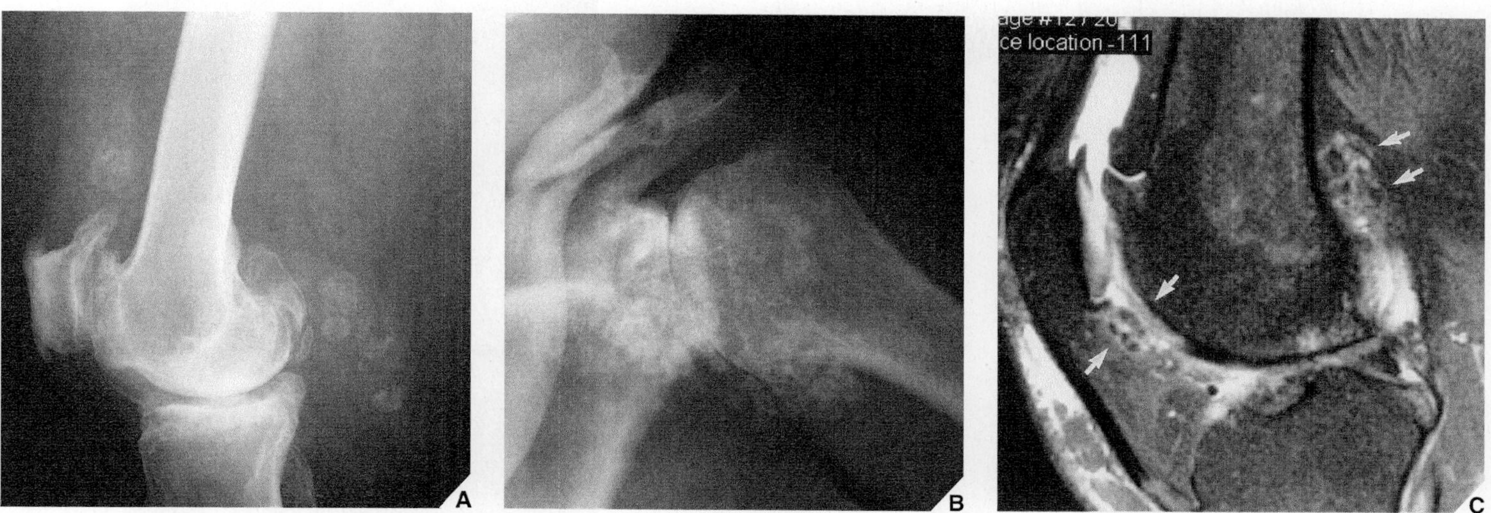

FIGURE 23.10 Secondary osteochondromatosis. **(A)** Lateral radiograph of the knee in a 58-year-old man with advanced osteoarthritis of the femoropatellar joint compartment shows multiple osteochondral bodies in the suprapatellar bursa and within the popliteal cyst. **(B)** Radiograph of the left shoulder in a 68-year-old woman with osteoarthritis of the glenohumeral joint shows multiple intraarticular osteochondral bodies. **(C)** Sagittal T2-weighted fat-suppressed MRI of the knee in a 54-year-old woman reveals osteoarthritis and numerous, various in size, osteochondral bodies *(arrows)*.

have been produced experimentally in animals by repeated injections of blood into the knee joint. Some investigators have suggested a disturbance in lipid metabolism as a causative factor. It has also been postulated by Jaffe and colleagues that these lesions may represent an inflammatory response to an unknown agent. Stout and Lattes contended that they are true benign neoplasms. Although the latter theory was presumed to be supported by pathologic studies indicating that the histiocytes present in PVNS may function as facultative fibroblasts and that foam cells may derive from histiocytes, thus relating PVNS to a benign neoplasm of fibrohistiocytic origin, these findings do not constitute definite proof that PVNS is a true neoplasm. They are rather indicative of a special form of a chronic proliferative inflammation process, as has already been postulated by Jaffe and colleagues.

Clinically, diffuse PVNS is a slowly progressive process that manifests as mild pain and joint swelling with limitation of motion. Occasionally, increased skin temperature is noted over the affected joint. The knee joint is most commonly affected, and 66% of patients present with a bloody joint effusion. In fact, the presence of a serosanguineous synovial fluid in the absence of a history of recent trauma should strongly suggest the diagnosis of PVNS. The synovial fluid contains elevated levels of cholesterol, and fluid reaccumulates rapidly after aspiration. Other joints may be affected, including the hip, ankle, wrist, elbow, and shoulder. There is a 2:1 predilection for females. Patients range from 4 to 60 years of age, with a peak incidence in the third and fourth decades (Fig. 23.11). The duration of symptoms can range from 6 months to as long as 25 years.

Although a few "malignant" PVNS have been reported in the literature, this diagnosis is still debatable (see later). Recently, attention has been drawn to the extraarticular form of diffuse PVNS, also referred to as *diffuse-type giant cell tumor*. This condition is characterized by the presence of an infiltrate, and extraarticular mass with or without involvement of the adjacent joint. This presentation of PVNS creates a real diagnostic challenge for both radiologist and pathologist because its extraarticular location, invasion of the osseous structures, and more varied histologic infiltrative pattern may suggest malignancy.

Imaging Features

Radiography reveals a soft-tissue density in the affected joint, frequently interpreted as joint effusion. However, the density is greater than that of simple effusion, and it reflects not only a hemorrhagic fluid but also lobulated synovial masses (Fig. 23.12). A marginal, well-defined erosion of subchondral bone with a sclerotic margin may be present (incidence reported from 15% to 50%), usually on both sides of the affected articulation. Narrowing of the joint space has also been reported. In the hip, multiple cyst-like or erosive areas involving non–weight-bearing regions of the acetabulum, as well as the femoral head and neck, are characteristic. Calcifications are encountered only in exceptional cases.

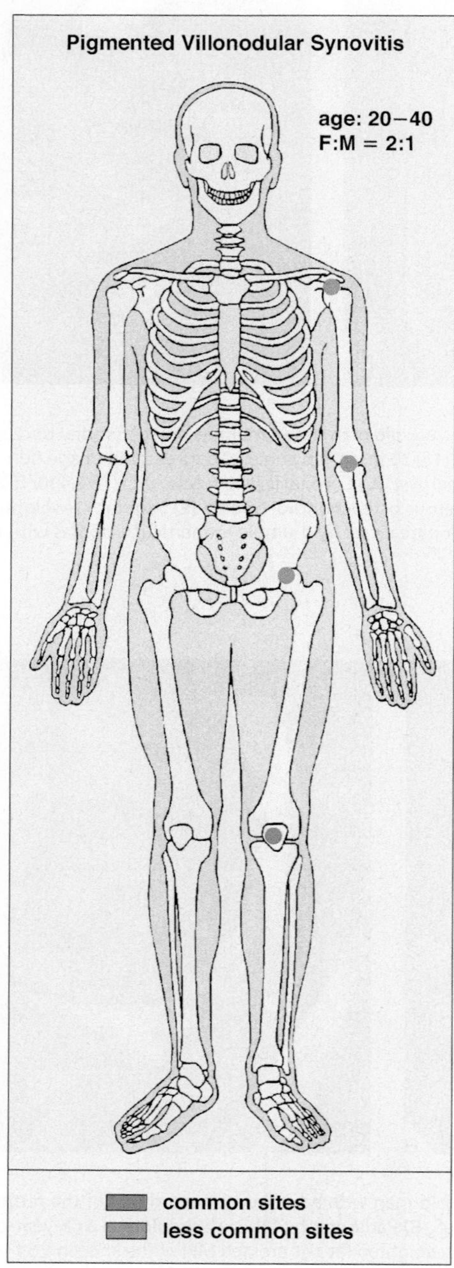

FIGURE 23.11 PVNS: sites of predilection, peak age range, and male-to-female ratio.

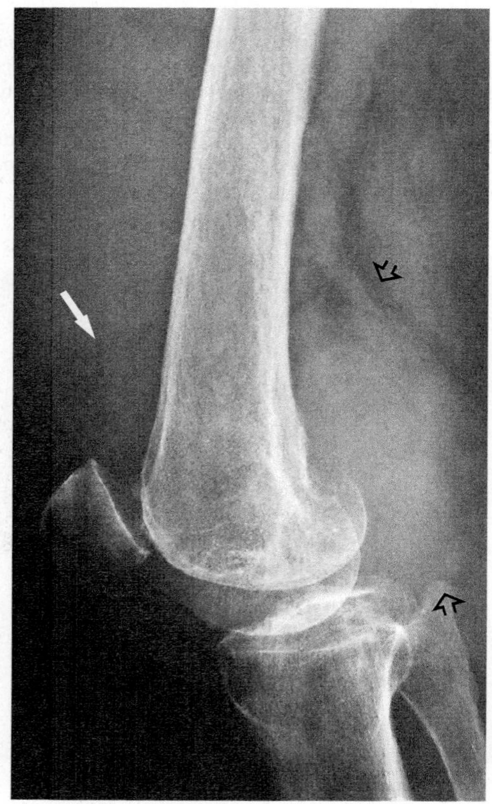

FIGURE 23.12 Pigmented villonodular synovitis (PVNS). Lateral radiograph of the knee of a 58-year-old man shows a large suprapatellar joint effusion *(arrow)* and a dense, lumpy soft-tissue mass eroding the posterior aspect of the lateral femoral condyle *(open arrows)*. These features suggest PVNS. Note that posteriorly the density is greater than that of a suprapatellar fluid.

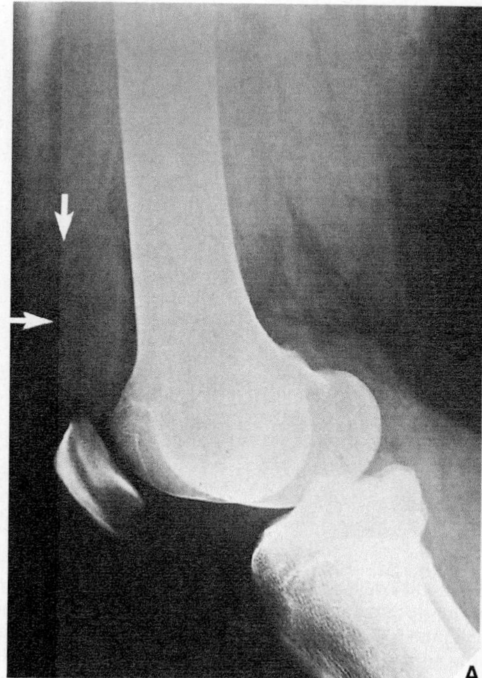

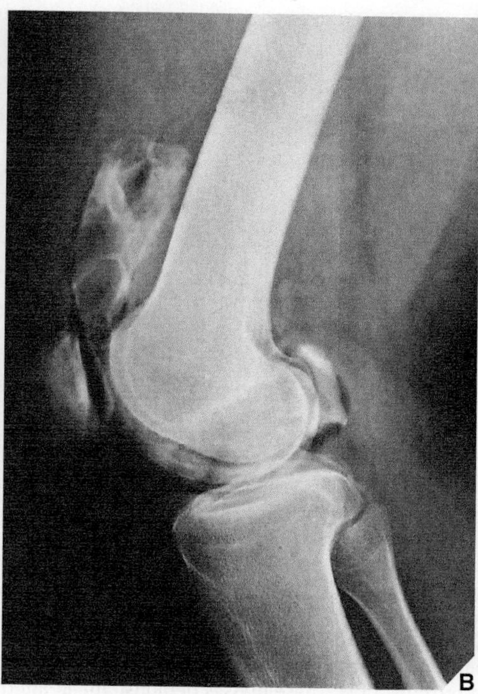

FIGURE 23.13 **Arthrography of PVNS.** **(A)** Lateral radiograph of another patient shows what appears to be a suprapatellar effusion *(arrows)*. The density of the "fluid," however, is increased, and there is some lobulation evident. **(B)** Contrast arthrogram of the knee shows lobulated filling defects in the suprapatellar pouch, representing lumpy synovial masses. Joint puncture yielded thick bloody fluid, which explains the increased density of the soft-tissue mass seen on the radiograph.

Arthrography reveals multiple lobulated masses with villous projections, which appear as filling defects in the contrast-filled suprapatellar bursa (Fig. 23.13). CT effectively demonstrates the extent of the disease. The increase in iron content of the synovial fluid results in high Hounsfield values, a feature that can help in the differential diagnosis. Ultrasound can demonstrate an intraarticular synovial mass or show diffuse involvement in the joint (Fig. 23.14). MRI is extremely useful in making a diagnosis, because on T2-weighted images, the intraarticular masses demonstrate a combination of high–signal intensity areas, representing fluid and congested synovium, interspersed with areas of intermediate to low signal intensity, secondary to random distribution of hemosiderin in the synovium (Fig. 23.15). In general, MRI shows a low signal on T1- and T2-weighted images because of hemosiderin deposition and thick fibrous tissue (Figs. 23.16 and 23.17). In addition, within the mass, signals consistent with fat can be noted, which are caused by clumps of lipid-laden macrophages. Other MRI findings include hyperplastic synovium and occasionally bone erosions. Administration of gadolinium in the form of gadolinium diethylenetriamine pentaacetic acid (Gd-DTPA) leads to a notable increase in overall heterogeneity, which tends toward an overall increase in signal intensity of the capsule and septae. This enhancement of

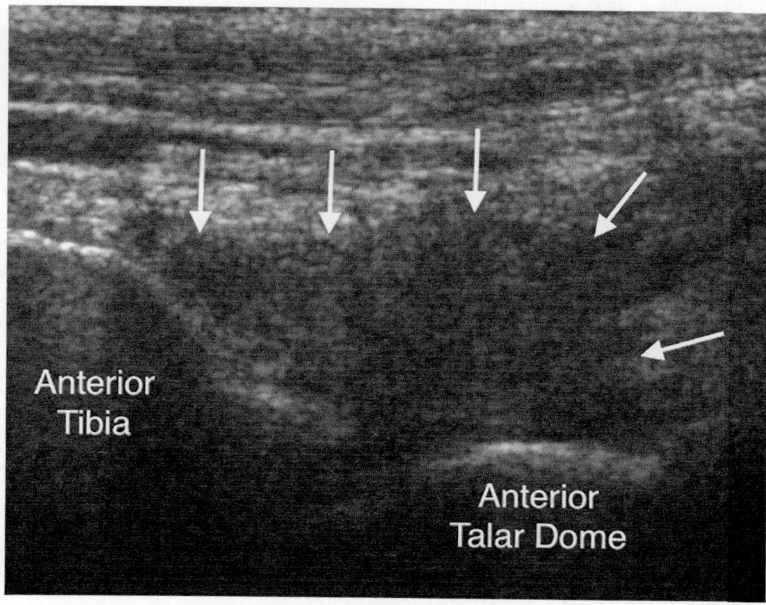

FIGURE 23.14 **Ultrasound of PVNS.** Longitudinal ultrasound image of the ankle of a 26-year-old woman demonstrates an intraarticular soft-tissue mass within the anterior aspect of the joint showing low reflectivity *(arrows)*. (Courtesy of Prof. Andrew J. Grainger, Cambridge, United Kingdom, from Greenspan A, Grainger AJ. Articular abnormalities that may mimic arthritis. *J Ultrason* 2018;18:212–223.)

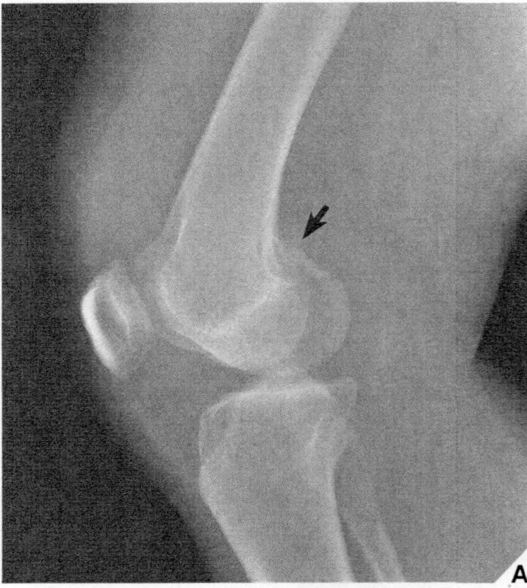
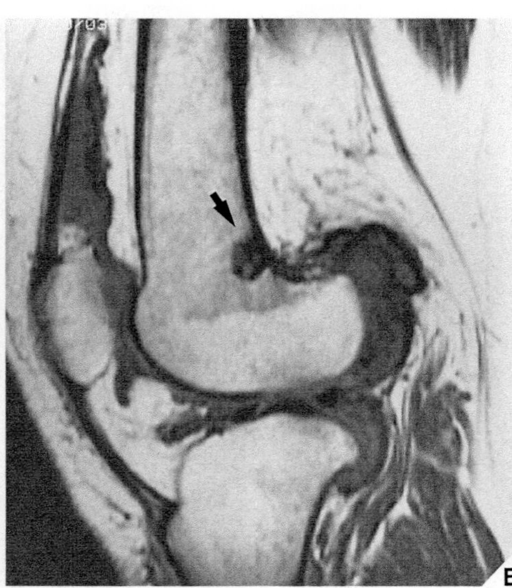
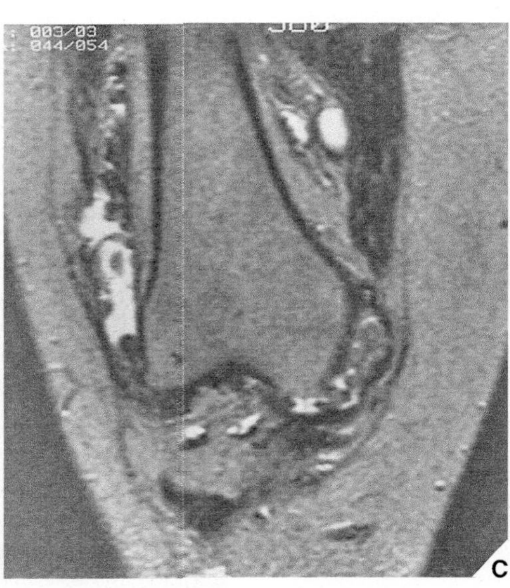

FIGURE 23.15 MRI of PVNS. A 22-year-old woman had several episodes of knee pain and swelling. Bloody fluid was aspirated from the knee joint on two occasions. **(A)** Lateral radiograph of the right knee shows fullness in the suprapatellar recess that was interpreted as "joint effusion." Note also the increased density in the region of the popliteal fossa and subtle erosion of the posterior aspect of the distal femur *(arrow)*. **(B)** Sagittal MRI (spin echo [SE]; repetition time [TR] 800/echo time [TE] 20 msec) shows a lobulated mass in the suprapatellar recess, extending into the knee joint and invading the infrapatellar fat. Note also the lobulated mass in the posterior aspect of the joint capsule, extending toward the proximal tibia. These masses demonstrate an intermediate-to-low signal intensity. The erosion at the posterior aspect of the distal femur (supracondylar) is clearly demonstrated by an area of low signal intensity *(arrow)*. **(C)** Coronal MRI (SE; TR 1,800/TE 80 msec) demonstrates areas of high signal intensity that represent fluid and congested synovium, interspersed with areas of intermediate to low signal intensity, characteristic of hemosiderin deposits.

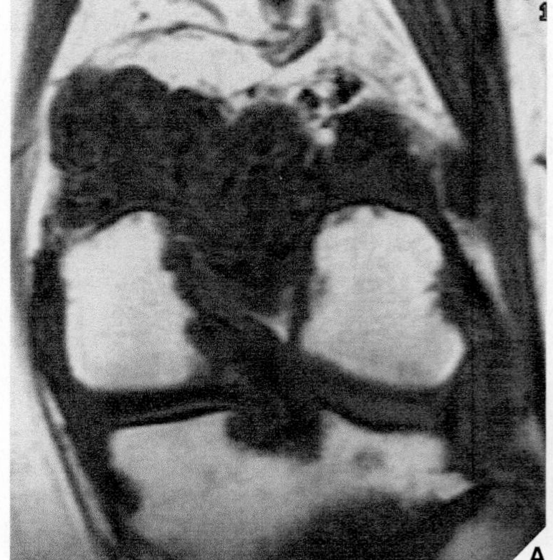
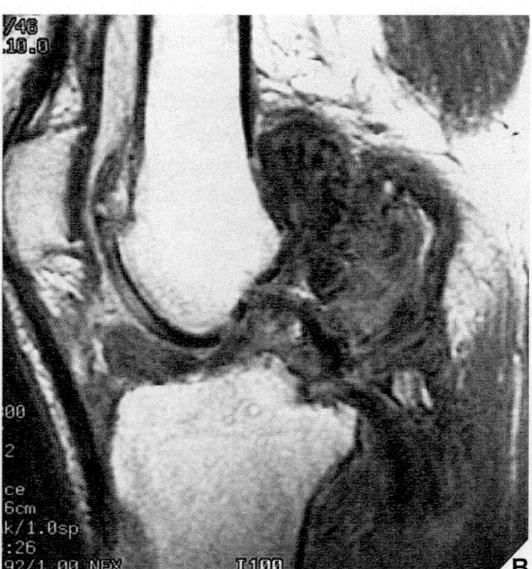
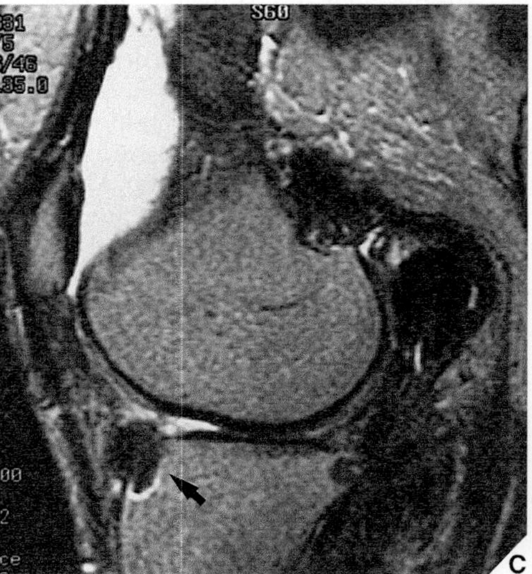

FIGURE 23.16 MRI of PVNS. **(A)** Coronal and **(B)** sagittal T1-weighted (spin echo [SE]; repetition time [TR] 600/echo time [TE] 12 msec) MR images of the knee of a 40-year-old man show lobulated low–signal intensity masses mainly localized to the popliteal fossa. **(C)** Sagittal T2-weighted (SE; TR 2,300/TE 80 msec) MR image shows high-intensity fluid in the suprapatellar recess. The lobulated masses of PVNS remain of low signal intensity. Note marginal erosion of the anterior tibia *(arrow)*.

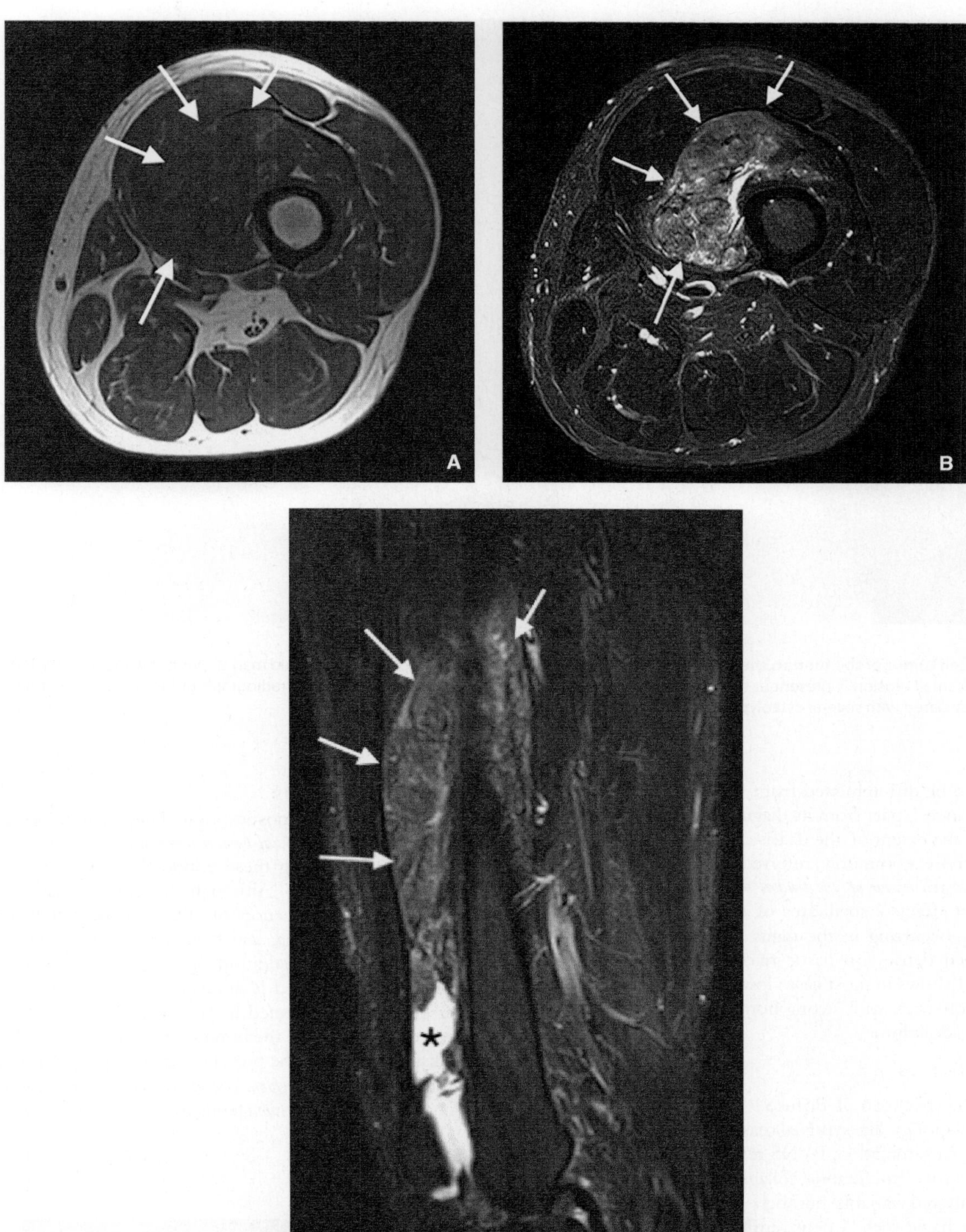

FIGURE 23.17 MRI of PVNS. **(A)** Axial T1-weighted MR image obtained at the level of suprapatellar recess of a 57-year-old man, who presented with a thigh mass, shows a mass arising from the suprapatellar recess exhibiting an intermediate signal intensity, isointense with skeletal muscles *(arrows)*. **(B)** Axial and **(C)** sagittal T2-weighted fat-suppressed MR images show the mass exhibiting intermediate-to-low signal with foci of high signal, representing synovium and fluid *(arrows)*. The sagittal image also reveals joint effusion *(asterisk)*. (Courtesy of Prof. Andrew J. Grainger, Cambridge, United Kingdom, from Greenspan A, Grainger AJ. Articular abnormalities that may mimic arthritis. *J Ultrason* 2018;18:212–223.)

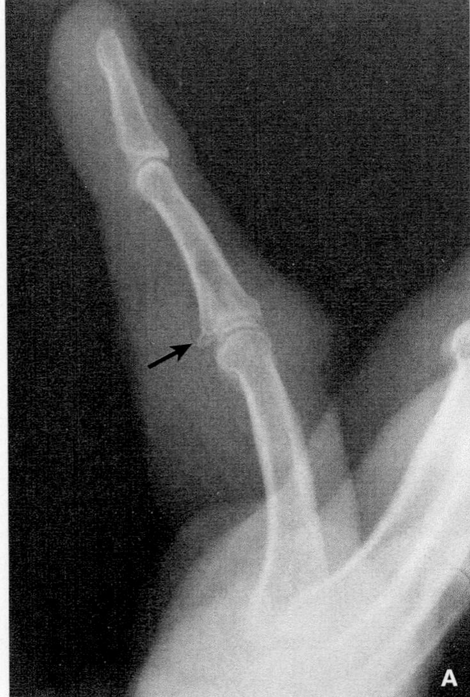

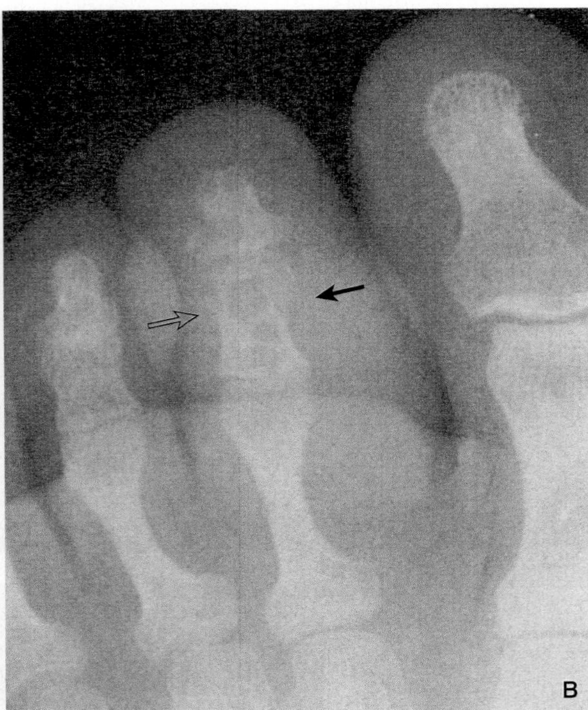

FIGURE 23.18 Giant cell tumor of the tendon sheath. **(A)** Lateral radiograph of the index finger of a 58-year-old man shows a soft-tissue mass at the site of the proximal interphalangeal joint. A small erosion is present at the base of the middle phalanx *(arrow)*. **(B)** Anteroposterior radiograph of the second toe of the middle-aged man shows a soft-tissue mass associated with several osteolytic defects in the middle phalanx *(arrows)*.

the synovium allows it to be differentiated from the fluid invariably present, which does not enhance. Apart from its diagnostic effectiveness, MRI is also useful in defining the extent of the disease.

Localized PVNS, more commonly referred to as *localized tenosynovial giant cell tumor* or *giant cell tumor of the tendon sheath,* presents as a well-circumscribed lesion that affects a small area of synovium or the tendon sheath, most commonly occurring in the digits. Radiography shows localized well-circumscribed dense soft-tissue mass often associated with erosion (Fig. 23.18). MRI shows in most cases low signal intensity on both T1- and T2-weighted sequences, with strong homogeneous enhancement after administration of gadolinium.

Pathology

Gross examination of the specimen of diffuse PVNS reveals tan-colored or reddish-brown firm or spongy-like synovial mass, with hypertrophic villi (Fig. 23.19). On histologic examination, PVNS reveals a tumor-like proliferation of the synovial tissue. Proliferating collagen-producing polyhedral cells are preset with scattered variable numbers of multinucleated giant cells surrounding hemorrhagic foci. A dense infiltration of mononuclear histiocytes is observed, accompanied by plasma cells, xanthoma cells, and lymphocytes. Mitotic figures are not uncommon. Variable amount of hemosiderin can be present. Long-standing lesions show fibrosis and hyalinization.

Gross specimen of a giant cell tumor of the tendon sheath demonstrates a well-circumscribed lobulated tumor, white-tan to gray in color with yellowish and brown foci, partially encased by a fibrous capsule. Invasion of bone or joint is commonly present (Fig. 23.20). Histopathology shows tissue composed of different proportions of small, round, or spindle-shaped mononuclear cells with pale cytoplasm and round or kidney-shaped frequently grooved nuclei, osteoclast-like multinucleated giant cells, foamy macrophages, and siderophages. Hemosiderin deposits are almost always present.

Immunochemistry, which is the same for both diffuse and localized forms, shows positivity for CD68, CD163, CD45, and some cases for CD34. Genetic abnormalities consist of translocation t(1;2)(p11;q37) with *COL6A3-CSF1* gene fusion. Rearrangements of the 1p11-13 region have also been reported.

Differential Diagnosis

The most common diagnostic possibilities include *hemophilic arthropathy*, *synovial chondromatosis*, *synovial hemangioma*, and *synovial sarcoma*. MRI is very effective in distinguishing these entities because it can reveal hemosiderin deposition in PVNS. Although this feature may also be present in *hemophilic arthropathy*, detection of diffuse hemosiderin clumps, synovial irregularity and thickening, and distention of the synovial sac favor the diagnosis of PVNS. In addition, hemophilia, unlike PVNS, commonly affects multiple joints and is associated with growth disturbance at the articular ends of the affected bones. *Synovial chondromatosis* may manifest with pressure erosions of the bone similar to those of PVNS. However, it can be distinguished by the presence of multiple joint bodies, calcified or uncalcified. *Synovial hemangioma* is commonly associated with the formation of phleboliths. *Synovial sarcoma* tends to have a shorter T1 and longer T2 on

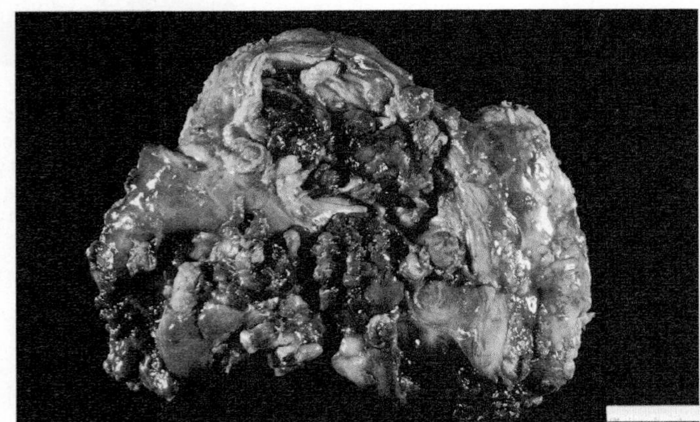

FIGURE 23.19 Pathology of PVNS. Photograph of the surgical specimen of the knee synovium shows plump papillary and villous projections of the lesion. The reddish-brown staining is due to hemosiderin deposition. (Courtesy of Michael J. Klein, MD, New York.)

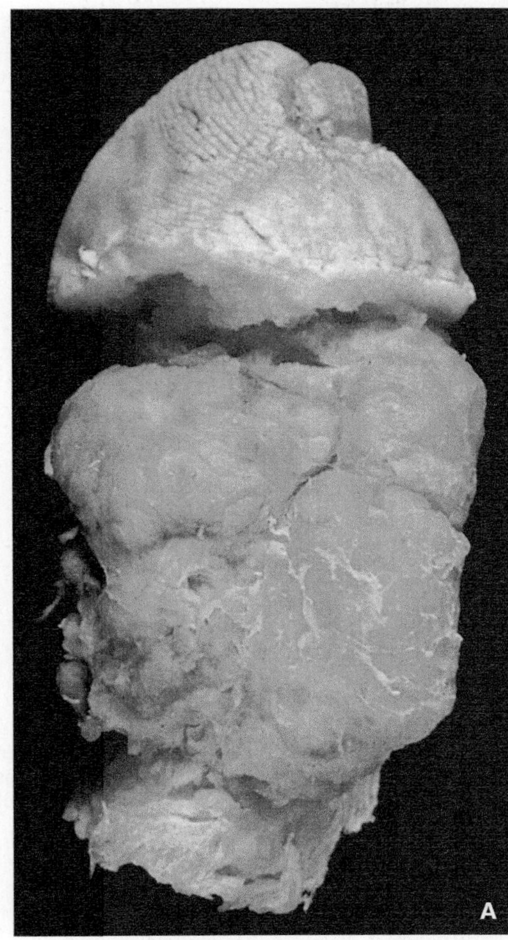

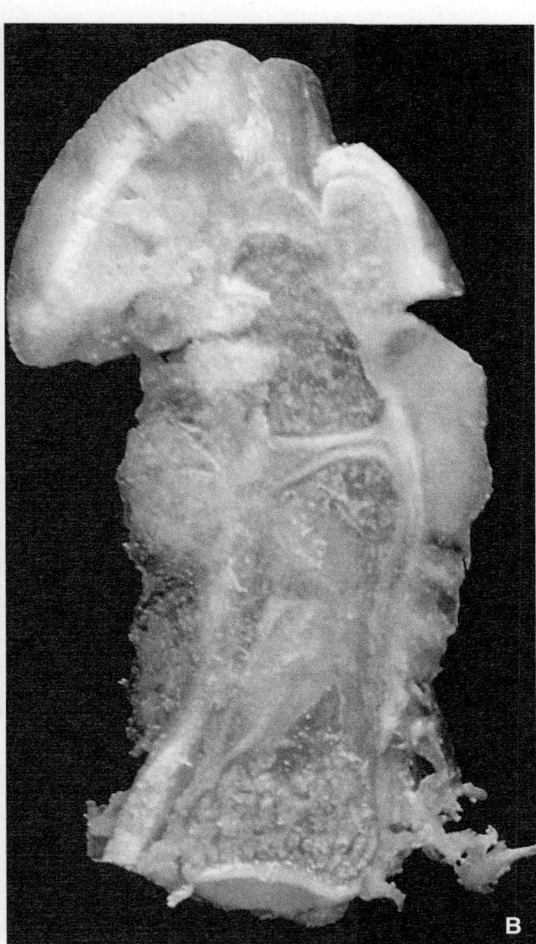

FIGURE 23.20 Pathology of giant cell tumor of the tendon sheath. **(A)** Photograph of the amputated second toe (same patient as depicted in Fig. 23.18B) shows a tan-reddish tumor encasing the middle phalanx. **(B)** Sagittal section through the specimen demonstrates soft-tissue tumor surrounding the middle phalanx and extending into the medullary cavity. It also invades the distal interphalangeal joint. (Modified from Bullough P. *Orthopaedic pathology*, 5th ed. Maryland Heights, MO: Mosby; 2009, with permission from Elsevier.)

MRI compared with PVNS, and when calcifications are present, the latter diagnosis can be excluded.

Differential diagnosis for localized giant cell tumor of the tendon sheath should include *enchondroma*, *soft-tissue chondroma*, and *gout*.

Treatment and Prognosis

Treatment usually consists of surgical open or arthroscopic synovectomy. Occasionally, intraarticular radiation synovectomy is used when the abnormal synovial tissue is less than 5 mm thick. Recently, reports appeared of postsynovectomy adjuvant treatment with external beam radiation therapy or intraarticular injection of radioactive material such as yttrium-90 (^{90}Y). Local recurrence is not uncommon and is reported in approximately 50% of cases.

Synovial Hemangioma

Clinical Features

Synovial hemangioma is a rare benign lesion that most commonly affects the knee joint, usually involving the anterior compartment. This lesion has also been found in the elbow, wrist, and ankle joints as well as in bursae and tendon sheaths. Most cases affect children and adolescents. Almost all patients with synovial hemangioma are symptomatic, frequently presenting with a swollen knee or with mild pain or limitation of movement in the joint. Sometimes patients report a history of recurrent episodes of joint swelling and various degrees of pain of several years' duration. Synovial hemangioma is often associated with an adjacent cutaneous or deep soft-tissue hemangioma. For this reason, some investigators classify knee joint lesions as intraarticular, juxtaarticular, or intermediate, depending on the extent of involvement. Synovial hemangioma is frequently misdiagnosed. According to one estimate, a correct preoperative diagnosis is made in only 22% of cases.

Imaging Features

Synovial hemangiomas used to be evaluated by a combination of conventional radiography, arthrography, angiography, and contrast-enhanced CT. Although radiographs appear normal in at least half of the patients, they may reveal soft-tissue swelling, a mass around the joint, joint effusion, or erosions (Fig. 23.21). Phleboliths, periosteal thickening, advanced maturation of the epiphysis, and arthritic changes are also occasionally noted on conventional radiographs. Arthrography usually shows nonspecific filling defects with a villous configuration. Ultrasound has limitations in assessing some joint recesses because it may be challenging to find a sonographic window. However, when the hemangioma is identified, it typically appears as a vascular mass of heterogenous hypoechogenicity. Phleboliths, when present, will be seen as brightly echogenic foci within the lesion. Vascular channels may be identified, depending on their size. Doppler examination may demonstrate flow within the vessels, which may be high or slow flow depending on the nature of the lesion (Fig. 23.22). Angiograms yield much more specific information than radiography or ultrasound. They can often reveal a vascular lesion and can demonstrate pathognomonic features of hemangioma. Contrast-enhanced CT of the joint typically reveals a heterogeneous-appearing soft-tissue mass that displays tissue attenuation approximating that of skeletal muscle and containing areas of decreased attenuation, some

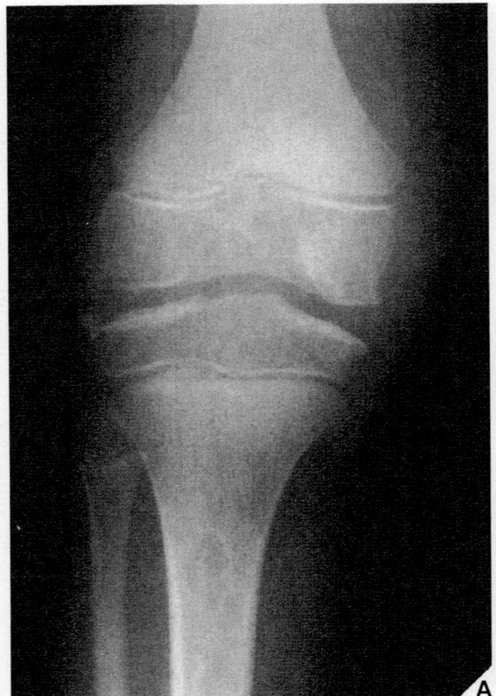

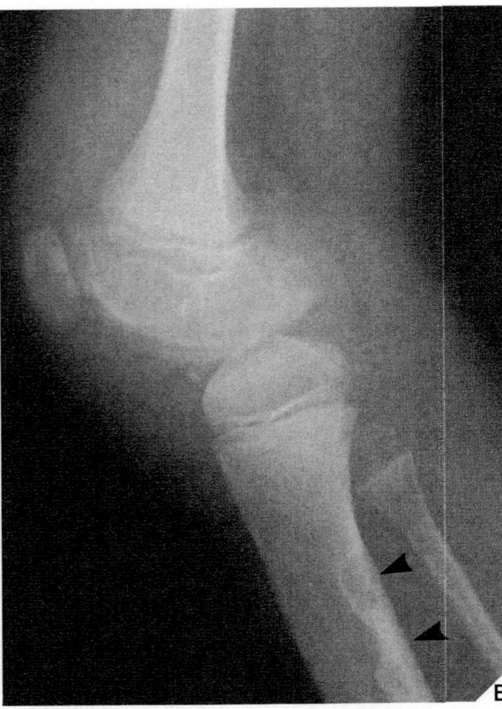

FIGURE 23.21 Synovial hemangioma. **(A)** Anteroposterior and **(B)** lateral radiographs of the right knee of a 7-year-old boy show articular erosions at femoropatellar and femorotibial joint compartments. Soft-tissue masses are seen anteriorly and posteriorly. An incidental finding is a nonossifying fibroma in the posterior tibia *(arrowheads)*. (Reprinted with permission from Greenspan A, Remagen W. *Differential diagnosis of tumors and tumor-like lesions*. Philadelphia: Lippincott-Raven Publishers; 1998.)

approaching that of fat. CT is effective for demonstrating phleboliths and revealing patchy enhancement around them as well as enhancement of tubular areas and contrast pooling within the lesion. In some cases, CT reveals enlarged vessels feeding and draining the mass, as well as enlarged adjacent subcutaneous veins.

At present, MRI has become the modality of choice for the evaluation of hemangiomas because with this modality, a presumptive diagnosis can be made. The soft-tissue mass typically exhibits an intermediate signal intensity on T1-weighted sequences, appearing isointense with or slightly brighter than muscle but much less bright than fat. The mass is usually much brighter than subcutaneous fat on T2-weighted images and on fat suppression sequences (Figs. 23.23 and 23.24; see also Fig. 23.22C,D) and shows thin, often serpentine, low-intensity septa within it. In general, the signal intensity characteristics of hemangiomas appear to be related to a number of factors, including slow flow, thrombosis, vessel occlusion, and stagnant blood that pools in larger vessels and dilated sinuses as well as to the variable amounts of adipose tissue in the lesion. After intravenous injection of gadolinium, there is evidence of enhancement of the hemangioma. In patients with a cavernous hemangioma of the knee, fluid–fluid levels are also observed (Fig. 23.24C), a finding recently reported also in soft-tissue hemangiomas of this type.

Pathology

Originating in the subsynovial layer mesenchyme of the synovial membrane, synovial hemangioma is a vascular lesion that contains variable amounts of adipose, fibrous, and muscle tissue as well as thrombi in the vessels. When the lesion is completely intraarticular, it is usually well circumscribed and apparently encapsulated, attached to the synovial membrane by a pedicle of variable size, and adherent to the synovium on one or more surfaces by separable adhesions. Grossly, the tumor is a lobulated soft, brown, doughy mass with overlying villous synovium that is often stained mahogany brown by hemosiderin (Fig. 23.25). On microscopic examination, the lesion exhibits arborizing vascular channels of different sizes and a hyperplastic overlying synovium, which may show abundant iron deposition in chronic cases with repeated hemarthrosis. Some lesions may show villous hyperplasia of the synovium.

Differential Diagnosis

The differential diagnosis of synovial hemangioma includes *PVNS* and *synovial chondromatosis*. All proliferative chronic inflammatory processes, such as rheumatoid arthritis, tuberculous arthritis, and hemophilic arthropathy, should also be considered in the differential diagnosis, but these conditions, when involving the knee, can usually be distinguished clinically. Because it is extremely uncommon, lipoma arborescens is rarely included in the differential diagnosis. MRI is diagnostic for the latter condition, showing typical frond-like projections of the lesion and fat characteristics (bright on T1- and intermediate on T2-weighted images). In *PVNS*, radiography commonly reveals findings similar to those of synovial hemangioma, such as joint effusion and a mass in the suprapatellar recess or popliteal fossa region. Radiographs may also demonstrate bone erosions on both sides of the joint. MRI, however, is usually diagnostic for PVNS, demonstrating that the synovium exhibits nodular thickening and masses of heterogeneous signal intensity. Most of the lesion will display a higher signal intensity than muscle on both T1- and T2-weighted sequences, with other portions exhibiting a low signal intensity on all sequences, reflecting the hemosiderin content of the tumor. *Synovial chondromatosis* can be distinguished from synovial hemangioma if radiography shows calcified bodies. Intraarticular osteochondral fragments of uniform size are almost pathognomonic for this condition. CT may be helpful in demonstrating faint calcifications not otherwise seen.

Treatment and Prognosis

Small lesions can be removed completely without risk of local recurrence. Prognosis is excellent in majority of cases.

Lipoma Arborescens

Clinical Features

Lipoma arborescens, also known as *villous lipomatous proliferation of the synovial membranes*, is a rare intraarticular disorder characterized by nonneoplastic lipomatous proliferation of the synovium. The term *arborescens* (from the Latin word *arbor*, meaning tree) describes the characteristic tree-like morphology of the hypertrophied synovium, which exhibits a frond-like appearance. The term *lipoma* is a misnomer because there is no focal mass.

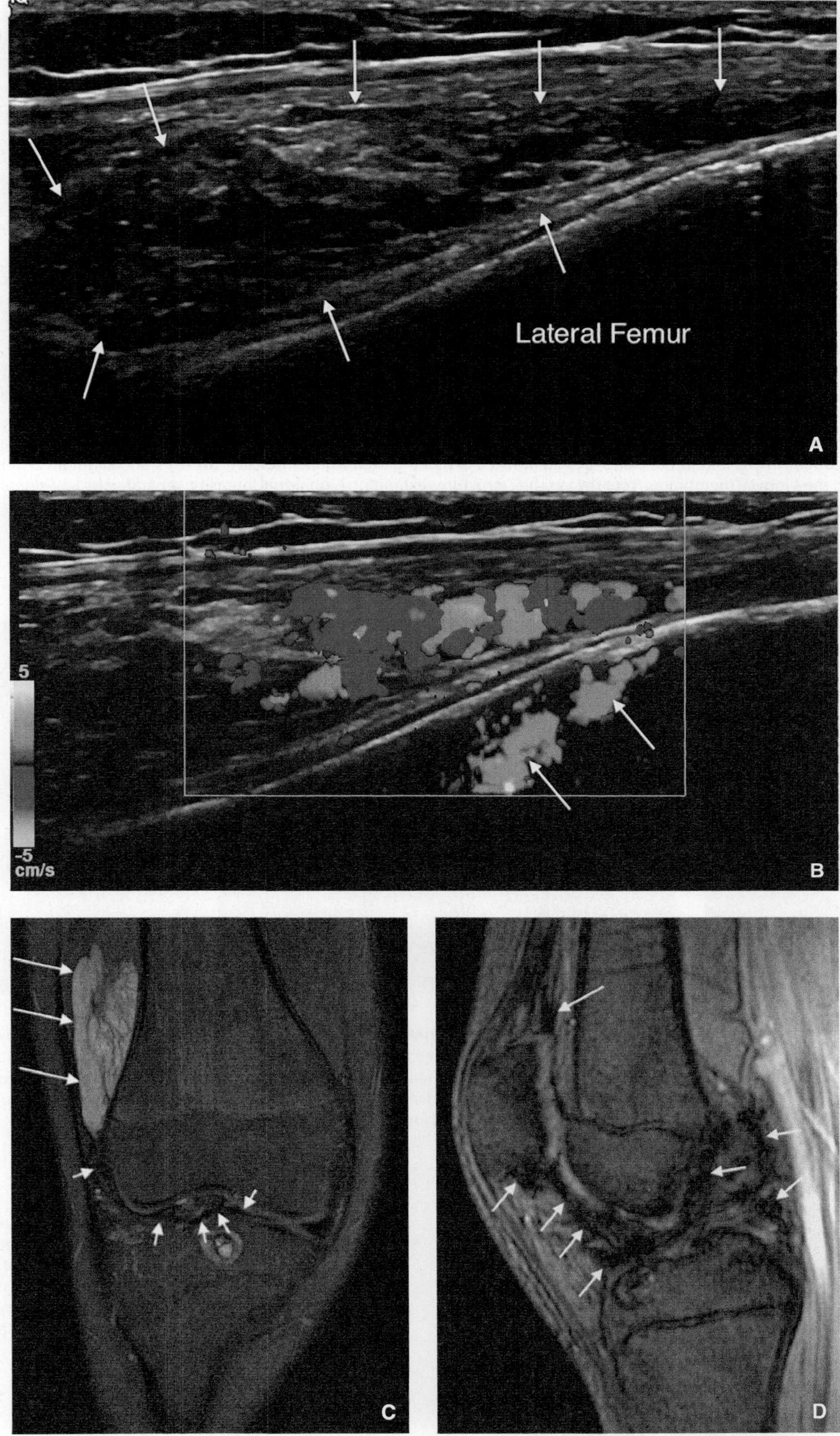

FIGURE 23.22 Ultrasound and MRI of synovial hemangioma. (A) Longitudinal ultrasound of the knee of a 17-year-old girl, who presented with a history of recurrent hemarthrosis and palpable mass over anterolateral aspect of the knee, shows a heterogenous predominantly hyporeflective mass alongside the lateral femoral metaphysis *(arrows)*. **(B)** Color Doppler examination demonstrates flow in the torturous vessels within the lesion. The apparent "flow" within the femur *(arrows)* is caused by reverberation artefact. **(C)** Coronal proton density–weighted fat-suppressed MR image of the knee shows the mass exhibiting high signal intensity with some internal low-signal septations and striation *(long arrows)*. Note also a low-signal foci in the joint *(short arrows)* due to hemosiderin-laden synovium from recurrent hemarthrosis. **(D)** Sagittal gradient-echo MR image shows a typical blooming artefact from the joint due to a susceptibility artefact from the hemosiderin *(arrows)*. (Courtesy of Prof. Andrew J. Grainger, Cambridge, United Kingdom, from Greenspan A, Grainger AJ. Articular abnormalities that may mimic arthritis. *J Ultrason* 2018;18:212–223.)

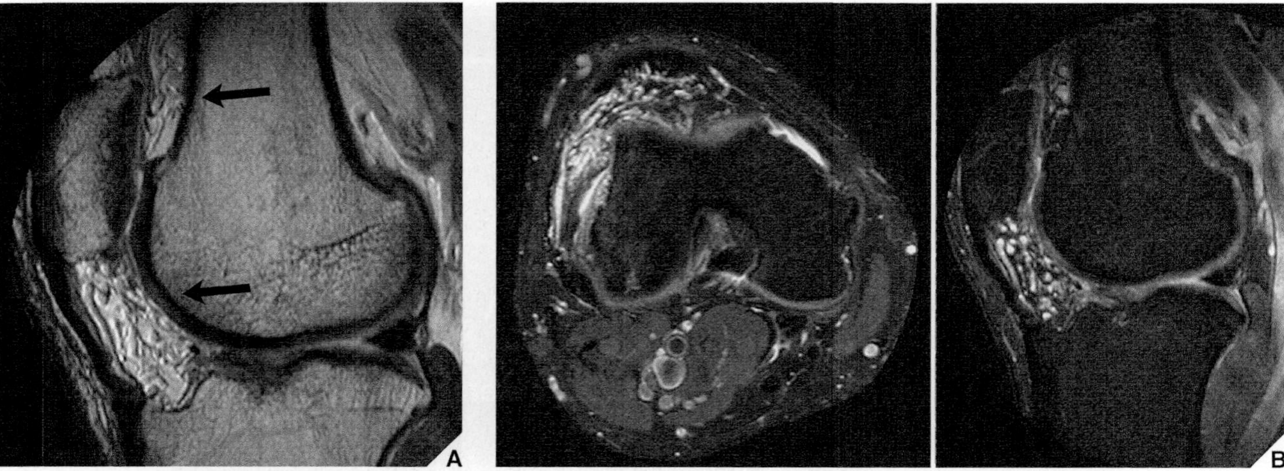

FIGURE 23.23 MRI of synovial hemangioma. **(A)** Sagittal T1-weighted MR image of the knee of a 34-year-old man shows lace-like pattern of several vascular channels within the femoropatellar joint compartment and in the Hoffa fat pad *(arrows)* exhibiting high signal intensity. **(B)** Axial and sagittal T2-weighted MR images confirm the presence of hemangiomas within the synovial membrane. Note the vascular structures exhibiting high signal intensity, separated by low-signal linear structures, representing fibro-fatty septa.

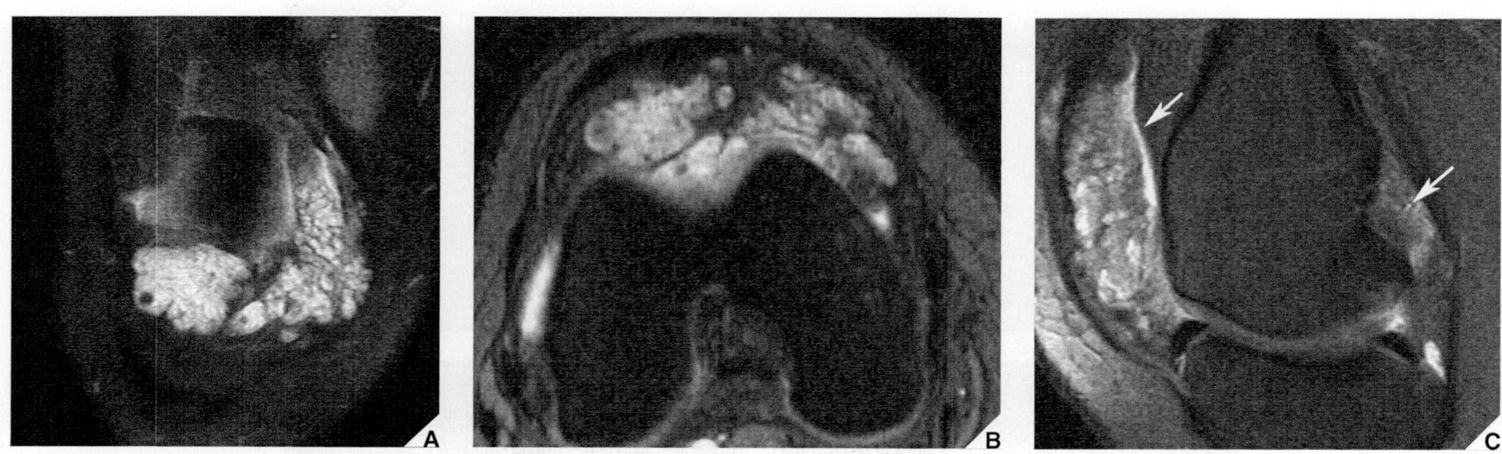

FIGURE 23.24 MRI of synovial hemangioma. **(A)** Coronal proton density–weighted MRI of the knee demonstrates an intraarticular hyperintense lesion with a lace-like pattern of multiple vascular channels extending from the medial aspect of the knee to the region of the infrapatellar fad pad. **(B)** Axial gradient recalled echo (GRE) MRI shows the multiple vascular channels separated by fibrous septa and extending to the infrapatellar fat pad. **(C)** Sagittal T1-weighted fat-saturated MRI obtained following intravenous administration of gadolinium demonstrates partial enhancement of the distended vascular channels and multiple small fluid–fluid levels corresponding to the "cavernous" nature of the tumor. Note the extension into the suprapatellar recess and into the posterior aspect of the joint *(arrows)*.

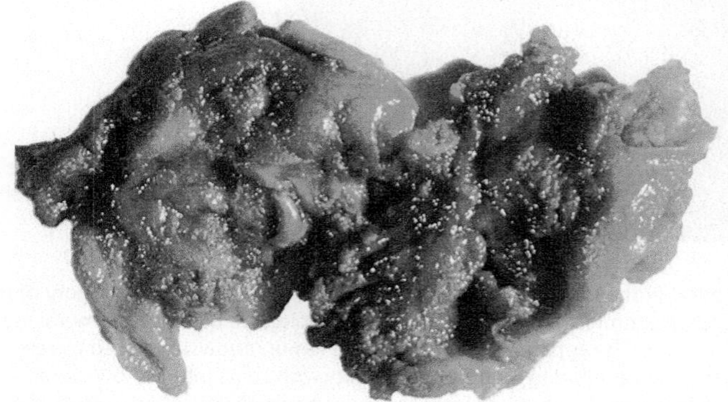

FIGURE 23.25 Pathology of synovial hemangioma. Surgical specimen removed from the knee joint shows strawberry-like appearance of the synovial lining and marked hemosiderin staining of the tissue. (Reprinted from Bullough P. *Orthopaedic pathology*, 5th ed. Maryland Heights, MO: Mosby; 2009, with permission from Elsevier.)

It has been suggested that a more appropriate term for this condition would be *synovial lipomatosis*. Lipoma arborescens may be monoarticular or polyarticular. The cause of this disorder remains uncertain, although association with osteoarthritis, rheumatoid arthritis, psoriasis, and diabetes mellitus has been postulated. This lesion most commonly affects the knee joint, although involvement of other joints, such as shoulder, hip, wrist, elbow, and ankle, has been sporadically reported by various authors. Occasionally, this condition may affect multiple joints. There have been also sporadic reports of bursae and tendon sheaths involvement. It is more prevalent in males, usually between the fourth and seventh decades. These patients present with slowly increasing but painless joint effusion accompanied by synovial thickening.

Imaging Features

Imaging studies, particularly MRI, are very characteristic and allow definite diagnosis of this condition. Joint effusion is invariably present, associated with frond-like masses arising from the synovium that have the signal intensity of fat on all imaging sequences (Figs. 23.26 and 23.27). Occasionally, a chemical shift artifact is present at the fat–fluid interface. Ultrasound typically shows lipoma arborescens as a synovial-based hyperechoic frond-like mass, associated with joint effusion (Fig. 23.28).

Pathology

Histopathologically, lipoma arborescens is characterized by hyperplasia of subsynovial fat, formation of mature fat cells, and the presence of proliferative villous projections. Osseous and chondroid metaplasia can occur.

Differential Diagnosis and Treatment

Differential diagnosis should include PVNS, synovial chondromatosis, synovial hemangioma, hemophilic arthropathy, and a variety of intraarticular inflammatory conditions.

Treatment usually consists of surgical open or arthroscopic synovectomy. Recurrences are uncommon.

Malignant Tumors

Synovial Sarcoma

Clinical Features

Synovial sarcoma (synovioma, synovioblastic sarcoma) is an uncommon mesenchymal neoplasm, comprising approximately 8% to 10% of soft-tissue sarcomas. Despite its name (which was designated because of histologic resemblance of synovial sarcoma to normal synovial tissue), it does not arise from synovium, although it may originate from any other structure, including joint capsules, bursae, and tendon sheaths. The tumor usually occurs before age 50, most commonly between ages 15 and 40 years. There is no gender predilection. The extremities account for 80% to 90% of synovial sarcomas, and the most common sites are around the knee and foot. In exceptional instances, the tumor may be intraarticular. Synovial sarcoma is usually slow growing, with an indolent course, although in late stages it may demonstrate aggressiveness. Metastases to the lung by the hematogenous route and to the soft tissue have been reported. Schajowicz cited a local recurrence rate of more than 50%. The clinical symptoms usually include soft-tissue swelling or a mass and progressive pain. On physical examination, a diffuse or discrete soft-tissue mass is present, usually tender on palpation.

Imaging Features

The imaging features of synovial sarcoma include a soft-tissue mass, usually in close proximity to a joint (Fig. 23.29A) and occasionally associated with bone invasion (Fig. 23.29B). A periosteal reaction may also be observed. The soft-tissue calcifications, usually amorphous in type, are present in approximately 25% to 30% of cases, commonly located at the periphery of the tumor. Less frequently, a central punctuate calcific pattern may be seen. Rarely, extensive calcifications or ossifications resembling an osteoid matrix or bone can be present. This presentation may lead to erroneous diagnosis including soft-tissue osteosarcoma or chondrosarcoma, synovial chondromatosis, myositis ossificans, or tumoral calcinosis.

Scintigraphic evaluation reveals increased uptake of radiopharmaceutical agent on blood flow and blood pool images consistent with increased vascularity of these tumors (Fig. 23.30).

CT effectively demonstrates the extent of the soft-tissue mass, calcifications, and bone invasion. This modality also is effective to assess the chest for pulmonary metastases. MRI shows the tumor to be heterogeneous, multilobulated septated mass of low-to-intermediate signal intensity with infiltrative margins on T1-weighted sequences, displaying a high signal on T2 weighting (Fig. 23.31), and diffuse but heterogenous enhancement after administration of gadolinium (Figs. 23.31E and 23.32). The most extensive to date MRI study of synovial sarcoma in 34 patients reported by Jones and associates showed that it tends to be deep, large (85% were greater than 5 cm in diameter), and located in the extremities, with epicenter close to the joint. The lesion was usually heterogeneous on T2-weighted images and was clearly delineated from surrounding tissues. Forty-four percent of the cases had a high signal on both T1- and T2-weighted sequences, consistent with hemorrhage within the tumor. Several investigators consider so-called *triple signal intensity sign*, due to a combination of cystic and solid elements, fibrous tissue, hemorrhage, and hemosiderin deposition, as the most characteristic for this tumor (see Figs. 23.31D and 23.32E). Some multilobulated tumors may contain septa and fluid–fluid levels, creating the "bowl of grapes" sign. During the slow growth phase, synovial sarcoma may exhibit a relatively "benign" appearance on MRI, with a low–signal intensity capsule and relatively uniform signal intensity of the tumor, resembling benign tumors such as schwannoma (Fig. 23.33).

Pathology

Gross specimen shows tan or gray commonly multinodular soft mass, occasionally multicystic, sometimes with areas of hemorrhage and necrosis (Fig. 23.34). On histopathologic examination, several subtypes of synovial sarcoma have been recognized. Among them are biphasic (fibrous and epithelial), monophasic (the most common subtype), purely glandular, calcifying, and poorly differentiated variants. The classical biphasic type exhibits distinct spindle-cell and epithelial components arranged in glandular or nest-like patterns. Spindle cells are small and fairly uniform with ovoid, pale-staining nuclei. The monophasic synovial sarcoma is composed of interdigitating fascicles and "ball-like" structures formed by the spindle cells. The calcifying variant shows spindle-cell elements and calcifications localized to areas of hyalinization.

Immunohistochemistry shows positivity for cytokeratins 7, 8, 14, and 19 and epithelial membrane antigen (EMA) in the epithelial areas. In addition, there is positivity for CD99 and BCL2, and negativity for CD34. A consistent finding, present in about 90% of tumors, is a cytogenetic aberration of translocation involving chromosomes X and 18 [t(x;18)(p11.2;q11.2)], resulting in fusion of *SYT* gene (also known as *SS18* or *SSXT*, encoding 55-kDa protein) to either *SSX1* or *SSX2*. A minority of cases have a gene rearrangement involving *SSX4*.

Differential Diagnosis

Differential diagnosis should include benign conditions, such as soft-tissue chondroma, myositis ossificans, tumoral calcinosis, and gout, and malignant tumors such as soft-tissue osteosarcoma and soft-tissue chondrosarcoma.

Treatment and Prognosis

Treatment includes a wide local resection, followed with adjuvant chemotherapy with combination of cisplatin, vincristine, doxorubicin, and ifosfamide. Postoperative radiation therapy is reserved for the patients in whom surgical intervention was not able to ascertain clear margins of resection. In some cases, amputation of a limb remains a treatment of choice. Local recurrences and metastatic spread of the tumor are common complications. Best prognosis is if tumors are smaller than 5 cm.

Synovial Chondrosarcoma

Clinical Features

Synovial chondrosarcoma is a rare tumor that originates from the synovial membrane. It may arise as a primary synovial tumor or it may develop as a malignant transformation of synovial (osteo)chondromatosis. The concept

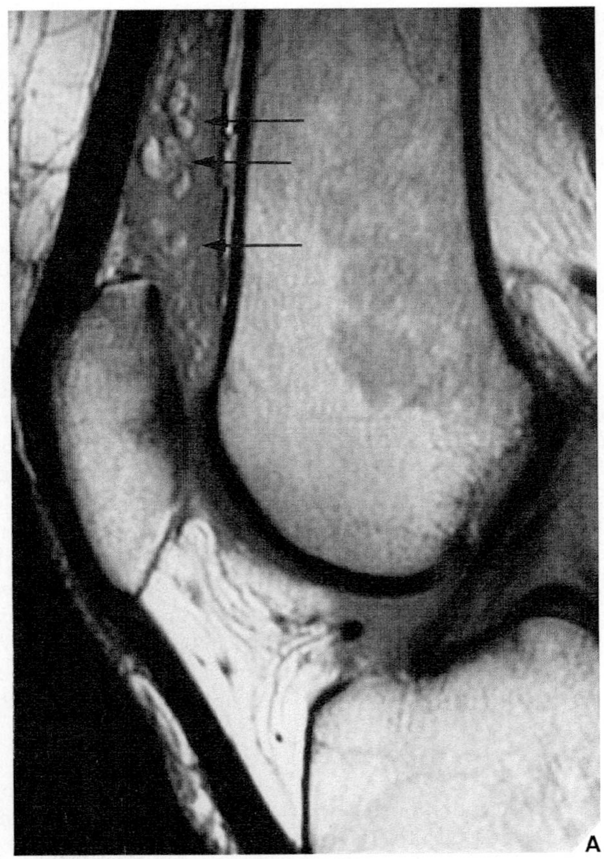

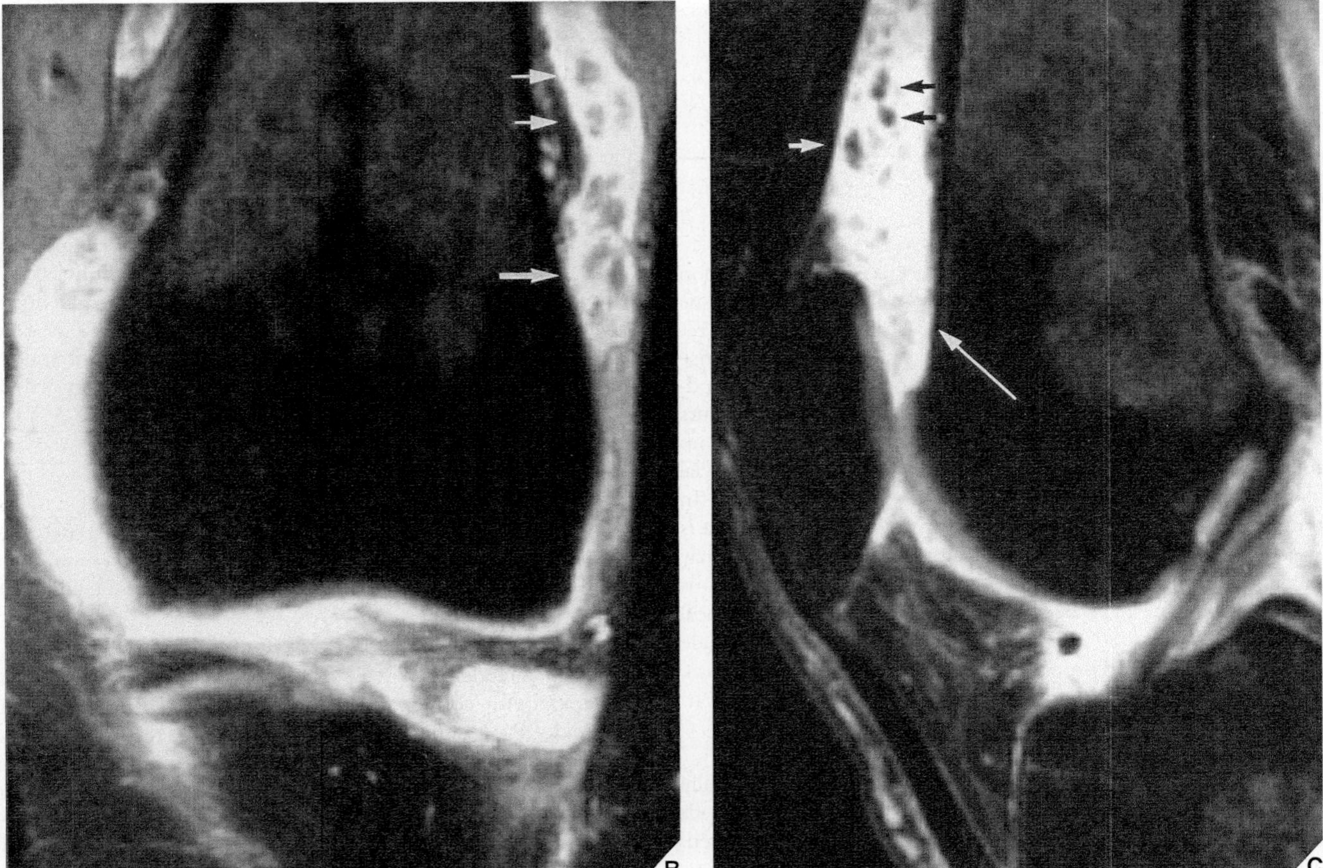

FIGURE 23.26 MRI of lipoma arborescens. A 54-year-old woman reports fullness in the left knee for the past 5 months. Conventional radiography (not shown here) revealed knee joint effusion. **(A)** Sagittal proton density MRI shows numerous structures within suprapatellar recess exhibiting signal intensity consistent with fat *(arrows)*. **(B)** Coronal and **(C)** sagittal T2-weighted fat-suppressed images demonstrate high–signal intensity joint effusion *(long arrow)*. Hypertrophic synovial villa *(short arrows)* again shows signal consistent with fat.

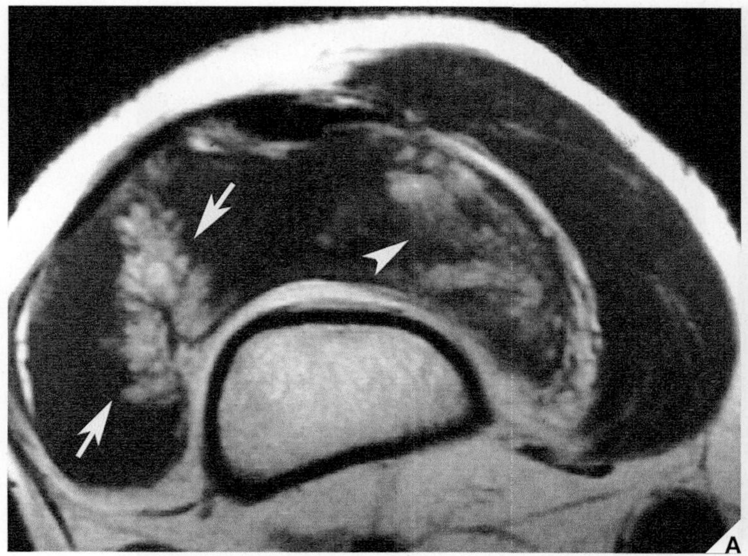

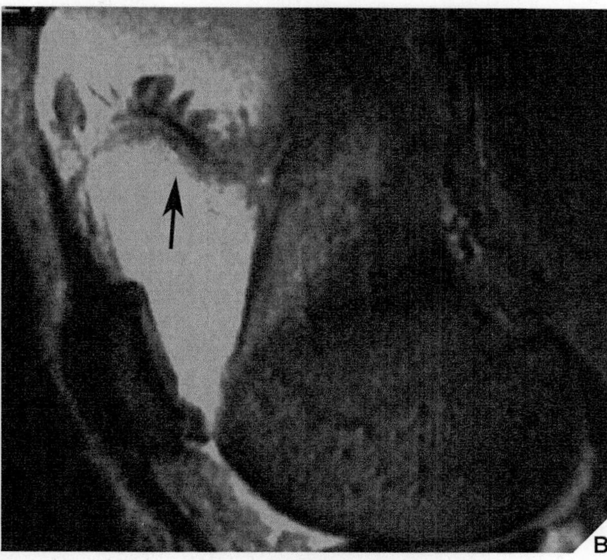

FIGURE 23.27 MRI of lipoma arborescens. **(A)** Axial T1-weighted MRI demonstrates an intraarticular "tree-like" lipomatous mass in the fluid-distended suprapatellar recess of the knee joint *(arrows)*. Note additional intraarticular lipomatous growths in the medial aspect of the suprapatellar recess *(arrowhead)*. **(B)** Sagittal T2-weighted MRI demonstrates the tree-like lipoma arborescens in the suprapatellar recess *(arrow)*.

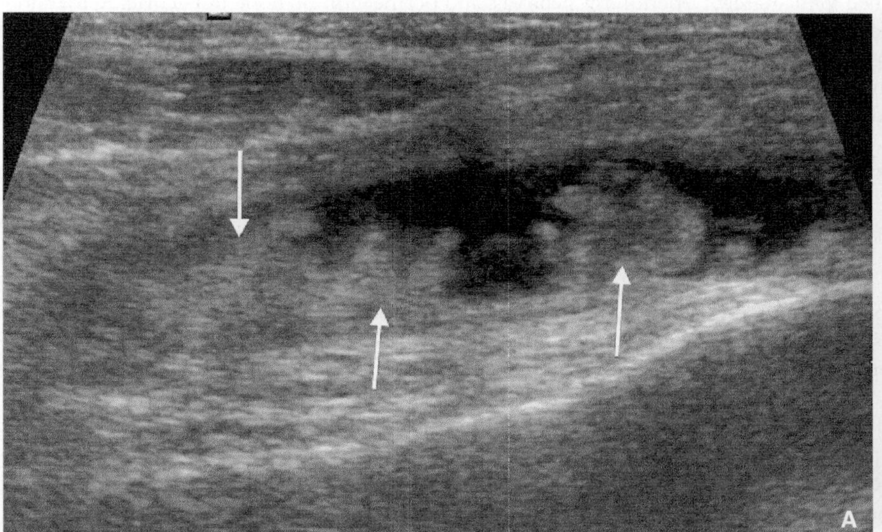

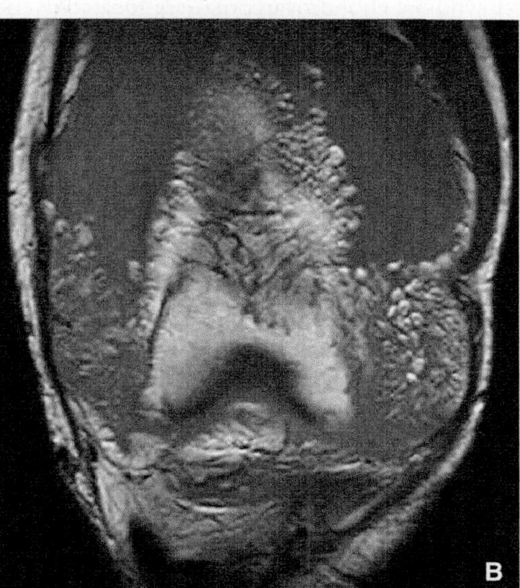

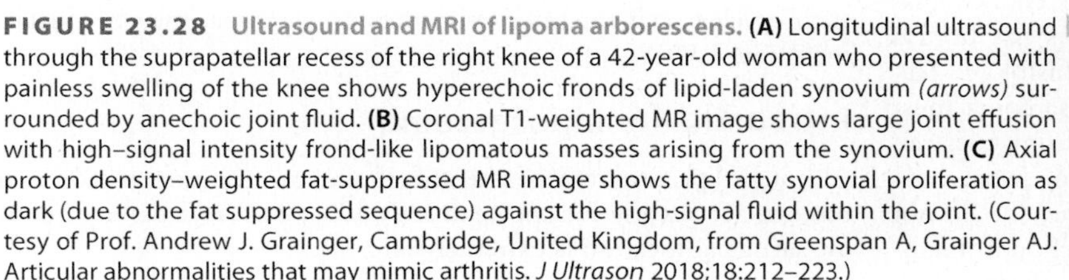

FIGURE 23.28 Ultrasound and MRI of lipoma arborescens. **(A)** Longitudinal ultrasound through the suprapatellar recess of the right knee of a 42-year-old woman who presented with painless swelling of the knee shows hyperechoic fronds of lipid-laden synovium *(arrows)* surrounded by anechoic joint fluid. **(B)** Coronal T1-weighted MR image shows large joint effusion with high–signal intensity frond-like lipomatous masses arising from the synovium. **(C)** Axial proton density–weighted fat-suppressed MR image shows the fatty synovial proliferation as dark (due to the fat suppressed sequence) against the high-signal fluid within the joint. (Courtesy of Prof. Andrew J. Grainger, Cambridge, United Kingdom, from Greenspan A, Grainger AJ. Articular abnormalities that may mimic arthritis. *J Ultrason* 2018;18:212–223.)

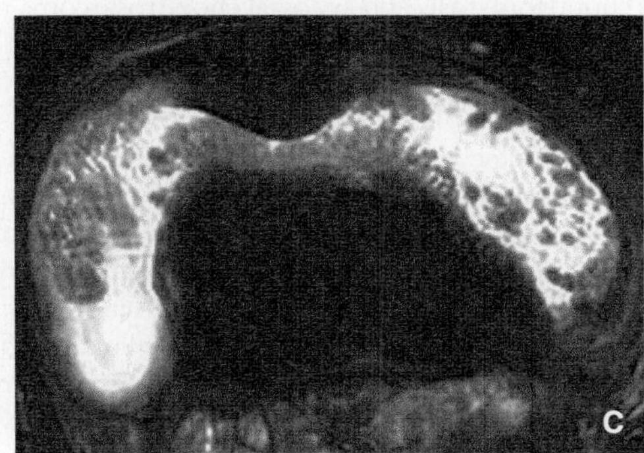

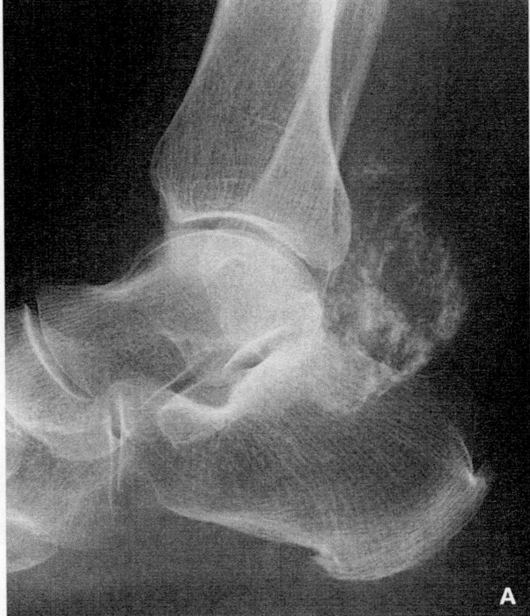

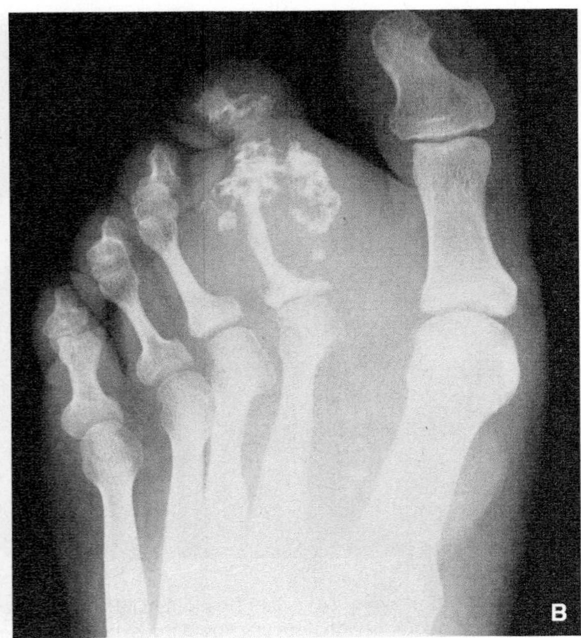

FIGURE 23.29 Synovial sarcoma. **(A)** Lateral radiograph of the left ankle of a 71-year-old woman shows a large calcified mass located in the soft tissues anteriorly to the Achilles tendon, not affecting the adjacent bones. **(B)** Dorsoplantar radiograph of the right foot of a 55-year-old woman shows a large soft-tissue mass with coarse calcifications, eroding the proximal phalanx of the second toe. (**B**, Reprinted with permission from Greenspan A, Borys D. *Radiology and pathology correlation of bone tumors: a quick reference and review*. Philadelphia: Wolters Kluwer; 2016:370, Fig. 8.26B.)

of malignant degeneration of synovial chondromatosis is still controversial and the entity is rare, with fewer than 40 well-documented cases on record.

Most synovial chondrosarcomas are located in the knee joint. Rarely, other joints such as the hip, elbow, or ankle are affected. Involvement of the small joints of the hands is exceedingly rare. These malignancies show a slight predominance in men, and patients range in age from 25 to 70 years. The symptoms include pain and swelling, with duration in most patients exceeding 12 months. In patients with primary synovial (osteo) chondromatosis, malignant transformation to synovial chondrosarcoma should be clinically suspected if there is development of soft-tissue mass at the site of the affected joint.

Imaging Features

Radiologically, the presence of chondroid calcifications within the joint, destruction of the adjacent bones, and a soft-tissue mass are highly suggestive of a synovial chondrosarcoma. In a few documented cases, MRI showed lobular soft-tissue masses within the joint exhibiting heterogenous but predominantly isointense to muscle signal on T1- and hyperintense signal on T2-weighted images. In patients with documented primary synovial (osteo)chondromatosis, a soft-tissue mass and destructive changes in the joint should suggest the development of a secondary synovial chondrosarcoma (Fig. 23.35). Note, however, that frequently both uncomplicated synovial chondromatosis and synovial chondrosarcoma may exhibit similar features on radiography and MRI.

Pathology

The histopathologic distinction between primary synovial chondromatosis and secondary malignancy in synovial chondromatosis has been a matter of dispute. Manivel and associates suggested that histologic features equivalent to those of grade 2 or 3 central chondrosarcoma must be present before chondrosarcoma arising in synovial chondromatosis can be diagnosed. Occasional foci of increased cellularity showing hyperchromatic atypical cells, consistent with grade 1 chondrosarcoma, should not be sufficient evidence for a malignant change in synovial chondromatosis. However, evidence of aggressive growth (invasion) and a lesion's lack of attachment to the synovial lining, combined with hypercellularity and pleomorphisms of the cells, should support the diagnosis of malignancy. Bertoni and coworkers have attempted to develop criteria for making this crucial distinction. They identified several microscopic features indicative of malignancy. The distinguishing features of synovial chondrosarcoma include the following: tumor cells arranged in sheets, myxoid changes in the matrix, hypercellularity with crowding and spindling of nuclei at the periphery, necrosis, and permeation of bone trabeculae. Remarking on the danger of misinterpreting synovial chondromatosis as chondrosarcoma on both radiographic and histopathologic examination, Bertoni and colleagues singled out pulmonary metastases as the only distinguishing feature.

Differential Diagnosis

The main differential diagnosis is between synovial chondrosarcoma and synovial (osteo)chondromatosis. Frequently, the imaging findings in both conditions are similar, although the development of destructive changes around the affected joint favors synovial chondrosarcoma. However, these destructive changes should be differentiated from periarticular erosions occasionally present in synovial chondromatosis. PVNS can usually be excluded without much difficulty because it does not exhibit calcifications and, in addition, shows rather characteristic MRI features (see previous text).

Malignant Pigmented Villonodular Synovitis

Kalil and Unni reported a case of malignancy in PVNS and cited eight other cases from the literature. Enzinger and Weiss defined malignant PVNS as a malignant lesion occurring with concomitant or previously documented benign PVNS at the same location. Bertoni and coworkers documented histologic evolution from benign to malignant PVNS in three cases. The malignancy in PVNS is an extremely rare occurrence, yet this is a controversial issue, mainly because other synovium-centered lesions, such as clear cell sarcoma or epithelioid sarcoma, may be mistaken for malignant PVNS.

Intraarticular Liposarcoma

Although liposarcomas of the soft tissues are not uncommon malignant tumors, accounting for approximately 16% of all soft-tissue sarcomas, the intraarticular location is extremely rare.

Intraarticular low-grade myxoid liposarcoma and high-grade intraarticular liposarcoma, both tumors located within the knee joint, have been reported. The MRI features of intraarticular tumors are quite similar to those in the extraarticular location, namely, heterogenous but mostly intermediate signal intensity on T1-weighted images, and heterogenous intermediate-to-high signal intensity on T2 weighting.

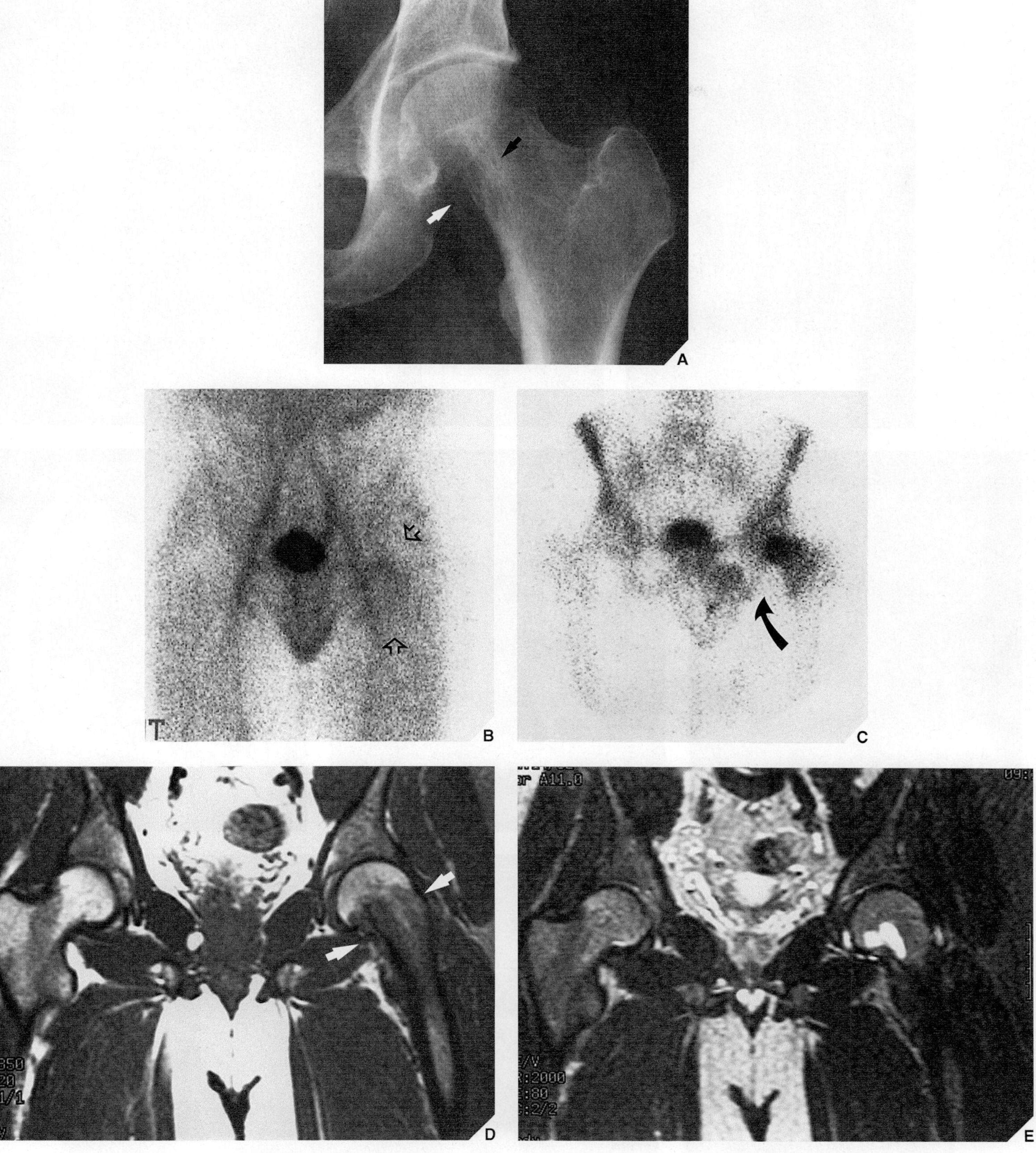

FIGURE 23.30 **Scintigraphy and MRI of synovial sarcoma. (A)** Anteroposterior radiograph of the left hip of a 37-year-old man shows an osteolytic lesion in the femoral neck bordered laterally by sclerotic margin *(arrows)*. **(B)** Scintigraphic (blood pool) examination demonstrates increased vascularity to the left hip joint *(open arrows)*. **(C)** Delayed radionuclide bone scan with technetium-99m (^{99m}Tc) methylene diphosphonate (MDP) shows increased uptake of the radiopharmaceutical tracer in the femoral head and neck and around the hip joint *(curved arrow)*. **(D)** Coronal T1-weighted (spin echo [SE]; repetition time [TR] 850/echo time [TE] 20 msec) MR image shows a low–signal intensity lesion affecting the medial aspect of the left femoral neck *(arrows)*. **(E)** Coronal T2-weighted (SE; TR 2,000/TE 80 msec) MR image demonstrates increased signal in the femoral neck and in the medial and lateral aspects of the hip joint. Excision biopsy revealed intraarticular synovial sarcoma.

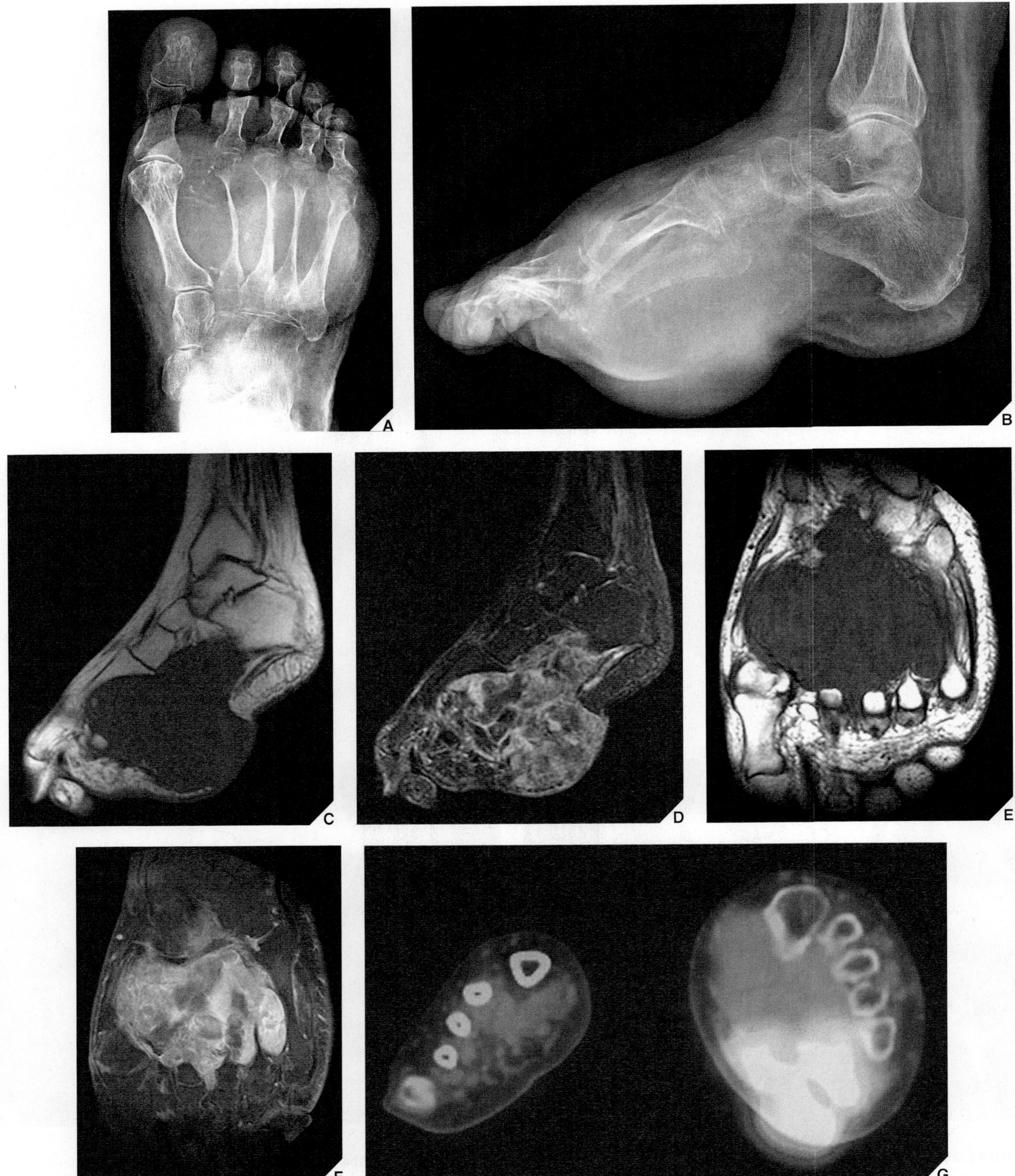

FIGURE 23.31 MRI and fluorodeoxyglucose (FDG) positron emission tomography (PET)/CT of synovial sarcoma. **(A)** Anteroposterior and **(B)** lateral radiographs of the left foot of a 57-year-old woman show a large soft-tissue mass containing calcifications, affecting mainly the plantar aspect of the foot. Observe erosions of the second, third, and fourth metatarsal bones. **(C)** Sagittal T1-weighted MRI shows the mass to be of intermediate-to-low signal intensity. **(D)** Sagittal inversion recovery (IR) MR image shows the heterogeneous mass exhibiting mixtures of low, intermediate, and high signal intensities (triple signal intensity sign). **(E)** Axial (long axis) T1-weighted MR image and **(F)** one obtained after intravenous administration of gadolinium demonstrate heterogenous enhancement of the tumor. **(G)** Axial fused FDG PET/CT image of both feet reveals a large hypermetabolic tumor in the soft tissues of the left foot. Excision biopsy confirmed the diagnosis of synovial sarcoma.

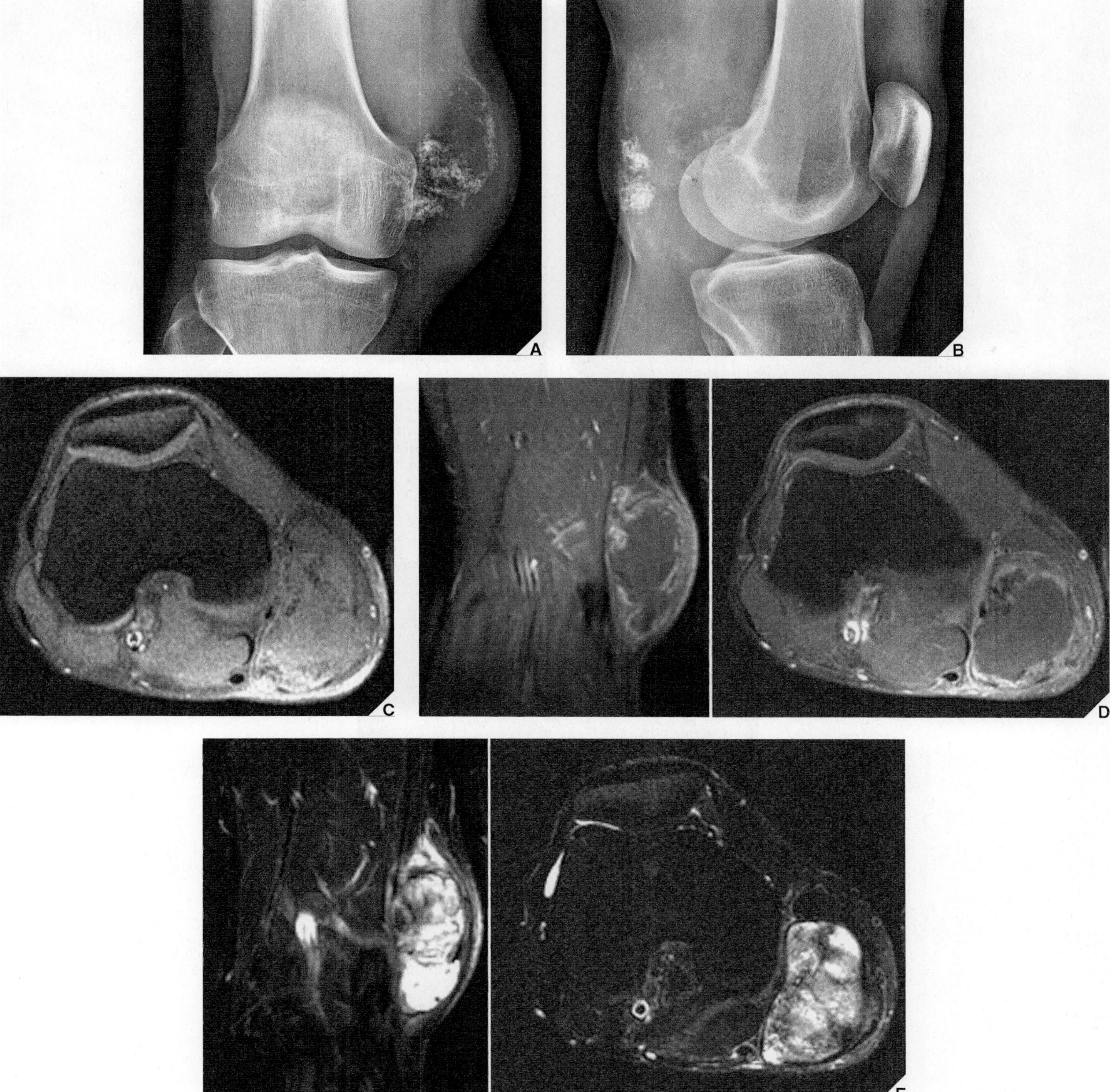

FIGURE 23.32 MRI of synovial sarcoma. **(A)** Anteroposterior and **(B)** lateral radiographs of the left knee of a 34-year-old man show a large soft-tissue mass adjacent to the posterolateral aspect of the medial femoral condyle containing calcifications. The osseous structures are not invaded. **(C)** Axial T1-weighted MRI shows the mass to be predominantly of intermediate signal intensity. **(D)** Coronal and axial T1-weighted MR images obtained after intravenous administration of gadolinium show peripheral enhancement of the tumor. **(E)** Coronal and axial T2-weighted MR images demonstrate heterogenous tumor exhibiting mixture of high, intermediate, and low signal intensity (triple signal intensity sign), characteristic of synovial sarcoma. The diagnosis was confirmed by excision biopsy.

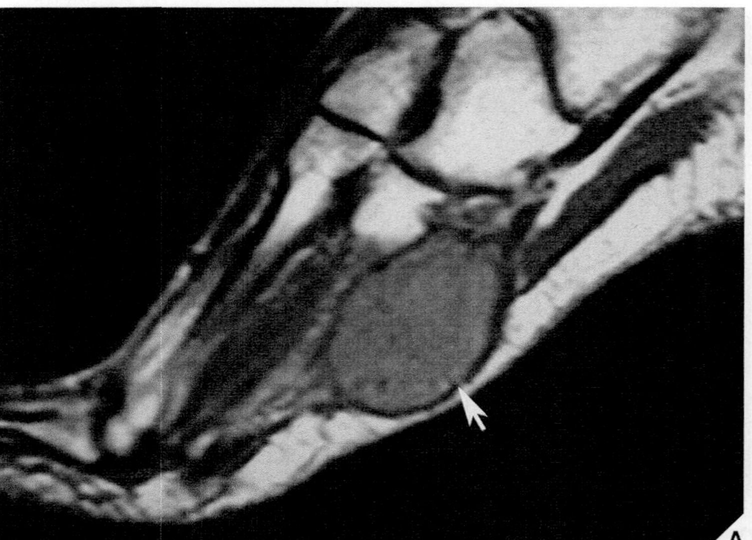

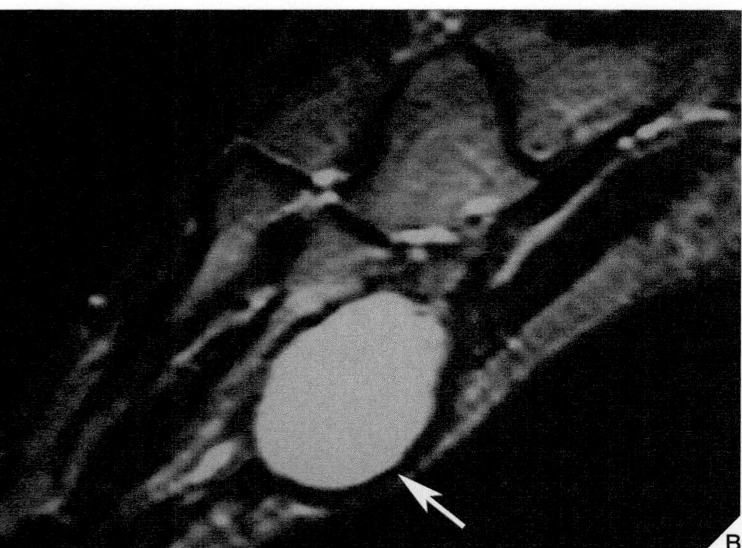

FIGURE 23.33 MRI of synovial sarcoma. **(A)** Sagittal T1-weighted MRI of the foot of a young man, who noticed a mass for over a year in the plantar lateral aspect of the foot, shows well-circumscribed hypointense tumor exhibiting a low–signal intensity capsule *(arrow)*. **(B)** Sagittal T2-weighted MR image demonstrates uniform high signal intensity of the well-encapsulated lesion *(arrow)*. The preoperative diagnosis was neurinoma or schwannoma. The final histologic diagnosis was synovial sarcoma.

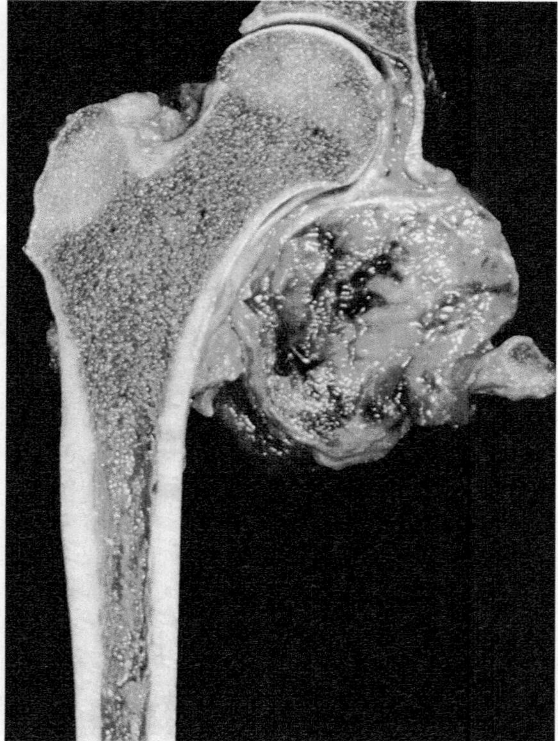

FIGURE 23.34 Pathology of synovial sarcoma. Coronal section of the specimen of the right hip joint and proximal femur shows a large well-circumscribed tan-yellowish juxtaarticular soft-tissue mass displaying foci of hemorrhage. (Modified from Bullough P. *Orthopaedic pathology*, 5th ed. Maryland Heights, MO: Mosby; 2009, with permission from Elsevier.)

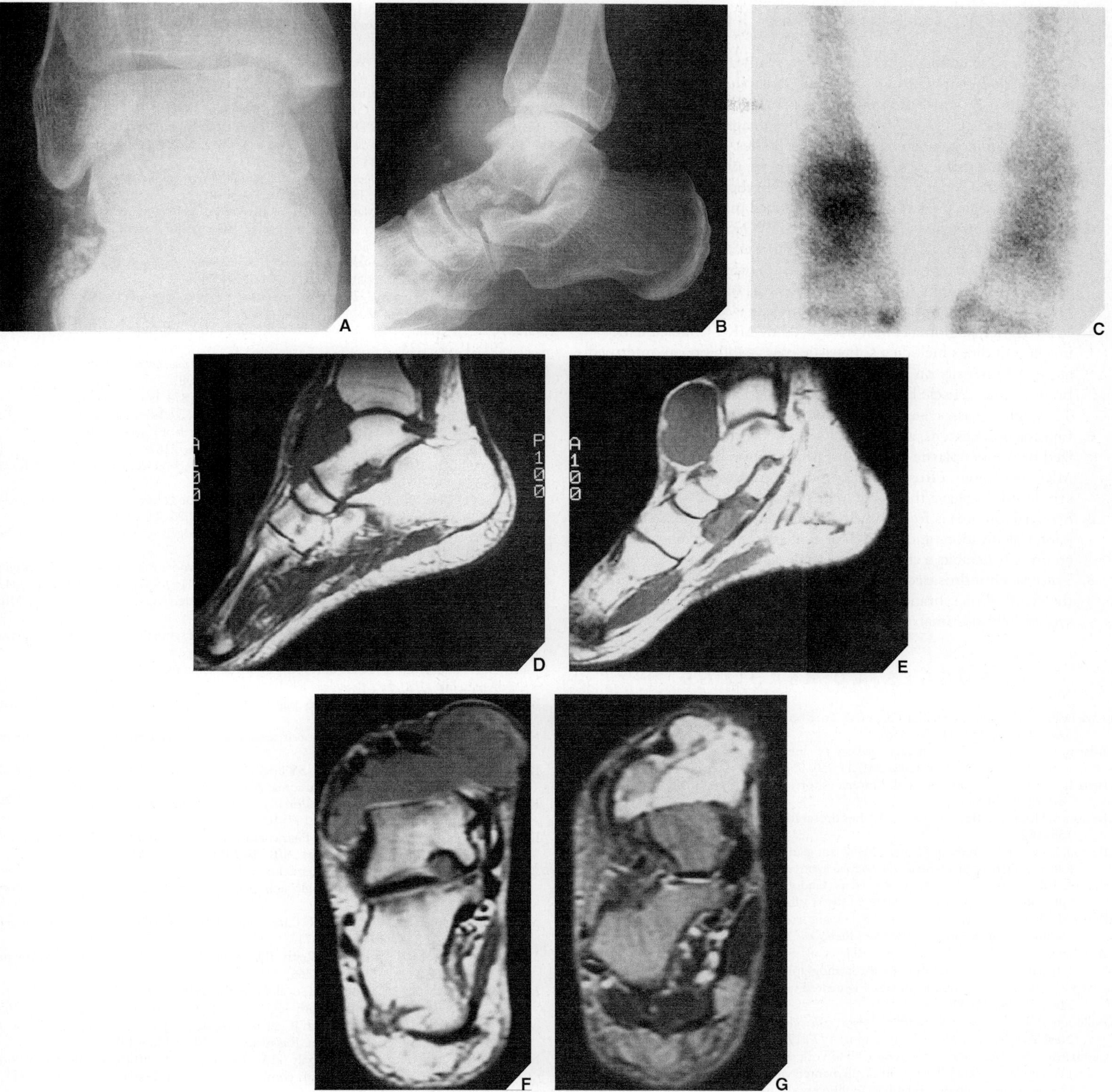

FIGURE 23.35 Scintigraphy and MRI of malignant transformation of synovial osteochondromatosis to synovial chondrosarcoma. **(A)** Anteroposterior and **(B)** lateral radiographs of the right ankle of a 64-year-old man with a long history of synovial chondromatosis show a large soft-tissue mass on the dorsal aspect of the ankle joint, eroding the talus. Multiple calcifications, uniform in size and shape, are noted laterally. **(C)** After injection of 15 mCi (555 MBq) of technetium-99m (^{99m}Tc)-labeled methylene diphosphonate (MDP), there is increased uptake of radiopharmaceutical tracer in the right ankle. **(D)** Sagittal T1-weighted (spin echo [SE]; repetition time [TR] 400/echo time [TE] 20 msec) MR image shows the mass displaying intermediate signal intensity, isointense with the muscles. **(E)** Parasagittal T1-weighted (SE; TR 400/TE 20 msec) MR image demonstrates the mass to be well encapsulated. **(F)** Coronal proton density (SE; TR 1,800/TE 29 msec) MR image shows that the mass is continuous with the ankle joint. **(G)** Coronal T2-weighted (SE; TR 2,000/TE 80 msec) MR image demonstrates the mass to be of high signal intensity. Punctuated areas of low signal intensity within the mass represent calcifications. (Reprinted with permission from Greenspan A, Remagen W. *Differential diagnosis of tumors and tumor-like lesions of bones*. Philadelphia: Lippincott-Raven Publishers; 1998.)

PRACTICAL POINTS TO REMEMBER

1. Characteristic radiographic findings of synovial (osteo)chondromatosis include joint effusion, numerous radiopaque osteochondral bodies (usually small and uniform in size), and bone erosions.
2. Arthrography, CT, and MRI are effective imaging modalities to demonstrate noncalcified intraarticular bodies.
3. PVNS is invariably accompanied by serosanguineous synovial fluid. Radiography reveals a soft-tissue density in the affected joint caused by hemorrhagic fluid and lobulated synovial masses.
4. MRI is very effective in the diagnosis of PVNS because on T2 weighting, the intraarticular masses demonstrate a characteristic combination of high–signal intensity areas representing fluid and congested synovium, interspersed with areas of intermediate to low signal intensity secondary to the presence of hemosiderin.
5. Synovial hemangioma is best diagnosed by MRI. Characteristic imaging findings include a soft-tissue mass exhibiting an intermediate signal intensity on T1-weighted images (isointense with or slightly brighter than muscle but not as bright as fat) and high signal on T2 weighting associated with serpentine low-intensity septa.
6. Lipoma arborescens, a very rare intraarticular disorder, is characterized by nonneoplastic lipomatous proliferation of the synovium. MRI shows joint effusion and frond-like masses arising from the synovium that have the signal intensity of fat on all sequences.
7. Synovial sarcoma is frequently located in close proximity to the joint. Calcifications and bone erosion are common findings. This tumor commonly exhibits a characteristic triple signal intensity sign on MRI.
8. Synovial chondrosarcoma, a very rare tumor that originates from the synovial membrane, may be primary lesion or may develop in synovial chondromatosis.

SUGGESTED READINGS

Abdelwahab IF, Kenan S, Steiner GC, et al. True bursal pigmented villonodular synovitis. *Skeletal Radiol* 2002;31:354–358.

Adams ME, Saifuddin A. Characterisation of intra-articular soft tissue tumours and tumour-like lesions. *Eur Radiol* 2007;17:950–958.

Bejia I, Younes M, Moussa A, et al. Lipoma arborescens affecting multiple joints. *Skeletal Radiol* 2005;34:536–538.

Bertoni F, Unni KK, Beabout JW, et al. Chondrosarcomas of the synovium. *Cancer* 1991;67:155–162.

Bertoni F, Unni KK, Beabout JW, et al. Malignant giant cell tumor of the tendon sheaths and joints (malignant pigmented villonodular synovitis). *Am J Surg Pathol* 1997;21:153–163.

Besette PR, Cooley PA, Johnson RP, et al. Gadolinium-enhanced MRI of pigmented villonodular synovitis of the knee. *J Comput Assist Tomogr* 1992;16:992–994.

Bixby SD, Hettmer S, Taylor GA, et al. Synovial sarcoma in children: imaging features and common benign mimics. *AJR Am J Roentgenol* 2010;195:1026–1032.

Blacksin MF, Ghelman B, Freiberger RH, et al. Synovial chondromatosis of the hip. Evaluation with air computed arthrotomography. *Clin Imaging* 1990;14:315–318.

Bravo SM, Winalski CS, Weissman BN. Pigmented villonodular synovitis. *Radiol Clin North Am* 1996;34:311–326.

Bullough PG. *Atlas of orthopaedic pathology: with clinical and radiologic correlations*, 2nd ed. New York: Gower Medical Publishing; 1992:17.25–17.28.

Campanacci M. *Bone and soft-tissue tumors*. New York: Springer; 1990:998–1012.

Chen DY, Lan JL, Chou SJ. Treatment of pigmented villonodular synovitis with yttrium-90: changes in immunologic features, Tc-99m uptake measurements, and MR imaging of one case. *Clin Rheumatol* 1992;11:280–285.

Cotten A, Flipo RM, Chastanet P, et al. Pigmented villonodular synovitis of the hip: review of radiographic features in 58 patients. *Skeletal Radiol* 1995;24:1–6.

Cotten A, Flipo RM, Herbaux B, et al. Synovial haemangioma of the knee: a frequently misdiagnosed lesion. *Skeletal Radiol* 1995;24:257–261.

Crotty JM, Monu JUV, Pope TL Jr. Synovial osteochondromatosis. *Radiol Clin North Am* 1996;34:327–342.

De Beuckeleer L, De Schepper A, De Belder F, et al. Magnetic resonance imaging of localized giant cell tumour of the tendon sheath (MRI of localized GCTTS). *Eur Radiol* 1997;7:198–201.

De St. Aubain Sommerhausen N, Dal Cin P. Diffuse-type giant cell tumour. In: Fletcher CDM, Unni KK, Mertens F, eds. *Pathology & genetics: tumours of soft tissue and bone*. Lyon, France: IARC Press; 2002:112–114.

De St. Aubain Sommerhausen N, Dal Cin P. Giant cell tumour of tendon sheath. In: Fletcher CDM, Unni KK, Mertens F, eds. *Pathology & genetics: tumours of soft tissue and bone*. Lyon, France: IARC Press; 2002:110–111.

Demertzis JL, Kyriakos M, Loomans R, et al. Synovial hemangioma of the hip joint in a pediatric patient. *Skeletal Radiol* 2014;43:107–113.

Devaney K, Vinh TN, Sweet DE. Synovial hemangioma: report of 20 cases with differential diagnostic considerations. *Hum Pathol* 1993;24:737–745.

Enzinger FM, Weiss SW. Benign tumors and tumor-like lesions of synovial tissue. In: *Soft tissue tumors*. St. Louis: Mosby; 1988:638–658.

Enzinger FM, Weiss SW. *Soft tissue tumors*, 3rd ed. St. Louis: Mosby; 1995:749–751, 757–786.

Eustace SE, Harrison M, Srinivasen U, et al. Magnetic resonance imaging in pigmented villonodular synovitis. *Can Assoc Radiol J* 1994;45:283–286.

Flanagan AM, Delaney D, O'Donnell P. The benefits of molecular pathology in the diagnosis of musculoskeletal disease: part I of a two-part review: soft tissue tumors. *Skeletal Radiol* 2010;39:105–115.

Fletcher CDM, Bridge J, Hogendoorn P, et al, eds. *Pathology and genetics of tumours of soft tissue and bone*. Lyon, France: IARC Press; 2013.

Greenspan A, Azouz EM, Matthews J II, et al. Synovial hemangioma: imaging features in eight histologically proven cases, review of the literature, and differential diagnosis. *Skeletal Radiol* 1995;24:583–590.

Greenspan A, Borys D. *Radiology and pathology correlation of bone tumors: a quick reference and review*. Philadelphia: Wolters Kluwer; 2018:353–380.

Greenspan A, Gershwin ME. *Imaging in rheumatology: a clinical approach*. Philadelphia: Wolters Kluwer; 2018:377–419.

Greenspan A, Grainger AJ. Articular abnormalities that may mimic arthritis. *J Ultrason* 2018;18:212–223.

Greenspan A, Remagen W. *Differential diagnosis of tumors and tumor-like lesions of bones and joints*. Philadelphia: Lippincott-Raven Publishers; 1998.

Grieten M, Buckwalter KA, Cardinal E, et al. Case report 873: lipoma arborescens (villous lipomatous proliferation of the synovial membrane). *Skeletal Radiol* 1994;23:652–655.

Haldar M, Randall RL, Capecchi MR. Synovial sarcoma: from genetics to genetic-based animal modeling. *Clin Orthop Relat Res* 2008;466:2156–2167.

Hermann G, Abdelwahab IF, Klein MJ, et al. Synovial chondromatosis. *Skeletal Radiol* 1995;24:298–300.

Hermann G, Klein MJ, Abdelwahab IF, et al. Synovial chondrosarcoma arising in synovial chondromatosis of the right hip. *Skeletal Radiol* 1997;26:366–369.

Hopyan S, Nadesan P, Yu C, et al. Dysregulation of hedgehog signaling predisposes to synovial chondromatosis. *J Pathol* 2005;206:143–150.

Huang G-S, Lee C-H, Chan WP, et al. Localized nodular synovitis of the knee: MR imaging appearance and clinical correlates in 21 patients. *AJR Am J Roentgenol* 2003;181:539–543.

Hughes TH, Sartoris DJ, Schweitzer ME, et al. Pigmented villonodular synovitis: MRI characteristics. *Skeletal Radiol* 1995;24:7–12.

Jaffe HL, Lichtenstein L, Sutro CJ. Pigmented villonodular synovitis, bursitis and tenosynovitis. *Arch Pathol Lab Med* 1941;31:731–765.

Jones BC, Sundaram M, Kransdorf MJ. Synovial sarcoma: MR imaging findings in 34 patients. *AJR Am J Roentgenol* 1993;161:827–830.

Kalil RK, Unni KK. Malignancy in pigmented villonodular synovitis. *Skeletal Radiol* 1998;27:392–395.

Karasick D, Karasick S. Giant cell tumor of tendon sheath: spectrum of radiologic findings. *Skeletal Radiol* 1992;21:219–224.

Kawai A, Woodruff J, Healey JH, et al. SYT-SSX gene fusion as a determinant of morphology and prognosis in synovial sarcoma. *N Engl J Med* 1998;338:153–160.

Khan AM, Cannon S, Levack B. Primary intra-articular liposarcoma of the knee. Case report. *J Knee Surg* 2003;16:107–109.

Lin J, Jacobson JA, Jamadar DA, et al. Pigmented villonodular synovitis and related lesions: the spectrum of imaging findings. *AJR Am J Roentgenol* 1999;172:191–197.

Llauger J, Palmer J, Rosón N, et al. Pigmented villonodular synovitis and giant cell tumors of the tendon sheath: radiologic and pathologic features. *AJR Am J Roentgenol* 1999;172:1087–1091.

Manivel JC, Dehner LP, Thompson R. Case report 460: synovial chondrosarcoma of left knee. *Skeletal Radiol* 1988;17:66–71.

Mendelhall WM, Mendelhall CM, Reith JD, et al. Pigmented villonodular synovitis. *Curr Opin Oncology* 2011;23:361–366.

Murphey MD, Gibson MS, Jennings BT, et al. From the archives of the AFIP: imaging of synovial sarcoma with radiologic-pathologic correlation. *Radiographics* 2006;26:1543–1565.

Murphey MD, Vidal JA, Fanburg-Smith JC, et al. Imaging of synovial chondromatosis with radiologic-pathologic correlation. *Radiographics* 2007;27:1465–1488.

Nassar WAM, Bassiony AA, Elghazaly HA. Treatment of diffuse pigmented villonodular synovitis of the knee with combined surgical and radiosynovectomy. *HSS J* 2009;5:19–23.

Ontell F, Greenspan A. Chondrosarcoma complicating synovial chondromatosis: findings with magnetic resonance imaging. *Can Assoc Radiol J* 1994;45:318–323.

Rubin BP. Tenosynovial giant cell tumor and pigmented villonodular synovitis: a proposal for unification of these clinically distinct but histologically and genetically identical lesions. *Skeletal Radiol* 2007;36:267–268.

Rybak LD, Khaldi L, Wittig J, et al. Primary synovial chondrosarcoma of the hip joint in a 45-year-old male: case report and literature review. *Skeletal Radiol* 2011;40:1375–1381.

Schajowicz F. Synovial chondromatosis. In: *Tumors and tumorlike lesions of bones and joints*. New York: Springer; 1981:541–545.

Shaerf DA, Mann B, Alorjani M, et al. High-grade intra-articular liposarcoma of the knee. *Skeletal Radiol* 2011;40:363–365.

Sheldon PJ, Forrester DM, Learch TJ. Imaging of intraarticular masses. *Radiographics* 2005;25:105–119.

Sommerhausen NSA, Fletcher CDM. Diffuse-type giant cell tumor: clinicopathologic and immunohistochemical analysis of 50 cases with extraarticular disease. *Am J Surg Pathol* 2000;24:479–492.

Stout AP, Lattes R. Tumors of the soft tissue. In: *Atlas of tumor pathology*, 2nd series, fascicle 1. Washington, DC: Armed Forces Institute of Pathology; 1967.

van Rijswijk CSP, Hogendoorn PCW, Taminiau AHM, et al. Synovial sarcoma: dynamic contrast-enhanced MR imaging features. *Skeletal Radiol* 2001;30:25–30.

Vergara-Lluri ME, Stohr BA, Puligandla B, et al. A novel sarcoma with dual differentiation: clinicopathologic and molecular characterization of a combined synovial sarcoma and extraskeletal myxoid chondrosarcoma. *Am J Surg Pathol* 2012;36:1093–1098.

White EA, Omid R, Matcuk GR, et al. Lipoma arborescens of the biceps tendon sheath. *Skeletal Radiol* 2013;42:1461–1464.

Wilkerson BW, Crim JR, Hung M, et al. Characterization of synovial sarcoma calcification. *AJR Am J Roentgenol* 2012;199:W730–W734.

Winnepenninckx V, De Vos R, Debiec-Rychter M, et al. Calcifying/ossifying synovial sarcoma shows t(x;18) with SSX2 involvement and mitochondrial calcifications. *Histopathology* 2001;38:141–145.

Wittkop B, Davies AM, Mangham DC. Primary synovial chondromatosis and synovial chondrosarcoma: a pictorial review. *Eur Radiol* 2002;12:2112–2119.

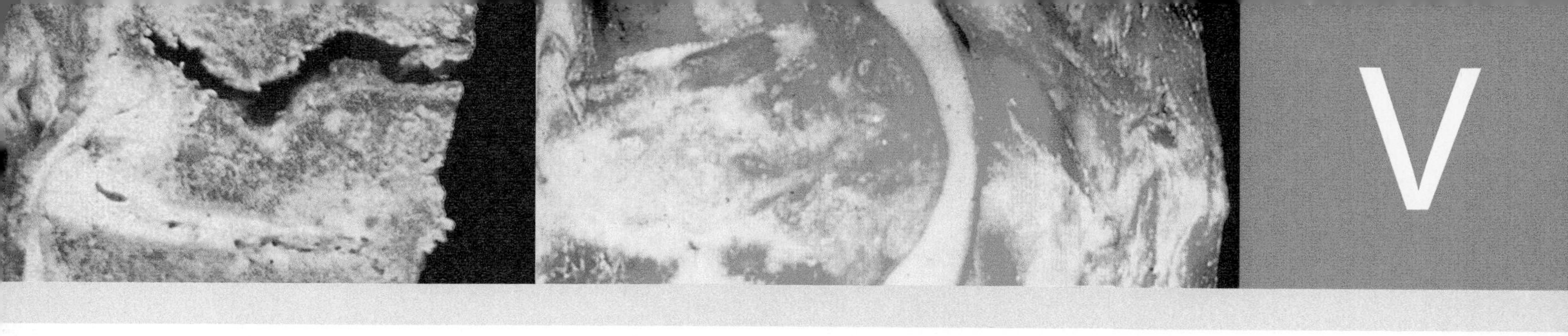

V

INFECTIONS

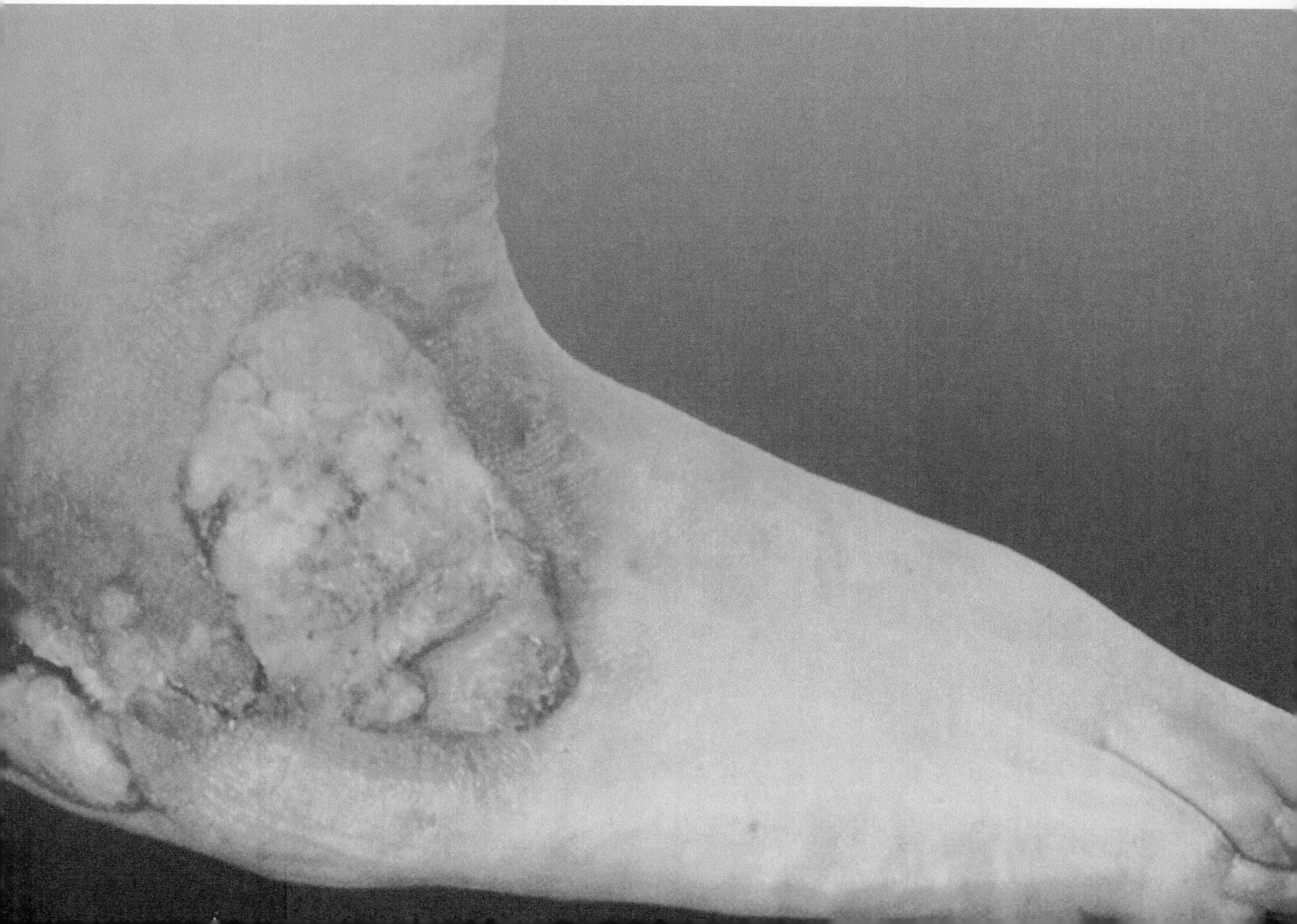

24

Imaging Evaluation of Musculoskeletal Infections

Musculoskeletal Infections

Infections of the musculoskeletal system can be subdivided into three categories: (a) those involving bones (osteomyelitis), (b) those involving joints (infectious arthritis), and (c) those involving soft tissues (cellulitis). Because of the complexity of the vertebrae and their soft-tissue structures, infectious processes of the spine are considered under a separate heading.

Osteomyelitis

Three basic mechanisms allow an infectious organism—whether bacterium, virus, mycoplasma, rickettsia, or fungus—to reach the bone: (a) *hematogenous spread* via the bloodstream from a remote site of infection, such as the skin, tonsils, gallbladder, or urinary tract; (b) spread from a *contiguous source* of infection, such as from the soft tissues, teeth, or sinuses; and (c) *direct implantation*, such as through a puncture or missile wound or an operative procedure (Fig. 24.1).

Hematogenous spread is common in children, and the usual focus of infection develops in the metaphysis. The metaphyseal location of infection in children is related to an osseous–vascular anatomy that differs in the infant, child, and adult (Fig. 24.2). In the child (ages 1 to 16 years), there is separation of the blood supply to the metaphysis and epiphysis, each having its own source. Moreover, the arteries and capillaries of the metaphysis turn sharply without penetrating the open growth plate; in the region where capillaries become venules, the rate of blood flow is sluggish. Also contributing to the greater incidence of metaphyseal osteomyelitis in children is secondary thrombosis of end arteries with bacteria during transient bacteremia. In the infant (up to 1 year), however, osteomyelitis may sometimes have its focus in the epiphysis because some metaphyseal vessels may penetrate the growth plate and reach the epiphysis (see Fig. 24.2). With obliteration of the growth plate in the adult, there is vascular continuity between the shaft and the articular ends of the bone; hence, the focus of osteomyelitis can develop in any part of a bone.

Contiguous spread and direct implantation are more common in adults. The sites of bone infection via either of these routes are directly related to the focus of soft-tissue infection or the location of the wound.

Infectious Arthritis

An infectious agent may enter the joint by the same basic routes as in osteomyelitis: by direct invasion of the synovial membrane, either secondary to a penetrating wound or after a joint-replacement procedure; from an infection of the adjacent soft tissues; or indirectly via a blood-borne infection. Infectious arthritis may also occur secondary to a focus of osteomyelitis in the adjacent bone (Fig. 24.3).

Cellulitis

Soft-tissue infections most commonly result from a break in the skin leading to direct introduction of an infectious agent. Some patients, such as those with diabetes, are particularly prone to cellulitis caused by a combination of factors, including skin breakdown and local ischemia.

Infections of the Spine

Infections in the spine may be located in a vertebral body, an intervertebral disk, the paravertebral soft tissues, or the epidural compartment; very rarely, an infection may involve the contents of the spinal canal or the spinal cord. The mechanisms of infection are the same as those of osteomyelitis and infectious arthritis. An intervertebral disk infection, for example, may result from a puncture of the canal or of the disk itself during a procedure as well as from a penetrating injury. It can also spread from a contiguous source of infection such as a paraspinal abscess. Most common, however, is hematogenous spread after surgical procedures such as laminectomy or spinal fusion, or during generalized bacteremia or sepsis (Fig. 24.4). Regardless of the primary location of the infectious process, *Staphylococcus aureus* is responsible for more than 90% of all infections of the spine.

Imaging Evaluation of Infections

The imaging modalities used to evaluate infections of the musculoskeletal system include the following:

1. Conventional radiography
2. Computed tomography (CT)
3. Arthrography
4. Myelography and diskography
5. Fistulography (sinogram)
6. Arteriography
7. Radionuclide imaging (scintigraphy, bone scan)
8. Ultrasound (US)
9. Magnetic resonance imaging (MRI)
10. Percutaneous aspiration and biopsy (fluoroscopy guided, CT guided, or US guided)

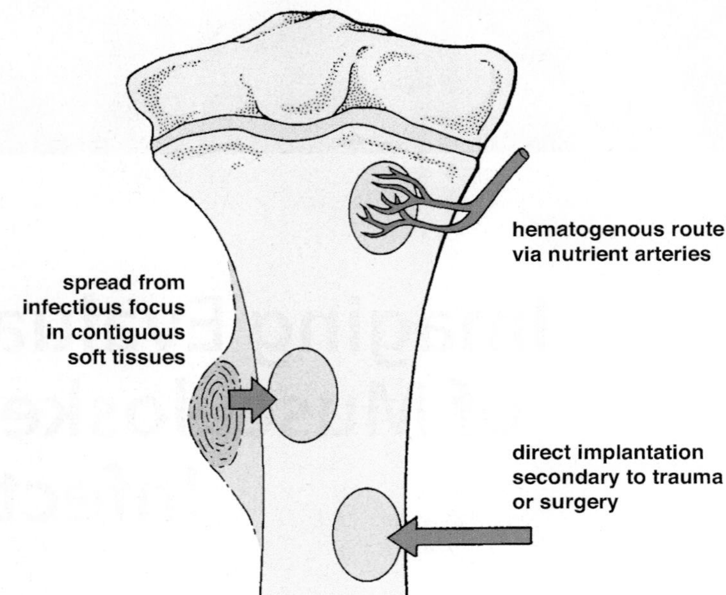

FIGURE 24.1 **Entry routes of an infectious organism into a bone.** Infectious agents may gain entry to a bone through hematogenous spread, a source of infection in the contiguous soft tissues, or through direct implantation secondary to trauma or surgery.

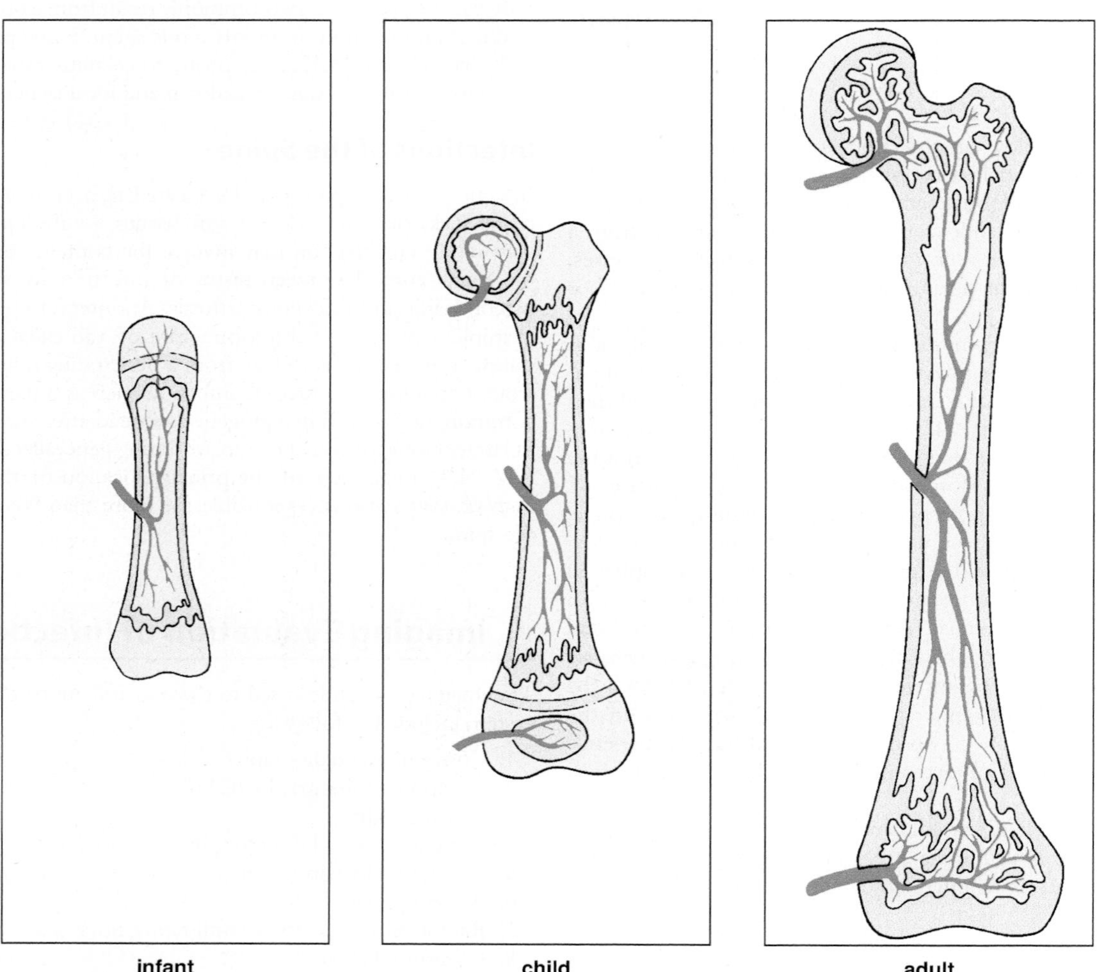

FIGURE 24.2 **Vascular anatomy of long bone.** The vascular anatomy of a long bone differs in an infant, a child, and an adult. These differences account for the various locations of infection in each age group. In an infant, nutrient, transphyseal, and foveal arteries are abundant. In a child, the physis becomes avascular when the foveal and transphyseal arteries recede. After the growth plate closes, the foveal arteries and periarticular arteries again become prominent.

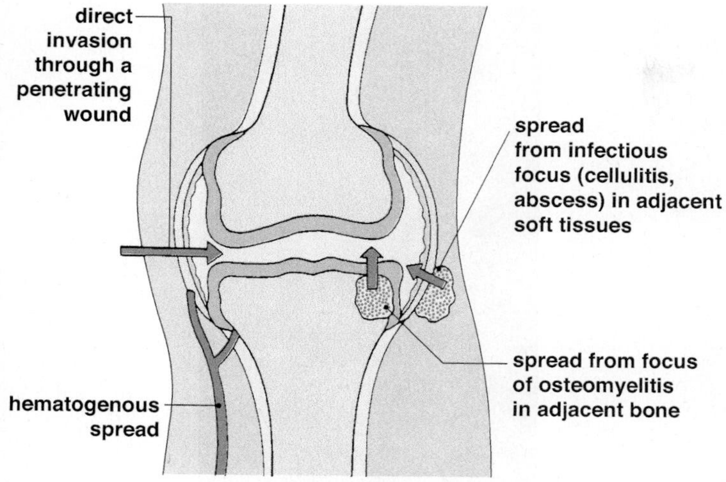

FIGURE 24.3 Entry routes of an infectious organism into a joint. The routes of infection in infectious arthritis are similar to those of osteomyelitis, which itself may be a source of spread.

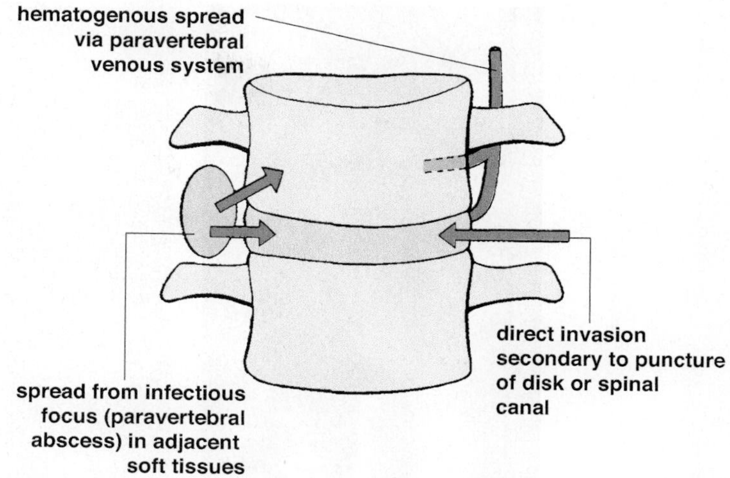

FIGURE 24.4 Entry routes of an infectious organism into a vertebra. The potential routes of infection of a vertebra or an intervertebral disk are direct invasion, hematogenous spread, and extension from a focus of infection in the adjacent soft tissues.

Conventional Radiography, Computed Tomography, and Arthrography

In most instances, radiography is sufficient to demonstrate the pertinent features of a bone or joint infection (Fig. 24.5; see also Figs. 4.74 and 4.75). Digital magnification in a Picture Archive and Communication System (PACS) work station is helpful in delineating subtle changes representing cortical destruction or periosteal new bone formation (Fig. 24.6). In the past, conventional tomography using multidirectional motion (trispiral tomography) was effective in demonstrating sequestra or subtle sinus tracts in the bone (Fig. 24.7) but at present has been almost completely replaced by CT (Fig. 24.8), which plays a determining role in demonstrating the extent of infection in bones and soft tissues and at times may be very helpful in making a specific diagnosis (Fig. 24.9). Arthrography has rather limited application in the diagnosis of joint infections (see Fig. 25.24B).

Radionuclide Imaging

Scintigraphy has a very prominent role in diagnosing bone and soft-tissue infections. In suspected osteomyelitis, radionuclide bone scan using technetium-99m (^{99m}Tc)-labeled phosphonates is routinely used because there is an accumulation of tracer in the infected areas. A three- or four-phase technique is particularly useful for distinguishing infected joint tissues from infected periarticular soft tissues if radiography is not diagnostic. With cellulitis, diffuse increased uptake is present in the first two phases, but there is no significant increase in uptake in the bone in the third and fourth delayed phases. Conversely, osteomyelitis causes focally increased uptake in all four phases (Fig. 24.10). In addition, the three-phase bone scan can accurately diagnose osteomyelitis within 3 days of the development of symptoms, much earlier than can be seen with conventional radiography. The three-phase bone scan can also be useful in diagnosing septic arthritis in situ or with extension into the adjacent bone.

Once the bone sustains an injury, such as surgery, fracture, or neuropathic osteoarthropathy, that causes increased bone turnover, routine scintigraphy with technetium-labeled phosphonate becomes less specific for infection. However, radionuclide studies using gallium (a ferric analog) and indium are more specific in these instances. There is still no general agreement on the exact mechanism of gallium localization in infected tissues. After intravenous injections of gallium, more than 99% is bound to various plasma proteins, including transferrin, haptoglobin, lactoferrin, albumin, and ferritin. At least five mechanisms of gallium transfer from the plasma into inflammatory exudates and cells have been suggested. These include direct leukocyte uptake, direct bacteria uptake, the protein-bound tissue uptake, increased vascularity, and increased bone turnover. Because gallium binds to the iron-binding molecule transferrin, the mechanism of gallium uptake in infectious processes is best explained by hyperemia and elevated permeability that increase delivery of the protein-bound tracer transferrin into the area of inflammation. Cells associated with the inflammatory response, particularly polymorphonuclear white cells in which lactoferrin is carried within intracytoplasmic granules, deposit iron-binding proteins extracellularly at the site of inflammation, serving to combat the infection by sequestering needed iron from bacteria. Lactoferrin, which has a high binding affinity for iron, takes the gallium away from the transferrin.

Gallium can also be used to assess the patient's response to therapy. Particularly in osteomyelitis, gallium concentrations enhance the specificity of an abnormal bone scan, and decreased gallium uptake closely follows a good response to therapy.

The other tracer used in infections is indium. Because indium-labeled white blood cells are usually not incorporated into areas of increased bone turnover, scintigraphy with indium-111 (^{111}In) oxine–labeled leukocytes is used as a sensitive and specific test in the general diagnosis of infection of the musculoskeletal system and in specific instances when infection complicates previous fracture or surgery. Like other imaging procedures in nuclear medicine, this test monitors the internal distribution of a tracer agent to provide diagnostic information. The inherent ability of white blood cells to accumulate at sites of inflammation makes their use in this test particularly effective in the diagnosis of infections. Merkel et al. reported the sensitivity of indium scintigraphy in detecting infections to be 83%, with a specificity of 94% and an accuracy of 88%.

It must be stressed, however, that because the ^{111}In-labeled leukocytes also accumulate in active bone marrow, the sensitivity for the detection of chronic osteomyelitis is reduced. To improve the diagnostic ability of this technique, a combined ^{99m}Tc-sulfur colloid bone marrow/^{111}In-labeled leukocyte study is advocated. A particularly difficult problem is the patient with diabetic foot neuropathy in whom superimposed infection is suspected. In this circumstance, radiography and even MRI are not very specific. Although soft-tissue infection can be detected by the latter technique, early changes of osteomyelitis may be missed. Often, no single imaging method can provide the correct diagnosis, and a combination of imaging techniques should be used. The traditional sequential use of gallium-67 (^{67}Ga) citrate in conjunction with the ^{99m}Tc-methylene diphosphonate (MDP) bone scan as an aid to diagnose osteomyelitis in the diabetic foot has been supplanted by the use of ^{111}In-labeled leukocytes. The drawback of this technique is that there remain difficulties in differentiating infection in the bone (osteomyelitis) from that in the adjacent tissue (cellulitis). A more recent attempt to improve this situation is the use of a combined ^{99m}Tc-bone scan/^{111}In-labeled leukocyte study to determine whether the leukocyte collection is in the bone or in the soft tissue. A new challenger to ^{111}In leukocyte scanning is the ^{99m}Tc-hexamethylpropylene amino oxine (HMPAO)-labeled leukocyte scan. At the time of this writing, other methods are being tested,

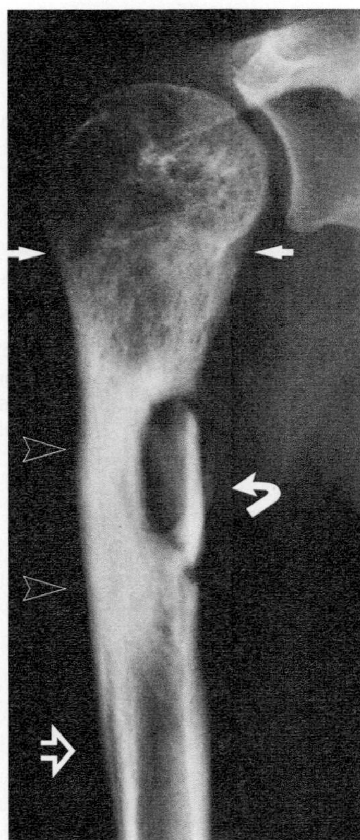

FIGURE 24.5 Chronic osteomyelitis. Anteroposterior radiograph of the right humerus demonstrates the classic features of chronic active osteomyelitis. There is destruction of the medullary portion of the bone *(arrows)*, reactive sclerosis *(arrowheads)*, and periosteal new bone formation *(open arrow)*. Note also a large sequestrum on the medial aspect of the humerus *(curved arrow)*, the hallmark of an active infectious process.

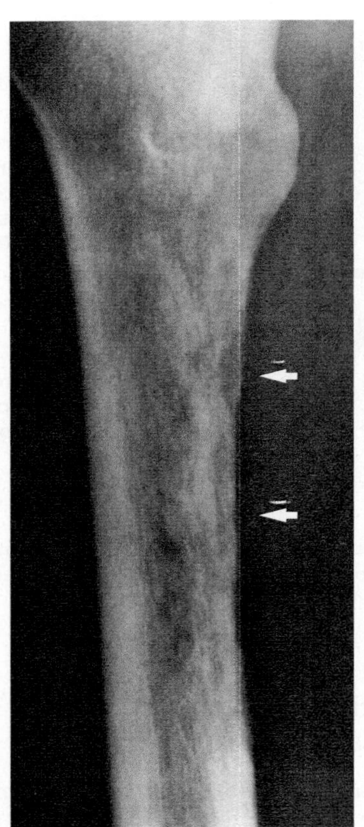

FIGURE 24.6 Acute osteomyelitis. Digital magnification study of the right femur demonstrates subtle changes representative of cortical destruction and formation of periosteal new bone in an early stage of osteomyelitis *(arrows)*. These findings were not well delineated on the conventional radiographs.

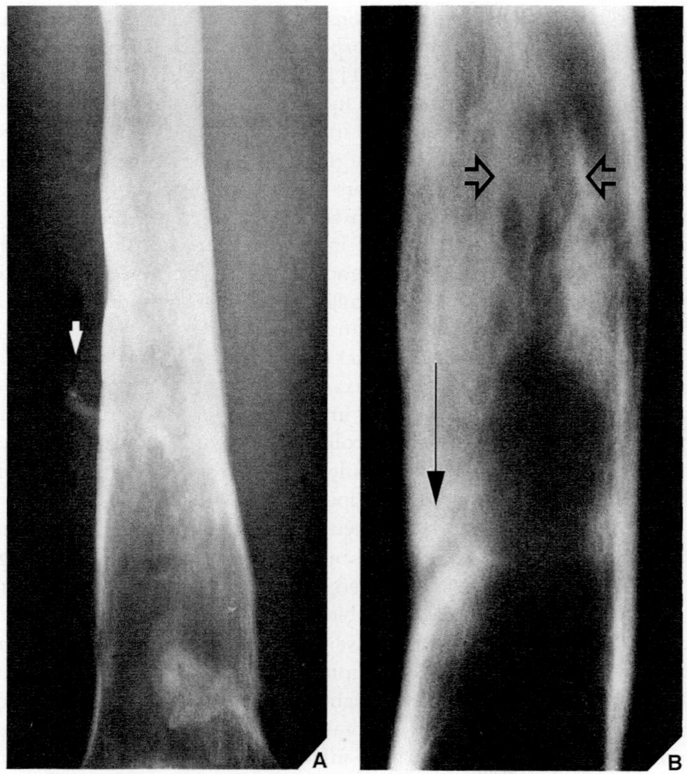

FIGURE 24.7 Tomography of active osteomyelitis. **(A)** Radiograph of the left femur shows thickening of the cortex, reactive sclerosis, and foci of destruction in the medullary cavity. Faint calcifications in the soft tissue *(arrow)* suggest the presence of a fistula. **(B)** Conventional tomogram enhanced by magnification clearly demonstrates a sequestrum *(open arrows)* and a sinus tract in the cortex *(long arrow)*, the characteristic features of active osteomyelitis.

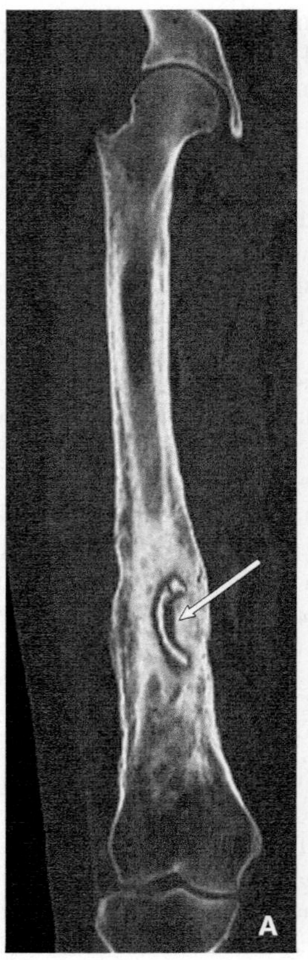

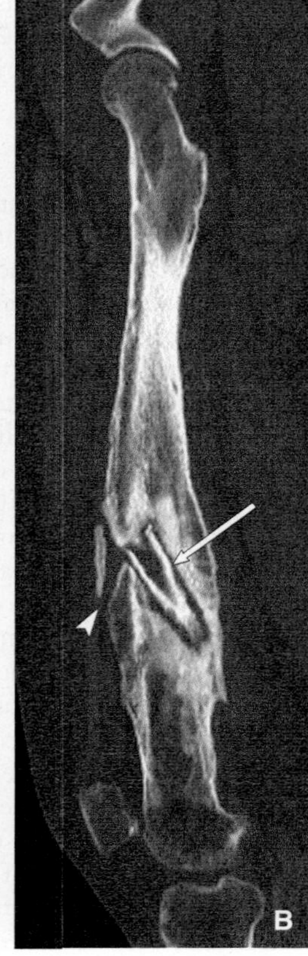

FIGURE 24.8 CT of sequestrum. A 42-year-old woman, who was diagnosed in the past with chronic osteomyelitis of the femur, presented with draining sinus above her right patella. **(A)** Coronal and **(B)** sagittal reformatted CT images of the femur show sequestrum *(arrows)* and sinus tract *(arrowhead)*.

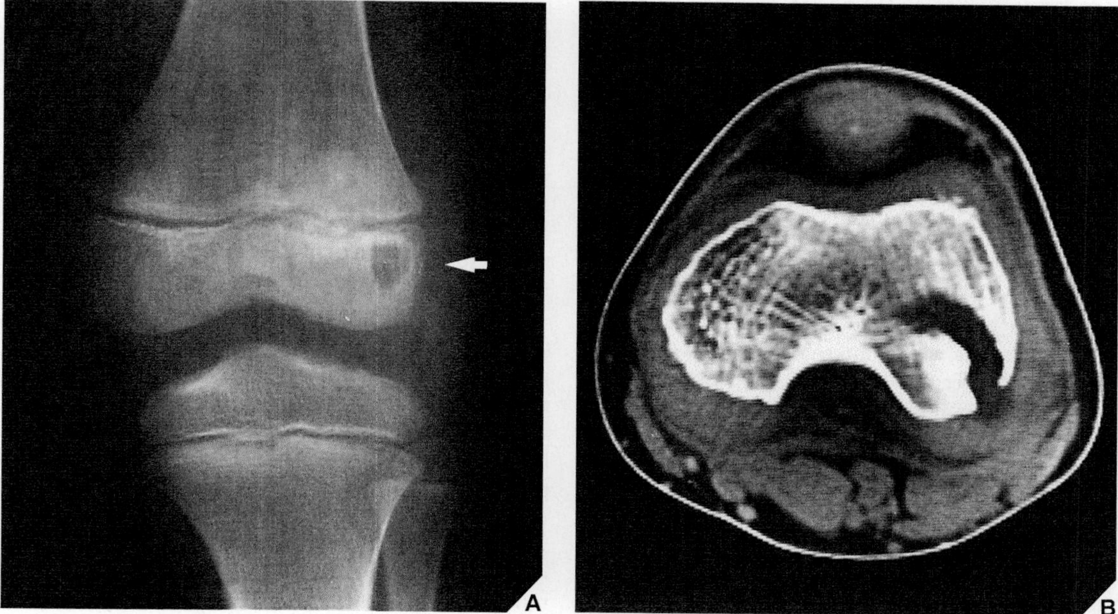

FIGURE 24.9 CT of bone abscess. A 7-year-old boy had intermittent pain in the left knee for 3 weeks; the pain was worse at night and was promptly relieved by salicylates. **(A)** Initial anteroposterior radiograph of the left knee demonstrates a radiolucent lesion with a well-defined, partly sclerotic border in the lateral portion of the distal femoral epiphysis *(arrow)*. Osteoid osteoma and chondroblastoma were considered in the differential diagnosis. **(B)** CT examination, however, reveals cortical disruption at the posterolateral aspect of the lateral femoral condyle, a finding not seen on the standard radiographs. The serpentine configuration of the radiolucent tract and its extension into the cartilage prompted a diagnosis of epiphyseal bone abscess, which was confirmed on bone biopsy.

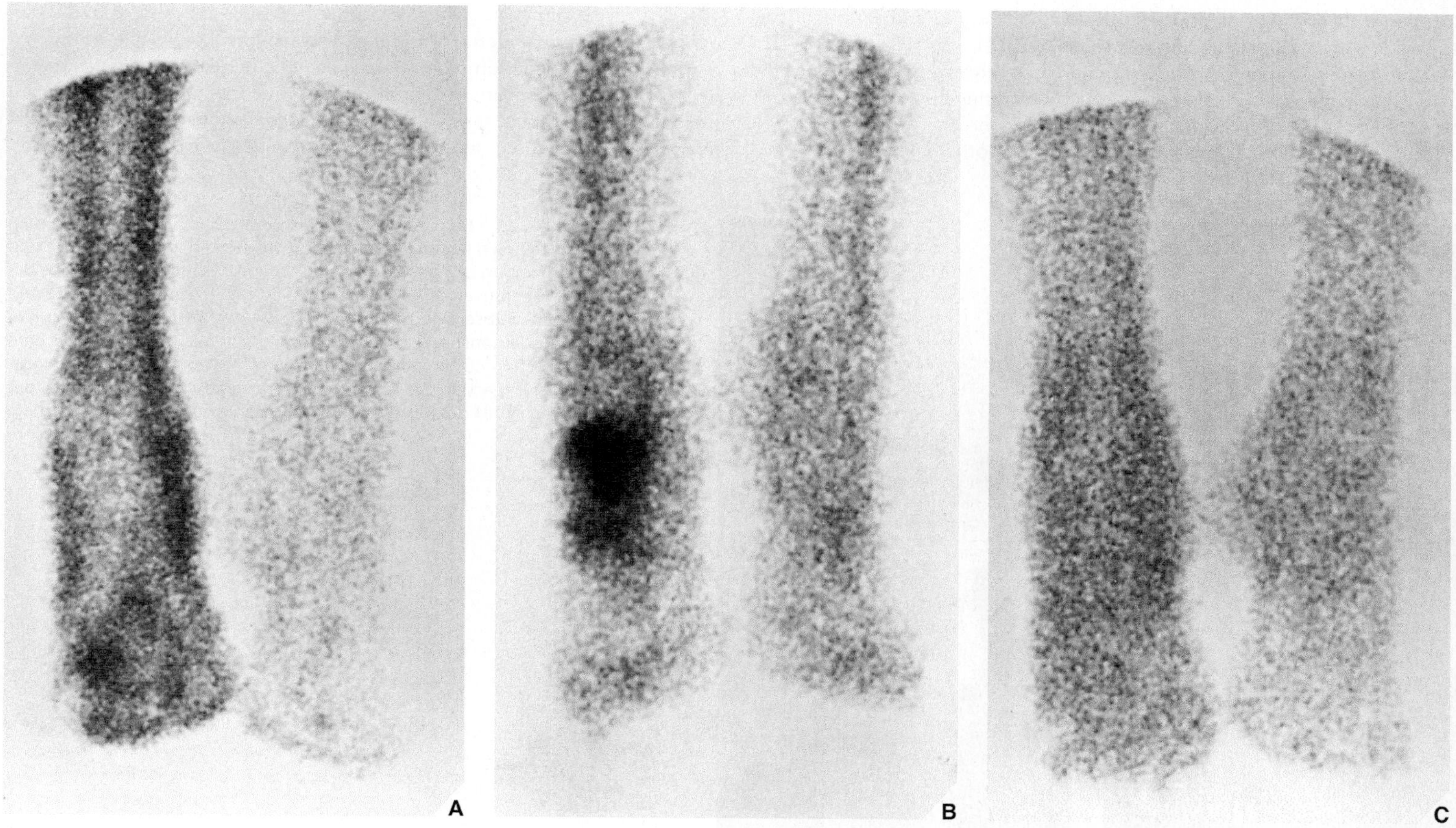

FIGURE 24.10 Application of radionuclide bone scan in infection. A 52-year-old woman with pain in her right ankle had cellulitis around the ankle joint. Although radiographs did not reveal changes in the joint suggestive of infectious arthritis, this possibility could not be ruled out clinically because early changes of infection may not be detected on standard radiographs. A three-phase radionuclide bone scan was performed. **(A)** In the first phase, 1 minute after intravenous injection of a 15 mCi (555 MBq) bolus of ^{99m}Tc-labeled MDP, there is increased activity in the major vessels of the right leg. **(B)** In the second phase, 3 minutes after injection, a blood pool scan demonstrates increased uptake in the area of the infected soft tissues. **(C)** In the third phase, 2 hours after injection, almost complete washout of the radiopharmaceutical agent, with no evidence of localization in the bones on both sides of the joint, excludes the diagnosis of infectious arthritis.
(Courtesy of R. Goldfarb, MD, New York.)

namely, isotope-labeled (^{99m}Tc, ^{111}In, or iodine-123 [^{123}I]) monoclonal antigranulocyte antibodies, isotope-labeled polyclonal immunoglobulin G (IgG), isotope-labeled monocytes, isotope-labeled chemotactic polypeptide analogs, and isotope-labeled specific antibodies against bacteria. Preliminary application of fluorodeoxyglucose positron emission tomography (FDG PET) for evaluation of infections yielded promising results.

Arteriography, Myelography, Fistulography, and Ultrasound

Arteriography is important in the evaluation of the patient's vascular supply, particularly if a reconstructive procedure is planned. Myelography is still useful in evaluating infections within the spinal canal as well as in vertebral osteomyelitis and disk infection (see Fig. 25.51). Fistulography (sinogram) is an important examination for outlining sinus tracts in the soft tissues and for evaluating their extension into the bone (Fig. 24.11). US can occasionally be used in diagnosing soft-tissue and joint infections as well as osteomyelitis. This modality has the advantage of being easily accessible and available at relatively reasonable cost. In addition, this technique does not expose the patient to ionizing radiation. Real-time capability of US is unique in providing a means to evaluate structures under dynamic conditions. In diffuse soft-tissue infection, US may be helpful in distinguishing primary disease from that associated with underlying abscess such as in pyomyositis or osteomyelitis. Furthermore, US plays an important role in the guidance of percutaneous biopsy and aspiration of infectious lesions as well as the therapeutic drainage of abscesses.

Magnetic Resonance Imaging

At the present time, MRI established its place in the evaluation of bone and soft-tissue infections. As several studies have indicated, osteomyelitis, soft-tissue abscesses, joint and tendon sheath effusions, and various forms of cellulitis are well depicted by this modality. MRI is as sensitive as ^{99m}Tc-MDP in demonstrating osteomyelitis and more sensitive and more specific than other scintigraphic techniques in demonstrating soft-tissue infections primarily because of its superior spatial resolution. The proper evaluation of musculoskeletal infections with MRI requires both T1- and T2-weighted images in at least two imaging planes. In anatomically complex areas such as the pelvis, spine, foot, and hand, three planes may be necessary. During the early phases of osteomyelitis, MRI findings include a poorly defined area of low signal intensity in the bone marrow cavity on short spin-echo repetition time (TR)/echo time (TE) sequences (T1 weighting) along with increased signal intensity in the bone marrow cavity on long TR/TE sequences (T2 weighting), associated with thin periosteal reaction and surrounding soft-tissue edema (Fig. 24.12). The periosteal reaction is seen on MRI shortly after the infection takes place, before it is demonstrated on conventional radiography or CT. In order to visualize periosteal reaction on conventional radiography or CT, calcium deposition is needed, and this takes place after several days from the beginning of the pathologic process causing the periosteal elevation (infection, trauma, or tumor). However, MRI can depict the periosteal elevation immediately because it does not require calcium deposition. In addition, the periosteum is a thin, low–signal intensity layer, and when it becomes separated from the underlying cortex, it is surrounded with hyperintense edema, blood, or tumoral tissue, depending on the causative process, allowing good visualization on T2-weighted MRI (Fig. 24.12C).

Once the focus of osteomyelitis becomes chronic, an intraosseous abscess is formed (Brodie abscess). A Brodie abscess represents a pus-filled cavity within the bone with an internal lining of granulation tissue, surrounded with reactive sclerosis fading away peripherally. Periosteal reaction is also a feature of chronic osteomyelitis. These pathologic features can be well demonstrated on MRI (Figs. 24.13 and 24.14). During the late stages of chronic, untreated osteomyelitis, thick, chronic periosteal reaction involves the infected bone (the "involucrum"), and fragments of necrotic bone (the "sequestrum") develops. As the infection progresses, the intraosseous abscess opens to the surface of the bone and creates a draining sinus ("cloaca") to the adjacent skin surface. Often, the sequestrum is extruded through the cloaca in this late stage of the infection. All these pathologic stages of chronic osteomyelitis are very well depicted with MRI (see Fig. 24.14).

Increased signal intensity of the soft tissues on long TR/TE sequences with poorly defined margins is considered indicative of edema and/or nonspecific inflammatory changes. Well-demarcated collections of decreased signal intensity on T1-weighted sequences and increased signal intensity surrounded by zones of decreased signal intensity on T2-weighted images are considered indicative of soft-tissue abscesses (Fig. 24.15).

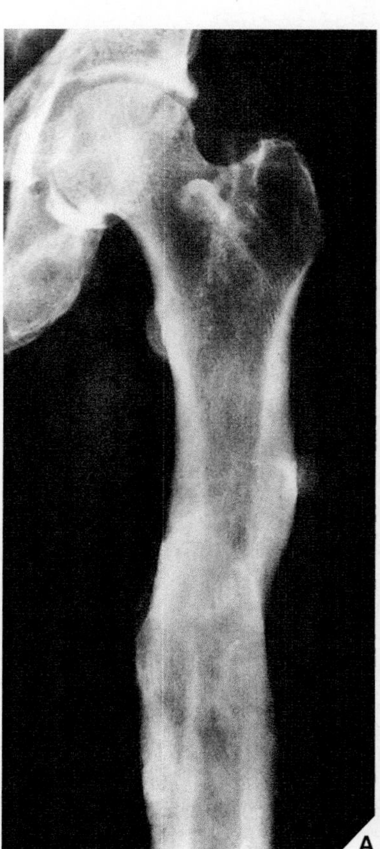

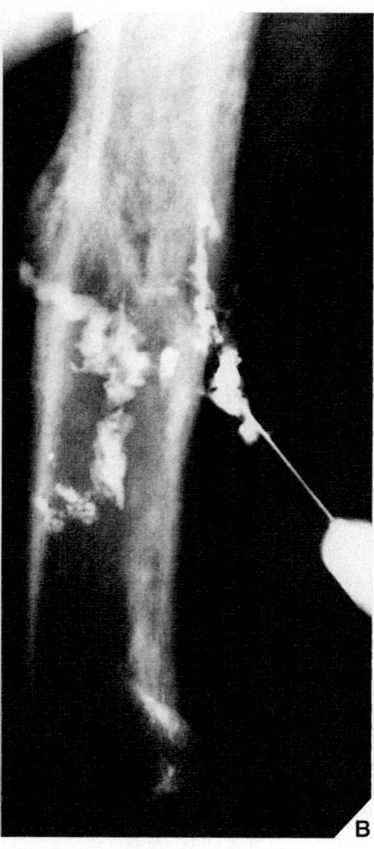

FIGURE 24.11 **Fistulography in osteomyelitis.** A 48-year-old man who had sustained a fracture of the femur was treated with open reduction and internal fixation using an intramedullary rod. Chronic osteomyelitis developed postoperatively. The rod was removed, and the infection was treated with antibiotics. Subsequently, a draining sinus developed. **(A)** Radiograph of the left femur demonstrates changes typical of chronic osteomyelitis. There is focal destruction of the medullary portion of the bone, reactive sclerosis, and a periosteal reaction. **(B)** A sinogram performed to evaluate the extent of the draining fistula demonstrates an intraosseous sinus tract with multiple ramifications.

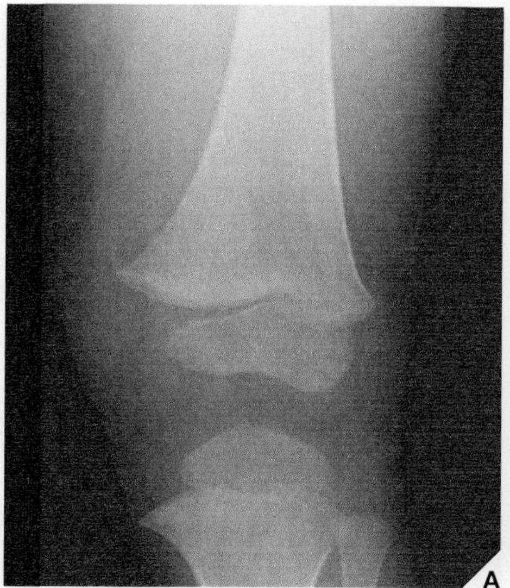

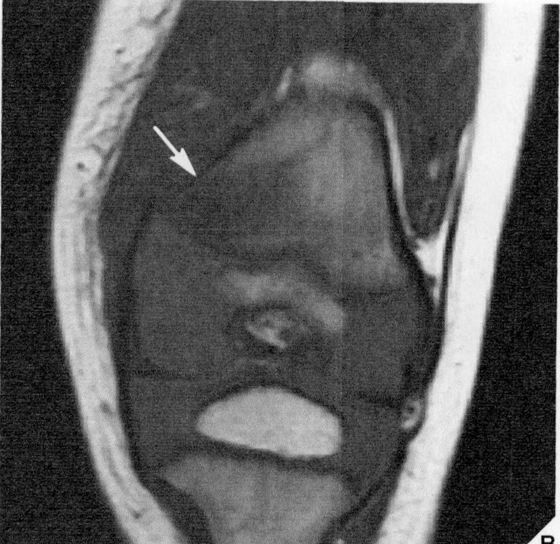

FIGURE 24.12 MRI of acute osteomyelitis. **(A)** Frontal radiograph of the knee of a 3-year-old child shows no abnormalities. **(B)** Coronal T1-weighted MRI demonstrates an ill-defined area of low signal intensity in the distal metaphysis of the femur *(arrow)*. **(C)** Axial T2-weighted MRI demonstrates high signal intensity in the same area *(arrow)*, with periosteal reaction *(arrowhead)* and soft-tissue edema.

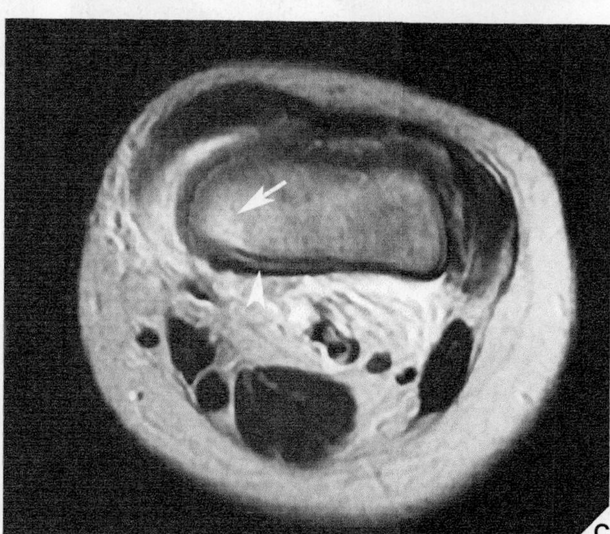

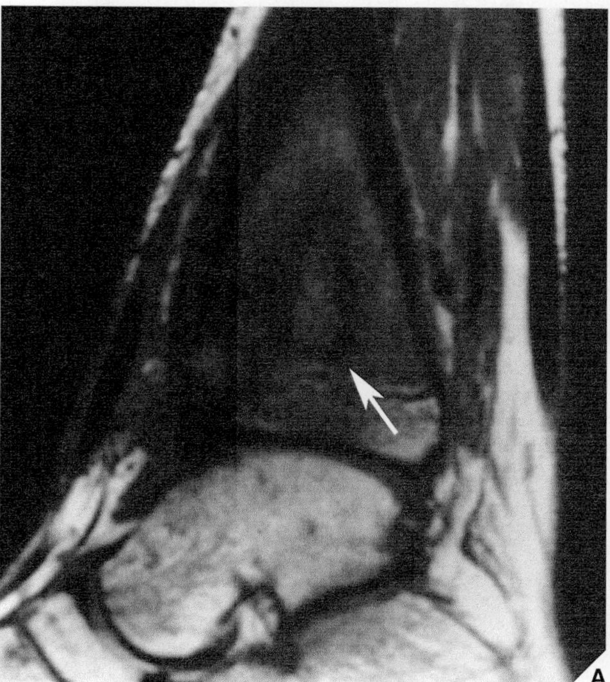

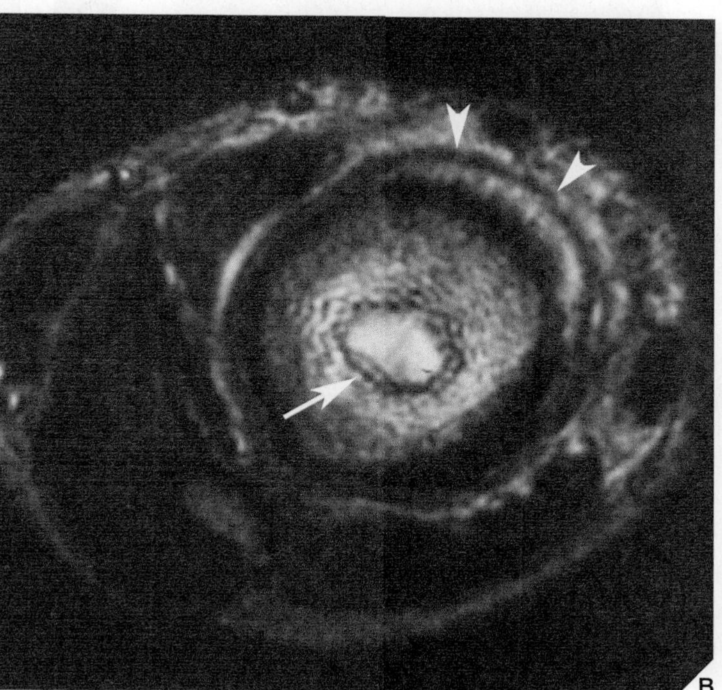

FIGURE 24.13 MRI of chronic osteomyelitis/Brodie abscess. **(A)** Sagittal T1-weighted MRI of the ankle of a 12-year-old girl shows an intramedullary abscess in the distal tibial metaphysis *(arrow)*, with surrounding low–signal intensity area corresponding to edema, and anterior periosteal reaction. **(B)** Axial T2-weighted MRI shows the hyperintense intramedullary abscess (Brodie abscess) *(arrow)* with surrounding hyperintense edema and anterior periosteal reaction *(arrowheads)*.

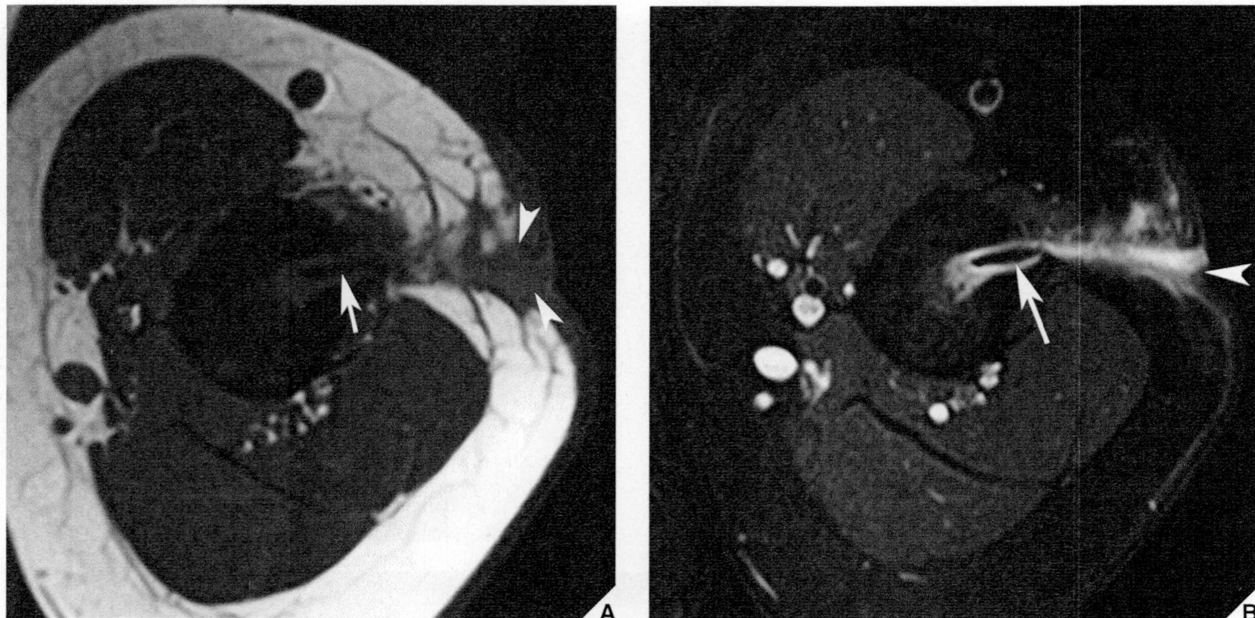

FIGURE 24.14 MRI of chronic osteomyelitis. **(A)** Axial T1-weighted MRI of the humerus demonstrates low signal intensity and thickening of the midshaft of the humerus with a lytic area penetrating the lateral cortex, representing a chronic abscess with surrounding sclerosis and a cloaca with a draining sinus that extends to the skin *(arrowheads)*. The low–signal intensity linear structure inside the cloaca represents the sequestrum being extruded *(arrow)*. Note the thick, chronic periosteal reaction of the humerus. **(B)** Axial short time inversion recovery (STIR) MRI demonstrates the sequestrum *(arrow)* being extruded through the cloaca and the draining sinus *(arrowhead)*.

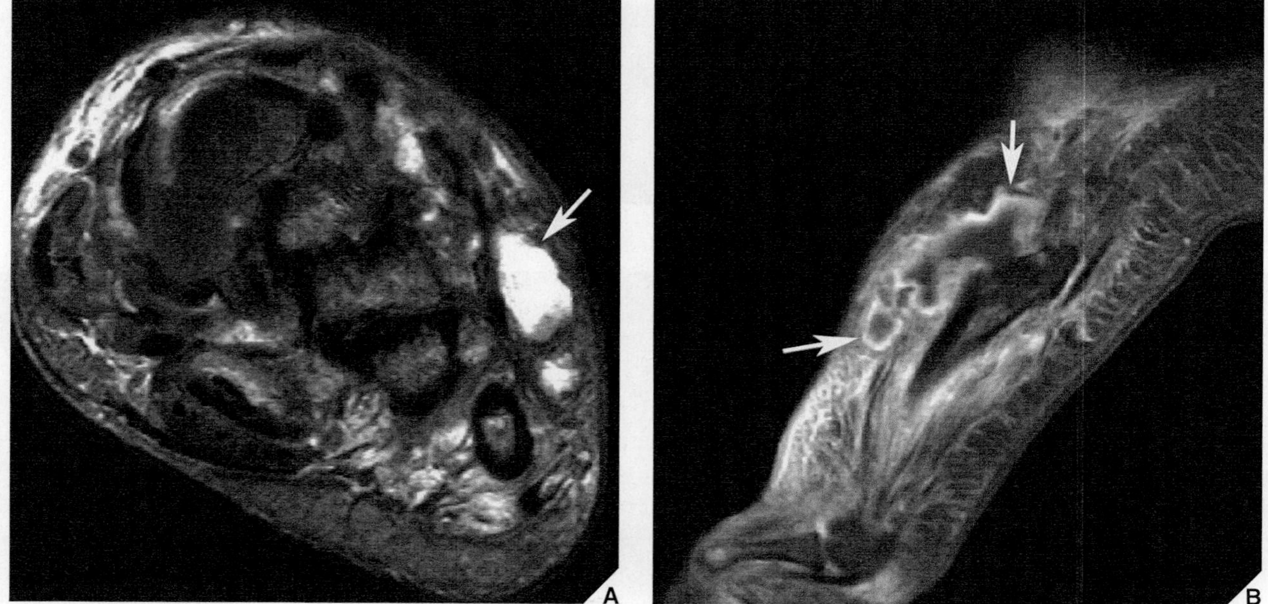

FIGURE 24.15 MRI of soft-tissue abscess. **(A)** Short axis T2-weighted image of the foot in a diabetic patient demonstrates a hyperintense fluid collection in the dorsal aspect of the foot *(arrow)*. **(B)** Sagittal T1-weighted fat-saturated MRI obtained after intravenous injection of gadolinium demonstrates the hypointense, irregular abscess in the dorsum of the foot with ring enhancement *(arrows)*, corresponding to the granulation hypervascular tissue in the inner wall of the abscess.

Decreased signal intensity on short TR/TE sequences and increased signal intensity on long TR/TE sequences in the area of the joint capsule or tendon sheath are consistent with synovial effusions and fluid in the tendon sheath.

Contrast enhancement using intravenous injection of gadolinium is routinely used for the diagnosis of musculoskeletal infections. This technique allows the differentiation of osteomyelitis from bone marrow edema or an abscess from cellulites or phlegmon in the soft tissues. The abscess demonstrates high–signal intensity enhancement of its capsule, whereas the central portion remains of low signal intensity. Conversely, cellulites and phlegmon exhibit diffuse contrast enhancement.

Invasive Procedures

Percutaneous aspiration and US-guided, CT-guided, or fluoroscopy-guided biopsy of a suspected focus of infection may be performed in the radiology suite. It can rapidly confirm a suspected diagnosis of infection and reveal the causative organism.

Monitoring the Treatment and Complications of Infections

Imaging plays an indispensable role in monitoring the treatment of infectious disorders of bone and associated soft tissues (Fig. 24.16). Follow-up radiographs and radionuclide bone scans should be obtained at regular intervals to evaluate the disease state (acute, subacute, chronic, or inactive) (Fig. 24.17) and any complications that may arise (Fig. 24.18). The differentiation of active from inactive osteomyelitis may, however, be extremely difficult by radiologic techniques. The extensive osteosclerotic changes in inactive infection may obscure small foci of osteolytic change signifying reactivation. CT may at times be helpful in delineating fluffy periostitis, poorly marginated areas of osteolysis, or sequestra.

The main complication of osteomyelitis in infants and children is growth disturbance if the focus of infection is in the vicinity of the growth plate (Fig. 24.19). Pathologic fracture is another common complication

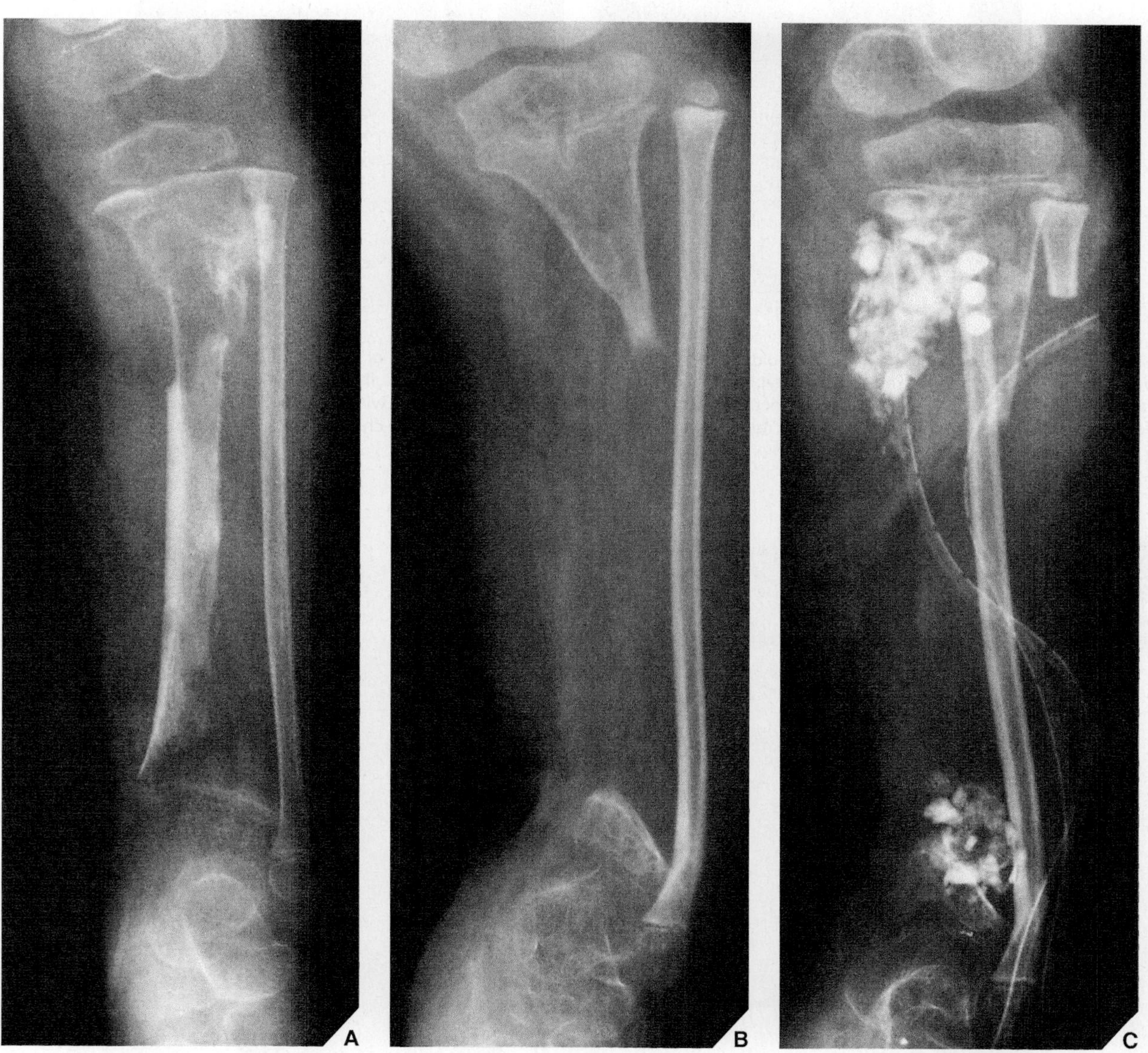

FIGURE 24.16 **Treatment of osteomyelitis.** A 3-year-old girl developed osteomyelitis of the left tibia after chronic tonsillitis. **(A)** Anteroposterior radiograph of the left leg shows extensive destruction of the tibia with sequestration of the diaphysis. Extensive and long-standing conservative treatment using broad-spectrum antibiotics failed to produce any improvement. **(B)** One year later, the dead sequestered segment of the tibial diaphysis was resected as a first stage in reconstruction of the limb. **(C)** Two months later, a fibular graft was attached to the proximal stump of the tibial diaphysis, and bone chips were applied proximally and distally to ensure bony union and stability.

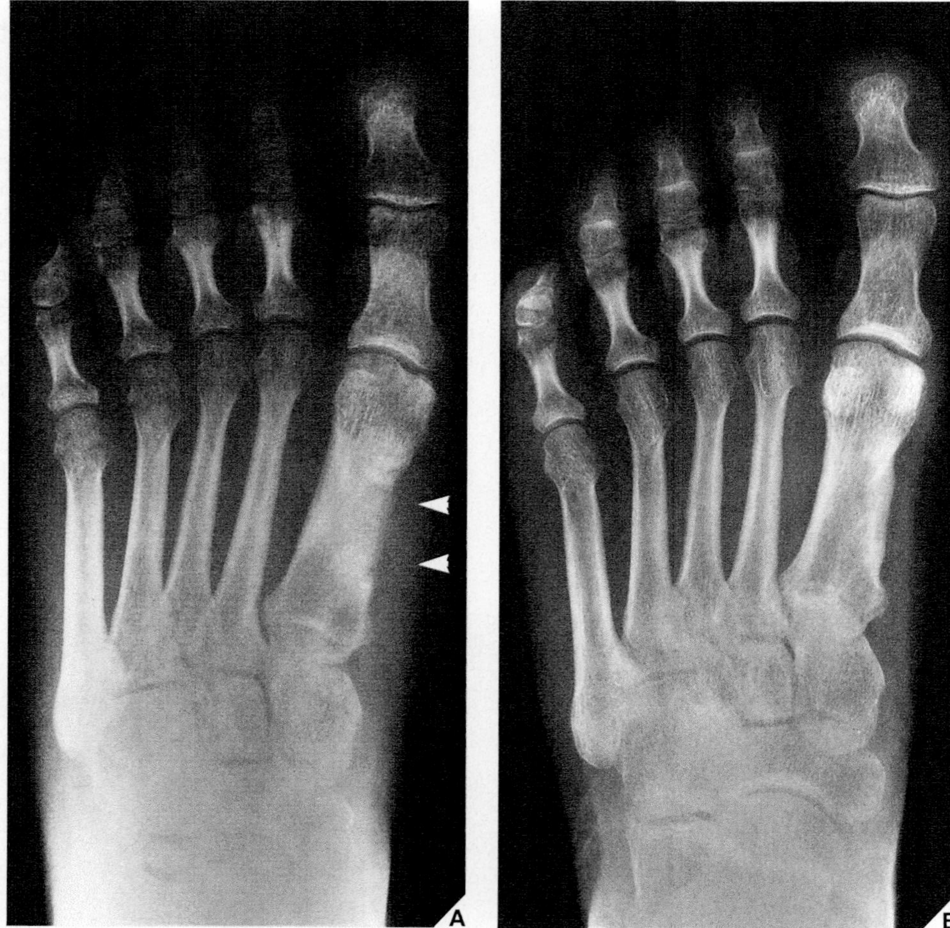

FIGURE 24.17 **Treatment of osteomyelitis.** A 17-year-old girl developed an acute pyogenic infection of the first metatarsal bone after a puncture injury of her right foot. **(A)** Anteroposterior radiograph demonstrates changes typical of active osteomyelitis: cortical and medullary bone destruction, a periosteal reaction, and diffuse soft-tissue swelling *(arrowheads)*. Note also the significant periarticular osteoporosis. After extensive treatment with antibiotics, a radiograph of the foot **(B)** shows complete healing of the infection, which is in an inactive phase. There is residual endosteal sclerosis, but no destructive changes are evident, and the soft-tissue planes are normal.

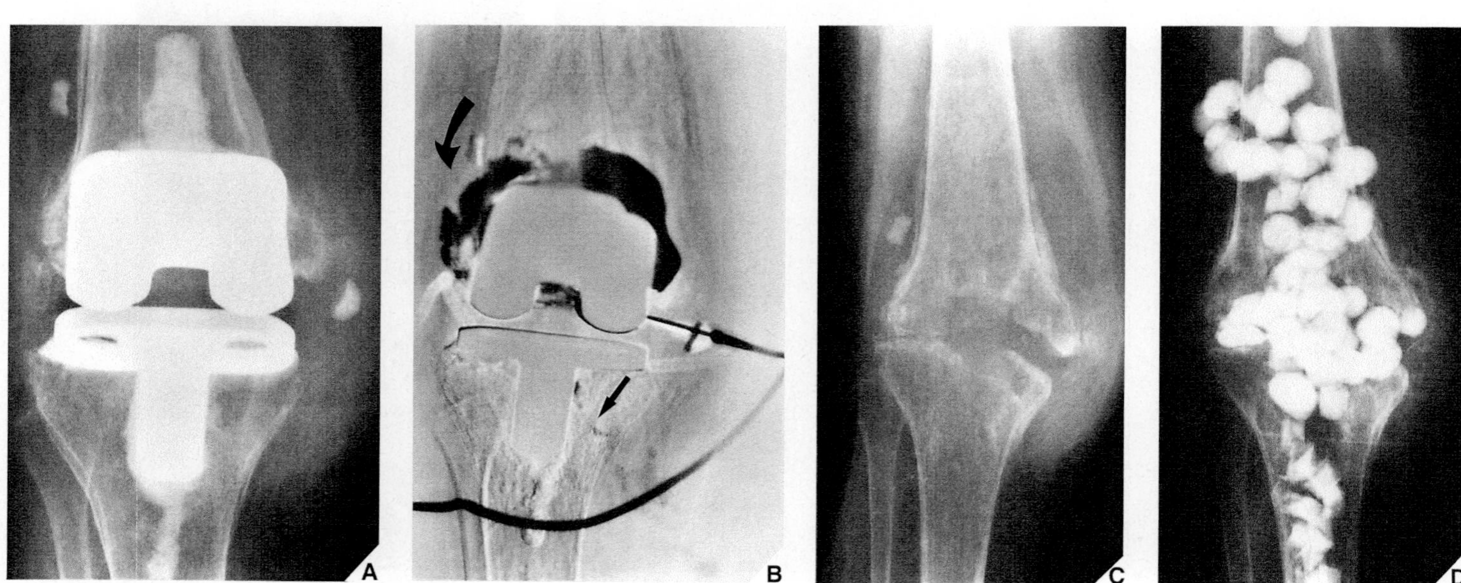

FIGURE 24.18 **Treatment of joint infection after a total knee arthroplasty.** A 62-year-old woman developed an infection of the right knee joint after total knee arthroplasty. **(A)** Anteroposterior radiograph shows the joint replacement with a condylar-type cemented prosthesis. Active infection is still evident, as demonstrated by the soft-tissue swelling, joint effusion, and periosteal reaction. Small foci of bone destruction are seen in the proximal tibia. **(B)** An aspiration arthrogram (subtraction study) demonstrates abnormal extension of contrast agent into osteolytic areas of the tibia *(arrow)*. The irregular outline on the lateral aspect of the joint *(curved arrow)* is caused by synovitis. Bacteriologic examination of the aspirated material yielded *S. aureus*. **(C)** After unsuccessful treatment of the infection with broad-spectrum antibiotics, the prosthesis had to be removed. Note the typical appearance of active osteomyelitis of distal femur and proximal tibia. **(D)** The treatment at this stage consisted of methylmethacrylate cement balls soaked with antibiotics and applied to the infected joint and medullary cavity of the femur and tibia.

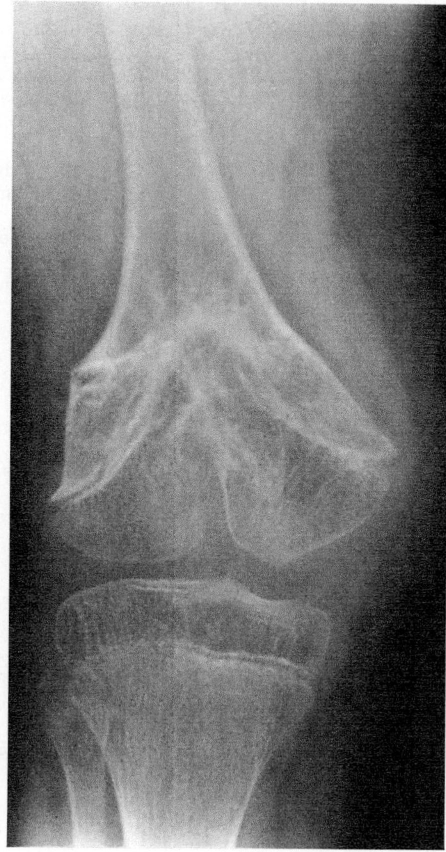

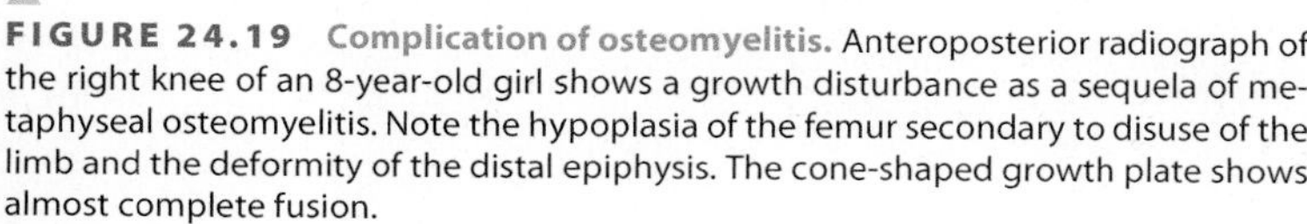

FIGURE 24.19 Complication of osteomyelitis. Anteroposterior radiograph of the right knee of an 8-year-old girl shows a growth disturbance as a sequela of metaphyseal osteomyelitis. Note the hypoplasia of the femur secondary to disuse of the limb and the deformity of the distal epiphysis. The cone-shaped growth plate shows almost complete fusion.

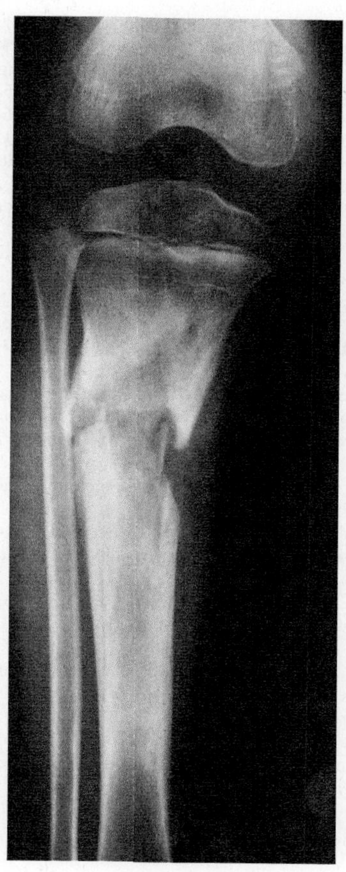

FIGURE 24.20 Complication of osteomyelitis. Radiograph of the right leg of a 6-year-old boy with chronic active osteomyelitis of tibia shows a pathologic fracture, a complication of the infectious process.

of osteomyelitis (Fig. 24.20). In adults, the most serious, although rare, complication is the development of a malignant neoplasm in a chronically draining sinus tract (see Fig. 22.61).

PRACTICAL POINTS TO REMEMBER

1. Three basic mechanisms allow an infectious organism to reach a bone or joint:
   - hematogenous spread
   - spread from a contiguous source
   - direct implantation.
2. The metaphysis is the most common site of an infectious focus in children, primarily because of the nature of the osseous–vascular anatomy at this stage of development, whereas the shaft of a long bone is a common site of infection in adult patients.
3. Radionuclide bone scan using ^{99m}Tc-labeled phosphonates is a very useful radiologic modality for distinguishing a joint infection from cellulitis of the periarticular soft tissues.
4. The scintigraphic radiopharmaceuticals most specific for detection of musculoskeletal infection are ^{67}Ga citrate and ^{111}In oxine.
5. MRI is more specific and more sensitive than scintigraphic techniques in demonstrating bone and soft-tissue infections, primarily because of its superior spatial resolution. Both T1- and T2-weighted sequences in at least two imaging planes should be obtained.
6. Percutaneous aspiration biopsy of a suspected focus of infection is the most direct route for confirming a diagnosis and identifying the causative organism.

SUGGESTED READINGS

Alazraki NP. Radionuclide imaging in the evaluation of infections and inflammatory disease. *Radiol Clin North Am* 1993;31:783–794.

Al-Sheikh W, Sfakianakis GN, Mnaymneh W, et al. Subacute and chronic bone infections: diagnosis using In-111, Ga-67 and Tc-99m MDP bone scintigraphy, and radiography. *Radiology* 1985;155:501–506.

Becker W, Goldenberg DM, Wolf F. The use of monoclonal antibodies and antibody fragments in the imaging of infectious lesions. *Semin Nucl Med* 1994;24:142–153.

Beltran J, McGhee RB, Shaffer PB, et al. Experimental infections of the musculoskeletal system: evaluation with MR imaging and Tc-99m MDP and Ga-67 scintigraphy. *Radiology* 1988;167:167–172.

Beltran J, Noto AM, McGhee RB, et al. Infections of the musculoskeletal system: high-field-strength MR imaging. *Radiology* 1987;164:449–454.

Bierry G, Huang AJ, Chang CY, et al. MRI findings of treated bacterial septic arthritis. *Skeletal Radiol* 2012;41:1509–1516.

Bläuenstein P, Locher JT, Seybold K, et al. Experience with the iodine-123 and technetium-99m labelled anti-granulocyte antibody MAb47: a comparison of labelling methods. *Eur J Nucl Med* 1995;22:690–698.

Butalia S, Palda VA, Sargeant RJ, et al. Does this patient with diabetes have osteomyelitis of the lower extremity? *JAMA* 2008;299:806–813.

Dagirmanjian A, Schils J, McHenry M, et al. MR imaging of vertebral osteomyelitis revisited. *AJR Am J Roentgenol* 1996;167:1539–1543.

Dangman BC, Hoffer FA, Rand FF, et al. Osteomyelitis in children: gadolinium-enhanced MR imaging. *Radiology* 1992;182:743–747.

Datz FL. The current status of radionuclide infection imaging. In: Freeman LM, ed. *Nuclear medicine annual.* New York: Raven Press; 1993:47–76.

Datz FL. Indium-111-labeled leukocytes for the detection of infection: current status. *Semin Nucl Med* 1994;24:92–109.

Datz FL, Morton KA. New radiopharmaceuticals for detecting infection. *Invest Radiol* 1993;28:356–365.

Demirev A, Weijers R, Geurts J, et al. Comparison of [18 F]FDG PET/CT and MRI in the diagnosis of active osteomyelitis. *Skeletal Radiol* 2014;43:665–672.

Erdman WA, Tamburro F, Jayson HT, et al. Osteomyelitis: characteristics and pitfalls of diagnosis with MR imaging. *Radiology* 1991;180:533–539.

Fox IN, Zeiger L. Tc-99m-HMPAO leukocyte scintigraphy for the diagnosis of osteomyelitis in diabetic foot infections. *J Foot Ankle Surg* 1993;32:591–594.

Gold RH, Hawkins RA, Katz RD. Bacterial osteomyelitis: findings on plain radiography, CT, MR, and scintigraphy. *AJR Am J Roentgenol* 1991;157:365–370.

Guhlmann A, Brecht-Krauss D, Suger G, et al. Chronic osteomyelitis: detection with FDG PET and correlation with histopathologic findings. *Radiology* 1998;206:749–754.

Harcke HT, Grissom LE. Musculoskeletal ultrasound in pediatrics. *Semin Musculoskelet Radiol* 1998;2:321–329.

Hopkins KL, Li KCP, Bergman G. Gadolinium-DTPA-enhanced magnetic resonance imaging of musculoskeletal infectious processes. *Skeletal Radiol* 1995;24:325–330.

Jacobson AF, Harley JD, Lipsky BA, et al. Diagnosis of osteomyelitis in the presence of soft-tissue infection and radiologic evidence of osseous abnormalities: value of leukocyte scintigraphy. *AJR Am J Roentgenol* 1991;157:807–812.

Jaramillo D, Treves ST, Kasser JR, et al. Osteomyelitis and septic arthritis in children: appropriate use of imaging to guide treatment. *AJR Am J Roentgenol* 1995;165: 399–403.

Kaim A, Maurer T, Ochsner P, et al. Chronic complicated osteomyelitis of the appendicular skeleton: diagnosis with technetium-99m labelled monoclonal antigranulocyte antibody-immunoscintigraphy. *Eur J Nucl Med* 1997;24:732–738.

Krznaric E, Roo MD, Verbruggen A, et al. Chronic osteomyelitis: diagnosis with technetium-99m-d, l-hexamethylpropylene amine oxime labelled leucocytes. *Eur J Nucl Med* 1996;23:792–797.

Lee SK, Suh KJ, Kim YW, et al. Septic arthritis versus transient synovitis at MR imaging: preliminary assessment with signal intensity alterations in bone marrow. *Radiology* 1999;211:459–465.

McGuinness B, Wilson N, Doyle AJ. The "penumbra sign" on T1-weighted MRI for differentiating musculoskeletal infection from tumour. *Skeletal Radiol* 2007;36: 417–421.

Merkel KD, Brown ML, Dewanjee MK, et al. Comparison of indium-labeled-leukocyte imaging with sequential technetium-gallium scanning in the diagnosis of low-grade musculoskeletal sepsis. A prospective study. *J Bone Joint Surg Am* 1985;67:465–476.

Miller TT, Randolph DA Jr, Staron RB, et al. Fat-suppressed MRI of musculoskeletal infection: fast T2-weighted techniques versus gadolinium-enhanced T1-weighted images. *Skeletal Radiol* 1997;26:654–658.

Morrison WB, Schweitzer ME, Bock GW, et al. Diagnosis of osteomyelitis: utility of fat-suppressed contrast-enhanced MR imaging. *Radiology* 1993;189:251–257.

Morrison WB, Schweitzer ME, Wapner KL, et al. Osteomyelitis in feet of diabetics: clinical accuracy, surgical utility, and cost-effectiveness of MR imaging. *Radiology* 1995;196:557–564.

Palestro CJ, Love C, Tronco GG, et al. Combined labeled leukocyte and technetium 99m sulfur colloid bone marrow imaging for diagnosing musculoskeletal infection. *Radiographics* 2006;26:859–870.

Palestro CJ, Roumanas P, Swyer AJ, et al. Diagnosis of musculoskeletal infection using combined In-111 labeled leukocyte and Tc-99m SC marrow imaging. *Clin Nucl Med* 1992;17:269–273.

Peters AM. The utility of [^{99m}Tc]HMPAO-leukocytes for imaging infection. *Semin Nucl Med* 1994;24:110–127.

Ruf J, Oeser C, Amthauer H. Clinical role of anti-granulocyte MoAb versus radiolabeled white blood cells. *Q J Nucl Med Mol Imaging* 2010;54:599–616.

Schauwecker DS. The role of nuclear medicine in osteomyelitis. In: Collier D Jr, Fogelman I, Rosenthall L, eds. *Skeletal nuclear medicine*. St. Louis: CV Mosby; 1996:183–202.

Schauwecker DS. The scintigraphic diagnosis of osteomyelitis. *AJR Am J Roentgenol* 1992;158:9–18.

Sorsdahl OA, Goodhart GL, Williams HT, et al. Quantitative bone gallium scintigraphy in osteomyelitis. *Skeletal Radiol* 1993;22:239–242.

Stöver B, Sigmund G, Langer M, et al. MRI in diagnostic evaluation of osteomyelitis in children. *Eur Radiol* 1994;4:347–352.

Tigges S, Stiles RG, Roberson JR. Appearance of septic hip prostheses on plain radiographs. *AJR Am J Roentgenol* 1994;163:377–380.

Turecki MB, Taljanovic MS, Stubbs AY, et al. Imaging of musculoskeletal soft tissue infections. *Skeletal Radiol* 2010;39:957–971.

Van Holsbeeck M, Introcaso JH. *Musculoskeletal ultrasound*. St. Louis: Mosby-Year Book; 1991:207–229.

Vartanians VM, Karchmer AW, Giurini JM, et al. Is there a role for imaging in the management of patients with diabetic foot? *Skeletal Radiol* 2009;38:633–636.

Wang A, Weinstein D, Greenfield L, et al. MRI and diabetic foot infections. *Magn Reson Imaging* 1990;8:805–809.

Zeiger LS, Fox IN. Use of indium-111-labeled white blood cells in the diagnosis of diabetic foot infections. *J Foot Surg* 1990;29:46–51.

25

Osteomyelitis, Infectious Arthritis, and Soft-Tissue Infections

Osteomyelitis

Osteomyelitis can generally be divided into pyogenic and nonpyogenic types. The former may be further classified, on the basis of clinical findings, as subacute, acute, or chronic (active and inactive), depending on the intensity of the infectious process and its associated symptoms. From the viewpoint of anatomic pathology, osteomyelitis can be divided into diffuse and localized (focal) forms, with the latter referred to as *bone abscesses*.

Pyogenic Bone Infections

Acute and Chronic Osteomyelitis

Clinical Features

The clinical course of osteomyelitis depends on the interaction between the infectious organism and the host tissue. The severity of infection is contingent on the virulence of the invading organism, the site of infection, the patient's general health, and patient's age.

The majority of patients with acute hematogenous osteomyelitis are children. The most common clinical presentation is high fever and local pain. The most frequent sites of infection are the areas of rapid growth including the distal femur, the proximal tibia, the proximal femur, the proximal humerus, and the distal radius. In most cases, the responsible organism is *Staphylococcus aureus*. In adults, acute hematogenous osteomyelitis is seen mainly in debilitated persons with chronic diseases, such as genitourinary infection, or in those with peripheral vascular insufficiency, in many cases associated with diabetes. In the latter group, the infection is usually affecting the small bones of the feet. The etiology is commonly polymicrobial and may be due to anaerobic organism. The separate group prone to infections consists of the drug addicts. In most of these patients, *Pseudomonas aeruginosa* and streptococcal species are the responsible organisms. The focus of osteomyelitis is usually in the spine or in the pelvis, although the infection may occur anywhere in the skeletal system, sometimes affecting unusual sites like clavicle, sternum, or symphysis pubis.

Osteomyelitis resulting from direct inoculation of bacteria from punctured wounds, traffic accidents, and iatrogenic infections currently has become a more common clinical problem. Usually the infection is polymicrobial in nature, with *Staphylococcus*, *Streptococcus*, and gram-negative organisms such as *Pseudomonas* being on top of the list. Iatrogenic infections are the result of surgical intervention involving open reduction and internal fixations of various fractures or related to joint replacement. The causative organisms commonly identified in such cases are *S. aureus*, *P. aeruginosa*, and some of the anaerobic organisms.

Imaging Features

The earliest radiographic signs of bone infection are soft-tissue edema and loss of fascial planes. These are usually encountered within 24 to 48 hours of the onset of infection. The earliest changes in the bone are evidence of a destructive lytic lesion, usually within 7 to 10 days after the onset of infection (Fig. 25.1), and a positive radionuclide bone scan. Within 2 to 6 weeks, there is progressive destruction of cortical and medullary bone, an increased endosteal sclerosis indicating reactive new bone formation, and a periosteal reaction (Fig. 25.2; see also Fig. 24.6). In 6 to 8 weeks, sequestra indicating areas of necrotic bone usually become apparent; they are surrounded by a dense involucrum, representing a sheath of periosteal new bone (Fig. 25.3). The sequestra, which can be effectively demonstrated with computed tomography (CT) (Fig. 25.4) or magnetic resonance imaging (MRI) (see Fig. 24.14), and involucra develop as the result of an accumulation of inflammatory exudate (pus), which penetrates the cortex and strips it of periosteum, thus stimulating the inner layer to form new bone. The newly formed bone is in turn infected, and the resultant barrier causes the cortex and spongiosa to be deprived of a blood supply and to become necrotic. At this stage, termed *chronic osteomyelitis*, a draining sinus tract often forms (Figs. 25.5 to 25.7; see also Figs. 24.7B and 24.11B). Small sequestra are gradually resorbed, or they may be extruded through the sinus tract.

The MRI manifestations of acute osteomyelitis before the formation of an intraosseous abscess are nonspecific. Bone marrow edema and early periosteal reaction may be the only findings (see Fig. 25.1C–E). However, if there is a soft-tissue infection, such as abscess or ulceration, adjacent to the area in question, the diagnosis of acute osteomyelitis is more likely (see Figs. 25.58 and 25.59). Another described MRI sign of acute osteomyelitis is the presence of fat globules in the bone marrow surrounded by edema (see Fig. 25.1F). The fat globules can also be seen in the adjacent soft tissues. This finding is probably related to increased intramedullary pressure leading to septic necrosis with death of the lipocytes and subsequent release of free fatty globules. Although this finding is not pathognomonic, it supports the diagnosis of osteomyelitis and excludes the presence of a bone tumor.

Pathology

The pathologic changes depend on the stage of infectious process, whether acute or chronic. In acute stage, bacterial growth evokes an acute inflammatory reaction consisting of polymorphonuclear leukocytes (neutrophils) infiltration, edema, and ischemic necrosis of bone trabeculae and bone marrow. Osteoclastic bone resorption is followed by reactive new bone formation. When the infectious process spreads through the bone marrow and Haversian systems to reach the subperiosteal space, a subperiosteal

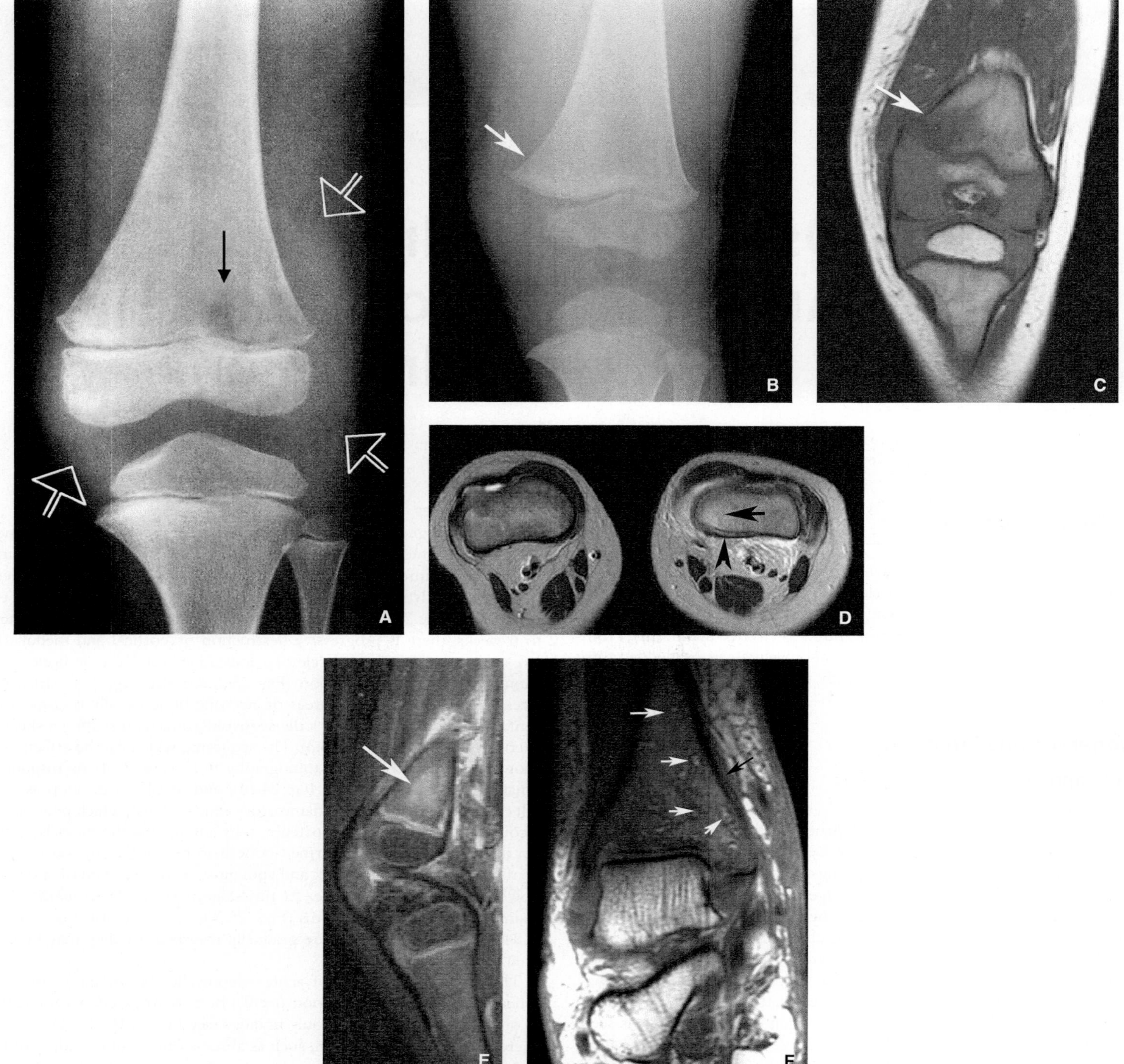

FIGURE 25.1 Acute osteomyelitis—early radiographic and MRI manifestations. (A) A 7-year-old boy had a fever and a painful knee for 1 week. Anteroposterior radiograph of the left knee demonstrates the earliest radiographic signs of bone infection: a poorly defined osteolytic area of destruction in the metaphyseal segment of the distal femur *(arrow)* and soft-tissue swelling *(open arrows)*. **(B)** Anteroposterior radiograph of the left knee of a 3-year-old boy with fever and painful knee shows subtle lucency in the distal metaphysis of the femur *(arrow)*. **(C)** Coronal T1-weighted, **(D)** axial T2-weighted, and **(E)** sagittal short time inversion recovery (STIR) MR images demonstrate an ill-defined area of abnormal signal intensity in the medial aspect of the distal metaphysis of the left femur *(arrows)* and periosteal reaction (*arrowhead* in **D**) with surrounding soft-tissue edema. **(F)** Coronal T1-weighted MR image of the right ankle of a 60-year-old woman with pain, redness, and swelling of the lower leg shows low–signal intensity bone marrow edema in the distal tibia with early periosteal reaction *(black arrow)*, representing acute osteomyelitis. Note the multiple small, hyperintense fat globules within the bone marrow of the distal tibia *(white arrows)*.

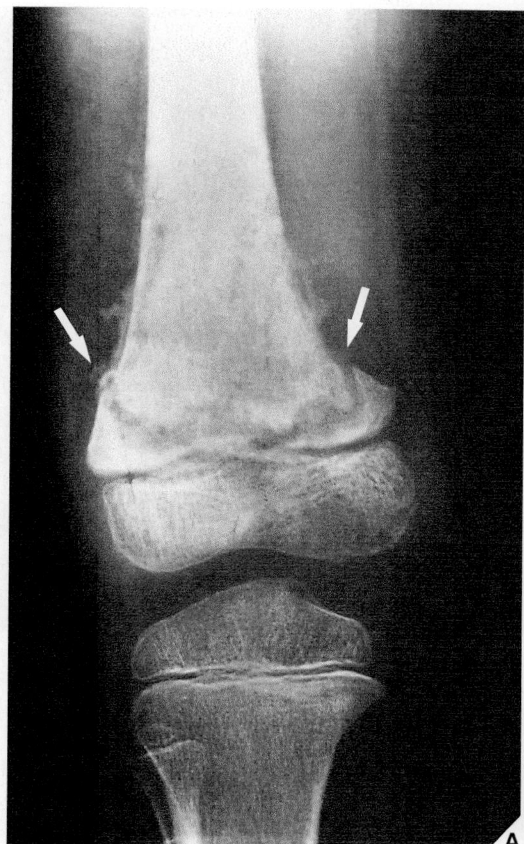

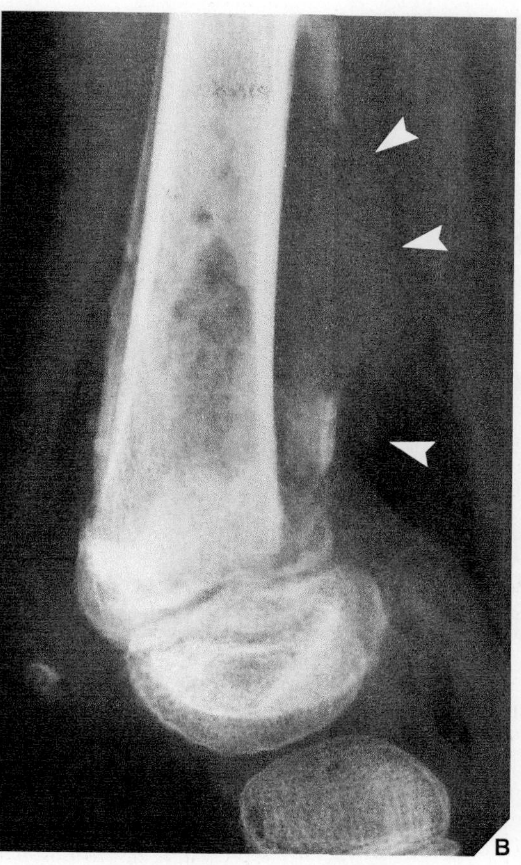

FIGURE 25.2 **Acute osteomyelitis.** **(A)** Anteroposterior and **(B)** lateral radiographs of the knee of an 8-year-old boy show widespread destruction of the cortical and medullary portions of the metaphysis and diaphysis of the distal femur, together with periosteal new bone formation. Note the pathologic fracture *(arrows)*. On the lateral view, a large subperiosteal abscess is evident *(arrowheads)*.

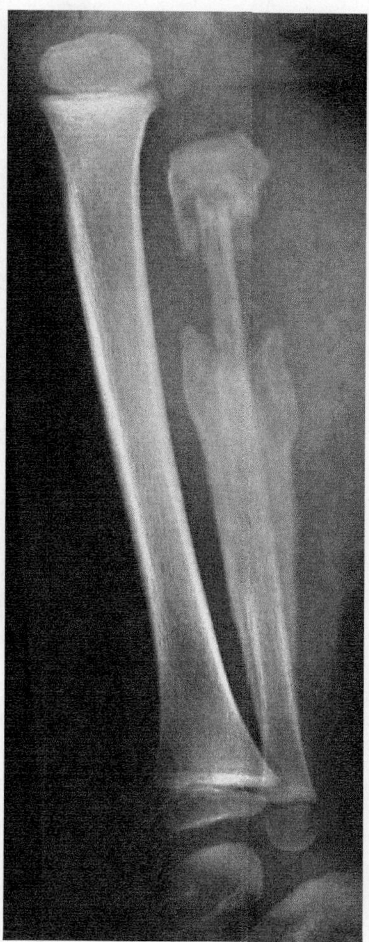

FIGURE 25.3 **Active osteomyelitis.** Sequestra surrounded by involucrum, as seen here in the left fibula of a 2-year-old child, is a feature of advanced osteomyelitis, usually apparent after 6 to 8 weeks of active infection. (Courtesy of Richard H. Gold, MD, Los Angeles, California.)

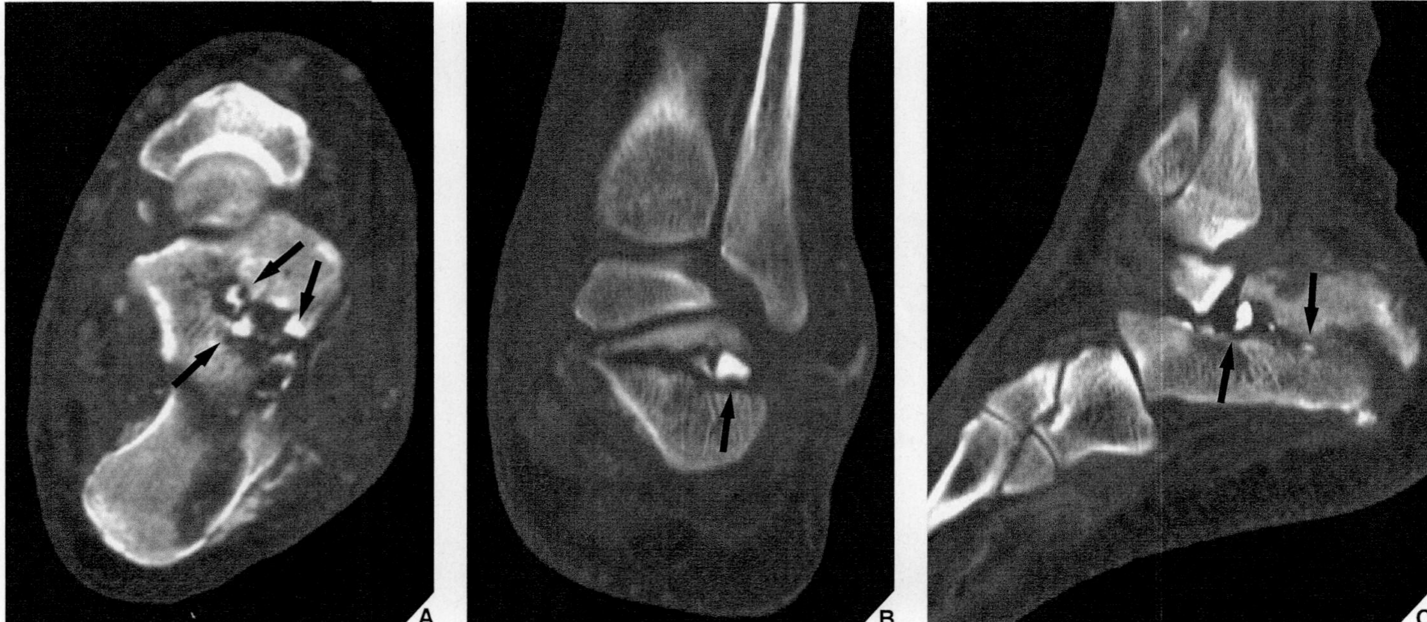

FIGURE 25.4 CT of active osteomyelitis. **(A)** Axial, **(B)** coronal reformatted, and **(C)** sagittal reformatted CT images of the left foot of a 72-year-old diabetic man demonstrate an active osteomyelitis of the calcaneus. Note several high-attenuation osseous fragments representing sequestra *(arrows).*

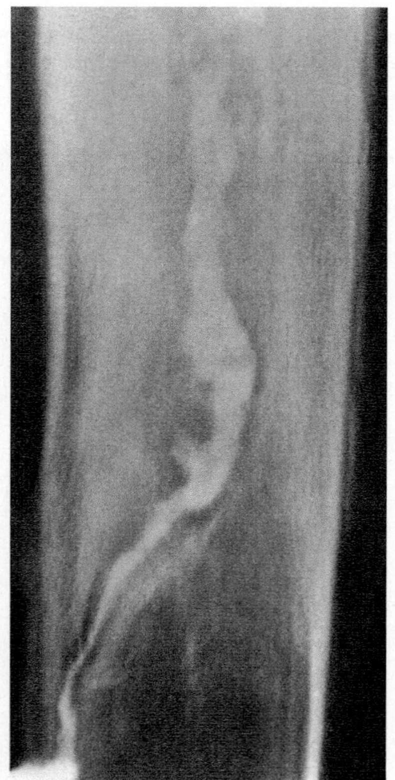

FIGURE 25.5 Chronic osteomyelitis. A 28-year-old man with sickle cell disease developed osteomyelitis, a frequent complication of this condition. A sinogram shows a draining sinus typical of chronic osteomyelitis. Note the extent of the serpentine tract in the medullary portion of the bone.

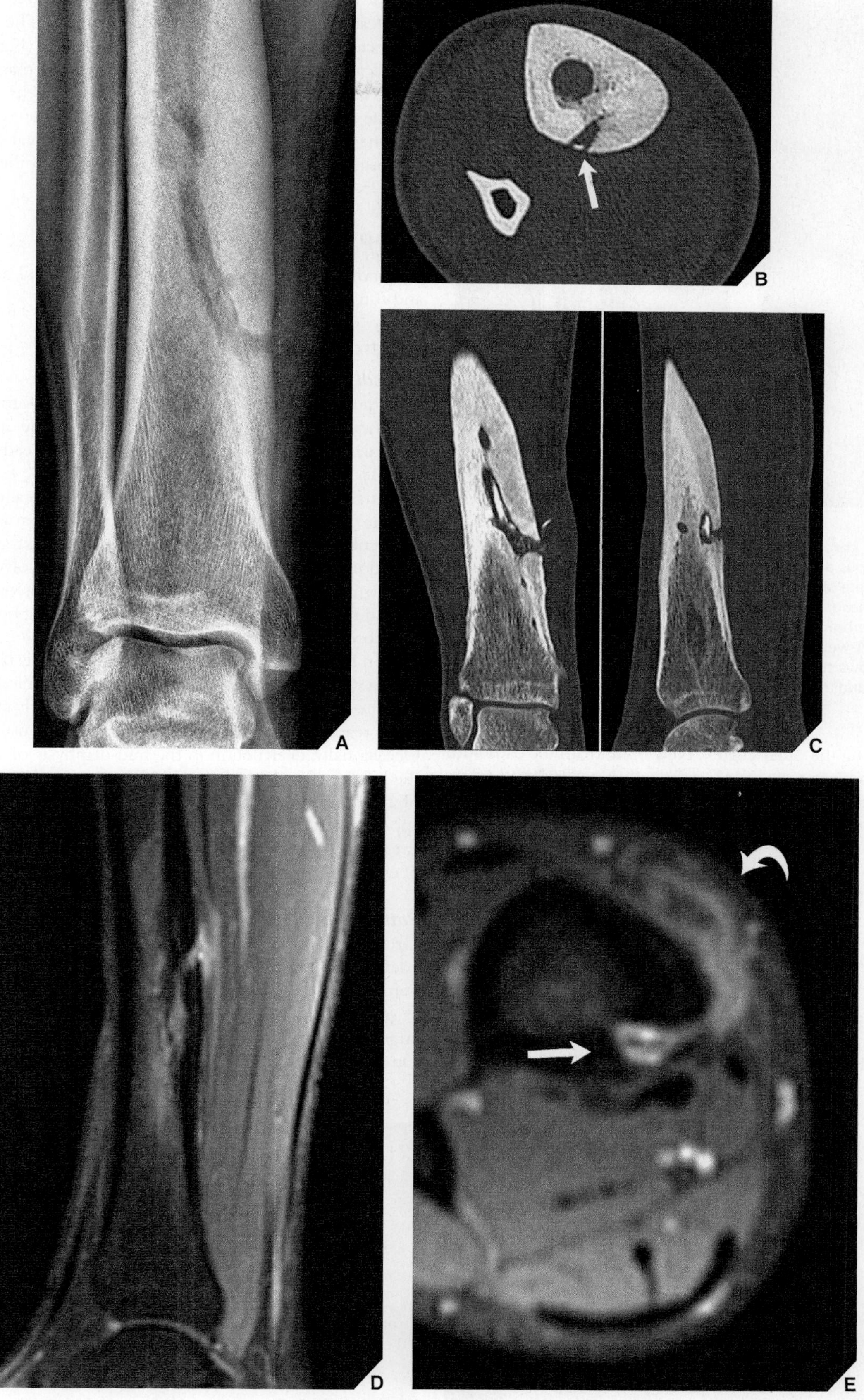

FIGURE 25.6 CT and MRI of chronic osteomyelitis. A 20-year-old man presented with a draining sinus in the lower right leg for the past 4 months. **(A)** Anteroposterior radiograph shows thickening of the medial cortex of tibia and a radiolucent tract extending from the medullary cavity to the soft tissues. **(B)** Axial CT section shows a sinus tract and a low-attenuation sequestrum *(arrow)*. **(C)** Coronal and sagittal reformatted CT images clearly demonstrate the intraosseous sinus containing several sequestra. **(D)** Sagittal and **(E)** axial T1-weighted MR images obtained after intravenous administration of gadolinium show enhancement of bone marrow indicative of osteomyelitis, sinus tract *(arrow)*, and soft-tissue abscess with ring enhancement *(curved arrow)*.

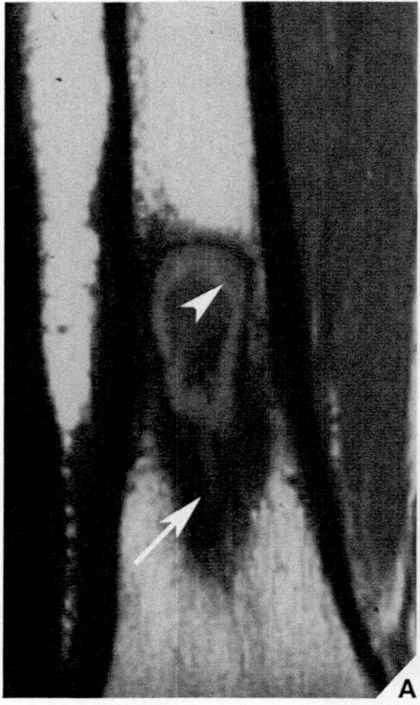

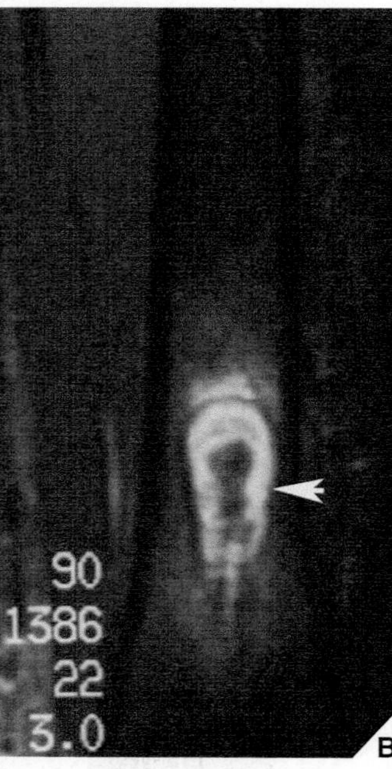

FIGURE 25.7 MRI of chronic osteomyelitis. **(A)** Coronal T1-weighted MRI demonstrates an intraosseous abscess displaying low signal intensity of its central portion and the intermediate signal intensity of the inner wall, which represents granulation tissue *(arrowhead)*. The low-signal intensity area surrounding the abscess represents reactive bone sclerosis. Note the early formation of a draining sinus *(arrow)*. **(B)** Coronal T1-weighted fat-saturated MRI obtained after intravenous injection of gadolinium shows strong enhancement of the granulation tissue in the wall of the abscess *(arrow)* and the enhancement of the draining sinus.

abscess may develop along the outer cortex. New bone from the cambium layer of periosteum produces a sleeve of reactive bone, which is known as an *involucrum*. When the abscess strips the periosteum from the cortex, the blood supply becomes compromised, resulting in formation of *sequestrum*. In the following weeks, the acute inflammation is gradually replaced by a lymphocyte and plasma infiltrate, leading to chronic osteomyelitis. At this stage the formation of draining sinus tracts is a common finding (Fig. 25.8).

Subacute Osteomyelitis

Brodie Abscess

This lesion, originally described by Brodie in 1832, represents a subacute localized form of osteomyelitis, commonly caused by *S. aureus*. The highest incidence (approximately 40%) is in the second decade. More than 75% of cases occur in male patients. Its onset is often insidious, and systemic manifestations are generally mild or absent. The abscess, which is usually localized in the metaphysis of the radius (Fig. 25.9), tibia, or femur, is typically elongated, with a well-demarcated margin and surrounded by reactive sclerosis. As a rule, sequestra are absent, but a radiolucent tract may be seen extending from the lesion into the growth plate (Fig. 25.10). A bone abscess may often cross the epiphyseal plate, but seldom does an abscess develop in and remain localized to the epiphysis or diaphysis (Fig. 25.11; see also Fig. 24.9).

Nonpyogenic Bone Infections

The most common nonpyogenic bone infections are tuberculosis, syphilis, and fungal infections.

Tuberculous Infections

Clinical and Imaging Features

Tuberculosis is a chronic necrotizing granulomatous infection caused by *Mycobacterium tuberculosis*. Tuberculous bone infection usually occurs secondarily as a result of hematogenous spread from a primary focus of infection such as the lung or genitourinary tract. About 50% of the patients with skeletal tuberculosis present clinically with active pulmonary disease. Skeletal tuberculosis represents approximately 3% of all cases of tuberculosis and approximately 30% of all extrapulmonary tuberculous infections. In 10% to 15% of cases, bone involvement without articular disease is encountered. In children, tuberculous osteomyelitis has a predilection for the metaphyseal segment of the long bones; in adults, the joints are more often affected.

In the long and short bones, progressive destruction of the medullary region with abscess formation is apparent on radiography. Typically, there is evidence of osteoporosis, but at least in the early stage of the disease, little or no reactive sclerosis or periosteal reaction is usually present (Fig. 25.12). Occasionally, destruction in the mid-diaphysis of a short tubular bone of the hand or foot (*tuberculous dactylitis*) may produce a fusiform enlargement of the entire diaphysis, a condition known as *spina ventosa* (Fig. 25.13). The appearance of multiple disseminated lytic lesions in short tubular bones is termed *cystic tuberculosis*, a form of skeletal tuberculosis seen particularly in children.

Pathology

Gross examination of the areas affected by tuberculosis shows thickened, edematous tissue having a caseous or toothpaste-like consistency, commonly studded with grayish small nodules with opaque centers, known as *granulomas*. These granulomas frequently become confluent and produce larger areas of white necrotic material, so-called *caseation (or cheesy) necrosis*. On microscopic examination, the typical tubercle consists of a central

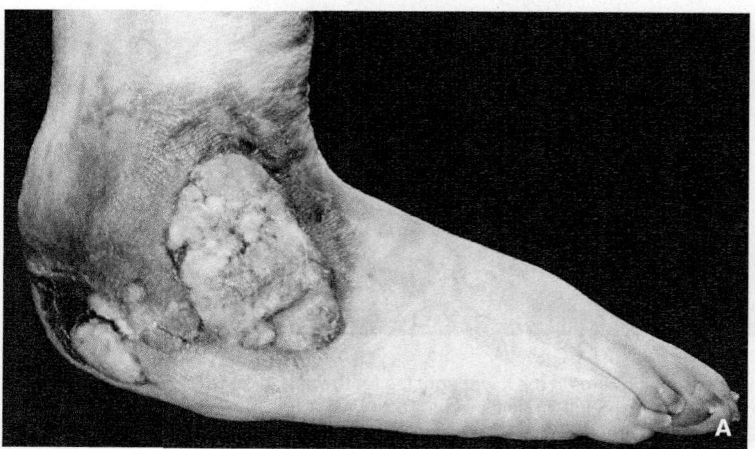

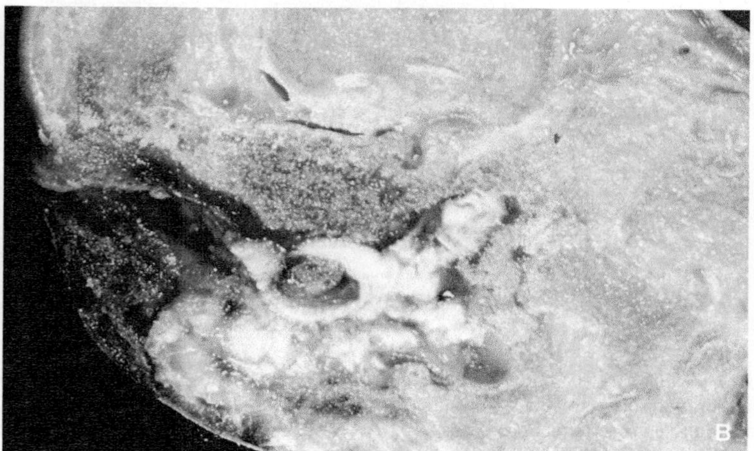

FIGURE 25.8 Pathology of chronic osteomyelitis. **(A)** Clinical photograph of the foot and ankle of a patient with long-standing osteomyelitis of the calcaneus shows overgrowth of partially ulcerated hyperkeratotic skin. **(B)** Sagittal section of the hindfoot shows a draining sinus extending from the infected bone to the ulcerated skin. Observe invasion of firm white tissue from the skin surface into the underlying soft tissue and bone. (Reprinted from Bullough P. *Orthopaedic pathology*, 5th ed. Maryland Heights, MO: Mosby; 2009, with permission from Elsevier.)

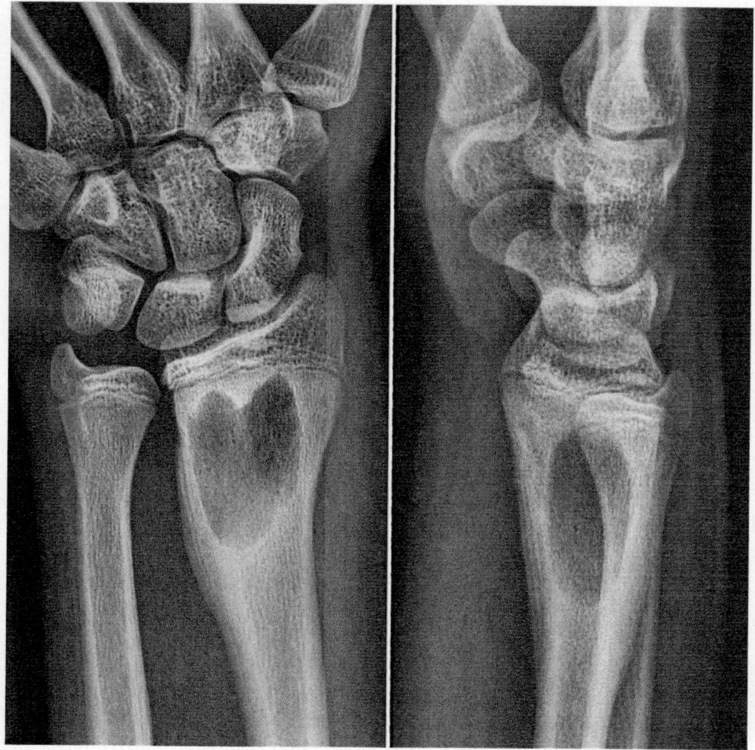

FIGURE 25.9 Bone abscess. A 13-year-old boy presented with chronic pain in right distal forearm. Dorsovolar and lateral radiographs of the wrist show a radiolucent lesion with narrow zone of transition in the metadiaphysis of the radius associated with well-organized lamellated periosteal reaction from the ulnar aspect of the bone.

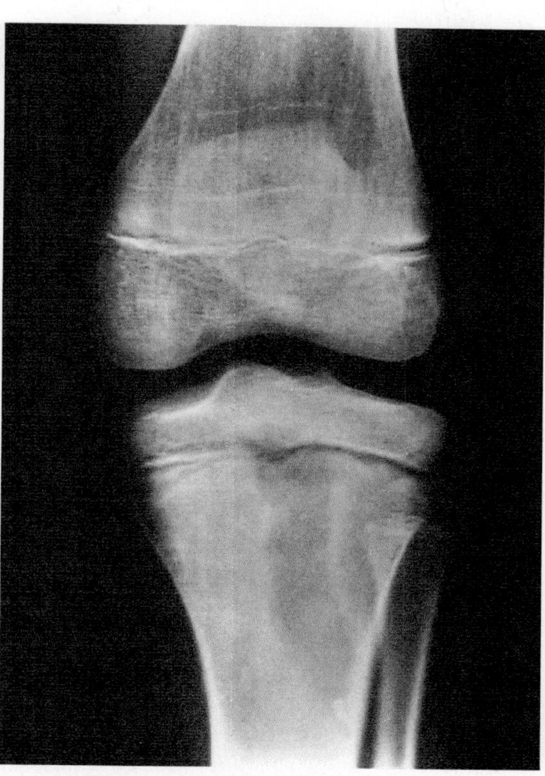

FIGURE 25.10 Bone abscess. Anteroposterior radiograph of the left knee of an 11-year-old boy with a subacute Brodie abscess in the proximal diaphysis and metaphysis of the tibia shows a radiolucent tract extending into the growth plate.

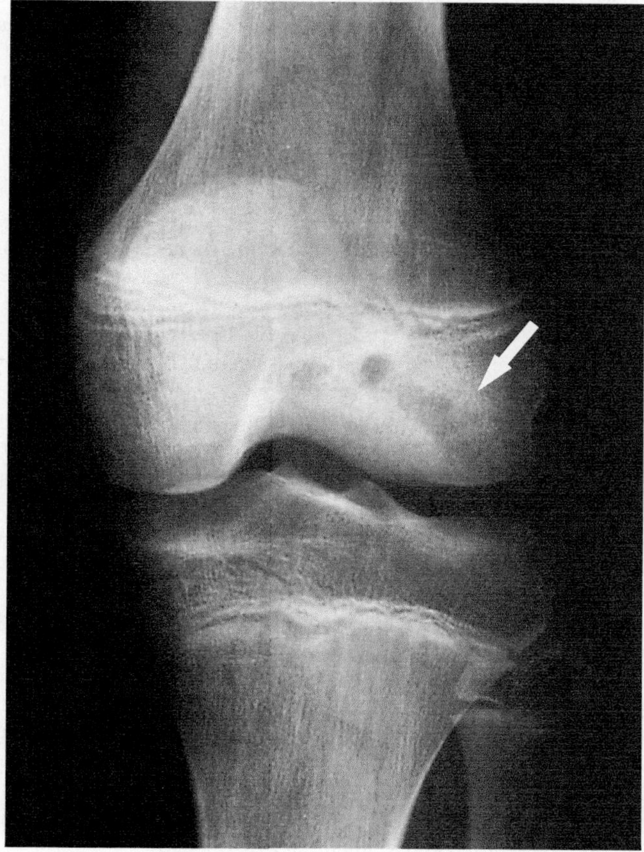

FIGURE 25.11 Bone abscess. Anteroposterior radiograph of the left knee of a 13-year-old boy demonstrates a well-defined osteolytic lesion surrounded by reactive sclerosis in the distal epiphysis of the femur *(arrow)*. This is a rare site for a bone abscess.

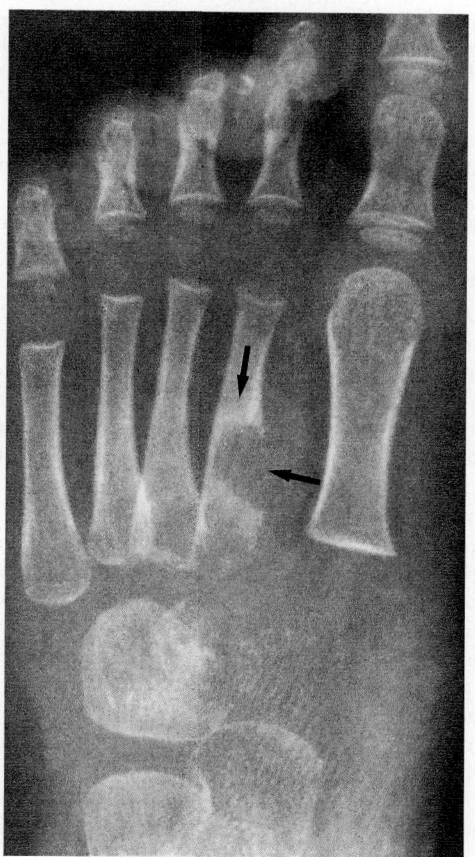

FIGURE 25.12 Tuberculosis of bone. A 20-month-old girl had progressive swelling of the right foot. Anteroposterior radiograph shows a well-defined lytic defect in the medial aspect of the second metatarsal *(arrows)*; there is no evidence of reactive sclerosis or periosteal new bone formation, but soft-tissue swelling is apparent. Aspiration of a lesion yielded 1 mL of pus-like fluid, which on bacteriologic examination revealed acid-fast bacteria. The causative agent proved to be *M. tuberculosis*.

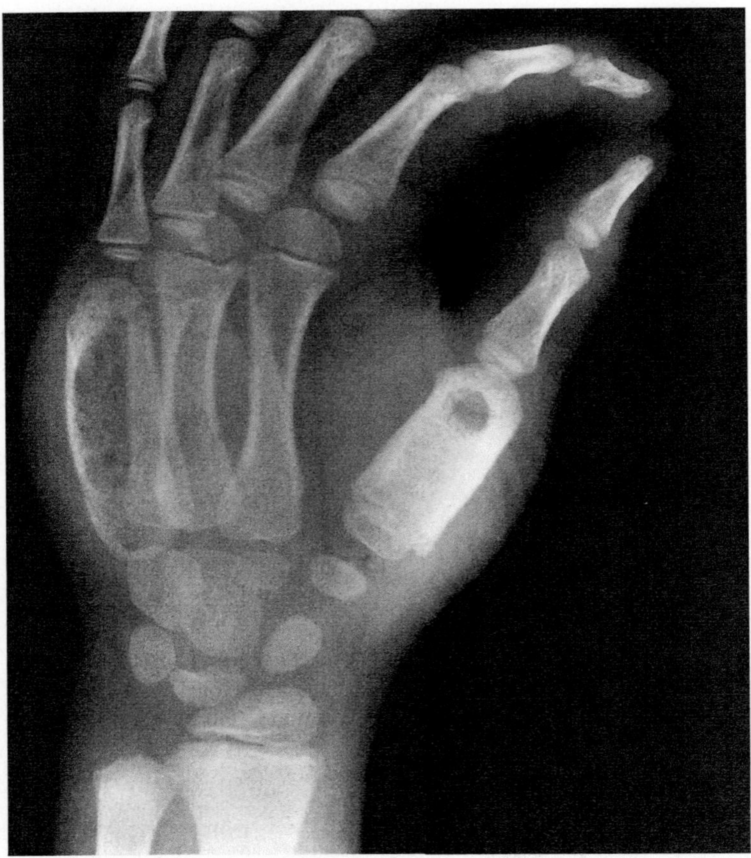

FIGURE 25.13 Tuberculosis of bone. Oblique radiograph of the right hand of a 7-year-old boy shows expansive fusiform lesions of the first and fifth metacarpals associated with soft-tissue swelling; there is no evidence of a periosteal reaction. Such diaphyseal enlargement secondary to tuberculosis is known as *spina ventosa*.

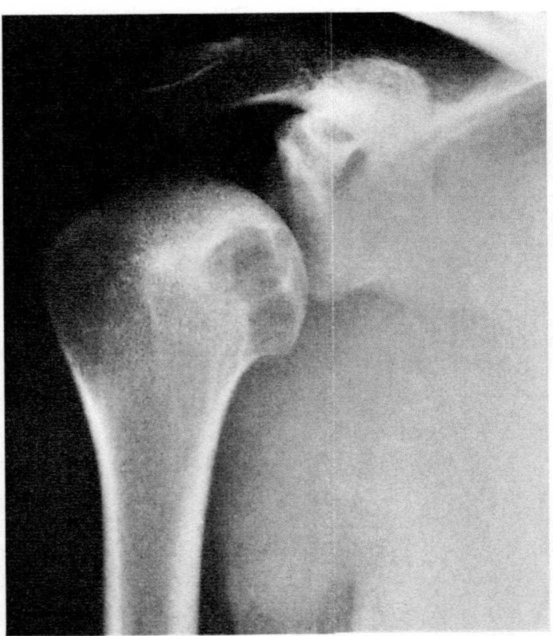

FIGURE 25.14 Cryptococcosis of bone. Anteroposterior radiograph of the right shoulder of an 18-year-old man demonstrates a destructive osteolytic lesion in the medial aspect of the humeral head, with minimal sclerosis and no periosteal reaction—the typical appearance of a fungal infection. Aspiration biopsy showed the abscess to be caused by a cryptococcal infection.

necrotic area surrounded by pale histiocytes (epithelioid cells) among which are scattered giant cells with peripherally arranged nuclei, known as *Langerhans giant cells*, all enclosed within a rim of fibrosis infiltrated by lymphocytes and plasma cells.

Fungal Infections

Clinical Features

Fungal bone infections are infrequent, the most common being coccidioidomycosis, blastomycosis, actinomycosis, cryptococcosis, and nocardiosis. The infection is usually low grade, with the formation of an abscess and a draining sinus. The lesion may resemble a tuberculous skeletal infection because the abscess is usually found in cancellous bone with little or no reactive sclerosis or periosteal response (Fig. 25.14). The location of a lesion at a point of bony prominence—such as along the edges of the patella, the ends of the clavicles, or in the acromion, coracoid process, olecranon, or styloid process of the radius or ulna—may also suggest a fungal infection. Solitary marginal lesions of the ribs and lesions involving the vertebrae in an indiscriminate fashion, including the body, neural arch, and spinous and transverse processes, also favor fungal infectious process.

Among the fungal infections, coccidioidomycosis is of particular importance, not only because of an increase in the number of these infections in recent years but also because it may closely resemble skeletal tuberculosis. It is a systemic disease caused by the soil fungus *Coccidioides immitis*. This infection is endemic throughout the southwestern United States and the bordering regions of northern Mexico. Infection occurs through inhalation of dust containing the organism. The primary site of infection is the lung, and disease is commonly asymptomatic. Dissemination of coccidioidomycosis is rare, but the incidence is increased in patients with specific risk factors. Those at increased risk include African Americans, Filipinos, Mexicans, males, pregnant women, children younger than 5 years, adults older than 50 years, and immunosuppressed patients. Patients with disseminated coccidioidomycosis usually present during the course of primary pulmonary infection. However, some patients with disseminated disease may have no clinical history or radiographic evidence of pulmonary disease. The skin and subcutaneous tissues are the most common sites of disseminated coccidioidal infection, followed by mediastinal involvement. The skeletal system is the third most common site of dissemination, and osseous manifestations occur in 10% to 50% of patients with disseminated disease.

Imaging Features

Radiographic presentation of the lesion of coccidioidomycosis is variable, but it is usually characterized by well-marginated, punched-out osteolytic lesions, typically involving long and flat bones. The lesions are typically unilocular (Fig. 25.15) but occasionally may be multifocal (Figs. 25.16 and 25.17). The other pattern frequently observed is a permeative type of bone destruction, only occasionally accompanied by periosteal reaction. Soft-tissue swelling and osteoporosis are much more common with the permeative pattern than with the punched-out lesions. The third most common pattern is joint involvement (septic arthritis), usually monoarticular and almost invariably associated with osseous involvement (see Fig. 25.17B,C). Changes typically seen in joints include periarticular osteoporosis, a permeative/destructive pattern involving both articular surfaces, soft-tissue swelling, and occasional periostitis. Joint involvement in coccidioidomycosis is indistinguishable from that seen with tuberculosis.

Scintigraphy is valuable in the evaluation of patients with disseminated coccidioidomycosis. Radionuclide scans using gallium-67 (^{67}Ga) citrate and technetium-99m (^{99m}Tc) methylene diphosphonate (MDP) have been used to localize disease and can identify disseminated lesions that are clinically unsuspected. No false-negative bone scans have been reported. CT and MRI are helpful in defining osseous involvement and in determining the extent of soft-tissue disease (see Figs. 25.16 and 25.17). The lesions exhibit low attenuation, often appearing bubbly and expansive. On MRI, the lesions show decreased signal on T1-weighted images, with a corresponding increase on T2-weighted and gradient-echo sequences.

Recently, osteomyelitis caused by *Nocardia asteroides* has been reported in patients with HIV infection who developed AIDS. The clinical and imaging manifestations of this infectious process closely resemble those of tuberculosis. The most cases of *Nocardia* osteomyelitis resulted from direct extension of soft-tissue infection; however, hematogenous dissemination has also been reported.

FIGURE 25.15 Coccidioidomycosis of bone. Anteroposterior radiograph of the left shoulder of a 22-year-old woman with pulmonary coccidioidomycosis shows destruction of the acromion *(arrow)*. Observe a soft-tissue abscess *(arrowhead)*.

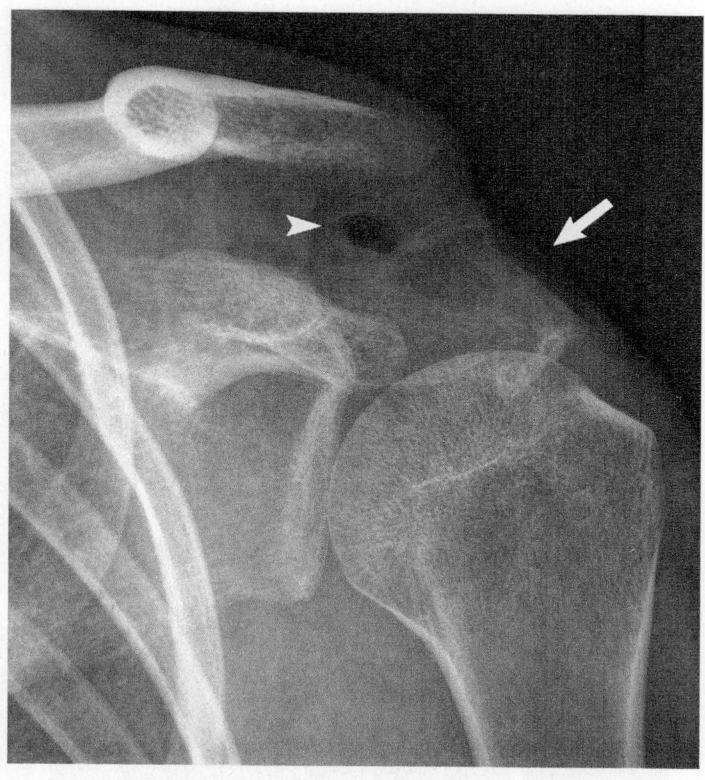

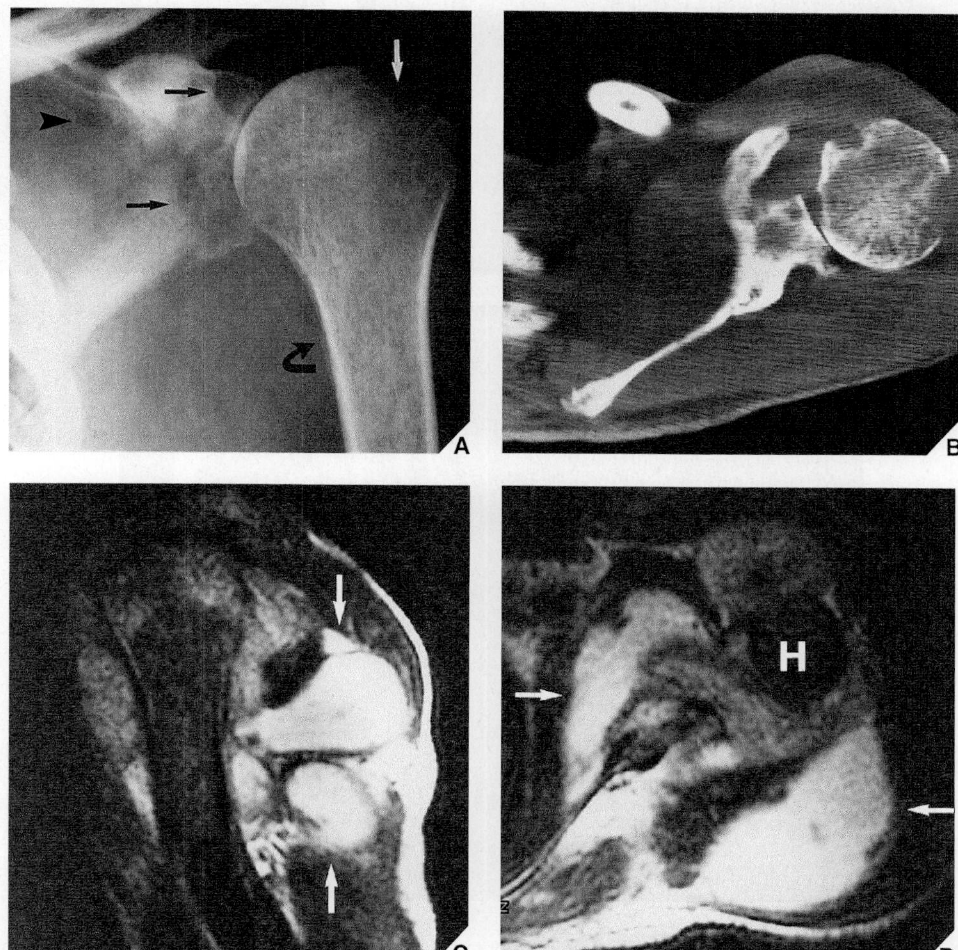

FIGURE 25.16 MRI of coccidioidomycosis of bone. A 42-year-old man presented with a 4-week history of pain and decreased range of motion in the left shoulder. He had been previously hospitalized for pulmonary coccidioidomycosis. **(A)** Anteroposterior radiograph shows several osteolytic lesions affecting the superolateral aspect of the humeral head and glenoid *(arrows)*. Small punched-out lesion is noted in the body of the scapula *(arrowhead)*. The *curved arrow* points to periosteal reaction along the medial humeral shaft. **(B)** CT section reveals erosions of the anterior and posterolateral aspects of the humeral head. Also apparent are destruction of the articular surfaces of the humeral head and glenoid and narrowing of the glenohumeral joint. **(C)** Sagittal and **(D)** axial fast spin echo (repetition time [TR] 4000/echo time [TE] 102 msec) MR images show multiple, well-defined soft-tissue abscesses displaying high signal intensity *(arrows)*. H, humeral head.

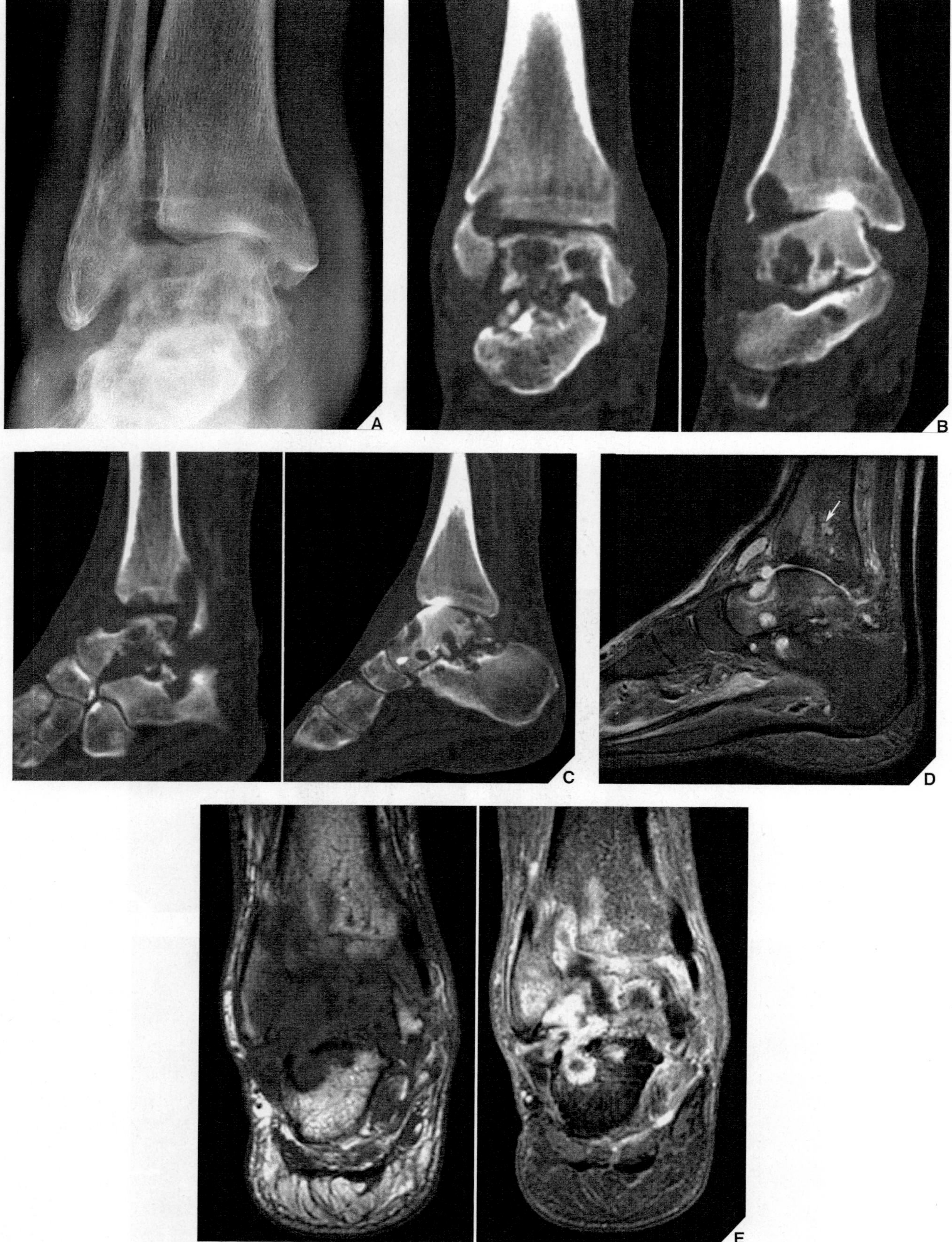

FIGURE 25.17 CT and MRI of coccidioidomycosis of bone. **(A)** Anteroposterior radiograph of the right ankle of a 69-year-old man shows destruction of the tibiotalar joint, several radiolucent lesions in the talus, deformity of the ankle mortise, and large soft-tissue swelling and edema. **(B)** Two coronal and **(C)** two sagittal CT sections demonstrate articular erosions of the ankle and subtalar joints and several osteolytic lesions within the talus and calcaneus. **(D)** Sagittal inversion recovery (IR) MR image shows multiple erosions of the talus and calcaneus with extensive bone marrow edema. Note also the tibial involvement *(arrow)*. **(E)** Coronal T1-weighted fat-suppressed MR images obtained before *(left)* and after *(right)* intravenous administration of gadolinium demonstrate diffuse signal abnormality of the talus, distal tibia, and fibula, with erosions in the calcaneus and inferior aspect of the talus. The bone marrow and the erosions show prominent enhancement.

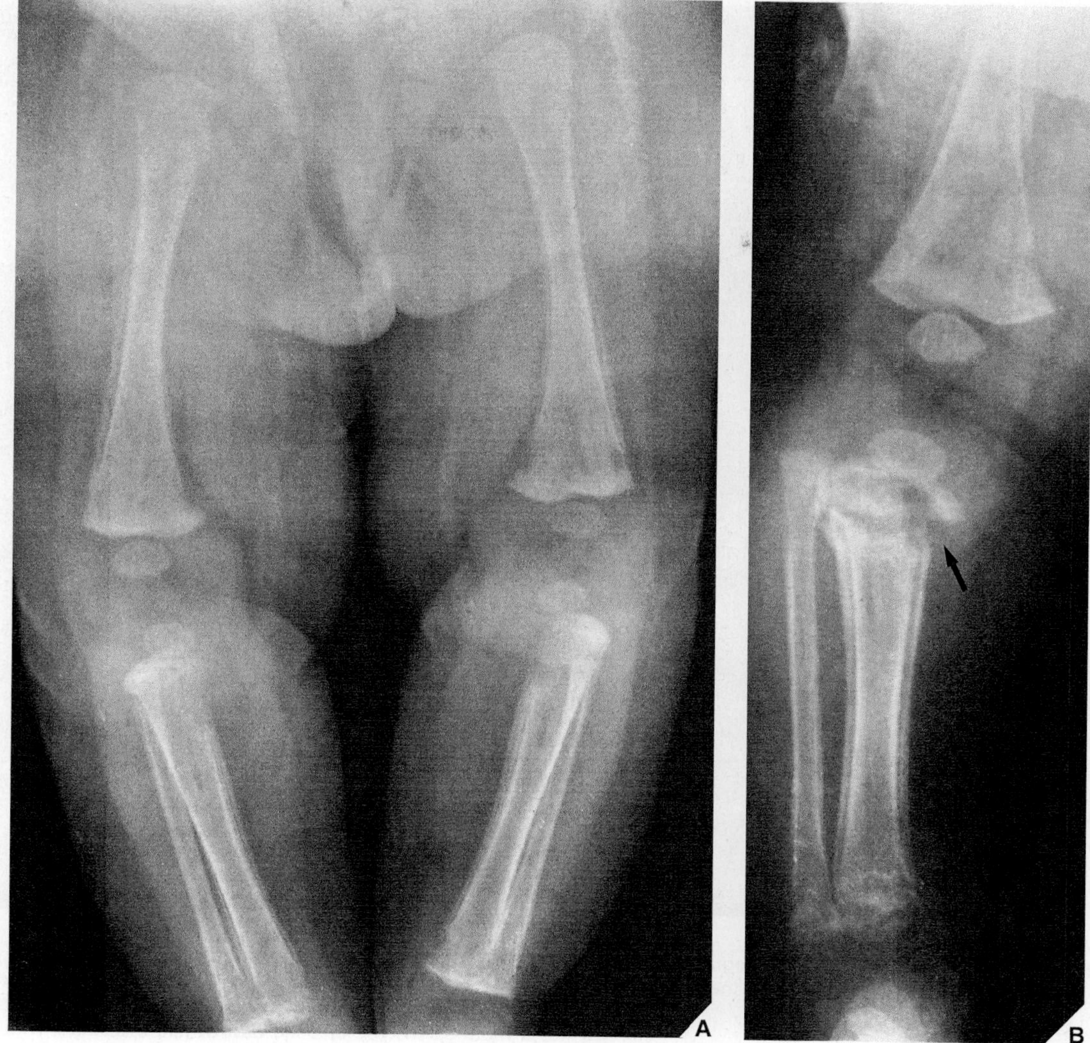

FIGURE 25.18 **Congenital syphilis of bone.** **(A)** Anteroposterior radiograph of the lower legs of a 7-week-old infant demonstrates characteristic periostitis affecting the femora and tibiae. In addition, destructive changes are evident in the medullary portion of the proximal tibiae. **(B)** Two months later, the infectious process has progressed, with destruction of the tibial metaphysis and marked periostitis. The characteristic erosion of the medial surface of the proximal tibial metaphysis is termed the *Wimberger sign (arrow)*.

Syphilitic Infection

Clinical and Imaging Features

Syphilis is a chronic systemic infectious disease caused by a spirochete, *Treponema pallidum*. *Congenital syphilis*, which is transmitted from mother to fetus, may manifest as a chronic osteochondritis, periostitis, or osteitis. The lesions, which most frequently involve the tibia, are characteristically widespread and symmetric in appearance; destructive changes are usually seen in the metaphysis at the junction with the growth plate, producing what is called the *Wimberger sign* (Fig. 25.18). In the later stages of disease, involvement of the tibia results in a characteristic anterior bowing known as *saber-shin deformity*.

Acquired syphilis may manifest either as a chronic osteitis exhibiting irregular sclerosis of the medullary cavity or as syphilitic abscesses known as *gumma* (Fig. 25.19). The latter form of the disease may simulate pyogenic osteomyelitis, but the absence of sequestra typically found in bacterial osteomyelitis allows the distinction to be made.

Pathology

The characteristic pathologic findings in all stages of syphilis is perivascular mononuclear cuffing, also referred to as *microangiitis*, due to invasion of the wall of small blood vessels by spirochetes. This leads to obliterative endarteritis with concentric endothelial proliferative thickening and luminal occlusion. In the skeleton, these changes predominantly affect the periosteal blood vessels. Due to vascular occlusion (endarteritis obliterans), variable in size destructive granulomatous-like nodular lesions known as *gummas* develop within the cortical bone and bone marrow.

Differential Diagnosis of Osteomyelitis

Usually, the radiographic appearance of osteomyelitis is so characteristic that the diagnosis is easily made with the clinical history, and ancillary radiologic examinations such as scintigraphy, CT, and MRI are rarely needed. Nevertheless, osteomyelitis may at times mimic other conditions. Particularly in its acute form, it may resemble Langerhans cell histiocytosis or Ewing sarcoma (Fig. 25.20). The soft-tissue changes in each of these conditions, however, are characteristic and different. In osteomyelitis, soft-tissue swelling is diffuse, with obliteration of the fascial planes, whereas Langerhans cell histiocytosis, as a rule, is not accompanied by significant soft-tissue swelling or a mass. The extension of an Ewing sarcoma into the soft tissues presents as a well-defined soft-tissue mass with preservation of the fascial planes. The duration of a patient's symptoms also plays an important diagnostic role. It takes a tumor such as an Ewing sarcoma from 4 to 6 months to destroy the bone to the same extent that osteomyelitis does in 4 to 6 weeks and that Langerhans cell histiocytosis does in only 7 to 10 days. Despite these differentiating features, however, the radiographic pattern of bone destruction, periosteal reaction, and location in the bone may be very similar in all three conditions (see Fig. 22.16).

A bone abscess, particularly in the cortex, may closely simulate a nidus of osteoid osteoma (see Fig. 17.22). In the medullary region, however, the presence of a serpentine tract favors the diagnosis of bone abscess over osteoid osteoma (Fig. 25.21).

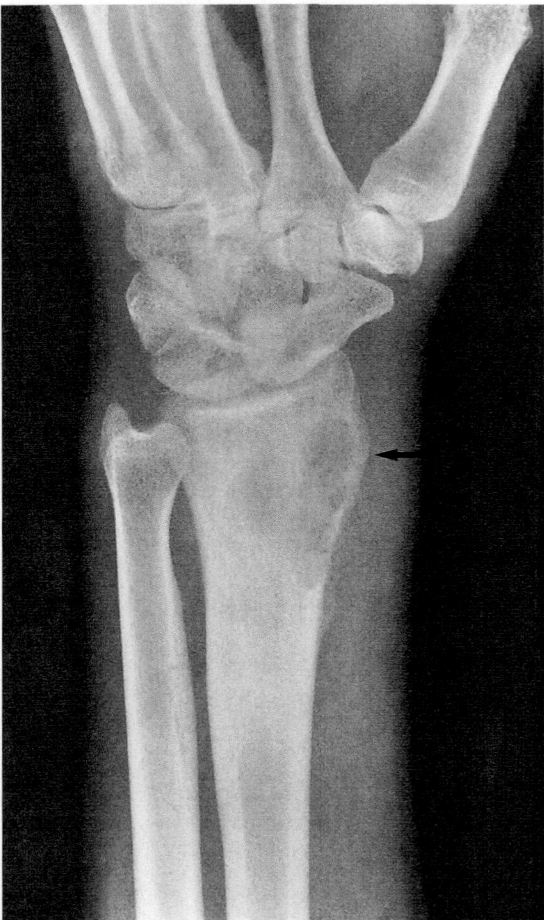

FIGURE 25.19 **Acquired syphilis of bone.** Oblique radiograph of the distal forearm of a 51-year-old man shows a lytic abscess (gumma) in the lateral aspect of the distal radius *(arrow)*.

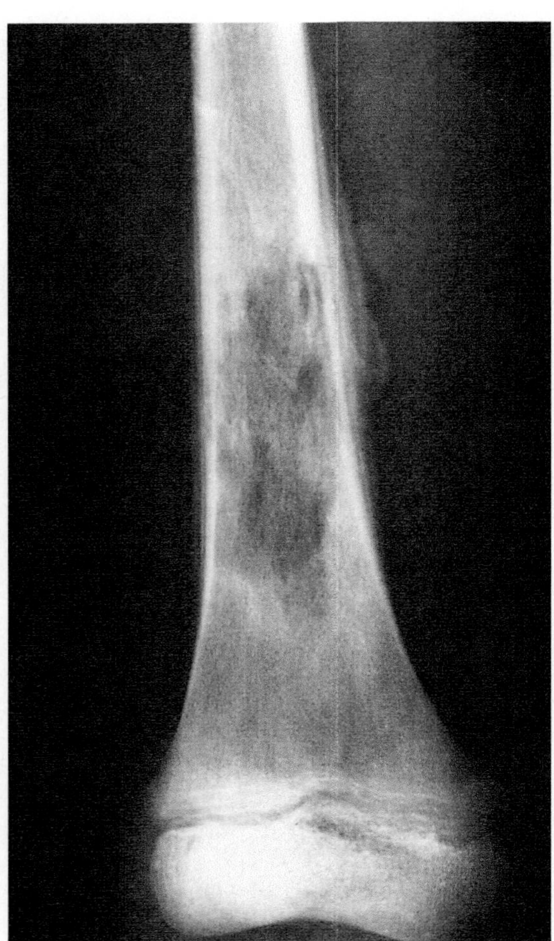

FIGURE 25.20 **Osteomyelitis resembling Ewing sarcoma.** A 7-year-old boy presented with pain in his right leg for 3 weeks. Anteroposterior radiograph demonstrates a lesion in the medullary portion of the distal femoral diaphysis with a moth-eaten type of bone destruction, associated with a lamellated periosteal reaction and a small soft-tissue prominence. These radiographic features suggest a diagnosis of Ewing sarcoma. The absence of a definite soft-tissue mass and the short symptomatic period, however, point to the correct diagnosis of osteomyelitis, which was confirmed by biopsy.

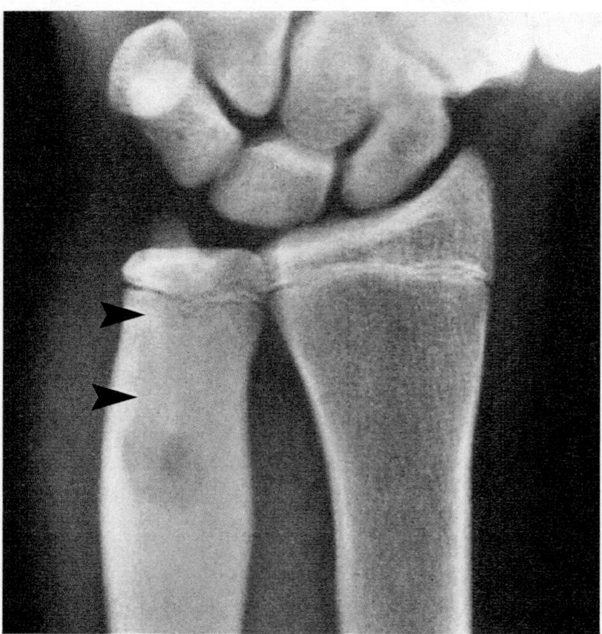

FIGURE 25.21 **Bone abscess resembling osteoid osteoma.** A 17-year-old boy had a typical history of osteoid osteoma: nocturnal bone pain relieved promptly by salicylates. Anteroposterior radiograph of the distal forearm demonstrates a radiolucent lesion in the distal ulnar diaphysis. The presence of a serpentine tract extending from the radiolucent focus into the growth plate *(arrowheads)* indicates a diagnosis of bone abscess.

Chronic Recurrent Multifocal Osteomyelitis

Chronic recurrent multifocal osteomyelitis (CRMO) is an acute inflammatory multifocal process affecting more than one bone, occurring mostly in children and adolescents with imaging and clinical manifestations similar to osteomyelitis but without infection and lack of known pathogen. CRMO is now considered an inherited autoinflammatory disease caused by immune dysregulation, without autoantibodies or antigen-specific T cells. Some investigators suggested a link between CRMO and a rare allele of marker D18S60, resulting in a haplotype relative risk of chromosome 18 (18q21.3-18q22). The condition is characterized by the insidious onset of pain with swelling and tenderness over the affected bones. Clavicular and sternal involvement is common, although the long and short tubular bones may also be affected (Fig. 25.22). The diagnosis is made by exclusion of other entities such as bacterial osteomyelitis, SAPHO syndrome (which is an acronym of condition manifested by a combined occurrence of **s**ynovitis, **a**cne, **p**ustulosis, **h**yperostosis, and **o**steitis), Langerhans cell histiocytosis, and variety of bone tumors. Treatment options include nonsteroidal antiinflammatory drugs, pamidronate, and bisphosphonates.

Related condition is the Majeed syndrome, an autoinflammatory disorder inherited in an autosomal recessive manner and caused by mutations in *LPIN2* gene, consisting of CRMO, congenital dyserythropoietic anemia, and neutrophilic dermatosis.

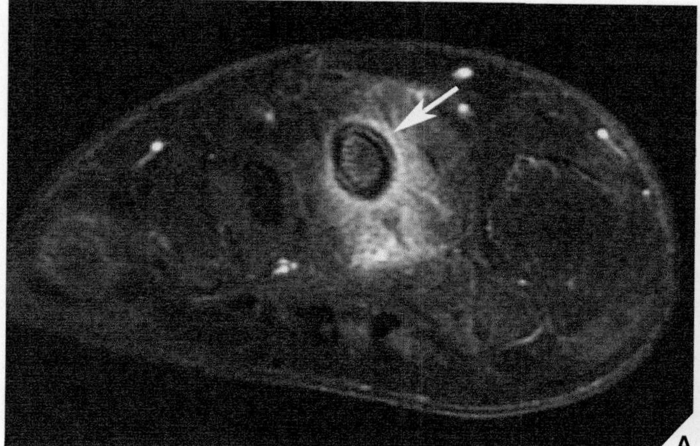

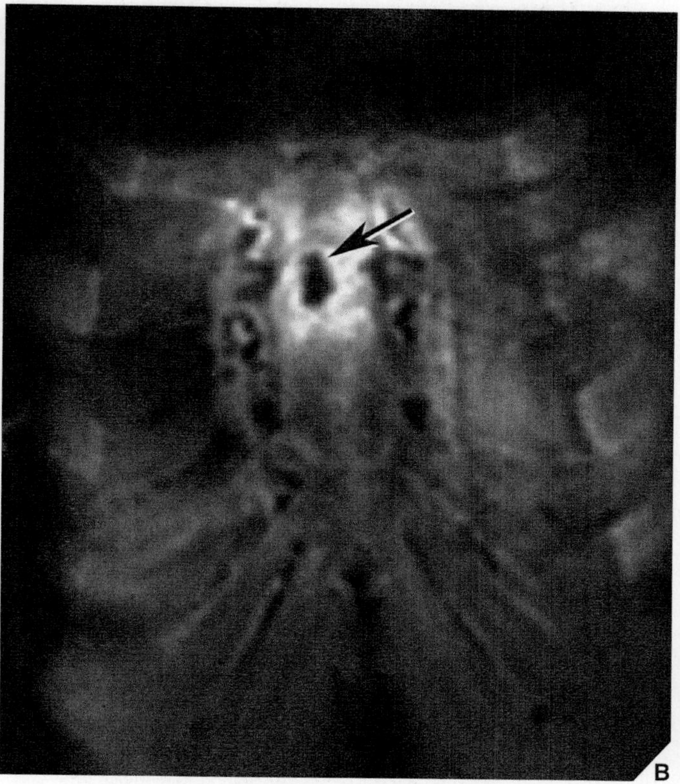

FIGURE 25.22 MRI of CRMO. A 12-year-old girl presented with history of chronic foot pain and anterior chest wall pain. **(A)** Short-axis T2-weighted fat-saturated MRI of the forefoot shows signal alteration of the second metatarsal with periosteal reaction *(arrow)* and surrounding soft-tissue edema. **(B)** Coronal T1-weighted fat-saturated MRI of the sternum obtained after intravenous injection of gadolinium demonstrates a focal area of low signal intensity in the body of the sternum *(arrow)* surrounded by enhancing edema.

Infectious Arthritides

Most infectious arthritides demonstrate a positive radionuclide bone scan and a very similar radiographic picture, including joint effusion and destruction of cartilage and subchondral bone with consequent joint space narrowing (see Fig. 12.44). However, certain clinical and radiographic features are characteristic of individual infectious processes as demonstrated at various target sites (Table 25.1).

Pyogenic Joint Infections

The clinical signs and symptoms of pyogenic (septic) arthritis depend on the site and extent of involvement as well as the specific infectious organism. Although most cases of septic arthritis are caused by *S. aureus* and *Neisseria gonorrhoeae*, other pathogens—including *P. aeruginosa*, *Enterobacter cloacae*, *Klebsiella pneumoniae*, *Candida albicans*, and *Serratia marcescens*—are being encountered with increasing frequency in joint

TABLE 25.1 Clinical and Radiographic Hallmarks of Infectious Arthritis at Various Target Sites

Type	Site	Crucial Abnormalities	Techniques/Projections
Pyogenic Infections[a]	Peripheral joints	Periarticular osteoporosis	Radionuclide bone scan (early)
		Joint effusion	Standard views specific for site of involvement
		Destruction of subchondral bone (on both sides of joint)	Aspiration and arthrography
			Magnetic resonance imaging (MRI)
	Spine	Narrowing of disk space	Anteroposterior and lateral views
		Loss of definition of vertebral end plate	
		Paraspinal mass	Computed tomography (CT), MRI
		Partial or complete obstruction of intrathecal contrast flow	Myelogram
		Destruction of disk	Diskogram and aspiration
Nonpyogenic Infections			
Tuberculosis	Large joints	Monoarticular involvement (similar to rheumatoid arthritis)	Radionuclide bone scan
		"Kissing" sequestra (knee)	Standard views
		Sclerotic changes in subchondral bone	CT
	Spine	Gibbous formation	Anteroposterior and lateral views
		Lytic lesion in vertebral body	
		Destruction of disk	Diskogram and aspiration
		Paraspinal mass	CT, MRI
		Soft-tissue abscess ("cold" abscess)	Myelogram
		Obstruction of intrathecal contrast flow	
Lyme disease	Knee	Narrowing of femoropatellar compartment	Lateral view
		Edematous changes in infrapatellar fat pad	CT, MRI

[a]In intravenous drug users, unusual sites of infection are encountered, including the vertebra; the sacroiliac, sternoclavicular, and acromioclavicular joints; and the pubic symphysis. The radiologic techniques used to evaluate infections at these sites, as well as the crucial radiographic abnormalities, are the same as those for the more common sites.

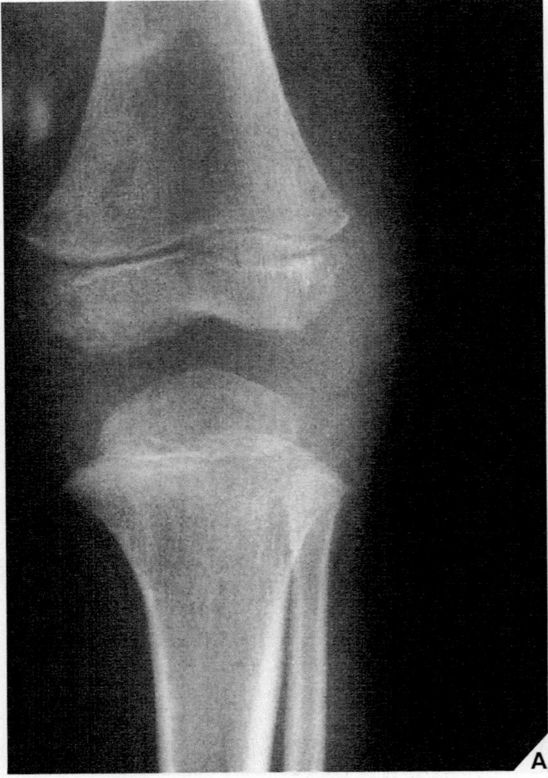

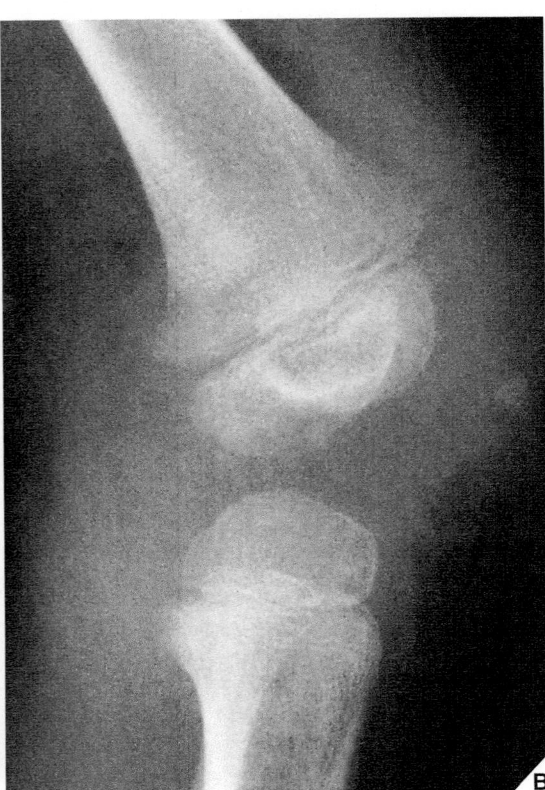

FIGURE 25.23 Septic arthritis. **(A)** Anteroposterior and **(B)** lateral radiographs of the left knee of a 4-year-old child demonstrate a significant degree of periarticular osteoporosis and a large joint effusion. Note the small erosions of the distal epiphysis of the femur and the preservation of the joint space. Aspiration revealed hematogenous spread of a staphylococcal urinary tract infection.

infections in drug users caused by the contamination of injected drugs or needles.

Any small or large joint can be affected by septic arthritis, and hematogenous spread in drug addicts is characterized by unusual locations of the lesion, such as the spine (vertebrae and intervertebral disks), sacroiliac joints, sternoclavicular and acromioclavicular articulations, and pubic symphysis.

Conventional radiography usually suffices to demonstrate septic arthritis. Certain characteristic radiographic features may be helpful in arriving at the correct diagnosis. Generally, a single joint is affected, most commonly a weight-bearing joint like the knee or hip. The early stage of joint infection may be seen simply as joint effusion, soft-tissue swelling, and periarticular osteoporosis, but "radiographic" joint space is usually preserved (Fig. 25.23).

In the later phase of pyogenic arthritis, articular cartilage is destroyed; characteristically, both subarticular plates are involved and the joint space narrows (Fig. 25.24). Arthrography, which is often performed after aspiration of the joint to obtain a fluid specimen for bacteriologic examination, helps determine the extent of joint destruction and demonstrate the presence of synovitis (Fig. 25.24B). Radionuclide bone scan is often effective in distinguishing a joint infection from a periarticular soft-tissue infection (see Fig. 24.10). It is also useful in monitoring the progress of treatment, although several weeks may be required before the scan demonstrates a completely normal appearance. The MRI manifestations of pyogenic arthritis include joint effusion with surrounding soft-tissue edema and bone marrow edema (Fig. 25.25). In more advanced stages, cartilage and bone destruction may be seen due to associated osteomyelitis (Figs. 25.26 and 25.27; see also Fig. 12.44B). "Lamellated" joint effusion demonstrated

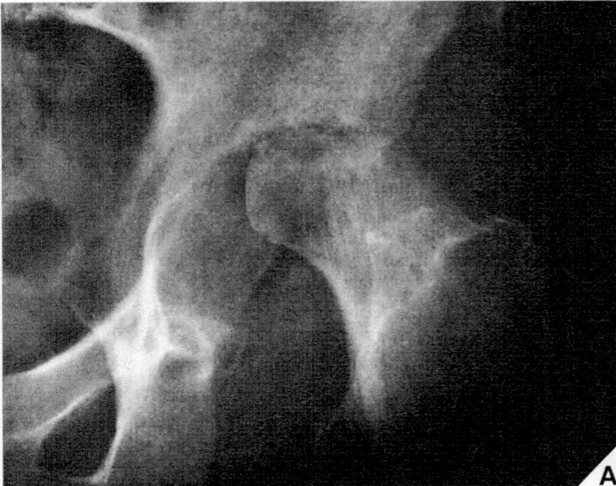

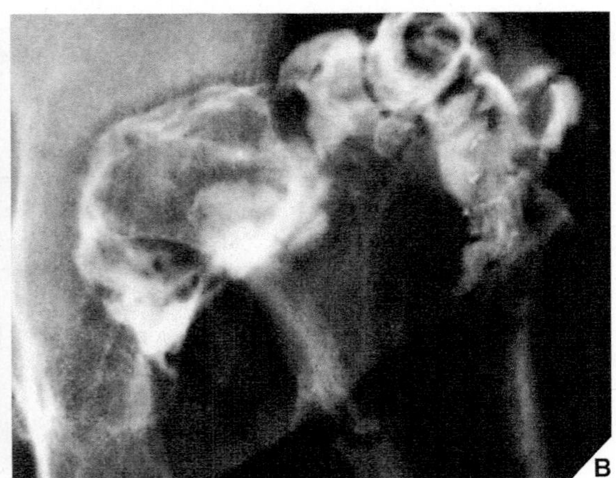

FIGURE 25.24 Septic arthritis. A 64-year-old woman had had an upper respiratory infection 6 months before pain developed in her left hip. **(A)** Anteroposterior radiograph of the hip demonstrates complete destruction of the articular cartilage on both sides of the joint and erosion of the femoral head. Note the significant degree of osteoporosis. **(B)** Contrast arthrography was performed primarily to obtain joint fluid for bacteriologic examination, which yielded *S. aureus*. The contrast agent outlines the destroyed joint, showing a synovial irregularity consistent with chronic synovitis.

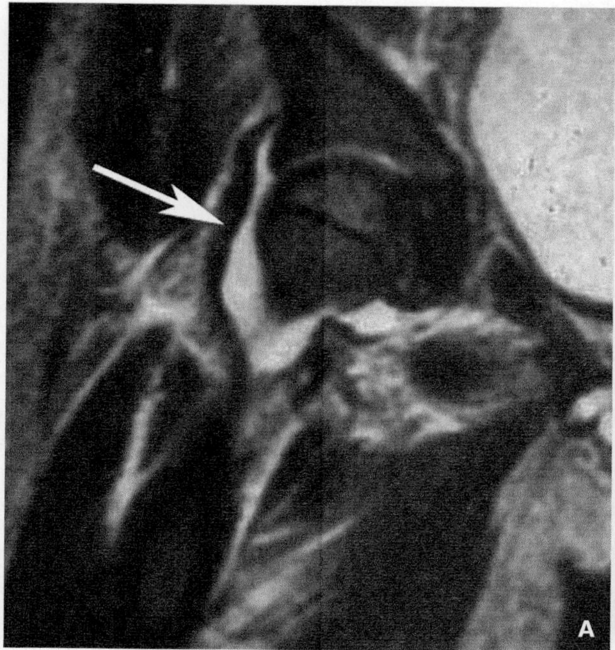

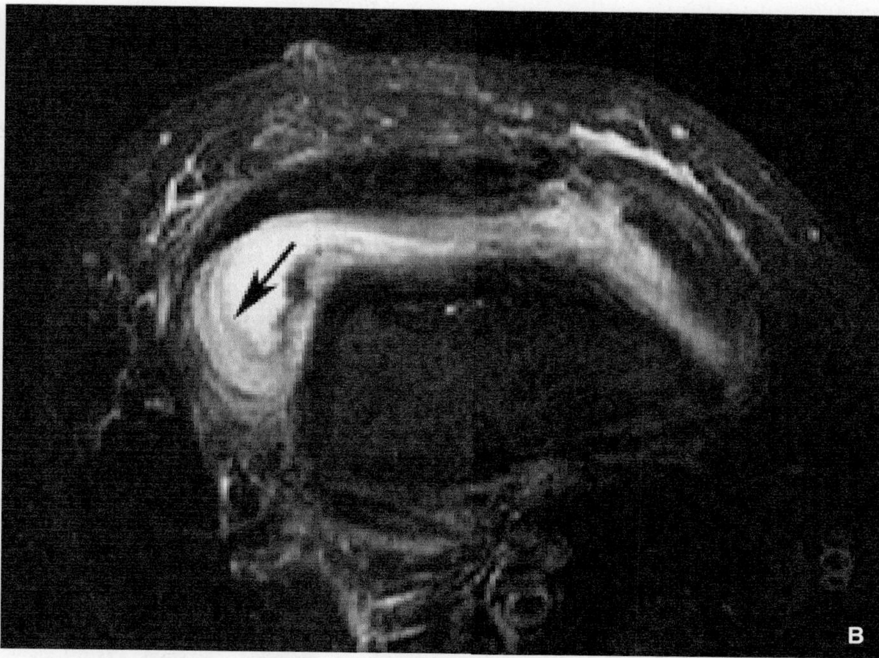

FIGURE 25.25 **MRI of septic arthritis.** **(A)** Coronal T2-weighted MRI of the right hip of a 12-year-old boy demonstrates a joint effusion with capsular distension *(arrow)*. There is edema of the surrounding muscles, suggesting the diagnosis of septic arthritis. There are no signs of osteomyelitis. **(B)** Axial T2-weighted fat-suppressed MR image of the knee in another patient with proven septic arthritis demonstrates a joint effusion with a "lamellated" appearance *(arrow)*.

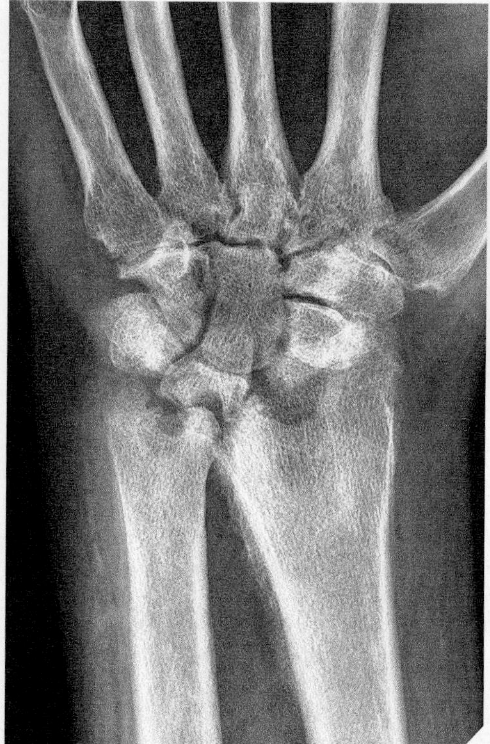

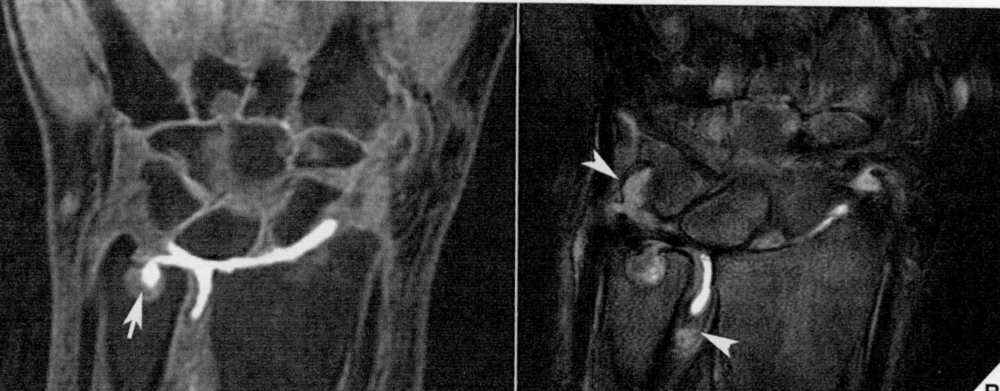

FIGURE 25.26 **MRI of septic arthritis.** **(A)** Dorsovolar radiograph of the right wrist of a 43-year-old man shows destruction of the radiocarpal joint and erosive changes of the distal radius, distal ulna, lunate, and scaphoid bones. Note also involvement of the carpometacarpal articulation. There is periosteal reaction of the distal radius and ulna and soft-tissue swelling. **(B)** Coronal three-dimensional gradient recalled echo (GRE) fat-suppressed **(left)** and coronal proton density–weighted fat-suppressed **(right)** MR images demonstrate an erosion of the distal ulna *(arrow)* with a radiocarpal joint effusion extending to the distal radioulnar joint through a complete tear of the triangular fibrocartilage. Note the intermediate-to-low signal intensity of most of the effusion and mild surrounding soft-tissue edema *(arrowheads)* consistent with synovitis due to septic arthritis.

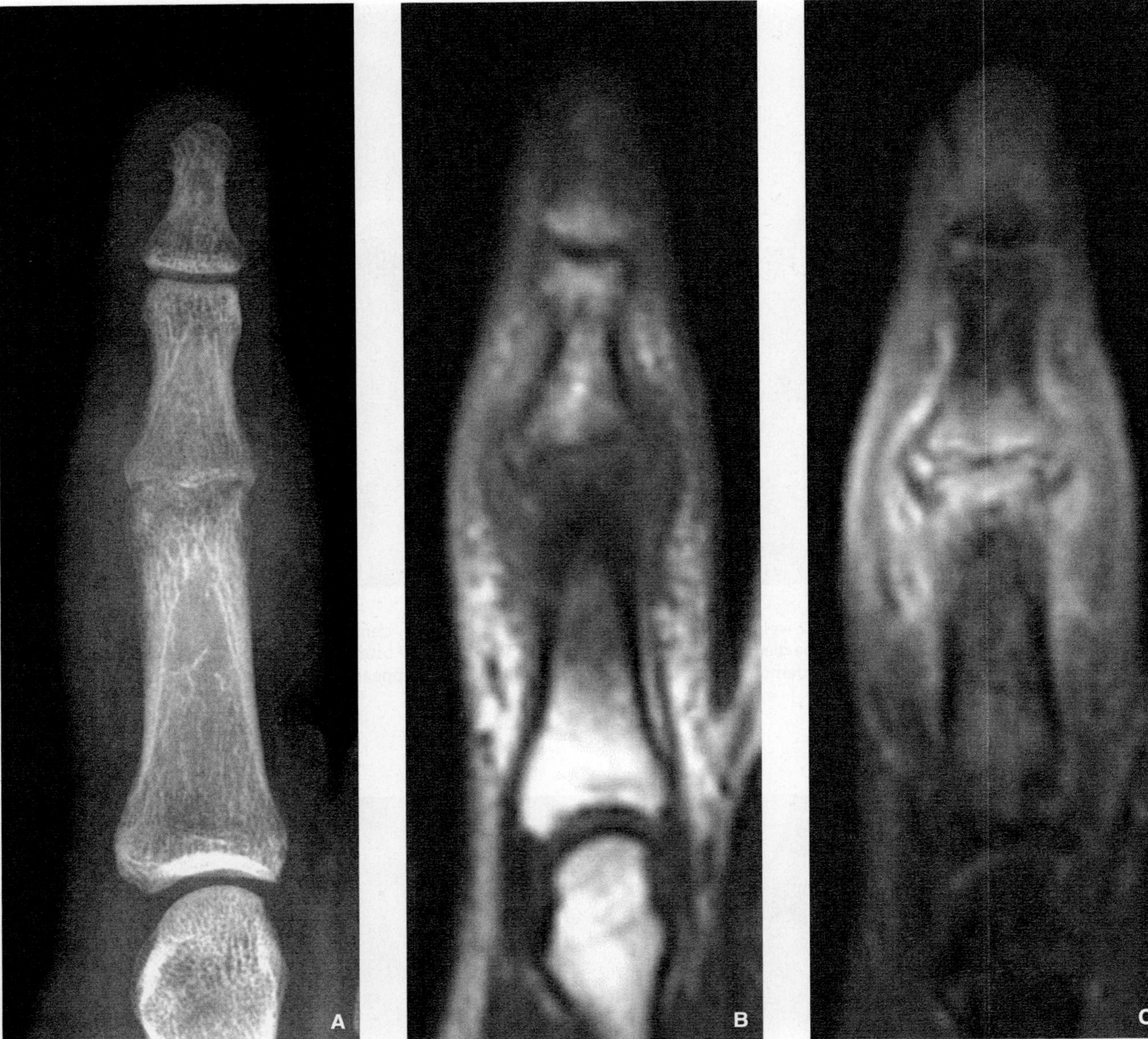

FIGURE 25.27 MRI of septic arthritis. **(A)** Radiograph of the index finger of a 26-year-old man shows narrowing of the proximal interphalangeal joint and a large soft-tissue swelling. **(B)** Coronal T1-weighted and **(C)** coronal T1-weighted fat-suppressed MR image obtained after intravenous administration of gadolinium show destruction of the joint, joint effusion, involvement of the subchondral bone, and diffuse soft-tissue edema.

with MRI has been described as a reliable sign of septic arthritis (see Fig. 25.25B). This finding was originally described in patient with infected knee arthroplasty but can also be seen in the joint of patients without prior arthroplasty, more often in the knee.

Complications

Infectious arthritis of peripheral joints in children may lead to the destruction of the growth plate, with resulting growth arrest (see Fig. 24.19). The infection may also spread to an adjacent bone, causing osteomyelitis. Degenerative arthritis and intraarticular bony ankylosis may also occur.

Nonpyogenic Joint Infections

Tuberculous Arthritis

Clinical Features

Tuberculous arthritis represents 1% of all forms of extrapulmonary tuberculosis, although the number of cases has recently been on the rise. The acid-fast tubercle bacilli *M. tuberculosis* and *Mycobacterium bovis* are the causative organisms. The infection may be found in all groups but more commonly in children and young adults. Predisposing factor such as trauma, alcoholism, drug abuse, intraarticular injection of steroids, or prolonged systemic illness is found in most patients with tuberculous arthritis. The joint infection usually is caused by either direct invasion from an adjacent focus of osteomyelitis or hematogenous dissemination of the tubercle bacillus. Large weight-bearing joints such as the hip or knee are most often affected, and monoarticular involvement is the rule.

Imaging Features

Conventional radiography is usually sufficient to demonstrate the identifying features of tuberculous arthritis, although its early radiographic appearance is often indistinguishable from that of monoarticular rheumatoid arthritis. However, the involvement of only one joint, as demonstrated by scintigraphy, favors an infectious process (Fig. 25.28). A triad of radiographic abnormalities (Phemister triad), composed of periarticular osteoporosis, peripherally located osseous erosions, and gradual diminution of the joint space, should suggest the correct diagnosis; CT examination, however, can be helpful in delineating subtle features (Fig. 25.29). Occasionally, wedge-shaped necrotic foci, so-called *kissing sequestra*, may be present on both sides of the affected joint, especially in the knee. At a later stage of the disease, there may be complete destruction of the joint, and sclerotic changes in adjacent bones are

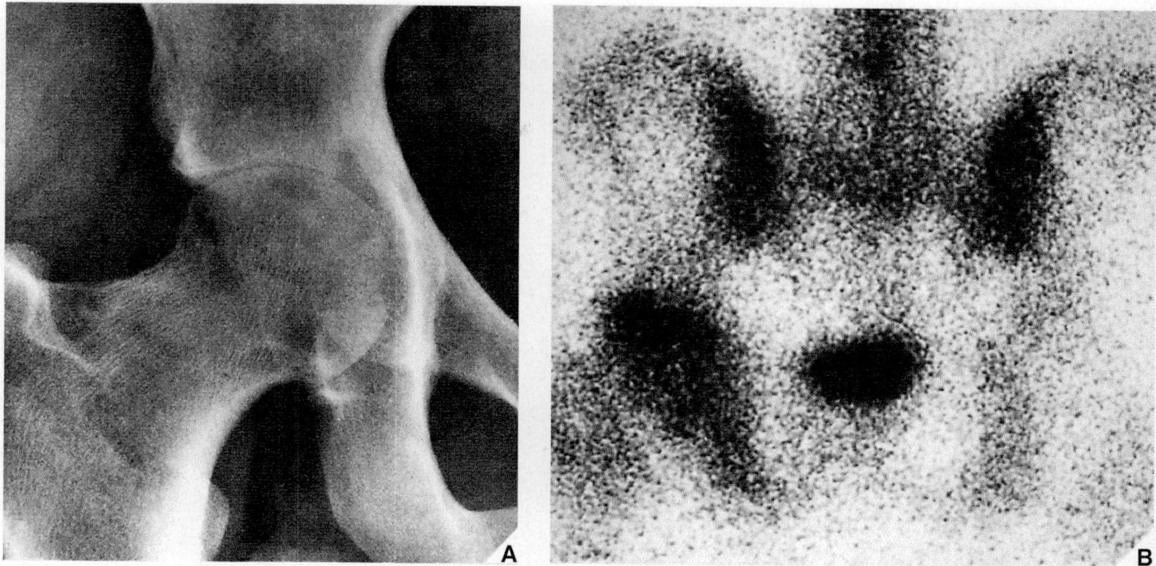

FIGURE 25.28 Tuberculous arthritis. A 29-year-old woman with chronic alcoholism presented with right hip pain. **(A)** Anteroposterior radiograph of the hip demonstrates diminution of the joint space, particularly in the weight-bearing region, as well as periarticular osteoporosis. **(B)** Radionuclide bone scan using ^{99m}Tc-labeled diphosphonate demonstrates increased uptake of radiopharmaceutical tracer only in the right hip. The increased activity at both sacroiliac joints is a normal finding. The diagnosis of tuberculous arthritis was confirmed by joint aspiration.

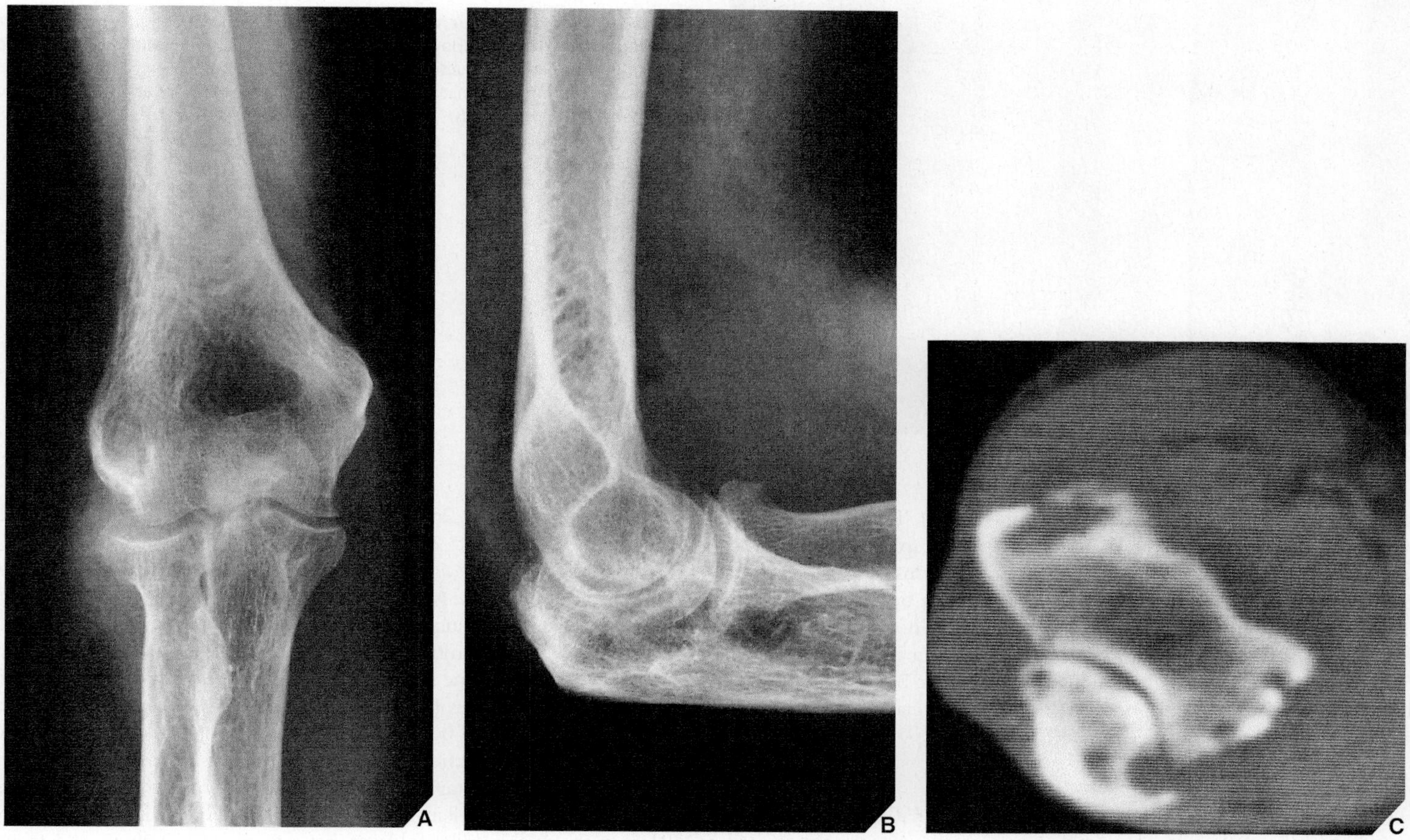

FIGURE 25.29 CT of tuberculous arthritis. A 70-year-old man from India presented with pain in the left elbow for 4 months. According to his daughter, he had been treated for chronic lung disease. **(A)** Anteroposterior and **(B)** lateral radiographs of the elbow demonstrate a large joint effusion, as indicated by positive anterior and posterior fat-pad signs on the lateral projection. Small periarticular erosions are not clear on these views. **(C)** CT section shows narrowing of the joint and peripheral erosions typical of tuberculous infection.

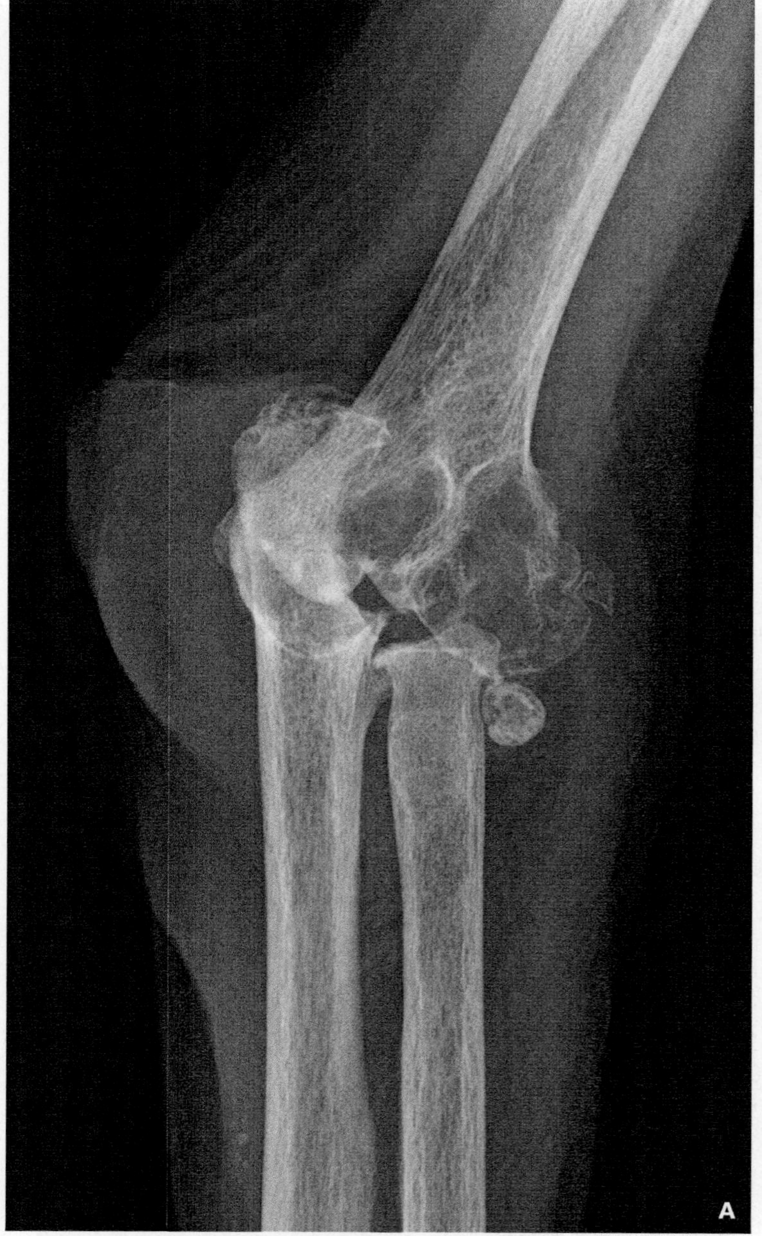

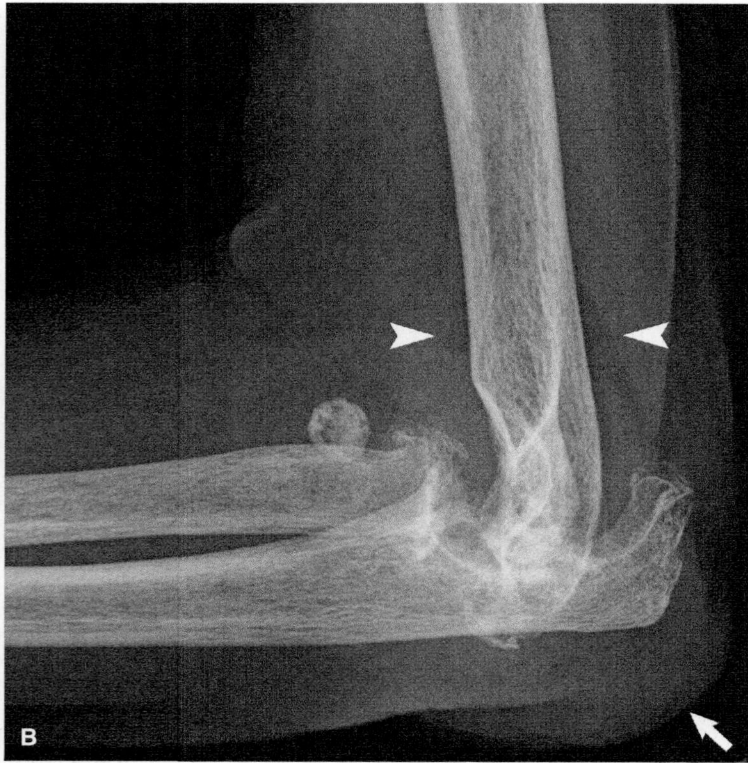

FIGURE 25.30 Tuberculous arthritis. **(A)** External oblique and **(B)** lateral radiographs of the left elbow of a 70-year-old woman with pulmonary tuberculosis show complete destruction of all compartments of the elbow joint associated with a large joint effusion, as demonstrated by the positive anterior and posterior fat-pad sign *(arrowheads)*. Soft-tissue mass at the site of olecranon *(arrow)* is secondary to bursitis.

more frequently encountered (Figs. 25.30 and 25.31). The MRI manifestations of tuberculous arthritis parallel the radiographic changes, with bone marrow edema, joint effusion, marginal erosions, and progressive cartilage loss. The presence of multiple intraarticular bodies ("rice" bodies) is characteristic of tuberculous arthritis, tenosynovitis, and bursitis (Fig. 25.32A), although they may be seen also in rheumatoid arthritis and synovial chondromatosis. Tuberculous bursitis is rare but should be considered in the differential diagnosis of bursitis, especially if the infected bursa is grossly distended (Fig. 25.32B,C).

Pathology

Grossly there is separation of the articular cartilage that is dissected from the underlying bone by granulomatous tissue. As the disease progresses, the articular cartilage and subchondral bone on both sides of the joint become completely destroyed (Fig. 25.33). In the later stage of untreated disease, ankylosis of the joint commonly occurs. The histopathology of tuberculous arthritis is identical to one of tuberculous osteomyelitis discussed in the previous text.

Other Infectious Arthritides

Less frequently encountered than pyogenic or tuberculous arthritis are joint infections caused by fungi (actinomycosis, cryptococcosis, coccidioidomycosis [Fig. 25.34], histoplasmosis, sporotrichosis, and candidiasis), viruses (smallpox), and spirochetes (syphilis, yaws).

Of interest is *Lyme arthritis*, an infectious articular condition caused by the spirochete *Borrelia burgdorferi*, which is transmitted by the tick *Ixodes dammini* or related ticks such as *Ixodes pacificus* and *Ixodes ricinus*. The illness usually begins in the summer with a characteristic skin lesion (erythema chronicum migrans) at the site of a tick bite, and flu-like symptoms; within weeks to months, a chronic arthritis develops that is characterized by erosions of cartilage and bone. The joint involvement has some similarities to juvenile idiopathic arthritis and reactive arthritis. A joint effusion may be present in the early stages of the disease, and characteristic edematous changes of the infrapatellar fat pad may be noted in the knee (Fig. 25.35). MRI may show ribbonlike folds of hypertrophied synovium and frondlike extensions of synovium and synovial fluid into infrapatellar fat pad (Fig. 25.36).

Parasitic disease of the musculoskeletal system due to infestation by the roundworms, flatworms, or tapeworms, such as hookworm disease, loiasis, filariasis, cysticercosis, or echinococcosis, is relatively uncommon in the western hemisphere, but in some endemic areas, parasitic infection needs to be considered in the differential diagnosis of bone and soft-tissue lesions, especially when there are unusual imaging findings. One of these conditions, hydatid cyst disease, also known as *echinococcosis* or *echinococcal*

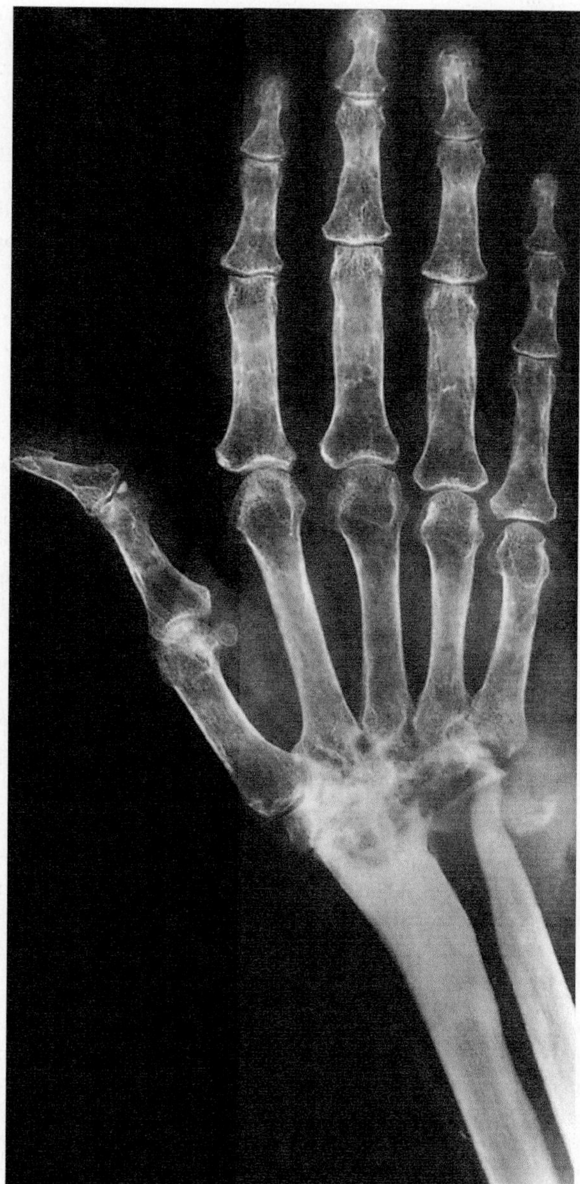

FIGURE 25.31 **Tuberculous arthritis.** Posteroanterior radiograph of the left wrist and hand of a 52-year-old woman with pulmonary tuberculosis shows advanced arthritis involving the left carpus. There is complete destruction of the radiocarpal, midcarpal, and carpometacarpal articulations as well as whittling and sclerotic changes in the distal radius and ulna. Note the osteoporosis distal to the affected joints and the soft-tissue swelling.

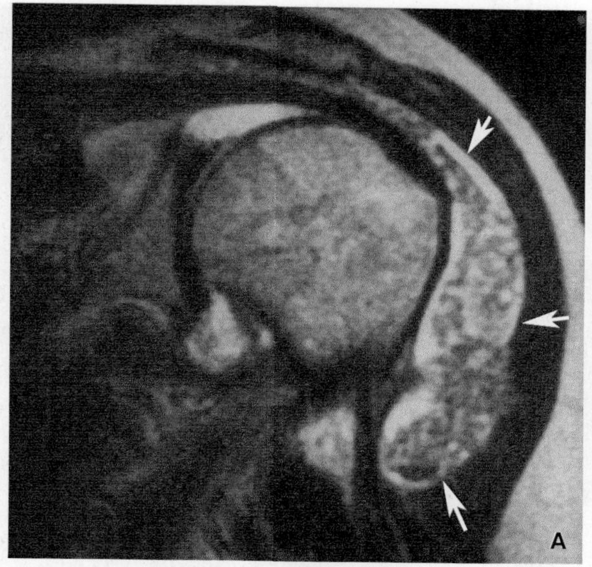

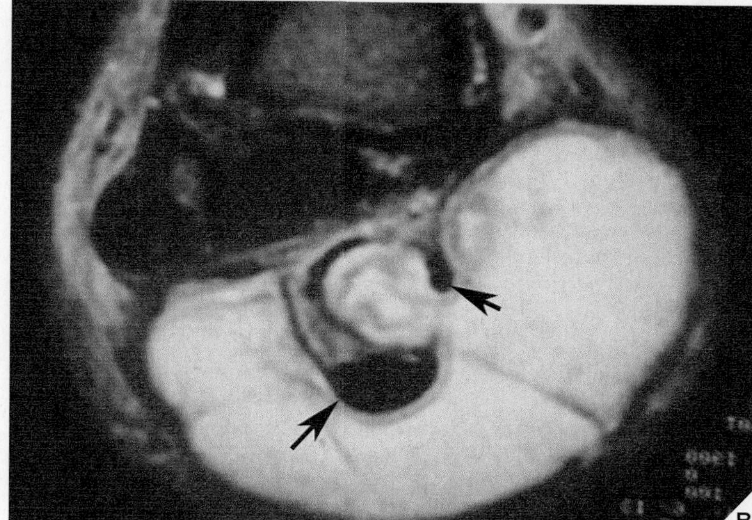

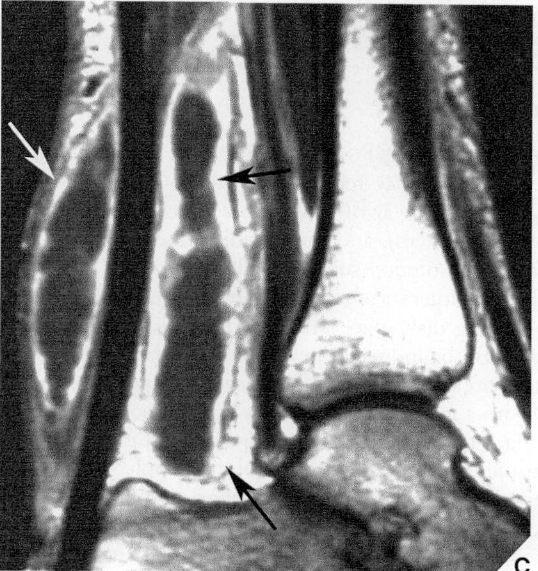

FIGURE 25.32 **MRI of tuberculous bursitis.** **(A)** Coronal T2-weighted MR image of the left shoulder of a patient with tuberculous subdeltoid bursitis shows multiple "rice bodies" within the fluid-distended bursa *(arrows)*. **(B)** Axial T2-weighted MRI of the ankle in another patient demonstrates a markedly distended retro-Achilles bursa surrounding posteriorly the Achilles and the plantaris tendons *(arrows)*. **(C)** Sagittal T1-weighted fat-saturated MRI obtained after intravenous administration of gadolinium demonstrates the enhancement of the wall of the bursa *(arrows)*. (**B,C**, Courtesy of Prof. Jose Marcos-Robles, Madrid, Spain.)

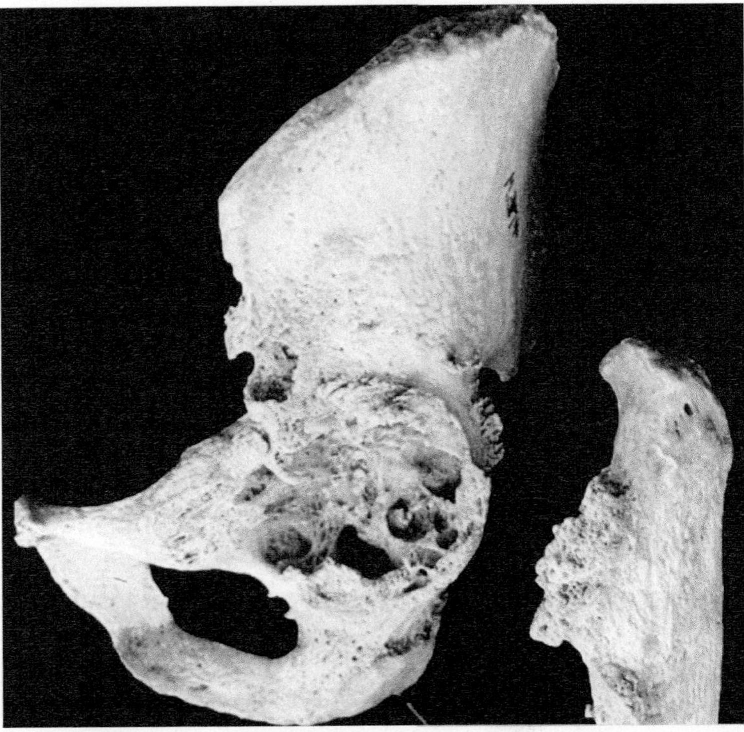

FIGURE 25.33 Pathology of tuberculous arthritis. Macerated bone specimen obtained at the autopsy shows destructive changes of the left hip joint. In addition, observe total destruction of the femoral head with only a stump of femoral neck remaining attached to the shaft of the femur. (Reprinted from Bullough P. *Orthopaedic pathology*, 5th ed. Maryland Heights, MO: Mosby; 2009, with permission from Elsevier.)

disease, a parasitic infection caused by a tapeworm *Echinococcus granulosus*, affects musculoskeletal system in about 1% to 4% of all reported cases. In the bones, expansive, bubble-like lytic lesions are encountered, and cyst formation in the various viscera (liver, lungs) and soft tissue is characteristic feature. MR is an effective modality to image the hydatid cysts within the soft tissues (Fig. 25.37).

Infections of the Spine

Pyogenic Infections

Clinical and Imaging Features

Infectious organisms may reach the spine by several routes. Hematogenous spread occurs by way of arterial and venous routes (the Batson paravertebral venous system), and the organism lodges in the vertebral body, commonly in the anterior subchondral region. This osteomyelitic focus can spread to the intervertebral disk through perforation of the vertebral end plate, causing disk space infection (diskitis) (Fig. 25.38). Disk space infection can also be induced directly by the implantation of an organism through puncture of the spinal canal, either during spinal surgery or, rarely, by spread from a contiguous site of infection such as a paravertebral abscess (see Fig. 24.4). Disk infection may also occur in children via a hematogenous route because there is still a blood supply to the disk.

Radiographically, disk infection is characterized by narrowing of the disk space, destruction of the adjacent vertebral end plates, and a paraspinal mass. Although most cases are obvious on standard anteroposterior and lateral radiographs of the spine (Fig. 25.39), CT (Fig. 25.40) may yield additional information. Radionuclide bone scan can detect early infection before any changes are noticed radiographically (Fig. 25.41). Occasionally, diskography is performed, but as in the use of arthrography in joint infections, the primary objective is obtaining a specimen for bacteriologic examination. A contrast study, however, may outline the extent of a disk infection (Fig. 25.42).

MRI has become the modality of choice in diagnosing and evaluating infections of the spine. Characteristic findings of disk space narrowing, disk destruction, paraspinal soft-tissue thickening, and edematous changes in the paraspinal musculature are well demonstrated by this technique (Figs. 25.43 and 25.44).

Pathology

Gross specimen of the spine with disk space infection reflects the imaging findings, showing irregularity of the vertebral end plates and sclerosis of the bone. At the early stage of infection, the disk space is narrowed. As the infectious process progresses, the intervertebral disk undergoes fragmentation and complete destruction associated with vertebral collapse leading to kyphosis (Fig. 25.45).

Nonpyogenic Infections

Tuberculosis of the Spine

Clinical and Imaging Features

Infection of the spine by the tubercle bacillus is known as *tuberculous spondylitis* or *Pott disease*. The vertebral body or intervertebral disk may be involved, with the lower thoracic and upper lumbar vertebrae being the preferred sites of infection. The disease constitutes 25% to 50% of all cases of skeletal tuberculosis. In most patients, the onset of symptoms is insidious and includes local pain and systemic signs of chronic debilitating illness. At the time of initial presentation, the patient may experience persistent back pain later associated with signs of nerve root compression and radiculopathy. Not infrequently, other neurologic symptoms such as lower extremity weakness, loss of reflexes, or even paraplegia may develop. This latter symptom is the most serious complication of tuberculous spondylitis, and it results from extension of the infectious process into the peridural space with resultant spinal cord compression (see Fig. 25.48).

The imaging features of tuberculous infection of the spine are similar to those seen in pyogenic infections. There is disk space narrowing, and the vertebral end plates adjacent to the involved disk show evidence of destruction. A paraspinal mass is common (Fig. 25.46). Rarely, the infectious process may destroy a single vertebra or part of a vertebra (pedicle) without invasion of the disk.

Pathology

The primary granulomatous abscesses may be located in the vertebral body either anteriorly, paradiskally, or centrally (Fig. 25.47). The anterior location accounts for about 20% of cases and leads to cortical bone destruction beneath the anterior longitudinal ligament. The paradiskal location, which accounts for over 50% of the cases, leads to destruction of the intervertebral disk and commonly the infectious process spreads to the adjacent vertebral body. Usually it also extends posteriorly into the subdural space. As the disease progresses, the abscesses may eventually compress the spinal cord. The central lesions, which account for the remaining cases, begin in the midportion of the vertebral body, and then spread to involve and destroy the entire vertebral body (Fig. 25.48) and the adjacent intervertebral disks (Fig. 25.49).The microscopic findings in tuberculous spondylitis are similar to those of tuberculous osteomyelitis discussed in the previous text.

Complications

Tuberculosis of the spine may cause collapse of a partially or completely destroyed vertebra, leading to kyphosis and a gibbous formation. Extension of infection to the adjacent ligaments and soft tissues is also rather frequent; the psoas muscles are often the site of secondary tuberculous infections, commonly called *cold abscesses* (Fig. 25.50). The most common complication of tuberculous spondylitis, however, is compression of the thecal sac and spinal cord with resulting paraplegia. Myelography (Fig. 25.51) and MRI are very helpful diagnostically if compression is suspected.

Coccidioidomycosis of the Spine

Involvement of the spine most commonly manifests as vertebral osteomyelitis or rarely as disk space infection (spondylodiskitis). In the former variant, both punched-out and permeated lesions are observed in the vertebral bodies. Cases with almost complete vertebral destruction have also been reported (Fig. 25.52). Coccidioidomycosis often involves the vertebral appendages, and paraspinal soft-tissue extension is common. Disk space narrowing and gibbous deformity, although previously reported, are unusual

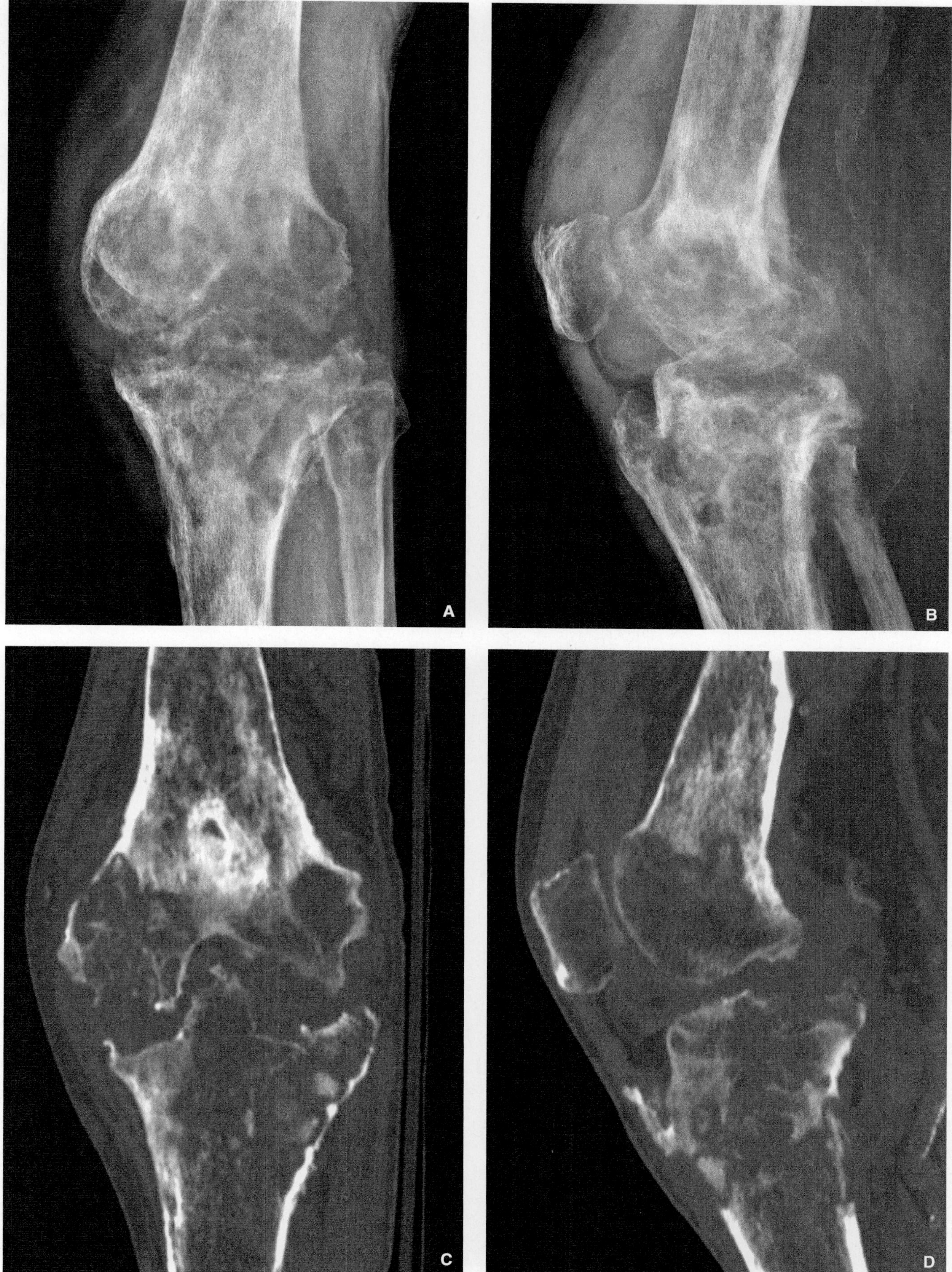

FIGURE 25.34 Coccidioidomycotic arthritis. **(A)** Anteroposterior and **(B)** lateral radiographs of the left knee of a 62-year-old man with pulmonary coccidioidomycosis show diffuse demineralization of osseous structures, destruction of the joint, and several osteolytic foci within the distal femur, proximal tibia, and proximal fibula. Observe also a large knee joint effusion. **(C)** Coronal and **(D)** sagittal reformatted CT images characterize better the extend of osseous and joint destruction.

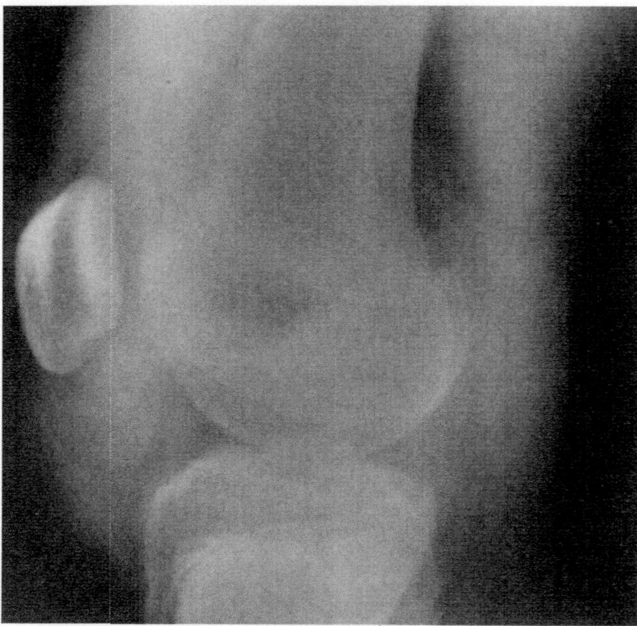

FIGURE 25.35 Lyme arthritis. Lateral radiograph of the right knee of a 13-year-old boy, who presented with intermittent soft-tissue swelling and knee effusion for several months, shows periarticular osteoporosis, joint effusion, soft-tissue swelling, and areas of mottled density at the site of infrapatellar fat pad. (Reprinted from Lawson JP, Rahn DW. Lyme disease and radiologic findings in Lyme arthritis. *AJR Am J Roentgenol* 1992;158:1065–1069. Copyright © 1992 American Roentgen Ray Society.)

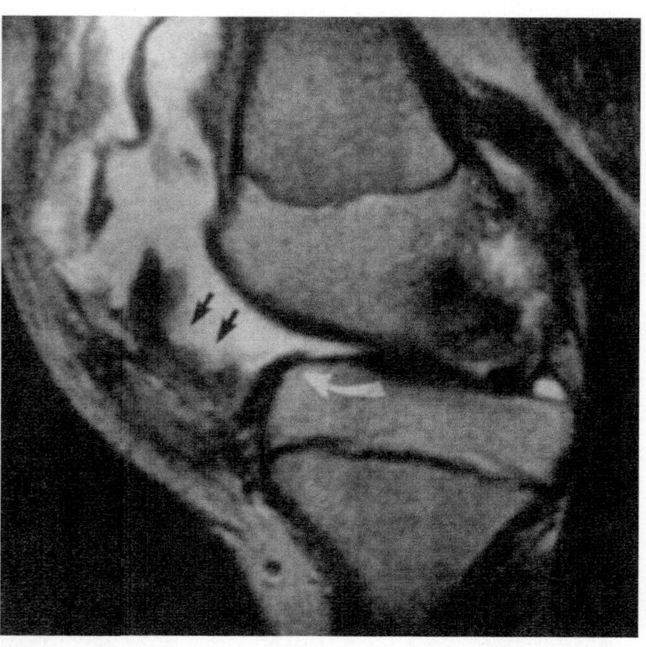

FIGURE 25.36 MRI of Lyme arthritis. Sagittal T2-weighted MRI of the left knee of a 17-year-old boy, who presented with knee swelling for 7 months, reveals joint effusion that displaced medial meniscus anteriorly *(curved white arrow)*. Note ribbon-like folds of hypertrophied synovium and frond-like extensions of synovium and synovial fluid into infrapatellar fat pad *(black arrows)*. (Reprinted from Lawson JP, Rahn DW. Lyme disease and radiologic findings in Lyme arthritis. *AJR Am J Roentgenol* 1992;158:1065–1069. Copyright © 1992 American Roentgen Ray Society.)

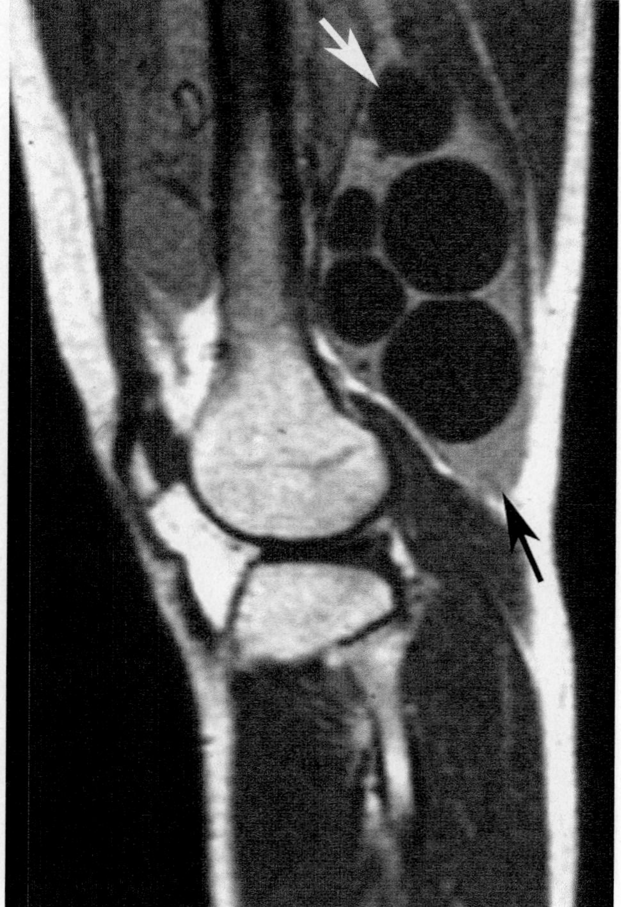

FIGURE 25.37 MRI of hydatid disease. Sagittal T1-weighted MRI of the knee shows a large fluid collection in the posterior aspect of the distal thigh *(arrows)* containing multiple smaller fluid collections, representing hydatid cysts.

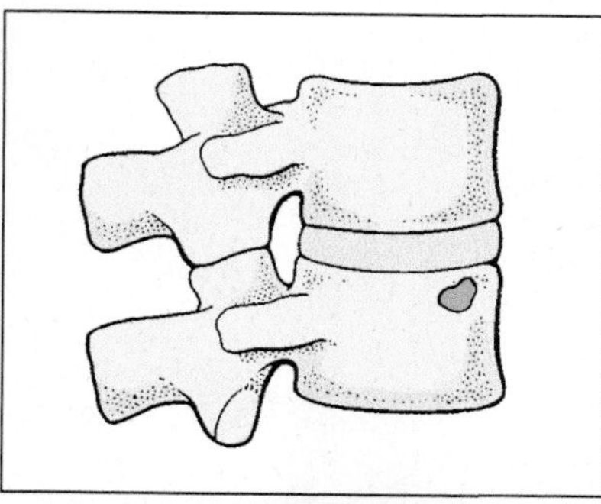

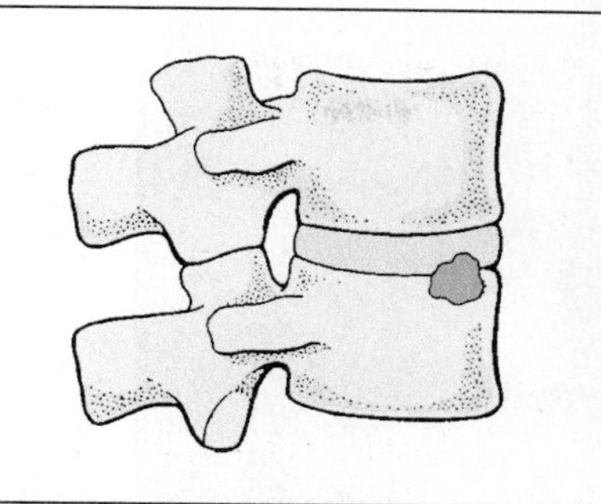

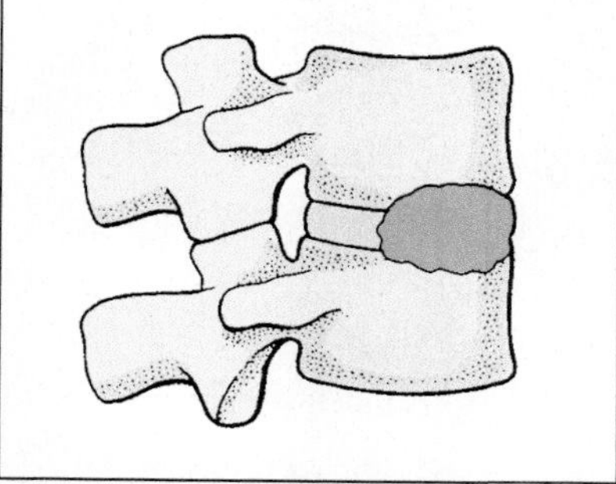

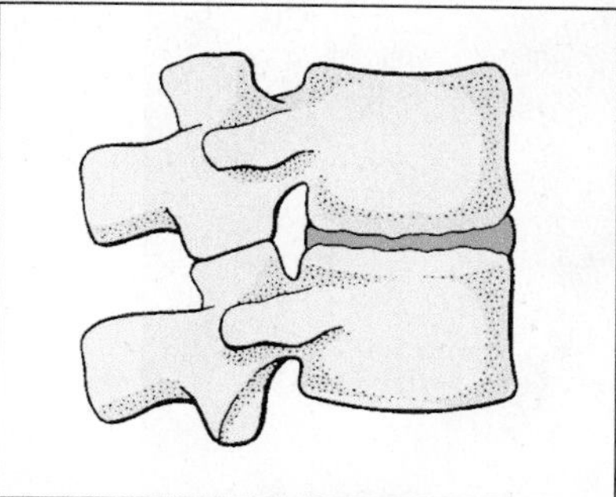

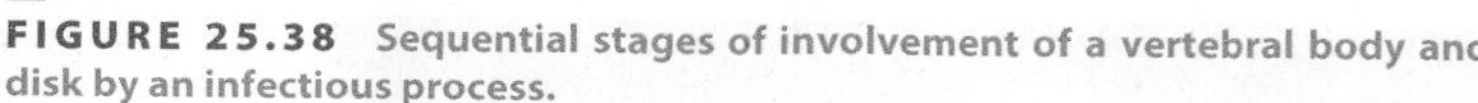

FIGURE 25.38 Sequential stages of involvement of a vertebral body and disk by an infectious process.

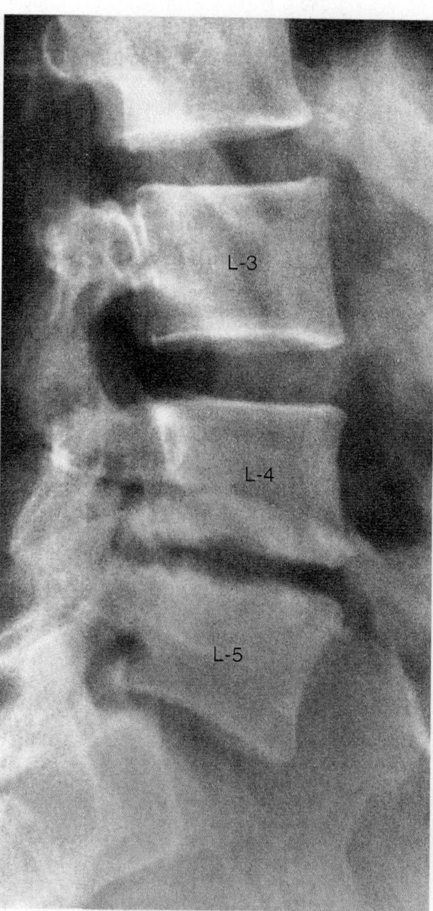

FIGURE 25.39 **Intervertebral disk infection.** Lateral radiograph of the lumbar spine of a 32-year-old man demonstrates the typical radiographic changes of disk infection. There is narrowing of the disk space at L4-5, and the inferior end plate of L4 and superior end plate of L5 are indistinctly outlined. Note the normal end plates at the L3-4 disk space.

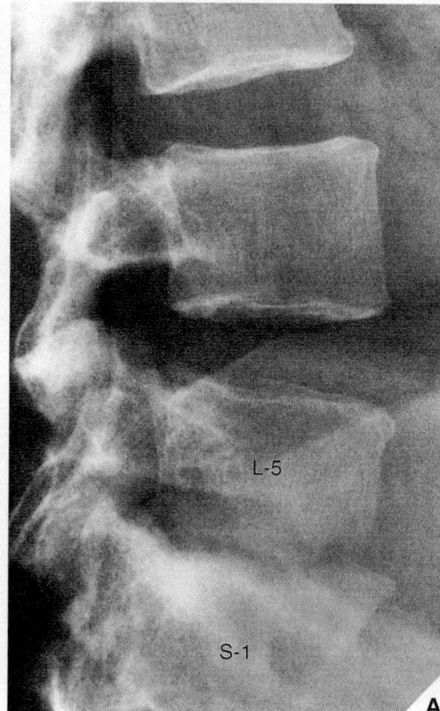

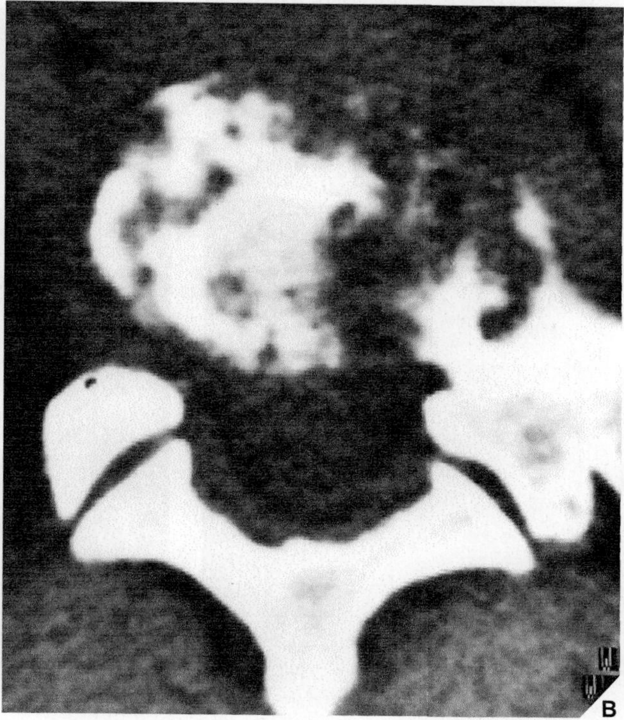

FIGURE 25.40 **CT of intervertebral disk infection.** A 40-year-old man presented with lower back pain for 8 weeks, which he attributed to lifting a heavy object. **(A)** Lateral radiograph of the lumbosacral spine shows narrowing of the L5-S1 disk space and suggests some fuzziness of the adjacent vertebral end plates. **(B)** CT section through the disk space clearly shows destructive changes of the disk and vertebral end plate characteristic of infection.

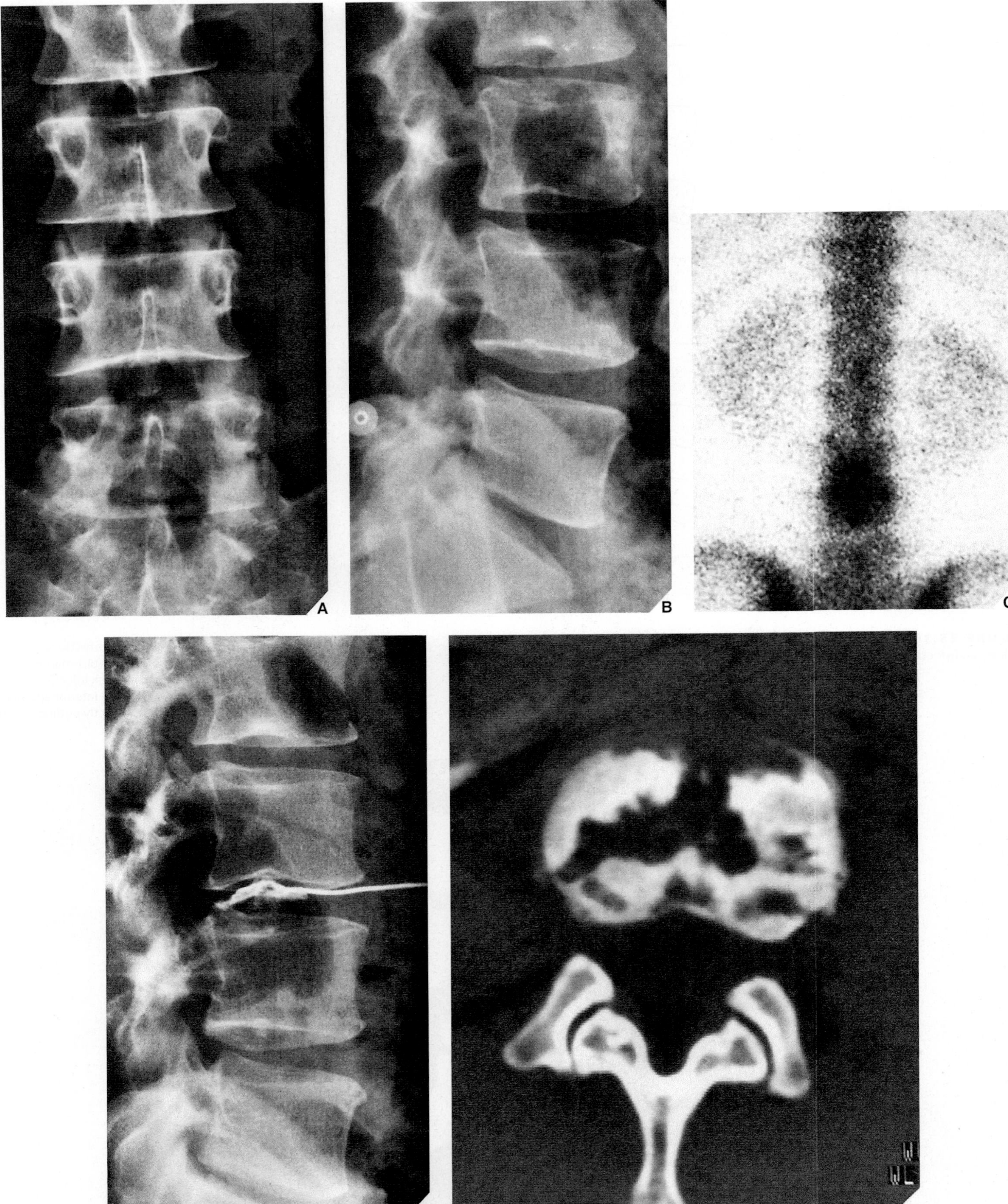

FIGURE 25.41 Scintigraphy and CT of intervertebral disk infection. **(A)** Conventional anteroposterior and **(B)** lateral radiographs of the lumbar spine of a 40-year-old man who had back pain for 4 weeks show no definite abnormalities. **(C)** Radionuclide bone scan, however, reveals an increased uptake of radiopharmaceutical tracer at the L3-4 level. **(D)** On a subsequent diskogram, using the oblique approach, partial disk destruction is evident. **(E)** The extent of destruction is revealed by CT. Bacteriologic examination of aspirated fluid yielded *Escherichia coli*.

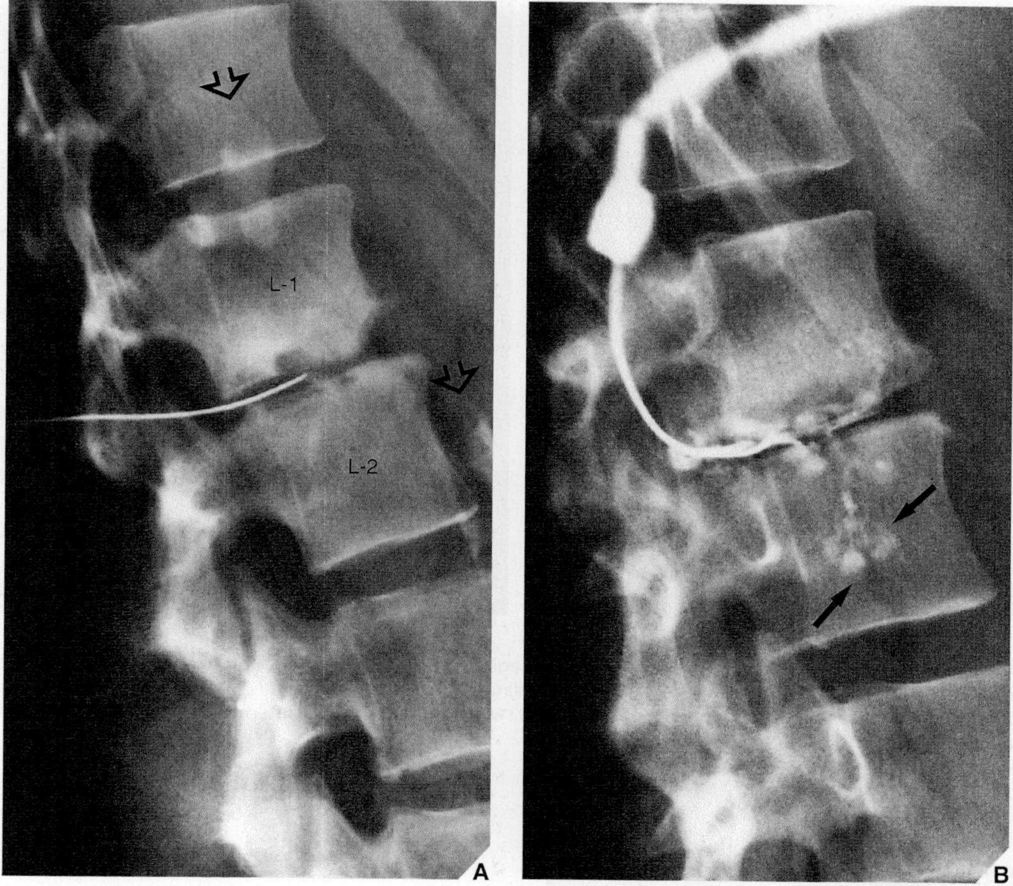

FIGURE 25.42 Diskography of disk space infection and vertebral osteomyelitis. A 22-year-old intravenous drug user with back pain for 2 months was diagnosed with an intervertebral disk infection. A diskogram was performed primarily to aspirate fluid for bacteriologic examination, which revealed *P. aeruginosa*. Before the puncture, the patient received an intravenous injection of iodine contrast agent to visualize the kidneys, as a precautionary step before spine biopsy at that level. **(A)** Lateral radiograph of the lumbar spine shows narrowing of the disk space at L1-2 and destruction of the adjacent vertebral end plates. The spinal needle is located in the center of the disk. The *open arrows* point to opacified calyces of kidney. **(B)** Lateral radiograph obtained during the injection of metrizamide demonstrates extension of the contrast into the body of L2 *(arrows)*, indicating the presence of vertebral osteomyelitis.

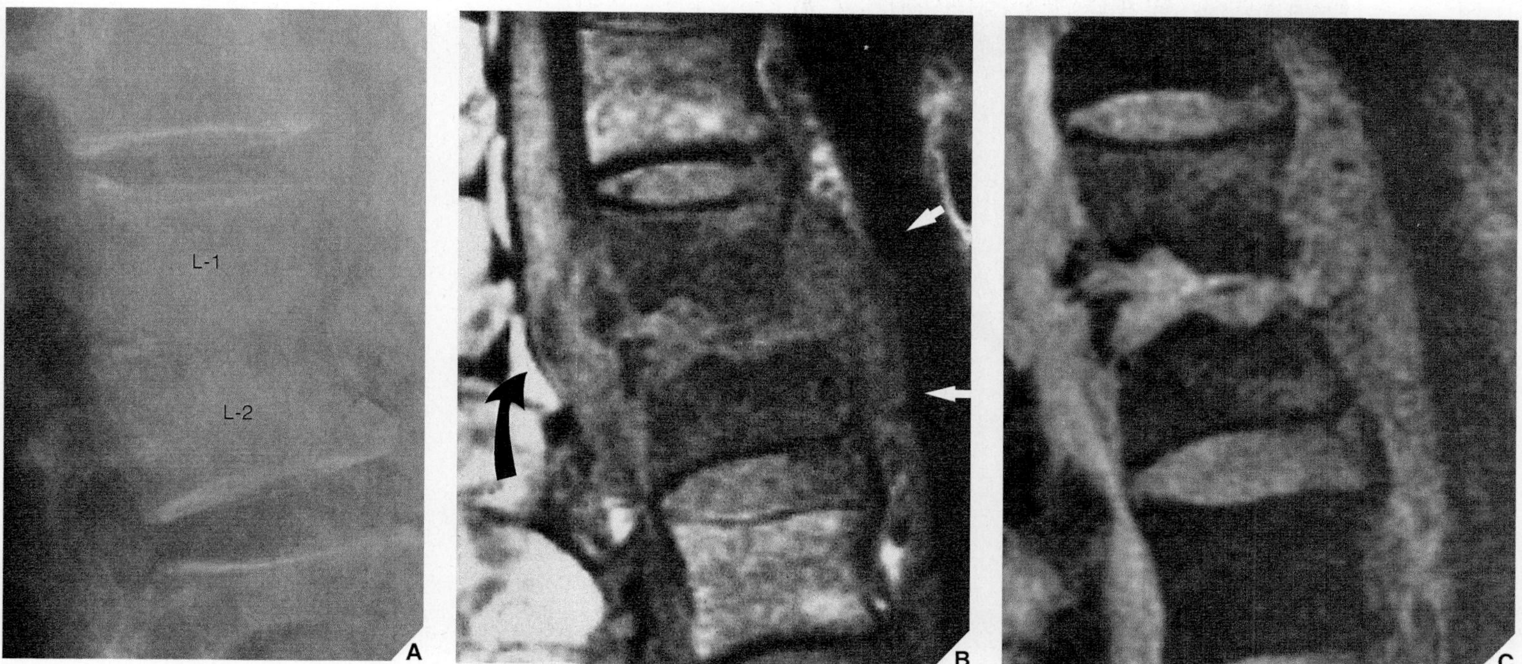

FIGURE 25.43 MRI of disk space infection and vertebral osteomyelitis. A 48-year-old man who is an intravenous drug user developed disk infection at L1-2. **(A)** Lateral radiograph demonstrates classic changes of disk infection: narrowing of the disk space and destruction of the vertebral end plates. **(B)** Sagittal spin echo T1-weighted MR image (TR 600/TE 20 msec) demonstrates, in addition to the destruction of the disk, a large inflammatory mass extending anteriorly *(arrows)*, destroying anterior longitudinal ligament and infiltrating paraspinal soft tissues. Posteriorly, it invades the content of spinal canal *(curved arrow)*. **(C)** Sagittal T2*-weighted gradient (multiplanar gradient recalled) MR image shows more clearly the fragmentation of the posterior aspect of adjacent vertebral bodies and compression of the thecal sac by a large abscess.

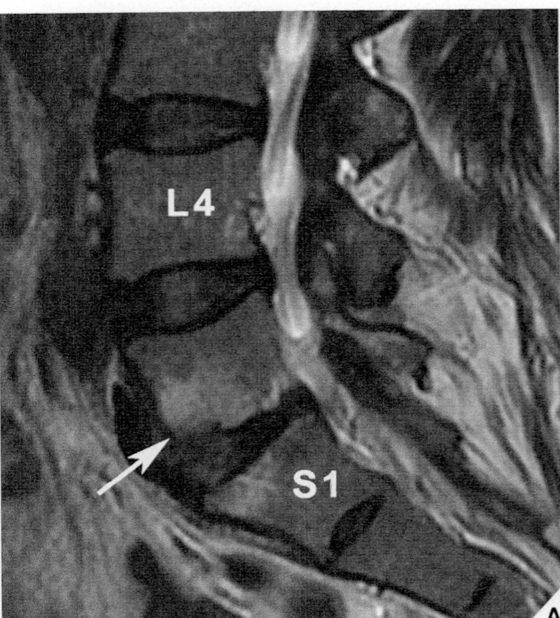

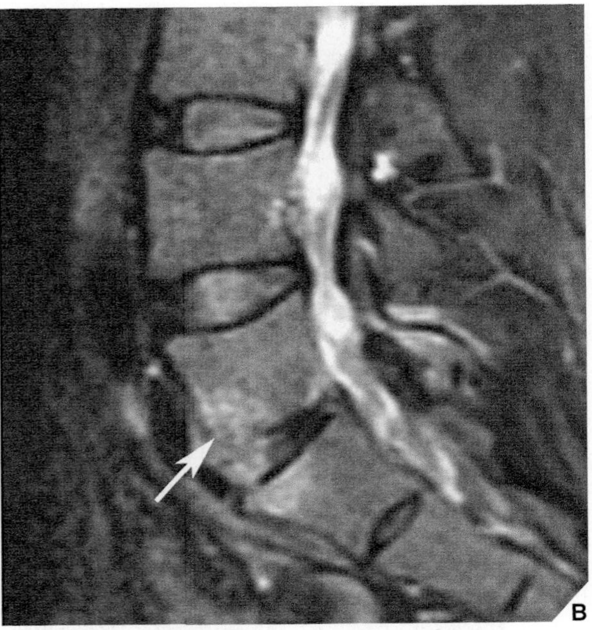

FIGURE 25.44 MRI of disk space infection and vertebral osteomyelitis. **(A)** Sagittal T2-weighted and **(B)** short time inversion recovery (STIR) MR images of the lumbar spine of a 53-year-old man show a focal area of decortication of the inferior end plate of L5 *(arrows)* representing osteomyelitis, with bone marrow edema of the inferior aspect of the L5 vertebral body and superior aspect of the S1 vertebral body. There is swelling and high signal intensity of the anterior aspect of the intervertebral disk with mild prevertebral soft-tissue edema. There are no signs of epidural abscess.

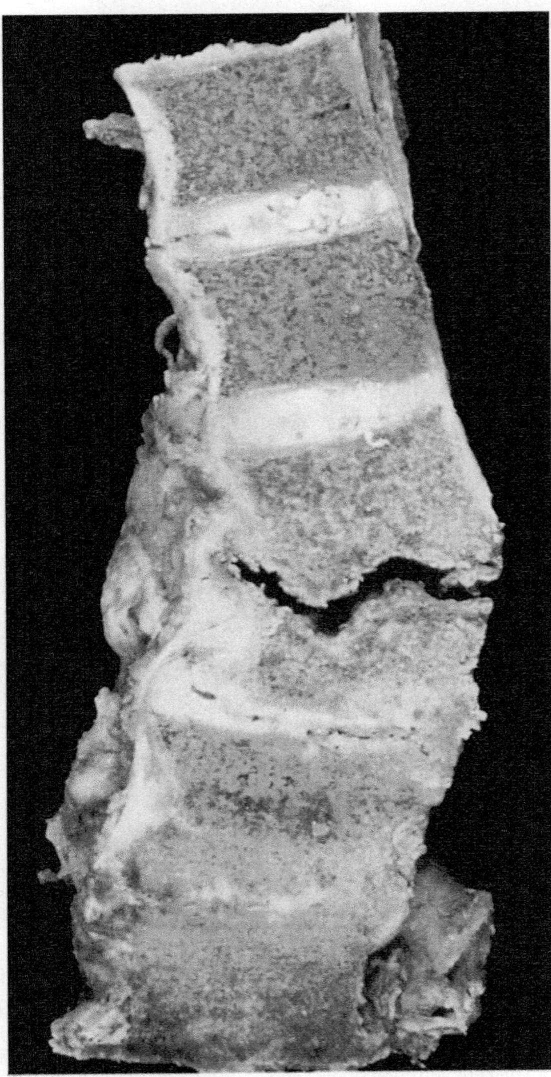

FIGURE 25.45 Pathology of disk space infection and vertebral osteomyelitis. Photograph of a sagittal section of thoracolumbar junction of the spine shows involvement of two vertebral bodies and intervening disk space. There is segmental collapse due to complete destruction of the intervertebral disk associated with kyphotic deformity. (Modified from Bullough P. *Orthopaedic pathology*, 5th ed. Maryland Heights, MO: Mosby; 2009, with permission from Elsevier.)

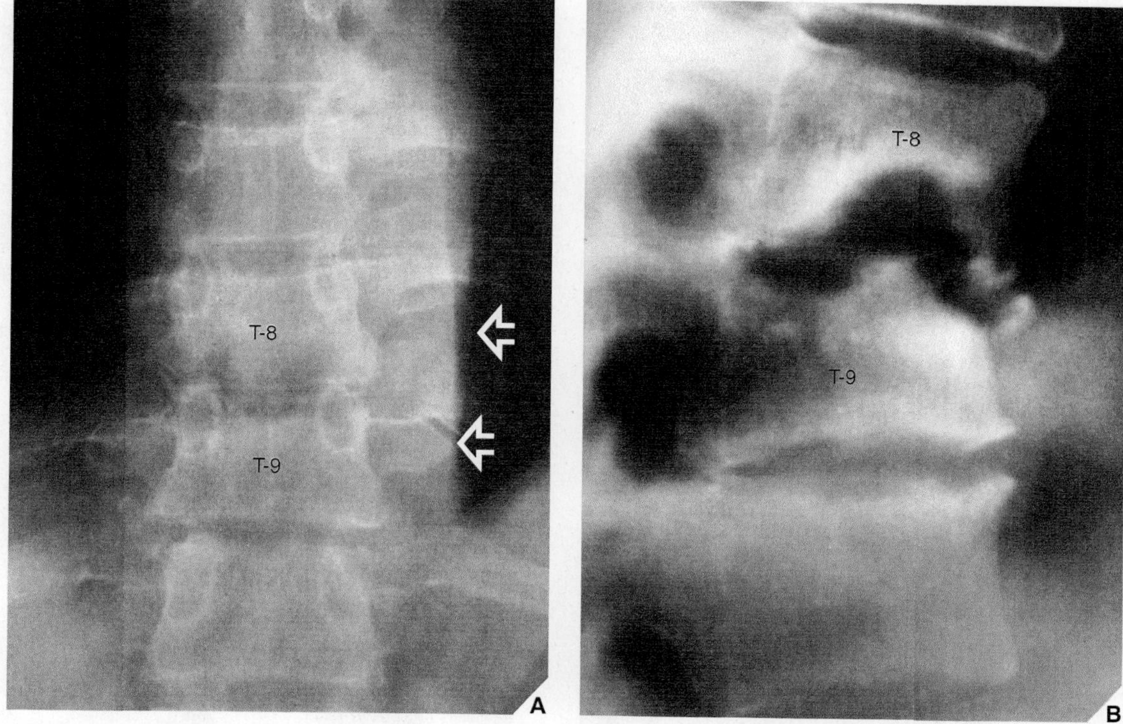

FIGURE 25.46 Tuberculous spondylitis. **(A)** Anteroposterior radiograph of the thoracic spine in a 50-year-old man shows narrowing of the T8-9 disk space, associated with a paraspinal mass on the left side *(open arrows)*. **(B)** Lateral conventional tomogram shows destruction of the disk and extensive erosions of the inferior aspect of the body of T8 and the superior end plate of T9.

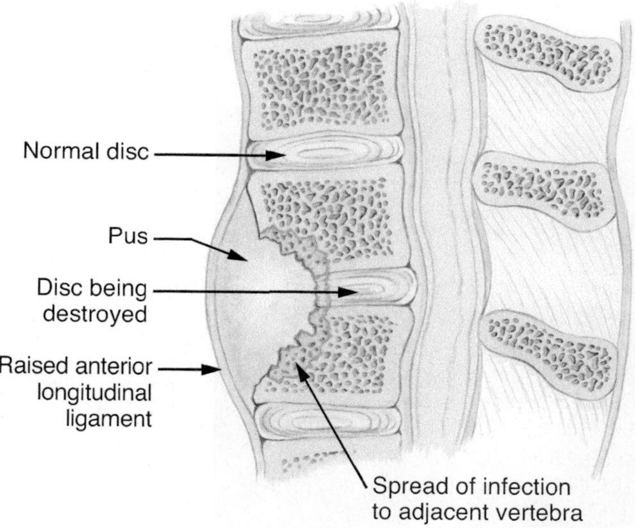

FIGURE 25.47 Pathology of tuberculous spondylitis. Schematic representation of the spread of tuberculosis of the spine. (Reprinted with permission from Vigorita JV, Ghelmsan B, Mintz D. *Orthopaedic pathology*, 3rd ed. Philadelphia: Wolters Kluwer; 2016:262.)

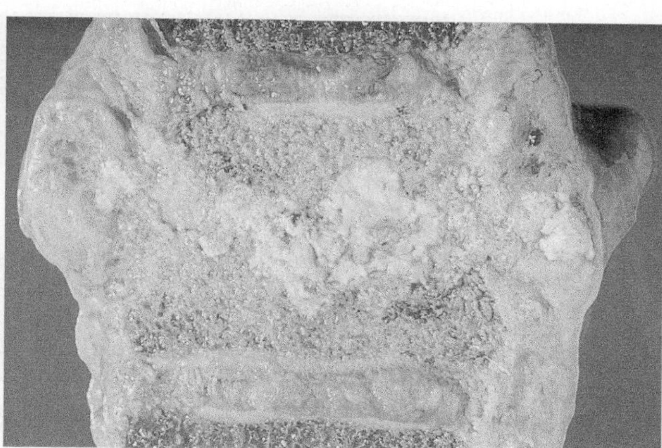

FIGURE 25.48 Pathology of tuberculous spondylitis. Photograph of the coronal section of the thoracic vertebra shows destruction of the vertebral body with classic yellow, cheese-like caseating necrosis. (Reprinted with permission from Vigorita JV, Ghelmsan B, Mintz D. *Orthopaedic pathology*, 3rd ed. Philadelphia: Wolters Kluwer; 2016:265.)

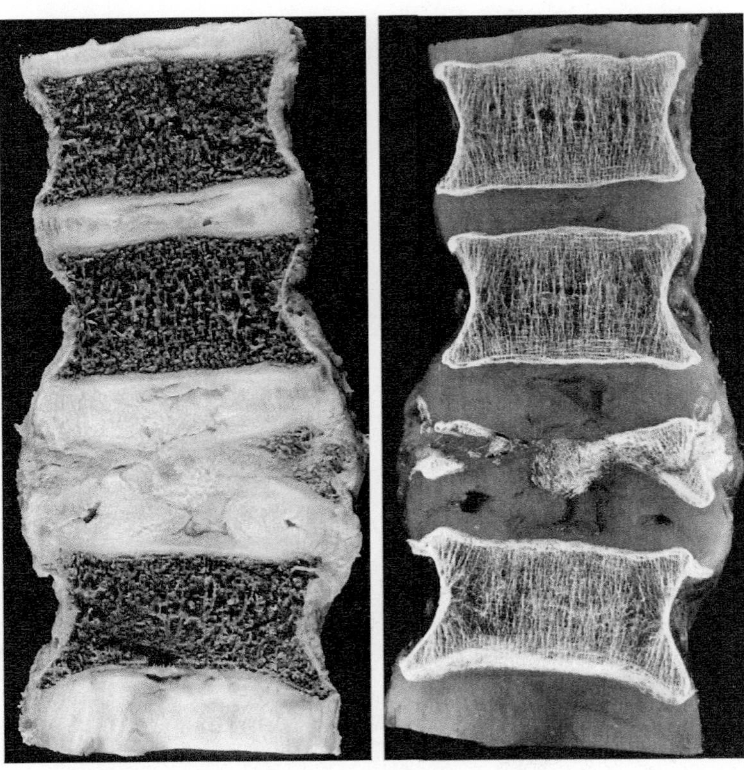

FIGURE 25.49 **Pathology of tuberculous spondylitis.** Photograph of a coronal section through the specimen of the lumbar spine of a 67-year-old man and radiograph of the specimen show complete destruction and collapse of L3. Observe involvement of the adjacent intervertebral disks. (Reprinted from Bullough P. *Orthopaedic pathology*, 5th ed. Maryland Heights, MO: Mosby; 2009, with permission from Elsevier.)

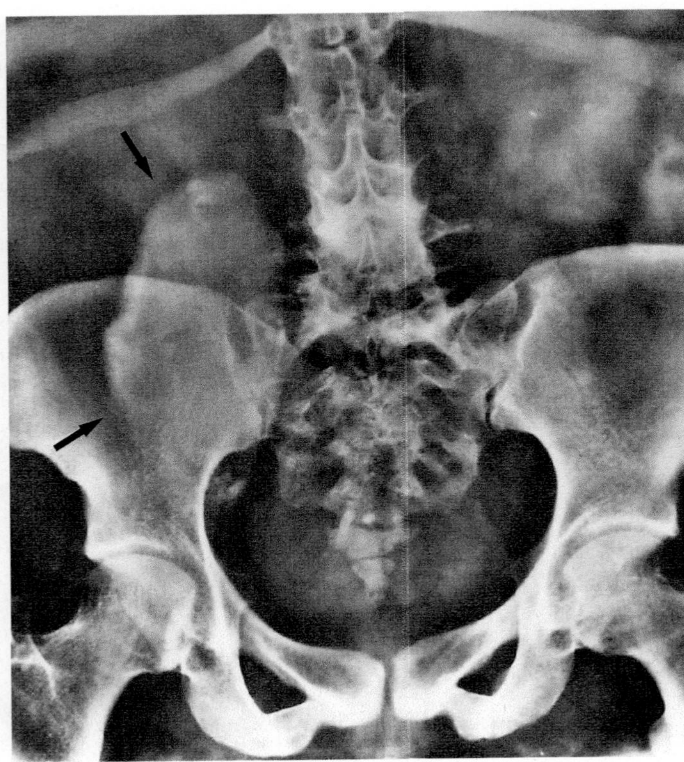

FIGURE 25.50 **Tuberculous cold abscess.** Anteroposterior radiograph of the pelvis in a 35-year-old woman with spinal tuberculosis shows an oval radiodense mass with spotted calcifications overlapping the medial part of the ilium and right sacroiliac joint (right psoas muscle) *(arrows)*. This is the typical appearance of a cold abscess.

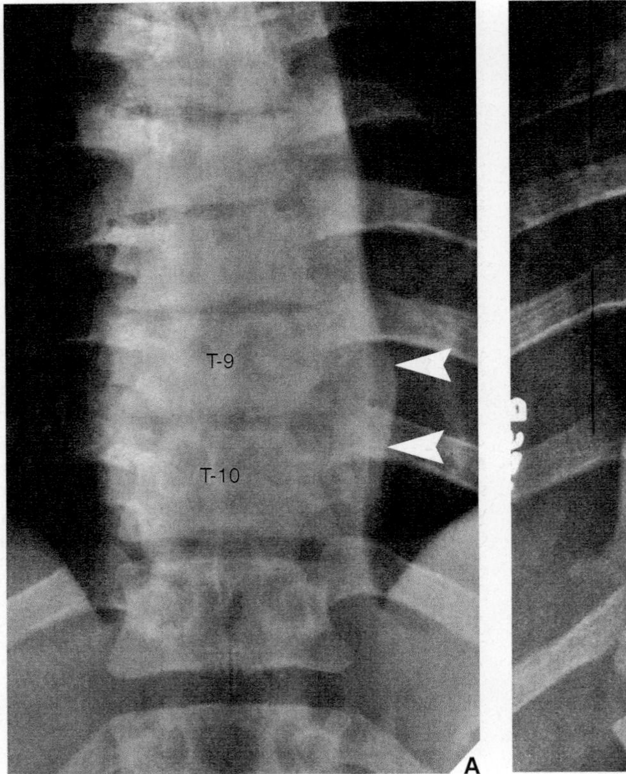

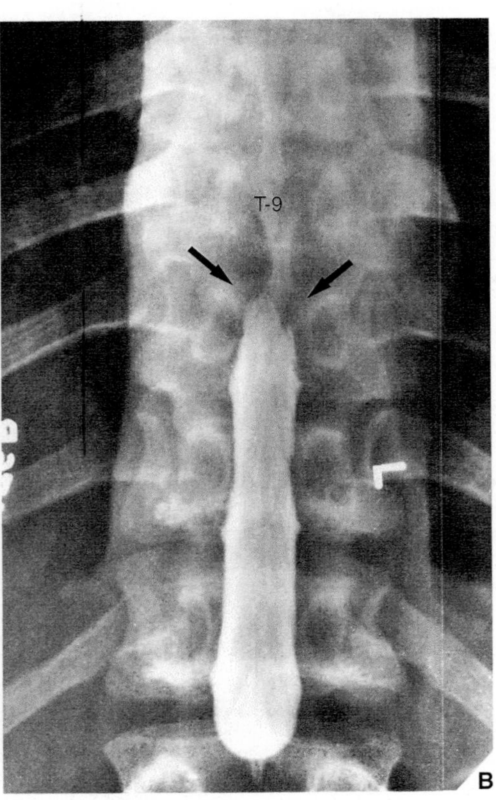

FIGURE 25.51 **Myelography of tuberculous diskitis.** A 39-year-old man with a history of pulmonary tuberculosis had neurologic symptoms of spinal cord compression. **(A)** Anteroposterior radiograph of the lower thoracic spine shows minimal disk space narrowing at T9-10 and a large left paraspinal mass *(arrowheads)*. **(B)** A myelogram shows complete obstruction of the flow of contrast in the subarachnoid space at the level of the disk infection *(arrows)*.

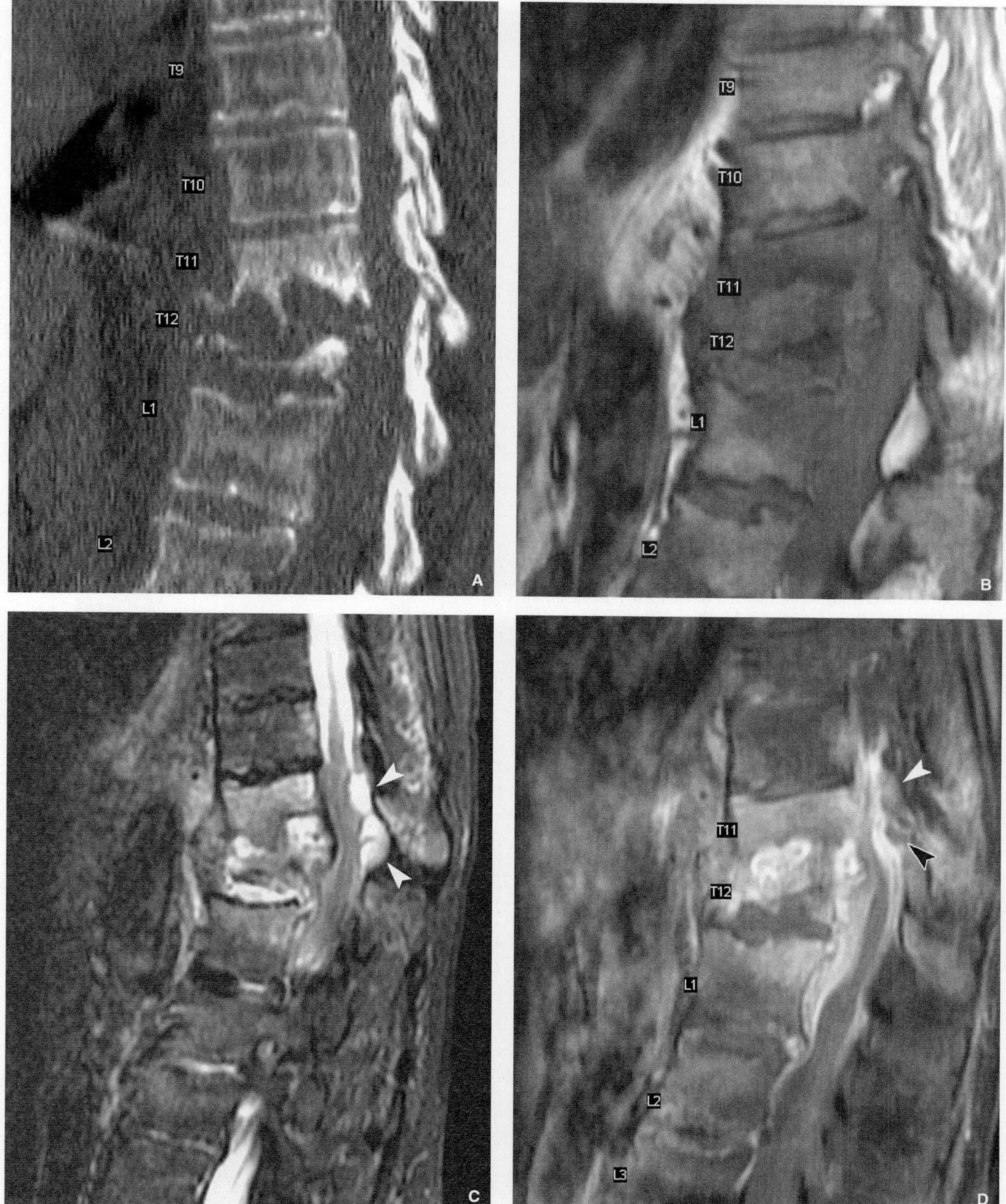

FIGURE 25.52 **CT and MRI of coccidioidomycosis of the spine.** **(A)** Sagittal reformatted CT image of thoracolumbar segment of the spine of a 66-year-old woman diagnosed with pulmonary coccidioidomycosis shows destruction of the T11, T12, and L1 vertebra associated with involvement of the intervening disk spaces. **(B)** Sagittal proton density-weighted, **(C)** sagittal short time inversion recovery (STIR), and **(D)** sagittal T1-weighted fat-suppressed MR image obtained after intravenous administration of gadolinium characterize the infectious process better. There is epidural thickening with dorsal bilobar abscess compressing the dorsal aspect of the spinal cord at the level T11-12 *(arrowheads)*. Also noted is edema of the spinal cord extending from T11 to L1.

findings in coccidioidomycosis, whereas both these findings are common in tuberculosis.

Soft-Tissue Infections

Soft-tissue infections (cellulitis) usually result from direct introduction of organisms through a skin puncture; they are also seen as a complication of systemic disorders such as diabetes. The most frequently encountered organisms are *S. aureus*, *Clostridium novyi*, and *Clostridium perfringens*. These gas-forming organisms may cause an accumulation of gas in the soft tissues that can easily be recognized on radiography as radiolucent bubbles or streaks in the subcutaneous tissues or muscles (Fig. 25.53). This finding usually indicates gangrene caused by anaerobic bacteria. Soft-tissue edema and obliteration of fat and fascial planes are also evident on the standard radiographic examination (Fig. 25.54). CT is effective in this respect (Figs. 25.55 and 25.56) and in addition can differentiate pure cellulitis from that associated with bone infection (Fig. 25.57).

Currently, MRI is considered to be a gold standard to evaluate soft-tissue infection. In particular, soft-tissue abscesses, as well as involvement of tendon sheaths and muscles, are accurately depicted with this modality. Soft-tissue abscesses appear as rounded or elongated—but always well-demarcated—areas of decreased signal intensity on T1-weighted images, changing to increased signal intensity on T2-weighted images (Fig. 25.58; see also Fig. 24.15). Occasionally, a peripheral band of decreased signal intensity is seen that represents the fibrous capsule surrounding the abscess. Infected fluid collection within the tendon sheath is always hyperintense on T2 weighting and hypointense on T1 weighting, but this cannot be differentiated from noninfected fluid.

Diabetic patients are at high risk to develop soft-tissue abscesses, septic arthritis, septic tenosynovitis, and osteomyelitis adjacent to skin ulcerations, more commonly at the level of the toes, first and fifth metatarsals, and calcaneus. MRI is considered the modality of choice to evaluate for the presence and extent of the infection (Fig. 25.59).

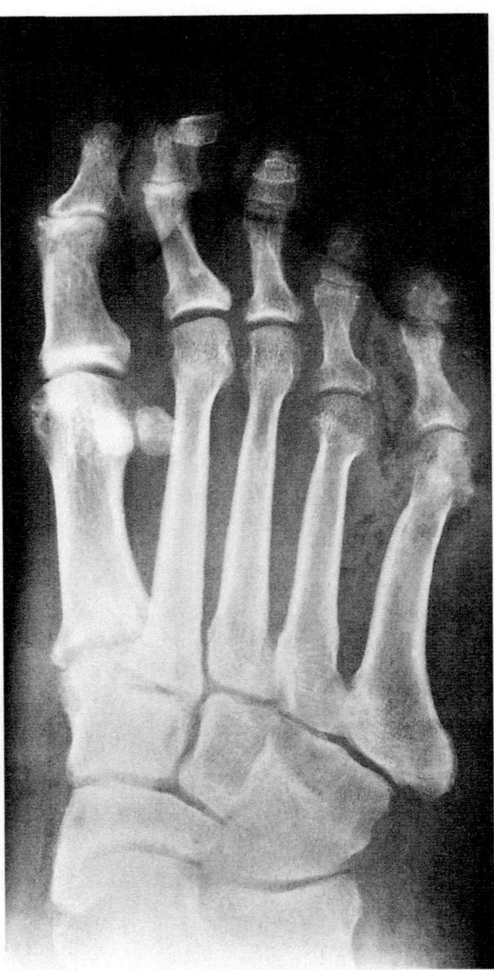

FIGURE 25.54 Gangrene of soft tissues. Oblique radiograph of the foot of a 59-year-old man with long-standing diabetes mellitus shows marked soft-tissue swelling and edema, particularly in the region of the fourth and fifth digits. Radiolucent streaks of gas are typical of gangrenous infection.

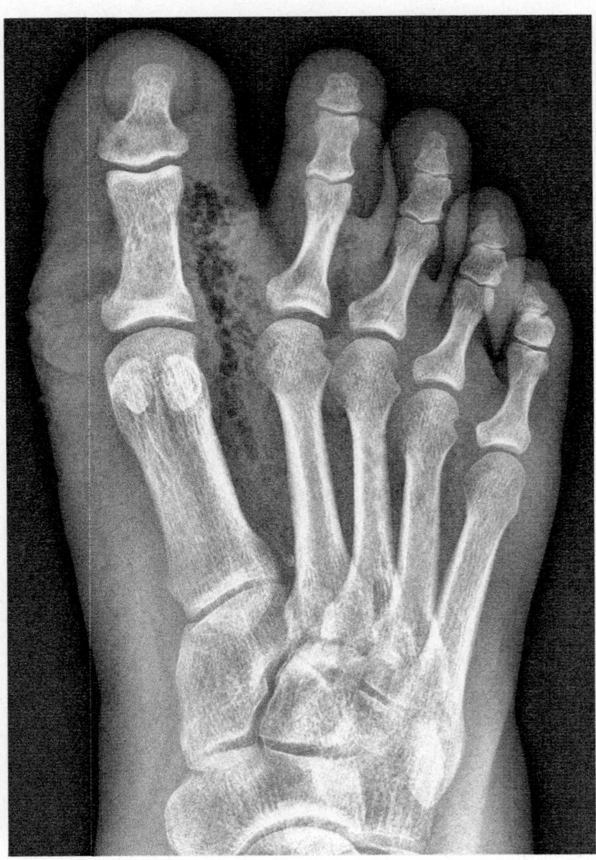

FIGURE 25.53 Soft-tissue infection. Anteroposterior radiograph of the left foot of a 34-year-old diabetic woman shows marked soft-tissue swelling and edema of the medial aspect of the forefoot associated with extensive formation of gas bubbles. The osseous structures are not affected.

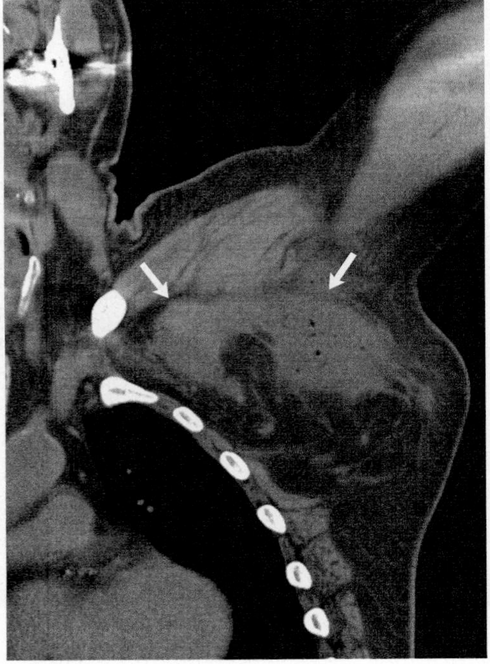

FIGURE 25.55 CT of soft-tissue abscess. Coronal reformatted CT image shows a large heterogenous soft-tissue mass with foci of gas in the left axilla, under the lateral aspect of the pectoralis major muscle *(arrows)*, in a 72-year-old man.

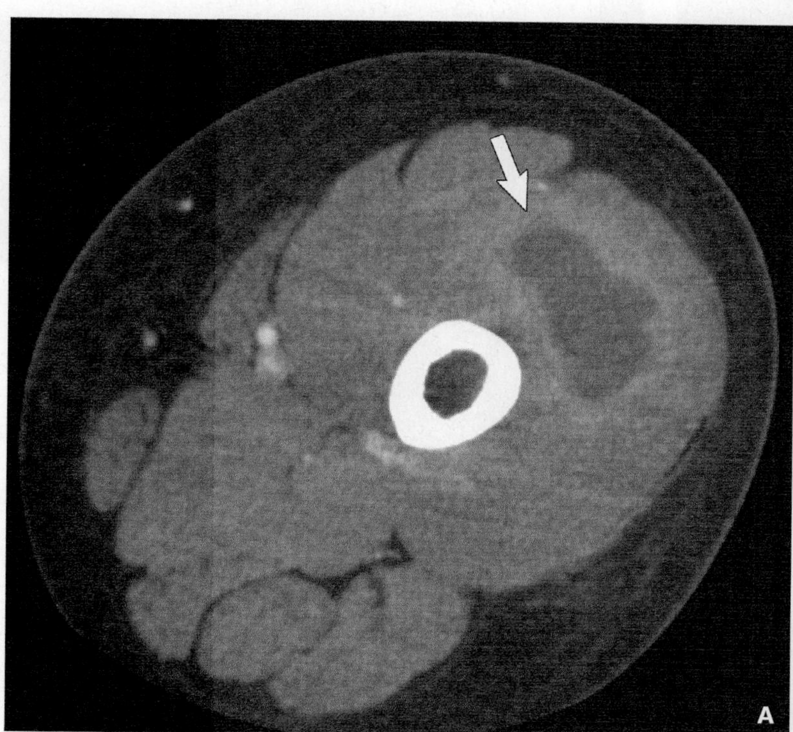

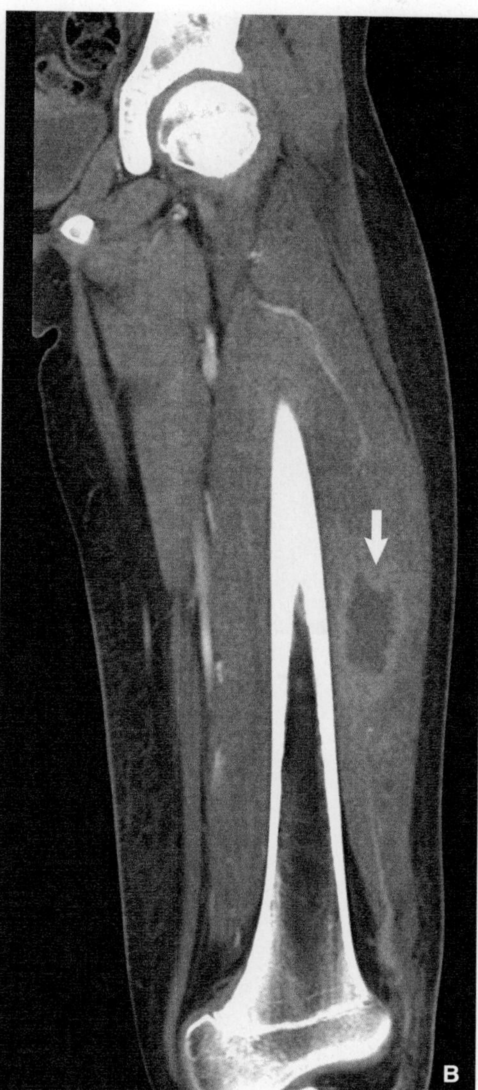

FIGURE 25.56 CT of soft-tissue abscess. **(A)** Axial and **(B)** coronal reformatted CT images of the left thigh of an 11-year-old girl with septicemia show a large abscess with a thick wall in *vastus lateralis (arrows)*.

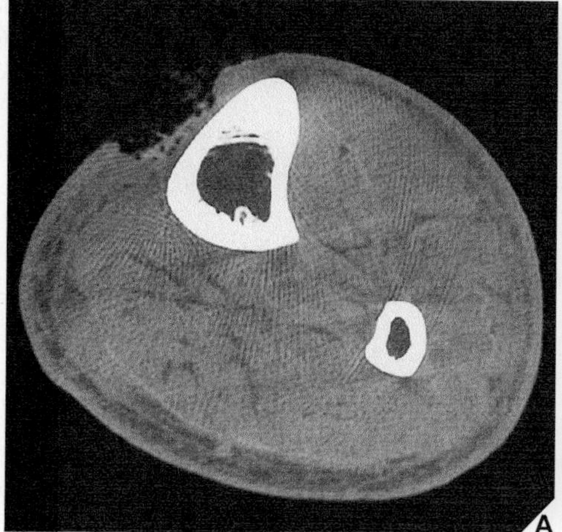

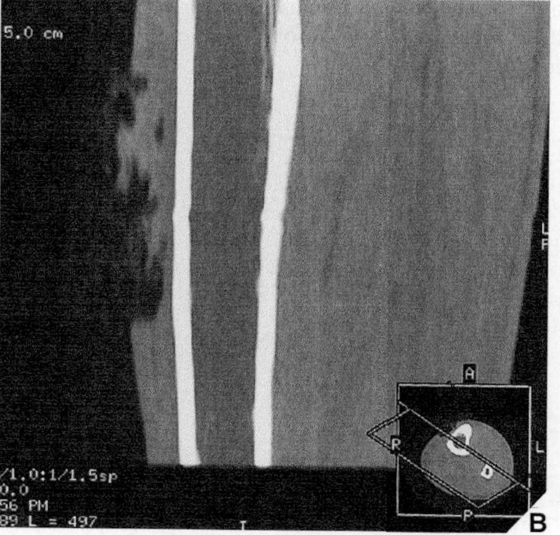

FIGURE 25.57 CT of soft-tissue abscess. A 26-year-old man developed an infection of the anterior aspect of the left lower leg. **(A)** Axial CT section and **(B)** oblique sagittal reformatted images show an abscess and its relation to the tibia. Note that the cortex is not affected.

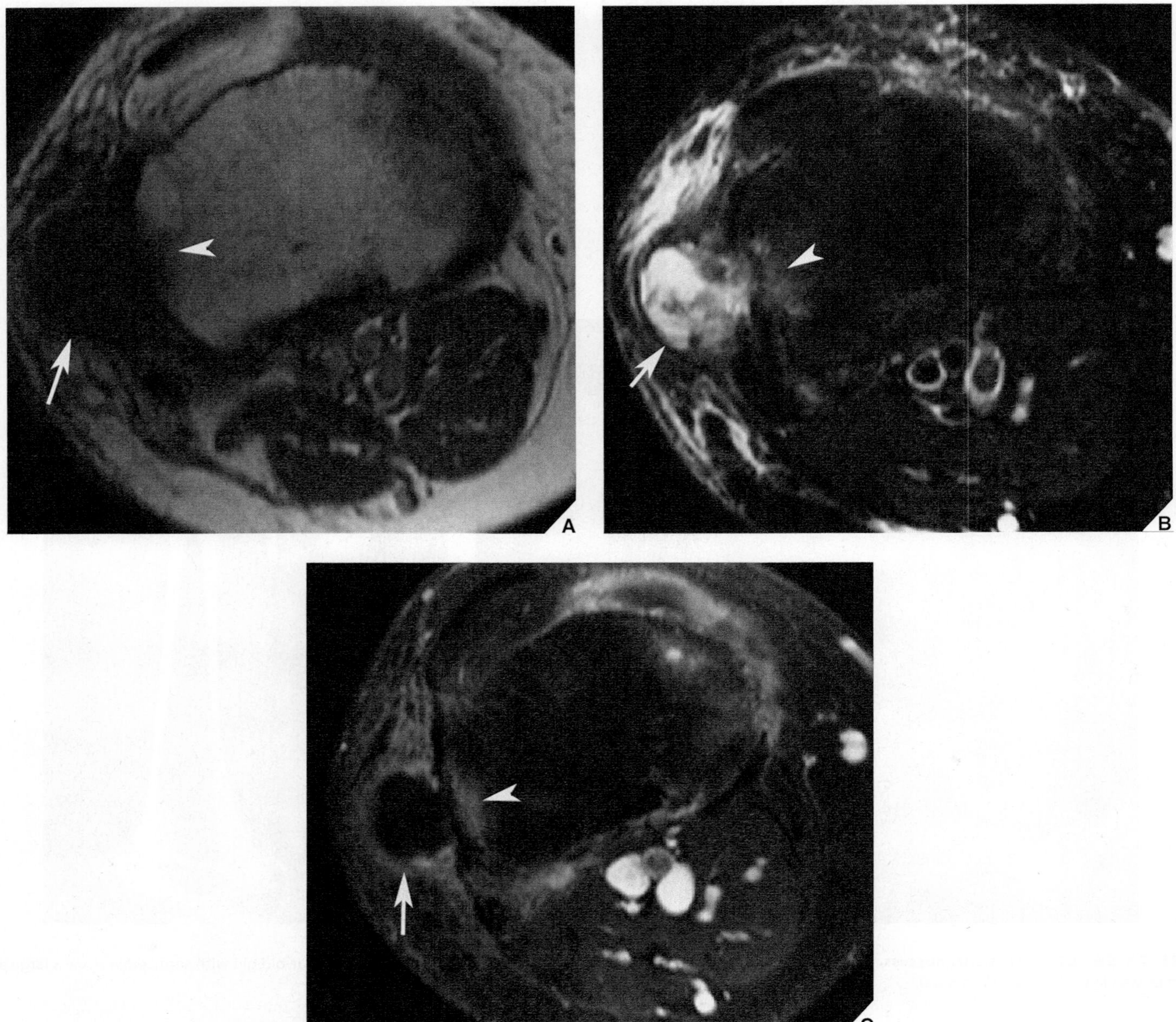

FIGURE 25.58 MRI of soft-tissue abscess. **(A)** Axial T1-weighted MRI of the knee demonstrates a low–signal intensity fluid collection in the lateral aspect of the knee *(arrow)* with reactive hypointense bone marrow edema of the adjacent tibia *(arrowhead)*. **(B)** Axial T2-weighted MRI shows the hyperintense fluid collection *(arrow)* with surrounding soft-tissue edema and bone marrow edema *(arrowhead)*. Note the small focal area of decortication of the tibia at this level, indicating osteomyelitis. **(C)** Axial T1-weighted fat-saturated MRI obtained after intravenous injection of gadolinium demonstrates enhancement of the wall of the abscess *(arrow)* and the adjacent tibial edema/osteomyelitis *(arrowhead)*.

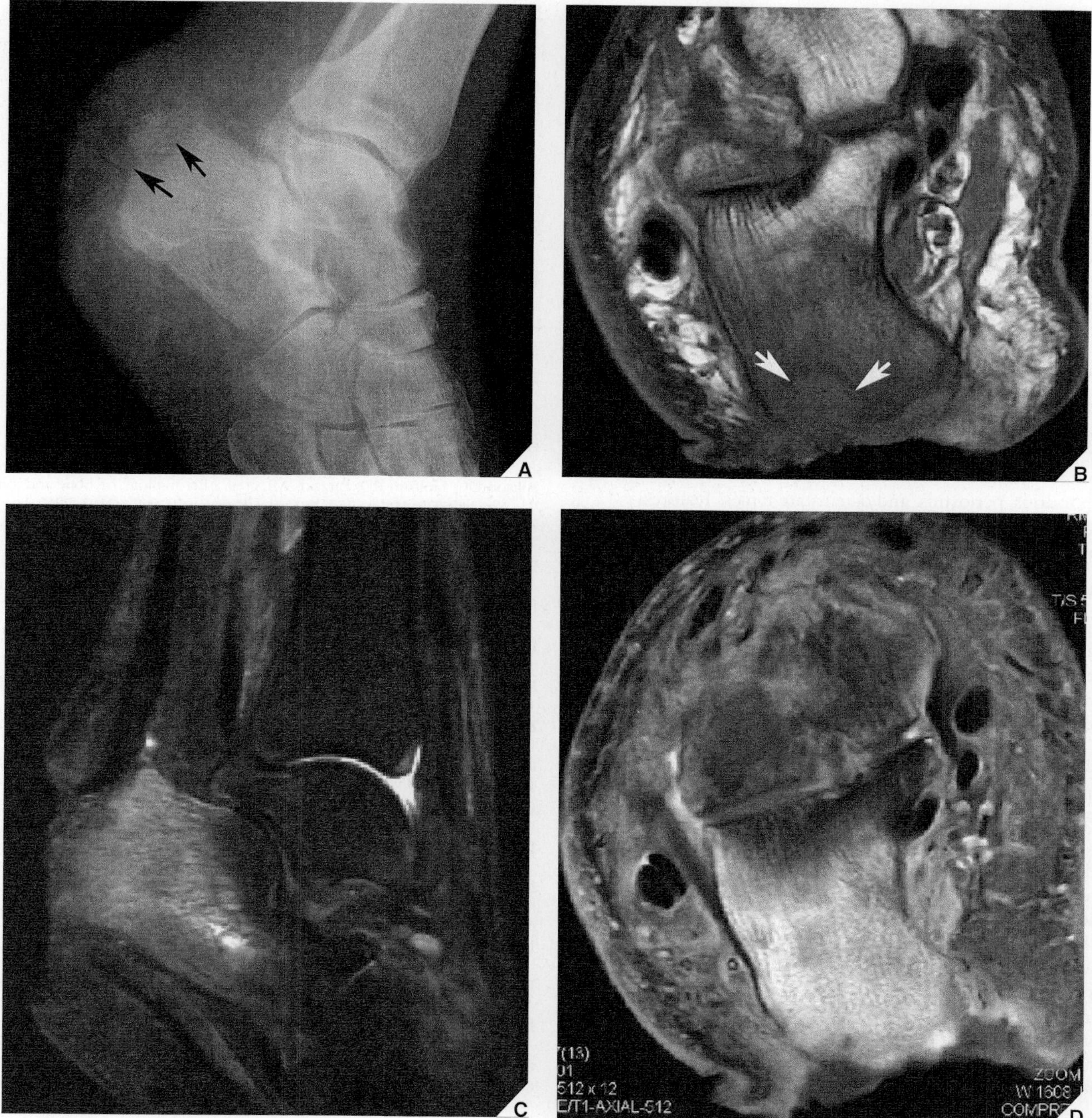

FIGURE 25.59 MRI of diabetic foot. **(A)** Lateral radiograph of the ankle demonstrates a large heel ulcer with decortication of the posterior process of the calcaneus *(arrows)* and extensive soft-tissue edema. **(B)** Axial T1-weighted MRI shows the large heel ulcer and a focal area of bone destruction in the posterior process of the calcaneus *(arrows)*. **(C)** Sagittal short time inversion recovery (STIR) MRI shows extensive edema of the calcaneus and the large heel ulcer. **(D)** Axial T1-weighted fat-saturated MRI obtained after intravenous administration of gadolinium demonstrates extensive enhancement of bone marrow of the calcaneus and the large heel ulcer.

PRACTICAL POINTS TO REMEMBER

Osteomyelitis

1. The imaging hallmarks of osteomyelitis include:
   - cortical and medullary bone destruction
   - reactive sclerosis and a periosteal reaction
   - the presence of sequestra and involucra.
2. The metaphysis is a characteristic site of osteomyelitis in children.
3. Acute osteomyelitis of a long bone frequently mimics Ewing sarcoma and Langerhans cell histiocytosis. The clinical history, especially the duration of symptoms before the discovery of bone changes, usually serves as a clue to the correct diagnosis.
4. A destructive metaphyseal lesion extending into the epiphysis usually indicates a bone abscess.
5. A Brodie abscess may clinically and radiographically mimic an osteoid osteoma. In the differential diagnosis, the presence of a radiolucent tract extending from the lesion into the growth plate favors an infectious process.
6. In congenital syphilis:
   - osteochondritis, periostitis, and osteitis are typical features
   - destruction at the medial aspect of the metaphysis of a long bone (Wimberger sign) is characteristic.

Infectious Arthritis

1. The characteristic radiographic features of septic arthritis of the peripheral joints include:
   - periarticular osteoporosis, joint effusion, and soft-tissue swelling (early phase)
   - destruction of cartilage and the subchondral plates on both sides of the joint (late phase).
2. In tuberculosis of a peripheral joint, which usually manifests as a monoarticular disease (strongly resembling rheumatoid arthritis), the Phemister triad of radiographic abnormalities is characteristic and includes:
   - periarticular osteoporosis
   - peripheral osseous erosions
   - gradual narrowing of the joint space.
3. Lyme arthritis exhibits some similarities to juvenile rheumatoid arthritis and reactive arthritis. Characteristic edematous changes of the infrapatellar fat pad and folds of hypertrophied synovium are demonstrated on MRI.
4. Parasitic infections of the musculoskeletal system are rare in the United States. MRI is very effective in demonstrating hydatid cysts within the soft tissues in patients affected by echinococcosis.

Infections of the Spine

1. In the imaging evaluation of spine infections:
   - radionuclide bone scan can detect disk infection prior to the appearance of any radiographic signs
   - the diskogram is a valid examination performed primarily to obtain aspirate fluid for bacteriologic study
   - MRI is the modality of choice to diagnose and evaluate spine infection.
2. Pyogenic infection of the spine is recognized radiographically by:
   - narrowing of the disk space
   - destruction of both vertebral end plates adjacent to the involved disk
   - a paraspinal mass.
3. The radiographic hallmarks of tuberculous infection of an intervertebral disk are:
   - narrowing of the disk space
   - loss of the sharp outline of the adjacent vertebral end plates.
4. Tuberculous infection of the spine may:
   - destroy the disk and vertebra, leading to kyphosis and a gibbus formation
   - extend into the soft tissues, forming a cold abscess.

Soft-Tissue Infections

1. Cellulitis caused by gas-forming bacteria in soft tissues (gangrene) is recognized radiographically by:
   - soft-tissue edema and swelling
   - radiolucent bubbles or streaks representing accumulations of gas.
2. Diabetic subjects are particularly prone to soft-tissue infections, the feet being common sites.
3. Scintigraphy using indium-111–labeled white cells is useful in detecting and localizing the site of infection, whereas MRI is ideal in evaluating the extent of infection in the soft tissues.
4. MRI using contrast enhancement with gadolinium allows the differentiation of abscess from cellulitis or phlegmon.

SUGGESTED READINGS

Abdelwahab IF, Present DA, Zwass A, et al. Tumorlike tuberculous granulomas of bone. *AJR Am J Roentgenol* 1987;149:1207–1208.

Alexander GH, Mansuy MM. Disseminated bone tuberculosis (so-called multiple cystic tuberculosis). *Radiology* 1950;55:839–842.

Allison DC, Holtom PD, Patzakis MJ, et al. Microbiology of bone and joint infections in injecting drug abusers. *Clin Orthop Relat Res* 2010;468:2107–2012.

Al-Shahed MS, Sharif HS, Haddad MC, et al. Imaging features of musculoskeletal brucellosis. *Radiographics* 1994;14:333–348.

Bayer AS, Guze LB. Fungal arthritis. Fungal arthritis. II. Coccidioidal synovitis: clinical, diagnostic, therapeutic, and prognostic considerations. *Semin Arthritis Rheum* 1979;8:200–211.

Behrman RE, Masci JR, Nicholas P. Cryptococcal skeletal infections: case report and review. *Rev Infect Dis* 1990;12:181–190.

Brodie BC. An account of some cases of chronic abscess of the tibia. *Med Chir Trans* 1832;17:238–239.

Brown R, Wilkinson T. Chronic recurrent multifocal osteomyelitis. *Radiology* 1988;166: 493–496.

Bruno MS, Silverberg TN, Goldstein DH. Embolic osteomyelitis of the spine as a complication of infection of the urinary tract. *Am J Med* 1960;29:865–878.

Chelboun J, Sydney N. Skeletal cryptococcosis. *J Bone Joint Surg Am* 1977;59A:509–514.

Cremin BJ, Fisher RM. The lesions of congenital syphilis. *Br J Radiol* 1970;43:333–341.

Crim JR, Seeger LL. Imaging evaluation of osteomyelitis. *Crit Rev Diagn Imaging* 1994;35:201–256.

Dalinka MK, Greendyke WH. The spinal manifestations of coccidioidomycosis. *J Can Assoc Radiol* 1971;22:93–99.

Davies AM, Hughes DE, Grimer RJ. Intramedullary and extramedullary fat globules on magnetic resonance imaging as a diagnostic sign for osteomyelitis. *Eur Radiol* 2005;15:2194–2199.

Duncan GJ, Tooke SM. Echinococcus infestation of the biceps brachii. A case report. *Clin Orthop Relat Res* 1990;(261):247–250.

Erdman WA, Tamburro F, Jayson HT, et al. Osteomyelitis: characteristics and pitfalls of diagnosis with MR imaging. *Radiology* 1991;180:533–539.

Ferguson PJ, Sandu M. Current understanding of the pathogenesis and management of chronic recurrent multifocal osteomyelitis. *Curr Rheumatol Rep* 2012;14:130–141.

Gilmour WM. Acute haematogenous osteomyelitis. *J Bone Joint Surg Br* 1962;44B:841–853.

Gold RH, Hawkins RA, Katz RD. Bacterial osteomyelitis: findings on plain radiography, CT, MR, and scintigraphy. *AJR Am J Roentgenol* 1991;157:365–370.

Golla A, Jansson A, Ramser J, et al. Chronic recurrent multifocal osteomyelitis (CRMO): evidence for a susceptibility gene located on chromosome 18q21.3-18q22. *Eur J Hum Genet* 2002;10:217–221.

Handly B, Moore M, Creutzberg G, et al. Bisphosphonate therapy for chronic recurrent multifocal osteomyelitis. *Skeletal Radiol* 2013;42:1741–1778.

Haygood TM, Williamson SL. Radiographic findings of extremity tuberculosis in childhood: back to the future? *Radiographics* 1994;14:561–570.

Hopkins KL, Li KC, Bergman G. Gadolinium-DTPA-enhanced magnetic resonance imaging of musculoskeletal infectious processes. *Skeletal Radiol* 1995;24:325–330.

Jain R, Sawhney S, Berry M. Computed tomography of vertebral tuberculosis: patterns of bone destruction. *Clin Radiol* 1993;47:196–199.

Jaovisidha S, Chen C, Ryu KN, et al. Tuberculous tenosynovitis and bursitis: imaging findings in 21 cases. *Radiology* 1996;201:507–513.

Kak V, Chandrasekar PH. Bone and joint infections in injection drug users. *Infect Dis Clin North Am* 2002;16:681–695.

Karchevsky M, Schweitzer ME, Morrison WB, et al. MRI findings of septic arthritis and associated osteomyelitis in adults. *AJR Am J Roentgenol* 2004;182:119–122.

Klein MJ, Bonar SF, Freemont T, et al, eds. *Atlas of nontumor pathology. Non-neoplastic diseases of bones and joints.* Washington, DC: American Registry of Pathology; 2011:411–543.

Lawson JP, Rahn DW. Lyme disease and radiologic findings in Lyme arthritis. *AJR Am J Roentgenol* 1992;158:1065–1069.

Lawson JP, Steere AC. Lyme arthritis: radiologic findings. *Radiology* 1985;154:37–43.

Lund PJ, Chan KM, Unger EC, et al. Magnetic resonance imaging in coccidioidal arthritis. *Skeletal Radiol* 1996;25:661–665.

Martin J, Marco V, Zidan A, et al. Hydatid disease of the soft tissues of the lower limb: findings in three cases. *Skeletal Radiol* 1993;22:511–514.

May DA, Disler DG. Case 50: primary coccidioidal synovitis of the knee. *Radiology* 2002;224:665–668.

McGahan JP, Graves DS, Palmer PES. Coccidioidal spondylitis: usual and unusual radiographic manifestations. *Radiology* 1980;136:5–9.

McGahan JP, Graves DS, Palmer PES, et al. Classic and contemporary imaging of coccidioidomycosis. *AJR Am J Roentgenol* 1981;136:393–404.

Merkle EM, Schulte M, Vogel J, et al. Musculoskeletal involvement in cystic echinococcosis: report of eight cases and review of the literature. *AJR Am J Roentgenol* 1997;168:1531–1534.

Moore SL, Jones S, Lee JL. *Nocardia* osteomyelitis in the setting of previously unknown HIV infection. *Skeletal Radiol* 2005;34:58–60.

Phemister DB, Hatcher CM. Correlation of pathological and roentgenological findings in the diagnosis of tuberculosis arthritis. *AJR Am J Roentgenol* 1933;29:736–752.

Pimprikar MV, Kekatpure AL. Subdeltoid bursa tuberculosis with rice bodies formation: case report and review of literature. *J Orthop Case Rep* 2014;4:57–59.

Plodkowski AJ, Hayter CL, Miller TT, et al. Lamellated hyperintense synovitis: potential MR imaging sign of an infected knee arthroplasty. *Radiology* 2013;266:256–260.

Resnick D, Niwayama G. Osteomyelitis, septic arthritis, and soft tissue infection: mechanisms and situations. In: Resnick D, ed. *Diagnosis of bone and joint disorders*, 3rd ed. Philadelphia: WB Saunders; 1995:2325–2418.

Resnick D, Niwayama G. Osteomyelitis, septic arthritis, and soft tissue infection: organisms. In: Resnick D, ed. *Diagnosis of bone and joint disorders*, 3rd ed. Philadelphia: WB Saunders; 1995:2448–2558.

Roderick MR, Ramanan AV. Chronic recurrent multifocal osteomyelitis. *Adv Exp Med Biol* 2013;764:99–107.

Schauwecker D. Osteomyelitis: diagnosis with In-111-labeled leukocytes. *Radiology* 1989;171:141–146.

Theodorou DJ, Theodorou SJ, Kakitsubata Y, et al. Imaging characteristics and epidemiologic features of atypical mycobacterial infections involving the musculoskeletal system. *AJR Am J Roentgenol* 2001;176:341–349.

Toledano TR, Fatone EA, Weis A, et al. MRI evaluation of bone marrow changes in the diabetic foot: a practical approach. *Semin Musculoskelet Radiol* 2011;15:257–268.

Zeppa MA, Laorr A, Greenspan A, et al. Skeletal coccidioidomycosis: imaging findings in 19 patients. *Skeletal Radiol* 1996;25:337–343.

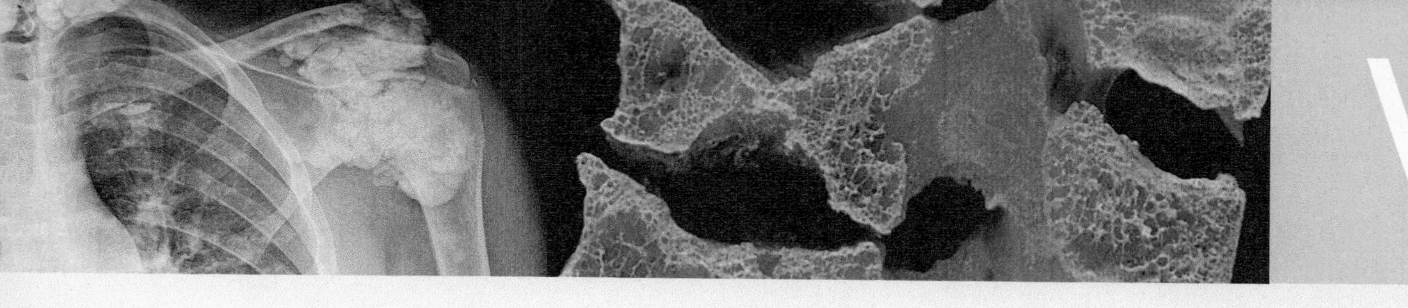

VI

METABOLIC, ENDOCRINE, AND MISCELLANEOUS DISORDERS

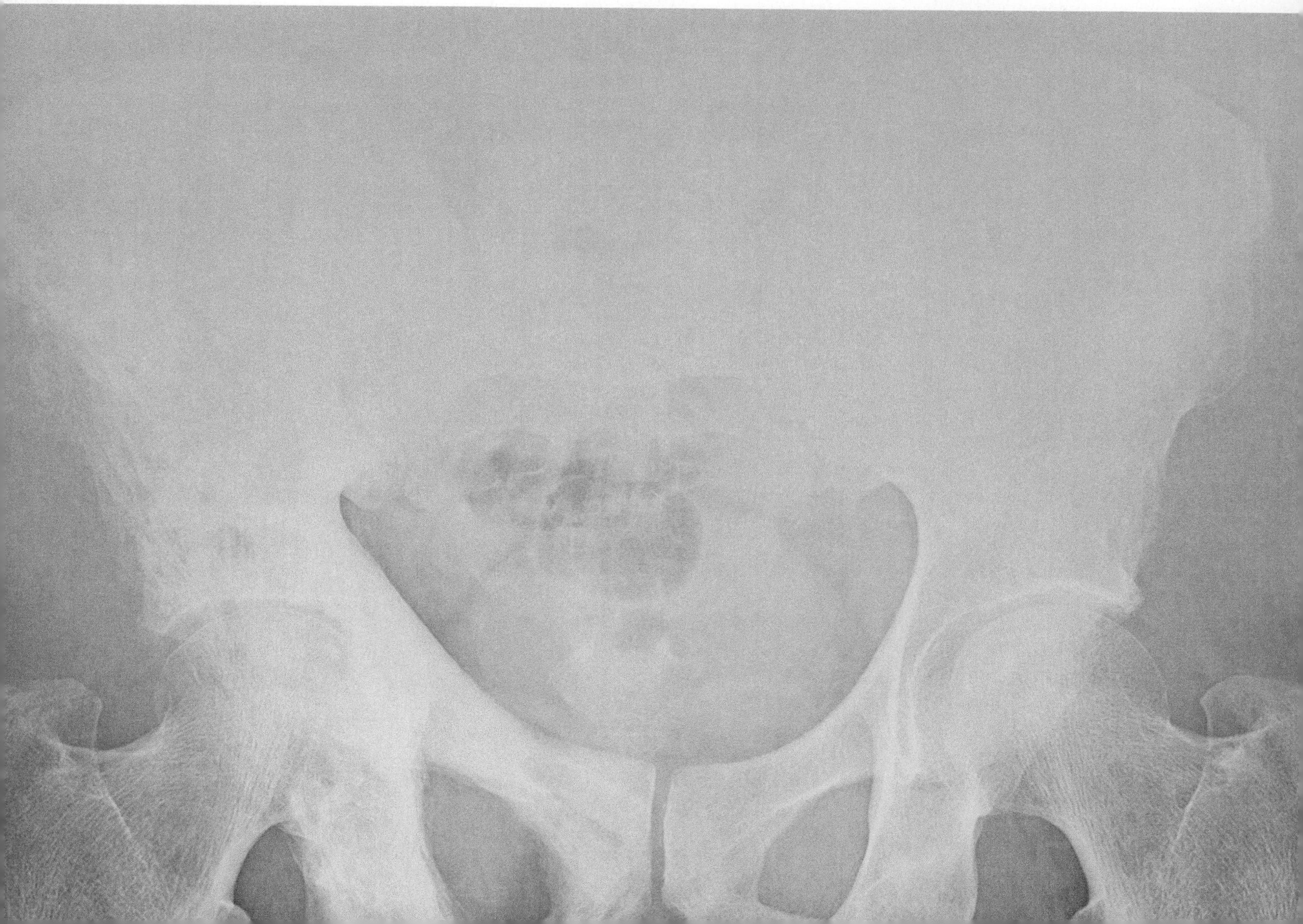

26

Imaging Evaluation of Metabolic, Endocrine, and Miscellaneous Disorders

Composition and Production of Bone

Bone tissue consists of two types of material: (a) an extracellular material, which includes *organic matrix* or *osteoid tissue* (collagen fibrils within a mucopolysaccharide ground substance) and an *inorganic crystalline component* (calcium phosphate or hydroxyapatite); and (b) a cellular material, which includes *osteoblasts* (cells that induce bone formation), *osteoclasts* (cells that induce bone resorption), and *osteocytes* (inactive cells).

Bone is a living, dynamic tissue. Old bone is constantly being removed and replaced with new bone. Normally, this continuous process of bone resorption and formation is in balance (Fig. 26.1A), and the mineral content of the bones remains relatively constant. In some abnormal circumstances, however, when the metabolism of the bone is disturbed, this balance may be upset. If, for example, osteoblasts are more active than usual, or if osteoclasts are less active, more bone is produced (a state known as *too much bone*) (Fig. 26.1B). If, however, osteoclasts are normal or overactive and osteoblasts underactive, then less bone is produced ("too little bone") (Fig. 26.1C). A generalized reduction in bone mass may also be caused by decreased mineralization of osteoid, with equilibrium in the rate of bone resorption and production (Fig. 26.1D).

The growth and mineralization of bone are influenced by a variety of factors, the most important of which are the levels of growth hormone produced by the pituitary gland, of calcitonin produced by the thyroid gland, and of parathormone produced by the parathyroid glands, along with the dietary intake, intestinal absorption, and urinary excretion of vitamin D, calcium, and phosphorus.

It should be remembered, however, that normal bone density changes with age, increasing from infancy until age 35 to 40 years, and then progressively decreasing at the rate of 8% per decade in women and 3% in men.

Evaluation of Metabolic and Endocrine Disorders

Most metabolic and endocrine disorders are characterized radiographically by abnormalities in bone density that are generally related to increased bone production, increased bone resorption, or inadequate bone mineralization. The bones affected by these conditions appear abnormally radiolucent (osteopenia) or abnormally radiodense (osteosclerosis) (Table 26.1).

Radiologic Imaging Modalities

The imaging modalities most often used to evaluate metabolic and endocrine bone disorders are

1. Conventional radiography
2. Computed tomography (CT)
3. Radionuclide imaging (scintigraphy, bone scan)
4. Magnetic resonance imaging (MRI)
5. Ultrasound (US)

Conventional Radiography

Radiography is the simplest method of evaluating bone density. This technique can easily detect even very small increases in bone density; however, it generally fails to detect decreases in overall skeletal mineralization unless the reduction reaches at least 30%. It must be pointed out that normal bone can easily acquire an abnormal radiographic appearance as a result of technical errors, such as improper settings for kilovoltage and milliamperage. Overexposure, for instance, creates the appearance of increased bone radiolucency, whereas underexposure creates an artificially increased bone radiodensity.

For these reasons, inspection of a standard radiograph should focus less on apparent increases or decreases in bone density but more on the thickness of the bone cortex. Cortical thickness is directly correlated with skeletal mineralization; it can be objectively measured and compared either with a normal standard or with subsequent studies in the same patient. The cortical thickness measurement is obtained by adding the width of the two cortices in the midpoint of a given bone, a sum that should be approximately one half of the overall diameter of the bone; it may also be expressed as an index of bony mass, derived by dividing the combined cortical thickness by the total diameter of the bone (Fig. 26.2). The second or third metacarpal bone is commonly used to obtain these measurements (Fig. 26.3).

A related method for assessing bone density that also uses radiography is the photodensitometry technique. This technique is based on the observation that the photographic density of a bone on a radiographic film is proportional to its mass. Through the use of a photodensitometer, the photographic density of a given bone can be compared with that of known standard wedges, giving an accurate assessment of the degree of bone density.

The appearance of relative increased bone radiolucency on standard radiographs should not be called *osteoporosis* because such a finding is not specific for osteoporosis, osteomalacia, or hyperparathyroidism. Most authorities agree that increased radiolucency is best termed *osteopenia* (poverty of bone). *Osteoporosis* refers specifically to a reduction in the amount of bone

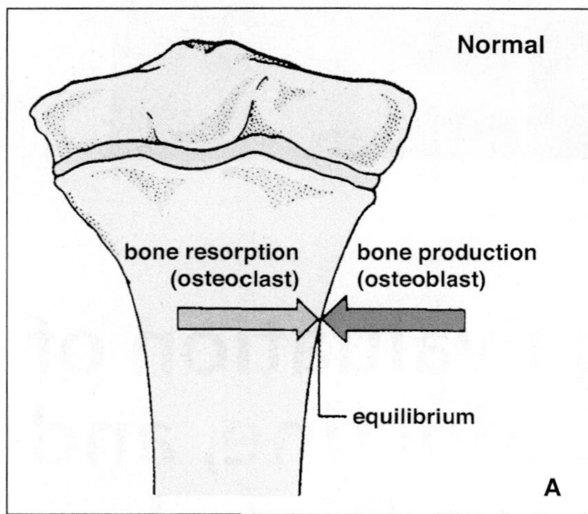

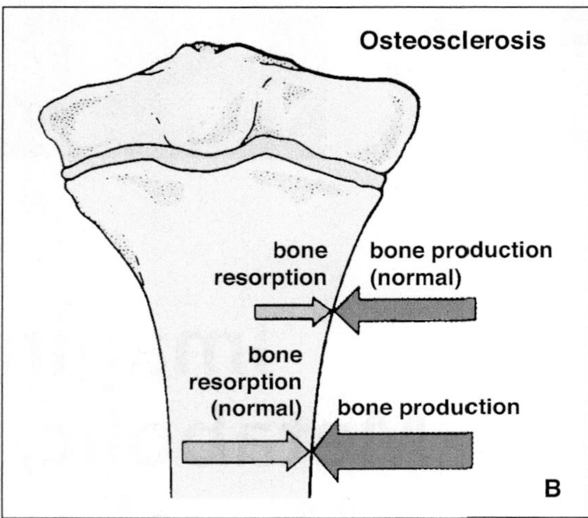

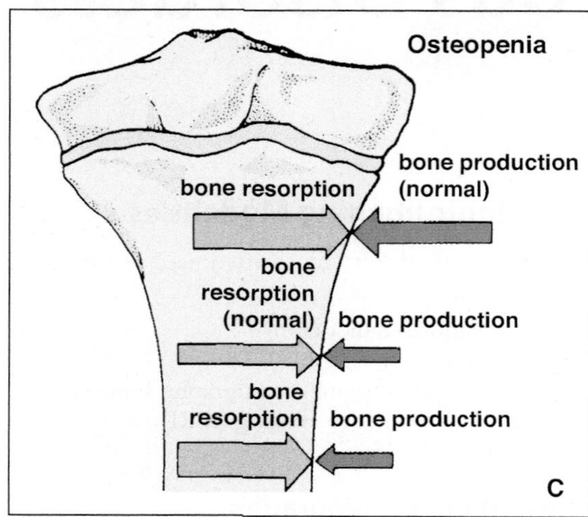

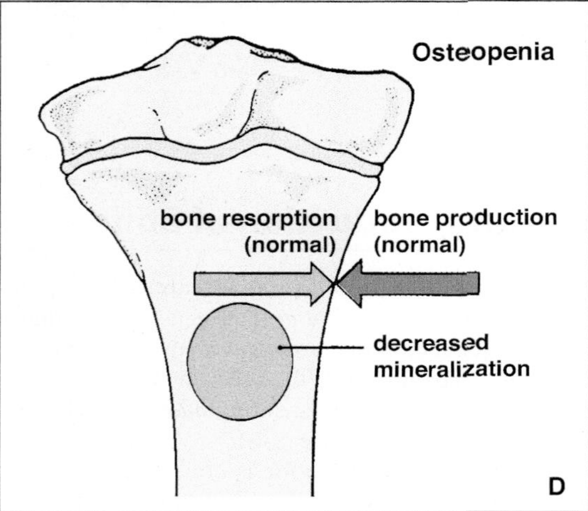

FIGURE 26.1 Bone production and bone resorption. **(A)** In normal bone, the relationship between bone resorption and bone production is in balance. **(B)** One abnormal state ("too much bone") is characterized by decreased bone resorption and normal bone production or by normal bone resorption and increased bone production. **(C)** The other abnormal state ("too little bone") is characterized by increased bone resorption and normal bone production, by normal bone resorption and decreased bone production, or by increased bone resorption and decreased bone production. **(D)** Too little bone may also be caused by a decrease in bone mineralization, with bone resorption and production in balance.

TABLE 26.1 Metabolic and Endocrine Disorders Characterized by Abnormalities in Bone Density

Increased Radiodensity	Increased Radiolucency
Secondary hyperparathyroidism	Osteoporosis
Renal osteodystrophy	Osteomalacia
Hyperphosphatasia	Rickets
Idiopathic hypercalcemia	Scurvy
Paget disease	Primary hyperparathyroidism
Osteopetrosis[a]	Hypophosphatasia
Pycnodysostosis[a]	Hypophosphatemia
Melorheostosis[a]	Acromegaly
Hypothyroidism	Gaucher disease
Mastocytosis	Homocystinuria
Myelofibrosis	Osteogenesis imperfecta[a]
Gaucher disease (reparative stage)	Fibrogenesis imperfecta
Fluorine poisoning	Cushing syndrome
Intoxication with lead, bismuth, or phosphorus	Ochronosis (alkaptonuria)
Osteonecrosis	Wilson disease (hepatolenticular degeneration)
Tuberous sclerosis	Hypogonadism

[a]These conditions are discussed in Part VII: "Congenital and Developmental Anomalies."

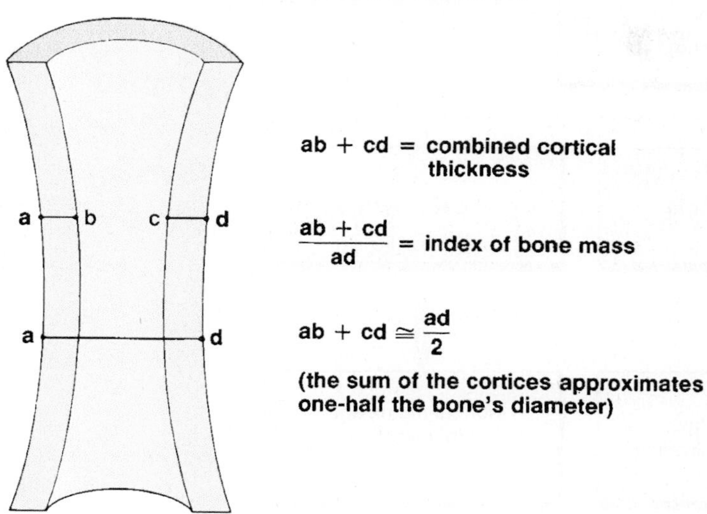

FIGURE 26.2 Measurement of cortical thickness. Determination of cortical thickness is based on the measurement of the cortices of the metacarpals (usually the second or third). It may be expressed either as the simple sum of the two cortices or as that sum divided by the total thickness of the bone, in which case it is considered an index of bony mass. Normally, the sum of the cortices should be approximately one half the overall diameter of the metacarpal bone.

tissue (deficient bone matrix) and *osteomalacia* refers to a reduction in the amount of mineral in the matrix (deficient mineralization); both conditions are characterized by increased bone radiolucency (Fig. 26.4). Any condition in which bone resorption exceeds bone formation results in osteopenia, regardless of the specific pathogenesis of the condition. In fact, diffuse osteopenia is found in osteoporosis, osteomalacia, hyperparathyroidism, neoplastic conditions such as multiple myeloma, and in a wide variety of other disorders.

Although osteopenia is a nonspecific finding, radiography can help detect other important radiographic features leading to a specific diagnosis. Among these are Looser zones, representing pseudofractures or insufficiency-type stress fractures that are characteristic of osteomalacia (Fig. 26.5); widening of the growth plate and flaring of the metaphysis, which are typical findings in rickets (Fig. 26.6); subperiosteal bone resorption, an identifying feature of hyperparathyroidism (Fig. 26.7); and focal areas of osteolytic destruction and endosteal scalloping, which are characteristic of multiple myeloma (Fig. 26.8).

Magnification radiography was in the past a useful technique applied to metabolic disorders for demonstrating the details of bone structure. Currently, digital magnification using picture archive and communication system (PACS) workstation allowing filmless high-resolution image-display format (already discussed in Chapter 2) is most effective in delineating the subperiosteal bone resorption characteristic of hyperparathyroidism, or cortical tunneling (Fig. 26.9), which may be seen in any process that causes increased bone resorption. Cortical tunneling occurs very early in a pathologic process and may be found even in the absence of other radiographic abnormalities.

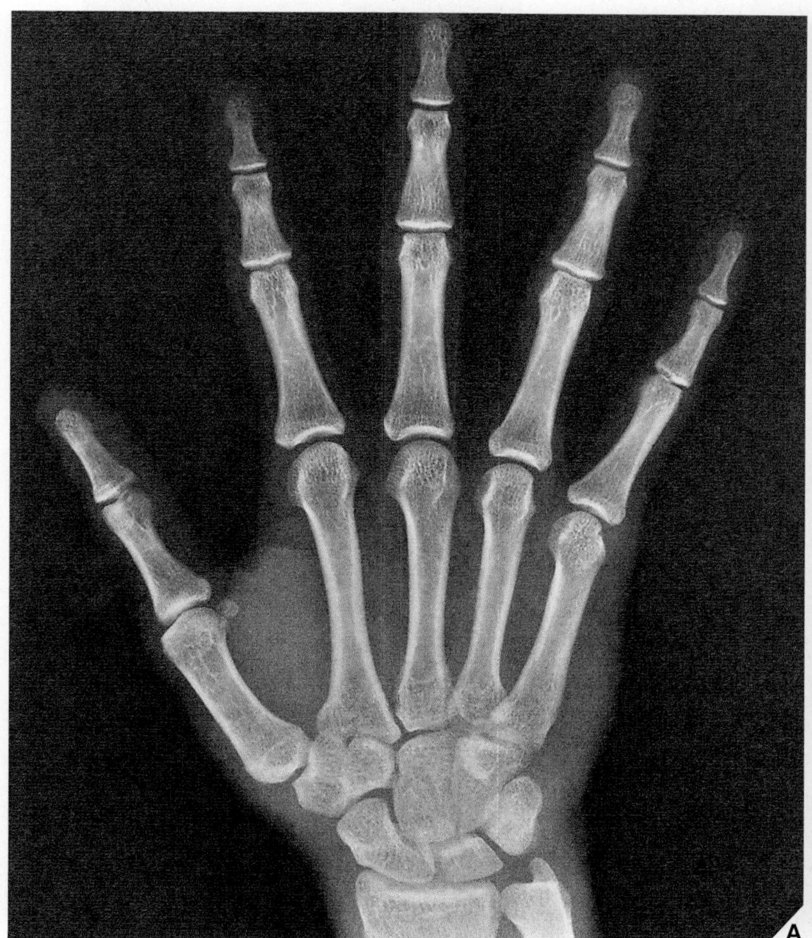

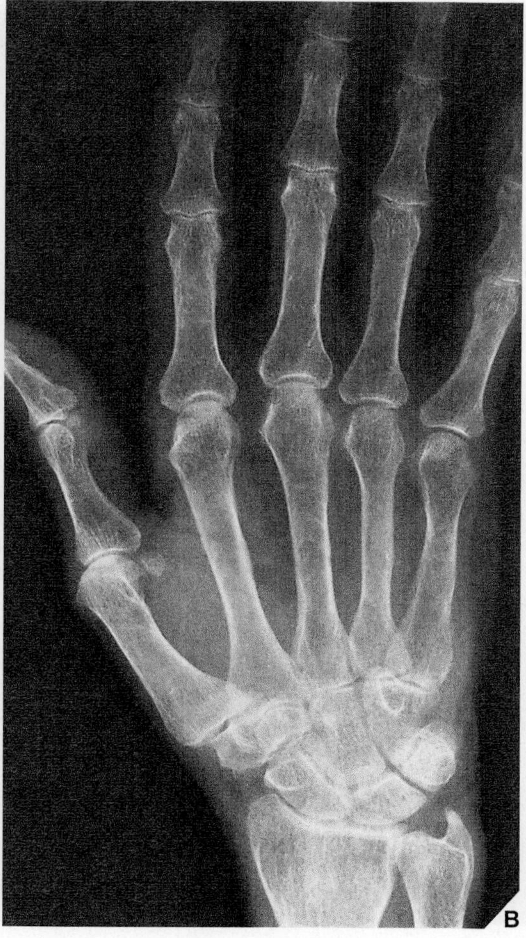

FIGURE 26.3 Cortical thickness of the hand. Dorsovolar radiographs of the hand show normal **(A)** and abnormal **(B)** thickness of the cortex of the second and third metacarpal bones.

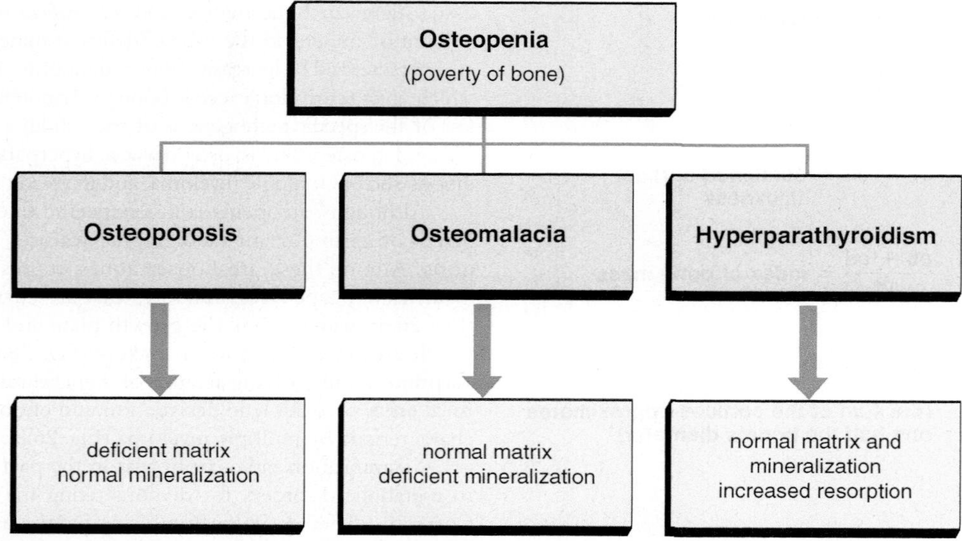

FIGURE 26.4 **Osteopenia.** Increased radiolucency of bone on a standard radiograph is best termed *osteopenia* or *bone rarefaction* rather than *osteoporosis*, and it is a typical feature not only of osteoporosis but also of osteomalacia and hyperparathyroidism, which are clinically distinct conditions.

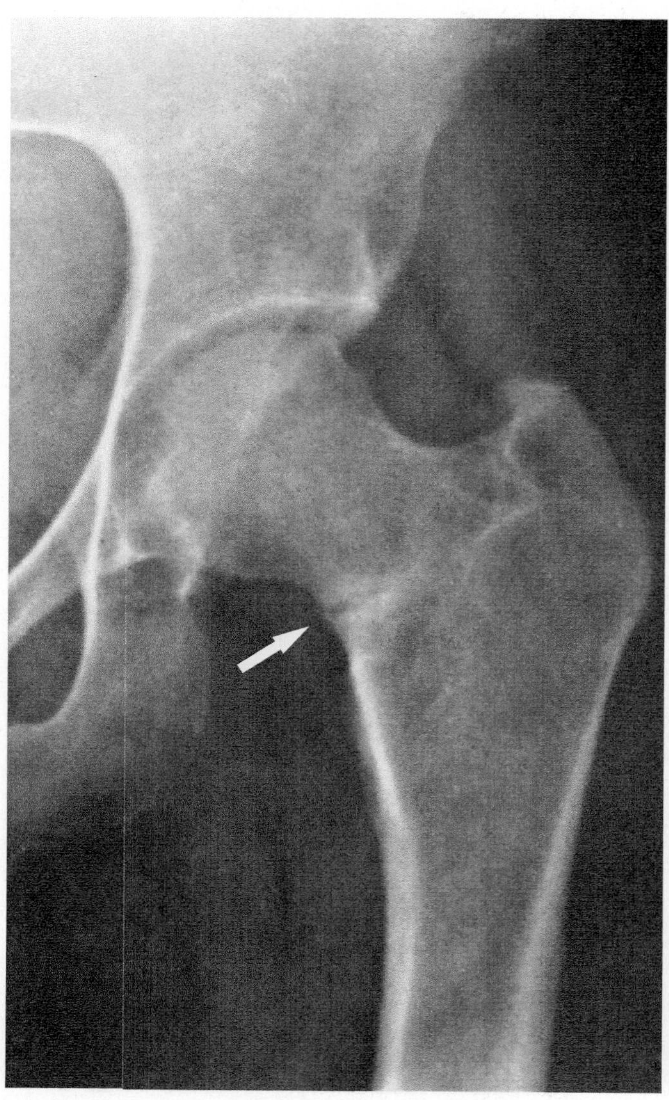

FIGURE 26.5 **Osteomalacia.** Looser zone or pseudofracture (or perhaps better called *insufficiency-type stress fracture*), seen here in the femoral neck *(arrow)*, is represented by a radiolucent defect in the cortical bone that reflects accumulation of nonmineralized osteoid tissue and is a characteristic finding in osteomalacia.

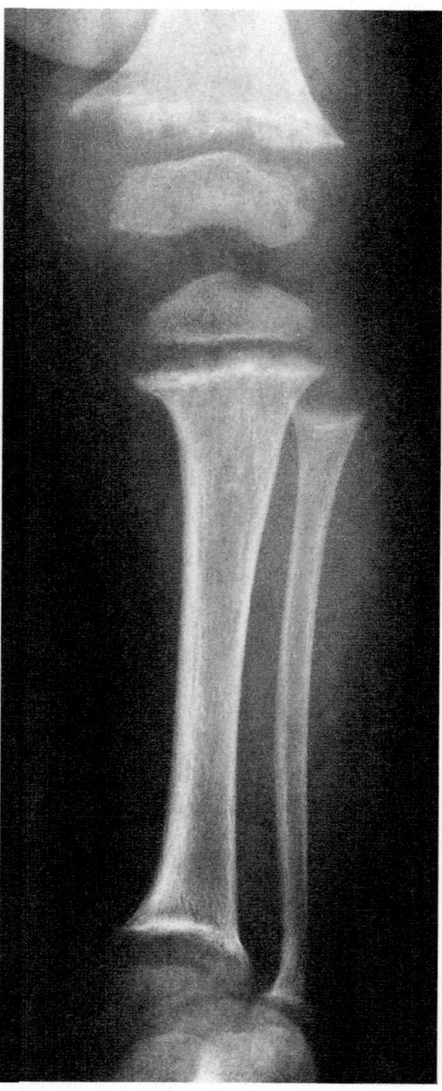

FIGURE 26.6 **Rickets.** Radiograph of the lower leg of a 2.5-year-old child shows the characteristic widening of the growth plate, specifically the zone of provisional calcification, and "cupping" of the metaphysis.

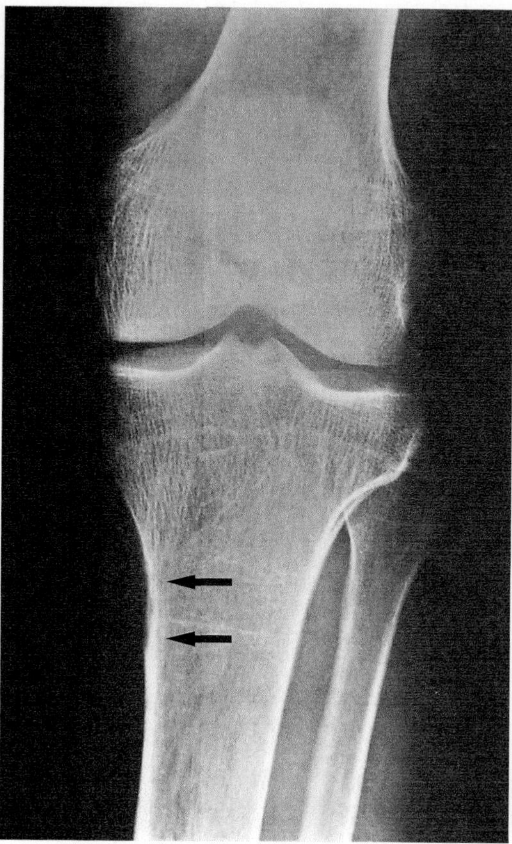

FIGURE 26.7 **Hyperparathyroidism.** Anteroposterior radiograph of the left knee of a 42-year-old woman with primary hyperparathyroidism caused by hyperplasia of the parathyroid glands demonstrates increased bone radiolucency and areas of subperiosteal bone resorption on the medial aspect of the proximal tibia *(arrows)*, characteristic of the condition.

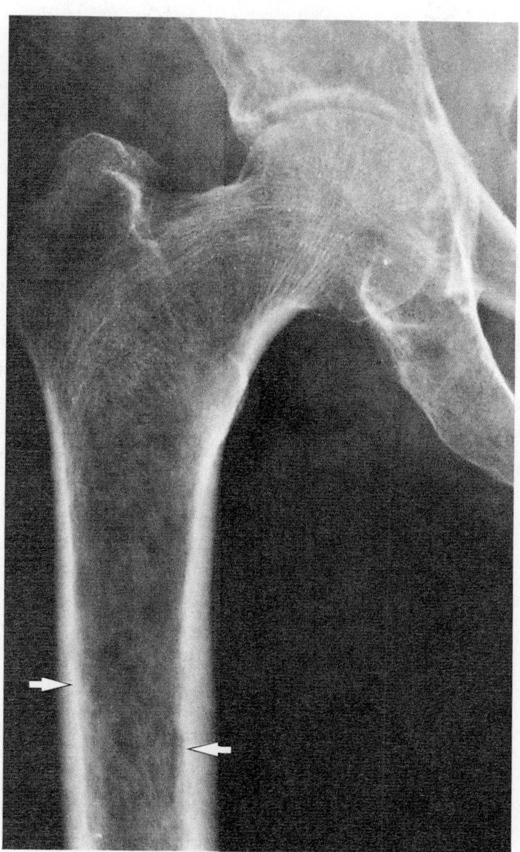

FIGURE 26.8 **Multiple myeloma.** Radiograph of the hip of a 58-year-old woman shows increased radiolucency of the bones. Focal radiolucencies and endosteal scalloping *(arrows)* can also be seen in the femur.

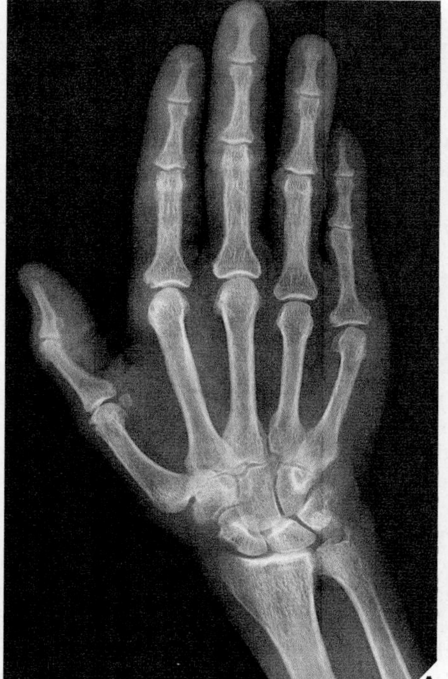

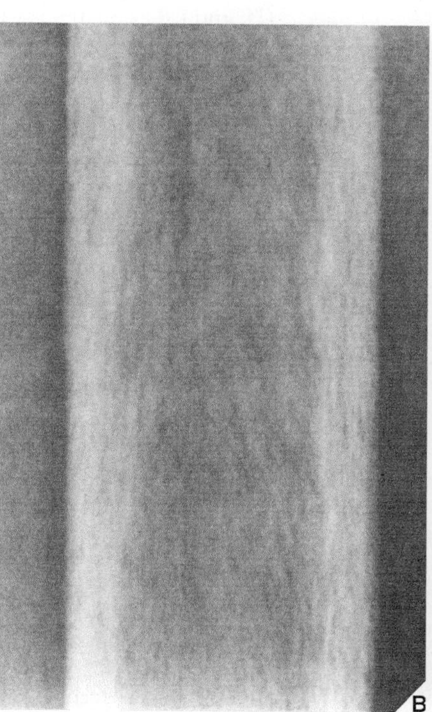

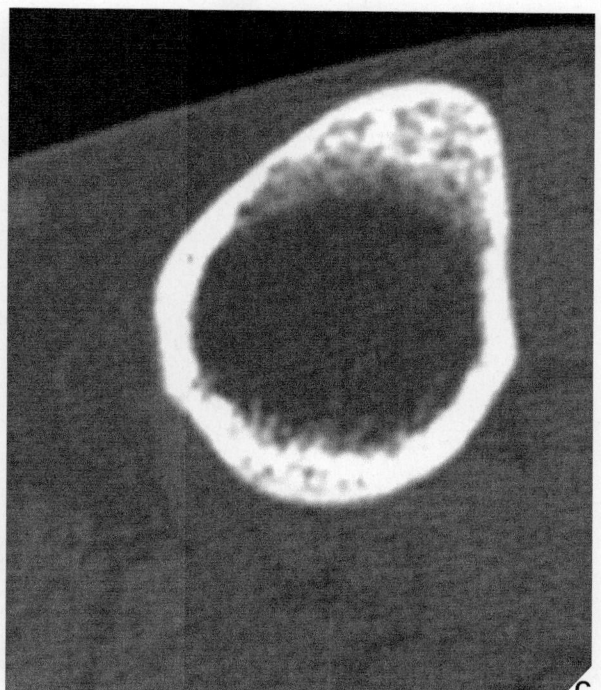

FIGURE 26.9 **Hyperparathyroidism.** **(A)** Dorsovolar radiograph of the hand of a 52-year-old woman demonstrates the typical changes of this condition: increased bone radiolucency (osteopenia); subperiosteal resorption best seen on the radial aspects of the middle phalanges of the index, middle, and ring fingers; acroosteolysis of the tufts of the index and middle fingers; loss of osseous trabeculae; and tunneling of the cortices, which reflects a rapid bone turnover. **(B)** Magnification study of the femur of the same patient obtained on PACS station shows the fine details of bone structure. The tunneling of the cortices is better appreciated. **(C)** Axial CT image demonstrates cortical tunneling in cross section.

Computed Tomography

CT was used in the past to obtain quantitative analysis of bone mineral content of the axial skeleton (QCT [quantitative CT]), however, due to its high radiation exposure, the technique has been mostly replaced by dual-energy x-ray absorptiometry (DEXA) scanning. CT, however, plays a significant role in the evaluation of osteoporosis-related fractures of the spine, pelvis, and lower extremities (insufficiency fractures).

Scintigraphy

Radionuclide imaging is a nonspecific modality, but it is a very sensitive detector of active bone turnover. For this reason, it is frequently effective in the evaluation of various metabolic diseases. It is particularly valuable in screening patients with Paget disease to determine the distribution of the lesion and activity of the disease (Fig. 26.10). The insufficiency-type stress fractures commonly seen in osteomalacia may be identified by this modality. In renal osteodystrophy, radionuclide bone scan may reveal the absence of renal images, confirming poor renal function. In hyperparathyroidism, it may detect silent sites of brown tumors. In the reflex sympathetic dystrophy syndrome, it may reveal abnormalities in the affected bone even before positive changes are seen on standard radiography. Similarly, in regional migratory osteoporosis, focal abnormalities may be present on the radionuclide bone scan long before radiographic changes become prominent.

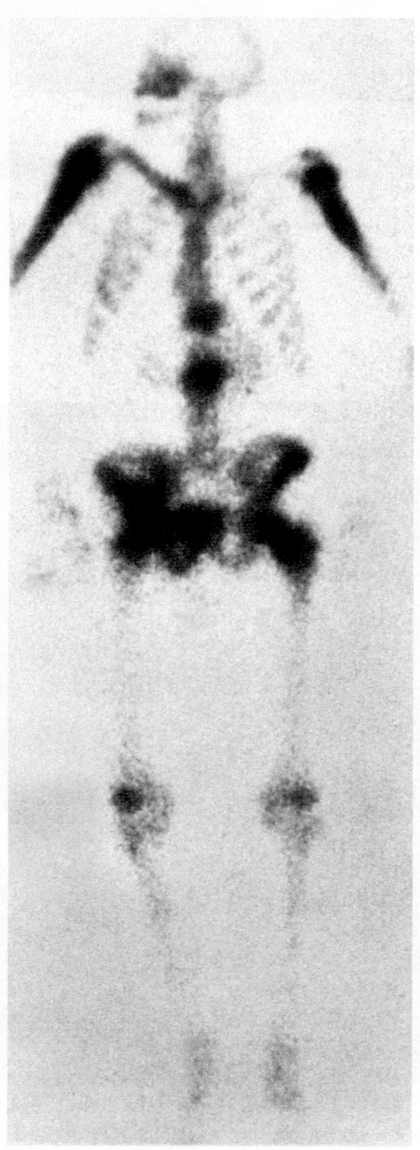

FIGURE 26.10 Scintigraphy of Paget disease. Radionuclide bone scan in this 72-year-old man with obvious clinical and radiographic evidence of Paget disease in the pelvis and proximal femora shows additional silent sites of involvement in patellae and humeri as well as in several thoracic and lumbar vertebrae.

Technetium-99m sestamibi (^{99m}Tc-MIBI) single-photon emission CT (SPECT) combined with image-fused CT (SPECT/CT) gained wide acceptance in localization of ectopic parathyroid adenomas causing primary hyperparathyroidism. Using a hybrid SPECT/CT instrument that couples a SPECT camera with CT camera in a single integrated unit affords the advantage of obtaining the three-dimensional (3D) functional information offered by SPECT with precise anatomic location provided by CT, thus improving the preoperative localization of parathyroid adenomas (Fig. 26.11). Trials using C-11 methionine positron emission tomography also confirmed the effectiveness of this technique to correctly localize abnormal parathyroid glands in patients with hyperparathyroidism.

Magnetic Resonance Imaging

MRI is occasionally helpful in evaluating metabolic and endocrine disorders. This technique may provide important information about bone marrow status in such disorders as transient regional osteoporosis (Fig. 26.12), regional migratory osteoporosis, and reflex sympathetic dystrophy syndrome (also known as *complex regional pain syndrome*, *reflex neurovascular dystrophy*, *amplified musculoskeletal pain syndrome*, *Sudeck atrophy*, and *causalgia*). It may effectively demonstrate bone marrow abnormalities in Gaucher disease, particularly medullary bone infarctions and osteonecrosis (Fig. 26.13). In osteomalacia, MRI may outline so-called *pseudofractures* or *Looser zones*. In Paget disease, MRI is very effective in revealing early stages of emerging complications, particularly the development of sarcoma in pagetic bone (see Fig. 29.29).

Imaging Techniques for Measurement of Bone Mineral Density

During the past few decades, the development of noninvasive technologies that allow accurate measurements of bone mass has revolutionized the study of osteoporosis and related disorders. Accurate detection and quantification of changes in bone mineralization became extremely valuable for the diagnosis and management of metabolic bone disorders. Several different techniques using different energy sources have been developed to measure bone mineral density, including radionuclide and x-ray methods, CT, and US.

Radionuclide and X-ray Techniques

Several radionuclide and x-ray techniques are used to determine bone mineral density. These include single-photon absorptiometry (SPA), dual-photon absorptiometry (DPA), single x-ray absorptiometry (SXA), and DEXA. These methods are used in clinical practice to assess patients with metabolic disease affecting the skeleton, to establish a diagnosis of osteoporosis or assess its severity, and to monitor response to therapy.

Single-Photon Absorptiometry

SPA is used to determine bone mineral density at peripheral sites, such as a finger or the radius, and measures primarily cortical bone. A single energy source is used, either iodine-125 or americium-241. The drawbacks of this technique include the need to replace decaying isotopes and inadequate spatial resolution. Moreover, the measurements are relatively insensitive to metabolic stimuli, and variations in thickness of soft tissue may lead to underestimation or overestimation of bone mineral density.

Dual-Photon Absorptiometry

DPA was introduced to overcome some of the limitations of SPA and to permit measurement of central bone sites such as the spine and the hip. The radionuclide source is gadolinium-153, which produces photons at two energy levels (44 and 100 KeV). The scans are obtained with a whole-body rectilinear scanner. The measurement reflects compact and trabecular bone in the scan path. The primary advantages of DPA are low radiation dose, diagnostic accuracy, and the availability of many accessible measurement sites. Its disadvantages include a relatively long scanning time.

Single X-ray Absorptiometry

SXA, unlike SPA and DPA, uses an x-ray system as a photon source. It is applicable mainly to peripheral bone sites such as the radius and calcaneus.

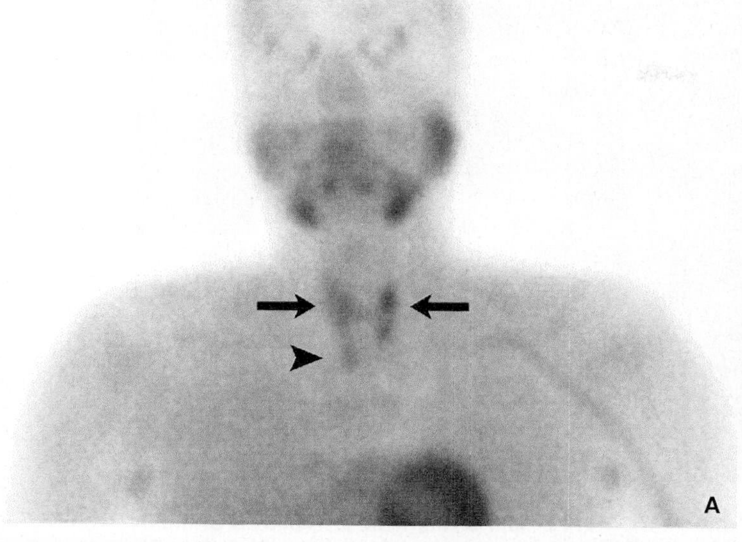

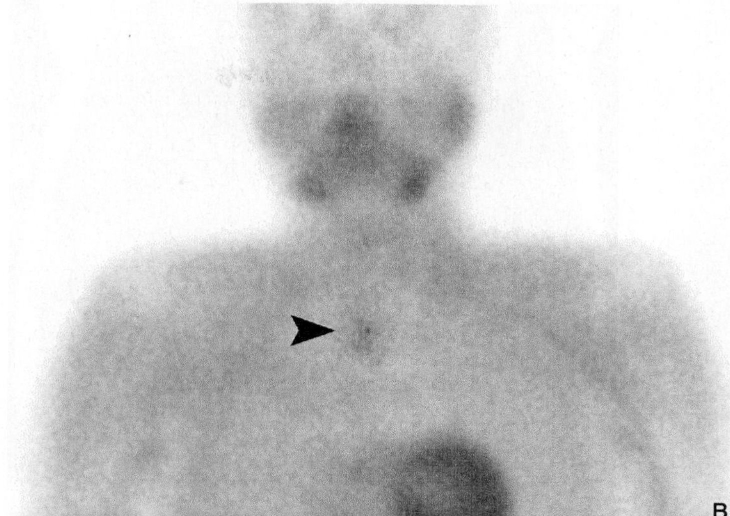

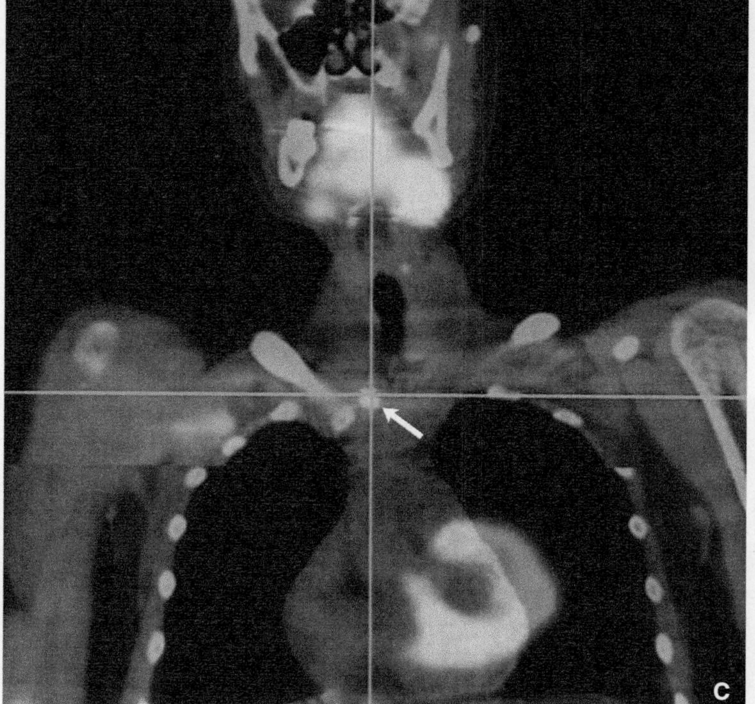

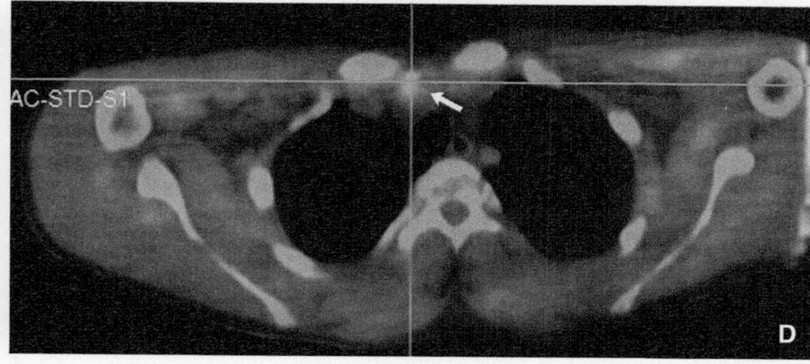

FIGURE 26.11 **SPECT/CT of ectopic parathyroid adenoma.** A 26-year-old man with a clinical and laboratory signs and imaging features of primary hyperparathyroidism was investigated for the presence of parathyroid glands abnormalities. After intravenous injection of 23.8 mCi of ^{99m}Tc-MIBI, the static planar early **(A)** and delayed **(B)** frontal images of the neck and chest were obtained. The early image shows increased uptake of ^{99m}Tc-MIBI in the thyroid gland *(arrows)* and in the parathyroid adenoma, located inferiorly to the thyroid *(arrowhead)*. The delayed image shows normal washout from the thyroid gland but persistent activity within the parathyroid adenoma, which is in ectopic location *(arrowhead)*. SPECT/CT color-fusion coronal **(C)** and axial (transverse) **(D)** images demonstrate at the cross-hairs focus of increased activity consistent with ectopic location of the parathyroid adenoma in the upper right mediastinum *(arrows)*. (Courtesy of David K. Shelton, MD, Sacramento, California.)

SXA has the advantages of being portable and inexpensive. Its disadvantages include the need for a water bath to determine soft-tissue equivalencies.

Dual-Energy X-ray Absorptiometry

At present, the most effective technique for measuring bone mineral density is DEXA, which uses photons produced from a low-dose energy source. The physical principles of DEXA are similar to those of DPA. However, the gadolinium source is replaced by an x-ray source with two energy levels that enable discrimination between bone and surrounding soft tissue. Therefore, an area-based two-dimensional (2D) image is generated, and measurements of bone mineral density can be calculated and compared with normal ranges matched for chronologic age (Fig. 26.14). Because of the increased flux from an x-ray tube rather than from an isotope source, scanning time and the collimation of the x-ray beam can be decreased. DEXA can be used for spine, hip, and whole-body measurements, enabling patients to be classified as normal, osteopenic, or osteoporotic.

Digital Computer-Assisted X-ray Radiogrammetry

Digital computer-assisted x-ray radiogrammetry (DXR) provides a bone mineral density calculation by a combined computerized radiogrammetric and textural analysis of the three middle metacarpal bones. The involved computer algorithms automatically define regions of interest around the narrowest parts of metacarpals and subsequently define the outer and inner cortical edges. The mean of the cortical thickness and overall bone cortical thickness are calculated. The acquisition technique and the analysis process itself have high reproducibility values, suggesting a high precision of the DXR method.

Quantitative Ultrasound Technique

US visualization is based on a mechanical wave vibrating at a frequency range from 20 kHz to 100 MHz. Passage of this wave through bone causes cortex and trabecular component to vibrate on a microscale. The physical and mechanical properties of the bone then progressively alter the shape, intensity, and speed of the propagating wave, which, as Hans et al. pointed out, allows characterization of bone tissue in terms of US velocity (speed of sound) and broadband US attenuation. These parameters allow the determination of bone mineral density, predominantly at the calcaneus. Although this method is not as accurate as the methods listed in the previous text, the absence of ionizing radiation with US, the portability of the equipment, and its cost-effectiveness make US assessment of bone mineral density an attractive option for screening patients suspected of having osteoporosis.

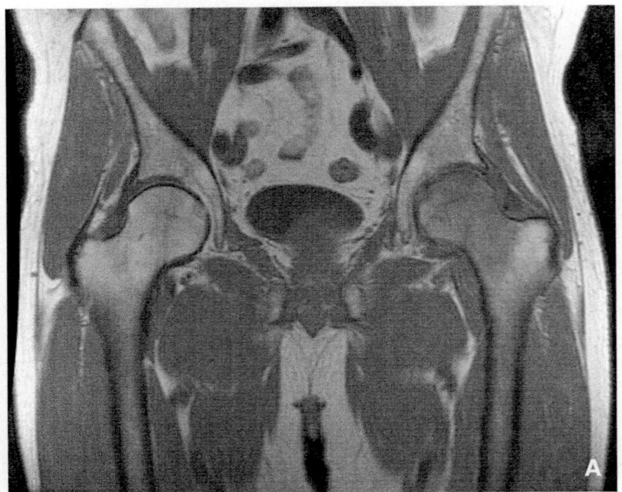

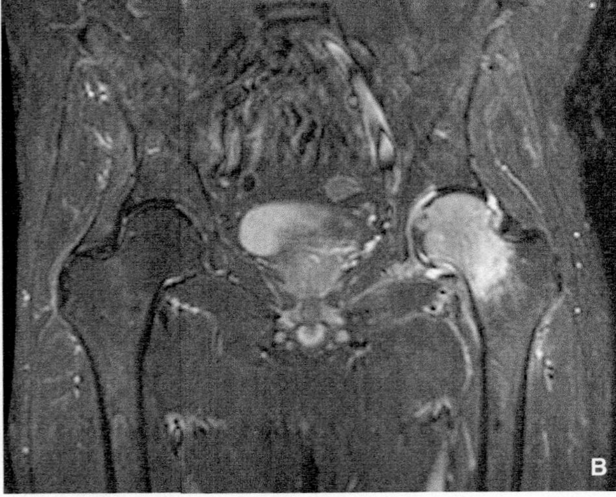

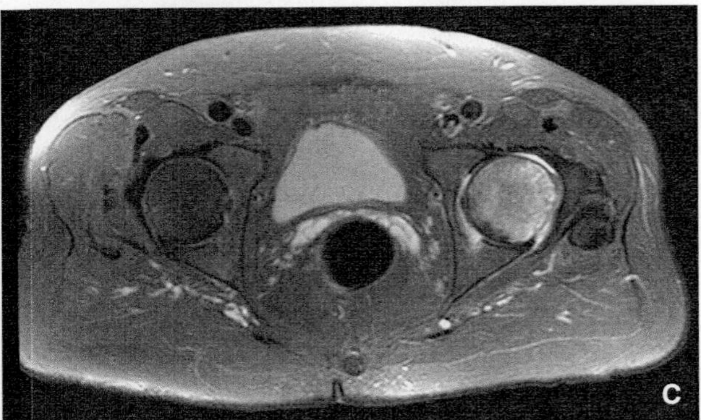

FIGURE 26.12 MRI of transient osteoporosis of hip. A 50-year-old man presented with left hip pain. **(A)** Coronal T1-weighted MRI shows decrease signal intensity in the left femoral head and neck. **(B)** Coronal short time inversion recovery (STIR) and **(C)** axial T2-weighted MR images demonstrate high signal in the same sites. In most patients, bone marrow edema subsides in several months, but some patients develop a small subchondral fracture of the femoral head, which is often visible after bone marrow edema had cleared.

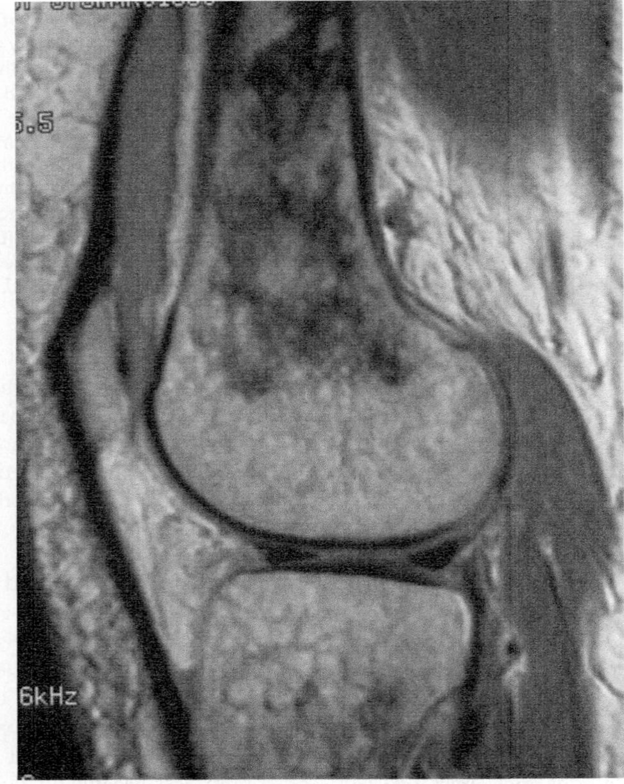

FIGURE 26.13 MRI of Gaucher disease. Sagittal T2-weighted MRI of the knee in a young patient demonstrates a "bubbly" pattern of the bone marrow of the distal femur and proximal tibia with areas of irregular low signal intensity in the distal femur related to the bone marrow infiltration by Gaucher cells and associated sclerosis and bone infarcts.

Name: NVM
Patient ID: 00011
Sex: Female
Ethnicity: White
Height: 63.7 in
Weight: 161.5 lb
Age: 69

Referring Physician: 0554

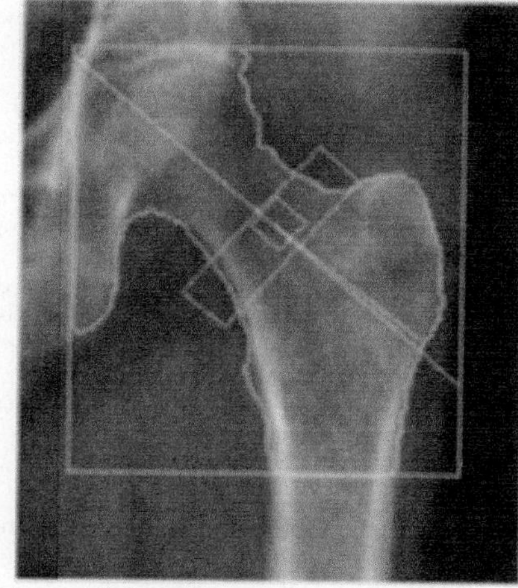

Image not for diagnostic use
99 x 111

Scan Information:

Scan Date: December 19, 2002 ID: K1219020L
Scan Type: a Left Hip
Analysis: December 19, 2002 12:07 Version 11.2
Left Hip
Operator: DSA
Model: QDR 4500A (S/N 45115)
Comment: 2301

DXA Results Summary:

Region	Area (cm²)	BMC (g)	BMD (g/cm²)	T-Score	PR (%)	Z-Score	AM (%)
Neck	5.07	2.68	0.528	-2.9	62	-1.1	81
Troch	11.31	5.31	0.469	-2.3	67	-1.0	82
Inter	16.59	12.79	0.771	-2.1	70	-0.9	85
Total	**32.96**	**20.77**	**0.630**	**-2.6**	**67**	**-1.1**	**83**
Ward's	1.15	0.38	0.335	-3.4	46	-0.9	76

Total BMD CV 1.0%
WHO Classification: Osteoporosis
Fracture Risk: High

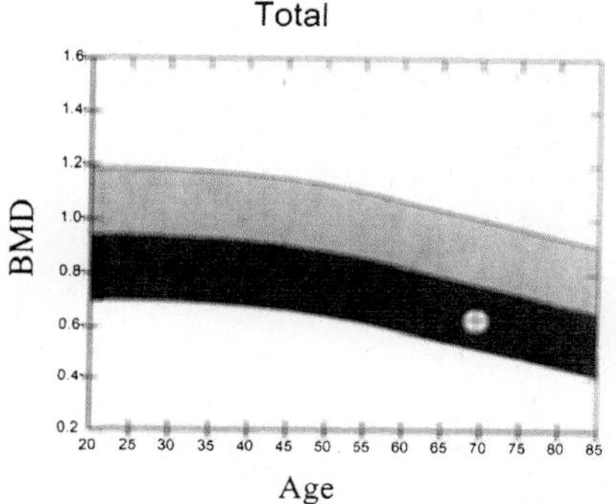

Reference curve and scores matched to White Female

FIGURE 26.14 DEXA measuring of bone mineral density. A 69-year-old woman was suspected of developing osteoporosis. DEXA scan of her left hip confirmed this diagnosis, indicating in addition high risk for a fracture.

PRACTICAL POINTS TO REMEMBER

1. On a standard radiograph, increased bone radiolucency (osteopenia) or increased bone density (osteosclerosis) is related to the process of bone formation and resorption, which under normal circumstances is in equilibrium:
   - if bone resorption exceeds bone production, either because of an increase in osteoclast activity or because of a decrease in osteoblast activity, or if there is insufficient mineral deposition in the matrix, then the result is increased radiolucency of the bone
   - if bone production surpasses bone resorption, either because of an increase in osteoblast activity or because of a decrease in osteoclast activity, then the result is increased radiodensity of the bone.
2. Instead of the specific term *osteoporosis*, the nonspecific descriptive term *osteopenia* is used to refer to any generalized or regional rarefaction of the skeleton, expressed radiographically as increased bone radiolucency, regardless of the specific pathogenesis. The main reason for this usage is that it is usually impossible to distinguish between the various causes of increased bone radiolucency. The term *osteosclerosis* refers to any increase in bone density, again regardless of the cause of the condition.
3. *Osteoporosis* is a specific term defining a state in which bone tissue (bone matrix) is reduced but mineralization of the organic matrix is normal. *Osteomalacia* is a specific term defining a state in which there is insufficient mineralization of osteoid tissue.
4. The important radiologic techniques used in the evaluation of various metabolic and endocrine conditions include:
   - conventional radiography
   - CT
   - radionuclide imaging (scintigraphy, bone scan)
   - MRI
   - US.
5. Scintigraphy is a nonspecific but highly sensitive modality to detect bone turnover in various metabolic and endocrine disorders.
6. ^{99m}Tc-MIBI SPECT/CT is an effective imaging method in evaluation of parathyroid adenomas in primary hyperparathyroidism.
7. MRI provides important information of the status of the bone marrow in such disorders as transient regional osteoporosis, regional migratory osteoporosis, idiopathic juvenile osteoporosis, and reflex sympathetic dystrophy syndrome. This technique is also effective in the evaluation of Gaucher disease and Paget disease.
8. Several methods have been developed for accurate assessment of mineral content of the bone, including SPA, DPA, DEXA, QCT, and DXR.
9. At present, DEXA is considered the most effective technique providing measurement of bone mineral density that can be compared with normal ranges matched for chronologic age.
10. Quantitative US technique for determining bone mineral density is an attractive method due to portability of the equipment, cost-effectiveness, and absence of ionizing radiation.

SUGGESTED READINGS

Adams JE. Single and dual energy x-ray absorptiometry. *Eur Radiol* 1997;7(suppl 2):S20–S31.

Baran DT, Faulkner KG, Genant HK, et al. Diagnosis and management of osteoporosis: guidelines for the utilization of bone densitometry. *Calcif Tissue Int* 1997;61:433–440.

Cann CE. Quantitative CT for determination of bone mineral density: a review. *Radiology* 1988;166:509–522.

Choi D, Kim D-Y, Han CS, et al. Measurements of bone mineral density in the lumbar spine and proximal femur using lunar prodigy and the new pencil-beam dual-energy x-ray absorptiometry. *Skeletal Radiol* 2010;39:1109–1116.

Crozier F, Champsaur P, Pham T, et al. Magnetic resonance imaging in reflex sympathetic dystrophy syndrome of the foot. *Joint Bone Spine* 2003;70:503–508.

DeMayo R, Haims AH, McRae MC, et al. Correlation of MRI-based bone marrow burden score with genotype and spleen status in Gaucher's disease. *AJR Am J Roentgenol* 2008;191:115–123.

Dhainaut A, Hoff M, Kälvesten, et al. Long-term in-vitro precision of direct digital x-ray radiogrammetry. *Skeletal Radiol* 2011;40:1575–1579.

Gamble CL. Osteoporosis: making the diagnosis in patients at risk for fracture. *Geriatrics* 1995;50:24–33.

Gayed IW, Kim EE, Broussard WF, et al. The value of 99mTc-sestamibi SPECT/CT over conventional SPECT in the evaluation of parathyroid adenomas or hyperplasia. *J Nucl Med* 2005;46:248–252.

Grampp S, Jergas M, Glüer CC, et al. Radiologic diagnosis of osteoporosis. Current methods and perspectives. *Radiol Clin North Am* 1993;31:1133–1145.

Grampp S, Steiner E, Imhof H. Radiological diagnosis of osteoporosis. *Eur Radiol* 1997;7(suppl 2):S11–S19.

Guglielmi G, Schneider P, Lang TF, et al. Quantitative computed tomography at the axial and peripheral skeleton. *Eur Radiol* 1997;7(suppl 2):S32–S42.

Hans D, Fuerst T, Duboeuf F. Quantitative ultrasound bone measurement. *Eur Radiol* 1997;7(suppl 2):S43–S50.

Kanis JA, Melton LJ III, Christiansen C, et al. The diagnosis of osteoporosis. *J Bone Miner Res* 1994;9:1137–1141.

Lai KC, Goodsitt MM, Murano R, et al. A comparison of two dual-energy x-ray absorptiometry systems for spinal bone mineral measurement. *Calcif Tissue Int* 1992;50:203–208.

Lang P, Steiger P, Faulkner K, et al. Osteoporosis. Current techniques and recent developments in quantitative bone densitometry. *Radiol Clin North Am* 1991;29:49–76.

Lomoschitz FM, Grampp S, Henk CB, et al. Comparison of imaging-guided and non-imaging-guided quantitative sonography of the calcaneus with dual x-ray absorptiometry of the spine and femur. *AJR Am J Roentgenol* 2003;180:1111–1116.

Lorberboym M, Minski I, Macadziob S, et al. Incremental diagnostic value of preoperative 99mTc-MIBI SPECT in patients with a parathyroid adenoma. *J Nucl Med* 2003;44:904–908.

Malich A, Boettcher J, Pfeil A, et al. The impact of technical conditions of x-ray imaging on reproducibility and precision of digital computer-assisted x-ray radiogrammetry (DXR). *Skeletal Radiol* 2004;33:698–703.

Miller PD, Bonnick SL, Rosen CJ. Consensus of an international panel on the clinical utility of bone mass measurements in the detection of low bone mass in the adult population. *Calcif Tissue Int* 1996;58:207–214.

Nelson DA, Brown EB, Flynn MJ, et al. Comparison of dual photon and dual energy x-ray bone densitometers in a clinic setting. *Skeletal Radiol* 1991;20:591–595.

Ng P, Lenzo NP, McCarthy MC, et al. Ectopic parathyroid adenoma localised with sestamibi SPECT and image-fused computed tomography. *Med J Aust* 2003;179:485–487.

Purz S, Kluge R, Barthel H, et al. Visualization of ectopic parathyroid adenomas. *N Engl J Med* 2013;369:2067–2069.

Rosenberg AE. The pathology of metabolic bone disease. *Radiol Clin North Am* 1991;29:19–36.

Roy M, Mazeh H, Chen H, et al. Incidence and localization of ectopic parathyroid adenomas in previously unexplored patients. *World J Surg* 2013;37:102–106.

Scientific Advisory Board of the Osteoporosis Society of Canada. Clinical practice guidelines for the diagnosis and management of osteoporosis. *CMAJ* 1996;155:1113–1133.

Staron RB, Greenspan R, Miller TT, et al. Computerized bone densitometric analysis: operator-dependent errors. *Radiology* 1999;211:467–470.

Tatoń G, Rokita E, Wróbel A, et al. Combining areal DXA bone mineral density and vertebrae postero-anterior width improves the prediction of vertebral strength. *Skeletal Radiol* 2013;42:1717–1725.

Weber T, Cammerer G, Schick C, et al. C-11 methionine positron emission tomography/computed tomography localizes parathyroid adenomas in primary hyperparathyroidism. *Horm Metab Res* 2010;42:209–214.

27

Osteoporosis, Rickets, and Osteomalacia

Osteoporosis

Osteoporosis is a generalized metabolic bone disease characterized by insufficient formation or increased resorption of bone matrix that results in decreased bone mass and microarchitectural deterioration of bone. Although there is a reduction in the amount of bone tissue, the tissue present is still fully mineralized. In other words, the bone is quantitatively deficient but qualitatively normal.

Osteoporosis has a variety of possible causes and consequently manifests in a number of different forms (Table 27.1). The basic distinction in osteoporosis is between those types that are *generalized* or *diffuse*, involving the entire skeleton, and those that are *localized* to a single region or bone (*regional*) (Fig. 27.1). The basic distinction between possible causes is between those that are *congenital* and those that are *acquired.*

Generalized Osteoporosis

Certain radiographic features are common to virtually all forms of osteoporosis regardless of their specific cause. There are always some diminution of cortical thickness and decrease in the number and thickness of the spongy bone trabeculae (Fig. 27.2). These changes are more prominent in non–weight-bearing segments and those not subject to stress. The first sites affected by osteoporosis, as well as the ones that are best demonstrated on radiographic study, are the periarticular regions, where the cortex is anatomically thinner (Fig. 27.3). In the long bones, the thickness of the cortices decreases, the bones become brittle, and there is increased clinical incidence of fractures, particularly of the proximal femur (Fig. 27.4), the proximal humerus, the distal radius, and the ribs.

Besides variety of methods evaluating osteoporosis (discussed in detail in Chapter 26), some simple methods using conventional radiography have been developed.

The analysis of the trabecular pattern of the bones has been emphasized as an effective method to evaluate osteoporosis because patterns of trabecular loss correlate well with increasing severity of osteoporosis. In the femur, these changes may be evaluated according to the pattern of the principal compressive group of trabeculae, the secondary compressive group of trabeculae, and the principal tensile group of trabeculae (Fig. 27.5 and Table 27.2). The trabecular pattern of the proximal end of the femur is an excellent indicator of the severity of the osteoporosis.

In early osteoporosis, both the compressive and tensile trabeculae are accentuated because of initial resorption of the randomly oriented trabeculae, and thus, the radiolucency of the Ward triangle becomes more prominent. With increasing severity of osteoporosis, the tensile trabeculae are reduced in number and regress from the medial femoral border to the lateral. When trabecular resorption increases, the outer portion of the principal tensile trabeculae opposite the greater trochanter disappears, opening the Ward triangle laterally. As osteoporosis increases in severity, resorption of all trabeculae occurs, with the exception of those in the principal compressive group. In advanced osteoporosis, the principal compressive component is the last to be involved, a process manifested by a decrease in the number and length of individual trabeculae. Eventually, the upper femur may be completely devoid of all trabecular markings.

The other major area in which osteoporotic changes are evaluated is the axial skeleton, particularly the spine. This is especially true in osteoporosis associated with aging, that is, *involutional* (senescent and postmenopausal) *osteoporosis*, in which the vertebral bodies are particularly vulnerable. Initially, there is a relative increase in the density of the vertebral end plates due to resorption of the spongy bone, causing what is called an *empty box appearance* (Fig. 27.6). Later, there is an overall decrease in density with a loss of any trabecular pattern, creating a "ground glass" appearance. A typical feature of vertebral involvement in osteoporosis is biconcavity of the vertebral body resulting from expansion of the adjacent disks, leading to arch-like indentations on both superior and inferior margins of the weakened vertebral bodies (Fig. 27.7). Terms used to describe this configuration in instances of severe osteoporosis included "fish vertebra", "codfish vertebra", "fish-mouth vertebra", "fish-tail vertebra", "fish-bone deformity", and "hourglass deformity". The term "fish vertebra", "codfish vertebra", and "fish-bone vertebra" were coined because of similarity with the vertebrae of some fish species. The term "fish-mouth vertebra", most commonly used, was coined because biconcave vertebral bodies resemble an open fish mouth. Occasionally this term is also used to describe step-like central depression of the end plates of the vertebral body in sickle cell disease, although more common expression for this appearance is H-shaped deformity (see Fig. 1.3). In advanced stages of osteoporosis, there is complete collapse of the vertebral body associated with a wedge-shaped deformity. In the thoracic spine, this leads to increased kyphosis.

Histopathologic examination of osteoporotic vertebrae reveals that there is selective loss of the horizontal trabeculae, with a consequent accentuation of the vertical trabeculae. This can be observed also on the gross specimen of the vertebral bodies (Fig. 27.8). Highly characteristic is also a change in vertebral shape including flattening, anterior wedging, and biconcavity (Fig. 27.9), as discussed earlier.

Of special interest in generalized osteoporosis are the three major varieties of *iatrogenic osteoporosis*. *Heparin-induced osteoporosis* may develop after long-term, high-dose daily heparin treatment (more than 10,000 units). Precisely how this type of osteoporosis is initiated and develops is not clearly understood, although osteoclastic stimulation and osteoblastic inhibition with suppressed endochondral ossification have been implicated as potential causes. Spontaneous fractures of the vertebrae, ribs, and femoral neck are noted on radiographic studies. *Dilantin-induced osteoporosis* occasionally develops after prolonged use of phenytoin (Dilantin). The vertebral column and ribs are usually affected, and fractures are a common complication.

Steroid-induced osteoporosis, occurring either during the course of Cushing syndrome or iatrogenically during treatment with various corticosteroids, is characterized by decreased bone formation and increased bone resorption.

TABLE 27.1 Causes of Osteoporosis

Generalized (Diffuse)		Localized (Regional)
Genetic (Congenital)	*Deficiency States*	*Miscellaneous (continued)*
Osteogenesis imperfecta	Scurvy	Immobilization (cast)
Gonadal dysgenesis:	Malnutrition	Disuse
Turner syndrome (XO)	Anorexia nervosa	Pain
Klinefelter syndrome (XXY)	Protein deficiency	Infection
Hypophosphatasia	Alcoholism	Reflex sympathetic dystrophy syndrome (Sudeck atrophy)
Homocystinuria	Liver disease	Transient regional osteoporosis
Mucopolysaccharidosis	*Neoplastic*	Transient osteoporosis of the hip
Gaucher disease	Myeloma	Regional migratory osteoporosis
Anemias	Leukemia	Idiopathic juvenile osteoporosis
Sickle cell syndromes	Lymphoma	Paget disease (hot phase)
Thalassemia	Metastatic disease	
Hemophilia	*Drug-induced*	
Christmas disease	Heparin-induced	
Endocrine	Dilantin-induced	
Hyperthyroidism	Steroid-induced	
Hyperparathyroidism	*Miscellaneous*	
Cushing syndrome	Involutional (senescent/ postmenopausal)	
Acromegaly	Amyloidosis	
Estrogen deficiency	Ochronosis	
Hypogonadism	Paraplegia	
Diabetes mellitus	Weightlessness	
Pregnancy	Idiopathic	

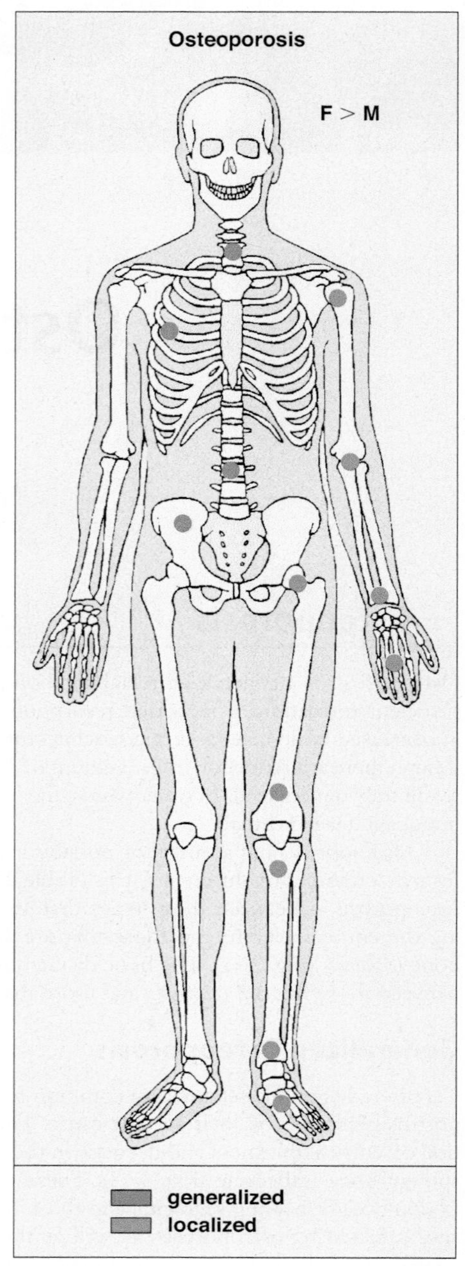

FIGURE 27.1 Target sites of osteoporosis.

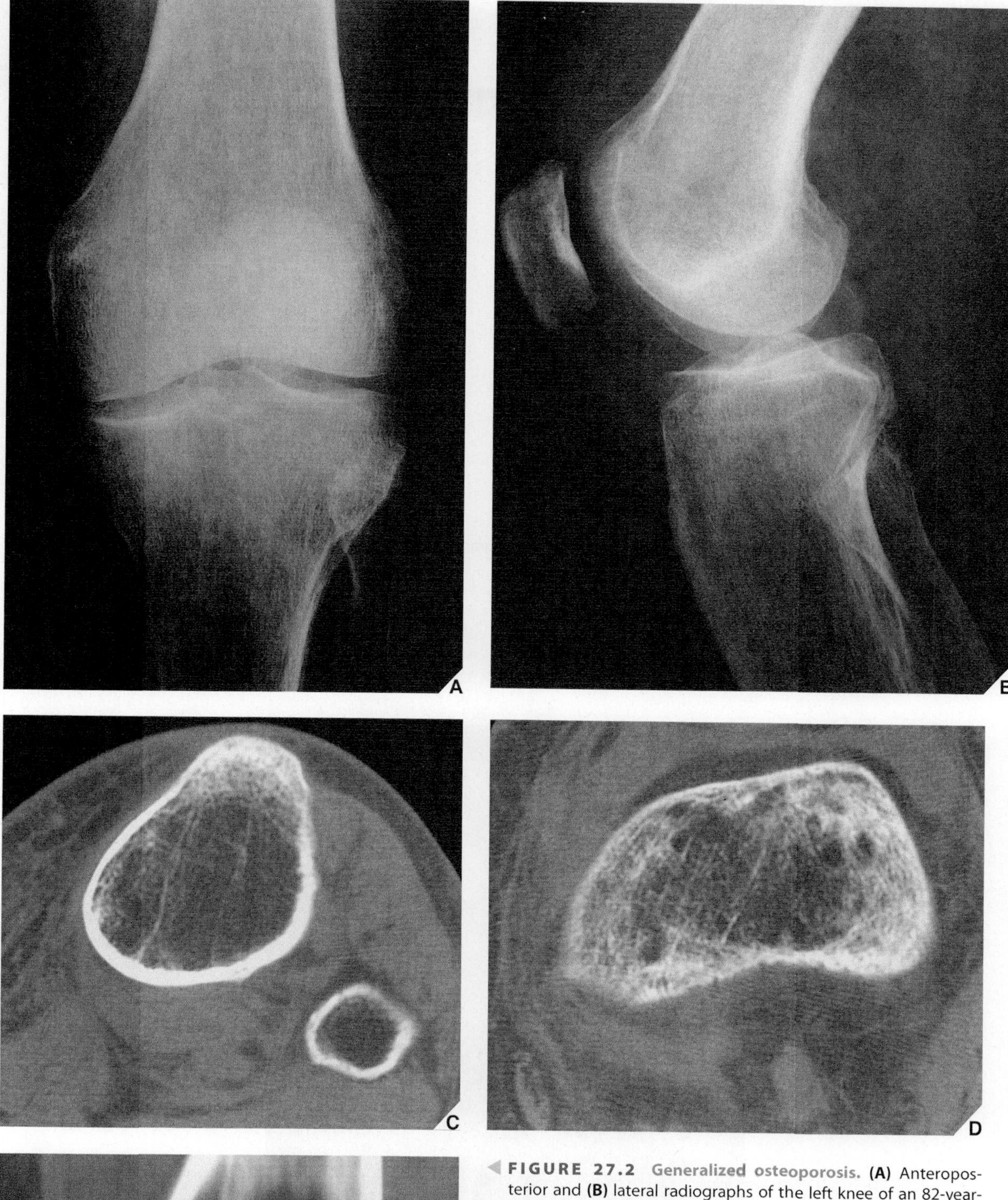

FIGURE 27.2 Generalized osteoporosis. **(A)** Anteroposterior and **(B)** lateral radiographs of the left knee of an 82-year-old man reveal increased radiolucency of bones, thinning of the cortices, and sparse trabecular pattern. These changes are more effectively demonstrated on axial computed tomography (CT) sections obtained through the proximal tibia **(C)** and distal femur **(D)** as well as on reformatted coronal image of the distal femur **(E)**.

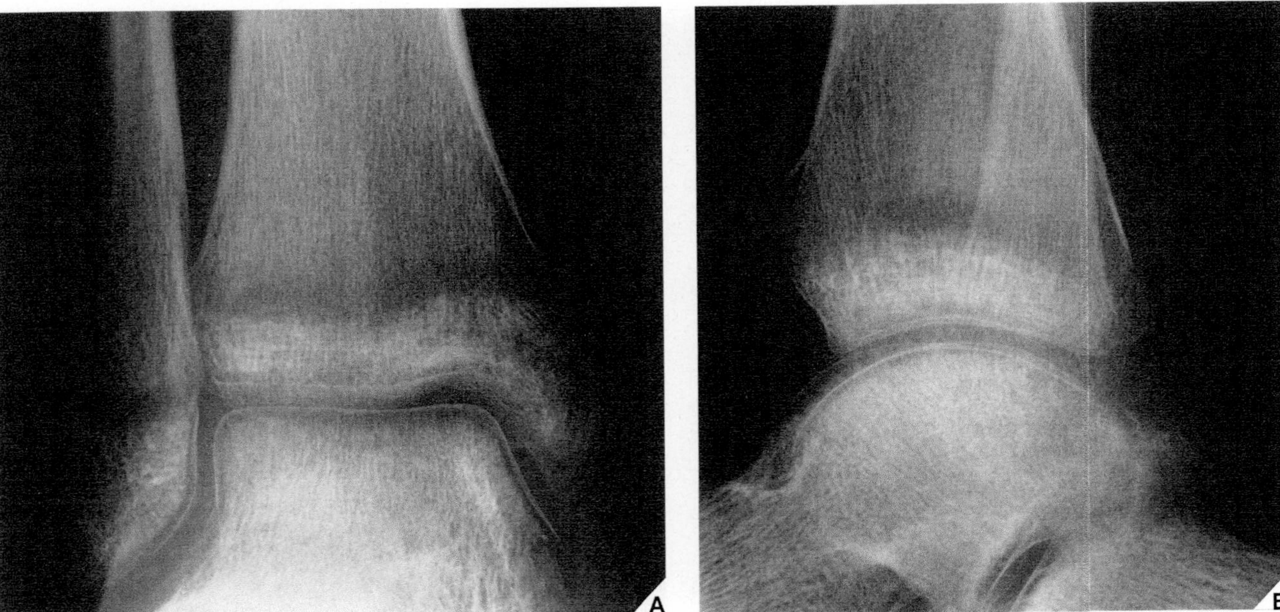

FIGURE 27.3 Periarticular osteoporosis. **(A)** Anteroposterior and **(B)** lateral radiographs of an ankle reveal sparse trabecular pattern and increase radiolucency in the subchondral areas.

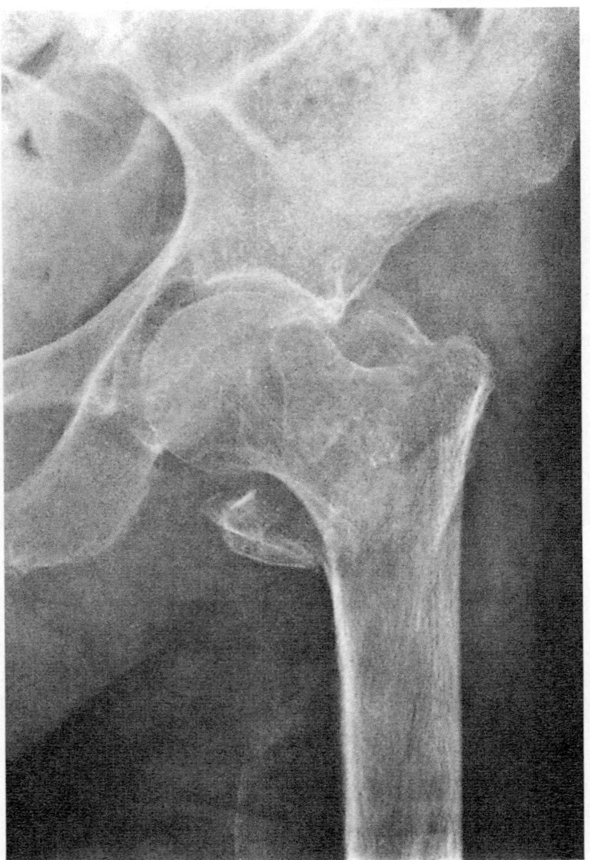

FIGURE 27.4 Osteoporosis complicated by a fracture. An 85-year-old woman with advanced postmenopausal osteoporosis sustained an intertrochanteric fracture of the left femur, as seen on this anteroposterior radiograph. Note the thinning of the cortex and the increased radiolucency of the bones.

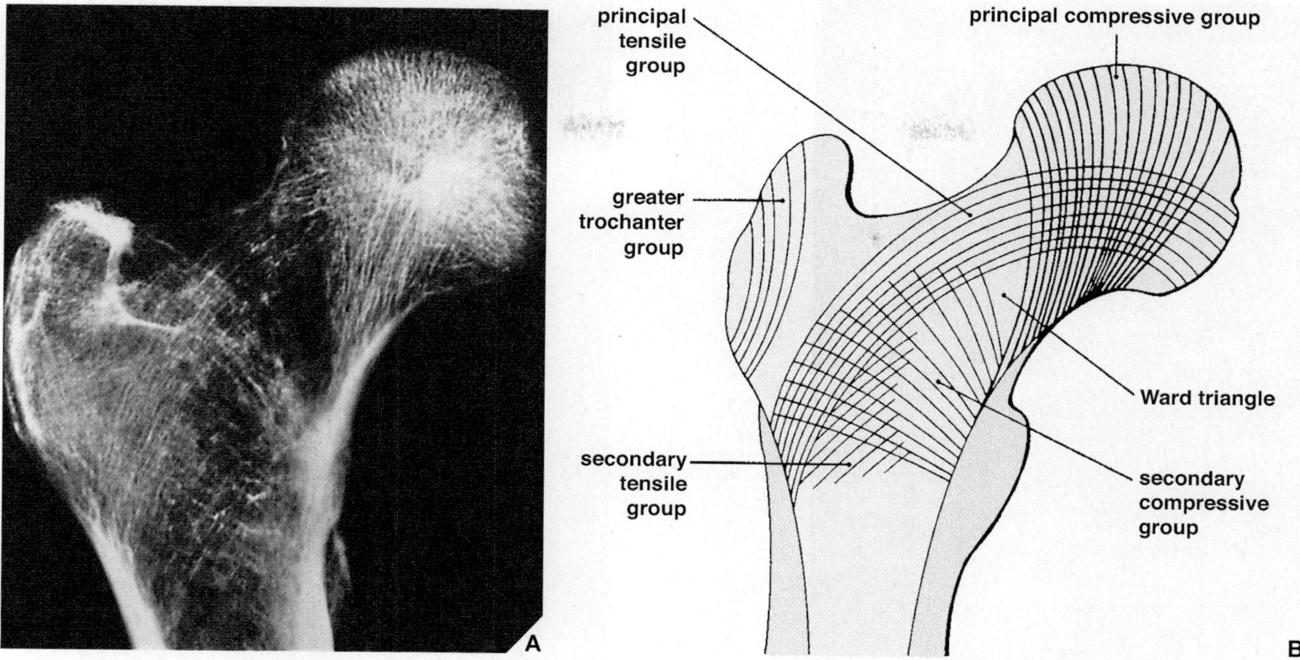

FIGURE 27.5 Trabecular pattern of the proximal femur. (A) The trabecular pattern of the proximal end of the femur is an excellent indicator of the severity of the osteoporosis. **(B)** Confluence of principal tensile, principal compressive, and secondary compressive trabeculae in the femoral neck forms a triangular region of radiolucency, the Ward triangle. The principal tensile trabeculae are more important than the secondary trabeculae; the compressive trabeculae are more important than the tensile trabeculae. Bone loss occurs in order of increasing importance.

TABLE 27.2 The Five Major Groups of Trabeculae

1. *Principal compressive group*
   - Extend from medial cortex of femoral neck to superior part of femoral head
   - Major weight-bearing trabeculae
   - In normal femur are the thickest and most densely packed
   - Appear accentuated in osteoporosis
   - Last to be obliterated
2. *Secondary compressive group*
   - Originate at the cortex, near the lesser trochanter
   - Curve upward and laterally toward the greater trochanter and upper femoral neck
   - Characteristically thin and widely separated
3. *Principal tensile group*
   - Originate from the lateral cortex, inferior to the greater trochanter
   - Extend in an arch-like configuration medially, terminating in the inferior portion of the femoral head
4. *Secondary tensile group*
   - Arise from the lateral cortex below the principal tensile group
   - Extend superiorly and medially to terminate after crossing the middle of the femoral neck
5. *Greater trochanter group*
   - Composed of slender and poorly defined tensile trabeculae
   - Arise laterally below the greater trochanter
   - Extend upward to terminate near the greater trochanter's superior surface

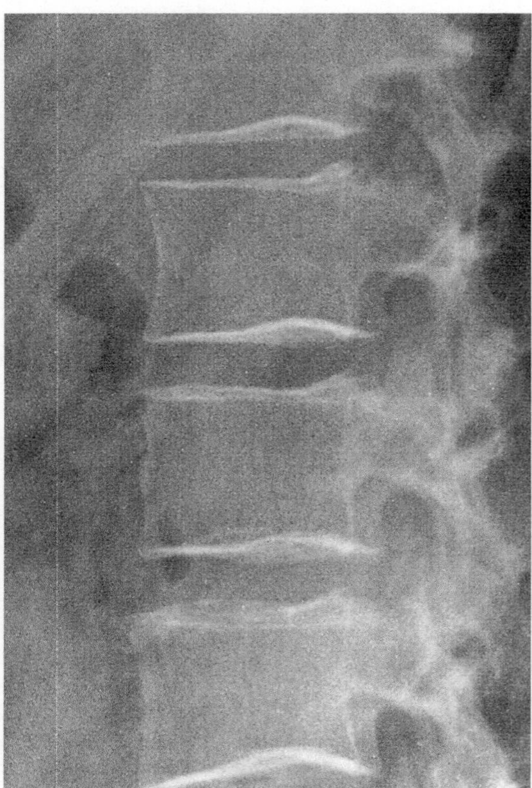

FIGURE 27.6 **Involutional osteoporosis.** Lateral radiograph of the lumbar spine of an 89-year-old woman demonstrates a relative increase in the density of the vertebral end plates and resorption of the trabeculae of spongy bone, creating an empty box appearance.

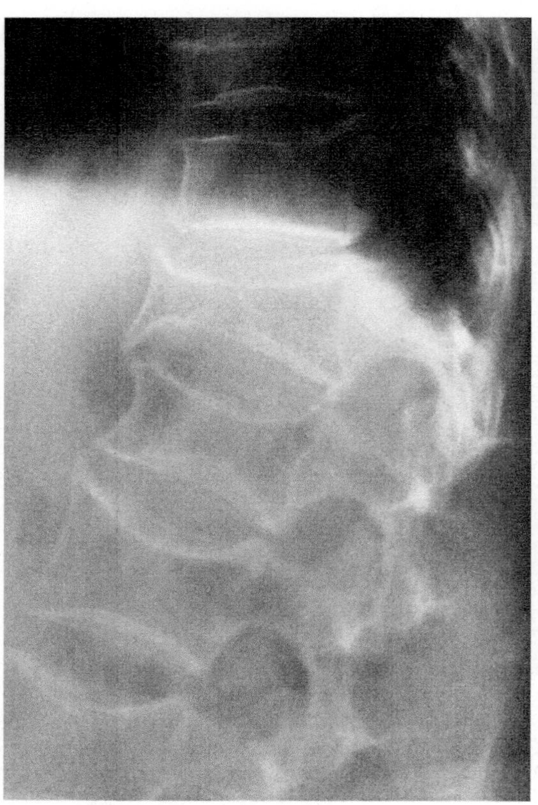

FIGURE 27.7 **Involutional osteoporosis.** Biconcavity, or codfish vertebrae, seen here on the lateral radiograph of the thoracolumbar spine in an 80-year-old woman, results from weakness of the vertebral end plates and intravertebral expansion of nuclei pulposi.

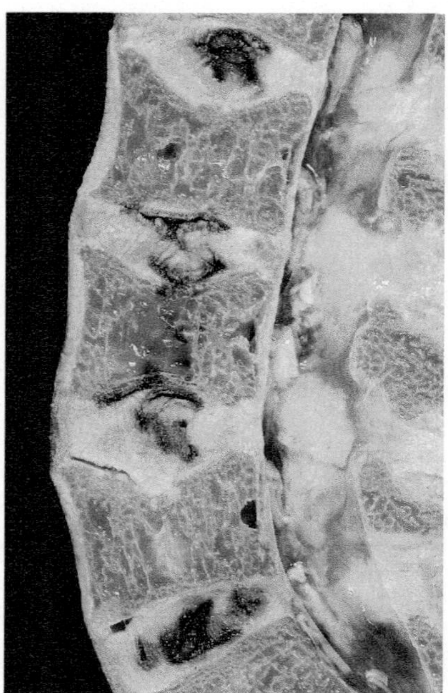

FIGURE 27.8 **Pathology of osteoporosis.** Photograph of sagittal section of the lower lumbar spine shows biconcavity of the vertebral bodies secondary to the central collapse of the vertebral end plates and intravertebral expansion of the intervertebral disks. (Reprinted with permission from Vigorita JV, Ghelmsan B, Mintz D. *Orthopaedic pathology*, 3rd ed. Philadelphia: Wolters Kluwer; 2016:125.)

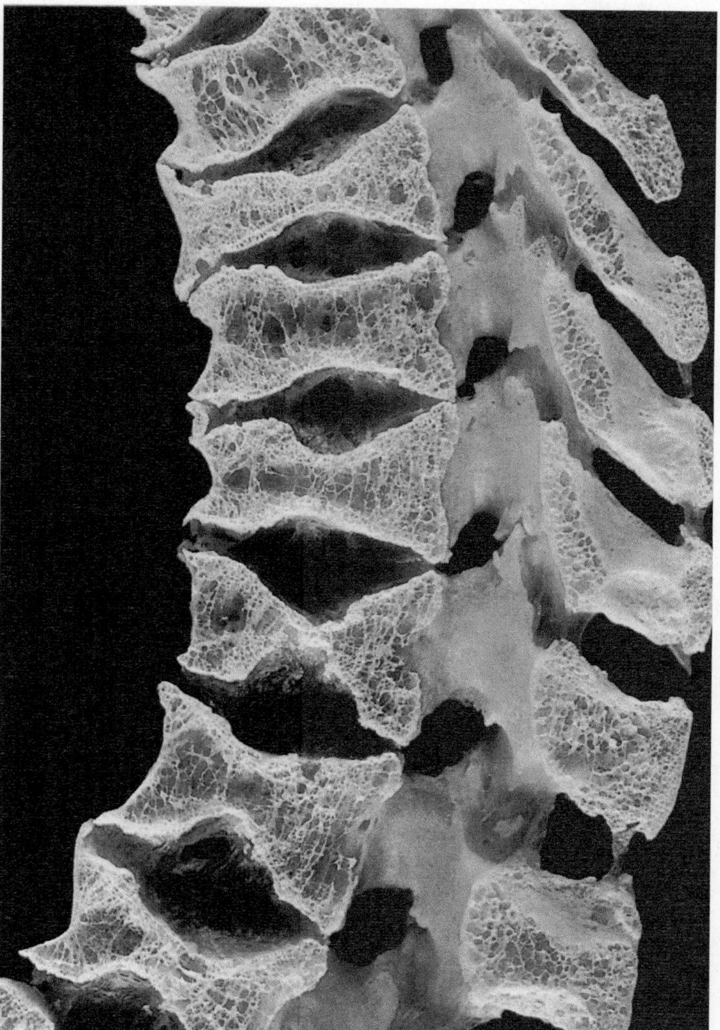

FIGURE 27.9 Pathology of osteoporosis. Photograph of a sagittal section of a macerated thoracic spine shows the various patterns and degrees of vertebral body collapse. In the upper segment, flattening of the vertebral bodies with some anterior wedging is present, whereas in the lower part, the more typical for osteoporosis biconcave compression fractures of the central portion of the end plates is seen, typical for so-called *fish-mouth vertebrae*. (Reprinted from Bullough P. *Orthopaedic pathology*, 5th ed. Maryland Heights, MO: Mosby; 2009, with permission from Elsevier.)

Although the axial skeleton is most often affected, the appendicular skeleton may also be involved. In the spine, considerable thickening and sclerosis of the vertebral end plates occur without a concomitant change in the anterior and posterior vertebral margins.

Osteoporosis associated with neoplastic processes is discussed in Chapter 16.

Localized Osteoporosis

Transient regional osteoporosis is a collective term for a group of conditions that have one feature in common: rapidly developing osteoporosis that usually affects the periarticular regions and has no definite etiology like trauma or immobilization. It is a self-limiting and reversible disorder, of which three subtypes have been described. *Transient osteoporosis of the hip* is seen predominantly in pregnant women and in young and middle-aged men. Its primary manifestation is local osteoporosis involving the femoral head and neck and the acetabulum (see Fig. 26.12). *Regional migratory osteoporosis*, which affects the knee, the ankle, and the foot, is mainly seen in men in their fourth and fifth decades. This migratory condition is characterized by pain and swelling around the affected joints. It develops rapidly and subsides in about 6 to 9 months; there may be subsequent recurrence and involvement of other joints. *Idiopathic juvenile osteoporosis* is commonly seen during or just before puberty and typically regresses spontaneously. Skeletal involvement is often symmetrical and is generally juxtaarticular in location. It is frequently associated with pain and the presence of vertebral body compression fractures.

Localized osteoporosis secondary to immobilization in a cast or due to disuse of a painful limb is discussed in Chapter 4. Sudeck atrophy (reflex sympathetic dystrophy syndrome) may also occur as a complication of fractures (see Fig. 4.77).

Rickets and Osteomalacia

Whereas in osteoporosis the fundamental change is decreased bone mass, in rickets (which occurs in children) and osteomalacia (which occurs in adults), the essential bone abnormality is faulty mineralization (calcification) of the bone matrix. If adequate amounts of calcium and phosphorus are not available, proper calcification of osteoid tissue cannot occur.

In the past, the most common cause of rickets (the term evolved from the old English word *wrick*, meaning "to twist") and osteomalacia was *deficient intake* of vitamin D, which is responsible for calcium and phosphorus homeostasis and for maintenance of proper bone mineralization. Now, however, the major causes include *inadequate intestinal absorption*, resulting in the loss of calcium and phosphorus through the gastrointestinal tract in patients who have gastric, biliary, or enteric abnormalities or have undergone gastrectomy or other gastric surgery; *renal tubular disorders* (proximal and/or distal tubular lesions frequently leading to renal tubular acidosis); and *renal osteodystrophy* secondary to renal failure, which results in loss of calcium through the kidneys. Several other conditions associated with osteomalacia have been identified, such as neurofibromatosis, fibrous dysplasia, and Wilson disease, but the exact relationship between the underlying disorder and osteomalacia is still unclear (Table 27.3).

Rickets

Infantile Rickets

Found mainly in infants between 6 and 18 months of age, infantile rickets is characterized by generalized demineralization of the skeleton, which leads to bowing deformities in weight-bearing bones when infants begin to stand and walk. Infants with early rickets are restless and sleep poorly. Closing of the fontanelles is delayed. The earliest physical sign is softening of the cranial

TABLE 27.3 Etiology of Rickets and Osteomalacia

Nutritional Deficiency
Vitamin D
Dietary
Insufficient sunlight
Impaired synthesis
Calcium
Phosphorus
Absorption Abnormalities
Gastric surgery
Intestinal surgery (bypass)
Gastric disorders (obstruction)
Intestinal disorders (sprue)
Renal Disorders
Renal tubular disorders
Proximal tubular lesions (failure of absorption of inorganic phosphate, glucose, amino acids)
Distal tubular lesions (renal tubular acidosis)
Combined proximal and distal tubular lesions
Renal osteodystrophy
Miscellaneous
Associated with
Wilson disease
Fibrogenesis imperfecta
Fibrous dysplasia
Neurofibromatosis
Hypophosphatasia
Neoplasm

vault (craniotabes). Enlargement of the cartilage at the costochondral junction produces a prominence known as *rachitic rosary*. The serum values of calcium and phosphorus are low and that of alkaline phosphatase is increased.

The key radiographic features are observed in the metaphysis and the epiphysis—the regions where growth is most active—particularly at the distal ends of the radius, ulna, and femur as well as at the proximal ends of the tibia and fibula (Fig. 27.10). Deficient mineralization in the provisional zone of calcification is reflected in widening of the growth plate and cupping and flaring of the metaphysis, which appears disorganized and "frayed" (Figs. 27.11 and 27.12; see also Fig. 26.6). In the secondary ossification centers of the epiphysis, similar changes are seen; the bone becomes radiolucent, with loss of sharpness at the periphery, and bowing deformities frequently occur (Fig. 27.13).

Vitamin D–Resistant Rickets

This condition is found in older children (those above 30 months of age), and four distinct types have been reported. *Classic vitamin D–resistant* (or hypophosphatemic) *rickets*, also known as *familial vitamin D–resistant rickets*, is a congenital disorder that is transmitted as a sex-linked dominant trait. Recent studies indicated that hypophosphatemic rickets occur as the result of mutation of *PHEX* gene found on the X chromosome. This gene

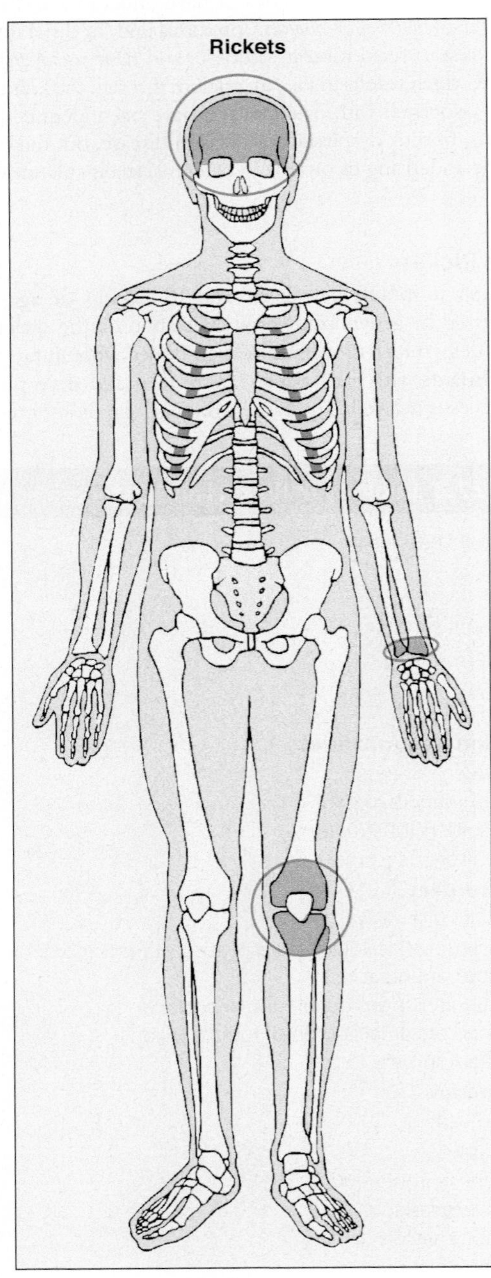

FIGURE 27.10 Target sites of rickets.

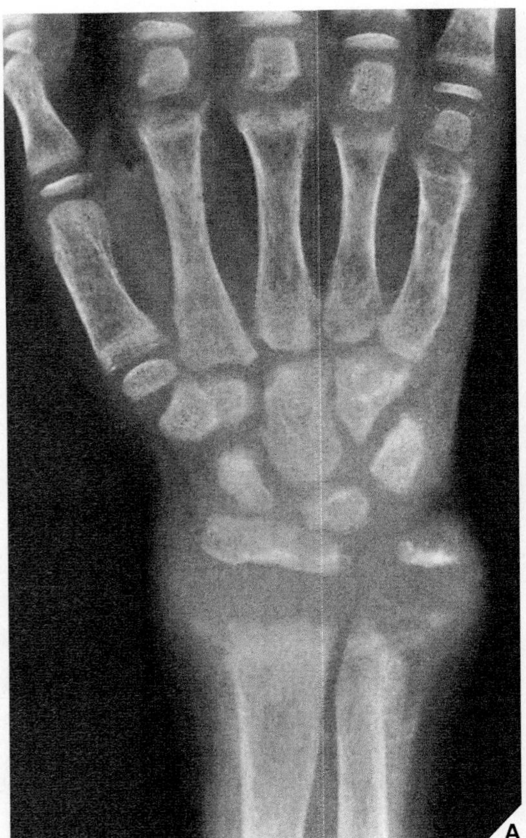

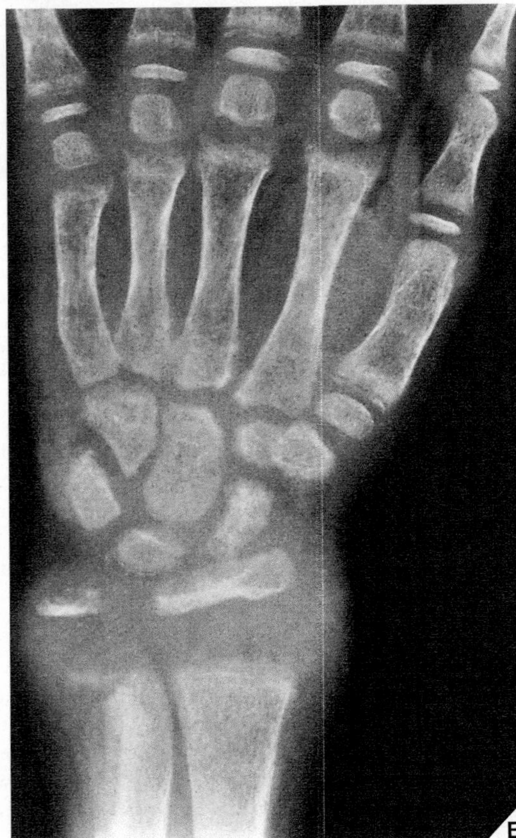

FIGURE 27.11 Rickets. **(A,B)** Anteroposterior radiograph of both hands of an 8-year-old boy with untreated dietary rickets shows osteopenia of the bones, widening of the growth plates of the distal radius and ulna, and flaring of the metaphyses, all typical features of this condition.

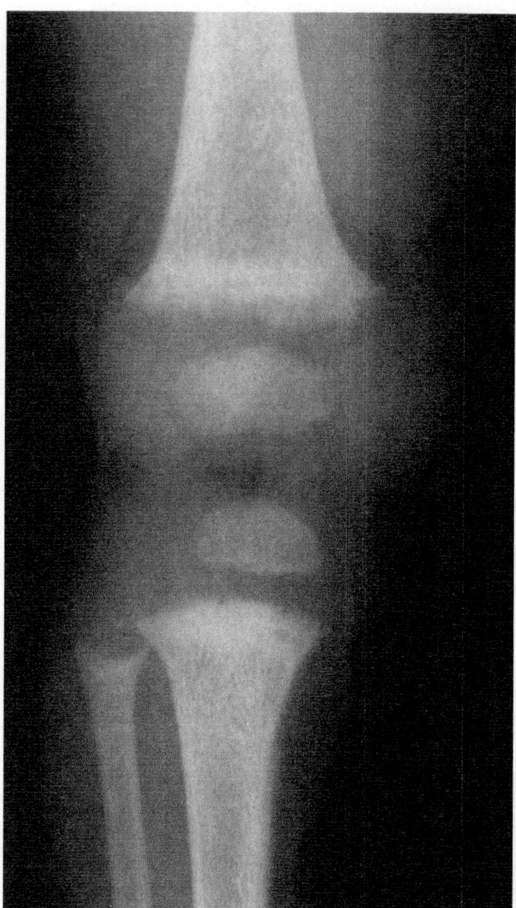

FIGURE 27.12 Rickets. Anteroposterior radiograph of the knee in a 4-year-old boy shows widening of the growth plates of the distal femur and proximal tibia secondary to lack of mineralization in the provisional zone of calcification. Note also cupping and flaring of the metaphyses.

normally produces an enzyme zinc-metallopeptidase. Loss of function of this gene results in circulatory clearance of fibroblast growth factor 23 (FGF-23) that acts on the kidneys to increase phosphate excretion and decrease alpha-1 hydroxylase activity. This results in hypophosphatemia but normal levels of serum calcium. Patients are short, stocky, and bowlegged. Ectopic calcifications and ossifications in the axial and the appendicular skeleton, along with occasional sclerotic changes, are among the identifying radiographic findings. *Vitamin D–resistant rickets with glycosuria* is characterized by an abnormal resorptive mechanism for glucose and inorganic phosphate. *Fanconi syndrome* (named after a Swiss pediatrician Guido Fanconi) is characterized by a defect in the proximal renal tubules and deficient resorption of phosphate, glucose, and several amino acids. The clinical features of this syndrome include hypokalemia, hyperchloremia, acidosis, polyuria, polydipsia, growth failure, and development of hypophosphatemic rickets in children and osteomalacia in adults. *Acquired hypophosphatemic syndrome* manifests in late adolescence or early adulthood; it is probably of toxic etiology.

The radiographic findings in all four types of vitamin D–resistant rickets are similar to those in infantile rickets. Bowing of the legs and shortening of the long bones, however, are more pronounced, and occasionally, the bones appear sclerotic (Fig. 27.14).

Osteomalacia

Osteomalacia, which results from the same pathomechanism as rickets, occurs only after bone growth has ceased, and hence, the term refers to changes in the cortical and trabecular bone of the axial and appendicular skeleton. It is most often caused by faulty absorption of fat-soluble vitamin D from the gastrointestinal tract secondary to malabsorption syndrome. It may also result from dysfunction of the proximal renal tubules, resulting in so-called *renal osteomalacia*. The most common clinical presentation of this condition is bone pain and muscle weakness.

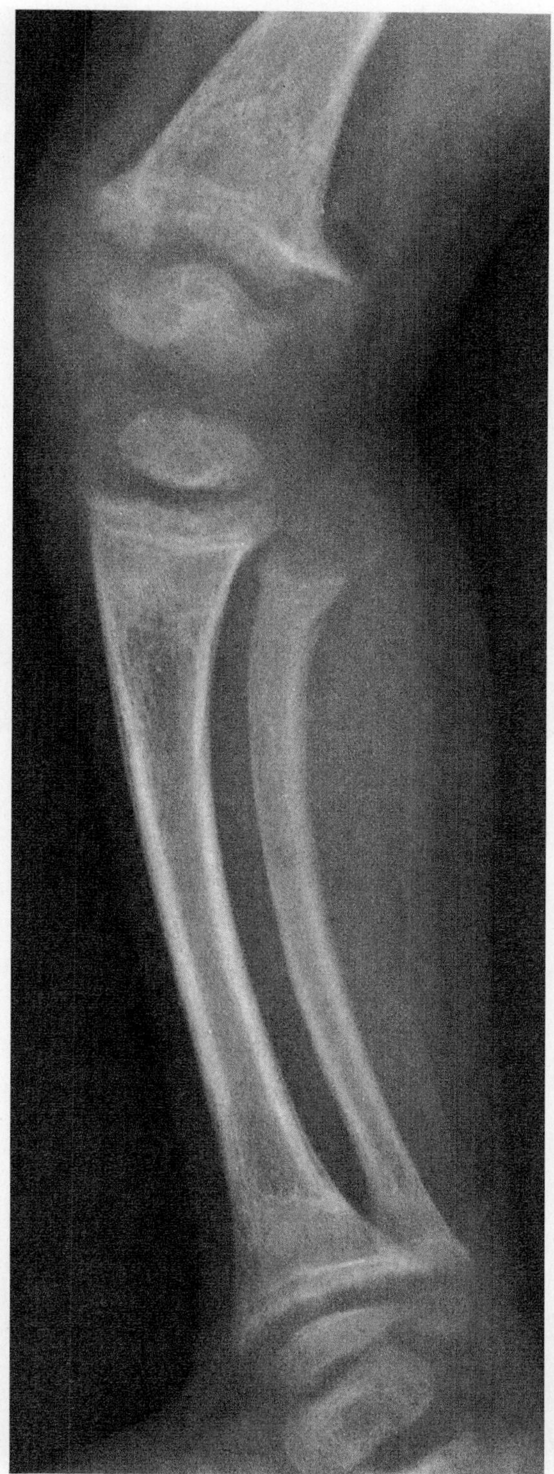

FIGURE 27.13 Rickets. Lateral radiograph of the lower leg of a 3-year-old girl with vitamin D–deficiency rickets shows increased bone radiolucency, widening of the growth plates, cupping and flaring of the metaphyses, and blurring of the outline of the secondary ossification centers, all radiographic hallmarks of this condition. Note also bowing of the tibia and fibula, a frequent feature of rickets.

Histologically, osteomalacia is characterized by excessive quantities of inadequately mineralized bone matrix (osteoid) coating the surfaces of trabeculae in spongy bone and lining the haversian canals in the cortex.

Radiographically, osteomalacia presents with generalized osteopenia, and multiple, bilateral, and often symmetric radiolucent lines are seen in the cortex perpendicular to the long axis of the bone; they are referred to as *pseudofractures* or *Looser zones* (Fig. 27.15; see also Fig. 26.5). These defects,

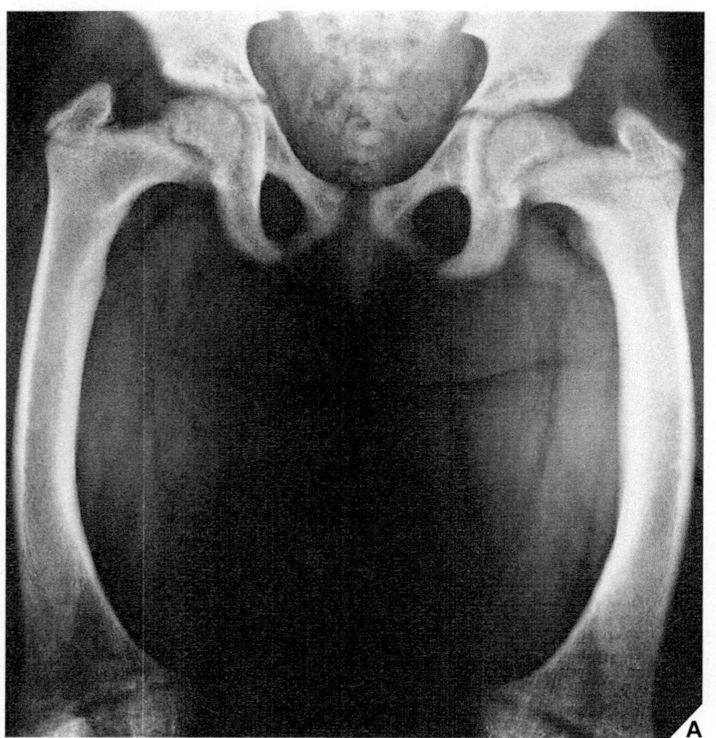

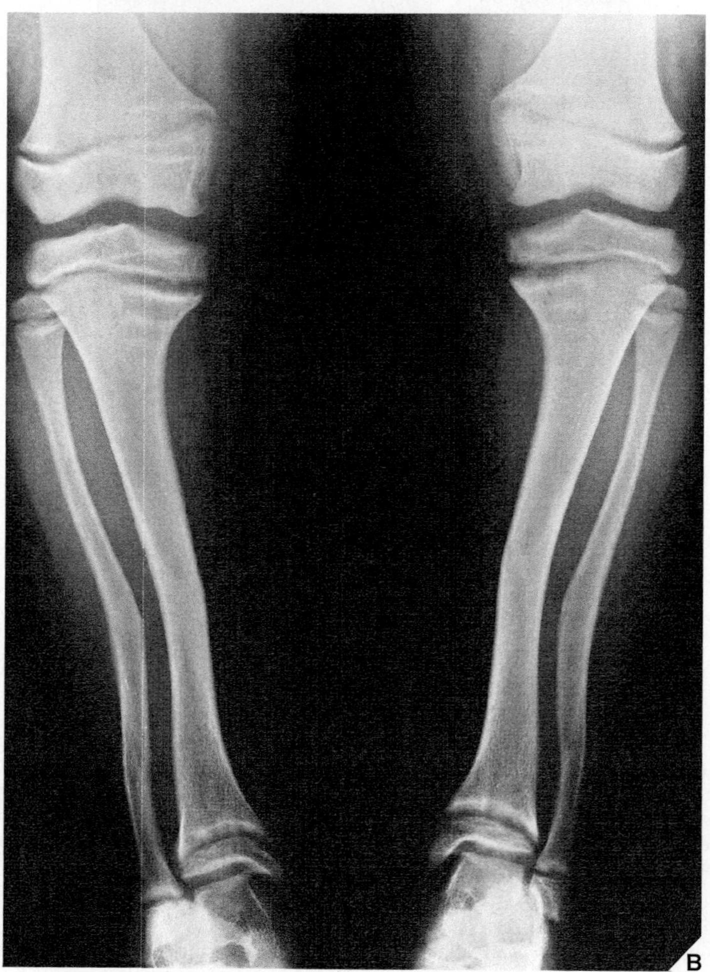

FIGURE 27.14 Vitamin D–resistant rickets. **(A)** Anteroposterior radiograph of the femora of a 9-year-old girl with vitamin D–resistant (hypophosphatemic) rickets shows lateral bowing and shortening of both bones. There is also evidence of sclerotic changes, which are occasionally seen in this condition. **(B)** The radiograph of the knees and lower legs of the same patient shows a bowing deformity of the tibiae and fibulae as well as widening and deformity of the growth plates about the knees and the ankles.

which represent cortical insufficiency stress fractures filled with poorly mineralized callus, osteoid, and fibrous tissue, are common along the axillary margins of the scapulae, the inner margin of the femoral neck, the proximal dorsal aspect of the ulnae, the ribs, and the pubic and ischial rami (Fig. 27.16). The condition, described by Milkman and known as *Milkman syndrome*, is a mild form of osteomalacia in which the pseudofractures are particularly numerous.

An interesting form of osteomalacia is *oncogenic osteomalacia* (also known as *tumor-induced osteomalacia* [TIO]), a paraneoplastic syndrome characterized by hypophosphatemia, hyperphosphaturia, and low levels of plasma 1,25-dihydroxyvitamin D (1,25[OH]$_2$D), caused by a bone and soft-tissue tumors or tumor-like lesions. The tumors commonly responsible for this syndrome are usually benign, slow-growing vascular lesions (such as hemangioma or hemangiopericytoma), osteoblastoma-like lesions, nonossifying fibroma-like lesions, and very rarely some malignant neoplasms. It has been suggested that similar to X-linked hypophosphatemia, mutations in FGF-23 are the etiologic factor in TIO. Tumors producing this syndrome secrete excessive amounts of phosphatonin, which impairs phosphate reabsorption, leading to hypophosphatemia and low levels of 1,25(OH)$_2$D. The clinical symptoms include muscle weakness, bone pain, and occasionally fractures. The condition is reversed when the inciting lesion is resected.

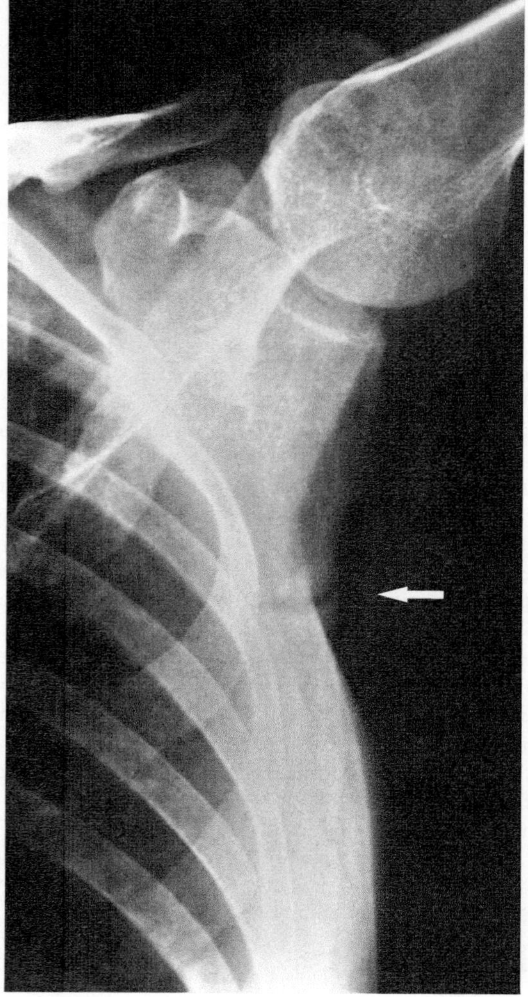

FIGURE 27.15 Osteomalacia. Anteroposterior radiograph of the left shoulder of a 25-year-old woman with osteomalacia caused by malabsorption syndrome shows a radiolucent cleft perpendicular to the cortex of the scapula *(arrow)*. Such defects, known as *pseudofractures* (*Looser zones*), are almost pathognomonic for osteomalacia (see also Fig. 26.5).

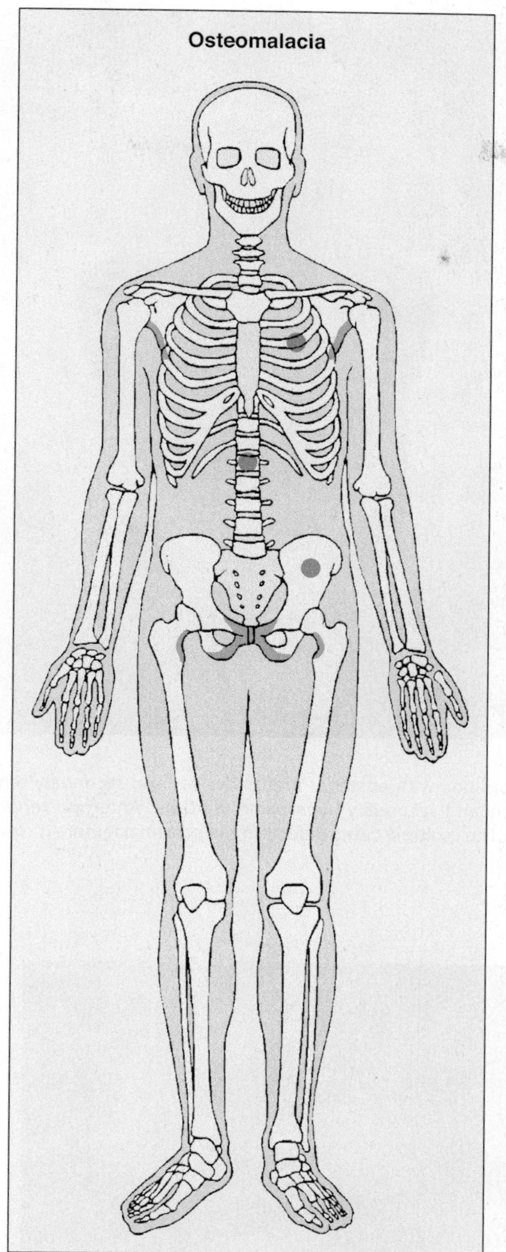

FIGURE 27.16 Target sites of osteomalacia.

Renal Osteodystrophy

A skeletal response to long-standing renal disease, renal osteodystrophy (also referred to as *uremic osteopathy*) is usually associated with chronic renal failure due to glomerulonephritis or pyelonephritis. The condition is also seen in patients who are on dialysis or who have undergone renal transplantation.

Two main mechanisms, acting in unison but varying in severity and proportion, are responsible for osseous changes associated with this condition: secondary hyperparathyroidism and abnormal vitamin D metabolism. The secondary hyperparathyroidism is provoked by phosphate retention and leads to depression of serum calcium, which in turn stimulates release of parathormone from parathyroid glands. The abnormal vitamin D metabolism is affected by renal insufficiency because the kidney is the source of an enzyme, 25-OH-D-1 α-hydroxylase, which converts the inactive vitamin D from 25-hydroxyvitamin D (25-OH-D) to active $1,25(OH)_2D$. Only this most potent, physiologically active form of vitamin D is responsible for calcium and phosphorus homeostasis and for the maintenance of proper bone mineralization.

The major imaging manifestations of renal osteodystrophy are those associated with rickets, osteomalacia, and secondary hyperparathyroidism. Rickets and osteomalacia secondary to renal osteodystrophy are seldom seen in its pure form; usually, there are superimposed changes typical of secondary hyperparathyroidism (Fig. 27.17). Increased bone radiolucency and cortical thinning may be present (Fig. 27.18), but Looser zones are very uncommon. In most patients, some sclerotic changes develop in the bones. Slipped epiphyses may be seen in advanced uremic disease. Soft-tissue calcifications are commonly encountered (Fig. 27.19).

Gross pathologic specimen of the spine shows loss of normal trabecular pattern of the vertebral body with increased sclerosis at the site of the vertebral end plates (Fig. 27.20), mirroring changes seen on the radiographs. Histopathologic examination reveals increased immature, woven bone formation on the surface of bone trabeculae very similar to one seen in the hyperparathyroidism and osteomalacia. There is diffuse paratrabecular fibrosis with prominent osteoclast activity, although some osteoblastic activity is also detected. As the disease progresses, tunneling bone resorption becomes a prominent feature.

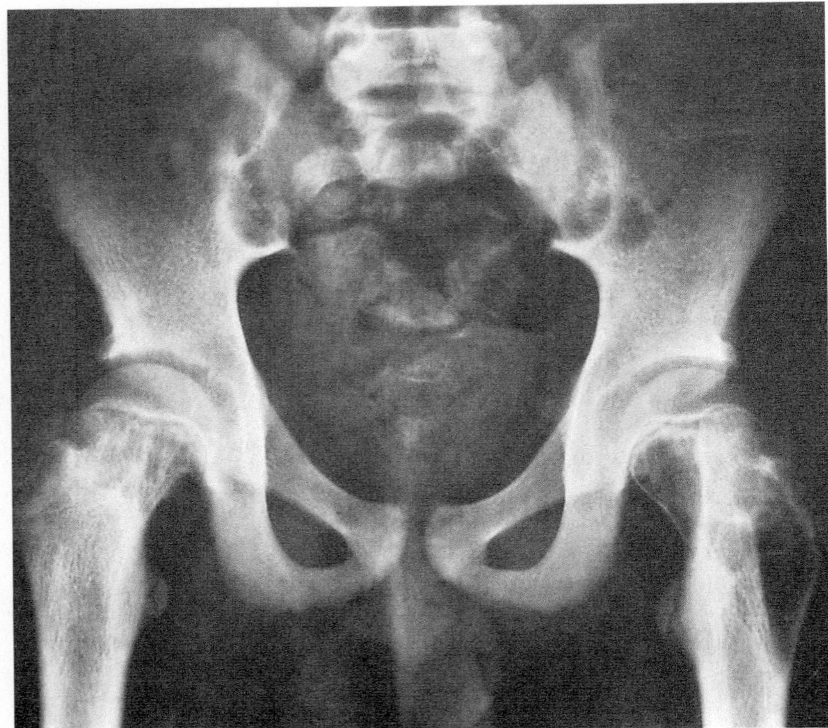

FIGURE 27.17 **Renal osteodystrophy.** A 13-year-old boy with posterior urethral valves and secondary renal failure exhibited radiographic changes typical of renal osteodystrophy, encompassing a mixture of osteomalacia and secondary hyperparathyroidism. Anteroposterior radiograph of the pelvis shows sclerotic changes in the bones and characteristic widening of the sacroiliac joints. The multiple cystic defects in the proximal femora (brown tumors) indicate secondary hyperparathyroidism.

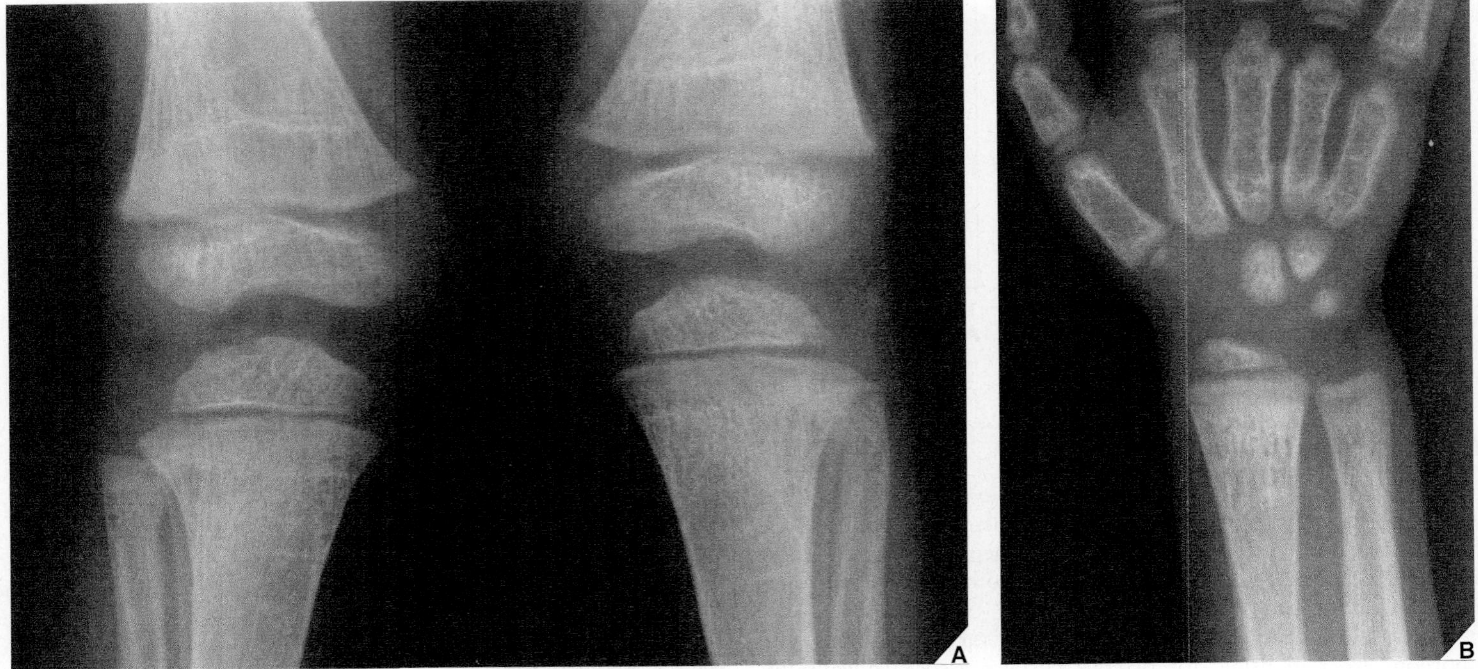

FIGURE 27.18 **Renal osteodystrophy.** **(A)** Anteroposterior radiograph of the knees and **(B)** dorsovolar radiograph of the wrist of a 6-year-old boy with chronic pyelonephritis reveals osteopenic bones and thin cortices. (Courtesy of Philip E. S. Palmer, MD, Davis, California.)

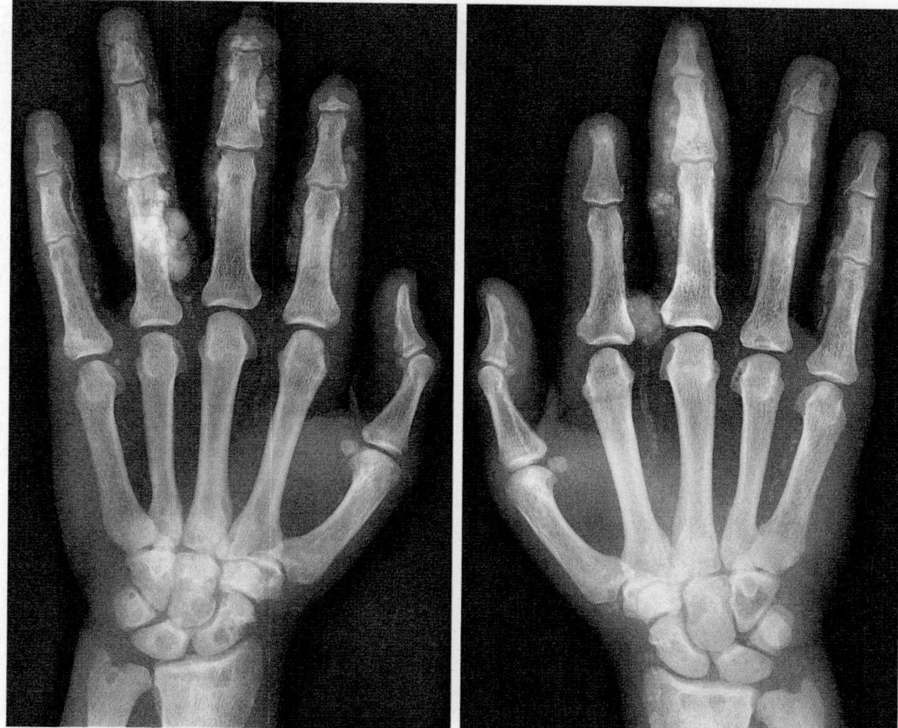

FIGURE 27.19 **Renal osteodystrophy.** Conventional radiographs of the hands of a 45-year-old man on dialysis because of an end-stage renal disease show extensive soft-tissue calcifications and acroosteolysis of the distal phalanges of the index and middle fingers of the right hand and the ring finger of the left hand. Note also several brown tumors in the carpal bones.

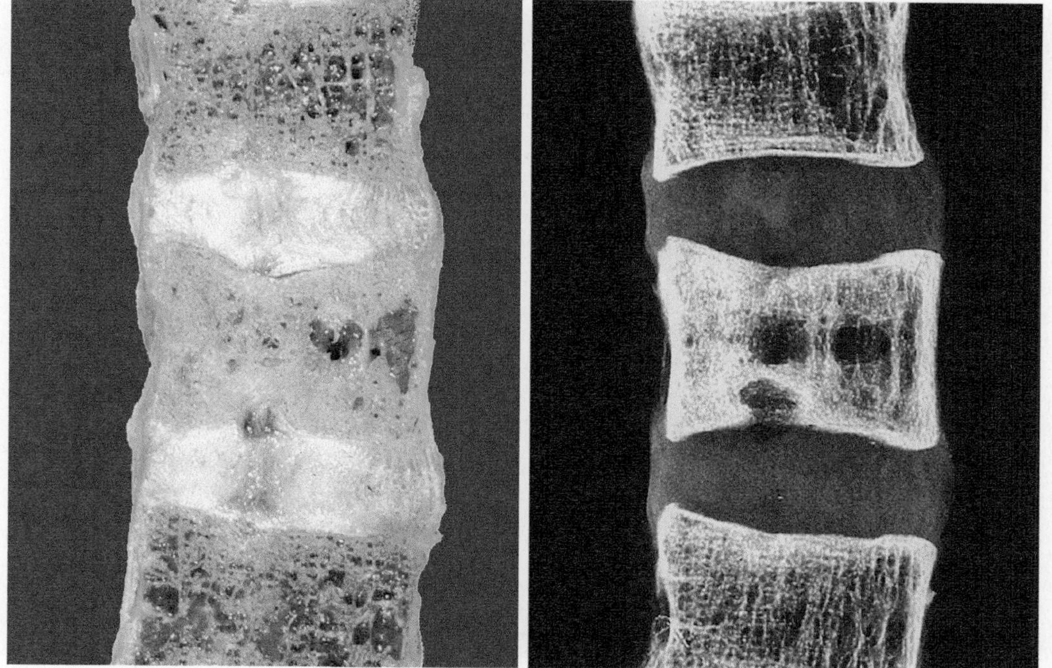

FIGURE 27.20 **Pathology of renal osteodystrophy.** Photograph of a sagittal section of a segment of the lower thoracic spine and specimen radiograph show loss of normal trabecular pattern of the vertebrae with partial collapse and increased sclerosis at the site of the vertebral end plates. (Reprinted from Bullough P. *Orthopaedic pathology*, 5th ed. Maryland Heights, MO: Mosby; 2009, with permission from Elsevier.)

PRACTICAL POINTS TO REMEMBER

Osteoporosis

1. Osteoporosis is characterized by:
   - insufficient formation or increased resorption of bone matrix, resulting in decreased bone mass
   - increased radiolucency of bone and thinning of the cortices on conventional radiography.
2. The target sites of osteoporotic changes are:
   - the axial skeleton (spine and pelvis)
   - the periarticular regions of the appendicular skeleton.
3. The analysis of the trabecular pattern in the proximal end of femur is an effective method of evaluating osteoporosis because patterns of trabecular loss correlate well with increasing severity of osteoporosis.
4. In the spine, characteristic radiographic features that indicate the severity of osteoporotic involvement are:
   - empty box appearance (early stage)
   - codfish vertebrae
   - multiple wedge-shaped fractures (advanced stage).
5. There are several noninvasive methods available that allow accurate measurements of bone mineral density in patients with osteoporosis. The most effective technique is dual-energy x-ray absorptiometry (DEXA), which uses photons produced from a low-dose energy source.

Rickets and Osteomalacia

1. Rickets (in children) and osteomalacia (in adults) are the result of faulty mineralization (calcification) of the bone matrix.
2. On radiographic examination, rickets is characterized by:
   - generalized osteopenia
   - bowing deformities of the long bones, particularly the femur and tibia
   - widening of the growth plate (secondary to deficient mineralization in the provisional zone of calcification) and cupping or flaring of the metaphysis, particularly in the proximal humerus, distal radius and ulna, and distal femur.
3. The radiographic findings in vitamin D–resistant rickets are similar to those in infantile rickets. Bowing deformities and shortening of the long bones are, however, more pronounced.
4. Radiographically, osteomalacia is characterized by:
   - generalized osteopenia
   - symmetric radiolucent lines in the cortex (Looser zones or pseudofractures).
5. Renal osteodystrophy, usually associated with chronic renal failure due to glomerulonephritis or pyelonephritis, represents a skeletal response to long-standing renal disease. The major radiographic manifestations are those associated with rickets, osteomalacia, and secondary hyperparathyroidism, with predominance of osteosclerosis, bone resorption, and bowing deformities.

SUGGESTED READINGS

Beaulieu JG, Razzano D, Levine RB. Transient osteoporosis of the hip in pregnancy. *Clin Orthop Relat Res* 1976;115:165–168.

Briggs AM, Wrigley TV, Tully EA, et al. Radiographic measures of thoracic kyphosis in osteoporosis: Cobb and vertebral centroid angles. *Skeletal Radiol* 2007;36:761–767.

Carpenter TO. Oncogenic osteomalacia—a complex dance of factors. *N Engl J Med* 2003;348:1705–1708.

Chong WH, Molinolo AA, Chen CC, et al. Tumor-induced osteomalacia. *Endocr Relat Cancer* 2011;18:R53–R77.

Gillespy T III, Gillespy MP. Osteoporosis. *Radiol Clin North Am* 1991;29:77–84.

Hesse E, Rosenthal H, Bastian L. Radiofrequency ablation of a tumor causing oncogenic osteomalacia. *New Engl J Med* 2007;357:422–424.

Hunder GG, Kelly PJ. Roentgenologic transient osteoporosis of the hip. A clinical syndrome? *Ann Intern Med* 1968;68:539–552.

Jones G. Radiological appearance of disuse osteoporosis. *Clin Radiol* 1969;20:345–353.

Jonsson KB, Zahradnik R, Larsson T, et al. Fibroblast growth factor 23 in oncogenic osteomalacia and X-linked hypophosphatemia. *N Engl J Med* 2003;348:1656–1663.

Lang P, Steiger P, Faulkner K, et al. Osteoporosis: current techniques and recent developments in quantitative bone densitometry. *Radiol Clin North Am* 1991;29:49–76.

Mayo-Smith W, Rosenthal DI. Radiographic appearance of osteopenia. *Radiol Clin North Am* 1991;29:37–47.

Milkman LA. Pseudofractures (hunger osteopathy, late rickets, osteomalacia). *Am J Roentgenol* 1930;24:29–37.

Murphey MD, Sartoris DJ, Quale JL, et al. Musculoskeletal manifestations of chronic renal insufficiency. *Radiographics* 1993;13:357–379.

Murphy WA Jr, DiVito DM. Fuller Albright, postmenopausal osteoporosis, and fish vertebrae. *Radiology* 2013;268:323–326.

Pitt MJ. Rickets and osteomalacia are still around. *Radiol Clin North Am* 1991;29:97–118.

Sundaram M. Founders lecture 2007: metabolic bone disease: what has changed in 30 years? *Skeletal Radiol* 2009;38:841–853.

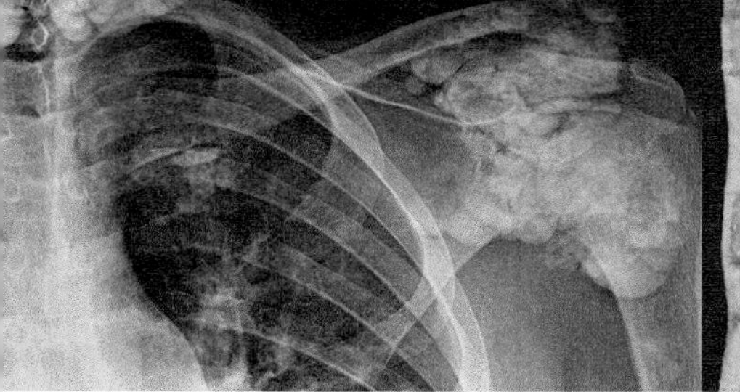
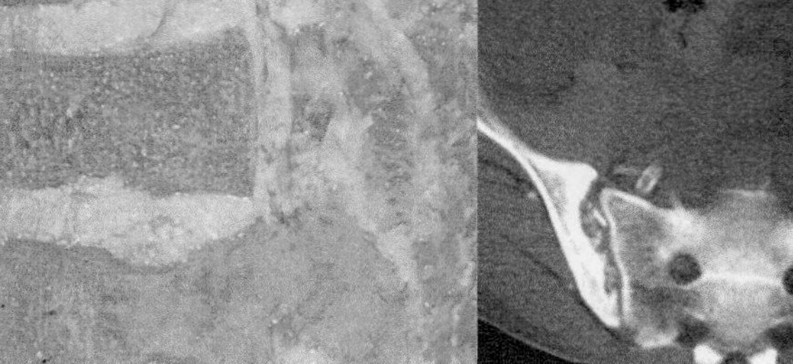

28

Hyperparathyroidism

Pathophysiology

Hyperparathyroidism, also known as *generalized osteitis fibrosa cystica* or *Recklinghausen disease of bone*, is the result of overactivity of the parathormone-producing parathyroid glands. Increased production of this hormone is secondary to either gland hyperplasia (9% of cases) or adenoma (90%); only in very rare instances (1%) does hyperparathyroidism occur secondary to parathyroid carcinoma. Excessive secretion of parathormone, which acts on the kidneys and on bone, leads to disturbances in calcium and phosphorus metabolism, resulting in hypercalcemia, hyperphosphaturia, and hypophosphatemia. Renal excretion of calcium and phosphate is increased, and serum levels of calcium are elevated, whereas those of phosphorus are reduced. Serum levels of alkaline phosphatase are also elevated.

Hyperparathyroidism can be divided into primary, secondary, and tertiary forms. The classic form of the disorder, *primary hyperparathyroidism*, is marked by an increased secretion of parathormone resulting from hyperplasia, adenoma, or carcinoma of the parathyroid glands. Primary hyperparathyroidism is usually associated with hypercalcemia. Women are affected about 3 times as often as men, and the condition is most commonly seen in the patient's third to fifth decade. Primary hyperparathyroidism is a genetically heterogenous disorder caused by mutations in the *MEN1*, *CDC73*, or *CASR* gene. The *MEN1* gene regulates production of a protein menin, which acts as a tumor suppressor. The *CDC73* gene provides instructions for making the parafibromin protein, another tumor suppressor. The loss of parafibromin's tumor suppressor function leads to the development of parathyroid adenoma, or parathyroid carcinoma. The *CASR* gene provides instructions for producing a protein called the *calcium-sensing receptor* (CaSR) responsible for regulating the amount of calcium in the body, in part by controlling the production of parathormone.

Secondary hyperparathyroidism is caused by an increased secretion of parathyroid hormone (PTH) in response to a sustained hypocalcemic state. Usually, the fundamental cause of parathyroid gland hyperfunction is impaired renal function. Hyperphosphatemia due to renal failure results in chronic hypocalcemia, which in turn promotes increased parathyroid secretion. Although secondary hyperparathyroidism is usually hypocalcemic, it may be normocalcemic as an adaptive response to the hypocalcemic state. *Tertiary hyperparathyroidism* represents a transformation from a hypocalcemic to a hypercalcemic state. The parathyroid glands "escape" from the regulatory effect of serum calcium levels. Patients in whom this escape occurs are usually receiving kidney hemodialysis; they are considered to have autonomous hyperparathyroidism.

Although primary hyperparathyroidism is traditionally synonymous with the hypercalcemic form of the disorder, some patients nonetheless may have normal or even reduced serum calcium levels. For this reason, Reiss and Canterbury proposed an alternative method of classifying hyperparathyroidism based on serum calcium levels. In this system, hyperparathyroidism is considered either hypercalcemic, normocalcemic, or hypocalcemic.

In order to understand the clinical, pathologic, and imaging manifestations of hyperparathyroidism, knowledge of the interrelated roles of PTH and vitamin D in the metabolism of calcium is essential.

Physiology of Calcium Metabolism

Serum concentrations of calcium are maintained within a narrow normal physiologic range (2.20 to 2.65 mmol per L or 8.8 to 10.6 mg per dL) by the intestines and kidneys, the major sites of classic negative feedback mechanisms that balance calcium intake and excretion. The bones also contribute to preserving calcium homeostasis and, because they represent approximately 99% of elemental calcium in the human body, are considered to be a calcium reservoir. Essential to these mechanisms involving a variety of hormones is the action of PTH, a polypeptide hormone whose secretion is induced by a decrease in the level of calcium in the extracellular fluid. In primary hyperparathyroidism, there is inappropriate oversecretion of PTH in the presence of elevated serum calcium levels, whereas secondary hyperparathyroidism is marked by appropriate PTH production in response to chronic hypocalcemia.

PTH works to increase serum calcium concentrations by several means. Predominant among these is conserving calcium in the kidneys by promoting both increased reabsorption of calcium and increased excretion of phosphates in the distal renal tubules. PTH also promotes release of calcium and phosphorus from bone by increasing the number and activity of osteoclasts, resulting in bone resorption, although the exact mechanism by which this occurs is not fully understood. Finally, although PTH has been shown to have no direct effect on intestinal calcium absorption, it plays a role in stimulating vitamin D metabolism, with subsequent increased absorption of calcium and phosphorus by the intestines.

Both forms of vitamin D in the human body—ergocalciferol (vitamin D_2), a synthetic compound and frequent food additive; and cholecalciferol (vitamin D_3), formed predominantly in the skin from 7-dehydrocholesterol by the action of ultraviolet light—are metabolized to 25-hydroxyvitamin D in the liver. The critical step in the metabolism of vitamin D occurs in the kidneys, where 25-hydroxyvitamin D undergoes hydroxylation to its most active form, 1,25-dihydroxyvitamin D, and an inactive metabolite, 24,25-dihydroxyvitamin D. This step is catalyzed by the renal enzyme 1-α-hydroxylase, which is synthesized in the kidneys under the stimulation of PTH in the presence of decreased serum calcium and phosphate levels. This gives the kidneys a unique central role in the metabolism of vitamin D. 1,25-Dihydroxyvitamin D is the primary mediator of calcium and phosphorus absorption in the small intestine. The kidneys also have the ability to switch between producing the active and inactive forms of vitamin D, yielding a fine control of calcium metabolism.

Clinical Features

Hyperparathyroidism is known as a *disease of stones and bones*. The symptoms of hyperparathyroidism are related to nephrolithiasis, skeletal abnormalities, and hypercalcemia. Hypercalcemia produces weakness, muscular hypotonia, nausea, anorexia, constipation, polyuria, and thirst. The skeletal abnormalities most commonly seen are generalized osteopenia and foci of bone destruction, which are commonly referred to as *brown tumors*. These pseudotumors represent areas of fibrous scarring in which osteoclasts collect, blood decomposes, and cysts form. The most common sites of involvement are the mandible, clavicle, ribs, pelvis, and femur. Also, subchondral and subperiosteal bone resorption is invariably present. Kidney involvement results in nephrocalcinosis, impairment of renal function, and uremia.

Imaging Features

The major target sites in the skeletal system for hyperparathyroidism are the shoulder, the hand, the vertebrae, and the skull (Fig. 28.1). Conventional radiography is usually sufficient to demonstrate its characteristic features: generalized osteopenia; subperiosteal, subchondral, and cortical bone resorption; brown tumors; and soft-tissue and cartilage calcifications (secondary tumoral calcinosis). Subperiosteal resorption is particularly well demonstrated on radiographs of the hands, where it usually affects the radial aspects of the middle phalanges of the middle and index fingers (Fig. 28.2; see also Figs. 26.7 and 26.9), although other bones can also be affected (Fig. 28.3). Commonly, subchondral bone resorption is present resulting in depression of overlying articular cartilage (Fig. 28.4). Also characteristic of this condition is resorption of the acromial ends of the clavicle (Fig. 28.5). Intracortical resorption is manifested by longitudinal striations, a finding known as *tunneling*, which can be most clearly appreciated on magnification studies (see Fig. 26.9B,C). Another characteristic feature is loss of the lamina dura around the tooth socket, which normally is seen as a thin sharp white line surrounding the peridental membrane that attaches the tooth to bone (Fig. 28.6). In the skull, there is a characteristic mottling of the vault, which yields a "salt-and-pepper" appearance (Fig. 28.7). Localized destructive changes in bones affected by hyperparathyroidism take the form of cyst-like lesions of various sizes, commonly referred to as *brown tumors*. The jaw, pelvis, and femora are the usual sites for these lesions, but they may be found in any part of the skeleton (Fig. 28.8).

In secondary hyperparathyroidism, other characteristic features may be present in addition to the imaging abnormalities just discussed. A generalized increase in bone density occurs, particularly in younger patients. In the spine, this change is reflected in dense sclerotic bands seen adjacent to the vertebral end plates, giving the vertebrae a sandwich-like appearance. This phenomenon is termed *rugger-jersey spine* because the sclerotic bands form horizontal stripes resembling those of rugby shirts (Figs. 28.9 and 28.10). However, it must be kept in mind in the evaluation of hyperparathyroidism

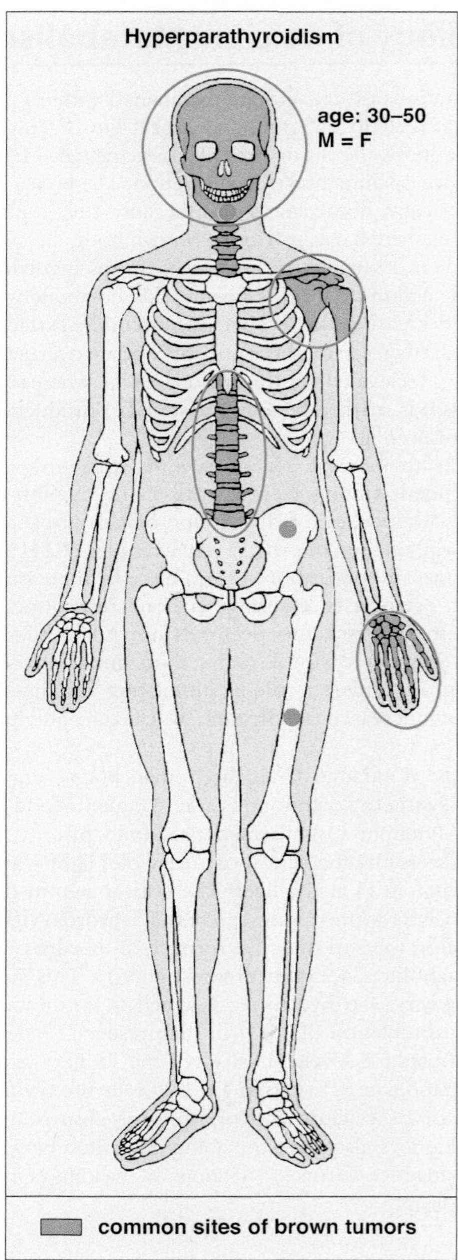

FIGURE 28.1 Major target sites of hyperparathyroidism.

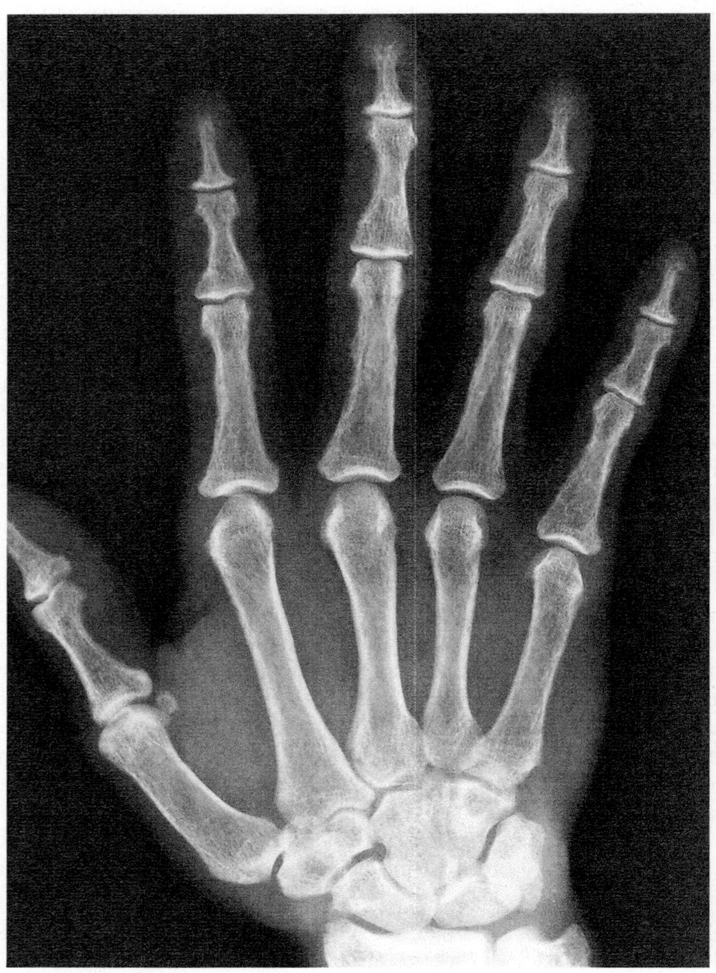

FIGURE 28.2 Primary hyperparathyroidism. Dorsovolar radiograph of the left hand of a 42-year-old man with primary hyperparathyroidism caused by hypertrophy of the parathyroid glands shows typical subperiosteal resorption affecting primarily the radial aspects of the middle phalanges of the middle and index fingers.

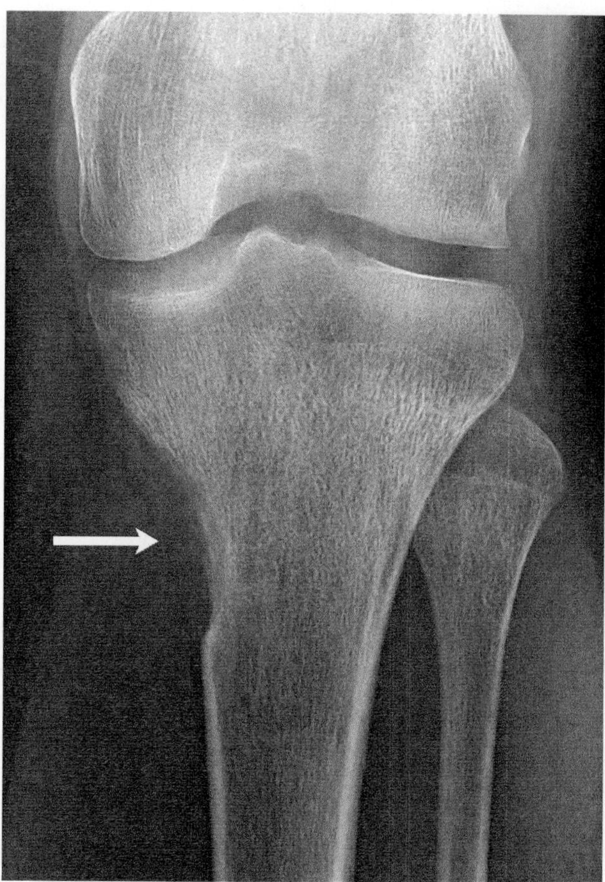

FIGURE 28.3 **Primary hyperparathyroidism.** Anteroposterior radiograph of the knee of a 32-year-old man shows a subperiosteal and cortical resorption at the medial aspect of the tibia *(arrow)*.

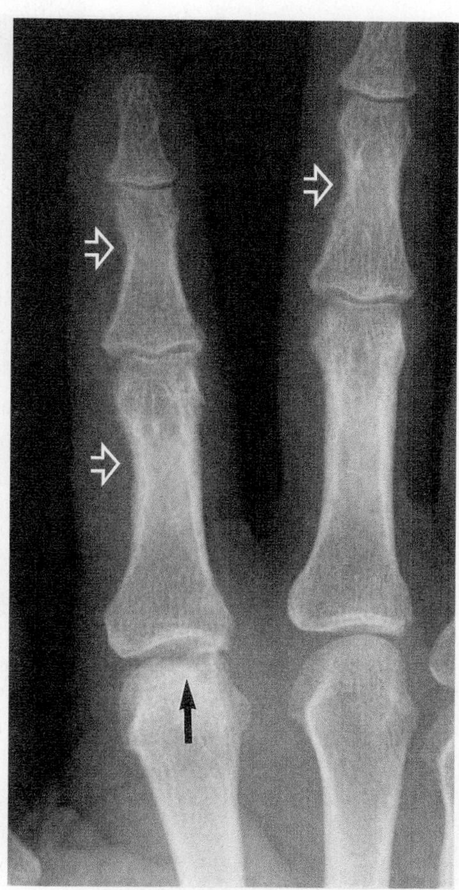

FIGURE 28.4 **Primary hyperparathyroidism.** Subchondral bone resorption is present at the head of the second metacarpal *(arrow)*. Note also subperiosteal resorption at the proximal and distal phalanges *(open arrows)*.

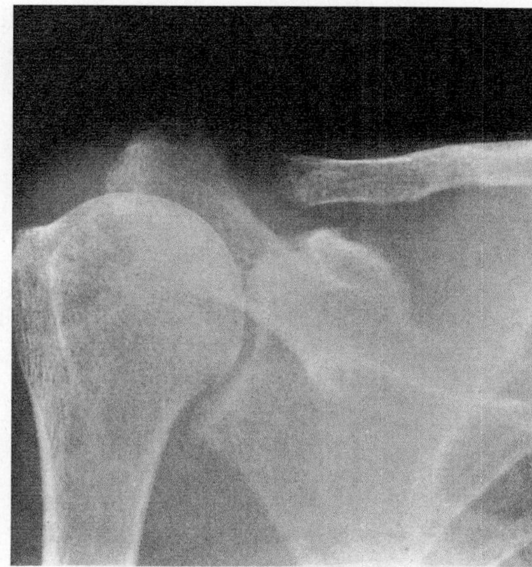

FIGURE 28.5 **Primary hyperparathyroidism.** Anteroposterior radiograph of the right shoulder of a 36-year-old woman shows resorption of the acromial end of the clavicle.

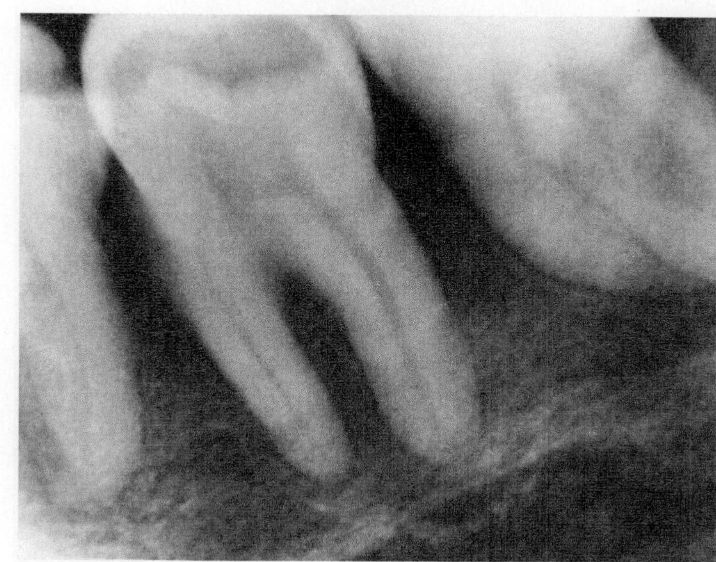

FIGURE 28.6 **Primary hyperparathyroidism.** Radiograph of the lower second molar tooth shows loss of the lamina dura around the tooth socket.

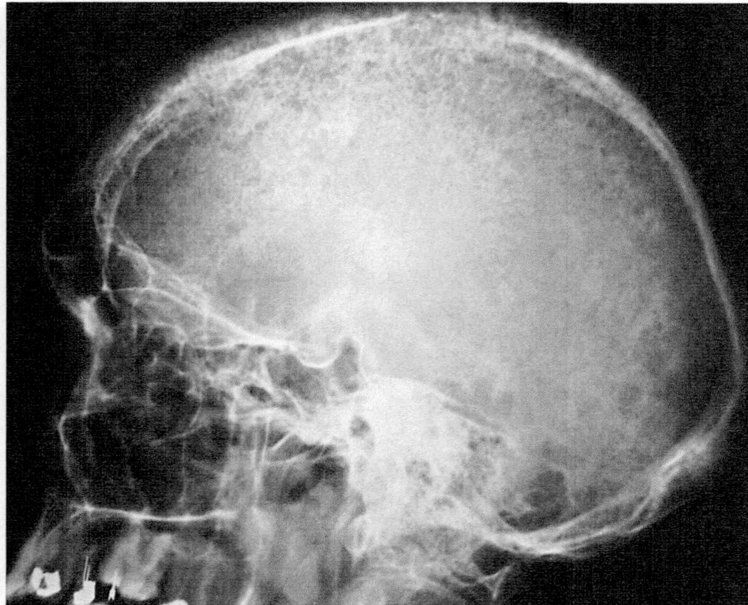

FIGURE 28.7 Primary hyperparathyroidism. Lateral radiograph of the skull of the patient seen in Figure 28.2 demonstrates a decrease in the overall density of the bone and a granular appearance of the cranial vault—the so-called *salt-and-pepper skull*.

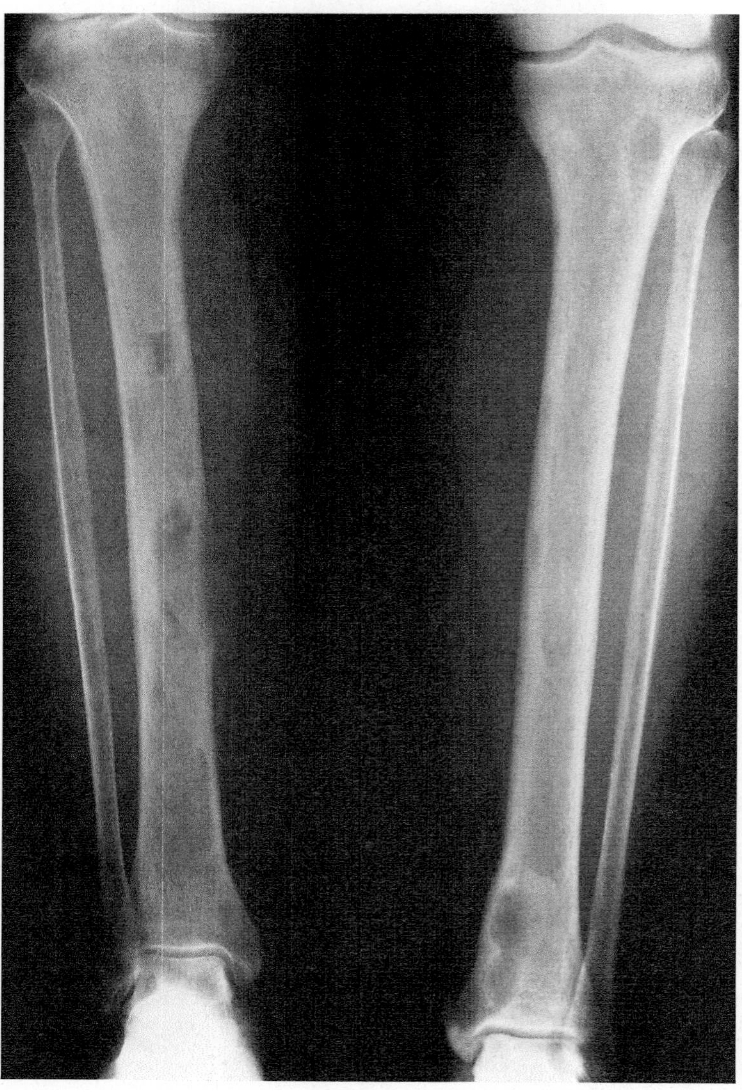

FIGURE 28.8 Primary hyperparathyroidism. Anteroposterior radiograph of the lower legs of the same patient seen in Figure 28.5 shows multiple lytic lesions (brown tumors) in both tibiae.

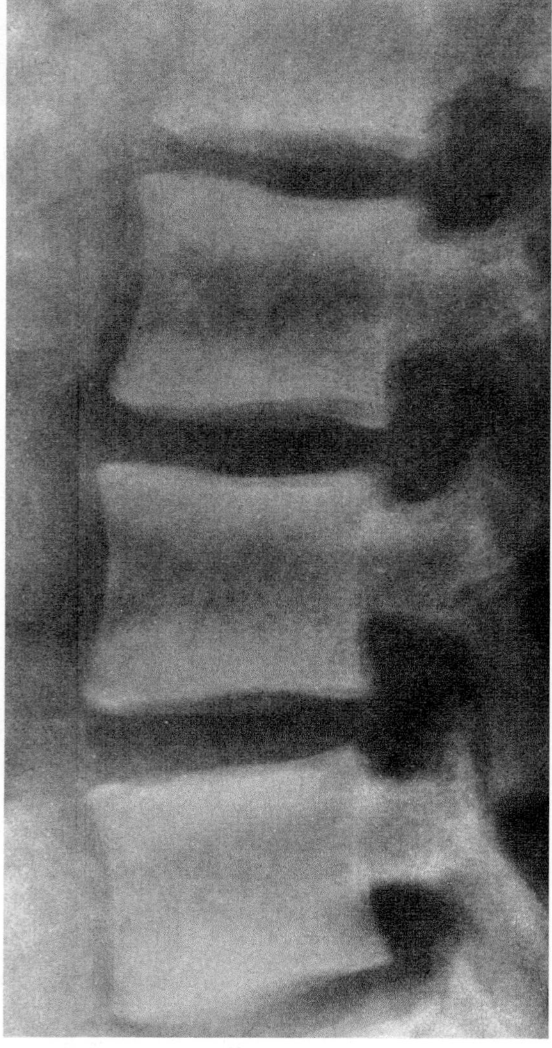

FIGURE 28.9 Secondary hyperparathyroidism. A 17-year-old boy with chronic renal failure developed secondary hyperparathyroidism. Lateral radiograph of the lumbar spine demonstrates sclerotic bands adjacent to the vertebral end plates—the so-called *rugger-jersey spine*.

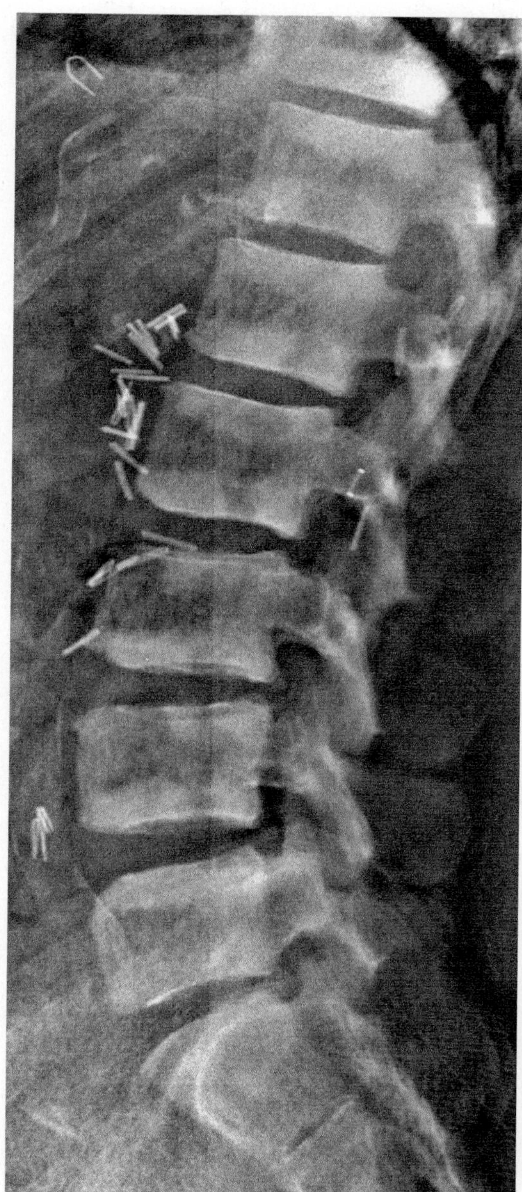

FIGURE 28.10 **Secondary hyperparathyroidism.** Lateral radiograph of the lumbar spine of a 68-year-old man with renal failure shows typical appearance of the so-called *rugger-jersey spine*.

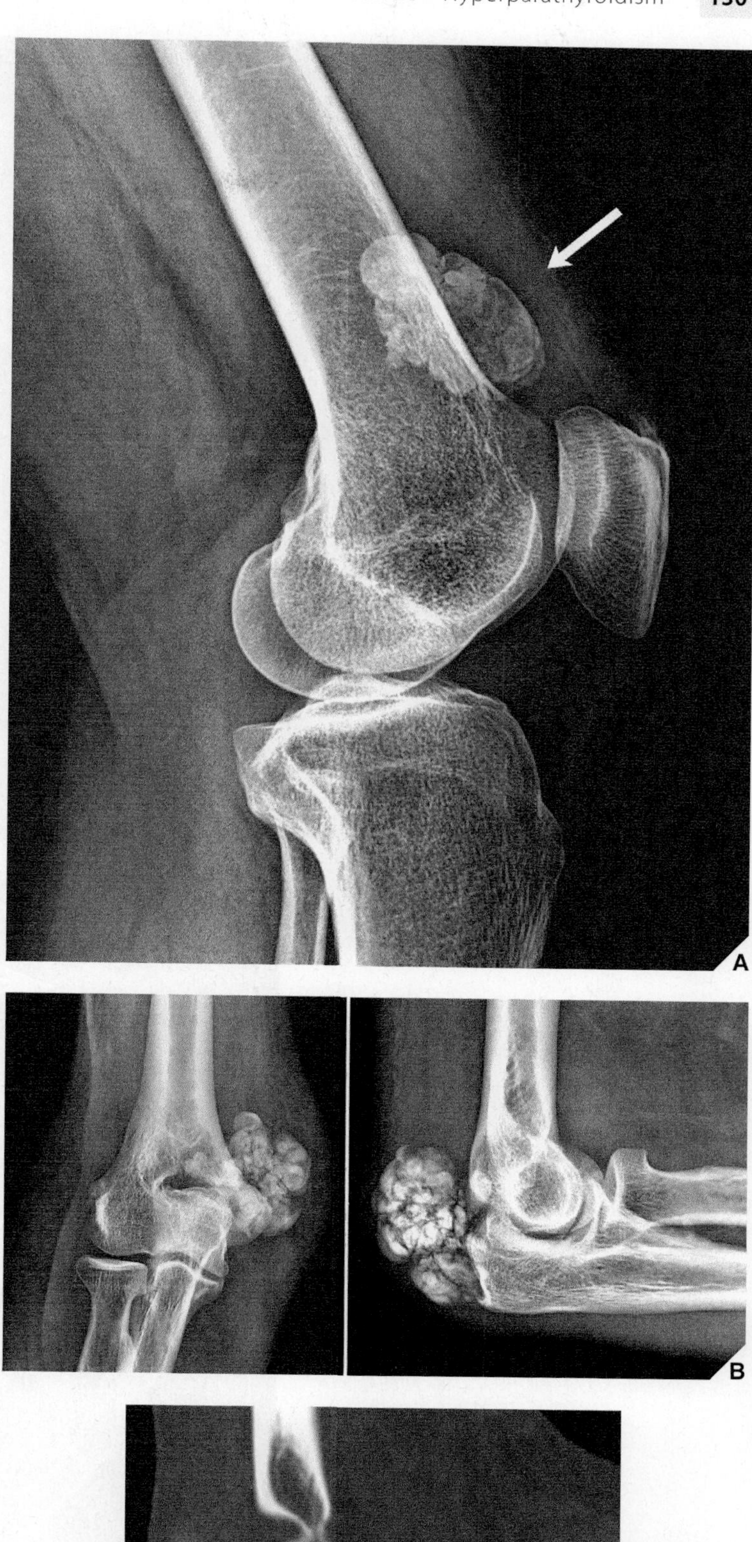

FIGURE 28.11 **Secondary hyperparathyroidism.** A 52-year-old man with clinical diagnosis of renal failure and secondary hyperparathyroidism presented with soft-tissue calcifications at several sites including **(A)** the knee *(arrow)* and **(B,C)** elbow.

that osteosclerotic changes may also occur as a manifestation of healing, either spontaneously or as a result of treatment. Deposition of calcium in fibrocartilage, articular cartilage, and soft tissue is common (Fig. 28.11), and vascular calcifications are much more frequent in patients with secondary hyperparathyroidism (Figs. 28.12 and 28.13). Bone resorption involving the subchondral bone may lead to pseudowidening of the affected joints, characteristically within the sacroiliac joints (Fig. 28.13D).

Pathology

Early histopathologic changes consist of fibrovascular proliferation that displaces the bone marrow in a paratrabecular distribution. This is accompanied by increased osteoclastic activity. The bone trabeculae become ragged and scalloped. Dissection of osseous trabeculae by groups of osteoclasts leave characteristic tunnels inside the bone. Cortical porosity is greatly increased in such a way that the compact bones comes to resemble cancellous bone. This process is known as *tunneling* or *dissecting resorption* and is characteristic of hyperthyroid bone disease. In addition, localized areas of massive bone resorption associated with hemorrhage leads to formation of "brown tumors" (Fig. 28.14).

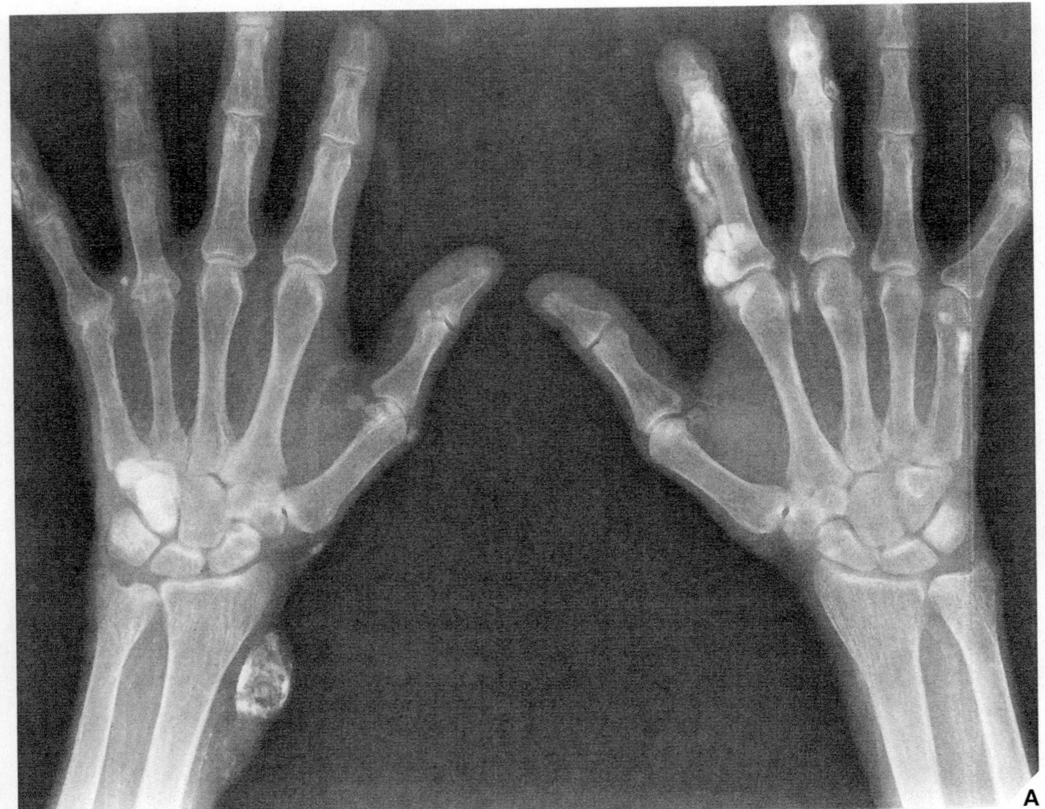

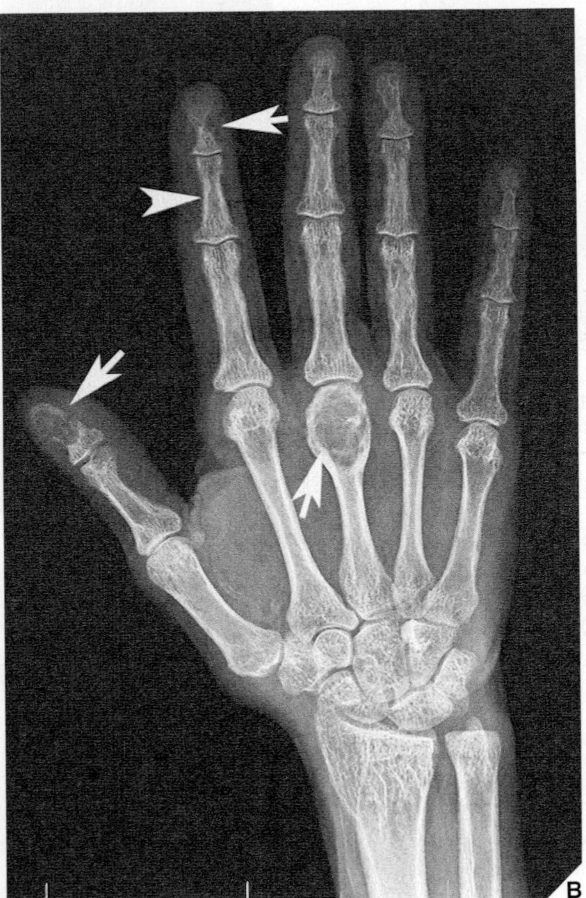

FIGURE 28.12 Secondary hyperparathyroidism. **(A)** Posteroanterior radiograph of the distal forearms and hands of a 48-year-old woman shows evidence of soft-tissue and vascular calcifications, characteristic findings in secondary hyperparathyroidism. Note also diffuse osteopenia. **(B)** Dorsovolar radiograph of the hand of another patient with secondary hyperparathyroidism due to chronic renal failure demonstrates multiple lytic lesions in the third metacarpal, distal first phalanx, and distal second phalanx, representing brown tumors *(arrows)*. Note the characteristic subperiosteal bone resorption involving multiple phalanges *(arrowhead)* and the presence of vascular calcifications.

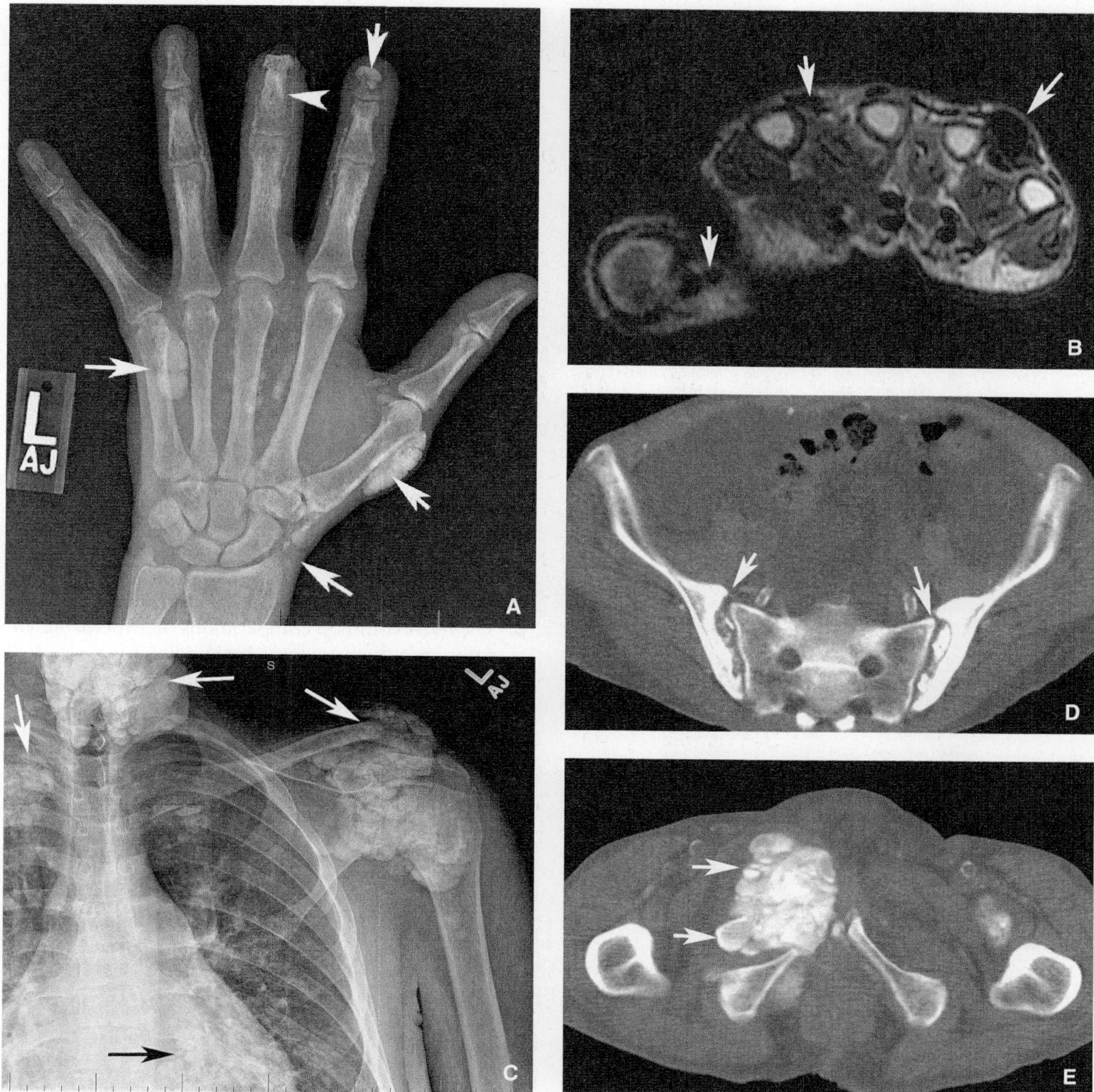

FIGURE 28.13 CT and MRI of secondary hyperparathyroidism. **(A)** Posteroanterior radiograph of the left hand of a 53-year-old woman with chronic renal disease and secondary hyperparathyroidism shows multiple calcific deposits in the soft tissues *(arrows)*, extensive vascular calcifications, and subperiosteal bone resorption better seen in the middle phalanx of the third digit *(arrowhead)*. The patient had a prior amputation of the distal phalanx of the third digit. **(B)** Axial T2-weighted magnetic resonance image of the left hand demonstrates hypointense foci in the subcutaneous tissue *(arrows)* corresponding to the calcific deposits seen on the radiographs. **(C)** Anteroposterior radiograph of the left shoulder shows multiple calcific deposits in the left shoulder, neck, and chest wall *(arrows)*. **(D)** Axial CT section of the pelvis demonstrates bone sclerosis and pseudowidening of the sacroiliac joints *(arrows)* due to subchondral bone resorption. **(E)** Axial CT of the lower pelvis shows a large calcific deposit (secondary tumoral calcinosis) with multiple calcium-fluid levels *(arrows)*.

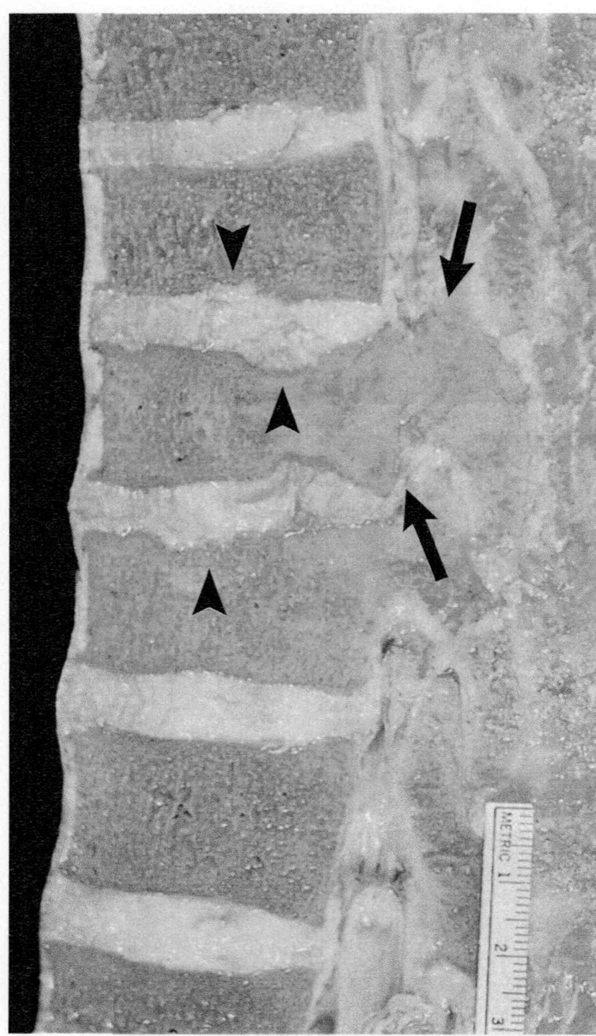

FIGURE 28.14 Pathology of hyperparathyroidism. Photograph of a sagittal section through a segment of thoracolumbar spine shows distortion of cancellous bone trabeculae and partial resorption of the vertebral end plates *(arrowheads)*. One of the vertebral bodies shows a large destructive lesion extending posteriorly into the spinal canal filled with brownish-tan tissue *(arrows)*. On microscopic examination, this proved to be a brown tumor. (Reprinted from Bullough P. *Orthopaedic pathology*, 5th ed. Maryland Heights, MO: Mosby; 2009, with permission from Elsevier.)

Complications

Both primary and secondary hyperparathyroidism may be complicated by pathologic fractures, which usually occur in the ribs and vertebral bodies. Hyperparathyroidism arthropathy, another frequent complication, has been discussed in more detail in Chapter 15. Slipped capital femoral or humeral epiphysis may also be observed on occasion. The involvement of ligaments and tendons results in capsular and ligamentous laxity, which may lead to joint instability. Occasionally, spontaneous tendon avulsion has been observed, a phenomenon attributed to the direct effect of PTH on connective tissue. Even less frequently, intraarticular crystal deposition (calcium pyrophosphate dihydrate) in cartilage, capsule, and synovium may occur, which may lead to the pseudogout syndrome.

PRACTICAL POINTS TO REMEMBER

1. The typical radiographic changes of primary (hypercalcemic) hyperparathyroidism include:
   - generalized osteopenia
   - subperiosteal, subchondral, and cortical resorption
   - resorption of the acromial end of the clavicle
   - a salt-and-pepper appearance of the skull
   - cyst-like lesions (brown tumors) of varying sizes.
2. Subperiosteal resorption of bone is best demonstrated on a dorsovolar radiograph of the hands because these changes characteristically occur on the radial aspects of the middle phalanges of the middle and index fingers.
3. Subchondral resorption of bone is most commonly seen in the sacroiliac, sternoclavicular, and acromioclavicular joints.
4. Cortical resorption (tunneling) is best appreciated on magnification radiography of the hand or long bones.
5. Secondary hyperparathyroidism (due to renal disease) is typified radiographically by:
   - a generalized increase in bone density
   - sclerotic bands adjacent to the vertebral end plates, known as *rugger-jersey spine*
   - soft-tissue calcifications.
6. The most common complications of hyperparathyroidism include pathologic fractures (vertebral bodies, ribs), metabolic arthropathies, and slipped epiphyses (femoral and humeral).

SUGGESTED READINGS

Beale MG, Salcedo JR, Ellis D, et al. Renal osteodystrophy. *Pediatr Clin North Am* 1976;23:873–884.

Brandi ML, Falchetti A. Genetics of primary hyperparathyroidism. *Urol Int* 2004;72(suppl 1):11–16.

Brecht-Krauss D, Kusmierek J, Hellwig D, et al. Quantitative bone scintigraphy in patients with hyperparathyroidism. *J Nucl Med* 1987;28:458–461.

Brown TW, Genant HK, Hattner RS, et al. Multiple brown tumors in a patient with chronic renal failure and secondary hyperparathyroidism. *AJR Am J Roentgenol* 1977;128:131–134.

de Graaf P, Schicht IM, Pauwels EKJ, et al. Bone scintigraphy in renal osteodystrophy. *J Nucl Med* 1978;19:1289–1296.

Genant HK, Heck LL, Lanzl LH, et al. Primary hyperparathyroidism. A comprehensive study of clinical, biochemical and radiographic manifestations. *Radiology* 1973;109:513–524.

Hooge WA, Li D. CT of sacroiliac joints in secondary hyperparathyroidism. *J Can Assoc Radiol* 1981;32:42–44.

Massry S, Ritz E. The pathogenesis of secondary hyperparathyroidism of renal failure. Is there a controversy? *Arch Intern Med* 1978;138:853–856.

Murphey MD, Sartoris DJ, Quale JL, et al. Musculoskeletal manifestations of chronic renal insufficiency. *Radiographics* 1993;13:357–379.

Olsen KM, Chew FS. Tumoral calcinosis: pearls, polemics, and alternative possibilities. *Radiographics* 2006;26:871–885.

Reiss E, Canterbury JM. Spectrum of hyperparathyroidism. *Am J Med* 1974;56:794–799.

Resnick D. Erosive arthritis of the hand and wrist in hyperparathyroidism. *Radiology* 1974;110:263–269.

Resnick D. The "rugger jersey" vertebral body. *Arthritis Rheum* 1981;24:1191–1192.

Resnick D, Niwayama G. Subchondral resorption of bone in renal osteodystrophy. *Radiology* 1976;118:315–321.

Roche CJ, O'Keeffe DP, Lee WK, et al. Selections from the buffet of food signs in radiology. *Radiographics* 2002;22:1369–1384.

Sundaram M, Joyce PF, Shields JB, et al. Terminal phalangeal tufts: earliest site of renal osteodystrophy findings in hemodialysis patients. *AJR Am J Roentgenol* 1979;133:25–29.

Teplick JG, Eftekhari F, Haskin ME. Erosion of the sternal ends of the clavicles. A new sign of primary and secondary hyperparathyroidism. *Radiology* 1974;113:323–326.

Wittenberg A. The rugger jersey spine sign. *Radiology* 2004;230:491–492.

29

Paget Disease

Pathophysiology and Clinical Features

Paget disease, a relatively common bone disorder, is a chronic, progressive disturbance in bone metabolism that primarily affects older persons. It is slightly more common in men than in women (3:2), with an average age of onset between 45 and 55 years, although the disease has been known to occur in young adults. The prevalence of Paget disease varies considerably in different parts of the world, reaching its greatest incidence in Great Britain, Australia, and New Zealand.

The precise nature of Paget disease and its etiology are still debatable. Sir James Paget named the disease *osteitis deformans* in the belief that the basic process was infectious in origin. Other etiologies have also been proposed, such as neoplastic, vascular, endocrinologic, immunologic, traumatic, and hereditary. The hereditary etiology was supported by identification of mutations in the gene *SQSTM1*, which encodes a protein p62 involved in regulating osteoclast functioning, in patients with familial and sporadic Paget disease. In addition, mutations at the *CSF1*, *OPTN*, and *TNFRSF11A* genes have been linked with risk factors for Paget disease. Patients with *SQSTM1* mutations tend to have more severe Paget disease and a high degree of penetrance with increasing age. More recently, the new associations were found within genes *PML* located on the chromosome 15q24, *RIN3* on 14q32, and *NUP205* on 7q33. Conversely, ultrastructural studies and the discovery of giant multinucleated osteoclasts containing microfilaments in the affected cytoplasm, as well as intranuclear inclusion bodies, suggest a viral etiology. Some investigators have obtained immunocytologic evidence identifying the particles as analogous to those from the measles group virus material. Other immunologic studies have demonstrated viral antigens in affected cells identical to those from the respiratory syncytial virus. The most recent research indicates a paramyxovirus as an etiologic factor.

Whatever the fundamental cause of Paget disease, its basic pathologic process has to do with the balance between bone resorption and appositional new bone formation. There is disordered and extremely active bone remodeling, secondary to both osteoclastic bone resorption and osteoblastic bone formation in a characteristic mosaic pattern, which is the histologic hallmark of this condition. Biochemically, the increase in osteoblastic activity is reflected in elevated levels of serum alkaline phosphatase, which can rise to extremely high values. Similarly, the increase in osteoclastic bone resorption is reflected in high urinary levels of hydroxyproline, which is formed as a result of collagen breakdown.

The skeletal abnormalities seen in Paget disease are frequently asymptomatic and may be an incidental finding on radiographic examination or at autopsy. When the changes are symptomatic, clinical manifestations are often related to complications of the disease, such as deformity of the long bones, warmth in the involved extremity, periosteal tenderness and bone pain, fractures, secondary osteoarthritis, neural compression, and sarcomatous degeneration. The distribution of a lesion varies from monostotic involvement to widespread disease. The following bones, in order of decreasing frequency, are most often affected: the pelvis, femur, skull, tibia, vertebrae, clavicle, humerus, and ribs (Fig. 29.1). The fibula is involved only in exceptional cases.

Imaging Features

The imaging features of Paget disease correspond to the pathologic processes in the bone and depend on the stage of the disorder. In the early phase, the *osteolytic* or *hot phase*, active bone resorption is evident as a radiolucent wedge or an elongated area with sharp borders that destroys both the cortex and cancellous bone as it advances along the shaft. The terms frequently used to describe this phenomenon are *advancing wedge*, *candle flame*, and *blade of grass* (Figs. 29.2 and 29.3). In flat bones such as the calvarium or the iliac bone, an area of active bone destruction known as *osteoporosis circumscripta* appears as a purely osteolytic lesion (Fig. 29.4). In the skull, most commonly affected sites are the frontal and occipital bones; both inner and outer calvarial tables are involved, but the former is usually more extensively affected.

In the *intermediate* or *mixed phase*, bone destruction is accompanied by new bone formation, with the latter process tending to predominate. Bone remodeling appears radiographically as thickening of the cortex and coarse trabeculation of cancellous bone (Fig. 29.5). In the pelvis, cortical thickening and sclerosis of the iliopectineal and ischiopubic lines are present. Pubic rami and ischia may enlarge. In the spine, the thin cortex of the vertebral body, which disappears in the hot phase, is later replaced by broad, coarsely trabeculated bone, forming what appears to be a "picture frame" around the body (Fig. 29.6). In the skull, focal patchy densities with a "cotton ball" appearance are characteristic (Fig. 29.7).

In the *cool* or *sclerotic phase*, a diffuse increase of bone density occurs together with enlargement and widening of the bone and marked cortical thickening, with blurring of the demarcation between cortex and spongiosa (Fig. 29.8). Bowing of long bones may become a striking feature (Fig. 29.9). In the pelvis obliteration of the demarcation between the cortex and spongy bone and sclerotic changes are the common findings (Fig. 29.10). Similar changes are observed in the skull, where obliteration of the diploic space is also a typical feature (Fig. 29.11).

It is important to remember that, because in the long bones Paget disease starts at one articular end and advances to the other, all three phases of the disorder may coexist in the same bone (Fig. 29.12A). Likewise, different phases may coexist in the flat bones or in the spine (Fig. 29.12B).

Computed tomography (CT) demonstrates characteristic features of Paget disease (Figs. 29.13 and 29.14). Magnetic resonance imaging (MRI) may be employed to demonstrate cortical and intramedullary involvement better, to exclude (or confirm) extension of the process into the soft tissues and to asses for potential malignant transformation. On T1-weighted sequences, intermediate-to-low signal intensity is usually noted. On T2 weighting, the signal may be high, intermediate, or low, depending

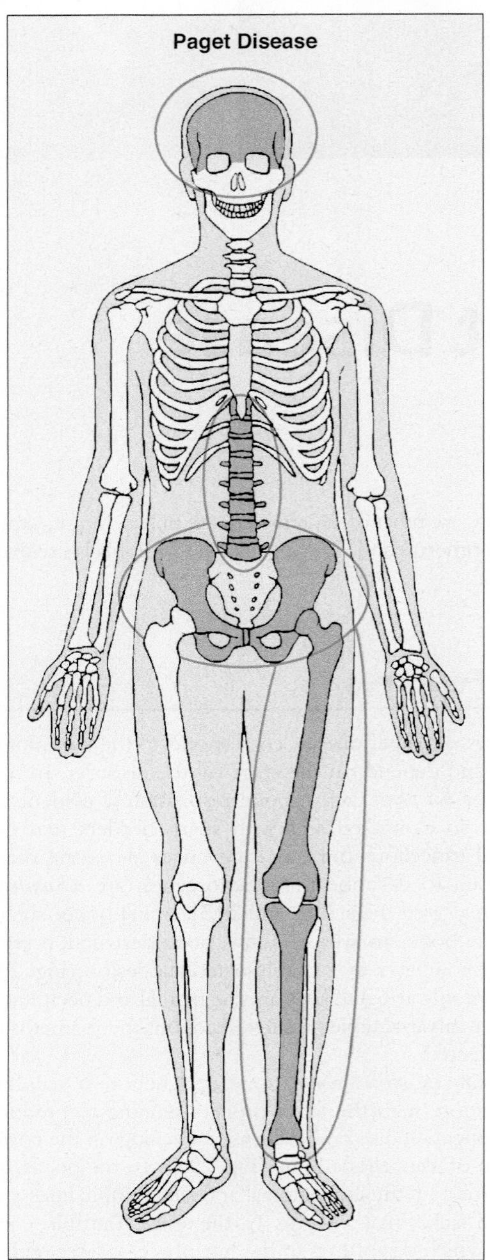

FIGURE 29.1 Major target sites of Paget disease.

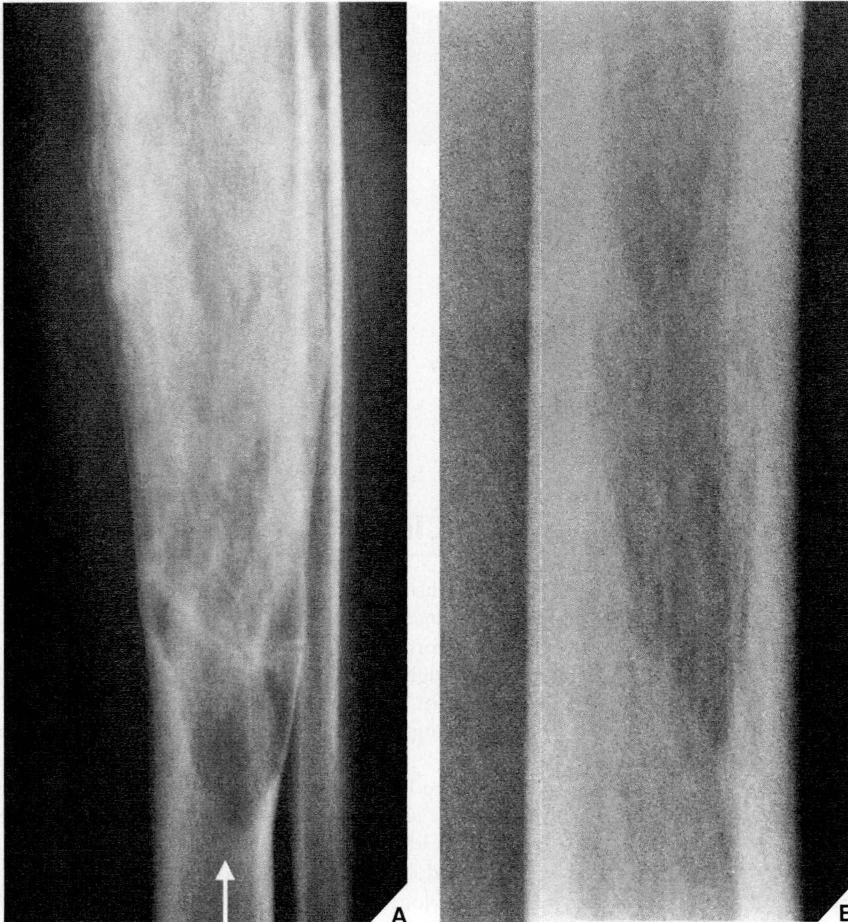

FIGURE 29.2 Osteolytic phase of Paget disease. **(A)** Anteroposterior radiograph of the lower leg of a 68-year-old woman shows an advancing wedge of osteolytic destruction in the midportion of the tibia *(arrow)*. **(B)** Magnification study of the midfemur in another patient shows the purely osteolytic phase of Paget disease. In both examples, the lesion resembles a blade of grass or a candle flame. (**A**, Reprinted with permission from Sissons HA, Greenspan A. Paget's disease. In: Taveras JM, Ferrucci JT, eds. *Radiology—imaging, diagnosis, intervention*, vol. 5. Philadelphia: JB Lippincott; 1986:1–14.)

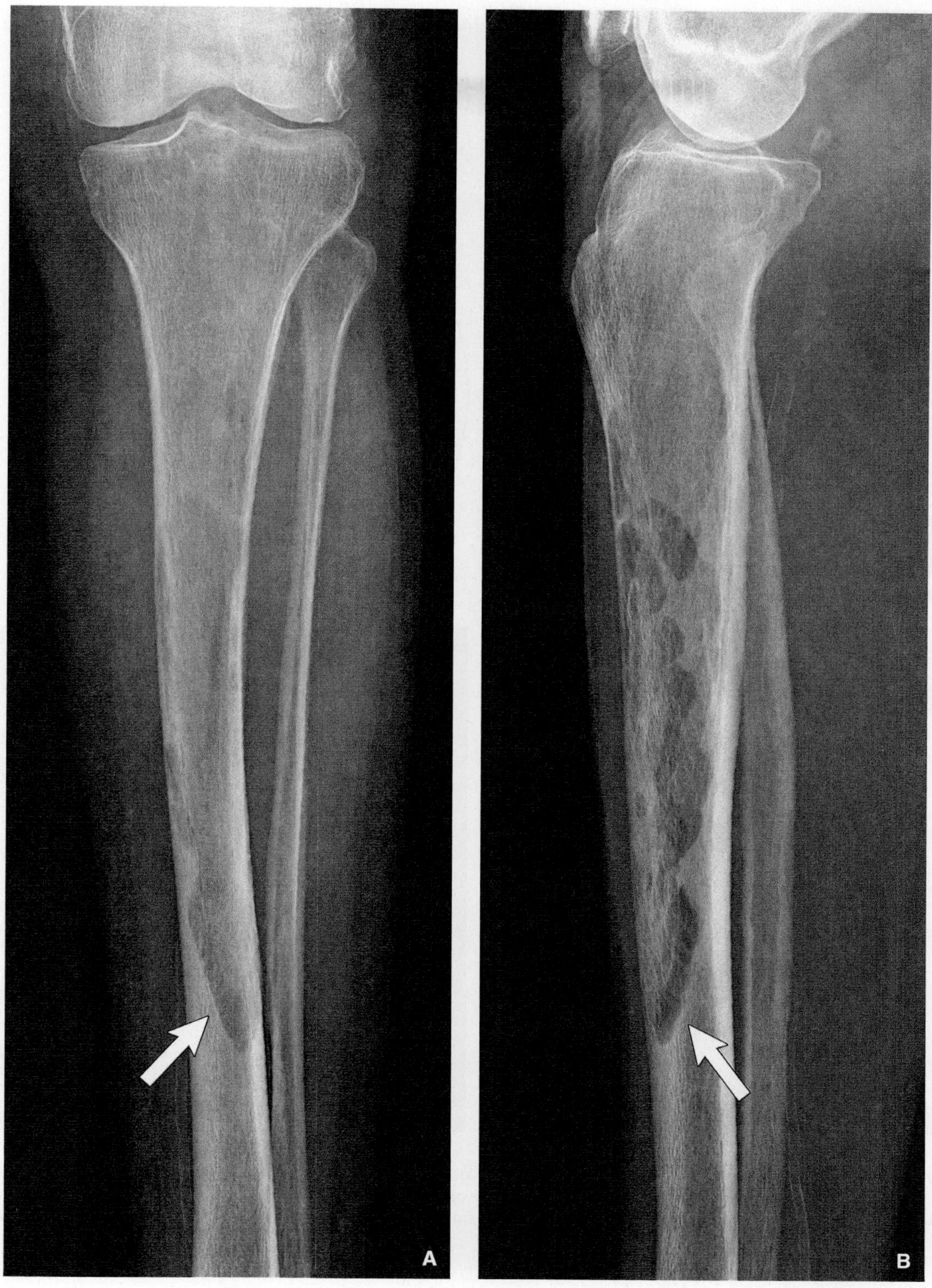

FIGURE 29.3 Osteolytic phase of Paget disease. **(A)** Anteroposterior and **(B)** lateral radiographs of the left leg of an 83-year-old man show acute phase of the disease with characteristic blade of grass appearance *(arrows)*.

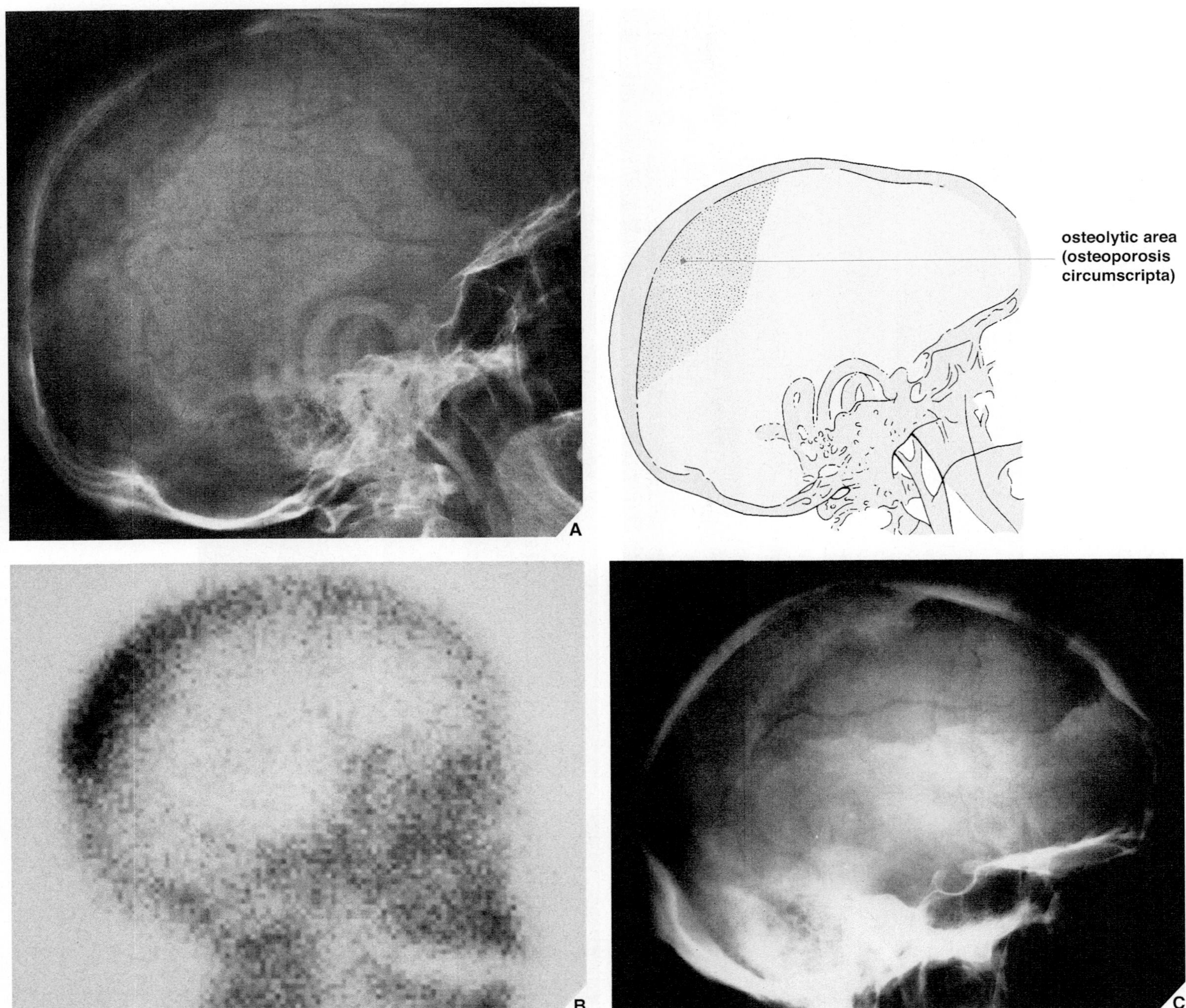

FIGURE 29.4 **Osteolytic phase of Paget disease.** **(A)** Lateral radiograph of the skull of a 60-year-old man shows an osteolytic lesion in the parietooccipital area. This sharply demarcated defect, known as *osteoporosis circumscripta*, represents a hot phase of the disease. **(B)** Radionuclide bone scan shows a characteristic localized increased uptake of the radiopharmaceutical tracer resulting in the appearance of a "yarmulke" sign. **(C)** Lateral radiograph of the skull of a 65-year-old woman reveals osteoporosis circumscripta in the frontoparietal area. *(Continued)*

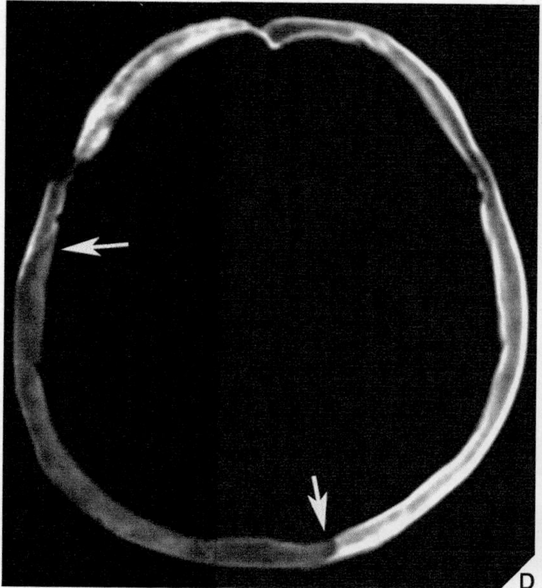

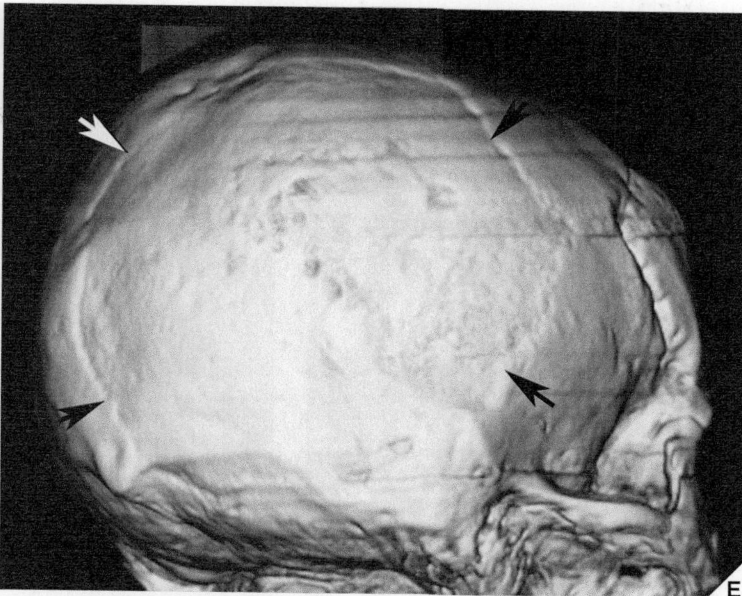

FIGURE 29.4 Osteolytic phase of Paget disease. ***(Continued)*** **(D)** Axial CT and **(E)** three-dimensional (3D) CT reconstruction image of the skull in shaded surface display of another patient with osteoporosis circumscripta show large sharply marginated lytic defect in the right temporal-occipital area *(arrows)*. (**C**, Courtesy of Evan Stein, MD, Brooklyn, New York.)

on the stage of the disease and degree of fibrosis and sclerosis (Figs. 29.15 and 29.16).

Scintigraphy displays increased uptake of bone-seeking radiotracer in all three phases of the disease, but particularly in the hot and intermediate, due to increased vascularity and osteoblastic activity in abnormal bone (Figs. 29.17 to 29.19; see also Figs. 26.10 and 29.11D,E).

Pathology

Gross specimen of pagetic bone shows prominent but disorganized trabecular pattern and areas of bone resorption (Fig. 29.20). The microscopic appearance, just like imaging appearance, depends on the stage of the disease. In the acute phase, there is combination of bone resorption, endosteal fibrosis, and prominence of vascular sinusoids. In cancellous bone, the trabeculae are slender and sparse; in cortical bone large resorption cavities are present. Pagetic osteoclasts are much larger than those associated with physiologic bone resorption and possess more nuclei with prominent nucleoli. In the intermediate phase, although there is still some osteoclastic activity present, also noted is increased osteoblastic activity and bone trabeculae become irregular in outline, some thinner and some thicker than normal. The increased rate of bone resorption and bone formation results in an increased number of reversal cement lines. This creates a characteristic mosaic pattern. In the cool phase, cell activity is less intense and vascularity diminishes. The histopathologic picture dominates by thickly reconstructed bone that demonstrates markedly increased numbers of prominent and irregular cement lines showing a bold mosaic pattern.

Differential Diagnosis

Several conditions may mimic Paget disease, while the disease itself may be mistaken for other pathologic processes; for example, involvement of a single bone can be mistaken for monostotic fibrous dysplasia, and a uniform increase in osseous density may mimic lymphoma or metastatic cancer. The rugger-jersey appearance of the spine in secondary hyperparathyroidism may resemble Paget vertebra (see Figs. 28.9 and 28.10). Vertebral hemangioma also looks very much like Paget vertebra on a radiograph, except that the vertebral body is not enlarged, and the vertebral end plates are well outlined (see Figs. 20.58, 20.60, and 20.62). However, the condition that bears the most striking resemblance to Paget disease is familial idiopathic hyperphosphatasia, also called *juvenile Paget disease* (see Figs. 30.1 and 30.2). In this condition, unlike Paget disease, the articular ends of the bone may not be affected.

Complications

Pathologic Fractures

Of the numerous complications observed in patients with Paget disease, the most common are pathologic fractures in the long bones. They may resemble partial or incomplete stress (insufficiency) fractures, appearing radiographically as multiple short horizontal radiolucent lines on the convex aspect of the cortex (Fig. 29.22). True complete fractures are referred to as *banana-type* because of the horizontal direction of the fracture line as it traverses the affected bone (Figs. 29.23 and 29.24), and they have also been compared with crushed rotten wood or chalk. Fractures are more likely to occur during the osteolytic or hot phase, and they are frequently the main presenting manifestation of Paget disease.

Degenerative Joint Disease

The development of degenerative joint disease is a common complication of Paget disease. This secondary form of osteoarthritis usually occurs in the knee and hip articulations, where the characteristic changes are present, including joint space narrowing and osteophyte formation. Involvement of the acetabulum may be complicated by acetabular protrusio (Fig. 29.25).

Neurologic Complications

The neurologic complications of Paget disease are secondary to involvement of the vertebral column and skull. Collapse of a vertebral body, for example, causes extradural spinal canal block, which may lead to paraplegia (Fig. 29.26). Severe involvement of the bony spinal canal may lead to spinal stenosis, the presence of which can be effectively demonstrated by CT (Fig. 29.27). Basilar invagination due to softening of the skull may lead to encroachment on the foramen magnum and neurologic deficit.

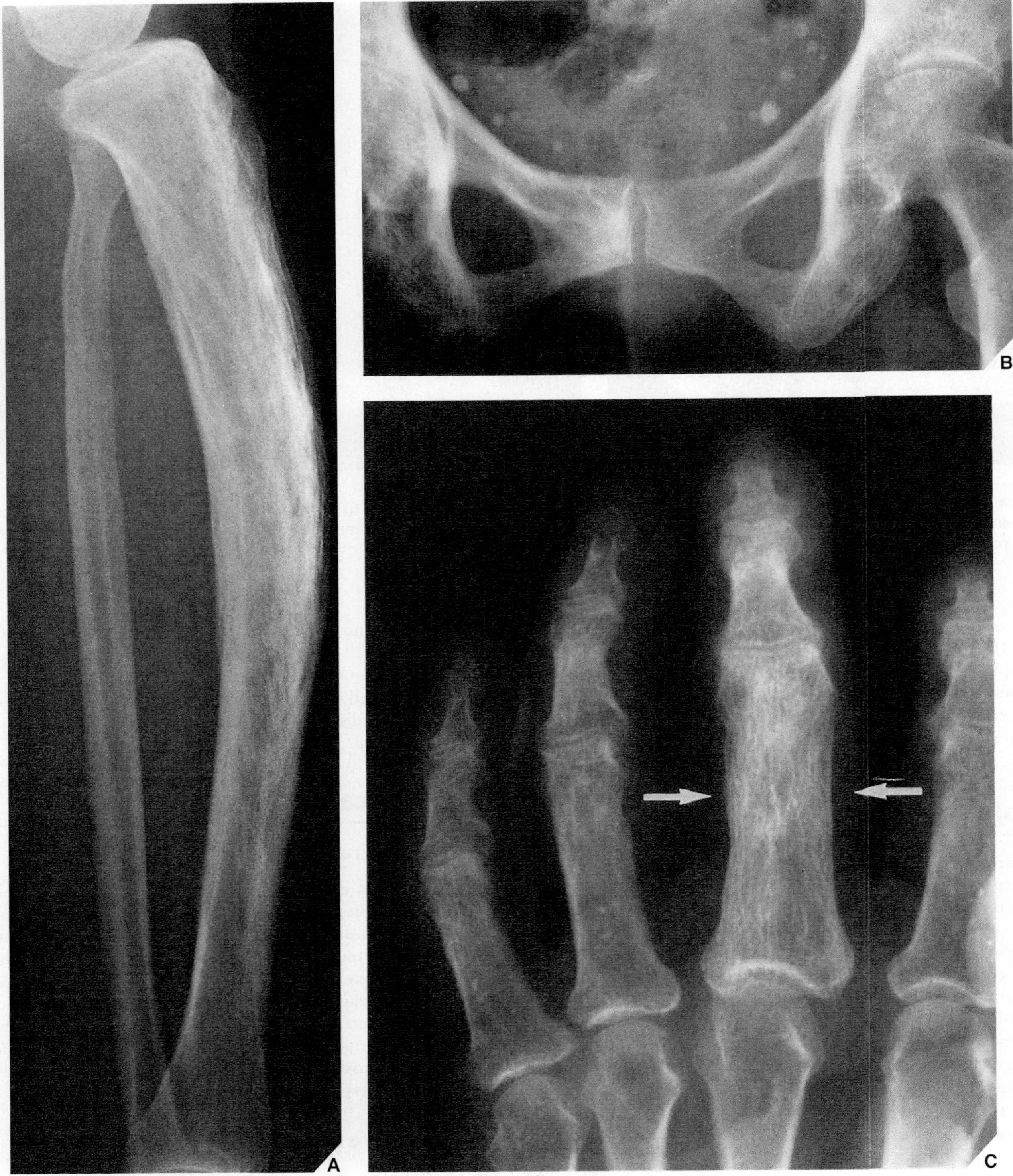

FIGURE 29.5 Intermediate phase of Paget disease. **(A)** In the intermediate phase, seen here affecting the tibia in a 62-year-old woman, thickening of the cortex and a coarse trabecular pattern in the medullary portion of the bone are characteristic features. Note the anterior bowing. **(B)** In another patient, an 81-year-old woman, intermediate phase is seen in the pubic and ischial bones. **(C)** Mixed phase affecting the proximal phalanx of the middle finger *(arrows)* is seen in a 67-year-old woman with monostotic form of the disease.

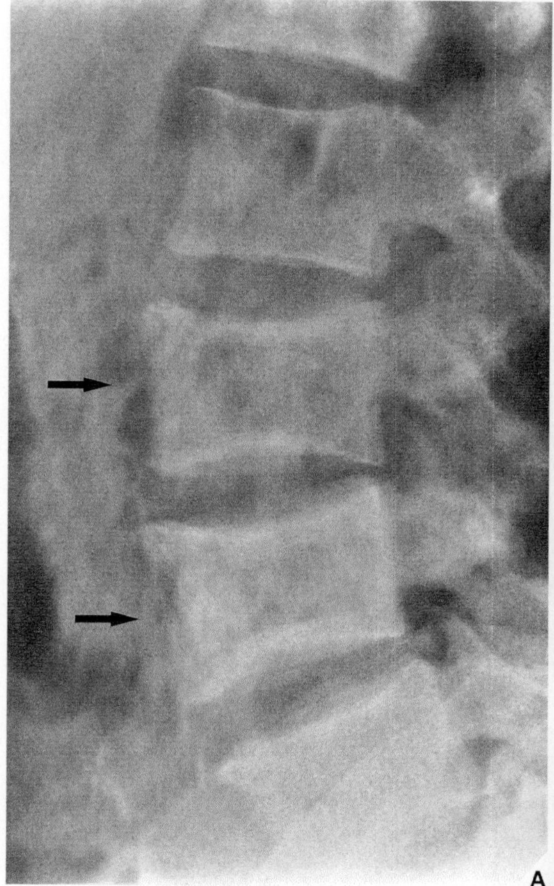

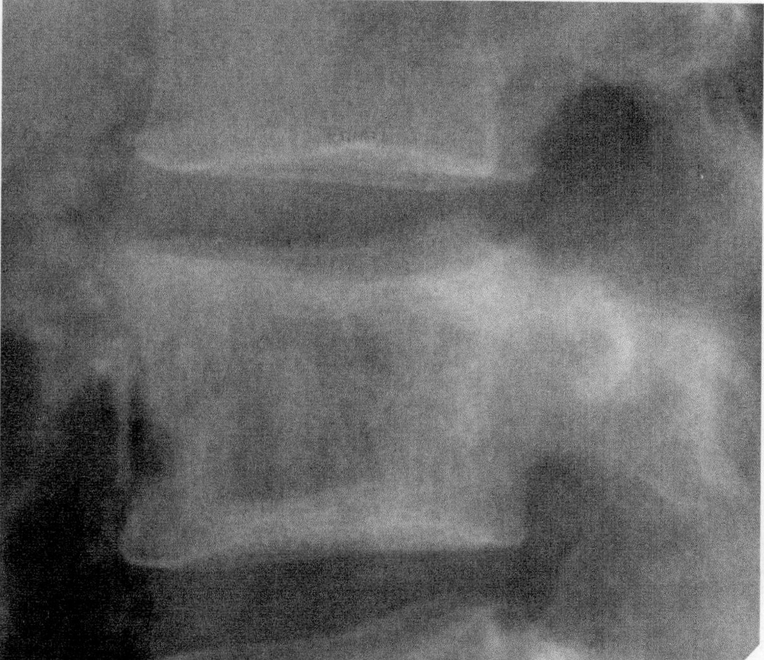

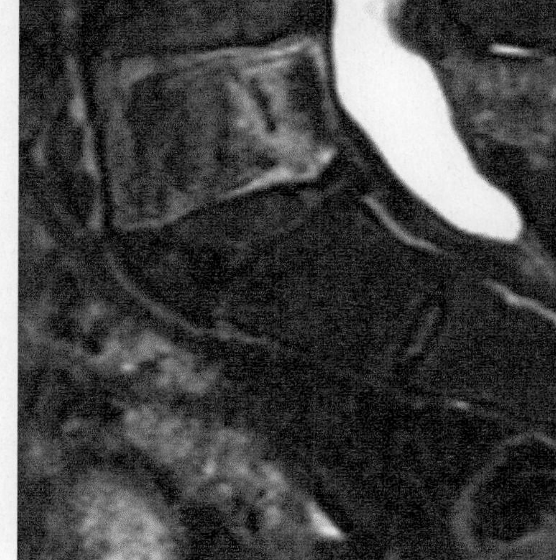

FIGURE 29.6 Intermediate phase of Paget disease. **(A)** Involvement of the lumbar spine in the mixed phase can be recognized by the "picture frame" appearance of the vertebral bodies *(arrows)* created by dense sclerotic bone on the periphery and greater radiolucency in the center. Note the partial replacement of vertebral end plates by coarsely trabeculated bone. **(B)** In another patient, the picture frame appearance of the vertebral body of L2 marks the intermediate phase of Paget disease. **(C)** Sagittal STIR MRI of the lumbar spine in another patient with Paget disease affecting the L5 vertebral body shows the MRI equivalent of picture frame. (**A**, Reprinted with permission from Sissons HA, Greenspan A. Paget's disease. In: Taveras JM, Ferrucci JT, eds. *Radiology—imaging, diagnosis, intervention*, vol. 5. Philadelphia: JB Lippincott; 1986:1–14; **C**, Courtesy of Oleg Opsha, MD, Brooklyn, New York.)

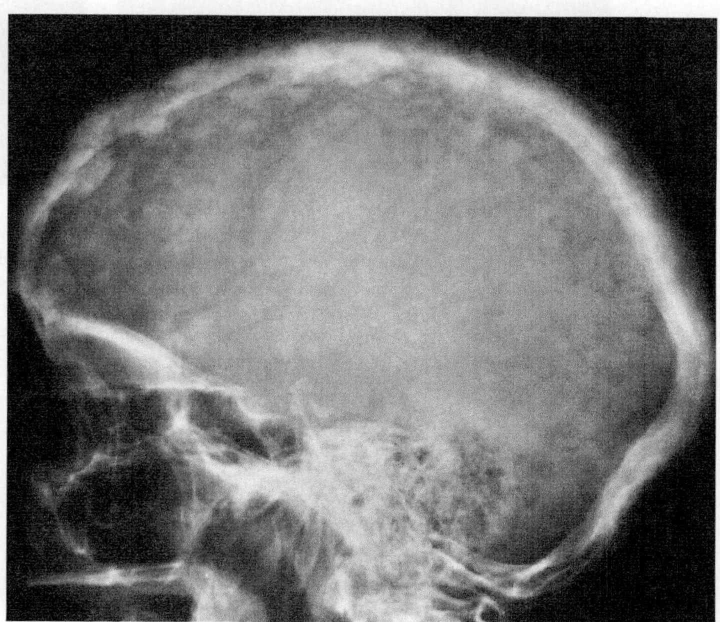

FIGURE 29.7 Intermediate phase of Paget disease. Focal patchy densities in the skull, having a "cotton ball" appearance, are typical of the intermediate phase of Paget disease as seen in this radiograph of a 68-year-old woman.

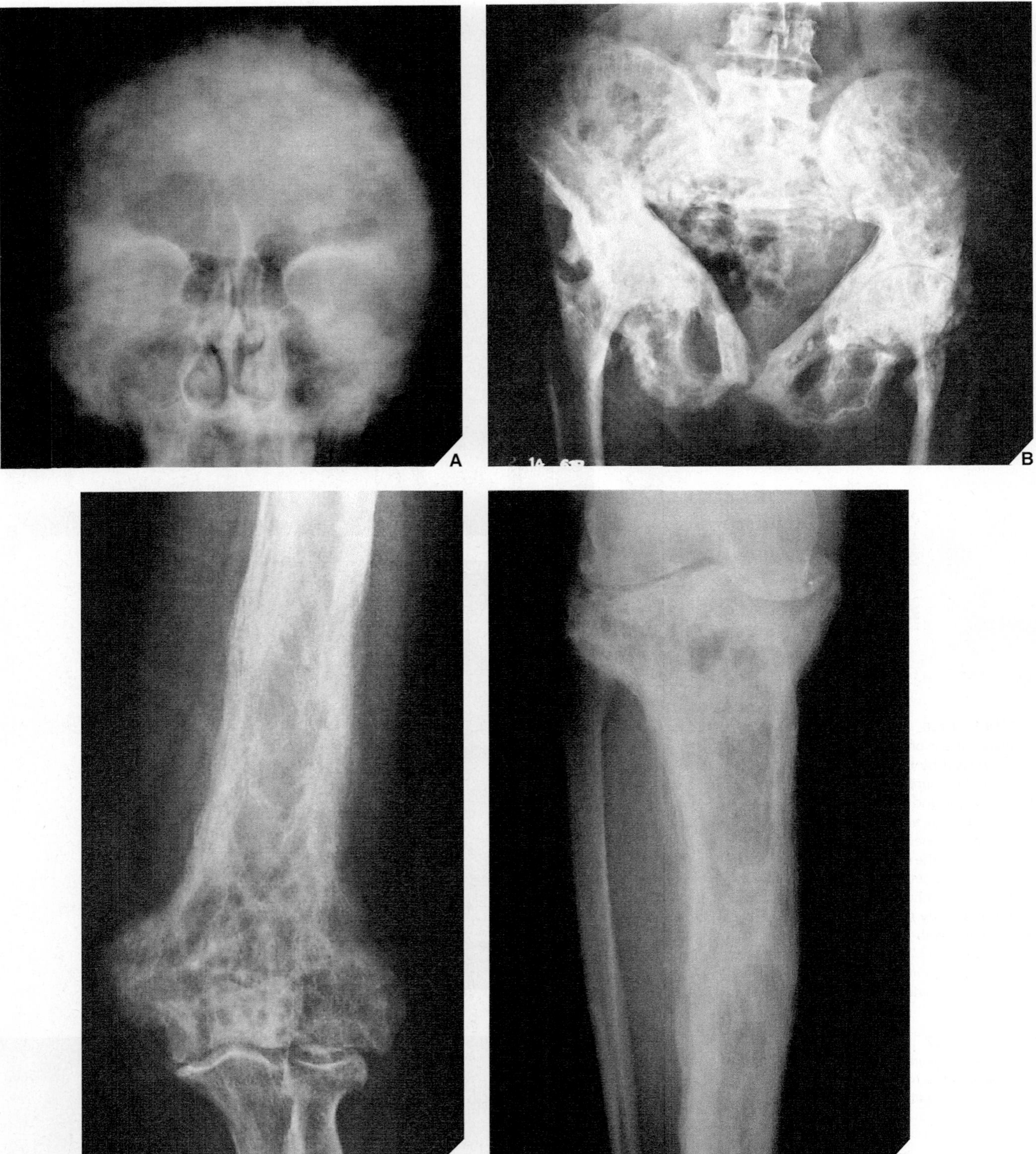

FIGURE 29.8 **Cool phase of Paget disease.** In the cool phase, there is considerable thickening of the cortex and bone deformity. **(A)** Anteroposterior radiograph of the skull of an 82-year-old woman reveals typical changes of the cool phase of Paget disease. **(B)** The pelvic cavity, seen here in an 80-year-old woman, assumed a triangular appearance. **(C)** Involvement of a long bone, in this case the distal humerus of a 60-year-old woman, exhibits marked cortical thickening, narrowing of the medullary cavity, and a coarse trabecular pattern. **(D)** Similar changes are present in the tibia in a 72-year-old man. (**A,B**, Reprinted with permission from Sissons HA, Greenspan A. Paget's disease. In: Taveras JM, Ferrucci JT, eds. *Radiology—imaging, diagnosis, intervention*, vol. 5. Philadelphia: JB Lippincott; 1986:1–14.)

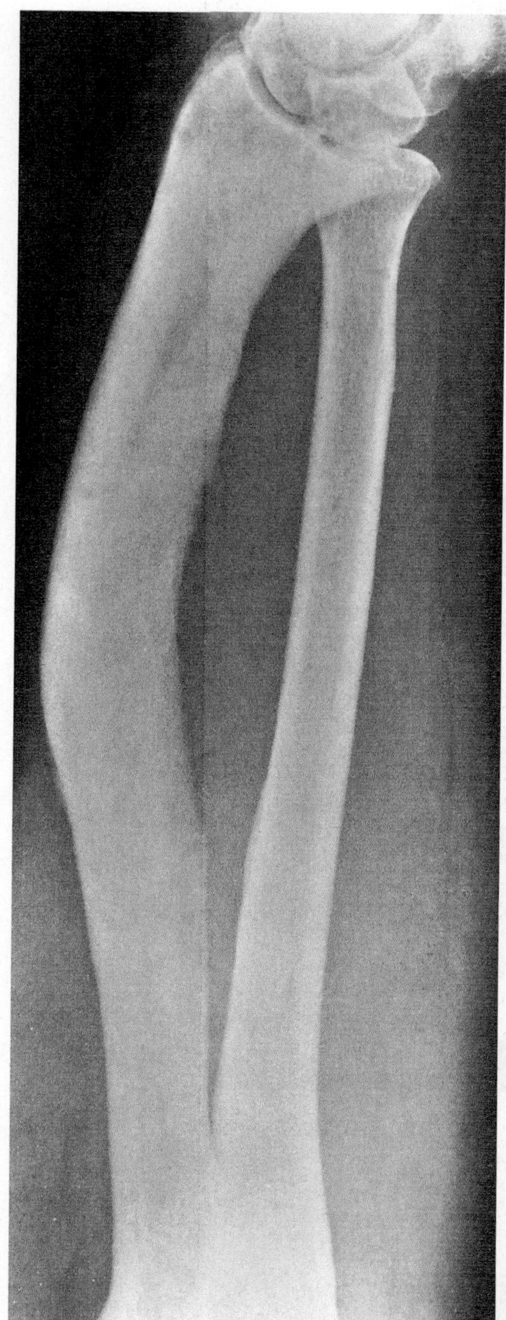

FIGURE 29.9 Cool phase of Paget disease. Anteroposterior radiograph of the forearm of a 57-year-old man with polyostotic Paget disease shows enlargement of the left radius with a marked bowing deformity. Other signs of the cool phase of the disease are seen in the diffuse sclerotic changes and the indistinct demarcation between the cortex and the spongiosa, also affecting the proximal ulna.

Neoplastic Complications

Benign or malignant giant cell tumors, single or multiple, may complicate Paget disease. The usual sites of these tumors are the calvarium and the iliac bone.

The development of a bone sarcoma is a serious but rare complication of Paget disease; the incidence is less than 1%. Osteosarcoma is by far the most common histologic type, followed by fibrosarcoma, malignant fibrous histiocytoma, chondrosarcoma, and lymphoma, with the pelvis, femur, and humerus at highest risk for the development of malignant transformation. The main radiographic features of this complication are development of a lytic lesion at the site of Paget disease, cortical breakthrough, and formation of a soft-tissue mass (Fig. 29.28A), which can be confirmed with CT (Fig. 29.28B) or MRI (Fig. 29.29); a periosteal reaction is rare. There is often a pathologic fracture as well. The radiographic appearance of Paget sarcoma must be distinguished from that of metastases of a primary carcinoma of the kidney (Fig. 29.30), breast, or prostate. The metastatic deposit may be lodged in either unaffected or pagetic bone. The prognosis for patients with sarcomatous degeneration of Paget disease is poor; the mean survival time usually does not exceed 6 to 8 months. Occasionally, an osteosarcoma in pagetic bone may metastasize to other bones and soft tissues, but metastases to the lung, liver, and adrenals are much more likely.

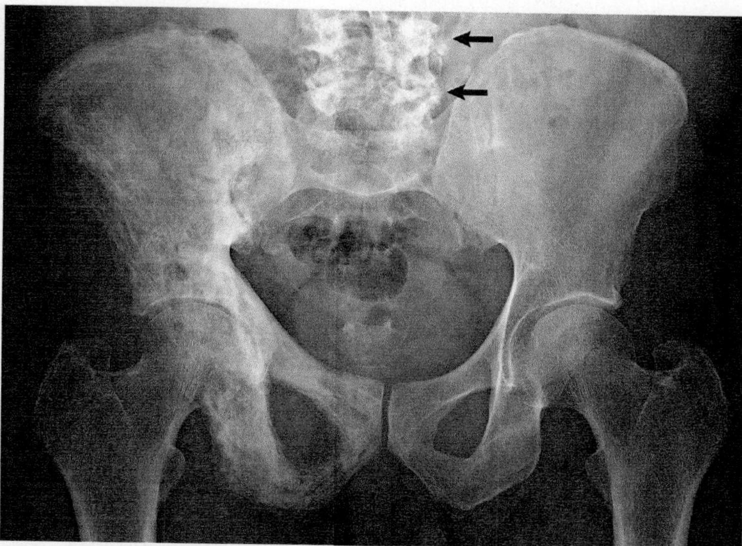

FIGURE 29.10 Cool phase of Paget disease. Anteroposterior radiograph of the pelvis of a 71-year-old man shows thickening of the cortex and coarse trabecular pattern of the right hemipelvis characteristic for cool phase of the disease. Observe also involvement of the L4 and L5 vertebrae *(arrows)*.

Orthopaedic and Medical Management

Orthopaedic treatment. Because of the variable clinical presentation of Paget disease, decisions regarding therapy must be based on the particular manifestations in each patient. The goal of the orthopaedic treatment is the control and relief of pain rather than restitution of normal bone quality. The role of the orthopaedic surgeon in the management of Paget disease is to evaluate and treat the cause of a patient's pain, to assess and manage any deformities, and to provide therapy for pathologic fractures and tumors developing in pagetic bone. The radiologist contributes to these aims by providing essential information. For example, CT is useful for demonstrating spinal stenosis, which frequently leads to neurologic symptoms in patients with Paget disease (see Fig. 29.19). Radionuclide imaging is also a valuable technique, particularly for determining the skeletal distribution of the disease (see Fig. 26.10). Surgical intervention is indicated for the treatment of pathologic fractures, advanced, disabling arthritis, and extreme bowing deformities of the long bones. Stress or insufficiency fractures, which occur most often in the tibia and proximal femur, are treated by bracing and protection from weight bearing for a period of several months. Complete fractures are treated either with intramedullary rods or with compression plates and screws. For arthritic complications, which are particularly frequent in the hip and knee articulations, total joint replacement is usually performed.

Medical treatment consists of inhibiting osteoclastic activity by subcutaneous or intramuscular injections of calcitonin, a 32-amino-acid hormone secreted by the C cells of the thyroid gland, and oral administration of bisphosphonates, which bind to areas of high bone turnover, decreasing bone resorption. The main action of bisphosphonates is decreasing osteoclastic activity. The most frequently used drugs in this group include etidronate, pamidronate, alendronate, risedronate, and tiludronate.

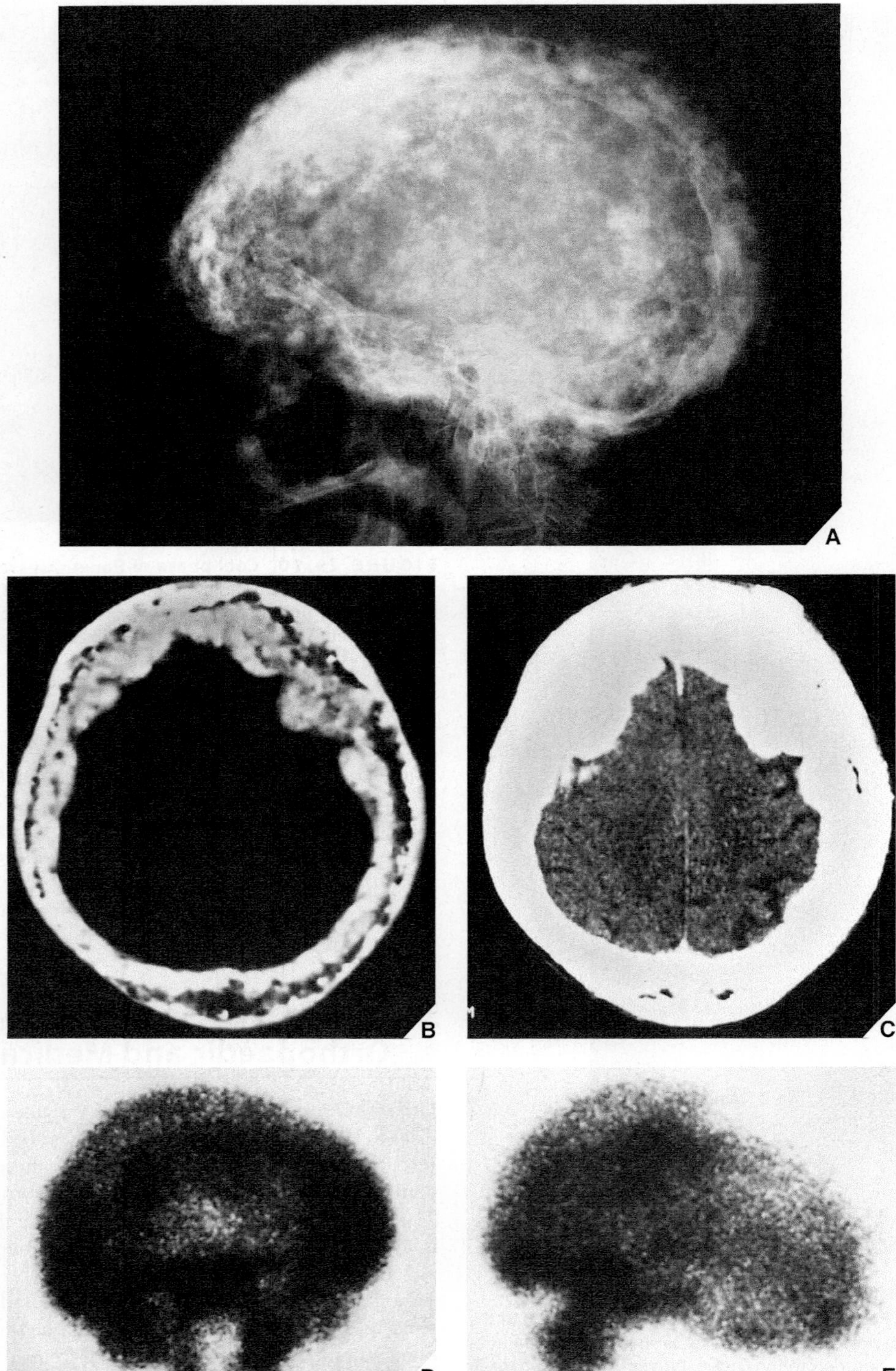

FIGURE 29.11 Cool phase of Paget disease. **(A)** Lateral radiograph of the skull of an 80-year-old woman demonstrates numerous coalescent densities associated with thickening and sclerosis of the cranial vault and base of the skull. CT sections clearly demonstrate predominant involvement of the inner table with marked diminution of the diploic space **(B)** and thickening of the cranial vault **(C)**. Scintigraphy in frontal **(D)** and lateral **(E)** projection demonstrates markedly increased uptake of radiopharmaceutical tracer.

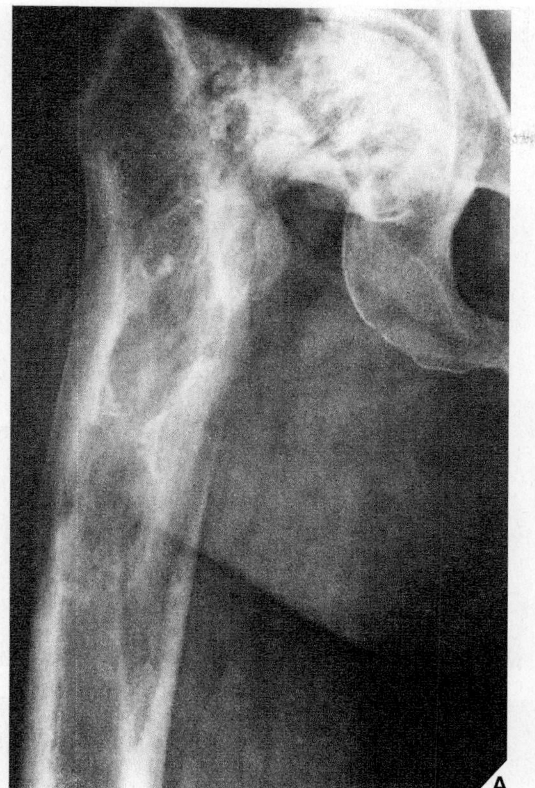

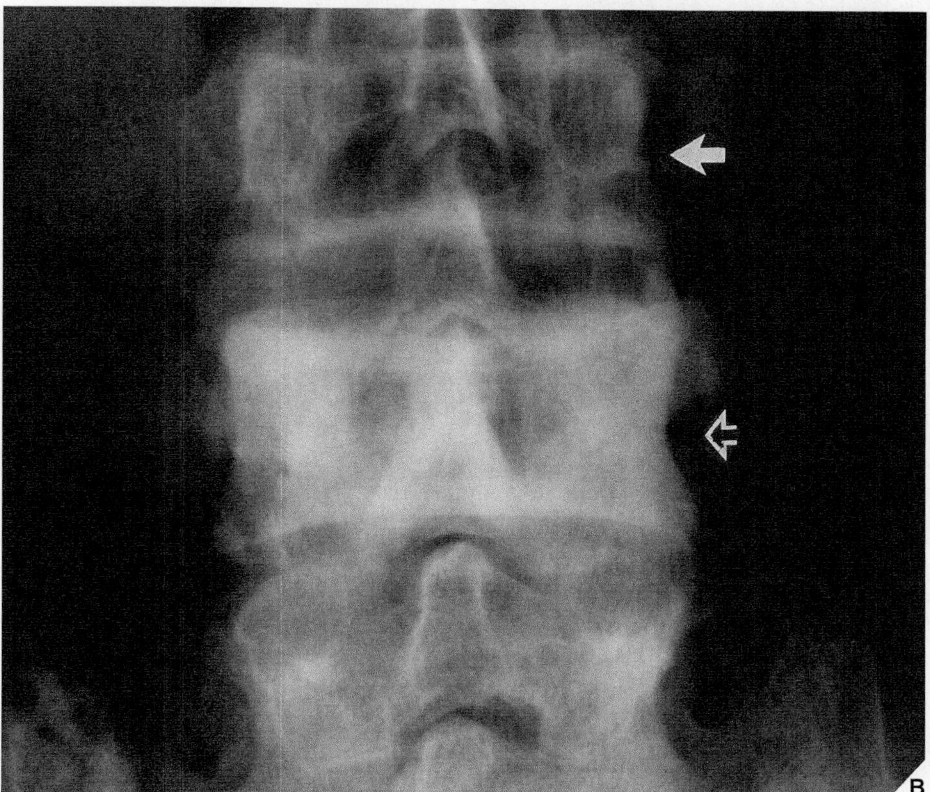

FIGURE 29.12 **Coexistence of different phases of Paget disease.** **(A)** Anteroposterior radiograph of the proximal half of the femur of a 77-year-old woman demonstrates all three phases of the disorder. The cool phase is seen in the femoral head, the intermediate phase in the proximal shaft, and the hot phase, represented by an osteolytic wedge of resorption, in the medial cortex more distally. **(B)** In another patient, a 54-year-old man, intermediate phase is seen in the vertebra L3 *(arrow)*, whereas the L4 reveals a cool phase *(open arrow)*.

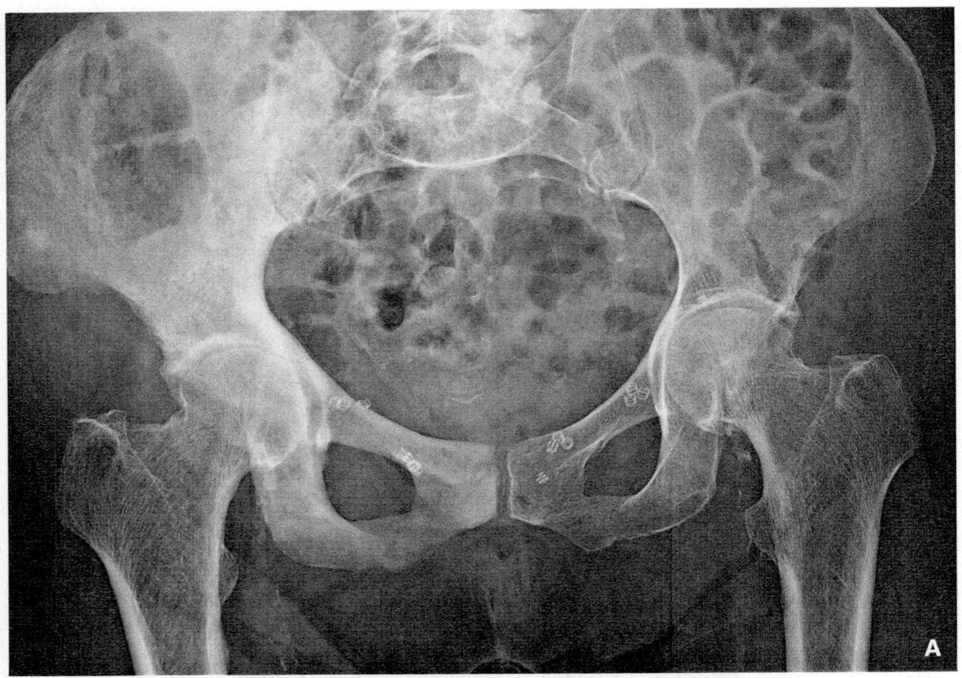

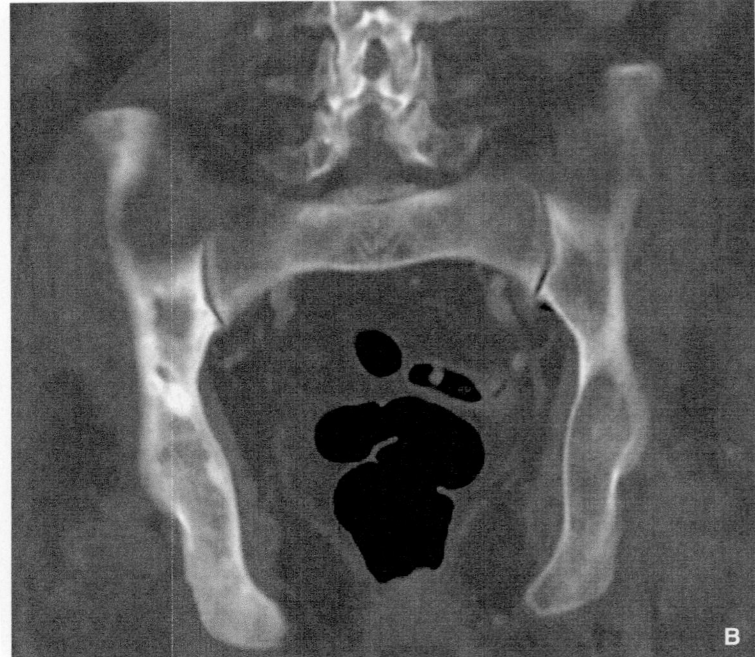

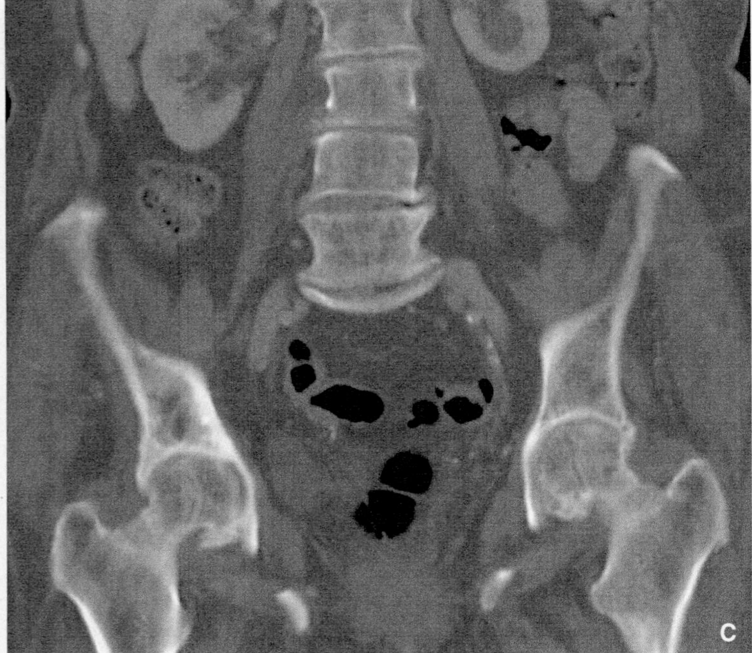

FIGURE 29.13 CT of Paget disease. **(A)** Anteroposterior radiograph of the pelvis of a 99-year-old woman shows sclerotic changes of the right hemipelvis. **(B,C)** Two coronal reformatted CT sections demonstrate thickening of the cortex and coarse trabecular pattern of the affected bones. Compare with normal left hemipelvis.

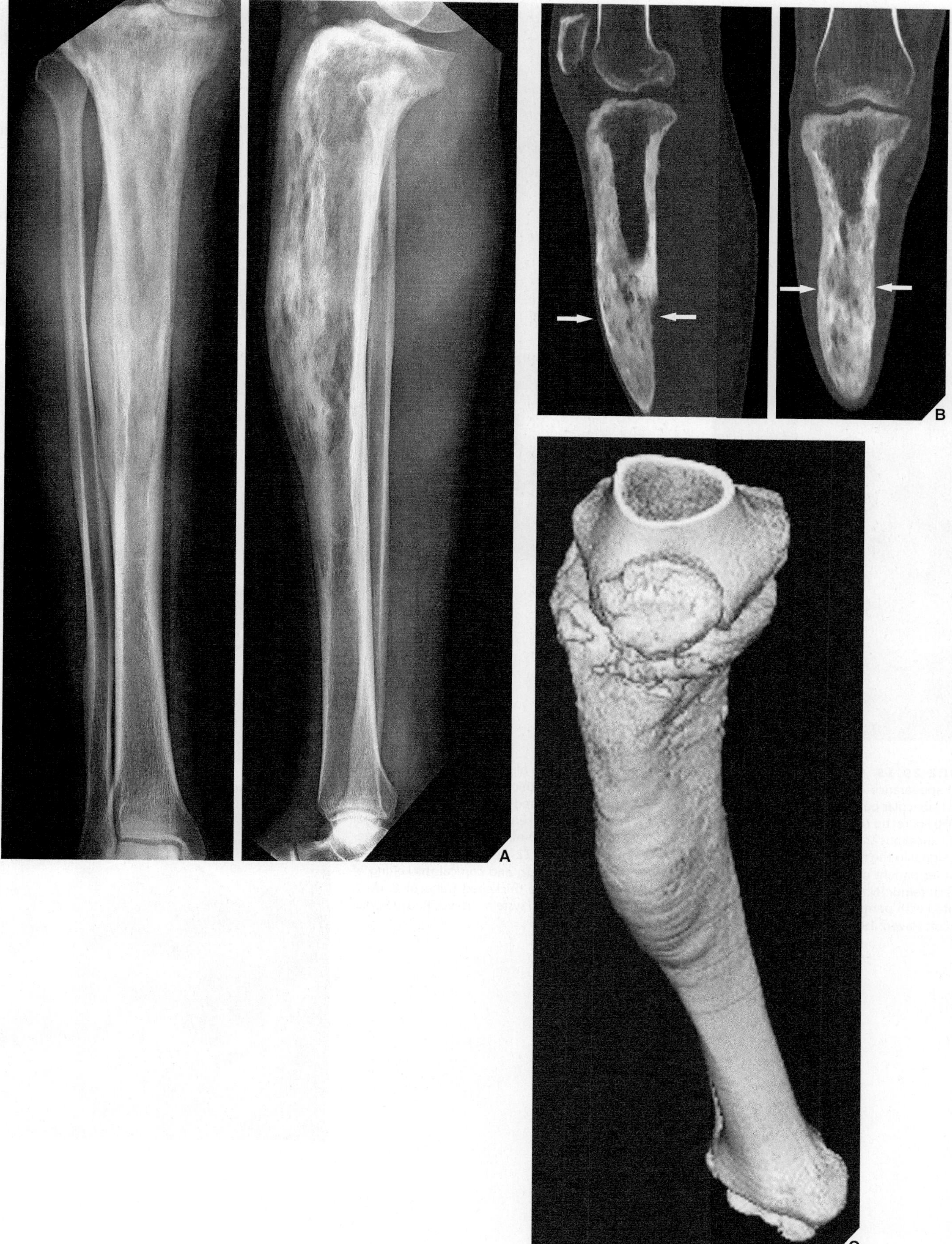

FIGURE 29.14 CT and three-dimensional (3D) CT of Paget disease. **(A)** Anteroposterior and lateral radiographs of the right leg of a 75-year-old man show thickening of the cortex and a coarse trabeculation of the proximal tibia. **(B)** Sagittal and coronal reformatted CT images demonstrate these abnormalities to the better advantage. Note lack of distinction between the cortex and the spongiosa *(arrows)*. **(C)** 3D CT reconstructed image shows deformity of the tibia and anterior bowing.

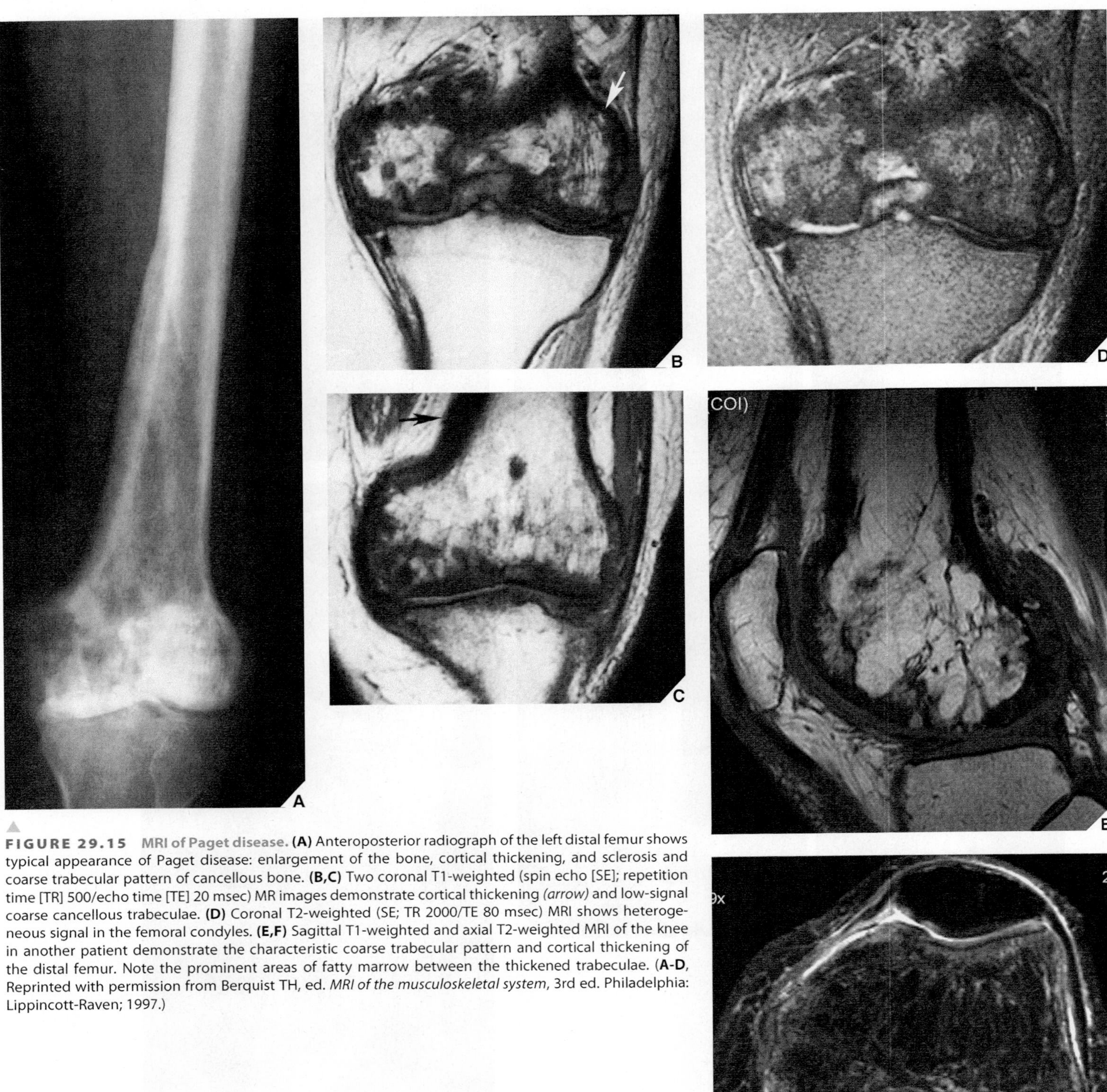

FIGURE 29.15 **MRI of Paget disease.** **(A)** Anteroposterior radiograph of the left distal femur shows typical appearance of Paget disease: enlargement of the bone, cortical thickening, and sclerosis and coarse trabecular pattern of cancellous bone. **(B,C)** Two coronal T1-weighted (spin echo [SE]; repetition time [TR] 500/echo time [TE] 20 msec) MR images demonstrate cortical thickening *(arrow)* and low-signal coarse cancellous trabeculae. **(D)** Coronal T2-weighted (SE; TR 2000/TE 80 msec) MRI shows heterogeneous signal in the femoral condyles. **(E,F)** Sagittal T1-weighted and axial T2-weighted MRI of the knee in another patient demonstrate the characteristic coarse trabecular pattern and cortical thickening of the distal femur. Note the prominent areas of fatty marrow between the thickened trabeculae. (**A-D**, Reprinted with permission from Berquist TH, ed. *MRI of the musculoskeletal system*, 3rd ed. Philadelphia: Lippincott-Raven; 1997.)

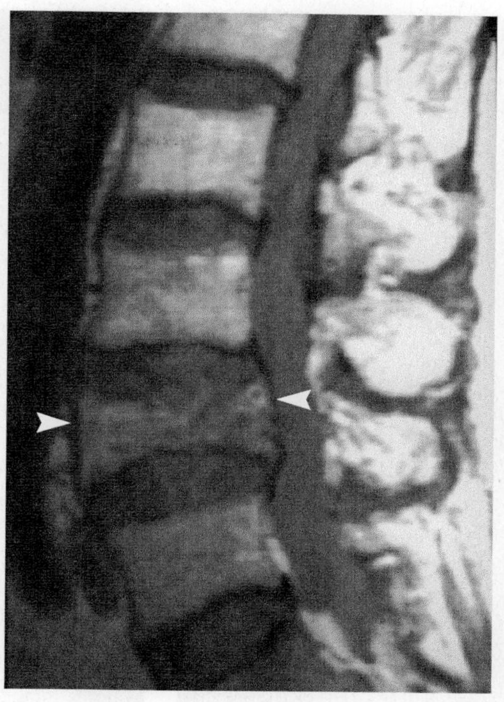

FIGURE 29.16 **MRI of Paget disease.** Sagittal T1-weighted (spin echo [SE]; repetition time [TR] 500/echo time [TE] 20 msec) MR image of the lumbar spine shows involvement of the vertebra by Paget disease *(arrowheads)*. (Reprinted with permission from Berquist TH, ed. *MRI of the musculoskeletal system*, 3rd ed. Philadelphia: Lippincott-Raven; 1997.)

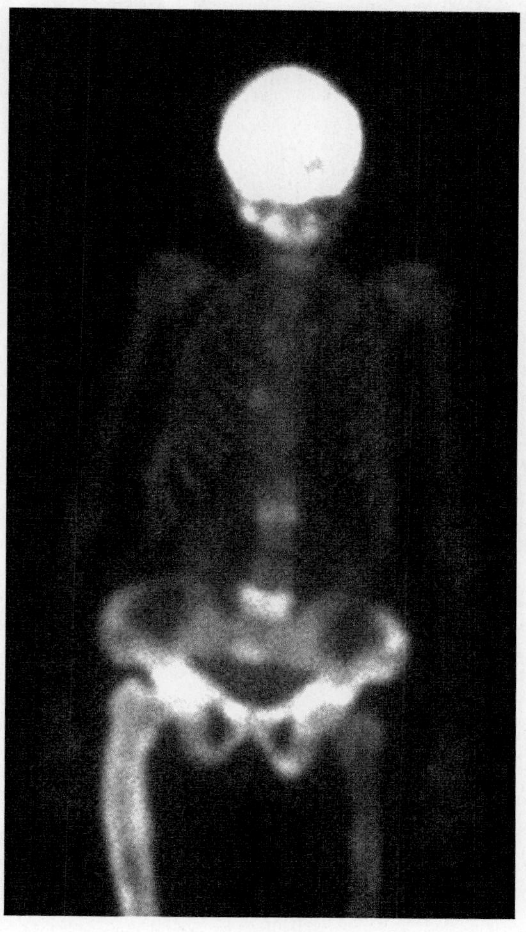

FIGURE 29.17 **Scintigraphy of polyostotic Paget disease.** After intravenous injection of 23mCi (851 MBq) of technetium-99 methylene diphosphonate (^{99m}Tc MDP), a total-body radionuclide bone scan that was obtained in an 82-year-old man demonstrates increased uptake of radiopharmaceutical tracer within the skull, lumbar vertebrae, pelvic bones, and both femora (right greater than left).

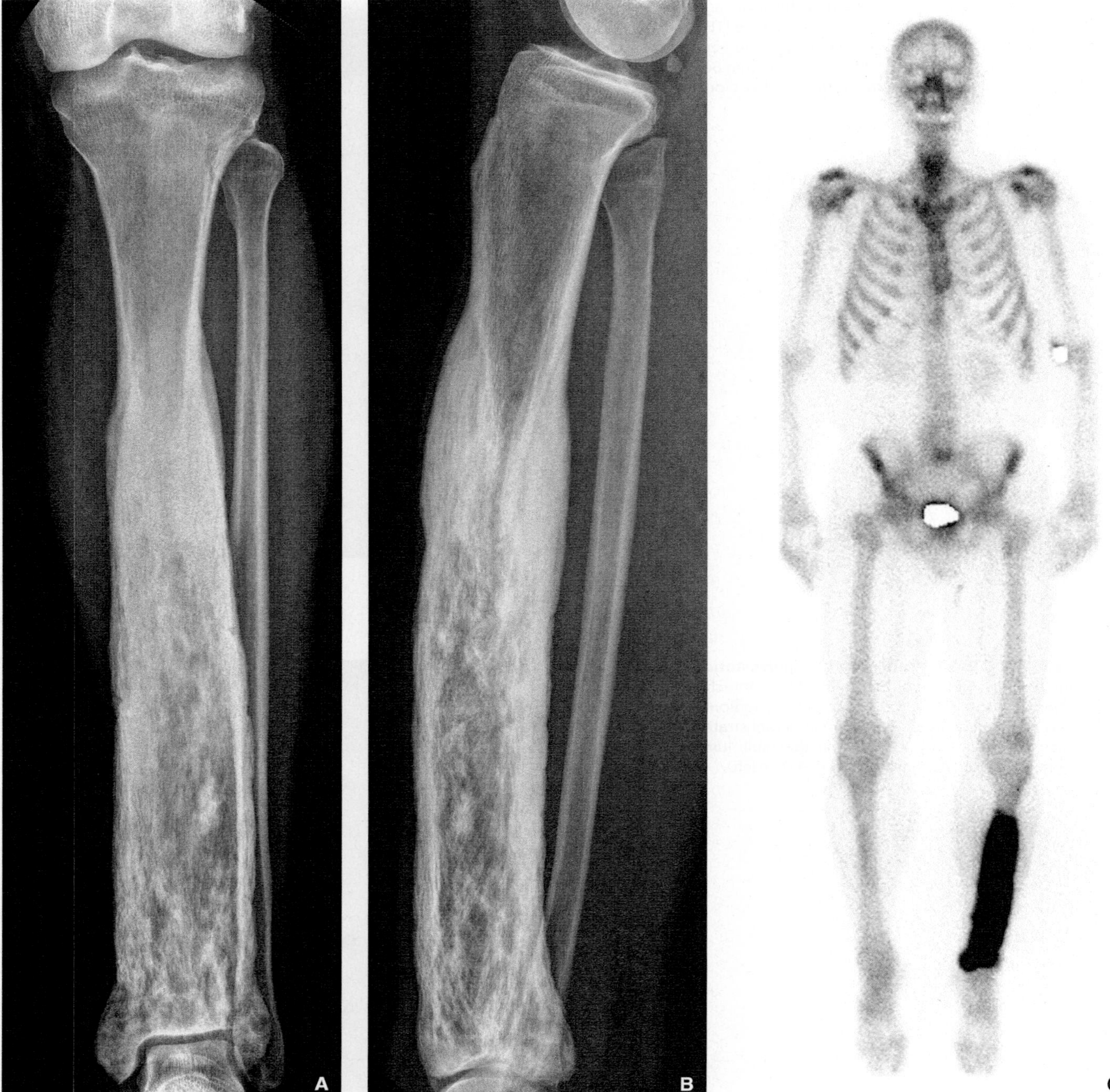

FIGURE 29.18 Scintigraphy of monostotic Paget disease. **(A)** Anteroposterior and **(B)** lateral radiographs of the left leg of a 60-year-old man show enlargement of the bone, thickening of the cortex, and coarse trabecular pattern of the tibia representing the cool phase of the disease. **(C)** Whole-body radionuclide bone scan obtained after intravenous administration of 15 mCi (555 MBq) technetium-99m methylene diphosphonate (^{99m}Tc MDP) shows markedly increased uptake of the radiopharmaceutical tracer within the tibia.

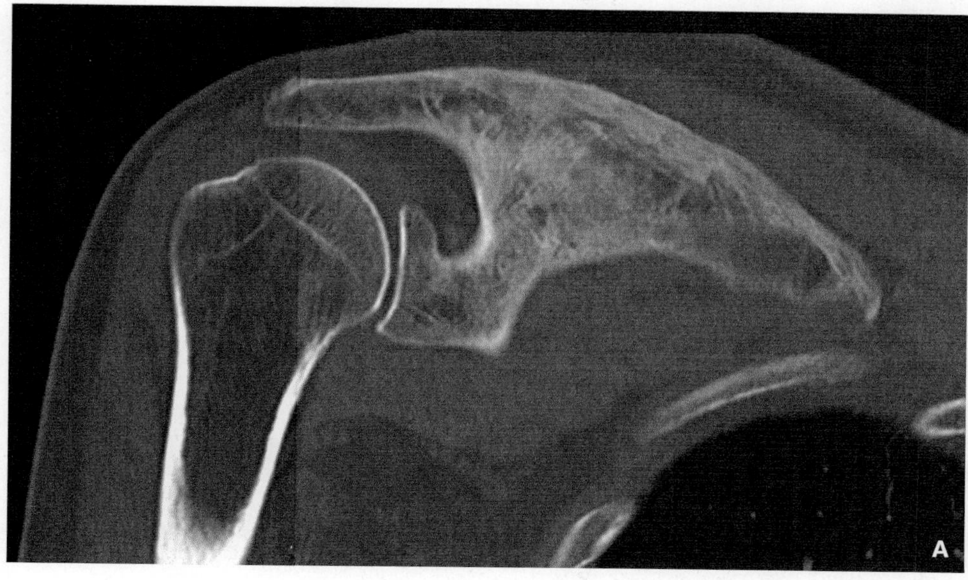

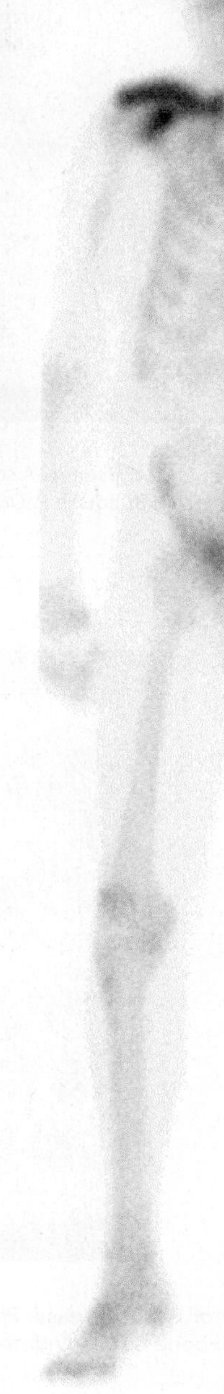

FIGURE 29.19 Scintigraphy and CT of monostotic Paget disease. **(A)** Coronal reformatted CT section of the right shoulder of an 88-year-old man shows sclerotic changes and coarse trabecular pattern affecting most of the he scapula. **(B)** Whole-body radionuclide bone scan obtained after intravenous administration of 15 mCi (555 MBq) technetium-99m methylene diphosphonate (^{99m}Tc MDP) shows markedly increased uptake of the radiopharmaceutical tracer limited to the right scapula.

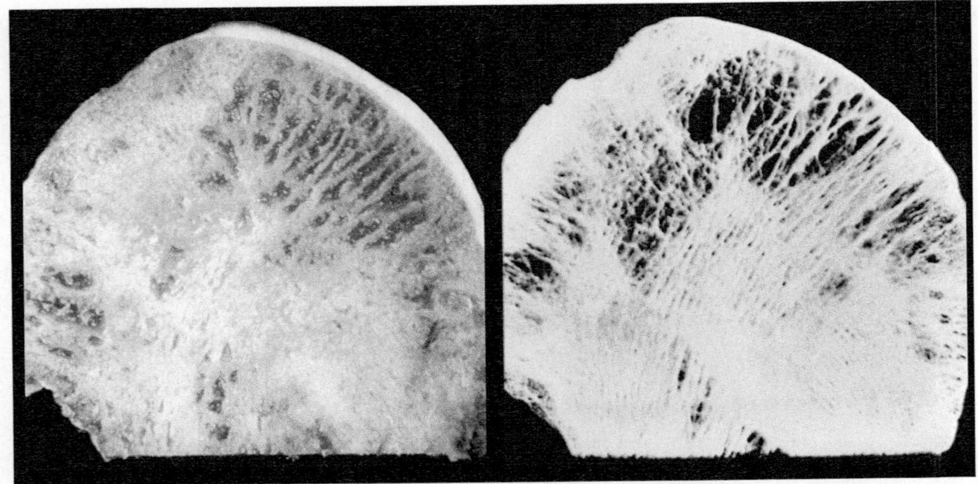

FIGURE 29.20 **Pathology of Paget disease.** A section through the resected femoral head and specimen radiograph shows disorganized trabecular pattern and focal area of bone resorption. (Modified from Bullough P. *Orthopaedic pathology*, 5th ed. Maryland Heights, MO: Mosby; 2009, with permission from Elsevier.)

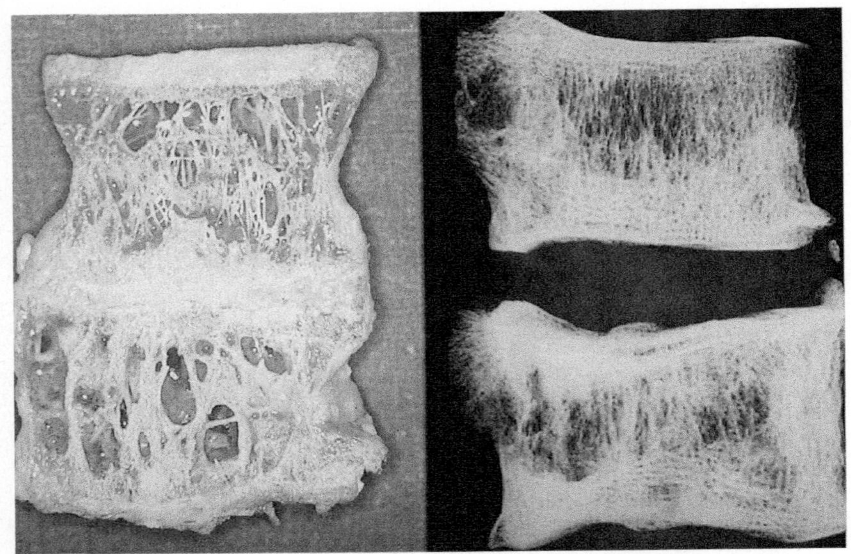

FIGURE 29.21 **Pathology of Paget disease.** Photograph and specimen radiograph of two vertebrae show characteristic coarsening of the trabeculae and patchy sclerosis. Internal architecture of bone is greatly distorted. (Reprinted with permission from Vigorita JV, Ghelmsan B, Mintz D. *Orthopaedic pathology*, 3rd ed. Philadelphia: Wolters Kluwer; 2016:185.)

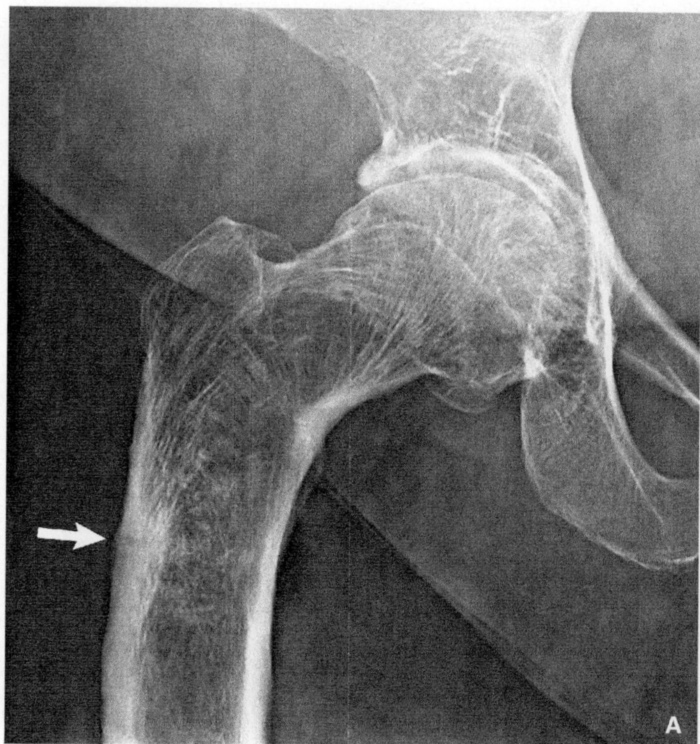

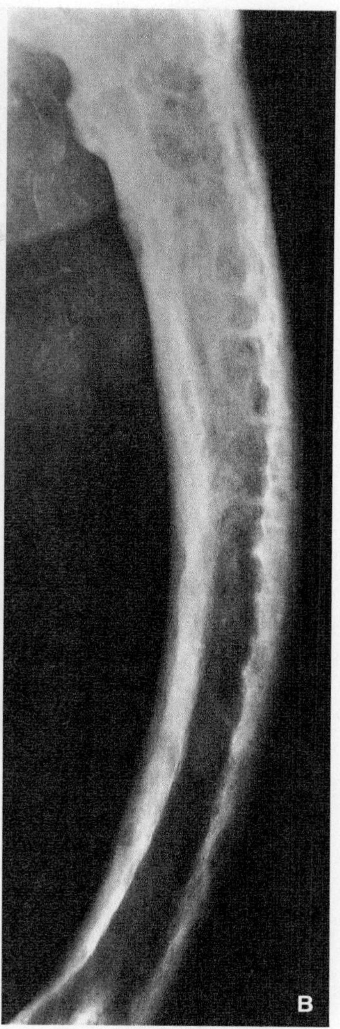

FIGURE 29.22 Stress/insufficiency fractures in Paget disease. **(A)** Anteroposterior radiograph of the right hip of a 70-year-old woman shows Paget disease affecting the proximal femur. Observe the insufficiency fracture within the lateral cortex *(arrow)*. **(B)** Numerous insufficiency fractures, seen in the lateral cortex of the femur in an 80-year-old man with advanced Paget disease, are the most common complications of this condition.

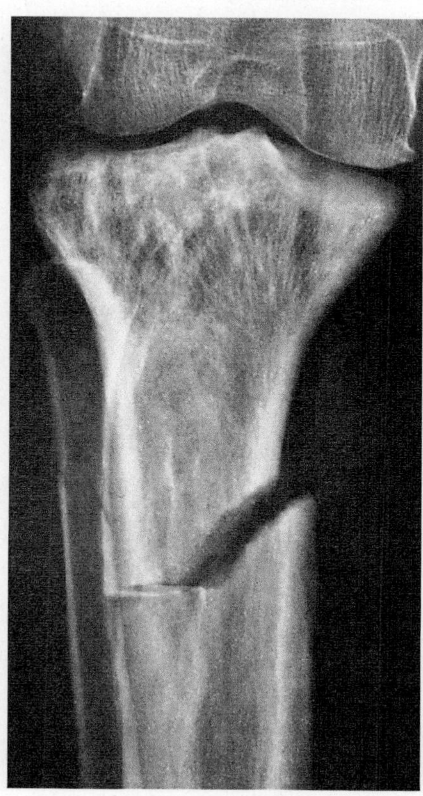

FIGURE 29.23 Pathologic fracture in Paget disease. A 62-year-old man with monostotic Paget disease affecting the right tibia sustained a pathologic fracture. Note that the fracture line traverses the area of active, osteolytic bone destruction. (Reprinted with permission from Sissons HA, Greenspan A. Paget's disease. In: Taveras JM, Ferrucci JT, eds. *Radiology—imaging, diagnosis, intervention*, vol. 5. Philadelphia: JB Lippincott; 1986:1–14.)

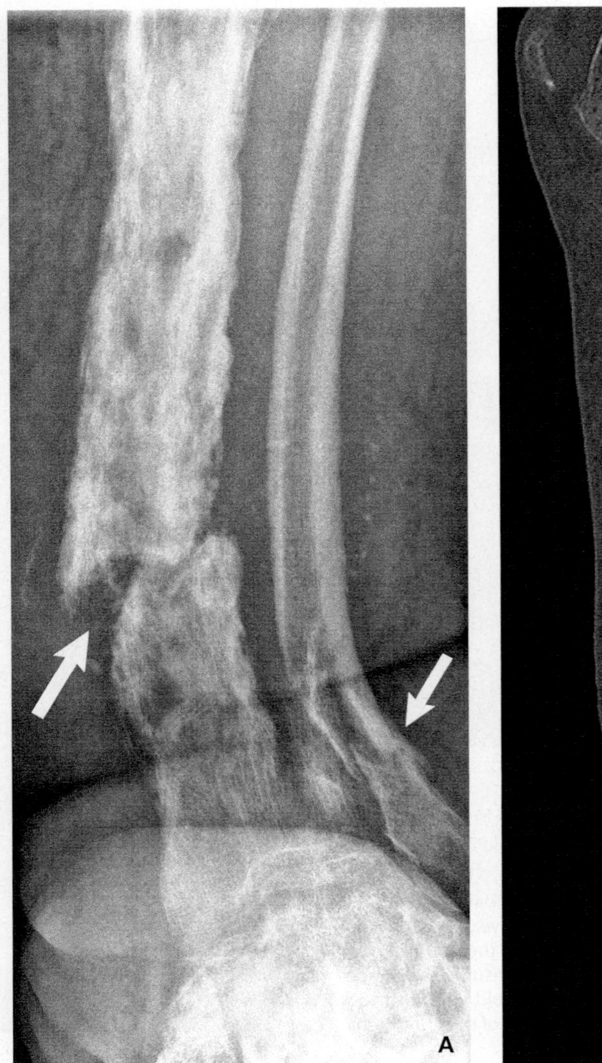

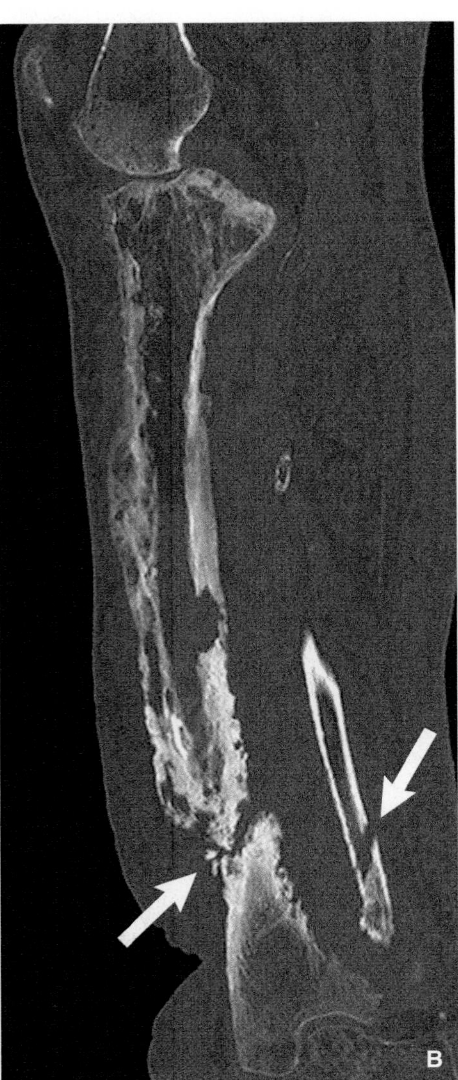

FIGURE 29.24 CT of pathologic fracture in Paget disease. **(A)** Anteroposterior radiograph of the distal left leg of an 89-year-old man and **(B)** sagittal reformatted CT image show a cool phase of the disease affecting the tibia and distal segment of the fibula, complicated by the pathologic fractures *(arrows)*.

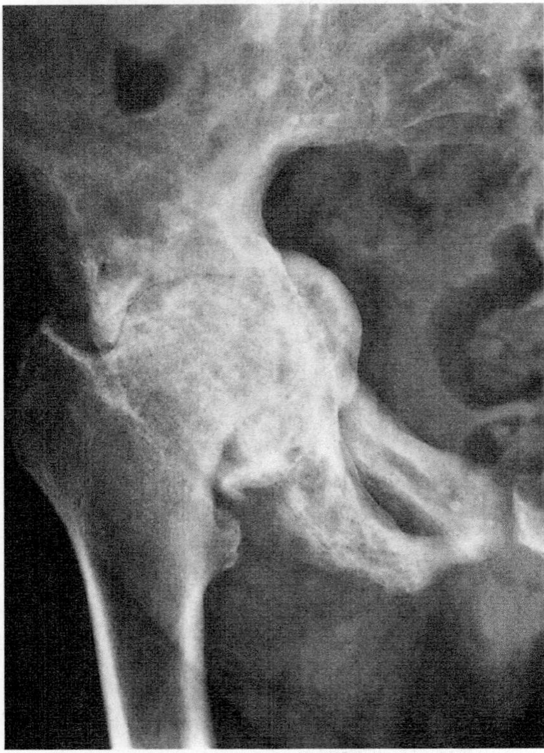

FIGURE 29.25 Secondary osteoarthritis in Paget disease. A 75-year-old woman with long-standing polyostotic Paget disease had been reporting progressive pain in her right hip for 1 year. Anteroposterior radiograph demonstrates advanced osteoarthritis associated with acetabular protrusio.

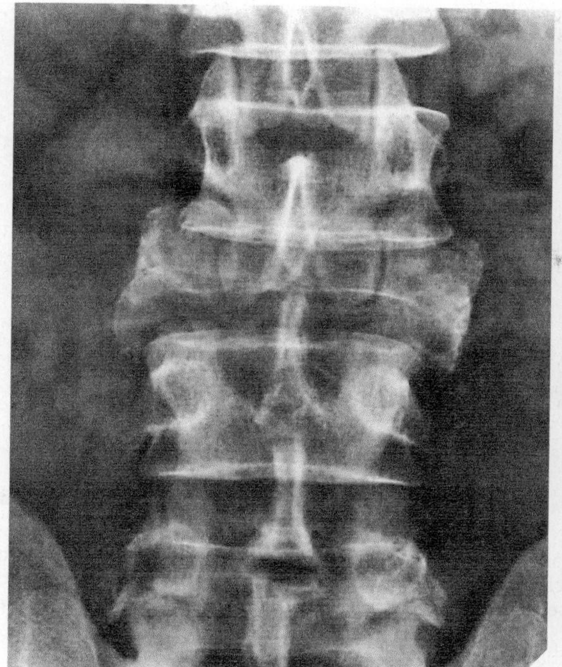

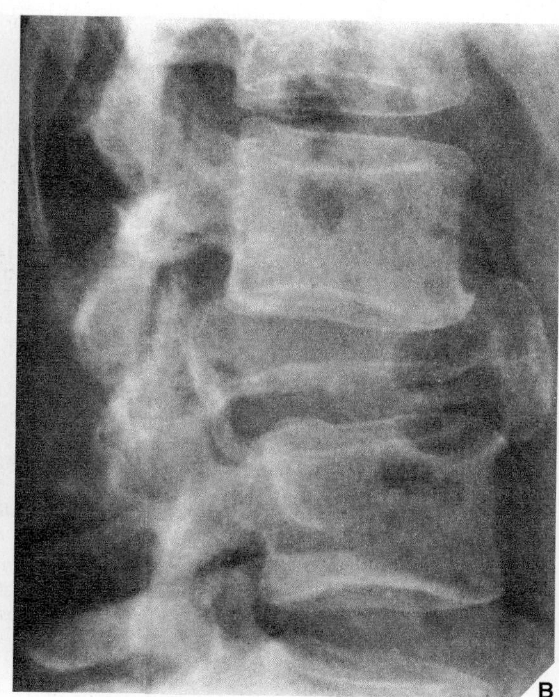

FIGURE 29.26 Pathologic fracture in Paget disease. A 60-year-old man with polyostotic Paget disease presented with lower back pain and neurologic symptoms. **(A)** Anteroposterior and **(B)** lateral radiographs of the lumbar spine show a pathologic burst fracture of L3 with encroachment on the spinal canal, which was the source of his symptoms. (Reprinted with permission from Sissons HA, Greenspan A. Paget's disease. In: Taveras JM, Ferrucci JT, eds. *Radiology—imaging, diagnosis, intervention*, vol. 5. Philadelphia: JB Lippincott; 1986:1–14.)

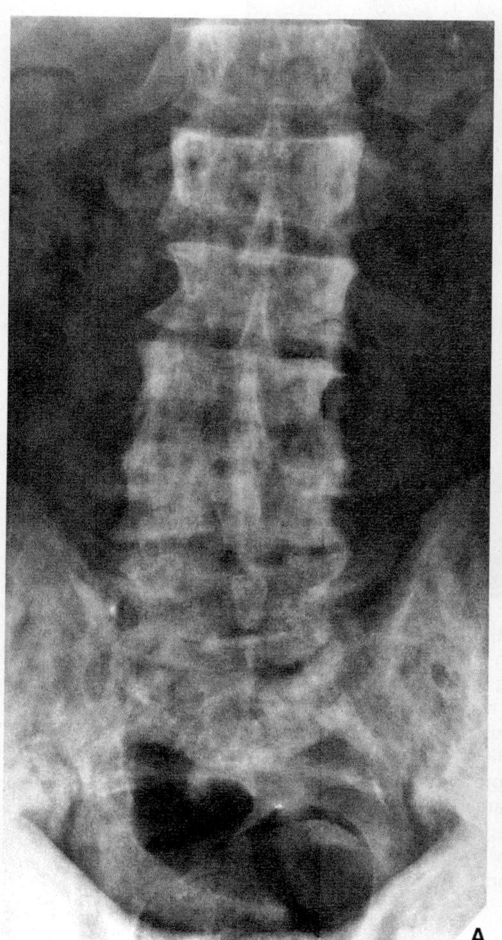

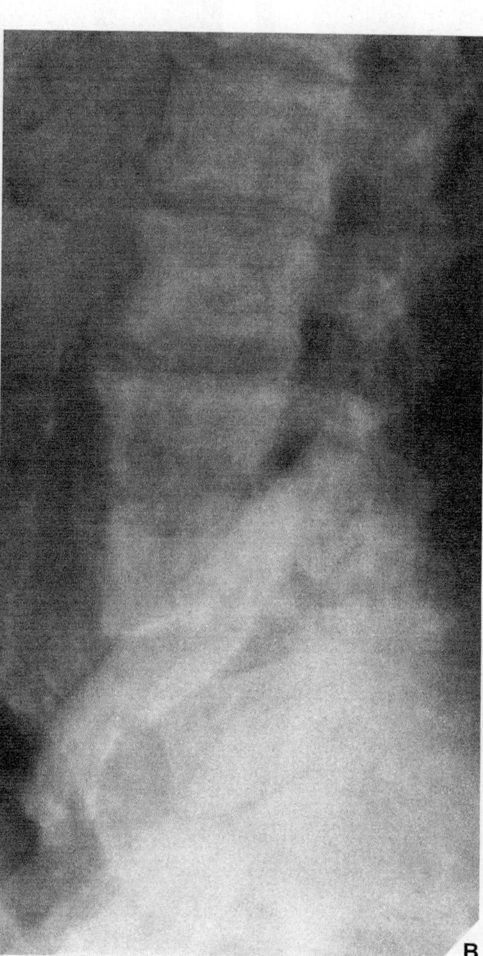

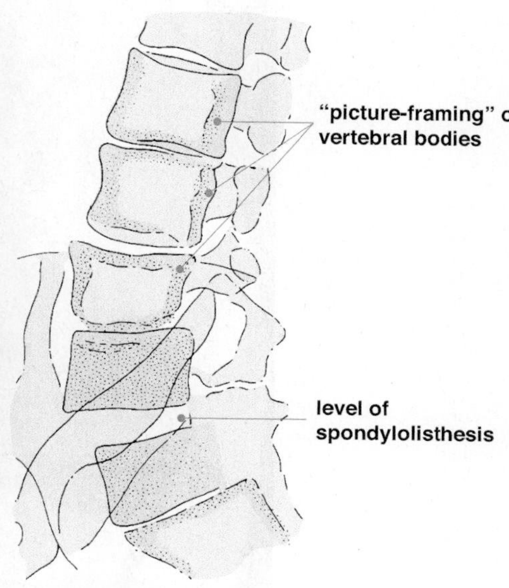

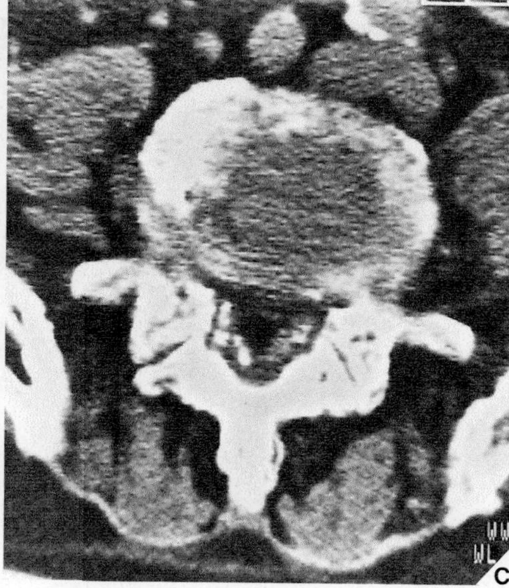

FIGURE 29.27 CT of spinal complications in Paget disease. An 84-year-old man with extensive polyostotic Paget disease for many years developed degenerative spondylolisthesis and spinal stenosis. **(A)** Anteroposterior and **(B)** lateral radiographs of the lumbar spine show Paget disease in the cool phase. Second-degree degenerative spondylolisthesis is seen at the L4-5 level. **(C)** CT section through L5 demonstrates narrowing of the spinal canal characteristic of spinal stenosis, the major cause of most neurologic symptoms in Paget disease.

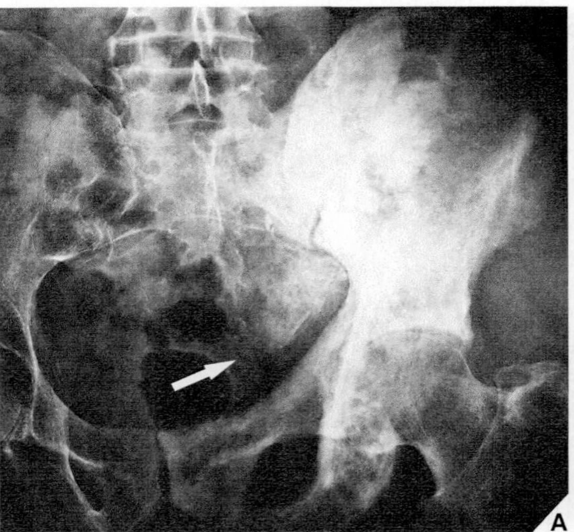

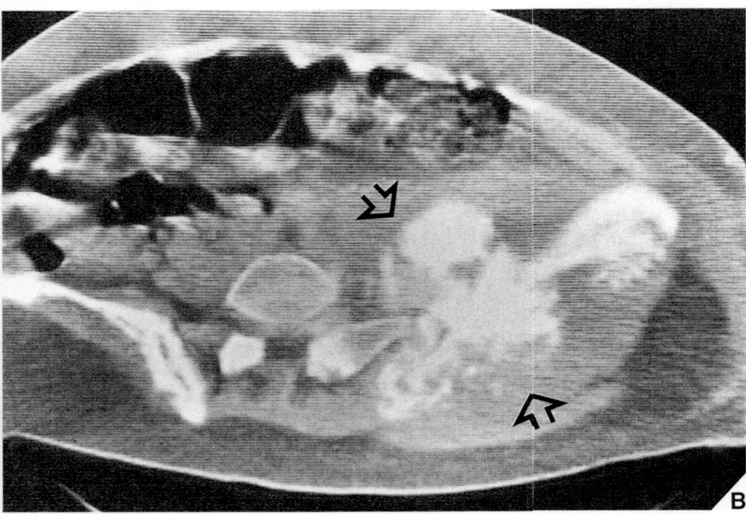

FIGURE 29.28 CT of Paget sarcoma. A 70-year-old woman with Paget disease affecting her left hemipelvis had a rare complication, sarcomatous degeneration. **(A)** Radiograph of the pelvis shows extensive involvement of the left ilium, pubis, and ischium by Paget disease. There is also destruction of the cortex and a large soft-tissue mass accompanied by bone formation *(arrow)*, typical findings for osteosarcoma. **(B)** CT scan demonstrates the soft-tissue mass more clearly *(open arrows)*.

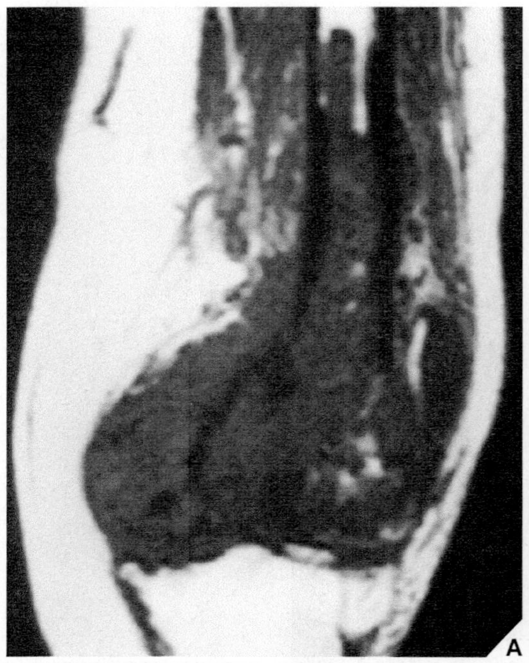

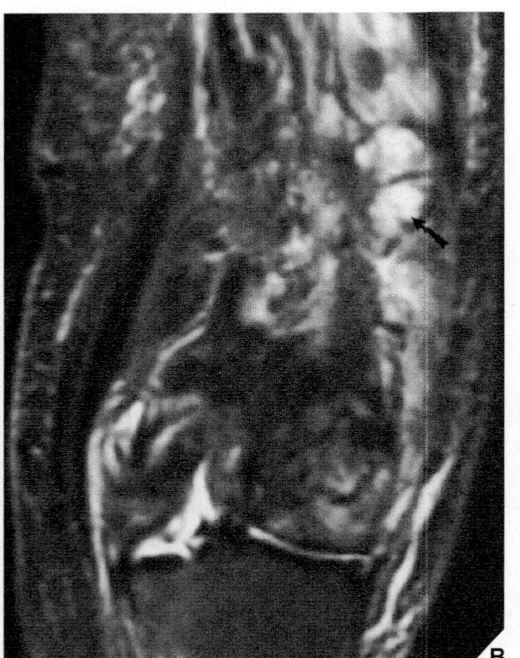

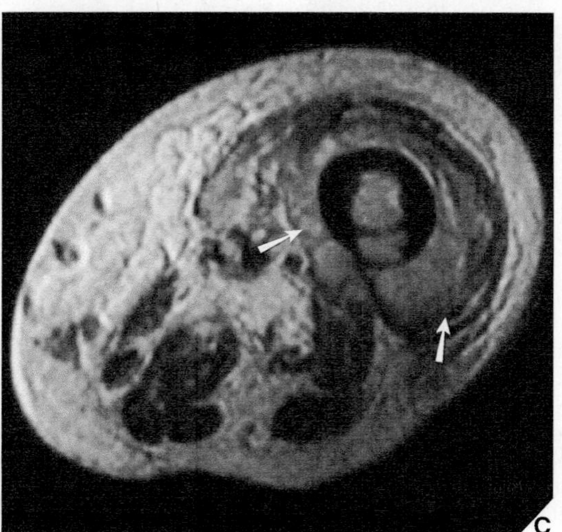

FIGURE 29.29 MRI of Paget sarcoma. **(A)** Coronal T1-weighted (spin echo [SE]; repetition time [TR] 500/echo time [TE] 20 msec) MR image shows Paget disease affecting the distal femur. Destruction of the cortex and soft-tissue mass are well demonstrated. **(B)** Coronal STIR and **(C)** axial T2-weighted sequences confirm the presence of a soft-tissue mass *(arrows)*, thus corroborating the diagnosis of malignant transformation. (Reprinted with permission from Berquist TH, ed. *MRI of the musculoskeletal system*, 3rd ed. Philadelphia: Lippincott-Raven; 1997.)

FIGURE 29.30 Metastases in Paget disease. Anteroposterior radiograph of the pelvis of a 55-year-old woman with Paget disease for 10 years shows extensive osteolytic destruction of the right ilium, ischium, and pubis secondary to metastatic renal cell carcinoma (hypernephroma). Note the typical involvement of the pelvis by Paget disease. This metastatic lesion should not be mistaken for Paget sarcoma.

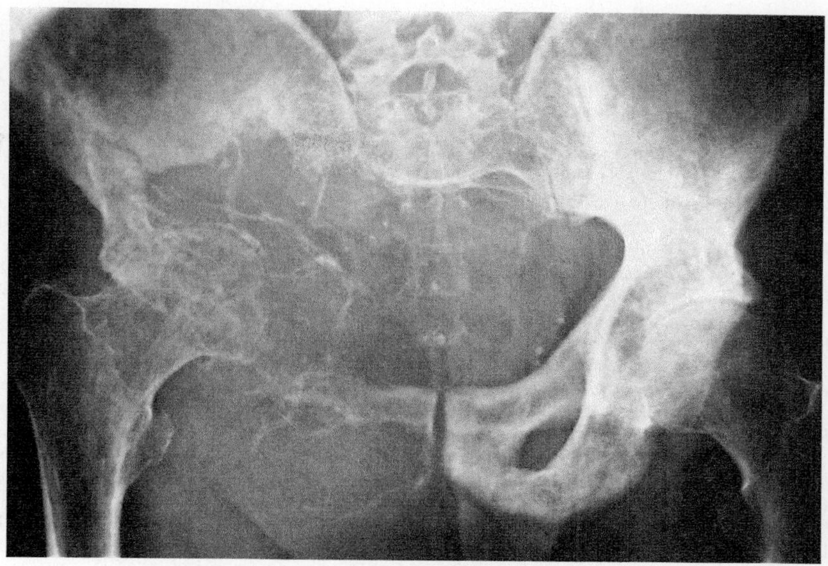

Recently, promising results were achieved with ibandronate and zoledronate. Administration of plicamycin, previously called *mithramycin*, inhibits RNA synthesis and has a potent cytotoxic effect on osteoclasts. The serum alkaline phosphatase determination and the 24-hour urinary hydroxyproline measurement were the main indicators of the response of the disease to medical treatment; however, the recently developed biochemical markers of bone resorption and formation allow a more accurate assessment of disease activity and response to therapy.

PRACTICAL POINTS TO REMEMBER

1. The histologic hallmark of Paget disease is a mosaic pattern of disorderly and active bone remodeling secondary to osteoclastic resorption and osteoblastic formation.
2. The characteristic radiographic features of Paget disease of bone include:
   - involvement of at least one articular end of a long bone
   - thickening of the cortex and enlargement of the affected bone
   - a coarse trabecular pattern to the spongiosa
   - bowing deformities of the long bones
   - a picture frame appearance of a vertebral body.
3. Particular radiographic changes in Paget disease are related to the stage of the disorder. In the acute (hot) phase, a radiolucent osteolytic area is seen:
   - in the calvarium or in a flat bone, where it is known as *osteoporosis circumscripta*
   - in a long bone, where it appears as an advancing wedge of active disease, resembling a candle flame or a blade of grass.
4. Radionuclide bone scan, which invariably shows an increased uptake of the tracer in bones affected by Paget disease, is effective in determining the distribution of the lesion.
5. The most frequent complication of Paget disease is pathologic fracture, either incomplete stress/insufficiency fractures or "banana-type" complete fractures.
6. The most serious complication of Paget disease is sarcomatous degeneration. Radiographically, it can be recognized by:
   - osteolytic bone destruction at the site of the pagetic lesion
   - cortical breakthrough
   - a soft-tissue mass.

   Malignant transformation must be distinguished from metastatic lesions to pagetic bone from a primary carcinoma of the lung, breast, kidney, gastrointestinal tract, or prostate.
7. Paget disease must be distinguished from:
   - "juvenile Paget disease" (familial idiopathic hyperphosphatasia)
   - van Buchem disease (hyperostosis corticalis generalisata)
   - vertebral hemangioma
   - rugger-jersey spine seen in secondary hyperparathyroidism
   - lymphoma
   - extensive osteoblastic metastases.

SUGGESTED READINGS

Adkins MC, Sundaram M. Radiologic case study: insufficiency fracture of the acetabular roof in Paget's disease. *Orthopedics* 2001;24:1019–1020.

Albagha OME, Wani SE, Visconti MR, et al. Genome-wide association identifies three new susceptibility loci for Paget's disease of bone. *Nat Genet* 2011;43:685–689.

Altman RD, Bloch DA, Hochberg MC, et al. Prevalence of pelvic Paget's disease of bone in the United States. *J Bone Miner Res* 2000;15:461–465.

Anderson DC. Paget's disease of bone is characterized by excessive bone resorption coupled with excessive and disorganized bone formation. *Bone* 2001;29:292–293.

Bahk YW, Parh YH, Chung SK, et al. Bone pathologic correlation of multimodality imaging in Paget's disease. *J Nucl Med* 1995;36:1421–1426.

Basle MF, Chappard D, Rebel A. Viral origin of Paget's disease of bone? *Presse Med* 1996;25:113–118.

Beaudouin C, Dohan A, Nasrallah T, et al. Atypical vertebral Paget's disease. *Skeletal Radiol* 2014;43:991–995.

Berquist TH, ed. *MRI of the musculoskeletal system*, 3rd ed. Philadelphia: Lippincott-Raven; 1996:920–922.

Birch MA, Taylor W, Fraser WD, et al. Absence of paramyxovirus RNA in cultures of pagetic bone cells and in pagetic bone. *J Bone Miner Res* 1994;9:11–16.

Brandolini F, Bacchini P, Moscato M, et al. Chondrosarcoma as a complicating factor in Paget's disease of bone. *Skeletal Radiol* 1997;26:497–500.

Brown JP, Chines AA, Myers WR, et al. Improvement of pagetic bone lesions with risedronate treatment: a radiologic study. *Bone* 2000;26:263–267.

Colarintha P, Fonseca AT, Salgado L, et al. Diagnosis of malignant change in Paget's disease by T1–201. *Clin Nucl Med* 1996;21:299–301.

Conrad GR, Johnson AW. Solitary adenocarcinoma metastasis mimicking sarcomatous degeneration in Paget's disease. *Clin Nucl Med* 1997;22:300–302.

Delmas PD, Meunier PJ. The management of Paget's disease of bone. *N Engl J Med* 1997;336:558–566.

Fenton P, Resnick D. Metastases to bone affected by Paget's disease: a report of three cases. *Int Orthop* 1991;15:397–399.

Frassica FJ, Sim FH, Frassica DA, et al. Survival and management considerations in postirradiation osteosarcoma and Paget's osteosarcoma. *Clin Orthop Relat Res* 1991;270:120–127.

Greditzer HG III, McLeod RA, Unni KK, et al. Bone sarcomas in Paget disease. *Radiology* 1983;146:327–333.

Greenspan A. A review of Paget's disease: radiologic imaging, differential diagnosis, and treatment. *Bull Hosp Jt Dis* 1991;51:22–33.

Greenspan A. Paget's disease: current concept, radiologic imaging, and treatment. *Recent Adv Orthop* 1993;1:32–48.

Greenspan A, Norman A, Sterling AP. Precocious onset of Paget's disease—a report of three cases and review of the literature. *J Can Assoc Radiol* 1977;28:69–72.

Hadjipavlou A, Gaitanis IN, Kontakis GM. Paget's disease of the bone and its management. *J Bone Joint Surg Br* 2002;84(2):160–169.

Hadjipavlou A, Lander P, Srolovitz H, et al. Malignant transformation in Paget disease of bone. *Cancer* 1992;70:2802–2808.

Hosking D, Meunier PJ, Ringe JD, et al. Paget's disease of bone: diagnosis and management. *BMJ* 1996;312:491–495.

Hutter RV, Foote FW Jr, Frazell EL, et al. Giant cell tumors complicating Paget's disease of bone. *Cancer* 1963;16:1044–1056.

Kang H, Park Y-C, Yang KH. Paget's disease: skeletal manifestations and effect of biphosphonates. *J Bone Metab* 2017;24:97–103.

Kaufmann GA, Sundaram M, McDonald DJ. Magnetic resonance imaging in symptomatic Paget's disease. *Skeletal Radiol* 1991;20:413–418.

Kilcoyne A, Heffernan EJ. Atypical proximal femoral fractures in patients with Paget disease receiving bisphosphonate therapy. *AJR Am J Roentgenol* 2011;197:W196–W197.

Kim CK, Estrada WN, Lorberboym M, et al. The "mouse face" appearance of the vertebrae in Paget's disease. *Clin Nucl Med* 1997;22:104–108.

Kumar A, Kumar PG, Prakash MS, et al. Paget's disease diagnosed on bone scintigraphy: case report and literature review. *Indian J Nucl Med* 2013;28:121–123.

Kunin JR, Strouse PJ. The "yarmulke" sign of Paget's disease. *Clin Nucl Med* 1991;16:788–789.

Lander PH, Hadjipavlou AG. A dynamic classification of Paget's disease. *J Bone Joint Surg Br* 1986;68B:431–438.

Laurin N, Brown JP, Morisette J, et al. Recurrent mutation of the gene encoding sequestome 1 (SQSTM1/p62) in Paget disease of bone. *Am J Hum Genet* 2002;70:1582–1588.

Leach RJ, Singer FR, Roodman GD. The genetics of Paget's disease of bone. *J Clin Endocrin Metab* 2001;86:24–28.

Meunier PJ, Vignot E. Therapeutic strategy in Paget's disease of bone. *Bone* 1995;17:489S–491S.

Mills BG, Frausto A, Singer FR, et al. Multinucleated cells formed in vitro from Paget's bone marrows express viral antigens. *Bone* 1994;15:443–448.

Mirra JM. Pathogenesis of Paget's disease based on viral etiology. *Clin Orthop Relat Res* 1987;217:162–170.

Mirra JM, Brien EW, Tehranzadeh J. Paget's disease of bone: review with emphasis on radiologic features. Part I. *Skeletal Radiol* 1995;24:163–171, 173–184.

Moore TE, Kathol MH, El-Koury GY, et al. Unusual radiologic features of Paget's disease of bone. *Skeletal Radiol* 1994;23:257–260.

Nicholas JJ, Srodes CH, Herbert D, et al. Metastatic cancer in Paget's disease of bone: a case report. *Orthopedics* 1987;10:725–729.

Paget J. On a form of chronic inflammation of bones (osteitis deformans). *Med Chir Trans* 1877;60:37–64.

Potter HG, Schneider R, Ghelman B, et al. Multiple giant cell tumors and Paget disease of bone: radiographic and clinical correlations. *Radiology* 1991;180:261–264.

Rosenbaum HD, Hanson DJ. Geographic variation in the prevalence of Paget's disease of bone. *Radiology* 1969;92:959–963.

Ryan PJ, Fogelman I. Paget's disease—five years follow-up after pamidronate therapy. *Br J Rheumatol* 1994;33:98–99.

Sissons HA, Greenspan A. Paget's disease. In: Taveras JM, Ferrucci JT, eds. *Radiology—imaging, diagnosis, intervention*, vol. 5. Philadelphia: JB Lippincott; 1986:1–14.

Smith SE, Murphey MD, Motamedi K, et al. From the Archives of the AFIP. Radiologic spectrum of Paget disease of bone and its complications with pathologic correlation. *Radiographics* 2002;22:1191–1216.

Sundaram MG, Khanna G, El-Khoury GY. T1-weighted MR imaging for distinguishing large osteolysis of Paget's disease from sarcomatous degeneration. *Skeletal Radiol* 2001;30:378–383.

Wallace E, Wong J, Reid IR. Pamidronate treatment of the neurologic sequelae of pagetic spinal stenosis. *Arch Intern Med* 1995;155:1813–1815.

Whyte MP. Paget's disease of bone. *N Engl J Med* 2006;355:593–600.

Wittenberg K. The blade of grass sign. *Radiology* 2001;221:199–200.

Yu T, Squires F, Mammone J, et al. Lymphoma arising in Paget's disease. *Skeletal Radiol* 1997;26:729–731.

30

Miscellaneous Metabolic and Endocrine Disorders

Familial Idiopathic Hyperphosphatasia

Clinical Features

Familial idiopathic hyperphosphatasia, also known as *hyperostosis corticalis deformans juvenilis*, *familial osteoectasia*, or *juvenile Paget disease*, is a rare autosomal recessive disorder affecting young children, generally within their first 18 months and exhibiting a striking predilection for those of Puerto Rican descent. The condition is associated with progressive bone deformities. Clinically, it is characterized by dwarfism, painful bowing of the limbs, muscular weakness, abnormal gait, acetabular protrusio, pathologic fractures, spinal deformities, loss of vision and hearing, elevation of serum alkaline phosphatase, and an increase in the amount of leucine aminopeptidase. Recent investigations suggest that this disorder is caused by mutations in the *TNFRSF11B* gene located on the long arm of chromosome 8 (8q24) that result in deficiency of osteoprotegerin (OPG). OPG is a cytokine receptor, also known as *osteoclastogenesis inhibitor factor* (OCIF), which normally suppresses bone resorption by regulating activity of osteoclasts.

Imaging Features

Increased turnover of bone and skeletal collagen demonstrated by radionuclide bone scan is a characteristic finding in familial idiopathic hyperphosphatasia. Its radiographic features are typical. Although this disorder has no relationship to classic Paget disease, it is often referred to as *juvenile Paget disease*, and it exhibits similar radiographic features. The long bones are increased in size, showing thickening of the cortex and a coarse trabecular pattern (Figs. 30.1 and 30.2). Likewise, bowing deformities are common, as are involvement of the pelvis and skull (Fig. 30.3). However, unlike Paget disease, the epiphyses are usually not affected.

Treatment consists of administration of bisphosphonates and calcitonins.

Differential Diagnosis

A few conditions exist similar to familial idiopathic hyperphosphatasia that belong to the general group of endosteal hyperostoses, or hyperostosis corticalis generalisata. In particular, an autosomal recessive form of these disorders, van Buchem disease, although classified as chronic hyperphosphatasia tarda, is in fact a distinct dysplasia. Its onset is later than that of congenital hyperphosphatasia, and the age of patients ranges from 25 to 50 years. The major radiographic finding is a symmetric thickening of the cortices of the long and short tubular bones. The femora are not bowed, and the articular ends are spared. The cranial bones show marked thickening of the vault and the base. Serum alkaline phosphatase levels are elevated, but calcium and phosphorus levels are normal. More detailed description of this dysplasia is provided in Chapter 33.

Acromegaly

Clinical Features

Increased secretion of growth hormone (somatotropin) by the eosinophilic cells of the anterior lobe of the pituitary gland, as a result of either hyperplasia of the gland or a tumor, leads to acceleration of bone growth. If this condition develops before skeletal maturity (i.e., while the growth plates are still open), then it results in gigantism; development after skeletal maturity results in acromegaly. The onset of symptoms is usually insidious, and the involvement of certain target sites in the skeleton is typical (Fig. 30.4). Gradual enlargement of the hands and feet as well as exaggeration of facial features are the earliest manifestations. The characteristic facial changes result from overgrowth of the frontal sinuses, protrusion of the jaw (prognathism), accentuation of the orbital ridges, enlargement of the nose and lips, and thickening and coarsening of the soft tissues of the face.

Imaging Features

Radiographic examination reveals a number of characteristic features of this condition. A lateral radiograph of the skull demonstrates thickening of the cranial bones and increased density. The diploe may be obliterated. The sella turcica, which houses the pituitary gland, may or may not be enlarged. The paranasal sinuses become enlarged (Fig. 30.5) and the mastoid cells become overpneumatized. The prognathous jaw, one of the obvious clinical features of this condition, is apparent on the lateral view of the facial bones.

The hands also exhibit revealing radiographic changes. The heads of the metacarpals are enlarged, and irregular bony thickening along the margins, simulating beak-like osteophytes, may be seen. Increase in the size of the sesamoid at the metacarpophalangeal joint of the thumb may be helpful in evaluating acromegaly. Values of the sesamoid index (determined by the height and width of this ossicle measured in millimeters) greater than 30 in women and greater than 40 in men suggest acromegaly; however, generally, the dividing line between normal and abnormal values is not sharp enough to allow individual borderline cases to be diagnosed on the basis of this index alone. Characteristic changes are also seen in the distal phalanges; their bases enlarge and the terminal tufts form spur-like projections. The joint spaces widen as a result of hypertrophy of articular cartilage (Fig. 30.6), and hypertrophy of the

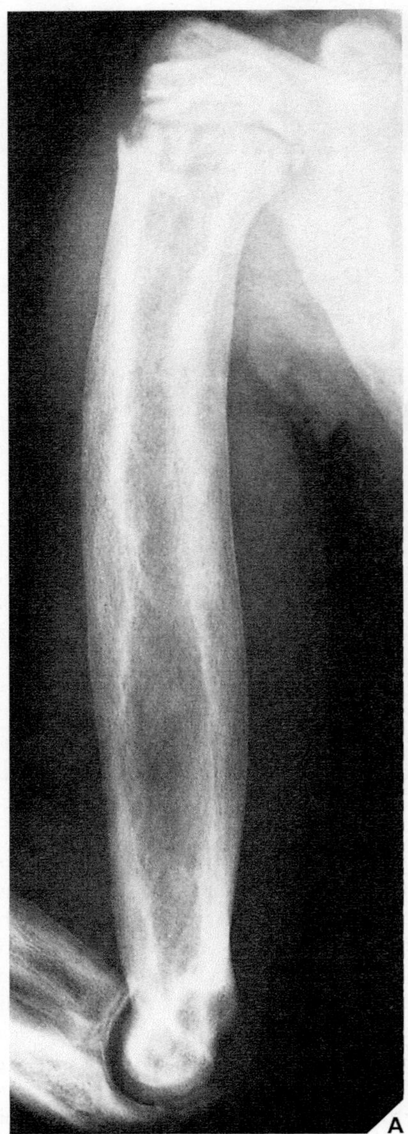

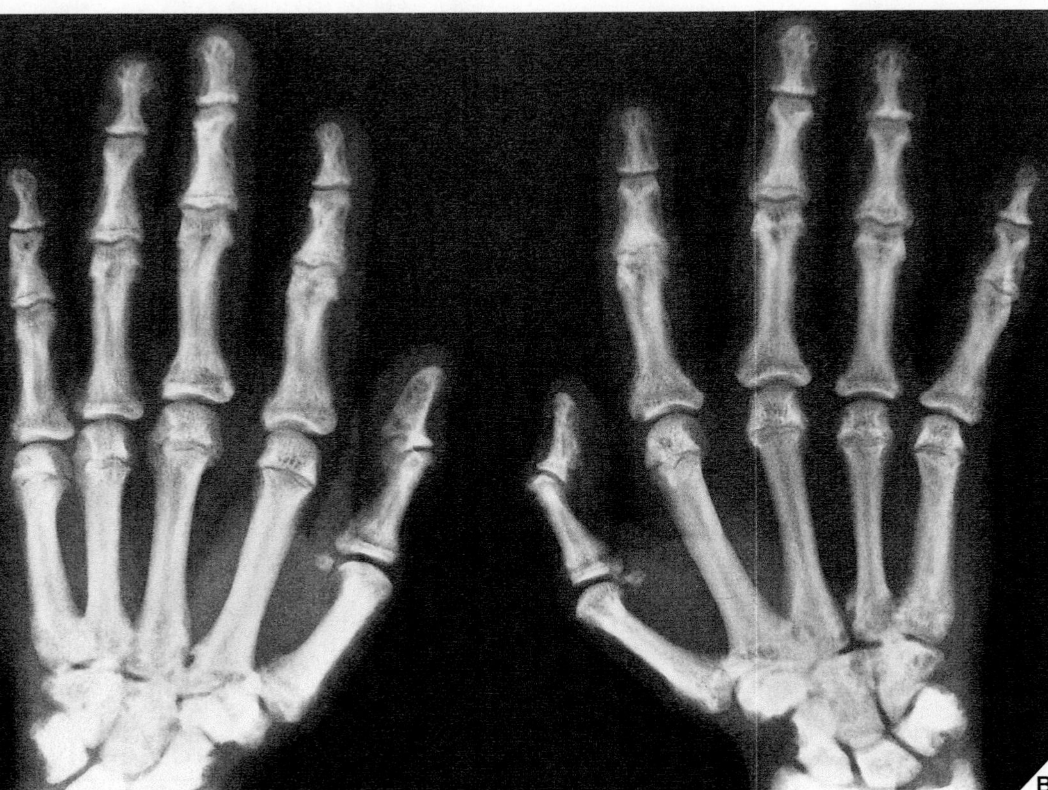

FIGURE 30.1 Familial idiopathic hyperphosphatasia. **(A)** Anteroposterior radiograph of the shoulder and arm of a 12-year-old Puerto Rican boy reveals marked thickening of the cortex of the humerus and coarsening of the bony trabeculae, resembling pagetic bone. **(B)** Radiograph of the hands shows sclerotic changes in the bones and a marked narrowing of the medullary cavity of the metacarpals and phalanges.

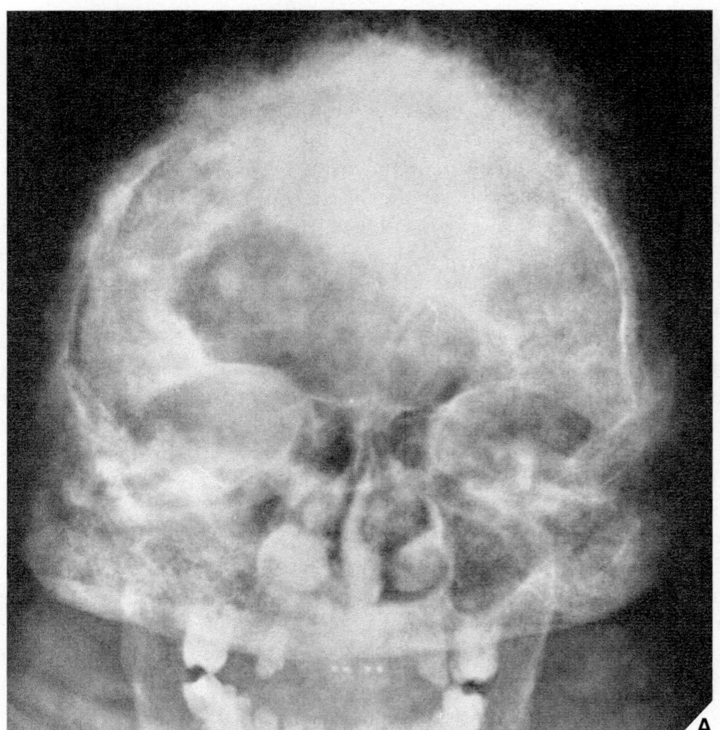

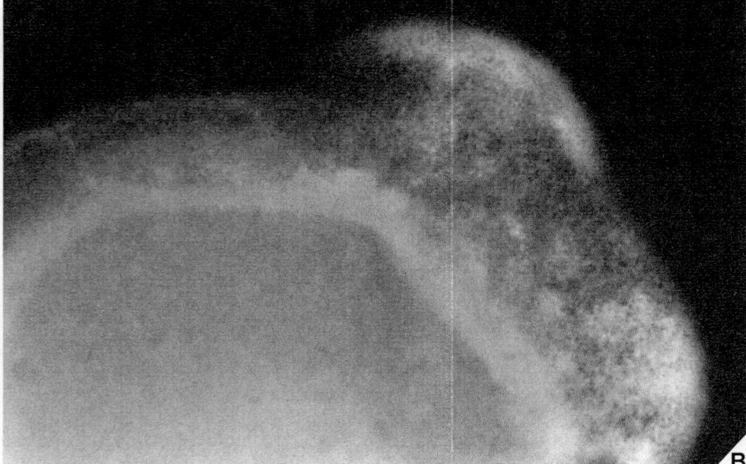

FIGURE 30.2 Familial idiopathic hyperphosphatasia. **(A)** Anteroposterior radiograph of the skull of a 30-year-old man shows calvarial thickening and sclerosis resembling that of Paget disease. **(B)** Magnification study reveals marked thickening of the inner table and widening of the diploe.

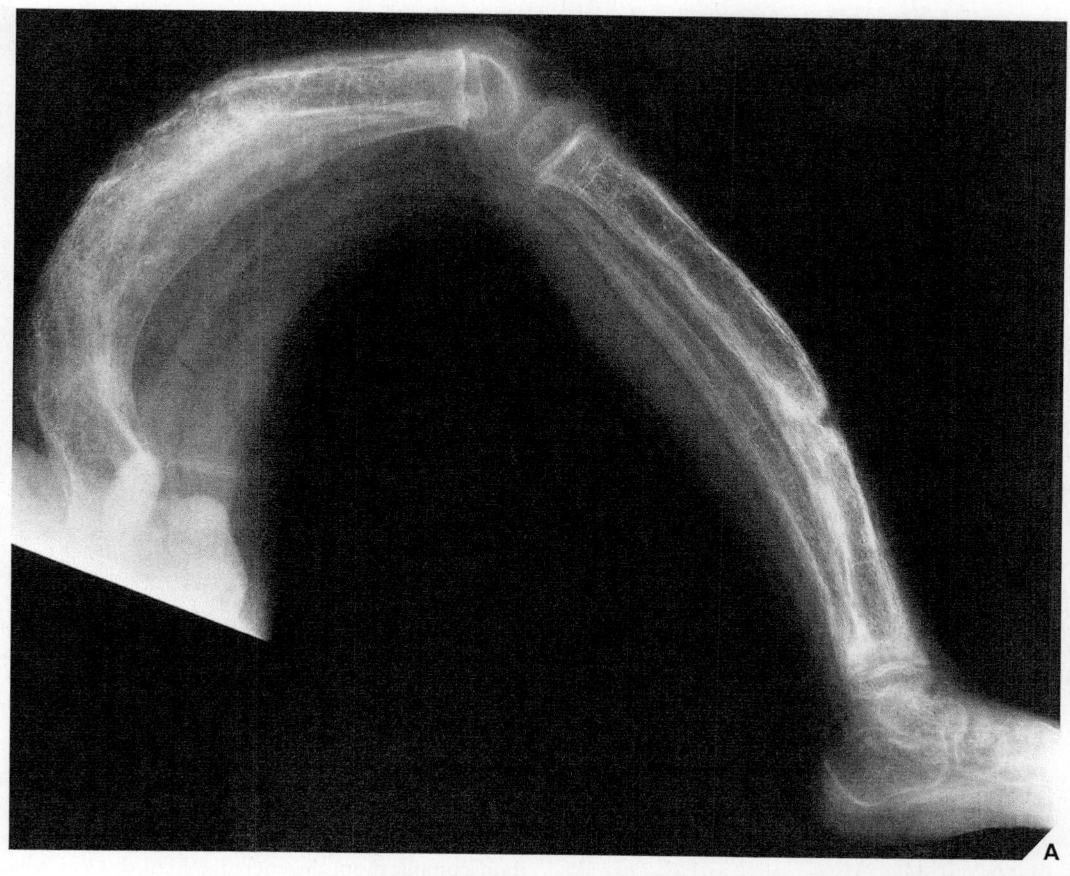

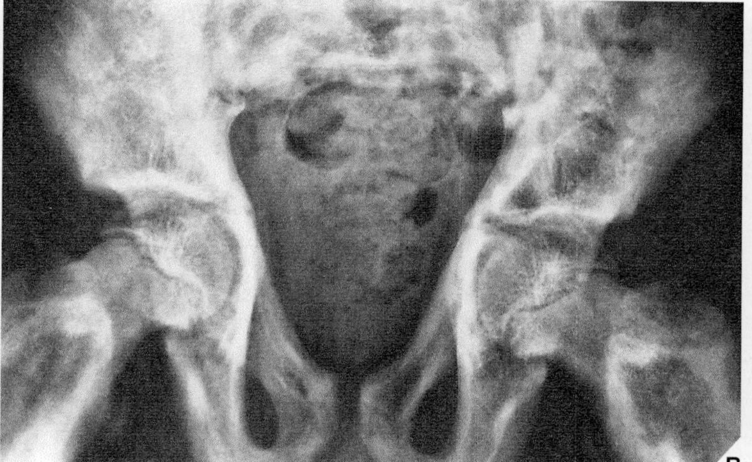

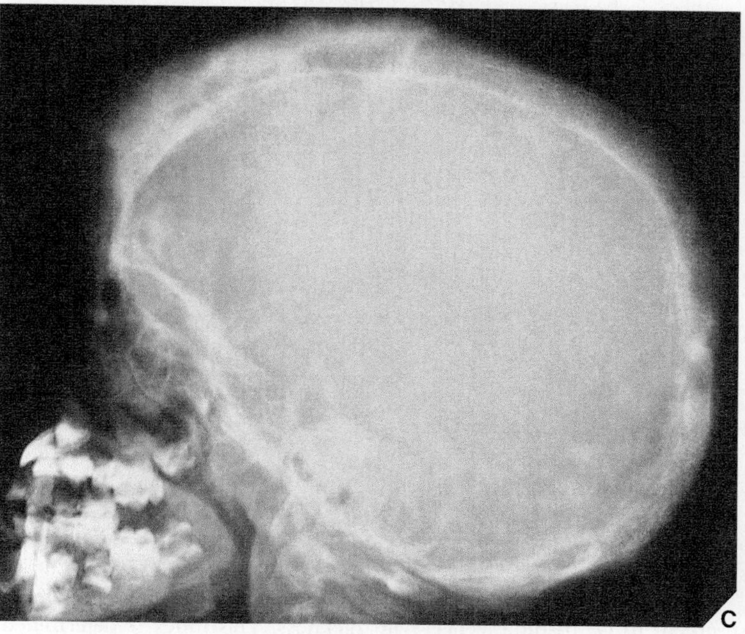

FIGURE 30.3 **Familial idiopathic hyperphosphatasia. (A)** Radiograph of a 4-year-old boy demonstrates marked bowing of the long bones of the lower extremity, a striking feature of this disorder. **(B)** Anteroposterior radiograph of the pelvis shows the coarse trabecular pattern and cortical thickening typical of this condition. Note that the epiphyses are not affected. **(C)** Lateral radiograph of the skull demonstrates thickening of the tables and a "cotton ball" appearance of the cranial vault, similar to that of Paget disease. (**B**, Reprinted with permission from Sissons HA, Greenspan A. Paget's disease. In: Taveras JM, Ferrucci JT, eds. *Radiology—imaging, diagnosis, intervention.* Philadelphia: JB Lippincott; 1986:1–14.)

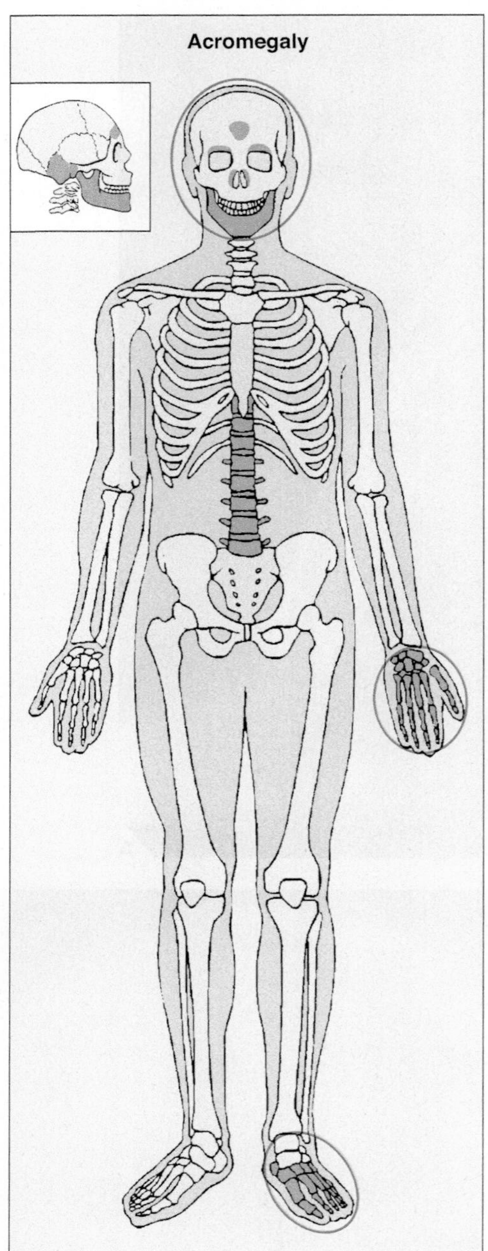

FIGURE 30.4 The most clearly revealing target sites of acromegaly.

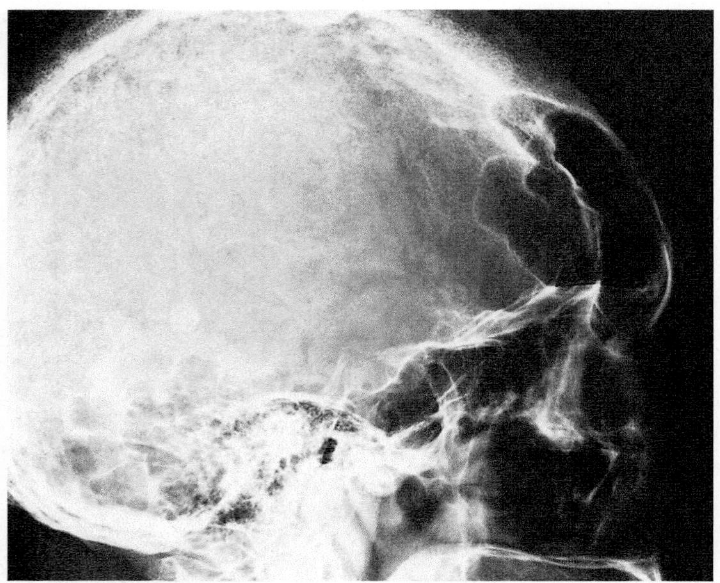

FIGURE 30.5 Acromegalic skull. Lateral radiograph of the skull of a 75-year-old woman shows marked enlargement of the frontal sinuses, prominent supraorbital ridges, and thickening of the frontal bones.

soft tissues may also occur, leading to the development of square, spade-shaped fingers.

Evaluation of the foot on the lateral view allows an important measurement to be made, the heel-pad thickness. This index is determined by the distance from the posteroinferior surface of the calcaneus to the nearest skin surface. In a normal 150-lb subject, the heel-pad thickness should not exceed 22 mm. For each additional 25 lb of body weight, 1 mm can be added to the basic value; thus, 24 mm would be the highest normal value for a 200-lb person. If the heel-pad thickness is greater than the established normal value, then acromegaly is a strong possibility (Fig. 30.7), and determination of growth hormone level by immunoassay is called for.

The spine in acromegaly may also reveal identifying features. A lateral radiograph of the spine may disclose an increase in the anteroposterior diameter of a vertebral body as well as scalloping or increased concavity of the posterior vertebral margin (Fig. 30.8). Although the exact mechanism of this phenomenon is not known, bone resorption has been implicated as a potential cause. Other conditions have also been associated with posterior vertebral scalloping (Table 30.1). In addition, thoracic kyphosis is often increased in spinal acromegaly and lumbar lordosis is accentuated. The intervertebral disk space may be wider than normal because of overgrowth of the cartilaginous portion of the disk.

The articular abnormalities seen in acromegaly are the result of a common complication, degenerative joint disease, which is in turn the result

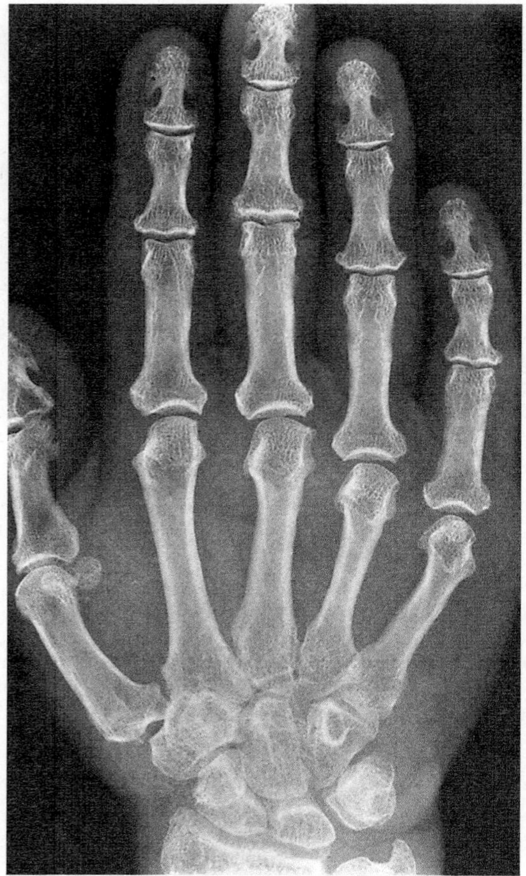

FIGURE 30.6 Acromegalic hand. Dorsovolar radiograph of the hand of a 38-year-old woman shows characteristic overgrowth of the terminal tufts and spur-like projections. The bases of the terminal phalanges are also enlarged, and the radiographic joint spaces are widened.

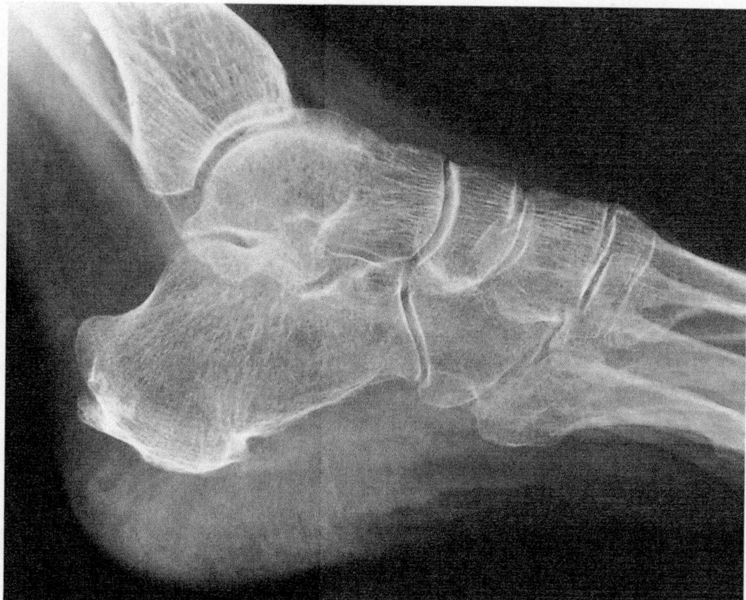

FIGURE 30.7 Acromegalic foot. Lateral radiograph of the foot of a 58-year-old man shows a heel-pad thickness of 38 mm, far above normal for this patient who weighs only 140 lb. This measurement corresponds to the shortest distance between the calcaneus and the plantar aspect of the heel.

of overgrowth of the articular cartilage and subsequent inadequate nourishment of abnormally thick cartilage. The combination of joint space narrowing, osteophytes, subchondral sclerosis, and formation of cyst-like lesions is similar to the primary osteoarthritic process. Acromegalic arthropathy was also discussed in Chapter 13.

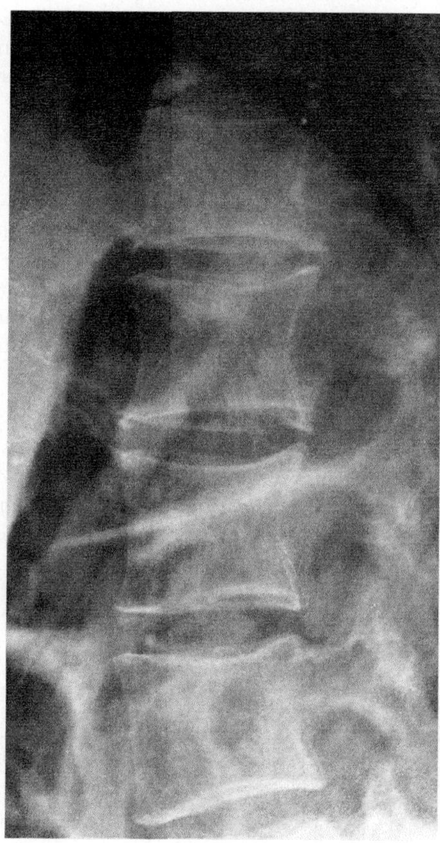

FIGURE 30.8 Acromegalic spine. Lateral radiograph of the thoracolumbar spine of a 49-year-old woman demonstrates posterior vertebral scalloping, a phenomenon apparently caused by bone resorption.

TABLE 30.1 Causes of Scalloping in Vertebral Bodies
Increased Intraspinal Pressure
Intradural neoplasms
Intraspinal cysts
Syringomyelia and hydromyelia
Communicating hydrocephalus
Dural Ectasia
Marfan syndrome
Ehlers-Danlos syndrome
Neurofibromatosis
Bone Resorption
Acromegaly
Congenital Disorders
Achondroplasia
Morquio disease
Hunter syndrome
Osteogenesis imperfecta (tarda)
Physiologic Scalloping

Reprinted from Mitchell GE, Lourie H, Berne AS. The various causes of scalloped vertebrae with notes on their pathogenesis. *Radiology* 1967;89:67–74. Copyright © 1967 by The Radiological Society of North America, Inc.

Gaucher Disease

Classification and Clinical Features

Gaucher disease is a familial inherited disturbance transmitted as an autosomal recessive trait, arising from numerous mutations at the genetic locus encoding the enzyme glucocerebrosidase (glucocerebrosidase cerebroside β-glucosidase) located on chromosome 1 (1q21), that leads to the defective activity of lysosomal hydrolase. It is a metabolic disorder characterized by the abnormal deposition of cerebrosides (glycolipids) in the reticuloendothelial cells of the spleen, liver, and bone marrow. These altered macrophages, called *Gaucher cells*, are the histologic hallmark of the disease. Gaucher disease is classified into three distinct categories (phenotypes):

Type I: The *nonneuronopathic*, or *adult type*, is the most common form, occurring mainly in Ashkenazi Jews. Onset is in the patient's first or second decade, and the individuals affected usually live normal life spans. Bone abnormalities and hepatosplenomegaly characterize this form of the disease, although some patients may not show any symptoms.

Type II: The *acute neuronopathic* form is lethal within the patient's first year. This type apparently has no predilection for any ethnic group. Hepatosplenomegaly is invariably present, in addition to brain damage and seizure disorder.

Type III: The *subacute juvenile neuronopathic* form, occurring mainly in Swedish nationality from the Norrbotten region begins in the latter part of the first year and follows a malignant course similar to that of type II. Patients present with hepatosplenomegaly, anemia, respiratory problems, mental retardation, and seizures and usually die by the end of their second decade of life.

The presenting clinical features of patients depend on the type of disease they have. The adult form of the disorder (type I) is the most common one and typically presents with abdominal distention secondary to splenomegaly. Recurrent bone pain is a sign of skeletal involvement, and acute severe bone pain together with swelling and fever suggests acute pyogenic osteomyelitis. This clinical complex, which is the result of ischemic necrosis of bone, has been called *aseptic osteomyelitis*. Pingueculae may be present in the eyes, and the skin may acquire a brown pigmentation. Epistaxis or other hemorrhages caused by thrombocytopenia may occur. The diagnosis is made by demonstrating characteristic Gaucher cells in bone marrow aspirate or in a biopsy specimen from the liver.

Imaging Features

The radiographic examination in Gaucher disease reveals characteristic findings. There is a diffuse osteoporosis that is frequently associated with

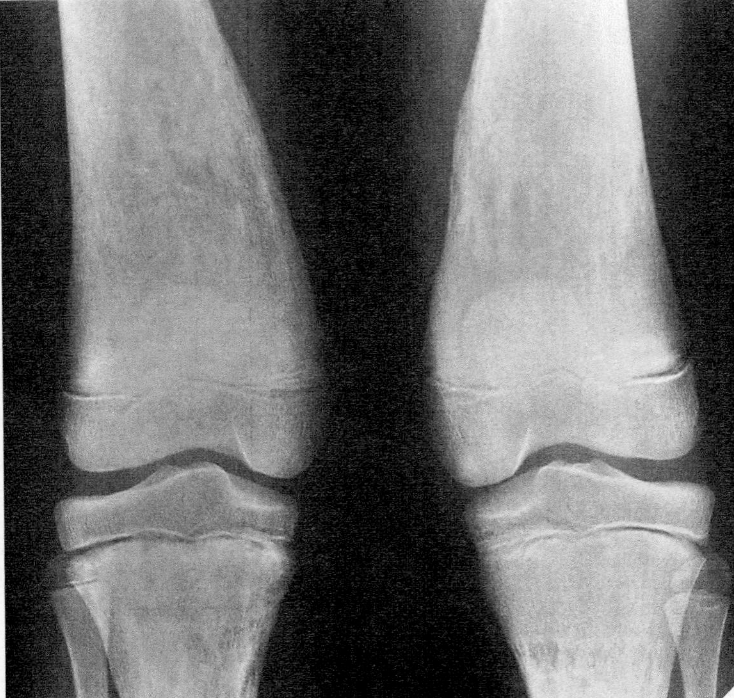

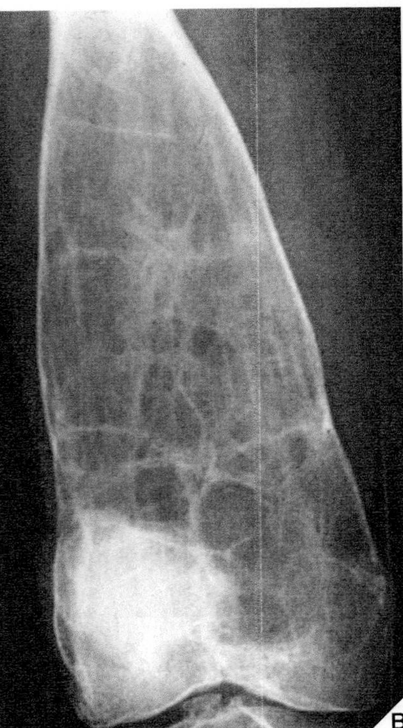

FIGURE 30.9 Gaucher disease. **(A)** Anteroposterior radiograph of a 12-year-old boy with adult-type of disease shows the Erlenmeyer flask deformity of both distal femora, secondary to medullary expansion. Note the thinning of the cortex caused by diffuse osteoporosis. **(B)** Anteroposterior radiograph of the distal femur in another patient demonstrates characteristic Erlenmeyer flask deformity. Note the enlarged spaces between trabeculae due to the accumulation of Gaucher cells, giving a "bubbly" appearance.

medullary expansion. In the ends of the long bones, this phenomenon is referred to as the *Erlenmeyer flask deformity* (Fig. 30.9 and Table 30.2). Localized bone destruction assuming a honeycomb appearance is also typically seen (Fig. 30.10); gross osteolytic destruction is usually limited to the shafts of the long bones and occasionally may be seen within the cortical bone. Moreover, sclerotic changes are common, occurring secondary to a repair process or bone infarctions (Fig. 30.11). Medullary bone infarction and a periosteal reaction may lead to a bone-within-bone phenomenon, which may resemble osteomyelitis (Fig. 30.12). Hermann and associates conducted a study of 29 patients with type I Gaucher disease using magnetic resonance imaging (MRI) to determine the usefulness of this technique in the evaluation of bone marrow involvement. The results of this investigation suggest that MRI is a valuable noninvasive modality in this respect to assess disease activity. Apparently, the patients with decreased signal intensity within bone marrow on both T1-weighted and T2-weighted images but showing a relative increase in signal intensity from T1 weighting to T2 weighting can be considered to have an "active process" that correlates well with their symptoms. More recently, quantitative MRI technique in form of quantitative chemical shift imaging (QCSI) was introduced. This technique quantifies the fat content in bone marrow by using the difference in resonant frequencies between fat and water, thus detecting the reduction in the fat fraction that occurs when Gaucher cells displace the normal triglyceride-rich adipocytes in bone marrow. Low bone marrow fat fractions as detected by QCSI have been shown to correspond to increased clinical activity of the disease and emerging osseous complications. This technique also can be effective as a tool for monitoring response to treatment.

TABLE 30.2 Causes of Erlenmeyer Flask Deformity

Gaucher disease
Niemann-Pick disease
Fibrous dysplasia
Sickle cell anemia
Thalassemia
Multiple cartilaginous exostoses
Ollier disease (enchondromatosis)
Albers-Schönberg disease (osteopetrosis)
Engelmann disease (progressive diaphyseal dysplasia)
Pyle disease (metaphyseal dysplasia)
Pycnodysostosis
Lead poisoning

Complications

The most common complication of Gaucher disease is osteonecrosis of the femoral head and occasionally of the femoral condyles (Fig. 30.13). Superimposition of degenerative changes is also a frequent finding that necessitates surgery. Pathologic fractures are common, and they may involve the long bones as well as the spine. The most serious complication (although fortunately a rare one) is malignant transformation at the site of bone infarcts.

Treatment

Enzyme replacement therapy using placental-derived alglucerase or recombinant (i.e., imiglucerase) preparations has resulted in hematologic improvement and resolution of hepatosplenomegaly. In some patients, signs of skeletal regeneration have been reported. Occasionally, splenectomy is performed. Bone marrow transplantation also has been tried with mixed results.

Tumoral Calcinosis

Pathophysiology and Clinical Features

First described by Inclan and coworkers in 1943, tumoral calcinosis is characterized by the presence of single or multiple periarticular lobulated cystic masses containing chalky material. Their formation is the result of the deposition of calcium salt in the soft tissues about the joints—the shoulders (particularly near the scapula), hips, and elbow joints—as well as on

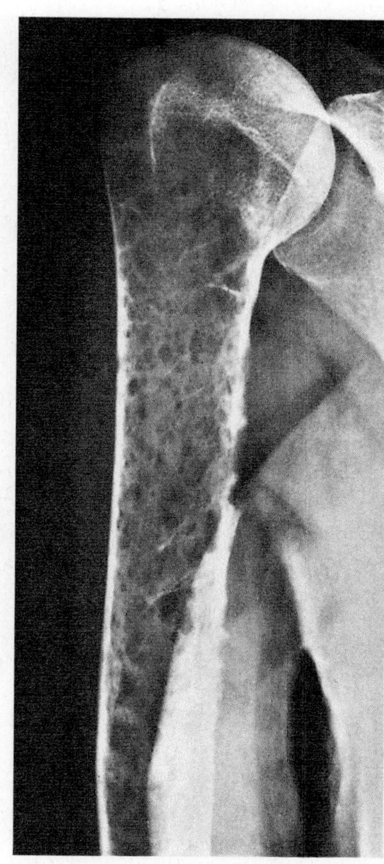

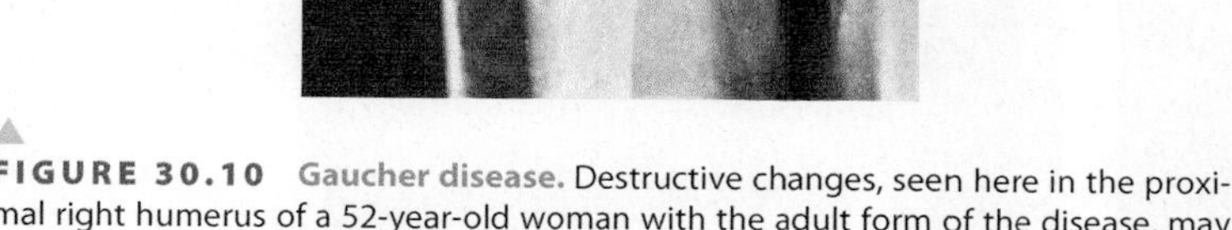

FIGURE 30.10 Gaucher disease. Destructive changes, seen here in the proximal right humerus of a 52-year-old woman with the adult form of the disease, may assume a honeycomb appearance.

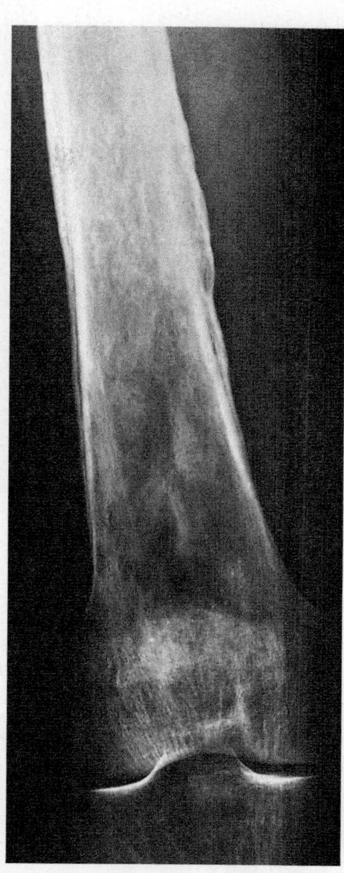

FIGURE 30.11 Gaucher disease. Anteroposterior radiograph of the right distal femur of a 29-year-old man demonstrates medullary infarction of the bone and endosteal and periosteal reactions secondary to reparative processes.

FIGURE 30.12 Gaucher disease. Lateral radiograph of the distal femur in a 28-year-old woman shows extensive medullary infarction and periosteal new bone formation, producing a bone-within-bone appearance.

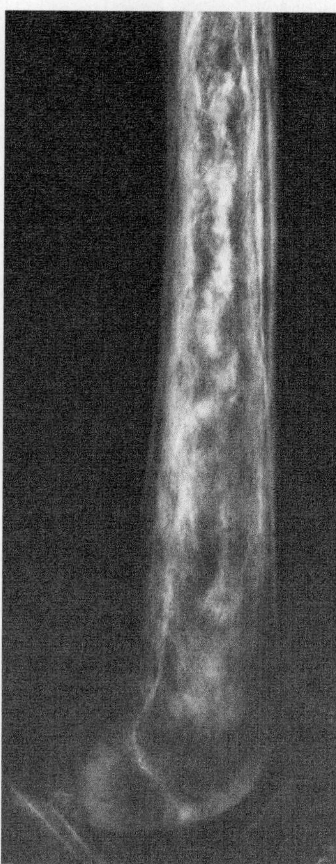

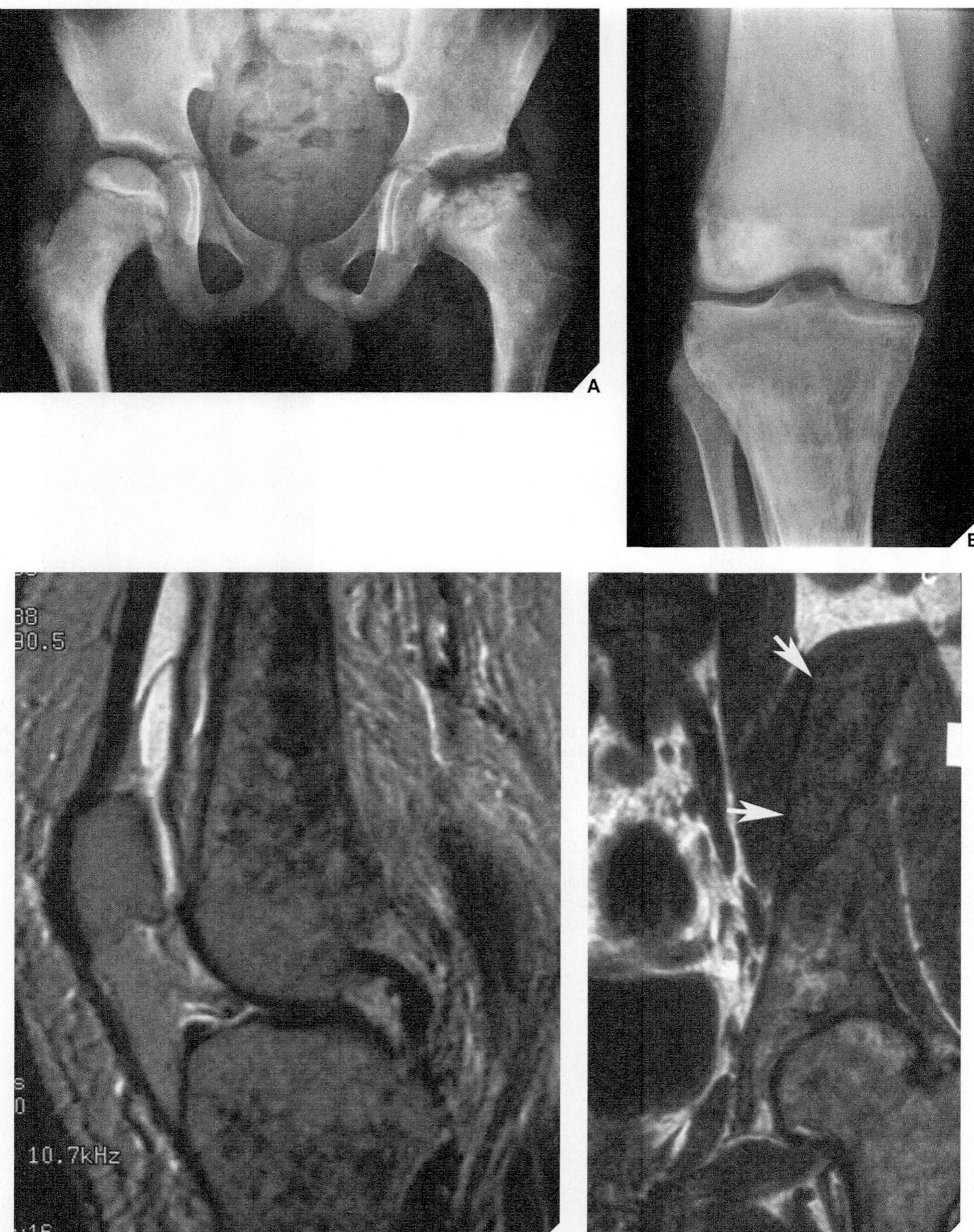

FIGURE 30.13 **Gaucher disease complicated by osteonecrosis.** **(A)** Anteroposterior radiograph of the pelvis of an 11-year-old Ashkenazi Jew with nonneuronopathic type of disease shows osteonecrosis of the left femoral head, a common complication of this disorder. **(B)** Anteroposterior radiograph of the right knee of a 25-year-old man demonstrates osteonecrotic changes of the medial and lateral femoral condyles. Note also the extensive bone infarction of the proximal tibia. **(C)** Sagittal T2-weighted MRI of the knee of another patient demonstrates extensive areas of low signal intensity in the bone marrow of the distal femur and proximal tibia representing fibrosis and bone infarcts. **(D)** Coronal T1-weighted MRI of the left hip of another patient shows multiple areas of low signal intensity of the bone marrow of the pelvis and left femur related to marrow fibrosis and bone infarcts. Note the soft-tissue extension of the Gaucher cell deposits in the pelvis *(arrows)*.

the extensile surfaces of the limbs. The masses are painless and usually occur in children and adolescents. Blacks are affected more frequently than other racial groups, with most cases of tumoral calcinosis reported from Africa and New Guinea. Because the cause is unknown, the diagnosis is one of exclusion. Other causes of soft-tissue calcifications, such as secondary hyperparathyroidism, hypervitaminosis D, gout and pseudogout, myositis ossificans, paraarticular chondroma, and calcinosis circumscripta, must be excluded before the diagnosis of tumoral calcinosis can be made. Recent studies have shown that individuals with familial tumoral calcinosis harbor mutations in either the *FGF23* or *GALNT3* genes. The *GALNT3* gene encodes GalNAc-T3, which prevents degradation of the phosphaturic hormone, fibroblast growth factor 23 (FGF23), that is required for normal renal phosphate reabsorption. Mutations in either *GALNT3* or *FGF23* result in hyperphosphatemic familial tumoral calcinosis or its variant, hyperostosis-hyperphosphatemia syndrome.

Imaging Features

Radiographic examination usually reveals well-demarcated and lobulated calcific masses that are circular or oval and located about the joints (Fig. 30.14). Less commonly extensive involvement of the soft tissues is encountered (Fig. 30.15). The soft-tissue masses vary in density; some are lacy and amorphous, and others are almost bone-like in appearance. Only in very rare instances is the calcific deposit located within the joint capsule. Cross-section imaging such as computed tomography (CT) provides better evaluation of the site and distribution of the calcific masses (see Fig. 30.15D,E).

Treatment

Surgical excision of the calcified masses is the most effective form of treatment, although attempts to treat this disorder with low-calcium and low-phosphate diets and phosphate-combining antacids have had some success.

Hypothyroidism

Pathophysiology and Clinical Features

Hypothyroidism is a syndrome encountered in infants and children, resulting from a deficiency of the thyroid hormones thyroxine and triiodothyronine, either during fetal life (cretinism) or early childhood (juvenile myxedema or juvenile hypothyroidism). The deficiency may be primary, caused by disease of the thyroid gland, or secondary, caused by

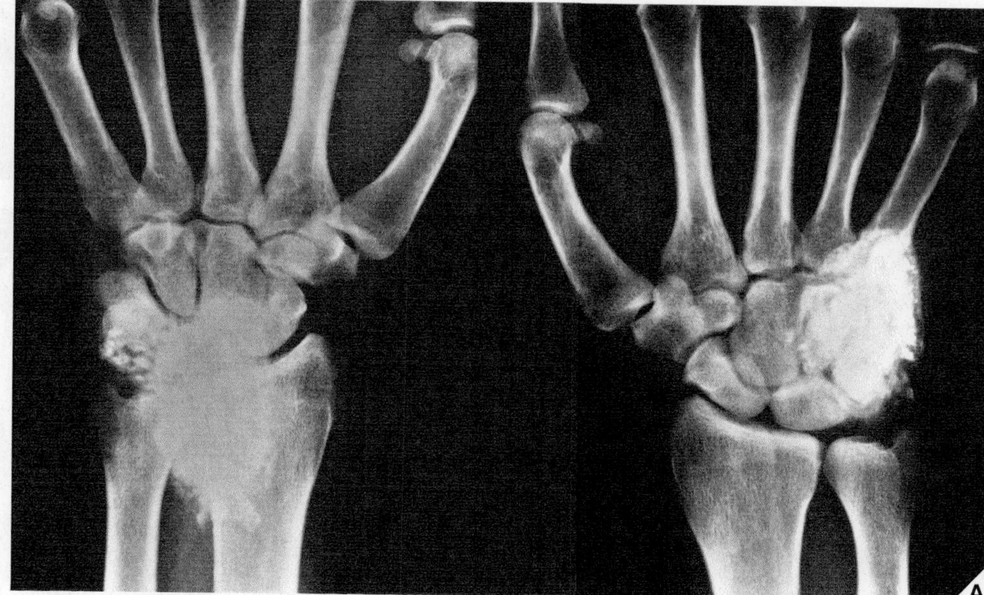

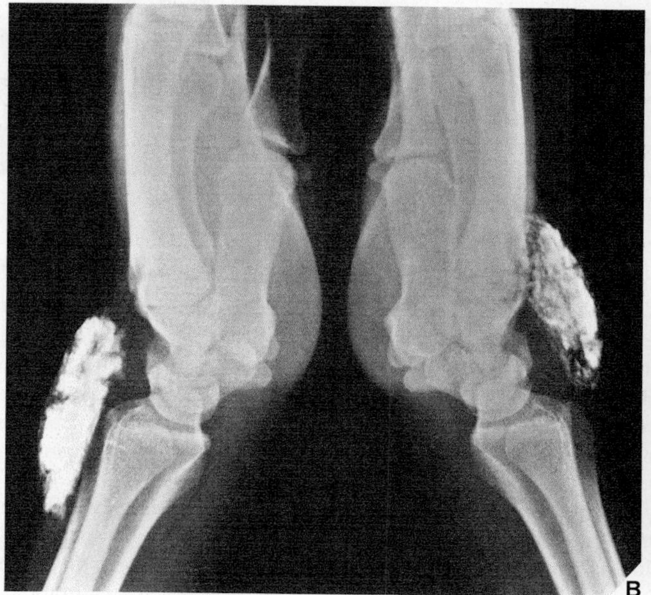

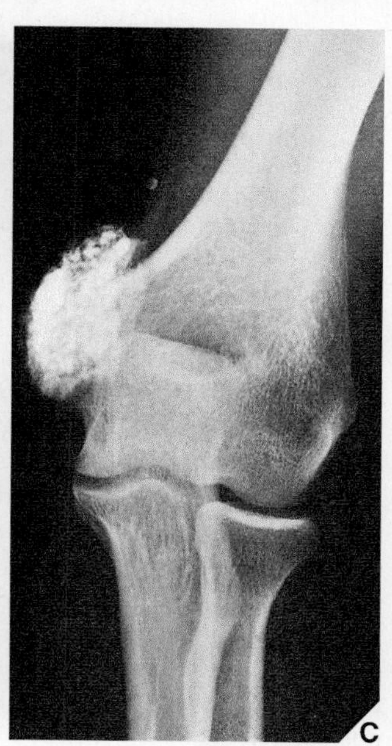

FIGURE 30.14 Tumoral calcinosis. A 66-year-old black patient, a native of New Guinea, had multiple bumps about the wrists and elbows since childhood. **(A)** Dorsovolar and **(B)** lateral radiographs of the wrists demonstrate calcific masses located on the dorsal aspect just beneath the skin. **(C)** Anteroposterior radiograph of the right elbow shows similar tumoral accumulation of calcium on the anteromedial aspect.

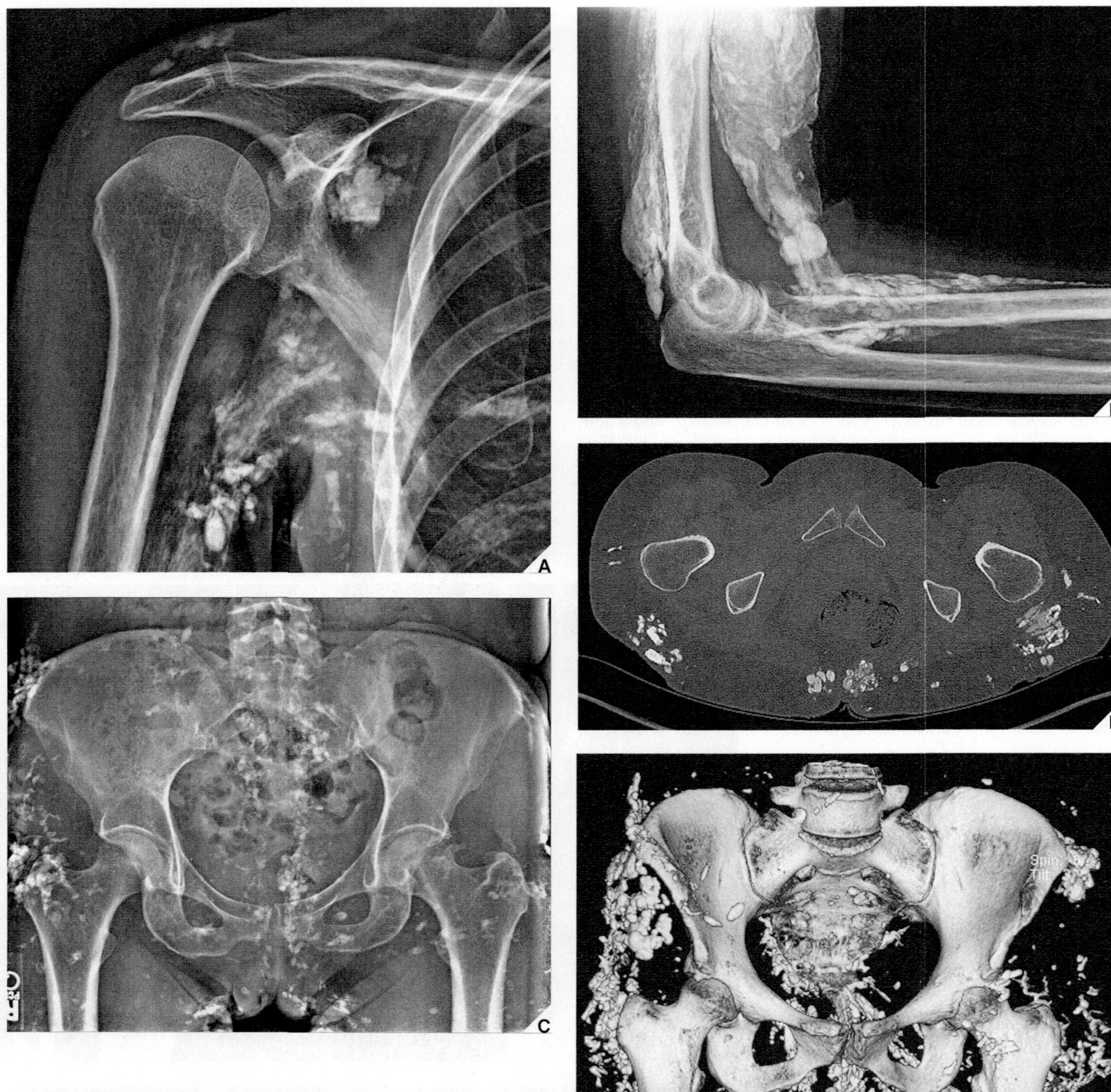

FIGURE 30.15 Tumoral calcinosis—extensive involvement of soft tissues. A 53-year-old African American woman without known underlying diseases and normal values of serum calcium, phosphorus, and alkaline phosphatase, presented with multiple calcified soft-tissue masses, around the shoulder girdle and axilla **(A)**, around the elbow including the biceps and triceps muscles **(B)**, and around the pelvis including upper thighs and the buttocks **(C–E)**.

lack of thyroid-stimulating hormone (TSH) produced by the pituitary gland. Mutations in the *DUOX2*, *PAX8*, *SLC5A5*, *TG*, *TPO*, *TSHB*, *TSHR*, and 2(*THOX2*) genes are responsible for congenital hypothyroidism by either preventing or disrupting normal development of the thyroid gland before birth (thyroid dysgenesis or thyroid agenesis), or, if the thyroid gland is present, by preventing the production of thyroid hormones. The major target sites are the growth plates and epiphyses, best demonstrated in the hands and the hips (Fig. 30.16). The key symptoms and signs include lethargy, constipation, an enlarged tongue, abdominal distention, and dry skin. The manifestations are typically less severe when the deficiency occurs in early childhood as an acquired disease than when it is congenital.

Imaging Features

The fundamental radiographic feature in both forms of hypothyroidism is delayed skeletal maturation with stunting of bone growth leading to dwarfism. In particular, the appearance of the secondary ossification centers is greatly delayed, as a dorsovolar radiograph of the hand may demonstrate (Fig. 30.17). Epiphyses ossify from numerous ossification centers, thereby acquiring a fragmented appearance and on occasion appearing abnormally dense (Fig. 30.18). This process may be mistaken for osteonecrosis, as seen in Legg-Calvé-Perthes disease (see Figs. 32.32A, 32.34, and 32.35), or for certain dysplasias, such as dysplasia epiphysealis punctata, also known as *Conradi disease*. Underpneumatization of the sinuses and mastoids are also typical radiographic findings associated with hypothyroidism.

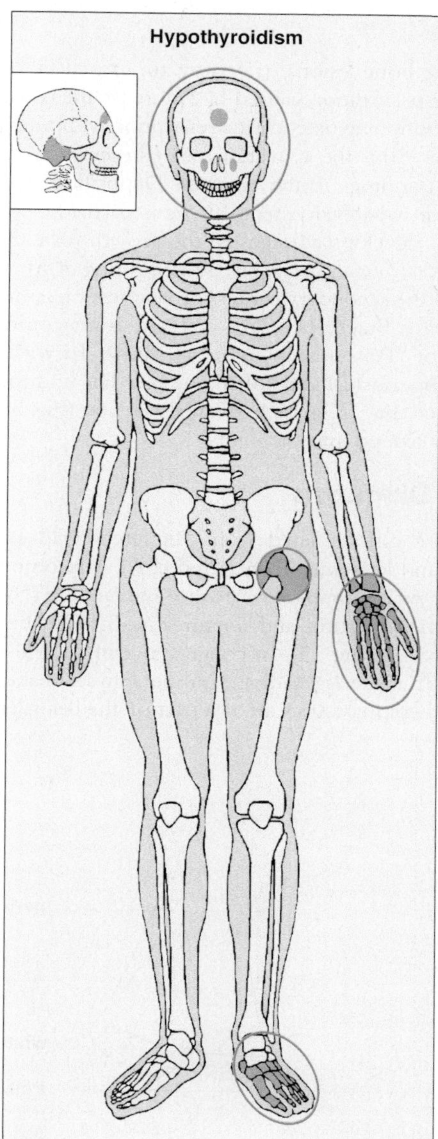

FIGURE 30.16 Target sites of hypothyroidism.

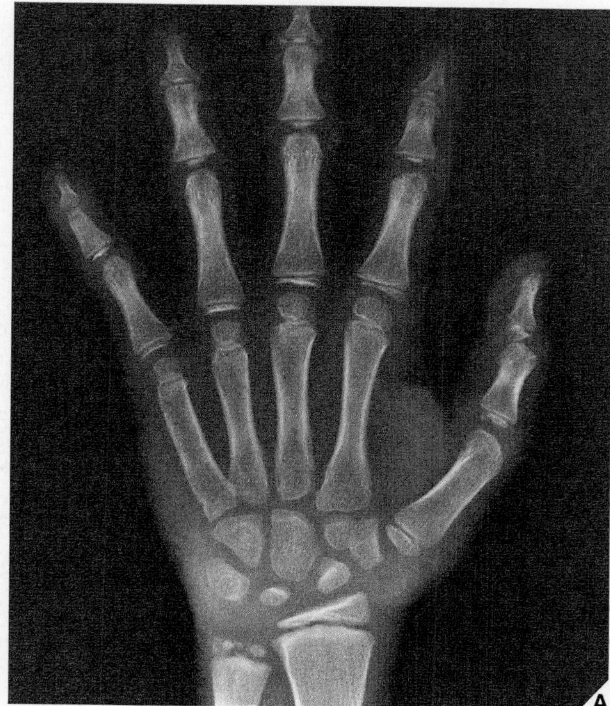

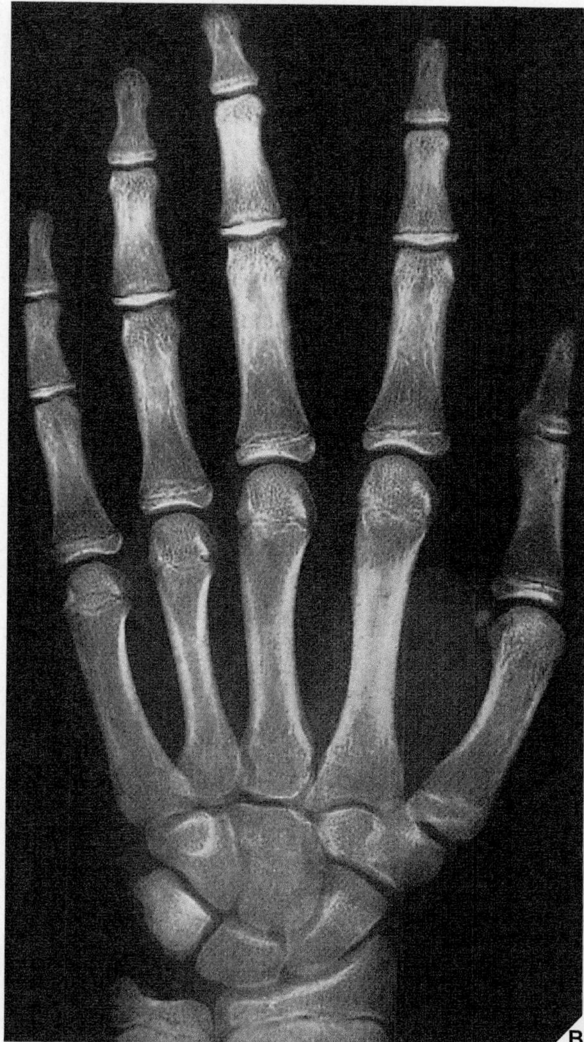

FIGURE 30.17 **Juvenile hypothyroidism. (A)** Dorsovolar radiograph of the right hand of a 13-year-old boy demonstrates skeletal immaturity; the bone age is approximately 8 years. Note the "fragmented" secondary ossification centers of the distal ulna and distal phalanges. In fact, they represent separated foci of ossification. **(B)** The hand radiograph of a healthy boy of the same age is shown for comparison.

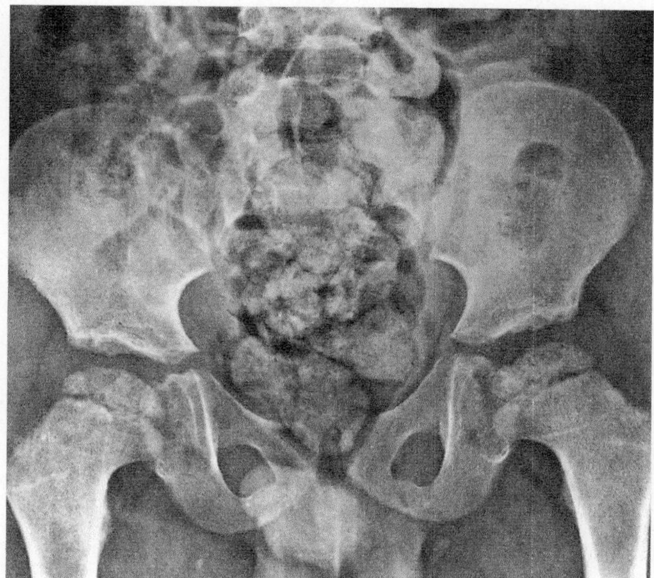

FIGURE 30.18 **Congenital hypothyroidism (cretinism).** Anteroposterior radiograph of the pelvis of a 5-year-old boy shows pseudofragmentation of both capital femoral epiphyses. This process may be mistaken for Legg-Calvé-Perthes disease.

Complications

One of the common complications of hypothyroidism is the development of slipped femoral capital epiphysis. The radiographic findings of this condition are described in Chapter 32.

Scurvy

Pathophysiology and Clinical Features

Barlow disease, as scurvy is also known, results from a deficiency of ascorbic acid (vitamin C). The function of vitamin C is to maintain intracellular substances of mesenchymal derivation, such as connective tissue, osteoid tissue in bones, and dentin in the teeth. In infants, primary deficiency is caused most commonly by failure to supplement the diet with vitamin C, whereas in adults, it is usually caused by food idiosyncrasies or an insufficient diet. Deficiency of vitamin C causes a hemorrhagic tendency, leading to subperiosteal bleeding and abnormal function of osteoblasts and chondroblasts. The latter results in defective osteogenesis.

Early clinical symptoms are nonspecific and include weakness, tiredness, irritability, loss of appetite, diarrhea, and occasionally a low-grade fever. Later, additional symptoms may developed such as swollen and bleeding gums, teeth loss, weight loss, tender and swollen joints, and shortness of breath.

Imaging Features

The characteristic bone lesions of scurvy are caused by cessation of endochondral bone ossification caused by failure of the osteoblasts to form osteoid tissue. Continuing osteoclastic resorption without adequate formation of new bone yields the appearance of osteoporosis, with generalized osteopenia and thinning of the cortices. Deposition of calcium phosphate continues in whatever osteoid tissue is formed, so that an area of increased density develops adjacent to the growth plate. Such areas have been called the *white lines of scurvy* (Fig. 30.19). A ring of increased density is also seen around the secondary centers of ossification, a finding known as a *Wimberger ring sign*. Fractures of the metaphysis are common, producing a "corner" sign or "Pelkan beak" (see Fig. 30.19). Increased capillary fragility leads to subperiosteal and soft-tissue bleeding and the formation of hematomas, which may trigger a periosteal reaction (Fig. 30.20). In adults, the bleeding may extend into the joints.

Differential Diagnosis

Scurvy should be differentiated from "battered child syndrome," congenital syphilis, and leukemia. In battered child syndrome (also known as *shaken baby syndrome* or *parent–infant trauma syndrome* [PITS]), characteristic metaphyseal corner fractures and fractures in different healing stages are characteristic (see Chapter 33). In congenital syphilis, the epiphyseal centers are normal. In leukemia, radiolucent metaphyseal bands are common, but fractures and epiphysiolysis are not part of the disorder.

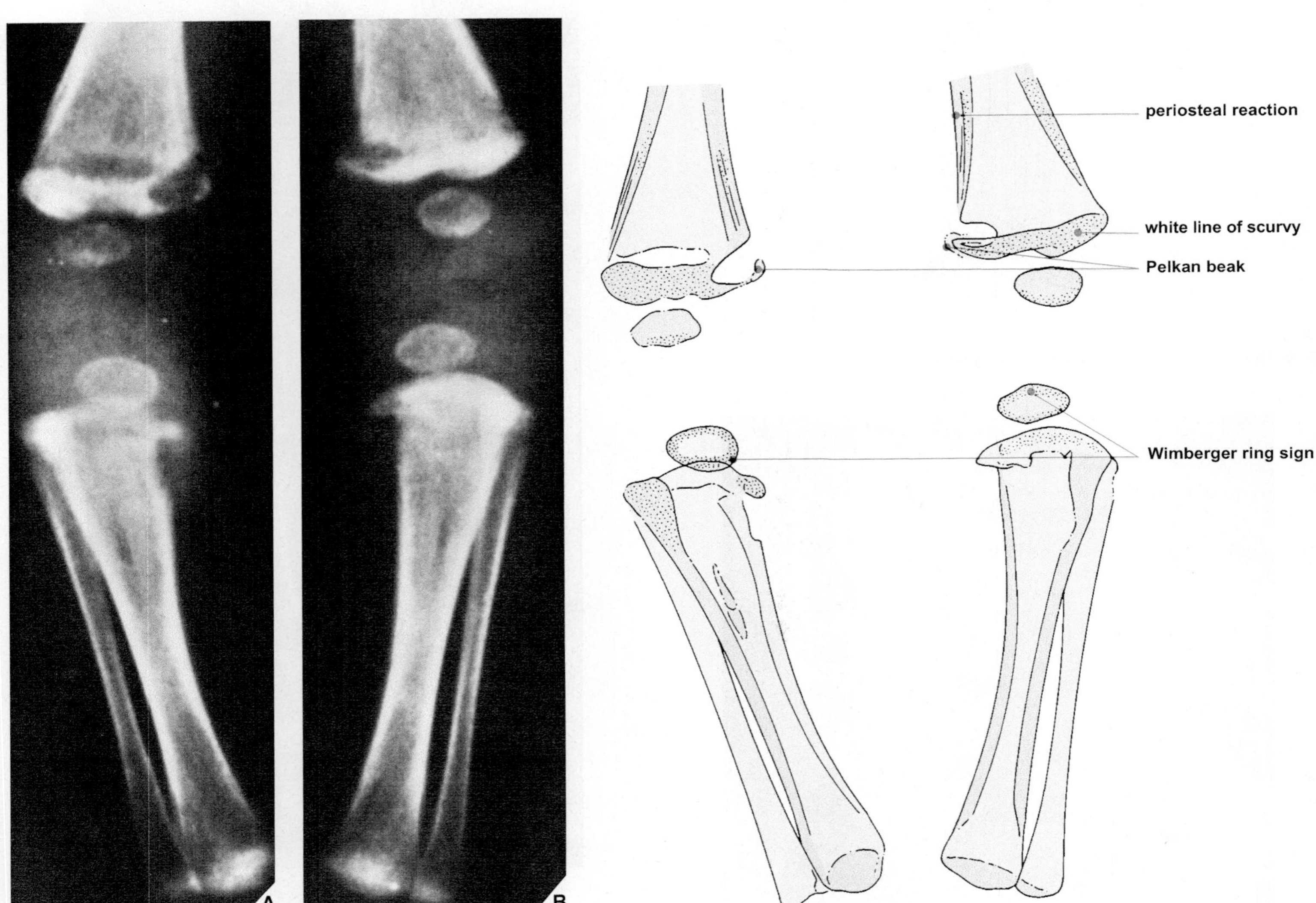

FIGURE 30.19 Scurvy. **(A,B)** Anteroposterior radiographs of the lower legs of an 8-month-old infant show the typical skeletal changes of scurvy. Note the dense segment adjacent to the growth plate (white line of scurvy), the ring of increased density around the secondary ossification centers of the distal femora and proximal tibiae (Wimberger ring sign), and the beaking of the metaphysis of both tibiae (Pelkan beak). A periosteal reaction secondary to subperiosteal bleeding is also noted.

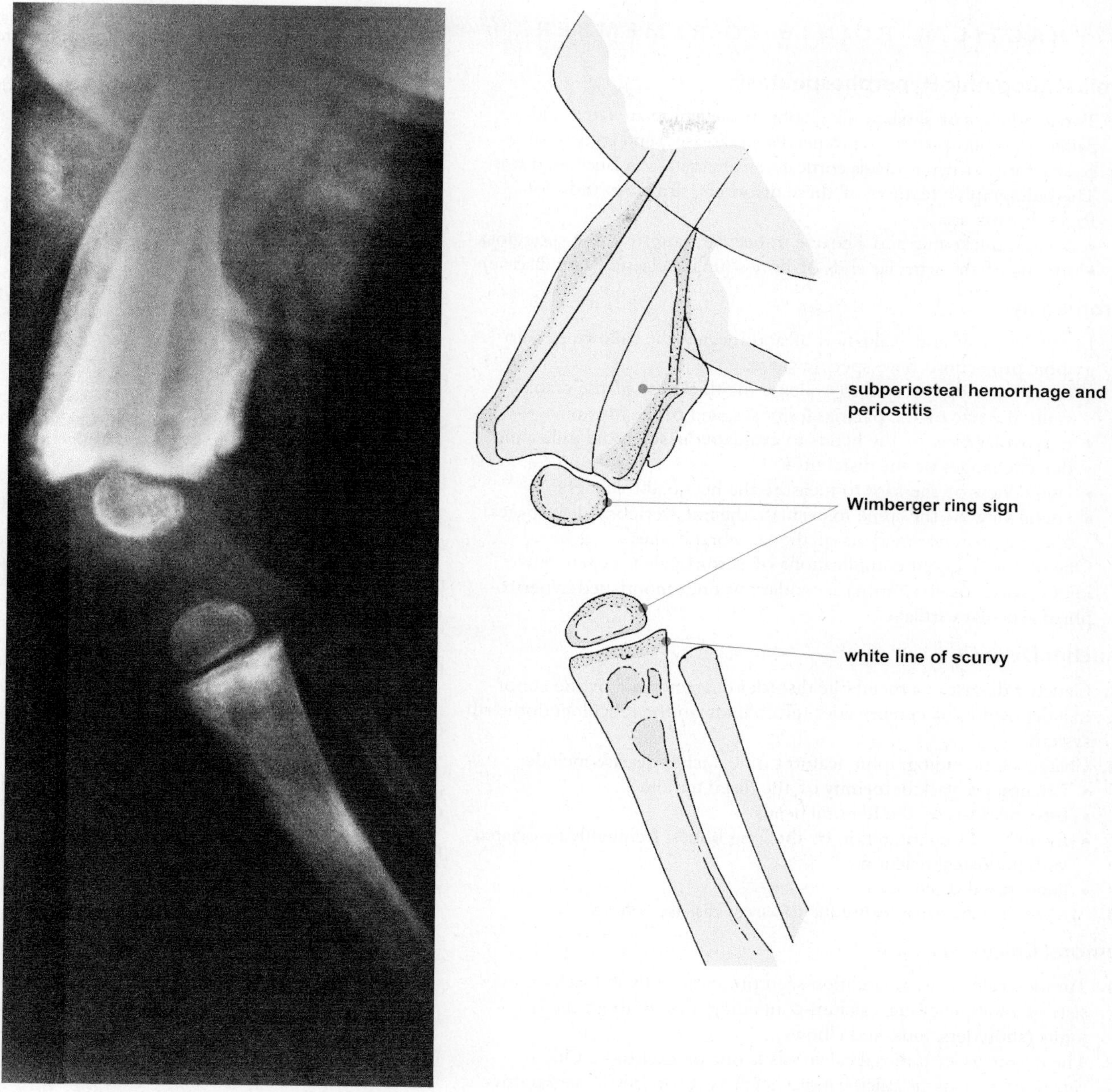

FIGURE 30.20 **Scurvy.** Lateral radiograph of the right leg of a 10-month-old infant with subperiosteal bleeding secondary to scurvy shows a marked periosteal reaction in the distal femoral diaphysis. A peripheral ring of increased density and central radiolucency, the Wimberger ring sign, is evident in the posteriorly displaced ossification center of the distal femoral epiphysis and in the proximal tibial epiphysis. Note also "white line" in the tibial metaphysis.

PRACTICAL POINTS TO REMEMBER

Familial Idiopathic Hyperphosphatasia

1. Two conditions of similar radiographic presentation are familial idiopathic hyperphosphatasia ("juvenile Paget disease") and autosomal recessive form of hyperostosis corticalis generalisata, van Buchem disease.
2. The radiographic features of these disorders, similar to those of Paget disease, are:
   - cortical thickening and a coarse trabecular pattern to the spongiosa
   - sparing of the articular ends of bones (unlike classic Paget disease).

Acromegaly

1. In the diagnosis and evaluation of acromegaly, the following radiographic projections have specific value:
   - lateral view of the skull to evaluate the thickness of the cranial vault, the size of the paranasal sinuses, and prognathism
   - dorsovolar view of the hands to evaluate the sesamoid index and detect changes of the distal tufts
   - lateral view of the foot to measure the heel-pad thickness
   - lateral view of the spine to evaluate the intervertebral disk spaces and the posterior margins of the vertebral bodies.
2. One of the frequent complications of acromegaly is degenerative joint disease (osteoarthritis) secondary to undernourished hypertrophied articular cartilage.

Gaucher Disease

1. Gaucher disease is a metabolic disorder characterized by the abnormal deposition of cerebrosides (glycolipids) in the reticuloendothelial system.
2. Characteristic radiographic features of Gaucher disease include:
   - Erlenmeyer flask deformity of the distal femora
   - osteonecrosis of the femoral heads
   - medullary bone infarction of the long bones, frequently associated with periosteal reaction
   - generalized osteopenia.
3. MRI is a noninvasive technique to assess disease activity.

Tumoral Calcinosis

1. Tumoral calcinosis, a condition seen predominantly in blacks, consists of multiple cystic, calcium-containing masses about the large joints (shoulders, hips, and elbows).
2. The diagnosis of tumoral calcinosis is one of exclusion: Other causes of soft-tissue calcifications, such as secondary hyperparathyroidism, hypervitaminosis D, and juxtacortical myositis ossificans, must be excluded.

Hypothyroidism

1. The fundamental radiographic feature of hypothyroidism (cretinism and juvenile myxedema) is retarded skeletal maturation, which is best demonstrated on a dorsovolar view of the hand.
2. Other characteristic radiographic features of hypothyroidism include:
   - a fragmented appearance of the ossification centers of the epiphyses
   - increased density of both epiphyses and metaphyses.
3. In the femoral heads, these features may mimic osteonecrosis (Legg-Calvé-Perthes disease) or dysplasia epiphysealis punctata (Conradi disease).

Scurvy

1. The characteristic radiographic changes seen in scurvy (deficiency of vitamin C) include:
   - generalized osteopenia
   - white lines of scurvy adjacent to the growth plate
   - Wimberger ring sign, representing increased density around ossification centers
   - the corner sign or Pelkan beak, representing metaphyseal fractures
   - periosteal reaction secondary to subperiosteal bleeding.
2. Conditions that should be differentiated from scurvy include:
   - battered child syndrome (shaken baby syndrome)
   - congenital syphilis
   - leukemia.

SUGGESTED READINGS

Albright F. Changes simulating Legg Perthes disease (osteochondritis deformans juvenilis) due to juvenile myxoedema. *J Bone Joint Surg* 1938;20:764–769.

Beutler E. Gaucher disease. Review article. *N Engl J Med* 1991;325:1354–1360.

Chong B, Hegde M, Fawkner M, et al. Idiopathic hyperphosphatasia and *TNFRSF11B* mutations: relationships between phenotype and genotype. *J Bone Miner Res* 2003;18:2095–2104.

Cremin BJ, Davey H, Goldblatt J. Skeletal complications of type I Gaucher disease: the magnetic resonance features. *Clin Radiol* 1990;41:244–247.

Cundy T, Hegde M, Naot D, et al. A mutation in the gene *TNFRSF11B* encoding osteoprotegerin causes an idiopathic hyperphosphatasia phenotype. *Hum Mol Genet* 2002;11:2119–2127.

Delanghe JR, Langlois MR, De Buyzere ML, et al. Vitamin C deficiency and scurvy are not only a dietary problem but are codetermined by the haptoglobin polymorphism. *Clin Chem* 2007;53:1397–1400.

Desnick RJ. Gaucher disease (1882–1982): centennial perspectives on the most prevalent Jewish genetic disease. *Mt Sinai J Med* 1982;49:443–455.

Duncan TR. Validity of sesamoid index in diagnosis of acromegaly. *Radiology* 1975;115: 617–619.

Feldman RH, Lewis MM, Greenspan A, et al. Tumoral calcinosis in an infant. A case report. *Bull Hosp Jt Dis Orthop Inst* 1983;43:78–83.

Frishberg Y, Topaz O, Bergman R, et al. Identification of a recurrent mutation in GALNT3 demonstrates that hyperostosis-hyperphosphatemia syndrome and familial tumoral calcinosis are allelic disorders. *J Mol Med* 2005;83:33–38.

Garringer HJ, Malekpour M, Esteghamat F, et al. Molecular genetic and biochemical analyses of FGF23 mutations in familial tumoral calcinosis. *Am J Physiol Endocrinol Metab* 2008;295:E929–E937.

Grabowski GA. Gaucher disease. *Adv Hum Genet* 1993;21:341–377.

Grabowski GA. Phenotype, diagnosis, and treatment of Gaucher's disease. *Lancet* 2008;372:1263–1271.

Hermann G. Skeletal manifestation of type 1 Gaucher disease—an uncommon genetic disorder. *Osteol Közlem* 2001;10:141–148.

Hermann G, Shapiro RS, Abdelwahab IF, et al. MR imaging in adults with Gaucher disease type I: evaluation of marrow involvement and disease activity. *Skeletal Radiol* 1993;22:247–251.

Horev G, Kornreich L, Hadar H, et al. Hemorrhage associated with bone crisis in Gaucher disease identified by magnetic resonance imaging. *Skeletal Radiol* 1991;20: 479–482.

Ichikawa S, Baujat G, Seyahi A, et al. Clinical variability of familial tumoral calcinosis caused by novel GALNT3 mutations. *Am J Med Genet A* 2010;152:896–903.

Inclan A, Leon P, Camejo MG. Tumoral calcinosis. *JAMA* 1943;121:490–495.

Johnson LA, Hoppel BE, Gerard EL, et al. Quantitative chemical shift imaging of vertebral bone marrow in patients with Gaucher disease. *Radiology* 1992;182:451–455.

Katz R, Booth T, Hargunani R, et al. Radiological aspects of Gaucher disease. *Skeletal Radiol* 2011;40:1505–1513.

Kho KM, Wright AD, Doyle FH. Heel pad thickness in acromegaly. *Br J Radiol* 1970;43: 119–125.

Kleinberg DL, Young IS, Kupperman HS. The sesamoid index. An aid in the diagnosis of acromegaly. *Ann Intern Med* 1966;64:1075–1078.

Mankin HJ, Rosenthal DI, Xavier R. Gaucher disease. New approaches to an ancient disease. *J Bone Joint Surg Am* 2001;83:748–760.

Masi L, Gozzini A, Franchi A, et al. A novel recessive mutation of fibroblast growth factor-23 in tumoral calcinosis. *J Bone Joint Surg Am* 2009;91:1190–1198.

Mass M, van Kuijk C, Stoker J, et al. Quantification of bone involvement in Gaucher disease: MR imaging bone marrow burden score as an alternative to Dixon quantitative chemical shift MR imaging—initial experience. *Radiology* 2003;229:554–561.

McNulty JF, Pim P. Hyperphosphatasia. Report of a case with a 30 year follow-up. *Am J Roentgenol Radium Ther Nucl Med* 1972;115:614–618.

Mitchell GE, Lourie H, Berne AS. The various causes of scalloped vertebrae with notes on their pathogenesis. *Radiology* 1967;89:67–74.

Oppenheim IM, Canon AM, Barcenas W, et al. Bilateral symmetrical cortical osteolytic lesions in two patients with Gaucher disease. *Skeletal Radiol* 2011;40:1611–1615.

Park SM, Chatterjee VKK. Genetics of congenital hypothyroidism. *J Med Genet* 2005;42:379–389.

Steinbach HL, Russell W. Measurement of the heel-pad as an aid to diagnosis of acromegaly. *Radiology* 1964;82:418–423.

Van Buchem FSP, Hadders HN, Ubbens R. An uncommon familial systemic disease of the skeleton: hyperostosis corticalis generalisata familiaris. *Acta Radiol* 1955;44:109–120.

Zimran A, Gelbart T, Westwood B, et al. High frequency of the Gaucher disease mutation at nucleotide 1226 among Ashkenazi Jews. *Am J Hum Genet* 1991;49:855–859.

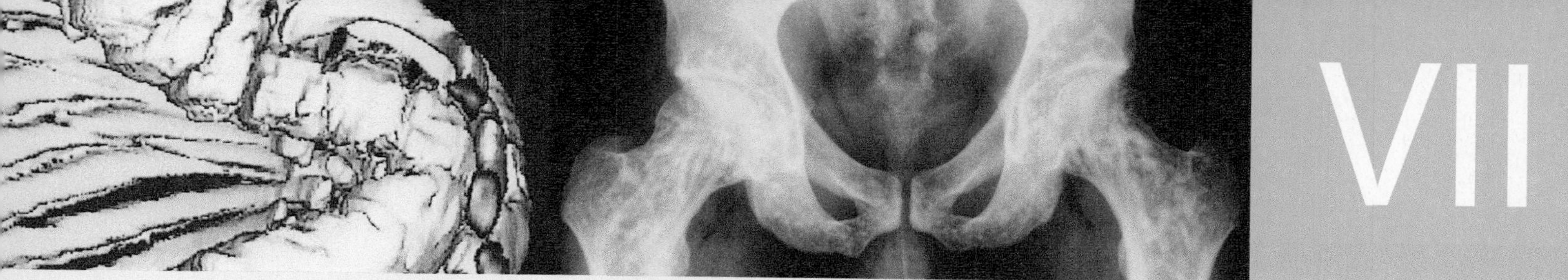

VII

CONGENITAL AND DEVELOPMENTAL ANOMALIES

31

Imaging Evaluation of Skeletal Anomalies

Classification

The conditions discussed in this part comprise disturbances in skeletal formation, development, growth, maturation, and modeling. Some of these anomalies arise during fetal development, such as congenital absence of a whole or part of a limb, supernumerary digits in a hand or foot, or fused digits, and are obvious at the time the baby is born. Some may begin to develop during fetal life but become apparent later in childhood, such as Hurler syndrome (gargoylism) or osteogenesis imperfecta tarda. Other anomalies, such as certain sclerosing dysplasias, develop after birth because of a genetic predisposition and become manifest later in life.

Congenital anomalies can be classified in various ways, but because of their complexity, a full and detailed classification of these disorders is beyond the scope of this chapter. To simplify the variety of classifications, which are constantly changing and expanding, the congenital anomalies may be divided from the pathologic point of view into those involving disturbances of bone formation, bone growth, and bone maturation and modeling (Table 31.1). Anomalies of bone formation include the *complete failure of a bone to form* and *faulty formation* of bones, which may manifest in a decreased number of bones (agenesis and aplasia) (Fig. 31.1A,B) or in the number of supernumerary bones (polydactyly) (Fig. 31.1C,D). Anomalies of formation may also be encountered in aberrations involving bone *differentiation*, which include pseudoarthroses (Fig. 31.2A) and bone fusions (syndactyly and synostosis) (Fig. 31.2B–E). Combined anomalies of faulty bone formation (agenesis and polydactyly) associated with anomalies of faulty bone differentiation (coalition and syndactyly) have also been recorded (Fig. 31.3). Disturbances in bone growth may lead to *aberrations in the size or shape* of bones. These may manifest in undergrowth (hypoplasia or atrophy) (Fig. 31.4A–C), overgrowth (hypertrophy or gigantism) (Fig. 31.3D), or deformed growth, such as congenital tibia vara (see Figs. 32.47 and 32.51). Anomalies related to bone growth may also be exhibited in abnormalities affecting the *motion in a joint*, such as contractures, subluxations, and dislocations (Fig. 31.5). Among the last group of congenital anomalies affecting the skeletal system are those exhibiting aberrations in bone *growth*, *maturation*, and *modeling*, as manifest in the various dysplasias (Fig. 31.6).

A second simple classification system is anatomic and based on the affected region of the body. This system comprises anomalies of the shoulder girdle and upper limb, pelvis and lower limb, spine, and the skeleton in general.

Imaging Modalities

Radiologic examination is essential for the accurate diagnosis of many congenital and developmental anomalies, which in some instances (such as osteopoikilosis or osteopathia striata) are totally asymptomatic and only revealed on radiographs obtained for other purposes. It also plays an important part in monitoring the progress of treatment. In many instances, the results of therapy, whether conservative or surgical, can be assessed only on the basis of the proper radiologic examination.

The imaging modalities most commonly used in diagnosing congenital malformations of the bones and joints are the following:

1. Conventional radiography, including standard and special projections
2. Arthrography
3. Myelography
4. Computed tomography (CT)
5. Radionuclide imaging (scintigraphy, bone scan)
6. Ultrasound (US)
7. Magnetic resonance imaging (MRI)

In most instances, the diagnosis can be made on the standard radiographic projections specific for the anatomic site under investigation. As in most other orthopaedic conditions, radiographs should be obtained in at least two projections at 90 degrees to one another (Fig. 31.7; see also Fig. 4.1). Supplemental views, however, are sometimes necessary for a full evaluation of an anomaly, particularly those affecting complex structures such as the ankle and foot (Fig. 31.8). Weight-bearing radiographs of the foot should be obtained whenever possible.

Ancillary imaging techniques play an important role in the evaluation of many congenital and developmental conditions. Myelography, for example, is still valuable for detecting anomalies of the spine (Fig. 31.9). In congenital dislocations, particularly in the hip, arthrography still plays a role showing the crucial abnormalities of this disorder (Fig. 31.10); it is also effective in demonstrating developmental anomalies affecting the articular cartilage and menisci of the knee, as in Blount disease (Fig. 31.11). CT examination is particularly valuable in the evaluation of congenital hip dislocations. Apart from providing important interpretive data about this complex anomaly, including demonstration of details of the relationship between the acetabulum and the femoral head, CT provides an accurate assessment of the degree of reduction of the head after treatment, often disclosing very subtle abnormalities not detected by radiography or arthrography of the hip (Fig. 31.12). A further application of CT is seen in its ability to measure the angle of anteversion of the femoral head, that is, the degree of anterior torsion of the femoral head and neck from the coronal plane (Figs. 31.13 and 31.14). Three-dimensional (3D) CT reconstructed images may be helpful in the global visualization of spinal deformities (Figs. 31.15 and 31.16).

Other ancillary techniques also have important functions in the evaluation of skeletal anomalies. Radionuclide bone scan, for instance, is particularly effective in detecting silent sites of skeletal abnormality in

TABLE 31.1 Simplified Classification of Congenital Anomalies of the Skeletal System

Anomalies of Bone Formation	*Anomalies of Bone Maturation and Modeling*
Complete failure of formation (agenesis, aplasia)	Failure of endochondral bone maturation and modeling
Partial failure of formation (hemimelia)	Failure of intramembranous bone maturation and modeling
Faulty formation	Combined failure of endochondral and intramembranous bone maturation and modeling
Decreased number of bones	*Constitutional Diseases of Bone*
Increased number of bones	Abnormalities of cartilage and/or bone growth and development (osteochondrodysplasias)
Faulty differentiation	Malformation of individual bones, isolated or in combination (dysostoses)
Pseudoarthrosis	Idiopathic osteolyses
Fusion (synostosis, coalition, syndactyly)	Chromosomal aberrations and primary metabolic abnormalities
Anomalies of Bone Growth	
Aberrant size	
Undergrowth (hypoplasia, atrophy)	
Overgrowth (hypertrophy, gigantism)	
Aberrant shape (deformed growth)	
Aberrant fit (subluxation, dislocation)	

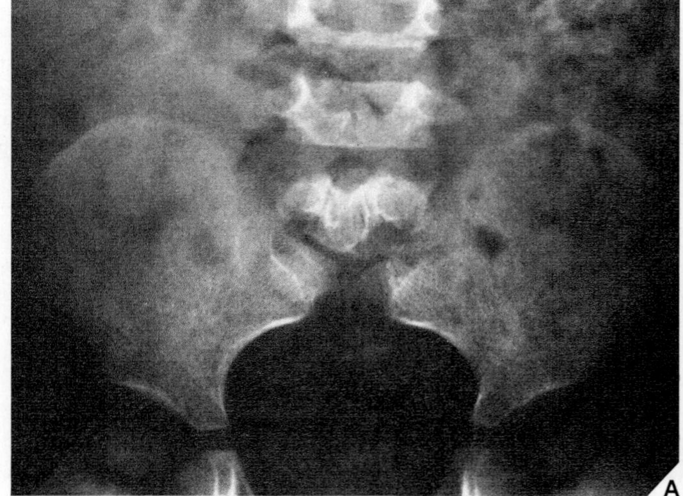
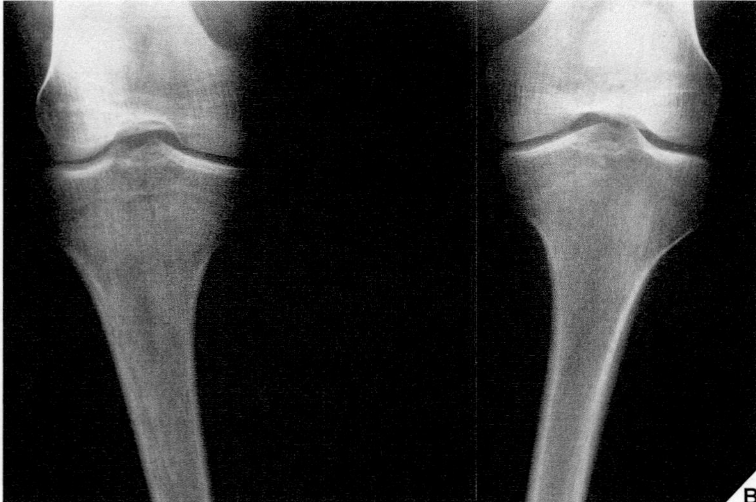
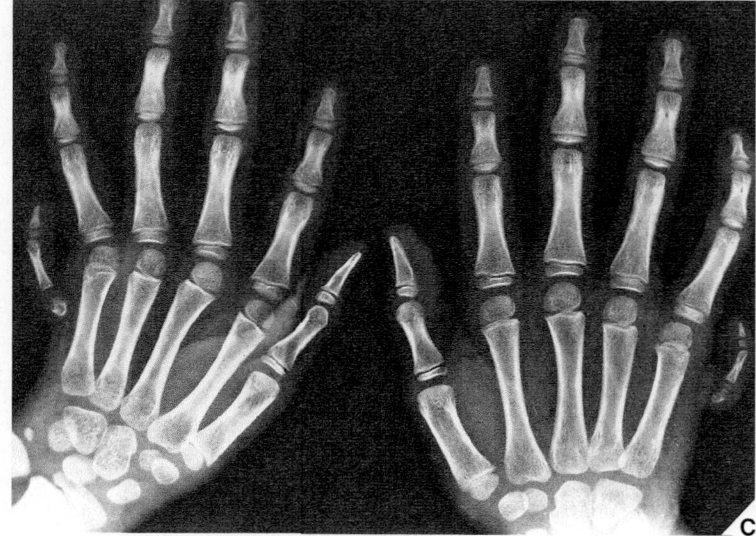
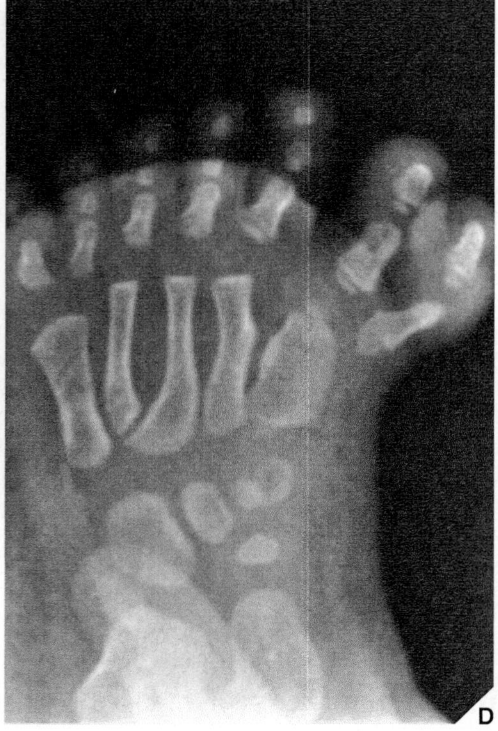

FIGURE 31.1 Anomalies of bone formation. Congenital anomalies related to disturbances in bone formation may be seen in the complete failure of a bone to form, as shown on this radiograph of the pelvis of a 1-year-old girl with sacral agenesis **(A)** and in a 26-year-old woman with bilateral agenesis of the fibulae **(B)**, or in formation of supernumerary bones, as seen in this 12-year-old boy with polydactyly in both hands **(C)** and in this 3-year-old girl with polydactyly in the right foot **(D)**.

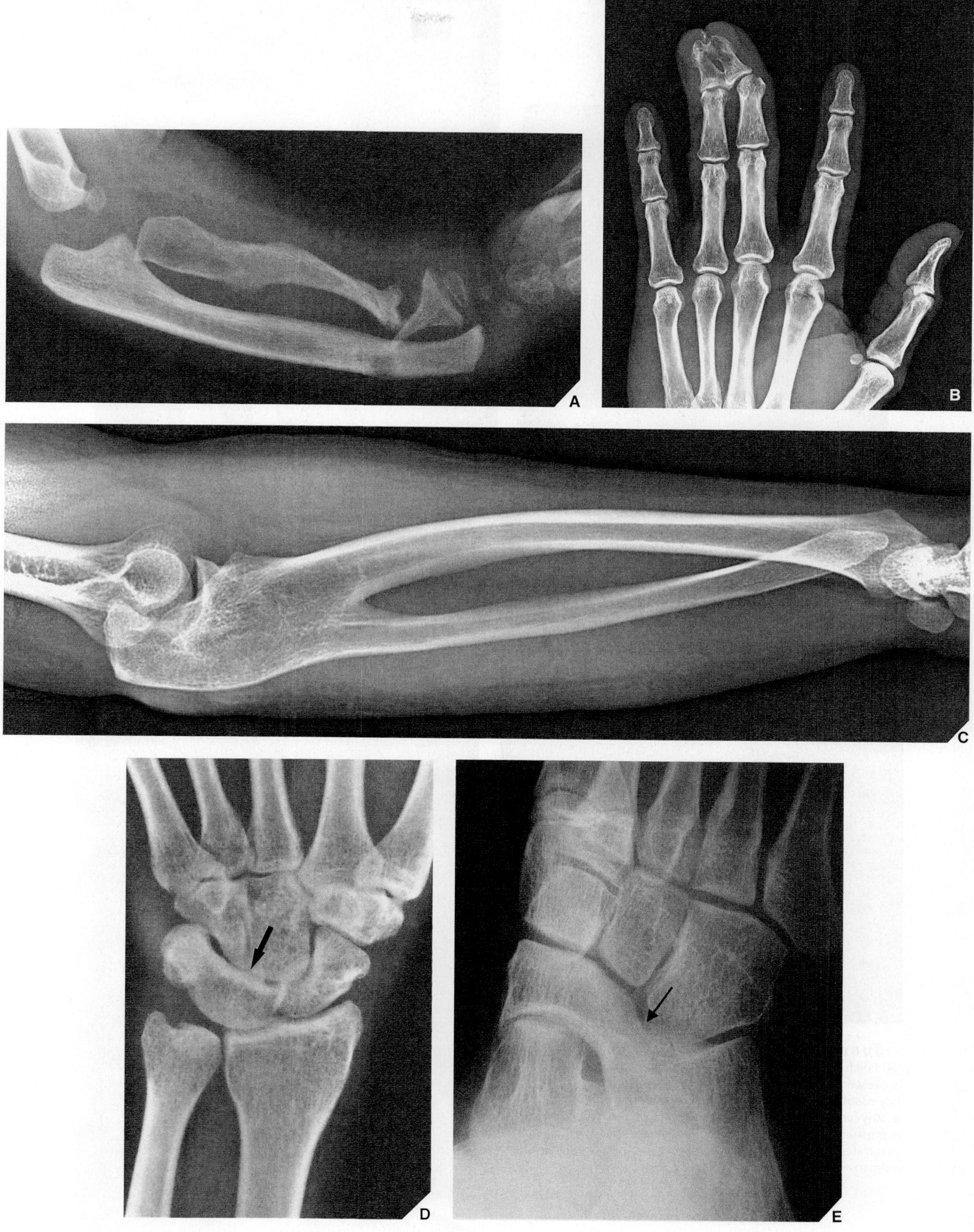

FIGURE 31.2 Anomalies of bone formation. Congenital anomalies related to bone division may manifest in congenital pseudoarthrosis, seen here involving the left radius in a 4-year-old boy **(A)**; in full fusion of the two digits (syndactyly) as in this 54-year-old man **(B)**, and partial fusion (synostosis) of two bones, seen here affecting the proximal radius and ulna in a 21-year-old woman **(C)**; or in coalition, manifested by complete fusion of the lunate and triquetrum bones *(arrow)* in a 33-year-old man **(D)** and in the fusion of the calcaneus and navicular bones *(arrow)* in a 21-year-old man **(E)**.

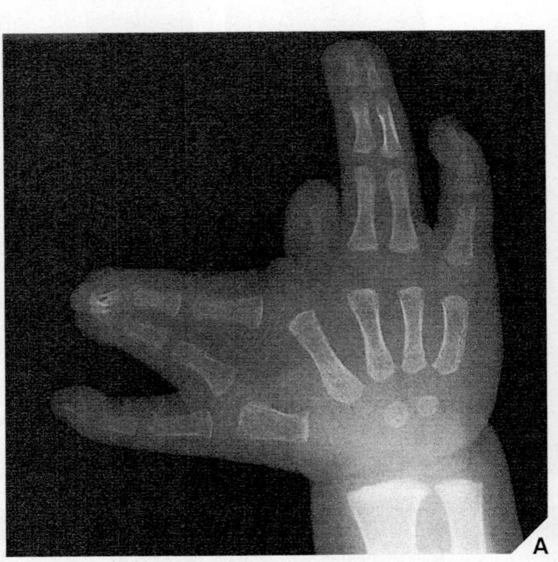

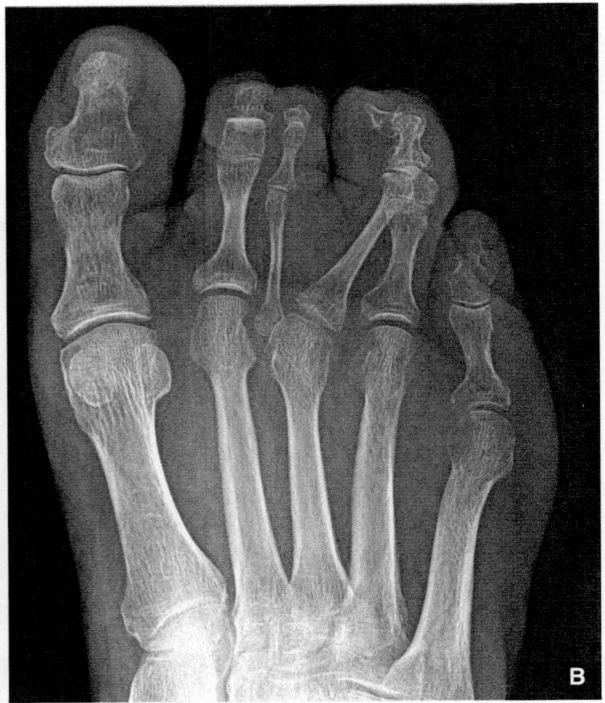

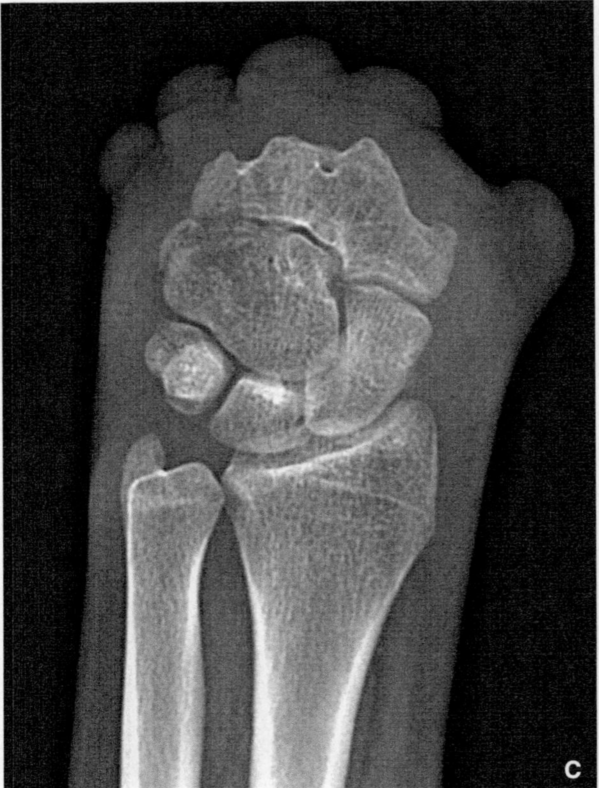

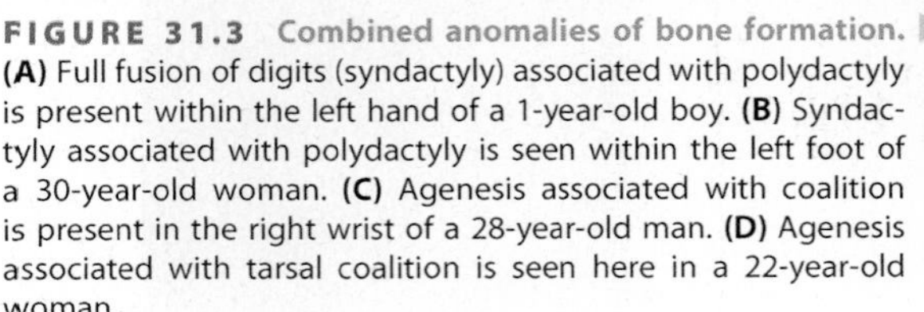

FIGURE 31.3 Combined anomalies of bone formation. **(A)** Full fusion of digits (syndactyly) associated with polydactyly is present within the left hand of a 1-year-old boy. **(B)** Syndactyly associated with polydactyly is seen within the left foot of a 30-year-old woman. **(C)** Agenesis associated with coalition is present in the right wrist of a 28-year-old man. **(D)** Agenesis associated with tarsal coalition is seen here in a 22-year-old woman.

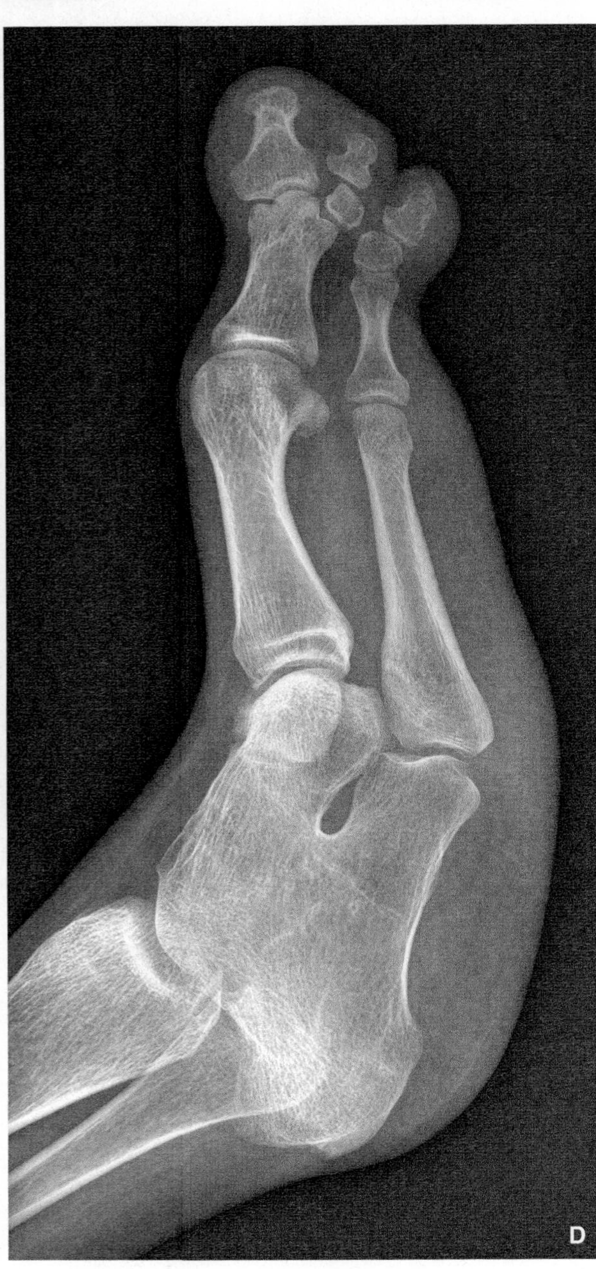

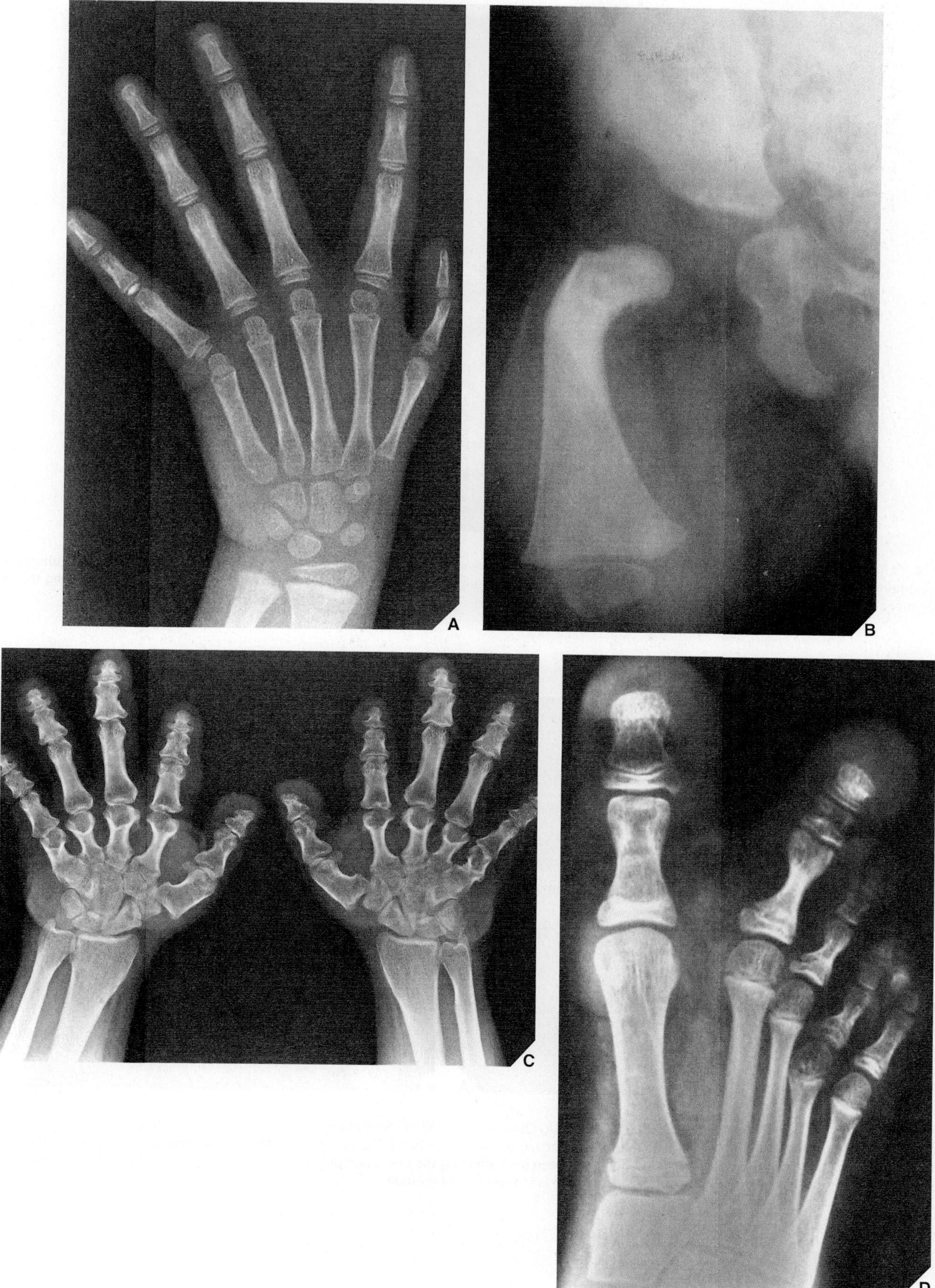

FIGURE 31.4 Anomalies of bone growth. Congenital anomalies related to the size of bones may manifest in hypoplasia, as seen here in the right thumb of a 4-year-old girl **(A)** and in the proximal femur of a 7-month-old boy with proximal femoral focal deficiency **(B)**, or in congenital brachydactyly, shown here in both hands of a 25-year-old woman **(C)**. Overgrowth may also be encountered, as in this case of macrodactyly (megalodactyly) involving the first two digits of the left foot of a 12-year-old girl **(D)**.

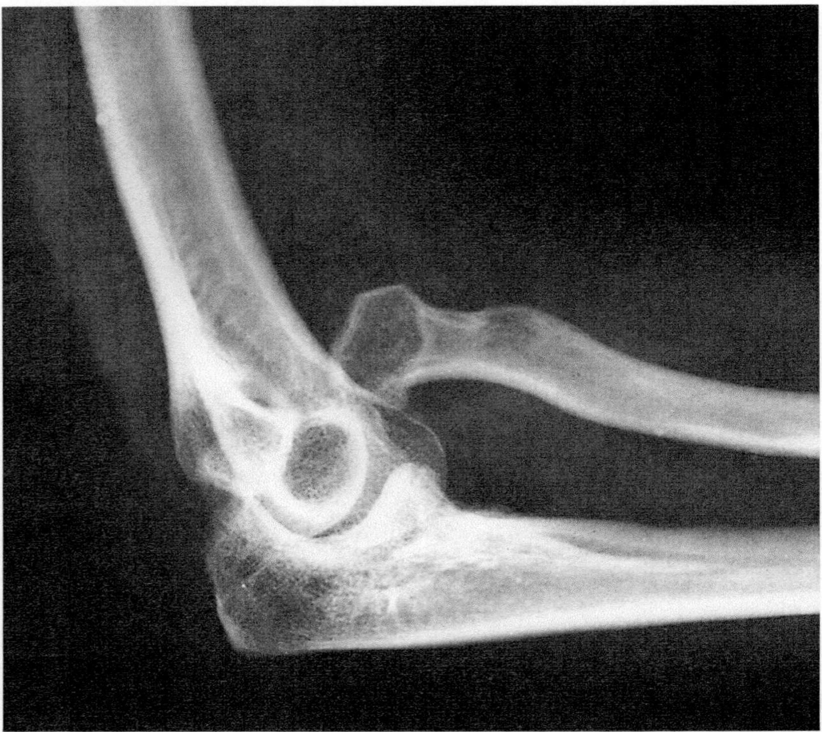

FIGURE 31.5 **Anomaly of bone growth.** Congenital dislocation of the radial head, seen here in a 35-year-old woman, is an anomaly related to aberrant bone growth leading to a condition affecting the motion of a joint. Note the hypoplasia and abnormal shape of the radial head, an important feature differentiating this condition from traumatic dislocation.

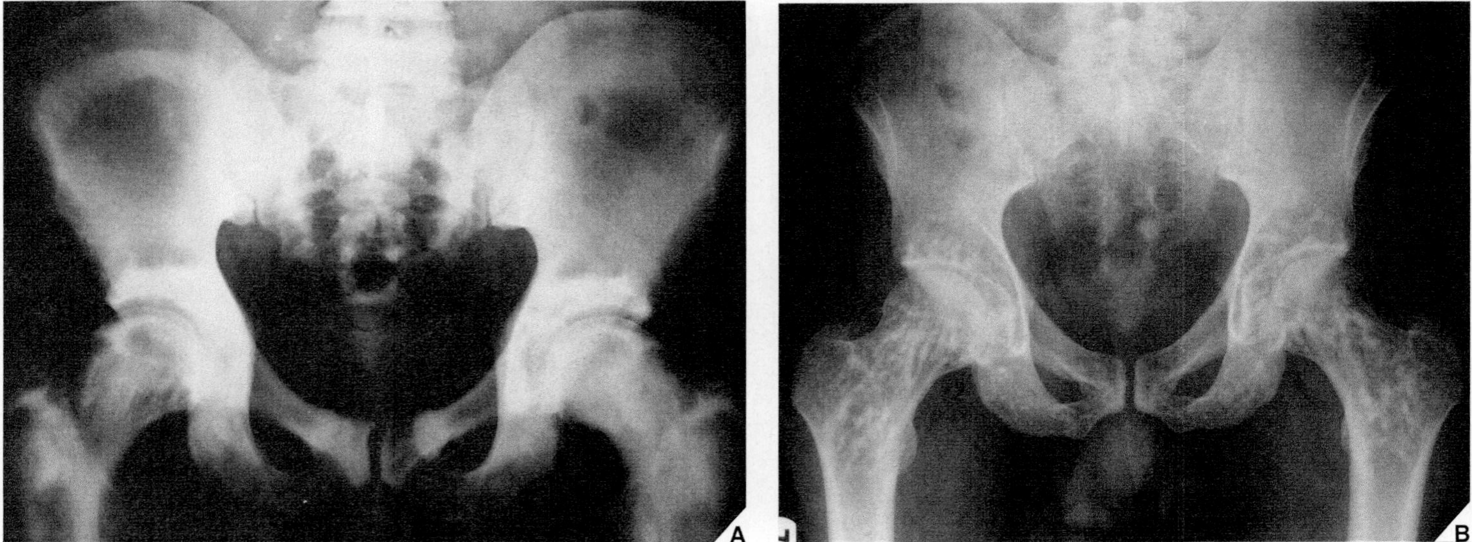

FIGURE 31.6 **Anomaly of bone development and maturation.** **(A)** Osteopetrosis (Albers-Schönberg disease), seen here affecting the spine, pelvis, and both femora of a 28-year-old man, is a congenital anomaly related to the development and maturation of bone. The persistence of immature spongiosa packing the marrow cavity results in the dense marble-like appearance of the bones. **(B)** Osteopoikilosis, seen here affecting the pelvis and proximal femora of a 21-year-old man, is a developmental anomaly of endochondral bone formation, where islands of secondary spongiosa fail to resorb and remodel.

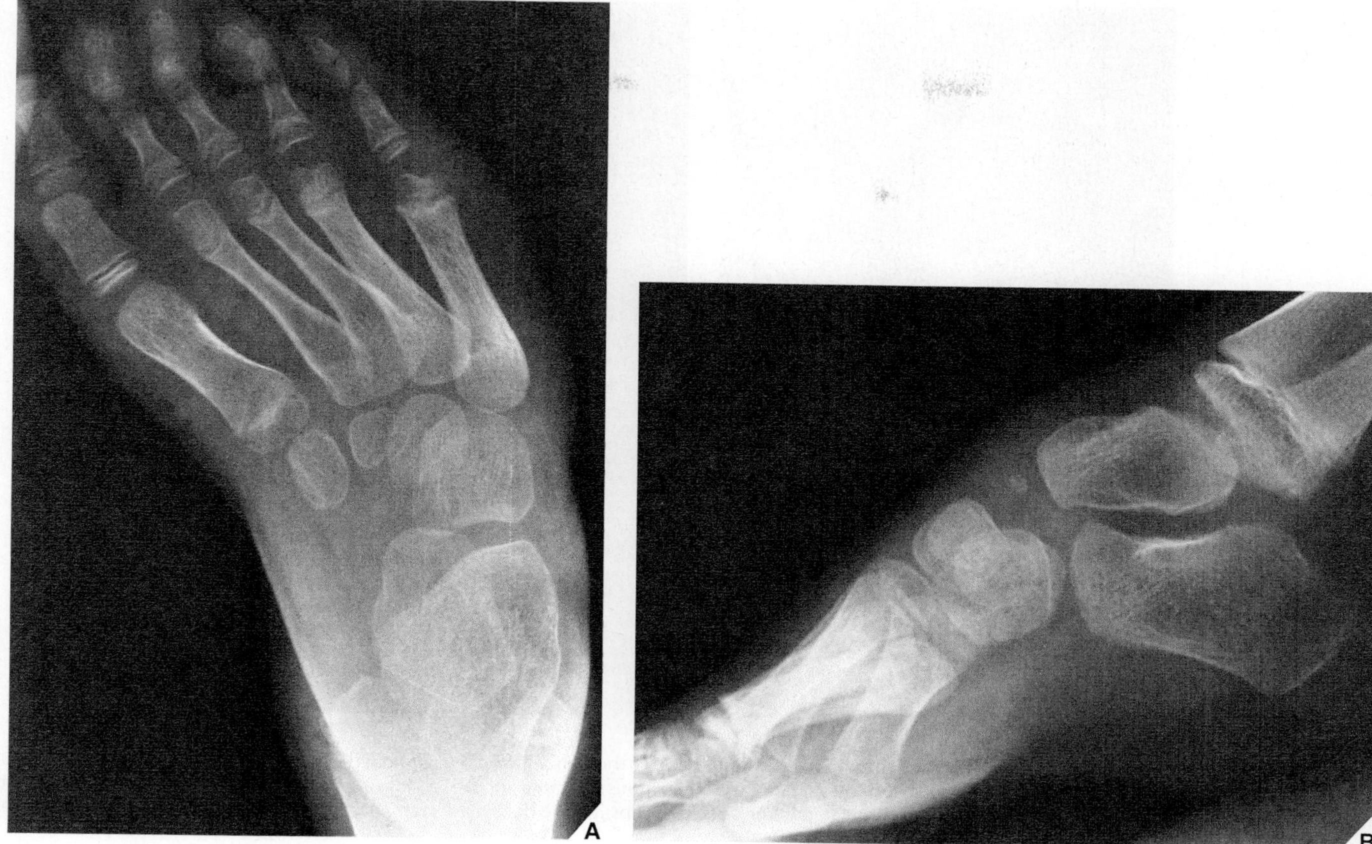

FIGURE 31.7 Clubfoot deformity. (A) Dorsoplantar and **(B)** lateral radiographs of the foot of a 7-year-old boy are sufficient to demonstrate all the components of congenital equinovarus deformity of the foot (clubfoot), namely, the equinus position of the heel, the varus position of the hindfoot, and the adduction and varus deformity of the forefoot.

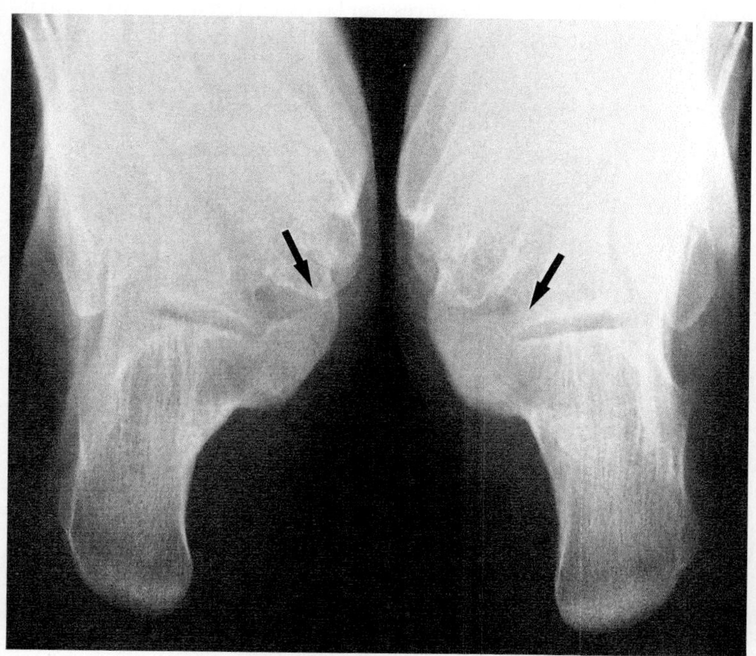

FIGURE 31.8 Talocalcaneal coalition. Posterior tangential (Harris-Beath) projection of both calcanei in a 23-year-old woman demonstrates bony fusion at the level of the middle facet of both subtalar joints *(arrows)*, a diagnostic feature of a talocalcaneal coalition.

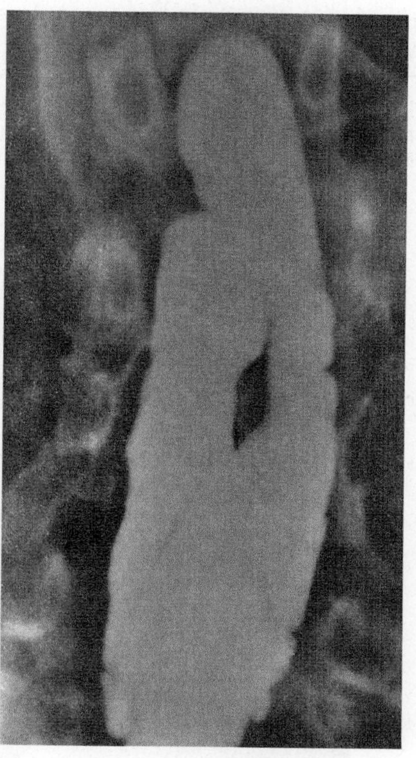

FIGURE 31.9 Diastematomyelia. A myelogram of a 9-year-old girl demonstrates a filling defect in the center of the contrast-filled thecal sac, caused by a fibrous spur attached to the vertebral body. This finding is diagnostic of diastematomyelia, a rare congenital anomaly of the vertebrae and spinal cord. Note the associated increase in the interpedicular distances.

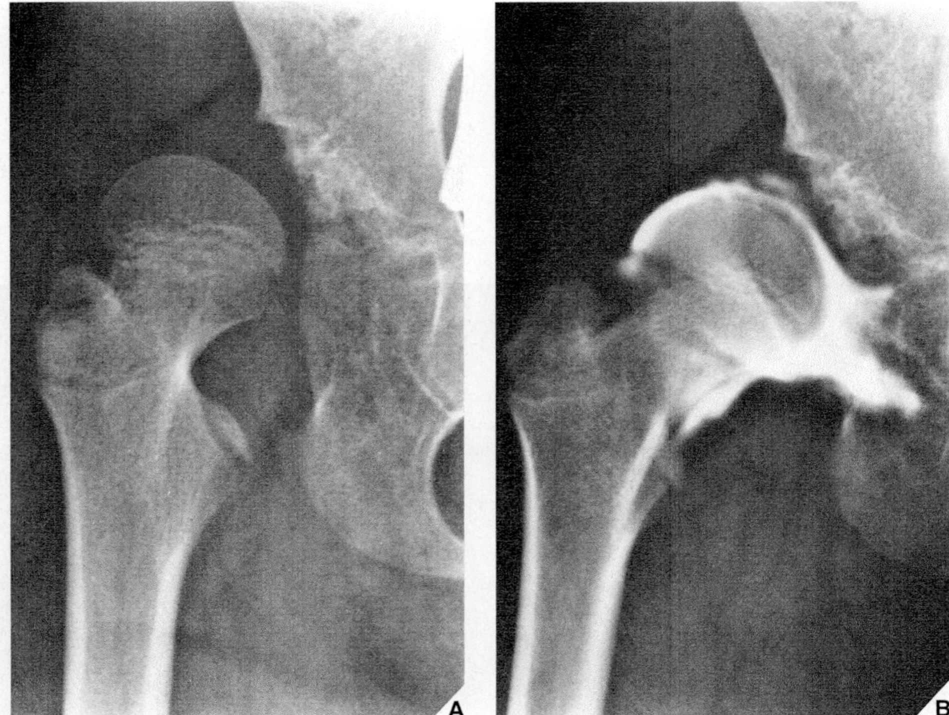

FIGURE 31.10 Congenital hip dislocation. **(A)** Standard anteroposterior radiograph of the right hip of a 7-year-old girl who was treated conservatively demonstrates persistent complete dislocation. **(B)** Arthrography was performed to evaluate the cartilaginous structures of the joint. In addition to a deformed cartilaginous limbus, the ligamentum teres appears thickened and contrast agent has accumulated in the stretched capsule. The thickened ligamentum teres frustrated several previous attempts at closed reduction.

various developmental dysplasias (Fig. 31.17). US is frequently used in the diagnosis of congenital skeletal abnormalities, including hip dysplasia and dislocation. It is effective in assessing the position of the femoral head in the acetabulum as well as the status of the cartilaginous acetabular roof and other cartilaginous structures such as the limbus that cannot be demonstrated on the standard radiographs (Fig. 31.18). This technique also offers a noninvasive method of examining the infant hip, which might otherwise require arthrography. In addition, US does not expose the patient to ionizing radiation.

MRI is ideally suited to evaluate congenital and development anomalies of the spine because all structures, including neural components, are shown simultaneously. Because MRI evaluation is mainly an assessment of neuroanatomic development, spin echo (SE) T1-weighted images are usually obtained (Fig. 31.19). However, anomalies affecting the spinal cord and thecal sac are best seen on T2-weighted images because of high contrast of the spinal fluid. These sequences can be quite effective in demonstrating, for example, tethered cord, spinal dysraphism, and diastematomyelia (Figs. 31.20 to 31.22).

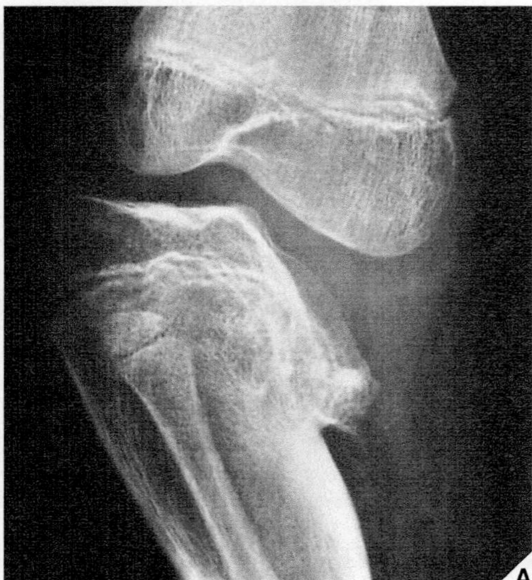

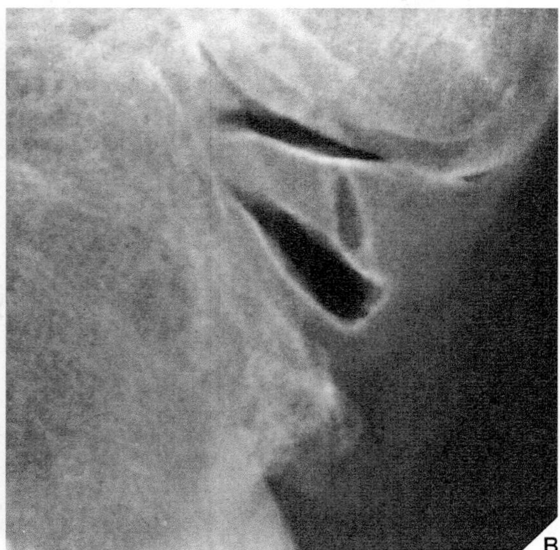

FIGURE 31.11 Blount disease. **(A)** Anteroposterior radiograph of the knee of a 4-year-old boy demonstrates congenital tibia vara (Blount disease). **(B)** Double-contrast arthrogram of the knee shows hypertrophy of the medial meniscus and thick nonossified cartilage at the medial aspect of the proximal tibial epiphysis.

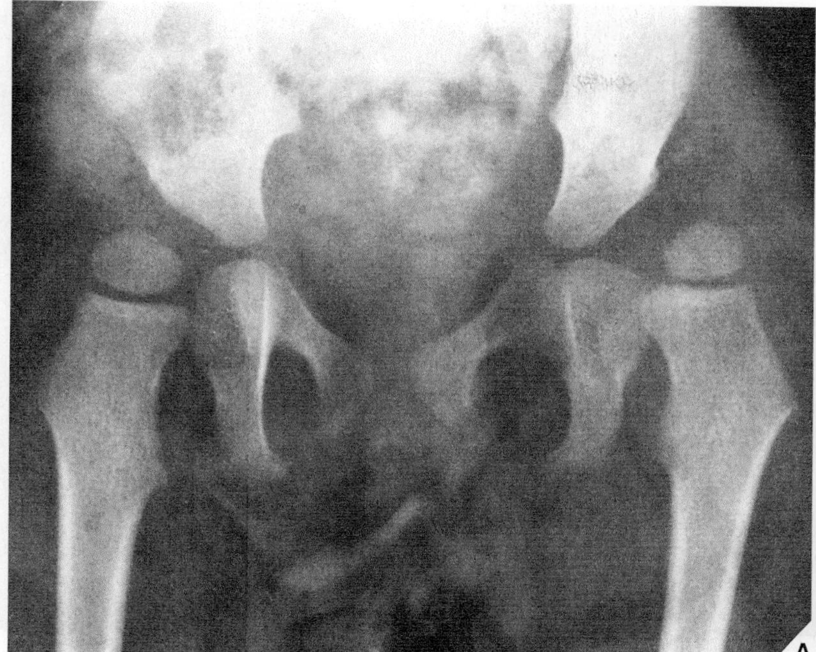

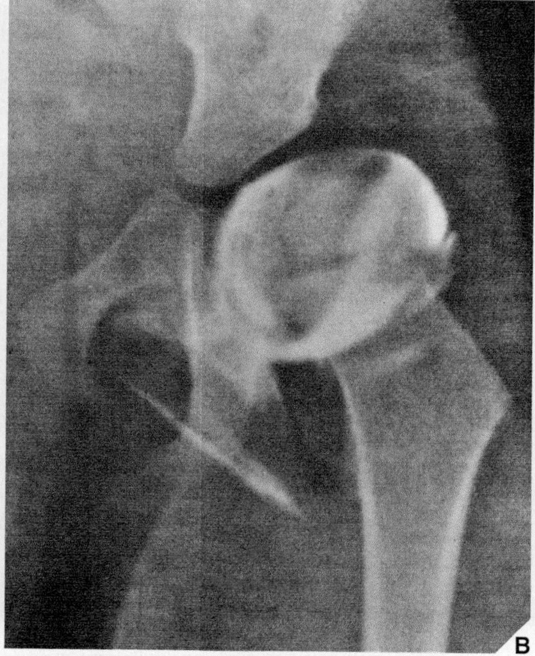

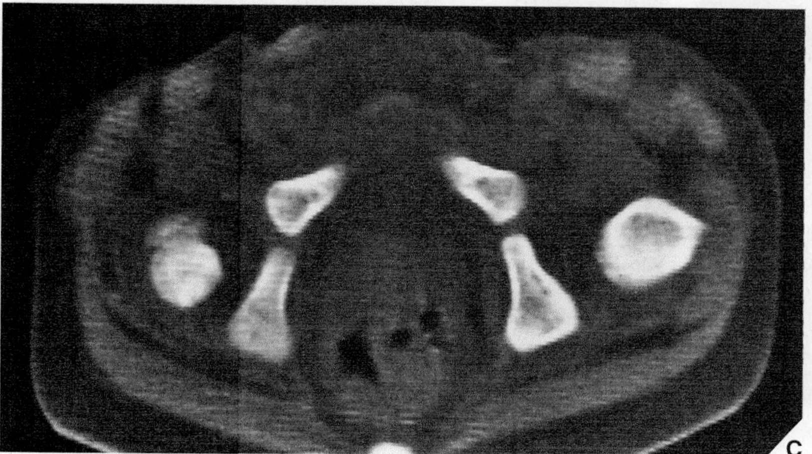

FIGURE 31.12 Congenital hip dislocation. **(A)** Anteroposterior radiograph of the pelvis in a 1-year-old girl demonstrates congenital dislocation of the left hip. After conservative management with a Pavlik harness, a contrast arthrogram **(B)** was performed to evaluate the results of treatment. The femoral head appears to be well seated in the acetabulum. Note the smoothness of the Shenton-Menard line (see Fig. 32.10A). **(C)** CT section, however, demonstrates persistence of posterolateral subluxation.

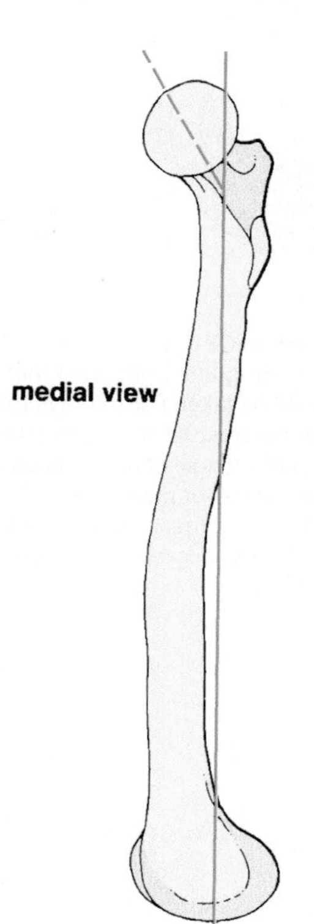

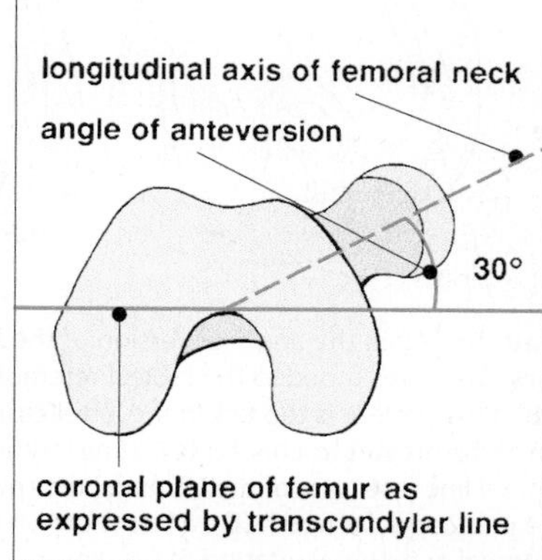

Age (years)	Normal Values of Angle of Anteversion
0–1	30°–50°
1–2	30°
3–5	25°
skeletal maturity	8°–15°

FIGURE 31.13 Anteversion of the femoral head. The angle of anteversion of the femoral head represents the degree of anterior torsion of the femoral head and neck from the coronal plane. It is determined by the angle formed between the longitudinal axis of the femoral neck and the coronal plane of the femur as expressed by a transcondylar line (see Fig. 31.14).

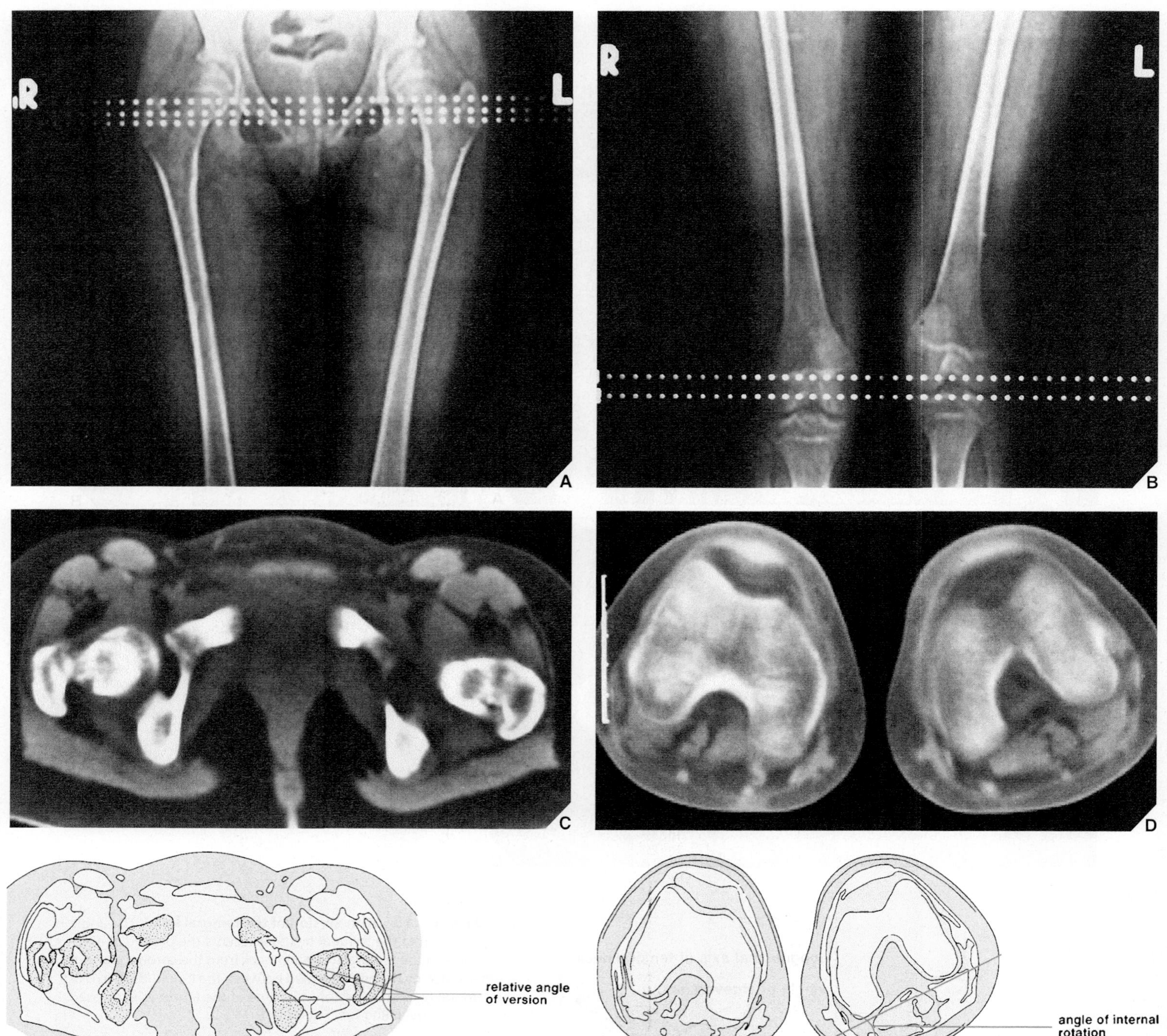

FIGURE 31.14 CT determination of the angle of version of the femoral head. To obtain the angle of version of the femoral head on CT examination, the patient is supine, with the lower extremities in the neutral position, the feet taped together, and the knees taped to the table. Preferably, a single scanogram is obtained that includes both hips and knees on the same film; however, separate films may be obtained **(A,B)** if the patient is too tall. In the latter case, care should be taken not to move the patient between the two takes. On a section through the femoral neck and the upper portion of the greater trochanter **(C)**, a line is drawn through the femoral neck, using the femoral head and greater trochanter as guides. The angle that this line forms with the horizontal line (the level of the CT table) determines the *relative* angle of anteversion (or retroversion) of the femoral head. On the CT section through the femoral condyles at the intercondylar notch **(D)**, a line is drawn through the posterior margins of the condyles, and the angle formed by this line and the horizontal line determines the degree of internal or external rotation of the extremities. From these two measurements, a *true* angle of version (anteversion or retroversion) is calculated. If the knee is in internal rotation, as in the present case, the sum of both angles yields the degree of anteversion. If the knee is in external rotation, the angle obtained at the knee must be subtracted from the angle at the hip, yielding the degree of version.

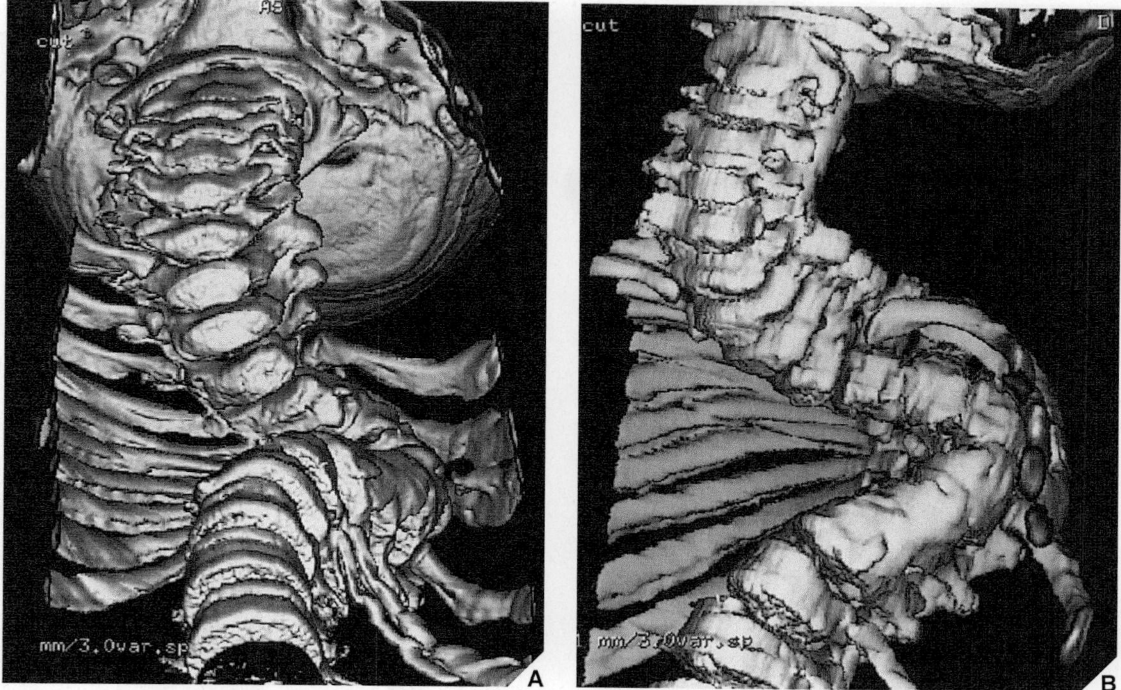

FIGURE 31.15 **3D CT of congenital kyphoscoliosis.** 3D CT reconstructed images of the spine of a 4-year-old boy with congenital kyphoscoliosis in frontal **(A)** and lateral **(B)** orientation are effective in global demonstration of spinal deformity.

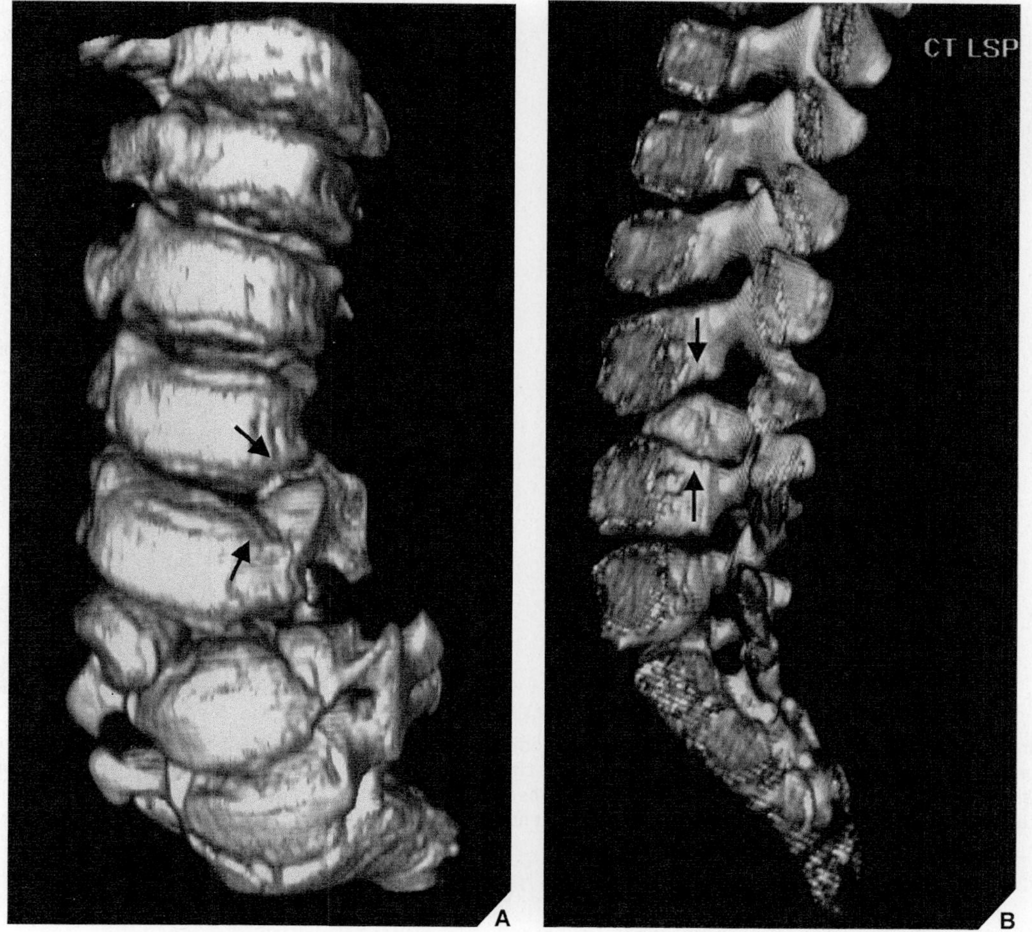

FIGURE 31.16 **3D CT of congenital hemivertebra.** **(A)** Frontal and **(B)** lateral views of 3D CT reconstructed images of the lumbar spine of a 5-year-old girl with congenital dextroscoliosis reveal a hemivertebra *(arrows)* wedged between L3 and L4.

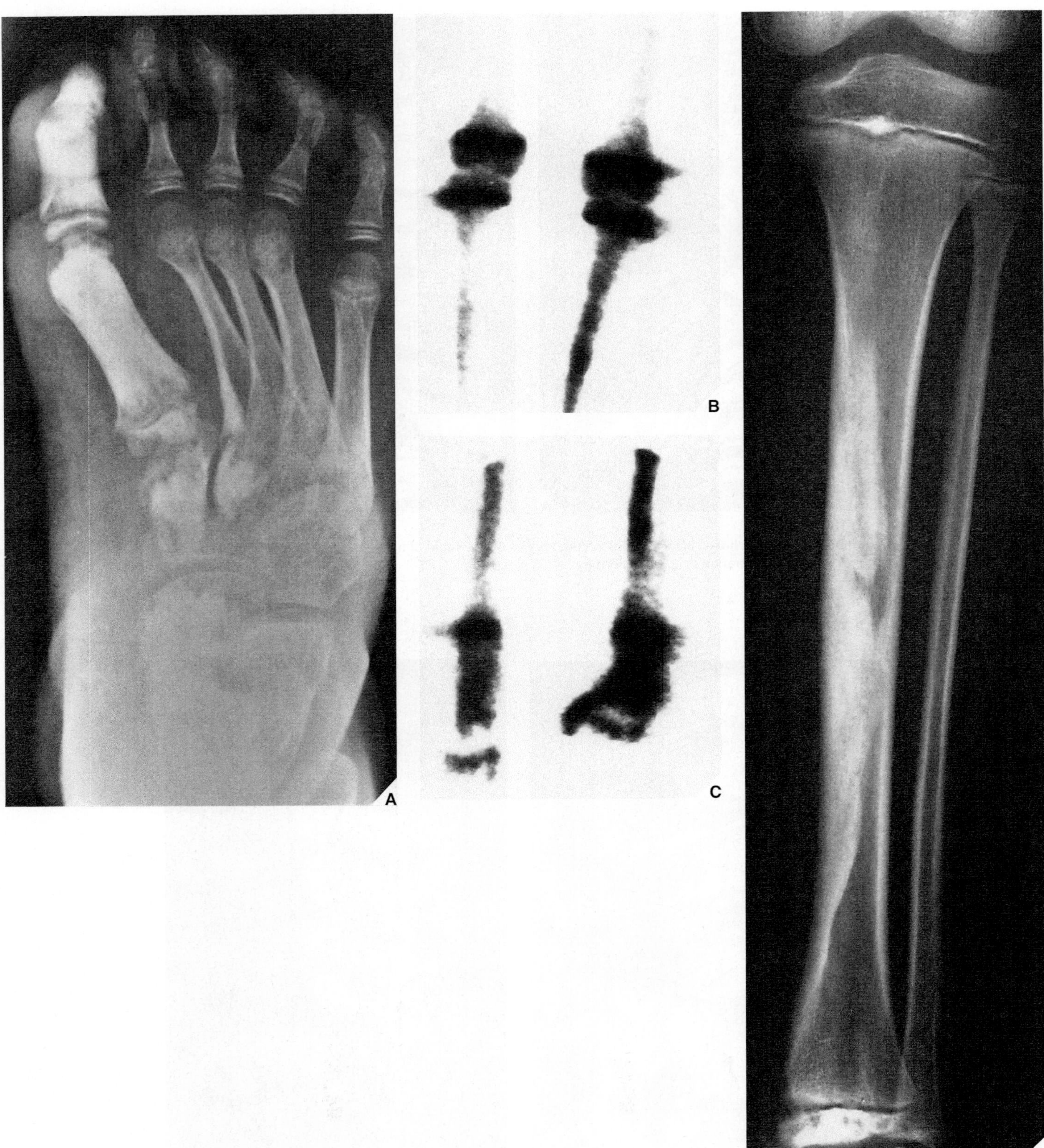

FIGURE 31.17 **Scintigraphy of melorheostosis.** A 9-year-old boy had a deformity of the left foot since birth, which was diagnosed as a clubfoot. **(A)** Dorsoplantar radiograph of the foot demonstrates the clubfoot deformity, together with sclerotic changes in the phalanges of the great toe, the first and second metatarsals, the first and second cuneiforms, the talus, and the calcaneus. Such changes are typical of melorheostosis, a form of sclerosing dysplasia. **(B,C)** On radionuclide bone scan, the extent of skeletal involvement is indicated by increased uptake of radiopharmaceutical agent not only in the foot but also in the left tibia, which is confirmed on a subsequent radiograph of the left leg **(D)**.

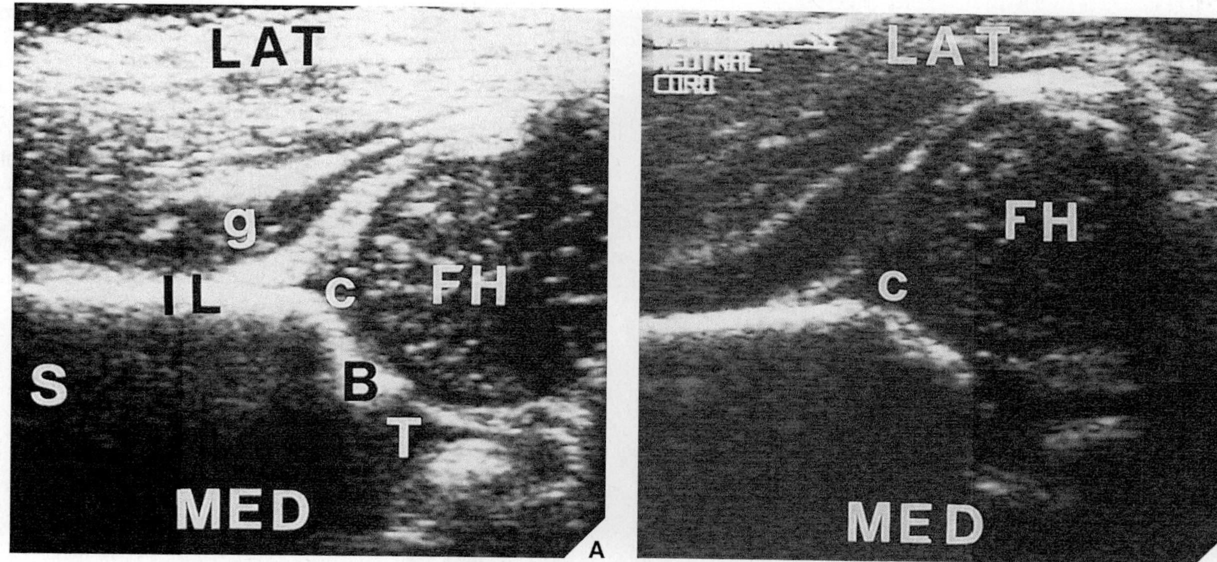

FIGURE 31.18 **US of congenital hip dysplasia.** **(A)** Coronal US of the left hip in a newborn boy shows normal relationship of the femoral head and acetabulum. **(B)** Coronal US of the left hip in a newborn girl shows dysplastic acetabulum and laterally subluxated femoral head. *LAT*, lateral; *g*, gluteus muscle; *IL*, ilium; *c*, cartilaginous acetabulum; *FH*, femoral head; *S*, superior; *B*, bony acetabulum; *T*, triradiate cartilage; *MED*, medial. (Courtesy of E. Gerscovich, MD, Sacramento, California.)

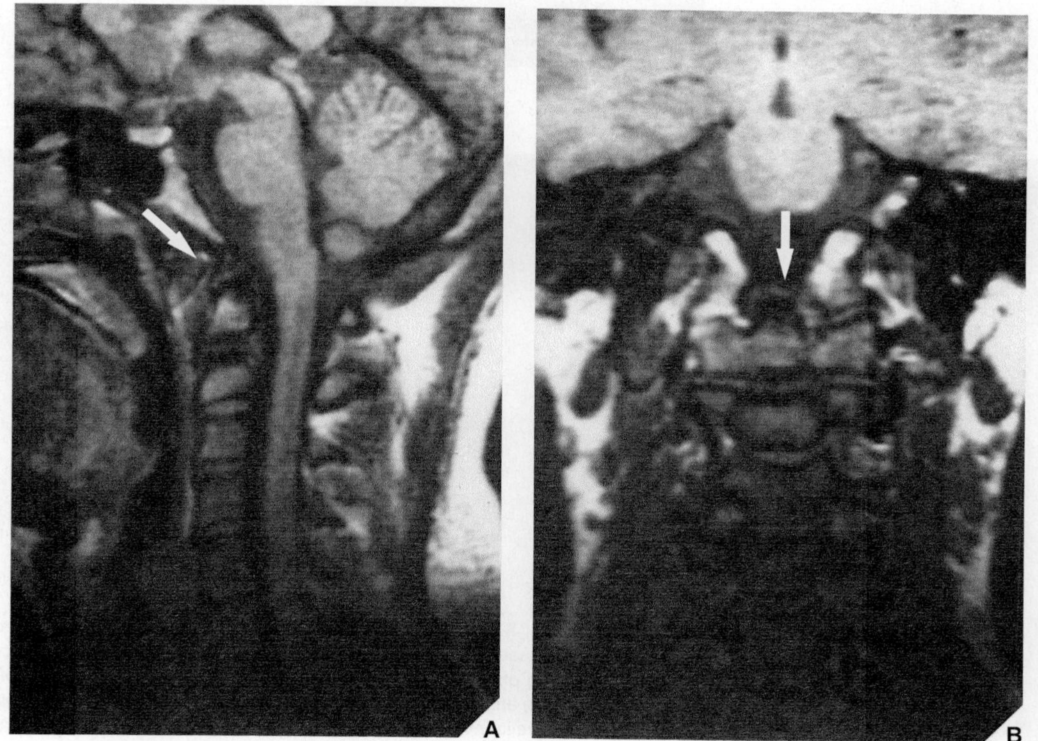

FIGURE 31.19 **MRI of hypoplasia of the odontoid.** **(A)** Sagittal T1-weighted MR image (SE; repetition time [TR] 800/echo time [TE] 20 msec) demonstrates a hypoplastic odontoid *(arrow)*, which arises from a normal second vertebral body. The anterior arch of the first cervical vertebra is not visualized because of fusion to the occiput. **(B)** Coronal T1-weighted (SE; TR 800/TE 20 msec) MR image confirms that the second cervical vertebral body is normal but only a rudimentary odontoid process has formed *(arrow)*. The atlas has fused with the occiput so that there are no occipital condyles. (Reprinted with permission from Beltran J. *MRI: musculoskeletal system*. Philadelphia: JB Lippincott; 1990.)

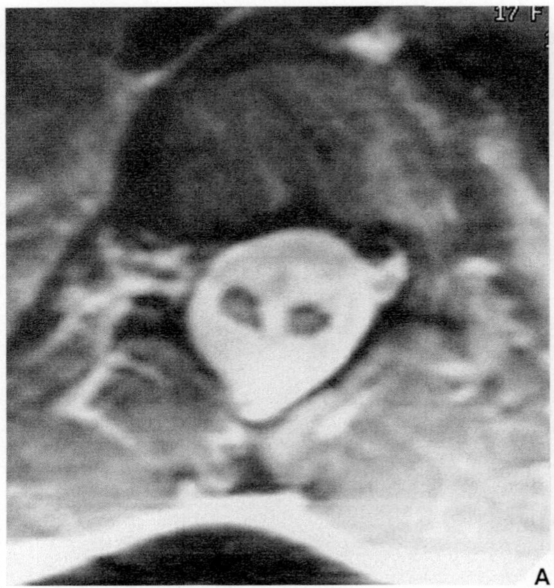

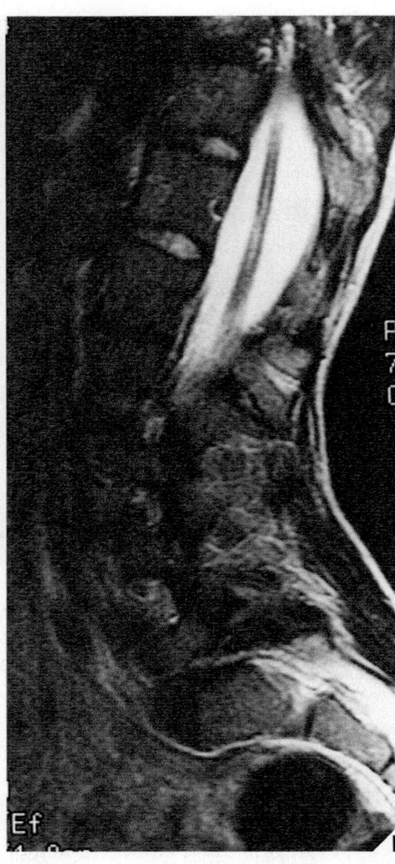

FIGURE 31.20 MRI of diastematomyelia. **(A)** Axial proton density–weighted (fast spin echo [FSE]; repetition time [TR] 5000/echo time [TE] 16 msec [Ef]) MR image in a 17-year-old girl with spina bifida and diastematomyelia shows a split spinal cord at the level of T12. **(B)** Sagittal T2-weighted (FSE; TR 3000/TE 133 msec [Ef]) MR image shows a low-signal fibrous septum within a markedly expanded thecal sac. The spinal fluid exhibits high signal intensity.

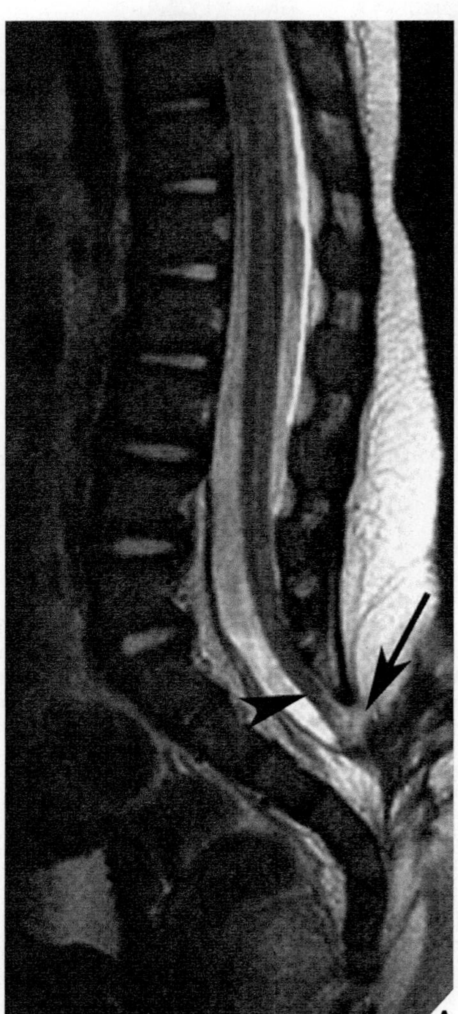

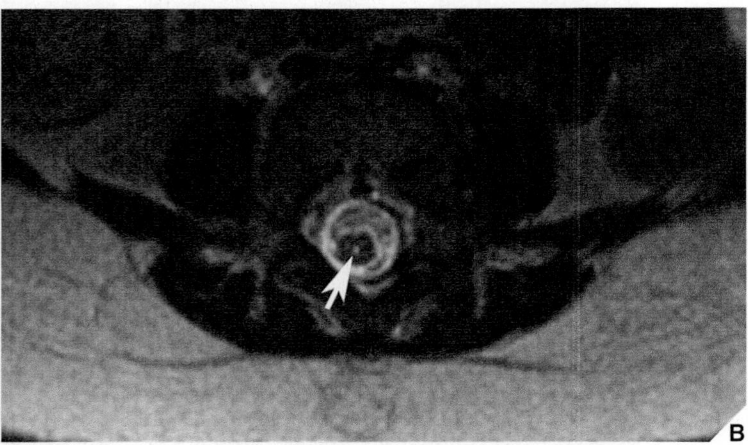

FIGURE 31.21 MRI of tethered cord. **(A)** Sagittal T2-weighted MRI of the lumbosacral spine of a newborn with a skin dimple over the sacrum shows thickening of the filum terminale *(arrowhead)* with a low position of the conus medullaris, anchored at the level of dysraphism of the sacrum *(arrow)*. There is syringomyelia involving the lumbar cord and visualized thoracic cord. Note the fibrous stranding in the subcutaneous fat over the sacrum. There is no associated meningomyelocele or lipoma. **(B)** Axial T2-weighted MRI at the level of L4 demonstrates syringomyelia *(arrow)*.

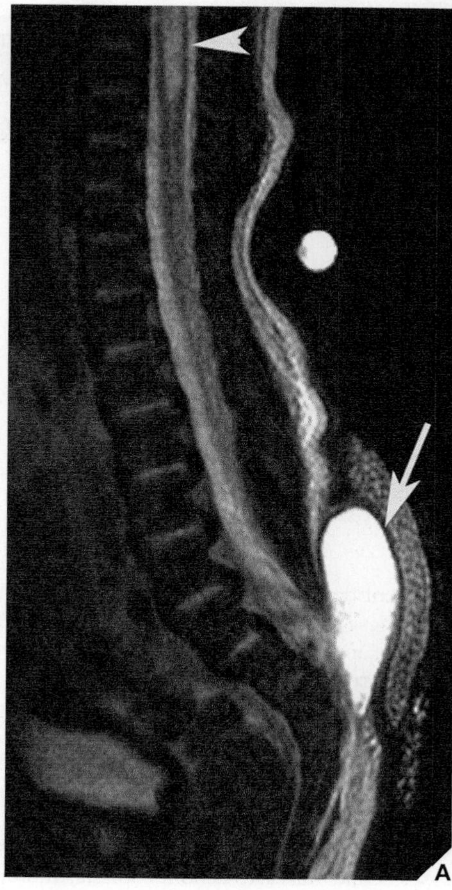

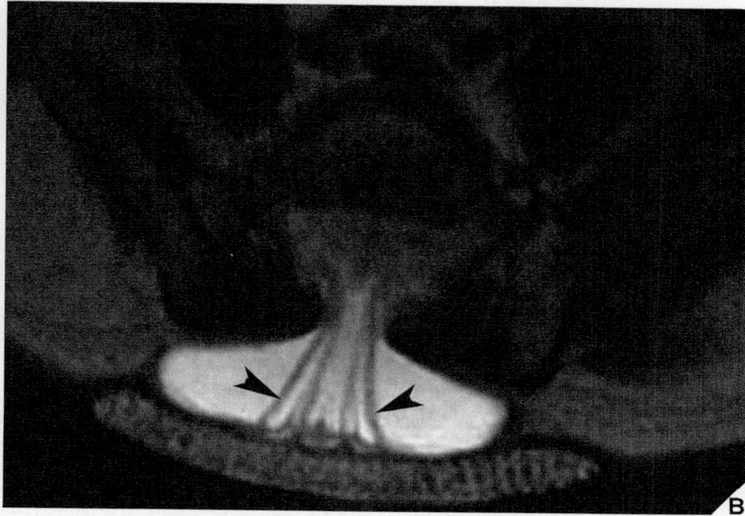

FIGURE 31.22 MRI of myelomeningocele and tethered cord. **(A)** Sagittal T2-weighted MRI of the thoracolumbar spine of a newborn demonstrates sacral dysraphism with myelomeningocele *(arrow)*, tethered cord, and syringomyelia of the lower thoracic cord *(arrowhead)*. **(B)** Axial T2-weighted MRI at the level of S1 demonstrates the meningocele through the sacral defect containing neural elements *(arrowheads)*. The patient also had tonsillar herniation, not shown. The final diagnosis was Chiari type I malformation.

PRACTICAL POINTS TO REMEMBER

1. Congenital anomalies comprise disturbances in bone formation, bone growth, and bone maturation and modeling.
2. Although most congenital and developmental anomalies can be diagnosed on standard radiographs, the use of ancillary techniques should be considered, such as:
   - radionuclide bone scan, particularly in determining the distribution of sites of involvement in various dysplasias
   - CT examination, particularly in the evaluation of congenital hip dislocation and determining the angle of version of the femoral head
   - 3D CT, particularly in the evaluation of spinal deformities
   - US, particularly in the evaluation of congenital hip dysplasia
   - MRI, particularly in the evaluation of abnormalities of the spine, thecal sac, and spinal cord.
3. Special projections may be required for the evaluation of anomalies of complex structures such as the ankle and foot.
4. The results and progress of treatment of various congenital disorders, especially congenital hip dislocation, can best be monitored by US and CT examinations.

SUGGESTED READINGS

Beighton P, Cremin B, Faure C, et al. International nomenclature of constitutional diseases of bone. *Ann Radiol* 1984;27:275.

Berkshire SB Jr, Maxwell EN, Sams BF. Bilateral symmetrical pseudarthrosis in a newborn. *Radiology* 1970;97:389–390.

Brower JS, Wootton-Gorges SL, Costouros JG, et al. Congenital diplopodia. *Pediatr Radiol* 2003;33:797–799.

Chung MS. Congenital differences of the upper extremity: classification and treatment principles. *Clin Orthop Surg* 2011;3:172–177.

Eich GF, Babyn P, Giedion A. Pediatric pelvis: radiographic appearance in various congenital disorders. *Radiographics* 1992;12:467–484.

Gerscovich EO. Infant hip in developmental dysplasia: facts to consider for a successful diagnostic ultrasound examination. *Appl Radiol* 1999;28:18–25.

Graf R. New possibilities for the diagnosis of congenital hip joint dislocation by ultrasonography. *J Pediatr Orthop* 1983;3:354–359.

International nomenclature of constitutional diseases of bone. *Am J Roentgenol* 1978;131: 352–354.

Kozin SH. Upper-extremity congenital anomalies. *J Bone Joint Surg Am* 2003;85(8): 1564–1576.

Kulik SA Jr, Clanfon TO. Tarsal coalition. *Foot Ankle Int* 1996;17:286–296.

Laor T, Jaramillo D, Hoffer FA, et al. MR imaging in congenital lower limb deformities. *Pediatr Radiol* 1996;26:381–387.

Newman JS, Newberg AH. Congenital tarsal coalition: multimodality evaluation with emphasis on CT and MR imaging. *Radiographics* 2000;20:321–332.

Reed MH, Genez B. Hands. In: Reed MH, ed. *Pediatric skeletal radiology*. Baltimore: Williams & Wilkins; 1992:584–625.

Rubin P. *Dynamic classification of bone dysplasias*. Chicago: Year Book Medical; 1972.

Sharma BG. Duplication of the clavicle with triplication of the coracoid process. *Skeletal Radiol* 2003;32:661–664.

Stanitski DF, Stanitski CL. Fibular hemimelia: a new classification system. *J Pediatr Orthop* 2003;23:30–34.

Wechsler RJ, Karasick D, Schweitzer ME. Computed tomography of talocalcaneal coalition: imaging techniques. *Skeletal Radiol* 1992;21:353–358.

Wechsler RJ, Schweitzer ME, Deely DM, et al. Tarsal coalition: depiction and characterization with CT and MR imaging. *Radiology* 1994;193:447–452.

32

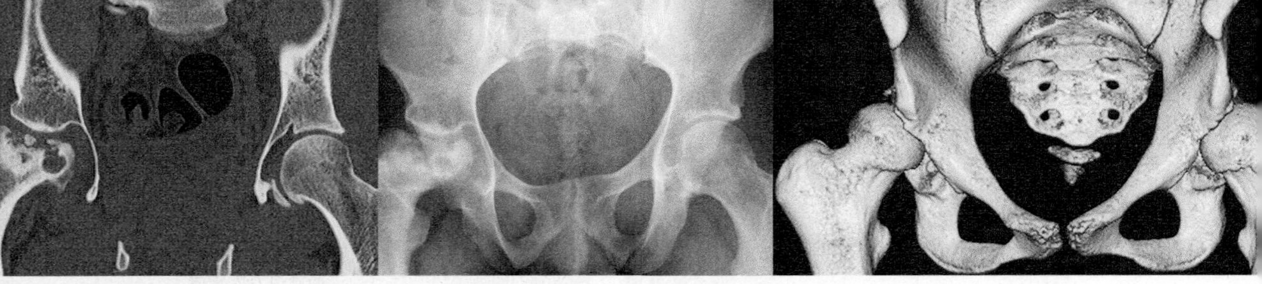

Anomalies of the Upper and Lower Limbs

Anomalies of the Shoulder Girdle and Upper Limbs

Congenital Elevation of the Scapula

Sprengel deformity, as congenital elevation of the scapula is also known, may be unilateral or bilateral. It is marked by the appearance of a scapula that is small, high in position, and rotated with its inferior edge pointing toward the spine—features that are easily identified on an anteroposterior radiograph of the shoulder or chest (Fig. 32.1). The left shoulder is the most commonly affected, and about 75% of all cases are observed in girls. Some cases of this anomaly are inherited in an autosomal dominant manner, although most cases are sporadic. A familial form of the Sprengel deformity is known as *Corno disease*. The finding of a congenitally elevated scapula is important because of this condition's frequent association with other anomalies, such as congenital scoliosis, fused ribs, spina bifida, and fusion of the cervical or upper thoracic vertebrae, the latter deformity known as *Klippel-Feil syndrome*, also a congenital disorder (Fig. 32.2) caused by mutations in the *GDF3* and *GDF6* genes. Furthermore, there is sometimes a bony connection between the elevated scapula and one of the vertebrae (usually the C5 or C6 vertebra), creating what is known as the *omovertebral bone* (Fig. 32.3).

Dentate Scapula

Dentate scapula, also known as *glenoid hypoplasia*, is a relatively rare congenital anomaly of the scapula due to underdevelopment of the ossification center of the inferior glenoid, leading to glenoid retroversion, small glenoid, and predisposition to early osteoarthritis of the glenohumeral joint. This condition is asymptomatic or mildly symptomatic in younger patients, but it becomes symptomatic in adult and elderly patients who present with limited range of motion, shoulder pain, and posterior glenohumeral instability leading to posterior dislocation. Imaging findings (Fig. 32.4) include undulating "dentate" appearance of the glenoid with widening of the inferior glenohumeral joint, posterior labral tear, and retroversion of the glenoid. Associated dysplastic changes can be seen, including hypoplasia of the proximal humerus, hooking of the distal clavicle, and hypertrophy of the coracoid process. In the adult patient, secondary osteoarthritis is a common complication, with chondral loss and osteophyte formation.

Madelung Deformity

This developmental anomaly of the distal radius and carpus, originally described by the German surgeon Otto Madelung in 1879, usually manifests in adolescent girls presenting with pain in the wrist and decreased range of motion but with no history of previous trauma or infection. Today, the term *Madelung deformity* is often used to describe a variety of conditions in the wrist marked by premature fusion of the distal physis of the radius, with consequent deformity of the distal ulna and wrist. From the etiologic viewpoint, these abnormalities can be divided into posttraumatic deformities, dysplasias, and idiopathic conditions. A genetic cause has also been proposed. Association with mesomelic dwarfism (e.g., Leri-Weill dyschondrosteosis, caused by deletion or duplication of the *SHOX* gene located within the band Xp22.3 of the chromosome X) and a mutation on the X chromosome (e.g., Turner syndrome) has also been described. The posttraumatic deformity may occur after repetitive injury or after a single event that disrupts the growth of the distal radius. Among the bone dysplasias associated with Madelung deformity are multiple hereditary cartilaginous exostoses, Ollier disease, achondroplasia, multiple epiphyseal dysplasia, and the mucopolysaccharidoses including Hurler and Morquio syndromes.

On physical examination, the hand is translated volarly to the long axis of the forearm and there is dorsal subluxation of the ulna. A decreased range of motion limits supination, dorsiflexion, and radial deviation, but pronation and palmar flexion are usually preserved.

The radiographic criteria for the diagnosis of Madelung deformity have been described in the world literature, and are summarized in Table 32.1. The posteroanterior and lateral projections of the distal forearm and wrist are sufficient to demonstrate any of the abnormalities associated with this deformity (Figs. 32.5 and 32.6).

Surgical treatment of Madelung deformity is indicated for pain relief and cosmetic improvement. A variety of procedures are available. These include ligament release (Vickers physiolysis), wedge osteotomy, Carter-Ezaki dome osteotomy, and radioscaphocapitate arthrodesis. Occasionally, a Darrach or a Suavé-Kapandji procedure is indicated.

Anomalies of the Pelvic Girdle and Hip

An overview of the most effective radiographic projections and radiologic techniques for evaluating the most common anomalies of the pelvic girdle and hip is presented in Table 32.2.

Congenital Hip Dislocation (Developmental Dysplasia of the Hip)

The hip joint is the most frequent site of congenital dislocations. The condition occurs with an incidence of 1.5 per 1,000 births and 8 times more often in girls than in boys. In unilateral dislocation, the left hip is involved twice as often as the right, and bilateral dislocation occurs in more than 25% of affected children. More commonly encountered in white than in black persons, the condition is very common in Mediterranean and Scandinavian countries; it is almost unknown in China, which may be explained in part by the Chinese custom of carrying the infant on the mother's back with its hips flexed and abducted.

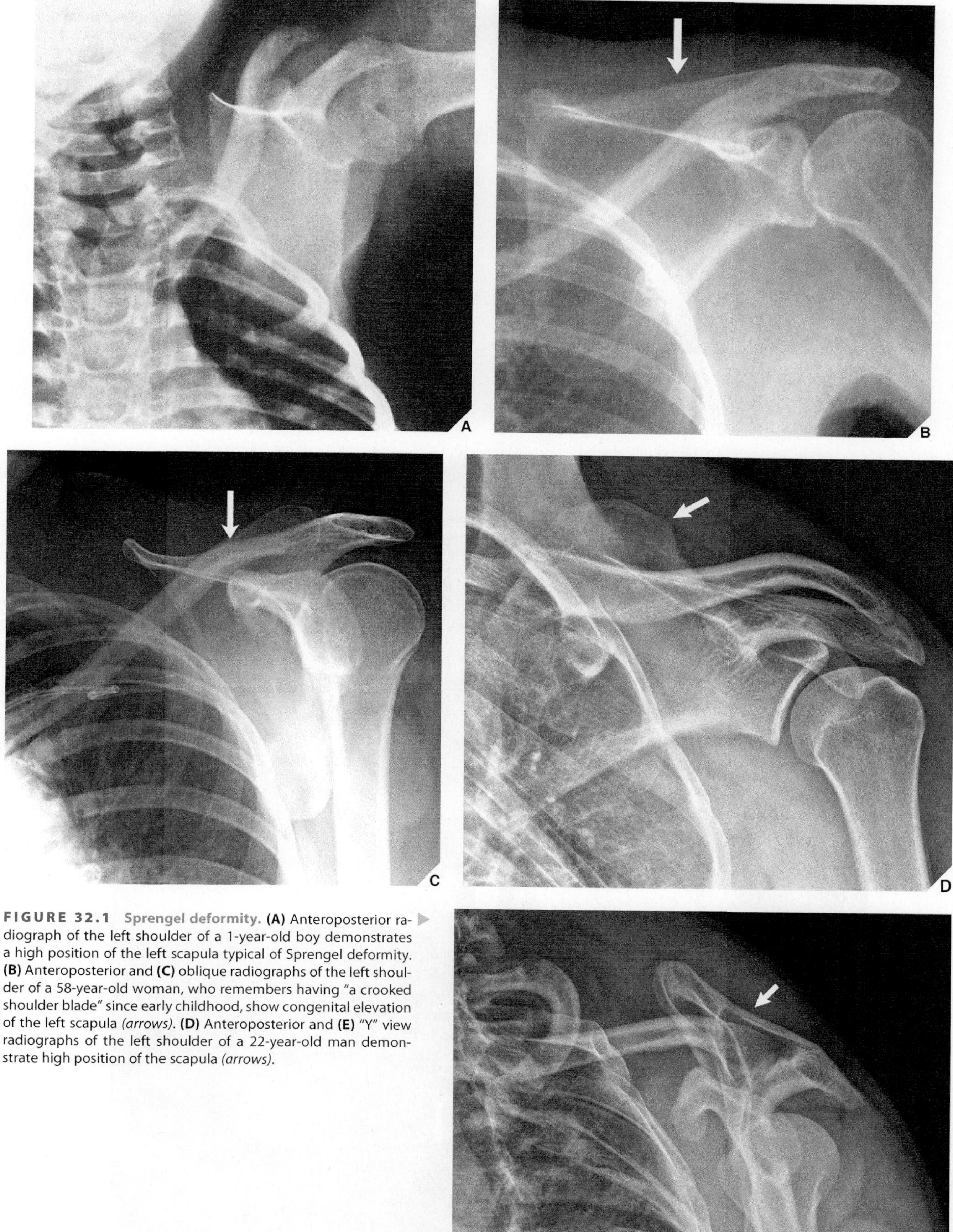

FIGURE 32.1 **Sprengel deformity.** **(A)** Anteroposterior radiograph of the left shoulder of a 1-year-old boy demonstrates a high position of the left scapula typical of Sprengel deformity. **(B)** Anteroposterior and **(C)** oblique radiographs of the left shoulder of a 58-year-old woman, who remembers having "a crooked shoulder blade" since early childhood, show congenital elevation of the left scapula *(arrows)*. **(D)** Anteroposterior and **(E)** "Y" view radiographs of the left shoulder of a 22-year-old man demonstrate high position of the scapula *(arrows)*.

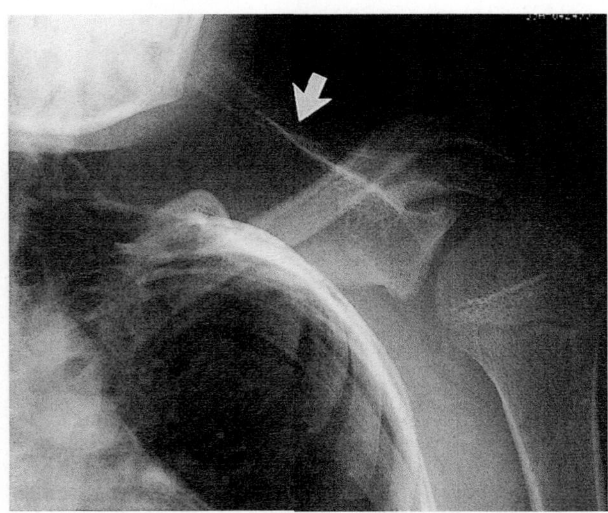

FIGURE 32.2 Klippel-Feil syndrome and Sprengel deformity. Anteroposterior radiograph of the left shoulder of a 13-year-old boy with Klippel-Feil syndrome shows an elevated scapula *(arrow)*.

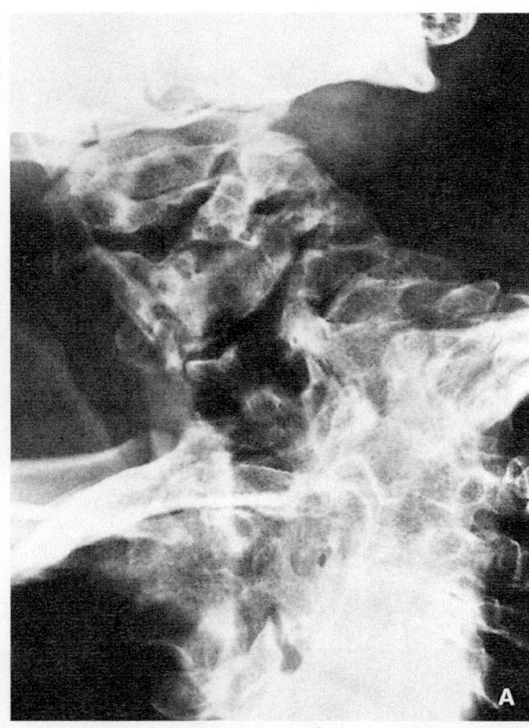

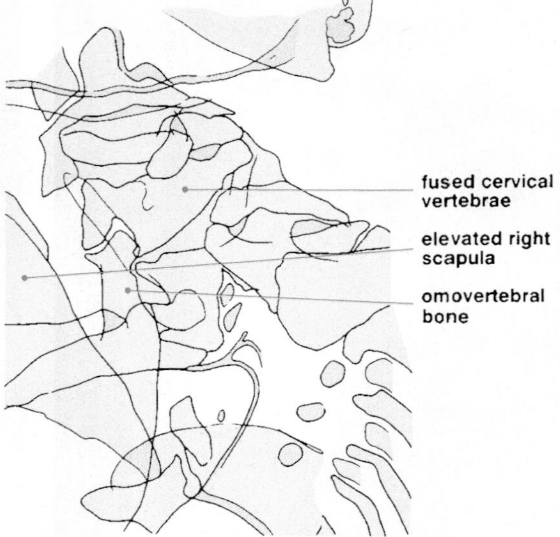

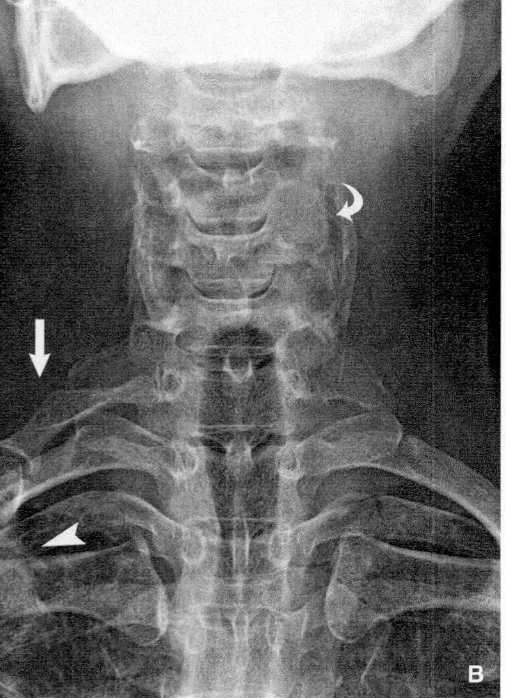

FIGURE 32.3 Klippel-Feil syndrome and Sprengel deformity. (A) Posteroanterior radiograph of the cervical and upper thoracic spine in a 37-year-old woman with Sprengel deformity associated with Klippel-Feil syndrome (fusion of the cervical vertebrae) shows the omovertebral bone connecting the elevated right scapula and the C5 vertebra. **(B)** Anteroposterior radiograph of the cervical and upper thoracic spine of a 66-year-old man shows a partial fusion of the lower cervical vertebrae *(curved arrow)* and omovertebral bone *(arrow)*. *Arrowhead* points to the elevated scapula.

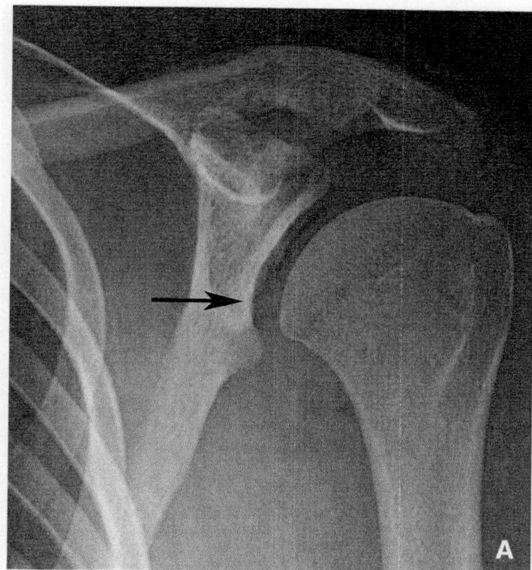

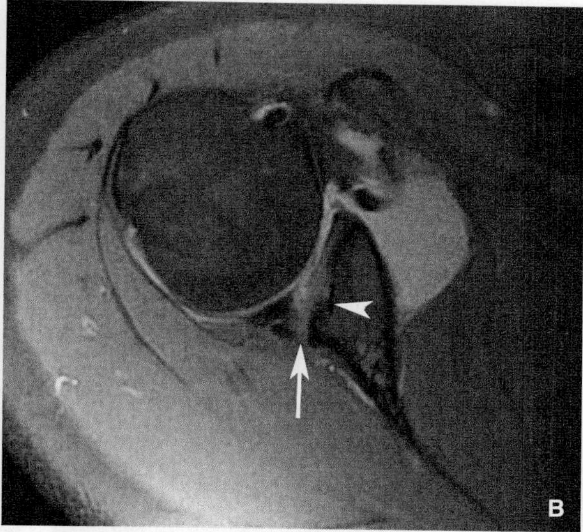

FIGURE 32.4 Dentate scapula (glenoid hypoplasia). **(A)** Anteroposterior radiograph of the left shoulder demonstrates hypoplasia of the inferior margin of the glenoid with an undulating margin *(arrow)*. **(B)** Axial T1-weighted fat-saturated MR arthrogram of the shoulder demonstrates the hypoplasia of the posterior inferior glenoid *(arrowhead)* associated with a posterior labral tear *(arrow)*.

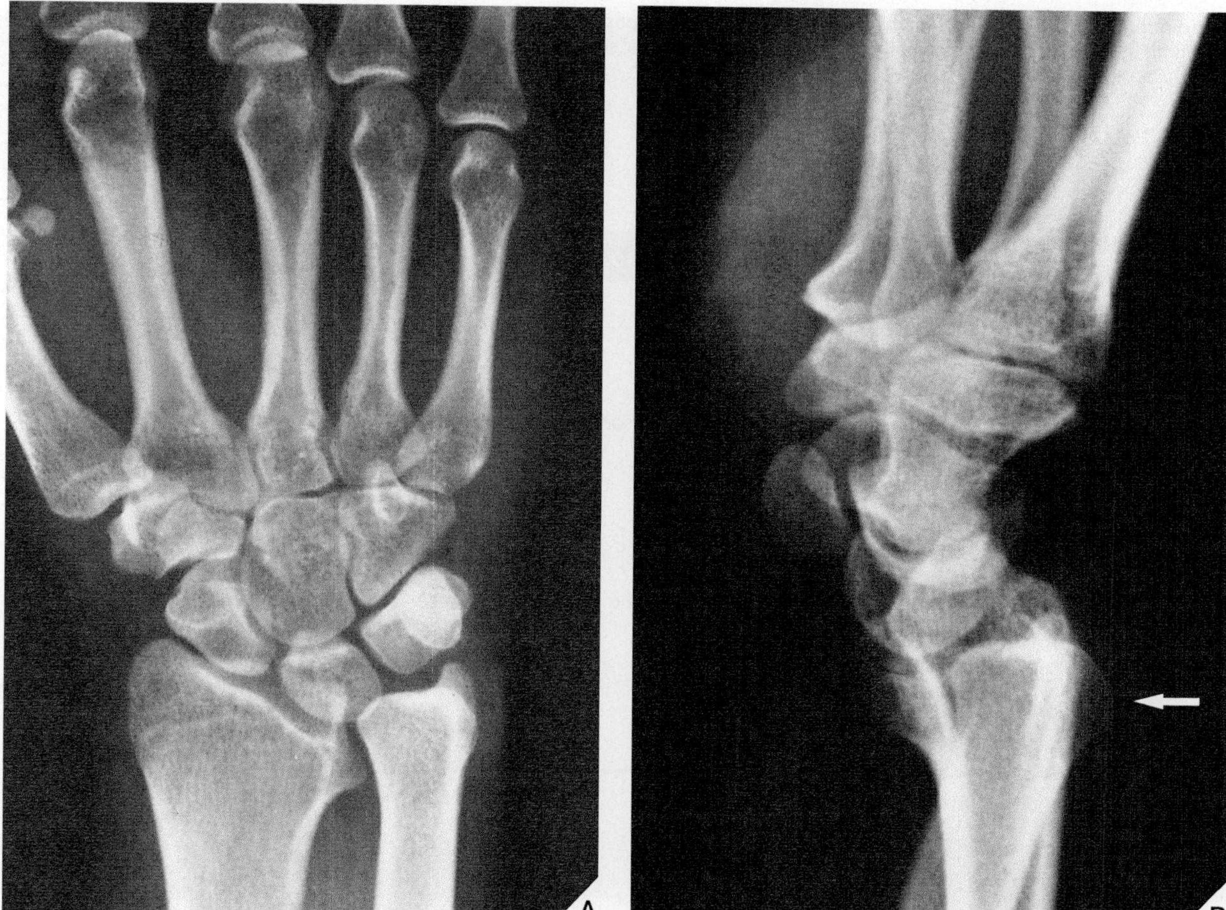

FIGURE 32.5 Madelung deformity. **(A)** Posteroanterior radiograph of the left wrist of a 21-year-old woman shows a decrease in the length of the radius, the distal end of which has assumed a triangular shape. This is associated with a triangular configuration of the carpus, with the lunate at the apex wedged between the radius and the ulna. **(B)** Lateral radiograph demonstrates dorsal subluxation of the ulna *(arrow)*.

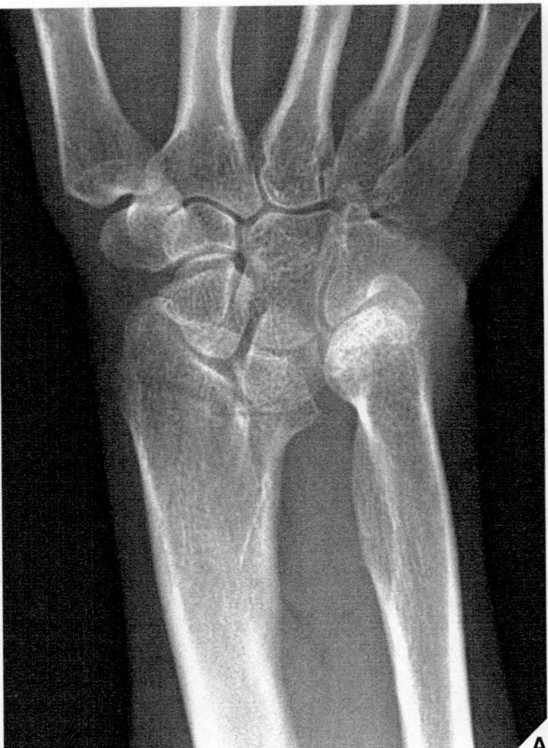

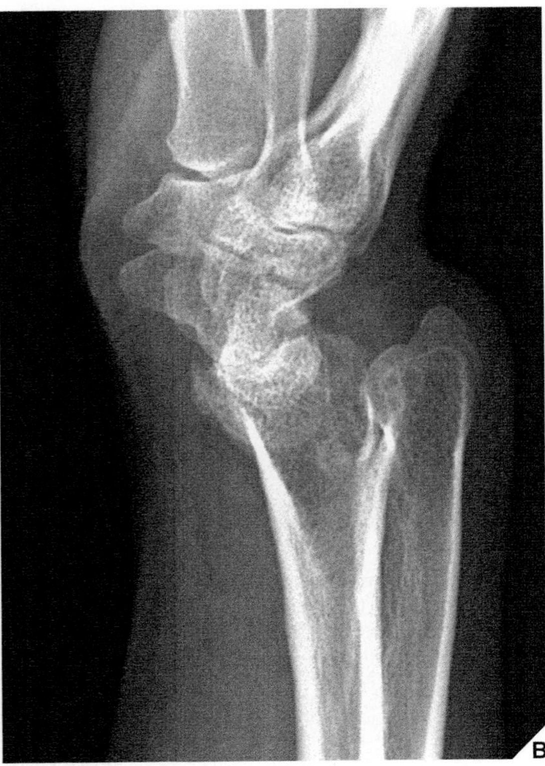

FIGURE 32.6 Madelung deformity. (A) Posteroanterior and **(B)** lateral radiographs of the left wrist of a 42-year-old woman show characteristic changes of this anomaly including decreased length of the radius, elongation of the ulna associated with dorsal subluxation, and triangular configuration of the carpus with lunate wedged between the radius and the ulna. (Courtesy of Robert M. Szabo, MD, Sacramento, California.)

TABLE 32.1 Radiographic Criteria for the Diagnosis of Madelung Deformity
Changes in the Radius
Double curvature (medial and dorsal)
Decrease in bone length
Triangular shape of the distal epiphysis
Premature fusion of the medial part of the distal physis, associated with medial and volar angulation of the articular surface
Focal radiolucent areas along the medial border of bone
Exostosis at the distal medial border
Changes in the Ulna
Dorsal subluxation
Increased density (hypercondensation and distortion) of the ulnar head
Increase in bone length
Changes in the Carpus
Triangular configuration with the lunate at the apex
Increase in distance between the distal radius and the ulna
Decrease in carpal angle

Data from Dannenberg M, Anton JI, Spiegel MB. Madelung's deformity. Consideration of its roentgenological diagnostic criteria. *Am J Roentgenol* 1939;42:671.

TABLE 32.2 Most Effective Radiographic Projections and Radiologic Techniques for Evaluating Common Anomalies of the Pelvic Girdle and Hip

Projection/Technique	Crucial Abnormalities
Congenital Hip Dislocation	
Anteroposterior of pelvis and hips	Determination of Hilgenreiner Y-line Acetabular index Perkins-Ombredanne line Shenton-Menard line (arc) C-E angle of Wiberg Ossification center of capital femoral epiphysis Relations of femoral head and acetabulum
Anteroposterior of hips in abduction and internal rotation	Andrén-von Rosen line
Arthrography	Congruity of the joint Status of Cartilaginous limbus (limbus thorn) Ligamentum teres Zona orbicularis
CT (alone or with arthrography)	Relations of femoral head and acetabulum
Ultrasound	Superior, lateral, or posterior subluxation Position of femoral head in acetabulum Status of Acetabular roof Cartilaginous limbus
Developmental Coxa Vara	
Anteroposterior of pelvis and hips	Varus angle of femoral neck and femoral shaft
Proximal Femoral Focal Deficiency	
Anteroposterior of hip and proximal femur	Shortening of femur Superior, posterior, and lateral displacement of proximal femoral segment
Arthrography	Nonossified femoral head
Legg-Calvé-Perthes Disease	
Anteroposterior and frog-lateral of hips	Osteonecrosis of femoral head as indicated by crescent sign and subchondral collapse Gage sign Subluxation of femoral head Horizontal orientation of growth plate Calcifications lateral to epiphysis Cystic changes in metaphysis Sagging rope sign
Arthrography	Incongruity of hip joint Thickness of articular cartilage
Radionuclide bone scan	Decreased uptake of isotope (earliest stage) Increased uptake of isotope (late stage)
CT and MRI	Incongruity of hip joint Osteonecrosis
Slipped Capital Femoral Epiphysis	
Anteroposterior of hips	Loss of Capener triangle sign Periarticular osteoporosis Widening and blurring of growth plate Decreased height of femoral epiphysis Absence of intersection of epiphysis by line tangent to lateral cortex of femoral neck Herndon hump Chondrolysis (complication)
Frog-lateral of hips	Absence of intersection of epiphysis by line tangent to lateral cortex of femoral neck Actual slippage (displacement) of femoral epiphysis
Radionuclide bone scan and MRI	Osteonecrosis (complication)

C-E, center-edge; CT, computed tomography; MRI, magnetic resonance imaging.

TABLE 32.3 Clinical Manifestations of Congenital Dislocation of the Hip

Limited abduction of the flexed hip (due to shortening and contraction of hip adductors)
Increase in depth or asymmetry of the inguinal or thigh skinfolds
Shortening of one leg
Allis or Galeazzi sign[a]—lower position of knee of affected side when knees and hips are flexed (due to location of femoral head posterior to acetabulum in this position)
Ortolani "jerk" sign ("clunk of entry" or reduction sign)
Barlow test ("clunk of exit" or dislocation sign)
Telescoping or pistoning action of thighs[a] (due to lack of containment of femoral head within acetabulum)
Trendelenburg test[a]—dropping of normal hip when child, standing on both feet, elevates unaffected limb and bears weight on affected side (due to weakness of hip abductors)
Waddling gait[a]

[a]This finding can occur in older children.

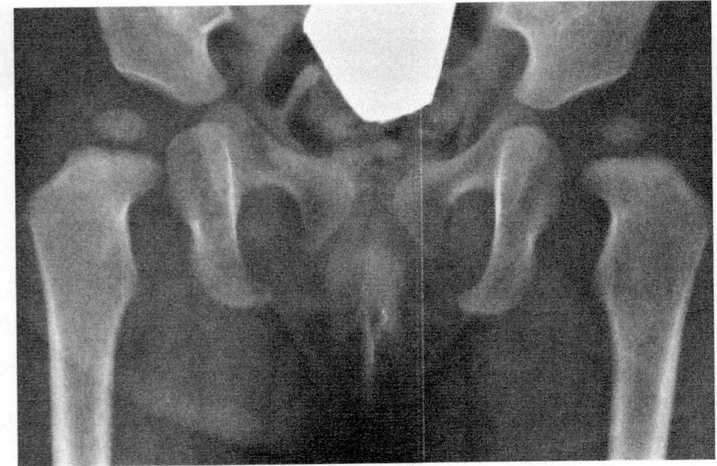

FIGURE 32.8 Congenital hip dysplasia. Anteroposterior radiograph of the pelvis of a 1-year-old girl shows congenital superolateral subluxation of the left hip. Note the slightly smaller size of the ossification center for the left femoral epiphysis.

The criteria for the diagnosis of congenital dislocation of the hip (CDH) include physical and imaging findings. Certain clinical signs have been identified that are helpful in the evaluation of newborns and infants for possible CDH (Table 32.3).

Radiographic Features

Each of the stages of CDH—dysplasia of the hip, subluxation of the hip, and dislocation of the hip—has a characteristic radiographic presentation. The term *congenital hip dysplasia*, first introduced by Hilgenreiner in 1925, refers to delayed or defective development of the hip joint leading to a deranged articular relationship between an abnormal acetabulum and a deformed proximal end of the femur (Fig. 32.7). The condition is considered a precursor of subluxation and dislocation of the hip, although some authorities use the term *developmental dysplasia of the hip* (DDH) to denote all stages of CDH. In *congenital subluxation of the hip*, there is an abnormal relationship between the femoral head and the acetabulum, but the two are in contact (Fig. 32.8). *Congenital dislocation of the hip*, however, is marked by the femoral head's complete loss of contact with the acetabular cartilage; the proximal femur is displaced most often superiorly, but lateral, posterior, and posterolateral dislocation may also be seen (Fig. 32.9).

Measurements

In contrast to an adult hip, the relationship between the femoral head and the acetabulum in a newborn's hip cannot be assessed by direct visualization because the femoral head is not ossified, and as a cartilaginous body, it is not visible on conventional radiographs. The ossification center first appears between the ages of 3 and 6 months, and a delay in its appearance should be viewed as an indication of congenital hip dysplasia. The neck of the femur must therefore be used for ascertaining this relationship. The anteroposterior radiograph of the pelvis serves as the basis for determining several indirect indicators of the relationship between the femoral head and the acetabulum. To obtain accurate measurements, however, proper positioning of the infant is imperative; the lower extremities should be extended in the neutral position and longitudinally aligned, whereas the central ray should be directed toward the midline, slightly above the pubic symphysis, to ensure the symmetry of both halves of the pelvis. The measurements used to evaluate the relation of the femoral head to the acetabulum are the following (Fig. 32.10):

1. The *Hilgenreiner line* or *Y-line*, which is drawn through the superior part of the triradiate cartilage, is itself a valuable indicator of femoroacetabular relations and serves as the basis for all other indicators.
2. The *acetabular index*, which is an angle formed by a line tangent to the acetabular roof and the Y-line, cannot alone be diagnostic of dislocation because it can occasionally exceed 30 degrees in normal subjects. Generally, however, values greater than 30 degrees are considered abnormal and indicate impending dislocation. Some investigators propose that only angles in excess of 40 degrees are significant.
3. The *Perkins-Ombredanne line*, which is drawn perpendicular to the Y-line through the most lateral edge of the ossified acetabular cartilage, is helpful in determining subluxation and dislocation of the hip. The intersection of this line with the Y-line creates four quadrants; normally, the medial aspect of the femoral neck or the ossified capital femoral epiphysis falls in the lower medial quadrant.

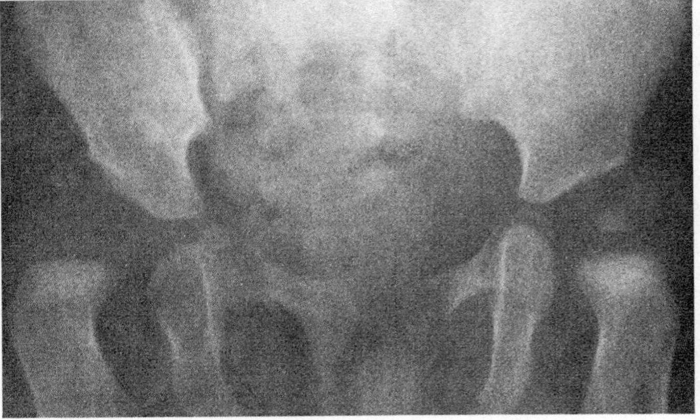

FIGURE 32.7 Congenital hip dysplasia. Anteroposterior radiograph of the pelvis of a 1-year-old boy shows a slightly flattened acetabulum and delayed appearance of the ossification center for the right femoral epiphysis; ossification center of the left femoral epiphysis is normally centered over the triradiate cartilage.

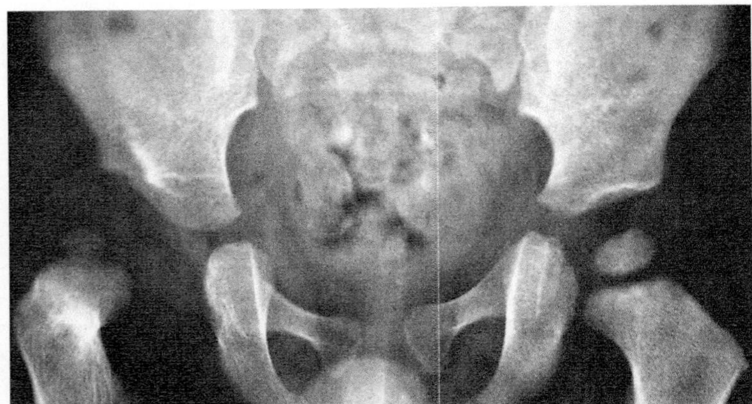

FIGURE 32.9 Congenital hip dislocation. Anteroposterior radiograph of the pelvis of a 2-year-old boy demonstrates complete superolateral dislocation of the right hip. Note the abnormal position of the center of ossification in relation to the acetabulum compared with the normal left hip.

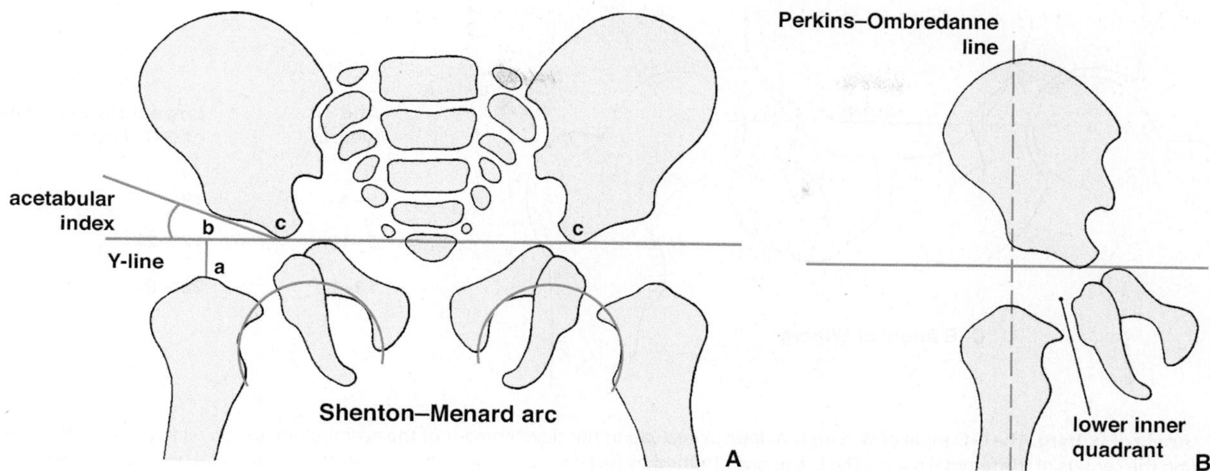

FIGURE 32.10 Measurements helpful to evaluate the relation of the femoral head to the acetabulum. **(A)** The *Hilgenreiner line* or *Y-line* is drawn through the superior part of the triradiate cartilage. In normal infants, the distance represented by a line *(ab)* perpendicular to the Y-line at the most proximal point of the femoral neck should be equal on both sides of the pelvis, as should the distance represented by a line *(bc)* drawn coincident with the Y-line medially to the acetabular floor. In infants aged 6 to 7 months, the mean value for the distance *(ab)* has been determined to be 19.3 ± 1.5 mm; the distance for *(bc)* is 18.2 ± 1.4 mm. The *acetabular index* is an angle formed by a line drawn tangent to the acetabular roof from point *(c)* at the acetabular floor on the Y-line. The normal value of this angle ranges from 25 to 29 degrees. The *Shenton-Menard line* is an arc running through the medial aspect of the femoral neck and the superior border of the obturator foramen. It should be smooth and unbroken. **(B)** The *Perkins-Ombredanne line* is drawn perpendicular to the Y-line through the most lateral edge of the ossified acetabular cartilage, which actually corresponds to the anteroinferior iliac spine. In normal newborns and infants, the medial aspect of the femoral neck or the ossified capital femoral epiphysis falls in the lower inner quadrant. The appearance of either of these structures in the lower outer or upper outer quadrant indicates subluxation or dislocation of the hip.

4. The *Shenton-Menard line*, which forms a smooth arc through the medial aspect of the femoral neck and the superior border of the obturator foramen, may be interrupted in subluxation or dislocation of the hip. Even under normal circumstances, however, the arc may not be smooth if the radiograph is obtained with the hip in external rotation and adduction.
5. The *Andrén-von Rosen line*, which is drawn on a radiograph obtained with the hips abducted 45 degrees and internally rotated, describes the relation of the longitudinal axis of the femoral shaft to the acetabulum (Fig. 32.11). In dislocation or subluxation of the hip, this line bisects or falls above the anterosuperior iliac spine.

After the capital femoral epiphysis achieves full ossification at approximately 4 years of age, a diagnosis of gross displacement can usually be made without difficulty. The evaluation of subtle hip dysplasias, however, can be aided by another parameter of the relation of the femoral head to the acetabulum, the *center-edge (C-E) angle of Wiberg* (Fig. 32.12). Determination of this angle is most useful after full ossification of the femoral head because its relationship to the acetabulum is then fully established.

Arthrography and Computed Tomography

Aside from conventional radiography, hip arthrography is the useful technique for evaluating CDH. During the procedure, radiographs are routinely obtained with the hip in the neutral (Fig. 32.13A) and frog-lateral positions (Fig. 32.13B) as well as in abduction, adduction, and internal rotation. In subluxation, the femoral head lies lateral to just below the margin of the acetabular cartilaginous labrum, and the joint capsule is usually loose (Fig. 32.14). In complete dislocation, the femoral head lies superior and lateral to the edge of the labrum (Fig. 32.15). Deformities may also be encountered in the cartilaginous limbus, a structure lying between the femoral head and the acetabulum. In advanced stages, it may be inverted and hypertrophied, thus making the reduction impossible. Moreover, the portion of the capsule lying medial to the femoral head is usually constricted to form an isthmus with a "figure-eight" appearance.

Computed tomography (CT), either alone (Fig. 32.16) or with arthrography, is also a frequently used modality in the evaluation of CDH. In subluxation or dislocation, the congruity of the acetabulum and the femoral head, which is normally centered over the triradiate cartilage, is disturbed (Fig. 32.17). CT has proved to be the most accurate technique for determining the degree of subluxation or dislocation. It is also an essential modality for monitoring the progress of CDH treatment. In the adult patient, it provides an effective method to evaluate the undercoverage of the femoral head by bony acetabulum (Fig. 32.18).

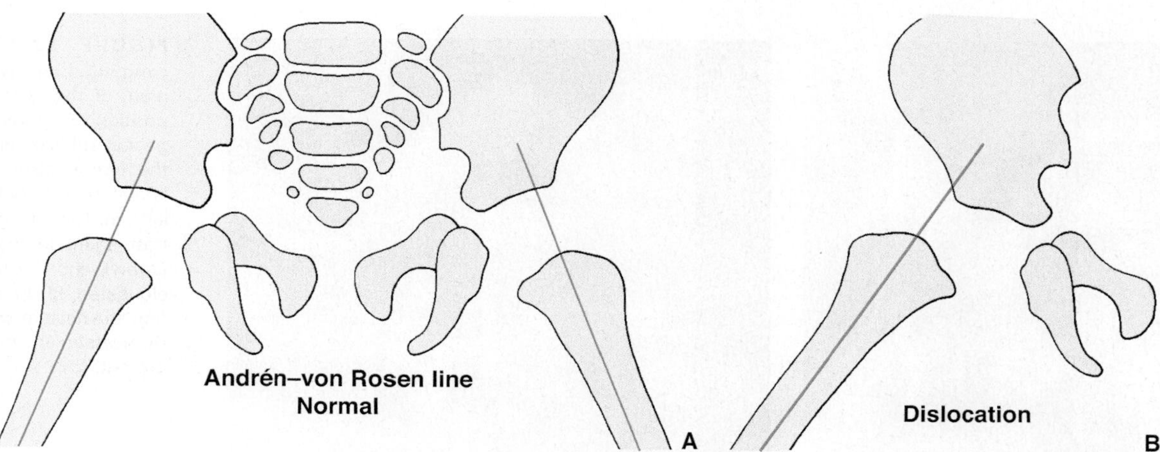

FIGURE 32.11 The Andrén-von Rosen line. **(A)** With at least 45 degrees of hip abduction and internal rotation, the line is drawn along the longitudinal axis of the femoral shaft. In normal hips, it intersects the pelvis at the upper edge of the acetabulum. **(B)** In subluxation or dislocation of the hip, the line bisects or falls above the anterosuperior iliac spine.

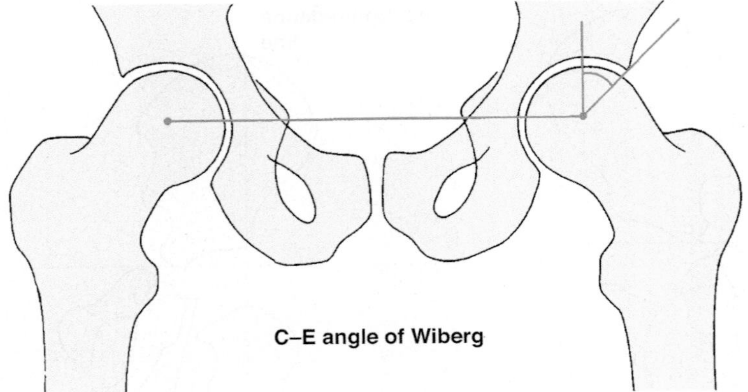

Age (years)	Lowest Normal Value of C–E Angle
5–8	19°
9–12	12°–25°
13–20	26°–30°

FIGURE 32.12 Angle of Wiberg. The C-E angle of Wiberg is helpful in evaluating the development of the acetabulum and its relation to the femoral head. A baseline is projected, connecting the centers of the femoral heads. The C-E angle is formed by two lines originating in the center of the femoral head, one drawn perpendicular to the baseline into the acetabulum, and the other connecting the center of the femoral head with the superior acetabular lip. Values below the lowest normal value given for each age group indicate hip dysplasia.

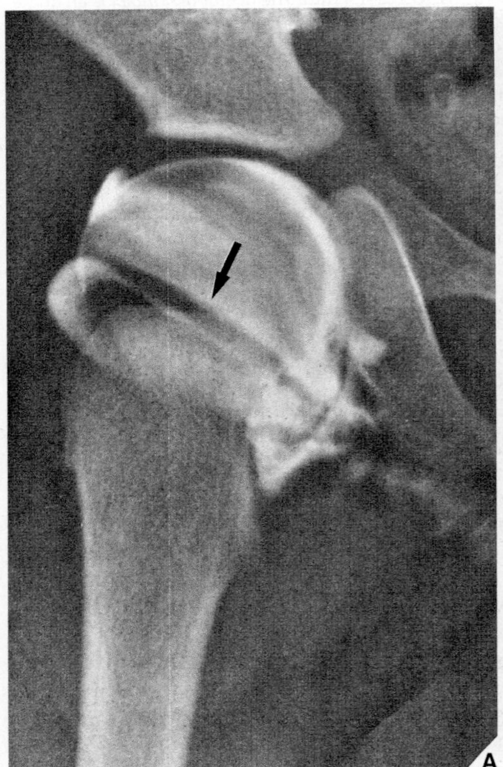

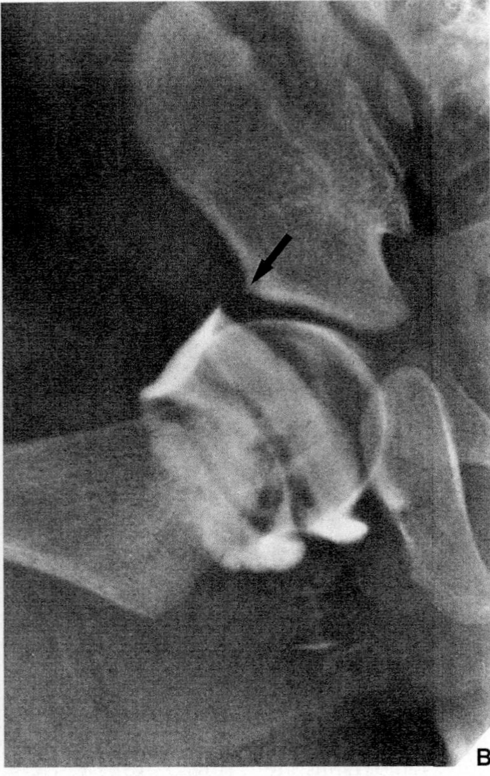

FIGURE 32.13 Arthrogram of a normal hip. **(A)** Arthrogram of the right hip in the neutral position in a 5-month-old boy shows contrast agent accumulating in the large recesses medial and lateral to the constriction produced by the orbicular ligament *(arrow)*. Note the smoothness and even thickness of the cartilage covering the femoral head. **(B)** On the frog-lateral view, contrast is seen outlining the edge of the cartilaginous labrum *(arrow)*. The ligamentum teres can be seen medial to the femoral head, extending from the inferior portion of the acetabulum.

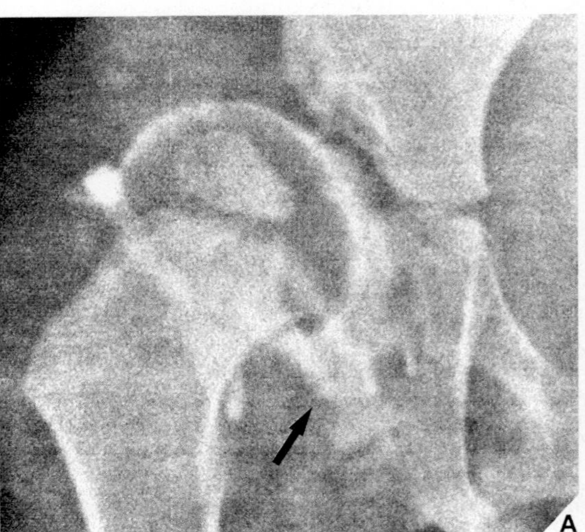

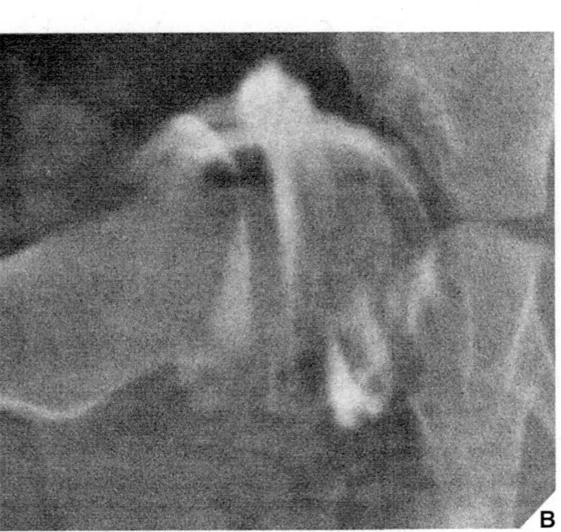

FIGURE 32.14 Arthrogram of congenital hip dysplasia. **(A)** Arthrogram of the right hip in the neutral position in a 1-year-old girl with congenital subluxation of the hip shows the typical displacement of the hip lateral to but below the acetabular labrum. There is accumulation of contrast agent in the stretched capsule *(arrow)*, and the ligamentum teres is elongated. **(B)** In the frog-lateral position, the head moves more deeply into the acetabulum, but subluxation is still present.

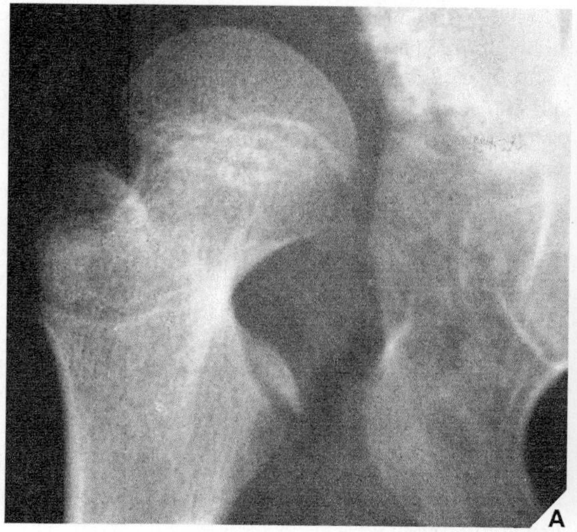

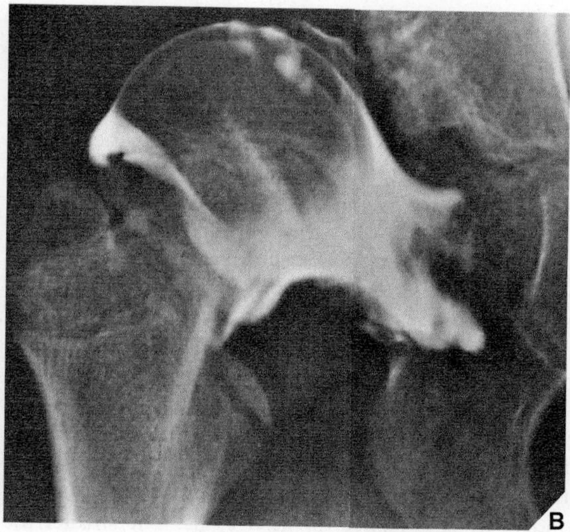

FIGURE 32.15 Arthrogram of congenital hip dislocation. **(A)** Anteroposterior radiograph of the right hip in an 8-year-old girl demonstrates complete superolateral dislocation of the femoral head. Note the shallow acetabulum. **(B)** Arthrogram of the hip shows a deformed cartilaginous limbus and stretching of the ligamentum teres. The femoral head lies superior and lateral to the edge of the cartilaginous labrum. Note the accumulation of contrast agent in the loose joint capsule.

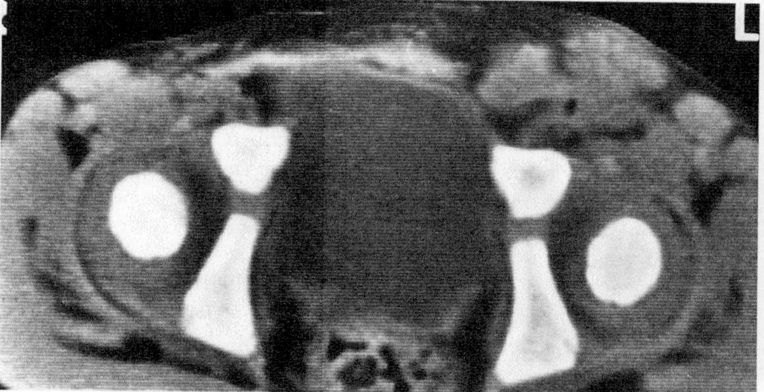

FIGURE 32.16 CT of the normal hips. Axial section of both hips in a 19-month-old infant shows good congruity of the acetabula and femoral heads, which are centered over the triradiate cartilage.

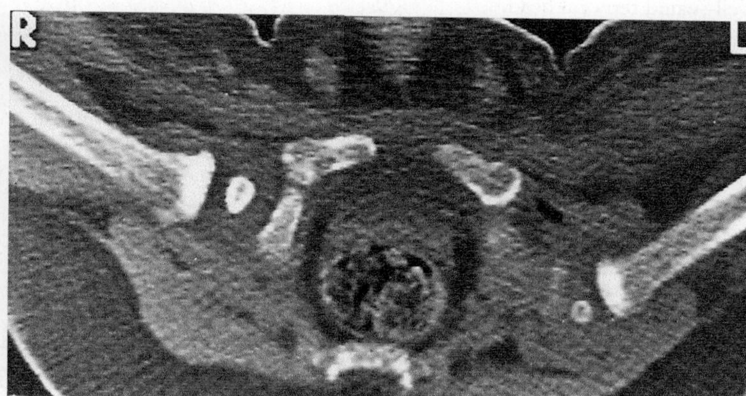

FIGURE 32.17 CT of congenital hip dislocation. Axial section through the proximal femora and hips of a 6-month-old boy shows posterolateral dislocation of the left hip. The right hip is normal.

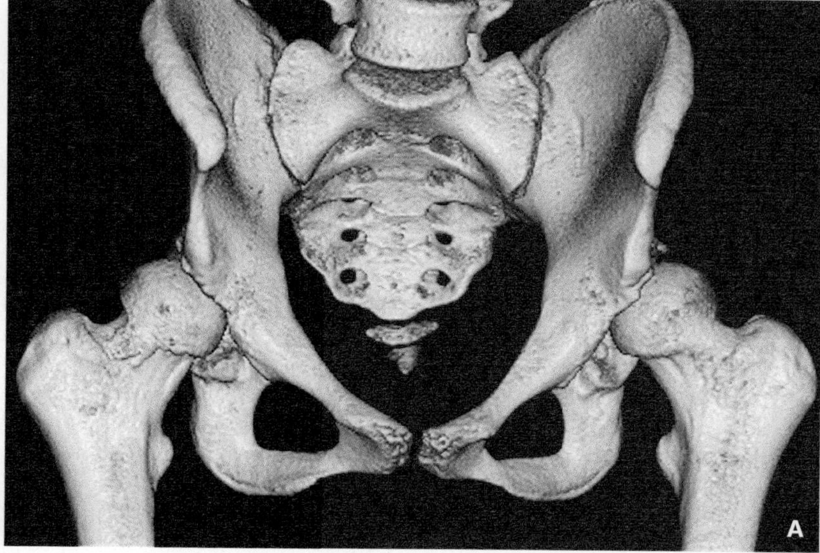

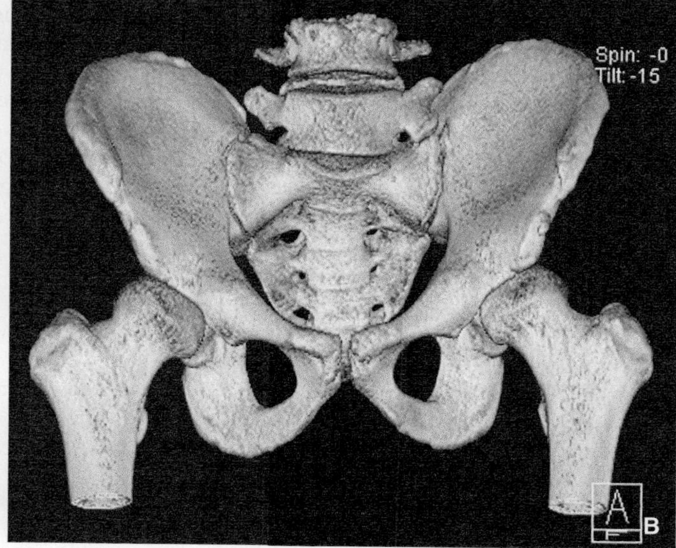

FIGURE 32.18 3D CT of congenital hip dysplasia. **(A)** 3D reconstructed CT image of the pelvis of a 15-year-old girl shows bilateral hip dysplasia associated with subluxation. **(B)** 3D reconstructed CT image of the pelvis of a 32-year-old man with congenital bilateral hip dysplasia shows undercoverage of the femoral heads by bony acetabula.

Ultrasound

Ultrasound has become one of the most effective techniques to diagnose and evaluate congenital hip dysplasia. It is performed with the patient at rest and during motion and stress. A lateral approach is widely used, with the infant supine or in the lateral decubitus position. Scanning is performed in the coronal plane with the hips extended or flexed (see Fig. 31.18). In the axial plane, the thighs are in 90 degrees of flexion, and images are obtained with and without stress. The osseous and cartilaginous components of the hip joint are well demonstrated on the displayed images, and acetabular coverage of the femoral head can be assessed. In addition, the slope of the acetabulum (α-angle) can be measured with respect to the iliac line. An angle of 60 degrees or more is normal. An angle 50 to 60 degrees is considered physiologic before age 3 months but needs to be followed up by repeat studies. Values less than 50 degrees are abnormal at any age. A second angle (β-angle) is formed by the iliac line and a line drawn from the labrum to the transition point between the iliac bone and the bony acetabulum. This measurement is indicative of the acetabular cartilaginous roof coverage and is secondary in significance to the α-angle. The smaller the β-angle, the less the cartilaginous coverage because of a better acetabular bony containment of the femoral head. The dynamic study, first described by Harcke in 1984, incorporates the use of real-time ultrasound visualization of the hip joint. The purpose of this technique is to demonstrate the instability. It is performed in the transverse flexion projection and consists of a Barlow maneuver to try to displace, sublux, or dislocate an apparently well-seated femoral head.

Three-dimensional (3D) sonographic evaluation of DDH has been attempted. This technique permits evaluation of the osseous and fibrocartilaginous acetabulum and its relationship to the femoral head in a global fashion (*gestalt*) without the need for detailed acetabular angle measurements. The information obtained can be stored for later review, analysis, and additional reconstructions with different parameters. The computer-generated sagittal plane image offers a unique view of the hip that is unobtainable with conventional sonography (Fig. 32.19). The generated spatial-revolving image likewise yields an informative craniocaudal (bird's eye) view of the infant hip (Fig. 32.20). The 3D appearance of the revolving image is enhanced by the transparency of the reconstruction, in contrast to the contour reconstructions available with 3D CT.

Magnetic Resonance Imaging

The role of magnetic resonance imaging (MRI) for evaluation of the developmental dysplasias of the hip has evolved. Although the various investigators do not recommend this technique for routine use, nevertheless, they point out the beneficial features of this modality such as qualitative information not available through radiography, particularly in the patients in whom the conservative treatment failed. Conversely, some authors suggest that MRI provides accurate anatomic information regarding the labrum, the ligamentum teres, the intraarticular fat pad (pulvinar), the transverse ligament, and the iliopsoas tendon. In addition, in some studies of the young adults, MRI studies demonstrated improved detection and characterization of DDH by providing morphologic information about acetabular deficiency. This technique also allowed evaluation of potential associated injuries to the articular cartilage, the labrum, and the ligamentum teres (Fig. 32.21).

Classification

Dunn has proposed a classification of CDH based primarily on the shape of the acetabular margins, the gross contour of the femoral head, and whether there is eversion or inversion of the limbus:

Type I: This is usually seen in neonates. The changes along the acetabular margins are mild. The femoral head, which is anteverted but spherically normal, is not completely covered by acetabular cartilage. This may lead to variable instability, particularly in extension and adduction of the hip. The labrum may also be deformed.

Type II: The hips are subluxed, and the cartilaginous labrum shows eversion. The femoral head is normally anteverted but shows a loss of sphericity. The acetabulum is shallower than in type I, and the failure of the acetabular roof to ossify laterally leads to an increased acetabular angle.

Type III: There is significant deformity of the acetabulum and femoral head, which is posterosuperiorly dislocated, leading to the formation of a false acetabulum by eversion of the labrum. The limbus is hypertrophied, and the ligamentum teres is elongated and pulled, bringing with it the transverse acetabular ligament. This situation compromises the acetabular space, precluding complete reduction.

In 1979, Crowe and colleagues proposed classification of congenital hip dislocation in the adults based on the extent of proximal migration of the femoral head. Grade I comprises those cases showing minimal abnormal development of the femoral head and acetabulum with less than 50% subluxation; grade II—those cases showing abnormal development of the acetabulum with 50% to 75% subluxation; grade III—when the acetabulum is developed without a roof and there is full dislocation in the hip joint (75% to 100%), with false acetabulum developing at the site of dislocated femoral head; and grade IV—when the femur is positioned high on the pelvis (high hip dislocation, 100% dislocation).

Treatment

The principle behind conservative treatment is to reduce the dislocation of the femoral head, by means of a flexion–abduction maneuver, for a period sufficient enough to permit proper growth of the head and acetabulum, which in turn ensures a congruent and stable hip joint. This approach is usually taken in the very early stages of CDH and in infants younger than age 2 years; it includes splinting, such as with the Frejka splint or Pavlik harness, as well as various traction procedures (Fig. 32.22). Colonna or buck skin traction is usually used in children 2 months to 12 years of age, with a well-padded spica cast applied simultaneously to the unaffected side. Interval radiographs are obtained to monitor the progress of the traction and the descent of the femoral head. A system for this purpose, composed of various traction "stations," has been described by Gage and Winter (Fig. 32.23). It has been reported that the achievement of "station +2" by means of skeletal traction, before further treatment by open or closed reduction, is associated with a far smaller frequency of osteonecrosis of the femoral head.

When the conservative approach fails, the child is too old for conservative treatment, or the abnormalities are too extensive, then surgical management is indicated. Imaging assessment of the hip, in which CT examination plays the leading role, is mandatory before surgical intervention because it provides the surgeon with excellent images of the anatomy of the hip, particularly the size of the femoral head, its relation to the acetabulum, and the acetabular configuration. The information regarding these structures may contraindicate the use of certain surgical procedures.

Several surgical techniques are now used for treatment of congenital hip dysplasia. Their common goal is to achieve better coverage of the femoral head. These surgical procedures can be divided into four categories: shelf operations, in which bone grafts are used to extend the acetabular roof; acetabuloplasties, in which the acetabular roof is mobilized and turned down; pelvic osteotomies, in which the acetabulum is redirected; and pelvic displacement osteotomies, in which the femoral head is positioned beneath the displaced bony portion of the pelvis. *Capsulorrhaphy* consists of removal of the excess of the stretched joint capsule, combined with a femoroplasty and/or acetabuloplasty. *Femoral varus derotational osteotomy* is performed to correct an excessive anteversion of the neck and valgus deformity. It involves a varus angulation of the proximal femur, with or without rotation, to redirect the femoral head into the acetabulum (Fig. 32.24). The most popular procedure is the *Salter osteotomy* of the innominate bone, which may be combined with simultaneous derotational varus osteotomy of the femoral neck. It is usually performed in children aged 1 to 6 years. The principle of this technique is to redirect the abnormal orientation of the acetabulum, which in children with CDH faces more anterolaterally, thus rendering the hip stable only in abduction, flexion, and internal rotation. This redirection is accomplished by displacing the entire acetabulum anterolaterally and downward, without changing its shape or capacity, by means of a triangular bone graft (Fig. 32.25). *Pemberton osteotomy* is an incomplete transiliac osteotomy, hinging the anterolateral acetabular roof on the flexible triradiate cartilage. This procedure is indicated when there is an elongated, dysplastic acetabulum; however, it should be performed only in children younger than age 7 years when there is flexibility

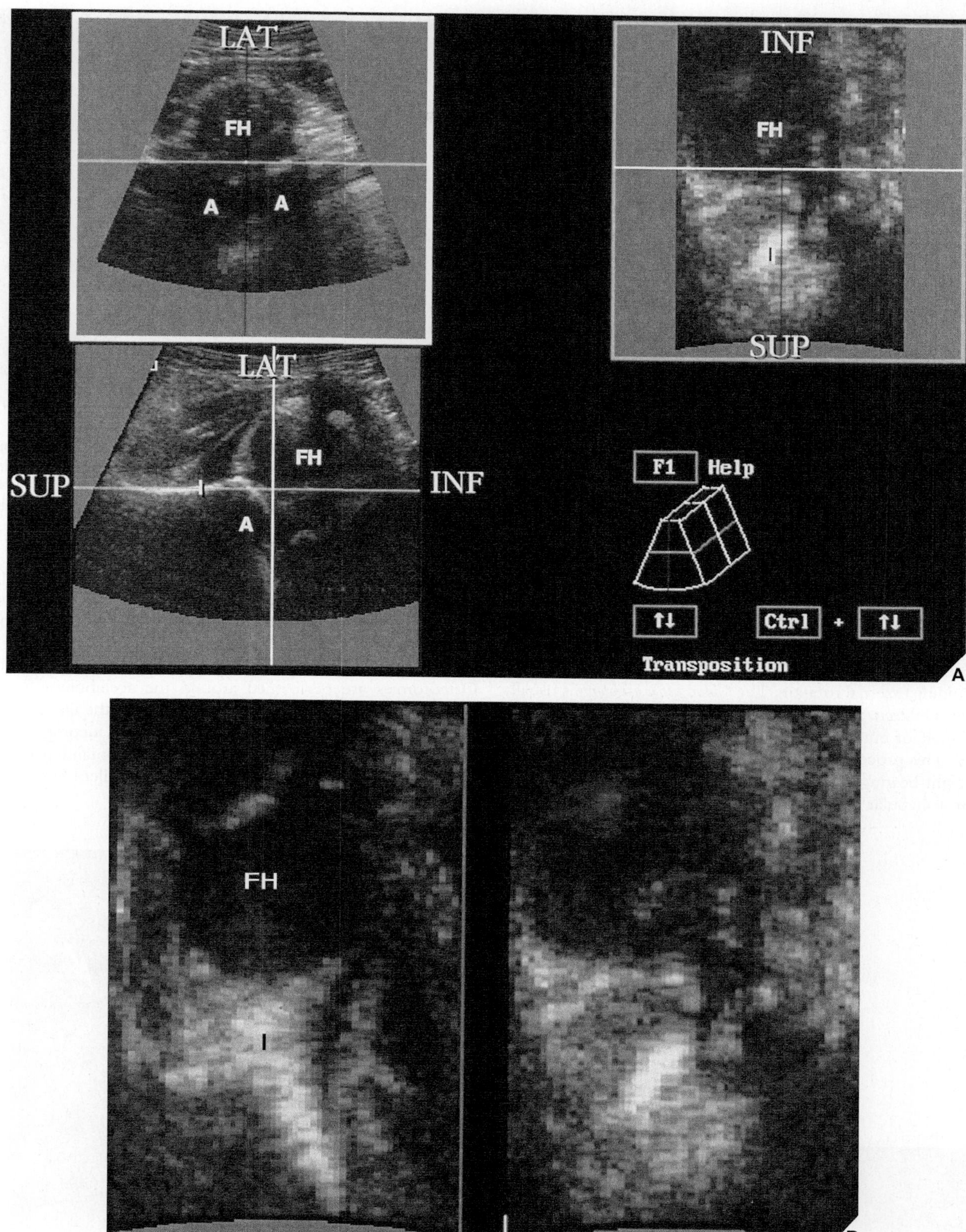

FIGURE 32.19 Ultrasound of congenital hip dysplasia. (A) On the coronal 3D ultrasound image of the left hip in a 3-day-old girl **(lower left)**, the acetabulum *(A)* appears shallow, and subluxation of the femoral head *(FH)* can be observed at the intersection of the ilium *(I)* line with the medial third of the FH. On the reconstructed axial image **(upper left)**, the FH is subluxated but still in contact with the A. On the sagittal image **(upper right)**, only the peripheral segment of FH is visualized. **(B)** A sagittal image of a normal left hip **(left)** is shown for comparison. Note that FH is centered over the I line. A sagittal image of a subluxated head **(right)** clearly shows distortion of FH–I line relationship. *LAT*, lateral; *INF*, inferior; *SUP*, superior. (Reprinted from Gerscovich EO, Greenspan A, Cronan MS, et al. Three-dimensional sonographic evaluation of developmental dysplasia of the hip: preliminary findings. *Radiology* 1994;190:407–410. Copyright © 1994 by The Radiological Society of North America, Inc.)

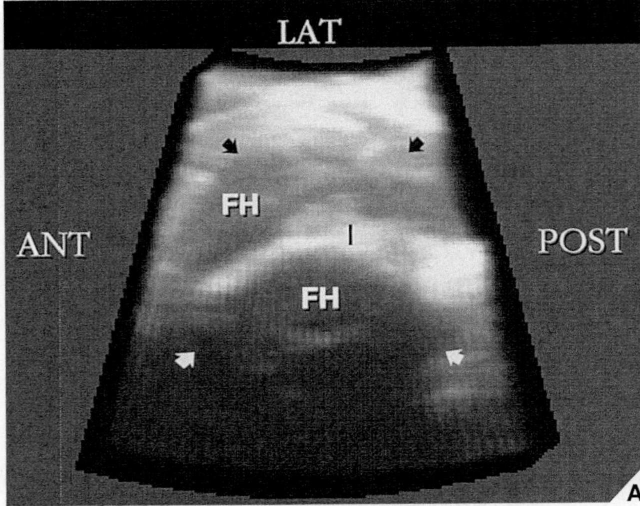

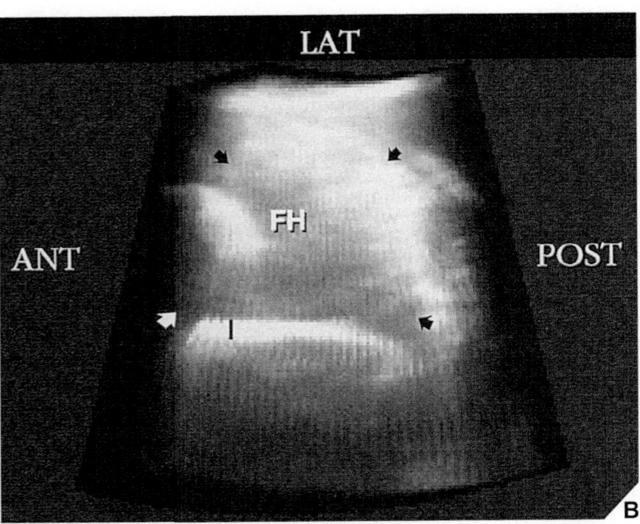

FIGURE 32.20 3D ultrasound of congenital hip dysplasia. **(A)** Craniocaudal projection (bird's eye view) of a normal left hip shows the ilium *(I)* projecting over the midportion of the femoral head *(FH)* (*arrows* outline its contour). **(B)** Craniocaudal projection of a subluxated left hip shows that the I projects over the medial portion of the FH (*arrows* outline its contour). The FH is laterally displaced. *LAT*, lateral; *ANT*, anterior; *POST*, posterior. (Reprinted from Gerscovich EO, Greenspan A, Cronan MS, et al. Three-dimensional sonographic evaluation of developmental dysplasia of the hip: preliminary findings. *Radiology* 1994;190:407–410. Copyright © 1994 by The Radiological Society of North America, Inc.)

in the triradiate cartilage and when growth remains for remodeling of the joint surfaces. *Steele triple innominate osteotomy* is usually indicated for children older than age 6 to 8 years who have an immobile symphysis pubis. In addition to Salter osteotomy, osteotomies of the inferior and superior pubic rami are performed. The acetabulum is brought forward and rotated in the frontal plane, avoiding external rotation. The *Chiari pelvic osteotomy* is usually reserved for older children. This is a displacement osteotomy that essentially provides a shelf or buttress to limit further proximal subluxation of the femoral head. This procedure displaces the femoral head medially and increases the weight-bearing surface of the head by producing an overhanging superior acetabular ledge. This technique may also be combined with a varus derotational osteotomy of the femoral neck. *Ganz osteotomy*, also known as *Bernese periacetabular osteotomy*, is usually performed in older children and adolescents and occasionally in adults. The principle behind the procedure is to allow anterior and lateral rotation and medialization of the hip without violation of the posterior column of the hemipelvis. Osteotomies are performed around the acetabulum (complete osteotomy of the pubis and biplanar osteotomy of the ilium); however, the cut through the posterior column of the ischium is incomplete. The acetabular fragment is rotated anteriorly and laterally (maintaining anteversion) and is then medialized. This procedure provides excellent femoral head coverage and acetabular mobility.

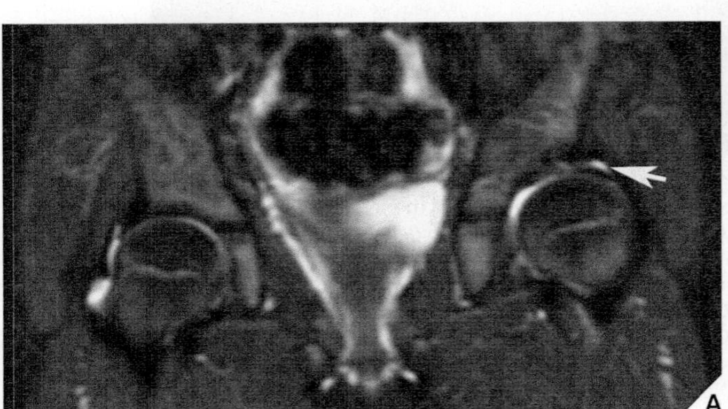

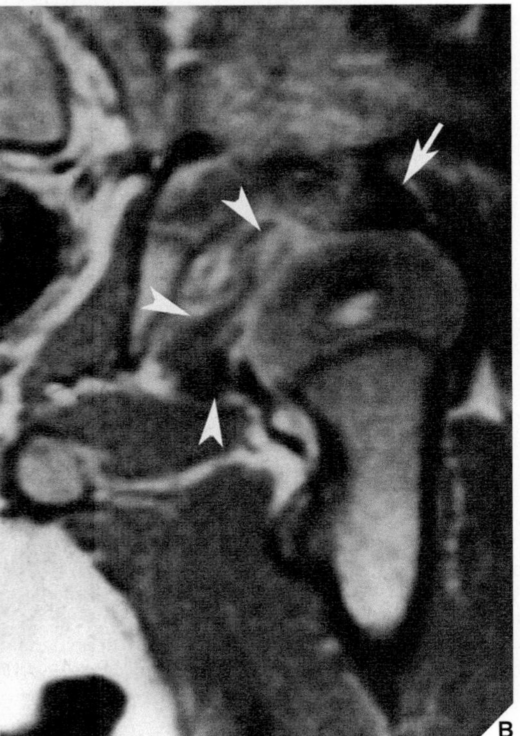

FIGURE 32.21 MRI of congenital hip dysplasia. **(A)** Coronal T2-weighted MRI of a 5-year-old boy with left DDH demonstrates a shallow left acetabulum, uncoverage of the femoral head, and a superiorly rotated and torn labrum *(arrow)*. **(B)** Coronal T1-weighted MRI of a 5-month-old boy with left DDH demonstrates lateral subluxation and uncoverage of the femoral head, a dysplastic and shallow acetabulum, an everted and hypertrophied labrum *(arrow)*, and hypertrophy of the pulvinar and transverse ligament *(arrowheads)*.

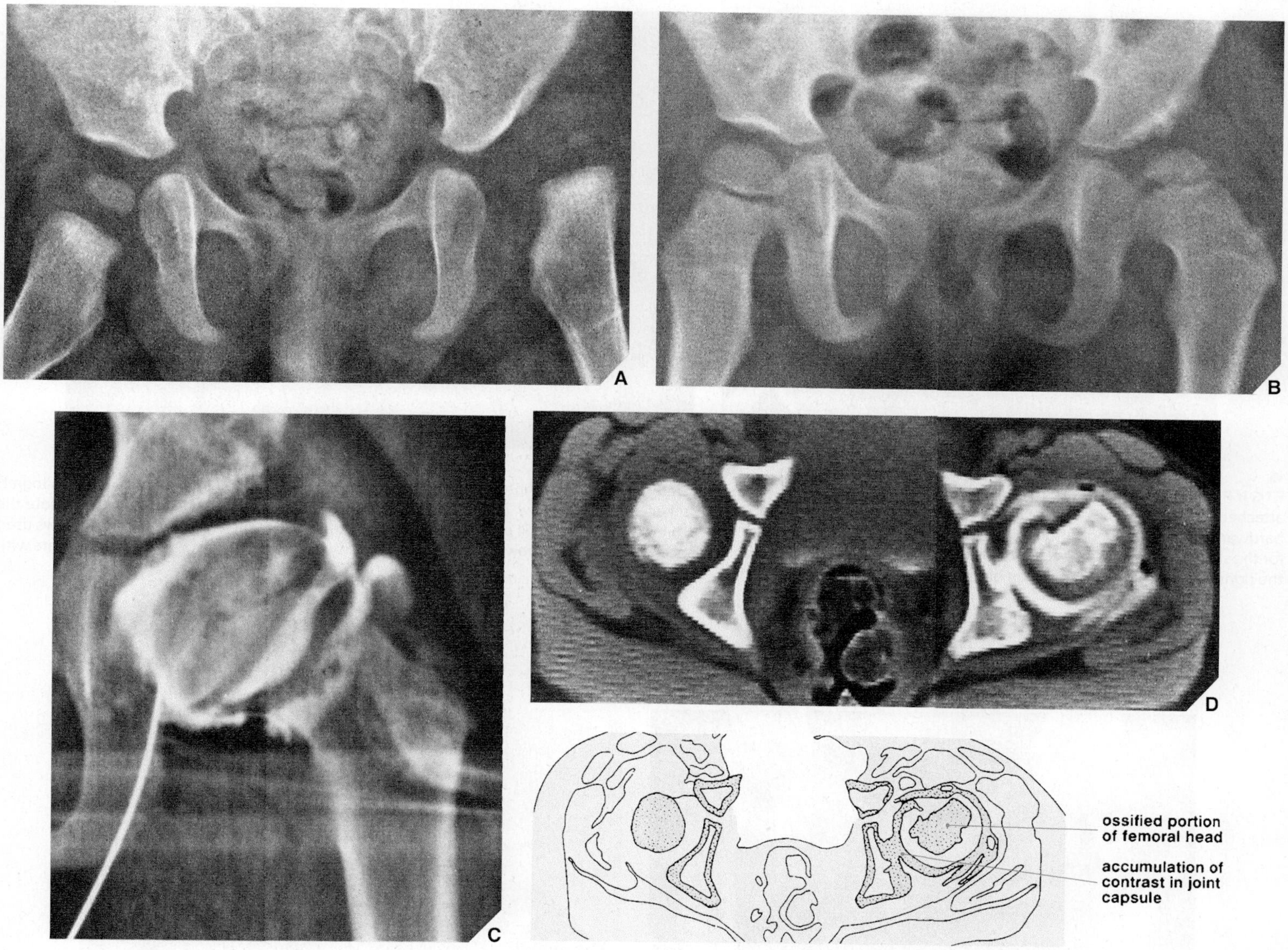

A

B

C

D

ossified portion of femoral head

accumulation of contrast in joint capsule

FIGURE 32.22 **Treatment of congenital hip dysplasia.** **(A)** Anteroposterior radiograph of the pelvis in a 1-year-old boy demonstrates the typical appearance of congenital dislocation of the left hip. **(B)** After conservative treatment with a Pavlik harness at age 2 years, there is still subluxation. Note the broken Shenton-Menard arc. At age 3 years, after further conservative treatment by skin traction and application of a spica cast, there is almost complete reduction of subluxation, as demonstrated by contrast arthrography **(C)**. **(D)** CT scan, however, demonstrates some minimal residual lateral displacement of the femoral head, as evidenced by the medial accumulation of contrast.

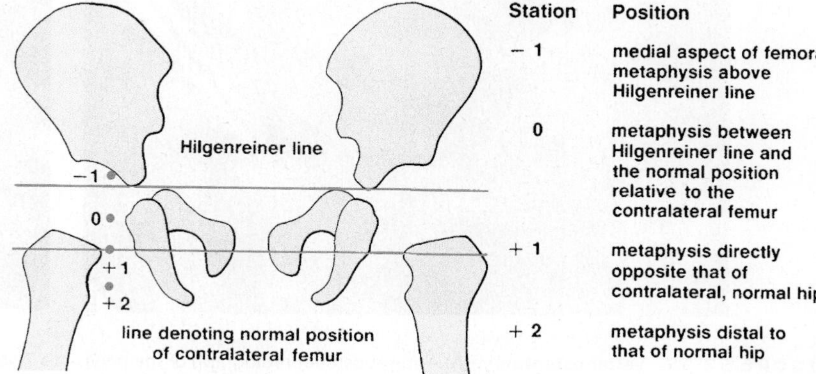

FIGURE 32.23 **The Gage and Winter system.** This measurement of stations for monitoring the progress of treatment by traction and the descent of the femoral head is based on the position of the proximal femoral metaphysis relative to the ipsilateral acetabulum and the contralateral normal hip.

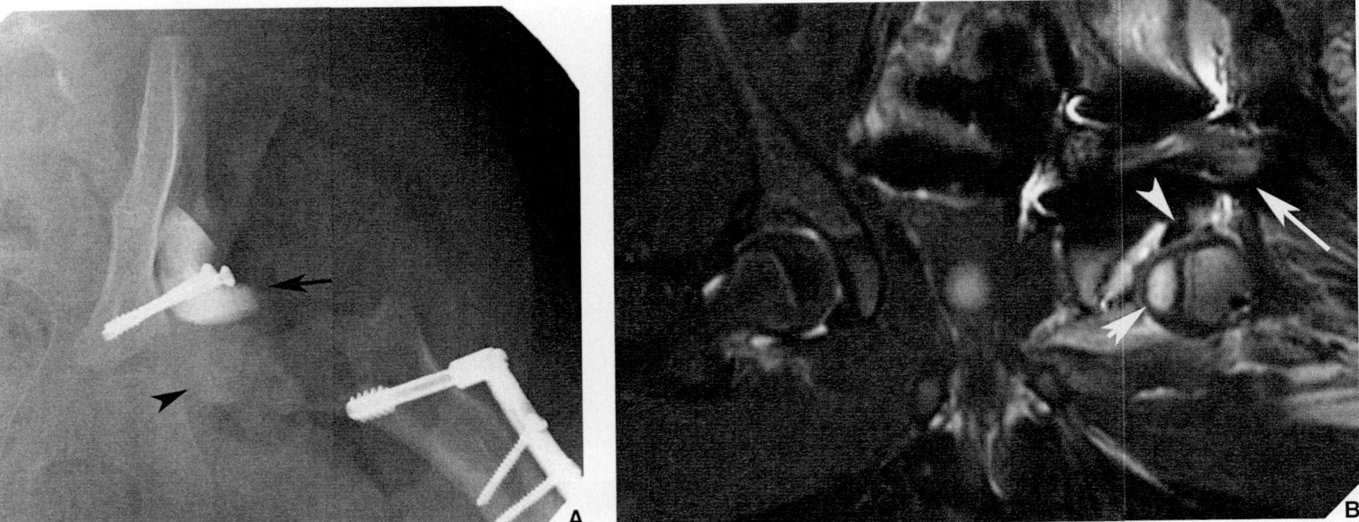

FIGURE 32.24 **Femoral varus derotational osteotomy and acetabular shelf procedure.** **(A)** Anteroposterior radiograph of the left hip demonstrates a bone allograft attached with two metallic screws in the superior lateral aspect of a dysplastic left acetabulum *(arrow)*, providing good coverage of the femoral head *(arrowhead)*. Note the hardware of the varus derotational osteotomy in the proximal left femur. **(B)** Coronal T2-weighted MRI of the same patient demonstrates the artifact due to the screws used for the shelf operation *(long arrow)*. The humeral head is still separated from the acetabulum *(short arrow)* due to the presence of infolded labrum *(arrowhead)*. Compare with the right side for the normal position of the femoral head within the acetabulum.

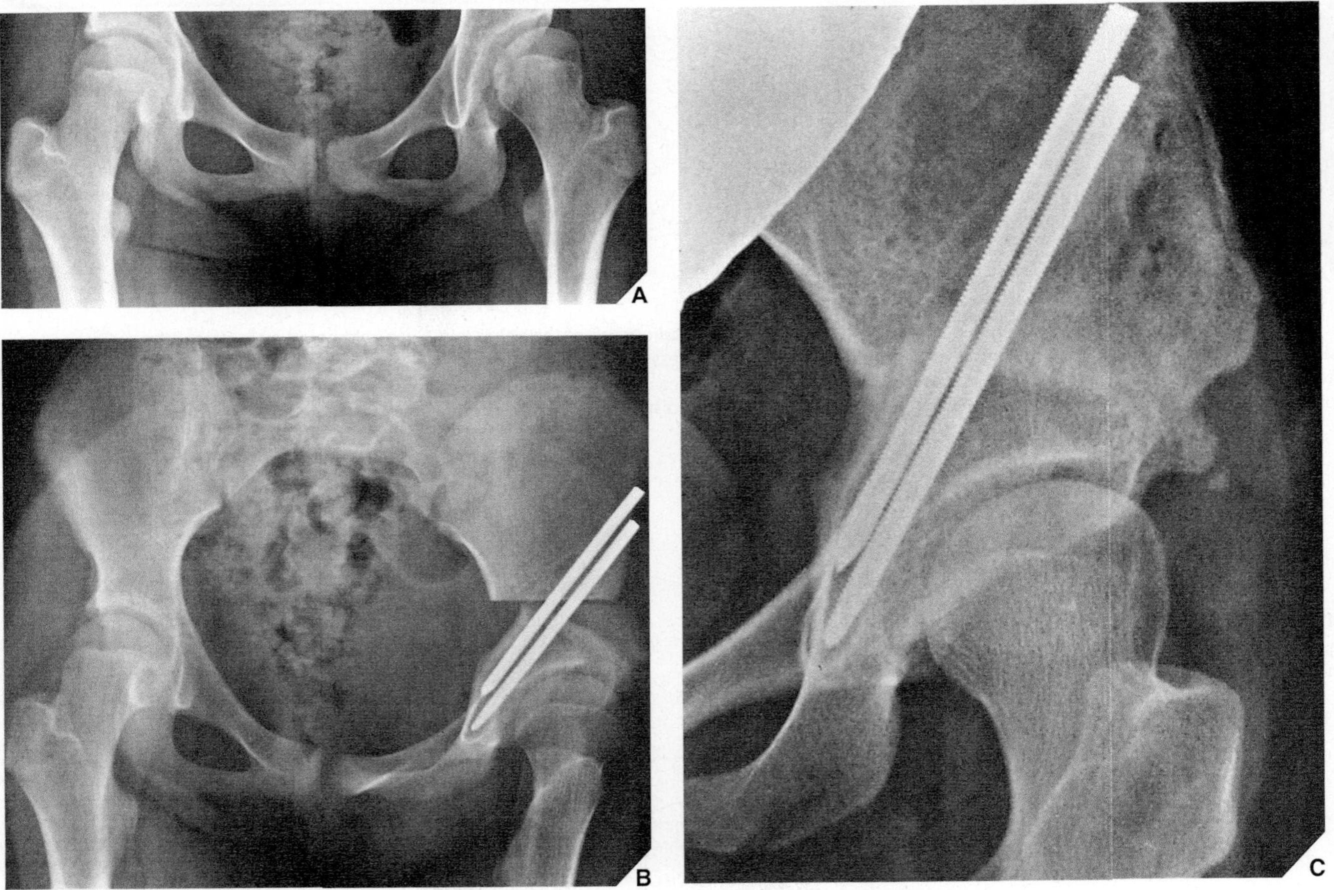

FIGURE 32.25 **Salter osteotomy.** **(A)** Anteroposterior radiograph of the pelvis in a 7-year-old girl with CDH shows persistent superolateral subluxation of the left hip following conservative treatment. Note the anterolateral orientation of the acetabulum in comparison with the normal right hip. **(B)** Postoperative radiograph after Salter osteotomy through the supraacetabular portion of the iliac bone shows the acetabulum displaced anterolaterally and downward; a triangular bone graft, taken from the anterolateral aspect of the ilium, is secured by two Steinmann pins at the site of the osteotomy. **(C)** Four years later, the femoral head is completely covered by the acetabulum. Because of a valgus configuration of the femoral neck, the patient may yet require a varus derotational osteotomy.

Complications

Conservative and surgical management of CDH may be complicated by osteonecrosis of the femoral head, redislocation, infection, sciatic nerve injury, or early fusion of the growth plate caused by prolonged casting. The most frequent late complication of untreated and treated CDH is degenerative joint disease.

Proximal Femoral Focal Deficiency

Proximal femoral focal deficiency (PFFD) is a congenital anomaly characterized by dysgenesis and hypoplasia of variable segments of the proximal femur. The defect ranges in severity from femoral shortening associated with a varus deformity of the neck to the formation of only a small stub of distal femur.

Classification and Imaging Features

Several classifications of PFFD have been proposed. The one offered by Levinson and colleagues, which is based on the severity of the abnormalities involving the femoral head, femoral segment, and acetabulum, is the most practical from the prognostic point of view:

Type A: The femoral head is present, and the femoral segment is short. There is a varus deformity of the femoral neck. The acetabulum is normal.

Type B: The femoral head is present, but there is an absence of bony connection between it and the short femoral segment. The acetabulum exhibits dysplastic changes.

Type C: The femoral head is absent or represented only by an ossicle. The femoral segment is short and tapered proximally. The acetabulum is severely dysplastic.

Type D: The femoral head and acetabulum are absent. The femoral segment is rudimentary, and the obturator foramen is enlarged.

Conventional radiography is usually sufficient to make a diagnosis of PFFD. The femur is short, and the proximal segment is displaced superior, posterior, and lateral to the iliac crest; ossification of the femoral epiphysis is invariably delayed (Fig. 32.26). Arthrography is useful in the evaluation of this anomaly, particularly in its classification, because early in infancy, the nonossified femoral head and acetabulum can be outlined adequately with a positive contrast agent (Fig. 32.26C). This technique is also helpful in distinguishing PFFD from the occasionally similar presentations of CDH. In severe cases of PFFD, MRI may be useful to establish the presence or absence of cartilaginous bridge between the proximal and distal femoral segments (Fig. 32.27).

Treatment

Several surgical procedures are used to correct this anomaly, including amputation. One limb-sparing procedure involves conversion of the knee to a hip joint by flexing it 90 degrees and fusing the femur to the pelvis. Another technique, developed by Borggreve in 1930 and called the *turn-about procedure* or *rotation-plasty* after an improvement by Van Nes, converts the foot into the knee joint; the limb is then fitted with a leg prosthesis.

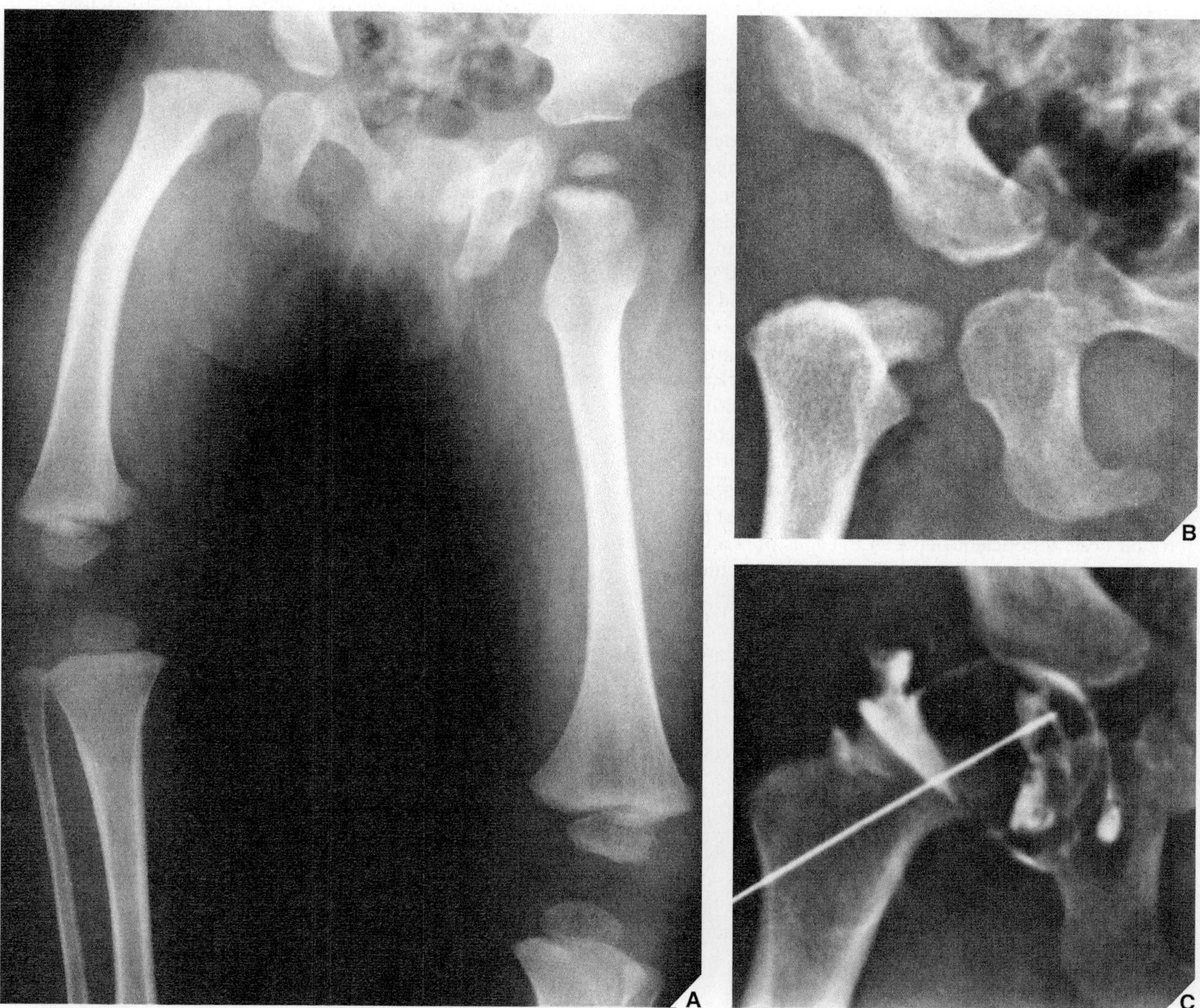

FIGURE 32.26 Proximal femoral focal deficiency. (A) Anteroposterior radiograph in an 18-month-old boy who had a short right leg demonstrates a varus configuration at the right hip joint, the absence of an ossification center for the proximal femoral epiphysis and shortening of the femur—the classic radiographic features of PFFD. **(B)** A coned-down view of the right hip shows superior, posterior, and lateral displacement of the proximal femoral segment in relation to the acetabulum. **(C)** Arthrography was performed to classify the abnormality, and the presence of the femoral head in the acetabulum and the absence of any defect in the femoral neck were found, making this a type A focal deficiency.

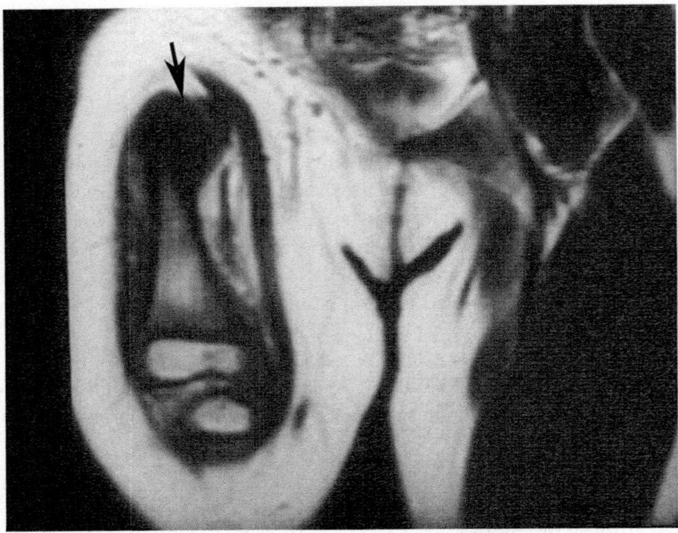

FIGURE 32.27 **MRI of proximal focal femoral deficiency.** Coronal T1-weighted MR image of the right femur of a young girl with PFFD demonstrates absent proximal right femoral shaft terminating in a blunted chondral surface *(arrow)*, which was not bridging with the hypoplastic proximal femoral head and neck (not shown).

Legg-Calvé-Perthes Disease

Legg-Calvé-Perthes disease, also known as *coxa plana*, is the name applied to osteonecrosis (ischemic necrosis) of the proximal epiphysis of the femur. Recent genetic studies suggest that beta fibrinogen gene *G-455-A* polymorphism is a risk factor for this condition. The anomaly occurs 5 times more often in boys than in girls, usually between the ages of 4 and 8 years. Its appearance at an early age is usually associated with a better prognosis. Either hip can be affected, and bilateral involvement, which is successive rather than simultaneous, is seen in approximately 10% of cases (Fig. 32.28). The clinical symptoms consist of pain, limping, and limitation of motion. Not infrequently, the pain is localized not to the involved hip but to the ipsilateral knee. It is a self-limiting disorder that eventually heals, but because of the progressive deformity it produces in the shape of the femoral head and neck, it often leads to precocious osteoarthritis of the hip joint. The cause of this anomaly has been the subject of debate. Some investigators consider it a type of idiopathic osteonecrosis, but trauma or repeated microtrauma may play a role in compromising the circulation of blood to the femoral capital epiphysis. Trueta has suggested that the blood supply to the femoral head is deficient between the ages of 4 and 8 years and that this might be a factor in the development of the condition.

Imaging Features

Radiologic examination is essential for diagnosing Legg-Calvé-Perthes disease and for identifying its prognostic signs. Conventional radiography is adequate for evaluating most of the features of the disease (see Fig. 32.28), whereas arthrography helps in the assessment of acetabular congruity, the thickness of the articular cartilage, and the degree of subluxation (Fig. 32.29). The earliest indication of Legg-Calvé-Perthes disease is demonstrated on radionuclide bone scan by a decreased uptake of tracer in the hips caused by a deficient blood supply. However, with progression of the disease, an increased uptake is seen, which reflects reparative processes.

The earliest radiographic sign of Legg-Calvé-Perthes disease is periarticular osteoporosis and periarticular soft-tissue swelling, with distortion of the pericapsular and iliopsoas fat planes. There may also be a discrepancy in the size of the ossification centers of the capital epiphyses. Later, lateral displacement of the affected ossification center produces widening of the medial aspect of the joint, the presence of the crescent sign (which at times may be detected only on the frog-lateral projection of the hip) (Fig. 32.30), or of radiolucent fissures in the epiphysis, indicates progression of the disease. At a more advanced stage, flattening and sclerosis of the capital epiphysis become apparent and are associated with an increased density of the femoral head secondary to necrosis of the bone, microfractures, and reparative changes known as *creeping substitution*. A vacuum phenomenon may occasionally be seen, caused by nitrogen gas released into the fissures in the capital epiphysis. Cystic changes may also be encountered in the metaphyseal segment. Later, there may be broadening of the femoral neck. Throughout the course of the disease, the joint space is remarkably well preserved because the articular cartilage is not affected. Only in the end stage of Legg-Calvé-Perthes disease, when secondary osteoarthritis develops, does the joint become compromised as in primary degenerative joint disease.

One of the radiographic features of advanced Legg-Calvé-Perthes disease is the so-called *sagging rope sign*. It consists of a thin, curved, U-shaped opaque line in the proximal femoral metaphysis, extending laterally from the inferior border of the femoral neck (Fig. 32.31).

The Moss technique is used to determine the degree of deformity of the femoral head. This consists of overlaying the anteroposterior radiograph of the hip with a template having concentric circles spaced 2 mm apart. If the concentricity of the femoral head deviates by more than two of the 2-mm circles, then the result is rated "poor"; deviation equal to one 2-mm circle is "fair," and no deviation is rated "good." Lateral subluxation can be measured by means of the C-E angle of Wiberg (see Fig. 32.12). It must be stressed that both measurements do not correlate well with development of secondary osteoarthritis, the main complication of Legg-Calvé-Perthes disease.

Several investigators have stressed the applicability of MRI for early detection of Legg-Calvé-Perthes disease and for evaluation of cartilaginous

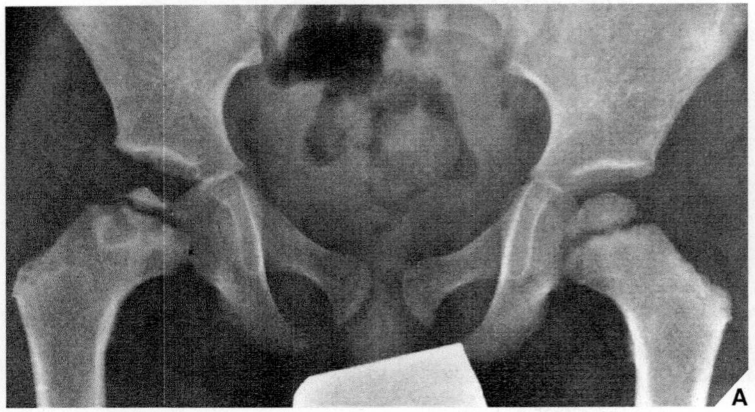

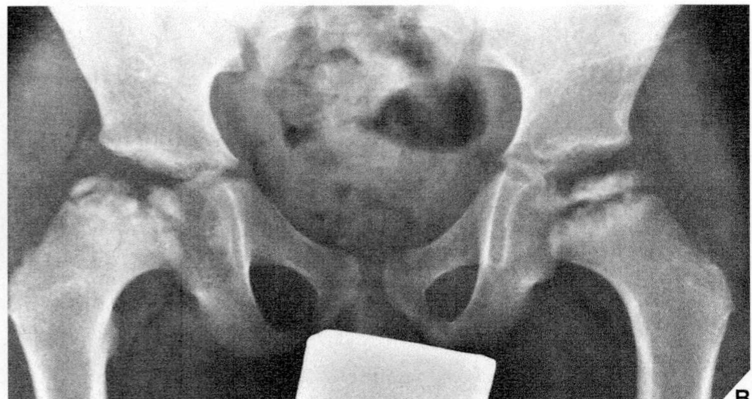

FIGURE 32.28 **Legg-Calvé-Perthes disease.** A 5-year-old boy presented with pain in the right hip for several months. **(A)** Anteroposterior radiograph of the pelvis and hips shows advanced stage of this condition affecting the right hip, where osteonecrosis and collapse of the capital femoral epiphysis are apparent, as are extensive changes in the metaphysis. Note the lateral subluxation in the hip joint. The left hip is normal. **(B)** Three years later, the left hip also became involved. Note the progression of osteonecrotic changes in the right femoral epiphysis.

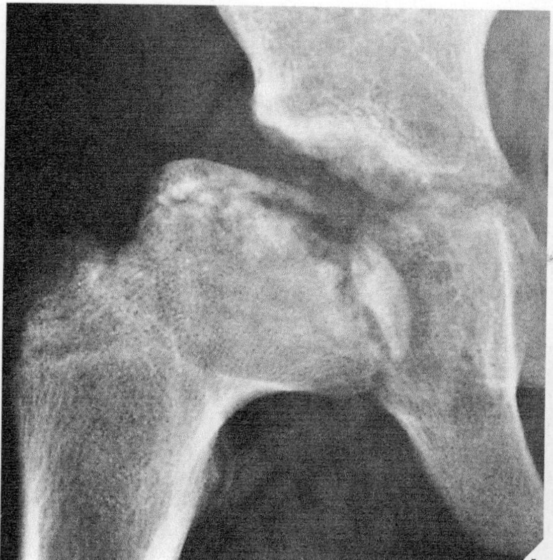

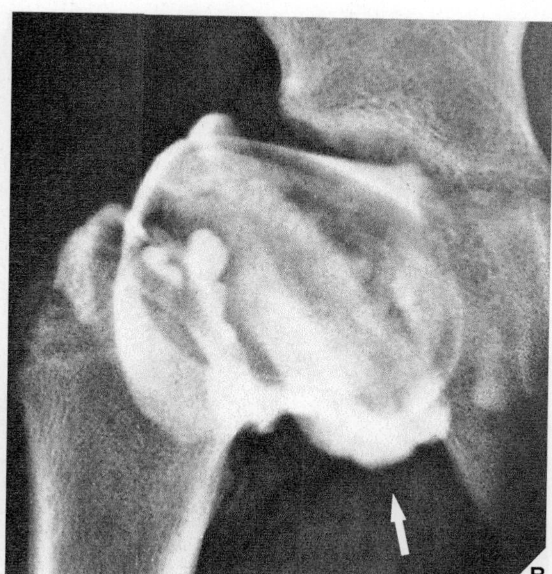

FIGURE 32.29 Arthrogram of Legg-Calvé-Perthes disease. A 6-year-old boy presented with progressive pain in the right hip joint and a limp for the previous 8 months. **(A)** Anteroposterior radiograph shows a dense, flattened, and deformed femoral epiphysis, with subchondral collapse and fragmentation, diffuse metaphyseal changes, broadening of the femoral neck, and lateral subluxation. **(B)** Contrast arthrogram demonstrates flattening of the articular cartilage at the lateral aspect of the femoral head and a relatively smooth contour of the cartilage at the anteromedial aspect. The pulling of the contrast medially *(arrow)* indicates lateral subluxation.

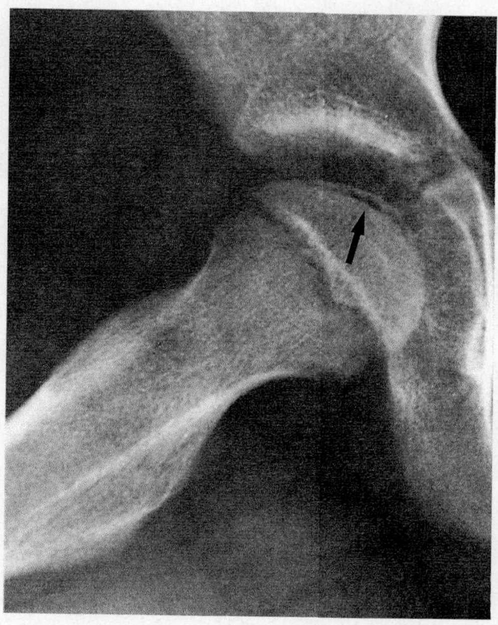

FIGURE 32.30 Legg-Calvé-Perthes disease. Frog-lateral view of the right hip of a 7-year-old girl shows the crescent sign *(arrow)*, one of the earliest radiographic features of osteonecrosis.

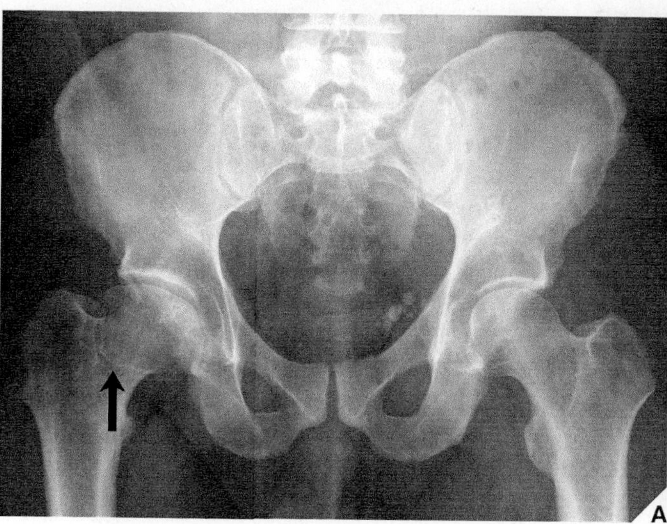

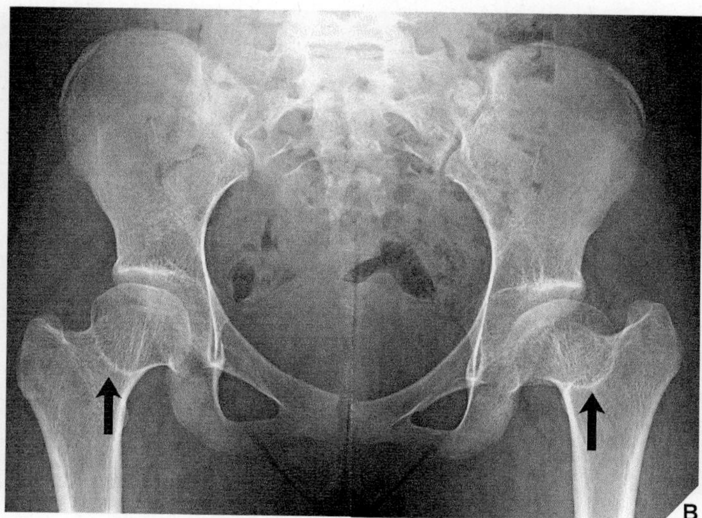

FIGURE 32.31 Legg-Calvé-Perthes disease. **(A)** Anteroposterior radiograph of the pelvis of a 30-year-old man shows enlargement of the right femoral head (coxa magna), flattening of the articular aspect, and deformity, consistent with osteonecrosis. The *arrow* points to the sagging rope sign. **(B)** Anteroposterior radiograph of the pelvis of a 17-year-old girl shows late stage of bilateral osteonecrosis of the femoral heads. Note bilateral sagging rope sign *(arrows)* characteristic of this condition.

and synovial changes. This technique has also proved valuable for determination of the cartilaginous shape of the femoral head. MRI allows preoperative and postoperative assessment of containment of the femoral head and enables its medial aspect to be visualized. The advantages of MRI over arthrography are noninvasiveness, the ability to obtain images in several imaging planes (i.e., axial, coronal, and sagittal), and lack of exposure to the side effects of radiation and injection of intraarticular contrast (Figs. 32.32 and 32.33).

Classification

Several classification systems and prognostic indicators have been developed for the evaluation of Legg-Calvé-Perthes disease. Waldenström proposed a three-stage system based on the progression of the osteonecrotic process. The first stage is marked by changes in the blood supply to the femoral epiphysis, with secondary alteration in the shape and density of the femoral head. In the second stage, revascularization takes place, and necrotic bone is replaced by new bone (creeping substitution). The third

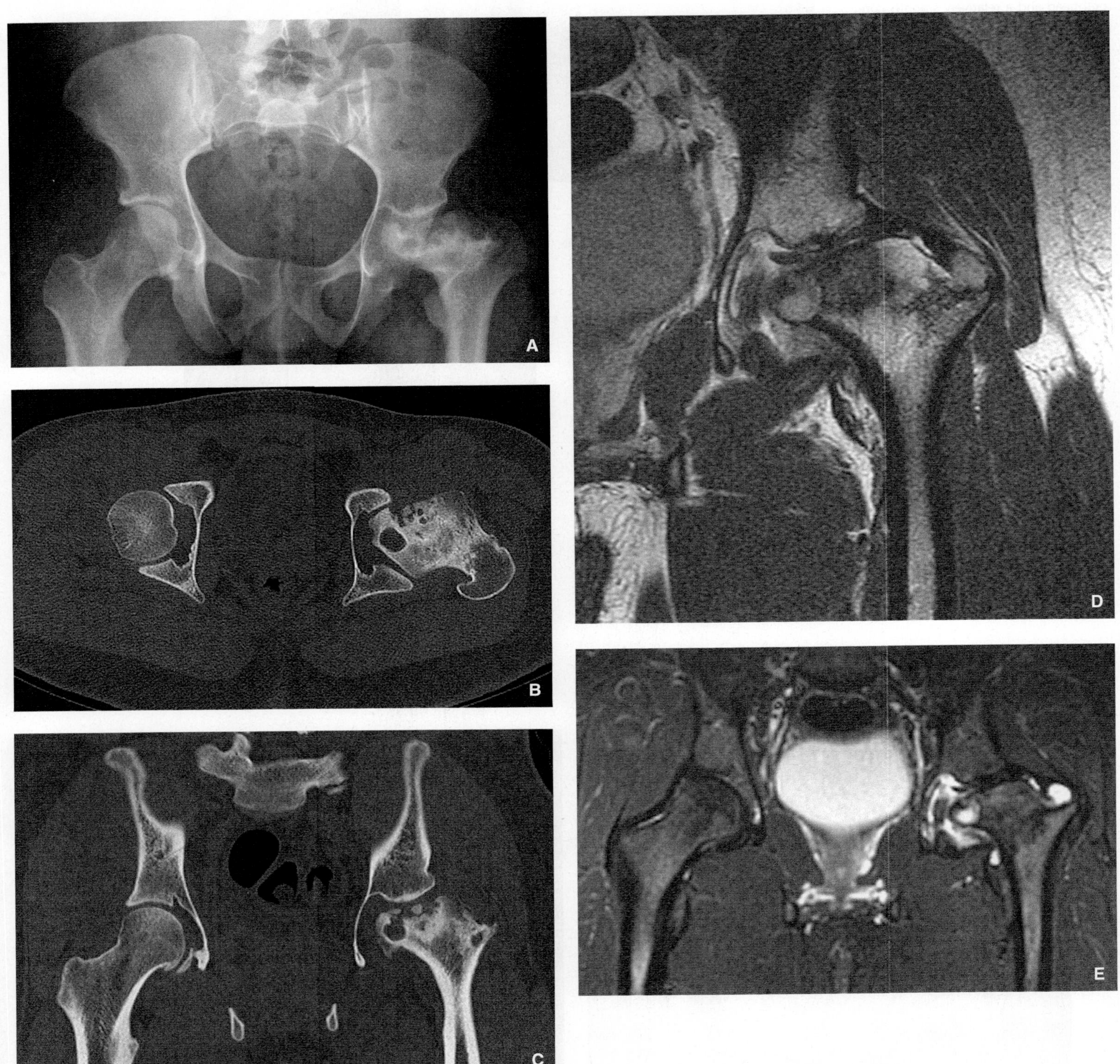

FIGURE 32.32 **CT and MRI of Legg-Calvé-Perthes disease.** **(A)** Anteroposterior radiograph of the pelvis of a 19-year-old man shows typical changes of this condition affecting the left hip. **(B)** Axial and **(C)** coronal reformatted CT images of the pelvis show osteonecrosis of the markedly deformed left femoral head with bone fragmentation. **(D)** Coronal proton density–weighted MR image of the left hip shows deformity and osteonecrosis of the femoral head associated with lateral subluxation and deformity of the acetabulum. **(E)** Short time inversion recovery (STIR) MR image of the pelvis shows in addition left hip joint effusion.

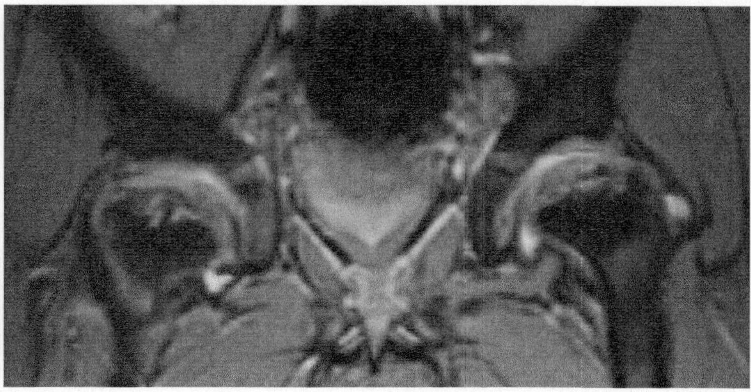

FIGURE 32.33 MRI of Legg-Calvé-Perthes disease. Coronal gradient recalled echo (GRE) MRI demonstrates bilateral involvement with flattening and fragmentation of the proximal femoral epiphysis and irregular growth plates.

stage represents a healing phase of the disease in which reconstruction of the femoral epiphysis may result either in congruency of the joint or in incongruency because of deformity of the femoral head (coxa magna), with a predisposition to degenerative changes.

The Catterall classification, which has better prognostic value, divides this anomaly into four groups based on radiographic findings:

Group 1: The anterior portion of the epiphysis is involved; there is no evidence of subarticular collapse or fragmentation of the femoral head. The prognosis is good, and patients do well even without treatment, particularly those younger than age 8 years.

Group 2: The anterior portion of the epiphysis is more severely affected, but the medial and lateral segments are still preserved (Fig. 32.34). Small cystic changes may be seen in the metaphysis. The prognosis is worse than that of patients in group 1, but healing may occur, particularly in children younger than 5 years.

Group 3: The entire epiphysis appears dense, yielding a "head-within-a-head" phenomenon. The changes are more generalized, and the neck becomes widened. The prognosis is poor, and more than 70% of patients require surgical intervention.

Group 4: There is marked flattening and "mushrooming" of the femoral head, eventually leading to its complete collapse; the metaphyseal changes are extensive (Fig. 32.35). The prognosis is much worse than in the previous groups.

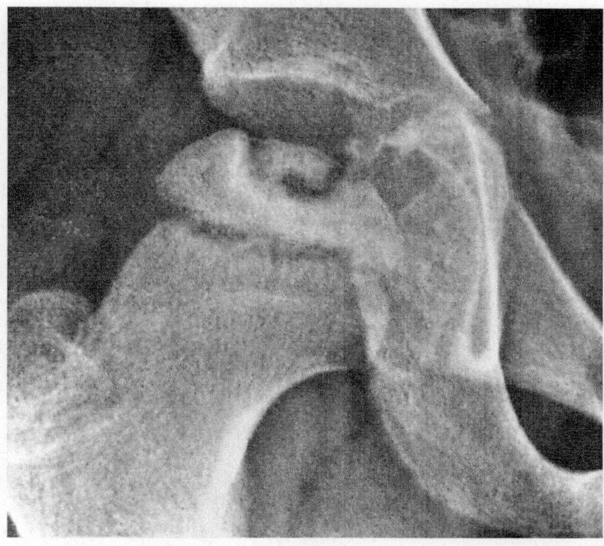

FIGURE 32.34 Legg-Calvé-Perthes disease. Anteroposterior radiograph of the right hip of a 9-year-old boy demonstrates a more advanced stage of disease (Catterall group 2). Note the central defect in the femoral head, with preservation of the lateral and medial buttresses.

Subsequently, Catterall improved this classification by introducing four "head-at-risk" signs that signify a poor prognosis; these features can be demonstrated on an anteroposterior projection of the hip joint:

1. Gage sign—a radiolucent, V-shaped osteoporotic segment in the lateral portion of the femoral head (Fig. 32.36)
2. Calcification lateral to the epiphysis, representing extruded cartilage and indicating pressure on the head from the lateral edge of the acetabulum (see Fig. 32.35)
3. Lateral subluxation of the femoral head (see Figs. 32.29A and 32.35)
4. Horizontal inclination of the growth plate, indicating physeal growth closure (see Fig. 32.28B)
5. Murphy and Marsh added a fifth sign to this group of indicators—diffuse metaphyseal changes (see Fig. 32.29A)

Patients in any of the four groups who have two or more "head-at-risk" signs have a significantly worsened prognosis. Moreover, the prognosis is poor when the disease is in a late stage at the time of diagnosis and when the patient is older than age 6 years.

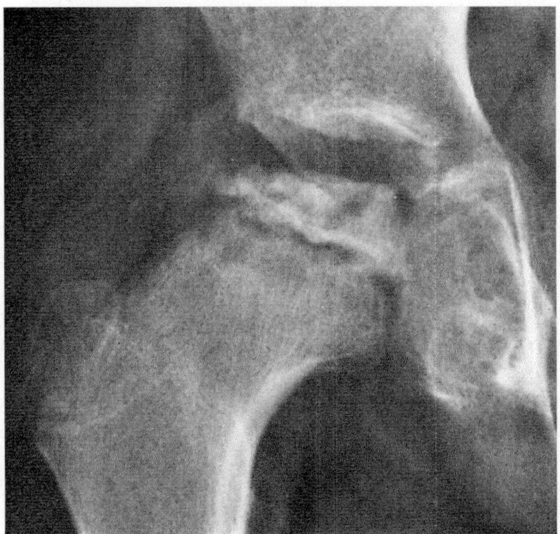

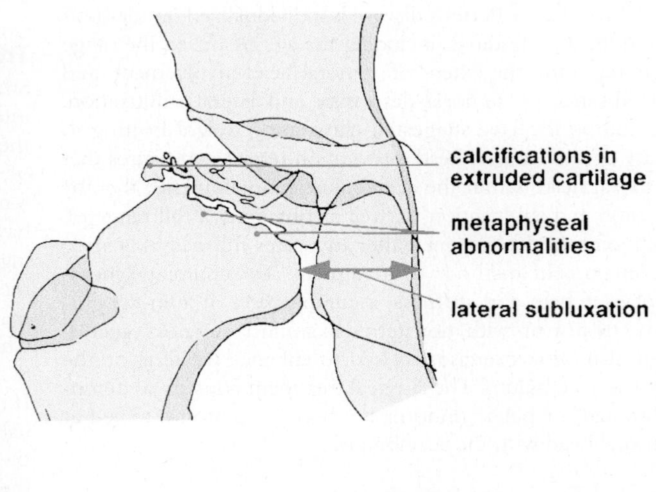

FIGURE 32.35 Legg-Calvé-Perthes disease. Anteroposterior radiograph of the right hip of an 8-year-old girl with advanced disease (Catterall group 4) shows increased density and fragmentation of the entire femoral head. "Head-at-risk" signs are apparent in the metaphyseal changes and the lateral subluxation. Calcifications lateral to the epiphysis represent extruded cartilage and indicate pressure on the head from the lateral edge of the acetabulum.

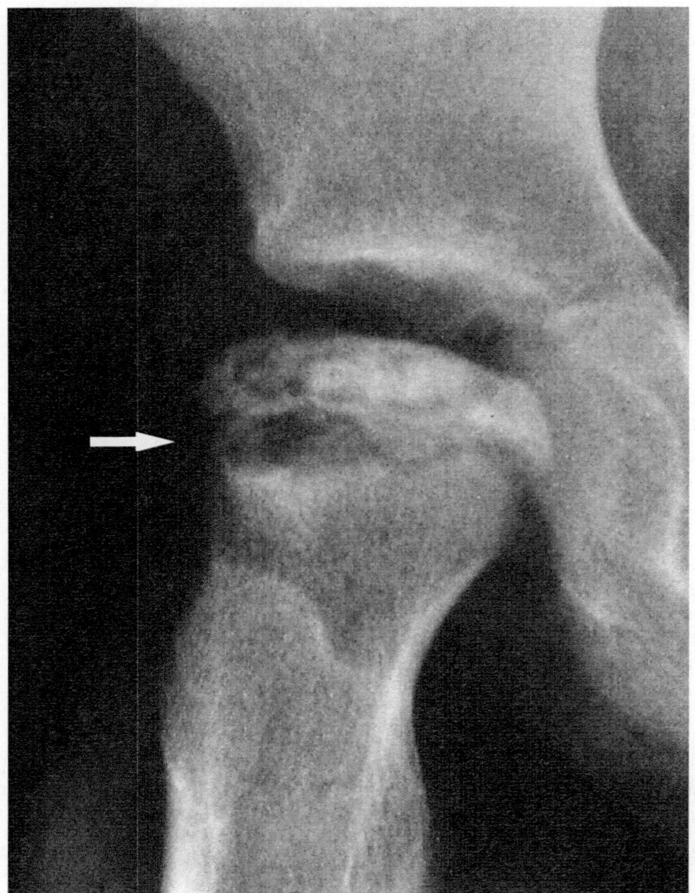

FIGURE 32.36 Legg-Calvé-Perthes disease. A V-shaped radiolucent defect in the lateral aspect of the physis, a Gage sign *(arrow)*, indicating a "head-at-risk," is demonstrated in this 7-year-old girl.

Differential Diagnosis

The differential diagnosis of this condition should include other causes of osteonecrosis and fragmentation of the femoral head, which may be seen, for example, in hypothyroidism, Gaucher disease, and sickle cell anemia.

Treatment

The treatment of Legg-Calvé-Perthes disease is individualized on the basis of the clinical and imaging findings, including the age of onset, the range of motion in the hip joint, the extent of femoral head involvement, and the presence or absence of femoral deformity and lateral subluxation. Although some authorities have suggested eliminating weight bearing to prevent deformity of the femoral head, prevention requires measures that maintain the femoral head within the acetabulum (containment), thereby preventing extrusion and subluxation, as well as obtaining a full range of motion in the hip joint. In this respect, Salter advocates full weight bearing together with containment methods of treatment. To minimize synovitis and its sequelae of pain and stiffness, a combination of non–weight-bearing, traction, treatment with nonsteroidal antiinflammatory agents, and gentle range-of-motion exercises is used to enhance molding of the femoral head by the acetabulum. The surgical treatment consists of femoral (varus derotational) or pelvic (innominate bone) osteotomy, aimed at covering the femoral head with the acetabulum.

Slipped Capital Femoral Epiphysis

Slipped capital femoral epiphysis (SCFE) is a disorder of adolescence in which the femoral head gradually slips posteriorly, medially, and inferiorly with respect to the neck. Boys are affected more often than girls are, and children of both sexes with this disorder are often overweight. In boys, the left hip is involved twice as often as the right, whereas in girls, both hips are affected with equal frequency. Bilateral involvement occurs in 20% to 40% of patients.

Although the specific cause of SCFE is obscure, its onset, which is usually insidious and without a history of trauma, commonly coincides with the growth spurt at puberty. Studies by Harris have suggested that an imbalance between growth hormone and sex hormones weaken the growth plate, rendering it more vulnerable to the shearing forces of weight bearing and injury.

Regardless of its cause, SCFE represents a Salter-Harris type I fracture through the growth plate of the proximal femur. This comes about through posterior, medial, and inferior displacement of the capital epiphysis, resulting in a varus deformity in the hip joint and external rotation and adduction of the femur. Pain in the hip, or occasionally the knee, is often the presenting symptom of this condition, and physical examination may reveal shortening of the involved extremity and limitation of abduction, flexion, and internal rotation in the hip joint.

Imaging Features

The radiographic abnormalities that may be seen in SCFE depend on the degree of displacement of the capital epiphysis. The anteroposterior radiograph of the hip, supplemented by a frog-lateral view, is usually sufficient to make a correct diagnosis. Several diagnostic indicators of SCFE have been identified on the anteroposterior radiograph of the hip (Fig. 32.37). The triangle sign of Capener may be of value in recognizing early SCFE. On conventional radiograph of the normal adolescent hip, an intracapsular area at the medial aspect of the femoral neck is seen overlapping the posterior wall of the acetabulum, creating a dense triangular shadow; in most cases of SCFE, this triangle is lost (Fig. 32.38). In a later stage, periarticular osteoporosis becomes apparent, as do widening and blurring of the physis and a decrease in height of the epiphysis (see Fig. 32.37). Moreover, as the disease progresses, slippage of the capital epiphysis can be identified by the absence of an intersection of the epiphysis with a line drawn tangent to the lateral cortex of the femoral neck (Fig. 32.39). The frog-lateral projection of the hip reveals slippage more readily (Fig. 32.39B), and comparison radiographs of the opposite side are helpful. Chronic stages of this disorder exhibit reactive bone formation along the superolateral aspect of the femoral neck, along with remodeling; this creates a protuberance and broadening of the femoral neck, which gives it a "pistol-grip" appearance known as a *Herndon hump* (Fig. 32.40). At times, SCFE occurs as a result of acute trauma, in which case it is known as a *transepiphyseal fracture* (Fig. 32.41).

MRI is useful in the evaluation of SCFE. This technique, in addition to findings revealed by radiography, may show bone marrow edema of the affected femur and early manifestation of SCFE or pre-SCFE (Figs. 32.42 and 32.43).

Treatment and Complications

SCFE is treated surgically by closed or open reduction of the slippage and internal fixation using various types of nails, wires, and pins to prevent further slippage and to induce closure of the physis. One of the complications of treatment is inadvertent penetration of the articular cartilage of the femoral head by a Knowles pin during placement. Lehman and colleagues have introduced a cannulated pin that prevents this complication by allowing contrast agent to be injected during surgery to determine proper placement of the pin in the femoral head on fluoroscopy. Other complications may be encountered that are not necessarily related to surgical treatment. Chondrolysis is observed in approximately 30% to 35% of patients with SCFE and is much more common in black patients than in white patients. It usually occurs within 1 year of the slippage and may be evident by gradual narrowing of the joint space (Fig. 32.44). Osteonecrosis secondary to the precarious blood supply to the femoral head and the vulnerability of the epiphyseal vessels has been reported in approximately 25% of patients with SCFE (Fig. 32.45). Secondary osteoarthritis may also occur, and it can be recognized by a typical narrowing of the joint space, subchondral sclerosis, and marginal osteophyte formation (Fig. 32.46; see also Fig. 32.40B). A severe varus deformity of the femoral neck, known as *coxa vara*, may also be encountered.

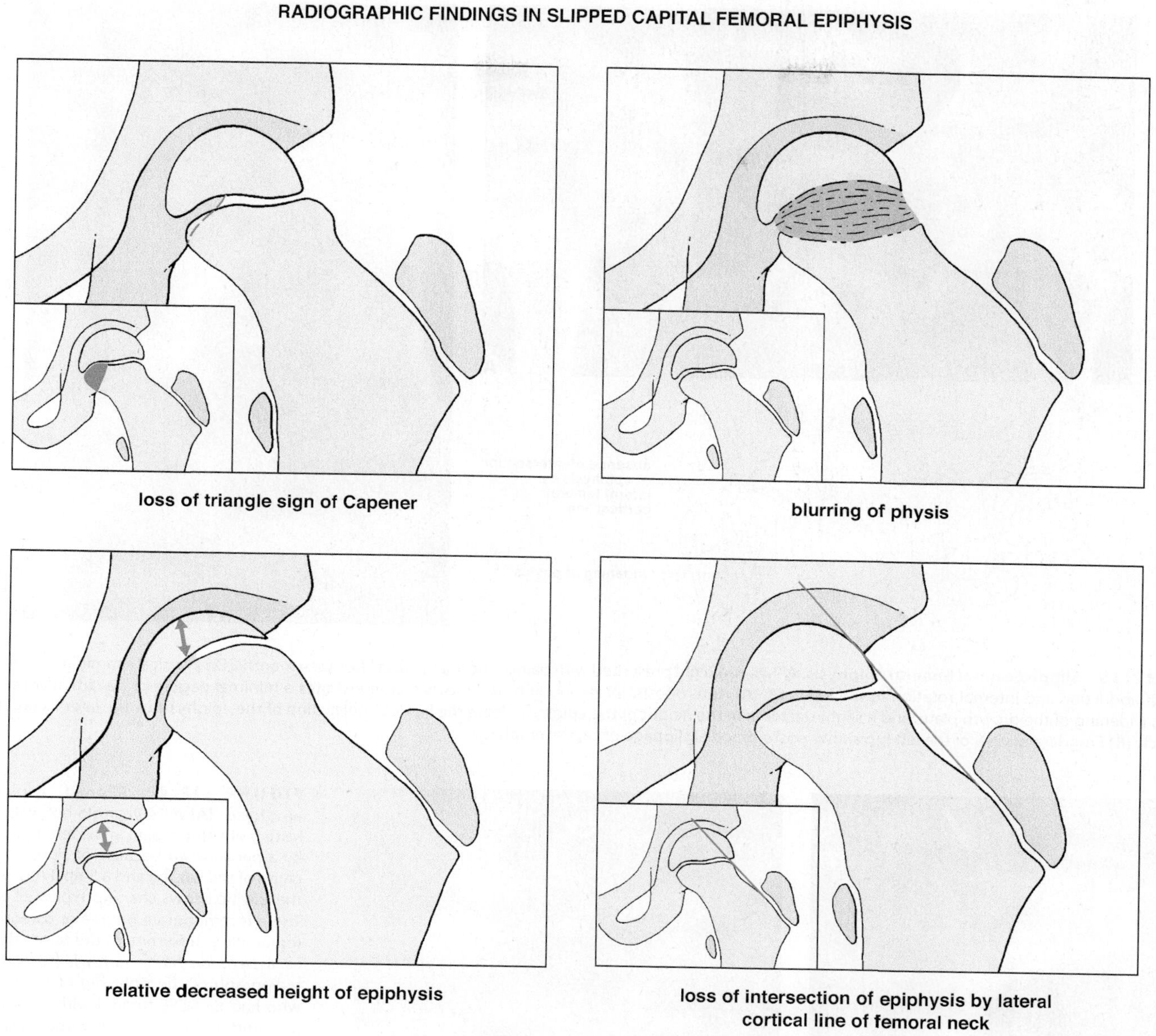

RADIOGRAPHIC FINDINGS IN SLIPPED CAPITAL FEMORAL EPIPHYSIS

loss of triangle sign of Capener

blurring of physis

relative decreased height of epiphysis

loss of intersection of epiphysis by lateral cortical line of femoral neck

FIGURE 32.37 **Slipped capital femoral epiphysis.** Various radiographic findings have been identified as diagnostic clues to SCFE. The *insets* show the normal appearance.

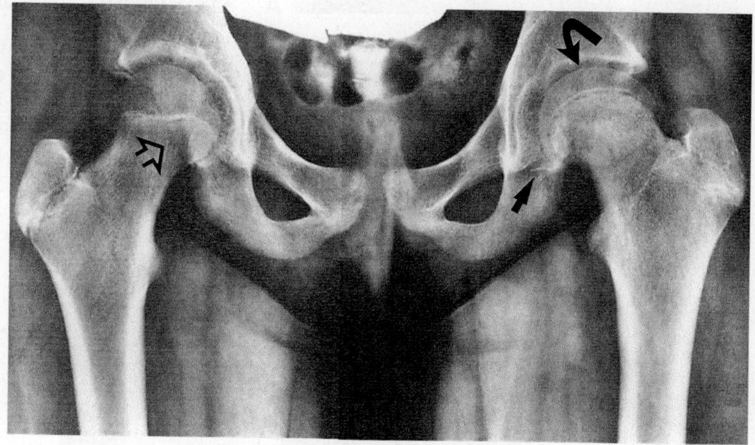

FIGURE 32.38 **Slipped capital femoral epiphysis.** Anteroposterior radiograph of the hips of a 12-year-old girl shows the absence of a triangular density in the area of overlap of the medial segment of the femoral metaphysis with the posterior wall of the acetabulum (Capener sign) *(black arrow)*. The triangle is clearly seen in the normal right hip *(open arrow)*. Note also relative decreased height of left femoral epiphysis *(curved arrow)*.

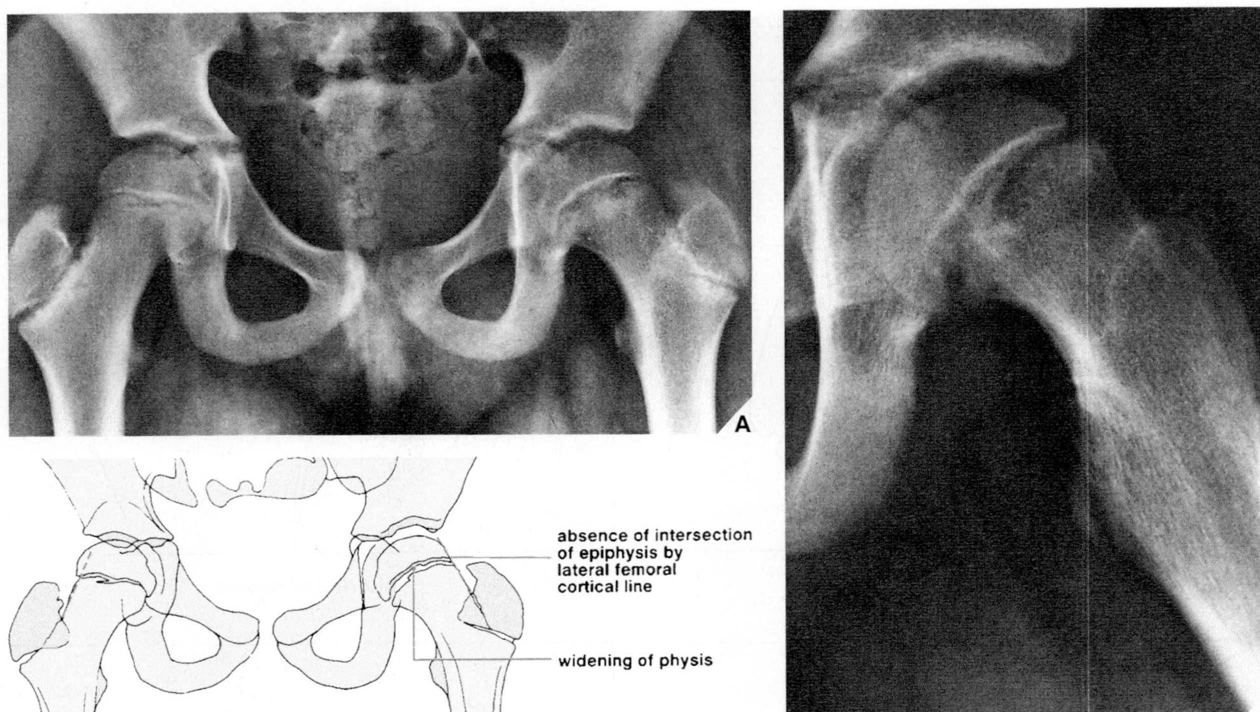

FIGURE 32.39 **Slipped capital femoral epiphysis.** A 9-year-old girl presented with pain in the left hip and knee for 4 months. On physical examination, there was slight limitation of abduction and internal rotation in the hip joint. **(A)** Anteroposterior radiograph of the pelvis demonstrates a minimal degree of periarticular osteoporosis of the left hip, widening of the growth plate, and a slight decrease in the height of the epiphysis. Note the lack of intersection of the epiphysis by the lateral cortical line of the femoral neck. **(B)** Frog-lateral view of the left hip shows posteromedial slippage of capital epiphysis.

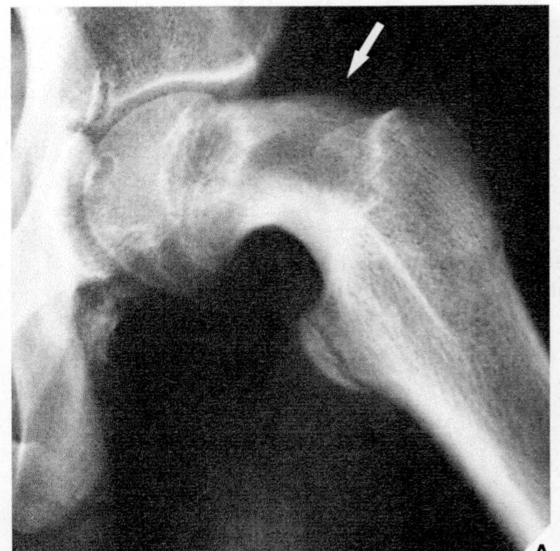

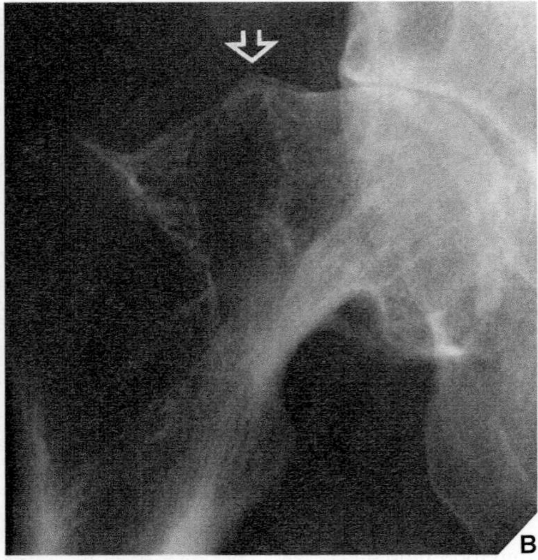

FIGURE 32.40 **Slipped capital femoral epiphysis.** **(A)** A 14-year-old boy with a 14-month history of chronic pain in the left hip was examined by a pediatrician because of significant foreshortening of the left leg and a limp. Frog-lateral view of the left hip shows changes typical of chronic SCFE. There is a moderate degree of osteoporosis and a remodeling deformity of the femoral neck, known as a *Herndon hump (arrow)*. **(B)** Anteroposterior radiograph of the right hip of a 20-year-old man who had an SCFE treated with pins demonstrates a Herndon hump *(open arrow)* and secondary osteoarthritis.

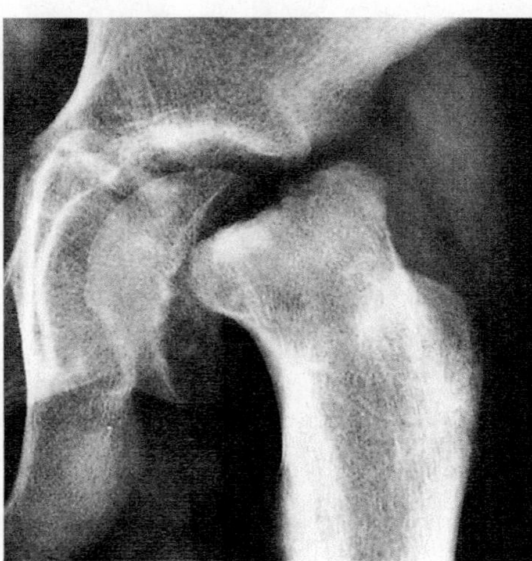

FIGURE 32.41 **Slipped capital femoral epiphysis.** Anteroposterior radiograph of the left hip of a 13-year-old boy who was thrown from a car in an automobile accident shows acute slippage of the femoral epiphysis. This injury represents a Salter-Harris type I fracture through the growth plate.

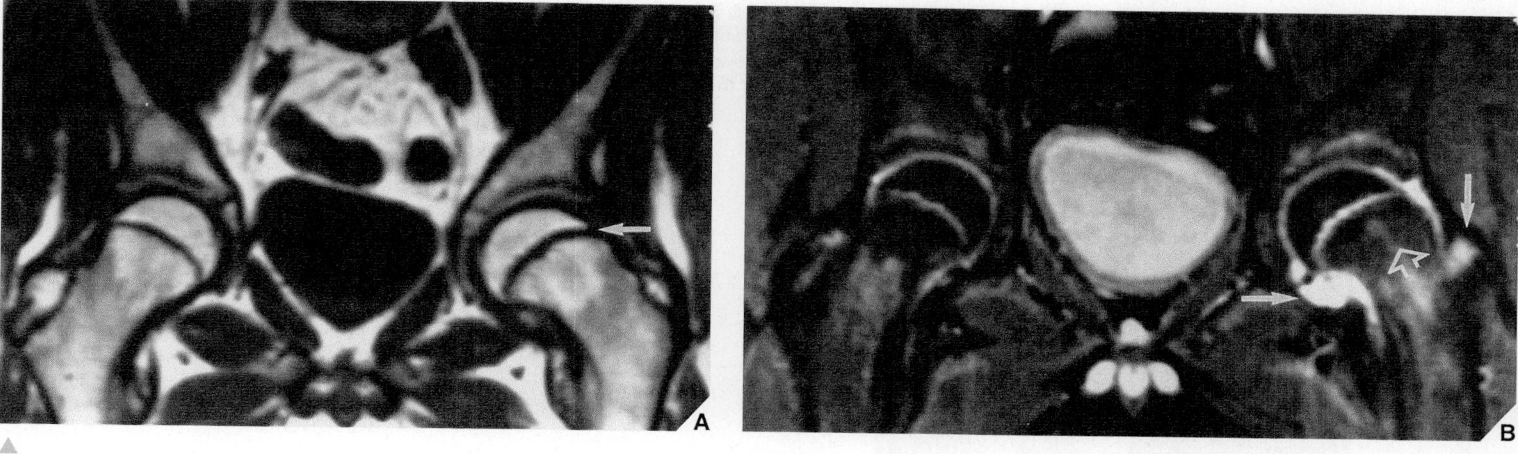

FIGURE 32.42 MRI of SCFE. **(A)** Coronal T1-weighted MRI of the hips in a 14-year-old boy shows slipped femoral epiphysis on the left side *(arrow)*. The right hip is normal. **(B)** Coronal T2-weighted fat-suppressed MR image reveals joint effusion *(arrows)* and marrow edema in the metaphysis *(open arrow)*.

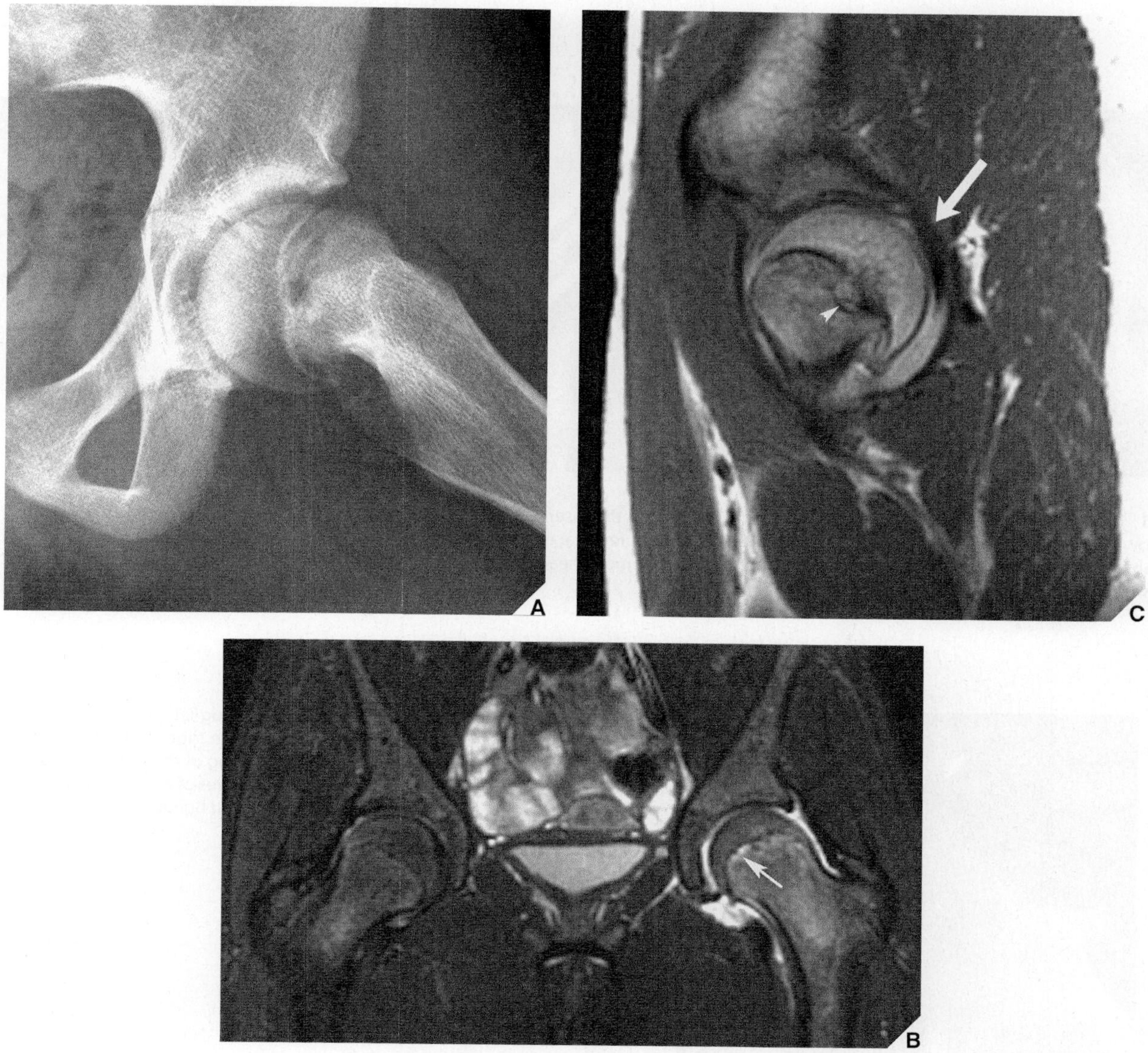

FIGURE 32.43 MRI of SCFE. **(A)** Frog-lateral view of the left hip of a 13-year-old girl shows medial displacement of the epiphysis of the femur. **(B)** Coronal short time inversion recovery (STIR) MRI of the pelvis demonstrates fluid in the left hip joint. Observe relative decrease in the height of the femoral epiphysis due to posterior displacement and bone marrow edema of the metaphysis extending to the intertrochanteric region. Note the irregularity and increased signal of the physis *(arrow)*. **(C)** Sagittal proton density–weighted MR image shows posterior displacement of the femoral epiphysis *(arrow)* and the focal widening of the physis *(arrowhead)*.

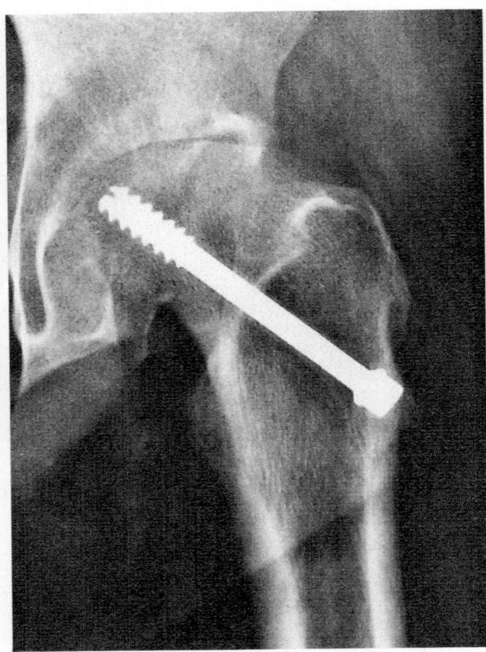

FIGURE 32.44 Complication of SCFE. Anteroposterior radiograph of the left hip of a 13-year-old girl, who 1 year earlier had been treated for SCFE, shows narrowing of the joint secondary to chondrolysis, a complication of this condition.

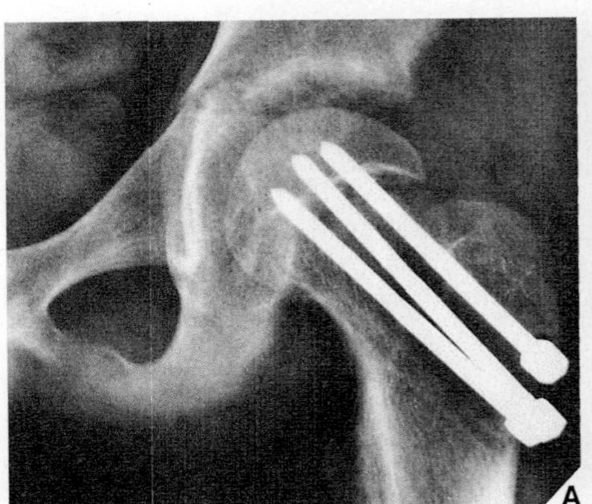

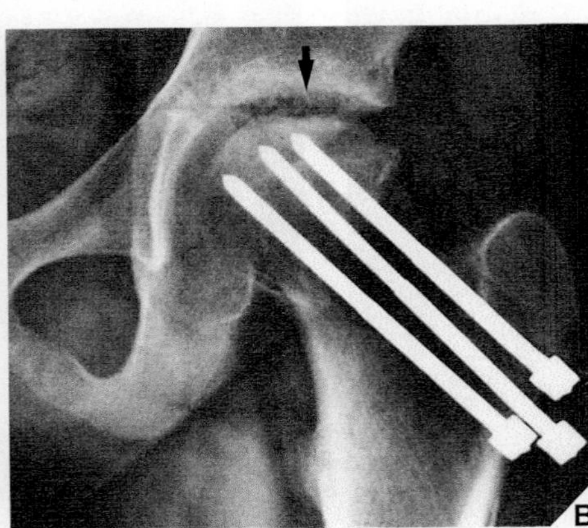

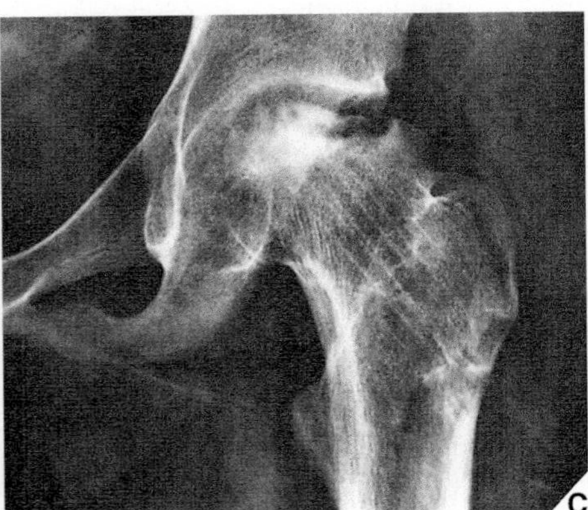

FIGURE 32.45 Complication of SCFE. A 12-year-old boy was treated by the insertion of three Knowles pins into the femoral head **(A)**. Six months later, a repeat radiograph **(B)** shows minimal flattening of the weight-bearing segment of the femoral epiphysis *(arrow)*, an early sign suggesting osteonecrosis. The pins were removed. **(C)** On a radiograph obtained 1 year later, there is an increase in density of the femoral head together with fragmentation of the epiphysis and subchondral collapse, features of advanced osteonecrosis.

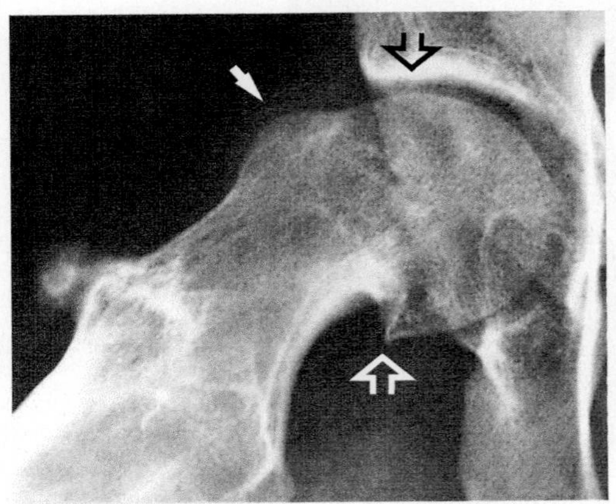

FIGURE 32.46 Complication of SCFE. Frog-lateral radiograph of the right hip of a 14-year-old boy who had acute slippage of the capital epiphysis at age 9 years demonstrates narrowing of the joint space and osteophytosis *(open arrows)*, characteristic features of a secondary osteoarthritic process. Note the presence of a Herndon hump *(arrow)*.

Anomalies of the Lower Limbs

An overview of the most effective radiographic projections and radiologic techniques for evaluating common anomalies of the lower limb and foot is presented in Table 32.4.

Congenital Tibia Vara

Congenital tibia vara, or *Blount disease*, as this developmental anomaly is also known, predominantly affects the medial portion of the proximal tibial growth plate, as well as the medial segments of the tibial metaphysis and epiphysis, resulting in a varus deformity at the knee joint. The cause of this condition is unknown, but it is probably a multifactorial disorder with genetic, humoral, biomechanical, and environmental factors. Bateson has demonstrated convincingly that Blount disease and physiologic bow-leg deformity are part of the same condition, which is influenced by early weight bearing and racial factors. On the basis of a study of South African black children, among whom there is an increased incidence of Blount disease (as there is in Jamaica), Bathfield and Beighton have suggested that its cause might be related to the custom of mothers carrying

TABLE 32.4 Most Effective Radiographic Projections and Radiologic Techniques for Evaluating Common Anomalies of the Lower Limb and Foot

Projection/Technique	Crucial Abnormalities
Congenital Tibia Vara	
Anteroposterior of knees	Depression of medial tibial metaphysis with beak formation Varus deformity of tibia Premature fusion of tibial growth plate
Arthrography	Hypertrophy of Nonossified portion of epiphysis Medial meniscus
Genu Valgum	
Anteroposterior of knees	Valgus deformity
Infantile Pseudoarthrosis of the Tibia	
Anteroposterior and lateral of tibia	Bowing of tibia Pseudoarthrosis
Dysplasia Epiphysealis Hemimelica	
Anteroposterior and lateral of ankle (or other affected joint)	Unilateral bulbous deformity of distal tibial (or any affected) epiphysis
Talipes Equinovarus	
Anteroposterior of foot	Varus position of hind foot Adduction and varus position of forefoot Kite anteroposterior talocalcaneal angle (less than 20 degrees) TFM angle (greater than 15 degrees) Metatarsal parallelism
Lateral of foot (weight-bearing or with forced dorsiflexion)	Equinus position of the heel Talocalcaneal subluxation Kite lateral talocalcaneal angle (less than 35 degrees)
Congenital/Developmental Planovalgus Foot	
Anteroposterior of foot	Medial projection of axial line through the talus
Lateral of foot	Flattening of longitudinal arch
Congenital Vertical Talus	
Lateral of foot	Vertical position of talus Talonavicular dislocation Boat-shaped or Persian-slipper appearance of foot
With forced plantar flexion	Possibility of reduction of dislocation
Anteroposterior of foot	Flat-foot deformity Medial displacement of talus Abduction of forefoot
Calcaneonavicular Coalition	
Lateral of foot	Anteater nose sign
Lateral or medial oblique (45 degrees) of foot and CT	Fusion of calcaneus and navicular bone
MRI	Fibrous or cartilaginous coalition
Talocalcaneal Coalition	
Medial oblique (15 degrees) of foot	Fusion of talus and calcaneus
Lateral of foot	Talar beak "C"-sign Obliteration of subtalar joint
Posterior tangential of calcaneus and CT	Fusion or deformity of middle facet of subtalar joint
Subtalar arthrography	Cartilaginous or fibrous bridge
Talonavicular Coalition	
Lateral of foot	Fusion of talus and navicular bones
CT	Same as above

TFM, talus–first metatarsal; CT, computed tomography; MRI, magnetic resonance imaging.

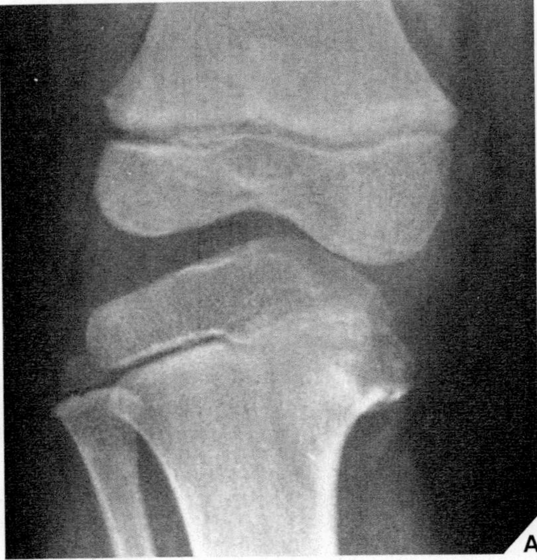

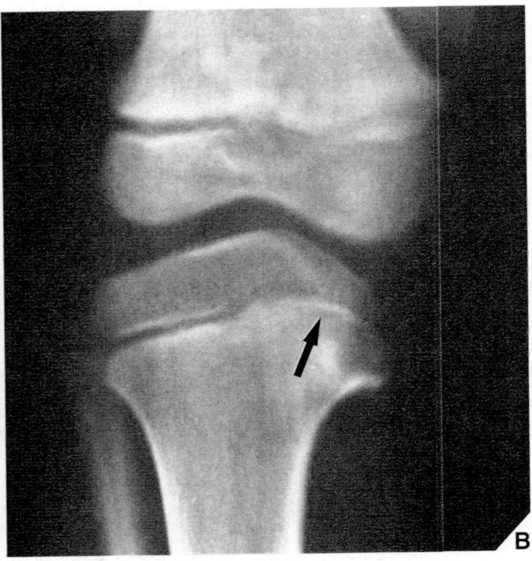

FIGURE 32.47 **Blount disease. (A)** Anteroposterior radiograph of the right knee of an 8-year-old girl shows the typical changes of congenital tibia vara. There is, in addition, a possible fusion of the medial portion of the growth plate. **(B)** Conventional tomogram confirms the presence of a bony bridge in the medial aspect of the physis *(arrow)*. Treatment of this condition would require either epiphysiodesis or bridge resection in addition to corrective valgus osteotomy of the tibia.

children on their backs. The child's thighs are abducted and flexed, and the flexed knees gripping the mother's waist are forced to assume a varus configuration.

Two forms of Blount disease have been identified: *infantile tibia vara*, which is usually bilateral and affects children younger than age 10 years, with onset most commonly between ages 1 and 3 years; and *adolescent tibia vara*, which is usually unilateral and occurs in children between the ages of 8 and 15 years. The course of the adolescent form of the disease is less severe and its incidence less frequent than in the infantile form. Regardless of its variants, Blount disease must be differentiated from other causes of tibia vara, such as those seen as sequelae to trauma.

Imaging Features and Differential Diagnosis

Radiologically, the early stages of Blount disease are marked by hypertrophy of the nonossified cartilaginous portion of the tibial epiphysis and hypertrophy of the medial meniscus, which represent compensatory changes secondary to growth arrest at the medial aspect of the physis. As the metaphysis and growth plate become depressed, the cartilage decreases in height. In advanced stages of the disease, there is premature fusion of the growth plate on the medial side (Fig. 32.47). The presence of fusion is important information for surgical planning because either resection of the bony bridge or epiphysiodesis (fusion of the physis) would be required in addition to the corrective osteotomy. Double-contrast arthrography is a valuable technique in the radiologic evaluation of Blount disease because it permits visualization of nonossified cartilage of the medial plateau (Fig. 32.48) and associated abnormalities of the medial meniscus (Fig. 32.49). MRI is also helpful to visualize the condition of the growth plate, the epiphyseal cartilage, and the degree of deformity of the epiphysis and menisci (Fig. 32.50). This information is valuable for preoperative assessment.

In most cases, it is also possible to distinguish Blount disease radiographically, particularly in its advanced stage, from developmental bowing of the legs. In Blount disease, the medial aspect of the tibial metaphysis is characteristically depressed, exhibiting an abrupt angulation

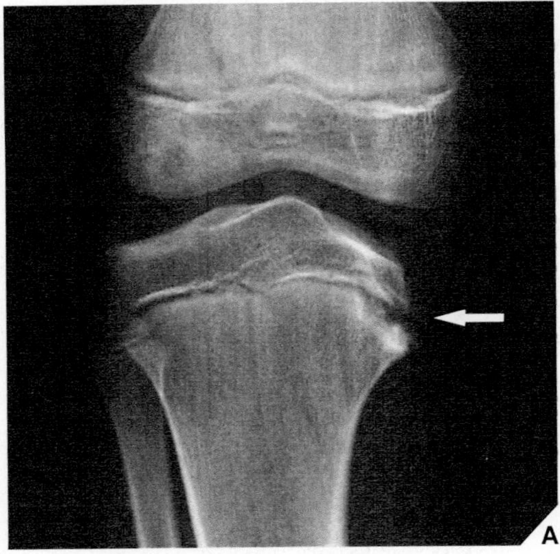

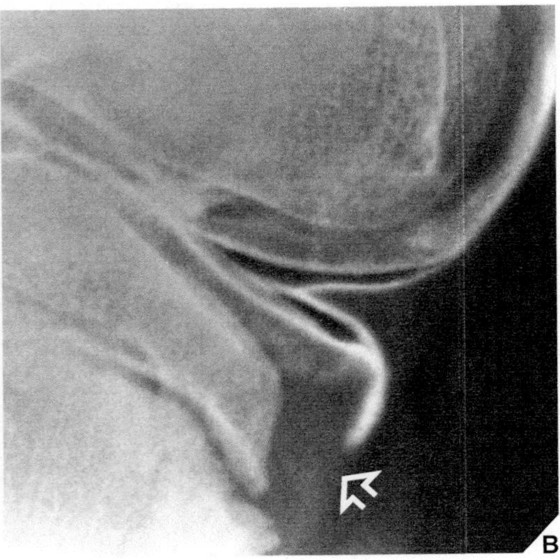

FIGURE 32.48 **Arthrography of Blount disease. (A)** Anteroposterior radiograph of the right knee of a 10-year-old boy demonstrates the classic appearance of this condition, as evident in the depression of the medial metaphysis associated with a beak formation and slanting of the medial tibial epiphysis *(arrow)*. **(B)** Spot film of an arthrogram shows contrast outlining the thickened nonossified cartilage of the medial tibial plateau *(open arrow)*. In this case, the medial meniscus shows no abnormalities.

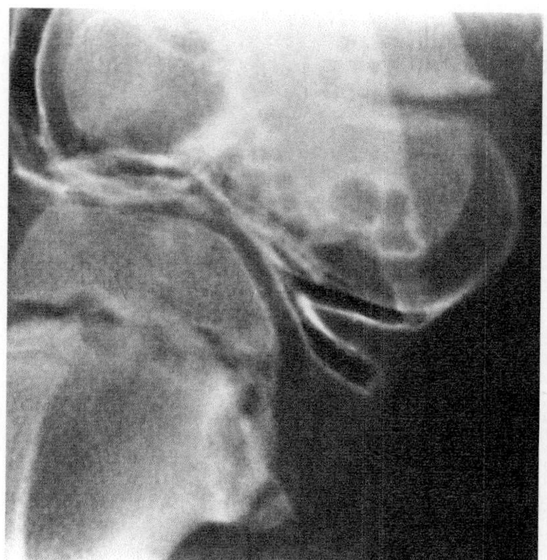

FIGURE 32.49 Arthrogram of Blount disease. Fluoroscopic spot film of a knee arthrogram in a 4-year-old girl shows hypertrophy of the medial aspect of the proximal tibial cartilage and an enlarged medial meniscus.

and formation of a beak-like prominence, which is associated with cortical thickening of the medial aspect of the tibia. Similar changes are seen in the medial aspect of the tibial epiphysis. Because of the sharp angulation of the metaphysis and adduction of the diaphysis, the tibia assumes a varus configuration (Fig. 32.51). In most instances, the lateral cortex of the tibia remains relatively straight. In developmental bowleg deformity, however, a gentle bilateral bowing is noted in the medial and lateral femoral and tibial cortices; the growth plates appear normal, and depression of the tibial metaphysis with a beak formation is absent (Fig. 32.52). Physiologic bowing resolves to straight alignment without treatment as ambulation increases, with the reversal usually beginning at approximately age 18 months. Both conditions, however, may be associated with internal tibial torsion. Developmental bowing usually persists for approximately 18 to 24 months, and in most affected children, it decreases progressively, although bowing may occasionally progress with skeletal maturation. Blount disease can be differentiated from rickets on the basis of ossification of the metaphyses and the absence of widening of the growth plate (see Figs. 27.12 and 27.13).

Classification

Based on the progression of radiographic changes in Blount disease, Langenskiöld divided congenital tibia vara into six stages as a guideline for prognosis and treatment:

Stage I: a varus deformity of the tibia, associated with irregularity of the growth plate and a small beak at the medial metaphysis; usually seen in children from 2 to 3 years of age

Stage II: a definite depression of the medial portion of the metaphysis, associated with slanting of the medial aspect of the epiphysis; usually seen in children from 2 to 4 years of age

Stage III: progression of the varus deformity and a very prominent beak, with occasional fragmentation of the medial portion of the metaphysis; seen in children between ages 4 and 6 years

Stage IV: marked narrowing of the growth plate and severe slanting of the medial aspect of the epiphysis, which shows an irregular border; usually seen in children between ages 5 and 10 years

Stage V: marked deformity of the medial epiphysis, which is separated into two parts by a clear band, the distal part having a triangular shape; seen in children between 9 and 11 years of age

Stage VI: an osseous bridge between the epiphysis and metaphysis and possible fusion of the triangular fragment of the separated medial epiphysis to the metaphysis; seen in children between ages 10 and 13 years

Stages V and VI represent phases of irreparable structural damage.

Smith introduced a simplified classification of Blount disease in an attempt to relate the grade of deformity to the need for treatment. His scheme comprises four grades: grade A, potential tibia vara; grade B, mild tibia vara; grade C, advanced tibia vara; and grade D, physeal closure.

Treatment

Blount disease is usually treated conservatively with braces. If the deformity continues to progress despite such treatment, a high valgus tibial osteotomy may be required to achieve normal alignment of the limb; usually, correction of a rotary deformity requires an osteotomy of the proximal fibula as well. Arthrography or MRI may be required before surgery to determine the status of the tibial articular cartilage, information helpful in planning the degree of angular correction necessary to eliminate the deformity.

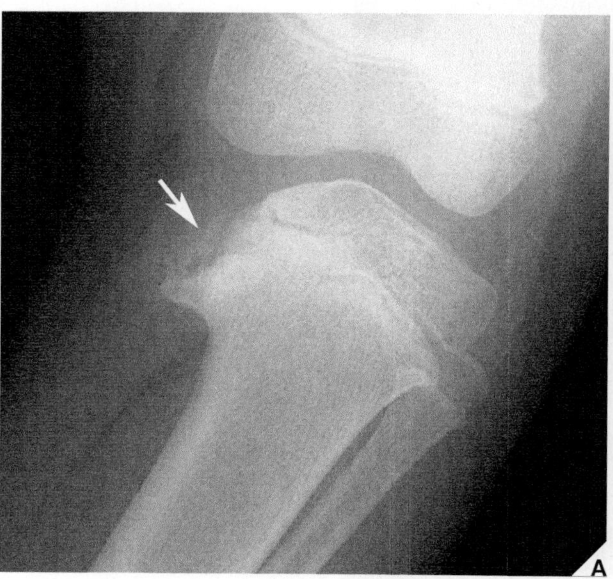

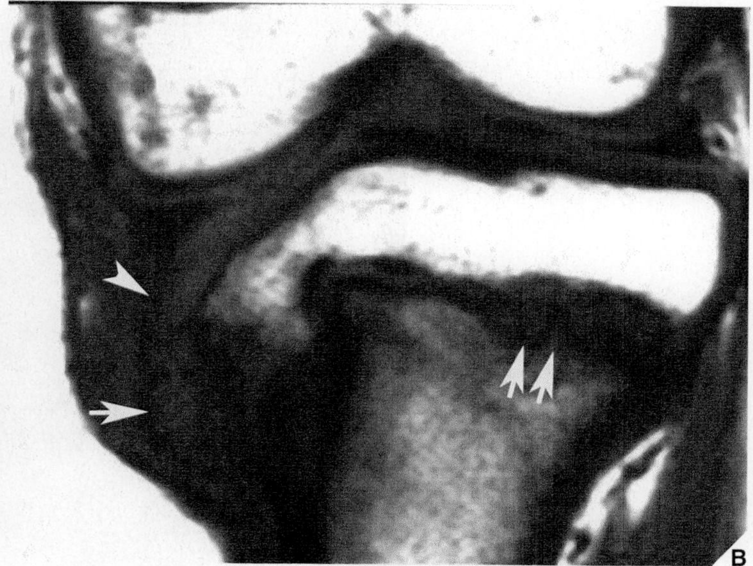

FIGURE 32.50 MRI of Blount disease. **(A)** Anteroposterior radiograph of the left knee demonstrates the characteristic depression of the medial tibial plateau and medial epiphyseal fragmentation *(arrow)*. **(B)** Coronal T1-weighted MR image demonstrates the irregular, depressed epiphyseal cartilage of the medial tibial plateau *(arrowhead)* with partial calcification and fragmentation of the depressed medial epiphyseal cartilage *(arrow)*. Note the irregularity and widening of the growth plate, not evident on the radiograph *(double arrows)*.

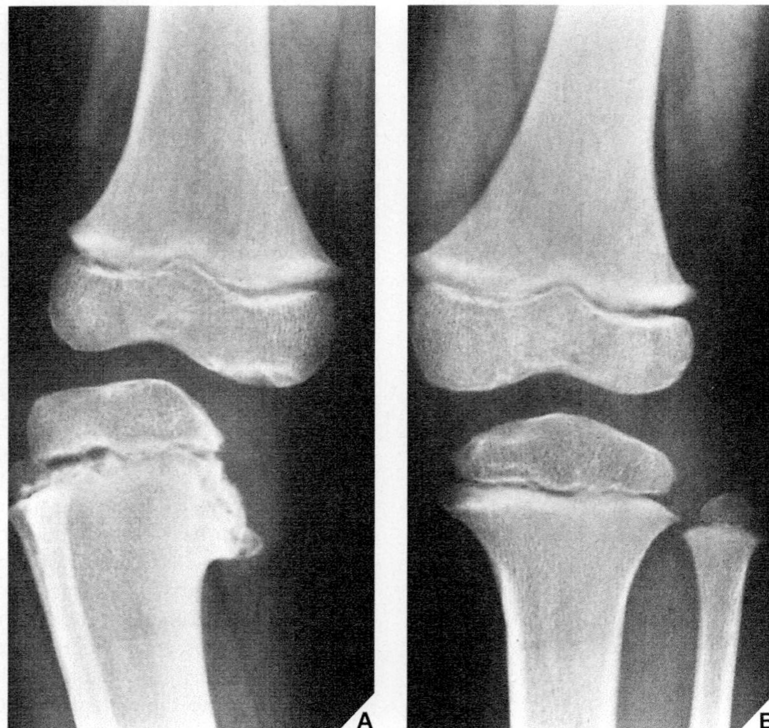

FIGURE 32.51 **Blount disease.** **(A)** Anteroposterior radiograph of the right knee of a 4-year-old girl with unilateral congenital tibia vara shows depression of the medial tibial metaphysis associated with a beak formation and medial slant of the tibial epiphysis. **(B)** The left knee is normal.

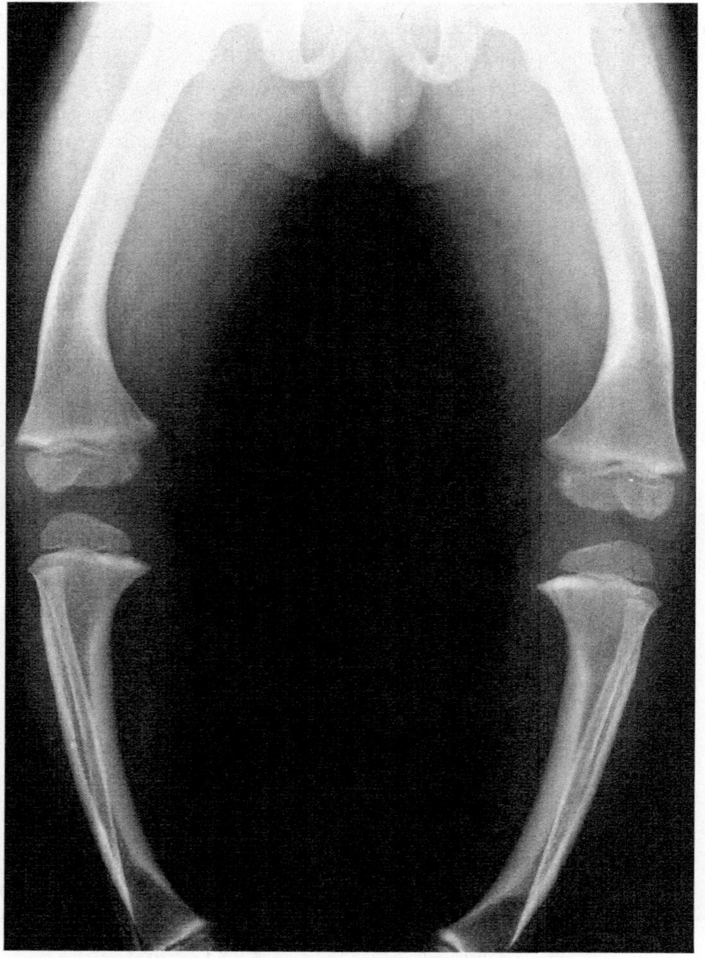

FIGURE 32.52 **Developmental bowleg deformity.** Weight-bearing (standing) anteroposterior radiograph of the legs of a 3-year-old boy demonstrates bowleg deformity of the femora and a varus configuration of the knees. However, there are no signs of Blount disease; both proximal tibial metaphyses and growth plates are normal, although there is associated internal torsion of both tibiae and thickening of the medial femoral and tibial cortices, which is frequently seen in this condition.

Dysplasia Epiphysealis Hemimelica

Also known as *Trevor-Fairbank disease*, this is a developmental disorder characterized by asymmetric cartilaginous overgrowth of one or more epiphyses in the lower extremity, with a decided preference for the distal tibial epiphysis and the talus. The lesion is characteristically found on one side of the affected limb, hence the name *hemimelica*. Mouchet and Belot in 1926 reported the first case and used the term *tarsomegalie*. Trevor in 1950 reviewed 10 cases and used the term *tarsoepiphyseal aclasis*, and finally in 1956, Fairbank reported 14 cases and coined the term *dysplasia epiphysealis hemimelica*. Its cause is unknown, and there is no definite familial or hereditary predilection. Males are affected 3 times as often as females. Pathologically, the lesion shows similarity to an osteochondroma, and for this reason, it is occasionally referred to as *epiphyseal* or *intraarticular osteochondroma*. Clinically, there is deformity and restricted motion of the affected joint, and pain, particularly around the ankle, is the most frequent presenting symptom in adults.

Imaging Features and Treatment

A diagnosis of Trevor-Fairbank disease can be established through radiographic and MRI examination. It typically presents with an irregular, bulbous overgrowth of the ossification center or epiphysis on one side, resembling an osteochondroma (Figs. 32.53 to 32.56). Occasionally, the other ossification centers, particularly at the knee, may be similarly affected in the same individual.

Treatment for the condition is individualized according to the amount of deformity and pain; usually, surgical resection of the lesion is required. Recurrence is common.

Talipes Equinovarus

Clubfoot is a congenital deformity comprising four elements: (a) an equinus position of the heel, (b) a varus position of the hindfoot, (c) adduction and a varus deformity of the forefoot, and (d) talonavicular subluxation. Before the ossification of the navicular bone at 2 to 3 years of age, only the first three elements can be verified radiographically.

Measurements and Radiographic Features

A sound knowledge of the anatomy of the foot is essential to understanding and properly describing the various foot abnormalities involved in this disorder (see Fig. 10.2). Certain lines and angles drawn on dorsoplantar and lateral radiographs of the foot are helpful in identifying the deformity. The most useful of these are the Kite angles and the talus–first metatarsal (TFM) angle (Fig. 32.57). In the clubfoot deformity, the Kite anteroposterior talocalcaneal angle is less than 20 degrees, the lateral angle is less than 35 degrees, and the TFM angle is greater than 15 degrees (Fig. 32.58). In addition to these measurements, there are other alignments in the normal infant's foot that are disrupted in the clubfoot deformity. For example, the anteroposterior view of the normal foot reveals the parallel alignment of the metatarsal bones, which in the clubfoot deformity converge proximally. Likewise, in the determination of the Kite anteroposterior talocalcaneal angle, the lines of the angle normally intersect the first and fourth metatarsals; in the clubfoot anomaly, these lines fall lateral to the normal points. It is important to note that rendering accurate measurements of these various angles requires a carefully standardized technique for obtaining the anteroposterior and lateral views of the foot because slight changes in position can alter the relationship of the bones. Whenever possible, both projections should be obtained in weight-bearing positions. With infants in whom this is not possible, an anteroposterior view is obtained with the infant seated and the knees held together; the sagittal plane of the leg must be at a right angle to the radiographic cassette, on which the infant's feet are secured. When a weight-bearing lateral view is not possible, the infant's knee should be held in flexion and the foot should be held in dorsiflexion.

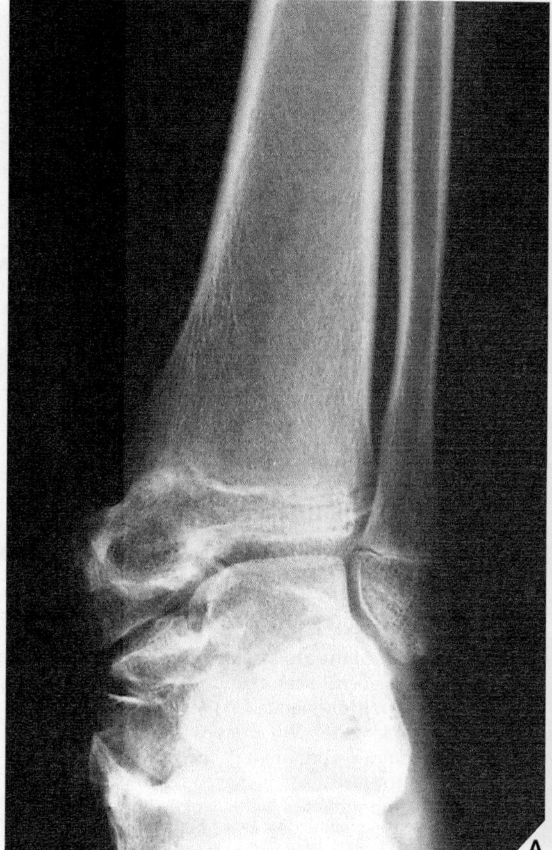

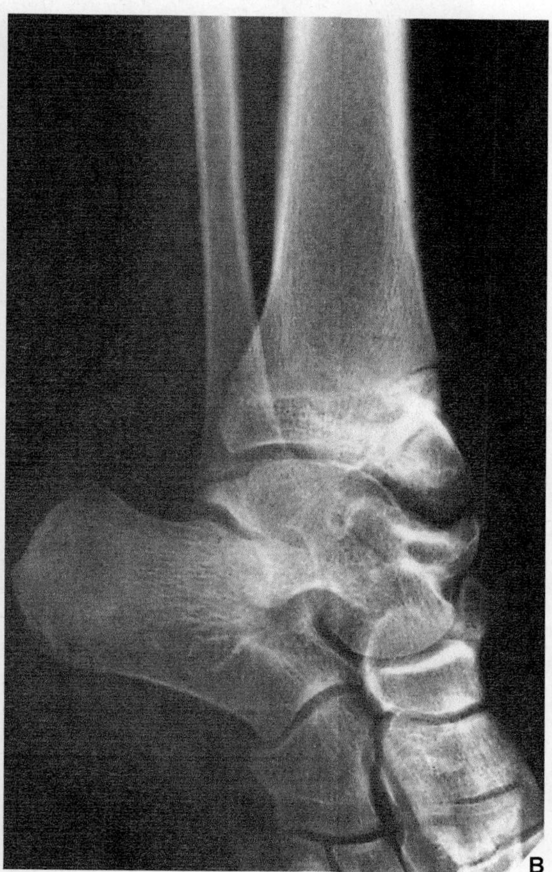

FIGURE 32.53 **Trevor-Fairbank disease of the ankle.** A 12-year-old girl presented with pain and limitation of motion in the ankle joint. **(A)** Anteroposterior and **(B)** lateral radiographs of the ankle demonstrate deformity and enlargement of the medial malleolus, talus, and navicular bone, features typical of dysplasia epiphysealis hemimelica. Note that the growth disturbance is limited to the medial side of the ankle and foot.

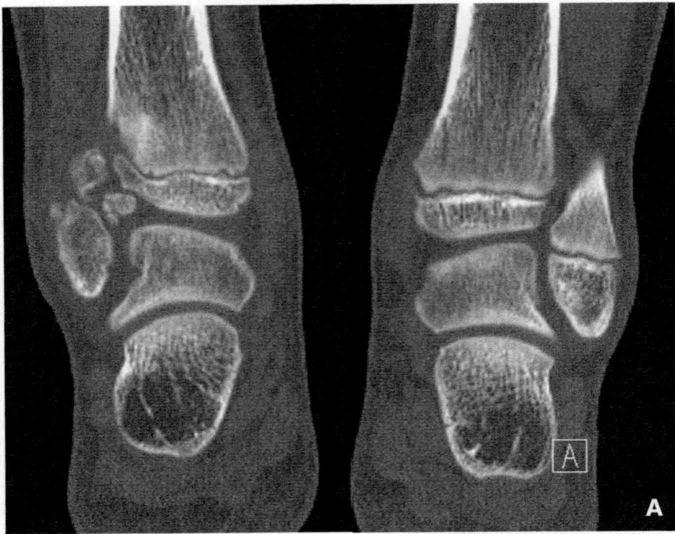
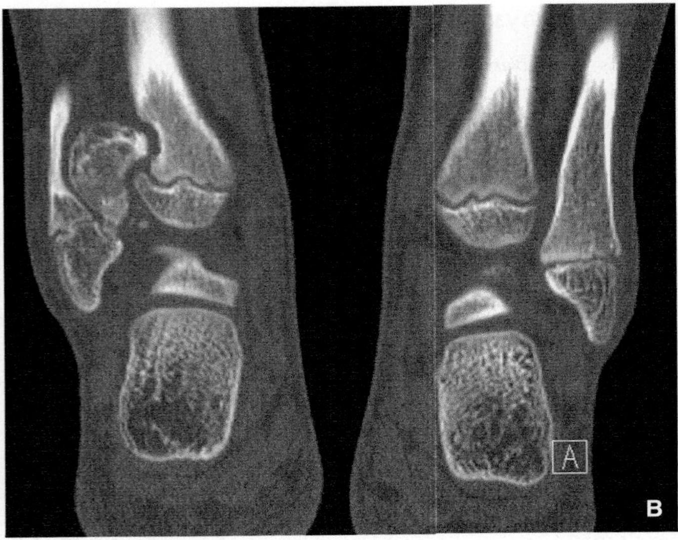

FIGURE 32.54 CT of Trevor-Fairbank disease of the ankle. **(A,B)** Two coronal reformatted CT images of both ankles of a 17-year-old girl show an osteochondroma-like mass arising from the epiphysis of the right tibia eroding the tibial metaphysis and distal metaphysis and epiphysis of the fibula. Observe marked deformity of the right ankle joint (compare with the normal left ankle).

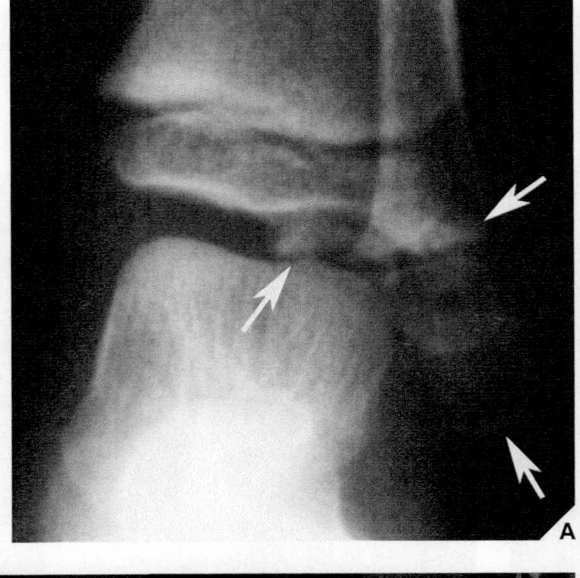
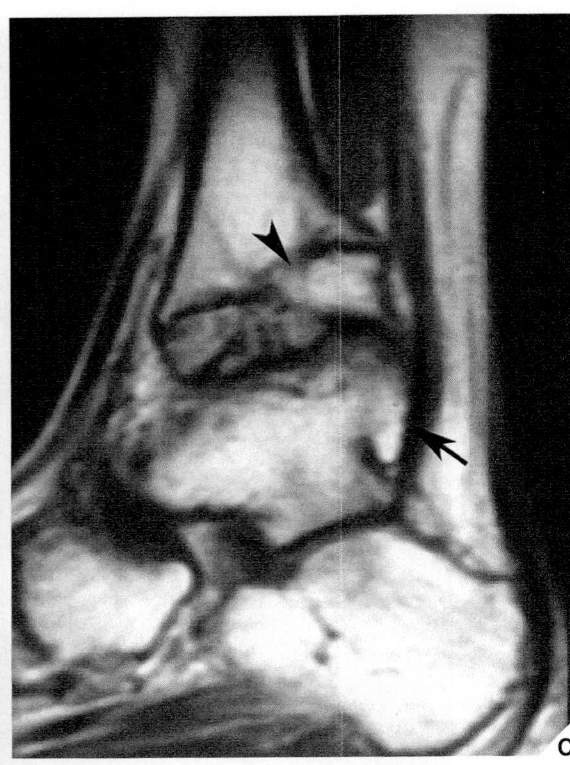
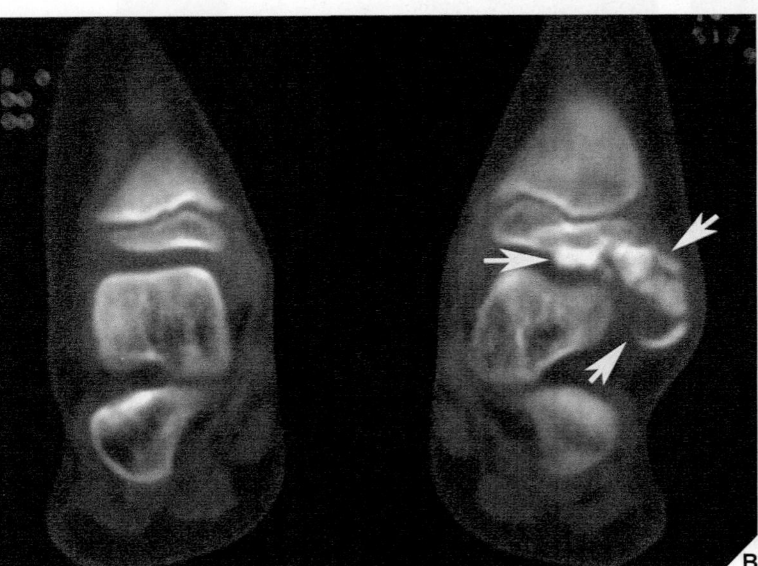

FIGURE 32.55 CT and MRI of Trevor-Fairbank disease of the ankle. **(A)** Anteroposterior radiograph of the left ankle of a 7-year-old boy demonstrates an osteochondroma-like mass originated in the distal tibial epiphysis, with intraarticular extension *(arrows)*. **(B)** Coronal CT of bilateral ankles confirms the origin of the tumor-like excrescence from the distal tibial epiphysis and demonstrates the intraarticular component *(arrows)*. Note the deformed and expanded medial malleolus and the chondroid-type calcifications. **(C)** Sagittal T1-weighted MRI of the ankle in another patient with Trevor-Fairbank disease demonstrates the osteochondroma-like mass originating from the posterior aspect of the talar dome *(arrow)*. Note the remodeling deformity of the distal tibial epiphysis *(arrowhead)*.

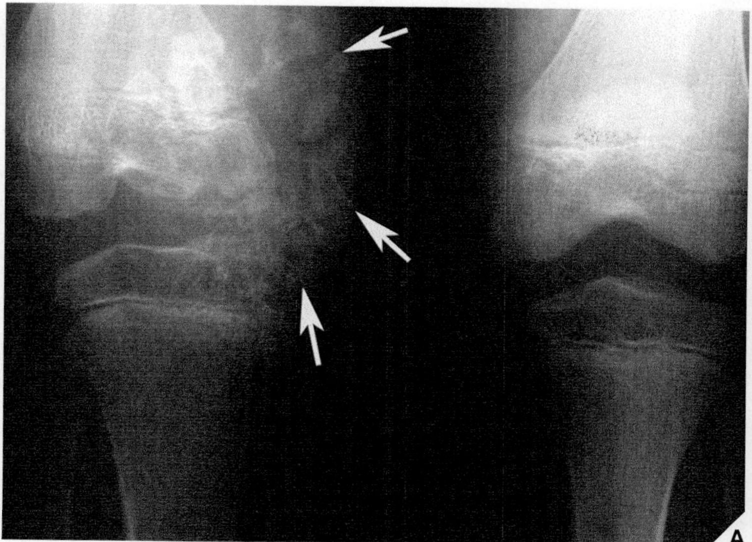

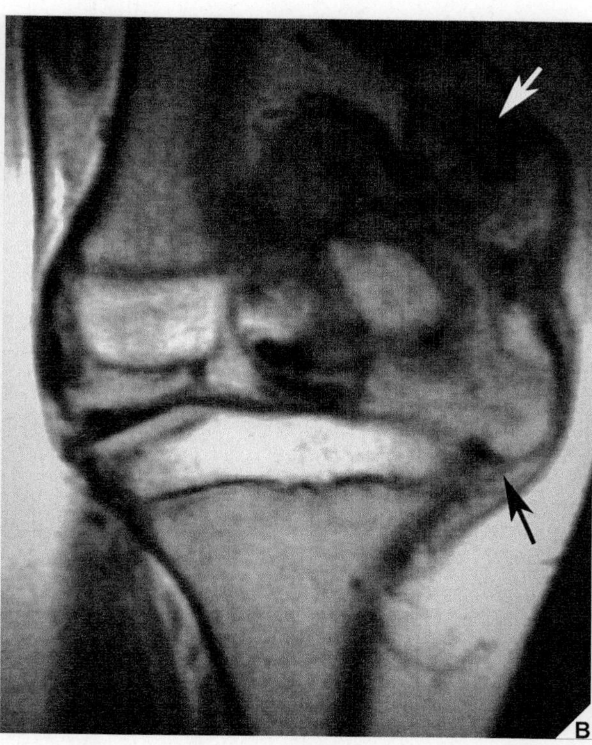

FIGURE 32.56 MRI of Trevor-Fairbank disease of the knee. **(A)** Anteroposterior radiograph of the knees demonstrates a calcified cartilaginous mass extending from the medial epicondyle and medial metaphysis of the right femur to the medial proximal tibial epiphysis *(arrows)*. **(B)** Coronal T1-weighted MRI of the right knee confirms the extent of involvement of the tumor, "bridging" from the femur to the tibia *(arrows)*.

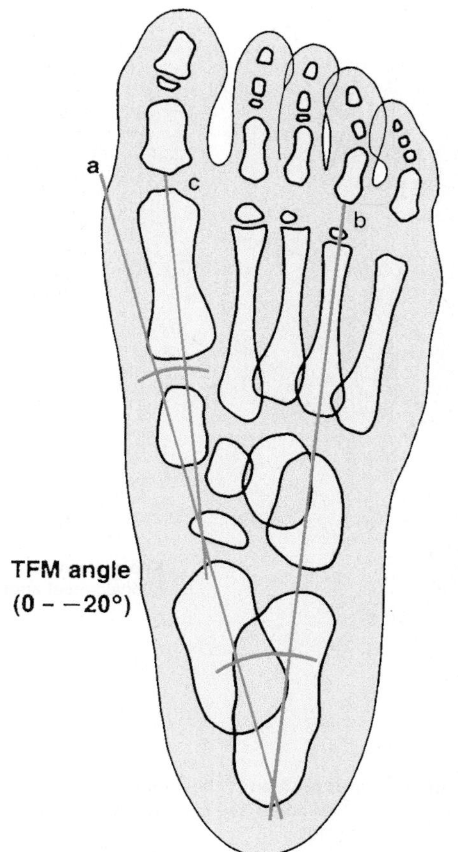

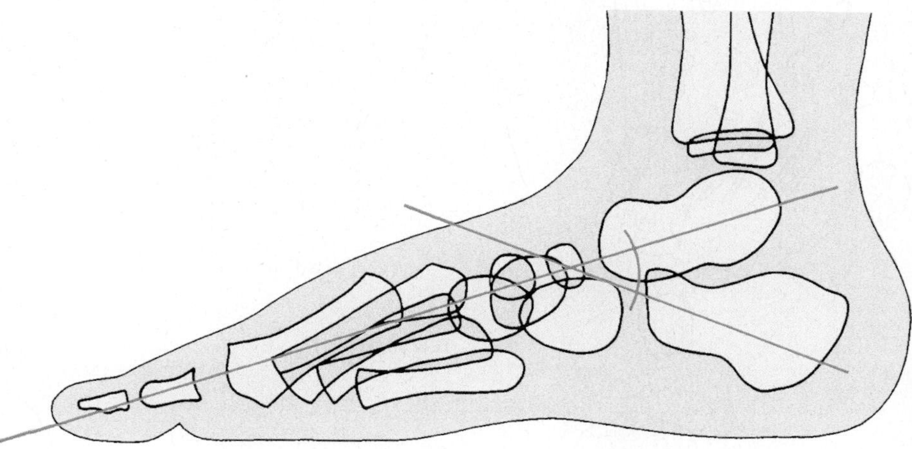

FIGURE 32.57 The Kite measurements. **(A)** The Kite anteroposterior talocalcaneal angle and the TFM angle are determined on a weight-bearing dorsoplantar radiograph of the foot. The Kite angle is the intersection of two lines: One line *(a)* drawn through the longitudinal axis of the talus normally intersects the first metatarsal bone; a second line *(b)* drawn through the longitudinal axis of the calcaneus usually intersects the fourth metatarsal. The angle of intersection of these lines normally ranges from 20 to 40 degrees; an angle less than 20 degrees indicates a varus position of the hindfoot. The TFM angle is determined on the same radiograph by a line *(c)* drawn through the longitudinal axis of the first metatarsal and intersecting line *(a)*. The values of this angle normally range between 0 and −20 degrees; positive values indicate adduction of the forefoot. **(B)** The Kite lateral talocalcaneal angle is determined on a weight-bearing lateral radiograph of the ankle and foot by the intersection of lines drawn through the longitudinal axes of the talus and calcaneus (lines parallel to the inferior borders of these two bones). Normally, this angle measures between 35 and 50 degrees; an angle less than 35 degrees indicates an equinus deformity of the heel.

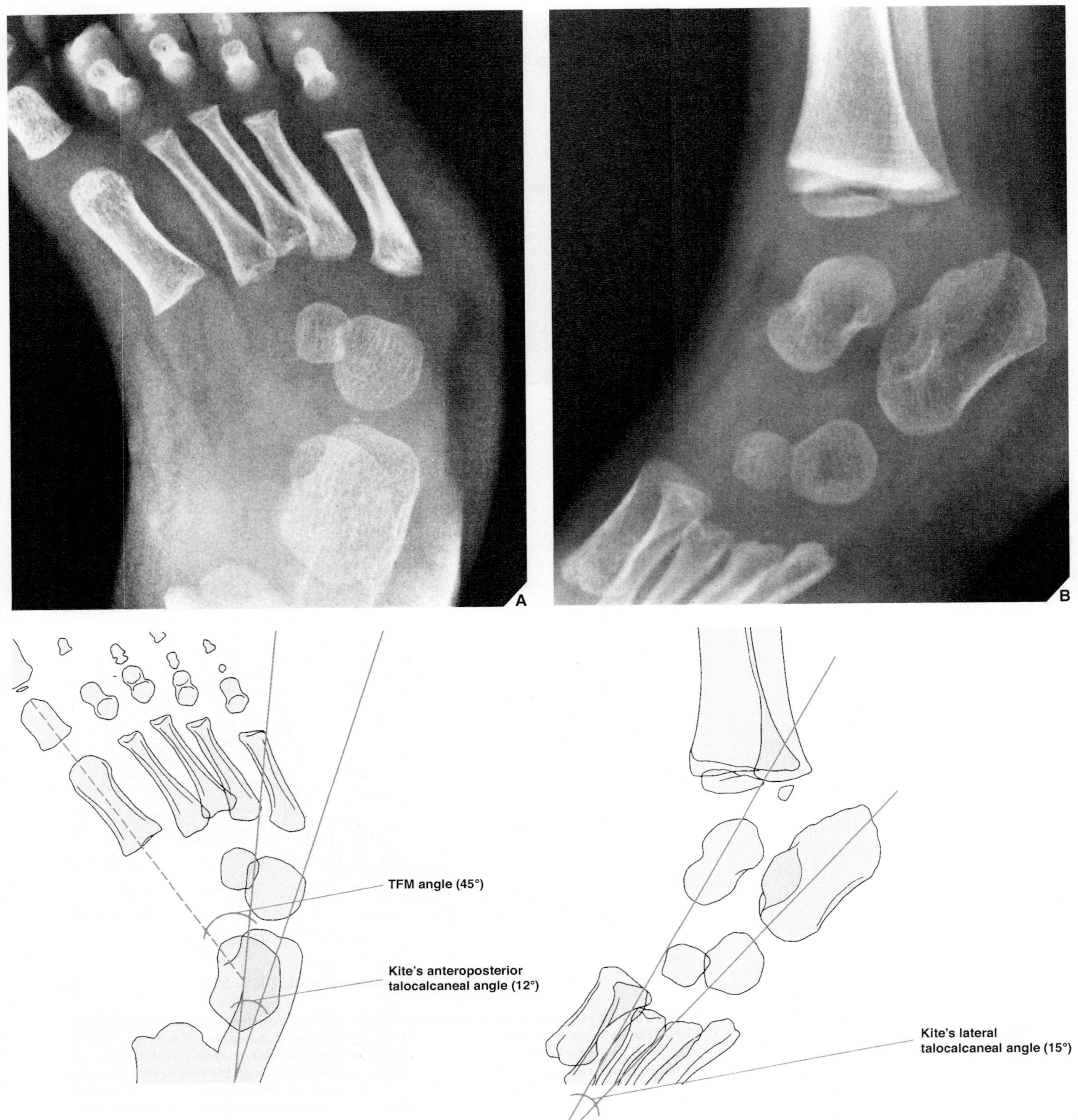

FIGURE 32.58 **Clubfoot deformity. (A)** Dorsoplantar radiograph of the left foot of a 2-year-old boy demonstrates a varus position of the hindfoot, as determined by the Kite anteroposterior talocalcaneal angle, as well as adduction of the forefoot, as indicated by the abnormal values of the TFM angle (see Fig. 32.57A). **(B)** On the lateral projection, an equinus position of the heel is evident from the determination of the Kite lateral talocalcaneal angle (see Fig. 32.57B).

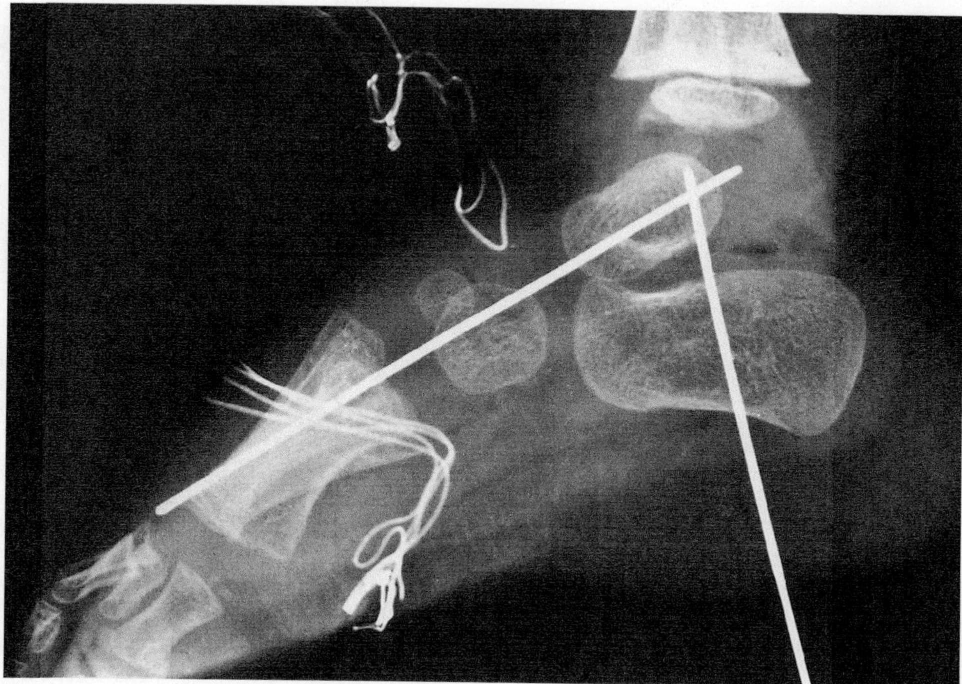

FIGURE 32.59 Treatment of the clubfoot deformity. Intraoperative radiograph of the foot of a 2-year-old girl was obtained to verify the degree of correction of a clubfoot. After soft-tissue release (Achilles tendon lengthening and a posterior ankle joint syndesmotomy), two Kirschner wires were passed across the talonavicular and subtalar joints to stabilize the hindfoot. Note the correction of the equinus deformity, as determined by the horizontal position of the calcaneus and the normal value of the Kite lateral talocalcaneal angle (compare with Fig. 32.58B).

Treatment

Most clubfoot deformities can be corrected with conservative treatment using various manipulations and casts. The necessary degree of correction can be determined from the lines and angles described previously. If complete correction cannot be achieved with conservative treatment, then surgical release is usually performed, and intraoperative radiography is used to confirm the results (Fig. 32.59). Radiographic evaluation is also essential after surgery to monitor the patient's progress. The most common complication of surgery for a clubfoot is related to overcorrection, which results in a rocker-bottom flat-foot deformity.

Congenital Vertical Talus

Congenital vertical talus, as its name denotes, consists of primary dislocations in the talonavicular and talocalcaneal joints, with the talus assuming a vertical position and pointing plantarly and medially. This anomaly, also known as *rocker-bottom foot*, occurs more often in males than in females and is usually diagnosed in the first few weeks after birth. This condition is usually associated with multiple other congenital anomalies and only rarely is an isolated deformity. The reported familial cases are inherited as an autosomal dominant mode with incomplete penetrance. Recent genetic investigations suggest that the mutation in the *HOXD10* gene located in chromosome 2q31 is a causative factor. The foot is usually in dorsiflexion, and a prominent bulge is present on the plantar surface in the midtarsal region. The entire foot may assume a "boat-shaped" or "Persian-slipper" configuration.

Imaging Features

Radiographic examination, particularly the lateral projection, is diagnostic. The talus is seen in a vertical position, and in children aged 2 to 3 years, the fully ossified navicular bone makes talonavicular dislocation obvious (Fig. 32.60). The presence of talonavicular dislocation differentiates this

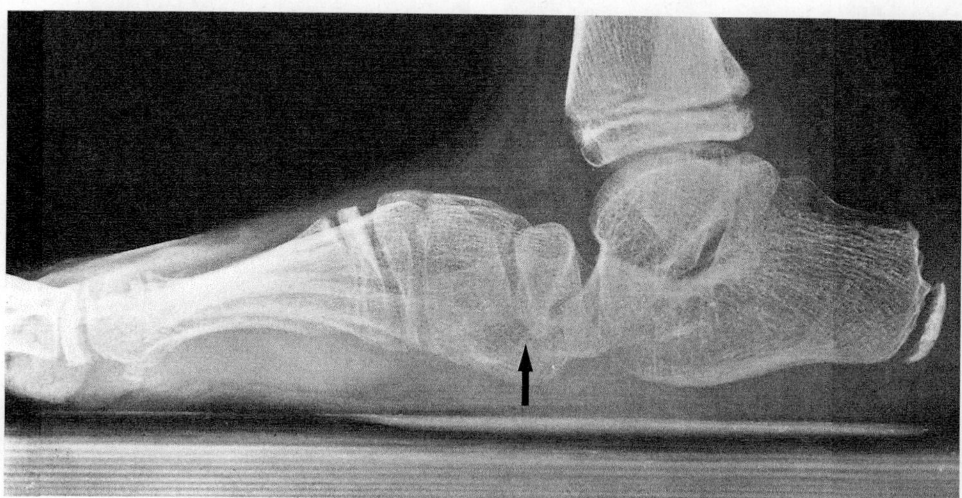

FIGURE 32.60 Congenital vertical talus. Lateral weight-bearing radiograph of the foot of a 12-year-old boy shows obvious dislocations in the talonavicular and talocalcaneal articulations. Note the hourglass deformity of the talus and the wedging of the navicular bone *(arrow)*.

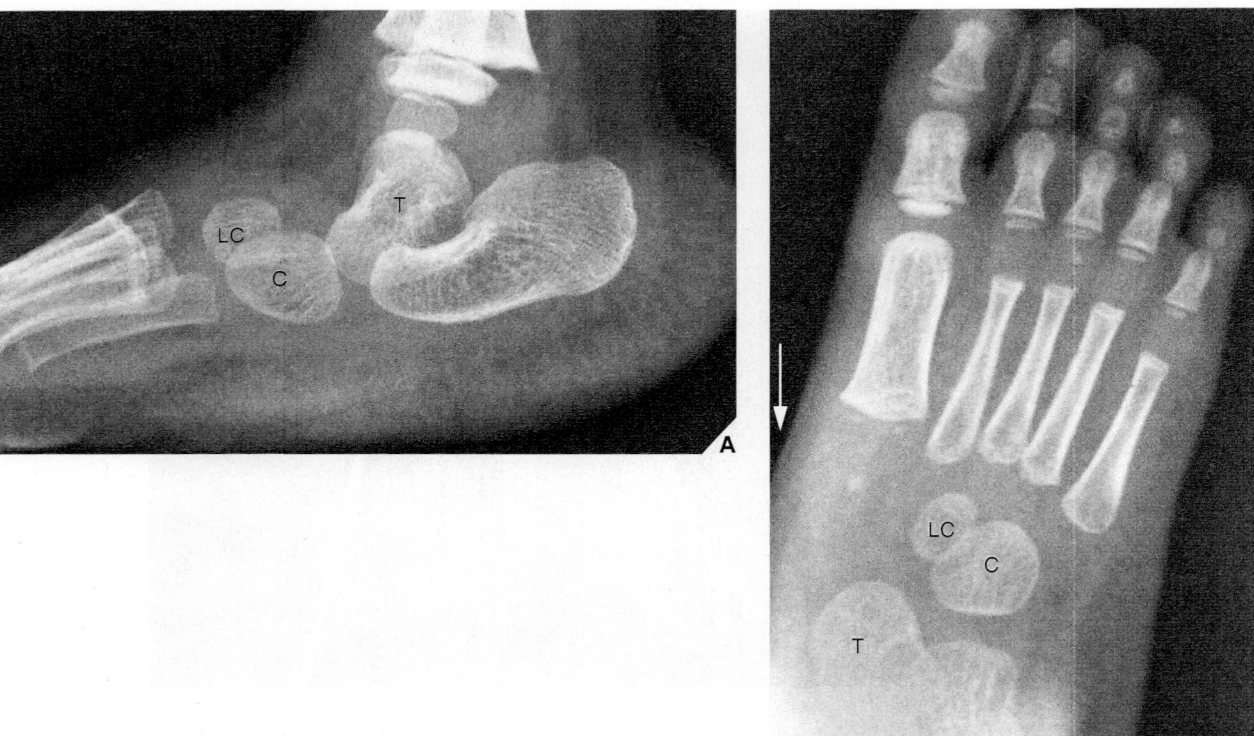

FIGURE 32.61 Congenital vertical talus. **(A)** Lateral radiograph of the foot of a 2-year-old boy demonstrates the vertical position of the talus and the equinus position of the calcaneus. Note the flattening of the longitudinal arch and the alignment of the lateral cuneiform bone with the talar neck. **(B)** Dorsoplantar radiograph shows the talus pointing medially; the navicular bone is not yet ossified. Note the soft-tissue bulge at the medial aspect of the foot *(arrow)*. *T*, talus; *C*, cuboid; *LC*, lateral cuneiform.

condition from the developmental flat-foot deformity. Before ossification of the navicular bone occurs, congenital vertical talus can be identified on the lateral radiograph by a slight equinus position of the calcaneus, by widening of the calcaneocuboid joint, and by a valgus position of the forefoot, which is dorsiflexed at the midtarsal joint. The longitudinal arch is reversed, and the entire foot assumes a "rocker-bottom" configuration (Fig. 32.61A). The dorsoplantar projection characteristically reveals medial displacement of the distal talus and abduction of the forefoot (Fig. 32.61B). It is important to obtain a lateral radiograph with the foot in forced plantar flexion to see whether the dislocation can be reduced (Fig. 32.62) because on the basis of this finding, the surgeon can decide not only between conservative and surgical treatment but also on the type of operation to perform.

Treatment

Most cases of congenital vertical talus require surgical correction of the deformity by soft-tissue release, reduction of the dislocation, and pinning of the talus to the navicular bone (Fig. 32.63). In children older than age 6 years, the navicular bone is resected. Radiographic confirmation of the correction is essential.

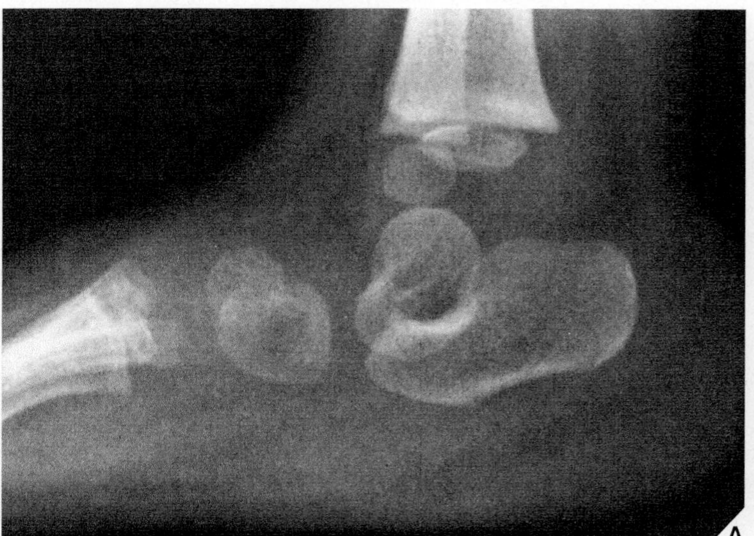

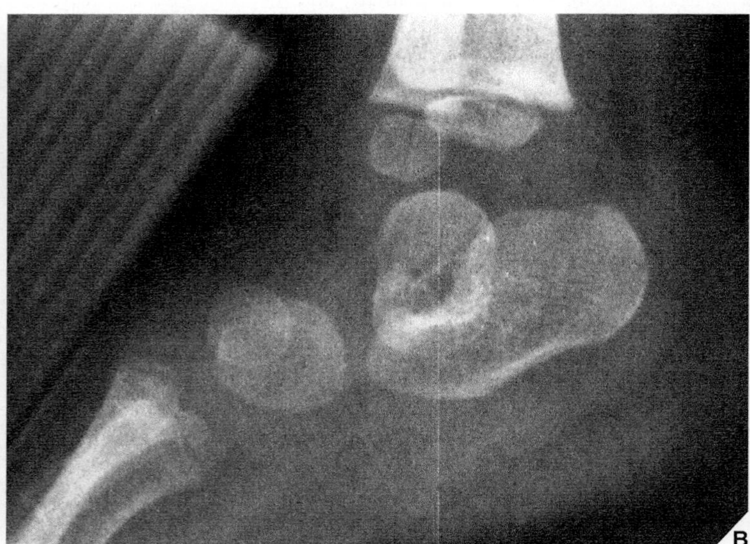

FIGURE 32.62 Congenital vertical talus. **(A)** Lateral radiograph of the foot of a 2-year-old girl shows the vertical orientation of the talus, as well as talonavicular dislocation, although the navicular bone is not ossified. **(B)** Forced plantar flexion of the foot does not reduce the dislocation.

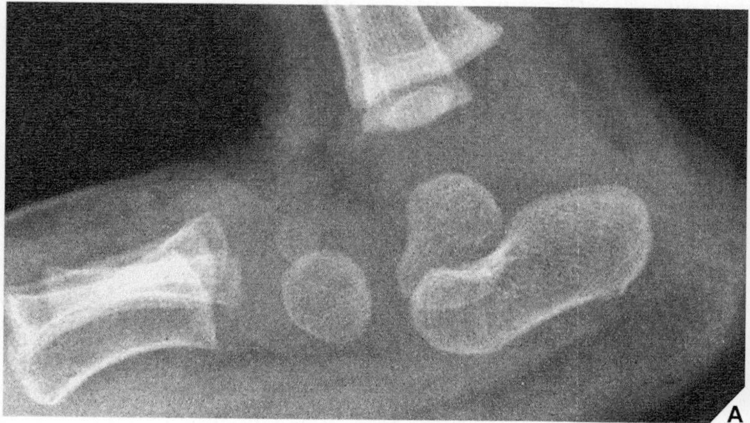

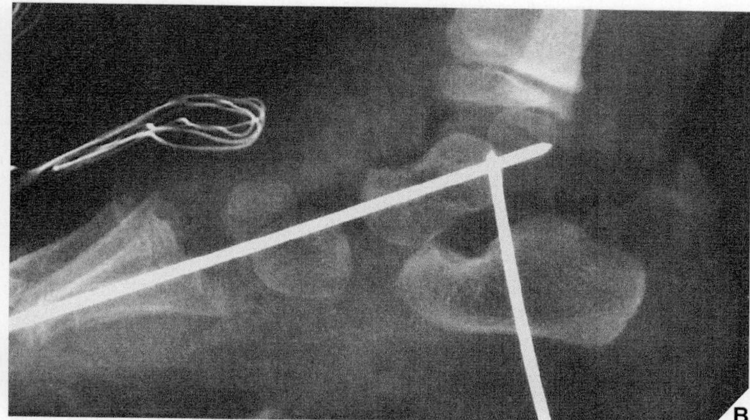

FIGURE 32.63 Congenital vertical talus. **(A)** Preoperative radiograph of the foot of a 2-year-old girl shows the longitudinal axis of the talus in continuity with that of the tibia. **(B)** Intraoperative film demonstrates satisfactory reduction of the talonavicular dislocation.

Tarsal Coalition

Tarsal coalition refers to the fusion of two or more tarsal bones to form a single structure. This fusion may be complete or incomplete, and the bridge may be fibrous (syndesmosis), cartilaginous (synchondrosis), or osseous (synostosis). Various bones may be affected, but most commonly, the coalition occurs between the calcaneus and navicular bone, less frequently between the talus and calcaneus, and least often between the talus and navicular and calcaneus and cuboid bones. At times, more than two bones may be affected. Despite its occurrence at birth, signs and symptoms of tarsal coalition rarely develop before the patient's second or third decade. Pain, particularly associated with prolonged walking or standing, is a typical presenting symptom. On physical examination, peroneal muscular spasm and restricted joint mobility (the so-called *peroneal spastic foot*) are revealed.

Although the clinical presentation usually suggests the correct diagnosis, radiologic examination is diagnostic. The primary sign of tarsal coalition is evidence of fusion. Secondary signs may also be present, such as dysmorphic sustentaculum tali, nonvisualization of the middle subtalar facet, the talar beak (see Figs. 32.69, 32.70, and 32.72), shortening of the talar neck, or ball-and-socket ankle joint (see Fig. 32.68), representing adaptive alterations of the affected and adjacent bones and articulations.

Calcaneonavicular Coalition

The best projection for demonstrating this type of fusion is either lateral or a 45-degree medial (internal) oblique view of the foot (Fig. 32.64), although CT may at times be useful. The anteater snout (nose) sign is characteristic for this anomaly. This sign, visible on the lateral radiograph of the ankle, is caused by a tubular elongation of the anterior process of the calcaneus that approaches or overlaps the navicular bone and resembles the snout of an anteater (Fig. 32.65). The secondary signs include hypoplasia of the talus head. MRI is effective in demonstrating cartilaginous or fibrous coalition (Fig. 32.66).

Talonavicular Coalition

This rare type of tarsal coalition is best seen on the lateral radiograph of the foot or on CT and MRI examinations (Figs. 32.67 and 32.68).

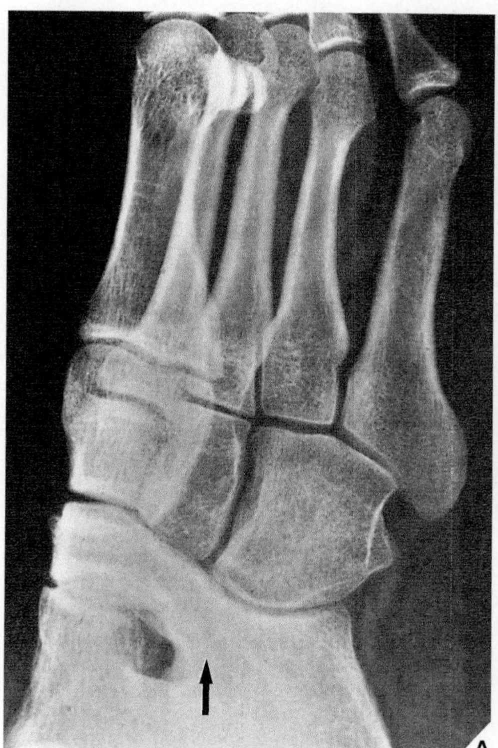

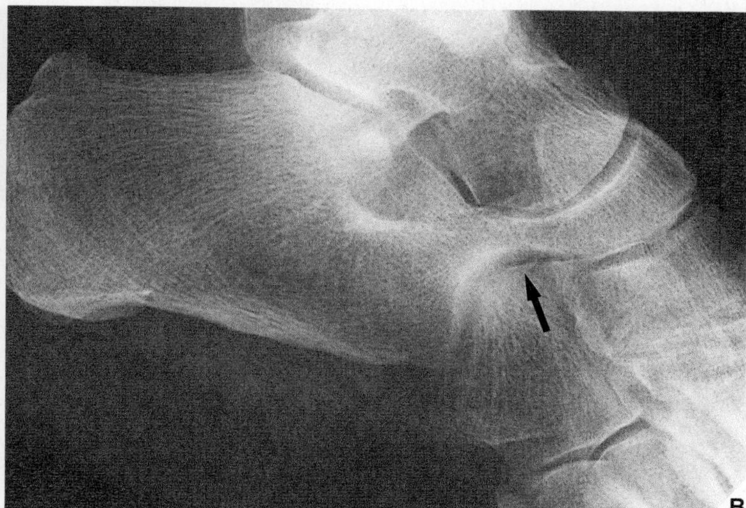

FIGURE 32.64 Calcaneonavicular coalition. **(A)** A 45-degree internal oblique projection of the foot of an 18-year-old man demonstrates solid osseous bridge between the calcaneus and navicular bones *(arrow)*. **(B)** In another patient, a lateral radiograph of the foot demonstrates a similar osseous fusion of these two bones *(arrow)*.

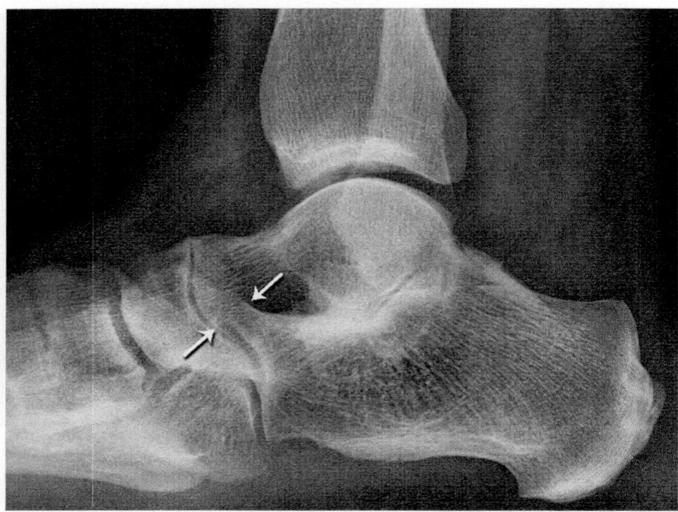

FIGURE 32.65 Calcaneonavicular coalition. Lateral radiograph of the foot of a 27-year-old woman shows characteristic for this anomaly, the anteater nose sign *(arrows)*.

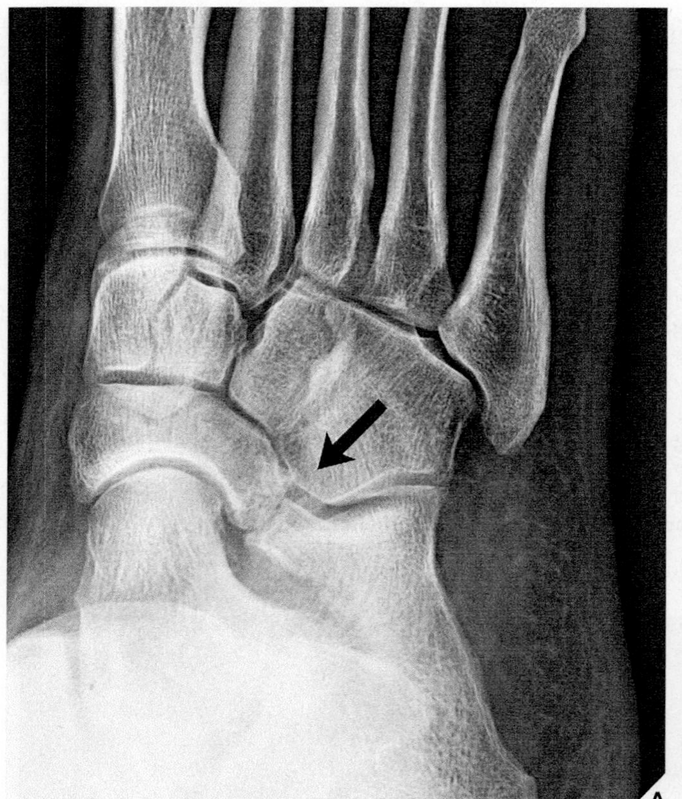

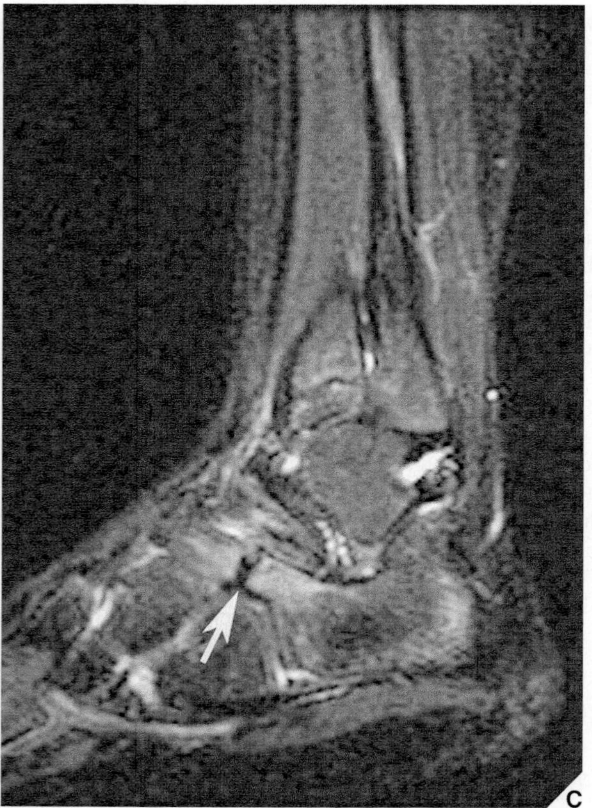

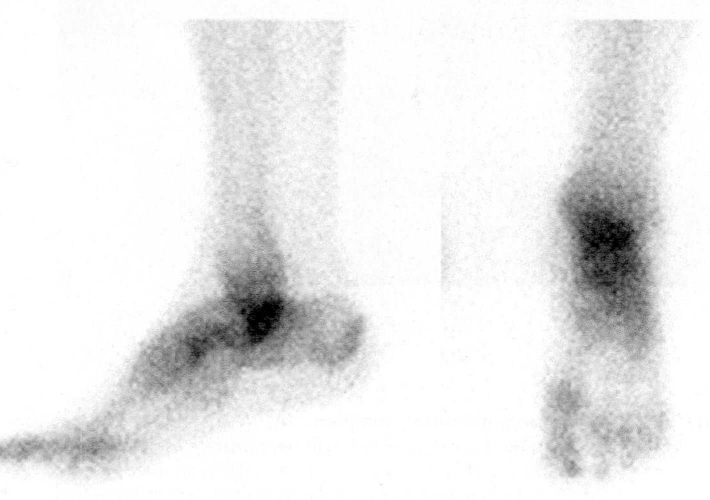

FIGURE 32.66 Scintigraphy and MRI of calcaneonavicular coalition. **(A)** Oblique radiograph of the left foot of a 38-year-old man shows decreased distance between the anterior process of the calcaneus and navicular bone *(arrow)*. **(B)** Radionuclide bone scan of the left foot obtained after intravenous injection of 25 mCi (925 MBq) of technetium-99m methylene diphosphonate (^{99m}Tc-MDP) shows increased uptake of the radiopharmaceutical tracer in the region of navicular bone and subtalar joint. **(C)** Sagittal short time inversion recovery (STIR) MR image demonstrates low–signal intensity band at the calcaneonavicular junction *(arrow)*, representing a fibrous coalition. Note the stress edema of the anterior process of the calcaneus and lateral pole of the navicular, due to altered biomechanics of the foot.

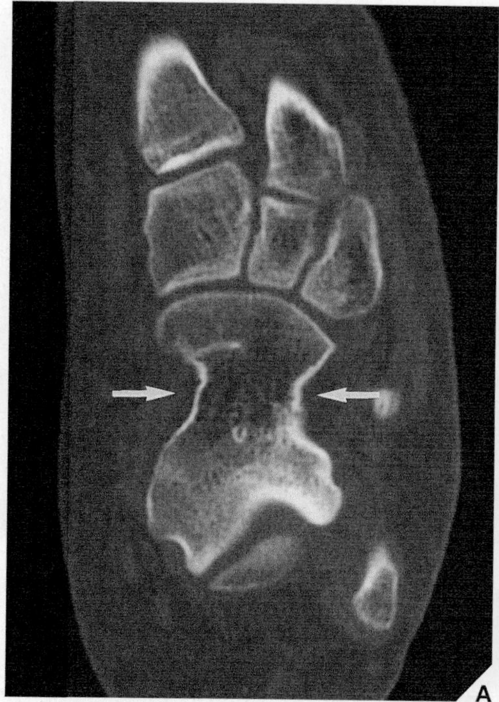

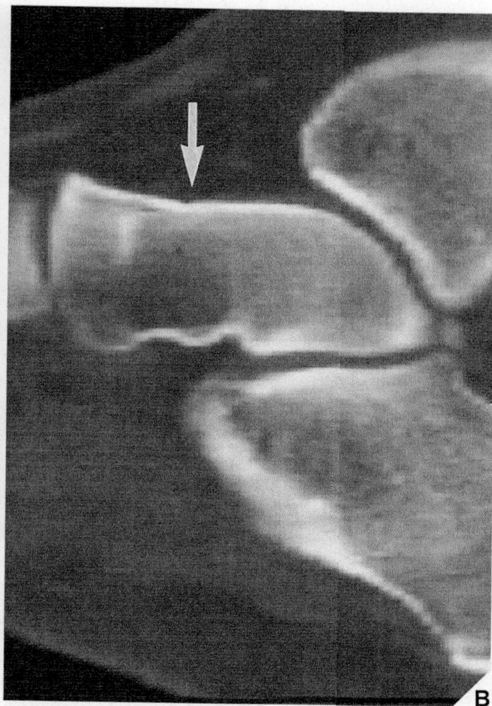

FIGURE 32.67 CT of talonavicular coalition. **(A)** Axial and **(B)** reformatted sagittal CT sections show a solid osseous fusion of the talus and navicular bones *(arrows)* in a 17-year-old boy.

Talocalcaneal Coalition

Because osseous fusion of the talus and calcaneus most often occurs at the level of the sustentaculum tali and the middle facet of the subtalar joint, it can effectively be demonstrated on oblique and Harris-Beath (posterior tangential) projections (Fig. 32.69); occasionally, CT or MRI examinations may also be useful (Figs. 32.70 to 32.74). In suspected cartilaginous or fibrous union that is not readily demonstrated on radiographs, secondary changes should be sought, such as close apposition of the articular surfaces of the middle facet of the subtalar joint, eburnation and sclerosis of the articular margins, and broadening or rounding of the lateral process of the talus. Moreover, a C-shaped continuous line extending from the talus to the sustentaculum tali (the so-called *C sign*, originally described by Lateur et al. in 1994) is visible on lateral radiographs of the ankle (see Figs. 32.72A, 32.73A, and 32.74A). This line is created by the combined shadows of the talar dome and the fused facets of the subtalar joint, together with a prominent inferior outline of the sustentaculum tali. In addition, the so-called *absent middle facet sign*, which refers to the lack of visualization of the middle facet of the subtalar joint on standing lateral view of the ankle and originally described by Harris in 1955, may be helpful in diagnosing this anomaly. A common secondary sign of talocalcaneal coalition is an osseous excrescence at the dorsal aspect of the talus, forming what is called a *talar beak* (see Figs. 32.69A and 32.70A), which is seen in the osseous, chondrus, and fibrous types of coalition. It is important to keep in mind, however, that a similar hypertrophy of the talar ridge may be seen in other conditions as well; for example, it may be related to abnormal capsular and ligamentous traction associated with degenerative changes in the talonavicular joint (Fig. 32.75). Demonstration of nonosseous forms of tarsal coalition may require subtalar arthrography or MRI (see Fig. 32.73). Similarly, when the clinical presentation is unclear and standard radiographs are equivocal, radionuclide bone scan may help localize the site of coalition by an increased uptake of radiopharmaceutical tracer, although this is a nonspecific finding.

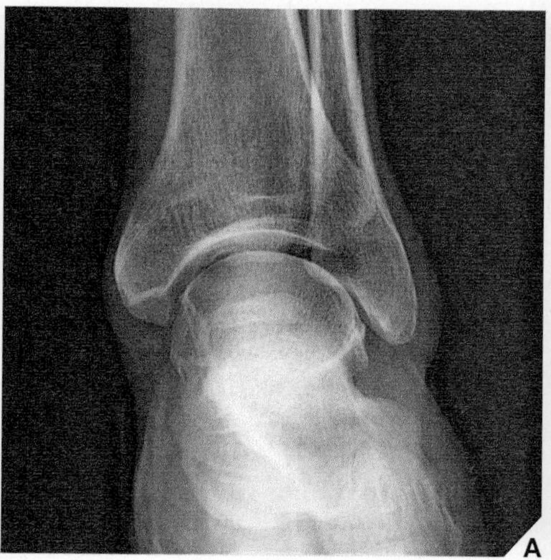

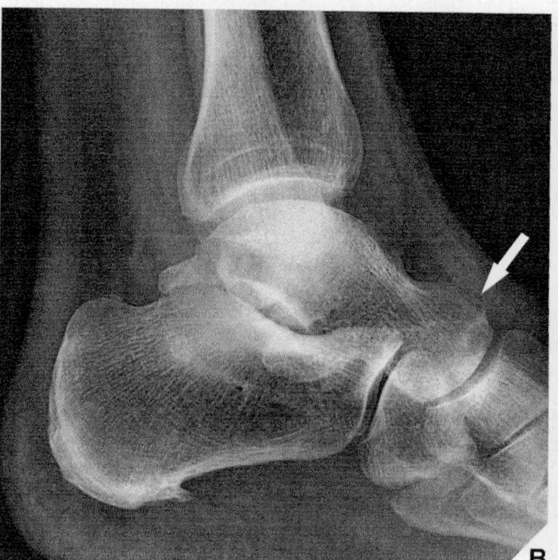

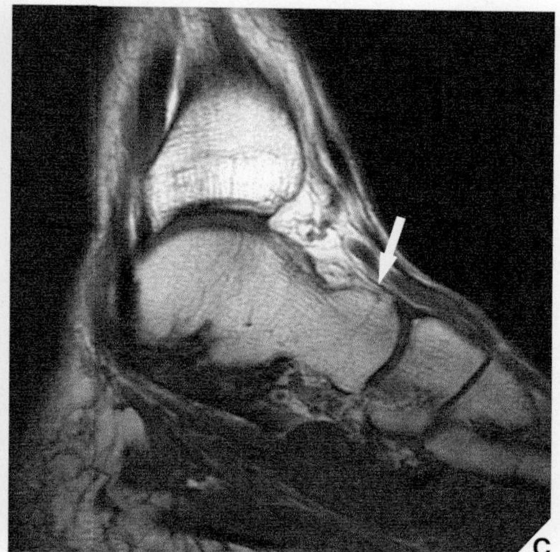

FIGURE 32.68 MRI of talonavicular coalition. **(A)** Anteroposterior radiograph of a 52-year-old man shows a ball-and-socket deformity of the ankle joint. **(B)** Lateral radiograph and **(C)** sagittal T1-weighted MR image show osseous fusion of the talus and navicular bones *(arrows)*.

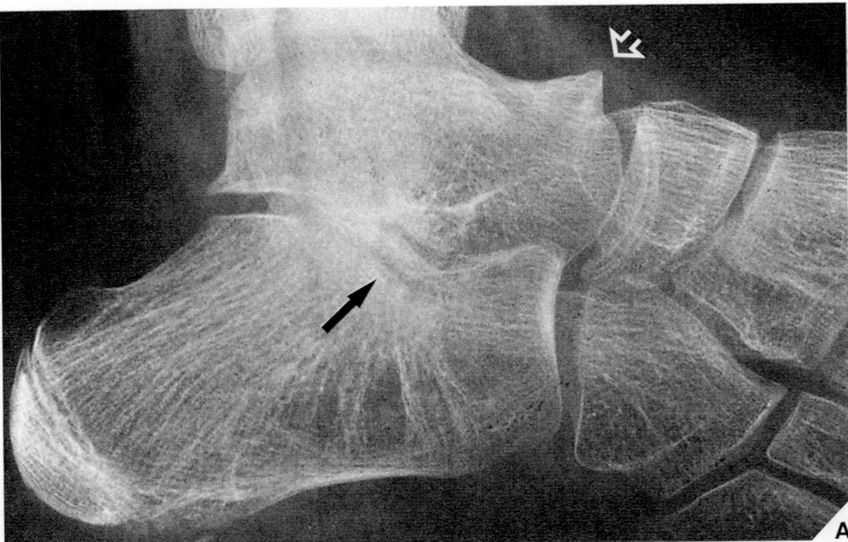

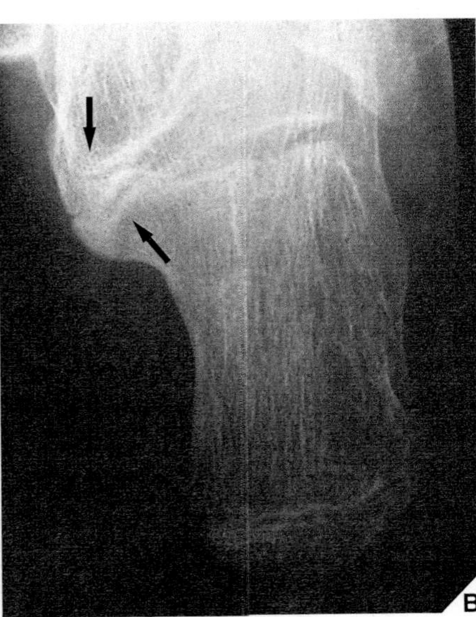

FIGURE 32.69 Talocalcaneal coalition. **(A)** Oblique radiograph of the hindfoot of a 12-year-old boy shows obliteration of the middle facet of the subtalar joint *(arrow)*. Note the prominent talar beak *(open arrow)*. **(B)** A Harris-Beath view confirms the osseous talocalcaneal coalition *(arrows)*.

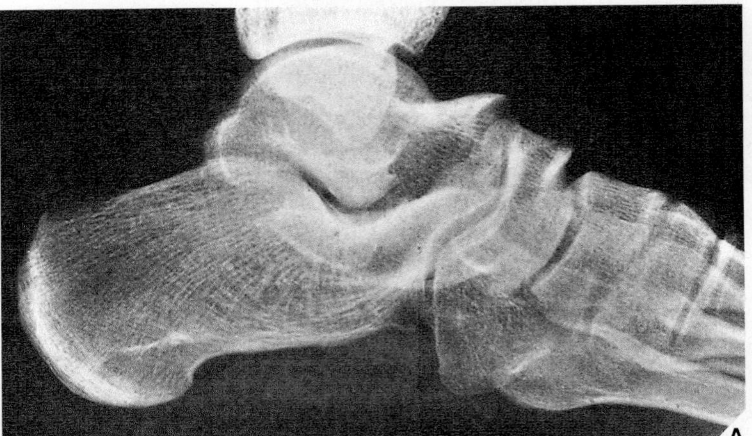

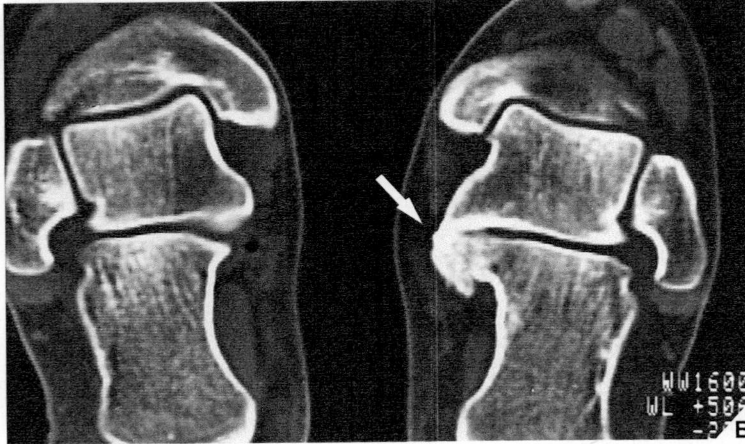

FIGURE 32.70 CT of talocalcaneal coalition. A 25-year-old man presented with pain in his left foot that was particularly pronounced after prolonged walking or standing. **(A)** Lateral radiograph of the left foot shows sclerotic changes in the middle facet of the subtalar joint, narrowing of the posterior talocalcaneal joint space, and a prominent talar beak—features suggesting tarsal coalition. **(B)** Coronal CT section clearly demonstrates narrowing of the middle facet joint space and an osseous bridge *(arrow)*. The normal right foot is shown for comparison.

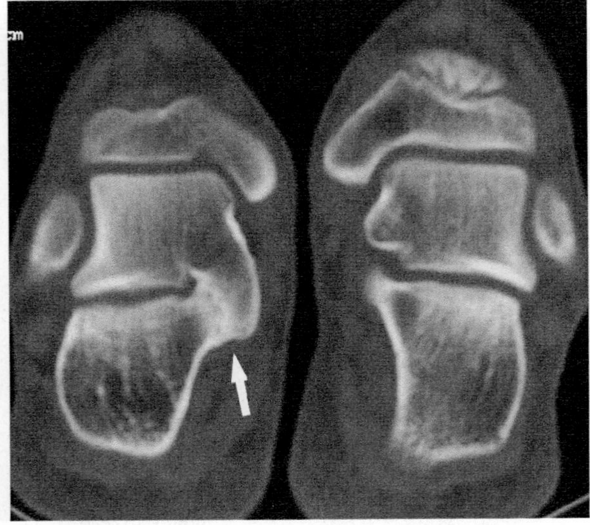

FIGURE 32.71 CT of talocalcaneal coalition. A coronal CT scan in a 12-year-old boy with right foot pain shows an osseous talocalcaneal coalition at the site of the middle subtalar facet *(arrow)*. The left foot is normal.

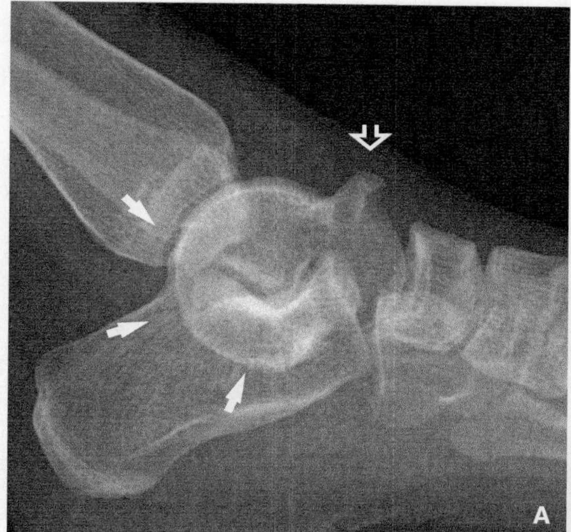

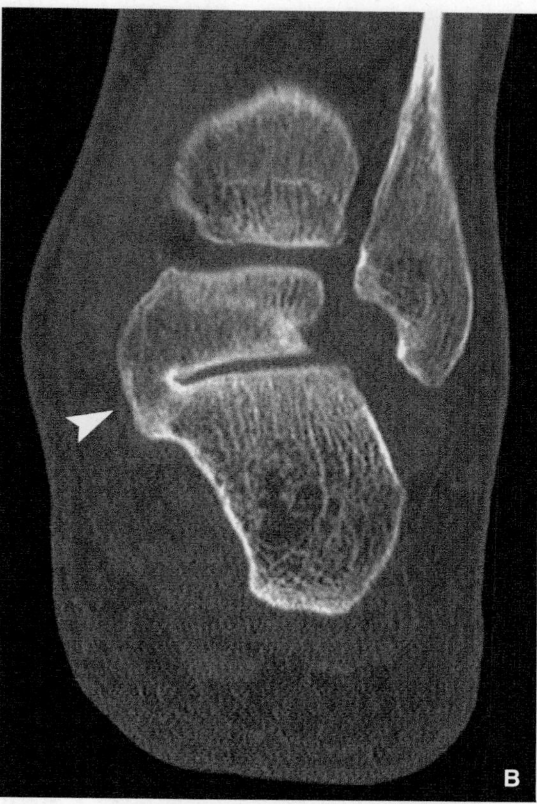

FIGURE 32.72 CT of talocalcaneal coalition. **(A)** Lateral radiograph of the ankle of a 19-year-old woman shows a prominent anterior talar beak *(open arrow)* and a "C" sign *(arrows)*, created by combined shadows of the talar dome and fused middle facet of the subtalar joint. **(B)** CT section confirms the osseous fusion at the site of the middle subtalar facet *(arrowhead)*.

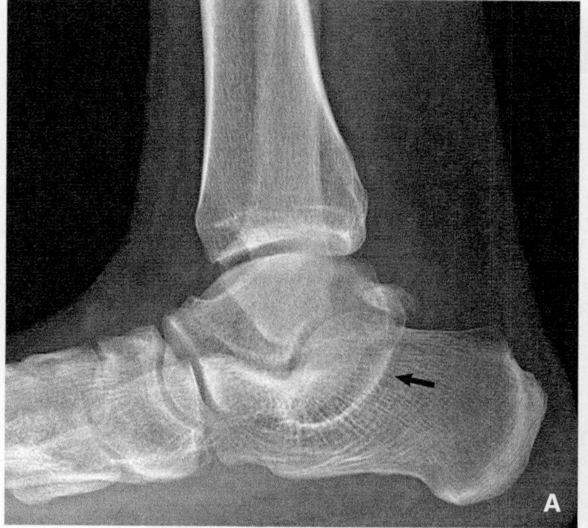

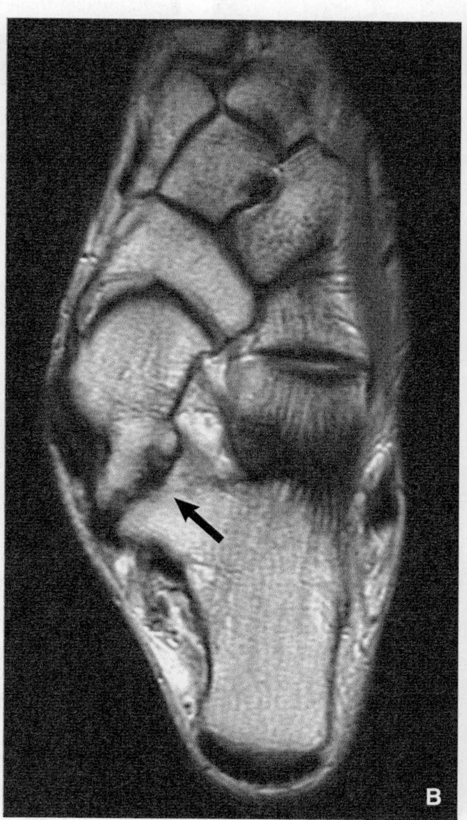

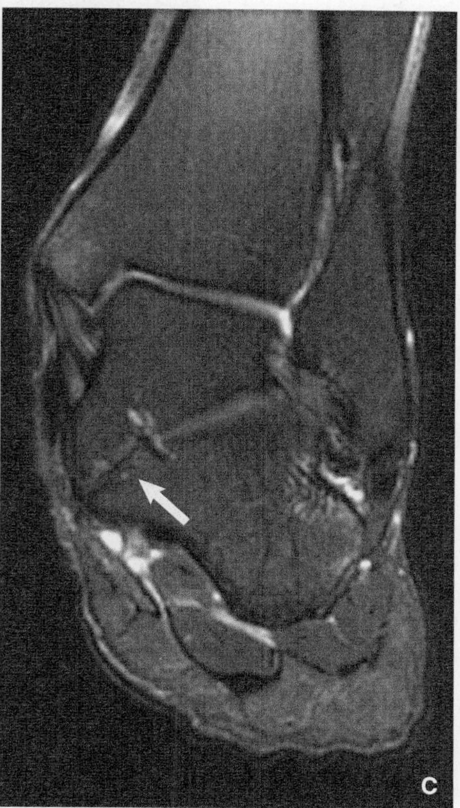

FIGURE 32.73 MRI of talocalcaneal coalition. **(A)** Lateral radiograph of the left ankle of a 35-year-old man shows flat foot deformity and typical "C"-sign *(arrow)*. **(B)** Axial proton density–weighted and **(C)** coronal T2-weighted MR images confirm fibrous talocalcaneal coalition *(arrows)*.

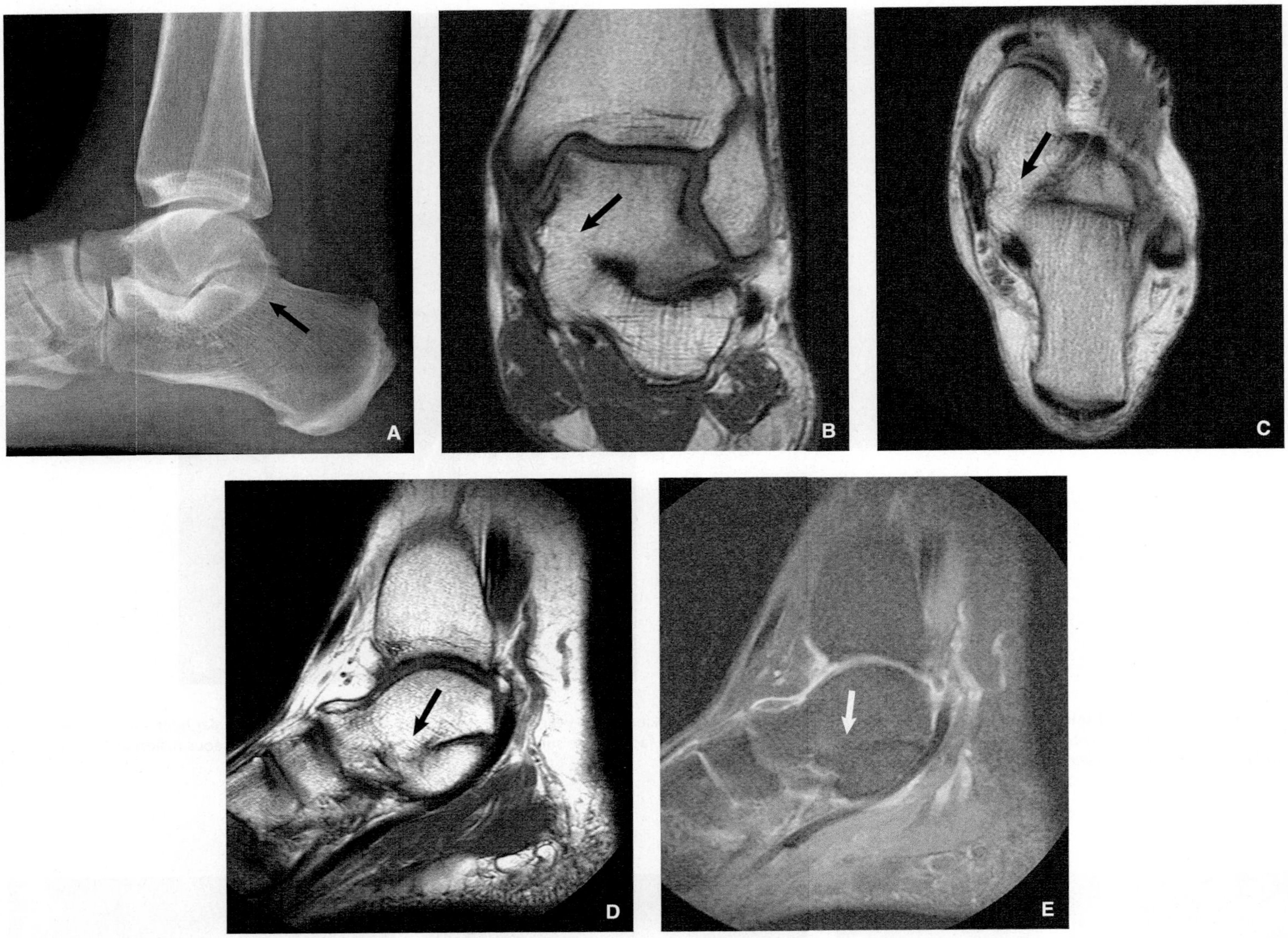

FIGURE 32.74 **MRI of talocalcaneal coalition.** **(A)** Lateral radiograph of the left ankle of a 61- year-old woman shows a "C"-sign *(arrow)*. **(B)** Coronal T1-weighted, **(C)** axial T1-weighted, **(D)** sagittal T1-weighted, and **(E)** sagittal proton density–weighted fat-suppressed MR images confirm the presence of solid osseous talocalcaneal coalition *(arrows)*.

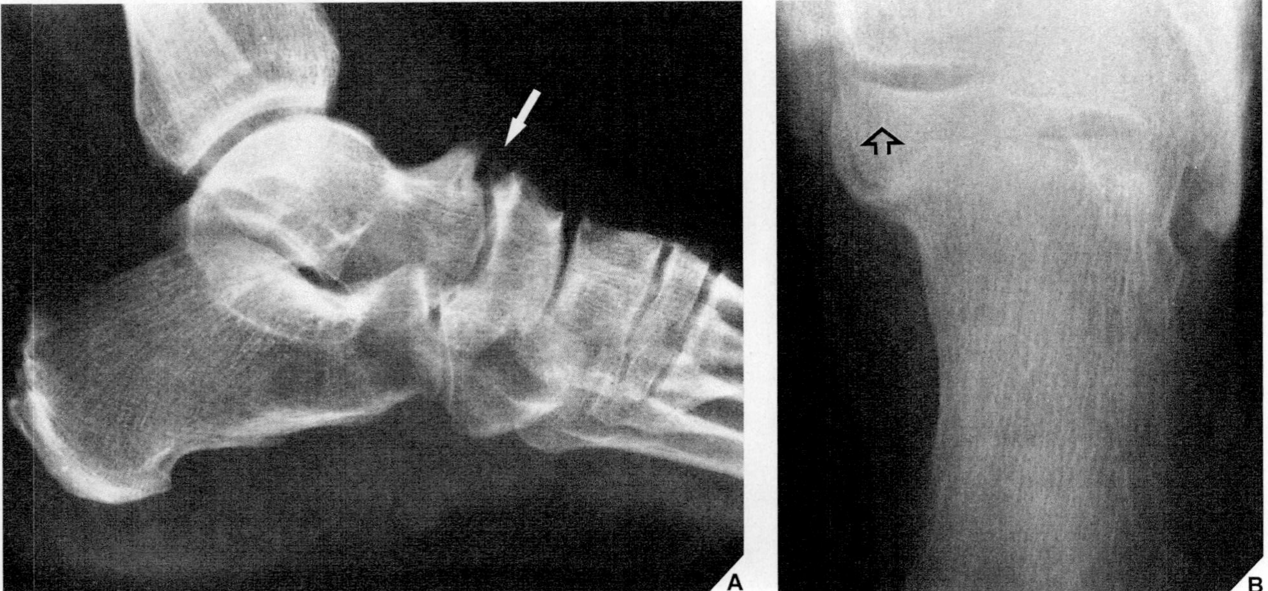

FIGURE 32.75 **Talonavicular osteoarthritis.** **(A)** Lateral radiograph of the foot of a 61-year-old woman demonstrates a talar beak and degenerative changes in the talonavicular joint *(arrow)*. The middle and posterior facets of the subtalar joint appear normal. **(B)** A Harris-Beath view shows normal middle facet of subtalar joint *(open arrow)* and no evidence of tarsal coalition.

PRACTICAL POINTS TO REMEMBER

Anomalies of the Shoulder Girdle and Upper Limbs

1. Congenital elevation of the scapula (Sprengel deformity) is frequently accompanied by other anomalies, most commonly Klippel-Feil syndrome (fusion of the cervical or upper thoracic vertebrae).
2. Dentate scapula, also referred to as *glenoid hypoplasia*, is a rare congenital anomaly due to underdevelopment of the ossification center for the inferior glenoid, leading to glenoid retroversion, small glenoid, and predisposition to precocious osteoarthritis of the glenohumeral joint.
3. A Madelung deformity can be effectively evaluated on the posteroanterior and lateral radiographs of the distal forearm and wrist. The constant findings include:
   - a decreased radial and an increased ulnar length
   - medial and dorsal bowing of the radius
   - a triangular configuration of the carpal bones with the lunate at the apex.

Anomalies of the Pelvic Girdle and Hip

1. CDH is bilateral in more than 25% of affected children; therefore, in apparently unilateral cases the unaffected hip should be carefully examined.
2. Several lines and angles can be drawn on an anteroposterior radiograph of the pelvis and hips to help determine CDH:
   - the Hilgenreiner Y-line
   - the Perkins-Ombredanne line
   - the Andrén-von Rosen line
   - the Shenton-Menard arc
   - the acetabular index
   - the C-E angle of Wiberg.
3. In addition to conventional radiography, the imaging evaluation of CDH requires arthrography and CT scan, which is particularly valuable in monitoring the results of treatment.
4. Ultrasound is a highly effective technique to diagnose and evaluate congenital hip dysplasia. The osseous and cartilaginous components of the hip joint are well demonstrated, and acetabular coverage of the femoral head can be assessed.
5. 3D ultrasound of the infant hip offers a unique image in the sagittal plane and allows evaluation of the joint from the craniocaudal (bird's eye) view.
6. Before conservative or surgical treatment, skin or skeletal traction is applied to bring the dislocated femoral head to "station +2" to avoid osteonecrosis of the femoral head.
7. The Gage and Winter traction stations are determined by the position of the proximal femoral metaphysis (femoral neck) relative to the ipsilateral acetabulum and contralateral normal hip.
8. PFFD can mimic congenital hip dislocation. Arthrography is helpful in distinguishing these anomalies by demonstrating:
   - presence of the femoral head in the acetabulum in type A
   - a defect in the femoral neck in type B
   - the absence of the femoral head in types C and D.
9. Legg-Calvé-Perthes disease (coxa plana) represents osteonecrosis (ischemic necrosis) of the proximal epiphysis of the femur. The imaging evaluation of this condition includes:
   - a radionuclide bone scan, particularly in the early stages
   - conventional radiography
   - contrast arthrography
   - MRI.
10. The most frequently encountered radiographic findings in Legg-Calvé-Perthes disease include:
    - periarticular osteoporosis
    - increased density and flattening of the capital epiphysis
    - a crescent sign
    - fissuring and fragmentation of the epiphysis
    - cystic changes in the metaphysis and broadening of the femoral neck
    - lateral subluxation in the hip joint.
11. A femoral "head-at-risk" in Legg-Calvé-Perthes disease is defined by five radiographic signs indicating a poor prognosis:
    - a radiolucent, V-shaped defect in the lateral portion of the femoral head (Gage sign)
    - calcifications lateral to the femoral epiphysis
    - lateral subluxation of the femoral head
    - a horizontal orientation of the growth plate
    - diffuse metaphyseal cystic changes.
12. Sagging rope sign is a characteristic feature of an advanced Legg-Calvé-Perthes disease.
13. An SCFE is a Salter-Harris type I fracture through the physis, which is best demonstrated on the frog-lateral projection. Important diagnostic clues include:
    - loss of the triangle sign of Capener
    - decreased height of the epiphysis
    - widening and blurring of the growth plate
    - lack of intersection of the epiphysis by the lateral cortical line of the femoral neck.

Anomalies of the Lower Limbs

1. Congenital tibia vara (Blount disease) can be differentiated from developmental bowing of the legs by its characteristic presentation with depression of the medial tibial metaphysis associated with abrupt angulation and the formation of a beak-like prominence on the metaphysis.
2. Dysplasia epiphysealis hemimelica (Trevor-Fairbank disease) most often affects the ankle joint. The radiographic hallmark of this lesion, which histologically resembles osteochondroma, is an irregular bulbous overgrowth of one side of the ossification center or epiphysis.
3. The clubfoot deformity is recognized radiographically by:
   - an equinus position of the heel
   - a varus position of the hindfoot
   - adduction and a varus position of the forefoot
   - talonavicular subluxation.
4. In the evaluation of the clubfoot deformity, certain angles and lines drawn on the anteroposterior and lateral radiographs of the foot are helpful:
   - the Kite anteroposterior and lateral talocalcaneal angles
   - the TFM angle
   - the extension of lines drawn through the longitudinal axis of the talus and the calcaneus.
5. Proper positioning of the feet is a crucial factor in the radiographic evaluation of infants and small children. Weight-bearing films should be obtained whenever feasible; in small infants, the foot should be pressed against the radiographic cassette.
6. Congenital vertical talus can be distinguished from developmental flat foot by the presence of dislocation in the talonavicular and talocalcaneal articulations.
7. In tarsal coalition, the most common cause of the so-called *peroneal spastic foot deformity*, fusion of the affected bones (usually the talus and calcaneus or calcaneus and navicular bone) may be:
   - fibrous (syndesmosis)
   - cartilaginous (synchondrosis)
   - osseous (synostosis).
8. The imaging evaluation of tarsal coalition includes:
   - conventional radiographs in the lateral projection (which reveals the most frequently encountered secondary sign of this condition, the formation of a talar beak) as well as in Harris-Beath and oblique projections
   - CT
   - subtalar arthrography
   - MRI, which may reveal cartilaginous or fibrous coalition.

SUGGESTED READINGS

Apley AG, Wientrob S. The sagging rope sign in Perthes disease and allied disorders. *J Bone Joint Surg Br* 1981;63-B:43–47.

Bahk W-J, Lee H-Y, Kang Y-K, et al. Dysplasia epiphysealis hemimelica: radiographic and magnetic resonance imaging features and clinical outcome of complete and incomplete resection. *Skeletal Radiol* 2010;39:85–90.

Bateson EM. Non-rachitic bowleg and knock-knee deformities in young Jamaican children. *Br J Radiol* 1966;39:92.

Bateson EM. The relationship between Blount's disease and bow legs. *Br J Radiol* 1968;41:107–114.

Bathfield CA, Beighton PH. Blount disease. A review of etiological factors in 110 patients. *Clin Orthop Relat Res* 1978;135:29–33.

Bellyei A, Mike G. Weight bearing in Perthes' disease. *Orthopedics* 1991;14:19–22.

Beltran LS, Rosenberg ZS, Mayo JD, et al. Imaging evaluation of developmental hip dysplasia in the young adult. *AJR Am J Roentgenol* 2013;200:1077–1088.

Bennett JT, Mazurek RT, Cash JD. Chiari's osteotomy in the treatment of Perthes' disease. *J Bone Joint Surg Br* 1991;73B:225–228.

Blount WP. Tibia vara. Osteochondrosis deformans tibiae. *J Bone Joint Surg* 1937;19:1–29.

Borggreve J. Kniegelenksersatz durch das in der Beinlangsachse um 180 Gedrehte Fussgelenk. *Arch Orthop Unfall-Chir* 1930;28:175–178.

Bos CF, Bloem JL, Obermann WR, et al. Magnetic resonance imaging in congenital dislocation of the hip. *J Bone Joint Surg Br* 1988;70-B:174–178.

Brown RR, Rosenberg ZS, Thornhill BA. The C sign: more specific for flatfoot deformity than subtalar coalition. *Skeletal Radiol* 2001;30:84–87.

Catterall A. *Legg-Calvé-Perthes' disease.* New York: Churchill Livingstone; 1982.

Catterall A. The natural history of Perthes' disease. *J Bone Joint Surg Br* 1971;53B:37–53.

Chapman VM. The anteater nose sign. *Radiology* 2007;245:604–605.

Cheema JI, Grissom LE, Harcke HT. Radiographic characteristics of lower-extremity bowing in children. *Radiographics* 2003;23:871–880.

Craig JG, van Holsbeeck M, Zaltz I. The utility of MR in assessing Blount disease. *Skeletal Radiol* 2002;31:208–213.

Crim JR, Kjeldsberg KM. Radiographic diagnosis of tarsal coalition. *AJR Am J Roentgenol* 2004;182:323–328.

Crowe JF, Mani VJ, Ranawat CS. Total hip replacement in congenital dislocation and dysplasia of the hip. *J Bone Joint Surg Am* 1979;61(1):15–23.

Dannenberg M, Anton JI, Spiegel MB. Madelung's deformity. Consideration of its roentgenological diagnostic criteria. *Am J Roentgenol* 1939;42:671.

Dillman JR, Hernandez R. MRI of Legg-Calve-Perthes disease. *AJR Am J Roentgenol* 2009;193:1394–1407.

Ducou le Pointe H, Mousselard H, Rudelli A, et al. Blount's disease: magnetic resonance imaging. *Pediatric Radiol* 1995;25:12–14.

Dunn PM. Perinatal observations on the etiology of congenital dislocation of the hip. *Clin Orthop Relat Res* 1976;(119):11–22.

Dunn PM. The anatomy and pathology of congenital dislocation of the hip. *Clin Orthop Relat Res* 1976;(119):23–27.

Egund N, Wingstrand H. Legg-Calvé-Perthes disease: imaging with MR. *Radiology* 1991;179:89–92.

Fairbank TJ. Dysplasia epiphysealis hemimelica (tarso-epiphysial aclasis). *J Bone Joint Surg Br* 1956;38-B:237–257.

Fisher R, O'Brien TS, Davis KM. Magnetic resonance imaging in congenital dysplasia of the hip. *J Pediatr Orthop* 1991;11:617–622.

Gage JR, Winter RB. Avascular necrosis of the capital femoral epiphysis as a complication of closed reduction of congenital dislocation of the hip. A critical review of twenty years' experience at Gillette Children's Hospital. *J Bone Joint Surg Am* 1972;54(2):373–388.

Ganz R, Klaue K, Vinh TS, et al. A new periacetabular osteotomy for the treatment of hip dysplasias. Technique and preliminary results. *Clin Orthop Relat Res* 1988;232:26–36.

Gerscovich EO. A radiologist's guide to the imaging in the diagnosis and treatment of developmental dysplasia of the hip. I. General considerations, physical examination as applied to real-time sonography and radiology. *Skeletal Radiol* 1997;26:386–397.

Gerscovich EO. A radiologist's guide to the imaging in the diagnosis and treatment of developmental dysplasia of the hip. II. Ultrasonography: anatomy, technique, acetabular angle measurements, acetabular coverage of femoral head, acetabular cartilage thickness, three-dimensional technique, screening of newborns, study of older children. *Skeletal Radiol* 1997;26:447–456.

Gerscovich EO, Greenspan A, Cronan MS, et al. Three-dimensional sonographic evaluation of developmental dysplasia of the hip: preliminary findings. *Radiology* 1994;190:407–410.

Ghatan AC, Hanel DP. Madelung deformity. *J Am Acad Orthop Surg* 2013;21:372–382.

Goldman AB, Schneider R, Martel W. Acute chondrolysis complicating slipped capital femoral epiphysis. *AJR Am J Roentgenol* 1978;130:945–950.

Greenhill BJ, Hugosson C, Jacobsson B, et al. Magnetic resonance imaging study of acetabular morphology in developmental dysplasia of the hip. *J Pediatr Orthop* 1993;13:314–317.

Harcke HT. Screening newborns for developmental dysplasia of the hip: the role of sonography. *AJR Am J Roentgenol* 1994;162:395–397.

Harcke HT, Kumar SJ. The role of ultrasound in the diagnosis and management of congenital dislocation and dysplasia of the hip. *J Bone Joint Surg Am* 1991;73(4):622–628.

Harper KW, Helms CA, Haystead CM, et al. Glenoid dysplasia: incidence and association with posterior labral tears as evaluated with MRI. *AJR Am J Roentgenol* 2012;184:984–988.

Harris RI. Rigid valgus foot due to talocalcaneal bridge. *J Bone Joint Surg Am* 1955;37:169–182.

Harris WR. The endocrine basis for slipping of the upper femoral epiphysis. An experimental study. *J Bone Joint Surg Br* 1950;32B:5–11.

Herring JA. The treatment of Legg-Calvé-Perthes disease. A critical review of the literature. *J Bone Joint Surg Am* 1994;76A:448–458.

Herring JA, Neustadt JB, Williams JJ, et al. The lateral pillar classification of Legg-Calvé-Perthes disease. *J Pediatr Orthop* 1992;12:143–150.

Ito H, Matsuno T, Hirayama T, et al. Three-dimensional computed tomography analysis of non-osteoarthritic adult acetabular dysplasia. *Skeletal Radiol* 2009;38:131–139.

Jawad MU, Scully SP. In brief: Crowe's classification: arthroplasty in developmental dysplasia of the hip. *Clin Orthop Relat Res* 2011;469:306–308.

Kim HT, Eisenhauer E, Wenger DR. The "sagging rope sign" in avascular necrosis in children's hip diseases—confirmation by 3D CT studies. *Iowa Orthop J* 1995;15:101–111.

Kim SH. Signs in imaging. The C sign. *Radiology* 2002;223:756–757.

Langenskiöld A. Tibia vara; (osteochondrosis deformans tibiae); a survey of 23 cases. *Acta Chir Scand* 1952;103:1–22.

Langenskiöld A, Riska EB. Tibia vara (osteochondrosis deformans tibiae): a survey of seventy-one cases. *J Bone Joint Surg Am* 1964;46A:1405–1420.

Lateur LM, Van Hoe LR, Van Ghillewe KV, et al. Subtalar coalition: diagnosis with the C sign on lateral radiograph of the ankle. *Radiology* 1994;193:847–851.

Legg AT. An obscure affection of the hip-joint. *Boston Med Surg J* 1910;162:202–204.

Lehman WB, Grant A, Rose D, et al. A method of evaluating possible pin penetration in slipped capital femoral epiphysis using a cannulated internal fixation device. *Clin Orthop* 1984;186:65–70.

Levinson ED, Ozonoff MB, Royen PM. Proximal femoral focal deficiency (PFFD). *Radiology* 1977;125:197–203.

Liu PT, Roberts CC, Chivers FS, et al. "Absent middle facet": a sign on unenhanced radiography of subtalar joint coalition. *AJR Am J Roentgenol* 2003;181:1565–1572.

Lowe HG. Necrosis of articular cartilage after slipping of capital femoral epiphysis. Report of six cases with recovery. *J Bone Joint Surg Br* 1970;52B:108–118.

Maldjian C, Patel TY, Klein RM, et al. Efficacy of MRI in classifying proximal focal femoral deficiency. *Skeletal Radiol* 2007;36:215–220.

Masciocchi C, D'Archivio C, Barile A, et al. Talocalcaneal coalition: computed tomography and magnetic resonance imaging diagnosis. *Eur J Radiol* 1992;15:22–25.

Meehan PL, Angel D, Nelson JM. The Scottish Rite abduction orthosis for the treatment of Legg-Perthes disease. A radiographic analysis. *J Bone Joint Surg Am* 1992;74(1):2–12.

Mouchet AA, Belot J. Tarsomegalie. *J Radiol Electrol* 1926;10:289–293.

Murphy RP, Marsh HO. Incidence and natural history of "head at risk" factors in Perthes' disease. *Clin Orthop Relat Res* 1978;132:102–107.

Newman JS, Newberg AH. Congenital tarsal coalition: multimodality evaluation with emphasis on CT and MR imaging. *Radiographics* 2000;20:321–332.

Nielsen JB. Madelung's deformity. A follow-up study of 26 cases and a review of the literature. *Acta Orthop Scand* 1977;48:379–384.

Oestreich AE, Mize WA, Crawford AH, et al. The "anteater nose": a direct sign of calcaneonavicular coalition on the lateral radiograph. *J Pediatr Orthop* 1987;7:709–711.

Ogden JA, Conlogue GJ, Phillips MS, et al. Sprengel's deformity. Radiology of the pathologic deformation. *Skeletal Radiol* 1979;4:204–211.

Pavlik A. Die funktionelle Behand-lungmethode mittels Riemenbügel als Prinzip der konservativen Therapie bei angeborenen Hüftgelenks verrenkungen der Säuglinge. *Z Orthop* 1958;8:341–352.

Phillips WE II, Burton EM. Ultrasonography of development displacement of the infant hip. *Appl Radiol* 1995;24:25–32.

Rab GT. Surgery for developmental dysplasia of the hip. In: Chapman MW, ed. *Operative orthopaedics*, 2nd ed. Philadelphia: JB Lippincott; 1993:3101–3112.

Resnick D. Talar ridges, osteophytes, and beaks: a radiologic commentary. *Radiology* 1984;151:329–332.

Sakellariou A, Sallomi D, Janzen DL, et al. Talocalcaneal coalition. Diagnosis with the C-sign on lateral radiographs of the ankle. *J Bone Joint Surg Br* 2000;82(4):574–578.

Salter RB. Etiology, pathogenesis and possible prevention of congenital dislocation of the hip. *Can Med Assoc J* 1968;98:933–945.

Salter RB. Legg-Perthes disease: the scientific basis for methods of treatment and their indications. *Clin Orthop Relat Res* 1980;150:8–11.

Salter RB. Role of innominate osteotomy in the treatment of congenital dislocation and subluxation of the hip in the older child. *J Bone Joint Surg Am* 1966;48:1413–1439.

Salter RB. The present status of surgical treatment for Legg-Perthes disease. *J Bone Joint Surg Am* 1984;66A:961–966.

Salter RB, Thompson GH. Legg-Calvé-Perthes disease. The prognostic significance of the subchondral fracture and a two-group classification of the femoral head involvement. *J Bone Joint Surg Am* 1984;66(4):479–489.

Scham SM. The triangular sign in the early diagnosis of slipped capital femoral epiphysis. *Clin Orthop Relat Res* 1974;103:16–17.

Shingade VU, Song H-R, Lee S-H, et al. The sagging rope sign in achondroplasia—different from Perthes' disease. *Skeletal Radiol* 2006;35:923–928.

Smith CF. Tibia vara (Blount's disease). *J Bone Joint Surg Am* 1982;64(4):630–632.

Sohn C, Lenz GP, Thies M. 3-Dimensional ultrasound image of the infant hip. *Ultraschall Med* 1990;11:302–305.

Sorge G, Ardito S, Genuardi M, et al. Proximal femoral focal deficiency (PFFD) and fibular A/hypoplasia (FA/H): a model of a developmental field defect. *Am J Med Genet* 1995;55:427–432.

Sprengel W. Die angeborne Verschiebung des Schulterblattes nach oben. *Arch Klin Chir* 1891;42:545.

Stevenson DA, Mineau G, Kerber RA, et al. Familial predisposition to developmental dysplasia of the hip. *J Pediatr Orthop* 2009;29:463–466.

Taniguchi A, Tanaka Y, Kadono K, et al. C sign for diagnosis of talocalcaneal coalition. *Radiology* 2003;228:501–505.

Terjesen T, Rundén TO, Johnsen HM. Ultrasound in the diagnosis of congenital dysplasia and dislocation of the hip joints in children older than two years. *Clin Orthop Relat Res* 1991;262:159–169.

Tönnis D. Normal values of the hip joint for the evaluation of x-rays in children and adults. *Clin Orthop Relat Res* 1976;119:39–47.

Trevor D. Tarso-epiphyseal aclasis: a congenital error of epiphyseal development. *J Bone Joint Surg Br* 1950;32-B(2):204–213.

Trueta J. The normal vascular anatomy of the human femoral head during growth. *J Bone Joint Surg Br* 1957;39-B(2):358.

Tyler PA, Rajeswaran G, Saifuddin A. Imaging of dysplasia epiphysealis hemimelica (Trevor's disease). *Clin Radiol* 2013;68:415–421.

Van Nes CP. Rotation-plasty for congenital defects of the femur: making use of the ankle of the shortened limb to control the knee joint of a prosthesis. *J Bone Joint Surg Br* 1950;32-B:12–16.

Waldenström H. The first stages of coxa plana. *J Bone Joint Surg* 1938;20:559–566.

Wechsler RJ, Karasick D, Schweitzer ME. Computed tomography of talocalcaneal coalition: imaging techniques. *Skeletal Radiol* 1992;21:353–358.

Wechsler RJ, Schweitzer ME, Deely DM, et al. Tarsal coalition: depiction and characterization with CT and MR imaging. *Radiology* 1994;193:447–452.

Wenger DR, Bomar JD. Human hip dysplasia: evolution of current treatment concepts. *J Orthop Sci* 2003;8(2):264–271.

Werner CML, Ramseier LE, Ruckstuhl T, et al. Normal values of Wiberg's lateral center-edge angle and Lequesne's acetabular index—a coxometric update. *Skeletal Radiol* 2012;41:1273–1278.

33

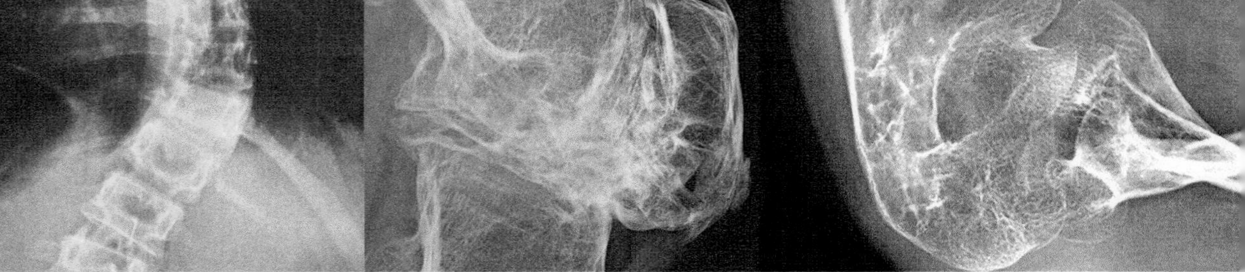

Scoliosis and Anomalies with General Affliction of the Skeleton

Scoliosis

Regardless of its cause (Fig. 33.1), *scoliosis* is defined as a lateral curvature of the spine occurring in the coronal plane. This fact differentiates it from kyphosis, a posterior curvature of the spine in the sagittal plane, and lordosis, an anterior curvature of the spine also in the sagittal plane (Fig. 33.2). If the curve occurs in both coronal and sagittal planes, then the deformity is called *kyphoscoliosis*. Besides a lateral curvature, scoliosis may also have a rotational component in which vertebrae rotate toward the convexity of the curve.

Idiopathic Scoliosis

Idiopathic scoliosis, which constitutes almost 75% of all scoliotic abnormalities, can be classified into three groups. The *infantile* type, of which there are two variants, occurs in children younger than age 4 years; it is seen predominantly in boys, and the curvature usually occurs in the thoracic segment with its convexity to the left. In the *resolving* (benign) variant, the curve commonly does not increase beyond 30 degrees and resolves spontaneously, requiring no treatment. The *progressive* variant carries a poor prognosis, with the potential for severe deformity unless aggressive treatment is initiated early in the process. *Juvenile idiopathic scoliosis* occurs equally in boys and girls from the ages of 4 to 9 years. By far, the most common type of idiopathic scoliosis, comprising 85% of cases, is the *adolescent* form, seen predominantly in girls from 10 years of age to the time of skeletal maturity. The thoracic or thoracolumbar spine is most often involved, and the convexity of the curve is to the right (Fig. 33.3). Although the cause of this type is unknown, it has been postulated that a genetic factor may be at work and that idiopathic scoliosis is a familial disorder. The results of cytogenetic investigations point to mutations in *SNTG1* gene encoding gamma-1-syntrophin located at chromosome 8q11.2, although the aberrations in the regions of chromosomes 6, 9, 16, and 17 may also be responsible for inheritance of this disorder.

Congenital Scoliosis

Congenital scoliosis is responsible for 10% of the cases of this deformity. It may generally be classified into three groups, according to MacEwen (Fig. 33.4): those resulting from a *failure in vertebral formation*, which may be partial or complete (Fig. 33.5); those caused by a *failure in vertebral segmentation*, which may be asymmetric and unilateral or symmetric and bilateral; and those resulting from a *combination* of the first two. The effects of congenital scoliosis on balance and support result in faulty biomechanics throughout the skeletal system.

Miscellaneous Scolioses

Several other forms of scoliosis having a specific cause may develop, including neuromuscular, traumatic, infections, metabolic, degenerative, and secondary to tumors, among others. Their discussion is beyond the scope of this text.

Imaging Evaluation

The radiographic examination of scoliosis includes standing anteroposterior and lateral radiographs of the entire spine; a supine anteroposterior radiograph centered over the scoliotic curve (see Figs. 33.3 and 33.5), which is used for the various measurements of spinal curvature and vertebral rotation (discussed later); and anteroposterior radiographs obtained with the patient bending laterally to each side for evaluation of the flexible and structural components of the curve. Care should be taken to include the iliac crests in at least one of these radiographs for a determination of skeletal maturity (see Figs. 33.14 and 33.15).

Ancillary techniques, such as computed tomography (CT), may be required for evaluating congenital lesions such as segmentation failures. Intravenous urography (intravenous pyelography, IVP) is essential in congenital scoliosis for evaluating the presence of associated anomalies of the genitourinary tract (Fig. 33.6). Magnetic resonance imaging (MRI) is the technique of choice to evaluate associated abnormalities of the spinal cord and the nerve roots.

An overview of the radiographic projections and radiologic techniques used in the evaluation of scoliosis is presented in Table 33.1.

Measurements

To evaluate the various types of scoliosis, certain terms (Fig. 33.7) and measurements must be introduced. Measurement of the severity of a scoliotic curve has practical application not only in the selection of patients for surgical treatment but also in monitoring the results of corrective therapy. Two widely accepted methods of measuring the curve are the Lippman-Cobb (Fig. 33.8) and Risser-Ferguson techniques (Fig. 33.9). The measurements obtained by these methods, however, are not comparable. The values yielded by the Lippman-Cobb method, which determines the angle of curvature only by the ends of the scoliotic curve, depending solely on the inclination of the end vertebrae, are usually greater than those given by the Risser-Ferguson method. This also applies to the percentages of correction as determined by the two methods; the more favorable correction percentage is obtained by the Lippman-Cobb method. The latter method, which has been adopted and standardized by the Scoliosis Research Society, classifies the severity of scoliotic curvature into seven groups (Table 33.2).

FIGURE 33.1 General classification of scoliosis on the basis of cause.

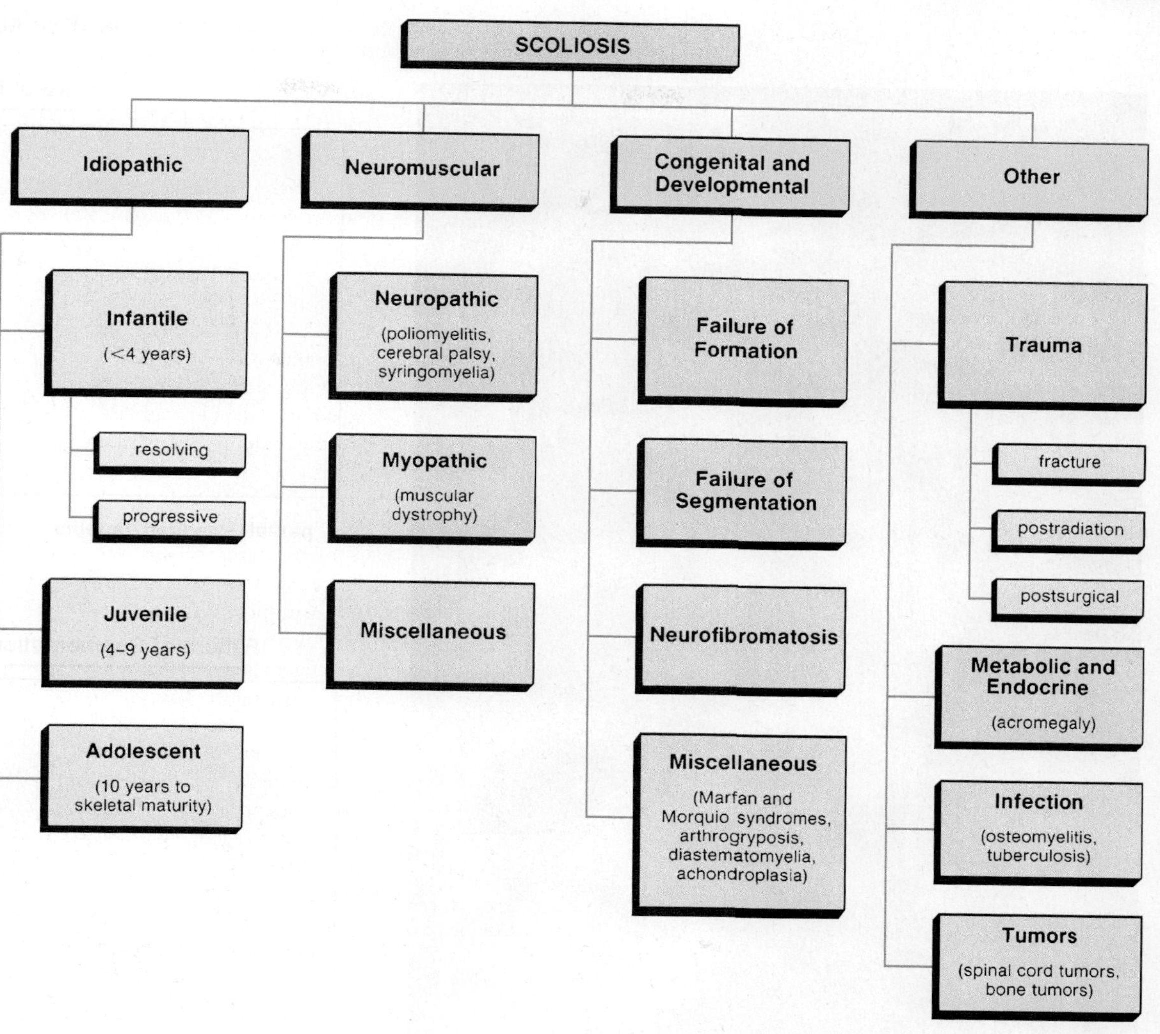

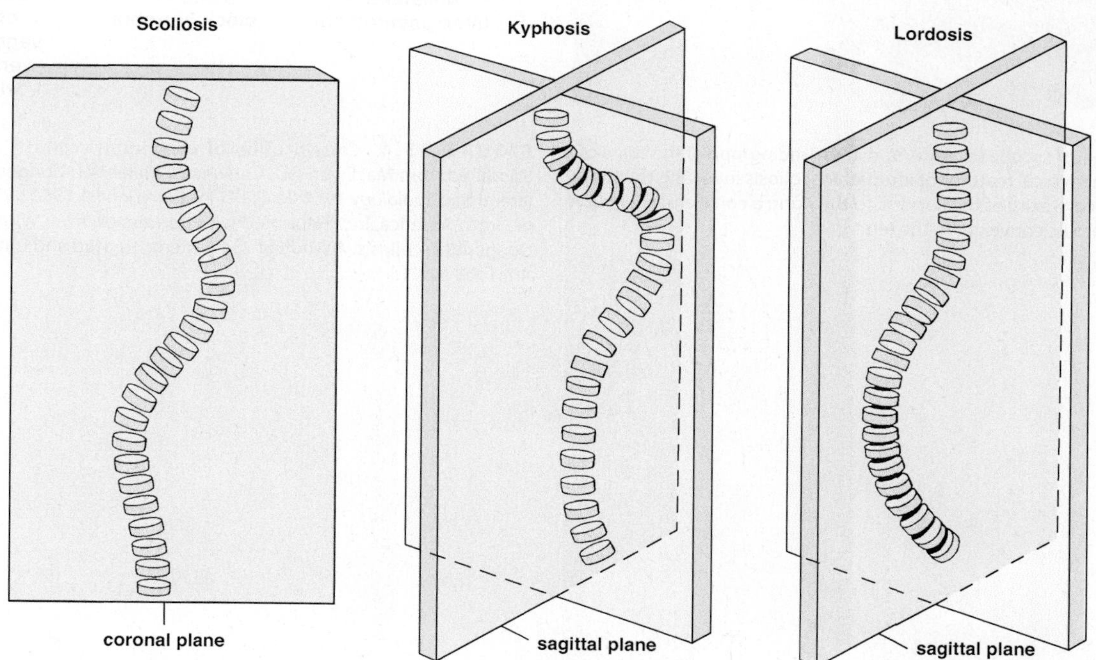

FIGURE 33.2 Definitions. Scoliosis is a lateral curvature of the spine in the coronal (frontal) plane. Kyphosis is a posterior curvature of the spine, and lordosis is an anterior curvature, both occurring in the sagittal (lateral) plane.

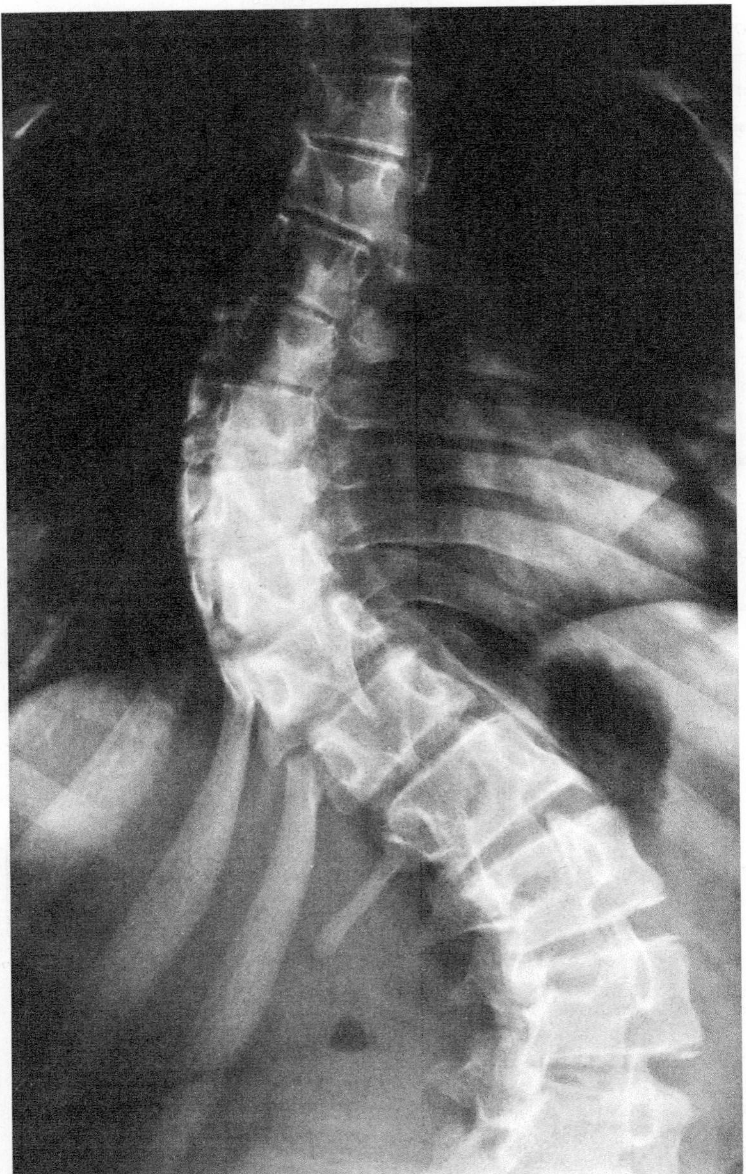

FIGURE 33.3 Idiopathic scoliosis. Anteroposterior radiograph of the spine of a 15-year-old girl shows the typical features of idiopathic scoliosis involving the thoracolumbar segment. The convexity of the curve is to the right; a compensatory curve in the lumbar segment has its convexity to the left.

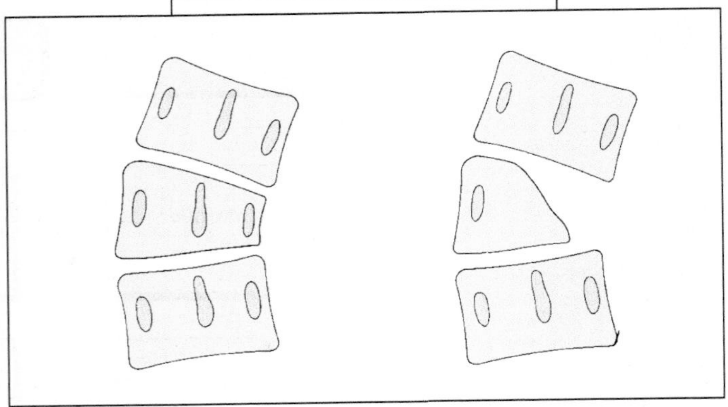

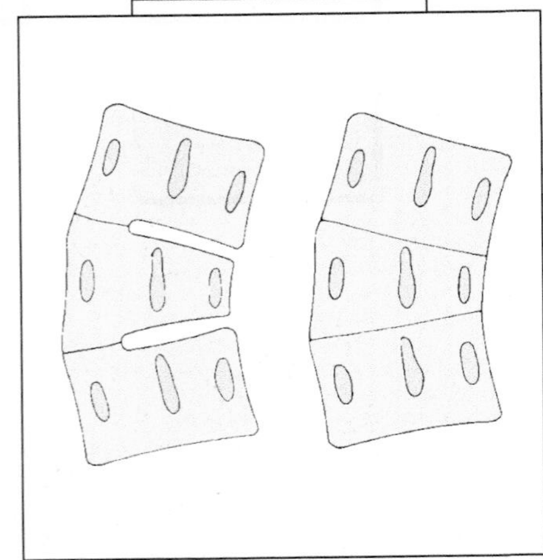

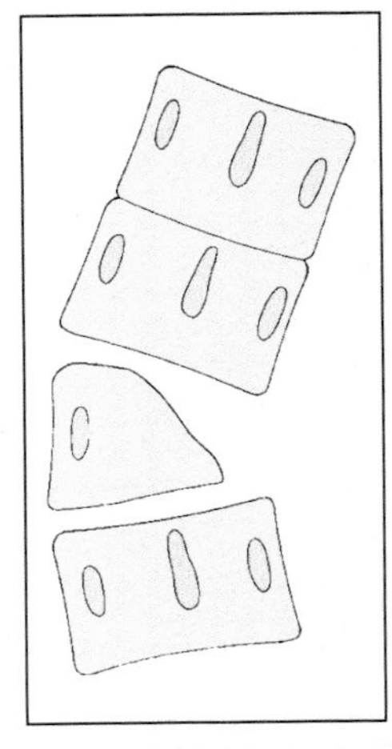

FIGURE 33.4 Classification of congenital scoliosis on the basis of cause. (Modified from MacEwen GD, Conway JJ, Miller WT. Congenital scoliosis with a unilateral bar. *Radiology* 1968;90:711–715. Copyright © 1968 by The Radiological Society of North America, Inc.; Reprinted with permission from Winter RB, Moe JH, Eilers VE. Congenital scoliosis. A study of 234 patients treated and untreated. *J Bone Joint Surg Am* 1968;50A:1.)

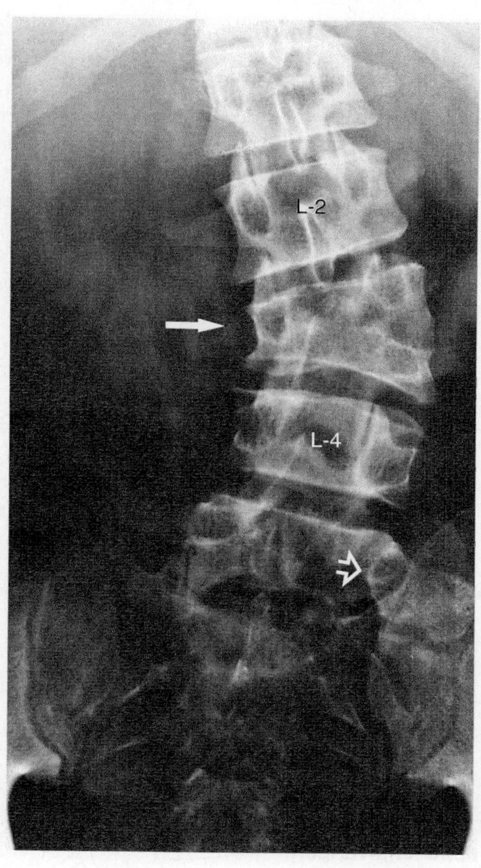

FIGURE 33.5 Congenital scoliosis. Anteroposterior radiograph of the lumbosacral spine of a 22-year-old man demonstrates scoliosis caused by hemivertebra, a complete unilateral failure of formation. Note the deformed L3 vertebra *(arrow)* secondary to the faulty fusion of the hemivertebra on the left side, where two pedicles are evident. The resulting scoliosis has its convex border to the left. An associated anomaly is also apparent from the presence of the so-called *transitional lumbosacral vertebra (open arrow).*

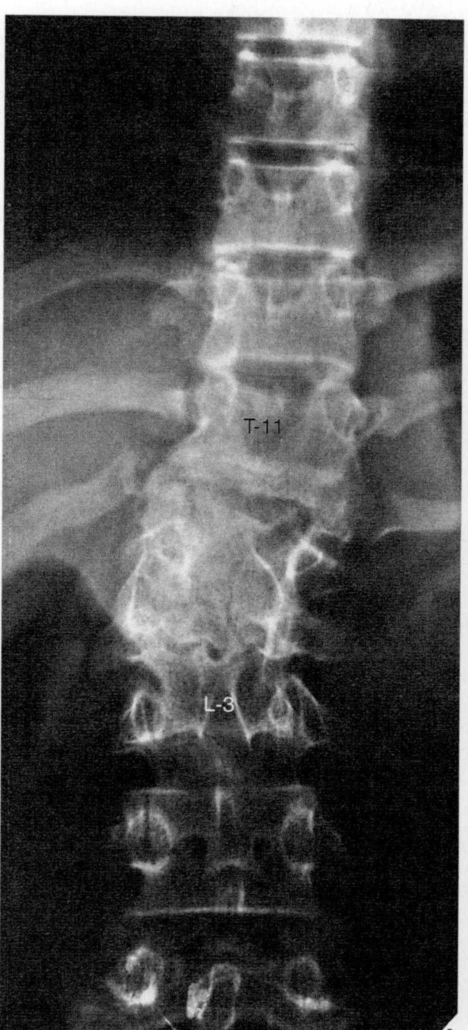

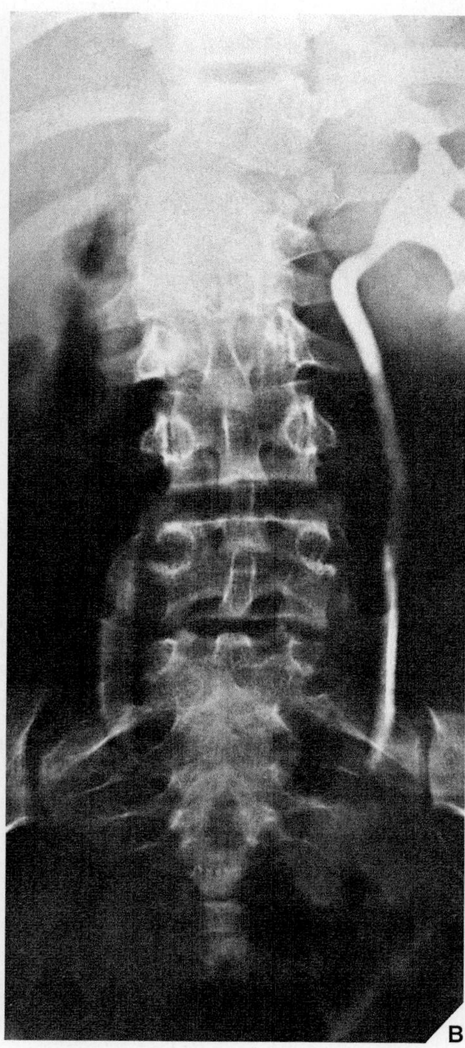

FIGURE 33.6 Congenital scoliosis. (A) Supine anteroposterior radiograph of the thoracolumbar spine of a 13-year-old girl shows congenital scoliosis secondary to block vertebrae consisting of a fusion of T12-L2. **(B)** IVP in the same patient demonstrates only the left kidney, an example of renal agenesis. Congenital scoliosis is frequently associated with urinary tract anomalies.

TABLE 33.1 Standard Radiographic Projections and Radiologic Techniques for Evaluating Scoliosis

Projection/Technique	Demonstration
Anteroposterior of spine	Lateral deviation Angle of scoliosis (by Risser-Ferguson and Lippman-Cobb methods and scoliotic index) Vertebral rotation (by Cobb and Nash-Moe methods)
Anteroposterior of pelvis	Ossification of ring apophysis as determinant of skeletal maturity Ossification of iliac crest apophysis as determinant of skeletal maturity
Lateral bending of spine	Flexibility of curve Amount of reduction of curve
Lateral of spine	Associated kyphosis and lordosis
Computed tomography (CT)	Congenital fusion of vertebrae Hemivertebrae
Myelography	Tethering of cord
Magnetic resonance imaging (MRI)	Abnormalities of nerve roots Compression and displacement of thecal sac Tethering of cord
Intravenous urography	Associated anomalies of genitourinary tract (in congenital scoliosis)
Ultrasound	

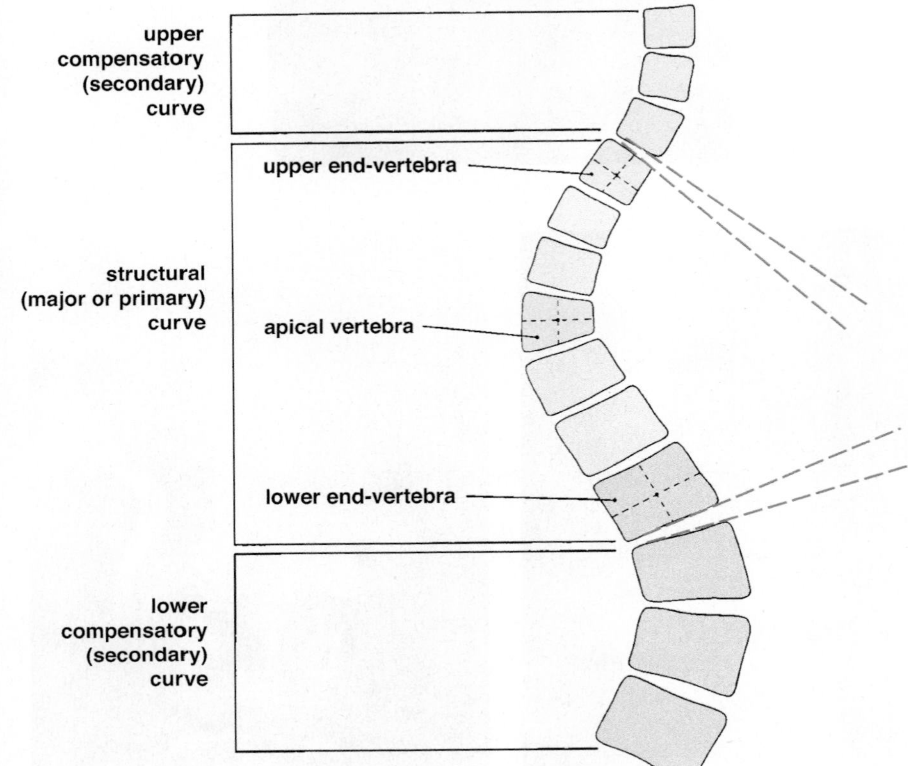

FIGURE 33.7 Terminology used in describing the scoliotic curve. The end vertebrae of the curve are defined as those that tilt maximally into the concavity of the structural curve. The apical vertebra, which shows the most severe rotation and wedging, is the one whose center is most laterally displaced from the central line. The center of the apical vertebra is determined by the intersection of two lines, one drawn from the center of the upper and lower end plates and the other from the center of the lateral margins of the vertebral body. The center should not be determined by diagonal lines through the corners of the vertebral body.

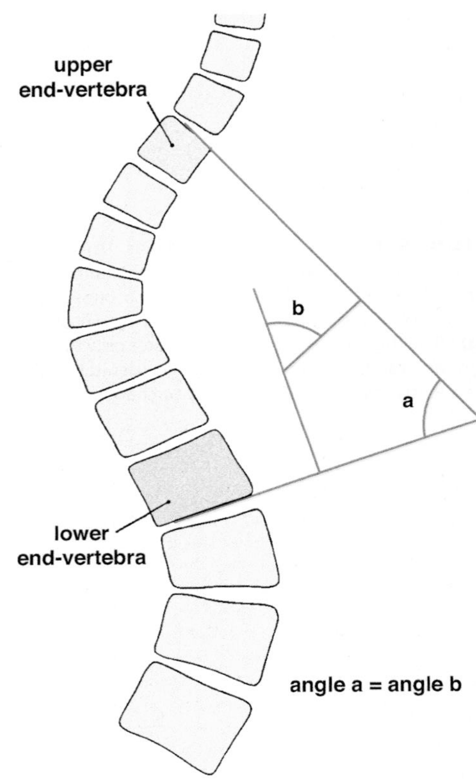

FIGURE 33.8 Lippman-Cobb method. In this method of measuring the degree of scoliotic curvature, two angles are formed by the intersection of two sets of lines. The first set of lines, one drawn tangent to the superior surface of the upper end vertebra and the other tangent to the inferior surface of the lower end vertebra, intersects to form angle *(a)*. The intersection of the other set of lines, each drawn perpendicular to the tangential lines, forms angle *(b)*. These angles are equal, and either may serve as the measurement of the degree of scoliosis.

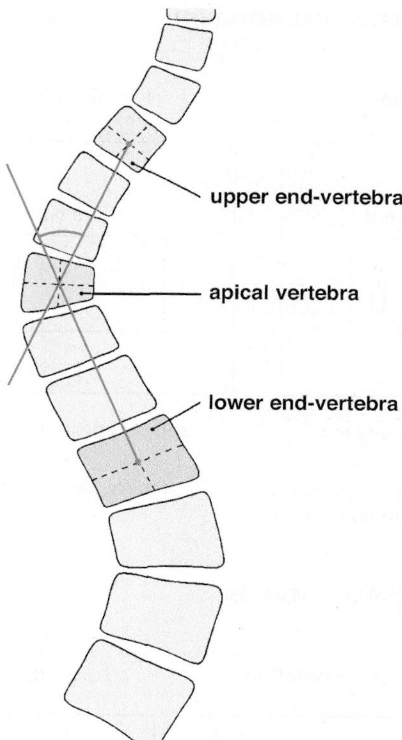

FIGURE 33.9 Risser-Ferguson method. In this method, the degree of scoliotic curvature is determined by the angle formed by the intersection of two lines at the center of the apical vertebra: the first line originating at the center of the upper end vertebra and the other at the center of the lower end vertebra.

Another technique for measuring the degree of scoliosis, introduced by Greenspan and colleagues in 1978, uses a "scoliotic index." Designed to give a more accurate and comprehensive representation of the scoliotic curve, this technique measures the deviation of each involved vertebra from the vertical spinal line as determined by points at the center of the vertebra immediately above the upper end vertebra of the curve and at the center of the vertebra immediately below the lower end vertebra (Fig. 33.10). Its most valuable feature is that it minimizes the influence of overcorrection of the end vertebrae in the measured angle, a frequent criticism of the Lippman-Cobb technique. Furthermore, short segments or minimal curvatures, often difficult to measure with the currently accepted methods, are easily measurable with this technique.

Computerized methods for measuring and analyzing the scoliotic curve have also been introduced. Although more accurate than the manual methods, they require more sophisticated equipment and are more time-consuming than the methods described earlier.

In addition to the measurement of scoliotic curvature, the radiographic evaluation of scoliosis also requires the determination of other factors. Measurement of the degree of *rotation of the vertebrae* of the involved segment can be obtained by either of two methods currently in use. The Cobb technique for grading rotation uses the position of the spinous process as a point of reference (Fig. 33.11). On the normal anteroposterior radiograph of the spine, the spinous process appears at the center of the vertebral body if there is no rotation. As the degree of rotation increases, the spinous process migrates toward the convexity of the curve. The Nash-Moe method, also based on the measurements obtained on the anteroposterior projection of the spine, uses the symmetry of the pedicles as a point of reference, with the migration of the pedicles toward the convexity of the curve determining the degree of vertebral rotation (Fig. 33.12).

The final factor in the evaluation of scoliosis is the determination of *skeletal maturity*. This is important for both the prognosis and treatment of scoliosis, particularly the idiopathic type, because there is a potential for significant progression of the degree of curvature as long as skeletal maturity has not been reached. Skeletal age can be determined by comparison of a radiograph of a patient's hand with the standards for different ages available in radiographic atlases. It can also be assessed by radiographic observation of the ossification of the apophysis of the vertebral ring (Fig. 33.13) or, as is often performed, from the ossification of the iliac apophysis (Figs. 33.14 and 33.15).

Treatment

Various surgical procedures are available for the treatment of scoliosis. The main objective of surgery is to balance and fuse the spine to prevent the deformity from progressing; its secondary objective is to correct the scoliotic curve to the extent of its flexibility. Determining the level of fusion depends on several factors, including the cause of the scoliosis and the age of the

TABLE 33.2 Lippman-Cobb Classification of Scoliotic Curvature

Group	Angle of Curvature (Degrees)
I	<20
II	21–30
III	31–50
IV	51–75
V	76–100
VI	101–125
VII	>125

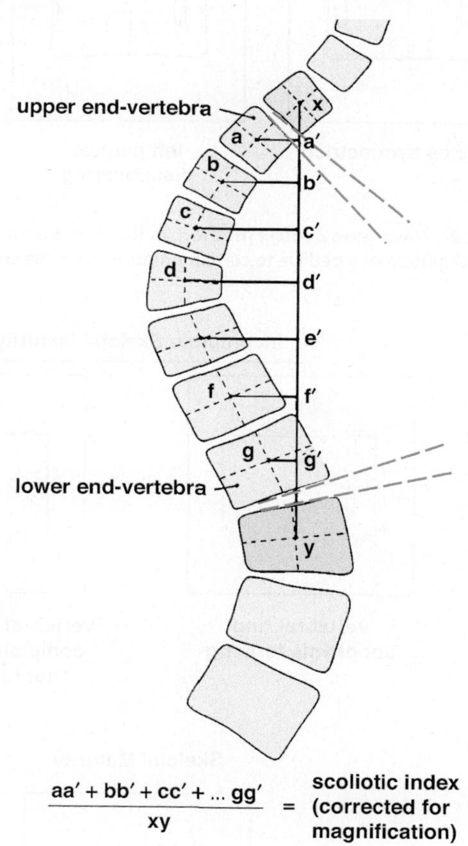

FIGURE 33.10 Scoliotic index—Greenspan method. In the measurement of scoliosis using the scoliotic index, each vertebra *(a–g)* is considered an integral part of the curve. A vertical spinal line *(xy)* is first determined whose endpoints are the centers of the vertebrae immediately above and below the upper and lower end vertebrae of the curve. Lines are then drawn from the center of each vertebral body perpendicular to the vertical spinal line *(aa', bb', ... gg')*. The values yielded by these lines represent the linear deviation of each vertebra; their sum, divided by the length of the vertical line *(xy)* to correct for radiographic magnification, yields the scoliotic index. A value of zero denotes a straight spine; the higher the scoliotic index, the more severe the scoliosis.

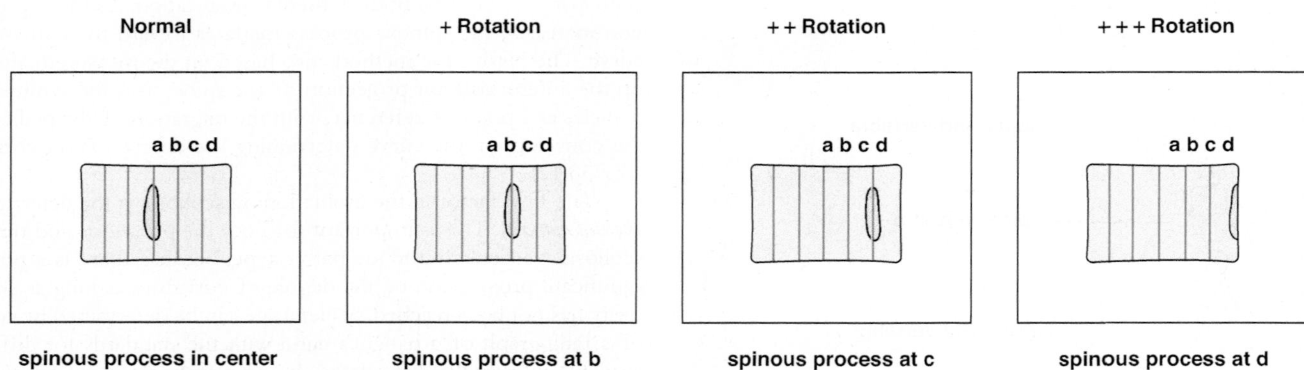

FIGURE 33.11 **Cobb spinous process method.** In this method for determining rotation, the vertebra is divided into six equal parts. Normally, the spinous process appears at the center. Its migration to certain points toward the convexity of the curve marks the degree of rotation.

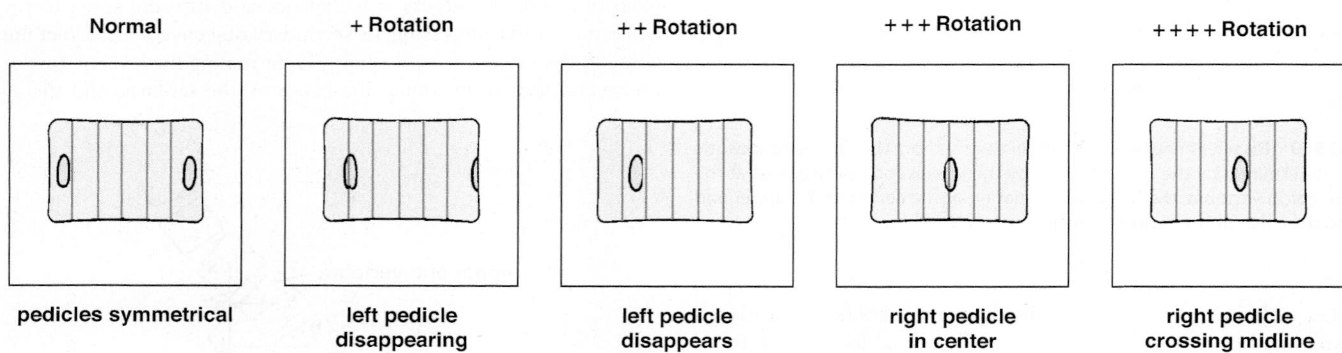

FIGURE 33.12 **Nash-Moe pedicle method.** In this method for determining rotation, the vertebra is also divided into six equal parts. Normally, the pedicles appear in the outer parts. Migration of a pedicle to certain points toward the convexity of the curve determines the degree of rotation.

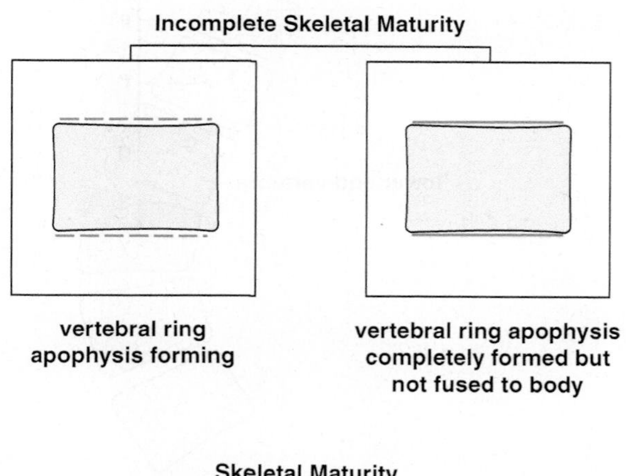

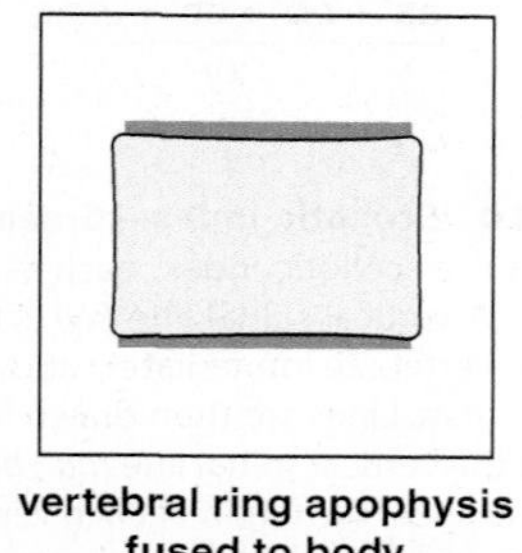

FIGURE 33.13 **Skeletal maturity.** Determination of skeletal maturity from ossification of the vertebral ring apophysis.

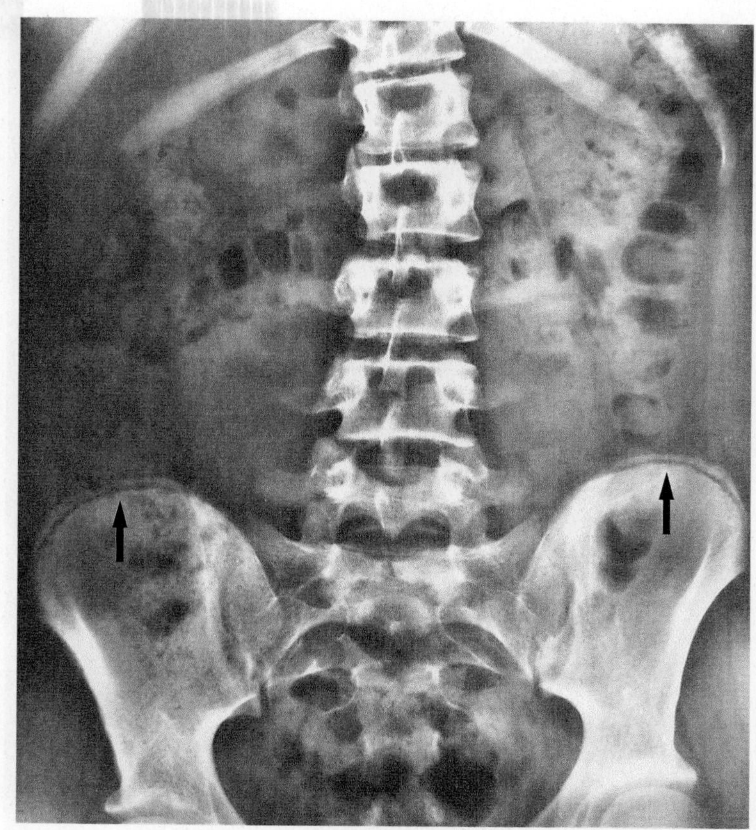

FIGURE 33.14 **Skeletal maturity.** The ossification of the iliac apophysis is helpful in determining skeletal age. Progression of the apophysis in this 14-year-old girl with idiopathic scoliosis has been completed, but the lack of fusion with the iliac crest *(arrows)* indicates continuing skeletal maturation.

patient as well as the pattern of the scoliotic curve and the extent of vertebral rotation as evaluated during the radiographic examination of the patient.

Spinal fusion is now commonly accompanied by internal fixation of the spine to provide stability. One of the most popular methods for internal fixation is the Harrington-Luque technique (Wisconsin segmental instrumentation), using square-ended distraction rods and wire loops inserted through the bases of the spinous processes and connected to two contoured paravertebral rods (Fig. 33.16). The procedure involves decortication of the laminae and spinous processes, obliteration of the posterior facet joints by removal of the cartilage, and the placement of an autogenous bone graft from the iliac crest along the concave side of the curve. The hooks of the distraction rods are inserted under the laminae at the upper and lower ends of the curve. The prebent stainless-steel paravertebral rods (Luque rods or L-rods) are anchored into the spinous process or pelvis, depending on the location of the curve; wires, passed through the base of the spinous process at each level of the spine to be fused, are then fixed to the L-rods. Variations in this technique have been used with L-rod instrumentation alone, which involves the use of sublaminar wires fixed to the rods, or a combination of Harrington distractors and wires fixed to them. Cotrel-Dubousset spinal instrumentation using knurled rods has also gained popularity. Fixation is achieved via pediculotransverse double-hook purchase at several levels. The two knurled rods are additionally stabilized by two transverse traction devices. The Dwyer technique, involving anterior fixation of the spine and obliteration of the intervertebral disks, is also used in the surgical treatment of scoliosis but more often in the paralytic types of the deformity.

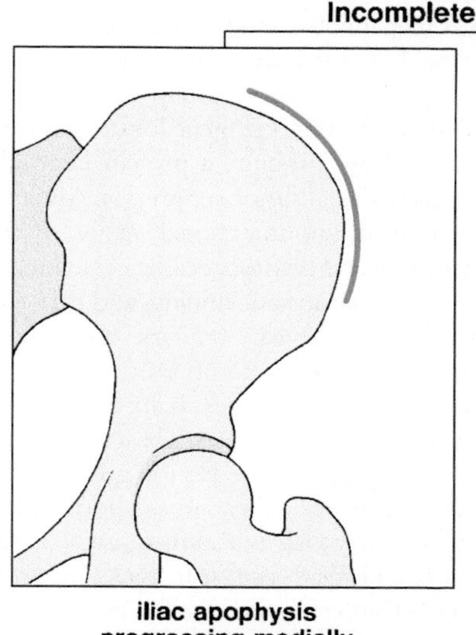

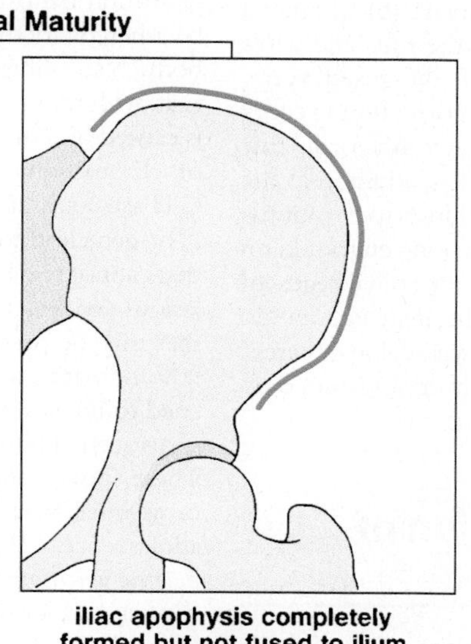

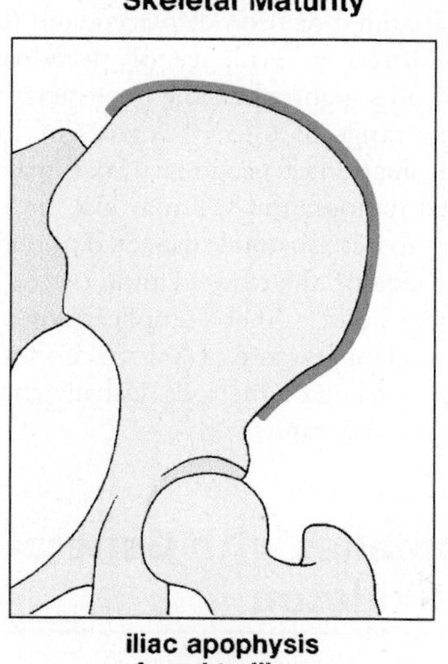

FIGURE 33.15 **Skeletal maturity.** Determination of skeletal maturity from the status of ossification of the iliac apophysis.

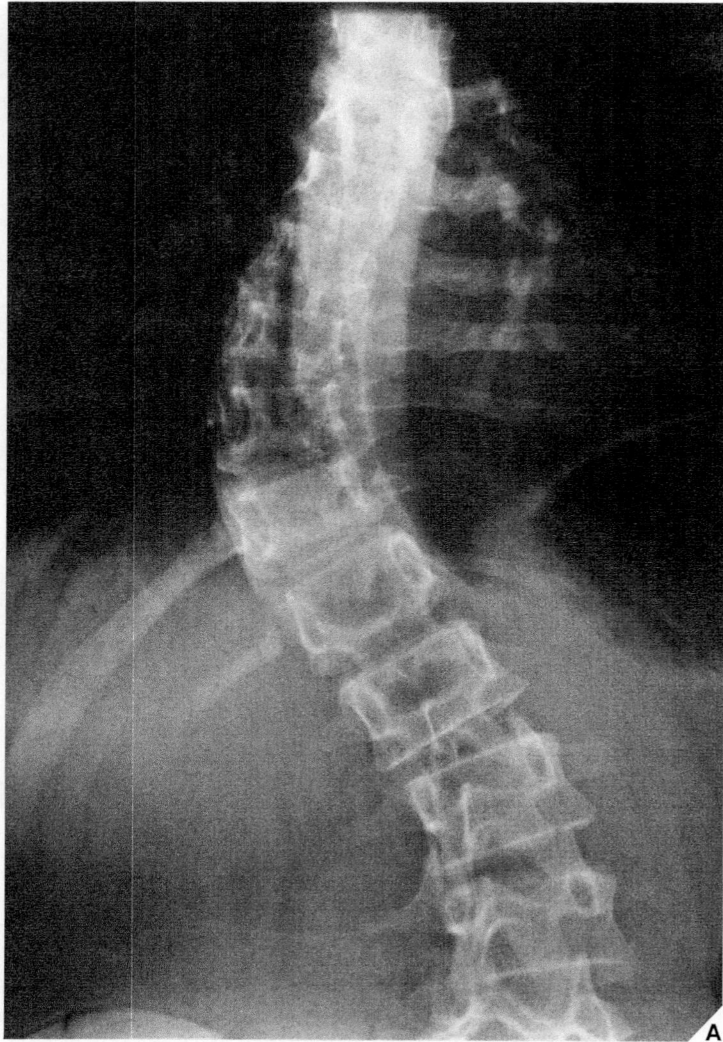

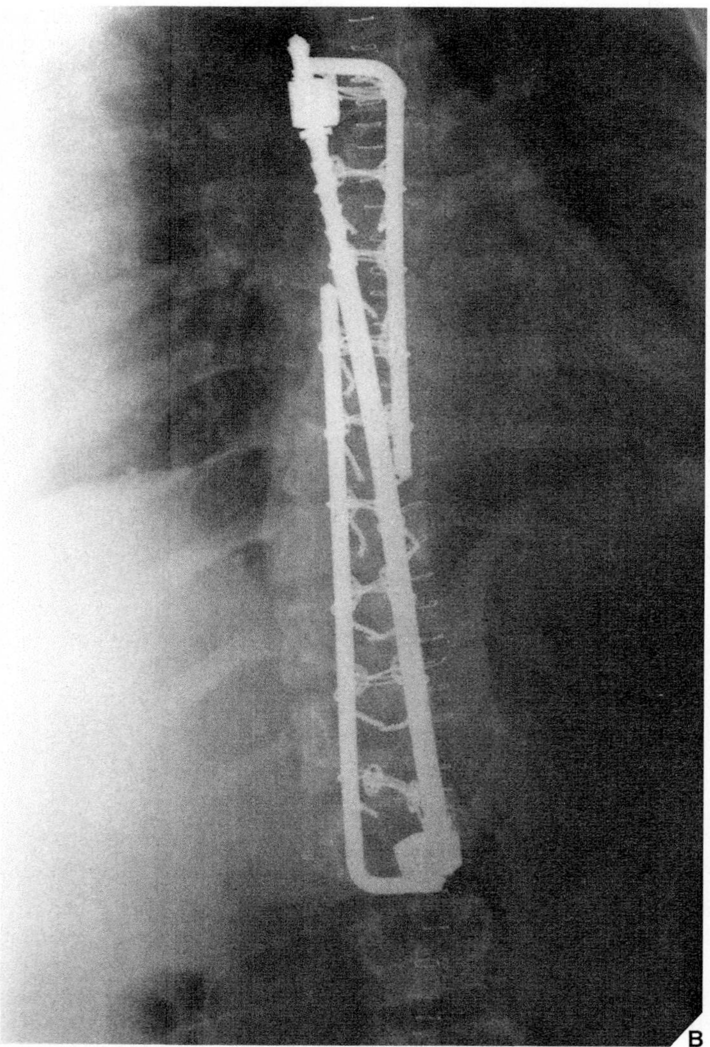

FIGURE 33.16 Treatment of scoliosis. **(A)** Preoperative anteroposterior radiograph of the lumbar spine in a 15-year-old girl shows idiopathic dextroscoliosis. **(B)** Postoperative radiograph shows the placement of the Harrington distractor and two L-rods. Note the multiple sublaminar wires fixed into the prebent L-rods.

The postoperative radiographic evaluation of internal fixation by the Harrington-Luque technique should focus on (a) whether the hooks of the Harrington rod are properly anchored with their brackets on the laminae of the superior and inferior vertebrae of the fused segment, (b) whether a hook has separated or been displaced, and (c) whether the rods and wires are intact. Moreover, evidence of pseudoarthrosis of the fused vertebrae should be sought when the postoperative loss of correction exceeds 10 degrees; a range of 6 to 10 degrees of loss of correction is ordinarily seen. The evaluation of pseudoarthrosis may require CT in addition to the conventional radiography. CT may also be needed within 6 to 9 months after surgery to demonstrate suspected nonunion of the bone engrafted on the concave side of the curve. Union of the graft with the spinal segment should appear solid. Other complications involving the instrumentation may occur, such as fracture of a distraction rod or of a wire cable or screw, or excessive bending of the rods. Usually, these are easily demonstrated on conventional radiographs.

Anomalies with General Affliction of the Skeleton

Table 33.3 presents an overview of radiographic projections and radiologic techniques most effective for evaluating congenital and developmental anomalies with general affliction of the skeleton.

Neurofibromatosis

Originally considered a disorder of neurogenic tissue (nerve-trunk tumors), neurofibromatosis (also called *von Recklinghausen disease*) is now believed to be a hereditary dysplasia that may involve almost every organ system of the body. Neurofibromatosis type 1 is transmitted as an autosomal dominant trait, with more than 50% of cases reporting a family history. The condition is caused by a mutation or deletion of the *NF1* gene located on the long arm of chromosome 17 (17q11.2) whose product, a protein neurofibromin (a GTPase-activating enzyme), serves as a tumor suppressor. Mutations in the *NF1* gene lead to the production of a nonfunctional version of this protein that cannot regulate the cell growth and division. Sessile or pedunculated skin lesions (*mollusca fibrosa*) are an almost constant finding, and café-au-lait spots that may be present at birth or may appear over time occur in more than 90% of patients. The latter lesions have a smooth border that has been likened to the coast of California; this distinguishes them from the café-au-lait spots seen in fibrous dysplasia, which have rugged "coast of Maine" borders. These spots increase in size and number as the person grows older. Axillary or inguinal freckles are rare at birth but appear throughout childhood and adolescence. Plexiform neurofibromatosis is a diffuse involvement of the nerves, associated with elephantoid masses of soft tissue (*elephantiasis neuromatosa*), and localized or generalized enlargement of a part or all of a limb (Fig. 33.17A–D). Other tumors associated with *NF1* include subcutaneous and intramuscular neurofibromas, spinal neurofibromas, optic gliomas, and cerebellar astrocytomas. Patients with *NF1* are prone to malignant tumors

TABLE 33.3 Most Effective Radiographic Projections and Radiologic Techniques for Evaluating Common Anomalies with General Affliction of the Skeleton

Projection/Technique	Crucial Abnormalities
Arthrogryposis	
Anteroposterior, lateral, and oblique of affected joints	Multiple subluxations and dislocations Fatlike lucency of soft tissues Cubital and popliteal webbing
Down Syndrome	
Anteroposterior	
of pelvis and hips	Hip dysplasia
of ribs	11 pairs of ribs
Dorsovolar of both hands	Clinodactyly and hypoplasia of fifth fingers
Lateral of cervical spine	Atlantoaxial subluxation
Tomography (lateral) of cervical spine (C1, C2)	Hypoplastic odontoid
Neurofibromatosis	
Anteroposterior, lateral, and oblique of long bones	Pitlike erosions Pseudoarthrosis of distal tibia and fibula
Anteroposterior	
of ribs	Rib notching
of lower cervical/upper thoracic spine	Scoliosis Kyphoscoliosis
Oblique of cervical spine	Enlarged neural foramina
Lateral of thoracic/lumbar spine	Posterior vertebral scalloping
Myelography	Intraspinal neurofibromas Increased volume of enlarged subarachnoid space Localized dural ectasia
Computed tomography (CT)	Complications (e.g., sarcomatous degeneration)
Magnetic resonance imaging (MRI)	Neurofibromas
Osteogenesis Imperfecta	
Anteroposterior, lateral, and oblique of affected bones	Osteoporosis Bowing deformities Trumpetlike metaphysis Fractures
Lateral of skull	Wormian bones
Anteroposterior and lateral of thoracic/lumbar spine	Kyphoscoliosis
Achondroplasia	
Anteroposterior	
of upper and lower extremities	Shortening of tubular bones, particularly humeri and femora
of pelvis	Rounded iliac bones Horizontal orientation of acetabular roofs Small sciatic notches
of spine	Narrowing of interpedicular distance
Lateral of spine	Short pedicles Posterior scalloping of vertebral bodies
Dorsovolar of hands	Short, stubby fingers Separation of middle finger (trident appearance)
CT	Spinal stenosis
Morquio-Brailsford Disease	
Anteroposterior and lateral of spine	Oval- or hook-shaped vertebrae with central beak
Anteroposterior	
of pelvis and hips	Overconstriction of iliac bodies Wide iliac flaring Dysplasia of proximal femora
Hurler Syndrome	
Anteroposterior and lateral	
of spine	Rounding and lower beaking of vertebral bodies Recessed hooked vertebra at apex of kyphoscoliotic curve
of skull	Frontal bossing Synostosis of sagittal and lambdoidal sutures Thickening of calvarium J-shaped sella turcica
Anteroposterior of pelvis	Flaring of iliac wings Constriction of inferior portion of iliac body Shallow, obliquely oriented acetabula
Osteopetrosis	
Anteroposterior and lateral	Increased density (osteosclerosis)
of long bones	Bone-in-bone appearance
of spine	"Rugger-jersey" vertebral bodies
Anteroposterior of pelvis	Ringlike pattern of normal and abnormal bone in ilium
Pyknodysostosis	
Anteroposterior and lateral of long bones	Increased density (osteosclerosis)
Dorsovolar of hands	Resorption of terminal tufts (acroosteolysis)
Lateral of skull	Wormian bones Persistence of anterior and posterior fontanelles Obtuse (fetal) angle of mandible
Osteopoikilosis	
Anteroposterior of affected bones	Dense spots at the articular ends of long bones
Osteopathia Striata	
Anteroposterior of affected bones	Dense striations, particularly in metaphysis
Progressive Diaphyseal Dysplasia	
Anteroposterior of long bones (particularly lower limbs)	Symmetric fusiform thickening of cortex Sparing of epiphyses
Endosteal Hyperostosis	
Anteroposterior of long bones, lateral of skull, anteroposterior and oblique of mandible	Symmetric endosteal thickening of the diaphyseal cortex of long bones (narrowing of the medullary canal) Osteosclerosis of skull, facial bones, and mandible
Dysosteosclerosis	
Anteroposterior of long bones, lateral of skull, anteroposterior and oblique of mandible	Generalized sclerosis of the skeleton Short stature and short limbs Small mandible Bulky forehead
Metaphyseal Dysplasia (Pyle Disease)	
Anteroposterior and lateral of knees	Erlenmeyer flask–like expansion of distal femur and proximal tibia
Lateral of skull	Widening of medial portions of clavicles Genu valgum Mild sclerosis of skull base
Craniometaphyseal Dysplasia	
Anteroposterior and lateral of long bones	Overgrowth of skull, prognathism, prominent forehead
Anteroposterior and lateral of skull	Leontiasis ossium (leonine facies) Sclerosis of skull base Thinning of the cortices of long and short tubular bones Juxtaarticular radiolucency of bones
Melorheostosis	
Anteroposterior and lateral of affected bones	Asymmetric, wavy hyperostosis (like dripping candle wax) Ossifications of periarticular soft tissues
Craniodiaphyseal Dysplasia	
Anteroposterior and lateral of skull	Hyperostosis and sclerosis of skull, spine, ribs
Lateral of spine	Defective remodeling of diaphyses and metaphyses of long bones
Anteroposterior ribs	Thinning of the cortices of long bones
Anteroposterior and lateral of long bones	
Hyperostosis Generalisata with Striations of Bones	
Anteroposterior and lateral of long bones	Widening of long bones, cortical thickening, coarse striations
Lateral of skull	Sclerosis of cranial vault

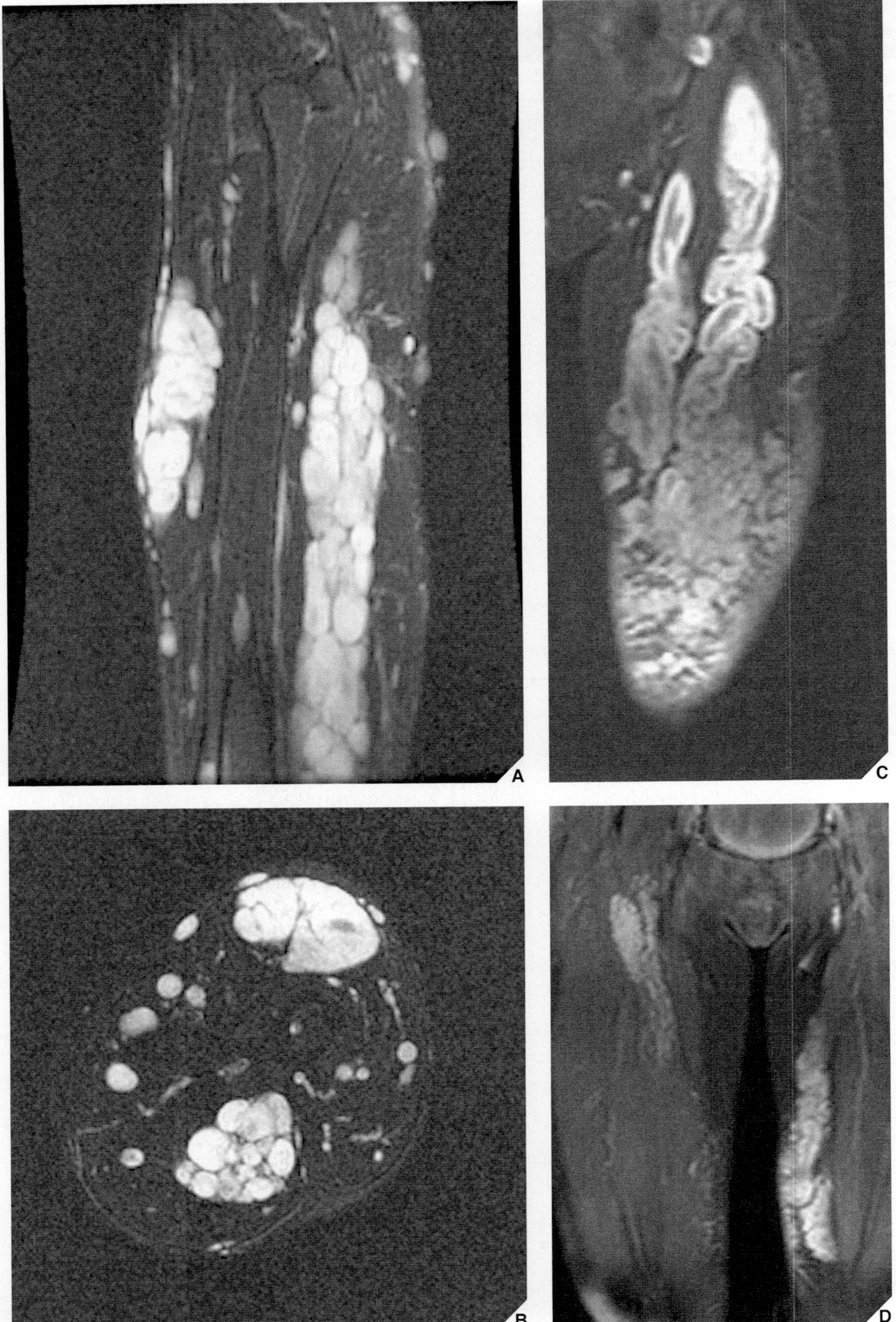

FIGURE 33.17 MRI of neurofibromatosis. A 19-year-old man presented with a history of slow but progressive enlargement of his left thigh. Clinical examination also revealed several café-au-lait spots. **(A)** Sagittal inversion recovery (IR) and **(B)** axial T2-weighted fat-suppressed MR images of the upper left thigh show numerous of large, lobulated bright masses representing neurofibromas, the largest involving the sciatic nerve, consistent with plexiform type of neurofibromatosis. Another patient, an 18-year-old woman with known *NF1* presented with sensory deficits in both thighs. **(C)** Postcontrast coronal T1-weighted fat-saturated MRI of the left thigh and **(D)** coronal postcontrast MRI of both thighs demonstrate bilateral plexiform neurofibromas involving the lateral and anterior femorocutaneous nerves, more prominent on the left. Note the characteristic "bull's-eye" enhancement of the neurofibromas of the left thigh, with peripheral pattern of enhancement. *(Continued)*

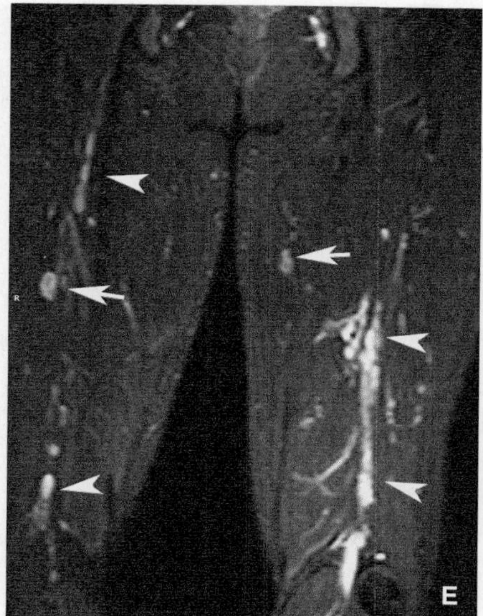

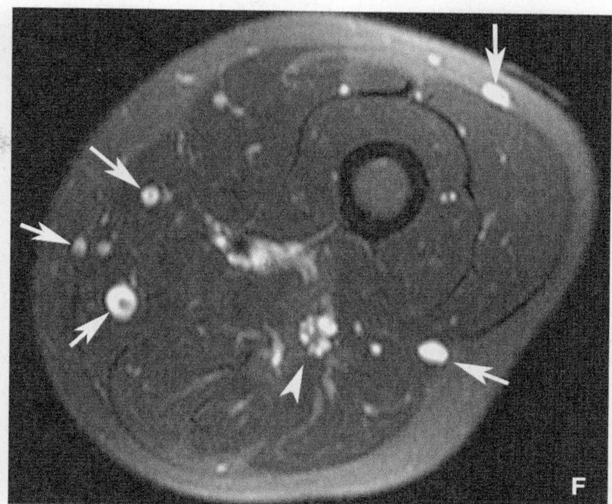

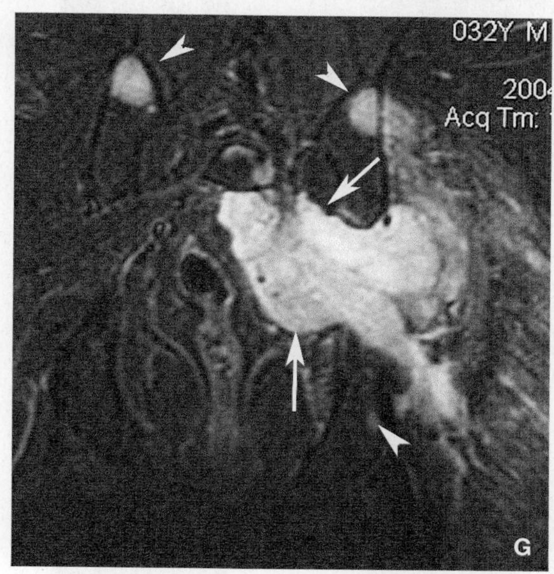

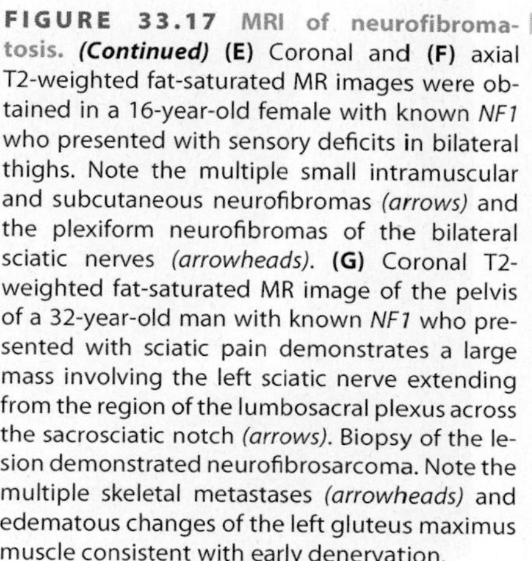

FIGURE 33.17 MRI of neurofibromatosis. ***(Continued)*** **(E)** Coronal and **(F)** axial T2-weighted fat-saturated MR images were obtained in a 16-year-old female with known *NF1* who presented with sensory deficits in bilateral thighs. Note the multiple small intramuscular and subcutaneous neurofibromas *(arrows)* and the plexiform neurofibromas of the bilateral sciatic nerves *(arrowheads)*. **(G)** Coronal T2-weighted fat-saturated MR image of the pelvis of a 32-year-old man with known *NF1* who presented with sciatic pain demonstrates a large mass involving the left sciatic nerve extending from the region of the lumbosacral plexus across the sacrosciatic notch *(arrows)*. Biopsy of the lesion demonstrated neurofibrosarcoma. Note the multiple skeletal metastases *(arrowheads)* and edematous changes of the left gluteus maximus muscle consistent with early denervation.

such as neurofibrosarcomas (Fig. 33.17E–G) or liposarcomas (see Fig. 22.62). Neurofibromas arising in the epineurium (plexiform neurofibromas) have over 10% probability of malignant transformation to neurofibrosarcomas.

Skeletal abnormalities are often encountered in neurofibromatosis; at least 50% of patients demonstrate some osseous changes, most commonly extrinsic, pitlike cortical erosions resulting from direct pressure by adjacent neurofibromas. This is commonly seen in the long bones (Fig. 33.18) and ribs. The long bones often exhibit bowing deformities, and pseudoarthroses, seen in approximately 10% of cases, most commonly occur in the lower tibia and fibula (Fig. 33.19). This type of false joint formation must be differentiated from congenital pseudoarthrosis. Moreover, the long bones are the site of lesions that were once considered to represent intraosseous neurofibromas; these cyst-like radiolucencies are now regarded as lesions representing fibrous cortical defects and nonossifying fibromas, associated with neurofibromatosis (see Fig. 19.10). Whittling of the bones is also a typical feature of neurofibromatosis (Fig. 33.20).

The spine is the second most common site of skeletal abnormalities in neurofibromatosis. Scoliosis or kyphoscoliosis, which characteristically involves a short segment of the vertebral column with acute angulation, commonly occurs in the lower cervical or upper thoracic spine. Widening of the intervertebral foramina in the cervical segment may also occur, resulting from dumbbell-shaped neurofibromas arising in spinal nerve roots (Fig. 33.21). In the thoracic and lumbar segments, scalloping of the posterior border of vertebral bodies is another characteristic feature (Fig. 33.22). Although most of these abnormalities can easily be diagnosed with conventional radiography, some ancillary techniques may be useful. CT-myelography and MRI are particularly valuable for demonstrating the increased volume of the enlarged subarachnoid space and the localized dural ectasia extending into the scalloped defects in the vertebral bodies. A characteristic MRI manifestation of neurofibromas is hypointensity in the center of the lesion and hyperintensity in the periphery (bull's-eye lesion) (see Fig. 33.17C,D). Prominent enhancement of these lesions is seen following intravenous administration of gadolinium.

Neurofibromatosis type 2 is autosomal dominant disorder with a high penetrance caused by mutation of an *NF2* gene located on the chromosome 22 (22q12.2), which regulates the production of a tumor-suppressor protein merlin (for *m*oesin-*e*zrin-*r*adixin-*l*ike prote*in*), also referred to as *schwannomin*. Type 2 of neurofibromatosis is characterized by multiple schwannomas, meningiomas, and ependymomas.

Osteogenesis Imperfecta

Osteogenesis imperfecta (OI), also known as *fragilitas ossium*, is a congenital, non–sex-linked, hereditary disorder that manifests in the skeleton as a primary defect in the bone matrix. It is characterized by bone fragility resulting from abnormal quality and/or quantity of type I collagen. Depending on the type of OI, the inheritance of the disorder can be autosomal dominant, autosomal dominant with new mutation, or autosomal recessive. It has been suggested that this disease results from mutations in the genes *COL1A1*, *COL1A2*, *CRTAP*, and *LEPRE1*. Looser, in 1906, divided this condition into two forms, "congenita" and "tarda," and suggested that they are expressions of the same disease. OI congenita (Vrolik disease) has been classified as the more severe form, which is evident at birth and marked by bowing of the upper and lower extremities in an infant who is either stillborn or does not survive the neonatal period. The more benign OI tarda (Ekman-Lobstein

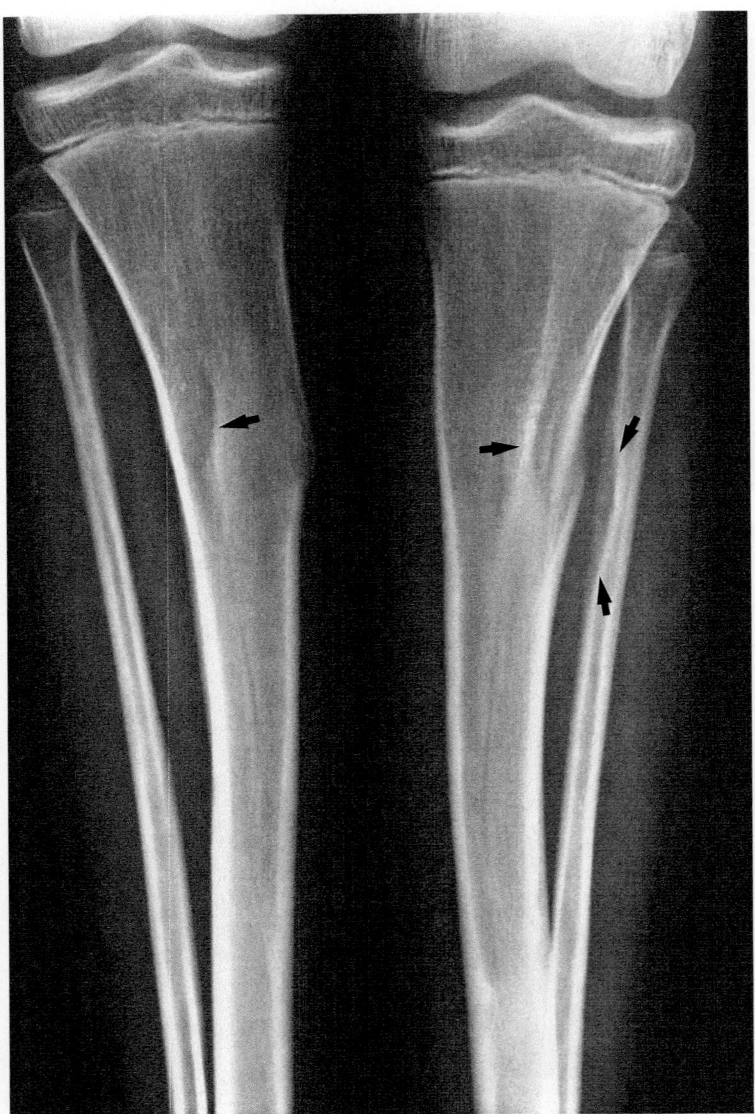

FIGURE 33.18 Neurofibromatosis. Anteroposterior radiograph of the lower legs of an 11-year-old girl shows pitlike erosions in the proximal tibiae and fibulae *(arrows)*, a common finding in this condition.

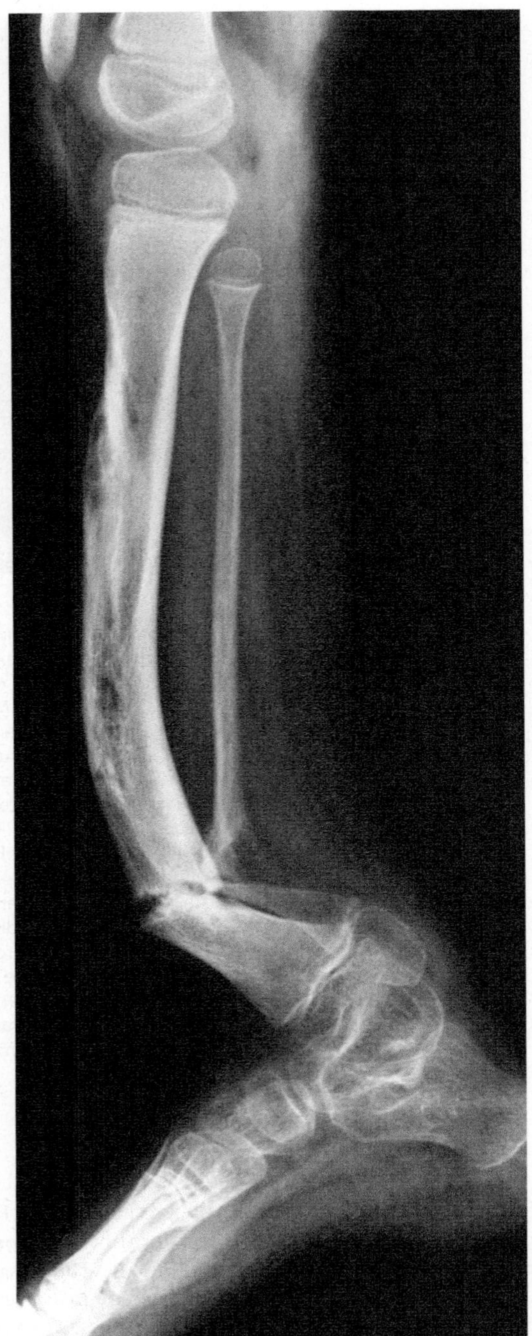

FIGURE 33.19 Neurofibromatosis. Lateral radiograph of the right lower leg of an 11-year-old boy with generalized disease demonstrates anterior bowing of the distal tibia and fibula associated with pseudoarthrosis. Note the pressure erosions in the middle third of the tibial diaphysis.

disease), in which there is a normal life expectancy, may show fractures present at birth, but these more often appear later in infancy. This condition is also associated with other manifestations, such as deformities of the extremities, blue sclerae, laxity of ligaments, and dental abnormalities.

Classification

In general, four major clinical features characterize OI: (a) osteoporosis with abnormal bone fragility, (b) blue sclera, (c) defective dentition (dentinogenesis imperfecta), and (d) presenile onset of hearing impairment. Other clinical features also may be seen, among them are ligamentous laxity and hypermobility of joints, short stature, easy bruising, hyperplastic scars, and abnormal temperature regulation. The earlier classification of OI into two types, congenita and tarda, failed to reflect the complexity and heterogenous nature of this disorder. The classification proposed by Sillence and colleagues in 1979, and later revised, is based on phenotypic features and the mode of inheritance. Currently, four major types of OI and their subtypes are recognized:

Type I: This most common type of the disorder is a relatively mild form, with autosomal dominant inheritance. Bone fragility is mild to moderate, and osteoporosis is invariably present. Sclerae are distinctly blue, and hearing loss or impairment is a common feature. Stature is normal or near-normal. Wormian bones are present. The two subtypes are distinguished by the presence of normal teeth (subtype IA) or dentinogenesis imperfecta (subtype IB).

Type II: This is the fetal or perinatal lethal form of the disorder. This form demonstrates an autosomal dominant inheritance with new mutation. The very severe nature of generalized osteoporosis, bone fragility, and severe intrauterine growth retardation results in death in the fetal or early perinatal period. Of those infants who survive, 80% to 90% die by 4 weeks of age. All patients in this group have radiologic features typical of OI. In addition, the sclerae are blue and the face has a triangle shape caused by soft craniofacial bones and a beaked nose. The calvarium is large relative to the face, and the skull shows a marked lack of mineralization as well as wormian bones. Limbs are short, broad, and angulated. Three subtypes, A, B, and C, are marked by differences in the appearance of the ribs

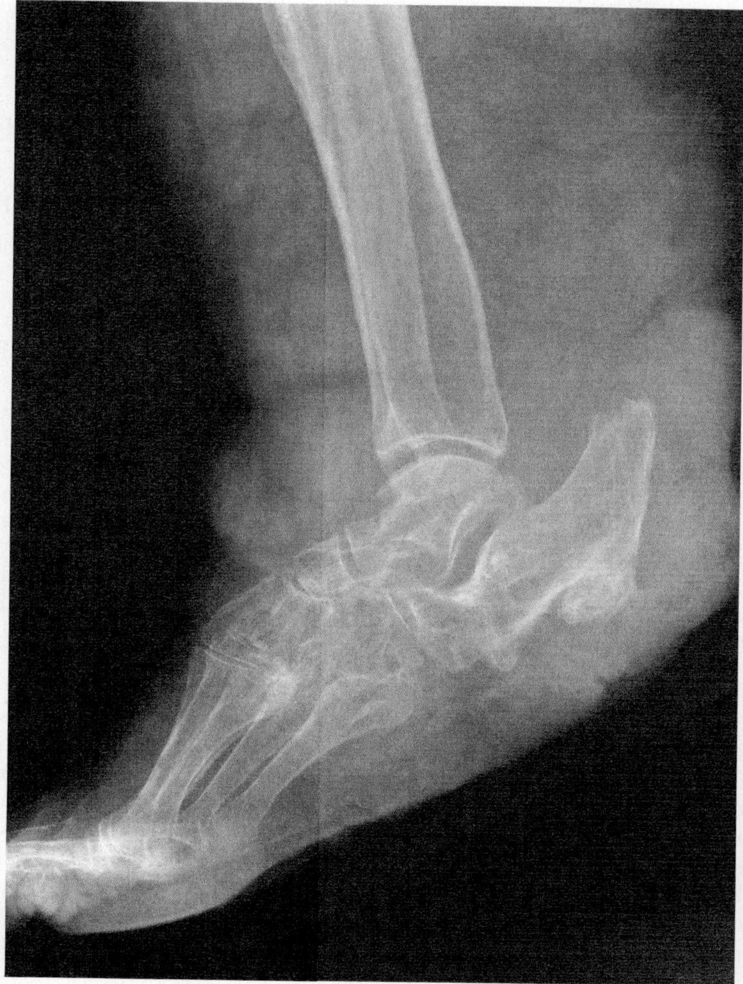

FIGURE 33.20 **Neurofibromatosis.** Lateral radiograph of the lower leg and foot of a 37-year-old woman shows whittling of the calcaneus and marked hypertrophy of the soft tissues (elephantiasis), typical for plexiform type of this condition.

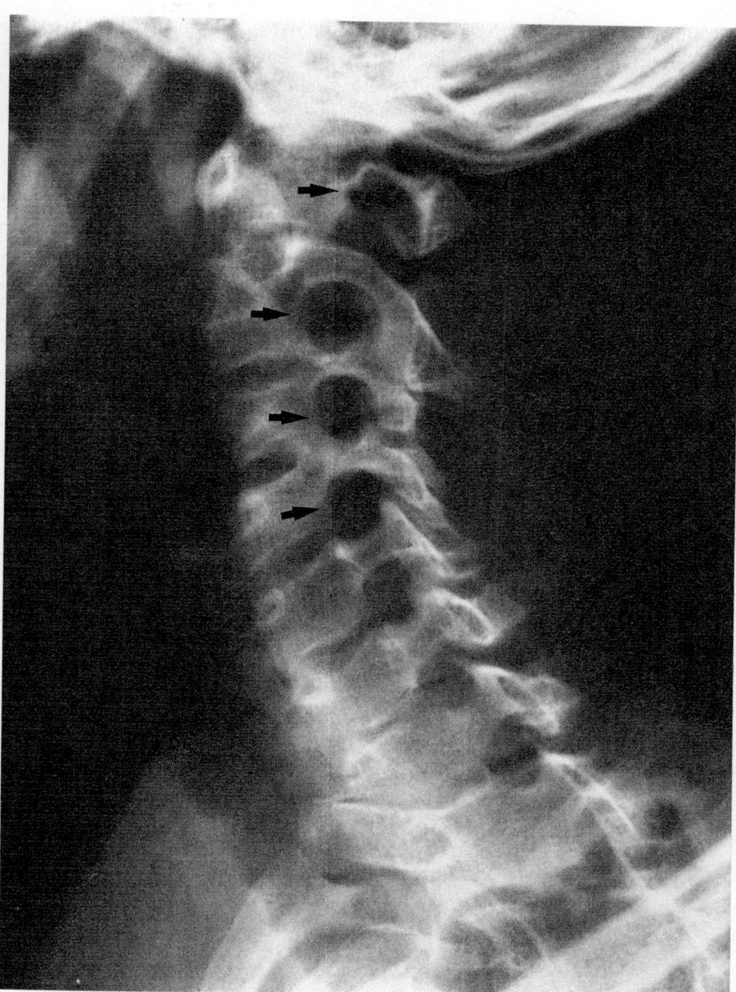

FIGURE 33.21 **Neurofibromatosis.** Oblique radiograph of the cervical spine of a 26-year-old man demonstrates widening of the upper neural foramina *(arrows)* secondary to "dumbbell" neurofibromas arising in the spinal nerve roots.

and the long bones. In subtype A, the long bones are broad and crumpled and the ribs are broad, with continuous beading. In subtype B, the long bones also are broad and crumpled, but the ribs show either discontinuous beading or no beading. Subtype C is characterized by thin fractured long bones and ribs that are thin and beaded.

Type III: This is a severe progressive form and represents a rare autosomal dominant inheritance with new mutations. Bone fragility and osteopenia are considerable, leading with age to multiple fractures and severe progressive deformity of the long bones and spine. Bone abnormalities are generally less severe than in type II and more severe than in type I or IV. Sclerae are normal, although pale blue or gray at birth, but the color changes through infancy and early childhood until it is normal by adolescence or adulthood. The calvarium is large, thin, and poorly ossified; wormian bones are present.

Type IV: This is also a rare type of OI and is inherited as an autosomal dominant trait. Characteristically, osteoporosis, bone fragility, and deformity are present, but they are very mild. Sclerae are usually normal. The incidence of hearing impairment is low and is even lower than in type I.

Glorieux and colleagues added two more types, V and VI, and Ward and associates described in details the rarest form of OI, type VII. Type V includes the patients who originally have been classified as type IV but had a discrete phenotype including hyperplastic callus formation without evidence of mutations in type I collagen. These patients also exhibit calcification of the radioulnar interosseous membrane and radiodense

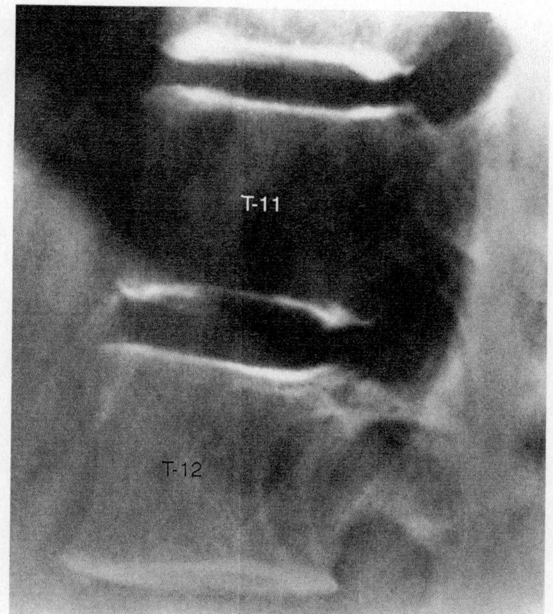

FIGURE 33.22 **Neurofibromatosis.** Lateral spot film of the lower thoracic spine in a 29-year-old woman shows scalloping of the posterior border of the T12 vertebra, a common manifestation of this condition.

metaphyseal bands adjacent to the growth plates. Histologically, this type is characterized by a mesh-like pattern of lamellation under polarized light microscopy. Type VI includes the patients who sustained more frequent fractures (particularly of the vertebrae) than those with type IV, first documented between 4 and 18 months of age. Sclerae of these patients were white or faintly blue, and dentinogenesis imperfecta was uniformly absent. Serum alkaline phosphatase levels were elevated compared with age-matched patients with OI type IV. The type VII is an autosomal recessive form, with moderate to severe phenotype, characterized by fractures at birth, blue sclerae, early deformity of the lower extremities, coxa vara, and osteopenia. Rhizomelia is a prominent clinical feature. This form of OI has been localized to chromosome 3p22-24.1, which is outside the loci for type I collagen genes.

Imaging Features

The imaging features of OI are easily identified on conventional radiographs. Severe osteoporosis, deformities of the bones, and thinning of the cortices are consistently observed features. The bones are also attenuated and gracile, with a trumpet-shaped appearance to the metaphysis (Fig. 33.23). The fractures are commonly observed (Fig 33.24). Other typical skeletal abnormalities are seen in the skull, where wormian bones are a recognizable feature (Fig. 33.25), and in the spine, where severe kyphoscoliosis may develop from a combination of osteoporosis, ligamentous laxity, and posttraumatic deformities (Fig. 33.26). In children with a severe degree of disorder, the metaphyses and epiphyses of the long bones may exhibit numerous scalloped radiolucent areas with sclerotic margins (Fig. 33.27). This appearance is referred to as *popcorn calcifications*, and it may be the result of traumatic fragmentation of the growth plate. The pelvis is invariably deformed, and acetabular protrusio is a common finding (Fig. 33.28).

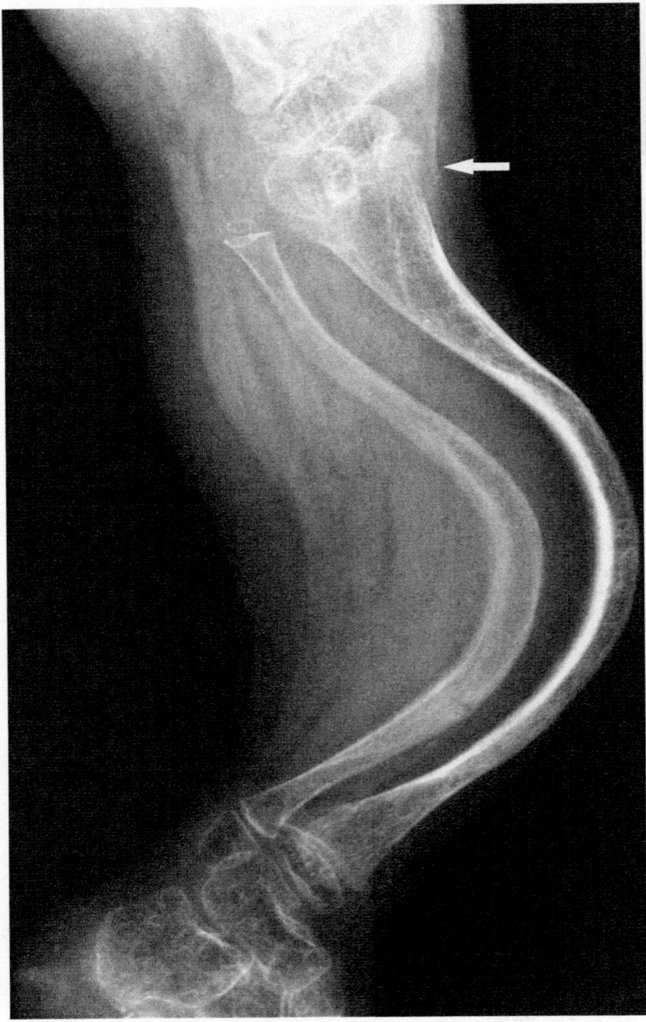

FIGURE 33.23 Osteogenesis imperfecta. Lateral radiograph of the leg of a 12-year-old boy with type III disease demonstrates thinning of the cortices and anterior bowing of the tibia and fibula. Note the trumpet-shaped appearance of the tibial metaphysis *(arrow)*.

Differential Diagnosis

Occasionally, OI may be misdiagnosed as child abuse and vice versa. Patient and family history, physical examination, diagnostic imaging, and the clinical course of the abnormalities all contribute to the distinction of this condition from child abuse. The keys to distinguishing OI from a battered child syndrome ("shaken baby syndrome," parent–infant trauma syndrome) are (a) the presence of blue sclera or abnormal teeth in OI, (b) investigation of clinical and family history (invariably positive in OI), (c) physical examination, and (d) radiologic examination for the detection of wormian bones and osteoporosis in OI and metaphyseal corner fractures and "bucket-handle" fractures that are highly specific and virtually pathognomonic features of child abuse. Several other features are also specific for child abuse, including multiple rib fractures, especially posterior rib fractures near or at the costovertebral junction; multiple fractures and/or multiple fractures showing different stages of healing; and sternal or scapular fractures, especially of the acromion. Transverse, oblique, or spiral fractures of a long bone with normal mineralization in the absence of any previous history, especially in a nonambulatory infant, are also highly suggestive of child abuse. The key to diagnosis of either condition is the correlation of clinical history, physical examination, family history, and imaging findings.

Treatment

There is no specific treatment for OI other than correction of the deformities it produces and the prevention of fractures. The condition, however, tends to improve spontaneously at puberty, with cessation or a decrease in the number of fractures. Some reports suggest a gradual increase in bone density after treatment with intravenous infusion of sodium pamidronate. The limb deformities are corrected by various types of osteotomies, with the popular method being the Sofield ("shish kabob") technique, in which the deformed bones are osteotomized in a fragmentation procedure, cut into short segments, and then realigned by threading them onto a rigid or expandable rod (Fig. 33.29). The most common complications of this treatment are rod breakage, refracture of the bone at the end of the metallic device, and pseudoarthrosis.

Achondroplasia

Clinical Features

Achondroplasia is a hereditary autosomal dominant anomaly that begins in utero caused by a failure in endochondral bone formation and affects the growth and development of cartilage. About 80% of cases result from a sporadic mutation in the fibroblast growth factor (FGF) receptor gene encoding *FGFR3*, located on the chromosome 4. There are two mutations in the gene, both involving a change of the amine acid glycine at position 380 to arginine. The most striking feature of achondroplasia is short-limb, rhizomelic (disproportional) dwarfism. The hands and feet are short and stubby; the trunk is relatively long, with the chest flattened in the anteroposterior dimension; and the lower limbs are often bowed, producing a characteristic waddling gait. The head is large, with prominent frontal bossing, a depressed nasal bridge, and a "scooped-out" facial appearance.

Imaging Features

Radiographically, achondroplasia exhibits distinctive features. As is typical in rhizomelic dwarfism, the tubular bones of the limbs are shortened, with the proximal segments (humeri and femora) more severely affected than the distal portions of the extremities (radius, ulna, tibia, and fibula); the growth plates assume a V-shaped configuration (Fig. 33.30). In the hand, the fingers are short and stubby, with the middle finger separated from the others, giving the hand a "trident" appearance (Fig. 33.31). Identifying features of this disorder may also be encountered in the spine and pelvis. The spine exhibits a characteristic narrowing of the interpedicular distance and short pedicles, which often result in spinal stenosis; scalloping of the posterior aspect of the vertebral bodies is also a common finding (Fig. 33.32). In the pelvis, which is short and broad, the iliac bones are rounded, lacking the normal flaring; the acetabular roofs are horizontally oriented; and the sciatic notches are small. These features together give the hemipelvis the appearance of a ping-pong paddle. The shape of the inner contour of the pelvis has also been likened to a champagne glass (Fig. 33.33).

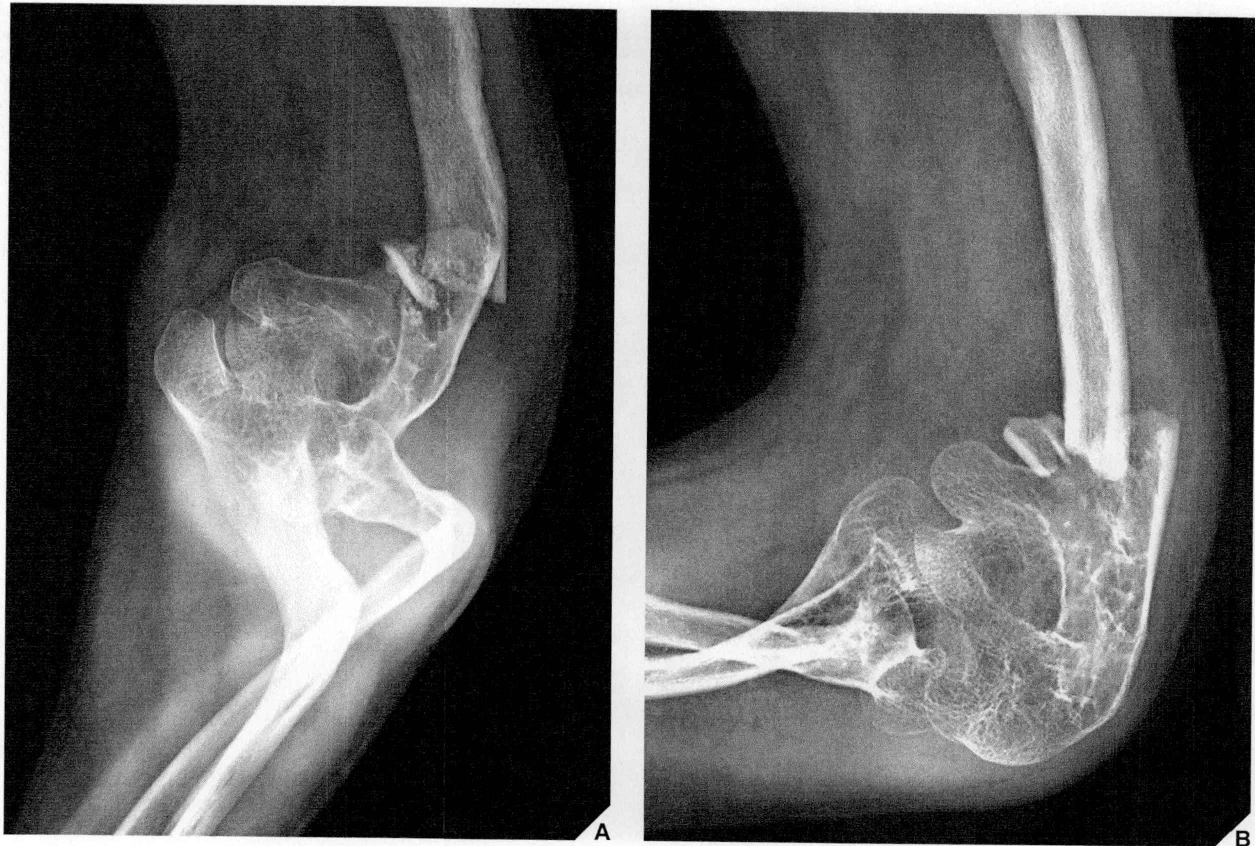

FIGURE 33.24 Osteogenesis imperfecta. **(A)** Anteroposterior and **(B)** lateral radiographs of the elbow of a 27-year-old man show typical appearance of bones in this condition. Note comminuted supracondylar fracture of the humerus.

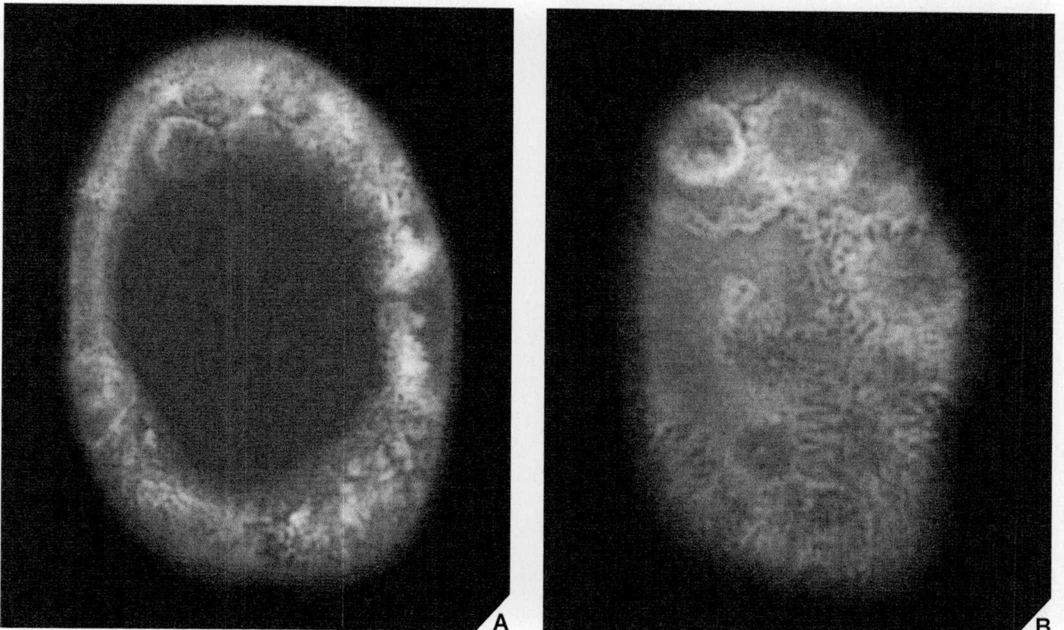

FIGURE 33.25 CT of osteogenesis imperfecta. Axial CT sections of the skull **(A)** through the frontal and parietal bones and **(B)** through the vertex show sutural (wormian) bones.

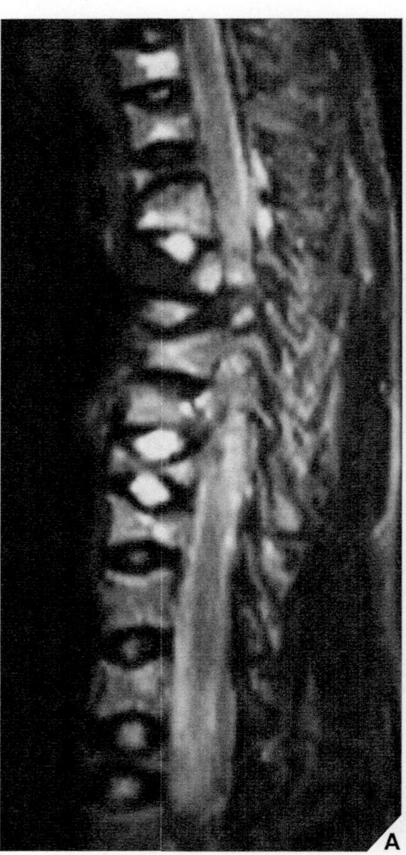

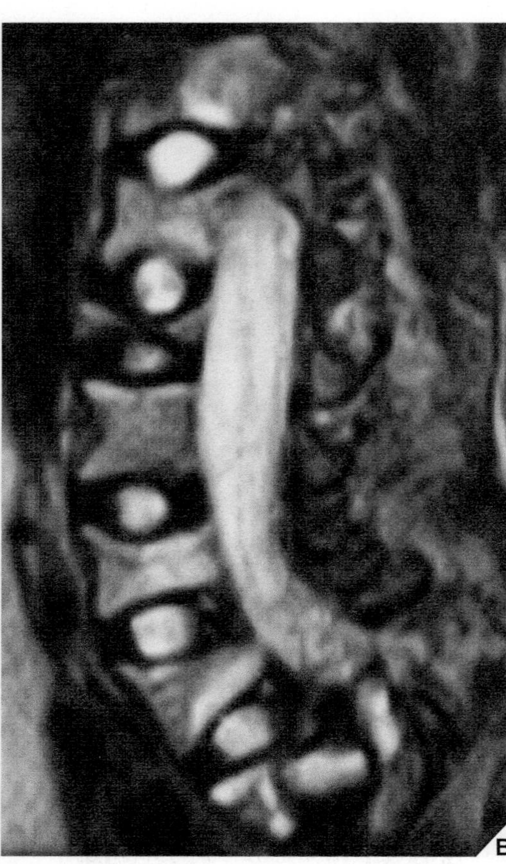

FIGURE 33.26 MRI of OI. **(A)** Sagittal T2-weighted MR image of the thoracic spine of a 13-year-old boy shows compression fractures of several vertebral bodies associated with kyphosis and compression of the spinal cord. **(B)** Sagittal T2-weighted MRI of the lumbar spine demonstrates multiple vertebral fractures and dural ectasia.

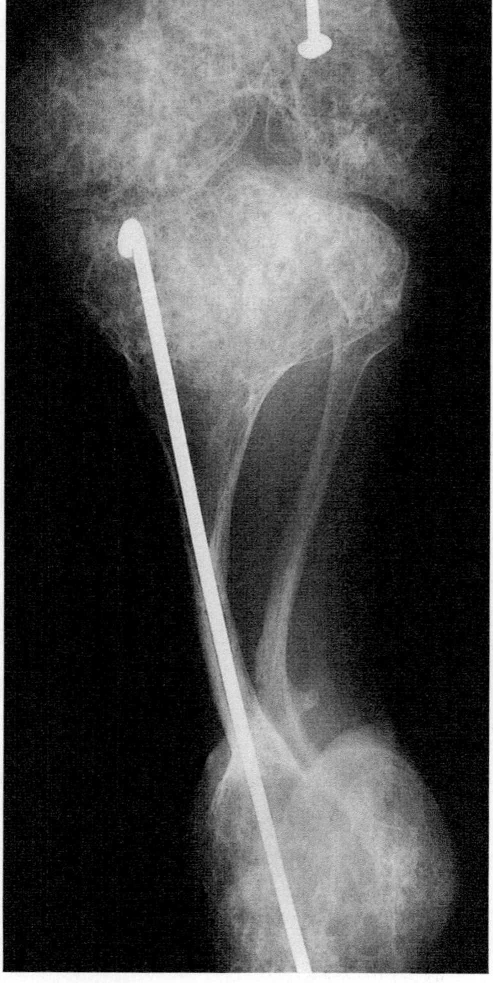

FIGURE 33.27 Osteogenesis imperfecta. Anteroposterior radiograph of the left leg of a 12-year-old boy with a type III disease shows "popcorn calcifications" at the articular ends of the long bones. A Rush pin has been placed in the tibia because of a pathologic fracture.

FIGURE 33.28 **Osteogenesis imperfecta.** Marked deformity of the pelvis, seen here in a 27-year-old woman, is a consistent finding in OI tarda. Note the bilateral acetabular protrusio and the pathologic fracture of the right femur *(arrow)*.

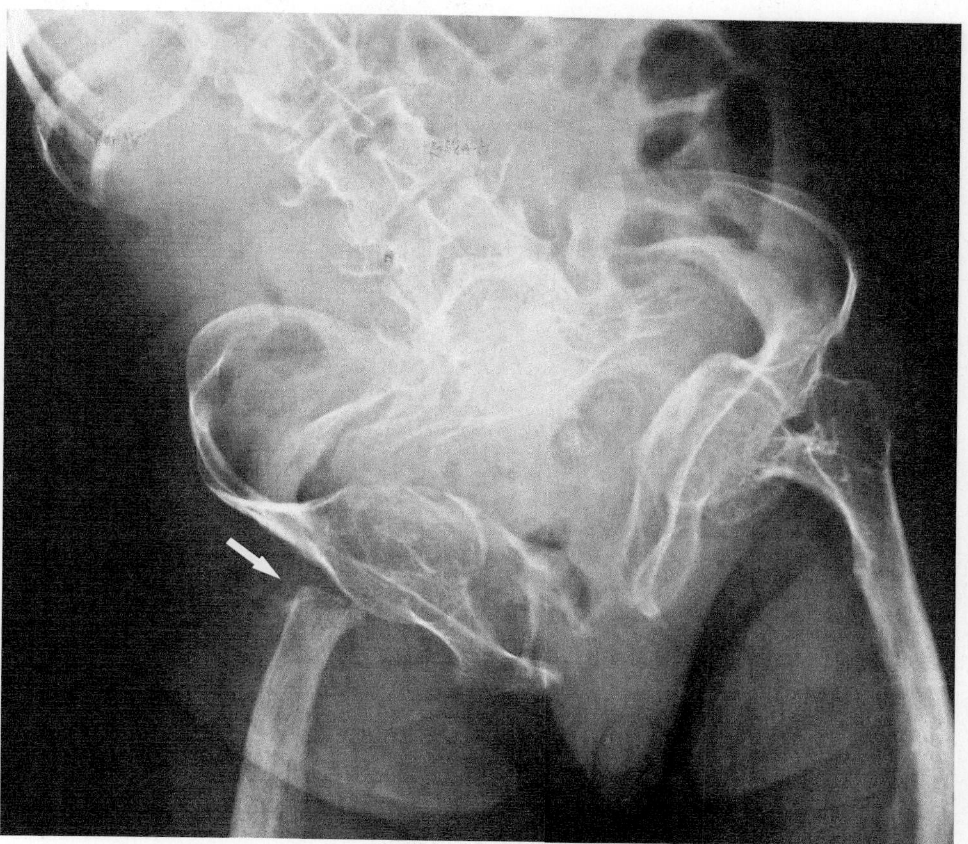

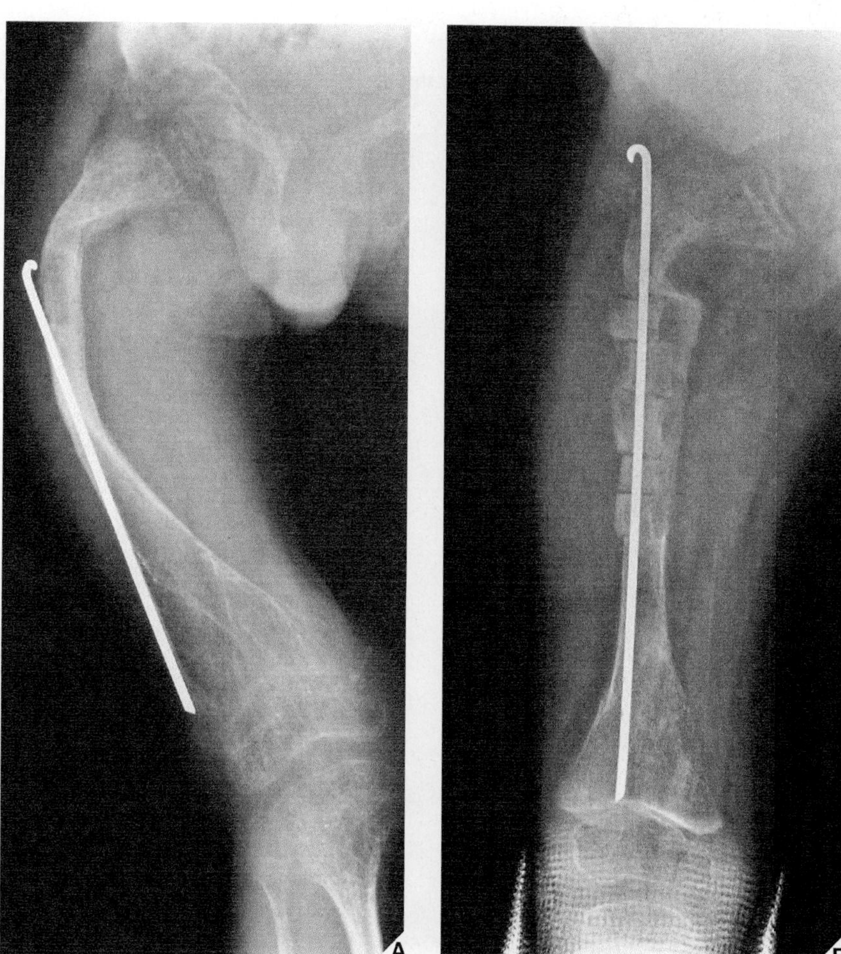

FIGURE 33.29 **Treatment of OI.** A 10-year-old boy with severe long bone deformities sustained a pathologic fracture of the right femur. **(A)** A single intramedullary Kirschner wire was inserted, and union was achieved. However, there is still marked lateral bowing of the femur. **(B)** Postoperative radiograph after a Sofield osteotomy shows the osseous segments of the femur realigned on a rigid rod.

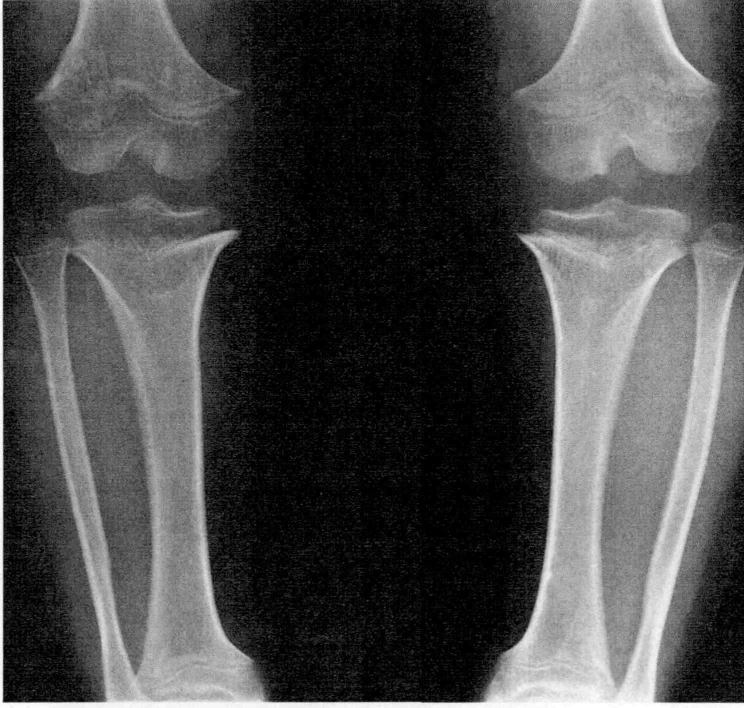

FIGURE 33.30 Achondroplasia. Anteroposterior radiograph of the lower legs of a 12-year-old boy shows the short, broad tibiae characteristic of this disorder; the fibulae are relatively longer. The epiphyses about the knee joints have a V-shaped configuration and appear recessed into the trumpetlike metaphyses.

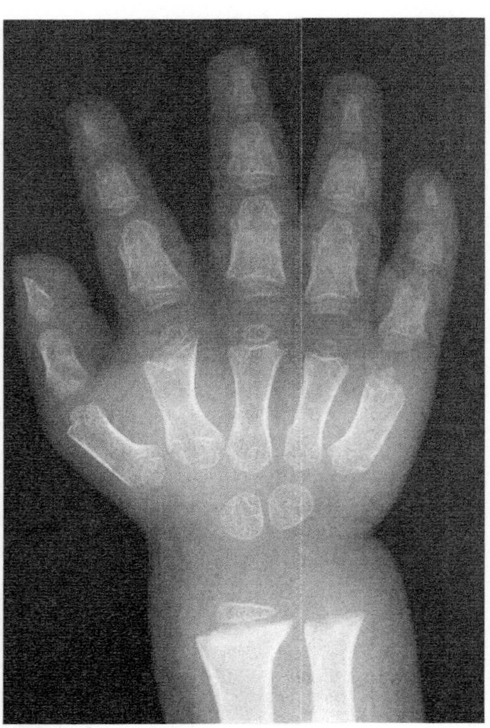

FIGURE 33.31 Achondroplasia. Typical trident appearance of a hand in a 3-year-old girl. Note short metacarpals and short phalanges of the fingers.

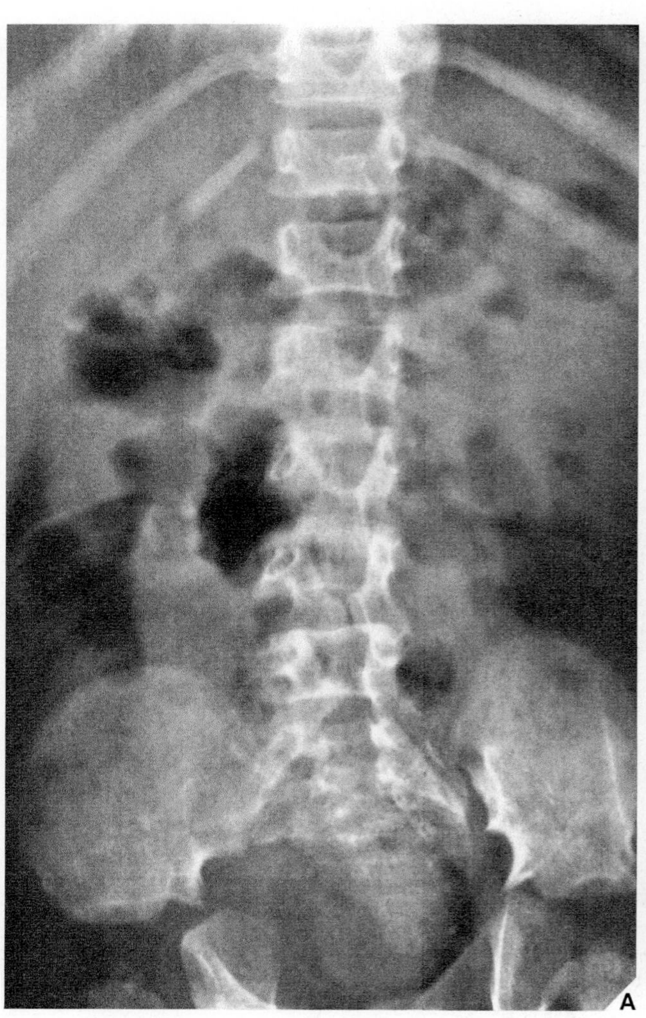

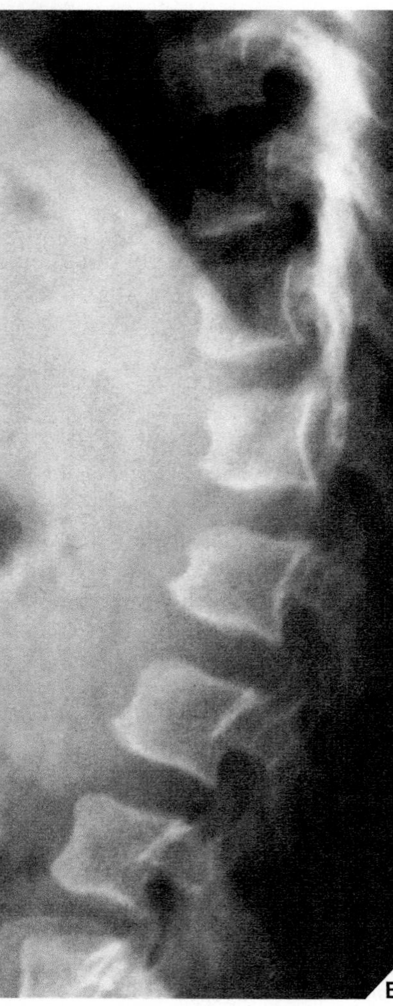

FIGURE 33.32 Achondroplasia. **(A)** Anteroposterior radiograph of the thoracolumbar spine of a 2-year-old boy shows progressive narrowing of the interpedicular distance of the lumbar vertebrae in a caudal direction. **(B)** Lateral radiograph reveals the short pedicles and posterior vertebral scalloping.

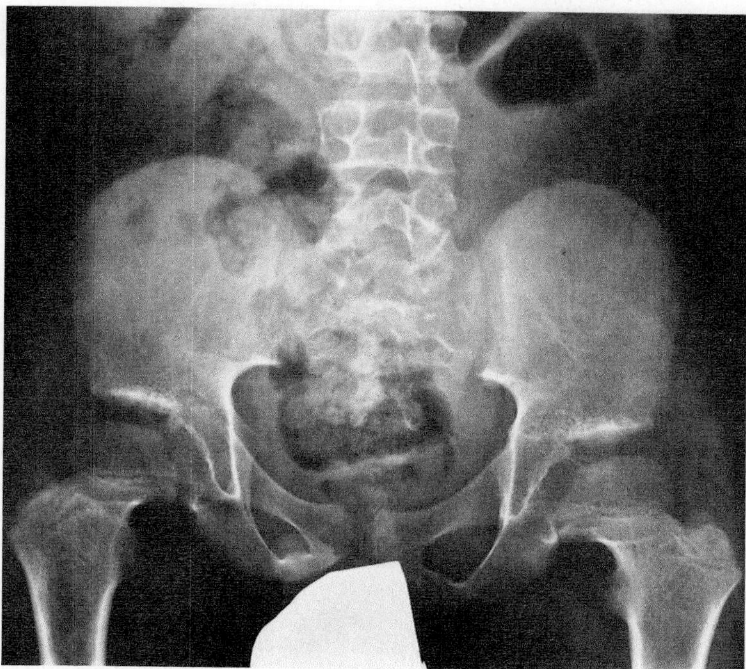

FIGURE 33.33 Achondroplasia. Anteroposterior radiograph of the pelvis of a 13-year-old boy shows the classic manifestations of this condition. The iliac bones are rounded, lacking their normal flaring, and the acetabular roofs are horizontal—features rendering the appearance of a ping-pong paddle. Note also the "champagne glass" inner contour of the pelvic cavity.

Complications

Most individuals with achondroplasia lead a normal life, with a life expectancy of about 10 years less than general population. The most serious complication of achondroplasia is related to the spinal stenosis secondary to the typically short pedicles. Narrowing of the foramen magnum predisposes to cervical cord and brainstem compression. Communicating hydrocephalus may also occur. Patients with the disease also occasionally have herniation of the nucleus pulposus. CT and MRI are the procedures of choice for confirming these two complications.

Differential Diagnosis

It is important to note that there are two other conditions resembling achondroplasia, but they differ from it in the severity of their symptoms and in radiographic presentation. *Hypochondroplasia* is a mild form of osteochondrodystrophy, in which the skeletal abnormalities are less severe than in achondroplasia. The skull is unaffected. *Thanatophoric dwarfism*, conversely, is thought to be a severe form of achondroplasia. It is lethal either in utero or within hours to days after birth.

Mucopolysaccharidoses

Mucopolysaccharidoses (MPS) constitute a group of hereditary disorders having in common an excessive accumulation of mucopolysaccharides (glycosaminoglycans) secondary to deficiencies in specific lysosomal enzymes. Although several distinctive types of MPS have been delineated (Table 33.4), each with distinctive clinical and radiologic features, a specific diagnosis of any of these conditions is made on the basis of the patient's age at onset, the level of neurologic stunting, the amount of corneal clouding, and other clinical features. With the exception of Morquio-Brailsford disease, all the MPS are marked by excessive urinary excretion of dermatan and heparan sulfate. Several cytogenetic studies clarified to certain degree the cause of these disorders. For instance, mutations in the *IDUA* gene is responsible for MPS type I; mutations in the *IDS* gene cause MPS II; mutations in the *SGSH*, *NAGLU*, *HGSNAT*, and *GNS* genes cause MPS III; and mutations in the *GALNS* and *GLBI* genes result in MPS IV. GALNS deficiency induces the accumulation of glycosaminoglycans (GAGs), keratin sulfate (KS), and chondroitin 6-sulfate (C6S) in various tissues, particularly bone, cartilage, ligaments, heart valves, and cornea.

The MPS exhibit common imaging findings. These include osteoporosis, oval- or hook-shaped vertebral bodies, and an abnormal configuration of the pelvis, with overconstriction of the iliac bodies and wide flaring of the iliac wings. The tubular bones are shortened, and dysplastic changes are evident in the proximal femoral epiphyses (Fig. 33.34). The joints are also deformed, and soft tissues are copious (Fig. 33.35). The MPS, however, do show variations in these radiographic abnormalities; Hurler syndrome, for example, exhibits a characteristic rounding of the vertebral end plates on the lateral projection; the vertebral bodies appear oval in shape, but frequently, there is a dorsolumbar gibbous with a hypoplastic hook-shaped, recessed vertebral body.

Fibrodysplasia Ossificans Progressiva (Myositis Ossificans Progressiva)

Fibrodysplasia ossificans progressiva is a rare systemic autosomal dominant disorder with variable expressivity and complete penetrance. The responsible *ACVR1* gene has recently been mapped to chromosome 17q21-22, and another study has localized it to chromosome 4q21-31. In most cases, only a single family member is affected. This suggests the involvement of a sporadic mutation.

Clinical Features

Most patients are affected early in life (from birth to age 5 years), and there is no gender predominance. The earliest clinical symptom is the appearance of painful nodules and masses in the subcutaneous tissue, particularly around the head and neck, with associated stiffness and limitation of movement. Subsequently, excessive ossification of muscles, ligaments, and fascia occur, with the predominant sites of involvement in the head and neck, the dorsal paraspinal muscles, the shoulder girdles, and the hips. Involvement of intercostal musculature interferes with respiration. Bilateral malformation of the great toes is a common finding.

Clinically, the condition progresses from the shoulder girdle to the upper arms, spine, and pelvis. The natural history is one of remissions and exacerbations; death secondary to respiratory failure caused by constriction of the chest wall is an almost inevitable outcome. No effective treatment is known to date.

Imaging Features

Abnormalities of the thumb and great toe are present at birth and precede the soft-tissue ossification. The characteristic radiologic changes consist of agenesis, microdactyly, or congenital hallux valgus, occasionally with fusion at the metacarpophalangeal or metatarsophalangeal joints (Figs. 33.36A and 33.37C). Short, big toes and short thumbs may be associated with clinodactyly

TABLE 33.4 Classification of the Mucopolysaccharidoses (MPS)

Designated Number	Eponym	Genetic and Clinical Characteristics
MPS I-H	Hurler syndrome (gargoylism)	Autosomal recessive, *IDUA* gene mutations Corneal clouding, mental retardation, micrognathia, hepatosplenomegaly, cardiomegaly Urinary excretion of dermatan and heparan sulfates Deficiency of α-l-iduronidase enzyme
MPS I-S	Scheie syndrome	Autosomal recessive Corneal clouding, retinal degeneration, glaucoma, normal mental development, pigeon chest, short neck, prominent clavicles and scapulae, stiff joints, carpal tunnel syndrome, deformities of hands and feet, flattening of the vertebral bodies, aortic valve disease, inguinal and umbilical hernias
MPS I-H/S	Hurler-Scheie compound syndrome	Moderate mental retardation, short stature, corneal clouding, hearing loss Urinary excretion of same product as in MPS I-H and same enzyme deficiency
MPS II	Hunter syndrome (mild and severe variants)	Sex chromosome–linked recessive disorder (males only) Mild mental retardation, absence of corneal clouding Urinary excretion of same product as in MPS I-H Deficiency of iduronate sulfatase
MPS III	Sanfilippo syndrome (A, B, C, and D variants)	Autosomal recessive Progressive mental retardation, motor overactivity, coarse facial features, death by second decade Urinary excretion of heparan sulfate Deficiency of heparan-*N*-sulfatase (A) Deficiency of α-*N*-acetylglucosaminidase (B) Deficiency of acetyl-CoAlpha-glucosaminide acetyltransferase (C) Deficiency of *N*-acetylglucosamine-6-sulfatase (D)
MPS IV	Morquio-Brailsford disease (type A, classic; type B, milder abnormalities)	Autosomal recessive Short-trunk dwarfism, characteristic posture with knock knees, lumbar lordosis, and severe pectus carinatum; hypoplasia of odontoid; corneal opacities; impaired hearing; hepatosplenomegaly; widely spaced teeth Urinary excretion of keratan sulfate Deficiency of *N*-acetylgalactosamine-6-sulfate sulfatase (A) Deficiency of beta-galactosidase (B)
MPS V	Redesignated MPS I-S	See above (MPS I-S)
MPS VI	Maroteaux-Lamy syndrome	Autosomal recessive Normal intelligence, short stature, lumbar kyphosis; hepatosplenomegaly, joint contractures, heart defects Urinary excretion of dermatan sulfate Deficiency of *N*-acetylgalactosamine-4-sulfatase
MPS VII	Sly syndrome	Autosomal recessive Growth and mental retardation, hydrocephalus, hepatosplenomegaly, inguinal and umbilical hernia, pulmonary infections, skeletal dysplasia, short stature Urinary excretion of heparan and dermatan sulfates Deficiency of β-glucuronidase
MPS VIII	DiFerrante syndrome	Probably genetic trait Short stature Urinary excretion of keratan and heparan sulfates Deficiency of glucosamine-6-sulfate sulfatase
MPS IX	Natowicz syndrome	Soft-tissue masses around joints, short stature, normal intelligence Deficiency of hyaluronidase

of the fifth finger as well as with brachydactyly. In the soft tissues, extensive ossifications are seen, along with bridging osseous masses in the cervical and thoracic spine, the thorax, and the extremities (Figs. 33.36B and 33.37A,B). Involvement of the insertions of ligaments and tendons occasionally produces osseous excrescences mimicking exostoses. Joint ankylosis results most often from ossification of the surrounding soft tissue, but a true intraarticular fusion may occur (Figs. 33.36C and 33.37B). CT provides accurate anatomic localization of preosseous lesions. MRI, particularly contrast-enhanced studies, may further characterize soft-tissue abnormalities. Early stage lesions exhibit low signal intensity on T1-weighted sequences and high signal intensity on T2-weighted images, accompanied by marked homogeneous enhancement on postgadolinium studies.

Pathology

The primary histopathologic abnormality is in the connective tissues. Occasionally, particularly in the early stages, the pathologic changes may resemble aggressive fibromatosis. Late-stage lesions consist of mature bone of lamellar structure having both compact and cancellous elements. The pathologic abnormalities are similar to those of myositis ossificans circumscripta, but the zoning phenomenon of centripetal ossification is absent. The earliest histologic changes consist of edema and inflammatory exudate, followed by mesenchymal proliferation and formation of a large mass of collagen. This collagen is capable of accepting the deposition of calcium salts. Eventually, the lesion is transformed into irregular masses of lamellar and woven bone.

Sclerosing Dysplasias of Bone

The sclerosing bone dysplasias are a group of developmental anomalies that reflect disturbances in the formation and modeling of bone, most commonly as a result of inborn errors in metabolism. A common defect in many of these disorders is reflected in a failure of cartilage and/or bone to resorb during the process of skeletal maturation and remodeling.

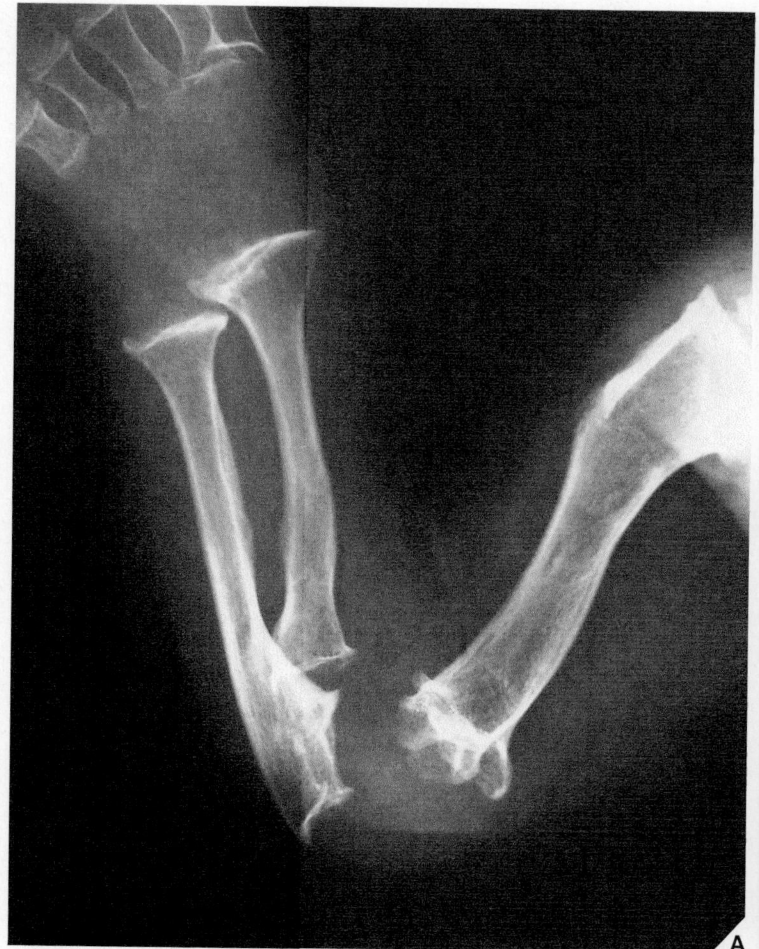

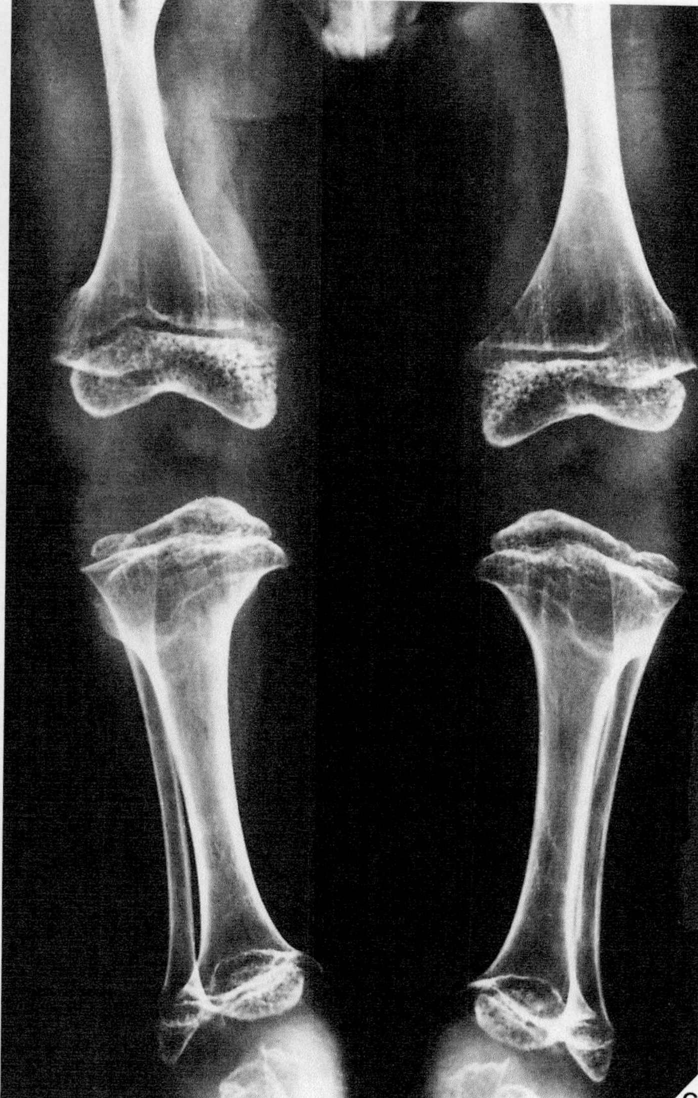

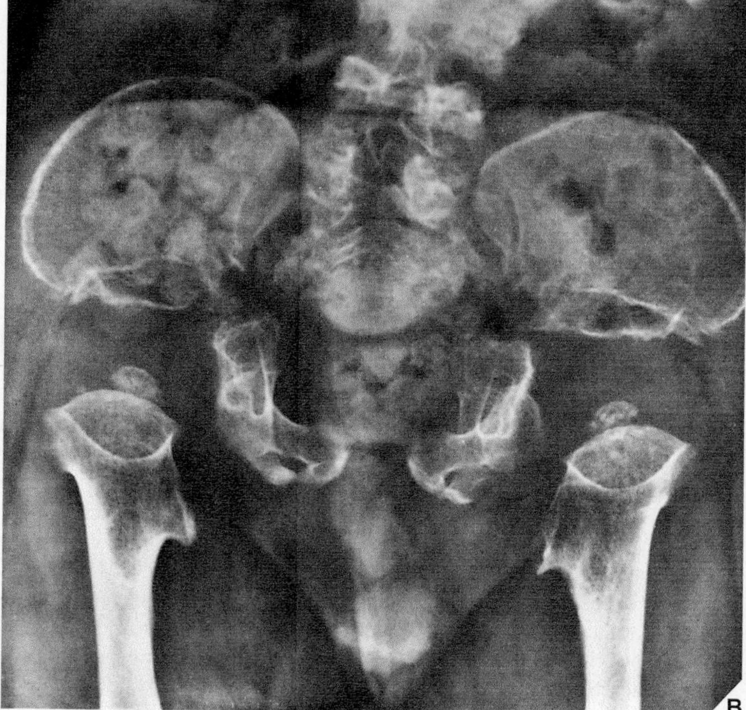

FIGURE 33.34 Morquio-Brailsford disease. The classic features of this disease are present in radiographic studies of a 3-year-old boy. **(A)** Radiograph of the right arm shows foreshortening and deformity of the humerus, radius, and ulna, with an irregular outline of the metaphyses. **(B)** Anteroposterior radiograph of the pelvis and hips shows flaring of the iliac wings and constriction of the iliac bodies. The narrowing of the pelvis at the level of the acetabula, which are distorted, produces a characteristic "wine glass" appearance. Note the fragmentation of the ossification centers in the femoral heads and the broadening of the femoral necks, with subluxation in the hip joints and a *coxa valga* deformity. **(C)** The legs show deformities in the epiphyses of the femora and tibiae as well as foreshortening of these bones. *(Continued)*

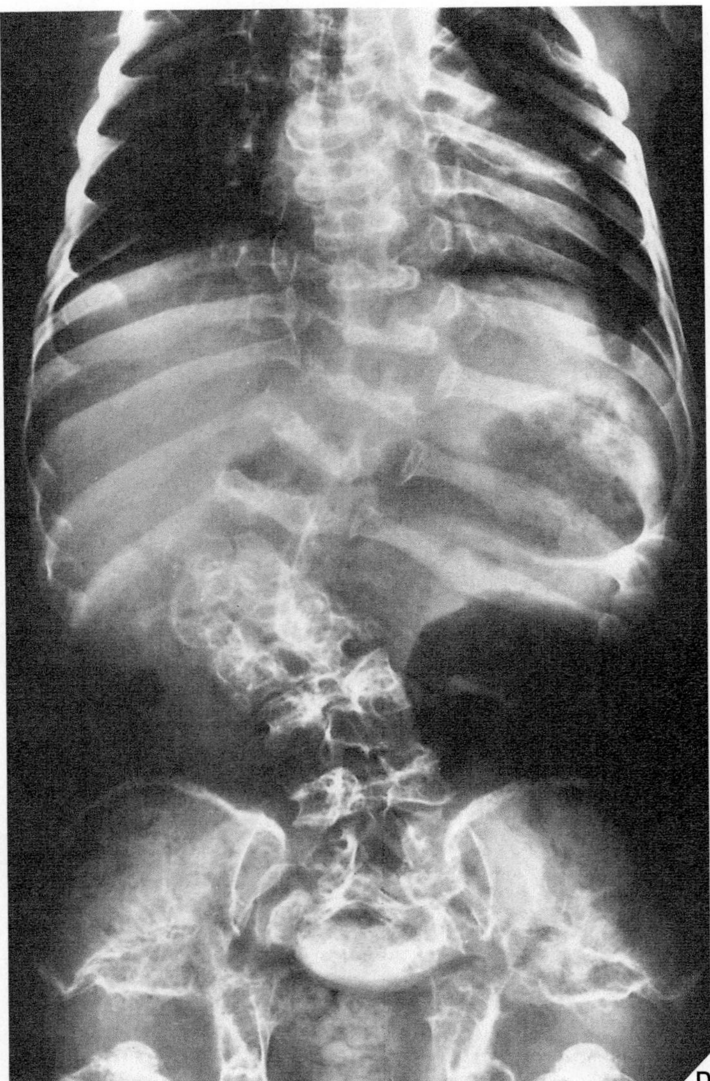

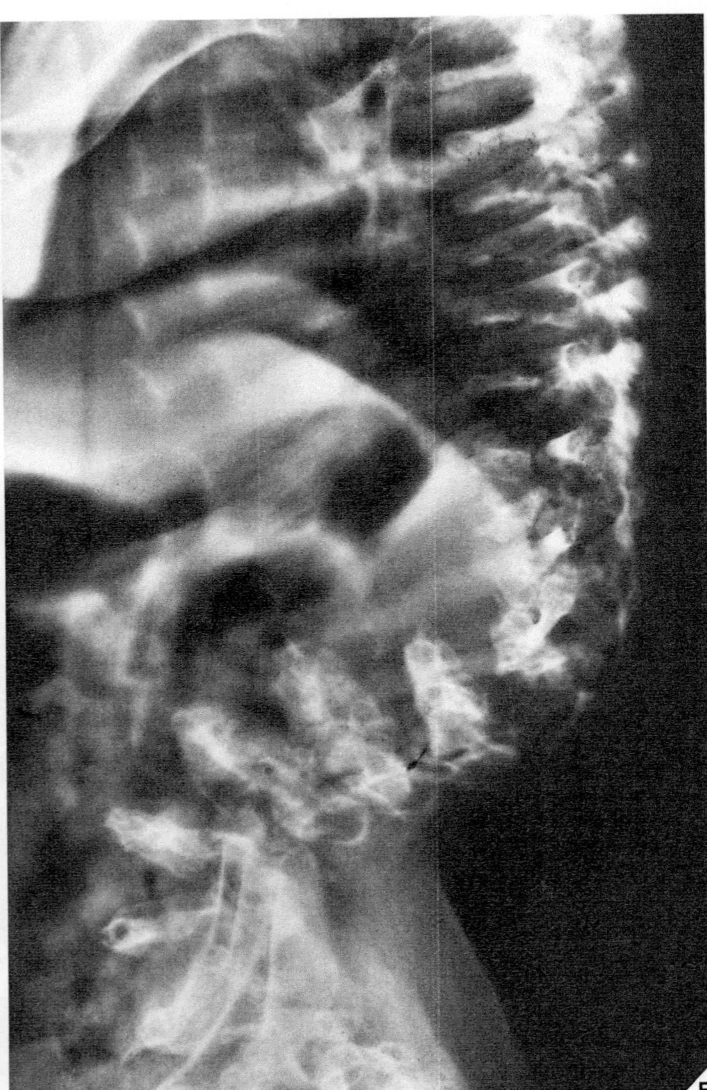

FIGURE 33.34 Morquio-Brailsford disease. ***(Continued)*** **(D)** Anteroposterior radiograph of the spine shows marked kyphoscoliosis. The vertebrae are grossly deformed and flat (platyspondylia), and the ribs are wide but with narrow vertebral ends, giving them a characteristic "canoe paddle" appearance. Note the pronounced osteoporosis. **(E)** Lateral radiograph of the spine demonstrates hyperlordosis in the lumbar segment and kyphosis at the thoracolumbar junction. Note the shape of the vertebral bodies, with the characteristic irregular outline of the end plates and central tonguelike or beak-like projections in the lumbar segment.

One defect in many cases involves the resorption capabilities of osteoclasts in the presence of normal osteoblastic activity. In other instances, the defect lies in excessive bone formation by osteoblasts, which may occur in the presence of normal or diminished osteoclastic activity. These basic errors in metabolism most commonly arise during the processes of endochondral and intramembranous ossification. All sclerosing dysplasias share the common feature of excessive bone accumulation resulting in the radiographic appearance of increased bone density. Norman and Greenspan have developed a classification of these disorders based on the site of failure, whether endochondral or intramembranous, in skeletal development and maturation. In 1991, Greenspan expanded and modified this classification (Table 33.5). The approach reflected in this classification is focused on target sites of involvement and pathomechanism of these dysplasias.

Osteopetrosis

An inherited disorder, osteopetrosis (also called *Albers-Schönberg disease* or *marble-bone disease*), involves a failure in resorption and remodeling of bone formed by endochondral ossification. The result is an excessive accumulation of primary spongiosa (calcified cartilage matrix) in the medullary portion of flat bones and long and short tubular bones as well as in the vertebrae. Although the etiology of this condition is still debatable, deficiency of the enzyme carbonic anhydrase in osteoclasts was attributed to the defective bone resorption by these cells. Moreover, mutations of the gene *SLC4A2* in calve and mouse models have been reported. Osteopetrosis is classified according to the mode of inheritance, severity, age of onset, and associated clinical features. Two variants of osteopetrosis have been described. The infantile "malignant" autosomal recessive form is recognized at birth or in early childhood, and if not treated by bone marrow transplantation, it is frequently fatal because of severe anemia secondary to substantial quantities of cartilage and immature bone packing the marrow cavity. The genetic failure of this variant has been assigned to chromosome 11q13 and is believed to involve the loss-of-function mutations in genes *TCIRG1*, *CLCN7*, *OSTM1*, *SNX10*, and *PLEKHM1*, leading to abundance of osteoclasts but with severe impaired resorptive function (defective osteoclast's ruffled border, hence inability to resorb bone and cartilage) as well as mutations in genes *TNFSF11* and *TNFRSF11A*, leading to decreased number of osteoclasts. The "benign" autosomal dominant adult form has been mapped to chromosome 1p21 and is marked by sclerosis of the skeleton, is compatible with a long life span. Some reports describe what appear to be additional variants of this developmental anomaly, which illustrate the heterogeneity of inheritance of osteopetrosis: intermediate recessive type; autosomal recessive type with renal tubular acidosis and cerebral calcifications; and X-linked osteopetrosis associated with severe immunodeficiency, lymphedema, and ectodermal changes.

Pathology

Gross examination of the bones usually shows widening in the region of the metaphysis and diaphysis, assuming Erlenmeyer flask–like deformity (Fig. 33.38). The affected bones have increased density, and on sectioning,

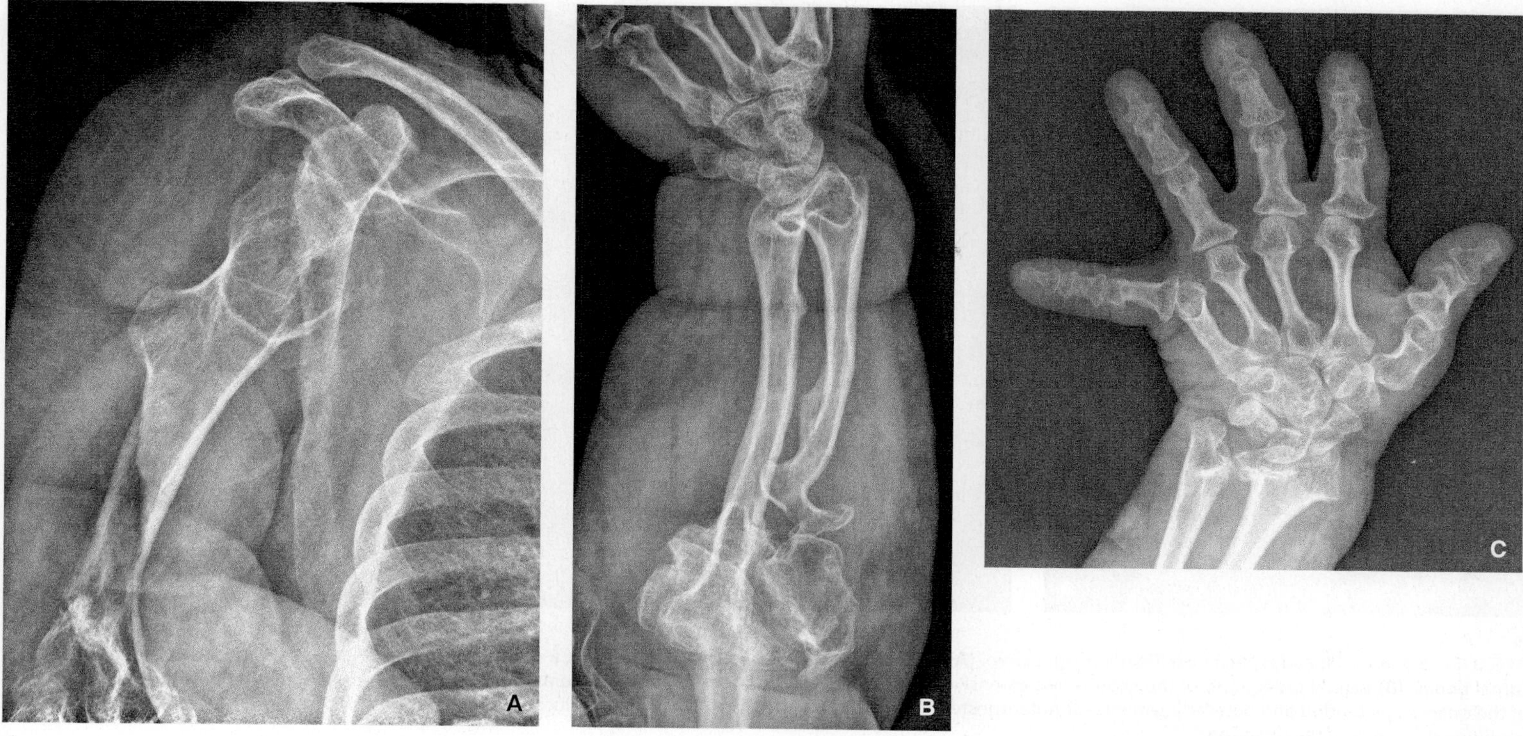

FIGURE 33.35 Morquio-Brailsford disease. **(A)** Anteroposterior radiograph of the right shoulder and humerus of a 54-year-old woman shows deformity of the shoulder joint and foreshortening of the humerus. **(B)** Anteroposterior radiograph of the right forearm shows similar foreshortening of the bones and deformity of the elbow joint. Observe also overabundance of the soft tissues. **(C)** Dorsovolar radiograph of the right hand shows dysplastic changes of the short tubular bones and deformities of the distal radius and ulna.

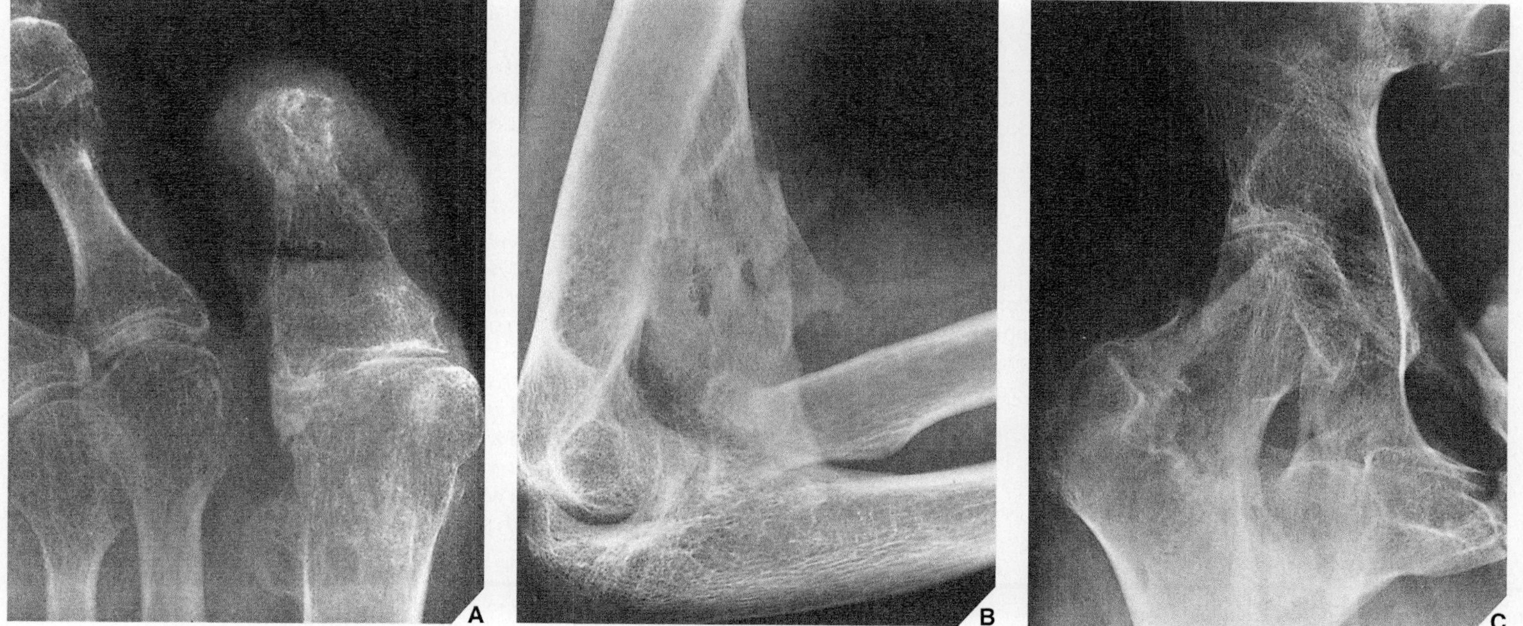

FIGURE 33.36 Fibrodysplasia ossificans progressiva. A 28-year-old man was diagnosed with fibrodysplasia ossificans progressiva at age 3 years. **(A)** Microdactyly of the great toe is a frequent feature of this disorder. **(B)** Lateral radiograph of the elbow shows extensive ossification in the soft tissues, bridging the distal humerus to the radius and ulna. **(C)** Massive ossification around the hip accompanies the ankylosis of the hip joint.

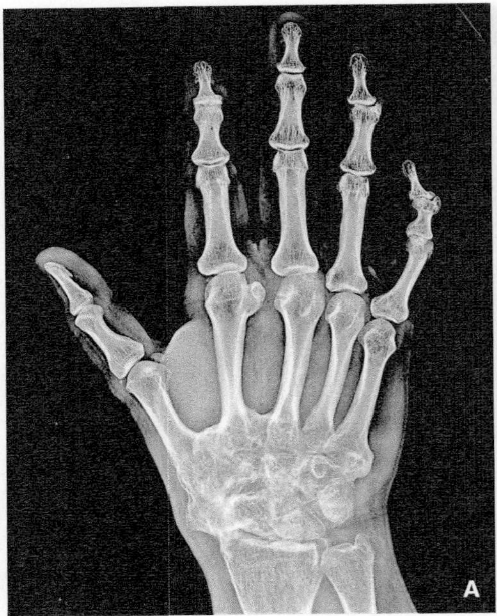

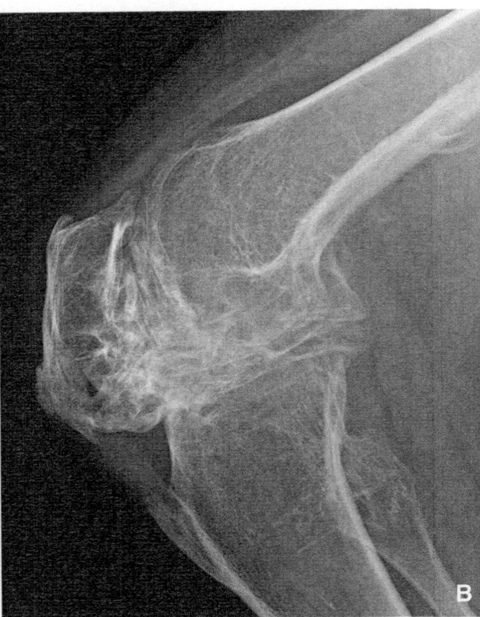

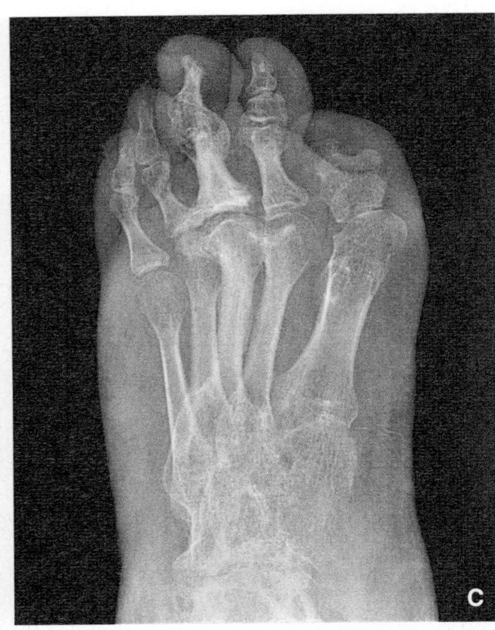

FIGURE 33.37 **Fibrodysplasia ossificans progressive.** **(A)** Dorsovolar radiograph of the left hand of a 41-year-old woman shows ossifications and bridging of the carpal bones. **(B)** Lateral radiograph of the knee shows extensive ossifications of the soft tissues with obliteration and ankylosis of the joint spaces. Note also ossification of the quadriceps tendon and patellar ligament. **(C)** Anteroposterior radiograph of the right foot shows ossifications and ankylosis of the third toe. Observe typical for this condition deformity of the great toe.

TABLE 33.5 Classification of Sclerosing Dysplasias of Bone

I. Dysplasias of Endochondral Bone Formation
- Affecting primary spongiosa (immature bone)
  - Osteopetrosis (Albers-Schönberg disease)
    - Autosomal recessive type (lethal)
    - Autosomal dominant type
    - Intermediate recessive type
    - Autosomal recessive type with tubular acidosis (Sly disease)
  - Pycnodysostosis (Maroteaux-Lamy disease)
- Affecting secondary spongiosa (mature bone)
  - Enostosis (bond island)
  - Osteopoikilosis (spotted bone disease)
  - Osteopathia striata (Voorhoeve disease)

II. Dysplasias of Intramembranous Bone Formation
- Progressive diaphyseal dysplasia (Camurati-Engelmann disease)
- Hereditary multiple diaphyseal sclerosis (Ribbing disease)
- Endosteal hyperostosis (hyperostosis corticalis generalisata)
  - Autosomal recessive form
    - van Buchem disease
    - Sclerosteosis (Truswell-Hansen disease)
  - Autosomal dominant form
    - Worth disease
    - Nakamura disease

III. Mixed Sclerosing Dysplasias (Affecting Both Endochondral and Intramembranous Ossification)
- Affecting predominantly endochondral ossification
  - Dysosteosclerosis
  - Metaphyseal dysplasia (Pyle disease)
  - Metaphyseal dysplasia (Braun-Tinschert type)
  - Craniometaphyseal dysplasia
- Affecting predominantly intramembranous ossification
  - Melorheostosis
  - Progressive diaphyseal dysplasia with skull base involvement (Neuhauser variant)
  - Craniodiaphyseal dysplasia
  - Hyperostosis generalisata with striations of bones (Fairbank disease)
- Coexistence of two or more sclerosing bone dysplasias (overlap syndrome)
  - Melorheostosis with osteopoikilosis and osteopathia striata
  - Osteopathia striata with cranial sclerosis (Horan-Beighton syndrome)
  - Osteopathia striata with osteopoikilosis and cranial sclerosis
  - Osteopathia striata with generalized cortical hyperostosis
  - Osteopathia striata with osteopetrosis
  - Osteopoikilosis with progressive diaphyseal dysplasia

Modified by permission from Springer: Greenspan A. Sclerosing bone dysplasias—a target-site approach. *Skeletal Radiol* 1991;20:561–583.

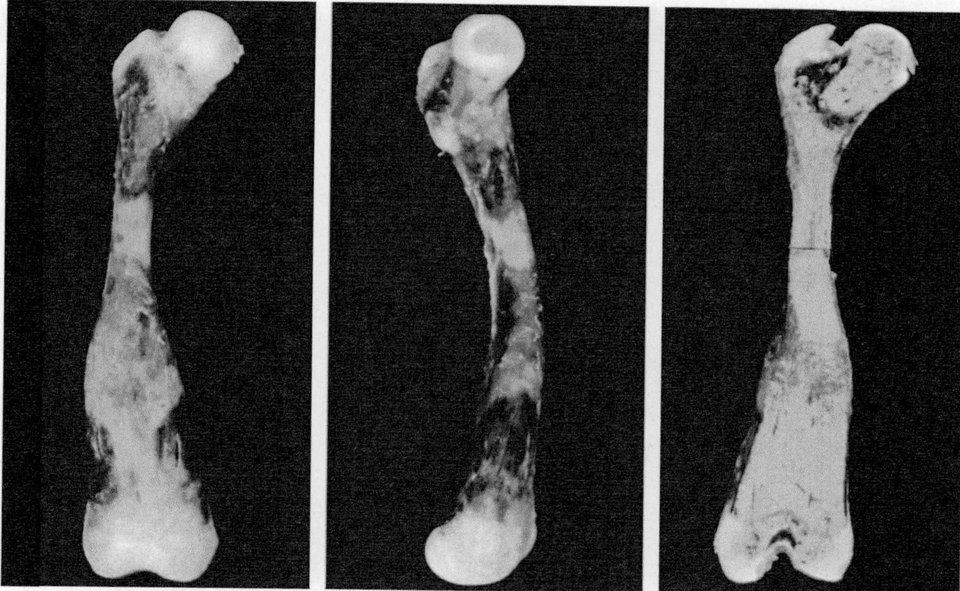

FIGURE 33.38 Pathology of osteopetrosis. Gross appearance of the femur removed from a child with autosomal recessive form of osteopetrosis, seen in frontal *(left)*, lateral *(center)*, and cut section *(right)*, show characteristic Erlenmeyer flask–like deformity of the distal end of the bone. Observe exaggerated anterior bowing, subperiosteal hemorrhage, and uniform density of the bone on cut section. (Reprinted from Bullough P. *Orthopaedic pathology*, 5th ed. Maryland Heights, MO: Mosby; 2009, with permission from Elsevier.)

the tissue is very compact with complete loss of normal architecture (Fig. 33.39). The characteristic histopathologic features of osteopetrosis is the persistence of calcified cartilage of the primary spongiosa with obliteration of the bone marrow cavity. This calcified cartilage is bordered by haphazardly distributed interconnected trabeculae of woven and lamellar bone in variable proportions and of variable thickness, often exhibiting prominent cement lines. In most forms of osteopetrosis, the osteoclasts are increased in number. Despite this, they lie loosely within the intertrabecular spaces and do not resorb bone. In fact, the electron microscopic studies have demonstrated that osteoclasts are defective—they lack ruffled borders and although the cells are in proximity to the bone, they do not appear to be functioning.

Imaging Features

The radiographic hallmark of this disorder, as of all sclerosing bone dysplasias, is increased bone density (Fig. 33.40). The radiographic examination also reveals a lack of differentiation between the cortex and the medullary cavity and occasionally a "bone-in-bone" appearance (Figs. 33.41 and 33.42). The long and short tubular bones exhibit a club-like deformity and splaying of their ends secondary to a failure in remodeling (Figs. 33.43 and 33.44). The same failure in the spine results in a characteristic "bone within bone" or sandwich-like appearance of the vertebral bodies (Figs. 33.45 and 33.46; see also Fig. 33.42A). Osteopetrosis may occur in a cyclic pattern, with intervals of normal growth. This produces alternating bands of normal and abnormal bone in a ringlike pattern, which is particularly well

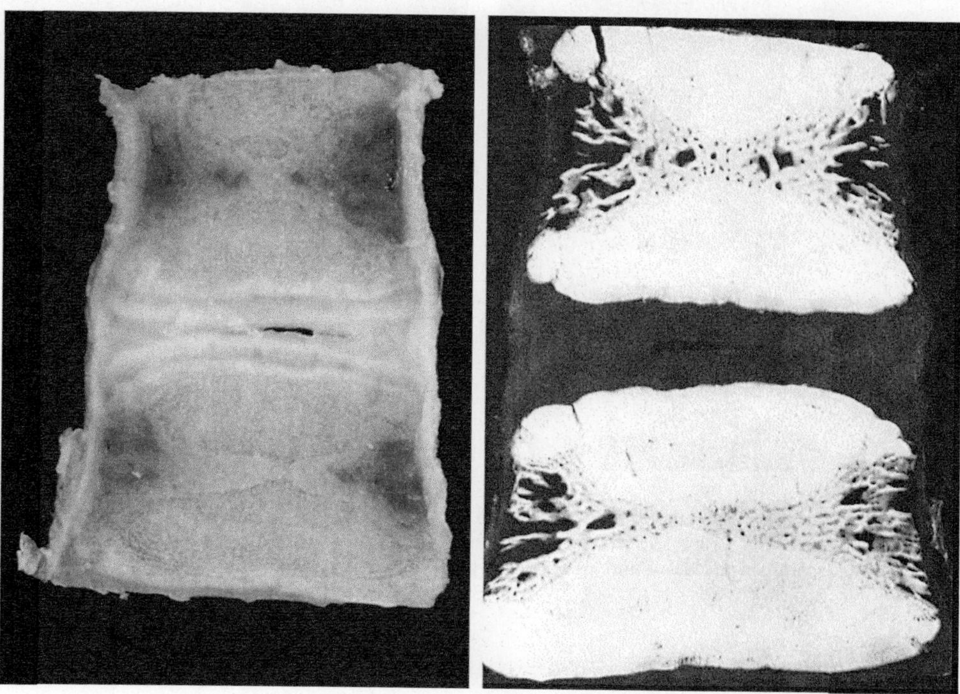

FIGURE 33.39 Pathology of osteopetrosis. Photograph *(left)* and the specimen radiograph *(right)* of the coronal section through two vertebrae of a newborn with autosomal recessive form of osteopetrosis show the extremely dense bone with marrow tissue confined only to the central peripheral portions. (Reprinted from Bullough P. *Orthopaedic pathology*, 5th ed. Maryland Heights, MO: Mosby; 2009, with permission from Elsevier.)

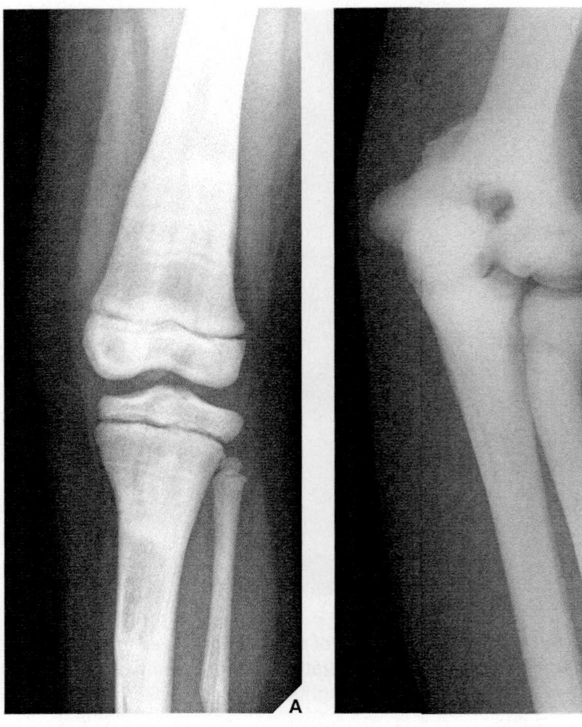

FIGURE 33.40 Osteopetrosis. **(A)** Anteroposterior radiograph of the knee of a 6-year-old girl and **(B)** anteroposterior radiograph of the elbow of a 24-year-old man show classic appearance of osseous structures in this dysplasia: The bones are homogenously dense, and there is lack of clear outline of the endocortex.

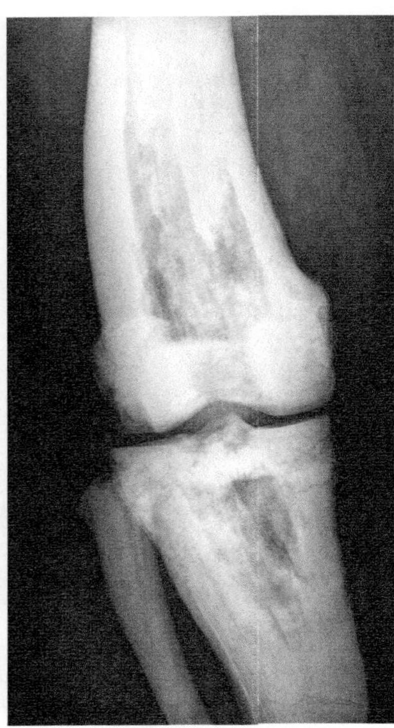

FIGURE 33.41 Osteopetrosis. Anteroposterior radiograph of the right knee of a 28-year-old man shows "bone-in-bone" appearance of the distal femur and proximal tibia.

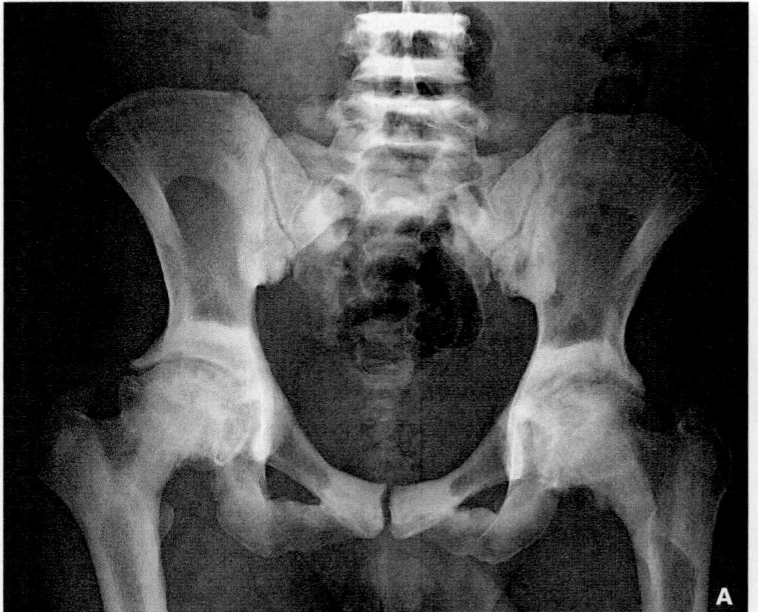

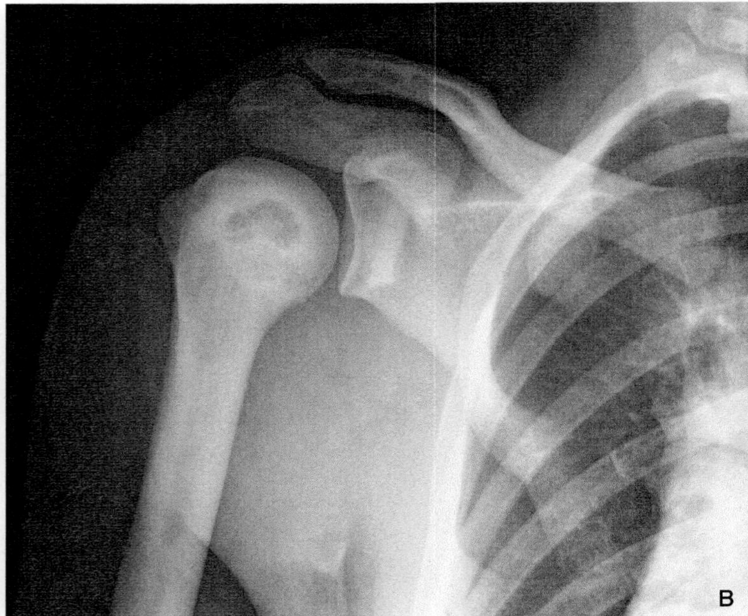

FIGURE 33.42 Osteopetrosis. **(A)** Anteroposterior radiograph of the pelvis of a 28-year-old man shows sclerosis of the iliac, ischial and pubic bones, acetabula, and proximal femora. Note sandwich-like appearance of the L4 and L5 vertebrae and "bone-within-bone" appearance of the iliac bones. **(B)** Anteroposterior radiograph of the right shoulder shows sclerosis of the humerus, scapula, and clavicle and "bone-within-bone" appearance of the humeral head.

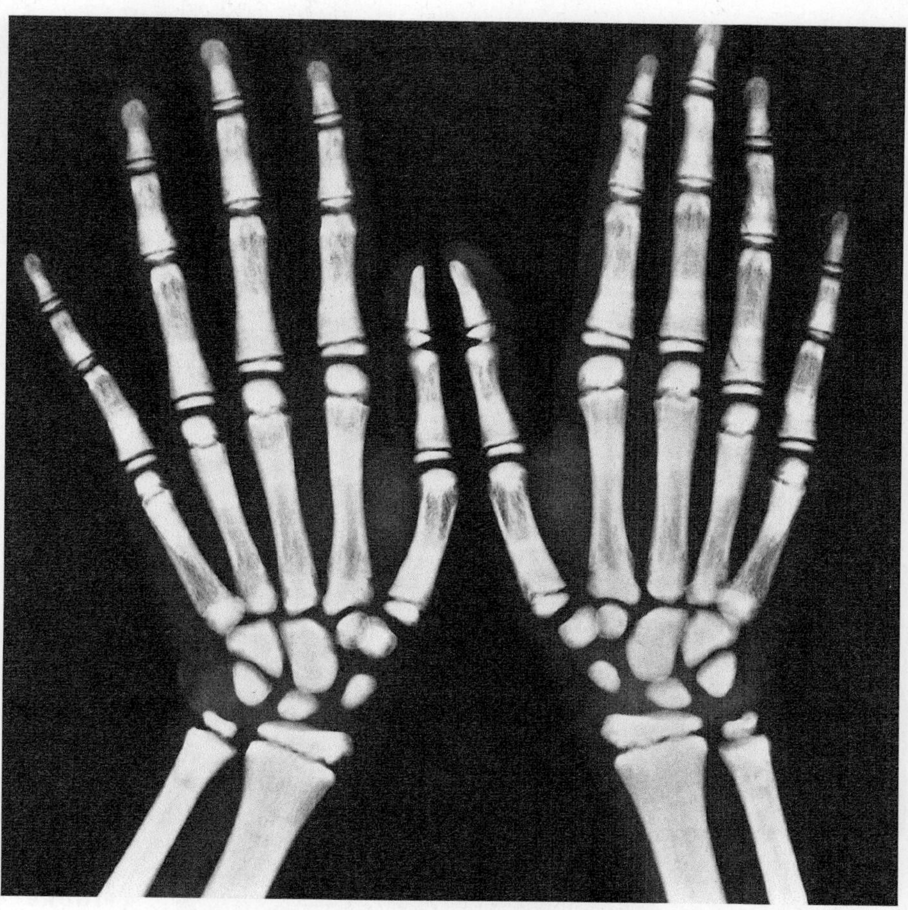

FIGURE 33.43 Osteopetrosis. Dorsovolar radiograph of both hands of a 7-year-old boy shows the dense sclerotic bones lacking differentiation between the cortex and medullary cavity that are characteristic of this condition. The metacarpals appear club-like because of a failure in bone remodeling.

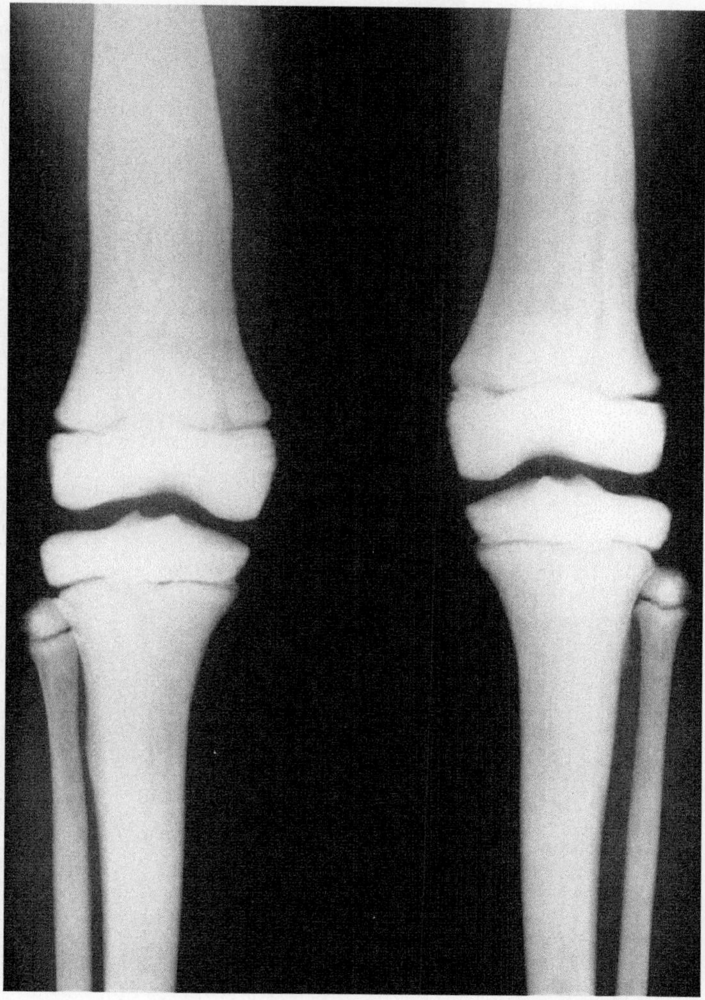

FIGURE 33.44 Osteopetrosis. Anteroposterior radiograph of the knees of a 10-year-old girl shows a uniform increase in bone density in the epiphyses, metaphyses, and diaphyses, with a lack of distinction between the cortical and medullary portions of the bones. The trabecular pattern is completely obliterated by the accumulation of immature bone. Note the splaying deformity of the distal femora and proximal tibiae as a result of remodeling failure.

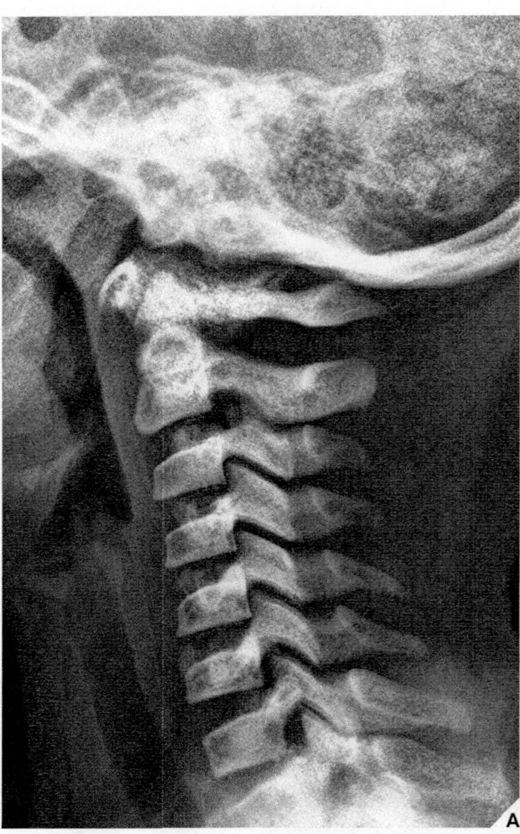

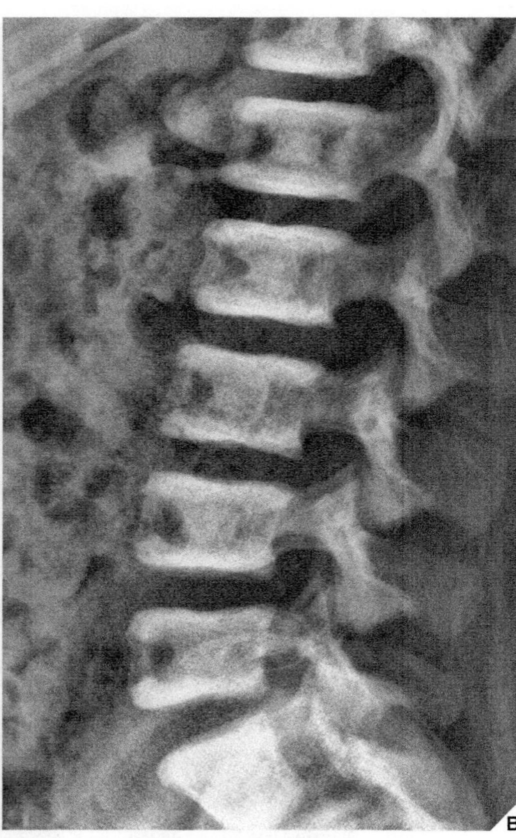

FIGURE 33.45 Osteopetrosis. Lateral radiographs of **(A)** cervical and **(B)** lumbar spine of a 6-year-old girl show characteristic sandwich-like appearance of the vertebral bodies.

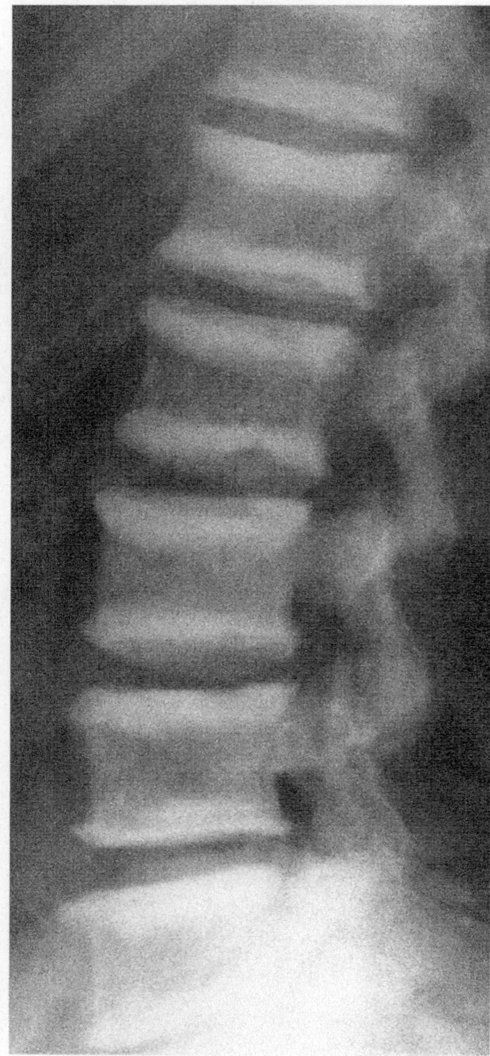

FIGURE 33.46 Osteopetrosis. Lateral radiograph of the thoracolumbar spine in a 14-year-old boy demonstrates the characteristic sandwich-like or "rugger-jersey" appearance seen in this disorder. Note the overall increase in bone density.

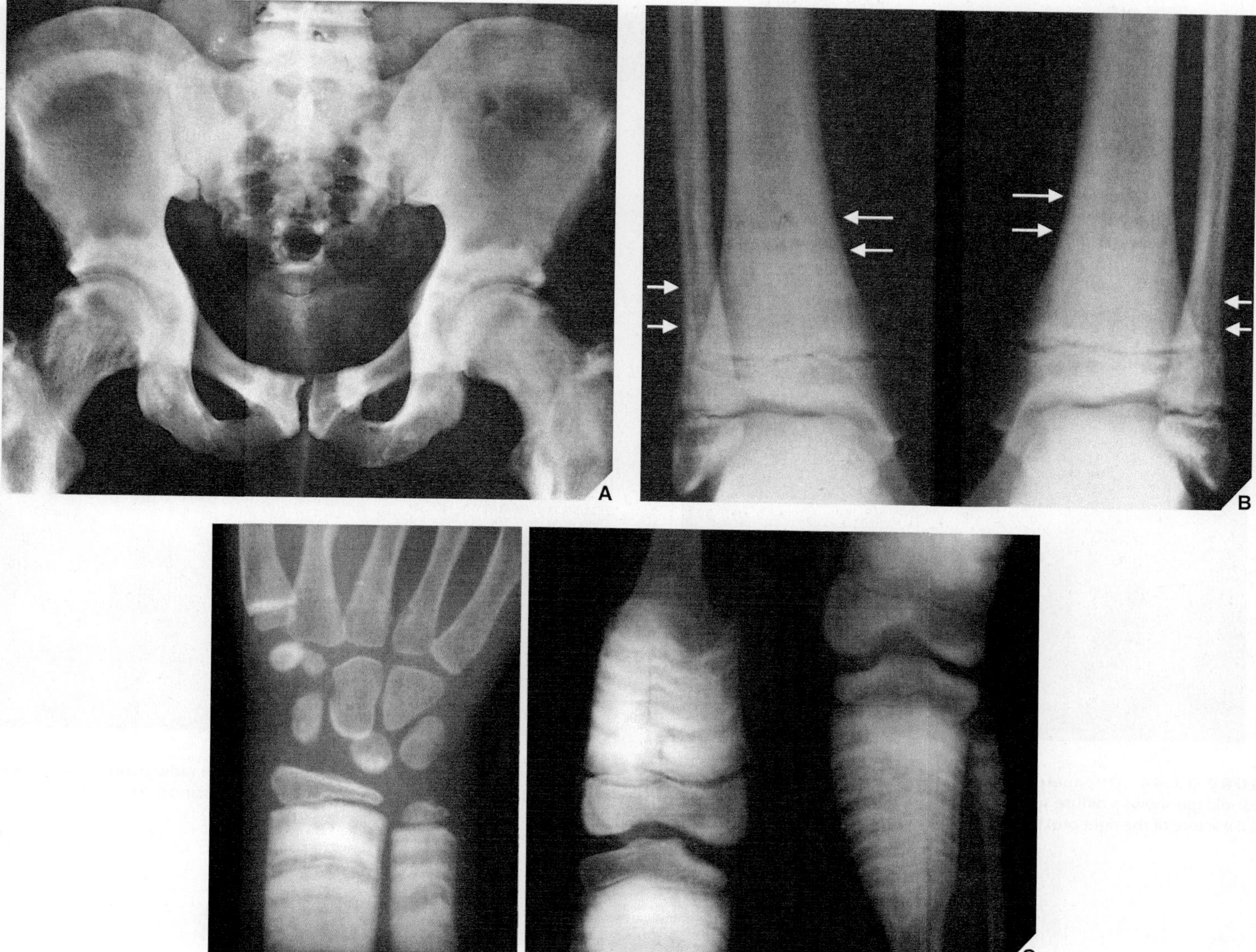

FIGURE 33.47 Osteopetrosis. Radiographic examination of a 12-year-old girl demonstrates the cyclic pattern of this dysplasia. In the pelvis **(A)**, alternating bands of normal (radiolucent) and abnormal (sclerotic) bone are arranged in a ringlike pattern in both iliac wings. In both legs **(B)**, the alternating sclerotic and radiolucent bands are seen in the distal diaphyses and metaphyses of the tibiae and fibulae *(arrows)*. **(C)** In another patient, a 3-year-old boy, the alternating sclerotic and radiolucent bands are present in the distal radius and ulna and around the knee joint.

demonstrated in the metaphysis of long bones and in flat bones such as the pelvis and scapula (Fig. 33.47).

Complications

Fractures are a common complication of osteopetrosis caused by brittle bones (Figs. 33.48 to 33.51). The expanding bone can narrow nerve foramina resulting in blindness, deafness, and facial palsy. Children are also at risk for developing hypocalcemia, tetanic seizures, and secondary hyperparathyroidism. The bone marrow suppression leads to pancytopenia and anemia. Osteopetrosis with renal tubular acidosis may be compatible with a long life span, however, many patients, particularly those who present in the first 2 years of life, develop acidosis, growth failure, increasing mental retardation, and cerebral calcifications.

Pyknodysostosis (Pycnodysostosis)

Pyknodysostosis (Maroteaux-Lamy disease) is an inherited autosomal recessive disorder caused by mutations in the cathepsin-K (*CTSK*) gene located on chromosome 1q21, which leads to the substitution of the arginine at position 122 by glutamine (R122Q) in a lysosomal cystine protease cathepsin K, the expression of which is the reduction of osteoclasts' abilities of bone resorption. Skeletal manifestations of this dysplasia result from a failure of resorption of primary spongiosa. Patients with this disease, like the French painter Toulouse-Lautrec, have a disproportionately short stature, which becomes evident in early childhood. Unlike patients with osteopetrosis, however, those with pyknodysostosis are usually asymptomatic; a pathologic fracture may be the occasion of its discovery.

Imaging Features

Radiographically, pyknodysostosis presents with the increased bone density common to all sclerosing bone dysplasias. In addition, in the skull, there is frontal and occipital bossing, persistence of the anterior and posterior fontanelles, wormian bones, and an obtuse angle to the ramus of the mandible (Fig. 33.52). Moreover, there is often a lack of pneumatization as well as hypoplasia of the paranasal sinuses. Osteolysis/erosions of the distal ends of the clavicle is a common finding. Spinal abnormalities may also occur: Failures in segmentation resulting in block vertebrae are occasionally present, especially in the upper cervical and lumbosacral regions. The feature distinguishing this disease from osteopetrosis is resorption of the terminal tufts of the distal phalanges of the fingers and toes (Fig. 33.53). The latter feature, known as *acroosteolysis* may be seen in a variety of other conditions (see Table 14.3). Some investigators argued, however, that this abnormality is in fact the result of partial agenesis/aplasia of terminal phalanges that simulates true acroosteolysis.

Pathology

Although histologically similar to one another, pyknodysostosis and osteopetrosis exhibit some differences on the microscopic and ultrastructural

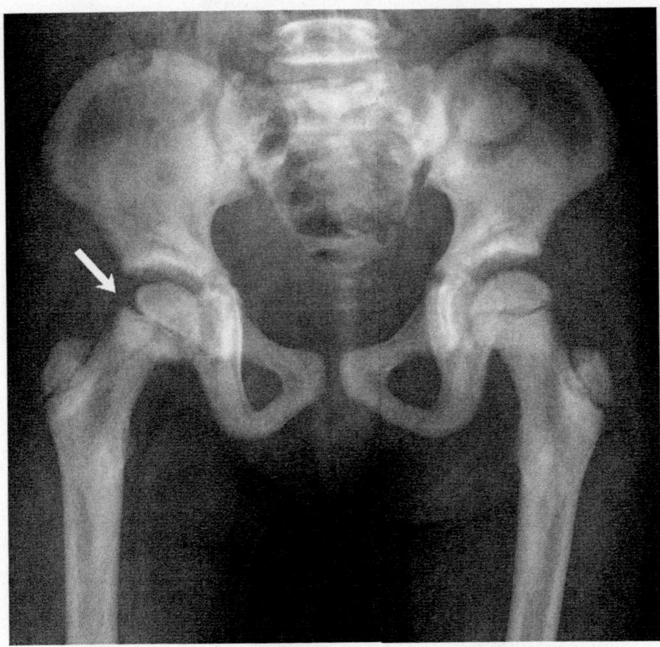

FIGURE 33.48 Osteopetrosis. Anteroposterior radiograph of the pelvis of a 6-year-old girl shows a diffuse sclerosis of the visualized bones. There is Salter-Harris type II fracture of the right proximal femur *(arrow)*.

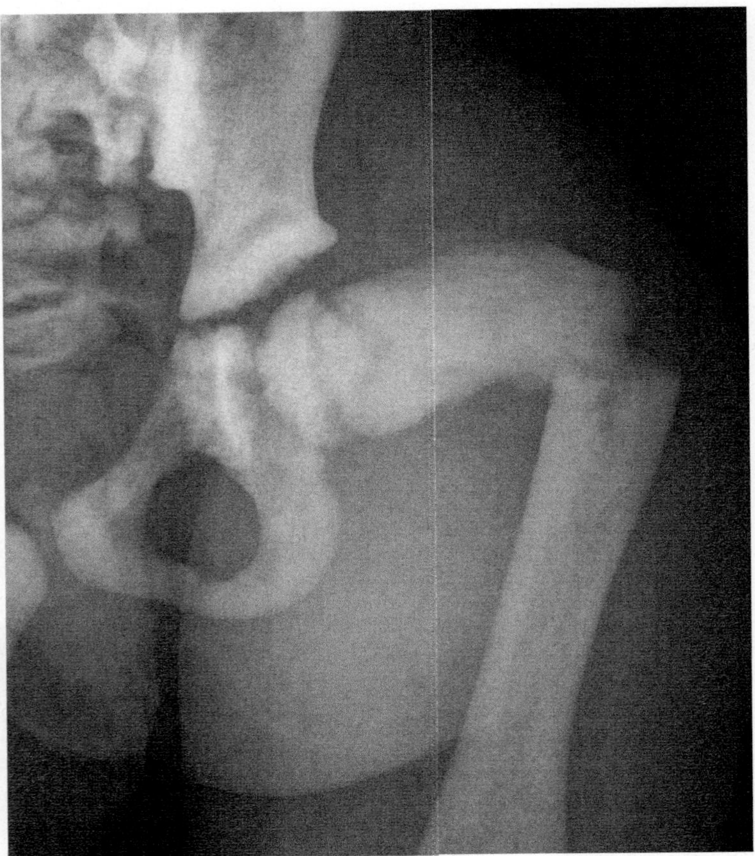

FIGURE 33.49 Osteopetrosis. Anteroposterior radiograph of the left hip of a 10-year-old boy shows sclerotic changes in the pelvis and the proximal femur associated with a pathologic fracture.

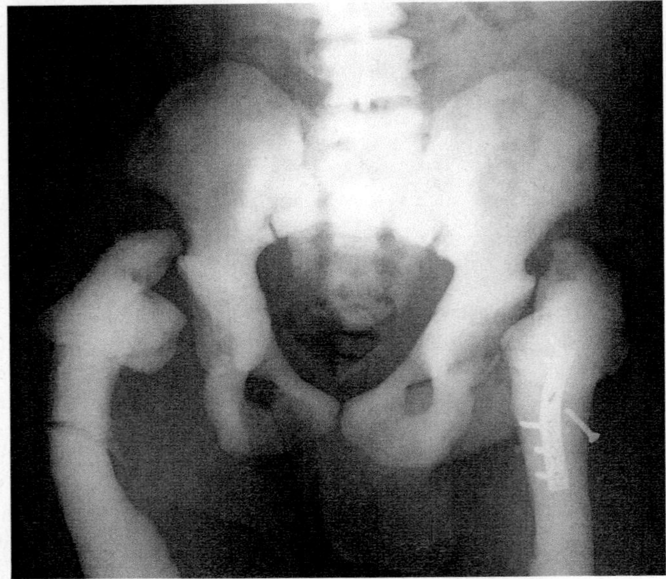

FIGURE 33.50 Osteopetrosis. Anteroposterior radiograph of the pelvis of a 33-year-old man shows numerous fractures involving bilateral proximal femora. Note also bilateral hip dislocation.

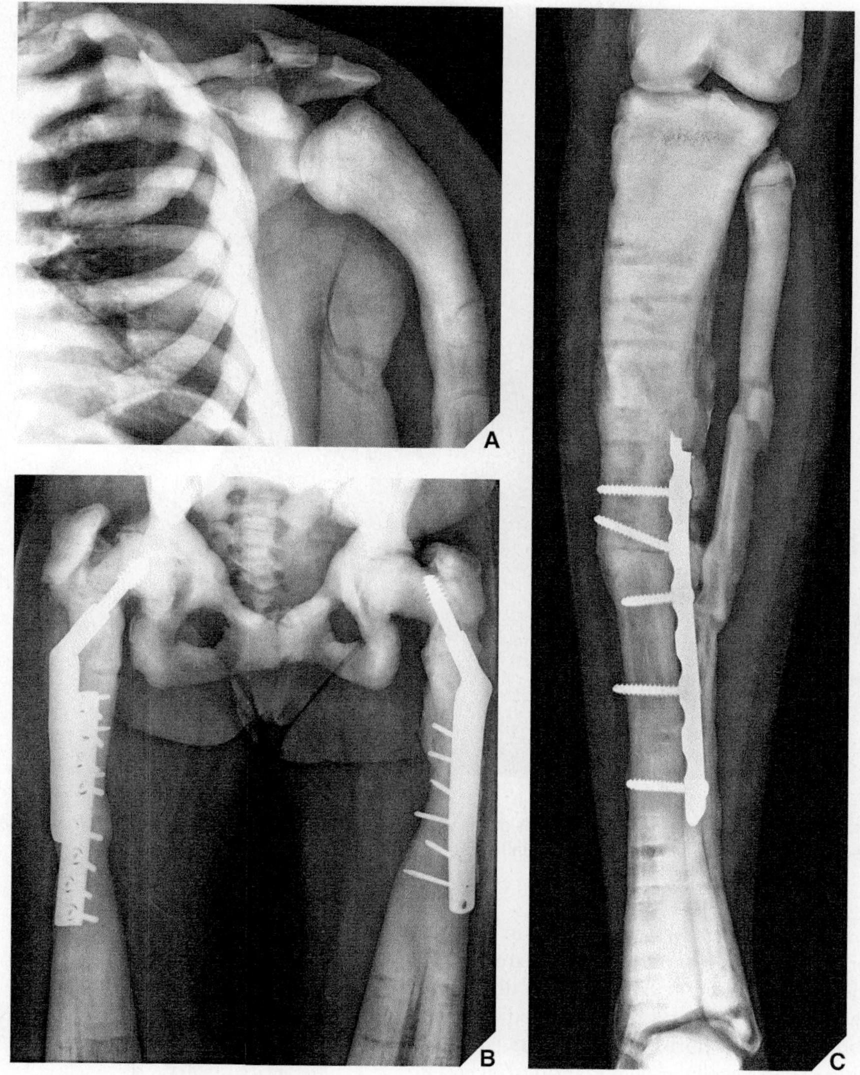

FIGURE 33.51 Osteopetrosis. **(A)** Anteroposterior radiograph of the left shoulder of a 54-year-old man with known osteopetrosis since his early childhood shows multiple fractures involving the ribs, clavicle, and proximal humerus. The fractures are also seen in the proximal femora **(B)** and left tibia and fibula **(C)**.

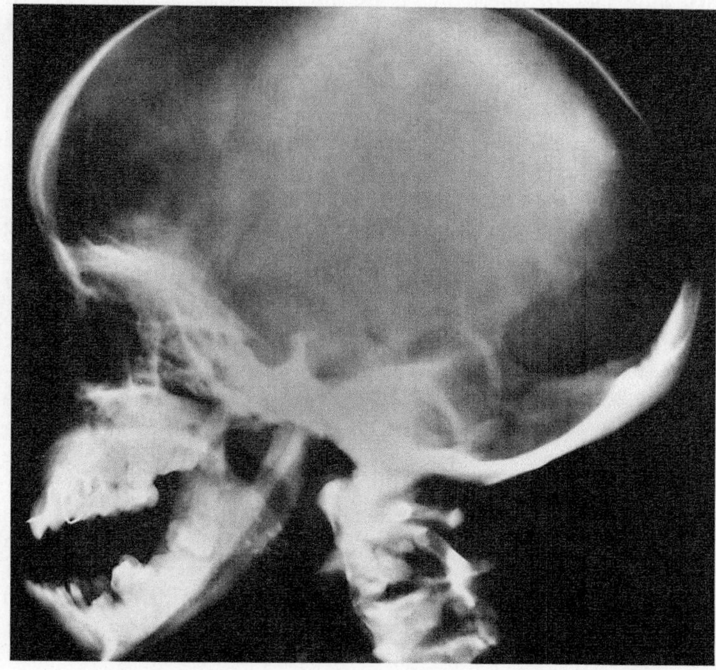

FIGURE 33.52 Pyknodysostosis. Lateral radiograph of the skull and facial bones of an 8-year-old boy shows persistence of the anterior and posterior fontanelles and the obtuse (fetal) angle of the mandible, common manifestations of this disorder. (Courtesy of W. E. Berdon, MD, New York.)

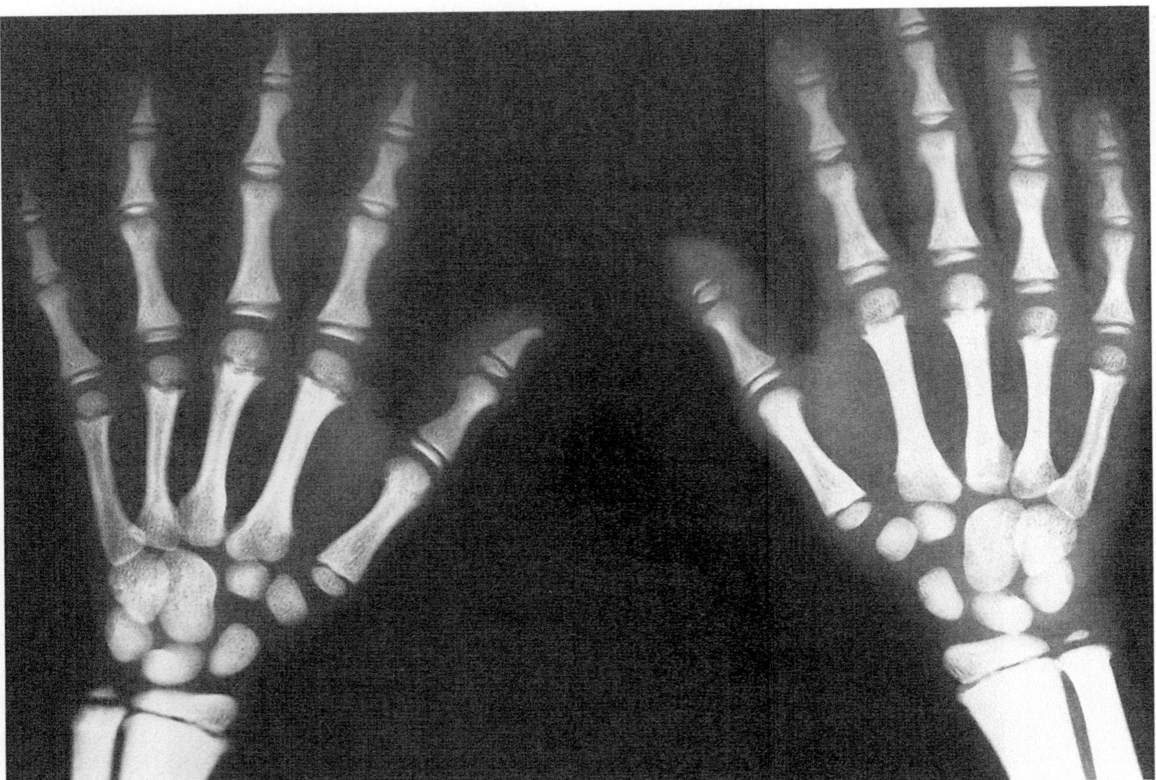

FIGURE 33.53 Pyknodysostosis. Dorsovolar radiograph of both hands of a 9-year-old boy shows resorption of the terminal phalangeal tufts (acroosteolysis), a feature differentiating this condition from osteopetrosis. (Courtesy of J. Dorst, MD, Baltimore.)

levels. Most significant among these is evidence of hematopoiesis in pyknodysostosis because the medullary canal, although narrowed in diameter, is still patent. Both osteoblastic and osteoclastic activity may be diminished. Electron microscopy of pyknodysostotic bone has identified large cytoplasmic vacuoles filled with bone collagen fibrils in osteoclasts. This finding suggests defective intracellular or extracellular degradation of skeletal collagen, perhaps due to an abnormality in the bone matrix or in the function of osteoclasts.

Enostosis, Osteopoikilosis, and Osteopathia Striata

When endochondral ossification proceeds normally, but mature bony trabeculae coalesce and fail to resorb and remodel, the resulting developmental anomalies are referred to as *enostosis* (*bone island*), *osteopoikilosis*, and *osteopathia striata*. The exact mode of inheritance of each is not known, but all three are probably transmitted as autosomal dominant traits.

The most common and mildest of the three is *enostosis*, which is asymptomatic; it is important, however, to differentiate this condition from an osteoid osteoma (see Figs. 16.26 and 17.7B) and from osteoblastic bone metastasis. Any bone in the skeleton may be affected. On imaging studies, the lesion appears as a homogeneously dense and sclerotic focus of compact bone within the cancellous bone. It may be ovoid, round, or oblong and is usually oriented with the long axis of the bone parallel to the cortex. In the majority of cases, bone islands measure 1 mm to 2 cm in greatest diameter, although "giant" bone islands (over 2 cm) have been observed, usually exhibiting the same imaging features as their smaller counterparts. A highly characteristic feature of the lesion is a pattern that has been described as *thorny radiation* or *pseudopodia*: Thickened mature bone trabeculae radiate in streaks through the lesion, aligned with the axes of surrounding uninvolved trabeculae and blending with them in a feathered or brushlike fashion (Figs. 33.54 to 33.57). Most bone islands represent completed episodes of bone remodeling and thus are not metabolically active. They usually do not grow or demonstrate activity on skeletal scintigraphy, although some may exhibit increased uptake of the radiopharmaceutical tracer. This phenomenon, according to the investigations conducted by Greenspan and colleagues, may be related to osteoblastic activity and higher degree of bone remodeling in some of the bone islands.

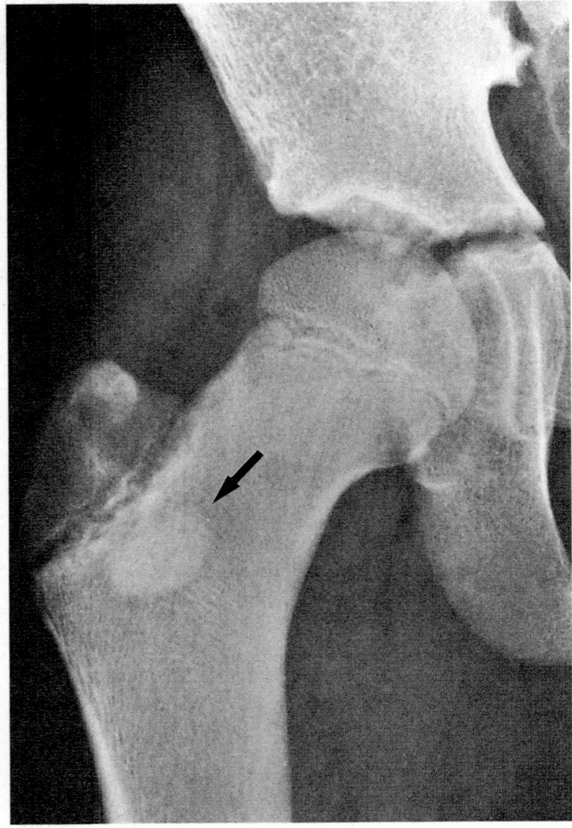

FIGURE 33.54 Enostosis. Anteroposterior radiograph of the right hip of a 10-year-old boy who was examined for an injury reveals, as an incidental finding, a giant bone island in the femoral neck *(arrow)*, which was completely asymptomatic.

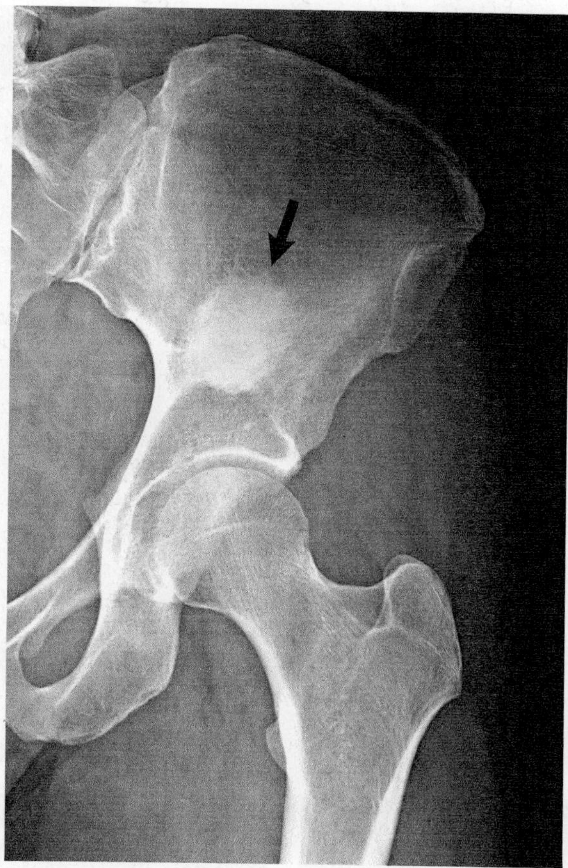

FIGURE 33.55 **Enostosis.** Anteroposterior radiograph of the pelvis of a 37-year-old woman shows a giant bone island in the ilium exhibiting typical rough border *(arrow)*.

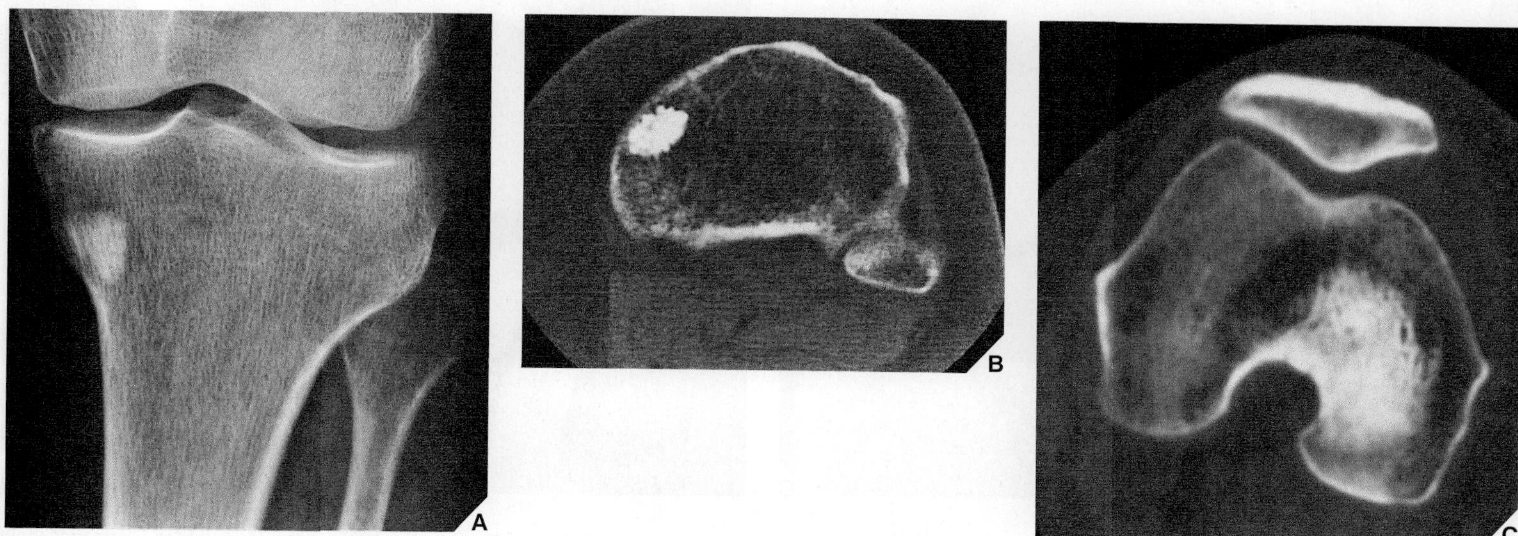

FIGURE 33.56 **CT of enostosis.** **(A)** Anteroposterior radiograph of the knee and **(B)** CT section through the proximal tibia demonstrate a bone island, displaying characteristic brush border. **(C)** In another patient, CT section through the knee joint shows a giant bone island in the medial femoral condyle.

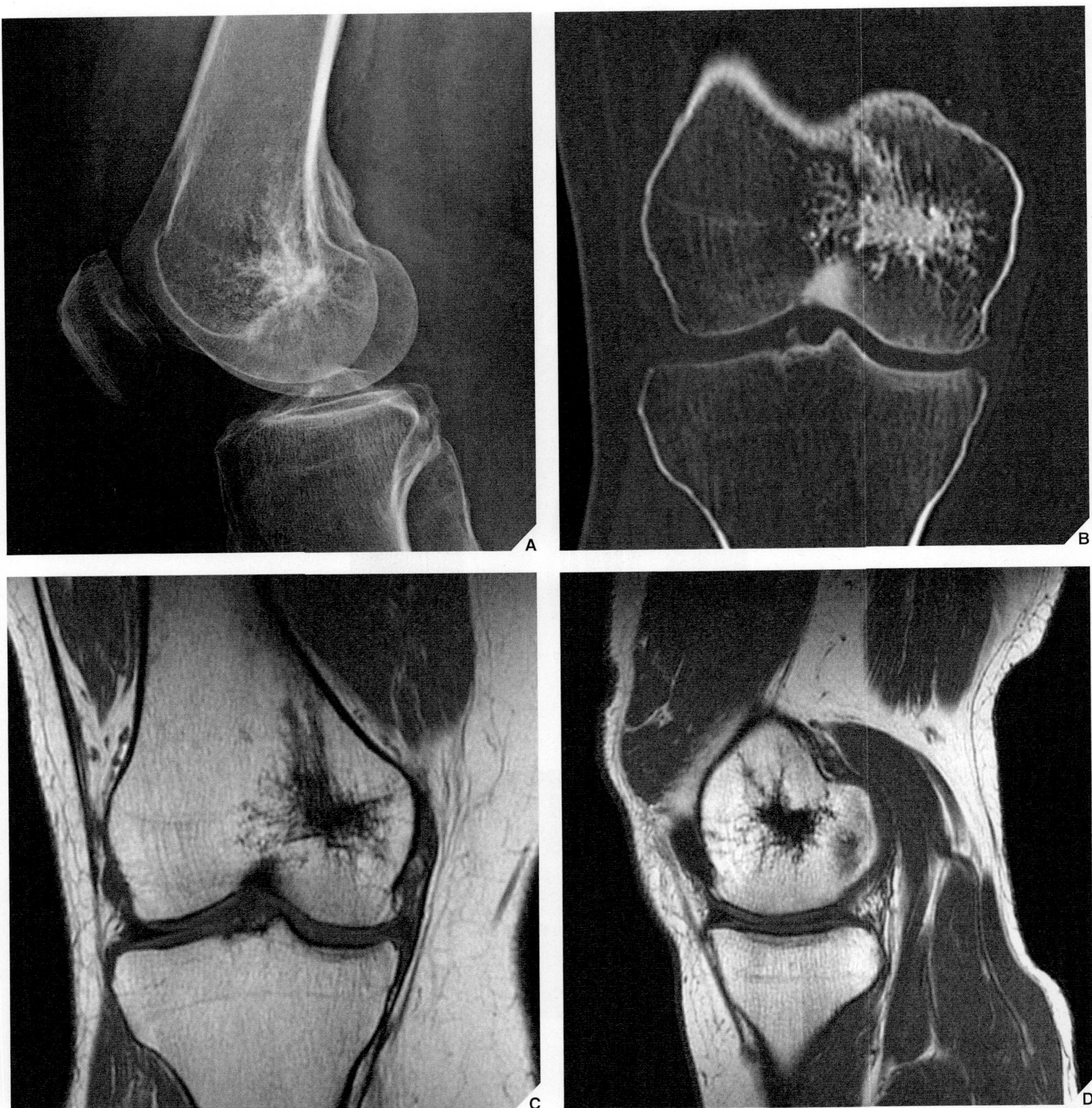

FIGURE 33.57 CT and MRI of enostosis. **(A)** Lateral radiograph of the knee, **(B)** coronal reformatted CT, and **(C)** coronal and **(D)** sagittal T1-weighted MR images show a giant bone island located in the medial femoral condyle, displaying classic pseudopodia.

Osteopoikilosis (osteopathia condensans disseminata or "spotted-bone" disease) is also an asymptomatic disorder, and it is characterized by multiple bone islands symmetrically distributed and clustered near the articular ends of a bone (Fig. 33.58). The condition, which is inherited as an autosomal dominant trait, is believed to result from loss-of-function heterozygous germline mutations in the *LEMD3* (also called *MAN1*) gene, which encodes an inner nuclear membrane protein. It is occasionally associated with the hereditary dermatologic condition, dermatofibrosis lenticularis disseminata (Buschke-Ollendorff syndrome), which is marked by the presence of connective tissue elastic-type nevi of the skin and papular fibromas over the back, arms, and thighs. This association suggests that osteopoikilosis may be a manifestation of a metabolic disorder of connective tissue reflected in a failure in remodeling of mature osseous trabeculae. The imaging studies demonstrate focal condensations of compact lamellar bone in the spongiosa, having characteristic roentgenographic features. They appear as small, symmetrically scattered radiopacities whose appearance at the articular ends of the long bones and in the small carpal and tarsal bones is pathognomic. The lesions may also be present in other areas

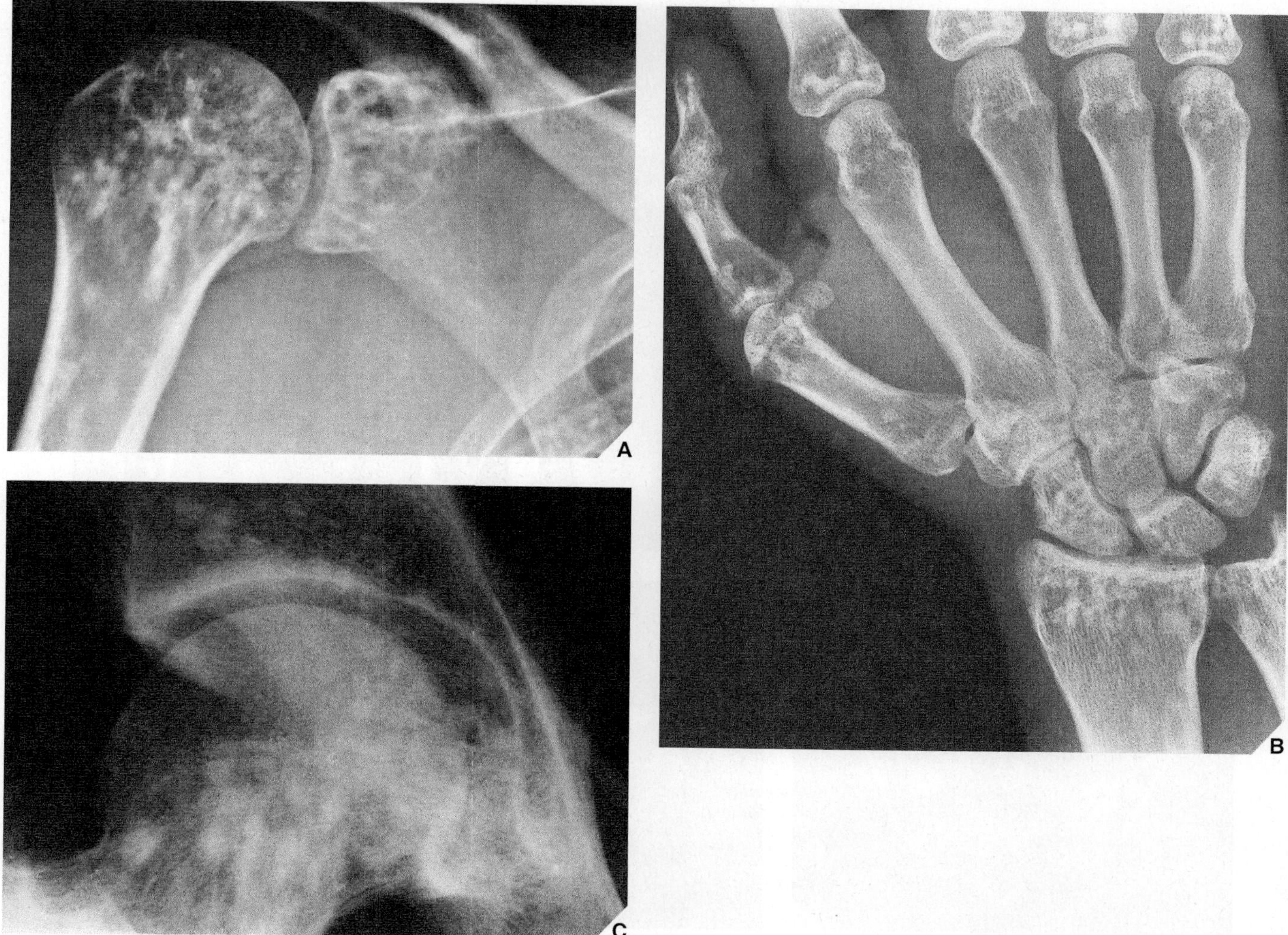

FIGURE 33.58 Osteopoikilosis. **(A)** Anteroposterior radiograph of the shoulder of a 34-year-old man who had pain in his right shoulder after an automobile accident shows no fracture or dislocation. However, multiple sclerotic foci representing lesions of osteopoikilosis are apparent, scattered near the articular ends of the scapula and humerus. A subsequent bone survey showed extensive involvement of the skeleton, especially the hands, wrists **(B)**, and hips **(C)**.

of articulation, for example, around the acetabulum and glenoid; the spine and ribs, although rare, may also be affected. In general, the lesions may exhibit one of three configurations: (a) lenticular-round, oval, or nodular; (b) linear-striated or oblong; and (c) mixture of the two. The last two configurations may not, however, represent the pure entity but rather the coexistence of osteopoikilosis and osteopathia striata. Although radiography is usually sufficient to make a diagnosis of osteopoikilosis, questionable cases may require radionuclide imaging, which is diagnostic. In osteopoikilosis, a bone scan is relatively normal, unlike in metastatic disease, which invariably shows an increased uptake of radiopharmaceutical tracer. CT is rarely required, but it shows cross-sectional distribution of the lesions (Figs. 33.59 and 33.60).

Histologically, both enostoses and the lesions of osteopoikilosis are characterized by foci of compact bone scattered in the spongiosa, with prominent cement lines and occasionally Haversian systems of nutrient canals. Clinically, osteopoikilosis must be distinguished from more severe disorders such as mastocytosis and tuberous sclerosis as well as from osteoblastic metastatic lesions.

Osteopathia striata, also an autosomal dominant disorder, the least common condition in this group, is an asymptomatic lesion marked by fine or coarse linear striations, chiefly in the long bones and at sites of rapid growth such as the knee (Figs. 33.61, 33.62A, and 33.63B), shoulder, and wrist (Fig. 33.62B), although the other sites may also be affected (Fig. 33.63A,C). Skeletal scintigraphy is invariably normal. Patients with the pure form of this disorder exhibit no known associated physical abnormalities or characteristic laboratory findings. Several authors postulate a relationship between this disorder and osteopoikilosis; some suggest that it is in fact a variant of osteopoikilosis. The association of osteopathia striata with cranial sclerosis (Horan-Beighton syndrome) has been described, as a rare X-linked dominant inherited bone dysplasia caused by mutations involving the *WTX* (also called *FAM123B* and *AMER1*) gene on the X chromosome (proximal Xq11), encoding an inhibitor of WNT signaling. Patients can be asymptomatic, but more commonly they present with typical facial dysmorphism, sensory defects, internal organ anomalies, and growth and mental retardation. Calvarial bones thickening, responsible for characteristic facies, and linear striations in the metaphyses of the long bones and pelvis represent the main features of this dysplasia. Limited study of individuals with focal dermal hypoplasia (Goltz-Gorlin syndrome) has revealed a high incidence of concomitant osteopathia striata, an association that may be more than coincidental. In addition, skin abnormalities (poikiloderma with focal dermal hypoplasia); papillomas of the mucous membranes; abnormalities of the eyes, kidneys, and teeth; as well as several osseous deformities including syndactyly, oligodactyly, polydactyly, and hypoplasia of the craniofacial bones have been recorded. The mode of inheritance of this condition is sporadic or X-linked dominant.

Progressive Diaphyseal Dysplasia (Camurati-Engelmann Disease)

Failure of bone resorption and remodeling at the sites of intramembranous ossification (such as the cortex of tubular bones, the vault of the skull, the mandible, or the midsegment of the clavicle) is the abnormality typically noted in progressive diaphyseal dysplasia, also called *osteopathia hyperostotica* and *Camurati-Engelmann disease*. The disorder usually manifests itself in the first decade of life, males being more frequently affected than

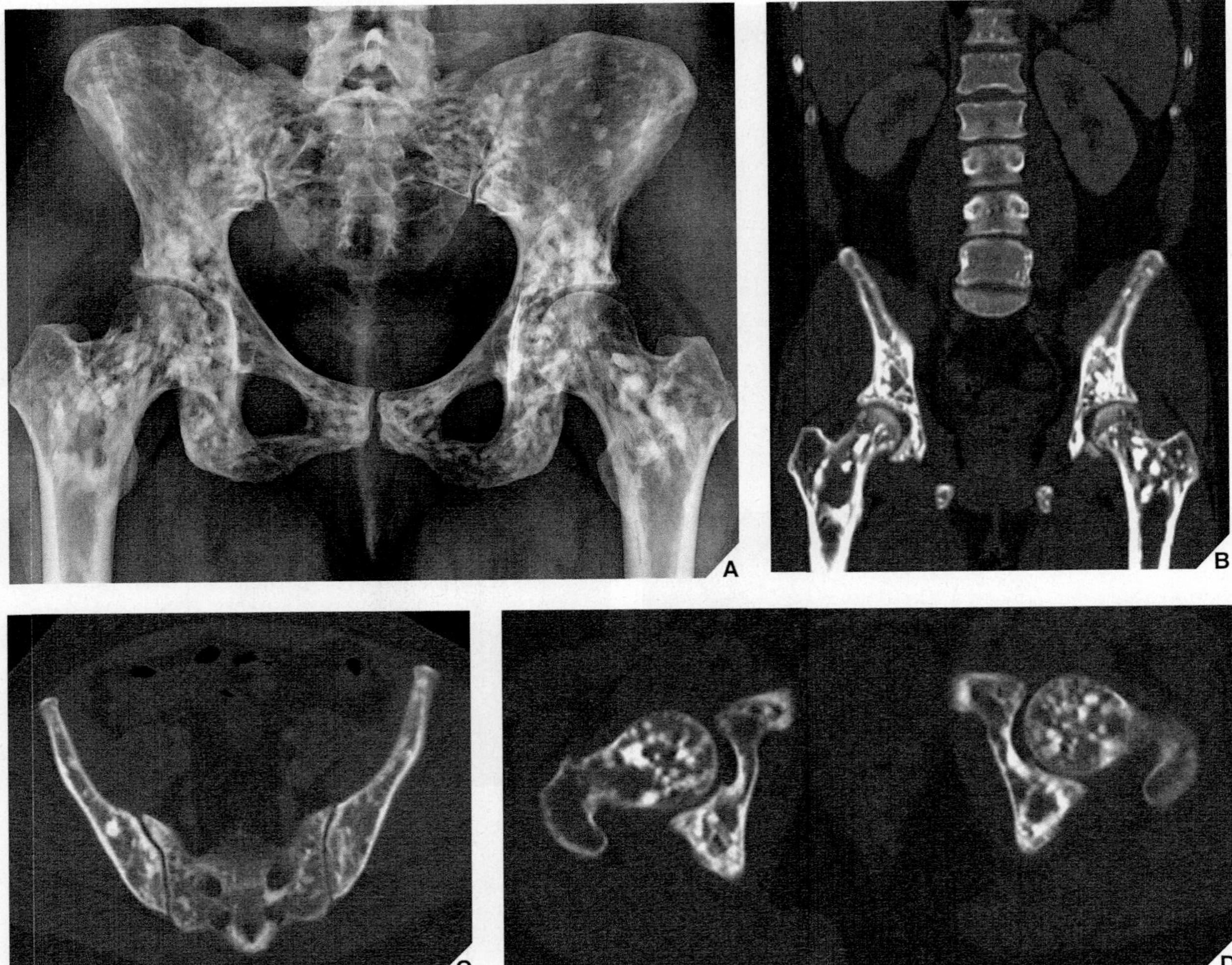

FIGURE 33.59 CT of osteopoikilosis. **(A)** Anteroposterior radiograph of the pelvis of a 38-year-old woman shows multiple sclerotic lesions in the pelvic bones and proximal femora. **(B)** Coronal CT reformatted image shows involvement of the iliac bones, femora, and several vertebral bodies. Axial CT sections obtained through the pelvis **(C)** and the hip joints **(D)** show cross-sectional distribution of the lesions.

females. Like enostosis, osteopoikilosis, and osteopathia striata, this is an autosomal dominant disorder with considerable variability of expression. Both sporadic and familial cases have been described. Some investigations suggest that this disease results from domain-specific mutations (*R218H*) in the transforming growth factor-β1 (*TGFB1*) gene with locus in the chromosome 19q13.1-q13.3. The majority are missense mutations in exon 4 leading to single amino acid substitutions in the encoded protein. Clinically, it is characterized by growth retardation, muscle wasting, joint contractures, pain and weakness in the extremities, and a waddling gait. The level of urinary hydroxyproline is normal, indicating normal bone turnover, and blood chemistry and marrow and peripheral blood elements are normal as well, although occasionally the erythrocyte sedimentation rate and C-reactive protein (CRP) levels may be increased. The condition is self-limiting and generally resolves by 30 years of age.

Because of its striking tendency toward symmetric involvement of the extremities, with characteristic sparing of the epiphysis and metaphysis (the sites of endochondral ossification), progressive diaphyseal dysplasia is recognized radiographically by symmetric fusiform thickening of the cortices of the long bone shafts, particularly in the lower extremities, although the upper extremities may also be affected (Fig. 33.64). The affected bone is usually sharply demarcated from normal bone. The thickening of the cortex, which represents both endosteal and periosteal accretion, progresses along the long axis of the bone both proximally and distally. The external contour of the bone is usually smooth. Occasionally, the skull shows hyperostosis of the calvaria, and some cases of frontal bossing and enlargement of the mandible have also been reported. In some cases described by Neuhauser, there were sclerotic changes at the base of the skull. This latter finding is curious because such changes at the skull base are typical for an error in endochondral ossification. Such a finding invites speculation that perhaps there are two forms of progressive diaphyseal dysplasia, one expressing a pure form of a failure of intramembranous ossification, and the other, a mixed form, showing an endochondral component as well.

The differential diagnosis should include chronic osteomyelitis, infantile cortical hyperostosis, pachydermatoperiostitis, hypertrophic osteoarthropathy, vitamin D intoxication, fluorosis, and peripheral vascular disease.

Hereditary Multiple Diaphyseal Sclerosis (Ribbing Disease)

A familial disorder similar to progressive diaphyseal dysplasia, described by Ribbing in 1949 and later by Paul in 1953, is generally asymptomatic and exhibits limited asymmetric involvement, usually only of the long bones, especially the tibia and the femur. This condition is generally believed to be the same disorder as Camurati-Engelmann disease (Fig. 33.65), although some authors suggest an autosomal recessive inheritance. It occurs after puberty and is more common in women. Serial studies have shown that lesions may slowly progress over the years, eventually becoming stationary. Radiography reveals focal sclerosis largely caused by the formation of endosteal and periosteal new bone. The medullary portions of the bones are constricted to varying degrees. These findings can be confirmed by CT. Limited studies using MRI showed cortical thickening and bone marrow edema with minimal edema of adjacent soft tissues. Scintigraphy shows an increased uptake of technetium-99m (^{99m}Tc) methylene diphosphonate at the sites of radiographic abnormalities, although markers for bone formation such as alkaline phosphatase and osteocalcin, and bone resorption, like N-telopeptide, pyridinoline, and deoxypyridinoline, are normal. Histopathologic features are not specific. Reactive cortical thickening is present, with variable formation

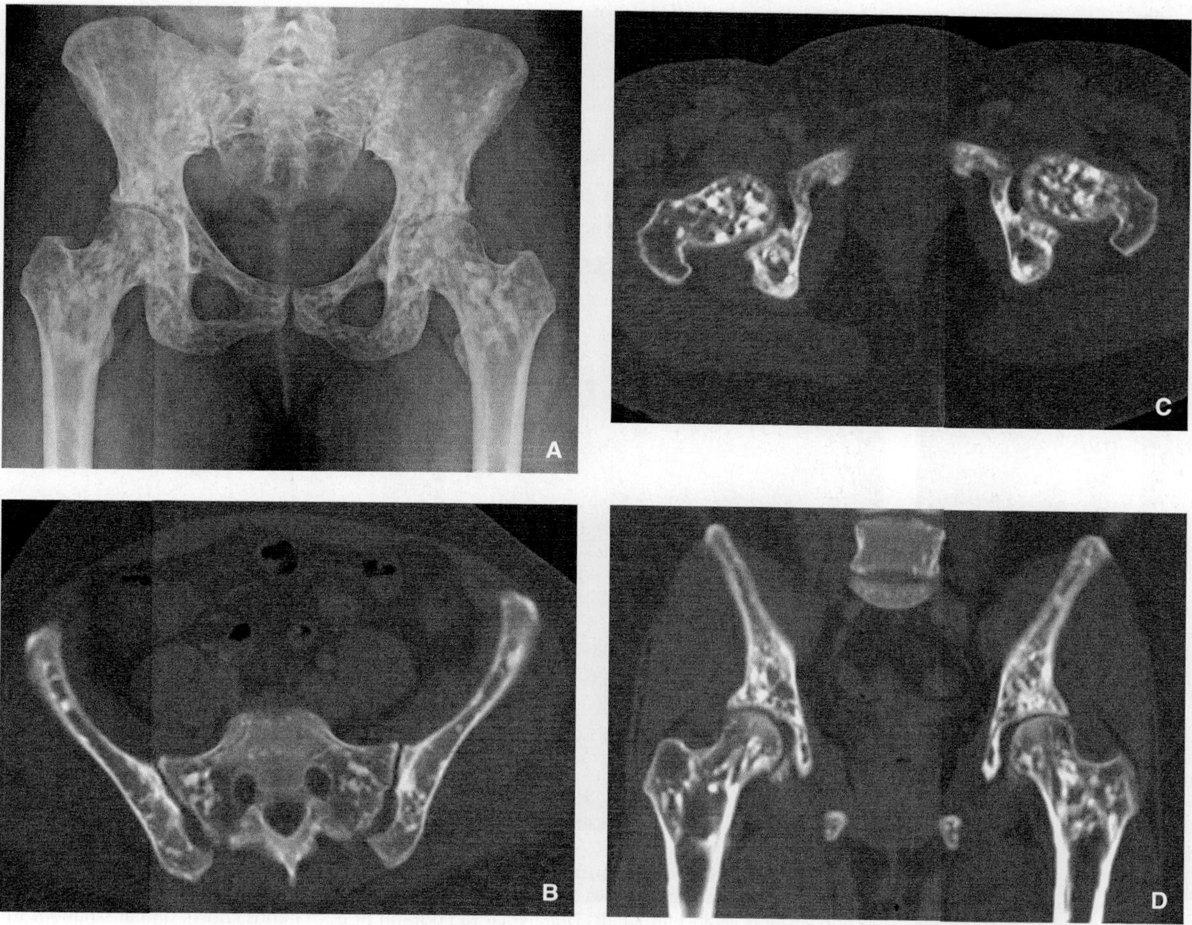

▲ **FIGURE 33.60** CT of osteopoikilosis. **(A)** Anteroposterior radiograph of the pelvis, **(B)** axial CT of the pelvis, **(C)** axial CT of the hips, and **(D)** coronal reformatted CT of the pelvis of a 48-year-old woman show classic appearance of this sclerosing dysplasia.

FIGURE 33.61 Osteopathia striata. Anteroposterior radiograph of the right knee of a 14-year-old girl who had a history of trauma reveals, as an incidental finding, fine linear striations in the diaphysis and metaphysis of the distal femur and proximal tibia; the epiphyses, however, are spared. ▶

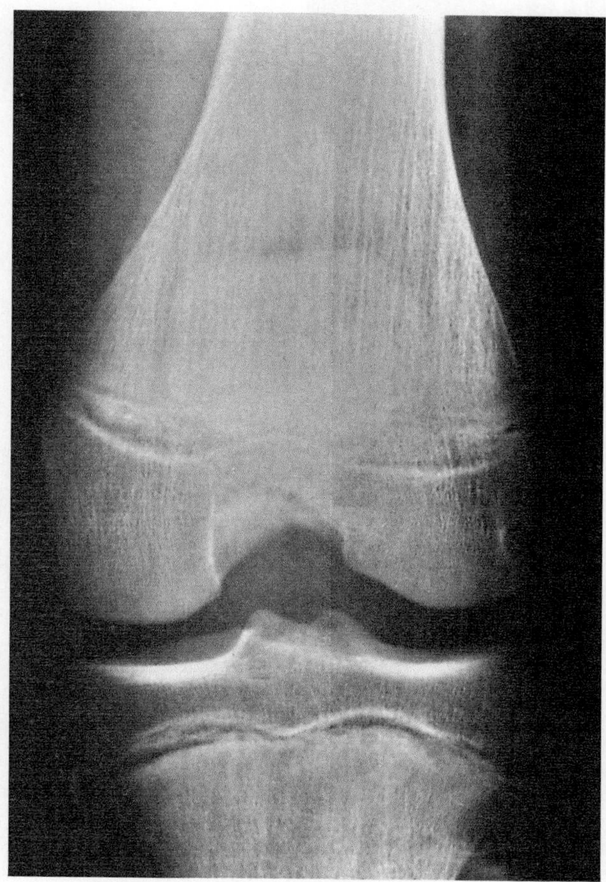

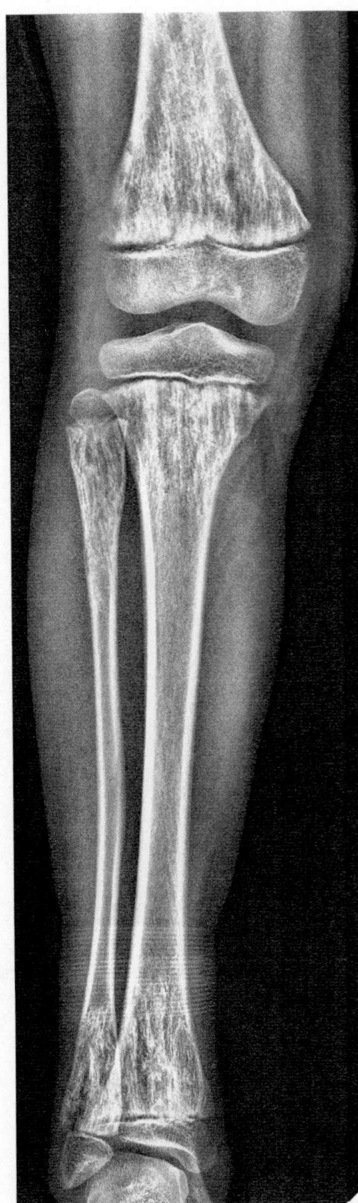

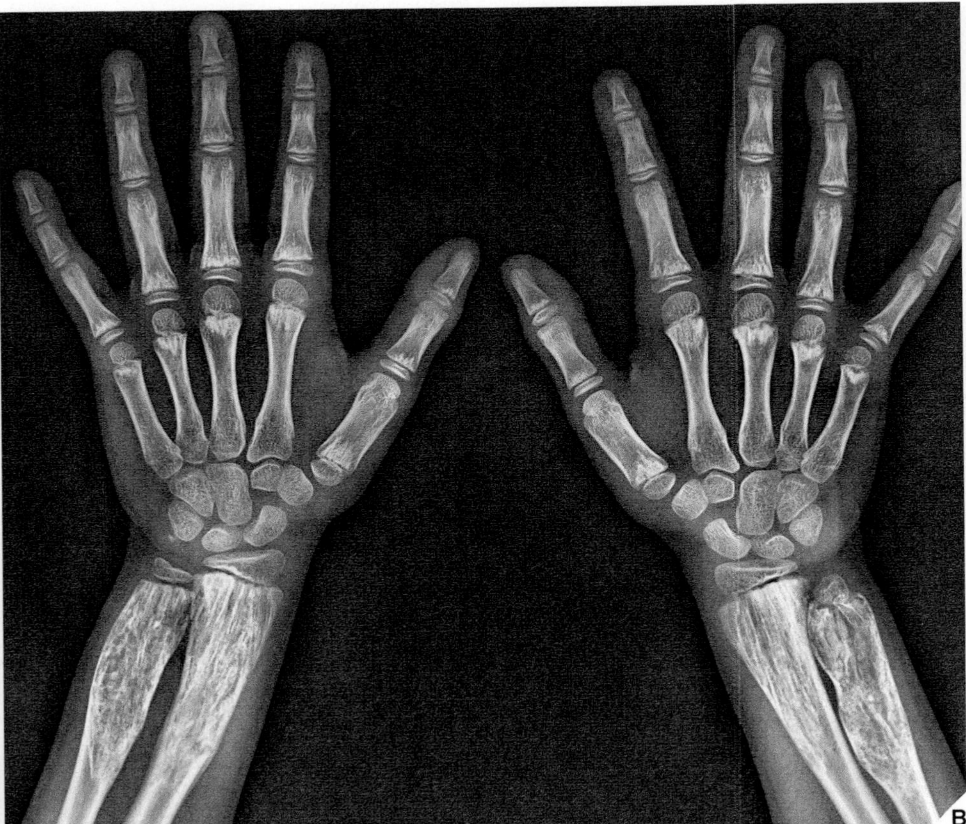

FIGURE 33.62 Osteopathia striata. (A) Anteroposterior radiograph of the right knee including the leg of a 6-year-old girl shows dense striations within the metaphyses of the distal femur and proximal and distal tibia and fibula. (B) Dorsovolar radiograph of both hands shows similar striations in the distal metaphyses of the radius and ulna.

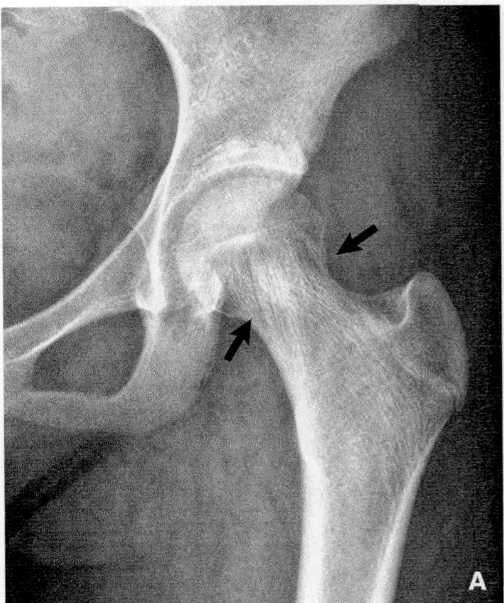

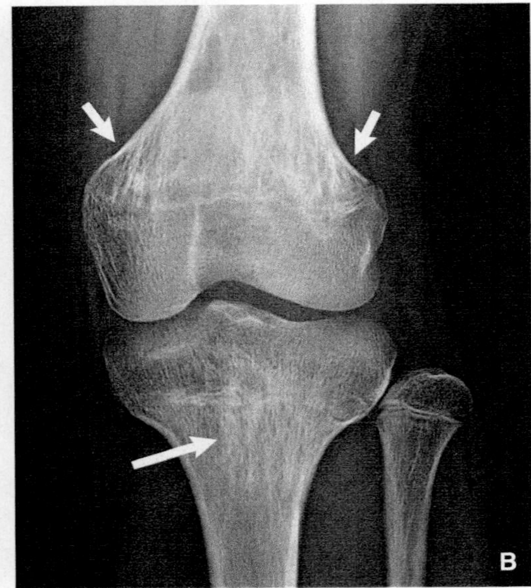

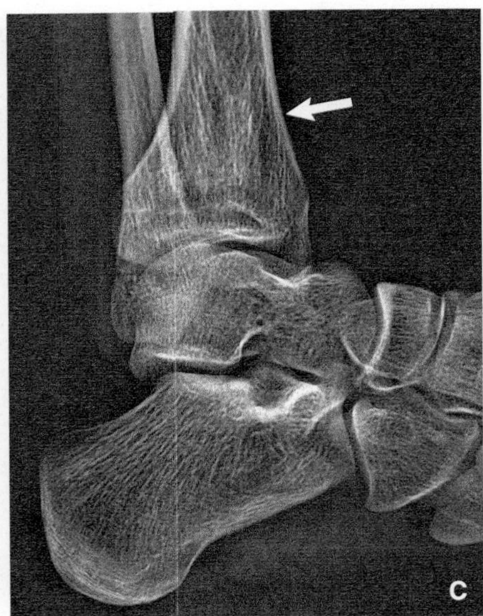

FIGURE 33.63 Osteopathia striata. (A) Lateral radiograph of the hip, (B) anteroposterior radiograph of the knee, and (C) lateral radiograph of the ankle of a 15-year-old girl show coarse striations within the metaphyseal portions of the affected bones *(arrows)*.

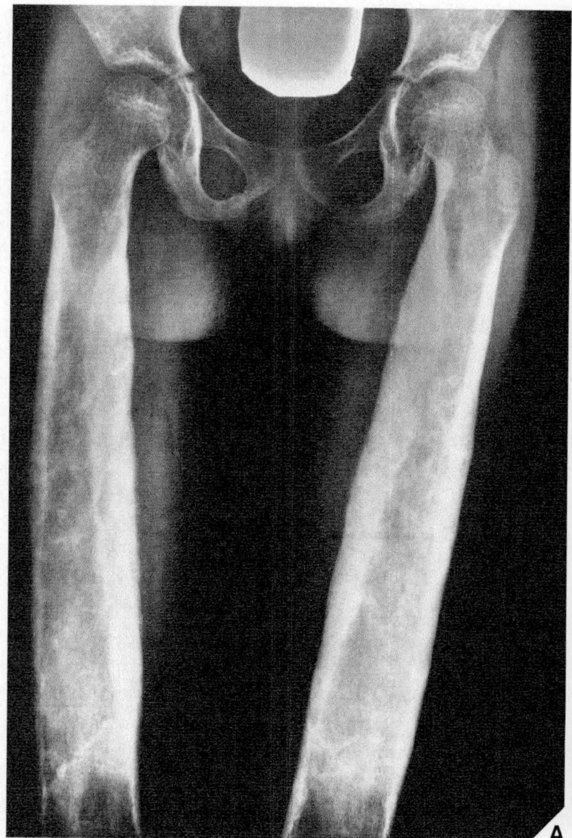

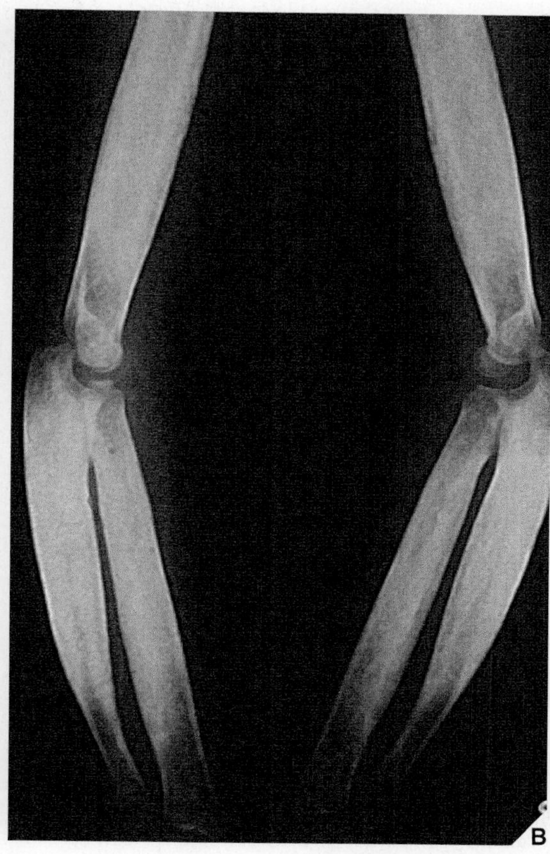

FIGURE 33.64 Camurati-Engelmann disease. **(A)** Anteroposterior radiograph of the hips and upper femora of an 8-year-old boy shows symmetric fusiform thickening of the cortices. Note that only the sites of intramembranous bone formation are affected, whereas the sites of endochondral bone formation are spared. **(B)** Anteroposterior radiograph of the upper extremities in another patient demonstrates similar findings with diffuse, symmetric fusiform sclerosis of the long bones, sparing the epiphyses. (**A**, Courtesy of W. E. Berdon, MD, New York.)

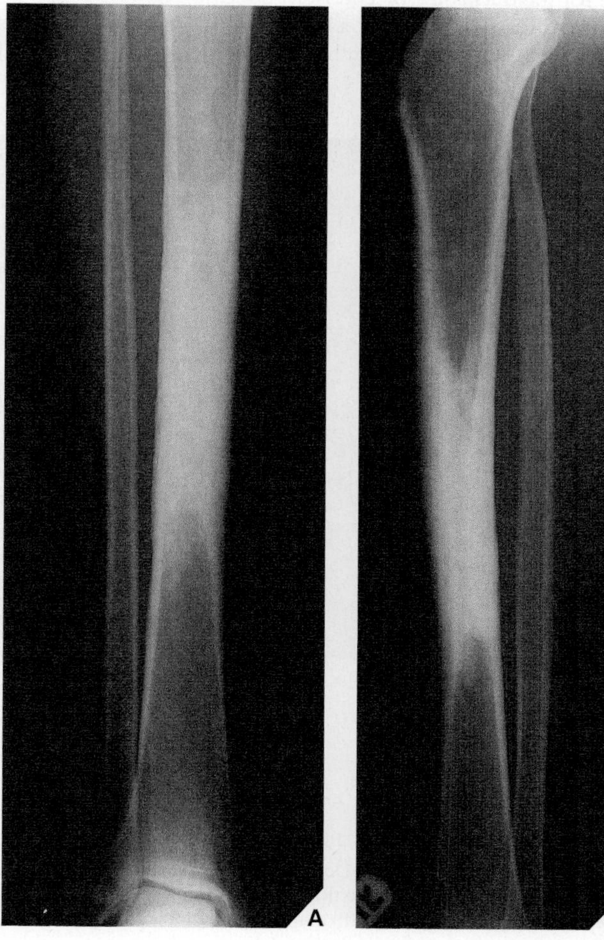

FIGURE 33.65 Ribbing disease. **(A)** Anteroposterior and **(B)** lateral radiographs of the right lower leg in an asymptomatic 32-year-old man show features of hereditary multiple diaphyseal sclerosis. Note the slightly irregular circumferential thickening of the cortex of midtibia associated with endosteal sclerosis.

of woven bone and fibrosis. One study revealed increased numbers of osteocytes per unit area compared with normal bone as well as focal increases in plump osteoblastic rimming. Haversian systems were normal to markedly reduced in size. In contrast to the histologic evidence of progressive, active bone resorption and new bone apposition in Camurati-Engelmann disease, Ribbing disease shows evidence of only new bone formation. Although they are usually nonspecific, pathologic findings can aid in excluding other diagnoses, for example, infection.

The differential diagnosis for the patient with Ribbing disease, in addition to infection (osteomyelitis), should include Chester-Erdheim disease, endosteal hyperostosis, intramedullary osteosclerosis, monomelic medullary osteosclerosis, and some metabolic disorders associated with increased bone density.

Endosteal Hyperostosis (Hyperostosis Corticalis Generalisata)

This rare dysplasia can be classified on the basis of mode of inheritance into two groups comprising four types. *Van Buchem disease* and *Truswell-Hansen disease* (also known as *sclerosteosis)* are autosomal recessive forms of endosteal hyperostosis, whereas *Worth disease* and *Nakamura disease* are autosomal dominant forms. In fact, a number of investigators have proposed viewing the autosomal dominant and autosomal recessive forms of endosteal hyperostosis as separate entities. The principal imaging features of these rare conditions is a generalized and symmetric endosteal thickening (osteosclerosis) of the diaphyseal cortex of the long bones, associated with thickening of the skull, facial bones including mandible, and all sites of intramembranous ossification. The thickening of the diaphyseal cortex is not associated with any apparent increase in the diameter of the affected bones, as in progressive diaphyseal dysplasia; rather, thickening results in narrowing of the medullary canal. Involvement of the mandible is a common but poorly described feature of this group of very different disorders. Bone biopsy has no value in differentiating these dysplasias because, other than endosteal thickening, the pathologic findings are nonspecific. However, in view of the fact that the formation of the medullary cavity is the result of endosteal resorption by osteoclasts, diminished activity of these cells may be responsible for the thickening of endosteal bone.

Van Buchem disease is caused by a noncoding deletion that removes an *SOST*-specific regulatory element in bone. In bone, *SOST* is expressed predominantly by osteocytes, and glycoprotein sclerostin suppresses bone formation by inhibiting the canonical Wnt signaling pathway. Sclerosteosis is caused by loss-of-function mutations of the *SOST* gene, which encodes a secreted sclerostin. Balemans and coworkers assigned the locus for this disease to 17q12-q21 chromosome, the same general region as the locus for van Buchem disease.

Van Buchem and Worth disease have similar imaging features, a fact that led to confusion with one another until Beals discovered their different mode of inheritance. As in the first case of a twin brother and sister described by van Buchem, both diseases demonstrate diffuse symmetric endosteal hyperostosis affecting the diaphyseal cortex of the long and short tubular bones (Fig. 33.66A) and mandible accompanied by sclerosis of the skull, shoulder girdle, pelvic girdle, and thoracic cage. However, two features of van Buchem disease help to distinguish it from Worth disease: more severe involvement of the mandible, which may greatly enlarge (Fig. 33.66B), and small periosteal excrescences arising from affected long bones. Clinical features differentiating these two dysplasias have also been observed. Unlike Worth disease, van Buchem disease is marked by progressive cranial nerve deficit, particularly of the facial nerves, and elevated levels of alkaline phosphatase.

Three cases of an autosomal dominant type of endosteal hyperostosis, different from the Worth type, have been reported in a Japanese family by Nakamura and associates, now referred to as *Nakamura disease*. What apparently distinguishes these cases from Worth disease are unusual manifestations of sclerosis of the jaw bones: the maxilla and mandible were enlarged, but sclerotic changes had a mottled appearance and the rami of the mandible were spared. The neurocranium showed endosteal sclerosis as well as loss of the diploe.

Sclerosteosis is an unusual autosomal recessive disorder, which exhibits homozygosity for the same genetic defect as van Buchem disease. The majority of patients have been of the Afrikaner community of South Africa. In early childhood, individuals with this disorder show sign of overgrowth and sclerosis of the skeleton, particularly the skull. The condition is progressive, and complications arise due to cranial nerve involvement. Height and weight often become excessive; adult males reach uncommonly tall stature. Overgrowth of the cranium, together with hypertrophy of the mandible and frontal regions leads to relative midfacial hypoplasia and distortion of the facies. Syndactyly of the index and middle fingers is a

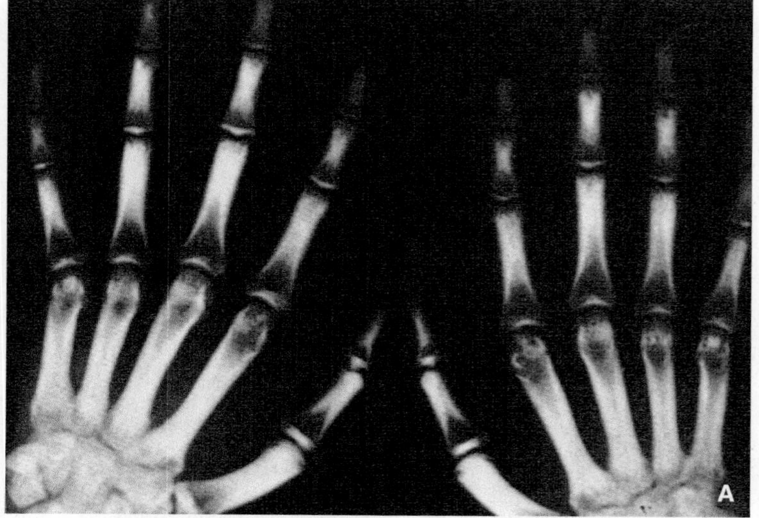

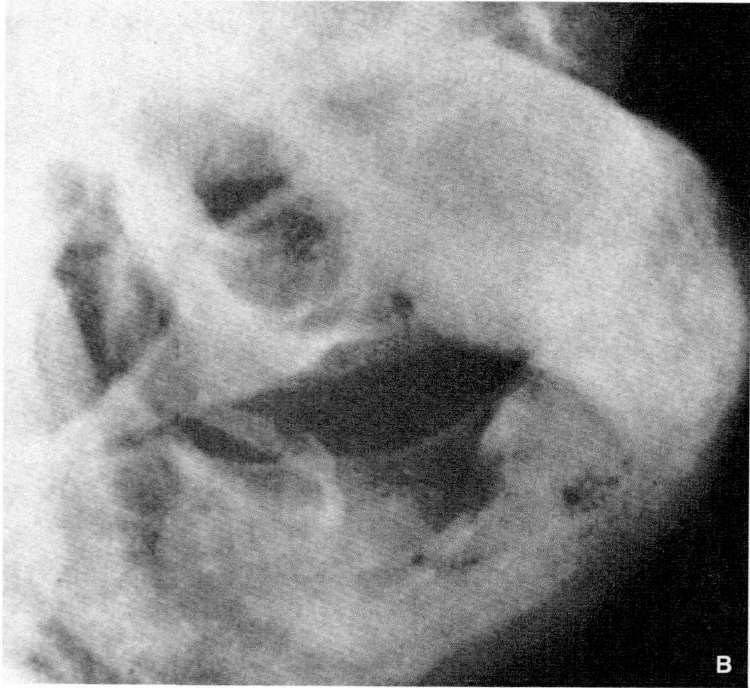

FIGURE 33.66 Van Buchem disease. **(A)** Dorsovolar radiograph of both hands shows endosteal thickening of the cortices of the short tubular bones with almost complete obliteration of the medullary canal. Observe that the articular ends of the bones, the site of endochondral ossification, are not affected. **(B)** Oblique radiograph of the mandible shows sclerotic changes associated with marked expansion. (Courtesy of Prof. P. Beighton, University of Cape Town, Rondebosch, Republic of South Africa.)

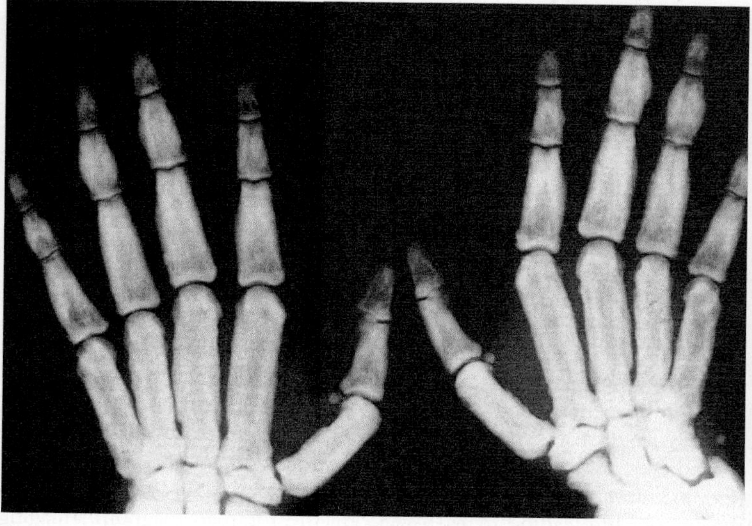

FIGURE 33.67 Sclerosteosis. Dorsovolar radiograph of both hands shows periosteal and endosteal hyperostosis and disturbance in modeling. (Courtesy of Prof. P. Beighton, University of Cape Town, Rondebosch, Republic of South Africa.)

frequent feature. Sclerosteosis is potentially a lethal disorder; death often occurs in early adulthood as a result of increased intracranial pressure. The distinguishing imaging features of sclerosteosis are a massive increase in size and density of affected parts of the skeleton, predominantly the cranium and tubular bones, and deformities throughout the skeleton, reflecting errors in bone modeling. Gross widening and sclerotic changes are often seen in the calvaria, which appears dense and thickened with obliteration of the diploic space. The body of the mandible may enlarge massively in adults, resulting in prognathism. General enlargement with thickening of the cortex and increase in density can be observed in the clavicles, ribs, and bones of the pelvic girdle. Vertebral changes are confined to the posterior elements, notably the pedicles and laminae of the lumbar and sacral vertebrae. The cortices of the long and short tubular bones show sclerosis and hyperostosis, with marked periosteal and endosteal thickening and evidence of disturbance in modeling (Fig. 33.67). A neurogenetic and pathophysiologic studies of sclerosteosis, which included histomorphometric analysis of calvarial tissue following in vivo tetracycline labeling, showed that dense, thickened trabeculae were associated with active-appearing osteoblasts, increased total bone volume, and increased linear extent of bone formation and appositional rate. Osteoclastic bone resorption appeared depressed. Thus, the changes observed in sclerosteosis appear to represent both osteoblastic hyperactivity and diminished activity of osteoclasts, resulting in a failure of bone resorption.

Dysosteosclerosis

First described by Spranger et al. in 1974, this sclerosing dysplasia is caused by mutations in *SLC29A33* gene, which encodes a nucleoside transporter. It is inherited as an autosomal recessive manner, but an X-linked pedigree has also been reported. Dysosteosclerosis is marked by short stature and bone fragility. Limb length is short relative to the trunk, the mandible is small, and the forehead and parietal regions are bulky. Expansion of the metaphyses of the long bones may result in Erlenmeyer flask–like deformity (Fig. 33.68A). Bone encroachment narrows the optic foramina, and compression of the optic nerves causes blindness. In general, dysplastic changes predominate at sites of endochondral bone formation. As in osteopetrosis, imaging reveals a generalized sclerosis of the skeleton, disturbed diaphyseal and metaphyseal modeling of the long bones, and thickening of the base of the skull. In addition, there is sclerosis of the mastoids and paranasal sinuses, with narrowing of the optical canals (Fig. 33.68B). Typically noted is platyspondylisis (vertebral flattening), hypoplasia of the pelvis, and thickening of the calvaria. Microscopic examination of biopsy specimens of metaphyses reveals unresorbed spicules of calcified cartilage, irregularly covered with a thin rim of immature osteoid, both of which appear to be heavily mineralized (hence the imaging appearance of osteosclerosis). In some areas, the matrix is poorly organized, suggesting woven bone. Cartilage, on the other hand, appears normal. These findings in the metaphysis closely resemble those seen in osteopetrosis and suggest an error in endochondral bone formation due to diminished osteoclastic resorption, subsequently leading to disturbance in bone formation. In a study of histologic heterogeneity in hyperostotic bone dysplasia,

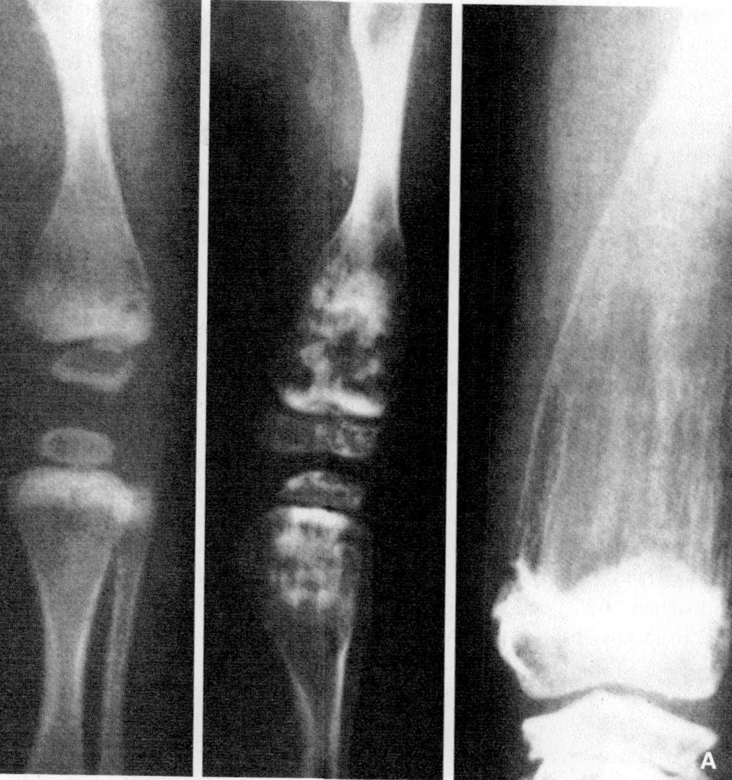

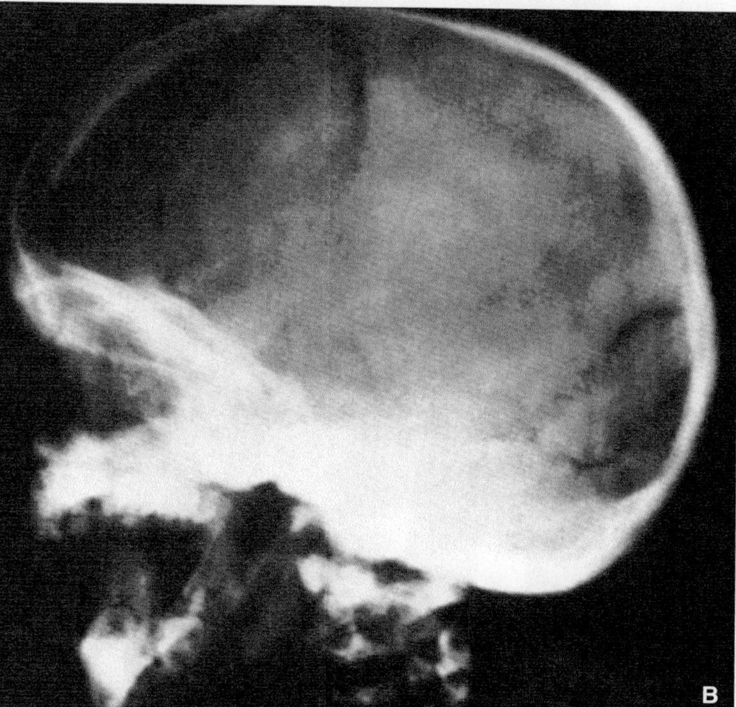

FIGURE 33.68 Dysosteosclerosis. **(A)** Anteroposterior radiographs of the lower limbs of a patient with dysosteosclerosis at 20 months of age *(left)*, 5 years *(middle)*, and 15 years *(right)*. Observe progression of metaphyseal widening, which has assumed an Erlenmeyer flask–like configuration by 15 years of age. **(B)** Lateral radiograph of the skull shows sclerosis of the base, obliteration of the frontal sinuses and mastoids, and mild thickening of the calvaria. (Courtesy of Prof. P. Beighton, University of Cape Town, Rondebosch, Republic of South Africa.)

investigators noted the similarity between the metaphyseal histopathology of dysosteosclerosis and lead intoxication, which suggested a deficiency of a lead-sensitive enzyme as the basic defect in this dysplasia. However, involvement of the membranous bones of the skull in dysosteosclerosis, which on histologic examination appears immature and woven rather than compact and lamellar, points to an additional defect in intramembranous ossification in the pathogenesis of this mixed sclerosing bone dysplasia.

Pyle Disease

Also known as *Pyle-Cohn syndrome* and *familial metaphyseal dysplasia*, this autosomal recessive disorder caused by mutation of the *SFRP4* (secreted frizzled related protein 4) gene on chromosome 7p14, belongs to the mixed sclerosing dysplasias with target site for both endochondral (predominantly) and intramembranous bone formation. In 1931, Edwin Pyle, an orthopaedic surgeon from Waterbury, Connecticut, first reported this condition in a 5-year-old boy who presented with *genu valgum*, mild limitation of extension in the elbow joints, and palpable widening of the clavicles, manifestations representing deficient modeling of the metaphyses of the tubular bones. This dysplasia is characterized by thinning of the cortices; broadening of the metaphyses of the long bones resulting in Erlenmeyer flask–like deformity (Fig. 33.69); expansion of the medial ends of the clavicles, pubic, and ischial bones; and sclerosis of the base of the skull. The nasal sinuses and mastoids may be poorly developed. In the spine, platyspondylisis is occasionally observed. In addition to those typical sites of endochondral bone formation, the calvaria, a site of intramembranous bone formation, are also affected. Mild *genu valgum* deformity presenting in childhood is the main clinical feature of this condition. Dental malocclusion and mild prognathism may also be observed. This sclerosing bone dysplasia is benign, general health is unimpaired, and life span is normal.

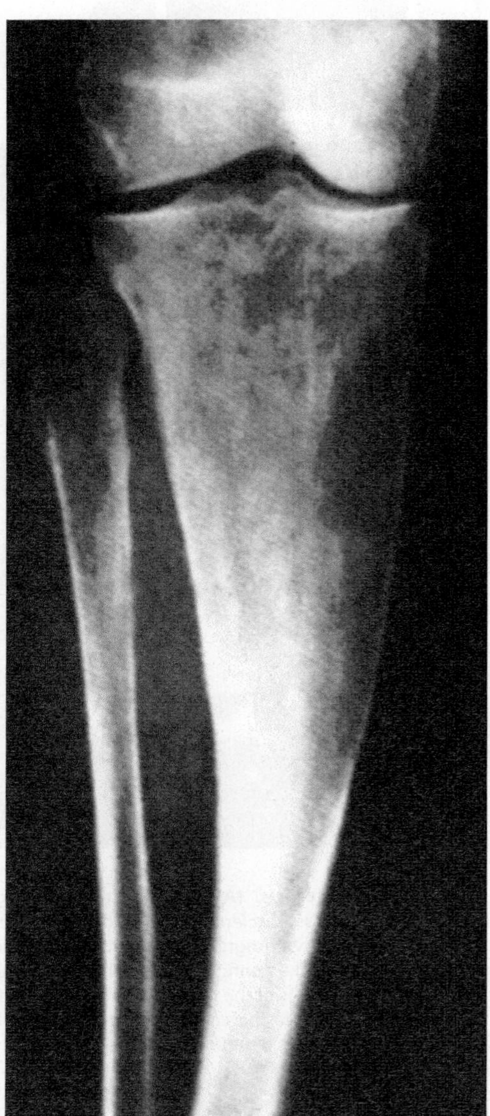

FIGURE 33.69 Pyle disease. Anteroposterior radiograph of the right proximal leg shows striking expansion of the metaphysis and proximal diaphysis of the tibia that resulted in Erlenmeyer flask–like deformity. Observe thinning of the cortices of the proximal tibia and fibula. (Courtesy of Prof. P. Beighton, University of Cape Town, Rondebosch, Republic of South Africa.)

Craniometaphyseal Dysplasia

This mixed sclerosing dysplasia affecting predominantly endochondral ossification, also referred to as *osteochondrodysplasia* or *Jackson type* of craniometaphyseal dysplasia, is a genetic autosomal dominant disorder caused by the mutation of *ANKH* gene located on the chromosome 5p15.2-p14.1. Some of the cases may have an autosomal recessive form of inheritance, in which case a potential locus is chromosome 6q21-q22. It is characterized by metaphyseal widening very similar to Pyle disease, prominent mandible, progressive diffuse hyperostosis of craniofacial bones, resulting in widely spaced eyes, broad and flat nasal bridge, and a "leonine" facial appearance (*leontiasis ossea*). Progressive thickening of craniofacial bones continues throughout life leading to narrowing of the foramen magnum. Imaging studies reveal thinning of the cortex and radiolucencies of the long bones; club-like flaring and broadening of the metaphyses (Erlenmeyer flask deformity); and overgrowth of the bones of the skull, facial bones, and mandible (Fig. 33.70). Bone compression of cranial nerves may result in facial paralysis, deafness, and blindness.

Melorheostosis

A rare condition of unknown cause, melorheostosis (Leri disease) shows no evidence of hereditary features. It belongs to a group of bone disorders called the *mixed sclerosing dysplasias*, which combine characteristics of both endochondral and intramembranous failure of ossification. It has been postulated that the disease develops due to a loss-of-function mutation in *LEMD3* gene. This gene, also known as *MAN1*, encodes for an integral protein of the inner nuclear membrane. Happle suggested that melorheostosis originates from an early mutation event with loss of the corresponding wild-type allele at gene locus of osteopoikilosis, however, some investigators concluded that mutation in the *LEMD3* gene does not cause isolated melorheostosis. Laboratory abnormalities affect osteoblastic-specific factor 2 (OSF-2), osteonectin, fibronectin, TGF-β, and FGF-23. Similar to osteopoikilosis, melorheostosis may also occasionally be associated with Buschke-Ollendorff syndrome.

Clinical Features

The presenting symptom is pain intensified by activity. Limitation of joint motion and stiffness are common, due to contractures, soft-tissue fibrosis, and periarticular bone formation in the soft tissues. There is no gender predilection, and the age of presentation ranges from 2 to 64 years. The condition may be monostotic (*forme fruste*), affecting only one bone; monomelic, affecting one limb; or polyostotic, with generalized affection of the skeleton. Long bones are most commonly affected, with other sites including the pelvis, and short tubular bones of the hands and feet. The lower extremities are affected more commonly than the upper extremities. The ribs and the bones of the skull are rarely affected. Melorheostosis affecting thoracic vertebrae complicated by involvement of the facet joints has also been reported.

Imaging Features

Conventional radiography is sufficient to make a diagnosis. The lesion is characterized by a wavy hyperostosis that resembles melted wax dripping down the side of a candle (*hyperostose en coulee*), the feature from which the disease derives its name (Greek *melos-* [member]; *rhein-* [flow], *osteon-* [bone]); moreover, only one side of the bone is usually involved (Figs. 33.71 to 33.73). Besides this typical pattern, other appearances have been described including osteoma-like (Fig. 33.74), osteopathia striata–like, and mixed type of presentation. Associated joint abnormalities are also well delineated on standard radiographs. The involvement of soft tissues is not rare, and the ossified masses resembling myositis ossificans are often present around the hip and knee joints (Fig. 33.75). CT effectively reveals involvement of the cortex and the medullary cavity and clear demarcation of normal from abnormal bone (Fig. 33.76A). MRI shows low signal intensity localized to the affected areas on all pulse sequences (Figs. 33.76B,C and 33.77).

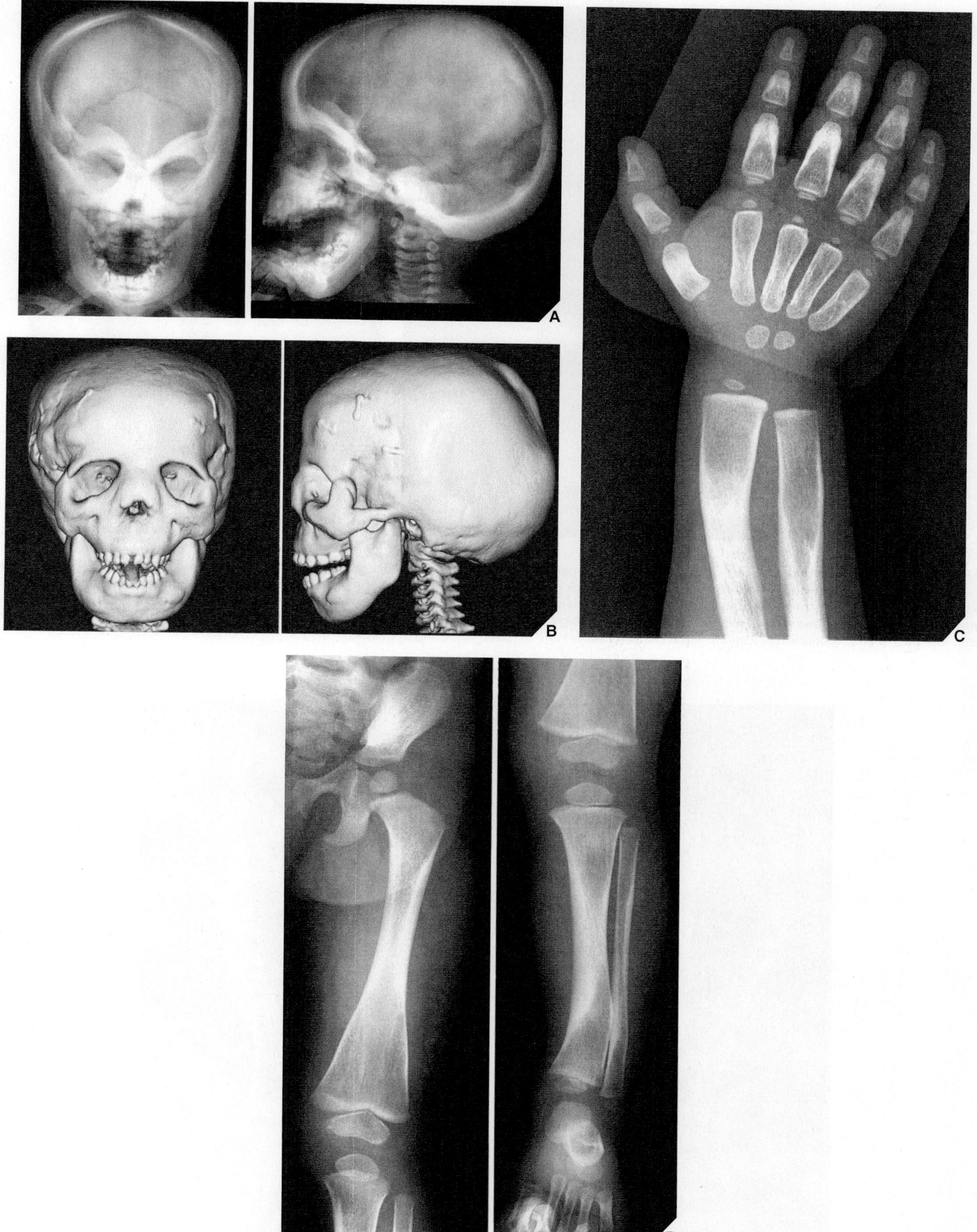

FIGURE 33.70 **Craniometaphyseal dysplasia.** **(A)** Anteroposterior and lateral radiographs of the skull of a 2-year-old girl, and **(B)** three-dimensional (3D) CT reconstructed images show hypertrophic changes of the facial bones and calvaria, giving a leonine facial appearance. Note mandibular hypertrophy and overgrowth of the zygomatic arches. Radiographs of **(C)** the hand and **(D)** lower extremity show thinning of the cortices, juxtaarticular radiolucency of the bones, and flaring of the metaphyses with Erlenmeyer flask–like deformity of the distal femur.

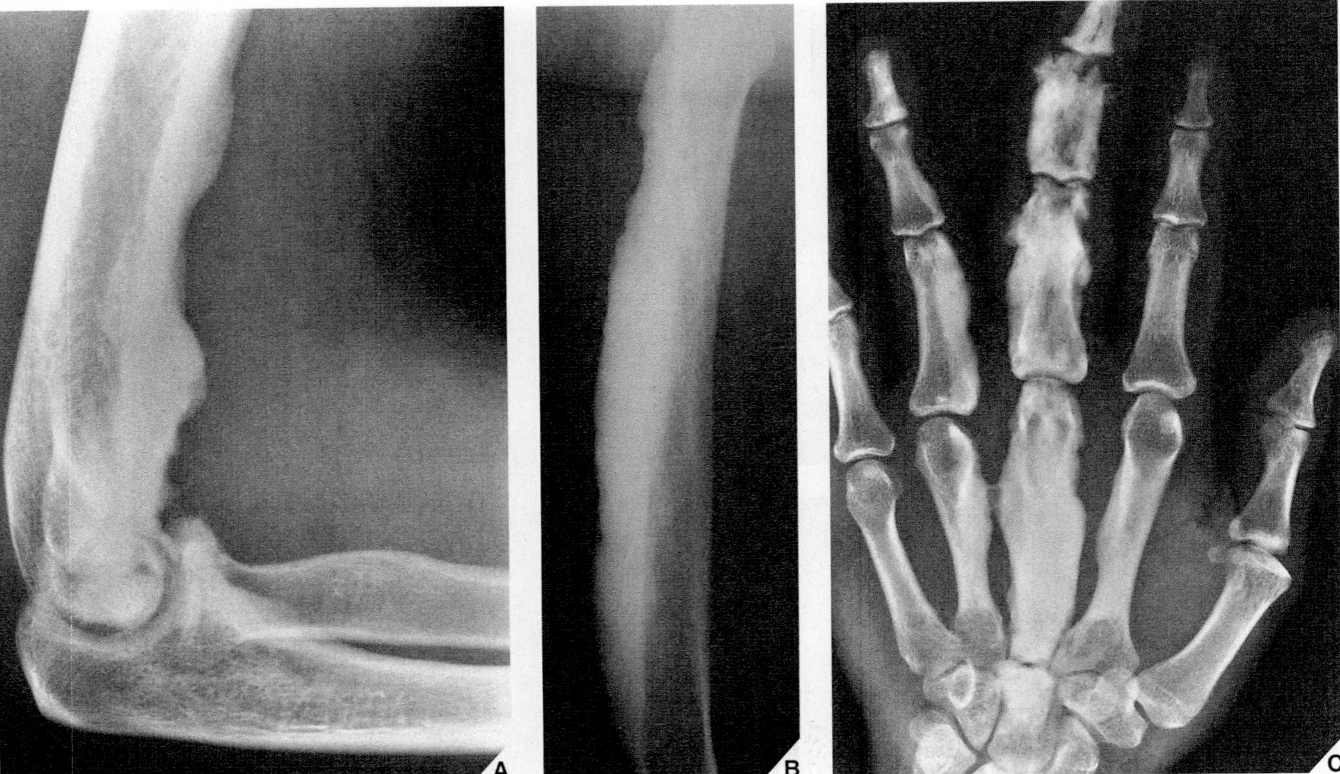

FIGURE 33.71 Melorheostosis. A 28-year-old man presented with pain in the right elbow and an enlargement of the middle finger of his right hand. **(A)** Lateral radiograph of the elbow demonstrates a flowing hyperostosis of the anterior cortex of the distal humerus, typical of melorheostosis. Note the bridging of the joint by the lesion and the involvement of the coronoid process of the ulna. **(B)** The radiograph of the right femur shows involvement of only the anterolateral aspect of the bone. **(C)** Dorsovolar radiograph of the right hand shows marked hypertrophy of the middle digit. The cortices (the sites of intramembranous ossification) are involved, as are the articular ends of the bones (the sites of endochondral ossification). This is characteristic feature of mixed sclerosing dysplasias.

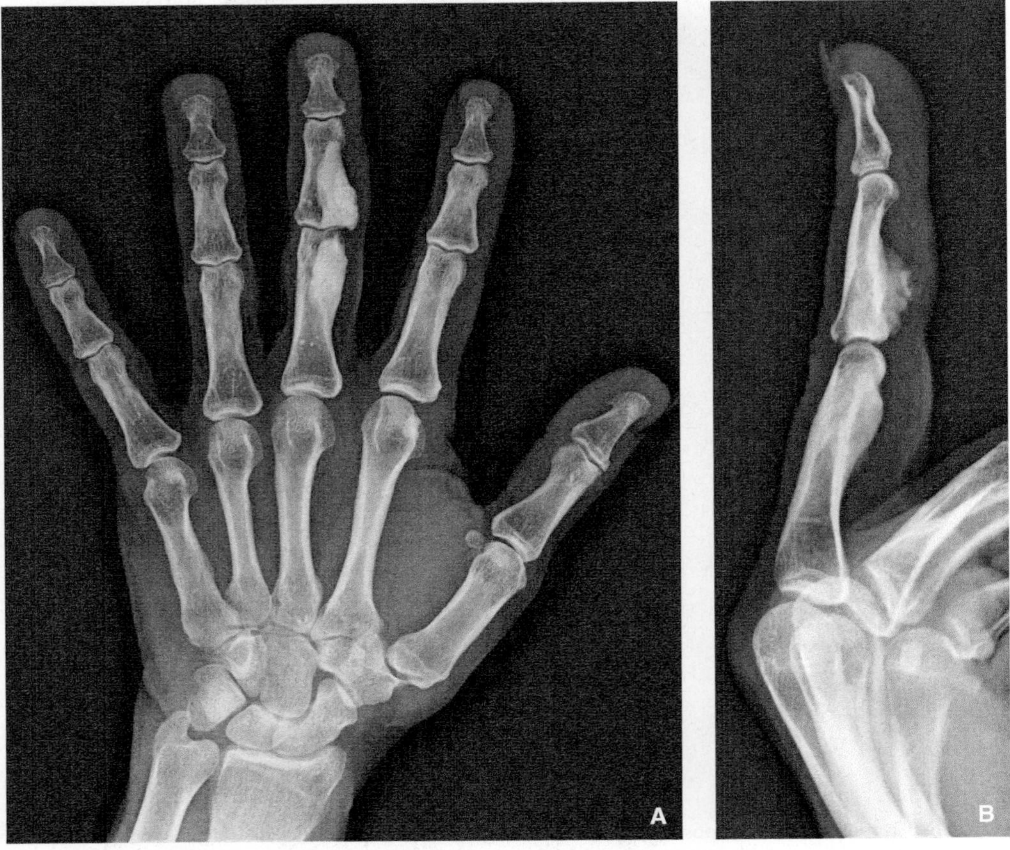

FIGURE 33.72 Melorheostosis. **(A)** Dorsovolar radiograph of the right hand and **(B)** lateral radiograph of the middle finger of a 60-year-old woman show flowing hyperostosis affecting the radial and volar aspects of the proximal and middle phalanges.

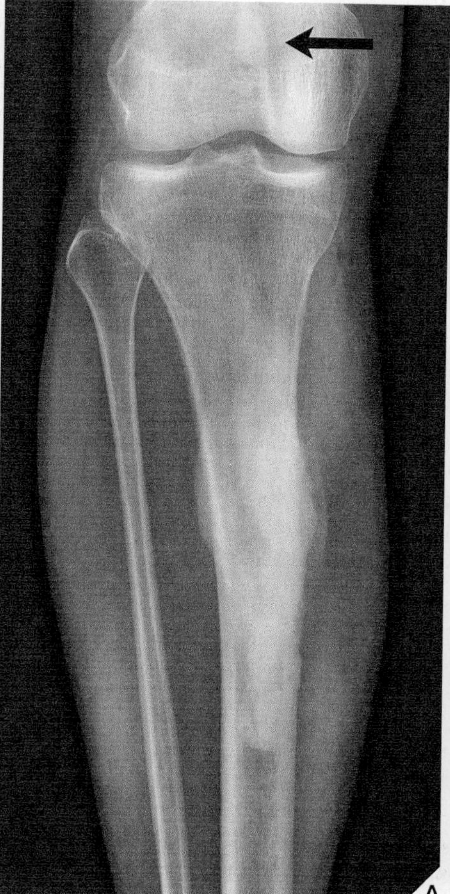

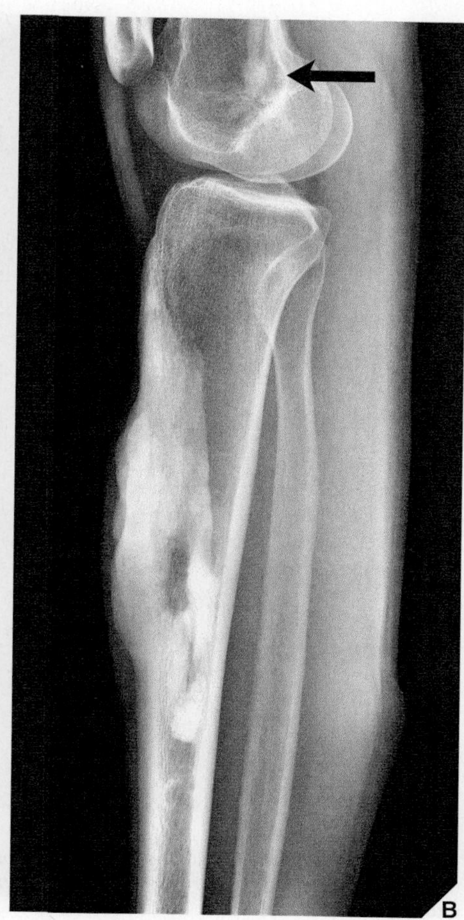

FIGURE 33.73 Melorheostosis. (A) Anteroposterior and **(B)** lateral radiographs of the right leg of a 31-year-old woman show sclerotic changes affecting predominantly anterior aspect of the tibia. Note also a medullary focus of melorheostosis in the distal femur *(arrows)*.

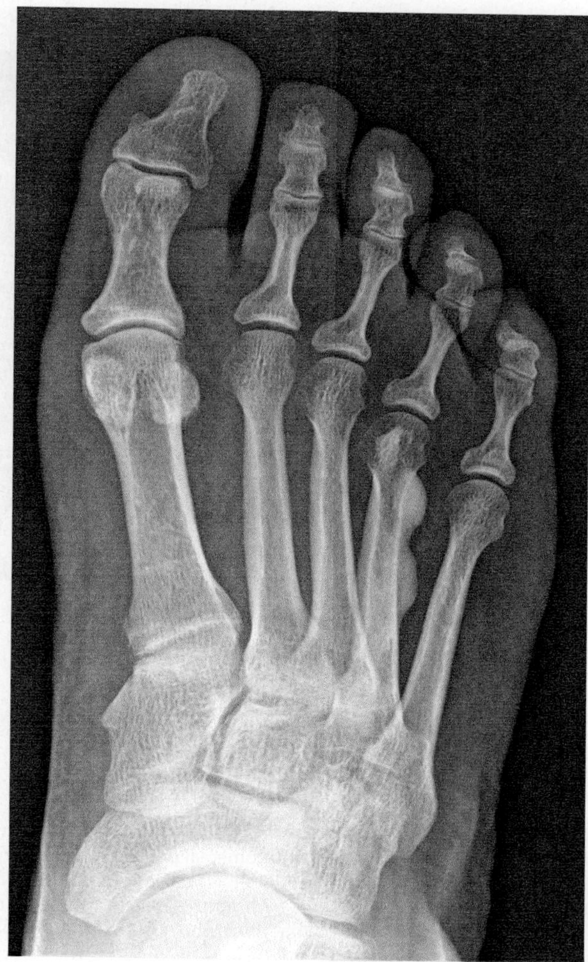

FIGURE 33.74 Melorheostosis. Anteroposterior radiograph of the left foot of a 65-year-old woman shows "osteoma-like" presentation of this lesion affecting the fourth metatarsal bone.

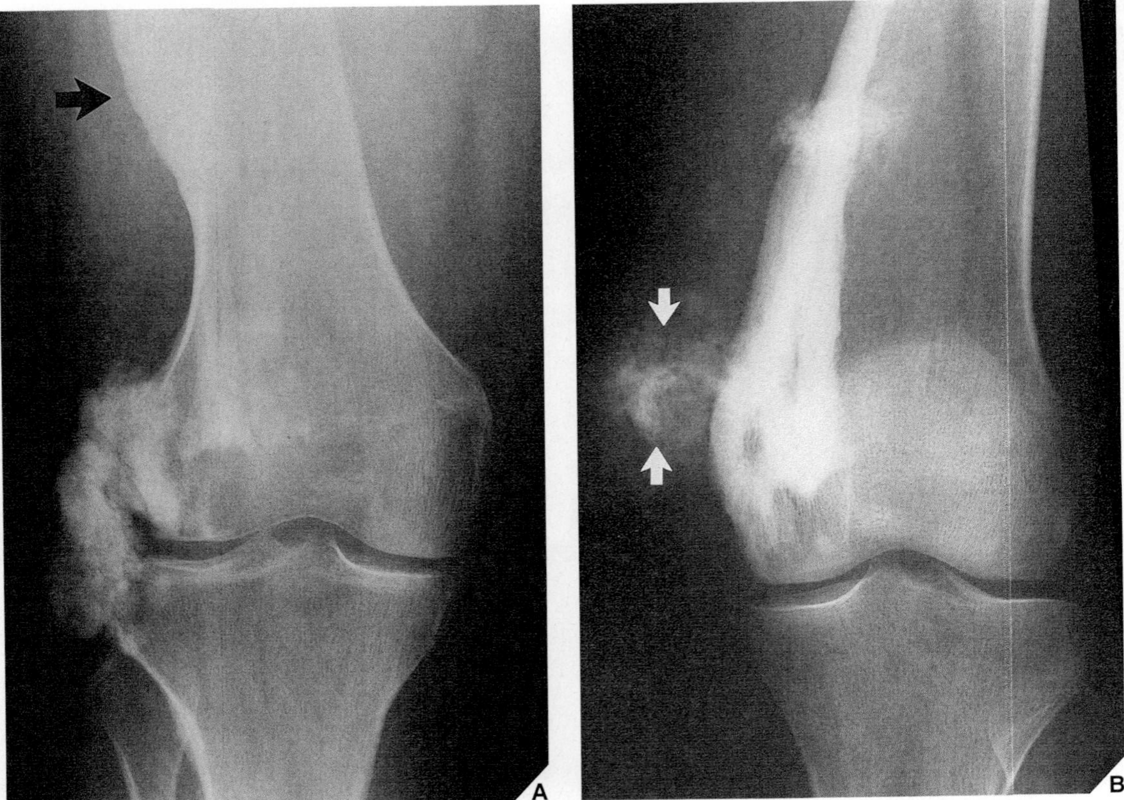

FIGURE 33.75 Melorheostosis. **(A)** Anteroposterior radiograph of the right knee in a 46-year-old woman shows ossifications of the soft tissues at the lateral aspect of the knee joint. The femoral cortex is also affected *(arrow)*. **(B)** A radiograph of the left knee in a 25-year-old woman shows involvement of the medial femoral cortex extending into the soft tissues *(arrows)*.

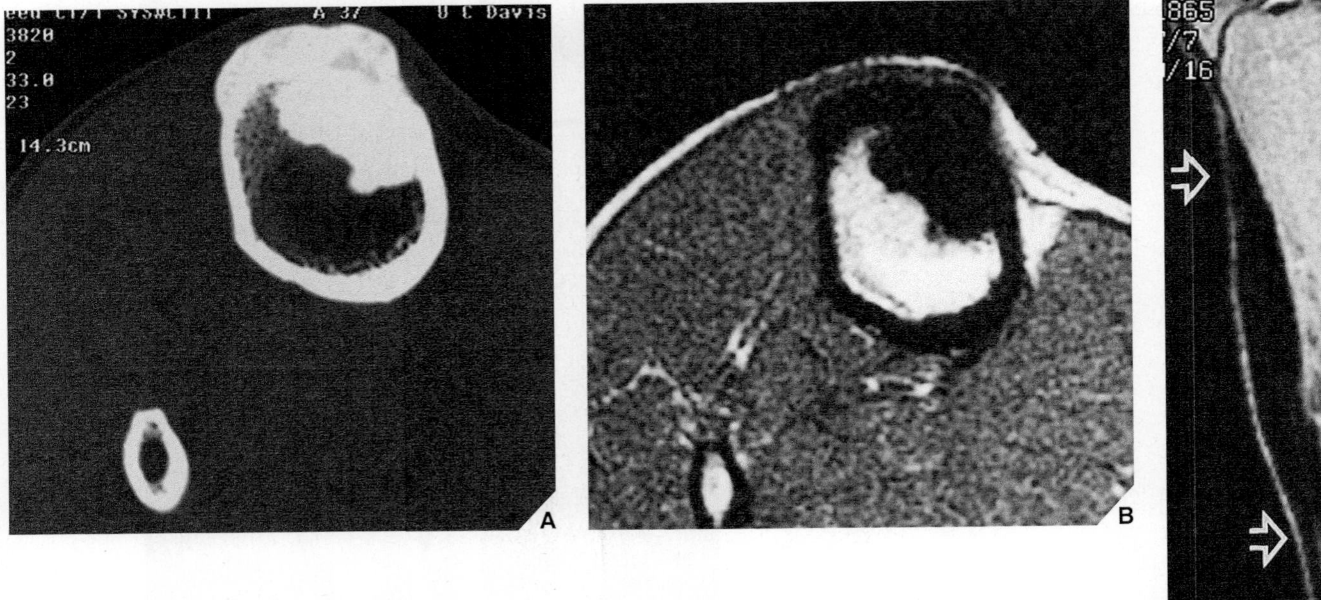

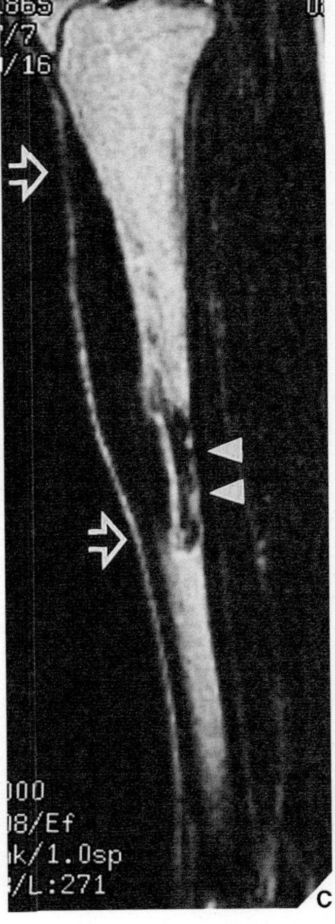

FIGURE 33.76 CT and MRI of melorheostosis. **(A)** CT section through the middle segment of tibia in a 30-year-old woman shows involvement of the anterior cortex and anteromedial portion of medullary cavity. **(B)** Axial T1-weighted (spin echo [SE]; repetition time [TR] 800/echo time [TE] 16 msec) MRI shows the lesion to be of low signal intensity, which is the same as the cortical bone. The uninvolved bone marrow exhibits high signal similar to the subcutaneous fat. **(C)** Sagittal T2-weighted (fast spin echo; TR 3000/TE 108 msec) MR image shows that the lesion remains of low signal intensity *(open arrows)*. *Arrowheads* point to the medullary involvement.

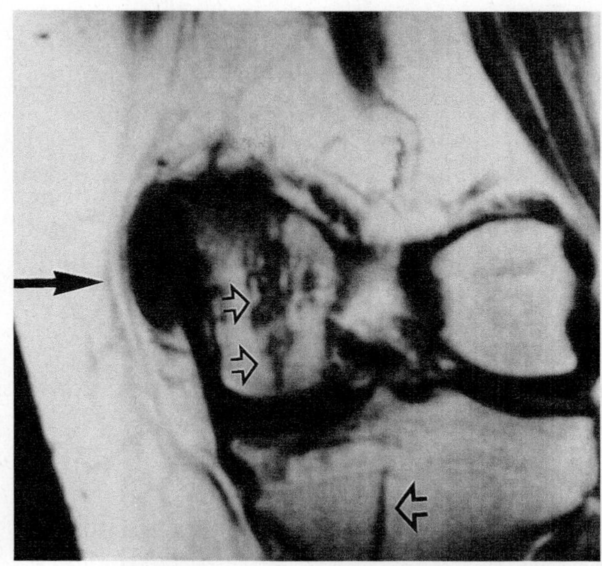

FIGURE 33.77 **MRI of melorheostosis.** Coronal T1-weighted (spin echo [SE]; repetition time [TR] 800/echo time [TE] 20 msec) MR image of the knee in a 20-year-old man shows decreased signal intensity of the ossific mass attached to the femoral condyle *(arrow)* as well as in the medullary foci of melorheostosis *(open arrows)*.

This technique is also helpful for imaging of soft-tissue involvement. In one study reported by Judkiewicz and associates, soft-tissue masses were heterogeneous on all MRI pulse sequences with signal void in areas corresponding to mineralization on conventional radiographs. Most of the soft-tissue masses exhibited ill-defined margins, were contiguous or adjacent to areas of osseous hyperostosis, and demonstrated enhancement after administration of gadolinium diethylenetriamine pentaacetic acid (Gd-DTPA). Radionuclide bone scan shows invariably an increased uptake of the radiopharmaceutical tracer (Fig. 33.78) and thus can determine other sites of skeletal involvement (see Fig. 31.17). The factors responsible for increased uptake include the increased mass of the cortex, osteoblastic activity, and local hyperemia. Microscopic examination of melorheostotic specimens reveals nonspecific, hyperostotic periosteal bone formation with thickened trabeculae and fibrotic changes in the marrow spaces. The bone appears primitive and consists largely of primary Haversian systems, particularly on the periosteal surface, that are almost completely obliterated by the deposition of sclerotic, thickened, and somewhat irregular lamellae. Islands of cartilage in periarticular lesions have been described, with evidence of both endochondral and intramembranous bone formation within the cellular fibrous tissue, and osteoblastic activity along the margins of osteons. Soft-tissue components usually consist of fibrovascular and fibroadipose tissue with variably distributed foci of chondroid and osseous metaplasia. Biochemical investigations revealed normal serum calcium, phosphorus, and alkaline phosphatase levels.

Differential diagnosis should include among others osteoma, parosteal osteosarcoma, and myositis ossificans.

Treatment

The disorder is chronic and occasionally debilitating. Conservative treatment with bisphosphonate (pamidronate) infusion has been tried occasionally, with mixed results. Surgical treatment consists of soft-tissue procedures such as tendon lengthening, excision of fibrous and osseous tissue, fasciotomy, and capsulotomy. Other procedures include corrective osteotomies, excision of hyperostotic bone, and even amputations in severely affected and painful limbs caused by vascular ischemia. Recurrences are common.

Craniodiaphyseal Dysplasia

This dysplasia represents a rare autosomal recessive disorder marked by hyperostosis and sclerosis involving mainly the skull, spine, and ribs. It is a progressive disease in which distortion of the face become apparent in early childhood, and blindness and deafness may occur due to compression of the second and eighth cranial nerves. The diaphyses and metaphyses of long bones show defective remodeling, appearing widened in diameter, sometimes with thinning of the cortex. Although the pelvis may be elongated, it is not sclerotic. The histopathologic features of this sclerosing bone dysplasia point to defect in both endochondral and intramembranous ossification. In addition, unlike craniometaphyseal dysplasia, this disorder exhibits an increased turnover of lamellar bone as well as hyperactivity of the osteoclast. Lamellar bone is more mature than is usually seen in early childhood, appearing very bright under polarized light, with well-developed, complex haversian systems.

Hyperostosis Generalisata with Striations of Bones

This dysplasia shows characteristic features of widening of the long bones, cortical thickening, and coarse striations in the cancellous bone. It was first described by Fairbank in 1951 in a 28-year-old man with coarse striations of the axial and appendicular skeleton, hyperostosis of the tubular bones, and sclerosis of the skull. It affects predominantly males in a wide range of ages at first presentation (the youngest reported patient was 6, the oldest 80). In some of the reported cases, a hereditary etiology was suggested, whereas some cases were sporadic. The imaging hallmarks of this sclerosing bone dysplasia include widening and cortical thickening of the long tubular bones, coarse striations of the cancellous bones, including epiphyses and vertebral bodies, and thickening of the skull base and sclerosis of the cranial vault. Microscopically noted is cortical hyperostosis, periosteal thickening, and capillary proliferation, without evidence of cellular proliferation of the osteoblasts or osteoclasts.

Other Mixed Sclerosing Dysplasias

Six general types of overlap syndrome (the coexistence of two or more osteosclerotic dysplasias) can be identified on the basis of their imaging patterns (see Table 33.5). The most common of these syndromes is the coexistence of melorheostosis, osteopathia striata, and osteopoikilosis. The radiographic features of this "overlap syndrome" are a combination of each of these three dysplasias (Fig. 33.79), a phenomenon suggesting a common pathogenetic mechanism. Although these conditions may not appear exactly as the classic description of the individual entities, the morphologic changes are sufficiently representative to designate them as a mixture of sclerosing bone dysplasias. The existence of these overlap syndromes affirms Abrahamson's observations that not all sclerosing dysplasias are distinct entities and that there are common factors in their development. In fact, nearly every investigator in the area of osteosclerotic dysplasias has speculated about a relationship among melorheostosis, osteopathia striata, and osteopoikilosis, or among other reported dysplasias. Osteopetrosis, osteopoikilosis, and osteopathia striata are clearly heritable disorders. Conversely, melorheostosis occurs only sporadically, although osteosclerotic changes consistent with melorheostosis, osteopathia striata, and dysplasia epiphysealis hemimelica have been reported in patients with no familial history of bone abnormalities. This combination of dysplasias represents not only the coexistence of two or more dysplasias but also an overlap of

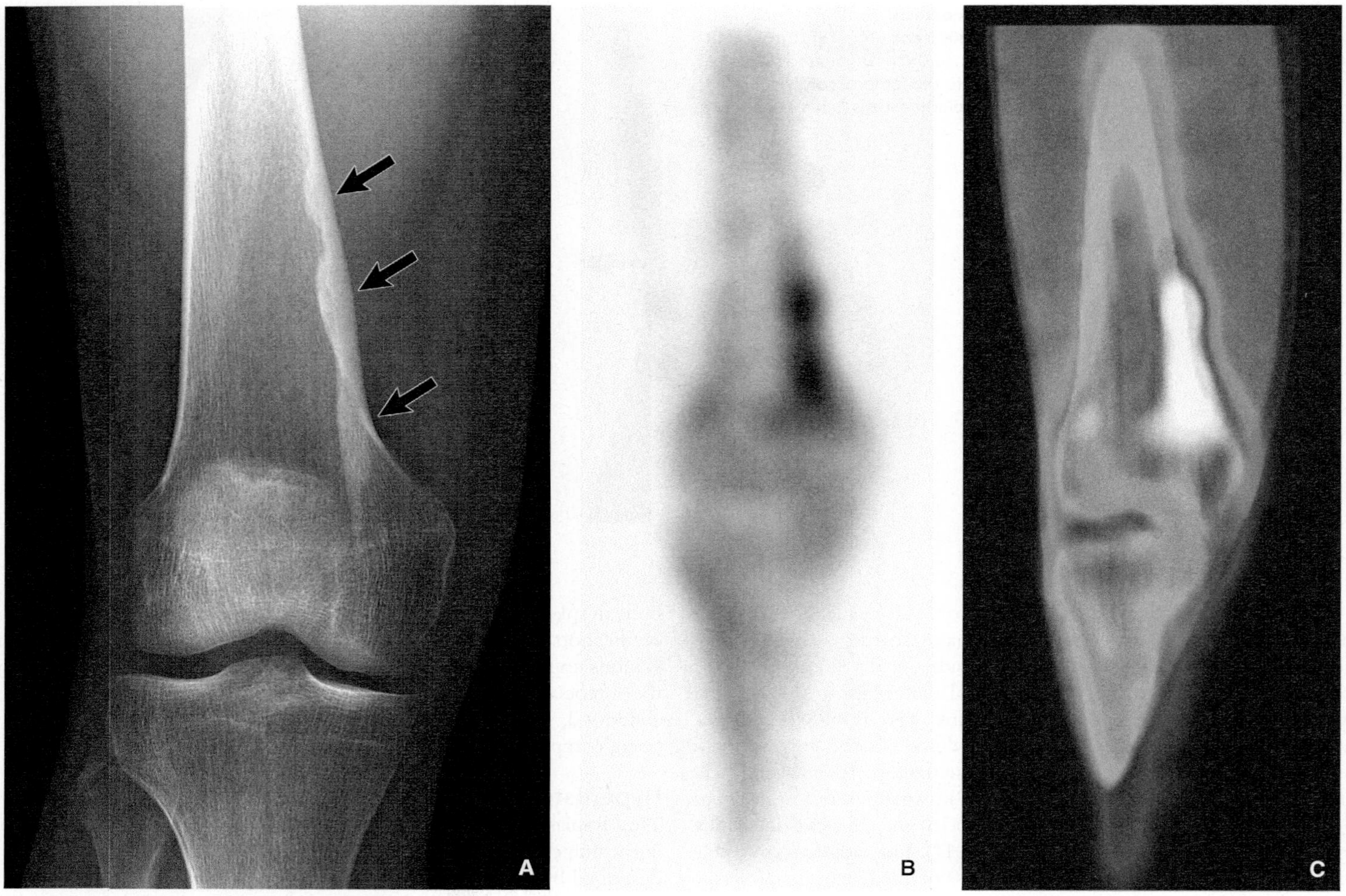

FIGURE 33.78 **Scintigraphy and single-photon emission computed tomography (SPECT) of melorheostosis.** **(A)** Anteroposterior radiograph of the right distal femur of a 21-year-old man shows a sclerotic lesion affecting the endosteal aspect of the medial cortex *(arrows)*. **(B)** Radionuclide bone scan and **(C)** fused SPECT image obtained after intravenous administration of 25 mCi ^{99m}Tc medronate shows increased radiotracer activity at the site of the lesion.

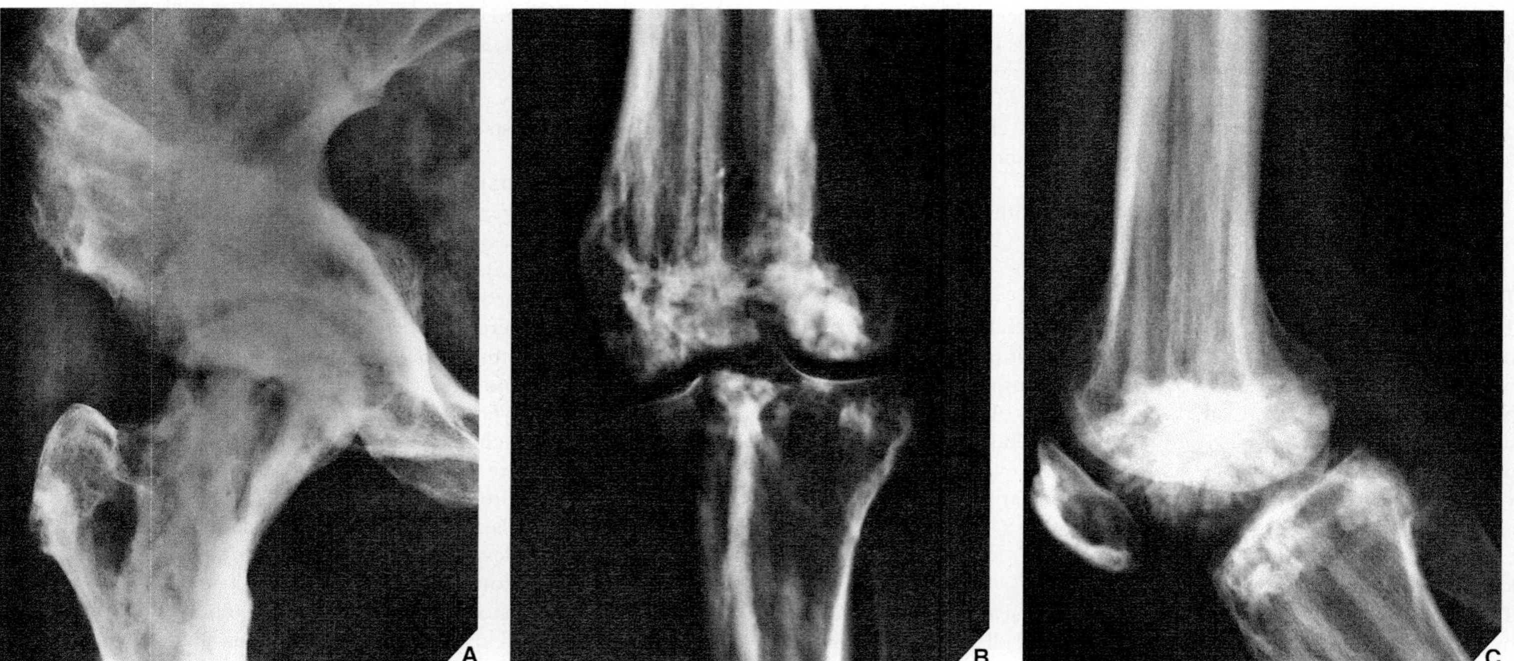

FIGURE 33.79 **Mixed sclerosing dysplasia ("overlap syndrome").** These radiographic studies in an 18-year-old male demonstrate the coexistence of melorheostosis with osteopoikilosis and osteopathia striata. **(A)** Anteroposterior radiograph of the right hemipelvis and hip shows the wavy hyperostosis typical of melorheostosis affecting the iliac bone and proximal femur. **(B)** Anteroposterior and **(C)** lateral radiographs of the knee demonstrate the linear striations characteristic of osteopathia striata in the distal femur and proximal tibia as well as the focal densities that are the identifying feature of osteopoikilosis. (Reprinted with permission from Greenspan A. Sclerosing bone dysplasias. In: Taveras JM, Ferrucci JT, eds. *Radiology: diagnosis, imaging, intervention*. Philadelphia: JB Lippincott; 1993:16; Fig. 13A,B.)

dysplasias, each showing evidence of a disturbance in endochondral or intramembranous bone formation, or both. If there is a common factor at some stage in the development of osteopathia striata, osteopoikilosis, and melorheostosis, that factor also points to a common mechanism affecting both endochondral and intramembranous ossification and thus suggests a common pathogenesis for most of sclerosing dysplasias of bone.

PRACTICAL POINTS TO REMEMBER

Scoliosis

1. Congenital scoliosis may result from:
   - a failure of vertebral formation, which may be unilateral and partial (wedged vertebra) or unilateral and complete (hemivertebra)
   - a failure of segmentation, which may be unilateral (unsegmented bar) or bilateral (block vertebra)
   - failures of both formation and segmentation.
2. Idiopathic scoliosis, the most prevalent type of scoliosis (70%), can be divided into infantile (male > female), juvenile (male = female), and adolescent (male < female) categories. In the last type, the structural (major) curve is located in the thoracic or thoracolumbar segment, with its convexity to the right.
3. In the evaluation of scoliosis, the shape of the curve usually indicates the variant, so that:
   - an S-shaped curve is common in idiopathic scoliosis
   - a C-shaped curve indicates the neuromuscular variant
   - scoliosis marked by a sharply angled short spinal segment is most commonly congenital in origin (e.g., neurofibromatosis, hemivertebra).
4. The scoliotic curve is described as composed of:
   - a structural (major or primary) curve demarcated by upper and lower (transitional) end vertebrae
   - compensatory (secondary) curves proximal and distal to the transitional vertebrae
   - an apical vertebra showing the most rotation and wedging and whose center is most displaced from the central spinal line.
5. Several methods for measuring the scoliotic curve are available:
   - the Lippman-Cobb method, in which the angle is determined only by the inclination of the end vertebrae of the curve
   - the Risser-Ferguson method, which uses three points as determinants of the curve—the centers of the upper and lower end vertebrae and of the apical vertebra
   - the scoliotic index method, which measures the deviation of each vertebra in the scoliotic curve from the central spinal line.
6. To ensure accuracy in determining the degree of correction of a scoliotic curve, the same measuring points should be used in comparing the pretreatment and posttreatment curvature, even if the end vertebrae have changed their locations.
7. The rotation of a vertebral body can be evaluated on the anteroposterior radiograph by:
   - the Cobb method, which uses the position of the spinous process as a point of reference
   - the Nash-Moe method, which uses the pedicles as points of reference.
8. The determination of skeletal maturity, an important factor in the prognosis and treatment of congenital scoliosis, may be made by:
   - comparison of a radiograph of a patient's wrist and hand with standards in radiographic atlases
   - evaluation of the ossification of the vertebral ring apophysis or iliac crest apophysis.

Anomalies with General Affliction of the Skeleton

1. The skeletal abnormalities frequently encountered in neurofibromatosis include:
   - extrinsic cortical erosions
   - pseudoarthroses, particularly in the tibia and fibula
   - short segment kyphoscoliosis marked by acute angulation in the lower cervical and upper thoracic spine
   - enlarged neural foramina and scalloping of the posterior aspect of vertebral bodies.
2. Malignant transformation to sarcoma is the most serious complication of the plexiform variant of neurofibromatosis.
3. The radiographic hallmarks of OI, a disorder characterized by excessive fragility of the bones, include:
   - severe osteoporosis
   - thinning of the cortices
   - sutural (wormian) bones
   - bone deformities, such as trumpet-shaped metaphyses
   - popcorn calcifications at the articular ends of long bones
   - kyphoscoliosis
   - multiple fractures.
4. Radiographically, achondroplasia is characterized by:
   - rhizomelic (disproportional) dwarfism
   - a configuration of the hemipelvis resembling ping-pong paddles and a champagne-glass appearance of the inner pelvic contour
   - narrowing of the interpedicular distance in the lumbar spine (spinal stenosis)
   - scalloping of the posterior aspect of vertebral bodies
   - trident appearance of the hand.
5. The various disorders constituting the MPS share common radiographic features:
   - osteoporosis
   - oval- or hook-shaped vertebral bodies
   - an abnormal configuration of the pelvis
   - shortened tubular bones.
6. Fibrodysplasia ossificans progressiva (myositis ossificans progressiva) is characterized by extensive ossifications of the muscular structures and subcutaneous tissues, leading to joint ankylosis and constriction of the chest wall. Congenital abnormalities of the thumb and great toe (agenesis, microdactyly, etc.) should alert the radiologist to the possibility of this severely crippling disorder.
7. The sclerosing bone dysplasias share the radiographic feature of increased bone density.
8. The radiographic hallmarks of osteopetrosis and pyknodysostosis, disorders related to the failure of endochondral ossification, are:
   - a uniformly increased bone density
   - the absence of remodeling
   - obliteration of the boundary between the medullary cavity and cortex.

   Pathologic fractures are common.
9. The specific changes characteristic of pyknodysostosis include:
   - acroosteolysis
   - obtuse angle of the mandible
   - lack of pneumatization and hypoplasia of paranasal sinuses
   - persistence of the fontanelles
   - wormian (sutural) bones.
10. Enostosis, osteopoikilosis, and osteopathia striata, conditions also related to a failure of endochondral ossification, are characterized radiographically by:
    - foci of sclerotic, mature bone in the medullary cavity (enostosis and osteopoikilosis)
    - fine linear striations (osteopathia striata) at sites of rapid bone growth.
11. Progressive diaphyseal dysplasia and hereditary multiple diaphyseal sclerosis, conditions related to the failure of intramembranous ossification, are recognized radiographically by thickening of the cortices of the long bones. The articular ends of the bones are, as a rule, not affected.
12. Craniometaphyseal dysplasia is characterized by cranial and facial bones hyperostosis, a leonine facial appearance (leontiasis ossea), and "club-like" flaring (Erlenmeyer flask–like deformity) of the metaphyses.
13. Melorheostosis, a mixed sclerosing bone dysplasia marked by failure of endochondral and intramembranous ossification, is recognized

radiographically by a flowing hyperostosis ("wax drippings") associated with involvement of the surrounding soft tissues and joint.

14. Overlap syndrome designation applies to the coexistence of two or more sclerosing bone dysplasias, most commonly melorheostosis, osteopoikilosis, and osteopathia striata.

SUGGESTED READINGS

Abi-Ghanem AS, Asmar K, Boulos F, et al. Osteoma-like melorheostosis: a rare type of skeletal dysplasia depicted on FDG PET/CT. *Skeletal Radiol* 2019;48:1299–1303.

Ablin DS, Greenspan A, Reinhart M, et al. Differentiation of child abuse from osteogenesis imperfecta. *AJR Am J Roentgenol* 1990;154:1035–1046.

Abrahamson MN. Disseminated asymptomatic osteosclerosis with features resembling melorheostosis, osteopoikilosis, and osteopathia striata. Case report. *J Bone Joint Surg Am* 1968;50:991–996.

Ahlawat S, Blakeley JO, Langmead S, et al. Current status and recommendations for imaging in neurofibromatosis type 1, neurofibromatosis type 2, and schwannomatosis. *Skeletal Radiol* 2020;49:199–219.

Artner J, Cakir B, Wernerus D, et al. Melorheostosis: current concepts in diagnosis and treatment—a review of literature (313 cases). *J Musculoskeletal Res* 2012;15:1230.

Ashish G, Shashikant J, Ajay P, et al. Melorheostosis of the foot: a case report of a rare entity with a review of multimodality imaging emphasizing the importance of conventional radiography in diagnosis. *J Orthop Case Rep* 2016;6:79–81.

Aström E, Söderhäll S. Beneficial effect of long term intravenous bisphosphonate treatment of osteogenesis imperfecta. *Arch Dis Child* 2002;86:356–364.

Balemans W, Patel N, Ebeling M, et al. Identification of a 52 kb deletion downstream of the SOST gene in patients with van Buchem disease. *J Med Genet* 2002;39:91–97.

Balemans W, Van den Ende J, Paes-Alves AF, et al. Localization of the gene for sclerosteosis to the van Buchem disease-gene region on chromosome 17q12-q21. *Am J Hum Genet* 1999;64:1661–1669.

Barbosa M, Perdu B, Senra V, et al. Osteopathia striata with cranial sclerosis. *Acta Med Port* 2010;23:1147–1150.

Barnes PD, Brody JD, Jaramillo D, et al. Atypical idiopathic scoliosis: MR imaging evaluation. *Radiology* 1993;186:247–253.

Bartuseviciene A, Samuilis A, Skucas J. Camurati-Engelmann disease: imaging, clinical features and differential diagnosis. *Skeletal Radiol* 2009;38:1037–1043.

Baser ME. The distribution of constitutional and somatic mutations in the neurofibromatosis 2 gene. *Hum Mutat* 2006;27:297–306.

Beals RK. Endosteal hyperostosis. *J Bone Joint Surg Am* 1976;58:1172–1173.

Behninger C, Rott HD. Osteopathia striata with cranial sclerosis: literature reappraisal argues for X-linked inheritance. *Genet Couns* 2000;11:157–167.

Beighton P. Pyle disease (metaphyseal dysplasia). *J Med Genet* 1987;24:321–324.

Beighton P, Barnard A, Hamersma H, et al. The syndromic status of sclerosteosis and van Buchem disease. *Clin Genet* 1984;25:175–181.

Beighton P, Cremin BJ, Hamersma H. The radiology of sclerosteosis. *Br J Radiol* 1976;49:934–939.

Beighton P, Durr L, Hamersma H. The clinical features of sclerosteosis. A review of the manifestations in twenty-five affected individuals. *Ann Intern Med* 1976;84:393–397.

Bhullar TPS, Portinaro NMA, Benson MKD. The measurement of angular deformity: an extended role for the "Cobbometer." *J Bone Joint Surg Br* 1995;77B:506–507.

Bridges AJ, Hsu K-C, Singh A, et al. Fibrodysplasia (myositis) ossificans progressiva. *Semin Arthritis Rheum* 1994;24:155–164.

Bridwell KH. Spinal instrumentation in the management of adolescent scoliosis. *Clin Orthop Relat Res* 1997;335:64–72.

Brien EW, Mirra JM, Latanza L, et al. Giant bone island of femur. Case report, literature review, and its distinction from low grade osteosarcoma. *Skeletal Radiol* 1995;24:546–550.

Brown RR, Steiner GC, Lehman WB. Melorheostosis: case report with radiologic-pathologic correlation. *Skeletal Radiol* 2000;29:548–552.

Brunkow ME, Gardner JC, Van Ness J, et al. Bone dysplasia sclerosteosis results from loss of the SOST gene product, a novel cystine knot-containing protein. *Am J Hum Genet* 2001;68:577–589.

Campos-Xavier AB, Saraiva JM, Savarirayan R, et al. Phenotypic variability at the TGF-β_1 locus in Camurati-Engelmann disease. *Hum Genet* 2001;109:653–658.

Camurati M. Di un raro caso di osteite simmetrica ereditaria degli arti inferiori. *Chir Organi Mov* 1922;6:662–665.

Caron KH, DiPietro MA, Aisen AM, et al. MR imaging of early fibrodysplasia ossificans progressiva. *J Comput Assist Tomogr* 1990;14:318–321.

Chanchairujira K, Chung CB, Lai YM, et al. Intramedullary osteosclerosis: imaging features in nine patients. *Radiology* 2001;220:225–230.

Chitayat D, Silver K, Azouz EM. Skeletal dysplasia, intracerebral calcifications, optic atrophy, hearing impairment, and mental retardation: nosology of dysosteosclerosis. *Am J Med Genet* 1992;43:517–523.

Cobb JR. Outline for the study of scoliosis. *AAOS Instr Course Lect* 1948;5:261–275.

Coccia PF, Krivit W, Cervenka J, et al. Successful bone-marrow transplantation for infantile malignant osteopetrosis. *N Engl J Med* 1980;302:701–708.

Connor J, Evans DA. Genetic aspects of fibrodysplasia ossificans progressiva. *J Med Genet* 1982;19:35–39.

D'Addabbo A, Macarini L, Rubini G, et al. Correlation between bone imaging and the clinical picture in two unsuspected cases of progressive diaphyseal dysplasia (Engelmann's disease). *Clin Nucl Med* 1993;18:324–328.

Damle NA, Patnecha M, Kumar P, et al. Ribbing disease: uncommon cause of a common symptom. *Indian J Nucl Med* 2011;26:36–39.

Davis DC, Syklawer R, Cole RL. Melorheostosis on three-phase bone scintigraphy. Case report. *Clin Nucl Med* 1992;17:561–564.

Del Fattore A, Cappariello A, Teti A. Genetics, pathogenesis and complications of osteopetrosis. *Bone* 2008;42:19–29.

De Vits A, Keymeulen B, Bossuyt A, et al. Progressive diaphyseal dysplasia (Camurati-Engelmann's disease). Improvement of clinical signs and of bone scintigraphy during pregnancy. *Clin Nucl Med* 1994;19:104–107.

Donáth J, Poór G, Kiss C, et al. Atypical form of active melorheostosis and its treatment with bisphosphonate. *Skeletal Radiol* 2002;31:709–713.

Dorst JP. Mucopolysaccharidosis IV. *Semin Roentgenol* 1973;8:218–219.

Drummond DS. Neuromuscular scoliosis: recent concepts. *J Pediatr Orthop* 1996;16:281–283.

Eastman JR, Bixler D. Generalized cortical hyperostosis (Van Buchem disease): nosologic considerations. *Radiology* 1977;125:297–304.

Elmore SM. Pycnodysostosis. A review. *J Bone Joint Surg Am* 1967;49A:153–158.

Engelmann G. Ein Fall von Osteopathia hyperostotica (sclerotisans) multiplex infantilis. *Fortschr Geb Rontgenstr* 1929;39:1101–1106.

Fairbank T, ed. Case 55: hyperostosis generalisata with striation of the bones. In: *An atlas of general affections of the skeleton*. Edinburgh, London: Livingstone; 1951:118–119.

Ferner RE. Neurofibromatosis 1. *Eur J Hum Genet* 2007;15:131–138.

Fotiadou A, Arvaniti M, Kiriakou V, et al. Type II autosomal dominant osteopetrosis: radiological features in two families containing five members with asymptomatic and uncomplicated disease. *Skeletal Radiol* 2009;38:1015–1021.

Fujimoto H, Nishimura G, Tsumurai Y, et al. Hyperostosis generalisata with striations of the bones: report of a female case and a review of the literature. *Skeletal Radiol* 1999;28:460–464.

Furia JP, Schwartz HS. Hereditary multiple diaphyseal sclerosis: a tumor simulator. *Orthopedics* 1990;13:1267–1274.

Gelb BD, Shi GP, Chapman HA, et al. Pycnodysostosis, a lysosomal disease caused by cathepsin K deficiency. *Science* 1996;273:1236–1238.

Gelman MI. Autosomal dominant osteosclerosis. *Radiology* 1977;125:289.

Ghai S, Sharma R, Ghai S. Mixed sclerosing bone dysplasia—a case report with literature review. *Clin Imaging* 2003;27:203–205.

Glorieux FH, Rauch F, Plotkin H, et al. Type V osteogenesis imperfecta: a new form of brittle bone disease. *J Bone Miner Res* 2000;15:1650–1658.

Glorieux FH, Ward LM, Rauch F, et al. Osteogenesis imperfecta type VI: a form of brittle bone disease with a mineralization defect. *J Bone Min Res* 2002;17:30–38.

Gorlin RJ, Glass L. Autosomal dominant osteosclerosis. *Radiology* 1977;125:547–548.

Greenspan A. Bone island (enostosis): current concept—a review. *Skeletal Radiol* 1995;24:111–115.

Greenspan A. Sclerosing bone dysplasias—a target-site approach. *Skeletal Radiol* 1991;20:561–583.

Greenspan A, Azouz EM. Bone dysplasia series. Melorheostosis: review and update. *Can Assoc Radiol J* 1999;50:324–330.

Greenspan A, Pugh JW, Norman A, et al. Scoliotic index: a comparative evaluation of methods for the measurement of scoliosis. *Bull Hosp Joint Dis* 1978;39:117–125.

Greenspan A, Stadalnik RC. Bone island: scintigraphic findings and their clinical application. *Can Assoc Radiol J* 1995;46:368–379.

Greenspan A, Steiner G, Knutzon R. Bone island (enostosis): clinical significance and radiologic and pathologic correlations. *Skeletal Radiol* 1991;20:85–90.

Greenspan A, Steiner G, Sotelo D, et al. Mixed sclerosing bone dysplasia coexisting with dysplasia epiphysealis hemimelica (Trevor-Fairbank disease). *Skeletal Radiol* 1986;15:452–454.

Hagiwara H, Aida N, Machida J, et al. Contrast-enhanced MRI of an early preosseous lesion of fibrodysplasia ossificans progressiva in a 21-month-old boy. *AJR Am J Roentgenol* 2003;181:1145–1147.

Happle R. Melorheostosis may originate as a type 2 segmental manifestation of osteopoikilosis. *Am J Med Genet A* 2004;125A:221–223.

Heanney C, Shalev H, Elbedour K, et al. Human autosomal recessive osteopetrosis maps to 11q13, a position predicted by comparative mapping of the murine osteosclerosis (oc) mutation. *Hum Mol Genet* 1998;7:1407–1410.

Hellemans J, Preobrazhenska O, Willaert A, et al. Loss-of-function mutations in LEMD3 result in osteopoikilosis, Buschke-Ollendorff syndrome and melorheostosis. *Nat Genet* 2004;36:1213–1218.

Hopwood JJ, Morris CP. The mucopolysaccharidoses. Diagnosis, molecular genetics and treatment. *Mol Biol Med* 1990;7:381–404.

Hui PKT, Tung JYL, Lam WWM, et al. Osteogenesis imperfecta type V. *Skeletal Radiol* 2011;40:1609, 1633.

Irie T, Takahashi M, Kaneko M. Case report 546: endosteal hyperostosis (Worth type). *Skeletal Radiol* 1989;18:310–313.

Jain VK, Arya RK, Bharadwaj M, et al. Melorheostosis: clinicopathological features, diagnosis, and management. *Orthopedics* 2009;32:512.

Janssens K, Gershoni-Baruch R, Van Hul E, et al. Localisation of the gene causing diaphyseal dysplasia Camurati-Engelmann to chromosome 19q13. *J Med Genet* 2000;37:245–249.

Joseph DJ, Ichikawa S, Econs MJ. Mosaicism in osteopathia striata with cranial sclerosis. *J Clin Endocrinol Metab* 2010;95:1506–1507.

Judkiewicz AM, Murphey MD, Resnik CS, et al. Advanced imaging of melorheostosis with emphasis on MRI. *Skeletal Radiol* 2001;30:447–453.

Kaitila L, Rimoin DL. Histologic heterogeneity in the hyperostotic bone dysplasias. *Birth Defects Orig Artic Ser* 1976;12:71–79.

Kaplan FS, McCluskey W, Hahn G, et al. Genetic transmission of fibrodysplasia ossificans progressiva. Report of a family. *J Bone Joint Surg Am* 1993;75:1214–1220.

Kennedy JG, Donahue JR, Aydin H, et al. Metastatic breast carcinoma to bone disguised by osteopoikilosis. *Skeletal Radiol* 2003;32:240–243.

Kerkeni S, Chapurlat R. Melorheostosis and FGF-23: is there a relationship? *Joint Bone Spine* 2008;75:486–488.

Kim H, Kim HS, Moon ES, et al. Scoliosis imaging: what radiologists should know. *Radiographics* 2010;30:1823–1842.

Kiper POS, Saito H, Gori F, et al. Cortical-bone fragility—insights from sFRP4 deficiency in Pyle's disease. *N Engl J Med* 2016;374:2553–2562.

Kleinman PK. Differentiation of child abuse and osteogenesis imperfecta: medical and legal implications. *AJR Am J Roentgenol* 1990;154:1047–1048.

Kobayashi H, Kotoura Y, Hosono M, et al. A case of melorheostosis with a 14-year-old follow-up. *Eur Radiol* 1995;5:651–653.

Korovessis PG, Stamatakis MV. Prediction of scoliotic cobb angle with the use of the scoliometer. *Spine (Phila Pa 1976)* 1996;21:1661–1666.

Kotwal A, Clarke BL. Melorheostosis: a rare sclerosing bone dysplasia. *Curr Osteoporos Rep* 2017;15:335–342.

Kozlowski K, Nicol R, Hopwood JJ. A clinically mild case of mucopolysaccharidosis type I—Scheie syndrome (case report). *Eur Radiol* 1995;5:561–563.

Lachman RS, Burton BK, Clarke LA, et al. Mucopolysaccharidosis IVA (Morquio A syndrome) and VI (Maroteaux-Lamy syndrome): under-recognized and challenging to diagnose. *Skeletal Radiol* 2014;43:359–369.

Lee RD. Clinical images of osteopathia striata. *Pediatr Radiol* 2004;34:753.

Leisti J, Kaitila I, Lachman RS, et al. Dysosteosclerosis (case report). *Birth Defects* 1975;11:349.

Lenke LG, Bridwell KH, Blanke K, et al. Radiographic results of arthrodesis with Cotrel-Dubousset instrumentation for the treatment of adolescent idiopathic scoliosis. A five to ten-year follow-up study. *J Bone Joint Surg Am* 1998;80:807–814.

Léri A, Joanny J. Une affection non décrite des os. Hyperostose en coulée sur toute la longeur d'un membre ou mélorhéostose. *Bull Mem Soc Med Hop Paris* 1922;46:1141.

Looser E. Zur Kenntnis der Osteogenesis Imperfecta Congenita et Tarda (sogenannte idiopatische Osteopsatyrosis). *Mittlg Grenzgebiete Med Chir* 1906;15:161–207.

MacEwen GD, Conway JJ, Miler WT. Congenital scoliosis with a unilateral bar. *Radiology* 1968;90:711–715.

Makita Y, Nishimura G, Ikegawa S, et al. Intrafamilial phenotypic variability in Engelmann disease (ED): are ED and Ribbing disease the same entity? *Am J Med Genet* 2000;91:153–156.

Marchesi DG, Transfeldt EE, Bradford DS, et al. Changes in vertebral rotation after Harrington and Luque instrumentation for idiopathic scoliosis. *Spine (Phila Pa 1976)* 1992;17:775–780.

Maroteaux P, Lamy M. La pycnodysostose. *Presse Med* 1962;70:999–1002.

Maroteaux P, Lamy M. The malady of Toulouse-Lautrec. *JAMA* 1965;191:715–717.

Menon AG, Anderson KM, Riccardi VM, et al. Chromosome 17p deletions and p53 gene mutations associated with the formation of malignant neurofibrosarcomas in von Recklinghausen neurofibromatosis. *Proc Natl Acad Sci U S A* 1990;87:5435–5439.

Motyckova G, Fisher DE. Pycnodysostosis: role and regulation of cathepsin K in osteoclast function and human disease. *Curr Mol Med* 2002;2:407–421.

Mumm S, Wenkert D, Zhang X, et al. Deactivating germline mutations in LEMD3 cause osteopoikilosis and Buschke-Ollendorff syndrome, but not sporadic melorheostosis. *J Bone Miner Res* 2007;22:243–250.

Murray RO, McCredie J. Melorheostosis and the sclerotomes: a radiological correlation. *Skeletal Radiol* 1979;4:57–71.

Nakamura K, Nakada Y, Nakada D. Unclassified sclerosing bone dysplasia with osteopathia striata, cranial sclerosis, metaphyseal undermodeling, and bone fragility. *Am J Med Genet* 1998;76:389–394.

Nakamura T, Yamada N, Nonaka R, et al. Autosomal dominant type of endosteal hyperostosis with unusual manifestations of sclerosis of the jaw bones. *Skeletal Radiol* 1987;16:48–51.

Nash CL Jr, Moe JH. A study of vertebral rotation. *J Bone Joint Surg Am* 1969;51:223–229.

Neuhauser EBD, Schwachman H, Wittenberg M, et al. Progressive diaphyseal dysplasia. *Radiology* 1948;51:11–22.

Norman A, Greenspan A. Bone dysplasias. In: Jahss MH, ed. *Disorders of the foot and ankle: medical and surgical management*, vol. 1, 2nd ed. Philadelphia: WB Saunders; 1991:754–770.

Ostrowski DM, Gilula LA. Mixed sclerosing bone dystrophy presenting with upper extremity deformities. A case report and review of the literature. *J Hand Surg Br* 1992;17:108–112.

Park HS, Kim JR, Lee SY, et al. Symptomatic giant (10-cm) bone island of the tibia. *Skeletal Radiol* 2005;34:347–350.

Paul LW. Hereditary multiple diaphyseal sclerosis (Ribbing). *Radiology* 1953;60:412–416.

Pyle EL. A case of unusual bone development. *J Bone Joint Surg* 1931;13:874–876.

Raad MS, Beighton P. Autosomal recessive inheritance of metaphyseal dysplasia (Pyle disease). *Clin Genet* 1978;14:251–256.

Reichenberger E, Tiziani V, Watanabe S, et al. Autosomal dominant craniometaphyseal dysplasia is caused by mutations in the transmembrane protein ANK. *Am J Hum Genet* 2001;68:1321–1326.

Rhys R, Davies AM, Mangham DC, et al. Sclerotome distribution of melorheostosis and multicentric fibromatosis. *Skeletal Radiol* 1998;27:633–636.

Ribbing S. Hereditary, multiple, diaphyseal sclerosis. *Acta Radiol* 1949;31:522–536.

Riccardi VM. The genetic predisposition to and histogenesis of neurofibromas and neurofibrosarcoma in neurofibromatosis type 1. *Neurosurg Focus* 2007;22:E3.

Rucker TN, Alfidi RJ. A rare familial systemic affection of the skeleton: Fairbank's disease. *Radiology* 1964;82:63–66.

Rutherford EE, Tarplett LJ, Davies EM, et al. Lumbar spine fusion and stabilization: hardware, techniques, and imaging appearances. *Radiographics* 2007;27:1737–1749.

Scott H, Bunge S, Gal A, et al. Molecular genetics of mucopolysaccharidosis type I: diagnostic, clinical, and biological implications. *Hum Mutat* 1995;6:288–302.

Sebastian A, Loots GG. Genetics of Sost/SOST in sclerosteosis and van Buchem disease animal models. *Metabolism* 2018;80:38–47.

Seeger LL, Hewel KC, Yao L, et al. Ribbing disease (multiple diaphyseal sclerosis): imaging and differential diagnosis. *AJR Am J Roentgenol* 1996;167:689–694.

Sillence DO. Osteogenesis imperfecta: an expanding panorama of variants. *Clin Orthop Relat Res* 1981;159:11–25.

Sillence DO, Senn A, Danks DM. Genetic heterogeneity in osteogenesis imperfecta. *J Med Genet* 1979;16:101–116.

Slone RM, MacMillan M, Montgomery WJ, et al. Spinal fixation. Part 2. Fixation techniques and hardware for the thoracic and lumbosacral spine. *Radiographics* 1993;13:521–543.

Sobacchi C, Schulz A, Coxon FP, et al. Osteopetrosis: genetics, treatment and new insights into osteoclast function. *Nat Rev Endocrinol* 2013;9:522–536.

Spieth ME, Greenspan A, Forrester DM, et al. Radionuclide imaging in forme fruste of melorheostosis. *Clin Nucl Med* 1994;19:512–515.

Spranger JW, Langer LO Jr, Wiederman HR. *Bone dysplasias. An atlas of constitutional disorders of skeletal development.* Philadelphia: WB Saunders; 1974.

Stein SA, Witkop C, Hill S, et al. Sclerosteosis: neurogenetic and pathophysiologic analysis of an American kinship. *Neurology* 1983;33:267–277.

Stokes IA. Three-dimensional terminology of spinal deformity. A report presented to the Scoliosis Research Society by the Scoliosis Research Society Working Group on 3-D terminology of spinal deformity. *Spine (Phila Pa 1976)* 1994;19:236–248.

Suresh S, Muthukumar T, Saifuddin A. Classical and unusual imaging appearances of melorheostosis. *Clin Radiol* 2010;65:593–600.

Thomsen MN, Schneider U, Weber M, et al. Scoliosis and congenital anomalies associated with Klippel-Feil syndrome types I-III. *Spine (Phila Pa 1976)* 1997;22:396–401.

Tomatsu S, Yasuda E, Patel P, et al. Morquio A syndrome: diagnosis and current and future therapies. *Pediatr Endocrinol Rev* 2014;12:141–151.

Truswell AS. Osteopetrosis with syndactyly: a morphological variant of Albers-Schönberg's disease. *J Bone Joint Surg Br* 1958;40-B:209–218.

van Buchem FSP. Hyperostosis corticalis generalisata. Eight new cases. *Acta Med Scand* 1971;189:257–267.

van Buchem FSP, Hadders HN, Hansen JF, et al. Hyperostosis corticalis generalisata. Report of seven cases. *Am J Med* 1962;33:387–397.

van Buchem FSP, Hadders HN, Ubbens R. An uncommon familial systemic disease of the skeleton: hyperostosis corticalis generalisata familiaris. *Acta Radiol* 1955;44:109–120.

van Dijk FS, Cobben JM, Kariminejad A, et al. Osteogenesis imperfecta: a review with clinical examples. *Mol Syndromol* 2011;2:1–20.

Vanhoenacker FM, Balemans W, Tan GJ, et al. Van Buchem disease: lifetime evolution of radioclinical features. *Skeletal Radiol* 2003;32:708–718.

Vanhoenacker FM, De Beuckeleer LH, Van Hul W, et al. Sclerosing bone dysplasias: genetic and radioclinical features. *Eur Radiol* 2000;10:1423–1433.

Van Hul W, Balemans W, Van Hul E, et al. Van Buchem disease (hyperostosis corticalis generalisata) maps to chromosome 17q12-q21. *Am J Hum Genet* 1998;62:391–399.

Voorhoeve N. L'image radiologique non encore decrit d'une anomalie du squelette; ses rapports avec la dyschondroplasie et l'osteopathia condensans disseminata. *Acta Radiol* 1924;3:407–411.

Wallace SE, Lachman RS, Mekikian PB, et al. Marked phenotypic variability in progressive diaphyseal dysplasia (Camurati-Engelmann disease): report of a four-generation pedigree, identification of a mutation in TGFB1, and review. *Am J Med Genet A* 2004;129A:235–247.

Ward LM, Rauch F, Travers R, et al. Osteogenesis imperfecta type VII: an autosomal recessive form of brittle bone disease. *Bone* 2002;31:12–18.

Whyte MP, Murphy WA. Osteopetrosis and other sclerosing bone disorders. In: Avioli LV, Krane SM, eds. *Metabolic bone disorders*, 2nd ed. Philadelphia: WB Saunders, 1990:616–658.

Whyte MP, Murphy WA, Fallon MD, et al. Mixed-sclerosing-bone-dystrophy: report of a case and review of the literature. *Skeletal Radiol* 1981;6:95–102.

Winter RB, Haven JJ, Moe JH, et al. Diastematomyelia and congenital spine deformities. *J Bone Joint Surg Am* 1974;56:27–39.

Wise CA, Gao X, Shoemaker S, et al. Understanding genetic factors in idiopathic scoliosis, a complex disease of childhood. *Curr Genomics* 2008;9:51–59.

Worth HM, Wollin DG. Hyperostosis corticalis generalisata congenita. *J Can Assoc Radiol* 1966;17:67–74.

Zhang Y, Castori M, Ferranti G, et al. Novel and recurrent germline LEMD3 mutations causing Buschke-Ollendorff syndrome and osteopoikilosis but not isolated melorheostosis. *Clin Genet* 2009;75:556–561.

Zheng H, Zhang Z, He JW, et al. A novel mutation (R122Q) in the cathepsin K gene in a Chinese child with pyknodysostosis. *Gene* 2013;521:176–179.

Zicari AM, Tarani L, Perotti D, et al. WTX R353X mutation in a family with osteopathia striata and cranial sclerosis (OS-CS): case report and literature review of the disease clinical, genetic and radiological features. *Ital J Ped* 2012;38:27.

Ziran N, Hill S, Wright ME, et al. Ribbing disease: radiographic and biochemical characterization, lack of response to pamidronate. *Skeletal Radiol* 2003;31:714–719.

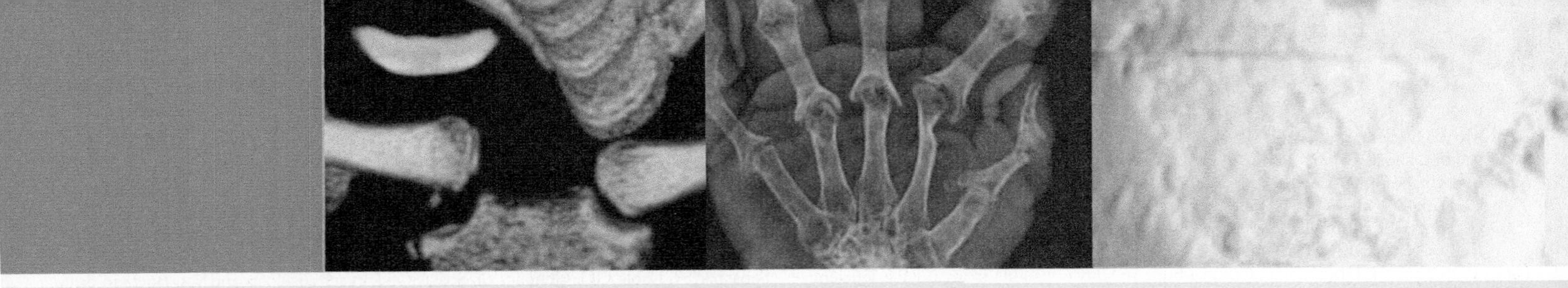

Index

Page numbers in *italics* denote figures; those followed by a "t" denote tables.

C

D

G

Q

R

T

U

V

W

X

Y

Z